GENERAL
THORACIC
SURGERY

fifth edition

GENERAL THORACIC SURGERY

fifth edition volume

1

Edited by

Thomas W. Shields, M.D., D.Sc. (Hon.)

Professor Emeritus of Surgery
Northwestern University Medical School
Chicago, Illinois

Joseph LoCicero III, M.D.

Associate Professor of Surgery
Harvard Medical School
Boston, Massachusetts

Ronald B. Ponn, M.D.

Assistant Clinical Professor of Surgery
Yale University School of Medicine
New Haven, Connecticut

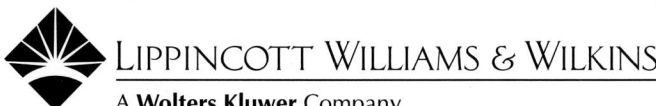

LIPPINCOTT WILLIAMS & WILKINS

A **Wolters Kluwer** Company

Philadelphia · Baltimore · New York · London
Buenos Aires · Hong Kong · Sydney · Tokyo

Acquisitions Editor: Lisa McAllister
Developmental Editor: Michelle M. LaPlante
Production Editor: Jane Bangley McQueen, Silverchair Science + Communications
Manufacturing Manager: Kevin Watt
Cover Designer: Christine Jenny
Compositor: Silverchair Science + Communications
Printer: Edwards Brothers

5th Edition

©2000 by LIPPINCOTT WILLIAMS & WILKINS
530 Walnut St.
Philadelphia, PA 19106 USA
LWW.com

Library of Congress Cataloging-in-Publication Data
General thoracic surgery / edited by Thomas W. Shields, Joseph
 LoCicero III, Ronald B. Ponn. -- 5th ed.
      p.   cm.
   Includes bibliographical references and indexes.
   ISBN 0-683-30619-7
   1. Chest--Surgery.   I. Shields, Thomas W., 1922-
II. LoCicero, Joseph, 1948-   . III. Ponn, Ronald B.
   [DNLM: 1. Thoracic Surgical Procedures.   WF 980 G326 1999]
RD536.G45   1999
617.5'4059--dc21
DNLM/DLC
for Library of Congress   99-34438
                                                          CIP

Care has been taken to confirm the accuracy of the information presented and to describe generally accepted practices. However, the authors, editors, and publisher are not responsible for errors or omissions or for any consequences from application of the information in this book and make no warranty, expressed or implied, with respect to the currency, completeness, or accuracy of the contents of the publication. Application of this information in a particular situation remains the professional responsibility of the practitioner.

The authors, editors, and publisher have exerted every effort to ensure that drug selection and dosage set forth in this text are in accordance with current recommendations and practice at the time of publication. However, in view of ongoing research, changes in government regulations, and the constant flow of information relating to drug therapy and drug reactions, the reader is urged to check the package insert for each drug for any change in indications and dosage and for added warnings and precautions. This is particularly important when the recommended agent is a new or infrequently employed drug.

Some drugs and medical devices presented in this publication have Food and Drug Administration (FDA) clearance for limited use in restricted research settings. It is the responsibility of health care providers to ascertain the FDA status of each drug or device planned for use in their clinical practice.

10 9 8 7 6 5 4 3 2

Contents

Volume I

The Lung, Pleura, Diaphragm, and Chest Wall

SECTION I. ANATOMY OF THE CHEST WALL AND LUNGS

SECTION II. PHYSIOLOGY OF THE LUNGS

SECTION III. THORACIC IMAGING

SECTION XVI. OTHER TUMORS OF THE LUNG

Volume II
The Esophagus

SECTION XVII. ANATOMY

SECTION XVIII. PHYSIOLOGY

SECTION XIX. DIAGNOSTIC STUDIES

SECTION XX. OPERATIVE PROCEDURES IN THE MANAGEMENT OF ESOPHAGEAL DISEASE

The Mediastinum

SECTION XXIV. ANATOMY

SECTION XXV. NONINVASIVE DIAGNOSTIC INVESTIGATIONS

SECTION XXVI. INVASIVE DIAGNOSTIC INVESTIGATIONS AND SURGICAL APPROACHES

SECTION XXVII. MEDIASTINAL INFECTIONS, OVERVIEW OF MASS LESIONS IN THE MEDIASTINUM, AND CONTROL OF VASCULAR OBSTRUCTING SYMPTOMATOLOGY

SECTION XXIX. MEDIASTINAL CYSTS

Contributing Authors

Homeros Aletras, M.D.
Professor and Chairman
Department of Surgery
Salonika University
Salonika, Greece

John C. Alexander, Jr., M.D.
Professor of Surgery
Northwestern University Medical School
Chicago, Illinois

Mark S. Allen, M.D.
Associate Professor of Surgery
Mayo Medical School
Rochester, Minnesota

Thomas A. Aloia, M.D.
Research Fellow
Department of General and Thoracic Surgery
Duke University Medical Center
Durham, North Carolina

Scott K. Alpard, M.D.
Research Fellow in Surgery
University of Texas Medical School at Galveston
Galveston, Texas

Robert W. Anderson, M.D.
Professor and Chairman
Department of Surgery
Duke University School of Medicine
Durham, North Carolina

William Scott Arnold, M.D.
Attending Physician
Cardiothoracic Service
Carilion Roanoke Memorial Hospital
Roanoke, Virginia

Carl L. Backer, M.D.
Associate Professor of Surgery
Northwestern University Medical School
Chicago, Illinois

Manjit S. Bains, M.B., B.S.
Clinical Professor of Surgery
Weill Medical College of Cornell University
New York, New York

Felix D. Battistella, M.D.
Associate Professor of Surgery
University of California, Davis, School
* of Medicine*
Sacramento, California

Ronald H. R. Belsey, M.D.
Former Visiting Professor
University of Chicago Pritzker School
* of Medicine*
Chicago, Illinois

John R. Benfield, M.D.
Professor Emeritus of Cardiothoracic Surgery
University of California, Davis, School
* of Medicine*
Sacramento, California

Akhil Bidani, M.D.
Professor of Internal Medicine
University of Texas Medical School at Galveston
Galveston, Texas

Charles E. Blevins, Ph.D.
Professor Emeritus of Anatomy
Indiana University School of Medicine
Indianapolis, Indiana

Jean-Philippe Bocage, M.D.
Assistant Professor of Thoracic Surgery
University of Medicine and Dentistry of New
* Jersey—Robert Wood Johnson Medical School*
New Brunswick, New Jersey

Anne Greth Bondeson
Professor of Surgery
Central Hospital
Skovde, Sweden

Christiana M. Brenin, M.D.
*Westchester Institute for the Treatment of Cancer
    and Blood Diseases*
Dickstein Cancer Treatment Center
White Plains, New York

Edward A. Brunner, M.D., Ph.D.
Professor of Anesthesiology
Northwestern University Medical School
Chicago, Illinois

Aart Brutel de la Rivière, M.D., Ph.D.
*Professor and Chairman of Cardiothoracic
    Surgery*
University Medical Center Utrecht
Utrecht, The Netherlands

Peter H. Burri, M.D.
Professor and Chairman of Anatomy
University of Berne
Berne, Switzerland

Robert J. Caccavale, M.D.
Associate Clinical Professor of Surgery
*University of Medicine and Dentistry of New
    Jersey—Robert Wood Johnson Medical School*
New Brunswick, New Jersey

Christian T. Campos, M.D.
Assistant Professor of Surgery
Harvard Medical School
Boston, Massachusetts

J. Jeffrey Carr, M.D., M.S.
*Assistant Professor of Radiology and Public
    Health Sciences*
Wake Forest University School of Medicine
Winston-Salem, North Carolina

C. James Carrico, M.D.
Professor and Chairman
Department of Surgery
University of Texas Southwestern Medical School
Dallas, Texas

Robert J. Cerfolio, M.D.
Associate Professor of Cardiothoracic Surgery
University of Alabama School of Medicine
Birmingham, Alabama

Martin H. Cohen, M.D.
Professor of Medicine
Temple University School of Medicine
Philadelphia, Pennsylvania

Juan A. Cordero, Jr., M.D.
Chief Resident in Surgery
*University of Rochester School of Medicine and
    Dentistry*
Rochester, New York

Yvon Cormier, M.D.
Professor of Medicine
Laval University Faculty of Medicine
Sainte-Foy, Quebec, Canada

James D. Cox, M.D.
Professor and Head of Radiation Oncology
*University of Texas M. D. Anderson Cancer
    Center*
Houston, Texas

Robert M. Craig, M.D.
Professor of Medicine
Northwestern University Medical School
Chicago, Illinois

Lawrence L. Creswell, M.D.
Assistant Professor of Surgery
Washington University School of Medicine
St. Louis, Missouri

Anne McB Curtis, M.D.
Professor of Diagnostic Radiology
Yale University School of Medicine
New Haven, Connecticut

Richard S. D'Agostino, M.D.
Attending Thoracic and Cardiovascular Surgeon
Lahey-Hitchcock Medical Center
Burlington, Massachusetts

Benedict D. T. Daly, M.D.
Professor of Cardiothoracic Surgery
Tufts University School of Medicine
Boston, Massachusetts

Thomas M. Daniel, M.D.
Professor of Thoracic Surgery
University of Virginia School of Medicine
Charlottesville, Virginia

Gail Darling, M.D.
Assistant Professor of Surgery
University of Toronto Faculty of Medicine
Toronto, Ontario, Canada

Philippe G. Dartevelle, M.D.
Professor of Thoracic and Vascular Surgery
Paris Sud University
Paris, France

Steven R. DeMeester, M.D.
Assistant Professor of Surgery
University of Southern California School
  of Medicine
Los Angeles, California

Tom R. DeMeester, M.D.
Professor and Chairman
Department of Surgery
University of Southern California School
  of Medicine
Los Angeles, California

Claude Deschamps, M.D.
Associate Professor of Surgery
Mayo Medical School
Rochester, Minnesota

Jean Deslauriers, M.D.
Professor of Surgery
Laval University Faculty of Medicine
Sainte-Foy, Quebec, Canada

Ronald B. Dietrick, M.D.
Formerly Director of Medical Services
Kwangju Christian Hospital
Kwangju, South Korea

Ali Dodge-Khatami, M.D.
Fellow in Pediatric Cardiac Surgery
Northwestern University Medical School
Chicago, Illinois

Donald B. Doty, M.D.
Clinical Professor of Surgery
University of Utah School of Medicine
Salt Lake City, Utah

John R. Doty, M.D.
Chief Resident in General Surgery
Johns Hopkins Hospital
Baltimore, Maryland

Robert J. Downey, M.D.
Assistant Professor of Surgery
Weill Medical College of Cornell University
New York, New York

Carolyn M. Dresler, M.D.
Associate Professor of Surgery
Temple University School of Medicine
Philadelphia, Pennsylvania

André C. H. Duranceau, M.D.
Professor of Surgery
University of Montreal Faculty of Medicine
Montreal, Quebec, Canada

Forrest C. Eggleston, M.D.
Formerly Professor and Head of Surgery
Christian Medical College
Ludhiana, Punjab, India

Nabil M. El-Baz, M.D.
Associate Professor of Anesthesiology
Rush Medical College of Rush University
Chicago, Illinois

John A. Elefteriades, M.D.
Professor and Chief
Department of Cardiothoracic Surgery
Yale University School of Medicine
New Haven, Connecticut

F. Henry Ellis, Jr., M.D.
Clinical Professor of Surgery, Emeritus
Harvard Medical School
Boston, Massachusetts

Bahman Emami, M.D.
Professor and Chairman
Department of Radiotherapy
Loyola University Chicago Stritch School
  of Medicine
Maywood, Illinois

Gary R. Epler, M.D.
Associate Clinical Professor of Medicine
Harvard Medical School
Boston, Massachusetts

L. Penfield Faber, M.D.
Professor of Surgery
Rush Medical College of Rush University
Chicago, Illinois

John A. Federico, M.D.
Assistant Clinical Professor of Surgery
Yale University School of Medicine
New Haven, Connecticut

Richard H. Feins, M.D.
Assistant Professor of Surgery
University of Rochester School of Medicine and
  Dentistry
Rochester, New York

Ronald Feld, M.D.
Professor of Medicine
University of Toronto Faculty of Medicine
Toronto, Ontario, Canada

Stanley C. Fell, M.D.
Professor of Thoracic Surgery
Albert Einstein College of Medicine
Bronx, New York

Pasquale Ferraro, M.D.
Assistant Professor of Surgery
University of Toronto Faculty of Medicine
Toronto, Ontario, Canada

Willard A. Fry, M.D.
Professor of Surgery
Northwestern University Medical School
Chicago, Illinois

Patrick J. Fultz, M.D.
Associate Professor of Radiology
University of Rochester School of Medicine and
    Dentistry
Rochester, New York

Henning A. Gaissert, M.D.
Assistant Professor of Surgery
Brown University School of Medicine
Providence, Rhode Island

Warren B. Gefter, M.D.
Professor of Radiology
University of Pennsylvania School of Medicine
Philadelphia, Pennsylvania

Gary G. Ghahremani, M.D.
Professor of Radiology
Northwestern University Medical School
Chicago, Illinois

Juan Gil, M.D.
Professor of Pathology
Mount Sinai School of Medicine
New York, New York

Robert J. Ginsberg, M.D.
Professor of Surgery
Weill Medical College of Cornell University
New York, New York

Jeffrey Glassroth, M.D.
George R. and Elaine Love Professor and Chair
Department of Medicine
University of Wisconsin Medical School
Madison, Wisconsin

Peter Goldstraw, Ch.M.
Consultant Thoracic Surgeon and Clinical Director
    of Surgery
Royal Brompton and Harefield National Health
    Service Trust
London, United Kingdom

Leo I. Gordon, M.D.
Professor of Medicine
Northwestern University Medical School
Chicago, Illinois

Richard M. Gore, M.D.
Professor of Radiology
Northwestern University Medical School
Chicago, Illinois

F. Anthony Greco, M.D.
Director of the Sarah Cannon–Minnie Pearl
    Cancer Center
Department of Medical Oncology
Centennial Medical Center
Nashville, Tennessee

Hermes C. Grillo, M.D.
Professor of Surgery
Harvard Medical School
Boston, Massachusetts

Sean C. Grondin, M.D.
Fellow in Thoracic Surgery
Harvard Medical School
Boston, Massachusetts

Jay L. Grosfeld, M.D.
Lafayette F. Page Professor and Chairman
Department of Surgery
Indiana University School of Medicine
Indianapolis, Indiana

Milton D. Gross, M.D.
Professor of Internal Medicine
University of Michigan Medical School
Ann Arbor, Michigan

Robert A. Gustafson, M.D.
Professor of Surgery
West Virginia University School
    of Medicine
Morgantown, West Virginia

Jeffrey A. Hagen, M.D.
Associate Professor of Surgery
University of Southern California School
of Medicine
Los Angeles, California

John D. Hainsworth, M.D.
Associate Professor of Medicine
Vanderbilt University School of Medicine
Nashville, Tennessee

David H. Harpole, Jr., M.D.
Associate Professor of Surgery
Duke University School of Medicine
Durham, North Carolina

Renee S. Hartz, M.D.
Professor of Surgery
Tulane University School of Medicine
New Orleans, Louisiana

Hiroto Hatabu, Ph.D., M.D.
Associate Professor of Radiology
University of Pennsylvania School of Medicine
Philadelphia, Pennsylvania

John H. Hay, M.B., B.Chir.
Clinical Associate Professor of Surgery
(Radiation Oncology)
University of British Columbia Faculty
of Medicine
Vancouver, British Columbia, Canada

Lauren D. Holinger, M.D.
Professor of Otolaryngology–Head and Neck
Surgery
Northwestern University Medical School
Chicago, Illinois

Babette J. Horn, M.D.
Assistant Professor of Anesthesiology
Northwestern University Medical School
Chicago, Illinois

Guo Jun Huang, M.D.
Professor of Thoracic Surgery
Chinese Academy of Medical Sciences
Beijing, China

C. Anthony Hughes, M.D.
Department of Otolaryngology
Children's Memorial Hospital
Chicago, Illinois

Alfred Jaretzki III, M.D.
Associate Professor of Clinical Surgery
Columbia University College of Physicians and
Surgeons
New York, New York

K. "Jay" Jeyasingham, M.B., Ch.M.
Honorary Clinical Lecturer in Surgery
University of Bristol
Bristol, United Kingdom

Larry R. Kaiser, M.D.
Eldridge Eliason Professor of Surgery
University of Pennsylvania School of Medicine
Philadelphia, Pennsylvania

Gregory P. Kalemkerian, M.D.
Clinical Associate Professor of Medicine
University of Michigan School of Medicine
Ann Arbor, Michigan

Rajeev Kapoor, M.B.B.S., M.S.
Reader in Surgery
Christian Medical College
Ludhiana, Punjab, India

Thomas J. Keane, M.B., B.Ch.
Professor and Chairman of Surgery (Radiation
Oncology)
University of British Columbia Faculty
of Medicine
Vancouver, British Columbia, Canada

Merrill S. Kies, M.D.
Professor of Medicine
Northwestern University Medical School
Chicago, Illinois

Timothy J. Kinsella, M.D.
Professor and Chair
Department of Radiation Oncology
Case Western Reserve University School of Medicine
Cleveland, Ohio

Thomas J. Kirby, M.D.
Professor of Surgery
Case Western Reserve University School of Medicine
Cleveland, Ohio

Paul A. Kirschner, M.D.
Professor of Cardiothoracic Surgery
Mount Sinai School of Medicine
New York, New York

Herbert Knight, M.D.
Assistant Clinical Professor of Medicine
Yale University School of Medicine
New Haven, Connecticut

Ritsuko Komaki, M.D.
Professor of Radiation Oncology
University of Texas M. D. Anderson Cancer Center
Houston, Texas

Michael J. Kornstein, M.D.
Professor of Pathology
Virginia Commonwealth University Medical
*   College of Virginia School of Medicine*
Richmond, Virginia

Robert J. Korst, M.D.
Assistant Attending Thoracic Surgeon
Memorial Sloan-Kettering Cancer Center
New York, New York

Mark J. Krasna, M.D.
Associate Professor of Surgery
University of Maryland School of Medicine
Baltimore, Maryland

Rodney J. Landreneau, M.D.
Professor of Surgery and Human Oncology
MCP Hahnemann University School of Medicine
Pittsburgh, Pennsylvania

Johanna M. LaSala, M.D.
Attending Physician
Hospital of St. Raphael
New Haven, Connecticut

Pierre Leblanc, M.D.
Professor of Chest Medicine
Laval University Faculty of Medicine
Sainte-Foy, Quebec, Canada

Ralph J. Lewis, M.D.
Clinical Professor of Surgery
University of Medicine and Dentistry of New
*   Jersey—Robert Wood Johnson Medical School*
New Brunswick, New Jersey

Claudia R. Libertin, M.D.
Clinical Professor of Medicine
Yale University School of Medicine
New Haven, Connecticut

Richard W. Light, M.D.
Professor of Medicine
Vanderbilt University School of Medicine
Nashville, Tennessee

Jeffrey C. Lin, M.D.
Department of Cardiothoracic Surgery
MCP Hahnemann Allegheny General Hospital
Pittsburgh, Pennsylvania

Michael J. Liptay, M.D.
Assistant Professor of Surgery
Northwestern University Medical School
Chicago, Illinois

Joseph LoCicero III, M.D.
Associate Professor of Surgery
Harvard Medical School
Boston, Massachusetts

Massimo Loda, M.D.
Associate Professor of Pathology
Harvard Medical School
Boston, Massachusetts

Susan R. Luck, M.D.
Professor of Surgery
Northwestern University Medical School
Chicago, Illinois

John C. Lucke, M.D.
Chief of Cardiothoracic Surgery
Department of Veterans Affairs Medical Center
Asheville, North Carolina

Jeffrey P. Ludemann, M.D.
Clinical Instructor in Otolaryngology
University of British Columbia Faculty of
*   Medicine*
Vancouver, British Columbia, Canada

Paolo Macchiarini, M.D., Ph.D.
Chair of Thoracic and Vascular Surgery
Hannover University Medical School
Hannover, Germany

Michael J. Mack, M.D.
Assistant Professor of Thoracic Surgery
University of Texas Southwestern Medical School
Dallas, Texas

James W. Mackenzie, M.D.
Professor of Surgery
University of Medicine and Dentistry of New
*   Jersey—Robert Wood Johnson Medical School*
New Brunswick, New Jersey

Kamal A. Mansour, M.D.
Professor of Surgery
Emory University School of Medicine
Atlanta, Georgia

Gilbert Massard, M.D.
Professor of Surgery
University of Strasbourg
Strasbourg, France

Douglas J. Mathisen, M.D.
Professor of Surgery
Harvard Medical School
Boston, Massachusetts

Richard A. Matthay, M.D.
Boehringer Ingelheim Professor of Medicine
Yale University School of Medicine
New Haven, Connecticut

Donna E. Maziak, M.D.C.M.
Assistant Professor of Thoracic Surgery
University of Ottawa Faculty of Medicine
Ottawa, Ontario, Canada

Robert J. McKenna, Jr., M.D.
Clinical Professor of Thoracic Surgery
University of California, Los Angeles, UCLA
  School of Medicine
Los Angeles, California

Joseph S. McLaughlin, M.D.
Professor of Surgery
University of Maryland School of Medicine
Baltimore, Maryland

Máirín McMenamin, M.D.
Resident in Pathology
Beth Israel Deaconess Medical Center
Boston, Massachusetts

Minesh P. Mehta, M.D.
Associate Professor of Human Oncology
University of Wisconsin Medical School
Madison, Wisconsin

Steven J. Mentzer, M.D.
Associate Professor of Surgery
Harvard Medical School
Boston, Massachusetts

Bryan F. Meyers, M.D.
Assistant Professor of Surgery
Washington University School of Medicine
St. Louis, Missouri

Daniel L. Miller, M.D.
Assistant Professor of Surgery
Mayo Medical School
Rochester, Minnesota

Joseph I. Miller, Jr., M.D.
Professor of Cardiothoracic Surgery
Emory University School of Medicine
Atlanta, Georgia

Wallace T. Miller, M.D.
Professor of Radiology
University of Pennsylvania School of Medicine
Philadelphia, Pennsylvania

Wallace T. Miller, Jr., M.D.
Assistant Professor of Radiology
University of Pennsylvania School of Medicine
Philadelphia, Pennsylvania

Darroch W. O. Moores, M.D.
Clinical Associate Professor of Surgery
Albany Medical College
Albany, New York

Donald G. Mulder, M.D.
Professor of Surgery
University of California, Los Angeles, UCLA
  School of Medicine
Los Angeles, California

Thomas Muley, Ph.D.
Department of Thoracic Surgery
Thoraxklinik Heidelberg-Rohrbach
Heidelberg, Germany

Gordon F. Murray, M.D.
Professor and Chairman
Department of Surgery
West Virginia University School of Medicine
Morgantown, West Virginia

Tsuguo Naruke, M.D.
Deputy Director and Chairman of Surgery
National Cancer Center Hospital
Tokyo, Japan

Keith S. Naunheim, M.D.
Professor of Surgery
St. Louis University School of Medicine
St. Louis, Missouri

Dao M. Nguyen, M.D.
Senior Investigator
Thoracic Oncology Section
National Cancer Institute, National Institutes
  of Health
Bethesda, Maryland

John L. Nosher, M.D.
Clinical Professor and Chair
Department of Radiology
University of Medicine and Dentistry of New
* Jersey—Robert Wood Johnson Medical School*
New Brunswick, New Jersey

Christopher J. O'Connor, M.D.
Assistant Professor of Anesthesiology
Rush Medical College of Rush University
Chicago, Illinois

Jemi Olak, M.D.
Attending Thoracic Surgeon
Lutheran General Hospital
Park Ridge, Illinois

Gerald N. Olsen, M.D.
Professor of Medicine
University of South Carolina School of Medicine
Columbia, South Carolina

Kenji Omura, M.D.
Gastrointestinal Surgical Section
Kanazawa University School of Medicine
Kanazawa, Japan

Mark B. Orringer, M.D.
John Alexander Distinguished Professor
* of Surgery*
University of Michigan Medical School
Ann Arbor, Michigan

Andranik Ovassapian, M.D.
Professor of Clinical Anesthesia and Critical
* Care*
University of Chicago Pritzker School of Medicine
Chicago, Illinois

Kerry Paape, M.D.
Attending Surgeon
Cardiovascular Institute of the South
Houma, Louisiana

Peter C. Pairolero, M.D.
Professor of Surgery
Mayo Medical School
Rochester, Minnesota

Harvey I. Pass, M.D.
Professor of Surgery and Oncology
Wayne State University School of Medicine
Detroit, Michigan

G. Alexander Patterson, M.D.
Professor of Surgery
Washington University School of Medicine
St. Louis, Missouri

David Payne, M.D.
Assistant Professor of Radiation Oncology
University of Toronto Faculty of Medicine
Toronto, Ontario, Canada

Carlos A. Perez, M.D.
Professor of Radiology
Washington University School of Medicine
St. Louis, Missouri

Marvin Pomerantz, M.D.
Professor of Surgery
University of Colorado School of Medicine
Denver, Colorado

Ronald B. Ponn, M.D.
Assistant Clinical Professor of Surgery
Yale University School of Medicine
New Haven, Connecticut

John Popp, M.D.
Professor and Chairman
Department of Surgery
Albany Medical College
Albany, New York

Joe B. Putnam, Jr., M.D.
Associate Professor of Thoracic and Cardiovascular
* Surgery*
University of Texas M. D. Anderson Cancer
* Center*
Houston, Texas

Jacquelyn A. Quin, M.D.
Fellow in Cardiothoracic Surgery
University of Texas Southwestern Medical School
Dallas, Texas

Carolyn E. Reed, M.D.
Professor of Surgery
Medical University of South Carolina College
* of Medicine*
Charleston, South Carolina

Frederick J. Rescorla, M.D.
Associate Professor of Surgery
Indiana University School of Medicine
Indianapolis, Indiana

Marleta Reynolds, M.D.
Associate Professor of Surgery
Northwestern University Medical School
Chicago, Illinois

Thomas W. Rice, M.D.
Head
General Thoracic Surgery
Cleveland Clinic Foundation
Cleveland, Ohio

Melanie L. Richards, M.D.
Assistant Professor of Surgery
University of Texas Medical School at
*   San Antonio*
San Antonio, Texas

Philip G. Robinson, M.D.
Assistant Professor of Clinical Pathology
University of Miami School of Medicine
Miami, Florida

Valerie W. Rusch, M.D.
Professor of Surgery
Weill Medical College of Cornell University
New York, New York

Steven A. Sahn, M.D.
Professor of Medicine
Medical University of South Carolina
Charleston, South Carolina

L. R. Scherer III, M.D.
Clinical Associate Professor of Surgery
Indiana University School of Medicine
Indianapolis, Indiana

Joachim Schirren, M.D.
Assistant Chief of Thoracic Surgery
Thoraxklinik Heidelberg-Rohrbach
Heidelberg, Germany

David S. Schrump, M.D.
Senior Investigator and Head
Surgery Branch, Thoracic Oncology Section
National Cancer Institute, National Institutes
*   of Health*
Bethesda, Maryland

Granger R. Scruggs
Research Assistant to Michael J. Mack, M.D.
University of Texas Southwestern Medical
*   School*
Dallas, Texas

William P. Sexauer, M.D.
Assistant Professor of Medicine
MCP Hahnemann University School of Medicine
Philadelphia, Pennsylvania

Robert C. Shamberger, M.D.
Associate Professor of Surgery
Harvard Medical School
Boston, Massachusetts

Farid M. Shamji, M.D.
Associate Professor of Thoracic Surgery
University of Ottawa Faculty of Medicine
Ottawa, Ontario, Canada

Brahm Shapiro, M.D., Ch.B., Ph.D.
Professor of Internal Medicine
University of Michigan Medical School
Ann Arbor, Michigan

Frances A. Shepherd, M.D.
Associate Professor of Medicine
University of Toronto Faculty of Medicine
Toronto, Ontario, Canada

Thomas W. Shields, M.D., D.Sc. (Hon.)
Professor Emeritus of Surgery
Northwestern University Medical School
Chicago, Illinois

Gerard A. Silvestri, M.D.
Associate Professor of Medicine
Medical University of South Carolina College
*   of Medicine*
Charleston, South Carolina

Sunil Singhal, M.D.
Resident
Johns Hopkins Hospital
Baltimore, Maryland

William G. Spies, M.D.
Associate Professor of Radiology
Northwestern University Medical School
Chicago, Illinois

Amit Srivastava, M.D.
Senior Attending Physician
MacNeal Hospital
Berwyn, Illinois

Robert D. Stewart, M.D.
Attending Cardiothoracic Surgeon
Beth Israel Deaconess Medical Center
Boston, Massachusetts

Alan H. Stolpen, M.D., Ph.D.
Associate Professor of Radiology
University of Iowa College of Medicine
Iowa City, Iowa

John M. Streitz, Jr., M.D.
Clinical Assistant Professor of Surgery
University of Minnesota—Duluth School of Medicine
Duluth, Minnesota

David J. Sugarbaker, M.D.
Professor of Surgery
Harvard Medical School
Boston, Massachusetts

Scott J. Swanson, M.D.
Assistant Professor of Surgery
Harvard Medical School
Boston, Massachusetts

Panagiotis N. Symbas, M.D.
Professor of Surgery
Emory University School of Medicine
Atlanta, Georgia

Lynn T. Tanoue, M.D.
Associate Professor of Medicine
Yale University School of Medicine
New Haven, Connecticut

Weike Tao, M.D.
Resident in Anesthesiology
University of Texas Medical School at Galveston
Galveston, Texas

Norman W. Thompson, M.D.
Henry King Ransom Professor of Surgery
University of Michigan Medical School
Ann Arbor, Michigan

Victor F. Trastek, M.D.
Professor of Surgery
Mayo Medical School
Rochester, Minnesota

Przemek W. Twardowski, M.D.
Medical Oncologist
City of Hope Comprehensive Cancer Center
Duarte, California

Hiroshi Urayama, M.D.
Vascular Surgical Section
Kanazawa University School of Medicine
Kanazawa, Japan

Harold C. Urschel, Jr., M.D., Ph.D.
Clinical Professor of Thoracic and Cardiovascular Surgery
University of Texas Southwestern Medical School
Dallas, Texas

Arvydas D. Vanagunas, M.D.
Associate Professor of Medicine
Northwestern University Medical School
Chicago, Illinois

Robert M. Vanecko, M.S., M.D.
Professor of Surgery
Northwestern University Medical School
Chicago, Illinois

Alexander Vasilakis, M.D.
Assistant Professor of Surgery
West Virginia University School of Medicine
Morgantown, West Virginia

Mohan Verghese, M.D.
Professor and Head
Department of Surgery and Cardiothoracic Surgery
Christian Medical College
Ludhiana, Punjab, India

Romeo A. Vidone, M.D.
Associate Clinical Professor of Pathology
Yale University School of Medicine
New Haven, Connecticut

Ingolf Vogt-Moykopf, M.D.
Professor of Thoracic Surgery
Heidelberg University
Heidelberg, Germany

Richard L. Wahl, M.D.
Professor of Internal Medicine and Radiology
University of Michigan Medical School
Ann Arbor, Michigan

Fady S. Wanna, M.D.
Chief Resident in Cardiothoracic Surgery
Emory University School of Medicine
Atlanta, Georgia

William H. Warren, M.D.
Associate Professor of Surgery
Rush Medical College of Rush University
Chicago, Illinois

Lacey Washington, M.D.
Attending Radiologist
MCP Hahnemann Allegheny General Hospital
Pittsburgh, Pennsylvania

Yoh Watanabe, D.M.Sc.
Professor and Chairman
Department of Surgery
Kanazawa University School of Medicine
Kanazawa, Japan

Ewald R. Weibel, M.D.
Professor of Anatomy
University of Berne
Berne, Switzerland

Jean-Marie Wihlm, M.D.
Thoracic and Cardiovascular Surgeon
University of Strasbourg
Strasbourg, France

Earle W. Wilkins, Jr., M.D.
Clinical Professor of Surgery, Emeritus
Harvard Medical School
Boston, Massachusetts

John G. Williams, M.D.
Assistant Professor of Surgery
University of Texas Southwestern Medical School
Dallas, Texas

Hak Yui Wong, M.D.
Assistant Professor of Anesthesiology
Northwestern University Medical School
Chicago, Illinois

Cameron D. Wright, M.D.
Associate Professor of Surgery
Harvard Medical School
Boston, Massachusetts

Manoel Ximenes III, M.D., Ph.D.
Professor and Head of Thoracic Surgery
University of Brasilia
Brasilia, Brazil

Anjana V. Yeldandi, Ph.D.
Associate Professor of Pathology
Northwestern University Medical School
Chicago, Illinois

Joseph B. Zwischenberger, M.D.
Professor of Surgery
University of Texas Medical School at Galveston
Galveston, Texas

Preface

The fifth edition of *General Thoracic Surgery* has been extensively expanded and revised to present comprehensive coverage of the ever-expanding field of general thoracic surgery. The pertinent information necessary for understanding and management of the many problems related to the thorax and its contents that may confront the general thoracic surgeon is presented in exquisite detail. To ensure the attainment of this goal, I have enlisted the aid of Dr. Joseph LoCicero III and Dr. Ronald B. Ponn as associate editors. Together, we have selected acknowledged experts from many fields of endeavor: the basic sciences; pulmonary medicine; radiology; nuclear medicine; pathology; bronchoesophagology; anesthesiology; endocrinology; medical, radiologic, and surgical oncology; and general thoracic surgery, as well as other surgical specialties, to contribute their expertise to this text.

There are 29 sections, as well as an appendix devoted to presentation of the basics of statistical analysis that has become so important in the evaluation of clinical trials. There are 190 chapters, of which 54 are new. The new chapters primarily present advances in the basic sciences, diagnostic procedures, and surgical techniques that are relevant to the general thoracic surgeon. The sections on Carcinoma of the Lung and Other Tumors of the Lung contain many of the new chapters to more extensively cover these important fields. Likewise, the sections on the Mediastinum have been greatly expanded and essentially present the detailed and updated coverage that was originally published in the text *Mediastinal Surgery* by the senior editor in 1991. A few of the chapters from the fourth edition remain unchanged, but the vast majority of the previous chapters have been rewritten by new authors or have been extensively revised by the previous authors to be current with the literature through 1998 and early 1999.

As with any text that becomes more inclusive, repetition and differences in opinion have become common. These, within bounds, are healthy, as each author frequently views the same subject from a different vantage point and adds additional references that are of value in understanding the subject under consideration. Cross-references again are in abundance. Effort has been made to further expand the index so that it appropriately reflects all the subjects included in the text.

My associates and I wish to thank the many contributors from here in North America and abroad in Europe, Asia, and South America for the effort that they have expended in preparation of their contributions to the fifth edition. Each is of inestimable value and enhances the validity and importance of the text. We believe this text should not only be of interest to the thoracic surgeon but also useful to our colleagues in other specialties who have an interest in the chest and its contents.

Thomas W. Shields
Senior Editor

Acknowledgment

The editors wish to acknowledge the outstanding effort and dedication of Ms. Diane April of the Department of Surgery of Northwestern Memorial Hospital in the preparation and editorial unification of the contributions to the text. Without her expertise in traveling the information highway of the present computer age, we truly could not have produced this outstanding text.

PART I

The Lung, Pleura, Diaphragm, and Chest Wall

SECTION I

Anatomy of the Chest Wall and Lungs

CHAPTER 1

Anatomy of the Thorax

Charles E. Blevins

The thorax is a flexible, airtight cage whose framework comprises the most continuously active combination of skeletal, muscular, and articulating tissues in the body. Its primary function is to produce movements responsible for ventilation of the lungs. It also affords protection for thoracic viscera and support for the upper extremities, but such responsibilities are secondary to the vital function of producing the alternating changes in pressure required for inflation and deflation of the lungs. Such pressure changes must be orderly, well coordinated, and accompanied by close compliance of the lungs with changes in thoracic dimensions. The volume and rate of air movement must be compatible with vital needs for oxygen under a variety of conditions. To meet such requirements, a uniquely functional anatomic apparatus is required.

RESPIRATORY MOVEMENTS

Movements of the thorax are the result of both active and passive events. During inspiration, the thorax is enlarged actively by coordinated muscle contractions. As a direct result of increased thoracic dimensions, intrathoracic, intrapleural, and intrapulmonic pressures are reduced sequentially so that atmospheric air is forced into the lungs. Expiration is a passive event, largely due to the relaxation of forces generated during inspiration. It is marked by the return of thoracic dimensions to resting levels and by increased pressure within the chest, pleural cavities, and lungs. Muscle activity may facilitate the expiratory phase of breathing, but it is not essential.

Inspiratory movements enlarge the thorax in all dimensions. They are a blend of efforts directed in the anteroposterior, bilateral, and superoinferior axes. An increase in anteroposterior dimensions is marked by forward and upward movement of the lower part of the sternum, which is called the *pump-handle* movement. The sternum is anchored more firmly at its upper extent by relatively short ribs and costal cartilages than at its lower limits where both

ribs and cartilages are longer. Because the points of pivot of the ribs are located at their vertebral articulations, elevation of the ribs lifts the body of the sternum outward and forward. The greatest excursion occurs at the level of the longest ribs—that is, ribs five to seven. The axis for such movement is on a line drawn through the head, neck, and tubercle of each rib (Fig. 1-1).

During normal quiet respiration, the ribs are elevated by contraction of the intercostal muscles. Taylor (1960) and Campbell (1955) reported that the scalene muscles also aid in elevation in some individuals. Jones and associates (1953) reported that the effect of muscles within individual intercostal spaces is apparently small, but synchronous contraction of all intercostal muscles is sufficient to elevate the rib cage as a unit. The resultant increase in anteroposterior dimension is greatest at the level of ribs five to seven (see Fig. 1-1).

Increase in bilateral dimensions is marked by upward and lateral excursion in the vicinity of the midaxillary line. The greatest degree of movement is noted in ribs 7 to 10, whose costal cartilages descend and then ascend before articulation with the sternum. Because the middle of each rib-cartilage unit is lower than either costovertebral or costosternal articulations, elevation swings each unit upward and laterally, much like the action of lifting a bucket handle upward toward the middle of its arc of swing (Fig. 1-2). This action is accomplished by contraction of intercostal muscles also, but Cherniack and Cherniack (1961) suggested that it is facilitated by muscle fibers of the diaphragm that are perpendicular to the costal margin.

The greatest increase in thoracic dimensions during inspiration is in the superoinferior dimensions. It is accomplished by contraction of the diaphragm, which is generally described as dome shaped. The dome, however, is uneven; its anterolateral attachments are at higher levels than its posterolateral attachments. Furthermore, the dome is indented by the heart and may present two domes, one related to the liver and one related to the stomach and spleen. Contraction of the majority of its muscle fibers flattens the diaphragm

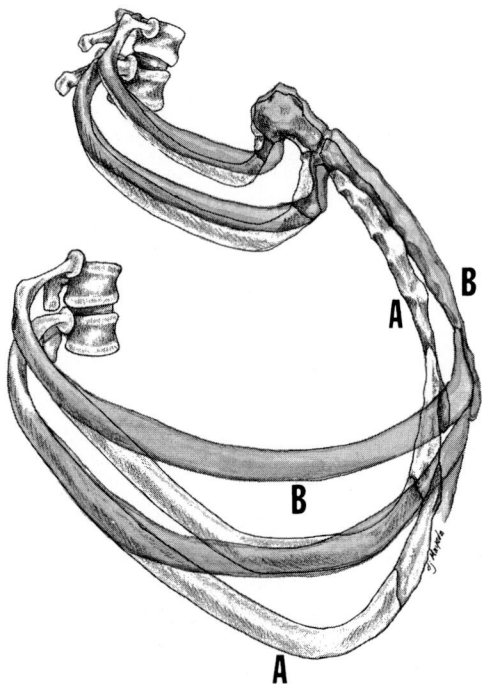

Fig. 1-1. The pump-handle movement in breathing. Compare the position of the sternum and ribs at (**A**) the beginning and (**B**) the end of inspiration. Note the increase in anteroposterior dimensions.

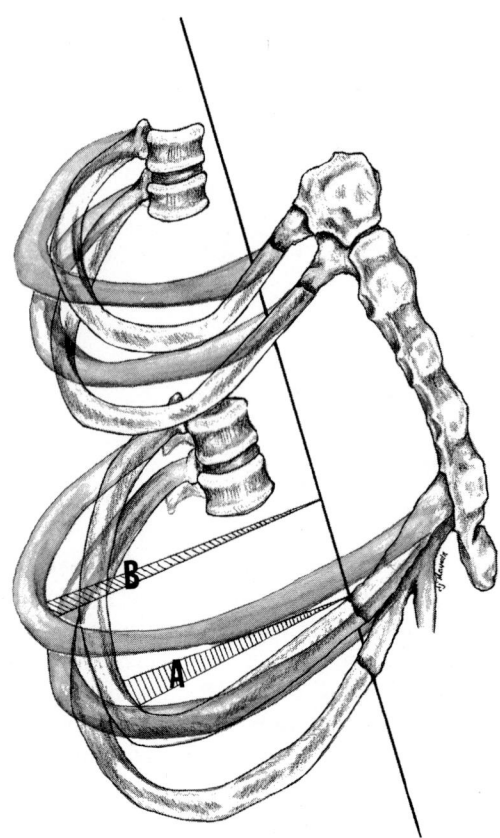

Fig. 1-2. The bucket-handle movement in breathing. Compare distance of the ribs from central axis of the thorax at (**A**) the beginning and (**B**) the end of inspiration. Note increase in lateral dimensions.

against the abdominal viscera, thereby increasing vertical intrathoracic dimensions. Contraction of its peripheral or costal muscle fibers also may produce an outward flaring of the lowest costal margin. During quiet respiration, the diaphragm undergoes an excursion of approximately 1 to 2 cm, but it may move as much as 6 to 7 cm during deep breathing. The lower ribs are believed to be helpful in resisting upward and medial pull of the diaphragm as a result of stabilization by the serratus posterior inferior muscles. The quadratus lumborum may stabilize the twelfth rib, but its effect on respiration is probably insignificant.

The diaphragm and intercostal muscles are therefore the primary muscles of inspiration. Movements of the diaphragm account for 75 to 80% of pulmonary ventilation during quiet respiration, compared with 20 to 25% contributed by the intercostal muscles, mainly the external intercostals and the anterior portions of the internal intercostals. During severe or labored breathing, however, other skeletal muscles may be used. The sternocleidomastoid, serratus posterior superior, and levatores costarum may be active in elevation of the ribs. Muscles of the extremities also may be helpful in moments of severe need. With the torso in fixed position, movement of the arms and shoulders away from the thorax may be sufficient to enlarge thoracic dimensions to a small but sometimes necessary degree. Deltoid, trapezius, pectoral, and latissimus dorsi muscles are involved in such activity.

Expiration can occur only when intrapulmonic pressure exceeds that of the atmosphere. At the end of inspiration, the lungs are inflated and stretched. Inspiratory muscles have reached optimal efficiency in expanding the rib cage against atmospheric pressure. At this point, elastic resistance of lung tissue is at first equal to and then greater than muscular forces that would retain the expanded state of the thorax. The lungs recoil elastically and the consequent increase in intrapulmonic pressure is sufficient to force air out of the lungs. Both soft and hard tissues of the thoracic wall comply passively with the reduction of lung volume, aided by atmospheric pressure directed against them. Expiration stops when intrapulmonic pressure is once again equal to atmospheric pressure. In quiet breathing, expiration is accomplished almost exclusively by elastic recoil of the lungs and rib cage. During vigorous or carefully controlled expiration, however, such as while singing, shouting, abdominal straining, or playing a wind instrument, muscles of the abdominal wall may aid in the reduction of thoracic dimensions by compression of abdominal viscera against the diaphragm.

Although the change from inspiratory to expiratory efforts thus represents a shift from active to passive events, the change in airflow is not a chaotic event. Rather, it is well regulated by the diaphragm, which continues to contract with decreasing efficiency but does not reach the zero point until the middle of expiration. In this respect, it is similar to the action of limb musculature, in which gradual relaxation of flexor muscles prevents uncoordinated movement of an extremity in the opposite direction by antagonistic extensors. As described by Agostini and Torri (1962), during maximal breathing efforts, the diaphragm also contracts toward the end of vigorous expiration, limiting the extent to which the lungs can collapse.

SURFACE LANDMARKS AND STRUCTURES SUPERFICIAL TO THE THORAX

The thoracic surgeon is primarily concerned with the thoracic wall and the thoracic contents; however, a few overall considerations of structures related to surface features are helpful in orientation to deeper structures of the thorax itself (Fig. 1-3). In all but the most obese subjects, the outline of the sternum can be visualized in the thoracic midline. Extending laterally and slightly upward from the jugular notch of the sternum, the clavicles curve forward and then backward toward the shoulders. From the lowermost margin of the body of the sternum, the lower margin of the rib cage diverges bilaterally to reach its lowest level at the midaxillary line.

The outline of the sternocleidomastoid muscles may be seen extending diagonally upward from the upper part of the anterior surface of the manubrium of the sternum and the medial one-third of the clavicle toward the base of the skull. Immediately below the clavicle, the outline of the

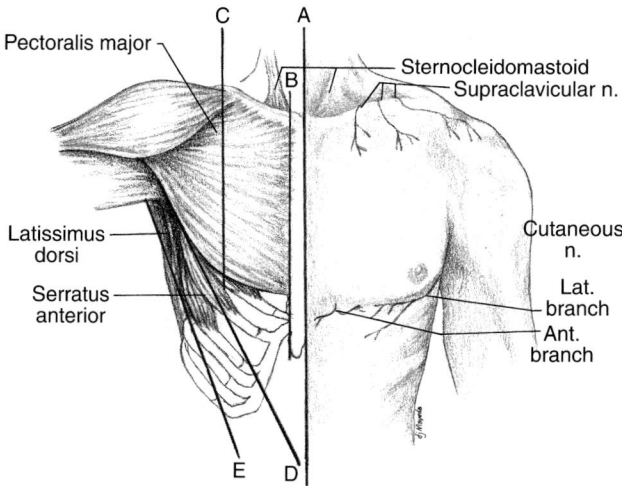

Fig. 1-3. Surface features and details of structures superficial to the thoracic wall in the pectoral region and the axilla. Musculoskeletal features are shown on the left. Surface features and cutaneous innervation are shown on the right. Cutaneous branches of the fifth intercostal space are illustrated as typical of other intercostal spaces not shown. Common lines of reference are shown. A, midsternal line; B, lateral sternal line; C, midclavicular line; D, anterior axillary fold; E, posterior axillary fold.

pectoralis major muscle is evident. These muscles extend bilaterally from broad clavicular, sternal, and costal origins, converge toward the axilla, and form a bilaminar, U-shaped tendon that attaches to the lateral lip of the intertubercular sulcus of the humerus. The lower margin of each pectoralis major muscle forms the anterior fold of the axilla. The pectoralis major muscles are supplied by medial and lateral pectoral nerves from the brachial plexus and are versatile in function. They adduct and rotate the arm medially and in addition may elevate it (clavicular portion) or depress it (sternocostal portion). If the shoulder girdle is held in fixed position, these muscles also may elevate the upper ribs in forced inspiration. During artificial respiration, pulling the flexed upper extremity toward the head may also force the pectoralis major muscles to elevate the upper ribs.

Deep to the pectoralis major muscles lie the pectoralis minor muscles. They originate by slips from the second to fifth ribs and converge upward to a tendon that inserts on the coracoid process of the scapula. Supplied also by the medial and lateral pectoral nerves, these muscles are active in depressing and rotating the shoulders downward.

In thin, muscular subjects, the serratus anterior muscles can be visualized along the anterolateral aspects of the thoracic wall. They originate by slips from the upper eight ribs. They are applied closely to the thoracic wall as they pass upward and laterally to attach to the anterior surface and medial border of the scapula on either side. They hold the scapulae toward the thoracic wall and are important in adduction and elevation of the arms above the horizontal position during scapulohumeral movement. On each side, the serratus anterior is supplied by the long thoracic nerve, which passes downward in the midaxillary line on the external surface of the muscle.

In men, the nipple lies near the lower border of the pectoralis major muscles, just lateral to the midclavicular line, over the fourth intercostal space or fourth or fifth ribs. Nipple position is inconsistent in women because of the variable size of the mammary gland, which lies generally over the second to sixth ribs. The axillary tail extends upward into the axilla along the lower border of the pectoralis major muscle.

Cutaneous innervation of the anterolateral thoracic wall is supplied by supraclavicular nerves and terminal filaments of thoracic spinal nerves. Skin above, overlying, and slightly below the clavicle is supplied by supraclavicular nerves, which arise as terminal filaments of spinal nerves C3 and C4. The remainder of the thoracic wall is supplied by anterior cutaneous and lateral cutaneous branches of thoracic spinal nerves.

The posterior aspect of the thorax is covered almost completely by superficial muscles of the back, but a few bony landmarks are either visible or palpable (Fig. 1-4). In the midline, the spinous process of the seventh cervical vertebra (vertebra prominens) stands out clearly. Below this process, the spine of the first thoracic vertebra may be equally visible. Spines of the remaining 11 thoracic verte-

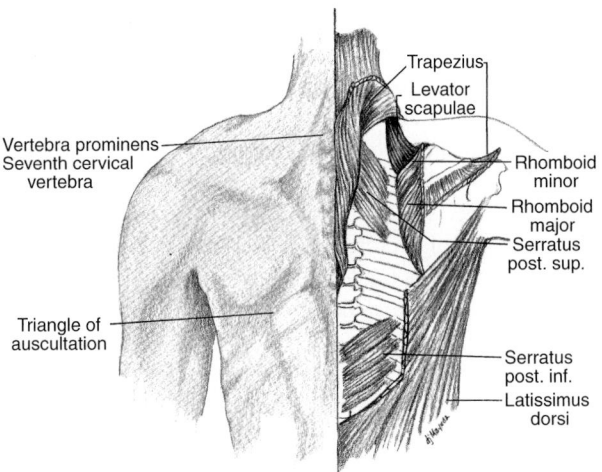

Fig. 1-4. Surface features and details of structures superficial to the posterior aspect of the thorax. The scapula has been displaced upward and laterally on the right side to permit a better view of muscles superficial to the thorax.

brae extend downward so that the tip of each overlies the body of the vertebra below. In the midthoracic levels, the vertebral spines may be sufficiently long to overlie the intervertebral disc below the subjacent vertebra. The medial border of each scapula lies lateral to the midline at the level of the second to seventh ribs. The spine of the scapula extends diagonally upward from the medial border at approximately the third thoracic vertebra to end in the acromion at the shoulder.

Surface contours of the back of the thorax are formed by muscles of the shoulder and scapular region; these muscles support and help move the upper extremity. Posterolateral margins of the neck and uppermost limits of the shoulder are marked by the trapezius muscles. Each of these arises from broad origins, including the superior nuchal line of the occipital bone, the ligamentum nuchae of the neck, the spine of the seventh cervical vertebra, and spines and supraspinous ligaments of all thoracic vertebrae. Fibers sweep downward, laterally, and upward toward the shoulder, where they insert on the spine and acromion of the scapula and on the lateral one-third of the clavicle. In lower cervical and upper thoracic levels, their aponeurotic origin is sufficiently devoid of muscle fibers to allow spines of thoracic vertebrae to be easily palpable. The trapezius muscles are supplied by spinal accessory nerves and by filaments from cervical spinal levels C3 and C4. They are powerful stabilizers of the scapulae and shoulders and can elevate, depress, or adduct the scapulae, thereby aiding in the entire spectrum of scapulohumeral movements.

Lower and lateral parts of the back of the thorax are covered by the latissimus dorsi muscles. These muscles arise by broad aponeurotic origins, from spines of lower thoracic vertebrae, the lumbodorsal fascia, and the iliac crests. Additional slips of muscle also arise from outer surfaces of the lower three or four ribs and blend with overlying com-

ponents. Muscle fibers converge upward to insert by tendons into the intertubercular groove of the humerus on each side. In their upper thirds, these muscles converge with the teres major muscles to form the posterior folds of the axillae. The latissimus dorsi muscles are adductors, extensors, and medial rotators of the arm. Each is supplied by a thoracodorsal nerve from the posterior cord of the brachial plexus. Because of attachment to the ribs, the latissimus dorsi muscles also can be considered accessory muscles of respiration.

The lower border of the trapezius muscle overlies the upper border of the latissimus dorsi. Near the point of overlap, a triangle is formed by the lateral border of the trapezius, the upper border of the latissimus dorsi, and the medial border of the scapula. Save for lower fibers of the rhomboid muscles, this area is free of an intervening mass of muscle tissue. Because a stethoscope placed over this triangle can detect respiratory sounds relatively free of distortion, it is called the *triangle of auscultation.*

Deep to the trapezius and latissimus dorsi muscles lies a layer of muscles involved in scapular movements and, to a lesser degree, movements of the ribs. Those related to the scapula are the levator scapulae, rhomboid major, and rhomboid minor muscles. The thin levator scapulae extend from the transverse processes of the first three or four cervical vertebrae diagonally downward to attach at the superior angle of the scapula on each side. The rhomboid minor may be fused with the rhomboid major. It extends from spines of the seventh cervical vertebra and first thoracic vertebra to the medial border of the scapula near the base of its spine. The rhomboid major arises from the spines of the second to fifth thoracic vertebrae and the supraspinous ligament between these vertebrae and is attached to the medial border of the scapula, usually below the spine of the scapula. The levator scapulae, rhomboid major, and rhomboid minor elevate, adduct, and retract the scapula. All are supplied by the dorsal scapular nerve, but the levator scapulae are supplied also by branches from C4 and C5.

The serratus posterior muscles are said to be inspiratory muscles and thus merit brief attention. The serratus posterior superior muscles arise by aponeuroses from the ligamentum nuchae and spinous processes of the seventh cervical vertebra and the first to third thoracic vertebrae and are attached to the upper borders of the first three to five ribs. They are supplied by ventral rami of segmental spinal nerves (intercostal nerves) and are said to be active in the elevation of the upper ribs. The serratus posterior inferior muscles take aponeurotic origins from spinous processes of the lower two thoracic and upper two lumbar vertebrae; they insert by muscular slips on the lower three or four ribs. They are supplied also by ventral rami of segmental spinal nerves and are presumably able to prevent upward displacement of their ribs during inspiration.

Innervation of skin over the back is provided by medial cutaneous branches of dorsal rami of C4, C5, C8, T1, and T2 and by medial and lateral cutaneous branches of T3–T10.

Considerable overlap and asymmetry of these nerves have been described by Johnston (1908).

ANATOMIC FEATURES

Firm structural support for the thorax is provided by the sternum, 10 pairs of costae: ribs and costal cartilages, two pairs of ribs without cartilage, and 12 thoracic vertebrae and their intervertebral discs. Collectively, these components surround a cavity that is reniform in cross-section, related to the neck above by a narrow thoracic inlet and to the abdominal cavity below by a larger thoracic outlet. The inlet is surrounded by the manubrium of the sternum, the first ribs, and the first thoracic vertebra. Its anterior boundaries lie approximately 1 inch below the posterior limits. The inlet is roofed by bilateral thickened endothoracic fascia (Sibson's fascia or suprapleural membrane) and subjacent parietal pleura, which project upward into the base of the neck. Additional details of soft tissue relations of the thoracic inlet are considered at the end of this chapter in the section on Surface Anatomy. The outlet is formed by the xiphoid process, fused costal cartilages of ribs 7 to 10, the anterior portions of the eleventh ribs, the shafts of the twelfth ribs, and the body of the twelfth thoracic vertebra. The anterior margin of the outlet is at the level of the tenth thoracic, the lateral limits at the second lumbar, and the posterior margin at the twelfth thoracic vertebra. The outlet is therefore higher at its anterior margin than at its posterior limit and reaches its lowest level in the lateral aspect near the midaxillary line. It is sealed off from the abdominal cavity by the diaphragm.

Sternum and Its Joints

The sternum is an elongated, flat bone that lies in the anterior midline. It is 15 to 20 cm long and is formed from cartilaginous precursors that ossify separately to form three components: the manubrium, body, and xiphoid process (Fig. 1-5).

The manubrium is approximately 5 cm wide in its upper half and 2.5 to 3.0 cm wide in its lower half. Its upper border is thickened and marked on either side by a notch for articulation with the clavicle. Centrally, an indentation is present, which together with the sternal ends of each clavicle forms the jugular, suprasternal notch. The widest portion of the manubrium is marked by bilateral indentations, the costal incisura, to accommodate articulation of the first costal cartilage. At the lower limits, each lateral margin of the bone is indented by a demifacet for articulation of the upper half of the second costal cartilage. The lower margin of the manubrium articulates with the body of the sternum.

The body or longest portion of the sternum is slightly more than twice the length of the manubrium. It is slanted at a steeper angle than the manubrium; hence its articulation with that bone forms an angle, called the *sternal angle*. The outer border of this angle is readily palpable and lies at the level of the fourth to fifth thoracic vertebrae or their intervening intervertebral disc. The joint is a synchondrosis:

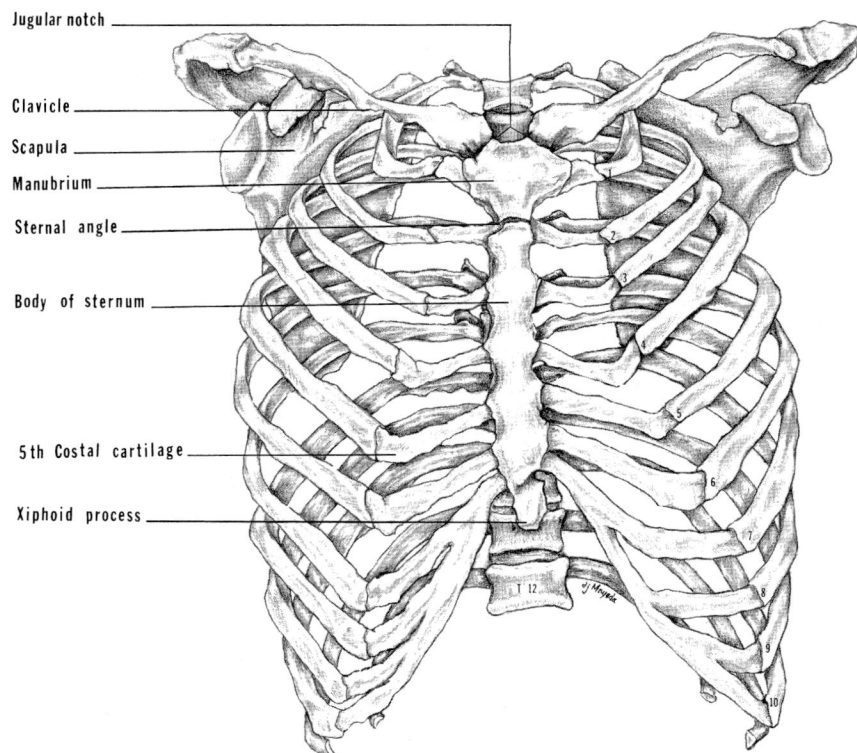

Jugular notch

Clavicle

Scapula

Manubrium

Sternal angle

Body of sternum

5th Costal cartilage

Xiphoid process

Fig. 1-5. Anterior view of the skeleton of the thorax and bones of the pectoral girdle. Bilateral asymmetry is evident in the body and xiphoid process of the sternum. The left subcostal arch is slightly higher than the right one.

Articular surfaces of each bone are covered with hyaline cartilage and are united by fibrocartilage. It is sufficiently flexible to allow movement of the body on the more stable manubrium during respiratory movements. Ossification of the joint may form a synostosis during adult years, thus limiting flexibility, but as noted by Trotter (1934), correlation is not observed between age and its incidence.

Lateral margins of the body exhibit segmental incisurae for articulation of costal cartilages two to seven. The incisura for the second costal cartilage is incomplete, for it represents only the lower half of the articulation surface that is completed by the demifacet on the lower margin of the manubrium. The body ends at approximately the level of the tenth to eleventh thoracic vertebrae, where it forms a cartilaginous joint with the xiphoid process.

The xiphoid is a cartilaginous process that is usually ossified by middle age. It is the shortest and thinnest part of the sternum and may occasionally be bifid or perforated. It extends downward for a variable distance to end in the sheath of the rectus abdominis muscle. Its posterior surface is even with that of the sternal body; its anterior surface is somewhat recessed. The xiphoid is flexible at the xiphisternal joint, but it moves with the sternum during respiratory movements. Supportive costoxiphoid ligaments, extending from its anterior surface to the front of the seventh costal cartilage, prevent its backward displacement by contractions of the diaphragm.

The midline of the sternum is almost completely subcutaneous and is therefore easily accessible for sternal puncture, sternal transfusion, or incision during thoracic surgery. Its lateral margins are covered by origins of the sternal components of the pectoralis major muscles.

Ribs and Their Joints

The size and shape of the thorax are largely determined by the ribs and costal cartilages. A rib and its associated cartilage are properly termed a *costa*. The costae form continuous arches that extend backward for a short distance in relation to the vertebrae, turn forward at the angle, and extend toward the sternum, with which all but two pairs of them articulate directly or indirectly. Developmentally, the costae arise as arched, cartilaginous struts extending serially and horizontally from their respective vertebral bodies to the sternum. As development proceeds, the vertebral ends of each costal pair migrate cephalad. This shift in position is more pronounced in costal pairs two to nine and, as a result, the head of each of these ribs becomes pressed against the body of the vertebra immediately above. At the end of the growth period, ribs two to nine articulate with both their own and the immediately supra-adjacent vertebrae. The tenth rib may migrate sufficiently to articulate with the ninth and tenth thoracic vertebrae, or it may remain low enough to articulate only with the body of the tenth thoracic vertebra. The eleventh and twelfth ribs migrate only slightly and thus form joints only with their own vertebrae. The angle of costal elements of the thoracic wall relative to the vertebrae and the sternum is therefore the result of cephalic migration of vertebral extremities and relative retention of sternal extremities at their original levels.

Ossification is initiated at the bend or angle of the costae. It spreads posteriorly toward the vertebrae and anteriorly toward the sternum. By the time bone deposition stops, the short vertebral portion is completely ossified. Because that part of the costa from the angle forward is longer, its ossification is not complete by the time bone formation ceases. The ossified portion of each costa becomes the rib proper and the unossified part remains as costal cartilage.

Relations of ribs and their costal cartilages to the sternum and to each other vary at different levels (Fig. 1-6; see Fig 1-5). The upper seven pairs of ribs articulate directly with the sternum by way of costal cartilages and are therefore called true or vertebrosternal ribs. In contrast, the lower five pairs are called false ribs, because they do not articulate with the sternum at all. Of the false ribs, three pairs (the eighth, ninth, and tenth) are called vertebrocostal because their associated cartilages articulate with immediately supradjacent cartilages. The remaining pairs, 11 and 12, terminate in cartilaginous tips, ending in muscles of the abdominal wall. Because their only articulation is with the vertebrae, they are called vertebral ribs.

The costal cartilages change sequentially in length and direction. The first and second costal cartilages are short and follow a slightly downward course. The third and fourth gradually increase in length and are horizontal, or nearly so. The fifth to seventh cartilages extend downward from the tip of their ribs and then turn upward to meet the sternum. Because both ribs and cartilages of these costae are the longest and most flexible, they are maximally involved in the bucket-handle rib movement. The fused cartilages of ribs 7 to 10 course diagonally upward to the lower end of the sternum to form the infrasternal angle.

Ribs exhibit many similar features, but their form is variable at different levels. They increase in length from the first to the seventh and then gradually shorten to the twelfth. The most common features are characteristic of ribs three to nine, which are frequently called *typical ribs*. From their vertebral to sternal ends, each of these ribs is formed by a head, a neck, and a shaft (Fig. 1-7). The head is enlarged and marked by two facets, separated by an interarticular crest. The upper facet articulates with a facet on the body of the supradjacent vertebra. A slightly larger inferior facet articulates with a facet on the body of the adjacent vertebra whose number corresponds with that of the rib. The joint formed between costal facets, supradjacent, and adjacent vertebral bodies is termed a *costovertebral joint*.

The neck of each rib extends dorsolaterally for approximately 2.5 cm and is marked by a crest on its upper border. The end of the neck and beginning of the shaft are marked by a tubercle. The tubercle bears a roughened elevation and a smooth articular surface. The elevation serves as an attachment for costotransverse ligaments. The articular surface

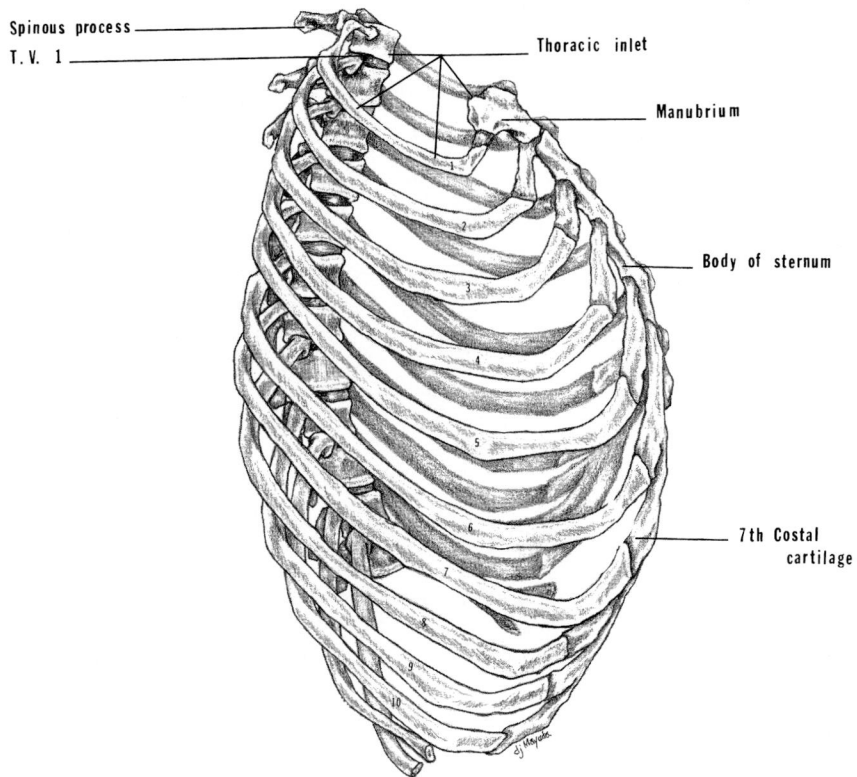

Fig. 1-6. Lateral view of the thoracic cage.

meets a facet on the transverse process of the corresponding vertebra to form the costotransverse joint.

The shaft of the rib extends dorsolaterally for an additional 5.0 to 7.5 cm and then turns gradually forward and downward. The accentuated portion of this forward curvature is called the angle of the rib. The angle marks the lateral extent of the erector spinae muscles of the back. Throughout its course, the shaft is twisted slightly so that its superolateral border is rounded and convex. The lower margin of the inferomedial surface is scored by a costal groove for the intercostal vessels and nerves. This groove is most clearly defined on the inner aspect of the posterior half of each rib. The shaft terminates in a small indentation, which forms a hyaline-cartilaginous joint with its costal cartilage.

The less typical ribs differ in the following respects. The first rib is shorter than the rest and, beyond its neck, is wider and more curved. The head is small and bears only one facet for articulation with the body of the first thoracic vertebra. The upper and lower surfaces of the shaft are flat and its edges are sharp. Near the middle of the shaft, a rounded tubercle is present that serves as an attachment for the anterior scalene muscle. Behind the tubercle is a depression where the first rib is crossed by the subclavian artery. A smaller depression for the subclavian vein may sometimes be noted in front of the tubercle.

The second rib is nearly twice the length of the first and articulates with the bodies of the first and second thoracic vertebrae. Its shaft is curved but not twisted and is marked

by a roughened tubercle for upper digitations of the serratus anterior muscle.

The eleventh and twelfth ribs are sequentially shorter than supradjacent ones and bear only one articular surface for

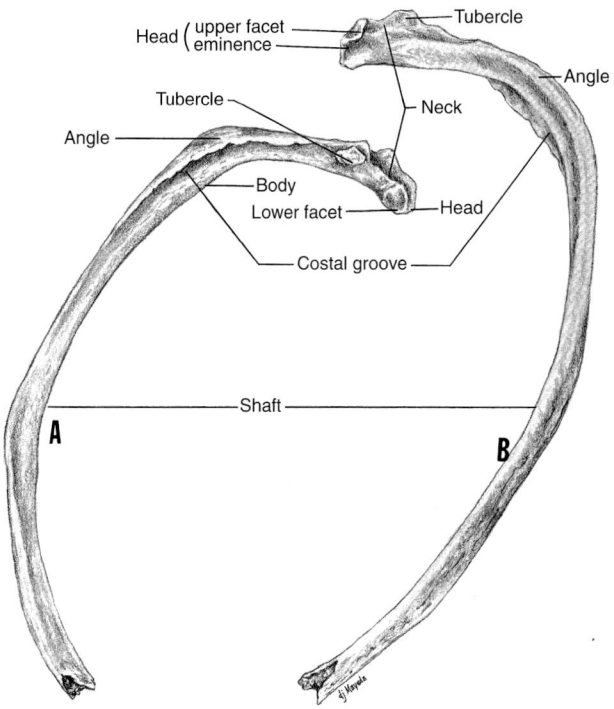

Fig. 1-7. A typical rib. **A.** Inferior view. **B.** Superior view.

their corresponding vertebrae. They exhibit poorly defined or completely absent necks, angles, and costal grooves. The length of the twelfth rib is of consequence in renal surgery. Although it is often shorter in a woman than in a man, Hughes (1949) has shown that longer ones, 11 to 14 cm, are more common than shorter ones, 1.5 to 6.0 cm. The posterior margin of parietal pleura normally crosses the twelfth rib at the lateral margin of the erector spinae muscles. If the twelfth rib is short, the surgeon may inadvertently palpate the lower border of the eleventh rib to determine the level for the initial incision. Such an incision risks entering the thoracic cavity instead of extraperitoneal tissue or renal fascia behind the kidneys.

Variations in rib structure may be of clinical significance. The first rib may be fused with the second at the scalene tubercle. This union is usually associated with other variations in the second rib, sternum, or associated thoracic vertebrae. The seventh cervical vertebra may bear a cartilaginous or ossified rib called a cervical rib. Such a rib may be short or it may be attached to the first costal cartilage or to the manubrium. Variations in the thoracic inlet or the presence of a cervical rib can produce compression of the subclavian artery and the brachial plexus, resulting in compromise of neurovascular supply to the upper extremity. Occasionally, the sternal extremity of the third or fourth rib may be bifid, and the eighth rib may reach the sternum on one or both sides. A lumbar rib may be associated with the first lumbar vertebra.

The structure of the heads of ribs two through nine and the associated vertebrae shows that the costovertebral joints consist of two joint cavities, each composed of costal and vertebral facets. The cavities are separated by a ligament extending from the interarticular crest of the rib to the intervertebral disc. Articular surfaces are covered with fibrous cartilage; joint cavities are surrounded by a synovial articular capsule. The capsule is thickened by radiate ligaments that fan out from the head of the rib to adjacent vertebral bodies.

Costotransverse joints, between the articular tubercle and the transverse process of the rib, are also synovial. Articular surfaces are covered with hyaline cartilage and the joint is enclosed by a fibrous capsule. The capsule is reinforced by costotransverse ligaments, which connect the neck and tubercle of the rib to the transverse process of its own vertebra and to that immediately above. Motions involved in both the bucket-handle and pump-handle movements of breathing are permitted by the flexibility of both the costovertebral and costotransverse joints. Fixation of these joints adversely affects pulmonary function.

Intercostal Spaces

The frequency with which the spaces between ribs are used in surgical approaches to the thorax prescribes an understanding of their muscular, fascial, and neurovascular features (Figs. 1-8 through 1-11). Lying deep to the skin,

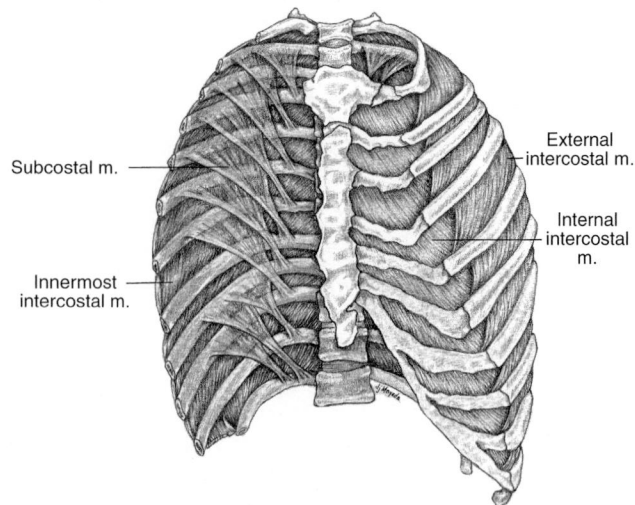

Fig. 1-8. Anterior view of the thoracic wall and muscles of the intercostal spaces. The left side of the thorax is intact. The anterior half of the right side has been removed to demonstrate the inner aspect of the posterolateral thoracic wall.

superficial fascia (tela subcutanea), and muscles related to the thoracic girdle and upper extremity, each intercostal space is traversed by three layers of muscle and their related deep fascia. Both muscles and fascia are attached to periosteum at the upper and lower borders of the ribs. During thoracoplasty, an incision over the body of the rib and subsequent retraction of its periosteum during removal of the rib do not violate the contents of the intercostal spaces.

From the surgical approach, the first layer of tissue to be encountered within the intercostal space is composed of the external intercostal muscles. Their fibers extend diagonally downward and forward from the lower margin of each rib to

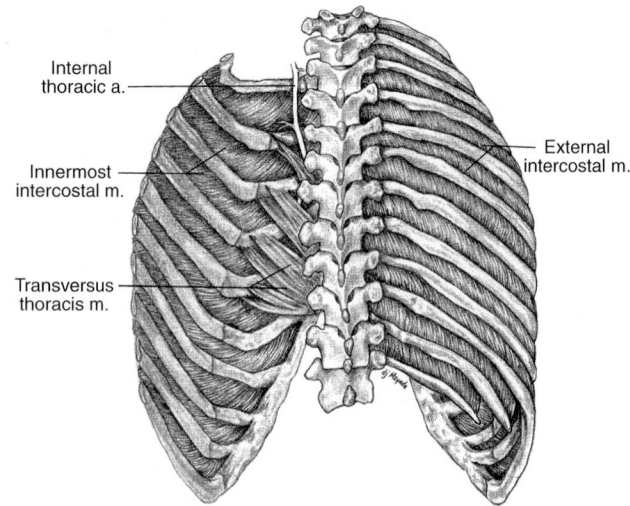

Fig. 1-9. Posterior view of the thoracic wall and muscles of the intercostal spaces. The right side of the thorax is intact. The posterior half of the left side has been removed to show the inner aspect of the anterior thoracic wall.

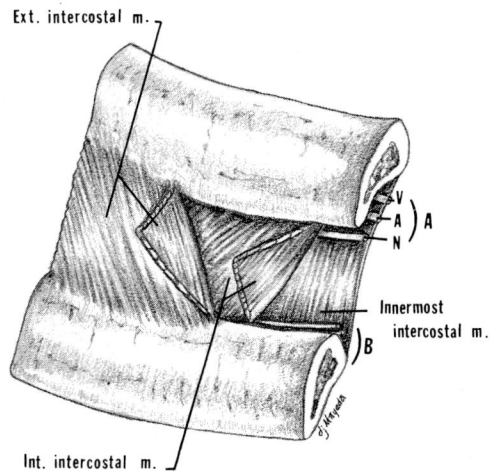

Fig. 1-10. Relations of structures within an intercostal space. **A.** Intercostal vessels and nerves are shown. **B.** Collateral vessels are shown. A, artery; N, nerve; V, vein.

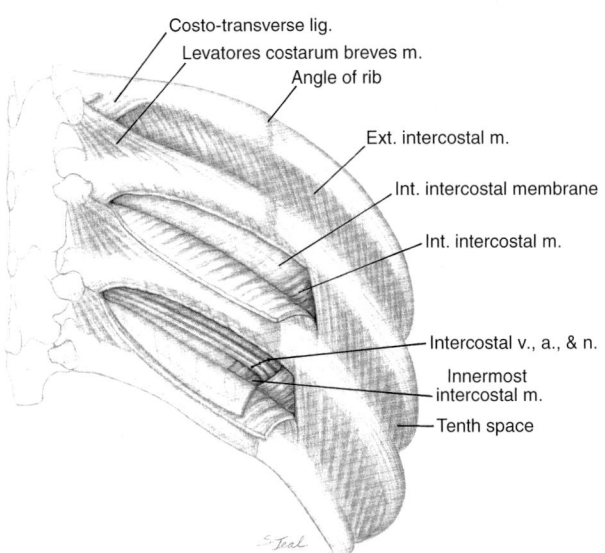

Fig. 1-11. Exposure of the posterior part of intercostal spaces 8, 9, and 10. Note that the intercostal vein (v.), artery (a.), and nerve (n.) lie between the internal intercostal muscle and the innermost intercostal muscle layers. From the intervertebral foramen to the angle of the rib, the intercostal vessels and nerves are covered by the internal intercostal membrane.

the upper margin of the subjacent rib. Musculature of this layer is continuous from a posterior position at the tubercle of the rib and posterior fibers of the costotransverse ligament (Fig. 1-12; see Figs. 1-9 and 1-11) to an anterior position at or near the costal cartilages. At this point, the investing fascia of the muscle continues further anteriorly to the sternum as the external, anterior intercostal membrane (Fig. 1-13; see Fig. 1-12). Intercostal muscles of the lower seven intercostal spaces interdigitate with the external oblique muscle of the abdominal wall. The next layer encountered consists of the internal intercostal muscles and their fascia. Muscle fibers extend downward and backward

between costal cartilages in the anterior-medial part of the intercostal space and between the ribs proper further laterally and posteriorly in the intercostal space. The reverse direction of these muscle fibers from those of the external intercostal muscle lends a cross-diagonal supportive force. Musculature of this layer extends from the sternum (see

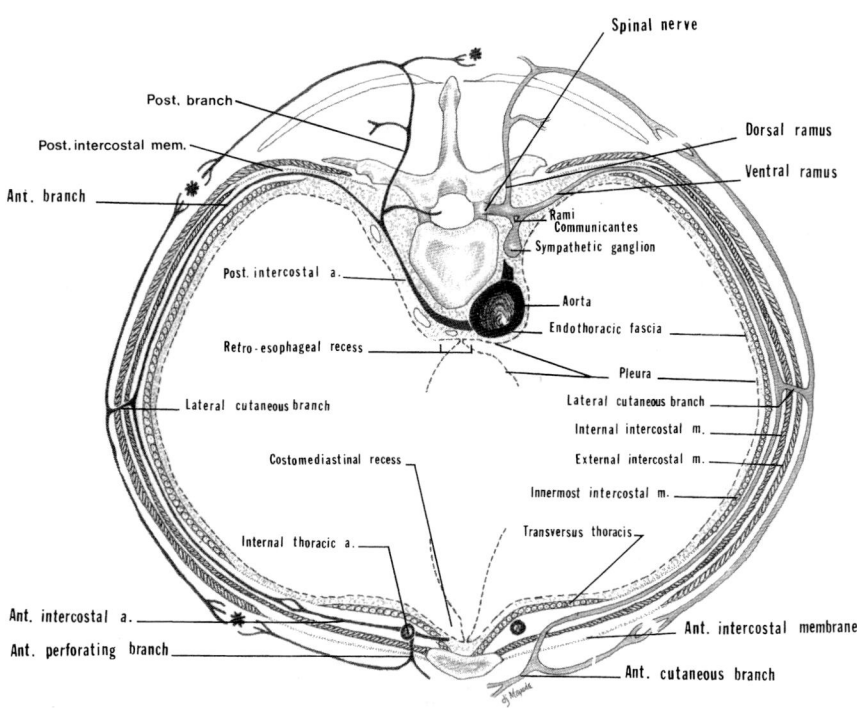

Fig. 1-12. Summary scheme of structures within an intercostal space. Arteries are shown on the left, nerves on the right.

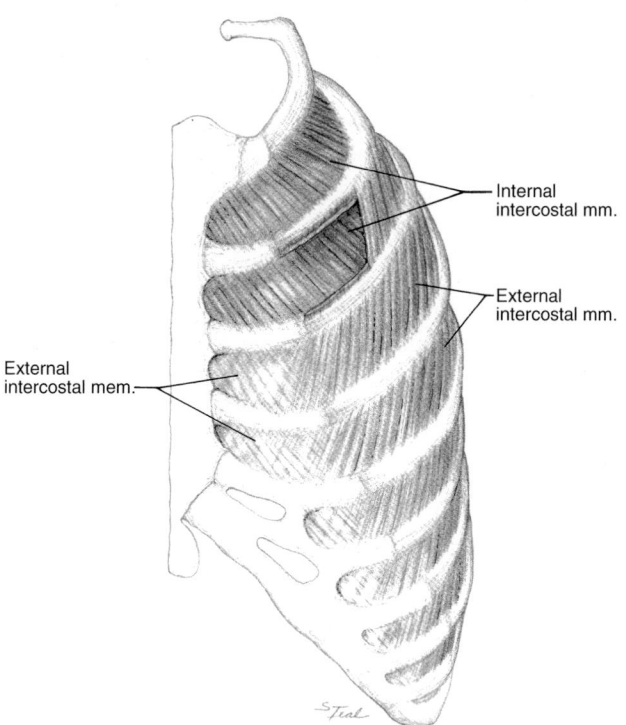

Internal
intercostal mm.

External
intercostal mm.

External
intercostal mem.

Fig. 1-13. Anterior view of the left half of the thorax. Note the opposing diagonal course of the external intercostal muscle fibers versus those of the internal intercostal muscle fibers. The external, anterior intercostal membrane extends from the costochondral junction to the sternum in the intercostal spaces.

Figs. 1-12 and 1-13) as far posteriad as the angle of the ribs (see Figs. 1-11 and 1-12). At this point, their investing fasciae form the internal-posterior-intercostal membrane, which attaches to the tubercle of each rib and the adjacent vertebra (see Fig. 1-11). Neurovascular components of the intercostal spaces are encountered immediately deep to these two layers. From above downward, the intercostal vein, artery, and nerve enter the posterior part of the intercostal space (see Figs. 1-11 and 1-12). In this region, they lie within the endothoracic fascia deep to the internal intercostal membrane and just superficial to parietal pleura (see Fig. 1-12). They remain in this position for a distance of 4 to 6 cm, at which point they gain the space between the internal and innermost intercostal muscles along the costal groove near the angle of the ribs (see Figs. 1-7 and Figs. 1-10 through 1-12). The neurovascular component therefore lies in the upper limits of the intercostal space, in contrast to the collateral branches, which lie in the lower limits. The origin and distribution of these neurovascular elements are considered in detail later. Their position with respect to the ribs is important during incision of the intercostal space. Because major intercostal vessels and nerves lie in close relation to the lower border of each rib, incisions near this level are to be avoided. A preferable site is along the upper margin of each rib. Although accessory nerves and vessels may be sectioned at this level, loss of function or sensitivity is negligi-

ble. It is equally important, however, to understand that the overlap of adjacent nerves is so great that paralysis and complete anesthesia are seldom produced within one intercostal space unless its nerve, the one above, and the one below are all severed.

The next layer of tissue encountered is less well defined. It consists of the innermost intercostal, subcostal, and transversus thoracis muscles and their fasciae. The innermost intercostals are best developed in the middle portion of the intercostal space (see Figs. 1-9 through 1-12) and may be absent completely in the upper regions of the thoracic wall. They extend between adjacent ribs in the same direction as the internal intercostal muscles. Davies and associates (1932) considered them inner laminae of the internal intercostal muscles. The subcostal muscles extend as a variable number of slips from the lower margin of the angle of the ribs, diagonally across more than one intercostal space to the upper margin of the second or third rib below. The transversus thoracis is a thin layer of muscle on the inner aspect of the anterior thoracic wall. Aponeurotic slips of this muscle extend diagonally upward from the body and xiphoid process of the sternum to costal cartilages. The lowermost fibers of the transversus thoracis are almost horizontal and are continuous with the transversus abdominis muscle of the abdominal wall.

Deep to the third layer of muscles is the endothoracic fascia. It consists of variable amounts of areolar connective tissue, affording a natural cleavage plane for separation of the subjacent pleura from the thoracic wall.

The arterial supply of the intercostal spaces consists of posterior and anterior intercostal arteries. The posterior intercostal arteries of the first and second intercostal spaces arise from the highest intercostal arteries, which are branches of the subclavian artery; those of the remaining nine intercostal spaces are branches of the thoracic aorta. These arteries supply most of their respective intercostal spaces except the anteriormost limits. Each gives rise to a posterior branch supplying the spinal cord and deep muscles and skin of the back, an anterior branch running between the vein and nerve in the costal groove, and a collateral branch arising near the angle of the rib and descending to the upper border of the rib below. In the midaxillary line, each anterior branch gives rise to a lateral cutaneous branch, which perforates the intercostal space to supply overlying skin. The posterior intercostal artery coursing below the twelfth rib is called the subcostal artery. It follows a course similar to those above but has no collateral branches.

The anterior intercostal arteries arise as segmental branches of the internal thoracic arteries in the first five or six intercostal spaces and as branches of the musculophrenic arteries in the lower intercostal spaces. Two such arteries are given off in each intercostal space, one passing toward the upper rib and one toward the lower. They continue laterally to anastomose with terminal branches of anterior and collateral branches of the posterior intercostal arteries.

The intercostal spaces are drained by 11 pairs of posterior intercostal veins and one pair of subcostal veins. These vessels follow the course of the posterior intercostal arteries and for the most part are tributary to the azygos or hemiazygos venous system. They lie above the nerve and artery throughout their course. Major blood flow is directed posteriorly by valves, but terminal vessels also may be tributary to the internal thoracic veins by way of small anterior intercostal veins. Posterior intercostal veins of the first intercostal space may be tributary to the brachiocephalic, vertebral, or superior intercostal veins. The second, third, and fourth posterior intercostal veins drain into the superior intercostal vein on each side; these in turn drain into the brachiocephalic vein on the left and into the azygos vein on the right. Right and left subcostal veins join the ascending lumbar veins on their respective sides of the thorax and ascend as the azygos and hemiazygos veins, respectively.

Lymphatic drainage of the anterior limits of the upper four or five intercostal spaces enters the sternal, internal thoracic nodes, which lie along the internal thoracic arteries. Their efferent vessels are tributary to a single vessel that joins the bronchomediastinal trunk. These nodes may be invaded commonly by metastases from breast carcinoma. Posterolateral portions of the intercostal spaces are drained by lymphatics that are tributary to one or two nodes near the vertebral ends of each intercostal space. Such nodes also receive lymphatic tributaries from the pleura. Nodes of upper intercostal spaces drain into the thoracic duct; those of the lower spaces are tributary to the cisterna chyli.

The thoracic wall is innervated segmentally by 12 pairs of thoracic spinal nerves. Upper thoracic spinal nerves also supply innervation to the axilla and upper extremity. Lower thoracic spinal nerves also supply portions of the abdominal wall and are called thoracoabdominal nerves. The midthoracic spinal nerves, T4–T6, exhibit the most common pattern and are considered typical nerves to the thoracic wall. Each spinal nerve is formed from a dorsal and a ventral root. The dorsal root contains sensory neurons that are distributed to posterior gray columns of the spinal cord. The ventral root contains somatic motor neurons originating in anterior gray columns of the spinal cord. Near the intervertebral foramen, the dorsal and ventral roots unite to form a mixed spinal nerve. Each spinal nerve gives rise to a small meningeal nerve and then passes out of the intervertebral foramen, to branch into a dorsal and ventral ramus (see Fig. 1-12).

The dorsal ramus of the thoracic spinal nerve passes backward to supply paravertebral back muscles and skin of the back. It forms medial and lateral cutaneous branches. Medial branches supply periosteum, ligaments, and joints of the vertebrae, as well as deep muscles of the back before terminating in cutaneous filaments. Lateral branches supply the small levator costae muscles and deep back muscles and follow a long descending course before becoming cutaneous. Extensive terminal overlap and anastomoses occur among medial and lateral cutaneous branches of dorsal rami from different spinal levels. Consequently, cutaneous pain is difficult to localize in this region.

Just lateral to the intervertebral foramen, the ventral ramus of the thoracic nerve establishes communications with the sympathetic chain by two branches or rami communicantes (see Fig. 1-12). The white ramus contains preganglionic sympathetic fibers, and the gray ramus contains postganglionic sympathetic fibers. Beyond this point, the ramus continues as the intercostal nerve and is responsible for segmental distribution to skin, muscle, and serous membranes of the thoracic wall. Each intercostal nerve passes backward below the rib in the vicinity of costotransverse ligaments and then gains the costal groove. It continues its course in the plane between the innermost intercostal and internal intercostal muscles. Near the angle of the rib, a collateral branch is given off. This branch passes laterally and then forward in the lower part of the intercostal space, terminating as a lower anterior cutaneous nerve.

Near the midaxillary line, a lateral cutaneous branch is given off. It pierces the intercostal muscles, passes through the serratus anterior muscles, and then forms anterior and posterior cutaneous branches.

Just lateral to the sternal margin, the intercostal nerve lies between transversus thoracis and internal intercostal muscles. At this point, it pierces overlying internal and external intercostal muscles, becomes subcutaneous, and forms anterior and median cutaneous branches.

Each segment of the thoracic wall is thus supplied circumferentially from behind and forward by branches of the dorsal ramus and collateral, lateral, and anterior branches of the ventral ramus. The ventral rami (intercostal nerves) supply the intercostal, subcostal, serratus posterior superior, and transversus thoracis muscles and the skin overlying the intercostal spaces. Although the pattern of innervation for each intercostal space is basically similar, considerable intersegmental overlap is characteristic. For that reason, complete paralysis or anesthesia in only one intercostal space does not occur unless the nerve of that space, as well as those of the intercostal spaces above and below, is sectioned.

Surface Anatomy

Knowledge of the surface relations of lobes and fissures of the lungs is important in percussion, auscultation, and radiographic evaluation of the pulmonary field. Although the lungs are in constant motion during respiration, the surface relations observed by Brock (1954) are essentially as described in Chapter 6. Knowledge of the topography of the various fissures of the lung is helpful in localizing abnormal pulmonary sounds as well as in localizing abnormal densities in radiographs of the chest (Figs. 1-14 and 1-15).

For surgical purposes, the lungs and pleura may be considered coextensive, with their respective costal, mediastinal, and diaphragmatic surfaces separated only by a film of serous fluid. In quiet respiration, those parts of the lung within the costomediastinal and costodiaphragmatic recesses

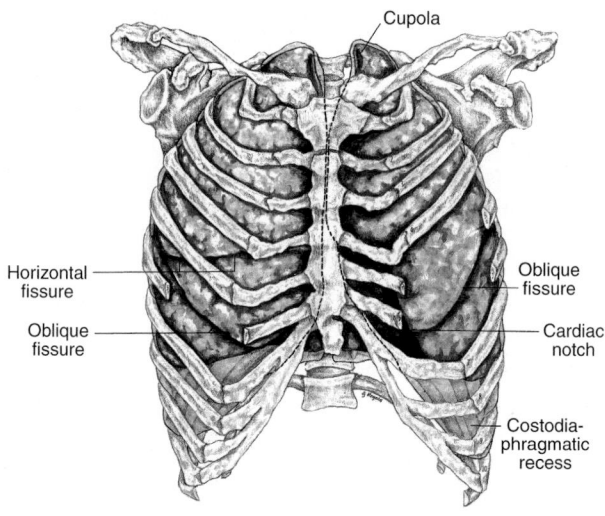

Fig. 1-14. Anterior view of the thorax showing surface relations of pleura and lungs. Pleural borders subjacent to bone are shown by interrupted lines.

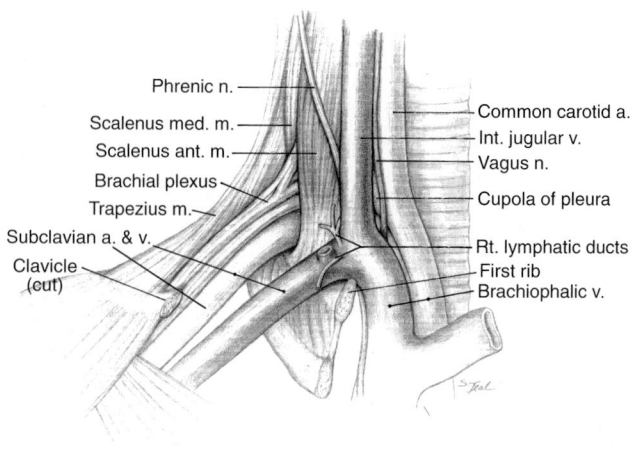

Fig. 1-16. Relations of the pleural cupola on the right side. Note the position of the cupola near the inferior and medial border of the scalenus anterior muscle, where it is crossed by the phrenic and vagus nerves. The subclavian artery passes anterior to the insertion of the scalenus anterior muscle on the first rib. The subclavian artery and the brachial plexus lie posterior and lateral to the muscle.

are inflated insufficiently to be identified by percussion. Percussible limits of the lower border of the lung normally lie at slightly higher levels than the lower limits of the pleura. The frequency with which indwelling lines or catheters are surgically inserted into the subclavian veins and the consequence of damaging nearby pleura or neurovascular structures require special knowledge of soft tissue relations at the thoracic inlet (Figs. 1-16 and 1-17). On both sides of the thorax, the subclavian vein lies deep to the clavicle and crosses the first rib anterior to the attachment of the serratus anterior

muscle on the scalene tubercle of the first rib. The second part of the subclavian artery passes posterior to the scalenus anterior muscle and its third part lies lateral to the attachment of muscle on the first rib. Likewise, components of the brachial plexus pass behind and then lateral to the scalenus anterior muscle. More important, in relation to pulmonary function, the cupola of the pleura is consistently related to the inferior and medial border of the scalenus anterior muscle. In this position, the cupola reaches its most superficial position

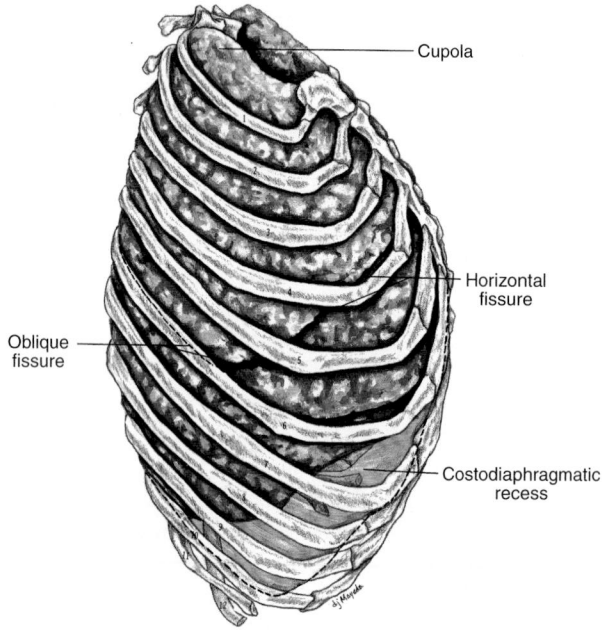

Fig. 1-15. Lateral view of the thorax showing surface relations of pleura and lungs.

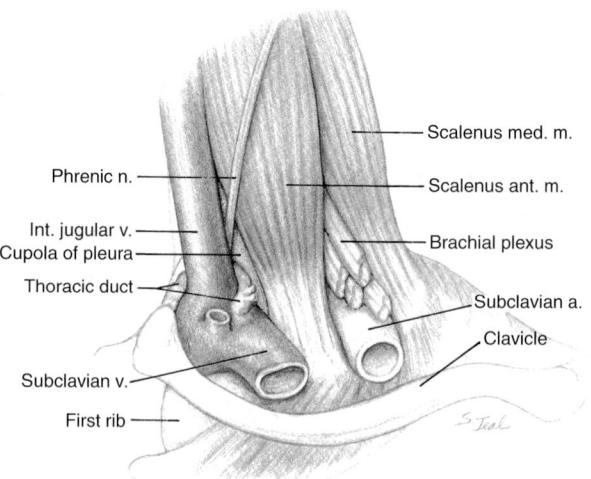

Fig. 1-17. Relations of the pleural cupola on the left side. Note the position of the cupola near the inferior and medial border of the scalenus anterior muscle. The cupola is crossed by the phrenic and vagus nerves. The vagus nerve lies between the internal jugular vein and the common carotid artery, but it is not visible in this dissection.

and therefore is susceptible to damage during invasive surgical procedures. This portion of the cupola also is crossed superficially by the phrenic nerve and the vagus nerve. On the right side, the vagus nerve descends within the carotid fascia between the internal jugular vein and the common carotid artery and subsequently crosses the first part of the subclavian artery to enter the thorax between the common carotid and subclavian arteries. On the left side, the vagus nerve lies on the cupola of the pleura between the internal jugular vein and the common carotid artery to enter the thorax between the common carotid and subclavian arteries.

REFERENCES

Agostini E, Torri G: Diaphragm contraction as a limiting factor to maximum expiration. J Appl Physiol 17:427, 1962.

Brock RC: The Anatomy of the Bronchial Tree: With Special Reference to the Surgery of Lung Abscess. 2nd Ed. London: Oxford University Press, 1954.

Campbell ETM: The role of the scalene and sternomastoid muscles in breathing in normal subjects. An electromyographic study. J Anat 89:378, 1955.

Cherniack RM, Cherniack L: Respiration in Health and Disease. Philadelphia: WB Saunders, 1961.

Davies F, Gladstone RJ, Stibbe EP: Anatomy of intercostal nerves. J Anat 66:323, 1932.

Hughes FA: Resection of twelfth rib in surgical approach to renal fossa. J Urol 61:159, 1949.

Johnston HM: The cutaneous branches of the posterior primary divisions of the spinal nerves and their distribution in the skin. J Anat Physiol 43:80, 1908.

Jones DS, Beargie RT, Pauly TE: Electromyographic study of some muscles of costal respiration in man. Anat Rec 117:17, 1953.

Taylor A: The contribution of the intercostal muscles to the effort of respiration in man. J Physiol (Lond) 151:390, 1960.

Trotter M: Synostosis between manubrium and body of sternum in Whites and Negroes. Am J Phys Anthropol 18:439, 1934.

READING REFERENCES

Basmajian JV: Grant's Method of Anatomy. 10th Ed. Baltimore: Williams & Wilkins, 1980.

Gardner E, et al: Anatomy. 3rd Ed. Philadelphia: WB Saunders, 1969.

Healy JE, Seybold WD: A Synopsis of Clinical Anatomy. Philadelphia: WB Saunders, 1969.

Hollinshead WH, Rosse C: Textbook of Anatomy. 4th Ed. Philadelphia: JB Lippincott, 1985.

Lachman E: Comparison of posterior boundaries of lungs and pleura as demonstrated on cadaver and on roentgenogram of the living. Anat Rec 83:521, 1942.

Mainland D, Gordon ET: Position of organs determined from thoracic radiographs of young adult males, with study of cardiac apex beat. Am J Anat 68:457, 1941.

Woodbourne RT: Essentials of Human Anatomy. 7th Ed. New York: Oxford University Press, 1983.

CHAPTER 2

Embryology of the Lung

David H. Harpole, Jr., and Thomas A. Aloia

BACKGROUND AND HISTORY

The field of embryology is rich with important investigators and scientific breakthroughs. Pulmonary embryology's history is no exception. As with other areas of human embryology, the first theories of lung development were derived from animal models. To place human lung development in perspective, embryologists including Krogh (1904), Pattle and Hopkinson (1963), and Hugues (1967) focused their early work on fish, amphibians, and birds. With a solid understanding of the evolution of air-breathing species, later work such as that of Witschi (1956) was focused on mammals and primates.

Many of the principles of animal embryology were directly applied to human lung development. Most of these principles furthered our understanding of human lung embryogenesis, but others were ultimately not applicable to the human model and stalled advancement in the field. For example, the fact that pulmonary development in the rhesus monkey is more rapid than that of the human led some to miscalculate the timing of important human embryologic milestones. In 1965, Lynne M. Reid commented that, "[w]ork on the human lung has been bedeviled for the last 50 years with unjustified extrapolations from animal work to man." Despite the setbacks to which Reid refers, we currently have a clear picture of pulmonary development in the human.

Important contributions to human pulmonary embryology have been made by a number of individuals. In 1936, Dubreuil and colleagues devised the first system of nomenclature for pulmonary development. Concurrently, Congdon and Streeter, working at the Carnegie Institute during the first half of this century, were able to systematically document pulmonary development in relation to development of the fetus as a whole. Over the next 20 years several embryologists, including Loosli and Potter (1951), Bucher and Reid (1961), Boyden and Tomsett (1965), and Hislop and colleagues (1972), made major contributions specific to pulmonary development. We are particularly indebted to Boyden for advancing the technique of wax modeling of the

bronchial tree and vasculature. More recently, Campiche and colleagues (1963) and Thurlbeck (1988) have made important advances in related fields.

Breakthroughs made by these and other researchers have not been made in a vacuum. Their contributions to clinical medicine have been pivotal to our understanding of both pediatric and adult lung function and pathology. For example, the discovery of surfactant and its role in lung function has led to the routine use of inhaled surfactant in the neonatal intensive care unit, substantially decreasing the morbidity and mortality of prematurity. As discussed at the end of this chapter, pulmonary embryology research continues to be a rich area of study with great translational potential. It is hoped that continued work on pulmonary development will yield many more meaningful therapeutic strategies for the treatment of both surgical and medical pulmonary disease.

This chapter provides a framework for subsequent chapters in this text by detailing embryonic pulmonary development. Clinical correlations are provided when relevant to intrauterine events. Although much of the chapter focuses on prenatal pulmonary development, it is important to note that pulmonary morphogenesis and differentiation do not end at birth. Significant alveolar remodeling and growth occur during childhood. The development of the lung in humans certainly extends to the age of 8 years and may continue beyond this mark in some individuals.

In this chapter significant events are marked using crown-rump length and Carnegie Stage after Streeter (1945a, 1945b, 1948, 1951). All dates given are timed from ovulation unless otherwise specified.

PULMONARY PARENCHYMAL EMBRYOGENESIS

Development of the pulmonary parenchyma has been thoroughly investigated and has been divided into a number of phases by various authors and governing bodies (Table 2-1). Dubreuil and associates (1936) divided prenatal pulmonary development into glandular and canalicular phases.

Table 2-1. Developmental Schema in Pulmonary Embryology and Their Authors

Dubreuil et al., 1936	Loosli and Potter, 1951	Boyden, 1972	Thurlbeck, 1988
Glandular: up to 6 mos	Glandular: week 5 to 4 mos	Pseudoglandular: week 5 to week 17	Embryonic: day 26 to day 52
Canalicular: 7 mos to birth	Canalicular: 4 mos to 6 mos	Canalicular: week 13 to week 25	Pseudoglandular: day 52 to week 16
Alveolar: postnatal	Alveolar: 6 mos to birth	Terminal sac period: week 24 to birth	Canalicular: week 17 to week 28 Saccular: week 29 to week 36 Alveolar: week 36 to term

Later Loosli and Potter (1951) modified this system, renaming the period from 6 months' gestation until birth as the alveolar period. In 1972, Boyden (1972a), based on his studies of histology and wax models, defined a pseudoglandular phase from 5 to 16 weeks, an overlapping canalicular phase from 13 to 24 weeks, and a terminal sac period from 25 weeks until birth. In this system the term *alveolar* is confined to postnatal pulmonary development. In 1970 the Commission on Embryological Terminology (1970) ratified Boyden's phase schema and added an embryonic period.

Thurlbeck (1988) described a system that divides Boyden's final stage, the terminal sac period, into a saccular period and an alveolar period based on late gestational alveolar maturation. In their most recent text, O'Rahilly and Müller (1996), taking into account the variability in the timing of events that define each stage, present a flexible schema of overlapping phases that is probably most accurate (Fig. 2-1). The system used in this chapter is that of the Commission on Embryological Terminology, with minor modification by the system introduced by Thurlbeck in 1988.

Embryonic Phase

Smith (1957) first identified the formation of the tracheoesophageal groove in the foregut of a 3-mm, Carnegie stage-10 fetus. This development, which begins early in week 4, is summarized in Figure 2-2. At this point the cranial ventral foregut has enlarged and an invaginating ridge of endodermal tissue has formed tracheoesophageal folds.

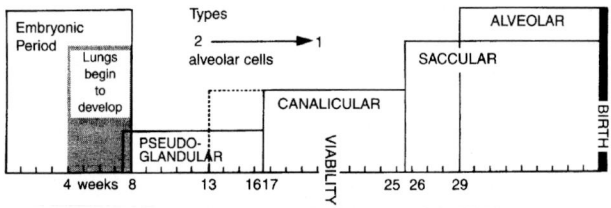

Fig. 2-1. Overlapping phases in the development of the lung according to current thought. From O'Rahilly R, Müller F: Human Embryology and Teratology. 2nd Ed. New York: Wiley-Liss, 1996, p. 266. With permission.

The folds meet in the midline, defining a dorsal esophageal lumen and a ventral laryngotracheal primordia. Fusion of the tracheoesophageal folds then progresses from caudad to cephalad. Subsequent necrosis and degeneration of intervening tissue allow separation of the esophagus and trachea. As the trachea and esophageal primordia separate, both are elongating. Complete separation is not achieved until approximately day 41 (stage 17, 11 to 14 mm). According to Zachary and Emery (1961), incomplete separation at this phase is the precursor for tracheoesophageal fistulae and their associated anomalies.

The primordial lung bud develops from the distal end of the newly formed trachea. O'Rahilly and Boyden (1973) first visualized the lung bud in a day-26, stage-12, 4-mm fetus, marking the beginning of the embryonic phase of lung development. The embryonic phase, which spans postovulatory days 26 to 52, focuses on the morphogenesis of the proximal airways and the early differentiation of adjacent mesenchymal tissue.

Shortly after the development of the lung bud, right and left lung primordia are seen. As the embryonic mediastinum develops the left lung main bronchus assumes a shorter and more horizontal orientation. This asymmetry appears to be independent of mechanical influences from the developing heart, which does not occupy its final position in the mediastinum until the seventh week. Axial growth as well as dichotomous division of the airways continues during the embryonic phase (Fig. 2-3). By 52 days postovulation (stage 22, 23 to 28 mm), secondary bronchi are visualized, marking the end of the embryonic phase and the beginning of the pseudoglandular phase of development.

Pseudoglandular Phase

As the pulmonary primordia move from the embryonic phase to the pseudoglandular phase, the bronchi continue to grow and mature. Histologically, the bronchi are lined with a glycogen-laden, cuboidal epithelium, giving the growing lung a glandular appearance. The period when this characteristic appearance of the lung is present spans weeks 5 through 17 of pulmonary embryogenesis and is termed the *pseudoglandular phase* by Boyden (1972a). Whereas the embryonic phase focused on tracheal and lung bud

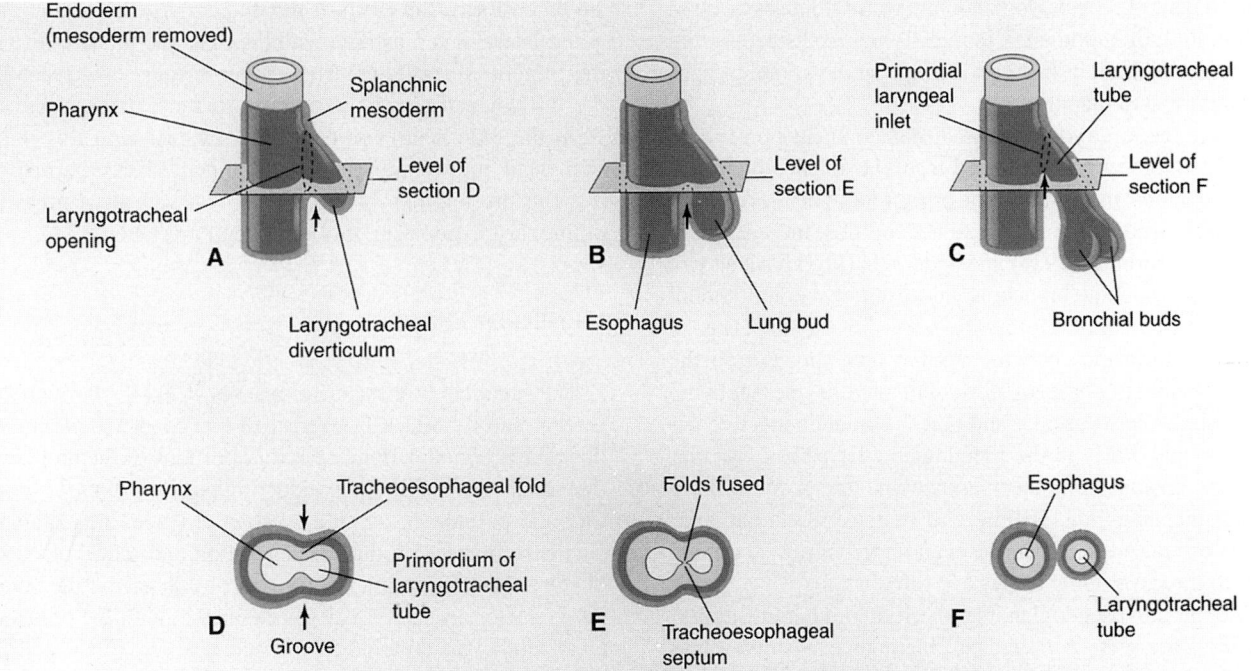

Fig. 2-2. Successive stages in the development of the tracheoesophageal septum during the fourth and fifth weeks. **A–C.** Lateral views of the caudal part of the primordial pharynx showing the laryngotracheal diverticulum and partitioning of the foregut into the esophagus and laryngotracheal tube. **D–F.** Transverse sections illustrating formation of the tracheoesophageal septum and showing how it separates into the laryngotracheal tube and esophagus. From Moore KL, Persaud TVN: The Developing Human: Clinically Oriented Embryology. 6th Ed. Philadelphia: WB Saunders, 1998, p. 259. With permission.

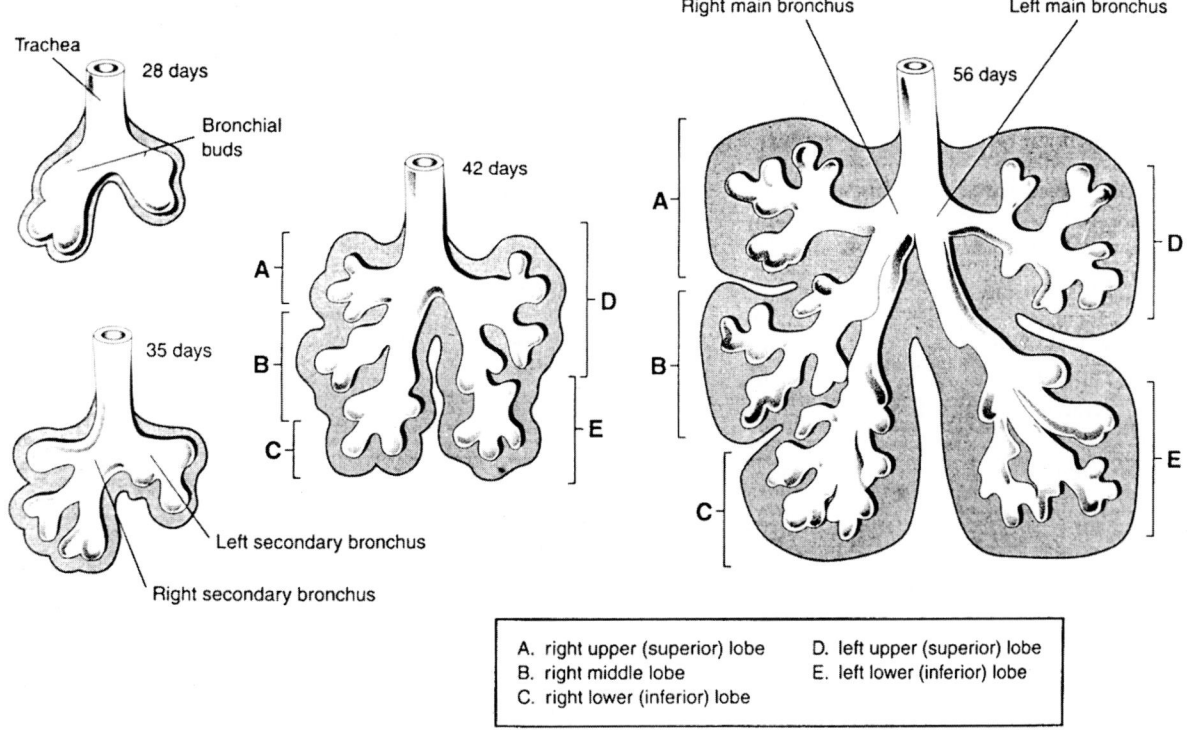

A. right upper (superior) lobe   D. left upper (superior) lobe
B. right middle lobe   E. left lower (inferior) lobe
C. right lower (inferior) lobe

Fig. 2-3. Successive stages in the development of the bronchi and lungs. From Moore KL, Persaud TVN: The Developing Human: Clinically Oriented Embryology. 6th Ed. Philadelphia: WB Saunders, 1998, p. 263. With permission.

development, the pseudoglandular phase focuses on the proliferation of endothelial, mesenchymal, and surrounding structures including the conducting airways, pulmonary vasculature, and diaphragm.

During the embryonic phase of development poorly differentiated mesenchyme derived from the splanchnic mesoderm envelops the pulmonary primordia. The developing lung is dependent on the presence of this mesenchyme. Studies by Rudnick (1933) and Taderera (1967) have shown that both bronchial branching and pulmonary endothelial development will not properly occur in the absence of species-specific mesenchyme. As the lung moves into the pseudoglandular phase of development, this mesenchyme differentiates into vascular and other stromal connective tissue elements. Early in the pseudoglandular period vascular plexuses arising from the mesenchyme are seen forming around the lung bud. By the end of the pseudoglandular phase, vascular development is well under way and connections to the developing heart have formed.

Late in the pseudoglandular period, bronchial support structures are seen. A ringed cartilaginous exoskeleton was visualized by Bucher and Reid (1961) at the level of the trachea by week 10 and around segmental bronchi by week 16. The bronchi are not only elongating throughout this phase but they are also branching. In the right chest the right main stem bronchus bifurcates twice, forming three secondary bronchi. These bronchi, along with their surrounding mesenchyme, form the right upper, middle, and lower lobes. On the left a single major dichotomous branching occurs, forming the upper lobar bronchus, whereas the main bronchus terminates as the left lower lobe. Another round of dichotomous branching leads to the development of 18 total tertiary branches called *bronchopulmonary segments*, 10 to the right and 8 to the left.

Dichotomous branching at the terminus of each tertiary bronchus proceeds throughout the remainder of the pseudoglandular phase. The majority of this branching takes place between weeks 10 and 16. By the end of the sixteenth week, Bucher and Reid (1961) were able to identify 4 to 25 generations of conducting airways depending on the location of the segment. This subsegmental branching continues into the beginning of week 17. At this point all nonrespiratory airway elements have formed, but the terminal bronchi, respiratory bronchi, and acinar units are difficult to delineate. These terminal sac structures are defined during the canalicular phase of development.

Beside conducting airway growth, the pseudoglandular phase also encompasses important developmental milestones for several surrounding structures including the chest wall, mediastinum, and diaphragm. During weeks 8 through 10 the diaphragm is developing through a complex set of mesenchymal layer fusions as pointed out by Boyden (1972b). As the lungs grow first dorsally and then inferiorly, the pleural spaces descend. Bremer (1943) observed that during this descent two layers of innermost chest wall musculature are burrowed from the chest wall. The first, a dor-

sal layer, forms the crura of the diaphragm. The second, an anterolateral layer, merges with the first, and the two fuse as the lumbocostal trigone. These fusions must take place by day 60 when the intestines return to the peritoneal cavity from the umbilical coelom. Failure of fusion at this point may lead to eventration or abdominal viscus herniation through the foramen of Bochdalek and various degrees of pulmonary hypoplasia, morbidity, and mortality.

Canalicular Phase

The canalicular phase encompasses weeks 17 through 26. Bucher and Reid (1961) confirmed that by the beginning of this phase, all axial, nonrespiratory portions of the bronchial tree are present. With the conducting portions of the respiratory and pulmonary vascular system in place, the canalicular phase focuses on the capillarization and morphogenesis of the pulmonary acini. By the end of this period the respiratory system is capable of gas exchange, with the potential to sustain an air-breathing existence.

Boyden (1974) showed that distal bronchioles in the week-17 fetus terminate in several generations of closely arranged buds. Histologically, the air spaces at this point are composed of large rounded areas, and the intervening connective tissue is abundant (Fig. 2-4A). During the canalicular phase the interstitial tissue between each air space thins. At the same time elastic tissue forms around the air spaces. The elastic tissue serves two functions. First, it lends elasticity to the lung, providing the source for passive expiratory force in postnatal life. Second, it helps to demarcate each saccular unit. As the saccular units become delineated, the acinus, composed of one terminal bronchiole, two to four respiratory bronchioles, and four to seven saccules per respiratory bronchiole, can be defined (Fig. 2-5).

During this phase capillaries move toward their adjacent air spaces as the air spaces enlarge and the saccular interstitium shrinks (Fig. 2-4B and C). Boyden (1974) showed that the apposition of capillaries to the air spaces begins first at the most distal respiratory units and bronchial branch points. Based on histologic studies it was first thought that the capillaries actually penetrated the lumen of the air spaces. Elegant studies first by Low (1953) using the electron microscope (Fig. 2-6) and later by Campiche and colleagues (1963) proved that the capillaries insert themselves between cuboidal epithelial cells and near the bronchial lumen, but a thin layer of cytoplasm always intervenes. This process progresses centripetally from the most distal respiratory elements finally capillarizing the respiratory bronchioles.

Simultaneous with saccular capillarization, the acinar endothelium, as shown by Policard and colleagues (1954), is differentiating into type I and II pneumocytes. Some of the acinar epithelial cells efface, allowing a microthin membrane for gas exchange between corpuscles and alveolar air spaces. These cells are termed *type I pneumocytes*, and they represent 80 to 90% of the alveolar surface area. They tend

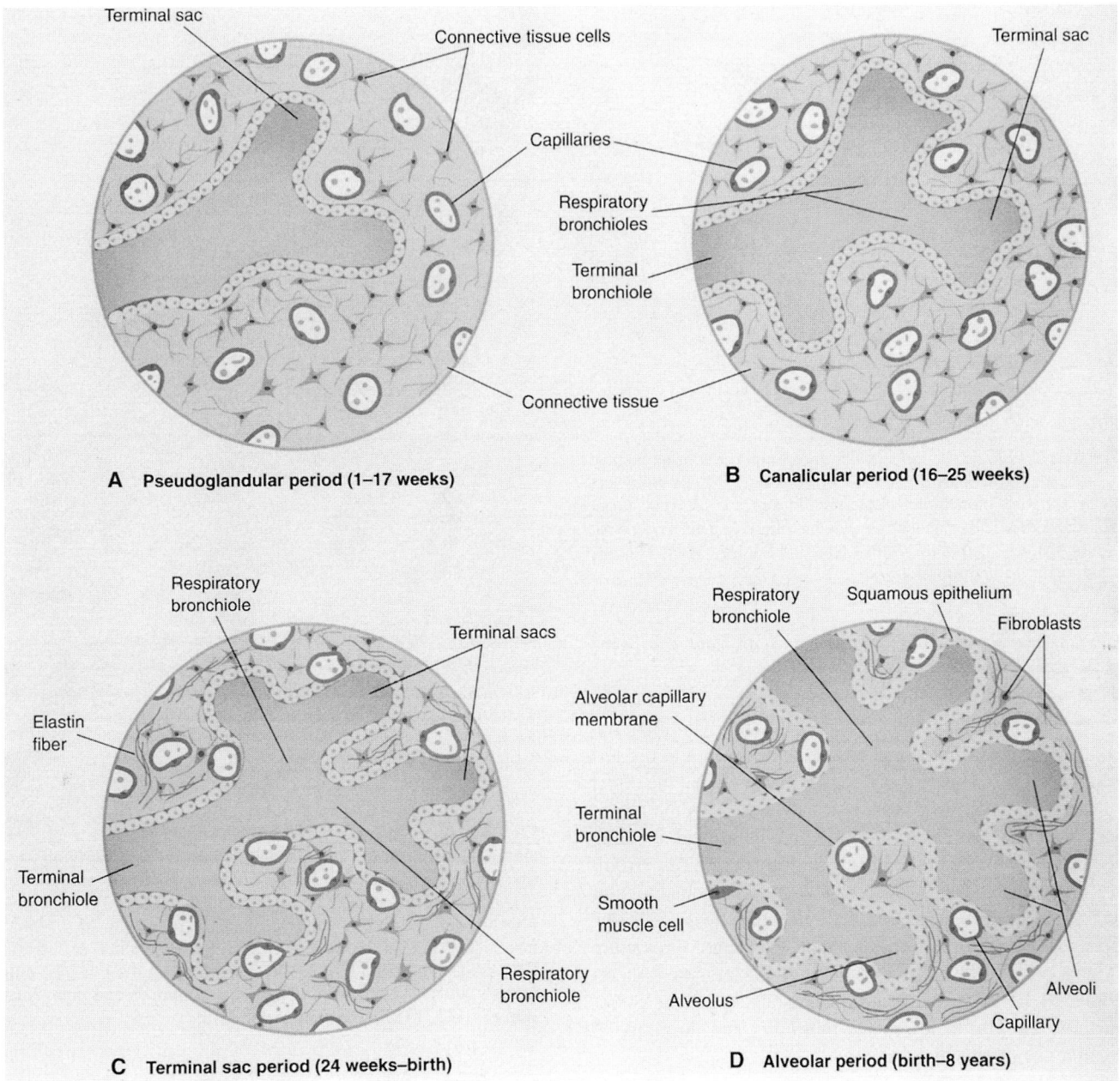

Fig. 2-4. Diagrammatic sketches of histologic sections, illustrating progressive stages of lung development. **A, B.** Note the rounded appearance of the air spaces, the abundance of interstitial tissue, and the distance from the capillaries to the air spaces. **C, D.** The alveolocapillary membrane is thin and some capillaries bulge into the terminal sacs (future alveoli). From Moore KL, Persaud TVN: The Developing Human: Clinically Oriented Embryology. 6th Ed. Philadelphia: WB Saunders, 1998, p. 264. With permission.

to be depleted of cytoplasmic glycogen and are specialized for gas exchange. At birth the thickness of the blood gas barrier formed by the fusion of the capillary wall and the type I pneumocyte is as little as 4 μm (Fig. 2-7).

In contrast to type I pneumocytes, type II pneumocytes retain the glycogen of their cuboidal precursors. Both Campiche and colleagues (1963) as well as Sorokin (1966) identified eosinophilic lamellar bodies, which form from the Golgi's apparatus and store phospholipid, in the cytoplasm

of these cells by the end of the second trimester (Fig. 2-8). Subsequently, Meyrick and Reid (1973) noted that the type II pneumocytes begin production of phosphatidylcholine, a precursor of the major surfactant phospholipid, dipalmitoyl phosphatidylcholine. In the mature lung, Farrell (1973) pointed out that this phospholipid is produced using the cytidine diphosphocholine pathway. The production of surface active material from this pathway is influenced by a number of neural and hormonal factors including the presence of

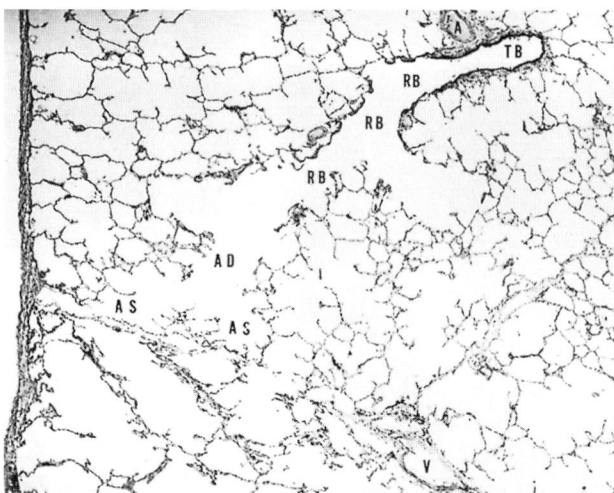

Fig. 2-5. Histologic section showing the components of an acinus. A, muscular pulmonary artery; AD, alveolar duct; AS, alveolar sac; RB, respiratory bronchiole; TB, terminal bronchiole; V, vein. From Thurlbeck WM: Normal anatomy and histology. *In* Thurlbeck WM, Churg AM, eds. Pathology of the Lung. 2nd Ed. New York: Thieme, 1995, p.15. With permission.

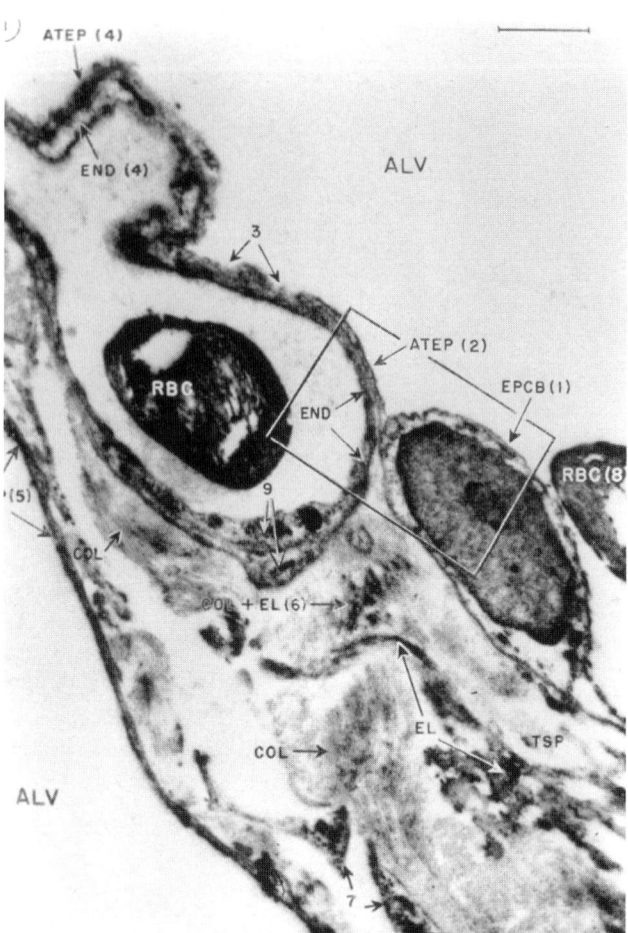

Fig. 2-6. Electron micrograph of the human alveolar wall. The epithelial cell body (1) attenuates (2) to cover the underlying capillary. The cellular duality of the blood-air barrier is obscured at (3), but these layers are again distinguishable at (4). Both unit fibers of collagen (COL) and elastin (EL) are visible. ALV, alveolus; ATEP, attenuated epithelium; EPBC, epithelial cell body; RBC, red blood cell; TSP, tissue space. From Low FN: The pulmonary alveolar epithelium of laboratory animals and man. Anat Rec *117*:241, 1953. With permission.

surrounding mesenchyme, corticosteroids, and thyroxine (Fig. 2-9).

Along with phospholipid, surfactant contains various apoproteins, carbohydrates, and cholesterol. This material coats the alveolus, creating a monolayer of fluid at the air-cell interface. Von Neergaard (1929) observed that the effect of this monolayer is to reduce surface tension in the alveolus, preventing its collapse during expiration, and reducing the elastic property of the lung by at least two-thirds. Brumley and colleagues (1967) noted that sufficient quantities of surfactant are produced by 24 to 26 weeks to provide the alveolar stability required for gas exchange. Premature infants born at this stage of pulmonary development therefore may be viable, although exogenous surfactant is frequently required to lessen the morbidity and mortality of hyaline membrane disease.

Terminal Sac Phase

The terminal sac phase, which lasts from week 24 until birth, focuses on respiratory saccule development. By the beginning of the third trimester three orders of respiratory bronchi can be seen clearly to originate from each terminal bronchiole. Loosely defined respiratory buds present at the beginning of the canalicular phase are now developed into several orders of distinct capillarized saccules. Throughout the terminal sac phase the saccules continue to become septated. The septations create thin-walled subsaccular structures that mature into true alveoli.

This transformation represents a continuum of development from saccule to alveolus. There is debate about the exact time when saccules become alveoli. Boyden (1967,

1972a) believed that the development of alveoli occurred postnatally and depended on the force of air movement within the lung. In his schema, therefore, the terminal sac phase was present until birth. Thurlbeck (1988) identified maturing alveoli prenatally during the third trimester and so divided the terminal sac phase into saccular and alveolar stages (Fig. 2-10). In either case it is clear that the majority of alveolar morphogenesis occurs postnatally. Based on lung morphometry studies by Weibel (1963) and Langston and colleagues (1984) it is estimated that only 20 million to 50 million alveoli, or 8% of alveoli present in adulthood, have formed by 40 weeks' gestation. A summary of the intrauterine development of the intrasegmental bronchial tree, including postnatal landmarks, is provided in Figure 2-11.

During the third trimester of gestation respiratory movements have been identified, although they are intermittent.

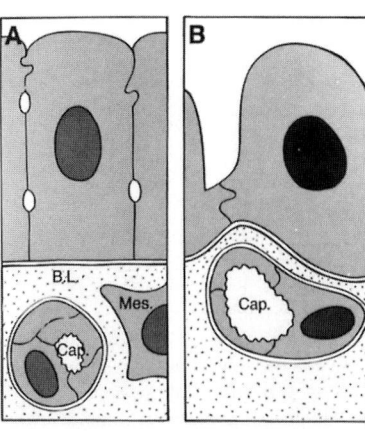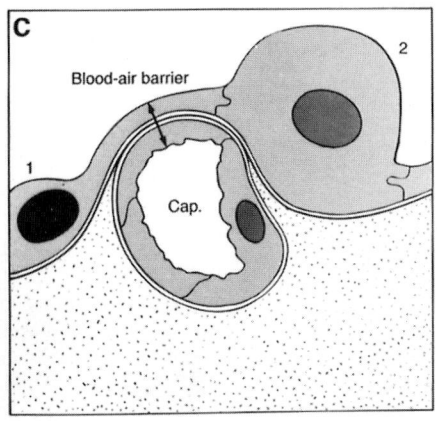

Fig. 2-7. Electron microscope studies of human lung. **A.** Pseudoglandular phase showing tall columnar cell rich in glycogen. **B.** A cell becoming cuboidal. The capillary is now closer. **C.** Canalicular phase showing types 1 and 2 alveolar cells. The blood-air barrier has formed. BL, basal lamina; Cap., capillary; Mes., mesenchymal cell. From O'Rahilly R, Müller F: Human Embryology and Teratology. 2nd Ed. New York: Wiley-Liss, 1996, p. 268. With permission.

There has been considerable debate about the triggers of these motions, their role in pulmonary alveolar development, and their role in amniotic fluid production. The embryonic diaphragm, innervated by the phrenic nerve, does contract, although in utero this action produces paradoxical respiratory movement with chest contraction and abdominal distention. Windle and colleagues (1939) believed that intrauterine respiratory movements were a response to abnormally low fetal oxygenation as sensed by peripheral chemoreceptors. Later, studies conducted by Biscoe and colleagues (1969) and by Woodrum and colleagues (1977) on the lamb fetus showed that these movements were centrally controlled and do not depend on input from the carotid body chemoreceptors. It is now clear that fetal lung movements are mediated at the level of the brainstem.

The role of fetal lung movements in alveolar development is still debated. At one time it was thought that these movements created a net inspiration of amniotic fluid and that this influx helped mold and form alveoli. It is now known that the net movement of fluid is from the lung to the amnion. DeBlasio and colleagues (1960) demonstrated that aspiration of amniotic fluid does not occur in utero prior to labor. This fact has important clinical significance. Gluck and coworkers (1971) noted that the presence of increasing levels of pulmonary surfactant expelled from the lungs into the amniotic milieu during the third trimester allows for calculation of a lecithin-sphingomyelin ratio in fluid drawn at amniocentesis. This ratio is an accurate measure of fetal

Fig. 2-8. Type II epithelial cell from a human lung. The alveolar surface is partially covered by flaps of cytoplasm from type I epithelial cells up to the intercellular junctions at the arrows. There are several lamellar bodies (LB) in the apical cytoplasm. Microvilli are present on the exposed apical surface (×19,000). From Thurlbeck WM: Normal Anatomy and Histology. In Thurlbeck WM, Churg AM, eds. Pathology of the Lung. 2nd Ed. New York: Thieme, 1995, p. 18. With permission.

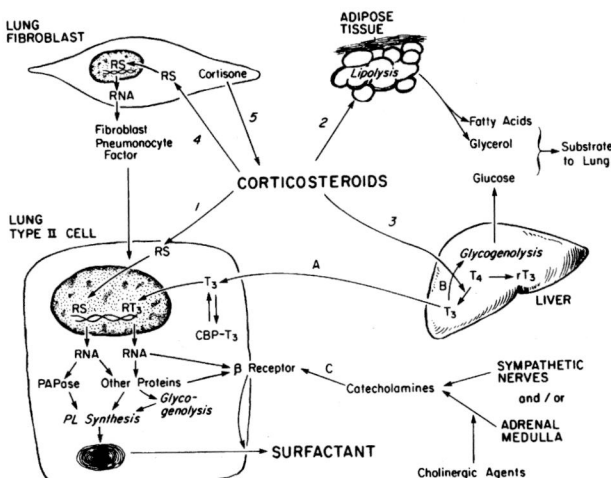

Fig. 2-9. Possible mechanisms by which glucocorticoids may influence fetal lung differentiation. β-receptor, β-adrenergic receptor; CBP, cytosol-binding protein [for thyroid hormone]; PL, phospholipid; RS, receptor-corticosteroid complex. From Ballard PL: Hormonal regulation of the surfactant system. In Monset-Couchard M, Minkowski A, eds. Physiological and Biochemical Basis for Perinatal Medicine. Basel: Karger, 1981, pp. 42–53. With permission.

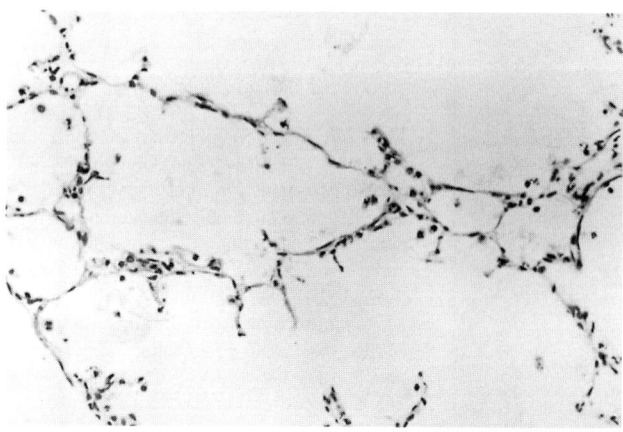

Fig. 2-10. Thirty-six weeks' gestation. Alveolar phase. Thin-walled alveoli are readily visible (hematoxylin and eosin, original magnification ×200). From Langston C, et al: Human lung growth in late gestation and in the neonate. Am Rev Respir Dis *129*:607, 1984. With permission.

lung maturity and correlates with postnatal resistance to hyaline membrane disease in premature infants.

Pediatric Lung Maturation

Boyden and Tompsett (1965) and Dunnill (1962) are credited with the most complete analysis of postnatal lung maturation. Studying models and reconstructions of lung specimens from infants and children at several ages from 2 days of life to 7 years, these researchers were able to detail

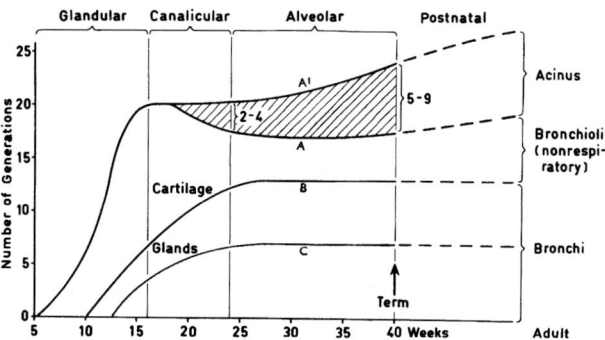

Fig. 2-11. Summary of intrauterine development of the intrasegmental bronchial tree. Line A represents the increase in the number of bronchial generations; shaded area between A and A[1] represents the respiratory part of the bronchial tree (i.e., respiratory bronchioles and alveolar ducts). Line B shows the extension of cartilage along the bronchial tree, and line C, the extension of mucous glands. The diagram includes adult values, showing the increase in total generations in the postnatal period. From Bucher U, Reid L: Development of the intrasegmental tree; the pattern of branching and development of cartilage at various stages of intrauterine life. Thorax *16*:207, 1961. With permission.

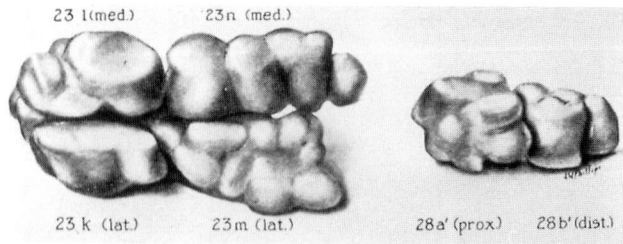

Fig. 2-12. Wax reconstructions of terminal air sacs in a 2-day-old infant (original magnification ×85). Note the shallowness and variations in size of the pulmonary alveoli that appear as smaller elevations on the surface of the terminal air sacs during the perinatal period. From Boyden EA, Tompsett DH: Changing patterns in the developing lungs of infants. Acta Anat *61*:182, 1965. With permission.

this important period of pulmonary development (Fig. 2-12). During the 1960s and 1970s these researchers published a number of papers recording the results of these experiments. In 1974, Hislop and Reid, uniting this research to their knowledge of prenatal lung development, summarized pulmonary acinar development from the embryonic phase to adulthood (Fig. 2-13).

During their studies, Boyden and Tompsett (1965) identified two types of alveolar development that occur during the first several months of life. First, saccule walls continue to septate and thin, transforming greater numbers of alveolar primordia into mature alveoli. Second, alveolar ducts are created as transitional ducts, which link distal respiratory bronchioles to the saccules, become alveolarized. Alveolar development then progresses centripetally from the alveolar ducts toward the terminal bronchioles. The individual alveoli grow in size, but this growth is overshadowed by the rapid increase in the number of alveoli that form via these two mechanisms. Studying lung tissue from a child 15 months of age, Dunnill (1962) estimated that 127 million alveoli had formed.

By age 3, a third and final mechanism for postnatal alveolar development is identified. Boyden (1967), studying the superior lingual segment of a child who was 3 years and 7 months old, found multiple diverticula arising from terminal bronchioles. The endothelium lining these new saccules was seen in various stages of metaplasia. The most mature of these saccules was lined with a thin epithelial layer that was invaginated by a new capillary network resembling the canalization process in the embryo. Other saccules were lined by a transitional, low cuboidal epithelium, whereas relatively less developed saccules were lined by bronchiolar cuboidal epithelium. These new alveoli continue to form and mature throughout early childhood, greatly increasing the total alveolar surface area for gas exchange.

Two other important histologic features of alveolar morphogenesis have been identified in the pediatric lung. Lambert ducts, named after the anatomist who described them in 1955, are cuboidal cell–lined tubes that connect alveolar units from

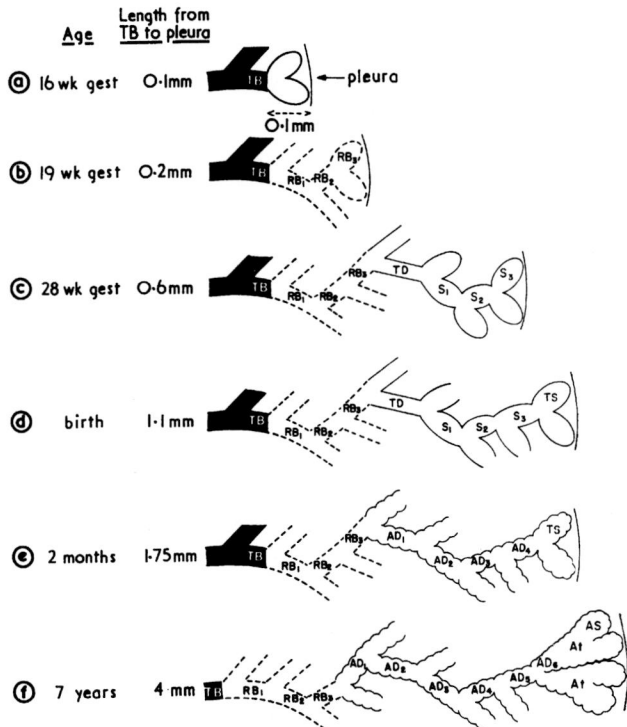

Fig. 2-13. Schematic representation of the growth of the acinus (subpleural). **a.** At 16 weeks' gestation, the airways terminate as a tubule close to the pleura. **b.** By 19 weeks' gestation, the last generation of airway shows thinned epithelium and forms the first respiratory bronchiolus (RB) and a second generation of respiratory bronchioli has formed by branching. **c.** By 28 weeks' gestation, three generations of respiratory bronchioli and one generation of transitional duct (TD) have arisen by further branching. The transitional duct gives rise to two primitive saccules (S). **d.** By birth, three generations of saccules are found, all ending in terminal saccules. No true alveoli are present, although indentations representing future alveoli are found. **e.** By 2 months, alveoli have developed in the walls of respiratory bronchioli, transitional ducts, and saccules. **f.** By 7 years, remodeling of respiratory bronchioli and alveolar ducts has occurred. Also, the terminal sac has formed the adult atrium (At), which has given rise to alveolar sacs (AS) that formed by budding. This pattern is similar to that found in the adult. Any further development is probably attributable to an increase in size. TB, terminal bronchiole. From Hislop A, Reid L: Development of the acinus in the human lung. Thorax 29:90, 1974. With permission.

adjacent respiratory segments. They have been identified in lung tissue from a child as young as 7 years. Inhaled gases can traverse these ducts, allowing accelerated diffusion of these gases and equalization of air pressure between alveoli supplied by different terminal bronchioles. Lambert ducts differ from the pores of Kohn, first identified in 1893 by Kohn, which are much smaller and connect adjacent alveoli from the same respiratory segment. This movement speeds the diffusion of gases, improving the efficiency of gas exchange.

From age 8 years to adulthood, alveolar units continue to develop de novo but at a slower pace. Dunnill (1962) esti-

mates that by age 9, 280 million alveoli are present. This is near to the number of alveoli found in the adult lung. The total surface area of the alveoli at this age measures 32 m^2. Throughout adolescence, individual alveolar size increases as the chest cavity increases in volume. Hislop and colleagues (1972) showed that the conducting airways keep pace during this period by both axial elongation and increased diameter. As the alveolar elements enlarge the area for gas exchange increases. Between 8 years and adulthood, the surface area of the lung doubles to 75 m^2.

PULMONARY VASCULAR AND STROMAL EMBRYOGENESIS

Vascular Development

Knowledge of the basic structure of the aortae and the forming heart is key to the understanding of pulmonary vascular embryology. At 22 days (stage 10, 2 mm), paired dorsal aortae and a ventral aortic sac exist. The ventral aortic sac is contiguous with the cranial end of the heart tube, the truncus arteriosus. The dorsal aortae are connected to the ventral aortic sac via a series of paired aortic arches. Each arch corresponds to a pharyngeal pouch that sits within and extends out from the triangle formed by the midline ventral aorta and the posterolateral paired dorsal aortae (Fig. 2-14).

The arches form progressively from craniad to caudad. At the 2-mm stage, only the first arch is present. At this point the first arch provides the only connection from the dorsal aortae to the ventral aortic sac. Over the next several days of development, some arches regress whereas others are transformed into more permanent structures. By the time the sixth arch appears at day 30 (stage 14, 6 mm), the first two arches have regressed. The third arch forms the common carotid arteries whereas the fourth arch forms the aortic arch proper. The fifth arch is vestigial and regresses. It is the destiny of the sixth arch to form the proximal pulmonary arterial circulation (Fig. 2-15).

Near day 32 of fetal development, the sixth arch vessels give off primordial right and left pulmonary arteries (Fig. 2-16A). Over the next 2 weeks, a complex set of transformations occur in the sixth arch region. First, the dorsal portion of the right arch thins. The ventral portion of the left arch becomes the primordial main pulmonary artery, absorbing the ventral portion of the right sixth arch (Fig. 2-16B). At the same time the truncus arteriosus is being divided by the aorticopulmonary septum, isolating the pulmonary arterial blood source to the right ventricle. By day 50 (stage 20, 18 mm), the dorsal right sixth arch has regressed completely and the ventral left sixth arch is firmly established as the main pulmonary artery. The dorsal left sixth arch remains, connecting the main pulmonary artery at its bifurcation to the left dorsal aorta as the ductus arteriosus (Fig. 2-16C). Intrauterine development of the intrapulmonary portion of

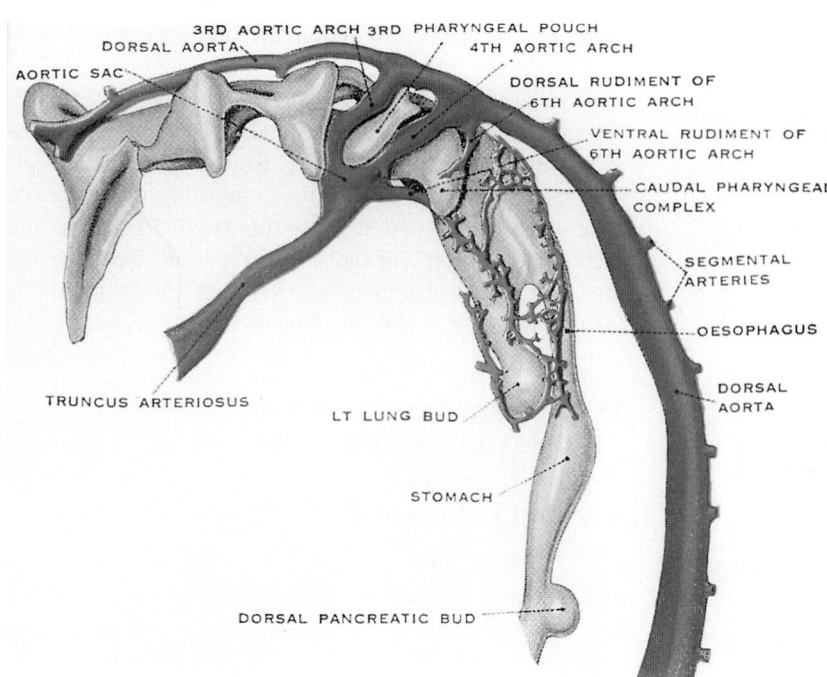

Fig. 2-14. The left lateral aspect of a model of the pharynx and branchial arch arteries in a 5-mm human embryo (after Congdon). The first and second arch arteries have retrogressed, the third and fourth arch arteries are complete, and the dorsal and ventral endothelial sprouts of the sixth (pulmonary) arch artery have nearly met. From the ventral sprouts, plexiform vessels pass to the lung bud.

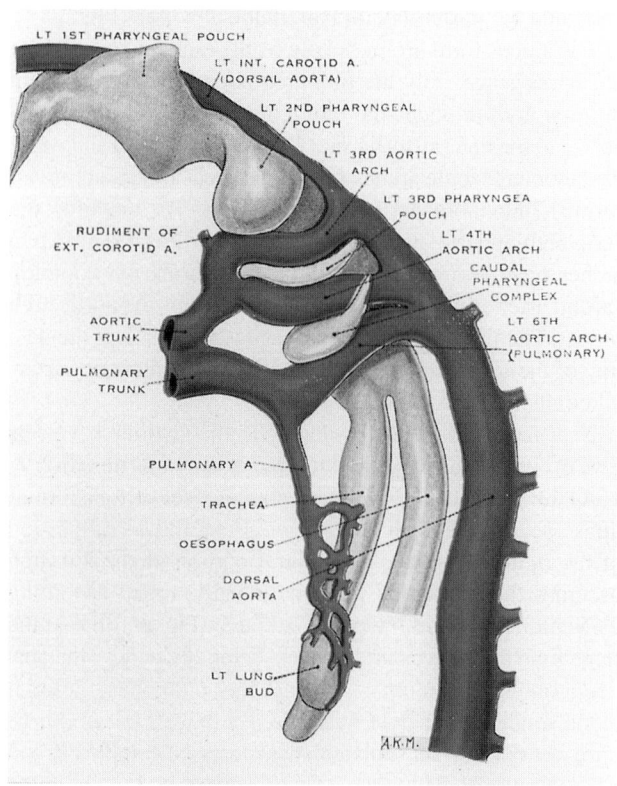

Fig. 2-15. The left lateral aspect of a model of the pharynx and branchial arch arteries in an 11-mm human embryo (after Congdon). The sixth (pulmonary) arch artery is complete and the third arch artery is bent cranially at its dorsal end and its stream is about to be deflected in that direction.

the pulmonary arterial system follows the branching pattern of the bronchi. By the completion of gestation the pulmonary arteries will supply all alveolar units and most of the pleura.

At birth, a rapid shift in pulmonary physiology occurs. Right ventricular blood is no longer shunted primarily through the ductus arteriosus. As the pulmonary vascular resistance decreases in response to high oxygen tension and vasoactive mediator release, as shown by Heymann and coworkers (1969), the pulmonary arteries receive the majority of the right ventricular output. At birth most of the fluid that filled the airways in utero is expelled. Respiratory movements become regular and air is inspired into the now patent airways. With perfusion of the pulmonary arteries and inspiration of air, gas exchange begins across the alveolar endothelium and respiration is initiated. During infancy and childhood the relative low-pressure state of the pulmonary arterial vasculature is preserved as the pulmonary arteries lose a considerable amount of their muscularity.

Development of the pulmonary venous system is only slightly less complex than that of the pulmonary arteries. Near day 22 (stage 11, 2.5 to 3.0 mm), bilateral primordial common pulmonary veins are seen exiting the sinoatrial region of the heart tube. By day 32 (stage 14, 6 to 7 mm), the pulmonary venous system is anastomosed to each lung bud vascular plexus bilaterally. The right and left main pulmonary veins then undergo a series of divisions. The most proximal of these divisions is resorbed, forming portions of the left atrium. Poddubnyi (1973) confirmed that by 9 weeks of development, the left atrium is well formed and paired left and right pulmonary venous orifices are present. He also showed that as in the pulmonary arterial system, arborization of the intrapulmonary portion of the pulmonary venous system follows the bronchial template.

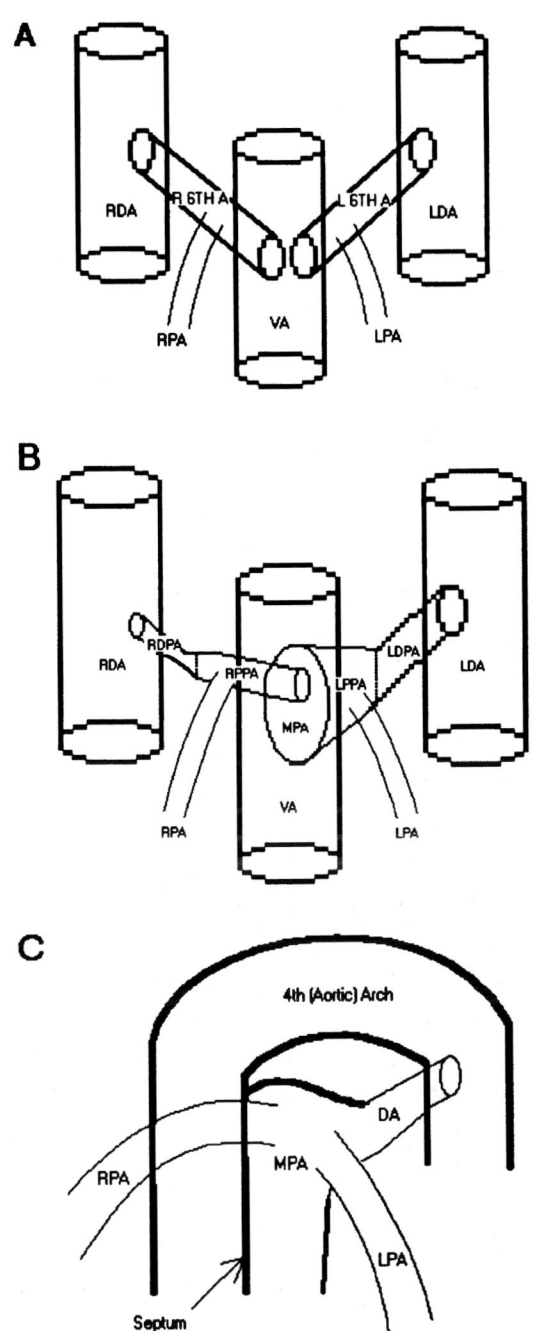

Before the formation of the pulmonary arteries and veins, both respiratory and nonrespiratory portions of the primordial lung are supplied by systemic connections that anastomose the aortae to vascular plexuses that have formed from the pulmonary mesenchyme surrounding each lung bud. As the nonrespiratory portions of the bronchial tree develop, they continue to be vascularized by this foregut plexus from the aorta, which drains into the subcardinal veins and vena cavi. These systemic connections are lost later in development when formal connections are created to the systemic circulation in the form of bronchial arteries and veins. From weeks 20 to 32, the bronchial arteries and veins mature. When fully developed, the bronchial arteries supply the airway walls, hilum, hilar pleura, and large blood vessel walls. The bronchial venous system drains a territory limited to the hilum, with the remainder of the lung and pleura draining to the pulmonary circulation.

Innervation of the Lung

Development of the pulmonary nerve supply parallels the development of the airways and pulmonary blood vessels. Ectodermally derived neural crest cells migrate into the undifferentiated mesenchyme of the week-4 embryo. Nerve development then continues from hilum to periphery as target tissues develop with contributions from the vagus nerve and the thoracic sympathetic plexus. By week 7 extrachondral nerve bundles are seen in proximal airway walls. Later subchondral plexuses are visualized in parallel with the extrachondral plexuses. In distal airways without cartilage, the two plexuses are seen to merge, finally terminating at the level of the terminal sacs, as noted by Larsell (1922).

By week 10 the extrapulmonary portions of the pulmonary arterial and venous trees are innervated. As intrapulmonary vascular connections mature, more peripheral arteries and veins are innervated. The nerves themselves receive a rich blood supply from the bronchial arteries. By 8 postnatal months, the entire nervous system is complete. At maturity the pulmonary nervous system innervation includes airways from the trachea to the alveolus, airway appendages and epithelium including mucous glands, and peripulmonary tissues including blood vessels, lymphatics, and the pleura.

Fig. 2-16. Diagrammatic representation of pulmonary artery development from the right and left sixth aortic arches. **A.** By day 32 of development the right and left sixth branchial arch arteries (R 6TH A, L 6TH A) have joined the respective dorsal aortae (RDA, LDA) to the ventral aortic sac (VA) and have given off primordial right and left pulmonary arteries (RPA, LPA). **B.** Near day 40 several changes are evident. The right distal sixth arch (RDPA) has thinned. The left proximal sixth arch (LPPA) has enlarged to include the right proximal pulmonary artery (RPPA), becoming the main pulmonary artery (MPA). **C.** By day 50, the transverse septum has divided the truncus arteriosus into right and left ventricular outflow tracts. The right dorsal aorta has regressed. The proximal left sixth arch has completed its transformation into the main pulmonary artery. The left distal pulmonary artery remains as the ductus arteriosus (DA), shunting the fetal right ventricular output away from the lungs into the systemic circulation.

Other Cell Types and Pulmonary Structures

Various cell types and structures not discussed previously are contributed to the developing lung by each embryologic dermal layer. Beside alveolar type I and II pneumocytes, the endoderm differentiates in the conducting airways into ciliated cells, secretory goblet cells, intermediate cells, Clara cells, and basal cells. In more proximal airways the cells take on a pseudostratified appearance and subepithelial bronchial glands develop. The distal airways demonstrate a

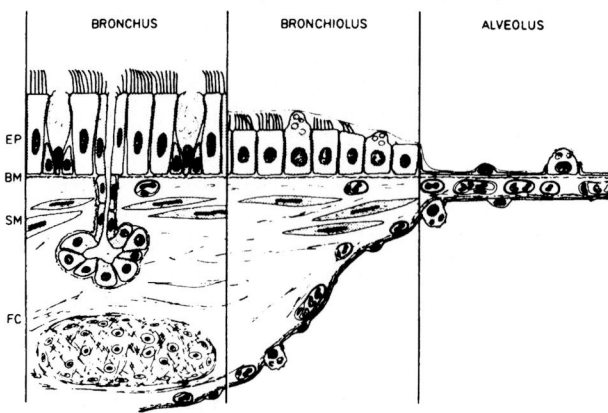

Fig. 2-17. The change of airway wall structure at the three principal levels. The epithelial layer (EP) gradually becomes reduced from pseudostratified to cuboidal and then to squamous but retains its organization as a mosaic of lining and secretory cells. The smooth muscle layer (SM) disappears in the alveoli. The fibrous coat (FC) contains cartilage only in bronchi and gradually becomes thinner as the alveolus is approached. BM, basement membrane. From Burri PH, Weibel ER. Funktionelle Aspekte der Lungenmorphologie. *In* Fuchs WA, Vogeli E (eds): Röntgendiagnostik der Lunge. Aktuelle Probleme der Röntgendiagnostik, 2nd Ed. Bern: Huber, 1973. With permission.

histologically simple epithelium and contain fewer secretory elements (Fig. 2-17). Beside blood vessels, the mesoderm contributes several structures including cartilage, muscle, connective tissue, and lymphatics. Ectodermal derivatives include the pulmonary nervous system as well as neuroendocrine derivatives including the Kulchitsky's cell and members of the amine precursor uptake and decarboxylation family of neuroendocrine cells. According to Jeffery and Reid (1977), all of these cell types can be seen as early as week 16 of fetal lung development. Later in development, hematologic elements including lymphocytes and mast cells infiltrate the bronchial epithelium and are seen in the submucosal pulmonary parenchyma.

FUTURE DIRECTIONS

The study of pulmonary embryology is ongoing. The field has progressed far beyond the level of wax model reconstructions and light microscopy. Technological advances have allowed current embryologists to view lung development at the molecular level. Much of the current work on lung development is focused on signaling pathways and the role of growth factors in morphogenesis and cytodifferentiation. For example, Shiratori and coworkers (1996) have implicated keratinocyte growth factor in a complex cascade of carefully timed events involved in lung morphogenesis. Epidermal growth factor and transforming growth factor-β_1 have been identified by Chinoy and colleagues (1988) as well as Minoo and colleagues (1995) as having important

regulatory roles in airway branching and bronchial development. As we gain a better understanding of these complex interactions, it is hoped that work at the molecular level will yield therapeutic strategies in neonates with pulmonary developmental abnormalities as well as in pediatric and adult patients with pulmonary parenchymal injury.

REFERENCES

Biscoe TJ, Purvis MJ, Sampson SR: Types of nervous activity which may be recorded from the carotid sinus nerve in the sheep fetus. J Physiol *190*:443, 1969.

Boyden EA, Tompsett DA: The changing patterns in the developing lungs of infants. Acta Anat *47*:185, 1965.

Boyden EA: Notes on the development of the lung in infancy and early childhood. Am J Anat *121*:749, 1967.

Boyden EA: Development of the human lung. *In* McQuarrie I (ed): Brennermann's Practice of Pediatrics. Vol. 4. Hagerstown, MD: Harper and Row, 1972a.

Boyden EA: The structure of compressed lungs in congenital diaphragmatic hernia. Am J Anat *134*:497, 1972b.

Boyden EA: The mode of origin of pulmonary acini and respiratory bronchioles in the fetal lung. Am J Anat *141*:317, 1974.

Bremer JL: The diaphragm and diaphragmatic hernia. Arch Pathol *36*:539, 1943.

Brumley GW, Hodson WA, Avery ME: Lung phospholipids and surface tension. Correlations in infants with and without disease, and in adults. Pediatrics *40*:13, 1967.

Bucher U, Reid L: Development of the intrasegmental tree; the pattern of branching and development of cartilage at various stages of intrauterine life. Thorax *16*:207, 1961.

Campiche MA, et al: An electron microscope study of the fetal development of the lung. Pediatrics *32*:976, 1963.

Chinoy MR, et al: Influence of epidermal growth factor and transforming growth factor beta-1 on patterns of fetal mouse lung branching morphogenesis in organ culture. Pediatr Pulmonol *25*:244, 1988.

DeBlasio A, Ambrosio G, D'Amora G: Sui movimenti respiratori endouterini del feto umano a termine. Pediatria *68*:1124, 1960.

Dubreuil G, et al: Observations sur le developpement du poumon humain. Bull Histol Technol Physiol *13*:235, 1936.

Dunnill MS: Postnatal growth of the lung. Thorax *17*:329, 1962.

Farrell PM: Regulation of pulmonary lecithin synthesis. *In* Villee CA, Villee DB, Zuckerman J (eds): Respiratory Distress Syndrome. New York: Academic Press, 1973.

Gluck L, et al: Diagnosis of the respiratory distress syndrome by amniocentesis. Am J Obstet Gynecol *109*:440, 1971.

Heymann MA, et al: Bradykinin production associated with oxygenation of the fetal lamb. Circ Res *25*:521, 1969.

Hislop A, et al: Postnatal growth and function of the pre-acinar airways. Thorax *27*:265, 1972.

Hislop A, Reid L: Development of the acinus in the human lung. Thorax *29*:90, 1974.

Hugues GM: Evolution between air and water. *In* De Reuck AVS, Potter R (eds): Ciba Foundation Symposium: Development of The Lung. Boston: Little, Brown and Co, 1967.

Jeffery PK, Reid L: Ultrastructural features of airway lining epithelium in the developing rat and human lung. J Anat *120*:295, 1977.

Kohn HM: Zur histologie der inderevenden fibrosen Pneumonie. Munch Med Wochenschr *40*:42, 1893.

Krogh A: On the cutaneous and pulmonary respiration of the frog: a contribution to the theory of gas exchange between the blood and the atmosphere. Skand Arch Physiol Leipz *15*:328, 1904.

Lambert MW: Accessory bronchioli-alveolar communications. J Pathol Bacteriol *70*:311, 1955.

Langston C, et al: Human lung growth in late gestation and in the neonate. Am Rev Respir Dis *129*:607, 1984.

Larsell O: The ganglia, plexuses and nerve terminations of the mammalian lung and pleura pulmonalis. J Comp Neurol *35*:97, 1922.

Loosli CG, Potter EL: The prenatal development of the human lung. Anat Rec *109*:320, 1951.

Low FN: The pulmonary alveolar epithelium of laboratory animals and man. Anat Rec *117*:241, 1953.

Meyrick B, Reid L: Electron microscope aspects of surfactant secretion. Proc R Soc Med *66*:386, 1973.

Minoo P, et al: TTF-1 regulates lung epithelial morphogenesis. Dev Biol *172*:694, 1995.

O'Rahilly R, Boyden EA: The timing and sequence of events in the development of the human respiratory system during the embryonic period proper. Z Anat Entwicklungsgesh *141*:237, 1973.

O'Rahilly R, Müller F: The respiratory system. *In* Human Embryology and Teratology. 2nd Ed. New York: Wiley-Liss, 1996.

Pattle RE, Hopkinson DAW: Lung lining in bird, reptile, and amphibia. Nature *200*:894, 1963.

Poddubnyi IG: Embryonic development of the pulmonary veins. Arch Anat Histol Embryol *64*:49, 1973.

Policard A, et al: L'alveole pulmonaire au microscope electronique. Presse Med *62*:1775, 1954.

Rudnick D: Developmental capacities of the chick lung in chorioallantoic grafts. J Exp Zool *66*:125, 1933.

Shiratori M, et al: Keratinocyte growth factor and embryonic rat lung morphogenesis. Am J Respir Cell Mol Biol *15*:328, 1996.

Smith EI: The early development of the trachea and esophagus in relation to atresia of the esophagus and tracheoesophageal fistula. Contrib Embrol Carnegie Inst Wash *36*:41, 1957.

Sorokin SP: A morphologic and cytochemical study on the great alveolar cell. J Histochem Cytochem *14*:884, 1966.

Streeter GL: Developmental horizons in human embryos: description of age group XI, 13 to 20 somites and age group XII, 21 to 29 somites. Contrib Embryol Carnegie Inst Wash *30*:211, 1945a.

Streeter GL: Developmental horizons in human embryos: description of age group XIII and XIV. Contrib Embryol Carnegie Inst Wash *31*:27, 1945b.

Streeter GL: Developmental horizons in human embryos: description of age group XI, 13 to 20 somites and age groups XV, XVI, XVII, and XVIII. Contrib Embryol Carnegie Inst Wash *32*:133, 1948.

Streeter GL: Developmental horizons in human embryos: description of age group XI, 13 to 20 somites and age groups XIX, XX, XXI, XXII, and XXIII, being the fifth issue of a survey of the Carnegie collection prepared for publication by Herser CH, Corner GW. Contrib Embryol Carnegie Inst Wash *34*:165, 1951.

Taderera JV: Control of lung differentiation in vitro. Dev Biol *16*:489, 1967.

Thurlbeck W: Lung growth. *In* Pathology of the Lung. New York: Thieme, 1988.

von Neergaard K: Neue Auffassungen uber einen Grundbergergriff der Atemmechanik, Die Retraktionskraft der Lunge, abhangig von der Oberflachenspannung in den Alveolen. Z Gestamte Exp Med *66*:373, 1929.

Weibel ER: Morphometry of the Human Lung. Berlin: Springer-Verlag, 1963.

Windle WF, et al: Aspiration of amniotic fluid by the fetus: an experimental roentgenological study in the guinea pig. Surg Gynecol Obstet *69*:705, 1939.

Witschi E: Development of Vertebrates. New York: Saunders, 1956.

Woodrum DE, et al: Initiation of breathing in the fetal lamb: response to cyanide, hypoxemia and hypercapnia following peripheral denervation. J Appl Physiol *42*:630, 1977.

Zachary RB, Emery JL: Failure of separation of larynx and trachea from the esophagus: persistent esophagotrachea. Surgery *49*:525, 1961.

CHAPTER 3

Ultrastructure and Morphometry of the Human Lung

Peter H. Burri, Juan Gil, and Ewald R. Weibel

ORGANIZATION OF THE LUNG

The application of electron microscopy and quantitative methods in morphology—morphometry—has widened the general understanding of lung structure and set the course for a more functional approach to the study of pulmonary architecture. It cannot be the aim of this chapter, however, to cover all aspects of lung microanatomy; in this respect, the reader is referred to the specialized literature. We would rather present the morphologic and quantitative background needed to understand the functioning of the gas-exchange apparatus.

The lung is composed of three phases: air, tissue, and blood. The tissue forms a complete barrier between air and blood; it is a stable structural framework, whereas air and blood are continuously exchanged. In describing the ultrastructure of the lung, we emphasize the specializations of the tissue in forming boundary spaces for air and blood. Morphometry deals with the quantitative relations among these three phases.

From the functional point of view, the organization of the lung may be defined in relation to the hierarchy of airways and blood vessels, from the trachea down to alveoli, or from the main stem of the pulmonary artery through the capillary network to the pulmonary veins entering the left atrium.

All of this is jointly considered in the scheme of Figure 3-1. Besides showing the three phases, the diagram introduces the three major functional zones of the lung; first, the conductive zone consisting of air channels and blood vessels, the function of which is to guide and distribute air and blood into the peripheral lung units; second, the respiratory zone comprised of alveoli and capillaries; and third, the intermediate or transitory zone containing elements of both.

FINE STRUCTURE OF THE LUNG

Fine Structure of Conducting Airways

The conducting airways are a system of tubes, which multiply toward the periphery by division according to the principle of irregular dichotomy. From the trachea to bronchi to bronchioles, the structure of the airway gradually changes. What is common to all is the general scheme of a three-layered wall made of a mucosa, a muscle layer, and a connective tissue sheath (Fig. 3-2) and the presence of a typical ciliated epithelium, which we describe first.

Lining Epithelium of Conductive Airways

The inspired air must be humidified and warmed before it reaches the delicate gas-exchange area; furthermore, air pollutants and dust, as well as airborne microorganisms, must be removed. Although the upper respiratory tract, in particular the nasal portion, is especially designed for these functions, the respiratory epithelium (Fig. 3-3), of all conducting airways, shows special features for the handling of airborne particles. The respiratory epithelium is a ciliated pseudostratified columnar epithelium with numerous scattered goblet cells. Ciliated cells occur from the trachea down to the last respiratory bronchiole, but their height decreases with the reduction of the airway diameter; ciliated cells of the trachea are columnar (Fig. 3-4), whereas those of the respiratory bronchioles are cuboidal (Fig. 3-5). The frequency of goblet cells also decreases toward the periphery; in bronchioles, they are replaced by Clara cells (see Fig. 3-5). These are complex exocrine cells known to be equipped with active P450 cytochrome metabolic pathways capable of actively participating in the detoxification of foreign substances. Understanding the nature of their secretory function has

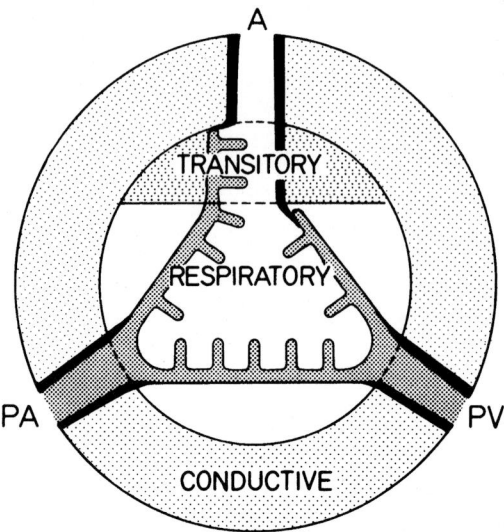

Fig. 3-1. Schematic representation of lung zones. A, airways; PA, pulmonary artery; PV, pulmonary vein.

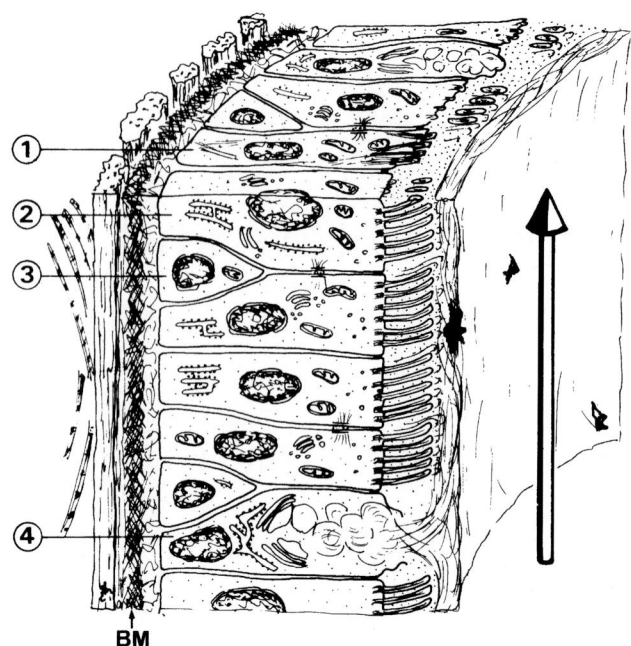

Fig. 3-3. Pseudostratified epithelium of bronchus with brush (1), ciliated (2), basal (3), and goblet cells (4). The cilia beat in a serous fluid that is topped by a mucous layer secreted partly by goblet cells. A strong basement membrane (BM) and a layer of longitudinal elastic fibers form the basis of the epithelium.

proved more difficult. Dierynck (1995), Hermans (1998), and Yao (1998a, b) and their colleagues have reported the presence of small (10 or in particular 16 kD) Clara cell proteins thought to be powerful immunosuppressants or anti-inflammatory substances active in the modulation of inflammatory responses. Cytologic, kinetic, and histochemical studies by Breeze and Wheeldon (1977), Jeffery and Reid (1977), Jeffery (1983), Spicer (1983), St. George (1985), and Plopper (1991) and their colleagues have provided insights into the cell types of the airway epithelium of various

species, including humans. In investigations, great emphasis also has been put on the neuroendocrine cells interspersed in the epithelium, often called Feyrter, Kulchitsky, amine precursor uptake and decarboxylation (APUD), or small granule cells. These neuroendocrine cells are present in the respiratory tract of all vertebrate species investigated so far. Lauweryns and Cokelaere (1973) found the neuroendocrine cells thinly scattered along the airways, either isolated or clustered in neuroepithelial bodies. Neuroepithelial bodies are assumed to function as chemoreceptors; they may act on pulmonary vascular or airway smooth muscle by secreting vasoactive substances. Sorokin and coworkers (1983) found them to represent a heterogeneous population of cells, and according to investigations by Hoyt and coworkers (1990) in the hamster lung, they are no more considered to be of neural crest origin.

The frequently found basal cells represent a proliferative pool of undifferentiated cells, which are thought to replace the overlying cells on differentiation and maturation. Less common are the brush cells and migratory cells. Finally, one should mention the occurrence of naked nerve endings between individual cells, more frequent in the trachea and large bronchi. They are thought to be irritant receptors.

Figure 3-3 shows a schematic representation of a portion of the respiratory epithelium of a bronchus. The function of this epithelium is to capture airborne particles in a sticky mucous layer and to remove them efficiently from the lung. For this purpose, cilia show a synchronized rhythmic beat

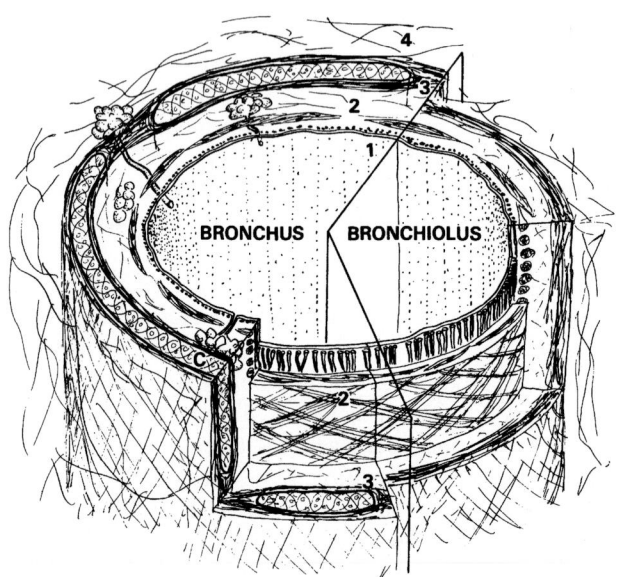

Fig. 3-2. Structure of bronchi and bronchioles. 1, mucosa with epithelium and elastic fibers; 2, smooth muscle layer; 3, fibrous layer contains cartilage (C) in the bronchi; 4, peribronchial sheath of loose connective tissue.

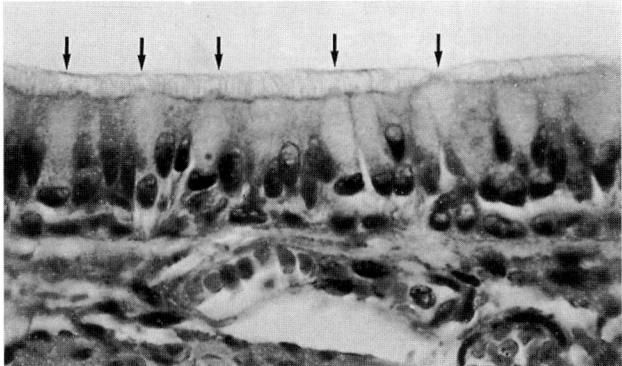

Fig. 3-4. Pseudostratified epithelium from bronchus. Note goblet cells (*arrows*) (original magnification ×600).

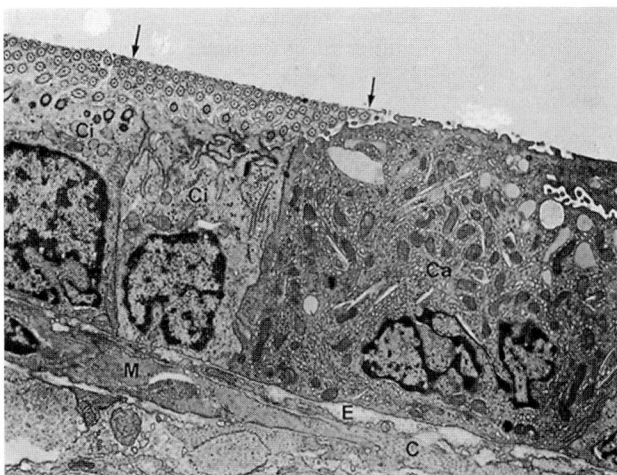

Fig. 3-5. Electron micrograph of bronchiolar wall with simple cuboidal epithelium made up of ciliated cells (Ci) and Clara cells (Ca). In place of the mucous layer is a fine osmiophilic film (*arrows*) at the air-liquid interface. A smooth muscle cell (M) and collagenous (C) and elastic (E) fibers are seen in the subepithelial tissue. Rat lung fixed by vascular perfusion (original magnification ×9200).

within a thin layer of low-viscosity fluid. On top, a blanket of mucus is moved in the direction of the pharynx, carrying intercepted particles. This cleaning mechanism can be compared with a conveyor belt and is often called the *mucociliary escalator*. The mechanism of mucus propulsion has been described in detail by Sleigh (1991). The mucous layer is secreted onto the epithelial surface by goblet cells and by seromucous glands located in the walls of trachea and bronchi (see Fig. 3-2). The small bronchioles are most likely devoid of mucus, as their wall contains neither goblet cells nor glands. As shown by the two of us (JG and ERW 1971), their surface is formed by a fluid layer of low viscosity that is sometimes topped by a thin osmiophilic film. Finally, the presence in the bronchial secretion of several humoral agents, which would protect the airways against infections, has been reported.

Trachea and Bronchi

Trachea and bronchi are characterized by the presence of cartilage within the fibrous sheath of their walls (see Fig. 3-2). In the trachea and stem bronchi, the cartilage is in the form of incomplete rings; in the trachea, these cover the ventral and lateral aspects, whereas the dorsal wall contains a strong layer of transverse smooth muscle. After approximately the second or third generation, these rings are gradually replaced by irregular cartilage plates, and a layer of smooth muscle appears between mucosa and cartilage.

All conducting airways are surrounded by an external, loose connective tissue sheath (see Fig. 3-2), which is continuous with the other connective elements of the lung. It is a structure of considerable physiologic significance, because it contains bronchial vessels to supply the bronchial wall with blood from the systemic circulation, as well as nerves and lymphatic vessels. Only a small part of the arterial bronchial flow, in some species as little as 25%, is drained by the bronchial veins. Most of it goes into the peribronchial venous plexus and from there into the pulmonary veins, forming a small right-to-left shunt. The bronchus is accompanied usu-

ally by a branch of the pulmonary artery, which is enveloped by connective tissue continuous with the peribronchial sheath.

Lymphatic vessels contained in these peribronchial and perivascular sheaths, as well as in the subpleural and septal connective tissue, constitute the main drainage path for the interstitial fluid.

Bronchioles

A bronchiole is an airway devoid of cartilage and seromucous glands; goblet cells are rare. Because airway structure does not change abruptly, either seromucous glands or goblet cells may still be present in transitional zones. Bronchioles are rather small conducting airways, measuring approximately 1 mm or less in diameter. Their added cross-sectional area is such, however, that they are not supposed to contribute substantially to the flow resistance of the airways in the normally breathing healthy individual. Their walls are generally thin and molded into the surrounding parenchyma. They are supplied with blood from the lesser circulation, rather than from bronchial arteries. The bronchiolar mucosa is lined by a simple cuboidal epithelium (see Fig. 3-5) composed of ciliated cells and Clara cells, which, as mentioned in the section discussing epithelial properties, have a dual detoxifying and secretory function. They are the object of intense study, and their exocrine secretory activity is being linked with a modulation of the inflammatory and immunologic response to injury. Their position as defensive cells is crucial because in the normal respiratory tidal range, bronchioles are the last conducting airways to receive bulk air in conjunction with inspiration. In bronchioles Clara cells take the place of goblet cells found in larger airways.

In bronchioles, the smooth muscle cells form a well-developed, relatively thick layer arranged in a geodesic network, capable of narrowing the airway.

Resistance to Airflow in Conducting Airways

The partition of airflow resistance between large and small airways both in health and disease has been controversial. It is universally accepted that, in the healthy lung, the major site of resistance is the large, central airways, whereas the bronchioles contribute less than 20%, but it is important to know that pathologic increases of resistance always occur in the bronchiolar region. Airflow in the trachea is turbulent; in the bronchioles it is laminar. In between, it is often referred to as transitional, implying an admixture of both, although experimental studies are difficult to perform. One of the major contributions to the understanding of the pathophysiology of emphysema was the clarification of the mechanisms of early airway closure. A priori, examination of the bronchiolar anatomy immediately reveals the factors that account for their active and passive narrowing: smooth muscle, compression by neighboring parenchyma during inflation, and internal surface tension. The elements that counteract the narrowing and act to cause bronchiolar dilatation are less evident, however, made possible only by the radial insertion of alveolar walls in their periphery and by the principle of mechanical interdependence. The integrity of alveolar walls is therefore essential in keeping bronchioles open during deflation. In conditions such as emphysema, in which alveolar walls are lost, the loss of bronchiolar support causes a calamitous early collapse of small bronchioles at the onset of expiration, with trapping of air in all areas of the parenchyma located behind the obstruction.

Fine Structure of Transitory Airways

Respiratory Bronchioles

The last generation of exclusively conducting bronchioles is the terminal bronchioles. These branch to form approximately three generations of respiratory bronchioles (Fig. 3-6), which have essentially the same structure as other bronchioles except that, here and there and increasingly toward the periphery, the continuity of their wall is interrupted by areas of typical gas-exchanging tissue. Contrary to common textbook descriptions, the cuboidal epithelial cells of respiratory bronchioles are in most cases ciliated; short cilia can even be demonstrated in close proximity to alveoli.

Alveolar Ducts and Sacs

The mammalian airways form a blind-ending system. Dichotomy as a branching pattern can be demonstrated up to the last ranks of the airway system, the alveolar ducts and alveolar sacs (see Fig. 3-6). These structures differ from the bronchioles described previously in that they lack a proper

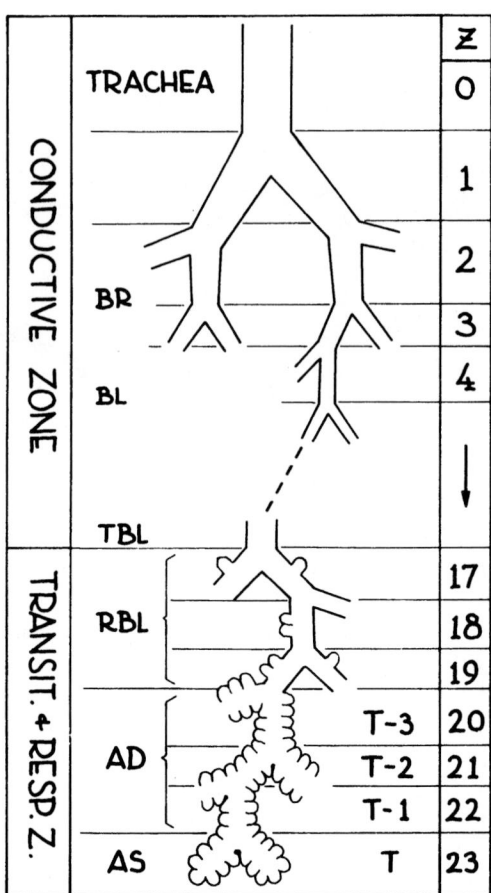

Fig. 3-6. Schematic representation of the sequence of airway branches as a function of generation z. Bronchi (BR), bronchioles (BL), terminal (TBL), and respiratory (RBL) bronchioles are followed by alveolar ducts (AD) and sacs (AS) in the terminal generation. T = 23. From Weibel ER: Morphometry of the Human Lung. Heidelberg: Springer, 1963, p. 111. With permission.

wall; instead, their wall is formed by the openings of alveoli (Fig. 3-7); their epithelial lining is nothing more than extensions of squamous alveolar epithelial cells. It is generally admitted that three generations of alveolar ducts immediately follow the last respiratory bronchioles. Finally, the last ducts give rise to two alveolar sacs. An alveolar sac represents the blind end of the airway branching system.

Fine Structure of the Gas-Exchange Region

In the respiratory zone of the lung, the blood is spread in capillaries in the walls of the alveoli. The air-blood contact becomes intimate and gas exchange can take place.

Alveoli

Alveoli are small pouches placed in groups around respiratory bronchioles, alveolar ducts, and alveolar sacs. They

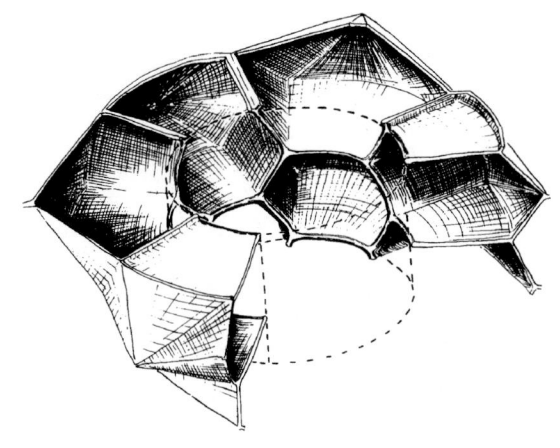

A

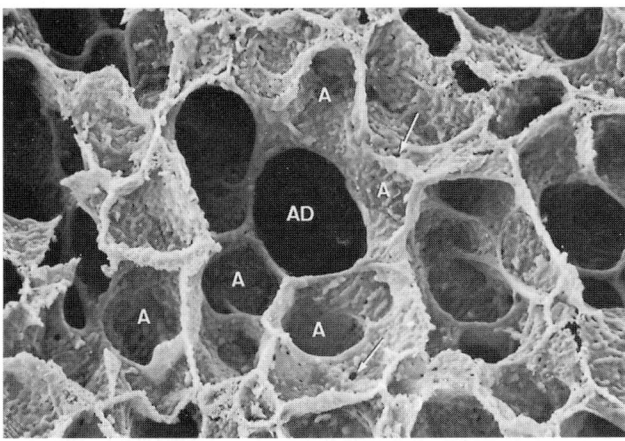

B

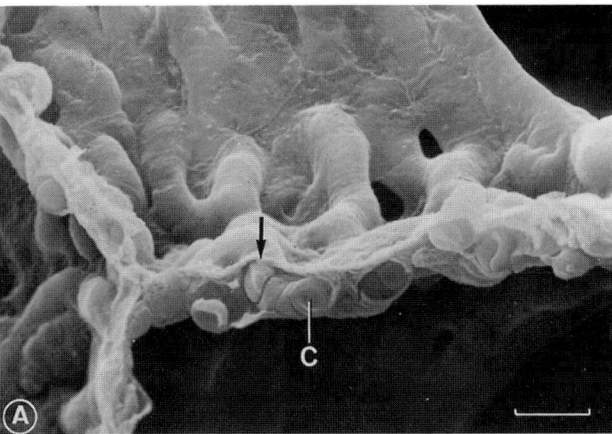

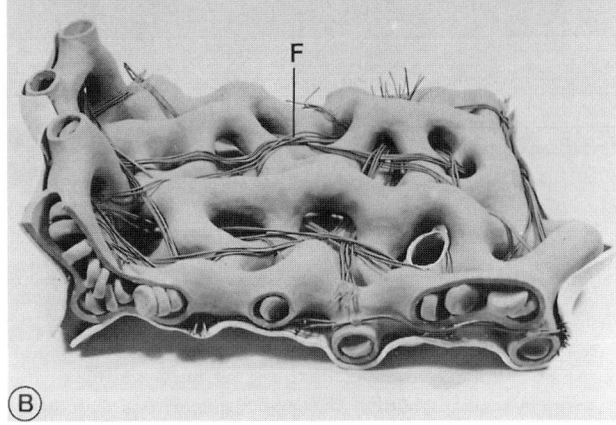

Fig. 3-7. A. Schematic representation of arrangement of alveoli around the alveolar duct. From Weibel ER: Morphometry of the Human Lung. Heidelberg: Springer, 1963, p. 57. With permission. **B.** Scanning electron micrograph of human lung (original magnification ×150). A, alveoli; AD, alveolar duct; *arrows* point to pores of Kohn.

Fig. 3-8. Capillaries in the alveolar wall of human lung are shown (**A**) in a scanning electron micrograph and (**B**) in a model. Note thin tissue barrier separating air and blood (*arrow*) and fibers (F) interwoven with capillary network (C) (scale marker = 10 μm). From Weibel ER: The Pathway for Oxygen. Cambridge: Harvard University Press, 1984. With permission.

are polyhedral structures lacking one side—the mouth, which opens into the airways—and they have been compared with the cells of a honeycomb (see Fig. 3-7) or with the air bubbles in a foam. A polygonal shape in general is economical, for it allows a close packing of the alveoli. The studies of Haefeli-Bleuer and one of us (E.R.W.) (1988) on human pulmonary acini revealed that the shape of alveoli is not simple and that often an *alveolus* appears like a cluster of several connected pouches, as in Figure 3-7B. Furthermore, alveolar shape also depends on the degree of lung inflation, according to one of us (J.G.) and coworkers (1979). Only in fully inflated lungs has the alveolar configuration some similarity to the cells of a honeycomb. At lower inflation degrees, alveoli are often cuplike.

The alveolar wall is always common to two adjacent alveoli and is called the *alveolar* or *interalveolar septum* (see Fig. 3-7B). The most conspicuous feature of the septum is a single but dense network of capillaries, which is shown in Figure 3-8 in face view. Sometimes, the septa are interrupted by pores of Kohn, which provide a path of com-

munication between adjoining alveoli. The septa also contain a skeleton of connective tissue fibers that is specially well developed around the mouth of the alveoli, where it forms a polygonal ring (see Fig. 3-7) and may contain smooth muscle fibers. The collagenous and elastic fibrous elements form a three-dimensional continuum that extends from the pleura to the hilus. This continuum ensures transmission of chest and diaphragmatic movements into the deeper regions of the lung, but it contributes only a smaller part to the retracting force of the lung, the major part being caused by surface forces. We (E.R.W. and J.G.) (1977) and one of us (E.R.W.) (1984) discussed the arrangement of the connective tissue in detail.

Alveolocapillary Tissue Barrier

Figure 3-9 shows a section of a small portion of an interalveolar septum with a capillary. The septum is lined on both sides by alveolar epithelial cells, which, in this instance, are thin. The capillary is lined also by a single squamous cell

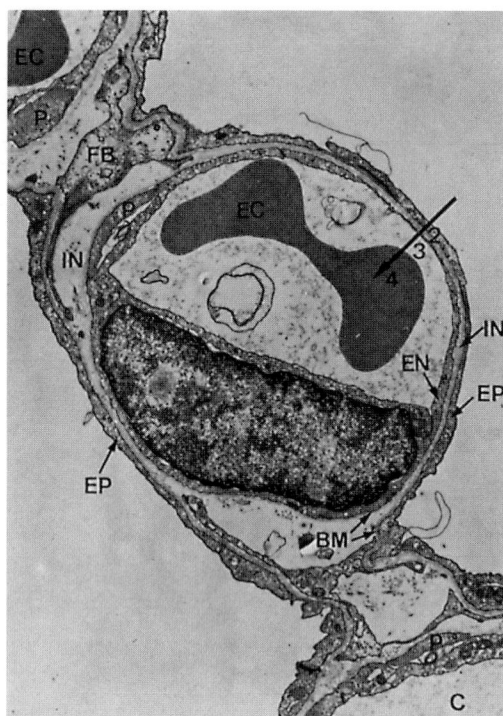

Fig. 3-9. Electron micrograph of alveolar capillary (C) from monkey lung with erythrocyte (EC). Note endothelial cell lining of capillary (EN), processes of pericytes (P), and the thin extensions of squamous alveolar epithelial cells (EP) covering the alveolar surface. The interstitial space (IN) is bounded by two basement membranes (BM) and contains some fibroblast processes (FB) as well as a few connective tissue fibrils. This lung was fixed by instillation of fixative into airways, resulting in a loss of the surface lining layer; hence only parts 2 (tissue barrier), 3 (blood plasma), and 4 (erythrocyte) of the gas exchange pathway are preserved (×8600). From Weibel ER: Morphometric estimation of pulmonary diffusion capacity. I. Model and method. Respir Physiol *11*:54, 1970–71. With permission.

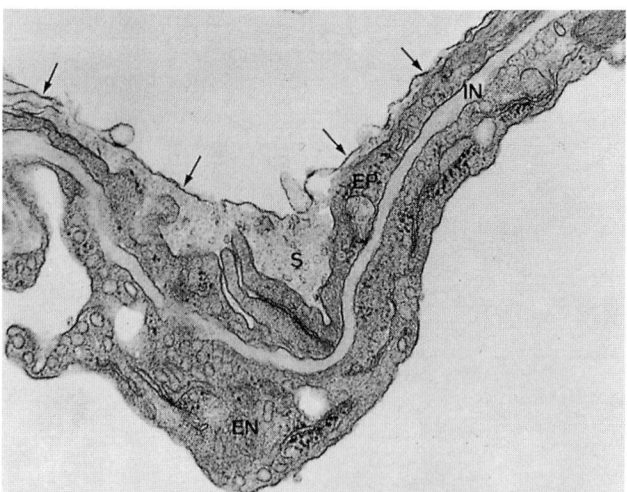

Fig. 3-10. Air-blood barrier of rat lung fixed by vascular perfusion to preserve surface lining layer (S) made up of base layer and osmiophilic surface film (*arrows*) (original magnification ×38,700). EN, endothelial cell lining of capillary; EP, squamous alveolar epithelial cells; IN, interstitial space. From Weibel ER: Morphometric estimation of pulmonary diffusion capacity. Respir Physiol *11*:54, 1970–71. With permission.

Although they are some 30 to 40% less numerous than the type II cells, they cover 92 to 95% of the total alveolar surface. The nuclei lie in depressions between two capillaries. These cells are poor in organelles, such as mitochondria or endoplasmic reticulum, which are confined to the perinuclear cytoplasm, whereas the cytoplasmic extensions essentially contain only pinocytotic vesicles. Crapo and associates (1982) found that in humans, a single type I cell covers some 5,000 μm^2 of the alveolar surface, on the average.

Alveolar cells type II are cuboidal (Fig. 3-13). These cells also have been called granular pneumocytes, septal cells,

layer, the endothelium. Together with the intercalated connective tissue, these two cell layers constitute the alveolocapillary tissue barrier, which is the structure separating air and blood in the pulmonary gas-exchange region. It is supplemented by an extremely thin extracellular lining layer that contains macrophages (Figs. 3-10 and 3-11). The morphometric characteristics of the cell population that constitutes this tissue barrier in the human lung are shown in Table 3-1.

Epithelium

The epithelium of the alveoli is continuous, although its thickness in places only reaches 0.1 to 0.3 μm, which is at the limit of resolution of the light microscope. The study by Low (1952) brought the first conclusive evidence for an uninterrupted epithelial lining of alveoli. It consists of the following cell types (see Table 3-1).

Alveolar epithelial cells type I (Fig. 3-12), also called *squamous cells*, send out broad, thin cytoplasmic extensions.

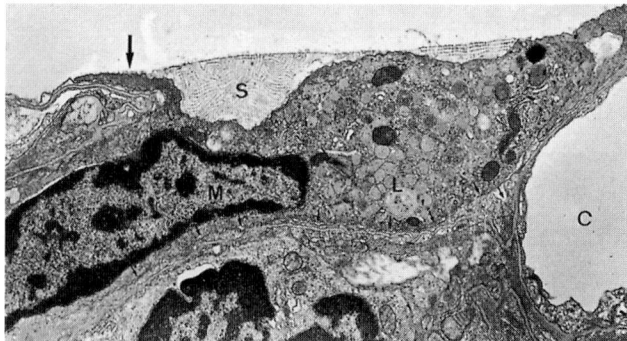

Fig. 3-11. Alveolar macrophage (M) with pseudopods and groups of lysosomal vesicles (L) in cytoplasm submerged beneath surface lining layer (S) and closely stuck to the alveolar epithelium (*arrows*). The base layer of the surface lining layer contains so-called tubular myelin figures. The capillary (C) is empty because of fixation by vascular perfusion (original magnification ×10,500). From Gil J: Ultrastructure of lung fixed under physiologically defined conditions. Arch Intern Med *127*:896, 1971. With permission.

Table 3-1. Morphometric Characteristics of Cell Population in the Human Alveolar Septal Tissue

	Cell Number		Average Cell	
	Absolute $n \times 10^9$	Relative %	Volume (μm^3)	Apical Surface (μm^2)
Pneumocytes I	19	8.3	1763	5098
Pneumocytes II	37	15.9	889	183
Endothelial cells	68	30.2	632	1353
Interstitial cells	84	36.1	637	—
Macrophages	23	9.4	2491	—

Modified from Crapo JD, et al: Cell numbers and cell characteristics of the normal human lung. Am Rev Respir Dis *126*:332, 1982.

alveolar cells, and great alveolar cells, although they are smaller than type I cells. They have no cytoplasmic extensions and typically are in niches between capillaries of the alveolar septum. Their free surface is covered by somewhat irregular microvilli. The cells occupy 5 to 8% of the alveolar surface and form junctional complexes with neighboring alveolar cells type I. Compared with alveolar cells type I, the granular pneumocyte is rich in mitochondria, endoplasmic reticulum, Golgi's apparatus, and multivesicular bodies. Their most distinctive morphologic feature, however, is the presence of lamellar osmiophilic inclusions, the lamellar bodies, unique organelles known for many years as the sites of storage of surface-active phospholipids as described by one of us (J.G.) and Reiss (1973). They have been shown, according to Dobbs (1989), to participate in the secretion of surfactant apoproteins. Less well understood but probably of great importance is the participation of these cells in the recycling of alveolar surface materials; as is discussed, this is achieved by way of receptor-mediated endocytosis

through SP-A binding protein (surfactant-specific glygoprotein), as shown by Wissel and coworkers (1996).

A third pneumocyte, the brush cell, was described by Meyrick and Reid (1968). In the rat, this cell can be found in terminal bronchioles; it is, however, rare in the gas-exchange zone. The brush cell is characterized by a spray of rather thick and regular cylindrical microvilli at the surface and by thick bundles of microfibrils in the cytoplasm. Brush cells are large, but only a small part of their membrane reaches the epithelial surface. Similar cells occur in larger airway epithelia and in other organs also; their significance is still obscure.

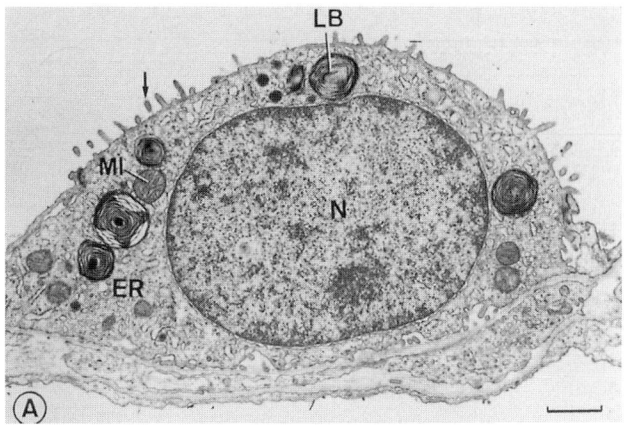

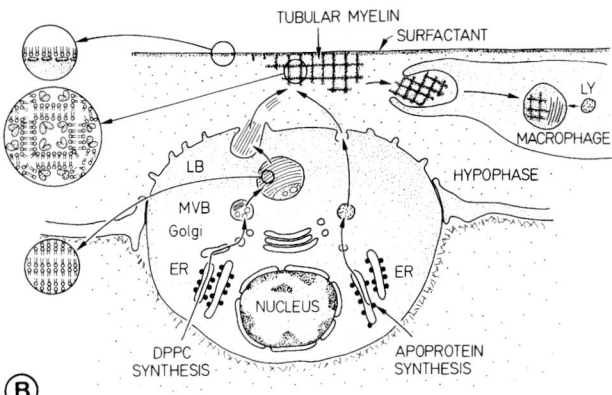

Fig. 3-13. A. In a type II epithelial cell, the abundant cytoplasm surrounding the nucleus (N) contains the characteristic osmiophilic lamellar bodies (LB), which store surfactant, and a rich complement of organelles such as endoplasmic reticulum (ER) and mitochondria (MI). The surface membrane carries microvilli (*arrow*) and junctions (J) with neighboring type I cells. From Weibel ER: Design and structure of the human lung. *In* Fishman AP (ed). Pulmonary Diseases and Disorders. New York: McGraw-Hill, 1971. With permission. **B.** Diagram of pathways for synthesis and secretion of surfactant dipalmitoylphosphatidyl chlorine (DPPC) and apoproteins by a type II cell, and for their removal by macrophages and by recycling. Note the arrangement of phospholipids in the lamellar bodies, tubular myelin, and surface film. Dashed line depicts possible alternative route of apoprotein secretion. MVB, multivesicular body. Modified from Weibel ER: The Pathway for Oxygen. Cambridge: Harvard University Press, 1984.

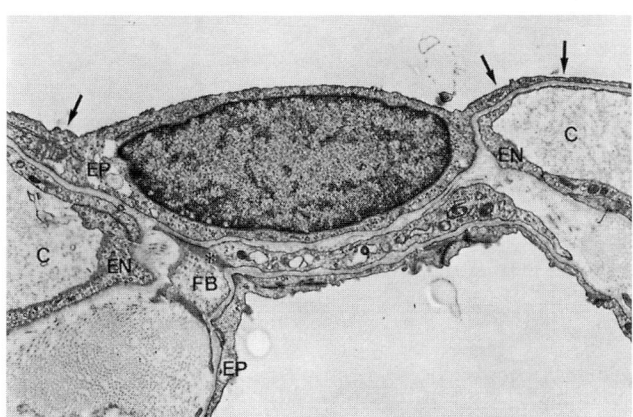

Fig. 3-12. Type I alveolar cell with thin cytoplasmic extensions (*arrows*) (original magnification ×8600). C, alveolar capillary; EN, endothelial cell lining of capillary; EP, squamous alveolar epithelial cells; FB, fibroblast process with an intracytoplasmic bundle of contractile filaments (*).

Alveolar macrophages (dust cells) are the cells of the alveolar lining layer (see Fig. 3-12). They are large cells exhibiting many vacuolar inclusions and lysosomes. Most of their phagosomes are filled with dark, lipid-rich inclusions. In their functional location, they are closely apposed to the alveolar epithelial surface and are submersed under the surfactant film of the lining layer (see Fig. 3-11); their bodies are in depressions of the alveolar wall and they send out large extensions. In conventional histologic preparations, they have been removed from their original position on the alveolar wall; they appear to float in the alveolar space and their surface is generally rounded off so that they acquire the appearance of large, spherical cells. Contrary to previous views that alveolar macrophages are derivatives of the epithelium, it has been shown convincingly that they derive from blood monocytes.

Interstitium

The interstitium is the space between the basal laminae of alveolar epithelium and capillary endothelium (see Fig. 3-9). It contains connective tissue and interstitial fluid. The connective tissue comprises cells, fibers, and amorphous substance containing proteoglycans, allegedly in a gel matrix. The distribution of connective tissue can vary considerably. In places where the air-blood barrier is thin, connective tissue may be reduced to a few isolated, fine fibrils or may even be absent, in which instance the adjoining basement membranes fuse. These latter regions are particularly important for gas exchange. In lung edema, they usually are not widened by interstitial fluid and can therefore be called *restricted* as opposed to those unrestricted, thicker portions of interstitium between capillaries, where interstitial fluid can accumulate under pathologic conditions. The interstitial fibroblasts have been demonstrated to contain contractile filaments (see Fig. 3-12), so Kapanci (1976) and coworkers (1974) suggested that they could regulate blood flow through the alveolar septum. In view of the interstitial structure described, one of us (E.R.W.) and Bachofen (1979) proposed an alternative function for these cells: They could control the compliance of the unrestricted interstitial regions by regulating the width of the septum. In the postnatal rat lung, the interstitial cells form two distinct populations of cells: a lipid-containing and a non–lipid-containing type. The lipid droplets of the lipid-containing type disappear, however, before weaning; the fate of the lipid-containing type remains unclear, according to Maksvytis and coworkers (1984). Lymphatic vessels are never found in alveolar septa. Nevertheless, a continuous path of the interstitial fluid toward the lymphatics of the subpleural space and of the peribronchial and perivascular connective sheaths has been postulated; the fluid probably follows connective fibers.

Endothelium

The endothelial cells form a capillary wall that is similar in structure to the endothelium in some other organs (Fig.

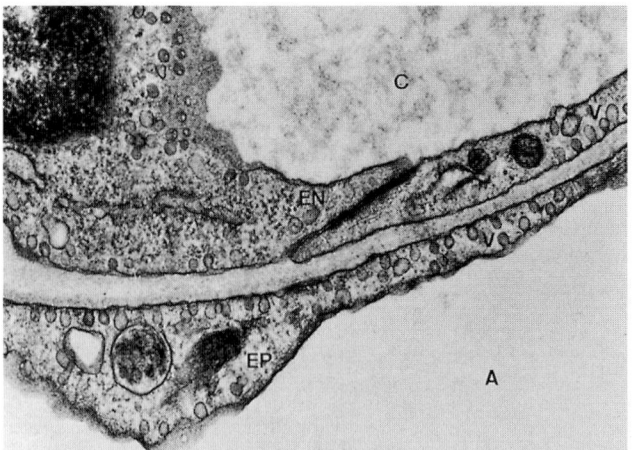

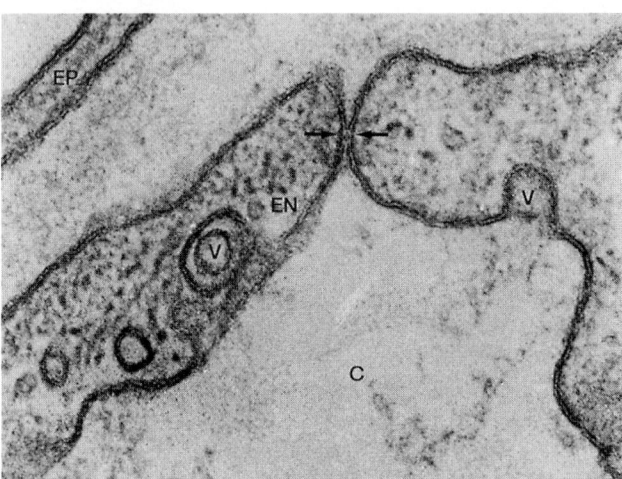

Fig. 3-14. A. Air-blood barrier showing thin cytoplasmic extensions of alveolar epithelium type I (EP) and endothelial cells (EN) with intercellular junction. Note abundance of pinocytotic vesicles (V) (original magnification ×37,000). **B.** High-power view of junction between two capillary endothelial cells. The triple-layered structure of the cell membranes is apparent. In the junction the membranes are closely apposed over a short stretch (*arrows*). Note pinocytotic vesicles (V) (original magnification ×184,800). A, alveolus; C, capillary.

3-14; see Figs. 3-9 and 3-10). The cells form thin cytoplasmic extensions and hence resemble the alveolar epithelial cells of type I. A single cell covers between 1,000 and 1,500 μm^2 of the capillary lumen. Lung capillaries have no fenestrations. Further details are discussed subsequently.

Extracellular Lining Layer and Pulmonary Surfactant

On the basis of theoretic considerations, as early as 1929, von Neergaard predicted that the alveolar surface must be lined by a layer of surface-active fluid, now commonly called *pulmonary surfactant*. It is an essential element, ensuring the stability of the air-filled lung. Its basic characteristics are twofold: first, it lowers the surface tension at the air-liquid interface of the alveoli; and second, its surface tension is variable with the degree of inflation of alveoli.

Morphologic demonstration of pulmonary surfactant is only possible with the electron microscope. In routine preparations, usually no traces of this material are found (see Fig. 3-9). In lungs fixed by vascular perfusion, an extracellular duplex lining layer on the alveolar surface can be preserved (see Fig. 3-10), which two of us (J.G. and E.R.W.) (1969 and 1970) supposed to contain the alveolar surfactant system fixed in situ. Much of this material forms pools in pits and irregularities of the alveolar wall, which smooths it out. These pools are polymorphous: Sometimes they are of moderate electron density with dark specks, or they may contain lipid micelles or tubular myelin, a liquid crystal made up of surface active lipoproteins.

The synthesis and secretion of pulmonary surfactant are the functions of the type II pneumocytes. Figure 3-13B shows how the organelles of this cell are involved in synthesizing, storing, and secreting the surfactant phospholipids and the specific apoproteins. The single most abundant component of surfactant is the phospholipid dipalmitoyl phosphatidylcholine. Four major proteins have been identified in alveolar surfactant. Two of these, SP-A and SP-D, are hydrophilic and members of the lectin superfamily, associated with immunoglobulins. SP-A strongly binds phospholipids, whereas SP-D does not; both are actively involved not only in lowering surface tension but also immediately associated with phospholipids, but the clarification of their exact roles is proving to be difficult, as noted by Johansson and Curstedt (1997). It appears that tubular myelin figures (see Fig. 3-11) are an extracellular reserve form of surfactant, which can spread on the surface when alveoli enlarge. For further details and references, see Weibel (1985), Mason and Williams (1991), and Hawgood (1991). As shown by one of us (JG) and Reiss (1972), the availability of Ca^{2+} is crucial for the stability of tubular myelin as a recognizable morphologic structure.

Fine Structure of Pulmonary Blood Vessels

Alveolar Capillaries

The dense capillary network (see Fig. 3-8) that is intercalated between adjoining alveoli and forms part of the interalveolar septa is lined by an uninterrupted endothelial cell layer (see Fig. 3-9). Characteristically, these endothelial cells are formed of two parts: 1) a region of cytoplasm surrounding the nucleus and containing the majority of cellular organelles, such as mitochondria, endoplasmic reticulum, Golgi's complex, and various granules; and 2) thin cytoplasmic extensions, which are 0.1 µm thick and virtually free of organelles. In the thinnest regions (<0.1 µm) they are composed of two cell membranes and some intercalated cytoplasm (see Fig. 3-9); the portions of average thickness contain numerous pinocytotic vesicles that are, in part,

attached to either of the cell membranes (see Figs. 3-9 and 3-14). These vesicles are involved in the transport of materials, mainly of proteins, across the endothelial cell. In connection with passage of macromolecules, the main problem, however, is the different permeability between endothelium and epithelium. General agreement exists that the epithelium represents the chief permeability barrier of the lung. Endothelium can be permeated under a variety of circumstances. The explanation for this difference was provided by comparative freeze-fracture studies of endothelial versus epithelial junctions. The epithelial tight junctions consist of a continuous network of three to five interconnected ridges and grooves; the endothelial junctions have only one to three rows of particles with few interconnections and even some discontinuities, as discussed by Schneeberger (1991). Because it is believed that an inverse correlation exists between the number of strands constituting a tight junction and its permeability, it follows that epithelial junctions are tight, whereas endothelial junctions are relatively leaky.

Alveolar capillaries are associated with pericytes. Pericytes seem to be less frequent in the alveolar capillaries than in the systemic capillaries and less densely branched. Their function is still debated: they are supposed to be contractile cells. In normal lungs they are α-smooth muscle and positive for actin, but negative for smooth muscle myosin heavy chain and desmin. Under pathologic conditions they seem to acquire the immunocytochemical characteristics of smooth muscle cells as reported by Nehls and Drenckhahn (1991).

Ultrastructure of Larger Pulmonary Vessels

The endothelial lining of pulmonary arteries and veins differs from that of alveolar capillaries in that the cytoplasmic extensions are thicker (Fig. 3-15). They are likewise rich in pinocytotic vesicles and may contain numerous cellular organelles. These endothelial cells also contain a characteristic rod-shaped granule (Fig. 3-16) known to occur in all vascular endothelia of all vertebrate species as originally described by one of us (E.R.W.) and Palade (1964). In the mammalian vascular system, these organelles are particularly numerous in medium-sized and larger branches of pulmonary arteries and veins, whereas they occur less frequently in systemic vessels of the same size. Based on indirect evidence, two of us (P.H.B. and E.R.W.) (1968) proposed that these organelles contain a procoagulative substance. This assumption proved to be correct. Wagner and associates (1982) and Warhol and Sweet (1984), using immunocytochemical techniques, demonstrated that the endothelial specific organelles contained factor VIII-related antigen, also called von Willebrand factor. More recently, Bonfanti and colleagues (1989) and McEver and colleagues (1989) showed that the granule membrane carries the leukocyte-binding protein P-selectin, also found in the α-granules of platelets.

The electron microscopic study of intima and media of pulmonary vessels does not reveal many features that are

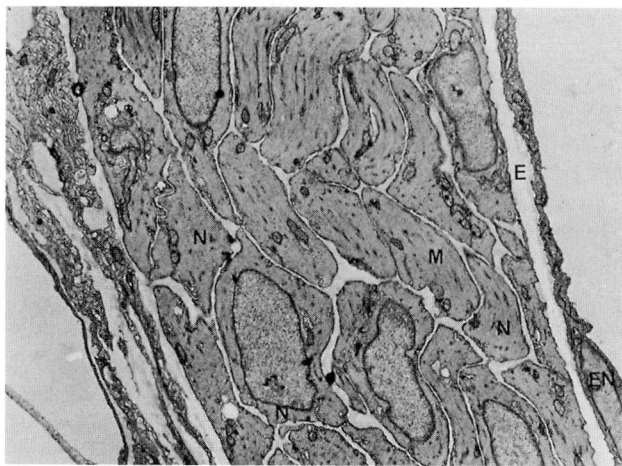

Fig. 3-15. Electron micrograph of longitudinal section of medium-sized pulmonary artery of muscle type. The endothelium (EN) lies over a strong elastic membrane (E). The smooth muscle fibers (M) are obliquely sectioned; their cytoplasm shows a fine filamentous structure. Some muscle cells (labeled N) show intercellular contacts (nexus), serving spread of excitation among the cells (original magnification ×5850).

not manifest by light microscopy. The circular smooth muscle cells of peripheral vessels of the muscular type are long, slender, and rather densely arranged (see Fig. 3-15). In elastic vessels (larger pulmonary arteries) the connective tissue elements prevail (see Fig. 3-16); the space between the prominent elastic laminae contains much collagenous tissue and relatively short smooth muscle cells, which extend from one elastic lamina to the next in an

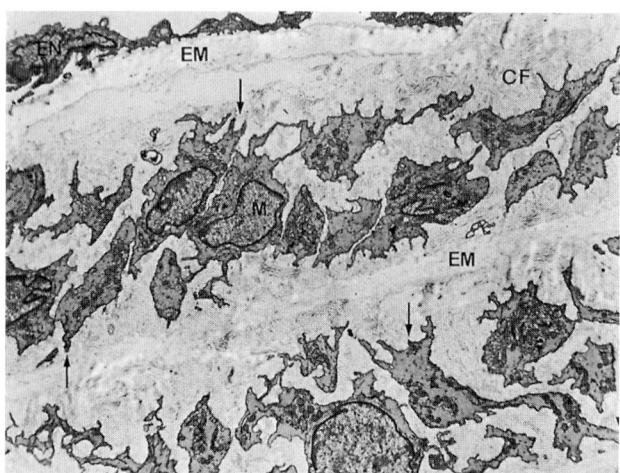

Fig. 3-16. Electron micrograph of pulmonary artery of elastic type. Note three strong elastic membranes (EM), paralleling the endothelium (EN), and ramified smooth muscle cells (M), which take an oblique course reaching from one elastic membrane to the next (*arrows*). Direction of muscle fibers alternates from one layer to the next. Collagen fibrils (CF) are abundant and mixed with elastic fibers (original magnification ×4850).

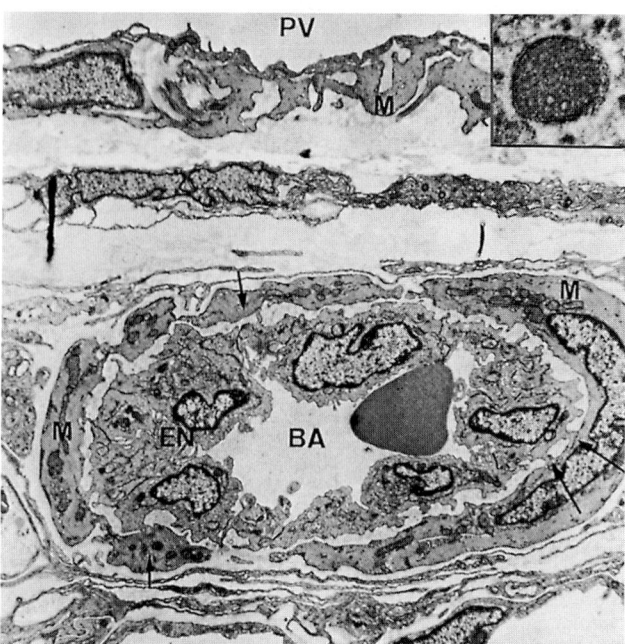

Fig. 3-17. Bronchial arteriole (BA) in a semicontracted state with thick endothelium (EN) and a simple layer of smooth muscle cells (M). Note numerous contacts between endothelial and muscle cells (*arrows*). At top, section of wall of small pulmonary vein (PV) with loose smooth muscle layer (M) and endothelium (original magnification ×4850). Inset shows sample of specific endothelial organelles (also called Weibel-Palade bodies) at higher power. Note membrane and internal tubules (original magnification ×83,200).

oblique course and appear to insert on the elastic laminae with ramified ends (see Fig. 3-16). In Figure 3-17, a portion of a longitudinal section of a medium-sized pulmonary vein is shown; its thin wall is made up of an endothelium, a few irregularly arranged smooth muscle fibers, and collagenous as well as elastic fibers. One interesting feature is that smooth muscle cells of these vessel walls not only form close intercellular contacts in the form of patches or nexus (see Figs. 3-15 and 3-16) but also have close cell-to-cell contact with endothelial cells by means of short extensions across the internal elastic membrane (see Fig. 3-17). It is assumed that cell-to-cell contacts between endothelial or epithelial cells and smooth muscle or interstitial cells are important in inducing and regulating various cell functions.

Bronchial Vessels

The arteries of the bronchial wall are of the muscle type. Figure 3-17 shows a small bronchial arteriole with one layer of circular smooth muscle and typically thick endothelial layer. Note the many contacts between muscle and endothelial cells. Bronchial arteries are often characterized by intimal longitudinal smooth muscle bundles that one of us (E.R.W.) (1959) found to be related to the stretch strain to

Table 3-2. Approximate Distribution of Total Lung Volume in Milliliters for Adult Human Lung at Three-fourths Total Lung Capacity[a]

Zones	Compartments			
	Air Channels	Tissue	Blood	
Conducting	Bronchi 170	Walls Septa Fibers	Arteries 150	Veins 150
Transition	Respiratory bronchioles Alveolar ducts 1500	Lymph 200	Arterioles 60	Venules 60
Respiratory	Alveoli 3150	Barrier 150	Capillaries 140	

[a]Total lung volume = 5.7 L.
From Weibel ER: Morphometry of the humanl lung. *In* Arcangeli P, et al (eds). Normal Values for Respiratory Function in Man. Milano: Panminerva Medica, 1970. p. 242.

which these vessels are frequently exposed rather than to a special regulatory function.

MORPHOMETRY OF THE LUNG

The application of morphometric methods in analyzing lung tissue has yielded new insights into lung structure and its dimensions and has opened the possibility of a morphologic approach to the study of lung function.

Compartmental Distribution of Lung Volume

Any morphologic analysis of the functional capacity of the gas-exchange apparatus involves exact knowledge of the total lung volume and of its compartmental distribution.

To illustrate the distribution of the lung volume among the various zones and constituents, we consider the lung of a medium-sized adult inflated to approximately three-fourths total lung capacity; the total lung volume would then amount to approximately 5.7 L. Table 3-2 gives the approximate distribution of this volume among the lung compartments as derived from morphometric analysis of fixed lungs. The greatest compartment is the air space, of which approximately two-thirds is in alveoli and only a small fraction in conductive airways, representing the anatomic dead space.

Number and Size of Alveoli and Capillaries

Alveoli

In spite of its ability to supply the organism with enough oxygen, the lung of the newborn is still immature structurally. Besides primitive air sacs, which have often been misinterpreted as alveoli, only a fraction of the final number of alveoli is present at birth. One of us (P.H.B.) (1974) and

coworkers (1974), as well as Kauffman and associates (1974), studied the postnatal development of alveoli using the rat lung as a model. It showed that alveoli were formed by outgrowth of new, so-called secondary septa from the sides of the primary ones present at birth. This occurrence transformed the smooth-walled channels and saccules of the newborn lung into alveolar ducts and alveolar sacs. This process was followed by an important remodeling of the septal structure. Indeed, in contrast to the mature septum containing a single capillary network interlaced with a fibrous skeleton, the primary and secondary septa presented a three-layered structure: A capillary network was found on both sides of a thick central sheet of connective tissue. The restructuring now consisted of a massive reduction of the interstitial tissue, probably accompanied by fusions of capillary segments. Zeltner and coworkers (1987) and Zeltner and one of us (P.H.B.) (1987) obtained similar findings in studies on human lung growth. At approximately 1 month of age, a human lung compared well structurally with the lung of a 1-week-old rat. Although alveolar formation in humans starts during late fetal life, according to Langston and coworkers (1984), more than 80% of all alveoli are formed postnatally. After alveolization, the septal structure is altered much in the same way as in the rat lung: A remodeling of the parenchymal microvasculature reduced the double capillary network to a single one. Figure 3-18 summarizes the findings of these studies and proposes a new staging and timing of lung development and growth. It appears that alveolization proceeds at a faster pace than assumed so far: Bulk alveolar formation seems to be terminated at approximately 1.5 years of age. It is further accompanied and followed, respectively, by a stage of microvascular maturation lasting from a few months after birth to the age of 2 or 3 years. This statement does not preclude that after the phase of obtrusive rapid alveolization some further alveoli may be added at much slower pace in immature regions and at the uttermost periphery of the lung parenchyma. One of us (E.R.W.) (1963) found that, in the adult, the number of alveoli aver-

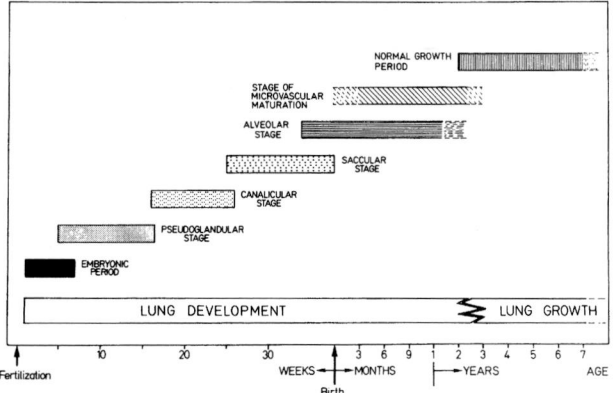

Fig. 3-18. Stages and timing of human lung development. Open-ended bars indicate that the exact start and end of the stages are still unknown. From Zeltner TB, Burri PH: The postnatal development and growth of the human lung. II. Morphology. Respir Physiol 67:269, 1987. With permission.

ages 300 million. According to Angus and Thurlbeck (1972), the number is related to body length and may vary largely between 200 and 600 million.

For a lung of an adult inflated to three-fourths of its maximal volume, one of us (E.R.W.). (1963) found that the average alveolar diameter lies between 250 and 290 μm. Glazier and associates (1967), however, demonstrated on dog lungs that alveolar size is not identical in all parts of the lung, but that in an erect lung, the upper parts contain larger alveoli than the dependent parts, because of the weight of the lung tissue.

Capillaries

As shown previously, capillaries form a dense network spreading over the surface of alveoli (see Fig. 3-8). This network is made up of hexagonal meshes, which means that usually three capillary segments are connected to each other at a junction point. The capillary network seems to be continuous over many interalveolar facets, perhaps even over a whole lobule or more. Terminal branches of arteries and veins connect to this vast network at points separated by approximately 5 mm. This determines microvascular fields that are approximately 0.5 mm in diameter and function like capillary microperfusion units but are not clearly demarcated by anatomic boundaries. In a morphometric analysis of eight normal human lungs by Gehr and coworkers (1978a), the total capillary volume varied between 125 and 387 mL (mean, 213 mL) and the capillary surface area from 74 to 189 m^2 (mean, 126 m^2).

During lung growth, capillary volume showed the steepest increase among all the parameters relevant for gas exchange. During the first 6 months, capillaries held only 22% of the volume of the interalveolar septa; this value reached 42% in adult lungs, according to Zeltner, one of us (P.H.B.), and coworkers (1987). Between 1 month of age and adulthood, capillary volume increases approximately 35 times and capillary surface area approximately 20 times in the human lung. With the capillary density being approximately equal, new capillaries have

to be continuously added to the existing network. Caduff, Fischer, and one of us (P.H.B.) (1986) and one of us (P.H.B.) and Tarek (1990) demonstrated by scanning electron microscopy and by ultrastructural analysis of serial sections that the pulmonary capillary network grows by formation of new intercapillary meshes rather than by sprouting new capillaries. The process has been termed by Paton and associates (1972) *intussusceptive microvascular growth*—growth within itself—in analogy to the growth of cartilage. It consists in the formation of transcapillary tissue pillars that divide existing capillary segments. The newly formed and originally small individual tissue pillars (diameter <1.5 μm) subsequently increase in diameter and thus give rise to new intercapillary meshes. In the meantime, Patan, one of us (P.H.B.), and coworkers (1992, 1996, 1997) could demonstrate various modes of pillar formation in intussusceptive growth and also prove that intussusceptive microvascular growth is not only present in the lung but represents a widespread and fundamental angiogenic process in vascularized organisms. This new angiogenic mechanism also has been demonstrated in tumor growth by Nagy and coworkers (1995).

Gas Exchange Surface and the Air-Blood Barrier

The alveolocapillary air-blood barrier is composed of a surface-lining layer, epithelium, interstitium, and endothelium that have to be crossed by the oxygen molecules on their way from air to blood. The following dimensions of this barrier are of greatest importance for gas exchange: first, the surface area of air-tissue interface; second, the surface area of tissue-blood interface; and third, the thickness of the barrier and of its components.

The alveolar surface area of the adult human lung has been found to vary between 97 and 194 m^2 (mean, 143 m^2). This range is in contrast to previously published results, where by light microscopic morphometry, values between 70 and 80 m^2 had been obtained. This discrepancy is because of the higher resolution of the electron microscope, which allows one to measure the complex free surface of the epithelial cells. With the light microscope, one could analyze only a smoothed surface of the alveolar wall.

In most species investigated, the total capillary surface area did not differ from the alveolar surface area by more than 10 to 12%. In the rat lung, the capillary-to-alveolar surface ratio is 1.05:1.1, which means that the capillary surface area of the rat lung is 5 to 10% higher than the alveolar surface. In the human and in the dog lung, where the capillaries are less dense, the quotient is approximately 0.88.

Thickness and Composition of the Alveolocapillary Barrier

From Figure 3-9, it is evident that the width of the alveolocapillary barrier can vary from approximately 0.3 to several microns. The thickness of this tissue barrier is important because it determines, together with other parameters, the diffusion resistance of the barrier that oxygen molecules moving from the alveolus to the capillary must overcome. This resistance is low in thin and higher in thick parts, so that the flux of gas at each point is inversely proportional to local barrier thickness. Hence, the thin parts of the barrier contribute most to gas exchange. In estimating an overall average thickness, this factor is best taken into account by determining the harmonic mean thickness of the air-blood barrier, i.e., the average of the reciprocal value of thickness, rather than the arithmetic mean, which estimates the tissue mass building the barrier. The arithmetic and harmonic mean thicknesses vary relatively little in various mammalian species. On average, the harmonic mean thickness is approximately one-third of the arithmetic mean thickness. Estimates on human lungs give values of approximately 0.6 μm for the harmonic mean barrier thickness, whereas the arithmetic mean thickness is approximately 2 μm.

Morphometric Estimation of Diffusing Capacity

The term *diffusing capacity of the lung* (DL) has been introduced by physiologists, as noted by Forster (1964), to estimate the conductance of the pulmonary gas exchange apparatus for gaseous diffusions between alveolar air and capillary blood. The physiologic definition uses Ohm's law and states that, for oxygen,

$$D_{L_{O_2}} = \dot{V}_{O_2}/\Delta P_{O_2}$$

in which $\dot{V}_{O_2}$ is the O_2 uptake and ΔP_{O_2} is the mean gradient of O_2 partial pressure between alveoli and capillaries.

It is implicit in the definition that a major part of DL is determined by structural properties of the lung, mainly by the available gas-exchange surfaces, by the thickness of the air-blood barrier, and by the capillary blood volume. One of us (E.R.W.) (1970, 1971) noted that refinements in morphometric methods have made it possible to estimate DL from measurements of lung structure performed on electron micrographs. To this end, the air-hemoglobin barrier must be subdivided into three partial resistances or conductances—that is, the reciprocal of the resistances, which are arranged in series, as shown in Figures 3-9 and 3-19. We then find DL from the sum of the partial resistances:

$$\frac{1}{D_L} = \frac{1}{D_t} + \frac{1}{D_p} + \frac{1}{D_e}$$

where D_t, D_p, and D_e are the diffusion conductances in tissue, plasma, and erythrocytes, respectively. This original model has been revised, because it turns out that the tissue and plasma layers cannot be easily separated; they act as a single barrier because the flow of plasma past the tissue barrier is slow compared with O_2 diffusion. In a new variant of the model, as described by one of us (E.R.W.) and colleagues (1993), the total diffusion barrier thickness τhb is

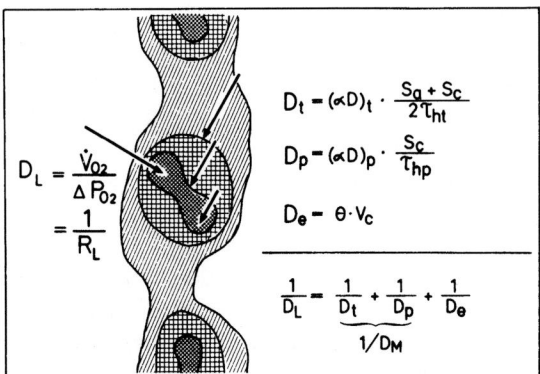

Fig. 3-19. Model for estimating pulmonary diffusing capacity from physiologic (left) and morphometric information (right).

estimated as extending from the alveolar to the erythrocyte surface (see Fig. 3-9). Together with an estimate of membrane surface, this yields the so-called membrane diffusing capacity (see Fig. 3-19), which is combined with D_e to calculate DL. DL can be calculated if we measure the alveolar and capillary surface areas (S_a and S_c), the capillary volume (V_c), and the harmonic mean thicknesses (τ_h) of tissue (t), plasma (p), and total barrier (b). In addition, we need to know appropriate values for the physical coefficients of permeability (αD) and of the rate of O_2 binding by the blood (τ_h). Table 3-3 presents the results obtained by Gehr and associates (1978a) in a morphometric study of adult human lungs. Using most reasonable estimates of the physical coefficients, one of us (E.R.W.) (1984) found $D_{L_{O_2}}$ to amount to approximately 160 mL O_2/minute per mm Hg.

For comparison, the currently available or accepted physiologic values of DL at rest amount to approximately 30 mL O_2/minute per mm Hg. This value is hence far below the morphometric estimates. It should be noted that two different things are measured: Morphometry estimates the size of the gas-exchange apparatus that is maximally available for gas exchange. Its values refer to a fully expanded lung. This can lead to an overestimation of DL by as much as 25 to 50%, because one of us (J.G.) and associates (1979) showed that in lungs inflated with air and fixed by vascular perfusion, parts of the diffusion barrier are folded away from the surface even

Table 3-3. Basic Morphometric Parameters and Diffusing Capacity in Human Lung

Weight	74	kg
Alveolar surface	143	m²
Capillary surface	126	m²
Capillary volume	213	mL
Tissue barrier	0.62	μm
Plasma barrier	0.15	μm
Total barrier	1.10	μm
$D_{L_{O_2}}$	205	mL O_2 / min/mm Hg

at highest inflation and thus do not contribute to gas exchange. Furthermore, we suppose that a gradient from air to blood exists at every point along the alveolar capillary. Under resting conditions, this is most certainly not the case; in fact, it is probable that the capillary blood is saturated before it leaves the capillary, as Karas and associates (1987) showed for the lungs of animals performing heavy exercise. We would therefore expect that the physiologic estimates of DL at rest should amount to only 20 to 40% of the maximal or true diffusing capacity. That this reasoning is probably correct is shown by the findings of Bitterli and coworkers (1971) in humans that, in exercise, physiologic estimates may yield values of DL between 70 and 100 mL O_2/minute per mm Hg. The morphometric estimate of pulmonary diffusing capacity in humans is therefore approximately two times larger than the physiologic estimate. One of us (E.R.W.) and colleagues (1983) confirmed this difference by direct measurement of the physiologic and morphometric values of DL in animals. We concluded from this that the lung provides a gas-exchange apparatus that is large enough to allow O_2 to diffuse to the blood in sufficient quantity when O_2 consumption is elevated due to work. Destruction of lung tissue, as occurs in emphysema, would tend to reduce the true diffusing capacity by reduction of the gas-exchange surfaces and, possibly, by thickening of the barrier.

Figure 3-20 shows the results of a comparative study of DL in mammalian species ranging from the smallest mammal, the Etruscan shrew, weighing only 2 g, to the horse. It is apparent that DL is related directly to body mass; in contrast, maximal O_2 consumption, $\dot{V}O_2$ mass, varies with the 0.8 power of body mass. Consequently, the lung's capacity for O_2 uptake is not matched to the body's need for O_2 when one compares animals of different body size.

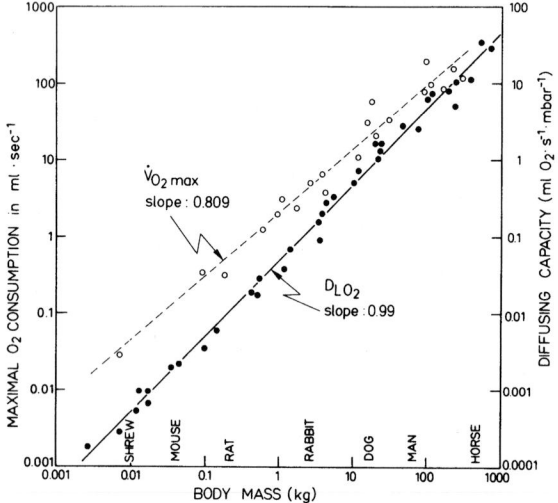

Fig. 3-20. The pulmonary diffusing capacity (*full dots*) and maximal O_2 consumption (*open circles*) scale with body mass at a different slope on a double-logarithmic plot. From Weibel ER: The Pathway for Oxygen. Cambridge: Harvard University Press, 1984. With permission.

On the other hand, the lung can respond to increased O_2 demands or to reduced environmental O_2 at high altitude by enlarging the pulmonary diffusing capacity, as we (P.H.B. and E.R.W.) (1971), Hugonnaud (1977), and Gehr (1978b) and their colleagues showed. One of us (E.R.W.) and colleagues (1987) found that athletic animals, such as dogs or horses, have a larger diffusing capacity than animals of the same size but lower O_2 needs. The question of how the lung's morphometric properties are related to the body's O_2 needs is still a matter of scientific debate, as one of us (E.R.W.) (1984) and Taylor and coworkers (1987) noted. Furthermore, numerous reports indicate that the perinatal and postnatal period of alveolization is a highly sensitive phase susceptible to disturbances induced by environmental, chemical, and hormonal factors. In particular, it was shown, first by Massaro and coworkers (1985) and then by others, that alveolization of the rat lung is seriously impaired by minute repeated postnatal doses of dexamethasone. Tschanz, one of us (P.H.B.), and coworkers (1995) demonstrated that glucocorticoids induced a precocious maturation of the lung microvasculature and, by this, prevented adequate septation of the peripheral air spaces, resulting in a lower number of alveoli.

Morphometry of Conducting and Transitory Airways and Blood Vessels

Figure 3-21 shows a plastic cast of a human lung; in the right lung, only the airways have been modeled, whereas in the left lung, pulmonary arteries and veins have been demonstrated also. It is apparent that the airways branch toward the periphery by systematically dividing in two—that is, by dichotomy. This dichotomy, however, is not regular; the two branches arising from a parent branch may differ considerably in both length and diameter. This is called irregular dichotomy. Figure 3-22 shows a similar cast of an acinus from a human lung in which the casting material, silicon rubber, has filled the airways to the most peripheral alveoli. On such preparations, Haefeli-Bleuer and one of us (E.R.W.) (1988) showed that the most peripheral airways, the respiratory bronchioles, and alveolar ducts also branch by irregular dichotomy.

The pattern of dichotomous branching provides a scheme with respect to which the systematic progression of the increase in the number of branches and of the reduction in dimensions can be described. If we first disregard the irregularities, we can estimate the average number of generations necessary to provide a sufficient number of terminal airway channels to carry alveoli for gas exchange—namely, alveolar ducts and sacs. One of us (E.R.W.) (1963) alone and with Haefeli-Bleuer (1988) estimated this average number of generations at 23. Figure 3-6 shows that the first 16 generations are purely conducting airways, leading from the trachea to the terminal bronchioles. From generation 17 on, alveoli are progressively incorporated into the airway wall

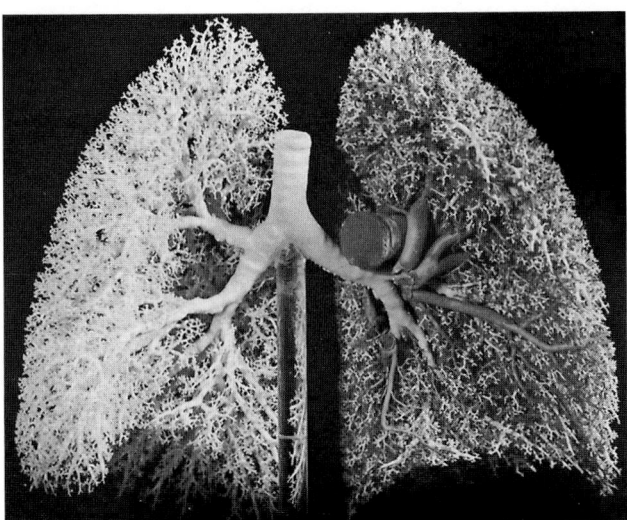

Fig. 3-21. Cast of human lung, showing airways in right lung and pulmonary arteries and veins in left lung. Note irregular dichotomy of all branches.

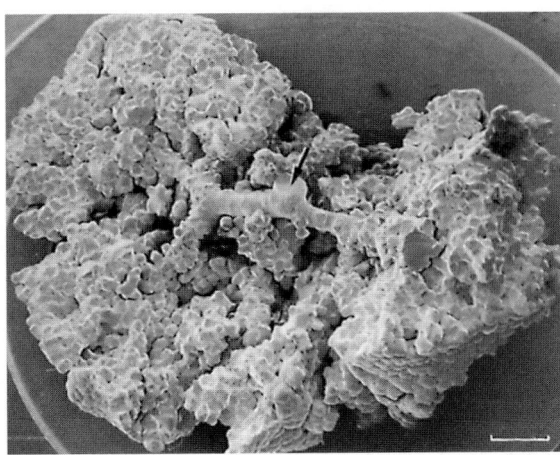

Fig. 3-22. Scanning electron micrograph of a silicon rubber cast of a human pulmonary acinus. Part of the alveolar ducts have been trimmed off to show the transitional bronchiole (*arrow*) and the first few orders of respiratory bronchioles. Note that alveolar ducts and sacs are densely covered by alveoli (scale marker = 1 mm).

until, in the twentieth generation, the entire wall is occupied by them. On the basis of more recent information, the transition from terminal to alveolated bronchioles may occur at generation 14, so that a total of nine generations carry alveoli. It must be stressed that these are average values and that, because of the irregularity, airways terminate in alveolar sacs anywhere from approximately generations 15 to 30.

This irregularity becomes apparent if length and diameter of the bronchial branches are measured on casts. Nevertheless, average dimensions can be calculated from these size distributions. If the average diameters (d) are plotted semilogarithmically against generations (z) (Fig. 3-23), we find them to follow an exponential function, namely,

$$d(z) = d_0 \cdot 2^{-z/3}$$

Therefore, with each generation, the average airway diameter is reduced by $\sqrt[3]{1/2}$, which, as pointed out by Thompson (1942), is known in hydrodynamics to be a function of optimal size relationship between parent and daughter branches. But Figure 3-23 also reveals that the diameters of peripheral or transitory airways that are provided with alveoli do not fit on this function; they are considerably larger than one would expect from their position in the bronchial tree. This difference can be explained by their different roles in conveying oxygen from ambient air to alveoli. In conducting airways, air is transported en masse—that is, a solution of O_2 in nitrogen is flowing through the tubes, and hydrodynamic principles prevail. Toward the periphery, however, O_2 molecules have to advance toward the alveolar surface by diffusion in the gas phase, and this, as emphasized by Gomez (1965), requires a greater cross-sectional area of the peripheral airways.

From this detailed information, we can construct a first model of the lung that may be useful for some general con-

siderations on the structure-function relationship in the airway system. The model assumes regular dichotomy over 23 generations. Its most pertinent dimensional properties are given in Table 3-4. It may be noted that the anatomic dead space of 150 mL, as estimated by physiologic methods, is reached at approximately generation 16, which corresponds to terminal bronchioles.

Irregular dichotomous models also can be constructed. Figure 3-24 reveals the numbers of generations necessary to arrive at airways of 2-mm diameters, as well as the distribution of distances from these branches to the trachea; these

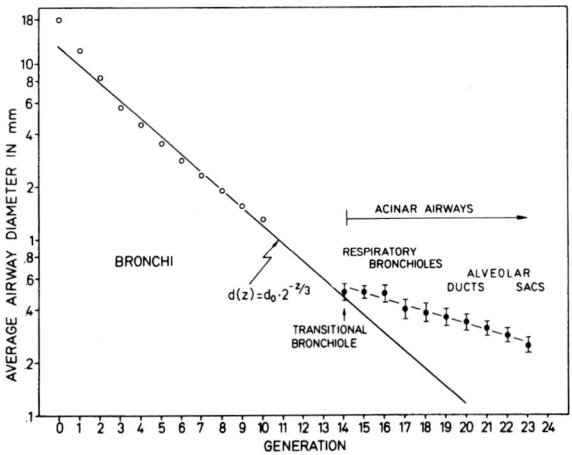

Fig. 3-23. Progressive reduction by cube root of one-half of average diameter of conducting airways in regularized dichotomy model contrasts with the slow decrease of diameter of acinar airways with progressive generations of branching. Compare text. From Haefeli-Bleuer B, Weibel ER: Morphometry of the human pulmonary acinus. Anat Rec *220*:401, 1988. With permission.

Table 3-4. Dimensions of Human Airway Model (Average Adult Lung with Volume 4800 mL at Approximately Three-fourths Maximal Inflation)

Generation	Number per Generation	Diameter	Length	Total Cross Section	Total Volume	Accumulated Volume
z	$n(z)$	$d(z)$	$l(z)$	$A(z)$	$V(z)$	$\sum_{i=0}^{z} V(i)$
		cm	cm	cm^2	cm^3	cm^3
0	1	1.8	12.0	2.54	30.50	30.5
1	2	1.22	4.76	2.33	11.25	41.8
2	4	0.83	1.90	2.13	3.97	45.8
3	8	0.56	0.76	2.00	1.52	47.2
4	16	0.45	1.27	2.48	3.46	50.7
5	32	0.35	1.07	3.11	3.30	54.0
6	64	0.28	0.90	3.96	3.53	57.5
7	128	0.23	0.76	5.10	3.85	61.4
8	256	0.186	0.64	6.95	4.45	65.8
9	512	0.154	0.54	9.56	5.17	71.0
10	1024	0.130	0.46	13.4	6.21	77.2
11	2048	0.109	0.39	19.6	7.56	84.8
12	4096	0.095	0.33	28.8	9.82	94.6
13	8192	0.082	0.27	44.5	12.45	106.0
14	16384	0.074	0.23	69.4	16.40	123.4
15	32768	0.066	0.20	113.0	21.70	145.1
16	65536	0.060	0.165	180.0	29.70	174.8
17	131072	0.054	0.141	300.0	41.80	216.6
18	262144	0.050	0.117	534.0	61.10	277.7
19	524288	0.047	0.099	944.0	93.20	370.9
20	1048576	0.045	0.083	1600.0	139.50	510.4
21	2097152	0.043	0.070	3220.0	224.30	734.7
22	4194304	0.041	0.059	5880.0	350.00	1084.7
23[a]	8388608	0.041	0.050*	11800.0	591.00	1675.0

[a]Adjusted for complete generation.

branches were located between generations 4 and 13 and at 18 to 31 cm from the root of the trachea. Each of these approximately 400 branches of 2-mm diameter leads through an average of 14 subsequent branchings until alveolar sacs are reached. The units of lung tissue that they supply have a volume of some 12 mL and contain approximately 740,000 alveoli each. This consideration of irregularity can be carried further, but one should refer to the original publications by one of us (E.R.W.) (1963) and Haefeli-Bleuer and one of us (E.R.W.) (1988) for additional information.

Different models of the airway tree have been proposed. Horsfield (1991) considers the airway tree as a system of confluent tubes originating in parenchymal airways and ending in the trachea; this minimizes the effects of branching irregularities but otherwise leads to the same conclusions on the physiologic effects of airway design. West and coworkers (1986) used the principles of fractal geometry to arrive at a different description of the airway branching pattern.

Another way of looking at airway design starts with the observation that the branching pattern of airways is similar at all levels from the main stems out to the peripheral bronchioles. This is an example of what is called *scale-invariant self-similarity*, and it results from lung development that progresses systematically by branching of the terminal tube combined with proportional growth of the airways, as

demonstrated by Kitaoka (1996) in collaboration with two of us (P.H.B. and E.R.W.). Self-similarity is the basic feature underlying a geometry of nature, called *fractal geometry*, as introduced by Mandelbrot (1977, 1983). The question obviously comes up: Are the airways designed like a fractal tree? If so, this would have interesting consequences on our interpretation of the relation between form and function in the lung as explored by one of us (E.R.W.) (1991, 1997).

The test for the fractal nature of the airway tree is to look at how the dimensions of the branches change along the tree. Self-similarity, or the scale-invariate constancy of proportions, leads to the prediction that the diameter of airways should be a power law function of the generation, as worked out by West and coworkers (1986). If the data plotted in Figure 3-23 are replotted on a double logarithmic scale (Fig. 3-25), it is seen that the data swing around the double log regression line. From this type of analysis, performed on several species, West and coworkers (1986) concluded that the airways have the basic properties of a fractal tree; the deviation of the data points from the straight line relationship may well have to do with the irregularities of branching imposed by the fact that the shape of the lung is determined by the shape of the space available in the chest.

The most interesting virtue of a fractal tree is that it fills, with its tips, the space homogeneously and densely, as shown

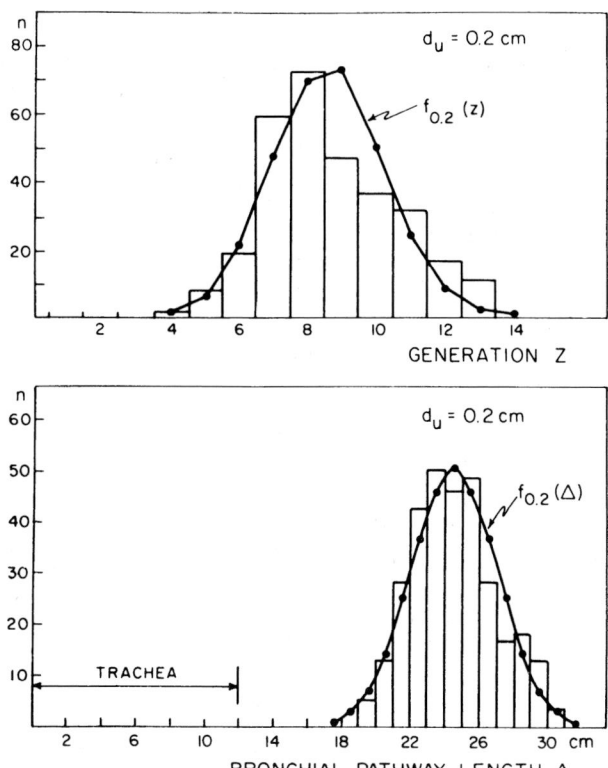

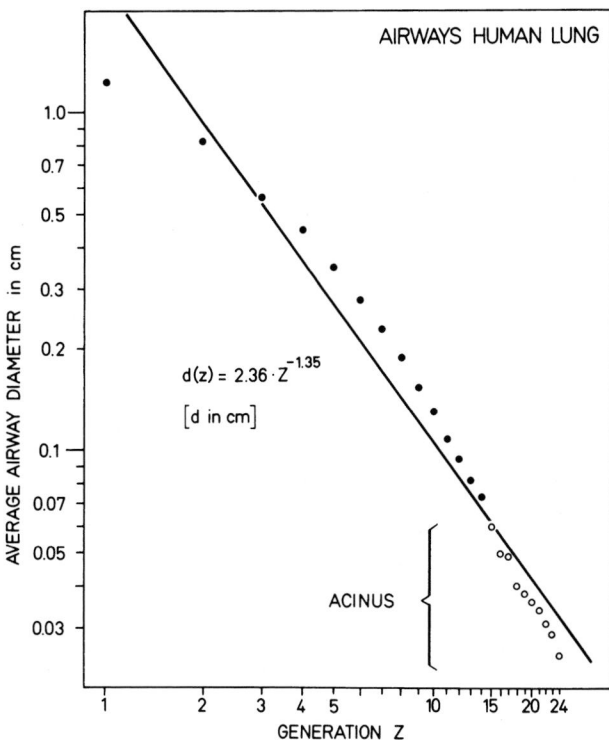

Fig. 3-24. Distribution of airways of 2-mm diameter with respect to generation z and distance from larynx Δ. Modified from Weibel ER: Morphometry of the Human Lung. Heidelberg: Springer, 1963, p. 126.

Fig. 3-25. The same data for airway diameter as in Figure 3-23 plotted as a power law against generation to test for fractal nature of airways. From Weibel ER: Fractal geometry: a design principle for living organisms. Am J Physiol 261:L361, 1991. With permission.

by Kitaoka and coworkers (1996). Furthermore, in an ideal fractal tree, the distance from each end tip to the origin is equal for all tips irrespective of whether they are close to the origin or at the outermost corner. Because the lung can be conceived of as a fractal tree, we predict that the pathway length for ventilation from the trachea to all the end tips of the airway tree are approximately equal by basic design. Figure 3-24 shows that the distribution of these distances is quite narrow.

The blood vessels undergo, in principle, the same sequence of branching as the airways, with some differences in detail. Pulmonary arteries are topographically closely associated with the airways (see Fig. 3-21); down to the respiratory bronchioles their branching would therefore seem to parallel that of the airways, but this is only partially true. It is well known that relatively large pulmonary arteries may send smaller branches to the capillary network of adjacent groups of alveoli. These accessory branches are called *supernumerary arteries* and cause, on the one hand, a more rapid progression of arterial branching and, on the other, greater irregularity in the arterial dimensions per generation.

At present, no extensive data on the morphometry of the pulmonary vascular tree are available. A preliminary model can be derived by comparing pulmonary arteries with airways and by determining the average generation number of dichotomous branching. The larger branches of the pul-

monary artery, perhaps down to a 2-mm diameter and reaching to the eighth generation on the average, have dimensions closely approximating those of the accompanying bronchi. In a first approximation, we may therefore use the measurements obtained on the bronchial tree to describe the major pulmonary arterial tree. We would therefore claim that these branches reduce their dimension with each generation to obey the hydrodynamic law of optimal size reduction described previously (see Fig. 3-23). Next, we may determine the total number of precapillaries—that is, of the terminal arterial branches that lead into the capillary network—and calculate from that the average generation number of dichotomous branching needed to reach this number; one of us (E.R.W.) and Gomez (1962) found this to be on the order of 28 generations, hence approximately five generations more than the airways. The diameter of these precapillaries is between 20 and 30 μm; if this range is plotted in Figure 3-23, it falls on the function for dimensional reduction by $\sqrt[3]{1/2}$ fitted to the major branches, which suggests that the pulmonary arterial tree reduces the dimension of its branches progressively following a hydrodynamic law for optimal reduction of diameters in a dichotomous branching system all the way out to the terminal branches. This seems logical, as mass flow of blood occurs throughout, the diffusion of gases in the blood phase playing a negligible role for transport along the vessel axis. All this is highly conjectural, however, as long as it is not substantiated by more extensive actual measurement.

REFERENCES

Angus GE, Thurlbeck WM: Number of alveoli in the human lung. J Appl Physiol 32:483, 1972.

Bitterli J, et al: Repeated measurements of pulmonary O_2 diffusing capacity in man during graded exercise. In Scherrer M (ed): Pulmonary Diffusing Capacity on Exercise. Stuttgart: H Huber, 1971, p. 139.

Bonfanti R, et al: PADGM (GMP140) is a component of Weibel-Palade bodies of human endothelial cells. Blood 73:1109, 1989.

Breeze RG, Wheeldon EG: The cells of the pulmonary airways. Am Rev Respir Dis 116:705, 1977.

Burri PH: The postnatal growth of the rat lung. III. Morphology. Anat Rec 180:77, 1974.

Burri PH, Dbaly J, Weibel ER: The postnatal growth of the rat lung. I. Morphometry. Anat Rec 178:711, 1974.

Burri PH, Tarek MR: A novel mechanism of capillary growth in the rat pulmonary microcirculation. Anat Rec 228:35, 1990.

Burri PH, Weibel ER: Beeinflussung einer spezifischen Cytoplasmischen Organelle von Endothelzellen durch Adrenalin. Z Zellforsch 88:426, 1968.

Burri PH, Weibel ER: Morphometric estimation of pulmonary diffusion capacity. II. Effect of PO_2 on the growing lung. Respir Physiol 11:247, 1971.

Caduff, JH, Fischer LC, Burri PH: Scanning electron microscope study of the developing microvasculature in the postnatal rat lung. Anat Rec 216:154, 1986.

Crapo JD, et al: Cell numbers and cell characteristics of the normal human lung. Am Rev Respir Dis 125:332, 1982.

Dierynck I, et al: Potent inhibition of both human interferon-gamma production and biologic activity by the Clara cell protein CC16. Am J Respir Cell Mol Biol 12:205, 1995.

Dobbs LG: Pulmonary surfactant. Annu Rev Med 40:431, 1989.

Forster RE: Diffusion of gases. In Fenn WD, Rahn H (eds): Handbook of Physiology, Section 3, Respiration. Vol. I. Washington, DC: American Physiological Society, 1964, p. 839.

Gehr P, Bachofen H, Weibel ER: The normal human lung: ultrastructure and morphometric estimation of diffusion capacity. Respir Physiol 32:121, 1978a.

Gehr P, et al: Adaptation of the growing lung to increase $\dot{V}O_2$. III. The effect of exposure to cold environment in rats. Respir Physiol 32:345, 1978b.

Gil J, Reiss OK: Isolation and characterization of lamellar bodies and tubular myelin from rat lung homogenates. J Cell Biol 58:152, 1973.

Gil J, Weibel ER: Improvements in demonstration of lining layer of lung alveoli by electron microscopy. Respir Physiol 8:13, 1969–70.

Gil J, Weibel ER: Extracellular lining of bronchioles after perfusion-fixation of rat lungs for electron microscopy. Anat Rec 169:185, 1971.

Gil J, et al: The alveolar volume to surface area relationship in air and saline-filled lungs fixed by vascular perfusion. J Appl Physiol 47:990, 1979.

Glazier JB, et al: Vertical gradient of alveolar size in lungs of dogs frozen intact. J Appl Physiol 23:694, 1967.

Gomez DM: A physico-mathematical study of lung function in normal subjects and in patients with obstructive pulmonary diseases. Med Thorac 22:275, 1965.

Haefeli-Bleuer B, Weibel ER: Morphometry of the human pulmonary acinus. Anat Rec 220:401, 1988.

Hawgood S: Composition, structure, and metabolism. In Crystal RG, West JB (eds): The Lung Scientific Foundation. Vol. 1. New York: Raven Press, 1991, p. 247.

Hermans C, et al: Determinants of Clara cell protein (CC16) concentration in serum: a reassessment with two different immunoassays. Clin Chim Acta 272:101, 1998.

Horsfield K. Pulmonary airways and blood vessels considered as confluent trees. In Crystal RG, West JB (eds): The Lung Scientific Foundation. Vol. 1. New York: Raven Press, 1991, p. 721.

Hoyt RF Jr, McNelly N, Sorokin SP: Dynamics of neuroepithelial bodies (NEB) formation in developing hamster lung: light microscopic autoradiography after 3H-thymidine labeling in vivo. Anat Rec 227:340, 1990.

Hugonnaud C, et al: Adaptation of the growing lung to increased oxygen consumption. II. Morphometric analysis. Respir Physiol 29:1, 1977.

Jeffery PK: Morphologic features of airway surface epithelial cells and glands. Am Rev Respir Dis 128:14S, 1983.

Jeffery PK, Reid LM: The respiratory mucous membrane. In Brain JD, Proctor DF, Reid LM (eds): Respiratory Defense Mechanisms. Part I. New York: Marcel Dekker, 1977.

Johansson J, Curstedt T: Molecular structures and interactions of pulmonary surfactant components. Eur J Biochem 244:675, 1997.

Kapanci Y: Location and function of contractile interstitial cells of the lungs. In Bonhuys A (ed): Lung Cells in Disease. New York: Elsevier North-Holland, 1976, p. 69.

Kapanci Y, et al: "Contractile interstitial cells" in pulmonary alveolar septa. J Cell Biol 60:375, 1974.

Karas RH, et al: Adaptive variation in the mammalian respiratory system in relation to energetic demand. VII. Flow of oxygen across the pulmonary gas exchanger. Respir Physiol 69:101, 1987.

Kauffman SL, Burri PH, Weibel ER: The postnatal growth of the rat lung. II. Autoradiography. Anat Rec 180:63, 1974.

Kitaoka H, Burri PH, Weibel ER: Development of the human fetal airway tree: analysis of the numerical density of airway endtips. Anat Rec 244:207, 1996.

Langston C, et al: Human lung growth in late gestation and in the neonate. Am Rev Respir Dis 129:607, 1984.

Lauweryns JM, Cokelaere M: Hypoxia sensitive neuroepithelial bodies. Intrapulmonary secretory neuroreceptors modulated by the CNS. Z Zellforsch 145:521, 1973.

Low FN: Electron microscopy of the rat lung. Anat Rec 113:437, 1952.

Maksvytis HJ, et al: In vitro characteristics of the lipid-filled interstitial cell associated with postnatal lung growth: evidence for fibroblast heterogeneity. J Cell Physiol 118:113, 1984.

Mandelbrot BB: The Fractal Geometry of Nature. San Francisco: Freeman, 1977.

Mandelbrot BB: The Fractal Geometry of Nature. 2nd Ed. San Francisco: Freeman, 1983.

Mason RJ, Williams MC: Alveolar type II cells. In Crystal RG, West JB (eds): The Lung Scientific Foundation. Vol. 1. New York: Raven Press, 1991, p. 235.

Massaro D, et al: Postnatal development of alveoli. Regulation and evidence for a critical period in rats. J Clin Invest 76:1297, 1985.

McEver RP, et al: GMP-140, a platelet α-granule membrane protein, is also synthesized by vascular endothelial cells and is localized in Weibel-Palade bodies. J Clin Invest 84:92, 1989.

Meyrick B, Reid L: The alveolar brush cell in rat lung: a third pneumocyte. J Ultrastruct Res 23:71, 1968.

Nagy JA, et al: Pathogenesis of ascites tumor growth: angiogenesis, vascular remodeling, and stroma formation in the peritoneal lining. Cancer Res 55:376, 1995.

Nehls V, Drenckhahn D: Heterogeneity of microvascular pericytes for smooth muscle type alpha-actin. J Cell Biol 113:147, 1991.

Patan S, Haenni B, Burri PH: Implementation of intussusceptive microvascular growth in the chicken chorio-allantoic membrane (CAM): 1. Pillar formation by folding of the capillary wall. Microvasc Res 51:80, 1996.

Patan S, Haenni B, Burri PH: Implementation of intussusceptive microvascular growth in the chicken chorio-allantoic membrane (CAM): 2. Pillar formation by capillary fusion. Microvasc Res 53:33, 1997.

Patan S, et al: Intussusceptive microvascular growth: a common alternative to capillary sprouting. Arch Histol Cytol 55:65, 1992.

Plopper CG, Hyde DM, Buckpitt AR. Clara cells. In Crystal RG, West JB (eds): The Lung Scientific Foundation. Vol. 1. New York: Raven Press, 1991, p. 215.

Schneeberger EE: Airway and alveolar epithelial cell junctions. In Crystal RG, West JB (eds): The Lung Scientific Foundation. Vol. 1. New York: Raven Press, 1991, p. 205.

Sleigh MA: Mucus propulsion. In Crystal RG, West JB (eds): The Lung Scientific Foundation. Vol. 1. New York: Raven Press, 1991, p. 189.

St. George JA, et al: An immunohistochemical characterization of Rhesus monkey respiratory secretions using monoclonal antibodies. Am Rev Respir Dis 132:556, 1985.

Sorokin SP, et al: Comparative biology of small granule cells and neuroepithelial bodies in the respiratory system: short review. Am Rev Respir Dis 128:26S, 1983.

Spicer SS, et al: Histochemical properties of the respiratory tract epithelium in different species. Am Rev Respir Dis *128*:20S, 1983.

Taylor CR, et al: Adaptive variation in the mammalian respiratory system in relation to energetic demand. VIII. Structural and functional limits to oxidative metabolism. Respir Physiol *69*:117, 1987.

Thompson D'Arcy W: Growth and Form. New York: Cambridge University Press, 1942, p. 448.

Tschanz SA, Damke BM, Burri PH: Influence of postnatally administered glucocorticoids on rat lung growth. Biol Neonate *68*:229, 1995.

Von Neergaard K: Neue Auffassungen über einen Grundbegriff der Atemmechanik. Die Retraktionskraft der Lunge, abhängig von der Oberflächenspannung in den Alveolen. Z Gesamte Exp Med *66*:373, 1929.

Wagner DD, Olmsted JB, Marder VJ: Immunolocalization of von Willebrand protein in Weibel-Palade bodies of human endothelial cells. J Cell Biol *95*:355, 1982.

Warhol MJ, Sweet JM: The ultrastructural localization of von Willebrand factor in endothelial cells. Am J Pathol *117*:310, 1984.

Weibel ER: Die Blutgefässanastomosen in der menschlichen Lunge. Z Zellforsch *50*:653, 1959.

Weibel ER: Morphometry of the Human Lung. Heidelberg: Springer, 1963.

Weibel ER: Morphometric estimation of pulmonary diffusion capacity. I. Model and method. Respir Physiol *11*:54, 1970–71.

Weibel ER: The Pathway for Oxygen: Structure and Function in the Mammalian Respiratory System. Cambridge, MA: Harvard University Press, 1984, pp. 1–425.

Weibel ER: Lung cell biology. *In* Fishman AP, Fisher AB (eds): Handbook of Physiology. Section 3, The Respiratory System. Vol. I. Bethesda: American Physiological Society, 1985, p. 47.

Weibel ER: Fractal geometry: a design principle for living organisms. Am J Physiol *261*:L361, 1991.

Weibel ER: Design of airways and blood vessels considered as branching trees. *In* Crystal RG, et al (eds): The Lung: Scientific Foundations. Vol. 1. 2nd Ed. Philadelphia: Lippincott-Raven Publishers, 1997, p. 1061.

Weibel ER, Bachofen H: Structural design of the alveolar septum and fluid exchange. *In* Fishman AP, Renkin EM (eds): Pulmonary Edema. Bethesda: American Physiological Society, 1979.

Weibel ER, Gil J: Structure function relationship at the alveolar level. *In* West JG (ed): Bioengineering Aspects of the Lung. New York: Marcel Dekker, 1977.

Weibel ER, Gomez DM: Architecture of the human lung. Science *137*:577, 1962.

Weibel ER, Palade GE: New cytoplasmic components in arterial endothelia. J Cell Biol *23*:101, 1964.

Weibel ER, et al: Maximal oxygen consumption and pulmonary diffusing capacity: a direct comparison of physiologic morphometric measurements in canids. Respir Physiol *54*:173, 1983.

Weibel ER, et al: Adaptive variation in the mammalian respiratory system in relation to energetic demand. VI. The pulmonary gas exchanger. Respir Physiol *69*:81, 1987.

Weibel ER, et al: Morphometric model for pulmonary diffusing capacity. I. Membrane diffusing capacity. Respir Physiol *93*:125, 1993.

West BJ, Bhargava V, Goldberg AL: Beyond the principle of similitude; renormalization in the bronchial tree. J Appl Physiol *60*:1089, 1986.

Wissel H, et al: SP-A-binding protein BP55 is involved in surfactant endocytosis by type II pneumocytes. Am J Physiol *271*:L432, 1996.

Yao XL, et al: Interferon-gamma stimulates human Clara cell secretory protein production by human airway epithelial cells. Am J Physiol *247*:L864, 1998a.

Yao XL, et al: Tumer necrosis factor-alpha stimulates human Clara cell secretory protein production by human airway epithelial cells. Am J Respir Cell Mol Biol *19*:629, 1998b.

Zeltner TB, Burri PH: The postnatal development and growth of the human lung. II. Morphology. Respir Physiol *67*:269, 1987.

Zeltner TB, et al: The postnatal development and growth of the human lung. I. Morphometry. Respir Physiol *67*:247, 1987.

READING REFERENCES

Ballard PL: Hormones and Lung Maturation. Berlin: Springer, 1986.

Burri PH: Development and growth of the human lung. *In* Fishman AP, Fischer AB (eds): Handbook of Physiology, Section 3, The Respiratory System. Vol. I. Bethesda: American Physiological Society, 1985, p. 1.

Burri PH: Development and regeneration of the lung. *In* Fishman AP (ed): Pulmonary Diseases and Disorders. Vol. 1. New York: McGraw-Hill, 1988, pp. 61–78.

Burri PH: Postnatal development and growth of the pulmonary microvasculature. *In* Motta PM, Murakami T, Fujita H (eds): Scanning Electron Microscopy of Vascular Casts: Methods and Applications. Boston: Kluwer Academic Publishers, 1992, pp. 139–156.

Gil J: Ultrastructure of lung fixed under physiologically defined conditions. Arch Intern Med *127*:896, 1971.

Gil J: Models of Lung Disease. Vol. 47. New York: Marcel Dekker, 1990.

Murray JF: The Normal Lung. 2nd Ed. Philadelphia: WB Saunders, 1986.

Scarpelli EM, Mantone AJ: The pulmonary surfactant system. *In* Robertson B, van Golde LMG, Batenburg JJ (eds): Pulmonary Surfactant. Amsterdam: Elsevier Science Publishers, 1984, p. 119.

Thurlbeck WM: Pathology of the Lung. New York: Thieme, 1988.

Von Hayek H: Die menschliche Lunge. 2. Auflage. Heidelberg: Springer, 1970.

Weibel ER: Functional morphology of lung parenchyma. *In* Macklem PT, Mead J (eds): Handbook of Physiology, Section 3, The Respiratory System. Vol. III. Part 1. Bethesda: American Physiological Society, 1986, p. 89.

Weibel ER: Design of biological organisms and fractal geometry. *In* Nonnenmacher T, Losa GA, Weibel ER (eds): Fractals in Biology and Medicine. Basel: Birkhäuser Verlag, 1994, p. 68.

CHAPTER 4

Cellular and Molecular Biology of the Lung

Steven J. Mentzer

The primary function of the lung is gas exchange to maintain aerobic metabolism. To sustain an active human adult, oxygen must be adsorbed and carbon dioxide removed. This process requires a mechanism for ventilation of large volumes of respiratory gases. The upper airways function to conduct gas into and out of the lung. When the respiratory gases reach the alveoli, a large alveolar surface area facilitates the efficient exchange of oxygen and carbon dioxide.

The ventilation of respiratory gases results in the exposure of the lung to a variety of airborne pathogens. A complex defense system uses mechanical and immunologic mechanisms to protect the host from biological pathogens. The importance of mechanical mechanisms of mucociliary clearance is illustrated by the heritable disease cystic fibrosis. In addition to biological threats, the ventilation of gases means that the lung is exposed also to a variety of environmental toxins. Cigarette smoke is a toxin that has effects on both gas exchange (emphysema) and the cells that line the airways (bronchial carcinoma). Similar environmental exposures may be responsible for other acquired genetic diseases of the lung.

LARGE CONDUCTING AIRWAYS

A variety of cells and their products ensure optimal gas exchange and limit the effect of airborne pathogens on lung function. The tracheobronchial tree is characterized by airway epithelium specialized for conductance and mucociliary clearance. A mixed population of epithelial cells lines the trachea and bronchi (Table 4-1). These epithelial cells include basal cells, goblet cells, and ciliated columnar epithelium. Characteristic of the proximal airways is the presence of ciliated columnar epithelial cells and goblet cells. Basal cells and so-called intermediate cells are present also. The function of basal cells is unclear, but basal cells may give rise to both goblet cells and ciliated epithelial cells. Specialized lymphoid tissues are located along the main airways and especially at the bifurcation of airways where particles and pathogen deposition are concentrated.

Mucous and Serous Glands

Mucous and serous glands are present in the large airways down to the bronchiolar level. The glands are located between the muscle and the cartilage layers of the large airways. The glands are composed of both serous and mucous tubules. Although there may be some mixture, separate areas of the gland are comprised by consistent serous or mucous tubules. These tubules end in collecting and ciliated ducts. The mucous cells are primarily restricted to mucous tubules. The myoepithelial cells that line part of the mucous glands are responsible for expelling mucus contents into the airway lumen. The mucous glands are supplied by the sympathetic nervous system. Serous cells can be found in serous tubules and have been identified to the level of the bronchioles. The main function of serous cells is to produce lysozyme and possibly aid in the transport of immunoglobulin A (IgA) across the glandular epithelium. IgA is produced by plasma cells, which are found in the region of bronchial glands.

Goblet Cells

The goblet cell is a surface mucus-secreting cell present throughout the bronchial airways. Goblet cells produce mucus. Respiratory airway mucus is composed of glycoproteins with unique viscoelastic properties. These glycoproteins are collectively called *mucins*. Mucins are heterogeneous macromolecules that have domains for the passive clearance of both proteins and lipids. Mucins may also actively bind micro-organisms. The mucin glycoproteins may function as ligands for lectinlike surface receptors of micro-organisms. The role of the goblet cell in mucin pro-

Table 4-1. Epithelial Cells

Cells	Location	Function
Basal cells	Tracheobronchial airways	Barrier, progenitor
Columnar secretory cells	Tracheobronchial airways	Mucus production
Ciliated cells	Tracheobronchial airways	Mucociliary clearance
Clara cells	Bronchioles	Secretory, progenitor
Alveolar type I	Alveoli	Air-blood barrier
Alveolar type II	Alveoli	Surfactant, progenitor

duction is particularly apparent after airway injury. Exposure to cigarette smoke, for example, leads to goblet cell metaplasia as well as glandular hypertrophy. Goblet cell metaplasia also may be observed in a variety of other inhalational injuries or in many conditions characterized by a chronic cough.

Ciliated Columnar Cells

The percentage of ciliated columnar epithelial cells is generally higher in the large airways than in the peripheral airways. Approximately 50% of the cells in the trachea are ciliated epithelium, whereas only 15% of cells in the fifth generation airways are ciliated. In humans, the ratio of ciliated cells to goblet cells is approximately 5:1. Ciliated cells propel mucus through the airways.

Approximately 250 cilia are located on the luminal surface of each ciliated cell. The cilia are composed of an array of longitudinal microtubules called an *axoneme*. The axoneme is arranged with a central doublet surrounded by nine outer doublets. A sliding movement of the microtubules past each other generates the movement of the cilia. The 9 + 2 arrangement of microtubules in human cilia is similar to the structure of axonemes in other plants and animals. The clinical importance of cilia is illustrated by the primary ciliary dyskinesia syndrome. Primary ciliary dyskinesia can involve bronchiectasis, chronic rhinosinusitis, and poorly motile spermatozoa. Kartagener's syndrome, which includes the diagnosis of situs inversus in addition to cilia dysfunction, is a subset of primary ciliary dyskinesia. The normal airway cilia function to propel both water and mucus. When the cilia propel mucus, the tip of the cilia penetrates the mucus and claws the mucus forward. At the end of the propulsive stroke, the cilia tip leaves the mucus and moves backward beneath the mucus in a recovery stroke. The average beat frequency of cilia ranges from 12 to 15 beats per minute, but is sensitive to both clinical and pharmacologic factors. Neurohormonal control of ciliary beat frequency appears to be regulated by a β-adrenergic mechanism. Ciliated epithelial cells also appear to be sensitive to environmental injury. Cigarette smoke is associated with a loss of ciliated epithelium and

Table 4-2. Factors Influencing Mucociliary Clearance

Factor	Effect on Mucus	Effect on Cilia
Smoke	Increase quantity	Decrease
Lidocaine	No effect	No effect
β-Adrenergic agonists	No effect	Increase
Expectorants	Mucolytic effect	No effect
Gravity	No effect	No effect
Hydration	Decrease viscoelasticity	No effect

replacement with squamous metaplasia. Ischemic injury of the airway, as seen after lung transplantation, also is associated with the loss of ciliated epithelium and an increase in squamous metaplasia.

Effective mucociliary clearance is critical for lung defense (Table 4-2). When ciliary activity is inadequate to remove all secretions from the airway, the physical presence of the mucus initiates a neural reflexive cough. The cough generates a high shear force that dislodges the mucus and expels it from the airway. In healthy persons, mucus transport in the airways does not require a cough. In contrast, when excess mucus resides in the airway, high expiratory air velocity can play an important role in the clearance of secretions.

Effective mucociliary clearance also depends on the viscoelastic properties of the mucus. In general, the viscosity and elasticity of the mucus varies inversely with the water content. When the water content of the mucus is high, the mucus is effectively cleared without a cough. When the water content of the mucus is low, the mucus is thick and tenacious. Mucus with high viscosity and elasticity can be effectively cleared by a cough. The clinical problem of high viscosity and elasticity occurs in the patient with a poor cough or impaired airflow. For example, the patient with a paretic vocal cord or chronic obstructive lung disease may not be able to generate sufficient airflow to expel the mucus with high viscoelasticity. The inability to clear the airway mucus may result in decreasing airflow and mucus impaction.

SMALL CONDUCTING AIRWAYS

The terminal bronchiole represents the most distal purely conducting portion of the tracheobronchial tree. Although there is some anatomic variation, bronchioles are generally distinguished from bronchi by the fact that bronchi contain cartilage in their walls, whereas bronchioles do not. Terminal bronchioles, like the proximal airways, have an epithelial lining that is specialized for conductance and mucociliary clearance.

The transitional zone between gas exchange areas and the conducting airways is termed *bronchioles*. Bronchioles are the most distal conducting airways proximal to the pulmonary acinus. The epithelial lining of bronchioles is largely comprised of Clara cells. These nonciliated and nonsquamous epithelial cells comprise 70 to 90% of the cells throughout the transitional bronchiolar zone.

Clara Cells

Clara cells appear to have multiple metabolic functions. The ultrastructure of the Clara cell is characterized by extensive apical projections into the airway lumen and prominent endoplasmic reticulum. A variety of functional studies have established Clara cells as a primary site of xenobiotic metabolism. The Clara cell may also function as a secretory cell for the terminal airways. Clara cell secretory granules may be a source of surfactant apoproteins in the human lung. Clara cells also may serve as a source of arachidonic acid metabolites and antileukoproteases.

The turnover of epithelial cell populations in the bronchiolar region of the lung is low. With injury, however, a dramatic increase occurs in epithelial proliferative activity. Clara cells appear to function as a progenitor of themselves as well as ciliated cells in the bronchioles. The bronchiolar ciliated cell appears to be a principal target of oxidant gases. As bronchiolar ciliated cells are injured, a proliferation of bronchiolar Clara cells occurs. The hyperplasia of Clara cells may effectively increase the number of respiratory bronchioles by several airway generations. The relationship of Clara cell hyperplasia to bronchiolitis and obliterative small airway processes is unknown.

ALVEOLAR CELLS

The terminal bronchioles give rise to respiratory bronchioles. The respiratory bronchioles are not only conducting airways, but also give rise to alveolar ducts that are studded with alveoli. Alveoli are the true gas-exchange surfaces of the lung. The alveoli are composed of specialized epithelial and endothelial cells separated by an interstitial matrix. Associated with these cells are alveolar macrophages. Alveolar macrophages are pivotal regulatory cells in the host defense of the distal airway.

Alveolar Type I Cell

The alveolar type I cells are the dominant component of a continuous layer of alveolar epithelium. The alveolar type I cell forms a thin membrane over 90% of the alveolar surface. The alveolar type I cell is broad and flat with highly branched cytoplasmic processes. Ultrastructural studies have shown that the alveolar type I cells have small nuclei and few mitochondria. This simplified cellular machinery is believed to be associated with terminal differentiation. Because of their inability to divide, alveolar type I cells are dependent on alveolar type II cells for their replacement.

The alveolar type I cells provide an important barrier to the leakage of water and solutes out of the blood and into the air spaces. This function is the result of tight junctions between alveolar cells. The alveolar tight junctions form a continuous seal between the luminal and abluminal compartments. In addition to serving a barrier function, tight junctions may regulate the polarity of the cell membrane.

Because the alveolar type I cell is incapable of mitosis and repair, these cells are sensitive to injury. In most models of acute lung injury, alveolar type I cells are the first cells to be damaged. Damaged alveolar type I cells detach from the epithelium, leaving behind denuded basement membrane. The basement membrane alone provides a poor mechanical barrier. The consequence of a loss of alveolar type I cells is edema and hemorrhage into the alveolar spaces. Subsequent impairment in gas exchange persists until the proliferation of the alveolar type II cells can replace the lost cell population.

Alveolar Type II Cells

Alveolar type II cells make up approximately 15% of the cells in the distal lung. Alveolar type II cells have a distinctive appearance by light microscopy. In contrast to the squamous alveolar type I cell, alveolar type II cells are cuboidal. The intracellular stores of surface-active material give the alveolar type II cells a distinctive granular appearance. This distinctive appearance has led to the description of alveolar type II cells as *granular pneumocytes*.

The primary function of alveolar type II cells is the synthesis and secretion of surface-active material. Alveolar type II cells contain unique organelles called *lamellar bodies*. Lamellar bodies contain layers of surfactant phospholipids surrounded by a limiting membrane. Lamellar bodies also contain lysosomal enzymes and surfactant proteins. The lipid contained in the lamellar bodies is secreted at the cellular apex. The lamellar body fuses with the apical cell membrane and the surfactant is released into alveolar space. After the release of surfactant lipids, the spheroid lamellar bodies appear to reorganize into a structure called *tubular myelin*. Tubular myelin may function to aid in adsorption and facilitate the distribution of surfactant along the alveolar surface.

Alveolar type II cells also may play an important role in the maintenance of the alveolar epithelium by their ability to differentiate into alveolar type I cells. The repair of injured alveolar epithelium occurs by the proliferation of alveolar type II cells. The proliferating type II cells appear to be capable of differentiating into either new alveolar type II cells or into squamous alveolar type I cells. The signals that regulate differentiation of the proliferating alveolar type of cells appear to be related to the extracellular matrix. The connective tissue that supports the alveolar epithelium may provide the signals that regulate differentiation.

Alveolar type II cells also appear to be important in disease. Alveolar type II cells are morphologically hyperplastic after lung injury. The appearance of alveolar type II cells by light microscopy has led to the term *reactive pneumocytes*. Reactive pneumocytes also express more major histocompatibility complex class I and class II antigens. The expression of increased levels of major histocompatibility complex suggests that alveolar type II cells may have an immunologic function or play a role in local autoimmune processes.

Surfactant

Surfactant plays an important role in modulating the surface forces in the alveolus. Surfactant forms a film at the surface of the alveolar lining fluid. The effect of surfactant on surface tension depends on alveolar surface area. Surface tension at the alveolar surface is reduced by the surfactant by promoting lung expansion on inspiration. On expiration, the reduction in surface tension at low transpulmonary pressures prevents atelectasis and lung collapse.

Surfactant is composed of several heterogeneous phospholipid-rich lipoproteins. In the alveolus, surfactant includes the surface phospholipid monolayer, tubular myelin, and an apoprotein component. The dominant component of surfactant is phospholipids (Table 4-3). Phospholipids are amphipathic molecules with a polar head attached to a glyceryl backbone. Acyl chains of variable length are attached to the glycerol backbone. In an aqueous environment, such as the alveolus, the phospholipids generally exist as a closed bilayer. Although the exact phospholipid composition can vary, the general characteristic of phospholipid mixtures is that they spontaneously form a surface film at an air-fluid interface. The formation of this surface film significantly lowers surface tension. When the surface area decreases, as in expiration, the phospholipid molecules are packed more tightly, further lowering surface tension.

The protein composition of surfactant appears to play an important role in surfactant function. The most abundant surfactant protein is SP-A. SP-A is a large collagenlike glycoprotein that makes up approximately 4% of the total mass of isolated surfactant. Surfactant is produced in the alveolar type II cells and perhaps also synthesized in Clara cells. The chemical interaction between SP-A and surfactant lipids is complex. SP-A may play a role in regulating the secretion and turnover of surfactant. Two additional surfactant apoproteins, SP-B and SP-C, have unusual chemical properties in that both are remarkably hydrophobic. Because of their hydrophobicity, these two apoproteins are often referred to as *surfactant proteolipids*. Both of these proteins are thought to play a role in the formation of the surfactant film.

The functional role of the surfactant system is illustrated in several pathologic conditions. Acute respiratory distress syndrome is respiratory failure secondary to atelectasis that accompanies premature birth. Premature birth is associated with a deficiency of the surfactant system. When these infants are treated with exogenous surfactant, a dramatic improvement in the mechanical properties of the lung occurs. The reduction in surface tension associated with the exogenous surfactant results in a pulmonary inflation and a dramatic improvement in ventilation.

ENDOTHELIAL CELLS

Endothelial cells in the lung form a continuous nonfenestrated vascular lining extending from the pulmonary arteries to the pulmonary veins with an intervening capillary meshwork. The blood vessels in the lung are unique vessels in the body because they are low-resistance vessels that carry deoxygenated blood on the arterial side and oxygenated blood on the venous side of the circulation. Endothelial cells make up 40% of all lung cells. The endothelial cells of the lung form a continuous sheet with an area of 130 m^3. In the alveolar capillaries, endothelial cells have specialized organelle-free cytoplasm to facilitate gas exchange. These endothelial cells have a thin avesicular zone that is only 35 to 55 nm thick.

Endothelial cells generally orient in the long axis of the vessel, suggesting a morphologic response to existing shear forces. Similar to epithelial cells, endothelial cells have both luminal and abluminal *domains* to the cell membrane. These cell membrane domains are separated by intercellular tight junctions. Luminal domains have distinct functional characteristics. Proteins that regulate a variety of metabolic functions are expressed on the luminal surface (Table 4-4). In addition, luminal domains appear to direct the secretion of cellular products, including von Willebrand's factor. The abluminal cell membrane interacts with extracellular matrix and directs transport of plasma molecules toward the interstitium.

The luminal membrane of endothelial cells is covered by a fuzzy coat or glycocalyx composed of glycosaminoglycans, oligosaccharide moieties of glycoproteins, glycolipids, and sialoconjugates. The cell membrane and its glycocalyx regulate a variety of cell functions. The luminal cell membrane mediates all cellular interactions and regulates recruit-

Table 4-3. Components of Surfactant

Component	Percent	Function
Lipids	95	
Phospholipids	78	Modify surface tension
Neutral lipids	10	Modify surface tension
Proteins	5–10	
Serum proteins	0–5	Variety of functions
Apoproteins	5	Regulate turnover

Table 4-4. Endothelial Cell Surface Proteins and Enzymes

Angiotensin-converting enzyme
Nucleotidases
Lipoprotein lipase
Thrombin
Fibrinolytic factors
Antifibrinolytic factors

ment of leukocytes into the lung. Enzymes, such as angiotensin-converting enzyme, lipoprotein lipase, as well as receptors for insulin and low-density lipoproteins, are expressed at the blood interface. Plasma proteins, such as immunoglobulin, fibrinogen, fibrin, α_2-macroglobulin and albumin are temporarily associated with the cell surface.

ALVEOLAR MACROPHAGE

The most common immune cell in the lung is the alveolar macrophage. The alveolar macrophage is 5 to 10 times more common in the lung than are T lymphocytes. Alveolar macrophage appears to have multiple functions in the lung. A primary function is their ability to scavenge particles and remove debris from the lung parenchyma. The ability of alveolar macrophages to phagocytize micro-organisms provides an important defense against airborne pathogens. The alveolar macrophage also appears to play an important role in the repair and maintenance of lung parenchymal tissue.

Macrophages are far more common in the lower respiratory tract than in the tracheobronchial tree. Alveolar macrophages are believed to be derived from blood monocytes that migrate from pulmonary capillaries into the lung. Alveolar macrophages are thought to have a limited potential to divide and proliferate. The significant increase in alveolar macrophage concentration in some conditions (e.g., granulomatous lung disease) suggests either active recruitment of blood monocytes or the ability of alveolar macrophages to divide in situ.

Although alveolar macrophages can have several different phenotypes, subpopulations of alveolar macrophages have not been defined clearly. The reason for this discrepancy is that alveolar macrophages can exist at a variety of different activation states. The activation states of alveolar macrophages appear to regulate the capacity to phagocytize, kill target cells, migrate, and release a broad range of secretory products. The activation signals for alveolar macrophages can include such diverse signals as the phagocytosis of inert particles, receptor binding of immunoglobulin, or exposure to cytokines.

Alveolar macrophages play an important role in maintaining the sterility of the airway. Alveolar macrophages are an important defense against airborne bacteria. The bacterial pathogens can be phagocytized as inert particles or by specific surface receptors on the alveolar macrophage membrane. Surface receptors may include membrane-bound immunoglobulin or receptors for terminal mannose sugars. Once the pathogen is phagocytized, the phagosome fuses with lysosome and the organism is killed by an oxidative burst. Alveolar macrophages also use nonoxidative mechanisms, including proteases, lysozymes, and a variety of other bacteriocidal proteins. An understanding of macrophage-dependent mechanisms of bactericidal activity holds the promise of novel antibacterial therapies.

The effectiveness of alveolar macrophages in the capacity to eliminate micro-organisms is varied. Some micro-organisms are susceptible to alveolar macrophages, whereas others are resistant. Some common bacterial pathogens such as *Staphylococcus aureus* are readily eliminated by alveolar macrophages. In contrast, *Pseudomonas aeruginosa* and *Klebsiella pneumoniae* are relatively resistant to alveolar macrophages and require the presence of neutrophils for elimination. The selectivity of alveolar macrophages can be of clinical importance. For example, patients who have neutropenia from chemotherapy have enhanced susceptibility to macrophage-resistant bacteria. Other resistant infectious agents include organisms such as *Mycobacterium tuberculosis* and *Toxoplasma gondii*. These organisms can continue to grow within alveolar macrophages. Activation of alveolar macrophages, with cytokines such as interferon-γ, can be effective in enhancing the growth suppression of these pathogens.

Alveolar macrophages also play an important role in eliminating damaged lung tissue or airway debris. The role of the alveolar macrophage in maintaining the normal structure of the lung is illustrated by two clinical examples. Alveolar proteinosis is a disease characterized by hypoxemia from large amounts of proteinaceous material found within the alveolar air spaces. The alveolar macrophages in these cases are filled with surfactantlike material. The normal macrophage regulation of surfactant turnover appears to be impaired in these patients. Another example is the anthracosis observed in long-term smokers. The anthracotic material found in bronchoalveolar lavage specimens as well as in the histologic examination of the peripheral lung is commonly found within alveolar macrophages. The macrophage appears to be the primary mode of elimination of airway debris.

Alveolar macrophages also may play an important role in directly modulating lung function. Alveolar macrophages have been found to secrete a variety of products that have a direct effect on pulmonary blood flow and vascular permeability. An example of this activity is the ability of alveolar macrophages to secrete nitric oxide. Alveolar macrophages also may secrete a variety of substances that affect airway resistance and hyperreactivity. Examples of these mediators include thromboxane A_2, platelet-derived growth factor, and platelet-activating factor.

LUNG LYMPHATICS

Individual lymphocytes can be located in the alveolar walls and on the epithelial surfaces of the airways. It is these cells that are recovered in the bronchoalveolar lavage specimens along with alveolar macrophages. In the normal bronchoalveolar lavage specimen, the mononuclear cells include lymphocytes, alveolar macrophages, and epithelial cells. The normal lavage lymphocyte composition is approximately 60% T cells, 10% B cells, and 30% null cells. Clinical conditions in which large numbers of T lymphocytes are obtained from bronchoalveolar lavage specimens include sarcoidosis and acute lung transplant rejection. The study of these T lymphocytes holds the promise of a minimally invasive diagnostic test for a variety of lung diseases. More organized lymphoid tissue, comprised of lymphoid aggregates and nodules, can be found along the bronchial tree. These so-called bronchus-associated lymphoid tissues (BALTs) are located beneath the airway epithelium and are most common at the bifurcation of airways. The lymphocytes found in BALTs are the B lymphocytes associated with humoral immunity. Although BALTs are common in experimental animals, the normal human lung has only rudimentary BALTs.

The anatomic distribution of lymphoid cells in the lung can be illustrated by a lymphomatous involvement of the lung. Lymphoma tissue in the lung generally predominates along the airways and subpleural surfaces of the lung. Work in lymphocyte trafficking suggests that lymphocytes "home" to these tissues. The predominance of lymphocytes along the airways appears to be a pathologic illustration of the normal trafficking of lymphocytes to mucosa-associated lymphoid tissue.

The airway-associated lymphoid tissues play an important role in the immune response to inhaled antigens. In humans, lymph nodes play a more important role in the response to inhaled antigens than in experimental animals. Most of the lymph node tissue is located in the hilum of the lung and in the mediastinum. Inhaled antigens are delivered to these lymph nodes via peribronchial afferent lymphatics. The course of these lymphatic channels is illustrated by the embolic spread of lung malignancies. Tumor emboli sequentially appear in hilar and mediastinal lymph nodes. Interruption of these hilar lymphatic channels can be of clinical importance in lung transplantation and in sleeve resections of the lung. Submucosal lymphatics do not recanalize for more than 3 weeks after interruption and can be associated with increased lung water and impaired immunity.

The lymph node provides the scaffolding that facilitates the interaction of the B and T lymphocytes as well as the antigen-presenting cells of the immune system. T lymphocytes are cells that constantly recirculate throughout the body. Recirculation provides a mechanism for distributing immune cells throughout the body as well as ensuring antigen-reactive diversity. B lymphocytes can be found leaving the antigen-stimulated lymph node, but generally are not found in the unstimulated efferent lymph. When the lymph node is stimulated by antigen, the cell output in the lymph decreases and the size of the lymph node increases dramatically. This type of antigen-induced lymph node enlargement is observed commonly in a variety of infectious conditions. The increase in lymph node size is caused by the rapid recruitment of lymphocytes from the blood. The lymphocytes recirculating in the blood bind to specialized lymph node endothelium called *high endothelial venules*. High endothelial venules are plump endothelial cells only found in specialized lymphatic tissue such as the lymph node. The recruited lymphocytes migrate to specific compartments within the lymph node. T cells are found in the paracortical

regions, whereas B cells and associated germinal centers are found in the cortex of the lymph node. The enlarged lymph node provides the ideal cellular and chemical microenvironment for the generation of antigen-specific immune responses.

GENETIC REGULATION IN THE LUNG

Genetic control of lung cells has important implications for normal growth and development of the lung. Some diseases of the lung, such as cystic fibrosis and α_1-antitrypsin deficiency, have a clear hereditary association. Genetic changes or mutations in these diseases occur in the germline. Because the genetic changes are inherited, the genetic abnormalities exist in every cell of the body.

More commonly, the genetic associations in lung diseases are sporadic. For example, most of the genetic changes leading to cancer in lung cells occur in cells that would otherwise be considered genetically normal. Environmental toxic or infectious exposures can lead to acquired or somatic mutations. These genetic changes exist only in the affected cells.

Multiple Genetic Hits of Carcinogenesis

The potential interaction of inherited and acquired genetic mutations was initially described by studying the epidemiology of retinoblastoma. Patients with retinoblastoma were found to have either a positive family history of the disease (i.e., inherited retinoblastoma) or no apparent family history (i.e., sporadic retinoblastoma). Statistical analysis by Knudson (1971) suggested that more than one genetic mutation, or *hit*, is required for either inherited or sporadic retinoblastoma. People born with a germline retinoblastoma gene (Rb) mutation already have one hit. Any retinal cell that acquires a second hit in the Rb gene can develop into a retinoblastoma tumor. People with this germline mutation are therefore more likely to develop cancer than those without this mutation. In the setting of this genetic predisposition, retinoblastoma tends to occur earlier in life and is commonly associated with other malignancies.

In contrast, retinal cells in people born without the Rb germline mutation must acquire two mutations to develop into the retinoblastoma tumor. Consistent with these enhanced requirements for tumorigenesis, patients with a sporadic form of retinoblastoma manifest the disease later in life, and the disease is less likely to be associated with other cancers. These observations suggest that the hits necessary to transform a cell toward malignancy can be both acquired and inherited.

The basic concept of multiple mutational hits has been supported with studies of the Rb tumor-suppressor gene. Cloning of the Rb gene has shown that in Rb tumors, both alleles of the Rb gene are inactivated, consistent with the two hits necessary for tumorigenesis (Fig. 4-1). The muta-

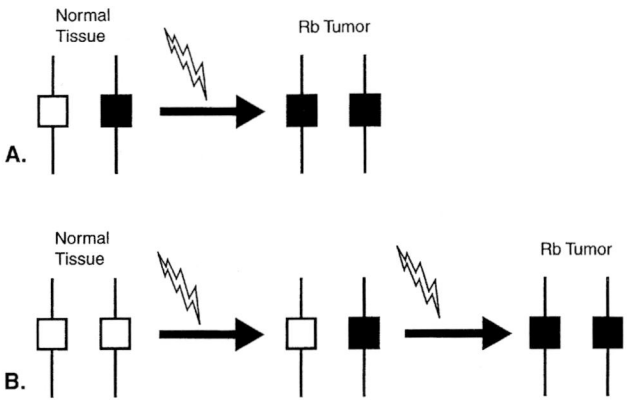

Fig. 4-1. Schematic of the *RB* gene and the *two-hit* hypothesis. **A.** An individual who inherits a mutation of the *RB* gene only requires one additional hit for the development of retinoblastoma. **B.** In contrast, an individual without a germline mutation of the *RB* gene requires mutational events affecting both genes to develop retinoblastoma.

tional hits described in tumorigenesis generally mean a change in the normal sequence of nucleotide base pairs. This change can involve a change as small as the deletion of one nucleotide base pair or as large as the elimination of the entire gene or group of genes. In non–small cell carcinoma of the lung, absent or abnormal Rb proteins have been observed in up to 30% of tumors. A correlation also may exist between the level of abnormal Rb protein expression and the stage of the non–small cell lung cancer. In one study, Xu and associates (1991) found abnormal Rb expression was present in 20% of stage I and II patients and 60% of stage III and IV patients.

Several potential mechanisms exist for the development of genetic mutations. In normal cells, the DNA of the 46 chromosomes is stably replicated during each mitotic cycle. When damage occurs in the DNA of the somatic cells, several DNA repair mechanisms exist to ensure the fidelity of DNA replication. Disruptions in the DNA repair mechanisms are observed naturally in aging. This genetic instability also is associated with prolonged exposure to occupational and environmental carcinogens. Cigarette smoke, for example, may play a role in disrupting DNA repair mechanisms.

A common feature of lung cancer is an abnormal number or arrangement of chromosomes in the tumor cells. Chromosomal aneuploidy is a gross manifestation of genetic instability. Aneuploidy is often detected by cytogenetic analysis or flow cytometry. Large segments of genetic information can be inverted, duplicated, deleted, or translocated onto another chromosome. These arrangements frequently result in the disruption of genes that can be associated with malignancy. The most common chromosomal abnormality identified in lung cancer is the loss of the chromosome 3p. The loss of 3p has been observed in more than 90% of small cell lung cancers and approximately 50% of non–small cell lung cancers. The loss of 3p may contribute to the development of lung cancers because as many as three tumor-suppressor genes reside on the 3p chromosome.

Another mechanism for the mutation of somatic genes is the insertion of viral DNA. DNA viruses incorporate themselves into genomic DNA. The presence of viral DNA frequently leads to cell death. On occasion, however, viral DNA can convert normal cells into cancer cells. Examples of viral induction include lymphomas associated with Epstein-Barr virus malignant mesothelioma associated with SV-40.

Oncogenes

Oncogenes are a class of genes that are expressed in normal cells. The overexpression or mutation of these genes, however, can be associated with uncontrolled growth and tumorigenesis (Table 4-5). In general, oncogenes are phenotypically dominant; a single mutation in one of the paired alleles is sufficient to promote carcinogenesis. An operational definition of an oncogene is a gene whose introduction into a cell results in the transformation of the cell (i.e., the cell takes on some of the phenotypic and growth characteristics of a cancer cell).

The original description of oncogenes came from the study of cancer-associated viruses. These viruses were associated with cellular transformation in animals such as monkeys, chickens, rodents, and cats. The classic definition of an oncogene is a cancer-causing gene carried by an acute transforming retrovirus that has a normal counterpart (homologue) referred to as a *proto-oncogene*. Investigations have shown that the oncogene in Rous' sarcoma virus was not a genuine viral gene, but a preexisting cellular gene, as identified by Stehelin and colleagues (1976), that was copied and modified by an ancestor of Rous' sarcoma virus. The copied and modified gene was used by the virus to transform animal cells. Oncogenes were identified, and are generally named, based on the virus in which they were originally carried. For example, RAS is an oncogene from the rat sarcoma virus and SRC is an oncogene from the Rous' sarcoma virus. Although the research into RNA tumor viruses has no causal link to human cancer, research on animal retroviruses has provided pivotal insights into the identity of cancer-causing genes.

Oncogenes generally have been found to encode proteins involved in signal transduction. Signal transduction proteins are responsible for the transmission of signals from the cell membrane to the replication machinery within the cell nucleus. The involvement of oncogenes in the transduction

Table 4-5. Common Oncogenes

Name	Tumor Associations
c-*erb*-b2-*neu*	Breast, ovary, gastric
myc	Lymphomas, carcinomas
RET	Thyroid carcinoma
K-*ras*	Lung, colon
H-*ras*	Bladder
N-*myc*	Neuroblastoma

RET, receptor-type tyrosine kinase.

Table 4-6. Oncogenes Associated with Human Lung Cancer

Name	Frequency (%)
K-*ras*	30
myc	10–40[a]
erb-2	25
bcl-2	25

[a]*myc* expression varies from 10% in non–small cell lung cancers to up to 40% in some series of small cell lung carcinomas.

Table 4-7. Common Tumor Suppressor Genes

Name	Tumor Association
DCC	Colon
APC	Colon, familial polyposis
BRCA-1, *BRCA*-2	Hereditary breast, ovarian
p53	Leukemia, multiple carcinomas
RB	Retinoblastoma
WT1	Wilms' tumor

of the signals provides clues for the understanding of normal growth and control as well as tumorigenesis. When functioning normally, proto-oncogenes promote cell growth and division. The mutations that transform these proto-oncogenes into oncogenes lead to a loss in normal cellular regulation and uncontrolled cell growth. The growth-promoting function of oncogenes in signal transduction explains the genetic dominance of the mutation. A mutated oncogene has a growth-promoting effect on the cell irrespective of the function of the other allele.

Of the 50,000 to 100,000 genes in the human genome, only approximately 50 genes have been found to transform cells in vitro. Even fewer genes have been found in mutant form in human cancers (Table 4-6). Only 20 of the proto-oncogenes capable of cellular transformation have actually been found in human tumors and even fewer have been associated with thoracic malignancies. An example of a clinically relevant oncogene is K-*ras*, homologous to Kirsten murine sarcoma virus oncogene. K-*ras* mutations are found in up to 30% of adenocarcinomas. Rosell and coworkers (1993) have shown that *ras* mutations and increased *ras* expression have been correlated with decreased survival in non–small cell lung cancer.

Tumor-Suppressor Genes

A common sense approach to cellular regulation would suggest that there are growth-suppressing as well as growth-promoting signals within the cell. The finding that only approximately 20% of human tumors are associated with oncogenes suggests that the mutation or loss of growth-suppressing genes might also be important in tumorigenesis. The discovery of the *RB* (retinoblastoma) gene has provided a model for this type of dysregulation. The normal *RB* gene product serves to constrain cell growth and division. When both alleles are mutated or lost, the normal cellular control mechanism is lost. The genes with these features have been collectively referred to as *antioncogenes* or *tumor-suppressor genes* (Table 4-7).

Tumor-suppressor genes are present in all normal cells. When these genes are missing or inactivated by mutation, the cells exhibit uncontrolled growth. This observation has led to the conclusion that tumor-suppressor genes normally function to restrain cell growth. In general, one normal allele of a tumor-suppressor genes pair is sufficient to prevent

malignant transformation. The loss of all or part of the chromosome containing the tumor-suppressor gene is commonly referred to as the *loss of heterozygosity*. If both copies of the gene are mutated or deleted, the function of the tumor-suppressor genes is lost.

In cancers with an inherited component, one copy of the tumor-suppressor gene is mutated at birth. With the acquired mutation of the remaining allele, cellular growth is no longer suppressed and tumorigenesis can occur. As heritable forms of retinoblastoma have demonstrated, people who inherit a mutated allele have a much higher risk of developing cancer because they have only one functioning gene in reserve. The molecular data from a variety of malignancies suggests that tumor-suppressor gene mutations contribute to the development of many cancers.

The most common tumor-suppressor gene mutations have been observed in the *p53* gene. Mutant versions of the *p53* gene have been found in DNA samples from more than one-half of human tumors examined. The reason that *p53* is so common in human tumors is partly related to its mode of action. When the *p53* gene is mutated, the mutated gene loses its ability to suppress cell growth. The mutated *p53* gene also acquires the ability to actively disrupt the function of the remaining intact gene. The consequence of this ability is that only one mutated gene copy is required to interfere with growth suppression; an effect that is described as a *dominant-negative* mode of action. Levine and associates (1991) have shown that the *p53* gene also appears to have several other unique functions that promote cellular proliferation and inhibit cell death (apoptosis).

In lung cancer, *p53* is associated with a point mutation in the *p53* gene. This point mutation appears to be related to chemicals from cigarette smoking. The overall frequency of *p53* mutations in non–small cell lung cancer is approximately 50% and 80% in small cell lung cancer. The expression of *p53* mutations has not yet been correlated with prognosis in lung cancer. Other tumor-suppressor genes are also found in human lung cancer (Table 4-8).

As more is learned about the function of these genes, tumor-suppressor genes will probably be found to encode proteins involved in transducing negative signals. Tumor-suppressor gene products will also probably be found to be involved in the receiving and processing signals from the cell membrane. Proteins that normally function to inhibit the replication machinery within the cell nucleus may be affected. An example of this processing is the growth-suppressing sig-

Table 4-8. Tumor Suppressor Genes in Human Lung Cancer

Name	Frequency (%)[a]
3p chromosome deletion	50–90
RB	15–90
p53	50–80
p16	60

[a]In almost all series, the higher frequency reflects findings in non–small cell lung cancer and the higher frequencies reflect small cell lung cancer.

nal provided by transforming growth factor-β (TGF-β). When TGF-β binds to the cell membrane, most cells stop growing. In contrast, when certain cells lose *RB* gene function, they lose the ability to respond to TGF-β. These cells grow unrestrained even when exposed to high doses of TGF-β.

The clinical relevance of any given tumor-suppressor gene most likely will depend on the condition of the entire tumor cell genome. The multiple-step model of carcinogenesis argues that a mutation or alteration in any given gene only serves to push a cell down the pathway to full-blown malignancy. The evolution of a clinically relevant cancer requires the presence of multiple successive changes in distinct genes (Fig. 4-2). The collective effect of these changes is required to push the cell from abnormal to malignant.

Cystic Fibrosis

Cystic fibrosis is a common genetic disease with 5% of white Americans carrying the mutant version of the gene. Approximately 1 in 2500 children of European descent carries two defective copies of the gene. These children have the disease of cystic fibrosis. The disease of cystic fibrosis causes impairment of the pancreas, intestines, and liver. Frequently, the most devastating consequence of the disease is the persistent infection in the lung and the subsequent damage to the airways.

For many years, clinicians recognized that children with cystic fibrosis have excessive salt in their sweat. This clini-

cal observation reflected both the pathogenesis and genetic basis for cystic fibrosis. Even the test for cystic fibrosis, the measurement of chloride content in the child's perspiration, remains the cornerstone of the clinical diagnosis. The observation of the excessive salt secretion of children with the disease also provides an important clue to its genetic origin.

In 1989, a large group of collaborators announced the identification of the gene responsible for cystic fibrosis. The product of this gene was called the *cystic fibrosis transmembrane conductance regulator* (CFTR) because of its probable regulation of chloride secretion. Sequencing of the gene revealed a mutation that was present in 70% of all cystic fibrosis patients. This gene is frequently referred to as the *δF508 mutation*. The mutation involves the deletion of three nucleotides from the gene with the resulting loss of a single amino acid (phenylalanine) at position 508 in the CFTR protein.

The CFTR protein appears to form a chloride-permeable channel in the outer membrane of many cells. The movement of chloride through the pore is regulated by the protein, depending on the metabolic condition of the cell. When the gene is mutated, the protein product is retained within the endoplasmic reticulum of the cell and is never expressed at the cell surface. If a normal gene exists, sufficient quantities of the CFTR reach the cell membrane to facilitate relatively normal chloride movement. Consistent with the recessive inheritance pattern of cystic fibrosis, the clinical disease is apparent only when both genes are mutant.

Although the genetic defect of cystic fibrosis is clear, the pathogenesis of the clinical syndrome remains unclear. The submucosal glands in the conducting airways appear to express a large amount of the CFTR protein. How the absence of normal CFTR leads to the hyperinflated lungs and recurrent *P. aeruginosa* infections is unknown. Further studies of the function of this protein may provide important clues regarding normal ventilation and host defense of the lung.

REFERENCES

Knudson AG Jr: Mutation and cancer: statistical study of retinoblastoma. Proc Natl Acad Sci U S A 68:820, 1971.
Levine AJ, Momand J, Finlay CA: The p53 tumour suppressor gene. Nature 351:453, 1991.
Rosell R, et al: Prognostic impact of mutated K-ras gene in surgically resected non-small cell lung cancer patients. Oncogene 8:2407, 1993.
Stehelin D, et al: DNA related to the transforming gene(s) of avian sarcoma viruses is present in normal avian DNA. Nature 260:170, 1976.
Xu HJ, et al: Absence of retinoblastoma protein expression in primary non-small cell lung carcinomas. Cancer Res 51:2735, 1991.

READING REFERENCES

Agostini C, Semenzato G: Immunology of idiopathic pulmonary fibrosis. Curr Opin Pulm Med 2:364, 1996.
Alam S, Chan KM: Noninfectious pulmonary complications after organ transplantation. Curr Opin Pulm Med 2:412, 1996.
Albelda SM: Gene therapy for lung cancer and mesothelioma. Chest 111:144S, 1997.

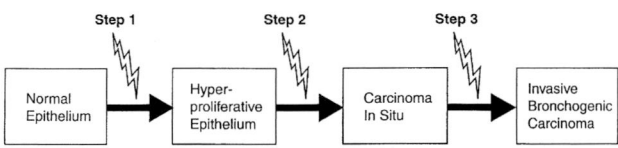

Fig. 4-2. Schematic of the *multiple hit* hypothesis of carcinogenesis. The specific mutations that lead to human lung cancer are unknown at this time. Based on observed abnormalities in lung cancer tumors, a schematized sequence of events is the following: Step 1. The deletion of the 3p chromosome results in the loss of several tumor suppressor genes, leading to dysregulated bronchial epithelial growth and possibly to adenoma. Step 2. The loss of the tumor suppressor gene *p53* results in cytologic changes consistent with carcinoma in situ. Step 3. The overexpression of the *ras* oncogene results in the development of invasive bronchial carcinoma.

Barbacid M: *ras* genes. Annu Rev Biochem 56:779, 1987.

Berg EL, et al: Homing receptors and vascular addressins: cell adhesion molecules that direct lymphocyte traffic. Immunol Rev *108*:5, 1989.

Bishop JM: Cellular oncogenes and retroviruses. Annu Rev Biochem 52:301, 1983.

Bishop JM: Viral oncogenes. Cell *42*:23, 1985.

Bowen LK, et al: Role of passenger leukocytes in allograft rejection: effect of depletion of donor alveolar macrophages on the local production of TNF-alpha, T helper 1/T helper 2 cytokines, IgG subclasses, and pathology in a rat model of lung transplantation. J Immunol *159*:4084, 1997.

Butcher EC, Picker LJ: Lymphocyte homing and homeostasis. Science *272*:60, 1996.

Carbone DP: The biology of lung cancer. Semin Oncol 24:388, 1997.

Carney DN, De Leij L: Lung cancer biology. Semin Oncol 15:199, 1988.

Cavenee WK, et al: Prediction of familial predisposition to retinoblastoma. N Engl J Med *314*:1201, 1986.

Coggins CR: A review of chronic inhalation studies with mainstream cigarette smoke in rats and mice. Toxicol Pathol 26:307, 1998.

Crestani B, Aubier M: Inflammatory role of alveolar epithelial cells. Kidney Int Suppl *65*:S88, 1998.

Crowell RE, Belinsky SA: Genetic changes in lung cancer: potential biomarkers for early detection and prevention. J Lab Clin Med *130*:550, 1997.

Dejana E, Corada M, Lampugnani MG: Endothelial cell-to-cell junctions. FASEB J *9*:910, 1995.

Dong XY, et al: Molecular cytogenetic alterations in the early stage at human bronchial epithelial cell carcinogenesis. J Cell Biochem Suppl *28*:74, 1997.

Dorreen MS: Role of biological markers and probes in lung carcinomas. Bull Eur Physiopathol Respir 22:137, 1986.

Downey GP, Granton JT: Mechanisms of acute lung injury. Curr Opin Pulm Med *3*:234, 1997.

Dunsmore SE, Rannels DE: Extracellular matrix biology in the lung. Am J Physiol *270*:L3, 1996.

Dziadziuszko R, Jassem E, Jassem J: Clinical implications of molecular abnormalities in lung cancer. Cancer Treat Rev 24:317, 1998.

Erickson HP: Gene knockouts of c-*src*, transforming growth factor beta 1, and tenascin suggest superfluous, nonfunctional expression of proteins. J Cell Biol *120*:1079, 1993.

Fearon ER, Vogelstein B: A genetic model for colorectal tumorigenesis. Cell *61*:759, 1990.

Floros J, Kala P: Surfactant proteins: molecular genetics of neonatal pulmonary diseases. Annu Rev Physiol 60:365, 1998.

Folkesson HG, et al: Alveolar epithelial clearance of protein. J Appl Physiol *80*:1431, 1996.

Fulkerson WJ, et al: Pathogenesis and treatment of the adult respiratory distress syndrome. Arch Intern Med *156*:29, 1996.

Gallatin M, et al: Lymphocyte homing receptors. Cell *44*:673, 1986.

Gerritsen ME, Bloor CM: Endothelial cell gene expression in response to injury. FASEB J 7:523, 1993.

Giaccone G: Oncogenes and antioncogenes in lung tumorigenesis. Chest *109*:130S, 1996.

Goerke J: Pulmonary surfactant: functions and molecular composition. Biochim Biophys Acta *1408*:79, 1998.

Graziano SL: Non-small cell lung cancer: clinical value of new biological predictors. Lung Cancer *17*(Suppl 1):S37, 1997.

Groeger AM, et al: Advances in the understanding of lung cancer. Anticancer Res 17:2519, 1997.

Hasday JD, McCrea KA: Inherited predisposition to lung cancer. Occup Med 7:227, 1992.

Hecht SS: Biochemistry, biology, and carcinogenicity of tobacco-specific N-nitrosamines. Chem Res Toxicol *11*:559, 1998.

Heldin CH, Westermark B: Growth factors: mechanism of action and relation to oncogenes. Cell 37:9, 1984.

Hermans C, Bernard A: Pneumoproteinaemia: a new perspective in the assessment of lung disorders. Eur Respir J *11*:801, 1998.

Hollingsworth RE Jr, Hensey CE, Lee WH: Retinoblastoma protein and the cell cycle. Curr Opin Genet Dev 3:55, 1993.

Jansen HM: The role of alveolar macrophages and dendritic cells in allergic airway sensitization. Allergy 51:279, 1996.

Ketai LH, Godwin JD: A new view of pulmonary edema and acute respiratory distress syndrome. J Thorac Imaging *13*:147, 1998.

Klein G, Klein E: Evolution of tumours and the impact of molecular oncology. Nature *315*:190, 1985.

Langer CJ, Rosvold E: Newer aspects in the diagnosis, treatment, and prevention of non-small cell lung cancer. Part II. Curr Probl Cancer *20*:217, 1996.

Ledermann JA, Souhami RL: Biology of lung cancer. Curr Opin Oncol *5*:294, 1993.

Lewis JF, et al: Physiologic responses and distribution of aerosolized surfactant (Survanta) in a nonuniform pattern of lung injury. Am Rev Respir Dis *147*:1364, 1993.

Luchtel DL, et al: Histological methods to determine blood flow distribution with fluorescent microspheres. Biotech Histochem 73:291, 1998.

Massague J: The transforming growth factor-beta family. Annu Rev Cell Biol 6:597, 1990.

McCormack FX: Structure, processing and properties of surfactant protein A. Biochim Biophys Acta *1408*:109, 1998.

Mentzer SJ, et al: Patterns of lung involvement by malignant lymphoma. Surgery 113:507, 1993.

Monton C, Torres A: Lung inflammatory response in pneumonia. Monaldi Arch Chest Dis 53:56, 1998.

Mossman BT, Kamp DW, Weitzman SA: Mechanisms of carcinogenesis and clinical features of asbestos-associated cancers. Cancer Invest 14:466, 1996.

Nakstad B, et al: Subpopulations of human lung alveolar macrophages: ultrastructural features. Ultrastruct Pathol 13:1, 1989.

Nelson S, Summer WR: Innate immunity, cytokines, and pulmonary host defense. Infect Dis Clin North Am 12:555, 1998.

Novick RJ, et al: Lung preservation: the importance of endothelial and alveolar type II cell integrity. Ann Thorac Surg 62:302, 1996.

Novick RJ, et al: Exogenous surfactant therapy in thirty-eight hour lung graft preservation. J Thorac Cardiovasc Surg *108*:259, 1994.

Nowell PC: Chromosomal and molecular clues to tumor progression. Semin Oncol 16:116, 1989.

Pabst R: Is BALT a major component of the human lung immune system? Immunol Today *13*:119, 1992.

Perry ME, Levine AJ: Tumor-suppressor p53 and the cell cycle. Curr Opin Genet Dev 3:50, 1993.

Peters-Golden M, Coffey M: Role of leukotrienes in antimicrobial defense of the lung. J Lab Clin Med *132*:251, 1998.

Pober JS, Cotran RS: Cytokines and endothelial cell biology. Physiol Rev 70:427, 1990.

Przygodzki RM: Molecular pathology of neoplastic lung diseases. Pathology 4:169, 1996.

Richardson GE, Johnson BE: The biology of lung cancer. Semin Oncol 20:105, 1993.

Richmond I, et al: Bronchus associated lymphoid tissue (BALT) in human lung: its distribution in smokers and non-smokers. Thorax 48:1130, 1993.

Roth JA: Gene replacement strategies for lung cancer. Curr Opin Oncol *10*:127, 1998.

Salgia R, Skarin AT: Molecular abnormalities in lung cancer. J Clin Oncol 16:1207, 1998.

Saumon G, Dreyfuss D: Role of distal airspace epithelium for resolving alveolar edema. Kidney Int Suppl 65:S84, 1998.

Schluger NW, Rom WN: The host immune response to tuberculosis. Am J Respir Crit Care Med *157*:679, 1998.

Sekido Y, Fong KM, Minna JD: Progress in understanding the molecular pathogenesis of human lung cancer. Biochim Biophys Acta *1378*:F21, 1998.

Semenzato G, et al: Lung lymphocytes: origin, biological functions, and laboratory techniques for their study in immune-mediated pulmonary disorders. Crit Rev Clin Lab Sci 33:423, 1996.

Shennib H, Nguyen D: Bronchoalveolar lavage in lung transplantation. Ann Thorac Surg 51:335, 1991.

Shimizu Y, et al: Lymphocyte interactions with endothelial cells. Immunol Today *13*:106, 1992.

Sminia T, et al: Structure and function of bronchus-associated lymphoid tissue (BALT). Crit Rev Immunol 9:119, 1989.

Smit EF, et al: New prognostic factors in resectable non-small cell lung cancer. Thorax 51:638, 1996.

Standiford TJ: Cytokines and pulmonary host defenses. Curr Opin Pulm Med *3*:81, 1997.

Vachtenheim J: Occurrence of ras mutations in human lung cancer. Minireview. Neoplasma *44*:145, 1997.

Van Zandwijk N, Van't Veer LJ: The role of prognostic factors and onco-genes in the detection and management of non-small-cell lung cancer. Oncology (Huntingt) *12*:55, 1998.

Vogelstein B, et al: Genetic alterations during colorectal-tumor development. N Engl J Med *319*:525, 1988.

Volm M, et al: Expression of oncoproteins in primary human non-small cell lung cancer and incidence of metastases. Clin Exp Metastasis *11*:325, 1993.

Volm M, Mattern J: Resistance mechanisms and their regulation in lung cancer. Crit Rev Oncog *7*:227, 1996.

Wang BM, et al: Diagnosing pulmonary alveolar proteinosis. A review and an update. Chest *111*:460, 1997.

Ward PA: Phagocytes and the lung. Ann N Y Acad Sci *832*:304, 1997.

Warner AE, Barry BE, Brain JD: Pulmonary intravascular macrophages in sheep. Morphology and function of a novel constituent of the mononuclear phagocyte system. Lab Invest *55*:276, 1986.

Weinberg RA: Tumor suppressor genes. Science *254*:1138, 1991.

Weintraub SJ: Inactivation of tumor suppressor proteins in lung cancer. Am J Respir Cell Mol Biol *15*:150, 1996.

Wiedemann HP, Stoller JK: Lung disease due to alpha 1-antitrypsin deficiency. Curr Opin Pulm Med *2*:155, 1996.

Wright JR: Immunomodulatory functions of surfactant. Physiol Rev *77*:931, 1997.

Zissel G, Muller-Quernheim J: Sarcoidosis: historical perspective and immunopathogenesis (Part I). Respir Med *92*:126, 1998.

CHAPTER 5

Surgical Anatomy of the Lungs

Thomas W. Shields

Until recent decades, the anatomy of the lungs was a little understood and seemingly unimportant subject. With the development of radiographic and endoscopic techniques and the advancement of pulmonary surgery, detailed anatomic knowledge of the lungs became a necessity.

The essential anatomic unit of the lung, the bronchopulmonary segment, was established as that portion of the lung substance that represents the total branching of a major, segmental subdivision of a lobar bronchus. These units are named for their topographic position in the lung.

LOBES AND FISSURES

The right lung is composed of three lobes—the upper, middle, and lower—and is the larger of the two lungs. The left is made up of only two lobes, the upper and lower. Two fissures are usually present on the right. The oblique (major) fissure separates the lower lobe from the upper and middle lobes, and the horizontal (minor) fissure separates the other two (Fig. 5-1). In life, the oblique fissure on the right begins posteriorly at the level of the fifth rib or intercostal space, runs downward and forward approximating the course of the sixth rib, and ends at the diaphragm in the vicinity of the sixth costochondral junction. The horizontal fissure begins in the oblique fissure in the region of the midaxillary line at the level of the sixth rib and runs anteriorly to the costochondral junction of the fourth rib. On the left, the oblique (major) fissure is found (Fig. 5-2). This begins at a somewhat higher level posteriorly, between the third and fifth ribs, and runs downward and forward to end in the region of the sixth or seventh costochondral junction.

Variations in the fissures do occur, and often part or all of a fissure fails to develop. This is seen commonly as a more or less complete fusion of the middle lobe and the anterior portion of the upper lobe in over 50% of lungs examined. Accessory fissures occur also, and certain portions of the lung may be demarcated into so-called accessory lobes. On occasion, such fissures are visible as linear shadows on the radiograph of the chest, and the accessory lobe may appear less radiolucent than the surrounding portions of the lung. The usual accessory lobes are the posterior accessory, inferior accessory, middle lobe of the left lung, and azygos lobe (Fig. 5-3). In contrast to the first three named, which are true accessory lobes made up of specific bronchopulmonary segments, the azygos lobe is not a true accessory lobe because it is formed of varying portions of one or two segments (apical and posterior) of the right upper lobe. The fissure is formed by an aberrant loop of the azygos vein and its mesentery of two layers of the parietal pleura and two of the visceral pleura (Fig. 5-4). On the radiograph, this fissure may appear as an inverted comma to the right of the mediastinum (Fig. 5-5). This anomaly is seen in 0.5 to 1.0% of the anatomic dissections and routine radiographs of the chest.

BRONCHOPULMONARY SEGMENTS

Each lobe of the right and left lungs is subdivided into several individual anatomic units, the bronchopulmonary segments. The general pattern is that of 18 segments, 10 in the right lung and eight in the left. Initially, there were many differences in the nomenclature for the various segments as the result of the publications of the individual investigators working in North America and in Europe. Sealy and associates (1993) presented an excellent review of this topic. The terminology suggested by Brock (1946) and Jackson and Huber (1943) and that adopted by the Ad Hoch International Committee on Nomenclature that was published for the latter by Brock in 1950 are shown in Table 5-1. Subsequently, in 1989, the latest Nomina Anatomica nomenclature for the lung segments was published and is essentially that suggested originally by Jackson and Huber (1943) (Table 5-2). However, the numerical designations, especially those for the segments and structures of the right and left upper lobes, are dissimilar. Most surgeons in America use the numbers suggested by Jackson and Huber

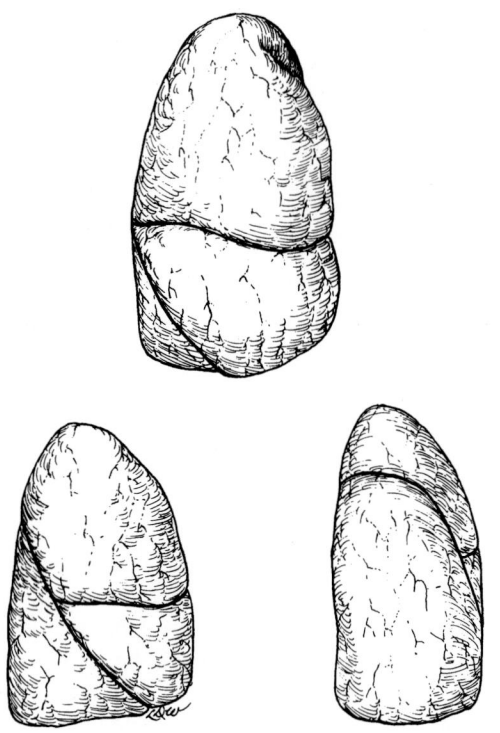

Fig. 5-1. Anterior, lateral, and posterior aspects of the right lung. Redrawn and modified from Anson BJ: Atlas of Human Anatomy. Philadelphia: WB Saunders, 1950, p. 199.

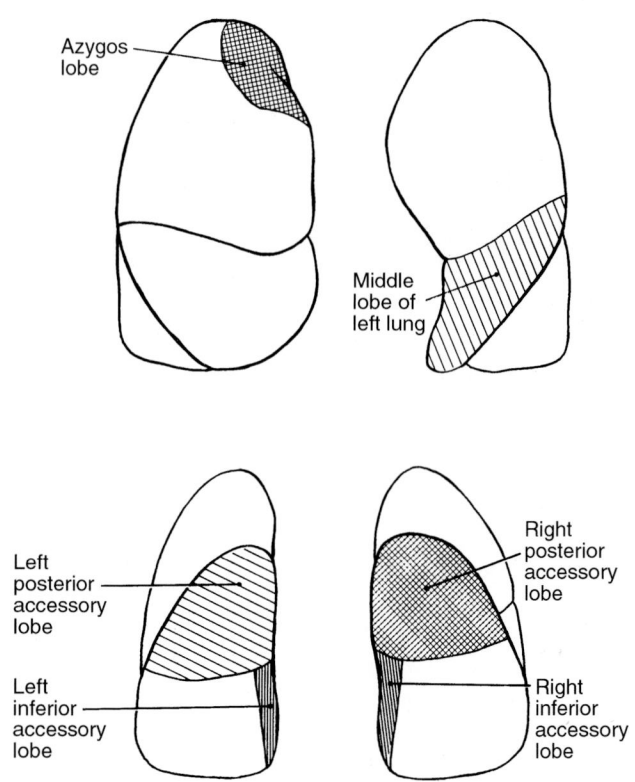

Fig. 5-3. Accessory lobes of the lungs.

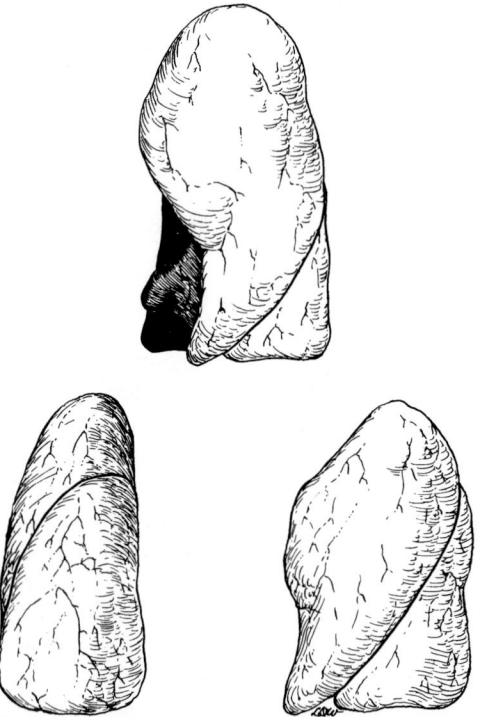

Fig. 5-2. Anterior, lateral, and posterior aspects of the left lung. Redrawn and modified from Anson BJ: Atlas of Human Anatomy. Philadelphia: WB Saunders, 1950, p. 199.

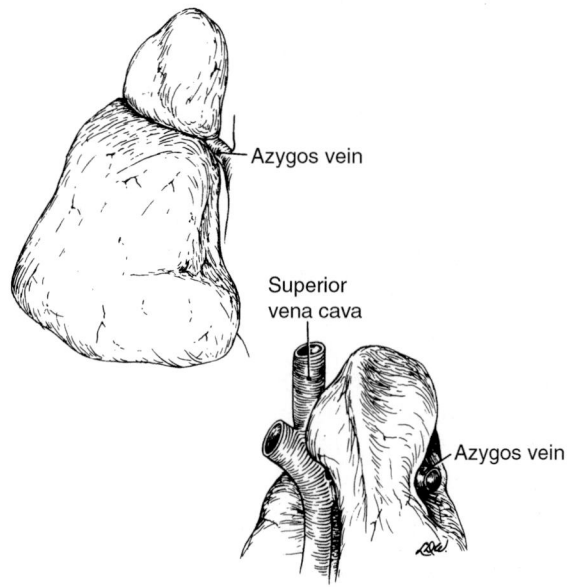

Fig. 5-4. Anterior and posterior views of the azygos lobe formed by an aberrant loop of the azygos vein. Redrawn and modified from Anson BJ: Atlas of Human Anatomy. Philadelphia: WB Saunders, 1950, pp. 203–204.

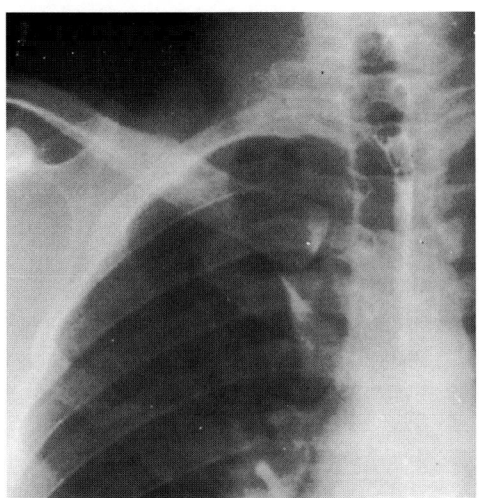

Fig. 5-5. Radiograph of the chest showing an azygos lobe.

(1993) and Boyden (1945, 1955) (see Table 5-2). However, Overholt and Langer (1947) and Beattie and colleagues (1992) have used the numerical designations adopted by the Nomina Anatomica (1989). Likewise, as noted by Wakabayashi (personal communication 1996), the Japanese surgeons use the Nomina Anatomica numerical designations as well. Therefore, one should be aware of the discrepancies in the literature relative to the numerical designations for the various segments and the structure contained therein (bronchi, veins, and arteries). In this text, the terms and numbers used throughout are those suggested by Jackson and Huber (1943) and Boyden (1945, 1955). The topographic positions of the segments are shown in Figure 5-6. Knowledge of the detailed anatomic features of the bronchial distribution and the vascular supply of each segment is essential for the surgeon. Although a general pattern exists in the anatomic features in each segment, variation is

Table 5-1. Nomenclature Adopted by the Ad Hoc International Committee Meeting at the Time of the International Congress of Otorhinolaryngology in 1949

International Nomenclature	Brock	Jackson and Huber
Right upper lobe bronchus		
Apical (1)	Pectoral	Anterior
Posterior (2)	Subapical	Posterior
Anterior (3)	Apical	Apical
Middle lobe bronchus		
Lateral (4)	Lateral	Lateral
Medial (5)	Medial	Medial
Right lower lobe bronchus		
Apical (6)	Apical	Superior
Medial basal (cardiac) (7)	Cardiac	Medial basal
Anterior basal (8)	Anterior basal	Anterior basal
Lateral basal (9)	Middle basal	Lateral basal
Posterior basal (10)	Posterior basal	Posterior basal
Left upper lobe bronchus		
Upper division	Apicopectoral	Upper division
Apical (1)	Apical	Apical
Apicoposterior 1 and 2	—	Apical-posterior
Posterior (2)	Subapical	Posterior
Anterior (3)	Pectoral	Anterior
Lingula	Lingula	Lower (lingular) division
Superior (4)	Upper	Superior
Inferior (5)	Lower	Inferior
Left lower lobe bronchus		
Apical (6)	Apical	Superior
Anterior basal (8)	Anterior basal	Anterior medial basal
Lateral basal (9)	Middle basal	Lateral basal
Posterior basal (10)	Posterior basal	Posterior basal

Note: Two of the five systems, those of Brock and Jackson and Huber, are included. The problem of the presence of a medial basal segment on the left was not resolved and was omitted entirely. Brock's apical instead of Jackson's and Huber's superior was adopted for the first branch of the lower lobe. From the Society of Thoracic Surgeons, Sealy WC, Connally SR, Dolton ML: Naming the bronchopulmonary segments and the development of pulmonary surgery. Ann Thoracic Surg 55:184, 1993. With permission.

Table 5-2. Bronchopulmonary Segmental Nomenclature and Numerical Designations

	Right lung			Left lung
		Upper lobe		
Apical	1 [1]		Superior division	
Anterior	2 [3]		Apical posterior	1 + 3 [1 + 2]
Posterior	3 [2]		Anterior	2 [3]
			Inferior division—lingula	
			Superior lingular	4 [4]
			Inferior lingular	5 [5]
		Middle lobe		
Lateral	4 [4]			
Medial	5 [5]			
		Lower lobe		
Superior	6 [6]		Superior	6 [6]
Medial basal [cardiac]	7 [7]		Anteromedial	7 + 8
			[medial basal-cardiac]	[7]
Anterior basal	8 [8]		[Anterior basal]	[8]
Lateral basal	9 [9]		Lateral basal 9 [9]	
Posterior basal	10 [10]		Posterior basal	10 [10]

Note: Terms and numerals in brackets are those of the Nomina Anatomica, 1989.

the rule. The usual pattern and the most common deviations from it are best portrayed by separate descriptions of the bronchial, arterial, and venous systems.*

---

*The described anatomic patterns and variations of the bronchi and pulmonary arteries and veins have been selected by the author primarily from the studies of Birnbaum (1954); Bloomer, Liebow, and Hales (1960); and Boyden (1955).

BRONCHIAL TREE

The trachea bifurcates at about the level of the seventh thoracic vertebra into the right and left main stem bronchi. Compared with the left bronchus, which arises at a sharper angle, the right bronchus arises in a more direct line with the trachea, an important factor in the localization of aspirated material.

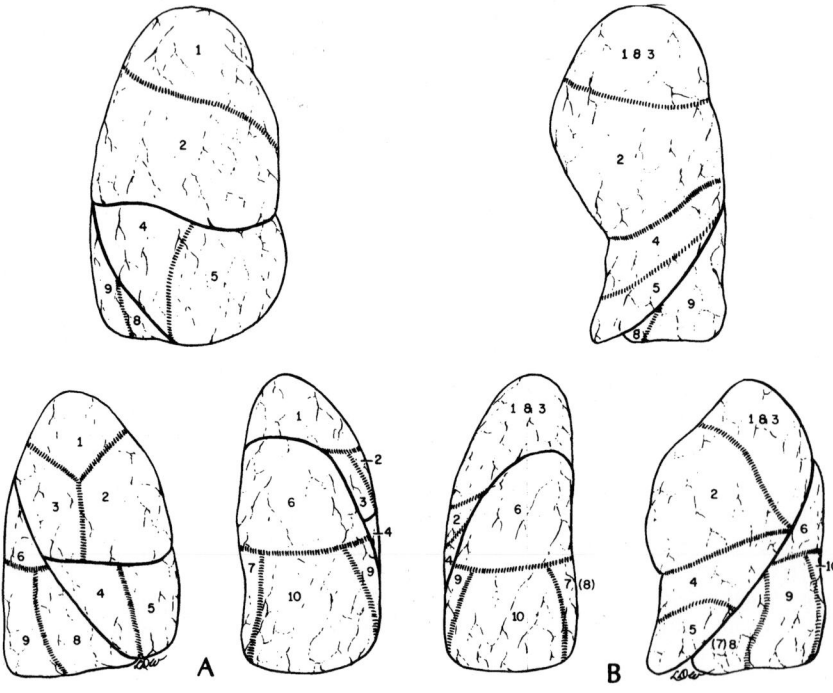

Fig. 5-6. A. Topographic positions of the bronchopulmonary segments of the right lung seen in anterior, lateral, and posterior views. **B.** Topographic positions of the bronchopulmonary segments of the left lung seen in anterior, lateral, and posterior views.

Right Bronchial Tree

The length of the right main bronchus from the trachea to the point where the right upper lobe bronchus branches from its lateral wall is approximately 1.2 cm. The upper lobe bronchus, approximately 1 cm in length, in turn gives off three segmental bronchi—one to the apical, one to the posterior, and one to the anterior segment. The branching may be a simple trifurcation or with varying combinations of the three major branches. The segmental bronchi further subdivide to supply the various portions of the segments.

Proceeding distally from the takeoff of the upper lobe bronchus, the primary bronchus is known as the *bronchus intermedius*, over which the main stem pulmonary artery crosses, thus giving rise to the term *eparterial bronchus* to designate the right upper lobe bronchus. After a distance of approximately 1.7 to 2.0 cm, the middle lobe bronchus arises from the anterior surface of the bronchus intermedius. It varies in length between 1.2 and 2.2 cm before it bifurcates into lateral and medial branches. The superior segmental bronchus of the lower lobe arises from the posterior wall of the bronchus intermedius, slightly distal to the middle lobe bronchus. The superior segment is called the *posterior accessory lobe* when a fissure is present. This bronchus most often arises as a single branch and divides into three rami, usually by bifurcation or rarely by trifurcation. Distal to the superior bronchus, the basal stem bronchus sends off segmental bronchi to the medial (the inferior accessory lobe when a fissure is present) anterior, lateral, and posterior basal segments. The medial basal bronchus arises anteromedially and is distributed to the anterior and paravertebral surfaces of the lower lobe. The anterior basal branch arises on the anterolateral aspect of the basal trunk approximately 2 cm distal to the superior segmental bronchus and divides into two major rami. The lateral basal bronchus and the posterior basal bronchus most often arise as a common stem. Each of these bronchi, in turn, divides typically into two major subdivisions (Fig. 5-7).

Numerous variations occur, but the basic pattern encountered is as described. Infrequently, the upper lobe bronchus on the right undergoes two separate bifurcations to form the three bronchopulmonary segments. Of more interest is the rare occurrence of a tracheal bronchus that arises most commonly 2 cm above, or at the level of, the tracheal carina. A tracheal bronchus is estimated to be present in 0.1 to 2.0% of human tracheobronchial trees, depending on the manner of diagnosis and the population group studied, as noted by Barat and Konrad (1987). The tracheal bronchus occurs for all practical purposes exclusively on the right. Two major types exist: one consists of the right upper lobe bronchus and its divisions, and the other consists only of the apical segmental bronchus (ectopic or supernumerary) (Fig. 5-8). These, as well as other less common variations, have been described in the report by McLaughlin and colleagues (1985). Le Roux (1962) and Atwell (1966, 1967) also discussed these anomalies. The diameter of the tracheal bronchus ranges between 0.5 and 1.0 cm and its length between 0.6 and 2.0 cm. Infrequently, an anomalous bronchus arises from the medial wall of the bronchus intermedius. It is found in 0.09 to 0.5% of the general population. It may occur at any level of the bronchus intermedius. Most often, however, it occurs at, or just distal to, the level and opposite to the orifice of the right upper lobe (Fig. 5-9). A few may arise more distally toward the level of the takeoff of the middle lobe bronchus. The anomalous bronchus, designated as the accessory cardiac bronchus by Brock (1946), may be only a short blind stump or diverticulum without any distal branches. In approximately one-half of the times it is present, according to McGuiness and associates (1993), the accessory cardiac bronchus may have a number of rudimentary or near normal branches associated with variable amounts of lung parenchyma. The length of this anomalous bronchus, according to Deskalakis (1983), may vary from 0.5 to 5.0 cm. On a rare occasion, two accessory cardiac bronchi may be present, as noted by Mangiulea and Stinghe (1968). These authors also noted that an accessory cardiac bronchus may be found in association with the occurrence of a tracheal bronchus. The clinical findings and significance of a tracheal bronchus and an accessory cardiac bronchus are presented subsequently in this chapter. The variations in the middle lobe bronchus and its branchings, other than an occasional superoinferior spatial relationship of the segments rather than lateral and medial arrangements, are of little interest. In the division of the lower lobe bronchus, the presence of a subsuperior or an accessory subsuperior bronchus is a frequent finding. One to three such bronchi may be identified.

Left Bronchial Tree

The left main bronchus is longer than the right and its first branch arises anterolaterally as the left upper lobe bronchus approximately 4 to 6 cm distal to the tracheal carina. This bronchus is approximately 1.0 to 1.5 cm long and divides into superior and inferior (lingular) branches. The superior division ascends and the inferior descends. The superior branch most often bifurcates into an apical posterior segmental bronchus and an anterior segmental bronchus. Occasionally, the anterior segment migrates inferiorly to create a trifurcate pattern. The inferior or lingular bronchus, the analog of the middle lobe, is variable in length (1 to 2 cm) and subsequently divides into superior and inferior divisions, the former of which in turn subdivides into posterior and inferior rami.

Approximately 0.5 cm distal to the left upper lobe orifice, the lower lobe stem bronchus gives off its first branch, the superior segmental bronchus. This bronchus arises posteriorly and bifurcates in most instances, but trifurcation does occur. After giving off the superior branch, the basal trunk

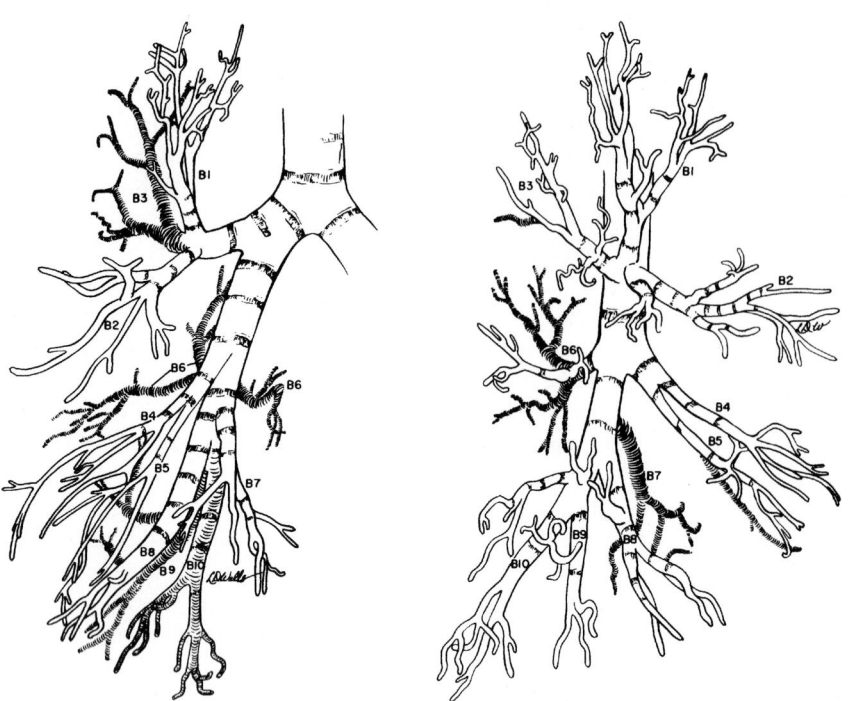

Fig. 5-7. Right bronchial tree, anterior and lateral views. Boyden's modification of numerical nomenclature used. Redrawn and modified from Brock RC: The Anatomy of the Bronchial Tree. 2nd Ed. London: Oxford University Press, 1954, pp. 190–191.

continues for an average distance of 1.5 cm as a single trunk. The bronchus then usually bifurcates into an anteromedial basal segmental bronchus and a common stem bronchus for the lateral basal and posterior basal bronchi. These branches further subdivide into numerous rami for their respective segments (Fig. 5-10).

On the left side, the common variations are in the distribution of the segmental bronchi from the superior and inferior divisions of the left upper lobe bronchus and the presence of a subsuperior or accessory subsuperior bronchus arising from the lower lobe bronchus. Many of these deviations from normal have little clinical importance but are sig-

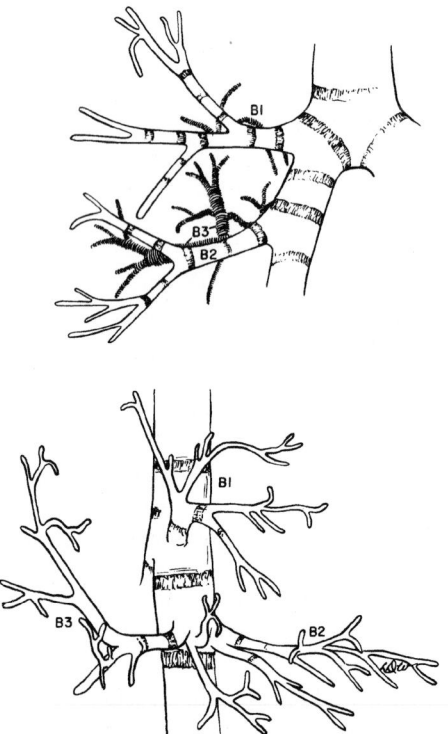

Fig. 5-8. Tracheal bronchus supplying the apical segment of the right upper lobe. Redrawn and modified from Bloomer WE, Liebow AA, Hales MR: Surgical Anatomy of the Bronchovascular Segments. Springfield, IL: Charles C. Thomas, 1960, p. 25.

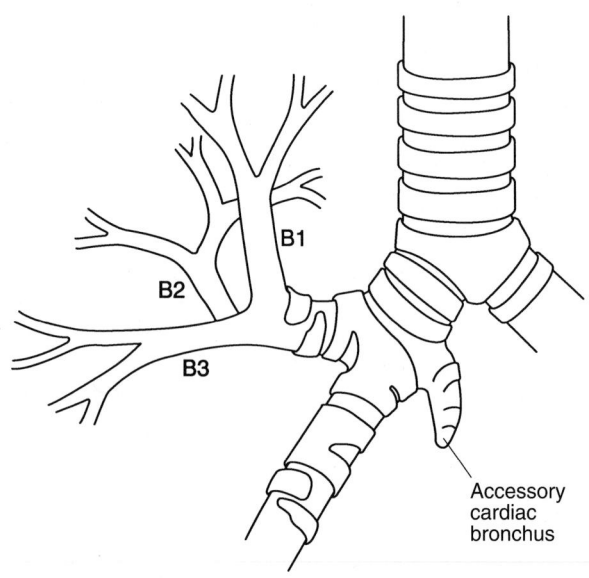

Fig. 5-9. Accessory cardiac bronchus arising from the medial wall of the bronchus intermedius at the level of and opposite to the orifice of the right upper lobe bronchus. Adapted from Keane MP, et al: Accessory cardiac bronchus presenting with haemoptysis. Thorax 52:490, 1997.

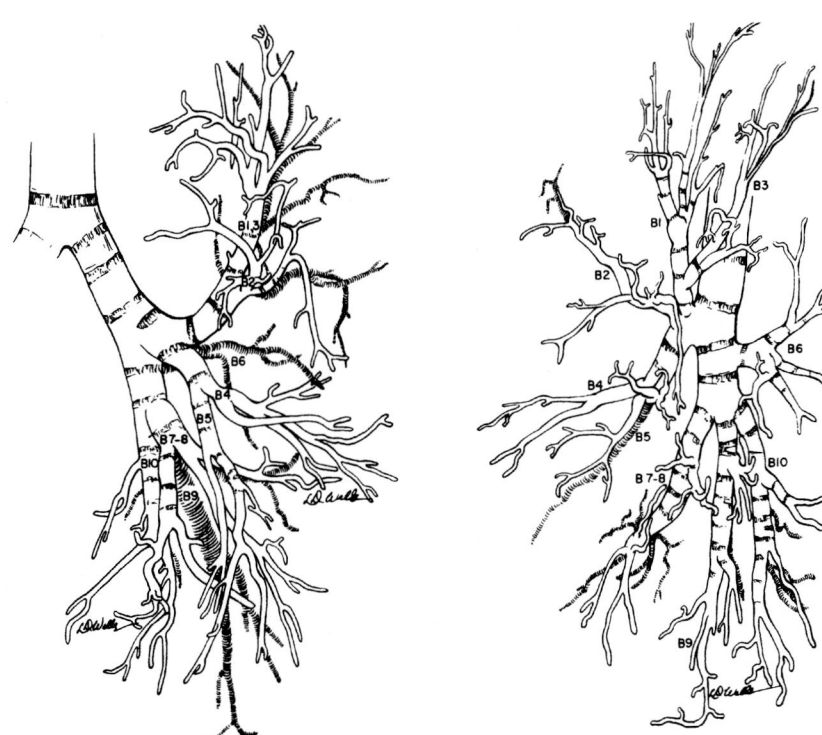

Fig. 5-10. Left bronchial tree, anterior and lateral views. Boyden's modification of numerical nomenclature used. Redrawn and modified from Brock RC: The Anatomy of the Bronchial Tree. 2nd Ed. London: Oxford University Press, 1954, pp. 191–192.

nificant at the time of surgical resection of the various portions of the lungs.

A rare anomaly—a so-called bridging bronchus—has been described on three occasions. The bridging bronchus arises from the left main stem bronchus and crosses the mediastinum to supply the right lower lobe and, at times, a portion of the middle lobe. This anomalous bronchus was first reported by Gonzalez-Crussi and associates in 1976. Subsequently, Starshak (1981) and Bertucci (1987) and their associates each reported a patient with this anomalous bridging bronchus (see the section on Clinical Findings and Significance of Tracheobronchial Anomalies, later in this chapter). This occurrence may be frequently associated with either a pulmonary venous or a pulmonary artery abnormality.

PULMONARY ARTERIAL SYSTEM

The main pulmonary artery arises to the left of the aorta and passes superiorly and to the left. It occupies a position anterior to the left main bronchus and divides into the right and left main pulmonary arteries. These two vessels lie in an oblique line that is parallel and slightly superior to the pulmonary veins. The right main pulmonary artery is longer than the left, but its extrapericardial length up to its first branch is less than that of the left. The branching pattern of the pulmonary arteries is more variable than that of the bronchi, although the arteries tend to lie closely adjacent to the segmental bronchi and to follow their branching. No one pattern for either the right or the left pulmonary artery may

be described as standard. A relatively typical distribution of the segmental arteries is often encountered, however, and from this, the multitude of variations may be readily understood (Figs. 5-11 and 5-12).

Right Pulmonary Artery

As it leaves the pericardial sac, the right pulmonary artery is anterior and inferior to the right main bronchus and posterior and superior to the superior pulmonary vein. The first branch is the truncus anterior, the major vessel carrying blood to the right upper lobe. It arises superolaterally and divides into two branches. The more superior branch of the truncus anterior again divides to form an apical branch that loops posteriorly over the upper lobe bronchus to supply a variable portion of the posterior segment. The latter vessel is known as the posterior recurrent artery. The more inferior branch of the truncus anterior goes to the anterior segment but also may give off a branch to the apical segment. The truncus anterior carries the entire blood supply to the right upper lobe in 1 of 10 individuals. In most persons, one or more ascending vessels from the interlobar portion of the pulmonary artery are present also. The interlobar portion crosses over the bronchus intermedius. Generally, only one ascending vessel to the upper lobe is present. This branch, frequently small in caliber, supplies almost exclusively the posterior segment and is referred to as the posterior ascending artery. At the same level, or even either slightly proximal or distal to the posterior ascending artery, the middle lobe artery arises anteromedially from the interlobar portion of

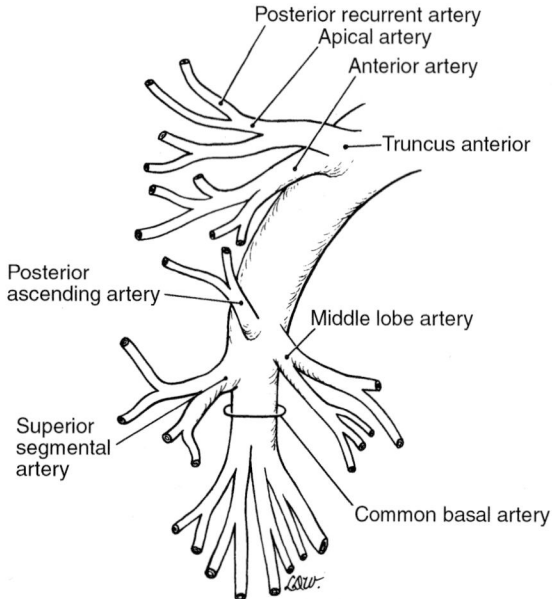

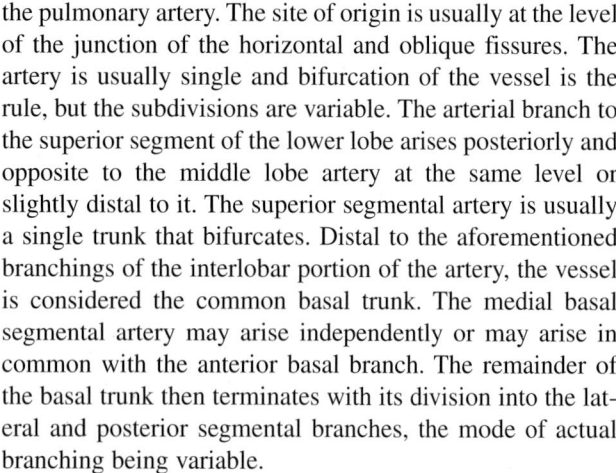

Fig. 5-11. Common pattern of branching of the right pulmonary artery.

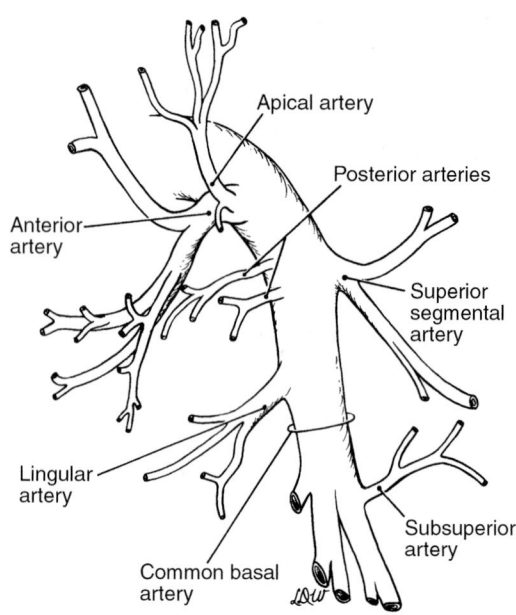

Fig. 5-12. Common pattern of branching of the left pulmonary artery.

the pulmonary artery. The site of origin is usually at the level of the junction of the horizontal and oblique fissures. The artery is usually single and bifurcation of the vessel is the rule, but the subdivisions are variable. The arterial branch to the superior segment of the lower lobe arises posteriorly and opposite to the middle lobe artery at the same level or slightly distal to it. The superior segmental artery is usually a single trunk that bifurcates. Distal to the aforementioned branchings of the interlobar portion of the artery, the vessel is considered the common basal trunk. The medial basal segmental artery may arise independently or may arise in common with the anterior basal branch. The remainder of the basal trunk then terminates with its division into the lateral and posterior segmental branches, the mode of actual branching being variable.

The major variations in the right arterial system occur with almost each of the aforementioned branchings. In as much as 20% of the population, two arteries arise from the anterior trunk. These vessels are designated as the truncus anterior superior and the truncus anterior inferior. When they are present, the recurrent posterior branch is almost always a branch of the truncus anterior superior. Infrequently, more than one ascending branch to the upper lobe arises from the interlobar portion of the artery; the more proximal branch supplies a portion of the anterior segment. On occasion, the posterior ascending artery arises from the superior segmental artery or, even more rarely, from the middle lobe artery. The middle lobe artery, as well as the superior segmental artery, although usually a single vessel, may be represented by two or, at times, even three vessels. Last, in addition to the variable branchings of the common basal trunk, a subsuperior or accessory

subsuperior artery may arise from either the common stem or the posterior basal branch.

Left Pulmonary Artery

The left pulmonary artery ascends to a higher level, passes more posteriorly, and has a greater extrapericardial length before giving off its first segmental branch to the lung than does the right pulmonary artery. The branches to the left upper lobe arise from the anterior, posterosuperior, and interlobar portions of the vessel. The number of branches may vary from two to seven, but four branches to the lobe form the most common pattern. Generally, the first branch arises from the anterior portion of the artery to supply the anterior segment, a part of the apical segment, and occasionally, the lingular division of the lobe. The first branch of this anterior segmental artery supplies the anterior segment and also may give off a lingular branch. Usually, it also branches to provide a vessel carrying blood to the apical segment. The second and, infrequently, a third branch from this first anterior trunk give rise to a vessel, or vessels, going to the anterior segment, to the apical segment, and, uncommonly, to the posterior segment. This anterior trunk is generally short, and often the branches may appear as separate vessels arising from a common opening from the main artery. A second branch from the main artery as it passes distally and posterosuperiorly over the left upper lobe bronchus and into the interlobar fissure is present in almost 80% of instances. This second arterial branch and, occasionally, a third is given off anterosuperiorly to the apical posterior segment. Posteriorly, as the artery passes into the interlobar fissure, it branches to form a vessel going to the superior segment of the lower lobe. This vessel usually is a single one that bifurcates or, infrequently, trifurcates at a variable distance from its takeoff from the main stem arterial trunk. Most often, the lingular artery originates from the interlobar portion of the pulmonary artery distal to the superior segmental artery and constitutes the lingular arterial supply in toto in 80% of persons. At a variable distance from the origin of the lingular vessel, the pulmonary stem artery, now the common basal trunk, most commonly divides into two major branches. The more anterior branch supplies the anteromedial basal segment, and the posterior one supplies the lateral basal and posterior basal segments. The patterns of branching of the common basal trunk and its major divisions are variable.

Likewise, major variations may occur in all the segmental branches of the left pulmonary artery. As mentioned, the first anterior branch may supply the lingular division as well as other portions of the upper lobe, and although it occurs in fewer than 1 in 10 individuals, this branch may carry all the blood supplying the lingular division. Another variation is that the first anterior branch may carry only the blood supplying the apical segment; the anterior segment in this situation receives its arterial supply from the interlobar portion of the artery. As noted, the superior segmental artery usually arises proximal to the branch, or branches, going to the lingula, but in as many as one in three persons, the superior segmental branch may be distal to the lingular artery take-

off. Both these vessels may be multiple. Again, in one of three persons, a branch of one of the lingular vessels or even a direct branch from the interlobar portion of the artery may supply some blood to the anterior segment of the left upper lobe. Rarely, this vascular branch carries the entire arterial supply to this segment. As on the right, branches to the subsuperior segmental region are often found arising as single or multiple vessels from the common basal stem or, more frequently, from the posterior basal branch. Last, a vessel may arise from the common basal stem or one of its branches to contribute to the lingular blood supply.

PULMONARY VENOUS SYSTEM

The venous drainage pattern of the lung reveals a greater number of variations than does the arterial pattern. The usual two major venous trunks from both lungs are the superior and inferior pulmonary veins. The tributaries of these veins are intersegmental and form various combinations to create the major trunks (Figs. 5-13 and 5-14).

Right Pulmonary Veins

The superior pulmonary vein lies anterior and somewhat inferior to the pulmonary artery. It usually is made up of four major branches, which drain the upper and middle lobes. The

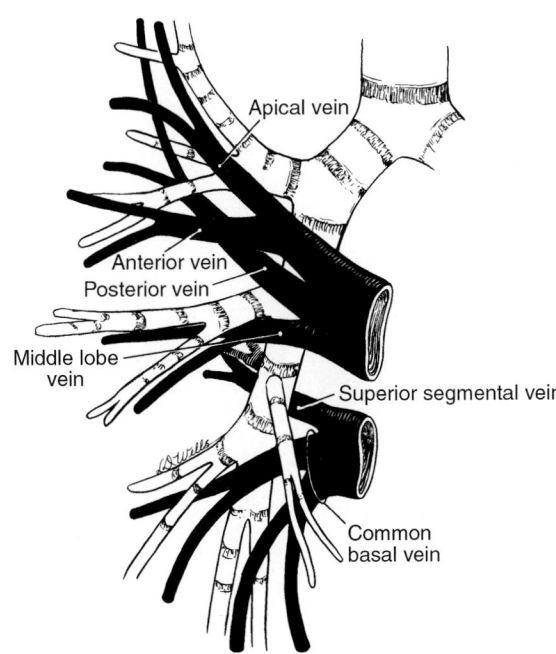

Fig. 5-13. Schematic representation of the tributaries of the right superior and inferior pulmonary veins. Adapted from Kubick S: Klinische Anatomie, Ein Farbfoto-Atlas der Topographie 2. Aufl (Band III-Thorax). Stuttgart: Georg Thieme, 1971, p. 97.

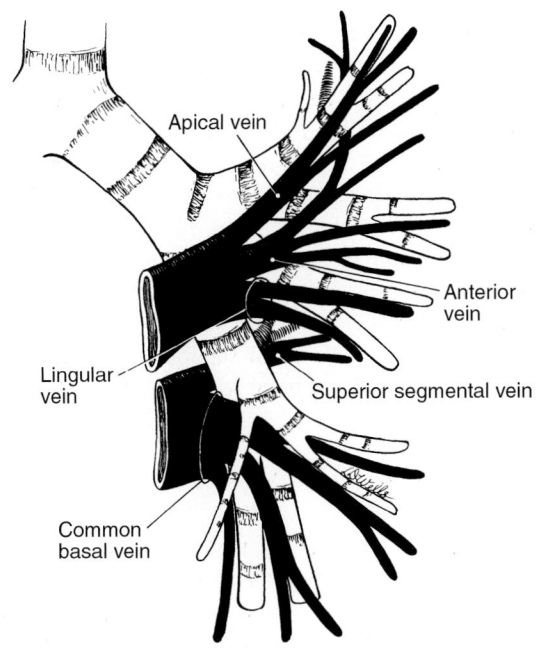

Fig. 5-14. Schematic representation of the tributaries of the left superior and inferior pulmonary veins. Adapted from Kubick S: Klinische Anatomie, Ein Farbfoto-Atlas der Topographie 2. Aufl (Band III-Thorax). Stuttgart: Georg Thieme, 1971, p. 97.

first three branches from above downward drain the upper lobe and are identified as the apical anterior, anterior-inferior, and posterior branches. The posterior branch is composed of central and interlobar divisions. The fourth and most inferior trunk drains the middle lobe and generally is made up of two branches. Although the middle lobe vein most often joins the superior pulmonary vein, on occasion, it may enter the pericardium and drain into the atrium as a separate vessel. Rarely, it becomes a tributary of the inferior pulmonary vein. This variant on the right side has been described in two patients by Sujimoto and colleagues (1998). Yamashita (1978) has reported that the incidence of this anomaly was 4.8% in 120 specimens of the right lung and only 2.5% of the left lung.

The inferior pulmonary vein is inferior and posterior to the superior vein. It drains the lower lobe and as a rule is made up of two major trunks. The first is the superior segmental vein, which drains the superior segment. The other branch, known as the common basal vein, is made up of superior basal and inferior basal tributaries, and these vessels drain the various basal segments of the lower lobe.

Left Pulmonary Veins

On the left, the superior pulmonary vein is applied closely to the anteroinferior aspect of the pulmonary artery, and, as a result, obscures the anterior branches of the artery. This vein is made up of three to four tributaries that drain the entire upper lobe. The first division, the apical posterior vein, is made up of an apical ramus and a posterior ramus. The second division represents the anterior vein, which may have three rami: superior, inferior, and posterior. The third and fourth divisions represent the superior and inferior lingular veins. A single trunk may represent these veins in approximately 50% of persons. This trunk, as seen with the middle lobe vein on the right, may drain into the inferior pulmonary vein; this variant occurs more commonly on the left than on the right, although, as noted previously, the data of Yamashita (1978) do not support this statement.

The inferior pulmonary vein, as on the right, is located inferior and posterior to the superior vein and has two similar tributaries: the superior segmental and the common basal veins. The latter is made up of superior and inferior basal divisions, which drain the basal segments of the lobe.

INTRAPERICARDIAL ANATOMY

The right pulmonary artery passes from the left to the right behind the ascending aorta and constitutes the superior border of the transverse sinus. It then lies behind the superior vena cava and forms the superior border of the postcaval recess of Allison (Fig. 5-15); the medial and inferior borders of this recess are the superior vena cava and right superior pulmonary vein. Although the right pulmonary artery is longer than the left pulmonary artery, it is not as accessible

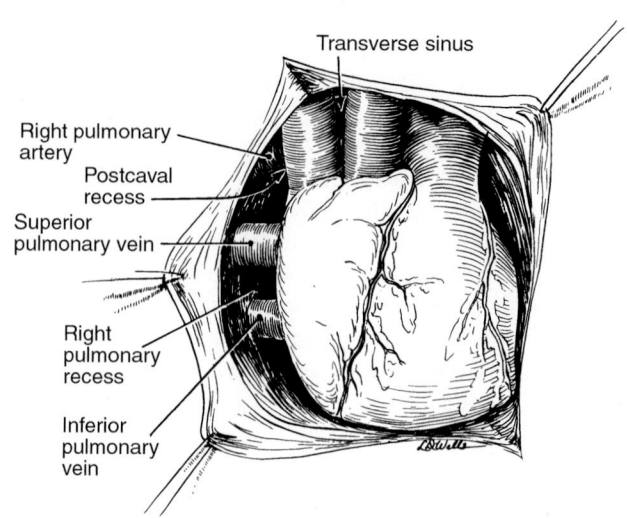

Fig. 5-15. Intrapericardial anatomy on the right. Redrawn from Healey JE Jr, Gibbon JH Jr: Intrapericardial anatomy in relation to pneumonectomy for pulmonary carcinoma. J Thorac Surg 19:864, 1950.

as the left. The left pulmonary artery passes inferior to the aortic arch and forms the superior border of the left pulmonary recess. The medial border of this recess is formed by the fold of Marshall (Fig. 5-16).

The superior and inferior pulmonary veins bulge into the pericardium and are invested to a greater or lesser extent by the pericardium's serous layer. On the right, these two vessels most often enter into the left atrium separately, although rarely they form one vessel. In contrast, on the left, the two veins form a common trunk in one in four persons. On rare occasions, either on the right or left, the superior and inferior pulmonary veins may join within the lung substance or in the fissure to form a single trunk draining the entire lung before entering the pericardial sac. Examples of this anomaly have

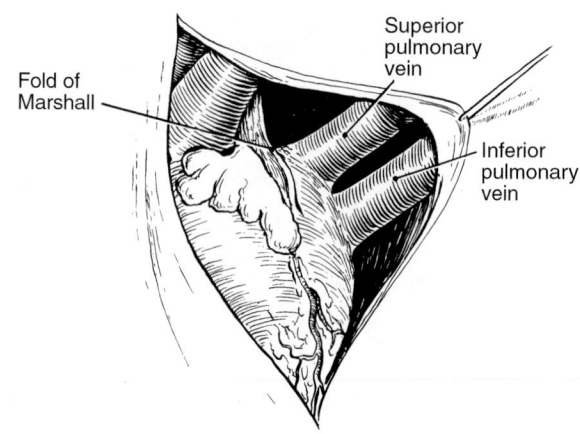

Fig. 5-16. Intrapericardial anatomy on the left. Redrawn from Healey JE Jr, Gibbon JH Jr: Intrapericardial anatomy in relation to pneumonectomy for pulmonary carcinoma. J Thorac Surg 19:864, 1950.

been reported by Benfield (1971), Tretheway (1974), Hasuo (1981), and Meguro (1998) and their associates.

The serous (parietal) pericardial investments of the vessels are important because these fibrous tissue layers must be divided to obtain free access to the entire circumference of the individual vessel. On the right, the serous layer leaves the lateral and posterior surfaces of the superior vena cava and comes to lie on the artery in the postcaval recess. At this point, only about one-fifth of the circumference of the vessel is free. In contrast, three-fourths of the circumference is free in the transverse sinus medial to the superior vena cava. From the artery, the serous layer passes inferiorly and reflects on the superior, anterior, and inferior surfaces of the superior vein; approximately one-third of this vessel is not free posteriorly. The layer then descends to cover most of the inferior pulmonary vein and then passes down to envelop the inferior vena cava. On the left, the reflection of the serous pericardium passes over the anterior and inferior surfaces of the left pulmonary artery, and approximately one-half of the vessel is free in the pericardial sac. The layer then descends inferiorly to the superior vein, so that only the posterior surface is not free in the sac. It then passes downward to envelop the inferior vein, which is subsequently almost totally free within the sac, except for a small surface located posteriorly.

BRONCHIAL ARTERIES AND VEINS

The bronchial arterial system arises from the systemic circulation and accounts for approximately 1% of the cardiac output. It empties mainly into the pulmonary veins and a lesser bronchial vein system that enters the azygos venous system on the right and the hemiazygos on the left. The origins of the arteries are variable from the aorta, intercostal arteries, and, occasionally, from the subclavian or innominate arteries. Rare origin from other systemic vessels of the chest (internal mammary artery) or even from a coronary artery has been recorded.

The most extensive anatomic study was reported by Caudwell and associates (1948). These investigators recorded nine patterns of origin. In 90% of the 150 cadaver specimens studied, the pattern was one of four types (Fig. 5-17), and the remaining 10% were distributed in five other less common variations (Table 5-3). Liebow (1965) performed corrosion casts of the bronchial arterial system in 50 cadavers, and his findings were in essential agreement with those of the aforementioned authors.

Caudwell and colleagues (1948) reported that the level of origin of the bronchial arteries was from the third to eighth vertebral bodies, most commonly between the levels of the fifth and sixth thoracic vertebrae, and arose from the descending thoracic aorta and rarely from the arch. Most of the bronchial vessels arose separately (74% of specimens), and only in 26% did two vessels have a common origin. The right bronchial arteries arose from the anterolateral or lateral surface of the aorta and rarely from its posterior aspect. In

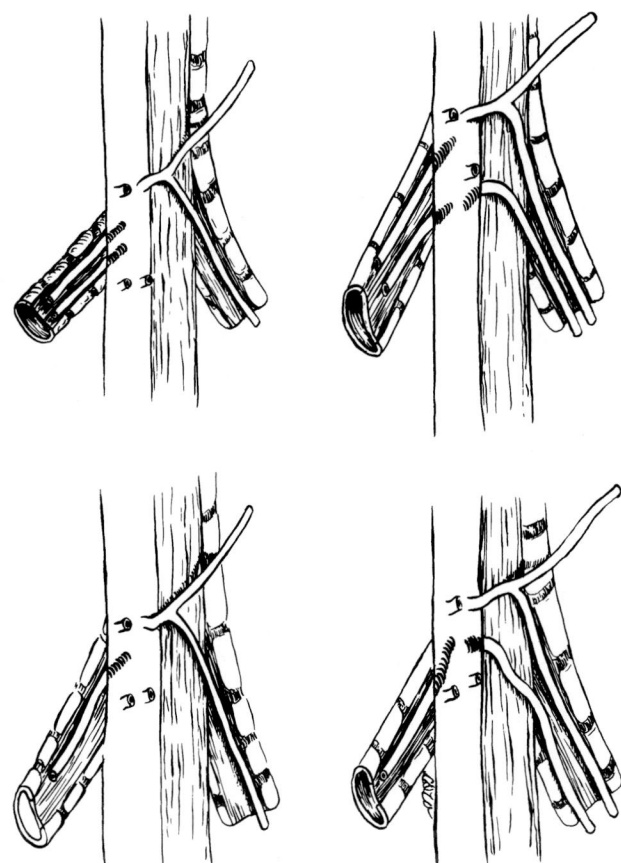

Fig. 5-17. The four most common sites of origin and numbers of bronchial arteries to the right and left lung (see Table 5-3 for percentage of occurrence of each). From Caudwell EW, et al: The bronchial arteries. An anatomic study of 150 human cadavers. Surg Gynecol Obstet *86*:395, 1948. With permission.

Table 5-3. Origins and Number of Bronchial Arteries in 150 Dissected Autopsy Specimens

Anatomic Variation	Number of Right Bronchial Arteries	Number of Left Bronchial Arteries	Percent Incidence
I	1	2	40.8
II	1	1	21.3
III	2	2	20.8
IV	2	1	9.7
V	1	3	4.0
VI	2	3	2.0
VII	3	2	0.6
VIII	1	4	0.6
IX	4[a]	1	0.6

[a]A branch from the left bronchial artery anterior to the esophagus passing to the right bronchus plus two right bronchial arteries from the aorta and one right bronchial artery from the subclavian artery.
From Caudwell EW, et al: The bronchial arteries. An anatomic study of 150 human cadavers. Surg Gynecol Obstet *86*:395, 1948. With permission.

88.7% of specimens, the right bronchial artery arose in common with an aortic intercostal vessel: 78% from the first, 7.3% from the second, and 1.3% from the third. Nathan and colleagues (1970) described the anatomy of this major right bronchial artery. They found that it arose anywhere from 0.5 to 5.0 cm from the origin of the intercostal artery from its origin from the aorta and courses upward and forward toward the right main stem bronchus. In its courses on the right anterolateral aspect of the vertebral column, it passes to the right of the thoracic duct and crosses the esophagus to terminate at the lower level of the trachea near the origin of the right main stem bronchus. At the level of the trachea, it crosses lateral to the vagus nerve. In its mediastinal course, the right bronchial artery generally runs parallel to the arch of the azygos vein by which it is overlapped.

On the left, the bronchial arteries are more variable in their courses to the bronchus and, according to Caudwell and associates (1948), 94% arise directly from the aorta. Only 4% are associated with an intercostal vessel, which invariably is a right intercostal artery. In most instances, the bronchial vessels that arise from the aorta pass in back of the trachea, and in only a few cases does one pass in front of the trachea. Rarely, such a branch to the right may be in close proximity to the tracheal carina. It is possible a branch of such an anatomically situated vessel could be injured during a mediastinoscopy as suggested by Miller and Nelems (1989).

These anatomic studies by the aforementioned investigators have been confirmed by the angiographic observations of Olson and Athanasoulis (1982) and other interventional radiologists. Deffebach and associates (1987) reviewed the distribution of the bronchial arteries once they entered the hilus of the lung and course within the bronchial tree. Essentially, the arteries to either side form a communicating arc around the main bronchus. From here, the main arterial divisions radiate along the major bronchi. These vessels are closely applied to the bronchial wall, with generally two divisions, an anterior and posterior branch, along each bronchus. The vessels follow the course of the bronchus and divide, as do the bronchi. Networks of intercommunicating vessels are often present on the bronchial walls. It has been assumed that two-thirds of this blood supply empties into the pulmonary veins and that the rest empties into the bronchial veins. The bronchial veins are present in the mucosa and also external to the bronchial cartilage. The direction of flow is to the venous plexus of the perihilar regions and then subsequently into either the azygos or hemiazygos systems.

CLINICAL FINDINGS AND SIGNIFICANCE OF TRACHEOBRONCHIAL ANOMALIES

Tracheal Bronchus

A tracheal bronchus may remain undetected throughout a person's life, but occasionally it is symptomatic in young children and less commonly in adults. McLaughlin and col-

leagues (1985) identified 18 tracheal bronchi in children under the age of 5 years; eight of them were diagnosed by bronchoscopy in 412 children with respiratory symptomatology. Five children underwent resection of the anomalous bronchus and its supplied lung tissue because of recurrent pneumonia. The tracheal bronchus often was associated with other congenital defects: tracheal stenosis, hypoplastic or fused first and second thoracic ribs, bilateral lumbar first ribs, and other minor vertebral anomalies. Down syndrome often is present. In adults, complications are rare. Of interest was the occurrence of a bronchial adenoma within a tracheal bronchus and causing hemoptysis that was reported by Epstein (1951) and the occurrence of a bronchial carcinoma in a tracheal bronchus reported by Kim and associates (1998).

On rare occasions, bilateral tracheal bronchi may be present, the right and left tracheal bronchi supplying a portion or all of the respective upper lobe of the right and left lung. Holinger and colleagues (1952) were the first to describe this anomaly in a living infant, who subsequently died of respiratory complications. Cope and associates (1986) also identified a 14-month-old infant with similar malformations who apparently had no difficulty because of their presence and was reported to be well at 2 years of age. Lastly, Holinger (1952) described an isolated left tracheal bronchus that curved posteriorly and medially to supply the right upper lobe.

Accessory Cardiac Bronchus

The presence of an accessory cardiac bronchus more often than not remains undetected until discovered on a diagnostic bronchoscopy or computed tomography of the lung; it is undetectable by standard chest radiography. Sotile and associates (1988) initially described the computed tomographic findings, and these were further defined by McGuinness and coworkers in 1993. Occasionally, most often in adults, this rare anomaly gives rise to symptoms as the result of infection within the anomalous bronchus. Hemoptysis from mucosal ulceration or persistent symptoms of unresolved pulmonary infection are the common clinical features, as noted by Keane and colleagues (1997), that lead to its identification. According to Deskalakis (1983), one patient developed a middle lobe syndrome because of the presence of this anomalous bronchus. In patients with a long accessory cardiac bronchus, pulmonary infection and subsequent pleural empyema may occur as one of the more serious complications. This has been reported by Suzuki and Hirata (1991) in the Japanese literature. Control of persistent symptomatology is achieved by resection of the offending accessory cardiac bronchus.

Bridging Bronchus

The three patients with a bridging bronchus were baby girls who demonstrated respiratory distress and pulmonary infection. All three had multiple congenital anomalies in addition to the bridging bronchus. Death occurred in each patient, in two after attempted surgical resection of the affected lobe.

REFERENCES

Atwell SW: An aberrant bronchus. Ann Thorac Surg 2:438, 1966.

Atwell SW: Major anomalies of the tracheobronchial tree: with a list of the minor anomalies. Dis Chest 52:611, 1967.

Barat M, Konrad HR: Tracheal bronchus. Am J Otolaryngol 8:118, 1987.

Beattie EJ, Bloom ND, Harvey JC: Thoracic Oncology. New York: Churchill Livingstone, 1992.

Benfield JR, Gots RE, Mills D: Anomalous single left pulmonary vein mimicking a parenchymal nodule. Chest 59:101, 1971.

Bertucci GM, et al: Bridging bronchus and posterior left pulmonary artery: a unique association. Pediatr Pathol 7:637, 1987.

Birnbaum, GL: Anatomy of the Bronchovascular System. Its Application to Surgery. Chicago: Year Book Medical Publishers, 1954.

Bloomer WE, Liebow AA, Hales MR: Surgical Anatomy of the Bronchovascular Segments. Springfield, IL: Charles C. Thomas, 1960.

Boyden E: The intrahilar and related segmental anatomy of the lung. Surgery 18:706, 1945.

Boyden EA: Segmental Anatomy of the Lungs. New York: McGraw-Hill, 1955.

Brock RC: The Anatomy of the Bronchial Tree. London: Oxford University Press, 1946.

Brock RC (reporter): The nomenclature of broncho-pulmonary anatomy: an international nomenclature accepted by The Thoracic Society. Thorax 5:222, 1950.

Caudwell EW, et al: The bronchial arteries. An anatomic study of 150 human cadavers. Surg Gynecol Obstet 86:395, 1948.

Cope R, Campbell JR, Wall M: Bilateral tracheal bronchi. J Pediatr Surg 21:443, 1986.

Deffebach ME, et al: The bronchial circulation, small but a vital attribute of the lung. Am Rev Respir Dis 135:463, 1987.

Deskalakis MK: Middle lobe syndrome due to accessory cardiac bronchus. South Med J 76:941, 1983.

Epstein I: Bronchial adenoma in supernumerary tracheal lobe; report of unusual case. J Thorac Surg 21:362, 1951.

Gonzalez-Crussi F, et al: "Bridging bronchus." A previously undescribed airway anomaly. Am J Dis Child 130:1015, 1976.

Hasuo K, et al: Anomalous unilateral single pulmonary vein mimicking pulmonary varices. Chest 79:602, 1981.

Holinger PH, et al: Congenital malformations of the trachea, bronchi, and lung. Ann Otol Rhinol Laryngol 61:1159, 1952.

Jackson CL, Huber JF: Correlated applied anatomy of bronchial tree and lungs with system nomenclature. Dis Chest 9:319, 1943.

Keane MP, et al: Accessory cardiac bronchus presenting with haemoptysis. Thorax 52:490, 1997.

Kim J, et al: Surgical resection of lung cancer originating in a tracheal bronchus. Ann Thorac Surg 66:944, 1998.

Le Roux BT: Anatomical abnormalities of the right upper lobe bronchus. J Thorac Cardiovasc Surg 44:225, 1962.

Liebow AA: Patterns of origin and distribution of the major bronchial arteries in man. Am J Anat 117:19, 1965.

Mangiulea VG, Stinghe RV: The accessory cardiac bronchus. Bronchoscopic aspect and review of the literature. Dis Chest 54:433, 1968.

McGuinness G, et al: Accessory cardiac bronchus: CT features and clinical significance. Radiology 189:563, 1993.

McLaughlin FJ, et al: Tracheal bronchus: association with respiratory morbidity in childhood. J Pediatr 106:751, 1985.

Meguro H, et al: A case of single left pulmonary vein with deficiency of left inferior pulmonary vein. J Jpn Assoc Chest Surg 12:539, 1998.

Miller RR, Nelems B: Mediastinal lymph node necrosis: A newly recognized complication of mediastinoscopy. Ann Thorac Surg 48:247, 1989.

Nathan H, Orda R, Barkay M: The right bronchial artery, anatomical considerations and surgical approach. Thorax 25:328, 1970.

Nomina Anatomica. 6th ed. New York: Churchill Livingstone, 1989.

Olson PR, Athanasoulis CA: Hemoptysis: Treatment with transcatheter embolizations of the bronchial arteries. In Athanasoulis CA, et al: Interventional Radiology. Philadelphia: WB Saunders, 1982, p. 196.

Overholt RH, Langer LA: New technique for pulmonary segmental resection. Its application in the treatment of bronchiectasis. Surg Gynecol Obstet 84:257, 1947.

Sealy WC, Connally SR, Dalton ML: Naming the bronchopulmonary segments and the development of pulmonary surgery. Ann Thorac Surg 55:184, 1993.

Sotile SC, Brady MB, Brogdon BG: Accessory cardiac bronchus: demonstration by computed tomography. J Comput Tomogr 12:144, 1988.

Starshak RJ, et al: Bridging bronchus. A rare airway anomaly. Radiology 140:95, 1981.

Sujimoto S, et al: Anatomy of inferior pulmonary vein should be clarified in lower lobectomy. Ann Thorac Surg 66:1799, 1998.

Suzuki M, Hirata S: A case of accessory bronchus with acute empyema treated by open drainage. Nippon Kyobu Shikkan Gakkai Zasshi 29:600, 1991.

Tretheway DG, et al: Single left pulmonary vein with normal pulmonary venous drainage: a roentgenographic curiosity. Am J Cardiol 34:237, 1974.

Yamashita H: Variations in the pulmonary segments and the bronchovascular tree. In Yamashita H (ed): Roentgenographic Anatomy of the Lung. Tokyo: Igakushoin, 1978, p. 70.

READING REFERENCES

Allison PR: Intrapericardial approach to the lung root in the treatment of bronchial carcinoma by dissection pneumonectomy. J Thorac Surg 15:99, 1946.

Barrett RJ, Day JC, Tuttle WM: The arterial distribution to the left upper pulmonary lobe. J Thorac Surg 32:190, 1956.

Barrett RJ, O'Rourke PV, Tuttle WM: The arterial distribution to the right upper pulmonary lobe. J Thorac Surg 36:117, 1958.

Brock RC: The Anatomy of the Bronchial Tree. 2nd Ed. London: Oxford University Press, 1954.

Cory RAS, Valentine EJ: Varying patterns of the lobar branches of the pulmonary artery. Thorax 14:267, 1959.

Cudkowicz L: The Human Bronchial Circulation in Health and Disease. Baltimore: Williams & Wilkins, 1968.

Harris JH Jr: The clinical significance of the tracheal bronchus. AJR Am J Roentgenol 79:228, 1958.

Healey JE Jr, Gibbon JH Jr: Intrapericardial anatomy in relation to pneumonectomy for pulmonary carcinoma. J Thorac Surg 19:864, 1950.

Kent EM, Blades B: The surgical anatomy of the pulmonary lobes. J Thorac Surg 12:18, 1942.

Kubik S, Healey JE: Surgical Anatomy of the Thorax. Philadelphia: WB Saunders, 1970.

Milloy FJ, Wragg LE, Anson BJ: The pulmonary arterial supply to the right upper lobe of the lung based upon a study of 300 laboratory and surgical specimens. Surg Gynecol Obstet 116:35, 1963.

Milloy FJ, Wragg LE, Anson BJ: The pulmonary arterial supply to the upper lobe of the left lung. Surg Gynecol Obstet 126:811, 1968.

CHAPTER 6

Lymphatics of the Lungs

Thomas W. Shields

The lung has an extensive network of lymphatic vessels that are situated in the loose connective tissue beneath the visceral pleura, in the connective tissue in the interlobular septa, and in the peribronchial vascular sheaths.

In the pulmonary parenchyma, the lymphatic capillaries form extensive plexuses within the connective tissue sheaths that surround the airways and the blood vessels. The origin of these channels is believed to be at the level of the terminal and respiratory bronchioles, and they do not extend into the interalveolar septa according to Leak and Jamuar (1983). The channels begin as blind-end tubes and saccules. As these channels extend proximally toward the hilar area associated with the enlarging airways and blood vessels, they have been designated as juxtaalveolar lymphatics by Lauweryns (1971) and Leak (1980). These networks drain into larger collecting vessels with thicker walls and contain monocuspid, conical valves that direct the flow of lymph toward the hilar area in a centripetal direction. The physiologic mechanisms controlling this lymphatic flow are little understood.

Lymphatic channels that also drain the periphery of the lung lobules run in the lobular septa along with the pulmonary veins. With the occurrence of extra-alveolar interstitial edema, some of these may be recognized as Kerley's B lines radiographically, as noted by Steiner (1973).

The extensive subpleural network drains primarily by the channels in the interlobular septa to the hilar area, but direct connections to the mediastinum have been recorded by Rouvière (1932), Borrie (1952, 1965), and Riquet and associates (1989). The channels in the lobular septa have multiple connections with the channels in the bronchovascular sheaths. These connecting channels are frequently up to 4 cm in length and lie midway between the hilus and the periphery of the lung. When distended, they are recognized as Kerley's A lines.

Collections of lymphatic cells may be seen along the course of the lymphatic channels and within the bronchial structures, but recognizable intrapulmonary lymph nodes are identified only infrequently in contrast to the common presence of bronchopulmonary lymph nodes.

PULMONARY LYMPH NODES

The pulmonary lymph nodes are divided into the intrapulmonary and bronchopulmonary nodes. The latter are subdivided into the lobar and hilar lymph nodes.

Intrapulmonary Lymph Nodes

The intrapulmonary lymph nodes are located infrequently just beneath the visceral pleura. Rarely, a peripheral lymph node may present as a solitary peripheral nodule as reported by Greenberg (1961). Trapnell (1964) was able to identify radiologically peripheral lymph nodes in only 1 of 92 inflated lungs obtained at autopsy, an incidence of just over 1%. With high-resolution computed tomography (CT), some of the small lesions identified in patients with multiple metastases to the lung are proved subsequently to be small peripheral lymph nodes.

In addition to these rare, radiographically identified intrapulmonary lymph nodes, Trapnell (1963) reported the identification of other intrapulmonary lymph nodes in the substance of the lung by a combined technique of injection of the subpleural lymphatics and subsequent radiologic evaluation of autopsy lung specimens. Intrapulmonary nodes were observed in 5 of 28 injected specimens, an incidence of 18%. The actual location of these nodes was undocumented.

Dail (1995) suggested that intraparenchymal lymph nodes could be identified in approximately 10% of resected lobes when they were looked for. Kradin and associates (1985) recorded that all such nodes were anthracotic and were not encapsulated. The identified lymph nodes were solitary in 65% of the cases and multiple in the remainder; in 22%, two lymph nodes were found and in 12% there were three or more identified. The multiple nodes may be in the same lobe in 40% of the cases in which they are found, but in 60%, the lymph nodes are located bilaterally. The size varies from less than 0.5 cm to 1.0 to 1.5 cm. Most are in the range of 0.5 to 1.0 cm; only rarely is a larger one present. All these intraparenchymal lymph nodes are within 1 cm of the pleura, adjacent to it or in an interlobular septum. With rare exception, these lymph nodes are found only in adults and are identified more commonly in individuals older than 50 years of age.

Bronchopulmonary Lymph Nodes

Nagaishi (1972) noted that segmental lymph nodes are related to the bifurcation of the segmental bronchi or may lie in the bifurcation of the branches of the associated pulmonary arteries and may extend out to the fifth- or sixth-order segmental bronchi.

The lobar bronchopulmonary lymph nodes are found at the angles formed by the origins of the various lobar bronchi and lie in close association with the bronchus or the adjacent pulmonary vessels. The hilar lymph nodes are situated alongside the lower portions of the main bronchi or the respective pulmonary artery and the pulmonary veins lying within the visceral pleural reflections.

The number of bronchopulmonary lymph nodes is variable. These lymph nodes more frequently are present in greater numbers in children than in adults. Borrie (1965) suggests that the maximal development of these nodes is reached by the end of the first decade of life, and then these lymph nodes gradually atrophy and disappear during adulthood. The presence of pulmonary infection or malignancy greatly affects the number of bronchopulmonary lymph nodes that may be identified.

In a study of 200 operative specimens of lungs containing lung cancer, Borrie (1965) identified lymph nodes in 13 locations in the right lung and 15 locations in the left lung that are now considered bronchopulmonary lymph nodes. These sites are listed in Table 6-1 and are shown schematically in Figures 6-1 and 6-2. The incidence of bronchopulmonary lymph nodes present in each location is listed in Table 6-2.

Hilar Lymph Nodes

The hilar lymph nodes are contiguous with the lobar lymph nodes distally as well as with the mediastinal lymph nodes proximally. The hilar lymph nodes lying superior to the right main stem bronchus classically have been considered to extend up to the inferior border of the azygos vein, but this concept was questioned by Tisi and associates (1983) in their recommendations about the location of the various mediastinal lymph node stations. The lymph nodes medial to the right main stem bronchus may be considered as hilar nodes when located away from the tracheal carina and within the visceral pleural sheath, but as they become subjacent to this structure, they are best termed *subcarinal lymph nodes* and thus belong to the lymph nodes of the mediastinal compartment.

On the left side, the anatomic separation between the hilar and the mediastinal lymph nodes proximally is at an imaginary plane connecting the lateral surfaces of the ascending

Table 6-1. Distribution of Bronchopulmonary Lymph Nodes

Right Lung	Left Lung
Between upper and middle lobe bronchi	Angle between left upper and lower lobe bronchi
Below middle lobe bronchus	Above upper lobe bronchus
Medial to upper lobe bronchus	Medial to left main bronchus
Above upper lobe bronchus	Medial to superior segmental bronchus
Junction of oblique and transverse fissure lying on right pulmonary artery	Medial to upper lobe bronchus
Medial to superior segmental bronchus	Above superior segmental bronchus
Behind upper lobe bronchus	Anterior to left main bronchus
Medial to middle lobe bronchus	Behind left main bronchus
Between superior segmental bronchus and lower lobe bronchus	Medial to lower lobe bronchus
Medial to lower lobe bronchi	Behind upper lobe bronchus
Above superior segmental bronchus	Lateral to left main bronchus
Between anterior and medial basal bronchi	Lateral to lower lobe bronchus
Lateral to lower lobe bronchus	Lateral to upper lobe bronchus
	Between segmental bronchi of left upper lobe
	Between superior segmental bronchus and basal bronchi

Note: Listed in order of decreasing frequency of the number of times lymph nodes identified in each location.
From Borrie J: Lung Cancer. Surgery and Survival. New York: Appleton-Century-Crofts, 1965. With permission.

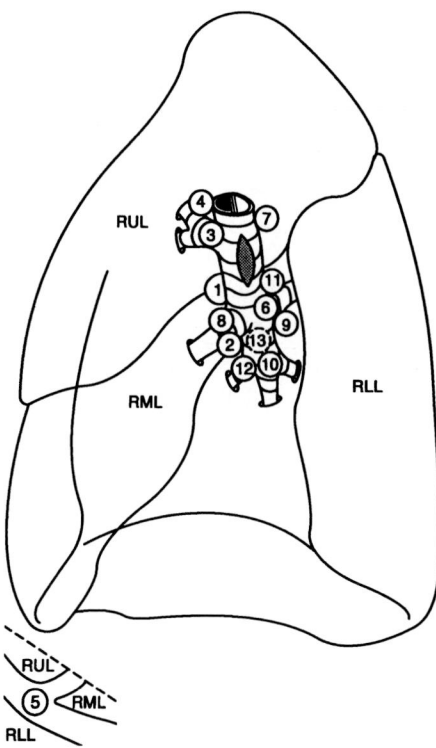

Fig. 6-1. Bronchopulmonary lymph nodes of the right lung. Drawing of the medial aspect of the right lung shows the 13 most common locations of lymph nodes identified in 93 specimens by Borrie. The sites are numbered in the order of decreasing frequency in which lymph nodes were identified in each respective site (see Tables 6-1 and 6-2). Inset at bottom shows the lateral view of the junction of the oblique and transverse fissures. At this site, lymph nodes are lateral to the origins of the middle and lower lobe branches of the right pulmonary artery. RLL, right lower lobe; RML, right middle lobe; RUL, right upper lobe. Redrawn from Borrie J: Lung Cancer. Surgery and Survival. New York: Appleton-Century-Crofts, 1965.

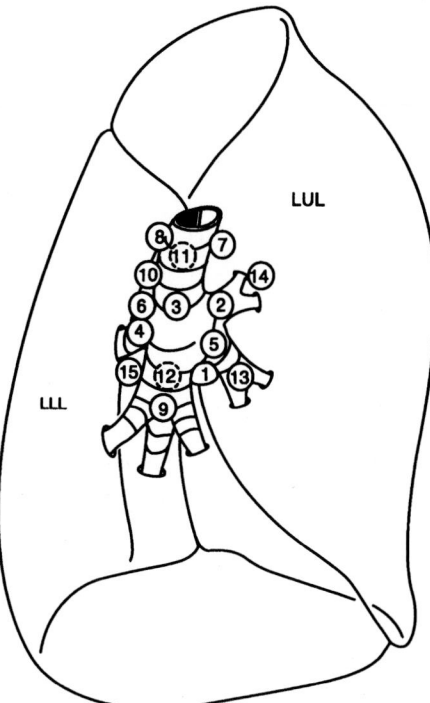

Fig. 6-2. Bronchopulmonary lymph nodes of the left lung. Drawing of the medial aspect of the left lung shows the 15 most common locations of bronchopulmonary lymph nodes identified in 101 specimens by Borrie. The sites are numbered in the order of decreasing frequency in which lymph nodes were identified in each respective site (see Tables 6-1 and 6-2). LLL, left lower lobe; LUL, left upper lobe. Redrawn from Borrie J: Lung Cancer. Surgery and Survival. New York: Appleton-Century-Crofts, 1965.

and descending portions of the thoracic aorta. The left hilar nodes are located medial, anterior, posterior, and lateral to the left main stem bronchus in order of decreasing frequency in number. The hilar nodes located anteriorly are found in relationship to the left main stem pulmonary artery. Proximally, these latter nodes are contiguous with the subaortic lymph nodes of the mediastinum, including the lymph node located at the site of the ligament arteriosum, the so-called Bartello's node. The nodes on the medial surface of the main stem bronchus, as their position advances upward, become subcarinal in location.

Lobar Lymph Nodes

The two most common locations in which lobar lymph nodes are found in the right lung are between the upper lobe bronchus and middle lobe bronchus: the area that Borrie (1952) termed the *right bronchial sump* (the superior inter-

Table 6-2. Bronchopulmonary Nodes

Right Lung Area	% Nodes Present[a]	Left Lung Area	% Nodes Present[b]
1	100	1	97
2	65.5	2	49
3	42	3	33
4	40	4	32
5	29	5	29
6	25	6	22
7	22.5	7	21
8	22.5	8	17
9	21.5	9	16
10	10	10	14
11	7.5	11	13
12	3	12	8
13	2	13	6
		14	6
		15	4

[a]Percent of 93 right lung specimens containing bronchopulmonary lymph nodes in each area.
[b]Percent of 101 left lung specimens containing bronchopulmonary lymph nodes in each area.
Adapted from Borrie J: Lung Cancer. Surgery and Survival. New York: Appleton-Century-Crofts, 1965.

lobar lymph node of Rouvière [1932]) and the region just below the middle lobe bronchus adjacent to the lower lobe bronchus (the inferior interlobar lymph node of Rouvière [1932]). In the left lung, the most common location is at the angle of the left upper lobe bronchus and the lower lobe bronchus. Borrie (1952) designated this area as the left lymphatic sump and the nodes found here correspond to the left interlobar node of Rouvière (1932).

Right Lymphatic Sump

The lymph nodes in the lymphatic sump of the right lung lie in relationship to the bronchus intermedius (Fig. 6-3). According to Nohl-Oser (1989), a constant lymph node is found at the upper posterior end of the major fissure in the angle between the right upper lobe bronchus and the bronchus intermedius. A branch of the bronchial artery coursing over the posterior aspect of the right main bronchus leads to it (Fig. 6-4). Another lymph node is found on the interlobar portion of the pulmonary artery where this vessel gives off the posterior ascending segmental branch to the posterior segment of the upper lobe and the superior segmental artery to the superior segment of the lower lobe. Inferiorly, this lymph node is contiguous with a constant node lying above the superior segmental bronchus of the lower lobe. Other lymph nodes of the sump are found at the base of the major fissure lying closely alongside the interlobar

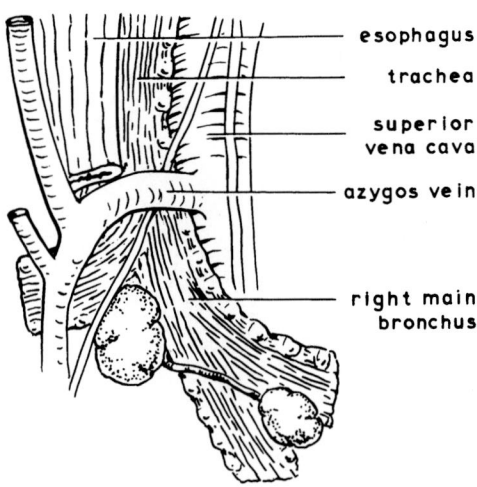

Fig. 6-4. The posterior aspect of the right main bronchus, as seen when the lung is pulled forward during dissection. The subcarinal lymph nodes and the node below the right upper lobe bronchus are seen. A constant bronchial artery leading to the latter node is shown. From Nohl-Oser HC: Lymphatics of the lung. *In* Shields TW, ed. General Thoracic Surgery. 3rd Ed. Philadelphia: Lea & Febiger, 1989. With permission.

portion of the pulmonary artery or in the bifurcations of its branches. Frequently, lymph nodes are identified more anteriorly, lying among the upper lobe branches of the superior pulmonary vein.

Other Interlobar Lymph Nodes of the Right Lung

In addition to the sump nodes, the other interlobar lymph nodes can be grouped, according to Borrie (1965), into those of the upper, middle, and lower lobes. The lymph nodes of the right upper lobe are located above the upper lobe bronchus, medial to it, and just behind it. Those lying above the bronchus merge with the hilar nodes of the distal portion of the right main stem bronchus. The lymph nodes of the middle lobe, in addition to the subjacent node below the middle lobe bronchus (the inferior interlobar node of Rouvière [1932]) are located lateral to the middle lobe bronchus near its confluence with the lower lobe bronchus, as well as medial to it. The right lower lobe lymph nodes, in addition to the aforementioned superior and inferior sump nodes, are found medial to the superior segmental bronchus or between it and the basal bronchi. Lymph nodes are present also in relationship to the basal stem of the lower lobe bronchus and lie on its medial aspect, lateral to it, and between the anterior and medial basal bronchi.

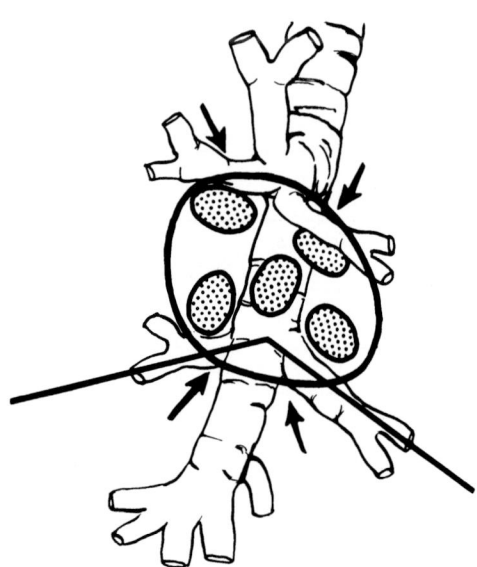

Fig. 6-3. The collection of lymph nodes lying within the right lymphatic sump. The line drawn through the axis of the superior segmental bronchus of the lower lobe and the middle lobe bronchus represents the level below which nodes are not involved by malignant disease in the upper lobe. Arrows indicate the tendency of lymphatic drainage. From Nohl-Oser HC: Lymphatics of the lung. *In* Shields TW, ed. General Thoracic Surgery. 3rd Ed. Philadelphia: Lea & Febiger, 1989. With permission.

Left Lymphatic Sump

The collection of lymph nodes described by Nohl (1956, 1962) and Nohl-Oser (1972) as comprising the left lym-

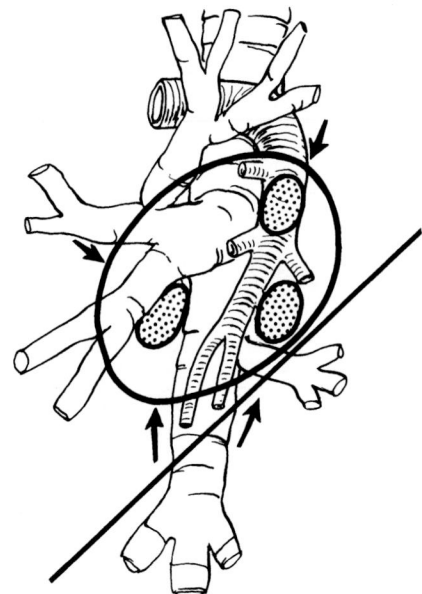

Fig. 6-5. The left lymphatic sump (see text), found by opening the main fissure. The straight line, drawn through the superior (apical) segmental bronchus of the left lower lobe, represents the level below which lymphatic drainage from the upper lobe does not occur. Arrows indicate tendency of lymphatic drainage. From Nohl-Oser HC: Lymphatics of the lung. *In* Shields TW, ed. General Thoracic Surgery. 3rd Ed. Philadelphia: Lea & Febiger, 1989. With permission.

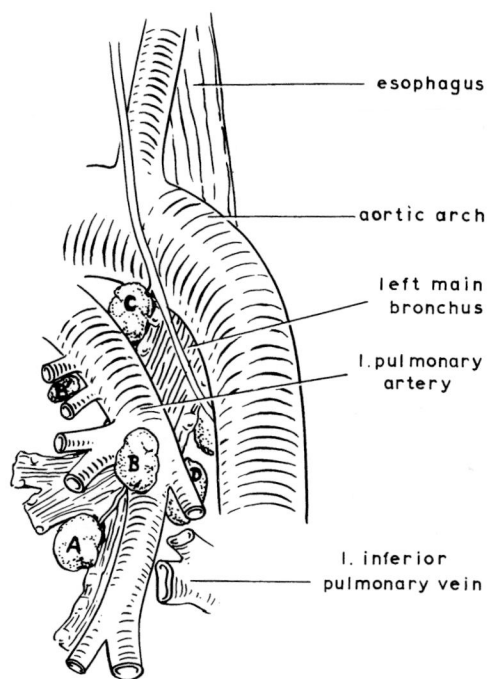

Fig. 6-6. The lymph nodes most frequently seen on opening the main fissure of the left lung. A constant node (A) lies in the angle between the upper and lower lobe bronchi, with a bronchial artery leading to it. Other lymph nodes (B and B') are found on the main pulmonary artery and in the angles of the branches. The constant node (C) behind and above the pulmonary artery, before it enters the fissure, is shown. Another node (D) above the inferior pulmonary vein is seen with its connections to the inferior tracheobronchial nodes higher up. From Nohl-Oser HC: Lymphatics of the lung. *In* Shields TW, ed. General Thoracic Surgery. 3rd Ed. Philadelphia: Lea & Febiger, 1989. With permission.

phatic sump lies between the upper and lower lobes in the main fissure (Fig. 6-5). A constant node is present in the bifurcation between the upper and lower lobe bronchi in close relationship to the origin of the lingular, inferior division, branch of the upper lobe (Fig. 6-6). A small bronchial arterial branch passing across the membranous portion of the left main bronchus leads to it. Other lymph nodes are found lying on the interlobar portion of the left pulmonary artery in the fissure and in the angles formed by its branches. Another constant node is described, which is found above and posterior to the left main stem bronchus. This node is contiguous with a node lying in the angle formed by the main stem bronchus and the takeoff of the bronchus to the superior segment of the lower lobe.

Other Interlobar Lymph Nodes of the Left Lung

In addition to the left lymphatic sump nodes, Borrie (1965) noted that lymph nodes of the left upper lobe are present medial, posterior, and lateral to the upper lobe bronchus. Lymph nodes are present also between the segmental divisions of this bronchus.

The lymph nodes of the left lower lobe are located more commonly in the vicinity of the superior segmental bronchus of the lobe. They are found medial, above, and inferior to it, between it and the basal bronchi. The other

lobar nodes of the lower lobe are found medial or lateral to the basilar stem of the lower lobe bronchus.

LYMPHATIC DRAINAGE OF THE LOBES OF THE LUNG TO THE BRONCHOPULMONARY LYMPH NODES

The lymphatic drainage of the lobes of the lungs is primarily to the bronchopulmonary nodes, although direct lymphatic drainage to the mediastinal lymph nodes was described by Rouvière (1932), Borrie (1952), Cordier (1958), and Riquet (1989) and their colleagues. This direct drainage is discussed subsequently.

The right upper lobe lymphatic drainage, as deduced from the study of Borrie (1956), is commonly to one of the superior interlobar lymph nodes (the sump nodes) on the lateral aspect of the bronchus intermedius, to the nodes above the right upper lobe bronchus and to those medial to it. Subsequent drainage is proximal to the azygos or subcarinal lymph nodes. Drainage has not been described as occurring to any lymph nodes below the level of the right lymphatic sump.

The middle lobe lymphatics drain to lymph nodes of the superior sump region, although drainage to the inferior sump node also occurs. Drainage from the right lower lobe is to the inferior interlobar node and to the superior sump nodes, primarily those lying on the medial surface of the bronchus intermedius.

Drainage of the left upper lobe from all segments may occur to the left sump nodes. Nodes about the upper lobe bronchus and the left main stem bronchus also receive drainage from this lobe. Lymphatic drainage of the lower lobe is to the subjacent peribronchial nodes and to the interlobar sump nodes. From here, drainage is proximal to the hilar or mediastinal lymph node groups, or both.

Lymphatic drainage from the middle and right lower lobes and the left lower lobe also occurs to the nodes in the respective pulmonary ligament. These lymph nodes are considered mediastinal. The incidence of nodes identified in Borrie's work (1965) was 12% in the right pulmonary ligament and 47% in the left.

MEDIASTINAL LYMPH NODES

The mediastinal lymph nodes that are important in the lymphatic drainage of the lungs can be divided into four distinct but interconnected groups: the anterior (prevascular) lymph nodes in the anterior mediastinal compartment, tracheobronchial lymph nodes, paratracheal lymph nodes, and posterior lymph nodes in the visceral compartment of the mediastinum.

Anterior Mediastinal Lymph Nodes

The anterior mediastinal lymph nodes are in the prevascular compartment of the mediastinum and override the upper portions of the pericardium and great vessels as these extend upward. On the right side, the nodes lie parallel and anterior to the right phrenic nerve. They extend upward to and along the superior vena cava to the area beneath the right innominate vein. On the left, they are in close proximity to the origin of the pulmonary artery and the ligamentum arteriosum. They extend upward near the left phrenic nerve to lymph nodes lying along the inferior border of the left innominate vein in the region where it is joined by the left superior intercostal vein.

Tracheobronchial Lymph Nodes

The tracheobronchial lymph nodes lie in three groups about the bifurcation of the trachea. The right and left superior tracheobronchial nodes are located in the obtuse angles between the trachea and the corresponding main stem bronchus. These nodes lie outside of the pretracheal fascia. The lymph nodes of the right superior tracheobronchial

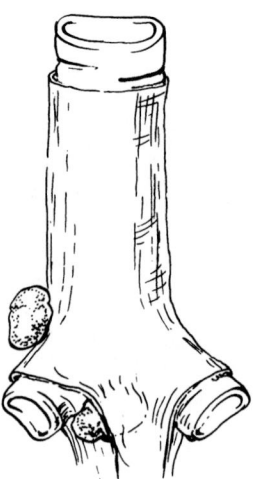

Fig. 6-7. The location of the inferior tracheobronchial nodes within the pretracheal fascial envelope and the superior tracheobronchial nodes outside this fascial layer. Redrawn from Sarrazin R, Voog R: La Mediastinoscopie. Paris: Masson, 1968.

group are medial (beneath) the arch of the azygos vein and above the right pulmonary artery. These nodes are contiguous with the right superior hilar nodes distally and the right paratracheal nodes proximally. On the left side, the superior tracheobronchial nodes lie deep within the concavity of the aortic arch. Some are closely related to the left recurrent laryngeal nerve; others are situated slightly more anteriorly and are contiguous with the node at the ligamentum arteriosum and the root of the left pulmonary artery. Their association with these nodes constitutes the link between the nodes in the visceral compartment and those in the anterior mediastinal lymph node group.

The inferior tracheobronchial nodes, more commonly referred to as the subcarinal nodes, lie in the angle of the bifurcation of the trachea (Fig. 6-7). Although these nodes, in contrast to the superior tracheobronchial groups, lie within the pretracheal fascial envelope, they lie outside the relatively dense bronchopericardial membrane. These nodes are contiguous with the hilar nodes on the medial aspect of both the right and left main stem bronchi. Some of the subcarinal lymph nodes lie more posteriorly in relationship to the tracheal bifurcation and are on the anterior surface of the esophagus and are thus connected with the posterior group of lymph nodes. In addition, Brock and Whytehead (1955) described a low anterior tracheal group lying in front of the lower end of the trachea, which constitutes a bridge between the right superior tracheobronchial lymph nodes and the subcarinal, inferior tracheobronchial lymph nodes.

Paratracheal Lymph Nodes

The paratracheal lymph nodes are situated on the right and left sides of the trachea above the respective superior tracheobronchial nodes and extend upward along the tra-

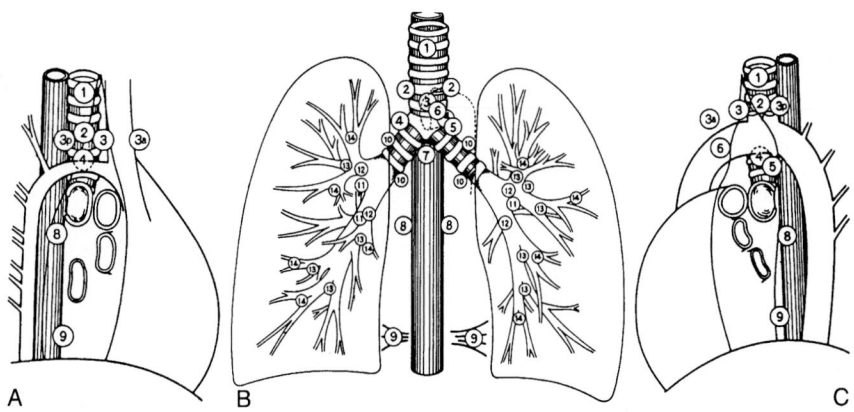

Fig. 6-8. Modified lymph node map of Naruke and the American Joint Committee (see Table 6-3 for definitions). **A.** Right lateral view. **B.** Frontal view. **C.** Left lateral view. From Naruke T, et al: Lymph node mapping and curability at various levels of metastasis in resected lung cancer. J Thorac Cardiovasc Surg 76:832, 1978. With permission.

chea. The right paratracheal lymph nodes lie anterolaterally to the trachea and to the right of the innominate artery. Inferiorly, these nodes are overlapped by the superior vena cava. More superiorly, these nodes lie behind and above the innominate artery to the right of the midline of the trachea and extend to the inlet of the chest. Inferiorly, the left paratracheal nodes lie above the tracheobronchial angle to the left of the midline of the trachea behind the aortic arch. More superiorly, they are situated above the arch but behind the great vessels and extend to the inlet of the chest. The left paratracheal lymph nodes are generally smaller in size and number compared with the right paratracheal lymph nodes.

Posterior Mediastinal Lymph Nodes

The posterior mediastinal lymph nodes may be separated into two groups: the paraesophageal nodes and those located in either pulmonary ligament. These posterior nodes are identified less commonly in the superior portion than in the inferior portion of the mediastinum. A paraesophageal node occasionally is found retrotracheally at the level of the arch of the azygos vein. The paraesophageal nodes as a group are more numerous in the inferior portion of the mediastinum and are found more frequently on the left than on the right side. The inferiorly located nodes have connections with the para-aortic nodes beneath the diaphragm. In the pulmonary ligament on either side, usually two or more small lymph nodes may be present. A relatively constant node, and usually the largest, lies in close proximity to the inferior border of the inferior pulmonary vein and is often termed the *sentinel node*.

Mediastinal Lymph Node Maps

Naruke and associates (1978) suggested the use of an anatomic map with the aforementioned conventional lymph node stations numbered so that the various lymph node stations involved by tumor could be uniformly recorded in

Table 6-3. American Joint Committee for Cancer Staging and End Results Reporting Classification of Regional Lymph Nodes

Mediastinal (N$_2$) Nodes	Bronchopulmonary (N$_1$) Nodes
Superior mediastinal nodes	10. Hilar
1. Highest mediastinal	11. Interlobar
2. Upper paratracheal	12. Lobar
3. Pre- and retrotracheal	13. Segmental
4. Lower paratracheal (including azygos nodes)	
Aortic nodes	
5. Subaortic (aortic window)	
6. Para-aortic (ascending aorta or phrenic)	
Inferior mediastinal nodes	
7. Subcarinal	
8. Paraesophageal (below carina)	
9. Pulmonary ligament	

patients with lung cancer (Fig. 6-8). This mapping scheme is used by most Japanese surgeons and has been used with minor modifications by the Sloan-Kettering Memorial group and others in North America. The American Joint Committee for Cancer Staging and End Results Reporting (AJC) published a similar map in its 1983 fascicle. The lymph node stations are defined in Table 6-3. The American Thoracic Society (ATS) in a report by Tisi and colleagues (1983), however, noted what they believed to be deficiencies in the commonly accepted specific anatomic definition of each nodal station when determined by mediastinoscopy, mediastinotomy, and CT examinations of the chest. Although some of the points were minor, a major area of conflict was the recommendation that the hilar stations, the right and left stations 10 of the Naruke and AJC maps, be deleted because of the ambiguity of the radiologic definition of these areas. It was suggested that these areas be redesignated as peribronchial on the left and tracheobronchial on the right and be assigned to the mediastinal compartments, both stations being outside of the pleural reflection. The ATS suggested the anatomic stations as listed in Table 6-4 and located as represented in Figure 6-9. The ATS map has

Table 6-4. Proposed Definitions of Regional Nodal Stations for Prethoracotomy Staging

X	Supraclavicular nodes
2R	Right upper paratracheal (suprainnominate) nodes: nodes to the right of the midline of the trachea between the intersection of the caudal margin of the innominate artery with the trachea and the apex of the lung. (Includes highest R mediastinal node.) (Radiologists may use the same caudal margin as in 2L.)
2L	Left upper paratracheal (supra-aortic) nodes: nodes to the left of the midline of the trachea between the top of the aortic arch and the apex of the lung. (Includes highest L1 mediastinal node.)
4R	Right lower paratracheal nodes: nodes to the right of the midline of the trachea between the cephalic border of the azygos vein and the intersection of the caudal margin of the brachiocephalic artery with the right side of the trachea. (Includes some pretracheal and paracaval nodes.) (Radiologists may use the same cephalic margin as in 4L.)
4L	Left lower paratracheal nodes: nodes to the left of the midline of the trachea between the top of the aortic arch and the level of the carina, medial to the ligamentum arteriosum. (Includes some pretracheal nodes.)
5	Aortopulmonary nodes: subaortic and para-aortic nodes, lateral to the ligamentum arteriosum or the aorta or left pulmonary artery, proximal to the first branch of the LPA.
6	Anterior mediastinal nodes: nodes anterior to the ascending aorta or the innominate artery. (Includes some pretracheal and preaortic nodes.)
7	Subcarinal nodes: nodes arising caudal to the carina of the trachea but not associated with the lower lobe bronchi or arteries within the lung.
8	Paraesophageal nodes: nodes dorsal to the posterior wall of the trachea and to the right or left of the midline of the esophagus. (Includes retrotracheal but not subcarinal nodes.)
9	Right or left pulmonary ligament nodes: nodes within the right or left pulmonary ligament.
10R	Right tracheobronchial nodes: nodes to the right of the midline of the trachea from the level of the cephalic border of the azygos vein to the origin of the right upper lobe bronchus.
10L	Left peribronchial nodes: nodes to the left of the midline of the trachea between the carina and the left upper lobe bronchus, medial to the ligamentum arteriosum.
11	Intrapulmonary nodes: nodes removed in the right or left lung specimen plus those distal to the main stem bronchi or secondary carina. (Includes interlobar, lobar, and segmental nodes.)

From Tisi GM, et al: Clinical staging of primary lung cancer. Am Rev Respir Dis *127*:659, 1983. With permission.

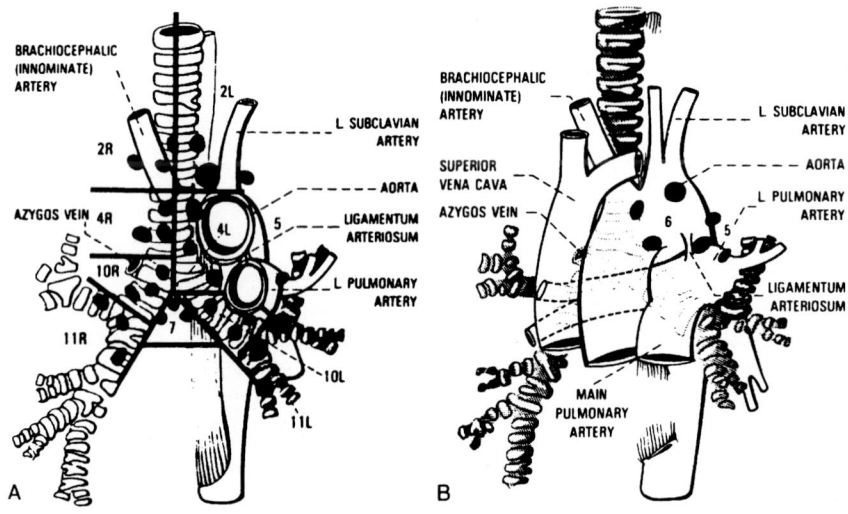

Fig. 6-9. **A.** American Thoracic Society map of regional pulmonary nodes (see Table 6-4 for definitions). **B.** American Thoracic Society map of regional nodes in stations 5 and 6. From Tisi GM, et al: Clinical staging of primary lung cancer. Am Rev Respir Dis *127*:659, 1983. With permission.

been adopted by many investigators in North America. The validity of one schema over the other is moot. In reviewing data presented in the literature, however, cognizance of the differences in the method of recording the data must be borne in mind for their proper interpretation.

In an attempt to resolve the confusion created by the two aforementioned classifications and maps of the lymph node stations, a committee representing both the American Committee on Cancer and the Union International Contre le Cancer decided to adopt a modified version of both the AJC and ATS classifications and lymph node maps. The adapted clas-

sification and map were published by Mountain and Dresler (1997) (Fig. 6-10 and Table 6-5). The recommended schema essentially resolves the problems between the two previous schemata by using anatomic landmarks that identify all lymph node stations within the mediastinal pleural reflection as N_2 nodes and anatomic landmarks that identify all lymph node stations distal to the pleural reflections and within the pleura as N_1 nodes. It is hoped that these will become the standards for recording mediastinal and pulmonary lymph nodes by the radiologic, pathologic, and thoracic surgical communities. Certainly, these should be used

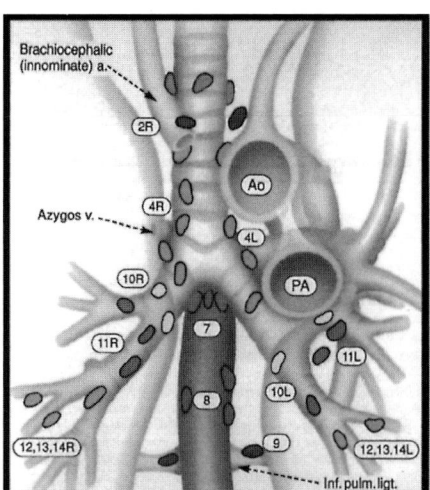
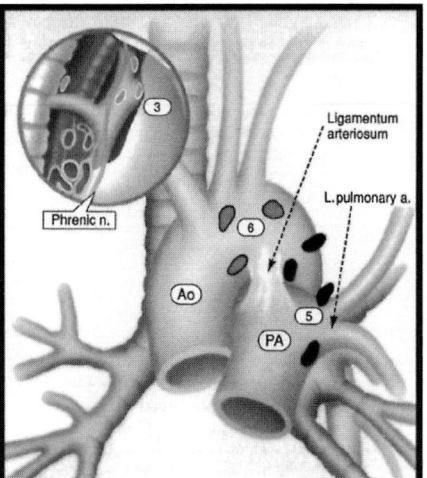

Fig. 6-10. Regional lymph node stations: (1) Superior mediastinal nodes are stations 1, 2, 3, and 4; (2) aortic nodes are stations 5 and 6; and (3) inferior mediastinal nodes are stations 7, 8, and 9. Intrapleural nodes are stations 10, 11, 12, 13, and 14. (See Table 6-4 for definitions.) Ao, aorta; PA, pulmonary artery. Adapted from Mountain CF, Dresler CM: Regional lymph node classification for lung cancer staging. Chest *111*:1718, 1997.

Table 6-5. Lymph Node Map Definitions

Nodal Station	Anatomic Landmarks
N2 nodes: All N2 nodes lie within the mediastinal pleural envelope	
1. Highest mediastinal nodes	Nodes lying above a horizontal line at the upper rim of the brachiocephalic (left innominate) vein where it ascends to the left, crossing in front of the trachea at its midline.
2. Upper paratracheal nodes	Nodes lying above a horizontal line drawn tangential to the upper margin of the aortic arch and below the inferior boundary of No. 1 nodes.
3. Prevascular and retrotracheal nodes	Prevascular and retrotracheal nodes may be designated 3A and 3P; midline nodes are considered to be ipsilateral.
4. Lower paratracheal nodes	The lower paratracheal nodes on the right lie to the right of the midline of the trachea between a horizontal line drawn tangential to the upper margin of the aortic arch and a line extending across the right main bronchus at the upper margin of the upper lobe bronchus, and contained within the mediastinal pleural envelope; the lower paratracheal nodes on the left lie to the left of the midline of the trachea between a horizontal line drawn tangential to the upper margin of the aortic arch and a line extending across the left main bronchus at the level of the upper margin of the left upper lobe bronchus, medial to the ligamentum arteriosum and contained within the mediastinal pleural envelope.
	Researchers may want to designate the lower paratracheal nodes as No. 4s (superior) and No. 4i (inferior) subsets for study purposes; the No. 4s nodes may be defined by a horizontal line extending across the trachea and drawn tangential to the cephalic border of the azygos vein; the No. 4i nodes may be defined by the lower boundary of No. 4s and the lower boundary of No. 4 as described above.
5. Subaortic (aortopulmonary window)	Subaortic nodes are lateral to the ligamentum arteriosum or the aorta or left pulmonary artery and proximal to the first branch of the left pulmonary artery and lie within the mediastinal pleural envelope.
6. Para-aortic nodes (ascending aorta or phrenic)	Nodes lying anterior and lateral to the ascending aorta and the aortic arch or the innominate artery, beneath a line tangential to the upper margin of the aortic arch.
7. Subcarinal nodes	Nodes lying caudal to the carina of the trachea but not associated with the lower lobe bronchi or arteries within the lung.
8. Paraesophageal nodes (below carina)	Nodes lying adjacent to the wall of the esophagus and to the right or left of the midline, excluding subcarinal nodes.
9. Pulmonary ligament nodes	Nodes lying within the pulmonary ligament, including those in the posterior wall and lower part of the inferior pulmonary vein.
N1 nodes: All N1 nodes lie distal to the mediastinal pleural reflection and within the visceral pleura	
10. Hilar nodes	The proximal lobar nodes, distal to the mediastinal pleural reflection and the nodes adjacent to the bronchus intermedius on the right; radiographically, the hilar shadow may be created by enlargement of both hilar and interlobar nodes.
11. Interlobar nodes	Nodes lying between the lobar bronchi.
12. Lobar nodes	Nodes adjacent to the distal lobar bronchi.
13. Segmental nodes	Nodes adjacent to the segmental bronchi.
14. Subsegmental nodes	Nodes around the subsegmental bronchi.

From Mountain CF, Dresler CM: Regional lymph node classification for lung cancer staging. Chest *111*:1718, 1997. With permission.

to designate the lymph node stations in all future randomized lung cancer protocols.

Number and Size of Lymph Nodes in the Various Mediastinal Locations

The first major report of the number of lymph nodes in the mediastinum was published by Beck and Beattie (1958). In cleared specimens of the mediastinum from five autopsies, they reported an average of three nodes in the anterior mediastinum and an average of 50 in the tracheobronchial area of the mediastinum. Of the latter, an average of 16 nodes were located in the peribronchial region, 11 in the subcarinal, and 23 in the paratracheal regions. These data were essentially nonspecific anatomically as were the data recorded by Genereux and Howie (1984). These authors, however, were among the first investigators, including Baron (1982), Osborne (1982), Ekholm (1980), and Moak (1982) and their colleagues, to record the size of normal mediastinal lymph nodes as identified by CT scanning. From 89 to 95% of normal lymph nodes identified in these studies were less than 11 mm. Genereux and Howie's data were essentially similar to those of the other early investigators.

Glazer and associates (1985) not only reported the size of normal nodes but also correlated the number of lymph nodes usually identified by CT and their size in each of the superior mediastinal stations and the subcarinal region as described by the ATS map (see Fig. 6-9A and B). The data were generated by a retrospective review of 56 CT scans of patients without primary inflammatory pulmonary disease or primary lung neoplasm. The largest normal mediastinal nodes were found in the subcarinal and right tracheobronchial regions and, as a rule, the nodes were larger on the right side than on the left side. The maximum number of nodes and the size above

Table 6-6. Normal Lymph Nodes in the Mediastinum as Identified on Computed Tomography Examination in 56 Patients

	% Patients with Nodes Present	Mean Number of Nodes Present[a]	Short Axis Measurement Above Which Node is Considered Enlarged (mm)
2R	95	2	7
2L	75	2	7
4R	100	3	10
4L	81	3	10
5	59	1	9
6	86	5	8
7	95	2	11
8R	57	1	10
10L	45	1	7
10R	100	3	10
11L	70	1	7

[a]Approximate mean without standard deviation.
Adapted from Glazer GM, et al: Normal mediastinal lymph nodes: number and size according to American Thoracic Society mapping. AJR Am J Roentgenol 144:261, 1985.

Table 6-7. Number of Mediastinal Lymph Nodes Dissection of the Mediastinum of 40 Cadavers

Node Station[a]	% with Nodes Present	Number of Nodes Max	Number of Nodes Mean	Short Transverse Diameter (mm) Maximum Standard[b]
2R	80	11	2.5	7.8
2L	68	7	2.1	5.6
4R	98	11	4.8	9.2
4L	98	16	4.5	9.2
5	58	6	1.1	8.5
6	85	15	4.7	7.2
7	100	6	2.9	12.3
8R	58	6	1.2	8.2
8L	50	5	1.1	6.1
9R	10	2	0.1	3.9
9L	35	3	0.5	6.5
10R	95	10	3.5	10.8
10L	90	7	2.4	6.8

[a]Stations as defined by the American Thoracic Society map.
[b]Maximum standard was set at +2 SD from mean.
From Kiyono K, et al: The number and size of normal mediastinal lymph nodes: A postmortem study. AJR Am J Roentgenol 150:771, 1988. With permission.

which a node was considered enlarged are listed in Table 6-6 for each of the mediastinal stations. From these data, it was suggested that 10 mm be considered the upper limit for the short axis of normal mediastinal lymph nodes. An anatomic study by Kiyono and associates (1988) in which the mediastinal lymph nodes were dissected in 40 cadavers produced similar results (Table 6-7). These authors suggested the normal size for the diameter of the short axis of the lymph nodes in stations 2, 5, 6, 8, 9, and 10L to be 8 mm; for stations 4 and 10R to be 10 mm; and for station 7 to be 12 mm.

Relative to the number of lymph nodes, it may be noted that CT examination may fail to identify all the nodes present, particularly in the subaortic and subcarinal regions, and does not demonstrate nodes present in either of the pulmonary ligaments or those in the inferior paraesophageal area. The use of endoscopic ultrasound examination, which is particularly sensitive for the detection of mediastinal nodes in these latter areas, was reported by Kondo and colleagues (1990). These investigators, although the patients studied had carcinoma of the lung, were able to identify lymph nodes in these latter areas, but the data are incomplete as to the actual number of normal nodes identified in the various regions (Table 6-8).

Table 6-8. Number of Nodes Identified in the Inferior Compartment of the Mediastinum[a] by Transesophageal Ultrasound (TEUS) versus Computed Tomography (CT)

	Stations 7, 8, and 10	R9	L9
TEUS	274	8	22
CT	96	1	2

[a]Naruke map.
Adapted from Kondo D, et al: Endoscopic ultrasound examination for mediastinal lymph node metastases of lung cancer. Chest 98:587, 1990.

Again, however, most lymph nodes considered normal were less than 10 mm (97%).

LYMPHATIC DRAINAGE OF THE LUNGS TO THE MEDIASTINAL LYMPH NODES

The lymphatic drainage of the lungs to the mediastinal lymph nodes has been studied extensively. Various techniques of injection of dyes into the lymphatic channels of lungs from autopsy specimens of stillborn infants and adults without pulmonary disease have been used in the studies of Rouvière (1932), Cordier and associates (1958), and Riquet and colleagues (1989). Borrie (1952, 1965) and Nohl (1962) studied the drainage patterns by dissection of the operative specimens from lungs of cancer patients, as have many investigators subsequently, including Naruke (1978), Martini (1983), Libshitz (1986), Watanabe (1990, 1991), and Ishida (1990) and their associates. In addition to these studies, Nohl-Oser (1972) and Greschuchna and Maassen (1973) published their findings from the evaluation of the superior mediastinum by mediastinoscopy in patients with lung cancer. Also in living patients, but without known pulmonary disease, the lymphatic drainage of the lungs was studied by the technique of lymphoscintigraphy using antimony sulfide colloid or rhenium colloid labeled with ^{99m}Tc injected into the various bronchopulmonary segments via the fiberoptic bronchoscope by Hata and associates (1981).

Although the terminology for the lung segments and the mediastinal lymph nodes, as well as their locations, varied considerably in these multiple studies, relatively consistent drainage patterns for each lung and its respective lobes and segments can be identified reasonably.

The patterns of normal lymphatic drainage from the lungs to the mediastinum are relatively consistent despite minor variations suggested by different workers, which may be the result of the methods of investigation used and the selection of the subjects studied. The dynamic study by lymphoscintigraphy in normal healthy subjects as reported by Hata and associates (1981) and summarized in 1990 appears to be a highly satisfactory schemata to recommend. The patterns of drainage from the right and left lung segments are seen in Figure 6-11. A summary of the findings is quoted from Hata and colleagues (1990).

Right Lung

The lymphatic drainage from the apical and posterior segments of the right upper lobe flows via the hilar nodes into the right superior tracheobronchial nodes and further into the paratracheal nodes and up into the neck in the right scalene nodes through ipsilateral upper paratracheal nodes. Approximately one-half of the lymph from the anterior segment of the upper lobe flows via the same route. The other one-half flows into the subcarinal nodes or into the right anterior mediastinal nodes. Lymph that passes through the subcarinal nodes may flow further into the right scalene nodes through the pretracheal and ipsilateral paratracheal nodes, and a small amount of lymph is observed to flow into the left paratracheal nodes. Lymph that goes to the right anterior mediastinal nodes flows along the left brachiocephalic vein into the left anterior mediastinal nodes and into the left scalene nodes.

The routes of lymphatic drainage from the bronchi of the middle lobe and the superior segment of the right lower lobe are similar. Most of the lymph from these segmental bronchi flows into the subcarinal or right superior tracheobronchial nodes and then to the right upper paratracheal nodes. Some of the lymph from the bronchi of the middle lobe also flows into the subcarinal and left paratracheal nodes, or into the right anterior mediastinal nodes, as mentioned for lymphatic drainage from the anterior segment of the right upper lobe.

A dominant flow of the lymphatic drainage occurs from the basal segments of the right lower lobe into the subcari-

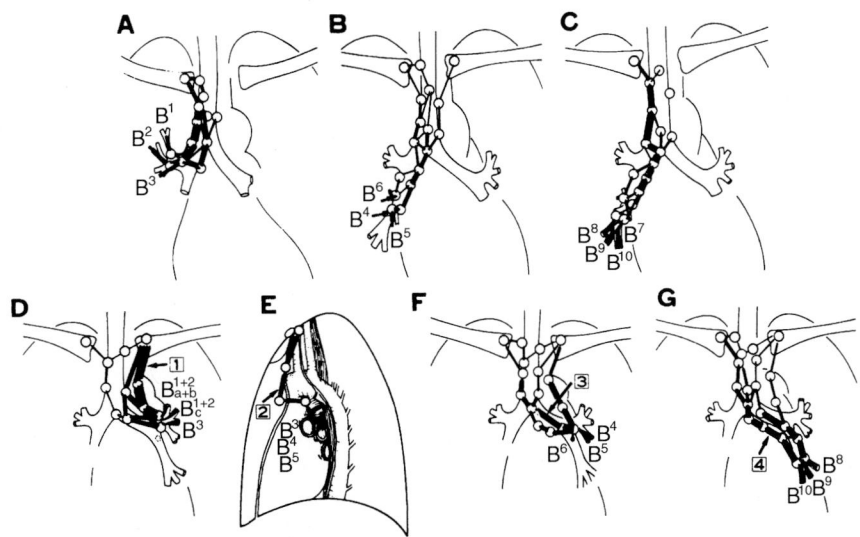

Fig. 6-11. Standard patterns of lymphatic drainage of the lungs. **A.** From segments of the right upper lobe. **B.** From segments of the middle lobe and superior segment of the right lower lobe. **C.** From basal segments of the right lower lobe. **D.** Route 1 from the left lung. **E.** Route 2 from the left lung. **F.** Route 3 from the left lung. **G.** Route 4 from the left lung. See text for explanation. From Hata E, et al: Rationale for extended lymphadenectomy for lung cancer. Theor Surg 5:191990. With permission.

nal nodes through the bronchopulmonary nodes. The lymph then flows into the ipsilateral lower and upper paratracheal nodes and further into the right scalene nodes.

Left Lung

Four major routes are described by Hata and associates (1990) for the lymphatic drainage from the segmental bronchi of the left lung. The first passes through the subaortic nodes. This route divides into two pathways. One runs along the left vagus nerve to the left scalene nodes, and the other runs along the left recurrent laryngeal nerve to the highest left mediastinal nodes. The second route runs through the para-aortic nodes upward along the left phrenic nerve via the anterior mediastinal nodes to the left scalene nodes. The third route runs along the left main bronchus to the left superior tracheobronchial nodes and the paratracheal nodes. From the left tracheobronchial nodes, this route divides into two branches. One extends to the right side of the mediastinum through the right upper pretracheal node, and the other runs upward along the left side of the trachea to the highest left mediastinal nodes. The fourth route runs under the left main bronchus to the subcarinal nodes. After passing the subcarinal nodes, this route extends to the right superior tracheobronchial nodes or through the lower pretracheal node to the right upper paratracheal nodes. Some branches extend upward along the left side of the trachea to the highest left mediastinal nodes.

As a consequence, the lymphatic drainage from the left lung is variable; however, the major routes of lymphatic drainage from each segment are as follows. The most important route of lymphatic drainage from the apicoposterior segmental bronchus of the upper lobe is the first route. Although the second route is the most common for lymphatic drainage from the anterior and lingular segments of the upper lobe, the other routes are used as well for lymphatic drainage from these segments. Lymph from the superior segmental bronchus of the lower lobe drains commonly along the first, third, and fourth routes. The most important route of drainage from the basal segmental bronchi of the lower lobe is the fourth route.

Significance of the Lymphatic Drainage Patterns

The routes described by Hata and associates (1990), mainly agree with the patterns described by Rouvière (1932) and Nohl (1956). In addition, other significant features of the lymphatic drainage from the various lobes of the lungs to the mediastinal lymph nodes, as well as reemphasis of some of the aforementioned observations, must be pointed out. The drainage from the right lung is essentially unilateral, and cross-over to lymph nodes in the contralateral mediastinum is infrequent. Hata and colleagues (1981) noted drainage from the right upper lobe into the left paratracheal nodes and sequentially from the right prevascular nodes into the left prevascular (anterior) nodes.

Similar pathways were observed infrequently from the middle lobe and superior segment of the lower lobe. Drainage from the basilar segments of the right lower lobe rarely progressed to the left side of the mediastinum, although Riquet and colleagues (1989) recorded the presence of one direct drainage channel from the right basal segments to the left pulmonary ligament. In patients with known carcinoma of the lung studied by prethoracotomy mediastinoscopy, contralateral drainage from the right lung to the mediastinum was likewise observed with minimal frequency. Nohl-Oser (1972) and Greschuchna and Maassen (1973) reported that the incidence of contralateral metastases from tumors of the right upper lobe with metastatic mediastinal node disease were 5% and 9%, respectively. From tumors of the right lower lobe with associated metastatic mediastinal node disease, the incidences of contralateral disease were 7% and 5%, respectively. When the total number of tumors of the right lung (less than one-half with metastatic mediastinal node involvement) is used as the denominator in the series reported by Nohl-Oser (1972), the incidences of crossover from the right upper and right lower lobes are reduced to 2% and 3%, respectively.

In contrast, contralateral mediastinal drainage from the left lung is relatively common, occurring most frequently via the subcarinal nodes, as initially pointed out by Rouvière (1932) and reconfirmed by all of the subsequent studies. Occasionally, crossover occurs by means of the lower pretracheal node in drainage from the left lower lobe. Again, Riquet and associates (1989) identified a direct channel from the left to a right paratracheal node. These workers also described direct channels from the left lower lobe to the opposite side of the lower portion of the inferior mediastinum. In the mediastinoscopy data of Nohl-Oser (1972) and Greschuchna and Maassen (1973), contralateral involvement from tumors of the left upper lobe to the right side of the mediastinum in patients with mediastinal node involvement was 22% and 21%, respectively. From the left lower lobe, the figures were 40% and 33%, respectively. Again, to put these data into perspective, 28% of the patients in Nohl-Oser's (1972) study had metastatic mediastinal nodal involvement from tumors of the left lung so that the 22% and 40% incidences represent an actual 6% and 11% incidence of crossover from the left upper and lower lobes to the right side of the mediastinum. These percentages are in agreement with the findings of Hata and associates (1990), who found 7% and 11% incidences, respectively, in patients who had undergone bilateral mediastinal node dissection for left lung tumors.

Drainage from the lower lobes on either side to the ipsilateral superior mediastinal lymph nodes is common.

Drainage to the inferior mediastinum, to the subcarinal lymph nodes, from the right upper lobe does occur. This finding was first observed by Rouvière (1932) and, although discounted by Nohl (1962) and Nohl-Oser (1972), it has been amply reconfirmed by the studies of Borrie (1965) and Hata (1981, 1990), Riquet (1989), and Watanabe (1990), and their associates. Watanabe and colleagues (1990) reported a 13% incidence of subcarinal lymph node involvement in 45 patients with right upper lobe tumors. Libshitz and coinvestigators reported a similar 14% incidence of such involvement.

Drainage of the superior division of the left upper lobe to the subcarinal area is unusual but, as noted by Hata and colleagues (1981), commonly occurs from the inferior (lingular) division of that lobe.

Direct lymphatic channels from either lung drain to the mediastinal lymph nodes, bypassing the bronchopulmonary nodes in a significant number of lungs. This phenomenon was observed previously and has been described as *skip* metastases in lung cancer patients by Martini (1987), Libshitz (1986), Ishida (1990), and their associates, among others. Skip metastases from the right upper lobe were seen in the superior tracheobronchial nodes most frequently; a few occurred in the paratracheal node group and infrequently to the subcarinal lymph nodes. Right lower lobe tumors exhibited skip metastases to the subcarinal nodes and to the inferior pulmonary nodes. On the left side, upper lobe lesions tended to show skip metastasis to the subcarinal and aortic window areas; the lower lobe lesion showed a similar pattern as seen on the right—that is, the subcarinal and inferior pulmonary ligament nodes. Riquet and colleagues (1989) used injection studies of the subpleural lymphatics of adult lungs obtained at autopsy to identify direct lymphatic channels running from the subpleural plexus of the lobar segments to the various mediastinal lymph nodes without passing through the bronchopulmonary nodes. Most of these channels were superficial, but a few penetrated the lung substance. On occasion, these direct but separate channels coexisted with other channels draining into the bronchopulmonary lymph nodes. These direct channels were observed in 22% of the segments injected in the right lung and 25% of the segments in the left lung. In all other specimens, the dye followed the classic patterns and filled the respective bronchopulmonary lymph nodes. A summary of the study by Riquet and colleagues (1989) is found in Table 6-9. Drainage to the ipsilateral pulmonary ligament nodes from the right and left lower lobes and subsequently to the inferior paraesophageal lymph nodes was pointed out by Borrie (1952) and others of the aforementioned investigators.

Drainage from the superior mediastinum continues to progress cephalad to the scalene lymph nodes in the neck, more often involving the right than the left scalene area.

Last, lymphatic drainage from the lower regions of the mediastinum may progress caudad to the para-aortic lymph nodes below the diaphragm. Riquet and associates (1988, 1990) described a direct channel from the basal segments of both lungs to juxtaceliac nodes. This drainage pathway also had been noted by Meyer (1958).

All of the aforementioned points must be remembered in the overall consideration of the lymphatic drainage from the lungs. The clinical relevance of the lymphatic drainage and the various lymph node groups are discussed in the respective chapters relating to infections and tumors of the lungs.

Table 6-9. Direct Pathways to Mediastinal Lymph Nodes from the Lungs

Site	Percent	Total % for Each Lung
Right upper lobe	36.3	
Middle lobe	18.6	22.2
Right lower lobe	22.3	
Left upper lobe	38.6	25.0
Left lower lobe	21.1	

Adapted from Riquet M, Hidden G, Debesse B: Direct lymphatic drainage of lung segments to the mediastinal nodes. An anatomic study of 260 adults. J Thorac Cardiovasc Surg 97:623, 1989.

REFERENCES

Baron RL, et al: Computed tomography in the preoperative evaluation of bronchogenic carcinoma. Radiology 145:727, 1982.
Beck E, Beattie EJ: The lymph nodes in the mediastinum. J Int Coll Surg 29:247, 1958.
Borrie J: Primary carcinoma of the bronchus: Prognosis following surgical resection (Hunterian Lecture). Ann R Coll Surg Engl 10:165, 1952.
Borrie J: Lung Cancer: Surgery and Survival. New York: Appleton-Century-Crofts, 1965.
Brock R, Whytehead LL: Radical pneumonectomy for bronchial carcinoma. Br J Surg 43:8, 1955.
Cordier G, et al: Les lymphatiques des bronches et des segments pulmonaires. Bronches 8:8, 1958.
Dail DH: Uncommon tumors. In Dail DH, Hammer SP, Colby TV (eds): Pulmonary Pathology Tumors. New York: Springer-Verlag, 1995.
Ekholm S, et al: Computed tomography in preoperative staging of bronchogenic carcinoma. J Comput Assist Tomogr 4:763, 1980.
Genereux GP, Howie JL: Normal mediastinal lymph node size and number: CT and anatomic study. AJR Am J Roentgenol 142:1095, 1984.
Glazer GM, et al: Normal mediastinal lymph nodes: number and size according to American Thoracic Society mapping. AJR Am J Roentgenol 144:261, 1985.
Greenberg HB: Benign subpleural lymph node appearing as a pulmonary "coin" lesion. Radiology 77:97, 1961.
Greschuchna D, Maassen W: Die lymphogenen Absiedlungswege des Bronchialkarzinoms. Stuttgart: Georg Thieme, 1973.
Hata E, Troidl H, Hasegawa T: In vivo Untersuchungen der Lymphdrainage des Bronchialsystems beim Menchen mit des Lympho-Szintigraphie: Eine neue diagnostische Technik. In Hamelmann H, Troidl H (eds): Behandlung des Bronchialkarzinoms. Stuttgart: Georg Thieme, 1981.
Hata E, et al: Rationale for extended lymphadenectomy for lung cancer. Theor Surg 5:19, 1990.
Ishida T, et al: Strategy for lymphadenectomy in lung cancer three centimeters or less in diameter. Ann Thorac Surg 50:708, 1990.
Kiyono K, et al: The number and size of normal mediastinal lymph nodes: a postmortem study. AJR Am J Roentgenol 150:771, 1988.
Kondo D, et al: Endoscopic ultrasound examination for mediastinal lymph node metastases of lung cancer. Chest 98:586, 1990.
Kradin RI, Spirn PW, Mark EJ: Intrapulmonary lymph nodes. Clinical, radiologic and pathologic features. Chest 87:662, 1985.
Lauweryns JM: The blood and lymphatic microcirculation of the lung. In Sommers SC (ed): Pathology Annual. New York: Appleton-Century-Crofts, 1971, p. 365.
Leak LV: Lymphatic removal of fluids and particles in the mammalian lung. Environ Health Perspect 35:55, 1980.
Leak LV, Jamuar MP: Ultrastructure of pulmonary lymphatic vessels. Am Rev Respir Dis 128:S59, 1983.
Libshitz HI, McKenna RJ, Mountain CF: Patterns of mediastinal metastases in bronchogenic carcinoma. Chest 90:229, 1986.
Martini N, Flehinger BJ: The role of surgery in N2 lung cancer. Surg Clin North Am 67:1037, 1987.
Martini N, et al: Results of resection in non-oat cell carcinoma of the lung with mediastinal lymph node metastases. Ann Surg 198:386, 1983.
Manual for Staging Cancer. Chicago: American Joint Committee for Cancer Staging and End-results Reporting, 1983.

Meyer KK: Direct lymphatic connections from the lower lobes of the lung to the abdomen. J Thorac Surg 35:726, 1958.

Moak GD, et al: Computed tomography vs. standard radiology in the evaluation of mediastinal adenopathy. Chest 82:69, 1982.

Mountain CF, Dresler CM: Regional lymph node classification for lung cancer staging. Chest 111:1718, 1997.

Nagaishi C: Functional Anatomy and Histology of the Lung. Baltimore: University Park Press, 1972.

Naruke T, Suemasu K, Ishikawa S: Lymph node mapping and curability at various levels of metastasis in resected lung cancer. J Thorac Cardiovasc Surg 76:832, 1978.

Nohl HC: An investigation into the lymphatic and vascular spread of carcinoma of the bronchus. Thorax 11:172, 1956.

Nohl HC: The Spread of Carcinoma of the Bronchus. London: Lloyd-Luke Ltd, 1962.

Nohl-Oser HC: An investigation of the anatomy of the lymphatic drainage of the lungs as shown by the lymphatic spread of bronchial carcinoma. Ann R Coll Surg Engl 51:157, 1972.

Osborne DR, et al: Comparison of plain radiography, conventional tomography and computed tomography in detecting intrathoracic lymph node metastases from lung carcinoma. Radiology 142:157, 1982.

Riquet M, Hidden G, Debesse B: Abdominal nodal connexions of the lymphatics of the lung. Surg Radiol Anat 10:251, 1988.

Riquet M, Hidden G, Debesse B: Direct lymphatic drainage of lung segments to the mediastinal nodes. An anatomic study of 260 adults. J Thorac Cardiovasc Surg 97:623, 1989.

Riquet M, et al: Direct metastasis to abdominal lymph nodes in bronchogenic carcinoma [letter to the editor]. J Thorac Cardiovasc Surg 100:153, 1990.

Rouvière H: Anatomie des Lymphatics de le Homme. Paris: Masson et Cie, 1932.

Steiner RE: The radiology of the pulmonary circulation. In Shanks CS, Kerley P (eds): A Textbook of X-Ray Diagnosis. London: HK Lewis, 1973, p. 121.

Tisi GM, et al: Clinical staging of primary lung cancer. Am Rev Respir Dis 127:659, 1983.

Trapnell DH: The peripheral lymphatics of the lung. Br J Radiol 36:660, 1963.

Trapnell DH: Recognition and incidence of intrapulmonary lymph nodes. Thorax 19:44, 1964.

Watanabe Y, et al: Mediastinal spread of metastatic lymph nodes in bronchogenic carcinoma. Mediastinal nodal metastases in lung cancer. Chest 97:1059, 1990.

Watanabe Y, et al: Mediastinal nodal involvement and the prognosis of non-small cell lung cancer. Chest 100:422, 1991.

SECTION II

Physiology of the Lungs

CHAPTER 7

Pulmonary Gas Exchange

William P. Sexauer and Jeffrey Glassroth

LOCUS OF BLOOD-GAS INTERFACE

The alveolar-capillary membrane is the place where inspired air and pulmonary blood meet and gas transfer occurs. This membrane is made up of the attenuated cytoplasm of an alveolar lining cell (alveolar type I cell) and its basement membrane, plus the attenuated cytoplasm of the capillary endothelial cell and its basement membrane. Divertie and Brown (1964) described a space of variable width between the two basement membranes, the interstitial space. The majority of disease processes that alter the alveolar-capillary membrane interfere with gas transport across this membrane and probably produce their deleterious effects by interfering with pulmonary ventilation, pulmonary blood flow, or the homogeneous distribution of blood and air, or by some combination of these distribution defects.

PHYSICS AND PHYSIOLOGY OF GASES

Pressure and temperature changes alter the volume of all gases in a predictable manner. Because of marked variation in solubility and chemical reaction rates in body fluids, the behavior of different gases in a liquid phase in vivo varies widely.

Laws Pertaining to Gases in the Gas Phase

At constant pressure, the volume of a gas is directly proportional to the temperature (Charles' law). At constant temperature, the volume is inversely proportional to the pressure (Boyle's law).

The combination of Charles' and Boyle's laws gives the relationship: $PV = nRT$, in which n is the number of moles of gas, R is a constant having the same value for all perfect gases, and T is the absolute temperature in degrees Kelvin (K). $T = t°C + 273$. At 0°C and 760 mm Hg pressure, 1 mole of any perfect gas has a volume of 22.41 L.

The partial pressure of one gas in a mixture of gases of volume (V) is equal to the pressure that the gas would exert if it occupied the same volume (V) in the absence of other gases (Dalton's law). The partial pressure of each gas in a mixture is proportional to the fraction of the mixture made up by that gas; for example, the fraction of oxygen in room air is 0.21, and the sum of the partial pressures of all the gases in a mixture equals the total pressure of the gas mixture. The partial pressure of any gas in a mixture is the product of the total or barometric pressure (P_B) multiplied by the fraction of the gas in the mixture (F): $P = P_B \times F$. If water vapor exists in the mixture, the partial pressure of water vapor must be subtracted from the barometric pressure. Water vapor pressure is assumed to equal 47 mm Hg when a gas is fully saturated at 37°C: $P = (P_B - 47) \times F$. For example:

$$\text{Barometric pressure} = 760 \text{ mm Hg}$$

$$\text{Oxygen concentration} = 20.93\%$$

$$P_{O_2} = (760 - 47) \times 0.2093 = 149 \text{ mm Hg}$$

Environmental Conditions and Measurement of Gases

Body Temperature and Pressure, Saturated with Water Vapor

Under the condition of body temperature and pressure, saturated with water vapor (BTPS), the temperature of the gas is 37°C and the partial pressure of water vapor is 47 mm Hg.

Ambient Temperature and Pressure, Saturated

Under most circumstances, the ambient temperature is lower than body temperature. A gas at ambient temperature and pressure, saturated (ATPS), usually contains less water vapor than under BTPS conditions, depending on ambient temperature and relative humidity.

Standard Temperature and Pressure, Dry

Oxygen, carbon dioxide, and carbon monoxide volumes are expressed at standard temperature and pressure, dry (STPD), conditions. This manner of expression is customary for any gas undergoing metabolic exchange. Lung volumes and ventilation are expressed at BTPS conditions. A minute ventilation of 10 L/minute STPD is equivalent to 12 or 13 L/minute BTPS.

Conversion from Ambient Temperature and Pressure, Saturated, Volumes to Body Temperature and Pressure, Saturated with Water Vapor, Volumes

As air temperature increases from ambient (ATPS) to BTPS conditions, gas volumes increase because of thermal expansion. If a fluid reservoir such as that within the lung is present, the water vapor pressure increases to 47 mm Hg. The expansion caused by heat and the increase in volume caused by the addition of water vapor are expressed in the formula:

$$V_{BPS} = V_{ATPS} \times \frac{273 + 37}{273 + t_A} \times \frac{P_B - P_{H_2O}}{P_B - 47}$$

273 = melting point of ice in °K
37 = body temperature in °C (degrees centigrade)
t_A = ambient temperature °C
P_B = barometric pressure, in mm Hg
P_{H_2O} = water vapor pressure at t_A
47 = water vapor pressure at 37°C (saturated)

Laws Pertaining to Gases in Liquids

Partial Pressure

A gas in contact with a liquid exchanges molecules with the liquid. When equilibrium is reached, the number of gas molecules entering the liquid phase equals the number leaving to enter the gas phase, and the partial pressures of the gas in both the liquid and the gas phase are equal.

Volume

The volume of a gas contained in a liquid is expressed in volumes percent (mL per 100 mL of liquid). These volumes are usually expressed under STPD conditions. The gas may be merely physically dissolved, in chemical combination, or both. For example, the oxygen content of the arterial blood of a healthy subject with a hemoglobin concentration of 14 g percent while breathing room air is approximately 19 volumes percent (19 mL oxygen STPD per 100 mL of whole blood). All but 0.3 volumes percent of the oxygen is in chemical combination with hemoglobin.

Unique Properties of Specific Gases

Different gases have special biological properties. Some gases (oxygen and carbon dioxide) undergo metabolic exchange, other gases are insoluble in the pulmonary membrane and remain in the gas phase, and other gases have specific effects on the body that make them valuable as anesthetic agents.

Gases That Undergo Metabolic Exchange

Oxygen

This essential component of cellular respiration is carried in the blood in two forms: in physical solution in the plasma and in chemical combination with hemoglobin. The quantity of oxygen that can be carried in physical solution is minimal, approximately 1.5% of the total, compared with the large amount of oxygen that exists in chemical combination with hemoglobin. The quantity of oxygen combined with hemoglobin depends on the partial pressure of oxygen in the blood. This relationship (Fig. 7-1), the oxyhemoglobin dissociation curve, has a sigmoid shape with a steep slope between 10 and 60 mm Hg P_{O_2}. The curve is comparatively flat between 70 and 100 mm Hg (see Fig. 7-1). The characteristics of this curve must be considered when treating hypoxemia.

Changes in P_{O_2} at the upper portion of the curve have little effect on the arterial oxygen saturation. At the lower end of the curve where the oxygen pressures are equivalent to the P_{O_2} in the capillaries, large quantities of oxygen are available for tissue metabolism. Both acidosis and tempera-

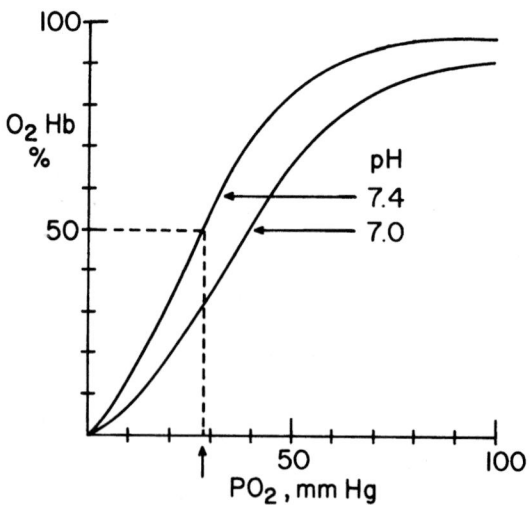

Fig. 7-1. Oxyhemoglobin (O_2 Hb) dissociation curve. The sigmoid relationship between P_{O_2} and percent saturation of hemoglobin with oxygen is shown together with the rightward shift of the curve that occurs with acidosis. The arrow denotes the p50 (see text).

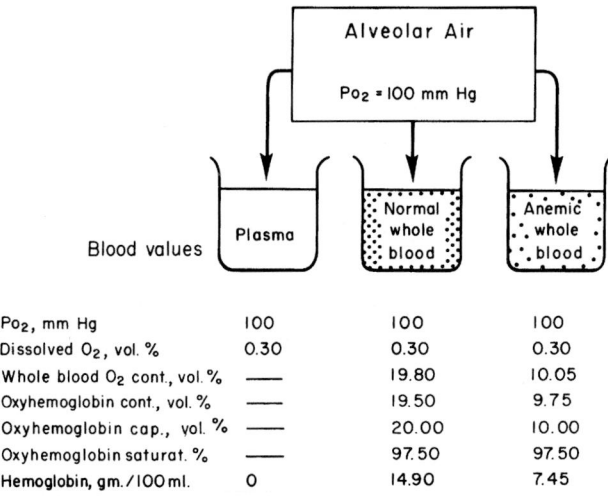

Fig. 7-2. Oxygen solubility and hemoglobin binding. Plasma in contact with oxygen contains only that amount of gas that can dissolve (0.00003 mL oxygen per mL plasma per mm Hg Po_2). Each gram per 100 mL blood of hemoglobin combines with 1.34 mL of oxygen. With 14.90 g percent hemoglobin, the oxygen capacity is 20.00 volumes percent. At a Po_2 of 100 mm Hg and with this hemoglobin, blood contains 19.50 volumes percent oxygen. When the oxygen dissolved in the plasma is added to the oxygen bound to hemoglobin, the total oxygen content becomes 19.80 volumes percent. Were this patient anemic with only 7.45 g percent of hemoglobin, the saturation at the same Po_2 would be identical. The whole blood oxygen content exceeds the oxyhemoglobin capacity in the anemic patient because of the relatively greater contribution of dissolved oxygen to the whole blood oxygen content. From Preston FW, Beal JM (eds): Basic Surgical Physiology. Chicago: Year Book, 1969. With permission.

ture elevation shift the oxyhemoglobin saturation curve to the right (see Fig. 7-1). This rightward shift makes oxygen more readily available in the more acid environment of the tissues. The quantity of dissolved oxygen is directly proportional to the partial pressure of oxygen in blood and equals 0.003 mL of oxygen per 100 mL of blood per mm Hg Po_2. With an arterial Po_2 of 90 mm Hg, the amount of dissolved oxygen in the blood is equal to 0.27 mL per 100 mL; but if the subject breathes 100% oxygen and achieves an arterial Po_2 of 600 mm Hg, the amount of dissolved oxygen would be 1.8 mL per 100 mL of blood.

Even during 100% oxygen breathing, the dissolved oxygen contributes little to the total blood oxygen content if hemoglobin values are near normal. One gram of hemoglobin combines chemically with 1.34 mL of oxygen. If the blood hemoglobin is 15 g/100 mL, then 20.1 mL of oxygen/100 mL of blood can be carried in association with hemoglobin at saturation. The actual quantity of oxygen in combination with hemoglobin depends on the partial pressure of oxygen and the amount of available hemoglobin (Fig. 7-2). The blood hemoglobin that is combined with oxygen (oxyhemoglobin) divided by the oxygen capacity of

the blood sample (hemoglobin concentration multiplied by 1.34) gives the percent saturation of the hemoglobin with oxygen. Oxygen partial pressures in excess of 60 mm Hg add comparatively little to the oxygen content of the blood (see Fig. 7-1).

The oxygen-combining characteristics of hemoglobin may be expressed in terms of the p50 (see Fig. 7-1). The p50 is the partial pressure of oxygen at which hemoglobin is 50% saturated. When measured under a temperature of 37°C, pH 7.40, and Pco_2 40 mm Hg, the p50 is normally 27 mm Hg. Certain diseases or conditions may change the p50. For example, as noted previously, an increase in hydrogen ion concentration, temperature, or both shifts the oxygen-hemoglobin dissociation curve to the right and increases the p50. An increase in carbon dioxide tension or in the enzyme 2,3 diphosphoglycerate (2,3 DPG) also shifts the curve to the right. The opposite change in temperature, hydrogen ion concentration, carbon dioxide tension, or 2,3 DPG shifts the curve to the left and lowers the p50 below 27 mm Hg. An increase in 2,3 DPG occurs in the presence of chronic hypoxemia (e.g., at high altitudes and in chronic severe anemia) and shifts the curve to the right. This action facilitates the release of oxygen in the tissues because rightward movement of the oxygen-hemoglobin dissociation curve results in a lower saturation of hemoglobin at higher partial pressures of oxygen. In addition to an increase in 2,3 DPG, other compensations for chronic hypoxemia improve the delivery of oxygen to the tissues, such as an increase in cardiac output and secondary polycythemia. Substantial carboxyhemoglobinemia, as in acute carbon monoxide poisoning, has a physiochemical effect on the oxygen-hemoglobin curve and shifts it to the left and up. This action lowers the p50, increases the affinity of hemoglobin for oxygen, and compounds the problem of tissue hypoxemia initially caused by the combination of a significant amount of hemoglobin with carbon monoxide. The shift in the oxygen-hemoglobin dissociation curve contributes to the acute lactic acidosis that often follows tissue hypoxia irrespective of the cause.

Carbon Dioxide

Contrary to its limited capacity for oxygen, blood can accommodate enormous quantities of carbon dioxide (Fig. 7-3). Carbon dioxide is carried in the blood as a dissolved gas, as bicarbonate ions, carbonic acid, carbaminohemoglobin, and as other carbamino compounds. Reduced, unoxygenated hemoglobin has a greater affinity for carbon dioxide than does oxyhemoglobin. This upward shift in the carbon dioxide dissociation curve at low Po_2 is called the *Haldane effect* and facilitates transfer of carbon dioxide from tissue to capillary blood, where the Po_2 is low, and facilitates transfer of carbon dioxide from the capillary into the pulmonary alveolus where the Po_2 is higher (see Fig. 7-3).

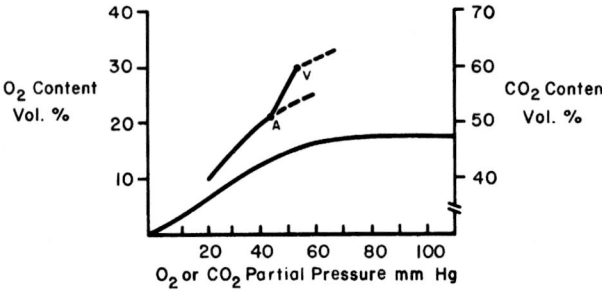

Fig. 7-3. Oxygen and carbon dioxide dissociation curves for whole blood. Oxyhemoglobin saturation of this blood at any P_{O_2} can be determined by dividing the corresponding oxygen content into the oxygen capacity (18.0 volumes percent in this case). The carbon dioxide dissociation curve is relatively linear over the range of partial pressures usually encountered in clinical practice. The difference in the carbon dioxide curve for the arterial (A) and venous (V) blood is caused by a greater carbon dioxide–carrying capacity of unoxygenated hemoglobin (Haldane effect). From Preston FW, Beal JM (eds): Basic Surgical Physiology. Chicago: Year Book, 1969. With permission.

Gases That Are Soluble but Metabolically Inactive

Carbon Monoxide

Coburn (1970) noted that carbon monoxide is produced by the body in small quantities and is therefore involved in metabolic exchange, but we consider it a foreign and inactive gas. Carbon monoxide is moderately soluble in the pulmonary membrane and has an affinity for hemoglobin 210 times greater than does oxygen. Because of these properties, carbon monoxide in low concentrations and for brief exposure periods is highly useful in the measurement of the diffusion capacity. Even brief exposure to high concentrations or prolonged exposure to relatively low levels of carbon monoxide can be highly toxic, because large amounts of carboxyhemoglobin, which is a stable compound, are produced and prevent hemoglobin from participating in oxygen transport.

Nitrogen

Nitrogen diffuses across the pulmonary membrane and is present in body tissues at the same partial pressure as in alveolar air. Inhalation of 100% oxygen rapidly eliminates nitrogen from the alveolar air, but a small amount of nitrogen continues to diffuse into the alveolar air from the large body tissue stores. Prolonged breathing of 100% oxygen eventually eliminates nitrogen stores from the body.

Gases That Are Insoluble in the Pulmonary Membrane

Helium and Neon

At low concentrations, helium and neon are essentially insoluble in tissue and within brief time intervals do not diffuse across the pulmonary membrane. Because they can be confined to the pulmonary gas compartment, concentration changes of these gases can be used to calculate the size of lung volume compartments.

Anesthetic Gases

All gases used for inhalation anesthesia are highly soluble in both blood and tissue and therefore diffuse rapidly through the pulmonary membrane. Nitrous oxide is a common example, and is the most widely used inorganic gas in anesthesia. The blood concentration required to produce surgical anesthesia in humans varies, but is approximately 23 volumes percent. To achieve this concentration, the inspired nitrous oxide percentage must be high, so an increased inspired oxygen concentration must be given along with it to avoid hypoxemia. Nitrous oxide is carried in solution in the blood, not in combination with hemoglobin, and is almost completely eliminated from blood and tissue promptly on termination of nitrous oxide inhalation. A minute quantity diffuses through the skin of anesthetized subjects.

MEASUREMENTS OF GAS EXCHANGE

Total pulmonary gas exchange may be measured by collecting expired air and calculating the amount of oxygen consumed and carbon dioxide produced per unit of time. The normal resting adult man consumes approximately 275 mL of oxygen and produces 230 mL of carbon dioxide per minute. Such measurements give little information about the actual efficiency of gas exchange.

Pulmonary Diffusing Capacity

Whether in the gas phase, dissolved in the plasma, or in chemical association, gases move from regions of higher to lower pressures. The diffusing capacity is a measure of the capacity of the pulmonary membrane to transfer gas between alveolar air and pulmonary capillary blood. Carbon dioxide diffuses from the pulmonary capillary blood into the alveolar air because the capillary P_{CO_2} is higher than the alveolar P_{CO_2}. Carbon dioxide is highly soluble in the pulmonary membrane, and its diffusion is rarely impaired despite extensive lung disease. Retention of carbon dioxide occurs whenever alveolar ventilation is ineffective, resulting in an increase in alveolar P_{CO_2} and a reduction of the gradient for carbon dioxide across the pulmonary membrane. Limitations of oxygen diffusion do result in clinically significant disease. Although oxygen diffusion can be determined, carbon monoxide is a more convenient agent for diffusion measurements.

Carbon monoxide diffusion can be measured by three basic methods: single breath, rebreathing, and steady state

Table 7-1. Blood Gases and Acid–Base Status in Various Conditions

Condition (clinical example)	Breathing pattern	Status	P_{O_2} (mm Hg)	P_{CO_2} (mm Hg)	pH	HCO_3^- (mEq/L)
Normal	—	—	75–90	38–42	7.38–7.42	20–28
Respiratory alkalosis (anxiety)	Hyperventilation	Acute	High	Low	High	Normal
Respiratory alkalosis (narcotic overdose)	Hyperventilation	Acute	Low	High	Low	Normal
Respiratory alkalosis (pulmonary fibrosis)	Hyperventilation	Chronic	Low or normal	Low	High normal	Low
Respiratory alkalosis (obstructive disease)	Hypoventilation[a]	Chronic	Low	High	Low normal	High
Metabolic acidosis (diabetic acidosis)	Hyperventilation	Acute	High	Low	Low	Low
Metabolic alkalosis (prolonged vomiting)	Hypoventilation[a]	Chronic	Low	High	High	High

[a]May not be clinically apparent.

or continuous breathing. The term *diffusion capacity* may well be a misnomer. Many processes are involved in the transfer of carbon monoxide from inspired air to pulmonary capillary blood. Diffusion is only one part of this system, and diffusion may not be measurable apart from other factors that influence gas transfer.

Results of measurements of the carbon monoxide diffusing capacity are influenced by the method used, the volume of blood in the pulmonary capillary bed, the blood hemoglobin level, and the breathing pattern. Finley and colleagues (1962) noted that abnormal carbon monoxide diffusion values may result from ventilation-perfusion imbalance. As an example of this concept, exaggerated to absurdity, consider a patient with completely normal lungs, one of which is perfused but not ventilated and the other ventilated with air containing trace amounts of carbon monoxide but not perfused. No carbon monoxide uptake occurs, even though the pulmonary membrane is normal. A reduction in the blood gas interface secondary to a loss of capillary surface area, as occurs when pulmonary capillary volume is reduced, is one basis for the impaired diffusion in some lung diseases. Because the diffusing capacity measures more than just gas diffusion, the term *transfer factor* has been adopted to describe the overall process. Irrespective of the gas used, the diffusion capacity or transfer factor calculation requires a determination of gas uptake per unit of time and a measurement of the pressure difference between the alveolus and the pulmonary capillary. The result is expressed in milliliters per minute per millimeters of mercury.

The diffusion defects noted in diffuse lung diseases are the result of a combination of factors, including a reduction in the pulmonary capillary bed volume, a decrease in the surface area of the blood gas interface, and imbalances in the ventilation and perfusion of the pulmonary parenchyma secondary to nonuniform distribution of the pathologic changes within the lung parenchyma. The classic concept of the alveolar capillary block, a uniform increase in the thickness of the pulmonary membrane that retards the movement of gas, is probably inaccurate, particularly in the resting state.

Arterial Blood Gases

An indirect but useful method of estimating the adequacy of pulmonary gas exchange is the measurement of arterial blood gas tensions and pH. In the normal resting state, with the subject breathing room air, blood gas and pH values are maintained within narrow limits. The arterial P_{O_2} is greater than 75 to 80 mm Hg, depending on the subject's age; the arterial P_{CO_2} is between 38 and 42 mm Hg; the pH is 7.38 to 7.42; and the plasma bicarbonate ion is 20 to 28 mEq/L. The position of the normal subject at the time the blood sample is taken has little effect on the results, but in persons with considerable abdominal obesity or diaphragmatic paralysis, significant changes in arterial blood gas composition may occur when the individuals move from the erect to the supine position. Hyperventilation reduces alveolar P_{CO_2}, increases alveolar P_{O_2}, and has similar effects on arterial blood gas composition. In the normal subject, mild exercise has no significant effect on the arterial P_{O_2}; a mild increase in the P_{O_2} occurs if the exercise is vigorous. In diseases associated with ventilation-perfusion imbalance, however, an acute decrease in the arterial P_{O_2} may occur with exercise. The arterial blood gas and pH in various states are illustrated in Table 7-1.

When interpreting arterial P_{O_2} (Pa_{O_2}) measurements, the alveolar oxygen tension (PA_{O_2}) should be estimated. This can be accomplished as follows:

$$PA_{O_2} = FI_{O_2} \times (P_B - 47) - \frac{(Pa_{CO_2})}{R}$$

in which FI_{O_2} is the inspired fraction or percentage of oxygen, P_B is barometric pressure (assume 760 mm Hg at sea level), 47 is water vapor pressure at 37°C, Pa_{CO_2} is the alveolar CO_2, which is assumed to equal the measured arterial CO_2 (Pa_{CO_2}), and R is the respiratory quotient, assumed to be 0.8.

The equation may be simplified to:

$$PA_{O_2} = FI_{O_2} - (Pa_{CO_2} \times 1.25)$$

The alveolar-arterial oxygen difference ($PA_{O_2} - Pa_{O_2}$) of a person breathing room air averages approximately 8 mm Hg in young persons and increases with age to values of more than 20 mm Hg in the eighth decade. Calculation of this difference corrects for changes in level of ventilation (i.e., Pa_{CO_2}). A $Pa_{O_2} - Pa_{O_2}$ value should never be negative or near zero. Such a calculation suggests a laboratory error.

Acid–Base Balance

An acute change in arterial P_{CO_2} is accompanied by an acute change in arterial pH in the opposite direction. The pH shift approximates 0.01 units per mm Hg change in P_{CO_2}. Under acute conditions, the serum bicarbonate concentration exerts little influence on the relationship of pH and P_{CO_2}. It takes from hours to days for the renal compensatory mechanisms to alter the bicarbonate level and thus correct the pH after an abrupt and persistent change in P_{CO_2}. Such compensation does not occur with brief changes in ventilation, but is present whenever hyperventilation or alveolar hypoventilation is chronic. Renal buffering mechanisms respond to chronic increases in arterial P_{CO_2} and concomitant decreases in pH by retaining bicarbonate. Chronic hyperventilation leading to sustained hypocapnia and an elevated pH stimulates compensatory renal bicarbonate excretion. Some examples of acid–base derangements are shown in Table 7-1. Acid–base balance and its relationship to pulmonary gas exchange are described further. It may be misleading to attempt an interpretation of arterial blood gas and pH changes without some knowledge of the status of the patient and prior treatment. Combined respiratory and metabolic acid–base problems may become complex and the acid–base status can be unraveled only with full knowledge of the clinical condition of the patient.

FACTORS AFFECTING PULMONARY GAS EXCHANGE

Partition of Ventilation

Each inspiration has a useful component that bathes the alveoli with fresh air and a component that "goes along for the ride" and ventilates only the conducting tubes—alveolar and dead-space fractions of the tidal volume. That portion of the ventilation distributed to alveoli where gas exchange occurs is the alveolar ventilation. Ventilation of lung regions with anatomically intact but nonfunctioning alveoli is equivalent to ventilation of the conducting airways (dead-space ventilation). The normal subject, breathing quietly at rest, has approximately 1 mL of dead-space volume per pound of body weight. The total minute ventilation measured at the mouth reveals little regarding effective alveolar ventilation. But if one also knows the respiratory rate, it is possible to estimate alveolar ventilation, assuming that most alveoli are functioning. For example, two patients breathe a total of 5 L/minute. One patient, however, breathes 25 times per minute with a tidal volume of 200 mL, whereas the other patient breathes 10 times a minute with a tidal volume of 500 mL. The patient with a 200-mL tidal volume mainly ventilates the dead space. The actual dead-space volume (VD) and the ratio between dead space and tidal volumes (VD/VT) can be measured if the alveolar and expired concentrations of a gas undergoing metabolic exchange and the tidal volume are known. Carbon dioxide is customarily used, and it is assumed that the arterial and alveolar P_{CO_2} are equivalent. The formula for these measurements, as shown, merely states that the ratio of dead-space volume to tidal volume is the same as the ratio of alveolar (arterial) CO_2 to expired CO_2.

$$VD/VT = \frac{P_{CO_2} \text{ (arterial)} - P_{CO_2} \text{ (expired)}}{P_{CO_2} \text{ (arterial)}}$$

Distribution of Ventilation

Several methods are available to evaluate the uniformity or nonuniformity of the distribution of inspired air. One method requires that the patient inhale 100% oxygen for 7 minutes, thereby washing out the nitrogen in the lungs. With a nitrogen meter and continuous sampling of the expired air stream, a continuous plot of the breath-by-breath exhaled nitrogen concentration is obtained. In the normal subject, a rapid decrease of nitrogen occurs within the first minute or two of oxygen breathing. Patients with gross alveolar hypoventilation or marked maldistribution of ventilation have a slow washout curve. When ventilation abnormalities are marked, the washout curve has an erratic pattern, with much variation in the breath-to-breath concentration of exhaled nitrogen. In the presence of localized areas of marked hypoventilation, as in bullous disease, the nitrogen concentration in the forced expiratory air sample delivered at the end of the 7-minute washout period is elevated. Another method for evaluating ventilation uniformity uses a single-breath nitrogen washout. The patient inspires 100% oxygen to total lung capacity and exhales completely while the nitrogen concentration and volume of the single expirate are monitored. The alveolar portion of the expiration should have a nearly constant nitrogen concentration if inspired oxygen is uniformly distributed within the lung.

A single-breath nitrogen washout curve is shown in Figure 7-4. The initial portion of the expirate contains no nitrogen as it consists solely of the terminal portion of the previous inhaled oxygen (phase 1). As expiration continues, the nitrogen concentration increases rapidly as the dead space is rinsed with alveolar gas (phase 2). A nitrogen plateau then appears, which increases slowly, at a rate of 1.0 to 1.5% nitrogen per L expired, in normal subjects (phase 3). A steep (concentration increase of greater than 1.5% N_2/L) or irregular phase 3 occurs whenever ventilation is nonuniform. In obstructive lung disease, values of 10% N_2/L or greater are not unusual. Most adults have a fourth phase.

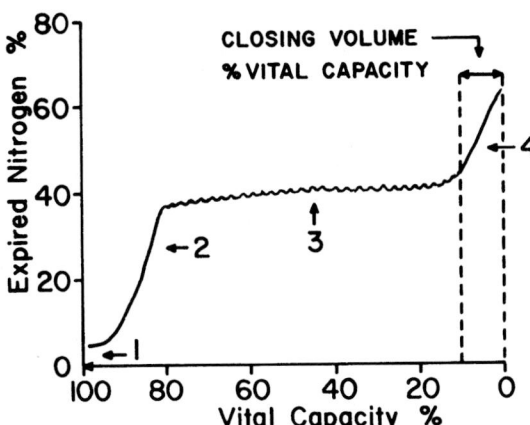

Fig. 7-4. Tracing of expired nitrogen concentration and expired volume from total lung capacity to residual volume. The four phases of the curve (see text) are shown. Oscillations of the nitrogen tracing during phase 3 are synchronous with the heartbeat and are caused by cardiac churning of gases in the airways.

The onset of phase 4 is apparent from an abrupt increase in nitrogen concentration. This sudden rise occurs when the lung volumes are small and airways to the dependent portions of the lung close. The lung volume corresponding with the onset of phase 4 is known as the *closing volume*. Because of a gradation of intrapleural pressure from apex to base in the upright subject, small airways in the dependent lung zones are subjected to higher transpulmonary pressures than those at the apex. The basal airways close at small lung volumes, producing the characteristic phase 3–4 junction that defines the closing volume. The increase in nitrogen concentration during phase 4 is attributable to the lesser dilution of upper zone nitrogen during the previous oxygen inhalation. Also, basal lung zones, with a lower N_2 concentration, cease contributing to expiration after the onset of phase 4. The closing volume enlarges and the phase 4 onset moves up in the vital capacity, toward total lung capacity with age and in the presence of small airway pathology. As the closing volume point increases progressively in the patient's lung volume, it eventually exceeds the resting end-expiratory lung volume, which is the functional residual capacity. Thus, some dependent airways close at the end of every breath. During normal resting tidal ventilation, ventilation of dependent lung zones is reduced, creating a ventilation-perfusion imbalance. This imbalance increases with age and is one of the factors responsible for a decline in the arterial oxygen tension of the elderly.

Distribution of Blood Flow

Pulmonary blood flow can be considered uniform in anatomic terms if every alveolus receives equivalent blood flow. In functional terms, physiologic uniformity exists when blood flow is distributed to each alveolus in proportion to its ventilation. Blood flow nonuniformity occurs to some degree in normal individuals. In an upright subject breathing normally at rest, the lung bases are perfused, whereas the apices are minimally perfused owing to gravity and the low hydrostatic pressures in the pulmonary circuit. The apical areas of the lung receive considerable ventilation but are poorly perfused. This mismatch is not sufficiently great to be physiologically significant in the normal individual.

The distribution of blood flow to various portions of the lung can be evaluated by several methods. Chest radiography may demonstrate relative hyperlucency of one parenchymal region, suggesting a local reduction in pulmonary blood flow as may occur with a pulmonary embolus. Perfusion scans using radioactive tagged macroaggregated albumin that lodges in the pulmonary capillaries provide good evidence of the gross distribution of blood flow within the pulmonary vascular bed (see Chapter 13). More precise visualization of pulmonary blood flow requires catheterization and contrast visualization of the vascular bed. Arterial blood gas determinations are not particularly useful for estimating abnormalities in the distribution of pulmonary blood flow. In most instances in which nonuniformity of blood flow is the sole functional abnormality, arterial blood gas values are within normal limits.

Relationship of Ventilation and Perfusion

Effective gas exchange within the lung requires a close approximation of the distribution of ventilation and pulmonary capillary blood flow. Major nonuniformity or mismatching between ventilation ($\dot{V}$) and perfusion ($\dot{Q}$) are reflected in arterial blood gas abnormalities. In normal individuals, the distribution of blood flow and ventilation to various areas of the lung is neither completely homogeneous nor equally matched. Some regions of lung, for example, tend to receive relatively more ventilation than blood flow. Normally, the development of such dead space has no adverse consequences that follow from this relationship. Physiologic disturbances occur primarily when blood flow to regions that are relatively underventilated (i.e., low $\dot{V}/\dot{Q}$) is substantial. This is seen in healthy obese individuals in whom ventilation is reduced or absent in the lower lung regions, whereas perfusion in these areas remains relatively intact. This is caused by basilar airway compression and closure in the paradiaphragmatic regions and may result in a reduced PaO_2. Atelectasis and pneumonitis are examples of pathologic abnormalities associated with a low $\dot{V}/\dot{Q}$ that may result in severe hypoxemia. Elimination of carbon dioxide tends to be unaffected because other, more normal, lung regions are usually overventilated in compensation. This allows maintenance of a normal or low arterial carbon dioxide tension. Compensation for a decrease in oxygen tension, on the other hand, is limited by the shape of the oxyhemoglobin dissociation curve (see Fig. 7-1).

Evidence suggests that local control of $\dot{V}/\dot{Q}$ matching is mediated, at least in part, by nitric oxide. Nitric oxide is a vasodilator that is produced and released in a controlled manner from the pulmonary vascular endothelium. Hypoxia reduces nitric oxide production, which may mediate hypoxic pulmonary vasoconstriction. The ability of inhaled nitric oxide to produce local pulmonary vasodilation without causing systemic vasodilation may have therapeutic implications in disease states such as adult respiratory distress syndrome.

Shunts and Venous Admixture

A right-to-left shunt exists whenever blood passing through the pulmonary capillaries is not exposed to ventilated alveoli and is not oxygenated. Thus, as noted by Robin and associates (1977), a shunt can be considered an area of lung in which $\dot{V}/\dot{Q}$ is zero. Shunts occur in such conditions as lobar pneumonia and with acute atelectasis of a lobe or entire lung. The fraction of total pulmonary blood flow that is shunted can be approximated by measurement of arterial Po_2. With minor degrees of shunting, the Po_2 with the subject at rest and breathing room air may be normal. Up to 6% right-to-left shunt occurs in healthy subjects, and this "physiologic" shunt results from venous blood normally entering the pulmonary veins, left atrium, or left ventricle. Whenever a greater than normal degree of shunting exists, hypoxemia is present, and inhalation of 100% oxygen for 10 to 20 minutes fails to increase the Po_2 above 550 mm Hg, which would be expected in normal individuals. The ratio of shunted to total pulmonary blood flow can be estimated as follows if the arterial Po_2 is greater than 150 mm Hg during 100% oxygen breathing:

$$\frac{\text{Shunt flow}}{\text{Total flow}} = \frac{[Po_2\,(\text{alveolar}) - Po_2\,(\text{arterial blood})] \times 0.003}{(\text{arterial-mixed venous } O_2 \text{ content}) + [Po_2\,(\text{alveolar}) - Po_2\,(\text{arterial})] \times 0.003}$$

Po_2 (alveolar) = the alveolar Po_2 while breathing 100% oxygen.
Alveolar Po_2 is estimated from the barometric pressure minus water vapor pressure (47 mm Hg) and alveolar Pco_2 (approximately 40 mm Hg).
Thus, Po_2 (alveolar) = (760 − 47) − 40 = 673 mm Hg.
0.003 = the solubility factor for converting Po_2 into oxygen content in volume percent (see Fig. 7-2).
Arterial-mixed venous O_2 content = the difference in oxygen content between mixed venous and arterial blood. It is usually from 4 to 6 volumes percent and can be assumed for the purpose of estimating shunt flow.

The assumed value for the difference between mixed venous and arterial oxygen content has a definite effect on the calculated shunt. The larger the difference between alveolar and arterial Po_2, the greater the effect of the assumed value of arterial-mixed venous difference on the calculated shunt flow.

Venous admixture is a variant of right-to-left shunt that involves a relative but not total lack of ventilation to the involved area (i.e., $\dot{V}/\dot{Q}$ is low but greater than zero). Ventilation of a lung region may be normal, but if blood flow is increased, ventilation may be relatively inadequate; or ventilation may be decreased in the presence of normal blood flow. Venous admixture results from relative ventilation-perfusion imbalances. Unlike a true shunt, the arterial Po_2 deficit of venous admixture can be corrected by 100% oxygen breathing in most instances. However, the use of high oxygen concentrations to measure shunt may cause absorptive atelectasis in those regions with a low $\dot{V}/\dot{Q}$ and, thereby, increase the shunt. Nevertheless, measurement of the *shunt fraction* has practical application (e.g., for monitoring the progress of acutely ill patients with adult respiratory distress syndrome). This practical usefulness is especially true when samples of mixed venous blood are available from a central (Swan-Ganz) catheter line, allowing accurate determination of the mixed venous and arterial oxygen content difference.

MANAGEMENT OF PATIENTS WITH IMPAIRED GAS EXCHANGE

Diagnosis and proper management of impaired gas exchange require accurate measurement of arterial blood gases and pH. Minimal or subclinical defects in gas transport or distribution may require measurements of diffusion, and alveolar and arterial Po_2 at rest and with exercise. It has been estimated that a 50% reduction in the exercise carbon monoxide diffusing capacity is needed before a significant reduction in the exercise arterial Po_2 is noted. Nevertheless, the majority of clinically significant problems can be evaluated by obtaining data from a careful history and physical examination supplemented by arterial blood measurements.

Proper interpretation of arterial blood gas and pH values requires a thorough knowledge of the patient's previous history of lung disease, or other medical and surgical problems that might alter pulmonary gas transport. Diuretics, corticosteroids, and sedative drugs are frequent causes of abnormal arterial blood gas composition. Knowledge of prior use of sedatives and analgesics is most important in evaluating blood gas data, particularly in patients with pulmonary disease, because they may be unduly sensitive to respiratory depression from small doses that are usually well tolerated. Calculation of the $Pao_2 - Pao_2$ difference assists the clinician in identifying aberrations in arterial blood gas values that are attributable to primary disturbances of ventilation without accompanying changes in the lung parenchyma. Patients with abnormal breathing patterns who are thought to have abnormal gas transport may have acid–base disturbances instead. For example, hypoventilation with an attendant increase in arterial Pco_2 and decrease in Po_2 may occur because of severe metabolic alkalosis.

Many therapeutic options are available for the management of patients with alterations in pulmonary gas exchange.

Selection of the appropriate program should be based on a careful evaluation of patients and their metabolic status, particularly their arterial blood gas measurements. Important goals include optimization of tissue oxygenation and maintenance of relatively normal acid–base balance. To achieve adequate oxygenation, oxygen-carrying capacity (hemoglobin concentration, cardiac output, and regional blood flow) must be maintained. Arterial P_{O_2} should, ideally, be at least 65 to 75 mm Hg to completely saturate hemoglobin. This value may be achievable with relatively low concentrations of F_{IO_2}. When gas exchange is seriously deranged, concentrations exceeding an F_{IO_2} of 0.50 may be needed, raising the possibility of pulmonary oxygen toxicity. As pointed out by Weisman and coworkers (1982), positive airway pressure, either as continuous positive airway pressure or positive end-expiratory pressure, may allow significant reductions in the amount of supplemental oxygen needed to maintain acceptable arterial P_{O_2} levels. Excessive levels of positive pressure, however, particularly in patients with volume depletion, may cause a reduction in cardiac output. Thus, careful monitoring of these patients is essential. In patients who appear unlikely to maintain adequate levels of ventilation, as indicated by an increasing arterial P_{CO_2} or an excessive degree of ventilatory effort, mechanical ventilation is advisable. Modes such as assist-control, intermittent mandatory ventilation, synchronized intermittent mandatory ventilation, and pressure support are available to facilitate optimal mechanical support. Noninvasive methods, such as bi-level positive airway pressure, also may be appropriate for certain patients.

For the patient in whom hypoxemia is the major problem, several other interventions may be helpful. If the patient has a primarily unilateral pulmonary process, positioning the patient with the uninvolved side down may improve $\dot{V}/\dot{Q}$ matching via gravitational effects on blood flow and thereby improve oxygenation. Likewise, positioning patients with established adult respiratory distress syndrome in the prone position, or alternating the supine with prone position, has been shown to improve oxygenation in some cases. Patients with hypoxemia and excessive secretions should receive therapies to assist secretion clearance. Hypoxemic patients with major atelectasis refractory to conservative measures may benefit from bronchoscopy to alleviate mucous plugging.

REFERENCES

Coburn RF: Current concepts: endogenous carbon monoxide production. N Engl J Med *282*:207, 1970.
Divertie MB, Brown AL Jr: The fine structure of the normal human alveolar-capillary membrane. JAMA *187*:938, 1964.
Finley TN, Swenson EW, Comroe JH Jr: The cause of arterial hypoxemia at rest in patients with "alveolar-capillary block syndrome." J Clin Invest *41*:618, 1962.
Robin ED, et al: A shunt is (not) a shunt is (not) a shunt. Am Rev Respir Dis *115*:553, 1977.
Weisman IM, Rinaldo JE, Rogers RM: Current concepts: positive end-expiratory pressure in adult respiratory failure. N Engl J Med *307*:1381, 1982.

READING REFERENCES

Bates DV: Respiratory Function in Disease. 3rd Ed. Philadelphia: WB Saunders, 1989.
Tobin MJ: Principles and Practice of Mechanical Ventilation. New York: McGraw-Hill, 1994.
West JB: Respiratory Physiology: The Essentials. 3rd Ed. Baltimore: Williams & Wilkins, 1985.

CHAPTER 8

Mechanics of Breathing

William P. Sexauer and Jeffrey Glassroth

The term *mechanics of breathing* refers to the elastic properties of the lung and chest wall and to airflow resistance. These properties are described and related to lung volume and airflow measurements, the standard tests of ventilatory function (Table 8-1). The subdivisions of the lung volume referred to are shown in Figure 8-1.

ELASTIC PROPERTIES OF THE LUNG

The inflated lung is an elastic structure that tends to deflate itself. The deflation force exerted by an expanded lung is the elastic recoil pressure. This recoil pressure increases with increasing lung volume, and the pressure required to maintain inflation equals the elastic recoil pressure. Irrespective of the manner in which it is measured, the recoil pressure of the lung is always considered positive because it is always directed toward deflation. The elastic recoil pressure is expressed as the pressure difference between the alveolar lumen and the pleural space. Alveolar pressure is equivalent to atmospheric pressure when the glottis and mouth are open and no airflow occurs. Therefore, under these conditions, the intrapleural pressure is equal but opposite in sign to the elastic recoil pressure.

Pleural pressure changes can be conveniently and reliably measured in the upright subject by placing a small tube with an attached balloon in the esophagus. Under static conditions (i.e., in the absence of airflow) a given degree of lung inflation is maintained either by inspiratory muscle contraction, by the elasticity of the chest wall resisting inward collapse, or both. The resting lung volume or functional residual capacity (FRC) is the result of the balance between equal but opposite forces generated by the inward elastic recoil of the lungs and the outward recoil of the chest cage.

A pressure-volume plot made under static conditions (Fig. 8-2) defines the elastic properties of the lung. Multiple measurements of the elastic recoil pressure or the intrapleural pressure and corresponding intrathoracic gas volume over the entire range of lung volumes are necessary to describe the entire pressure-volume curve of the lung. The pressure-volume relationship of the lung is often described in terms of lung compliance. If measured over the tidal volume portion of the curve, it is almost linear and is expressed as the change in volume per unit change in pressure (milliliter per centimeter H_2O).

The pressure-volume relationship is basic to an understanding of the fundamental relation between the work of breathing and lung mechanics. The "stiffer" lung displays a more horizontal curve (Fig. 8-2C), meaning that it takes a greater pressure to achieve the same inflation volume compared with a normal lung (Fig. 8-2A). These lungs are called *less compliant*. At lung volumes approaching total lung capacity (TLC), considerably more pressure per liter of inspired volume is required than at smaller lung volumes. In both health and disease, the tidal volume occurs on the steepest part of the pressure-volume curve where the largest volume change is accomplished with a minimal pressure change. For any given ventilatory requirement, every person has an optimal pattern of tidal volume and breathing frequency at which the work of breathing is minimal. When the lungs are stiff, a pattern of rapid, shallow breathing is adopted, and this pattern minimizes the work of breathing. Even so, more effort than normal is required to ventilate stiff lungs (see Fig. 8-2C). Although it would appear that the patient with emphysema is at an advantage because less effort is required to deform the lungs (Fig. 8-2B), work of breathing is increased because of obstruction to airflow and because hyperinflation requires that tidal breathing be shifted to a less advantageous position on the pressure-volume curve.

Hyperinflation also increases the inward elastic recoil of the chest wall, a force that must be overcome by the respiratory muscles before alveolar ventilation can occur. In addition, hyperinflation places the inspiratory muscles at a mechanical disadvantage from which they are less efficiently able to perform the work required to overcome this added load. Lung volume reduction surgery, advocated for patients with severe emphysema, entails the surgical

Table 8-1. Subdivisions of Lung Volume

Gas volumes commonly reported
 Vital capacity is the maximum volume that can be expired after a maximal inspiration.
 Total lung capacity is the volume in the lungs after a maximal inspiration.
 Residual volume is the volume remaining in the lungs after a maximal expiration. In normal individuals, residual volume is approximately 25 to 30% of total lung capacity.
 Functional residual capacity is the volume in the lungs at the end of a normal expiration.
 Tidal volume is the volume of a spontaneous breath.
Other volumes
 Inspiratory capacity is the maximal volume that can be inspired from the resting end-expiratory position to total lung capacity.
 Expiratory reserve volume is the volume that can be expired from a spontaneous end-expiratory position (i.e., from functional residual capacity to residual volume).
 Inspiratory reserve volume is the volume that can still be inspired from a spontaneous end-inspiratory position.

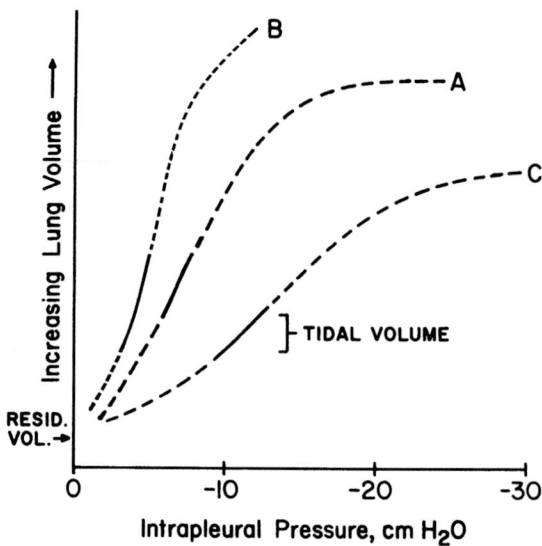

Fig. 8-2. Pressure-volume curves: A, normal; B, emphysema; and C, pulmonary fibrosis. The solid line represents the tidal volume in these three conditions. Resid. Vol., residual volume.

removal of the portions of the lung that function least well, thereby reducing intrathoracic volume. This may theoretically provide benefit by reducing elastic load, increasing lung elastic recoil pressure, and restoring the respiratory muscles toward a more advantageous mechanical position.

The elastic properties of the lung reside mainly in the alveolar walls and their liquid lining. The walls contain a network of collagen, elastic, and reticular fibers in addition to their capillary network and epithelial lining. The thin liquid film on the luminal surface of the alveolar epithelium creates a surface tension that accounts in part for lung elasticity. Surface tension forces tend to reduce the surface to the smallest possible area. In the bubblelike alveolus, surface tension increases as the size of the bubble decreases, and, if unopposed, leads to alveolar collapse. A lipid substance in the alveolar lining fluid reduces surface tension at

the gas–liquid interface, thereby protecting the lungs against alveolar collapse. This substance, surfactant, can be extracted from normal lung tissue and is absent or reduced in persons with pulmonary atelectasis, hyaline membrane disease, or infarction. Surfactant maintains relatively constant surface-tension forces despite varying degrees of lung inflation and alveolar size.

Although pressure changes in the lung are similar everywhere during inflation, ventilation is not evenly distributed throughout the normal organ. At successive horizontal levels of the lung, from apex to base, the volume change produced by a given pressure change becomes progressively greater. The most dependent portions of the lung receive more ventilation per unit of lung tissue than the uppermost levels. The reason for this discrepancy is the effect of gravity. Although pressure changes producing inflation are essentially the same over the normal lung surface, the absolute pressure is not. In the upright position, the weight of the lung makes the intrapleural pressure at the lung base less negative than it is at the apex. With a less negative intrapleural pressure at the bases, the elastic recoil pressure and the volume of each alveolus at the base are less than in higher regions at the onset of inspiration (Fig. 8-3). With inflation, the pressure change transmitted to all lung tissue is the same, but different regions inflate to different volumes depending on where, on the pressure-volume curve, inflation commences. A dependent portion has a lesser recoil pressure to begin with; therefore, a normal breath inflates a basal region more than other areas because its behavior is confined to a steeper portion of the pressure-volume curve. Perfusion of the normal lung is similarly affected by gravity so that a fairly good match between ventilation and perfusion is maintained throughout the lung.

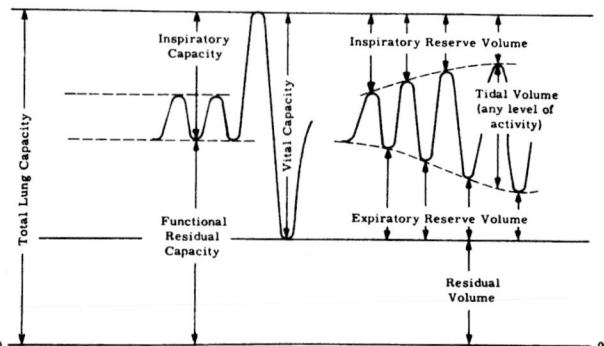

Fig. 8-1. Lung volumes. From Standardization of definitions and symbols in respiratory physiology. Fed Proc 9:602, 1950. With permission.

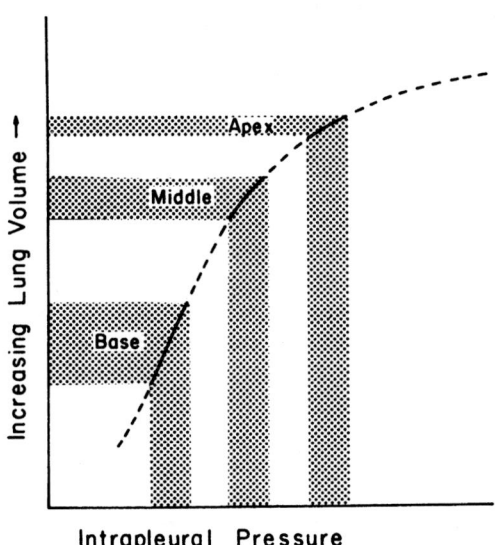

Fig. 8-3. Effect of gravity in the upright position. As one approaches the base of the lung, there is a greater volume change per unit of lung tissue for the same pressure change.

In diseases of the lungs in which the elastic properties are not uniformly the same, regional ventilation becomes nonuniform. Adjacent lung regions, even neighboring alveoli, have different pressure-volume characteristics. Thus, the same pressure change, even when beginning at the same absolute level of intrapleural pressure, produces different volume changes in neighboring areas. The pressure-volume characteristics as measured with an esophageal balloon are those of the whole lung and are averages that may obscure regional differences. Diffuse infiltrative disease, such as diffuse pulmonary fibrosis, produces inequalities not only in inspired gas distribution, but also in the distribution of blood flow, resulting in abnormal gas exchange. The overall adverse effects of these diseases can best be assessed by measurements of gas exchange and arterial blood gas content (see Chapter 7).

ELASTIC AND MECHANICAL PROPERTIES OF THE CHEST WALL

Lung inflation and deflation are accomplished by changes in the dimensions of the chest wall. These dimensional changes are determined by the elastic properties of the bony and soft tissue structures of the thorax and by the muscle forces that impart motion to the respiratory system. Like the lung, the chest wall exerts a recoil pressure proportional to its volume of expansion. This recoil pressure is measured as the difference between pleural pressure and body surface pressure under static conditions when the muscles of respiration are completely relaxed. By plotting this pressure against the thoracic gas volume, one obtains the pressure-volume relationship of the chest wall. The compliance of the chest wall, as described by the slope of this relationship, is

normally high enough so that the rib cage and soft tissue structures do not restrict respiratory movement.

Certain factors, however, may restrict movement of the chest wall and reduce its compliance. An increase in the longitudinal dimension of the thorax is primarily determined by movement of the diaphragm. Diaphragmatic movement may be restricted by conditions that increase intra-abdominal pressure, such as pregnancy, obesity, ascites, and intra-abdominal tumors. Changing from the erect to the supine position also may restrict the diaphragm by shifting the weight of the abdominal contents toward the diaphragm. These conditions generally reduce vital capacity, TLC, and FRC.

Changes in the anteroposterior and transverse dimensions of the chest wall are primarily affected by the intercostal muscles and accessory muscles of respiration, and depend on the mobility of the rib cage. Thus, conditions that result in deformation or fixation of the thorax, such as kyphoscoliosis or ankylosing spondylitis, also may restrict expansion. Obesity also may reduce chest wall compliance by increasing the soft tissue mass of the thorax. Moreover, because respiratory movement ultimately depends on the action of the respiratory muscles, conditions that result in paralysis or weakness of the respiratory muscles severely limit ventilation and often cause respiratory failure. Because of the difficulties of measuring chest wall compliance, muscle strength, and leverage, as well as intra-abdominal pressure and gravitational forces, it is customary to rely on measurements of their consequences, such as changes in lung volumes, gas exchange, ventilation, and perfusion. The results of these tests plus knowledge of the clinical status of the patient are usually adequate to determine whether the chest wall or underlying lung disease is at fault.

LUNG VOLUME MEASUREMENTS

An isolated decrease in a lung volume does not affect health as long as adequate volume remains to permit normal ventilation of the alveoli. Although the tidal volume normally increases with exercise, the ventilation necessary for a given level of exercise can be achieved by increasing either tidal volume or breathing frequency. Thus, compensation for a limited lung volume can be attained by increasing the breathing frequency. In the presence of lung diseases characterized by airway obstruction, however, ventilation is maintained by a relatively greater increase in tidal volume than in frequency. This interrelation between tidal volume and frequency is further considered in the section Work of Breathing, later in this chapter.

The reduction of lung volumes occurring with diseases of the chest wall, lungs, or pleura provides a crude guide to the severity of the disease. Thus, volume measurements may be useful for deciding when therapeutic intervention is appropriate or in judging the response or lack of response to therapy. Lung volume measurements are made easily, and their reproducibility renders them useful for longitudinal studies in a given patient. For example, a loss of 500 mL on serial testing of a patient with an initial vital capacity of 4 or 5 L would be significant. However, a single measurement is not a sensitive indicator of early disease because of an approximately 20% variation in lung volumes among persons of the same age, height, and sex.

Although no specific diagnosis is suggested by a lung volume decrease, simple volume measurements, particularly the vital capacity, are just as sensitive an index of disease as the direct measurement of mechanical factors that determine static lung volumes, such as the lung compliance.

Vital Capacity

The vital capacity can be determined either by adding separate measurements of the maximal expired volume and maximal inspired volume starting from the resting lung volume, or by using a single expiratory effort starting from TLC (see Fig. 8-1). The maneuver may be performed in a leisurely or slow manner as distinct from the forced vital capacity. In the forced maneuver, the patient empties the lungs as rapidly as possible starting from TLC. In patients with obstructive lung disease, this forced maneuver may increase expiratory obstruction and produce a spuriously low measurement of vital capacity (see Airway Resistance during Expiration, later in this chapter).

Functional Residual Capacity

The FRC is the volume of gas remaining in the lungs at the end of normal expiration. Two methods are used for measurements of FRC: inert gas dilution or washout and body plethysmography. Nitrogen, argon, and helium are the inert gases customarily used. For an accurate determination, the gas must be evenly distributed or washed out from all air-containing units of the lung. This may not occur or may occur only slowly, in the presence of bullous disease, airway obstruction, or other conditions in which portions of the lung are poorly ventilated.

For the plethysmographic method of measuring FRC, the subject sits in an airtight cabinet, the body plethysmograph. Measurements of changes in alveolar pressure and lung volume are made simultaneously while the patient is panting against an obstruction to airflow that is interposed briefly at the mouth. Alveolar pressure is equivalent to the pressure at the mouth under these circumstances. With this method, all of the gas within the chest, even in the presence of airway obstruction or bullous disease, is measured. The test is simple to perform but relatively elaborate, and costly equipment is required. The same apparatus can be used, however, for the direct measurement of airway resistance. Discrepancies between plethysmographic and inert gas volume determinations may reflect the volume of poorly ventilated lung that is present.

Residual Volume

The residual volume, air remaining in the lungs after complete expiration, is calculated by subtracting the expiratory reserve volume (see Fig. 8-1) from the FRC determined by any of the preceding methods and is therefore no more accurate than the FRC.

Total Lung Capacity

The TLC is usually computed by merely adding the separately determined vital capacity and residual volume. It is less reproducible than the vital capacity because the variability in the separately measured volume components may be additive. The TLC also can be calculated from chest radiography and includes all the gas within the lungs, similar to the plethysmographic measurements.

AIRFLOW RESISTANCES

To generate airflow, the bellows action of the chest wall must overcome the elastic properties of the lungs and chest wall plus frictional resistances to motion. These frictional resistances consist of pressure losses from air flowing through the airways and to friction within the tissues of the lung and chest wall during breathing movements. Unlike measurements of elastic recoil pressures made under static conditions, resistances are a dynamic property and must be measured while there is airflow. The components of total airflow resistance within the lungs and thorax are airway resistance, lung tissue resistance, and chest wall resistance. The sum of the last two resistances is approximately equal to the airway resistance. The resistances of lung tissue and chest wall tend to be minimally affected by disease and are overshadowed by the magnitude of the changes in airway resistance. The majority of airway resistance occurs in large airways, those 2 mm or larger in diameter.

Increases in airflow resistance are attributable primarily to increases in airway resistance; thus, indirect measurements of airflow resistance, such as the maximum midexpiratory flow rate, volume expelled in the first second of the forced vital capacity maneuver, and maximum voluntary ventilation, may be used as an index of airway resistance.

Measurements of airflow resistance provide an average value for the entire system of airways. In any generalized obstructive lung disease, some airways have a higher resistance to airflow than others, and flow is greater into alveoli whose conducting airways have the lowest resistance. The

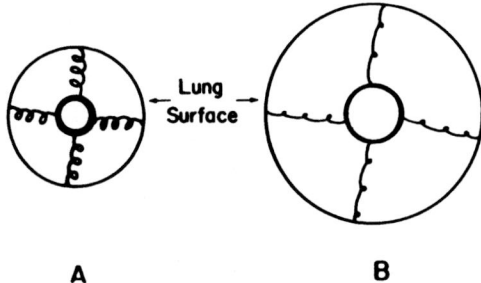

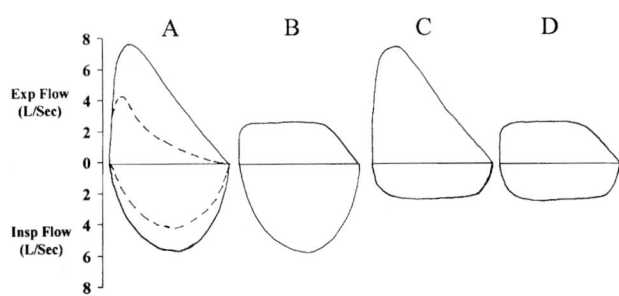

Fig. 8-4. Effect of inspiration on an intrapulmonary airway. **A.** End-expiration. **B.** End-inspiration. The inner circle also could represent an alveolus.

Fig. 8-5. Schematic representation of normal and abnormal flow volume loops. Flow is on the ordinate and volume on the abscissa, with residual volume to the right and total lung capacity to the left. (A) The solid line represents a normal flow volume loop. The dashed line represents a typical loop from a patient with obstructive airway disease, in which the greatest reduction in airflow occurs in the mid and low ranges of the vital capacity. (B) Flow volume loop shows a truncated expiratory (Exp) limb with normal inspiration, indicative of a variable intrathoracic obstruction such as an eccentric endotracheal tumor. (C) The truncated inspiratory (Insp) limb with a normal appearing expiratory limb is consistent with a variable extrathoracic upper airway obstruction (e.g., laryngeal lesions, vocal cord paralysis). (D) Reduced maximal flows during both inspiration and expiration are characteristic of a fixed upper airway obstruction, usually seen with circumferential airway lesions.

result is a nonuniform distribution of inspired air creating a mismatch between ventilation and perfusion and impairment of gas exchange.

Airway Resistance during Inspiration

Airway diameter varies depending on the gradient between intraluminal and extraluminal airway pressures. These gradients function in an opposite manner for intrathoracic and extrathoracic airways. The extrathoracic airway diameter increases during expiration, whereas the intrathoracic airway increases in diameter on inspiration. An exception is a fixed orifice type of obstruction such as occurs in association with a tumor completely encircling an airway. Airway dilatation on inspiration is produced by radial traction provided by elastic forces of the lung tissue surrounding the airway (Fig. 8-4). A loss of elastic recoil, such as that occurring in emphysema, results in a decrease of airway caliber. Conversely, an increase in elastic forces increases traction on the airway, enlarging airway dimensions.

Inspiratory airflow increases in direct proportion to the force or effort applied. Patients with chronic obstructive pulmonary disease, in whom impaired expiratory airflow is invariably present, may have decreased inspiratory flow as well. Inspiratory flow is reduced in patients with chronic bronchitis and in those with asthma because the bronchial lumen is narrowed by secretions and edema, bronchospasm, or both. Inspiratory flow is reduced also when airways become stiff and less expansile because of inflamed bronchial walls or become narrow owing to decreased radial traction (see Fig. 8-4). Inspiratory flow measurements, usually made from an inspiratory flow-volume loop (Fig. 8-5), are primarily useful in unusual, but often remedial, localized obstructions of major airways, because limitation of inspiratory flow may equal or exceed expiratory flow limitation. In patients with the usual types of obstructive lung diseases, inspiratory flow limitation is not clinically important, whereas expiratory flow limitation is invariably severe.

Airway Resistance during Expiration

Unlike inspiratory flow, which depends to a major extent on the muscular effort generated, expiratory flow depends primarily on the mechanical properties of the lungs and is related to effort only up to a certain point. Beyond this point, further increases in effort do not increase expiratory flow and in some instances may decrease it. This concept is illustrated in the isovolume pressure-flow curves in Figure 8-6. These curves are obtained by performing a series of active expirations with increasing effort at a particular lung volume and by plotting flow rates against corresponding pleural pressure. In this instance, pleural pressure represents the driving pressure or force related to muscular effort. In Figure 8-6 curves obtained at three different lung volumes are represented. Between TLC and 75% of TLC, flow increases with effort and depends not only on effort but also on the patency of airways and high elastic recoil of the lung at high volumes. At volumes below approximately 75% of TLC, expiratory flow increases with effort up to a point, at which further increases in effort do not lead to a higher flow rate. Flow reaches a maximal level at this point because further increases in pleural pressure resulting from effort tend to compress airways and limit flow to the same extent that they tend to drive flow. This dynamic compression occurs because intrathoracic airways are exposed to pleural pressures. This concept is illustrated by the model in Figure 8-7. In this model, the lung or alveolus and airway are suspended in a box representing the thorax. The lung is separated from the chest wall for descriptive purposes only, and the space

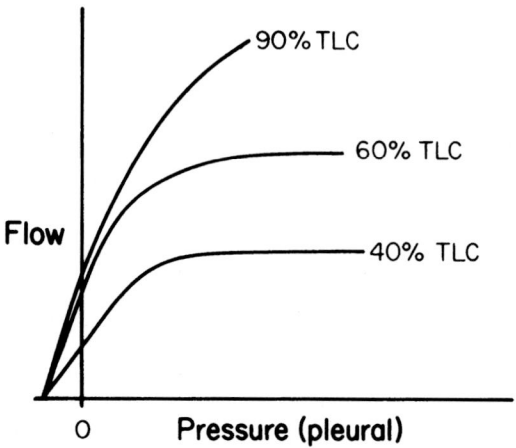

Fig. 8-6. Isovolume pressure flow plot at three different lung volumes. TLC, total lung capacity.

between the lung and chest wall should be considered the airless pleural space. The numbers represent pressure in centimeters of water. In Figure 8-7A, the pleural pressure is equal to the pressure surrounding the airways. At this level of lung inflation, the pleural pressure is equal and opposite in sign to the elastic recoil pressure of the lung (+10; no pressure gradient is present to produce airflow), and net alveolar pressure is atmospheric, or zero. During active expiration (Fig. 8-7B), pleural pressure becomes less negative. Because alveolar pressure is equal to the sum of pleural pressure and lung recoil pressure, it increases by an amount equal to the increase in pleural pressure. At this point, the difference between alveolar pressure (+20) and airway opening pressure (0) represents the total pressure producing

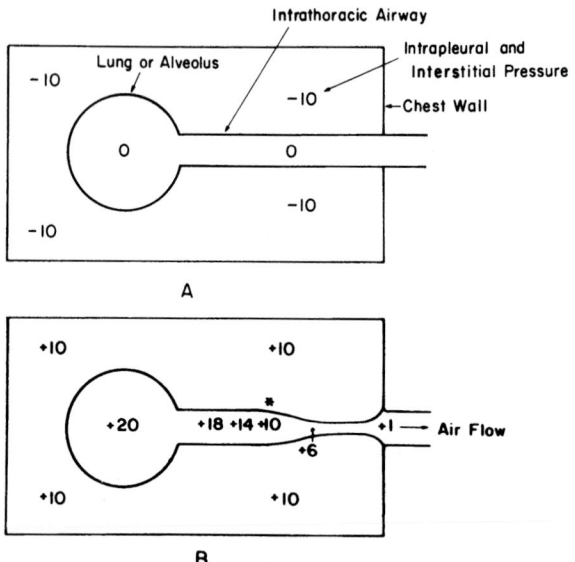

Fig. 8-7. See text for discussion. Static recoil pressure is +10 cm H_2O. **A.** Static conditions. **B.** Dynamic conditions. Airway is compressed downstream from point marked by asterisk.

expiratory flow. It follows that at some point between the alveolus and the airway opening, airway intraluminal pressure is equal to pleural pressure, and intraluminal pressures downstream from this point are less than pleural pressure. This downstream segment tends to collapse and limits flow. With any further increase in effort, the downstream segment tends to collapse even further. In this case, any additional increase in driving pressure resulting from greater effort is merely dissipated in keeping the collapsed segment open.

Maximal flow over most of the vital capacity is thus effort independent, but it is dependent on the lung recoil pressure and the resistance of peripheral airways upstream from the collapsible segment. Therefore, diseases such as emphysema that reduce the elasticity of airways and lung tissue tend to produce flow limitation by reducing the driving pressure and by making airways more collapsible. Diseases such as chronic bronchitis and asthma produce flow limitation by increasing the resistance of upstream or peripheral airways. Because maximal expiratory flow over the effort-independent range of the vital capacity (below 75% of TLC) depends on the resistance of peripheral airways, tests of forced expiration have become a useful means of detecting airway disease in its early stages.

Because of the pressure, volume, and flow relationships of the lung, the presence of airway obstruction can be determined by measuring maximal expiratory flow. Because maximal flow is relatively independent of effort and primarily dependent on the recoil pressure of the lung, and because the recoil pressure of the lung is dependent on lung volume, one need only relate the measured flow to the lung volume at which it is measured; this relationship is called a *flow-volume curve* (see Fig. 8-5).

The initial acceleration phase of the expiratory half of the loop represents the inertia of the system. Thereafter, maximal flow decreases as lung volume decreases. The initial portion of the curve between TLC and approximately 75% of TLC is the effort-dependent portion. Beyond this point, maximal flow is relatively independent of effort and dependent on lung recoil and the resistance of airways upstream from the collapsible segment. By measuring flow at a particular volume, such as 50% or 25% of the vital capacity, and comparing it with established normal standards, one can detect the presence of airflow limitation. Measurements made from the maximal expiratory flow-volume curve can identify patients with early expiratory airflow limitation before abnormalities occur in their timed vital capacity measurements. Although such measurements are more sensitive, they are neither as reproducible nor as specific as spirometric tests of forced expiration that relate expired volume to the time of expiration, such as the timed vital capacity.

Timed Vital Capacity

Timed vital capacity is obtained from the conventional spirogram, a graph of expired volume and time. The patient

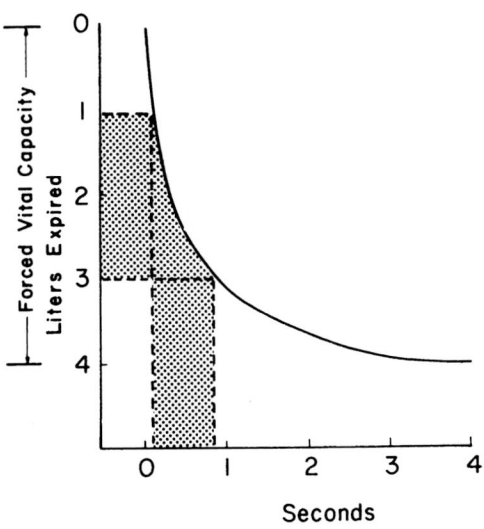

Fig. 8-8. The forced vital capacity curve. Both the mid-half of the forced vital capacity and the time required to deliver this mid-half volume are shaded.

makes a forced expiration from TLC (Fig. 8-8). Because the effort must be maximal, the patient must be cooperative and the technician must be able to coax the patient to do his or her best. The slope of a tangent to the volume-time curve at any point represents airflow at that point. Because airflow is maximal as long as a certain minimal effort is exceeded, portions of the forced vital capacity curve are reproducible, provided the patient exerts his or her best effort. Both reproducibility and appearance of the tracing can be used to judge the dependability of the results obtained.

Other analyses from the timed vital capacity include the volume expired in the first second of the forced vital capacity maneuver. It includes the earliest part of expiration, which is effort dependent, and a later portion, which is less so. If airflow is diminished because of disease, flow tends to decrease throughout expiration. Measurement of airflow in the first 2 and first 3 seconds of the expiratory effort helps verify the 1-second value. If the 1-second volume is low but the 2- and 3-second volumes are normal, one suspects poor performance. Some laboratories report the volume expired at 0.75 or even 0.5 seconds. These volumes have the same significance as the 1-second volume. Reduced 1-second volumes are particularly meaningful when the patient's total vital capacity is normal, because airflow obstruction is then likely. If the total vital capacity is reduced, then the forced 1-second volume may be reduced also, whether or not airflow obstruction is present. Therefore, it is useful to report the 1-second volume, or other timed fractional volumes, as a percentage of the total forced vital capacity, the so-called forced expiratory volume in 1 second to forced vital capacity ratio.

Another derived index of airflow is the forced expiratory flow between 25% and 75% of vital capacity, also called the *maximum midexpiratory flow rate.* This rate is calculated by

measuring the time required to expire the middle 50% of the vital capacity. Because it is an estimate of the average rate of airflow over the middle half of the vital capacity, it is expressed in units of flow. Hence, the middle 50% of the vital capacity in liters is divided by the time taken to expire it (see Fig. 8-8). Because this measurement is derived from the effort-independent portion of the forced vital capacity, it primarily reflects the flow characteristics in peripheral airways upstream from or proximal to the collapsible segment. For this reason, the forced expiratory flow between 25% and 75% of vital capacity is considered a useful test of small airway function.

Peak Flow

Peak flow can be measured either from the flow-volume loop (see Fig. 8-5) or with a simple hand-held anemometer type of device such as the Wright Peak Flow Meter. These two methods do not give comparable results and both depend on patient effort. Despite these limitations, determination of peak flow is one test that young children are often able to perform well and may be the only way of measuring their airflow. Measurement of peak expiratory flow rate with a portable device is a simple but objective measure of airway obstruction in asthmatic patients. Subjects typically measure peak expiratory flow rate once or twice daily and compare these values with their personal best peak expiratory flow rate; values less than 80% of an individual's best value may indicate an exacerbation and the need for more aggressive therapy or medical evaluation.

Maximum Voluntary Ventilation

Maximum voluntary ventilation is determined by having the patient breathe as fast and as deeply as possible for a fraction of a minute. The expired volume is measured and the ventilation is expressed in liters per minute. The determination depends on both adequate inspiratory and expiratory airflow plus considerable endurance and patient cooperation. When properly performed, it provides an excellent index of overall ventilatory ability. It also serves as an alternate test of airflow and as a check on the results of other expiratory flow measurements. Because the maximum midexpiratory flow rate and timed fractions of the forced vital capacity are calculated from the same volume-time curve (see Fig. 8-8), both will be spuriously low if the performance is poor.

Relation of the Functional Residual Capacity and Residual Volume to Airflow Obstruction

FRC and residual volume may increase in obstructive lung disease by two mechanisms. First, there may be a loss of lung tissue and therefore lung elasticity. The chest wall

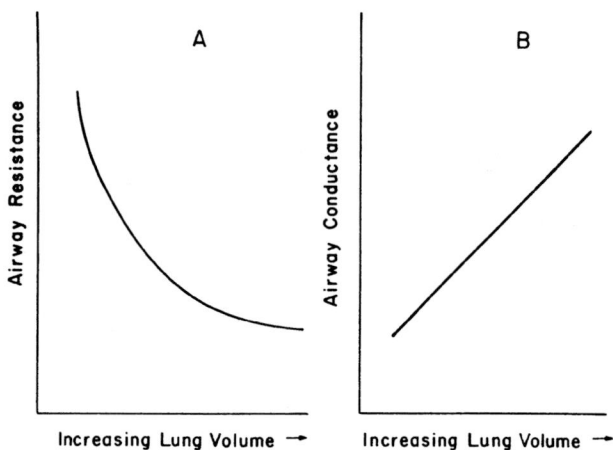

Fig. 8-9. A. The airway resistance is dependent on the lung volume at which it is measured and is nonlinear. **B.** The reciprocal of airway resistance, airway conductance, is linearly related to lung volume. The slope of this line is the specific conductance.

forces that counterbalance lung elastic recoil are less opposed and expand the thorax to a larger volume. The loss of lung elastic recoil also results in dynamic airway compression and sometimes airway closure during expiration, resulting in air trapping behind these high-resistance airway segments. Second, if airway resistance is increased to such a degree that the patient cannot exhale the inspired volume before inspiring the next breath, the patient increases the intrathoracic gas volume until expiratory resistance has decreased sufficiently to allow satisfactory exhalation (Fig. 8-9).

Measurements of Airway Resistance and Airflow

The pressure drop from the alveoli to the mouth and the airflow at the mouth can be measured and provide a direct measure of airway resistance (resistance = pressure/flow). Airway resistance depends on the lung volume at which it is measured, as would be expected because airways narrow at decreasing lung volumes (see Fig. 8-4) independent of the dynamic narrowing previously described. Proper interpretation of an airway resistance value requires knowledge of the lung volume at which it was measured, particularly in the presence of airflow obstruction, because lung volumes are often increased. Lung volumes range so widely among normal subjects that both airway resistance and the corresponding lung volume must be measured. With the body plethysmography method, both volume and resistance are determined simultaneously. The relationship between airway resistance and lung volume (Fig. 8-9A) is curvilinear, whereas the relationship between the reciprocal of airway resistance, airway conductance, and lung volume is nearly linear (Fig. 8-9B). The slope of this conductance-lung volume plot is the specific conductance. The specific conduc-

tance is relatively insensitive to changes of resistance in the peripheral airways until it has increased severalfold, because changes in small airway resistance are masked by the relatively higher resistance of the upper airways. Direct resistance or conductance measurements are seldom more sensitive for defining airway obstruction than is a well-performed forced vital capacity determination.

WORK OF BREATHING

Breathing requires that the respiratory muscles or a mechanical ventilator generate a pressure (force) sufficient to move the volumes of air required for ventilation. Force is required to stretch tissue, to counteract gravity, and to overcome frictional resistances of tissues and airways. An optimal combination of breathing frequency and tidal volume exists at which the work of breathing is minimal. This combination varies between subjects and for specific metabolic requirements. If tidal volume is increased, the pressures required become disproportionately large (see pressure-volume curve in Fig. 8-2). If breathing frequency increases, the airway resistance increases owing to additional flow turbulence and to increased expiratory airway narrowing because of dynamic airway compression. Attempts to drive the respiratory system faster than it will respond, using pressures greater than those required for maximum expiratory airflow, represent wasted effort. In both health and disease, each person spontaneously selects whatever combination of tidal volume and breathing frequency achieves the required ventilation at a minimal work of breathing. In normal humans, the work of breathing requires little energy, approximately 1 mL of oxygen per L of ventilation. In disease, the oxygen cost of breathing increases greatly and may represent a large portion of the metabolic needs of the patient, thereby limiting the proportion of total oxygen uptake available for muscles not involved in ventilation. Thus, exercise capacity is limited when lung disease causes a substantial increase in the work of breathing.

In clinical practice, the work of breathing may be increased by factors other than intrinsic disease of the respiratory system. This is commonly encountered in mechanically ventilated patients, in whom the added resistance to airflow imposed by the endotracheal tube increases the work of breathing during spontaneous respiration. The resistance increases with increasing flow rate and decreasing endotracheal tube diameter in a nonlinear fashion (Fig. 8-10). This may be of critical importance when attempting to wean the patient with marginal pulmonary reserve. In addition, some patients with airway obstruction develop endogenous increases in end-expiratory pressure, so-called *auto–positive end-expiratory pressure (auto-PEEP)* or *intrinsic PEEP*, which may increase their work of breathing because auto-PEEP must be overcome to trigger ventilatory airflow in certain modes. Strategies used to minimize or overcome these added respiratory loads include use of

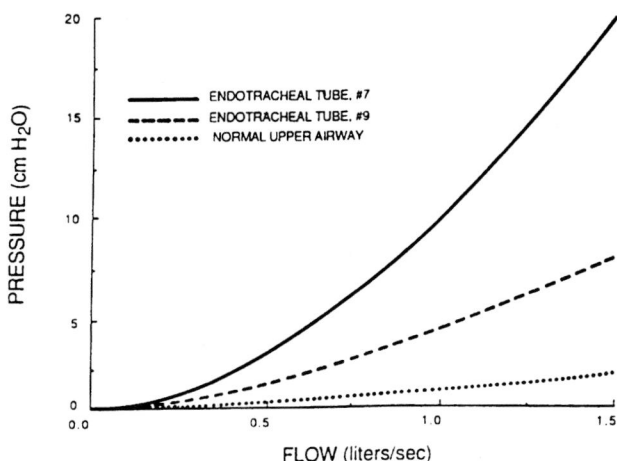

Fig. 8-10. The relationship between flow rate and pressure gradient across two different diameter endotracheal tubes compared with the normal upper airway. Resistance to airflow, defined as pressure divided by flow rate, increases as the tube diameter decreases. From Kreit JW, Eschenbacher WL: The physiology of spontaneous mechanical ventilation. Clin Chest Med 9:19, 1988. With permission.

larger diameter endotracheal tubes and the application of low levels of ventilator support sufficient to overcome the resistance of the tube and, for auto-PEEP, application of external PEEP.

PRACTICAL APPLICATION OF PULMONARY MECHANICS

An understanding of pulmonary mechanics is extremely useful when applied to the management and monitoring of ventilated patients. Ventilation depends on volume changes driven by pressure gradients, and it does not matter whether the force is generated by respiratory muscles or by a mechanical ventilator.

In ventilated patients, for example, it is useful to evaluate and monitor maximal dynamic, or peak pressure, and static, or plateau pressure (PS). Peak pressure is that required to distend the entire respiratory system at a given inspiratory flow and tidal volume. In ventilated patients, this system includes the machine circuitry and tubing in addition to the lung and chest wall. Therefore, increases in peak pressure may be related to a variety of conditions that either decrease respiratory system compliance or increase resistance to gas flow, including parenchymal lung disease or fluid or air in the pleural space, or increased airway resistance (e.g., airway secretions, kinked tubing, and so forth). Plateau pressure is that required to distend the respiratory system at peak inspiration in the absence of gas flow. Any additional pressure that has been added to the system (PEEP) is subtracted; PS is measured by imposing a transient airway occlusion, or inspiratory pause, of approximately 1 second. Under these no-flow conditions, PS

reflects alveolar pressure rather than the entire respiratory system and thus is not influenced by conditions such as bronchospasm or airway secretions.

Respiratory system or static compliance characterizes the pressure-volume relationship of the lung and can be determined in a mechanically ventilated patient once plateau pressure is measured.

$$\text{Compliance} = \frac{\text{Tidal volume}}{\text{PS-PEEP}}$$

Normal = 60 to 100 mL/cm H_2O

Measuring respiratory system compliance is worthwhile in diseases such as adult respiratory distress syndrome, which is characterized by severely reduced compliance. Compliance can be used to monitor progress or modify PEEP therapy in adult respiratory distress syndrome. For example, compliance should improve with increases in PEEP as alveoli are recruited, but it may be reduced when PEEP is increased to the point of overdistention. Additionally, the difference between the peak and static (no-flow) pressures provides an estimate of the pressure required to overcome airflow resistance. Increases in peak-static pressure difference suggest increasing resistance to airflow. A firm understanding of the mechanics of breathing can be valuable in optimizing the management of critically ill patients.

READING REFERENCES

General

Bates DV: Respiratory Function in Disease. Philadelphia: WB Saunders, 1989.
Chusid EL: The Selective and Comprehensive Testing of Adult Pulmonary Function. Mt. Kisco, NY: Futura Publishing, 1983.
Murray JF: The Normal Lung. 2nd Ed. Philadelphia: WB Saunders, 1986.
West JB: Respiratory Physiology: The Essentials. 3rd Ed. Baltimore: Williams & Wilkins, 1985.
Wilson AF: Pulmonary Function Testing—Indications and Interpretations. Orlando: Grune & Stratton, 1985.

Chest Wall and Lung Elasticity

Gibson GJ, Pride NB: Lung distensibility. Br J Dis Chest 70:143, 1976.
Rahn H, et al: The pressure-volume diagram of the thorax and lung. Am J Physiol 146:161, 1946.
Turner JM, Mead J, Wohl ME: Elasticity of human lungs in relation to age. J Appl Physiol 25:664, 1968.

Airflow Resistance

Fry DQ, Hyatt RE: Pulmonary mechanics: a unified analysis of the relationship between pressure, volume and gasflow in the lungs of normal and diseased human subjects. Am J Med 29:672, 1960.
Hogg JC, Macklem PT, Thurlbeck WM: Site and nature of airway obstruction in chronic obstructive lung disease. N Engl J Med 278:1355, 1968.
Hyatt RE, et al: Expiratory flow limitation. J Appl Physiol 55:169, 1983.
Mead J, et al: Significance of the relationship between lung recoil and maximum expiratory flow. J Appl Physiol 22:95, 1967.
Pride NB, et al: Determinants of maximum expiratory flow from the lungs. J Appl Physiol 23:646, 1967.

Work of Breathing

Kreit JW, Eschenbacher WL: The physiology of spontaneous and mechanical ventilation. Clin Chest Med 9:11, 1988.

Ranieri VM, et al: Auto-positive end-expiratory pressure and dynamic hyperinflation. Clin Chest Med 17:379,1996.

Practical Application of Pulmonary Mechanics

Marini JJ: Lung mechanics determinations at the bedside: Instrumentation and clinical application. Resp Care 35:669, 1990.

Suter PM, Fairley HB, Isenberg MO: Optimal end-expiratory airway pressure in patients with acute pulmonary failure. N Engl J Med 292:284, 1975.

SECTION III

Thoracic Imaging

CHAPTER 9

Radiographic Evaluation of the Lungs and Chest

Anne McB Curtis and Wallace T. Miller

For the physician interested in diseases of the chest, chest radiography is of paramount importance in identifying the presence of such disease and in providing clues about its nature.

ROUTINE EXAMINATION

Adequate radiographic examination of the chest necessitates at least two projections to provide a three-dimensional view of the thorax: posteroanterior (PA) and lateral projections.

High-kilovoltage technique is now generally accepted practice. This technique involves the use of x-rays at the 129-kilovolt (peak) range with a fine-line grid, which increases the information on the radiograph by providing less contrast but more penetration. Information about the mediastinum and retrocardiac areas is increased compared with films done at a lower kilovoltage. An added advantage of this high-kilovolt technique is the decreased time required for exposure, reducing patient motion. If at all possible, chest films should be performed on a dedicated chest radiographic unit, allowing for the best and most consistent technique.

If the high-kilovolt technique for standard films is not available, a grid radiograph with higher kilovolt or milliampere, or both, and a fixed or moving grid allow better visualization of the mediastinum and lesions behind the heart and diaphragm. This technique, however, is not optimal for imaging of the pulmonary parenchyma (Fig. 9-1).

The lateral radiograph is of considerable importance in the routine examination of the chest, because some lesions in the chest are apparent only in the lateral view. Examples include small mediastinal lesions, some masses in the anteromedial portions of the lung adjacent to the mediastinum (Fig. 9-2), lesions in the vertebral column, lesions behind the heart and diaphragm on the PA view, and small pleural effusions. For routine screening films, in the absence of apparent chest disease, Sagel and associates (1974) found

that a lateral view may not be indicated, because the yield of information is low. In all other situations, a lateral examination should be included.

SUPPLEMENTARY RADIOGRAPHIC VIEWS

Occasionally, views in addition to the PA and lateral may be useful to establish the parenchymal nature of a lesion. This may be done with 9-degree oblique PA films or apical lordotic films. The oblique radiograph is designated right or left anterior or right or left posterior on the basis of the patient's relationship to the film cassette. In a right anterior oblique position, the right side of the patient is closer to the film and the patient is facing the film cassette. In the shallow oblique projections, the patient is rotated slightly, approximately 5 degrees to the right and left. The slight change in position of the patient between the two films allows separation of overlapping structures that have produced a *confluence* of shadows or pseudonodule, while a parenchymal nodule is seen in both positions (Fig. 9-3). Of course, computed tomography (CT) can clarify whether a nodule is seen. However, if CT is not readily available or if expense is a consideration, the oblique technique may be useful.

It is helpful when examining oblique radiographs to remember that posteriorly placed lesions in the lung maintain a constant relationship with the spine and anteriorly placed lesions in the lung maintain a constant relationship with the heart.

Figure 9-4 demonstrates some of the normal anatomic structures seen on the oblique radiograph. Note that these are not shallow obliques.

The lordotic and reverse lordotic views are based on the same principles as the shallow oblique views: a change in position separates overlapping structures. These views are used frequently in evaluation of the pulmonary apices where lesions may be obscured by overlying ribs and clavicles in the PA projection. In the lordotic view, anteriorly placed lesions appear to move upward and those located posteriorly

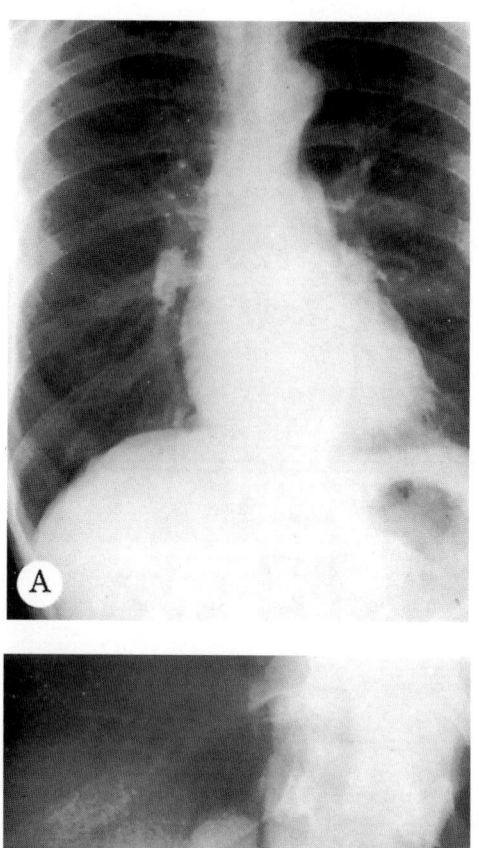

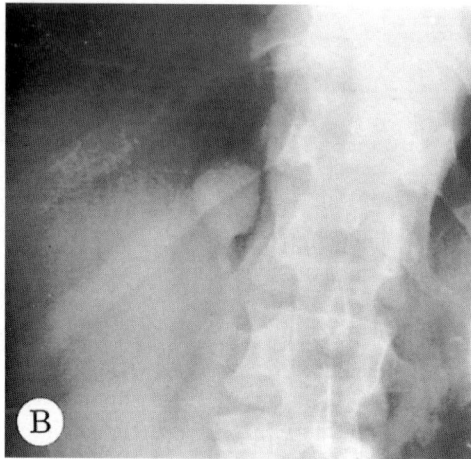

Fig. 9-1. Pulmonary granuloma. **A.** The routine posteroanterior radiograph at a low-kilovoltage technique appears normal. **B.** An overpenetrated grid radiograph demonstrates a pulmonary nodule in the right lung seen through the right hemidiaphragm.

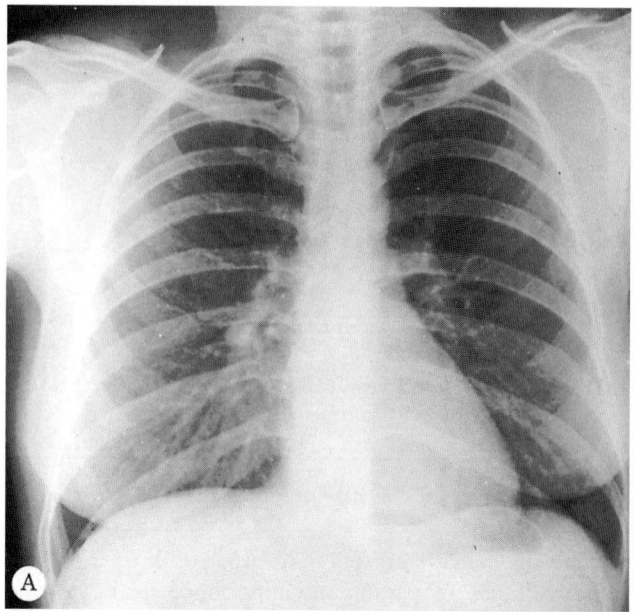

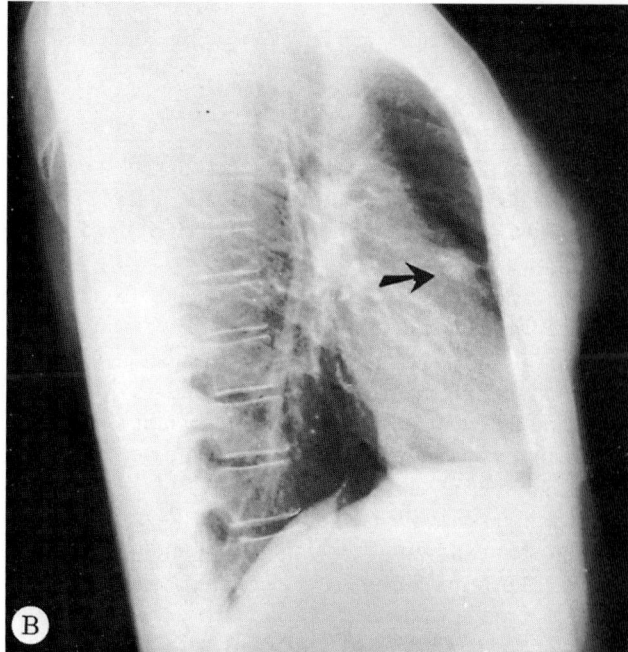

Fig. 9-2. Carcinoma of the lung. **A.** The posteroanterior radiograph demonstrates a subtle increase in density at the inferior portion of the right hilum that would probably be unobserved without the lateral film. **B.** The lateral view demonstrates an obvious retrosternal abnormality (*arrow*). The mass was in the right upper lobe and was a primary lung cancer.

move downward (Fig. 9-5). A full chest lordotic view demonstrates middle lobe collapse or consolidation if a lateral film is not obtainable.

Lateral decubitus radiographs are extremely important in the investigation of suspected pleural effusion or of air-fluid levels in pulmonary or pleural cavities. The decubitus radiograph is made with the x-ray beam projected in a horizontal plane and the patient lying on his or her side. In a left lateral decubitus view, the patient lies on the left side and free pleural fluid forms a layer along the left lateral chest wall (Fig. 9-6). Amounts of fluid as small as 50 to 100 mL can be identified in the lateral decubitus position. If a pneumothorax is present and the examination is being made to investigate the air-outlined pleura, the x-ray beam should be centered on the elevated rather than the recumbent side of

the patient. If effusion and pneumothorax, hydropneumothorax, are present, an air-fluid level is seen on the lateral decubitus projection.

It is critical to remember that a fluid level, and particularly an air-fluid level, is not visible unless the beam is in a horizontal projection, regardless of the patient's position; the beam must be tangential to the fluid or air-fluid interface. With the patient in a supine position with a vertical beam or in a semi-

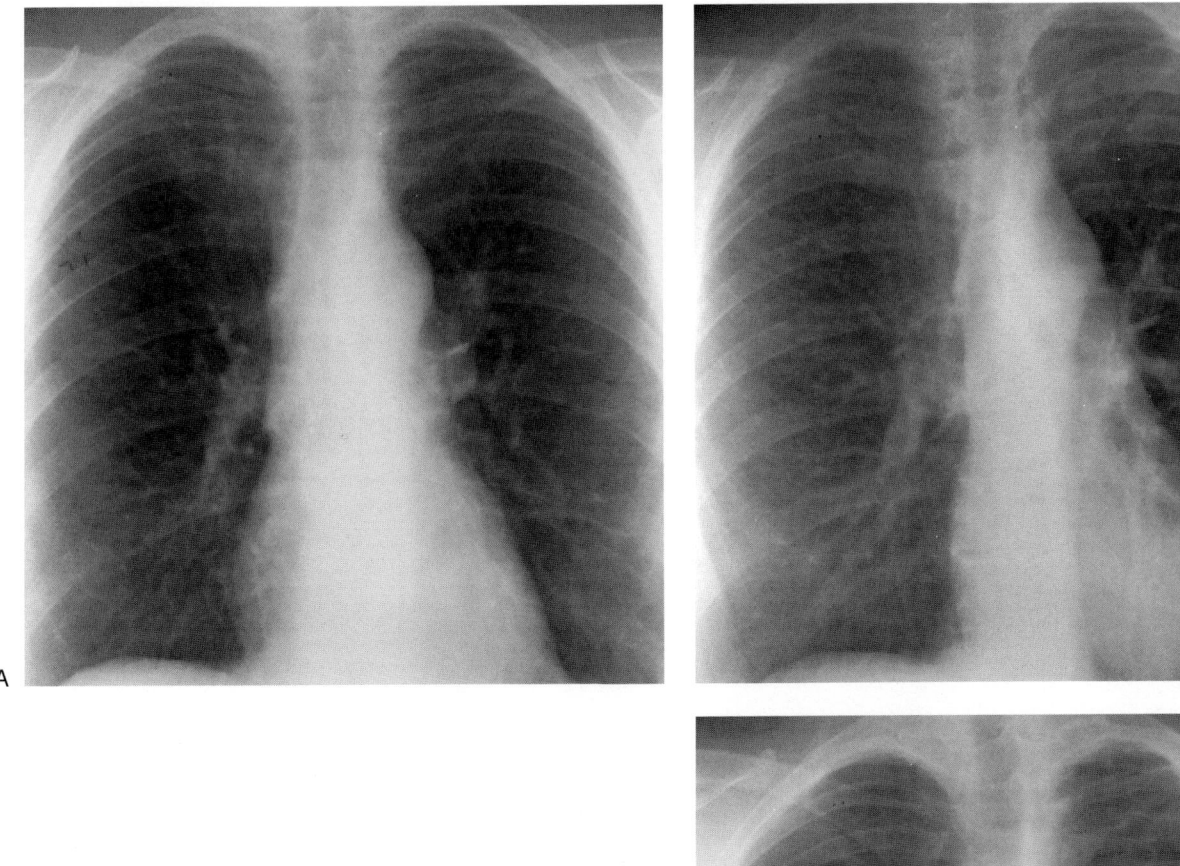

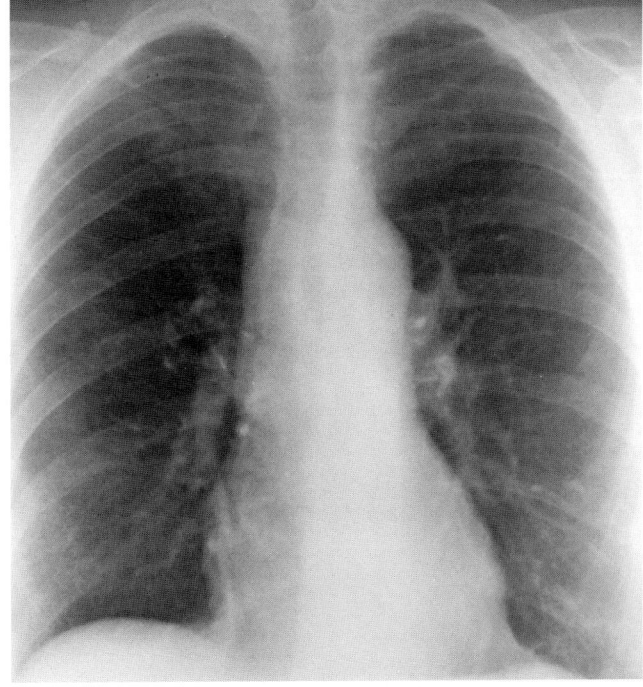

Fig. 9-3. Posteroanterior (**A**) and shallow oblique views (**B, C**). A nodule was questioned behind the right anterior second rib and in the fourth to fifth intercostal space posteriorly. On oblique views, no nodule is appreciated.

erect position with a nonhorizontal beam, the air-fluid level is not visualized (Figs. 9-7 and 9-8).

Lateral decubitus views are useful also when air trapping is suspected, usually when an inhaled endobronchial foreign body is suspected. Normally, the dependent lung decreases in size (see Fig. 9-6). If obstructed, the obstructed lung fails to decrease in size when placed in the dependent or down side position (Fig. 9-9). Both decubitus views are helpful for comparison if available. Note that expiratory radiography also may be helpful in

assessing pulmonary air trapping, either local or diffuse. They can be helpful in the investigation of endobronchial neoplasms or particularly in the localization of inhaled endobronchial foreign bodies in children. A foreign body usually results in an emphysematous lobe or lung so that on the expiratory radiograph the mediastinum shifts to the side opposite the foreign body or obstructed bronchus. Fluoroscopy also demonstrates the mediastinal shift with air trapping. In very small children, the decubitus views are the easiest to obtain.

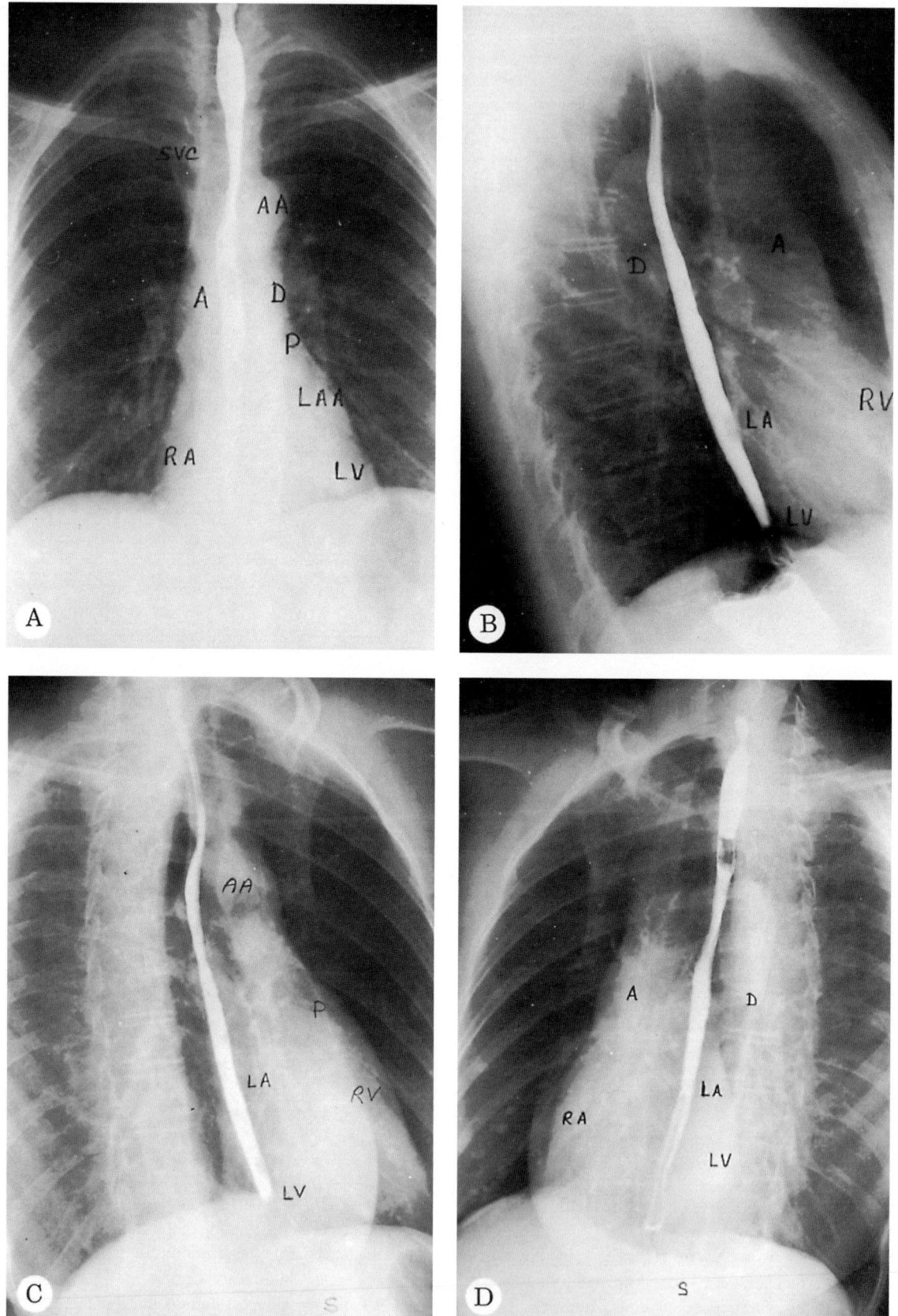

Fig. 9-4. Normal posteroanterior (**A**), lateral (**B**), right anterior oblique (**C**), and left anterior oblique (**D**) radiographs. A, ascending aorta; AA, aortic arch; D, descending aorta; LA, left atrium; LAA, left atrial appendage; LV, left ventricle; P, main pulmonary artery; RA, right atrium; RV, right ventricle; S, stomach; SVC, superior vena cava. Tharium is in the esophagus.

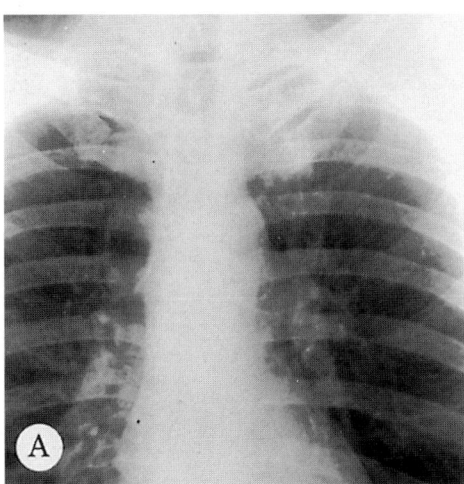
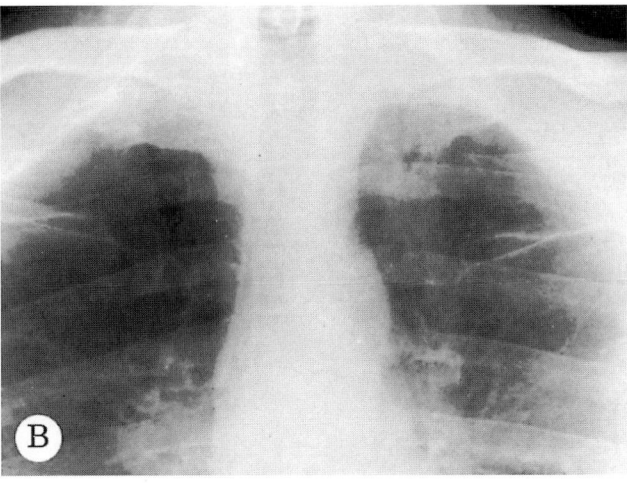

Fig. 9-5. Carcinoma of the lung. A subtle increase in density is seen to the left anterior first rib in comparison with the right, which raises suspicion of a mass on the posteroanterior radiograph (**A**). An apical lordotic view (**B**) demonstrates a definite mass in the left apex below the left first rib. Note asymmetry when compared with the right apex.

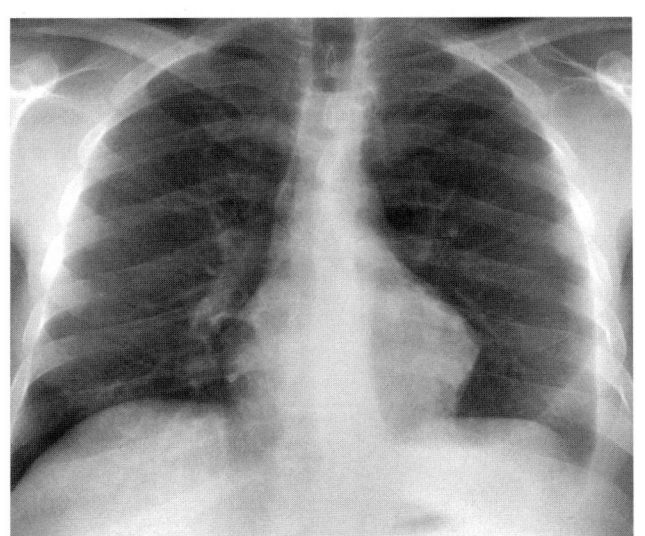

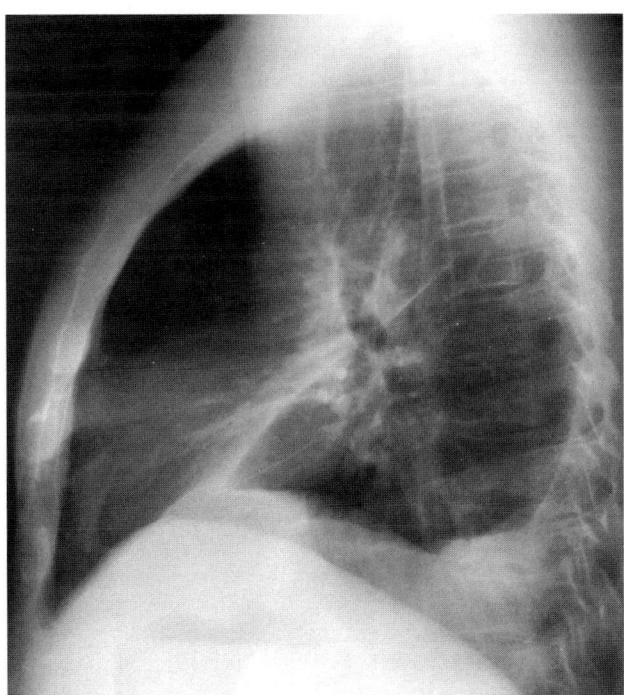

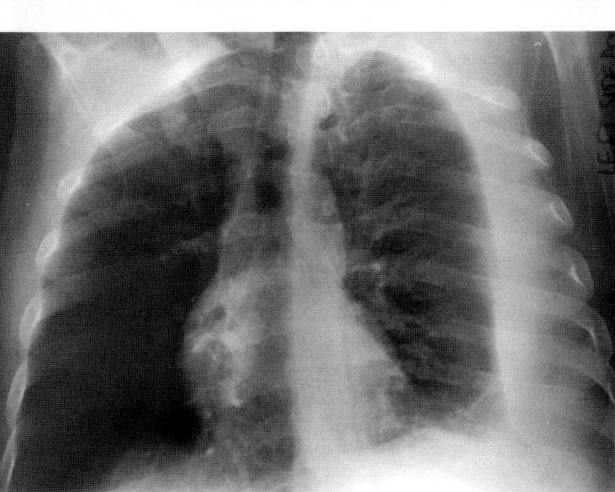

Fig. 9-6. Pleural effusion. Posteroanterior (**A**) and lateral (**B**) views demonstrate blunting of the left costophrenic angle. Left lateral decubitus view (**C**) demonstrates a large layering pleural effusion against the left chest wall. Note on the posteroanterior view (**A**) the increased distance between gastric bubble and left hemidiaphragm (compare with Fig. 9-2A), indicating a subpulmonic component of the pleural fluid.

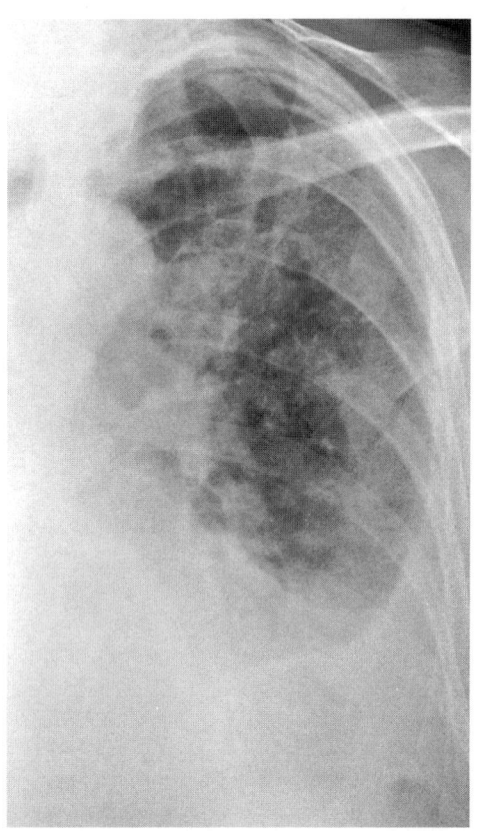

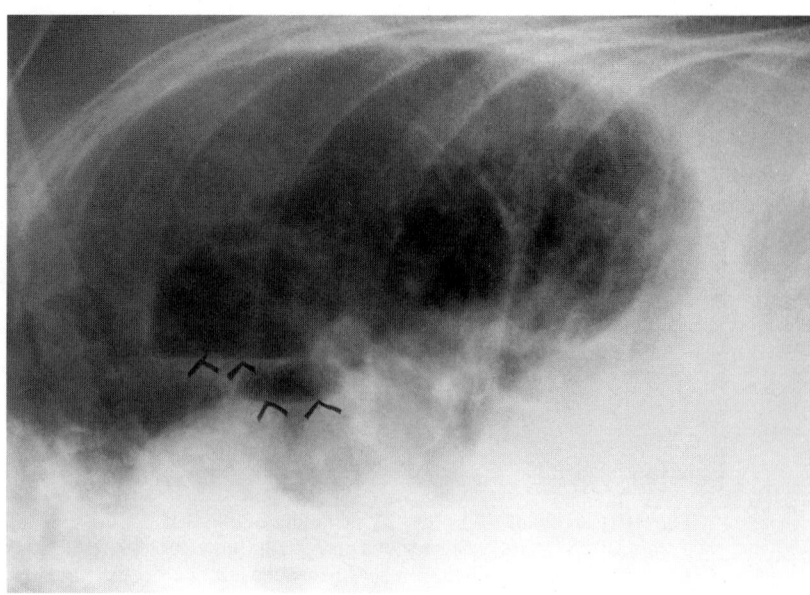

A

B

Fig. 9-7. Pyopneumothorax. **A.** No air-fluid level is seen on the posteroanterior supine view. **B.** Left lateral decubitus radiograph with horizontal projection of the x-ray beam shows multiple air-fluid levels (*arrowheads*) consistent with unsuspected empyema and pneumothorax.

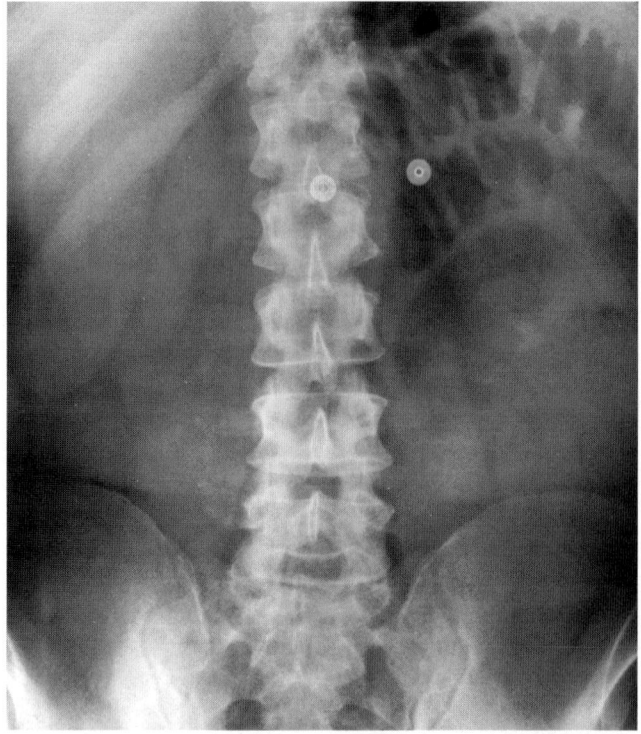

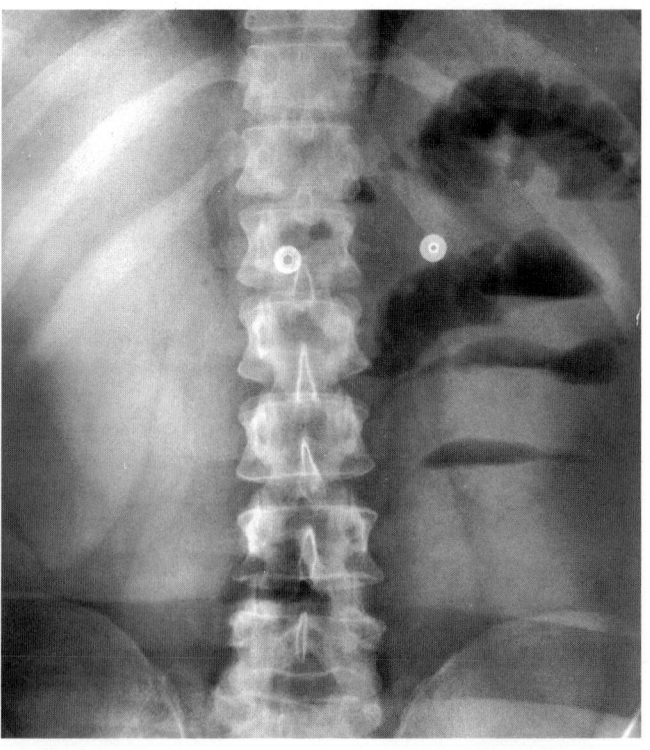

A

B

Fig. 9-8. Air-fluid levels. **A.** Supine abdomen demonstrates a few dilated loops of bowel in the left upper quadrant. **B.** With the erect position and a horizontal beam, multiple air-fluid levels are identified, indicating small-bowel obstruction.

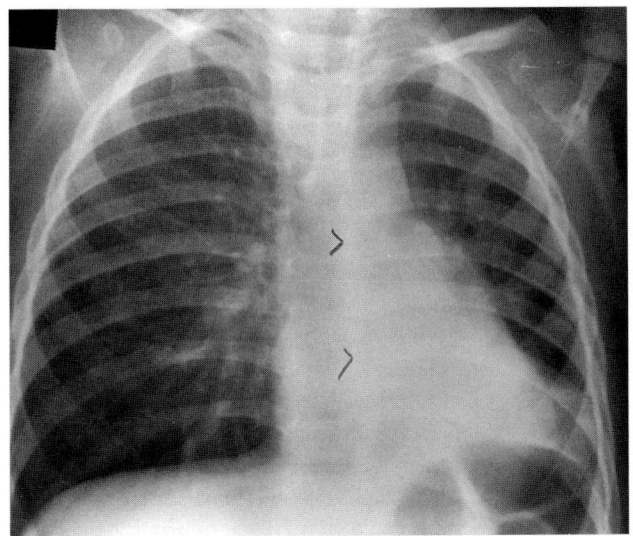

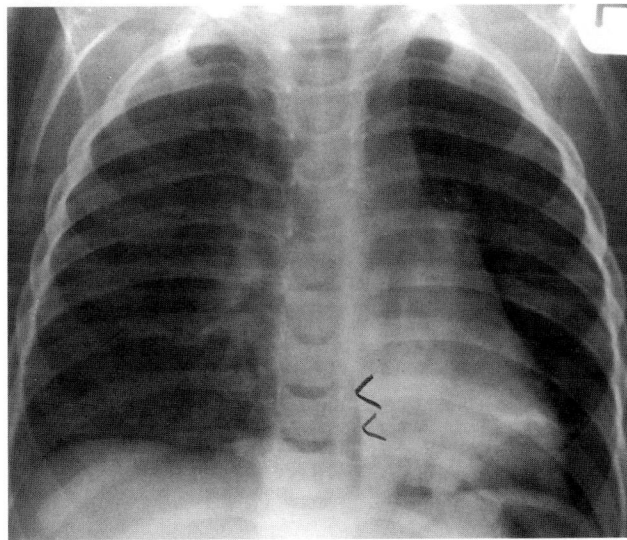

Fig. 9-9. Obstructed right main stem bronchus from inhaled peanut. **A.** Erect posteroanterior radiograph demonstrates signs of air trapping with shift of the mediastinum and the azygoesophageal (AE) recess to the left (*arrowheads*). **B.** A right lateral decubitus view shows no collapse of right lung and persistent shift to the left (*arrowheads*), indicating airway obstruction (compare with Fig. 9-6).

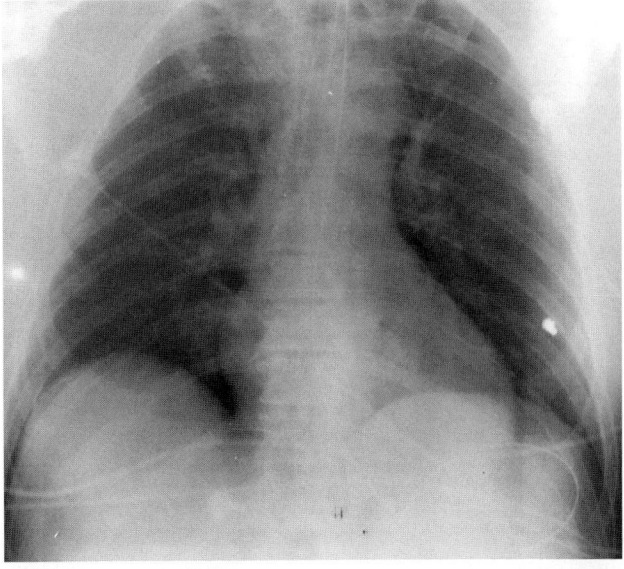

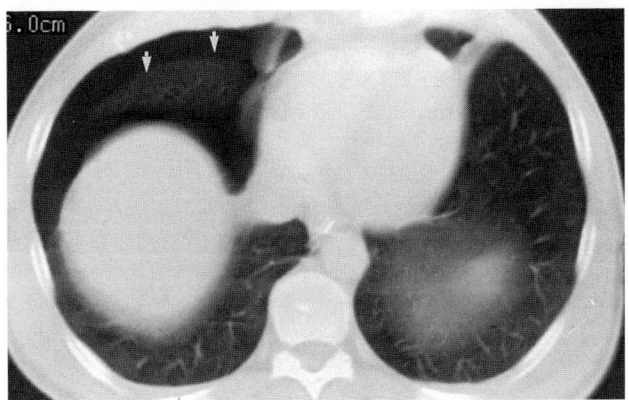

Fig. 9-10. Pneumothorax on supine films. **A.** The right costophrenic angle is deeper and more lucent than the left as a result of anterior location of pleural air in the supine position. **B.** Computed tomographic scan confirms location anteriorly (*arrows*).

The expiratory radiograph is also useful in investigating a suspected pneumothorax that may be poorly visualized with routine inspiration. The pneumothorax is better demonstrated with expiration because the volume of air in the lungs decreases, whereas that in the pleural space remains the same. In addition, contrast between the pleural air and the collapsed lung is increased, as the lung becomes denser in expiration.

The supine radiograph is made when the patient is unable to sit or stand and is the routine projection for infants, because it is difficult to obtain satisfactory erect images in young infants. Portable films, done primarily in the intensive care unit (ICU), account for 50% of chest films as reported by one of us (W.T.M., 1997). Limitations of imaging imposed by the medical conditions of the patients, as well as the portable imaging modality, require meticulous technique. Portable films may be done in the erect position, but patients in the ICU are frequently unable to sit up. Tocino (1996) notes that a supine position is preferred to the semierect position for reproducibility of technique from day to day. When possible, all foreign objects that are superimposed on the patient should be removed to avoid confusion. Milne (1986) cautions that the interpretation of the supine radiograph should take into consideration the magnification of the cardiomediastinal structures as a result of the anteroposterior projection. The supine position also results in engorgement of mediastinal veins, producing mediastinal widening and increasing the upper lobe pulmonary vessels. This should not be confused with the vascular engorgement of congestive failure.

Both pleural effusions and pneumothoraces distribute differently in the thorax when the patient is in a supine position as demonstrated by Tocino and Westcott (1996). Added lucency may be seen anteromedially and laterally above the hemidiaphragms with a supine pneumothorax. The anterolateral location of a pneumothorax results in asymmetric costophrenic angles (deep sulcus sign) (Fig. 9-10). Pleural

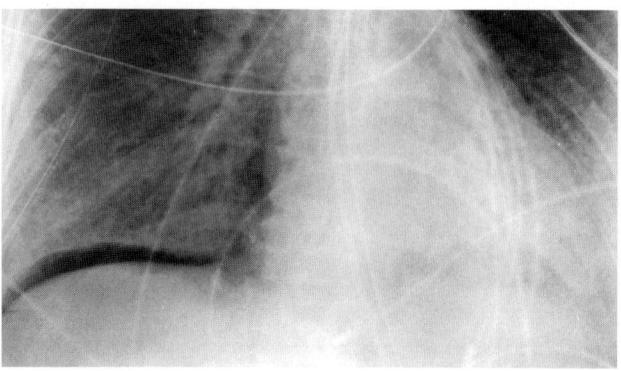

Fig. 9-11. Subpulmonic pneumothorax on supine film. Intrapleural air outlines base of right lung.

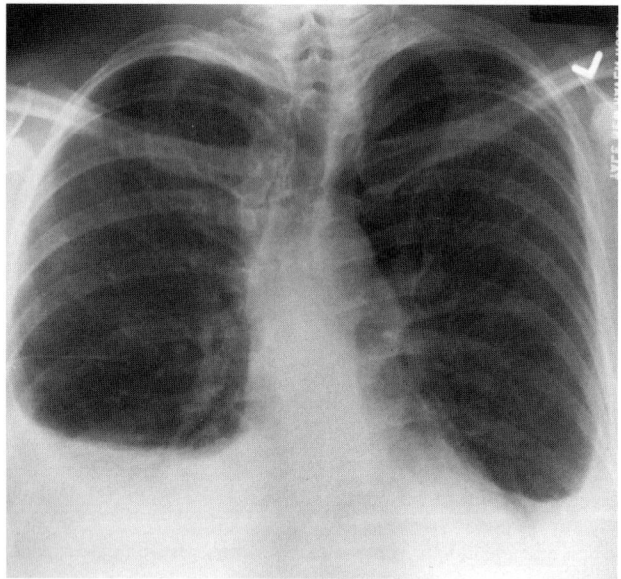

A

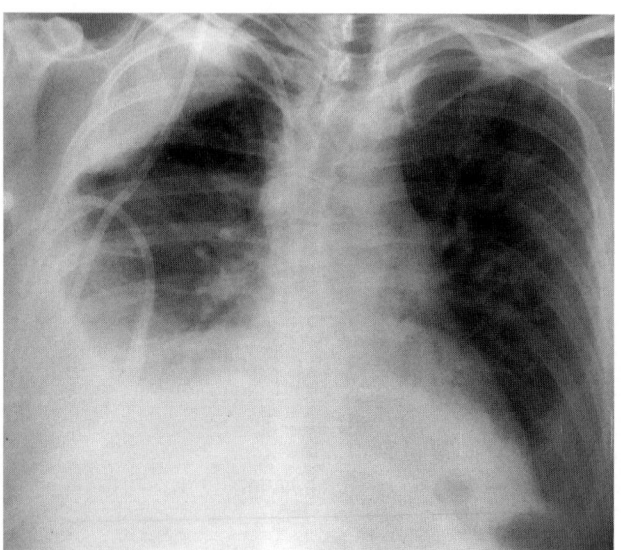

B

Fig. 9-12. Pleural effusion on erect (**A**) and supine (**B**) films. Fluid layers over right apex from the right costophrenic angle when patient is supine.

air also may be seen beneath the lung in a subpulmonic location (Fig. 9-11). In the supine position, pleural effusions may redistribute from the costophrenic angles to the apices of the thorax (Fig. 9-12).

DIGITAL RADIOGRAPHY

Digital radiography is a technique in which storage systems other than film are used to record the radiographic image. The most widely used is the photostimulable phosphor plate storage system. When the phosphor plate is radiated, energy is stored in the form of trapped electrons. When the phosphor plate is scanned with laser light, visible light is emitted, and the analog signal converted to a digital signal for further analysis. Obvious advantages to this method are efficient image storage and image transmission. As Ravin and Chotas (1997) note, digital image receptors have a wide range of sensitivity and a linear response to radiation over that range. The detected image is therefore independent of the exposure level. This decreases the need for repeat radiography, particularly when a portable technique is used.

Image processing of the wide range of densities obtained can accentuate the visibility of structures superimposed over the mediastinum. Schaefer and colleagues (1989) demonstrated improved visibility of these structures in comparison with standard screen film combinations. This is also advantageous in the ICU when looking for tubes and catheters.

Image processing also can enhance noise, which in turn may decrease conspicuity of low-contrast objects. In addition, the appearance of interstitial lung disease may be created if edge enhancement is overused. One has to allow for a learning curve when working initially with computed radiography as compared with film-screen images.

COMPUTED TOMOGRAPHY

CT has changed markedly since it was introduced in the 1970s, both in improved image quality and the development of slip-ring gantry technology that eliminates the need for electric cables and allows continuous rotation of the gantry for data acquisition. Spiral-helical CT (volumetric data acquisition) has significant advantages over conventional CT as described by Leung (1997). The thorax can be imaged in a single breath-hold, which decreases respiratory misregistration of lesions, and minimizes motion artifacts. Images may be displayed in the conventional fashion or in a multiplanar or three-dimensional mode. Nonionic contrast with increased speed of injection, efficient use of scanning time, overlapping reconstructions, and decreased reconstruction time are also significant developments according to Zeman and colleagues (1998). Three-dimensional reconstruction and manipulation of the three-dimensional images may be particularly useful to the chest surgeon when evaluating

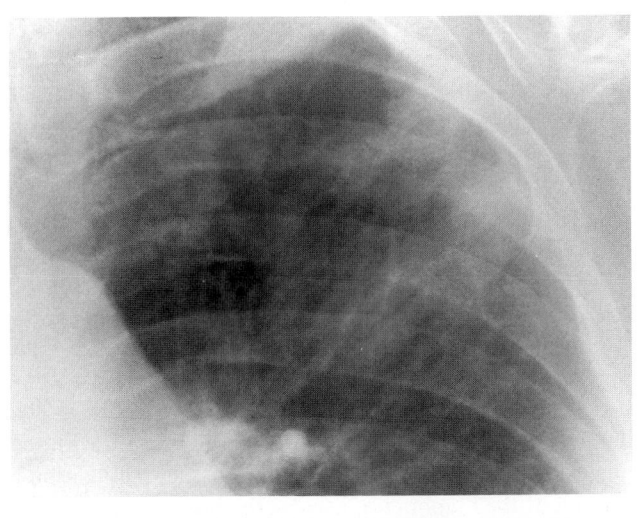

A

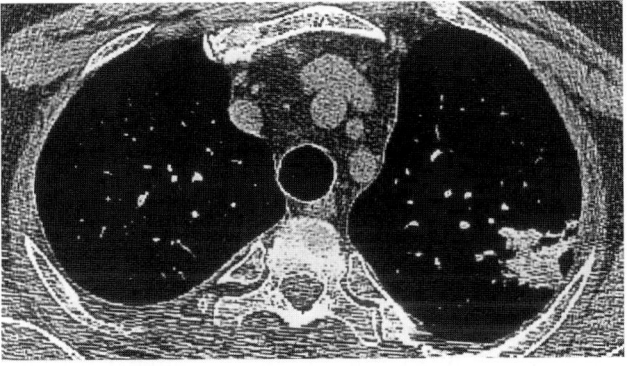

B

Fig. 9-13. Amiodarone toxicity. **A.** Poorly marginated focal opacity in the left upper lobe. Patient had no pulmonary symptoms. **B.** On computed tomography, opacity measures 127 Hounsfield units compatible with iodine accumulation in the lung, a sign of amiodarone toxicity.

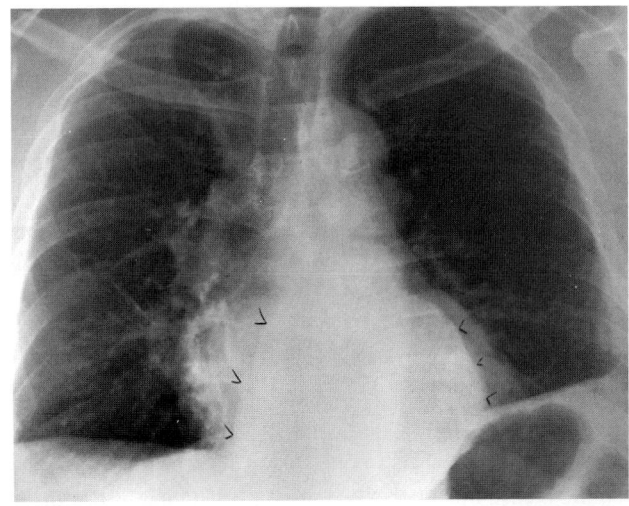

A

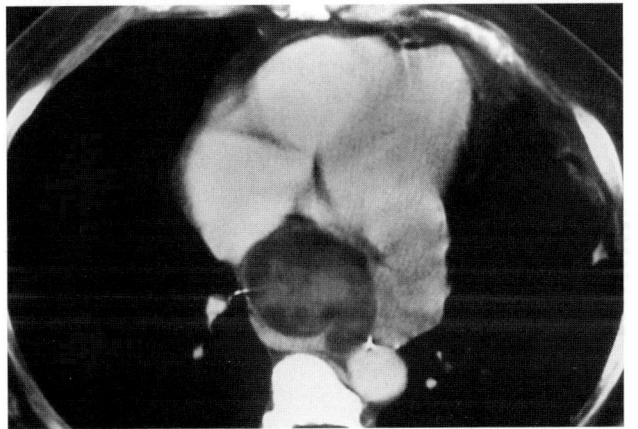

B

Fig. 9-14. Liposarcoma of the mediastinum. **A.** Posteroanterior chest view shows mediastinal mass (*arrowheads*) of indeterminate origin. **B.** Computed tomography demonstrates heterogeneous mass with some low densities compatible with fat.

involvement of mediastinal structures, particularly the great vessels, by malignant lymphadenopathy.

CT is far more sensitive in the detection of density differences: differences of 0.5% can be recognized by this technique, whereas density differences of 4 to 5% are necessary for recognition on the usual radiograph. Subtle differences in density may be accentuated by changing the scale of contrast and the center point (i.e., window width and level). An example of abnormal increase in density in the lung may be seen with amiodarone therapy. This may result in an accumulation of iodine within the pulmonary macrophages. Although the increase in density is not appreciated on plain film, it may be seen on CT scan and indicates pulmonary toxicity (Fig. 9-13).

CT scanning is particularly useful in identifying mediastinal nodes when the routine chest radiograph is equivocal or normal. Unfortunately, size criteria for enlargement do not allow complete separation of malignant from benign lymphadenopathy. McCloud and colleagues (1992) noted a sensitivity of 64% and a specificity of 62% when results of CT scanning of the mediastinum in patients with lung cancer

were correlated with surgical findings. This may not obviate mediastinoscopy but does provide guidelines for further surgical staging or may identify patients who are candidates for adjunct chemotherapy. In addition, CT scanning is useful in the mediastinum, where absorption characteristics of various masses may yield useful information (Fig. 9-14).

CT scanning demonstrates many more nodules than does plain film radiography. Unfortunately, differentiation of benign from malignant nodules is frequently not possible, and more than one-half of the nodules detected may be benign. Swensen and colleagues (1996) have demonstrated that benign and malignant nodules have different contrast enhancement patterns on CT that reflect different vascular supplies. After intravenous injection of nonionic contrast—the amount determined by the patient's size—thin sections are taken through the lesion in question every minute for 4 to 5 minutes. The CT numbers, reflecting degree of enhancement, are compared with those before contrast injection. This protocol separated benign from malignant nodules with a sensitivity of 98% and a specificity of 73% when 20 Hounsfield units were used as the threshold above which malignancy was identified. In this way surgery may be obviated in some cases.

Careful radiographic follow-up is indicated even if the nodule enhances in an apparently benign fashion, because the sensitivity is not 100%.

MAGNETIC RESONANCE IMAGING

Magnetic resonance (MR) imaging uses radio waves modified by a magnetic field to produce images that contain somewhat different information than that obtained in the standard radiograph or CT scan. Intravenous contrast is also not required. MR imaging in the chest is particularly useful in studying mediastinal structures: Lymph nodes are distinguished easily from mediastinal fat. The great vessels are readily imaged in a multiplanar fashion, and no contrast is required for the evaluation of thoracic aortic disease. MR imaging is superior to CT in imaging the brachial plexus in the case of a suspected Pancoast's or apical tumor (see Chapter 11).

FLUOROSCOPY

Air trapping is readily identified using fluoroscopy. Limitation or absence of diaphragmatic motion can be evaluated with fluoroscopy when an elevated hemidiaphragm is seen on routine chest radiography. Evaluation of diaphragmatic motion fluoroscopically must be done with the subject in the supine position in both PA and lateral projections. True paralysis of the diaphragm may be overlooked if fluoroscopy is done with the patient breathing quietly or if the fluoroscopy is performed with the patient in the erect position. Asking the supine patient to sniff quickly demonstrates elevation or paradoxic motion of the paralyzed diaphragm.

Partial eventration of the diaphragm is a common finding. It may be misinterpreted as diaphragmatic paralysis if the patient is fluoroscoped only in the PA position. The dome of the diaphragm may move paradoxically with the patient in this position. However, in the lateral position a portion of the diaphragm, usually the posterior portion, is seen to move normally. This finding indicates a localized diaphragmatic weakness—eventration—rather than true paralysis.

Fluoroscopy is useful to demonstrate air trapping, particularly when an inhaled foreign body is suspected. On expiration, bronchial obstruction prevents decrease in volume of the obstructed lung and results in shift of the mediastinum away from the obstructed side. In young children correlation of mediastinal motion with the phase of respiration may be difficult to evaluate. Decubitus views produce similar results: The obstructed side fails to collapse in the dependent position, indicating obstruction

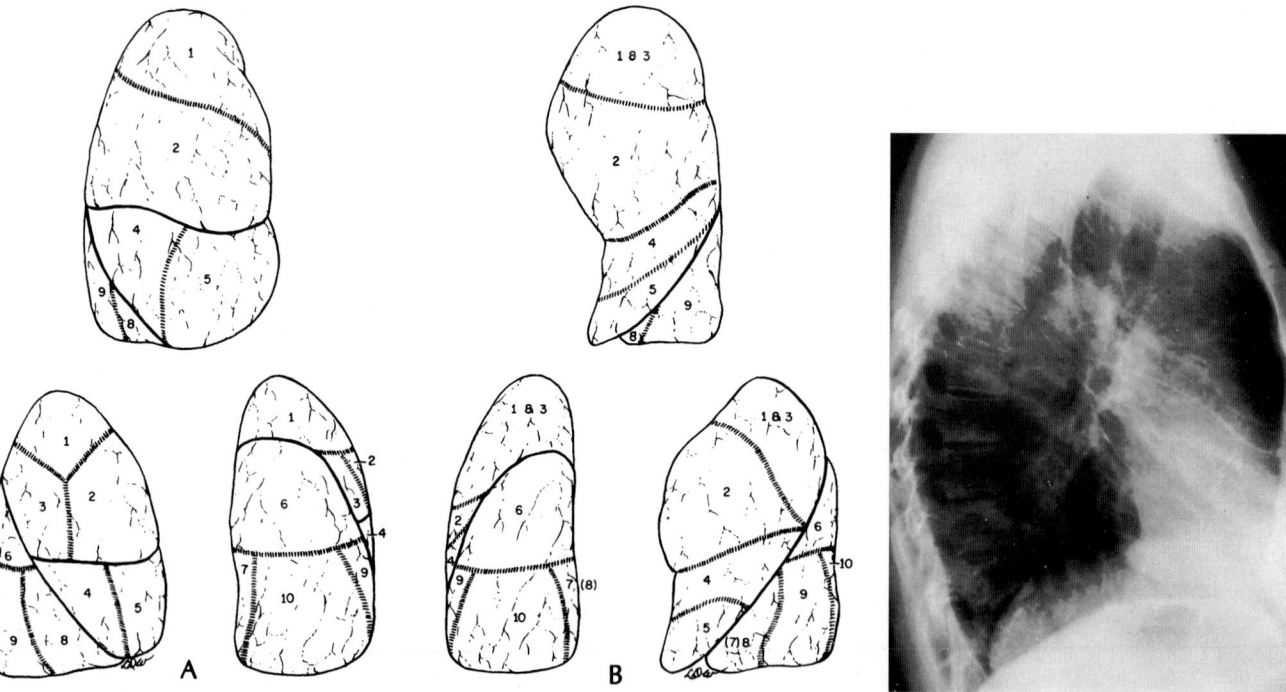

Fig. 9-15. A. Topographic positions of the bronchopulmonary segments of the right lung seen in the anterior, lateral, and posterior views. **B.** Topographic positions of the bronchopulmonary segments of the left lung seen in the anterior, lateral, and posterior views. **C.** Radiograph revealing the major fissures bilaterally and minor fissure on the right. Patient had interstitial edema and fluid in the fissures.

(see Supplementary Radiographic Views, previously in this chapter).

Fluoroscopy is an excellent technique for transthoracic needle aspiration biopsy of pulmonary lesions. Being able to visualize the lesion in real time is a significant advantage over CT-guided biopsy and decreases the time of the biopsy considerably. However, small lesions may not be evident in two projections on fluoroscopy, and CT guidance is needed. Real-time CT guidance systems are becoming available. This allows biopsy of small "moving" lesions adjacent to vital structures.

LUNG

The anatomic positions of the lung and the normal fissures are described in Chapter 5. The interlobar septa or major fissures are frequently visible on chest radiography (Fig. 9-15) and are of great help in assessing loss of volume in any of the lobes. Anomalous septa are not uncommon. Any pulmonary segment may have an anomalous fissure between that segment and the remainder of the lobe, resulting in an accessory lobe. The most common anomalous fissures are the superior and inferior accessory fissures. The superior accessory fissure occurs in 5% of anatomic specimens and separates the superior segment of the lower lobe from the basilar segments. The inferior accessory fissure occurs in approximately 30% of anatomic specimens and separates the medial basal segment of the right lower lobe from the remainder of the right lower lobe. Another commonly seen anatomic fissure is the azygos fissure, which extends superolaterally from the azygos vein to the apex of the right lung. This fissure is seen in 1% of specimens and does not create a true accessory lobe, as do most other anomalous fissures. More often than not, the fissures are incomplete. This allows collateral air drift between lobes of the lung. It also may account for peripheral distribution of pleural effusions as they are prevented from uniform distribution through the incomplete fissure (see Fig. 9-15).

Each lobe of the lung is divided into several pulmonary segments, each of which is supplied by a segmental bronchus. Various names have been applied to the pulmonary subsegments. The widely used classification of

Jackson and Huber (1943) and the numeric classification of Boyden (1955) are presented in Table 9-1 and are illustrated in Figure 9-15. The pulmonary segments may undergo consolidation or atelectasis. The characteristic configuration of pulmonary consolidation of the various segments is schematically presented in Figures 9-16 through 9-20. Occasionally, consolidation of an anomalous pulmonary segment can be recognized on routine radiography. Identification of a segmental distribution of an opacity is helpful in developing a differential diagnosis.

The pulmonary arteries accompany the bronchial tree and exhibit a segmental distribution similar to that of the bronchial tree. The pulmonary veins are slightly larger than the arteries and lie lateral to them in the upper lobes and somewhat more horizontal in the lower lobes. The pulmonary veins run in the intralobular septa, whereas the arteries and bronchi are distributed centrally in the pulmonary lobules. It frequently is possible to distinguish between the arteries and veins on routine radiography of the chest.

Table 9-1. Bronchopulmonary Segments

	A. Right lung	C. Upper lobe	B. Left lung
Apical	1	Superior division	
Anterior	2	Apical posterior	1 + 3
Posterior	3	Anterior	2
		1. Inferior division, lingula	
		Superior lingular	4
		Inferior lingular	5
		D. Middle lobe	
Lateral	4		
Medial	5		
		E. Lower lobe	
Superior	6	Superior	6
Medial basal	7	Anteromedial basal	7 + 8
Anterior basal	8	Lateral basal	9
Lateral basal	9	Posterior basal	10
Posterior basal	10		

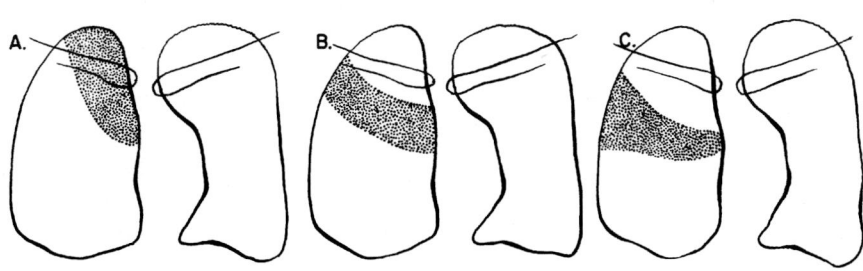

Fig. 9-16. Consolidation of the right upper lobe. A. Apical segment. B. Posterior segment. C. Anterior segment.

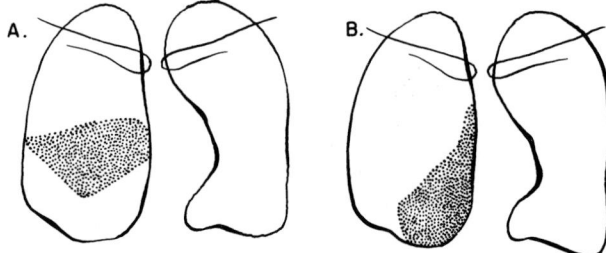

Fig. 9-17. Consolidation of the right middle lobe. **A.** Lateral segment. **B.** Medial segment.

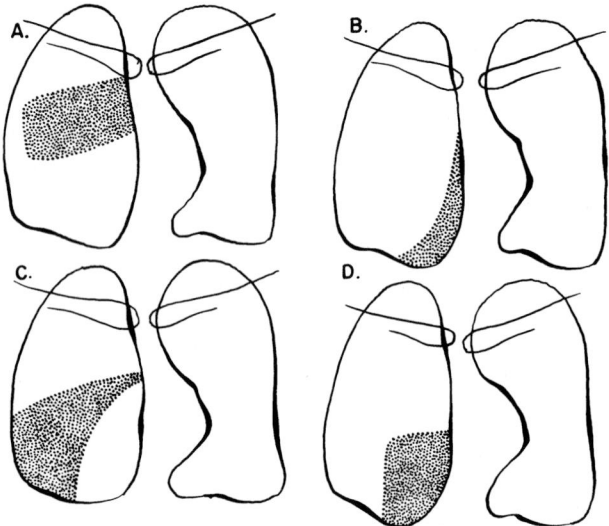

Fig. 9-18. Consolidation of the right lower lobe. **A.** Superior segment. **B.** Medial basal segment. **C.** Lateral basal segment. **D.** Posterior basal segment.

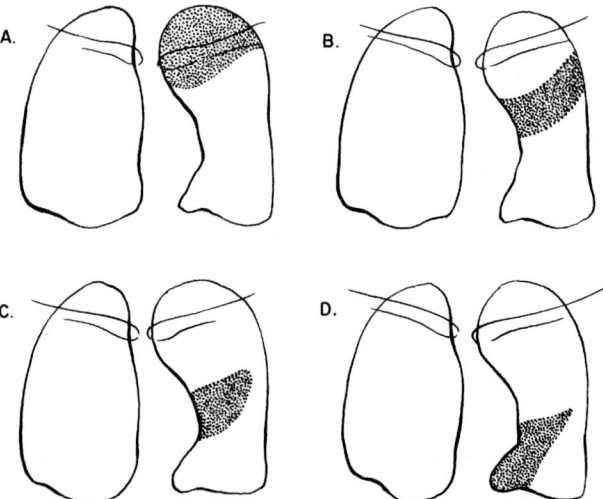

Fig. 9-19. Consolidation of the left upper lobe. **A.** Apical posterior segment. **B.** Anterior segment. **C.** Lingular segment, superior division. **D.** Lingular segment, inferior division.

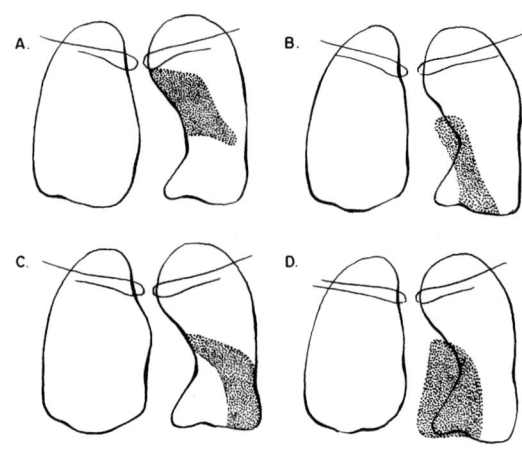

Fig. 9-20. Consolidation of the left lower lobe. **A.** Superior segment. **B.** Lateral basal segment. **C.** Anteromedial basal segment. **D.** Posterior basal segment.

MEDIASTINUM

The heart occupies the major part of the lower half of the mediastinum anterior to the spine. On the PA radiograph, the transverse diameter of the heart is normally one-half or less of the maximum transverse diameter of the chest. Detailed discussion of the anatomy and pathology of the heart is beyond the scope of this text. Figure 9-4 demonstrates the normal position of the cardiac chambers and the great vessels in the PA and lateral projections.

Anatomists divide the mediastinum into the superior and inferior mediastinum and into anterior, middle, and posterior compartments. For the surgeon, designation of superior and inferior compartments is of little importance. What is important, however, is the division of the mediastinum into three compartments: the anterior, middle (visceral), and posterior or paravertebral compartments, as seen on the lateral radiograph (see Chapter 148).

In the anatomic division of the mediastinum, the heart, aorta, and brachiocephalic vessels bound the anterior compartment posteriorly and the sternum bounds it anteriorly. The middle mediastinum contains the heart, ascending aorta, great vessels, trachea, main stem bronchi, and esophagus. The *posterior mediastinum* in reality is nonexistent and should be considered to be the two paravertebral sulci. The radiologic classification of mediastinal lesions becomes simple when one includes the descending aorta and the esophagus in the middle (visceral) compartment, and those structures that lie posterior to the anterior spinal ligament in the paravertebral areas or posterior compartments. Thus, arbitrary divisions can be made on the lateral radiograph (Fig. 9-21) to divide the mediastinum into these three compartments.

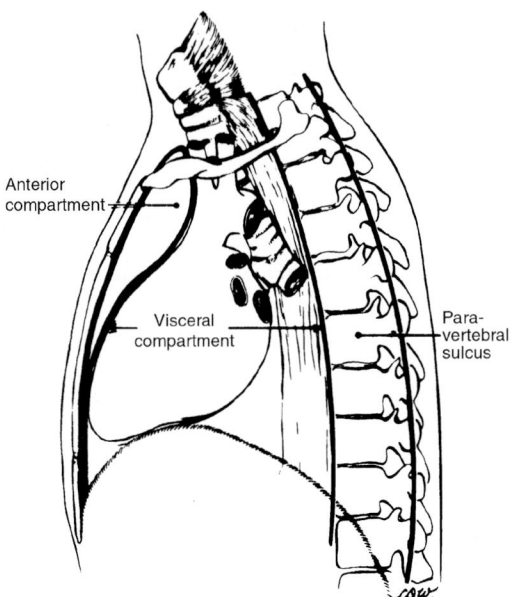

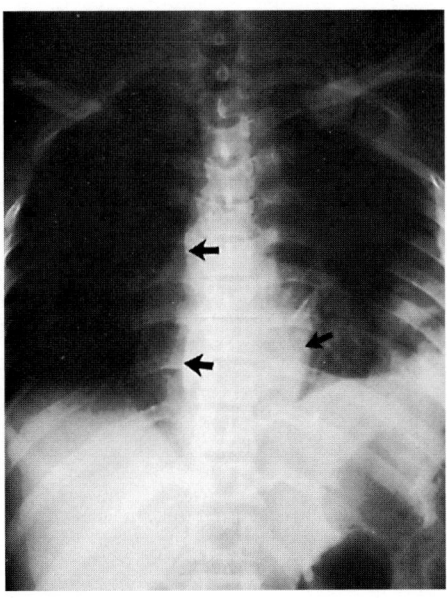

Fig. 9-21. The mediastinal compartments. The anterior compartment is defined by an imaginary line from the anterior border of the trachea extended to the xiphoid. The middle or visceral compartment is defined by the posterior margin of the anterior mediastinum and posteriorly by the anterior border of the spine. The posterior or paravertebral compartment lies behind the anterior margin of the spine.

Various lines or stripes occur about the mediastinum on the PA radiograph. Displacement of these stripes is often indicative of mediastinal pathology. These stripes are described by Groskin (1993) in Heitzman's *The Lung, Radiographic-Pathologic Correlations.*

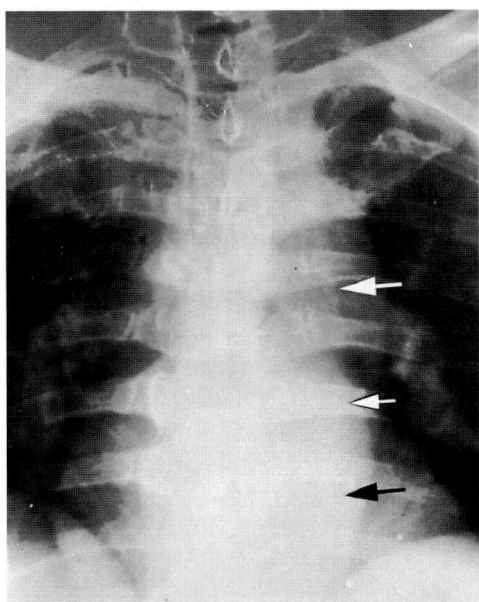

Fig. 9-22. Paraspinal line is seen only on the left in most patients. It increases in width with ectasia or tortuosity of the aorta, as in this patient (*arrows*).

Fig. 9-23. Tuberculosis of the spine. Displacement of paraspinal line (*arrows*) on the right secondary to tuberculous abscess.

The paraspinal line, as Brailsford (1943) described, is a longitudinal density lying to the left of the thoracic spine (Fig. 9-22). The paraspinal line is related to the left-sided position of the descending aorta and is seen on the right side if the descending aorta is present on the right. Ordinarily, no paraspinal line is seen on the right, but in patients with large hypertrophic spurs, the spurs may push the paraspinal line out, making it visible. Tumors or inflammatory processes involving the vertebral bodies and paravertebral space characteristically displace the paraspinal line (Fig. 9-23). The line is ordinarily less than 1 cm from the left border of the vertebral column, but in some people, it may lie normally as far as 3 cm to the left of the vertebral column (see Fig. 9-22). This is usually the result of a tortuous or ectatic aorta.

The anterior junction line is an oblique linear density presenting from right to left downward over the trachea for a distance of several centimeters (Fig. 9-24). The line is produced by the contiguous pleura of the right and left upper lobes as they touch anterior to the great vessels. The posterior junction line results similarly from contiguous pleura behind the trachea and above the transverse aorta. This line is differentiated from the anterior junction line by the fact that it extends above the clavicles.

The inferior esophageal pleural interface represents the medial border of the right lung in the azygoesophageal recess and lies posterior to the heart and anterior to the azygos vein. The lung in the recess outlines the right side of the distal esophagus (see Fig. 9-24). The superior esophageal pleural stripe is slightly higher than the anterior junction line and is slightly to the left. It represents the apposition of the two lungs against the esophagus in the retrotracheal area of the upper mediastinum. All of these mediastinal lines and interfaces can be displaced by lesions in the adjacent mediastinum.

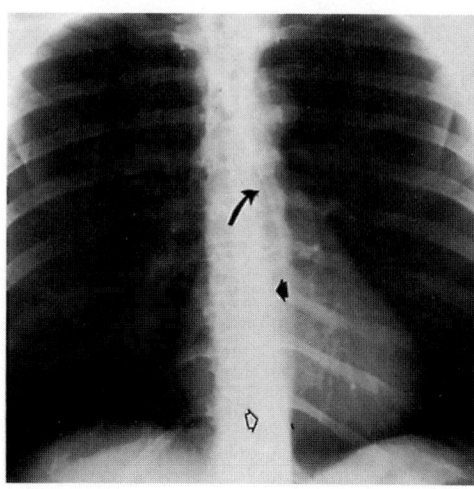

Fig. 9-24. Mediastinal lines and interfaces. Anterior junction line (*curved arrow*); paraspinal stripe (*short closed arrow*); and azygoesophageal recess (*open arrow*).

DIAPHRAGM AND CHEST WALL

The diaphragm is a musculotendinous structure that separates the thorax from the abdomen. It is divided into right and left hemidiaphragms. The hemidiaphragm is usually lower on the side where the heart is anatomically placed in the absence of displacement caused by some pathologic process. Thus, the right hemidiaphragm is usually higher than the left. Felson (1973) found, in a series of 500 normal chests, that the left hemidiaphragm was at a level even with or higher than the right in 9% of the subjects.

Variations of diaphragmatic contour are frequent. Most commonly, a segment of the diaphragm is elevated because of a lack of muscle in the segment (localized eventration). Fluoroscopy is helpful in distinguishing between eventration and paralysis.

The chest wall is composed of the bones and muscles of the thoracic cage. The bones are readily identifiable on radiography because of their increased radiographic density. The muscular shadows are not readily identifiable except when absent or occasionally hypertrophied. In a well-positioned chest radiograph, the overall lucency of both hemithoraces should be the same. If they are discrepant, the differential diagnosis includes either added soft tissue density as in pleural effusion or chest wall hematoma, as well as decreased soft tissue density, which is frequently the result of mastectomy.

ABNORMAL CHEST

Abnormalities of the Lung

Radiographic images result from the differential absorption or attenuation of the x-ray by various body tissues.

Bone, soft tissue, fat, and air absorb different amounts of energy from the x-ray beam and thus can be distinguished radiographically. The chest is admirably suited for detection of pathology for one major reason: The lung contains air in the bronchi and alveoli, producing excellent contrast between the lung and the adjacent structures or soft tissue densities. The lungs are involved frequently with local or systemic diseases that may appear on radiography as abnormally increased density and increased grayness, but occasionally as increased lucency or blackness to the lungs. It is important for the radiologist and the surgeon to recognize certain primary patterns of abnormal density occurring in the lungs as these patterns often indicate the nature of the patient's illness.

Atelectasis

Atelectasis, or collapse, is loss of volume of the lung, lobe, or segment from any cause. Fraser and Paré (1989) list five mechanisms of atelectasis. Resorption atelectasis occurs secondary to obstruction of a major bronchus or multiple small bronchi. For the surgeon, this type of atelectasis is the most important because it is often secondary to obstruction of a major bronchus either by tumor, foreign body, or bronchial mucus plug. Passive atelectasis occurs secondary to a space-occupying process in the thorax, particularly pneumothorax or hydrothorax. Compression atelectasis is a localized parenchymal collapse contiguous to a space-occupying pulmonary mass or bulla. Adhesive atelectasis denotes collapse occurring in the presence of patent bronchi, presumably secondary to abnormalities of surfactant. The most frequent presentation of this is subsegmental or platelike atelectasis as described by Westcott and Cole (1985). This form of atelectasis occurs in association with pneumonia. Cicatrization atelectasis results from pulmonary fibrosis or scarring, either localized or general.

Several radiographic signs suggest atelectasis. The most reliable sign of collapse is displacement of interlobar fissures. Localized increase in density of the collapsed lobe is another reliable sign of atelectasis. Indirect signs of atelectasis include elevation of the hemidiaphragm of the ipsilateral side; deviation of the trachea and other mediastinal structures toward the involved side; compensatory hyperaeration of the rest of the ipsilateral lung, and sometimes of the contralateral lung, with herniation of the contralateral upper lobe across the mediastinum; displacement of the hilus toward the collapsed lobe or segment; and decrease in size of the bony hemithorax of the involved side. These indirect signs are ordinarily seen only with atelectasis of major segments of the lung. They are less reliable than the direct signs and can occasionally be simulated by normal anatomic variations.

Certain fundamental observations can be made about lobar collapse. The proximal portion of the lobe is teth-

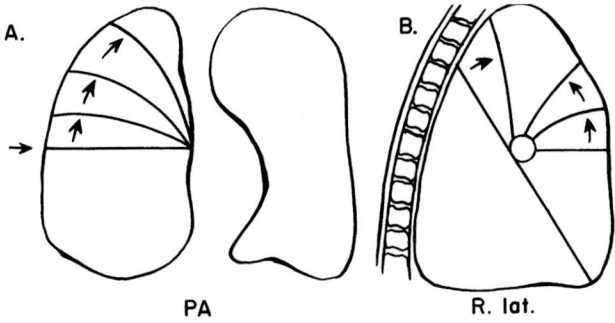

Fig. 9-25. Lobar collapse of the right upper lobe. PA, posteroanterior; R. lat., right lateral. From Lubert M, Crause GB: Patterns of lobar collapse as observed radiographically. *Radiology* 56:165, 1951. With permission.

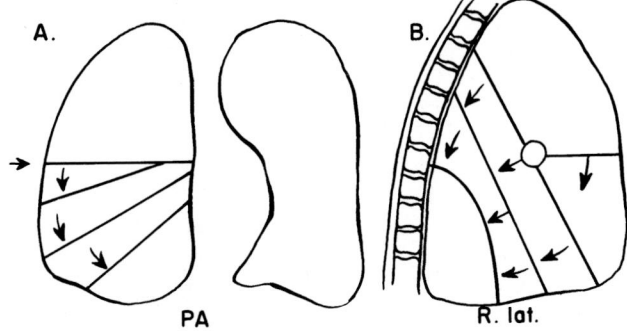

Fig. 9-27. Lobar collapse of the right lower lobe. PA, posteroanterior; R. lat., right lateral. From Lubert M, Crause GB: Patterns of lobar collapse as observed radiographically. *Radiology* 56:165, 1951. With permission.

ered to the hilus and consequently the radiographic shadow of the collapsed lobe always points toward the hilus. Lobar collapse always occurs toward the mediastinum on the PA view. On the lateral radiograph, the upper lobe collapses anteriorly, the lower lobe collapses posteriorly, and the middle lobe symmetrically decreases in volume.

Lubert and Krause (1951) described the radiographic patterns of lobar collapse, and Woodring and Reed (1996) correlated this with CT scans. The patterns of lower lobe collapse are similar on the right and left sides, whereas the patterns of upper lobe collapse are slightly different. Figures 9-25 through 9-29 show schematic representations of lobar collapse, as described by Lubert and Krause (1951).

Recognition of the presence of a collapsed lobe is frequently difficult, particularly if the collapse is almost complete (Figs. 9-30 through 9-37). Of great help in identifying the presence of atelectasis is the silhouette sign, popularized by Felson (1973). The sign is based on the premise that consolidation of a segment or lobe of a lung contiguous with the border of the heart, aorta, diaphragm,

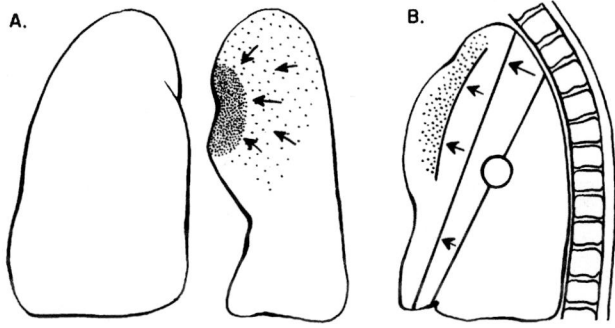

Fig. 9-28. Lobar collapse of the left upper lobe. **A.** Posteroanterior view. **B.** Lateral view. From Lubert M, Crause GB: Patterns of lobar collapse as observed radiographically. *Radiology* 56:165, 1951. With permission.

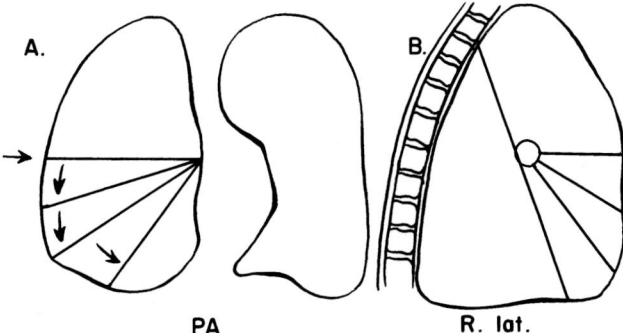

Fig. 9-26. Lobar collapse of the right middle lobe. PA, posteroanterior; R. lat., right lateral. From Lubert M, Crause GB: Patterns of lobar collapse as observed radiographically. *Radiology* 56:165, 1951. With permission.

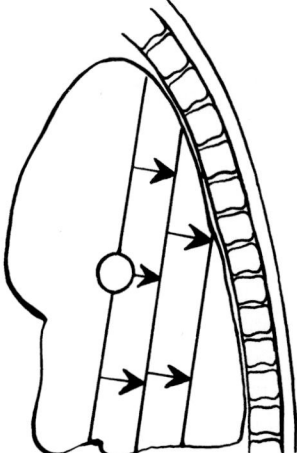

Fig. 9-29. Lobar collapse of the left lower lobe lateral view. From Lubert M, Crause GB: Patterns of lobar collapse as observed radiographically. *Radiology* 56:165, 1951. With permission.

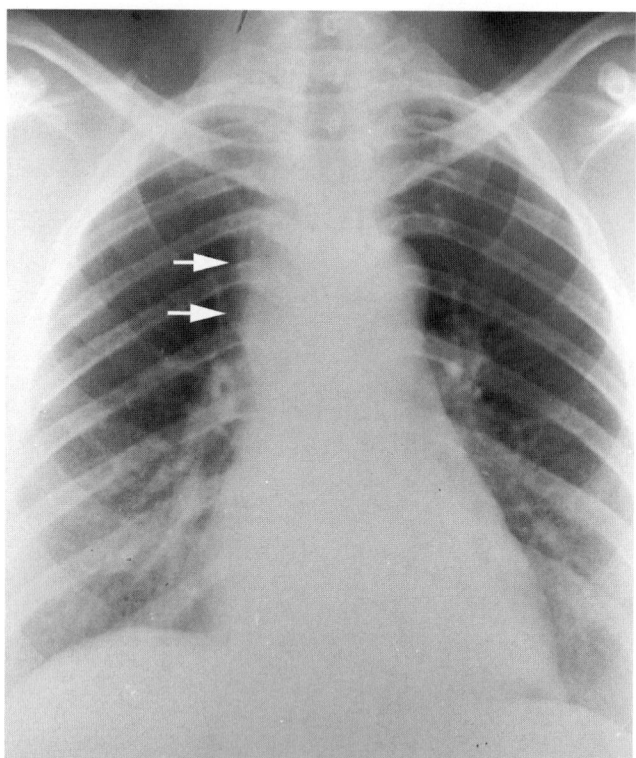

A

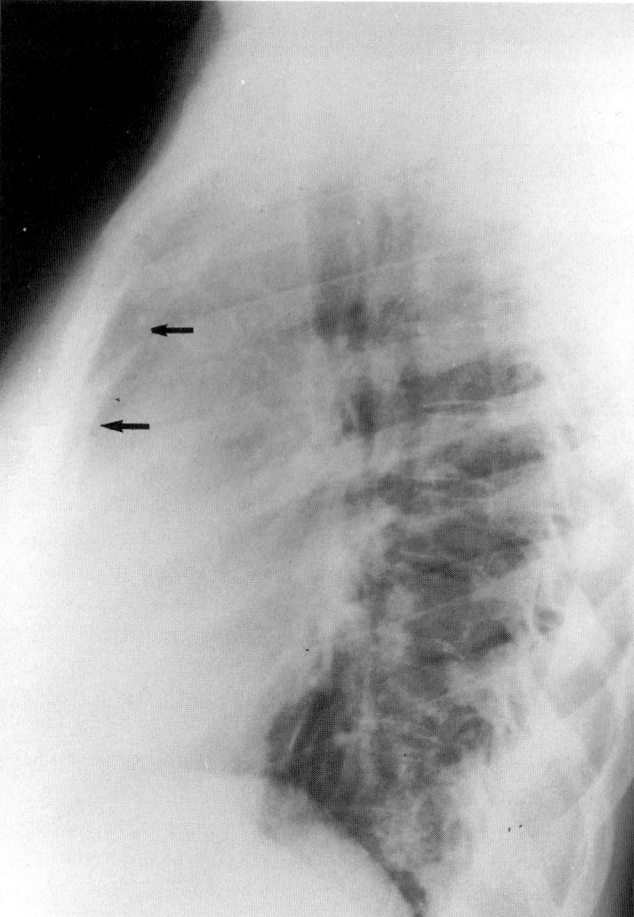

B

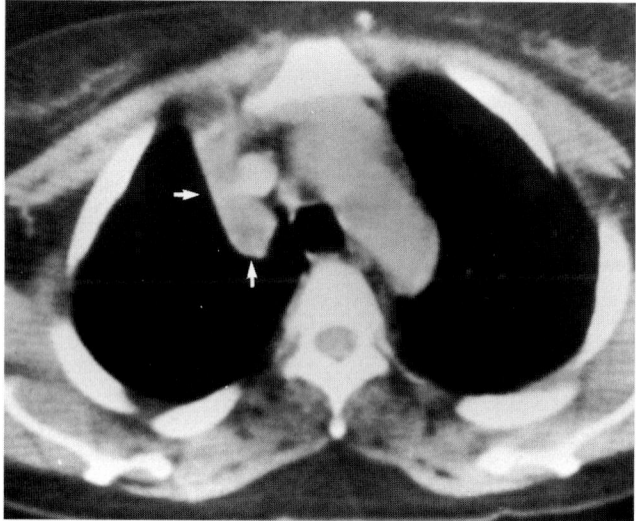

C

Fig. 9-30. Right upper lobe atelectasis. **A.** Posteroanterior view demonstrates the collapsed right upper lobe causing haziness and widening of the right upper mediastinal border (*arrows*). **B.** Lateral view shows retrosternal soft tissue density (*arrows*) that is the collapsed right upper lobe. **C.** Computed tomographic scan shows wedge-shaped collapsed right upper lobe to the right of the mediastinum (*arrows*).

or mediastinum obliterates that portion of the border of the radiograph. Frequently, this obliteration of a heart border or a fuzziness of the diaphragm is the first clue to the presence of atelectasis. The observation of atelectasis is important because it may indicate an endobronchial tumor or acutely may be the explanation for a sudden decrease in oxygenation, particularly in the ICU (see Fig. 9-36). Occasionally the whole lung collapses. In the acute setting the cause is usually mucus plugging (Fig. 9-37A).

It is important to distinguish this from pleural effusion or surgical absence of the lung (Fig. 9-37B). Decrease in the volume of the opaque hemithorax and shift of the mediastinum to the opaque side are reliable indicators that the lung is absent or collapsed, and thoracentesis or chest tube placement is not indicated. On the other hand, shift of the mediastinum away from the opaque hemithorax indicates space-occupying tissue, either fluid or tumor (Fig. 9-37C).

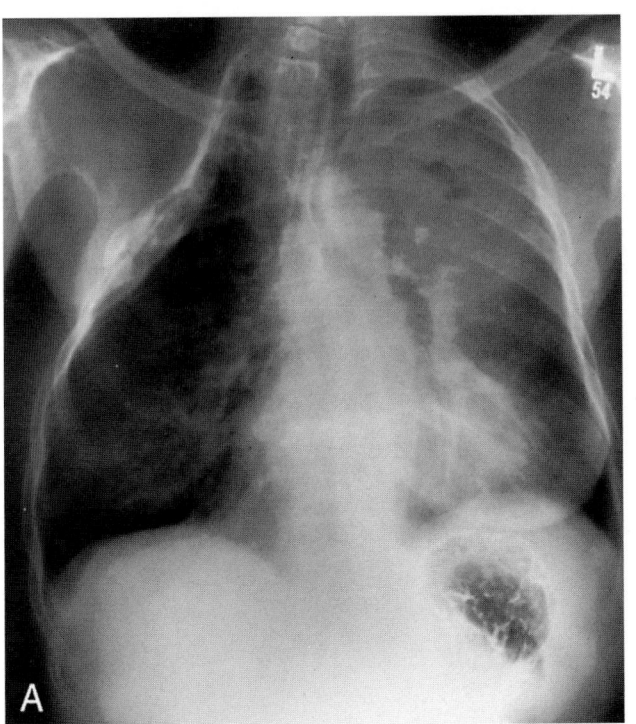
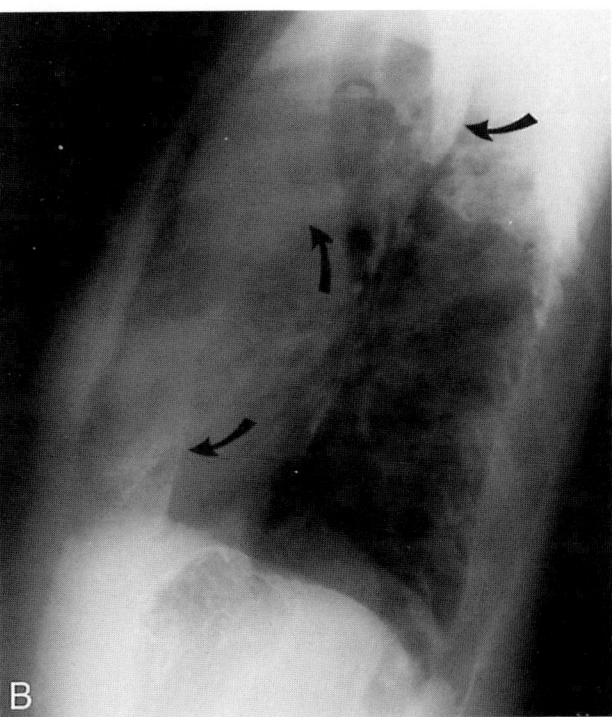

Fig. 9-31. Left upper lobe atelectasis related to tumor. **A.** Posteroanterior radiograph shows an old thoracoplasty on the right. On the left, note hazy density over the left upper lung field with loss of definition of the left cardiac border, characteristic of left upper lobe atelectasis. A small collection of air can be seen over the left second anterior rib, representing a cavity within necrotic tumor. **B.** Lateral view shows the left major fissure (*arrows*) to be pulled forward in its lower portion but bulging in its upper portion. This characteristic *s* sign is seen when a lobe collapses around a tumor. The tumor is a large cavitary mass in the upper lobe but not involving the lingula, which collapses anteriorly.

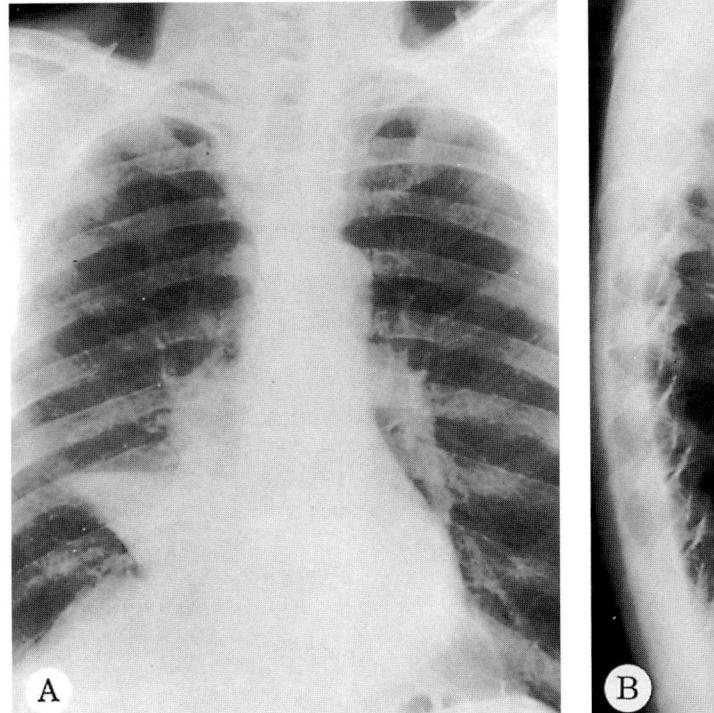
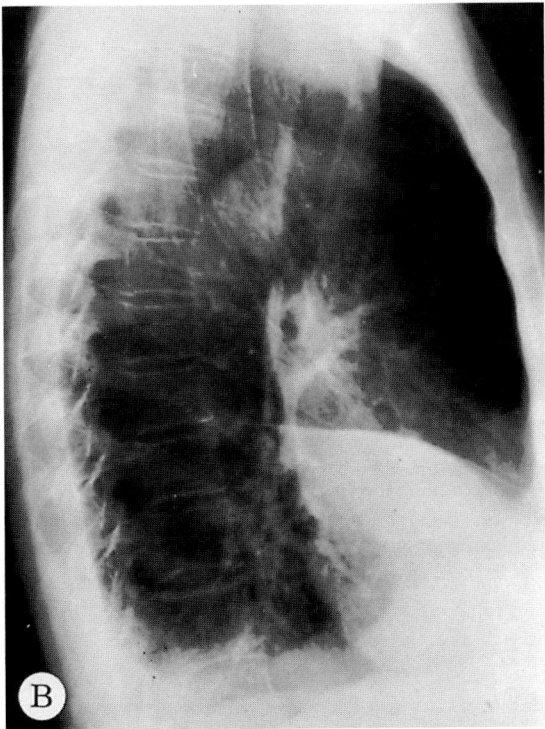

Fig. 9-32. Carcinoma with right middle lobe collapse. **A.** Posteroanterior radiograph shows obliteration of the right cardiac border by the collapsed right middle lobe (silhouette sign) with an associated mass in the right hilus. **B.** The approximation of major and minor fissures can be noted on the lateral view.

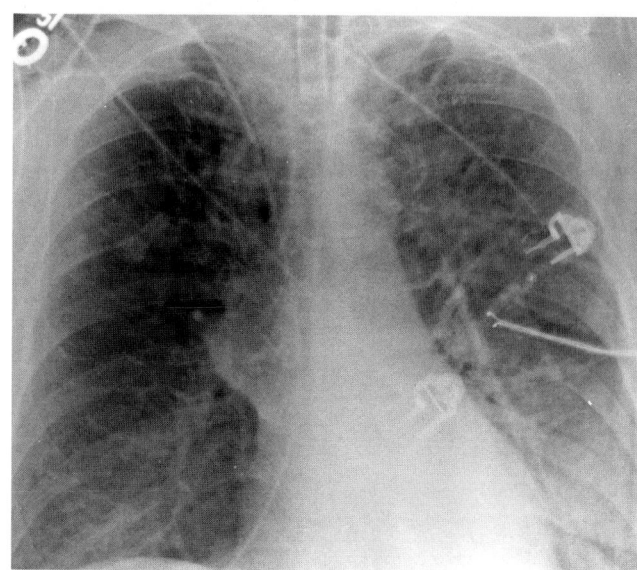

A

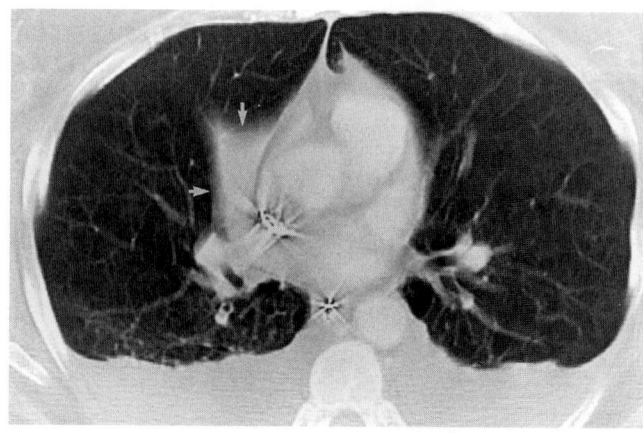

B

Fig. 9-33. Right middle lobe collapse simulating mass at the right hilum. **A.** Anteroposterior view of chest demonstrates mass opacity at right hilum that appeared in 1 day. **B.** Computed tomographic scan demonstrates mass to be result of collapsed middle lobe.

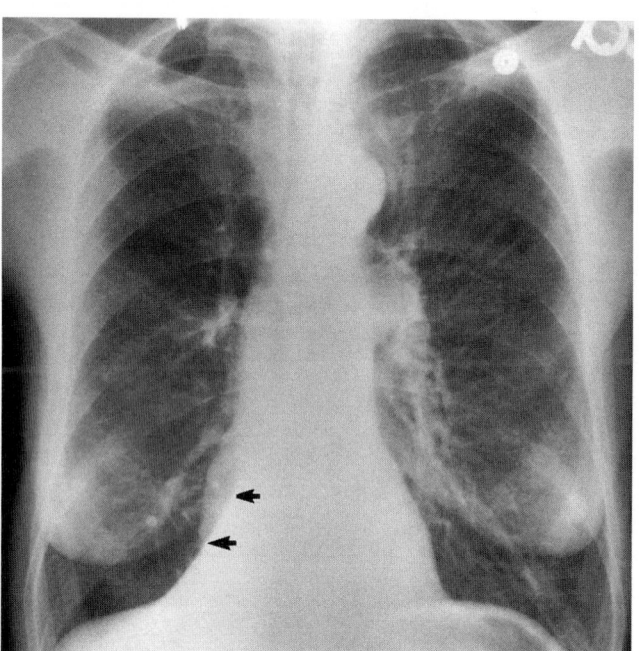

A

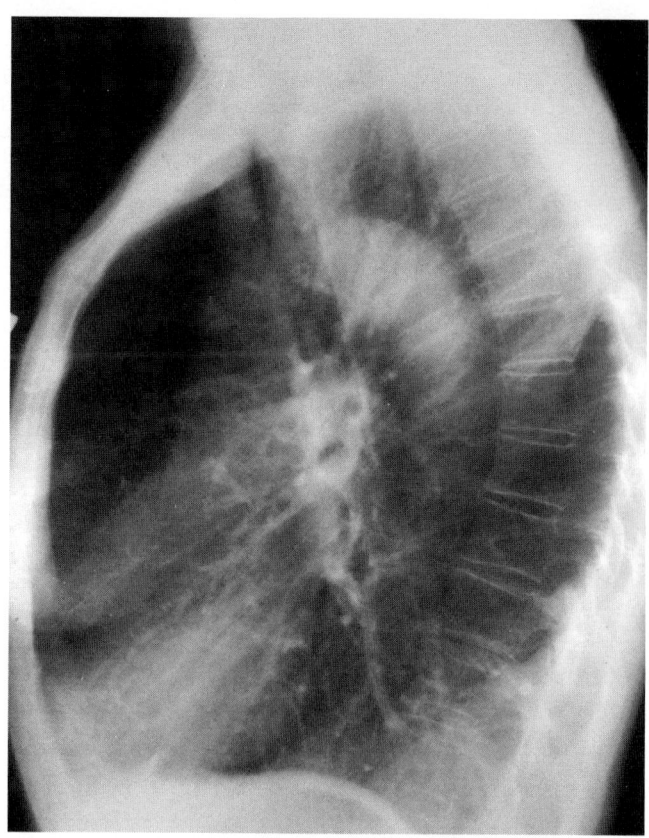

B

Fig. 9-34. Right lower lobe atelectasis. **A.** Posteroanterior film demonstrates triangular opacity superimposed over right-sided heart border that obliterates the medial right hemidiaphragm (*arrows*); this is the collapsed right lower lobe. **B.** Lateral film shows only one diaphragm, left, as the right is obscured by non-aerated right lower lobe (silhouette sign).

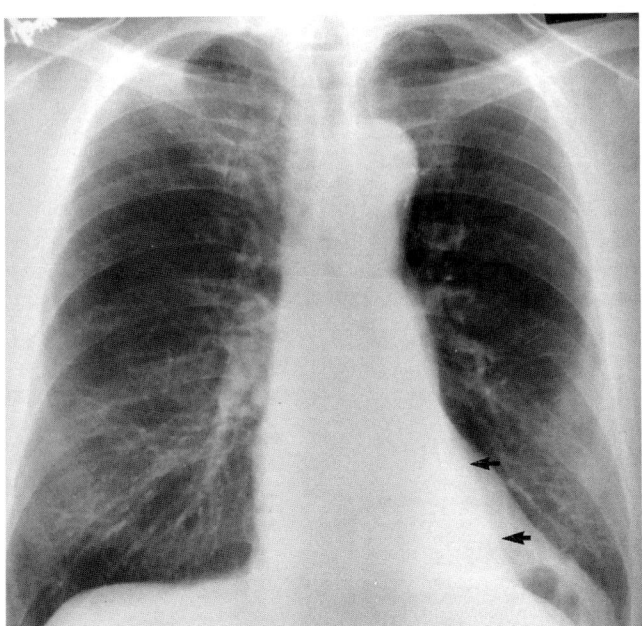

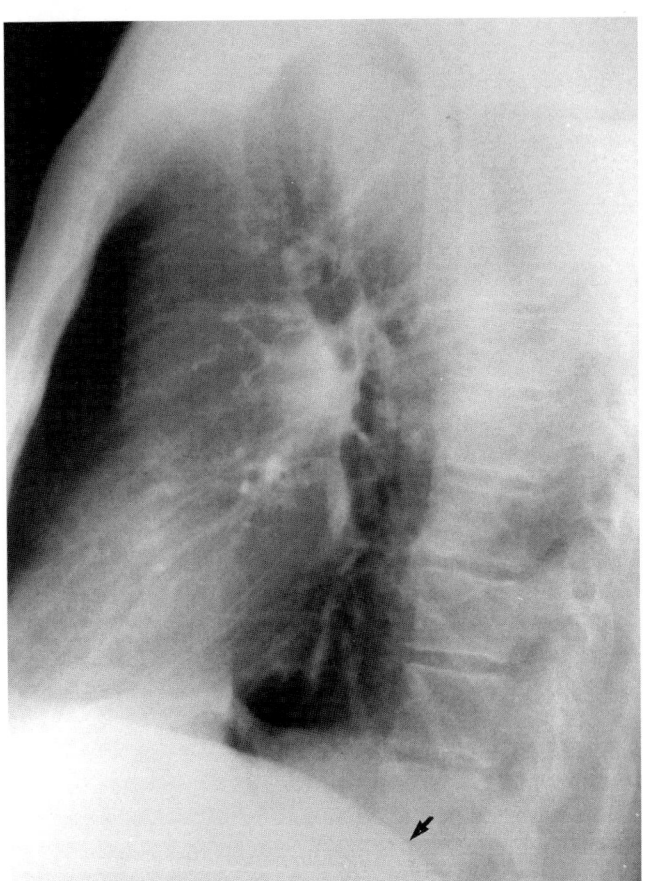

Fig. 9-35. Left lower lobe atelectasis. **A.** Posteroanterior film demonstrates triangular opacity seen over left-sided heart (*arrows*), obliterating left hemidiaphragm medially. Note also small left hilus as interlobar artery is shifted down with the collapsed left lower lobe. **B.** Lateral view shows obliteration of posterior left hemidiaphragm secondary to collapsed left lower lobe (*arrow*). Note similarity to findings of right lower lobe atelectasis (see Fig. 9-34).

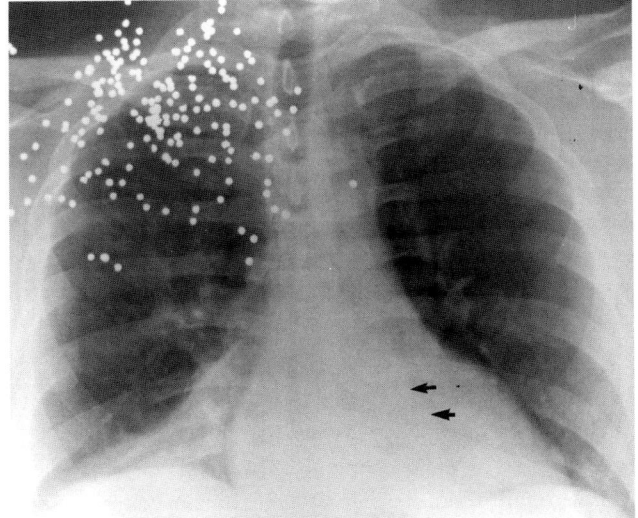

Fig. 9-36. Bilateral lower lobe collapse. Anteroposterior supine portable chest view shows bilateral triangular opacities at bases from collapse of both right and left lower lobes (*arrows*). This occurred postoperatively and the patient's resulting shortness of breath was thought to be from pulmonary embolism, as the atelectasis was not appreciated. No evidence of pulmonary embolus existed on ventilation-perfusion scan.

Diffuse Pulmonary Disease

The air spaces and vessels are enveloped and supported by the connective tissue skeleton of the lung. The basic unit of lung function is the secondary pulmonary lobule, which is composed of three to five terminal bronchioles. The terminal bronchiole is the smallest purely air-conducting bronchus in which no gas exchange takes place (Fig. 9-38). Each of these secondary lobules is separated from its neighboring secondary lobules by connective tissue envelopes or septa that are continuous with the pleural surface of the lung. The pulmonary veins and lymphatics run in these connective tissue septa. The peripheral connective tissue is contiguous with the axial connective tissue that acts as a sheath about the bronchovascular bundles, as stated by Weibel and Gil (1977), and provides structural support for the lung. Passages for gas exchange exist between secondary lobules, the pores of Kohn, and between peribronchial alveoli, the canals of Lambert. The intralobular septa are also incomplete. This arrangement, according to Groskin (1993), accounts in part for the radiographic appearance of peribronchial disease and nonuniform air space disease. The aforementioned author also notes that the distribution of the interstitial connective

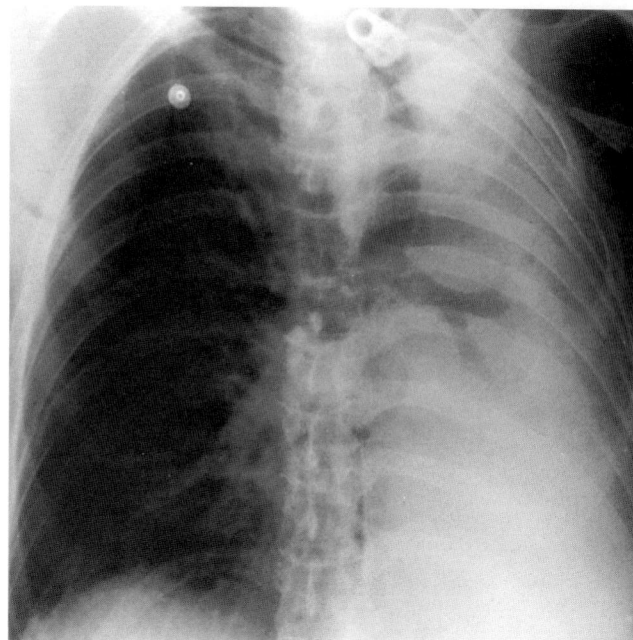

A

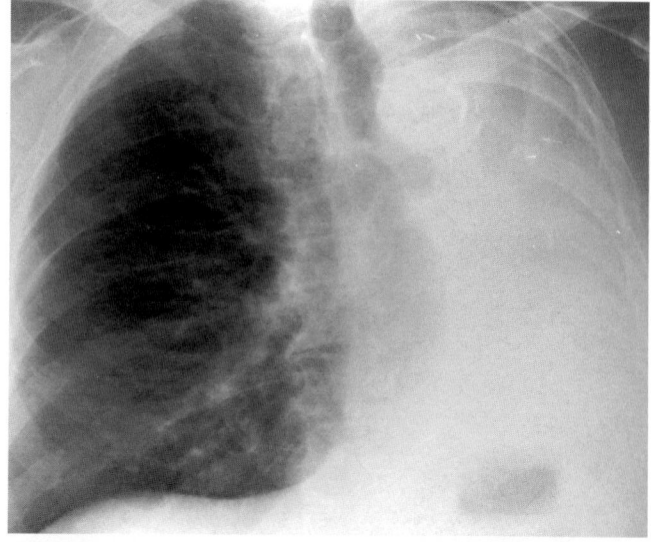

B

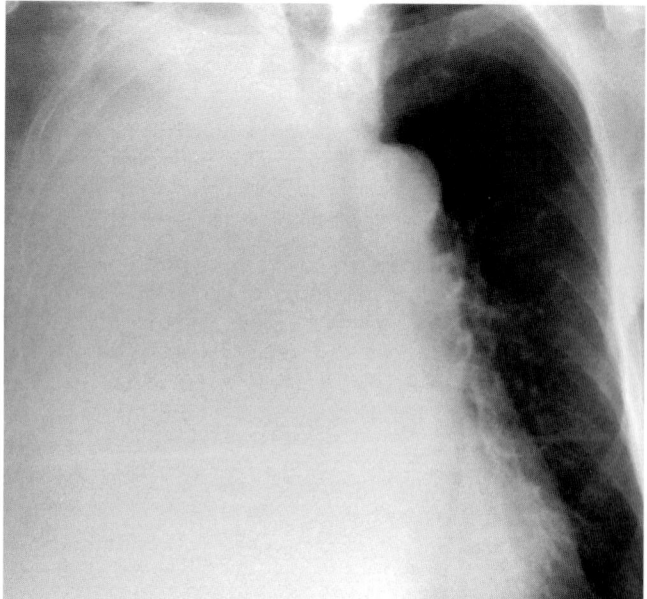

C

Fig. 9-37. Complete opacification of a hemithorax. **A.** An opaque left hemithorax with shift of the mediastinum to the left is shown. This occurred over 1 day in the intensive care unit. Note the patent bronchi on the left to the left upper and lower lobes. This is the result of collapse from mucus plugging as found at bronchoscopy. **B.** Opaque left hemithorax with mediastinum shifted to the left ipsilateral side is demonstrated. Surgical clips on the left and cut-off of left main stem bronchus indicate that patient has had a pneumonectomy. **C.** An opaque right hemithorax with shift *away* from the opaque thorax to the left, the contralateral side, is seen. This indicates mass effect of fluid, tumor, or both. An endobronchial lesion cannot be inferred in this situation.

tissues accounts for the appearance of interstitial processes. Recognition of these resulting patterns, air space, interstitial, and nodular, enables the physician to limit the differential diagnosis in an individual patient to one that is appropriate to that particular clinical setting (Table 9-2).

Recognition of a pattern as alveolar (air space, interstitial, or reticulonodular) is helpful in directing further clinical evaluation of the patient.

The radiographic findings suggesting alveolar disease as enumerated by Groskin (1993) are 1) a lobar or segmental distribution, 2) poor margination of the opacity, 3) a tendency to coalesce, 4) the presence of air bronchograms (Fig. 9-39), and 5) a butterfly or batwing distribution (Fig. 9-40). The air bronchogram was described originally by Fleischner (1948) and has been popularized by Felson (1973). The air

bronchogram is a result of replacement of air in the distal alveolar spaces by fluid of any kind (e.g., blood, pus, or edema). In the normal lung, air in the bronchi both centrally and peripherally is not visible because the surrounding alveoli are filled with air and the bronchial walls are too thin to be visualized on plain radiography. When the alveolar air is replaced with fluid, the intrabronchial air becomes visible. Finally, rapidly changing pulmonary lesions favor alveolar disease over interstitial disease, which tends to change more slowly. Occasionally, pneumonia may present as a mass lesion (round pneumonia). This is more common in children than adults. Clinical history should suggest the diagnosis (Fig. 9-41).

Common causes of a diffuse alveolar pattern are pneumonia, pulmonary edema, bleeding into the alveoli, or aspira-

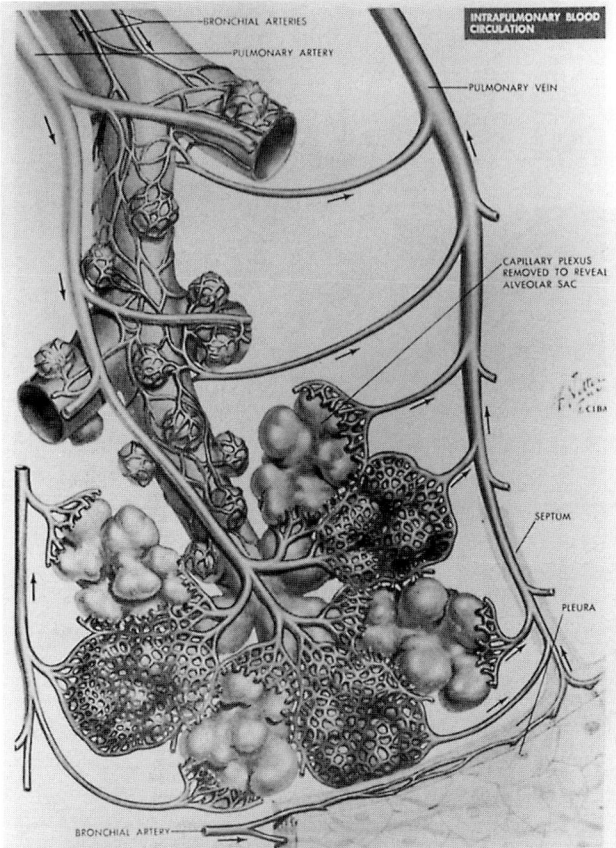

Fig. 9-38. Structure of terminal pulmonary air spaces. Note origin of two respiratory bronchioles from terminal bronchiole. Alveoli are seen to bud directly from respiratory bronchiole. Also demonstrated is primary pulmonary lobule composed of alveolar duct and lung subtended by it. Modified from Groskin SA: Heitzman's The Lung, Radiographic-Pathologic Correlations. St. Louis: Mosby–Year Book, 1993.

tion of blood or gastric contents into the alveoli. Less common causes of diffuse alveolar consolidation include parenchymal sarcoidosis, pulmonary alveolar proteinosis, metastatic carcinoma from many causes but especially breast carcinoma, and occasionally bronchioloalveolar cell carcinoma (see Table 9-2).

Interstitial disease is suggested when a reticulolinear pattern is seen. It results from thickening of the connective tissues of the lungs. Involvement of the peripheral connective tissue, intralobular septa, and subpleural space results in Kerley's lines as described in Shanks and Kerley's *Textbook of X-ray Diagnosis* (1951). Kerley's lines also may be seen in subpleural edema. All the Kerley's lines—A, B, and C—represent thickening of the intralobular septa from any cause: fluid, blood, cells, or fibrosis. The most frequent and easy to recognize are the Kerley's B lines. Kerley's B lines are linear shadows up to 1 cm in length, extending perpendicular to the pleural surfaces of the costophrenic angles (Fig. 9-42). Kerley's A lines radiate superiorly from the hila, and Kerley's C lines result in a reticulate appearance to the parenchyma, particularly at the lung bases. Involvement of

Table 9-2. Radiographic Patterns Produced by Pulmonary Disease

Disseminated alveolar diseases
  Acute
    Common
      Pulmonary edema
      Pneumonia
      Hemorrhage, including pulmonary infarction
      Hyaline membrane disease
  Chronic
    Common
      Alveolar proteinosis
      Alveolar cell carcinoma
      Lymphoma
      Sarcoid
    Rare
      Tuberculosis
      Fungus disease
      Alveolar microlithiasis
      Lipoid pneumonia
Pseudoalveolar appearance
  Interstitial pneumonia in an exudative phase
  Cellular filling of the air space
  Replacement of lung structure by interstitial process
    Granulomatous
    Cellular
    Fibrotic
Disseminated interstitial diseases
  Acute
    Common
      Interstitial pulmonary edema of any phase
  Chronic
    Common
      Idiopathic pulmonary fibrosis (chronic interstitial pneumonia)
      Tuberculosis
      Fungus disease
      Adult respiratory distress syndrome
      Radiation reaction in lung
      Scleroderma
      Pneumoconiosis
      Sarcoidosis
      Histiocytosis X
      Hodgkin's disease
    Rare
      Obstructed anomalous pulmonary venous return
      Pulmonary dysmaturity
      Rheumatoid lung
Disseminated nodular disease
  Acute
    Common
      Viral pneumonia
      Miliary tuberculosis
      Pulmonary edema
      Hyaline membrane disease
    Rare
      Metastases
      Miliary fungus disease
      Septic emboli
  Chronic
    Common
      Metastases
      Sarcoidosis
      Tuberculosis
      Fungus disease
      Pneumoconiosis
      Alveolar cell carcinoma
    Rare
      Lymphoma
      Histiocytosis X (early)
      Silo filler's disease

Adapted from Groskin SA: Heitzman's the Lung: Radiographic-Pathologic Correlations. St. Louis: Mosby–Year Book, 1993.

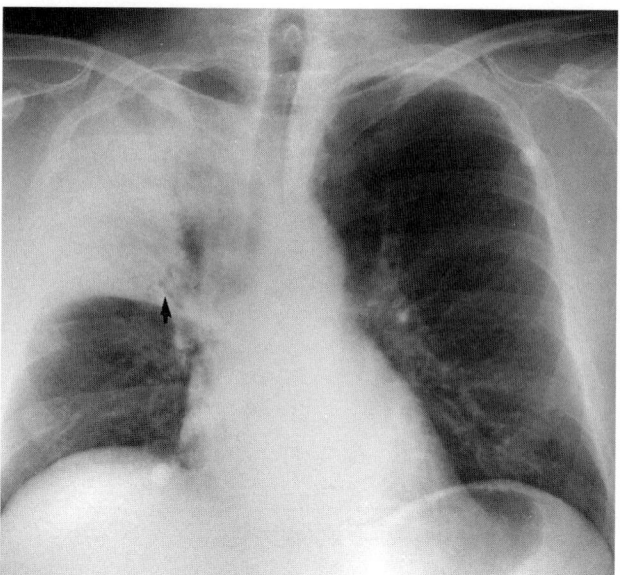

Fig. 9-39. Right upper lobe pneumonia. Note air bronchograms (*arrow*), branching radiolucencies, and lobar distribution indicative of air space disease.

the central connective tissue results in increased bronchovascular markings, hilar haze, and peribronchial cuffing as noted by Groskin (1993). Although these may be difficult to identify initially, recognition of Kerley's lines greatly aids in the differential diagnosis (see Table 9-2).

Common diseases causing a diffuse interstitial pattern include interstitial pulmonary edema, pneumoconiosis, sarcoidosis, metastatic tumor (both nodular and lymphangitic forms), diffuse interstitial pneumonia, collagen disease (e.g.,

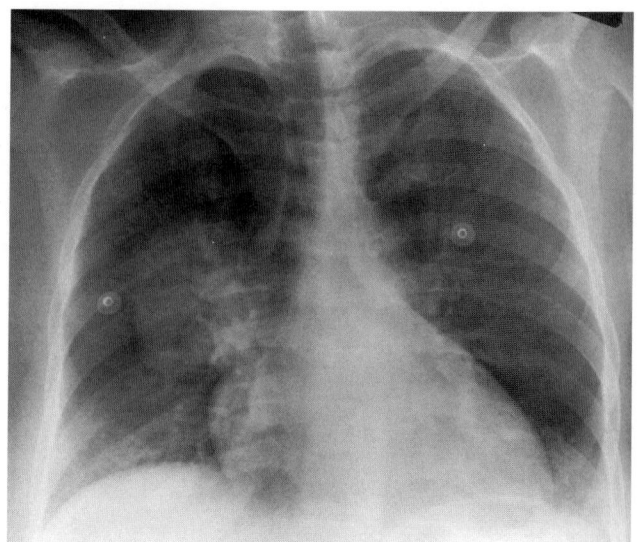

A

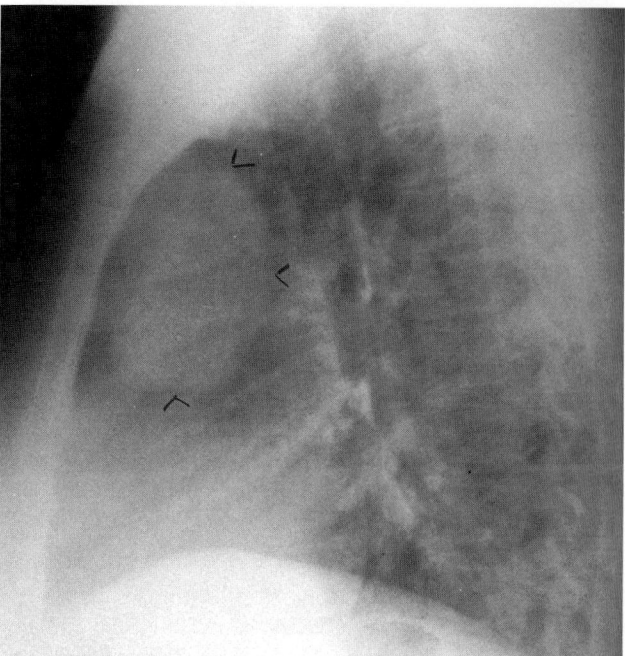

B

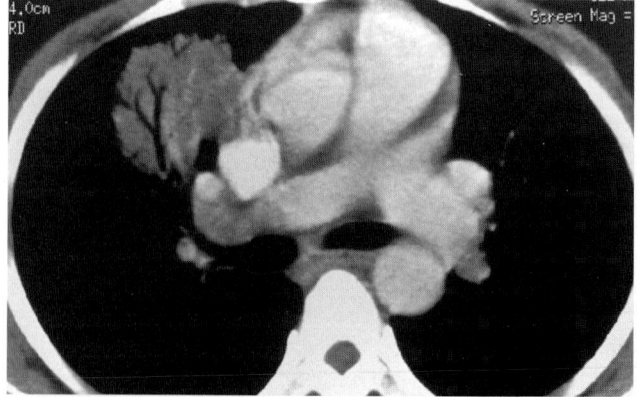

C

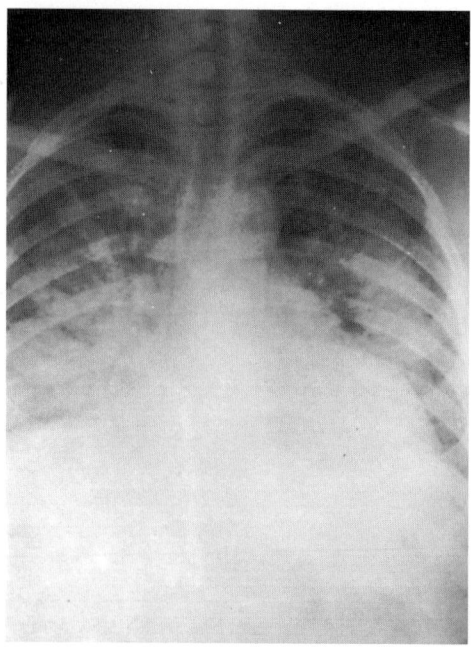

Fig. 9-40. Pulmonary edema. Note the patchy confluence of the diffuse alveolar pattern with a butterfly wing distribution.

Fig. 9-41. Round pneumonia. **A.** Posteroanterior view demonstrates a mass at the right hilum. **B.** This is anterior to the hilum on the lateral view (*arrowheads*). **C.** Computed tomography shows the presence of air bronchograms. Organism identified on culture was *Haemophilus influenzae*.

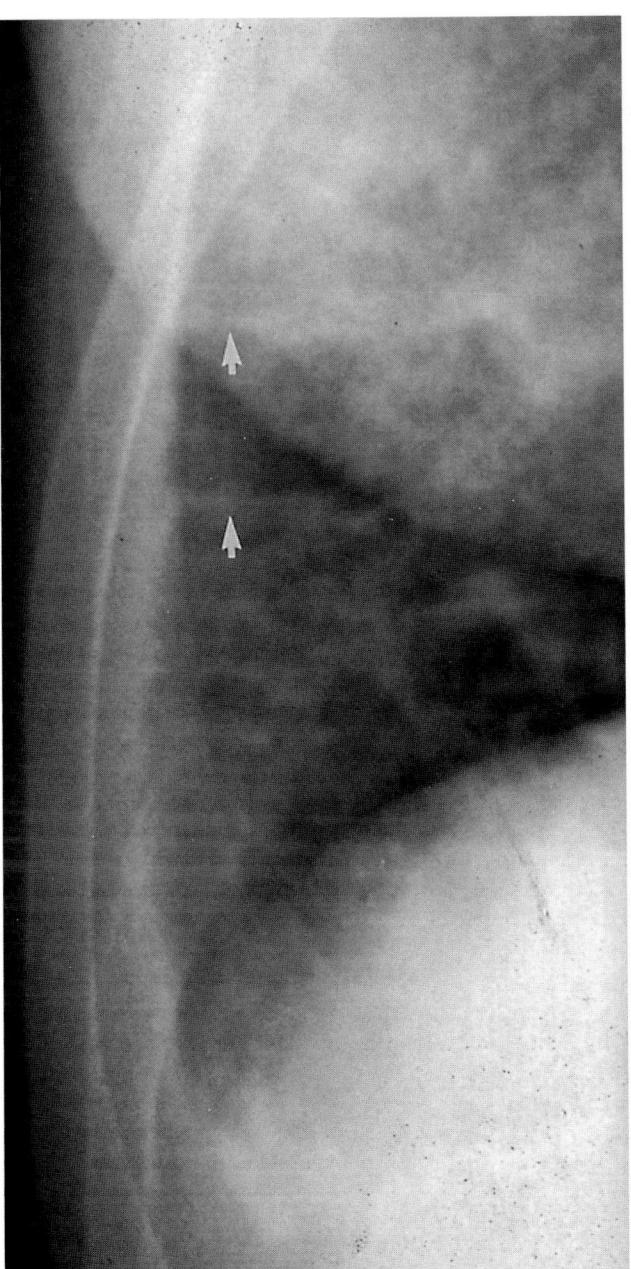

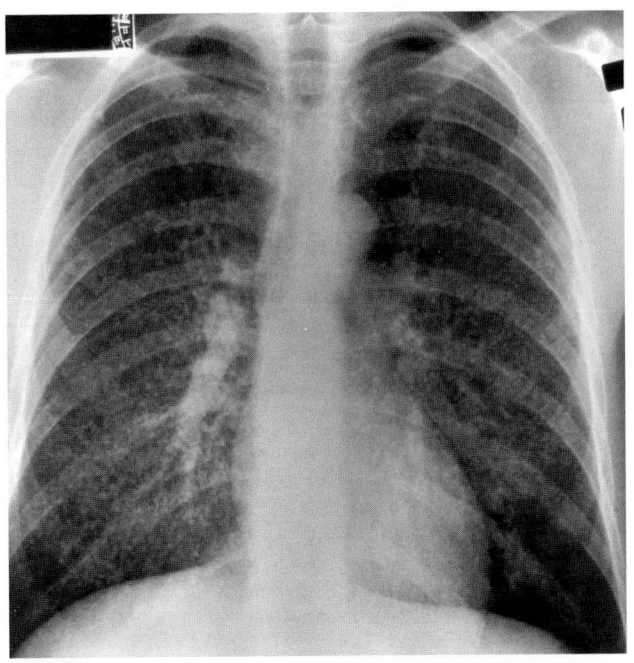

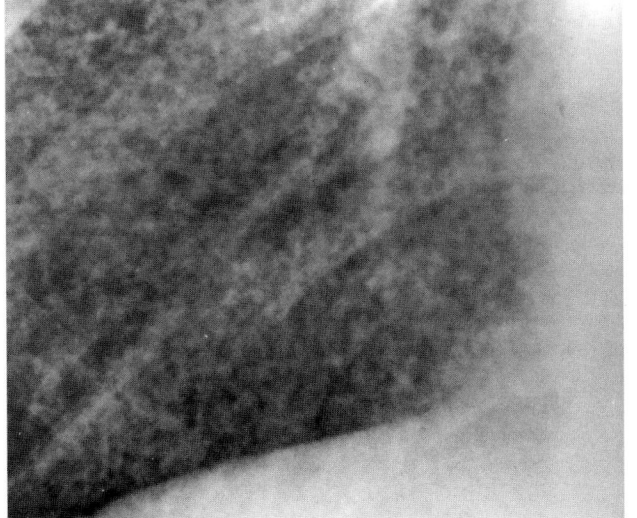

Fig. 9-42. Lymphangitic metastases from renal cell carcinoma. Posteroanterior view of the right costophrenic angle demonstrates perpendicular linear opacities extending from the pleura of the right costophrenic angle (Kerley's B lines) (*arrows*).

Fig. 9-43. Miliary histoplasmosis. Posteroanterior (**A**) and cone down (**B**) views. Fine nodular or miliary pattern compatible with interstitial process.

scleroderma and rheumatoid lung), eosinophilic granuloma of the lung, and idiopathic pulmonary fibrosis.

Discrete nodules of varying sizes are also indicative of interstitial disease. These nodules may vary from minute to large and usually show a lack of confluence and have sharply defined margins (Fig. 9-43). A reticulonodular pattern also may be present in interstitial disease. A slow rate of change of a diffuse process favors interstitial over alveolar disease.

High-resolution or thin-slice CT scanning provides additional information about anatomic distribution and extent of interstitial lung disease, which is well described by Colby and Swensen (1996). This technique is discussed in detail in Chapter 10.

Localized Pulmonary Densities

Localized pulmonary densities may have poorly circumscribed or discrete margins. If the margins are poorly circumscribed, a solitary density most likely denotes pneumonia or pulmonary infarction. Primary lung tumors may present

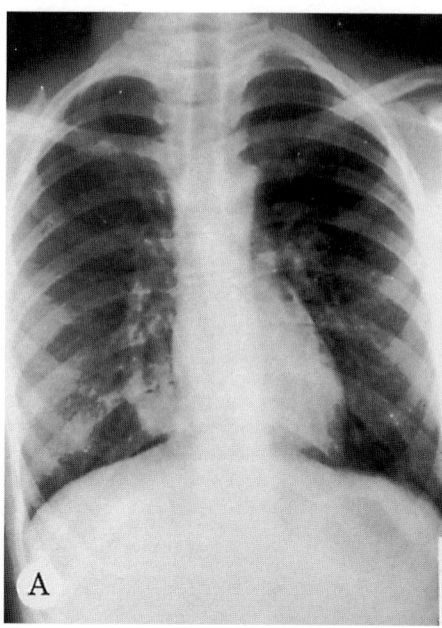

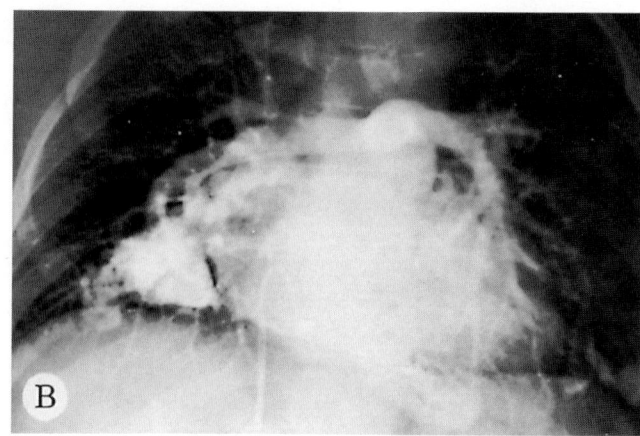

Fig. 9-44. Pulmonary arteriovenous malformation. **A.** Serpiginous lobulated density next to the right heart border. **B.** A pulmonary angiogram demonstrates multiple malformations. These malformations are now easily identified on computed tomography.

in this fashion so that it is important to follow a poorly circumscribed density to complete clearing to be certain that it does not represent a tumor with postobstructive pneumonic changes. Pulmonary tuberculosis and other chronic inflammatory diseases also manifest as poorly localized pulmonary densities. A chronic infiltrate in the apical or posterior segment of the upper lobe or in the superior segment of the lower lobe should make one suspect tuberculosis. Cavitation is also suggestive of tuberculosis. Without

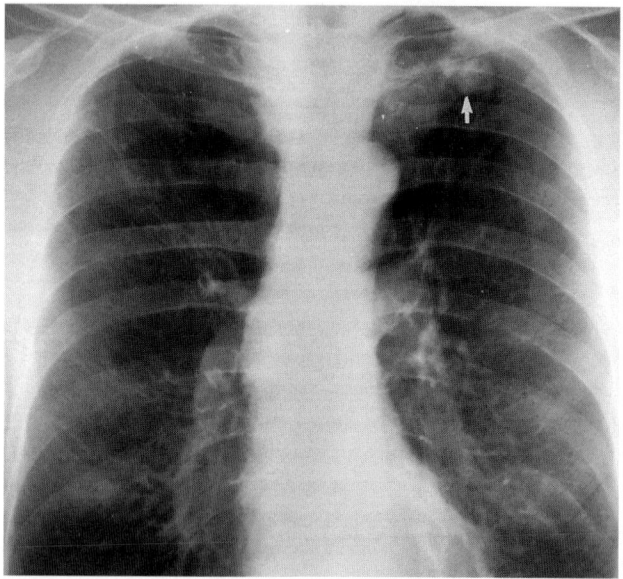

Fig. 9-45. Carcinoma. Single eccentric calcification at inferior aspect of mass (*arrow*). This pattern does not indicate benign disease in this instance.

old films, tuberculosis must always be considered active, regardless of radiographic appearance, as demonstrated by one of us (W.T.M.) and MacGregor (1978).

The sharply circumscribed pulmonary density most likely is a tumor or a granuloma. Primary or metastatic carcinoma commonly manifests in this fashion. Tuberculous granulomata, histoplasmosis and other fungal diseases, benign pulmonary tumors, and occasionally pneumoconiosis may present as a sharply circumscribed pulmonary density. Also to be considered are pulmonary infarct, pneumonia, arteriovenous malformation (Fig. 9-44), bronchial cyst, and bronchial adenoma. New techniques such as contrast-enhanced CT scanning and positron-emission tomographic scanning may offer promising alternatives to surgery. The characteristics of a solitary nodule occasionally lead to identification. Calcification, solid, popcorn, or laminated indicates benign disease. Eccentric calcification indicates a malignant process until proven otherwise (Fig. 9-45). Old films are the most important clue to etiology: If a nodule is present unchanged for 2 years, it is behaving in a biologically benign fashion and no further intervention is needed. Absent old films, further evaluation is warranted for diagnosis. It is sometimes possible to ascertain the nature of a solitary pulmonary nodule by appropriate clinical tests, but a transthoracic lung biopsy or video-assisted thoracoscopic surgery is usually necessary to make a definitive diagnosis. Positron-emission tomographic scanning as well as contrast-enhanced CT offer possible alternatives to surgery (see Chapters 10 and 12).

Multiple sharply circumscribed densities almost invariably indicate metastatic malignant disease. Occasionally, however, rheumatoid nodules, fungal disease, Wegener's granulomatosis, or alveolar sarcoidosis may produce a sim-

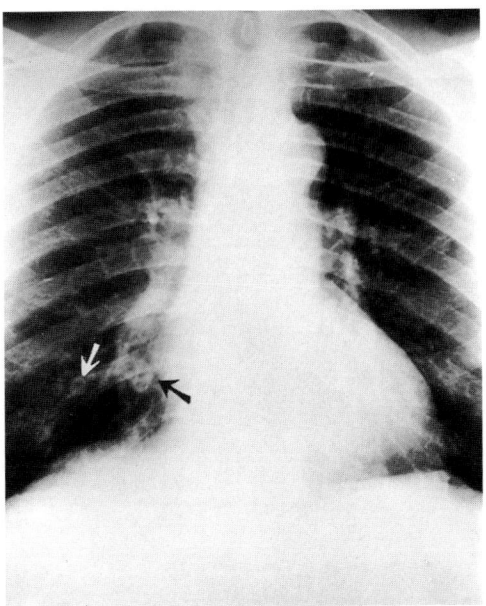

Fig. 9-46. Septic emboli. Several pulmonary nodules are present in both lungs with cavitation of two right lower lobe nodules (*arrows*).

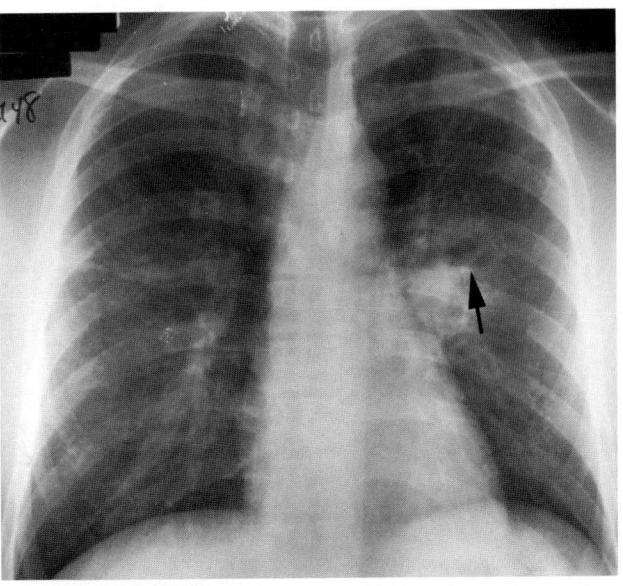

A

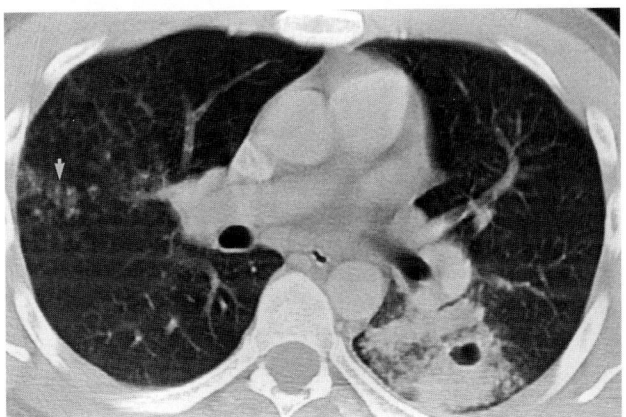

B

Fig. 9-47. *Mycobacterium tuberculosis.* **A.** Posteroanterior view demonstrates opacity at left hilus with an air-fluid level (*arrow*) indicating cavitation; possible nodular changes in the right mid-lung zone indicating endobronchial spread. **B.** Computed tomography of cavity on the left and nodular endobronchial spread on the right (*arrow*).

ilar pattern. Septic emboli may appear as multiple pulmonary nodules, but these are usually cavitary (Fig. 9-46).

Cavitation of a solitary pulmonary density usually indicates a lung abscess, primary bronchial carcinoma, tuberculosis (Fig. 9-47), or fungal disease. Tumors and lung abscesses ordinarily have thick, shaggy walls, whereas fungal disease and tuberculosis often have thin, smooth walls. If a lung abscess is chronic, the wall that initially was thick and shaggy generally becomes thin and smooth. Multiple cavitary lesions in the chest suggest septic emboli, metastatic tumor, tuberculosis, fungal disease, or Wegener's granulomatosis.

Calcification within a solitary pulmonary nodule can help to point to its etiologic basis. Certain types of calcification are strong evidence of benign disease. Central calcification or concentric ringlike calcification suggests granuloma. Multiple punctate calcifications throughout the lesion suggest granuloma or hamartoma. Eccentric calcification may be seen in a granuloma, but it also can be seen in primary lung carcinoma (see Fig. 9-45). Thus, an eccentric calcification cannot be taken as an indication of benign disease. Multiple pulmonary calcifications usually indicate healed pulmonary infections such as histoplasmosis, tuberculosis, or varicella pneumonia.

Determination of the rate of change of a pulmonary density is also important. If previous radiographs can be obtained for comparison, they may reveal that the lesion is changing rapidly, slowly, or not at all. If prior radiographs cannot be obtained, follow-up examination in 1 week or several weeks may reveal the growth rate of the pulmonary process.

Abnormalities of the Pleura

Pleural Effusion

A collection of fluid within the pleural space is the most common pleural abnormality. Fluid in the pleural cavity appears radiographically as a homogeneous opacity that is ordinarily in a dependent position in the pleural cavity. The fluid may be exudate, transudate, blood, pus, or chyle. Small amounts of free pleural fluid may be difficult to detect radiographically. Careful observation of the posterior costophrenic sulcus on the lateral radiograph often shows minor blunting of the sulcus with as little as 50 to 100 mL of fluid. A lateral decubitus view may confirm the presence of free pleural fluid (see Fig. 9-6).

With larger pleural effusions, the lateral costophrenic sulcus is blunted also. On occasion, the fluid may remain infra-

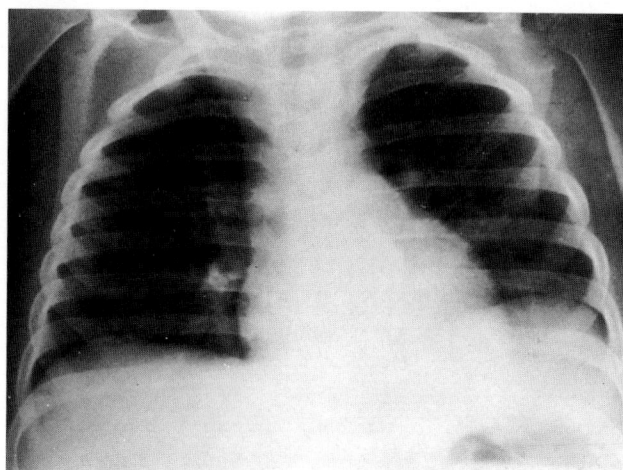

Fig. 9-48. Left pleural effusion. The separation of the stomach bubble from the lung is caused by a large left pleural effusion in this child with nephrosis. Another sign of a subpulmonic effusion is displacement of the apex of the left hemidiaphragm. Note that the costophrenic angle is not blunted. A decubitus view would confirm the diagnosis with layering of fluid.

pulmonary and displace the lung upward so that the lateral costophrenic angle remains sharp (Fig. 9-48). This infrapulmonary location of fluid can be suspected if the apparent hemidiaphragm is elevated; if the costophrenic sulcus is blunted posteriorly; or if the gas bubble in the gastric fundus lies some distance below the dome of the apparent hemidiaphragm, if the apparent apex of the involved hemidiaphragm is displaced laterally, or both. Decubitus views demonstrate that fluid is free and not loculated. CT scanning commonly identifies pleural effusions not seen on routine radiography.

As the amount of pleural effusion increases, passive atelectasis occurs in the underlying lung, and eventually the mediastinum may be displaced to the contralateral side (see Fig. 9-37C).

Fluid may become loculated in the pleural space, in which instance it may be difficult to differentiate from localized pleural thickening. Loculated pleural fluid generally has a convex border toward the hilus (Fig. 9-49). Pleural thickening is more likely to have a concave border toward the hilus. Loculated pleural effusion may appear in the interlobar fissure, where it assumes a cigar-shaped configuration. This is referred to as a *pseudotumor*. Localized pleural tumor may masquerade as localized pleural thickening or pleural fluid. On occasion, loculated fluid may assume a lobar shape (Fig. 9-50) or simulate a mass (Fig. 9-51).

Common causes of pleural effusion are tuberculosis, pneumonia, viral pleural infection, metastatic tumor, primary lung or primary pleural tumor, lymphoma and leukemia, pulmonary infarction, chest trauma, collagen vascular disease, congestive heart failure, and intra-abdominal problems such as subphrenic abscess or pancreatitis.

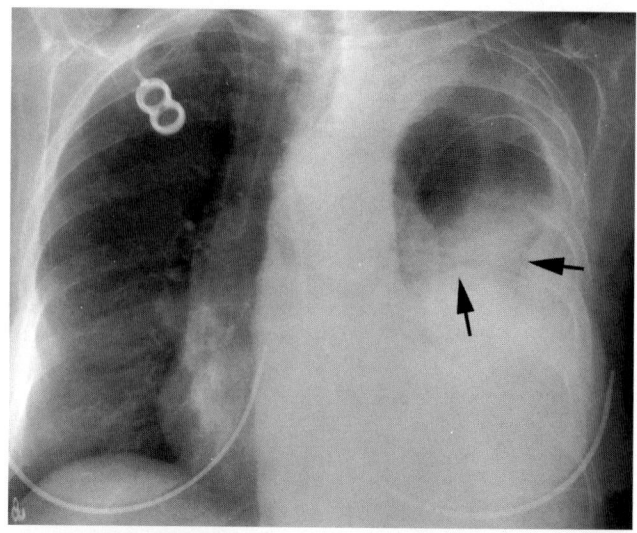

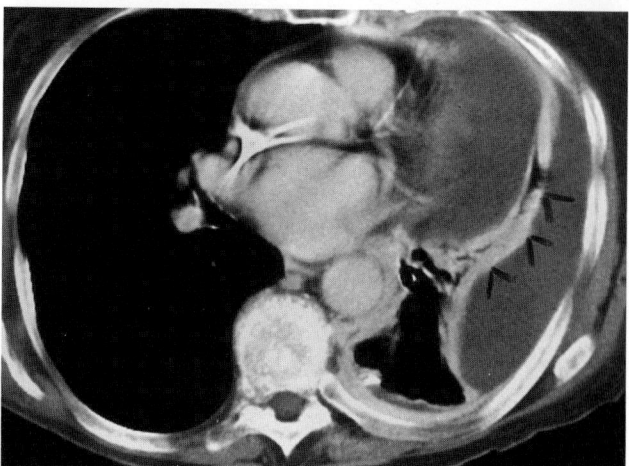

Fig. 9-49. Empyema and loculated pleural effusion. **A.** Lobulated contour (*arrows*) of peripheral opacity on posteroanterior chest view suggests loculation. **B.** Computed tomographic scan demonstrates two locules of fluid separated by contrast-enhanced lung (*arrowheads*).

Pleural Thickening

Pleural thickening represents a localized fibrosis of the pleura that may be secondary to several causes. It is commonly seen at both apices, at the costophrenic angles, and occasionally along the lateral chest wall. It can be distinguished from free pleural fluid in a radiograph made with the subject in the decubitus position. Distinguishing pleural thickening from loculated pleural fluid may be more difficult. CT scan, with intravenous contrast if necessary, distinguishes between fluid and soft tissue. The lack of change over a long period of time suggests pleural thickening rather than loculated fluid.

Causes of localized pleural thickening are usually old infection, particularly tuberculosis, or remote pulmonary infarction. Generalized pleural thickening occurs following the healing of hemothorax or pyothorax and commonly is associated with tuberculosis. Asbestosis or talc pneumoco-

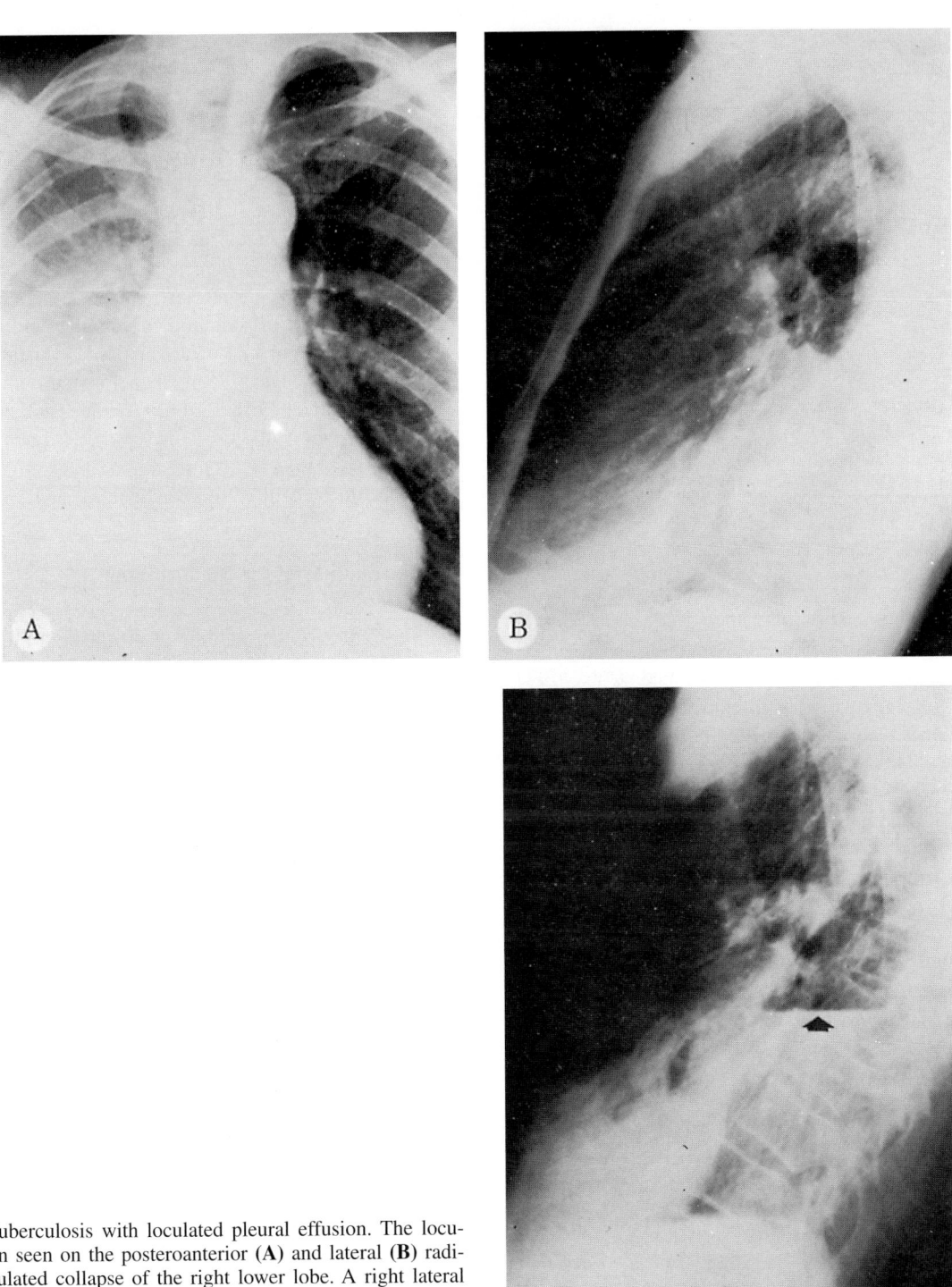

Fig. 9-50. Tuberculosis with loculated pleural effusion. The loculated effusion seen on the posteroanterior (**A**) and lateral (**B**) radiographs simulated collapse of the right lower lobe. A right lateral decubitus radiograph showed no evidence of free effusion. After thoracentesis, however, a large collection of loculated fluid with an air-fluid level (*arrow*) was apparent (**C**).

niosis also may cause either focal or diffuse pleural thickening. Diffuse pleural mesothelioma (Fig. 9-52) may be difficult to distinguish from benign pleural thickening, although pleural effusion and pleural nodulation are often present with mesothelioma as well as contraction of the involved hemithorax. CT demonstrates the pleural changes, particularly the nodularity and contraction of the pleural space. Video-

assisted thoracoscopy or open biopsy is frequently necessary, because the transthoracic needle biopsy sample generally is too small for pathologic identification of mesothelioma.

Apical pleural thickening may be difficult to distinguish from superior sulcus tumor. O'Connell and colleagues (1983) have demonstrated that asymmetry of the apices should suggest a superior sulcus tumor. Rib destruction adjacent to the

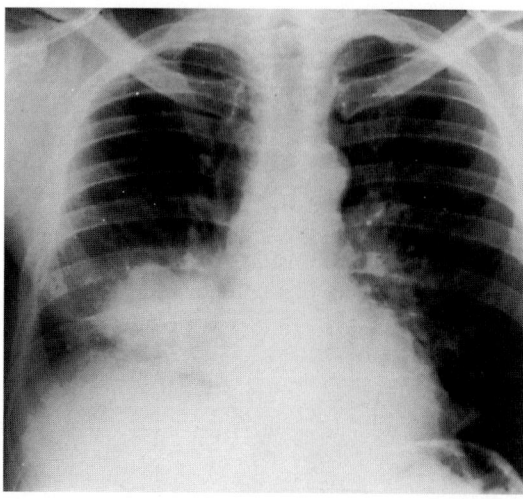

Fig. 9-51. Loculated empyema. This loculated collection of fluid near the border of the right side of the heart simulates a lung mass.

apical thickening or significant change over a short period of time suggests a malignant process. Symmetric apical thickening may be a normal variant, as demonstrated by Vix (1977). MR imaging is particularly useful in identifying or excluding a superior sulcus tumor. Calcification of the pleura is usually secondary to old hemothorax, pyothorax, or tuberculosis. Calcified plaques are seen with asbestos exposure. These occur on the hemidiaphragms, parietal pleura of the chest walls, mediastinum, and pericardium.

Pneumothorax

The presence of air within the pleural cavity is easily detected radiographically by identifying a thin line of visceral pleura surrounding the partially collapsed lung. This feature is best seen at the apex of the lung when the patient

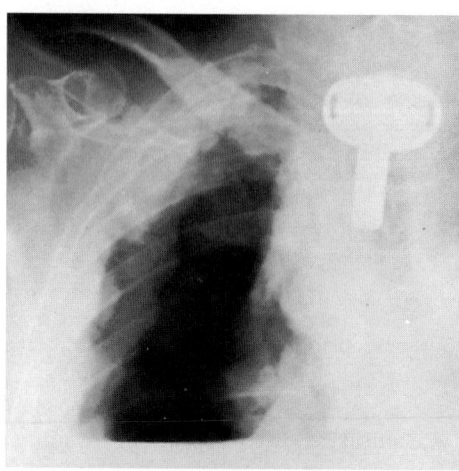

Fig. 9-52. Pleural mesothelioma. Diagnostic pneumothorax demonstrates diffuse pleural involvement by mesothelioma.

is upright but sometimes is seen only laterally or at the lung base, particularly if the patient is supine. It may be necessary to obtain a radiograph in expiration to be absolutely certain that a small pneumothorax is present. The expiratory image accentuates the pneumothorax because the volume of air in the lung decreases while the air in the pleural space remains the same, thus increasing the apparent size of the pneumothorax. In addition, the density of the lung in expiration increases, which accentuates the difference in contrast between pleural air and less aerated lung. Fluid in the pleural space in association with pneumothorax demonstrates the straight line of an air-fluid level rather than the curved line (meniscus) seen when no pneumothorax is present. A straight air-fluid level may on occasion be the finding that makes the radiologist aware that a pneumothorax is present (see Fig. 9-7). Again, a horizontal projection of the x-ray beam is required to appreciate an air-fluid level.

Abnormalities of the Mediastinum

The radiographic features of mediastinal tumors are discussed in detail in Chapter 152. Several aspects of mediastinal disease might be emphasized, however. In all mediastinal lesions, it is important to determine the location of the mass because the differential diagnosis varies considerably for each of the three mediastinal compartments. The one mass that commonly occurs in all three compartments is lymph node enlargement. It is often possible to determine the probable etiologic basis for the enlargement of lymph nodes by using certain helpful radiographic criteria.

Sarcoidosis has a characteristic pattern when it causes enlarged nodes. This pattern has been called the *1-2-3 sign* because three prominent areas of enlarged nodes are identified, in both hila and in the right paratracheal area. In sarcoidosis, the hilar nodes also tend to be more peripherally situated or peribronchial with discrete nodes identifiable rather than one large amorphous mass tight against the mediastinum as is more commonly seen in association with metastatic tumor or lymphoma. CT demonstrates more extensive lymphatic involvement in all these processes than is seen on chest radiography.

Lymphoma usually presents in only one node-bearing area rather than in several, and this area is commonly the anterior mediastinum. Lymph node enlargement in one nodal area alone or in one hilus and the mediastinum in a younger individual should make the clinician suspect lymphoma. In an older person, this same pattern should make one suspect a small cell carcinoma of the lung.

Middle mediastinal node enlargement may be identifiable only on films exposed during barium swallow or by CT scanning. Enlargement of nodes in the middle mediastinum is usually indicative of metastatic tumor, most commonly from the lung.

Primary tuberculosis commonly manifests as node enlargement in one hilus or in the mediastinum. It is more common in children and commonly is associated with a parenchymal pulmonary lesion. It occurs frequently in the immunocompromised adult, in which case the pattern is similar to that seen with lymphoma. The radiologic presentation varies with the CDC count.

Early lymph node enlargement may be difficult to detect. The importance of previous radiographs for comparison must be emphasized once again. A slightly widened mediastinum that has not changed for several years is not significant, whereas a minor alteration of mediastinal outline can be important if not present on radiographs made at an earlier date. CT is invaluable in demonstrating mediastinal adenopathy if any reason exists to suspect it.

Masses occurring in the anterior cardiophrenic angle are almost invariably benign, except in a patient with known lymphoma or abdominal malignancy, and so probably do not merit further investigation. These masses include pericardial cysts, foramen of Morgagni hernia, prominent pericardial fat pad, and pericardial fat necrosis.

Abnormalities of the Diaphragm and Chest Wall

The radiographic features of abnormalities of the diaphragm are covered in Chapters 47 to 53 and are not discussed here.

The most common chest wall abnormalities identifiable radiographically involve the ribs. Abnormalities of the chest wall that protrude into the thorax create a characteristic radiographic appearance that has been labeled the extrapleural sign by Felson (1973). These extrapleural lesions are smooth; are seen well in only one projection, in which they are tangential to the x-ray beam; and usually have an oblique angle at their borders, where the parietal pleura is being stripped from the thoracic cage. Whenever an extrapleural lesion is observed, the underlying rib should be examined carefully. Metastatic malignant disease of the rib is the most common cause of the extrapleural sign. Myeloma, primary rib tumor, fractures, or osteomyelitis may be responsible for this finding. Primary tumor of the chest wall or extrapleural hematoma also may present in this fashion.

Abnormalities of the soft tissues of the chest also may be discernible on the radiograph of the chest but are better visualized by CT scanning. The nipple of the breast frequently creates a shadow simulating a pulmonary nodule and must be considered when the nodule overlies the breast area. Extraparenchymal nodules or shadows such as a nipple shadow tend to have incomplete margins; the edges are not seen all the way around the nodule.

CONTRAST EXAMINATIONS

Air in the bronchi and pulmonary alveoli provides an excellent contrast medium and makes the plain film exami-

nation of the chest fruitful. CT affords excellent delineation of mediastinal structures with or without oral and intravenous contrast. This has replaced the barium swallow for delineation of mediastinal masses. As demonstrated in several articles, high-resolution and CT scanning have replaced bronchography for visualization of the tracheobronchial tree.

ANGIOGRAPHY

Opacification of the vasculature of the chest is often helpful in the investigation of a pulmonary or mediastinal abnormality. It is currently used when CT or MR imaging yields an equivocal diagnosis and of course when a percutaneous invasive procedure is contemplated.

Many congenital abnormalities, such as arteriovenous malformations, sequestrations, and anomalous venous structures, are diagnosed using intravenous contrast and helical CT techniques. Aortic lesions are readily demonstrated with MR imaging, which has the advantage of obtaining images in multiple planes.

The primary indication for pulmonary intravascular contrast in the thorax is for the diagnosis of pulmonary emboli. This has remained the standard definitive examination. However, with the advent of high-speed acquisition of data with CT (i.e., helical CT scanning) and the development of nonionic contrast to diminish motion artifacts, CT is used increasingly as a method of diagnosing pulmonary emboli. This is the CT pulmonary angiogram. A wide range of sensitivity (63 to 100%) and of specificity (55 to 96%) has been reported. Visualization of large central clots is at least equal to that of pulmonary angiography. Peripherally, most studies include fourth-order vessels, branches to the pulmonary segments. The reported demonstration of subsegmental clots, those beyond fourth-order branches, is extremely variable, and the clinical significance of these peripheral emboli has yet to be defined. Drucker and colleagues (1998) report a sensitivity of 53% and a specificity of 97% with experienced CT angiogram readers. They note that the observed low sensitivity suggests that the CT pulmonary angiogram may be used to confirm a ventilation-perfusion lung scan but not replace it as a screening test for pulmonary embolism. Currently, multicenter studies are underway to examine the accuracy of CT in the diagnosis of pulmonary emboli and the relation of CT contrast angiography to ventilation-perfusion scanning for the diagnosis of pulmonary emboli (see Chapter 13).

REFERENCES

Boyden EA: Segmental Anatomy of the Lungs. A Study of the Patterns of the Segmental Bronchi and Related Pulmonary Vessels. New York: McGraw-Hill, 1955.

Brailsford JF: The radiographic posteromedial border of the lung or the linear thoracic paraspinal shadow. Radiology *41*:34, 1943.

Colby TV, Swensen SJ: Anatomic distribution and histopathologic patterns in diffuse lung disease: correlation with HRCT. J Thorac Imaging *11*:1, 1996.

Drucker EA, et al: Acute pulmonary embolism: assessment of helical CT for diagnosis. Radiology 209:235, 1998.

Felson B: Chest Roentgenology. Philadelphia: WB Saunders, 1973.

Fleischner FG: The visible bronchial tree: a roentgen sign in pneumonic and other pulmonary consolidations. Radiology 5:184, 1948.

Fraser RG, Paré JAP: Diagnosis of Diseases of the Chest. 3rd Ed. Philadelphia: WB Saunders, 1989.

Groskin SA: Heitzman's The Lung Radiographic-Pathologic Correlations. St. Louis: Mosby–Year Book, 1993.

Jackson CL, Huber JF: Correlated applied anatomy of the bronchial tree and lungs with a system of nomenclature. Dis Chest 9:319, 1943.

Leung AN: Spiral CT of the thorax in daily practice: optimization of technique. J Thorac Imaging 12:2.1997.

Lubert M, Krause GR: Patterns of lobar collapse as observed radiographically. Radiology 56:165, 1951.

McCloud TC, et al: Bronchogenic carcinoma: analysis of staging in the mediastinum with CT by correlative lymph node mapping and sampling. Radiology 182:319, 1992.

Miller WT: The radiologist in the intensive care unit. Semin Roentgenol 32:86,1997.

Miller WT, MacGregor RR: Tuberculosis: frequency of unusual radiographic findings. AJR Am J Roentgenol 130:867, 1978.

Milne EN: A physiological approach to reading critical care unit films. J Thorac Imaging 1:60, 1986.

O'Connell RS, McLoud TC, Wilkins EW: Superior sulcus tumor: radiographic diagnosis and workup. AJR Am J Roentgenol 140:25, 1983.

Ravin CE, Chotas HG: Chest radiography. Radiology 204:593, 1997.

Sagel SS, et al: Efficacy of routine screening and lateral chest radiographs in a hospital-based population. N Engl J Med 291:1001, 1974.

Schaefer CM, et al: Improved control of image optical density with low dose digital and conventional radiography in bedside imaging. Radiology 173:713, 1989.

Shanks SC, Kerley P: A Textbook of X-ray Diagnosis. Vol 2. Philadelphia: WB Saunders, 1951.

Swensen SJ, et al: Lung nodule enhancement at CT: prospective findings. Radiology 201:447, 1996.

Tocino I: Chest imaging in the intensive care unit. Eur J Radiol 23:46, 1996.

Tocino I, Westcott JL: Barotrauma. Radiol Clin North Am 34:59, 1996.

Vix VA: Roentgenographic manifestations of pleural disease. Semin Roentgenol 12:277,1977.

Weibel ER, Gil J: Structure function relationship at the alveolar level. In West JG (ed): Bioengineering Aspects of the Lung. New York: Marcel Dekker, 1977.

Westcott JL, Cole S: Plate atelectasis. Radiology 155:1,1985.

Woodring JH, Reed JC: Radiographic manifestations of lobar atelectasis. J Thorac Imaging 11:109, 1996.

Zeman RK, et al: Helical body CT: evolution of scanning protocols. AJR Am J Roentgenol 170:1427, 1998.

READING REFERENCES

Genereaux GP: Radiologic assessment of diffuse lung disease. In Tavaras JM, Ferrucci JT: Radiology: Diagnosis Imaging, Intervention. Philadelphia: JB Lippincott, 1986.

Heitzman ER: The Mediastinum: Radiologic Correlations with Anatomy and Pathology. St. Louis: CV Mosby, 1977.

Niklason LT, et al: Portable chest imaging: comparison of storage phosphor digital, asymmetric screen-film, and conventional screen-film systems. Radiology 186:387, 1993.

Parkes WR: Occupational Lung Disorders. London: Butterworths, 1982.

Renner RR, Pernice NJ: The apical cap. Semin Roentgenol 12:299, 1977.

CHAPTER 10

Computed Tomography of the Lungs, Pleura, and Chest Wall

Lacey Washington and Wallace T. Miller, Jr.

Computed tomography (CT) is now firmly established as an indispensable radiologic modality for the evaluation of the chest. The advantages of CT over plain radiography include resolution of smaller differences in density and the provision of greater anatomic detail. CT may be used for the detection of abnormalities in the mediastinum, lungs, pleura, and chest wall and in many cases is helpful for further characterization of processes seen in the mediastinum, lungs, and pleura on plain chest radiographs.

INDICATIONS FOR CHEST COMPUTED TOMOGRAPHY

Thoracic CT is not a screening procedure. The high radiation dose of CT (compared with that of chest radiography) should limit its use to patients in whom specific clinical questions must be addressed. Although an institution may have a standard CT protocol, multiple operator-dependent variables need to be selected on each CT examination to optimize the information acquired in light of the particular clinical question. Variables that need to be addressed include slice thickness, slice spacing, field of view, and the timing of intravenous (IV) contrast administration (when indicated).

Multiple long-accepted indications for chest CT and a variety of indications that are more experimental or are gaining acceptance exist. Indications for CT to evaluate mediastinal abnormalities are discussed in Chapter 152.

Lungs

CT is most commonly used to evaluate the lungs in several settings. In the evaluation of primary neoplasms of the lung, CT is used in the staging of bronchial carcinoma or is used to attempt to identify a primary neoplasm in a patient with positive sputum cytology and negative chest radiograph and

bronchoscopy. In patients with primary neoplasms elsewhere, CT may be used to look for occult pulmonary metastases when surgery is planned for a primary neoplasm with a high rate of metastasis to the lung or to look for additional nodules when a chest radiograph demonstrates a single pulmonary nodule in this setting, as noted by Fraser and colleagues (1994) and the Society for Computed Body Tomography (1979). CT is used in primary lung and metastatic neoplasms to assess response to treatment. When a solitary pulmonary nodule is identified on plain radiograph, CT is the established technique to assess for diffuse or central calcification. More recently, Swensen and colleagues (1995, 1996) and Yamashita and colleagues (1995) have suggested that dynamic contrast administration may be used to distinguish lesions that have a greater vascular supply in the hope that this will distinguish malignant from benign nodules.

In the setting of pneumonia, CT can be used to evaluate for complications of infection that may explain a poor response to treatment. A special technique known as *high-resolution CT* (HRCT) is used for the detection and characterization of pulmonary emphysema, bronchiectasis, and interstitial lung disease, including interstitial pneumonias. Interest in using CT to evaluate for pulmonary emboli has been increasing.

Pleural Space

CT can be used to evaluate for a pleural effusion when its detection is made difficult by overlying pulmonary opacities and especially when ultrasound is confusing, as identified by Fraser and colleagues (1994) and the Society for Computed Body Tomography (1979). CT is particularly useful when a pleural effusion contains multiple locules or is loculated in a medial or subpulmonic location. CT is also helpful in the detection of pleural-based neoplasms and can be used to identify pleural plaques.

Chest Wall

CT can be used to identify osseous destruction and soft tissue masses in the evaluation of neoplastic involvement of the chest wall caused by chest wall primary tumors or by metastases. In the absence of bony destruction, however, CT can be inaccurate in assessing direct chest wall extension of primary lung tumors. CT can be used to detect the involvement of the chest wall by infection, particularly when osseous destruction occurs.

Clinical Settings

Mirvis and colleagues (1987) advocate the use of CT in critically ill and ventilator-dependent patients who can only be imaged by portable radiography whenever an unexplained clinical deterioration that may be caused by an abnormality within the chest is present. As Naidich and colleagues (1990) indicate, another common clinical question that may be addressed by CT is the evaluation of hemoptysis, which most commonly results from either a malignancy or bronchiectasis, both of which may be seen on CT.

Interventions

A wide variety of interventions in the chest may be performed under CT guidance as reviewed by Klein (1995) and Giron (1996) and their colleagues. Most commonly, CT can be used to guide percutaneous biopsy of small lung nodules and masses for the diagnosis of malignancy and infection. Drainage of pleural empyemas and, less commonly, lung abscesses and pneumothoraces can also be performed with CT guidance.

TECHNIQUE

Standard and Helical Computed Tomography

A CT image is acquired using the same physical principles as plain radiography: the passage of x-ray beams through tissue, allowing the detection of differences in "density" or attenuation of x-ray beams, based on different atomic numbers. CT passes multiple, highly collimated x-ray beams at various angles through an anatomic plane; the attenuation is then measured by an array of detectors opposite the x-ray source. The geometry of the arrangement of source and detectors has evolved since the original CT scanners were developed, allowing for decreased scan times and therefore improved images. The information acquired by the array of detectors is then reconstructed with complex computer algorithms to create an image of the plane through which the beams have passed. This image is essentially a map of tissue densities. As Curry and associates (1990) indicate, density differences of only 0.5% can be recognized with CT, instead of the 10% density differences required for visualization on plain radiographs.

Although early CT scanners acquired one slice of data at a time, more recent technology has allowed scanners to acquire spiral or helical data sets. With helical or spiral scanners, the table moves continuously as the data are acquired. The computer then reconstructs axial images, which appear similar to images that are acquired axially. Vock (1990) and Kalender (1990) and their associates have reviewed the mechanism of spiral CT scanning. The entire chest can usually be imaged in one or two breath-holds, reducing or eliminating the problem of respiratory misregistration. One distinct advantage of this technique, as Remy-Jardin and coworkers (1993) point out, is that small pulmonary nodules are less likely to be missed. This type of acquisition also allows for three-dimensional reconstruction of complex anatomy, which sometimes may help elucidate the answers to specific clinical questions. For fine detail in the three-dimensional structures, thinner sections should be acquired through the area of interest; the specific indication for the study should therefore be known in advance. This technique is most commonly used in a dedicated examination of the airways, which may be performed to evaluate for a central airway mass (e.g., in a patient presenting with hemoptysis or evidence of airway obstruction) or airway stenoses.

The calculated tissue densities are converted into a scale of CT numbers or Hounsfield units, named after the inventor of the original CT scanner. The scale is designed such that the CT number for air is –1000 and the CT number for dense bone is +1000, with water having a CT number of 0. On this scale, fat has a CT number of approximately –100. The wide range of density values detected by CT cannot be displayed on a single set of images; therefore, multiple windows are used to display a single scan. In the chest, a set of mediastinal windows with relatively high contrast is used to demonstrate the narrow density differences in the mediastinum between fat and soft tissue, whereas a set of lung windows is used to display the lung parenchyma; a third set of bone windows should be examined to assess for osseous abnormalities. A window is specified by a level (the density that is approximately average for the tissue being displayed; displayed as a medium shade of gray) and a width (used to determine the range of CT numbers that will be displayed in gray between the values assigned to black and white). Different viewers and therefore different institutions have different preferences for the exact levels and window widths at which images are displayed.

Images acquired on CT are usually printed on film and stored as hard copy. However, CT data are essentially digital and may be stored on a variety of electronic media. Images that are stored electronically and recovered may be displayed in any window. Although lung, mediastinal, and bone windows should all be examined, bone windows are not usually filmed unless a specific bony abnormality is present; the images can be recalled and displayed if this is necessary.

Intravenous Contrast Media

Iodinated contrast media increase the density within the vessels when given intravenously, allowing a distinction to be made between vessels and soft tissue. They also increase the density of any tissue in proportion to the blood supply to that tissue, allowing soft tissue structures that are otherwise the same density to be distinguished. This can be particularly striking when tissue necrosis with an absent blood supply is contrasted with adjacent enhancing tissue. In evaluating mediastinal structures, IV contrast is not always necessary. Distinguishing between blood vessels and soft tissue structures such as enlarged lymph nodes is frequently possible by using the expected position of the blood vessels and their continuous nature on multiple images. However, IV contrast media are very important in evaluation of hilar structures. Hilar lymph nodes can be very difficult to distinguish from blood vessels in the absence of IV contrast media; therefore, using IV contrast (if possible) is important in any patient in whom hilar lymphadenopathy may be expected (Fig. 10-1).

Special uses of IV contrast that are currently under investigation include CT for pulmonary emboli and CT of pulmonary nodules. Incidental central pulmonary emboli can be seen against a background of IV contrast; more recently, an attempt has been made to tailor CT for the detection of emboli. The studies reported in the literature sometimes use an initial small bolus of IV contrast to assess the correct timing of contrast administration with respect to imaging. Diagnostic images are obtained with thin section imaging in a caudocranial direction during the rapid administration of IV contrast.

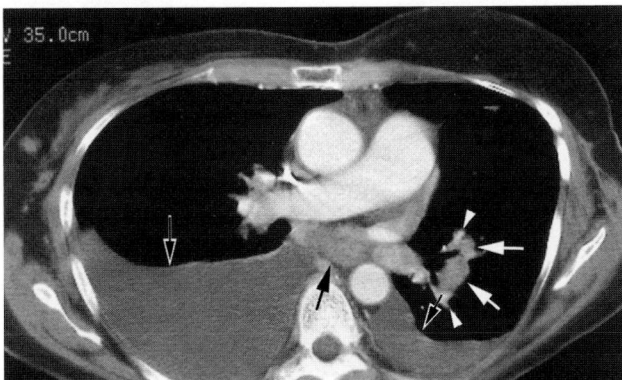

Fig. 10-1. Metastatic breast carcinoma. Intravenous contrast administration makes the hilar vessels (*arrowheads*) more dense than surrounding lymph nodes, allowing the detection of hilar lymphadenopathy (*straight arrows*) in this patient with metastatic breast carcinoma. Subcarinal lymphadenopathy (*black arrows*) and bilateral pleural effusions (*open arrows*) are also present.

When IV contrast is used to evaluate pulmonary nodules, serial images through the nodule are obtained over an interval of approximately 5 minutes. The change in attenuation is measured over time.

High-Resolution Computed Tomography

HRCT imaging of the chest was developed to allow improved diagnostic accuracy, sensitivity, and specificity in the evaluation of diffuse lung disease compared with images obtained by plain radiography. As Webb and colleagues (1996) state, when compared with conventional CT, thinner collimation is used to acquire images, resulting in marked improvement in spatial resolution. The algorithm by which the images are reconstructed is modified; specifically, HRCT uses a high-spatial frequency reconstruction algorithm. HRCT images are similar in appearance to macroscopic pathologic specimens. Other modifications that may be used include an increased kVp or mA technique, a large matrix size, and targeted image reconstruction.

Continuous scanning throughout the lungs with such thin sections would be prohibitive in terms of dose to the patient, time of scanning, and tube current; thus, discontinuous slices are acquired. Most commonly, 1.0- to 1.5-mm thick sections are obtained at 10-mm intervals through the lungs. No IV contrast is administered with a dedicated HRCT; however, some HRCT images are sometimes obtained in conjunction with a conventional CT or other protocol, depending on the clinical setting. Before any attempt is made to characterize pulmonary nodules with IV contrast administration, the simpler and more accepted technique of HRCT through the nodule should be performed to evaluate for calcification or fat as will be discussed later.

Electron-Beam Computed Tomography

Electron-beam CT is an uncommonly used form of CT that eliminates all motion of the x-ray tube and detectors and uses an electron gun to produce an x-ray beam from a tungsten target ring. This technique allows the acquisition of images in as little as 100 ms. Its primary uses are in the mediastinum, specifically in cardiac imaging; centers that have these machines, however, may use them for other applications in which a short scan time is helpful (e.g., in dynamic imaging of the airways, to see the change in airway caliber over time, or in the evaluation of pulmonary emboli).

LUNG PARENCHYMA

Diseases involving the lung parenchyma may be divided into those that primarily involve the air spaces, such as bacterial pneumonias, and those that involve predominantly the interstitium. Diseases may also be divided by their morphology into those that are nodular or masslike and those that are more infiltrative. The margins of any focal abnormality may be evaluated. Diseases may also be focal or diffuse.

CT is best for determining the extent of air space disease and may be helpful for evaluation of the relationship of a given parenchymal abnormality to structures such as the bronchi, vessels, mediastinum, pleura, or chest wall. When characterization of diffuse lung disease is required, HRCT is most helpful.

Pulmonary Nodules

A wide variety of pathologic conditions can present as a solitary pulmonary nodule or mass. According to the Fleischner Society glossary of terms for CT of the lungs by Austin and colleagues (1996), a nodule is less than 3 cm in diameter; rounded opacities greater than this size are usually called *masses*. The differential diagnosis for any given focal lung nodule depends in part on the clinical setting in which it is discovered and on its appearance (see Chapter 90).

If a nodule is discovered on plain radiography as part of a workup for metastatic disease, the first step in further evaluation should be the administration of a CT scan to identify additional nodules. If multiple nodules are seen throughout both lungs at CT, the probability that the nodule represents metastatic disease increases, although biopsy is required for definitive diagnosis. CT is very sensitive for the detection of pulmonary nodules. In geographic areas endemic for histoplasmosis, however, granulomas or subpleural lymph nodes may constitute up to 25% of lung nodules; these are indistinguishable from metastases unless they are calcified. In some series, such as that of Munden and associates (1997), as many as 40 to 50% of solitary pulmonary nodules less than 1 cm have been reported to represent carcinoma of the lung; however, this number may be lower in patient populations with a high incidence of granulomatous disease. Frequently, after a nodule is discovered, comparison with older films shows that the nodule was present in retrospect and is stable. It is widely accepted, based on knowledge of tumor doubling times, that a nodule that remains stable for 2 years is benign. According to Nathan and colleagues (1962), malignant pulmonary nodules double in volume between 20 and 400 days. Nodules that double more quickly than this are usually infectious in nature, whereas those that double more slowly usually represent such benign lesions as a hamartoma or granuloma.

If a nodule is truly solitary, evaluating its margins is important. As Huston and Muhm (1987) note, a nodule with spiculated margins suggests malignancy, with a high probability (approximately 90%) (Fig. 10-2).

In a solitary nodule less than 3 cm in diameter, with smooth margins, it is helpful to evaluate for calcification. Contiguous HRCT images should be obtained through the nodule; the use of this technique prevents partial-volume averaging of surrounding lung. A nodule with central, popcorn-shaped con-

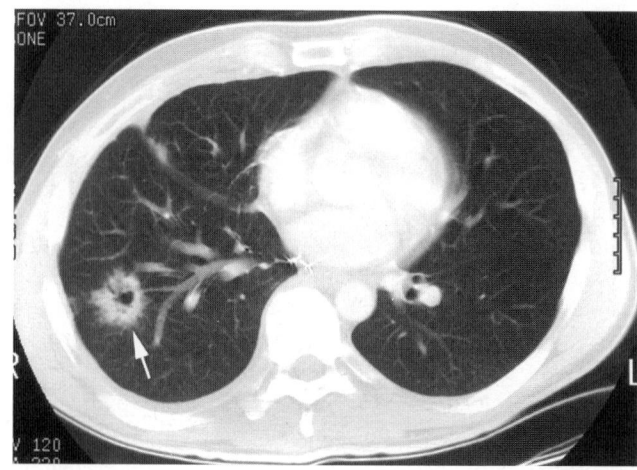

Fig. 10-2. Cavitary lung carcinoma. A cavitary mass (*arrow*) in the right lower lobe with spiculated margins representing a lung carcinoma.

centric rings or diffuse calcification may be confidently diagnosed as benign (Fig. 10-3). Eccentric calcification may be seen in some carcinomas; therefore, the presence of calcification alone does not specifically indicate a benign process. The presence of fat within a nodule is considered virtually diagnostic of benignity and specific for the diagnosis of a hamartoma. Historically, a technique used to help with the diagnosis of solitary pulmonary nodules was the CT reference phantom. This was developed to evaluate for calcification that was not visually obvious; the phantom was scanned and, based on the

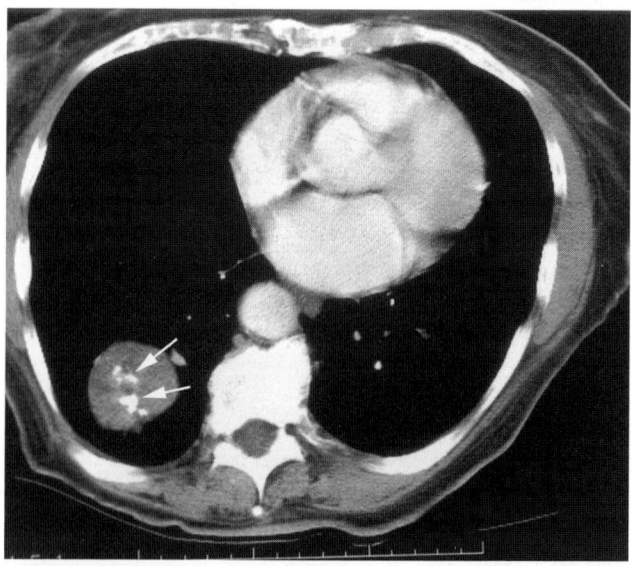

Fig. 10-3. Pulmonary hamartoma. Popcorn calcifications (*arrows*) in this right lower lobe mass are suggestive of cartilaginous calcifications. No fat was identified. Because lung carcinoma may contain foci of calcification, the patient underwent percutaneous biopsy, which demonstrated benign cartilage and mesenchymal tissue, supporting the diagnosis of a hamartoma.

work of Zerhouni and associates (1983), CT numbers higher than those of the phantom were considered diagnostic of calcification. This technique has fallen into disuse as the need for a reference phantom with modern CT scanners is not as clear as with older scanners, and a higher rate of false-benign diagnoses than originally reported may exist, according to Swensen and colleagues (1991).

A nodule without calcification but otherwise meeting the criteria mentioned is sometimes followed with serial CT examinations to evaluate for growth. This has become less common, because excisional biopsy has become a less invasive procedure with the increasing use of video-assisted thoracoscopic biopsy. Fine-needle aspiration biopsy may also be performed using CT or fluoroscopic guidance; Klein and coworkers (1996) note, however, that the yield of a confident diagnosis is lower for benign etiologies than for malignancy.

Occasionally specific morphologic features allow for confident characterization of a solitary pulmonary nodule or mass based on a single CT examination. Specifically, a nodule may be diagnosed as representing a pulmonary arteriovenous malformation or rounded atelectasis. Remy (1992) has suggested that CT may be superior to the more traditional angiography for the diagnosis of arteriovenous malformations. These can frequently be diagnosed based on the demonstration of a feeding arterial vessel and a large draining vein. Administration of IV contrast may not be necessary, but if performed, it should demonstrate arterial-phase dense enhancement unless the malformation is thrombosed (Fig. 10-4). Schneider and colleagues (1980) described the imaging features of rounded atelectasis, an abnormality that occurs in the lung adjacent to an area of pleural thickening, most commonly in patients with asbestos-related pleural disease. It also occurs in patients with pleural thickening of other etiologies. The mass is rounded and abuts the pleura; bronchovascular markings in the adjacent lung appear to curl into it, creating a "comet tail" sign.

Two new techniques have shown some promise in the evaluation of solitary pulmonary nodules; both need wider validation before they come into common practice. Swensen (1995, 1996) and Yamashita (1995) and their colleagues have suggested that CT with IV contrast administration as described with multiple images obtained over time through the nodule may distinguish between benign and malignant nodules on the basis of the more vascular nature of malignant processes. A nuclear medicine technique [fluorodeoxyglucose positron emission tomography (FDG-PET); see Chapter 12] has also shown some promise in distinguishing malignant from benign nodules on the basis of higher activity in the malignancies, as shown by Dewan (1993), Gupta, (1992), Hagberg (1997), and Patz (1993) and their associates.

Bronchial Carcinoma

CT of the chest has become a routine part of preoperative staging for lung carcinoma. Except when a contraindication to the use of iodinated contrast media exists, contrast-

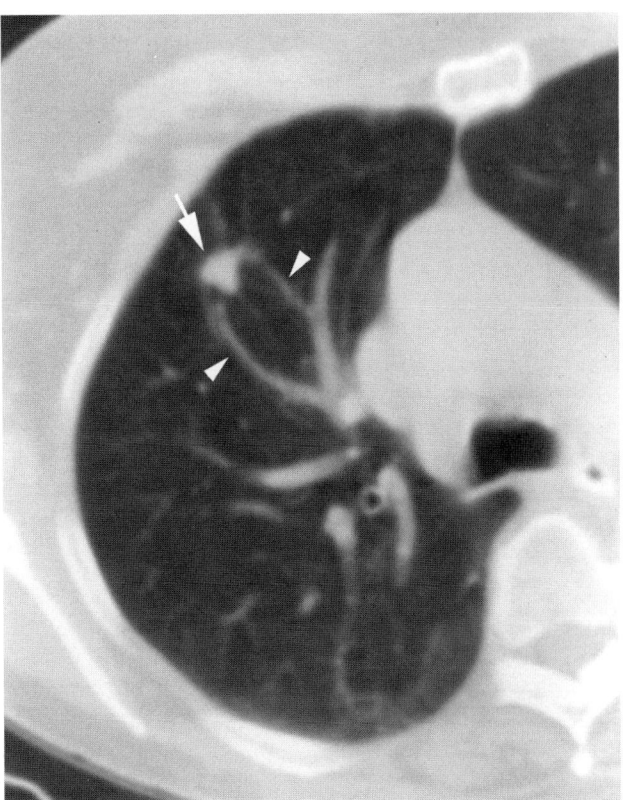

Fig. 10-4. An arteriovenous malformation in the right lung, manifested by a nodule (*arrow*) with feeding arteries (*arrowheads*). Draining veins were appreciated on other images. The vessels are incompletely visualized on this image; therefore, their continuous nature is not entirely appreciated, although a large portion of their course is demonstrated because they run very horizontally. Three-dimensional reconstructions may be very helpful in other cases.

enhanced CT should be obtained, because it aids in the detection of mediastinal and hilar lymph nodes and may help delineate the relationship of a centrally invading tumor to the aorta or pulmonary vessels. CT provides information about the size of the primary lesion and may suggest the possibility of direct extension of tumor to the contiguous structures of the chest wall, mediastinum, and diaphragm. CT is also used to evaluate for enlarged hilar and mediastinal lymph nodes and hematogenous dissemination of tumor elsewhere within the lungs or to the liver, adrenals, and bones. Webb and colleagues (1991) have shown that CT and magnetic resonance (MR) imaging have similar overall accuracy in the staging of lung carcinoma.

Establishing the presence of a tumor in the setting of postobstructive consolidation and atelectasis can be difficult, as can defining its size. Onitsuka and coworkers (1991) noted that rapid scanning after administration of IV contrast material may help with the distinction of tumor from surrounding consolidated lung, as tumors tend to show less enhancement than normal lung.

A number of studies demonstrated, however, that CT is neither sensitive nor specific for invasion by lung carcinoma of mediastinal structures or the chest wall. Pennes and colleagues (1985) found that CT had an accuracy of only 39%. Glazer and associates (1985) found better results: In a study of chest wall invasion, CT was shown to have an 87% sensitivity, 59% specificity, and 68% accuracy. In this study, however, localized chest wall pain was shown to be more specific (94%) and more accurate (85%) for the detection of chest wall invasion. CT signs of chest wall invasion that are very specific include bony destruction and presence of a soft tissue mass in the chest wall; Ratto and colleagues (1991) also found that obliteration of the extrapleural fat plane was 85% sensitive and 87% specific. This same study also suggested that a ratio of tumor-pleura contact to tumor diameter of greater than 0.9 was moderately sensitive and specific for chest wall invasion. Although the overall accuracy of CT and MR imaging in the staging of lung carcinoma are similar, when contiguity of tumor to chest wall or mediastinum is seen at CT, MR imaging may be better than CT in assessment of local invasion. This is particularly true in the case of superior sulcus (Pancoast) tumors, in which the axial orientation of CT slices limits evaluation of chest wall extension at the apex; the multiplanar capability of MR imaging allows for much better visualization in this region.

Like chest wall invasion, contiguity of tumor with the mediastinum cannot be equated with mediastinal invasion. However, displacement or compression of mediastinal vessels, trachea, or esophagus or obliteration of normal fat planes usually indicates mediastinal invasion.

Although the greatest contribution of CT to evaluation of lung carcinoma has been the detection of mediastinal lymphadenopathy, limitations of the sensitivity and specificity of CT exist for metastasis and mediastinal lymph nodes. The difficulty with the CT staging of bronchial carcinoma is that enlarged nodes may be negative for tumor, and normal-size lymph nodes (i.e., <1 cm) may contain microscopic metastases, as shown by Libshitz (1984) and Arita (1995) and their associates. Nevertheless, CT is useful for directing biopsy and can allow the appropriate nodes to be evaluated before definitive surgery is attempted. CT can identify the precise mediastinal location of these lymph nodes and can therefore influence the staging procedure used.

Staging CT of the chest may also detect hematogenous metastases to the adrenal glands, liver, contralateral lung, and bones. Because of the high propensity of lung carcinoma to metastasize to the adrenals, CT in lung cancer is routinely obtained through the level of the adrenal glands, to evaluate for masses. Unfortunately, benign adrenal masses (usually adrenal adenomas) are very common. On the routine contrast-enhanced CT of the chest, adrenal masses can be detected but cannot be characterized as benign or malignant.

Several imaging strategies for the characterization of adrenal masses have been developed. Mitchell and colleagues (1992) were the first researchers to recognize that adenomas could be distinguished from metastasis on the basis of lipid content. They performed MR chemical-shift imaging to show that masses that lose signal on out-of-phase sequences compared with in-phase sequences are highly likely to represent adenomas. Masses that do not meet these criteria require biopsy. This research has been confirmed by other groups, such as Bilbey (1995), Reinig (1994), and Tsushuma (1993) and their associates.

Because lipid content also reduces CT attenuation, unenhanced CT can be used to distinguish between benign and malignant adrenal masses. On unenhanced images a region of interest is placed over the mass and the Hounsfield unit measurement of the mass is obtained. According to Lee and colleagues (1991), a value of less than 10 Hounsfield units has a high positive predictive value for an adenoma, whereas a higher value indicates that the lesion may be a metastasis and should be biopsied.

Because unenhanced CT and MR imaging require a patient to return for a second study after the initial contrast-enhanced CT has been performed, other authors have attempted to use delayed CT imaging after the initial contrast injection to characterize adrenal masses. Brodeur and colleagues (1995) suggest that imaging after a delay of 1 hour could be used to characterize these masses, whereas Boland and associates (1997) suggest that imaging as soon as 12 to 18 minutes after the initial injection might be used.

As with the evaluation of pulmonary nodules, the nuclear medicine technique FDG-PET has shown some promise in the staging of lung cancers. PET imaging has the additional advantage over CT of allowing whole body imaging, which increases the detection of occult distant metastasis. In the evaluation of adrenal masses, Erasmus and colleagues (1998) reported a sensitivity of 100% and a specificity of 80%. The technique, however, is not widely available, and over time, the reported specificity can possibly decrease.

Air Space Disease

Air space disease can have a variety of manifestations on CT, as described by Naidich and associates (1985). Findings include: 1) air space nodules, which appear as poorly marginated opacities ranging up to 1 cm in size, caused by sublobular accumulations of fluid, hemorrhage, or cells; 2) coalescent densities that are usually the result of confluence of air space nodules (Fig. 10-5); 3) air bronchograms and air alveolograms; and 4) ground-glass opacity (Fig. 10-6). *Ground-glass opacity* is defined by Austin and colleagues (1996) in the Fleischner Society glossary as an area of increased lung density through which the vessels and bronchial margins are still distinguishable; this is presumably caused by focal hypoaeration. Air space patterns at CT are usually not specific for the etiology, and a wide variety of diseases can produce such patterns, including pneumonia, aspiration, hemorrhage, pulmonary edema, alveolar proteinosis, and alveolar cell carcinoma. CT adds little to the characterization of these diverse disease processes. However, CT may be used to define the extent of disease, which it can do more accurately than plain radiography. The extent and distribu-

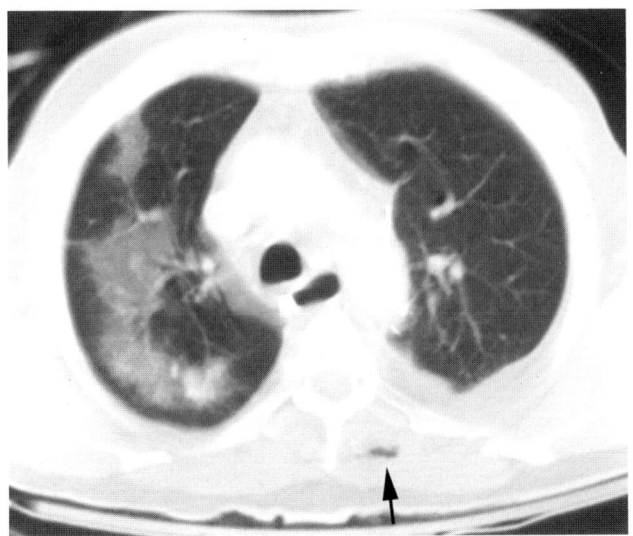

Fig. 10-5. Aspiration pneumonia and necrotizing fasciitis. Patchy right lung infiltrate is completely nonspecific; this represents aspiration pneumonia in this intensive care unit patient. Air is seen in the paraspinous muscles (*arrow*), due to necrotizing fasciitis; this finding of a life-threatening infection was not visible on plain radiographs.

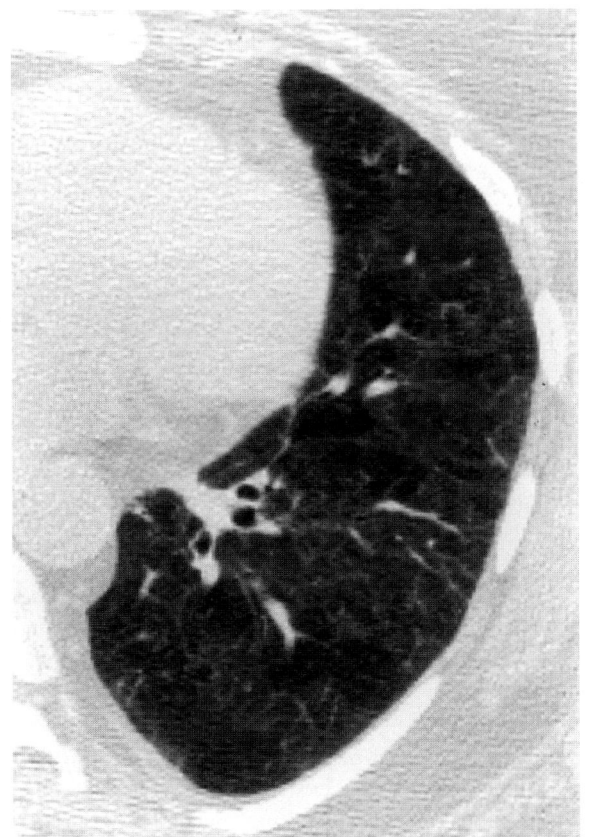

Fig. 10-6. Pneumocystis pneumonia. The chest radiograph on this person (*not shown*) was interpreted as normal. Note the inhomogeneous attenuation in this high-resolution computed tomography scan of the left lung. The higher attenuation is known as *ground-glass opacities*. This represented *Pneumocystis carinii* pneumonia.

tion of disease may influence the differential diagnosis: Diseases such as pulmonary edema and hemorrhage and pulmonary alveolar proteinosis are more likely to involve the pulmonary parenchyma diffusely. Multifocal involvement with areas of sparing is more likely to be caused by diseases such as bronchiolitis obliterans with organizing pneumonia, vasculitis, alveolar sarcoid, and chronic eosinophilic pneumonia, alveolar cell carcinoma, and lymphoma. Some forms of pneumonia are more likely to be diffuse, such as mycoplasma pneumonia, whereas most bacterial pneumonias are more likely to be unifocal or multifocal. As Epstein and colleagues (1982) pointed out, careful demonstration of the extent of disease is particularly important for patients with alveolar cell carcinoma.

CT may also limit or direct a differential diagnosis by demonstrating some features either not seen or not well delineated on plain film. A common example is occult cavitation in air space disease. Rare, more specific features that may be seen at CT include a halo sign, described by Kuhlman and coworkers (1985), ground-glass opacity surrounding an area of denser consolidation, suggesting hemorrhage (possibly on the basis of aspergillosis); or high density within an area of focal consolidation, suggesting the possibility of amiodarone toxicity. Another use of CT in air space disease is to identify the areas of most severe involvement, which may help guide transbronchial biopsy.

Cavitary Lung Disease

CT may be helpful in identifying cavities within areas of known lung disease. These are distinguished from areas of low attenuation scattered diffusely through the lungs, which usually represent diffuse lung disease and, like most diffuse lung diseases, are best characterized on HRCT.

Focal areas of low attenuation within areas of abnormal lung usually represent areas of cavitation. The presence of cavitation in an irregular area of consolidation, particularly when a known preexisting pneumonia is present, suggests certain pathogens, particularly gram-negative bacteria, anaerobic bacteria, and tuberculosis. This appearance can also be seen in vasculitis and, rarely, lymphoma. An intracavitary mass frequently represents a mycetoma or a focus of necrotic lung; this sign is classically described in aspergillosis, as noted by Gefter (1992), but has been reported in other infections including mucormycosis, nocardiosis, and bacterial abscess.

Localized thin-walled cavities may represent pneumatoceles or bullae. Bullae are usually seen in the setting of emphysema, whereas pneumatoceles can be seen in pneumonia or occasionally in cases of trauma.

Pneumonia

CT usually adds very little diagnostic information in uncomplicated pneumonia. In this setting, the most common use of CT is to assess for complications that may be producing a poor response to treatment. These include empyema, lung abscess, and bronchopleural fistula. Additional reasons for a poor response to treatment include infection with an atypical organism or one that is resistant to the antibiotics being used, postobstructive pneumonia, and noninfectious pulmonary abnormalities that may mimic pneumonia on plain radiographs. Of these, CT is most likely to be helpful in identifying a central lesion that is associated with a postobstructive pneumonia.

USE OF HIGH-RESOLUTION COMPUTED TOMOGRAPHY

The very thin sections obtained with HRCT allow for an anatomically accurate depiction of the fine structure of the lung parenchyma; this is of value in the characterization of many lung diseases, particularly diffuse lung diseases. Interstitial lung disease, emphysema, and bronchiectasis are evaluated well with HRCT. However, the acquisition of noncontiguous sections means that large portions of the lung parenchyma are not imaged; thus, small nodules can easily be missed. In addition, distinguishing small pulmonary vessels from nodules on HRCT may be more difficult, because thin sections through vessels usually appear rounded, whereas thick sections may demonstrate more of the linear shape of the vessel.

Interstitial Lung Disease

HRCT has become an important modality for the evaluation of interstitial lung disease, both in patients with confusing clinical findings and patients with questionable abnormalities on chest radiography. HRCT was developed to help address the weaknesses of the chest radiograph, which , as Hansell and Kerr (1991) point out, may be normal in up to 10% of patients with biopsy-proven lung disease and may give false-positive impressions of diffuse lung disease particularly in obese patients.

Diffuse lung diseases are best characterized on CT by their distribution within the anatomic unit of lung known as the *secondary pulmonary lobule*. This anatomic unit is the smallest unit of lung divided by connective tissue septa and varies in size from approximately 1.0 to 2.5 cm in diameter. The surrounding septa measure approximately 0.1 mm in thickness and are usually below the limits of HRCT resolution. When the septa are seen, they are usually abnormally thickened, and certain disease processes are suggested. The secondary pulmonary lobules each contain a centrilobular artery and bronchiole; other diseases tend to affect this centrilobular region.

As Webb and associates (1996) state, the basic patterns of interstitial lung disease at HRCT include centrilobular or peribronchovascular interstitial thickening, thickening of the interlobular septa, intralobular interstitial thickening, small nodules, and ground-glass opacities. Small nodules can be

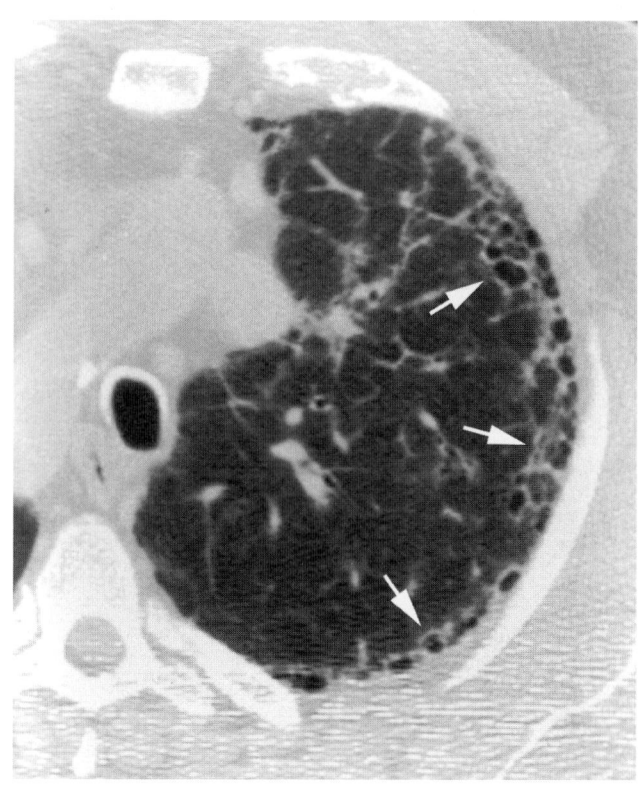

Fig. 10-7. Idiopathic pulmonary fibrosis. Intralobular septal thickening in usual interstitial pneumonitis or idiopathic pulmonary fibrosis. High-resolution computed tomography demonstrates the fine, netlike peripheral cysts (*arrows*) characteristic of this disease.

distributed randomly throughout the lung or can be found in a predominantly centrilobular distribution.

Webb and colleagues (1996) analyze the most common HRCT patterns of diffuse lung disease as follows:

1) Peribronchovascular thickening is most commonly seen in lymphangitic carcinomatosis, pulmonary edema, and sarcoidosis; interlobular septal thickening is also frequently seen in these diseases.
2) Intralobular septal thickening is manifested by a fine, peripheral netlike or reticular pattern and is most commonly seen in usual interstitial pneumonitis or asbestosis or in lung disease caused by collagen vascular diseases, such as scleroderma or rheumatoid arthritis (Fig. 10-7).
3) Small nodules distributed randomly are likely to be seen in miliary tuberculosis, fungal infections, or hematogenous metastases.
4) Small nodules in a peribronchovascular distribution are seen in sarcoidosis, silicosis, lymphangitic carcinomatosis, and lymphocytic interstitial pneumonitis in patients with acquired immunodeficiency syndrome.
5) Centrilobular nodules are primarily seen in endobronchial spread of tuberculosis, nontuberculous mycobacterial infections, bronchopneumonia, histiocytosis X, and hypersensitivity pneumonitis.

6) Last, ground-glass opacities have been stated to be a manifestation of air space disease and interstitial lung disease. Diseases that are likely to cause ground-glass opacity include usual interstitial pneumonitis; sarcoidosis; hypersensitivity pneumonitis; pulmonary alveolar proteinosis; acute interstitial pneumonias, such as *Pneumocystis carinii* and cytomegalovirus; and, most commonly, pulmonary edema (see Fig. 10-6).

The pattern of abnormality on CT can be used to assess the optimal way to obtain tissue for diagnosis of a lung disease. For example, diseases that produce abnormalities in a predominantly peribronchovascular pattern affect the lung tissue adjacent to the bronchi; transbronchial biopsy therefore has a high diagnostic yield for these diseases. Additionally, Leung and colleagues (1993) have shown that ground-glass opacity may indicate the presence of an ongoing active disease; biopsy directed toward areas of ground-glass opacity may therefore have a higher yield (see also Chapter 91).

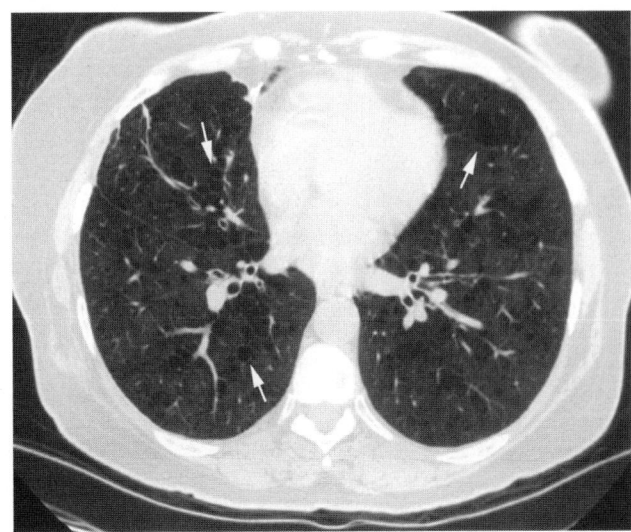

Fig. 10-8. Centrilobular emphysema. High-resolution computed tomography shows scattered small areas of low attenuation (*blacker areas*). This is characteristic of centrilobular emphysema. Some of the many areas of emphysema are indicated by the arrows.

Emphysema

A variety of diseases can lead to diffusely distributed areas of decreased lung attenuation on CT. These include relatively uncommon diseases, such as histiocytosis X and lymphangiomyomatosis; airway diseases, such as bronchiectasis; small airway diseases, such as bronchiolitis obliterans; and interstitial diseases with associated honeycombing. By far the most common disease to lead to decreased pulmonary parenchymal attenuation, however, is emphysema (see Chapter 83).

Three major subtypes of emphysema exist: 1) centrilobular emphysema, 2) panlobular emphysema, and 3) paraseptal emphysema. According to Webb and colleagues (1996), the chief CT characteristic that distinguishes these from diseases such as histiocytosis X or lymphangiomyomatosis is the absence of walls around the low-attenuation areas. The subtypes of emphysema are distinguished by their predominant location within the structure of the lung. In their milder forms, they are readily distinguished from one another; as they become more severe, however, the findings become more similar. Centrilobular emphysema is the most common type of emphysema and is most strongly associated with cigarette smoking; it is characterized by small, round areas of low attenuation grouped near the centers of secondary pulmonary lobules. Although the margins of the secondary pulmonary lobule are not always seen discretely, the presence of small scattered areas of emphysema is diagnostic of centrilobular emphysema (Fig. 10-8). Panlobular emphysema is the type of emphysema usually associated with alpha$_1$-antitrypsin deficiency and creates larger less well-defined areas of low attenuation. Centrilobular emphysema tends to be most severe in the upper lobes of the lungs, whereas panlobular emphysema is more severe in the lower lobes. A third kind of emphysema, paraseptal emphysema, can be seen either as an isolated phenomenon in young patients or in association with centrilobular emphysema. In young patients, it is often seen in association with spontaneous pneumothoraces.

Bullae are defined as sharply demarcated areas of emphysema measuring 1 cm or more in diameter with thin walls; these can become very large. Although most strongly associated with paraseptal emphysema, they can be seen in association with other types of emphysema. In patients for whom bullectomy is planned, HRCT can be used to define the extent of emphysema in the underlying lung.

HRCT can be useful in making the diagnosis of emphysema in patients who present with confusing clinical findings that may have suggested interstitial lung disease (e.g., an isolated low diffusing capacity on pulmonary function tests). A finding of significant emphysema may obviate a lung biopsy. Because HRCT can be used to assess the severity and distribution of emphysema, it is also being evaluated as a tool by Kazerooni and associates (1997) to assess patients who are being considered for lung volume reduction surgery.

Bronchiectasis

Bronchiectasis is best evaluated with HRCT, although it can be seen on conventional CT examinations. CT has replaced the older technique of bronchography in establishing this diagnosis. Criteria for the diagnosis of bronchiectasis include an airway with a diameter 1.5 or more times the diameter of the adjacent pulmonary artery, an airway seen to extend into the outer one-third of the lung, and an airway

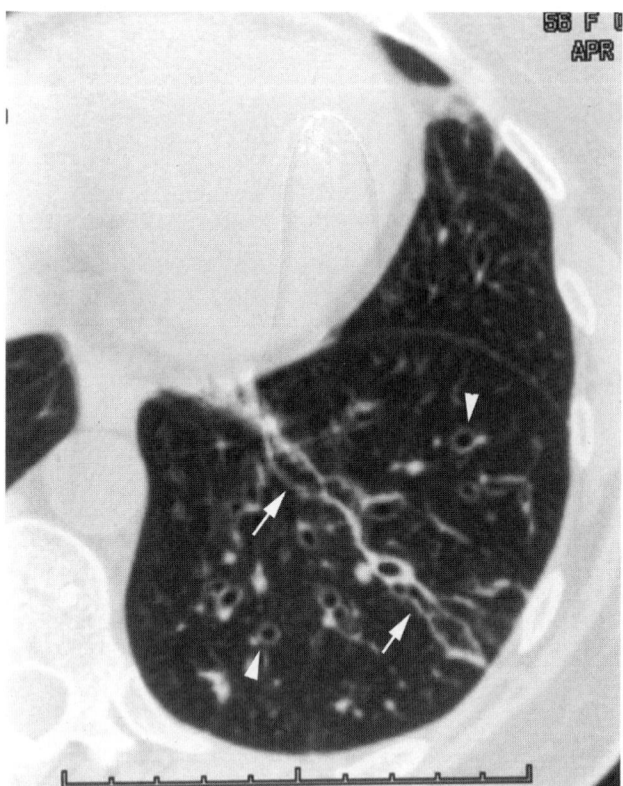

Fig. 10-9. Bronchiectasis manifested by the signet-ring sign (*arrowheads*) of bronchi more than 1.5 times the diameter of the accompanying artery, by bronchial wall thickening, and by a lack of tapering of the airways, known as *tram tracking* (*arrows*) seen along their long axis.

imaged along the long axis that either fails to taper as it becomes more distal or actually becomes larger in diameter (Fig. 10-9). The airway dilation should be irreversible; because bronchi may become transiently dilated during an episode of acute pneumonia, the diagnosis should not be made at that time.

The most common cause of bronchiectasis is acute, chronic, or recurrent infection. Diffuse bronchiectasis is most likely to occur in patients with underlying immune system abnormalities, such as cystic fibrosis, dyskinetic cilia syndrome (Kartagener's syndrome), or abnormalities of the immunoglobulin system. Focal bronchiectasis, however, may be caused by disorders such as mycobacterial infection or a single episode of severe acute pneumonia; it is also seen in allergic bronchopulmonary aspergillosis. The finding of focal bronchiectasis in a patient who presents with hemoptysis may allow for treatment of the hemoptysis by resection of the area of involved lung. Similarly, chronic infection with associated bronchiectasis may be treated by local resection of the involved area.

On a CT scan, large, solid-appearing branching structures usually represent areas of bronchiectasis with mucoid impaction. Tiny branching peripheral structures may represent dilated bronchioles with inflammatory bronchiolar wall thickening (known as *tree-in-bud opacities*), which indicate bronchiolectasis.

EVALUATION OF NONPARENCHYMAL LESIONS

Pulmonary Vascular Lesions

CT can be extremely useful in the noninvasive diagnosis of vascular lesions of the lung, including pulmonary arteriovenous malformation, pulmonary varix, scimitar syndrome, partial anomalous pulmonary venous return, and sequestration. Contrast-enhanced studies can demonstrate the vascular nature of these lesions. Arteriovenous malformations present as a pulmonary nodule or mass. Pulmonary varix and partial anomalous pulmonary venous return have distinct morphologic appearances. In patients with a chronic lower-lobe paravertebral mass or focal consolidation suspected of representing sequestration, the diagnosis may be established by CT if the abnormal systemic artery supplying the lesion is identified. This may obviate the need for more invasive conventional aortography.

Interest in using CT to test for pulmonary emboli has been increasing. This interest has developed largely because of dissatisfaction with ventilation perfusion scintigraphy. As Mayo and colleagues (1997) note, at the typical tertiary-care referral center, only 34% of cases imaged with ventilation-perfusion ($\dot{V}/\dot{Q}$) imaging have a combination of clinical suspicion and findings on $\dot{V}/\dot{Q}$ scans that give a high enough predictive value to obviate further imaging. Clinicians are often reluctant to order pulmonary angiograms because of the morbidity and mortality of the procedure, even when it is theoretically indicated, as noted by Sostman (1982) and Henschke (1995) and their associates. A widespread desire exists, therefore, for a better noninvasive examination for pulmonary embolism.

CT examinations tailored to detect pulmonary emboli have been performed with spiral and electron-beam CT. Studies must be tailored for this indication, with a rapid infusion of IV contrast; this technique is still in development. Central pulmonary emboli can be identified to the segmental arterial level with CT (Fig. 10-10). Mayo and colleagues (1997) found a higher sensitivity with this test than with $\dot{V}/\dot{Q}$ scanning. However, as Goodman (1995) and Teigen (1995) and their colleagues have shown, the sensitivity for subsegmental emboli is lower than for more central emboli. The significance of exclusively subsegmental emboli in pulmonary thromboembolic disease is still controversial. In addition, as Goodman and associates (1995) note, angiography is also less reliable in the detection of subsegmental emboli, with agreement among two angiographers of only 66% in the Prospective Investigation of Pulmonary Embolism Diagnosis (PIOPED) study. Whether CT for pulmonary embolism will come to replace $\dot{V}/\dot{Q}$ scanning (at least in the evaluation of some patients) or will become an intermediate step in the workup of some

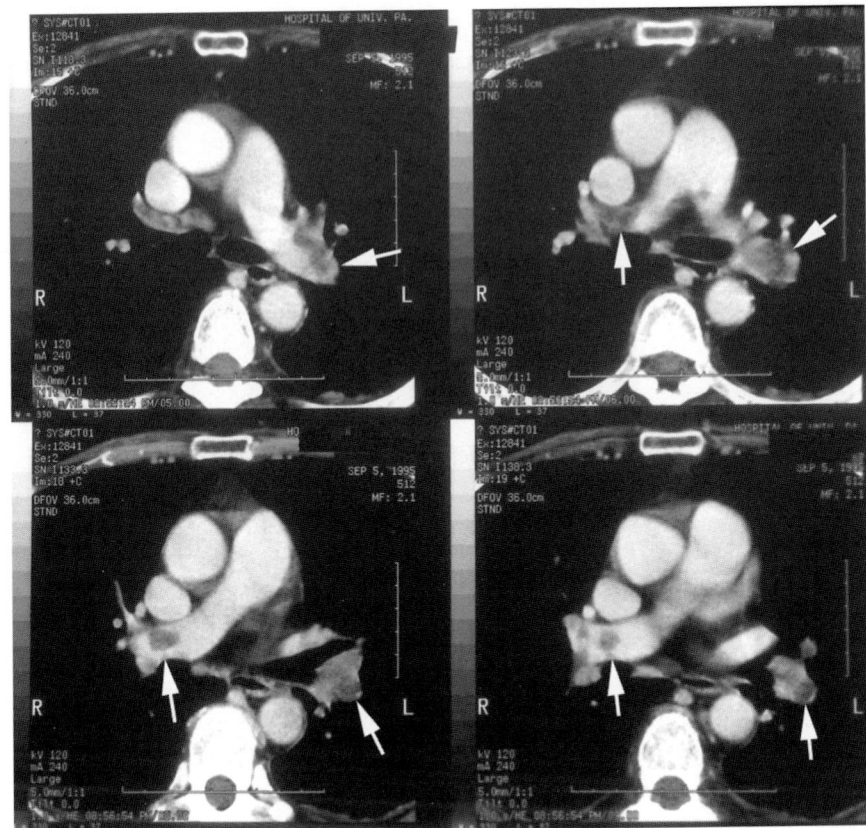

Fig. 10-10. Acute pulmonary embolism manifested by filling defects (*arrows*), darker areas within the enhancing lumens of the main right and left pulmonary arteries.

patients, partially replacing pulmonary arteriography, remains uncertain (see Chapter 13).

As with angiography, findings on CT in patients with chronic pulmonary thromboembolic disease are different from those in patients with acute pulmonary emboli. In this disorder, acute emboli fail to undergo normal lysis, become organized and fibrotic, and may ultimately become incorporated within the walls of the pulmonary arteries. Such chronic thromboemboli may lead to the development of pulmonary arterial hypertension, which may be treated with surgical thromboendarterectomy. Only patients with clots in the proximal pulmonary arteries are candidates for surgery. Remy-Jardin and colleagues (1992) have shown that the presence and extent of such central mural clots may be underestimated on conventional pulmonary arteriograms; CT may demonstrate them without the risks of the pulmonary arteriogram.

Pleural Processes

Much smaller abnormalities of the pleura are likely to be visible on CT compared with other imaging modalities, particularly when abnormalities within the lung parenchyma that may mask a pleural process are present. CT is also useful for patients with pleural effusions who are too ill to cooperate with lateral decubitus radiographs. Pneumotho-

races are similarly more difficult to detect in patients in whom erect radiographs cannot be obtained.

Ascites versus Pleural Effusion

Distinction of pleural fluid from ascites is not always straightforward with CT; a number of CT signs have been described to help with this differentiation. Specifically, the following criteria suggest ascites: 1) fluid is present inside the curved lines created by axial sections through the diaphragm and therefore below the diaphragm; 2) fluid does not elevate the crus of the diaphragm; 3) the interface between the fluid and liver or spleen is sharply defined, implying the absence of intervening diaphragmatic tissue; and 4) the fluid is posterior or medial to the liver at the level of the bare area. If the alternate conditions are met, the fluid is probably within the pleural space. Used individually, each of these signs may be indeterminate or misleading; if all four criteria for either pleural fluid or ascites are met, however, accurate distinction of one from the other may be made, as pointed out by Dwyer (1978), Griffin (1984), Halvorsen (1986), Naidich (1983), and Teplick (1982) and their colleagues among others. With a helical technique, sagittal or coronal reconstructions may also occasionally be used to help distinguish ascites from pleural fluid.

Although the distinction of exudative effusion from transudative effusion is definitively made only by thoracentesis, several CT signs have been reported to suggest that an effusion is exudative. Pleural thickening suggests an exudative effusion, with a specificity in a series reported by Aquino and associates (1994) of 96%; it is much less sensitive than specific, however, particularly in the setting of malignancy. As McLoud and Flower (1991) note, a large acute hemorrhage in the pleural space can sometimes by identified on CT by high attenuation within the pleural space or a fluid-hematocrit level.

Parapneumonic Effusion versus Empyema

Pleural fluid seen in a patient with pneumonia may represent a simple parapneumonic effusion, a complicated parapneumonic effusion, or empyema. The distinction is made by sampling the pleural fluid. Some CT features, however, may suggest that an effusion does not represent a simple parapneumonic effusion. Thickening of the visceral and parietal pleura, enhancement of these surfaces with IV contrast administration, and inflammation of the extrapleural fat may suggest either a complicated effusion or frank infection. The split pleura sign strongly suggests an exudative effusion, which is likely to be either empyema or complicated effusion in the presence of infection. This sign, as described by Stark and colleagues (1983), consists of demonstration of fluid that has relatively low attenuation between enhancing visceral and parietal pleura.

The presence of air in the pleural space can be caused by gas-forming organisms (although this is very rare), by recent instrumentation, or by empyema associated with bronchopleural fistula.

Bronchopleural Fistula

The term *bronchopleural fistula* indicates a communication between the lung parenchyma or airway and the pleural space. The presence of a bronchopleural fistula is often inferred on imaging studies from the presence of an air-fluid level in the pleural space, either in the absence of any intervention that might have introduced air into this space or persisting after such introduced air might have been expected to resolve.

As Hsu and colleagues (1972) noted, bronchopleural fistulae can be divided into central fistulae, which most commonly occur as a postoperative event (particularly after lobectomy or pneumonectomy) and peripheral bronchopleural fistulae. According to McManigle and coworkers (1990), central bronchopleural fistulae arise from the large airways and are best evaluated and characterized with bronchoscopy.

Peripheral bronchopleural fistulae are most frequently seen in the settings of tumor, infection, or bronchiectasis. CT can be used to characterize the abnormality in the underlying lung that might cause the fistula. Additionally, Westcott and Volpe (1995) demonstrated that if the monitoring

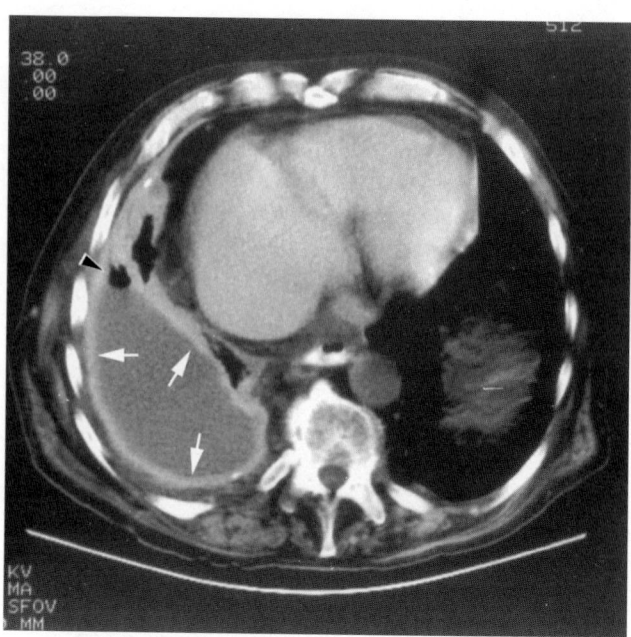

Fig. 10-11. Empyema. Air-fluid level (*arrowhead*) in the pleural space in this patient with an empyema and bronchopleural fistula. An elliptical fluid collection is present, and the inner margin of the collection is smooth and thin. The inner margin also appears dense (*arrows*), indicating enhancement with a split-pleura sign.

physician is alerted to the specific clinical question, thin-section CT through an area of abnormality may be able to demonstrate the communication or fistula between the abnormal lung and pleural space.

Abscess versus Empyema

Sometimes distinguishing a lung parenchymal abscess from an empyema with a bronchopleural fistula can be difficult. Both abnormalities may occur in association with pneumonia and demonstrate an air-fluid level on plain radiographs and CT. Shape and location should help distinguish between the two entities.

Empyemas are enclosed within the pleural cavity and conform to the shape of the chest wall, whereas lung abscesses arise within the lung parenchyma; for this reason, CT may help to make the distinction by providing greater spatial information. Empyemas are more commonly elliptical and usually have thin, smooth walls, especially along their inner margins (Fig. 10-11). Abscesses, in contrast, are more spherical, because they originate within the pulmonary parenchyma and destroy the adjacent lung. Most abscesses tend to have thickened, irregular walls and margins. Compression and crowding of the adjacent pulmonary parenchymal markings also suggest a pleural process rather than a lung abscess (in which the bronchi and vessels of the adjacent lung appear to be truncated abruptly at the edge of the abscess) at the margins of the destroyed lung, as pointed out by Stark and associates (1983).

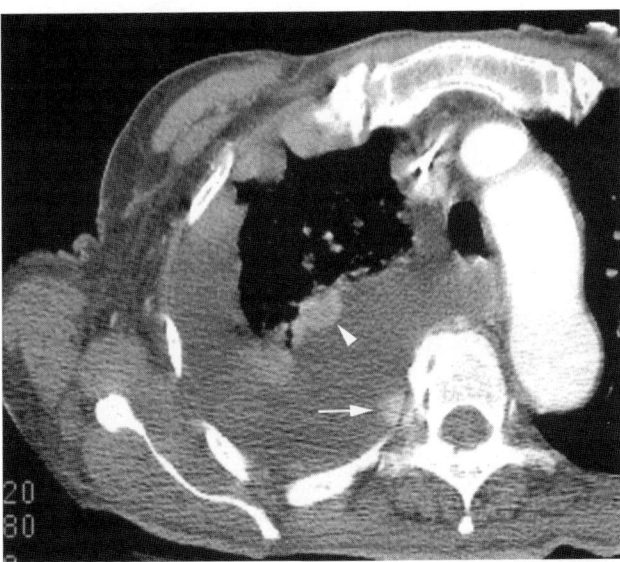

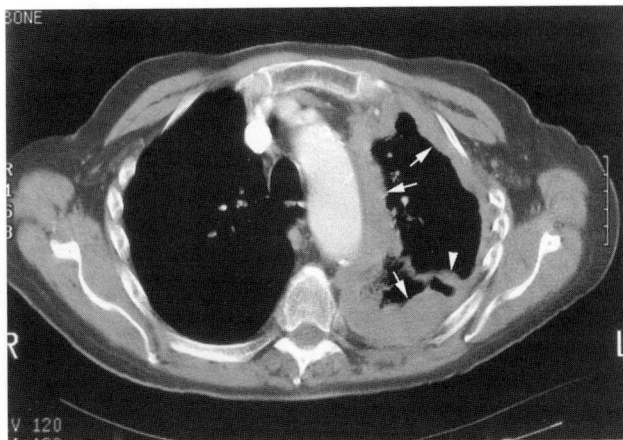

Fig. 10-13. Malignant mesothelioma. Soft tissue extending over all the pleural surfaces (*arrows*) of the left hemithorax in this patient with malignant mesothelioma. Note that the tumor extends into the major fissure (*arrowhead*).

Fig. 10-12. Metastatic breast carcinoma to the pleura. Enhancing nodules on the visceral (*arrow*) and parietal (*arrowhead*) pleural surfaces are seen in the presence of a malignant pleural effusion in a patient with metastatic breast carcinoma.

Pleural Soft Tissue Processes

CT is superior to plain film for distinguishing a pleural mass from a subpleural mass; however, even with CT, this distinction is not always easy to make. Soft tissue processes that can involve the pleura include neoplastic processes, such as metastatic disease, malignant mesothelioma, and benign tumors. Non-neoplastic soft tissue processes that can be seen in the pleural space include asbestos-related pleural plaques, postinflammatory or post-traumatic pleural thickening, and subpleural fat deposition.

When a new pleural effusion of unclear etiology is discovered, the effusion is often suspected to be malignant. The definitive diagnosis of a malignant pleural effusion requires a pathologic diagnosis. CT findings that suggest that an effusion is malignant include irregular pleural thickening and, particularly, the presence of enhancing pleural nodules or masses (Fig. 10-12). As Kuhlmand (1997) notes, other features that have been described in association with malignant effusions include pleural thickening that exceeds 1 cm and involvement of the mediastinal pleura. Malignant pleural effusions with pleural thickening or masses may be seen with pleural metastases from a wide variety of tumors or in malignant mesothelioma.

Malignant mesothelioma appears on a CT scan as a thick, pleurally based rind of soft tissue encasing the lung (Fig. 10-13). A variable quantity of fluid, usually loculated, is generally present. The density of this fluid is usually less than that of the rind of soft tissue; this difference is increased if IV contrast is administered. Malignant mesothelioma may spread directly to involve the mediastinum, pericardium, contralat-

eral lung, or chest wall. It may also spread through the diaphragm to involve the abdominal and retroperitoneal viscera. CT is generally considered the optimal study to identify the extent of involvement with mesothelioma, although MR imaging may also be used, particularly to evaluate the extent of diaphragmatic and transdiaphragmatic involvement.

Only two types of benign tumors commonly involve the pleura: benign localized fibrous tumors of the pleura (formerly known as *benign mesotheliomas*) and lipomas. Pleural fibromas appear as a mass of soft tissue attenuation, similar to muscle, without effusion. A diagnosis of pleural lipoma can be made with confidence when a mass of uniform fatty density is seen at CT as reported by McLoud and Flower (1991) (Fig. 10-14).

Asbestos-related pleural plaques appear as plateau-shaped pleural soft tissue masses. These are usually seen bilaterally and are predominantly located in the mid- to lower chest and over the diaphragms. They are frequently calcified, which adds to the confidence in making the diagnosis. Distinguishing noncalcified plaques over the diaphragms from pulmonary nodules may be difficult, particularly when the plaques are noncalcified. Occasionally asbestos-related plaques may simulate a pulmonary nodule on plain radiographs; if oblique radiographs are not helpful, CT may demonstrate the absence of nodules and show the plaques that explain the radiographic abnormality.

Chest Wall

Abnormalities of the chest wall for which cross-sectional imaging may be indicated include benign and mesenchymal tumors, primary and secondary malignancies, and inflammatory and infectious diseases. As with lung carcinoma, MR imaging is better for evaluating abnormalities near the

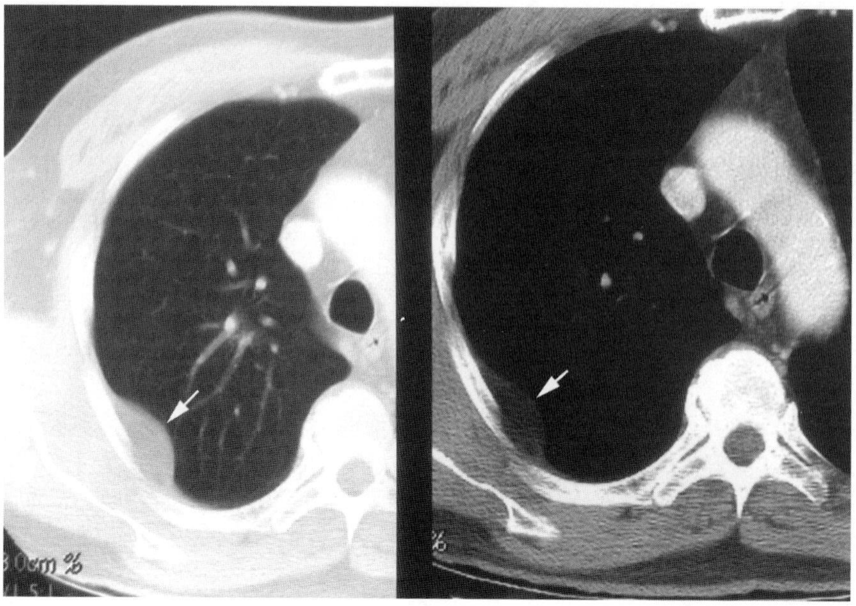

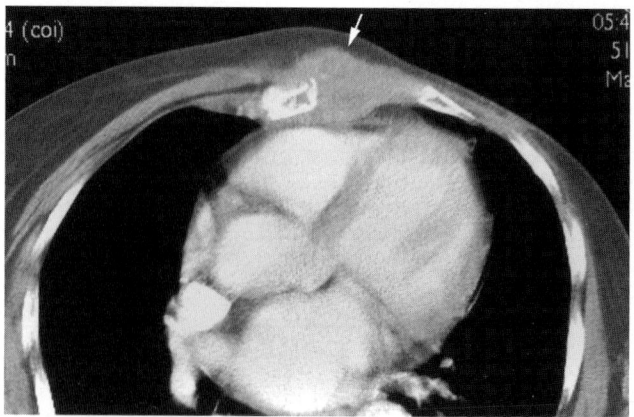

Fig. 10-14. Pleural mass of uniform fat density (*arrows*), indicating a pleural lipoma. The mass is readily seen on lung windows (**A**) but is almost invisible on mediastinal windows (**B**). Note that the attenuation of the mass changes in parallel with the subcutaneous fat.

A,B

lung apex; this particularly applies to lesions of the brachial plexus and for abnormalities of the diaphragm.

As with the pleural space, demonstration of a mass with homogeneous low attenuation of –100 to –160 Hounsfield units allows for the diagnosis of a lipoma. As Kuhlman and associates (1994) noted, liposarcoma usually is inhomogeneous with areas of soft tissue attenuation and fat attenuation.

Masses of soft tissue density are much less likely to be specifically characterized with CT or MR imaging. The primary use of CT in other chest wall neoplasms is to assess the extent of disease. Masses can arise from any of the soft tissues that make up the chest wall, including fibrous connective tissue, nerves, muscles, blood vessels, breast tissue, lymphatics, cartilage, and bone. Associated bony changes are often seen with chest wall masses. Tumors of neural origin in the costovertebral sulci are very common and include neurofibromas, schwannomas, neurofibrosarcomas, neuromas, neuroblastomas, ganglioneuromas, and ganglioneuroblastomas. Tumors of blood vessels include hemangiomas, which encompass a variety of subtypes; focal calcifications within these, known as *phleboliths*, may suggest the diagnosis. Lymphangiomas are frequently low in attenuation at CT; however, as Kuhlman and colleagues (1994) have stated, differentiation from surrounding muscle may be very difficult, particularly if no IV contrast is administered.

Of the malignant soft tissue tumors that may arise in the chest wall, breast carcinoma is by far the most common. CT has very little role to play in the diagnosis of breast carcinoma; however, advanced tumors may be incidentally identified, and CT can detect local recurrence after mastectomy (Fig. 10-15). Other malignancies that may arise in the chest wall include soft tissue sarcomas and lymphoma.

Tumors that are centered in bone on CT may include osseous metastases and tumors that are primary to cartilage or bone (Fig. 10-16). The most common primary tumor of bone in adults is multiple myeloma. Less common tumors include osteosarcoma, chondrosarcoma, and fibrosarcoma and benign tumors and tumorlike lesions, including fibrous dysplasia, enchondroma, and aneurysmal bone cyst. Although the appearance of all of these tumors at CT is likely to be fairly nonspecific, some of them have characteristic findings on plain film.

Infections in the chest wall are somewhat rare but may be life-threatening. As Kuhlman and associates (1994) noted, organisms that can cause such infections include pyogenic bacteria, actinomycetes, blastomycetes, *Nocardia*, *Aspergillus*, and *M. tuberculosis*. Some of these agents tend to involve the chest wall via extension from an underlying pulmonary infection. Other mechanisms by which chest wall infection may arise include infection of a surgical incision or other direct trauma. CT may demonstrate areas of bone destruction and

Fig. 10-15. Chest wall metastasis. Soft tissue mass (*arrow*) is present in the chest wall, adjacent to a left costal cartilage, indicating local recurrence of breast carcinoma in this patient who has undergone previous left mastectomy. Bone scans and plain radiographs of the ribs and sternum were negative.

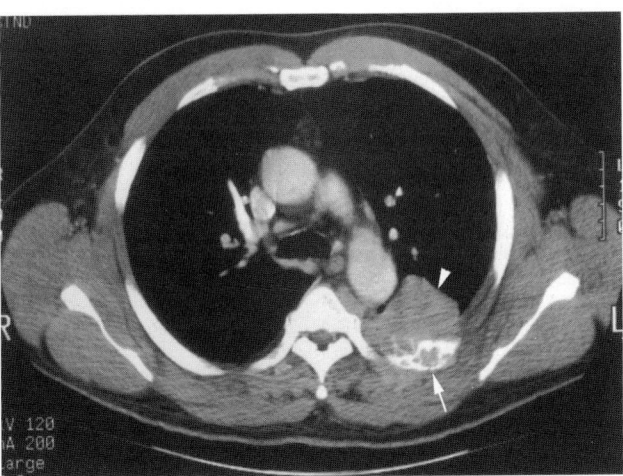

Fig. 10-16. Multiple myeloma involving a posterior rib, with bony destruction (*arrow*) and a soft tissue mass (*arrowhead*) projecting into the left lung.

skin fistulae. In the setting of necrotizing fasciitis, CT is probably the most sensitive imaging technique for the detection of gas within the soft tissues (see Fig. 10-5). Detection of discrete abscess collections, however, may not be easy on CT, particularly if no IV contrast is administered.

POSTOPERATIVE EVALUATION AND CRITICALLY ILL PATIENTS

The normal posteroanterior and lateral examination of the chest provides a great deal of spatial information about abnormalities within the chest, as they can be localized in two planes. However, critically ill patients and many postoperative patients are unable to undergo a standard radiographic examination of the chest. Portable radiography is much more limited, especially when imaged in a supine position.

In particular, pneumothoraces, pleural effusions, and parenchymal opacities at the lung bases may be very difficult to identify on supine radiographs (Fig. 10-17). Pleural fluid may be difficult to distinguish from parenchymal opacification at the bases on portable films. Air-fluid levels are also difficult to detect on portable films, and thus lung abscesses may also be missed on these radiographs. All of these abnormalities are easily detected on CT. Several series, including one by one of us (W.T.M.) and colleagues (1998), as well as those by Mirvis (1987) and Golding (1988) and their associates, show a contribution to the management of selected patients in whom CT was performed to assess for an explanation of clinical deterioration or failure to respond to therapy. In our series, the most commonly detected abnormalities were unsuspected fluid collections, previously undetected foci of pneumonia, and malignancies.

When CT is performed in postoperative patients, trauma patients, or other critically ill patients, thoracostomy tube position can be assessed. Cameron and col-

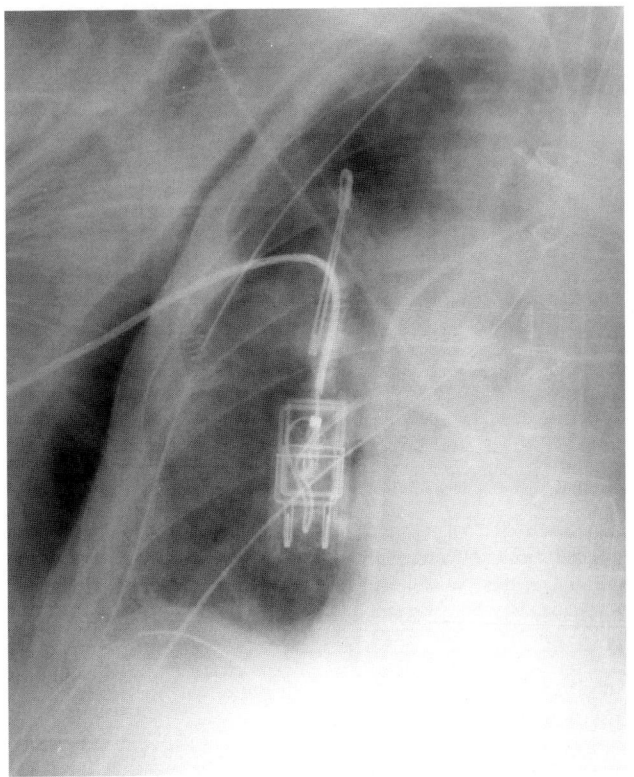

A

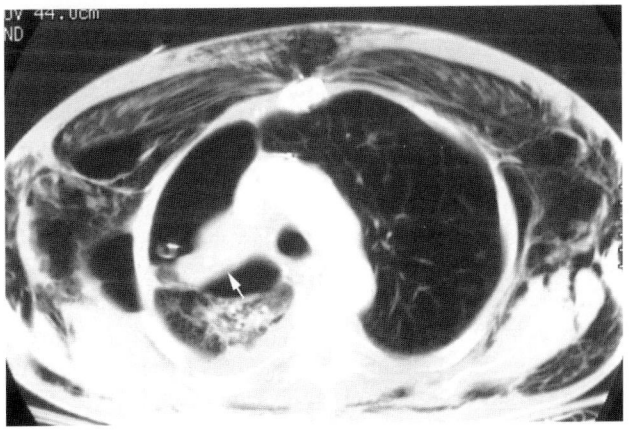

B

Fig. 10-17. Radiographically occult pneumothorax. **A.** Portable radiograph demonstrates subcutaneous emphysema but no definite pneumothorax in this patient with right-sided thoracostomy drains. **B.** A computed tomography scan again shows subcutaneous emphysema but also demonstrates a large anterior right pneumothorax, seen as an absence of lung markings anteriorly and as an atelectatic lung (*arrow*) posteriorly.

leagues (1997) have shown that a number of abnormalities in thoracostomy drain placement are visible on CT. These drains may terminate within the lung parenchyma, indicating that the pleura has been violated. Intraparenchymal placement, however, can be difficult to distinguish from placement within a fissure. Drains may also be placed with their tips abutting the mediastinum, which over time may lead to erosion of mediastinal structures or to contusion. Occasionally, the tubes may be placed entirely out-

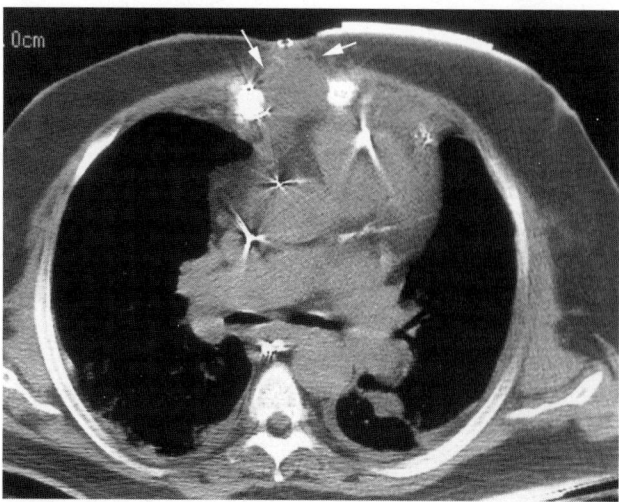

Fig. 10-18. Sternal osteomyelitis. Computed tomography demonstrates a fluid collection (*arrows*) separating the two halves of the sternum in this patient with a sternal wound infection. Widening was caused by bony erosion.

side the thoracic cavity, either in the chest wall or transdiaphragmatically into the abdomen.

Templeton and Fishman (1992) note that CT is an important part of evaluation of patients with suspected sternal wound infections after median sternotomy. CT can demonstrate fluid collections, which may be seen postoperatively both superficial and deep to the sternum. The identification of a fluid collection alone is not diagnostic of abscess. Collections may be sterile or infected; the fluid must be sampled for definitive diagnosis. If large amounts of gas are present in a collection, the probability that infection is present is increased, but small amounts of gas are normal in at least the first postoperative week. Bony destruction is very suggestive of sternal wound infection (Fig. 10-18). Mediastinitis, a life-threatening postoperative complication, can be difficult to diagnose. Soft tissue density obliterating the normal mediastinal fat can suggest this diagnosis; gas collections are also suggestive.

Templeton and Fishman (1992) note that CT has only a small role to play in the evaluation of sternal dehiscence, which is usually detectable on clinical grounds. Nevertheless, rotation of the sternal wires, displacement or fracture, and apparent widening of the transparency between the sternal fragments may be seen in such a dehiscence.

Kopka and colleagues (1996) have noted that retained surgical sponges are not always easily detected on CT. The dense markers on surgical sponges may be mistaken for calcifications, and small gas bubbles are frequently—but not always—present. Small gas bubbles may represent retained air in these sponges and should not be considered a sign of infection.

REFERENCES

Aquino SL, Webb WR, Gushiken BJ: Pleural exudates and transudates: diagnosis with contrast-enhanced CT. Radiology 192:803, 1994.

Arita T, et al: Bronchogenic carcinoma: incidence of metastases to normal sized lymph nodes. Thorax 50:1267, 1995.
Austin JH, et al: Glossary of terms for CT of the lungs: recommendations of the Nomenclature Committee of the Fleischner Society. Radiology 200:327, 1996.
Bilbey JH, et al: MR imaging of adrenal masses: value of chemical-shift imaging for distinguishing adenomas from other tumors. AJR Am J Roentgenol 164:637, 1995.
Boland GW, et al: Adrenal masses: characterization with delayed contrast-enhanced CT. Radiology 202:693, 1997.
Brodeur FJ, et al: Delayed enhanced CT: a method of differentiating adrenal adenomas from nonadenomas [abstract]. Radiology 197P:185, 1995.
Cameron EW, et al: Computed tomography of malpositioned thoracostomy drains: a pictorial essay. Clin Radiol 52:187, 1997.
Curry TS, et al: Christensen's Physics of Diagnostic Radiology. Media, PA: Williams & Wilkins, 1990.
Dewan NA, et al: Diagnostic efficacy of PET-FDG imaging in solitary pulmonary nodules. Chest 104:997, 1993.
Dwyer A: The displaced crus: a sign for distinguishing between pleural fluid and ascites on computed tomography. J Comput Assist Tomogr 2:598, 1978.
Epstein DM, et al: Lobar bronchioloalveolar cell carcinoma. AJR Am J Roentgenol 139:463, 1982.
Erasmus JJ, et al: Thoracic FDG PET: state of the art. Radiographics 18:5, 1998.
Fraser RS, et al (eds): Synopsis of Diseases of the Chest. Philadelphia: WB Saunders, 1994.
Gefter WB: The spectrum of pulmonary aspergillosis. J Thorac Imaging 7:56, 1992.
Giron J, et al: Interventional chest radiology. Eur J Radiol 23:58, 1996.
Glazer HS, et al: Pleural and chest wall invasion in bronchogenic carcinoma: CT evaluation. Radiology 157:191, 1985.
Golding RP, et al: Computed tomography as an adjunct to chest x-rays of intensive care unit patients. Crit Care Med 16:211, 1988.
Goodman LR, et al: Detection of pulmonary embolism in patients with unresolved clinical and scintigraphic diagnosis: helical CT versus angiography. AJR Am J Roentgenol 164:1369, 1995.
Griffin DJ, et al: Observation on CT differentiation of pleural and peritoneal fluid. J Comput Assist Tomogr 8:24, 1984.
Gupta NC, et al: Solitary pulmonary nodules: detection of malignancy with PET with 2-[F-18]-fluoro-2-deoxy-D-glucose. Radiology 184:441, 1992.
Hagberg RC, et al: Characterization of pulmonary nodules and mediastinal staging of bronchogenic carcinoma with F-18 fluorodeoxyglucose positron emission tomography. Eur J Cardiothorac Surg 12:92, 1997.
Halvorsen RA, et al: Ascites or pleural effusion? Radiographics 6:135, 1986.
Hansell DM, Kerr IH: The role of high resolution computed tomography in the diagnosis of interstitial lung disease. Thorax 46:77, 1991.
Henschke CI, et al: Changing practice patterns in the workup of pulmonary embolism. Chest 107:940, 1995.
Hsu JT, et al: Radiologic assessment of bronchopleural fistula with empyema. Radiology 103:41, 1972.
Huston J, Muhm JR: Solitary pulmonary opacities: plain tomography. Radiology 163:481, 1987.
Kalender WA, et al: Spiral volumetric CT with single-breath-hold technique, continuous transport, and continuous scanner rotation. Radiology 176:181, 1990.
Kazerooni EA, et al: Imaging of emphysema and lung volume reduction surgery. Radiographics 17:1023, 1997.
Klein JS, et al: Interventional radiology of the chest: image-guided percutaneous drainage of pleural effusions, lung abscess, and pneumothorax. AJR Am J Roentgenol 164:581, 1995.
Klein JS, Salomon G, Stewart E: Transthoracic needle biopsy with a coaxially placed 20-gauge automated cutting needle: results in 122 patients. Radiology 198:715, 1996.
Kopka L, et al: CT of retained surgical sponges (textilomas): pitfalls in detection and evaluation. J Comput Assist Tomogr 20:919, 1996.
Kuhlman JE: Complex disease of the pleural space: the 10 questions most frequently asked of the radiologist—new approaches to their answers with CT and MR imaging. Radiographics 17:1043, 1997.
Kuhlman JE, et al: Invasive pulmonary aspergillosis in acute leukemia: characteristic findings on CT, the CT halo sign, and the role of CT in early diagnosis. Radiology 157:611, 1985.

Kuhlman JE, et al: CT and MR imaging evaluation of chest wall disorders. Radiographics *14*:571, 1994.

Lee MJ, et al: Benign and malignant adrenal masses: CT distinction with attenuation coefficients, size and observer analysis. Radiology *179*:415, 1991.

Leung AN, et al: Parenchymal opacification in chronic infiltrative lung diseases: CT-pathologic correlation. Radiology *188*:209, 1993.

Libshitz HI, et al: Mediastinal evaluation in lung cancer. Radiology *151*:295, 1984.

Mayo JR, et al: Pulmonary embolism: prospective comparison of spiral CT with ventilation-perfusion scintigraphy. Radiology *205*:447, 1997.

McLoud TC, Flower CDR: Imaging the pleura: sonography, CT, and MR imaging. AJR Am J Roentgenol *156*:1145, 1991.

McManigle JE, et al: Bronchoscopy in the management of bronchopleural fistula. Chest *97*:1235, 1990.

Miller WT Jr, Tino G, Friedburg JS: Thoracic CT in the intensive care unit: assessment of clinical usefulness. Radiology *209*:491, 1998.

Mirvis SE, et al: Thoracic CT in detecting occult disease in critically ill patients. AJR Am J Roentgenol *148*:685, 1987.

Mitchell DG, et al: Benign adrenocortical masses: diagnosis with chemical-shift imaging. Radiology *185*:345, 1992.

Munden RT, et al: Small pulmonary lesions detected at CT: clinical importance. Radiology *202*:105, 1997.

Naidich DP, et al: Computed tomography of the diaphragm: peridiaphragmatic fluid localization. J Comput Assist Tomogr *7*:641, 1983.

Naidich DP, et al: Computed tomography of the pulmonary parenchyma. Part I. Distal air-space disease. J Thorac Imaging *1*:39, 1985.

Naidich DP, et al: Hemoptysis: CT-bronchoscopic correlations in 58 cases. Radiology *177*:357, 1990.

Nathan MH, Collins VP, Adams RA: Differentiation of benign and malignant pulmonary nodules by growth rate. Radiology *79*:221, 1962.

Onitsuka H, et al: Differentiation of central lung tumor from postobstructive lobar collapse by rapid sequence computed tomography. J Thorac Imag *6*:28, 1991.

Patz EF, et al: Focal pulmonary abnormalities: evaluation with F-18 fluorodeoxyglucose PET scanning. Radiology *188*:487, 1993.

Pennes DR, et al: Chest wall invasion by lung cancer: limitations of CT evaluation. AJR Am J Roentgenol *144*:507, 1985.

Ratto GB, et al: Chest wall invasion by lung cancer: computed tomographic detection and results of operation. Ann Thorac Surg *51*:182, 1991.

Reinig JW, et al: Differentiation of adrenal masses with MR imaging: comparison of techniques. Radiology *197*:41, 1994.

Remy J: Pulmonary arteriovenous malformations: evaluation with CT of the chest before and after treatment. Radiology *182*:808, 1992.

Remy-Jardin M, et al: Central pulmonary thromboembolism: diagnosis with spiral volumetric CT with single breath-hold technique: comparison with pulmonary angiography. Radiology *185*:381, 1992.

Remy-Jardin M, et al: Pulmonary nodules: detection with thick-section spiral CT versus conventional CT. Radiology *187*:513, 1993.

Schneider HJ, et al: Rounded atelectasis. AJR Am J Roentgenol *134*:225, 1980.

Society for Computed Body Tomography. Special report: new indications for computed body tomography. AJR Am J Roentgenol *133*:115, 1979.

Sostman HD, et al: Use of pulmonary angiography for suspected pulmonary embolism: influence of scintigraphic diagnosis. AJR Am J Roentgenol *139*:673, 1982.

Stark D, et al: Differentiating lung abscess and empyema: radiography and computed tomography AJR Am J Roentgenol *141*:163, 1983.

Swensen SJ, et al: CT evaluation of solitary pulmonary nodules: value of 185-H reference phantom. AJR Am J Roentgenol *156*:925, 1991.

Swensen SJ, et al: Pulmonary nodules: CT evaluation of enhancement with iodinated contrast material. Radiology *194*:393, 1995.

Swensen SJ, et al: Lung nodule enhancement at CT: prospective findings. Radiology *201*:447, 1996.

Teigen CL, et al: Pulmonary embolism: diagnosis with contrast-enhanced electron-beam CT and comparison with pulmonary angiography. Radiology *194*:313, 1995.

Templeton PA, Fishman EK: CT evaluation of poststernotomy complications. AJR Am J Roentgenol *159*:45, 1992.

Teplick JG, et al: The interface sign: a computed tomographic sign for distinguishing pleural and intra-abdominal fluid. Radiology *144*:359, 1982.

Tsushuma Y, Ishizaka H, Matsumoto M: Adrenal masses: differentiation with chemical-shift, fast low angle shot MR imaging. Radiology *186*:705, 1993.

Vock P, et al: Lung spiral volumetric CT with single breath-hold technique. Radiology *176*:864, 1990.

Webb WR, Muller NL, Naidich DP: High-Resolution CT of the Lung. Philadelphia: Lippincott-Raven, 1996.

Webb WR, et al: CT and MR imaging in staging non-small cell bronchogenic carcinoma: report of the Radiologic Diagnostic Oncology Group. Radiology *178*:705, 1991.

Westcott JL, Volpe JP: Peripheral bronchopleural fistula: CT evaluation in 20 patients with pneumonia, empyema or postoperative air leak. Radiology *196*:175, 1995.

Yamashita KS, et al: Solitary pulmonary nodule: preliminary study of evaluation with incremental dynamic CT. Radiology *194*:399, 1995.

Zerhouni EA, et al: A standard phantom for quantitative CT analysis of pulmonary nodules. Radiology *149*:767, 1983.

CHAPTER 11

Magnetic Resonance Imaging of the Thorax

Alan H. Stolpen, J. Jeffrey Carr, Hiroto Hatabu, and Warren B. Gefter

Chest radiography is almost always the first imaging study for evaluating known or suspected thoracic disease. Subsequent imaging may include computed tomography (CT), conventional contrast angiography, or echocardiography. Magnetic resonance (MR) imaging has been used primarily as a problem-solving tool: It clarifies the findings of other imaging modalities. However, MR imaging is also beginning to establish itself as the primary modality for evaluating a limited set of diseases. Unique strengths of MR imaging include high soft tissue contrast, multiplanar imaging, and noninvasive vascular imaging. From a technical standpoint, the thorax presents a challenge for MR imaging. Image quality is degraded by pulsatile blood flow, cardiac and respiratory motions, and the heterogeneous magnetic susceptibility of lung. Numerous technical innovations have remedied some of these problems. Yet physicians have been slow to embrace MR imaging. The relatively high cost and limited availability of MR imaging may be contributing factors. Clinical outcome studies will be needed to determine if MR imaging is cost effective for patients with thoracic disease. The goal of this chapter is to introduce the principles and practice of thoracic MR imaging and familiarize the reader with the strengths and weaknesses of this rapidly evolving modality.

Flexibility is both a strength and weakness of MR imaging. The number of ways to image the thorax with MR imaging is virtually unlimited, but not all imaging sequences can be applied to every patient. The MR imaging examination should be tailored to answer a specific clinical question or evaluate a specific pathologic entity. Thoracic MR imaging is poorly suited to an unfocused survey or "search and destroy" type examination. The referring clinician should provide a relevant clinical history to help the radiologist perform a proper MR study. Additional clinical information may be obtained by the technologist or radiologist by interviewing the patient before the examination. Excellent communication between the surgeon and

radiologist helps ensure that MR examinations will be appropriate, focused, and efficient.

THEORY AND TECHNIQUE

General Principles

To the uninitiated, MR images are enigmatic. The appearance and physical basis of soft tissue contrast are different for MR imaging and CT. Likewise, the mechanism of soft tissue enhancement by exogenous contrast materials is different for these two studies. In addition, the artifacts that must be understood to render a correct diagnostic interpretation differ between MR imaging and CT. These phenomena and others can be understood with a modicum of basic MR imaging theory. Although a complete theoretical description of MR imaging lies in quantum mechanics, many important concepts can be understood with simple analogies from classical physics.

MR imaging represents an interaction between certain atomic nuclei, an external magnetic field, and applied radio frequency (rf) waves. Atomic nuclei with an odd number of protons or neutrons exhibit a property called *spin*, a quantum mechanical phenomenon that does not connote a spinning motion. However, for heuristic purposes, it can be helpful to consider spin in the ordinary sense of a spinning top. In the human body the most abundant nuclear species with spin is the hydrogen nucleus or proton. The two tissues with the highest proton concentrations or proton densities are fat and water; pure water has a proton concentration of 110 M. Tissue proton density is proportional to MR signal intensity and is therefore a source of soft tissue contrast. Other nuclei in the human body, such as fluorine, phosphorus, and sodium, also exhibit spin but are present at much lower concentrations. Noble gases such as helium 3 and xenon 129 exhibit spin and can be hyperpolarized for use as inhalational contrast agents. Currently, hydrogen is the only nucleus routinely used in clinical MR imaging, although this could change in the future.

Spin

The spin of the positively charged hydrogen nucleus creates a small magnetic moment, analogous to a tiny bar magnet. In MR parlance, magnetic moments are called *spins*. The magnitude and direction of a spin can be represented by a small vector. An ensemble of spins is randomly oriented in the absence of an external magnetic field. However, in the presence of an external magnetic field (designated B_0 and oriented in the +Z direction), spin one-half nuclei establish a thermal equilibrium distribution in which they align either parallel or antiparallel to B_0. A slight excess of spins aligns with B_0 because this is a lower energy condition. At a magnetic field strength of 1.5 tesla, typical for a high field MR imaging scanner, only seven excess spins per million are aligned with B_0. MR signal intensity is proportional to the tissue density of excess spins. Although pure water has a total spin density of 110 M, the excess spin density is considerably lower at 0.8 mM. The stronger the external magnetic field, the greater the excess spin density. This explains why higher field strength MR imaging scanners usually produce better (i.e., less noisy) images.

Hyperpolarization

If the distribution of spins between the parallel and antiparallel states could somehow be altered from the thermal equilibrium distribution, it would be possible to increase MR signal intensity. In fact, a nonequilibrium spin distribution has been achieved with the noble gases helium 3 and xenon 129 using optical pumping to *hyperpolarize* the spins. Hyperpolarization increases the net magnetization by almost 100,000-fold. Despite the relatively low concentration of spins in a noble gas (approximately 45 mM under ordinary conditions), the MR signal is comparable with that of nonhyperpolarized water. Hyperpolarized noble gases offer the intriguing possibility of directly imaging air-containing spaces in the body such as the lungs (Fig. 11-1), tracheobronchial tree, and paranasal sinuses.

Nuclear Precession

A key concept is that spins precess about the axis of the external magnetic field in a manner similar to the wobble of a spinning top. The precession frequency is directly proportional to the strength of B_0 and is called the *Larmor frequency*. The proton Larmor frequency in a 1.5-tesla MR

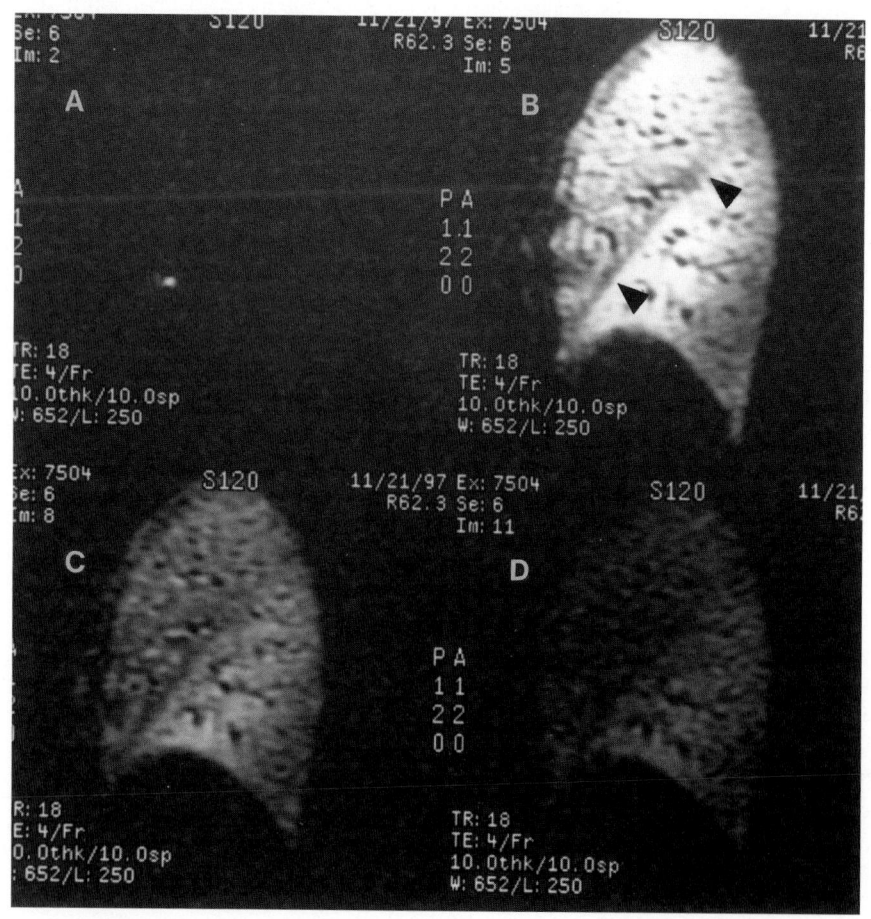

Fig. 11-1. Normal magnetic resonance (MR) pulmonary ventilation scan with hyperpolarized ^{3}He gas. Sagittal MR images were acquired through the same location in the right lung before **(A)** and after **(B–D)** inhalation of hyperpolarized gas (left is anterior, right is posterior). MR signal arises from hyperpolarized gas in the bronchoalveolar spaces. The MR signal intensity decreases as the section of right lung is reimaged **(B–D)** because of loss of magnetization. The major fissure **(B,** *arrowheads*) is seen as a signal void. Courtesy of Dr. Rahim R. Rizi.

imaging scanner is approximately 64 MHz, similar to the frequency of an FM radio station. Water protons precess slightly faster than fat protons, 220 Hz faster at 1.5 tesla. This small frequency difference can be exploited in *chemical shift* techniques such as opposed phase MR imaging and frequency-selective fat suppression.

The vector sum of all spin magnetic moments is called *net magnetization*. Only excess spins contribute to net magnetization: All other spins sum to zero. At equilibrium the net magnetization points in the +z direction, where it is called *longitudinal magnetization*. Longitudinal magnetization does not produce an MR signal. The plane perpendicular to the Z-axis is the XY-plane, and magnetization that lies in this plane is called *transverse magnetization*. At equilibrium no transverse magnetization occurs. MR signal is derived exclusively from transverse magnetization. Transverse magnetization produces a time-varying magnetic field that induces a tiny alternating current in a wire loop receiver placed near the source. These tiny currents are digitized, amplified, combined, and Fourier transformed to yield the MR image.

Coils

Receivers or coils are the physical entities that detect the faint signal emanating from the patient's tissues. Coils also transmit rf, thereby delivering rf energy into the patient. Coils can be specially configured to receive signal from anatomic regions of various sizes and shapes. The two most frequently used coils for thoracic imaging are the body coil and phased array torso coil. The body coil is built into the bore of most superconducting MR imaging scanners and can be used for imaging large anatomic regions, such as the entire thorax. The maximum craniocaudal *field of view* of the body coil is limited to approximately 48 cm. The phased array torso coil is used for imaging slightly smaller anatomic regions, such as the heart or thoracic aorta, but with better signal-to-noise and higher spatial resolution than the body coil. Special surface coils can be used for imaging small, well-defined regions, such as a portion of a rib, with high spatial resolution. In selecting a particular coil, one makes a tradeoff between anatomic coverage and spatial resolution.

Resonance

Radio frequency waves interact with spin magnetic moments when the rf frequency is tuned to the spin precession frequency. This concept is called *resonance* and is so important that it has been incorporated into the name MR imaging. Short rf pulses are used to change the orientation of or *tip* the net magnetization. For example, a 90-degree rf pulse, or 90-degree *flip angle*, tips longitudinal magnetization into the transverse plane, where it will generate a signal. A 180-degree rf pulse rotates transverse magnetization from the +x to the –x direction, in which case it is called a 180-degree refocusing pulse. Spin echo and fast spin echo sequences use both 90-degree and 180-degree rf pulses. Gradient echo sequences, such as those used in MR angiography, generally use rf pulses smaller than 90 degrees. Unlike spin echo sequences, gradient echo sequences do not use 180-degree refocusing pulses.

T_1 and T_2 Relaxation

A major source of soft tissue contrast in MR imaging is the varied relaxation behavior of hydrogen nuclei in different tissues. The two parameters that describe tissue relaxation are T_1 and T_2. MR imaging sequences can be designed to accentuate differences in T_1 or T_2, but not both at the same time. Images that accentuate tissue T_1 differences are called *T_1-weighted*, whereas those that accentuate T_2 differences are called *T_2-weighted*. It is often possible to characterize a tissue based on its relaxation behavior. The T_1 and T_2 behavior of a tissue may vary with magnetic field strength. Thus, soft tissues may appear somewhat different when they are imaged on MR imaging scanners having different magnetic field strengths.

T_1 is the characteristic time for spins to reestablish a thermal equilibrium distribution. At equilibrium no transverse magnetization occurs—only longitudinal magnetization. A 90-degree rf pulse, for example, temporarily disturbs the equilibrium by tipping all longitudinal magnetization into the transverse plane. Over time, the longitudinal magnetization increases exponentially from zero to the equilibrium value, which, under ordinary conditions, is also the maximum value. T_1 relaxation processes involve an exchange of energy between spins and their environment (the *lattice*), which is why T_1 is also called *spin-lattice* relaxation.

Proton T_1 values vary among tissues, and these differences generate soft tissue contrast on T_1-weighted MR images. Tissues with a short T_1 appear bright and those with a long T_1 appear dark. Many strategies exist for introducing T_1-weighting. Consider, for example, the behavior of longitudinal magnetization, initially at equilibrium, acted on by a train of 90-degree pulses separated by a repetition time of TR. If TR is much longer than T_1, the longitudinal magnetization returns to equilibrium before the next 90-degree pulse arrives. However, if TR is shorter than T_1, the longitudinal magnetization never reaches equilibrium. Instead, it reaches a steady state level that is less, sometimes much less, than its maximum value. And after the 90-degree pulse, the transverse magnetization, and the MR signal it produces, is also less than its maximum value. Fat protons have a shorter T_1 than water protons. To create T_1 contrast between fat and water, choose a TR that is longer than the T_1 of fat but shorter than the T_1 of water. The result is that fat appears brighter than water. Conversely, a very long TR virtually eliminates T_1 contrast from an image. The image acquisition time increases directly with TR, so long TR pulse sequences are lengthy.

T_2 is the characteristic time for decay of transverse magnetization. T_2^* is similar to T_2 but includes spin *dephasing* caused by magnetic field gradients and inhomogeneities. After an rf pulse creates transverse magnetization, all spins are *in phase*, which is to say that their magnetic moments all point in the same direction. At this time the vector sum, the transverse magnetization, assumes a maximum value. Subsequently, as the spins begin to interact with one another and with their environment, they fan out or *dephase* in the transverse plane. Eventually, the spins become randomly oriented and the vector sum vanishes. Any process that increases the rate of spin dephasing also increases the T_2 relaxation rate or, equivalently, shortens T_2. In the human body, T_2 relaxation processes are either intrinsic to a tissue, related to tissue interfaces, or caused by external causes such as magnetic field inhomogeneity. Intrinsic T_2 relaxation arises from the mutual interactions of spins within a tissue. It is generally true that greater interaction leads to T_2 shortening. This is why T_2 is also called *spin-spin* relaxation. Water protons have a long T_2 because water molecules move so rapidly, on an MR imaging time scale, that the spins cannot interact effectively with one another.

Like T_1, proton T_2 values also vary among tissues, and these differences generate soft tissue contrast on T2-weighted MR images. Tissues with a short T_2 appear dark and those with a long T_2 appear bright. Thus, water protons, which have a long T_2, appear bright on T_2-weighted images. In the lung, heterogeneous magnetic susceptibility markedly shortens T_2 and T_2^*. The complex architecture of the lung juxtaposes magnetically dissimilar tissues (i.e., those with different magnetic susceptibilities), specifically water in the lung interstitium and air in the bronchoalveolar tree. Consequently, normal lung parenchyma appear as a black signal void on most MR images. The low proton density of lung tissue also contributes to its MR appearance.

Echoes

Transverse magnetization decays rapidly, especially when magnetic gradients are on. The MR signal produced by the rapidly decaying transverse magnetization, which is called a *free induction decay*, cannot be used to make an ordinary MR image because it occurs too soon after the rf pulse. To introduce a temporal separation between the rf pulse and the MR signal, one forms an *echo* of the initial free induction decay. Echoes occur when dephasing spins are refocused. Refocusing causes the transverse magnetization and MR signal to pass through a second maximum, the echo. The delay between the initial rf pulse and the echo is called the *echo time* (TE). The maximum signal from the first echo is always less than that of the free induction decay. The signal decrement reflects T_2 decay over the period TE. Thus, TE can be used to control the amount of soft tissue T_2 contrast. A short TE decreases T_2 contrast, whereas a long TE increases it.

Many strategies exist for producing an echo, but only two are used routinely in clinical MR imaging: the 180-degree refocusing pulse and magnetic gradient reversal. These two types of echoes, and the MR imaging sequences based on them, are called *spin echo* and *gradient echo*. The strategy used to form the first echo can be repeated to form a second echo and a third echo and so on. *Fast spin echo* sequences use multiple, equally spaced 180-degree refocusing pulses, whereas *echo planar* sequences employ multiple magnetic gradient reversals. Hybrid spin echo/gradient echo sequences also exist, but are not widely used. The tradeoffs between spin echoes and gradient echoes relate to speed, image noise, soft tissue contrast, and suitability for vascular imaging.

IMAGING

Spatial Encoding

During each echo the receiver coil detects a cacophony of MR signals from billions and billions of hydrogen nuclei. The spatial location of these signals must be determined to make an image, a concept known as *spatial localization* or *spatial encoding*. MR imaging uses magnetic field gradients to localize spins in space. A magnetic field gradient, or simply a *gradient*, is a magnetic field whose strength varies linearly with position. MR imaging scanners are equipped with X, Y, and Z gradients. These can be used alone or in combination to produce a resultant gradient with any oblique orientation. The gradients add or subtract a small amount of magnetic field from the much larger B_0 field. As the magnetic field changes, so does the precession frequency of the hydrogen nuclei. In effect, the gradient sets up a map between spatial location and precession frequency. Exogenous metals, such as surgical clips, prosthetic joints, and vascular stents, may distort the gradient and the map and thereby produce substantial image artifact.

MR image data can be spatially encoded in two (2D) or three dimensions (3D). In 2D imaging, a specially constructed rf pulse *excites* spins (i.e., creates transverse magnetization) in a thin slice of tissue while a magnetic gradient is on. The thickness and orientation of the excited slice are controlled by the strength and orientation of the gradient as well as the rf pulse. MR images can be acquired in any plane: axial, sagittal, coronal, or oblique. In contrast, the orientation of CT images is physically constrained by the position of the patient within the gantry. By exciting hydrogen nuclei only within a single slice, the spatial encoding problem is reduced to two dimensions. These two dimensions are spatially mapped using *frequency encoding* in one direction and *phase encoding* in the other. The number of phase (N_p) and frequency encoding steps is called the *matrix* and this, in combination with the field of view, determines the in-plane spatial resolution of the MR image. The effect is to divide the imaged slice into N_p multiplied by number of frequency rectangular picture elements called *pixels*. A *voxel* is a 3D volume element whose face is a pixel and whose height is the slice thickness. The dimensions of the voxel determine the spatial resolution of an MR image.

Frequency encoding steps are time efficient so little penalty exists for increasing spatial resolution in this direction. However, phase encoding steps are time inefficient: Each additional step requires an additional TR period. The acquisition time for a conventional 2D spin echo or gradient echo imaging sequence is $TR \times N_p \times$ # signal averages. A typical matrix for a thoracic MR imaging is 256 frequency encoding steps and 128 to 192 phase encoding steps; the larger matrix element is assigned to the time efficient frequency encoding direction.

In 3D imaging, the rf pulse excites a rectangular volume of tissue, rather than a single slice, also in the presence of a magnetic gradient. The volume may be oriented in any plane or obliquity. The excited spins are spatially localized in three dimensions using frequency encoding in one direction and phase encoding in each of the other two directions. The acquisition time for a 3D imaging sequence is $TR \times N_{P-1} \times N_{P-2} \times$ # signal averages. To keep acquisition times reasonably brief, 3D imaging almost always uses a short TR fast gradient echo sequence. 3D imaging finds its greatest application in MR angiography.

Anatomy of a Pulse Sequence

A pulse sequence is the series of rf pulses and magnetic gradients that produces MR images at a specified location, in a specified anatomic plane, and with a specified soft tissue contrast. A pulse sequence is considered MR software, as opposed to the superconducting magnetic, the gradient coils, and the rf coils, which are MR hardware. Consider the organization of a commonly used pulse sequence: the 2D axial spin echo sequence with a 256 × 128 matrix. The sequence consists of a train of 128 nearly identical units, one unit for each phase encoding step. A unit begins with a slice selective 90-degree rf pulse that plays out while a gradient is on. Next, a 180-degree refocusing pulse plays out at time TE/2 and forms an echo at TE after the 90-degree pulse. The echo is acquired in the presence of a frequency encoding gradient, also called a *readout gradient*. The electronics of the MR imaging scanner digitize the echo into 256 data points. While the echo is evolving, a phase encoding gradient is turned on for a brief period. The strength of this gradient is stepped, with one step for each phase encode, from negative to positive values. The next unit begins with a 90-degree pulse at time TR after the previous 90-degree pulse. The pulse sequence ends after 128 units of 90-degree pulse, 180-degree pulse-echo are completed.

The 2D spin echo sequence can be T_1- or T_2-weighted by selecting the appropriate TR and TE. A short TR and short TE produce a T_1-weighted image, whereas a long TR and long TE produce a T_2-weighted image. Proton density or spin density weighting is obtained with a long TR and short TE. Proton density weighting is rarely used in the thorax because it provides little additional diagnostic information. Because acquisition times for a conventional T_2-weighted spin echo sequence are 10 minutes or longer, this sequence is being supplanted by the faster T_2-weighted fast spin echo sequence. Spin echo and fast spin echo sequences can be acquired in any plane. These sequences are used primarily to identify normal and abnormal soft tissue structures, assess tissue T_1 and T_2 signal intensity, and determine anatomic relationships.

Gradient echo sequences generally sacrifice soft tissue contrast for imaging speed. Many of the technological advances in MR imaging, such as stronger and faster gradients, faster receivers, and more time-efficient pulse sequences, are manifest in a variety of ultrafast gradient echo sequences. Ultrashort TR (<4 ms) and TE (<2 ms) gradient echo sequences are now standard on most commercially available, high-performance, clinical MR imaging scanners. Short acquisition times allow gradient echo images to be acquired during suspended respiration. Gradient echo images can be T_1-weighted by using a short TR/TE, a large flip angle (60 to 90 degrees), and spoiling of residual transverse magnetization. T_1-weighted fast gradient echo sequences are particularly useful for detecting soft tissue enhancement by gadolinium-based (Gd) contrast agents. For example, breath-hold, Gd-enhanced 3D MR angiography is based on a heavily T_1-weighted ultrafast 3D gradient echo sequence. 2D and 3D gradient echo sequences, particularly when used with flow compensation gradients, make flowing blood appear bright, but without administration of exogenous contrast materials. Cine MR imaging is similarly based on 2D gradient echo sequences.

Cardiac and Respiratory Gating

Cardiac and respiratory motions can degrade MR image quality in the thorax. Strategies such as cardiac gating, respiratory compensation, and respiratory gating have been devised to minimize image degradation. Cardiac gating synchronizes the MR image acquisition with an electrocardiographic (ECG) tracing derived from four ECG leads placed on the precordium or back. A cardiac gated T_1-weighted spin echo sequence uses the R-R interval as the TR. By contrast, a cardiac gated T_2-weighted spin echo sequence uses a multiple of the RR interval, such as $RR \times 3$ or $RR \times 4$, as the TR. Adjusting the trigger delay between the R wave and the 90-degree pulse allows imaging to be performed anywhere between systole and diastole. Cardiac gating is most effective when the RR interval is nearly constant, such as in normal sinus rhythm. Conversely, cardiac gating is less effective when the RR interval is highly variable, such as in atrial fibrillation. Frequent ectopic beats also diminish the success of cardiac gating. Pericardial effusion may cause low ECG voltage and poor cardiac gating. Bradycardia increases the image acquisition time but does not adversely affect image quality, although a long RR interval may cause

T$_1$-weighted images to appear proton density–weighted. Cardiac gating is standard in spin echo and fast spin echo imaging of the thorax.

Respiratory motion blurs images and causes ghosting artifact in the phase encoding direction. The simplest remedy is a breath-hold acquisition, but only certain fast gradient echo and fast spin echo acquisitions are amenable to breath holding. For longer acquisitions, such as 2D spin echo, an option called *respiratory compensation* can reduce image degradation. Respiratory compensation refers to any of several methods of reordering phase encoding steps to minimize the effects of respiratory motion. A bellows placed around the patient's chest or upper abdomen senses the respiratory excursion and transmits the information to the MR imaging scanner. Respiratory compensation is only moderately effective and functions poorly when respirations are irregular. Respiratory triggering is a recent innovation. With this technique, image data are collected only during the quiet period of expiration. A drawback of respiratory triggering is that it increases image acquisition times. Apneic periods and irregular respirations may interfere with the proper functioning of respiratory triggering. Another new respiratory gating method called *MR navigator echo* monitors diaphragmatic position. This method is not yet widely available on clinical MR imaging scanners.

Cine

Cine MR imaging creates a series of images at a single location at multiple time points in the cardiac cycle. The name *cine MR imaging* derives from the movielike appearance of the images when displayed consecutively in a loop. Using the ECG tracing, cine sequences divide the R-R interval into 8 to 24 time intervals and then acquire image data during each interval using a 2D gradient echo sequence. Laminar blood flow appears bright on cine images. Turbulent or abruptly accelerating flow produces signal loss within bright blood. This feature makes cine MR imaging useful for detecting flow abnormalities associated with stenotic and incompetent heart valves, ventricular septal defects, and vascular and anastomotic stenoses. Cine MR imaging is also used to study cardiac motion, the motion of intracardiac masses, and blood flow within an aortic dissection. However, for many of these conditions, echocardiography remains the primary imaging modality. A new version of cine MR imaging, which permits imaging during suspended respiration, uses an ultrafast gradient echo sequence and segmented k-space acquisition. Although ultrafast breath-hold cine MR imaging reduces respiratory artifact, its short TE may decrease the conspicuity of turbulent blood flow. Another innovation, spatial modulation of magnetization, has augmented the capabilities of cine MR imaging and permits detailed analysis of cardiac wall motion. Gradient echo cine MR imaging also can be combined with velocity encoding gradients along one or three orthogonal directions. This pulse sequence can be used to quantify flow velocity

and volume flow rates in blood vessels. New ultrafast versions of this pulse sequence permit velocity and flow measurements to be performed during one or several breath holds. Important differences exist between the flow data acquired with velocity-encoded cine MR imaging and Doppler ultrasound: Doppler interrogates the velocity spectrum from a small sample volume whereas MR imaging provides a flow velocity for each pixel in the image. Doppler also has higher temporal resolution.

Magnetic Resonance Contrast Agents

The intravenous MR contrast agents used in routine clinical examinations are low-molecular-weight chelates of the paramagnetic rare earth metal Gd. These agents are highly water soluble and rapidly equilibrate with the extracellular fluid compartment, except in the central nervous system, where the blood-brain barrier limits permeability. The chelator can be charged or uncharged, linear and flexible, or planar and rigid. Gd chelates are excreted by the kidneys, but otherwise exhibit no tissue or organ selectivity. Their safety profile is excellent, especially compared with the iodinated contrast materials used in CT and conventional angiography. Allergic reactions are quite rare, and only a single published report of Gd chelate–associated nephrotoxicity exists.

Gd-containing contrast agents increase the signal intensity of perfused tissues on T$_1$-weighted images. The kinetics of contrast enhancement are complex and reflect tissue perfusion, vascular permeability, and the interstitial volume fraction of the tissue. Although tissue enhancement may appear similar on MR imaging and CT, the mechanism of enhancement is different. Gd chelates interact with extracellular water to shorten the T$_1$ of the water protons. The Gd itself produces no MR signal. Thus, Gd acts indirectly. The iodine in iodinated contrast media directly attenuates x-rays. Gd chelates are more sensitive than iodinated contrast media, producing tissue enhancement at lower concentrations. A mass that does not enhance on CT may well enhance on MR imaging, which may lead to errors in lesion characterization. Caution is advised when extrapolating to MR imaging the lessons learned from CT.

Novel MR contrast agents are undergoing clinical testing in the United States and abroad. Among these are blood pool agents, which have potential application in thoracic MR angiography. Blood pool agents include large macromolecular polygadolinium complexes, small hydrophobic Gd chelates that bind to serum albumin, and colloidal iron oxide nanoparticles. Unlike ordinary Gd chelates, which rapidly equilibrate with the extracellular space, blood pool agents remain intravascular for long periods. These agents hold promise for improved MR pulmonary and coronary angiography. Colloidal iron oxide also has potential for improving the accuracy of lung cancer staging. This agent is phagocytosed by cells of the reticuloendothelial system. In particular, normal and reactive lymph nodes accumulate colloidal iron oxide, whereas lymph nodes replaced by malignant cells do not. Iron oxide–enhanced MR imaging represents an intriguing strategy for distinguishing benign and malignant adenopathy and may play an important role in the future.

Magnetic Resonance Angiography

MR angiography is rapidly becoming a noninvasive alternative to conventional contrast angiography. MR angiography techniques are categorized as *black blood* and *bright blood*, depending on the signal intensity of flowing blood. Spin echo is the classic black blood pulse sequence. Spatial saturation bands, cardiac gating in systole, and increased TE (approximately 20 ms) help suppress signal from flowing blood. Black blood spin echo MR angiography images also depict nonvascular soft tissue structures. Drawbacks to black blood MR angiography include long acquisition times, poor spatial resolution, and difficulty displaying the data as an angiogramlike projection image. Another drawback of black blood MR angiography is that slowly flowing blood may appear bright. This can lead to confusion in distinguishing intraluminal solid tissue, such as thrombus or tumor, from slowly flowing blood. Such confusion may be obviated with a promising new black blood MR angiography technique called *double inversion recovery fast spin echo*, used with or without cardiac gating.

Bright blood MR angiography techniques include time-of-flight (TOF) MR angiography, phase-contrast (PC) MR angiography, and Gd-enhanced 3D MR angiography. The three techniques use different strategies to make vessels appear brighter than surrounding soft tissues. It is important to understand that most bright blood MR angiography imaging sequences are inadequate for evaluating soft tissue structures; to obtain this information, additional imaging sequences must be appended to the MR imaging examination. TOF and PC MR angiography use *flow-related enhancement* to increase the signal intensity of flowing blood relative to that of the stationary background tissues. In addition, PC MR angiography develops vessel contrast from velocity-associated phase shifts in flowing blood.

TOF and PC MR angiography are infrequently used in the thorax because they are slow and not especially robust. They are best suited to imaging blood flow that is laminar and of constant velocity. Artifacts arise when blood flow is slow, turbulent, pulsatile, or in plane. Cardiac gating can reduce pulsatility artifact but increases acquisition times. For optimal results, 2D TOF sequences should be prescribed with the imaging slices oriented orthogonal to the direction of blood flow, a requirement that is not easily satisfied in the superior mediastinum. TOF MR angiography uses flow compensation gradients, also called *gradient moment nulling*, to maintain the phase coherence of flowing blood. In 3D TOF and PC MR angiography, vessels may become *saturated* as the blood flows within the imaging volume. These and other artifacts may cause signal loss that can simulate vascular disease. The long acquisition times preclude using these 3D MR angiography techniques during suspended respiration. Nonetheless, 2D TOF MR angiography, acquired during repeated breath holding, is useful for evaluating the superior vena cava.

The workhorse of thoracic MR angiography is Gd-enhanced 3D MR angiography, a technique originally developed by Prince and coworkers in 1993. An intravenous bolus of Gd chelate is used to create intravascular high signal on a heavily T_1-weighted fast 3D gradient echo sequence. Because flow-related enhancement plays almost no role in developing intravascular contrast, Gd-enhanced 3D MR angiography is more robust than TOF and PC MR angiography. Acquisition times are so short that images can be acquired in a single 15- to 30-second breath hold. The delay between contrast administration and imaging determines which vascular beds contain contrast agent and appear bright. Several data sets are usually collected to ensure adequate opacification of the desired vascular bed. The arterial phase MR angiography images are essentially a vascular luminogram, similar to that obtained with conventional angiography. These images do not adequately depict the true outer arterial wall, nor do they adequately depict nonvascular soft tissue structures. Such information is better appreciated on delayed postcontrast images, after contrast has enhanced many soft tissue structures, including the vasa vasorum. The image data from a Gd-enhanced 3D MR angiography study is easily postprocessed and displayed as an angiogramlike maximum intensity projection (MIP). Limited regions of vascular anatomy or pathology can be displayed with subvolume MIPs. Intriguing new display options include surface rendering and virtual intraluminal endoscopy.

Gd-enhanced 3D MR angiography is widely used to image the thoracic aorta, proximal great vessels, and central pulmonary arteries. In many medical centers this technique has supplanted conventional contrast angiography and CT for assessing the thoracic aorta in the setting of known or suspected aneurysm or dissection. Although transesophageal echocardiography is more widely available and widely used than MR angiography, transesophageal echocardiography is more invasive and suffers from artifacts and blind spots. However, in the operating room, transesophageal echocardiography will continue to be the imaging modality of choice.

Low-dose Gd-enhanced 3D MR venography represents the conceptual union of conventional contrast venography and Gd-enhanced 3D MR angiography. Instead of injecting iodinated contrast material to opacify upper extremity and superior mediastinal veins, a 60-mL intravenous bolus of Gd chelate diluted 1:20 in saline is injected. The 3D MR angiography pulse sequence is acquired during the contrast injection. The Gd chelate must be diluted because commercially available contrast materials are too concentrated and would cause the veins to appear dark rather than bright. This MR venography technique shows promise for evaluating suspected superior vena cava (SVC) syndrome as well as deep venous thrombosis of the subclavian and brachiocephalic veins. The dilute Gd bolus clears after a few minutes and

causes little residual intravascular or soft tissue enhancement. A standard, high-dose Gd-enhanced 3D MR angiography can be performed after the low-dose 3D MR venography.

Tissue Characterization

Thoracic imaging is performed to define anatomy or to
identify and characterize pathology. High soft tissue contrast
makes MR imaging well suited to these tasks. Soft tissues
are characterized on MR imaging according to signal intensity on T_1- and T_2-weighted images and degree of contrast
enhancement. Pulsation artifacts and flow voids are helpful
for identifying blood vessels with moderate to high flow.
Techniques such as fat and water suppression and opposed
phase imaging are used to increase the conspicuity of specific tissues. Normal lung parenchyma and small soft tissue
calcifications are poorly depicted on MR imaging. Abnormal lung parenchyma and pulmonary masses are seen on
MR imaging but are usually better characterized on CT.
Among the MR imaging techniques for detecting larger calcifications, long TE gradient echo and T_2-weighted conventional spin echo sequences are most sensitive, whereas
T_1-weighted spin echo and all fast spin echo are least sensitive. Normal lung parenchyma has been imaged using a
custom-designed ultrashort (<1 ms) TE, breath-hold, gradient echo pulse sequence; the images, although intriguing,
were inferior to high-resolution or conventional CT. Bone
appears black on all MR pulse sequences because it contains
few mobile protons. However, bone marrow is very well
depicted on MR imaging. Despite excellent soft tissue contrast, MR imaging is frequently unable to characterize a
mass as benign or malignant, although it may help to narrow
the differential diagnosis. Localizing a mass to one of the
three mediastinal compartments also helps to limit the differential diagnosis for MR imaging, just as it does for CT
and plain radiography.

Tissues that appear bright on T_1-weighted images include
fat, subacute blood products, and proteinaceous fluid, as
well as Gd-enhanced tissues. Fat- or water-suppressed T_1-
weighted images can help to unambiguously distinguish
macroscopic fat from hemorrhagic or proteinaceous fluid.
Opposed phase gradient echo imaging is sensitive for detecting microscopic fat within a mass lesion such as an adrenal
adenoma. On postcontrast T_1-weighted images it is incorrect
to assume that all bright tissues have been enhanced. Comparison must be made with the precontrast appearance of the
tissue. The rate, pattern, and degree of contrast enhancement
are helpful for characterizing a tissue or mass.

Tissues that appear bright on T_2-weighted images include
fat, water, and many tumors. Water is ubiquitous in the
human body. It is responsible for the vast majority of MR
signal in nonfatty tissues, organs, masses, and so forth. Not
all tissue water exhibits high T_2 signal, only free water. This
imprecise concept connotes water that is not bound to other
substances or surfaces. Certainly, watery fluid within a simple cyst qualifies as free. But intracellular water that is not

appreciably bound to subcellular elements or plasma membranes can also be free. For reasons that are largely obscure,
tumors often contain large amounts of free water and consequently exhibit higher T_2 signal intensity than nonneoplastic
tissues. Still, considerable overlap exists in the T_2 appearance of neoplastic and nonneoplastic tissues. Inflamed,
edematous, and necrotic tissues, for example, may appear
bright on T_2-weighted images. Granulation tissue may also
appear bright on T_2-weighted images but, unlike water, it
enhances brightly.

Pathologic conditions can result in visualization of abnormal areas of lung. Newer techniques are emerging that make
MR imaging of pulmonary parenchymal disease and pulmonary vascular abnormalities more feasible.

PATIENT COMPATIBILITY

Five to 10% of patients are unable to complete the MR
imaging examination because of claustrophobia. Many of
these patients are helped by conscious sedation. Some
patients are helped simply by a calm and reassuring radiologist or MR technologist. MR imaging is contraindicated in
patients with cardiac pacemakers, certain types of metallic
brain aneurysm clips, cochlear implants, and several other
devices that either do not function or are strongly deflected
by the magnetic field in the MR imaging scanner. Continually updated lists of MR-incompatible devices and materials
are published.

CLINICAL APPLICATIONS OF THORACIC MAGNETIC RESONANCE IMAGING

Anterior Mediastinum

Thyroid

Substernal thyroid masses are commonly noted as being
in the anterior mediastinal compartment, but actually the
majority are located in the pretracheal space behind the
innominate vessels and thus are in the visceral compartment
of the mediastinum (see Chapter 162).

The thyroid can extend caudally from the neck to a substernal location in the superior mediastinum of either the
anterior or visceral compartment, the latter being the most
common location. Thyroid goiters are the most common
masses extending from the neck into the chest. Multiplanar
MR imaging can demonstrate the extent of a goiter and its
anatomic relationships with the trachea, esophagus, and
great vessels. Goiters appear heterogeneous on T_1- and T_2-
weighted images and are usually hypointense to normal thyroid on T_1-weighted images. A multinodular appearance
may be appreciated. Goiters frequently contain multiple cystic nodules with high T_1 signal intensity, an indication that
the cysts contain proteinaceous (i.e., colloid cysts) or hem-

orrhagic fluid. Benign goiters are well encapsulated, whereas thyroid carcinoma may show aggressive spread and regional adenopathy. The T_1 and T_2 appearance of a thyroid mass is not sufficiently characteristic on MR imaging to distinguish benign from malignant disease. Moreover, MR imaging does not reliably demonstrate calcifications within a thyroid mass, nor does it depict lymphangitic spread of thyroid carcinoma in the lungs.

Parathyroid

Most individuals have four parathyroid glands, arranged as upper and lower pairs at the posterior aspect of the thyroid. Fewer than four parathyroid glands exist in approximately 10% of the population. Whereas the upper pair of parathyroid glands is usually orthotopic, the lower glands can be ectopic and located virtually anywhere in the mediastinum. The parathyroid glands frequently come to surgical attention because of primary hyperparathyroidism. The three most common causes of primary hyperparathyroidism, in decreasing order of frequency, are parathyroid adenomas (75 to 80%), primary parathyroid hyperplasia (10 to 15%), and parathyroid carcinoma (less than 5%).

The primary imaging modalities for the parathyroid glands are ultrasound and scintigraphy. Preoperative imaging is infrequent for surgical treatment of primary hyperparathyroidism. Recurrent or persistent hyperparathyroidism after surgical exploration of the neck suggests the presence of ectopic parathyroid tissue. In these patients, MR imaging or scintigraphy can help to locate an ectopic parathyroid adenoma before surgical reexploration. On MR imaging, ectopic parathyroid adenomas most commonly exhibit low T_1 signal, high T_2 signal, and avid contrast enhancement. This appearance is altered if hemorrhage is present within the adenoma. Imaging should be performed from the thyroid to the base of the heart to cover the potential locations of an ectopic gland. Although its sensitivity is high, MR imaging has two notable limitations: Lymph nodes can simulate ectopic parathyroid adenomas, and parathyroid carcinomas may be indistinguishable from adenomas. In clinical practice, MR imaging is used as a problem-solving tool when scintigraphy is inconclusive or nondiagnostic.

Thymus

The thymus gland is located in the anterior superior mediastinum and is composed of two fused pyramidal lobes. The thymus undergoes marked changes in size and shape between childhood and adulthood but ultimately undergoes fibrofatty involution. In patients under 30 years of age, the normal thymus is well depicted on T_1-weighted MR images because it is outlined by mediastinal fat, which has a higher signal intensity. The contrast between normal thymus and fat decreases with progressive fibrofatty involution. Thymic lesions include cysts, hyperplasia, benign and malignant thymomas, thymic carcinomas, thymic carcinoids, and thy-

molipomas. The thymus may also harbor lymphoma and germ cell tumors. In thymic hyperplasia, the bipyramidal architecture of the thymus is preserved. Among patients with thymoma, 50% come to clinical attention because of symptoms related to myasthenia gravis; however, only 10 to 15% of patients with myasthenia gravis have thymomas. Invasive, malignant thymoma is the most common primary malignancy of the mediastinum but is much less common than metastatic disease to the mediastinum. Compared with normal thymus, thymomas demonstrate lower T_1 and higher T_2 signal intensity. Thymomas also disrupt the normal pyramidal thymic morphology and appear as round or multilobulated masses. The diagnosis of invasive thymoma depends on aggressive imaging features, such as gross capsular invasion, mediastinal extension, vascular encasement, regional adenopathy, and pleural metastases. Benign and invasive thymomas are not reliably distinguished on T_1- and T_2-weighted MR images alone. The multiplanar imaging capabilities of MR imaging may provide an advantage over CT in accurately depicting extraglandular extension of malignant thymoma. Thymolipomas are benign tumors composed almost entirely of fat. They can grow to a large size and envelop the pericardium. On MR imaging, they exhibit the characteristic high T_1 and T_2 signal intensity of fat.

Germ Cell Tumors

More than 80% of mediastinal germ cell tumors are benign, with the great majority of these being dermoid cysts and benign teratomas. The malignant teratoma is the most common malignant germ cell tumor. Other less common germ cell tumors include seminomas and nonseminomatous germ cell tumors, choriocarcinomas, embryonal carcinomas, and endodermal sinus tumors. On MR imaging, T_1 and T_2 signal heterogeneity in an anterior mediastinal mass suggests the diagnosis of germ cell tumor. The high soft tissue contrast of MR imaging helps to identify specific components, such as cysts and fat, which are characteristic of dermoid cysts and teratomas. MR imaging techniques such as fat and water suppression and opposed phase imaging may help to unambiguously characterize microscopic or macroscopic fat within a lesion. MR imaging is also effective at characterizing cystic lesions. Simple fluid in a cyst exhibits low T_1 and high T_2 signal intensity, whereas complex, proteinaceous, or hemorrhagic fluid typically exhibits higher T_1 and variable, but generally lower, T_2 signal intensity. On CT, the high density of hemorrhagic or proteinaceous cysts may cause them to be mistaken for solid tumors. Gd chelate–enhanced MR images reliably demonstrate solid components or mural nodules within a complex cystic lesion. MR signal intensity alone does not reliably distinguish benign from malignant teratoma. Aggressive imaging features, such as mediastinal extension, regional adenopathy, and distant metastases, are needed to support a diagnosis of malignant teratoma. Tumoral calcification, often present in dermoid cysts and teratomas, is not reliably seen on MR imaging and is best depicted on noncontrast CT. Multiplanar MR images may help in preoperative planning by defining the vascular relationships of mediastinal germ cell tumors.

Lymphoma

Lymphomas are malignant neoplasms of lymphoid tissue that are classified as either Hodgkin's disease or non-Hodgkin's lymphoma. The preponderance of mediastinal lymphomas are Hodgkin's disease, and a majority of patients with Hodgkin's disease have mediastinal disease. An exception is the posterior mediastinum, paravertebral sulcus, where lymphomatous involvement almost always represents non-Hodgkin's lymphoma. CT is the primary imaging modality for the staging and surveillance of lymphoma. However, on CT, the morphology of individual benign and malignant lymph nodes is usually indistinguishable. Massive, confluent lymphadenopathy should suggest the diagnosis of lymphoma. Serial CT examinations are used to follow regression or progression of disease as determined by changes in the size of the nodal mass. Although this approach is adequate for many patients, it has pitfalls. The chief problem is assessing disease status in the residual mediastinal mass after initiation or completion of therapy. A residual mass may contain fibrotic tissue, but no viable tumor, whereupon it is called *sterilized lymphoma*. Alternatively, a residual mass may contain islands or larger amounts of viable tumor. CT cannot distinguish between viable tumor and sterilized lymphoma in a residual mass that initially shows a decrease in size. Treatment failures are not detected on CT until the residual mass enlarges, thus delaying further therapy.

MR imaging shows promise in evaluating residual mediastinal masses after chemotherapy or radiation therapy for lymphoma. As for CT, MR evaluation of the residual mass should include an assessment of interval size change. But in addition, several MR signal intensity patterns have predictive value for disease activity. Viable tumor contains moderate amounts of intracellular water and appears bright on T_2-weighted images. In contrast, the fibrotic tissue in sterilized lymphoma contains little water and appears dark on both T_1- and T_2-weighted images. This simple scheme is complicated by radiation-induced inflammation and tumor necrosis, two conditions that produce high T_2 signal and can be mistaken for viable tumor in the residual mass, especially during the first 6 months after therapy. If surrounding fat, which exhibits high T_1 and T_2 signal, is drawn into the fibrotic sterilized lymphoma, the residual mass may exhibit a complex MR appearance. However, careful comparison of the T_1- and T2-weighted images often reveals whether fat or tumor is the cause of the high T_2 signal. The same information can be obtained more simply with fat-suppressed T_2-weighted images. In summary, low T_2 signal in a shrinking residual mass indicates a good response to therapy, whereas high T_2 signal more than 6 months after therapy suggests tumor recurrence. Besides T_2 signal intensity, the degree of

Gd contrast enhancement may also predict disease activity in a residual mass. In more recent studies, low and decreasing levels of enhancement on serial MR studies correlated with a good response to therapy, whereas high and increasing levels of enhancement correlated with tumor recurrence. The relative merits of assessing disease activity with T_2 signal intensity or contrast enhancement remains to be determined. Radionuclide imaging with ^{67}Ga has also demonstrated value in detecting recurrent disease. The role of positron emission tomography (PET) is also being evaluated.

MR imaging and MR angiography are well suited to evaluating the relationship of mediastinal lymphoma to airways and vascular structures. Low-dose Gd-enhanced 3D MR venography offers a fast and noninvasive method for assessing superior mediastinal veins. Compression and thrombosis of deep veins, as well as collateral venous drainage, are readily depicted. The relative merits of this technique versus conventional contrast venography and duplex ultrasound remain to be determined. The multiplanar imaging capabilities of MR imaging can help demonstrate lymphomatous involvement of the chest wall, pleura, and pericardium. However, CT is superior for assessing lymphomatous involvement of the lung.

Middle Visceral Compartment

The visceral mediastinal compartment contains blood vessels, lymph nodes and lymphatics, the trachea and esophagus, and a variety of neural structures. The two most common pathologies in the middle compartment are lymphadenopathy and vascular lesions. Mediastinal adenopathy is either reactive or neoplastic. MR imaging and CT are comparably sensitive in detecting mediastinal lymph nodes. On MR imaging, bright mediastinal fat increases the conspicuity of lymph nodes, which are of lower signal intensity on T_1-weighted images. Higher soft tissue contrast and multiplanar imaging capabilities should provide an advantage for MR imaging over CT in identifying lymph nodes and distinguishing them from adjacent vascular structures. Cardiac and respiratory gating should be used routinely to decrease MR artifacts that might otherwise obscure lymph nodes. Because the spatial resolution of MR imaging is inferior to that of CT, MR imaging may incorrectly identify a cluster of small lymph nodes as a single enlarged node. Also, MR imaging is insensitive to nodal calcification. In patients with a contraindication to iodinated contrast agents, MR imaging should be the primary imaging modality for evaluating suspected mediastinal and hilar adenopathy.

Both CT and MR imaging use lymph node enlargement as a surrogate for pathology. Unfortunately, size is an imperfect indicator: Enlarged nodes can be reactive and small nodes can be malignant. Analysis of T_1 and T_2 signal intensities does not improve the accuracy of MR imaging because significant overlap exists between benign and malignant nodes. The limitations of CT and MR imaging support the primacy of lymph node sampling in staging lung cancer, although cross-sectional imaging may direct the mediastinoscopist to specific enlarged lymph nodes. PET scan with ^{18}F-fluorodeoxyglucose uses increased metabolic activity to identify malignant lymph nodes. The exact role of this imaging modality in staging and monitoring mediastinal and hilar adenopathy is currently under investigation.

Paracardiac and Intracardiac Masses

MR imaging is highly efficacious in demonstrating paracardiac and intracardiac masses. The most frequently encountered paracardiac masses are enlarged pericardial fat pads, pericardial cysts, and Morgagni hernias. Atrial myxoma is the most common primary intracardiac mass (50%) but occurs much less frequently than intracardiac mural thrombus. Thymolipoma is a rare fat-containing mass that often extends to the heart. Primary paracardiac and intracardiac malignancies are rare. Mediastinal lesions such as teratoma and lymphoma may extend to a paracardiac location. Similarly, bronchial carcinomas may involve the pericardium by direct extension or via malignant adenopathy. Malignant neoplasms can also metastasize to paracardiac and intracardiac sites.

Conventional ECG gated T_1-weighted spin echo images delineate the cardiac chambers, myocardium, epicardial fat, pericardium, and paracardiac fat and permit precise anatomic localization of mass lesions. T_1- and T_2-weighted MR images can define specific tissue characteristics, such as fat, hemorrhage, and cystic spaces. Cine MR imaging scans can demonstrate the movement of a mass relative to the heart, providing information about the site of attachment. Cine MR imaging may help differentiate a mobile mass such as atrial myxoma from a fixed mass such as mural thrombus. Cine images can also demonstrate compromised valve function. Post-Gd images are useful in differentiating solid vascular masses from avascular masses such as thrombus. Although echocardiography is usually the primary imaging modality for paracardiac masses, MR imaging may better define the location, origin, and extent of such masses. But like other imaging modalities, MR imaging frequently fails to provide a specific tissue diagnosis.

Mediastinal Cysts

Benign cystic lesions in the mediastinum can be congenital or acquired. They include bronchogenic cysts, pericardial cysts, neurenteric cysts, meningoceles, esophageal duplication cysts, thymic cysts, cystic hygromas, colloid cysts related to thyroid goiter, pancreatic pseudocysts, abscesses, and hematomas. Specific diagnosis requires careful evaluation of anatomic relationships and convincing evidence that the mass is cystic. Cystic mediastinal masses are often first identified on chest radiography, although their exact nature may be unknown. Noncontrast CT helps define the anatomic relationships of a cystic mass in the axial plane. Both precontrast and postcontrast CT are required to prove that a mass is cystic and

does not enhance. CT findings can be equivocal when the cyst contents are hyperdense on precontrast images.

MR imaging is used primarily as a problem-solving tool when the CT is equivocal. However, in patients with a contraindication to iodinated contrast material, MR imaging should be the primary imaging modality. Multiplanar MR images superbly depict the anatomic relationships of a cystic mediastinal mass. This information helps narrow the differential diagnosis. T_1- and T_2-weighted images confirm the cystic nature of most lesions and also characterize the cyst contents. For problematic complex cysts, Gd-enhanced MR imaging, sometimes in several imaging planes, can be used to exclude the presence of solid enhancing tissue within a cyst, a feature that portends malignancy. However, even simple benign cysts often demonstrate a thin, smooth rim of enhancement within the cyst wall. Bronchogenic cysts are either intrapulmonary or mediastinal, with the latter being more common. Mediastinal bronchogenic cysts are generally located near the carina but do not communicate with the bronchial tree. They are usually asymptomatic unless they compress critical adjacent structures such as airways or blood vessels. The cyst contents can vary from serous to proteinaceous and may contain blood products from prior hemorrhage. Serous fluid exhibits low T_1 signal, whereas hemorrhagic, proteinaceous, or mucinous fluid exhibits intermediate to high T_1 signal (Fig. 11-2). Enteric duplication cysts are usually posterior lesions that abut the esophagus or reside within the esophageal wall. Location provides the key to the correct diagnosis. Neurenteric cysts and meningocele are also paraspinal posterior mediastinal lesions. Their diagnosis is suggested by associated vertebral anomalies. The cerebrospinal fluid in a meningocele appears similar to pure water on MR imaging, exhibiting low T_1 and high T_2 signal intensity.

Posterior Compartment: Paravertebral Space

The abundance of paravertebral neural tissue explains the high frequency of neurogenic tumors in the paravertebral spaces. These tumors are classified according to the nerve of origin: neurofibromas, schwannomas, and malignant peripheral nerve sheath tumors from peripheral nerves; neuroblastomas, ganglioneuromas, and ganglioneuroblastomas from sympathetic nerves; and paragangliomas and pheochromocytomas from neuroectodermal cells closely associated with autonomic nerves. Other paravertebral masses include paraspinal abscesses, commonly related to tuberculosis; lymphoma, usually non-Hodgkin's lymphoma; extramedullary hematopoiesis; and primary and metastatic vertebral body neoplasms.

Neurofibromas can be intradural, extradural, or both, in which case they often assume a dumbbell shape and expand the neural foramina. Multiplanar MR imaging delineates the extent of tumor and depicts compression of adjacent soft tissue structures. CT is superior to MR imaging at depicting bony erosions. On MR imaging, nerve sheath tumors exhibit low to intermediate T_1 signal, high T_2 signal, and marked contrast enhancement. MR imaging does not reliably distinguish

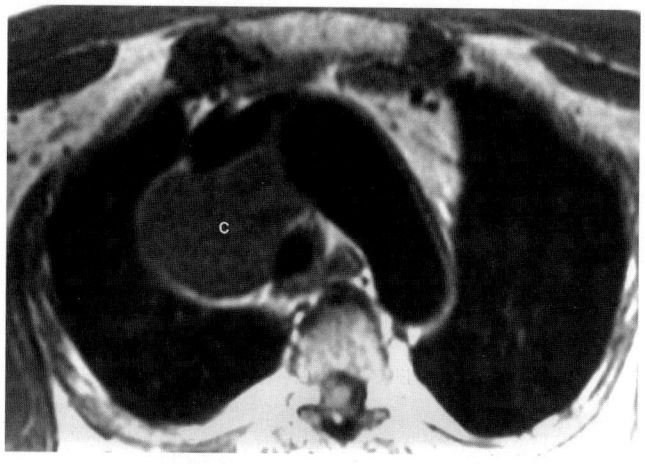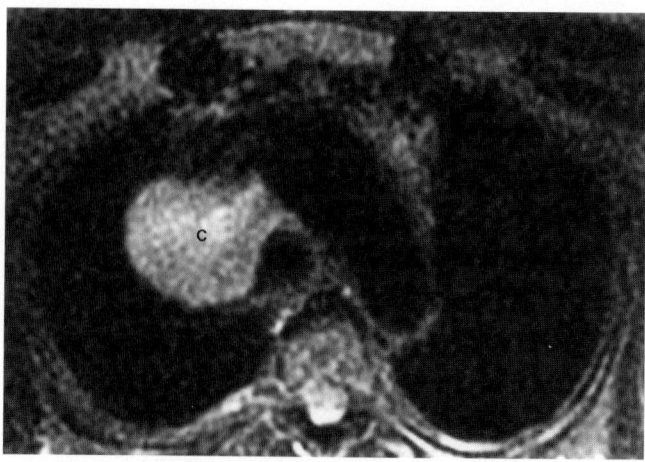

A   B

Fig. 11-2. Bronchogenic cyst. Axial, electrocardiogram gated T_1-weighted spin echo (**A**) and T_2-weighted fast spin echo (**B**) magnetic resonance images demonstrate a smooth, well-marginated cystic mass (c) in the right paratracheal space. The contents of the mass did not enhance (not shown).

benign from malignant tumors. Imaging features that usually connote a benign etiology, such as well-defined borders, are not helpful: Plexiform neurofibromas have an aggressive, invasive appearance, whereas early peripheral nerve sheath tumors can have a nonaggressive appearance. Of course, regional adenopathy and distant metastases would suggest the malignant nature of an otherwise indeterminate mass.

Lymphoma in the posterior mediastinum can encase the aorta and mimic an aortic dissection or aneurysm. Periaortic lymphoma is further suggested by a mass interposed between the vertebra and aorta, as well as adenopathy in other locations. These imaging features, although suggestive, are not diagnostic. Careful evaluation of aortic morphology on precontrast and postcontrast images may provide a clue to the correct diagnosis.

Ten percent of pheochromocytomas are extra-adrenal and 1% are located in the mediastinum, most commonly in the paravertebral sympathetic nerves. Another rare site for this tumor is the pericardium, particularly near the aortopulmonary window (see Chapter 184). Mediastinal pheochromocytomas can be difficult to detect. The primary imaging modality for tumor localization is the ^{131}I-metaiodobenzylguanidine scan. Although these scans have high sensitivity and specificity, they suffer from low anatomic resolution. MR imaging can be used as an adjunct, providing more precise anatomic localization of lesions identified on ^{131}I-metaiodobenzylguanidine scans. Pheochromocytomas are often highly conspicuous on MR imaging because they exhibit high T_2 signal and marked contrast enhancement. However, intratumoral hemorrhage can change the classic MR appearance.

THORACIC AORTA

In many institutions MR imaging is becoming the modality of choice for evaluating thoracic aortic aneurysm and

dissection. The standard MR examination of the thoracic aorta varies considerably according to institutional preferences. At our hospital the MR imaging consists of an axial ECG gated T_1-weighted spin echo sequence, an axial cine gradient echo sequence, a Gd-enhanced 3D MR angiography, and a postcontrast axial T_1-weighted sequence. The spin echo sequence provides black blood MR angiography and a survey of thoracic soft tissues. Cine MR imaging helps identify the intimal flap in aortic dissection, presence of flow in the true and false lumina, and aortic valvular insufficiency. Gd-enhanced 3D MR angiography assesses the presence and full extent of aneurysm or dissection and branch vessel involvement. Postcontrast axial images provide a second opportunity to evaluate thoracic soft tissues, identify the true outer wall of an aneurysmal vessel, and reveal active contrast extravasation from a ruptured aneurysm, pseudoaneurysm, or dissection.

The thoracic aorta is an elastic artery composed of an intima, media, and adventitia. The intima is covered with a thin layer of endothelial cells that contact blood flowing in the vessel lumen. The media contains vascular smooth muscle cells and elastin fibers. The adventitia is a layer of loose connective tissue that contains blood vessels (the vasa vasorum) and nerves. The vasa vasorum enhances and is easily identified on delayed postcontrast MR images, allowing accurate identification of the true outer wall. This is particularly helpful when the vessel lumen and true outer wall are separated by atherosclerotic plaque or mural thrombus.

Congenital anomalies of the aorta include variations in the branching of the great vessels. These anomalies are frequently asymptomatic and discovered incidentally on imaging studies. A common variant is a two-vessel aortic arch with a common trunk supplying the brachiocephalic and left common carotid arteries (bovine arch). Another common variant is a left vertebral artery, which takes origin directly from the aortic arch at a site between the ori-

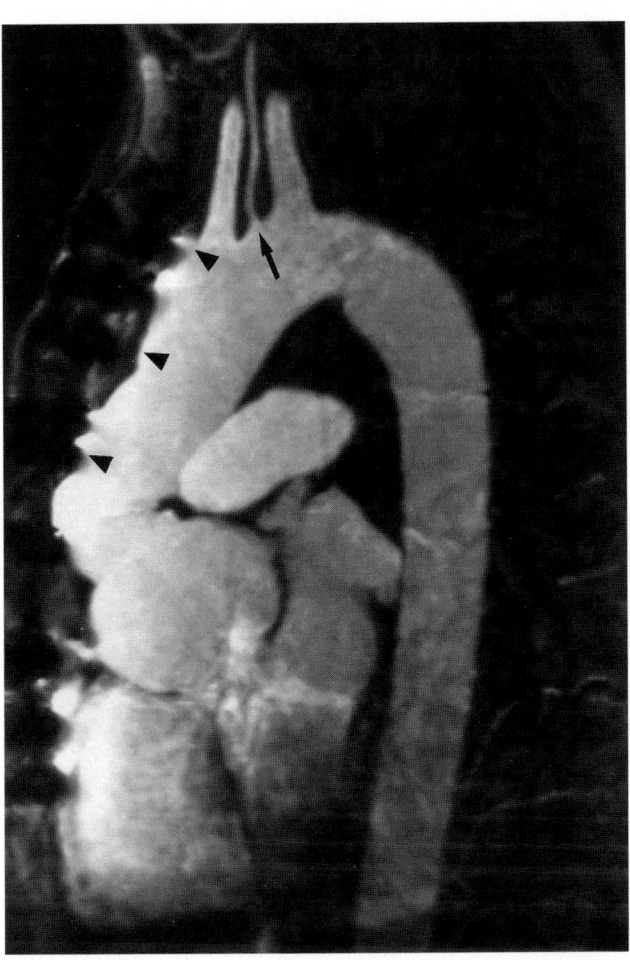

right aortic arch and mirror image branching. Conventional ECG gated spin echo MR images, often acquired in several imaging planes, can identify and characterize congenital vascular anomalies in the thorax. Gd-enhanced 3D MR angiography with multiplanar reformations and subvolume MIP is particularly helpful at depicting the origins and courses of branch vessels. Conventional angiography may fail to adequately delineate branch vessels because only a limited number of projections are obtained.

Coarctation and Aortic Dissection

Although MR imaging is useful in evaluation of aortic coarctation and is ideally suited to evaluate suspected aortic dissection, these subjects are not germane to this text. The reader is referred to the Reading References for this chapter.

Aortic Aneurysm

An aneurysm can be defined as an inappropriate dilatation of an artery. Atherosclerosis is the most common cause. Aneurysms can be classified according to morphology as fusiform or saccular. Fusiform aneurysms encompass the entire circumference of the vessel wall and exhibit a spindle shape. Saccular aneurysms involve only a portion of the vessel wall and manifest as an eccentric outpouching (Fig. 11-5). Aneurysms are classified as true if all three layers of the vessel, intima, media, and adventitia are intact, or as false or pseudoaneurysm if disruption of one or more layers occurs. Alternatively, a false aneurysm can be considered as a contained rupture.

The first steps in evaluating and managing an aneurysm are to define its location and extent. Knowing the rate of growth of an aneurysm is also important but requires previous imaging studies. Thoracic aneurysms can involve the ascending aorta, aortic arch, or descending aorta. The latter may extend below the diaphragm. Ascending aortic aneurysms that involve the aortic root may cause valvular dysfunction, most commonly aortic insufficiency. MR imaging is ideally suited to showing the anatomic relationships of an aneurysm with respect to vascular and nonvascular structures in the thorax. Large thoracic aortic aneurysms can become symptomatic from congestive heart failure caused by aortic insufficiency, from compression of the trachea or esophagus, from hoarseness caused by compression of the recurrent laryngeal nerve, or from erosion of bony structure bodies with subsequent pain.

Trauma can result in aortic transection or disruption. Traumatic injuries to the aorta are rapidly fatal, with most victims dying at the scene of injury. In a review of 275 cases of nonpenetrating aortic trauma, 87% of patients died within the first hour. Posttraumatic aneurysms of the thoracic aorta are distinctive by their locations. The two most common sites are the proximal ascending aorta and the aortic isthmus, the site of

Fig. 11-3. Variant aortic arch anatomy. Oblique sagittal maximum intensity projection image from a gadolinium-enhanced three-dimensional magnetic resonance angiography shows the left vertebral artery arising directly from the aortic arch (*arrow*) between the left common carotid and left subclavian arteries. Artifact anterior to the ascending aorta (*arrowheads*) is caused by metallic surgical clips from prior repair of a type A aortic dissection.

gins of the left common carotid and left subclavian arteries (Fig. 11-3). Less common is an aberrant right subclavian artery with a left aortic arch. In this variant, four vessels originate from the aortic arch. The aberrant right subclavian artery arises from the aorta distal to the left subclavian artery. The aberrant vessel can originate directly from the aorta or from an outpouching called the diverticulum of Kommerell. Rarely, the diverticulum becomes aneurysmal (Fig. 11-4). The aberrant right subclavian artery courses obliquely behind the esophagus from inferior left to superior right and leaves a characteristic impression on the esophagus on a barium esophagogram. An aberrant left subclavian artery with a right aortic arch is a much less common variant, but it is the most likely arch anatomy in an asymptomatic patient with a right aortic arch. This variant is infrequently associated with congenital heart disease. In contrast, congenital heart disease is present in the vast majority of patients with a

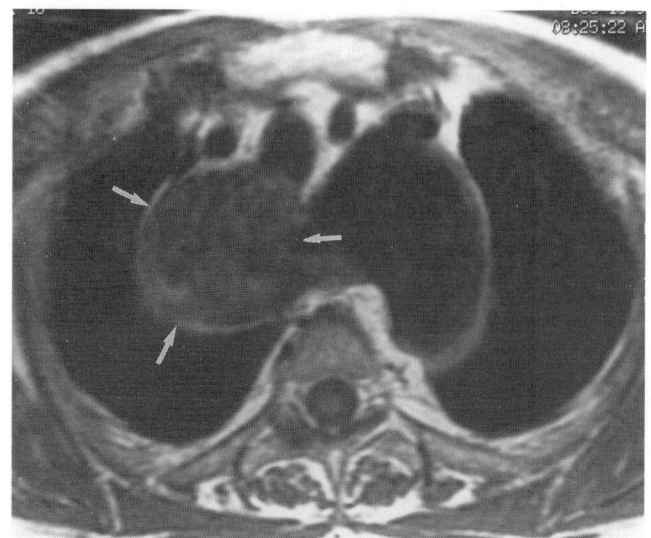

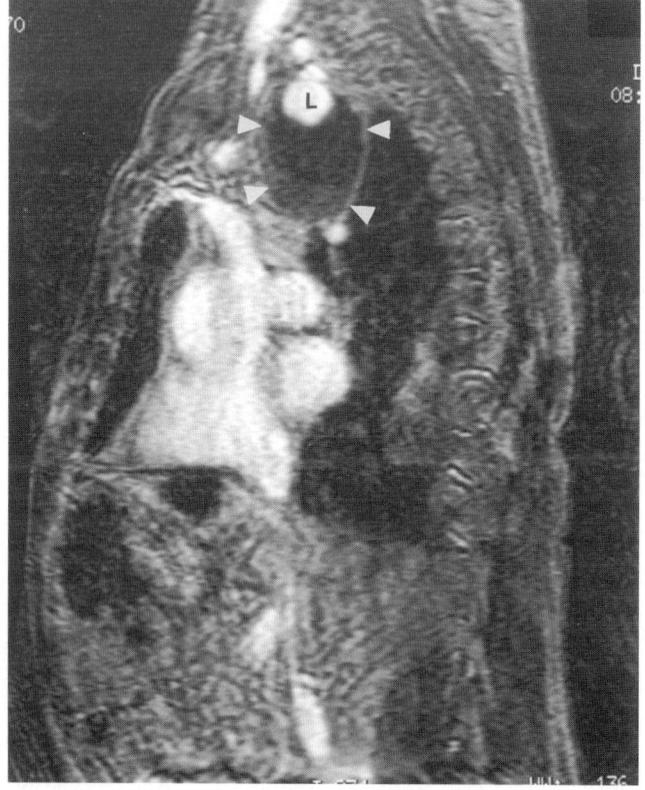

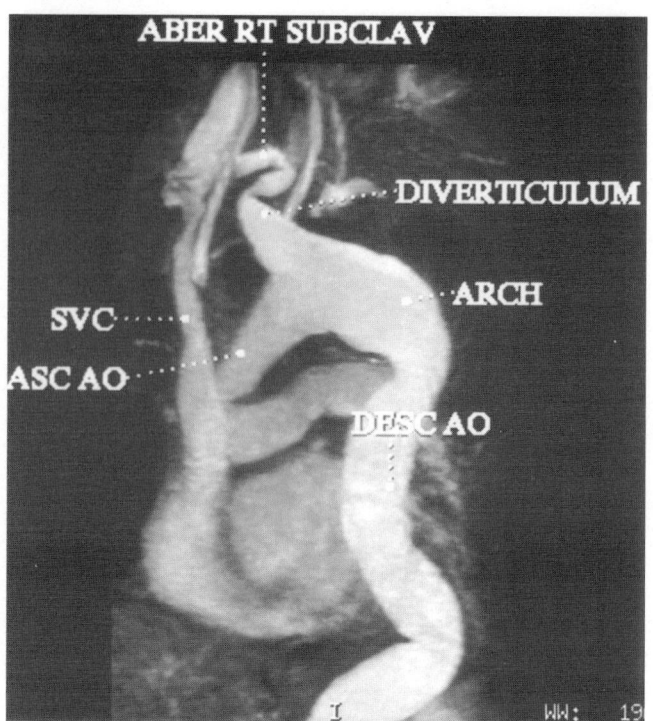

Fig. 11-4. Aberrant right subclavian artery with aneurysm of diverticulum of Kommerell. Axial, electrocardiogram gated, T_1-weighted spin echo MR image (**A**) demonstrates a rounded mediastinal mass (*arrows*) contiguous with the distal aortic arch. Intermediate T_1 signal intensity within the mass could represent slow blood flow or thrombus or both. An oblique coronal maximum intensity projection image from gadolinium-enhanced three-dimensional (3D) magnetic resonance (MR) angiography (**B**) shows an aberrant right subclavian (ABER RT SUBCLAV) artery arising from a diverticulum of Kommerell; the aneurysm is not appreciated. A sagittal reformatted image from the same 3D MR angiography, but acquired 1 minute later (**C**), shows that the mediastinal mass is actually an aneurysm with extensive mural thrombus (*arrowheads*). Whereas the arterial phase MR angiography image (**B**) depicts only the vascular lumen, similar to conventional contrast angiography, the delayed postcontrast MR angiography image (**C**) also depicts the wall of the aneurysm, thereby improving assessment of mural thrombus and residual lumen (L). ASC AO, ascending aorta; DESC AO, descending aorta; SVC, superior vena cava.

insertion of the ligamentum arteriosum. These sites of maximal aortic fixation are believed to be most susceptible to mechanical injury, especially deceleration injury. Among patients who survive traumatic aortic injury and reach medical care, approximately 95% have an injury of the aortic isthmus. Undiagnosed and untreated traumatic aortic injuries can result in a chronic aneurysm or pseudoaneurysm. These pseudoaneurysms generally have a saccular appearance and occur in a younger age group than do atherosclerotic aneurysms. The accepted standard for evaluating patients with suspected traumatic aortic injury is contrast angiography. Multiple projections may be required to identify subtle aortic lacerations. The

angiography suite is an excellent site for closely monitoring potentially unstable trauma patients. Trauma patients often undergo helical CT examinations because of concomitant injuries. The experience with MR imaging in traumatic aortic injury is limited. Current experience suggests that normal MR imaging does not completely exclude traumatic aortic injury, especially when the clinical suspicion is high. MR imaging and CT can identify blood in the mediastinal fat about the site of an aortic laceration. And the absence of such blood decreases the likelihood of traumatic aortic injury. In chronic traumatic aortic aneurysms, MR imaging can be used for follow-up and to determine the need for surgical intervention.

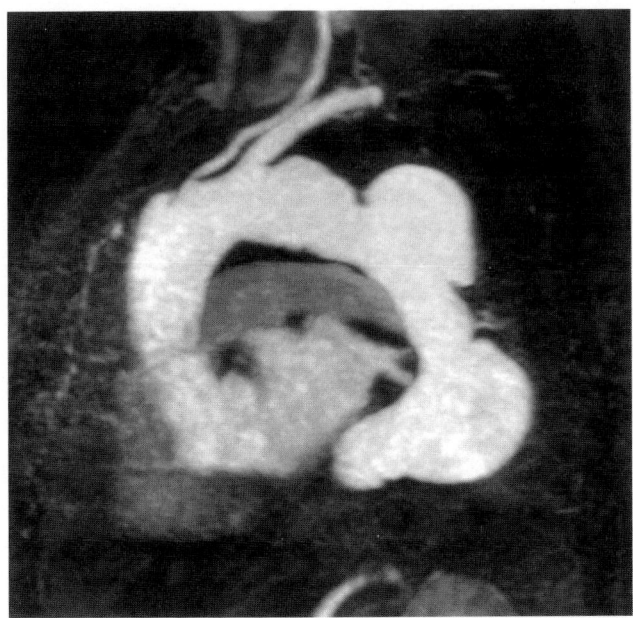

Fig. 11-5. Saccular aneurysms. Oblique sagittal maximum intensity projection image from a gadolinium-enhanced three-dimensional magnetic resonance angiography shows one small and two large saccular aneurysms of the proximal descending thoracic aorta. The distal descending aorta was not included in the volume used to create the maximum intensity projection image.

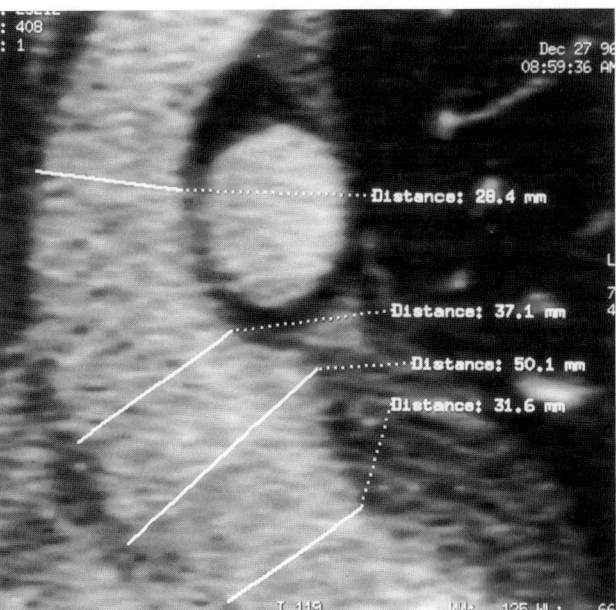

Fig. 11-6. Ascending aortic aneurysm in Marfan's disease. Oblique coronal maximum intensity projection image from gadolinium-enhanced three-dimensional magnetic resonance angiography shows aneurysmal dilatation of the ascending aorta that is most pronounced at the aortic sinus, giving the characteristic "tulip bulb" appearance. Vessel diameters were measured at four levels (from proximal to distal): aortic root, aortic sinus, sinotubular junction, and midascending aorta. This patient had aortic insufficiency (not shown), most likely from a dilatated aortic root.

Further studies are needed to define the role of MR imaging in the evaluation of these patients.

Accurate and reproducible measurement of an aneurysm is important for several reasons. The natural history of untreated thoracic aneurysms is progressive enlargement with increasing risk of rupture and death. In a series of 107 patients, the 5-year survival rate for untreated thoracic aortic aneurysms was 50%. Deaths were attributable to aneurysm rupture in 32%. Surgical intervention is based, in part, on the size and location of an aneurysm and on its rate of enlargement. Transaxial images, such as those obtained with conventional CT, may overestimate the diameter of an aneurysm that courses obliquely through the imaging plane. Aortic tortuosity also can complicate accurate measurement of an aneurysm on contrast angiography. Ideally, measurements should be made in a plane perpendicular to the long axis of the aneurysm. Three-dimensional reformations of MR imaging or CT data are helpful in this regard (Fig. 11-6). The presence of mural thrombus within an aneurysm leads to two different measurements: one for the diameter of the patent lumen and a second for the true wall-to-wall diameter. Imaging modalities such as contrast angiography and arterial phase Gd-enhanced 3D MR angiography depict only the lumen of the aneurysm. In contrast, CT, MR imaging, and ultrasound depict the entire aneurysm including the mural thrombus. Caution is warranted when comparing aneurysm measurements derived from different imaging modalities.

Atherosclerosis is by far the most common cause of thoracic aortic aneurysms. Atherosclerotic aneurysms are more common in men than in women and increase in frequency after the fourth decade of life. Within the thorax, the majority of atherosclerotic aneurysms are found in the descending aorta. Atherosclerosis is also the most common cause of aneurysms in the ascending aorta and aortic arch. However, an isolated aneurysm of the ascending aorta, especially in a younger patient, should prompt a search for another etiology, such as Marfan's syndrome (see Fig. 11-6) or a bicuspid aortic valve. Tertiary syphilis also can produce an isolated ascending aortic aneurysm (luetic aneurysm).

Aortic pseudoaneurysms can form secondary to penetrating trauma, as a surgical complication, or as a complication of an untreated aneurysm (Fig. 11-7). Common locations for postoperative aortic pseudoaneurysms include the cannulation site, the aortotomy site, and the graft suture line. Acute and subacute pseudoaneurysms are generally considered a surgical emergency. Their natural history is continued enlargement. Pseudoaneurysms become symptomatic as a result of compression of adjacent structures. Rupture of a thoracic aortic pseudoaneurysm is generally fatal. Conventional angiography is the standard for imaging pseudoaneurysms. However, the arguments for using MR imaging and MR angiography are quite persuasive. Gd-enhanced 3D MR angiography with multiplanar reformations and subvolume MIP images can depict the presence, location, and neck of a pseudoaneurysm, features that might otherwise be obscured by overlapping vessels on conventional angiography. Spin echo and delayed postcontrast MR images can detect throm-

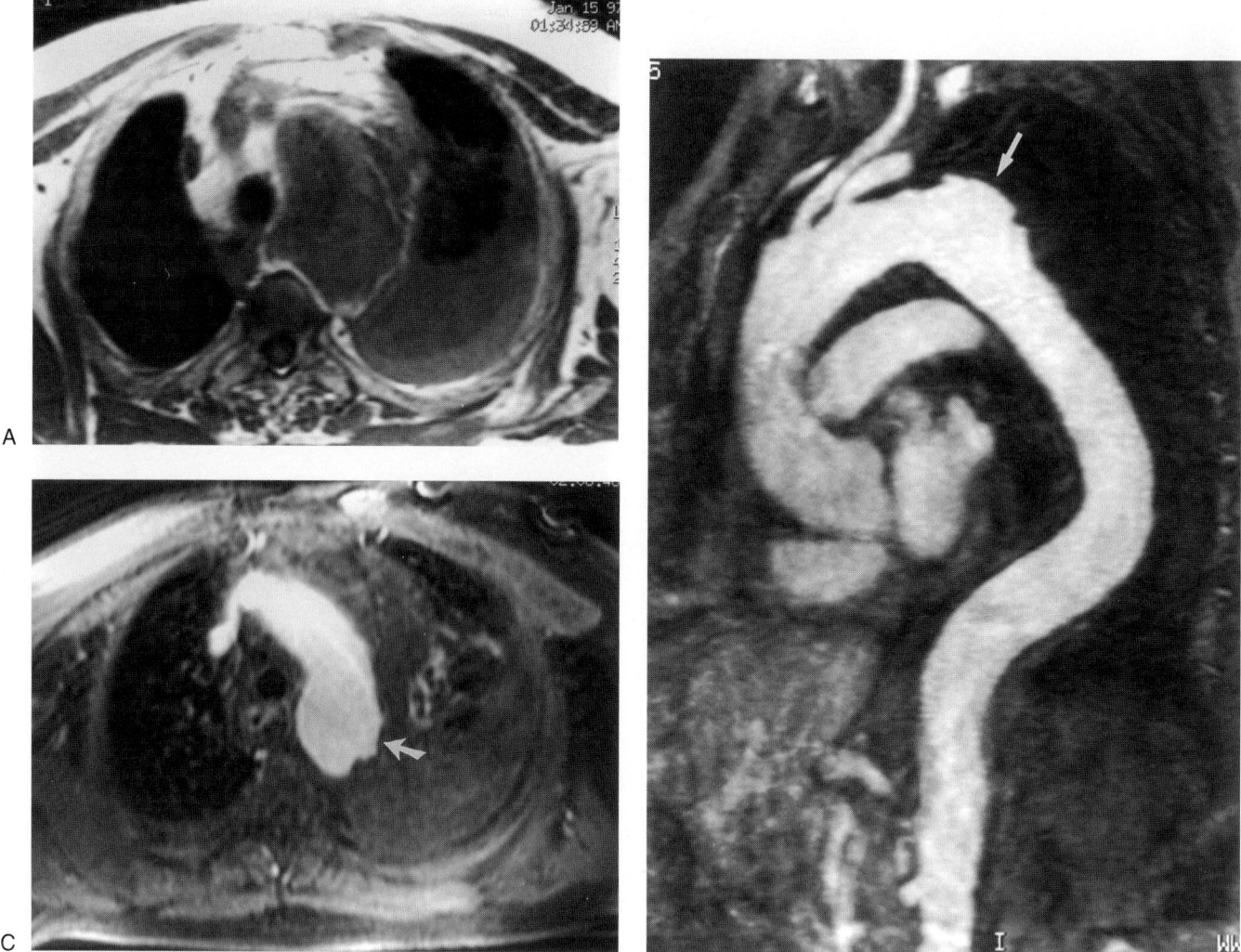

Fig. 11-7. Ruptured aortic aneurysm. Axial, electrocardiogram gated, T_1-weighted spin echo magnetic resonance (MR) image **(A)** shows mediastinal hemorrhage adjacent to the aortic arch and a large hemorrhagic left pleural effusion. Oblique sagittal maximum intensity projection image from a gadolinium-enhanced three-dimensional MR angiography **(B)** demonstrates a saccular aneurysm (*arrow*) of the proximal descending aorta. Axial post-contrast gradient-echo image **(C)** shows the aneurysm as a subtle luminal protrusion arising from the posterolateral aspect of the distal arch (*arrow*); at surgery, this was thought to represent the site of rupture.

bus within a pseudoaneurysm, complications related to a leaking pseudoaneurysm, and compression of adjacent anatomic structures. In the future MR imaging will likely play a greater role in preoperative planning of pseudoaneurysm repair.

For patients unable to tolerate surgical repair of thoracic and abdominal aortic aneurysms, covered endovascular stent grafts now offer a nonsurgical alternative. Stent grafts are custom designed for each patient. To determine if a patient is a candidate for stent graft therapy, the aneurysm must be evaluated for size, shape, location, and relationship to branch vessels. Most of the early evaluations have been performed using helical CT and CT angiography. Multiplanar reformations are important for making highly accurate measurements of the aneurysm and the lengths of the proximal and distal aneurysm necks. Measurements based solely on transaxial images may be inaccurate because of fore-

shortening. MR imaging and Gd-enhanced 3D MR angiography in particular offer an alternative to CT. In fact, MR may be the only suitable imaging modality for patients with impaired renal function or allergies to iodinated contrast media. Many commercially available stent grafts are constructed with Nitinol support struts, which, unlike most metals, produces little MR artifact. MR can also be used to evaluate patients for complications of stent graft placement such as endoleak. Studies are underway to assess the utility of MR imaging for thoracic aortic stent grafts.

PULMONARY VASCULATURE

MR imaging offers a noninvasive method for imaging the pulmonary vasculature (Figs. 11-8 and 11-9). The precise

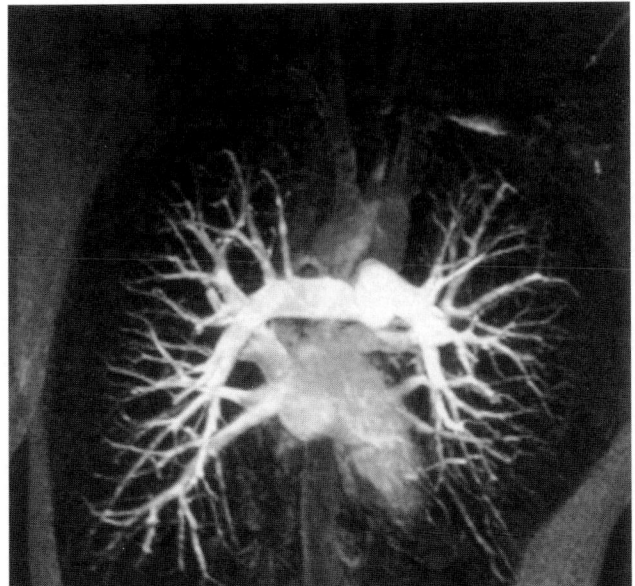

Fig. 11-8. Normal pulmonary magnetic resonance (MR) angiogram. Oblique coronal maximum intensity projection image from a gadolinium-enhanced three-dimensional MR angiography shows central, lobar, and segmental pulmonary arteries and overlapping pulmonary veins. The MR angiography was acquired during a single 25-second breath hold. The intravenous contrast bolus has not yet opacified the aorta.

role of MR imaging versus other image modalities remains to be established and certainly depends on the clinical circumstances. Conventional pulmonary angiography remains the standard, but research efforts have been aimed at identifying alternative modalities that are less invasive and do not expose patients to iodinated contrast materials. Radionuclide imaging of pulmonary ventilation and perfusion is widely used but suffers from limited specificity and anatomic localization. Contrast-enhanced helical CT shows promise for evaluating pulmonary vessels but, like MR imaging, its accuracy and ultimate clinical role remain to be determined.

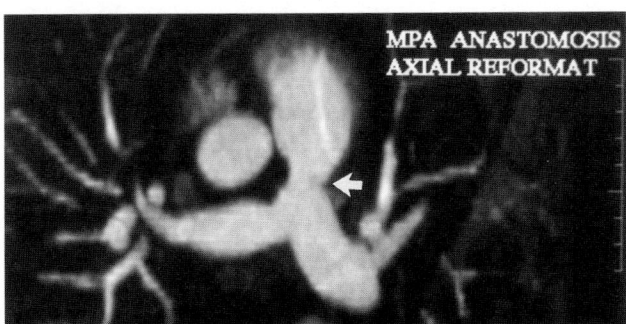

Fig. 11-9. Anastomotic stricture of main pulmonary artery. Axial maximum intensity projection image from gadolinium-enhanced three-dimensional magnetic resonance (MR) angiography shows moderate focal narrowing of the main pulmonary artery anastomosis (*arrow*). MR angiography was ordered to evaluate low blood oxygen saturation in a patient who recently underwent heart transplantation. MPA, mean pulmonary artery.

Pulmonary Hypertension

Pulmonary hypertension connotes abnormal increased pulmonary arterial pressure and increased pulmonary vascular resistance. The most common causes of pulmonary hypertension are recurrent pulmonary emboli, chronic lung diseases that increase pulmonary vascular resistance, and congenital or acquired heart diseases that increase pulmonary blood flow or vascular resistance (Fig. 11-10). Pulmonary hypertension is

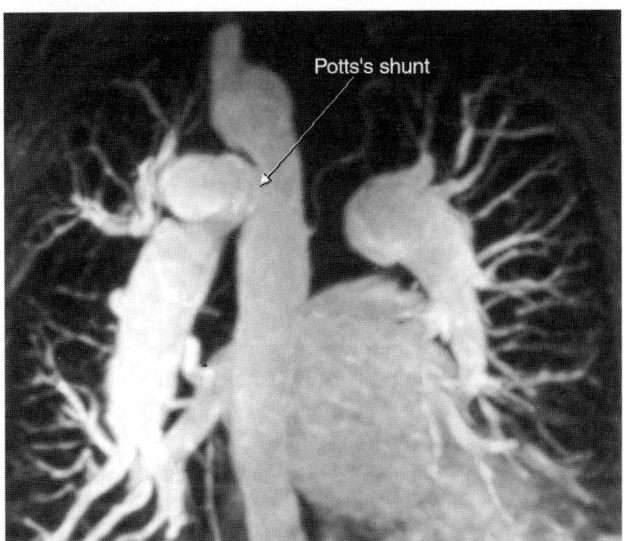

A

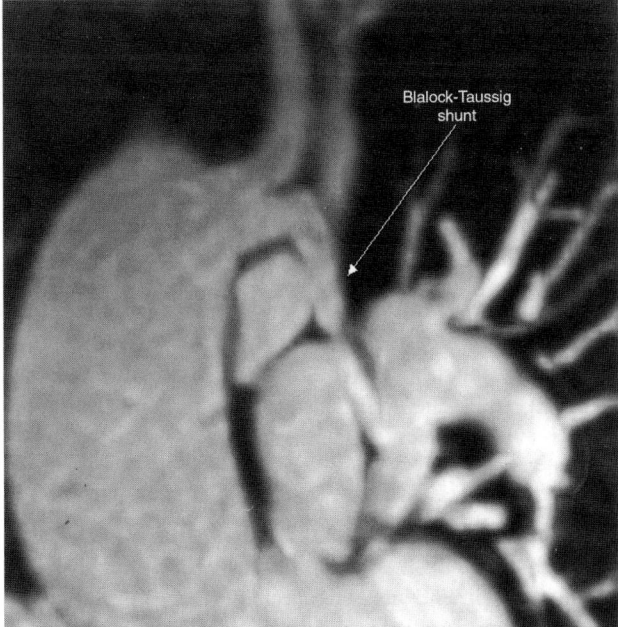

B

Fig. 11-10. Severe pulmonary hypertension in surgically treated pentalogy of Fallot with right aortic arch. Oblique coronal reformatted images from gadolinium-enhanced three-dimensional magnetic resonance (MR) angiography shows a widely patent Potts's shunt from the right descending aorta to a massively dilatated right pulmonary artery (**A**) and a patent Blalock-Taussig shunt constructed from the left subclavian artery to a less severely dilatated left pulmonary artery (**B**). The MR angiogram was obtained to evaluate the pulmonary circulation before right lung transplantation.

called *primary* or *idiopathic* when all known etiologies have been excluded. The risks associated with conventional pulmonary angiography increase in patients with elevated pulmonary artery and right-sided heart pressures.

Anatomic changes associated with pulmonary hypertension include dilated central pulmonary arteries, tapered or pruned peripheral pulmonary arteries, right ventricular hypertrophy, and reverse curvature of the interventricular septum. The size of the central pulmonary arteries correlates with the degree of pulmonary hypertension, although the correlation is imperfect. Mild pulmonary hypertension may produce no enlargement of the central pulmonary vessels. Conversely, central pulmonary arteries may be enlarged without concomitant pulmonary hypertension, such as occurs in poststenotic dilatation from pulmonary valvular stenosis.

Both MR imaging and CT are more accurate than plain chest radiography in assessing pulmonary artery size. ECG gated T_1-weighted MR spin echo images in the axial plane usually provide adequate black blood images for measuring the central pulmonary arteries. Alternatively, bright blood cine gradient echo or Gd-enhanced 3D MR angiography images can be used.

The severity of pulmonary hypertension has been correlated with increased intraluminal signal intensity in the pulmonary arteries on spin echo images. Signal intensity changes are most pronounced during systole and early diastole when, in normal patients, high flow velocities usually produce a signal void. Slow blood flow during late diastole leads to increased intraluminal signal intensity in both normal subjects and patients with pulmonary hypertension.

Pulmonary Embolism

Acute pulmonary embolism (PE) is a common but frequently undiagnosed and potentially life-threatening disorder. Two-thirds of patients with suspected PE prove to have another diagnosis. The etiology of PE is usually deep venous thrombosis (DVT), most commonly from the lower extremities. However, the frequent use of central venous catheters has increased the incidence of upper extremity DVT. The diagnostic workup of PE should include a search for DVT. Conceptually, PE and DVT should be considered two components of the same disorder, namely venous thromboembolic disease.

Chronic PE represents an uncommon complication of acute PE. Acute emboli become organized and incorporated into the pulmonary arterial wall, essentially forming mural thromboemboli. Patients with chronic PE often develop progressive pulmonary hypertension. Chronic PE can be treated with thromboendarterectomy if the thromboemboli are centrally located. However, centrally located mural thrombus may be difficult to detect on conventional pulmonary angiography because the resulting luminal narrowing may be subtle. Cross-sectional imaging techniques such as MR imaging and CT can visualize both the luminal narrowing and the mural thickening, thus increasing the conspicuity of central

thromboemboli (Fig. 11-11). In selected presurgical patients with central thromboemboli, cross-sectional imaging may obviate the need for conventional pulmonary angiography.

Disagreement exists concerning the optimal imaging strategy for suspected acute PE (see also Chapter 13). The choices include conventional pulmonary angiography, radionuclide ventilation-perfusion ($\dot{V}/\dot{Q}$) lung scan, CT, and MR imaging. The standard is conventional pulmonary angiography, yet this modality is underused because clinicians perceive, incorrectly, that it is risky. The $\dot{V}/\dot{Q}$ lung scan is commonly the first imaging examination after a chest radiograph in patients with suspected acute PE. A normal or low-probability $\dot{V}/\dot{Q}$ scan and a low clinical suspicion effectively excludes PE. Conversely, a high-probability $\dot{V}/\dot{Q}$ scan and a high clinical suspicion is sufficient to establish a diagnosis of PE and begin treatment; no further imaging studies are required. The weakness of the $\dot{V}/\dot{Q}$ scan relates to the large number of intermediate-probability (i.e., indeterminate) results, a situation that occurs in a majority of patients with lung consolidation on their chest radiograph. Also, a low-probability $\dot{V}/\dot{Q}$ scan coupled with a high clinical suspicion does not exclude acute PE. Unfortunately, many patients with an inconclusive $\dot{V}/\dot{Q}$ scan, who should undergo pulmonary angiography and a search for DVT, receive no further imaging. The clinical criteria for diagnosing acute PE are notoriously unreliable, and anticoagulation therapy carries a nontrivial morbidity. Outcome studies suggest that it may be possible to forego pulmonary angiography and anticoagulation therapy in a subset of patients with intermediate probability $\dot{V}/\dot{Q}$ lung scans who have normal cardiopulmonary reserve and no evidence of DVT.

The role of MR imaging and CT in evaluating suspected acute PE has yet to be established. Pulmonary vasculature imaging presents a formidable technical challenge for both modalities, but especially for MR imaging. Central pulmonary vessels are affected by cardiac and respiratory motions and pulsatile blood flow. For MR imaging, peripheral pulmonary vessels are affected by susceptibility artifact from air-filled lung. Advances in MR hardware and software have led to improved image quality. Cardiac and respiratory gating and spatial presaturation pulses are mandatory for non–breath-held black blood imaging sequences, such as T_1-weighted spin echo. Double inversion recovery fast spin echo is a newer pulse sequence that can be acquired during suspended respiration and that appears to produce more robust black blood MR angiography images, even without ECG gating. However, the relatively long minimum TE used in these pulse sequences exacerbates susceptibility-related signal loss in peripheral vessels. Therefore, only central pulmonary vessels are reliably evaluated by these techniques. Emboli appear as foci of increased intraluminal signal on spin echo images. Acute emboli, which likely contain methemoglobin, exhibit high T_1 signal, whereas chronic emboli exhibit lower T_1 signal. The conspicuity of emboli on spin echo images depends on differences between the high signal intensity of emboli and the low signal intensity of flowing blood. Slow pulmonary

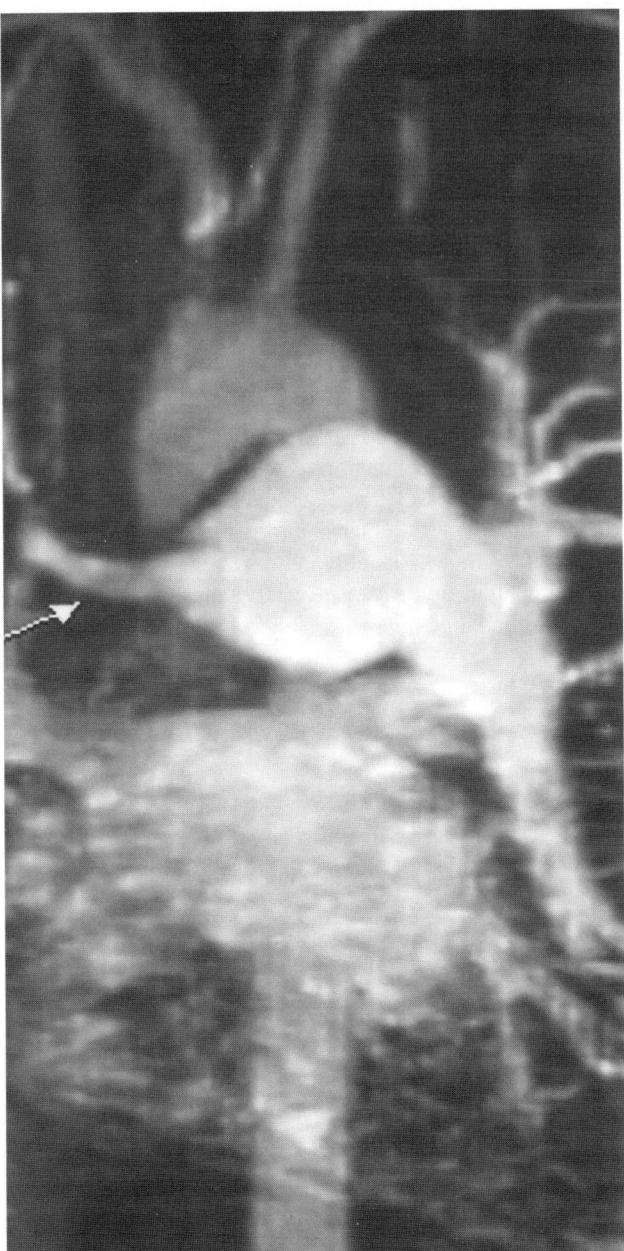

A

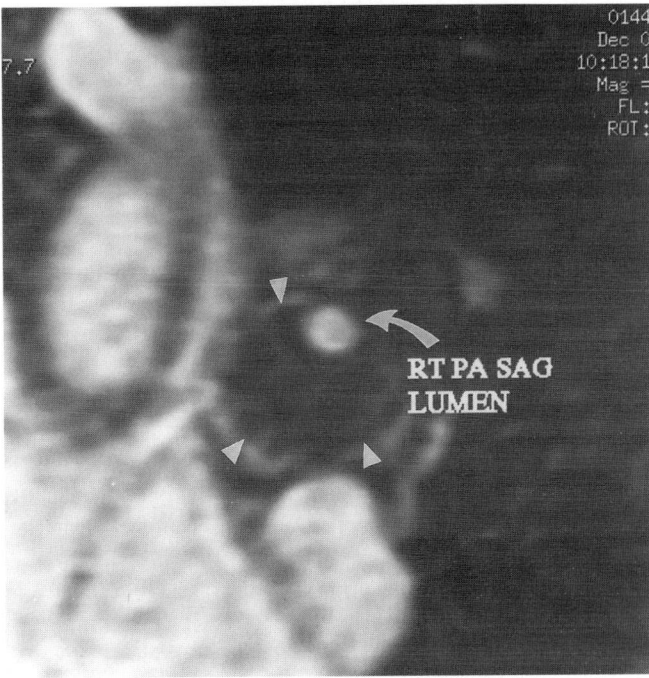

B

Fig. 11-11. Central pulmonary artery thrombosis. Coronal maximum intensity projection image from gadolinium-enhanced three-dimensional magnetic resonance angiography (**A**) shows marked dilatation of the main and left pulmonary artery from long-standing pulmonary hypertension. The right pulmonary artery is narrowed (*arrow*). A magnified sagittal (SAG) maximum intensity projection image (**B**) demonstrates a thick rind of mural thrombus (*arrowheads*) causing severe narrowing of right pulmonary artery (RT PA) lumen (*curved arrow*).

blood flow, which is characteristic of chronic pulmonary hypertension, decreases the conspicuity of central PE. Thus, the diagnosis of central PE can be excluded only if the pulmonary arteries appear entirely normal on black blood MR images. If intraluminal signal is present, the black blood MR angiography sequence should be considered inconclusive.

Cine gradient echo MR imaging is a bright blood technique that does not require exogenous contrast material. It is useful for distinguishing between slow blood flow and solid intraluminal masses such as emboli. On this imaging sequence, emboli appear as low signal foci surrounded by the higher signal of flowing blood. Cine MR imaging with spatial modulation of magnetization tagging increases the conspicuity of immobile structures within blood vessels, such as the mural

thrombus associated with chronic PE. However, susceptibility artifact and turbulent blood flow can introduce signal artifacts that simulate embolic disease on gradient echo images. Also, long image acquisition times impose a practical limit on the anatomic coverage achievable with standard cine MR imaging. Newer ultrafast cine gradient echo pulse sequences, which use a segmented k-space acquisition, permit greater anatomic coverage during a period of several breath holds. Although its exact role has yet to be determined, cine MR imaging is probably best used as a problem-solving technique for inconclusive spin echo images of central pulmonary arteries in patients with suspected central thromboembolic disease.

Gadolinium-enhanced 3D MR angiography is one of the most important techniques in MR imaging of the pulmonary vasculature. The entirety of both lungs and the mediastinum can now be imaged with 3- to 4-mm spatial resolution during a single 25- to 30-second breath hold on a state-of-the-art MR scanner. Postprocessing the MR angiography image data using multiplanar reformations and subvolume MIP helps to identify emboli that might otherwise be obscured by overlapping vessels. And efforts are underway to create image processing software that separates pulmonary arteries and veins. Gd-enhanced 3D MR angiography does have several drawbacks: 1) the state-of-the-art hardware and software that are desirable for 3D MR angiography are not widely available, 2) the duration of the breath hold may prove excessive for severely tachypneic or dyspneic patients, and 3) the spatial resolution of MR imaging and CT is inferior to that of conventional pulmonary angiography. To achieve a high degree of pulmonary vascular enhancement with extracellular Gd chelates, the time delay between contrast injection and MR imaging must be chosen carefully. Intravascular MR contrast agents, which remain in the intravascular compartment for hours, should obviate the need for precise timing. These expectations have proved correct in preliminary studies with several different intravascular MR contrast agents.

MR imaging and CT have demonstrated high sensitivity for detecting emboli in central and segmental pulmonary arteries; however, both modalities fall short of conventional pulmonary angiography in detecting subsegmental emboli. Questions remain about the clinical significance of subsegmental emboli in patients without evidence of DVT. Clinical outcome studies are needed to resolve these questions. MR imaging and CT offer an advantage over pulmonary angiography and V̇/Q̇ lung scans: "one-stop shopping." In patients with suspected acute PE, MR imaging and CT examinations can be easily augmented to include a search for DVT. Studies have shown that MR venography in particular has a high sensitivity and specificity for detection of DVT in the pelvis and lower extremities. Another advantage of MR imaging and CT is that they can identify many nonembolic causes of symptoms that mimic those of acute PE.

MR perfusion imaging is a new technique for evaluating blood flow in the lung. It is conceptually similar to a radionuclide perfusion scan but with higher spatial resolution and better anatomic localization. The goal of MR perfusion imaging is to identify regions of pulmonary parenchyma with decreased or absent perfusion. Although no attempt is made to image the pulmonary arteries directly or identify individual thromboemboli on these scans, the technique can supplement a pulmonary MR angiography study. It is assumed that peripheral wedge-shaped perfusion defects are caused by embolic narrowing or occlusion of the feeding artery. Pulmonary perfusion imaging is, in general, more sensitive than angiographic imaging for detecting peripheral emboli because the perfusion defect resulting from a subsegmental embolus is much larger than the embolus itself. Currently, two basic categories of MR pulmonary perfusion imaging exist. One version uses an intravenous bolus of Gd chelate to opacify the pulmonary parenchyma; the other uses arterial spin tagging. Subtraction images (postcontrast/tagged, precontrast/tagged) are used to increase the conspicuity of pulmonary perfusion abnormalities.

Pulmonary Arteriovenous Malformations

On chest radiography, pulmonary arteriovenous malformations (AVMs) are distinguished by their predilection for the periphery of the lower lobes and their large feeding arteries and draining veins. Multiple pulmonary AVMs are seen in one-third of patients and in association with hereditary hemorrhagic telangectasia (Osler-Weber-Rendu syndrome). More than one feeding artery is present in 20% of patients. The experience with MR imaging of pulmonary AVM is limited but promising. The key imaging sequence is Gd-enhanced 3D MR angiography. Multiplanar reformations and MIP reconstructions of 3D MR angiography data can demonstrate the enhancing nidus of the AVM as well as the course and size of all feeding and draining vessels (Fig. 11-12). This information

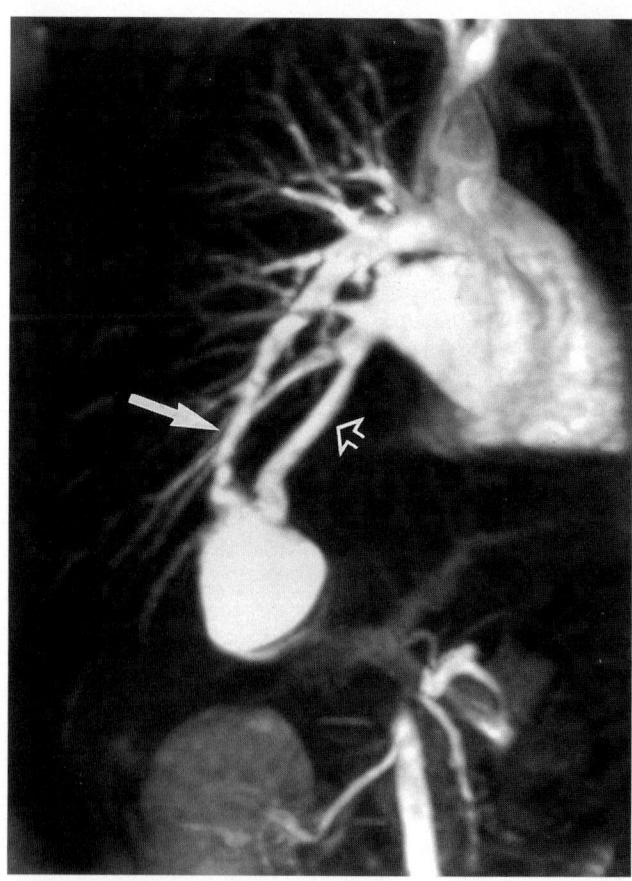

Fig. 11-12. Pulmonary arteriovenous malformation (AVM). Oblique sagittal maximum intensity projection image from gadolinium-enhanced three-dimensional magnetic resonance angiography shows a large, solitary AVM in the right lower lobe. The patient came to medical attention because of a brain abscess, a well-known complication of pulmonary AVM. The feeding artery (*closed arrow*) and draining vein (*open arrow*) are well depicted.

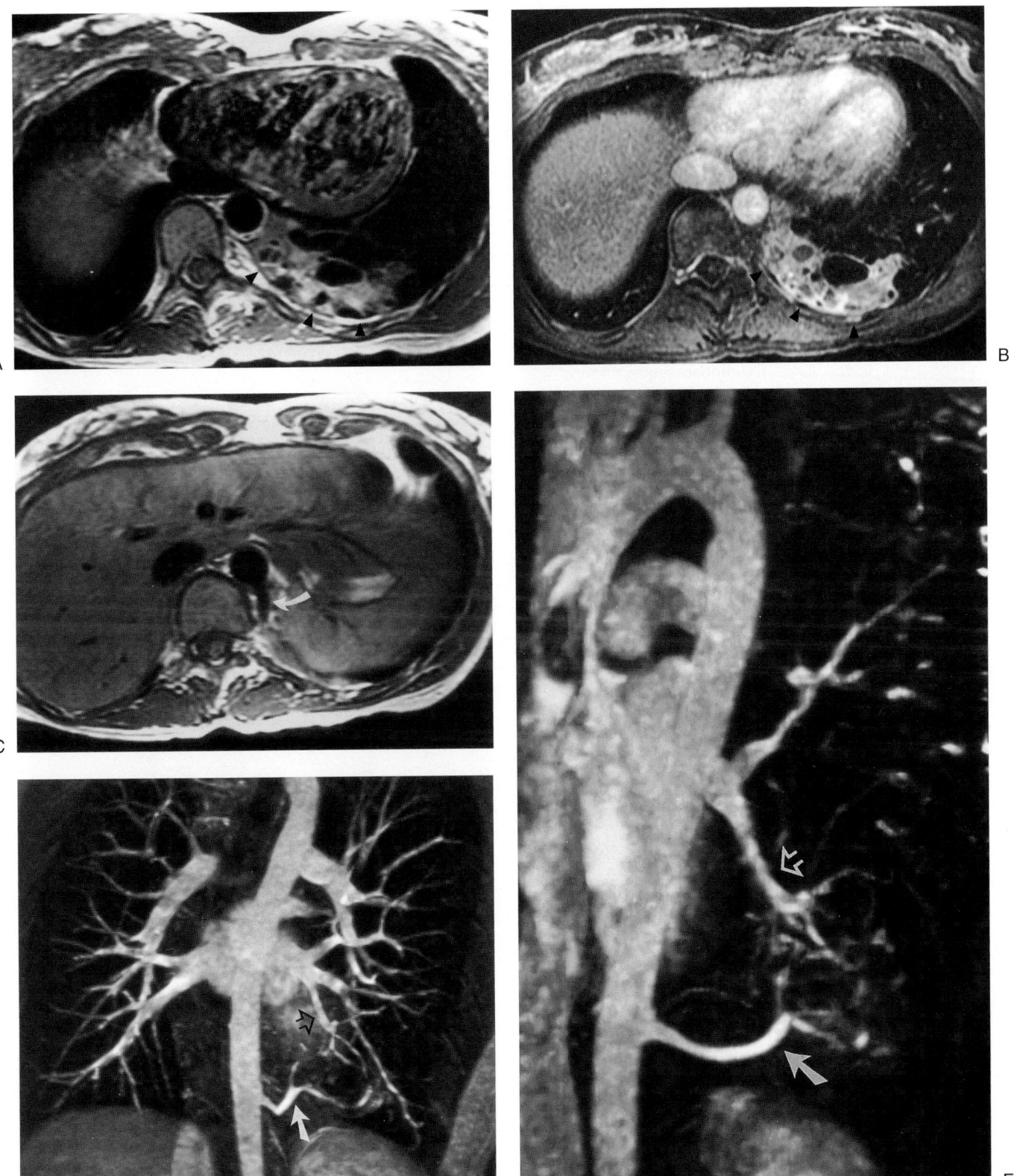

Fig. 11-13. Intralobar pulmonary sequestration in a 22-year-old woman with recurrent pulmonary infections. Precontrast (**A**) and postcontrast (**B**) axial T$_1$-weighted images show an enhancing solid and cystic mass (*arrowheads*) in the posterior basal segment of the left lower lobe. Axial T$_1$-weighted image at a level caudal to (**A**) shows a large feeding artery (*curved arrow*) arising from the aorta (**C**). Coronal (**D**) and oblique sagittal (**E**) maximum intensity projection images from gadolinium-enhanced three-dimensional magnetic resonance (MR) angiography demonstrate to better advantage the systemic arterial supply arising from the distal thoracic aorta (*solid arrow*) and left lower lobe pulmonary venous drainage (*open arrow*). The MR imaging was requested for preoperative planning.

can be used to help plan surgical repair or percutaneous embolization of the feeding vessel(s) (see Chapter 81).

Pulmonary Sequestrations

Pulmonary sequestrations are rare congenital malformations of lung that have no communication with the tracheobronchial tree. Two types occur: intralobar and extralobar. Intralobar sequestrations are surrounded by the visceral pleura, whereas extralobar sequestrations are surrounded by their own pleura. Intralobar sequestrations appear as a mass with solid and cystic components and are usually asymptomatic, unless they become infected. The most common location is the posterior segment of the left lower lobe, followed by the right lower lobe. Extralobar sequestrations are located near the left hemidiaphragm in 90% of patients and are sometimes infradiaphragmatic. They are usually asymptomatic. Both types of sequestrations derive their arterial supply from aorta or its branches, most commonly the descending thoracic aorta. The venous drainage of intralobar sequestrations is usually to the left atrium but may be to the right atrium. The venous drainage of extralobar sequestrations is always systemic, most commonly the inferior vena cava or azygous hemiazygous system. Although experience is limited, MR imaging appears to be an excellent modality for depicting sequestrations and their anatomic relationships and for identifying their vascular supply (Fig. 11-13). MR imaging can be useful for planning the surgical resection of a symptomatic sequestration.

MEDIASTINAL VEINS

MR is an excellent modality for the evaluation of mediastinal veins and can obviate the need for conventional contrast venography of the upper extremities. MR can delineate venous obstructions in the internal jugular, subclavian, and brachiocephalic veins and SVC (Fig. 11-14). Furthermore, MR can usually differentiate intraluminal thrombus or tumor from extrinsic compression. In contrast to conventional venography, MR can fully depict a mass lesion responsible for extrinsic venous compression. Axial 2D TOF MR venography is most useful for evaluating the internal jugular veins and SVC because their course is straight and directed perpendicular to the axial imaging plane. Sagittal 2D TOF MR venography can be used to study the subclavian veins, but we prefer a more versatile technique called low-dose Gd-enhanced 3D MR venography. This technique is analogous to conventional contrast venography and requires establishing intravenous access in the affected upper extremity or extremities. Image data from 3D MR venography can be postprocessed using multiplanar reformations and MIPs to extract the maximum amount of useful clinical information. Our standard MR venography exami-

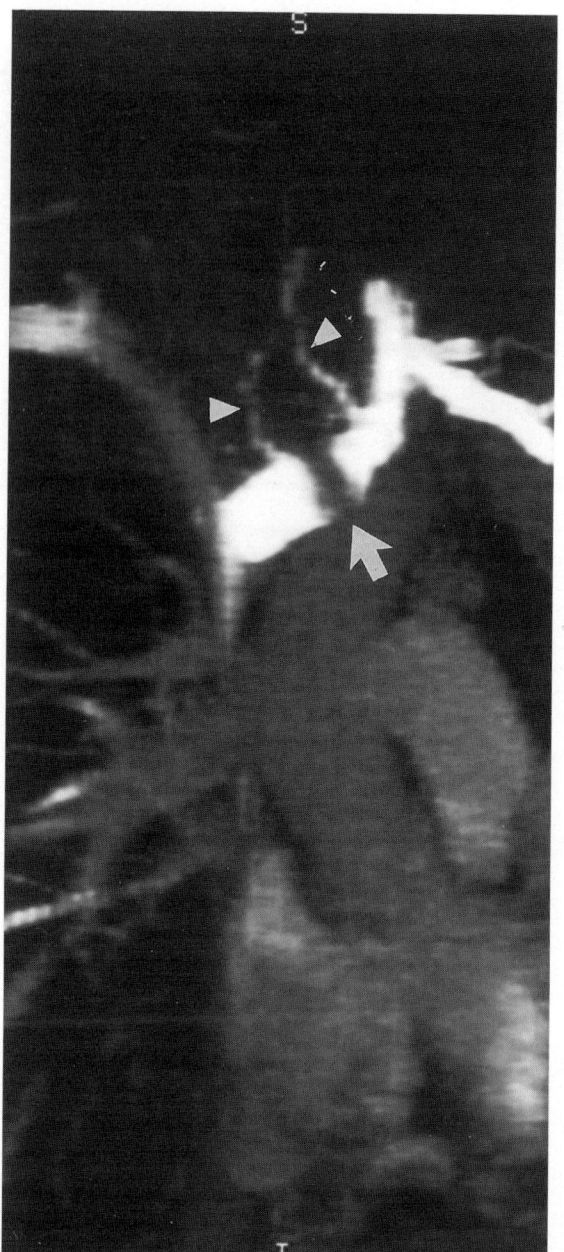

Fig. 11-14. Central venous thrombosis after left pneumonectomy and radiation therapy for squamous cell carcinoma of lung. Coronal (A) and axial (B) maximum intensity projection images from a bilateral upper extremity, low-dose gadolinium-enhanced three-dimensional (3D) magnetic resonance (MR) venogram demonstrate a tight, focal stenosis of the left brachiocephalic vein (A, arrow) and nonocclusive thrombus in the superior vena cava (B, arrow). Note the wishbone-shaped collateral veins, which permit flow around the stenosis (A, arrowheads). Oblique sagittal maximum intensity projection image from standard dose gadolinium-enhanced 3D MR angiography obtained during the venous phase (C) shows collateral flow in a prominent azygous vein (thick arrow) and enlarged intercostal veins (arrowheads). Nonocclusive thrombus is seen in the superior vena cava (SVC) (thin arrows). The thrombus did not enhance and was thought to be bland. MR venography was obtained to evaluate swelling of the left upper extremity and neck. Symptoms improved after balloon angioplasty and stenting of the SVC.

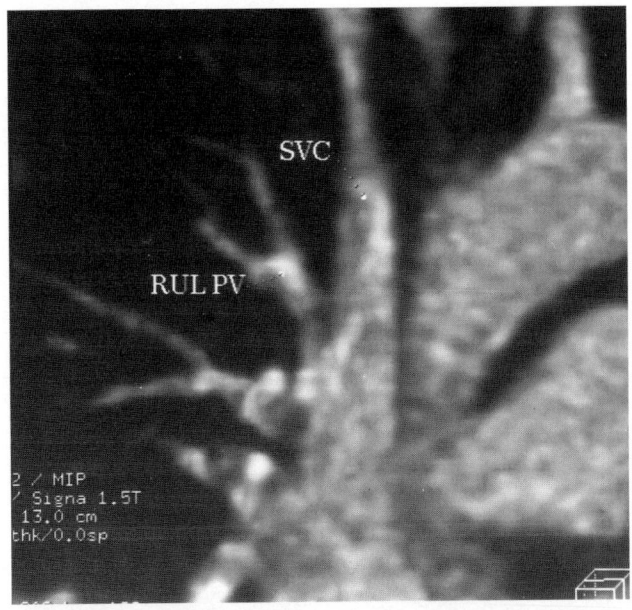

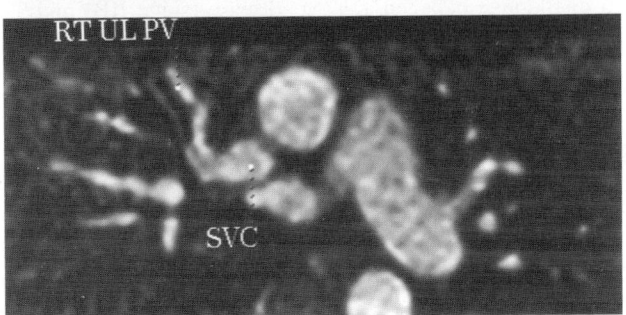

Fig. 11-15. Partial anomalous pulmonary venous return. Coronal (A) and axial (B) maximum intensity projection images from the venous phase of gadolinium-enhanced three-dimensional magnetic resonance angiography show a right upper lobe pulmonary vein (RT ULPV) draining into the superior vena cava (SVC). This patient also had a sinus venosus type atrial septal defect (not shown).

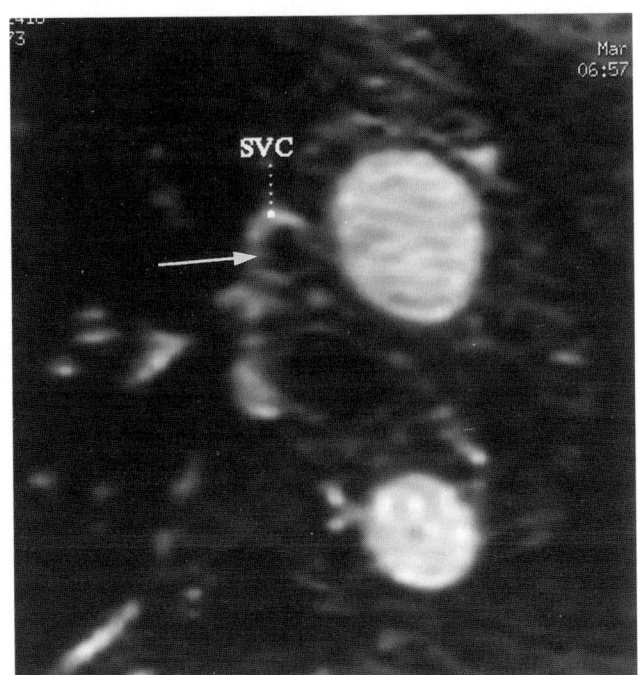

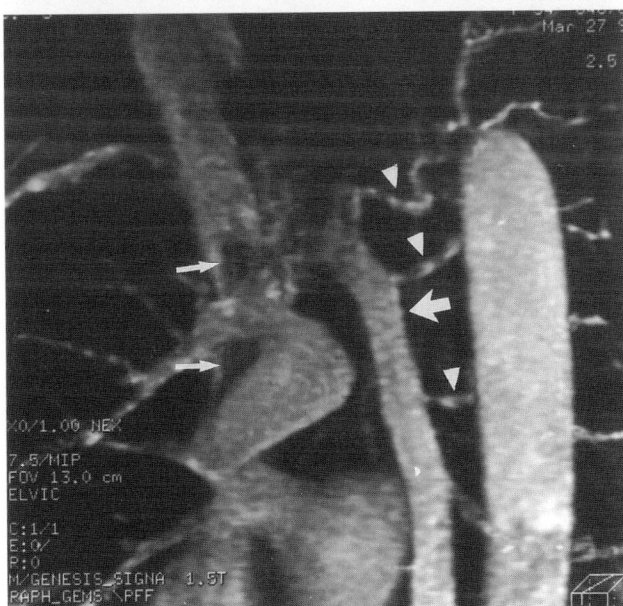

nation also includes ECG gated axial T_1-weighted spin echo images to evaluate the soft tissue anatomy of the thorax.

The demand for thoracic venography is increasing and likely reflects the ever-increasing use of central venous catheters. Vein searches are commonly requested to determine available sites for new central venous catheters. MR venography has been useful for the aforementioned indications as well as for the diagnosis of congenital venous anomalies such as persistent left SVC, anomalous pulmonary venous return (Fig. 11-15) and scimitar syndrome, and interruption of the inferior vena cava with azygos or hemiazygos continuation.

BRONCHIAL CARCINOMA

Lung cancer is the leading cause of cancer-related deaths in women and men. Surgical resection offers the only chance for a complete cure. The staging of lung cancer helps determine prognosis and therapeutic options including suitability for surgery. CT remains the cross-sectional imaging method of choice for staging most patients with lung cancer. CT offers many advantages over MR imaging including superior imaging of lung parenchyma to detect lymphangitic spread of tumor, higher sensitivity for detection of small (<5 mm) lung nodules, better spatial resolution, lower cost, shorter imaging times, and wide availability. CT can also readily detect calcifications in mediastinal lymph nodes and lung nodules. MR imaging should not be used to establish the initial diagnosis of lung cancer. Significant overlap exists between the T1, T2, and contrast enhancement characteristics of benign and malignant lung masses on MR imaging. However, MR imaging may provide certain benefits over CT in specific circumstances. The advantages of MR imaging are based on multiplanar imaging capabilities, superb depiction of vascular anatomy and blood flow, and high soft tissue contrast. Although destruction of rib cortex is more easily identified by CT, MR can identify tumor infiltration of rib bone marrow. MR imaging is probably best used as a problem-solving tool for inconclusive CT scan results. MR imaging has been particularly valuable in determining the resectability of superior sulcus (Pancoast's) tumors and assessing tumor invasion of mediastinal structures, chest wall, and spine. In patients who cannot receive iodinated contrast media for CT, MR imaging should be used as the primary imaging modality for staging lung cancer.

A study by the Radiologic Diagnostic Oncology Group showed no significant difference in the accuracy of CT and MR in staging lung cancers. The primary role of imaging is to distinguish between $T_3N_0M_0$ disease (stage IIB) and T_4 disease (stage IIIB). $T_3N_{0-1}M_0$ disease, which is potentially resectable, is characterized by direct tumor extension into the chest wall, diaphragm, mediastinal pleura, pericardium, or to within 2 cm of the carina. Stage IIIB disease, which is unresectable, is characterized by tumor invasion of the mediastinum, heart, great vessels, trachea, esophagus, carina, or vertebral bodies. Stage IIIB disease also includes cases with malignant adenopathy in the contralateral mediastinal or hilar nodal groups and those with malignant pleural effusions.

MR and CT have similar accuracy in evaluating hilar masses and adenopathy. Occasionally, on CT it is difficult to distinguish a hilar mass from an adjacent pulmonary vessel. In these instances MR imaging may be of value. Flowing blood usually produces a signal void (i.e., flow void) in the pulmonary vessels on spin echo MR images, allowing the vessels to be differentiated from hilar nodes and masses. Unfortunately, slow flow can lead to significant intravascular signal and negate the advantage of MR imaging. Tumors in the hilum can cause postobstructive atelectasis and pneumonitis. CT is superior to MR imaging for identifying obstructive endobronchial lesions. However, MR imaging can often differentiate atelectatic or pneumonitic lung from obstructing tumor. T_2-weighted MR images can identify fluid-filled air spaces in the postobstructive lung (*drowned lung*).

Although acquisition of CT images of the thorax is limited to the axial plane, MR images can be acquired in any orthogonal or oblique plane. This feature may provide an advantage for MR imaging in assessing tumor invasion. For tumor adjacent to the heart, MR imaging is valuable in distinguishing invasion of the pericardium from invasion of the cardiac muscle. The distinction is often best made on T_1-weighted images, where the pericardium is seen as a discrete low-signal structure that is separated from cardiac muscle by

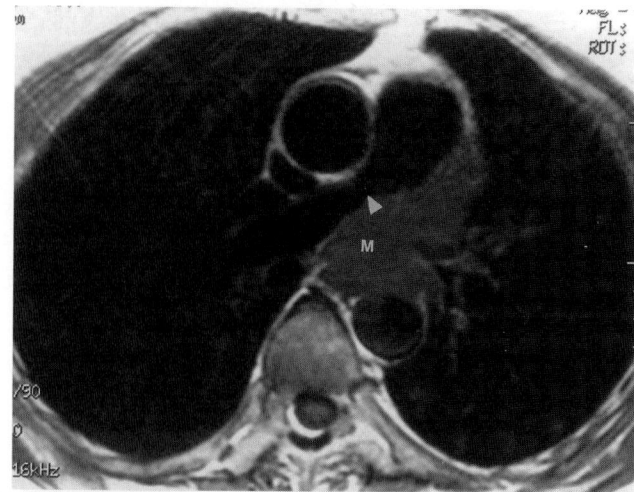

A

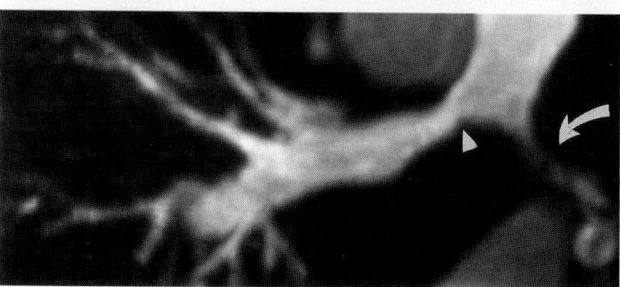

B

Fig. 11-16. Small cell lung cancer invading the mediastinum. Axial, electrocardiogram gated, T_1-weighted spin echo magnetic resonance (MR) image (**A**) shows a soft tissue mass (M) of intermediate signal intensity that obliterates the left pulmonary artery and left main stem bronchus and narrows the right pulmonary artery (*arrowhead*). An axial maximum intensity projection image from gadolinium-enhanced three-dimensional MR angiography (**B**) shows to greater advantage the severe segmental narrowing of the proximal left pulmonary artery (*curved arrow*) and milder, focal narrowing of the proximal right pulmonary artery (*arrowhead*). A prior radionuclide ventilation-perfusion lung scan revealed severely decreased left lung perfusion (not shown).

high-signal pericardial fat. MR imaging also can depict tumor extending to or encasing the carina, aorta, and pulmonary arteries. If vascular encasement is present, Gd-enhanced 3D MR angiography can assess the degree of luminal narrowing (Fig. 11-16). A combination of spin echo and MR angiography imaging often suffices to identify narrowing of the SVC and distinguish extrinsic compression from direct tumor invasion.

Adrenal Metastases

MR can help to characterize adrenal masses in patients with lung cancer. CT is currently the primary modality for evaluating the abdomen for metastases. Adrenal masses are discovered incidentally on 21% of CT examinations for staging lung cancer, and more than two-thirds of these are benign adrenal adenomas. However, CT is unable to characterize the adrenal mass as benign or malignant in approximately 40% of cases. Chemical shift MR imaging is a powerful technique that detects microscopic fat within an adrenal mass with greater specificity than CT. Approximately 90% of adrenal adenomas contain significant amounts of microscopic fat, whereas adrenal metastases from lung contain none. Chemical shift imaging consists of a pair of gradient echo MR images that are identical in all respects except for different TE values. The specific TE values depend on the magnetic field strength of the MR scanner. At 1.5 tesla these values are 2.1 and 4.2 ms. The TE of 2.1 ms is said to be "out-of-phase" or opposed phase, and the TE of 4.2 ms is "in-phase" because of the relative direction of the magnetization vectors for fat and water protons. If the signal intensity of an adrenal mass on the in-phase image is arbitrarily set to 100%, then the vast majority of adrenal adenomas lose signal on the out-of-phase image; adrenal metastases show no signal loss. Approximately 10% of adrenal adenomas cannot be characterized as benign using chemical shift imaging. However, chemical shift imaging has proved to be more reliable for evaluating adrenal masses than other MR-based methods, such as calculating T_1 and T_2 values or following dynamic contrast enhancement.

Superior Sulcus Tumors

Superior sulcus (Pancoast's) tumors arise from the apex of the lung close to the visceral pleural surface. These lesions show a propensity for invading the chest wall and may involve the brachial plexus, subclavian vessels, and spine (see Chapters 35 and 36). Treatment depends on which structures are involved. Gross involvement of the brachial plexus, encasement of the subclavian artery, and involvement of a large portion of a vertebral body or extension into the spinal canal generally render these cancers unresectable. CT is usually the first cross-sectional imaging study obtained for staging superior sulcus tumors. However, the axial plane can be suboptimal for assessing local tumor invasion. The multiplanar capabilities of MR imaging make it uniquely suited for evaluating these lesions. Three imaging planes—axial, coronal, and sagittal—are often required to assess all anatomic relationships. All of the important structures that can be invaded by these tumors are well visualized by MR, allowing for a more accurate determination of the resectability. MR pulse sequences on which fat appears bright, such as T_1-weighted spin echo, are useful for assessing chest wall invasion. Invasion is suspected on T_1-weighted pulse sequences when tumor, which exhibits low signal intensity, violates the subpleural fat plane. A similar approach can be used to assess tumor invasion of the brachial plexus and subclavian vessels, because these structures are also surrounded by fat. Gd-enhanced 3D MR angiography also can be used to evaluate arteries and veins for tumor invasion.

Posttreatment Evaluation

The early detection of recurrent tumor after surgery or radiation therapy may be difficult by chest radiography or CT. Granulation tissue and fibrosis in the postsurgical or postradiation bed can simulate or obscure tumor foci. This distinction can be difficult on MR imaging as well. One exception is mature fibrosis, which characteristically exhibits low signal intensity on T_1- and T_2-weighted images. Unfortunately, significant overlap occurs in the MR appearances of active fibrosis, inflammation, and recurrent tumor. Efforts to differentiate these entities based on T_1 and T_2 signal characteristics or the kinetics of contrast enhancement have proved unreliable. ^{18}F-fluorodeoxyglucose positron emission tomographic scanning appears more promising in this regard (see Chapter 12).

LUNG PARENCHYMA

MR imaging will probably never image lung parenchyma as well as CT. Conventional and high-resolution CT provide exquisite anatomic detail of lung parenchyma and air spaces. This detail is often critical for correctly diagnosing lung pathology on CT. In stark contrast, normal lung parenchyma usually appears as a signal void on conventional MR images. Standard spin echo pulse sequences also do not depict the pulmonary vasculature, except for the central vessels. The poor signal intensity of lung is caused by low intrinsic proton density and strong magnetic susceptibility gradients that cause intravoxel dephasing and signal loss. Work with ultrashort TE (0.7 ms) gradient echo pulse sequences and high-speed gradients, both of which minimize magnetic susceptibility effects, has produced modest success in imaging lung interstitium and small lung nodules. However, neither the specialized pulse sequence nor the scanner hardware are widely available. Thus, MR imaging currently should not be used to evaluate lung parenchyma.

MR imaging may play a limited role in evaluating space-occupying lesions of lung because these are less affected by magnetic susceptibility artifact. In one study, MR imaging detected all lung nodules greater than 5 mm in diameter but failed to detect several smaller (2 to 4 mm) nodules that were identified by CT. Sometimes the inability of conventional MR imaging to detect intrapulmonary blood vessels offers an advantage over CT by increasing the conspicuity of small pulmonary nodules that are adjacent to blood vessels. MR imaging falls short of CT in characterizing pulmonary nodules. Nodule characterization is often based on the pres-

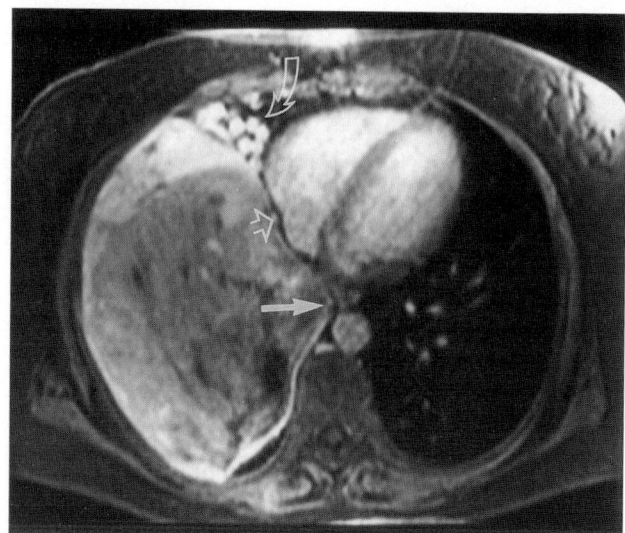

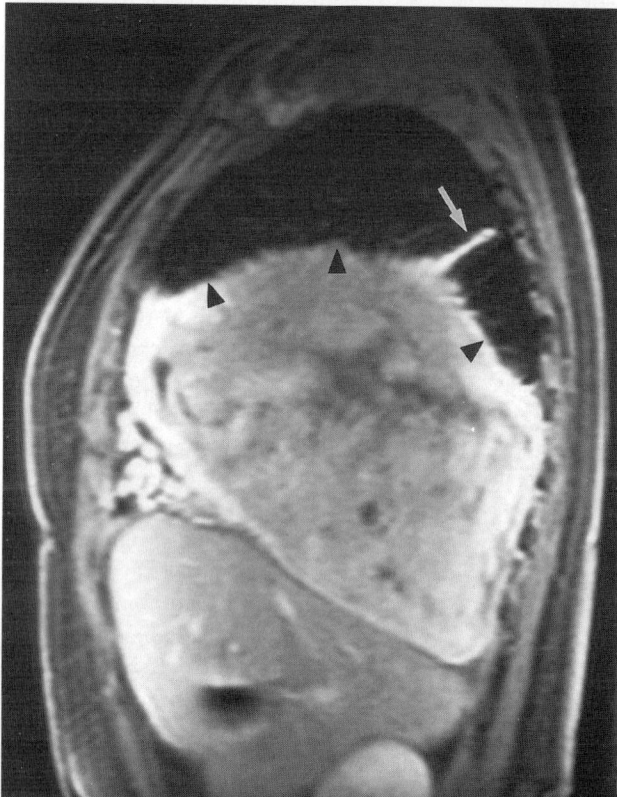

Fig. 11-17. Benign fibrous tumor of pleura. Axial (**A**) and sagittal (**B**) gadolinium-enhanced T_1-weighted magnetic resonance images demonstrate a large, nonaggressive, pleural-based mass that occupies almost the entire mid and lower right pleural cavity. Note the smooth interface between the mass and lung parenchyma (**B**, *arrowheads*) and how the mass extends into the major fissure (**B**, *arrow*). The mass abuts the pericardium (**A**, *open arrow*) and azygoesophageal recess (**A**, *closed arrow*), but does not invade either structure. The sagittal image (**B**) clearly shows that the mass is separate from the liver. Dilatated pulmonary vessels in the right pericardiophrenic angle (**A**, *open curved arrow*) are probably the result of impaired pulmonary venous return.

ence and distribution of calcium, which MR imaging cannot detect. MR imaging cannot reliably distinguish benign from malignant pulmonary nodules. Efforts to characterize nodules based on their T_1 and T_2 appearance or dynamic contrast enhancement have proved unrewarding.

CHEST WALL

The majority of primary neoplasms of the chest wall, except for skin, are of mesenchymal origin. The most common soft tissue tumor of the chest wall is a lipoma. Lipomas are benign lesions; however, they can appear aggressive when they extend between muscles or into a subpleural location. Lipomas have a characteristic appearance on MR imaging: They are homogeneously bright on T_1-weighted images and become dark on fat-suppressed images. Although other benign lesions of the chest wall occur, most cannot be proved to be benign by MR imaging. Malignancies of the chest wall may be caused by primary neoplasms, contiguous spread from mediastinal or lung neoplasms, or metastatic disease. Malignant lesions often have areas of necrosis, hemorrhage, or both. They usually exhibit a heterogeneous appearance on both T_1- and T_2-weighted images and enhance after intravenous contrast administration. It is usually impossible to offer a specific tissue diagnosis for a malignant chest wall mass based on its MR appearance. Furthermore, considerable overlap exists in the MR appearance of benign and malignant lesions. The strength of MR imaging lies in its ability to define the anatomic relationships between a chest wall mass and surrounding structures.

PLEURAL DISEASES

Pleural pathology is adequately delineated by either chest radiography or CT, although MR imaging can be useful in selected situations. Early work suggests that MR imaging may be able to noninvasively classify pleural fluid collections as transudative, exudative, or complex. The high signal intensity of lipids and subacute blood products on T_1-weighted sequences allows the identification of chylothorax and hemothorax, respectively. The multiplanar capability of MR can be useful for determining if a pathologic process is located in the lung parenchyma, pleura, or extrapleural space (Fig. 11-17). The high soft tissue contrast of MR imaging, especially after Gd enhancement, can be helpful in distinguishing complex fluid collections from solid neoplasms.

Malignant mesothelioma is an aggressive neoplasm of the pleura with a poor prognosis. The staging of mesothelioma helps determine the appropriate therapy, including surgery. Although CT is the primary imaging modality for staging this disease, MR imaging may play an adjunctive role when CT findings are equivocal. Multiplanar MR imaging may be useful for demonstrating invasion of the mediastinum, pericardium, chest wall, and diaphragm (Fig. 11-18).

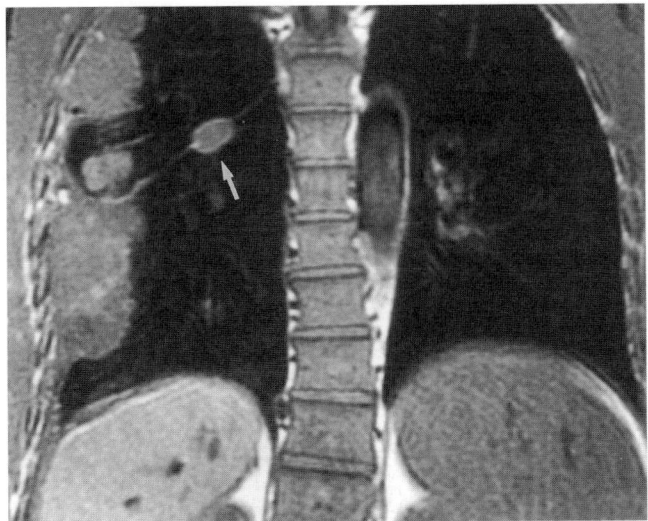

A

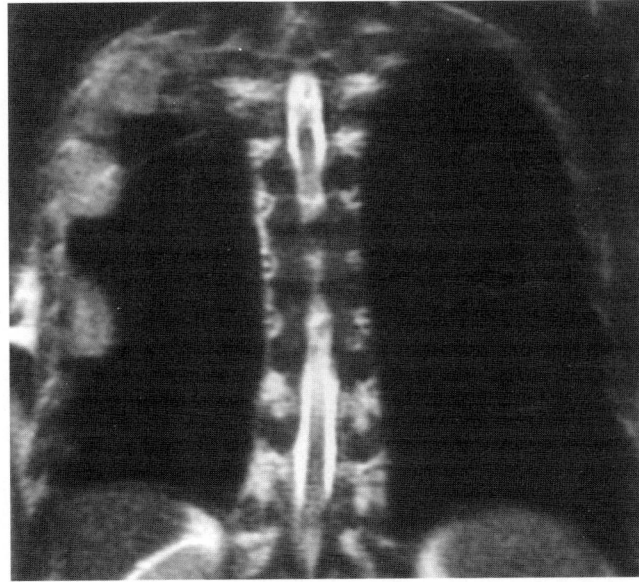

B

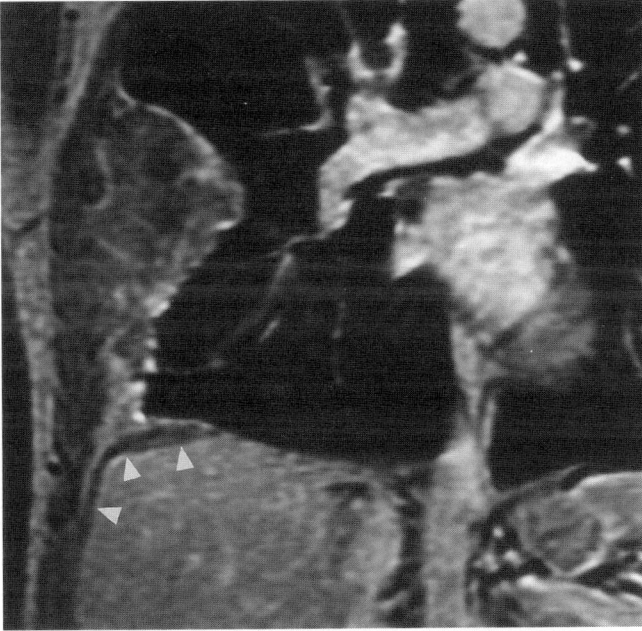

C

Fig. 11-18. Thoracic mesothelioma. Coronal magnetic resonance images demonstrate a bulky, lobulated, pleural-based soft tissue mass in the right hemithorax that demonstrates intermediate T_1 signal (A) and high T_2 signal (B). Mesothelioma extends into the major fissure (A, *arrow*). The mesothelioma shows predominantly peripheral enhancement on a fat-suppressed, gadolinium-enhanced, T_1-weighted image (C). The tumor invades the upper surface of the right hemidiaphragm but does not invade the liver. Note that the fat plane between the diaphragm and liver is preserved (C, *arrowheads*).

DIAPHRAGM

The complex shape of the diaphragm makes it difficult to assess on axial images. Moreover, on axial images it may be difficult to determine the location and extent of juxtadiaphragmatic pathology. MR imaging in the sagittal and coronal planes can determine if a mass is above or below the diaphragm or invades the diaphragm. Breath-hold imaging techniques, such as fast gradient echo and single-shot fast spin echo, eliminate respiratory motion artifact while providing adequate soft tissue contrast. Currently, clinical experience with MR imaging of the diaphragm is limited but increasing. Multiplanar MR imaging may be useful in the preoperative planning for repair of traumatic diaphragmatic rupture and congenital diaphragmatic hernias. More recently, MR imaging has been used to study diaphragmatic motion in lieu of fluoroscopy. This may be of

value in assessing phrenic nerve paralysis, as well as determining suitability for lung reduction surgery.

FUTURE OF MAGNETIC RESONANCE IMAGING

Radiologists and surgeons will be challenged to stay abreast of new developments in MR imaging. MR angiography may eventually replace conventional angiography for evaluation of the thoracic aorta. Ultrafast pulse sequences and hyperpolarized noble gases will provide better images of lung parenchyma and air spaces, respectively. The pulmonary V̇/Q̇ scans of the future could well be an MR image. New MR contrast agents will improve lesion detection and characterization. With these many advances, MR imaging will begin to provide functional as well as anatomic information. It is a mistake, however, to become mesmerized by technology. Although MR imaging can produce dazzling images of many thoracic disease processes, our mandate as health care providers is to choose the safest, most accurate, and most cost-effective imaging modality for our patients.

READING REFERENCES

Alley MT, et al: Ultrafast contrast-enhanced three-dimensional MR angiography: state of the art. Radiographics 18:273, 1998.

Alsop DC, et al: Multi-slice imaging of lung parenchyma in a single breath-hold using a sub-millisecond echo time fast gradient-echo sequence. Magn Reson Med 33:678, 1995.

Aronberg DJ, et al: The superior sinus of the pericardium: CT appearance. Radiology 153:489, 1984.

Axel L, Dougerty L: MR imaging of motion with spatial modulation of magnetization. Radiology 171:841, 1989.

Axel L, Dougherty L: Heart wall motion: improved method of spacial modulation of magnetization for MR imaging. Radiology 172:349, 1989.

Amundsen T, et al: Pulmonary embolism: detection with MR perfusion imaging of lung. A feasibility study. Radiology 203:181, 1997.

Auffermann W, et al: Diagnosis of recurrent hyperparathyroidism: comparison of MR imaging and other imaging techniques. AJR Am J Roentgenol 150:1027, 1988.

Bachert P, et al: Nuclear magnetic resonance imaging of airways in humans with use of hyperpolarized ³He. Magn Reson Med 36:192, 1996.

Bailes DR, et al: Respiratory ordered phase encoding (ROPE): a method for reducing respiratory motion artifacts in MR imaging. J Comput Assist Tomogr 9:835, 1985.

Bank ER: Magnetic resonance of congenital cardiovascular disease. Radiol Clin North Am 31:553, 1993.

Bergin CJ, Glover GH, Pauly JM: Lung parenchyma: magnetic susceptibility in MR imaging. Radiology 180:845, 1991.

Bergin CJ, et al: MR imaging of lung parenchyma: a solution to susceptibility. Radiology 183:673, 1992.

Bergin CJ, et al: MR evaluation of chest wall involvement in malignant lymphoma. J Comput Assist Tomogr 14:928, 1990.

Berlin SC: Magnetic resonance imaging of the cardiovascular system and airway. Pediatr Clin North Am 44:659, 1997.

Berthezene Y, et al: Magnetic resonance imaging detection of an experimental pulmonary perfusion deficit using a macromolecular contrast agent. Polylysine-gadolinium-DTPA40. Invest Radiol 27:346, 1992.

Berthezene Y, et al: Safety aspects and pharmacokinetics of inhaled aerosolized gadolinium. J Magn Reson Imaging 3:125, 1993.

Berthezene Y, et al: Lung perfusion demonstrated by contrast enhanced dynamic MR imaging. Application to single lung transplantation. Invest Radiol 32:351, 1997.

Bittner RC, Felix R: Magnetic resonance imaging of the chest: state-of-the-art. Eur Respir J 11:1392, 1998.

Bock JC, et al: Gd-DTPA-polylysine-enhanced pulmonary time-of-flight MR angiography. J Magn Reson Imaging 4:473, 1994.

Boiselle PM, et al: Imaging of mediastinal lymph nodes: CT, MR, and FDG PET. Radiographics 18:1061, 1998.

Bonomo L, et al: Lung cancer staging: the role of computed tomography and magnetic resonance imaging. Eur J Radiol 23:35, 1996.

Bourgouin PM, et al: Differentiation of bronchogenic carcinoma from postobstructive pneumonitis by magnetic resonance imaging: histopathologic correlation. J Thorac Imaging 6:22, 1991.

Cantoni S, et al: Enhancement of pleural effusions on MR images obtained after intravenous administration of Gd-DTPA. Radiology 193(P):148, 1994.

Castellino RA: The non-Hodgkin lymphomas: practical concepts for the diagnostic radiologist. Radiology 178:315, 1991.

Castellino RA: Hodgkin disease: practical concepts for the diagnostic radiologist. Radiology 159:305, 1986.

Chang YC, et al: Magnetic resonance angiography in the diagnosis of thoracic venous obstruction. J Formos Med Assoc 97:38, 1998.

Chong VF: Imaging thoracic malignancy. Ann Acad Med Singapore 24:254, 1995.

Cigarroa JE, et al: Diagnostic imaging in the evaluation of suspected aortic dissection: old standards and new directions. N Engl J Med 328:35, 1993.

Coady MA, et al: Penetrating ulcer of the thoracic aorta: what is it? how do we recognize it? how do we manage it? J Vasc Surg 27:1015, 1998.

Cooke JP, Kazmier FJ, Orszulak TA: The penetrating aortic ulcer: patho-

logic manifestations, diagnosis, and management. Mayo Clin Proc 63:718, 1988.

Cotran RS, Kumar V, Robbins SL: Robbins Pathologic Basis of Disease. 5th Ed. Philadelphia: WB Saunders, 1994.

Davis CP, et al: Postprocessing techniques for gadolinium-enhanced three-dimension MR angiography. Radiographics 17:1061, 1997.

Davis SD, et al: MR imaging of pleural effusions. J Comput Assist Tomogr 14:192, 1990.

De Bakey ME, Cooley DA, Creech O Jr: Surgical considerations of dissecting aneurysm of the aorta. Ann Surg 142:586, 1955.

De Bakey M, et al: Surgical management of dissecting aneurysms of the aorta. J Thorac Cardiovasc Surg 49:130, 1965.

de Lange EE, et al: Lung air spaces: MR imaging evaluation with hyperpolarized ³He gas. Radiology 210:851, 1999.

Deutsch HJ, et al: Chronic aortic dissection: comparison of MR imaging and transesophageal echocardiography. Radiology 192:645, 1994.

Doyle AJ: Demonstration of blood supply to pulmonary sequestration by MR angiography. AJR Am J Roentgenol 158:989, 1992.

Erdman WA, et al: Pulmonary embolism: comparison of MR images with radionuclide and angiographic studies. Radiology 190:499, 1994.

Evans AJ, et al: Detection of deep venous thrombosis: prospective comparison of MR imaging with contrast venography. AJR Am J Roentgenol 161:131, 1993.

Falaschi F, et al: MR signal as a predictive index of malignant pleural disease. Radiology 193(P):147, 1994.

Felson B: Chest Roentgenology. Philadelphia: WB Saunders, 1973.

Ferguson ER, et al: Evaluation of complex mediastinal masses by magnetic resonance imaging. J Cardiovasc Surg 39:117, 1998.

Feuerstein IM, et al: Pulmonary metastases: MR imaging with surgical correlation—a prospective study. Radiology 182:123, 1992.

Finn JP, et al: Central venous occlusion: MR angiography. Radiology 187:245, 1993.

Fisher MR, Higgins CB, Andereck W: MR imaging of an intrapericardial pheochromocytoma. J Comput Assist Tomogr 9:1103, 1985.

Fisher MR, Higgins H, Higgins CB: Magnetic resonance imaging of developmental venous anomalies. AJR Am J Roentgenol 145:705, 1985.

Flamm SD, VanDyke CW, White RD: MR imaging of the thoracic aorta. Magn Reson Imaging Clin N Am 4:217, 1996.

Foo TK, et al: Pulmonary vasculature: single breath-hold MR imaging with phased-array coils. Radiology 183:473, 1992.

Fortier M, et al: MR imaging of chest wall lesions. Radiographics 14:597, 1994.

Fraser RG, et al: Synopsis of Diseases of the Chest. 2nd Ed. Philadelphia: WB Saunders, 1994.

Fujimoto K, et al: Gd-DTPA-enhanced dynamic MR imaging in pulmonary disease: evaluation of usefulness in differentiating benign from malignant disease. Radiology 189(P):438, 1993.

Galli R, et al: Surgical indications and timing of repair of traumatic ruptures of the thoracic aorta. Ann Thorac Surg 65:461, 1998.

Gaubert JY, et al: Type A dissection of the thoracic aorta: use of MR imaging for long-term follow-up. Radiology 196:363, 1995.

Gefter WB, et al: Pulmonary vascular cine MR imaging: a noninvasive approach to dynamic imaging of the pulmonary circulation. Radiology 176:761, 1990.

Gefter WB: Magnetic resonance imaging in the evaluation of lung cancer. Semin Roentgenol 25:73, 1990.

Gefter WB, Hatabu H: Evaluation of pulmonary vascular anatomy and blood flow by magnetic resonance. J Thorac Imaging 8:122, 1993.

Gefter WB, Kundel H, Hatabu H: Magnetic resonance imaging in chest medicine. In Fishman AP (ed): Update: Pulmonary Diseases and Disorders. New York: McGraw-Hill, Inc, 1992.

Gefter WB, et al: New Directions in MR Research in the Lung. In Cutillo AG (ed): Application of Magnetic Resonance to the Study of Lung. Armonk, NY: Futura, 1995.

Gefter WB, et al: Pulmonary thromboembolism: recent developments in diagnosis using computed tomography and magnetic resonance imaging. State-of-the-Art Radiology 197:561, 1995.

Gierada DS, et al: Diaphragmatic motion: fast gradient-recalled-echo MR imaging in healthy subjects. Radiology 194:879, 1995.

Gomori JM, Grossman RI: Mechanisms responsible for the MR appearance and evolution of intracranial hemorrhage. Radiographics 8:427, 1988.

Grist TM, et al: Pulmonary angiography with MR imaging: preliminary clinical experience. Radiology 189:523 , 1993.

Groch MW, Turner DA, Erwin WD: Respiratory gating in magnetic resonance imaging: improved image quality over non-gated images for equal scan time. Clin Imaging 15:196, 1991.

Grover FL: The role of CT and MR imaging in staging of the mediastinum. Chest *106*:3915, 1994.

Gupta A, et al: Acute pulmonary embolism: diagnosis with MR angiography. Radiology *210*:353, 1999.

Haacke EM, Lenz GW: Improving image quality in the presence of motion by using rephasing gradients. AJR Am J Roentgenol *148*:1251, 1987.

Haggar AM, Froelich JW: MR imaging strategies in primary and metastatic malignancies. Radiol Clin North Am *26*:689, 1988.

Hartnell GG: Magnetic resonance angiography of the thoracic aorta. Magn Reson Imaging Clin N Am *1*:313, 1993.

Hartnell GG, et al: MR imaging of the thoracic aorta: comparison of spin-echo, angiographic, and breath-hold techniques. Radiology *191*:697, 1994.

Hartnell GG, et al: Magnetic resonance angiography of the central chest veins. Chest *107*:1053, 1995.

Hata A, Numano F: Magnetic resonance imaging of the vascular changes in Takayasu arteritis. Int J Cardiol *52*:45, 1995.

Hatabu H, Gefter WB: Clinical Applications of Magnetic Resonance in the Pulmonary Vasculature. *In* Cutillo AG (ed): Application of Magnetic Resonance to the Study of Lung. Armonk, NY: Futura, 1995.

Hatabu H, et al: Magnetic resonance approaches to the evaluation of pulmonary vascular anatomy and physiology. Magn Reson Q *7*:208, 1991.

Hatabu H, et al: MR imaging with spatial modulation of magnetization in the evaluation of chronic central pulmonary thromboembolism. Radiology *190*:791, 1994.

Hatabu H, et al: MR imaging and T2* measurement of lung parenchyma using a new submillisecond TE gradient echo sequence. Radiology *193*:147, 1994.

Hatabu H, et al: Pulmonary perfusion: qualitative assessment with dynamic contrast-enhanced MR imaging using ultra-short TE and inversion recovery turboflash. Magn Reson Med *36*:503, 1996.

Hatabu H, et al: Pulmonary perfusion and angiography: evaluation with breath-hold enhanced three-dimensional fast imaging steady state precession MR imaging with short TR and TE. AJR Am J Roentgenol *167*:653, 1996.

Heelan RT, et al: Superior sulcus tumors: CT and MR imaging. Radiology *170*:637, 1989.

Heelan RT, et al: Magnetic resonance imaging of the postpneumonectomy chest: normal and abnormal findings. J Thorac Imag *12*:200, 1997.

Henning J, Naverth A, Friedburg H: RARE imaging: fast imaging method for clinical MR. Magn Reson Med *3*:823, 1986.

Higgins CB: Role of magnetic resonance imaging in hyperparathyroidism. Radiol Clin North Am *31*:1017, 1993.

Higgins CB, Auffermann W: MR imaging of thyroid and parathyroid glands: A review of current status. AJR Am J Roentgenol *151*:1095, 1988.

Hill SL, Berry RE: Subclavian vein thrombosis: a continuing challenge. Surgery *108*:1, 1990.

Ho VB, Prince MR: Thoracic MR aortography: imaging techniques and strategies. Radiographics *18*:287, 1998.

Holland GA, et al: Prospective comparison of pulmonary MR angiography and ultrafast CT for diagnosis of pulmonary thromboembolic disease. Radiology *189(P)*:234, 1993.

Holmvang G: Usefulness of MR imaging in aortic dissection. N Engl J Med *326*:1670, 1992.

Horattas MC, Wright DJ, Fenton AH: Changing concepts of deep venous thrombosis of the upper extremity: report of a series and review of the literature. Surgery *104*:561, 1988.

Hsu BY, Edwards DK, Trambert MA: Pulmonary hemorrhage complicating systemic lupus erythematosus: role of MR imaging in diagnosis. AJR Am J Roentgenol *158*:519, 1992.

Hughes JP, Ruttley MS, Musumeci F: Case report: traumatic aortic rupture: demonstration by magnetic resonance imaging. Br J Radiol *67*:1264, 1994.

Im J-G, et al: MR imaging of the transverse sinus of the pericardium. AJR Am J Roentgenol *150*:79, 1988.

Ionescu AA, et al: Periaortic fat pad mimicking an intramural hematoma of the thoracic aorta: lessons for transesophageal echocardiography. J Am Soc Echocardiogr *11*:487, 1998.

Jelinek JS, et al: Small cell lung cancer: staging with MR imaging. Radiology *177*:837, 1990.

Johansen K: Infected and other unusual aneurysms. *In* Bergan JJ, Yao JST (eds): Aortic Surgery. Philadelphia: WB Saunders, 1989.

Joyce JW, et al: Aneurysms of the thoracic aorta: a clinical study with special reference to prognosis. Circulation *29*:176, 1964.

Kang YS, et al: Localization of abnormal parathyroid glands of the mediastinum with MR imaging. Radiology *189*:137, 1993.

Katz ES, et al: Tortuosity of the descending thoracic aorta simulating dis-

section on transesophageal echocardiography. J Am Soc Echocardiogr *10*:83, 1997.

Kauczor H, Surkau R, Roberts T: MR imaging using hyperpolarized gases. Eur J Radiol *8*:820, 1998.

Kawamoto S, et al: Thoracoabdominal aorta in Marfan syndrome: MR imaging findings of progression of vasculopathy after surgical repair. Radiology *203*:727, 1997.

Kawashima A, Fishman EK, Kuhlman JE: CT and MR evaluation of posterior mediastinal masses. Crit Rev Diagn Imaging *33*:311, 1992.

Kersting-Sommerhoff BA, et al: MR imaging of the thoracic aorta in Marfan patients. J Comput Assist Tomogr *11*:633, 1987.

Kersting-Sommerhoff BA, et al: Aortic dissection: sensitivity and specificity of MR imaging. Radiology *166*:651, 1988.

Kessler R, et al: Magnetic resonance imaging in the diagnosis of pulmonary infarction. Chest *99*:298, 1991.

Klein JS, Webb WR: The radiologic staging of lung cancer. J Thorac Imaging *7*:29, 1991.

Ko SC, et al: Diagnosis of pulmonary sequestration by magnetic resonance imaging. J Formos Med Assoc *97*:220, 1998.

Ko SF, et al: Dissection of retroesophageal aortic diverticulum and descending aorta in a patient with a right aortic arch. Cardiovasc Intervent Radiol *19*:438, 1996.

Krinsky GA, et al: Thoracic aorta: comparison of gadolinium-enhanced three-dimensional MR angiography with conventional MR imaging. Radiology *202*:183, 1997.

Kuhlman JE, et al: CT and MR imaging evaluation of chest wall disorders. Radiographics *14*:571, 1994.

Laurent F, et al: T2-weighted MR imaging of chest: advantages of turbo SE technique. Radiology *189(P)*:123, 1993.

Lepore V, et al: Magnetic resonance imaging in the follow-up of patients after aortic root reconstruction. Thorac Cardiovasc Surg *44*:188, 1996.

Lesko NM, Link KM: Mediastinum and lung. *In* Stark DD, Bradley WG (eds): Magnetic Resonance Imaging. Vol. 1. 3rd Ed. St. Louis: CV Mosby, 1999.

Leung DA, Debatin JF: Three-dimensional contrast-enhanced magnetic resonance angiography of the thoracic vasculature. Eur J Radiol *7*:981, 1997.

Li W, et al: Three-dimensional low dose gadolinium-enhanced peripheral MR venography. J Magn Reson Imaging *8*:630, 1998.

Lindsay J Jr: Diseases of the Aorta. Philadelphia: Lea & Febiger, 1994.

Link KM, Lesko NM: The role of MR imaging in the evaluation of acquired diseases of the thoracic aorta. AJR Am J Roentgenol *158*:1115, 1992.

Link KM, et al: Magnetic resonance imaging of the mediastinum. J Thorac Imaging *8*:34, 1993.

Liu YL, et al: A monitoring, feedback, and triggering system for reproducible breath-hold MR imaging. Magn Reson Med *30*:507, 1993.

Lorigan JG, Libshitz HI: MR imaging of malignant pleural mesothelioma. J Comput Assist Tomogr *13*:617, 1989.

Loubeyre P, et al: Dynamic contrast-enhanced MR angiography of pulmonary embolism: comparison with pulmonary angiography. AJR Am J Roentgenol *162*:1035, 1994.

Loubeyre P, et al: Magnetic resonance imaging evaluation of the ascending aorta after graft-inclusion surgery: comparison between an ultrafast contrast-enhanced MR sequence and conventional cine-MR imaging. J Magn Reson Imaging *6*:478, 1996.

Mai VM, Berr SS: MR perfusion imaging of pulmonary parenchyma using pulsed arterial spin labeling techniques: FAIRER and FAIR. J Magn Reson Imaging *9*:483, 1999.

Masani ND, et al: Follow-up of chronic thoracic aortic dissection: comparison of transesophageal echocardiography and magnetic resonance imaging. Am Heart J *131*:1156, 1996.

Matsunaga N, et al: Takayasu arteritis: protean radiologic manifestations and diagnosis. Radiographics *17*:579, 1997.

Mayo JR: Thoracic magnetic resonance imaging: physics and pulse sequences. J Thorac Imaging *8*:1, 1993.

Mayo JR, Mackey A, Müller NL: MR imaging of the lungs: value of short TE spin-echo pulse sequences. AJR Am J Roentgenol *159*:951, 1992.

McDermott VG, et al: Preoperative MR imaging in hyperparathyroidism: results and factors affecting parathyroid detection. AJR Am J Roentgenol *166*:705, 1996.

McLoud TC, Flower CDR: Imaging the pleura: sonography, CT, and MR imaging. AJR Am J Roentgenol *156*:1145, 1991.

McLoud TC, et al: MR imaging of superior sulcus carcinoma. J Comput Assist Tomogr *13*:233, 1989.

McMurdo KK, et al: Normal and occluded mediastinal veins: MR imaging. Radiology *159*:33, 1986.

Meaney JFM, et al: Diagnosis of pulmonary embolism with magnetic resonance angiography. N Engl J Med 336:1422, 1997.

Mendelsohn AM, et al: Is echocardiography or magnetic resonance imaging superior for precoarctation angioplasty evaluation? Cathet Cardiovasc Diagn 42:26, 1997.

Meza MP, Benson M, Slovis TL: Imaging of mediastinal masses in children. Radiol Clin North Am 31:583, 1993.

Milas BL, Savino JS: Pseudoaneurysm of the ascending aorta after aortic valve replacement. J Am Soc Echocardiogr 1:303, 1998.

Mitchell DG, et al: Benign adrenocortical masses: diagnosis with chemical shift MR imaging. Radiology 185:345, 1992.

Mohiaddin RH, et al: Magnetic resonance characterization of pulmonary arterial blood flow after single lung transplantation. J Thorac Cardiovasc Surg 101:1016, 1991

Müller NL, Mayo JR, Zwirewich CV: Value of MR imaging in the evaluation of chronic infiltrative lung diseases: comparison with CT. AJR Am J Roentgenol 158:1205, 1992.

Müller NL: Imaging of the pleura. Radiology 186:297, 1993.

Murayama S, et al: Signal intensity characteristics of mediastinal cystic masses on T1-weighted MR imaging. J Comput Assist Tomogr 19:188, 1995.

Murray JG, et al: Intramural hematoma of the thoracic aorta: MR image findings and their prognostic implications. Radiology 204:349, 1997.

Naidich DP, et al: Intralobar pulmonary sequestration: MR evaluation. J Comput Assist Tomogr 11:531, 1987.

Naidich DP, et al: Congenital anomalies of the lungs in adults: MR diagnosis. AJR Am J Roentgenol 151:13, 1988.

Naidich DP, Zerhouni EA, Siegelman SS: Computed Tomography and Magnetic Resonance of the Thorax. 2nd Ed. New York: Raven Press, 1991.

Nienaber CA, et al: The diagnosis of thoracic aortic dissection by noninvasive imaging procedures. N Engl J Med 328:1, 1993.

Nienaber CA, et al: Comparison of conventional and transesophageal echocardiography with magnetic resonance imaging for anatomical mapping of thoracic aortic dissection: a dual noninvasive imaging study with anatomical and/or angiographic validation. Int J Card Imaging 10:1, 1994.

Nienaber CA, et al: Intramural hemorrhage of the thoracic aorta. Diagnostic and therapeutic implications. Circulation 92:1465, 1995.

Nyman RS, et al: Residual mediastinal masses in Hodgkin disease: prediction of size with MR imaging. Radiology 170:435, 1989.

Olson EM, et al: Fast SE MR imaging of the chest: parameter optimization, and comparison with conventional SE imaging. J Comput Assist Tomogr 19:167, 1995.

Padovani B, et al: Chest wall invasion by bronchogenic carcinoma: evaluation with MR imaging. Radiology 187:33, 1993.

Panegyres PK, et al: Thoracic outlet syndromes and magnetic resonance imaging. Brain 116:823, 1993.

Poon PY, et al: Mediastinal lymph node metastases from bronchogenic carcinoma: detection with MR imaging and CT. Radiology 162:651, 1987.

Prince MR, et al: Dynamic gadolinium-enhanced three-dimensional abdominal MR arteriography. J Magn Reson Imaging 3:877, 1993.

Pugatch RD: Radiologic evaluation in chest malignancies: a review of imaging modalities. Chest 107:2945, 1995.

Quint LE, et al: Pheochromocytoma and paraganglioma: comparison of MR imaging with CT and I-131 MIBG scintigraphy. Radiology 165:89, 1987.

Rahmouni A, et al: Lymphoma: monitoring tumor size and signal intensity with MR imaging. Radiology 188:445, 1993.

Rehn SM, et al: Non-Hodgkin lymphoma: predicting prognostic grade with MR imaging. Radiology 176:249, 1990.

Remy-Martin M, et al: Diagnosis of pulmonary embolism with spiral CT: comparison with pulmonary angiography and scintigraphy. Radiology 200:699, 1996.

Rich S, Levitsky S, Brundage BH: Pulmonary hypertension from chronic pulmonary thromboembolism. Ann Intern Med 108:425, 1988.

Robbins RC, et al: Management of patients with intramural hematoma of the thoracic aorta. Circulation 88:1, 1993.

Rofsky NM, et al: Aortic aneurysm and dissection: normal MR imaging and CT findings after surgical repair with the continuous-suture graft-inclusion technique. Radiology 186:195, 1993.

Rosado-de-Christenson ML, et al: Extralobar sequestration: radiologic–pathologic correlation. Radiographics 13:425, 1993.

Rosado-de-Christenson ML, et al: Thymolipoma: analysis of 27 cases. Radiology 193:121, 1994.

Rubin E, et al: Diagnostic imaging and staging of primary lung cancer. Semin Surg Oncol 9:85, 1993.

Rubin GD, et al: Single breath-hold pulmonary magnetic resonance angiography. Optimization and comparison of three imaging strategies. Invest Radiol 29:766, 1994.

Schiebler ML, Listerud J: Common artifacts encountered in thoracic magnetic resonance imaging: recognition, derivation, and solutions. Top Magn Reson Imaging 4:1, 1992.

Schiebler ML, et al: Suspected pulmonary embolism: prospective evaluation with pulmonary MR angiography. Radiology 189:125, 1993.

Seelos K, et al: T2-weighted turbo-SE MR imaging with electrocardiogram gating for assessment of intra-, peri-, and paracardial masses at 0.5T. Radiology 185(P):118, 1992.

Semelka RC, et al: Single-breath whole-thorax Gd-DTPA-enhanced MR imaging of pulmonary nodules and interstitial disease: comparison with CT. Radiology 181(P):305, 1991.

Shields TW: Screening, staging, and diagnostic investigation of non-small cell lung cancer patients. Curr Opin Oncol 3:297, 1991.

Siegel MJ: Chest applications of magnetic resonance imaging in children. Top Magn Reson Imaging 3:1, 1990.

Soler R, et al: MR imaging of pseudocoarctation of the aorta: morphological and cine-MR imaging findings. Comput Med Imaging Graph 19:431, 1995.

Soler R, et al: Magnetic resonance imaging of congenital abnormalities of the thoracic aorta. Eur J Radiol 8:540, 1998.

Solomon SL, et al: Thoracic aortic dissection: pitfalls and artifacts in MR imaging. Radiology 177:223, 1990.

Spring BI, Schiebler ML: Normal anatomy of the thoracic inlet as seen on transaxial MR images. AJR Am J Roentgenol 157:707, 1991.

Spritzer CE, et al: Detection of deep venous thrombosis by magnetic resonance imaging. Chest 104:54, 1993.

Stanson AW, et al: Penetrating atherosclerotic ulcers of the thoracic aorta: Natural history and clinicopathologic correlations. Ann Vasc Surg 1:15, 1986.

Stock KW, et al: Demonstration of gravity-dependent lung perfusion with contrast-enhanced magnetic resonance imaging. J Magn Reson Imaging 9:557, 1999.

Taylor AM, et al: Magnetic resonance navigator echo diaphragm monitoring in patients with suspected diaphragm paralysis. J Magn Reson Imaging 9:69, 1999.

Teh BT: Thymic carcinoids in multiple endocrine neoplasia type 1. J Intern Med 243:501, 1998.

Turetschek K, et al: Double inversion recovery imaging of the brain: initial experience and comparison with fluid attenuated inversion recovery imaging. Magn Reson Imaging 16:127, 1998.

Vesely TM, et al: MR imaging of partial anomalous pulmonary venous connections. J Comput Assist Tomogr 15:752, 1991.

Webb WR, Golden JA: Imaging strategies in the staging of lung cancer. Clin Chest Med 12:133, 1991.

Webb WR, Sostman HD: MR imaging of thoracic disease: clinical uses. Radiology 182:621, 1992.

Webb WR, et al: CT and MR imaging in staging non-small cell bronchogenic carcinoma: report of the Radiologic Diagnostic Oncology Group. Radiology 178:705, 1991.

Weinreb JC, Mootz A, Cohen JM: MR imaging evaluation of mediastinal and thoracic inlet venous obstruction. AJR Am J Roentgenol 146:679, 1986.

Weinreb JC, Naidich DP: Thoracic magnetic resonance imaging. Clin Chest Med 12:33, 1991.

Wielopolski PA: Pulmonary arteriography. MR Imaging Clin North Am 1:295, 1993.

Wielopolski PA, Haacke EM, Adler LP: Three-dimensional MR imaging of the pulmonary vasculature: preliminary experience. Radiology 183:465, 1992.

Winer-Muram HT, et al: Primitive neuroectodermal tumors of the chest wall (Askin tumors): CT and MR findings. AJR Am J Roentgenol 161:265, 1993.

Wolffe KA, et al: Aortic dissection: atypical patterns seen at MR imaging. Radiology 181:489, 1991.

Wolffe KA, et al: Accuracy of MR angiography in depicting chronic pulmonary thromboembolic disease: evaluation at the segmental and lobar levels. Radiology 193(P):311, 1994.

Wolffe KA, et al: Utility of MR imaging in distinction between chronic pulmonary thromboembolic disease and primary pulmonary hypertension. Radiology 193(P):312, 1994.

Wyttenbach R, Vock P, Tschappeler H: Cross sectional imaging with CT and/or MR imaging of pediatric chest tumors. Eur J Radiol 8:1040, 1998.

Yamada I, Numano F, Suzuki S: Takayasu arteritis: evaluation with MR imaging. Radiology 188:89, 1993.

Yankelevitz DF, et al: Lung cancer: evaluation with MR imaging during and after irradiation. J Thorac Imaging 9:41, 1994.

CHAPTER 12

Positron Emission Tomography in Chest Diseases

Richard L. Wahl

For many years, positron emission tomography (PET) existed as a somewhat arcane research tool used most commonly for probing the function of the human brain. Making positron-emitting isotopes was complicated and generally required a cyclotron located near a specialized PET scanner and costing several million dollars. Because of the short half-life of PET tracers (2 minutes to 2 hours) the technique was not viewed as clinically practical for most hospital settings. However, in the 1990s, it has become apparent that the PET method has rather general usefulness in cancer imaging, and in particular in imaging known and suspected lung cancers. The increased feasibility of performing PET in more and more academic centers and larger community hospitals can be traced to improvements in computers, cyclotrons, distribution networks for radiopharmaceuticals, and an improved knowledge base regarding how PET can play a role in cancer imaging. It is now possible for medical centers to purchase a PET scanner for approximately the cost of a computed tomography (CT) scanner, or less, and to purchase needed PET radiotracers from regional cyclotrons, rather than invest in the operation of their own cyclotrons, making the PET tracers generally available in metropolitan areas across the United States. Approval by Medicare in the United States for several lung cancer-related applications has dramatically increased interest in this method.

GENERAL PRINCIPLES

Although chest radiography, CT, and, to a lesser extent, magnetic resonance imaging are well-established methods for lung cancer imaging, they are based on anatomic changes that, by their nature, can be nonspecific. By contrast, PET imaging can simplistically be thought of as a *metabolic CT scan* that displays anatomy in the body, but more important, displays aspects of the function or metabolism of the body at the same time in a precise anatomic framework. This is clinically relevant because the earliest changes in disease are those in physiology and not in anatomy. Thus, PET provides a look at more fundamental aspects of the disease process than is possible with anatomic imaging. This ability to look inside of lymph nodes, lung nodules, and postoperative and postradiation scars, and indeed, anywhere in the body, enables PET to provide unique functional imaging information about the body.

PET imaging is somewhat similar in concept to most nuclear medicine techniques, such as bone scanning. In nuclear imaging, a radiotracer is injected intravenously that homes to a specific tissue or organ based on its physical properties. As an example, in the commonly used bone scan, remodeling bone accumulates a diphosphonate analogue technetium 99m (^{99m}Tc) that can then be imaged using a special camera found in nuclear medicine departments called a *gamma camera*, which detects the gamma rays emitted from the patient by the ^{99m}Tc. The principle for PET is similar, in that a radioactive tracer that preferentially accumulates in tumor tissue because of altered tumor metabolism is used. Rather than a gamma ray–emitting isotope, the radiotracer used is a positron emitter. The positron is a positively charged electron, which is essentially antimatter. The positron travels a short distance in tissue and then encounters an electron. The two combine and then annihilate, giving off two 511-keV photons that travel in opposite directions. These photons can then be detected by the PET scanner. The PET scanner and its computers can determine the line on which the disintegration occurred, and then, with multiple decays and measurements, determine the point of origin of the decays using reconstruction methods such as those used to generate CT scans. The term *PET imaging* is actually a misnomer, because the positrons are not really imaged with a PET scanner; rather, the images obtained are of 511-keV photons from annihilation of the positron. A full review of the physics and instrumentation of PET is beyond the scope of this chapter, but interested readers are referred to the author's report in 1997. The most critical points regarding PET are that it is a method that is anatomically precise, quantitative, and that images a variety of potential physiologic processes, depending on the choice of the radiotracer injected.

Physiologic Basis of the Use of Radiotracer Fluoro-2-Deoxy-D-Glucose

Although a wide variety of physiologic processes can be imaged with PET, the one that is of the greatest practical significance for this clinical review is the increased glucose metabolism typically seen in malignant lung tumors. This increased glucose metabolism can be imaged using the radiotracer [18F] fluoro-2-deoxy-D-glucose (FDG). Increased metabolism of glucose by the tumor cell is in part caused by increased expression of glucose transporter messenger RNA and increased glucose transport proteins that result in greater glucose uptake and metabolism as shown by Flier and colleagues (1987). FDG is a D-glucose analogue and is recognized as D-glucose in its transport through the cell membrane and phosphorylation by hexokinase in the normal glycolytic pathway. However, once FDG is phosphorylated, structural changes created by a hexose-phosphate bond prevent FDG from being catabolized or transported out of the cell. Thus, not only is there increased uptake, but also accumulation of FDG occurs in the abnormally metabolizing tumor cells as described by Gallagher and associates (1978). Thus, the radiotracer FDG in the actively metabolizing cancer cells can be recognized by PET from that in normal tissues by the greater emission of 511 keV from the tumor tissue.

POSITRON EMISSION TOMOGRAPHY IN LUNG CANCER

The role of PET in imaging lung cancer can be divided into three general areas: 1) characterizing solitary pulmonary nodules as malignant or benign, 2) staging lung cancer both locoregionally and systemically, and 3) assessing response to treatment.

Positron Emission Tomography Imaging of Lung Cancer

The imaging of lung cancer was first reported by Kubota and coworkers (1985), who showed in eight patients that lung cancers accumulated more of the amino acid L-methio-

nine, with C11 as a label, than normal lung. This was confirmed in 16 more patients a few years later by Fujiwara and associates (1989). Although methionine uptake is of interest, and these studies showed feasibility for PET imaging of lung cancer, the 20-minute half-life of C11 made the use of C11-labeled tracers rather impractical in most clinical practice settings.

The first use of the more easily usable tracer FDG in lung cancer imaging (18F has a 109-minute half-life) was in a series of 12 lung cancers in which all were successfully imaged using FDG, regardless of histology. Nolop and colleagues (1987) reported that mean tumor to nontumor ratios of greater than 6:1 were seen, which is an adequate signal for PET imaging. Studies by Kubota and associates (1990) with C11 methionine and with FDG showed that benign solitary pulmonary nodules generally had considerably lower FDG uptake than malignant lesions. Tracer uptake in lesions, as estimated using the standardized uptake value (SUV), a semiquantitative index of tracer accumulation normalized to injected dose and body weight, was higher in malignant lesions than in benign. Gupta and colleagues (1992) showed in 20 patients that FDG uptake into primary lung cancers was significantly greater than that seen in benign pulmonary lesions, with an SUV of 5.63 ± 2.38 standard deviation (SD) in malignant and 0.56 ± 0.27 (SD) in benign lesions ($P < .001$). Patz and coworkers (1993) demonstrated that FDG PET was generally effective in separating primary lung cancers from inflammatory processes in the lung based on the lesion SUV. In a series of 51 patients with focal pulmonary abnormalities, of which 38 were solitary pulmonary nodules, it was noted that the 33 malignant lesions had an SUV of 6.5 ± 2.9 (SD), whereas benign lesions had an SUV of 1.7 ± 1.2 (SD). Thus, an excellent separation between benign and malignant lesions by SUV was observed in this early study.

Imaging of the Solitary Pulmonary Nodule

A prospective multicenter trial by Lowe and associates (1998) assessed solitary pulmonary nodules in 89 patients with FDG PET. The trial showed that PET with FDG had an overall sensitivity and specificity for detection of malignant nodules of 92% and 90%, respectively; using quantitative analysis, it was 98% sensitive and 69% specific. Some trends in differences in sensitivity were seen with smaller lesions, so that for the smaller lesions (smaller than 1.5 cm) visual analysis, as opposed to quantitative analysis, was of greater sensitivity (98%), but of lower specificity than quantitative analysis. Lesions as small as 7 mm were characterized correctly as malignant or benign. A trial from Germany conducted by Prauer and colleagues (1998) studied 54 pulmonary lesions 3 cm or smaller in diameter and showed PET to be 90% sensitive and 83% specific in lesion characterization as malignant or benign. False-negative results included two bronchial carcinomas and one metastasis. Some series

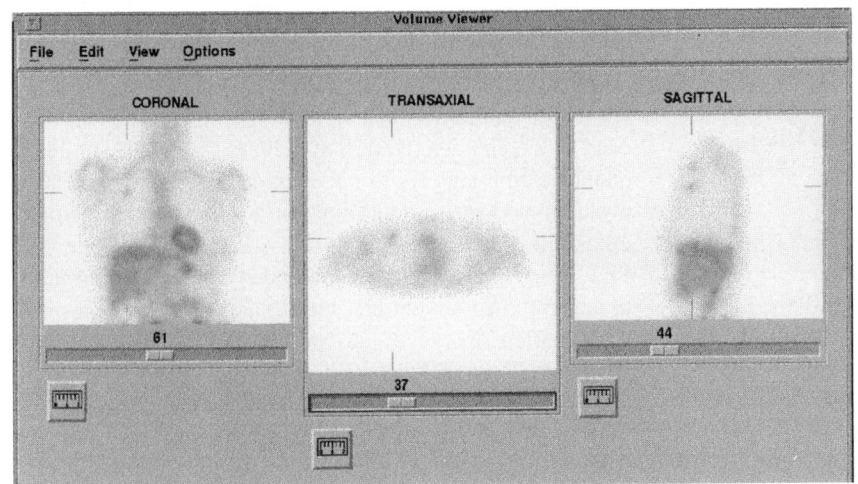

Fig. 12-1. [18F] Fluoro-2-deoxy-D-glucose (FDG) positron emission tomography scans of the thorax in a patient with a right upper lobe nodule that was considered suspicious for cancer. Coronal, transaxial, and sagittal images are provided that show moderate FDG uptake in the right upper lobe lesion. The normal heart and liver are also well visualized. This level of tracer uptake, slightly more than blood activity, is considered worrisome for lung cancer. Thus, this scan pattern would require biopsy for confirmation.

have had up to 10% false-negative rates, especially for small nodules if quantitative analysis is used, so a clear risk of missing tumors exists if PET is the only test performed on a solitary pulmonary nodule. It would seem prudent to recommend follow-up anatomic imaging tests of solitary pulmonary nodules after a negative PET result to exclude tumor growth, because a small percentage of patients with negative PET scan results of a solitary pulmonary nodule have malignant tumors that are not avid for FDG. Kim and coworkers (1998) have reported that this seems to occur with greater frequency in bronchioloalveolar carcinomas, for example, which have considerably lower uptake of FDG than other lung cancers. It is suggested that CT always be examined along with the PET study to be certain that bronchioloalveolar carcinomas are not missed on PET because of this lower tracer uptake. Nonetheless, PET is an accurate, although not perfect, method for evaluating solitary pulmonary nodules noninvasively. An example of a positive PET scan result is shown in Figure 12-1.

Because PET is an accurate test for evaluating a solitary pulmonary nodule, does PET have a clinically useful role in lesion assessment? The answer is still in evolution, but in the author's practice, the patients referred for PET of a solitary pulmonary nodule are often those patients who carry increased risk of complications caused by invasive procedures, especially a thoracotomy, to obtain tissue from nodules. These can include patients with severe emphysema in whom biopsy can be expected to impair function, patients with a propensity to bleed, patients with multiple nodules, and patients who are not inclined to accept biopsy. The practice of using PET in managing indeterminate pulmonary nodules varies depending on the referring physician's familiarity with the test, the expertise of the medical center in PET imaging, the reimbursement pattern at the medical center, the surgeon's experience, especially in minimally invasive surgery, as well as other factors. In some centers, PET is being used in the assessment of a majority of solitary pulmonary nodules. In others, however, it may be reserved for the more difficult cases. At our

medical center, the use has continued to increase as it is more available, experience grows, and reimbursement is growing. It must be understood, though, that PET is a good but not 100% sensitive test. Also, because the specificity of the test is less than 100%, not all *hot* solitary pulmonary nodules seen on PET represent cancers. Thus, biopsy or surgical removal of such hot nodules is required to ascertain their etiology.

The other issue important for referring physicians is that not all PET scanners are identical. There are two basic types of PET scanners. Dedicated PET scanners are designed and optimized to only perform PET imaging, and hybrid PET–single photon emission CT (SPECT) cameras are capable of performing both PET and SPECT, depending on how the camera is set up. Single photon imaging is the method used for bone scanning, for instance. However, at present, virtually all of the literature regarding the accuracy of PET imaging has been developed using dedicated PET scanners. The literature on the accuracy of the PET/SPECT hybrid devices is much more limited, but it is clear that major decrements occur in the PET, but not the SPECT, performance of such devices. All of the hybrid cameras sold to date have much lower count detection efficiencies and lower contrast resolution than dedicated PET scanners according to Shreve and associates (1998). In practice, this means that smaller lesions are generally not as well detected with the PET/SPECT hybrid devices as with a dedicated PET scanner. Thus, at present, it is probably most prudent to have PET imaging in patients with lung cancer or solitary pulmonary nodules performed using dedicated PET scanners until a sufficient base of published evidence is developed to show that the coincidence or hybrid PET/SPECT devices are performing satisfactorily in a given imaging question. Data to date suggest that for solitary pulmonary nodules larger than 1.5 to 2.0 cm, such devices may be adequate, but for smaller lesions and lesions outside of the thorax, as noted by Shreve and colleagues (1998), concerns exist that the hybrid devices may often be too inaccurate. This area is in rapid flux, but at present not all PET scanners are created equally, and the data reported in this chapter are virtually all from dedicated PET devices.

Positron Emission Tomography Evaluation of Hilar and Mediastinal Lymph Node Involvement

In addition to characterizing a solitary pulmonary nodule as malignant or benign, PET can address the important question of whether a lung cancer has spread from the primary site to regional hilar or mediastinal lymph nodes or systemically. This question is of obvious and critical importance in non–small cell lung cancer, in which cure is generally possible only with complete excision of all viable tumor from the thorax. With non–small cell lung cancer, it has been recognized that if tumor involves the mediastinum at the time of initial diagnosis, the patient's probability of survival for 5 years is reduced to just 5 to 10%. By contrast, if no mediastinal lymph node is involved, the 5-year survival is increased to a 40 to 50% probability. Thoracotomy may be inappropriate if there is a high likelihood of mediastinal tumor involvement at the time of diagnosis. Data in this area are emerging rapidly, but it is clear that CT alone has not done a good job of assessing tumor spread to the mediastinum noninvasively (i.e., sensitivity 52% and specificity 69%) as Webb and associates (1991) have pointed out.

In a study by Miyazawa and colleagues (1992), PET staging of the mediastinum was assessed in 25 patients evaluated with 11C methionine. PET showed higher 11C uptake in the tumor-involved lymph nodes than in the tumor-negative nodes (3.89 versus 2.38 mean SUV, $P < .001$). Furthermore, with retrospective setting of the discriminant threshold, a nearly 90% accuracy in characterizing the presence or absence of mediastinal metastases could be defined.

A prospective trial performed at the University of Michigan by the author and associates (1994) showed FDG PET to be significantly more accurate than CT in staging presumed primary non–small cell lung cancer. In this study of 23 patients, PET was significantly more accurate than CT (82% versus 52%, $P < .05$). In this study, PET was able to detect tumor involvement in normal-sized lymph nodes in some cases. In fact, in many cases it was possible to exclude tumor involvement in enlarged lymph nodes. A report by Knopp and coworkers (1992) from Heidelberg, Germany, has shown even better accuracy for FDG PET, but was performed with a PET scanner that had a limited field of view, and thus was not able to evaluate the entire mediastinum at risk for metastases, making pathologic correlation more challenging because not all nodal areas were imaged. Many studies, such as that of Sasaki and colleagues (1996), using PET for mediastinal staging have been reported in the 1990s showing PET to be more accurate than CT for mediastinal staging. For example, Vansteenkiste and coworkers (1998) showed the accuracy of CT and PET for mediastinal staging to be 68 and 94%, respectively. A meta-analysis of the PET and CT literature

by Dwamena and associates (1999) has shown a sensitivity and specificity of 79 and 91%, respectively, for PET, which is considerably higher than that for CT at 60 and 77%. Although qualitative and quantitative analysis have been used in the characterization of solitary pulmonary nodules, quantification appears to have less of a role in mediastinal evaluations. Precise determination of the quantity of tracer uptake in mediastinal lymph nodes is not easily done with PET. This is because lesions in nodes can be heterogeneous in makeup (i.e., not entirely tumor) and because the lesions, which often are small, do not have all of their counts "recovered" by PET because of limitations of PET resolution. Thus, to date, most studies of PET in mediastinal staging have been performed using qualitative analysis. Although this is currently the best method for interpreting PET images of the mediastinum, it remains to be seen whether integration of the CT findings with the PET can improve the accuracy of interpretations. This is an area of active study, but at present, it is prudent to read the PET scan with a recent CT available for correlation. Whether digital fusion of the CT and PET data will be a necessity for optimal clinical care, or just an interesting method of making attractive pictures, remains uncertain.

At present, hot nodes on PET in the mediastinum of a patient with non–small cell lung cancer are considered suspicious for metastatic tumor. At our medical center, and many others in the Midwest, hot nodes are not invariably caused by involvement with malignant tumors, however. Lymph nodes reactive to infections, nodes with sarcoid or tuberculosis, and nodes that have active granulomas can have increased tracer uptake and give false-positive results on PET. Similarly, small nodes can contain tumor foci that are too small to be seen on PET imaging. At our center, we believe that a negative PET scan result of the mediastinum in a patient with known non–small cell lung cancer indicates that operation for cure is feasible. By contrast, if a PET scan result is positive in the mediastinum, tissue confirmation of the etiology of the hot nodes should ideally be obtained to exclude the possibility of nonmalignant inflammatory disease. Although this practice may vary by locale and prevalence of nonmalignant inflammatory disease, this is likely the most prudent approach to this clinical setting, because it is obvious that surgery should not be denied patients because they have inflammatory nodal disease. However, the vast majority of cases of hot mediastinal lymph nodes on PET are nodes with tumor involvement. In studies from Europe, where it would seem inflammatory conditions such as histoplasmosis are not prevalent, positive mediastinal uptake of FDG has been reported to be quite consistently associated with the presence of metastatic tumor. The exact patterns of FDG uptake in the mediastinum most predictive of tumor involvement at PET are still under evaluation. However, based on the accuracy of PET reported from multiple clinical studies, PET for mediastinal staging of non–small cell lung cancer is now routinely provided by Medicare in the United States. As mentioned for solitary

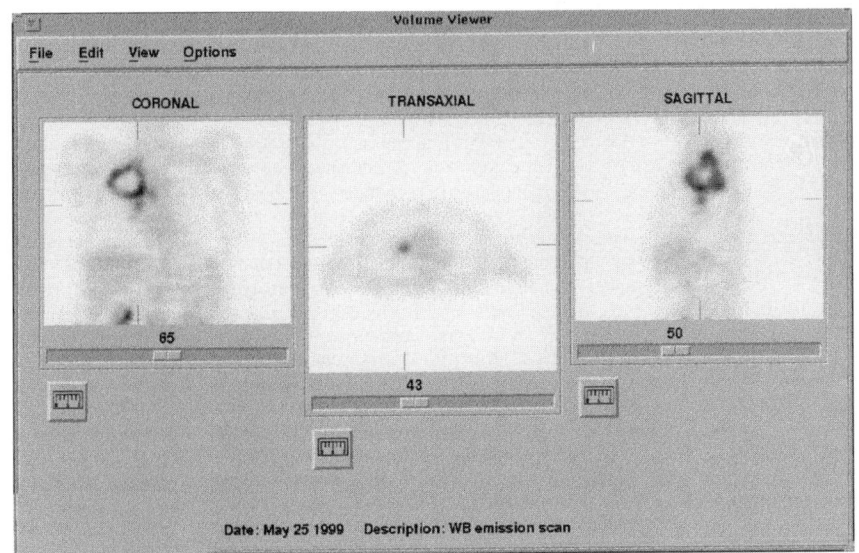

Fig. 12-2. [18F] Fluoro-2-deoxy-D-glucose (FDG) positron emission tomography scans of the thorax in a patient with a known right upper lobe lung carcinoma and mediastinal lymph nodes on computed tomography that were of uncertain significance. The findings are consistent with a large necrotic right upper lobe lung cancer, with FDG-avid mediastinal metastases in both the right and left mediastinum. No evidence of additional metastatic disease exists. The intense activity seen on the coronal view in the right upper abdomen is the right kidney, a normal organ of excretion for FDG.

pulmonary nodules, nearly all the literature available to date is for dedicated PET scanning devices. The use of coincidence or PET/SPECT hybrid devices in this setting is less well developed and less well supported by the literature. An example of a PET scan of the mediastinum is shown in Figure 12-2.

Although PET has been shown to be accurate in evaluating solitary pulmonary nodules for the presence or absence of malignancy and for mediastinal staging, few data exist on the accuracy of PET for assessing chest wall invasion or invasion of other structures. The author's opinion is that, at present, PET is not the optimal test for such determinations.

Whole Body Positron Emission Tomography Imaging

Although PET is a useful method in the thorax, the uptake of FDG into lung cancers is higher than into most normal tissues, including those in the abdomen and elsewhere in the body. For this reason, it is often possible to detect metastatic lung cancer remote from the thorax with PET. An accuracy of 96 and 66%, respectively, for PET and bone scanning in the evaluation of suspected metastatic osseous involvement in 110 consecutive patients with non–small cell lung cancer was reported. Bury and colleagues (1998) noted that the superior accuracy of PET was because of a much lower false-positive rate than in bone scanning. A 14% rate of finding additional metastases beyond the thorax during lung cancer staging was reported by Weder and associates (1998), suggesting PET should be performed on the whole body before a major surgical procedure is undertaken. Adrenal nodules, which are benign, as well as adrenal metastases, occur commonly in patients with non–small cell lung cancer. Benign adrenal nodules should be left alone and are not contraindications to surgical cure of the primary lung cancer. However, malignant adrenal nodules are generally a contraindication to surgery.

In specific evaluation of adrenal masses in patients with bronchial carcinoma, PET has shown a sensitivity of 100% with a specificity of 80% in a study of 33 patients conducted by Erasmus and coworkers (1997). Although these results need to be confirmed, PET appears to have a growing role in the study of adrenal nodules. Indeed, if PET was used for whole body staging instead of CT, such benign nodules would not be detected, which is a considerable advantage. Other studies, such as those by Valk (1995) and Lewis (1994) and their associates, have shown PET to be accurate at whole body staging. Reports by Gambhir (1998) and Scott (1998) and their colleagues have shown that by decision or economic analysis, management algorithms using PET to characterize pulmonary nodules or to stage lung cancer are cost-effective.

PET is a generally useful method for staging the entire body. The literature, however, does not support it to be equivalent to CT or magnetic resonance imaging for evaluating the brain for metastases. Griffeth and coworkers (1993) have noted that failure to detect brain metastases can occur because the uptake can be comparable with that of the normally glycolytically active brain, meaning lesions can be hidden by normal background brain. Thus, anatomic imaging is recommended for suspected brain lesions.

Value of Positron Emission Tomography in Patients with Small Cell Lung Cancer

Despite the considerable clinical experience in non–small cell lung cancer imaging with PET, much less experience exists with imaging small cell lung cancer. Our limited experience shows excellent images of this disease, but the available literature is small, so the precise role of PET with FDG in this disease is still in evolution. It is likely, however, that PET will be of considerable value in this tumor, although the role of PET may be more in treatment response monitoring than for staging, as small cell lung cancer is not a surgically managed disease in most instances.

Evaluation of Response to Therapy by Positron Emission Tomography

Evidence in support of FDG PET's role in characterizing solitary pulmonary nodules and in locoregional and systemic staging of non–small cell lung cancer is quite firm. Data on using the quantitative aspects of PET to assess the response to therapy are promising, but still emerging. According to the study of Patz and associates (1994) and one by the author and coworkers (1993), low FDG uptake after cancer treatment is considered a good sign. Data, such as that of Hebert and colleagues (1996), are emerging to suggest that PET plays a unique role in treatment management, both for chemotherapy and radiation therapy, but larger studies are needed to determine the precise role of PET in treatment response assessment. As an example, using quantitative methods FDG PET was 97% sensitive and 100% specific in assessing the presence or absence of cancer after non–small cell lung cancer treatment in 35 patients in a study by Patz and associates (1994). Some FDG uptake can occur in inflammation, as recorded by Jones and coworkers (1991), however, which can be a problem. Although FDG has been used in treatment monitoring, C11 methionine also has been used. For example, in lung cancer treatment monitoring, declines in methionine uptake into tumors were commonly seen by Kubota and coworkers (1993) with effective therapy. In some instances, the decline in methionine uptake was more predictive of the long-term survival of the patient than the change in tumor size.

REFERENCES

Bury T, et al: Fluorine-18 deoxyglucose positron emission tomography for the detection of bone metastases in patients with non-small cell lung cancer. Eur J Nucl Med 25:1244, 1998.

Dwamena B, et al: Mediastinal staging of non-small cell lung cancer (NSCLC) in the nineteen nineties: a meta-analytic comparison of positron emission tomography and x-ray computed tomography. Radiology, in press.

Erasmus JJ, et al: Evaluation of adrenal masses in patients with bronchogenic carcinoma using 18F-fluorodeoxyglucose positron emission tomography. AJR Am J Roentgenol 168:1357, 1997.

Flier JS, et al: Elevated levels of glucose transport and transporter messenger RNA are induced by ras or src oncogenes. Science 235:1492, 1987.

Fujiwara T, et al: Relationship between histologic type of primary lung cancer and carbon-11-L-methionine uptake with positron emission tomography. J Nucl Med 30:33, 1989.

Gallagher BM, et al: Metabolic trapping as a principle of radiopharmaceutical design: some factors responsible for the biodistribution of [18F] 2-deoxy-2-fluoro-D-glucose. J Nucl Med 19:1154, 1978.

Gambhir SS, et al: Analytical decision model for the cost-effective management of solitary pulmonary nodules. J Clin Oncol 16:2113, 1998.

Griffeth LK, et al: Brain metastases from non-central nervous system tumors: evaluation with PET. Radiology 186:37, 1993.

Gupta NC, et al: Solitary pulmonary nodules: detection of malignancy with PET with 2-[F-18]-fluoro-2-deoxy-D-glucose. Radiology 184:441, 1992.

Hebert ME, et al: Positron emission tomography in the pretreatment evaluation and follow-up of non-small cell lung cancer patients treated with radiotherapy: preliminary findings. Am J Clin Oncol 19:416, 1996.

Jones HA, et al: Positron emission tomography of 18 FDG uptake in localized pulmonary inflammation. Acta Radiol Suppl 376:148, 1991.

Kim BT, et al: Localized form of bronchioloalveolar carcinoma: FDG PET findings. AJR Am J Roentgenol 170:935, 1998.

Knopp MV, et al: Forschungsschwerpunkt Radiologische Diagnostik und Therapie, Deutsches Krebsforschungszentrum, Heidelberg. Positronenemissionstomographie des Thorax. Derzeitiger klinischer Stellenwert. Radiologe 32:290, 1992.

Kubota K, et al: Lung tumor imaging by positron emission tomography using C-11 L-methionine. J Nucl Med 26:37, 1985.

Kubota K, et al: Differential diagnosis of lung tumor with positron emission tomography: a prospective study. J Nucl Med 31:1927, 1990.

Kubota K, et al: Evaluation of the treatment response of lung cancer with positron emission tomography and L-[methyl-11-C]methionine: a preliminary study. Eur J Nucl Med 20:495, 1993.

Lewis P, et al: Whole-body 18F-fluorodeoxyglucose positron emission tomography in preoperative evaluation of lung cancer. Lancet 344:1265, 1994.

Lowe VJ, et al: Prospective investigation of positron emission tomography in lung nodules. J Clin Oncol 16:1075, 1998.

Miyazawa H, et al: Detection of mediastinal lymph node metastasis from lung cancer with positron emission tomography (PET) using 11-C-methionine. Nippon Kyobu Geka Gakkai Zasshi 40:2125, 1992.

Nolop KB, et al: Glucose utilization in vivo by human pulmonary neoplasms. Cancer 60:2682, 1987.

Patz EF Jr, et al: Focal pulmonary abnormalities: evaluation with F-18 fluorodeoxyglucose PET scanning. Radiology 188:487, 1993.

Patz EF Jr, et al: Persistent or recurrent bronchogenic carcinoma: detection with PET and 2-[F-18]-2-deoxy-D-glucose. Radiology 191:379, 1994.

Prauer HW, et al: Controlled prospective study of positron emission tomography using the glucose analogue [18f]fluorodeoxyglucose in the evaluation of pulmonary nodules. Br J Surg 85:1506, 1998.

Sasaki M, et al: The usefulness of FDG positron emission tomography for the detection of mediastinal lymph node metastases in patients with non-small cell lung cancer: A comparative study with X-ray computed tomography. Eur J Nucl Med 23:741, 1996.

Scott WJ, Shepherd J, Gambhir SS: Cost-effectiveness of FDG-PET for staging non-small cell lung cancer: a decision analysis. Ann Thorac Surg 66:1876, 1998.

Shreve PD, et al: Oncologic diagnosis with 2-[fluorine-18]fluoro-2-deoxy-D-glucose imaging: dual-head coincidence gamma camera versus positron emission tomographic scanner. Radiology 207:431, 1998.

Valk PE, et al: Staging non-small cell lung cancer by whole-body positron emission tomographic imaging. Ann Thorac Surg 60:1573, 1995.

Vansteenkiste JF, et al: Lymph node staging in non-small-cell lung cancer with FDG-PET scan: a prospective study on 690 lymph node stations from 68 patients. J Clin Oncol 16:2142, 1998.

Wahl RL: Clinical oncology update: the emerging role of PET. In DeVita VT, Hellman S, Rosenberg SA (eds): Principles and Practice of Oncology. 5th Ed. Philadelphia: Lippincott–Raven, 1997.

Wahl RL, et al: Metabolic monitoring of breast cancer chemohormonotherapy using positron emission tomography: initial evaluation. J Clin Oncol 11:2101, 1993.

Wahl RL, et al: Staging of mediastinal non-small cell lung cancer with FDG PET, CT, and fusion images: preliminary prospective evaluation. Radiology 191:371, 1994.

Webb WR, et al: CT and MR imaging in staging non-small cell bronchogenic carcinoma: report of the radiologic diagnostic oncology group. Radiology 178:705, 1991.

Weder W, et al: Detection of extrathoracic metastases by positron emission tomography in lung cancer. Ann Thorac Surg 66:886, 1998.

CHAPTER 13

Radionuclide Studies of the Lung

William G. Spies

Ventilation-perfusion ($\dot{V}/\dot{Q}$) imaging of the lungs remains the most commonly performed radionuclide procedure of the chest in most nuclear medicine laboratories, most often performed for the detection of pulmonary thromboembolism. Since the introduction of this technique in the early 1960s, considerable refinements of the method have been developed, in terms of new radiopharmaceuticals, newer instrumentation and techniques, and more sophisticated methods of interpretation.

$\dot{V}/\dot{Q}$ imaging also has been used for a variety of other clinical indications, such as the detection and quantification of obstructive airways disease, quantitation of right-to-left cardiac shunts, assessment of pulmonary trauma and inhalation injury, and monitoring of therapy in childhood asthma. The technique also has been used for the preoperative assessment of resectability of pulmonary neoplasms and prediction of postoperative pulmonary function. It also may be used in other clinical situations in which lung resection is contemplated in patients with compromised pulmonary function.

Gallium imaging of the chest is a sensitive method for the detection of a variety of neoplastic and inflammatory disorders. In the detection and staging of neoplasms, such as bronchial carcinoma and lymphomas, it is used in conjunction with other techniques, including chest radiography, computed tomographic (CT) scanning, and lymphangiography. Gallium imaging also has assumed an important role in the assessment of acute opportunistic infections, such as *Pneumocystis carinii* pneumonia, in patients who have positive test results for human immunodeficiency virus (HIV), and other entities associated with decreased immunocompetence. It also can be used for the quantification of pulmonary involvement with sarcoidosis, tuberculosis, and pneumoconioses.

Iodine 131 whole-body imaging is used to assess the presence of functioning metastases in patients with well-differentiated thyroid carcinomas. Iodine 131 (^{131}I) is also used therapeutically to ablate pulmonary and other metastases.

Radionuclide angiography is a useful noninvasive technique for evaluating vascular disorders of the chest, such as

superior vena cava syndrome, and for assessment of the vascularity of intrathoracic masses.

Experimental methods of pulmonary radionuclide imaging have focused on the assessment of function and metabolism, such as alveolar-capillary permeability, amine receptor function, and pulmonary fluid balance. Radiolabeled monoclonal antibodies have been developed for the detection and treatment of a variety of intrathoracic neoplasms, both primary and metastatic.

New peptide radiotracers are being developed for the specific detection of certain neoplasms. Somatostatin analogues of octreotide are in routine clinical use for the evaluation of patients with known or suspected neuroendocrine tumors, such as carcinoid, islet cell carcinoma, medullary carcinoma of the thyroid, and others. The most exciting development in radionuclide imaging is the use of positron emission tomography (PET) for the staging and follow-up of many thoracic and extrathoracic neoplasms, including bronchial carcinoma, colorectal carcinoma, brain tumors, breast carcinoma, melanoma, lymphoma, head and neck neoplasms, and others.

VENTILATION-PERFUSION IMAGING

Perfusion Imaging

Pulmonary perfusion imaging is performed by intravenously injecting radioactive particles that are large enough to be trapped in the pulmonary vasculature, specifically in the pulmonary arterioles and capillaries. The distribution of these particles is proportional to regional pulmonary blood flow. Technetium 99m (^{99m}Tc) is the radionuclide of choice for these studies, because of its favorable gamma energy for imaging with a nuclear medicine gamma scintillation camera (140 keV, low radiation dose to the patient, and short half-life of 6 hours).

The most commonly used radiopharmaceutical for pulmonary perfusion imaging is macroaggregated albumin (MAA) labeled with ^{99m}Tc. This agent is available commercially in kit form and provides particles in the range of approximately 10 to 60 μm in diameter. Human albumin microspheres also can be labeled with ^{99m}Tc, resulting in a more uniform particle size, but are associated with a longer biological half-life and greater cost and are not readily available at present. The usual dose of ^{99m}Tc-MAA given to an adult patient is 2 to 4 mCi of activity, which corresponds to approximately 200,000 to 500,000 particles injected. At this dose range, Harding and colleagues (1973) have shown that less than 0.1% of the pulmonary arterioles are temporarily occluded, and therefore no physiologic effects are anticipated. In patients known to have severe preexisting pulmonary arterial hypertension or having undergone prior pneumonectomy, the dose may be lowered to 1 to 1.5 mCi. Doses of more than 1 million particles are avoided to increase the margin of safety, as are doses less than 100,000 particles, at which point the images may show areas of inhomogeneity on the basis of poor count statistics, in the absence of actual perfusion abnormalities. The particles are broken down and leave the pulmonary vasculature with a biological half-life of 6 to 8 hours and are phagocytized by the reticuloendothelial system.

Adverse reactions, such as allergic responses to the radiopharmaceutical, have been reported, but are extremely rare. In addition to severe pulmonary arterial hypertension, other relative contraindications to pulmonary perfusion imaging with particulate radiopharmaceuticals include large right-to-left intracardiac shunts and pregnancy. None of these is an absolute contraindication, and in fact these agents are even used clinically to quantitate known right-to-left shunts. Rhodes and coworkers (1971) have reported several occurrences of transient ischemic episodes after injection of radiolabeled MAA, but not with human albumin microspheres. In pregnancy, a lower dose is used to minimize the radiation dose to the fetus, which is well within acceptable limits under these circumstances. In most cases, a lung scan may be performed appropriately and safely despite any of the aforementioned circumstances, provided that the previously mentioned precautions are taken and it is determined that the study is indeed clinically indicated.

^{99m}Tc-MAA is injected intravenously with the patient in the supine position, to minimize gravitational effects on the distribution of the particles in the pulmonary vasculature. After injection, the patient may be moved without affecting particle distribution. Imaging may be performed in either the upright or supine position. Eight views are routinely obtained: anterior, posterior, right and left posterior oblique, right and left anterior oblique, and right and left lateral. Both Caride (1976) and Nielsen (1977) and their associates have shown that the posterior oblique views are particularly important in detecting and localizing lower lobe perfusion defects, the most common site of involvement in pulmonary embolism (PE).

Imaging is performed with a gamma scintillation camera, most often using a large field of view camera with a low-energy parallel hole collimator, or a smaller standard field of view camera with a low-energy diverging collimator in the case of portable examinations. Each image is generally

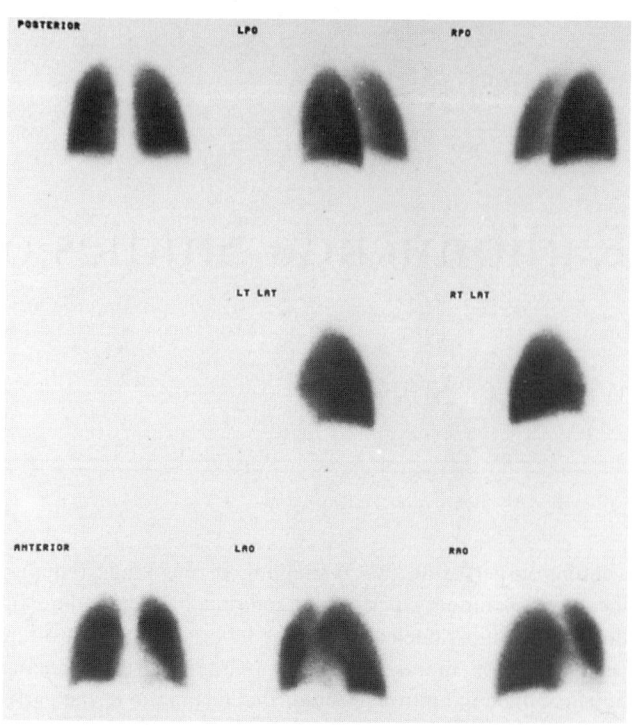

Fig. 13-1. Normal technetium 99m macroaggregated albumin-labeled perfusion study. (Top row, left to right) Posterior, left posterior oblique, and right posterior oblique views. (Middle row) Left lateral and right lateral views. (Bottom row) Anterior, left anterior oblique, and right anterior oblique views.

obtained for 500,000 to 1 million counts. A normal perfusion lung scan is illustrated in Figure 13-1. In some laboratories, single-photon emission computed tomography (SPECT) cross-sectional tomographic images are obtained also in the transaxial, sagittal, and coronal planes, although it is not commonly used clinically. Although SPECT imaging provides improved detection of smaller perfusion defects, it has not been shown clearly to improve the overall diagnostic accuracy of the study to date and may be difficult to obtain in some acutely ill patients.

Ventilation Imaging

Ventilation imaging is performed by having the patient inhale either a radioactive inert gas or a fine, uniform radiolabeled aerosol. The most widely used agent is xenon 133 (^{133}Xe) gas. Standard spirometric apparatus may be used for the study, but a system for venting and trapping the exhaled gas must be used because of the relatively long half-life of the radionuclide (5.3 days).

The ^{133}Xe ventilation study is usually performed in three phases. The patient first inhales deeply as 10 to 20 mCi of ^{133}Xe is injected into the intake port of the spirometer. The patient holds his or her breath as long as possible while a posterior image of the lungs is obtained for 25,000 to 250,000 counts. This single breath image reflects regional ventilatory rates. Areas of lung that are well ventilated accumulate activity, and areas that are poorly ventilated appear as photopenic ("cold") defects. This image may not be obtainable in patients who are extremely dyspneic. The patient then breathes a mixture of ^{133}Xe and oxygen in a closed system with a carbon dioxide absorber for 3 to 5 minutes to achieve an equilibrium in the distribution of the radioactive gas in the lungs. A 300,000 to 600,000 count equilibrium wash-in image is obtained at the conclusion of this phase. This image reflects the total ventilated lung volume, and all areas of lung that are ventilated show activity on the image. In some laboratories, serial images are obtained also during the wash-in phase.

The final and most important phase is the wash-out, during which the patient breathes room air and the exhaled ^{133}Xe gas is trapped in a charcoal system or vented away by an exhaust system. Serial wash-out images are obtained, typically at intervals of 30 seconds to 1 minute, for at least 5 minutes. On these images, the activity normally disappears from the lungs within 3 to 4 minutes, in a symmetric fashion. Areas of obstructive airways disease appear as focal or diffuse zones of ^{133}Xe retention or asymmetric washout. Many nuclear medicine physicians include posterior oblique images in the wash-out study if feasible, to better localize ventilatory abnormalities in the anteroposterior dimension. Normal and abnormal ventilation studies are shown in Figure 13-2. Alderson and colleagues (1974, 1976, 1980) and Alderson and Line (1980) showed that the ventilation study is nearly twice as sensitive as routine chest radiography and at least as sensitive as spirometric pulmonary function tests for the detection of obstructive airways disease. The wash-out portion of the study is the most sensitive part of the examination, and the duration of ^{133}Xe retention is qualitatively related to the severity of obstructive airways disease, as measured by pulmonary function studies.

^{133}Xe imaging has certain disadvantages. Ventilation studies with ^{133}Xe are normally performed before perfusion scans, because the energy of the photopeak of ^{133}Xe is lower

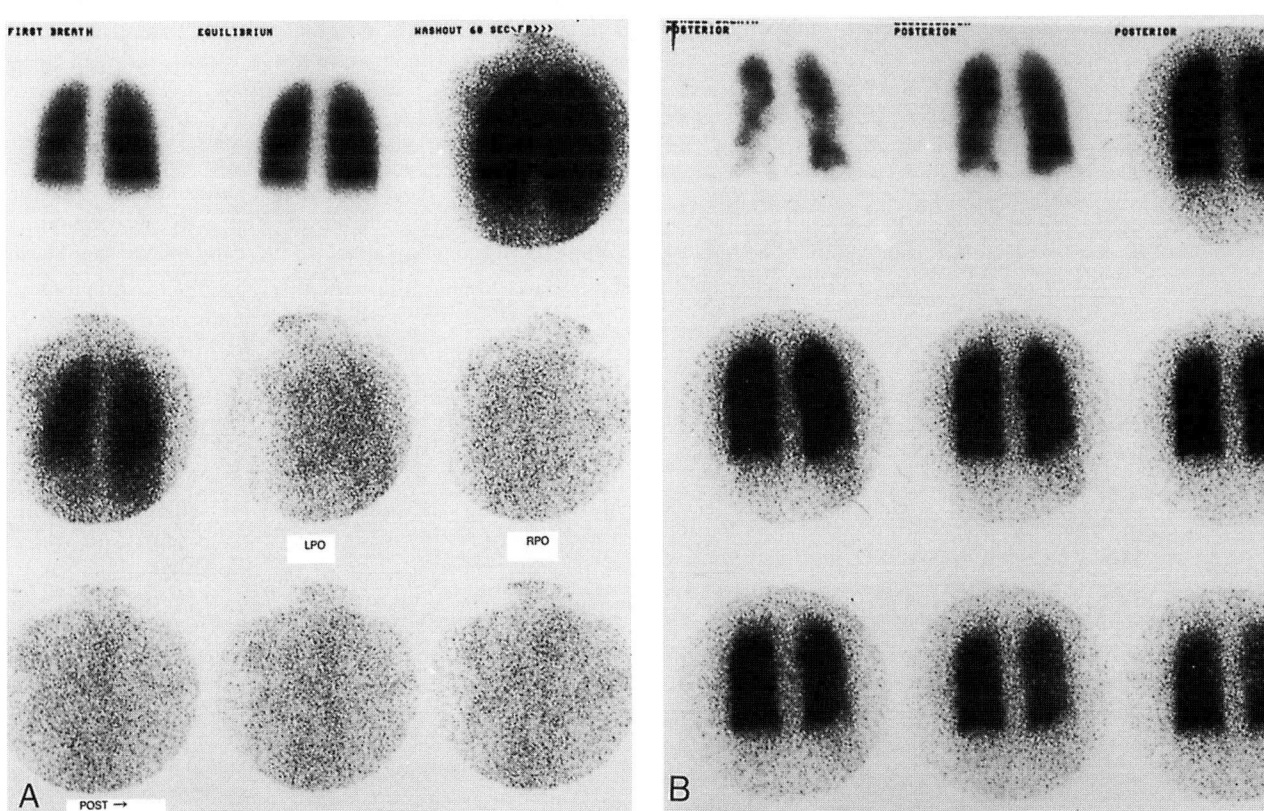

Fig. 13-2. A. Normal xenon 133 (^{133}Xe) ventilation study. (Top row) Posterior single breath image, posterior equilibrium wash-in image, 0- to 1-minute posterior wash-out image. (Middle row) One- to 2-minute posterior wash-out image, 2- to 3-minute left posterior oblique wash-out image, 3- to 4-minute right posterior oblique wash-out image. (Bottom row) Four- to 5-, 5- to 6-, and 6- to 7-minute posterior wash-out images. There is uniform, symmetric ventilation noted on the single breath and equilibrium wash-in images and normal wash-out, with complete clearance by 4 minutes. **B.** Abnormal ^{133}Xe ventilation study in a 65-year-old woman with chronic asthma and long-term ventilator dependency. Same views as shown in **A,** except that all images are in the posterior projection. Diffusely irregular ventilation is seen on the single-breath image, especially in the mid- and lower lung zones, left greater than right. More uniform uptake is noted on the equilibrium wash-in image. The wash-out study demonstrates diffuse, severe ^{133}Xe retention up to the final 6- to 7-minute wash-out view.

(81 keV) than the ^{99m}Tc photopeak (140 keV). If the perfusion study is performed first, then degradation of the ventilation images results from downscatter of ^{99m}Tc photons into the ^{133}Xe window. This effect is most detrimental to the relatively count-poor wash-out portion of the study, which is the most sensitive phase of the ventilation scan for the detection of obstructive airways disease. However, some advocates of postperfusion ^{133}Xe ventilation imaging argue that this approach allows ventilation studies to be tailored to the projection best showing the greatest perfusion defect(s) and obviated in the case of a normal perfusion scan. The feasibility of this approach has been discussed by Kipper and Alazraki (1982), but it has not been widely accepted, especially because most laboratories have relatively few normal perfusion studies. Another disadvantage of ^{133}Xe gas as a ventilation agent is the fact that the low energy of the ^{133}Xe photopeak is not optimally suited to imaging with the gamma camera, resulting in relatively low-resolution images. In addition, the long half-life requires the use of special disposal techniques and usually precludes the performance of portable ventilation studies. Finally, because of the dynamic nature of the study, multiple projections are not routinely obtainable, with the exception of the oblique wash-out views as described.

Other ventilatory agents have been used in an attempt to overcome these shortcomings. ^{127}Xe is another isotope of xenon gas having the advantage of higher gamma energies (172, 203, and 375 keV), enabling ventilation imaging to be performed after perfusion imaging. This capability allows for selection of the best projection for the ventilation study (i.e., the view that best shows the perfusion abnormality on the perfusion scan). Also, because the perfusion scan is done first, the ventilation study need not be obtained in patients whose perfusion scan result is normal. The longer half-life of 36.4 days allows for longer shelf-life of the radiopharmaceutical, and the radiation dose to the patient is also lower because of the absence of beta decay. The major limitations to the use of ^{127}Xe are its limited availability and greater cost, which result from its being a cyclotron-produced radionuclide.

Another gas that has been used for ventilation imaging is krypton 81m (^{81m}Kr), also a cyclotron-produced radionuclide. Unlike ^{127}Xe, ^{81m}Kr is available from a generator system that may be used to deliver multiple doses throughout a given day. ^{81m}Kr has a 190-keV photopeak, which is suitable for imaging and permits the ventilation study to be performed after the perfusion scan, or as is more often done, concurrently. The ultrashort half-life of 13 seconds eliminates disposal problems and allows portable studies to be performed without traps or exhaust systems and without undue radiation exposure to hospital personnel.

Goris (1977) and Rosen (1985) and their associates have shown how this study may be performed in conjunction with the perfusion study, obtaining multiple ventilation and perfusion views sequentially, alternately switching between the ^{99m}Tc and ^{81m}Kr photopeaks. This sequence may be performed without moving the patient, resulting in corresponding sets of ventilation and perfusion images in all eight projections. The ventilation images are obtained by having the patient breathe a ^{81m}Kr/oxygen mixture during tidal respiration. These images are nearly equivalent to single-breath ^{133}Xe images, with areas of abnormal ventilation appearing as zones of decreased activity. Schor (1978) and Susskind (1981) and their coworkers have demonstrated overall good agreement between ^{81m}Kr and the xenon ventilation scans, although it does appear that xenon studies are somewhat more sensitive for the detection of mild obstructive airways disease. This difference is probably mainly because a wash-out study cannot be performed with the ultrashort 13-second half-life of ^{81m}Kr. Other disadvantages of ^{81m}Kr include its high cost and limited availability, which have largely limited its clinical use. The parent half-life of the rubidium 81/^{81m}Kr generator is 4.6 hours. From a practical standpoint, the generator is only good for 1 day and usually is no longer usable by evening or obtainable on weekends for emergency $\dot{V}/\dot{Q}$ scans.

A popular alternative approach to ventilation imaging has been the use of ^{99m}Tc-labeled aerosols. Actually an older technique introduced by Taplin and Poe (1965), it regained popularity as a result of improved nebulizer technology, allowing for the production of a fine, uniform aerosol spray containing particles in the 1-to-2-μm or less size range. These aerosols are inhaled by the patient during tidal respiration and are deposited in the small airways. Alderson and colleagues (1984) have shown that this technique is usable in the clinical setting, as an alternative to gas ventilation studies. Good agreement with ^{133}Xe and ^{81m}Kr ventilation studies was found. It is particularly useful in situations in which gases are not available or cannot be used, such as portable examinations and studies on critically ill or uncooperative patients. A potential pitfall is the occurrence of marked deposition of the aerosol in the large central airways in patients with severe obstructive airways disease, which may lead to uninterpretable studies in approximately 6% of cases. Cabahug and associates (1996) demonstrated the superiority of ^{81m}Kr over ^{99m}Tc diethylenetriaminepentaacetic acid (DTPA) aerosol in assessing regional ventilation in patients receiving mechanical ventilation. Extensive central deposition of the aerosol in the trachea and central bronchi and the associated poor peripheral penetration of the aerosol resulted in a poor correlation between aerosol deposition and regional ventilation in these patients compared with the gas study. Examples of normal and abnormal ^{99m}Tc-DTPA aerosol images are shown in Figure 13-3.

More recently, Burch and colleagues (1986) in Australia have investigated the use of a ^{99m}Tc-labeled ventilation agent called *pseudogas* or *technegas*. This agent essentially consists of radioactive soot, an ultrafine, near-monodispersed carbon particle radioaerosol (0.12-μm diameter) produced by burning a spray of ^{99m}Tc pertechnetate with graphite in a specialized furnace containing argon gas. The smaller particle size compared with conventional nebulizer-produced aerosols results in a more uniform distribution throughout

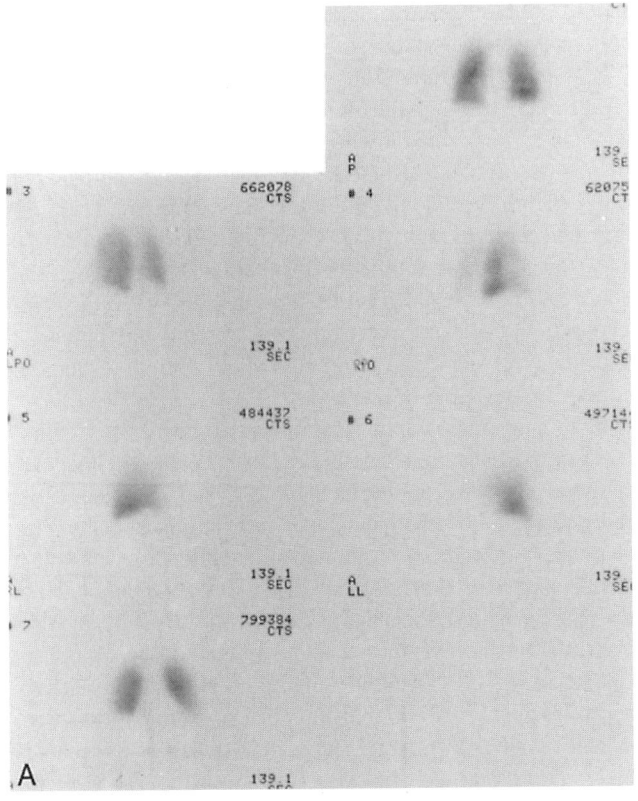

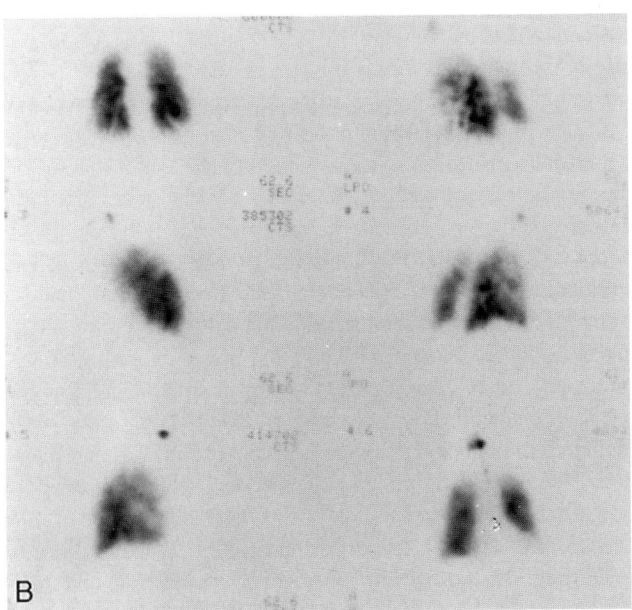

Fig. 13-3. A. Normal technetium 99m-diethylenetriaminepenta-acetic acid aerosol ventilation study. (Clockwise from upper right) Posterior, right posterior oblique, left lateral, anterior, right lateral, and left posterior oblique views. The activity inferior to the left lung represents swallowed aerosol in the stomach. **B.** Abnormal aerosol study in a 67-year-old woman with chronic congestive heart failure and obstructive airways disease. (Clockwise from upper left) Posterior, left posterior oblique, right posterior oblique, anterior, right lateral, and left lateral views. Note the central deposition of aerosol in the central airways and diffusely irregular ventilation, especially in the upper lobes. The activity superior to the lungs is aerosol adherent to the mask and tubing system.

the lungs, both in normal subjects and patients with obstructive airways disease, more closely approximating the distribution of a gas rather than an aerosol. In addition, less patient cooperation is required, because a sufficient amount of aerosol may be inhaled within one or two breaths in normal individuals and within 1 minute even in critically ill patients. Sullivan and coworkers (1988) found overall good correlation with ^{133}Xe gas and higher patient compliance when comparing the two agents in a limited pilot evaluation of patients having normal studies. Bellomo and associates (1994) reported a favorable 1-month outcome in patients with V̇/Q̇ lung scans obtained using technegas as the ventilation radiopharmaceutical that were interpreted as low probability for PE. A related agent was discovered as a variant in the production of technegas, as described by Mackey and coworkers (1997). This agent, named *pertechnegas*, possesses similar ventilatory properties as technegas, but also clears from the lungs with a biological half-life of approximately 7 to 10 minutes. Advantages of pertechnegas include less residual ventilatory activity after the study, resulting in less interference with the perfusion images, and less patient cooperation needed, because fewer breaths are taken, as discussed by Ashburn and associates (1993). On the other hand, the relatively rapid clearance results in deterioration in lung visualization and increase in background on the images obtained during the latter portion of the ventilation study. These radiopharmaceuticals are not approved by the U.S. Food and Drug Administration (FDA) and therefore are not available for general use in the United States at present.

VENTILATION-PERFUSION IMAGING IN THE DIAGNOSIS OF PULMONARY EMBOLISM

By far the most common application of V̇/Q̇ imaging is in the evaluation of patients with suspected PE. PE is a common cause of death in the United States, with an estimated annual incidence of more than 600,000 cases. A review by Rosenow and colleagues (1981) reported that more than 90% of PE originate in the deep venous system of the pelvis and thighs. Goldhaber (1998) emphasized that PE and lower extremity deep venous thrombosis (DVT) should be considered as part of the same pathologic process. Thus, the predisposing factors for lower extremity DVT are also factors that increase the risk of PE. These factors include prolonged bed rest, congestive heart failure, recent myocardial infarction, malignancy, shock, prior thromboembolic disease, and hypercoagulable states such as pregnancy, oral contraceptives, and polycythemia vera. Recent surgery is an important risk factor, particularly pelvic, abdominal, and thoracic procedures and orthopedic procedures such as total hip replacement. Dorfman and coworkers (1987) reported in a prospective evaluation that of 49 patients with venography-proven proximal DVT, 35% had high-probability V̇/Q̇ scan results and only 21% had normal scan results. Huisman and associates (1989) reported a 51% prevalence of asymptomatic

PE in patients with proven DVT undergoing V̇/Q̇ scans, as compared with a prevalence of only 5% in comparable patients suspected but proven not to have DVT on subsequent objective testing. Foley and coworkers (1989) found that serial V̇/Q̇ scintigraphy demonstrating new perfusion defects postoperatively after hip or knee replacement surgery was associated also with a significant number of cases of asymptomatic PE. Moser and associates (1994) found that nearly 40% of patients with DVT who had no symptoms of PE had evidence of PE based on V̇/Q̇ scans and chest radiographic findings. Conversely, Turkstra and coworkers (1997) found that 29% of patients with proven PE had DVT based on compression ultrasound study results.

Dalen and Alpert (1975) estimated that approximately 89% of patients experiencing PE survive longer than 1 hour after the initial event, but even in these patients, the correct diagnosis is made in less than one-third. The mortality of untreated PE is approximately 30%, whereas 92% of treated patients survive. Furthermore the signs, symptoms, and laboratory findings in PE are quite nonspecific. Thus, because the clinical diagnosis is difficult, and because effective therapy is available but not without risk to the patient, the availability of an accurate, noninvasive diagnostic test is highly desirable. One laboratory test that has been advocated for the evaluation of both suspected PE and DVT is measurement of D-dimer, a specific fibrin degradation product, using enzyme-linked immunosorbent assay or latex agglutination assay, as discussed by Ginsberg (1993) and Goldhaber (1993) and their associates. Quantitative D-dimer plasma levels are usually elevated in patients with acute PE. The enzyme-linked immunosorbent assay measurement is a sensitive but nonspecific test for the presence of acute PE. The latex agglutination is less sensitive but more specific and also is more rapidly performed. A relatively large range of reported sensitivity and specificity exists for these assays in the literature, as well as differing recommended diagnostic cutoff values. Goldhaber's group (1993) found D-dimer levels less than 500 ng/mL to be strongly predictive of a normal pulmonary angiogram, although there were some patient population biases present in their study. Ginsberg and associates (1993) suggest that the latex agglutination method may be better because of its higher specificity, but suggested larger clinical trials because of a relatively wide range of variability. In addition, because this test is less sensitive, a normal result cannot be reliably used to exclude the presence of PE, as described by the American College of Chest Physicians Consensus Committee on Pulmonary Embolism (1996). A review by Becker and associates (1996) interjects a note of caution, pointing out wide variability in assay performance, patient populations studied, and criteria for final diagnoses between 29 analyzed published studies. Based on review of prior studies, they estimated representative sensitivity and specificity of the latex assay for PE to be approximately 86% and 51%, respectively. They concluded that, given the present state of the art, D-dimer assays as yet

should not be used as routine screening diagnostic tests for venous thromboembolism.

Standard chest radiography is neither as sensitive nor specific for PE. Diagnostic findings are rarely seen, and most patients demonstrate only nonspecific abnormalities such as subsegmental atelectasis, elevation of a hemidiaphragm, or small pleural effusions. Often the chest radiograph is normal. Chest radiography is nevertheless important, because it may reveal other causes for the patient's symptoms and plays an important role in the interpretation of V̇/Q̇ scans. The radiograph is normally obtained immediately before or after the V̇/Q̇ scan, and in no case should be more than 24 hours from the time of the scan.

Pulmonary angiography is considered to be the most definitive test for PE, but is an invasive, expensive procedure that may be associated with significant morbidity and mortality, especially in inexperienced hands or in critically ill patients. Furthermore, the accuracy of pulmonary angiography varies with the techniques used and method of interpretation, and it is not a simple binary test. Stein and associates (1999), analyzing data from the Prospective Investigation of Pulmonary Embolism Diagnosis (PIOPED) study found conventional angiography not to be precise for the diagnosis of PE confined to subsegmental vessels. Considerable interobserver variability exists in such studies, and techniques to augment visualization of the smaller vessels are needed, such as superselective studies, balloon-occlusion angiography, or cineangiography. Angiography is most often reserved for patients having equivocal V̇/Q̇ scans; in whom a major discrepancy exists between the prescan clinical suspicion for PE and the V̇/Q̇ scan results; or those in whom heroic measures, such as pulmonary embolectomy or thrombolytic therapy, are contemplated. When necessary, pulmonary angiography should be performed preferably within 24 hours or sooner after the lung scan to avoid a false-negative angiogram result secondary to clot lysis. In experienced hands, using the V̇/Q̇ scan as a guide, pulmonary angiography is a safe and accurate procedure for the confirmation or exclusion of significant PE in selected cases. However, pulmonary angiography has been challenged by other less invasive imaging modalities, including digital subtraction angiography, spiral CT, and magnetic resonance (MR) imaging techniques; detailed discussion of these techniques in assessing PE is beyond the scope of this chapter (see Reading References, later in this chapter).

Despite the significant advances in spiral CT and MR imaging that have occurred since the mid-1980s, most authorities agree that at present, V̇/Q̇ imaging remains the screening procedure of choice for the evaluation of suspected PE, as noted by Goldhaber (1998). The system of interpretation devised by Biello and coworkers (1979) and refined by Alderson and colleagues (1981) and Biello (1987) became the de facto standard for evaluating these studies before 1990. The principles on which this system is based include the overwhelming incidence of multiple emboli in patients with PE (greater than 85% of cases) and the observation that PE usually produces perfusion defects in areas of normal ventilation (i.e., V̇/Q̇ mismatch). Although transient ventila-

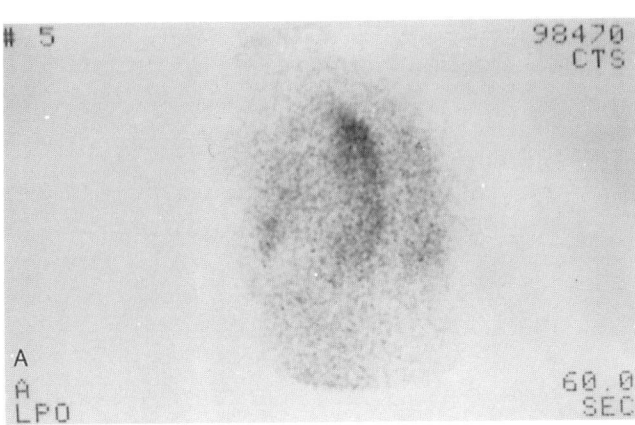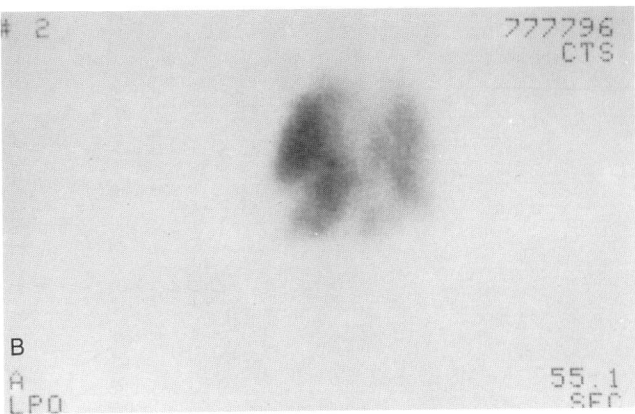

Fig. 13-4. Low-probability ventilation-perfusion (V̇/Q̇) scan with matched V̇/Q̇ abnormalities. **A.** Two- to 3-minute left posterior oblique xenon 133 wash-out image demonstrating focal areas of retention in the lingula, posterior segment of the left upper lobe, and posterior basal segment of the left lower lobe. **B.** Corresponding left posterior oblique technetium 99m perfusion image demonstrates matching perfusion defects in the same segments. The chest radiography result was normal.

tory abnormalities are demonstrated in experimental PE, such findings are fleeting, and Alderson and associates (1978) have shown that they are rarely observed clinically, except in the case of PE with infarction. Pulmonary infarction occurs in less than 10% of cases and is usually associated with radiographic abnormalities.

Perfusion defects are categorized by number, size, and location. Large defects constitute 75 to 100% of a bronchopulmonary segment, moderate subsegmental defects 25 to 75% of a segment, and small defects less than 25% of a segment. By convention, no single defect is larger than a whole segment; thus, any defect larger than a single segment is considered to constitute multiple defects. A common practice is to consider two moderate subsegmental defects to be essentially equivalent to a single segmental defect, although this is obviously an approximation. Nonsegmental defects are those that do not correspond to segmental pulmonary vascular anatomy, such as defects caused by the position of the diaphragm, the heart or great vessels, or other normal or pathologic structures. V̇/Q̇ scan findings are typically reported as being either normal or indicative of a high probability (greater than 90%), low probability (less than 5 to 15%), or intermediate to moderate probability for PE.

Normal perfusion images essentially exclude PE, regardless of the findings on chest radiography or ventilation scanning. Low-probability studies demonstrate limited areas of V̇/Q̇ match in radiographically normal lung zones or areas of mismatched perfusion defects in regions with substantially more extensive radiographic abnormality. Small subsegmental perfusion defects are associated rarely with angiographically demonstrable PE, even if unmatched and also constitute findings consistent with a low probability for PE. Less than 5% of patients with low probability scans had PE on angiography in the original Biello retrospective studies (Fig. 13-4).

High-probability scans demonstrate two or more unmatched defects in radiographically normal regions that are moderate or large in size or unmatched defects that correspond to radiographic abnormalities but are substantially larger. Approximately 90% of these scans are associated with PE on angiography (Fig. 13-5). The significance of a single segmental mismatch is controversial.

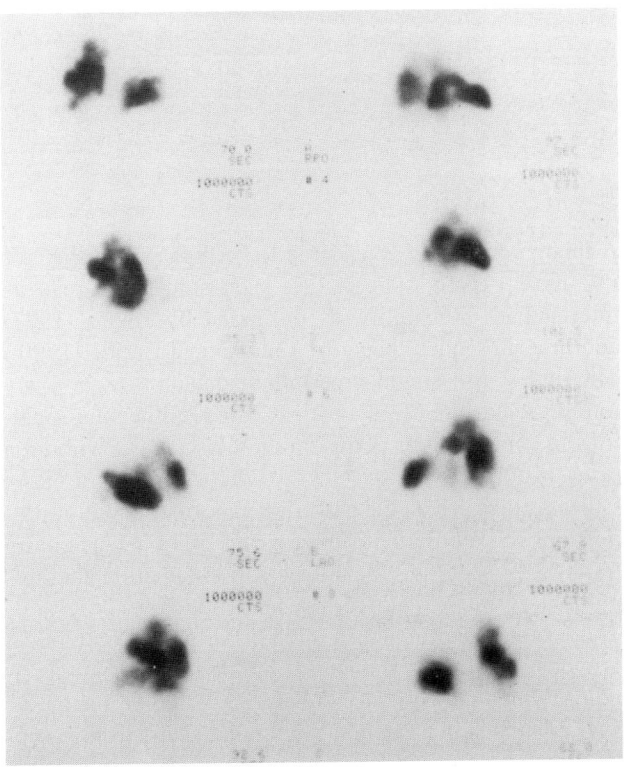

Fig. 13-5. High-probability ventilation-perfusion scan in a 48-year-old man with lymphoma and acute onset of shortness of breath and hypoxia. Technetium 99m perfusion study demonstrates multiple segmental perfusion defects bilaterally. The ventilation study (not shown) was essentially normal, and the chest radiograph demonstrated only small bibasilar pleural effusions.

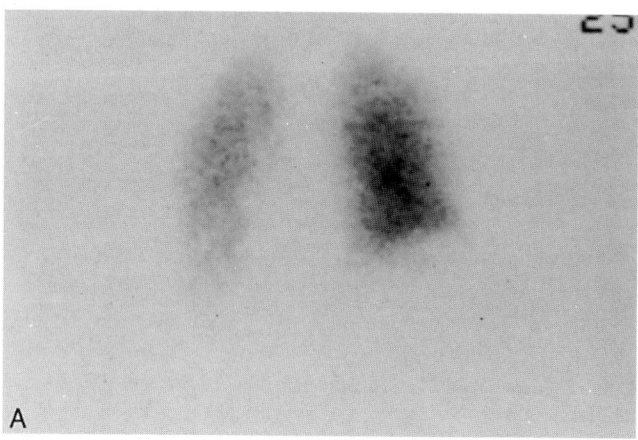

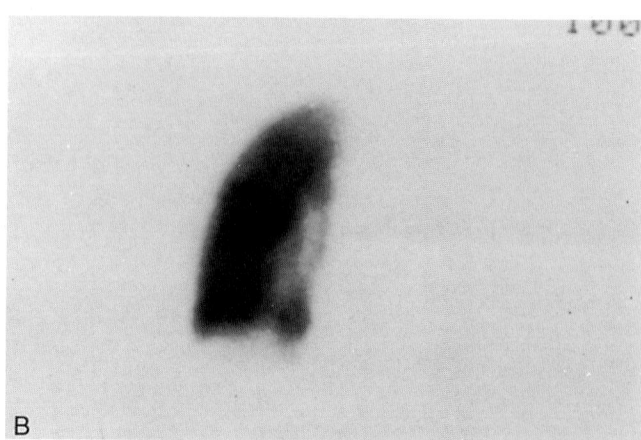

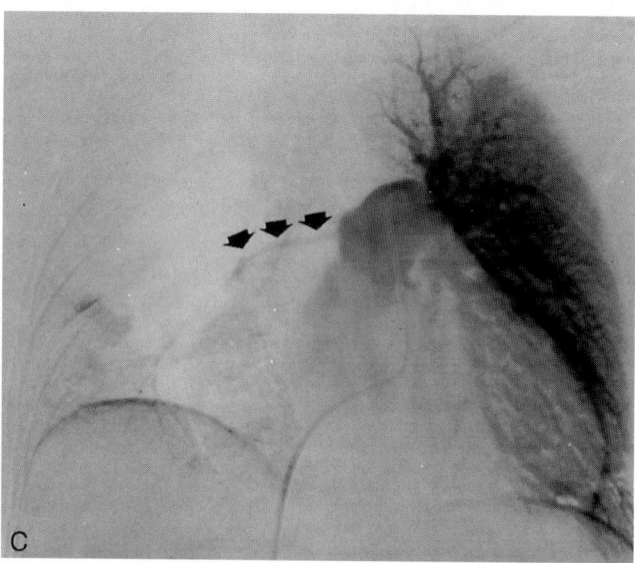

Fig. 13-6. Whole-lung ventilation-perfusion mismatch in a 28-year-old woman with known Takayasu's arteritis and acute chest pain and dyspnea. **A.** Posterior single-breath xenon 133 ventilation image demonstrates ventilation to both lungs, right greater than left. **B.** Posterior technetium 99m perfusion image demonstrates normal perfusion to the left lung with a prominent hilar defect and complete absence of perfusion to the right lung. **C.** Subtraction angiographic image from a main pulmonary artery injection demonstrates severe stenosis of the main right pulmonary artery (*arrows*) secondary to severe arteritis. Other views showed multiple areas of aneurysmal dilatation of the proximal left pulmonary artery branches. No pulmonary emboli were identified. From Spies WG, et al: Ventilation-perfusion scintigraphy in suspected pulmonary embolism: correlation with pulmonary angiography and refinement of criteria for interpretation. Radiology *159*:383, 1986. With permission.

Although originally considered to be high probability for PE, most experts suggest that such studies be read as intermediate probability, as discussed by Biello (1987) and in a subsequent paper by Catania and Caride (1990). The finding of a single large $\dot{V}/\dot{Q}$ mismatch is more likely to represent acute PE in a patient without other abnormalities in ventilation or perfusion on the scan and without a prior history of PE or other cardiopulmonary disease. Other entities producing perfusion abnormality out of proportion to ventilatory abnormality may occasionally mimic PE, such as vasculitides, prior radiation therapy, pulmonary artery stenoses, and some infectious processes. These other conditions can often be suspected on clinical grounds. The most common PE mimic is bronchial carcinoma, which may produce either $\dot{V}/\dot{Q}$ match or mismatch. $\dot{V}/\dot{Q}$ mismatch in bronchial carcinoma results from vascular compression or invasion by tumor, without significant bronchial obstruction. This possibility should especially be considered in the case of a whole-lung $\dot{V}/\dot{Q}$ mismatch. On the other hand, an endobronchial tumor may produce a lobar or whole-lung $\dot{V}/\dot{Q}$ match, because of airway obstruction with secondary reflex vasoconstriction and

shunting of pulmonary blood flow away from that region of the lung. A case of whole-lung mismatch secondary to pulmonary vasculitis associated with Takayasu's arteritis is illustrated in Figure 13-6.

Intermediate probability is assigned to cases in which extensive obstructive airways disease involves greater than 50% of the lung fields, perfusion defects correspond to radiographic abnormalities of comparable size, in cases in which only a single unmatched defect (moderate or large) in a radiographically normal region is present, or in any other cases not fitting into low-probability or high-probability categories (Fig. 13-7). In such cases, the $\dot{V}/\dot{Q}$ scan does not provide definitive evidence for or against the presence of PE. The post-test likelihood of PE in these patients lies somewhere in the large range between 10% and 90%, and the decision regarding further workup or therapy must be based on the level of pretest clinical suspicion and the clinical status of the patient. In those patients with intermediate-probability $\dot{V}/\dot{Q}$ scans and high pretest suspicion for PE, treatment with anticoagulants may proceed, with a repeat $\dot{V}/\dot{Q}$ scan often obtained in 10 to 14 days to assess resolution. In patients with low pretest suspicion, the $\dot{V}/\dot{Q}$

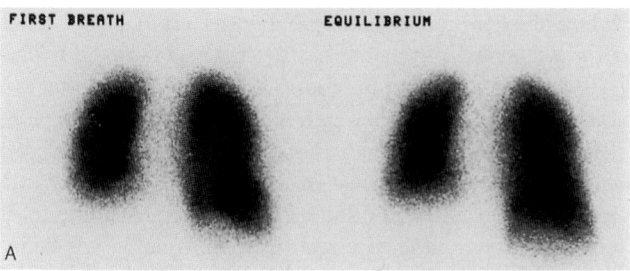

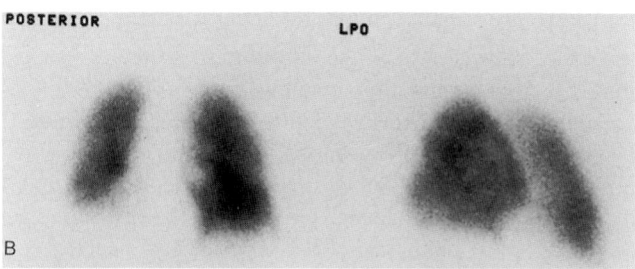

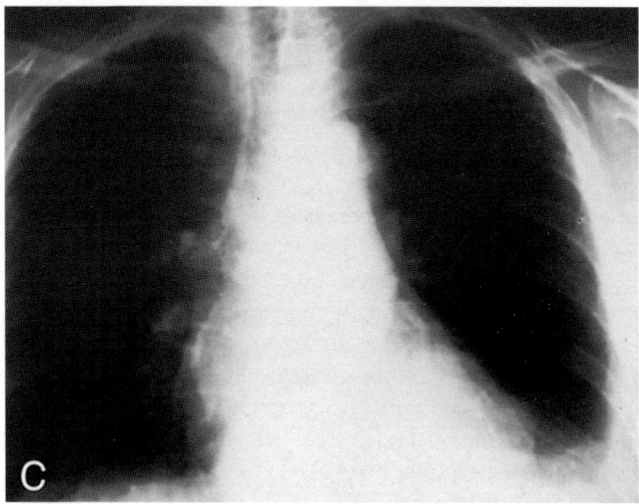

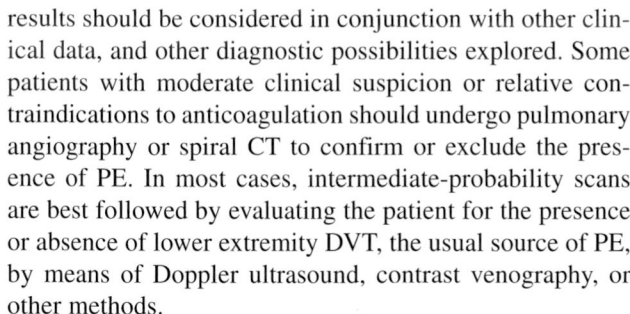

Fig. 13-7. Intermediate-probability ventilation-perfusion scan with a perfusion defect corresponding to a radiographic abnormality. The patient is a 64-year-old man with an acute left pleural effusion. **A.** Posterior single-breath (left) and equilibrium wash-in ventilation images demonstrate absent ventilation at the left lung base. **B.** Posterior (left) and left posterior oblique (LPO) perfusion images demonstrate a corresponding perfusion defect in the posterior basal segment of the left lower lobe. **C.** The anteroposterior chest radiograph shows a corresponding left basilar pleural effusion. Even though the ventilation and perfusion defects are matched, the findings are indicative of intermediate probability of pulmonary embolism because of the corresponding radiographic abnormality. Although pulmonary embolism is not highly likely, particularly with only one area of involvement, an embolus with associated infarction in the left lower lobe cannot totally be excluded. This type of finding is probably the most common variety of intermediate-probability lung scan.

results should be considered in conjunction with other clinical data, and other diagnostic possibilities explored. Some patients with moderate clinical suspicion or relative contraindications to anticoagulation should undergo pulmonary angiography or spiral CT to confirm or exclude the presence of PE. In most cases, intermediate-probability scans are best followed by evaluating the patient for the presence or absence of lower extremity DVT, the usual source of PE, by means of Doppler ultrasound, contrast venography, or other methods.

In most centers, the vast majority of pulmonary angiograms are performed in patients having intermediate probability scans. Patients with high-probability or low-probability scans generally do not require angiographic confirmation, unless overwhelming clinical suspicion exists to the contrary, or a contraindication to anticoagulation exists, in the case of a high-probability scan. Angiographic proof is also usually obtained in cases of contemplated heroic measures such as pulmonary embolectomy or thrombolytic therapy. I and my associates (1986a) found that less than 15% of patients referred for lung scans at a university medical center ultimately went on to angiography over nearly a 6-year period. Jacobson and associates (1997) assessed the clinical outcome of patients with intermediate-probability V̇/Q̇ scans using criteria similar to the modified Biello criteria. They found a 22% prevalence of thromboembolic disease at presentation in these patients, and only a 2% incidence of recurrent thromboembolic disease in these patients during a 6-month follow-up period.

The use of V̇/Q̇ scintigraphy in the diagnosis of PE has not been without controversy. Robin (1977) severely criticized lung scanning, claiming that it grossly overdiagnosed PE, especially in young, previously healthy patients, leading to unnecessary and potentially dangerous overuse of anticoagulants. These remarks came at a time when lung scans were usually performed without ventilation studies, and frequently comprised only two to four views, including data from the Urokinase Pulmonary Embolism Trial, as well as other studies described by Robin. No distinctions were made at that time regarding the size or number of perfusion defects, nor was consideration given to the findings on chest radiography. The nonspecificity of perfusion-only lung scanning is well known, because virtually all cardiopulmonary diseases may produce perfusion defects, including pneumonia, pleural effusion, congestive heart failure, and so forth. The limited accuracy of the diagnosis of PE with perfusion-only imaging has been demonstrated by McNeil (1976) and by me and my associates (1986a). This issue has been revisited by Miniati and associates (1996) in the Prospective Investigative Study of Acute Pulmonary Embolism Diagnosis trial.

In short, these early criticisms of lung scanning voiced by Robin (1997) and others have largely become irrelevant with the advent of modern techniques for radionuclide lung imaging, including the routine use of ventilation imaging, comparison with chest radiography, and use of the Biello criteria or related methods for interpretation. Comparisons between the Biello criteria and other interpretive schemes by

Carter (1982), Sullivan (1983), and Webber (1990) and their associates showed it to be the overall most accurate system for V̇/Q̇ scan interpretation up to that time.

Additional refinements were introduced by several investigators during the 1980s to further improve the accuracy of lung scanning in PE. Examples of such refinements include the stripe sign of Sostman and Gottschalk (1982); obtaining follow-up chest radiography, as suggested by Vix (1983); assessing the age of radiographic abnormalities that correspond with perfusion defects, as evaluated by me and my coworkers (1986a); and comparison of V̇/Q̇ scans with prior scans, as described by Alderson and colleagues (1983) and by me and coworkers (1986a). Use of these refinements resulted in a further slight improvement in diagnostic accuracy and decrease in the number of equivocal or intermediate-probability scans. The technique of SPECT has been evaluated in conjunction with lung scanning. This technique involves acquiring data using a rotating gamma camera that gradually circles the patient in a series of 64 to 128 graded steps. Tomographic images are then reconstructed in multiple planes, as in conventional transmission x-ray CT. This approach has met with great success in other areas of nuclear medicine, such as myocardial and cerebral perfusion imaging, and can provide more accurate detection and localization of V̇/Q̇ abnormalities, as suggested by Touya and coworkers (1986b). However, to date SPECT lung imaging has not been adopted widely or shown to significantly improve the diagnostic accuracy of V̇/Q̇ scintigraphy. Subsequent criticisms of V̇/Q̇ imaging centered around the fact that the data used to validate the Biello criteria were all derived from retrospective studies. Hull and associates (1983, 1985) and Hull and Raskob (1991) conducted prospective clinical trials of the diagnosis of PE in patients referred for impedance plethysmography for suspected DVT. This group obtained significantly poorer results with V̇/Q̇ imaging. Although they found that 86% of high-probability scans were associated with PE at angiography, they claimed that at least 25% of low-probability scans occurred in patients subsequently proven to have PE or DVT. These data have been the subject of considerable debate in the literature, the full extent of which is beyond the scope of the current discussion.

The many controversies relative to the value of V̇/Q̇ scanning and its role in the diagnosis of PE provided the impetus to the National Institutes of Health to sponsor a large, prospective multicenter trial of PE diagnosis that has come to be known as the PIOPED trial. The initial results of this study were reported by the PIOPED investigators (1990).

From an initial 5587 requests for lung scans, a total of 1493 patients ultimately gave consent for entry into the PIOPED study. The largest and most thoroughly evaluated group was the PIOPED angiographic pursuit arm of the study, consisting of 931 patients in whom V̇/Q̇ scans were obtained, with chest radiography and, if possible, pulmonary angiography performed within 24 hours. Another entire arm of the PIOPED study, consisting of patients in whom the decision for angiography was left to the discretion of the referring physician, has not been as thoroughly analyzed and reported to date and is not discussed further. A total of 755 angiograms were obtained in 931 patients in the PIOPED angiographic pursuit group (81%). All studies were performed using state-of-the-art techniques, and studies were interpreted in blinded fashion by two central readers from different institutions than the one in which the study was performed. Third readers, and if necessary, consensus groups were used in the event of disagreements. Although overall interobserver agreement was relatively high, disagreements occurred in some cases, particularly in borderline V̇/Q̇ scans and angiograms with questionable emboli in smaller branch vessels. Again, the occurrence of some disagreement in the reading of the pulmonary angiograms, although not frequent, underscores the fact that angiography is a tarnished gold standard, and not simply a binary positive or negative test, as it is often assumed to be, as noted by Stein and coworkers (1999). Juni and Alavi (1991) have pointed out that uncertainties in angiography interpretation tended to occur in the same cases in which the V̇/Q̇ scans were equivocal, namely the low- to intermediate-probability group.

It is noteworthy that the criteria used to interpret the V̇/Q̇ scans in the PIOPED trial, although in general similar to the modified Biello criteria, had some differences. High-probability scans required more extensive V̇/Q̇ mismatch than the Biello criteria, with a minimum of two segmental equivalent mismatches (i.e., two large, one large and two moderate, or four moderate mismatches) in radiographically normal sites necessary. The low-probability group was subdivided into low and very low categories, with very low including cases having three or fewer small subsegmental defects in radiographically normal areas. Inclusion of a single moderate mismatch in a radiographically normal region in the low-probability group proved to be an error, with roughly one-third of these cases being positive for PE at angiography. (Note that this finding is correctly designated as intermediate probability by the Biello criteria.) Additionally, the criteria for extensive obstructive airways disease on xenon ventilation scans varied somewhat from the modified Biello approach. Finally, the PIOPED V̇/Q̇ scan interpretations also included a separate personal probability estimate or gestalt interpretations performed independent of any formalized criteria, based solely on the personal experience and subjective impressions of the individual interpreter. Perhaps not surprisingly, in the hands of the experienced observers who participated in PIOPED, these personal probability estimates slightly outperformed the objective criteria.

Despite these differences, the summary results of the PIOPED study reported by the PIOPED investigators (1990) tended to support the earlier work of Biello and associates (1979). Of patients with high-probability scans and angiographic correlation, 88% had PE. Low-probability cases had a prevalence of PE of 12% and intermediate-probability studies a prevalence of 33%. The authors of the study and others, such as Bone (1990) in an editorial accompanying the original PIOPED data summary, have pointed out that the sensitivity of high-probability scans was only 41%, although the specificity was 97%. This result is not unexpected, because it is widely known by nuclear medicine physicians that many patients with PE tend to have intermediate probability scans, often caused either by perfusion defects corresponding to radiographic infiltrates or to areas of mismatch not sufficiently extensive to warrant a high-probability designation. Bone went on to claim that the study showed that 4% of "normal or near-normal" V̇/Q̇ studies proved to have PE, a conclusion that apparently is erroneous, because none of the actually normal study results in the PIOPED trial proved to be associated with PE, as reported by Worsley and Alavi (1995) in a more detailed analysis of the PIOPED data.

Of patients diagnosed as having PE in PIOPED, 24% died within 1 year, but only 2.5% died of PE and 8% had clinically apparent recurrent PE within 1 year. Most deaths resulted from associated conditions, such as cancer, infection, and cardiac disease, and occurred most often in patients with underlying cancer, left-sided congestive heart failure, or chronic lung disease, as reported by Carson and associates (1992). Stein and associates (1991) reported that although clinical evaluation again proved to be somewhat nonspecific in PIOPED, nevertheless, there were a number of extremely common clinical manifestations of PE in the trial, including dyspnea or tachypnea, pleuritic chest pain, decreased partial pressure of oxygen in arterial blood, radiographic findings, and signs of lower extremity DVT.

Areas that led to proposed modifications of the original PIOPED criteria included the extent of V̇/Q̇ mismatch needed for a high-probability interpretation and its relationship to the presence or absence of prior cardiopulmonary disease, the significance of matching perfusion and radiographic findings, the significance of cases with obstructive airways disease and pleural effusions, and issues related to the use of the PIOPED criteria in different patient populations. The finding of a single moderate V̇/Q̇ mismatch was incorrectly classified as low probability for PE, as discussed previously, and in fact, 36% of patients with this pattern in PIOPED had higher probability; therefore, it was correctly reclassified as intermediate probability, as in the Biello criteria, as noted by Gottschalk and associates (1993) and by Worsley and Alavi (1995). Stein and coworkers (1993a) found that in patients without prior cardiopulmonary disease, as few as one or more segmental equivalent V̇/Q̇ mismatches were sufficient to achieve a positive predictive value of greater than 85% for the presence of PE. On the other hand, in those patients with a history of prior cardiopulmonary disease, as many as 2.5 or greater segmental equivalent mismatches were necessary to achieve the same result. In other words, there was no discrete cutoff for high probability, but rather a continuum of gradually increasing specificity and positive predictive value as the number of V̇/Q̇ segmental equivalent mismatches increased. This finding was also true

for the other arm of the PIOPED study, in which the referring physician decided whether the patient required pulmonary angiography following the V̇/Q̇ scan. Borrowing from the concept of Morrell and associates (1993) that perfusion defect sizes are often underestimated, Stein and coworkers (1993b) suggested the use of "mismatched vascular defects" as opposed to moderate or large V̇/Q̇ mismatches, finding that both moderate and large mismatches considered as being vascular mismatched defects of equal significance resulted in nearly equal predictive value for PE as did using their previous concept of dividing the large and moderate defects into separate groups. This concept, in fact, returns to the original modified Biello criteria's equivalence between moderate and large defects, further unifying the two interpretive schemes. Subsequently, Gottschalk and associates (1996a) analyzed the data from the PIOPED consensus gestalt interpretations, finding that in patients with prior cardiopulmonary disease, experienced interpreters could accurately assess the likelihood of PE, whereas in those without such a history, they tended to underestimate the likelihood. This result underscores the concept that less V̇/Q̇ mismatch is required to diagnose PE in patients without a history of prior cardiopulmonary disease, without any sacrifice in the specificity or positive predictive value of the study. On the other hand, Worsley and coworkers (1996) found diagnostic performance of the PIOPED criteria to be similar in patients of varying ages, radiographic findings, and history of prior thromboembolism or cardiopulmonary disease. With respect to small subsegmental defects, Stein and colleagues (1996) found from PIOPED data that one to three small defects had a positive predictive value for PE of less than 10%, consistent with a low probability for PE, whereas more than three small defects were compatible with a low probability for PE (i.e., less than 20% positive predictive value).

As previously discussed, the most common cause for an intermediate probability V̇/Q̇ scan is the presence of corresponding perfusion defects and radiographic infiltrates or pleural effusions of comparable size, often with an associated ventilatory defect as well, the so-called triple match sign. Detailed analysis of such cases from PIOPED by Worsley and coworkers (1993b) revealed that the prevalence of PE is substantially higher in those cases in which the triple match occurs in the lower lung zones (33%) than if it occurs in the upper (11%) or middle (12%) lung zones, suggesting that triple matches in the latter two zones should be interpreted as low probability for PE. Gottschalk and associates (1996b) performed a similar analysis, excluding cases in which V̇/Q̇ mismatches or pleural effusions were present elsewhere, finding the positive predictive value of the triple match to be 23% in the lower lung zones versus 4% in the upper and middle zones. They also found that triple matches involving 25 to 50% of a zone had a higher predictive value than larger or smaller ones.

Sostman and Gottschalk (1992) found that the stripe sign was also a reliable sign for the absence of PE in that segment as it had been in previous studies and incorporated it into the modified PIOPED criteria. Based on a small number of cases, it was suggested by Gottschalk and coworkers (1993) that any number of matched V̇/Q̇ defects could be considered as low probability for PE, provided that the chest radiograph result was normal or nearly normal in those regions. This modification is in conflict with the Biello criteria and remains somewhat controversial at present. With respect to pleural effusions with corresponding perfusion defects, traditionally this finding has been interpreted as intermediate probability for PE. Bedont and Datz (1985) found that only 2 of 53 patients with matched V̇/Q̇ defects corresponding to a pleural effusion had documented thromboembolic disease, suggesting a low-probability interpretation. Worsley (1993a) and Gottschalk (1993) and their associates suggested that PIOPED data suggest that large pleural effusions with corresponding perfusion defects should be interpreted as low probability for PE, but smaller ones (i.e., blunting of a costophrenic angle with an associated defect) should remain intermediate probability. Goldberg and coworkers (1996) performed a retrospective analysis of cases interpreted according to the PIOPED criteria, found PE to be associated with pleural effusions of all sizes, and suggested that all such effusions with matching perfusion defects remain intermediate probability for PE. Thus, this issue remains unresolved. Finally, Gottschalk and associates (1993) also reported that V̇/Q̇ scans demonstrating a single V̇/Q̇ matching defect in less than 75% of a segment had a 24% prevalence of PE, based on a small group of 21 patients, and suggested that this category also should be interpreted as intermediate probability. This proposed change, based on a small number of cases, and in conflict with previous data, has not been adopted widely. Two similar versions of the suggested modified PIOPED criteria are described by Gottschalk (1993) and Worsley (1993a) and their colleagues.

Sostman and associates (1994) evaluated a revised set of PIOPED criteria including modifications similar to those discussed previously in a group of 104 consecutive patients undergoing V̇/Q̇ scintigraphy for suspected PE who also underwent pulmonary angiography. Using receiver operating characteristic analysis, they found the revised PIOPED criteria to be superior to the original PIOPED criteria, and again found the gestalt criteria to be superior to either of the two sets of defined criteria. Freitas and associates (1995) also reported a superior performance of the so-called modified PIOPED criteria compared with the original criteria in a prospective study of 1000 lung scans, in which postperfusion aerosol ventilation studies were used in all patients with abnormal perfusion scans. The use of the PIOPED criteria in different patient populations was reported by Lowe and coworkers (1995). They found a significantly different distribution between diagnostic categories when comparing data from a university medical center versus a community hospital. The university medical center had significantly more intermediate-probability studies (39% versus 10% at the community hospital) and high-probability studies (13% versus 4%) and fewer low-probability and normal studies. The

authors concluded that post-test probability data from the PIOPED study may not be directly applicable to V̇/Q̇ imaging for PE at community hospitals.

A final interesting set of data was provided in the Prospective Investigative Study of Acute Pulmonary Embolism Diagnosis (PISA-PED), as reported by Miniati and associates (1996). In this unique study, a series of 890 consecutive patients were prospectively evaluated with perfusion-only lung scintigraphy, followed by pulmonary angiography or clinical follow-up for 1 year for abnormal cases. Highly modified interpretive criteria for the lung scans were used, consisting of four distinct categories: normal, near normal, abnormal compatible with PE (PE+), and abnormal but not consistent with PE (PE–). Unlike any of the foregoing studies, in PISA-PED only the character of the perfusion defects, namely whether wedge-shaped or not, was considered, not their size, number, or correspondence to radiographic findings. Because of the nature of these unique criteria, both excellent interobserver and intraobserver agreement was obtained. More important, the sensitivity of the PE+ scan pattern was 92% and the specificity of the PE– pattern was 87%. Combining the perfusion scan probabilities with a three-point scale pretest clinical probability (i.e., PE likely, possible, or unlikely) produced excellent positive predictive values of 99% and 92%, respectively, for PE+ scans with likely or possible clinical likelihood. Conversely, the negative predictive value of a PE– study coupled with an unlikely clinical presentation was 97%. This study was strengthened by inclusion of one of the original PIOPED investigators in the lung scan interpretations. It suffers from potential patient selection biases because of the relatively high percentage of normal or near normal studies (25%) relative to PIOPED and other series and by virtue of the fact that angiography was obtained in only 62% of patients with abnormal perfusion scans and was omitted entirely in all cases of normal or near normal perfusion scans. Nevertheless, the results of the PISA-PED trial have breathed new life into the concept of perfusion-only lung scintigraphy, and will no doubt result in subsequent studies attempting to confirm or rebut its findings.

In summary, the PIOPED trial was an ambitious and largely successful attempt to prospectively evaluate the utility of V̇/Q̇ scintigraphy and pulmonary angiography in the diagnosis of PE. The results of the study support the continued use of the V̇/Q̇ scan as the noninvasive screening test of choice for this purpose, but underscore the fact that it must be used in conjunction with other clinical data and when necessary, follow-up pulmonary angiography, noninvasive or invasive studies, or both for the detection of DVT. At present, the revised PIOPED criteria and the revised Biello criteria are quite similar in most respects, and both represent valid approaches to the interpretation of V̇/Q̇ studies for suspected PE. For experienced observers, the addition of some form of fine-tuning or gestalt interpretation may significantly add to the overall accuracy and clinical usefulness of the study. The role of perfusion-only lung scintigraphy, as used in the PISA-PED study described by Miniati and coworkers (1996), requires further evaluation before it can be recommended for general clinical use.

OTHER APPLICATIONS OF VENTILATION-PERFUSION IMAGING

Bronchial Carcinoma

Although $\dot{V}/\dot{Q}$ scan results are frequently abnormal in patients with bronchial carcinoma, the scan is now rarely used for purposes of diagnosis or staging. Secker-Walker and Provan (1969) demonstrated perfusion defects associated with bronchial carcinoma, quantitated them using digital computers, and found that if the perfusion defect resulted in the abnormal lung providing less than 33% of total pulmonary perfusion, that the lesion was always unresectable. Subsequent exceptions to this rule have been reported. Ventilation also can be quantitated for various lung zones, allowing calculation of regional $\dot{V}/\dot{Q}$ ratios. Abnormalities in regional $\dot{V}/\dot{Q}$ ratio are associated also with nonresectability in most cases. It should be noted that these are indirect approaches to the assessment of tumor extent. Furthermore, these techniques are not sensitive enough to detect small or peripheral lesions. Fiberoptic bronchoscopy, CT of the chest, and more recently, PET imaging, in conjunction with standard chest radiography, are now the procedures of choice for the staging of bronchial carcinoma.

$\dot{V}/\dot{Q}$ imaging, however, in conjunction with quantitation using digital computers, can be useful in predicting postoperative pulmonary function. This determination may be of critical importance, because many patients with bronchial carcinoma have underlying chronic lung disease and may not be able to tolerate extensive pulmonary resection. Quantitation of pulmonary perfusion is typically performed in both the anterior and posterior projections, with either the geometric or arithmetic mean used to determine the relative percent perfusion received by each lung. In addition, dividing the lungs into upper, middle, and lower zones can provide simplified regional quantitative data. Quantitation of ventilation is more problematic, especially when dynamic ^{133}Xe ventilation imaging is performed. These measurements may also be made with ^{81m}Kr gas, technegas, or ^{99m}Tc-labeled aerosols, but central deposition of aerosol makes the latter less useful. Overall, quantitation of perfusion is generally regarded as being more clinically useful than quantitation of regional ventilation. Both Kristersson (1974) and Olsen and coworkers (1974) demonstrated a good correlation between relative pulmonary perfusion, assessed by prepneumonectomy perfusion lung scans, and postoperative pulmonary function, as measured by forced vital capacity and other pulmonary function indices. Kristersson (1974) and Boysen and associates (1977) recommended pneumonectomy in patients with bronchial carcinoma and compromised lung function when the predicted postoperative forced expiratory volume in 1 second

(FEV_1) is 800 mL/minute or more. Moldofsky and associates (1988) applied quantitative lung scintigraphy to predict postradiation therapy pulmonary function, finding that the posttherapy FEV_1 tended to be equal or greater than the predicted value in this setting, providing a useful lower limit estimate. A widely used rule states that patients require a postoperative or postradiation FEV_1 of greater than 700 mL/minute to avoid respirator dependence.

Lung Reduction Surgery

Such quantitation also may be used before resection of benign pulmonary lesions, such as bullae. Lung reduction surgery has been reintroduced as an alternative to conventional bullectomy or lung transplantation, as reviewed by Snider (1996). The rationale for lung reduction surgery is to reduce dyspnea and provide improved exercise tolerance by resecting hyperinflated, nonfunctional areas of the lungs, resulting in improved mechanical function of the lungs and reduced shunting of pulmonary blood flow from poorly ventilated lung zones. Pulmonary scintigraphy can assess the extent of disease preoperatively by localizing the sites of greatest involvement and identifying sites of shunting. In addition, quantitative $\dot{V}/\dot{Q}$ scintigraphy can help predict postoperative pulmonary function. Wang and associates (1997) evaluated the role of perfusion lung scintigraphy in the preoperative evaluation of patients referred for lung reduction surgery. They found that the quantitative lung perfusion imaging provided some limited prognostic information in these patients. They undertook blinded evaluation of perfusion lung images for the presence of heterogeneity of disease distribution, the percentage of lung that was maximally perfused and upper versus lower lobe predominance. Specifically, they found that upper lobe predominance and heterogeneity were the best predictors for a postoperative increase in the FEV_1.

Pulmonary Transplantation

Another application of quantitative radionuclide lung imaging has been in the preoperative and postoperative evaluation of patients undergoing unilateral pulmonary transplants, as described by the Toronto Lung Transplant Group (1986) and reviewed by me (1992). Preoperative studies may reveal asymmetry in lung perfusion that may dictate which lung to transplant, with the most severely affected lung usually being the one replaced. In addition, preoperative assessment can detect unsuspected PE in these patients. More important, changes in perfusion, ventilation, or both, to the transplanted lung may be useful in monitoring pulmonary rejection and other complications. As discussed in my review (1992), the transplanted lung usually receives significantly greater perfusion than the remaining native lung postoperatively, especially in patients with severe primary pulmonary hypertension as their underlying disorder, with relative ventilation being variable. The etiology of the chronic lung disease leading to transplantation may affect this relative pulmonary perfusion. In patients with chronic obstructive pulmonary disease, the relative perfusion may vary, in large part dependent on the pulmonary vascular resistance of the native lung. Medina and coworkers (1992) found the highest relative perfusion in the transplant in patients with primary pulmonary hypertension, compared with patients with chronic obstructive airways disease or idiopathic pulmonary fibrosis. Immediate postoperative studies may reveal considerable heterogeneity of perfusion in the transplanted lung, but focal defects are not normally present. The amount of perfusion to the transplant may again vary subsequently, tending to decrease over time in patients with primary pulmonary hypertension and to increase in those with chronic obstructive lung disease. Rejection usually produces significant decreases in perfusion to the transplant that may be reversible with successful treatment. Other complications are less likely to produce this finding, but it can occur also with inflammatory processes, and the correlation between decreases in graft perfusion and rejection is imperfect. In the case of double-lung transplants, Royal and associates (1992) found that the second lung received less relative perfusion than the first in proportion to increasing ischemic time, a finding that persisted for the first 3 postoperative months.

Other Applications of Ventilation-Perfusion Imaging

In primary airway obstruction caused by foreign bodies, mucous plugging, or endobronchial masses, $\dot{V}/\dot{Q}$ scans show striking ventilatory abnormalities. Often corresponding but less severe reductions in perfusion also exist, secondary to reflex vasoconstriction. These findings usually revert to normal when the airway obstruction is relieved, provided that irreversible lung damage has not resulted.

$\dot{V}/\dot{Q}$ imaging also may be useful in the evaluation of lung injury, as reviewed by Lull and associates (1983). Perfusion defects may be identified in patients having undergone blunt or penetrating trauma, and in some cases may precede radiographic changes. Both perfusion and ventilation defects may be observed in patients with pneumothorax or hemothorax, although such entities are usually diagnosed by chest radiography.

[133]Xe ventilation studies are useful in the evaluation of inhalation injuries. Inhalation injuries often occur in conjunction with burns and may result in a twofold to fivefold increase in mortality, depending on the extent of the burn. In the early hours after the injury, the patient may be asymptomatic and have normal chest radiographic findings. Within several days, edema and inflammation of the airways may result in progressive airway obstruction, leading to atelectasis, infection, or adult respiratory distress syndrome (ARDS). Intravenous administration of ^{133}Xe in saline solution during the early stages of inhalation injury demonstrates areas of abnormal wash-out corresponding to sites of early obstructive airways involvement. In this regard, ^{133}Xe is superior to

fiberoptic bronchoscopy in evaluating the distal airways, whereas bronchoscopy is better for the trachea and proximal bronchi. Agee and associates (1976) have reported that both proximal and distal involvement occurs in most cases; thus either test alone is diagnostic in approximately 90% of cases, and both tests together detect virtually all cases. The results of these studies are used in conjunction with clinical probability factors to help guide patient management.

Another application for ventilation imaging with radiolabeled aerosols involves the evaluation of lung disorders associated with alterations in alveolar-capillary membrane permeability. Examples of such disorders include various interstitial lung diseases, hyaline membrane disease in neonates, and ARDS. Damage to the pulmonary capillary membrane or a change in the Starling forces may result in increased alveolar-capillary permeability. Radioaerosols are normally cleared from the alveoli into the circulation and excreted by the kidneys with a pulmonary clearance half-time of approximately 90 minutes. In the presence of ARDS or other interstitial lung disease, this half-time may be substantially shortened. By measuring ^{99m}Tc-DTPA aerosol wash-out using digitally acquired images, time-activity wash-out curves can be generated readily. Coates and O'Brodovich (1986) reviewed this technique. Smokers have been found to have faster aerosol clearance rates than nonsmokers. Clearance rates are normal in patients with asthma or pneumonia, but may be prolonged in patients with interstitial edema. This technique is simple and noninvasive and has a potential role in the evaluation of patients at risk for developing ARDS or hyaline membrane disease, before the onset of clinical disease, and in the detection and monitoring of patients with other forms of interstitial lung disease or alveolitis. Susskind and associates (1997) evaluated this technique for the assessment of radiation-induced lung injury in patients undergoing radiation therapy for lung or breast carcinoma. Their results indicate significantly greater decreases in the clearance half-time of ^{99m}Tc-DTPA aerosol in patients who subsequently developed symptoms or radiographic evidence of radiation pneumonitis, occurring 1 to 3 months before the onset of clinically apparent disease. They suggested that this method could serve as a sensitive technique for the monitoring of these patients and facilitation of early treatment for radiation pneumonitis. However, to date this technique has not achieved widespread clinical use.

Whole-body imaging with pulmonary perfusion agents is used also to detect and quantitate right-to-left cardiac shunts. In the presence of a shunt, some particles bypass the pulmonary vascular bed via the shunt and enter the systemic circulation, where they are trapped in end organs in proportion to blood flow. ^{99m}Tc-human albumin microspheres were once frequently used for this application, because they are more stable in vivo than MAA, resulting in less potentially confusing activity in the kidneys and bladder secondary to the presence of free pertechnetate. Because human albumin microspheres are no longer commercially available, ^{99m}Tc MAA serves as an adequate substitute. In patients with significant shunts, the images demonstrate deposition of particles in the brain, kidneys, and extremities (Fig. 13-8). The data are acquired on a

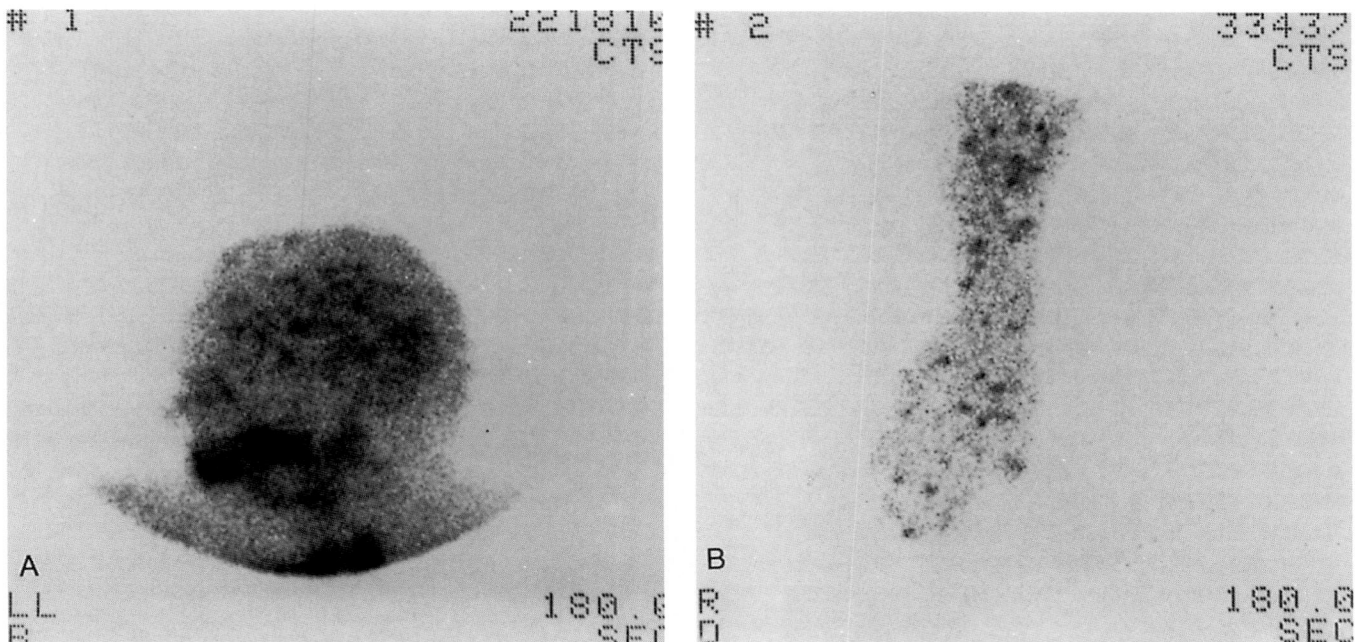

Fig. 13-8. Large right-to-left shunt. Technetium 99m (^{99m}Tc) human albumin microspheres study. **A.** Left lateral skull image demonstrates marked particle deposition in the brain. Some free ^{99m}Tc pertechnetate is present in the saliva in the mouth, salivary glands, and thyroid. **B.** Image of the right forearm and hand shows diffuse particle deposition. Quantitative analysis revealed a 49% right-to-left shunt.

computer and quantitated, expressing the shunt as a percentage. Normal subjects have approximately a 4% physiologic right-to-left shunt. Gates and associates (1974) obtained a good correlation with results obtained using the Fick oxygen technique at cardiac catheterization.

GALLIUM IMAGING

Gallium-67-citrate is a radiopharmaceutical used for the evaluation of inflammatory and certain neoplastic diseases. It is a cyclotron-produced radionuclide with a half-life of 78 hours and several gamma photopeaks, of which three are commonly used for imaging, including 93, 184, and 296 keV. An iron analogue, it is largely bound to serum transferrin after intravenous injection. Gallium imaging is a sensitive but nonspecific procedure, with increased activity noted in many inflammatory and neoplastic processes. Normal sites of uptake include the liver, skeleton, salivary glands, kidneys, spleen, breasts, and large bowel. Simon and Hoffer (1980) have demonstrated that faint diffuse lung uptake may be present in approximately 50% of normal individuals at 24 hours, which should not be confused with a diffuse pulmonary inflammatory process. For this reason, gallium imaging of the chest is usually performed at 48 to 72 hours after injection, although diagnostic findings may be seen on earlier images, and earlier imaging is often performed in cases of suspected acute thoracic infection, to facilitate earlier diagnosis and treatment. In children, prominent uptake may be seen in the normal thymus gland, limiting the usefulness of

gallium scanning for the evaluation of mediastinal masses in the pediatric age group. During the first 24 hours after injection, 10 to 25% of the dose is excreted, primarily by the kidneys. Subsequent excretion is primarily via the colon.

Hoffer (1980a) and Palestro (1994) have reviewed the mechanisms of gallium uptake in disease processes. Gallium accumulation in infectious processes is related to several factors, including uptake in white blood cells, primarily bound to lactoferrin in lysosomes and other cytoplasmic organelles; increased blood flow and capillary permeability at sites of inflammation, with binding to tissue lactoferrin; and direct bacterial uptake within iron-binding organelles called *siderophores*. Uptake in neoplastic processes is less well understood, but may involve hyperpermeability of tumor vessels, increased extracellular fluid spaces in tumors; uptake within the cytoplasm, associated with lysosomes and possibly the endoplasmic reticulum; iron-binding proteins; tumor cell surface receptors; or possibly other, as yet unknown, mechanisms.

Tumors having a high affinity for gallium include bronchial carcinoma, malignant mesothelioma, hepatocellular carcinoma, Hodgkin's disease, large cell lymphoma, HIV-associated lymphoma and Burkitt's lymphoma, melanoma, and certain testicular neoplasms, as reviewed by Hoffer (1980b). Gallium scanning in the staging of Hodgkin's disease is highly sensitive in the detection of mediastinal involvement, with a sensitivity of 90% or greater, particularly in the nodular-sclerosing type. Evaluation of the abdomen and pelvis is less accurate, because of interfering normal colonic activity, which may obscure sites of lymphadenopathy or simulate abnormalities. CT is usually

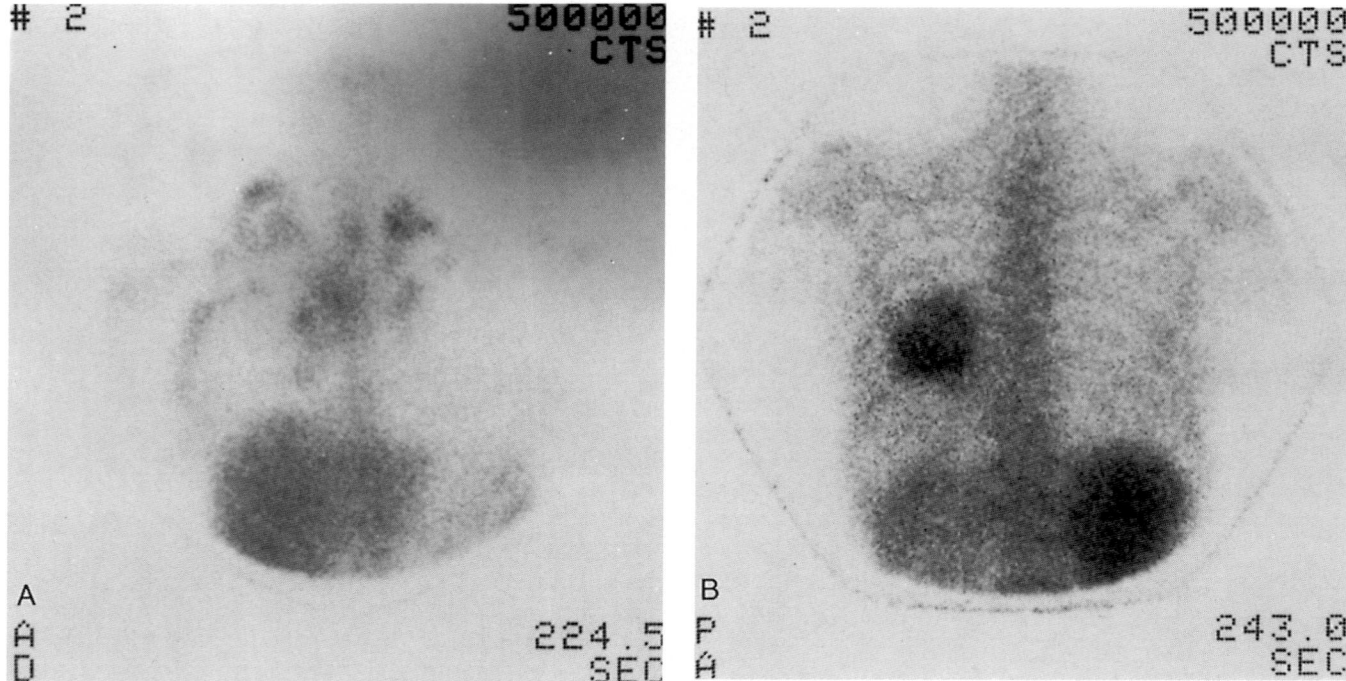

Fig. 13-9. Gallium uptake in thoracic neoplasms. **A.** A 72-hour anterior chest image demonstrates gallium uptake in bilateral supraclavicular, right hilar, superior mediastinal, and right axillary lymphadenopathy in a 39-year-old woman with Hodgkin's disease. The activity at the inferior aspect of the image is caused by normal hepatic and splenic gallium uptake. **B.** A 72-hour posterior chest image demonstrates increased gallium activity in a left lower lobe adenocarcinoma in a 50-year-old woman. From Spies WG, et al: Radionuclide imaging in diseases of the chest (part 2). Chest *83*:250, 1983. With permission.

used for evaluation of abdominal or pelvic lymphadenopathy. Gallium imaging has the advantage over CT of being able to detect active tumor involvement in normal-sized nodes and to correctly identify the absence of disease in successfully treated large nodal masses, in which persistent residual soft tissue masses of fibrotic tissue remain on CT. Gallium imaging is also sensitive for the detection of large cell non-Hodgkin's lymphoma, HIV-associated lymphoma, and Burkitt's lymphoma. Gallium scintigraphy may be used for the assessment of the response to therapy, both in non-Hodgkin's lymphoma and in Hodgkin's disease, as reported by Janicek (1997) and Front (1999) and their associates, respectively.

The overall sensitivity of gallium imaging in the staging of bronchial carcinoma is approximately 80 to 90%, without significant differences in different cell types, except for a possibly slightly lower sensitivity for adenocarcinoma. In general, primary lesions as small as 2 cm in diameter can be detected by planar imaging. The usefulness of gallium imaging in the assessment of mediastinal spread of tumor is controversial. Although it appears that gallium imaging is superior to standard chest radiography and plain tomography in this regard, the results of clinical trials have been variable. Alazraki and colleagues (1978) suggested that the absence of gallium uptake in the mediastinum in patients whose primary lesion concentrated gallium may obviate the need for preoperative mediastinoscopy. Other investigators, such as DeMeester and associates (1976), have had less impressive results. Savage

and coworkers (1976) have pointed out that because gallium uptake is nonspecific, false-positive results related to inflammatory disorders and sarcoidosis in the mediastinum may occur. The sensitivity of gallium imaging may be improved by using tomographic techniques, such as SPECT imaging. Nevertheless, as previously discussed, CT of the chest has become the primary imaging modality for the staging of bronchial carcinoma in most centers, although it has been challenged by another radionuclide technique, PET imaging, which is discussed later in this chapter and in Chapter 12. As mentioned previously in the case of lymphoma, pitfalls in CT staging include false-positive results caused by nonneoplastic enlargement of nodes and false-negative results caused by tumor involvement in normal-sized nodes. The search for metastases outside of the chest is best approached using other radionuclides, such as bone and liver–spleen scanning agents, and other techniques, such as CT of the abdomen. Examples of tumor uptake on gallium scans are shown in Figure 13-9.

Gallium imaging of the chest has also assumed an important role in the evaluation of infectious and other inflammatory disorders. Although standard chest radiography remains the primary imaging modality for the detection of pulmonary inflammatory disease, gallium scanning plays a complementary role. It is more sensitive for the detection of early infectious processes, better delineates mediastinal involvement, and allows for better follow-up of the response to therapy.

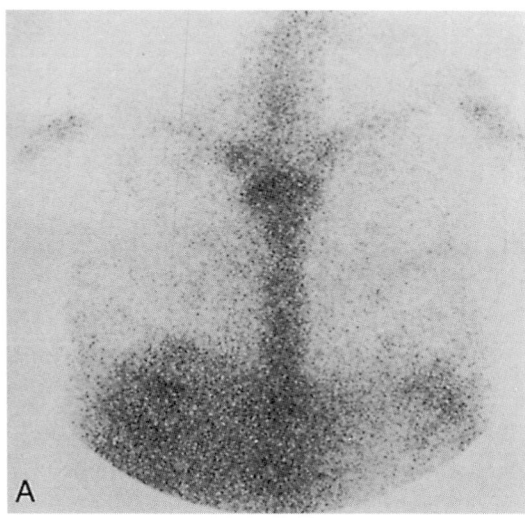

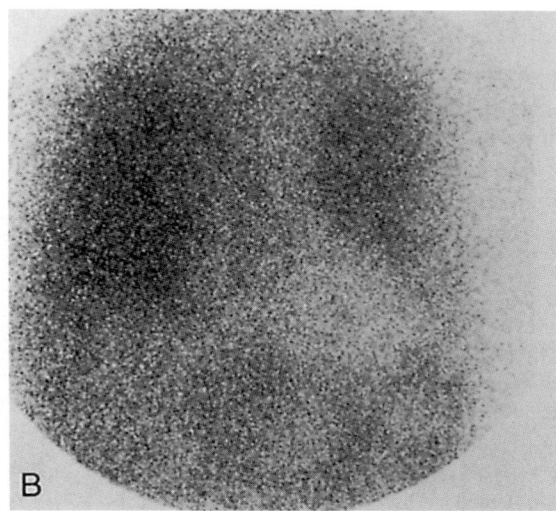

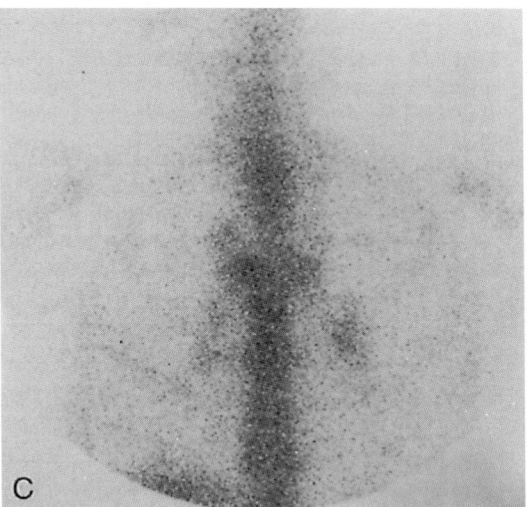

Fig. 13-10. Gallium imaging in immunocompromised patients. **A.** Normal 48-hour anterior gallium image of the chest. **B.** A 72-hour anterior chest image demonstrates diffuse bilateral increased pulmonary uptake in a 61-year-old man with acquired immunodeficiency syndrome and fever. Note the negative cardiac silhouette. The abnormality was also evident on 24-hour images. Initial chest radiography results were negative, but later films showed perihilar infiltrates. Bronchial aspirates were positive for *Pneumocystis carinii* pneumonia. **C.** A 72-hour anterior chest image shows bilateral hilar and right paratracheal lymphadenopathy in a 36-year-old male patient with acquired immunodeficiency syndrome who presented with nonproductive cough and fever. The patient proved to have *Mycobacterium avium-intracellulare* infection, which also involved the liver and bone marrow.

Diffusely increased pulmonary uptake is seen in opportunistic infections in immunocompromised hosts, such as *P. carinii* pneumonia or cytomegalovirus pneumonia, before the appearance of radiographic changes. Although previously a problem encountered mainly in patients with leukemia or lymphoma, this indication has assumed great importance in the past few years, with the proliferation of acquired immunodeficiency syndrome (AIDS). Barron and associates (1985) confirmed the usefulness of gallium imaging in AIDS patients with suspected *P. carinii* pneumonia, particularly in those with normal or equivocal chest radiographs. I and my associates (1989) reported a high sensitivity of 24-hour gallium images in the detection of *P. carinii* pneumonia, which makes the study more valuable for rapid clinical decision making. Kramer and colleagues (1989) described their experience with gallium imaging in a large series of AIDS patients presenting with acute fever or respiratory symptoms. In addition to confirming the usefulness of gallium imaging in the diagnosis of *Pneumocystis* and other opportunistic pneumonias, they also pointed out the additional patterns of focal lymph node uptake, seen primarily in cases of atypical tuberculosis (e.g., *Mycobacterium avium-intracellulare*) and lymphoma, and focal pulmonary uptake, often seen with acute bacterial pneumonias. Negative findings were associated with Kaposi's sarcoma or the absence of identifiable infection. In fact, the finding of a normal gallium scan in an HIV-positive patient with soft tissue chest masses is strong evidence for the presence of Kaposi's sarcoma. Abdel-Dayem and associates (1996) reported the usefulness of sequential thallium and gallium scans of the chest in AIDS patients with suspected Kaposi's sarcoma or other AIDS-related inflammatory and neoplastic processes. The pattern of a thallium-positive/gallium-negative study suggested the presence of Kaposi's sarcoma, although the sensitivity was reduced in patients who had coexisting opportunistic infections as well. Examples of normal and abnormal gallium image results of the chest are shown in Figure 13-10. Hattner and coworkers (1986) emphasized the favorable economic impact of gallium scanning in this clinical setting, in which they realized a potential cost savings of

38%, as a result of not needing bronchoscopy in cases of negative gallium scan results. Although diffuse pulmonary uptake is highly suspicious for the presence of acute opportunistic infection in this clinical setting, the finding is nonetheless nonspecific. The differential diagnosis of diffuse pulmonary uptake of gallium includes other diffuse bacterial and viral pneumonias, such as cytomegalovirus, tuberculosis, sarcoidosis, pulmonary toxicity from chemotherapeutic agents or other drugs, idiopathic pulmonary fibrosis, lymphangitic metastases, pneumoconiosis, and chemical pneumonitis after lymphangiography. Bronchoscopy and biopsy are therefore generally obtained in positive cases to establish the specific diagnosis.

Atypical patterns of gallium uptake in *P. carinii* pneumonia may occur, as noted by Kramer and associates (1987) and myself (1989). Perihilar uptake may occur before diffuse pulmonary uptake in some patients, analogous to the progression of findings noted on chest radiography. Upper lobe predominance may occur, possibly as the result of relative sparing of the lower lobes in patients receiving prophylactic aerosolized pentamidine therapy, which better penetrates the lung bases.

Although not of major importance in surgical practice, gallium imaging also has been used in the diagnosis and follow-up of granulomatous processes, such as tuberculosis and sarcoidosis, and pulmonary fibrotic disorders. Increased activity correlates with the presence of histologically active disease. Pulmonary uptake can be quantitated using a computer, resulting in excellent correlation with more invasive techniques, such as bronchoalveolar lavage in sarcoidosis, as described by Fajman and coworkers (1984). However, correlation with clinical symptoms and assessment of therapy is weaker.

IODINE 131 IMAGING

[131]I whole-body imaging is a standard procedure for the postoperative evaluation of patients with well-differentiated thyroid carcinoma. The whole-body scan detects the presence of residual normal thyroid tissue and functioning metastases in the thyroid bed, regional lymph nodes, lungs, or skeleton. Uptake of ^{131}I in pulmonary metastases may be demonstrated even in the absence of identifiable lesions on chest radiography (Fig. 13-11). The scan findings are used to determine whether a therapeutic dose of ^{131}I should be administered for the ablation of residual thyroid tissue, as well as the dose required. Ideally, according to Beierwaltes (1978), the scan is performed approximately 4 to 6 weeks after total thyroidectomy without thyroid hormone replacement to induce maximal endogenous thyroid-stimulating hormone stimulation of ^{131}I uptake by any metastases. Typical therapy doses for functioning pulmonary metastases range from approximately 175 to 200 mCi, with follow-up whole-body scanning performed 1 year later. In many cases, patients given doses in this range must be hospitalized until

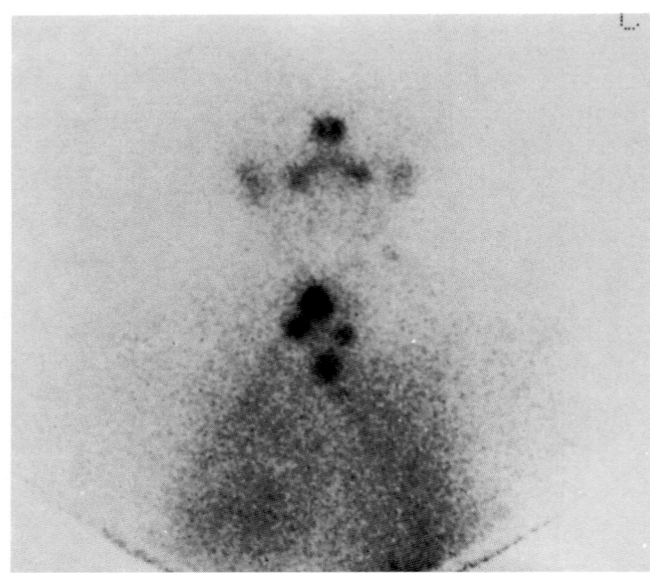

Fig. 13-11. Metastatic thyroid carcinoma. The patient is a 14-year-old girl post total thyroidectomy for well-differentiated mixed papillary-follicular thyroid carcinoma. An anterior iodine 131 image of the head and chest demonstrates four foci of metastatic disease in the thyroid bed and diffuse bilateral pulmonary uptake, consistent with lung metastases. A subtle focus of activity in the left neck may represent a cervical lymph node metastasis. The activity in the nasal region and mouth represents normal uptake by the nasal mucosa and salivary glands.

the retained dose drops below 30 mCi or in accordance with other local regulations.

The Nuclear Regulatory Commission has adopted new policies that permit outpatient ^{131}I therapy for thyroid carcinoma if certain radiation safety criteria can be met. Posttherapy repeat whole-body images are now obtained routinely at most institutions between 5 and 7 days after the therapeutic administration of ^{131}I and may provide additional diagnostic information in up to 50% of cases, as reported by me and my associates (1986b). If necessary, repeat therapy may be given, typically at yearly intervals as needed. With this dosing schedule, the incidence of toxicity related to radiation-induced pulmonary fibrosis or significant bone marrow suppression is low. On occasion, in cases of widespread, rapidly progressive metastatic disease, therapy may be repeated as frequently as 6 months apart. Follow-up scans may be obtained at longer intervals in patients with no evidence of recurrent disease. In some centers, use of quantitative dosimetry estimates in conjunction with diagnostic whole-body ^{131}I imaging permits administration of single-therapy doses larger than 200 mCi, which may potentially result in superior success rates and allow for more individualized treatment plans, as reported by Maxon and associates (1992). This approach is based on calculation of the delivered radiation dose to the tumor and to normal tissues, such as the lungs and bone marrow. In earlier work,

Maxon and associates (1983) estimated that doses of at least 30,000 rads to thyroid remnants and 8000 rads to metastases resulted in significantly increased rates of response to therapy. The review of Maxon and Smith (1990) indicates that approximately one-half of patients with functioning pulmonary metastases show resolution after ^{131}I therapy, one-quarter have some benefit, and the remaining one-quarter have no appreciable effect. The highest response rate (approximately 80% complete response) occurs in patients in whom the lesions are detectable only on ^{131}I whole-body scans. The 5-year mortality is significantly lower for patients whose lung metastases accumulate ^{131}I compared with those who do not (38% versus 69% mortality). Mortality is significantly higher in cases in which the pulmonary metastases are accompanied by metastases elsewhere. Empirical use of ^{131}I therapy in patients with negative whole-body scan results but suspected metastases based on elevated serum thyroglobulin levels has gained wide acceptance. Many patients managed in this fashion demonstrate lung uptake, or other sites of metastatic disease, or both on follow-up posttherapy ^{131}I whole-body scans, confirming that metastases were present.

RADIONUCLIDE ANGIOGRAPHY

Radionuclide angiography is a simple, safe, noninvasive method for evaluating blood flow to various organs. It can be used to delineate vascular anatomy and patency and to evaluate the vascularity of masses, as reviewed by Muroff and Freedman (1976). Radionuclide angiography is performed by obtaining a rapid sequence of images (0.5 to 3.0 seconds per image) over an area of interest, immediately after the intravenous injection of a radiopharmaceutical. It is a routine part of many nuclear medicine procedures, such as renal scans and bone scans performed for suspected osteomyelitis, acute fractures, or heterotopic ossification. In the case of the chest, such studies may be obtained alone or in conjunction with other standard nuclear medicine examinations. Almost any radiopharmaceutical may be used except MAA or human albumin microspheres, which would be trapped in the pulmonary vasculature. The examination is most often performed for evaluation of suspected vascular obstruction, as in superior vena cava syndrome (Fig. 13-12). The data may be quantitated using a digital computer. Radionuclide angiography may obviate the need for more invasive procedures, such as contrast venography or arteriography. Other potential diagnostic uses include the noninvasive demonstration of aortic aneurysms and vascular masses, such as hemangiomas and arteriovenous malformations. The major limitation of radionuclide angiography relates to its relatively poor spatial resolution compared with standard radiographic techniques, such as contrast angiography and digital subtraction angiography. Technically inadequate studies occur in a small percentage of cases, caused by poor bolus geometry or poor patient positioning.

FUTURE DEVELOPMENTS IN PULMONARY NUCLEAR MEDICINE

New developments in nuclear medicine have been directed toward more sophisticated evaluation of physiologic processes. Major advances usually result from the development of new radiopharmaceuticals, with the introduction of newer instrumentation then following. Pulmonary nuclear medicine has been no exception in this regard. Several approaches to improvement of the scintigraphic diagnosis of PE have already been discussed. Another technique is the use of indium 111-labeled autologous platelets. This technique is useful in the detection of DVT in the lower extremities, the precursor of PE. Investi-

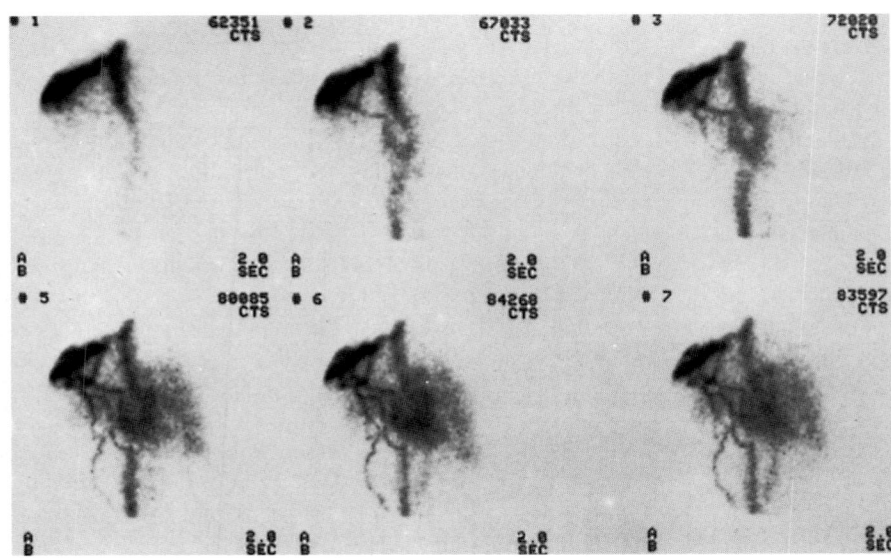

Fig. 13-12. Radionuclide angiography in superior vena cava syndrome. This 65-year-old man had poorly differentiated adenocarcinoma of the lung, with brain and liver metastases, and clinical signs suggestive of superior vena cava obstruction. Selected anterior images of the chest from a radionuclide angiogram performed after injection of technetium 99m diethylenetriamine-penta-acetic acid in a right antecubital vein demonstrate high-grade partial obstruction of the superior vena cava, with marked flow into dilatated collateral veins in the right axilla and anterior chest wall. Mild reflux into the right internal jugular vein and early visualization of the inferior vena cava via collateral flow are noted also. A small amount of activity is shown directly entering the superior vena cava and right heart.

gations led by Davis (1980) and Moser (1980) and their associates have suggested that imaging of PE in humans by this technique may be limited to emboli less than 12 hours old, and only in patients not on heparin. Murine monoclonal antibodies directed against platelets or components of fibrin blood clots have been developed. Line and associates (1997) reported a case in which a ^{99m}Tc-labeled Fab' antifibrin antibody demonstrated emboli in the hila, right atrium, and the region of the aortic arch in a patient with a high probability for PE V̇/Q̇ scan but negative Doppler ultrasound results of the lower extremities. A subsequent CT scan confirmed the presence of central PE. A potential pitfall of this technique is the potential for impaired delivery of tracer to the site of clot in patients with markedly reduced pulmonary blood flow. A related development is the peptide radiopharmaceutical Acutect, a ^{99m}Tc-labeled synthetic peptide shown in animal studies to bind preferentially to the glycoprotein IIb/IIIa adhesion-molecule receptors found on activated platelets, as described by Becker (1996) and in the Acutect prescribing information package insert (1998). This agent, which was recently approved by the FDA for use in humans, demonstrates focal hot spots or asymmetry at sites of acute lower extremity DVT, but not in sites of chronic thrombi. Its clinical usefulness relative to the other existing modalities for the detection of DVT is still uncertain. Hot spot imaging of PE may be accomplished using radioactive gases labeled with positron-emitting radionuclides of carbon or oxygen as reported by Nichols and associates (1978). In this case, inhaled radioactive gases diffuse across the alveolar-capillary membrane and are cleared from the lungs via pulmonary blood flow. As a result of decreased blood flow, the gas is retained in areas of PE, resulting in easily identified hot spots. Although apparently quite sensitive, this technique remains impractical for widespread use at present, because it requires not only a PET scanner but also an onsite cyclotron for production of these extremely short-lived radiopharmaceuticals.

PET imaging has experienced a rapid explosion of use as an exquisitely sensitive examination for the detection, staging, and follow-up of a number of neoplasms, using the radiopharmaceutical fluorine 18-labeled fluorodeoxyglucose. Fluorodeoxyglucose imaging has proven to be both a more sensitive and more cost-effective method for evaluation compared with CT and MR imaging in a variety of lesions, including bronchial carcinoma, as reviewed by Al-Sugair and Coleman (1998). PET is useful for differentiating between benign versus malignant solitary pulmonary nodules, staging of lung tumors, identifying benign pulmonary lesions, and differentiating between recurrent neoplasm and posttreatment fibrosis. Other tumors for which fluorodeoxyglucose PET imaging may assume a greater clinical role in the near future include colorectal carcinoma, breast carcinoma, melanoma, lymphoma, and others. PET imaging of the chest is covered in detail in Chapter 12.

Investigations have been conducted using other radiopharmaceuticals for evaluation of pulmonary metabolic functions, as reviewed by Touya and associates (1986a) and earlier by Budinger and colleagues (1982). In addition to its respiratory function, the lung is involved in the regulation of a number of circulating vasoactive substances, including the activation, deactivation, release, or removal of such substances as amines, hormones, drugs, and polypeptides. Examples of such substances include bradykinin, serotonin, prostaglandins, angiotensin I, histamine, and many others. One such line of research involves measuring the pulmonary uptake, extraction, and wash-out of ^{123}I-isopropyl-p-iodoamphetamine, an iodoamphetamine derivative. Pulmonary uptake of this agent is a passive, saturable process, as reported by Touya and associates (1985), whereas the agent ^{123}I-meta-iodobenzylguanidine (MIBG) is dependent on oxidative metabolism in the lung, as investigated by Slosman and coworkers (1986). Metabolic functions of the lung also may be studied in a more quantitative fashion using PET imaging with radioactive carbon (C) 11-labeled amines. Such studies may lead to better understanding of pulmonary metabolic functions and the ability to quantitate pulmonary amine endothelial receptors. Schuster (1998) reviewed the use of a variety of positron-emitting radiotracers for the evaluation of such lung functions as pulmonary blood flow, ventilation, pulmonary edema, pulmonary vascular permeability, and receptor and enzyme systems. Potential clinical applications include the diagnosis and treatment follow-up of hypertension, adult and neonatal respiratory distress syndrome, interstitial lung disease, pulmonary trauma, cystic fibrosis, asthma, and even certain psychiatric disorders. These approaches involve ultrashort-lived radiopharmaceuticals such as ^{11}C albumin microspheres, ^{15}O-labeled H_2O and CO and ^{13}N N_2,which require on-site cyclotrons for preparation, and thus have not to date led to clinical use.

Slutsky and Higgins (1984) evaluated the use of thallium 201 chloride, a radiopharmaceutical widely used for myocardial perfusion imaging, in the evaluation of pulmonary extracellular fluid balance, as related to the development of pulmonary edema. Lung permeability and fluid balance also may be evaluated by measuring the clearance of inhaled radiolabeled aerosols from the lungs, a process dependent on the state of the alveolar-capillary membrane permeability, as discussed earlier in this chapter.

Imaging with radiolabeled leukocytes may allow detection of changes in kinetics and distribution of leukocytes that may occur after exposure to toxins, such as high oxygen tension, or in ARDS, as suggested by the work of Suttorp and Simon (1982) involving leukocyte-mediated lung cell cytotoxicity after sustained hyperoxia.

A final area of research not limited to pulmonary nuclear medicine is the continued evaluation of radiolabeled monoclonal antibodies for the detection and treatment of various neoplasms and the detection of thromboemboli, as reviewed by Keenan and associates (1985) and more recently by Schlom (1991). This technique was applied by Zimmer and colleagues (1985) to the detection of small cell lung carcinoma, using a ^{131}I-labeled antibody developed in mice. Our group (1988) also performed a pilot evaluation of a ^{111}In-labeled monoclonal antibody directed against non–small cell lung carcinoma in patients with advanced primary lesions. These studies demonstrated good visualization of the primary tumors, but relative insensitivity for mediastinal involvement or other metastases in a small group of patients, in part because of high background activity in the liver and blood pool. Overall, monoclonal antibody studies in thousands of patients with various primary tumors have proven to be safe, with detection sensitivities in the 60 to 90% range, as noted by Goldenberg (1991). Usually, lesions greater than 1 to 2 cm are detected, although lesions as small as 4 to 5 mm may be detected with SPECT imaging, and in some cases lesions missed by anatomic imaging methods such as CT can be detected. During the 1990s, the FDA has approved several murine monoclonal antibodies labeled with ^{111}In and ^{99m}Tc for use in imaging several human neoplasms, including colorectal carcinoma, ovarian carcinoma, and prostate carcinoma. Ongoing investigations in this field include attempts to develop more tumor-specific and tumor-avid antibodies, including antibody fragments, attempts to decrease immunologic responses to murine antibodies (development of human antimouse antibodies), and the use of human rather than mouse monoclonal antibodies. In addition, newer labeling techniques allow tagging of monoclonal antibodies to ^{99m}Tc rather than ^{111}In or ^{131}I, resulting in better imaging characteristics. Monoclonal antibodies labeled with other beta or alpha emitters, such as yttrium 90, may permit radionuclide ablation of the various tumors, such as certain non-Hodgkin's lymphomas. The ultimate roles of radiolabeled monoclonal antibody imaging and therapy remain uncertain at present.

REFERENCES

Abdel-Dayem HM, et al: Evaluation of sequential thallium and gallium scans of the chest in AIDS patients. J Nucl Med 37:1662, 1996.
Acutect Prescribing Information. Diatide, Inc. And Nycomed Amersham, September 1998.
American College of Chest Physicians Consensus Committee on Pulmonary Embolism: Special report. Opinions regarding the diagnosis and management of venous thromboembolic disease. Chest 109:233, 1996.
Agee RN, et al: Use of 133-xenon in early diagnosis of inhalation injury. J Trauma 16:218, 1976.
Alazraki NP, et al: Reliability of gallium scan chest radiography compared to mediastinoscopy for evaluating mediastinal spread in lung cancer. Am Rev Resp Dis 117:415, 1978.
Alderson PO, Line BR: Scintigraphic evaluation of regional pulmonary ventilation. Semin Nucl Med 10:218, 1980.
Alderson PO, Secker-Walker RH, Forrest JV: Detection of obstructive pulmonary disease. Radiology 111:643, 1974.
Alderson PO, et al: The role of ^{133}Xe ventilation studies in the scintigraphic detection of pulmonary embolism. Radiology 120:633, 1976.
Alderson PO, et al: Ventilation-perfusion lung imaging and selective pulmonary angiography in dogs with experimental pulmonary embolism. J Nucl Med 19:164, 1978.
Alderson PO, et al: Comparison of ^{133}Xe single-breath and washout imaging in the scintigraphic diagnosis of pulmonary embolism. Radiology 137:481, 1980.
Alderson PO, et al: Scintigraphic detection of pulmonary embolism in patients with obstructive pulmonary disease. Radiology 138:661, 1981.
Alderson PO, et al: Serial lung scintigraphy: utility in diagnosis of pulmonary embolism. Radiology 149:797, 1983.
Alderson PO, et al: Tc-99m-DTPA aerosol and radioactive gases compared as adjuncts to perfusion scintigraphy in patients with suspected pulmonary embolism. Radiology 153:515, 1984.
Al-Sugair A, Coleman RE: Applications of PET in lung cancer. Semin Nucl Med 28:303, 1998.
Ashburn WL, et al: Technetium-99m labeled micro aerosol "pertechnegas": a new agent for ventilation imaging in suspected pulmonary emboli. Clin Nucl Med 18:1045, 1993.
Barron TF, et al: Pneumocystis carinii pneumonia studied by gallium-67 scanning. Radiology 154:791, 1985.
Becker DM, et al: D-dimer testing and acute venous thromboembolism. A shortcut to accurate diagnosis? Arch Intern Med 156:939, 1996.
Becker RC: Antiplatelet therapy. Sci Med 12, 1996.
Bedont RA, Datz FL: Lung scan perfusion defects limited to matching pleural effusions: low probability of pulmonary embolism. AJR Am J Roentgenol 145:1155, 1985.
Beierwaltes WH: The treatment of thyroid carcinoma with radioactive iodine. Semin Nucl Med 8:79, 1978.
Bellomo R, et al: The one month outcome of patients with a low probability technegas ventilation/perfusion lung scan. Nucl Med Commun 15:505, 1994.
Biello DR, et al: Interpretation of indeterminate lung scintigrams. Radiology 133:189, 1979.
Biello DR: Radiological (scintigraphic) evaluation of patients with suspected pulmonary thromboembolism. JAMA 257:3257, 1987.
Bone RC: Ventilation/perfusion scan in pulmonary embolism. "The Emperor is incompletely attired." JAMA 263:2794, 1990.
Boysen PG, et al: Prospective evaluation for pneumonectomy using the ^{99m}technetium quantitative perfusion lung scan. Chest 72:422, 1977.
Budinger TF, McNeil BJ, Alderson PO: Perspectives in nuclear medicine: pulmonary studies. J Nucl Med 23:60, 1982.
Burch WM, et al: Lung ventilation studies with technetium-99m pseudogas. J Nucl Med 27:842, 1986.
Cabahug CJ, et al: Utility of technetium-99m-DTPA in determining regional ventilation. J Nucl Med 37:239, 1996.
Caride VJ, et al: The usefulness of the posterior oblique views in perfusion lung imaging. Radiology 121:669, 1976.
Carson JL, et al: The clinical course of pulmonary embolism. N Engl J Med 326:1240, 1992.
Carter WD, et al: Relative accuracy of two diagnostic schemes for detection of pulmonary embolism by ventilation-perfusion scintigraphy. Radiology 145:447, 1982.
Catania TA, Caride VJ: Single perfusion defect and pulmonary embolism: angiographic correlation. J Nucl Med 31:296, 1990.
Coates G, O'Brodovich H: Measurement of pulmonary epithelial permeability with ^{99m}Tc-DTPA aerosol. Semin Nucl Med 16:275, 1986.
Dalen JE, Alpert JS: Natural history of pulmonary embolism. Prog Cardiovasc Dis 17:259, 1975.
Davis HH, et al: Scintigraphy with ^{111}In-labeled autologous platelets in venous thromboembolism. Radiology 136:203, 1980.
DeMeester TR, et al: Gallium-67 scanning for carcinoma of the lung. J Thorac Cardiovasc Surg 72:699, 1976.
Dorfman GS, et al: Occult pulmonary embolism: a common occurrence in deep venous thrombosis. AJR Am J Roentgenol 148:263, 1987.
Fajman WA, et al: Assessing the activity of sarcoidosis: Quantitative ^{67}Ga-citrate imaging. AJR Am J Roentgenol 142:683, 1984.
Foley M, et al: Pulmonary embolism after hip or knee replacement: postoperative changes on pulmonary scintigrams in asymptomatic patients. Radiology 172:481, 1989.
Freitas JE, et al: Modified PIOPED criteria used in clinical practice. J Nucl Med 36:1573, 1995.
Front D, et al: Hodgkin disease: prediction of outcome with ^{67}Ga scintigraphy after one cycle of chemotherapy. Radiology 210:487, 1999.
Gates GF, Orme HW, Dore EK: Cardiac shunt assessment in children with macroaggregated albumin technetium-99m. Radiology 112:649, 1974.
Ginsberg JS, et al: D-dimer in patients with clinically suspected pulmonary embolism. Chest 104:1679, 1993.
Goldberg SN, et al: Pleural effusion and ventilation/perfusion scan interpretation for acute pulmonary embolus. J Nucl Med 37:1310, 1996.

Goldenberg DM: Current status of cancer imaging with radiolabeled antibodies. Antibody Immunoconjugates Radiopharmaceuticals 4:517, 1991.

Goldhaber SZ: Medical progress: pulmonary embolism. N Engl J Med 339:93, 1998.

Goldhaber SZ, et al: Quantitative plasma D-dimer levels among patients undergoing pulmonary angiography for suspected pulmonary embolism. JAMA 270:2819, 1993.

Goris ML, et al: Applications of ventilation lung imaging with ⁸¹ᵐkrypton. Radiology 122:399, 1977.

Gottschalk A, Stein PD, Henry JW: Patient stratification by cardiopulmonary status in the diagnosis of pulmonary embolism. J Nucl Med 37:570, 1996a.

Gottschalk A, et al: Ventilation-perfusion scintigraphy in the PIOPED study. Part II. Evaluation of the scintigraphic criteria and interpretations. J Nucl Med 34:1119, 1993.

Gottschalk A, et al: Matched ventilation, perfusion and chest radiographic abnormalities in acute pulmonary embolism. J Nucl Med 37:1636, 1996b.

Harding LK, et al: The proportion of lung vessels blocked by albumin microspheres. J Nucl Med 14:579, 1973.

Hattner RS, Golden JA, Fugate K: Cost/benefit of real versus "ideal" management strategies of AIDS patients suspected of P. carinii pneumonia: effect of Ga-67 pulmonary imaging. J Nucl Med 27:914, 1986.

Hoffer P: Gallium: mechanisms. J Nucl Med 21:282, 1980a.

Hoffer P: Status of gallium-67 in tumor detection. J Nucl Med 21:394, 1980b.

Huisman MV, et al: Unexpected prevalence of silent pulmonary embolism in patients with deep venous thrombosis. Chest 95:498, 1989.

Hull RD, Raskob GE: Low-probability lung scan findings: a need for change. Ann Intern Med 114:142, 1991.

Hull RD, et al: Pulmonary angiography, ventilation lung scanning, and venography for clinically suspected pulmonary embolism with abnormal perfusion lung scan. Ann Intern Med 98:891, 1983.

Hull RD, et al: Diagnostic value of ventilation-perfusion lung scanning in patients with suspected pulmonary embolism. Chest 88:819, 1985.

Jacobson AF, Patel N, Lewis DH: Clinical outcome of patients with intermediate probability lung scans during six-month follow-up. J Nucl Med 38:1593, 1997.

Janicek M, et al: Early restaging gallium scans predict outcome in poor-prognosis patients with aggressive non-Hodgkin's lymphoma treated with high-dose CHOP chemotherapy. J Clin Oncol 15:1631, 1997.

Juni JE, Alavi A: Lung scanning in the diagnosis of pulmonary embolism: the emperor redressed. Semin Nucl Med 21:281, 1991.

Keenan AM, Harbert JC, Larson SM: Monoclonal antibodies in nuclear medicine. J Nucl Med 26:531, 1985.

Kipper MS, Alazraki N: The feasibility of performing ¹³³Xe ventilation imaging following the perfusion study. Radiology 144:581, 1982.

Kramer EL, et al: Gallium-67 scans of the chest in patients with acquired immunodeficiency syndrome. J Nucl Med 28:1107, 1987.

Kramer EL, et al: Diagnostic implications of Ga-67 chest-scan patterns in human immunodeficiency virus-seropositive patients. Radiology 170:671, 1989.

Kristersson S: Prediction of lung function after lung surgery. A ¹³³Xe-radiospirometric study of regional lung function in bronchial cancer. Scand J Thorac Cardiovasc Surg 18(Suppl):5, 1974.

Line BR, et al: Cardiopulmonary thromboembolism detected by Tc-99m MH-1 antifibrin antibody. Clin Nucl Med 22:376, 1997.

Lowe VJ, Bullard AG, Coleman RE: Ventilation/perfusion lung scan probability category distributions in university and community hospitals. Clin Nucl Med 20:1079, 1995.

Lull RJ, et al: Radionuclide evaluation of lung trauma. Semin Nucl Med 13:223, 1983.

Mackey DWJ, et al: Physical properties and use of pertechnegas as a ventilation agent. J Nucl Med 38:163, 1997.

Maxon HR, Smith HS: Radioiodine-131 in the diagnosis and treatment of metastatic well differentiated thyroid cancer. Endocrinol Metab Clin North Am 19:685, 1990.

Maxon HR, et al: Relation between effective radiation dose and outcome of radioiodine therapy for thyroid cancer. N Engl J Med 309:937, 1983.

Maxon HR, et al: I-131 therapy for thyroid cancer: quantitative dosimetric approach—outcome and validation in 85 patients. J Nucl Med 33:894, 1992.

McNeil BJ: A diagnostic strategy using ventilation-perfusion studies in patients suspect for pulmonary embolism. J Nucl Med 17:613, 1976.

Medina LS, et al: Postoperative evaluation of single-lung transplant patients with quantitative ventilation-perfusion imaging. Radiology 185(P):283, 1992.

Miniati M, et al: Value of perfusion lung scan in the diagnosis of pulmonary embolism: results of the prospective investigative study of acute pulmonary embolism diagnosis (PISA-PED). Am J Respir Crit Care Med 154:1387, 1996.

Moldofsky P, et al: Quantitative lung scans for prediction of post-radiotherapy pulmonary function. Clin Nucl Med 13:644, 1988.

Morrell NW, et al: The underestimation of segmental defect size in radionuclide lung scanning. J Nucl Med 34:370, 1993.

Moser KM, et al: Study of factors that may condition scintigraphic detection of venous thrombi and pulmonary emboli with indium-111-labeled platelets. J Nucl Med 21:1051, 1980.

Moser KM, et al: Frequent asymptomatic pulmonary embolism in patients with deep venous thrombosis. JAMA 271:223, 1994.

Muroff LR, Freedman GS: Radionuclide angiography. Semin Nucl Med 6:217, 1976.

Nichols AB, et al: Scintigraphic detection of pulmonary emboli by serial positron imaging of inhaled ¹⁵O-labeled carbon dioxide. N Engl J Med 299:279, 1978.

Nielsen PE, Kirchner PT, Gerber FH: Oblique views in lung perfusion scanning: clinical utility and limitations. J Nucl Med 18:967, 1977.

Olsen GN, Block AJ, Tobias JA: Prediction of postpneumonectomy pulmonary function using quantitative macroaggregate lung scanning. Chest 66:13, 1974.

Palestro CJ: The current role of gallium imaging in infection. Semin Nucl Med 24:128, 1994.

The PIOPED Investigators: Value of the ventilation/perfusion scan in acute pulmonary embolism. Results of the prospective investigation of pulmonary embolism diagnosis (PIOPED). JAMA 263:2753, 1990.

Rhodes BA, et al: Lung scanning with ⁹⁹ᵐTc-microspheres. Radiology 99:613, 1971.

Robin ED: Overdiagnosis and overtreatment of pulmonary embolism: the Emperor may have no clothes. Ann Intern Med 87:775, 1977.

Rosen JM, et al: Kr-81m ventilation imaging: clinical utility in suspected pulmonary embolism. Radiology 154:787, 1985.

Rosenow EC III, Osmundson PJ, Brown ML: Pulmonary embolism. Mayo Clin Proc 56:161, 1981.

Royal HD, Trulock EP, Ettinger NA: Effects of ischemic time on relative perfusion and ventilation in double-lung transplant patients. Radiology 185(P):282, 1992.

Savage P, Carmody R, Highman J: Evaluation of gallium-67 in the diagnosis of bronchial carcinoma. Clin Radiol 27:197, 1976.

Schlom J: Monoclonal antibodies: they're more and less than you think. In Broder S (ed): Molecular Foundations of Oncology. Chapter 6. Baltimore, MD: Williams & Wilkins, 1991.

Schor RA, et al: Regional ventilation studies with Kr-81m and Xe-133: A comparative analysis. J Nucl Med 19:348, 1978.

Schuster DP: The evaluation of lung function with PET. Semin Nucl Med 28:341, 1998.

Simon TR, Li J, Hoffer PB: The nonspecificity of diffuse pulmonary uptake of ⁶⁷Ga on 24-hour images. Radiology 135:445, 1980.

Slosman D, et al: Pulmonary accumulation of ¹³¹I-MIBG in the isolated perfused rat lung. J Nucl Med 27:1076, 1986.

Slutsky RA, Higgins CB: Thallium scintigraphy in experimental toxic pulmonary edema: relationship to extravascular pulmonary fluid. J Nucl Med 25:581, 1984.

Snider GL: Reduction pneumoplasty for giant bullous emphysema. Implications for surgical treatment of nonbullous emphysema. Chest 109:540, 1996.

Sostman HD, Gottschalk A: The stripe sign: a new sign for diagnosis of nonembolic defects on pulmonary perfusion scintigraphy. Radiology 142:737, 1982.

Sostman HD, Gottschalk, A: Prospective validation of the stripe sign in ventilation-perfusion scintigraphy. Radiology 184:455, 1992.

Sostman HD, et al: Evaluation of revised criteria for ventilation-perfusion scintigraphy in patients with suspected pulmonary embolism. Radiology 193:103, 1994.

Spies WG: Gallium-67 citrate imaging in acquired immunodeficiency syndrome. J Nucl Med Technol 17:23, 1989.

Spies WG: Diagnostic procedures for thoracic diseases: nuclear techniques. Chest Surg Clin N Am 2:521, 1992.

Spies WG, et al: Ventilation-perfusion scintigraphy in suspected pulmonary embolism: correlation with pulmonary angiography and refinement of criteria for interpretation. Radiology 159:383, 1986a.

Spies WG, Wojtowicz CH, Spies SM: Value of posttherapy whole-body scans in the evaluation of patients with thyroid carcinoma having undergone high-dose I-131 therapy. Radiology 161(P):224, 1986b.

Spies WG, et al: Monoclonal antibody imaging with In-111-labeled B72.3 in human non-small cell lung carcinoma. Radiology 169(P):74, 1988.

Spies WG, et al: Utility of 24 hour gallium images in the detection of acute pulmonary inflammatory processes in patients with acquired immunodeficiency syndrome. J Nucl Med 30:888, 1989.

Stein PD, Henry JW, Gottschalk A: Mismatched vascular defects. An easy alternative to mismatched segmental equivalent defects for the interpretation of ventilation/perfusion lung scans in pulmonary embolism. Chest 104:1468, 1993b.

Stein PD, Henry JW, Gottschalk A: Small perfusion defects in suspected pulmonary embolism. J Nucl Med 37:1313, 1996.

Stein PD, Henry JW, Gottschalk A: Reassessment of pulmonary angiography for the diagnosis of pulmonary embolism: relation of interpreter agreement to the order of the involved pulmonary arterial branch. Radiology 210:689, 1999.

Stein PD, et al: Clinical, laboratory, roentgenographic, and electrocardiographic findings in patients with acute pulmonary embolism and no pre-existing cardiac or pulmonary disease. Chest 100:598, 1991.

Stein PD, et al: Stratification of patients according to prior cardiopulmonary disease and probability assessment based on the number of mismatched segmental equivalent perfusion defects. Approaches to strengthen the diagnostic value of ventilation/perfusion lung scans in acute pulmonary embolism. Chest 104:1461, 1993a.

Sullivan DC, et al: Lung scan interpretation: effect of different observers and different criteria. Radiology 149:803, 1983.

Sullivan PJ, et al: A clinical comparison of technegas and xenon-133 in 50 patients with suspected pulmonary embolus. Chest 94:300, 1988.

Susskind H, et al: Sensitivity of Kr-81m and Xe-127 in evaluating nonembolic pulmonary disease. J Nucl Med 22:781, 1981.

Susskind H, et al: Impaired permeability in radiation-induced lung injury detected by technetium-99m-DTPA lung clearance. J Nucl Med 38:966, 1997.

Suttorp N, Simon LM: Lung cell oxidant injury: enhancement of polymorphonuclear leukocyte-mediated cytotoxicity in lung cells exposed to sustained in vitro hyperoxia. J Clin Invest 70:342, 1982.

Taplin GV, Poe ND: A dual lung-scanning technic for evaluation of pulmonary function. Radiology 85:365, 1965.

Thyrogen® Complete Prescribing Information. Genzyme Therapeutics, Genzyme Corporation and Knoll Pharmaceutical Company, 1998.

Toronto Lung Transplant Group: Unilateral lung transplantation for pulmonary fibrosis. N Engl J Med 314:1140, 1986.

Touya JJ, et al: A noninvasive procedure for in vivo assay of a lung amine endothelial receptor. J Nucl Med 26:1302, 1985.

Touya JJ, et al: The lung as a metabolic organ. Semin Nucl Med 16:296, 1986a.

Touya JJ, et al: Single photon emission computed tomography in the diagnosis of pulmonary thromboembolism. Semin Nucl Med 16:306, 1986b.

Turkstra F, et al: Diagnostic utility of ultrasonography of leg veins in patients suspected of having pulmonary embolism. Ann Intern Med 126:775, 1997.

Vix VA: The usefulness of chest radiographs obtained after a demonstrated perfusion scan defect in the diagnosis of pulmonary emboli. Clin Nucl Med 8:497, 1983.

Walker RH, Provan JL: Scintillation scanning of lungs in preoperative assessment of carcinoma of bronchus. BMJ 1:327, 1969.

Wang SC, et al: Perfusion scintigraphy in the evaluation for lung volume reduction surgery: correlation with clinical outcome. Radiology 205:243, 1997.

Webber MM, et al: Comparison of Biello, McNeil, and PIOPED criteria for the diagnosis of pulmonary emboli on lung scans. AJR Am J Roentgenol 154:975, 1990.

Worsley DF, Alavi A: Comprehensive analysis of the results of the PIOPED study. J Nucl Med 36:2380, 1995.

Worsley DF, Alavi A, Palevsky HI: Role of radionuclide imaging in patients with suspected pulmonary embolism. Radiol Clin North Am 31:849, 1993a.

Worsley DF, et al: Detailed analysis of patients with matched ventilation-perfusion defects and chest radiographic opacities. J Nucl Med 34:1851, 1993b.

Worsley DF, et al: Comparison of diagnostic performance with ventilation-perfusion lung imaging in different patient populations. Radiology 199:481, 1996.

Zimmer AM, et al: Radioimmunoimaging of human small cell lung carcinoma with I-131 tumor specific monoclonal antibody. Hybridoma 4:1, 1985.

READING REFERENCES

General References

Line BR: Scintigraphic studies of nonembolic lung disease. In Sandler MP, et al (eds): Diagnostic Nuclear Medicine. 3rd Ed. Chapter 31. Baltimore: Williams & Wilkins, 1996.

Mettler FA Jr, Guiberteau MJ: Essentials of Medicine Imaging. 4th Ed. Philadelphia: WB Saunders Co, 1998.

Royal HD: Pulmonary imaging for non-thrombotic disease. In Henkin RE, et al (eds): Nuclear Medicine. Chapter 91. St. Louis: Mosby, 1996.

Sostman HD, Neumann RD, Gottschalk A: Evaluation of patients with suspected venous thromboembolism. In Sandler MP, et al (eds): Diagnostic Nuclear Medicine. 3rd Ed. Chapter 30. Baltimore: Williams & Wilkins, 1996.

Spies WG: Ventilation/perfusion scintigraphy. In Henkin RE, et al (eds): Nuclear Medicine. Chapter 90. St. Louis: Mosby, 1996.

Other Less Invasive Modalities for Detection of Pulmonary Emboli

Alderson PO, Martin EC: Pulmonary embolism: diagnosis with multiple imaging modalities. Radiology 164:297, 1987.

Baldt MM, et al: Spiral CT evaluation of deep venous thrombosis. Semin Ultrasound CT MRI 18:369, 1997.

Black RD, et al: In vivo He-3 MR images of guinea pig lungs. Radiology 199:867, 1996.

Ferretti GR, et al: Acute pulmonary embolism: role of helical CT in 164 patients with intermediate probability at ventilation-perfusion scintigraphy and normal results at duplex US of the legs. Radiology 205:453, 1997.

Goodman LR, et al: Detection of pulmonary embolism in patients with unresolved clinical and scintigraphic diagnosis: helical CT versus angiography. AJR Am J Roentgenol 164:1369, 1995.

Goodman PC, Brant-Zawadzki M: Digital subtraction pulmonary angiography. AJR Am J Roentgenol 139:305, 1982.

Kim K, Muller NL, Mayo JR: Clinically suspected pulmonary embolism: utility of spiral CT. Radiology 210:693, 1999.

Mayo JR, et al: Pulmonary embolism: prospective comparison of spiral CT with ventilation-perfusion scintigraphy. Radiology 205:447, 1997.

Meaney JFM, et al: Diagnosis of pulmonary embolism with magnetic resonance angiography. N Engl J Med 336:1422, 1997.

Musset D, et al: Acute pulmonary embolism: diagnostic value of digital subtraction angiography. Radiology 166:455, 1988.

Piers DB, et al: A comparative study of intravenous digital subtraction angiography and ventilation-perfusion scans in suspected pulmonary embolism. Chest 91:837, 1987.

Portman MA: Cardiothoracic magnetic resonance angiography. Semin Ultrasound CT MR 13:274, 1992.

Posteraro RH, et al: Cine-gradient-refocused MR imaging of central pulmonary emboli. AJR Am J Roentgenol 152:465, 1989.

Remy-Jardin M, et al: Central pulmonary thromboembolism: diagnosis with spiral volumetric CT with the single-breath-hold technique—comparison with pulmonary angiography. Radiology *185*:381, 1992.

Remy-Jardin M, et al: Diagnosis of pulmonary embolism with spiral CT: comparison with pulmonary angiography and scintigraphy. Radiology *200*:699, 1996.

Rosso J, et al: Intravenous digital subtraction angiography and lung imaging: compared value in the diagnosis of pulmonary embolism. Clin Nucl Med *14*:183, 1989.

van Erkel AR, et al: Spiral CT angiography for suspected pulmonary embolism: a cost-effectiveness analysis. Radiology *201*:29, 1996.

Clinical Validity of "Low Probability" on Normal Ventilation-Perfusion Scans

Hull RD, et al: Clinical validity of normal perfusion lung scan in patients with suspected pulmonary embolism. Chest *97*:23, 1990.

Kahn D, et al: Clinical outcome of patients with a "low probability" of pulmonary embolism on ventilation-perfusion lung scan. Arch Intern Med *149*:377, 1989.

Kipper MS, et al: Long-term follow-up of patients with suspected pulmonary embolism and a normal lung scan. Chest *82*:411, 1982.

Lee ME, et al: "Low-probability" ventilation-perfusion scintigrams: clinical outcomes in 99 patients. Radiology *156*:497, 1985.

SECTION IV

Diagnostic Procedures

CHAPTER 14

Laboratory Investigations in the Diagnosis of Pulmonary Diseases

Romeo A. Vidone and Claudia R. Libertin

The practice of pathology continues to evolve with the development of new techniques. In the chest, and in the lung in particular, the pathologist is being asked to increase diagnostic skills with smaller specimens, as newer techniques such as immunohistochemistry, DNA probes, x-ray microanalysis, flow cytometry, and polymerase chain reaction (PCR) are added to the traditional pathologic, cytologic, and microbiological methods. Also, a population of immunosuppressed patients with resultant opportunistic infections who require a rapid and accurate diagnosis is challenging diagnostic methods. Rosai (1996a) provides a summary of the many special techniques currently available in surgical pathology.

TISSUE SPECIMENS

Tissue specimens for diagnostic purposes are obtained from three general categories of procedures: open lung biopsy, and at times anatomic resection; video-assisted thoracic surgical or thoracoscopic lung biopsy; and bronchoscopic transbronchial lung biopsy or transthoracic needle biopsy. Each approach has advantages and disadvantages, and each requires the careful selection of patients to provide the most effective results with the least risk.

A coordinated approach among physicians is required in the diagnosis of chest diseases. A synthesis of the radiologic and clinical findings generates a differential diagnosis and helps the surgeon determine the method and site of tissue acquisition. The pathologist depends on the input of the radiologist, pulmonologist, and surgeon to provide basic clinical information. This information guides proper handling of the specimen and an assessment of the representative nature of the material received so that a correct diagnosis can be made expeditiously.

Frozen Section

Frozen section diagnosis may be helpful and necessary in a number of situations. In confirmed or suspected neoplastic disease, accurate intraoperative diagnosis and staging guide the surgeon in determining the optimal operative strategy. This information determines the extent of the resection and the need for additional biopsy material, as discussed by Miller (1995), Miller and Evans (1995), and Rosai (1996b). In the nonneoplastic case, an immediate, specific diagnosis may be important for the acutely ill patient, especially the immunocompromised host, because of the potential for a rapidly progressive, life-threatening, acute pneumonic process. Stains for infectious organisms can be done on frozen section material or tissue smears and may allow prompt institution of specific antimicrobial therapy. The frozen section also aids in determining the need for additional studies and the selection of appropriate fixation and processing in special cases, as recommended by Katzenstein and Askin (1997).

Open Lung Biopsy and Video-Assisted Thoracic Surgical Lung Biopsy

Among the three methods for lung biopsy (i.e., open lung biopsy, video-assisted thoracic surgical, and transbronchial lung biopsy) open lung biopsy has the highest diagnostic yield but is the most invasive. Video-assisted thoracic surgical biopsy is gaining in favor because it results in less morbidity and is reliable for sampling peripheral diffuse lung diseases. Reports indicate that tissue can be obtained equivalent to that obtained in open lung biopsy, and the diagnostic yield appears to rival open lung biopsy, as reported by Miller (1992), Bensard (1993), Kadokura (1995), and Allen (1996) and their associates.

Biopsy Site

The question of the appropriate site of biopsy has created controversy since the report of Gaensler and Carrington (1980) who maintained that the lingula and middle lobe tip should be avoided. Studies by Wetstein (1986) and Miller and associates (1987) have shown no reason to avoid the lingula and right middle lobe. In fact, Gianoulis and Wright (1990) and Neuman and associates (1985) suggest avoiding the tip of any lobe other than the lingula (see Chapter 91). Mathieson and colleagues (1989) have pointed out that conventional and high-resolution computed tomography (CT) of the chest has proved to be highly effective in selecting the appropriate biopsy site in all forms of chronic interstitial and infiltrative lung disease, especially in the immunocompromised host.

The samples selected by the surgeon should cover different degrees of involvement by the disease process; moderately abnormal sites in diffuse lung disease, and the most abnormal regions with localized or patchy lung or pleural disease. When nodular densities are present, the surgeon should remove the entire nodule rather than removing a biopsy from the edge. A good general rule regarding the number of biopsies is to select two or three samples of approximately 3×2×1 cm.

Handling of the Specimen

The specimen should be sent to the laboratory immediately. When received in the laboratory, the tissue should be carefully handled because the handling of unfixed tissue can result in confusing artifacts. A new scalpel or new razor blade should be used for sectioning. The first consideration is frozen section. This is done for diagnosis, to determine the adequacy of the specimen, or for special techniques. Portions of the tissue should be sent to the microbiology laboratory for culture, if indicated. Direct smears can be made for immediate use or saved to be assessed later. If sufficient tissue is available, a portion can be placed in glutaraldehyde for electron microscopy or quick frozen in liquid nitrogen. The remainder is immediately fixed in formalin. Additional studies, such as special stains, immunohistochemistry, immunofluorescence, and electron microscopy, can be considered after review of the frozen and permanent sections. It cannot be emphasized too strongly that sufficient tissue should be available for routine light microscopy.

Ideally, lung tissue should be inflated before fixation, because the difference between collapsed and distended lung often materially aids in the interpretation of the specimen. With wedge lung biopsies this is difficult to achieve, but a simple technique is to inject the specimen with fixative using a thin-gauge needle, being careful not to overdistend the tissue. The tissue is then submerged in fixative for an appropriate period. Methods to accomplish this have been described by Dail (1994), Carrington and Gaensler (1978),

Churg (1983), Miller and Evans (1995), Thurlbeck (1995), and Katzenstein and Askin (1997).

TRANSBRONCHIAL LUNG BIOPSY

Transbronchial biopsy via bronchoscopy is the least invasive of the biopsy procedures. The bronchoscopist usually submits three to five pieces of tissue, each measuring approximately 1 to 2 mm in size, placed immediately in fixative and sends material for culture directly to the microbiology laboratory. All of the tissue fragments are embedded for permanent sections. Usually no attempt is made to provide aliquots for special studies because of the small volume of tissue available. The bronchoscopist should also biopsy any visible bronchial lesion or unusual appearing bronchial mucosa because this may provide valuable information. In addition, diagnostic accuracy can be improved when bronchial brushings and washings are added. The greatest yield with this technique is in patients with specific histologic features in a bronchovascular distribution, as described by Miller and Evans (1995). The highest yield is found with conditions such as sarcoidosis, malignancy, and some infections. However, Mathieson and associates (1989) have pointed out that with proper selection of patients based on CT findings, diagnostic material can be obtained in many cases of diffuse infiltrative disease.

Although important in all lung biopsies, the clinical and radiographic findings are essential in the interpretation of the small amount of material available for examination. Multiple sections of this material must be examined and, when indicated, appropriate stains for microorganisms should be applied. Brown-Brenn, Ziehl-Neilsen, Grocott's, Gomori's methenamine silver, and a variety of others can be equally informative. The interpretation of this material requires that the pathologist be familiar with common artifacts associated with this procedure, as has been described by Katzenstein and Askin (1997).

An important consideration is the determination of the adequacy of the specimen. Katzenstein and Askin (1997) consider at least one fragment of alveolated lung parenchyma as adequate, but Fraire and associates (1992) have suggested that 20 alveoli are necessary to consider the biopsy adequate.

ANATOMIC LUNG RESECTION

Resected specimens of segments, lobes, or lungs are handled in several ways depending on the diagnostic considerations, as discussed by Spencer (1985), Miller (1995), and Wang (1994). The majority of these specimens are obtained when neoplasm is suspected or proven. Communication between the surgeon and the pathologist is essential for the proper handling of the specimen so that any special considerations can be given to the examination of the specimen. If a diagnosis has not been established and neoplasm is suspected, a frozen section may be requested. If the lesion is malignant, additional material may be obtained from the margins of resection, lymph nodes, and any other areas of concern. If the lesion may be infectious, sterile cultures must be obtained before any possible contamination of the specimen occurs.

If the diagnosis is not clear, cultures and special procedures may be necessary. If asbestosis is a consideration, tissue samples for asbestos digestion should be taken; 3 to 5 g of tissue per site should be adequate. The routine fixative is formalin, which is satisfactory for general use; however, under special circumstances other fixatives should be considered as discussed by Rosai (1996b), Miller and Evans (1995), Dail (1994), and Schmidt (1983).

For routine studies, inflation of the lung, lobe, or segment should be carried out. Inflation of the lung provides the best pathologic description, tissue sampling, and photographs. The method of fixation and cutting we follow is the one used by the late A. A. Liebow at Yale, and used by one of us (R.A.V.) (1955, personal communication) and many of Liebow's former trainees in their subsequent practices. The method consists of placing a large container of formalin approximately 1.0 to 1.5 ft above the specimen with an attached tube. This gravity flow method allows for a pressure 3040 mm of water, which does not significantly affect the structure of the lung. The tube is placed in the proximal bronchus, held in place with a loose tie, and formalin is allowed to flow into the specimen until maximally inflated. It may be necessary to use a smaller catheter inserted into more distal bronchi or other inflation techniques to fill certain regions of lung beyond bronchial obstructions or areas compromised by prior incisions. The specimen is then placed in a pan of formalin and covered with formalin-soaked cotton or paper towel to protect the exposed areas. We recommend fixation for 24 hours; however, several hours of fixation may be adequate if same-day processing is necessary. After adequate fixation, metal probes are placed in two adjacent bronchi in the plane of the significant lesion. A long sharp knife is placed at a 45-degree angle against the probes. Pressure is applied and the cut is made using clean steady sweeps of the knife extending through the pleura. This results in the bronchi being bisected, and the intervening lung tissue is cut in a flat plane. The process is repeated until all of the bronchi have been opened and the pertinent lesion is exposed. For photography, the tissue can be placed in absolute alcohol for 10 to 20 minutes to enhance the color. Another equally satisfactory method is to cut down the two bronchi with scissors. The intervening lung tissue is then planed off with a sharp knife, giving a flat surface. This process is then repeated in the adjacent bronchi and intervening lung tissue.

An alternative method of sectioning, which may be preferred for correlation with radiographs, is to cut the lung with a sharp knife at 1-cm intervals producing sagittal sections. This process may go from lateral to medial, corresponding to a lateral chest film, or coronal slices from anterior to posterior corresponding to a posteroanterior chest radiograph, or horizontal slices corresponding to a CT scan. The choice of technique depends on the clinical and radiologic findings and special interest in the result.

Special techniques are available for demonstrating vascular and bronchial abnormalities. These methods are applied in unfixed lobectomy and pneumonectomy specimens and are adequately described by Spencer (1985) and Dail (1994). One technique, originally described by Liebow and associates (1947), using plastic with subsequent corrosion of tissues to study pulmonary, bronchial, and coronary arteries and their relationships was used by one of us (R.A.V.) and Liebow (1957) to study the collateral circulation of the lung. A disadvantage is the loss of tissue for routine processing. Another method using radiopaque material with colored gelatin has been used in our laboratory with some success to fill vessels and other hollow structures. This technique does not interfere with the specimen because it can be inflated with formalin through the bronchi, and routine sectioning and processing can be carried out. Many of these special techniques are used mainly on autopsy material.

CYTOPATHOLOGY AND DIAGNOSIS OF INFECTIOUS DISEASE

Sputum

Sputum consists of a mixture of mucus, exfoliated epithelial cells from the upper and lower respiratory tract, inflammatory cells, and debris. An adequate specimen must contain alveolar macrophages. Clinicians traditionally rely on the results of routine microscopy and culture of sputum to establish an etiologic diagnosis in pneumonia. A consensus impression is that management of pulmonary infections is simplified and optimal when an etiologic agent is identified, although considerable controversy exists regarding what extent diagnostic resources should be used to establish this goal, especially with invasive techniques that are performed at some risk to the patient. With the advent of bronchoscopy and fine-needle aspiration (FNA), the use of sputum for the diagnosis of cancer has declined. Therefore, the discussion of bronchoscopic techniques mainly centers on the diagnosis of pneumonias.

When neoplasm is suspected, however, sputum samples should be deep cough specimens taken in the early morning and collected over several days. In many cases, induced specimens may be necessary, which contain more and better preserved cells and increase the yield of cancer cells. The specimen can be sent directly to the laboratory or placed in an alcohol-based preservative. In the laboratory, two or more sets of slides are made and stained with the Papanicolaou's technique. We also stain with hematoxylin and eosin and Wright-Giemsa, and when sufficient material is available a cell block preparation is also made that is processed as tissue. The latter increases the cost but allows for special stains to be carried out and subsequently increases the yield.

Bronchial Brushings and Bronchial Lavage

Both in the immunocompetent and in the immunocompromised host, fiberoptic bronchoscopy is the preferred method for diagnosing a wide variety of localized and diffuse lung diseases (see Chapter 91). Bronchial brushings should be performed before bronchial biopsy to avoid contamination of the specimen with blood. The usual method consists of brushing the bronchial mucosa with the brush and rolling the brush over the central two-thirds of a microscopic slide and fixing it immediately in 95% alcohol or other suitable fixative. The slides are sent to the laboratory in fixative to be processed as for sputum.

For the diagnosis of infections (pneumonias), Bartlett and associates (1998) favor the use of bronchoscopic techniques in patients with fulminant clinical courses who require admission to the intensive care unit, patients who have complex pneumonias that are unresponsive to antimicrobial therapy, and in severely immunosuppressed patients. The two diagnostic procedures most frequently used to obtain lower respiratory tract secretions during bronchoscopy in evaluating a patient with an infiltrate are the protected specimen brush and bronchoalveolar lavage (BAL), as advocated by Allen and associates (1994).

Protected Specimen Brush

As pointed out by Meduri and Baselski (1991), bronchoscopy itself may cause contamination of the lower respiratory tract. Specialized procedures have been continuously under investigation to minimize bacterial contamination of bronchoscopic samples. Fiberoptic bronchoscopy technique uses a protected specimen brush to obtain lower airway secretions for microbial culture. The protected specimen brush consists of a telescoping double catheter that houses a sterile brush that can be extended beyond the distal end of the telescoped catheter. The outer cannula is occluded distally by a gelatin or wax plug that is expelled, as the brush is extended into the infected lung segment; thus, contamination of the brush by upper airway flora is minimized. The apparatus is applied through the operating channel of a standard fiberoptic bronchoscope as described by Allen and associates (1994).

Because the protected brush also may be somewhat contaminated by oropharyngeal bacteria, studies by Baker (1995) and Pollock (1983) and their colleagues used quantitative cultures to differentiate oropharyngeal contamination from pneumonia. Pulmonary pathogens were present in concentrations greater than 10^3 CFU/mL among patients diagnosed with pneumonia, based on clinical response to antibiotics or positive blood culture results. Because less invasive measures are often more practical, available, and less expensive for nonintubated patients, the focus of this

technique has centered on intensive care unit patients, particularly for the diagnosis of ventilator-associated pneumonia.

Bronchoalveolar Lavage

Clinicians have used BAL for many decades to diagnose a variety of pulmonary diseases (see Chapter 16). As pointed out by Allen and associates (1994), BAL samples a larger and more representative volume of respiratory secretions than does the protected specimen brush and allows for an immediate specimen for analysis. Special stains of the cytocentrifuged specimen allow for early evaluation of the clinical material. Pingleton and coworkers (1992) propose other testing that includes the percentage of inflammatory cells (macrophages and neutrophils) containing intracellular organisms (percent), the percentage of squamous epithelial cells as an indicator of oropharyngeal contamination, stains for recognition of specific microorganisms (Gram's stain, acid-fast stain, potassium hydroxide stain and methenamine-silver stain), as well as cytologic evaluation. Other potential advantages of BAL include avoidance of the expense of specialized equipment and minimal risk of pneumothorax and alveolar hemorrhage, as compared with the protected specimen brush.

For the diagnosis of lower respiratory tract infections per se, the role of BAL has been best defined in diagnosing *Pneumocystis carinii* pneumonia in patients with acquired immunodeficiency syndrome (AIDS) and in patients with pulmonary tuberculosis (see Chapter 91). Thorpe and colleagues (1987), as well as Kahn and Jones (1987), have found a use for BAL in conducting research and in the diagnosis of bacterial pneumonias. Unlike the generally accepted protocol using the protected brush specimen, less standardization exists for the lavage technique and processing of the BAL specimen.

Protected Specimen Brush versus Bronchoalveolar Lavage: Which Procedure Is Better for the Diagnosis of Bacterial Pneumonia?

In determining which procedure has a greater diagnostic accuracy in the diagnosis of bacterial pneumonia, studies that directly compare quantitative cultures obtained by both methods are most relevant (Table 14-1). However, no large definitive study has established the protected specimen brush or BAL to be superior over the other for the diagnosis of bacterial pneumonia. Baker and associates (1995) believe that current data do not suggest that either technique offers greater diagnostic accuracy. The comparative advantages of the procedures are shown in Table 14-2.

It should be emphasized that the routine use of quantitative invasive diagnostic techniques to retrieve lower respiratory tract secretions in the evaluation of patients with suspected pneumonia remains an area of controversy. Routine fiberoptic bronchoscopy and quantitative culture is not necessary for the majority of cases of community-acquired pneumonia in immunocompetent patients. On the other hand, the Infectious

Table 14-1. Studies that Compare Protected Specimen Brush and Bronchoalveolar Lavage in Ventilator-Associated Pneumonia

Study	No. with Pneumonia	Protected Specimen Brush Sensitivity/ Specificity; Threshold	Bronchoalveolar Lavage Sensitivity/ Specificity; Threshold	Accepted Standard
Chastre and Fagon (1994)	5	100/100; 10^3	60/85; 10^4	Positive pleural culture; cavitation by radiography, histology
Sole-Violan et al. (1993)	25	64/100; 10^3	76/100; 10^5	Quantitative cultures from either procedure
Timsit et al. (1995)	65	74/88; 10^3	82/88; 10^4	Clinical, positive fluid or lung cultures, cavitation by radiography, histology
Chastre et al. (1995)	11	82/89; 10^3	91/78; 10^4	Quantitative biopsy culture
Marquette et al. (1995)	19	57/88; 10^3	47/100; 10^4	Autopsy
Papazian et al. (1995)	18	42/95; 10^3	58/95; 10^4	Autopsy

Diseases Society of America (1998), as reported by Bartlett and colleagues (1998), proposes that quantitative bronchoscopy cultures be considered in patients with fulminant clinical courses, patients who are unresponsive to antimicrobial therapy, and patients who are severely immunosuppressed, irrespective of whether the pneumonia was community or nosocomially acquired or whether patients are mechanically ventilated or spontaneously breathing.

These procedures should not be performed and applied in isolation. The significance of the cultures should always be interpreted in the clinical context of the patient. The use of a specific threshold to define the presence of pneumonia does not take into account the fact that lung infections occur along a bacteriologic continuum. As noted by the American Thoracic Society (1996), diagnostic thresholds therefore may not be met with patients during early infection and patients who are receiving or who have recently received antibiotics. It also may be unacceptable to withhold therapy from patients when the clinical suspicion of infection is high, even if invasive methods show less than 10^3 CFU/mL by the protected specimen brush or less than 10^4 CFU/mL by BAL.

Precise methodology should be closely followed for specimen procurement by the bronchoscopist and specimen processing by the microbiologist. Adhering to these principles probably has the best influence on the diagnostic accuracy of these procedures. Finally, the majority of these techniques have been studied in severely ill, mechanically ventilated patients with nosocomial pneumonia. Extrapolating these findings to other patient populations may not be valid.

Pleural Fluid

When a pleural effusion is associated with a pulmonary process, examination of the fluid may provide a unifying malignant or infectious diagnosis (Fig. 14-1). As in other biopsy and aspiration procedures, basic clinical information and the differential diagnosis along with clinical laboratory findings, such as specific gravity, protein content, and any other chemistry values, improve efficiency and allow for the optimal use of resources. Fluid obtained by thoracentesis should be collected in a sterile container and sent directly to the laboratory. Aliquots are centrifuged. The supernatant is discarded and the sediment is used to prepare direct smears, cytocentrifuged preparations, or monolayer slides. A set of at least six slides is useful. The slides are alcohol fixed and

Table 14-2. Protected Specimen Brush Versus Bronchoalveolar Lavage: Quantitative Cultures for the Diagnosis of Bacterial Pneumonia

Relative advantages of bronchoalveolar lavage
  Samples a larger area with less risk for pneumothorax or alveolar hemorrhage
  Immediate specimen for analysis
    Specimens also may be processed for opportunistic pathogens such as *Pneumocystis carinii*, *Mycobacterium tuberculosis*, and nontuberculous mycobacteria
Relative advantages of the protected specimen brush
  Greater standardization of the procurement and processing of respiratory specimens
  Optimal threshold of quantitative cultures to diagnose pneumonia better defined

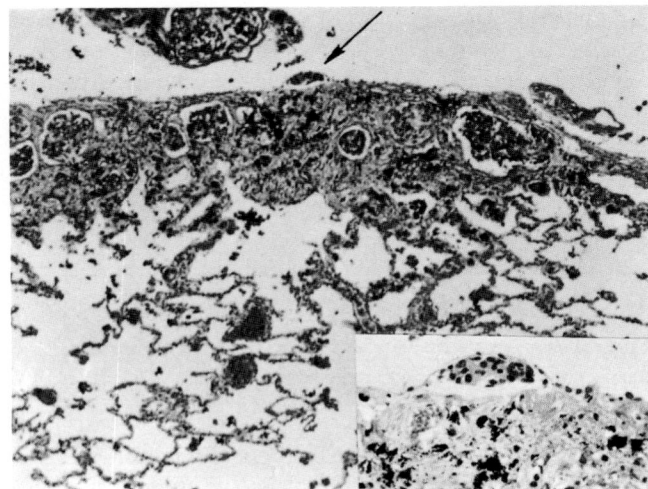

Fig. 14-1. Secondary carcinoma in subpleural lymphatics (*arrow*). Groups of tumor cells shed from this surface can be identified from centrifuged pleural fluid. (Inset) Clump of tumor cells immediately beneath pleural mesothelial membrane.

stained with Papanicolaou's technique, hematoxylin and eosin, and with Wright-Giemsa, especially if hematologic malignancy is suspected. Additional slides are also prepared for possible bacterial, fungal, and acid-fast stains. The remaining buttons of material are fixed and submitted as cell block preparations for histologic study.

Fine-Needle Aspiration Biopsy

Since the 1960s, the application of transthoracic FNA biopsy has steadily increased. FNA is especially useful in the evaluation of focal nodules or masses of the lung and pleura. The history and development of this technique and excellent results have been the subject of many reports. Of special interest are those of Tao (1988), Austin and Cohen (1993), Westcott (1980), and Stevens and Jackman (1984). FNA of the lung is most beneficial in patients who are spared a more invasive surgical procedure, such as when a nonresectable malignancy, metastases, or a nonsurgical disease is found, or establishing the diagnosis in a patient who refuses surgery or for whom surgery is medically contraindicated. The most common complication of this procedure is pneumothorax, which was reported to occur in 21 to 34% of patients by Austin and Cohen (1993), with only some 10% requiring treatment as noted by Stevens and Jackman (1984), Austin and Cohen (1993), and Westcott (1980).

Using CT, fluoroscopy, or ultrasound guidance, FNA is usually performed by radiologists. Early excellent results in the diagnosis of neoplasm as well as infectious diseases have been confirmed by many reports, as summarized by Tao (1988) and Das and associates (1992). Qadri and Ali (1991) have reported its value in the diagnosis of tuberculosis and Raab and colleagues (1993) for pulmonary coccidioidomycosis.

The value of a cytopathologist or cytotechnologist in attendance during the procedure has been emphasized by Austin and Cohen (1993). This allows for the immediate evaluation of the material for adequacy and one can then proceed with processing for any additional studies such as culture. After the smears are prepared, the material is rinsed in fixative; the sample can be processed as cytospins, thin layer preparations, and formalin-fixed cell blocks. The cell blocks are routinely examined histologically and in our experience can prove invaluable, in some cases, in improving diagnostic accuracy and providing material for special stains and immunohistochemistry.

SEROLOGIC TECHNIQUES FOR ESTABLISHING PRESENCE OF INFECTION*

Serologic methods are classified broadly into those techniques that detect microbial antigens and those that detect

the host antibody response to microbial infection. Serologic techniques depend on the use of immunoglobulins for the detection of antigens, as well as identification of circulating host antibody. Examples of an antigenic assay would be the latex agglutination assay used in the detection of cryptococcal antigen in the cerebral spinal fluid of patients with cryptococcal meningitis. Quantification of antigen assays is not imperative; in most cases, the demonstration of microbial antigen is sufficient to make a diagnosis of infection.

In contrast, quantitative serologic assay of patient antibody status is vitally important to distinguish active from past infection. Quantification is usually performed by serial dilution and reported as titers (i.e., 1:4, 1:256). Active infection usually results in high titer, such as 1:256, and an increase in titer, typically fourfold or greater in a patient previously exposed to the microbe. Two time points are necessary to make this determination, and serum is taken during the active phase and the convalescence phase for this comparison. Furthermore, assay of the class of antibody can be important, because immunoglobulin M (IgM) class antibodies are typical of the early humoral immunologic response, whereas IgG antibody response indicates long-standing immunity from previous encounter with the microbial antigen.

A daunting number of assays are used for the evaluation of the humoral response to microbial infection. The most commonly performed include complement fixation, indirect hemagglutination, direct and indirect immunofluorescence, enzyme-linked immunosorbent assay, radioimmunoassay, and immunodiffusion. The relative merits of each of these specific techniques are not particularly important to the clinician except insofar as they all represent tools to evaluate the humoral status of the patient vis-à-vis a specific microbe.

MOLECULAR BIOLOGICAL METHODS IN ESTABLISHING THE ORIGIN OF DISEASE

The application of these methods to clinical microbiology is revolutionizing the field. Some familiarity with the basic concepts behind these techniques enhances the clinician's understanding and interpretation of test results derived from these methods. DNA hybridization is the technique whereby DNA probes consisting of genetic material complementary to that of a specific organism are annealed to the native DNA of the organism of interest. Probes consist of oligonucleotides complementary to a segment in the microbe's genome and are extremely specific for each microbial species. The probe is tagged to allow detection, usually with a radioactive isotope, but attention is focusing on the development of nonradiometric probes that are more convenient and safer to use. Hybridization with DNA probes finds two primary applications in the clinical microbiology laboratory. Traditionally, hybridization has been used to speciate organisms from culture, such as mycobacteria. More recently, DNA probes have been applied with success directly to clinical specimens, including blood cultures.

*The remainder of the text has been added by the Senior Editor from a revision and update of Chapter 15 by Herbert B. Sommers and K. Eric Sommers in the fourth edition.

PCR is the process whereby minute quantities of genetic material can be expanded literally a billion-fold. The technique of PCR is actually easy to understand in concept, if not application. The specimen containing the organism of interest, and, obviously, its DNA, is incubated with 1) a DNA primer specific to the organism; 2) the building blocks of DNA, the nucleotide bases; and 3) a heat-sensitive polymerase that replicates DNA, given the right conditions and primer. Each cycle of PCR involves the replication of the DNA segment encoded by the primer, a process analogous to DNA replication during cell division. Because the polymerase is heat sensitive, the process can be halted and restarted simply by raising and lowering the incubation temperature. Thus, the process is easily cycled, and with each cycle, the DNA is replicated; events quickly assume a geometric quality, hence the chain reaction. Therein lies the enormous potential for expansion of the genetic material.

Restriction fragment length polymorphism, or DNA fingerprinting, is another technique that is applied to the identification and speciation of organisms. In this technique, DNA is cleaved with a specific restriction endonuclease and the resulting fragments are separated by gel electrophoresis. The pattern of fragment lengths is remarkably specific between species and even between individuals. Restriction fragment length polymorphism has been used in forensic medicine and has been used to identify attackers in rape cases. Molecular biology techniques and their application to infectious disease have been reviewed by Figueroa and Rasheed (1991).

Thus, molecular techniques are impressive by virtue of their remarkable sensitivity and specificity. These qualities, however, give rise to new problems relating to the interpretation of such exquisitely sensitive data. This problem is illustrated by Delgado and colleagues (1992), who prospectively studied blood samples from 24 liver transplant recipients using PCR and standard viral cultures for cytomegalovirus (CMV). They found that PCR was able to detect CMV DNA in the blood of all eight patients who developed symptomatic CMV illness, but PCR also detected CMV viremia in 9 of 24 patients who did not show evidence of virus from blood culture and did not have symptomatic disease. Thus, the sensitivity of PCR compared with culture was 100%, the specificity was 76%, but the positive predictive value was only 25%. The significance of PCR-positive culture and symptom-negative result is not known, and it is likely that such interpretive problems will be encountered as PCR gains wider clinical use.

SPECIFIC LABORATORY IDENTIFICATION OF VARIOUS INFECTIOUS AGENTS

Legionella

In July 1976, a strange and virulent form of pneumonia struck 182 members of the Pennsylvania branch of the American Legion during their annual meeting in Philadelphia; 18 legionnaires died. During the next 6 months, an intensive investigation resulted in the isolation of a new, completely different bacterial organism, now known as *Legionella pneumophila*. This organism differs from other medically significant bacteria in that it does not stain by Gram's method and is unique in having an absolute growth requirement for cysteine. An adequate amount of this compound to grow *Legionella* is not present in blood agar, chocolate agar, or other types of primary culture media. The organism also requires an increased concentration of CO_2 for growth and may take 7 to 12 days to appear on artificial culture media. The organism grows best on buffered charcoal yeast extract supplemented with α-ketoglutarate.

Stout and coworkers (1982) showed that the isolation of *L. pneumophila* and related species initially from the water in air-conditioning cooling towers and subsequently from the faucets, shower heads, and hot water storage tanks in hospitals emphasizes the ubiquitousness of this group of organisms. Because the organisms are widespread, it is clear that mere exposure to contaminated water is an insufficient condition for the occurrence of legionnaire's disease; host susceptibility is undoubtedly a critical factor. Patients undergoing immunosuppression for organ transplantation or other therapeutic reasons are at high risk and should be followed carefully for the sudden onset of severe and rapidly developing pneumonia.

Clinically, the disease may occur in epidemics, such as was seen in Philadelphia, or as sporadic cases acquired in the community. As noted by Balows and Fraser (1979), it has been recognized as a major cause of serious or fatal pneumonia in immunosuppressed or immunodefective patients, many of whom develop the disease while in the hospital.

The laboratory diagnosis of *Legionella* is based on rapid methods, culture, and serology. The serologic diagnosis of *Legionella* depends on development of convalescent titers and thus is not useful for diagnosis of acute disease. An exception is the demonstration of high titers (i.e., 1:256 or greater) during the acute disease that is indicative of active infection, particularly because symptomatic carriage does not occur, and reinfection with *Legionella* does not appear to be common. Culture is the most specific diagnostic method, but it has limited sensitivity and requires at least 2 days and maybe more.

Thus, to guide therapy, rapid methods for the diagnosis of *Legionella* have evolved. The technique used most widely is direct fluorescence antibody staining of sputum specimens; direct fluorescence antibody staining is rapid but suffers from a lack of sensitivity, usually approximately 60 to 75%. Other rapid methods include nucleic acid hybridization probes and detection of antigen in urine, sputum, or serum. Hybridization probes are specific and are considered by Rodgers and Pascule (1985) as acceptable alternatives to the direct fluorescence antibody. A nonradiometric hybridization technique has been developed by Fain and coworkers (1991). Assays for *Legionella* antigen in urine, sputum, and serum samples include enzyme-linked immunosorbent assay, latex agglutination, and radioimmunoassay techniques. These methods continue to be evaluated and may be used more widely in the future.

Nocardia

Nocardia is an aerobic filamentous bacterium belonging to the order Actinomycetales. Because they exhibit many of the morphologic characteristics of fungi in culture, such as aerial hyphae, they have been classified in the past as fungi. *Nocardia asteroides*, the predominant pathogenic species, is recognized as a significant opportunistic pathogen in immunosuppressed patients. The lung is the usual site of introduction for *Nocardia*, where it can cause a wide spectrum of histologic injury from minimal infiltration to abscess formation and necrotizing pneumonitis. Disseminated disease can follow lung infection and can progress to abscess formation in the brain. Sinus tract formation is a characteristic trait of disseminated *Nocardia* infection, with tracts forming from the mediastinum or from satellite abscesses in subcutaneous tissue and skin from hematogenous spread. *Nocardia* is a relatively more common opportunistic pathogen in cardiac transplant patients in particular, but is seen rarely in patients with AIDS for unknown reasons.

Diagnosis of this bacterial infection is based on demonstration of the organism in culture or by staining. Figure 14-2 illustrates a Gram-stained section of material taken from a pulmonary abscess caused by *N. asteroides*. Because *N. asteroides* is not stained by hematoxylin or eosin or the periodic acid–Schiff stain, it cannot be recognized unless Gram's stain or a methenamine silver stain is used. Although some stains of *Nocardia* may show an ability to retain an acid-fast or auramine stain, smears or sections have to be decolorized by a milder solution of acid, 1% sulfuric versus 3% hydrochloric. The ability to identify *Nocardia* in acid-fast and auramine-stained specimens varies considerably between different strains. *Nocardia* grows well on media for bacteria, fungi, and mycobacteria, and no special media are required for its recovery. Serologic assays are under development. Kjelstrom and Beaman (1993) developed a serologic panel to identify *N. asteroides* infection in a murine model, and Salinas-Carmona and colleagues (1993) developed a solid-phase enzyme-linked immunosorbent assay to confirm the diagnosis of *Nocardia brasiliensis* in human mycetoma cases. At present, however, serologic testing for *Nocardia* is not widely used in clinical practice.

Mycobacteria

Before the discovery of streptomycin and other chemotherapeutic agents, the diagnosis of tuberculosis was made on the basis of the clinical picture, a radiograph of the

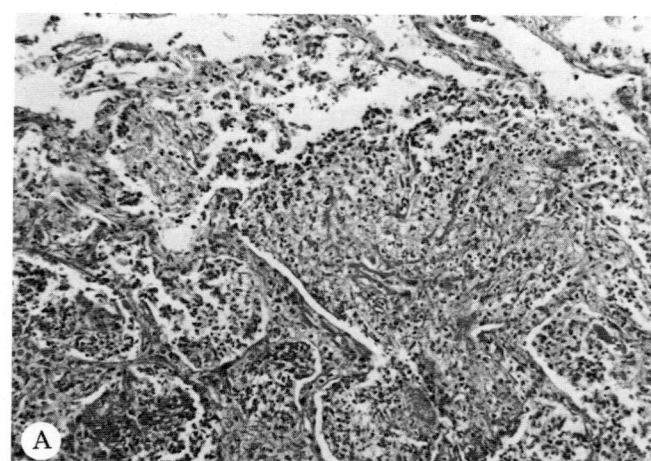

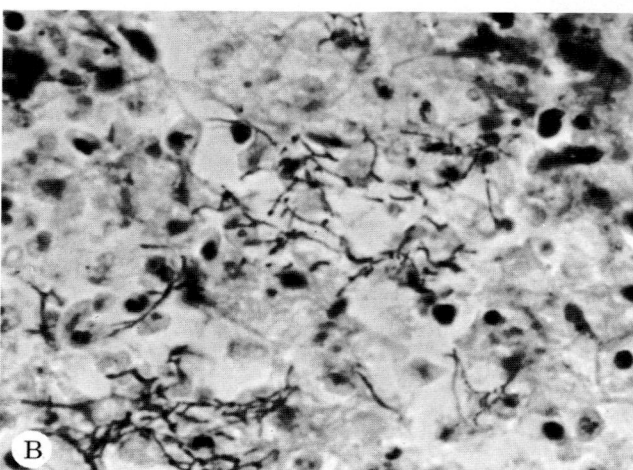

Fig. 14-2. Pulmonary abscess caused by *Nocardia asteroides*. The nocardial infections cause suppuration with abscess formation. **A.** Section stained with hematoxylin and eosin or periodic acid–Schiff does not demonstrate the organism. **B.** Gram-stained section shows thin, branching rods (original magnification ×650).

chest compatible with that of tuberculosis, and the demonstration of acid-fast bacilli in the sputum. With the development of antituberculous drugs, however, it became necessary to isolate the organism so that drug susceptibility studies could be made and resistance could be detected. As more cultures were made, variant strains from the typical type of organism (i.e., *Mycobacterium tuberculosis*) responsible for tuberculosis in human beings were found. In 1954, Timpe and Runyon described 100 such stains, proposing a grouping for atypical organisms. At present, these organisms are referred to as *mycobacteria other than tuberculosis*, popularized by Woods and Washington (1987), or as *nontuberculous mycobacteria* (NTM), used by Chester and Winn (1986), Contreras (1988), Fournier (1988), and their colleagues, among others, including Heifets (1997). The pathogenic or potentially pathogenic species of NTM are listed in Table 14-3.

Table 14-3. Major Pathogenic and Potentially Pathogenic Nontuberculous Mycobacteria

Photochromogens
    Mycobacterium kansasii
    Mycobacterium marinum
    Mycobacterium simiae
    Mycobacterium asiaticum
Scotochromogens
    Mycobacterium scrofulaceum
    Mycobacterium xenopi
    Mycobacterium szulgai
    Mycobacterium gordonae
Nonchromogens
    Mycobacterium avium
    Mycobacterium intracellulare
    Mycobacterium malmoense
    Mycobacterium ulcerans
    Mycobacterium paratuberculosis
    Mycobacterium haemophilum
    Mycobacterium genavense
Rapid growers
    Mycobacterium fortuitum
    Mycobacterium peregrinum
    Mycobacterium chelonei

Adapted from Heifets L: Mycobacteriology laboratory. Clin Chest Med *18*:35, 1997.

Specimen Collection in Pulmonary Tuberculosis

Sputum is the specimen most easily collected for use in making the diagnosis of pulmonary tuberculosis. A series of three to five early morning specimens is recommended because experience shows that the number of bacilli shed varies from day to day in patients excreting low numbers of organisms. This variation is probably related to intermittent focal ulceration of the bronchial mucosa, releasing different numbers of tubercle bacilli in the bronchi over irregular periods. Krasnow and Wayne (1969) showed that specimens collected by heated aerosol or nebulization after the patient arises in the morning produce positive culture results after shorter incubation times and with fewer contaminants than do specimens collected over 24 hours. The 24-hour specimens yielded more positive culture results, although they required longer incubation times and were more likely to be contaminated. Both types of specimens are of value. Collection at bronchoscopy of secretions for culture is best done by using bronchial washings or bronchial lavage, but these specimens should be processed immediately if local anesthetics have been used to facilitate passage of the bronchoscope. Bronchial brushes, used in collecting specimens for cytology, provide good specimens for culture. Note that after bronchoscopy, recovery of *Mycobacteria* increases in sputum specimens collected over the succeeding 24 to 48 hours. Early morning gastric aspiration for organisms swallowed during the night is recommended only for infants or children or for those patients whose sputum cannot be obtained naturally or by heated aerosol. The recovery of saprophytic, nonpathogenic species of *Mycobacteria* from

gastric aspirates can mislead the clinician until such time as identification of the organism is complete. In early stages of disseminated miliary tuberculosis, sputum specimens may not show the organism before invasion and ulceration of the bronchial tree. Demonstration or isolation of the organism in miliary tuberculosis may best be accomplished by liver biopsy, bone marrow aspiration, or, possibly, cerebrospinal fluid examination. Lung biopsy frequently is helpful.

Isolation of *M. tuberculosis* and other mycobacteria from sputum and other types of contaminated clinical specimens is facilitated by a digestion procedure to release mycobacteria from mucin, kill contaminating bacteria, and concentrate the number of mycobacteria to a smaller volume.

Inoculation of the concentrated specimen should be made to a minimum of two and preferably three different types of culture media, with an egg base (Lowenstein-Jensen) and an agar base (Middlebrook 7H11 agar), currently the most popular. Use of a third culture medium containing one or more antibiotics is strongly recommended to suppress nonmycobacterial organisms. Incubation of all media in 5 to 10% CO_2 results in an increased yield and rate of growth.

Stained smears of the concentrate should be made to search for the organism and to observe the numbers shed, an indication of the activity of the infection. Sputum smear results are positive for *Mycobacteria* in approximately 60 to 70% of specimens yielding positive culture results. Smears may be stained by one of the classic acid-fast techniques (e.g., Ziehl-Neelsen) or by a fluorochrome (e.g., auramine or a combination of auramine and rhodamine). The advantage of the fluorochrome stain is that it enables the microscopist to scan a larger field in a shorter period without loss of specificity. Although experienced microscopists may be able to tell different species of *Mycobacteria* by their shape on a stained smear, identifying characteristics are subtle and usually not dependable unless the observer sees many smears from patients with different species of *Mycobacteria*.

The complete identification of all mycobacterial isolates is almost mandatory, as the distinction between organisms known to cause disease and those not associated with disease is important in selecting proper therapy. Species identification can usually be accompanied by determining relatively few characteristics. Although the incidence of *M. tuberculosis* has continued to decline, except for a temporary increase in incidence during the mid-1980s until 1990, the incidence of disease from NTM is becoming more common.

The proper determination of antimycobacterial drug susceptibility is a highly technical and expensive procedure. Primary drug resistance of *M. tuberculosis*, defined as resistance by an organism to one or more drugs in a previously untreated patient, was thought to be less than 5%. Kopanoff and associates (1978), however, noted that a more widely selected group of patients has shown primary drug resistance of *M. tuberculosis* in 8 to 20% of isolates, depending on geographic location and ethnic group sampled. This previously unrecognized primary drug resistance of *M. tuberculosis* has suggested the need for more frequent routine determination of susceptibility studies than was considered necessary in the past. It is further emphasized that most patients with reactivation of *M. tuberculosis* who were previously treated may harbor resistant organisms. Last, NTM are primarily resistant to one or more of the standard mycobacterial agents.

New Methods for Identification of Mycobacteria

BACTEC Culture Technique

Development of radiometric procedures for the culture and identification of mycobacteria has revolutionized the field of mycobacteriology. Traditional techniques of identification relied on culture of the organism, often a painstakingly slow undertaking, and then the use of a battery of biochemical tests to elucidate the species to which an isolate would be assigned. In 1977, Middlebrook and associates described a broth culture medium (7H12) containing 1-^{14}C palmitic acid (i.e., BACTEC culture) that could be used for the detection of the growth of *M. tuberculosis*. The method relies on the measurement of ^{14}C-labeled CO_2 released during the metabolism of palmitic acid by mycobacteria in an ion chamber system (BACTEC, Johnston Laboratories, Towson, MD). Initial studies with the BACTEC system indicated that an inoculum of 200 viable units of *M. tuberculosis* could be detected in 12 to 14 days. The results led to further studies for the application of the technique to routine laboratory procedures to include detection, identification, and susceptibility testing with primary antituberculosis drugs by Siddiqi and associates (1981). A multicenter, collaborative study reported by Snider and colleagues (1981) found that although the results of drug susceptibility tests of *M. tuberculosis* with the radiometric and standard methods were similar, agreement was better with the BACTEC and the agar dilution procedure when comparing drug-susceptible strains than with drug-resistant strains. Overall, Siddiqi and associates (1981) found results with the new procedure were better when determined in a specialty laboratory for mycobacteria than in a routine clinical laboratory. Agreement for drug susceptibility testing between radiometric and standard agar dilution methods for *M. tuberculosis* was 95%. In addition, results were reportable on 98% of the tests in 5 days.

Using the BACTEC, *M. tuberculosis* usually can be detected rapidly in decontaminated clinical specimens by inoculation to a selective Middlebrook 7H12, a medium containing polymyxin B, amphotericin B, carbenicillin, and trimethoprim. Damato and colleagues (1983) showed that 70% of smear-positive specimens are culture positive in the radiometric procedure within 14 days, with or without the addition of polymyxin B, amphotericin B, carbenicillin, and trimethoprim to the medium, compared with 21 days by the standard procedure. Similarly, Morgan and associates (1983) found that detection times for recovery of *M. tuberculosis* from smear-negative specimens with radiometric

and conventional culture systems were 13.7 and 26.3 days, respectively. Radiometric and conventional culture procedures were approximately equivalent for the recovery of *M. tuberculosis* from 5375 clinical specimens, but Takahashi and Foster (1983) found the recovery of *Mycobacterium avium* complex was better using the radiometric procedure. In another collaborative study reported by Roberts and associates (1983) involving five laboratories, recovery and drug susceptibility tests of *M. tuberculosis* were completed in 18 days using the radiometric procedure, as opposed to 38.5 days for the conventional method.

Para-Nitro-α-Acetilamino-β-Hydroxy-Propiophonone Differentiation Test

Laszlo and Siddiqi (1984) described the use of para-nitro-α-acetilamino-β-hydroxy-propiophonone (NAP) to inhibit the growth of *M. tuberculosis* complex, but it does not inhibit the growth of NTM. This is a part of the BACTEC technology. Increase in the growth index in a NAP-free vial and its inhibition in a vial containing NAP indicates the presence of *M. tuberculosis*. Growth in both vials without any significant difference indicates the presence of NTM.

Cell-Wall Lipid Analysis

Three chromatographic methods have been proposed for speciation of mycobacteria on the basis of their cell-wall lipids: 1) gas-liquid chromatography reported by Tisdall and associates (1982), 2) high-performance high-pressure liquid chromatography described by Butler and colleagues (1991), and 3) thin-layer chromatography suggested by Jiminez and Larsson (1986). The techniques of these chromatographic methods as well as the pros and cons have been succinctly presented by Heifets (1997).

Nucleic Acid Probe

A commercially available probe (AccuProbe, Gen-Probe, San Diego, CA) for the identification of *M. tuberculosis* complex, *M. avium* complex, *Mycobacterium kansasii*, and *Mycobacterium gordonae* uses chemiluminescent acridinium ester-labeled single-stranded DNA probe complementary to the ribosomal RNA of the target bacteria. Again, the essential details have been described by Heifets (1997).

Polymerase Chain Reaction and Other Amplification Methods

The aforementioned PCR was suggested for the detection of *M. tuberculosis* by Eisenach and colleagues (1991), Forbes and Hicks (1993), and Shinnick and Jonas (1994), among others. According to Heifets (1997) the Roche Amplicon test includes four phases: 1) release of the DNA from bacteria in the specimen, 2) amplification, 3) hybridization of the amplified DNA sequences to the specific *M. tuberculosis* single-stranded DNA probe, and 4) detection. The process can result in a billion-fold amplification from each copy of a target DNA. The test, however, as pointed out by Heifets (1997), can only be used on new patients, has a false-negative result in 7% of patients and a false-positive result in 2%, and is limited to smear-positive sputum only because the sensitivity for smear-negative sputum can be only 70% or less. Thus, the use of PCR in the laboratory diagnosis of *M. tuberculosis* is actually quite limited.

The bacteriologic diagnosis of NTM (the photochromogens, scotochromogens, slowly growing nonchromogens, and rapidly growing mycobacteria), drug susceptibility testing, and the future trends in the laboratory investigation of mycobacteria are presented in Heifets' (1997) excellent review.

Fungal Infection of the Lung

The spectrum of fungal infection of the lung is shifting from the endemic, deep-seated infection, such as blastomycosis, to opportunistic infection with usually low pathogenic species, such as *Candida* and *Aspergillus*.

Fungal infection of the lung is best established by recovery of the infecting organism by culture. Morphologic changes in tissue biopsy specimens may be adequate to establish a diagnosis without culture. Histochemical staining, with periodic acid–Schiff, methenamine silver, mucicarmine, or Gram's stain, of histologic sections is helpful and may afford specific identification of different fungi. Monteagudo and associates (1995) have described an immunohistochemical staining method using a specific monoclonal antibody to identify *Candida albicans*. All too often, however, it is not possible to find pathognomonic organisms in the stained specimens and only a presumptive diagnosis can be made. Perhaps the two best stains for demonstration of fungi in tissue are periodic acid–Schiff and methenamine silver, but no one stain demonstrates all organisms.

Cultures of fungi can be made from tissues, sputum, pleural fluid, bronchial aspirates, or other clinical specimens. For optimal recovery, all specimens should be inoculated on several different types of culture media. Sabouraud's dextrose agar is an excellent general purpose culture medium. It is able to inhibit many strains of contaminating bacteria because its high dextrose content (4%) reduces the pH to 5.6. Specimens also should be inoculated to a second medium containing antibiotics and cycloheximide to suppress less fastidious bacteria and the contaminating molds. Because the cycloheximide and antibiotics in the second medium also inhibit certain pathogenic fungi, such as *Cryptococcus neoformans* and *Aspergillus fumigatus*, use of Sabouraud's or a similar noninhibitory agar should not be omitted. Sabouraud's medium should be incubated at both 25°C and 37°C, because different fungi may have varying rates of growth and different morphologic forms when grown at different temperatures. Fungi with more than one form are dimorphic, showing a yeastlike morphology at 37°C and a mycelial growth when incubated at

room temperature (i.e., 25°C). Examples of dimorphic fungi are *Histoplasma capsulatum*, *Blastomyces dermatitidis*, and *Sporothrix schenckii*. Growth of pathogenic fungi may take from 2 to 14 days, depending on the number of organisms present in the specimens and characteristics of the individual organism. For some fungi, unique growth requirements have led to special media. Any clinical information that may indicate the most likely organism helps in selecting the medium most likely to produce growth in the minimal time.

Members of the *Candida* and *Cryptococcus* species are easily identified by fermentation and carbohydrate assimilation tests. The use of several other biochemical tests in the speciation of fungi is helpful, but most pathogenic fungi are identified by morphologic characteristics noted on culture, such as septate or nonseptate mycelia, unique macroconidia or microconidia, and the gross and microscopic appearance of the growth nurtured on different types of media at 37°C and at room temperatures. Identification is usually made by examining portions of the culture under the microscope and by preparing small growing mounts, where the developing pattern of growth is followed by microscopic examination over several days. Some fungi lose certain of their specific features in culture, however, with the result that identification may take a prolonged period.

Serologic Tests

Many patients have had subclinical infections with different fungi, so a positive reaction to a serologic test for a fungal antigen in a random specimen may have little significance. To differentiate between an old and a current fungal infection on the basis of serologic tests, antibody titers are determined on serum obtained early in the course of the illness (i.e., acute phase) and at least 2 to 3 weeks later (i.e., convalescent phase). Laboratory precision in most serologic tests is seldom better than one dilution (twofold change) so that the results of most serologic tests should not be considered significant without an increase or decrease of at least two dilutions (fourfold change) such as any from ¼ to ¹⁄₁₆. In some patients, fungal infections may develop during immunosuppressive therapy for tumors or organ transplants. Both humoral and cellular immune responses may then be modified by drugs so that these responses to serologic tests may not be valid. Because of the infrequent need for such tests in most hospitals, requests for fungal serologic analysis are usually forwarded to municipal or state public health laboratories, resulting in some delay in obtaining the report. Direct communication with the reference laboratory usually hastens receipt of the report.

Of serologic tests for all the so-called deep fungal infections, those for blastomycosis are the least satisfactory. Cross-reactions with other antigens are most prone to occur. The immunodiffusion test for blastomycosis is specific, and a positive reaction can result in immediate treatment of the patient. The test has a sensitivity of approximately 80% and detects more blastomycosis than the complement fixation test. Negative test results do not exclude a diagnosis. In contrast to blastomycosis, the serologic diagnosis of histoplasmosis can be made by either of two types of serologic tests, depending on the stage of the illness. In the early phase of the disease, reaction to a latex agglutination test may be positive, probably because an IgM antibody is present. As the infection progresses, the reaction to the agglutination test fades and becomes negative. Somewhat later in the infection, complement-fixing antibodies develop; these correlate well with the activity of the disease. Titers of 1:8 and 1:16 may be considered presumptive evidence of histoplasmosis, whereas titers of 1:32 are highly suggestive of this infection. Cross-reactions with antigens from other fungi can occur in the complement fixation test and be misleading. In some patients, the antigenic stimulation from a skin test with histoplasmin may be sufficient to stimulate an increase in complement-fixing antibody titer, but usually not before 15 days. For this reason, the initial or acute serum for complement fixation studies should be obtained before skin tests are performed. Kaufman and Reiss (1985) found that if reaction to a skin test is positive in 72 hours, serum drawn for complement fixation does not reflect any change in titer at this time, although the possibility of an increase in the convalescent serum should be considered. Under these conditions, at least a fourfold or greater change in titer is needed to establish the diagnosis of active infection.

A microimmunodiffusion procedure is also recommended for detecting infection by *Histoplasma capsulatum*. The results are qualitative. Two precipitin bands have diagnostic value. One, designated *h*, is not influenced by skin testing and is consistently found in the serum of patients with active histoplasmosis. The second, designated *m*, is found in both acute and chronic histoplasmosis and also appears after normal, sensitized individuals have been skin tested with histoplasmin. The m band has been considered presumptive evidence of infection with *H. capsulatum*. Finding only m antibodies in sera may be attributed to active or inactive disease or to skin testing. Therefore, if the patient has not had a recent histoplasmin skin test, detection of an m band may serve as an indicator of early disease, because this band appears before the h band and disappears more slowly. Kaufman and Reiss (1985) stated that the demonstration of both bands is highly suggestive of active histoplasmosis, regardless of other serologic results.

In coccidioidomycosis, reaction to a precipitin test may be positive in early stages of the infection. As in histoplasmosis, the complement fixation antibody titer tends to increase as the disease becomes more advanced and decreases with control of the infection. Should the infection disseminate, a state of anergy may develop with a loss of all serologic evidence of the disease. In contrast to histoplasmin, skin testing with coccidioidin does not appear to stimulate humoral antibody formation.

Cryptococcosis is one of the most common fungal infections of the lung, although in most of its subjects, it may be present in a subclinical form. The disease usually becomes

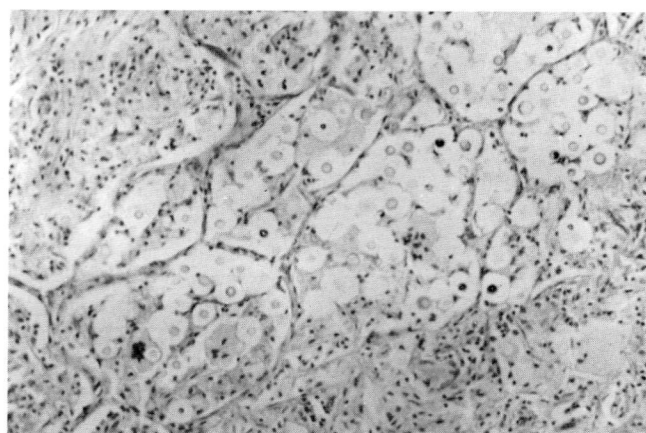

Fig. 14-3. Pneumonia from *Cryptococcus neoformans*. Note the large number of encapsulated cells filling the alveoli. The prominent capsule is well shown. In the early phase of the disease, circulating capsular polysaccharide may be demonstrated in the serum, urine, or cerebrospinal fluid before the appearance of antibodies (periodic acid-Schiff stain, original magnification ×450).

apparent in patients who have some defect in their host defense mechanism, particularly those who are receiving therapy for malignant lymphomas and those who have experienced immune suppression. The causative organism may proliferate in large numbers in the lung or brain. In many instances, the cellular reaction is minimal (Fig. 14-3), and the detection of circulating polysaccharide antigen is possible before the formation of circulating antibodies. When the infection appears to be controlled, either spontaneously or as a result of therapy, the polysaccharide antigen disappears, and circulating antibodies may be demonstrated by the indirect immunofluorescence antibody test or a cryptococcal yeast-cell agglutination procedure. An inverse relationship apparently exists in the time between the appearance of antigen in the serum or in the spinal fluid, during the early or acute stage of the disease, and the appearance of antibodies in the serum as the infection is brought under control. Using indirect fluorescence antibody, tube agglutination for antibody, and latex agglutination for antigen tests, Kaufman and Blumer (1968) were able to show serologic evidence of cryptococcosis in 92% of 66 patients.

Parasitic Infections of the Lung

Parasitic infections of the lungs are uncommon in the United States. When found, they usually are present in patients who are immunosuppressed or who have previously spent time in some part of the world in which echinococcosis, schistosomiasis, or amebiasis is endemic. Identification of the parasite in sputum, pleural fluid, or other clinical specimens is difficult, and recovery by culture is difficult or impossible, depending on the organism. Biopsy or excision of suspected lesions may be the most rapid and definitive procedure.

Intestinal nematodes, such as *Ascaris lumbricoides*, hookworm, and *Strongyloides stercoralis*, may incite a severe inflammatory reaction in the lung during passage from the pulmonary circulation into the bronchi. Sputum specimens may reveal the filarial form of the worms.

Development of serologic procedures to detect antibodies to different types of parasites that can be found in the lung has been of great help in establishing and confirming the presence of active infection with different parasites. Because many of these tests were developed and standardized only relatively recently, most are available only through public health laboratories. Walls (1985) summarized many of the tests available and methods for their performance.

The indirect hemagglutination test for pleuropulmonary amebiasis is sensitive and specific and is particularly valuable in the detection of tissue invasion by amebae. In contrast to its sensitivity in patients with hepatic and pulmonary involvement, Healy (1968) found the test less sensitive in those with acute amebic dysentery and relatively insensitive for asymptomatic intestinal carriers.

In hydatid disease, patients with echinococcal cysts in the liver have better serologic correlation than do those with cysts in the lung. Kagan and associates (1966) found that serologic tests for echinococcal cysts do not correlate well with pulmonary involvement. The reason for this discrepancy in the reliability of serologic tests between infection in the lungs and that in the liver is not known, but it may be that pulmonary cysts are not as closely associated with an active blood supply as are hepatic cysts.

Pulmonary schistosomiasis may develop as a further manifestation of intestinal and hepatic infection and usually is associated with pulmonary hypertension (Fig. 14-4). Although lung biopsy is a useful means of establishing the diagnosis and assessing the pulmonary vascular disease,

various serologic tests are available to help establish the diagnosis. Kagan and colleagues (1962) found the cholesterol lecithin cercarial slide flocculation test to be sensitive in 77% of patients with confirmed disease; however, the test cannot be performed on contaminated or chylous sera. A bentonite flocculation test was developed to overcome this difficulty, but Kagan (1968) found this test to be sensitive in only 70% of patients, reporting false-positive reactions in 15% of sera from patients without schistosomiasis.

Occasional instances of infection with the oriental lung fluke *Paragonimus westermani* are found in persons from the Far East. This infection may be mistaken for other types of chronic disease in the lung. Although complement fixation and other serologic tests have been described for detection of this parasite, they generally are not available in the United States due to the infrequent need for such procedures. A more detailed discussion on the different serologic procedures that have been described for parasitic agents has been presented by Walls (1985).

Pneumonitis Associated with *Pneumocystis carinii*

P. carinii is a small, unicellular organism producing a rapid, consolidating pneumonitis in debilitated patients, usually after prolonged periods of therapy with antimetabolites, corticosteroids, and antibiotics (Fig. 14-5); it is a frequent complication in patients with AIDS. Attempts to isolate and culture the organism have been unsuccessful. Although the disease was first recognized in malnourished infants and children in orphanages in Europe and Korea after World War II, infection with *P. carinii* occurs in this country in patients with AIDS, in patients with a compromised immune response, or in persons with complications caused by pro-

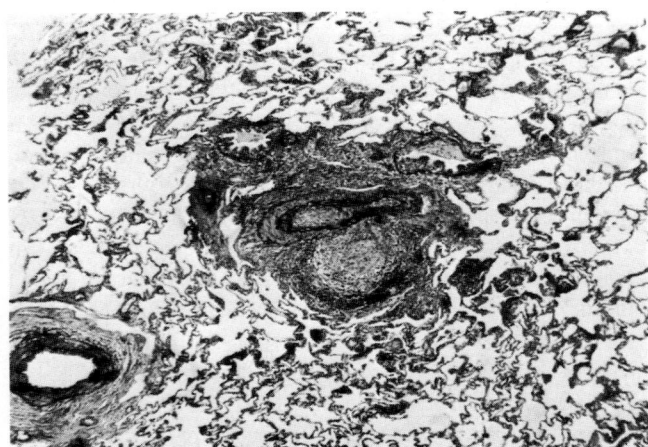

Fig. 14-4. Perivascular granuloma from *Schistosoma mansoni*. Note thickening of pulmonary vessels reflecting pulmonary hypertension. Lung biopsy is a useful means of establishing the diagnosis of schistosomal lung disease and assessing the degree of pulmonary vessel change (original magnification ×260).

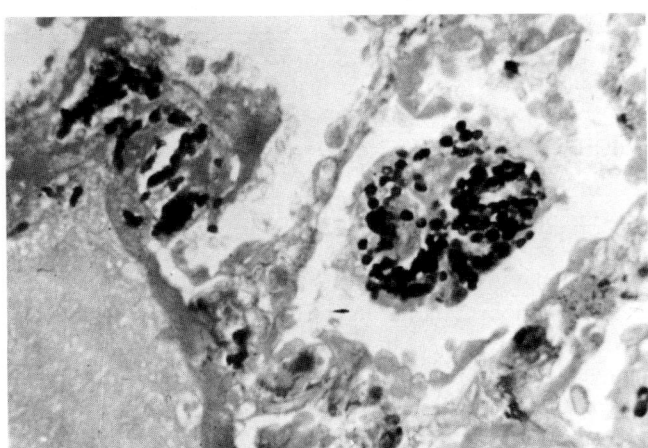

Fig. 14-5. *Pneumocystis carinii*. Large numbers of organisms are embedded in fibrin within alveoli. Tissue sections stained with hematoxylin and eosin do not show the organisms, best demonstrated with the Gomori's methenamine silver stain (original magnification ×650).

longed drug therapy for malignant tumors. Yale and Limper (1996) at the Mayo Clinic reviewed the occurrence of *P. carinii* pneumonia in 116 patients without AIDS. They found that 30.2% had hematologic malignancies, 25% had had an organ transplant, 22.4% had an underlying inflammatory disease process, 12.9% had solid tumors, and 9.5% had various other miscellaneous conditions. Prior corticosteroid therapy was also an important factor and had been administered in 90.5% of the patients within 1 month of the onset of the pneumonia.

The disease is more common than it was in the past. Well over 50% of patients with AIDS present with this infection. The percentage varies depending on whether the patients are intravenous drug abusers or homosexual men; the status of the patient's T-cell population also plays a role in its incidence.

Although the organism has been found in sputum smears and tracheal aspirates, dependence on this finding to establish the diagnosis is unreliable because few organisms are shed and many similar-appearing objects may be present on the smear. Most centers obtain an induced-sputum sample initially and then rapidly move to bronchoscopy and BAL if induced sputum is nondiagnostic. Transbronchial biopsy or even open biopsy may become necessary when BAL is nondiagnostic.

Three popular stains for cysts and trophozoite forms are methenamine silver, toluidine O, and Giemsa. According to Bartlett (1987), the Giemsa stain should not be used exclusively. The organism is not visible on sections stained by hematoxylin and eosin. Because the methenamine stain requires special reagents, the laboratory should be alerted to the possibility of a *Pneumocystis* infection before biopsy so that sections can be stained without delay. Good results within a period of 5 to 10 minutes have been obtained with a rapid staining procedure using toluidine O. An immunofluorescence stain, using monoclonal antibody, for sputum and BAL specimens has been developed and appears to be quite sensitive, as reported by Kovacs and colleagues (1988).

Attempts to develop an immunologic test have been hampered by the inability to grow the organism in the laboratory, and still no reliable serologic assay is available.

Viral Infections of the Lung

Although viral infections of the upper and lower respiratory tract are among the most frequent illnesses in humans, most of these infections are benign and self-limited. The most common etiologic agents are the influenza, parainfluenza, adenoviruses, and respiratory syncytial viruses. The situation is different in the immunosuppressed patient, in whom any of these agents can cause serious life-threatening infection. Viral infections of the lung account for the majority of opportunistic viral infections in immunosuppressed patients. In patients with AIDS, Klatt and Shibata (1988) found that CMV pneumonitis was present at autopsy in approximately 30% of patients, and evidence of the virus was present in most lung tissue examined. CMV is rarely the cause of death in these patients, however, but the development of CMV in the lungs of a patient infected with another pathogen, *Pneumocystis* for instance, portends a poor prognosis. The other herpesvirus, herpes simplex virus (HSV), varicella-zoster virus (VZV), and the Epstein-Barr virus (EBV), are also important pathogens in the immunosuppressed host. Only the herpesviruses are presented here.

Herpesviruses

The family of herpesviruses is unique because exposure to them is common in the general population, and these agents subsequently enter a latent state in virus-specific privileged areas within the body (i.e., lymphocytes for EBV and nerve ganglia for VZV). In the immunocompromised patient, reactivation of virus can lead to serious opportunistic infection; moreover, primary infection in the unexposed, immunosuppressed patient can manifest as overwhelming disseminated disease. CMV and EBV are also strongly immunomodulating, particularly in immunosuppressed individuals. These features of herpesviruses make them fascinating and a particular challenge in the immunosuppressed patient.

The demonstration that ganciclovir is an effective agent in the treatment of CMV infection in immunosuppressed patients by Kortz and Buhles (1986) and others has stressed the importance of early and accurate diagnosis. Whether infection in the transplant patient represents primary or secondary infection is of great importance in patients who receive organ transplant, because mortality from primary infection is far greater when compared with reactivation of latent infection. Primary infection in these patients usually represents receipt of an organ from a CMV-positive donor or blood products contaminated with the virus. Thus, serologic status is crucial in the pretransplant evaluation of these patients. Demonstration of IgM class antibodies or an increase in antibody titers is confirmatory evidence of reactivation, but these events occur relatively late in the course of illness and are not generally helpful in the diagnosis of acute disease.

Early diagnosis of CMV infection can be made in a variety of ways. The spin amplification shell vial technique is the most widely used rapid detection method for CMV. It features concentration of the virus using centrifugation, culture, and the use of monoclonal antibody assays for viral antigens. A result can be returned within 24 hours. In situ hybridization also has been used in place of monoclonal antibodies in conjunction with the shell vial culture. The use of direct immunofluorescence monoclonal antibodies to CMV antigens is rapid but less sensitive than the shell vial assay, and it has been supplanted by the shell vial technique. PCR has been used successfully in the rapid detection of CMV DNA in blood and other tissues, but its use in this setting is confounded by the interpretation of positive results. Histopathologic examination of tissue specimens using Wright-Giemsa staining can demonstrate typical cytopathic appearance (Fig. 14-6), but this method is relatively insensitive and usually requires invasive procedures to obtain tissue. Routine culture

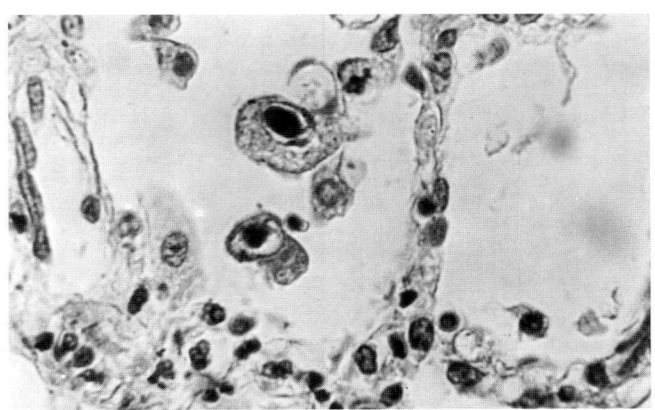

Fig. 14-6. Cytomegalovirus intranuclear inclusion body in alveolar macrophage. Not all viral diseases produce inclusion bodies, but those of the herpes-cytomegalovirus groups show well-formed intranuclear inclusions (original magnification ×650).

of CMV is done on human fibroblast cultures that are examined for characteristic cytopathic effect; this effect usually appears within 2 weeks, depending on the inoculum, and may occur sooner if specimen titers are high.

Lung involvement with primary VZV is not common in immunocompetent persons. In immunosuppressed individuals, however, primary VZV infection and pneumonia can be life threatening. Reactivation of VZV (i.e., shingles) in recipients of organ transplants also can progress to invasive pulmonary disease. The diagnosis of VZV is usually not difficult because of the characteristic exanthem in primary cases and the presence of shingles in reactivation cases. Serology, however, does play an important role, especially in transplant patients, because pretransplant seronegativity should lead to administration of soon-to-be-released vaccine. In addition, postexposure varicella-zoster immune globulin can be administered and is effective in decreasing morbidity in immunocompromised patients, as demonstrated by Zaia and coworkers (1983). Serum titers for VZV to confirm seroconversion or the presence of IgM are done. It is important to note that cross-reactivity is substantial, up to 33%, between antibody assays for HSV and VZV, and the absence of a similar titer increase to HSV may be necessary in these situations. In case of diagnostic uncertainty, materials from lesions or biopsy specimens can be submitted for routine culture, shell vial culture, and immunofluorescence staining, the latter being the most efficient method.

EBV is a ubiquitous pathogen that causes the usually self-limited clinical syndrome of infectious mononucleosis in younger patients. It only rarely causes pulmonary disease, but in transplant patients, EBV pneumonitis can be a manifestation of posttransplantation lymphoproliferative disease. Posttransplantation lymphoproliferative disease is associated with a wide spectrum of symptoms with outcome ranging from frankly malignant lymphoma to benign expansion of lymphoid tissue that responds to reduction of immunosuppression. The virus can be cultured from throat wash-

ings, but culture of shed virus is usually not helpful diagnostically, so the diagnostic approach is based primarily on serology and examination of tissue. Although detection of heterophile antibodies is sufficient in making the diagnosis in uncomplicated infectious mononucleosis, considerably greater information can be gained from measuring the serologic status of patients to four antigens: viral capsid antigen (VCA), EBV-induced nuclear antigen, early antigen (EA)-diffuse component, and the EA-restricted component. Five clinical states of EBV infection are recognized based on the evaluation of the humoral response to these antigens: 1) susceptible, if anti-VCA is absent; 2) current primary infection, if anti-VCA is positive and anti-EBVCA is absent, and anti-EA components are negative; 3) recent active infection, if anti-VCA is positive, anti-EBVCA is negative but anti-EA is positive; 4) past infection, if both anti-VCA and EBVCA are positive; and 5) reactivated infection shows both anti-VCA and anti-EBVCA are present and one of the anti-EA components is positive. The determination of reactivated versus primary infection can be of prognostic importance when dealing with posttransplantation lymphoproliferative disease, as demonstrated by Armitage and colleagues (1991). Tissue can be examined for viral antigens with an indirect immunofluorescence stain or in situ DNA hybridization.

HSV usually only causes invasive infection in immunosuppressed patients with transplanted organs or malignancies under treatment with cytotoxic medications. Pulmonary disease usually manifests as tracheobronchitis, but rarely pneumonia can occur. Orolabial or genital lesions are usually present concurrently. The finding of HSV in tracheal secretions is therefore difficult to interpret, and lung tissue is usually required to render a certain diagnosis of HSV pneumonia. Tissue is cultured and, depending on the concentration of virus in the specimen, can be positive as soon as 24 hours or as late as 5 days. A variety of rapid detection techniques are available, including in situ hybridization, shell vial assay, and an immunofluorescence technique. Serology is limited in the diagnosis of HSV infection.

REFERENCES

Allen MS, et al: Video-assisted thoracic procedures: the Mayo experience. Mayo Clinic Proc *71*:351, 1996.

Allen RM, Dunn WR, Limper AM: Diagnosing ventilator-associated pneumonia: the role of bronchoscopy. Mayo Clinic Proc *69*:962, 1994.

American Thoracic Society: Hospital-acquired pneumonia in adults: diagnosis, assessment of severity, initial antimicrobial therapy, and preventive strategies. Am J Respir Crit Care Med *153*:1711, 1996.

Armitage JM, et al: Posttransplant lymphoproliferative disease in thoracic organ transplant patients: ten years of cyclosporine-based immunosuppression. J Heart Transplant *10*:877, 1991.

Austin JHM, Cohen MB: Value of having a cytopathologist present during percutaneous fine-needle aspiration biopsy of lung: report of 55 cancer patients and meta-analysis of the literature. Am J Radiol *160*:175, 1993.

Baker AM, Bowton DL, Haponik EF: Decision making in nosocomial pneumonia: an analytic approach to the interpretation of quantitative bronchoscopic cultures. Chest *107*:85, 1995.

Balows A, Fraser DWE: International Symposium on Legionnaires' Disease. Ann Intern Med *90*:489, 1979.

Bartlett JG: Diagnosis of bacterial infections of the lung. Clin Chest Med 8:119, 1987.

Bartlett JG, et al: Community-acquired pneumonia in adults: guidelines for management. The Infectious Diseases Society of America. Clin Infect Dis 26:811, 1998.

Bensard DB, et al: Comparison of video thoracoscopic lung biopsy to open lung biopsy in the diagnosis of interstitial disease. Chest 103:7651, 1993.

Butler WR, Jost KC Jr, Kilburn JO: Identification of mycobacteria by high-performance liquid chromatography. J Clin Microbiol 29:2468, 1991.

Carrington CB, Gaensler EA: Clinical-pathologic approach to diffuse infiltrative lung disease. In Thurlbeck W, Abell M (eds): The Lung: Structure and Function. Baltimore: Williams and Wilkins, 1978, pp. 58–87.

Chastre J, Fagon JY: Invasive diagnostic testing should be routinely used to manage ventilated patients with suspected pneumonia. Am J Respir Crit Care Med 150:570, 1994.

Chastre J, et al: Evaluation of bronchoscopic techniques for the diagnosis of nosocomial pneumonia. Am J Respir Crit Care Med 152:231, 1995.

Chester AC, Winn WC Jr: Unusual and newly recognized patterns of non-tuberculous mycobacterial infection with emphasis on the immunocompromised host. Pathol Annu 21 (Pt 1):251, 1986.

Churg A: An inflation procedure for open lung biopsies. Am J Surg Pathol 30:411, 1983.

Contreras MA, et al: Pulmonary infection with nontuberculous mycobacteria. Am Rev Respir Dis 137:149, 1988.

Dail DH: Tissue sampling. In Dail DH, Hammer SP (eds): Pulmonary Pathology. 2nd ed. New York: Springer-Verlag, 1994, pp. 1–19.

Damato JJ, et al: Detection of mycobacteria by radiometric and standard plate procedures. J Clin Microbiol 17:1066, 1983.

Das DK, et al: Superficial and deep seated tuberculosis lesions: fine needle aspiration cytology diagnosis of 547 cases. Diagn Cytopathol 8:211, 1992.

Delgado R, et al: Low predictive value of polymerase chain reaction for diagnosis of cytomegalovirus disease in liver transplant recipients. J Clin Microbiol 30:1876, 1992.

Eisenach KD, et al: Detection of Mycobacterium tuberculosis in sputum samples using a polymerase chain reaction. Am Rev Respir Dis 144:1160, 1991.

Fain JS, et al: Rapid diagnosis of legionella infection by a nonisotopic in situ hybridization method. Am J Clin Pathol 95:719, 1991.

Figueroa ME, Rasheed S: Molecular pathology and diagnosis of infectious disease. Am J Clin Pathol 95:S8, 1991.

Forbes BA, Hicks KE: Direct detection of Mycobacterium tuberculosis in respiratory specimens in a clinical laboratory by polymerase chain reaction. J Clin Microbiol 31:1688, 1993.

Fournier AM, et al: Tuberculosis and nontuberculous mycobacteriosis in patients with AIDS. Chest 93:772, 1988.

Fraire AE, et al: Transbronchial lung biopsy: histopathologic and morphometric assessment of diagnostic utility. Chest 102:748, 1992.

Gaensler EA, Carrington CB: Open biopsy for chronic diffuse infiltrative lung disease: clinical, roentgenographic, and physiologic considerations in 502 patients Ann Thorac Surg 30:411, 1980.

Gianoulis M, Wright JL : An autopsy study of the structure of the small vessels in biopsies from the lingula and upper and lower lobes: implications for vascular assessment. Mod Pathol 3:567, 1990.

Healy GR: The use of and limitations to the indirect hemagglutination test in the diagnosis of intestinal amebiasis. Health Lab Sci 5:174, 1968.

Heifets L: Mycobacteriology laboratory. Clin Chest Med 18:35, 1997.

Jiminez J, Larsson L: Heating cells in acid methanol for 30 minutes without freeze-drying provides adequate yields of fatty acids and alcohols for gas chromatographic characterization of mycobacteria. J Clin Microbiol 24:844, 1986.

Kadokura M, et al: Pathologic comparison of video-assisted thoracic surgical lung biopsy with traditional open lung biopsy. J Thorac Cardiovasc Surg 109:494, 1995.

Kagan IG: Serologic diagnosis of schistosomiasis. Bull N Y Acad Med 44:262, 1968.

Kagan IG, et al: A clinical, parasitologic, and immunologic study of schistosomiasis in 103 Puerto Rican males residing in the United States. Ann Intern Med 56:457, 1962.

Kagan IG, et al: Evaluation of intradermal and serologic tests for the diagnosis of hydatid disease. Am J Trop Med 15:172, 1966.

Kahn FW, Jones JM: Diagnosing bacterial respiratory infection by bronchoalveolar lavage. J Infect Dis 155:862, 1987.

Katzenstein A-LA, Askin FB: Surgical Pathology of Non-Neoplastic Lung Disease. 3rd Ed. Philadelphia: WB Saunders, 1997.

Kaufman L, Blumer S: Value and interpretation of serological tests for the diagnosis of cryptococcosis. Appl Microbiol 16:1907, 1968.

Kaufman L, Reiss E: Serodiagnosis of fungal disease. In Lennette EH, et al: Manual of Clinical Microbiology. 4th Ed. Washington, DC: American Society of Microbiology, 1985.

Kjelstrom JA, Beaman BL: Development of a serologic panel for the recognition of nocardial infections in a murine model. Diagn Microbiol Infect Dis 16:291, 1993.

Klatt EC, Shibata D: Cytomegalovirus infection in the acquired immunodeficiency syndrome: clinical and autopsy findings. Arch Pathol Lab Med 112:540, 1988.

Kopanoff DE, et al: A continuing survey of tuberculosis primary drug resistance in the United States: March 1975 to November 1977. Am Rev Respir Dis 118:835, 1978.

Kortz SH, Buhles WC: Collaborative DHPG study group: treatment of serious cytomegalovirus infections with DHPG in patients with AIDS and other immunodeficiencies. N Engl J Med 314:801, 1986.

Kovacs JA, et al: Diagnosis of Pneumocystis carinii pneumonia: improved detection in sputum with use of monoclonal antibiotics. N Engl J Med 318:589, 1988.

Krasnow I, Wayne LG: Comparison of methods for tuberculosis bacteriology. Appl Microbiol 18:915, 1969.

Laszlo A, Siddiqi SH: Evaluation of a rapid radiometric differentiation test for the Mycobacterium tuberculosis complex by selective inhibition with p-nitro-alpha-acetylamino-beta-hydroxypropiophenone. J Clin Microbiol 19:694, 1984.

Liebow AA, et al: Plastic demonstration of pulmonary pathology. Bull Int Assoc Med Museums 27:116, 1947.

Marquette CH, et al: Diagnostic tests for pneumonia in ventilated patients: prospective evaluation of diagnostic accuracy using histology as a diagnostic gold standard. Am J Respir Crit Care Med 15:1878, 1995.

Mathieson JR, et al: Chronic diffuse infiltrative lung disease: comparison of diagnostic accuracy of CT and chest radiography. Radiology 171:111, 1989.

Meduri GU, Baselski V: The role of bronchoalveolar lavage in diagnosing nonopportunistic bacterial pneumonia. Chest 100:179, 1991.

Middlebrook G, Reggiardo Z, Tigert WD: Automatable radiometric detection of growth of Mycobacterium tuberculosis in selective media. Am Rev Respir Dis 115:1066, 1977.

Miller DL, et al: Video-thoracoscopic wedge excision of the lung. Ann Thorac Surg 54:410, 1992.

Miller RR: Gross examination of lung resection specimens. In Thurlbeck WM, Churg AM (eds): Pathology of the Lung. 2nd Ed. Stuttgart: Thieme, 1995, p. 117.

Miller RR, Evans KG: Lung biopsy. In Thurlbeck WM, Churg AM (eds): Pathology of the Lung. 2nd ed. Stuttgart: Thieme, 1995, pp. 107–115.

Miller RR, et al: Lingular and right middle lobe biopsy in the assessment of lung disease. Ann Thorac Surg 44:269, 1987.

Monteagudo C, et al: Specific immunohistochemical identification of Candida albicans in paraffin-embedded tissue with a new monoclonal antibody (1B12). Am J Clin Pathol 103:130, 1995.

Morgan MA, et al: Comparison of a radiometric method (BACTEC) and conventional culture media for recovery of mycobacteria from smear-negative specimens. J Clin Microbiol 18:384, 1983.

Neuman SL, Michel RP, Wang NS: Lingular lung biopsy: is it representative? Am Rev Respir Dis 132:1804, 1985.

Papazian L, et al: Bronchoscopic or blind sampling techniques for the diagnosis of ventilator-associated pneumonia. Am J Respir Crit Care Med 152:1982, 1995.

Pingleton SK, Faggon JY, Leeper KV: Patient selection for clinical investigation of ventilator-associated pneumonia: criteria for evaluating diagnostic techniques. Chest 102:553S, 1992.

Pollock HM, et al.: Diagnosis of bacterial pulmonary infections with quantitative protected catheter cultures obtained during bronchoscopy. J Clin Microbiol 17:255, 1983.

Qadri SM, Ali MA: Sensitivity of fine needle aspiration biopsy in the detection of mycobacterial infections. Diagn Cytopathol 7:142, 1991.

Raab SS, Silverman JF, Zimmerman KG: Fine needle aspiration biopsy of pulmonary coccidioidomycosis: spectrum of cytologic findings in 73 patients. Am J Clin Pathol 99:582, 1993.

Roberts GD, et al: Evaluation of the BACTEC radiometric method for recovery of mycobacteria and drug susceptibility testing of Mycobac-

terium tuberculosis from acid-fast smear-positive specimens. J Clin Microbiol 18:689, 1983.

Rodgers FG, Pascule AW: Legionella. *In* Lennette EH, et al (eds): Manual of Clinical Microbiology. 4th Ed. Washington, DC: American Society of Microbiology, 1985.

Rosai J: Special techniques in surgical pathology. *In* Rosai J (ed): Ackerman's Surgical Pathology. 8th Ed. St. Louis: CV Mosby, 1996a, pp. 29–62.

Rosai J: Gross techniques in surgical pathology. *In* Rosai J (ed): Ackerman's Surgical Pathology. 8th Ed. St. Louis: CV Mosby, 1996b, pp. 13–28.

Salinas-Carmona MC, Welsh O, Casillas SM: Enzyme-linked immunosorbent assay for serological diagnosis of *Nocardia brasiliensis* and clinical correlation with mycetoma infections. J Clin Microbiol 31:2901, 1993.

Schmidt WA: The chest. *In* Anonymous (ed): Principles and Techniques of Surgical Pathology. Vol 1. Menlo Park, CA: Addison-Wesley, 1983, pp. 389–411.

Shinnick TM, Jonas V: Molecular approach to the diagnosis of tuberculosis. *In* Bloom BR (ed): Tuberculosis: Pathogenesis, Protection, and Control. Washington, DC: ASM Press, 1994.

Siddiqi SH, Libonati JP, Middlebrook G: Evaluation of a rapid radiometric method for drug susceptibility testing of Mycobacterium tuberculosis. J Clin Microbiol 13:908, 1981.

Snider DE Jr, et al: Rapid drug susceptibility testing of *Mycobacterium tuberculosis*. Am Rev Respir Dis 123:402, 1981.

Sole-Violan J, et al: Comparative efficacy of bronchoalveolar lavage and telescoping plugged catheter in the diagnosis of pneumonia in mechanically ventilated patients. Chest 103:386, 1993.

Spencer H (ed): Pathology of the Lung. Oxford: Pergamon Press, 1985, pp. 1–77, 1097–1107.

Stevens GM, Jackman RJ: Outpatient needle biopsy of the lung: its safety and utility. Radiology 151:301, 1984.

Stout J, et al: Ubiquitousness of *Legionella pneumophila* in the water supply of a hospital with endemic Legionnaires' disease. N Engl J Med 306:466, 1982.

Takahashi H, Foster V: Detection and recovery of mycobacteria by a radiometric procedure. J Clin Microbiol 17:380, 1983.

Tao LC: Lung, Pleura, and Mediastinum. New York: Igaku-Shoin, 1988.

Thorpe JE, et al: Bronchoalveolar lavage for diagnosing acute bacterial pneumonia. J Infect Dis 155:855, 1987.

Thurlbeck WM: Examination of the lung: autopsy. *In* Thurlbeck WM, Churg AM (eds): Pathology of the Lung. Stuttgart, Germany: Thieme, 1995, pp. 129–136.

Timpe A, Runyon EH: The relationship of "atypical" acid-fast bacteria to human disease. J Lab Clin Med 44:202, 1954.

Timsit JF, et al: Effect of previous antimicrobial therapy on the accuracy of the main procedures used to diagnose nosocomial pneumonia in patients who are using ventilation. Chest 108:1036, 1995.

Tisdall PA, et al: Identification of clinical isolates of mycobacteria with gas-liquid chromatography: a 10-month follow-up study. J Clin Microbiol 16:400, 1982.

Vidone RA, Liebow AA: Anatomical and functional studies of the lung deprived of pulmonary arteries and veins, with an application in the therapy of transposition of the great vessels. Am J Pathol 33:539, 1957.

Walls KW: Serodiagnostic tests for parasitic diseases. *In* Lennette EH, et al: Manual of Clinical Microbiology. 4th Ed. Washington, DC: American Society of Microbiology, 1985.

Wang N-S: Anatomy. *In* Dail DH, Hammer SP (eds): Pulmonary Pathology. 2nd ed. New York: Springer-Verlag, 1994, pp. 21–44.

Westcott JL: Direct percutaneous needle aspiration of localized pulmonary lesions: results in 422 patients. Radiology 137:31, 1980.

Wetstein L: Sensitivity and specificity of lingular segmental biopsies of the lung. Chest 90:383, 1986.

Woods GL, Washington JA: Mycobacteria other than Mycobacterium tuberculosis: review of microbiologic and clinical aspects. Rev Infect Dis 9:275, 1987.

Yale SH, Limper AH: *Pneumocystis carinii* pneumonia in patients without acquired immunodeficiency syndrome: associated illness and prior corticosteroid therapy. Mayo Clin Proc 71:5, 1996.

Zaia JA, et al: Evaluation of varicella zoster immune globulin: Protection of immunosuppressed children after household exposure. J Infect Dis 147:737, 1983.

READING REFERENCES

Colby TV, Koss MN, Travis WD: Specimen Handling and Special Techniques in Tumors of the Lower Respiratory Tract. Washington, DC: Atlas of Tumor Pathology, AFIP, 1994.

Dail DH, Hammer SP (eds): Pulmonary Pathology. 2nd ed. New York: Springer-Verlag, 1994.

Feldman PS, Covell JL: Fine Needle Aspiration Cytology and its Clinical Applications: Breast and Lung. Chicago: American Society Clinical Pathologists Press, 1985.

Frable WJ: Thin Needle Aspiration Biopsy. Philadelphia: WB Saunders, 1983.

Homer KS, et al: Monoclonal antibody to *Pneumocystis carinii*. Comparison with silver stain in bronchial lavage specimens. Am J Clin Pathol 97:619, 1992.

Katzenstein A-LA, Askin FB: Surgical Pathology of Non-Neoplastic Lung Disease. 3rd Ed. Philadelphia: WB Saunders, 1997.

Kline TS: Handbook of Fine Needle Aspiration Biopsy Cytology. 2nd ed. New York: Churchill Livingstone, 1988.

Malese SC, Naryshkin S: Diagnosis of *Pneumocystis carinii* by cytologic examination of Papanicolaou-stained sputum specimens. Diagn Cytopathol 7:111, 1991.

Oda Y, et al: Detection of human cytomegalovirus, Epstein-Barr virus, and herpes simplex virus in diffuse interstitial pneumonia by polymerase chain reaction and immunohistochemistry. Am J Clin Pathol 102;495, 1994.

Rosai J: Ackerman's Surgical Pathology. 8th Ed. St. Louis: CV Mosby, 1996.

Solans EP, et al: Early diagnosis of cytomegalovirus pneumonitis in lung transplant patients. Arch Pathol Lab Med 119:33, 1995.

Spencer H (ed): Pathology of the Lung. Oxford: Pergamon Press, 1985.

Thurlbeck WM, Churg AM (eds): Pathology of the Lung. 2nd Ed. Stuttgart, Germany: Thieme, 1995.

Torres A, et al: Diagnostic value of quantitative cultures of bronchoalveolar lavage and telescoping plugged catheters in mechanically ventilated patients with bacterial pneumonia. Am Rev Respir Dis 140:306, 1989.

CHAPTER 15

Molecular Diagnostic Studies in Pulmonary Disease

Máirín McMenamin and Massimo Loda

Tremendous progress has been made in the elucidation of the complex molecular processes responsible for the maintenance, transmission, and expression of genetic information. Central to molecular biology are the processes of replication, transcription, and translation and the new experimental technologies involved in the manipulation of DNA, RNA, and protein. Medical treatment is increasingly based on new information regarding the mechanisms of action of diverse genes that are implicated in disease processes. As a result, those involved in patient care and treatment should have at least a basic understanding of molecular biology and related techniques to choose the best test for obtaining the information needed to guide management.

Discoveries in molecular pathogenetic mechanisms have had a major impact in the area of pulmonary disease. These developments are not only limited to the research arena but are also important in the screening and diagnosis of diverse pulmonary diseases, including those of genetic, infectious, and neoplastic etiologies. In addition, molecular biology has had profound effects on the development of new and safe products, including vaccines, therapeutic agents, and novel gene therapies, and is the basis of the evolving field of pharmacogenomics—the study of genes or chromosomal loci that are involved in determining the responsiveness of an individual to a given drug.

This chapter provides an introduction to basic molecular biology principles and selected molecular diagnostic techniques and demonstrates their application in specific pulmonary disease entities, including cancer, infections, and interstitial lung disease. Animal models of disease are reviewed, and gene therapy, with particular reference to its application in cystic fibrosis (CF) and as a prospective anticancer therapy, is discussed.

PRINCIPLES OF RECOMBINANT DNA TECHNOLOGY

General Principles

DNA and RNA are designed to retain, store, and express genetic information in the form of proteins. DNA comprises two antiparallel strands of nucleotide bases wound around each other in a right-handed double helix and aligned on a sugar-phosphate backbone. The negatively charged sugar-phosphate molecules are on the outside, and the planar bases of each strand stack one above the other in the center of the helix. The strands are joined noncovalently by means of hydrogen bonding between pairs of bases on opposite strands such that two hydrogen bonds join adenine to thymine and one hydrogen bond joins guanine to cytosine. The sequence of one DNA strand uniquely specifies the sequence of the other strand; this complementarity underlies the ability for in vitro manipulation of nucleic acids. DNA is organized into highly compact, regular units called *chromosomes*. An extraordinarily stable molecule, DNA loses its normal conformational structure only at extremes of heat or pH or in the presence of destabilizing agents. RNA, in contrast, is much less stable than DNA because of its single-stranded, more random structure; its susceptibility to alkaline hydrolysis; and its rapid degradation by ubiquitous enzymes called *RNAses*.

A gene is a section of DNA that contains the amino acid sequence code for a protein. Protein synthesis begins with the activation of the appropriate gene. A copy of the gene is made by the process of *transcription*, which is the synthesis of complementary single-stranded messenger RNA (mRNA). Before export to the cytoplasm, mRNA undergoes post-transcriptional modification. Pre-mRNA contains amino acid coding sequences called *exons* and noncoding sequences called *introns*. The introns are excised from mRNA by a process called *splicing*. mRNA is subsequently transported from the nucleus to the cytoplasm where its linear sequence of nucleotide triplets or codons is translated on the ribosomes to form a linear sequence of amino acids. The final product of a gene is the assembly of the constituent amino acids into functional proteins.

Control of the process of gene expression ultimately influences the activity or amount of protein product. Gene regulation takes place at the transcriptional and translational levels. Before transcription can be initiated, RNA polymerase—the enzyme responsible for stitching together the mRNA polymer—attaches initially on to DNA at a sequence termed the *promoter*. Certain genes, called *transcription factors*, together with coactivators and corepressors, can influence mRNA production of other genes, because they enable RNA polymerase to recognize the promoter. Transcription factors are regulated either by other upstream proteins or by phosphorylation. RNA transcription is capable of significant amplification of the signal it encodes.

The vast majority of the human genome is composed of noncoding DNA, the function of which has not been fully elucidated. Most of the variability among individuals occurs in noncoding DNA; this variability is termed *genetic polymorphism*. Repetitive noncoding sequences are present in multiple copies throughout the genome in tandem arrays called *satellites* or *microsatellites*, according to their length. The length of a set of satellites is unique to each individual. Because alleles at these sites are stably inherited, microsatellites are now one of the most useful classes of genetic polymorphic sequences used in the process of linkage analysis. Alterations of microsatellite sequences, a phenomenon known as *microsatellite instability*, is often due to malfunctioning of DNA repair enzymes. Microsatellite instability has been described in several tumor types, particularly in colon cancer but also in lung cancer.

Hybridization Assays

The ability to manipulate nucleic acids in vitro is based on molecular hybridization, which is the complementary base pairing between the target nucleic acids and a DNA or RNA probe. The process of hybridization can be accomplished on solid support, such as nitrocellulose or nylon membranes in Southern blotting, in solution as in the polymerase chain reaction (PCR), or at the cellular or subcellular levels, as for in situ hybridization (ISH).

Probes may be labeled either radioisotopically or with a variety of nonisotopic reporter molecules that can subsequently be revealed by means of a color reaction. In routine molecular diagnostics, particularly in commercially available kits, nonisotopic probes are rapidly replacing radiolabeled ones. The types of probes that can be used include short, single-stranded, synthetic DNA oligonucleotides; single-stranded antisense/complementary RNA probes of interme-

diate size; and long, double-stranded DNA probes. DNA oligonucleotide probes are primarily used in PCR reactions and for viral detection by ISH. The narrow window between specific signal and loss of it and the limited number of reporter molecules that can be tagged on these oligonucleotides are some of the disadvantages of using these probes. RNA probes, also known as *riboprobes*, are synthesized in vitro using RNA polymerase from either cloned DNA templates or PCR products. They are particularly suited for use in ISH and are sometimes used in Northern hybridization. DNA probes are especially suitable for use in solid support hybridization assays and fluorescent in situ hybridization (FISH).

In filter hybridization, probes target DNA or RNA sequences that have been previously bound to a solid substrate. Southern blot hybridization is a technique whereby DNA is cut at specific sites by enzymes called *restriction endonucleases* before gel electrophoresis and then transferred onto nitrocellulose or nylon filters. This permits determination of the size of the restriction fragment to which the probe hybridizes. This technique requires intact genomic DNA obtained from either fresh or snap-frozen tissue. Northern hybridization or blotting is a related technique that is used to detect RNA.

PCR involves the exponential in vitro amplification of a segment of DNA. It also involves a repetitive cycle of heat denaturation of DNA, annealing of sequence-specific oligonucleotide primers flanking the selected DNA fragment to be amplified, and synthesis of the target sequence by heat-stable DNA polymerases. The reaction results in the preferential amplification of the target sequence on the background of extraneous DNA, producing virtually unlimited amounts of the target. The scant availability of starting material (e.g., from bronchial brushings) is thus less of an obstacle when this technique is used for diagnostic purposes. Short segments of DNA extracted from formalin-fixed, paraffin-embedded tissues can also be amplified using PCR. Reverse-transcriptase PCR (RT-PCR) is a technique that can quantify gene expression by using PCR amplification of target RNA that has been previously converted to complementary DNA (cDNA) by reverse transcriptase, an enzyme present in retroviruses. These fragments of isolated DNA can also be inserted into highly replicating bacterial plasmids to obtain infinite copies of a single gene of interest from a background of unrelated DNA. RT-PCR offers several advantages over Northern blotting because only minute tissue samples are required (e.g., from microdissection) and the technique is much less labor intensive and can be quantitative. Several modifications of the basic PCR technique also suit specific needs. Examples include competitive PCR for gene dosage assays, nested PCR to increase the sensitivity of the reaction when targeting low–copy number genes, multiplex PCR in which multiple primer sets are used in the same reaction to simultaneously amplify several targets, and more recent technologies that allow accurate automated gene quantification studies (e.g., the quantification of c-erb-b2/*HER* 2/*neu* amplification as demonstrated by Gelmini and colleagues [1997] and the assessment of cytomegalovirus DNA copy number as demonstrated by Pappas and associates [1997]).

To perform Southern, Northern, and solution phase PCR assays, nucleic acid extraction is required, which necessitates the destruction of tissue architecture. In contrast, ISH involves the localization in specific cells of labeled RNA or DNA molecules that hybridize with complementary target DNA or RNA sequences on tissue sections or cytologic preparations. FISH is a cytogenetic technique that allows identification of translocations, deletions, structural rearrangements, loss of heterozygosities (LOHs), and gene amplification assessment in interphase nuclei. FISH is especially effective when performed on touch imprints but can also be performed on formalin-fixed and paraffin-embedded tissue. Computerized, bar code–controlled instruments are available that perform fully automated ISH, including FISH, immunohistochemistry, or a dual-staining combination of ISH and immunohistochemistry. Capodieci and colleagues (1998) reported that with the use of this instrument, conditions can be tightly controlled, resulting in increased reproducibility, reduced hybridization time, and diminished labor.

Pease and colleagues (1994) demonstrated a novel technology involving the merging of molecular biology and computer technology involves oligonucleotide arrays or DNA chips that carry cDNA microarrays. Thousands of synthetic oligonucleotide probes are constructed to portions of the target on a support grid that measures approximately 1 cm^2, and chemical reactions are activated by light. The bound sequences are then hybridized to nucleic acids extracted from the specimen of interest. After hybridization, a reading device scans the entire chip. DNA chips enable the expression level of hundreds of genes to be determined in a single experiment. Genetic mutations can also be detected by this technology. Gingeras and associates (1998) report an assay for *Mycobacterium tuberculosis* strains to detect mutations in the *rpoB* gene that results in rifampicin resistance. Systematic sequencing of cDNA libraries constructed from tumor RNAs is likely to exponentially increase the number of genes that can be screened simultaneously within one tumor. Kononen and colleagues (1998) have developed an array-based, high-throughput technique that facilitates analysis of gene expression at the cellular level in a large number of tumors. Up to 1,000 cylindrical tissue biopsies from individual tumors can be distributed in a single microarray. Sections of the paraffin block containing the microarray provide targets for parallel in situ detection of DNA, RNA, and protein targets in each specimen on the array, and consecutive sections allow the rapid analysis of hundreds of molecular markers in the same set of specimens. The use of FISH in studies of large numbers of clinical specimens is limited by the requirement to hybridize, stain, and interpret tumor specimens one slide at a time. However, when FISH is combined with tumor array technology, the analysis of hundreds of specimens per day can be achieved. This technology is capable of handling the influx of novel candidate cancer genes identified by RNA expression profile analyses.

APPLICATIONS OF MOLECULAR DIAGNOSTICS IN PULMONARY DISEASE

Linkage Analysis

Restriction fragment length polymorphisms are particularly well suited for genetic linkage studies in humans. Assessment of the statistical significance of linkage is made by calculating the ratio of the likelihood of linkage to the likelihood of random assortment. These genetic markers exploit the DNA sequence variations that exist between individuals and open up the entire human genome to genetic analysis. CF is an autosomal recessive disorder with an incidence of approximately 1 in 2,000 white births that results from mutations in the CF transmembrane conductance regulator (CFTR) gene. The disease is characterized by abnormal mucus production, concomitant recurrent pulmonary infection, and pancreatic insufficiency. The CF gene was discovered by identifying initially the inherited chromosomal region by linkage analysis. Whereas inheritance of the diseased gene can be traced by polymorphic markers, molecular testing, usually by PCR, and sequencing of the over 200 disease-associated mutations is now possible. A single mutation may account for 85% of CF in the northern European and North American white populations.

In Situ Hybridization

ISH can identify cells that make specific RNA for that protein, conclusively demonstrating production of the protein by the tumor cells. ISH is useful to distinguish nonspecific uptake of hormones from genuine hormone synthesis that may prove to be of diagnostic value in small cell carcinomas of the lung (SCLC), which frequently produce neuroendocrine markers. Hamid and coworkers (1989) used ISH to study the expression of the human bombesin (gastrin-releasing peptide) gene at the cellular level in SCLC. ISH has also been used to detect specific viral nucleic acids within tissues and tumors, because such DNA or RNA is present as many copies within a given infected cell. Fain and associates (1991) demonstrated that *Legionella* infection can be rapidly diagnosed by ISH detection of DNA. Cellular DNA or RNA that is overexpressed in some manner, as in oncogene amplification or unregulated protein transcription, can also be detected using this technique. Noguchi and colleagues (1990) used ISH to show heterogeneous amplification of the oncogene *myc* in SCLC. ISH, however, fails to detect oncogenes activated by means other than dysregulated transcription, such as point mutations that result in constitutive activation.

Quantitative Polymerase Chain Reactions

Quantitative PCR and RT-PCR have a variety of diagnostic applications that range from the assessment of oncogene overexpression to viral load in pneumonitis. DeMuth and colleagues (1998) described a gene expression index combining the expression levels of *c-myc*, *E2F-1*, and *p21* to discriminate all cultured and primary normal lung from malignant lung carcinoma cell lines and tumor specimens using quantitative RT-PCR. Kotsimbos and associates (1997) described an efficient, highly sensitive, quantitative PCR assay for human cytomegalovirus load detection in lung transplant recipients using competitive PCR and fluorescently labeled primers in transbronchial biopsies, bronchioloalveolar lavage specimens, and peripheral blood leukocytes.

DISEASE ENTITIES

Cancer

Landis and associates (1998) estimated that in 1998, 171,500 people in the United States were diagnosed with lung cancer; 160,100 deaths resulted, making lung cancer the leading cause of cancer-related death in the United States. For the purpose of therapy, lung cancer is divided into two groups comprising the four main histologic types. Non–small cell lung carcinoma (NSCLC) comprises approximately 75% of all lung tumors and includes squamous cell, adeno cell, and large cell carcinomas. The fourth type is SCLC, which constitutes the remaining 25% (see Chapter 95).

The role of molecular pathology in cancer diagnosis is focused on assessing clonality; assessing mutations in oncogenes and tumor suppressor genes (TSGs), both somatic and germline; determining overexpression of oncogenes or loss of function of TSGs; assessing cytogenetic abnormalities; and determining susceptibility to cancer by tracing genes or chromosomal regions closely linked to as yet unidentified genes by means of linkage analysis.

Oncogenes and Tumor Suppressor Genes

Proto-oncogenes are highly conserved cellular genes that are important in cellular pathways involved in growth and differentiation. Only one of the two alleles in a cell needs to be mutated to confer dominant oncogenic properties by altering the normal structure, expression pattern of the proto-oncogene, or both. Thus, oncogenes are genes that, when mutated in a critical area, act in a positive way to promote carcinogenesis. The activation of an oncogene may be associated with increased expression of its protein products.

Overexpression of an oncogene can occur because of genomic amplification, juxtaposition to strong viral or tissue-specific promoters controlling its transcription (e.g., after a translocation event), or by constitutive deregulated expression that follows a mutational event. Rearrangements of chromosomes, resulting in truncations, insertions, or deletions, may also result in oncogene activation or inactivation of TSGs. The majority of oncogenes identified are part of the cell's growth regulatory pathways and include growth factors, growth factor receptors, intracellular signal transducers, cell cycle proteins, and nuclear transcription factors. Many oncogenes are tyrosine kinases—enzymes that phosphorylate tyrosine residues of proteins.

TSGs code for proteins whose loss of function results in transformation in contrast to the activating mutations that generate oncogenic alleles from proto-oncogenes. Both alleles of a TSG must be inactivated. Similar to those of the proto-oncogenes, the normal functions of TSGs are diverse. When one allele is inactivated in the germline, such a genotype is transmitted to all somatic cells, rendering them more susceptible to a second mutational event affecting the remaining functional allele. This results in a greater predisposition to cancers in families carrying such germline mutations. Studies determining LOH play an important role in the discovery of such genes and in genetic linkage analysis.

Inherited Predisposition to Lung Cancer

Less is probably known regarding the contribution of hereditary factors to lung cancer development than for any of the other common solid tumors. No distinct familial forms of the common types of lung cancers have been defined as have been defined for colon and breast cancers. Specific genetic loci responsible for a predisposition to lung cancer development have therefore not been elucidated. Tsuji and colleagues (1994), however, have shown that lung adenocarcinoma may be the histologic type that is most linked to definite familial occurrence.

Lung cancer has been documented in some genetic syndromes that have an increased predisposition to other cancers. Li and associates (1988) showed that lung cancer may occur with increased frequency in the Li-Fraumeni syndrome that results from a germline mutation in the *p53* TSG. In addition, Donehower and colleagues (1992) showed that knock-out mice for the *p53* gene can develop lung adenocarcinomas. Lung cancers have also been described in carriers of the inactivating mutation in the retinoblastoma TSG.

Mattson and associates (1987) showed that only 10% of smokers develop lung cancer. Evidence from Sellers and colleagues (1990) and others have implied an important role for genetic predisposition in determining risk of lung cancer development among smokers. A growing body of data exists linking genetic differences in the capacity to metabolize tobacco carcinogens with risk for developing lung cancer. Caporaso and associates (1989) showed that male smokers who extensively metabolized the antihypertensive drug debrisoquine were at a fourfold-increased risk of developing lung cancer compared to slow metabolizers. Certain enzymes can influence lung cancer risk by catalyzing detoxification reactions that enhance the elimination of the toxic products. To-Figueras and colleagues (1996) linked low or absent activity of the M1 isoform of glutathione-S–transferase to high lung cancer risk. The existing PCR assays for detecting the genetic status of each important metabolizing enzyme require refinement. A genetic profile of each of the factors might define a significant indicator of risk status in a person who smokes.

Genetic Alterations in Sporadic Lung Cancer

Bos (1989) and Clements (1995) and their coworkers showed that when sensitive PCR-based methods are used for detection, K-ras mutations occur in 30 to 50% of lung adenocarcinomas. K-ras mutations are more common in adenocarcinomas than in squamous cell carcinomas, are very rare in bronchioloalveolar carcinomas, and have not been described in SCLC. Ras proteins have been implicated in the transduction of growth and differentiation signals from activated transmembrane receptors to downstream protein kinases. The major defect when ras is mutated is a marked decrease in its ability to interact with the GTPase-activating protein, termed RAS-GAP. Hence, the ras protein remains in the GTP-bound or active state, and normal cell growth regulation is disturbed. Slebos and colleagues (1990) and others have shown that mutated K-ras gene confers a worse prognosis to lung adenocarcinomas.

DePinho and coworkers (1991) demonstrated that approximately 30 to 40% of SCLC cases have activation of c-myc, n-myc, or l-myc by DNA amplification. Amplification of c-myc appears to be a negative prognostic factor in SCLC. A number of investigators, including Sklar and Prochownik (1991) and Niimi and colleagues (1991), have suggested that the reason for this poor prognosis is that increased c-myc protein modifies tumor response to certain treatment modalities. Persons (1993) and Capodieci (1998) and their colleagues reported that FISH can be used to detect c-myc and c-erb-b2/HER-2/neu amplification in formalin-fixed, paraffin-embedded tissue. Figure 15-1 (see Color Fig. 15-1) shows gene amplification of c-erb-b2/HER-2/neu in a cell line and normal complement of the gene in normal cells.

Amplification and overexpression of c-erb-b2/HER-2/neu oncogene, a receptor tyrosine kinase, has been found in many different human primary tumors, including NSCLC, and appears to be important in human carcinogenesis. Kern and colleagues (1990) found overexpression in approximately 35% of adenocarcinomas and slightly less frequently in squamous cell carcinomas. Yu and coworkers (1994) demonstrated that the protein product c-erb-b2/HER-2/neu (p185neu) can enhance metastatic potential in human lung cancers. Overexpression of p185neu by immunohistochemistry has been shown by Kern (1990) and Harpole (1995) and their colleagues to correlate with poor prognosis in

NSCLC. Figure 15-2 (see Color Fig. 15-2) shows immunohistochemical staining of p185neu in NSCLC, metastatic to a lymph node. Overexpression of c-erb-b2/HER-2/neu confers chemoresistance to NSCLC; Zhang and Hung (1996) showed that they could sensitize NSCLC cells to chemotherapeutic drugs by using a tyrosine kinase inhibitor. Thus, estimation of overexpression of this oncogene may influence therapeutic options.

Because many proto-oncogenes are tyrosine kinases, the function of such proteins can be modulated by reversible phosphorylation by phosphatases. Several oncogenes, including c-erb-b2 and epidermal growth factor receptor, the latter of which has been implicated in the pathogenesis of lung cancer, transmit signals through the proto-oncogene ras, leading to the activation by phosphorylation of mitogen-activated protein (MAP) kinases. MAP kinase activation is thus a central step in tumor growth stimulation by the most widely expressed and activated human oncogenes. A novel family of phosphatases called MAP kinase phosphatases (MKPs) that inactivate MAP kinase by dephosphorylation has been identified. The human prototype of MKP, MKP-1, is the product of immediate early genes induced by the same agents that, in fact, regulate MAP kinase activity. One of us (M.L.) and colleagues (1996) have shown that MKP-1 is overexpressed early in the carcinogenic pathway in lung cancer and in indolent lung tumors, such as bronchioloalveolar carcinomas, and progressive loss of expression with increasing grade and stage occurs. Figure 15-3 (see Color Fig. 15-3) shows expression of MKP-1 by ISH in a case of bronchioloalveolar carcinoma. Because MKP-1 has been shown to inhibit apoptotic MAP kinase, its overexpression may result in inhibition of programmed cell death with resultant advantages to tumor cell growth.

Many common sites of LOH exist in lung cancer, suggesting the presence of alterations in TSGs. Testa and colleagues (1994) demonstrated an average of 31 clonal karyotypic abnormalities in NSCLC primary tumors. Several well-described TSGs are known to be altered in lung cancers and almost certainly play a role in their evolution. The most well-defined TSG change in lung cancer is mutation of the p53 gene, which is the single most common genetic alteration observed in human cancer, often occurring late in carcinogenesis. Lane (1992) termed p53 the guardian of the genome because of its critical role in the control of the cell cycle. p53 protein is normally expressed at low levels, is unstable (rapidly degraded), and is thus not normally detectable by immunohistochemistry. When the gene is mutated, the p53 protein has a longer half-life, accumulating to levels detectable by immunohistochemistry. Normal growth control function may also be inactivated due to binding by proteins of DNA viruses [e.g., human papillomaviruses and subsequent degradation by the ubiquitin-proteosome pathway, as shown by Scheffner (1994) and Rolfe (1995) and their colleagues]. However, loss of gene function in lung cancers appears to be the major correlate to the very frequent LOH of chromosome 17p13.1 in all

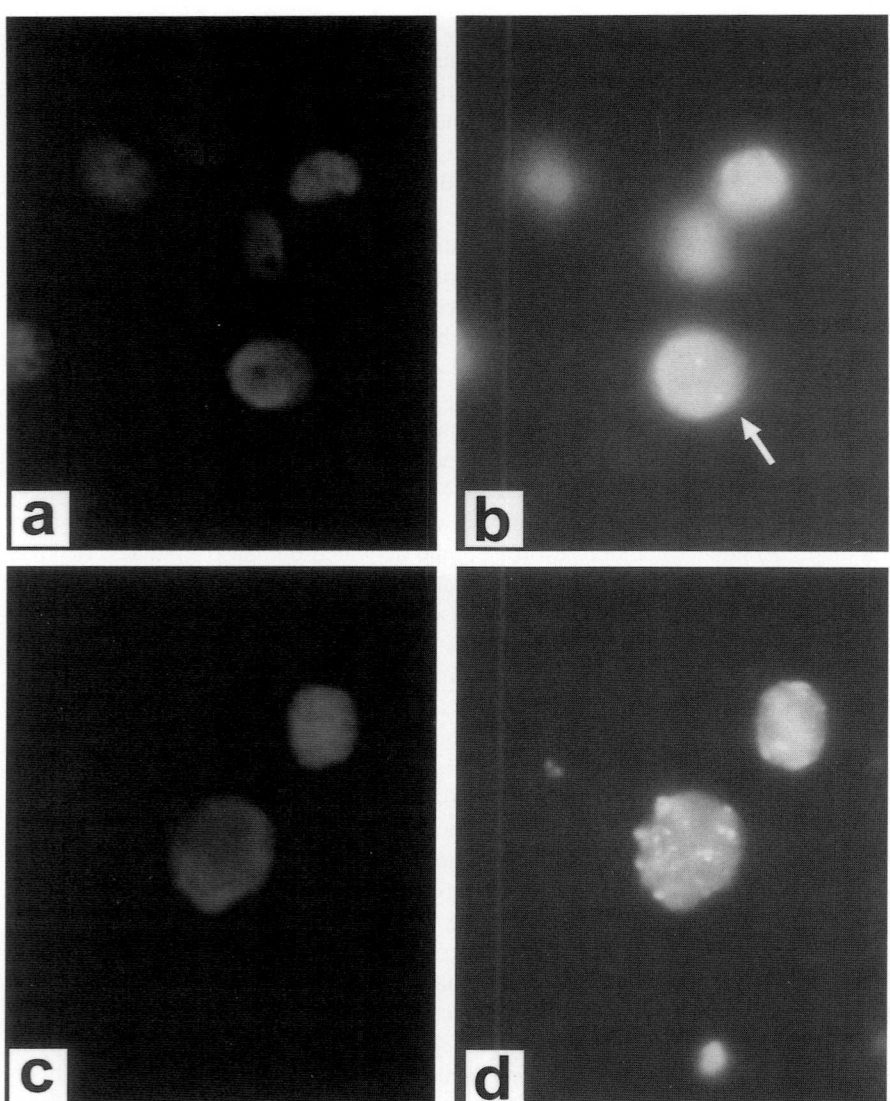

Fig. 15-1. Fluorescent in situ hybridization (FISH) demonstrating diploid complement of c-*erb*-b2/*HER2*/*neu* in normal cells. **a.** DAPI staining of cells. **b.** FISH (*arrow* designates diploid signal) and cancer cell line with amplification of c-*erb*-b2/*HER2*/*neu*. **c.** DAPI staining of cells. **d.** FISH. (See Color Fig. 15-1.) Courtesy of Dr. Paula Capodieci.

subtypes of lung carcinoma. Iggo and associates (1990) found *p53* mutations in approximately 50% of NSCLC and almost 100% of SCLC. Denissenko and colleagues (1996) found that benzo[a]pyrenediolepoxide, a tobacco carcinogen, directly binds to the hot spots for the *p53* mutations found in lung carcinomas. In studies of *p53* expression by immunohistochemistry in lung adenocarcinomas, Caamano and associates (1991) showed that overexpression of *p53* protein was associated with advanced stage; two other groups, Quinlan (1992) and McLaren (1992) and their colleagues, showed that overexpression of *p53* was associated with poor prognosis in lung cancers. Husgafvel-Pursiainen and associates (1997) used an enzyme-linked immunosorbent assay for estimating serum levels of mutant *p53* protein in a cohort of individuals with workplace exposure to asbestos or silica and subsequent lung cancers or mesotheliomas and compared serum *p53* levels with *p53* mutations and tissue accumulations of the mutant protein. They sug-

gested that serum *p53* levels are reasonably accurate in reflecting tissue alterations in *p53* at either the gene level, protein level, or both and can thus serve as early biomarkers of disease risk.

Yokota and colleagues (1987) showed that 13q LOH occurs in 75% of SCLC and 15% of NSCLC. This locus includes the site of the retinoblastoma gene (Rb) in chromosome region 13q14, which plays a critical role in cell cycle control. The Rb TSG is altered in nearly all SCLC tumors and in 30 to 40% of NSCLC, as shown by Hensel (1990) and Xu (1991) and their coworkers.

LOH of chromosome 3p occurs in 90 to 100% of SCLC and in 50 to 80% of NSCLC. Brauch (1990) and Hibi (1991) and their colleagues showed that chromosome areas within 3p21 are lost in NSCLC, and more distal regions at 3p25–p26 and more proximal regions at 3p12–p14 are more characteristically lost in SCLC. Intense efforts are being undertaken to identify TSGs in these areas. The fragile histidine triad gene

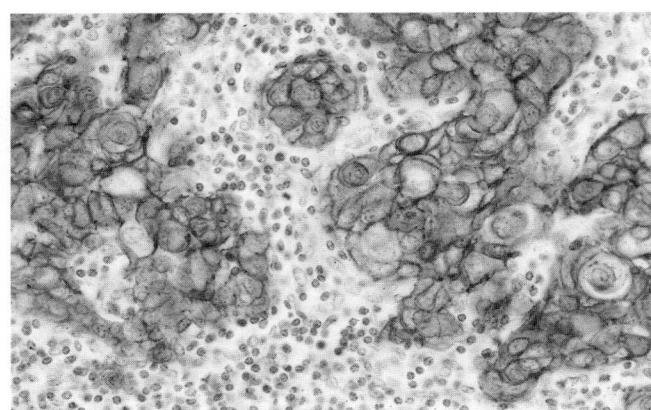

Fig. 15-2. Metastatic squamous cell carcinoma to a lymph node with positive staining of c-*erb*-b2/*HER2*/*neu*/*p185^neu* by immunohistochemistry. (See Color Fig. 15-2.)

(*FHIT*) located at chromosome 3p14.2 is another candidate TSG linked to lung cancer. Sozzi and associates (1996) showed that altered transcription splice products for the *FHIT* gene was a frequent characteristic of lung cancers. Fong and colleagues (1997) showed that allelic loss of this gene was common in lung cancer and preneoplastic bronchial lesions. Burke and coworkers (1998) demonstrated that loss of *FHIT* was a negative prognostic indicator in NSCLC, independent of tumor stage, size, tumor differentiation, and *p53* mutation status. The published data support a role for *FHIT* loss in the molecular pathogenesis of lung cancer.

Cytogenetic abnormalities of 9p are frequent in NSCLC. This site is the locus of two separate cyclin-dependent kinase inhibitors *p15* and *p16*. Kamb and colleagues (1994) showed that alterations of *p16* occur frequently in lung cancers. Loss of *p16* gene function occurs frequently via homozygous deletions in cell culture lines. Homozygous deletions of *p16* were also demonstrated in microdissected primary NSCLC by Packenham and associates (1995). Merlo and colleagues (1995) showed that transcriptional silencing associated with abnormal DNA methylation of the transcription start site region is another mechanism of loss of *p16* function. Absence of expression of the *p16* gene product is commonly observed in mesothelioma tumors and cell lines.

Mutations of *p27*, another cyclin-dependent kinase inhibitor, are rare in human tumors. Because of gene regulation occurring predominantly at the protein level, *p27* detection by immunohistochemistry is the method of choice for assessing its status in lung cancers. Esposito and coworkers (1997) demonstrated that *p27* loss is associated with poor prognosis in NSCLC and that this loss was a result of tumor-specific degradation of *p27*, as one of us (M.L.) and colleagues (1997) have demonstrated in colorectal carcinomas. Figure 15-4 (see Color Fig. 15-4) provides an example of a NSCLC with high *p27* expression and one with low *p27* expression by immunohistochemistry. In esophageal cancers, Singh and colleagues (1997) implicated cytoplasmic localization in *p27* inactivation. Catzavelos and colleagues (personal communication, 1998) found reduced levels of *p27* in 85% of NSCLC by immunohistochemistry and

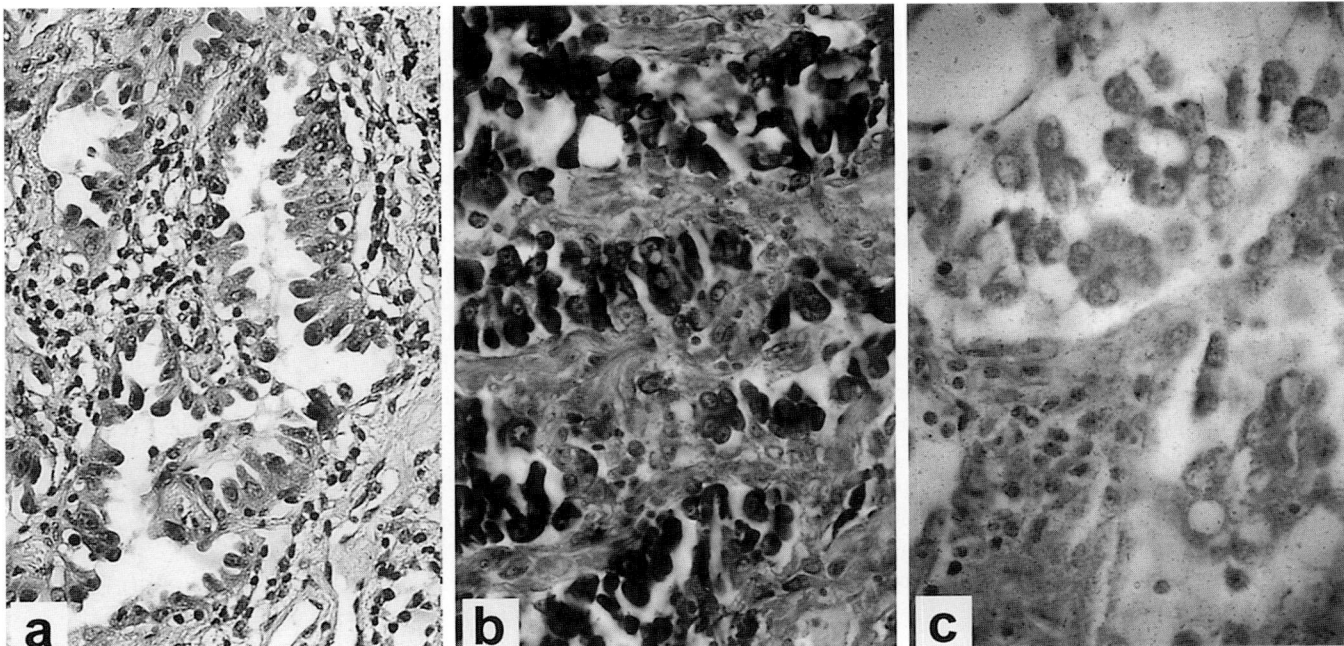

Fig. 15-3. a. Bronchioalveolar carcinoma stained by hematoxylin and eosin. **b.** In situ hybridization with antisense probe for mitogen-activated protein kinase phosphatase-1 demonstrating positive signal in the tumor cells. **c.** Control sense probe with absent signal in the tumor cells. (See Color Fig. 15-3.)

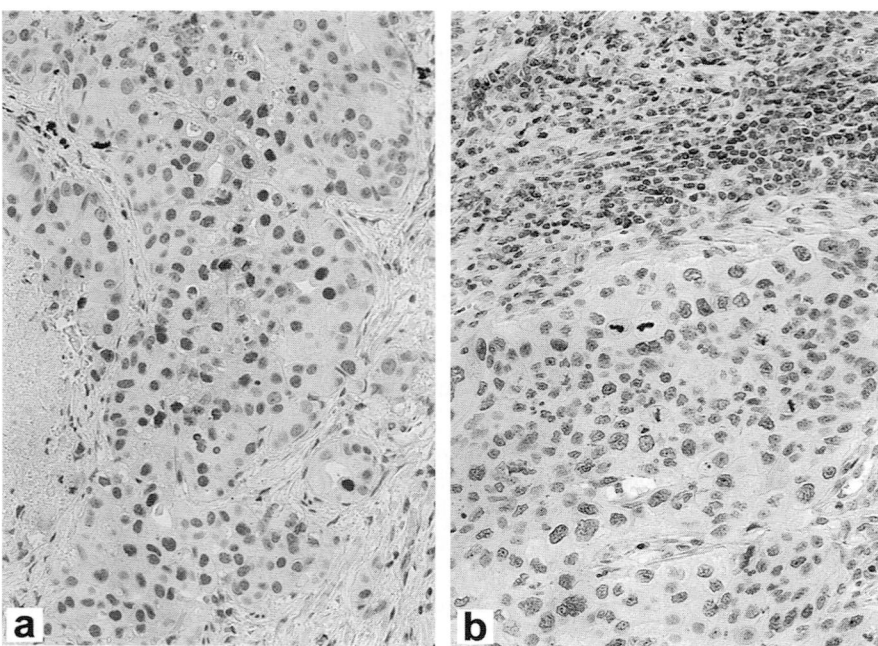

Fig. 15-4. *p27* expression by immunohisto-chemistry in non–small cell lung carci-noma. **a.** High expression of *p27* in tumor cells. **b.** Low expression of *p27* in tumor cells with lymphocytes serving as positive internal control. (See Color Fig. 15-4.) Courtesy of Dr. Michael Murphy.

showed a significant inverse correlation between *p27* level and tumor grade. They found that *ras* mutations were located exclusively in adenocarcinomas and showed no rela-tionship to *p27* levels. Confirmation of the involvement of the proteosome-mediated proteolysis in *p27* degradation should stimulate potential new strategies of nonsurgical treatments of NSCLC.

Malignant mesothelioma is one of the few extrarenal neo-plasms in which the Wilms' TSG (WT 1) expression is lost. Kleymenova and colleagues (1998) identified a site in intron 1 of WT 1 in rat mesothelioma cell lines that is frequently methylated. Renal cell carcinoma cell lines that did not express WT 1 were also methylated at the same site.

Wang and associates (1998) have described alterations in a candidate TSG, *PPP2RIB*, in lung and colon cell lines and solid tumors, corresponding to a high frequency of LOH on chromosome 11q23.

Cytogenetic analysis has been extended from the well-studied hematopathologic field to carcinomas, sarcomas, and melanomas. Fresh tissue is sent for short-term culture, from which metaphase chromosome spreads are plated on glass slides. Specific chromosomal abnormalities can be detected in many benign and malignant neoplasms. Distinct translocations in hematologic and solid tumors result either in the activation of proto-oncogene products or, more fre-quently, in the translation of novel tumor-specific fusion proteins. Because these fusion proteins are specific markers for individual subtypes of neoplasias, they are ideal indica-tors for the detection of disease and potential targets for therapy design. Genetic changes in carcinomas are gener-ally very complex, more so than those seen in a variety of lymphoid or mesenchymal tumors. Peripheral neuroecto-

dermal tumor (PNET) encompasses the family of lesions characterized by a specific and reproducible reciprocal chromosome translocation t(11;22) (q24;q12) and which show, to a varying degree, evidence of neuroectodermal dif-ferentiation. Demonstration of the cloned fusion gene prod-ucts of this translocation by the use of RT-PCR now allows accurate diagnosis at the molecular level. Askin and col-leagues (1979) originally described the clinical subset of PNET lesions that arise on the chest wall, often with involvement of the ribs, pleura, and lung, which have come to be known as *Askin tumors*. All PNETs show immunohis-tochemical positivity for the MIC-2 protein, best demon-strated by the antibodies HBA-71 or O-13, in addition to evidence of neuroectodermal differentiation. SCLC classi-cally has deletions of chromosome 3p14-23; mesothelioma has deletions of 3p13-23. The use of FISH technology has changed cytogenetics from a specialized and expensive technique reserved for special situations to the routine diag-nostic assessment of tumors. Assessing gene amplification and translocation in formalin-fixed tissue specimens is now possible. As more clinically useful distinctions are isolated, this technology will likely find an expanded role in diag-nostic pathology.

Screening and Molecular Markers

Successful therapies for NSCLC focus on early surgery with reported 5-year survival rates of approximately 50%, as shown by Williams and colleagues (1981). With the eluci-dation of the best genetic markers, they can be incorporated into diagnostic strategies that are already available for early diagnosis of lung cancer (e.g., sputum analysis). Mao and coworkers (1995) reported the detection of *p53* and *ras* gene mutations in sputum DNA months to years before clinical signs of tumor have been reported. These were retrospective studies in which the precise mutations that appeared in the tumors were known; prospective studies are needed to validate such approaches. Qi Chen and associates (1996) demonstrated microsatellite alterations in plasma DNA of patients with SCLC. In the future, germline DNA changes that reflect increased risk for the development of lung cancer might also play a role in population screening.

Sundaresan (1992) and Hung (1995) and their colleagues showed that *3p* loss occurs early in NSCLC and is detectable in preinvasive lesions. Fong (1997) and Tornielli (1997) and their colleagues detected loss of *FHIT* in preneoplastic bronchial lesions, suggesting that loss of this gene might be useful as a genetic marker. Kishimoto and colleagues (1995) showed *9p* and *17p* loss in preneoplastic lesions. Loss of function of *p16* may play a very early role, because LOH and homozygous deletions of chromosome 9p21 have been found in early lung cancer lesions. The timing of genetic events in lung carcinogenesis requires additional study and will help to define genes responsible for tumor initiation, provide targets to facilitate early lung cancer screening, and provide clues to genes involved in genetic predisposition to lung cancer.

DNA Mismatch Repair Genes

Highly conserved DNA repair genes play an important role in the maintenance of genetic integrity in normal cells. Inactivating mutations in the DNA repair genes leads to an increased rate of mutations in a variety of cellular genes in affected cells, including proto-oncogenes and TSGs. The accumulation of mutations in these growth-regulatory genes appears to be the rate-limiting step in tumorigenesis; therefore, inactivation of DNA damage recognition and repair genes greatly accelerates tumor progression. Microsatellites are highly polymorphic, short, tandem repeat sequences dispersed throughout the genome. Instability of these repeat sequences at multiple genetic loci result from mismatch repair errors caused by defective mismatch repair genes. The fundamental role of mismatch repair enzymes in human cancer is underscored by two findings: 1) by the fact that inherited cancer syndromes such as the autosomal dominant hereditary nonpolyposis colon cancer have been found to harbor defects in mismatch repair genes and are characterized by alteration of microsatellite sequences or microsatellite instability (MI); and 2) by the frequency with which MI is demonstrated in several human cancers of diverse tissue origin. Instability in microsatellite markers in lung cancer has been studied by several groups. Microsatellite instability is frequently observed in NSCLC, and the replication error phenotype is more common in clinically advanced disease and metastases.

Merlo and colleagues (1994) detected alterations of microsatellite loci consisting of deletions or expansions of (CA)n dinucleotide repeats in 45% of primary small cell lung cancers. Cancers that showed MI contained widespread allelic loss and had a uniformly poor prognosis. Fong and associates (1995) demonstrated MI in only 6.5% of cases of NSCLC and found it to be associated with extensive, concurrent molecular changes, including K-*ras* and *p53* mutations and frequent LOH at chromosomal regions 5q, 8p, 9p, 11p, and 17p. Wieland and colleagues (1996) detected MI at one or more loci in 29% of NSCLC. They found LOH of the mismatch repair gene hMLH1 at 3p21 in 82% of the tumors with MI, suggesting that defects in this gene may be important. Benachenhou and coworkers (1998) also revealed frequent allelic losses at the DNA mismatch repair locus hMSH3 in addition to hMLH1 in NSCLC.

Clonality

Assessment of clonality is especially useful when evaluating borderline lesions, such as atypical lymphoid proliferations in the lung, and the nature of a pleural effusion in a patient with a history of lymphoproliferative disease when flow cytometry is unhelpful, as in the case of recurrent/concurrent T-cell lymphoma. In these settings, a polyclonal population of cells indicates benign polyclonal hyperplasia, whereas clonal cells point to a neoplastic process. Many methods have been used to demonstrate clonality in tissues, including analysis of karyotypic abnormalities; gene rearrangements or translocations; point mutations in oncogenes and TSGs; viral sequences, such as the terminal repeat episomal sequence of the Epstein-Barr virus (EBV); microsatellite instability; loss of heterozygosity; and dosage compensation. Dosage compensation is a process in which the level of X-linked gene expression is equalized between the sexes by methylation of either the maternal or paternal allele. X-chromosome inactivation assays (which can be used only in females) use methylation-dependent restriction fragment length polymorphisms and probe to certain genes that are located on the X-chromosome, including glucose-6-phosphate dehydrogenase, phosphoglycerate kinase 1, and androgen receptor genes. To be clinically useful, the choice of a gene in the assessment of clonality must take into account the degree of polymorphism of the locus in the population. Signoretti and colleagues (1998) described a novel nonradioactive PCR single-strand conformational polymorphism (SSCP) technique to assess T-cell clonality in paraffin-embedded tissues of hyperplastic and neoplastic lymphoid populations. Consensus primers, generated against variable and joining regions, are used for TCR-γ gene rearrangement amplification. The SSCP imprint of PCR products that are generated is specific for each TCR-γ gene rearrangement and may be used to evaluate recurrent lesions in the same patient. Murphy and colleagues (1998) describe how the technique can be adapted for cytology preparations, such as pleural fluid. Figure 15-5 (see Color Fig. 15-5) shows T-lymphoblastic lymphoma in a lymph node, the subsequent pleural effusion with atypical lymphoid population, and the

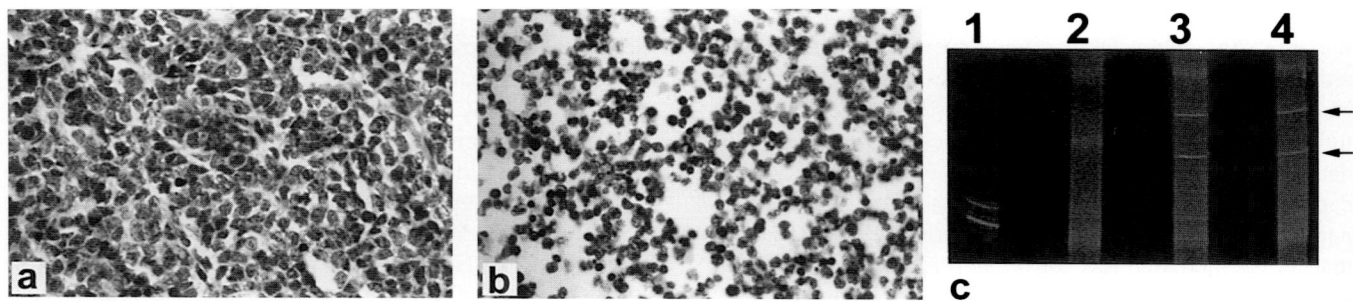

Fig. 15-5. T-lymphoblastic lymphoma in a lymph node (**a**) and subsequent pleural effusion with atypical lymphoid population (**b**), producing identical monoclonal banded patterns by polymerase chain reaction single-strand conformational polymorphism–based TCR-γ gene rearrangement analysis (**c**; lanes 3 and 4, *arrows*). (See Color Fig. 15-5.) Courtesy of Dr. Michael Murphy.

identical monoclonal banded patterns in both specimens by PCR-SSCP–based TCR-γ gene rearrangement analysis.

Body Cavity–Based Lymphomas

Diagnostic molecular hematopathology takes advantage of two events that take place in hematopoietic oncogenesis: gene rearrangements and chromosomal translocations. The former has been used as a marker of clonality, whereas the latter results in activation of proto-oncogenes with the production of chimeric oncoproteins. Techniques aimed at identifying these genetic events provide additional clinically relevant data for the diagnosis and classification of lymphoid neoplasms beyond the knowledge that can be obtained with immunophenotyping. The immunoglobulin, T-cell receptor genes, or both rearrange at the DNA level before clonal expansion in lymphoid cells. Because a given rearrangement is unique to a committed cell and its derivative clone, Southern blotting or PCR techniques are used to detect clonal populations in either fresh or archival tissues, otherwise undetectable by immunohistochemical methods. This is particularly useful for the analysis of T-cell neoplasms, because no immunophenotypic markers are available for assessment of clonality. Even though clonality is most often associated with cancer, clonal populations of lymphoid cells can be detected in patients with immune deficiencies, such as post–organ transplantation immunosuppression or acquired immunodeficiency syndrome (AIDS), in the absence of overt malignancy. In the interpretation of results of gene rearrangement studies, analyzing the results in the context of morphologic, immunophenotypic, and clinical data is extremely important.

Malignant lymphomas frequently arise in the pleural cavities of patients with long-standing tuberculous pyothorax or AIDS. These are known as *body cavity lymphomas* or *pyothorax-associated lymphomas*. Tumor cells frequently express EBV and human herpesvirus type 8 (HHV-8). Detection of the genome of these viruses may be used for diagnostic purposes; for the assessment of clonality as if

coupled to gene rearrangement as noted by Rockman (1997) and Purtilo (1984) or to monitor recurrence as demonstrated by Sasajima (1993), Szekely (1998), and Kanno (1998) and their colleagues.

Infectious Diseases Affecting the Lungs

Diagnostic molecular microbiology applies the principles of nucleic acid hybridization to the detection and characterization of pathogenetic microorganisms associated with infectious disease. PCR-based methods are replacing media-based biological amplification, and this is perhaps the area that has had the greatest impact in pulmonary disease. Fastidious organisms or viruses that cannot be cultured are now targets of molecular techniques. In addition, new organisms are being identified by molecular methods, and their association with human diseases are being elucidated. Molecular techniques have contributed to our understanding of the biology of pulmonary opportunists. Wakefield and associates (1994) showed that induced sputum could be used to detect *Pneumocystis carinii* in the lung of immunocompromised patients with a diagnostic sensitivity and specificity exceeding 95%. Proviral load evaluation by the DNA-PCR technique has been used to detect the presence of human immunodeficiency virus (HIV) in the lung parenchyma and to demonstrate its capability to infect different types of immunocompetent cells in dimercaprol. HHV-8 can be detected in early Kaposi's sarcoma lesions, which may occur in the lung by in situ PCR techniques.

Molecular identification of micro-organisms is especially useful in several ways: to avoid misinterpretation of false-positive serology due to the presence of cross-reacting antibodies to host antigens or to antigens of related organisms; to identify pathogenic organisms before seroconversion; to follow response to therapy; to identify mutations responsible for drug resistance; to subtype different strains; and for the rapid and accurate identification of organisms that require elaborate and long media-based cultures. Although detailed discussions of molecular microbiology are beyond the scope of this chapter, mycobacterial infections and EBV are discussed briefly.

Mycobacterial Infections

Mycobacterial infections have resurfaced as diseases with significant clinical impact and have a mortality of 60% if untreated. The frequency of mycobacterial infections in immunocompromised patients has increased. Inadequate treatment of many patients has led to an increase in the proportion of patients with drug-resistant strains of *M. tuberculosis*. Microscopic diagnosis of acid-fast bacilli is time consuming, not species specific, and insensitive, especially in treated patients. Culture of such organisms requires weeks, which can result in delays in therapy or inappropriate treatment of unaffected individuals. Molecular diagnostics can play an important role in adequate and timely treatment and in patient follow-up. Species-specific PCR for mycobacteria can be performed on a variety of samples, including sputum and paraffin-embedded tissue. PCR is sensitive and specific when results are compared with bacteriologic and clinical data. These tests can be performed in as few as 4 to 5 hours, permitting same-day reporting of results. Telenti and colleagues (1997) showed that genotyping can be performed using PCR-SSCP. Mutations in the *rpoB* gene (encoding the b subunit of the RNA polymerase) were identified in one study in all of the rifampin-resistant isolates and none of the susceptible strains.

Strain-specific differentiation of *M. tuberculosis* is complex, but it may be important to differentiate between whether an individual infection represents reactivation or exogenous reinfection or whether an unexpected positive culture result was due to possible contamination in the laboratory. Attention has focused on the insertion sequence IS*6110*, one of a number of mycobacterial, mobile genetic elements. IS*6110* is a naturally occurring transposable genetic element that appears to be detectable only in species belonging to the *M. tuberculosis* complex. Each strain contains a different number of identical copies of this transposable element. The number of copies of IS*6110* elements and the size of the restriction fragments containing these elements vary such that no two unrelated strains produce identical patterns when hybridized with a labeled IS*6110* probe. This forms the basis for a unique genetic fingerprint. Thus, molecular epidemiology can identify numerous suspected and unsuspected transmission links. Another promising technology for clinical tuberculosis laboratories involves oligonucleotide arrays or DNA chips. Gingeras and colleagues (1998) demonstrated that DNA arrays could be used for genotyping and species identification and for the detection of *rpoB* gene mutations.

Epstein-Barr Virus Infections

EBV is a double-stranded DNA herpesvirus that can persist in latent form in epithelial cells and B lymphocytes. In the majority of cases, EBV infection results in a self-limiting, transient lymphoproliferative disorder. In an immunosuppressed state, however, such as HIV infection or in therapeutic immunosuppression after organ transplantation, reactivation of latent infection may contribute to the development of full-blown malignancies. EBV immortalizes the cell and blocks differentiation, thus committing the cell to indefinite T-cell independent proliferation. EBV has thus been implicated in the pathogenesis of several neoplasms, including lymphoepithelioma-like carcinomas that have been described in many sites, including the lung. The role of EBV in body cavity-associated lymphomas has already been described. As is the case for most micro-organisms, a variety of techniques, including ISH and PCR, can be used to assess the presence of the actively replicating virus. The terminal repeat regions of the virus have been used as markers of clonality in angiocentric immunoproliferative lesions. Nonisotopic ISH for Epstein-Barr early RNA can be easily accomplished in paraffin-embedded tissues using oligonucleotide probes.

Interstitial Lung Disease

Diffuse interstitial lung diseases are triggered by diverse factors in an individual with a genetic predisposition. Certain genetic traits are emerging as risk factors for development of pulmonary fibrosis. Identification of patients with genetic susceptibility would theoretically allow improved monitoring of disease progression.

Pathogenesis of pulmonary fibrosis is linked to induction of some cytokines, such as tumor necrosis factor-α (TNF-α), transforming growth factor-β (TGF-β), interleukin 1B (IL-1B), and platelet-derived growth factor (PDGF). TNF-α is considered to be a key cytokine, because it stimulates growth of fibroblasts and increases collagen deposition; anti–TNF-α antibody prevents development of bleomycin or silica-induced interstitial pneumonitis in mice. TNF-α transgenic mice that overexpress TNF-α only in the lungs develop interstitial pneumonitis resembling idiopathic pulmonary fibrosis in humans. TNF-α transgenic mice have been studied by Sueoka and colleagues (1998) to analyze the sequential process of interstitial pneumonitis serving as a model of the inflammatory stage of idiopathic pulmonary fibrosis in humans. The pattern of cytokine gene expressions and synthesis as detected by semiquantitative RT-PCR and Northern blot analysis changed with the progression of histologic features. Clarifying the molecular pathogenesis of idiopathic pulmonary fibrosis in relation to histologic changes and cytokine expression with the aim of developing new treatments may be important. Because TNF-α and TGF-β have been implicated in the pathogenesis of interstitial fibrosis, early diagnosis might result in the initiation of early and more effective therapy, including anticytokine therapy. Inhibiting interactions between lung cells and extracellular matrix that lead to intracellular signal transduction (including *ras*) and MAP kinase pathways may also prove beneficial.

Although the etiology of sarcoidosis is still unknown, it is suspected to be the result of an antigen-driven process. Molecular biology techniques have led to clues toward the partial elucidation of pathogenetic mechanisms associated with this disease. Molecular diagnostic tests are not available; however, the detection using PCR by Popper (1994) and Ghossein (1994) and their colleagues of *M. tuberculosis* DNA in some patients with sarcoid suggests that at least in some cases the disease may be initiated by a mycobacterial infection. In the majority of patients with sarcoidosis, T-cell DNA recovered from bronchoalveolar lavage gives rise to a pattern on Southern blotting that can also be observed in other immune-mediated lung disorders, including hypersensitivity pneumonitis and lymphocytic interstitial pneumonia, which suggests that this finding represents a feature of lung T cells rather than the result of a specific rearrangement typical of a distinct disorder. Klein and associates (1995) have studied the diversity of the TCR repertoire in the granulomatous response occurring in the Kveim-Siltzbach (KS) skin test and have demonstrated an oligoclonal response. Cloning of the T cells that accumulate at sites of positive KS tests may lead to the detection of sarcoid antigens and thereby lead to an improved diagnostic test for sarcoidosis.

ANIMAL MODELS

Animal models can prove invaluable for clarifying genetic determinants of human cancer where little is known about the initial molecular steps underlying tumorigenesis. Animal models of human disease form the basis of experimental pathology and provide the best paradigm for the assessment of molecular findings in routine pathology practice. Multiple animal types, including dogs, mice, and rats, are susceptible to development of either spontaneous lung cancers or lung neoplasms induced by exposure to carcinogens. These may be particularly valuable for determining genetic changes that contribute to predisposition to lung neoplasia. Two models for the study of gene function relating to human diseases are transgenic and knock-out animals.

Transgenic animals are defined as those in which foreign DNA, usually a human gene, is introduced into fertilized cells and is subsequently inherited in the progeny of the host. By virtue of the way in which the construct is designed, it can be overexpressed in all tissues when transcription is driven by a strong constitutive promoter; equally, its expression can be restricted by tissue-specific or developmentally regulated promoters. Transgenic overexpression of TNF-α and TGF-β was shown by Miyazati (1995) and Lee (1995) and their colleagues to induce interstitial fibrosis, confirming the role of these growth factors in the pathogenesis of interstitial fibrosis.

Knock-out mice provide the ideal experimental setting when assessing the consequences of loss of function of a gene is important. Standard knock-out mice are made by specifically inactivating the gene of choice in embryonic stem cells. These are then injected into the mouse embryo where they have the potential to develop into the different cell types. As in transgenic mice, the inactivated gene is carried in the germline and passed to the progeny. To overcome early embryonic death as a result of absolute necessity for the gene of interest in development, genes may be selectively knocked out using cell type-specific gene targeting.

GENE THERAPY

Molecular techniques are identifying novel targets for the development of new treatment approaches to treatment for an expanding range of pulmonary diseases. Targeting of intracellular signal transduction pathways or cell cycle regulatory proteins is one approach to therapy. Gene therapy aims to induce or abolish the expression of proteins (depending on the target) by introducing or targeting the destruction of their coding genes in tumor cells. Delivery systems for therapeutic genes include viral vectors, particularly retroviruses; adenoviruses; adeno-associated viruses; herpesviruses; cationic liposomes; and anaerobic, genetically modified, clostridial organisms. Potential applications of gene therapy include the treatment of single-gene defects (such as CF) and more complex conditions, including cancer and inflammatory lung conditions (such as asthma, chronic obstructive airways disease, and adult respiratory distress syndrome). Molecular diagnostic tests will be used with increasing frequency to monitor novel genetic approaches in the treatment of pulmonary diseases. In CF, encouraging preliminary studies by Alton (1993), Zabner (1993), Caplen (1995), and Crystal (1995) and their associates have been published on topical delivery of the CFTR to the nasal epithelium or airways with overall encouraging results in the correction of the transepithelial chloride transport defect. Knowles and coworkers (1995), however, demonstrated no correction of the defective chloride secretion using adenoviral vector–mediated gene transfer to the nasal epithelium of 12 patients with CF. Only 6 to 10% of cells need to be corrected to counter the chloride transport defect, and only 5% of normal CFTR mRNA needs to be expressed to markedly increase chloride transport.

Genetic modification of critical elements of the inflammatory process may prove beneficial in complex pulmonary conditions characterized by lung inflammation, including adult respiratory distress syndrome, chronic obstructive pulmonary disease, and asthma. Examples of possible targets include overexpression of genes encoding anti-inflammatory cytokines, such as IL-10, and of inhibitors of inflammatory transcription factors (e.g., IB, the inhibitor of NF-B). The effectiveness of these treatments depends on selection of the appropriate cellular target, high enough stable expression of the introduced gene, and refinements in delivery vectors and suppression of host immune response. Monitoring of gene therapy with molecular diagnostic techniques is of paramount importance.

The strategy frequently used in cancer patients is to insert in tumor cells genes expressing molecules that induces a natural immune attack against the transfected neoplastic cells. Cells can also be driven to express thymidine kinase (a herpesvirus protein) and subsequent treatment with antiviral agents, such as ganciclovir, results in tumor cell death. Some of the genetic changes that frequently occur in established lung cancers are also potential therapeutic targets. Roth and colleagues (1996) demonstrated regression of lung tumors after injection with a retrovirus for expression of the wild-type *p53* gene. Esandi and associates (1997) reported the use of gene therapy in experimental malignant mesothelioma. Sterman and coworkers (1998) demonstrated that intrapleural administration of adenoviral-mediated herpes simplex virus thymidine kinase/ganciclovir gene therapy in patients with mesothelioma resulted in detectable gene transfer that was well tolerated by patients. Frizelle and colleagues (1998) demonstrated that adenovirus-mediated re-expression of p16INK4a in mesothelioma cells results in tumor regression. Hallahan and associates (1995) used a radiation-inducible promoter ligated to the TNF-α gene and demonstrated increased tumor cell death after irradiation. Dachs and colleagues (1997) demonstrated that transfection of cells in vitro with a hypoxia response element could be used to transcriptionally regulate gene expression in vivo under hypoxic conditions. Potentially, this approach allows the activation of a nontoxic prodrug to its toxic metabolite selectively in tumors with low oxygen levels. Certain species of the genus *Clostridium* can selectively germinate and grow in the hypoxic regions of solid tumors after intravenous injection of spores, as demonstrated by Malmgren and Flanagan (1995). Lemmon and colleagues (1997) genetically engineered *Clostridium beijerinkii* by introducing a plasmid that expressed nitroreductase that can convert CB1954 into a potent bifunctional alkylating agent. After the spores were injected into mice, nitroreductase protein and activity could be detected in tumors but not in normal tissue in the same mice.

CONCLUSION

Understanding the molecular events that underlie the pathogenesis of disease is creating a fundamental change in the way in which disease should be approached. The clinical application of molecular diagnostic techniques has allowed a more precise and rapid assessment of neoplastic and non-neoplastic pulmonary disease processes. Molecular diagnostic tests in addition to immunohistochemistry can be used in the identification and quantification of genes and gene products with potential prognostic value and those involved in chemoresistance, including *p53* and c-erb-b2/*HER*-2/*neu*. A specific tumor profile can be generated for an individual patient to assist in the selection of therapeutic management; with microarray technology, this is likely to become routine. More precise and timely therapeutic interventions are possible in diverse types of pulmonary diseases. The path to complete understanding of the molecular basis of disease, however, is still far from complete. Only a fraction of the estimated number of human genes has been identified and sequenced, and the function of only a few is known. Molecular biology is increasingly being used to elucidate the various steps of tumor initiation, progression, and metastasis. In addition, technical advances in recombinant DNA technology have resulted in the identification of tumor markers that are of prognostic importance and that may aid in early diagnosis. As other gene alterations important in the various stages of lung cancer progression are discovered, they will present more potential molecular targets for new and novel therapeutic strategies for lung cancer. Monitoring of gene therapy will require refined molecular diagnostic techniques to guide these novel therapeutic regimens. Understanding the molecular events underlying neoplastic transformation will translate into improved patient survival and prevention of cancer.

REFERENCES

Alton EW, et al: Non-invasive liposome-mediated gene therapy can correct the ion transport defect in cystic fibrosis mutant mice. Nat Genet 5:135, 1993.

Askin F, et al: Malignant small cell tumor of the thoracopulmonary region in childhood. A distinctive clinicopathologic entity of uncertain histogenesis. Cancer 43:2438, 1979.

Benachenhou N, et al: High resolution deletion mapping reveals frequent allelic losses at the DNA mismatch repair loci hMLH1 and hMSH3 in non-small cell lung cancer. Int J Cancer 77:173, 1998.

Bos JL: *Ras* oncogenes in human cancer: a review. Cancer Res 49:4682, 1989.

Brauch H, et al: Molecular mapping of deletion sites in the short arm of chromosome 3 in human lung cancer. Genes Chromosomes Cancer 1:240, 1990.

Burke L, et al: Allelic deletion analysis of the *FHIT* gene predicts poor survival in non-small cell lung cancer. Cancer Res 58:2533, 1998.

Caamano J, et al: Detection of p53 in primary lung tumors and non-small cell lung carcinoma cell lines. Am J Pathol 139:839, 1991.

Caplen NJ, et al: Liposome-mediated CFTR gene transfer to the nasal epithelium of patients with cystic fibrosis. Nat Med 1:39, 1995.

Capodieci P, et al: Automated in situ hybridization: diagnostic and research applications. Diagn Mol Pathol 7:69, 1998.

Caporaso NE, et al: Lung cancer risk, occupational exposure, and the debrisoquine metabolic phenotype. Cancer Res 49:3675, 1989.

Clements NC, et al: Analysis of K-ras gene mutations in malignant and nonmalignant endobronchial tissue obtained by fiberoptic bronchoscopy. Am J Respir Crit Care Med 152:1374, 1995.

Crystal RG, et al: Administration of an adenovirus containing the human CFTR cDNA to the respiratory tract of individuals with cystic fibrosis. Nat Genet 8:42, 1994.

Dachs GU, et al: Targeting gene expression to hypoxic tumor cells. Nat Med 3:515, 1997.

DeMuth JP, et al: The gene expression index c-myc x E2F-1/p21 is highly predictive of malignant phenotype in human bronchial epithelial cells. Am J Respir Cell Mol Biol 19:18, 1998.

Denissenko MF, et al: Preferential formation of benzo[a]pyrene adducts at lung cancer mutational hot spots in p53. Science 274:430, 1996.

DePinho RA, et al: Myc family oncogenes in the development of normal and neoplastic cells. Adv Cancer Res 57:1, 1991.

Donehower LA, et al: Mice deficient for p53 are developmentally normal but susceptible to spontaneous tumors. Nature 356:215, 1992.

Esandi MC, et al: Gene therapy of experimental malignant mesothelioma using adenovirus vectors encoding the HSVtk gene. Gene Ther 4:280, 1997.

Esposito V, et al: Prognostic role of the cyclin-dependent kinase inhibitor p27 in non-small cell lung cancer. Cancer Res 57:3381, 1997.

Fain JS, Bryan RN, Cheng L: Rapid diagnosis of Legionella infection by a nonisotopic in situ hybridization method. Am J Clin Pathol 95:719, 1990.

Fong KM, Zimmerman PV, Smith PJ: Microsatellite instability and other molecular abnormalities in non-small cell lung cancer. Cancer Res 55:28, 1995.

Fong KM, et al: FHIT and FRA3B 3p14.2 allele loss are common in lung cancer and preneoplastic bronchial lesions and are associated with cancer-related FHIT cDNA splicing aberrations. Cancer Res 57:2256, 1997.

Frizelle SP, et al: Re-expression of p16INK4a in mesothelioma cells results in cell cycle arrest, cell death, tumor suppression and tumor regression. Oncogene 16:3087, 1998.

Gelmini S, et al: Quantitative polymerase chain reaction-based homogeneous assay with fluorogenic probes to measure c-erbB-2 oncogene amplification. Clin Chem 43:752, 1997.

Ghossein RA, et al: A search for mycobacterial DNA in sarcoidosis using the polymerase chain reaction. Am J Clin Pathol 101:733, 1994.

Gingeras TR, et al: Simultaneous genotyping and species identification using hybridization pattern recognition analysis of generic Mycobacterium DNA arrays. Genome Res 8:425, 1998.

Hallahan DE, et al: Spatial and temporal control of gene therapy using ionizing radiation. Nat Med 1:786, 1995.

Hamid QA, et al: Detection of human probombesin mRNA in neuroendocrine (small cell) carcinoma of the lung. In situ hybridization with cRNA probe. Cancer 63:266, 1989.

Harpole DH, et al: A prognostic model of recurrence and death in stage I non-small cell lung cancer utilizing presentation, histopathology, and oncoprotein expression. Cancer Res 55:51, 1995.

Hensel CH, et al: Altered structure and expression of the retinoblastoma susceptibility gene in small cell lung cancer. Cancer Res 50:2735, 1990.

Hibi K, et al: Three distinct regions involved in 3p deletion in human lung cancer. Oncogene 7:445, 1992.

Hung J, et al: Allele-specific chromosome 3p deletions occur at an early stage in the pathogenesis of lung carcinoma. JAMA 273:558, 1995.

Husgafvel-Pursiainen K, et al: Mutations, tissue accumulations, and serum levels of p53 in patients with occupational cancers from asbestos and silica exposure. Environ Mol Mutagen 30:224, 1997.

Iggo R, et al: Increased expression of mutant forms of p53 oncogene in primary lung cancer. Lancet 335:675, 1990.

Kamb A, et al: A cell cycle regulator potentially involved in genesis of many tumor types. Science 264:436, 1994.

Kanno H, et al: Appearance of a different clone of Epstein-Barr virus genome in recurrent tumor of pyothorax-associated lymphoma (PAL) and a minireview of PAL. Leukemia 12:288, 1998.

Kern JA, et al: p185neu expression in human lung adenocarcinomas predict shortened survival. Cancer Res 50:5184, 1990.

Kishimoto Y, et al: Allele loss in chromosome 9p loci in preneoplastic lesions accompany non-small-cell lung cancers. J Natl Cancer Inst 87:1224, 1995.

Klein JT, et al: Selection of oligoclonal V-b specific T cells in the intradermal response to Kveim-Siltzbach reagent in individuals with sarcoidosis. J Immunol 154:1450, 1995.

Kleymenova EV, et al: Identification of a tumor-specific methylation site in the Wilms tumor suppressor gene. Oncogene 16:713, 1998.

Knowles MR, et al: A controlled study of adenoviral-vector-mediated gene transfer in the nasal epithelium of patients with cystic fibrosis. N Engl J Med 333:823, 1995.

Kononen J, et al: Tissue microarrays for high-throughput molecular profiling of tumor specimens. Nature Med 4:844, 1998.

Kotsimbos AT, et al: Quantitative detection of human cytomegalovirus DNA in lung transplant recipients. Am J Respir Crit Care Med 156:1241, 1997.

Landis SH, et al: Cancer statistics, 1997. CA Cancer J Clin 48:6, 1998.

Lane DP: p53, guardian of the genome. Nature 358:15, 1992.

Lee M-S, et al: Accumulation of extracellular matrix and developmental dysregulation in the pancreas by transgenic production of transforming growth factor-1. Am J Pathol 147:42, 1995.

Lemmon ML, et al: Anaerobic bacteria as a gene delivery system that is controlled by the tumor microenvironment. Gene Ther 4:791, 1997.

Li FP, et al: A cancer family syndrome in twenty kindreds. Cancer Res 48:5358, 1988.

Loda M, et al: Expression of mitogen-activated protein kinase phosphatase-1 in the early phases of human epithelial carcinogenesis. Am J Pathol 149:1553, 1996.

Loda M, et al: Increased proteosome-dependent degradation of the cyclin-dependent kinase inhibitor p27 in aggressive colorectal carcinomas. Nat Med 3:231, 1997.

Malmgren RA, Flanigan CC: Localization of the vegetative form of Clostridium tetani in mouse tumors following intravenous spore administration. Cancer Res 15:473, 1955.

Mao L, et al: Detection of oncogene mutations in sputum precedes a diagnosis of lung cancer. Cancer Res 54:1634, 1994.

Mattson ME, Pollack ES, Cullen JW: What are the odds that smoking will kill you? Am J Public Health 77:425, 1987.

McLaren R, et al: The relationship of p53 immunostaining to survival in carcinoma of the lung. Br J Cancer 66:735, 1992.

Merkel D, McGuire W: Ploidy, proliferative activity and prognosis: DNA flow cytometry of solid tumors. Cancer 65:1194, 1990.

Merlo A, et al: Frequent microsatellite instability in primary small cell lung cancer. Cancer Res 54:2098, 1994.

Merlo A, et al: 5' CpG island methylation is associated with transcriptional silencing of the tumor suppressor p16/CDKN2/MTS1 in human lung cancers. Nat Med 1:686, 1995.

Miyazaki Y, et al: Expression of a tumor necrosis factor-alpha transgene in murine lung causes lymphocytic and fibrosing alveolitis. J Clin Invest 96:250, 1995.

Murphy M, et al: Detection of recurrent non-Hodgkin's lymphoma in serous effusions by PCR [abstract]. Mod Pathol 11:41A, 1998.

Niimi S, et al: Resistance to anticancer drugs in NIH3T3 cells transfected with c-myc and/or c-H-ras genes. Br J Cancer 63:237, 1991.

Packenham JP, et al: Homozygous deletions at chromosome 9p21 and mutation analysis of p16 and p15 in microdissected primary non small cell lung cancers. Clin Cancer Res 1:687, 1995.

Pappas J, et al: A comparison of CMV DNA copy number in patient samples by qualitative and quantitative (TaqMan) PCR procedures [Abs197]. Abstr Gen Meet Am Soc Microbiol 97:154, 1997.

Pease AC, et al: Light-generated oligonucleotide arrays for rapid DNA sequence analysis. Proc Natl Acad Sci U S A 91:5022, 1994.

Persons DL, et al: Interphase molecular cytogenetic analysis of epithelial ovarian carcinomas. Am J Pathol 142:733, 1995.

Popper HH, Winter E, Hofler G: DNA of Mycobacterium tuberculosis in formalin-fixed, paraffin-embedded tissue in tuberculosis and sarcoidosis detected by polymerase chain reaction. Am J Clin Pathol 101:738, 1994.

Purtilo DT: Clonality of EBV-induced lymphoproliferative diseases in immune-deficient patients. N Engl J Med 19:191, 1984.

qi Chen X, et al: Microsatellite alterations in plasma DNA of small cell lung cancer patients. Nat Med 2:1033, 1996.

Quinlan DC, et al: Accumulation of p53 protein correlates with a poor prognosis in human lung cancer. Cancer Res 52:4828, 1992.

Rockman SP: Determination of clonality in patients who present with diagnostic dilemmas: a laboratory experience and review of the literature. Leukemia 11:852, 1997.

Rolfe M, et al: Reconstitution of p53-ubiquitinylation reaction from purified components: the role of human UBC4 and E6AP. Proc Natl Acad Sci U S A 92:3264, 1995.

Roth JA, et al: Retrovirus wild p53 gene transfer to tumors of patients with lung cancer. Nat Med 2:985, 1996.

Sasajima Y, et al: High expression of the Epstein-Barr virus latent protein EB nuclear antigen-2 on pyothorax-associated lymphomas. Am J Pathol 143:1280, 1993.

Scheffner M, et al: Identification of a human ubiquitin-conjugating enzyme that mediates the E6-AP-dependent ubiquitination of p53. Proc Natl Acad Sci U S A 91:8797, 1994.

Sellers TA, et al: Evidence for mendelian inheritance in the pathogenesis of lung cancer. J Natl Cancer Inst 82:1272, 1990.

Signoretti S, et al: Detection of clonal T-cell receptor gamma gene rearrangements in paraffin-embedded tissue by polymerase chain reaction and nonradioactive single-strand conformational polymorphism analysis. Am J Pathol 154:67, 1999.

Singh SP, et al: Loss or altered subcellular localization of p27 in Barrett's associated adenocarcinoma. Cancer Res 58:1730, 1998.

Sklar MD, Prochownik EV: Modulation of cis resistance in Friend erythroleukemia cells by c-myc. Cancer Res *51*:2118, 1991.

Slebos RJ, Kibdelaar RE, Dalesio O: K-ras oncogene activation as a prognostic marker in adenocarcinoma of the lung. N Engl J Med *323*: 561, 1990.

Sozzi G, et al: The FHIT gene at 3p14.2 is abnormal in lung cancer. Cell *85*:17, 1996.

Sterman DH, et al: Adenovirus-mediated herpes simplex virus thymidine kinase/ganciclovir gene therapy in patients with localized malignancy: results of a phase I clinical trial in malignant mesothelioma. Hum Gene Ther *9*:1083, 1998.

Sueoka N, et al: Molecular pathogenesis of interstitial pneumonitis with TNF-alpha transgenic mice. Cytokine *10*:124, 1998.

Sundaresan V, et al: p53 and chromosome 3 abnormalities, characteristic of malignant lung tumors, are detectable in preinvasive lesions of the bronchus. Oncogene *7*:1989, 1992.

Szekely L, et al: Restricted expression of Epstein-Barr virus (EBV)-encoded, growth transformation-associated antigens in an EBV- and human herpesvirus type 8-carrying body cavity lymphoma line. J Gen Virol *79*:1445, 1998.

Telenti A, et al: Genotypic assessment of isoniazid and rifampin resistance in *Mycobacterium tuberculosis*: a blind study at reference laboratory level. J Clin Microbiol 35:*719*, 1997.

Testa JR, et al: Cytogenetic analysis of 63 non small cell lung carcinomas: Recurrent chromosome alterations amid frequent and wide-spread genomic upheaval. Genes Chromosomes Cancer *11*:178, 1994.

To-Figueras J, et al: Glutathione-*S*-transferase MI and codon 72 *p53* polymorphisms in a northwestern Mediterranean population and their relation to lung cancer susceptibility. Cancer Epidemiol Biomarkers Prev *5*:337, 1996.

Tornielli S, et al: Analysis of *FHIT* gene alterations in primary tumors, bronchial mucosa biopsies and sputum specimens from lung cancer patients. Lung Cancer *18*:139, 1997.

Tsuji H, et al: Bilateral bronchioloalveolar carcinoma, showing familial aggregation of lung cancer. Nippon Kyobu Geka Gakkai Zasshi *42*:1061, 1994.

Wakefield AE, et al: Granulomatous *Pneumocystis carinii* pneumonia: DNA amplification studies on bronchoscopic alveolar lavage samples. J Clin Pathol *47*:664, 1994.

Wang SS, et al: Alterations of the *PPP2R1B* gene in human lung and colon cancer. Science *282*:284, 1998.

Wieland I, et al: Microsatellite instability and loss of heterozygosity at the hMLH1 locus on chromosome 3p21 occur in a subset of non-small cell lung carcinomas. Oncol Res *8*:1, 1996.

Williams DE, et al: Survival of patients surgically treated for stage I lung cancer. J Thoracic Cardiovasc Surg *82*:70, 1981.

Xing Z, et al: Overexpression of granulocyte-macrophage colony-stimulating factor induces pulmonary granulation tissue formation and fibrosis by induction of transforming growth factor-b1 and myofibroblast accumulation. Am J Pathol *150*:59, 1997.

Xu HJ, et al: Absence of retinoblastoma protein expression in primary non-small cell lung carcinomas. Cancer Res *51*:2735, 1991.

Yokota J, et al: Loss of heterozygosity of chromosome 3 in adenocarcinoma of the lung. Proc Natl Acad Sci U S A *84*:9252, 1987.

Yu D, et al: c-*erb*B-2/*neu* overexpression enhances metastatic potential of human lung cancer cells by induction of metastasis-associated properties. Cancer Res *54*:3260, 1994.

Zabner J, et al: Adenovirus-mediated gene transfer transiently corrects the chloride transport defect in nasal epithelia of patients with cystic fibrosis. Cell *75*:207, 1993.

Zhang L, Hung M-C: Sensitization of *HER-2/neu*-overexpressing non-small cell lung cancer to chemotherapeutic drugs by tyrosine kinase inhibitor emodin. Oncogene *12*:571, 1996.

CHAPTER 16

Bronchoscopic Evaluation of the Lungs and Tracheobronchial Tree

William H. Warren and L. Penfield Faber

The advent of fiberoptic technology has revolutionized endoscopy. Nowhere is this change more evident than in bronchoscopy in which the flexible bronchoscope has almost replaced the rigid bronchoscope as a diagnostic and therapeutic tool. Bronchoscopy, once dominated by only a few specialists, is now performed by pulmonologists, anesthesiologists, otolaryngologists, critical care specialists, and thoracic surgeons in a variety of clinical settings, including the hospital ward, intensive care unit, and operating room. A thoracic surgeon must have a clear understanding of all aspects of flexible and rigid bronchoscopy, including anesthetic techniques, instrument options, and the management of complications.

FACILITIES FOR BRONCHOSCOPY

Ideally, an area of the hospital or outpatient facility should be dedicated to endoscopic procedures. Because bronchoscopy is performed routinely as an outpatient procedure with intravenous sedation, recovery areas are needed also. In the best scenario, such suites would allow clinicians to perform procedures with fluoroscopic guidance and administer general anesthesia. Patients routinely have intravenous access and receive supplemental oxygen, as documented by Prakash and associates (1991a). Pulse oximetry and electrocardiographic monitoring are standard, according to Albertini and colleagues (1975). The examination room must be large enough to store all equipment, supplies, and accessories.

A storage area adjacent to the endoscopic room is ideal. Special holding racks and storage cases should be used routinely to minimize the risk of breakage. A portable cart supplied with a light source, bronchoscope, and accessories is a convenient way to perform bedside examinations. It can be returned to the storage area for cleaning and may be reused several times a day.

FLEXIBLE FIBEROPTIC BRONCHOSCOPY

Flexible bronchoscopy is a safe and reliable technique for evaluation of the tracheobronchial tree, providing valuable visual information and diagnostic specimens. Tracheobronchial, segmental, and subsegmental anatomy should be visualized easily. Currently available flexible bronchoscopes range from 6.2 mm in outer diameter (3.2-mm working channel to aspirate inspissated secretions and blood clots) to 3.5 mm in outer diameter (1.2-mm working channel) for pediatric patients (Table 16-1). One of the most often used adult bronchoscopes has an external diameter of 5.8 mm and a 2.2-mm working channel, allowing clear visualization and specimen retrieval of the entire tracheobronchial tree down to the fourth- or fifth-order bronchi (Fig. 16-1). A forward field of view is 120 degrees; the angle of deflection is 180 degrees upward and 130 degrees downward. A narrower instrument with an external diameter of 4.9 mm easily passes through a bronchus narrowed by stricture or tumor, and its 180-degree upward deflection facilitates examination of the often difficult to reach apical subsegment.

Flexible bronchoscopy can be accomplished in the pediatric patient using an instrument with a 3.5-mm external diameter and a working channel of 1.2 mm. It can be passed through a small endotracheal tube or alongside a jet ventilation catheter. The active endoscopist should have a variety of flexible bronchoscopes available for diagnostic and therapeutic versatility (Fig. 16-2).

The many advantages of flexible bronchoscopy over rigid bronchoscopy are listed in Table 16-2. Diagnostic brushings and biopsies of peripheral lesions can be performed with minimal risk. Examination is usually performed using topical anesthesia and intravenous sedation, avoiding the risks of general anesthesia. Retained secretions can be aspirated at the bedside in the ward or in the intensive care unit. Patients receiving ventilator support can be examined without compromise using a side-arm adaptor. The scope can be passed

Table 16-1. Fiberoptic Bronchoscope Specifications

Outer Diameter (mm)	Instrument Channel (mm)	Field of View (degrees)	Angle of Deflection (up–down, degrees)
3.5	1.2	90	160–100
4.9	2.2	120	180–130
5.8	2.2	120	180–130
5.9	2.8	120	180–130
5.9	2.0 + 1.5 (dual channel)	90	160–100
6.2	3.2	90	160–100

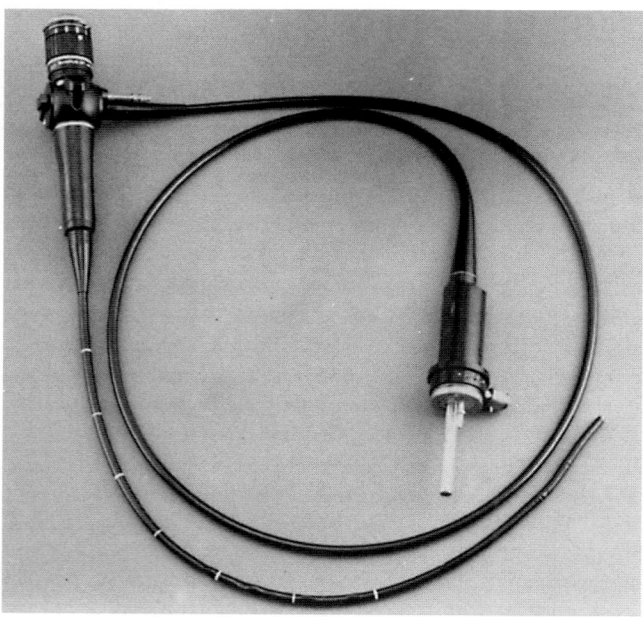

Fig. 16-1. Flexible fiberoptic bronchoscope (Olympus BF-10, Melville, NY).

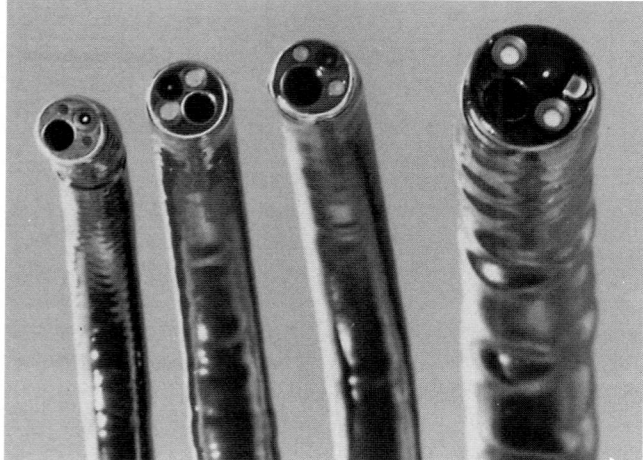

Fig. 16-2. Flexible fiberoptic bronchoscopes viewed on end. From left to right: 4.9-mm bronchoscope with 2.2-mm channel, 5.7-mm bronchoscope with 2.2-mm channel, 5.8-mm bronchoscope with 2.8-mm instrument channel, and 6.3-mm bronchoscope with 3.2-mm channel.

Table 16-2. Flexible Fiberoptic Bronchoscopy

Advantages
Patient comfort
Segmental visualization
Segmental biopsy
Peripheral biopsy
Transbronchial needle aspiration
Bedside aspiration
Bronchoscopy on ventilator
Bypass distortion
Photography
Increased cancer diagnosis
Brachytherapy
Laser bronchoscopy

Disadvantages
Small channel
Breakdown
Sterilization

through narrowed and distorted airways. Still or videophotography is easily used to document findings (Fig. 16-3).

Transbronchoscopic bronchial biopsies, brushing cytology, transbronchial needle aspirates (TBNA) and bronchoalveolar lavage (BAL) are readily performed, and the endoscopist should be familiar with indications and techniques for each.

RIGID BRONCHOSCOPY

The rigid, open-tube bronchoscopes commonly used in adults have an internal diameter of 6, 7, or 8 mm and are 40 cm in length (Fig. 16-4). Standard models provide only a tunnel view, but with experience, the endoscopist becomes accustomed to this view of the bronchi. Illumination is supplied from a halogen light source; a fiberoptic cable is attached to a light carrier that passes down the side wall of the bronchoscope. A ventilating side port permits assisted

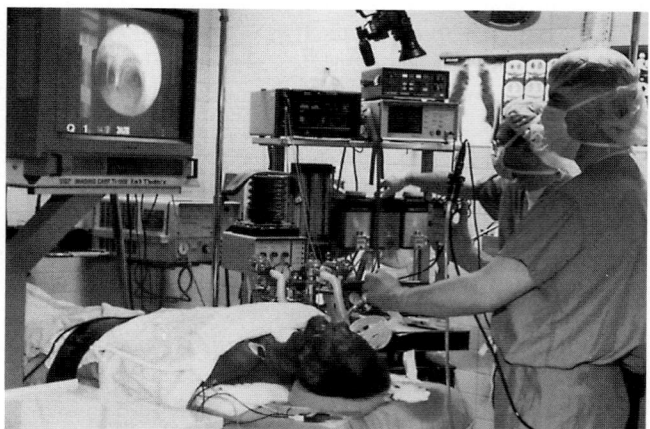

Fig. 16-3. Flexible bronchoscopy using a video-assisted technique.

Fig. 16-4. Standard 8-mm rigid bronchoscope with light carrier, rigid biopsy forceps, and glass eyepiece.

Table 16-3. Rigid Bronchoscopy

Advantages
Foreign body removal
Massive hemoptysis
Infant endoscopy
Dilate strictures
Tracheal obstruction
Laser bronchoscopy

Disadvantages
General anesthesia
Visualize segment
Biopsy segment
Peripheral biopsy upper lobe

ventilation; a glass eyepiece is placed over the end to convert the ventilating circuit to a nearly closed system. Visualization is significantly enhanced with 0-degree, 30-degree, and 90-degree telescopes. The flexible fiberoptic bronchoscope may be passed down an appropriately sized rigid bronchoscope to view fourth- and fifth-order bronchi and is of particular advantage in assessing upper lobe and distal airways when retrieving foreign bodies in children or assessing the airway beyond an obstructing lesion.

Rigid bronchoscopes have been designed to accept a Hopkins telescope, which provides optimal illumination and visualization. Using these telescopes, large but precise biopsy specimens can be obtained, in contrast to standard rigid bronchoscopy, during which visualization may be compromised by the insertion of the biopsy forceps (Fig. 16-5).

Rigid bronchoscopy is almost always performed under general anesthesia, but with all of its attendant risks. Despite the clearer view provided with angled telescopes, brushings and biopsies cannot be easily accomplished at the segmental level with the rigid bronchoscope. This major disadvan-

tage can be overcome by passing a flexible bronchoscope through a rigid bronchoscope. The advantages and disadvantages of rigid bronchoscopy are listed in Table 16-3.

INDICATIONS

Diagnostic and therapeutic indications for bronchoscopy are listed in Table 16-4. The suspicion of foreign body aspiration is an indication for bronchoscopy for both diagnosis and attempted removal. Flexible bronchoscopic techniques have been described for the removal of foreign bodies using grasping and basket forceps. The endoscopist, however, must be absolutely certain that a more complicated problem does not result from either losing sight of the foreign body or impacting it distally in the tracheobronchial tree. In this regard, the rigid bronchoscope remains the instrument of choice, allowing good exposure and airway control, especially in removing foreign bodies from the airways of

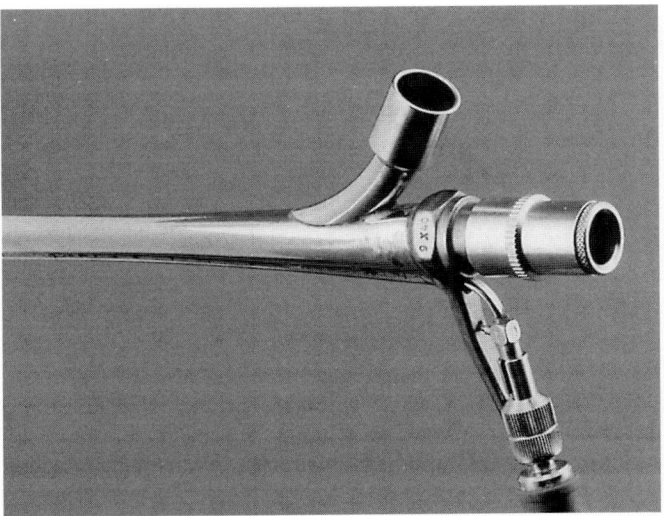

A

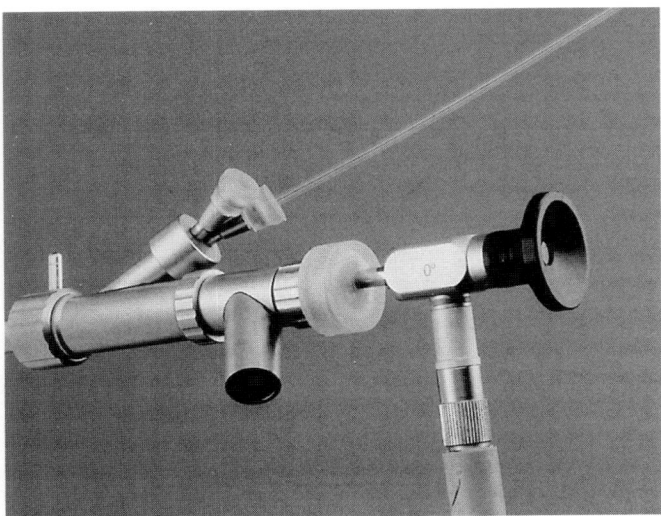

B

Fig. 16-5. A. Jackson ventilating rigid bronchoscope with eyepiece in place. The patient is ventilated through the side port. **B.** Dumon-Harrel rigid bronchoscope. The surgeon looks down the Hopkins rod and can simultaneously suction and obtain a biopsy through the various side ports.

Table 16-4. Indications for Bronchoscopy

Diagnostic
Severe cough
Change in cough
Abnormal chest radiograph findings
Hemoptysis
Wheeze
Unresolved pneumonia
Abnormal sputum cytology
Diffuse lung disease
Opportunistic infection
Bacteriologic sampling
Metastatic malignancy
Smoke inhalation
Pediatric airway obstruction
Bronchoalveolar lavage
Upper esophageal cancer

Therapeutic
Atelectasis
Lung abscess
Foreign body
Stricture
Laser

Other indications
Prolonged intubation
Difficult intubation
Bronchography
Gastric aspiration
Lobar gas sampling
Management of massive hemoptysis

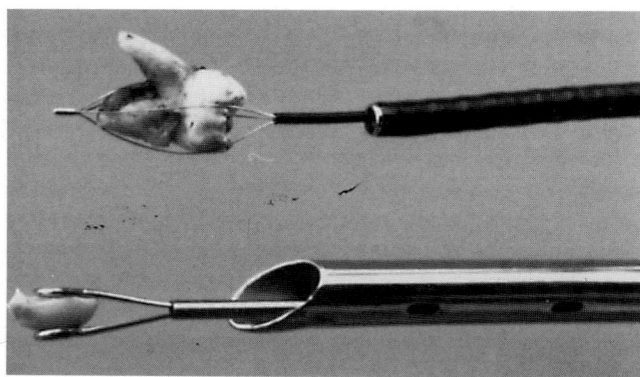

Fig. 16-6. Flexible bronchoscope with a foreign body basket retrieving a tooth, and a rigid bronchoscope with foreign body forceps grasping a peanut.

infants and children. Although, according to Lan and coworkers (1989), foreign bodies in adult patients can be retrieved with various types of snares passed down the working channel of the fiberoptic bronchoscope, Pasaoglu and colleagues (1991), as well as Weissberg and Schwartz (1987), reported that most foreign bodies can be removed easily and quickly with a rigid bronchoscope, especially in the pediatric population.

Inglis and Wagner (1992) reported the advantages of combining flexible and rigid bronchoscopy in such cases to improve the detection and retrieval rate, especially when fragments of the foreign body are lodged in the distal airway or in the upper lobe bronchi (Fig. 16-6). Clearly, endoscopists engaged in the art of foreign body retrieval must be facile with both rigid and flexible bronchoscopy according to Kelly and Marsh (1996).

A rigid bronchoscope should always be available when tracheal lesions are examined. Bleeding from biopsy sites or edema from tissue trauma can obstruct a narrowed lumen, which can be forcibly dilated with a rigid instrument.

A new and persistent cough, or a change in the cough pattern of a smoker, warrants a bronchoscopic examination. Furthermore, a wheeze, particularly one that is unilateral and fails to clear with coughing, should be investigated. Neoplasms can be diagnosed, even in the absence of radiologic findings. Sputum cytology is less commonly used as a screening tool as it has been in the past, because a flexible

bronchoscopic examination is much more successful in establishing the diagnosis and can localize the pathology.

When sputum cytology is used to screen high-risk patients for malignancy, patients with a normal chest radiography results and abnormal cytologic findings may be identified occasionally. In such cases, the mouth, pharynx, larynx, and entire tracheobronchial tree must be examined carefully to identify the site of the early carcinoma.

Autofluorescence bronchoscopy has been particularly valuable in this setting. Using a helium-cadmium laser for illumination, in vivo spectroscopy with an optical multichannel analyzer is performed during the bronchoscopic examination. Areas of severe dysplasia and carcinoma can be easily recognized by their decrease in autofluorescence intensity, whereas normal tissues autofluoresce predominantly in the short (green) wavelengths of the visible spectrum as documented by Lam and associates (1994). Preferential horizontal diffusion of longer wavelength fluorescent light from adjacent normal submucosa causes the premalignant and malignant epithelium to appear red (Fig. 16-7; see Color Fig. 16-7).

Sputum can be obtained in a sterile fashion to assess for opportunistic infections, especially in the immunocompromised patient. Endoscopic lobar and segmental lavage has proved to have therapeutic benefit in patients with cystic fibrosis and in postoperative patients unable to clear their secretions, which, on occasion, can be thick and tenacious. Retained bronchial secretions are easily suctioned at the bedside with minimal patient discomfort.

Although the most common cause of hemoptysis is chronic bronchitis, carcinoma is common in patients with abnormal chest radiograph results. Even if the radiography result is normal, according to Jackson (1985) and Poe (1988) and their associates, malignancy should be considered seriously if the patient is 40 years of age or older, has a significant smoking history, or has repeated episodes of hemoptysis more than 1 week in duration. In addition to a central lung cancer, hemoptysis associated with a wheeze or

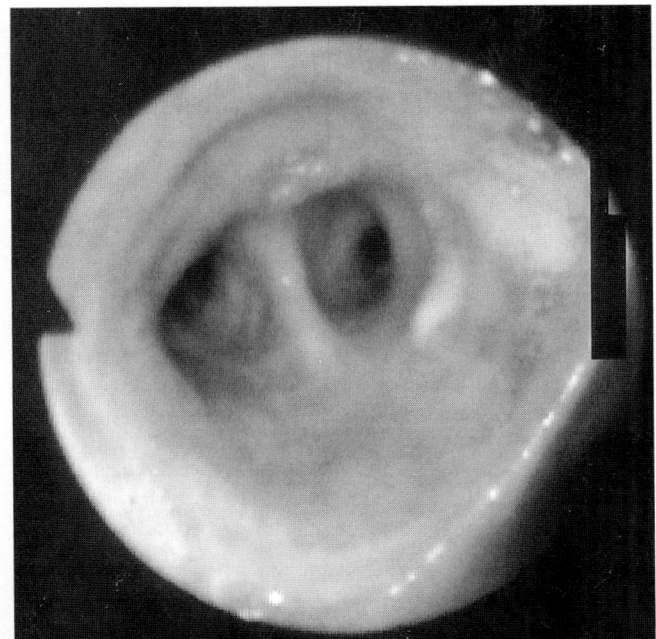

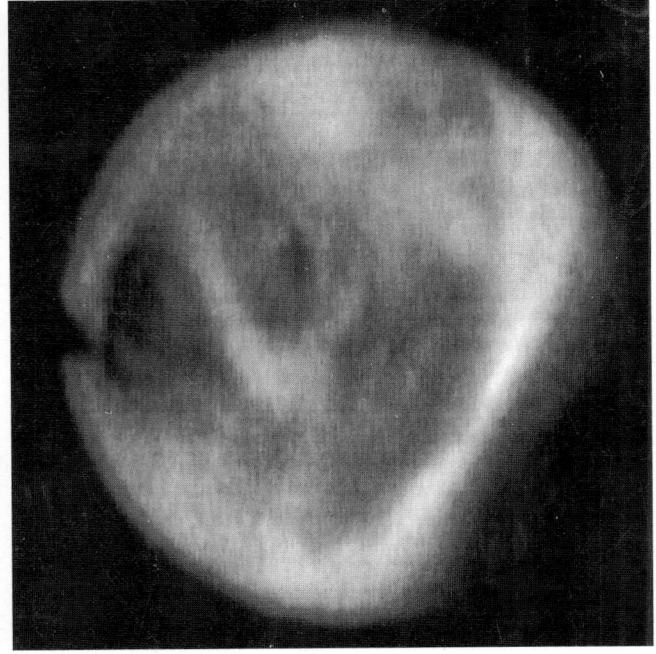

Fig. 16-7. A. Photograph of a normal-appearing bronchial mucosa using a white light source. **B.** Photograph of the same bronchial mucosa using a helium-cadmium laser light source to induce autofluorescence. (See Color Fig. 16-7.)

atelectasis may be caused by a bronchial carcinoid or an inflammatory bronchial stenosis.

Massive hemoptysis (600 mL in 24 hours) should be assessed with a rigid bronchoscope immediately. Airway control with rapid and repeated suctioning is readily accomplished, and a major bronchus can be packed with an epinephrine-soaked pledget. Massive hemoptysis can be assessed initially using a flexible bronchoscope through a cuffed endotracheal tube, but clots are not easily removed, and they often obscure visualization. The site of massive hemoptysis must be localized to prepare adequately for possible surgical excision, yttrium-aluminum-garnet (YAG) laser photoablation, endobronchial tamponade, or bronchial artery embolization as described by Saw and coworkers (1976).

When using YAG laser photoablation, rigid bronchoscopes permit photoablation and rapid débridement of an obstructing or a bleeding lesion while simultaneously maintaining control of the airway and providing a suction channel for evacuation of clots and secretions. Clinical experience with placing endobronchial stents almost exclusively involves using the rigid bronchoscope.

An abnormal chest radiograph result suggesting carcinoma warrants a careful evaluation of the tracheobronchial tree. Clinical judgment should always be used in deciding when to use bronchoscopy, but the physician should err on the side of an endoscopic evaluation to rule out a neoplasm. An obstructing carcinoma may be the underlying cause of an unresolving pneumonia, and an upper lobar infiltrate should be viewed with particular suspicion. Bronchoscopy also may be used to assess for metastatic tumors. According to Mohsenifar and colleagues (1978), bronchoscopy could confirm the diagnosis 54% of the time in patients undergoing flexible bronchoscopy for lesions suspected to be pulmonary metastases.

Bronchoscopy is indicated in the diagnosis and management of lung abscess. The passage of brushes and biopsy forceps into the abscess cavity can promote bronchial drainage, and sometimes an obstructing neoplasm or foreign body is discovered.

The therapeutic value of bronchoscopy to remove aspirated gastric contents remains in question, but a rapid and efficient bronchoscopy can support the diagnosis and may have therapeutic benefit, particularly if particulate matter is retrieved.

After inhalation of smoke or caustic fumes, bronchoscopy is a safe and expeditious way of assessing damage to the tracheobronchial mucosa. In these compromised patients, the airways frequently need repeated bronchoscopy to débride necrotic mucosa and inspissated secretions. Furthermore, the inflammatory response to this injury may progress for days, leading to delayed airway obstruction. Patients with cystic fibrosis may also, on occasion, require aspiration of persistently thick and tenacious secretions, but this step frequently is avoided by the routine use of vigorous physiotherapy and mucolytic agents.

The role of bronchoscopic examination of a patient with a fever of unknown origin or a pulmonary infiltrate after lung transplantation is widely accepted, as presented by Higenbottam and colleagues (1987). However, the need for surveillance biopsies in lung transplant recipients is controversial. According to Trulock (1995), routine surveillance bronchoscopies with random biopsies should be performed 2 to 3 weeks, 6 to 8 weeks, 9 to 12 weeks, 6 months, and 1 year after transplant, and annually thereafter. The most frequent unsuspected finding has been acute rejection and silent cytomegalovirus pneumonia. Early detection and treatment of these entities are thought to decrease the risk of chronic rejection according to Steinhoff and associates (1991). Others, such as Stillwell and colleagues (1995) maintain that, in asymptomatic patients, early stages of acute rejection or viral infection pose little risk of leading to serious consequences.

Another indication for bronchoscopic assessment of the tracheobronchial tree is the suspicion of airway trauma. Wheezing, hemoptysis, and the presence of subcutaneous, mediastinal, or both kinds of emphysema are classic findings, but injury to the airway is often overshadowed by concomitant injuries such as aortic rupture or myocardial contusion. Even when suspected, the findings of a torn bronchus can be remarkably subtle. Early diagnosis and repair of these injuries are of the utmost importance.

Evaluation and management of the obstructed airway in infants, as in adults, must be performed using rigid bronchoscopy. Subglottic stenosis, vascular rings, webs, tracheomalacia, and cysts are some of the many conditions encountered.

Developments since the early 1980s have included many interventional techniques coupled with bronchoscopy. These include YAG and CO_2 laser bronchoscopy, photodynamic therapy using chemical tissue sensitizers, such as porphyrin compounds, the placement of radioactive brachytherapy sources in the form of seeds or catheters, and the placement of endobronchial stents. These topics are discussed elsewhere (see Chapter 101).

TECHNIQUE FOR RIGID BRONCHOSCOPY

Rigid bronchoscopy is generally performed under general anesthesia, using the ventilation port on the side of the bronchoscope and capping the end of the scope with an eyepiece to convert the procedure to a nearly closed system. The eyepiece is removed for biopsy and aspiration (Fig. 16-8). Some loss of tidal volume around the bronchoscope is inevitable, but this can be minimized by packing the hypopharynx with gauze or by compression of the supraglottic area by the fingers of an assistant. The anesthesiologist must monitor the adequacy of the ventilation continuously; increased minute ventilation and tidal volumes are required. This method is safe for procedures lasting up to 20 minutes, but if longer periods are needed, other anesthetic techniques should be considered.

Jet ventilation through a rigid bronchoscope is a satisfactory method for delivering general anesthesia. A nitrous oxide gas and oxygen mixture can be delivered with an increased pressure that provides adequate oxygenation and a decreased arterial CO_2. Jet ventilation, however, is associated with unique complications and the anesthesiologist must be experienced with its use. The performance of rigid bronchoscopy under local anesthesia, while maintaining patient comfort, has become a lost art. The patient is placed

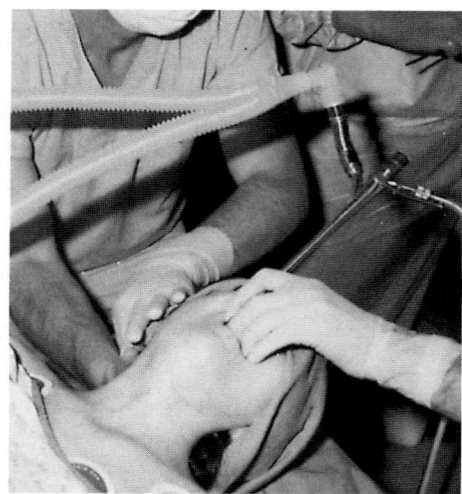

Fig. 16-8. Rigid ventilating bronchoscopy with biopsy performed using general anesthesia and open tube technique.

in a supine position with an assistant positioning the head so that the neck is slightly flexed and the chin is extended. The endoscopist elevates the epiglottis with the tip of the bronchoscope and passes the lubricated instrument through the glottis, into the upper trachea. The telescope system provides a magnified field of vision at 0 degrees, 30 degrees, and 90 degrees. If angle-viewing telescopes are not available, the flexible bronchoscope can be passed through the rigid bronchoscope to view upper lobe orifices and all segmental bronchi.

Examination of the trachea is accomplished after the bronchoscope passes through the glottis, and the carina is assessed for sharpness and mobility during ventilation. Widening or fixation suggests the involvement of the subcarinal nodes by tumor or an inflammatory process. Biopsy of the carina is obtained if it is widened or if submucosal extension of malignancy is suspected.

TECHNIQUE FOR FLEXIBLE BRONCHOSCOPY

Sedation

Sedation should be administered to provide patient comfort and cooperation. In several studies, however, 50% of the life-threatening complications from bronchoscopy stemmed from hypoxemia, hypercapnia, and respiratory depression secondary to oversedation. Therefore, the agents and their dosages must be individualized and may not be necessary in every case.

Preoperative opiates are given for their analgesic and antitussive properties. Meperidine is the most commonly administered agent according to an American College of Chest Physicians survey presented by Prakash and associates (1991b). It has an elimination half-life of 3.2 hours, but clearance is decreased in patients with renal, hepatic, or both renal

---

and hepatic failure. It, like all opiates, can cause respiratory depression and hypotension. Naloxone, a specific opioid antagonist, must be available whenever opioids are administered.

Intravenous benzodiazepines (diazepam and midazolam) are often administered, providing anxiolysis and antegrade amnesia. Midazolam has become the preferred agent. It is water soluble, with rapid onset, short duration of action, and an elimination half-life of only 2 hours in normal subjects. Renal failure does not alter the distribution, elimination, or clearance, but liver disease is associated with prolonged sedation. The recommended dose is 0.07 mg/kg. Diazepam is not water soluble and can cause significant, if only transient, phlebitis. Its elimination half-life is 24 to 57 hours in normal patients.

Both agents should be used with caution, especially in elderly patients and those with limited pulmonary reserve. Respiratory depression is a major side effect of both benzodiazepines; the degree of respiratory depression is similar with both drugs. Flumazenil is a specific benzodiazepine antagonist and should be available any time these agents are used. Because its elimination half-life is only 1 hour, repeat doses or a continuous infusion may be needed.

Antisialagogues

Most patients are premedicated with antisialagogue, such as atropine or glycopyrrolate, to reduce secretions and inhibit vasovagal responses as documented by Williams and colleagues (1998). These medications also make topical anesthesia more effective.

Topical Anesthesia

Topical anesthesia is preferred for fiberoptic bronchoscopy, but general anesthesia may be considered, particularly for prolonged examinations required to identify a carcinoma in situ in a patient with normal chest radiography findings.

The most common agents for topical anesthesia are lidocaine (2% and 4%) and tetracaine (0.5%, 1.0%, and 2.0%). Complications from topical anesthesia usually result from the administration of excessive amounts, as documented by Credle (1974), Suratt (1976), and Pereira (1978) and their associates. If carefully measured amounts are given and the endoscopist is always aware of the total milligram dosage instilled, reactions are minimized.

Lidocaine is a safe agent with a recommended adult dose up to 400 mg, but larger amounts have been given without serious side effects. The first sign of toxicity is usually central nervous system excitation or seizure before cardiovascular collapse; the duration of action is short. Lidocaine, however, does not provide the depth of anesthesia necessary for rigid bronchoscopy.

Tetracaine is another effective topical anesthetic, but side effects frequently occur when a dose of 80 mg is exceeded. The duration of action is prolonged, and the first sign of toxicity may be sudden cardiovascular collapse.

Combination of benzocaine-tetracaine is a popular topical anesthetic agent with rapid onset of action useful in rapid intubation. It is often administered in a propellant spray with a tolerance dose delivered in only 2 seconds. Dosing is therefore difficult to regulate, and this agent should be avoided when performing flexible bronchoscopy.

Several satisfactory methods are available to administer topical anesthesia. Using the nasotracheal route, the nasopharynx is anesthetized initially using an atomized topical agent, and the flexible bronchoscope is then passed through the nares to a level just proximal to the false cords. With the larynx in clear view, additional topical anesthetic is administered directly onto the vocal cords and into the trachea. The bronchoscope is then passed through the glottis and additional topical anesthesia is instilled down the tracheobronchial tree.

A second method of delivering topical anesthesia consists of initial spraying of the hypopharynx with 2% or 4% lidocaine using an atomizer. Five milliliters of 4% lidocaine is then injected transtracheally through the cricothyroid membrane using a short 21-gauge needle to minimize the risk of lacerating the posterior wall of the trachea. Slight bleeding often occurs with this technique, so it should be avoided when a patient is being examined for hemoptysis of unknown origin. Care is taken to confirm the position of the needle in the tracheal lumen by aspirating air before injecting, because it is possible to inject directly into the false cords, precipitating laryngospasm. Anesthesia of the larynx is achieved as the patient coughs out the medication. Supplemental 2% lidocaine is then instilled into the tracheobronchial tree while advancing the flexible bronchoscope. Because topical anesthetic agents inhibit bacterial growth, care should be taken to minimize the amount aspirated into collection traps for microbiological studies.

Flexible bronchoscopy is accomplished easily using general anesthesia. In the adult, a swivel adaptor is attached to the endotracheal tube, and ventilation is maintained through the side arm of the adaptor. The bronchoscope is passed through a tight-fitting plastic diaphragm on the adaptor. As large an endotracheal tube as possible should be selected.

In children, a 5.8-mm flexible bronchoscope can be passed down a 7.0-mm endotracheal tube, but the procedure must be interrupted intermittently to provide adequate ventilation. If a long procedure is anticipated, blood gas analysis or capnography monitoring is mandatory. The pediatric 3.5-mm bronchoscope is currently the best choice among the flexible instruments for use in children.

Examination

The first phase of a diagnostic bronchoscopy is clear visualization of the larynx and the vocal cords. Unsuspected leukoplakia, carcinoma in situ, and invasive carcinoma may

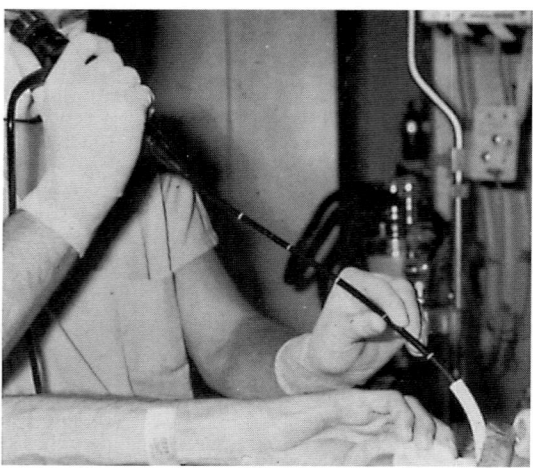

Fig. 16-9. Flexible fiberoptic bronchoscope is inserted through an oral endotracheal tube.

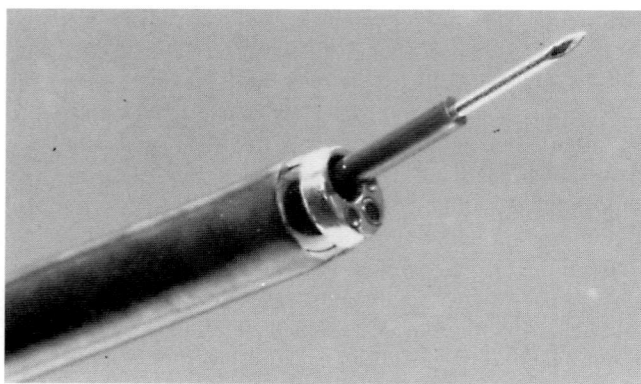

Fig. 16-10. Transbronchial needle for aspiration of mediastinal and hilar lymph nodes and masses.

be found. Vocal cord mobility must be assessed, because recurrent laryngeal palsy secondary to carcinoma of the lung generally is considered a sign of inoperability. The larynx also should be examined before passing the rigid bronchoscope.

The flexible fiberoptic bronchoscope can be inserted through either the nose or mouth into the hypopharynx and then through the glottis into the trachea. Passage of the instrument through the nares does not permit easy withdrawal and reinsertion for cleaning of the lens and clearing the channel of thick mucus. Biopsy and brushing cytology specimens must be withdrawn through the channel, and some of the specimen may be lost, decreasing the yield of diagnostic material.

An alternative technique involves passing an uncuffed 8.0-mm endotracheal tube through the orotracheal route as described by Sanderson and McDougall (1978) (Fig. 16-9). The patient breathes around and through an uncuffed endotracheal tube, providing rapid access to the airway while minimizing trauma to the larynx and subglottic region. Airway access is provided and the endotracheal tube allows rapid insertion and withdrawal of the bronchoscope. Brushing and biopsy specimens are retrieved by leaving the brush or forceps beyond the tip of the bronchoscope, avoiding loss of the specimen in the working channel. In addition, airway suctioning using a large-caliber catheter can be performed in the event of significant airway bleeding. Airflow resistance has been shown to increase significantly when a 5.8-mm bronchoscope is passed through an endotracheal tube smaller than an 8.5-mm outer diameter. According to Perry (1978), use of a smaller endotracheal tube could lead to hypercapnia and respiratory distress.

Since the mid-1980s, the technique of transbronchial needle aspiration cytology, championed by Wang (1986, 1989, 1995) and Shure and Fedullo (1983, 1984, 1985), has found increasing favor in sampling subcarinal and paratracheal lymph nodes and for examining widened spurs endoscopi-

cally. An 18-gauge needle is passed through the working channel of the bronchoscope and directed through the wall of the airway into the suspicious area. A histologic core is obtained.

Cytologic and histologic specimens are obtained by passing an ensheathed 21-gauge needle down the working channel of the bronchoscope (Fig. 16-10). Failure to withdraw the needle into the protective outer sheath has led to serious and costly repairs of flexible bronchoscopes as documented by Mehta and coworkers (1990). Once the sheath is advanced beyond the tip of the scope, the 1.5-cm needle is advanced beyond the sheath, through the wall of the trachea or bronchus, and into the mediastinal mass or suspicious lymph nodes (Fig. 16-11). The needle can be reinserted into this region several times, applying gentle suction each time the needle is advanced; suction must be avoided once the needle is completely withdrawn. Five milliliters of saline is then flushed through the needle to obtain an optimal cytologic sample, which is immediately centrifuged; the resulting pellet is resuspended in 1 mL of saline. The supernatant cell suspension is fixed in 95% ethanol, and prepared with Papanicolaou's stain. Tissue fragments are fixed in Bouin's solution and submitted for a cell block.

In 1986, Wang reported that 50% of patients judged to be surgical candidates had positive mediastinal node results when assessed by TBNA. Shure and colleagues (1985) described increased diagnostic accuracy when TBNA is used with bronchoscopic evidence of submucosal or peribronchial tumor. It should be noted, however, that TBNA has at least a 15% false-negative rate when assessing mediastinal nodes, according to Wang (1986); this number has been much higher in the hands of most less experienced bronchoscopists. TBNA should be performed before brushing or lavaging to avoid contaminating the airway, which could lead to an increased false-positive rate, according to Cropp (1984) and Schenk (1984) and their associates.

Mediastinal infection and bleeding are rare complications of TBNA of the mediastinum. Preoperative computed tomographic or magnetic resonance scanning is imperative to

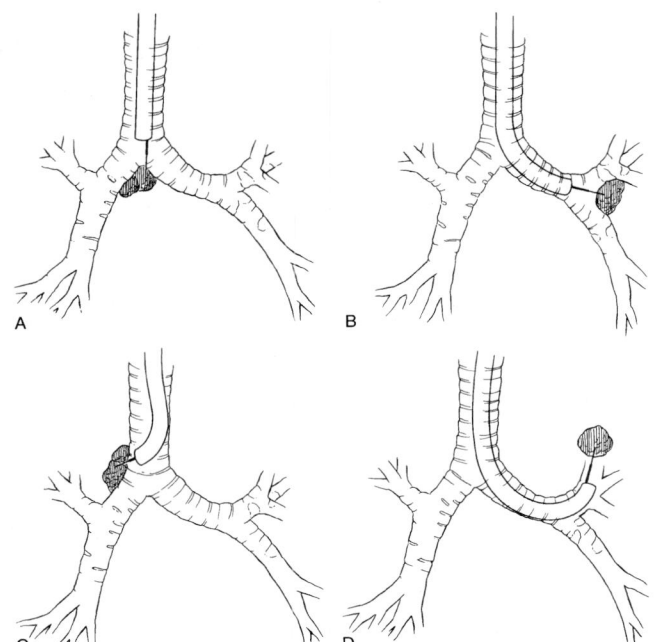

Fig. 16-11. Transbronchial needle aspirate of **(A)** subcarinal lymph nodes, **(B)** a mass at the bifurcation of the left main stem bronchus, **(C)** a nodal mass at the right tracheobronchial angle, and **(D)** a central mass in the left upper lobe.

define precisely the lesion in question, as well as to assess the proximity of major vessels. A more recent technique to localize and assess peribronchial and paratracheal pathology is ultrasound-assisted bronchoscopy. Using this technique, a 2-mm diameter, 95-cm long catheter containing a single ultrasound transducer is passed down the working channel of the bronchoscope and attached to an ultrasound unit. The motor of the ultrasound unit continuously rotates the transducer to obtain a real-time cross-sectional image of that area in contact with the probe. The side of the catheter is placed against the tracheobronchial mucosa in the proximity of the lesion in question to produce a cross-sectional image 2 cm in depth. However, using the criteria of size, echo density, homogeneity in structure, or demarcation of the nodal tissue from surrounding anthrasilicotic changes in the nodes produces the same echo pattern as tumor infiltration. Therefore, although ultrasound can be used as an imaging technique, it has limited diagnostic value. After selection and evaluation of the biopsy site, the ultrasound catheter is withdrawn and the needle apparatus is inserted. Biopsy is sometimes performed under fluoroscopic control. Experience with this technique in the United States is limited, but preliminary results are encouraging as reported by Goldberg (1994), Schuder (1991), and Naidich (1994) and their associates. Its ultimate value will rest in its cost-effectiveness in directing TBNA and thereby increasing the yield. Silvestri and associates (1996) have used esophageal ultrasound to visualize transbronchial needle biopsies of mediastinal nodes.

All lobar and segmental bronchi must be examined carefully and systematically, because a second lesion not visible on the chest radiography is occasionally identified. The bronchus leading to the known area of disease is then examined. The character of secretions and the bronchial mucosa are clues to the nature of the underlying pathologic condition. Subtle mucosal abnormalities associated with carcinoma include mucosal thickening, irregular bronchial folds or corrugation, and increased submucosal vascularity. Stradling (1981) documented that these findings may be associated with a loss of definition of the cartilaginous rings or circular folds, endobronchial stenosis, or extrinsic bronchial compression. The extent of the endoscopic findings must be examined carefully when anticipating a possible surgical resection.

Areas in which malignancy is suspected should undergo brushing and biopsy with a diagnostic yield higher than 90%, according to Popovich and associates (1982). Biopsies should be attempted, even when the lesion is suspected to be a bronchial carcinoid, because lung-sparing resections can be accomplished with minimal resection margins with this pathologic entity. Bleeding can be controlled with topical 1/10,000 epinephrine. Small fragments of tissue are obtained with 1.5-mm biopsy forceps, and multiple biopsies are often necessary to provide diagnostic material. Biopsy specimens of segmental lesions beyond the field of vision are often obtained under fluoroscopic control. Biopsy through the flexible bronchoscope requires persistence and practice, especially when the lesion is in the apical segments of the upper lobes. After each biopsy, the forceps is placed in saline, and concentrated formalin solution is added at the conclusion of the procedure to give a final dilution of 10%.

Kvale and associates (1976) reported that the accuracy of establishing the diagnosis of carcinoma increases with the number and types of specimens obtained. Many lesions have large necrotic areas, which do not provide diagnostic material if a biopsy is performed. Bronchial brushings are generally performed after the biopsy tissue has been obtained. A 7-mm brush is recommended for routine use because more cellular material is obtained (Fig. 16-12); 1.7-mm brushes have the advantage that they can be ensheathed and withdrawn through the working channel of the bronchoscope, but the yield of material is smaller as documented by Elkus (1994) and Lundgren (1983) and their associates. The bronchial brush may be inserted into narrowed segmental bronchi to provide a positive cytologic diagnosis. The brush is passed vigorously over the surface of the lesion and is then quickly stroked onto the surface of glass slide, which is immersed immediately in 95% ethanol (Fig. 16-13). Improved results are achieved if four separate brush specimens are obtained and sent to the laboratory.

Endobronchial findings may not be detected in peripheral lesions. Under these circumstances, fluoroscopic guidance is invaluable. Ideally, the lesion seems to move when it is sampled. When the lesion is beyond the field of vision, the diagnostic yield by biopsy alone is 46%; however, the yield

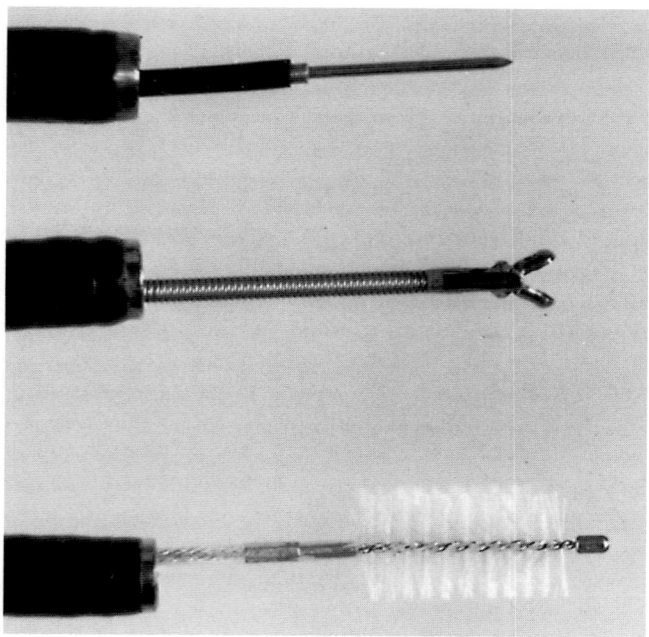

Fig. 16-12. Flexible fiberoptic bronchoscope with (from top to bottom) a 21-gauge transbronchial needle, a flexible cup biopsy forceps, and a 7-mm nylon brush.

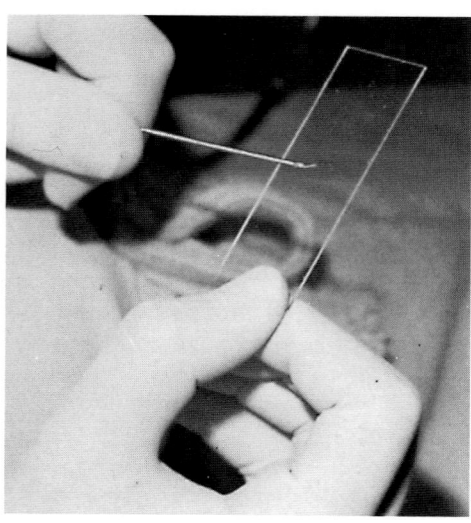

Fig. 16-13. Bronchial brush is rapidly smeared onto a glass slide, which is immediately immersed in 90% ethanol to fix the material for cytologic examination.

increases to 60% when combined with bronchial brushings, according to Cortese and McDougall (1979). Shure and Fedullo (1983) reported use of TBNA to establish the diagnosis of peripheral primary lung carcinoma presenting as a peripheral nodule or mass.

Transbronchial brushings and biopsies also may be used to assess pulmonary infiltrates according to Zavala (1978). The diagnoses of sarcoidosis, tuberculosis, bronchioloalveolar carcinoma, or pulmonary alveolar proteinosis can all be established bronchoscopically. The flexible bronchoscope is wedged initially in the segmental bronchus, and the biopsy forceps is advanced to the periphery of the diseased region. The forceps is then drawn back 3 to 4 mm, and the jaws are opened and advanced slightly to obtain the sample of the lung. The bronchoscope is left wedged in the segmental bronchus in the event of bleeding to allow irrigation with 1/10,000 epinephrine. Five to seven transbronchial biopsies have been found to provide the optimal diagnostic yield, and these samples should all be taken from the same lung to avoid the complication of bilateral pneumothorax and help to localize the bleeding site in the event of massive hemoptysis. Under fluoroscopic guidance, placement of the biopsy forceps near, but not at, the lung surface minimizes the risk of causing a pneumothorax. Coagulation studies (i.e., platelet count) should be obtained preoperatively to identify patients at high risk for bleeding. Uremic patients are also known to be at high risk for significant hemoptysis and precautions must be taken.

BAL is a useful technique to diagnose opportunistic infections, including cytomegalovirus, and bacterial, fungal, and *Pneumocystis carinii* pneumonia. BAL is performed by wedging the tip of the flexible bronchoscope into a subsegmental bronchus and irrigating and aspirating the segment with 20- to 50-mL aliquots of sterile saline. A total volume of 100 to 300 mL of saline is instilled and 40 to 70% of this volume is recovered as a specimen. In patients who have loss of elastic recoil, recovery of fluid is less, according to Helmers and Hunninghake (1989), because the subsegmental bronchiolar walls collapse when suction is applied. In addition to microbiological studies, lavage specimens have been used to diagnose malignancies and to obtain inflammatory cells and pneumocytes for research studies as discussed by Kvale and colleagues (1996).

BAL is a useful technique for obtaining microbiological specimens, especially in immunosuppressed patients. Fungal, bacterial, and viral culture specimens are easily acquired. In patients with acquired immunodeficiency syndrome the diagnosis of *P. carinii* pneumonia also can be made with a diagnostic yield exceeding 85%, according to Martin (1987), Ognibene (1984), and Pisani (1992) and their associates.

Cytologic specimens also can be obtained to establish the diagnosis in a variety of noninfectious, diffuse interstitial pulmonary diseases, including lipoid pneumonitis, histiocytosis, and berylliosis, all of which are uncommon entities, as documented by Daniele and associates (1985). BAL is of more limited value in the diagnosis of fibrosing alveolitis, sarcoidosis, and hypersensitivity pneumonitis, as noted by Stoller and colleagues (1987). Levy and associates (1988) reported that BAL has been used to establish the diagnosis of peripheral primary lung carcinoma. Rennard (1990) and Pirozynski (1992) also noted this fact, but BAL has not been widely advocated as a step in the diagnosis of cancer in North America, and it should not be considered a routine diagnostic procedure.

Potential complications of BAL include bronchospasm, hypoxia, fever, and transient decline in pulmonary function.

Patients must therefore be observed carefully after the procedure. The safety of BAL in patients with symptomatic asthma or with a forced expiratory volume in 1 second of less than 60% of predicted value has not been established, according to a National Heart, Lung, and Blood Institute workshop report (1985).

CONTRAINDICATIONS AND COMPLICATIONS

No absolute contraindications exist for bronchoscopy. Even severely ill and debilitated patients can undergo bronchoscopy safely if it is performed in an appropriate facility by an experienced endoscopist. Despite the relatively low risk, the benefits of performing bronchoscopy must be weighed against the potential for complication in each patient. Credle and colleagues (1974) reported a complication rate of 0.08% and a mortality of 0.01% in more than 24,000 flexible bronchoscopies. Premedication and topical anesthesia were responsible for 11 of the 22 major complications. More dilute solutions of the topical anesthetic agent provide a wider margin of safety. Intravenous diazepam counteracts the systemic effects of excessive amounts of lidocaine and should be readily available. Elderly and debilitated patients should receive minimal premedication, and topical anesthesia must be administered in carefully measured amounts. Respiratory depression is a frequent complication of intravenous sedation in this patient population as emphasized by Herf and associates (1977).

Careful evaluation and preparation of the patient as well as adequate facilities to monitor the patient are required to minimize complications. Pulse oximetry, continuous electrocardiography monitoring, and intermittent cuff blood pressure readings are all important parameters. Supplemental oxygen is supplied to minimize the risk of hypoxemia. Respiratory depression has been documented in the recovery period. According to Peacock and associates (1989), topical anesthesia may be responsible for prolonged periods of respiratory depression. Belen (1981) and Matsushima (1984) and their associates recommend that patients should not undergo pulmonary function testing for at least 8 hours after bronchoscopy. General anesthesia may be indicated if the patient has a history of intolerance to topical anesthetic agents or of difficult endoscopies under local anesthesia.

Massive bleeding is a recognized complication of bronchoscopy, as documented by Suratt and associates (1977). Bleeding disorders must be corrected by anticoagulant reversal or by the infusion of platelets either during or immediately before the procedure. A brushing or biopsy should not be done unless the prothrombin time is higher than 40% of normal and the platelet count is greater than 50,000. Patients with uremia or pulmonary hypertension also bleed easily, and, according to Zavala (1976), brushings and biopsies in these patients should be avoided. Topical epinephrine solution of 1/100,000 can be instilled into the segmental bronchus before brushing to minimize bleeding or to control established bleeding. In the event of endobronchial hemorrhage, Zavala (1976) recommended wedging the scope in the segmental bronchus to tamponade the lumen by the clot.

According to Pereira and colleagues (1978), pneumothorax can occur in up to 5% of patients undergoing a transbronchial lung biopsy. When lung biopsies are performed for diffuse lung disease, it is important to perform this procedure under fluoroscopic control to avoid perforation of the lung. Patients may complain of sharp chest pain if the parietal pleura is irritated.

Bronchoscopy should not be performed in a patient with bilateral vocal cord paralysis. The passage of the bronchoscope through the glottis can lead to edema, causing life-threatening airway obstruction and necessitating emergent intubation or tracheostomy. Patients with a tracheal obstruction should be examined cautiously, and biopsy or dilation of the tracheal lesion should be avoided if the airway is severely compromised, unless one is prepared to proceed directly to definitive tracheal surgery.

Bronchospasm is a potential complication in patients with known asthma, but it also may occur in patients with severe chronic obstructive lung disease. Asthmatics should be premedicated with corticosteroids and bronchodilators. Laryngospasm is the direct consequence of inadequate topical anesthesia; it can be avoided if the topical agent is placed precisely onto the vocal cords and into the tracheobronchial tree.

Patients with hepatitis, human immunodeficiency virus, or suspected active tuberculosis can undergo bronchoscopy if special care is taken by all personnel in the handling of the specimens and all instruments used are appropriately sterilized. Infections transmitted after properly cleaning instruments are rare, according to Suratt and coworkers (1977). Sepsis after bronchoscopy is uncommon, but fever is seen occasionally. Patients with underlying valvular heart disease should receive prophylactic antibiotics before bronchoscopy to minimize the risk of bacterial endocarditis.

PEDIATRIC BRONCHOSCOPY

Bronchoscopy in infants and small children requires expertise and familiarity with all available instrumentation as emphasized by Wood (1996). Examination of the infant airway using smaller Storz rigid instruments with viewing telescopes is usually performed using general anesthesia (Fig. 16-14). A 3.0- or 3.5-mm sheath permits passage of the 2.7-mm optical telescope that provides a good view of the infant's bronchi. A small suction catheter can be passed down the barrel. Secretions are removed readily for microbiological studies. Small biopsy and foreign body forceps can be manipulated through this small channel with the viewing telescope in place. Muntz and associates (1992) reported their experience performing transbronchial lung biopsies in the pediatric population through a rigid bronchoscope.

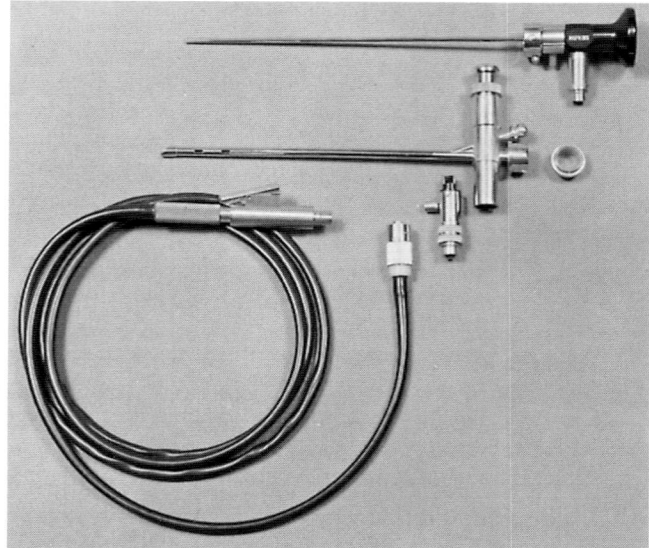

A

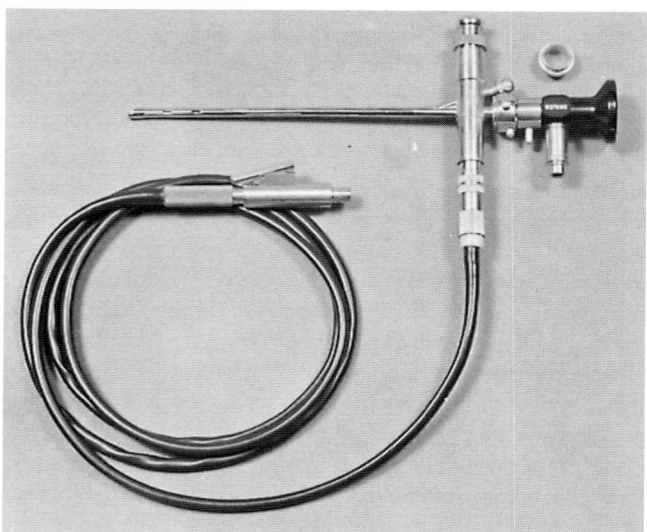

B

Fig. 16-14. Infant rigid bronchoscope (Storz), 3.5-mm diameter, with fiberoptic lighting. **A.** Components (from top to bottom): forward-viewing endoscopic telescope (Hopkins); bronchoscope with detachable window plus side channels for connection to anesthesia equipment, suctioning, and insertion of proximal light; proximal prismatic light carrier; and fiberoptic lighting cable. **B.** The bronchoscope after assembly.

Flexible fiberoptic bronchoscopy has become a practical tool in pediatrics with the development of a bronchoscope with an external diameter of 3.5 mm and a channel of 1.2 mm. It has found favor in clearing secretions, as well as aiding in localizing and retrieving foreign bodies. Examination of infants may be performed using sedation and topical anesthesia, provided the procedure is brief. Airway stenosis and obstruction are contraindications to flexible instrumentation.

Complications related to pediatric bronchoscopy can be life-threatening. Laryngospasm, subglottic edema, and bron-chospasm from manipulation may all compromise the airway. Stridorous breathing after the procedure is an indication for humidification of supplemental oxygen and the administration of systemic corticosteroids. A small bronchus may be perforated with resultant pneumothorax or pneumomediastinum.

REFERENCES

Albertini RE, Harrell JH, Moser KM: Management of arterial hypoxemia induced by fiberoptic bronchoscopy. Chest 67:134, 1975.

Belen J, et al: Modification of the effect of fiberoptic bronchoscopy on pulmonary mechanics. Chest 79:516, 1981.

Cortese DA, McDougall JC: Biopsy and brushing of peripheral lung cancer with fluoroscopic guidance. Chest 75:141, 1979.

Credle WF, Smiddy JF, Elliot RC: Complications of fiberoptic bronchoscopy. Am Rev Respir Dis 109:67, 1974.

Cropp AJ, Dimarco AF, Lankerani M: False-positive transbronchial needle aspiration in bronchogenic carcinoma. Chest 85:696, 1984.

Daniele RP, et al: Bronchoalveolar lavage: role in the pathogenesis, diagnosis and management of interstitial lung disease. Ann Intern Med 102:93, 1985.

Elkus RL, et al: A comparison of withdrawn and nonwithdrawn brushes in the diagnosis of lung cancer. J Bronchol 1:269, 1994.

Goldberg BB, et al: US-assisted bronchoscopy with use of miniature transducer-containing catheters. Radiology 190:233, 1994.

Helmers RA, Hunninghake GW: Bronchoalveolar lavage. In Wang KP (ed): Biopsy Techniques in Pulmonary Disorders. New York: Raven Press, 1989.

Herf SM, Suratt PM, Arora NS: Deaths and complications associated with transbronchial lung biopsy. Am Rev Respir Dis 115:708, 1977.

Higenbottam T, et al: The diagnosis of lung rejection and opportunistic infection by transbronchial lung biopsy. Transplant Proc 19:3777, 1987.

Inglis AF, Wagner DV: Lower complication rates associated with bronchial foreign bodies over the last 25 years. Ann Otol Rhinol Laryngol 101:61, 1992.

Jackson CV, Savage PJ, Quinn DL: Role of fiberoptic bronchoscopy in patients with hemoptysis and a normal chest roentgenogram. Chest 87:142, 1985.

Kelly SM, Marsh BR. Airway foreign bodies. Chest Surg Clin N Am 6:253, 1996.

Kvale PA, Bode FR, Kini S: Diagnostic accuracy in lung cancer. Comparison of techniques used in association with flexible fiberoptic techniques. Chest 69:752, 1976.

Kvale PA: Bronchoscopic biopsies and bronchoalveolar lavage. Chest Surg Clin N Am 6:205, 1996.

Lam A, et al: Early localization of bronchoscopic carcinoma. Diagn Ther Endosc 1:75, 1994.

Lan RS, et al: Use of fiberoptic bronchoscopy to retrieve bronchial foreign bodies in adults. Am Rev Respir Dis 140:1734, 1989.

Levy H, Horak DA, Lewis MI: The value of bronchial washings and bronchoalveolar lavage in the diagnosis of lymphangitic carcinomatosis. Chest 94:1028, 1988.

Lundgren R, Bergman F, Angstrom T: Comparison of transbronchial fine needle aspiration biopsy, aspiration of bronchial secretion, bronchial washing, brush biopsy and forceps biopsy in the diagnosis of lung cancer. Eur J Respir Dis 64:378, 1983.

Martin WJ, et al: Role of bronchoalveolar lavage in the assessment of opportunistic pulmonary infections: utility and complications. Mayo Clin Proc 62:549, 1987.

Matsushima Y, et al: Alterations in pulmonary mechanics and gas exchange during routine fiberoptic bronchoscopy. Chest 86:184, 1984.

Mehta AC, et al: The high price of bronchoscopy. Maintenance and repair of the flexible fiberoptic bronchoscope. Chest 98:448, 1990.

Mohsenifar Z, Chopra SK, Simmons DH: Diagnostic value of fiberoptic bronchoscopy in metastatic pulmonary tumors. Chest 74:369, 1978.

Muntz H, Wallace M, Lusk RP: Pediatric transbronchial lung biopsy. Ann Otol Rhinol Laryngol 101:135, 1992.

Naidich D, Harkin TJ: US-assisted bronchoscopy: is seeing believing? Radiology 190:18, 1994.

National Heart, Lung, and Blood Institute Workshop Summaries: Summary and recommendations of a workshop on the investigative use of fiberoptic bronchoscopy and bronchoalveolar lavage in asthmatics. Am Rev Respir Dis *132*:180, 1985.

Ognibene FP, et al: The diagnosis of *Pneumocystis carinii* pneumonia in patients with acquired immunodeficiency syndrome using subsegmental bronchoalveolar lavage. Am Rev Respir Dis *129*:929, 1984.

Pasaoglu I, et al: Bronchoscopic removal of foreign bodies in children: retrospective analysis of 822 cases. Thorac Cardiovasc Surg *39*:95, 1991.

Peacock AJ, Benson-Mitchell R, Godfrey R: Effect of fiberoptic bronchoscopy on pulmonary function. Thorax *45*:38, 1990.

Pereira W, Kovnat DM, Snider GL: A prospective cooperative study of complications following flexible fiberoptic bronchoscopy. Chest *73*:813, 1978.

Perry LB: Topical anesthesia for bronchoscopy. Chest *73S*:691, 1978.

Pirozynski M: Bronchoalveolar lavage in the diagnosis of peripheral, primary lung cancer. Chest *102*:372, 1992.

Pisani RJ, Wright AJ: Clinical utility of bronchoalveolar lavage in immuno-compromised hosts. Mayo Clin Proc *76*:221, 1992.

Poe RH, et al: Utility of fiberoptic bronchoscopy in patients with hemoptysis and a nonlocalizing chest roentgenogram. Chest *92*:70, 1988.

Popovich J Jr, et al: Diagnostic accuracy of multiple biopsies from flexible bronchoscopic biopsy: a comparison of central versus peripheral carcinoma. Am Rev Respir Dis *125*:521, 1982.

Prakash UBS, Stubbs SE: The bronchoscopy survey. Some reflections. Chest *100*:1660, 1991.

Prakash UBS, Offord KP, Stubbs SE: Bronchoscopy in North America: the ACCP survey. Chest *100*:1668, 1991.

Rennard SI: Future direction for bronchoalveolar lavage. Lung *168*:1050, 1990.

Sanderson DR, McDougall JC: Transoral bronchoscopy. Chest *73*:701, 1978.

Saw EC, et al: Flexible fiberoptic bronchoscopy and endobronchial tamponade in the management of massive hemoptysis. Chest *70*:589, 1976.

Schenk DA, et al: Potential false positive mediastinal transbronchial needle aspiration in bronchogenic carcinoma. Chest *86*:649, 1984.

Schuder G, et al: Endoscopic ultrasonography of the mediastinum in the diagnosis of bronchial carcinoma. Thorac Cardiovasc Surg *39*:299, 1991.

Silvestri GA, et al: Endoscopic ultrasound with fine-needle aspiration in the diagnosis and staging of lung cancer. Ann Thorac Surg *61*:1441,1996.

Shure D, Fedullo PF: Transbronchial needle aspiration of peripheral masses. Am Rev Respir Dis *128*:1090, 1983.

Shure D, Fedullo PF: The role of transcranial needle aspiration in the staging of bronchogenic carcinoma. Chest *86*:693, 1984.

Shure D, Fedullo PF: Transbronchial needle aspiration in the diagnosis of submucosal and peribronchial bronchogenic carcinoma. Chest *88*:49, 1985.

Steinhoff G, et al: Early diagnosis and effective treatment of pulmonary CMV infection after lung transplantation. J Heart Lung Transplant *10*:9, 1991.

Stillwell PC, Mehta AC, Arroliga AC: Is surveillance bronchoscopy indicated in lung transplant patients? Con surveillance. J Bronchol *2*:74–76, 1995.

Stradling P: Diagnostic Bronchoscopy. 4th Ed. New York: Churchill Livingstone, 1981.

Stoller JK, Rankin JA, Reynolds HY: The impact of bronchoalveolar lavage analysis on clinicians' diagnostic reasoning about interstitial lung disease. Chest *92*:839, 1987.

Suratt PM, Smiddy JF, Gruber B: Deaths and complications associated with fiberoptic bronchoscopy. Chest *69*:747, 1976.

Suratt PM, et al: Absence of clinical pneumonia following bronchoscopy with contaminated and clean bronchoscopes. Chest *71*:52, 1977.

Trulock EP: Is surveillance bronchoscopy indicated in lung transplant recipients? Pro surveillance. J Bronchol *2*:69, 1995.

Wang KP: Flexible transbronchial needle aspiration biopsy for histologic specimens. Chest *88*:860, 1986.

Wang KP: Flexible bronchoscopy with transbronchial needle aspiration: biopsy for cytology specimens. *In* Wang KP: Biopsy Techniques in Pulmonary Disorders. 1st Ed. New York: Raven Press, 1989.

Wang KP: Transbronchial needle aspiration and percutaneous needle aspiration for staging and diagnosis of lung cancer. Clin Chest Med *16*:535, 1995.

Weissberg D, Schwartz I: Foreign bodies in the tracheobronchial tree. Chest *91*:730, 1987.

Williams T, Brooks T, Ward C: The role of atropine premedication in fiberoptic bronchoscopy using intravenous midazolam sedation. Chest *113*:1394, 1998.

Wood RE: Pediatric bronchoscopy. Chest Surg Clin N Am *6*:237, 1996.

Zavala DC: Pulmonary hemorrhage in fiberoptic transbronchial biopsy. Chest *70*:584, 1976.

Zavala DC: Transbronchial biopsy in diffuse lung disease. Chest *73*:727, 1978.

READING REFERENCES

Fulkerson WJ: Fiberoptic bronchoscopy. N Engl J Med *311*:511, 1984.

Harrow EM, Wang KP: The staging of lung cancer by bronchoscopic transbronchial needle aspiration. Chest Surg Clin North Am *6*:223, 1996.

Kvale PA: Flexible bronchoscopy with brush and forceps biopsy. *In* Wang KP (ed): Biopsy Techniques in Pulmonary Disorders. New York: Raven Press, 1989.

Kvale PA: Bronchoscopic biopsies and bronchoalveolar lavage. Chest Surg Clin N America *6*:205, 1996.

Lindholm C-E, et al: Cardiorespiratory effects of flexible fiberoptic bronchoscopy in critically ill patients. Chest *74*:362, 1978.

Miller MB, Kvale PA: Diagnostic bronchoscopy. Chest Surg Clin North Am *2*:599, 1992.

Radke JR, et al: Diagnostic accuracy in peripheral lung lesions. Factors predicting success with flexible fiberoptic bronchoscopy. Chest *76*:176, 1979.

CHAPTER 17

Invasive Diagnostic Procedures

Jean-Philippe Bocage, James W. Mackenzie, and John L. Nosher

When primary malignancy of the lung is suspected, careful examination of the patient and radiologic studies may reveal other lesions that require biopsy to document metastatic disease. Invasive diagnostic procedures range from percutaneous ones, such as thoracentesis and percutaneous needle biopsy, to more invasive interventions as exemplified by scalene node biopsy, mediastinoscopy, bronchoscopy (Chapter 16), and video-assisted thoracic surgical (VATS) procedures (Chapter 18).

SCALENE NODE BIOPSY

Daniels (1949) recommended excision of lymph nodes in the scalene fat pad to diagnose intrathoracic disease. Before the introduction of mediastinoscopy, this procedure was used widely for evaluation of patients with suspected bronchial carcinoma or other neoplasms, such as esophageal cancer and intra-abdominal malignancies. Certainly, palpable scalene lymph nodes require biopsy. For many of these patients, needle biopsy may be a better choice than open scalene node biopsy. Phillips and Barker (1985) reported success in 86% of 42 such patients. Rohwedder and colleagues (1990) were successful in all 55 patients with palpable supraclavicular nodes, although two required repeat needle biopsy. Controversy still exists about the use of scalene node biopsy in patients with nonpalpable nodes. Wide variation exists in the reported yield from scalene node biopsy in such patients. In the report by Brantigan and colleagues (1973), 20% of 2254 patients with carcinoma of the lung had a positive biopsy result. Bernstein and colleagues (1985) found only 3.5% positive results. As pointed out by Leckie and colleagues (1963), partial explanation of the discrepancy between literature reports may be found in the accuracy of cervical palpation. It is, however, hard to reconcile the wide variation on this basis alone given the large size of the series reported by Brantigan and colleagues (1973). Nevertheless, as the mortality from mediastinoscopy is no greater than that from scalene node biopsy, the choice

between the two procedures centers on the expected yield. In the report of Ashraf and associates (1980), 27% of patients with cancer of the lung who were otherwise surgical candidates were found to have involved mediastinal lymph nodes, and Maassen (1985) found 36%. Therefore, mediastinoscopy has replaced scalene node biopsy for most patients in most centers. A notable exception, however, is the occasional patient with N_2 disease who is being considered for resection. In these patients, documentation of spread outside the thorax should preclude consideration of thoracotomy. Lee and Ginsberg (1996) have advocated the use of scalene node biopsy at time of mediastinoscopy for appropriate staging.

The same reasoning applies to patients suspected of having sarcoidosis. In the report by Greschuchna and Maassen (1971), results of mediastinoscopy were positive in 98% of cases, whereas results of scalene node biopsy were positive in only 75%. The use of scalene node biopsy for nonthoracic disease also has generated interest. It has been advocated for the staging of tumors in the pancreas, prostate, stomach, and cervix. Subsequent reports, such as that by Perez-Mesa and Spratt (1976), of patients with carcinoma of the cervix with nonpalpable nodes question the usefulness of scalene node biopsy for intra-abdominal disease with nonpalpable nodes. No clear-cut conclusions are to be drawn from the data available.

Procedure

Local anesthesia is used unless this operation is combined with other procedures. The incision is made on the side of palpable nodes. If they are not palpable, the incision is made on the right, except for those pulmonary lesions confined to the left upper lobe or if disease metastatic from the abdomen or pelvis is under consideration. A 5-cm incision is made in the skin crease approximately 2 cm above the clavicle, extending approximately 2 cm over the lateral border of the sternocleidomastoid muscle (Fig. 17-1). The sternocleido-

273

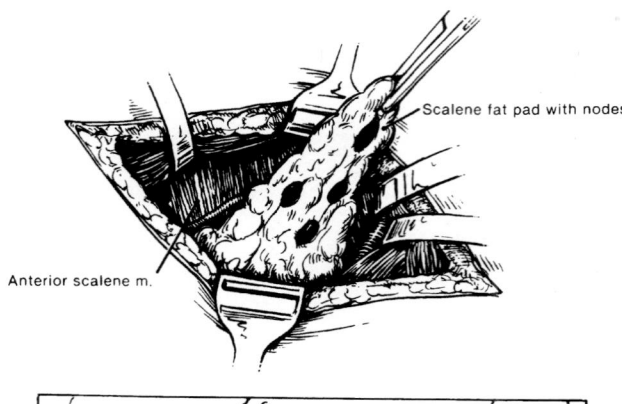

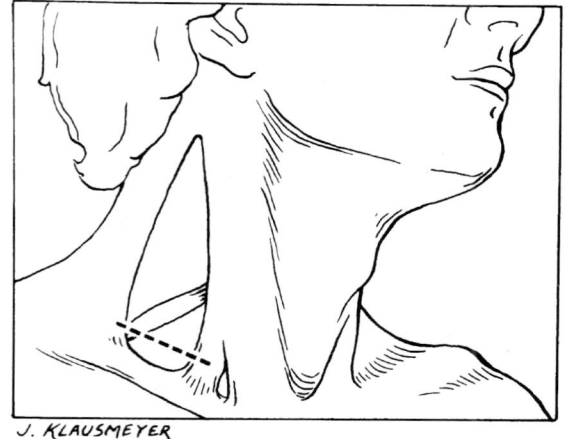

J. KLAUSMEYER

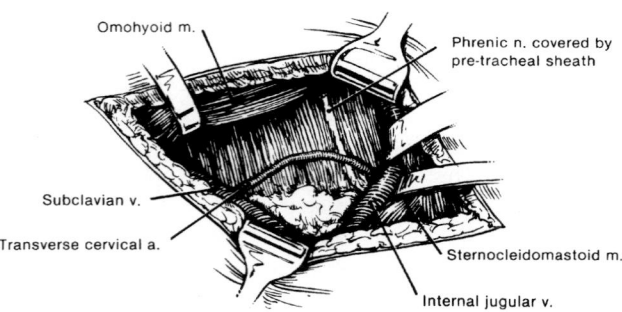

Fig. 17-1. Scalene node biopsy.

The transverse cervical artery often requires division, and the phrenic nerve should be avoided as it runs from lateral to medial in its position under the pretracheal fascial sheath. The thoracic duct must be ligated with nonabsorbable ligature if severed, as should its counterpart on the right.

Complications

Rare complications include air embolism, pneumothorax, arteriovenous fistula, and damage to the phrenic nerve. Mortality from this procedure should be negligible.

MEDIASTINOSCOPY

Although Harken and associates (1954) suggested a way to explore the nodes in the superior mediastinum from a lateral approach after excision of the scalene fat pad, it was the development of cervical mediastinoscopy by Carlens (1959) that led to the widespread use of this procedure. Its key features were general anesthesia and the development of a pretracheal tunnel through a small single cervical incision that combined with a specifically designed lighted speculum, the mediastinoscope, that permitted nodal sampling on each side of the trachea and more inferiorly.

Use of the Carlens' procedure spread from Sweden to North America with the strong support of Pearson (1968, 1980, 1986) and colleagues (1982). Cervical mediastinoscopy has become an integral part of the evaluation and staging of patients with suspected lung cancer. For reasons noted previously, it has usually replaced scalene node biopsy unless cervical nodes are palpable. It was an important advance in the management of lung cancer by providing for the first time a reliable prethoracotomy evaluation of the existence and extent of metastatic disease within the mediastinum. It established a practical method for determining the N status of the tumor, node, and metastasis (TNM) classification.

The prime indication for mediastinal lymph node biopsy is for prethoracotomy staging of lung cancer. The nodes accessible to standard cervical mediastinoscopy are levels two, three, and four (paratracheal), level seven (subcarinal), and sometimes level ten (tracheobronchial angle) (Fig. 17-2). Mediastinoscopy is also useful in the diagnosis of nodes involved with lymphoma l Hodgkin's disease, and granulomatous conditions such as sarcoidosis.

As demonstrated by Kirschner (1971a), Lewis and colleagues (1981), and Jahangiri and Goldstraw (1995), even advanced superior vena caval obstruction is not a contraindication to the operation. A report by Meersschaut and colleagues (1992) of 140 patients subjected to repeat mediastinoscopy citing no mortality, a sensitivity of 74%, and an accuracy of 94%, proves mediastinoscopy is a safe and reliable procedure even in this group of patients. For the ordinary patient, the risks of mediastinoscopy are extremely

mastoid muscle is retracted medially. Occasionally, it is necessary to divide a portion of the clavicular head of the muscle or to extend the incision between the two heads in obese or muscular patients. The omohyoid muscle is identified and retracted superiorly and laterally. The borders of the dissection are the internal jugular vein medially and the omohyoid superiorly and laterally. The subclavian vein at the inferior border of the dissection is often not identified clearly. The entire fat pad is excised unless obviously abnormal nodes are present; in which case it is not necessary to excise the entire fat pad. Unless frozen section confirms the presence of carcinoma, a portion of the lymph nodes should be sent for special stains and cultures.

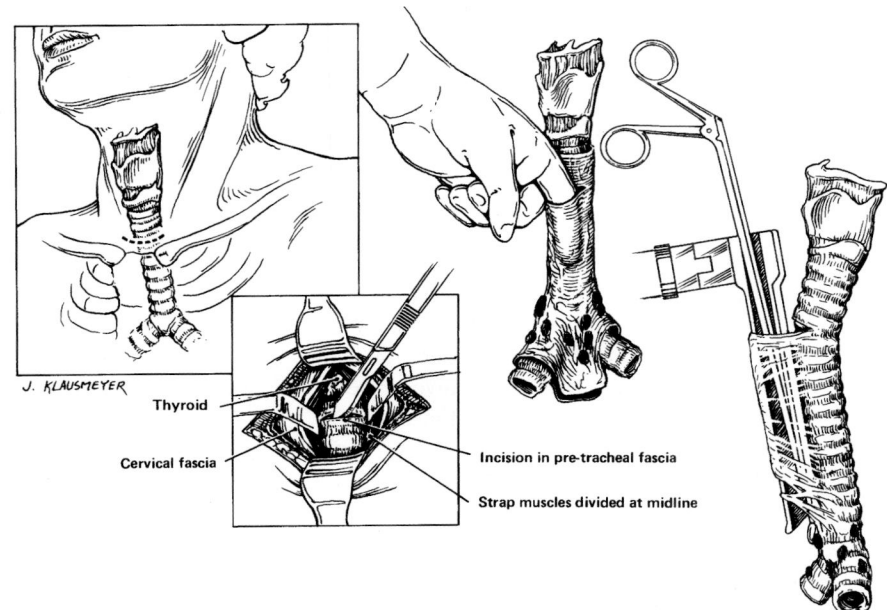

Fig. 17-2. Mediastinoscopy.

small. Mortality reported by Specht (1971) in more than 11,000 mediastinoscopic procedures compiled was 0.15%. In the prospective study of 1000 cases reported by Luke and colleagues (1986), the mortality was zero. On the Robert Wood Johnson Thoracic Surgery Service, our group has performed more than 3600 mediastinoscopic procedures with one mortality. Therefore, the safety of the procedure in experienced hands is well established.

Critics of this procedure have raised several questions about it. The first is cost. Certainly, mediastinoscopy does increase the cost of the evaluation of many patients. Nevertheless, when weighed against unnecessary thoracotomies and unnecessary mortality, the cost is insignificant. Furthermore, the report by Vallieres and associates (1991) of 138 mediastinoscopies carried out on an ambulatory basis without any mortality and the need for admission for medical observation in only eight of these patients, points the way for significant reduction in cost. The second concern is the advisability of the application of this technique to all patients being evaluated for carcinoma of the lung who are otherwise operable. Maassen (1985), in his experience of approximately 2000 mediastinoscopic procedures, demonstrated that even in 292 patients with peripheral T_1 lesions (less than 3 cm) the yield was 11%; the yield for central tumors in stages I and II was 23%; and that for peripheral tumors in stages I and II was 19%. These data make a strong case for performing cervical mediastinoscopy in all patients suspected of having carcinoma of the lung who are otherwise operable. Other authors with smaller series advocate mediastinoscopy only in cases of central lesions, those with hilar involvement, or those with mediastinal node involvement, suspected on radiographic examination. In a prospective study of 1000

patients subjected to mediastinoscopy, Luke and colleagues (1986) found tumor-bearing lymph nodes in 296 patients (29.6%). In 72% of these patients, no abnormality was noted on review of the chest radiographs.

Early reports of the use of computed tomographic (CT) scanning suggested that it could be used to select patients for mediastinoscopy. The reports of Brion (1985) and Daly (1987) and their colleagues demonstrated a 90% negative predictive index.

$$\text{Negative predictive index} = \frac{\text{Number of true negative}}{\text{Number of true negative} + \text{Number of false negative}} \times 100$$

In a prospective study of 170 patients with non–small cell disease reported by Webb and colleagues (1991), however, the sensitivity of CT imaging in detecting node metastasis was 52% and the specificity was 69%. The report by Izbicki and colleagues (1992) cast even greater doubt on the ability of CT scanning to stage carcinoma of the lung preoperatively. In this prospective study of 108 patients with carcinoma of the lung, on a patient-by-patient basis, CT scanning correctly predicted the nodal status in only 58% of patients. CT scanning apparently should not be used to exclude patients from mediastinoscopy. Backer and associates (1987) also questioned the routine use of mediastinal exploration, particularly in individuals with small peripheral lesions. They retrospectively evaluated 92 consecutive patients who had both CT scans and mediastinal exploration. Using a threshold of 1 cm for positive nodes, all scans and chest radiographs were reevaluated in a blinded fashion. In patients with peripheral lesions and a radiographically normal appearing mediastinum, the CT scan accurately predicted all positive nodes. In patients in whom the hilum or mediastinum was abnormal, the CT scan overevaluated the nodes but accurately identified all but one affected mediastinum. They recommended CT scan as a preliminary test to decrease the number of unnecessary mediastinoscopies. Patterson and coworkers (1987a) pointed out that metastatic disease might be found in 7% of patients in whom nodes were smaller than 1 cm on CT scan, particularly when the histologic cell type is adenocarcinoma. In reviewing their operative staging, Watanabe and Shimizu (1990) noted that metastatic disease could skip nodal stations with foci present in the mediastinum. This happened more frequently on the right (13%) than the left (8%), but with equal frequency among cell types.

Similarly, Gdeedo and colleagues (1997) have advocated routine cervical mediastinoscopy. One hundred consecutive patients with non–small cell lung carcinoma without distant metastases underwent staging by CT and cervical mediastinoscopy and the overall sensitivity and specificity of CT were 63% and 57%, respectively, and of mediastinoscopy 89% and 100%, respectively. Positive and negative predictive values of CT were 41% and 77%, respectively, and of mediastinoscopy were 100% and 96%, respectively. Accuracy of CT was 59% and of mediastinoscopy 97%. Accuracy of CT was lowest for left-sided and centrally located tumors and for lymph node station 7.

Therefore, we are persuaded that mediastinoscopy is an appropriate procedure for essentially all patients before planned resection. If the likelihood is high that the cervical mediastinal exploration will be negative, it is scheduled for the same day as the proposed resection. This technique adds but 20 to 30 minutes to the operative procedure.

If one does not accept the presence of mediastinal nodes as a contraindication to operation, the procedure loses much of its appeal. Reports by Kirsh (1971), Martini (1980), and Naruke (1988) and their colleagues documented reasonable survivorship of patients with N_2 disease discovered at operation. This apparently is a different set of patients than those in whom the nodes are discovered at cervical mediastinoscopy. Patterson and associates (1987b) reported 34 patients who had disease in the subaortic lymph nodes (station 5), but no metastatic disease in other mediastinal stations. The 3- and 5-year survival rates of the entire group were 44% and 28%, respectively. It was pointed out by Shields (1990) that, in general, a 5-year survival rate of approximately 2% can be expected in patients in whom N_2 disease is clinically recognizable or is identified by standard radiographic study or is discovered at mediastinoscopy. In those patients in whom N_2 disease is recognized only at thoracotomy, the 5-year survival rates are better. Nevertheless, surgical resection can be expected to salvage only 3 to 6% of patients with N_2 disease. Like others, we subject patients to thoracotomy if they are good risks for operation, have N_2 nodes low in the ipsilateral region and no evidence of extranodal growth at mediastinoscopy, or have isolated, mobile subaortic (station 5) metastases.

Lesions of the left upper lobe merit special considerations. Classical anatomic studies suggest that cervical mediastinoscopy would not be productive for these lesions. Nevertheless, clinical studies reported by Maassen (1985) note that 29% of lesions of the left upper lobe were positive at cervical mediastinoscopy. It is for this reason that we use standard cervical mediastinoscopy as the initial procedure for all patients. If a lesion is in the left upper lobe and the cervical mediastinoscopy result is negative, one may choose to follow, while the patient is still anesthetized, with anterior mediastinoscopy or the extended mediastinoscopic procedure of Ginsberg and colleagues (1987), particularly if the CT scan suggests involvement of station 5 or station 6 (anterior mediastinal) nodes.

Increasingly, however, we terminate this procedure and schedule the patient for VATS. At that time, the subaortic and anterior mediastinal nodal areas are explored and a decision is made to deem the patient unresectable or to proceed with resection, usually with VATS or, rarely, standard thoracotomy. We agree with Mentzer and associates (1997) that although imaging studies are sensitive in detecting abnormalities, specific staging usually requires a tissue biopsy. The mediastinoscope, bronchoscope, and three-chip thoracoscope (VATS) complement each other to provide appropriate staging while limiting morbidity.

An often contentious problem is the proper treatment of a patient with known small cell carcinoma on the basis of results of a needle biopsy. Although most of these patients do have widespread mediastinal involvement, it is important to document metastases by needle biopsy or by mediastinoscopy. In the rare patient with small cell carcinoma without nodal involvement (N_0) disease, the 5-year survivorship is more than 50%, as reported by Shah and colleagues (1992).

Technique

The CT scans are carefully reviewed before the operation. The operating table is adjusted to decrease obvious venous distention but not enough to increase the possibility of air embolism. The patient's neck should be slightly extended; but extensive hyperextension decreases the space between the sternum and the trachea and increases the possibility of compression of the innominate artery. The 4-cm transverse incision is centered over the trachea and made approximately 1 cm above the sternal ends of the clavicles and deepened through the platysma muscle (Fig. 17-3). The strap muscles are divided vertically in the midline, vigorous lateral traction is applied, the thyroid isthmus is retracted superiorly if in the field, and the pretracheal fascia is incised. With index-finger dissection, a tunnel is created within the pretracheal fascia immediately anterior and lateral to the trachea. Approaching the lower portion of this dissection, the envelope of pretracheal fascia is opened by blunt dissection. The index finger is withdrawn and the mediastinoscope is inserted within the tunnel created. A video mediastinoscope provides an excellent view and allows others to simultaneously observe the procedure. Closed biopsy forceps and a metal suction device are used to improve exposure of the lymph nodes previously identified by palpation. If none has been identified, the nodes in the paratracheal regions, tracheobronchial angles, and anterior subcarinal stations are sought. As shown in Figure 17-3, the nodes of station 5 and 6 (subaortic and para-aortic) are not accessible by standard cervical mediastinoscopy. Occasionally, aspiration biopsy may be helpful. Hemostasis is obtained primarily by coag-

ulation and packing, although application of a clip occasionally is necessary. Extreme care should be taken using electrocautery on the left to avoid injury to the recurrent laryngeal nerve. If significant bleeding occurs, the mediastinoscope is left in place and the area is packed with gauze for at least 10 minutes; the packing is then gently removed. If the bleeding is still significant, the packing is reapplied and preparation is made for thoracotomy. If hemostasis is achieved, the wound is closed.

Complications

The incidence of serious bleeding, as reported by Specht (1971), is 0.1 to 0.2%; the complications of vocal cord paralysis and pneumothorax occur slightly more frequently. Infrequent complications include damage to the esophagus, thoracic duct, bronchus, and trachea. Cardiac arrhythmias may occur. Wound seeding by tumor has been an extremely rare complication.

MODIFIED MEDIASTINOSCOPY

Occasionally, standard cervical mediastinoscopy does not provide appropriate access. This situation may occur in patients with lesions of the left upper lobe in whom standard cervical mediastinoscopy results are negative and in patients with lesions of the prevascular (anterior) space that is directly underneath the sternum. Ginsberg and colleagues (1987) devised a method for access to the anterior mediastinal (station 6) and aortopulmonary (station 5) nodes that are not accessible by standard cervical mediastinoscopy. This approach is through a tunnel created between the innominate artery and the left carotid artery (Fig. 17-4).

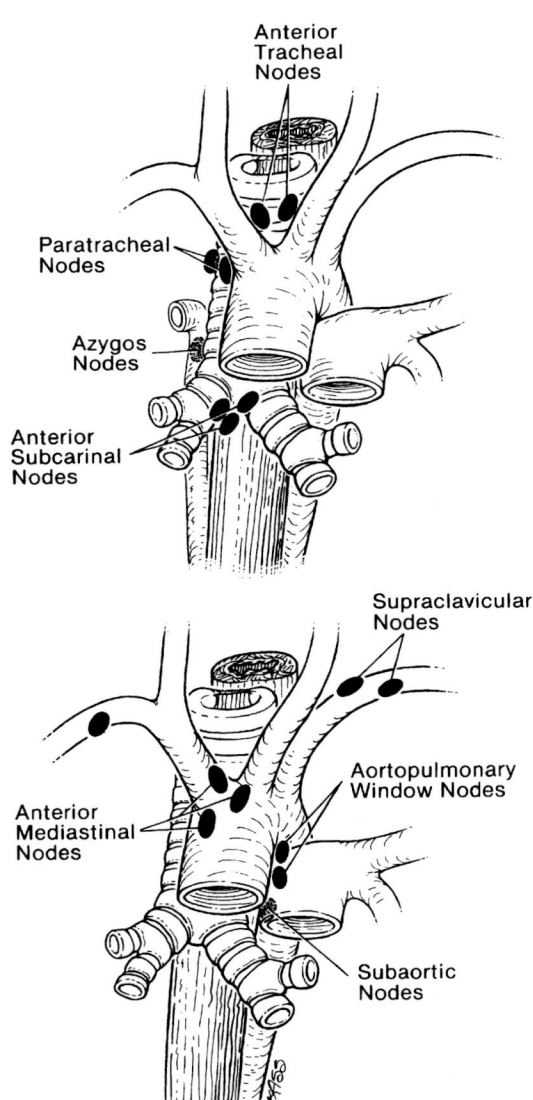

Fig. 17-3. Nodes accessible during surgical mediastinal exploration. Nodes that can be reached by the standard cervical mediastinoscopy are depicted on the left. Anterior mediastinal nodes and aortopulmonary window nodes depicted on the right require an extended mediastinoscopy, anterior mediastinotomy, videoassisted thoracic surgery, or needle biopsy.

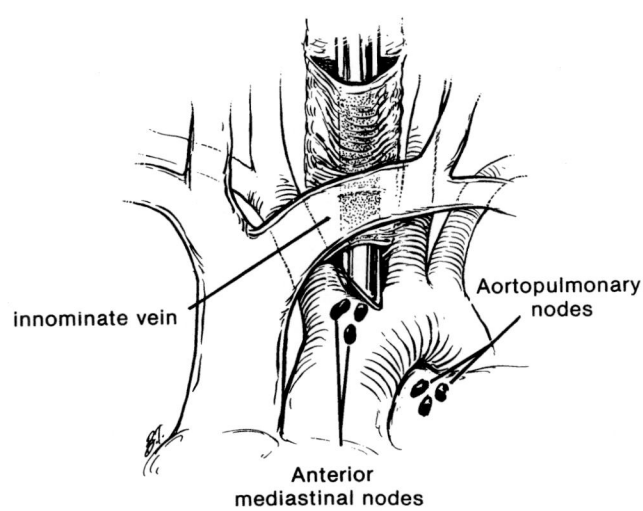

Fig. 17-4. Extended mediastinoscopy.

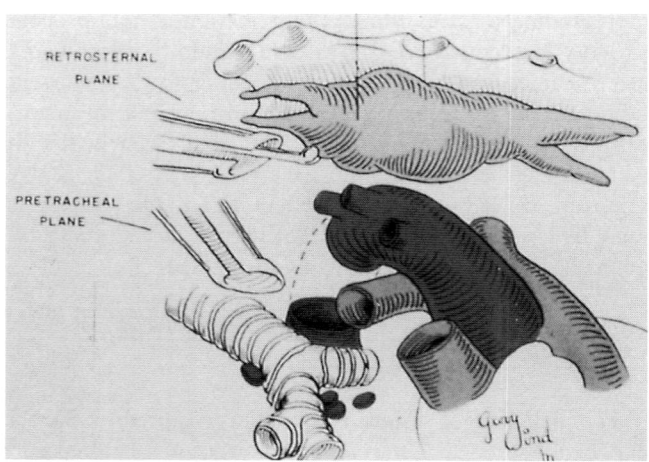

Fig. 17-5. Superior portion of the mediastinum shows the separate access with the mediastinoscopy into the anterior (prevascular) and visceral (retrovascular) compartments. Note the change in angle of the mediastinoscopy. From Shields TW: Mediastinal Surgery. Philadelphia: Lea & Febiger, 1991. With permission.

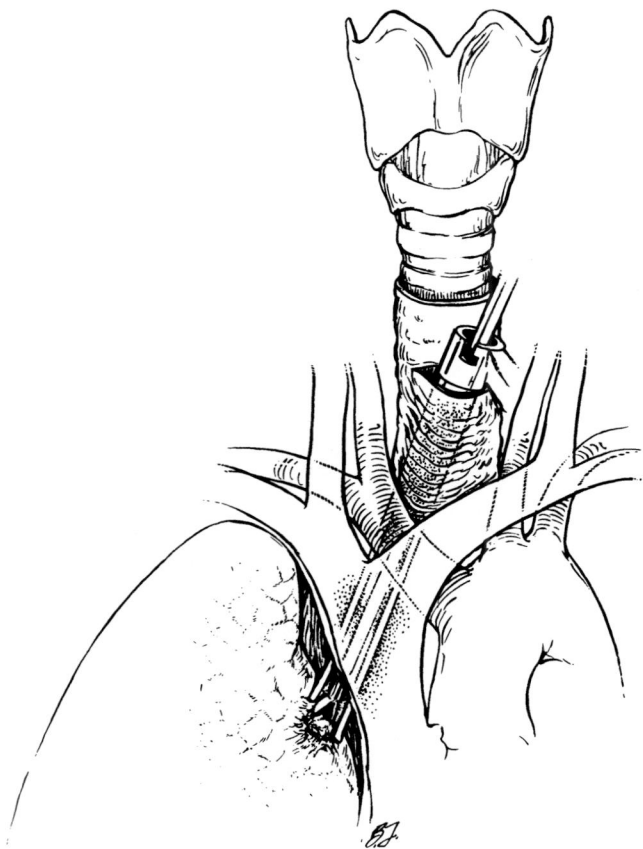

Fig. 17-6. Combined mediastinoscopy and right lung biopsy. From Baue AE: Glenn's Thoracic and Cardiovascular Surgery. 5th ed. Norwalk, CT: Appleton and Lange, 1991. With permission.

Kirschner (1971b) described a technique to provide access to this anterior space through the standard cervical mediastinoscopy incision in which the scope is passed into the mediastinum anterior to the great vessels (Fig. 17-5). Arom and associates (1977) described a subxiphoid approach to the anterior mediastinum. Also, Deslauriers and coworkers (1976) described a method for biopsy of the lung after digital opening of the mediastinal pleura (Fig. 17-6).

ANTERIOR MEDIASTINOTOMY AND ANTERIOR MEDIASTINOSCOPY

As previously noted, standard cervical mediastinoscopy does not provide access to the anterior mediastinal nodes (station 6) or to the aortopulmonary window nodes (station 5). Many authors, therefore, advocate anterior mediastinotomy as their primary choice for left upper lobe lesions. For reasons noted previously, we prefer cervical mediastinoscopy for all lesions as the primary procedure because it is a simpler procedure, is probably safer, and does not interfere with early radiation therapy. In the past, if the results were inconclusive from cervical mediastinoscopy for lesions of the left upper lobe, an anterior mediastinotomy was performed. As noted, the development of VATS would currently make this the choice for this situation rather than anterior mediastinotomy or the extended mediastinoscopy procedure of Ginsberg.

Technique

McNeill and Chamberlain (1966) described what has become a popular approach for anterior mediastinotomy. The second or third costal cartilage is excised subperichondrially and the posterior perichondrium is incised. The first and second intercostal bundles are divided. Alternately, an incision may be made through the second interspace without removing cartilage (Fig. 17-7). The internal mammary artery and vein are ligated individually. The pleura is mobilized laterally and the anterior mediastinal and aortopulmonary nodes are evaluated, as is the pulmonary hilum. A headlight is helpful and a mediastinoscope is often useful. Fine-needle aspiration occasionally makes this operation easier and safer. Appropriate samples are obtained and frozen section is often used. If the pleural cavity is entered for lung biopsy or evaluation of the hilum, or inadvertently, it is drained with an intercostal tube brought through a separate incision and attached to underwater seal suction.

Firmly matted nodes in the aortopulmonary window (station 5) or spread to the anterior mediastinal nodes (station 6) preclude thoracotomy. Nodes restricted to the aortopulmonary window that are easily resectable as judged by palpation would not preclude thoracotomy, as noted in the section on mediastinoscopy.

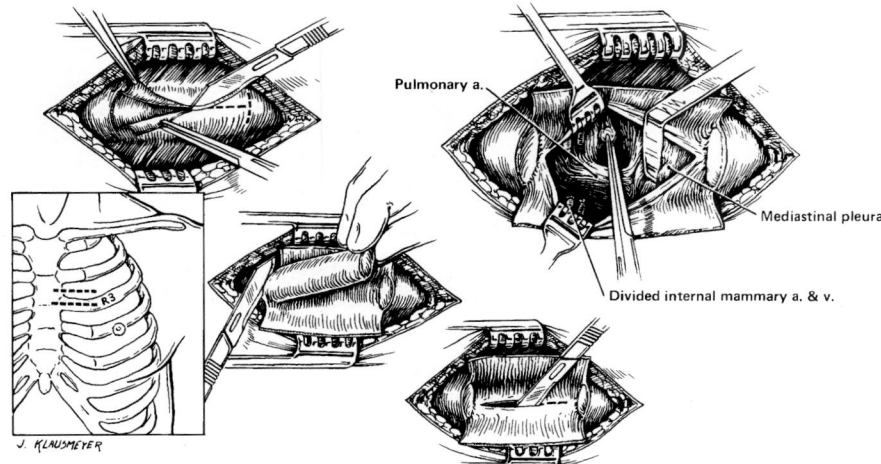

Fig. 17-7. Mediastinotomy. a., artery; v., vein.

THORACENTESIS

Accumulation of fluid in the pleural cavity is a major manifestation of pleural disease. When systemic disease, such as congestive heart failure, renal failure, or both, is suspected as the etiology of an effusion, treatment is recommended and its effect recorded before proceeding to thoracentesis. Smyrnois and associates (1990) noted that 60% of patients with a significant effusion may be asymptomatic. Pleural fluid should be removed for diagnostic thoracentesis when the etiology is unknown. Sahn (1988) reported that analysis can be diagnostic in 75% of patients. Usually, 100 mL of fluid is removed for examination. As noted in a report by the Health and Public Policy Committee of the American College of Physicians (1985) larger amounts may be associated with a higher rate of complications. To allow reexpansion and better visualization of the lung parenchyma, larger amounts of fluid can be removed as a therapeutic thoracentesis, but Sokolowski and coworkers (1989) reported that removal of more than 1.5 L may be associated with increased risks such as reexpansion edema. When performing therapeutic thoracentesis, the patient should be carefully monitored, and the procedure terminated if the patient complains of chest discomfort.

Classically, an effusion appears as a convex opacity on an upright chest radiograph. Two hundred fifty milliliters is usually necessary to visualize an effusion. A lateral decubitus film is useful in determining if the fluid is free flowing. As reported by McLoud and Flower (1991), newer modalities, such as ultrasonography, CT, and magnetic resonance imaging, have increased the sensitivity and accuracy of the diagnosis of pleural effusions. The radiologic and physical findings determine the site of aspiration. Usually, the best site is 2 in. below the superior aspect of the dullness. Small effusions can be aspirated with ultrasound guidance, as reported by Harnsberger (1983) and Grogan (1990) and their associates. CT scan is useful in managing a complex loculated effusion.

Technique

After the instillation of a local anesthetic, an 18-gauge needle is introduced close to the superior border of the rib to avoid the intercostal vessels and nerve. The needle is placed just inside the pleural space and the fluid aspirated. This reduces the incidence of parenchymal injury. As reported by Krausz and Manny (1976) a catheter also can be placed over the needle and threaded into the pleural space.

Examination of the fluid is critical. The appearance, odor, color, and character of the fluid provide diagnostic clues (Table 17-1). Most effusions are odorless; hence, a putrid effusion can be diagnostic of an empyema.

Cytologic examination is mandatory when a malignant process is part of the differential diagnosis. Cultures and sensitivity are obtained when bacterial infection is suspected. Chemical analyses require measurement of the pH, specific gravity, glucose, protein, and lactic dehydrogenase (see Chapter 68). The concentration of the last two substances in the pleural fluid is directly related to their level in the plasma. A blood sample is needed at the time of the thoracentesis to determine the relative serum and pleural fluid concentrations. A primary concern is whether the process is an exudate or transudate. Infection and neoplasm are the major causes of exudative effusions. Transudative effusions occur as a result of interference with absorption, excessive production, or both. Usually, a spe-

Table 17-1. Effusion and Related Diseases

Effusion	Disease
Red (hemorrhagic)	Tuberculosis, malignancy, trauma, embolism
White (milky)	Chyle, cholesterol
White (thick, viscous, cloudy)	Empyema, fistula(?)
Brown	Amebic

Table 17-2. Classification of Effusion

Differentiation	Transudate	Exudate
Lactate dehydrogenase (U/L)	<200	>220
Ratio of pleural/serum lactate dehydrogenase	<0.6	>0.6
Ratio pleural/serum protein (g/10 mL)	<0.5	>0.5

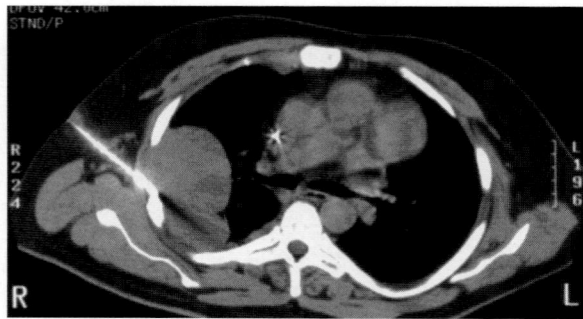

Fig. 17-8. Biopsy of this pulmonary parenchymal mass was performed with a 14-gauge cutting needle and confirmed the diagnosis of recurrent Hodgkin's disease.

cific gravity below 1.015 indicates a transudate. According to Sokolowski and associates (1989), further indication of an exudate may be noted by determining the ratio of pleural fluid protein to serum protein to be greater than 0.5, the pleural fluid lactate dehydrogenase (LDH) to serum LDH ratio to be greater than 0.6, and the pleural fluid LDH greater than two-thirds of the upper limits of normal for serum LDH. Table 17-2 may be helpful in the determination. Low sugar levels are suggestive of rheumatoid disease or tuberculosis. To reiterate, cytologic evaluation in suspected neoplastic effusions and culture for suspected bacterial infections are clearly indicated.

PERCUTANEOUS LUNG BIOPSY

The first percutaneous lung biopsy was reported by Leyden in 1883. In the 1940s and 1950s, considerable experience in percutaneous biopsy using fine needles was gained in Europe but only since the 1970s has this procedure gained wide acceptance in the United States.

Contributing to the acceptance of image-guided needle biopsy is the availability of modern radiologic imaging, which facilitates precise needle placement in large and small pulmonary nodules and mediastinal masses. Experienced cytopathologists armed with special stains, immunohistochemistry, and flow cytometry provide a means for definitive diagnoses from small biopsy specimens.

Percutaneous image-guided biopsy of the lung and mediastinum is performed using needles of 14 to 22 gauge. Needle designs range from the thin-walled spinal needles, needles with a variety of cutting edges, to automated cutting needles. Coaxial biopsy systems consist of a 17- to 20-gauge outer needle cannula that is placed adjacent to the lesion. Through the cannula, an 18- to 22-gauge cutting needle is passed into the lesion, thus providing the opportunity for multiple biopsy samples through a single pleural puncture. Biopsy of mediastinal, pleural, chest wall, and parenchymal masses that can be accomplished without traversing aerated lung may be performed safely with larger needle sizes ranging from 14 to 17 gauge, with resultant increase in specimen size (Fig. 17-8). For pulmonary nodules likely to represent bronchial carcinoma or metastatic disease, aspiration biopsy with 22-gauge spinal needles provides adequate material for definitive cytologic diagnosis as well as some material for cell block and histologic analysis. When Hodgkin's or non-Hodgkin's lymphoma is suspected, core biopsy with 14- to

20-gauge cutting needles increases the diagnostic yield. A specific diagnosis of benign disease is also more likely to be obtained using larger gauge cutting needles.

Planning the biopsy route to minimize the number of pleural surfaces crossed, minimize the length of the biopsy path, and avoid major vascular structures is accomplished by review of the posteroanterior and lateral chest radiographs and enhanced by a preprocedural CT scan. Fluoroscopic guidance can be used for biopsy of parenchymal, pleural, and mediastinal lesions easily identified on standard chest radiography. Although fluoroscopic guidance is economical, minimizes the requirement for patient cooperation, and minimizes procedure time, it is less frequently used in favor of CT guidance, which is less dependent on the operator. CT guidance provides a precise display of the lesion and relevant anatomic association, including pleural surfaces, vascular structures, and adjacent bullae. As reported by van Sonnenberg and associates (1992), it is particularly helpful for mediastinal biopsy and biopsy of nodules not readily apparent at fluoroscopy. In addition to being more costly than fluoroscopy, CT scanning increases the time required for performance of the procedure and, in the experience of van Sonnenberg and associates (1992), results in a higher incidence of pneumothorax. Sonography may be used to guide biopsy of pleural, mediastinal, and pulmonary parenchymal masses that extend to the chest wall, as described by Yang (1997).

An important part of preprocedural diagnostic planning is consideration of the special handling of specimens, especially flow cytometry, which enhances the diagnosis and subtyping of lymphoma. Austin and Cohen (1993) as well as Padhani and associates (1997) reported that the presence of a cytologist for immediate review of the biopsy material and assessment of specimen adequacy increases the yield of the procedure and may diminish the number of needle passes performed.

Indications and Contraindications

The indications for image-guided biopsy of parenchymal nodules include diagnosis of possible metastatic disease to lung in patients with known primary tumors, diagnosis of multiple pulmonary nodules, and diagnosis of solitary pulmonary nodules in patients who are either not surgical candidates or who refuse a thoracotomy without a preoperative diagnosis. As described by Weisbrod and associates (1984), pulmonary nodules and mediastinal disease can be diagnosed and staged by mediastinal fine-needle aspiration biopsy (FNAB). Biopsy of solitary pulmonary nodules in patients who are surgical candidates may provide a diagnosis of benign disease, identify lesions, such as small cell carcinoma or lymphoma, that are more appropriately treated by nonsurgical means, or provide a preoperative diagnosis of malignancy, eliminating the need for intraoperative biopsy before resection. In the experience of Yang (1997), FNAB, complemented when necessary by large-needle biopsy, is an accurate method of diagnosing infectious processes when bronchoscopic methods fail. Lesions suspected of being endobronchial or involving the air spaces are preferably diagnosed by transbronchial biopsy or bronchial washing. At some institutions, image-guided needle biopsy provides a minimally invasive method for diagnosing and subtyping Hodgkin's and non-Hodgkin's lymphoma.

Contraindications to FNAB are primarily uncorrectable coagulopathy or inability of the patient to cooperate during the biopsy procedure. Although emphysema increases the risk of pneumothorax, this condition does not diminish the usefulness of FNAB when the information rendered affects patient management and less invasive diagnostic procedures have failed.

Complications

The most common significant complication of FNAB is pneumothorax, which occurs in 8 to 61% of patients. Up to 40% of patients developing pneumothorax require chest tube placement. In the large experience of Weisbrod and coworkers (1984), pneumothorax occurred in 32% of 2421 FNABs, with chest tube placement required in 8%. This complication increases with needle size, the number of needle passes through the pleura, the use of CT guidance, and the presence of emphysema. According to Kazerooni and coworkers (1996), the most significant determinant of the risk of pneumothorax has been reported to be the depth of the lesion from the pleural surface (Fig. 17-9). Greater than 90% of pneumothoraces are diagnosed on the postprocedure radiograph or a radiograph routinely obtained 2 hours after the procedure. If these results are negative for pneumothorax, the patient can be safely discharged with specific instructions to return to the nearest facility should symptoms of pneumothorax occur. The presence of emphysema predicts prolonged air leak in patients requiring chest tube placement. Bleeding after FNAB occurs in 5% of patients, and in the absence of a bleeding diathesis is usually not clinically significant. Air embolism has been reported as a rare

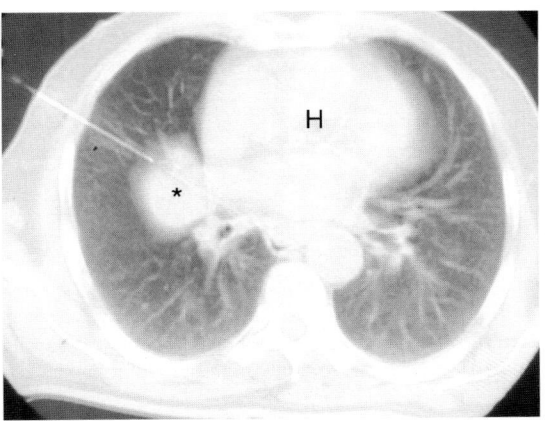

Fig. 17-9. Computed tomographically directed biopsy precisely demonstrates the needle location with respect to the mass (*) and heart (H). This biopsy could just as well have been performed using fluoroscopy. The biopsy revealed squamous carcinoma of lung. Biopsy of central lesions such as this may carry a greater risk of pneumothorax than peripheral lesions.

complication, as has tumor seeding of the biopsy tract. Tumor seeding occurs in less than 0.1% of FNAB but is almost certainly underdiagnosed; it was seen in 2 of 4000 biopsies reported by Nordenstrom and Bjork (1973) and none of almost 1500 biopsies reported by Lalli and associates (1978). Furthermore, Sinner and Sandstedt (1976) saw no diminution in survival in patients undergoing FNAB.

Results

FNAB is an accurate method of diagnosing bronchial carcinoma with a sensitivity of 77 to 95% in the experience of Westcott (1981) and Lalli and associates (1978), and a specificity approaching 100%. Sensitivity varies significantly with the skill and experience of the operator. Although Li and coworkers (1996) report diminished accuracy of diagnosis for small lesions, Westcott reported an accuracy of 93% in the diagnosis of lesions 15 mm or less in size (Fig. 17-10). Characterization of cell type is less accurate than the diagnosis of malignancy. Differentiation of small cell from non–small cell carcinoma, however, is reliable and, as reported by Koss and colleagues (1984), carries a specificity of 95%. Failure to diagnose malignancy on FNAB does not exclude its presence. Sampling error, necrotic specimens, and needle misdirection account for the 5 to 25% of false-negative diagnoses of malignancy with FNAB. To exclude malignancy on FNAB reliably, a specific alternative diagnosis of benign disease, such as granuloma or hamartoma, must be rendered. The use of larger diameter cutting needles increases the probability of a specific diagnosis of a benign lesion.

The role of image-guided biopsy of Hodgkin's and non-Hodgkin's lymphoma is evolving. Using fine needles to pro-

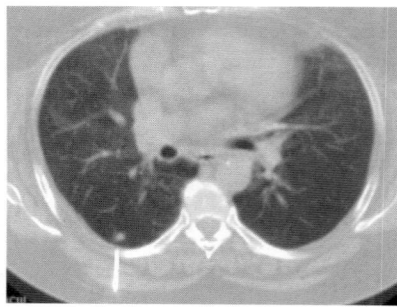

Fig. 17-10. Biopsy of this 5-mm adenocarcinoma of lung was successfully performed using computed tomographic guidance.

vide material for cytology and small cores for histologic evaluation; a diagnosis on which therapy can be based is reported to be rendered in less than 50% of patients. The addition of immunohistochemical staining and flow cytometry, along with the use, in appropriate cases, of 14- and 16-gauge cutting needles, increases the diagnostic yield to greater than 80% according to Quinn and associates (1995).

FNAB is an excellent way to diagnose metastatic disease to the mediastinum. Results of mediastinal biopsy have shown some variability. Westcott (1981) diagnosed primary or metastatic carcinoma in 94% of 72 patients with mediastinal involvement (Fig. 17-11). Herman and associates (1991) reported 143 mediastinal biopsies and correctly diagnosed 70% of metastases to the mediastinum, 91% of germ cell tumors, and 71% of thymomas, but only 42% of lymphomas and 20% of Hodgkin's disease (Fig. 17-12).

With proper patient selection, FNAB is a relatively safe and highly accurate method of diagnosing benign and malignant processes involving the chest wall, pleura, lung, and mediastinum. Because the results of this procedure depend on the skills of the radiologist and cytopathologist, results may vary significantly between institutions.

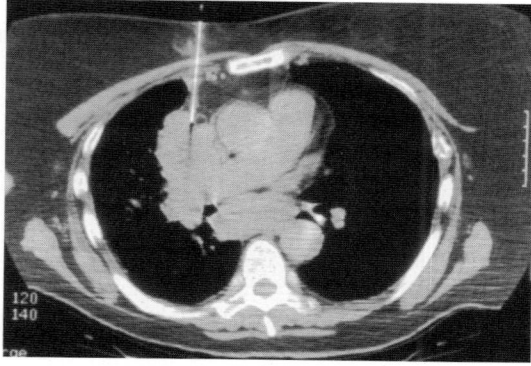

Fig. 17-11. Biopsy of mediastinal adenopathy in this patient under computed tomographic guidance revealed small cell carcinoma of lung.

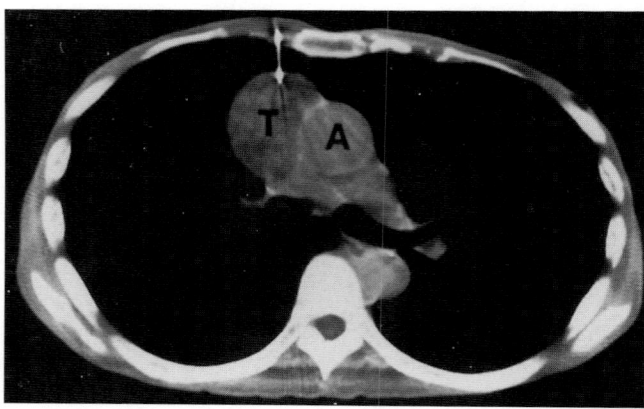

Fig. 17-12. Computed tomographically directed biopsy demonstrates this mass (T) to reside in the anterior and middle mediastinum. Computed tomography clearly demonstrates the location of the biopsy needle with respect to the mass and the thoracic aorta (A). The diagnosis determined from the biopsy of this mass was thymoma.

NEEDLE BIOPSY OF THE PLEURA

Pleural biopsy is indicated when pleural fluid analysis fails to provide the diagnosis in patients suspected of having a tuberculous or malignant effusion. Even without the presence of effusion, pleural biopsy may be helpful. In a report of 750 consecutive biopsies, Cowie and colleagues (1983) obtained adequate specimens in 79% of patients with pleural disease without pleural effusion. If empyema is suspected, pleural biopsy is contraindicated because of the risk of infection along the needle track. Also, pleural biopsy is not indicated if the effusion is thought to be associated with such diseases as pancreatitis, collagen vascular disease, or pulmonary emboli. As reported by Prakash and Reiman (1985) and Salyer and colleagues (1975), pleural biopsy may show evidence of malignant disease even when the pleural fluid cytology is not diagnostic. Similarly, the diagnosis of tuberculosis may be rendered from cultured biopsy material and from demonstration of caseating granulomas in 60 to 80% of cases of pleural tuberculosis, as documented by Feinsilver and associates (1986) and Von Hoff and LiVolsi (1975). As reported by Feinsilver and colleagues (1986), a second biopsy sometimes establishes a diagnosis if the first biopsy result is negative.

In general, a backward-biting needle, such as that designed by Cope or Abrams, is preferable. If the mass is large and without fluid, a forward-biting needle, such as the Vim-Silverman, may be used and has the advantage of providing a greater amount of tissue.

Technique

Adequate preoperative medication should be administered before needle biopsy of the pleura. Atropine is probably helpful to prevent the occasional vagal response to the procedure. After an appropriate amount of local anesthesia is given, the skin is punctured with a No. 11 blade and the needle is then inserted into the pleural space just above the selected rib. Usually, a definite popping sensation is noted. Care should be taken to prevent accidental penetration of the needle beyond the pleural space. The hook is impinged on the pleura, the cutting unit is then advanced over the hook, and the entire unit is withdrawn. The intercostal vessels and nerves in the superior aspect of the interspace are to be avoided.

THORACOSCOPY

Thoracoscopy is covered in Chapter 18. Open tube thoracoscopy or VATS can be used as a primary diagnostic and therapeutic procedure in the management of pleural disease, but traditionally is restricted to those patients in whom thoracentesis and needle biopsy are not diagnostic.

PERICARDIAL BIOPSY

Most symptomatic cases of chronic pericardial effusions are well treated by cardiologists with pericardiocentesis directed by two-dimensional echocardiography as described by Callahan and colleagues (1985). As reported by Jansen and colleagues (1986), 87% of these patients are managed successfully with catheter decompression. Occasionally, however, surgical biopsy and drainage are required. Under these circumstances, a decision must be made whether to perform the operation using the simpler subxiphoid approach as advocated by Naunheim and colleagues (1991) or through the left anterior lateral approach, which does require general anesthesia but probably gives better long-term results, as reported by Piehler and colleagues (1985).

Technique

The subxiphoid approach in pericardial biopsy is made using either local or general anesthesia. The vertical, upper abdominal midline incision extends over the xiphoid. The linea alba is divided and the xiphoid is retracted superiorly. The pericardium is identified after dissection of the diaphragm from the inner surface of the sternum. Fluid is aspirated and sent for cytologic and bacteriologic study. A window is made by excision of the pericardium as widely as can be done conveniently. Digital palpation can identify nodules and break up loculations for effective drainage. The pericardial tissue is also sent for bacteriologic and histologic study. The pericardial space is drained with a soft tube connected to underwater seal.

VATS is used to perform a biopsy of the pericardium to create a window and drain related effusions, as described by Lewis and colleagues (1992).

The transthoracic approach involves an anterior lateral left thoracotomy through the fifth or sixth interspace. The pericardial window is excised anterior to the phrenic nerves. Again, the fluid and pericardium are sent for appropriate culture and histologic and cytologic study. Two tubes brought out through separate stab wounds and attached to an underwater seal drain the left pleural space.

Results

Most patients respond well to pericardial biopsy, although as reported by Piehler and associates (1985), approximately 10% have recurrent symptoms from effusion and constriction. Most recurrences are noted in patients with the subxiphoid approach; in those patients, a more extensive pericardial resection should be done.

REFERENCES

Arom KV, et al: Subxiphoid anterior mediastinal exploration. Ann Thorac Surg 24:289, 1977.

Ashraf MH, Milsom PL, Walesby RK: Selection by mediastinoscopy and long-term survival in bronchial carcinoma. Ann Thorac Surg 30:208, 1980.

Austin JH, Cohen MB: Value of having a cytopathologist present during percutaneous fine-needle aspiration of lung: report of 55 cancer patients and meta-analysis of the literature. AJR Am J Roentgenol 160:175, 1993.

Backer CL, et al: Selective preoperative evaluation for possible N₂ disease in carcinoma of the lung. J Thorac Cardiovasc Surg. 93:337, 1987.

Bernstein MP, Ferrara JJ, Brown L: Effectiveness of scalene node biopsy for staging of lung cancer in the absence of palpable adenopathy. J Surg Oncol 29:46, 1985.

Brantigan JW, Brantigan CO, Brantigan OC: Biopsy of nonpalpable scalene lymph nodes in carcinoma of the lung. Am Rev Respir Dis 107:962, 1973.

Brion JP, et al: Role of computed tomography and mediastinoscopy in preoperative staging of lung carcinoma. J Comput Assist Tomogr 9:480, 1985.

Callahan JA, Seward JB, Tajik AJ: Cardiac tamponade: pericardiocentesis directed by two-dimensional echocardiography. Mayo Clin Proc 60:344, 1985.

Carlens E: Mediastinoscopy: a method for inspection and tissue biopsy in the superior mediastinum. Dis Chest 36:343, 1959.

Cowie RL, et al: Pleural biopsy. A report of 750 biopsies performed using Abram's pleural biopsy punch. S Afr Med J 64:92, 1983.

Daly BDT Jr, et al: Mediastinal lymph node evaluation by computed tomography in lung cancer. An analysis of 345 patients grouped by TNM staging, tumor size, and tumor location. J Thorac Cardiovasc Surg 94:664, 1987.

Daniels AC: A method of biopsy useful in diagnosing certain intrathoracic diseases. Dis Chest 16:360, 1949.

Deslauriers J, et al: Mediastinopleuroscopy: a new approach to the diagnosis of intrathoracic diseases. Ann Thorac Surg 22:265, 1976.

Feinsilver SH, Barrows AA, Braman SS: Fiberoptic bronchoscopy and pleural effusion of unknown origin. Chest 90:516, 1986.

Gdeedo A, et al: Prospective evaluation of computed tomography and mediastinoscopy in mediastinal lymph node staging. Eur Respir J 10:1547, 1997.

Ginsberg RJ, et al: Extended cervical mediastinoscopy. A single staging procedure for bronchial carcinoma of the left upper lobe. J Thorac Cardiovasc Surg 94:673, 1987.

Greschuchna D, Maassen W: Results of mediastinoscopy and other biopsies in sarcoidosis and silicosis. In Jepsen O, Sorensen HR (eds): Mediastinoscopy. Denmark: Odense University Press, 1971, pp. 79–82.

Grogan DR, et al: Complications associated with thoracentesis: a prospective, randomized study comparing three different methods. Arch Intern Med 150:873, 1990.

Harken DE, et al: A simple cervicomediastinal exploration for tissue diagnosis of intrathoracic disease. N Engl J Med 251:1041, 1954.

Harnsberger HR, Lee TG, Mukuno DH: Rapid, inexpensive real-time directed thoracentesis. Radiology 146:545, 1983.

Health & Public Policy Committee, American College of Physicians: Diagnostic thoracentesis and pleural biopsy in pleural effusions. Ann Intern Med 103:799, 1985.

Herman SJ, et al: Anterior mediastinal masses: utility of transthoracic needle biopsy. Radiology 180:167, 1991.

Izbicki JR, et al: Accuracy of computed tomographic scan and surgical assessment for staging of bronchial carcinoma. A prospective study. J Thorac Cardiovasc Surg 104:413, 1992.

Jahangiri M, Goldstraw P: The role of mediastinoscopy in superior vena caval obstruction. Ann Thorac Surg 59:453, 1995.

Jansen EW, et al: Treatment of pericardial effusion. J Thorac Cardiovasc Surg 90:795, 1986.

Kazerooni EA, et al: Risk of pneumothorax in CT-guided transthoracic needle aspiration biopsy of the lung. Radiology 198:371, 1996.

Kirschner PA: Mediastinoscopy in superior vena cava obstruction. In Jepsen O, Sorensen HR (eds): Mediastinoscopy. Denmark: Odense University Press, 1971a, pp. 40–42.

Kirschner PA: "Extended" mediastinoscopy. In Jepsen O, Sorensen HR (eds): Mediastinoscopy. Denmark: Odense University Press, 1971b, p. 131.

Kirsh MM, et al: Treatment of bronchogenic carcinoma with mediastinal metastases. Ann Thorac Surg 12:11, 1971.

Koss LG, Woyke S, Olszewski W: Aspiration Biopsy: Cytologic Interpretation and Histologic Bases. New York: Igaku-Shoin, 1984.

Krausz M, Manny J: A safe method of thoracentesis. J Thorac Cardiovasc Surg 72:323, 1976.

Lalli AF, et al: Aspiration biopsy of chest lesions. Radiology 239:36, 1978.

Leckie WJ, McCormack RJM, Walbaum PR: The case against routine scalene node biopsy in bronchial carcinoma. Lancet 1:853, 1963.

Lee JD, Ginsberg RJ: Lung cancer staging: the value of ipsilateral scalene lymph node biopsy performed at mediastinoscopy. Ann Thorac Surg 62:338, 1996.

Lewis RJ, Sisler GE, Mackenzie JW: Mediastinoscopy in advanced superior vena cava obstruction. Ann Thorac Surg 32:458, 1981.

Lewis RJ, et al: One hundred consecutive patients undergoing video-assisted thoracic operations. Ann Thorac Surg 54:421, 1992.

Leyden H: Uber infectiose pneumonie. Dtsch Med Wochenschr 9:52, 1883.

Li H, et al: Diagnostic accuracy and safety of CT-guided percutaneous needle aspiration biopsy of the lung: comparison of small and large pulmonary nodules. AJR Am J Roentgenol 167:105, 1996.

Luke WP, et al: Prospective evaluation of mediastinoscopy for assessment of carcinoma of the lung. J Thorac Cardiovasc Surg 9:53, 1986.

Maassen W: The staging issue-problems: accuracy of mediastinoscopy. In Delarue NC, Eschapasse H (eds): International Trends in General Thoracic Surgery. Lung Cancer. Vol. 1. Philadelphia: WB Saunders, 1985, pp. 42–53.

Martini N, et al: Prospective study of 445 lung carcinomas with mediastinal lymph node metastases. J Thorac Cardiovasc Surg 80:390, 1980.

McLoud TC, Flower DR: Imaging the pleura: sonography, CT, MR imaging. Am J Radiol 156:1145,1991.

McNeill TM, Chamberlain JM: Diagnostic anterior mediastinotomy. Ann Thorac Surg 2:532, 1966.

Meersschaut D, et al: Repeat mediastinoscopy in the assessment of new and recurrent lung neoplasm. Ann Thorac Surg 53:120, 1992.

Mentzer SJ, et al: Mediastinoscopy, thoracoscopy, and video-assisted thoracic surgery in the diagnosis and staging of lung cancer. Chest 112(4 Suppl):239S, 1997.

Naruke T, et al: The importance of surgery to non-small cell carcinoma of lung with mediastinal lymph node metastasis. Ann Thorac Surg 46:603, 1988.

Naunheim KS, et al: Pericardial drainage: subxiphoid vs transthoracic approach. Eur J Cardiothorac Surg 5:99, 1991.

Nordenstrom B, Bjork VO: Dissemination of cancer cells by needle biopsy of the lung. J Thorac Cardiovasc Surg 65:671, 1973.

Padhani AR, et al: The value of immediate cytologic evaluation for needle aspiration lung biopsy. Invest Radiol 32:453, 1997a.

Patterson GA, et al: A prospective evaluation of magnetic resonance imaging, computed tomography and mediastinoscopy in the preoperative assessment of mediastinal node status in bronchogenic carcinoma. J Thorac Cardiovasc Surg 94:679,1987a.

Patterson GA, et al: Significance of metastatic disease in subaortic lymph nodes. Ann Thorac Surg 43:155, 1987b.

Pearson FG: An evaluation of mediastinoscopy in the management of presumably operable bronchial carcinoma. J Thorac Cardiovasc Surg 55:617, 1968.

Pearson FG: Use of mediastinoscopy in selection of patients for lung cancer operations. Ann Thorac Surg 30:205, 1980.

Pearson FG: Lung cancer. The past twenty five years. Chest 89:200S, 1986.

Pearson FG, et al: Significance of positive superior mediastinal nodes identified at mediastinoscopy in patients with resectable cancer of the lung. J Thorac Cardiovasc Surg 83:1, 1982.

Perez-Mesa C, Spratt JS Jr: Scalene node biopsy in the pretreatment staging of carcinoma of the cervix uteri. Am J Obstet Gynecol 125:93, 1976.

Phillips MS Barker V: Extrathoracic lymph node aspiration in bronchial carcinoma. Thorax 40:398, 1985.

Piehler JM, et al: Surgical management of effusive pericardial disease. Influence of extent of pericardial resection on clinical course. J Thorac Cardiovasc Surg 90:506, 1985.

Prakash UBS, Reiman HM: Comparison of needle biopsy with cytologic analysis for the evaluation of pleural effusion: analysis of 414 cases. Mayo Clin Proc 60:158, 1985.

Quinn SF, et al: The role of percutaneous needle biopsies in the original diagnosis of lymphoma: a prospective evaluation. J Vasc Interv Radiol 6:947, 1995.

Rohwedder JJ, Handley JA, Kerr D: Rapid diagnosis of lung cancer from palpable metastases by needle thrust. Chest 98:1393, 1990.

Sahn SA: State of the art—The pleura. Am Rev Respir Dis 138:183, 1988.

Salyer WR, Eggleston JC, Erozan YS: Efficacy of pleural needle biopsy and pleural fluid cytopathology in the diagnosis of malignant neoplasm involving the pleura. Chest 67:536, 1975.

Shah SS, Thompson J, Goldstraw P: Results of operation without adjuvant therapy in the treatment of small cell lung cancer. Ann Thorac Surg 54:498, 1992.

Shields TW: The significance of ipsilateral mediastinal lymph node metastasis (N$_2$ disease) in non–small cell carcinoma of the lung. J Thorac Cardiovasc Surg 99:48, 1990.

Sinner WN, Sandstedt B: Small-cell carcinoma of the lung. Cytological, roentgenologic, and clinical findings in a consecutive series diagnosed by fine-needle aspiration biopsy. Radiology 121:269, 1976.

Smyrnois NA, Jederlinic PH, Irwin RS: Special report. Pleural effusion in an asymptomatic patient. Spectrum and frequency of causes and management considerations. Chest 97:192, 1990.

Sokolowski JW Jr, et al: Guidelines for thoracentesis and needle biopsy of the pleura. Am Rev Respir Dis 140:257, 1989.

Specht G: Discussion by Carlens. In Jepsen O, Sorenson HR (eds): Mediastinoscopy. Denmark: Odense University Press, 1971, p. 130.

Vallieres E, Page A, Verdant A: Ambulatory mediastinoscopy and anterior mediastinotomy. Ann Thorac Surg 52:1122, 1991.

van Sonnenberg, et al: Interventional radiology in the chest. Chest 102:608, 1992.

Von Hoff DD, LiVolsi V: Diagnostic reliability of needle biopsy of the parietal pleura. A review of 272 biopsies. Am J Clin Pathol 64:200, 1975.

Watanabe Y, Shimizu J: Mediastinal spread of metastatic lymph nodes in bronchogenic carcinoma. Chest 97:1059, 1990.

Webb WR, et al: CT and MR imaging in staging non-small cell bronchogenic carcinoma: report of the Radiologic Diagnostic Oncology Group. Radiology 178:705, 1991.

Weisbrod G, et al: Percutaneous fine needle aspiration biopsy of mediastinal lesions. Am J Radiol 143:525, 1984.

Westcott J: Percutaneous needle aspiration of hilar and mediastinal masses. Radiology 141:323, 1981.

Yang PC: Ultrasound-guided transthoracic biopsy of peripheral lung, pleural, and chest-wall lesions. J Thorac Imaging 12:272, 1997.

CHAPTER 18

Video-Assisted Thoracic Surgery as a Diagnostic Tool

Robert J. Caccavale and Ralph J. Lewis

Since we first demonstrated the success of video-assisted thoracic surgery (VATS) in 1990, the procedure has quickly demonstrated the magnitude of its potential (1992a). Although any dramatic change in widely accepted practice should not be embraced with abandon, the advent of video optics and compatible instrumentation has created the opportunity for thoracic surgeons to offer a powerful new alternative to their patients. VATS has evolved from a limited procedure, used primarily for simple pleural biopsies, into an important option for the diagnosis of intrathoracic disease and an increasingly preferable alternative for many thoracic resections. A vast array of standard thoracic surgical procedures that once required an open thoracotomy can now be performed successfully and safely using endoscopic techniques. VATS is superior to a standard thoracotomy in that it reduces surgical trauma, decreases postoperative pain and narcotic use, and preserves pulmonary function. These attributes, in turn, result in a reduced incidence of perioperative complications, shorter hospital stays, and a decreased need for intensive care services. The use of VATS instead of an open thoracotomy offers lower costs, better outcomes, and increased patient satisfaction.

The most common use of VATS is for the diagnosis of intrathoracic disease. Common indications for diagnostic VATS are listed in Table 18-1. As a diagnostic tool, VATS provides clear visualization of the thoracic cavity and superb access to the lung, pleura, mediastinum, and pericardium for specimen retrieval, while avoiding the morbidity of traditional open thoracotomy. A small, early study by the authors (1992b) documented the use of VATS for lung biopsy in 11 patients. All of the biopsies were successful and resulted in significantly less postoperative pain and earlier return to normal function than would have been expected with standard thoracotomy. In 1997, Mack and associates surveyed members of the General Thoracic Surgical Club concerning their use of VATS. The survey, with responses from 200 members, showed that the most common indications for

VATS were the diagnosis of the indeterminate pleural effusion (155), diagnosis of the indeterminate pleural mass (138), and lung biopsy for interstitial lung disease (134). The survey also showed that VATS was the preferred approach to these clinical problems. Additionally, review of the literature shows consistently successful use of VATS as a diagnostic tool (Table 18-2).

TECHNIQUE

All VATS procedures are performed under general anesthesia with an endotracheal tube capable of maintaining one-lung ventilation. Fiberoptic bronchoscopy confirms the correct position of the tube in all cases. Monitoring consists of pulse oximetry, electrocardiography, end-tidal CO_2, and pneumatic blood pressure measurement. Video optics consist of a 10-mm, 0-degree Panoview diagnostic telescope, a three-chip camera and camera head, and two medical-grade video monitors (Fig. 18-1). All patients are placed in a lateral decubitus position as for standard thoracotomy with the table flexed in its center to lower the hip and allow free movement of the diagnostic telescope. In addition, a small inflatable bag is placed under the patient's thorax to open the intercostal spaces (Fig. 18-2). With few exceptions, four intercostal incisions are made in a grid iron pattern, with two incisions along the anterior and two along the posterior axillary line, each measuring 2 cm in length (Fig. 18-3). The incisions are generally made through the fifth and eighth intercostal spaces, respectively. The initial pleural incision is always made bluntly, and digital exploration is performed to define adhesions. One 12-mm port is used to allow clear passage of the diagnostic telescope into the thorax (Ethicon Endosurgery, Cincinnati, OH).

The authors (1992a) have found that complications from VATS occur in less than 9% of patients, and persistent air leaks account for the majority of complications. At the time

285

Table 18-1. Common Indications for Diagnostic Video-Assisted Thoracic Surgery

Undiagnosed pleural effusion
Interstitial lung disease
Indeterminate lung nodule
Mediastinal staging and biopsy
Evaluation of pericardial disease
Trauma

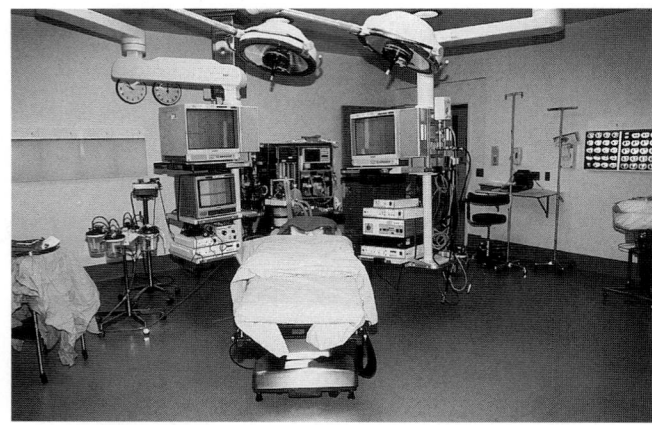

Fig. 18-1. Operating room setup for video-assisted thoracic surgery.

of the 1992 study, the use of VATS was believed to be contraindicated in patients with low oxygen saturations or when the pleural space was completely obliterated because of dense adhesions. However, further experience has shown that most patients, even those with extremely low oxygen saturations, tolerate one-lung ventilation and VATS remarkably well. Also, successful results can be achieved using VATS in patients with dense pleural adhesions.

UNDIAGNOSED PLEURAL EFFUSION

Pleural disease provided the first indication for thoracoscopy and remains today a common indication for VATS. Pleural effusions are common and clinically significant problems that often remain undiagnosed even after a thoracentesis and a closed pleural biopsy are performed. Boutin and

associates (1990) reported a series of 1000 pleural effusions of which more than one-fifth (215) remained undiagnosed after thoracentesis and needle biopsy of the pleura. For such patients, VATS has been a valuable tool for diagnosis with a high degree of accuracy. Yim and associates (1996) reported their experience with 46 patients with an indeterminate pleural effusion despite thoracentesis with or without blind pleural biopsy. All these patients underwent VATS exploration with biopsy with a diagnostic yield of 100%. Twenty-

Table 18-2. Summary of Studies Using Video-Assisted Thoracic Surgery as a Diagnostic Tool

Study	Asamura et al.	Bensard et al.	Lewis et al.	Lewis et al.	Liu et al.	Mack et al.	Yim et al.
Date	1997	1993	1992	1992	1997	1993	1996
Number of patients	135	22	11	113	50	242	69
Mean age/range	N/A	46 + 4 yrs	Range, 21–77 yrs	61 yrs (range, 17–85 yrs)	36.7 + 14.3 yrs (range, 17–71 yrs)	69 yrs (range, 21–87 yrs)	Range, 38–76 yrs
Mortality (%)	0.0	0.0	0.0	0.0	0.0	0.0	0.0
Morbidity (%)	0.0	9.1	9.1	8.8	0.0	3.6	0.0
Indications for video-assisted thoracic surgery	Nodules of unknown histology; exploration for final pretreatment staging; pleural effusion; pleural dissemination; nodal sampling	Pathologic diagnosis for interstitial lung disease	Diffuse interstitial pulmonary infiltrates; massive bullous disease; suspected metastatic breast carcinoma	Metastatic lung nodule; benign lung nodule; pleural effusion; diffuse lung disease; primary pulmonary malignancy; pericardial effusion; mediastinal mass	Penetrating injury; inadequate drainage of hemothorax; hemothorax with active bleeding; posthemothorax chylothorax; posthemothorax empyema	Indeterminate solitary pulmonary nodule	Management of indeterminate pleural effusions
Diagnostic accuracy (%)	100	100	100	100	100	100	91.3

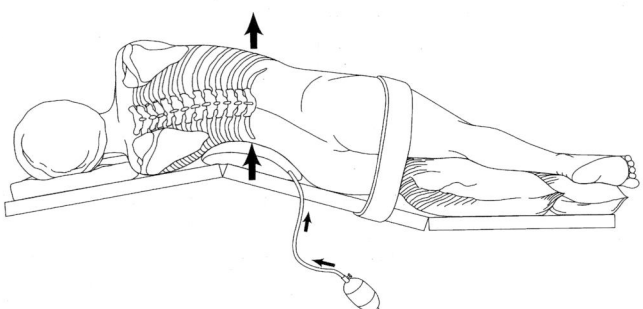

Fig. 18-2. Table flexed and bag inflated to lower hip and widen rib interspaces.

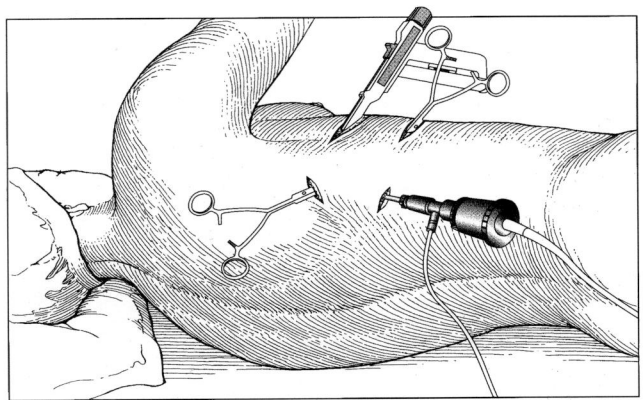

Fig. 18-3. Four incisions for improved access and visualization.

five of 46 patients were found to have a malignancy. The authors currently use VATS to provide a diagnosis in those patients with an undiagnosed pleural effusion after a nondiagnostic thoracentesis. Another group of patients who can benefit from VATS are those who have malignant cells in their pleural fluid but in whom a definitive diagnosis cannot be made between a poorly differentiated adenocarcinoma and a mesothelioma (Fig. 18-4; see Color Fig. 18-4).

Procedure

The aforementioned standard VATS technique is used to perform a pleural biopsy. The diagnostic telescope is brought into the thorax through the lower anterior port and a survey of the entire thorax is performed. Adhesions are

lysed, residual pleural fluid drained, and loculations are lysed. A portion of pleura is selected for biopsy based on its appearance. The pleura is incised and elevated with blunt dissection and cut with a scissors (Fig. 18-5; see Color Fig. 18-5). A frozen section is obtained and other areas are biopsied as needed. If indicated, pleurodesis can be accomplished by completing the parietal pleurectomy and insufflating talc into the pleural space.

Results

We reviewed the records of all our patients who underwent VATS over a 3-year period of January 1994 through

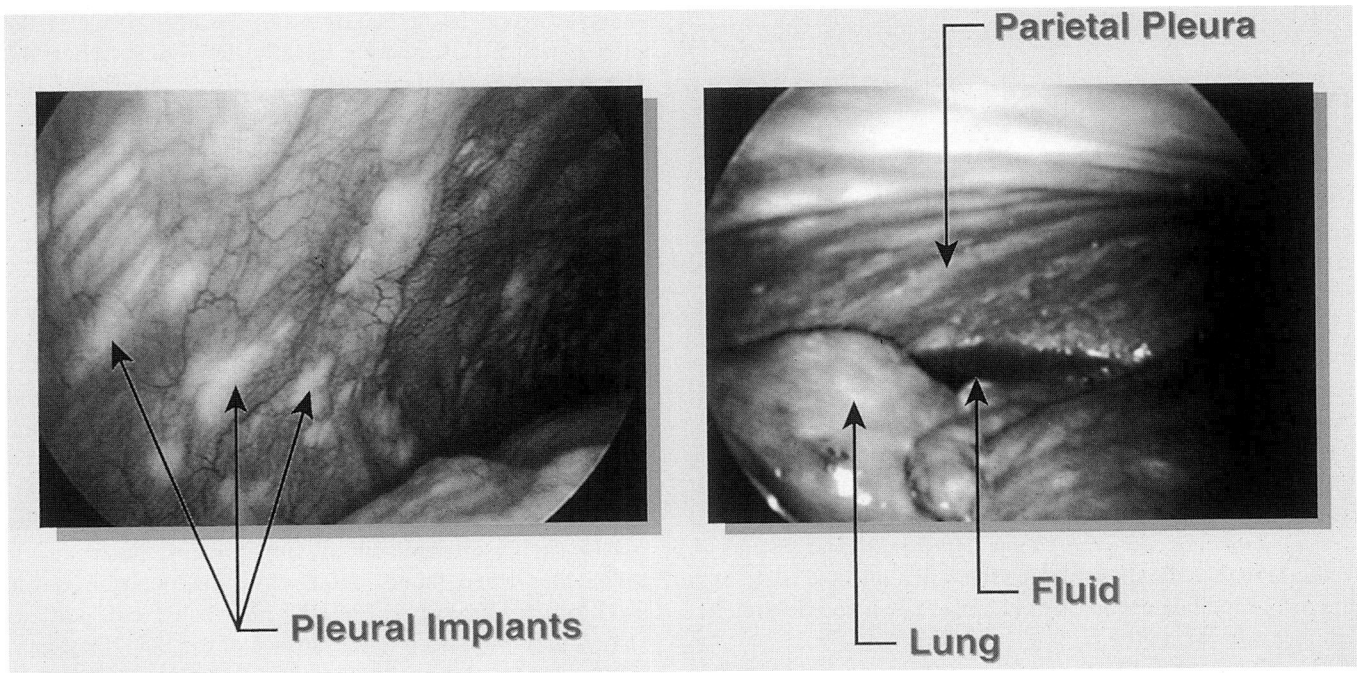

Fig. 18-4. Malignant pleural disease. (See Color Fig. 18-4.)

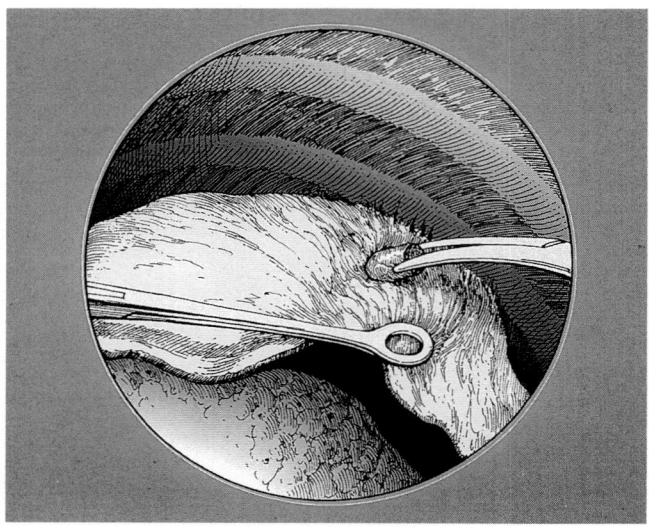

Fig. 18-5. Elevating pleura from chest wall. (See Color Fig. 18-5.)

December 1997. All information was prospectively gathered and entered into a database. One hundred eleven VATS pleural biopsies were performed on patients with an undiagnosed pleural effusion. The average age was 62 years (range, 19 to 86 years) with an average operative time of 35 minutes (range, 20 to 110 minutes). All procedures were diagnostic; 85 patients had a malignant diagnosis and 26 patients had a benign diagnosis. During the same operative procedure, all patients underwent pleurodesis with pleurectomy, talc poudrage, or both. Length of stay in the hospital was 3.2 days (range, 0 to 18 days). There were six postoperative complications, including one arrhythmia and five air leaks, which all resolved spontaneously.

INDETERMINATE LUNG NODULE

Considerable interest is generated by the solitary, circumscribed pulmonary nodule because many of these lesions are primary carcinomas. Lillington (1991) found 40% of the resected nodules were malignant, and the majority were primary malignancies. Although over 85% of patients with lung cancer die from their disease, current opinion maintains that survival rates can be improved if the carcinoma is removed when its size is less than 2 cm, making early diagnosis critically important to survival. History, physical examination, radiographic characteristics of the nodule, and old radiographs are important in determining proper management. A report by Trunk and associates (1974) found that nonsmokers under 35 years of age with a pulmonary nodule had less than a 1% chance of having a malignancy, whereas the risk of malignancy in older patients with a nodule over 3 cm is greater than 90%.

Diagnostic procedures such as bronchoscopy and sputum cytology are usually of little value in the investigation of a solitary lung nodule and are particularly ineffective at establishing a benign diagnosis. The diagnostic yield of flexible bronchoscopy varied between 20% and 80% in reports by Wallace and Deutsch (1982) and Cortese and McDougall (1979). It established specific benign diagnoses in only 10% of patients. Transthoracic fine-needle aspiration (FNA) has a reported sensitivity of 77 to 95% for diagnosing carcinoma in the experience of Westcott and colleagues (1981); however, a specific benign diagnosis was made in only 14% of cases as reported by Shulkin (1993). Failure to diagnose a malignancy with FNA does not exclude a neoplasm. Sampling errors, necrotic tissue, and missed lesions can account for a false-negative diagnosis when malignancy is present in up to 25% of FNAs. Therefore, a negative FNA result is of little help in the management of patients with pulmonary nodules.

VATS has become a popular procedure for resecting pulmonary nodules. It has an extremely high sensitivity and specificity as well as a low morbidity. Using VATS wedge resection for 242 patients with indeterminate lung nodules, Mack and associates (1993) established a definitive diagnosis in all patients. Benign lesions were found in 127 patients (52%) and a malignancy in 113 patients (48%). The mean hospital length of stay was 2.4 days and a 3.6% complication rate was reported.

Procedure

The standard VATS technique is used to resect pulmonary nodules, regardless of where the lesion is located. The upper anterior incision can be made longer, depending on the size of the nodule to be removed. The specimen is removed from the thorax from this location, because the interspaces in this area are usually the widest. Often the lesion is either visible or easily palpable by inserting a finger in the upper anterior intercostal incision (Fig. 18-6; see Color Fig. 18-6). Simultaneously, a soft sponge on a ring forceps is passed through one of the posterior incisions and used to push the lung into the palpating finger. To palpate the entire lung thoroughly, all adhesions must be lysed, and the inferior pulmonary ligament is divided to allow maximum mobility of the lung. Although palpation of the lung can be performed through any of the four ports depending on the location of the nodule, the upper anterior port works best in the majority of cases. Every effort is made to avoid grasping the lung with a clamp when trying to locate a small lesion, because crushing the nodule makes it extremely difficult to locate it and remove it completely. Therefore, most lung manipulation is performed with the use of small soft sponges on ring forceps. Early in our VATS experience, the technique of needle localization was used to help locate small lesions less than 1 cm, particularly if they were deep to the surface of the lung. However, using the palpation technique as described, this procedure is no longer necessary in the majority of cases, thus avoid-

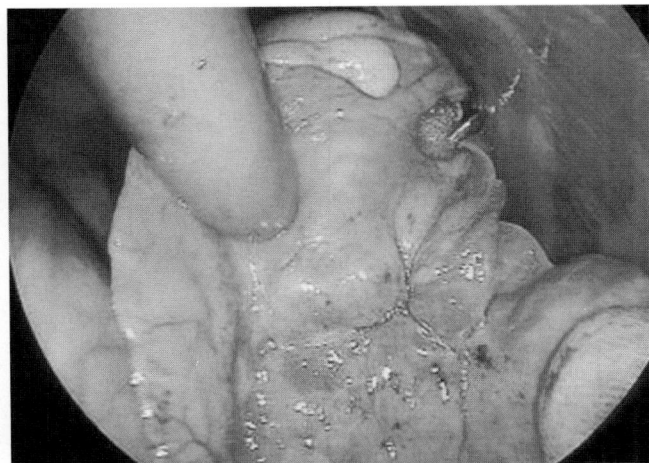

Fig. 18-6. Finger palpation of lung nodule. (See Color Fig. 18-6.)

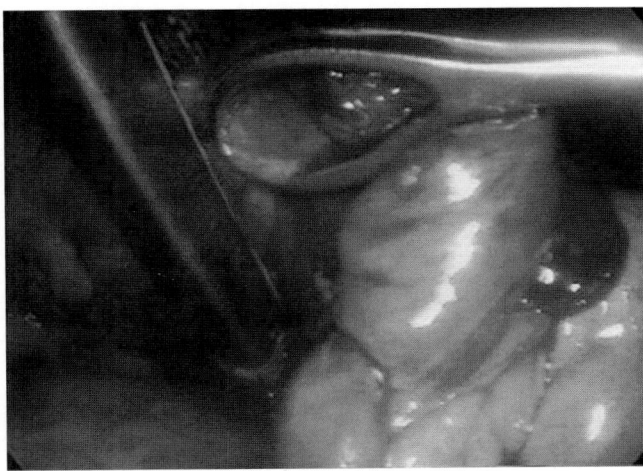

Fig. 18-8. Nodule within ring forceps with linear stapler in position. (See Color Fig. 18-8.)

ing needless cost, time, and discomfort to the patient. When the nodule is identified, depending on its size and location, it is either grasped gently within the rings of the forceps or, for larger lesions, a curved, atraumatic clamp is applied directly below the lesion (Figs. 18-7 and 18-8; see Color Fig. 18-8). In either case minimal manipulation and handling of the lesion occur, and complete removal is assured. By placing the ring forceps or curved clamp in the manner described, stapling the tissue below the lesion is easily accomplished using an endoscopic stapler (Endopath Thoracic ELC-Endoscopic Linear Cutter, Ethicon Endosurgery, Cincinnati, OH). By using all of the intercostal incisions, the proper angle and position of the stapler are more accurately attained. We believe that these types of strategic maneuvers have resulted in a marked reduction in air leaks even after the most complex wedge

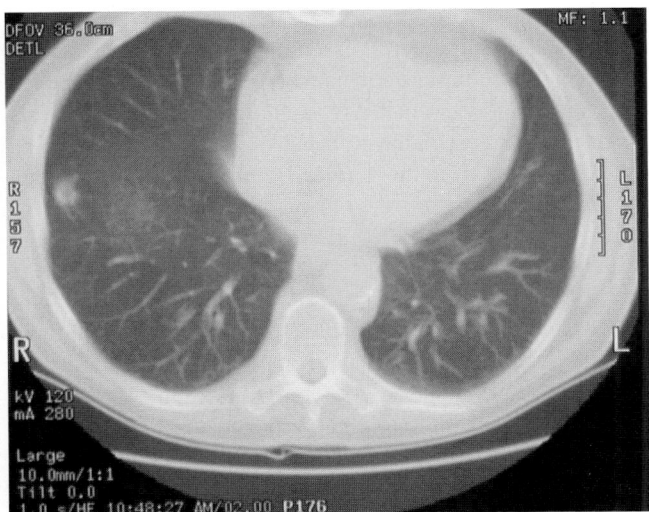

Fig. 18-7. Small lung nodule at right lung base.

resections. A 1-cm margin is always maintained around the lesion. Once the nodule is successfully resected, it is placed in a sterile rubber glove and removed from the thorax. A frozen section is performed to determine if further resection is necessary.

Results

Review of all our VATS cases over the previously mentioned 3-year period revealed 142 VATS wedge resections for indeterminate lung nodule. The procedure was diagnostic in all patients with 88 (62%) malignant and 54 (38%) benign. Of the malignant lesions, 51 were primary and 37 metastatic carcinomas. The average hospital stay was 1.7 days (range, 0 to 10 days). There was no hospital mortality and minimal minor morbidity (6.3%). Prolonged air leak was the most common complication and occurred in seven patients; however, the air leak resolved spontaneously in each patient without further treatment. Four of these patients had significant emphysema.

INTERSTITIAL LUNG DISEASE

Diffuse infiltrative diseases of the lung remain a diagnostic challenge, because they comprise a large and diverse group of diseases that produce a similar radiographic appearance. Over 100 different pathologic entities remain in the differential diagnosis of interstitial lung disease, which makes it difficult to identify the treatable causes. Tissue samples are usually needed to diagnose basic connective tissue problems and to rule out an infectious or neoplastic cause. A review of 502 patients with diffuse infiltrative lung disease by Gaensler and Carrington (1980) noted that an open lung biopsy was required in up to one-third of the patients to establish a diagnosis. In the past, because of a reluctance to subject these patients to the morbidity of open thoracotomy, biopsies were often not performed until late in the course of the disease. Less invasive procedures such as bronchoscopy with bronchoalveolar lavage, transbronchial biopsy, and transthoracic needle biopsy have been used in an attempt to avoid open lung biopsy, but have a low diagnostic yield. Burt and associates (1981) found a diagnostic yield of 59% for transbronchial biopsy and 94% for open lung biopsy when 20 patients underwent both procedures. VATS now offers a minimally invasive method for obtaining adequate lung tissue for diagnosis without the trauma of a limited thoracotomy. Numerous published reports comparing VATS lung biopsy to open lung biopsy have found comparable diagnostic accuracy and operating times. However, VATS had better results for morbidity, mortality, and length of hospital stay. The results published by Bensard and associates (1993) of a retrospective review of 43 patients who underwent diagnostic lung biopsy clearly favored the VATS approach. Twenty-one patients underwent open lung biopsy whereas 22 underwent a VATS lung biopsy. The diagnostic accuracy was equivalent, but the complication rate was higher (4 of 21 versus 2 of 22), the duration of chest tube drainage was longer (3.2 days versus 1.4 days), and the length of hospital stay was longer (5.7 days versus 2.6 days) in the open lung group. VATS has a number of advantages over open lung biopsy, including the absence of muscle and rib injury, vastly improved visualization of the entire thoracic cavity, and access to any part of the lung for biopsy. It should be noted, however, that patients who are dependent on ventilators are not good candidates for VATS lung biopsy, because it is often difficult or impossible to maintain one-lung ventilation during the procedure. The benefits of the VATS approach—for example, shortened hospital stay—are less important in this group of patients.

Procedure

Again, the standard VATS approach is used for a lung biopsy with the diagnostic telescope entering the thorax through the lower anterior incision. Using the preoperative radiograph as a guide, three sites are selected for biopsy, and these areas are directly inspected and palpated. If possible, one specimen is obtained from an area of lung that appears normal; a second specimen is taken from a transitional area; and the third from a heavily diseased region. Wedge resections are taken using the endoscopic linear stapler (Endopath Thoracic ELC-Endoscopic Linear Cutter, Ethicon Endosurgery, Cincinnati, OH), with care taken to orient the stapler appropriately through one of the four intercostal incisions. In this manner, the length of the staple line is minimized and minimal trauma occurs from twisting, turning, and pulling the lung tissue. In cases in which the lung tissue is friable and inflamed, this procedure helps to prevent parenchymal tears and air leaks.

Results

Over a 3-year period, 61 patients with interstitial lung disease underwent a VATS lung biopsy. The population included 30 men and 31 women with an average age of 57 years. Average operating time was 38 minutes. All procedures resulted in a definitive diagnosis. There was no surgical mortality, and only two patients had complications, which consisted of prolonged air leaks. The average length of the hospital stay was 1.5 days.

VATS is clearly changing the approach to patients with interstitial lung disease by providing a less invasive technique that achieves earlier tissue diagnosis. The increased use of VATS to perform a lung biopsy should lead to earlier and more specific treatment that may improve the patient's long-term outcome.

MEDIASTINAL STAGING AND BIOPSY OF LUNG CANCER

VATS is an excellent modality for staging patients with lung cancer. It offers an unmatched ability to visualize and biopsy every lymph node station in the ipsilateral thorax, which includes those unapproachable by traditional mediastinoscopy. Additional benefits of VATS exploration, when assessing resectability, include the opportunity to examine the tumor to rule out direct mediastinal invasion, the ability to find unsuspected pleural implants of tumor, and the discovery of small pleural effusions that may harbor malignant cells. Asamura and associates (1997) reported a series of 116 patients with documented lung cancer who underwent VATS staging. Findings confirming unresectability were identified in seven patients (6%). These included N_2 nodal metastasis in two patients, malignant pleural effusion in three patients, and pleural dissemination in two patients.

The majority of our patients who had proved or suspected lung cancer underwent VATS exploration for staging and assessment of resectability, because far more information can be obtained from this minimally invasive technique than from other staging procedures such as mediastinoscopy or parasternal mediastinotomy. If the VATS result is negative, a definitive procedure can be performed immediately, or, if metastatic disease is encountered, a number of therapeutic options are available, such as pleurectomy and talc poudrage if a malignant pleural effusion or pleural dissemination is found. Presently, mediastinoscopy is used only for patients whose computed tomographic scans show enlarged lymph nodes or those likely to require a pneumonectomy. These same principles of lymph node biopsy and assessment of tumor spread and dissemination also can be applied to carcinoma of the esophagus.

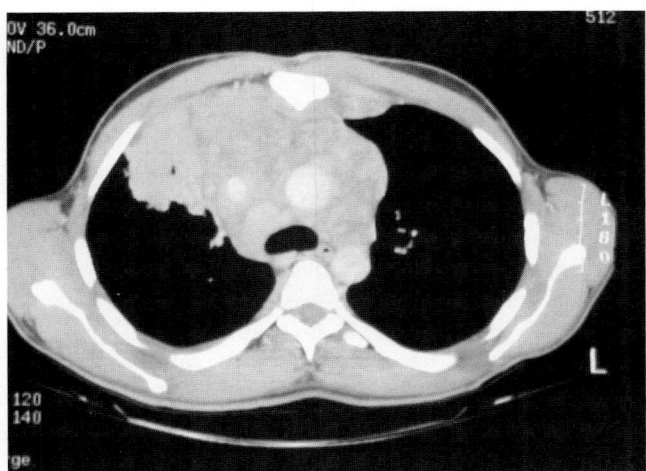

Fig. 18-9. Undiagnosed mediastinal mass.

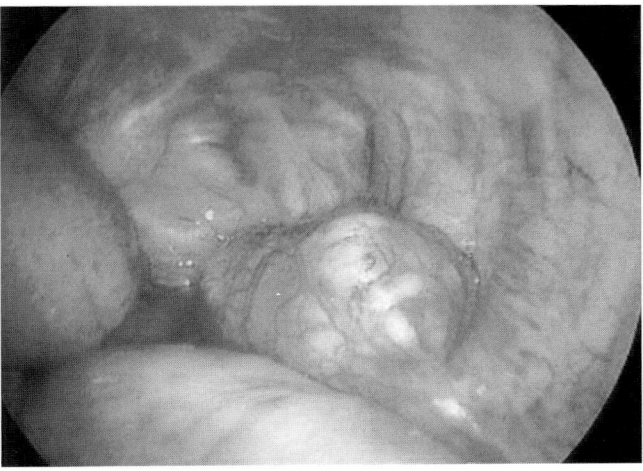

Fig. 18-10. Appearance of mediastinal mass as seen from right thorax. (See Color Fig. 18-10.)

VATS provides excellent exposure to all compartments of the mediastinum for evaluation of primary masses (Fig. 18-9). Lesions in all locations are readily accessible for biopsy or complete excision (Figs. 18-10 and 18-11; see Color Figs. 18-10 and 18-11). VATS is particularly useful in cases of suspected lymphoma in which large pieces of tissue are necessary for the pathologist to render an accurate diagnosis.

Procedure

The mediastinum is examined using the standard four-incision VATS technique. When evaluating mediastinal lymph nodes for the presence of metastasis caused by primary lung cancer, the mediastinal pleura is opened circumferentially around the hilum using a right-angled clamp and scissors. Blunt dissection with a peanut sponge is used to sweep the soft tissue from the hilar and mediastinal lymph nodes. A sample can be taken with a biopsy forceps or the entire node can be excised. Any bleeding from the vascular pedicle can be controlled using endoscopic clips, electrocautery, or the harmonic scalpel (Ethicon Endosurgery, Cincinnati, OH). When the inferior pulmonary ligament is divided, lymph nodes within the ligament and at the base of the inferior pulmonary vein are exposed and can be easily biopsied or excised. The dissection is continued cephalad along the esophagus, exposing nodes at American Thoracic Society level 8. Subcarinal lymph nodes are readily identified from either side by dissection under the main stem bronchus. Paratracheal nodes can be identified by dividing the mediastinal pleura over the trachea and bluntly dissecting in the plane between the trachea and the superior vena cava. The aortopulmonary window nodes can be exposed easily by identifying the area where the phrenic and vagus nerves cross the aortic arch. In addition to mediastinal lymph node sampling, the entire hemithorax is carefully surveyed to determine if evidence exists of metastatic spread of disease or direct spread of the tumor into adjacent structures.

A similar technique is used to expose and biopsy a mediastinal mass of unknown etiology. The majority of these cases, in our experience, are suspected lymphomas in which case a generous amount of tissue is necessary to accurately confirm the diagnosis. VATS provides clear visualization of the mass and the important local structures, which helps avoid inadvertent injury. After identification of the mass, the mediastinal pleura, if present, is opened. Specimens are then obtained either with a biopsy forceps, scalpel, or electrocautery. The lung and pleural surface are examined carefully for any unsuspected abnormalities. At the conclusion of the procedure, a small tube is placed in the thorax; it is often

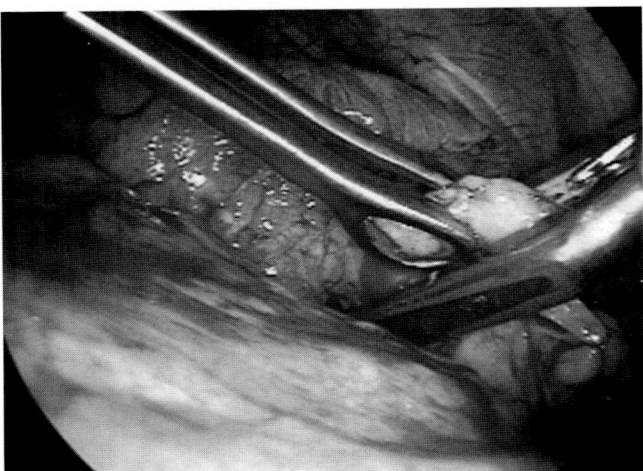

Fig. 18-11. Biopsy being performed using linear stapler for hemostasis (pathology: nodular sclerosing Hodgkin's lymphoma). (See Color Fig. 18-11.)

removed in the recovery room. Many patients are ready for discharge later that day.

Results

All patients with a proved or suspected carcinoma of the lung undergo VATS exploration and mediastinal lymph node sampling. Those found to have metastatic N_2 disease do not have resections performed and are referred to the medical oncologist for appropriate treatment. In some patients, parietal pleurectomy and talc insufflation are done to prevent intractable malignant effusions. Those with N_2 lymph nodes that have negative results proceed to surgical resection. In a group of 231 patients who underwent VATS exploration for a proven or suspected carcinoma of the lung, N_2 lymph nodes that had positive results were identified in 18 patients. For 32 patients who underwent mediastinal exploration for an undiagnosed mass, a diagnosis was made for each patient, with the most common findings being lymphoma, metastatic carcinoma, or benign lymph nodes. The average operating time was 60 minutes, with an average length of stay of 2.1 days. There was no morbidity or mortality.

PERICARDIAL DISEASE

Effusive pericardial disease remains a common and challenging problem. Pericardial resection has been effective as a diagnostic and therapeutic procedure. Subxiphoid pericardial resection remains the most appropriate approach for patients who have a malignant pericardial effusion with an advanced malignancy and a short expected survival. However, VATS has certain advantages over other methods for pericardial drainage. It can be approached from either thorax, provides excellent visibility of a broad area of pericardium, and allows for a more extensive pericardial resection. Coexisting pathology of the lung and pleura can be evaluated simultaneously, thereby increasing the diagnostic yield of the procedure. VATS pericardial resection is minimally invasive, well tolerated, and associated with a low recurrence rate.

Procedure

The standard four-incision VATS technique is used for pericardial resection. The pericardium is approached from either side, depending on associated pathology, otherwise the right side is preferred. After inserting the 0-degree diagnostic telescope, the pericardium is identified and a site anterior to the phrenic nerve is selected for pericardial resection. The pericardium is grasped with a clamp and incised with a scissors. At times, the pericardium can be

distended and extremely difficult to grasp because of the effusion. Under these circumstances, it is helpful to aspirate the pericardial sac to reduce the tension on the pericardium, which makes it easier and safer to open the pericardial sac. After the pericardium is opened and the fluid drained and collected, the interior of the pericardial sac is examined carefully. A generous portion of pericardium is removed using scissors or a harmonic scalpel. Both pericardium and pericardial fluid are sent for pathologic and microbiological assessment. If no other abnormalities are identified, a small chest tube is inserted. The tube is removed when the drainage subsides, usually within 24 to 48 hours after surgery.

Results

Over 3 years, 17 VATS procedures were performed for undiagnosed pericardial disease. There were 15 pericardial resections for effusive disease and two pericardial cysts were excised. All procedures were well tolerated and resulted in a diagnosis in all patients.

EVALUATION OF TRAUMA

VATS has been used as a diagnostic tool in patients suffering traumatic injuries to the thorax and upper abdomen. Liu and associates (1997) reported a series of 50 patients with chest trauma over an 18-month period who underwent exploratory VATS. Penetrating injury (38%), inadequate drainage of hemothorax (36%), and control of bleeding (22%) were the most common indications for VATS exploration. Among the 19 patients with penetrating injuries, four were found to have pulmonary lacerations, 13 had pleural tears, and two had diaphragmatic tears. Of 31 patients with blunt trauma who underwent VATS, 19 were found to have an unresolved blood clot, five had active bleeding from intercostal vessels, four had diaphragmatic tears, and one each had an inferior pulmonary ligament tear, traumatic chylothorax, and post-traumatic empyema. Overall, VATS was successful in all 50 patients, and no morbidity or mortality occurred.

REFERENCES

Asamura H, et al: Thoracoscopic evaluation of histologically/cytologically proven or suspected lung cancer: a VATS exploration. Lung Cancer 16:183, 1997.

Bensard DD, et al: Comparison of video thoracoscopic lung biopsy to open lung biopsy in the diagnosis of interstitial lung disease. Chest 103:765, 1993.

Boutin V, Astroul P, Seitz B: The role of thoracoscopy in the evaluation and management of pleural effusions. Lung 168:1113, 1990.

Burt ME, et al: Prospective evaluation of aspiration needle, cutting needle, transbronchial and open lung biopsy in patients with pulmonary infiltrates. Ann Thorac Surg 32:146, 1981.

Cortese DA, McDougall JC: Biopsy and brushing of peripheral lung cancer with fluoroscopic guidance. Chest 75:141, 1979.

Gaensler EA, Carrington CB: Open biopsy for chronic diffuse infiltrative lung disease: clinical, roentgenographic and physiological correlations in 502 patients. Ann Thorac Surg 30:411, 1980.

Lewis RJ, Caccavale RJ, Sisler GE: Special report: video-endoscopic thoracic surgery. N J Med 88:473, 1991.

Lewis RJ, et al: One hundred consecutive patients undergoing video-assisted thoracic operations. Ann Thorac Surg 54:421, 1992.

Lewis RJ, Caccavale RJ, Sisler GE: Imaged thoracoscopic lung biopsy. Chest 102:60, 1992.

Lillington GA, et al: Management of solitary pulmonary nodules. Dis Mon 37:271, 1991.

Liu DW, et al: Video-assisted thoracic surgery in treatment of chest trauma. J Trauma 42:670, 1997.

Mack MJ, et al: Video-assisted thoracic surgery: has technology found its place? Ann Thorac Surg 64:211, 1997.

Mack MJ, et al: Thoracoscopy for the diagnosis of the indeterminate solitary pulmonary nodule. Ann Thorac Surg 56:825, 1993.

Shulkin AN: Management of the indeterminate solitary pulmonary nodule: a pulmonologist's view. Ann Thorac Surg 56:743, 1993.

Trunk G, et al: The management and evaluation of the solitary pulmonary nodule. Chest 66:236,1974.

Wallace JM, Deutsch AL: Flexible fiberoptic bronchoscopy and percutaneous needle lung aspiration for evaluating the solitary pulmonary nodule. Chest 81:685, 1982.

Westcott JL, et al: Direct percutaneous needle aspiration of localized pulmonary lesions. Radiology 137:31, 1980.

Yim APC, et al: Thoracoscopic management of malignant pleural effusions. Chest 109:1234, 1996.

SECTION V

Assessment of the Thoracic Surgical Patient

CHAPTER 19

Pulmonary Physiologic Assessment of Operative Risk

Gerald N. Olsen

Surgical procedures inherently carry risks and benefits. Identification and amelioration of the risks preoperatively enhance postoperative outcome. In the arena of preoperative evaluation and its scientific literature, the definition of the term *complication* is important. A *complication* is an unplanned and unwanted second disease. This definition is crucial, because the studies that purport to evaluate for and treat postoperative complications often report such items as mild hypoxemia, asymptomatic decrement in lung function, radiographic discoid atelectasis, or transient arrhythmias. If the complication does not lengthen recovery room, intensive care unit, or hospital stay or increase care costs or mortality, describing an outcome as a true complication is not warranted. Generally accepted postoperative complications are listed in Table 19-1. Postoperative bronchitis that leads to lobar atelectasis, pneumonia, sepsis, respiratory failure, ventricular tachycardia, and death constitutes a progression of abnormalities that fits the criteria of complications because it lengthens the hospital stay, increases hospital costs, and causes mortality. Factors identifying patients at increased risk are outlined in Table 19-2.

Cardiopulmonary complications can occur after any surgical procedure but are particularly common after major operations on the upper abdomen and thorax. This is not to say that procedures such as craniotomy, thyroidectomy, and hip replacement are free of these complications, but they tend to be somewhat less frequent and are difficult to predict by preoperative assessment. In hip surgery, preoperative and postoperative anticoagulation may obviate the problem of pulmonary thromboembolism. Likewise, close postoperative observation may detect abnormalities that may progress to overt complications.

UPPER ABDOMINAL SURGERY

Much investigative work involving the upper abdomen has occurred since the rediscovery of the seminal studies of Pasteur (1908). Pasteur postulated that postoperative pulmonary collapse was related to diaphragmatic dysfunction. The observations of Ford and coworkers (1983) have tended to support this concept. The postoperative diaphragmatic dysfunction is primarily manifest in 50 to 60% reductions in vital capacity that last from a few hours to 5 days (Fig. 19-1). The etiology of this dysfunction remains unclear; although incisional pain is a factor, some data suggest that it is not related entirely to pain or muscle fatigue and may be overcome by voluntary efforts of the patient. These findings have led to the hypothesis of a pathologic reflex. This phenomenon has also been seen in animals whose upper abdominal viscera have been operatively manipulated. The ability of the patient to overcome the reduced vital capacity with voluntary deep breaths has been demonstrated by Chuter and colleagues (1990). Voluntary deep breaths appear to support the use of incentive spirometry as first proposed by Bartlett and associates (1973). However, a major study by Hall and colleagues (1991) showed no reduction in hospital stay or mortality associated with the routine use of postoperative incentive spirometry. Because this therapeutic modality is used in many hospitals in the United States, it may now be as firmly entrenched in postoperative therapy as was intermittent positive pressure breathing in the 1950s.

Evidence exists that the symptomatic and physiologic effects of upper abdominal surgery (e.g., cholecystectomy) are lessened significantly by the use of the laparoscopic technique. This development that has reduced postoperative recovery time may also reduce the need for extensive postoperative support. Laparoscopic upper abdominal surgery in a patient with chronic obstructive pulmonary disease (COPD) has not been studied extensively.

Based on the meta-analyses of Lawrence and colleagues (1990) and Zibrak and coworkers (1990), preoperative pulmonary function testing with spirometry remains unproven as a reliable predictor of increased postoperative pul-

297

Table 19-1. Postoperative Cardiopulmonary Complications

Atelectasis requiring specific therapy
Arrhythmias requiring therapy
Bronchitis
Death
Hypotension/shock
Myocardial infarction
Pneumonia
Pulmonary edema
Pulmonary embolism
Respiratory failure

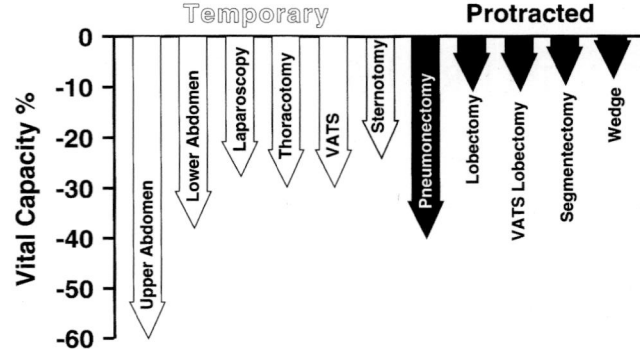

Fig. 19-1. Effect of surgical procedures on vital capacity. VATS, video-assisted thoracoscopic surgery.

monary risk for upper abdominal surgery. However, these investigators supported the use of these tests before lung resectional surgery.

LUNG RESECTIONAL SURGERY

Thoracotomy was originally performed for drainage of empyema. The 1940s and early 1950s are viewed by some as the halcyon days of general thoracic surgery. During this time, procedures such as plombage, thoracoplasty, and segmentectomy were developed for the management of pulmonary tuberculosis. Although the development of isoniazid led to a reduction in surgical indications, resection is still an option for management of some drug-resistant forms of *Mycobacterium tuberculosis* as well as that due to drug-resistant *Mycobacterium avium-intracellulare* (see Chapter 85).

Much of the experience in dealing with the pulmonary function effects of surgery date to the benchmark study of Gaensler and associates (1955). Current indications for thoracotomy for pulmonary resection include lung cancer, diagnostic lung biopsy, lung volume reduction surgery (LVRS), lung transplantation, and thoracotomy for the management of thoracic trauma.

Approximately 10 years after the post–World War II rise in cigarette consumption came the current epidemic of bronchogenic carcinoma. Graham and Singer published the first report of a successful pneumonectomy for lung cancer in 1933. Subsequently, lobectomy became the more com-

mon procedure and virtually the only hope for cure for those 25% of patients who presented without obvious metastases. Complicating the surgical approach to lung cancer was the rise in cases of COPD that occurred approximately 10 years after the rise in lung cancer (Fig. 19-2). Of those patients who present with bronchogenic carcinoma, approximately 90% have signs and symptoms of concomitant COPD. Approximately 20% of these patients have such severe pulmonary dysfunction as to potentially compromise the safety of the resection. Complicating this fact is the knowledge that nonoperative therapy of lung cancer is not often curative.

Lung resection in patients with lung cancer may be curative in 10 to 90% of cases, depending on the stage of the disease. The wide difference in the ends of this spectral range are related to the presence or absence of local or distant metastases. The preoperative search for the metastases constitutes the process known as *staging*. A complete discussion of this process can be found in Chapter 98. For the purposes of this discussion, the inability to remove (anatomically) all the tumor from the patient is called *unresectability*.

If a lung cancer patient is adequately staged and is presumed to be resectable, can surgery proceed forthwith? When lung tissue is removed from a patient, several physiologic effects occur. First is the thoracotomy effect. Even if no lung is resected, vital capacity declines approximately 25% in the early postoperative period, only normalizing after 4 to 6 weeks. Overall, the degree of pulmonary dysfunction is somewhat correlated with the volume of lung tissue removed (see Fig. 19-1). The use of video-assisted thoracoscopic surgery and muscle-sparing incisions to perform segmentectomy or lobectomy has not consistently resulted in a lessening of postoperative decrements in pulmonary function.

Since the report by Cooper and coworkers (1995), multiple studies have demonstrated significant symptomatic and physiologic improvement in selected patients after LVRS. Combining LVRS and lung cancer resection has been reported by McKenna and associates (1996). This study actually demonstrated improvements in pulmonary function

Table 19-2. Factors Increasing Postoperative Risk

American Society of Anesthesiologists class greater than 2
Advanced age
Complicated cardiac valvular replacement
Coronary artery disease
Chronic obstructive pulmonary disease
Emergency procedure
Extensive lung resection
Immune compromise
Morbid obesity
Prolonged operative duration
Smoking
Transplantation of major organs
Upper abdominal procedure

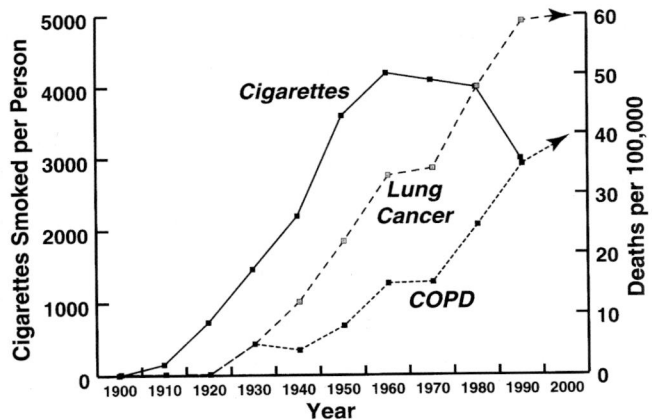

Fig. 19-2. Cigarette consumption, lung cancer, and chronic obstructive pulmonary disease (COPD) mortality.

after combined LVRS and cancer resection. No postoperative deaths occurred in this small study of 11 patients with severe COPD with a mean preoperative forced expired volume in 1 second (FEV_1) of 0.654 L.

When normal lung tissue is removed, two major consequences occur. The first is reduction of the pulmonary capillary bed. This reduction has little consequence in a patient with normal lungs, even after pneumonectomy. If pulmonary dysfunction already exists, however, postoperative pulmonary hypertension may lead to cor pulmonale and death. Although this outcome was a major concern in the early days of surgery for tuberculosis, it seems to be less frequently a problem in lung cancer surgery. The second undesirable effect of lung resection involves the removal or reduction of ventilatory capacity. In a patient with underlying COPD, this further reduction by pneumonectomy can precipitate acute and chronic respiratory failure and death. The inability of the patient to tolerate physiologically the loss of functional lung tissue is called *inoperability* in this discussion.

The mortality rate for pneumonectomy in a patient with normal lungs averages less than 5%. In the past, this figure was as high as 25% in those with severe COPD. Producing a ventilator-dependent respiratory cripple who has had a curative resection of his lung cancer is a disaster for the patient and a nightmare for the surgeon. Hence, a patient with resectable lung cancer but who is potentially inoperable from his COPD constitutes a frequent diagnostic and management conundrum.

Physiologic Assessment of the Lung Resection Candidate

According to the seminal study of Gaensler and coworkers (1955), a severe reduction of ventilatory function preoperatively could be used to predict mortality. If the maximum breathing capacity—now called *maximum voluntary ventilation* (MVV)—was less than 50% of predicted and the

forced vital capacity was less than 70% of predicted for the patient's age, height, and sex, mortality was 50% after pneumonectomy for tuberculosis.

In approaching these patients, a philosophical position is helpful. Each resectable patient should be considered to be a potential pneumonectomy candidate. The reasoning for this position is obvious. If the patient is physiologically acceptable for pneumonectomy, performance of a lesser resection has an even less detrimental effect on lung function. Likewise, if during the exploratory thoracotomy the tumor crosses the major fissure or extends to the hilum and a pneumonectomy is needed, the opportunity for an extensive physiologic evaluation is generally too late. An important question when dealing with a disease as deadly as lung cancer is "In whom is it too dangerous to attempt a curative resection?"

Routine Pulmonary Function Studies

Pulmonary function studies are performed to assess airflow, lung volume, lung mechanics, and gas exchange. Most of these studies require good cooperation and are thus effort-dependent. Because lung resection is primarily performed for lung cancer, underlying severe COPD should be ruled out or quantified. In the distant past, these routine studies were used to reject patients for resection. This rejection, based on routine studies, is no longer tenable, as knowledge about these problems has increased. These routine pulmonary function studies are now primarily used to either approve a patient for resection or indicate that further testing is advisable. Table 19-3 outlines those studies and criteria indicating a need for further evaluation. Many early studies espoused spirometric lung volume criteria, such as FEV_1 more than 2 L, as required for resection. This now appears to be unwise. For example, an FEV_1 of 2 L could be 50% of normal for a 6-ft-tall, 40-year-old man but virtually normal for a 5-ft-tall, 70-year-old woman. Thus, it is preferable to think in terms of percent of predicted normal for the

Table 19-3. Pulmonary Function Criteria for Lung Resection

Spirometry	Operable	Further Study Suggested
Forced vital capacity (FVC)	>60% predicted	<60% predicted
Forced expired volume in 1 second (FEV_1)	>60% predicted	<60% predicted
FEV_1:FVC ratio	>50%	<50%
Maximum voluntary ventilation	>50% predicted	<50% predicted
Gas exchange		
Diffusing capacity for carbon monoxide	>60% predicted	<60% predicted
Arterial carbon dioxide tension	<45 mm Hg	>45 mm Hg

patient's age, height, and sex. Race may also be included, but normal prediction equations are more frequently based on populations of healthy, nonsmoking whites. The MVV is an interesting test as it reflects airflow, lung mechanics, respiratory muscle strength and endurance. However, it is sensitive to suboptimal cooperation and pain and is thus facetiously called the *SED rate of pulmonary function studies*. It is performed by having the patient breathe into and out of the spirometer as deeply and fast as possible for 12 seconds. Some laboratories estimate or calculate this value by taking the FEV_1 in liters and multiplying by 40. A normal measured MVV does, however, tend to suggest good ventilatory function.

The diffusing capacity measures the volume of a dilute sample of carbon monoxide that is taken up by the lungs, generally during a single breath held for 10 seconds. The test evaluates the integrity of the alveolar capillary membrane and the pulmonary capillary blood volume. The single breath-hold test is also sensitive to reduced lung volume. Thus, it can be said that diffusing capacity of the lung for carbon monoxide (DLCO) reveals a decreased surface area available for gas exchange. Ferguson and colleagues (1988) found in a retrospective study of 237 lung resection patients that the preoperative DLCO was the best predictor of postoperative pulmonary complications.

The primary reason why these routine pulmonary function tests should not be used to reject a patient for resection is that these tests only reflect the function of both lungs working together at rest. For example, what if an adult man with lung cancer had an FEV_1 of 1.8 L or MVV of 49% of predicted? Should he be rejected for pneumonectomy? Further testing might reveal that the lung containing the tumor was not functioning owing to airway obstruction by the tumor. The patient has, therefore, already tolerated an autopneumonectomy, and little further functional loss would accompany the therapeutic procedure.

As shown by the classic report of Stein and associates (1962), a preoperative arterial PCO_2 ($PaCO_2$) of more than 45 mm Hg signifies chronic respiratory insufficiency; physiologic inoperability was automatically assumed. This assumption was proved false by the reports of Morice and colleagues (1992) and Kearney and colleagues (1994), who described multiple hypercapnic patients who survived lung resectional surgery.

Split Lung Function Studies

In the 1950s, a technique known as *bronchospirometry* was developed to assess unilateral lung function. In this procedure, a double-lumen endotracheal tube was passed to the tracheal carina. Each lumen was connected to a spirometer filled with 100% O_2. On breathing, the amount of O_2 uptake was a reflection of each lung's perfusion, and the volume of air exchanged during a vital capacity or MVV maneuver was a reflection of each lung's ventilation. Neuhaus and Cherniack (1968), the first to use this technique, developed

the following equation to predict the function remaining after pneumonectomy:

$$
\begin{array}{ccc}
\text{Predicted} & \text{Total} & \text{Percentage of function} \\
\text{postoperative} = \text{preoperative} \times & \text{contributed by lung} \\
\text{function} & \text{function} & \text{destined to remain}
\end{array}
$$

Example:

$$
\begin{array}{l}
\text{Postpneumo-} \\
\text{nectomy } FEV_1
\end{array} = 2\,L \times \begin{array}{l} \text{75\% function from} \\ \text{the non-tumor lung} \end{array} = 1.5\,L
$$

This simple equation achieved importance with the development and perfection of radiospirometry in the 1970s. In these less invasive studies of regional lung function, a nuclear medicine gamma camera and a radionuclide are used. Unilateral ventilation is assessed using inhalation of xenon 133 gas, and perfusion is measured using intravenously administered technetium 99m-labeled albumin macroaggregates. This methodology is available in most hospitals and is used routinely for the diagnosis of pulmonary embolism by detecting perfusion defects and areas of ventilation-perfusion mismatch. The addition of a computer to the gamma camera allows quantification of the radioactive counts emanating from each lung region and thus conversion into percent (Fig. 19-3). Kristersson and colleagues (1972) from Sweden first published their experience using the assessment of unilateral ventilation to calculate postpneumonectomy function. This report was followed by that of my colleagues and me (1974) in which we used measurements of unilateral perfusion. Subsequently, we also showed a good agreement in those patients with COPD and lung cancer between unilateral ventilation and perfusion, thus making measurement of both unnecessary. Mistakenly believing that hypercapnia and chronic respiratory failure are always associated in COPD with an FEV_1 less than 0.8 L, we suggested this value as a lower limit of operability. We modified this position, however, to correct for age, height, and sex by suggesting that the predicted value for postpneumonectomy FEV_1 be compared to the normal value predicted for the patient. If the calculated postpneumonectomy FEV_1—also called the *predicted postoperative* (ppo) FEV_1—was less than 35% of the normal value predicted for the patient, the patient was suggested to be inoperable. A subsequent prospective study of Markos and colleagues (1989) also suggested the less than 35% of normal value as being associated with an unacceptably high risk.

Wernly and associates (1980) extended the radiorespirometric technique to the prediction of postlobectomy pulmonary function. They developed and tested the following equation:

$$
\begin{array}{cccc}
\text{Expected} & \text{Preop-} & \text{\% of function} & \dfrac{\begin{array}{c}\text{Number of} \\ \text{segments of} \\ \text{the lobe to} \\ \text{be resected}\end{array}}{\begin{array}{c}\text{Total number} \\ \text{of segments} \\ \text{of the lung}\end{array}} \\
\text{loss} = \text{erative} \times & \text{of tumor-} \times \\
\text{in } FEV_1 & FEV_1 & \text{containing lung}
\end{array}
$$

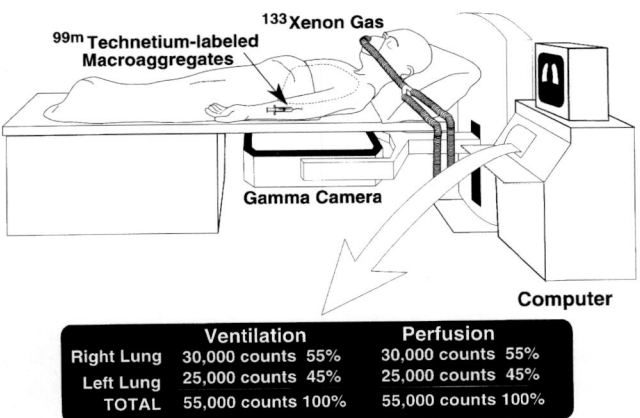

Fig. 19-3. Quantitative lung radiospirometry.

Example:

$$\frac{\text{Post–right upper}}{\text{lobectomy}} \times \frac{\text{Preoperative}}{\text{FEV}_1} = \frac{2.0\ \text{L} - \text{Loss}}{\text{in FEV}_1} =$$

$$2.0\ \text{L} \times \frac{40\% \text{ of perfusion}}{\text{from right lung}} \times \frac{\begin{array}{c}3 \text{ segments in}\\ \text{right upper lobe}\end{array}}{\begin{array}{c}10 \text{ segments in}\\ \text{entire right lung}\end{array}} = 0.24\ \text{L}$$

Thus, post–right upper lobectomy FEV$_1$ = 2 − 0.24 L = 1.76 L.

Juhl and Frost (1975) reported a technique of estimating postoperative function similar to that of Wernly but that did not require radiospirometry. In this technique, each lung segment is estimated to contribute ¹⁄₁₉—or 0.0526—of total lung function. Thus, one can estimate ppo function using the following equation:

$$\frac{\text{ppo}}{\text{function}} = \frac{\text{Preoperative}}{\text{function}} \times \frac{1 - (0.0526 \times \text{number}}{\text{of segments to be resected})}$$

Example:

$$\begin{array}{l}\text{Right upper}\\ \text{lobectomy} \\ \text{ppo FEV}_1\end{array} = \begin{array}{l}\text{Preopera-}\\ \text{tive FEV}_1 \\ \text{of 2 L}\end{array} \times \begin{array}{l}1 -\\ (0.0526 \times 3 \\ \text{segments})\end{array} = \frac{2 \times}{0.842} = 1.684\ \text{L}^*$$

Questions about the accuracy of lung scan prediction of postoperative lung function were raised by Ladurie and Ranson-Bitker (1986). These investigators reported a very large series of 159 pneumonectomy patients assessed by this technique. Their data showed that approximately 75% of the patients, when studied postoperatively, differed in their measured postoperative FEV$_1$ by 180 to 400 mL from what had been predicted preoperatively. This is an excessive error, especially if 0.8 L was chosen as a cut-off of operability. This report has been supported by the report of Zeiher and associates (1995), who used the segment-counting method of Juhl and Frost. This raises questions and uncertainty

---

*In both equations, nonfunctioning obstructed segments to be resected should be subtracted from both the numerator and denominator.

about the accuracy of the radiorespirometric or segment-counting estimates of ppo function.

The radionuclide lung scan, however, remains a valuable tool to assess what might be termed *regional anatomic physiology*. This technique simply allows the surgeon to assess radiologically the function of the lung to be removed as compared with the other lung regions.

Hemodynamic Studies

As stated, in the 1950s concern arose over the development of pulmonary hypertension and cor pulmonale after lung resection or thoracoplasty for tuberculosis. Carlens and associates (1951) introduced a cardiac catheter that could be passed to the pulmonary artery (PA). This catheter had an inflatable balloon much like that of a Swan-Ganz catheter—but much larger. Inflation of the 50-mL balloon in the main PA occluded it and produced a physiologic pneumonectomy. Measurements of PA pressure proximal to the balloon could be made at rest and on supine exercise to detect the presence of occult pulmonary hypertension. This technique, known as *temporary unilateral pulmonary artery occlusion* (TUPAO) was used effectively in a study by Uggla (1956). In this retrospective study, the author divided the patients into three groups based on postoperative outcome. These groups were identified as *fit for work, cardiorespiratory cripples*, or *dead*. The TUPAO pressure in the PA, along with the systemic arterial O$_2$ tension (PaO$_2$) seem to predict postoperative mortality the best. This procedure is technically demanding and had a failure rate of approximately 25% in a prospective study by our group (1975).

Fee and colleagues (1975) reported their experience using a Swan-Ganz catheter passed to the pulmonary artery before treadmill exercise. The exercise was used to increase cardiac output and thus uncover pulmonary hypertension not obvious at rest. In this report, the calculated pulmonary vascular resistance (PVR) seemed to be most predictive of postoperative death. A PVR of more than 190 dyne-sec-cm^{-5} seemed to be a predictor of postoperative mortality. However, these findings were not supported by a prospective study by our group (1989). We did not find differences in PVR helpful for identifying patients with severe COPD who were intolerant of lung resection as evidenced by death within 30 days or permanent ventilator dependency. These hemodynamic studies are technically challenging to perform and appear to be needed rarely in preoperative assessment.

Exercise Testing

Complications of lung resection may be technical, as in postoperative bronchopleural fistula or hemorrhage, and physiologic, as in cardiorespiratory failure. Few tests have the ability to predict the former, and many have been proposed to predict the latter. A brief report by Eugene and coworkers (1982) began a new area of investigation. Previous studies used exercise added to hemodynamic studies, such as

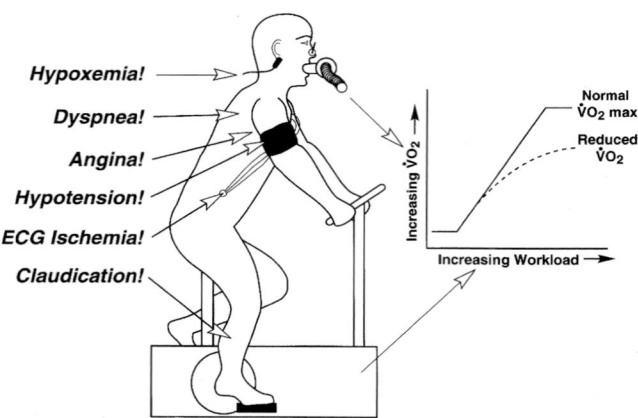

Fig. 19-4. Physiologic assessment by cycle exercise. ECG, electrocardiogram; $\dot{V}O_2$, oxygen consumption.

cardiac catheterization, to uncover pulmonary hypertension or were simply performed to assess the presence of unacceptable dyspnea preoperatively. The results of these previous studies were mixed at best. However, Eugene found that measurement of maximum oxygen consumption ($\dot{V}O_2$max) on incremental cycle ergometer exercise was a strong predictor of postoperative mortality. In this study, 75% of the patients whose preoperative exercise $\dot{V}O_2$max was less than 1 L died after lung resection, and none of those with a $\dot{V}O_2$max more than 1 L died. These patient groups were not significantly different from each other in their ventilatory function. Maximal oxygen consumption is the highest oxygen uptake measured during intense incremental workload exercise. At the point of $\dot{V}O_2$max, a further increase in work will not lead to a further increase in $\dot{V}O_2$, suggesting that the complete oxygen transport chain of lungs-heart-vessels-muscle is stressed to its limit (Fig. 19-4). Those patients with problems in the oxygen delivery system, such as heart or lung disease, do not achieve true plateau of $\dot{V}O_2$max. However, their lesser peak exercise $\dot{V}O_2$ is called *symptom-limited maximum* and is often confusingly abbreviated $\dot{V}O_2$max, just like maximal $\dot{V}O_2$. As exercise workload is increased incrementally, at some point (usually termed the *anaerobic threshold*) lactate production occurs. This lactate release signals greater O_2 utilization by the muscles than that supplied by the cardiopulmonary-vascular transport system.

Multiple studies have been published in follow-up to that of Eugene and colleagues (1982). These studies have, however, used different exercise protocols (e.g., submaximal steady state versus incremental maximal exercise in diverse patient groups). Results, therefore, have been variable. However, the preponderance of studies thus far seems to favor the measured $\dot{V}O_2$ as being a valuable postoperative predictor. For example, the study of Smith and coworkers (1984) found that a true $\dot{V}O_2$max of less than 15 mL/kg/min was predictive not only of death, but also of potentially survivable complications such as cardiac arrhythmias, pneumonia, and atelectasis. This study also found that the exercise

$\dot{V}O_2$ data were superior predictors to the calculation of ppo FEV_1 using the quantitative radionuclide lung scan discussed. Markos and colleagues (1989), however, reported exactly the opposite, noting that the $\dot{V}O_2$ on exercise did not discriminate postoperative outcome as well as the scan prediction. A possible explanation as to why these studies had such divergent results is that the patients were not preselected by any pulmonary function criteria as being at increased risk. The reduced $\dot{V}O_2$ on exercise is perhaps best predictive of postoperative mortality in patients with severe underlying lung disease but may suggest an increased postoperative morbidity when used in healthier patients. This concept seems to be supported by the report of my colleagues and me (1989) and that of Nakagawa and associates (1992). The Nakagawa study is of interest in that these investigators used flow-directed cardiac catheterization and exercised the patients to a blood lactate level of 20 mg/dL. Fatal postoperative complications were best predicted by the calculated oxygen delivery—arterial O_2 content × cardiac output—per meter of body surface area. An O_2 delivery of less than 500 mL/min/m² on exercise was present in all four patients who died postoperatively and in none of the 27 patients who survived. This study used invasive methodology to suggest the predictive value of assessing the oxygen transport system under the stress of submaximal exercise.

Corris and colleagues (1987) found in a small study that an accurate prediction of exercise $\dot{V}O_2$max was possible. Bolliger and associates (1995) confirmed the ability to predict exercise ppo $\dot{V}O_2$max using radiospirometry to determine the fraction of lung function contributed by the lung to be resected and multiplying this value by the preoperative exercise $\dot{V}O_2$max (Fig. 19-5). The equation for this procedure is as follows:

$$ppo\ \dot{V}O_2max = \frac{\text{Preoperative}}{\dot{V}O_2max} \times \frac{1 - \text{fraction of function}}{\text{from lung to be resected}}$$

Example:

$$\text{Preoperative } \dot{V}O_2max = 20 \text{ mL/kg/min}$$

From radiospirometry, the right upper lobe contributes 16% of total function.

$$\begin{array}{l} \text{Post–right} \\ \text{upper lobec-} \\ \text{tomy ppo} \\ \dot{V}O_2max \end{array} = \begin{array}{l} 20 \text{ mL/kg/min} \\ \times (1 - 0.16) \end{array} = 20 \times 0.84 = 16.8 \text{ mL/kg/min}$$

In a study of 25 patients with severely abnormal pulmonary function, those three patients with a ppo $\dot{V}O_2$max less than 10 mL/kg/min all died postoperatively.

A "low-tech" method of exercise testing that is virtually free of invasive or sophisticated technologic requirements has been described. Van Nostrand and coworkers (1968) reported that those patients who were unable to climb two flights of stairs because of unacceptable dyspnea failed to survive pneumonectomy. Stair climbing is a highly stressful exercise generally requiring a higher $\dot{V}O_2$ than cycle ergometry performed

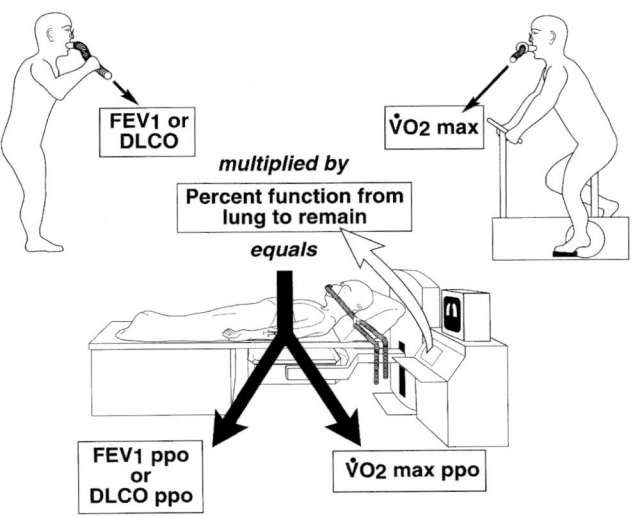

Fig. 19-5. Determination of predicted postoperative function. DLCO, diffusing capacity of the lung for carbon monoxide; FEV_1, forced expired volume in 1 second; ppo, predicted postoperative; $\dot{V}O_2$max, maximum oxygen consumption.

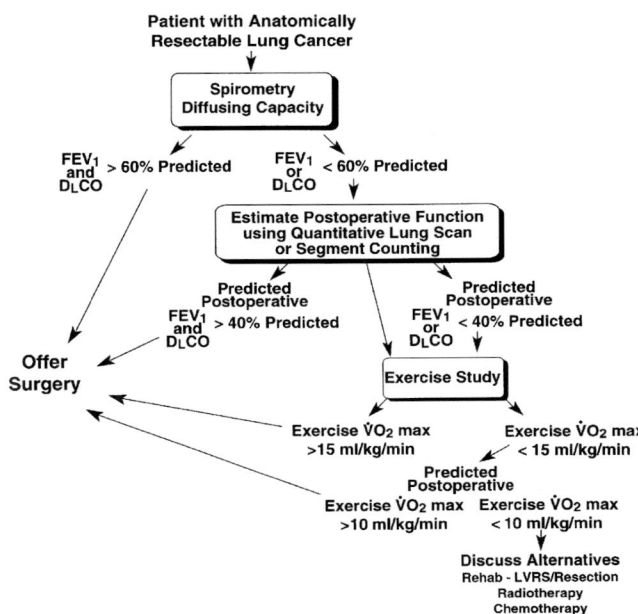

Fig. 19-6. Physiologic assessment algorithm. DLCO, diffusing capacity of the lung for carbon monoxide; FEV_1, forced expired volume in 1 second; LVRS, lung volume reduction surgery; $\dot{V}O_2$max, maximum oxygen consumption.

to the same symptom limit. Bolton and coinvestigators (1987) reported acceptable correlations between steps climbed and routine pulmonary function parameters in elderly male veterans. In a follow-up retrospective report, my colleagues and I (1991) reported that in elderly Veterans Administration patients not preselected by abnormal spirometry, successful climbing of three flights—76 steps—of stairs best separated patients after lung resection as to the length of postoperative intubation and hospital stay and the number of postoperative complications. The study was limited, however, by its retrospective design and the few reported postoperative deaths.

A patient with severe limitations of O_2 transport owing to heart, lung, or vascular disease is not able to climb stairs rapidly. The onset of chest pain, dyspnea, or claudication may signal these underlying problems. Thus, stair climbing may, after further study, prove to be a valuable preoperative screening test.

NONSURGICAL THERAPY

Gauden and associates (1995) reported a 27% 5-year survival rate in elderly patients with stage I non–small cell lesions treated with 50-Gy external beam radiotherapy. This report, coupled with some reports suggesting enhanced survival with chemotherapy, offers the physiologically inoperable patient more attractive options.

SUMMARY

Patients may be evaluated preoperatively in an attempt to predict the occurrence of pulmonary complications postop-

eratively. This effort may be performed using a history and physical examination to detect the existence of underlying heart or lung disease. Follow-up physiologic tests to confirm the degree of impairment have been reported extensively. Routine pulmonary function tests appear to play a minor role in upper abdominal and open heart surgery. Their primary value appears to be highest as screening tests before lung resection. No patients, however, should be summarily rejected for potentially curative surgery for lung cancer based solely on a spirometric finding. Further testing with quantitative radionuclide split function lung scans or segment counting permits an estimation of post–lung resection pulmonary function. Testing of exercise endurance and oxygen transport preoperatively and predicting postoperative $\dot{V}O_2$max appear to be the best final arbiter of physiologic operability. An algorithmic approach to the evaluation of the lung cancer patient is illustrated in Figure 19-6.

- Patients whose FEV_1 and DLCO exceed 60% of their predicted normal value may undergo resection up to and including pneumonectomy without further routine testing.
- Patients with lower FEV_1 and DLCO results should be subjected to a quantitative ventilation or perfusion radionuclide lung scan or segment-counting estimate of regional function. From these data, a predicted postpneumonectomy—or postlobectomy—FEV_1 or DLCO should be calculated and compared to the predicted normal value for the patient. If the ppo FEV_1 exceeds 40% of normal for that patient, an attempt at the indicated resection is warranted.

- For those patients whose ppo FEV_1 is less than 40% of their normal value, an exercise study with measured $\dot{V}O_2$ may be useful. If the measured $\dot{V}O_2$ on the maximum tolerated exercise is more than 15 mL/kg/min or ppo $\dot{V}O_2max$ is more than 10 mL/kg/min, surgical resection may be offered.
- If the measured exercise $\dot{V}O_2$ is less than 15 mL/kg/min, or ppo $\dot{V}O_2max$ is less than 10 mL/kg/min, one need not absolutely preclude an attempt at a surgical cure. Lung volume reduction surgery coupled with resection of the cancer is now an option. However, any resection should be preceded (as always) with an earnest discussion with the patient of the risks of disability, permanent ventilator dependency, and death.
- For those patients who are physiologically inoperable by all criteria or are reluctant to accept the risk of postoperative disability or death, chemotherapy and external beam radiation therapy may offer a 5-year survival.

REFERENCES

Bartlett RH, et al: Studies on the pathogenesis and prevention of postoperative pulmonary complications. Surg Gynecol Obstet 137:925, 1973.
Bolliger CT, et al: Lung scanning and exercise testing for the prediction of postoperative performance in lung resection candidates at increased risk for complications. Chest 108:341, 1995.
Bolton JWR, et al: Stair climbing as an indicator of pulmonary function. Chest 92:783, 1987.
Carlens E, Hanson HE, Nordenstrom B: Temporary unilateral occlusion of the pulmonary artery. J Thorac Surg 22:527, 1951.
Chuter TAM, et al: Diaphragmatic breathing maneuvers and movement of the diaphragm after cholecystectomy. Chest 97:1110, 1990.
Cooper JD, et al. Bilateral pneumectomy (volume reduction) for chronic obstructive pulmonary disease. J Thorac Cardiovasc Surg 109:106, 1995.
Corris PA, et al: Use of radionuclide scanning in the preoperative estimation of pulmonary function after pneumonectomy. Thorax 42:285, 1987.
Eugene J, et al: Maximum oxygen consumption: a physiologic guide to pulmonary resection. Surg Forum 33:260, 1982.
Fee JH, et al: Role of pulmonary vascular resistance measurements in preoperative evaluation of candidates for pulmonary resection. J Thorac Cardiovasc Surg 75:519, 1975.
Ferguson MK, et al: Diffusing capacity predicts morbidity and mortality after pulmonary resection. J Thorac Surg 86:894, 1988.
Ford GT, et al: Diaphragm function after upper abdominal surgery in humans. Am Rev Respir Dis 127:431, 1983.
Gaensler EA, et al: The role of pulmonary insufficiency in mortality and invalidism following surgery for pulmonary tuberculosis. J Thorac Cardiovasc Surg 29:163, 1955.
Gauden S, Ramsay J, Tripcony L: The curative treatment by radiotherapy alone of stage I non–small cell carcinoma of the lung. Chest 108:1278, 1995.
Graham EA, Singer JJ: Successful removal of an entire lung for carcinoma of the bronchus. JAMA 101:1371, 1933.
Hall JC, et al: Incentive spirometry versus routine chest physiotherapy for prevention of pulmonary complications after abdominal surgery. Lancet 337:953, 1991.
Juhl B, Frost N: A comparison between measured and calculated changes in the lung function after operation for pulmonary cancer. Acta Anaesth Scand Suppl 57:39, 1975.
Kearney DJ, et al. Assessment of operative risk in patients undergoing lung resection. Chest 105:753, 1994.
Kristersson S, Lindell S, Strandberg L: Prediction of pulmonary function loss due to pneumonectomy using ^{133}Xe-radiospirometry. Chest 62:696, 1972.
Ladurie M-L, Ranson-Bitker B: Uncertainties in the expected value for forced expiratory volume in one second after surgery. Chest 90:222, 1986.
Lawrence VA, Page CP, Harris GD: Preoperative spirometry before abdominal operations. Arch Intern Med 149:280, 1990.
Markos J, et al: Preoperative assessment as a predictor of mortality and morbidity after lung resection. Am Rev Respir Dis 139:902, 1989.
McKenna RJ, et al: Combined operations for lung volume reduction surgery and lung cancer. Chest 110:885, 1996.
Morice RC, et al: Exercise testing in the evaluation of patients at high risk for complications from lung resection. Chest 101:358, 1992.
Nakagawa K, et al: Oxygen transport during incremental exercise load as a predictor of operative risk in lung cancer patients. Chest 101:1369, 1992.
Neuhaus H, Cherniack NS: A bronchospirometric method of estimating the effect of pneumonectomy on the maximum breathing capacity. J Thorac Cardiovasc Surg 55:144, 1968.
Olsen GN, Block AJ, Tobias JA: Prediction of postpneumonectomy pulmonary function using quantitative macroaggregate lung scanning. Chest 66:13, 1974.
Olsen GN, et al: Pulmonary function evaluation of the lung resection candidate: a prospective study. Am Rev Respir Dis 111:379, 1975.
Olsen GN, et al: Submaximal invasive exercise testing and quantitative lung scanning in the evaluation for tolerance of lung resection. Chest 95:267, 1989.
Olsen GN, et al: Stair climbing as an exercise test to predict the postoperative complications of lung resection. Chest 92:587, 1991.
Pasteur W: Massive collapse of the lung. Lancet 2:1351, 1908.
Smith TP, et al: Exercise capacity as a predictor of post-thoracotomy morbidity. Am Rev Respir Dis 129:730, 1984.
Stein ME, et al: Pulmonary evaluation of surgical patients. JAMA 181:765, 1962.
Uggla LG: Indications for and results of thoracic surgery with regard to respiratory and circulatory function tests. Acta Chir Scand 111:197, 1956.
Van Nostrand D, Kjelsberg MD, Humphrey EW: Pre-resectional evaluation of risk from pneumonectomy. Surg Gynecol Obstet 127:306, 1968.
Wernly JA, et al: Clinical value of quantitative ventilation-perfusion lung scans in the surgical management of bronchogenic carcinoma. J Thorac Cardiovasc Surg 80:535, 1980.
Zeiher BG, et al: Predicting postoperative pulmonary function in patients undergoing lung resection. Chest 108:68, 1995.
Zibrak JD, O'Donnell CR, Marton, K: Indications for preoperative pulmonary function testing. Ann Intern Med 112:763, 1990.

CHAPTER 20

Preoperative Cardiac Evaluation of the Thoracic Surgical Patient and Management of Perioperative Cardiac Events

John C. Alexander, Jr., and Robert W. Anderson

Preoperative cardiac evaluation of patients undergoing thoracic surgery is important because thoracic surgery is associated with significant cardiac mortality and morbidity. Respiratory problems are the most common postoperative complication of thoracic surgery, but the problems associated with the highest mortality and most severe morbidity are cardiovascular in nature. These problems range from benign atrial arrhythmias to myocardial infarction, pulmonary emboli, and death. The incidence of cardiac complications increases with the patient's age. They occur more frequently in patients who undergo more extensive procedures such as pneumonectomy or esophagogastrectomy. A postoperative myocardial infarction after a major thoracic surgery procedure carries a mortality of nearly 50%.

General thoracic surgical procedures often have more profound effects on the cardiopulmonary system than cardiac surgery. A major lung resection decreases the pulmonary vascular bed and therefore may result in an acute increase in right ventricular and pulmonary artery pressure leading to right ventricular failure. Other physiologic changes associated with thoracic surgery include a decrease in lung compliance and diffusion capacity, with a resulting increase in the work of breathing, which increases myocardial workload and results in an increase in myocardial oxygen consumption, which may aggravate preexisting cardiac disease or lead to new onset ischemia in the patient with stable coronary artery disease.

Thoracic surgery is associated with an acute chest wall injury resulting in involuntary respiratory guarding and an increased work of breathing and decreased efficiency of respiration. Chest wall effects of thoracic surgery are associated with an acute decrease in forced expiratory volume in 1 second and vital capacity. In patients with diminished respiratory reserve, the acute ventilatory changes after surgery can lead to respiratory decompensation requiring prolonged mechanical ventilation and setting the stage for pneumonia. Minimally invasive thoracic surgical approaches have in some cases reduced the importance of acute chest wall–related problems; however, even in patients with the most minimal incisions, demonstrable changes in ventilatory mechanics can lead to significant complications. Thoracic surgery results in a planned reduction in physiologic reserve of the lungs, whereas cardiac surgery usually improves physiologic reserve of the heart.

Thoracic surgical procedures and upper abdominal vascular surgical procedures have the highest incidence of perioperative arrhythmias, myocardial infarction, and heart failure when compared with other general surgical procedures, as noted by Detsky (1986), Goldman (1977), and Steen (1978), and their associates.

EVALUATION OF OPERATIVE RISK: CARDIAC FACTORS

Operative risk is defined as the probability of morbidity or mortality after an operation because of the patient's preoperative condition, anesthesia, the surgical procedure itself, or the circumstances of the required postoperative convalescence. The decision to proceed with any therapeutic intervention, whether medical or surgical, must be made by weighing the potential risks against the hoped for benefits of the intervention, compared with the likely outcome of the natural history of the disease being considered for treatment. The heart is particularly important in the risk portion of the evaluation, because myocardial ischemia and infarction, arrhythmias, and heart failure are important and common complications that occur in thoracic surgical patients.

The greatest cardiac risk for a patient undergoing a thoracotomy is the presence of known coronary artery disease. Based on extensive data of Leppo (1995), Freeman (1989), Goldman (1977), Steen (1978), and Tarhan (1972) and their associates who studied more than 50,000 patients, the likelihood of a perioperative myocardial infarction was observed to be only 0.15% in patients without prior evidence of clinical heart disease. In patients with a documented prior infarction, however, the incidence of reinfarction during a major noncardiac procedure ranged from 2.8 to 17.7%, with a mean of approximately 6%. The mortality for perioperative myocardial infarction is high and averages approximately 50% despite aggressive treatment.

The risk of perioperative infarction is inversely related to the time interval between the original myocardial infarction and the surgical procedure. This risk follows a curvilinear, rather than a linear, relationship. Major noncardiac surgical procedures performed within 3 months of an acute myocardial infarction have been associated with a reinfarction rate of approximately 30%, whereas at 3 to 6 months after an infarction, the corresponding rate of reinfarction is approximately 14% and falls to 4% after 6 months. The institution of aggressive and comprehensive perioperative management guided by invasive hemodynamic monitoring, introduced by Rao and colleagues (1983), has produced a significant decrease in reinfarction rates; but when the postoperative period is complicated by an infarction, it is still associated with high mortality.

Postoperative infarctions are significantly more lethal than infarctions in general. The postoperative time frame is associated with increased cardiac workload because of the stress associated with surgery. Patients with postoperative infarcts must keep up with the increased myocardial workload during the postoperative period, which may result in progressive infarction and heart failure.

The acute changes in coagulation associated with the systemic inflammatory response to surgery make patients hypercoagulable in the early period postoperatively. Pulmonary embolus, deep vein thrombosis, and coronary thrombosis are potentiated by the hypercoagulable state, which partially explains the high incidence of these problems in the postoperative period.

Paul and Eagle (1995) have noted that interventional cardiology has added a dimension to the diagnosis and treatment of cardiac conditions that is important in the perioperative period. Patients with a positive cardiac history of infarction or angina should be considered for stress testing before surgery. A patient with clearly positive results from physiologic stress testing should undergo diagnostic testing and possibly interventions to correct cardiac problems before elective thoracic surgery. The occasional patient may need angioplasty or even a coronary artery bypass before or in conjunction with thoracic surgery to reduce the probability of a postoperative cardiac event. It is hoped that aggressive cardiology evaluation and treatment before surgery will lower operative risk in the select group of high-risk patients.

In patients who develop acute postoperative infarctions, aggressive interventional cardiology using percutaneous transluminal coronary angioplasty and stents may be life saving. Lytic therapy is relatively contraindicated in most acute coronary artery emergencies that occur early after major surgery. Angiography and catheter-based interventions are the procedures of choice for unstable angina in these patients.

INTERVENTIONAL CARDIOLOGY

A thorough cardiovascular history is vital in the preoperative evaluation of thoracic surgical patients and the findings must then be correlated with physical findings and laboratory testing. The factors associated with cardiac risk in thoracic surgical patients are summarized in Table 20-1. The presence of any of the risk factors noted in Table 20-1 should arouse suspicion of significant cardiac disease and, as suggested by Leppo (1995), should lead to a more comprehensive evaluation and possible presurgical intervention.

The clinical findings must be correlated with chest radiography and electrocardiography. The chronology and clinical course of prior myocardial infarction should be elucidated and evidence of left ventricular dysfunction as manifested by symptoms of congestive heart failure should be sought carefully. Attention also should be paid to the presence, severity, and pattern of angina pectoris and to the efficacy and appropriateness of the current medical regimen. Patients who are completely asymptomatic, have an active lifestyle, and have no significant risk factors for coronary artery disease, regardless of age, need not undergo further cardiac testing. Patients with symptomatic heart disease or baseline laboratory abnormalities suggestive of cardiac disease need further assessment. If symptoms of ischemic heart disease are present, stress testing should be considered before a major intrathoracic surgical procedure is recommended, particularly if the patient has a history of myocardial infarction, demonstrates symptomatic left ventricular dysfunction, or has diabetes mellitus.

The preoperative cardiac evaluation of thoracic surgical patients requires making important and reasonable decisions in a cost-effective manner. Some authors suggest that all patients older than a certain age undergo an extensive noninvasive, and possibly even an invasive, evaluation to determine the presence of coexistent coronary artery disease. The intent is to electively revascularize those patients in whom significant disease is identified. This approach, as noted by Abraham and Eagle (1994), is gaining support because evidence is accumulating that prophylactic revascularization by any technique provides greater protection from ischemic events after surgery and is more successful than intensive medical therapy during the postsurgical period.

Table 20-1. Cardiac Risk Factors in Thoracic Surgical Patients

Historical factors
    Myocardial infarction (especially within past 3 months)
    Congestive heart failure
    Angina pectoris
    Poorly controlled hypertension
    Symptomatic cardiac rhythm disturbance
    Family history of premature coronary disease
    Longstanding diabetes mellitus
    Pulmonary hypertension
Physical examination findings
    Presence of S_3 gallop or venous distention
    Abnormal cardiac rhythm
    Pulmonary rales
    Significant valvular murmur
    Hypertension
Laboratory findings
    Cardiomegaly on chest radiography
    Ischemic changes on electrocardiography (rest or stress)
    Ventricular ectopy on electrocardiography
    Abnormal cardiac rhythm on electrocardiography
    Hypotension induced by stress

A variety of stress test methods have been used to evaluate cardiac reserve. Each has its own characteristics and is particularly useful for certain types of patients. The underlying principle, however, is the same independent of methodology. Stress testing can determine the cardiac reserve in a controlled manner before the patient is subjected to the stress associated with surgery and the period following. The concept of *no time-outs* after a major surgical procedure emphasizes the importance of an adequate cardiac reserve to endure the stress of the perioperative period. Paul and Eagle (1995) believe that stress testing is the most useful screening procedure for patients during the planning phase of thoracic surgery if they have historical or physical findings suggestive of cardiac disease.

Transthoracic echocardiography and, when indicated, transesophageal echocardiography are useful noninvasive modalities to assess overall ventricular function and to detect any evidence for valvular pathology. Echocardiography is an excellent first-line screening examination in patients with any suggestive history or physical finding associated with heart failure.

Cardiac catheterization and coronary arteriography should be considered if the patient is unable to exercise to an adequate workload required in stress testing. Nonexercise stress testing [dobutamine echo or dipyridamole (Persantine) infusion] can be used if a physical limitation to exercise exists. The demonstration of significant anatomic coronary artery disease or physiologic ischemia or valvular disease during noninvasive and invasive testing requires consideration of revascularization or valve surgery in certain instances when severe dysfunction is present.

Thoracic surgical patients should be evaluated clinically for the presence of preexisting pulmonary hypertension that may be aggravated by resection of lung tissue leading to acute right ventricular failure. Persons thought to have pulmonary hypertension may require further noninvasive testing or a right-sided catheterization to evaluate the degree of pulmonary vascular disease. Echocardiography is also useful in estimating right ventricular performance and pulmonary pressures.

MANAGEMENT OF SURGICAL PATIENTS WITH CARDIOVASCULAR DISEASE

Since the 1970s, a substantial decrease has occurred overall in "premature" mortality from cardiovascular diseases. Some authors have suggested that modifications in dietary habits and an increased awareness of physical fitness are primarily responsible for these improvements in cardiovascular health. Good evidence also exists, however, that the use of modern drug therapy to control hypertension and reduce cholesterol also have played an important role in lowering cardiovascular disease morbidity and mortality. Consequently, many patients are surviving the ravages of cardiovascular disease only to be seen by surgeons later in their lives for problems, both cardiovascular and noncardiovascular, that require surgical treatment. Logically, one can expect to be faced with patients bringing an ever increasing set of cardiovascular problems to the operating room.

Because of their older age and multiple associated illnesses, these patients present risks that must be carefully considered in the design of their overall surgical management plan.

The cardiovascular diseases that are most frequently encountered in the thoracic surgical patient fall into four general categories: 1) hypertension, 2) chronic congestive heart failure, 3) angina pectoris secondary to ischemic heart disease, and 4) arrhythmias. Considerable overlap exists between these categories, from a physiologic standpoint and with regard to the pharmacologic agents used to treat them.

Hypertension

Hypertension is a common finding in surgical patients. The number of patients treated for this disorder has increased substantially since the 1970s. In approximately 95% of these patients, no single cause for the elevation in blood pressure can be identified. Although many popular theories exist to explain the increased peripheral vascular resistance seen in hypertension, the possibility that a single etiology is responsible for all essential hypertension is unlikely.

It is well recognized from therapeutic trials that many of the vascular complications that occur as a result of hypertension can be ameliorated by pharmacologic intervention to control hypertension. This finding has resulted in the widespread use of antihypertensive agents. These agents may have a profound influence on a patient's ability to appropriately respond to the stresses associated with surgery.

Diuretics

Diuretics, including the thiazides and furosemide, are recommended first-line agents used in the treatment of mild or moderate hypertension. Because these drugs increase urinary excretion of salt and water, relative hypovolemia may be of particular concern in surgical patients. Relative hypovolemia may result in tachycardia and hypotension with the administration of anesthetics. Hypovolemia may interfere with the ability of normal reflex tachycardia to increase cardiac output, a normal homeostatic response to decreasing cardiac output and blood pressure. As a result, minor blood loss during an operative procedure may result in profound hypotension and a severe decrease in cardiac output if preexisting intravascular and extracellular volume deficits are present because of prolonged diuretic administration. Obtaining a full history and observation of clinical signs of volume depletion, such as orthostatic hypotension or resting tachycardia, allow the clinician to recognize this situation and to take appropriate measures to restore volume preoperatively. Loop diuretics work by increasing delivery of sodium to the distal renal tubal. Sodium-potassium exchange occurs, resulting in a net potassium loss and hypokalemia following prolonged administration of most diuretic agents. In the presence of hypokalemia, the arrhythmogenic effects of digitalis, anesthetic agents, and stress of surgery may result in a cardiac rhythm disturbance and lead to premature ventricular contractions or ventricular fibrillation. Repletion of diminished total body potassium stores before major surgical procedures is essential to reduce the incidence of cardiac rhythm disturbances.

Adrenergic Blockers

A second class of agents used to manage hypertension is the adrenergic inhibitors. These drugs inhibit the function of the sympathetic nervous system and are classified according to the site at which they inhibit the sympathetic reflex arc. Each class of drug exhibits different forms of potential toxicity and may produce problems in surgical patients. The peripherally acting agents, such as reserpine and guanethidine, which are not commonly used today, produce profound sympathoplegia by either blocking or inhibiting biogenic amine functions in both peripheral and central neurons. The problems of depressed cardiac output and hypotension from blunted sympathetic responses in the presence of volume depletion or exposure to anesthetic agents are often seen in surgical patients who have received these agents before surgery. It is advisable to discontinue peripherally acting adrenergic blocking agents before any elective surgical procedure. Substitution of a more rapidly

acting and easily managed agent, such as a β-blocker or calcium channel antagonist, may be required.

The centrally acting adrenergic inhibitors, such as clonidine and methyldopa, reduce sympathetic outflow from vasopressor centers in the brainstem. These agents are also seldom used today. Because they allow these centers to retain their sensitivity to baroreceptor control, these drugs do not depress normal cardiovascular reflexes and do not depress cardiac output or produce orthostatic hypotension seen with peripherally acting agents. Abrupt withdrawal of clonidine may result in hypertensive crises or other evidence of profound sympathetic overactivity, and this drug should therefore be continued throughout the perioperative period or gradually withdrawn while other antihypertensive therapy is substituted.

Although β-blocking agents were used initially in patients with angina pectoris, it soon became apparent that they were extremely effective agents for the treatment of a variety of other disorders, such as hypertension, thyrotoxicosis, migraines, arrhythmias, glaucoma, and essential tremors. Most treatment programs in patients with mild or moderately severe hypertension include a β-blocker. β-Blockers are well tolerated in surgical patients and appear to offer a significant degree of protection from postoperative rhythm disturbances in addition to blood pressure control if continued without interruption throughout the postoperative period. Bronchospasm may be a problem with β-blockers in thoracic surgery patients, but usually patients can be managed with these agents in the postoperative period. Abrupt withdrawal of β-blockers has been associated with the onset of atrial arrhythmias and even acute myocardial infarction and should be avoided.

Vasodilators

Peripheral vasodilators, initially used in the management of hypertension only if a diuretic and adrenergic blocker do not control the blood pressure, are being used much more frequently. Hydralazine is the only drug used routinely as an oral agent. Intravenous nitroprusside, a potent vasodilator, is the agent of choice for the control of acute hypertension in the operating room or during the postoperative period. It is rapid acting and easily titrated under conditions of proper monitoring to achieve excellent control of the patient's blood pressure.

Angiotensin-Converting Enzyme Inhibitors

Captopril was the first orally effective inhibitor of angiotensin-converting enzyme (ACE), the enzyme responsible for conversion of inactive angiotensin I to the pressor peptide angiotensin II. Many new ACE inhibitor drugs are now available. This class of drugs, ACE inhibitors, is a group of potent and specific antihypertensive agents that lower total peripheral resistance; cause little change in cardiac output, heart rate, or pulmonary wedge pressure; and are particularly effective in hypertensive patients with elevated renin levels. They do not appear to interfere with normal cardiovascular homeostatic responses even when administered simultaneously with a diuretic. If significant volume depletion occurs as a result of a concomitantly administered diuretic, however, hypotension may develop. Abrupt withdrawal of ACE inhibitors may result in hypertension that is difficult to manage. These drugs should be continued throughout the perioperative period.

Uncontrolled hypertension in any postoperative surgical patient is a serious problem. It is essential to formulate a plan for the management and control of blood pressure in the operating room and postoperatively before discontinuing any form of antihypertensive therapy. This planning should include the surgeon, anesthesiologist, and cardiologist. After passing the period of hemodynamic instability surrounding the immediate operative period, the patient's normal antihypertensive regimen should be reinstituted to make the postoperative management less complex. Rapidly acting agents, such as intravenous nitroprusside, a potent vasodilator, or esmolol, an ultrashort-acting intravenous β-blocker, are the agents of choice for severe hypertension during the intraoperative or immediate postoperative period. These agents should be administered only under carefully monitored conditions because of their ability to rapidly produce profound hypotension.

Congestive Heart Failure

Traditional treatment for patients with evidence of cardiac failure has consisted of salt restriction, diuretics, and the administration of a digitalis preparation for cardiac rate control and an inotropic effect. Cohn (1982) and Cohn and associates (1986) recognized that an increase in impedance to left ventricular ejection is an important factor in producing the left ventricular dysfunction that characterizes cardiac failure. Increased impedance to ejection or afterload is the result of a complex series of peripheral vascular events produced by increased activity of the sympathetic system and the renin-angiotensin system. The final result of this abnormal activity is narrowing of the arterioles, decreased arterial compliance, and a reduction in venous compliance. An important conceptual change has occurred in the treatment of heart failure. Instead of vigorously stimulating the failing heart with inotropic agents, attempts are now made to reduce the cardiac afterload by the use of peripheral vasodilators. The concept of afterload reduction by pharmacologic means is well established in the treatment of hypertension and has been extended to other disease states that produce severe congestive heart failure such as aortic or mitral valve incompetence, ischemic heart disease, and the cardiomyopathic states that produce cardiac failure.

Drugs that produce vasodilatation can favorably affect the performance of the heart in two ways, according to Chatterjee

and Parmley (1983) and Ribner and colleagues (1982). First, by decreasing peripheral vascular resistance through the mechanism of arteriolar relaxation, the ventricular ejection fraction increases, stroke volume improves, and end-systolic volume decreases. Second, the relaxation of venous smooth muscle shifts blood from the central circulation into the peripheral venous capacitance bed, thereby decreasing the preload or end-diastolic volume, which results in a reduction in myocardial wall stress and consequent lowering of myocardial oxygen requirements and a decrease in left ventricular end-diastolic pressure and a decrease in pulmonary venous pressure and relief of pulmonary congestion. Improved diastolic perfusion of the myocardium as a result of lowering the transmyocardial pressure gradient between epicardial and endocardial blood vessels improves ventricular performance.

The surgical management of patients with concomitant congestive heart failure has been improved with the addition of vasodilator drugs to the therapeutic regimen. This improvement has been particularly evident in cardiovascular and thoracic surgical patients, who can be optimized preoperatively and brought to the operating room in a more stable state than was previously possible. The short- and long-term deleterious effects of uncontrolled hypertension are well recognized, and drugs that are currently available allow precise regulation of cardiac function and blood pressure both preoperatively and during the intraoperative period.

Any patient with cardiac disease severe enough to produce symptoms or findings of congestive heart failure represents a substantial risk for any thoracic surgical operation. A comprehensive evaluation of the patient's underlying cardiac pathology and the institution or continuation of appropriate therapy, coupled with the judicious use of intraoperative monitoring of cardiac function are mandatory to reduce surgical risk to an acceptable level. In almost all instances, drugs that have successfully controlled symptoms of cardiac failure before surgery should be continued throughout the preoperative, operative, and postoperative periods.

Arrhythmias

Bailey and Betts (1943) and Currens and associates (1943) first called attention to the incidence of both supraventricular and ventricular arrhythmias after thoracotomy for pulmonary and esophageal disease. Krosnick and Wasserman (1955) first drew attention to an association between the occurrence of postoperative arrhythmias and postoperative mortality. This argument was strengthened by Shields and Ujiki (1968) when they reported a series of 125 patients undergoing thoracotomy. The findings of their non-randomized study suggested that prophylactic digitalization reduced mortality related to arrhythmias. Since that time, considerable controversy regarding the incidence, importance, etiology, methods for treatment, and usefulness of prophylaxis for these arrhythmias has been present in the thoracic surgical literature. Ferguson (1992) carefully reviewed and documented the relationship between cardiac arrhythmias and thoracic surgery and concluded that the etiology of these arrhythmias is multifactorial. The propensity for arrhythmias in surgery is superimposed on a patient population already at high risk for arrhythmic complications. Ferguson concluded that despite the high incidence of arrhythmogenic complications after thoracotomy, adequate preoperative evaluation and a thorough understanding of the principles of postoperative management of rhythm disturbances suffice in almost all instances to keep the morbidity associated with this complication to a minimum.

The perioperative management of patients with cardiac arrhythmias and conduction disturbances is an important part of the care of thoracic surgical patients. Knowledge of the preoperative medication history, electrocardiography, echocardiography, and the patient's cardiovascular history are mandatory and should be combined with an understanding of the intraoperative and postoperative factors that facilitate the occurrence of cardiac rhythm disturbances. A number of factors may be identified perioperatively that predispose to the development of arrhythmias: 1) ventilatory problems that produce hypoxia or respiratory alkalosis, 2) hypokalemia and other electrolyte abnormalities, 3) toxicity to cardioactive anesthetics and other drugs, 4) hypotension, 5) hypertension, 6) reduced cardiac output, 7) anemia, 8) myocardial infarction, and 9) the vagal irritation and sympathetic increase associated with postthoracotomy pain that invariably are associated with thoracic surgical procedures. The most important predictor of postoperative arrhythmias is a history of preoperative arrhythmias. These factors must be considered in the evaluation of a surgical patient with cardiac rhythm disturbance, and initial treatment should always be directed toward correction of these abnormalities.

The aim of modern antiarrhythmic therapy is to reduce ectopic pacemaker activity. The indications for the use of antiarrhythmic drugs in surgical patients is based on a knowledge of the natural history of the rhythm disturbance and whether it is of physiologic significance in the overall management of the patient. Careful documentation and precise diagnosis of the type of rhythm disturbance are essential. Harrison (1985) suggested a limited role for the prophylactic use of drug therapy in an attempt to prevent the development of arrhythmias, because all antiarrhythmic drugs have proarrhythmic effects and therefore may actually precipitate a rhythm disturbance. In general, all cardiac rhythm disturbances that are potentially life-threatening, that cause hemodynamic compromise, or that result in symptoms should be diagnosed precisely and treated specifically. Patients with no known structural heart disease usually do not require specific drug therapy for benign rhythm disturbances such as sinus tachycardia, premature atrial beats, or unifocal premature ventricular beats. The most prudent approach may be to define underlying etiologic factors, such as fever, hypoxia, pain, or anxiety, and attempt to eliminate them. In some patients, the presence of heart disease

may complicate the use of antiarrhythmic therapy. Heart failure and conduction system disease are the most serious problems. Most of the antiarrhythmic drugs depress left ventricular function to a variable and dose-related degree. Patients with left ventricular dysfunction may tolerate these agents poorly. Drug therapy for patients with atrioventricular nodal disease or with conduction blocks below the atrioventricular node should be monitored carefully because of the potential for profound depression of cardiac conduction heart block and serious side effects.

Bradyarrhythmias

Sinus bradycardia in the surgical patient is usually caused by increased vagal tone related to direct stimulation of the carotid sinus, stimulation of the vagus nerves, or pain-induced increases in vagal tone. Myocardial ischemia should always be excluded as a cause for sudden cardiac slowing.

Sinus bradycardia is best treated by administering atropine intravenously in 0.5-mg boluses, up to 2.0 mg over a 30-minute period. If atropine therapy is unsuccessful, a continuous infusion of isoproterenol may be administered at a rate of 1 to 10 μg/min titrated to achieve the desired heart rate responses. If pharmacologic therapy is unsuccessful, a temporary transvenous pacemaker should be placed.

Ventricular Arrhythmias

Ventricular arrhythmia is a complex and changing subject that is not easily simplified. The criteria for instituting therapy are not clear, although patients with episodes of prolonged ventricular tachycardia and those with symptomatic or hemodynamically compromising ventricular dysrhythmia require treatment.

Intraoperative or postoperative ventricular ectopy is often precipitated by hypoxia, hypercarbia, hypokalemia, anxiety, fever, or drug excess, and correction of these problems often leads to cessation of the ectopy without resorting to specific drug therapy. Ventricular ectopic activity that occurs in the absence of clinical heart disease is generally benign and well tolerated.

In patients with a history of ischemic heart disease or with electrocardiographic or clinical evidence of perioperative ischemia or infarction in whom ventricular ectopic activity in the form of frequent multifocal ventricular beats or ventricular couplets develops, lidocaine therapy should be administered as a 50- to 100-mg intravenous bolus followed by continuous infusion at a rate of 1 to 3 mg/min titrated to control the ectopy. If lidocaine fails to control the rhythm, amiodarone, a newer antiarrhythmic drug, shows great promise for rapid and effective control of not only ventricular but also atrial arrhythmias.

Supraventricular Tachyarrhythmias

Development of supraventricular tachyarrhythmias in the thoracic surgical patient is usually associated with identifiable risk factors such as myocardial infarction or ischemia; congestive heart failure; electrolyte derangements; hypoxia; pulmonary embolism; administration of arrhythmogenic drugs, such as catecholamines; or fever associated with a major infection. Correction of these problems obviates the need for specific drug therapy in approximately one-third of patients.

Atrial fibrillation is the most common supraventricular arrhythmia observed in thoracic surgical patients. The first goal of treatment is to control the rapid ventricular response rate, which usually is done best by administering digoxin or β-blockers. For patients who have not taken digoxin previously, a total intravenous loading dose of 1.0 mg should be administered over 4 to 12 hours, usually beginning with 0.5 mg intravenously and then repeating 0.25-mg doses at 2-hour intervals to lower the ventricular rate to below 90 beats per minute. In patients with a rapid ventricular response to atrial fibrillation and no evidence of depressed ventricular function, verapamil can be given in doses of 2.5 to 5.0 mg intravenously every 15 minutes until a total dose of 10 mg is delivered. For severe cardiac compromise because of tachycardia, synchronized cardioversion remains the treatment of choice.

Treatment of the underlying medical problems driving atrial fibrillation and control of the ventricular response to atrial fibrillation usually result in conversion to normal sinus rhythm. If the patient remains in atrial fibrillation for 48 hours despite adequate control of the ventricular response, a specific antiarrhythmic drug, such as quinidine, procainamide, or amiodarone, should be considered in an attempt to achieve conversion into sinus rhythm.

Control of the ventricular rate in patients with atrial flutter is often more difficult than in patients with atrial fibrillation. Although the treatment approach has traditionally been to administer digitalis, good clinical evidence suggests that verapamil as the first drug may be more efficacious. Also, it is well known that atrial flutter is uniquely treatable by cardioversion, cardioversion should be used in any patient with evidence of hemodynamic compromise secondary to atrial flutter.

Other forms of supraventricular tachyarrhythmia, including atrioventricular nodal reentry tachycardia, sinus node reentry tachycardia, intra-atrial tachycardia, automatic junctional tachycardia, or a reentrant conduction pathway, may occur in surgical patients and require pharmacologic treatment. In some instances, these arrhythmias may be terminated by vagotonic maneuvers, but if this effort is unsuccessful, intravenous administration of verapamil in the same dosage recommended for atrial fibrillation is the agent of choice. Verapamil should be successful in approximately 80% of cases, but in those patients in whom rate reduction is not achieved, the administration of a β-blocker is indicated.

Esmolol is an ultrashort-acting cardioselective β-blocker. Esmolol is rapidly converted to inactive metabolites by blood esterases, and full recovery from β-blockade occurs rapidly, usually in less than 30 minutes in patients with a normal cardiovascular system. The indications for esmolol are situations in which a rapid β-blockade onset and termination are desired, such as in supraventricular tachycardia, perioperative tachycardia, or perioperative hypertension. The dose range is 50 to 400 μg/kg per minute intravenously.

Low Cardiac Output Syndromes

Low cardiac output syndrome in surgical patients must be recognized and treated promptly before severe cellular and organ damage occurs. The syndrome is secondary to inadequate perfusion at the tissue level, which may occur for a variety of reasons. The clinical picture is characterized by evidence of decreased organ perfusion with decreasing urinary output and an altered mental state in the awake patient. Acidosis ultimately results because of decreased tissue perfusion. In the postsurgical state, the body lacks the ability to efficiently reduce metabolic demand, leading to metabolic acidosis. Compromised cardiac output at this point, which cannot keep up with demand, can quickly result in death.

Low cardiac output in a surgical patient is best managed by a methodic and physiologic approach. Careful clinical observation and serial monitoring of hemodynamic parameters, such as heart rate, arterial blood pressure, cardiac filling pressures, and cardiac output, are mandatory. The metabolic status of the patient should be followed by serial arterial blood gas measurements and mixed venous oxygen content analysis. Electrolyte abnormalities should be sought and corrected as required. Monitoring with a Swan-Ganz catheter is important in these critically ill patients.

The most common cause of the low cardiac output state in surgical patients is hypovolemia, because of unreplaced blood or fluid losses that occur as a result of both the basic underlying disease process and the losses incurred at the time of any surgical procedure and third spacing of fluid. The typical feature in these patients is reduced filling pressures, particularly as noted from the measurement of pulmonary artery diastolic pressure as a measure of pulmonary capillary wedge pressure, representing left-sided filling pressures. Decrease in urine output and concentrated urine are present. Because of sympathetic compensatory efforts, the peripheral circulation is profoundly vasoconstricted, and the peripheral vascular resistance is elevated. The blood pressure is maintained until near collapse and cardiac output is profoundly decreased.

Management of the low cardiac output state associated with hypovolemia is relatively straightforward and begins with recognition of blood and fluid loss and is treated by judiciously replacing deficits with appropriate solution, blood products, or both. Therapy is best guided by Swan-Ganz catheter measurements of left-sided filling pressures and repeated determinations of cardiac output.

A second and more ominous cause of low cardiac output is primary myocardial dysfunction. The most frequent cause of primary myocardial dysfunction in thoracic surgical patients is ischemic heart disease with associated myocardial dysfunction related to severe ischemia or infarction. This type of dysfunction may be related to preexisting cardiac disease, myocardial infarction, or the residual effects of ischemia associated with the surgical procedure. Regardless of the etiology, the principles of diagnosis and the approach to management of this entity are the same. The left-sided filling pressures must be carefully optimized to take maximal advantage of the Frank-Starling mechanism without causing pulmonary edema. Cardiac rate and synchrony between atrium and ventricle are important factors in the maintenance of optimal cardiac pump function, and every attempt should be made to return them to normal, including the use of pacing devices.

The impaired myocardium functions best when the afterload against which it must function is reduced. Afterload reduction is best achieved by the use of short-acting peripheral vasodilators such as nitroprusside administered intravenously under carefully monitored conditions and titrated to maintain a systemic vascular resistance in the low to normal range. Additional support for the poorly functioning myocardium can be achieved by the use of an inotropic agent that improves cardiac contractility without producing a pronounced increase in cardiac rate or significant increases in peripheral vascular resistance. The inotropic agents that appear to achieve these goals most ably are dopamine, dobutamine, and amrinone, used either alone or in combination. If pharmacologic and fluid therapy are unsuccessful in restoring myocardial function, revascularization or mechanical support with a device such as the intra-aortic balloon pump must be considered, but the prognosis in this subgroup is guarded.

An increasingly recognized cause of the low cardiac output syndrome in thoracic surgical patients is the presence of systemic sepsis. A wide range of microbial agents can cause profound cardiovascular alterations leading to septic shock and death. The treatment of septic shock is more controversial than either hypovolemic or cardiogenic shock, and the mortality remains greater than 50% in almost all reported series.

The most important aspect of the management of a surgical patient who is septic is prompt recognition of the problem and careful monitoring of the hemodynamic status while commencing a thorough search for the source of the sepsis. Surgical drainage of sources of infection and the institution of antibiotics are crucial. In many instances, intravascular volume deficits are present and should be corrected. The hemodynamic interventions instituted in septic shock should augment cardiac output when demands for increased perfusion exist. In nonsurvivors, it is common for cardiac output to be high but ineffective at the tissue level because of shunting.

When perfusion cannot be improved further by expanding the intravascular volume, increasing the preload and reducing afterload should be considered. In some forms of septic shock, the primary hemodynamic alteration appears to be intense peripheral vasoconstriction that eventually produces tissue and organ damage. In this setting, the use of a vasodilator, such as nitroprusside or nitroglycerin, may be indicated under conditions of careful monitoring. Blood pressure commonly decreases when these agents are used, despite an increase in cardiac output. Some degree of hypotension is usually well tolerated by younger patients without preexisting coronary artery or cerebrovascular disease, but the fixed and stenotic lesions often present in the coronary and cerebral circulation of older patients place them at substantial risk for myocardial infarction or stroke.

When afterload reduction fails to improve cardiac output and tissue perfusion, the use of inotropic agents should be considered. The sympathomimetic agents dopamine, dobutamine, and amrinone can provide inotropic support in association with the dose-related peripheral vascular effects previously discussed. The objective is to increase cardiac output enough to achieve adequate tissue perfusion.

One of us (R.W.A.) and Visner (1990) noted that patients with septic shock appear to have a unique problem that presents a dilemma in management. Their cardiac output is usually more than sufficient to meet the peripheral metabolic demands of the body for the delivery of oxygen and substrate. Septic patients are often refractory to pharmacologic interventions, and by sustaining a high cardiac output, they eventually outrun their cardiac reserves. The use of a vasoconstricting agent may seem to be physiologically appropriate, but this type of intervention can severely depress cardiac output and tissue perfusion and is not recommended. Treatment of patients remains controversial.

Acute Congestive Heart Failure and Pulmonary Edema

Acute pulmonary edema in the thoracic surgical patient is often the result of relative fluid overload in the presence of chronically compromised cardiac function or the occurrence of a recent myocardial infarction. Therapy involves the use of oxygen and a diuretic intravenously, such as furosemide. Morphine, a narcotic possessing both venodilatory and vasodilatory properties, may be of benefit and may also alleviate the anxiety often seen in these patients. In some situations, it may be necessary to aid the failing ventricle by the use of intravenous vasodilators, such as nitroprusside or nitroglycerin, and treat with inotropic agents.

In the event that a rapid diuresis occurs, aggressive replacement of potassium is necessary to prevent hypokalemia. This task is best accomplished by the intravenous route; however, care must be taken to avoid hyperkalemia, which also may result in life-threatening arrhythmias. For patients who develop pulmonary edema in association with renal insufficiency, aggressive therapy with ultrafiltration or dialysis may be needed.

Thoracic surgical patients are uniquely susceptible to acute right ventricular failure because of sudden right ventricular pressure overload resulting from pulmonary artery hypertension, exacerbated by intraoperative pulmonary manipulation or resection of sufficient pulmonary tissue to limit the pulmonary vascular bed. This problem is best addressed by anticipating and avoiding it; however, acute pharmacologic treatment with oxygen, nitroprusside, and prostaglandin may be required.

REFERENCES

Abraham SA, Eagle KA: Preoperative cardiac risk assessment for noncardiac surgery. J Nucl Cardiol *1*:389, 1994.

Anderson RW, Visner M: Shock and circulatory collapse. *In* Sabiston DC, Spencer FJ (eds): Surgery of the Chest. Philadelphia: WB Saunders, 1990.

Bailey CC, Betts RH: Cardiac arrhythmias following pneumonectomy. N Engl J Med *229*:356, 1943.

Chatterjee K, Parmley WW: Vasodilator therapy for acute myocardial infarction and chronic congestive heart failure. J Am Coll Cardiol *1*:133, 1983.

Cohn JN: Physiologic basis of vasodilator therapy for heart failure. Am J Med *71*:135, 1982.

Cohn JN, et al: Effect of vasodilator therapy on mortality and chronic congestive heart failure. N Engl J Med *314*:1547, 1986.

Currens JH, White PD, Churchill ED: Cardiac arrhythmias following thoracic surgery. N Engl J Med *229*:360, 1943.

Detsky AS, et al: Predicting cardiac complications in patients undergoing non-cardiac surgery. J Gen Intern Med *1*:211, 1986.

Ferguson TB: Arrhythmias associated with thoracotomy. *In* Wolfe WG (ed): Complications in Thoracic Surgery. St. Louis: Mosby–Year Book, 1992.

Freeman WK, Gibbons RJ, Shub C: Preoperative assessment of cardiac patients undergoing non-cardiac surgical procedures. Mayo Clin Proc *64*:1105, 1989.

Goldman L, et al: Multifactorial index of cardiac risk in noncardiac surgical procedures. N Engl J Med *297*:845, 1977.

Harrison DC: Antiarrhythmic drug classification: new science and practical applications. Am J Cardiol *56*:185, 1985.

Krosnick A, Wasserman F: Cardiac arrhythmias in the older age group following thoracic surgery. Am J Med Sci *230*:541, 1955.

Leppo JA. Preoperative cardiac risk assessment for noncardiac surgery. Am J Cardiol *75*:42D, 1995.

Paul SD, Eagle KA: A stepwise strategy for coronary risk assessment for noncardiac surgery. Med Clin North Am *79*:1241, 1995.

Rao TLK, Jacobs KH, El-Etr AA: Reinfarction following anesthesia in patients with myocardial infarction. Anesthesiology *59*:499, 1983.

Ribner HS, Bresnahan D, Hsieh AM: Acute hemodynamic responses to vasodilator therapy in congestive heart failure. Prog Cardiovasc Dis *25*:1, 1982.

Shields TW, Ujiki GT: Digitalization for prevention of arrhythmias following pulmonary surgery. Surg Gynecol Obstet *126*:743, 1968.

Steen PA, Tinker JH, Tarhan S: Myocardial reinfarction after anesthesia and surgery. JAMA *239*:2566, 1978.

Tarhan S, et al: Myocardial infarction after general anesthesia. JAMA *220*:1451, 1972.

READING REFERENCES

American College of Cardiology/American Heart Association Task Force Report: Guidelines for perioperative cardiovascular evaluation for noncardiac surgery. J Am Coll Cardiol *27*:910, 1996.

Daoud EG, et al: Preoperative amiodarone as prophylaxis against atrial fibrillation after heart surgery. N Engl J Med *337*:1785, 1997.

Epstein SK, et al: Inability to perform bicycle ergometry predicts increased morbidity and mortality after lung resection. Chest *107*:311, 1995.

Izbicki JR, et al: Risk analysis and long-term survival in patients undergoing extended resection of locally advanced lung cancer. J Thorac Cardiovasc Surg *110*:386, 1995.

Krupski WC, Bensard DD: Preoperative cardiac risk management. Surg Clin North Am *75*:647, 1995.

Mangano DT: Preoperative risk assessment: many studies, few solutions. Anesthesiology *83*:897, 1995.

Opie LH: Drugs for the Heart. Philadelphia: WB Saunders, 1987.

Pomposelli JJ, et al: Surgical complication outcome (SCOUT) score: a new method to evaluate quality of care in vascular surgery. J Vasc Surg *25*:1007, 1997.

Potyk D, Raudaskoski P: Preoperative cardiac evaluation for elective noncardiac surgery. Arch Fam Med *7*:164, 1998.

Rose SD, Corman LC, Mason DT: Cardiac risk factors in patients undergoing noncardiac surgery. Med Clin North Am *63*:1271, 1979.

SECTION VI

Anesthetic Management of the General Thoracic Surgical Patient

CHAPTER 21

Preanesthetic Evaluation and Preparation

Hak Yui Wong and Edward A. Brunner

The development of modern surgery, and thoracic surgery in particular, was closely linked to the development of anesthesia and artificial ventilation. Until relatively recently, the feasibility of an operation was often limited by the patient's ability to survive the anesthesia. With advances in anesthetic knowledge and techniques, this is now seldom the case. Surgical procedures and demands are becoming increasingly complex, however, and patients who present for thoracic surgery are older and demonstrate greater complexity of their medical problems. Moreover, the economic demands imposed by managed care providers require that presurgical preparations previously performed on an inpatient basis be performed before hospital admission. The anesthesiologist's responsibility now consists not only of providing a complicated anesthetic but also of becoming an integral part of the continuum of medical care that the patient has hitherto received as an inpatient and now requires on an outpatient basis. The concept of the anesthesiologist as a perioperative physician involved in the preanesthetic evaluation and preparation of the patient, the postoperative care of the patient, and the intraoperative provision of the anesthetic is developing. To be able to discharge this function, the anesthesiologist must be thoroughly familiar with the patient's medical problems and the proposed operation.

Although a thorough history and physical examination by the primary physician provides much of the factual information sought by the anesthesiologist, it is no substitute for a preanesthetic evaluation that, in addition to general assessment, focuses on specific areas of the patient's condition in the context of the proposed operation. Thoracic operations often interfere physically with the function of vital structures, and each operation has unique features. Thus, it is important that the person performing the evaluation knows the nature of the operation, the degree and manner by which it and the anesthetic will stress the patient intraoperatively, and the residual physiologic defects that will exist postoperatively. Current standard of care, in addition, calls for explanation of the procedure and risks to the patient and obtaining a specific informed consent for the care provided by the

anesthesia team. Preanesthetic evaluation, therefore, cannot be relegated to the uninitiated.

ANESTHESIA PREOPERATIVE EVALUATION CLINIC

Preanesthetic evaluation should be initiated as far in advance of the operation as possible. This allows time to conduct additional tests and evaluations (if unsuspected abnormalities are uncovered), for consultations between specialists, and to initiate necessary diagnostic and corrective therapy. In addition, the patient is allowed time to absorb and adjust to the newly acquired information and to explore any questions that arise. With the trend toward ambulatory care, this may be difficult to achieve. Many hospital departments of anesthesia have established an anesthetic outpatient clinic staffed by anesthesiologists and nurse anesthetists to serve in this regard for patients not requiring preoperative hospitalization. Today, many patients scheduled for elective major surgical procedures, including major lung surgery and coronary artery bypass grafting, may have their workup completed on an ambulatory basis and not be admitted to the hospital until the morning of operation. The anesthesia preoperative evaluation clinic serves as a centralized location to integrate and coordinate admission, registration, insurance authorization, and laboratory and electrocardiographic facilities. Shuttling patients among services is minimized and cancellations and delays on the day of operation are virtually eliminated.

SCOPE OF PREANESTHETIC EVALUATION

The purpose of preanesthetic evaluation is to fulfill four objectives: 1) detection of problems and factors in the patient's physical condition that can compromise the ability to cope with perioperative stress or that can be aggravated by such stress, 2) appraisal of the impact of the specific pathology necessitating the surgery, 3) appraisal of several concerns peculiar to the practice of anesthesia, and 4) an assessment of the risk/benefit ratio of anesthetic management.

General Medical Condition

Describing general history taking, physical diagnosis, and laboratory investigations is beyond the scope of this text. Because of their impact on surgical and anesthetic outcome, several conditions that occur fairly commonly in thoracic surgical patients warrant meticulous search and emphasis. These include coronary heart disease, which may present as previous myocardial infarction, angina, arrhythmia, or congestive heart failure; aortic valve stenosis; cor pulmonale; obstructive airway disease; symptomatic cerebrovascular disease; electrolyte imbalance, particularly hypokalemia; diabetes mellitus; thyroid disorder; and polycythemia. Because many patients with chronic conditions have fixed and permanent abnormalities, evaluation should focus on determining if optimal treatment has been achieved and establishing the baseline for the particular patient.

Impact of Specific Pathology

Every surgical condition poses unique stress on the body and presents a different set of problems to the anesthesia team. This is particularly true in thoracic surgery, because the pathologic abnormalities often involve or impinge on the vital life-sustaining organs. From the standpoint of pathophysiology and anesthetic implications, general thoracic surgical conditions can be categorized into three groups: 1) esophageal diseases, 2) surgical diseases of the lungs, and 3) diseases of the mediastinum and pleura. Esophageal diseases include obstructive disorders predisposing patients to preoperative dehydration and malnourishment and refluxing and obstructive disorders predisposing patients to aspiration (either chronically or preoperatively), leading to pneumonitis. Surgical diseases of the lungs include abnormal sources of fluids, such as abscess and hemoptysis, leading to contamination of the normal lung tissues; abnormal solid tissues, such as tumors and consolidation, leading to right-to-left shunting; and obstructive lesions, preventing air flow. Diseases of the mediastinum and pleura include obstruction of airways or large veins, such as the superior vena cava syndrome; abnormal paths of communication, such as bronchopleural fistula; and abnormal collections of fluid, such as empyema (Table 21-1).

Anesthetic Concerns

Aside from the assessment of specific medical and surgical conditions, such as those discussed, the preanesthetic evalua-

tion addresses a set of issues best described as of unique concern to the practice of anesthesia.

Anesthetic History

The anesthetic history begins with a review of the patient's experience with previous anesthetics and an examination of old anesthetic records (if possible). Taking note of previous difficulties, such as difficult endotracheal intubation, prolonged apnea, or postoperative jaundice, can avert potential disasters. Careful and pertinent family history may alert one to the possibility of malignant hyperpyrexia or pseudocholinesterase deficiency.

Drug History

Polypharmacy is an integral part of modern medicine, including modern anesthesia. It is particularly important in older patients presenting for thoracic surgery, who may take up to five or six medications daily. To avoid adverse drug interaction, acquiring a drug history is mandatory (Table 21-2). This step also provides the opportunity to advise the patient on the continuation or discontinuation of medications preoperatively and to assess special precautions dictated by the intercurrent drug therapy.

Status of the Upper Airway

Evaluation of the status of the upper airway includes evaluation of the temporomandibular joints, the cervical spine, and the vertebrobasilar arteries. Because many thoracic surgical patients are at higher risk for pulmonary aspiration caused by full stomach and many patients have coexisting heart and lung disease that causes limited oxygen reserve, unexpected difficulty in maintaining airway patency or endotracheal intubation is best avoided. Many thoracic surgical procedures call for special airway instrumentation, such as endobronchial tubes, making attention to the state of the upper airway even more important. Results of upper airway evaluation may lead to the decision to use special equipment, such as the flexible fiberoptic bronchoscope, to assist in endotracheal intubation at the time of induction of anesthesia. Special studies, such as tomograms or computed tomography of the airway, occasionally are necessary to achieve a complete evaluation.

Intravascular Access

The ease of intravenous access should be assessed in relation to the extent and site of the proposed operation. Patients with inadequate peripheral access should be prepared for central venous cannulation. Potential arterial cannulation sites are examined and tested for the presence of adequate collaterals.

Postoperative Ventilation

The need for mechanical ventilation after the operation is often predictable, based on the nature of the operation, the

Table 21-1. Anesthetic Classification of General Thoracic Surgical Pathologic Conditions

Pathologic Condition	Implications
I. Esophageal disorders	
A. Obstructive disorders	Predispose patients to preoperative dehydration and malnourishment
B. Refluxing disorders	Predispose patients to chronic or perioperative aspirations and pneumonitis
II. Surgical disorders of lungs	
A. Abnormal collection of fluid (e.g., abscess, hemoptysis)	Contamination of normal lung tissues
B. Abnormal solid tissue (e.g., tumor, consolidation)	Right-to-left shunting
C. Obstructive lesions	Airflow obstruction, lung collapse
D. Abnormal lung tissue (e.g., bullous emphysema)	Risk of barotrauma and pneumothorax
III. Disease of the mediastinum and pleura	
A. Obstruction of large airway (e.g., subcarinal tumor)	Airflow obstruction unrelieved by endotracheal intubation
B. Obstruction of large vessels (e.g., superior vena cava syndrome)	Hemodynamic compromise
C. Abnormal paths of communication (e.g., broncho pleural fistula)	Difficult ventilation
D. Abnormal collection of fluid (e.g., empyema, pleural effusion)	Contamination of lung tissue Compression of lung tissue

anticipated impairment of the patient's respiratory reserve, the condition of the cardiovascular system, and the anesthetic technique used. In addition to advising the patient of this possibility, one may consider altering the choice of endotracheal tube; use of low-pressure, high-volume cuffs; the route of intubation; and the dose of respiratory depressant drugs.

Postoperative Pain Relief

At the time of preanesthetic evaluation, all patients should be apprised of the extent of anticipated postoperative discomfort and the types of pain relief available. Patient-controlled analgesia and intraspinal opioid administration are analgesic techniques that are superior to traditional intramuscular injections. Although patient-controlled analgesia is simple and noninvasive, it requires a great degree of patient motivation and physical participation. Spinal opioid administration may not require patient activity, but it involves careful assessment of the patient's anatomy, ruling out contraindications, and it places high demand on the technical skill of the provider. Opioids with or without local anesthetic can be administered into the intradural or epidural space either by pump driven infusion or by patient-controlled infusion. If patient participation is required, a period of patient instruction is essential in the preoperative period to ensure familiarity with the equipment. An honest appraisal regarding postoperative discomfort and reassurance that adequate analgesia will be provided can greatly reduce the patient's apprehension at this juncture.

Assessment of Risk

Risk is defined as the chance of adverse outcome, including death and serious morbidity. Pure anesthetic or surgical mishaps rarely occur, and adverse outcome after surgical procedures is largely multifactorial. Assignment of risk to anesthesia or surgery per se is nearly impossible. Thus, as summarized by Goldstein and Keats (1970), epidemiologic studies of anesthetic risk have widely varying results and severe limitations. One of us (E.A.B., 1975) found that at least four factors contribute to anesthetic risk: 1) physical status of the patient, 2) drugs used for anesthesia, 3) site and requirements of the operation, and 4) the skill of the medical personnel involved.

More pragmatically, from the standpoint of preanesthetic evaluation and intervention to minimize risks, adverse outcomes after thoracic surgery can be divided broadly into two groups. The first group of adverse events is mostly unrelated to the preoperative state of the patient and depends only on the nature of the surgery and the skill of the personnel. The thoracic site of operation confers a higher risk for postoperative complication. In addition, four intraoperative threats are constantly present during thoracic surgery: 1) sudden hemorrhage, 2) cardiac arrhythmia, 3) mechanical interference with the mediastinum, and 4) ventilation or oxygenation difficulties. Risks not unique to thoracic surgery include adverse drug interaction, anaphylaxis, and rare occurrences such as malignant hyperpyrexia.

The second group of adverse events is reasonably predictable from the preoperative state of the patient and the nature of the operation. Interventions that change the patient's preoperative state may, therefore, affect the occurrence of these events. They include pulmonary complications, such as atelectasis, infection, and respiratory failure, and cardiac conditions, including cor pulmonale, myocardial ischemic events, heart failure, and serious arrhythmias. An extensive literature concerning attempts at predicting these events, the associated mortality, and the effect of preoperative interventions is available.

Table 21-2. Drugs Associated with Significant Interaction during Anesthesia

Drug Class and Examples	Interact with	Interaction	Comment
Theophylline			
Aminophylline	Cimetidine	↑ Serum theophylline level	Substitute with ranitidine
Oxtriphylline	Ketamine		
	Halothane and/or pancuronium	Jointly reduce seizure threshold Predispose to cardiac arrhythmias when theophylline level is high	Check theophylline level before anesthesia
α-Adrenergic blockers			
Prazosin	Alpha agonists	↓↑ α-Adrenergic effects	Chronic use of α-blockers upregulates number of alpha-receptors
Phenoxybenzamine			
Labetalol			Exaggerated alpha response if α-blockers are acutely withdrawn
Clonidine			
β-Adrenergic blockers			
Propranolol	Beta agonists	↓ β-Adrenergic effect	May need up to 20× usual doses of beta agonists
Timolol			
Metoprolol	Ketamine	↓ Sympathetic stabilization of circulation	Chronic use upregulates number of beta receptors
Nadolol			
Atenolol	Enflurane	↑ Cardiac depression and reduced response to hypovolemia	Do not abruptly withdraw beta-blockade perioperatively
			High-dose beta blockade may be reduced to equivalent of 360 mg propranolol per day preoperatively
Calcium channel blockers			
Verapamil	β-blockers	Additive cardiac depression	
Diltiazem	Digitalis	↑↓ Blood digitalis level	
Nifedipine			
Nicardipine	Volatile anesthetics	Additive cardiac depression	
Central antihypertensives			
Reserpine	Volatile anesthetics	↓ Anesthetic requirement	
Guanabenz	Direct-acting sympathomimetics	↑ Sympathomimetic response	Antihypertensives should be maintained throughout perioperative period
Methyldopa	Indirect-acting sympathomimetics	↓ Sympathomimetic response	
	Propranolol	May cause hypertension (caused by beta$_2$-receptor blockade)	Reported with methyldopa only
Diuretics			
Furosemide	Antihypertensives	Potentiates hypotensive effect	
Bumetanide	Volatile anesthetics	Potentiates hypotensive effect	
Chlorthiazide	Digitalis	Hypokalemia ↑ toxicity	
	Muscle relaxants	Hypokalemia ↑ muscle weakness	
	Aminoglycosides	Potentiates ototoxicity	Especially with ethacrynic acid
Vasodilators and angiotensin-converting enzyme inhibitors			
Captopril			
Enalapril	Volatile anesthetics	↑ Hypotensive effect	
Hydralazine			
Monoamine oxidase inhibitors			
Pargyline	Meperidine	Excitement, agitation, hypertension, tachycardia, rigidity, convulsion, coma	May be related to ↑ serotonin level
Isocarboxazid			
Phenelzine	Indirect-acting sympathomimetics	Hypertensive crisis	Monoamine oxidase inhibitors should be withdrawn for 2 weeks before elective surgery
Tranylcypromine	Tricyclic antidepressants		
	Opioids	↑ Sedation	Reported with phenelzine only
	Succinylcholine	↑ Paralysis	Reported with phenelzine only
Tricyclic antidepressants			
Amitriptyline	Barbiturates	↑ Sleeping time	
Desipramine	Anticholinergics	↑ Central and peripheral cholinergic effects	
Imipramine			

(continued)

Table 21-2. *Continued*

Drug Class and Examples	Interact with	Interaction	Comment
Doxepin Nortriptyline	Direct-acting sympatho-mimetics	↑ Adrenergic response	
Phenothiazines and butyrophenones			
Chlorpromazine	Volatile anesthetics	↑ Hypotensive effect	Promethazine may have anti-analgesic effect
Fluphenazine	Opioid drugs	↑ Sedation and respiratory depression	
Promethazine			
Haloperidol	Barbiturates	↑ Sleeping time	
	Anticholinergics	↑ Anticholinergic effects	Chronic phenothiazine therapy may cause myocardial toxicity
	Sympathomimetics	↓ Adrenergic response	
Lithium	Barbiturates	↑ Sleeping time	
	Muscle relaxants	↑ Duration of relaxation	
	Diuretics	↑ Lithium level	
Digitalis	Succinylcholine	May induce ventricular dys-rhythmias	
	Volatile anesthetics	May ↓ digitalis-induced dys-rhythmias	
Organophosphates			
Echothiophate Isoflurophate	Succinylcholine	Prolonged apnea	Systemic absorption inhibits plasma cholinesterase
Antiarrhythmics			
Quinidine	Volatile anesthetics	↑ Cardiac depression	
Procainamide	Muscle relaxants	↑ Neuromuscular blockade	
Amiodarone	Vasodilators	↑ Hypotension	May be related to alpha-blocking action
Bretylium	Direct-acting sympatho-mimetics	↑ β-Adrenergic response	Only reported with bretylium

↑, increased; ↓, decreased.

One of the simplest and earliest rating scales for preoperative state is the American Society of Anesthesiologists (ASA) Physical Status classification (Table 21-3). Although the scale was originally conceived simply as a classification of a patient's physical status at the time of preanesthetic evaluation, Dripps and colleagues (1961), Vacanti and colleagues (1970), Marx and colleagues (1973), Brunner (1975), and Forrest and colleagues (1992) showed it to be a fairly good predictor of general outcome after surgery. Note that this classification is not a predictor of intraoperative risks unrelated to the patient's preoperative state, such as hemorrhage and cardiac arrhythmias.

Disposition

After careful review of the medical record, laboratory tests, patient interview, and examination and after taking into consideration the nature and demand of the proposed operation, a patient can usually be assigned to one of the fol-

Table 21-3. American Society of Anesthesiologists Classification of Physical Status

Status	Physical Attributes
I	Patients with no organic, physiologic, biochemical, or psychological disturbance. The pathologic process for which the operation is to be performed is localized and not related to a systemic disturbance. Examples are the physically fit for elective inguinal herniorrhaphy or hysterectomy.
II	Patients with mild systemic disturbance caused by the condition to be treated surgically or by other pathophysiologic processes. Examples are patients with mild diabetes or mild hypertension.
III	Patients with moderate systemic disturbance from whatever cause even though it may not be possible to define the degree of disability with finality. Examples are patients with previous myocardial infarction or persistent cardiac arrhythmias.
IV	Patients with severe systemic disorder already life-threatening and not always correctable by the operative procedure. Examples are patients with cardiac insufficiency or advanced pulmonary disease.
V	Moribund patients who have little chance for survival and are subject to operation in desperation. Examples are moribund patients with a ruptured aortic aneurysm or a mesenteric thrombosis.

lowing three categories: 1) the patient is in optimal condition and not at excessive risk, and anesthesia and surgery can proceed; 2) the patient's condition is questionable in some areas, and specialist consultation and investigation are needed; 3) the patient is obviously undertreated, and further preoperative treatment and follow-up evaluation are needed.

INTERDISCIPLINARY CONSULTATION

Because the anesthesiologist approaches the patient-operation complex from a perspective slightly different from that of other physicians, he or she frequently uncovers problems that may have been overlooked or ignored. It is important that the anesthesia and surgical teams maintain open and equitable communication so that such problems can be satisfactorily resolved before surgery.

When diagnostic or therapeutic uncertainty exists outside the defined expertise of both the surgeon and the anesthesiologist, specific specialist consultation is indicated. Examples are evaluation of chest pain and borderline electrocardiogram, diagnosis of complex arrhythmias, testing of pacemakers, and control of severe bronchospasm. Occasionally, a consultation may be needed in anticipation of a likely postoperative problem that will require specialist management, such as renal failure or total parenteral nutrition. A consultation is most rewarding when all who are involved maintain open communication and address specific questions. The traditional *carte blanche* "medical clearance" type of consultation is patronizing, misleading, and seldom helpful to the anesthesia and surgical teams in their patient management. Moreover, the anesthesiologist alone has to shoulder the responsibility for the stress of anesthesia and surgery on the patient and therefore must make the final judgment, together with the surgeon, on the patient's suitability for the procedure and the anesthetic technique of choice. Del Guercio and Cohn (1980) presented data that indirectly support this position. Of 148 elderly patients who had been cleared medically for surgery, subsequent invasive hemodynamic data showed 23.5% to have had increased risks. All who were in this group and had surgery died. Of special interest, these patients were readily identified by experienced anesthesiologists using ASA Physical Status classification (see Table 21-3).

Pulmonary Complications

Pulmonary complications are common after thoracic and abdominal surgical procedures. Anderson and associates (1963) have shown the well-known relationship between the site of operation and the incidence of complication. Thoracic surgery is the highest risk. One particular complication (respiratory insufficiency because of loss of lung tissue by surgical resection) is fairly predictable based on preoperative pulmonary function and the extent of surgical intervention. This topic is discussed in detail in Chapter 19.

Pulmonary complications not directly caused by lung resection are related to the effect of surgery and anesthesia on various aspects of the respiratory system: mucociliary transport, mechanics of breathing, and decrease in the functional reserve volume and forced vital capacity. Atelectasis is said to affect 10 to 50% of all surgical patients. Estimation of risk based on early epidemiologic studies is less than helpful: Patients and case mix were often undefined, varying end points were used in morbidity measurement, the bias of preoperative treatment was ignored, and the effects of retrospective and prospective design were often not delineated in such reports. The presence of chronic respiratory disease, cigarette smoking, and age older than 70 years, however, have been cited as risk factors for postoperative pulmonary complications. The focus of thoracic surgical literature itself has been on tuberculosis and cancer; the risk of other types of thoracic surgical procedures therefore has to be extrapolated from data collected from these conditions.

Based on the existing literature, an abnormal expiratory spirogram is clearly a strong predictor of postoperative complication, but no agreement exists about the cut-off point for prohibitive risk. Grossly abnormal forced vital capacity, maximum voluntary ventilation of less than 50% of the predicted value, and forced-expired volume in 1 second of less than 1 L have been shown to be a sensitive predictor of death. Gracey and colleagues (1979) found that response to bronchodilators is another index, with good response indicating a favorable outcome. Forrest and associates (1992) found that cardiac failure, myocardial ischemia, and obesity are predictive of pulmonary complications. Based on the expiratory spirogram and findings in the cardiovascular system, central nervous system, arterial blood gas measurement, and expected postoperative course, Shapiro and associates (1994) proposed a scoring system for predicting the risks of postoperative pulmonary complications and the need for intensive postoperative support. This is a step toward quantifying the risks and providing a basis for measurement of effects of the preoperative intervention. To date, however, no data verifying the score have been reported.

The benefit of preoperative treatment of chronic obstructive lung disease in reducing postoperative pulmonary complications has been shown by Stein and colleagues (1962), Tarhan and colleagues (1973), and Gracey and colleagues (1979). Conditions amenable to such treatment include infection, acute exacerbation of bronchospasm, bronchorrhea, and cigarette smoking.

Cardiac Complications

Because of the age of the thoracic surgical population, predisposing risk factors common to lung and heart disease, and the nature of thoracic surgery (especially lung resection), cardiovascular events are leading causes of mortality and morbidity, led only by pulmonary complications.

Predicting and modifying the risk of perioperative cardiovascular morbidity and mortality have been the center of much attention. Reports from Topkins and Artusio (1964), Tarhan and colleagues (1972), and Steen and colleagues (1978) emphasized the impact of coronary artery disease using previous myocardial infarction as a marker. The risk of sustaining a perioperative myocardial infarction after a previous infarction is approximately 6%, in contrast to 0.7% without previous myocardial infarction. History of a recent (less than 3 months old) myocardial infarction increases the risk five- to sixfold. Furthermore, mortality rate from perioperative reinfarction has been uniformly high (36 to 70%). Reports by Wells and Kaplan (1981), Rao and colleagues (1983), Foster and colleagues (1986), and Shah and colleagues (1990) indicate a lower rate of reinfarction in the perioperative period. Although Rao and associates (1983) attribute this improvement to aggressive monitoring and early correction of identified physiologic abnormalities, other yet unidentified factors may be involved. Of note is the frequency of perioperative myocardial infarction during the second and third postoperative days, when many patients have already been discharged from the intensive care unit. A longer period of intensive postoperative observation may be indicated for high-risk patients.

Besides previous myocardial infarction, signs of congestive heart failure, valvular heart disease, and abnormal cardiac rhythm are consistent and powerful predictors of

perioperative cardiovascular complications. Goldman and associates (1977) constructed the Cardiac Risk Index, which incorporates these and other less-weighted factors (Tables 21-4 and 21-5). Although the statistical method and universal applicability of this index have been questioned, it nevertheless highlights factors that are potentially amenable to preoperative treatment—such as congestive heart failure—and may therefore reduce morbidity and mortality.

PREANESTHETIC TREATMENT

Preanesthetic treatment of coexisting diseases uncovered during preanesthetic evaluation must be considered in the time-frame of urgency of the proposed surgery. In the best of circumstances, the objective would be to treat acute reversible disorders, return the patient with a chronic disorder to an optimal baseline, and act to minimize the postoperative functional derangement. Although the primary responsibility for implementing treatment rests with the primary physician and the surgeon, the anesthesiologist has a vested interest, because the result of such treatment may have a significant impact on the patient's intraoperative course.

The benefit of preoperative treatment of chronic obstructive lung disease in reducing postoperative pulmonary complications has been shown by Gracey and colleagues (1979), Tarhan and colleagues (1973), and Stein and colleagues (1962). Conditions amenable to such treatment include infection, acute exacerbation of bronchospasm, bronchorrhea, and cigarette smoking. Congestive heart failure as a result of cor pulmonale or ischemic heart disease is another situation in which adequate preoperative treatment may have a significant impact on postoperative mortality. Shields and Ujiki (1968) and Deutsch and Dalen (1969) discussed preoperative digitalization for thoracic surgery patients. Our current practice is not to use digitalization routinely to prevent cardiac arrhythmias caused by thoracic surgery. Data from Mahar and colleagues (1978), Hertzer and colleagues (1984), Foster and colleagues (1986), and Reul and colleagues (1986), how-

Table 21-5. Correlation of Cardiac Risk with Total Points

Total Points	% Cardiac Death[b]	% with Life-Threatening Complications[a,b]	% with No or Minor Complications[b]
0–5 (class I)	0.2 (1)	0.7 (4)	99 (532)
6–12 (class II)	2.0 (5)	5.0 (16)	93 (295)
13–25 (class III)	2.0 (3)	11.0 (15)	86 (112)
>26 (class IV)	56.0 (10)	22.0 (4)	22 (4)

Adapted from Goldman L, et al: Multifactorial index of cardiac risk in noncardiac surgical procedures. N Engl J Med 297:845, 1977.
[a]Intraoperative or postoperative myocardial infarction, pulmonary edema, or ventricular tachycardia without progression to cardiac deaths.
[b]Figures in parentheses denote number of patients.

Table 21-4. Factors Correlated with Cardiac Risk in Surgical Patients

Factor	Weighted Points
History	
Age >70 years	5
Myocardial infarction in previous 6 months	10
Physical examination	
S_3 gallop or jugular venous distention	11
Important valvular aortic stenosis	3
Electrocardiogram	
Rhythm other than sinus rhythm or premature atrial contractions on last preoperative electrocardiogram	7
>5 Premature ventricular contractions per minute at any time	7
General status	3
Pao_2 <60 or $Paco_2$ 50 mm Hg	
K <3 or HCO_3 <20 mEq/L^{-1}	
Blood urea nitrogen = 50 or creatinine 3 mg/dL^{-1}	
Abnormal serum glutamic–oxaloacetic transaminase, signs of liver disease, or bedridden patient	
Operation	
Intraperitoneal, intrathoracic, or aortic	3
Emergency	4
Total possible points	**53**

Adapted from Goldman L, et al: Multifactorial index of cardiac risk in noncardiac surgical procedures. N Engl J Med 297:845, 1977.

ever, indicate that coronary artery bypass graft surgery, when otherwise indicated, confers protection against postoperative infarction in patients undergoing noncardiac surgery. Whether percutaneous transluminal angioplasty confers the same protection is yet to be determined.

Occasionally, preanesthetic treatment may call for invasive monitoring of the patient and involvement of other medical specialists. For example, a patient with unstable angina needs extensive evaluation and treatment options, such as coronary artery bypass surgery and intraaortic balloon counterpulsation, may have to be explored by a team, including the cardiologist, the thoracic surgeon, and the anesthesiologist, before thoracic surgery is undertaken.

PSYCHOLOGICAL PREPARATION OF THE PATIENT

Evaluation of the patient's preoperative psychological state is an important part of the preanesthetic evaluation. For the patient, the impending operation is an anxiety-generating event. The anesthesiologist, because of his or her ability to modify that anxiety and to offer psychological support, can establish a close rapport with the patient in a short period. Such support and rapport have a calming effect on an otherwise anxious patient. Egbert and colleagues (1964) noted that an informative and reassuring approach from the anesthesiologist engenders patient confidence and reduces apprehension and anxiety. The patient should be encouraged to discuss fears and to explore events that will occur on the day of operation. Frank discussion of postoperative pain and assurance of the availability of adequate doses of analgesic drugs are helpful. This assurance can be augmented by appropriate drug therapy, helping to ensure that the patient arrives in the operating room calm, confident, and cooperative. The induction of anesthesia is safer, more controllable, and more pleasant for the calm patient than for one who is excited.

Egbert and associates (1963, 1964) emphasized that the need for strong postoperative narcotic analgesics, the incidence of postoperative complications, and the duration of hospital stay may be reduced significantly by an informative preoperative visit by the anesthesiologist.

INFORMED CONSENT

Before seeking consent to a particular course of anesthesia, the anesthesiologist has an obligation to inform the patient adequately of the potential benefits and risks of such a course and other available options. The difficulty lies in striking a balance between providing enough information and unduly alarming the patient, given the inherent risks of any anesthetic and surgery. Furthermore, the specific risks of thoracic surgery discussed and possible preventive and corrective measures must be honestly disclosed when applicable. This task may be eased in part by highlighting problems

and risks that are amenable to preoperative correction, advising the patient in general terms that any anesthetic poses risks, and then inquiring if the patient wishes to know the specifics of all the possible risks. Many patients would then guide the anesthesiologist as far as their coping would allow. The essence of such discussion should be documented and forms are needed as part of the proof of informed consent. On occasion, a patient may decline any discussion of risks, or the physician may find the patient in a state unsuitable to bear such an ordeal. These also should be documented.

PREANESTHETIC MEDICATION

The aim of preanesthetic medication is to decrease anxiety without producing excessive drowsiness; facilitate a smooth, rapid induction without prolonged emergence; provide amnesia for the perioperative period while maintaining cooperation before loss of consciousness; and relieve preoperative pain. The classes of drugs commonly used for this purpose include 1) sedatives, hypnotics, and tranquilizers; 2) opioids; 3) anticholinergics; and 4) antihistamines and antacids. The appropriate drugs and doses can be chosen only after the psychological and physiologic conditions of the patient have been evaluated. The type and extent of the operation, the expected postoperative course, and the anesthetic technique to be used also should be taken into consideration. In addition, Egbert and associates (1963) found that a good preanesthetic visit may be as effective as administration of sedatives in decreasing the level of anxiety. Several categories of patients should only rarely receive preanesthetic medication before arriving in the operating room. These are patients without informed consent and those with marginal cerebral function; uncorrected hypovolemia; or severe heart disease, lung disease, or both whose respiratory and sympathetic drives are crucial.

CONCLUSION

Preanesthetic evaluation and preparation are integral parts of good anesthetic practice. It is essential for establishing physician–patient rapport and ensuring that the patient is in an optimal state for the proposed operation. By being thoroughly familiar with the patient and the operation, the anesthesiologist can take steps to minimize intraoperative risk and postoperative problems and facilitate the performance of surgery. The choice of monitoring and anesthetic technique follows rationally and provides optimal safety for the patient.

REFERENCES

Anderson WH, Dossett BE, Hamilton GE: Prevention of postoperative pulmonary complications. JAMA 186:766, 1963.
Brunner EA: Factors related to anesthesia risk. Surg Gynecol Obstet 141:761, 1975.

Del Guercio LRM, Cohn JD: Monitoring operative risk in the elderly. JAMA *243*:1350, 1980.

Deutsch S, Dalen JE: Indications for prophylactic digitalization. Anesthesiology *30*:648, 1969.

Dripps RD, Lamont A, Eckenhoff JE: The role of anesthesia in surgical mortality. JAMA *178*:261, 1961.

Egbert LD, et al: The value of the preoperative visit by an anesthetist. JAMA *185*:553, 1963.

Egbert LD, et al: Reduction of postoperative pain by encouragement and instruction of patients. N Engl J Med *270*:825, 1964.

Forrest JB, et al: Multicenter study of general anesthesia. III. Predictors of severe perioperative adverse outcomes. Anesthesiology *76*:3, 1992.

Foster ED, et al: Risk of noncardiac operation in patients with defined coronary disease: the Coronary Artery Surgery Study (CASS) registry experience. Ann Thorac Surg *41*:42, 1986.

Goldman L, et al: Multifactorial index of cardiac risks in noncardiac surgical procedures. N Engl J Med *297*:845, 1977.

Goldstein A, Keats AS: The risk of anesthesia. Anesthesiology *33*:130, 1970.

Gracey DR, Divertie MB, Dider EP: Preoperative pulmonary preparation of patients with chronic obstructive pulmonary disease. Chest *76*:123, 1979.

Hertzer NR, et al: Coronary artery disease in peripheral vascular patients. A classification of 1,000 coronary angiograms and results of surgical management. Ann Surg *199*:223, 1984.

Mahar LJ, et al: Perioperative myocardial infarction in patients with coronary artery disease with and without aorta-coronary bypass grafts. J Thorac Cardiovasc Surg *76*:533, 1978.

Marx GF, Mateo CV, Orkin LR: Computer analysis of postanesthetic deaths. Anesthesiology *39*:54, 1973.

Rao TLK, Jacobs KH, El-Etr AA: Re-infarction following anesthesia in patients with myocardial infarction. Anesthesiology *59*:499, 1983.

Reul GJ Jr, et al: The effect of coronary bypass on the outcome of peripheral vascular operations in 1,093 patients. J Vasc Surg *3*:788, 1986.

Shah KB, et al: Reevaluation of perioperative myocardial infarction in patients with prior myocardial infarction undergoing noncardiac operations. Anesth Analg *71*:231, 1990.

Shapiro BA, et al: Clinical Application of Respiratory Care. 5th Ed. Chicago: Year Book Medical, 1994.

Shields TW, Ujiki GT: Digitalization for prevention of arrhythmias following pulmonary surgery. Surg Gynecol Obstet *126*:743, 1968.

Steen PA, et al: Myocardial reinfarction after anesthesia and surgery. JAMA *239*:2566, 1978.

Stein M, et al: Pulmonary evaluation of surgical patients. JAMA *181*:765, 1962.

Tarhan S, et al: Myocardial infarction after general anesthesia. JAMA *199*:318, 1972.

Tarhan S, et al: Risk of anesthesia and surgery in patients with chronic bronchitis and chronic obstructive disease. Surgery *74*:720, 1973.

Topkins MJ, Artusio JF: Myocardial infarction and surgery: a five year study. Anesth Analg *43*:715, 1964.

Wells PH, Kaplan JA: Optimal management of patients with ischemic heart disease for noncardiac surgery by complementary anesthesiologist and cardiologist interaction. Am Heart J *102*:1029, 1981.

Vacanti CJ, VanHouten RT, Hill RC: A statistical analysis of the relationship of physical status to postoperative mortality in 68,388 cases. Anesth Analg *49*:564, 1970.

SUGGESTED READING

Bendixen HH, et al: Respiratory Care. St. Louis: CV Mosby, 1965.

Editorial views: The ASA classification of physical status—a recapitulation. Anesthesiology *49*:233, 1978.

Eisen N, Reich DL: The patient with valvular heart disease. Problems Anesth *9*:153, 1997.

Fisher SP: Medical and economic issues in starting a preoperative screening clinic. Problems Anesth *9*:262, 1997.

Fleisher LA: Preoperative cardiac evaluation. Problems Anesth *9*:143, 1997.

Fleisher LA, ed: Preoperative evaluation in an era of cost containment. Problems Anesth *9*:143, 1997.

Forrest WH, Brown CR, Brown BW: Subjective responses to six common preoperative medications. Anesthesiology *47*:241, 1977.

Mangano DT: Perioperative cardiac morbidity. Anesthesiology *72*:153, 1990.

Rock P: The patient with lung disease. Problems Anesth *9*:165, 1997.

Smith NT, Corbascio AN: Drug Interactions in Anesthesia. 2nd Ed. Philadelphia: Lea & Febiger, 1986.

CHAPTER 22

Conduct of Anesthesia

Andranik Ovassapian

One-lung ventilation (OLV) is preferred during conventional intrathoracic operations but is necessary during thoracoscopic procedures performed in anesthetized patients. Pulmonary function tests and perfusion-ventilation studies are critical for selection of patients for lung resection to avoid a disastrous outcome. In addition to routine anesthetic problems, anesthesia for thoracic surgery is complicated by several factors: opening the chest produces a pneumothorax; manipulation of the lung, heart, and major vessels by the surgeon may interfere with ventilatory exchange and cardiovascular stability; and the lateral decubitus position changes the distribution of blood flow and pattern of ventilation and exposes the lower lung to the danger of contamination by secretions from the operative lung. Thus, for safe conduct of anesthesia for thoracic surgery, the anesthesiologist should be knowledgeable about the physiology of OLV and be skillful in techniques for isolation of the lungs.

The introduction of double-lumen endobronchial tubes for one-lung anesthesia by Bjork and Carlens in 1950 represented a major advance in thoracic anesthesia. In 1958, Jenkins and Clark advocated the routine use of double-lumen tubes for all intrathoracic operations. Yet the difficulty in blindly positioning these tubes and the resulting possibility of life-threatening complications discouraged their use by many anesthesiologists.

Several advances have made one-lung anesthesia safer and the double-lumen tube more popular. These include the availability of disposable—and in many ways superior—double-lumen tubes; the introduction of the bronchofiberscope (fiberscope) by Shinnick and Freedman (1982) and me and my colleagues (1983) for precise positioning of endobronchial tubes; and use of different treatment methods for management of hypoxemia during OLV and application of arterial blood gas or pulse oximetry for monitoring of blood oxygenation.

CHOICE OF ANESTHESIA

After thorough preoperative assessment and preparation of the patient, the anesthesiologist should choose an anesthetic plan that is both safe for the patient and suitable for the needs of the surgeon. An appropriate preoperative medication should be prescribed to relax and free the patient of apprehension. Narcotics minimize patient discomfort during placement of arterial cannulae and large intravenous lines. The respiratory depression caused by narcotics in patients with advanced pulmonary disease, however, should be kept in mind. Judicious use of intravenous narcotics such as fentanyl while the patient is in the operating room and before any procedures provides the necessary analgesia. Oxygen (2 to 3 L) through a nasal cannula should be instituted if conscious sedation is provided for placement of various lines and an epidural catheter. Respiratory depression and hypoxemia are common with intravenous sedation.

Anticholinergic agents such as atropine or glycopyrrolate are prescribed with the premedication to decrease secretions during airway instrumentation and to facilitate visualization of the airways when a fiberscope is used. Thornburn and colleagues (1986) showed that anticholinergic agents also improve pulmonary mechanics before general anesthesia. Because of the lower incidence of undesirable side effects, glycopyrrolate is the anticholinergic agent of choice.

General endotracheal and endobronchial anesthesia with controlled ventilation is an ideal anesthetic technique for most intrathoracic surgical procedures. A variety of high-frequency ventilation (HFV) techniques have been developed and recommended for operations performed on the airway and for intrathoracic procedures. During HFV, ventilatory excursions of the lungs are of low amplitude, which may facilitate surgical exposure and resection during intrathoracic operations. HFV has been used successfully in situations in which access to the airway is impaired. The success or failure of HFV and its advantages and disadvantages compared with conventional mechanical ventilation depend on the following: the type of HFV used, whether one-lung or two-lung ventilation is applied, and the type of surgical procedure. The three basic forms of HFV are high-frequency positive pressure ventilation (HFPPV), high-frequency jet ventilation (HFJV), and high-frequency oscillation (HFO). El-Baz and associates (1981, 1982) used one-lung HFPPV successfully for sleeve pneumonectomy and surgical procedures on large airways. Smith and colleagues (1981) reported successful use of HFPPV for pulmonary lobectomy. Hildebrand and coworkers (1984) applied HFJV for intrathoracic surgery, providing satisfactory operating conditions and ventilatory exchange. They indicated, however, that OLV using a double-lumen tube provides the optimal conditions if the difficulties associated with placement of double-lumen tubes and related complications can be avoided. Glenski and coworkers (1986) demonstrated that HFO resulted in adequate pulmonary gas exchange and excellent surgical conditions for peripheral lung procedures; however, for procedures on the major airways or mediastinal structures, surgical conditions were unsatisfactory during HFO. They believe that the disadvantages of HFO outweigh the advantages during intrathoracic surgery.

A unique feature of thoracic anesthesia is the use of OLV. The selection of an anesthetic technique and agent is influenced by whether OLV is used and whether a high concentration of inspired oxygen can be delivered to the patient. The volatile halogenated anesthetic agents such as isoflurane, sevoflurane, and halothane permit the administration of a high inspired concentration of oxygen. Sevoflurane is a newer volatile anesthetic agent that offers smooth induction of anesthesia and rapid recovery from anesthesia, a combination that is desirable for patients with lung disease. Abe and associates (1998) demonstrated that arterial oxygen tension during OLV with sevoflurane anesthesia was similar to that of isoflurane. Halogenated agents depress the airway reflexes, cause bronchodilation, and can be eliminated through the lungs. The high concentration of inhalation anesthetic agents may interfere with hypoxic vasoconstriction, however, diverting blood flow from the ventilated to the nonventilated lung, increasing intrapulmonary shunting, and decreasing Pao_2. Another disadvantage of inhalation agents is the ease with which they may depress the myocardium and decrease the cardiac output. When narcotic analgesics are added to the anesthetic regimen, the concentration of inhalation agent is lowered. This adjustment helps alleviate the aforementioned problems associated with halogenated agents.

Induction of anesthesia is achieved by the intravenous administration of 5 µg/kg fentanyl and 2 to 3 mg/kg of sodium thiopental or by propofol 2 to 3 mg/kg. Anesthesia is maintained with 50% nitrous oxide and 0.5 to 0.8% of isoflurane, or 1.0 to 1.5% sevoflurane. An additional 10 to 15 µg/kg of fentanyl is given before and during OLV when N_2O is discontinued and anesthesia is maintained with a low concentration of inhalation agent and oxygen. At the conclusion of OLV, nitrous oxide is started again and no additional narcotic is given thereafter. If necessary, higher concentrations of an inhalation agent are used to maintain adequate depth of anesthesia. Muscle relaxants are used for intubation of the trachea and preventing diaphragmatic movement during the operation.

Weinrich and associates (1980) recommended a combination of ketamine, nitrous oxide, and muscle relaxant as an anesthetic for thoracic surgery. Ketamine has sympathomimetic properties; therefore, it supports the cardiovascular system and causes bronchodilation. It is a useful drug for the induction of general anesthesia in hypovolemic patients with an unstable cardiovascular system.

The use of epidural anesthesia to supplement a light general anesthesia is another approach that warrants consideration. It offers the advantage of decreasing the use of neuromuscular blocking drugs or narcotic analgesics intraoperatively. This technique may receive more attention as epidural narcotics are used increasingly for the management of postsurgical pain. Training and experience in this technique, especially when a high or midthoracic approach is used, is needed. The technique should be used regularly to help sustain the expertise needed for its safe conduct.

During thoracic operations, it may be necessary to give various additional drugs for the control of cardiac dysrhythmias, systemic blood pressure, cardiac output, or acid–base balance. Their dosage is similar to that used in other types of anesthesia. Caution should be exercised, however, in the use of vasodilators and vasopressors during OLV. Vasodilators such as sodium nitroprusside and nitroglycerin interfere with hypoxic pulmonary vasoconstriction. The vasopressors exert more vasoconstriction in oxygenated vessels than in hypoxic vessels. Consequently, both groups of drugs may divert blood flow from the ventilated to the nonventilated hypoxic lung, which may then increase shunt and hypoxemia.

MONITORING

Various devices have been introduced to improve patient monitoring during anesthesia. Monitoring requirements differ among individual patients because of their general physical conditions, the presence or absence of cardiopulmonary disease, and the nature of their operative procedures. Monitoring of patients who are healthy and undergoing minor intrathoracic operations may be limited to routine monitors used in all patients undergoing general anesthesia. For most intrathoracic operations and during OLV, monitoring of beat-to-beat arterial blood pressure and the arterial blood oxygenation is essential. Direct arterial monitoring of blood pressure not only provides beat-to-beat measurement of pressure but also permits analysis of arterial blood gases and acid–base status during and after the operation. The pulse oximeter provides a noninvasive, continuous monitoring of the hemoglobin saturation and the heart rate. Improvement in the design of pulse oximeters, especially of the sensors, and introduction of an earlobe oximeter probe have made the pulse oximeter reliable and easy to use. The pulse oximeter displays the percentage of oxyhemoglobin. Over a wide range of arterial blood oxygen tension, the percentage of oxyhemoglobin does not change. Continuous monitoring of arterial blood gases and pH, which is now available, provides a better continuous monitoring method during OLV. The pulse oximeter also should be used postoperatively in postanesthesia and intensive care units.

The measurement of central venous pressure (CVP) is indicated in hypovolemic patients, when large volume shifts are anticipated, in patients with trauma and multiple injuries, and in patients with right ventricular dysfunction. Continuous or serial measurements are useful in the management of fluid and blood replacement when venous tone and myocardial function remain stable. The response of the CVP to a rapid volume infusion is a useful test of right ventricular function. The CVP is subject to mechanical interference, however, especially during thoracic surgery.

The internal jugular and subclavian veins are common sites for central venous cannulation. It is wise to use the vein ipsilateral to the thoracotomy, because pneumothorax is a known complication of deep vein cannulation. In patients with left ventricular dysfunction, the CVP may not provide accurate information about left ventricular filling pressure. Under these circumstances, a pulmonary capillary wedge pressure should be measured by using a flow-directed pulmonary artery catheter. In most patients, the pulmonary capillary wedge pressure corresponds well with the left atrial pressure. The pulmonary artery catheter allows measurements of pulmonary artery systolic, diastolic, and mean pressures, along with the pulmonary capillary wedge pressure, CVP, and cardiac output. In addition, mixed venous blood can be sampled and the shunt can be calculated. Peripheral and pulmonary vascular resistance can be calculated. Serial measurements of cardiac output can help to assess the status of the circulation and guide any necessary supportive therapy. Information derived from centrally placed catheters indicates how the myocardium manages the fluid load; however, the CVP and pulmonary wedge pressure reflect changes in blood volume when depth of anesthesia and myocardial performance are unchanged. The combination of a decrease in CVP or pulmonary wedge pressure and systemic arterial pressure suggests hypovolemia, whereas a high CVP and pulmonary wedge pressure with a low arterial pressure may indicate poor myocardial performance.

New anesthesia machines are equipped with monitors and alarm systems; these include an inspired oxygen concentration monitor and a spirometer to measure expired tidal volume, a low and high airway pressure, and an apnea alarm system. The use of muscle relaxants is monitored by a peripheral nerve stimulator, and the body temperature is measured by an esophageal or a tympanic membrane probe. The availability of mass spectrometry or end-tidal CO_2 analysis provides additional monitoring of the patient's ventilation and confirms the proper placement of an endotracheal tube. The addition of pulse oximetry, used to monitor arterial oxygen saturation noninvasively, permits the early detection of impaired oxygenation, especially during OLV.

ONE-LUNG ANESTHESIA

One-lung anesthesia is absolutely required under certain circumstances and provides safety for the patient and better operative conditions for the surgeon. Because of its complexity, however, it adds to anesthetic difficulties. The most common indication for one-lung anesthesia to provide the

surgeon with a quiet operating field. A bronchopleurocutaneous fistula, communicating empyema, bronchial hemorrhage, lung abscess, and giant air cyst and operations performed through video-assisted thoracoscopy are absolute indications for isolating the individual lungs. This measure prevents the spread of secretions to the healthy lung and helps to ensure adequate ventilation. Thoracoscopy, although not a new surgical technique, has gained popularity in recent years with the development of appropriate video equipment and is applied for many diagnostic and therapeutic intrathoracic operations, such as drainage of empyema, evacuation of hemothorax, bleb resection, and mediastinal lymph node and lung biopsy. Deflation of the operative lung is mandatory during video-assisted thoracoscopy.

Methods of Obtaining One-Lung Ventilation

Four categories of bronchial catheters or blockers are used to achieve separation of the lungs. These are single-lumen tubes with one or two cuffs, bronchial blockers, double-lumen tubes of several types, and the Univent tube (Fuji Systems Corp., Tokyo, Japan).

Single-Lumen Endotracheal Tubes

Single-lumen endotracheal tubes with one or two inflatable cuffs were the first tubes used for one-lung anesthesia. They are introduced into the bronchus of the healthy nonoperative lung. Their major disadvantage is that the operative lung cannot be inflated or suctioned without losing the separation of the lungs. These tubes are rarely used today.

Bronchial Blockers

Bronchial blockers are introduced into the bronchus of the diseased lung while the healthy nonoperative lung is ventilated through a tracheal or contralateral bronchial tube. Fogarty arterial embolectomy catheters have been used in children by Vale (1969) and Hogg and Lorhan (1970), as well as by Cay and associates (1975). They may be positioned blindly or, more usually, through a conventional bronchoscope or with the help of a bronchofiberscope under topical or general anesthesia. Ginsberg (1981) advocated the use of Fogarty catheters in adults, whereas Dalens and colleagues (1982) used Swan-Ganz pulmonary artery catheters in children. Aspiration of secretions or temporary ventilation of the diseased lung is not possible without losing the separation of the lungs. Dislodgment of blockers is common with coughing, changing from the supine to the lateral position, or during surgical manipulation.

Fiberscopic-Aided Placement of Balloon-Tipped Catheters as Bronchial Blockers

The fiberscope can be used to place a Fogarty or similar balloon-tipped catheter into the desired bronchus. As suggested by Ginsberg (1981), the distal end of the Fogarty catheter is angled to 30 degrees to facilitate advancement into either main stem bronchus. After the patient is anesthetized and paralyzed, rigid laryngoscopy is performed, and first a Fogarty catheter and then a tracheal tube are passed through the larynx into the trachea. A swivel adapter with an endoscopy port is placed on the tracheal tube connector and mechanical ventilation is begun. The fiberscope is passed through the swivel adapter into the trachea to expose the catheter and the carina. The tip of the catheter is then advanced under direct vision into the desired main stem bronchus.

For left-lung blockade, the tip of the Fogarty catheter is advanced into the lower lobe bronchus so that the balloon of the catheter is positioned just above the orifice of the left upper lobe bronchus. For blockade of the right lung, the balloon is placed against the orifice of the right upper lobe bronchus. Once the catheter is positioned correctly, the balloon is inflated with air to occlude the main stem bronchus. Rao and associates (1981) placed a Fogarty catheter in the diseased lung and tracheal tube in the main stem bronchus of the healthy lung in children to achieve the same objective as the double-lumen tube achieves in adults. If the Fogarty catheter fails to block the diseased bronchus, the dependent lung may still be protected by the presence of the bronchial tube. Baraka and colleagues (1982) reported a high incidence of right upper lobe collapse with blind intubation of the right main stem bronchus. This complication can be avoided by accurately positioning the tracheal tube with a fiberscope.

Double-Lumen Endobronchial Tubes

Double-lumen endobronchial tubes with two cuffs, consisting of two completely separate lumens, have their proximal ends separated into two connector limbs. A tracheal cuff is located proximal to the opening of the tracheal lumen, and a bronchial cuff is located at the tip of the bronchial tube. Tubes designed for intubation of the right main stem bronchus have an opening in the bronchial cuff (bronchial cuff slit) to permit ventilation of the right upper lobe. When a double-lumen tube is positioned properly and the bronchial and tracheal cuffs are inflated, a separate airway is formed for each lung. The main advantage of double-lumen bronchial tubes is that, although isolation of the lungs is preserved, one or both lungs can be ventilated. The Carlens double-lumen tube described in 1949, which has a carinal hook, and the Robertshaw double-lumen tube described in 1962, which has no carinal hook, are used most commonly. Edwards and Hatch (1965) reviewed their clinical experience with them. Burton and associates (1983) demonstrated the advantages of the disposable polyvinyl double-lumen tubes. The advantages of these tubes include a softer and more flexible structure, thin-walled tracheal and bronchial cuffs, a gentler distal curve, and a greater inside-to-outside diameter ratio. These clear plastic, disposable tubes also allow observation of the humidity of exhaled air during the respiratory cycle.

After the patient is anesthetized and paralyzed, the double-lumen tube is inserted into the trachea using a rigid laryngoscope. The left-sided tube is held 90 degrees rotated clockwise (to the right) and the right-sided tube is held 90 degrees rotated counterclockwise (to the left) so the tip of the bronchial lumen faces anteriorly. After the tip is advanced beyond the vocal cords, the left-sided tube is rotated 90 degrees counterclockwise and the right-sided tube is rotated 90 degrees clockwise, to situate the tube in its normal position in the trachea—that is, the bronchial lumen facing toward the intended bronchus. With the Carlens (left-sided) and White (right-sided) double-lumen tubes with a carinal hook, as the tip of the bronchial lumen passes the vocal cords, the Carlens tube is rotated 180 degrees counterclockwise and the White tube is rotated 180 degrees clockwise to bring the carinal hook anteriorly to negotiate the vocal cords. After the carinal hook passes beyond the vocal cords, the Carlens tube is rotated 90 degrees clockwise and the White tube is rotated 90 degrees counterclockwise to have the bronchial lumen face the intended bronchus.

If rigid laryngoscopy proved difficult for tracheal intubation with a double-lumen tube, a fiberscope may be used for this purpose, as described by the author (1996). The fiberscope is passed through the bronchial lumen of the tube. After exposure of the vocal cords, the fiberscope is advanced into the lower trachea. The double-lumen tube is maneuvered such that the tip of the tube faces posteriorly to pass beneath the epiglottis and then is rotated 180 degrees to bring the tip anteriorly to pass through the vocal cords. After entering the trachea, the tube is rotated 90 degrees right or left to position the tube such that the bronchial lumen faces toward the intended bronchus.

Once the double-lumen tube is placed in the trachea, the tracheal cuff is inflated. Mechanical ventilation is then initiated, with a tidal volume of 10 mL/kg and a rate of 8 breaths per minute. The rate of ventilation is adjusted to maintain a Pa_{CO_2} between 35 and 40 mm Hg. The fiberscope is then used to evaluate the bronchial tree and to position the double-lumen tube.

Fiberscopic Positioning of Left-Sided Double-Lumen Endobronchial Tubes

While mechanical ventilation continues, the fiberscope is introduced into the bronchial lumen. The fiberscope is rotated 90 degrees to the left and is advanced into the left main stem bronchus to evaluate its patency and length. Two techniques can be used for positioning the left endobronchial tube:

1) After inspection of the left main stem bronchus, the fiberscope is pulled back to position its tip 2 mm beyond the distal end of the endobronchial tube lumen. The fiberscope is rotated 90 degrees to the left and the tip is angulated to view the lateral wall of the trachea. The tracheal cuff is deflated and the fiberscope and double-lumen tube

are held together and advanced into the left main stem bronchus. The orifice of the left upper lobe bronchus comes into view when the fiberscope reaches 10 to 15 mm above this opening. The tube and fiberscope are advanced further until the distal end of the tube is positioned 5 mm above the opening of the left upper lobe bronchus (Fig. 22-1).

2) After evaluating the anatomy of the left main stem bronchus, the tip of the fiberscope is positioned 10 mm above the orifice of the left upper lobe bronchus. The tracheal cuff is deflated and the tube alone is advanced over the stationary fiberscope into the left main stem bronchus until it passes approximately 5 mm beyond the tip of the fiberscope. If the fiberscope is carefully stabilized during this maneuver, the tip of the endobronchial tube should lie 5 mm above the orifice of the left upper lobe bronchus. To confirm this positioning, the fiberscope is advanced beyond the endobronchial tube lumen to visualize both the upper and lower lobe bronchi.

After positioning the left endobronchial tube with either technique, the fiberscope is withdrawn from the bronchial lumen and inserted into the tracheal lumen. The relationship of the tracheal lumen distal opening to the tracheal wall and the position of the bronchial cuff and the opening of the right main stem bronchus is evaluated. If the endobronchial tube cuff is seen outside the left main stem bronchus, the tracheal cuff is deflated and the tube is advanced further until the proximal edge of the bronchial cuff lies 3 to 5 mm inside the left main stem bronchus. This placement ensures separation of the lungs and stability of the tube and prevents herniation of the bronchial tube cuff into the trachea. Any blockade of the distal lumen of the tracheal lumen may interfere with right lung ventilation. The bronchial and tracheal cuffs are then inflated using the minimal leak technique (Fig. 22-2).

Fiberoptic Positioning of Right-Sided Double-Lumen Endobronchial Tubes

Proper positioning of right-sided double-lumen tubes is technically more difficult because of the short, variable length of the right main stem bronchus. Rigg (1980) reported a high incidence of failure when these tubes were positioned blindly. I (1987) applied the following techniques successfully. The fiberscope is passed through the bronchial lumen of the tube into the right main stem bronchus. The patency, length, and anatomy of the right main stem bronchus, as well as the bronchus intermedius, are evaluated. If the right main stem bronchus is 15 mm or longer, placement of a right-sided double-lumen tube is possible. Either of the following two techniques can then be applied:

1) After inspection of the right main stem bronchus, the fiberscope is withdrawn inside the lumen of the endobronchial tube, the fiberscope is rotated 90 degrees to the

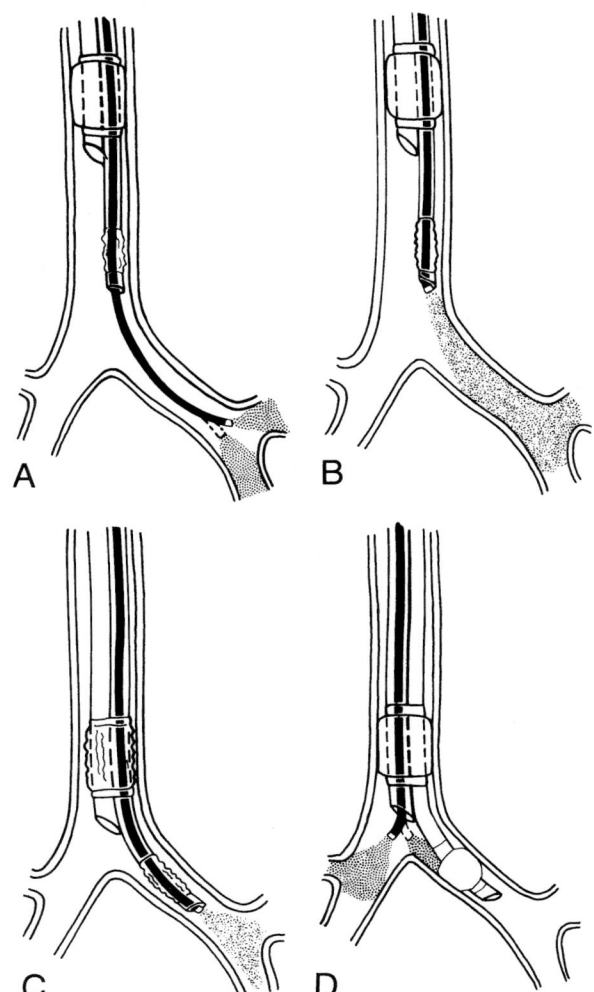

Fig. 22-1. Fiberscopic placement and positioning of left-sided, double-lumen endobronchial tube. **A.** The fiberscope is passed through the bronchial lumen into the left main stem bronchus. The patency, length, and anatomy of the left main stem bronchus and the position of the orifice of the left upper lobe bronchus are evaluated. **B.** The fiberscope is pulled back to position its tip 2 mm beyond the distal end of the bronchial lumen. The fiberscope is positioned 90 degrees rotated to the left with the tip angulated anteriorly toward the lateral wall of the trachea. **C.** The tracheal cuff is deflated, and the tube and fiberscope are advanced together inside the left main stem bronchus until the orifice of the left upper lobe comes into view. At this point, the tip of fiberscope is 10 to 15 mm above the left upper lobe orifice. The tube is advanced further to position the distal end of the tube approximately 5 mm above the orifice of left upper lobe bronchus. **D.** The fiberscope is passed through the tracheal lumen to check the position of the bronchial cuff and the opening of the right main stem bronchus.

right, and the tip is flexed anteriorly to position the tip of the fiberscope at the proximal end of the slit (*Murphy eye*) in the endobronchial tube. The tracheal cuff is deflated and the tube and fiberscope, while being held together, are advanced toward the right main stem

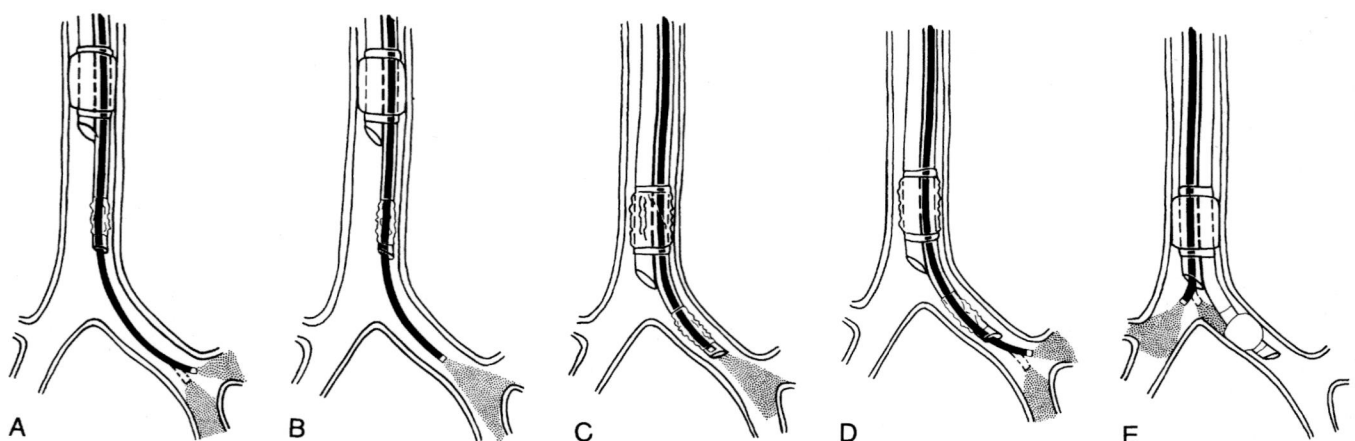

Fig. 22-2. Alternate approach to fiberscopic placement and positioning of left-sided, double-lumen endobronchial tube. **A.** The fiberscope is passed through the bronchial lumen into the left main stem bronchus. The patency, length, and anatomy of the left main stem bronchus and the position of the orifice of the left upper lobe bronchus are evaluated. **B.** The fiberscope is withdrawn, and its tip is positioned 10 mm above the origin of the left upper lobe bronchus. **C.** The tracheal cuff is deflated, and the tube is advanced over the fiberscope into the left main stem bronchus until it comes into view beyond the tip of the fiberscope. **D.** The fiberscope is advanced beyond the bronchial lumen to visualize the left upper lobe bronchus. **E.** The fiberscope is passed through the tracheal lumen to check the position of the bronchial cuff and the opening of the right main stem bronchus.

bronchus. The view through the endobronchial tube slit is the red mucosa of the tracheal and right main stem bronchial walls. The first indication of approaching the opening of the right upper lobe bronchus is a dark area at the distal end of the endobronchial tube slit—the termination of the bronchial wall and the beginning of the orifice to the right upper lobe bronchus. This view is seen when the proximal end of the endobronchial tube slit is approximately 10 to 15 mm above the opening to the right upper lobe bronchus. The tube and fiberscope are advanced further until the orifice of the right upper lobe bronchus comes into full view through the endobronchial tube slit (Fig. 22-3). If necessary, the fiberscope can be advanced through the endobronchial tube slit into the right upper lobe bronchus to visualize the three segments of the right upper lobe. The fiberscope is then rotated 90 degrees counterclockwise to its neutral position and is advanced beyond the tip of the endobronchial tube to check the opening of the right middle and lower lobe bronchi. The fiberscope is then withdrawn from the endobronchial tube lumen and is passed through the tracheal lumen to check the position of the bronchial cuff and the opening of the left main stem bronchus (see Fig. 22-3).

2) After inspection of the right main stem bronchus and bronchus intermedius, the fiberscope is pulled back and rotated 90 degrees clockwise, and its tip is flexed anteriorly to visualize the orifice of the right upper lobe bronchus. While the fiberscope is held stationary, the tip of the fiberscope is returned to the neutral position. The tracheal cuff is deflated, and the double-lumen tube is advanced over the fiberscope into the right main stem bronchus. When the distal end of the endobronchial tube comes into view through the fiberscope, advancement of the tube stops (Fig. 22-4). At this position, the endobronchial tube slit would be at the level of the orifice for the right upper lobe bronchus. It is critical that during advancement of the tube, the fiberscope is stabilized. The fiberscope is then withdrawn a few millimeters inside the bronchial lumen and its tip is flexed anteriorly to visualize the orifice of the right upper lobe bronchus through the slit in the endobronchial tube. Minor adjustments of the tube often are necessary to have a clear view of the right upper lobe orifice. The asymmetric design of the bronchial cuff in right-sided tubes makes it possible to position the tube correctly when the right main stem bronchus is as short as 15 mm. The upper border of the bronchial cuff often is just at the level of the carina. As a result, air leak around the bronchial cuff is encountered more often with a right-sided tube than with a left-sided double-lumen tube after the patient is placed in the lateral position. Advancing the tube and fiberoptic repositioning are achieved easily while the patient is in the lateral decubitus position.

Blind Positioning of Left-Sided Double-Lumen Tube

If the fiberscope is not available, a left-sided double-lumen tube can be positioned blindly with a high degree of success. After the tube is placed in the trachea, it is advanced to the depth of 28 to 31 cm at teeth level, depending on the size of the patient. Both the tracheal and bronchial cuffs are inflated to separate the lungs. With clamping the tracheal

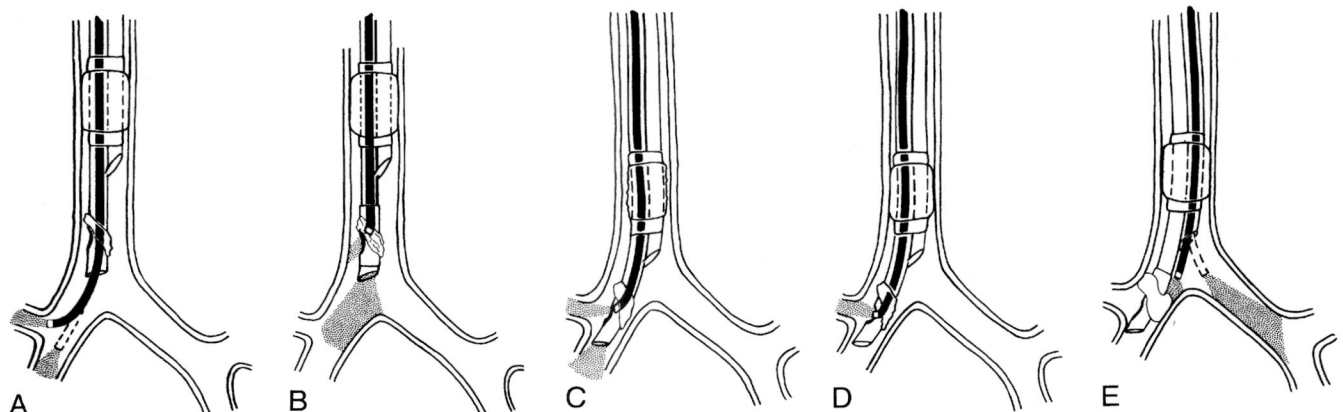

Fig. 22-3. Fiberscopic placement and positioning of right-sided, double-lumen tube. **A.** The fiberscope is passed through the bronchial lumen into the right main stem bronchus. The patency, length, and anatomy of the right main stem bronchus are evaluated. **B.** The fiberscope is withdrawn inside the bronchial lumen. The tip of the fiberscope is placed at the proximal end of the slit of the bronchial cuff 90 degrees rotated to the right and the tip is angulated anteriorly toward the lateral wall of the trachea. **C.** The tube and the fiberscope are then advanced together inside the right main stem bronchus until the orifice of the right upper lobe comes into view through the slit of the bronchial cuff. **D.** The fiberscope is advanced 2 to 3 mm through the bronchial slit inside the right upper lobe bronchus to visualize the three segments of the right upper lobe bronchus. **E.** The fiberscope is passed through the tracheal lumen to check the position of the bronchial cuff and the opening of the left main stem bronchus.

lumen, the breath sounds should now only be present on the left lung. If the breath sound is present on the right lung but is absent on the left lung, the bronchial tube has entered the wrong (right) bronchus. After ensuring the proper bronchial intubation, tracheal and bronchial tubes are clamped sequentially to confirm proper position (depth) of the tube. Placing the bronchial tube too deep blocks the left upper lobe bronchus, causing atelectasis, and may prevent air entry into the right lung. If the bronchial tube is not advanced far enough, the bronchial cuff herniates from left main stem bronchus, causing partial or complete occlusion of the right main stem bronchus, preventing ventilation of the right lung. Separation of the lungs will not be achieved if the bronchial tube remains above the carina.

Bahk and Oh (1998) have described another approach for blind positioning of the left-sided double-lumen tube using bronchial cuff pressure as a guide. The double-lumen tube is inserted deeply until resistance is felt. The pilot of the bronchial cuff is connected to a pressure gauge and the cuff is inflated with 1 to 2 mL of air until a pressure close to 30 cm H$_2$O is obtained. The double-lumen tube is slowly withdrawn until the intracuff pressure decreases to 15 cm. The bronchial cuff is deflated, and the tube is advanced 1 cm. This technique allowed Bahk and Oh to position the tube correctly 97.5% of the time.

Verifying the Functional Status of Double-Lumen Endobronchial Tubes

The following procedures help to determine whether the separation of the lungs has been achieved and adequate ven-

tilation can be applied through each lung. With a mechanical ventilator set at a tidal volume of 10 mL/kg of ideal body weight and a rate of eight breaths per minute, the exhaled tidal volume and the peak and plateau airway pressures are measured, and the expiratory flow rate on the respirometer and the humidification of both lumens by exhaled air are observed. After the tracheal connector tube is clamped, the breath sounds should only be present on the bronchial side, and the respirometer may show a 10 to 15% decrease in the exhaled tidal volume, whereas the expiratory flow rate should remain the same. The peak airway pressure should increase by no more than 50% when compared with two-lung ventilation. The clamp is then moved to the bronchial connector tube. Breath sounds should be present on the tracheal side. Tidal volume, expiratory flow rate, and peak airway pressure should change little from one lung to another. The clamp is then removed and the tube is secured. After the patient assumes the lateral position, the measurements of tidal volume and airway pressures are repeated with each lumen sequentially occluded.

Placement is considered unsatisfactory if separation of the lungs is incomplete; if when changing from two-lung ventilation to OLV, the tidal volume decreases by more than 15%; if the expiratory flow rate of either lung slows dramatically; or if the peak airway pressure increases by more than 50%.

If tube placement is unsatisfactory, the fiberscope is used to check the position of the bronchial cuff and to ensure that the tip of the bronchial or tracheal lumen is neither pressed against the bronchial or tracheal walls nor is blocking the orifice to the left upper lobe bronchus. For right-sided tubes,

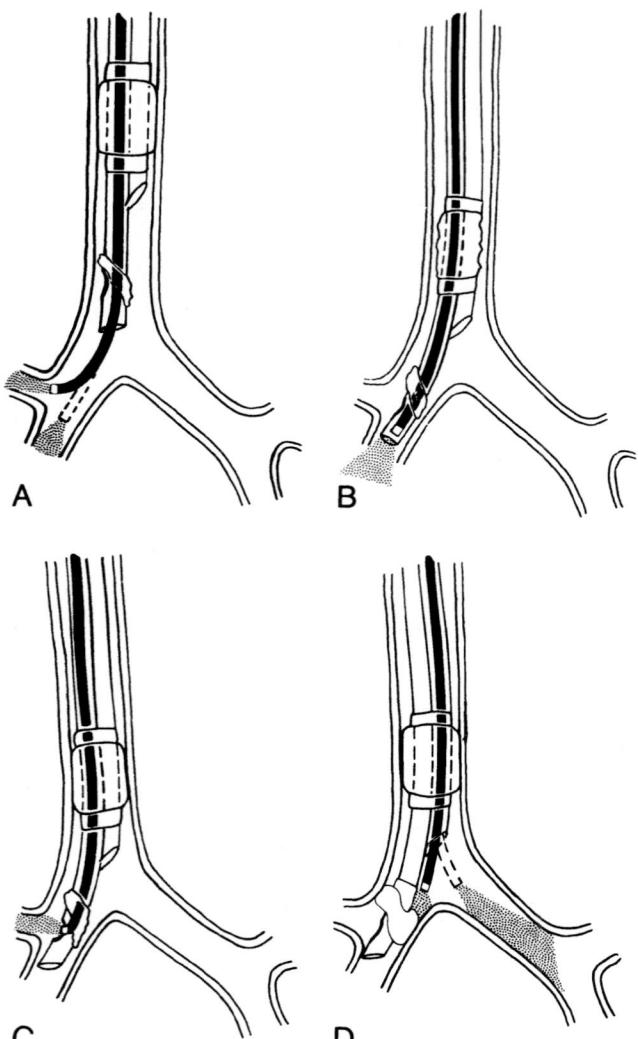

Fig. 22-4. Alternate approach to fiberscopic placement and positioning of right-sided, double-lumen endobronchial tube. **A.** The fiberscope is passed through the bronchial lumen into the right main stem bronchus. The patency, length, and anatomy of the right main stem bronchus are evaluated. The fiberscope is then rotated 90 degrees to the right and the tip of the fiberscope is flexed anteriorly to visualize the right upper lobe bronchus. While the fiberscope is held stationary, its tip is returned to the neutral position. **B.** The tracheal cuff is deflated, and the tube is advanced over the fiberscope into the right main stem bronchus until it comes into view beyond the tip of the fiberscope. **C.** The fiberscope is withdrawn inside the bronchial lumen to visualize the orifice of the right upper lobe bronchus through the slit of the bronchial cuff. **D.** The fiberscope is passed through the tracheal lumen to check the position of the bronchial cuff and the opening of the left main stem bronchus.

the position of the slit in the bronchial cuff with respect to the orifice of the right upper lobe must be rechecked as well as the patency of the right middle and lower lobes. In the presence of advanced lung disease with loss of lung tissue, empyema, or atelectasis, more exaggerated changes in the

preceding variables are expected when switching from two-lung ventilation to diseased lung ventilation. Bronchospasm may occur after bronchial intubation in lightly anesthetized patients or in patients with a reactive airway. In the presence of bronchospasm, more exaggerated changes in the variables are expected. These changes can be lessened by deepening anesthesia. The peak airway pressure and tidal volume measurement during OLV are presented in Table 22-1.

Univent Tubes

Introduced by Inoue and associates in 1984, the Univent tube is an endotracheal tube with two lumens, a larger lumen for ventilation and a smaller lumen that encloses the endobronchial blocker (Fig. 22-5). The endobronchial blocker has a hollow core that may be used for insufflation of oxygen, suctioning of secretions, and possibly jet ventilation.

The bronchial blocker has a high-volume cuff at its tip. A movable cap on the shaft of the bronchial blocker is incorporated to seal the leak between the shaft of the blocker and its housing lumen and to keep the blocker from moving. This cap is mounted over the blocker housing lumen as soon as the blocker is placed in the bronchus. An attached plug at the proximal end of the blocker is provided to close the internal lumen of the blocker. After tracheal intubation, the endobronchial blocker may be placed in either main stem bronchus. Inflating the tracheal and bronchial cuffs provides separation of the lungs and allows OLV. The Univent tube has a relatively larger external diameter for its internal diameter relative to a standard single-lumen tracheal tube.

The tip of the blocker is hard and repeated attempts during blind placement may traumatize the tracheobronchial tree. Arai and Hatano (1987) reported dislodgment of the tip of the bronchial blocker cap. If a Univent tube is left in place for postoperative ventilation, precaution should be taken to avoid inadvertent inflation of the bronchial blocker cuff; acute airway obstruction occurs if the blocker is moved into the trachea. One such incident was reported by Dougherty and Hannallah in 1992. MacGillivray (1988) reported that herniation of the bronchial cuff is common with the Univent tube because the Univent bronchial blocker cuff requires a larger volume of air (6 to 8 mL) compared with double-lumen tubes (2 to 3 mL). Herniation of the bronchial blocker cuff with the Univent tube is more likely when the blocker is placed inside the right main stem bronchus. Incomplete separation of the lungs is encountered also, although the incidence of such complications needs to be studied.

Positioning

First, the bronchial blocker is lubricated and moved a few times in and out of its housing lumen to ensure free movement of the blocker. The blocker is then retracted inside the housing lumen before the Univent tube is placed inside the trachea using a conventional intubation technique. The blocker can be advanced up to 8 cm beyond the tip of the main tube. For

Table 22-1. Tidal Volumes and Peak Airway Pressures during One-Lung Ventilation

	Supine		Lateral	
	TV	PAP	TV	PAP
Left-sided tube (N = 25)				
Two-lung ventilation	813 ± 71	22 ± 3	817 ± 76	23 ± 4
Left-lung ventilation	740 ± 81	34 ± 5	746 ± 62	35 ± 5
Right-lung ventilation	763 ± 71	32 ± 4	761 ± 65	33 ± 5
Right-sided tube (N = 8)				
Two-lung ventilation	818 ± 81	23 ± 4	821 ± 90	23 ± 4
Left-lung ventilation	750 ± 76	36 ± 5	759 ± 69	35 ± 3
Right-lung ventilation	722 ± 69	35 ± 7	758 ± 58	34 ± 4

TV, tidal volume of 10 to 12 mL/kg; PAP, peak airway pressure (cm H_2O).

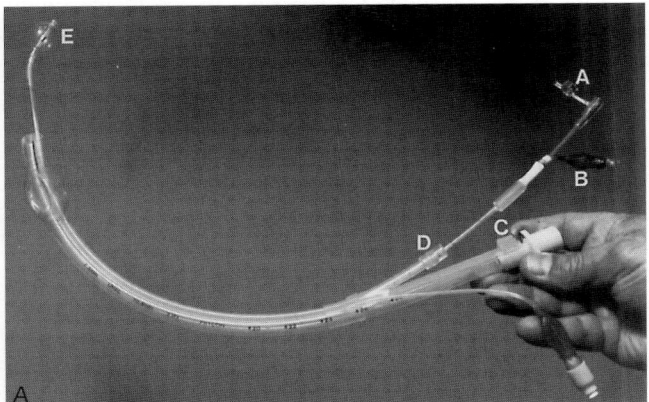

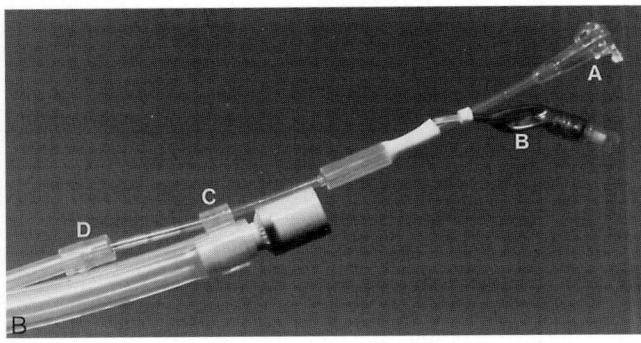

Fig. 22-5. Univent tube. **A.** The Univent tube with bronchial blocker is advanced outside the lumen of the tube and the balloon is inflated. A, attached plug to close the internal lumen of the blocker when one-lung ventilation is not applied. This cap should not be engaged (bronchial blocker lumen open) during one-lung ventilation. B, bronchial blocker inflation balloon. C, hand stopper secures the bronchial blocker and prevents its movement. D, movable cap on the shaft of the bronchial blocker to seal off the leak between the blocker and its housing lumen. It also keeps blocker from moving. E, inflated bronchial blocker cuff. **B.** Close-up of the proximal end of the Univent tube. A, plug that closes the lumen of the blocker. B, bronchial blocker balloon. C, hand stopper secures the bronchial blocker. D, movable cap on the shaft of bronchial blocker.

blind placement of the endobronchial catheter (blocker), the Univent tube is rotated 90 degrees toward the operative lung—the side to be blocked—and is taped in this position. The endobronchial blocker is then advanced several centimeters to enter the intended main stem bronchus.

After proper positioning of the endobronchial blocker, the shaft of the bronchial blocker is secured to the main tube with the cap and hand stoppers. Karwande (1987) reported successful blind placement of the blocker in 45 of 50 (90%) consecutive cases. For five patients, blocker placement had to be done under fiberscopic guidance. In two cases, the blocker was dislodged after it was positioned. Fiberscopic positioning was possible with the patient in the lateral decubitus position. Suctioning of the operative lung is possible through the lumen of the blocker, and, if necessary, the operative lung can be ventilated with HFV. Hultgren and coworkers (1986) reported successful use of Univent tubes in 30 consecutive patients, but in one patient, the blocker entered the wrong side. MacGillivray (1988) reported successful seal of the intended bronchus only in one of eight patients. Fiberscopic manipulation resulted in successful placement in another four patients, but a good seal could not be obtained in three patients and the Univent tube was replaced by a double-lumen tube.

Fiberscopic Positioning

After the Univent tube is placed in the trachea, the tube is rotated 90 degrees toward the operative side and taped. A bronchoscopic swivel adapter is connected to the tube. The fiberscope is passed through the Univent tube to identify the bronchial anatomy and to assist in bronchial blocker placement under fiberscopic observation. If the blocker enters the intended bronchus, the fiberscope is used for proper placement of the cuff inside the bronchus. If the blocker is not entering the intended bronchus, the fiberscope is used to guide the blocker toward the bronchus. The blocker is left in the desired position with the cuff deflated. Before going to OLV, the tube is disconnected from the anesthesia machine and the surgeon compresses the lung to collapse it. After the lung is collapsed, the blocker balloon is inflated to block the main stem bronchus. The listed advantages of the Univent tube include easier placement than occurs with double-lumen tubes and no need to change it for fiberoptic bronchoscopy or for postoperative ventilatory support. The functional status of OLV is checked as described in the section concerning double-lumen endobronchial tubes.

One-Lung Ventilation

Larsson and associates (1987) demonstrated that functional residual capacity (FRC), compliance, and fraction of total ventilation decrease slightly in the dependent lung when the anesthetized patient is placed in the lateral position. The FRC decreases further when the pleural cavity is opened, presumably because of further downward shift of the mediastinum. These findings are similar to those described by Froese and Bryan (1974), who attributed these changes in the lower dependent lung to compression of the lung by the weight of the mediastinum and to the elevation of the diaphragm. General anesthesia and muscle relaxation further decrease the FRC and cause atelectasis in the dependent lung. This decrease in FRC with maldistribution of ventilation in relation to perfusion results in further decrease in Pao_2. To avoid atelectasis of the dependent lung, tidal volume of 10 mL/kg is used. Kerr and associates (1973) showed that if minute ventilation is not decreased during OLV, the arterial carbon dioxide tension is maintained at a similar level to that of two-lung ventilation. The use of a large tidal volume to ventilate one lung results in increased peak airway pressure by approximately 50%. When airway pressure increases, Cote and colleagues (1983) showed that a larger proportion of the delivered total volume may be wasted because of the compression effect on gases, distention of the anesthesia machine breathing circuit, or both. The result may be a slight decrease in alveolar ventilation and increase in $Paco_2$.

The factors contributing to hypoxemia during OLV are shunting in the nonventilated lung, demonstrated by Kerr and associates (1973); ventilation-perfusion abnormalities in the ventilated lung; and reduction in the cardiac output. To counteract hypoxemia, the nonoperative lung should be ventilated with 100% oxygen with large tidal volume. In a small percentage of patients, however, the Pao_2 may still remain suboptimal. Various techniques have been applied to improve the arterial Pao_2 under these circumstances. One such technique is insufflation of oxygen into the nonventilated lung. Results are inconclusive; Rees and Wansbrough (1982) showed improvement, whereas Capan and associates (1980) showed that it is ineffective without application of continuous positive airway pressure (CPAP). The use of CPAP to the nonventilated lung improves arterial oxygenation, but it leads to overdistention of the operative lung and suboptimal surgical conditions. Applying HFJV with low driving pressure to the operative lung, Wilks and coworkers (1985) demonstrated improved oxygenation during OLV while maintaining a good surgical field. Nakatuska and associates (1988) compared the effect of CPAP and HFJV with the nondependent lung on the cardiac output and Pao_2 during OLV. The application of HFJV to the nondependent lung caused a significant increase in Pao_2 compared with deflation of the lung to atmosphere pressure and also maintained better cardiac output compared with CPAP. In addition, HFJV provides a quiet surgical field and satisfactory surgical exposure by delivering small tidal volumes with a low airway pressure in spite of vibratory movement of the surgical field. Malmkvist (1989) reported that intermittent reinflation of the upper lung with 2 L of oxygen every 5 minutes improved Pao_2 during OLV. It seems logical that gentle independent ventilation of the operative lung with small tidal volumes coordinated with the surgeon's movements would be a simple, inexpensive approach to improving Pao_2.

In the dependent lung, compression by the mediastinum and cephalad movement of the paralyzed diaphragm result in a decrease in FRC. This results in underventilation of well-perfused alveoli and an increase in airway closure. Trapped gas comes into equilibrium with mixed venous blood, contributing to arterial desaturation. Application of positive end-expiratory pressure to the dependent, ventilated lung may improve the situation. Khanam and Branthwaite (1973), however, observed that application of positive end-expiratory pressure to the ventilated lung may increase not only FRC, but also intra-alveolar pressure, shifting a higher proportion of pulmonary blood flow to the nonventilated lung, and contributing to a reduction in cardiac output.

Ashton and Cassidy (1985) showed that decreased cardiac output and systemic vascular resistance is induced by cardiac depressor reflexes as a result of stimulation of pulmonary stretch receptors. The magnitude of this cardiac depressor reflex is proportional to the magnitude of lung inflation. The effect of the reflex is antagonized by arterial baroreceptors, and a large tidal volume can reduce baroreceptor activity. This decrease in cardiac output in the face of systemic hypoxemia may lead to a significant decrease in oxygen transport. Depending on the degree of increased intra-alveolar pressure during application of positive end-expiratory pressure and its effect on the pulmonary circulation and cardiac output, the Pao_2 may increase, decrease, or remain the same, according to Katz and associates (1982). Pulmonary vascular congestion, interstitial edema of lower lung, hypovolemia, dysrhythmia, myocardial depression, and surgical manipulation can all decrease the cardiac output and contribute to arterial desaturation. Ligation of the branches of the pulmonary artery to the collapsed section of lung reduce the shunt and improve the arterial blood oxygenation.

Kerr (1973) and Flacke (1976) and their associates have shown that the shunt through the nonventilated lung is approximately 20 to 25% of the cardiac output. This degree of shunt is less than one would expect from complete collapse of the entire lung. Several factors are responsible.

First, the effect of gravity and hydrostatic pressure in the lateral decubitus position increases the blood flow to the dependent lung. Second, the operative lung may have decreased pulmonary blood flow, because of underlying pathologic conditions. Hurford and associates (1987) showed that in many patients, the degree of preoperative perfusion and ventilation of the operative lung correlated inversely with intraoperative oxygenation during OLV. Many patients with normal perfusion of the operative lung, however, did have an adequate level of oxygenation during OLV. This diminishes the value of operative lung ventilation perfusion as a predictor of hypoxemia during OLV. Third, Benumof (1978) showed that hypoxic pulmonary vasoconstriction increases pulmonary vascular resistance in the operative lung, which diverts blood flow away from the operative lung and toward the nonoperative, dependent lung.

Anesthetic concentrations of inhalation agents may abolish hypoxic pulmonary vasoconstriction, thereby increasing the blood flow to the nonventilated lung, and consequently decreasing the Pao$_2$. Rogers and Benumof (1983) showed that halothane and isoflurane cause an insignificant change in the amount of shunted blood when used in a concentration of one minimum alveolar concentration or less. To avoid the possible inhibition of hypoxic pulmonary vasoconstriction from higher concentrations of inhalation anesthetics and to minimize the respiratory depressant effect of high doses of narcotics, a combination of a narcotic and inhalation anesthetics may be particularly useful for intrathoracic operations.

Complications

Complications related to the isolation of lungs and application of OLV fall into two categories: technical and physiologic (Table 22-2). Because of the shape and large size of double-lumen tubes, the incidence of difficult tracheal intubation is higher than with the use of single-lumen tubes. The

Table 22-2. Complications of Bronchial Intubation and One-Lung Ventilation

Technical
  Unsuccessful or difficult intubation
  Trauma of the airway
    Minor trauma
    Rupture of tracheobronchial tree
  Improper position of the bronchial tube
    Tube not inserted far enough
    Intubation of wrong bronchus
    Tube inserted too far into the bronchus
  Tube dislodgement
Physiologic
  Hypoxemia
    Increased venous admixture
    Alteration of hypoxic pulmonary vasoconstriction
    Increased intra-alveolar pressure
    Atelectasis of dependent lung
    Decreased cardiac output

practical difficulties encountered with Robertshaw tubes were reviewed by Black and Harrison (1975). Complications included laceration of the tracheobronchial tree and malposition of the tube. The site of laceration is usually the posterior membranous wall of the trachea or a main stem bronchus. The diagnosis may be difficult to make, but it can be confirmed by fiberoptic bronchoscopy. Improper positioning of double-lumen endobronchial tubes reported by Read and associates (1977) includes failure to advance the tube far enough down the intended bronchus. Difficulties resulting from improperly positioned endobronchial tubes include incomplete isolation of the lungs; failure to collapse the operative lung; difficulty in ventilating one or both lungs; air entry into the wrong lung; and air trapping and unsatisfactory deflation of the lung. If not recognized, air trapping can eventually cause rupture of the lung and tension pneumothorax. If any of these circumstances arises, two-lung ventilation should be resumed, and the cause of the problem should be identified and corrected before OLV is attempted once again. The physiologic complication of OLV is hypoxemia.

BLOOD AND FLUID REPLACEMENT

Blood and fluid replacement during thoracic surgery is a delicate task and an extremely important part of the anesthetic management. Great care must be taken not to overload the circulation, especially in patients undergoing lobectomy or pneumonectomy, because the pulmonary venous capacitance is greatly reduced. Blood loss during most intrathoracic operations does not necessitate a transfusion, but major bleeding can occur at any time. A large intravenous cannula that allows blood and fluid to be administered rapidly is essential, as is the ready availability of blood. All fluids, especially blood, should be warmed during administration.

The perioperative fluid regimen recommended by Giesecke and Egbert (1986) is to replace insensible loss occurring while the patient receives nothing by mouth with a maintenance-type solution of 5% dextrose in water, or 5% dextrose in 0.45% saline at a rate of 2 mL/kg per hour. During surgery, in addition to 2 mL/kg per hour of insensible loss, an additional 6 mL/kg per hour of replacement-type solution lactated Ringer's, 5% dextrose in lactated Ringer's or saline, is recommended.

This regimen is followed only for the first 1 or 2 hours of the operation to avoid overhydration. Hutchin and associates (1969) discussed the danger of overhydration of patients during pneumonectomy. Infusion of large volumes of fluids may improve the urine output and circulatory dynamics, but at the risk of developing pulmonary edema and impaired lung mechanics. Twigley and Hillman (1985) stated that crystalloid solutions given intraoperatively go to the interstitial space. Baek and associates (1975) noted that excessive amounts of crystalloid solutions increase interstitial fluid, which causes peripheral and pulmonary edema without correcting the plasma volume deficit. To maintain an adequate blood volume and urine output and to avoid over-hydration and congestion of the tissues, including the lungs, Twigley and Hillman (1985) suggested using colloid solutions perioperatively. This suggestion is based on the fact that most intraoperative cardiovascular changes are secondary to an absolute or relative change in intravascular circulating volume, caused by bleeding and vasodilatory effects of anesthetic drugs. These changes are ideally corrected with a colloid. Colloid solutions are useful to expand plasma volume and should be considered for replacing blood and fluid loss when the patient's blood pressure and pulse rate reflect signs of hypovolemia. The controversy of crystalloid or colloid use for blood and fluid replacement continues unresolved. In addition to monitoring of blood pressure, pulse rate, and urine output, monitoring of CVP and pulmonary artery occlusive pressure is helpful in guiding appropriate fluid therapy, especially in patients with poor general health and during operations with major blood and fluid losses. As indicated by Wittnich and colleagues (1986), however, care is needed in techniques of measurement and interpretation of pulmonary artery occlusive pressure. They have shown that after pneumonectomy, inflation of the balloon of the pulmonary artery catheter can result in considerable occlusion of the remaining cross-sectioned area of pulmonary circulation. This increase in right ventricular afterload results in reduced cardiac output and reduced left atrial pressure. Therefore, pulmonary artery occlusive pressure may reflect the correct pressure of left atrial pressure, although this is a result of an acute change in cardiac output. Measuring pulmonary wedge pressure by advancing the catheter to peripheral vessels and without inflation of the balloon provides more accurate reading of the existing pressures.

Continuous measurement of CVP and pulmonary artery wedge pressures is helpful in patients with myocardial disease or advanced pulmonary disease. In a patient with a healthy heart, however, a serious overload of crystalloid solutions is possible without significant elevation of the CVP or pulmonary artery wedge pressure, particularly if infusion of fluid is constant over several hours. Soft tissue edema and increased urine output are the best signs of overload with intravenous fluids. Edema is seen most easily in the scleral conjunctiva. Congestion and edema of tissues caused by overhydration are also position dependent. In the lateral decubitus position, the nonoperative, healthy lung is dependent and accumulates more fluids. A moderate fluid overload can result in decreased Pao_2 intraoperatively and moderate to severe hypoxemia in the immediate postoperative period.

The shortage of blood, together with transfusion hazards, has stimulated a search for alternatives to the use of homologous blood since the 1970s. Transmission of acquired immunodeficiency syndrome through blood transfusion has further increased the public's fear of accepting blood transfusion. Autologous transfusion by aspiration from the surgi-cal field was reported by Bergman and coworkers (1974). Brewster and associates (1979) showed that intraoperative autotransfusion significantly reduced the use of homologous blood transfusion. Normovolemic hemodilution is possible on the day of the operation if the physical condition of the patient permits.

SPECIFIC PROCEDURES AND SUGGESTED MANAGEMENT

Bronchoscopy

A new airway device, the laryngeal mask airway (LMA), has become the technique of choice for fiberoptic bronchoscopy performed under general anesthesia or under topical anesthesia in critically ill patients. The LMA has made sharing of the airway by the surgeon and anesthesiologist an easy task, without compromising the patient's ventilation. The LMA was developed by Brain (1983) of England and consists of a silicone rubber tube with a distal end opening at a 30-degree angle into an elliptical-shaped mask (Fig. 22-6). Two bars are incorporated into the junction of the tube and mask, preventing the epiglottis from herniating into the tube. Before use, the cuff is deflated so that the edge of the cuff appears smooth and faces away from the mask inlet.

The tube of the LMA is held between index finger and thumb, with the tip of the index finger placed at the anterior aspect of the tube, at the junction of the tube and mask. The patient's head is extended in sniffing position and the LMA is placed into the mouth (Fig. 22-7). The tip of the LMA is pressed upward against the hard palate and advanced as deep as possible toward the hypopharynx using the index finger. As the index finger is withdrawn, the LMA is advanced further until resistance is felt. The cuff is inflated with the recommended volume of air (20, 30, and 40 mL for sizes 3, 4, and 5, respectively) and the LMA is secured with tape. With perfect positioning, the laryngeal inlet is in full view through the LMA (Fig. 22-8). Ferson and colleagues (1997) have reported that the LMA, in contrast to the endotracheal tube, allows a complete fiberoptic bronchoscopic survey of the larynx and trachea.

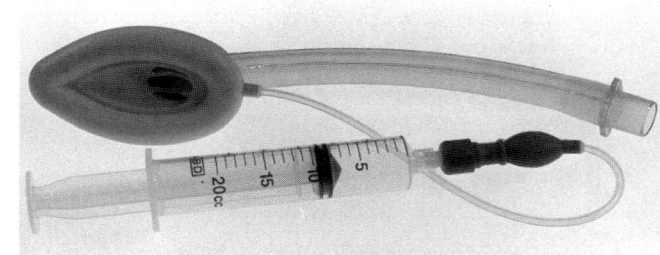

Fig. 22-6. The laryngeal mask airway with cuff inflated.

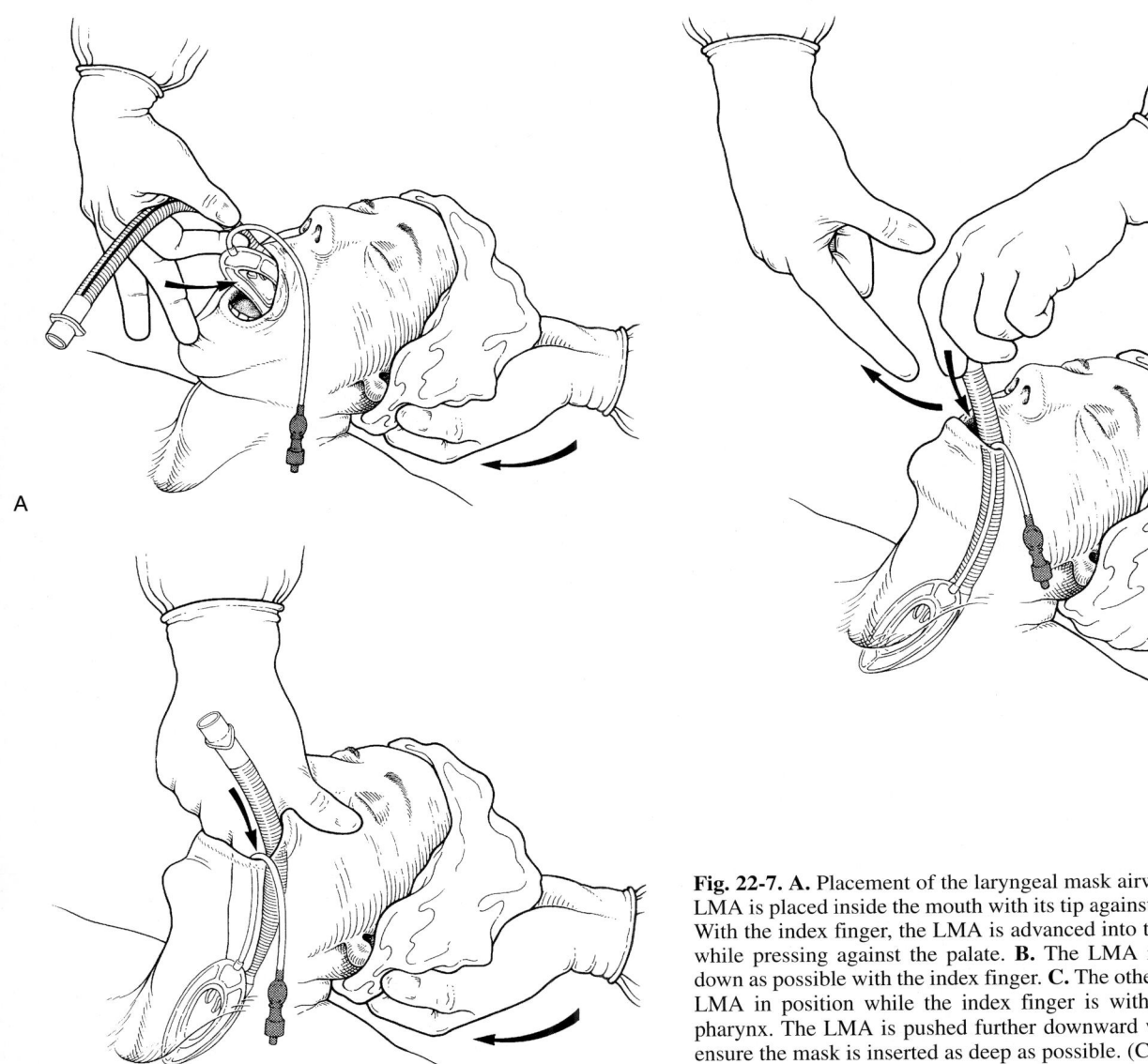

A

B

C

Fig. 22-7. A. Placement of the laryngeal mask airway (LMA). The LMA is placed inside the mouth with its tip against the hard palate. With the index finger, the LMA is advanced into the hypopharynx while pressing against the palate. **B.** The LMA is pushed as far down as possible with the index finger. **C.** The other hand holds the LMA in position while the index finger is withdrawn from the pharynx. The LMA is pushed further downward with the hand to ensure the mask is inserted as deep as possible. (Courtesy of LMA North America, Inc., San Diego, CA.)

Fiberoptic Bronchoscopy under Topical Anesthesia

Brimacombe and colleagues (1992, 1997) reported the use of LMA for fiberoptic bronchoscopy under topical anesthesia. Administration of glycopyrrolate, 0.3 to 0.4 mg intramuscularly, 30 minutes before bronchoscopy, or 0.2 to 0.3 mg intravenously, 10 minutes before bronchoscopy, is essential, because the airway must be dry for the topical anesthesia to be effective. After sedation, 10% aerosolized lidocaine is sprayed on the base of the tongue and tonsillar fossae; after 1 minute, lidocaine jelly is spread on the base of the tongue with a tongue blade. Lidocaine, 3 mL of 4%, is injected through the cricothyroid membrane to provide anesthesia of the larynx and trachea. If injection of local anesthetic through the cricothyroid membrane is undesirable or contraindicated, laryngotracheal anesthesia

is achieved by spraying local anesthetic through the fiberscope working channel ("spray as you go" technique). Graham and associates (1992) have shown that injection of lidocaine through the cricothyroid membrane provides a better topical anesthesia of the larynx and trachea, causes less cough, and is as acceptable to the patient as the spray as you go technique.

The LMA is placed, and the bronchoscopy swivel adapter is mounted on the LMA to allow passage of the bronchoscope. The LMA is connected to the anesthesia breathing system, which allows assistance and monitoring of the patient's ventilation.

If LMA is not available, an Ovassapian (1987) intubating airway (Fig. 22-9) is used, which keeps the tongue in an anterior position, facilitates exposure of the larynx, and protects the bronchofiberscope from being bitten by the patient.

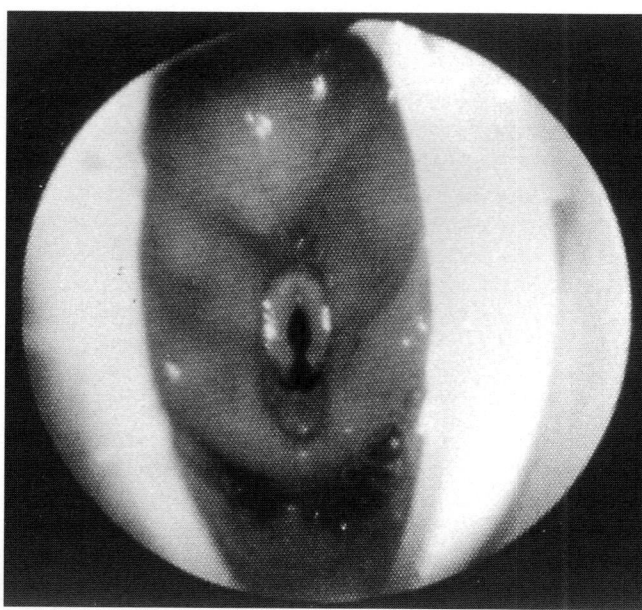

Fig. 22-8. Fiberscopic view of the larynx through a perfectly positioned laryngeal mask airway (LMA). The epiglottis is pushed upward and outside of the LMA, allowing complete exposure of the laryngeal inlet. In most cases, the tip of the epiglottis remains inside of the LMA, blocking 25 to 50% of the laryngeal view. (Courtesy of LMA North America, Inc., San Diego, CA.)

The bronchofiberscope is advanced through the intubating airway to expose the larynx.

Fiberoptic Bronchoscopy under General Anesthesia

When general anesthesia is required for fiberoptic bronchoscopy, traditionally the anesthesia is provided by an endotracheal tube or a face mask. The ratio of the external diameter of the bronchofiberscope to that of the internal diameter of the endotracheal tube is critical because the instrument reduces the effective ventilatory area of the endo-

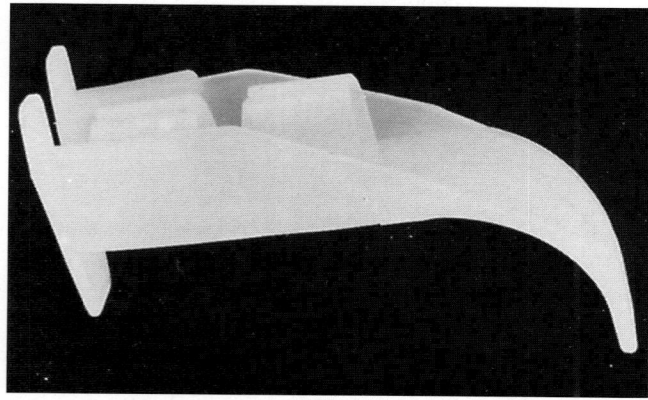

Fig. 22-9. The Ovassapian fiberoptic intubating airway.

tracheal tube lumen. A 5-mm fiberoptic bronchoscope reduces the internal diameter of an 8-mm endotracheal tube to such a degree that effective positive pressure ventilation is impossible, which limits the time for bronchoscopy.

Using a face mask for administration of anesthesia also limits the time of bronchoscopy because ventilation is interrupted during bronchoscopy. Modification of the face mask to provide an entry port for fiberoptic bronchoscopy allows bronchoscopy without interruption of ventilation, but the maintenance of the airway and ventilation of the patient could be difficult or impossible in some patients. The LMA not only provides an excellent airway for the patient but also allows unhurried examination of the larynx, vocal cord, upper trachea, and bronchial tree. The LMA permits the use of a larger fiberoptic bronchoscope without compromising airway resistance or effective ventilation.

Rigid Bronchoscopy

For rigid bronchoscopy in an anesthetized and paralyzed patient, ventilation can be carried out by intermittent positive pressure ventilation (IPPV) using a ventilating bronchoscope; by manual jet ventilation using a Venturi injector device described by Sanders (1967); by HFJV, as introduced by Erickson and Sjostrand (1977); or by positive-negative external compression or HFPPV reported by Hayek (1985). Manual jet ventilation can be achieved through a rigid bronchoscope or a fiberoptic bronchoscope, as described by Satyanarayana (1980). Vourc'h and coworkers (1983) compared manual jet ventilation with HFJV during bronchoscopy in patients with tracheobronchial stenosis. Arterial blood gas tensions were identical during both manual jet ventilation and HFJV at a rate of 150 per minute. From the endoscopist's point of view, HFJV is preferable to manual jet ventilation because the tracheobronchial wall remains immobile. During HFPPV, no air entrainment occurs, so that anesthetic gases can be delivered at known concentrations. With Hayek external positive-negative internal compression, the airway is not intubated and the surgeon has access to the airway without interference.

Mediastinoscopy

Mediastinoscopy can be performed using local anesthesia, but endotracheal general anesthesia is more pleasant for the patient, provides more flexibility for the surgeon, and facilitates management of a major complication that may occur during this procedure. Compression of the innominate artery by the mediastinoscope can diminish or block blood flow to the right carotid and subclavian arteries. Lee and Salvatore (1976) reported a sudden loss of pulse and blood pressure in the right arm during mediastinoscopy, which was misdiagnosed as a cardiac arrest. The right radial artery pulse should therefore be monitored by palpation or finger plethysmography to detect compression of the innominate artery. Sudden hypotension, bradycardia, or dysrhythmia may occur as a result of mechanical stimulation or compression of the trachea, vagus nerve, or great vessels. Repositioning of the mediastinoscope and intravenous administration of atropine or ephedrine may be necessary to restore the pulse rate and blood pressure. Massive bleeding caused by accidental injury to a major vessel is a distinct but rare possibility. The management of such bleeding necessitates thoracotomy and major surgical intervention. The anesthesiologist should be ready for massive replacement of fluids and blood. An intraoperative tension pneumothorax manifested by increased peak airway pressure, hypotension, and cyanosis is uncommon but requires immediate diagnosis and treatment, as stated by Furgang and Saidman (1972). Other reported complications associated with mediastinoscopy, reported by Ashbaugh (1970), include injury to the recurrent laryngeal nerve, phrenic nerve, or esophagus; transient hemiparesis; and air embolism.

Cysts of the Lung

IPPV or vigorous coughing might result in a dangerous increase in alveolar pressure and rupture of a cyst. Ting and associates (1963) reported that the size of a cyst increases if it is in communication with the bronchus and has a valve-type action so that air may enter but not leave the cyst during IPPV. In a closed cyst, administration of nitrous oxide should be avoided, as was suggested by Isonhower and Cucchiara (1976), because it could rapidly increase the volume of and pressure within the cyst. As the size of the cyst increases, it may cause compression atelectasis and mediastinal shift and interfere with adequate gas exchange. Ventilation also may become inadequate if a significant portion of the tidal volume enters and leaves the communicating cyst without participating in gas exchange. Overinflation and rupture of the cyst may cause tension pneumothorax and cardiopulmonary insufficiency.

If the disease is confined to one lung, Isonhower and Cucchiara (1976) suggested that isolation of the lungs with a double-lumen endobronchial tube avoids IPPV to the diseased side. Bilateral air cysts represent a difficult problem because of the possible increase in their size and their interference with gas exchange in the dependent lung while the surgeon operates on the upper lung. Bilateral thoracotomy may be necessary. Normandale and Feneck (1985) successfully applied HFJV for the anesthetic management of patients with bullous cystic lung disease.

Bronchopleural Fistula

The complications associated with a large bronchopleural fistula are loss of ventilation, contamination of the contralateral lung, and development of pneumothorax when IPPV is applied. These complications are best avoided by the passage of an endobronchial tube before induction of general anesthesia. Securing the airway with a double-lumen endobronchial tube in a conscious patient is a safe, but not always easy, approach. Placing patients in a head-up lateral decubitus position with the affected side down minimizes the chance of secretions moving into the tracheobronchial tree during intubation of the trachea. Francis and Smith (1962) indicated that the double-lumen endobronchial tube permits IPPV of the healthy lung, without the loss of minute ventilation through the fistula, and prevents soiling of the healthy lung. If tracheal intubation is difficult or not desirable in the conscious patient, general anesthesia with spontaneous ventilation can be used until the airway is secured with a double-lumen endobronchial tube. If a double-lumen tube cannot be applied and a single-lumen tube is placed, Baker and coworkers (1971) suggested maintaining spontaneous ventilation until the chest is opened. During surgery, the air leak can be minimized by manually packing the lung. Carlon and coworkers (1980) successfully applied high-frequency positive pressure and carbon dioxide removal in a patient with a large bronchopleural fistula. Hildebrand and associates (1984) indicated that HFJV at 100 cycles per minute was unsuitable during lobectomy with an open bronchus and resulted in a rapid deterioration in PaO_2 and an increase in $PaCO_2$. Their results conflict with those of Moulaert and Rolly (1983), who claimed that ventilation with an open bronchus was possible with HFJV at a rate of 250 cycles per minute.

Pneumothorax and Hemothorax

An important feature in the anesthetic management of these conditions is to drain them during local anesthesia before inducing anesthesia or administering IPPV.

Tracheal Resection

A thorough preoperative evaluation and understanding of the airway problem is essential. Good rapport must be established for the patient, and heavy premedication should be avoided. Close communication between the surgeon and anesthesiologist is essential during tracheal reconstruction, and each one should be fully aware of the other's plan, approach, and readiness before induction of anesthesia.

Various methods of maintaining adequate ventilation have been applied during operations on the trachea or bronchi. Use of a single-lumen endotracheal tube placed above the tracheal lesion preoperatively and advanced inside the trachea or bronchi below the tracheal lesion during surgery has been described by Belsey (1950) and Geffin and associates (1969). It is safer to secure the airway while the patient is awake.

If an awake intubation is not possible, a slow inhalation induction with a halogenated anesthetic agent with oxygen should be performed, with spontaneous ventilation maintained until tracheal intubation is achieved. The bronchofiberscope can be used to apply topical anesthesia to the larynx and trachea, to evaluate the site and degree of tracheal stenosis, and to intubate the trachea. The instrument enables the anesthesiologist to place the tip of the tube above the stenotic area and to avoid any trauma. After exposure of the trachea, as the surgeon starts resecting the lesion, the orotracheal tube is advanced beyond the lesion into the lower section of the trachea. The surgeon completes the resection and anastomosis in the presence of the endotracheal tube. To avoid the presence of an endotracheal tube in the surgical field, Akdikmen and Landmesser (1965) and Geffin (1969) described the use of two separate endotracheal tubes. The first endotracheal tube is placed orally above the tracheal lesion. The second sterile, armored endotracheal tube is inserted by the surgeon into the distal trachea or one of the main stem bronchi after cutting the trachea distal to the lesion. The second endotracheal tube is then connected to the anesthesia machine using sterile corrugated tubing and a Y-piece, and anesthesia is continued. After resection of the lesion and placement of sutures in the posterior tracheal wall, the surgeon removes the endotracheal tube placed in the distal trachea. The original orotracheal tube is advanced beyond the suture line into the lower trachea, or one of the main stem bronchi, until the surgeon completes the repair of the trachea.

A third approach is the use of HFJV through a small catheter, as described by Erickson (1975) and Rogers (1985) and their coworkers; manual jet ventilation, as reported by Lee and English (1974); and HFPPV as applied by El-Baz and colleagues (1982). Scamman and Choi (1986) used a sterile nasogastric tube for application of low-frequency jet ventilation and measurement of end-tidal CO_2 during tracheal resection. The distal end of the nasogastric tube was cut off above the highest side hole and placed 2 cm into the distal stump of the trachea. The larger lumen was connected to a Sander's jet apparatus and the smaller to a CO_2 analyzer. Normal arterial and end-tidal gas tensions were maintained while the surgeon completed the posterior and lateral wall anastomosis. Neuman and associates (1984) described successful use of HFJV for tracheal resection in a 7-year-old child.

To avoid contamination of the operating room from inhalation agents, intravenous anesthetics are used during HFPPV or jet ventilation. Early extubation is highly desirable to minimize the compromise of blood flow to the trachea. Woods (1961) and Coles (1976) and their associates applied extracorporeal circulation for management of tracheobronchial resection.

Laser Surgery

Laser surgery of the airway presents several potential anesthetic problems. These include ventilation and oxygenation through a compromised and shared airway and hazards introduced by the laser beam. The major hazards from laser surgery are fires and destruction of normal tissues. Fire can occur when the laser strikes a rubber or plastic endotracheal tube in an oxygen-rich anesthetic mixture. Nitrous oxide, like oxygen, supports combustion, whereas halogenated anesthetic agents are not flammable and do not support combustion. To minimize the danger of fire, Brutinel and associates (1983) recommended using 50% oxygen or less in nitrogen, whereas Eisenman and Ossoff (1986) favor a mixture of oxygen and helium during general anesthesia. The use of metallic or noncombustible disposable endotracheal tubes and protection of standard rubber or plastic endotracheal tubes by wrapping them with aluminum or copper tape have been thoroughly reviewed by Hermens and coworkers (1983). Endotracheal tubes wrapped with metallic tape may cause pharyngeal and laryngeal injury because of rough edges, and pieces of tape can loosen, break off, and be aspirated. All oil-based ointments and lubricants should be avoided because they are combustible and can be ignited. In case of fire, the procedure should be stopped and the endotracheal tube should be removed immediately. The lungs as well as the trachea may be injured by either smoke inhalation or a direct thermal burn.

Using a Hayek (1985) positive and negative external compressor allows air exchange without intubation. This device is in its early stages of experimental use. If proved safe and effective, it will eliminate the need for intubation, and therefore during total intravenous anesthesia, the surgeon will have sole access to the airway.

The surgical field should be immobile to minimize the chance of laser damage of normal tissue. Choice of anesthesia for bronchoscopic laser surgery depends on the surgical technique and the age and condition of the patient. Rontal and associates (1986) favor topical anesthesia with sedation whenever possible, but particularly in patients with higher grade airway obstruction. General anesthesia is the method of choice for most children and for adults who cannot tolerate local anesthesia. Dumon and associates (1984) favor spontaneous ventilation, whereas Brutinel (1983) and Vourc'h (1983) and their coworkers recommend controlled ventilation. If jet ventilation is chosen, scavenging of inhalation anesthetic agents is difficult, and total intravenous anesthesia must be provided. Prolonged respiratory depression, causing the need for postoperative ventilatory support, is a potential complication of total intravenous anesthesia. Whatever the anesthetic technique, the basic principle of anesthetic management of patients with a compromised airway should be followed. Communication between the anesthesiologist and the surgical team is essential, and a plan for management of total airway obstruction must be decided before induction of anesthesia. All routine safety precautions during laser surgery, both for the patient and the operating room personnel, should be observed. A sign noting that a laser is in use should be placed on the outside of the door. Finally, postoperative care is extremely important, as respiratory depression, laryngospasm, bronchospasm, airway obstruction, and hemorrhage can all occur and require immediate treatment.

REFERENCES

Abe K, et al: Arterial oxygenation and shunt fraction during one-lung ventilation: a comparison of isoflurane and sevoflurane. Anesth Analg 86:1266, 1998.

Akdikmen S, Landmesser CM: Anesthesia for surgery of the intrathoracic portion of the trachea. Anesthesiology 26:117, 1965.

Arai T, Hatano Y: Yet another reason to use a fiberoptic bronchofiberscope to properly site a double-lumen tube. Anesthesiology 66:581, 1987.

Ashbaugh DG: Mediastinoscopy. Arch Surg 100:586, 1970.

Ashton JH, Cassidy SS: Reflex depression of cardiovascular function during lung inflation. J Appl Physiol 58:137, 1985.

Baek SM, et al: Plasma expansion in surgical patients with high central venous pressure: the relationship of blood volume to hematocrit, CVP, pulmonary wedge pressure and cardiorespiratory changes. Surgery 78:304, 1975.

Bahk JH, Oh YS: A new and simple maneuver to position the left-sided double-lumen tube without the aid of fiberoptic bronchoscopy. Anesth Analg 86:1271, 1998.

Baker WL, et al: Management of bronchopleural fistulas. J Thorac Cardiovasc Surg 62:393, 1971.

Baraka A, et al: One lung ventilation of children during surgical excision of hydatid cysts. Br J Anaesthesiol 54:523, 1982.

Belsey R: Resection and reconstruction of the intrathoracic trachea. Br J Surg 38:200, 1950.

Benumof JL: Mechanism of decreased blood flow to atelectatic lung. J Appl Physiol 46:1047, 1978.

Bergman D, et al: Intraoperative autotransfusion during emergency thoracic and elective open heart surgery. Ann Thorac Surg 18:590, 1974.

Bjork VO, Carlens E: The prevention of spread during pulmonary resection by the use of a double-lumen catheter. J Thorac Cardiovasc Surg 20:151, 1950.

Black AMS, Harrison GA: Difficulties with positioning Robertshaw double-lumen tubes. Anaesth Intensive Care 3:299, 1975.

Brain AIJ: The laryngeal mask—a new concept in airway management. Br J Anaesth 55:801, 1983.

Brewster DC, et al: Intraoperative autotransfusion in major vascular surgery. Am J Surg 137:507, 1979.

Brimacombe J, et al: A potential new technique for awake fiberoptic bronchoscopy—use of the laryngeal mask airway. Med J Aust 156:876, 1992.

Brimacombe JR, Brain AIJ, Berry AM: The Laryngeal Mask Airway: A Review and Practical Guide. London: WB Saunders, 1997.

Brutinel WM, et al: Bronchoscopic therapy with neodymium-yttrium-aluminum-garnet laser during intravenous anesthesia. Chest 84:518, 1983.

Burton NA, et al: Advantages of a new polyvinyl chloride double lumen tube in thoracic surgery. Ann Thorac Surg 36:78, 1983.

Capan LM, et al: Optimization of arterial oxygenation during one-lung anesthesia. Anesth Analg 59:847, 1980.

Carlens E: A new flexible double-lumen catheter for bronchospirometry. J Thorac Cardiovasc Surg 18:742, 1949.

Carlon GC, et al: High frequency positive pressure ventilation in management of a patient with bronchopleural fistula. Anesthesiology 52:60, 1980.

Cay DL, et al: Selective bronchial blocking in children. Anaesth Intensive Care 3:127, 1975.

Coles JC, et al: A method of anesthesia for imminent tracheal obstruction. Surgery 80:379, 1976.

Cote CJ, et al: Wasted ventilation measured in vitro with eight anesthetic circuits with and without inlet humidification. Anesthesiology 59:442, 1983.

Dalens B, et al: Selective endobronchial blocking vs selective intubation based on 10 variables. Crit Care Med 10:643, 1982.

Dougherty P, Hannallah M: A potentially serious complication that resulted from improper use of the Univent tube. Anesthesiology 77:835, 1992.

Dumon JF, et al: Principles for safety in application of neodymium-YAG laser in bronchology. Chest 86:163, 1984.

Edwards EM, Hatch DJ: Experiences with double-lumen tubes. Anaesthesia 20:461, 1965.

Eisenman TS, Ossoff RH: Anaesthesia for bronchoscopic laser surgery. Otolaryngol Head Neck Surg 94:45, 1986.

El-Baz N, et al: One-lung high frequency positive pressure ventilation for sleeve pneumonectomy: an alternative technique. Anesth Analg 60:638, 1981.

El-Baz N, et al: One-lung frequency ventilation for tracheoplasty and bronchoplasty: a new technique. Ann Thorac Surg 34:564, 1982.

Erickson I, Sjostrand I: High frequency positive pressure ventilation and the pneumatic valve principle in bronchoscopy under general anesthesia. Acta Anesthesiol Scand (Suppl) 64:83, 1977.

Erickson I, et al: High frequency positive pressure ventilation during transthoracic resection of tracheal stenosis and during preoperative bronchoscopic examination. Acta Anaesthesiol Scand 19:13, 1975.

Ferson DZ, et al: The laryngeal mask airway: a new standard for airway evaluation in thoracic surgery. Ann Thorac Surg 63:768, 1997.

Flacke JW, et al: Influence of tidal volume and pulmonary artery occlusion on arterial oxygenation during endobronchial anesthesia. South Med J 69:617, 1976.

Francis JG, Smith KG: An anesthetic technique for the repair of bronchopleural fistula. Br J Anaesth 34:817, 1962.

Froese AB, Bryan AC: Effects of anesthesia and paralysis on diaphragmatic mechanics in man. Anesthesiology 41:242, 1974.

Furgang FA, Saidman LJ: Bilateral tension pneumothorax associated with mediastinoscopy. J Thorac Cardiovasc Surg 63:329, 1972.

Geffin B, et al: Anesthetic management of tracheal resection and reconstruction. Anesth Analg 48:884, 1969.

Giesecke AH, Egbert LD: Perioperative fluid therapy; crystalloids. In Miller RD (ed): Anesthesia. 2nd Ed. New York: Churchill Livingstone, 1986, p. 1313.

Ginsberg RJ: New technique for one-lung anesthesia using an endobronchial blocker. J Thorac Cardiovasc Surg 82:542, 1981.

Glenski JA, et al: High frequency, small volume ventilation during thoracic surgery. Anesthesiology 64:211, 1986.

Graham DR, et al: Comparison of three different methods used to achieve local anesthesia for fiberoptic bronchoscopy. Chest 102:704, 1992.

Hayek Z, et al: External high frequency ventilation without intubation. Crit Care Med 19:406A, 1985.

Hermens JM, et al: Anesthesia for laser surgery. Anesth Analg 62:218, 1983.

Hildebrand PJ, et al: High frequency jet ventilation: a method for thoracic surgery. Anaesthesia 39:1091, 1984.

Hogg CE, Lorhan PH: Pediatric bronchial blocking. Anesthesiology 33:560, 1970.

Hultgren BL, et al: A new tube for one lung ventilation: experience with Univent tube [abstract]. Anesthesiology 65:A481, 1986.

Hurford WE, et al: The use of ventilation/perfusion lung scans to predict oxygenation during one-lung anesthesia. Anesthesiology 67:841, 1987.

Hutchin P, et al: Pulmonary congestion following infusion of large fluid loads in thoracic surgical patients. Ann Thorac Surg 8:339, 1969.

Inoue J, et al: Endotracheal tube with movable blocker to prevent aspiration of intratracheal bleeding. Ann Thorac Surg 37:497, 1984.

Isonhower N, Cucchiara RF: Anesthesia for vanishing lung syndrome: report of a case. Anesth Analg 55:750, 1976.

Jenkins VA, Clark G: Endobronchial anesthesia with the Carlens catheter. Br J Anaesth 30:12, 1958.

Karwande S: A new tube for single lung ventilation. Chest 92:761, 1987.

Katz JA: Pulmonary oxygen exchange during endobronchial anesthesia: effects of tidal volume and PEEP. Anesthesiology 56:164, 1982.

Kerr JH, et al: Observations during endobronchial anesthesia. I. Ventilation and carbon dioxide clearance. Br J Anaesth 45:159, 1973.

Khanam T, Branthwaite MA: Arterial oxygenation during one-lung anesthesia. Anaesthesia 28:280, 1973.

Larsson A, et al: Variation in lung volume and compliance during pulmonary surgery. Br J Anesth 59:585, 1987.

Lee J, Salvatore A: Innominate artery compression simulating cardiac arrest during mediastinoscopy: a case report. Anesth Analg 55:748, 1976.

Lee P, English IC: Management of anesthesia during tracheal resection. Anaesthesia 29:305, 1974.

MacGillivray RG: Evaluation of a new tracheal tube with a movable bronchial blocker. Anesthesia 43:687, 1988.

Malmkvist G: Maintenance of oxygenation during one-lung ventilation effect of intermittent reinflation of the collapsed lung with oxygen. Anesth Analg 68:763, 1989.

Moulaert P, Rolly G: High frequency of jet ventilation for pulmonary resection. In Sheck PA, Sjostrand NH, Smith RB (eds): Perspectives in High Frequency Ventilation. Boston: Martinus-Nijhoff, 1983, p. 227.

Nakatuska M, et al: Unilateral high-frequency jet ventilation during one-lung ventilation for thoracotomy. Ann Thorac Surg 44:654, 1988.

Neuman CG, et al: High-frequency jet ventilation for tracheal resection in a child. Anesth Analg 63:1039, 1984.

Normandale JP, Feneck RO: Bullous cystic lung disease: its anesthetic management using high frequency jet ventilation. Anaesthesia 40:1182, 1985.

Ovassapian A: A new fiberoptic intubating airway. Anesth Analg 66:S132, 1987.

Ovassapian A: Fiberoptic aided bronchial intubation. In Ovassapian A (ed): Fiberoptic Endoscopy and the Difficult Airway. Philadelphia: Lippincott-Raven, 1996, p. 117.

Ovassapian A, Schrader S: Fiberoptic-aided bronchial intubation. Semin Anesth 6:133, 1987.

Ovassapian A, et al: Endobronchial intubation using flexible fiberoptic bronchoscope. Anesthesiology 59:A501, 1983.

Rao CC, et al: One-lung pediatric anesthesia. Anesth Analg 60:450, 1981.

Read RC, et al: Prospective study of the Robertshaw endobronchial catheter in thoracic surgery. Ann Thorac Surg 24:156, 1977.

Rees D, Wansbrough SR: One-lung anesthesia: percent shunt and arterial oxygen tension during continuous insufflation of oxygen to the nonventilated lung. Anesth Analg 61:507, 1982.

Rigg D: A comparison of the Robertshaw and Carlens-type double-lumen tubes for thoracic anesthesia. Anaesth Intensive Care 8:460, 1980.

Robertshaw FL: Low resistance double-lumen endobronchial tubes. Br J Anaesth 34:576, 1962.

Rogers RC, et al: High frequency jet ventilation for tracheal surgery. Anaesthesia 40:32, 1985.

Rogers SN, Benumof JL: Halothane and isoflurane do not impair arterial oxygenation during one-lung ventilation to patients undergoing thoracotomy. Anesthesiology 59:A532, 1983.

Rontal M, et al: Anesthetic management for tracheobronchial laser surgery. Ann Otol Rhinol Laryngol 95:556, 1986.

Sanders RD: Two ventilating attachments for bronchoscopes. Del Med J 39:170, 1967.

Satyanarayana T, et al: Bronchofiberscope jet ventilation. Anesth Analg 59:350, 1980.

Scamman FL, Choi WW: Low frequency jet ventilation for tracheal resection. Laryngoscope 96:678, 1986.

Shinnick JP, Freedman AP: Bronchofiberoptic placement of a double-lumen endotracheal tube. Crit Care Med 10:544, 1982.

Smith RB, et al: High frequency ventilation during pulmonary lobectomy: three cases. Respir Care 26:437, 1981.

Thornburn JR, et al: Comparison of the effects of atropine and glycopyrrolate on pulmonary mechanics in patients undergoing fiber-optic bronchoscopy. Anesth Analg 65:1285, 1986.

Ting EY, et al: Mechanical properties of pulmonary cysts and bullae. Am Rev Respir Dis 87:538, 1963.

Twigley AJ, Hillman KM: The end of the crystalloid era? Anaesthesia 40:860, 1985.

Vale R: Selective bronchial blocking in a small child. Br J Anaesth 41:453, 1969.

Vourc'h G, et al: High frequency jet ventilation versus manual jet ventilation during bronchoscopy in patients with tracheo-bronchial stenosis. Br J Anaesth 55:969, 1983.

Weinrich A, et al: Continuous ketamine infusion for one-lung anesthesia. Can J Anaesth 27:485, 1980.

Wilks D, et al: Selective high frequency jet ventilation of the operative lung improves oxygenation during thoracic surgery. Anesthesiology 63:A586, 1985.

Wittnich C, et al: Misleading "pulmonary wedge pressure" after pneumonectomy: its importance in postoperative fluid therapy. Ann Thorac Surg 42:192, 1986.

Woods F, et al: Resection of the carina and mainstem bronchi with extracorporeal circulation. N Engl J Med 254:492, 1961.

CHAPTER 23

High-Frequency Jet Ventilation

Christopher J. O'Connor and Nabil M. El-Baz

High-frequency ventilation (HFV), a method of mechanical ventilation, was first described in 1969 by Öberg and Sjöstrand, who observed that positive-pressure ventilation produced circulatory disturbances that interfered with hemodynamic measurements. To reduce the impact of mechanical ventilation on hemodynamics, they reduced tidal volumes to values approximating dead space volumes and simultaneously increased respiratory rates to 100 breaths per minute (BPM) to maintain minute volume and adequate ventilation. In 1967, Sanders demonstrated the first clinical application of HFV by using intermittent jets of compressed gas during bronchoscopic surgery. Heijman and colleagues (1972) extended these basic features of HFV by demonstrating adequate ventilation and oxygenation in surgical patients using jet ventilation at very high respiratory rates. Since these early experimental and clinical investigations, HFV has assumed a prominent place in the ventilatory management of critically ill neonates and during laryngoscopy, bronchoscopy, microlaryngeal surgery, and major airway surgery. The primary appeal of HFV during major airway surgery is its ability to maintain adequate gas exchange via small catheters while allowing unrestricted access to the open surgical airway. This chapter focuses on the use of HFV during tracheal and carinal resection, sleeve pneumonectomy, and routine pulmonary resection.

PRINCIPLES OF GAS DELIVERY

High-frequency ventilation is a general term encompassing several types of ventilation that use tidal volumes equal to or less than the volume of anatomic dead space delivered at high respiratory rates. Standiford and Morganroth (1989) have described three types of HFV: 1) high-frequency positive-pressure ventilation (HFPPV); 2) high-frequency jet ventilation (HFJV); and 3) high-frequency oscillation ventilation (HFO). HFPPV, which is similar to HFJV, uses a ventilator with reduced internal volumes and noncompliant ventilatory circuits to deliver tidal volumes of 1 to 5 mL/kg

at respiratory rates of 60 to 100 BPM. Because no gas entrainment occurs, the fractional inspired concentration of oxygen (FIO_2) in the delivered gas determines the oxygen content delivered to the patient. As with HFJV, exhalation is a passive process. HFJV involves the delivery of small jets of fresh gas from a high-pressure source (i.e., 50 psi) through a small, noncompliant catheter placed either through an endotracheal tube, through an additional lumen of the endotracheal tube, or into the airway directly. Gas flow is interrupted at periodic intervals by an electromagnetic solenoid valve to produce respiratory rates of 60 to 1600 BPM, although the usual frequency is 100 to 200 BPM (Fig. 23-1). A reducing valve that regulates the pressure of the gas supply produces the driving gas pressure (DGP) of the system. Optimally, the gas is humidified at the distal tip of the jet catheter. When the catheter is placed through an endotracheal tube, additional gases may be introduced at the proximal end of the endotracheal tube using a side port adapter. During major airway or laryngeal surgery, exhalation is passive and expired gases exit either through the opened endotracheal tube or through the open airway. During HFJV in the nonoperative critical care setting, unidirectional valves allow expiration through a separate expiratory line where positive end-expiratory pressure (PEEP) can be added to enhance oxygenation.

The high velocity of the jet entrains gas from the surrounding airway and produces a tidal volume comprised of the volume of the jet and the volume of the entrained gas. Because the amount of entrainment is difficult to quantify, the precise tidal volume and FIO_2 of the delivered gas are unknown, although typical tidal volumes are 3.0 to 4.5 mL/kg. The FIO_2 of the jet gas source—usually 1.0—and that of the entrained gas determine the final oxygen content of the gas delivered to the patient.

HFO uses a piston pump to oscillate gas in the airway at tidal volumes well below anatomic dead space volumes and at frequencies of 60 to 3600 BPM. In contrast to HFPPV and HFJV, inspiration and expiration are active processes. As noted by Clark and Gerstmann (1998), HFO is primarily

345

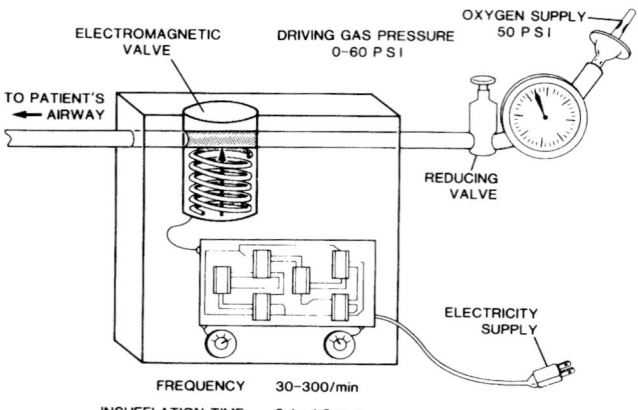

Fig. 23-1. A schematic of the high-frequency ventilator developed by the Department of Anesthesiology at Rush Medical College. The electromagnetic valve interrupts the driving gas pressure flow at a set frequency. The essential features of this system are similar to other high-frequency ventilators. From El-Baz N: One-lung high-frequency ventilation for tracheoplasty and bronchoplasty: a new technique. Ann Thorac Surg *34*:565, 1982. With permission.

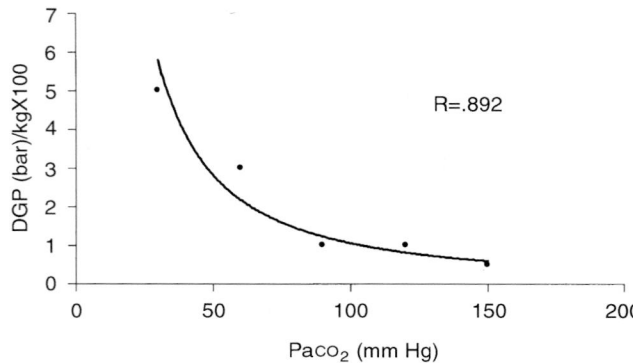

Fig. 23-2. The relationship between driving gas pressure (DGP) and $Paco_2$. At a frequency of 100 breaths per minute, the higher the DGP, the greater the tidal volume and minute ventilation and therefore the more effective elimination of CO_2. Hence, $Paco_2$ decreases with increased DGP. Modified from Klain M: Gas exchange in high frequency ventilation: an experimental study. *In* Scheck PA, Sjostrand UH, Smith RB (eds): Perspectives in High Frequency Ventilation. Boston: Martinus Nijhoff, 1983, p. 158. With permission.

used in the management of neonatal respiratory failure and is rarely used during thoracic surgery.

PRINCIPLES OF GAS EXCHANGE DURING HIGH-FREQUENCY JET VENTILATION

The precise mechanism by which gas transport and gas exchange occurs during HFJV is unknown. During conventional mechanical ventilation, gas transport in the major airways occurs by convection, or bulk flow, while gas exchange at the alveolocapillary membrane occurs by molecular diffusion. Consistent with the simple clinical observation of chest wall movement during HFJV, Klain (1985), Rouby and colleagues (1985), and Spoelstra and Tamsma (1987) documented that convective flow is also important during HFJV. Rouby and colleagues (1985) established the important role of bulk gas flow during HFJV by demonstrating a close relationship between tidal volume and $Paco_2$. Other mechanisms must be invoked, however, because tidal volumes as low as dead space volumes cannot support conventional convective gas transport. A process termed *augmented diffusion* has been described by Fredberg and colleagues (1980), who observed that the high velocity of gas flow during HFJV produces increased turbulence in the large conducting airways. These turbulent flows produce eddy currents that may enhance mixing of gas particles and partly account for gas transport not achieved by convection.

Although the mechanism of gas transport remains ill defined, the determinants of oxygenation and ventilation have been more thoroughly investigated. As shown by Klain (1985) and Calkins and colleagues (1985), the elimination of CO_2 during HFJV is dependent on minute ventilation and

is thus similar to conventional mechanical ventilation. During HFPPV, however, minute ventilation is more dependent on tidal volume and less dependent on respiratory rate. Tidal volume is primarily increased by increasing the DGP (Fig. 23-2). Although tidal volume may also be augmented by increasing either the inspiratory time or the size of the injection catheter, these are comparatively less important interventions. During HFJV, CO_2 elimination decreases and $Paco_2$ increases as ventilatory rates exceed 200 to 300 BPM (Fig. 23-3). This apparent paradox has been explained by air trapping at high frequencies that decreases tidal volume and impairs gas flow and CO_2 elimination.

Oxygenation is dependent on lung volume and mean airway pressure, both a function of the DGP. In addition, increasing inspiratory times (and thus tidal volume) and adding PEEP can also improve oxygenation. Benhamou and coworkers (1984) demonstrated a close relationship between Pao_2 and increases in mean airway pressure during HFJV in patients with acute respiratory failure. This increase in lung volume and recruitment of alveoli produces a PEEP effect that is largely responsible for the maintenance of oxygenation during HFJV. Although oxygenation is maintained with HFJV in a manner similar to standard mechanical ventilation, it does so with lower peak airway pressures and less overdistention of alveoli. Hazardous levels of auto-PEEP may, however, be produced by excessive jet frequencies (i.e., more than 200 to 300 BPM) or high inspiratory times (i.e., more than 40%) that limit the time for exhalation and may lead to gas trapping. This should be avoided in patients with chronic obstructive lung disease or asthma in whom inhomogeneous regional time constants for alveolar emptying and increased lung compliance may enhance the risk of gas trapping.

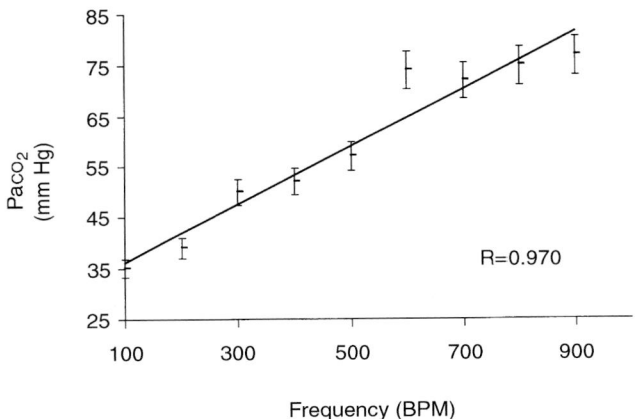

Fig. 23-3. The relationship between Pa_{CO_2} and ventilator frequency in anesthetized dogs. For a constant driving gas pressure and inspiratory time, a near linear relationship exists between Pa_{CO_2} and jet ventilator frequency. BPM, breaths per minute. Modified from Calkins JM, et al: Effects of high frequency jet ventilation design and operational variables upon arterial blood gas tensions. *In* Scheck PA, Sjostrand UH, Smith RB (eds): Perspectives in High Frequency Ventilation. Boston: Martinus Nijhoff, 1983, p. 72. With permission.

INTRAOPERATIVE APPLICATIONS OF HIGH-FREQUENCY VENTILATION

Laryngoscopy and Microlaryngeal Surgery

Endoscopic microlaryngeal laser surgery presents a challenge to the anesthesiologist and surgeon because the airway has to be shared for the control of ventilation and for instrumentation and excision of the lesion. HFJV with narrow caliber tubes or catheters permits satisfactory oxygenation and ventilation yet also provides unobstructed surgical access to the operative field. Eriksson and colleagues (1975), Carden (1973), one of us (N.E.B.) and colleagues (1985), and Giunta and colleagues (1989) have described the successful use of HFJV for endoscopic laryngeal laser surgery. One of us (N.E.B., 1985) used a 2-mm internal-diameter catheter for HFJV during laser excision of stenotic lesions of the larynx, trachea, and bronchi using an air-oxygen mixture with an F_{IO_2} below 0.3. This low F_{IO_2} minimizes the risk of catheter and airway fires, and the continuous outflow of gases prevents the contamination of the lungs by blood and debris, while simultaneously eliminating the smoke of tissue vaporization. Giunta and colleagues (1989) modified this approach in 228 adults undergoing laryngeal surgery by positioning a second rigid catheter distal to the jet catheter to measure airway pressure and to sample end-tidal CO_2. More recently, Strashnov and coworkers (1995) reported their experience with HFJV during 296 laryngeal procedures using smaller diameter catheters (1.4 to 1.8 mm) with elastic fixators attached to their distal end. These fixators stabilize the catheter in the center of the tracheal lumen and minimize

catheter "whip," a phenomenon that may lead to catheter displacement and ultimately contribute to tracheal mucosal injury. During HFJV for resection of stenotic laryngeal and tracheal lesions, an unobstructed path must be provided for the outflow of expiratory gases to prevent gas trapping and barotrauma.

Tracheal Resection and Sleeve Pneumonectomy

As with laryngeal surgery, HFJV provides optimal surgical access to the entire circumference of the transected airway and facilitates the construction of an airtight anastomosis while supporting ventilation and oxygenation. Early clinical reports by Lee and English (1974) and Eriksson and coworkers (1975) demonstrated the feasibility of HFJV using small catheters during tracheal resection. Dartevelle and colleagues (1988) reported the utility of HFJV in a larger series of 55 patients undergoing sleeve pneumonectomy. One of us (N.E.B.) and colleagues (1982) described the use of HFJV for six patients undergoing tracheal and carinal resection and sleeve pneumonectomy. The method of HFJV ventilation described in that report remains similar to our current approach. After anesthetic induction, a standard 6.5- to 7.5-mm internal diameter endotracheal tube is placed either above or through the tracheal stenosis, depending on the diameter of the lesion. Standard ventilation through the endotracheal tube is discontinued and the tube withdrawn to a more proximal position when the trachea is opened. A sterile, 45-cm long, 2-mm internal diameter catheter with a single opening at the tip is then passed through the endotracheal tube and positioned by the surgeon below the tracheal opening (Fig. 23-4). Any narrow-diameter catheter can be used, and several have been reported in the literature, including 14F suction catheters [as described by Perera and colleagues (1993)] and small-bore manometer tubing [as used by McKinney and coworkers (1988)]. For high tracheal lesions, the catheter tip is placed just above the carina. After completion of the anastomosis, the catheter is removed, the endotracheal tube is advanced, and conventional ventilation is resumed. The continuous outflow of gases from the distal airway prevents contamination of the lung with blood and debris, and the opened airway allows for egress of expired gases. In addition, the small tidal volume prevents significant mediastinal movement. For patients with critically stenotic tracheal lesions, the trachea can be directly intubated with the 2-mm catheter and HFJV maintained from the induction of anesthesia until the completion of the procedure. In these instances, placing a nasogastric tube to prevent gastric distention resulting from continuous positive airway pressure in the pharynx is useful.

For distal tracheal resections or sleeve pneumonectomies in which part of the carina is resected, several modifications of the aforementioned technique of HFJV are required to maintain oxygenation and ventilation. With distal tracheal resections, the distance between the incision and the carina

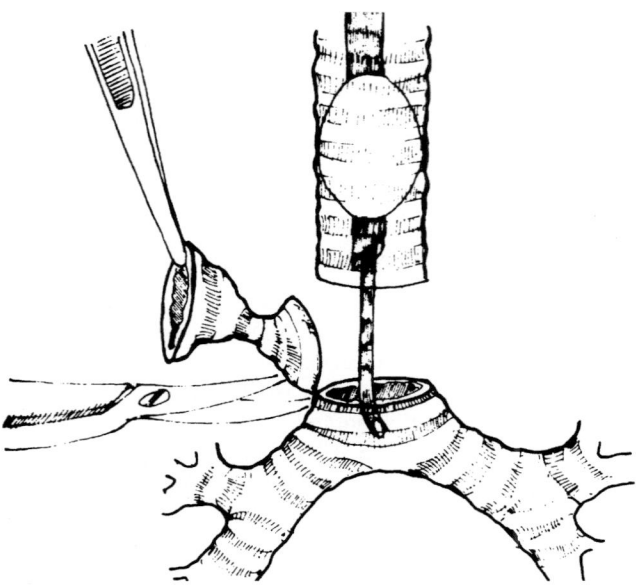

Fig. 23-4. High-frequency jet ventilation during tracheal resection. The catheter tip is placed through the withdrawn endotracheal tube to a position just below the tracheal incision but above the carina. From Giunta F, et al: Clinical uses of high frequency jet ventilation in anaesthesia. Br J Anaesth *63*:102S, 1989. With permission.

is too short to allow reliable catheter placement above the carina. In this instance, a catheter can be placed in each bronchus and bilateral HFJV performed using two jet ventilators as described by Watanabe and colleagues (1988) and McClish and coworkers (1985) (Fig. 23-5). Alternatively,

both catheters can be connected by a Y-piece to a single jet ventilator, as described by McKinney and colleagues (1988). Finally, a single catheter may be passed into the left main stem bronchus for one-lung ventilation (Fig. 23-6). Although oxygenation may be impaired owing to intrapulmonary shunt through the collapsed right lung, the gas jet emerging from the left main stem bronchus may partially ventilate the right upper lobe. One of us (N.E.B., 1982) achieved a mean PaO_2 of 230 mm Hg using this single jet catheter technique in patients undergoing carinal resection. Because of its simplicity, the single catheter technique may

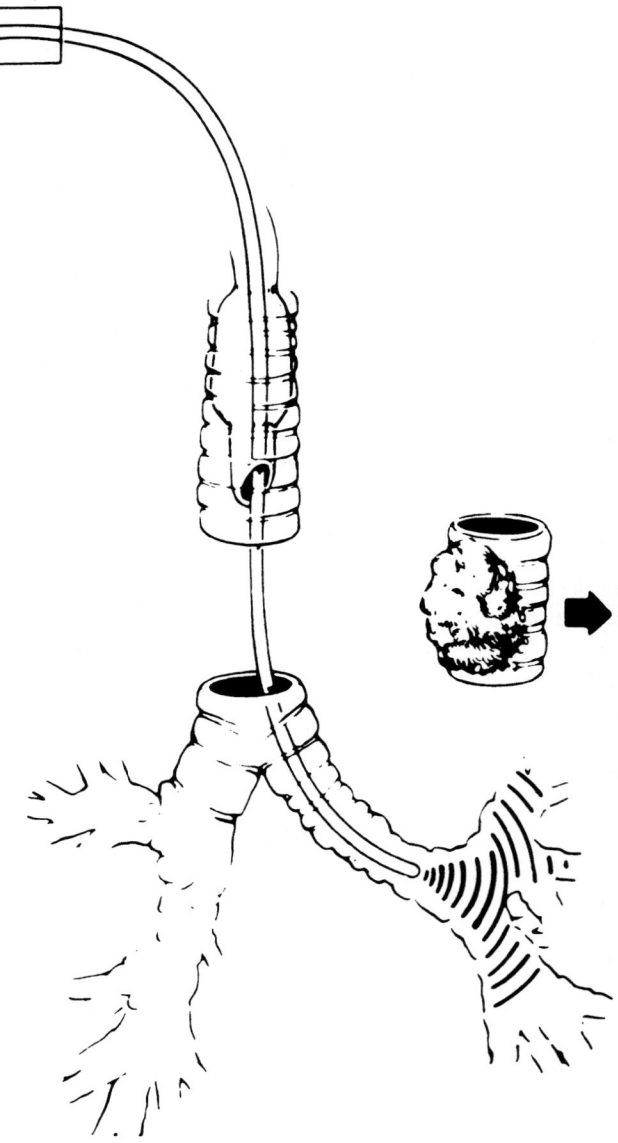

Fig. 23-6. High-frequency jet ventilation catheter placement for distal tracheal resections. The catheter is placed through an endotracheal tube into the left main stem bronchus for high-frequency jet ventilation of the left lung. With this technique, some ventilation of the right upper lobe occurs, minimizing shunt through the collapsed right lung.

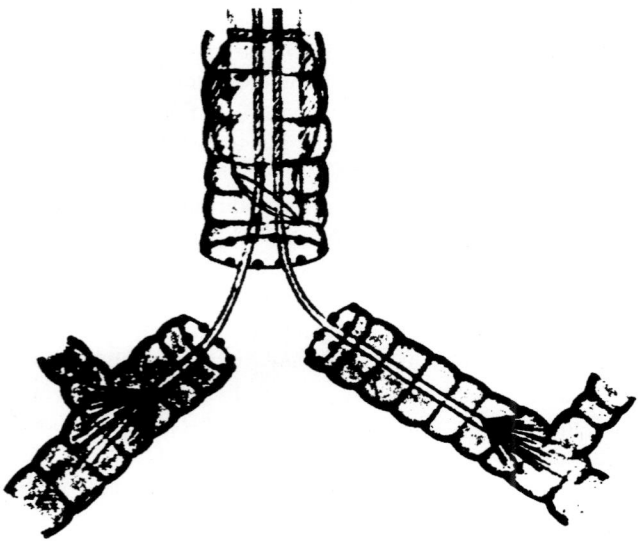

Fig. 23-5. High-frequency jet ventilation catheter position during carinal or low tracheal resections. Bilateral high-frequency jet ventilation is performed via a catheter placed in each main stem bronchus. From McClish A, et al: High-flow catheter ventilation during major tracheobronchial reconstruction. J Thorac Cardiovasc Surg *89*:508, 1985. With permission.

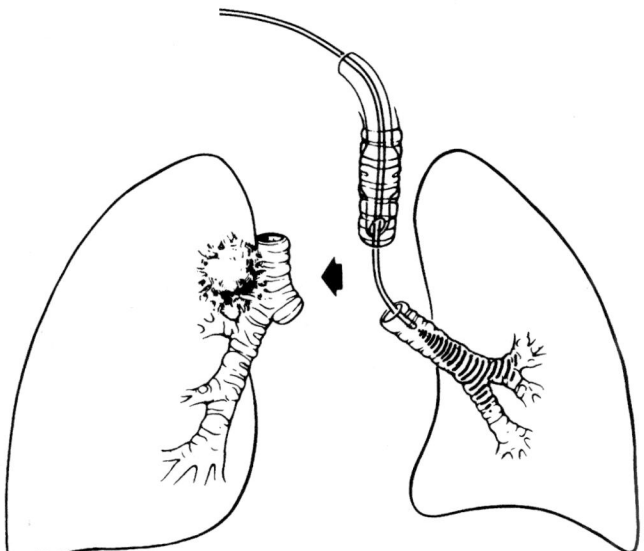

Fig. 23-7. High-frequency jet ventilation catheter in the left main stem bronchus during right sleeve pneumonectomy. The catheter is placed through an endotracheal tube and positioned in the left main stem bronchus just below the carina.

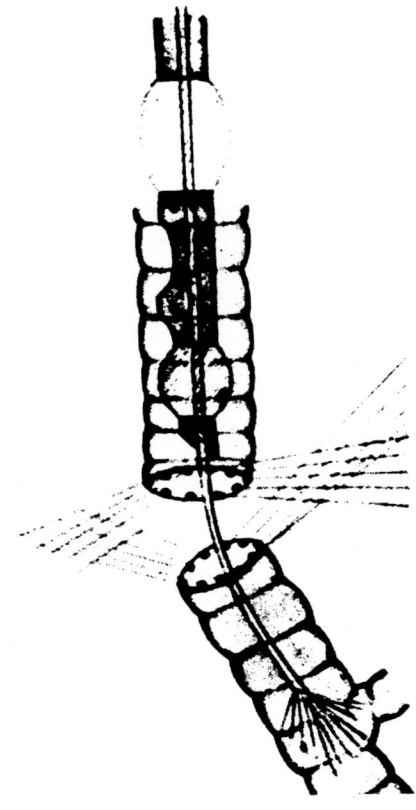

Fig. 23-8. High-frequency jet ventilation via a jet catheter placed through the bronchial lumen of a left endobronchial tube into the left main stem bronchus during right sleeve pneumonectomy. From McClish A, et al: High-flow catheter ventilation during major tracheobronchial reconstruction. J Thorac Cardiovasc Surg 89:508, 1985. With permission.

be the most sensible approach for distal tracheal or carinal resections. Bilateral catheter use can be reserved for patients who develop refractory hypoxemia during one-lung ventilation or when two jet ventilators are available.

HFJV is also an effective ventilatory technique during sleeve pneumonectomy. The catheter can be passed into the nonoperative main stem bronchus via a single-lumen endotracheal tube and one-lung jet ventilation performed as previously described (Fig. 23-7). Alternatively, a double-lumen endobronchial tube can be placed in the nonoperative bronchus and conventional one-lung ventilation performed until transection of the carina. At this point, the endobronchial tube is withdrawn into the proximal trachea and the jet catheter passed through the bronchial lumen into the dependent lung for one-lung HFJV (Fig. 23-8). Disadvantages of this approach are the potential problems of double-lumen endobronchial tube placement because of encroachment of the tumor near the carina and the expected hypoxemia resulting from one-lung ventilation. Ransom and colleagues (1996) provided a novel approach to this problem by using the bronchial blocker of a Univent tube (see Chapter 22) to collapse the right lung during the initial dissection phase of a right sleeve pneumonectomy. Immediately before resection of the airway, the blocker was repositioned in the left main stem bronchus and the left lung was ventilated using HFJV via the blocker lumen (Fig. 23-9).

HFJV overcomes many of the obstacles associated with ventilation during major airway surgery and provides a simple and effective alternative to conventional ventilation with single-lumen endotracheal tubes.

Other Areas of Thoracic Surgery

In contrast to airway surgery, HFJV has a limited role during routine pulmonary resection because of the effectiveness of conventional ventilation using double-lumen endobronchial tubes and continuous positive airway pressure applied to the nonventilated lung. Several authors, including Nevin and colleagues (1987) and Hildebrand and colleagues (1984), have documented the efficacy of HFJV as the sole ventilatory technique for thoracic surgery. Glenski and colleagues (1986) and Howland and colleagues (1987), however, observed that, despite adequate gas exchange during thoracotomy, HFJV produced lung hyperinflation that interfered with surgical exposure. A more logical application of HFJV during pulmonary resection, as documented by El-Baz and colleagues (1982), Nakatsuka and colleagues (1988), Godet and colleagues (1994), and Dikmen and colleagues (1997), is HFJV of the collapsed lung to maintain or improve oxygenation. Typically, an F_{IO_2} of 1.0 and low DGPs (i.e., 10 to 15 psi) provide adequate oxygenation without significant lung distention.

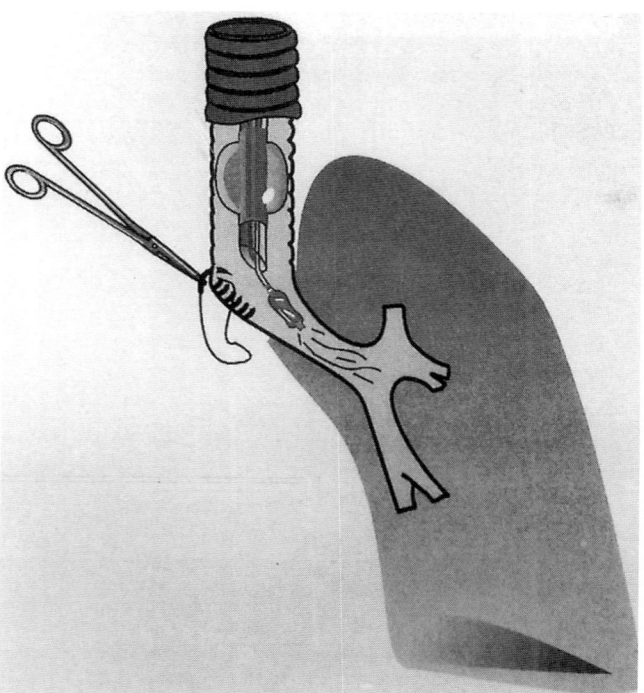

Fig. 23-9. Use of the bronchial blocker of a Univent tube for high-frequency jet ventilation of the left lung during right sleeve pneumonectomy. After one-lung ventilation of the left lung with the bronchial blocker in the right lung, the blocker is repositioned in the left main stem bronchus for high-frequency jet ventilation of the left lung during right pneumonectomy. From Ransom E, et al: Univent tube provides a new technique for jet ventilation. Anesthesiology 84:724, 1996. With permission.

Other Applications

Reports by Payne and colleagues (1990) and Wippermann and colleagues (1995) and others have suggested a role for HFJV in the management of bronchopleural fistulae because of a reduction in peak airway pressures. However, controlled trials comparing conventional ventilation and HFJV have not been performed to confirm the potential advantage of HFJV for patients with significant air leak. Smith and colleagues (1996) used percutaneous transtracheal jet ventilation for airway resuscitation during failed intubation while Sivarajan and coworkers (1995) demonstrated effective jet ventilation through the suction channel of a fiberoptic bronchoscope as an aid in difficult intubations. Cooper and Cohen (1994) also described the use of jet ventilation catheters for the elective management of difficult airways.

Guidelines for Intraoperative High-Frequency Jet Ventilation

The following are suggested guidelines for initial jet ventilator settings when using HFJV during major airway or thoracic surgery: 1) a DGP of 20 psi, 2) an inspiratory time of 30%, 3) an FIO_2 of 1.0, and 4) a frequency of 100 to 150 BPM. If these settings result in hypoxemia, the first step should be to ensure correct catheter position above the carina for tracheal resections or above the orifice of the upper lobe for carinal or sleeve resections. If catheter position is satisfactory, then the DGP should be increased in 5-psi increments to a maximum of 40 psi, although adequate oxygenation is almost always achieved with DGPs of 20 to 30 psi. Higher pressures may occasionally be required for patients with low lung compliance in whom a higher DGP is necessary to deliver an adequate tidal volume. If these maneuvers fail to improve oxygenation, the inspiratory time may be increased to 35 to 40%. If hypercarbia develops after confirmation of correct catheter position, the same sequence of changes used to improve oxygenation also improves CO_2 elimination. If hypercarbia develops despite increased DGPs and inspiratory times, the frequency may be increased in 10-BPM increments to a maximum of 250 BPM, although higher frequencies may produce unpredictable increases in $PaCO_2$.

LIMITATIONS OF HIGH-FREQUENCY JET VENTILATION

Important limitations to the intraoperative use of HFJV include the unavailability of jet ventilators in many operating rooms, unfamiliarity with the equipment required, and confusion over the principles of gas exchange and gas delivery during jet ventilation. A further drawback of HFJV during major airway surgery is the requirement for total intravenous anesthesia, as volatile anesthetics cannot be reliably and safely administered in the presence of an opened airway. In addition, several complications of HFJV occur that the physician must be aware of before initiating this ventilatory mode in the operating room. Barotrauma has been reported by Bunting and Allen (1995) and others and is most frequently encountered during laryngeal surgery when the tip of the jet catheters can become malpositioned, producing submucosal injection of air under high pressure. Displacement of the catheter into the stomach during laryngeal surgery may also produce gastric rupture as reported by Gilbert (1998). Theoretically, tracheobronchial disruption from an excessively mobile catheter tip may occur during major airway or thoracic surgery. However, the risk of barotrauma from a catheter impacting in a bronchus, producing locally high airway pressures, may be of greater concern during these procedures. Inadequate humidification of airway gases has also been implicated as a possible etiologic factor in these complications.

Although HFJV can be used in patients with obstructive lung disease, caution must be exercised to ensure an adequate expiratory pathway and time to prevent gas trapping and barotrauma. Although aspiration is a potential complication during HFJV, Jawan and Lee (1996) have convincingly demonstrated that aspiration is rare during transtracheal jet ventilation owing to a continuous outflow of gases away from the lung and up through the larynx, a similar observation made by one of us (N.E.B.) and associates (1982) during HFJV for tracheal and carinal resections.

CONCLUSION

The efficiency of gas exchange with HFJV and the unobstructed access provided by small catheters has established HFJV as an essential aspect of ventilatory management during major airway and thoracic surgery.

REFERENCES

Benhamou D, et al: Impact of changes in operating pressure during high-frequency jet ventilation. Anesth Analg 63:19, 1984.

Bunting HE, Allen RW: Barotrauma during jet ventilation for microlaryngeal surgery. Anaesthesia 50:374, 1995.

Calkins JM, et al: Effects of high frequency jet ventilation design and operational variables upon arterial blood gas tensions. In Scheck PA, Sjöstrand UH, Smith RB (eds): Perspectives in High Frequency Ventilation. Boston: Martinus Nijhoff, 1983, p. 72.

Carden E, et al: A comparison of venturi and side-arm ventilation in anaesthesia for bronchoscopy. Can J Anaesth 20:569, 1973.

Clark RH, Gerstmann DR: Controversies in high-frequency ventilation. Clin Perinatology 25:113, 1998.

Cooper RM, Cohen DR: The use of an endotracheal ventilation catheter for jet ventilation during a difficult intubation. Can J Anaesth 41:1196, 1994.

Dartevelle P, et al: Tracheal sleeve pneumonectomy for bronchogenic carcinoma: report of 55 cases. Ann Thorac Surg 46:68, 1988.

Dikmen Y, et al: Unilateral high frequency jet ventilation during one-lung ventilation. Eur J Anaesthiol 14:239, 1997.

El-Baz N, et al: High frequency ventilation through a small catheter for laser surgery of laryngotracheal and bronchial disorders. Ann Otol Rhinol Laryngol 94:483, 1985.

El-Baz N, et al: High-frequency positive-pressure ventilation for major airway surgery. In Scheck PA, Sjostrand UH, Smith RB (eds): Perspectives in High Frequency Ventilation. Boston: Martinus Nijhoff, 1983, p. 216.

El-Baz N, et al: One-lung high-frequency ventilation for tracheoplasty and bronchoplasty: a new technique. Ann Thorac Surg 34:564, 1982.

Eriksson, et al: High-frequency positive-pressure ventilation (HFPPV) during transthoracic resection of tracheal stenosis and during preoperative bronchoscopic examination. Acta Anaesth Scand 19:113, 1975.

Fredberg JJ, et al: Augmented diffusion in the airways can support pulmonary gas exchange. J Appl Physiol 49:232, 1980.

Gilbert TB: Gastric rupture after inadvertent esophageal intubation with a jet ventilation catheter. Anesthesiology 88:537, 1998.

Giunta F, et al: Clinical uses of high frequency jet ventilation in anaesthesia. Br J Anaesth 63:102S, 1989.

Glenski JA, et al: High frequency, small volume ventilation during thoracic surgery. Anesthesiology 64:211, 1986.

Godet G, et al: High-frequency jet ventilation vs continuous positive airway pressure for differential lung ventilation in patients undergoing resection of thoracoabdominal aortic aneurysm. Acta Anaesthesiol Scand 38:562, 1994.

Heijman K, et al: High frequency positive pressure ventilation during anaesthesia and routine surgery in man. Acta Anaesthesiol Scand 16:176, 1972.

Hildebrand PJ, et al: High frequency jet ventilation. A method for thoracic surgery. Anaesthesia 39:1091, 1984.

Howland WS, et al: High-frequency jet ventilation during thoracic surgical procedures. Anesthesiology 67:1009, 1987.

Hunsaker DH, et al: Anesthesia for microlaryngeal surgery: the case for subglottic jet ventilation. Laryngoscope 104:1, 1994.

Jawan B, Lee JH: Aspiration in transtracheal jet ventilation. Acta Anaesthesiol Scand 40:684, 1996.

Klain M: Gas exchange in high frequency ventilation: an experimental study. In Scheck PA, Sjostrand UH, Smith RB (eds): Perspectives in High Frequency Ventilation. Boston: Martinus Nijhoff, 1983, p. 158.

Lee P, English ICW: Management of anaesthesia during tracheal resection. Anaesthesia 29:305, 1974.

McClish A, et al: High-flow catheter ventilation during major tracheobronchial reconstruction. J Thorac Cardiovasc Surg 89:508, 1985.

McKinney M, et al: A new technique for sleeve resection and major bronchial resection using twin catheters and high frequency jet ventilation. Anaesthesia 43:25, 1988.

Nakatsuka M, et al: Unilateral high-frequency jet ventilation during one-lung ventilation for thoracotomy. Ann Thorac Surg 59:1610, 1995.

Nevin M, et al: A comparative study of conventional versus high-frequency jet ventilation with relation to the incidence of postoperative morbidity in thoracic surgery. Ann Thorac Surg 44:526, 1987.

Öberg PA, Sjöstrand U. Studies of blood pressure regulation: common carotid artery clamping in studies of the carotid-sinus baroreceptor control of the systemic blood pressure. Acta Physiol Scand 75:276, 1969.

Payne DK, et al: Tracheoesophageal fistula formation in intubated patients. Risk factors and treatment with high-frequency jet ventilation. Chest 98:151, 1990.

Perera ER, et al: Carinal resection with two high-frequency jet ventilation delivery systems. Can J Anaesth 40:59, 1993.

Ransom E: Univent tube provides a new technique for jet ventilation. Anesthesiology 84:724, 1996.

Rouby JJ, et al: Factors influencing pulmonary volumes and CO_2 elimination during high-frequency jet ventilation. Anesthesiology 63:473, 1985.

Rouby JJ, Viars P: Clinical use of high frequency ventilation. Acta Anaesthesiol Scand 33:134, 1989.

Sanders RD: Two ventilating attachments for bronchoscopes. Del Med J 39:170, 1967.

Sivarajan M, et al: Jet ventilation using fiberoptic bronchoscopes. Anesth Analg 80:384, 1995.

Sjostrand UH, Eriksson IA: High rates and low volumes in mechanical ventilation—Not just a matter of ventilatory frequency. Anesth Analg 59:567, 1980.

Smith RB, Alabin MS, Williams RL: Percutaneous transtracheal jet ventilation. J Clin Anesth 8:689, 1996.

Spoelstra AJG, Tamsma JA: High frequency jet ventilation: the influence of gas flow, inspiration time and ventilatory frequency on gas transport in healthy anaesthetized dogs. Br J Anaesth 59:1298, 1987.

Standiford TJ, Morganroth ML: High-frequency ventilation. Chest 96:1380, 1989.

Strashnov VI, et al: High-frequency jet ventilation in endolaryngeal surgery. J Clin Anesth 7:19, 1995.

Watanabe Y, et al: The clinical value of high-frequency jet ventilation in major airway reconstructive surgery. Scand J Thorac Cardiovasc Surg 22:227, 1988.

Wippermann CF, et al: Independent right lung high frequency and left lung conventional ventilation in the management of severe air leak during ARDS. Paediatr Anaesth 5:189, 1995.

CHAPTER 24

Anesthesia for Pediatric General Thoracic Surgery

Babette J. Horn

Conditions requiring thoracic surgery may affect children of any age. Anesthetic considerations in the older child and adolescent are similar to those in the adult patient. It is in the newborn that the pediatric anesthesiologist encounters the greatest challenge. Besides the technical problems created by the newborn's small size, unique anatomic, physiologic, and pharmacologic differences make neonatal anesthesia a field unto itself.

PHYSIOLOGIC CONSIDERATIONS IN THE NEONATE

Cardiovascular Adaptation

The cardiovascular system undergoes several changes during the transition to extrauterine life. Closure of the ductus venosus and foramen ovale converts the circulatory system from a parallel circuit to a series circuit (Figs. 24-1 to 24-3). Hypoxia, hypercarbia, sepsis, and hypothermia can cause undesirable right-to-left shunting of blood through the foramen ovale and ductus arteriosus, the anatomic closure of which may not be complete until 2 weeks after birth. Pulmonary resistance, elevated during fetal life and immediately after birth, decreases rapidly at first and attains adult values by 2 months of age (Fig. 24-4). During this time, however, the pulmonary vascular resistance is labile, and considerable constriction and dilatation can result from physiologic, pharmacologic, and environmental manipulations. The syndrome of persistent pulmonary hypertension of the newborn, characterized by refractory hypoxemia, hypercarbia, and acidosis, is common in patients with diaphragmatic hernias but can occur in virtually any stressed term infant.

Because it must work against increased resistance in utero, the right ventricle is hypertrophied and dominant in the newborn. Waugh and Johnson (1984) reported that both ventricles are noncompliant; their myocardial tissue has 30% fewer contractile elements than that of the adult.

Increases in preload cannot increase stroke volume because of the diminished contractility of the newborn myocardium (Fig. 24-5). Thornburg and Morton (1983) suggested that the infant is functioning on an unfavorable portion of the Starling curve; only a modest increase in filling pressure can precipitate congestive heart failure. The anesthesiologist must scrupulously avoid overzealous administration of intravenous fluids.

The cardiac output of a newborn (180 to 240 mL/kg per minute) is two to three times the adult value relative to size. This difference reflects the greater oxygen consumption and metabolic rate in this age group. Increases in cardiac output are achieved primarily by increases in heart rate (normal, 120 to 160 beats per minute) because the infant's myocardial contractility is relatively fixed. Sympathetic innervation of the heart is incomplete, as noted by Zaritsky and Chernow (1984), further impairing the ability to increase stroke volume. Systemic blood pressure is low in the newborn period (Table 24-1). Awareness of normal values is essential for the appropriate diagnosis and treatment of hypotension.

Respiratory Adaptation

Sarnaik and Preston (1982) reported the anatomic, mechanical, and functional peculiarities of the newborn respiratory system that increase the risk of arterial desaturation and hypoxemia. The trachea has an incompletely developed cartilaginous framework. Any extrathoracic obstruction, such as postextubation mucosal edema, causes tracheal collapse distally. Even a 1-mm ring of tracheal narrowing can cause severe respiratory distress because of the already small airway caliber (Fig. 24-6). The infant has a highly compliant chest wall because of a horizontally oriented rib cage. In diseases of poor lung compliance—for example,

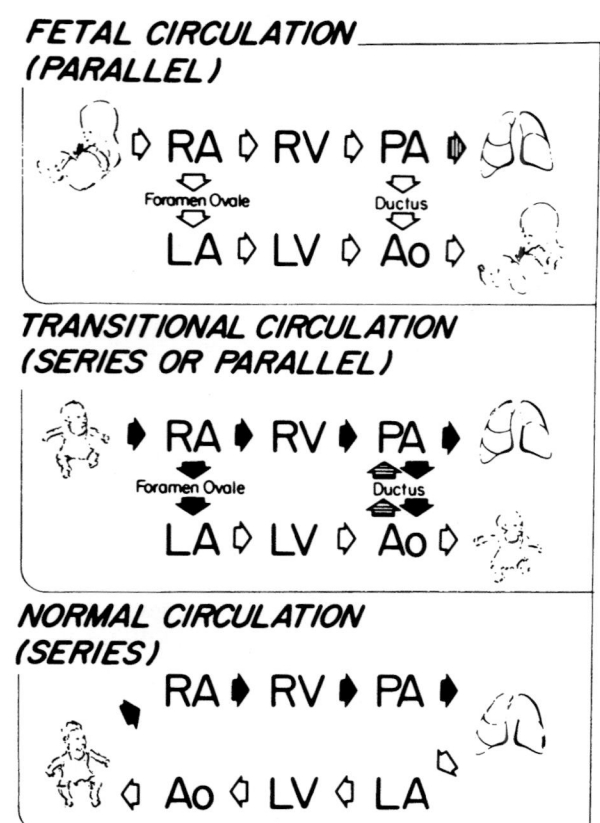

Fig. 24-1. Course of circulation during transition from fetal type circulatory pattern to adult type circulatory pattern. (Ao, aorta; LA, left atrium; LV, left ventricle; PA, pulmonary artery; RA, right atrium; RV, right ventricle.) From Ryan JF, et al (eds): A Practice of Anesthesia for Infants and Children. Orlando, FL: Grune & Stratton, 1986, p. 176. With permission.

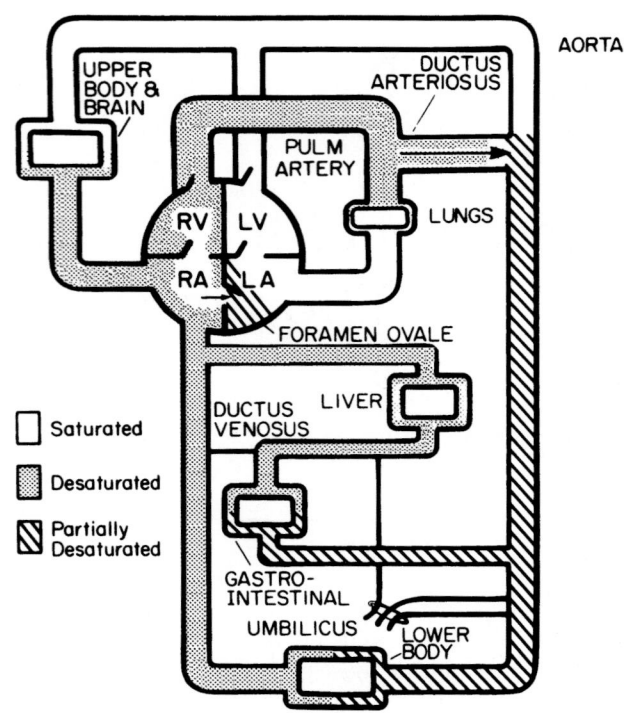

Fig. 24-2. Transitional circulation of the neonate when pulmonary vascular resistance is high. Desaturated blood is shunted from the right atrium (RA) across the foramen ovale to partially desaturate the left atrial (LA) blood. LV, left ventricle; RV, right ventricle. From Ryan JF, et al (eds): A Practice of Anesthesia for Infants and Children. Orlando, FL: Grune & Stratton, 1986, p. 176. With permission.

pulmonary edema and atelectasis—excessive lung recoil results in greater retraction of the soft chest wall and more loss of functional residual capacity than would occur in older children with stiffer chest walls.

When supine, the newborn's closing capacity impinges on tidal volume breathing. The resulting small airway collapse leads to atelectasis, ventilation-perfusion mismatch, and hypoxia. To prevent this situation from occurring intraoperatively, the anesthesiologist can use controlled ventilation and positive end-expiratory pressure.

Because of their high oxygen consumption and increased work of breathing, infants breathe at rapid rates of 30 to 50 breaths per minute. Cook (1981) reported that the diaphragm of infants has a preponderance of fast twitch muscle fibers that are prone to early fatigue. Conditions causing increased work of breathing are therefore not tolerated for long periods of time, and hypercarbia and respiratory failure occur.

Chemical and neural control of breathing are different in the newborn. The response to hypoxia is paradoxic, characterized by a brief period of hyperpnea, followed by apnea. The central chemoreceptors have a diminished sensitivity to Pco_2 compared with those of adults, that is, a higher Pco_2 is

needed to effect a similar increase in minute ventilation. Periodic breathing and apneic spells are common in the newborn, making close monitoring of respiratory function mandatory in the postoperative period.

Oxygen unloading at the tissue level is made more difficult by the high percentage of fetal hemoglobin in newborn erythrocytes. Because of its lower p50, hemoglobin F "holds on" to oxygen more tenaciously than does adult hemoglobin. The generally high hemoglobin concentration at birth (15 to 18 g/dL) is beneficial in increasing oxygen delivery to the cells (Fig. 24-7).

Metabolic Adaptation

Maintenance of normothermia is essential in the newborn. Adverse effects of hypothermia include apnea, hypoglycemia, metabolic acidosis, and increased oxygen consumption. Because of decreased subcutaneous tissue, a low surface area to volume ratio, and small body mass, the neonate has increased environmental heat losses. Nonshivering thermogenesis, mediated by catecholamine effects on brown fat deposits, is the primary heat-generating process in

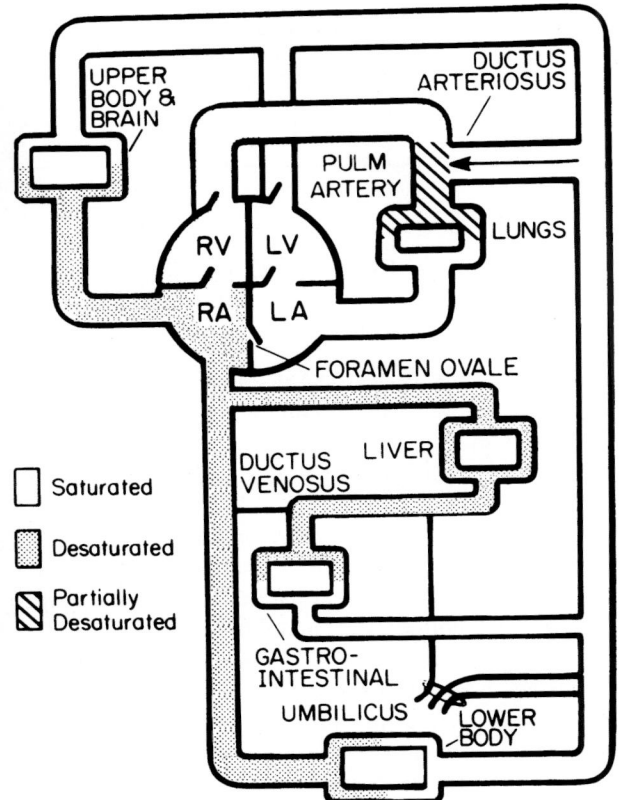

TRANSITIONAL CIRCULATION
LOW PULMONARY VASCULAR RESISTANCE

Fig. 24-3. Transitional circulation of the neonate when the pulmonary vascular resistance has fallen. Foramen ovale is closed and no intracardiac shunting can occur at that point. Left-to-right shunting of fully saturated blood from the aorta across the patent ductus arteriosus into the pulmonary artery arterializes blood flowing to the lungs. LA, left atrium; LV, left ventricle; RA, right atrium; RV, right ventricle. From Ryan JF, et al (eds): A Practice of Anesthesia for Infants and Children. Orlando, FL: Grune & Stratton, 1986, p. 176. With permission.

the newborn. This process increases oxygen consumption by as much as 200-fold. Methods of preventing heat loss intraoperatively include increasing ambient temperature and the use of radiant warmers, heating blankets, intravenous fluid warmers, and humidification of anesthetic gases. Baumgart and associates (1987) showed that covering the top of the head and extremities with plastic wrap effectively minimized evaporative heat losses during surgical procedures.

The use of forced-air warming covers and passive heat- and moisture-exchanging filters has significantly diminished heat loss in pediatric surgical patients. Bissonnette and Sessler (1989), as well as Kurz and colleagues (1993), have corroborated the efficacy of these newer technologies for improved thermoregulation.

Hypoglycemia occurs frequently in this age group, especially in the premature or small-for-gestational-age infant or in the infant of a diabetic mother. Causative factors in the

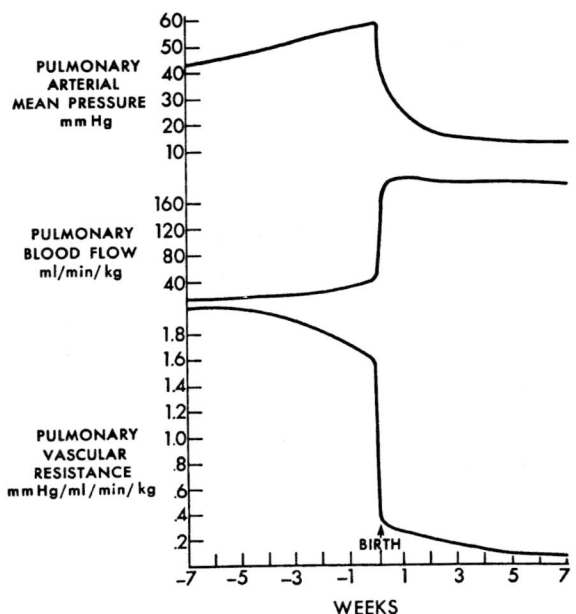

Fig. 24-4. The changes in pulmonary vascular resistance during the 7 weeks preceding birth, at birth, and in the 7 weeks postnatally. Prenatal data derived from lambs. From Rudolph AM: Congenital Diseases of the Heart. Chicago: Year Book, 1974, p. 31. With permission.

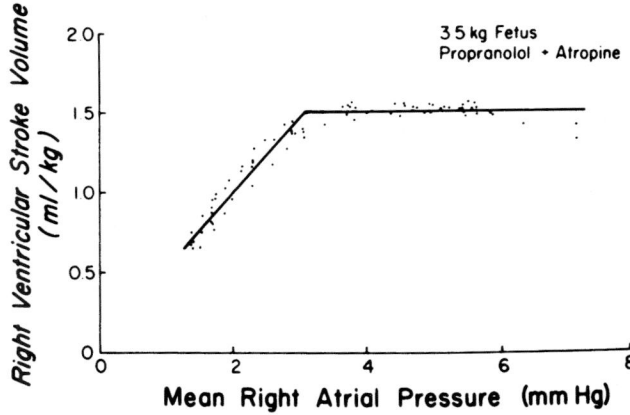

Fig. 24-5. Right ventricular stroke volume and right atrial pressure relationships in a sheep fetus. From Ryan JF, et al (eds): A Practice of Anesthesia for Infants and Children. Orlando, FL: Grune & Stratton, 1986, p. 176. With permission.

Table 24-1. Relationship of Age to Blood Pressure

Age	Normal Blood Pressure (mm Hg)	
	Mean Systolic	Mean Diastolic
0–12 hrs (preterm)	50	35
0–12 hrs (full term)	65	45
4 days	75	50
6 wks	95	55
1 yr	95	60
2 yrs	100	65
9 yrs	105	70
12 yrs	115	75

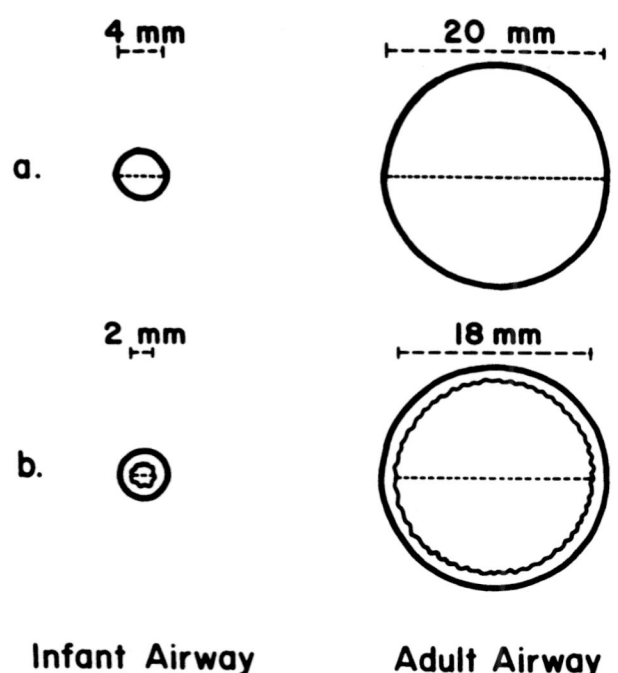

Fig. 24-6. Diagram of relative cross-sectional area of infant and adult trachea. **a.** No tracheal edema. **b.** 1 mm of edema encircling tracheal lumen.

development of neonatal hypoglycemia include diminished hepatic glycogen stores, decreased gluconeogenetic capabilities, and decreased response to glucagon secretion. Blood glucose values should be monitored frequently, adjusting the intravenous dextrose concentration accordingly. Normal blood glucose values in the newborn are listed in Table 24-2.

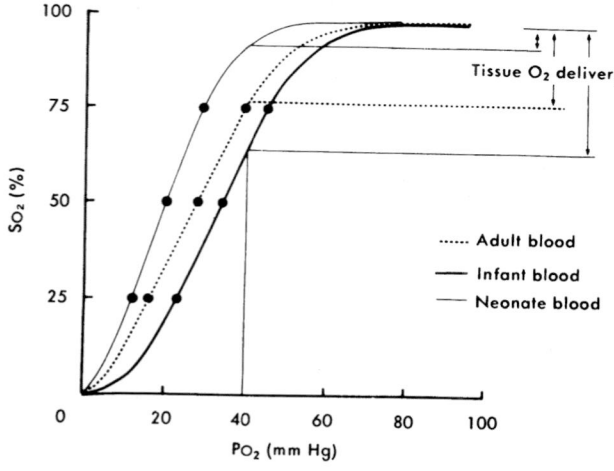

Fig. 24-7. Oxygen-hemoglobin dissociation curves with different oxygen affinities. In neonates with a lower p50 (20 mm Hg) and higher oxygen affinity, tissue oxygen unloading at the same tissue P_{O_2} is reduced. From Motoyama EK, Cook DR: Respiratory physiology. In Smith RM (ed). Anesthesia for Infants and Children. St. Louis: CV Mosby, 1980, p. 67. With permission.

Table 24-2. Normal Blood Glucose Values

Age	Blood Glucose (mg/dL)
Newborn (premature)	>30
Newborn (term)	>40
Adult	60–100

PHARMACOLOGIC CONSIDERATIONS IN THE NEONATE

Virtually all drugs used in the practice of adult anesthesia have been safely used in pediatric anesthesia. Because of the physiologic characteristics of the newborn, however, drug dosages are altered and target organ responses are monitored carefully.

Muscle relaxants such as succinylcholine and the nondepolarizing agents supplement almost all newborn anesthetics. Goudsouzian (1986) noted that infants require a larger dose of succinylcholine calculated on a per kilogram basis because of their increased extracellular fluid compartment. Goudsouzian and Standaert (1986), in an excellent review of the infant myoneural junction, discussed both the pharmacodynamic (immature neuromuscular junction) and pharmacokinetic (delayed excretion, increased diaphragm fatigue) reasons behind the abnormal response of newborns to nondepolarizing agents such as pancuronium. The intermediate-acting nondepolarizers atracurium/cisatracurium, vecuronium, and rocuronium have been used extensively in pediatric patients. Because of the shorter duration of action of all of these drugs and the rapid onset of paralysis in rocuronium, they are probably preferable to pancuronium for shorter procedures in very young patients.

Inhalation anesthetics such as nitrous oxide, halothane, and isoflurane are used frequently in pediatric thoracic surgical patients. Friesen and Henry (1986), as well as Schieber (1986) and Brett (1987) and their associates, reported that all these agents cause dose-dependent depression of cardiac function. Wear (1982) and Duncan (1987) and their colleagues noted that their use impaired baroreceptor reflexes. Hypotension and bradycardia commonly occur when the potent inhalation agents are administered in high concentrations. Because halothane has a low therapeutic index in infants, it must be used sparingly, with close attention paid to blood pressure and heart rate. Waugh and Johnson (1984) and Eisele and associates (1986) reported that nitrous oxide can increase pulmonary vascular resistance, which in theory is undesirable in neonates with the potential for persistent pulmonary hypertension of the newborn. Clinical studies reported by Hickey and coworkers (1986), however, have shown that nitrous oxide can be used in infants without significant increase in right-to-left shunting.

Fentanyl, a synthetic short-acting potent narcotic, has been used extensively in neonatal anesthesia. Hickey and associates (1985) noted its beneficial effects in attenuating the pulmonary vasoconstrictive response to tracheal stimulation. Schieber and colleagues (1985), as well as Robinson and Gregory (1981), observed cardiovascular stability with fentanyl analgesia. Yaster (1987) achieved a satisfactory anesthetic state in newborns presenting for a variety of surgical emergencies with doses of fentanyl in the 10.0 to 12.5 μg/kg range. Administration of greater than 5 μg/kg of fentanyl, a modest dose, usually precludes tracheal extubation at the conclusion of surgery, because this agent is a potent respiratory depressant. The newer, more potent narcotic sufentanil has been studied in pediatric patients undergoing cardiovascular surgical procedures. Extremely high doses in newborns were used by Anand and Hickey (1992) with positive results. The lower doses used by Moore and associates (1985) proved unsatisfactory when sufentanil was the sole anesthetic agent. For most pediatric thoracic surgical patients, sufentanil has no clear-cut benefit over the more familiar, less expensive fentanyl.

Barbiturates such as thiopental can be used as induction agents in newborns, but low doses should be used (2 to 3 mg/kg). Both immaturity of the blood-brain barrier and a relatively high cerebral blood flow combine to deliver a large fraction of the injected drug to the brain, thus allowing a lower dose to be used with equal efficacy. In addition, the barbiturates are myocardial depressants, and unacceptable degrees of hypotension may result from use of large doses.

Ketamine is a potent amnesic and analgesic agent that can be given intravenously (1 to 2 mg/kg) or intramuscularly (5 mg/kg) for the induction of general anesthesia. White and coworkers (1982) noted cardiovascular hemodynamics and spontaneous respirations are maintained because of sympathetic nervous system stimulation, accounting for the popularity of the drug in pediatric anesthesia. Ketamine causes copious salivation, so prior or concurrent administration of an antisialagogue (atropine, 20 μg/kg intramuscularly or 10 μg/kg intravenously) is necessary.

Propofol is a relatively new drug that has gained widespread use for induction and maintenance of anesthesia in adults. Its clinical efficacy in pediatric patients is being established as well. Age-dependent induction doses of 2 to 3 mg/kg were found effective based on work published by Westrin (1991). For maintenance of anesthesia propofol is usually administered by infusion; Smith and coworkers (1994) report on the higher infusion rate required by children as compared with adults. Dose-dependent decreases of heart rate and mean arterial blood pressure can be seen after propofol administration. An editorial written by Meakin (1995) cautions that the long-term use of propofol for sedation in the intensive care unit has been associated with metabolic acidosis, bradyarrhythmia, heart failure, and death.

Atropine is used in pediatric anesthesia for its anticholinergic properties. In the aforementioned dose range, it counteracts undesirable bradycardia associated with halothane and succinylcholine administration, vagal stimulation during laryngoscopy, and intraoperative visceral traction. Slow heart rates can lead to a decrease in cardiac output because

the newborn cannot compensate by increasing his or her stroke volume.

MONITORING

The purpose of monitoring any variable during an operation is to identify adverse trends before they become catastrophic events. Because of their diminished cardiopulmonary and metabolic reserves, infants require close intraoperative monitoring. Confounding the goal of vigilant invasive and noninvasive monitoring is the infant's small size, which can make even the simplest of procedures, such as applying electrocardiography leads, frustrating.

Standard Monitors

The following monitors are considered the standard of care in pediatric anesthesia.

Temperature Probe

Rectal or esophageal temperatures most closely approximate core temperature and are preferred over skin and axillary monitoring sites.

Electrocardiography

Cardiac rate and rhythm are the primary data obtained from this monitor. Ischemia detection is not as important in this age group because coronary artery disease is uncommon. Smaller electrodes are available for placement on the trunk, as well as limb leads designed for use around the wrists and ankles.

Precordial or Esophageal Stethoscope

The thin chest wall of infants permits auscultation of both heart and breath sounds with a precordial stethoscope. According to Smith (1980), this monitor is one of the most useful and important in pediatric anesthesia, especially during tracheoesophageal fistula (TEF) repair, when continuous use of an esophageal stethoscope is not possible.

Blood Pressure Cuff

Sizes to fit even the premature infant are now available. Usually the arm is not big enough to permit placement of a stethoscope, so only the systolic blood pressure is measured by looking for the "to and fro" movement of the sphygmomanometer needle.

Oxygen Analyzer

The oxygen analyzer is inserted in the inspiratory limb of the anesthesia circuit. The American Academy of Pediatrics

(1983), in its guidelines for perinatal care, and Lucey and Dangman (1984) emphasized that inspired oxygen concentrations must be measured carefully, because prolonged hyperoxia can lead to retinopathy in the infant whose postconceptual age is less than 46 weeks, in whom the retina has not completely matured.

Pulse Oximeter

Pulse oximetry has become an integral part of anesthesia care in the United States. The American Society of Anesthesiologists has mandated its use in all anesthetics and in the postanesthetic care unit. Excellent detailed reviews of the theory and technology behind pulse oximetry have been published by Tremper and Barker (1989), Alexander and colleagues (1989), and Severinghaus and Keller (1992). In the operating room, pulse oximetry is used primarily for detection of hypoxemia, although the plethysmographic tracing of the pulse oximeter saturation also can be used to monitor the circulation. Whether the use of pulse oximetry has resulted in improved patient outcome as a result of better detection of hypoxic events is still the subject of intense investigation, both by outcome studies, such as that of Moller and associates (1993), and closed claims analysis. One study by Coté and colleagues (1991) of pulse oximetry in pediatric patients underscores the ability of this monitor to detect clinically unrecognized hypoxemia in both the operating room and the recovery room. For operations associated with a high risk of intraoperative hypoxemia, such as TEF repair, the use of pulse oximetry, as noted by Bautista and associates (1986), has made early detection of impaired oxygenation possible.

Capnography and Capnometry

Capnography and capnometry make possible the monitoring of end-tidal CO_2 concentrations in exhaled gases of an anesthetized patient. Important intraoperative applications of this noninvasive technique, as summarized by Bhavani-Shankar and colleagues (1992), are 1) detection of esophageal intubation, circuit disconnect, and hypoventilation; 2) monitoring of CO_2 production; and 3) detection of abnormal alveolar ventilation and respiratory patterns. Presumably, the universal use of capnography will result in improved clinical outcome by virtue of earlier detection of dangerous respiratory problems.

Effective capnographic monitoring of pediatric patients is complicated by their small tidal volumes. Contamination with fresh gas flow is a problem, especially when the CO_2 sensor is placed too far from the endotracheal tube. Badgwell (1991) studied the accuracy of capnography as a function of sensor location in pediatric breathing circuits. The end tidal CO_2 approximated $Paco_2$ most closely when the sensor was positioned within the endotracheal tube itself using a small aspirating catheter. For trending purposes,

however, the sensor worked well when positioned conventionally, placed as close to the endotracheal tube as possible.

Additional Monitors

Additional monitoring devices are frequently used in pediatric thoracic surgery.

Indwelling Arterial Pressure Line

An indwelling arterial pressure line is an invaluable intraoperative aid. Beat-to-beat display of the blood pressure facilitates early detection of hypotension, which can result from hypovolemia or decreased venous return related to great vessel compression. Samples for blood gas, hemoglobin, and glucose analyses are obtained easily from an indwelling arterial catheter. Several sites for cannulation exist, each with its own advantages and drawbacks. The right radial artery provides access to preductal blood, but insertion of even a 22-gauge catheter may be technically difficult in a newborn. Umbilical artery catheterization is relatively easy in the first 24 hours of life, but it carries the risks of lower extremity vasospasm and embolization of particulate matter to other major arterial vessels.

Doppler Ultrasonic Flow Detector

The Doppler device provides auscultatory confirmation of systolic pressures when placed over the radial or brachial artery and used in conjunction with a blood pressure cuff. Whyte and associates (1975) reported excellent agreement between Doppler readings and transduced blood pressure values.

SPECIFIC PROBLEMS REQUIRING THORACOTOMY IN NEWBORNS

Congenital Diaphragmatic Hernia

Although repair of a congenital diaphragmatic hernia is not accomplished by thoracotomy (see Chapter 50), it traditionally has been included in discussions of neonatal thoracic surgical emergencies. Based on innovative investigation, the term *emergency* may no longer be correct. Work done by Nakayama (1991) and Sakai (1987) and their associates demonstrates a deterioration in pulmonary mechanics after emergent surgery in babies with congenital diaphragmatic hernia. Both groups of authors recommend a period of stabilization before operative treatment. During this stabilization period, the infant may receive pharmacologic treatment for pulmonary hypertension (tolazoline, dobutamine) as described by Ein (1980) and Drummond (1981) and their colleagues. Unconventional modes of ventilatory support (e.g., extracorporeal membrane oxygenation, high-frequency ventilation) have been used successfully by Bohn (1991) and O'Rourke and associates (1991). Because of the growing realization that the degree of pulmonary hypoplasia is an important determinant of ultimate survival, Bohn and colleagues (1987) made an attempt to quantitate disease severity so that treatment may be stratified based on predictors of outcome.

Proper airway management is essential to ensure the best possible outcome. Endotracheal intubation should be preceded by oxygenation with a bag and mask. Positive pressure ventilation is contraindicated to avoid distending intrathoracic bowel and thereby increasing the infant's respiratory distress. Once an artificial airway is established, vigorous hyperventilation (PaCO$_2$ 25 to 30 mm Hg) can be instituted.

Tracheoesophageal Fistula

Anesthetic management of infants with TEF may be complicated in the presence of prematurity, coexisting malformations, and aspiration pneumonia. Premature infants can have hyaline membrane disease, which may make intraoperative oxygenation and ventilation difficult. Additional malformations are commonly seen in neonates with TEF. VACTERL is one common grouping of malformations including *v*ertebral, *a*nal, *c*ardiac, *t*racheo*e*sophageal, *r*enal, and *l*imb anomalies in varying combinations. Aspiration pneumonitis, if it has occurred preoperatively, may complicate intraoperative ventilatory management and cause postoperative morbidity.

Preoperative evaluation of infants with TEF should include a complete blood count and chest radiography. The lung fields are inspected for infiltrates suggestive of aspiration pneumonia or for air bronchograms and reticular granular densities consistent with hyaline membrane disease. Cardiomegaly, increased pulmonary vascularity, or a right-sided aortic arch may indicate the presence of significant congenital heart disease. Our patients are evaluated by a neonatologist preoperatively, and a cardiologist is consulted if evidence of congenital heart disease exists.

Over a period of years, the surgical management of TEF has been modified. Gastrostomy under local anesthesia followed by right thoracotomy for TEF repair is not being performed as frequently. Rather, a single anesthetic is administered for TEF repair. Gastrostomy is done only for those cases in which the anatomy or medical condition warrant it.

Induction techniques and airway management are important controversial issues in the anesthetic care of infants having TEF repair. The relative merits and drawbacks of available induction techniques are hotly debated by pediatric anesthesiologists. Awake endotracheal intubation has the advantage of maintaining spontaneous breathing. Should intubation prove problematic, the patient will still be able to ventilate spontaneously and, it is hoped, will not become hypoxic. In vigorous term infants, however, awake intubation can be difficult to perform and may be associated with intraventricular hemorrhage. Critics also contend that the

procedure is inhumane and that some anesthesia should be provided before manipulating the airway. Many advocate an intravenous rapid-sequence induction using muscle relaxants. This technique results in ideal intubating conditions because the patient is paralyzed; however, use of paralysis necessitates the use of positive pressure ventilation. Care must be taken to avoid gastric distention by using rapid respiratory rates and low tidal volumes, and hypoxia can occur if the endotracheal tube cannot be expediently positioned appropriately. Buchino and associates (1986) reported severe respiratory compromise and death from persistent wedging of the endotracheal tube in the fistula. To avoid this catastrophe, Andropoulos and colleagues (1998) advocate prethoracotomy bronchoscopy for all patients to evaluate the size and location of the fistula. High-risk lesions (low-lying, large fistulae) that might predispose the patient to intraoperative ventilatory problems can be identified and managed appropriately. Reeves and associates (1995) report their experience with preoperative bronchoscopy in two infants with TEF. A Fogarty embolectomy catheter was inserted into the fistula, thereby occluding it and preventing loss of ventilation through it.

The ideal endotracheal tube tip position is just above the carina but below the fistula. Because the distance between the carina and the TEF may be only several millimeters, proper positioning of the endotracheal tube requires meticulous care. One way to achieve proper position of the endotracheal tube is by deliberate endobronchial intubation, verified by loss of breath sounds over the left hemithorax, with subsequent withdrawal of the tube until bilateral breath sounds are detected. If a gastrostomy tube is present, the end is placed under water and the absence of bubbling is verified. If bubbling occurs, then the endotracheal tube lies above the fistula and has been withdrawn too far.

Anesthesia can be maintained by the combination of inhalational agents and judicious use of narcotics. Intraoperative problems include hypotension from great vessel compression, hypoxia, and hypercarbia from lung retraction and endotracheal tube obstruction from secretions and clotted blood. In the otherwise healthy newborn without preoperative cardiopulmonary problems, extubation is usually possible at the conclusion of the operation. Premature infants, infants with serious associated anomalies, and those whose intraoperative courses have been complicated are usually brought back to the high-risk nursery with their endotracheal tubes in place. Some centers have been using caudal epidural catheters to deliver postoperative analgesia to these patients.

Congenital Lobar Emphysema

Although infants with congenital lobar emphysema may develop respiratory distress immediately after birth, most children are diagnosed after 1 month of age. Tachypnea, cyanosis, and diminished breath sounds over the affected side are the usual presenting symptoms and signs. The degree of respiratory distress is occasionally so severe that endotracheal intubation is performed before arrival in the operating room. Regardless of where the intubation is done, it is important to begin any airway manipulation with several minutes of preoxygenation with bag and mask. Positive pressure ventilation further distends the hyperinflated lobe and should be avoided if at all possible. Gupta and colleagues (1998) have successfully managed two infants with congenital lobar emphysema requiring thoracotomy with selective bronchial intubation. However, the benefit of avoiding hyperinflation of the emphysematous lobe must be balanced against the risk of hypoxemia should a right-sided endotracheal tube bypass the right upper lobe bronchus.

Thoracotomy for removal of the emphysematous lobe is the usual surgical management of this problem. If the cardiopulmonary status allows, anesthesia is induced by having the infant breathe a mixture of halothane in 100% oxygen. Nitrous oxide and positive pressure ventilation are avoided to prevent further increases in the size of the affected lobe. Clinically unstable or rapidly deteriorating infants are best managed by emergent awake intubation. If possible, anesthesia is maintained with halothane, oxygen, and spontaneous ventilation. Arterial blood gas analysis, however, often shows progressive hypoventilation and respiratory acidosis after the patient is placed in the lateral position. In this case, it may be necessary to provide gentle manual positive pressure until the chest is opened and compression of the good lung is relieved. At this point, pulmonary status improves substantially. After lobectomy, most infants show complete return to normal of the arterial blood gas values. Tracheal extubation at the conclusion of the surgical procedure is routine. Goto and associates (1987) mentioned the possible role of high-frequency jet ventilation in the intraoperative management of patients with congenital lobar emphysema.

THE OLDER CHILD

In general, anesthetic considerations for thoracic surgery in the older child are no different from those in the adult. One exception is the child with cystic fibrosis (CF). Because of its early onset and chronic course, CF is managed primarily by pediatric subspecialists. Failure of medical therapy to control pulmonary problems such as bronchiectasis and recurrent pneumothoraces may necessitate surgery. The excellent discussion of CF by Maclusky and Levison (1990) provides background knowledge to ensure a safe perioperative course.

CF is the most common lethal inherited disorder of whites. This autosomal recessive disease occurs in 1 in 2000 live births. Generalized exocrine gland dysfunction is the hallmark of this disease. Involvement of the pulmonary, cardiovascular, and gastrointestinal systems is of greatest concern for the anesthesiologist.

The pulmonary exocrine glands of CF patients secrete an abnormally tenacious mucus. Impaired mucociliary clearance of this mucus plus a predisposition to chronic endobronchial bacterial colonization causes progressive pulmonary damage. Bronchiectasis develops as a result of peribronchial inflammation and leads to airway collapse and air trapping. Shunting of blood through large bronchopulmonary collateral vessels may occur, with the potential for massive hemoptysis should these vessels rupture. Repeated cycles of infection, especially with *Pseudomonas* species, and pulmonary damage leads to chronic hypoxemia and ultimately cor pulmonale. Although, as noted by FitzSimmons (1993), improved medical management in the past 20 years has resulted in doubling of the mean survival age to 28 years, most CF patients die of chronic pulmonary disease and secondary cardiac failure.

Gastrointestinal involvement in CF occurs as a result of exocrine pancreatic insufficiency. Malnutrition and malabsorption are present to a variable extent in most patients. Inadequate levels of fat-soluble vitamins, especially vitamin K, can be problematic. Hypovitaminosis K can contribute to severe bleeding problems perioperatively.

Medical management of the patient with CF consists of the following: chest physiotherapy to aid in mobilization of secretions, antibiotic therapy for prevention and treatment of infection, bronchodilator therapy for airway hyperreactivity, and aggressive nutritional support. Situations that may require surgical intervention include severe bronchiectasis, recurrent pneumothoraces, and life-threatening hemoptysis.

Marmon and associates (1983) emphasized that preoperative optimization of the patient's medical condition is essential. This effort requires cooperation among the surgeon, pediatrician, and anesthesiologist. CF patients ideally are hospitalized several days before elective thoracic surgery to institute aggressive chest physiotherapy and antibiotic coverage. Nutritional status should be made optimal as well, including hyperalimentation if necessary. Preoperative laboratory studies establish the patient's baseline pulmonary status. These include hemoglobin, chest radiography, coagulation profile, pulmonary function tests, and arterial blood gas analysis; pulse oximetry and transcutaneous CO_2 are acceptable substitutes. If the patient has cor pulmonale or is receiving diuretics, additional information from echocardiography or serum electrolytes may be indicated.

Regional anesthesia is preferable to general anesthesia in patients with CF, but this technique is usually not suitable for thoracic surgical procedures. Use of a general anesthetic with volatile agents such as halothane or isoflurane has been successful in these cases. Avoidance of nitrous oxide permits use of high inspired oxygen tension and prevents expansion of air-containing pulmonary bullae by the more diffusible N_2O. The use of intravenous agents such as narcotics and benzodiazepines is discouraged to minimize postoperative respiratory depression. Although a review article by Lamberty and Rubin (1985) cited a high perioperative complication rate of 10%, the current complication rate may be lower, in part because of better patient selection, preoperative preparation, and intraoperative monitoring.

It is essential to avoid soiling the contralateral lung during pulmonary resection for bronchiectasis. Use of a double-lumen endotracheal tube is helpful if the patient's size permits. Experience with bronchial blockers has been limited in smaller patients.

Patients with CF may require intensive care after a long, difficult procedure, especially if their preoperative medical condition was poor or if unexpected intraoperative problems arose. Most patients, however, can be extubated in the operating room after thorough tracheal suctioning. They should receive oxygen therapy with pulse oximetry monitoring throughout their stay in the postanesthesia care unit and for 24 hours postoperatively.

Postoperative pain relief is an important aspect of the patient's care. Administration of narcotics is usually not recommended because of the risk of hypoventilation with subsequent hypercarbia and hypoxia. Alternative methods of postoperative analgesia include intercostal nerve block performed by the surgeon in the operating room, epidurally administered local anesthetic, or intravenous nonnarcotic medications such as ketorolac. Ideally, pain control is managed by or with the assistance of a hospital-based pain service.

VIDEO-ASSISTED THORACOSCOPY

Video-assisted thoracoscopic surgery is being used with increased frequency in a variety of pediatric surgical cases including lung biopsy, excision of mediastinal masses, and management of pleural fluid and air collections. This approach is also gaining popularity in the surgical management of scoliosis. Video-assisted exposure of the anterior thoracic spine for scoliosis correction has the theoretical advantages of decreased blood loss, postoperative pain, and shoulder dysfunction.

For the pediatric anesthesiologist caring for a patient having a minimally invasive thoracoscopic procedure, the greatest challenge lies in obtaining safe, effective one-lung anesthesia. The smallest size mass-produced double-lumen endotracheal tube routinely used for one-lung anesthesia in adults is No. 26F (5.5-mm internal diameter). In general, patients weighing less than 40 kg do not have tracheal lumens large enough to allow passage of this size endotracheal tube. Univent tubes (Fuji Systems Corporation, Tokyo, Japan), which are single-lumen endotracheal tubes with a self-contained movable bronchial blocker, are available in sizes suitable for small infants and children. Alternative techniques to isolate the lungs include selective bronchial intubation and use of an embolectomy catheter as a bronchial blocker. Because endobronchial intubation with a single-lumen tube often blocks the right upper lobe, modification of the endotracheal tube (notching of the distal end after removal of the Murphy eye) has been advocated by Tan

and coworkers (1999) in an effort to decrease this risk. Successful isolation of the lungs can be a time-consuming process in the smaller patient. An otolaryngologist's presence is often necessary for proper placement of a bronchial blocker, which, according to Borchardt and associates (1998), is associated with a risk of bronchial tear. The actual operating time may be increased for video-assisted thoracoscopic surgery compared with open thoracotomy in the pediatric population because of technical difficulties in achieving satisfactory one-lung anesthesia.

POSTOPERATIVE ANALGESIA

Schechter and associates (1986) noted that interest in postoperative pediatric pain control has dramatically increased in recent decades. Research in the areas of neonatal pain perception and narcotic administration in children, as reported by McGrath and Johnson (1988), has heightened physician awareness that these patients experience postoperative pain and that adequate relief of pain may improve overall outcome, especially in children undergoing thoracotomy.

Coe and colleagues (1991) and Craig (1981) summarize the well-described decrease in pulmonary function testing results after these operations, believed to result in part from poor respiratory effort caused by pain. Adequate analgesia was found by Shulman and coworkers (1984) and Conacher (1990) to ameliorate this problem. A more extensive meta-analysis of the effects of postoperative analgesic therapies on pulmonary outcome was published by Ballantyne and associates (1998). Their analysis showed that adequate relief of pain with epidural opioids, local anesthetics, or both significantly decreased morbidity from pulmonary infections, hypoxia, and atelectasis after thoracotomy in adults; however, successful analgesia did not prevent decreases in pulmonary function tests, specifically forced expiratory volume in 1 second, vital capacity, and peak expiratory flow.

Asantila and associates (1986) emphasized that a variety of options exist for the management of postoperative thoracotomy pain. Studies performed by Kambam (1989) and Ferrante (1991) and their colleagues evaluated the safety and efficacy of interpleural postoperative analgesia. Logas and associates (1987) described the use of thoracic epidural infusions for pain relief. Lumbar epidural infusions of local anesthetic alone or with morphine were used by some investigators including Guinard (1992), Salomaki (1991), Badner (1990), and Sandler (1992) and their coworkers. In general, these regional techniques provided better analgesia with fewer side effects (e.g., pruritus, nausea, urinary retention, and hypoventilation) than more traditional techniques such as parenteral narcotics. Nonnarcotic parenteral agents such as ketorolac and indomethacin have been used successfully in the management of postthoracotomy pain both in adults and children, as reported by Pavy (1990) and Watcha (1992) and their associates. Regional techniques for postoperative analgesia in children were shown by Desparmet (1987) and Dalens (1986) and their colleagues to be effective and safe after orthopedic and urologic procedures, and every reason exists to expect that children undergoing thoracotomy would derive similar benefit. Intrapleural analgesia was used successfully by McIlvaine and associates (1988), but the technique has not gained widespread popularity. Use of patient-controlled analgesia, as described by Berde and colleagues (1991), has become commonplace in the postoperative pediatric population. This technique provides greater patient satisfaction with a lower incidence of side effects when compared with intramuscular injections.

Use of these less traditional, more invasive methods of analgesia requires close patient monitoring and supervision of both the family and nursing staff. Many hospitals offer an anesthesiology-based multidisciplinary pain service to implement appropriate postoperative analgesia and to ensure its safety and efficacy. Ready (1988) and Shapiro (1991) and their colleagues have reported the successes of their respective pain services.

REFERENCES

Alexander CM, Teller LE, Gross JB: Principles of pulse oximetry: theoretical and practical considerations. Anesth Analg 68:368, 1989.

Anand KJ, Hickey PR: Halothane-morphine compared with high-dose sufentanil for anesthesia and postoperative analgesia in neonatal cardiac surgery. N Engl J Med 326:1, 1992.

American Academy of Pediatrics and American College of Obstetrics and Gynecology: Guidelines for Perinatal Care. Evanston, IL: American Academy of Pediatrics, 1983, pp. 212–213.

Andropoulos DB, Rowe RW, Betts JM: Anesthetic and surgical airway management during tracheo-esophageal fistula repair. Paediatr Anaesth 8:313, 1998.

Asantila R, Rosenberg PH, Scheinin B: Comparison of different methods of postoperative analgesia after thoracotomy. Acta Anaesthesiol Scand 30:421, 1986.

Badgwell JM: Oximetry and capnography monitoring. Anesth Clin North Am 9:821, 1991.

Badner NH, et al: Lumbar epidural fentanyl infusions for post-thoracotomy patients: analgesic, respiratory, and pharmacokinetic effects. J Cardiothorac Anesth 4:543, 1990.

Ballantyne JC, et al: The comparative effects of postoperative analgesic therapies on pulmonary outcome: cumulative meta-analyses of randomized, controlled trials. Anesth Analg 86:598, 1998.

Baumgart S, et al: Effect of heat shielding on convective and evaporative heat losses and on radiant heat transfer in the premature infant. J Pediatr 99:948, 1987.

Bautista MJ, Kuwahara BS, Henderson CU: Transcutaneous oxygen monitoring in an infant undergoing tracheoesophageal fistula repair. Can J Anaesth 33:505, 1986.

Berde CB, et al: Patient-controlled analgesia in children and adolescents: a randomized, prospective comparison with intramuscular administration of morphine for postoperative analgesia. J Pediatr 118:460, 1991.

Bhavani-Shankar K, Moseley H, Kumar AY: Capnometry and anesthesia. Can J Anaesth 39:617, 1992.

Bissonnette B, Sessler DI: Passive or active inspired gas humidification increases thermal steady-state temperatures in anesthetized infants. Anesth Analg 69:783, 1989.

Bohn DJ: Congenital diaphragmatic hernia. Anesth Clin North Am 9:899, 1991.

Bohn D, et al: Ventilatory predictors of pulmonary hypoplasia in congenital diaphragmatic hernia, confirmed by morphologic assessment. J Pediatr 111:423, 1987.

Borchardt RA, et al: Bronchial injury during lung isolation in a pediatric patient. Anesth Analg 87:324, 1998.

Brett CM, et al: The cardiovascular effects of isoflurane in lambs. Anesthesiology 67:60, 1987.

Buchino JJ, et al: Malpositioning of the endotracheal tube in infants with tracheoesophageal fistula. J Pediatr 109:524, 1986.

Coe A, et al: Pain following thoracotomy. Anaesthesia 46:918, 1991.

Conacher ID: Pain relief after thoracotomy. Br J Anaesth 65:806, 1990.

Cook DR: Muscle relaxants and children. Anesth Analg 60:335, 1981.

Coté CJ: A single-blind study of combined pulse oximetry and capnography in children. Anesthesiology 74:980, 1991.

Craig DB: Postoperative recovery of pulmonary function. Anesth Analg 60:46, 1981.

Dalens B, Tanguy A, Haberer JP: Lumbar epidural anesthesia for operative and postoperative pain relief in infants and young children. Anesth Analg 65:1069, 1986.

Desparmet J, et al: Continuous epidural infusion of bupivacaine for postoperative pain relief in children. Anesthesiology 67:108, 1987.

Drummond WH, et al: The independent effects of hyperventilation, tolazoline, and dopamine on infants with persistent pulmonary hypertension. J Pediatr 98:603, 1981.

Duncan PG, Gregory GB, Wade JG: The effect of nitrous oxide on baroreceptor function in newborn and adult rabbits. Can J Anaesth 28:339, 1987.

Ein SH, et al: The pharmacologic treatment of newborn congenital diaphragmatic hernia—a 2-year evaluation. J Pediatr Surg 15:384, 1980.

Eisele JH, Milstem MM, Goetzmann BW: Pulmonary vascular responses to nitrous oxide in newborn lambs. Anesth Analg 65:62, 1986.

Ferrante FM, et al: Intrapleural analgesia after thoracotomy. Anesth Analg 72:105, 1991.

FitzSimmons SC: The changing epidemiology of cystic fibrosis. J Pediatr 122:1, 1993.

Friesen RH, Henry DB: Cardiovascular changes in preterm neonates receiving isoflurane, halothane, fentanyl and ketamine. Anesthesiology 64:238, 1986.

Goto H, et al: High-frequency jet ventilation for resection of congenital lobar emphysema. Anesth Analg 66:684, 1987.

Goudsouzian NG: Muscle relaxants in children. In Ryan JF, et al: A Practice of Anesthesia for Infants and Children. Orlando, FL: Grune & Stratton, 1986, pp. 108–109.

Goudsouzian NG, Standaert FG: The infant and the myoneural junction. Anesth Analg 65:1208, 1986.

Guinard JP, et al: A randomized comparison of intravenous versus lumbar and thoracic epidural fentanyl for analgesia after thoracotomy. Anesthesiology 77:1108, 1992.

Gupta R, et al: Management of congenital lobar emphysema with endobronchial intubation and controlled ventilation. Anesth Analg 86:71, 1998.

Hickey PR, et al: Blunting of stress responses in the pulmonary circulation of infants by fentanyl. Anesth Analg 64:1137, 1985.

Hickey PR, et al: Pulmonary and systemic hemodynamic effects of nitrous oxide in infants with normal and elevated pulmonary vascular resistance. Anesthesiology 65:374, 1986.

Kambam JR, et al: Intrapleural analgesia for post-thoracotomy pain and blood levels of bupivacaine following intrapleural injection. Can J Anaesth 36:106, 1989.

Kurz A, et al: Forced-air warming maintains intraoperative normothermia better than circulating water mattresses. Anesth Analg 77:89, 1993.

Lamberty JM, Rubin BK: The management of anaesthesia for patients with cystic fibrosis. Anaesthesia 40:448, 1985.

Logas WG, et al: Continuous thoracic epidural analgesia for postoperative pain relief following thoracotomy: a randomized prospective study. Anesthesiology 67:787, 1987.

Lucey JF, Dangman B: A re-examination of the role of oxygen in retrolental fibroplasia. Pediatrics 73:82, 1984.

Maclusky I, Levison H: Disorders of the respiratory tract in children. In Chernick J (ed): Kendig's Disorders of the Respiratory Tract in Children. 5th Ed. Philadelphia: WB Saunders, 1990, pp. 692–730.

Marmon L, et al: Pulmonary resection for complications of cystic fibrosis. J Pediatr Surg 18:811, 1983.

McIlvaine WB, et al: Continuous infusion of bupivacaine via intrapleural catheter for analgesia after thoracotomy in children. Anesthesiology 69:261, 1988.

McGrath PJ, Johnson GD: Pain management in children. Can J Anaesth 35:107, 1988.

Meakin G: Role of propofol in paediatric anaesthetic practice. Paediatr Anaesth 5:147, 1995.

Moller JT, et al: Randomised evaluation of pulse oximetry in 20,802 patients: I and II. Anesthesiology 78:436, 1993.

Moore RA, et al: Hemodynamic and anesthetic effects of sufentanil as the sole anesthetic for pediatric cardiovascular surgery. Anesthesiology 62:725, 1985.

Nakayama DK, Motoyama EK, Tagge EM: Effect of preoperative stabilization on respiratory system compliance and outcome in newborn infants with congenital diaphragmatic hernia. J Pediatr 118:793, 1991.

O'Rourke PP, et al: The effect of extracorporeal membrane oxygenation on the survival of neonates with high-risk congenital diaphragmatic hernia. J Pediatr Surg 26:147, 1991.

Pavy T, Medley C, Murphy DF: Effect of indomethacin on pain relief after thoracotomy. Br J Anaesth 65:624, 1990.

Ready LB, et al: Development of an anesthesiology-based postoperative pain management service. Anesthesiology 68:100, 1988.

Reeves TS, Burt N, Smith CD: Is it time to reevaluate the airway management of tracheoesophageal fistula? Anesth Analg 81:866, 1995.

Robinson S, Gregory GD: Fentanyl-air-oxygen anesthesia for ligation of patent ductus arteriosus in preterm infants. Anesth Analg 60:331, 1981.

Sakai H, et al: Effect of surgical repair on respiratory mechanics in congenital diaphragmatic hernia. J Pediatr 111:432, 1987.

Salomaki TE, Laitinen JO, Nuutinen LS: A randomized double-blind comparison of epidural versus intravenous fentanyl infusion for analgesia after thoracotomy. Anesthesiology 75:790, 1991.

Sandler AN, et al: A randomized, double-blind comparison of lumbar epidural and intravenous fentanyl infusions for post-thoracotomy pain relief. Anesthesiology 77:626, 1992.

Sarnaik BP, Preston C: Physiologic peculiarities of the respiratory system in neonates. Anesth Rev 9:31, 1982.

Schechter NL, Allen A, Hanson K: Status of pediatric pain control: a comparison of hospital analgesic usage in children and adults. Pediatrics 77:11, 1986.

Schieber RB, Stiller RL, Cook DR: Cardiovascular and pharmacodynamic effects of high-dose fentanyl in newborn piglets. Anesthesiology 63:166, 1985.

Schieber RB, et al: Hemodynamic effects of isoflurane in the newborn piglet: comparisons with halothane. Anesth Analg 65:633, 1986.

Severinghaus JW, Keller JF: Recent developments in pulse oximetry. Anesthesiology 76:1018, 1992.

Shapiro BS, et al: Experience of an interdisciplinary pediatric pain service. Pediatrics 88:1226, 1991.

Shulman M, et al: Post-thoracotomy pain and pulmonary function following epidural and systemic morphine. Anesthesiology 61:569, 1984.

Smith I, et al: Propofol. An update on its clinical use. Anesthesiology 81:1005, 1994.

Smith RM: Anesthesia for Infants and Children. 4th Ed. St. Louis: CV Mosby, 1980, pp. 192–215.

Tan PPC, et al: A modified endotracheal tube for infants and small children undergoing video-assisted thoracoscopic surgery. Anesth Analg 86:1212, 1999.

Thornburg KL, Morton MJ: Filling and arterial pressure as determinants of RV stroke volume in the sheep fetus. Am J Physiol 244:H656, 1983.

Tremper KK, Barker SJ: Pulse oximetry. Anesthesiology 70:98, 1989.

Watcha MF, et al: Comparison of ketorolac and morphine as adjuvants during pediatric surgery. Anesthesiology 76:368, 1992.

Waugh R, Johnson GG: Current considerations in neonatal anesthesia. Can J Anaesth 31:700, 1984.

Wear R, Robinson S, Gregory GB: The effect of halothane on the baroresponses of adult and baby rabbits. Anesthesiology 56:188, 1982.

Westrin P: The induction dose of propofol in infants 1–6 months of age and in children 10–16 years of age. Anesthesiology 74:455, 1991.

White PF, Way WI, Trevor BJ: Ketamine: its pharmacology and therapeutic uses. Anesthesiology 56:119, 1982.

Whyte RK, et al: Assessment of Doppler ultrasound to measure systolic and diastolic pressures in infants and young children. Arch Dis Child 50:542, 1975.

Yaster M: The dose response of fentanyl in neonatal anesthesia. Anesthesiology 66:433, 1987.

Zaritsky B, Chernow B: Use of catecholamines in pediatrics. J Pediatr 105:341, 1984.

READING REFERENCES

Anand KJS, Hickey PR: Halothane-morphine compared with high-dose sufentanil for anesthesia and postoperative analgesia in neonatal cardiac surgery. N Engl J Med 326:1, 1992.

Kavanagh BP, Katz J, Sandler AN: Pain control after thoracic surgery. Anesthesiology 81:737, 1994.

Truog RD, et al: Repair of congenital diaphragmatic hernia during extracorporeal membrane oxygenation. Anesthesiology 72:750, 1990.

Vacanti JP, et al: The pulmonary hemodynamic response to perioperative anesthesia in the treatment of high-risk infants with congenital diaphragmatic hernia. J Pediatr Surg 19:672, 1984.

SECTION VII

Pulmonary Resections

CHAPTER 25

Thoracic Incisions

Willard A. Fry

The most popular incision for open general thoracic surgical procedures is the lateral thoracotomy, sometimes also called the axillary thoracotomy. For years, the posterolateral thoracotomy was considered the incision of choice for most operations involving the lung and esophagus. With increased use of double-lumen endotracheal tubes and refinement of instrumentation, particularly the stapling devices, however, the traditional posterolateral incision is reserved for difficult operations in which wide exposure is mandatory. Likewise, interest in using median sternotomy for operations on the lung has waned, although median sternotomy is still considered the incision of choice for most anterior mediastinal lesions. With increasing use of video-assisted thoracic surgical procedures (VATS), small accessory incisions, as suggested by Lewis and colleagues (1992), are becoming more popular (see Chapter 32).

When the patient is positioned for thoracotomy, especially in the lateral decubitus position, pressure points should be padded about the elbows using foam pads, an axillary roll should be placed under the dependent axilla to take pressure off the brachial plexus, and one or two pillows should be placed between the legs. Measures to discourage venous thrombosis in the lower extremities, such as tight elastic hose and a sequential compression device, should be considered. These measures, if used, should be in effect at the beginning of the operation. Salzman (1985) and Scurr (1987) suggested that external pneumatic compression with sequential compression sleeves connected to a sequential compression device is the safest and most cost-effective prophylaxis against venous thromboembolic disease. If the patient has a number of risk factors toward developing deep vein thrombosis, the perioperative use of heparin should be considered, as described by Hyers (1999).

The use of prophylactic antibiotics for general thoracic surgical procedures remains controversial. Cameron (1981) and Ilves (1981) and their associates reported conflicting results in controlled trials. In general, a first- or second-generation cephalosporin is used, and the main emphasis is on prophylaxis of the wound from *Staphylococcus aureus*

infections. On the basis of the work of Olak and associates (1991), I cannot recommend giving more than a single intravenous dose before making the skin incision. This recommendation is supported by Meakins (1998) writing on behalf of the American College of Surgeons.

POSTEROLATERAL THORACOTOMY

The posterolateral thoracotomy incision is made with the patient in the lateral decubitus position, with proper padding to the elbows, knees, and dependent axilla. Various maneuvers are available to hold the patient in an appropriate lateral position, including placing a sandbag under the operating table mattress, rolled sheets front and back, and bean bags. Two straps of 2-inch adhesive tape are used as well. The dependent arm is flexed at the elbow. The superior arm can be flexed similarly and appropriately padded, obtaining the so-called praying position, or it can be extended on a padded Mayo stand (Fig. 25-1A).

Only hairy portions of the skin that will be directly in the line of the incision or the chest tubes or their taping should be shaved, and if shaving is necessary, it should be done immediately before the operation, as recommended by Cruse and Foord (1973). My colleagues and I often find shaving is not necessary at all.

It is helpful to outline the proposed incision with a felt-tipped marking pen. Most pulmonary operations are best performed through a fifth interspace incision.

As shown in Figure 25-1B, the incision starts in front of the anterior axillary line, curves 4 cm under the tip of the scapula, and then takes a vertical direction between the posterior midline over the vertebral column and the medial edge of the scapula. It is usually not necessary to go farther cephalad than the level of the spine of the scapula.

The electrosurgical unit is used for hemostasis and musculofascial dissection. It is not generally recommended for dissection in the skin or subcutaneous tissues, and I usually reserve its use for cutting until I have reached the muscular

367

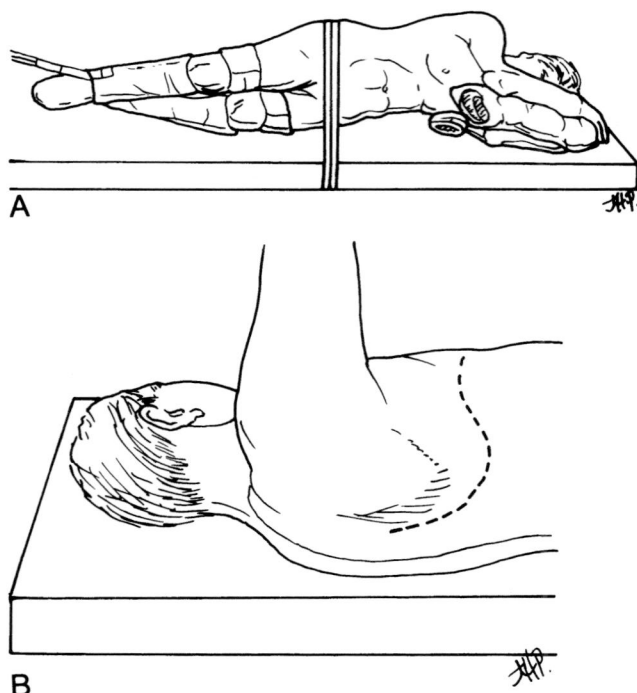

Fig. 25-1. Posterolateral thoracotomy. **A.** The patient is positioned in the "praying position" with pillows between the knees and padding under the elbows. Wide adhesive tape secures the position. Note the axillary roll and the sequential compression device. **B.** The incision curves in an S shape, passing 4 cm under the tip of the scapula over in the fifth interspace anteriorly.

fascia, based on the extensive wound healing studies of Cruse and Foord (1973). Glover and associates (1978) emphasized that use of the cutting current destroys less tissue than constant use of the coagulation current. On the other hand, my colleagues and I use the electrosurgical unit more frequently when operating on patients who have positive test results for human immunodeficiency virus or hepatitis. The lower portion of the trapezius muscle is divided, and, in the same plane more anteriorly, the latissimus dorsi muscle is divided also. Next, the lower portion of the rhomboid muscle, if the thoracotomy is high, and the continuous plane with the serratus anterior muscle are divided.

The desired interspace is located by placing a large right-angle retractor beneath the scapula and passing the hand up paraspinally. Sometimes, the first rib is obscured to easy palpation, but attachments of the serratus posterior superior muscle to the second rib serve as an added guide.

Rib section at the costovertebral angle level is recommended for patients over 40 years of age to decrease the incidence of rib fracture (Fig. 25-2). Generally, small portions of the superior and inferior rib are excised subperiosteally to prevent the cut edges from overriding in the postoperative period. Although some recommend section over clips or ligatures of the neurovascular bundle, it is

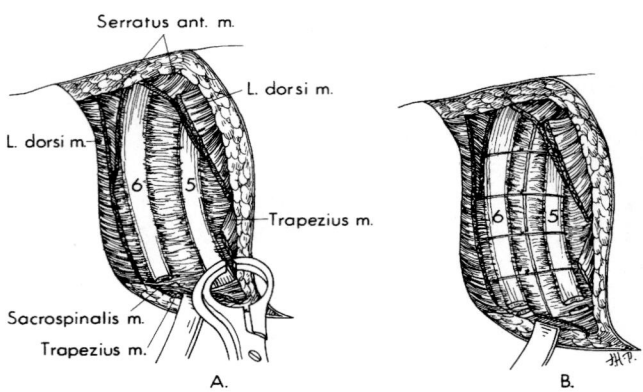

Fig. 25-2. Posterolateral thoracotomy. **A.** One or two ribs are sectioned at the costovertebral angle. A small portion of bone is removed to prevent overriding of the fragments at the time of closure. **B.** Four or more sutures of heavy absorbable suture are placed as pericostal sutures. The interspace distance is maintained. It is not necessary to suture the divided intercostal muscles except when a tight seal is desired for pneumonectomy.

not necessary. It is unusual to resect a long segment of rib for a routine thoracotomy, although it was usually done in the past. For repeat thoracotomies, however, it is often advisable to resect a long rib segment subperiosteally and to approach the pleural space through the bed of the resected rib, as extensive adhesions are often encountered on such reoperations, and the wider entry into the pleural space through the bed of a resected rib can be beneficial (Fig. 25-3).

The intercostal muscle incision down to the parietal pleura is made carefully in the lower portion of the interspace to avoid injury to the neurovascular bundle. The surgeon pauses to see if the lung moves freely under the pleura. If it does move freely, then few adhesions in the area of the

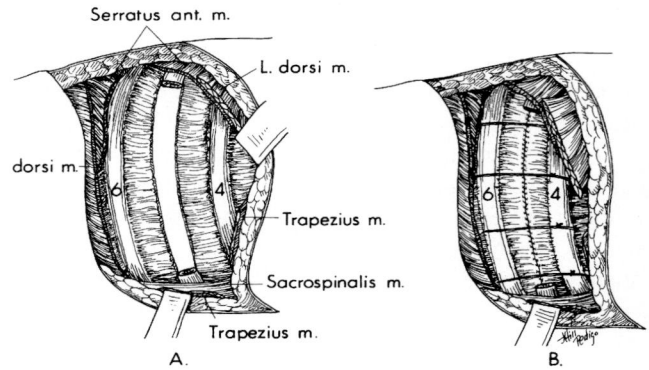

Fig. 25-3. Posterolateral thoracotomy. **A.** The fifth rib is resected subperiosteally and the pleural cavity is entered through an incision in the rib bed. Long rib resection is recommended for repeat thoracotomy. **B.** The rib bed is closed with running absorbable suture. The retained periosteum regenerates rudimentary bone. The interspace distance is maintained.

interspace can be expected. If the lung does not move freely, the surgeon must anticipate a significant number of adhesions and the need to divide them with care, particularly when the operation is a repeat thoracotomy. A large Finochietto-type rib spreader is inserted, placing the large superior blade behind the scapula. If desired, a smaller, Tuffier-type rib spreader can be placed more anteriorly to ensure a wide surgical field. The rib spreader is opened slowly and in stages to minimize the chance for rib fracture.

Closure of the incision is begun by inserting one or two chest tubes through a separate stab incision inferior to the skin incision in the anterior and midaxillary lines. The tract for the tube is tunneled for several centimeters to direct the tube, low and posterior for the back tube to drain fluid and high and anterior for the front tube to remove air. Tunneling the tube tract also reduces the chance for a pleurocutaneous fistula in the event that the tubes must remain in place for a long time, as in the case of a prolonged postoperative air leak. Generally, two tubes are used if a significant resection has been performed, as the operator can expect both air and fluid accumulation. In selected cases, such as a local excision of a lung lesion when no air leak exists or an esophageal operation in which the lung has not been cut, a single tube suffices. The size of the chest tube to be used depends on the preference of the operating surgeon, the size of the patient, and the nature of the particular operation. In general, it is not necessary to use a posterior tube larger than No. 32F or an anterior tube larger than No. 28F. Tubes smaller than No. 24F tend to kink. Plastic tubes are preferred over rubber, because they are less likely to clot. The chest tubes should be secured, when inserted, with a heavy suture; our preference is for No. 1 nylon to prevent slippage. The tubes are attached to a Y-tube connector, which is in turn affixed to an appropriate chest drainage system.

In the past, my colleagues and I (1990) preferred a continuous epidural analgesia (CEA) for our posterolateral and axillary thoracotomy patients. More recently, we have used an extrapleural, paravertebral catheter (PARA), with a continuous infusion of fentanyl (5 μg/mL) with bupivacaine 0.1% as described by Bimston and colleagues (1999) from our group. We initially described a fentanyl concentration of 10 μg/mL, but we believe that the lower dose of 5 μg/mL lessens some of the side effects such as drowsiness and nausea. Kaiser and associates (1998) also have described an experience in which they prefer the PARA over CEA. In instances of repeat thoracotomy or upper chest wall resection in which denuding or removal of the paravertebral parietal pleura is anticipated, the surgeon would be advised to have the anesthesiologist place a CEA catheter before induction of anesthesia. In the event that CEA or PARA is not feasible, we would recommend an intercostal nerve block with a long-acting local anesthetic such as 0.5% bupivacaine with epinephrine at the time of chest wall closure. Gallo and colleagues (1983) emphasized that an intercostal vascular injection must be avoided, because the intravascular injection of such compounds can have dire cardiovascu-

lar consequences. Generally, we block from the second to the seventh interspace. The injection should be at least 8 cm off the midline to avoid a subdural injection that would produce spinal anesthesia.

Pericostal sutures, usually four, of heavy absorbable material such as No. 2 polyglycolic acid are then placed. Each of the two musculofascial planes is closed with running suture of a similar material, usually size 1 or 0, the subcutaneous tissues with a size 2-0 running suture of the same material, and the skin with the surgeon's preferred material. Sadighi and Woodworth (1998) recommend placing a transcostal suture to minimize postoperative pain. We have not found it necessary to drill such holes in the rib.

The main advantage of the posterolateral thoracotomy is the superb exposure for most general thoracic procedures. The main disadvantages are the time expended because of the length of the incision and the amount of muscle and soft tissue transected.

AXILLARY THORACOTOMY

The axillary thoracotomy was originally developed for operations on the upper thoracic sympathetic nerve system. It was modified for first rib resection for thoracic outlet syndromes. Jensik (personal communication, 1993) used it preferentially for many years for pulmonary resections. Siegel and Steiger (1982) described how it has been rediscovered for more extensive general thoracic surgical procedures. Mitchell (1990) and Ponn and associates (1992) report several large series of axillary or lateral incisions with excellent results, although the largest series with which I am familiar comes from Noirclerc's group (1973). Some groups refer to it as a *lateral thoracotomy* to avoid confusion with small, high axillary incisions for first rib resections or apical bleb resections. Other groups refer to it as a *minithoracotomy* or *muscle-sparing thoracotomy*, but such nonspecific terminology should be discouraged. I prefer this incision for uncomplicated and straightforward pulmonary operations. It is not recommended for bulky tumors, sleeve resections, radical pneumonectomies, or repeat thoracotomies. This incision is particularly useful when a double-lumen endotracheal tube is used, as the controlled atelectasis combined with the ability of the anesthesiologist to elevate the mediastinum toward the operative field by applying positive end-expiratory pressure of 5 to 10 cm to the dependent lung provides favorable operating conditions. The chief advantages are the speed of opening and closing, the reduced blood loss from minimal muscle transection, and the resulting reduced postoperative discomfort. As shown in Figure 25-4, the only muscle group that is actually transected is the intercostals.

Upper lobe lesions are best approached through the fourth interspace. Middle and lower lobe lesions are easily handled through the fifth interspace. The patient is placed in a lateral decubitus position with the arm abducted at 90 degrees and positioned on an armrest. The antecubital fossa over the

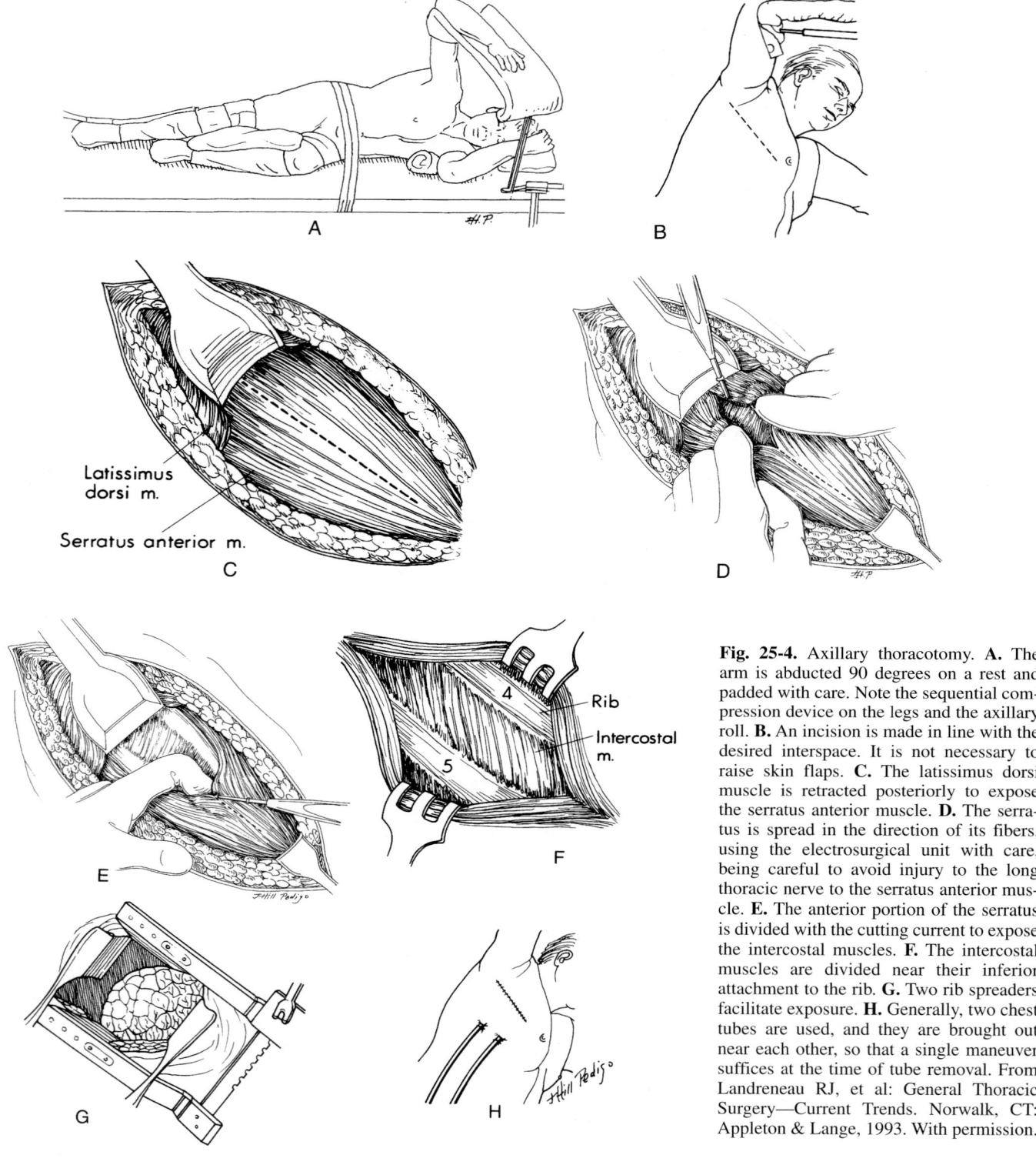

Latissimus dorsi m.

Serratus anterior m.

C

4
Rib
Intercostal
m.
5

Fig. 25-4. Axillary thoracotomy. **A.** The arm is abducted 90 degrees on a rest and padded with care. Note the sequential compression device on the legs and the axillary roll. **B.** An incision is made in line with the desired interspace. It is not necessary to raise skin flaps. **C.** The latissimus dorsi muscle is retracted posteriorly to expose the serratus anterior muscle. **D.** The serratus is spread in the direction of its fibers, using the electrosurgical unit with care, being careful to avoid injury to the long thoracic nerve to the serratus anterior muscle. **E.** The anterior portion of the serratus is divided with the cutting current to expose the intercostal muscles. **F.** The intercostal muscles are divided near their inferior attachment to the rib. **G.** Two rib spreaders facilitate exposure. **H.** Generally, two chest tubes are used, and they are brought out near each other, so that a single maneuver suffices at the time of tube removal. From Landreneau RJ, et al: General Thoracic Surgery—Current Trends. Norwalk, CT: Appleton & Lange, 1993. With permission.

armrest is padded. The skin incision is made over the desired interspace, the latissimus dorsi muscle is elevated bluntly for a short distance and retracted posteriorly, and the serratus anterior muscle is split in the direction of its fibers. The surgeon should not divide the muscle too far posteriorly to avoid injuring the long thoracic nerve to the serratus anterior muscle. The intercostal muscles are divided in a way similar to that described for a posterolateral thoracotomy, and the pleural space is entered. The incision is so limited that wound towels and intercostal towels are not used. The intercostal muscle incision is carried forward to the anterior curve of the ribs and posteriorly to the level of the sacrospinalis muscle group. A Finochietto rib spreader is placed between the ribs, and a Tuffier rib spreader is placed in the opposite direction to retract the skin and latissimus dorsi muscle.

Closure of the axillary thoracotomy is accomplished with three pericostal sutures of No. 2 polyglycolic acid after the placement of one or two chest tubes and usually the placement and positioning of a PARA catheter. Generally, traction on the pericostal sutures suffices to close the chest wall, because it is difficult to use a ratchet-type rib approximator through the small axillary thoracotomy incision. If a problem with rib approximation develops, a towel clip can be used to bring the ribs together. The serratus anterior muscle is closed with a running absorbable suture, as is the subcutaneous fascial layer. Skin closure technique is again at the surgeon's discretion.

The axillary thoracotomy is not recommended for the occasional thoracic surgeon or for a difficult operation, because the exposure is more limited than that of a posterolateral thoracotomy. However, it is a useful incision that deserves wider application than it has received in recent years. The axillary thoracotomy is associated with less postoperative discomfort than is noted with either the posterolateral thoracotomy or the median sternotomy. Kirby and coworkers (1995) have emphasized how little difference exists between a muscle-sparing thoracotomy and a VATS approach for lobectomy in terms of length of chest tube drainage, postoperative stay, and postoperative discomfort.

MEDIAN STERNOTOMY

The development of cardiac surgery has made median sternotomy the most common thoracic incision. It is the incision of choice for most cardiac operations and is used by preference by many thoracic surgeons for anterior mediastinal lesions, bilateral procedures such as the surgical treatment of bilateral spontaneous pneumothorax, and resection of multiple pulmonary lesions. Urschel and Razzuk (1986) wrote that they prefer it for many elective pulmonary resections, except for left lower lobe pulmonary resections. Cooper and colleagues (1978) demonstrated less alteration in pulmonary function by median sternotomy than by posterolateral thoracotomy. Median sternotomy was recommended by Baldwin and Mark (1985) and Perelman (1987) for anterior transpericardial repair of postpneumonectomy bronchopleural fistula. Orringer (1984) described a partial median sternotomy for exposure of the lower cervical and upper thoracic esophagus.

The patient is positioned supine, with one or both arms extended, at the preference of the surgeon and the anesthesiologist. Both arms are often placed at the patient's side. The vertical skin incision is made from just below the suprasternal notch to a point between the xiphoid process

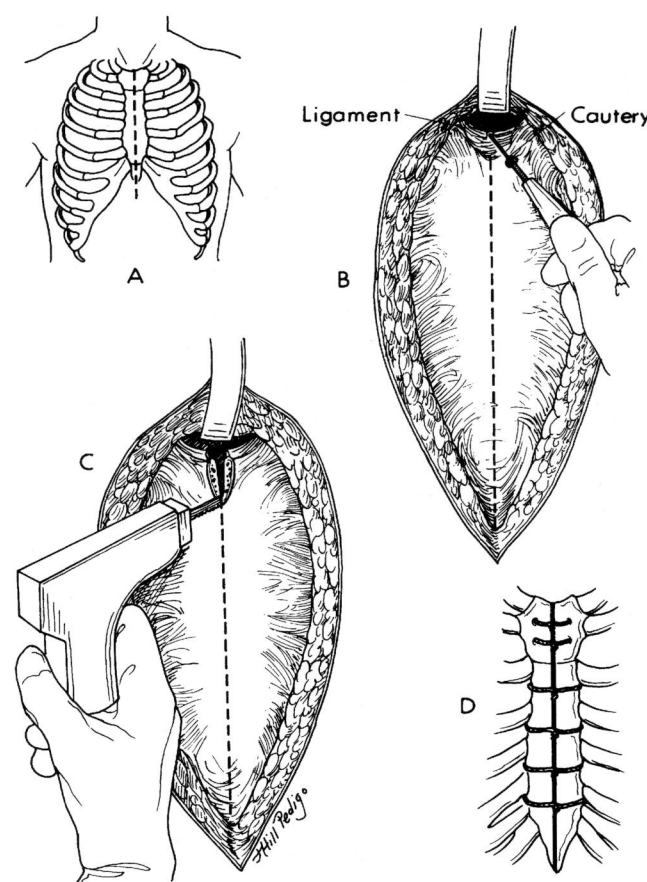

Fig. 25-5. Median sternotomy. **A.** The incision is made from the suprasternal notch to a point between the xiphoid process and umbilicus. **B.** The interclavicular ligament is divided with care. **C.** The sternal saw can be used in either direction. The anesthesiologist should not ventilate the lungs while the sternum is being divided. **D.** The upper two wires of No. 5 monofilament steel are passed through the manubrium.

and the umbilicus (Fig. 25-5). The pectoral fascia is divided and the periosteum is scored with the electrosurgical unit. Care is needed when mobilizing tissues off of the area of the manubrium and dividing the tough interclavicular ligament. The tissues just to one side of the xiphoid process are mobilized and the sternum is divided with a power saw, from the top down or from the bottom up. The anesthesiologist should cease ventilatory efforts as the sternum is being cut to lessen the chance of injury to the lung. Once the sternum is split, the two edges are gently but firmly retracted, and periosteal bleeding points are controlled with the electrosurgical unit. Bone wax is often not necessary in general thoracic surgical procedures, because the patient is not anticoagulated, as is usual for patients undergoing cardiac procedures. Robicsek and colleagues (1981) suggested that the foreign body effect of bone wax can have a deleterious effect on wound healing. A sternal spreader is placed low in the incision to minimize excessive traction on the upper ribs, with attendant occult fracture and neurologic insult, as described by Van der Salm and associates (1980). The use of the Lebsche sternal blade should be familiar to the thoracic surgeon so that sternotomy can be performed if the power saw fails or is unavailable.

Chest tubes or mediastinal drains, if the pleural space has not been entered, are passed through separate stab incisions. Sternotomy closure is accomplished with four to seven parasternal sutures of No. 5 stainless steel wire, the ends of which are securely twisted and buried in the sternal tissues. The pectoral fascia is closed with a running polyglycolic acid suture, as is the linea alba. The subcutaneous tissues are closed with running absorbable suture and the skin is closed with the surgeon's preferred material.

The scar from the usual vertical median sternotomy incision is a source of concern to some patients, especially young women. Various alternatives have been proposed, and the transverse submammary skin incision described by Laks and Hammond (1980) appears to have definite cosmetic advantages for certain patients. Those authors do caution about skin flap viability for prolonged operations, as rather extensive undermining of the skin flaps is required.

The main advantages of median sternotomy for general thoracic surgical procedures are its speed in opening and closing, its familiarity to many surgeons, and its outstanding exposure for anterior mediastinal lesions. The major disadvantage is poor exposure of posterior hilar structures, especially those of the left lower lobe. My colleagues and I think that a median sternotomy is more painful in the postoperative period than an axillary thoracotomy and that it is similar in the degree of postoperative discomfort to a posterolateral thoracotomy, although others disagree. I prefer to have the anesthesiologist place a CEA catheter before making the skin incision for a sternotomy. Many cardiac surgeons

eschew the CEA. When effective pain control following sternotomy is mandatory, such as after thymectomy for myasthenia gravis, CEA is an asset to good patient care.

ANTERIOR THORACOTOMY

The anterior thoracotomy has the distinct advantage of allowing the patient to remain supine, with a resulting improvement in cardiopulmonary function. It has been used with decreasing frequency because of improvement of anesthetic techniques and management, the option of median sternotomy, the development of mediastinal staging procedures such as mediastinoscopy and mediastinotomy, and the rapid development of VATS for lung biopsy. It remains the incision of choice of some surgeons for open lung biopsy. It is occasionally used in the Ivor Lewis procedure for carcinoma of the esophagus to eliminate the need for repositioning the patient after the intra-abdominal portion of the operation. Its main disadvantage is the limited exposure it provides.

The patient is positioned with a roll under the back and hips to elevate the operated side. The ipsilateral arm is placed under the back, on an elevated arm board, or on an over armrest at the preference of the surgeon. An incision is made over the fourth or fifth interspace from the midaxillary line to curve parasternally (Fig. 25-6). In women, the incision is made in the inframammary crease. The pectoral muscles are divided with an electrosurgical unit, and the intercostal incision is made in the usual fashion. If a major resection is expected, one or two costal cartilages may be divided parasternally to facilitate exposure of the surgical field. If the cartilages are divided, the neurovascular bundles

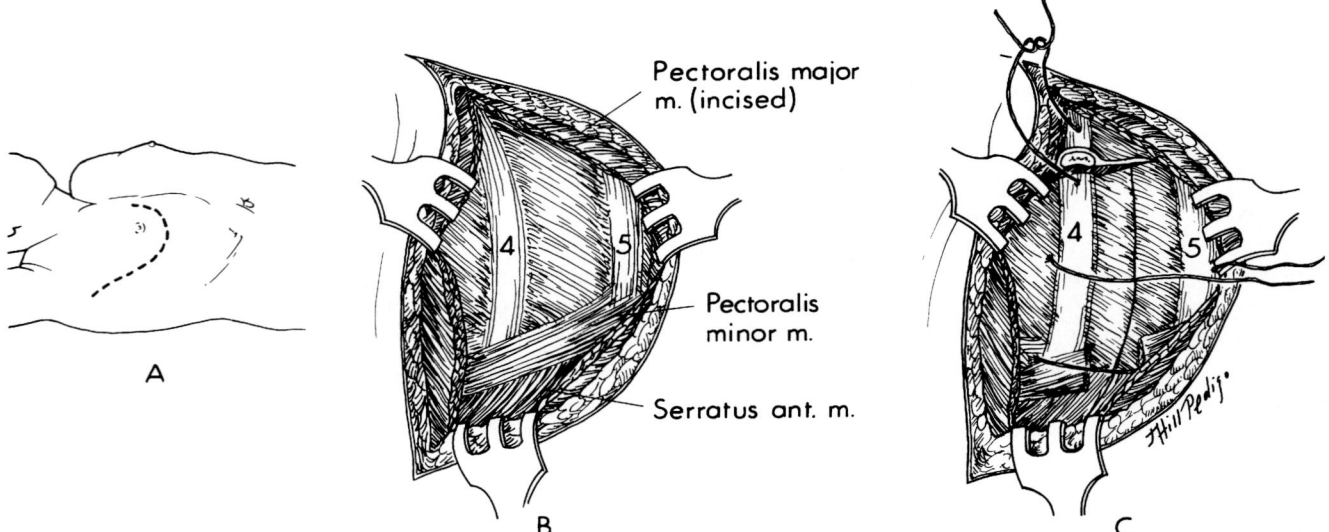

Fig. 25-6. Anterior thoracotomy. **A.** Outline of skin incision. **B.** Pectoralis major muscle divided over the fourth interspace. **C.** Closure of the intercostal incision by placement of pericostal sutures of heavy polyglycolic acid as well as sutures of the same material through the sectioned costal cartilage.

are divided over clamps and ligated to avoid tearing and excessive stretching of the blood vessels.

Closure of the anterior thoracotomy is similar to that of the other thoracotomy incisions. A heavy absorbable suture is placed through each end of the cartilage parasternally, if it has been divided.

A limited anterior thoracotomy should receive strong consideration when open lung biopsy is needed in the critically ill patient. In such a patient, the traditional VATS type of lung biopsy might be inappropriate, as it would require a double-lumen endotracheal tube and single-lung ventilation for a period of time. A small incision combined with the use of VATS-designed staples can be efficacious.

TRANSVERSE THORACOSTERNOTOMY

Cooper (1991) and Pasque and associates (1990) redescribed the transverse thoracosternotomy and many refer to it now as the *clamshell* or *crossbow* incision. Its primary role in recent years has been for bilateral lung transplantation. I, however, recommend it as an alternative to median sternotomy for bilateral general thoracic surgical procedures, such as the resection of bilateral metastatic lesions to the lungs and bilateral simultaneous treatment of spontaneous pneumothorax.

Bains and coworkers (1994) have emphasized its usefulness in thoracic oncology interventions.

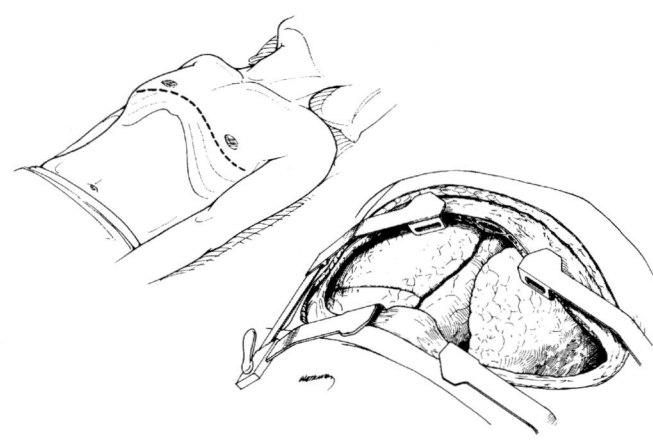

Fig. 25-7. Clamshell incision has become popular for bipulmonary lung transplantation and also for bilateral procedures on the lung when excellent exposure is mandatory. Patterson and colleagues believe that having the patient's arms at the side does not compromise the exposure.

The incision is made over the fourth or fifth interspace, and the sternum is transected with an oscillating saw (Fig. 25-7). Closure is accomplished with pericostal sutures of heavy polyglycolic acid, with a figure-of-eight maneuver about the sternum. I recommend placement of several Kirschner wires in the reapproximated sternum to reduce override and shift of the sternal ends (Fig. 25-8).

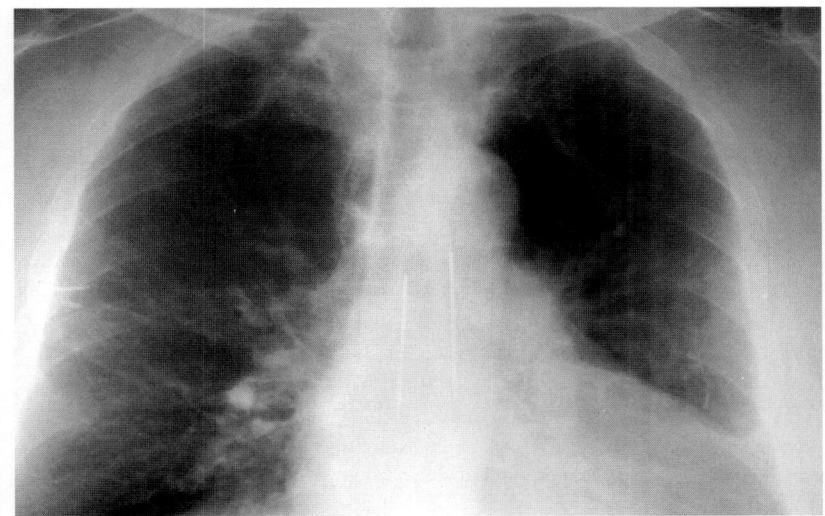

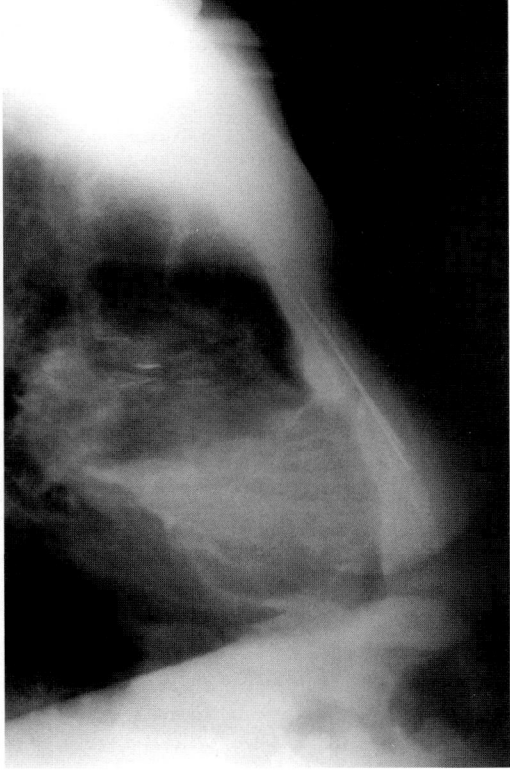

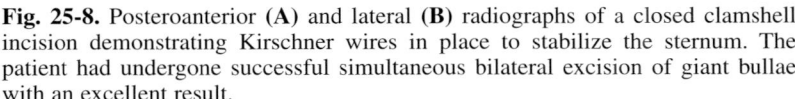

Fig. 25-8. Posteroanterior (A) and lateral (B) radiographs of a closed clamshell incision demonstrating Kirschner wires in place to stabilize the sternum. The patient had undergone successful simultaneous bilateral excision of giant bullae with an excellent result.

B

THORACOABDOMINAL INCISION

The thoracoabdominal incision provides extended exposure, particularly for operations in the lower thorax and upper abdomen. It has been used less frequently in the past and has been maligned more by hearsay perhaps than by actual fact. It can be particularly useful for difficult operations involving the lower esophagus. A seventh or eighth interspace incision is extended on the same oblique line into the upper quadrant over toward the midline. The costal margin is cut with a knife. Ginsberg (personal communication, 1993) recommended not excising a segment of cartilage and placing pericostal closure sutures securely on either side of the transected costal margin but not through the cartilage. He suggested that the incision results in a stable thorax with no significant increase in discomfort or dysfunction over a standard posterolateral thoracotomy. A curvilinear or radial incision can be made in the diaphragm to facilitate exposure. The diaphragm is closed with a running nonabsorbable suture such as No. 0 Prolene. Costochondritis has been reported in some series. Its incidence is low, but if it occurs, it is a troublesome complication. Heitmiller (1988) gave an excellent review of the incision.

REFERENCES

Bains M, et al: The clamshell incision: an improved approach to bilateral pulmonary and mediastinal tumors. Ann Thorac Surg 58:30, 1994.

Baldwin JC, Mark JBD: Treatment of bronchopleural fistula after pneumonectomy. J Thorac Cardiovasc Surg 90:813, 1985.

Bimston D, et al: Continuous extrapleural paravertebral infusion for postthoracotomy pain control. Surgery (submitted for publication – 1999).

Cameron JL, et al: Prospective clinical trial of antibiotics for pulmonary resections. Surg Gynecol Obstet 152:156, 1981.

Cooper JD, in discussion of Patterson GA, et al: Comparisons of outcomes of double and single lung transplantation for obstructive lung disease. J Thorac Cardiovasc Surg 101:623, 1991.

Cooper JD, Nelems JF, Pearson FG: Extended indications for median sternotomy in patients requiring pulmonary resection. Ann Thorac Surg 26:413, 1978.

Cruse PJE, Foord R: A five-year prospective study of 23,649 surgical wounds. Arch Surg 107:206, 1973.

Fry WA, Kehoe TJ, McGee JP: Axillary thoracotomy. Am Surg 56:40, 1990.

Gallo JA Jr, et al: Complications of intercostal nerve blocks performed under direct vision during thoracotomy. J Thorac Cardiovasc Surg 86:628, 1983.

Glover JL, Bendick PJ, Link WJ: The use of thermal knives in surgery: electrosurgery, lasers, plasma scalpel. Curr Probl Surg 15:26, 1978.

Heitmiller RF: The left thoracoabdominal incision. Ann Thorac Surg 46:250, 1988.

Hyers TM: Venous thromboembolism. Am J Respir Crit Care Med 159:1, 1999.

Ilves R, et al: Prospective, randomized, double-blind study using prophylactic cephalothin for major, elective general thoracic operations. J Thorac Cardiovasc Surg 81:813, 1981.

Kaiser AM, et al: Prospective, randomized comparison of extrapleural versus epidural analgesia for postthoracotomy pain. Ann Thorac Surg 66:367, 1998.

Kirby TJ, et al: Lobectomy–video-assisted thoracic surgery versus muscle-sparing thoracotomy. J Thorac Cardiovasc Surg 104:997, 1995.

Laks H, Hammond GL: A cosmetically acceptable incision for the median sternotomy. J Thorac Cardiovasc Surg 79:146, 1980.

Lewis RJ, et al: One hundred consecutive patients undergoing video-assisted thoracic operations. Ann Thorac Surg 54:421, 1992.

Meakins JL: American College of Surgeons Scientific American Surgery VI. Perioperative Care. 3. Prophylactic Antibiotics. New York: Scientific American, 1998, pp. 1–9.

Mitchell RL: The lateral limited thoracotomy incision: standard for pulmonary operations. J Thorac Cardiovasc 99:590, 1990.

Noirclerc M, et al: La thoracotomie latérale large sans section musculaire. Ann Chir Thorac Cardiovasc 12:181, 1973.

Olak J, et al: Randomized trial of one dose versus six-dose cefazolin prophylaxis in elective general thoracic surgery. Ann Thorac Surg 51:956, 1991.

Orringer MB: Partial median sternotomy: anterior approach to the upper thoracic esophagus. J Thorac Cardiovasc Surg 87:124, 1984.

Pasque MK, et al: Improved technique for bilateral lung transplantation: rationale and initial clinical experience. Ann Thorac Surg 49:785, 1990.

Perelman MJ, Rymko LP, Ambatiello GP: Bronchopleural fistula: surgery after pneumonectomy. In Eschapasse H, Grillo H (eds): International Trends in General Thoracic Surgery. Vol. 2. Philadelphia: WB Saunders, 1987, p. 407.

Ponn RB, et al: Comparison of late pulmonary function after posterolateral and muscle sparing thoracotomy. Ann Thorac Surg 53:675, 1992.

Robicsek F, et al: The embolization of bone wax from sternotomy incision. Ann Thorac Surg 31:357, 1981.

Sadighi PJ, Woodworth CS: Muscle-splitting thoracotomy. Am Surg 64:370, 1998.

Salzman EW: Physical techniques for prevention of venous thrombosis. In Bergan JJ, Yao JST (eds): Surgery of the Veins. Orlando: Grune & Stratton, 1985, pp. 519–528.

Scurr JH, Coleridge-Smith PD, Hasty JH: Regimen for improved effectiveness of intermittent pneumatic compression in deep venous thrombosis prophylaxis. Surgery 102:816, 1987.

Siegel T, Steiger Z: Axillary thoracotomy. Surg Gynecol Obstet 155:725, 1982.

Urschel H, Razzuk M: Median sternotomy as the standard approach for pulmonary resection. Ann Thorac Surg 41:130, 1986.

Van der Salm TJ, Cereda JM, Cutler BS: Brachial plexus injury following median sternotomy. J Thorac Cardiovasc Surg 80:447, 1980.

READING REFERENCES

Ashour M: Modified muscle sparing posterolateral thoracotomy. Thorax 45:1935, 1990.

Bethencourt DM, Holmes EC: Muscle-sparing posterolateral thoracotomy. Ann Thorac Surg 45:337, 1988.

Dart CH, Braitman HE, Larab S: Supraclavicular thoracotomy for diagnosis of apical lung and superior mediastinal lesions. Ann Thorac Surg 28:90, 1979.

Dartevelle P, et al: L'intéret de la voie combinée cervicale et thoracique dans la chirurgie des syndromes de Pancoast et Tobias d'origine tumorale. Chirurgie 109:399, 1983.

Lemmer JH, et al: Limited lateral thoracotomy. Arch Surg 125:873, 1990.

Mathey J, Aigueperse J, Lalardrie JP: La voie axillaire rétro-péctorale en chirurgie thoracique: technique et indications. Ann Chir 15:1115, 1961.

Murray KD, et al: A limited axillary thoracotomy as primary treatment for recurrent spontaneous pneumothorax. Chest 103:137, 1993.

Ravitch MM, Steichen FM: Atlas of General Thoracic Surgery. Philadelphia: WB Saunders, 1988, pp. 111–146.

CHAPTER 26

General Features of Pulmonary Resections

Thomas W. Shields

Resections of the lungs may vary from a minimal incision of the visceral pleura and enucleation of a hamartoma to a pneumonectomy. Most resections are unilateral, but synchronous bilateral excisions may be carried out. The standard procedures (Table 26-1) may be extended to include excision of a part of the chest wall, one of the thoracic parietes (pleura, pericardium, or diaphragm), an adjacent vascular structure (portion of the atrium or vena cava), and, rarely, part of the esophagus. Some pulmonary resections may be accomplished using local anesthesia (e.g., open lung biopsy), but most are performed with general endotracheal anesthetic management (see Chapter 22).

OPERATIVE POSITIONS AND THORACIC INCISIONS

Although each operative procedure has its own unique features, the standard operations are performed with the patient in the lateral decubitus, supine, or prone position. The selection of which position in which to place the patient is determined by the operation planned and, in part, the patient's physiologic condition. The supine position is associated with fewer physiologic changes in the patient's cardiopulmonary function than are noted with the other positions.

Lateral Decubitus Position

The lateral position permits the best access to the hilus of the lung. The structures contained within the hilus may be approached from either the anterior or posterior aspect, and thus the operator has greater control of the various structures than is afforded by the other approaches. The major disadvantage of the lateral position is that ventilation of the dependent lung is more difficult than in the posterior or supine position; however, perfusion of the dependent lung is increased as a result of the gravitational changes.

Prone Patient

The posterior approach while the patient is prone has a major advantage in that the bronchial secretions do not flood the trachea because of the superior position of the main stem bronchus. Also, the main stem bronchus is the most accessible structure and may be isolated and divided as the initial stage in the dissection of the hilar structures. The major disadvantages are that the access to the entire hilus is limited initially and that the vascular structures are the most distant from the operator.

Supine Patient

The anterior approach is now used commonly. The anterior thoracotomy approach, except for the more minor operative procedures, is used infrequently in North America. The disadvantage of poor access to the hilus and to contained structures generally outweighs the physiologic considerations. In many European clinics, however, this incision is still used for lobectomies and even occasionally for pneumonectomies. On the other hand, a median sternotomy incision for various types of pulmonary resections has become popular throughout the world. With controlled deflation of the lung and appropriate packing to elevate the lung anteriorly, the hilar structures are readily accessible on the right side. A left pneumonectomy, a left lower lobectomy, or other procedures on this lobe are difficult because of the position of the hilar structures, particularly that of the inferior pulmonary vein, behind the heart. As a consequence, a median sternotomy approach is not recommended for these procedures.

The multiple incisions and modifications thereof for the various intrathoracic operations have been described in

Table 26-1. Pulmonary Resections

Pneumonectomy
    Pleuropneumonectomy
    Tracheal sleeve pneumonectomy
Lobectomy
    Bilobectomy
    Sleeve lobectomy
Segmentectomy
Lung volume reduction surgery
Lesser resections
    Wedge excision
    Precision excision
    Blebectomy or bullectomy
    Enucleation

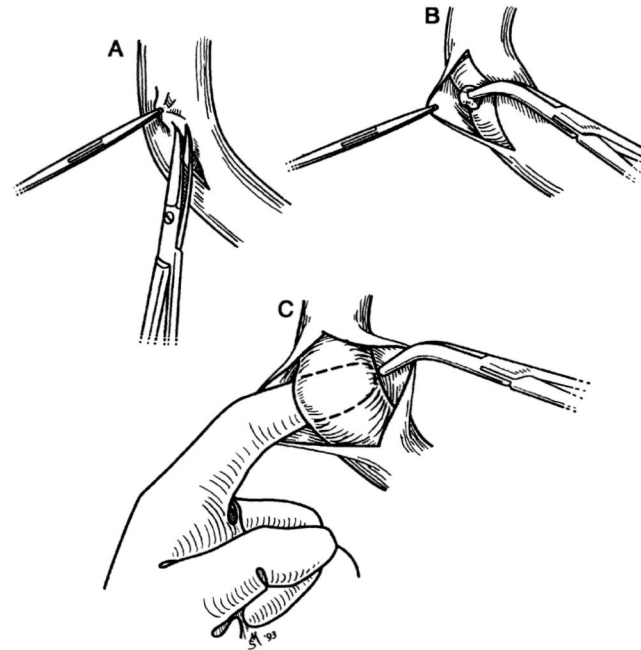

Fig. 26-1. Technique of dissection of a major pulmonary artery. **A.** Fascial envelope is elevated and incised longitudinally. **B.** Fascial layer is grasped and the vessel is bluntly dissected from it in the opposite direction. **C.** After freeing the vessel, the index finger is passed beneath the vessel between the fascial layer and the arterial wall, and a clamp is passed beneath the vessel using the finger as a guide.

Chapter 25. The trend is to use shorter posterolateral incisions and to spare the division of the major thoracic muscles as much as is compatible with appropriate operative exposure. The subperiosteal resection of a rib is done infrequently, although I believe better and tighter closure of the thoracic wall and pleural space can be accomplished and is indicated when a pneumonectomy is to be performed. Division or excision of a small posterior portion of a rib or ribs adjacent to the intercostal incision to improve exposure and to prevent a possible fracture of the rib as the intercostal space is retracted is practiced on an individual basis. If a fracture of one or more ribs occurs, control of any bleeding is mandatory and fixation of the fracture site by sutures is indicated to prevent overriding of the fractured ends to prevent further vascular injury or the occurrence of severe postoperative pain on chest wall movement.

GENERAL TECHNIQUES

The specific techniques of the various standard pulmonary resections are discussed in their respective chapters. The technique of video-assisted thoracoscopic resection is discussed in detail in Chapters 32 and 33. As an introduction, however, a discussion of the general features of the dissection and management of the bronchi, large vessels, and lung surfaces is appropriate.

Dissection and Control of the Major Arteries

Dissection of a major pulmonary artery is carried out with care. The vessel is thin walled and easily injured. Simultaneous traction and countertraction on the vessel wall once the proper plane has been established are to be avoided, although the fascial envelope can be retracted as the vessel wall is dissected away from it (Fig. 26-1). Pulling on a branch of the artery is also best avoided because the branch may easily be partially or completely avulsed from the main vessel wall. Both sharp and blunt dissection should be used, and finger mobilization of the posterior

aspect of the larger vessels is helpful. In dissecting the main pulmonary artery on the right side, the truncus anterior of the artery may be isolated and divided to obtain greater length of the main stem vessel. On the left side, the pulmonary artery may be isolated up to, or even proximal to, the ligamentum arteriosum, although one must guard against injury to the recurrent laryngeal nerve as it passes underneath the aortic arch from the front to the back of the aorta at this point.

The ligation of a major artery is accomplished in several ways. If it is long enough, the vessel may be doubly ligated with No. 00 or 0 nonabsorbable suture. The proximal end is then suture ligated between the two ligatures before division of the vessel. A simple transfixion suture is not sufficient, but a figure-of-8 suture through the center of the vessel and tied around it is satisfactory. Peterffy and Henze (1983) recommend the use of a pursestring suture. The vessel is then divided. If the vessel is too short to ligate safely in this manner, the artery may be held with two vascular clamps and divided, and the proximal cut end is closed with a continuous suture of No. 4-0 or 5-0 nonabsorbable monofilament suture. Some surgeons prefer to treat the pulmonary artery in this manner as a routine procedure. A third method of controlling the vessel is the use of a mechanical stapling device such as a TA 30 instrument using 3.5-mm or V staples.

The smaller branches of the artery may be satisfactorily controlled by triple ligation and division between the two most distal ligatures. With moderate-sized vessels, a transfixation suture is appropriate. Tension on any of these ligatures should be avoided, for even back bleeding from the lung side, if a ligature is pulled off, is troublesome.

If injury to the vessel occurs, the bleeding should be controlled initially by pressure with a gauze sponge, guarding against any maneuver that might further tear the vessel. Next, adequate exposure is ensured and proximal and distal control beyond the injury is obtained, or, when possible, a fine vascular clamp is applied directly to control the injured site. Repair is accomplished with an over and over fine vascular suture material.

Dissection and Control of the Major Veins

The major pulmonary veins and their branches are managed in a manner not dissimilar to that described for the pulmonary artery. The walls of the veins are stronger than those of the arteries, and injuries to them are less likely to occur. Occasionally, it is necessary to enter the pericardium to obtain sufficient length of the superior or inferior pulmonary vein. Once the vessel is free of the pericardial reflections (see Chapter 5), the vein is usually divided between vascular clamps and closed with a fine continuous vascular suture. Even a portion of the left atrial wall may be included in the excision and the atrial incision is closed in the standard manner. The pericardial defect, if small, is closed. If the opening is too large to close without compromise of the pericardial space, one of two maneuvers must be done to prevent postoperative herniation of the heart through the pericardial defect, with potential strangulation of the vessels and subsequent cardiac arrest. On the left side, the pericardium is opened down to the diaphragm; on the right side, because this maneuver does not prevent herniation, the cut edges of the pericardium are tacked to the surface of the heart or the defect is closed with a prosthetic soft tissue patch. Piccione and Faber (1991) suggest closing all large defects, either right- or left-sided, routinely with a soft tissue patch. Harvey and colleagues (1995) suggest that fenestration of the soft tissue patch be made to avoid the possibility of a pericardial tamponade.

Ligation of the veins as the initial step in a pneumonectomy for carcinoma has been advocated to lessen the possibility of spilling tumor cells into the circulation. The routine use of this maneuver, however, has not been shown to be beneficial, and the maneuver probably is not important. It has been suggested that initial ligation of the veins leads to overfilling of the vascular bed, resulting in an overdistended lung, which would be difficult to manipulate during the operative procedure, as well as resulting in the loss of an excessive amount of blood when the lung is removed. Miller and associates (1968) showed experimentally, however, that with initial ligation of the veins, reflex shunting of the blood

from the lung occurs promptly, and thus distention of the vascular bed does not occur.

Dissection and Closure of the Bronchus

Main Stem Bronchus

The main stem bronchus is usually the last hilar structure isolated in a pulmonary resection. However, it should be noted that Grismer and Read (1995) have recommended that the older technique of isolation and division of the bronchus be the first step in controlling the hilar structures in the performance of a pneumonectomy, a right upper lobectomy, or a right apical posterior segmentectomy. Regardless, whether the bronchus is the first or last structure mobilized, the technique of handling the bronchus remains essentially the same. On the right side, the dissection can be carried up to the tracheal carina without difficulty, but care is taken, even during lymph node dissection, not to completely denude the bronchus of its investing adventitial tissue and the contained blood supply. On the left side, the main stem bronchus should likewise be freed to the tracheal bifurcation, but this effort is more tedious because of its position within the aortic window. The proximal site of division of a main stem bronchus should be close to the bifurcation and the line of division should be placed across the bronchus to avoid a blind pocket on its lateral side. Moreover, the residual stump should be as short as possible. As a general rule, a clamp need not be placed proximal to the proposed line of division when a manual suture closure of the stump is to be done. Similarly, it is unnecessary if a stapling device is to be used to secure closure.

Takaro (1987) summarized the use and advantages of the mechanical stapler in bronchial closure. Hood (1985) recommended the TA 35 device with a staple size of 4.8 mm if a mechanical stapler is used. Both authors, among others, believe that the use of the stapler has reduced the incidence of breakdown of the bronchial closure. Peterffy and Calabrese (1979) reported the decreased incidence of a bronchopleural fistula with the use of a stapler versus the use of a chromic catgut suture closure. Such a comparison is not germane, because few would recommend catgut as the suture material of choice; a nonabsorbable suture such as silk, a fine monofilament stainless steel wire suture, or synthetic monofilament suture such as Vicryl or Prolene are the presently acceptable suture materials for closure of a bronchus. Furthermore, the recently noted decrease in incidence of a bronchial stump breakdown is more likely the result of a different selection of patients undergoing operations. In a discussion of Takaro's report, Vanetti and Bazelly (1987) reported better results with manual closure of the bronchial stump than with the use of a mechanical device. In fact, they were critical of the use of the Premium TA 55 clip, with which Hakim and Milstein (1985) recorded an alarming 15% incidence of bronchial fistula. With the use of the standard stapler, however, Vester and associates (1991) reported only a 1.6% incidence of bronchial leak.

In the manual closure of the bronchus, an occluding clamp is placed distal to the line of division to prevent soiling of the operative field from any contained material within the distal bronchial tree. A suture is placed in each lateral side of the bronchus just proximal to the line of excision and the bronchus is divided, either completely before closure or in sequence to avoid a completely open stump. With either method, the posterior membranous wall is approximated to the anterior cartilaginous wall with interrupted single or mattress 00 or 000 sutures of the operator's choice. Before complete closure, the proximal stump and trachea should be aspirated by means of a sterile catheter. Once the closure is complete, the stump is tested for any persistent air leaks by covering the stump with a sterile solution and having the anesthesiologist apply or increase inspiratory pressure to that side of the tracheobronchial tree. Any areas of leakage are controlled by additional sutures as necessary. Fibrin sealant has been used successfully by many surgeons to seal small leaks of the suture or staple line, as reported by Jensen and Sharma (1985) and Matthew and associates (1990). The technique of application of the glue is discussed in detail by the latter authors. Mouritzen and associates (1993) suggested the use of the sealant routinely on all bronchial closures.

Occasionally, a small tear in the membranous wall of the closed stump is identified. A buttress of adjacent tissue or a pledget of synthetic material should then be incorporated into a mattress suture closure of the area.

Frequently, one or two bronchial arteries need to be ligated after the bronchus has been divided. If bleeding is not controlled, these vessels may serve as a significant source of postoperative blood loss; the bronchial arterial system carries approximately 1% of the cardiac output.

After closure of the proximal end, the bronchial stump is covered with adjacent tissue, such as a pleural flap, the azygos vein, a pedicle graft of pericardial fat, or adjacent pericardium, to provide the stump with a viable tissue cover to help prevent the possible development of a leak from the stump, which normally heals by secondary intention. This cover is particularly important on the right side, because no natural coverage for the stump is available. On the left side, the short proximal stump recedes into the depth of the aortic window and is surrounded by the adjacent tissues.

Further precautions to protect the stump to ensure healing are indicated in the patient who has received preoperative irradiation; who has an active inflammatory process, such as positive acid-fast organisms in the sputum; who has an underlying multidrug-resistant mycobacterial infection; who is undergoing a completion pneumonectomy for a recurrent or continuing inflammatory process after a previous lesser resection; or in whom a bronchopleural fistula is being closed. In all these situations, the risk of bronchial dehiscence is increased. McGovern and associates (1988) have stressed the increased morbidity and problems with the

bronchial stump in patients undergoing a completion pneumonectomy for an inflammatory disease. As prophylaxis against bronchial dehiscence, coverage of the stump is recommended using a transplanted muscle flap, as described by Pairolero and Payne (1983). Brown and Pomerantz (1995) have extensively used these muscle flaps in patients with multiple drug-resistant mycobacterial tuberculosis who undergo major pulmonary resections. A pericardial fat pad, as described by Brewer and colleagues (1953, 1955), also has been used by Anderson and Miller (1995) as well as Saitoh and associates (1996) to achieve protection of a potentially compromised bronchial stump. The use of an omental flap is also satisfactory in these situations.

Lobar and Segmental Bronchi

The surgical closure of the divided lobar or segmental bronchi entails the same principles and techniques of management as for the main stem bronchi. As a general rule, however, it is unnecessary to cover these bronchial stumps with additional tissue when sufficient pulmonary parenchymal tissue is present, which, on inflation, surrounds the bronchial stump. If one is unsure that this will occur, simple coverage with a freed pleural flap is sufficient. When multiple drug-resistant mycobacterial organisms are present in the sputum or when preoperative neoadjuvant therapy including irradiation has been used, a more secure coverage of a lobar bronchial stump is indicated. A transposed muscular flap, a vascularized pericardial flap, or even an omental flap should be added to support the closure.

Lesser Bronchi

The small subsegmental branches of the bronchial tree need only be ligated to obtain adequate and satisfactory closure of the stump. It is important to stress that when an incomplete fissure has been dissected or a segmentectomy has been done, small bronchial openings should be sought carefully and ligated to prevent any major postoperative air leak.

Raw Surface of the Lung

Any parenchymal raw surfaces that are present after a resection should be thoroughly inspected, and any significant bleeding should be controlled. A moist sponge is applied to the surface and the lung is expanded. After 5 to 10 minutes, the sponge is removed and the lung surface is reinspected. If the dissection of the intersegmental plane has been done carefully, only small alveolar air leaks will be present. These tend to seal over promptly with reexpansion of the lung during the postoperative period. Any leakage from small bronchi, however, must be recognized and controlled; otherwise, the leak will persist and predispose to serious postoperative difficulties. Jensik (1986) advocated covering the raw surfaces with pleural flaps or reconstituting the lung by bringing the adjacent segments together. Such a step is generally unnecessary and may even lead to increased postoperative problems.

Matthew and associates (1990) suggested the use of fibrin glue to control air leaks and bleeding from parenchymal raw surfaces, but no data were given as to its efficacy in this particular situation. In a study by Mouritzen and colleagues (1993), the use of fibrin glue applied to the raw lung surfaces reduced the incidence and the persistence of postoperative air leakage as compared with a control group in which the glue was not applied. Wong and Goldstraw (1997), however, reported that the use of fibrin glue was not helpful in controlling moderate to severe alveolar air leaks after pulmonary resections.

When a stapler has been used for carrying out a wedge resection in a patient with essentially normal pulmonary parenchyma, a troublesome air leak is infrequent. If it occurs, the use of fibrin glue is a good solution. However, with the advent of lung volume reduction surgery in patients with emphysematous lungs by multiple nonanatomic stapled wedge excisions, serious persistent air leaks have occurred (see Chapter 83). With either unilateral or bilateral procedures, an incidence of prolonged air leaks of 30 to over 50% has been noted by Naunheim (1996), Cooper (1995), and Miller (1996) and their associates, as well as many others. In an effort to reduce this high incidence of air leaks, Cooper (1994) suggested the use of bovine pericardial strips placed on the stapling device to buttress the staple lines and thus reduce the incidence of air leaks. Although this technique has been less effective in bilateral than in unilateral procedures, Hazelrigg and colleagues (1997), in a controlled randomized study found the use of bovine buttressing strips to be more effective in controlling and reducing the duration of air leaks than not using the strips. Vaughn and associates (1997) have suggested the use of polytetrafluoroethylene sleeves as the buttressing material. Nomori and Horio (1997) have suggested the use of a gelatin-resorcinol-formaldehyde-glutaraldehyde glue spread stapler, and Horsley and Miller (1997) have used cyanoacrylate glue with a bovine pericardial patch to control these air leaks. Each of the aforementioned techniques must be evaluated by additional studies to confirm its usefulness.

MANAGEMENT OF THE PLEURAL SPACE

The management of the pleural space is fundamentally different after a pneumonectomy than after a lobectomy or a lesser resection procedure. After a pneumonectomy, the major concern is to have the space slowly obliterated by the subsequent anatomic changes in the position of the heart, mediastinal structures, diaphragm, contraction of the intercostal spaces, and accumulation of fluid, without the occurrence of infection. After a lobectomy or a lesser resection, reexpansion of the remaining lung tissue to obliterate the

pleural space without any major fluid collections is the desired clinical goal.

Postpneumonectomy Pleural Space

After removal of the specimen, the pleural space is irrigated and the chest wall is inspected for any sites of continued bleeding. When present, these are controlled with cautery or suture ligation as necessary. Special care is required in the event of persistent bleeding from an intercostal vessel or continued oozing at the posterior angle of the intercostal incision (see Chapter 37).

It is of major importance that the pleural space be dry (i.e., absence of continued bleeding) because the development of an acute massive hemothorax that necessitates reexploration is associated with a higher mortality and an increased incidence of a bronchopleural fistula, as noted by Peterffy and Henze (1983). After control of any bleeding sites, the pleural space is irrigated once again. Many surgeons instill a broad-spectrum antibiotic in a small amount of sterile solution into the space just before closure. No prospective data support this practice, but its use is reassuring in that the fluid that accumulates within the space is an excellent culture medium.

The postpneumonectomy pleural space usually is closed without drainage. If the development of an infection within the space is likely, a thoracotomy tube is placed into the space along the chest wall just above the hemidiaphragm. This is connected to an underwater seal drainage system. However, the drainage tube is clamped and only opened periodically to drain the accumulated fluid. Some surgeons (J.R. Pellett, personal communication, 1992) routinely drain the space for 24 hours to prevent too rapid accumulation of fluid in the space and to enable the detection of excessive postoperative bleeding if it occurs. Balanced pleural drainage to maintain the mediastinum in a normal midline position as suggested by Laforet and Boyd (1964) is not recommended.

After closure of the incision, the pressure within the space is adjusted as necessary to approximate a negative pressure of 2 to 4 cm of water on inspiration and a positive pressure of 2 to 4 cm of water on exhalation. Adjustment may be made simply by thoracentesis and removal of air until the trachea is in the midline at the sternal notch, or the actual pressures may be measured using a manometer.

Some authors advocate daily adjustment of the intrapleural pressure within the pneumonectomy space for 4 to 5 days after the pneumonectomy. When this is done, antibiotics may be placed within the cavity. Others, including myself, have found this procedure unnecessary and meddlesome, preferring to check the pressure only if clinical signs indicate its need.

Fate of the Pleural Space

After pneumonectomy, elevation of the ipsilateral leaf of the diaphragm, shift of the mediastinum toward the operated

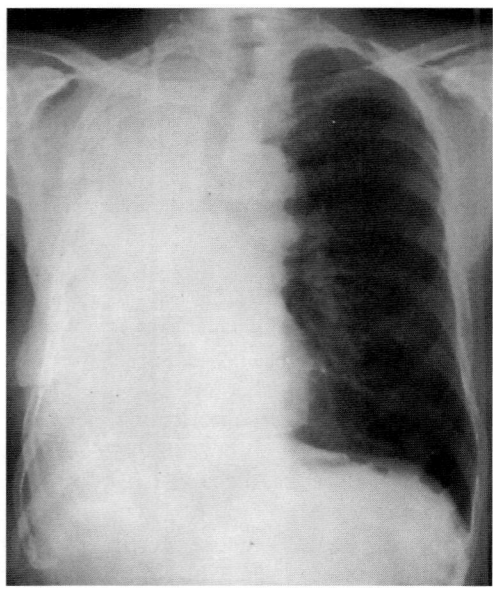

Fig. 26-2. Chest radiograph 2 weeks after right pneumonectomy.

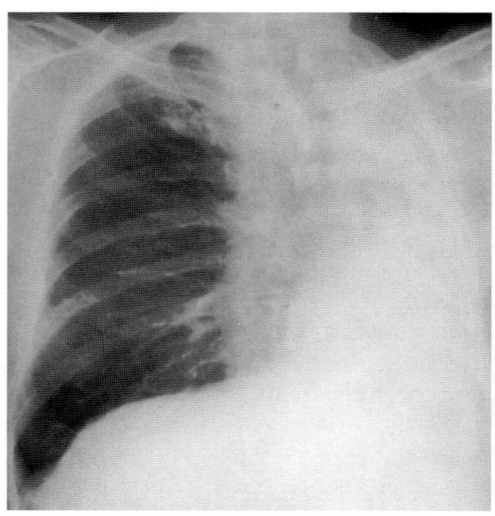

Fig. 26-3. Chest radiograph 3 years after left pneumonectomy.

side, and narrowing of the intercostal spaces of the ipsilateral side occur. In addition, serosanguinous fluid accumulates in the empty pleural space to fill the residual volume. The rate of accumulation of the fluid and the complete absorption of the air from the space are variable. Generally, the process is completed within 3 to 4 weeks, but it may take as long as 7 months (Fig. 26-2).

In the past, the phrenic nerve on the side of the pneumonectomy was crushed to obtain a prompter and higher elevation of the diaphragmatic leaf to reduce the residual volume of the postpneumonectomy space. The resultant paralysis of the ipsilateral leaf of the diaphragm, however, permits paradoxical movement of this portion of the thoracic cage. Although this effect is of no real consequence during normal breathing, the paradoxical movement of this paralyzed leaf does interfere with the efficacy of the cough mechanism. Thus, it is not recommended as a routine procedure.

A thoracoplasty often was performed postoperatively to obliterate the residual pleural space, thereby preventing the overdistention of the remaining contralateral lung as well as possibly reducing the incidence of infection of the space. Overdistention of the contralateral lung, however, is in itself not detrimental to lung function, and a standard thoracoplasty does adversely affect the function of the contralateral lung. Gaensler and Strieder (1989) showed a loss of approximately 25 to 30% of the preoperative vital capacity and approximately 20% of the maximum voluntary ventilation in the contralateral lung after a standard thoracoplasty was performed over a nonfunctioning lung. A plombage type of thoracoplasty is followed by less functional loss, but the foreign body frequently becomes associated with infection and consequently its use is not advised.

The fluid within the pleural space is gradually absorbed so that only a potential space remains. As absorption takes place, the heart and mediastinum shift farther toward the ipsilateral side, and the remaining contralateral lung herniates anteriorly and partially into the postpneumonectomy space to fill this residual thoracic volume (Fig. 26-3). Spirn and colleagues (1988) noted that this anterior herniation occurs after either a left or right pneumonectomy to a variable degree in all cases. Posteroprevertebral lung herniation occurs in approximately 50% of patients after a left pneumonectomy; its occurrence is not observed after a right pneumonectomy.

Complete absorption of the fluid is uncommon. Suarez and colleagues (1969) found complete absorption occurred in only 10 of 37 patients who died at varying time intervals after pneumonectomy. In the other 27 individuals, variable amounts of air or fluid remained in simple or loculated spaces. This early observation (that in only one-third of postpneumonectomy patients does the space become obliterated completely) was confirmed by the computed tomographic evaluation of the postpneumonectomy space by Biondetti and associates (1982). In the latter study, two-thirds of the postpneumonectomy spaces contained a unilocular fluid-filled space of varying size surrounded by thick fibrous margins.

Postlobectomy Pleural Space

After a lobectomy, the pleural space is drained routinely. Two thoracostomy tubes are used, one near the apex and one at the base, along the costal margin of the hemidiaphragm. These tubes are connected to an underwater seal drainage system. Supplemental negative suction may be used according to the preference of the operator. The tubes are kept in the pleural space until no air leak is present and the drainage is less than 50 mL per 24 hours. Care is needed to maintain patency of the drainage system as long as the thoracostomy tubes are in place.

With the re-expansion of the remaining lung, elevation of the diaphragmatic leaf, and shift of the mediastinum toward the ipsilateral side, the pleural space is usually obliterated within several days to a week. An asymptomatic persistent air space may remain, however, for a longer period.

Approximately 10% of persistent spaces become complicated, and Conlan (1990) reported that in 3%, the complication is of serious import (e.g., empyema or bronchopleural fistula). In patients in whom insufficient lung to fill the pleural space is anticipated, especially those with inflammatory disease processes, Lynn (1960) and Tamimi and colleagues (1976) recommend a preresection apical tailoring thoracoplasty to reduce the size of the pleural space and thus prevent the high incidence of serious morbidity seen in these patients. This procedure is rarely done at present, however, and is not recommended. If such a problem is anticipated, the chest wall incision should be performed so that the chest wall muscles are preserved for a possible transplant if one becomes necessary. Intraoperatively, if it is recognized that insufficient lung tissue is present to fill the pleural space, Brewer (1956) and Miscall (1956) and their associates suggested the use of a pleural partition or construction of a pleural tent to reduce the size of the space. Conlan (1990) discussed the technique of constructing the tent and its fate. Although this procedure was believed to have had advantages in reducing space complications when resections for inflammatory diseases were more common, there appear to be few indications for its use at present. However, Robinson and Preksto (1998) reported in an uncontrolled study that the creation of a pleural tent after an upper lobectomy resulted in a significantly shorter mean period of an air leak versus untented procedures: 1.6 ± 0.3 days versus 3.9 ± 1.2 days. The chest tubes could be removed sooner and hospital stay was shorter. Whether the tent should be created routinely or only if problems are anticipated remains a question. Deslauriers (personal communication, 1992), however, is a strong advocate for its use when it appears that insufficient lung volume remains to fill the pleural space after an upper lobectomy. He reports the value of a postoperative pneumoperitoneum to reduce the volume of the ipsilateral hemithorax, particularly if a basilar space is anticipated. He also suggests temporary paralysis of the ipsilateral leaf of the diaphragm, which I believe is contraindicated, however, because of the adverse effects of paradoxical motion of this leaf on the diaphragm, especially with coughing.

Adjunctive or concomitant tailoring thoracoplasty also has been suggested to reduce the size of the pleural spaces, but its use has been abandoned because of the deranged chest wall physiology postoperatively. Conlan (1990) suggested the use of an osteoplastic thoracoplasty to prevent the chest wall instability. Talamonti and colleagues (1989)

favored a modified plombage thoracoplasty using an inflatable prosthesis to fill the space. Most surgeons, however, recommend a muscle transplant to fill a potentially hazardous residual pleural space.

Postsegmentectomy Pleural Space

The pleural space after a segmentectomy or other lesser resectional procedure should be managed in a fashion similar to that described for the postlobectomy space. Air leaks for a greater or lesser period of time are the major problem in these patients.

Management after Minimal Resections

In most situations, even if minimal or no pulmonary tissue is resected, it is best to drain the pleural space as is done for a lobectomy or a segmentectomy. An exception may be the patient who has had only a lung biopsy or in whom the pleural space was entered by a limited anterior or occasionally a small axillary thoracotomy. In these instances, simple aspiration of the pleural space by use of a small catheter just before complete closure of the incision is all that is necessary. On the other hand, in patients with a standard posterolateral thoracotomy in whom only an exploratory procedure was performed, adequate postoperative thoracostomy tube drainage is indicated; usually, only one lower thoracostomy tube is necessary. Significant amounts of fluid may collect, necessitating subsequent thoracentesis if proper drainage has not been effected.

ANTIBIOTIC PROPHYLAXIS IN LUNG RESECTION

Intrapleural Antibiotic

Intrapleural antibiotic after resection is generally not recommended. Complete hemostasis and pleural irrigation are essential. At times a broad-spectrum antibiotic is instilled into the postpneumonectomy space, but proof that this is of value is lacking.

Systemic Antibiotic

Olak and colleagues (1991) conducted a randomized trial of one-dose versus six-dose cefazolin prophylaxis in elective general thoracic surgery and found no difference in the incidence of infectious complications. However, Bernard and associates (1994), in a double-blind trial of two doses of 1.5 g of cefuroxime, one at the time of induction of anesthesia and the second 2 hours later, versus the same regimen followed by a 1.5-g dose of the drug every 6 hours after the second dose for a total of 48 hours found that the latter regimen resulted in fewer cases of postoperative empyema and pneumonia than did the former. Obviously, additional studies are necessary before any conclusion can be reached as to the value of the use of prophylactic antibiotics in patients undergoing lung resection.

PHYSIOLOGIC EFFECTS

Ventilatory Changes

Postpneumonectomy

Early after a pneumonectomy, the ventilation of the remaining lung may be improved by a compensatory increase in the depth and rate of breathing. The lung becomes stiffer, however, and the elastic recoil pressure at total lung capacity increases. As a result, the work of breathing is increased. Diffusion capacity (DLCO) is decreased also. As the remaining lung adjusts to the changes in the thoracic volume available to it, the lung becomes hyperinflated. The result is an increase of 10 to 30% in its vital and total capacities.

Van Mieghem and Demedts (1989) found an overall 35 to 40% reduction of the preoperative forced vital capacity (FVC), forced expiratory volume in 1 second (FEV$_1$), and DLCO after pneumonectomy. These observations are similar to those of Ladurie and Ranson-Bitker (1985), who found that the vital capacity was over 50% of the predicted value 5 years after pneumonectomy in 98 patients.

In children, the late functional loss after pneumonectomy is less than that observed in the adult. Gas exchange is normal when the child is at rest. The total lung capacity and vital capacity are increased well above that predicted for one lung, and the maximum voluntary ventilation (maximum breathing capacity) is generally normal. DLCO is normal if the pneumonectomy is performed before puberty; this is probably the result of growth of the remaining lung in the young child. Cagle and Thurlbeck (1988) presented a thorough review of the experimental and clinical observations relative to postpneumonectomy compensatory lung growth. Many facets of the mechanisms stimulating this occurrence remain to be elicited, but stretch of the remaining lung is thought to be the initial stimulus for the compensatory growth of the remaining lung tissue.

If pneumonectomy is performed after puberty, reduction of the DLCO occurs, as is noted in the adult. After pneumonectomy in children, pulmonary hypertension is not a significant development.

Postlobectomy

With resection of a lobe of the lung, a part of the total alveolar, bronchial, and vascular masses is removed. Overinflation of the contralateral as well as of the remaining ipsilateral lung tissue results.

The remaining lung parenchyma is subjected to increased perfusion, despite an absolute reduction in the diffusion surface. The ratio of the dead space to the total lung volume increases, but a decrease of the dead space with respect to the tidal volume occurs. As a result, ventilatory efficiency is actually improved.

Ali and associates (1980) reported an early disproportionate functional loss after lobectomy that was greater than the predicted loss. They reported a mean decrease of approximately 30% in the FVC and FEV$_1$ when only a 25% reduction was predicted. Markos and colleagues (1989), however, did not observe this disproportionate loss; in fact, the observed mean losses in FVC and FEV$_1$ were less than had been predicted. The reasons for these discrepancies are unresolved. Van Mieghem and Demedts (1989) reported only a 15% decrease in the FVC after lobectomy. Berend and associates (1980) noted similar findings, a decrease of 12% and 10%, respectively, in the total lung capacity and vital capacity after lobectomy. They observed only a slight reduction of the FEV$_1$ and no change in the DLCO.

The loss may vary in the individual patient, however, and is influenced by the degree of functional loss present preoperatively and the presence or absence of postoperative complications. The occurrence of hemorrhage, effusion, air leak, empyema, fibrothorax, or bronchopleural fistula exerts a serious adverse effect on postoperative pulmonary function.

Werner and associates (1993) reported that late endurance testing and lung volumes in children and adolescents who had undergone lobectomy in infancy confirmed lung growth as well as lung distention. Good functional recovery was observed, but changes in regional ventilation and perfusion suggested dysplastic parenchyma and vascular bed in the lung that occupied the area of the previous resection.

Postsegmentectomy and Lesser Procedures

The physiologic changes after a segmentectomy are the same as those noted after a lobectomy. The late functional loss is related to the number of segments removed as well as to the occurrence of postoperative complications. The functional gain by the preservation of a segment of lobe is generally less than expected from its volume. The parenchymal tissue saved, however, may play a valuable role in helping to fill the pleural space. Unfortunately, even this is relative, because the incidence of postoperative complications occasionally is greater after segmentectomy than after a lobectomy. In the prospective study of the North American Lung Cancer Groups reported by Ginsberg and Rubenstein (1991), those patients who underwent a segmentectomy or a lesser resection exhibited an initial ventilating functional advantage over those who underwent a lobectomy. This functional advantage was lost, however, after the first year of observation.

The physiologic changes subsequent to a wedge resection in the absence of postoperative pleural complications are minimal. Those seen are more directly related to the thoracotomy incision than to the removal of the small part of lung. Early in the postoperative period, the lung volume is restricted. Inspiratory capacity and the expiratory reserve volume are decreased. The end-expiratory position is depressed as the result of pain in the chest wall. Alveolar hypoventilation with carbon dioxide retention and some degree of respiratory acidosis occurs. Oxyhemoglobin desaturation occurs and is greatest on the second and third postoperative days; it may persist for as long as 10 days. Compliance is reduced, resulting in an increased work of breathing. This reduction is most remarkable the first few hours after the operation and returns gradually to near normal within the first postoperative week.

Hemodynamic Changes

After a pneumonectomy, the pulmonary artery pressure is usually normal at rest. As noted by Van Mieghem and Demedts (1989), however, maximum effort tolerance decreases after pneumonectomy and an increase in both the pulmonary artery pressure and pulmonary vascular resistance occurs with effort. Cardiac output and stroke volume decrease during effort. These changes are accompanied with an increase in the peripheral arterial blood pressure as well as in the peripheral vascular resistance. Oxygen saturation decreases on effort, possibly because of an absolute decrease in the DLCO. After a lobectomy, similar hemodynamic changes are seen, but to a lesser degree.

Van Mieghem and Demedts (1989) suggested that the cardiovascular changes can be explained by the hypothesis that the removal of a substantial part of the vascular bed may result in an increase in the afterload of the right ventricle, which may interfere with the emptying of this ventricle. The increased afterload increases both the end-systolic and end-diastolic volumes of the right ventricle, which may in turn cause a shift of the interventricular septum to the left, with resultant changes that effect a decreased cardiac output.

The function of the right ventricle after pulmonary resection has been assessed by thermodilution methods and by right-sided heart pressure studies by both Reed (1992) and Okada (1994) and their associates. From these studies it was documented that the right ventricular ejection fraction decreases and the right ventricular end-diastolic volume index is increased, whereas the right ventricular stroke volume index is decreased as of the first day postoperatively; this continues for a variable length of time postoperatively. At rest the pulmonary artery pressure, pulmonary vascular resistance index, central venous pressure, and left ventricular function remain unaffected. However, with exercise the pulmonary artery pressure and the pulmonary vascular resistance index increase with further change in the right ventricular afterload. Okada and associates (1994) believe that at rest the changes noted in the right ventricular function compensate for the increase in right ventricular volume but cannot with exercise. Furthermore, they suggest that the

changes in the right ventricular afterload may be the major cause of right ventricular dysfunction after either a lobectomy or a pneumonectomy. Whether a shift of the interventricular septum to the left occurs, with resultant deleterious effect on left ventricular function as suggested by Van Mieghem and Demedts (1989), remains unresolved.

Of clinical interest is that, according to Ladurie and Ranson-Bitker (1985), sinoauricular tachycardia is present in over 75% of the late survivors of a pneumonectomy; in one-fourth of the patients, over 100 beats per minute were recorded. A functional, persistent systolic murmur at the right-sided heart base was observed in 12% of the patients. Right-sided heart overload, determined electrocardiographically, was present in 6% of the patients in their study.

The older the patient at the time of pneumonectomy or the greater the degree of preexistent chronic obstructive airway disease in the remaining lung, the greater the likelihood of functional incapacity. In evaluating the functional capacity, a direct relationship to the pulmonary artery pressure apparently exists; as the functional reserve decreases, the pulmonary artery pressure increases. The reduction in the functional capacity appears to be related more directly to the pulmonary artery pressure and pulmonary blood flow relationships in the remaining lung than to arterial saturation per se. The functional capacity appears to be governed and limited by the expansibility of the remaining vascular bed. When the limit of the bed is reached or exceeded, persistent pulmonary hypertension occurs and cor pulmonale results.

REFERENCES

Ali MK, et al: Predicting loss of pulmonary function after pulmonary resection for bronchogenic carcinoma. Chest 77:337, 1980.

Anderson TM, Miller JI Jr: Surgical technique and application of pericardial fat pad and pericardiophrenic grafts. Ann Thorac Surg 59:1590, 1995.

Berend N, Woolcock AJ, Marlin GE: Effects of lobectomy on lung function. Thorax 35:145, 1980.

Bernard A, et al: Antibiotic prophylaxis in pulmonary surgery. A prospective randomized double-blind trial of flash cefuroxine versus forty-eight-hour cefuroxine. J Thorac Cardiovasc Surg 107:896, 1994.

Biondetti PR, et al: Evaluation of post-pneumonectomy space by computed tomography. J Comput Assist Tomogr 6:238, 1982.

Brewer LA III, Bai AF: Surgery of the bronchi and trachea. Experience with the pedicled pericardial fat graft reinforcement. Am J Surg 89:331, 1955.

Brewer LA, Bai AF, Jones WM: The development of the pleural partition to prevent overexpansion of the lung following partial pulmonary resection. J Thorac Surg 31:165, 1956.

Brewer LA III, et al: Bronchial closure in pulmonary resection. A clinical and experimental study using a pedicled pericardial fat graft reinforcement. J Thorac Surg 26:507, 1953.

Brown J, Pomerantz M: Extrapleural pneumonectomy for tuberculosis. Chest Surg Clin North Am 5:289, 1995.

Cagle PT, Thurlbeck WM: Postpneumonectomy compensatory lung growth. Am Rev Respir Dis 138:1314, 1988.

Conlan AA: Prophylaxis and management of postlobectomy infected spaces. In Deslauriers J, Lacquet LK (eds): Thoracic Surgery: Surgical Management of Pleural Diseases. St. Louis: CV Mosby, 1990, p. 279.

Cooper JD: Technique to reduce air leaks after resection of emphysematous lung. Ann Thorac Surg 57:1038, 1994.

Cooper JD, et al: Bilateral pneumonectomy (volume reduction) for chronic obstructive pulmonary disease. J Thorac Cardiovasc Surg 109:106, 1995.

Gaensler EA, Strieder JW: Progressive changes in pulmonary function after pneumonectomy. J Thorac Surg 22:1, 1951.

Ginsberg RJ, Rubinstein L, for the Lung Cancer Study Group: Patients with T_1N_0 non-SCLC lung cancer. Lung Cancer 7(Suppl):83(Abstract 304), 1991.

Grismer JT, Read RC: Evolution of pulmonary resection techniques and review of the bronchus-first method. Ann Thorac Surg 60:1133, 1995.

Hakim M, Milstein BB: Role of automatic staplers in the etiology of bronchopleural fistula. Thorax 40:27, 1985.

Harvey JC, Erdman C, Beattie EJ: Pneumonectomy. Chest Surg Clin North Am 5:253, 1995.

Hazelrigg SR, et al: Effect of bovine pericardial strips on air leaks after stapled pulmonary resection. Ann Thorac Surg 63:1573, 1997.

Hood RM: Operations involving the lungs. In Hood RM (ed): Techniques in General Thoracic Surgery. Philadelphia: WB Saunders, 1985.

Horsley WS, Miller JI Jr: Management of the uncontrollable pulmonary air leak with cyanoacrylate glue. Ann Thorac Surg 63:1492, 1997.

Jensen C, Sharma P: Use of fibrin glue in thoracic surgery. Ann Thorac Surg 39:521, 1985.

Jensik RJ: The extent of resection for localized lung cancer: segmental resection. In Kittle CF (ed): Current Controversies in Thoracic Surgery. Philadelphia: WB Saunders, 1986.

Ladurie M L, Ranson-Bitker B: Quality of life following resection for lung cancer. In Delarue NC, Eschapasse H (eds): Lung Cancer. International Trends in General Thoracic Surgery. Vol. I. Philadelphia: WB Saunders, 1985, p. 296.

Laforet EG, Boyd TF: Balanced drainage of the pneumonectomy space. Surg Gynecol Obstet 118:1051, 1964.

Lynn RB: The prevention of postresection spaces following resection for pulmonary tuberculosis. Surg Gynecol Obstet 111:647, 1960.

Markos J, et al: Preoperative assessment as a predictor of mortality and morbidity after lung resection. Am Rev Respir Dis 139:902, 1989.

Matthew TL, et al: Four years' experience with fibrin sealant in thoracic and cardiovascular surgery. Ann Thorac Cardiovasc Surg 50:40, 1990.

McGovern EM, et al: Completion pneumonectomy: indications, complications, and results. Ann Thorac Surg 46:141, 1988.

Miller GE, Aberg THJ, Gerbode F: Effect of pulmonary vein ligation on pulmonary artery flow in dogs. J Thorac Cardiovasc Surg 55:668, 1968.

Miller JI Jr, Lee RB, Mansour KA: Lung volume reduction surgery: lessons learned. Ann Thorac Surg 61:1464, 1996.

Miscall LD, Duffy RW, Nolan RB: The pleural tent as a simultaneous tailoring procedure in combination with pulmonary resection. Am Rev Respir Dis 73:831, 1956.

Mouritzen C, Dromer M, Keinecke HO: The effect of fibrin glueing to seal bronchial and alveolar leakages after pulmonary resections and decortications. Eur J Cardiothorac Surg 7:75, 1993.

Naunheim KS, et al: Unilateral video assisted thoracoscopic surgery lung reduction. Ann Thorac Surg 61:1092, 1996.

Nomori H, Horio H: Gelatin-resorcinol-formaldehyde-glutaldehyde glue spread stapler prevents air leakage from the lung. Ann Thorac Surg 63:352, 1997.

Okada M, et al: Right ventricular dysfunction after major pulmonary surgery. J Thorac Cardiovasc Surg 108:503, 1994.

Olak J, et al: Randomized trial of one dose versus six dose cefazolin prophylaxis in elective general thoracic surgery. Ann Thorac Surg 51:956, 1991.

Pairolero PC, Payne WS: Postoperative care and complications in the thoracic surgical patient. In Glenn WWL, et al (eds): Thoracic and Cardiovascular Surgery. 4th Ed. Norwalk, CT: Appleton-Century-Crofts, 1983, p. 338.

Peterffy A, Calabrese E: Mechanical and conventional manual sutures of the bronchial stump. Scand J Thorac Cardiovasc Surg 13:87, 1979.

Peterffy A, Henze A: Haemorrhagic complications during pulmonary resection. A retrospective review of 1428 resections with 113 haemorrhagic episodes. Scand J Thorac Cardiovasc Surg 17:283, 1983.

Piccione W Jr, Faber LP: Management of complications related to pulmonary resection. In Waldhausen JA, Orringer MB (eds): Complications in Cardiothoracic Surgery. St. Louis: Mosby-Year Book, 1991, p. 336.

Reed CE, Spinale FG, Crawford FA Jr: Effect of pulmonary resection on right ventricular function. Ann Thorac Surg 53:578, 1992.

Robinson LA, Preksto D: Pleural tenting during upper lobectomy decreases chest tube time and total hospitalization days. J Thorac Cardiovasc Surg 115:319, 1998.

Saitoh Y, et al: Prevention of main bronchial fistula after pneumonectomy; wrapping with a pedicled pericardial flap containing the pericardiophrenic artery. J Jpn Assoc Chest Surg 10:778, 1996.

Spirn PW, et al: Radiology of the chest after thoracic surgery. Semin Roentgenol 23:9, 1988.

Suarez J, Clagett OT, Brown AL Jr: The postpneumonectomy space. J Thorac Cardiovasc Surg 57:539, 1969.

Takaro T: Use of staplers in bronchial closure. In Grillo HC, Eschapasse H (eds): International Trends in General Thoracic Surgery. Vol. 2. Philadelphia: WB Saunders, 1987.

Talamonti MS, et al: A new method of extraperiosteal plombage for atypical pulmonary tuberculosis. Chest 96:237S, 1989.

Tamimi TM, et al: The value of thoracoplasty before extensive unilateral resection for pulmonary tuberculosis. Am Surg 42:71, 1976.

Van Mieghem W, Demedts M: Cardiopulmonary function after lobectomy or pneumonectomy for pulmonary neoplasm. Respir Med 83:199, 1989.

Vanetti A, Bazelly B: Discussion of use of staples in bronchial closure. In Grillo HC, Eschapasse H (eds): International Trends in General Thoracic Surgery. Vol. 2. Philadelphia: WB Saunders, 1987.

Vaughn CC, et al: Prevention of air leaks after pulmonary wedge resection. Ann Thorac Surg 63:864, 1997.

Vester SR, et al: Bronchopleural fistula after stapled closure of the bronchus. Ann Thorac Surg 52:1253, 1991.

Werner HA, et al: Lung volumes, mechanics and perfusion after pulmonary resection in infancy. J Thorac Cardiovasc Surg 105:737, 1993.

Wong K, Goldstraw P: Effect of fibrin glue in the reduction of postthoracotomy air leaks. Ann Thorac Surg 64:979, 1997.

CHAPTER 27

Technical Aspects of Lobectomy

Stanley C. Fell and Thomas J. Kirby

Lobectomy by hilar dissection, first reported by Blades and Kent in 1940 for the surgical treatment of bronchiectasis, is now performed most commonly for the definitive treatment of lung cancer. The incision for lobectomy is usually a posterolateral thoracotomy, because it allows greater exposure and maneuverability for the surgeon. Anterolateral thoracotomy, median sternotomy, except for the left lower lobe, and muscle-sparing lateral thoracotomy are used also. Posterior thoracotomy, developed during the era of surgery for pulmonary tuberculosis and bronchiectasis, as described by Overholt and Langer (1951), and generally performed on a special operating table with the patient prone, is now of historic interest. Video-assisted thoracoscopic lobectomy, as reported by Lewis and associates (1992), is currently in the investigational stage and is not yet recommended as an acceptable alternative. Key points in performance of lobectomy are mobilization of the lobe, fissure dissection, and management of the vessels and bronchus.

MOBILIZATION OF THE LOBE

The pleural cavity is entered through the fifth intercostal space or through the bed of the fifth rib, often subperiosteally resected. If adhesive pleuritis is anticipated, entrance through the bed of the resected fifth rib allows for more expeditious mobilization of the lung, either in the intrapleural or extrapleural plane. Weblike avascular adhesions are managed by finger dissection and a sponge stick; cautery is applied for vascular adhesions. Inflammatory and cavitary lesions adherent to the parietal pleura are mobilized in the extrapleural plane.

The need for chest wall resection for tumors adherent to the parietal pleura is controversial. Trastek and associates (1984) advocate en bloc resection of lung and chest wall in this situation. McCaughan and colleagues (1985) recommend attempting extrapleural dissection if extrapleural extension is not documented preoperatively. If an extrapleural plane is readily achieved, chest wall resection is not performed, because these tumors often involve only visceral pleura. If the tumor is determined to be fixed to the chest wall intraopera-

tively, the extrapleural approach is abandoned and en bloc resection is performed. This approach does not adversely influence the survival rate.

After mobilization of the lung, the mediastinal pleura is incised about the hilum, the pathology is evaluated, and node sampling is performed as indicated.

FISSURE DISSECTION

Incomplete fissures result from congenital fusion of lung substance, inflammation, or extension of the pathologic process to the adjacent lobe. Combined sharp and blunt dissection along the interlobar plane is generally sufficient to separate the lobes. Application of a stapling device, or dividing lung parenchyma by clamp and suture, may be required. The interlobar arterial branches must be visualized during these efforts. Fused lobes also may be separated by retrograde dissection and traction on the divided bronchus using the intersegmental vein as a guide. Small blood vessels and air leaks require suture; if clamps or a stapler are used, diminution of lung volume and distortion of the remaining lobes should be kept to a minimum.

Single lung anesthesia and stapling devices have facilitated lobectomy, but total reliance on these methods is to be decried. The double-lumen endotracheal tube may be unavailable, unable to be placed properly, or become displaced. The surgeon must be able to dissect the lobar hilum and the fissures of a partially inflated lung, preferably manually ventilated.

MANAGEMENT OF LOBAR VESSELS

The key to an orderly lobectomy is thorough knowledge of the anatomy of the pulmonary artery, variations in its branching, and its proper dissection (see Chapter 5). In contrast to the fragile pulmonary segmental arteries, located deep within the fissures and intimately related to the segmental bronchi, the pulmonary veins and their tributary trunks have relatively strong walls and are easily accessible at the anterosuperior

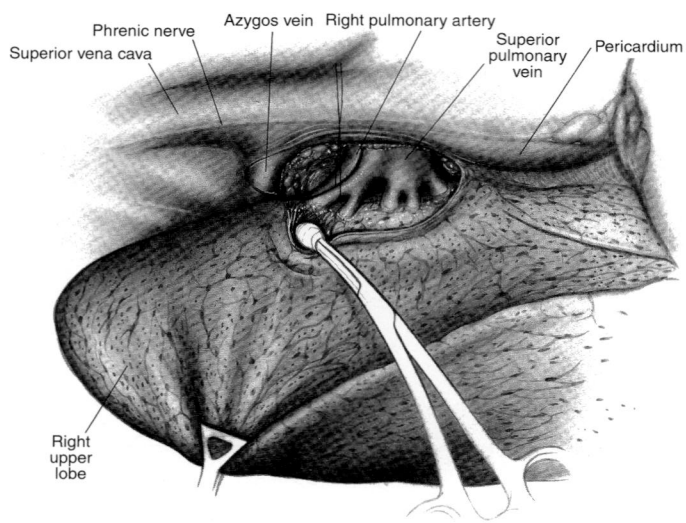

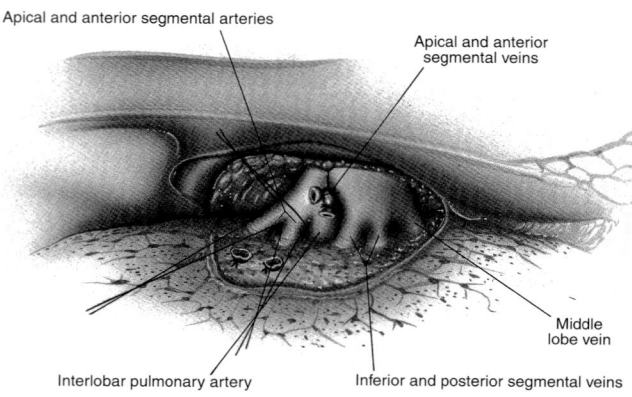

Fig. 27-1. A. Anterior aspect of the right hilum. Division of the apical segmental vein facilitates dissection of the superior trunk of the pulmonary artery. **B.** The superior arterial trunk before ligation. The anterior as well as the apical segmental vein has been divided to demonstrate the interlobar trunk of the pulmonary artery.

and posteroinferior aspects of the hilum. Occasionally, a common extrapericardial pulmonary vein is encountered.

The pulmonary arteries are best dissected from their fibrous sheath using scissors in the long axis of the vessel. Once a sufficient length of the vessel has been exposed, the sheath is grasped on either side and the artery is then rolled out of its sheath, allowing the passage of a right-angle clamp to encircle the vessel and to draw a ligature beneath it. Dissection of the artery with a clamp without prior sharp dissection invites hemorrhage. If segmental branches are short, additional length may be obtained by dissecting into lung parenchyma and dividing the lung substance with cautery.

Bronchial closure is generally performed with a 3.5- or 4.8-mm stapling device, depending on the compliance of the bronchus. Manual sewing of the bronchus may be indicated in some circumstances, an example being to ensure that the bronchial resection is proximal to an endobronchial tumor. Suture materials currently used include silk, polyglactin, and polypropylene. Manual closure proceeds as follows. A suitably sized toothed bronchus clamp is applied to the specimen side of the bronchus, and stay sutures are inserted in the upper and lower borders of the bronchus. With the underlying vascular structures protected by a Semb's clamp, the bronchus is transected. Bronchial sutures are placed approximately 3 mm apart and 3 mm from the cut edge. In the absence of single lung ventilation, placing the first suture at the midpoint of the bronchus reduces air leak. Surgeons' knots reduce tension on the cartilage, the knots being placed over the suture hole in the membranous portion to seal possible air leak from this area. The traction sutures may be tied in place or over the cut end. Repleuralization of the bronchial stump is of dubious value after a lobectomy, the stump being readily covered by the remaining parenchymal tissue within the hemithorax.

After removal of the specimen, the integrity of the bronchial closure is tested by the application of positive pressure to the endotracheal tube with a saline-filled hemithorax. Parenchymal air leaks also are localized and

repaired. Two thoracostomy tubes are placed through stab wounds in the anterior axillary line. The lower tube extends posteriorly on the diaphragm and the upper tube lies anteriorly to reach the apex of the pleura. An absorbable suture from the tip of the anterior tube to the apical pleura ensures its proper position. After closure of the chest, negative suction from 10 to 20 cm of water is applied to the drainage systems. The tubes are removed serially once drainage is less than 60 mL in 24 hours and the air leak has ceased.

RIGHT UPPER LOBECTOMY

The anatomy of the hilar structures of the right upper lobe is more complex than that of any other lobe, and arterial anomalies are more common. In approximately 80% of individuals, the anterior segment of the right upper lobe is partially or completely fused to the middle lobe, and a segmental dissection of this area is required.

The mediastinal pleura is incised about the hilum of the right lung, lateral to the superior vena cava, inferior to the azygos vein, continuing posteriorly over the bronchus, anterior to the vagus nerve that is visible subpleurally, to the level of the bronchus intermedius. Anteriorly, the incision is carried to the level of the superior pulmonary vein, posterior to the phrenic nerve (Fig. 27-1A). A pledget dissector is used to push the azygos vein superiorly, demonstrating the upper border of the right main bronchus and the upper lobe bronchus originating from it. Inferior to the azygocaval junction, a lymph node is found. Just below this lymph node is the upper border of the pulmonary artery. The areolar tissue overlying the pulmonary artery is dissected and the superior arterial trunk is visualized. This artery and its apical and anterior segmental branches are dissected. The apical segmental vein crosses the anterior segmental artery, and it is often convenient to ligate and divide this vein before dealing with the artery (Fig. 27-1B). The superior arterial trunk is doubly tied with 0 silk; the apical and

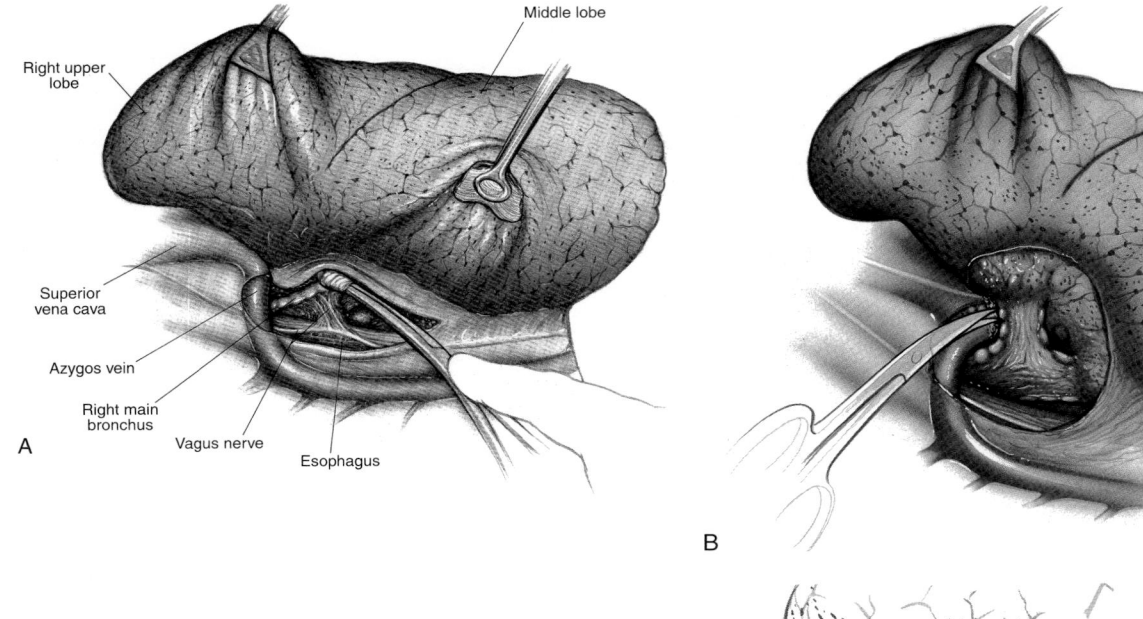

Fig. 27-2. A. Posterior aspect of the right upper lobe hilum after division of the mediastinal pleura. Vagal branches posterior to the bronchus are not yet divided. **B.** The right upper lobe bronchus is dissected. **C.** Finger dissection separates the bronchus from the interlobar pulmonary artery.

segmental branches are tied and then divided. If the segmental arteries are short, additional length may be obtained by dissecting with a right-angle clamp into the pulmonary parenchyma overlying the branches, dividing the parenchyma with cautery. Suture ligatures or clips are then applied, and the segmental arteries are divided.

After division of the superior trunk of the pulmonary artery, the common stem of the apical and anterior segmental veins is dissected and divided. The interlobar trunk of the pulmonary artery lies directly beneath the upper and middle stems of the superior pulmonary vein, and this dissection must be performed cautiously.

The remaining arterial supply to the right upper lobe is the posterior ascending artery, present in 90% of patients. Dissection of this artery can be the most formidable task in the procedure. Three approaches have been described: an anterior approach, approach through the oblique fissure, and a retrograde approach.

The anterior approach requires prior division of the posterior and inferior venous tributaries of the middle stem of the

superior vein, which is closely applied to the anterior surface of the inferior trunk of the pulmonary artery. Further dissection of the interlobar artery is required, because the posterior segmental artery arises from the anterior aspect of the interlobar artery just above the superior segmental artery. Isolation of the right pulmonary artery may be required because laceration of the posterior ascending artery or the interlobar artery from which it arises may occur during this dissection.

An approach to the posterior segmental artery via the oblique fissure is acceptable provided the oblique fissure is virtually complete. Otherwise, the artery is again at risk of injury. The retrograde method for completion of the dissection is both safe and expeditious.

Retrograde exposure of the posterior ascending artery proceeds as follows. Attention is directed to the posterior aspect of the hilum. The vagus nerve is grasped with an Allis clamp and retracted, thus demonstrating its branches to the right upper lobe. The branches are divided (Fig. 27-2A). Deep to the vagal branches, the bronchial artery may be observed; it is clipped and divided. The lower border of the upper lobe

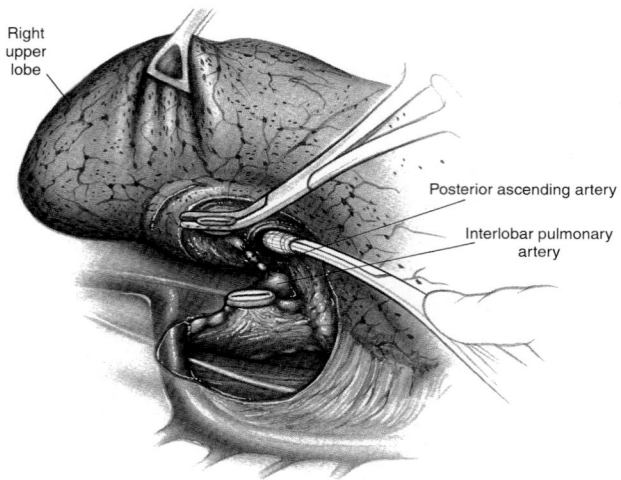

Fig. 27-3. The bronchus has been stapled and divided. Medial traction on the specimen facilitates dissection of the posterior ascending artery.

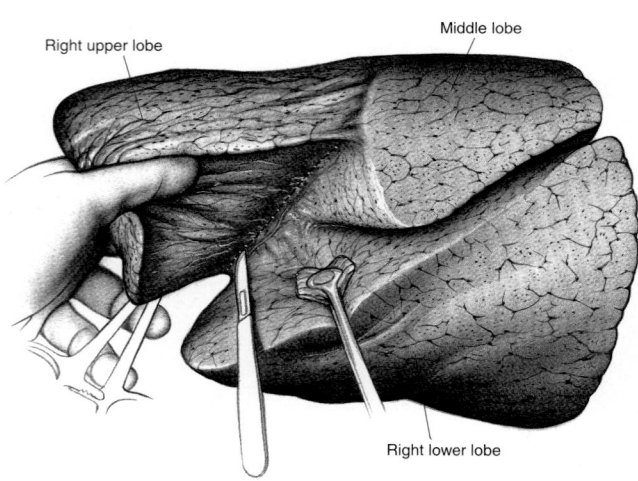

Fig. 27-4. The oblique fissure is completed by a sharp and blunt dissection and is stapled where required.

bronchus is dissected. In the crotch between the upper lobe bronchus and the intermediate bronchus is a constant lymph node. This node is dissected toward the specimen, clearing the inferior border of the right upper lobe bronchus. It is not advisable to pass a clamp from the lower border of the right upper lobe bronchus medially to encircle the bronchus, because the posterior ascending artery may be lacerated. Rather, scissor dissection of the medial surface of the bronchus is performed, sweeping areolar tissue and nodes toward the specimen (Fig. 27-2B). The bronchus is not denuded of its fascia, which supplies the vascularity required for healing. An index finger can then be inserted along the anterior aspect of the bronchus to reach its lower border (Fig. 27-2C). A right-angle clamp may then be passed safely about

the right upper lobe bronchus. A Semb's clamp is used to widen the peribronchial space, allowing for the passage of a 4.8-mm stapling device. The bronchus is either stapled and divided, or manually sutured. If stapled, the staple line generally includes the bronchial artery to the right upper lobe. The cut edge of the specimen side of the bronchus is grasped with an Allis clamp. Traction is placed on the Allis clamp, a toothed bronchus clamp is applied, and the Allis clamp is removed. By turning the handle of the bronchus clamp medially, thus elevating the cut bronchus, the fissure dissection is facilitated. With gentle medial traction on the bronchus clamp, the areolar tissue and nodes are readily dissected off the interlobar pulmonary artery and the posterior ascending artery is identified, ligated, and divided (Fig. 27-3). Occa-

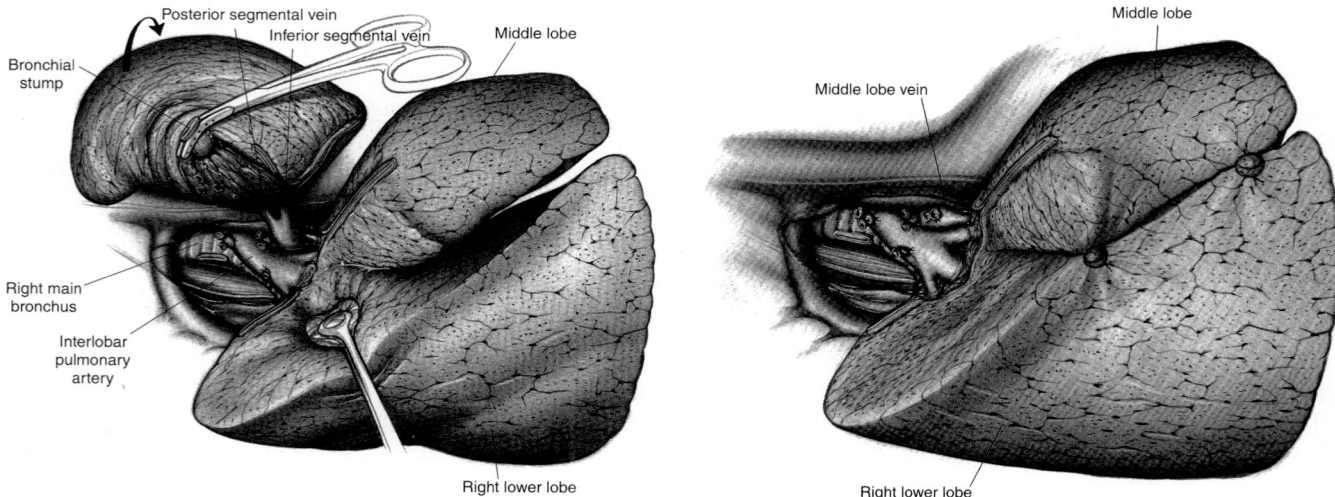

A

B

Fig. 27-5. A. Retracting the lobe medially and stapling the minor fissure exposes the middle trunk of the superior pulmonary vein. Note the relationship of this trunk to the underlying interlobar pulmonary artery. The middle lobe vein has been identified and preserved. **B.** Edges of the middle and lower lobes are approximated with silk ties to prevent middle lobe torsion.

sionally, an additional arterial branch to the anterior segment originates from the interlobar artery. Rarely, the posterior segmental artery originates from the superior segmental artery.

Attention is next directed to the fissures, which may be managed by sharp dissection along the intersegmental vein using partial inflation of the middle and lower lobes against the now airless upper lobe, by stapled division, or by a combination of both methods (Fig. 27-4). With the bronchus divided and the posterior segmental artery transected, it is safe to pass a stapling device to divide the posterior aspect of the oblique fissure. The minor fissure is similarly completed. We emphasize that attempts to divide fissures without prior identification of the segmental arteries may lead to hemorrhage. Medial traction of the bronchus clamp and further dissection with the interlobar artery under direct vision lead immediately to the middle trunk of the superior pulmonary vein and its posterior and inferior tributaries. At this point, the operator can appreciate the intimate relationship of these branches to the inferior trunk of the pulmonary artery (Fig. 27-5A). The common stem of the posterior and inferior veins is identified and the site of insertion of the middle lobe vein into the superior pulmonary vein is identified and preserved. The venous stem is doubly ligated, as are the posterior and inferior veins, which are then divided. The stapling device generally is not useful for managing the right superior pulmonary vein. The importance of minimizing air leak from the middle lobe cannot be overemphasized. The intersegmental vein defines the proper plane of dissection.

After the specimen is removed, the pleural cavity is irrigated and the bronchial closure is tested. The inferior pulmonary ligament is divided, allowing rotation of the lower lobe to facilitate complete filling of the pleural space. Because the fissure between the middle and lower lobes is generally complete, torsion of the middle lobe is possible. To prevent such torsion, the edges of the partially expanded middle and lower lobes are grasped with an Allis clamp, and a silk tie is used to approximate these edges along the

course of the fissure (Fig. 27-5B). A single application of a TA 30 stapling device accomplishes the same results, at much greater cost.

MIDDLE LOBECTOMY

Middle lobectomy is not commonly performed as an isolated procedure. In years past, it was performed for middle lobe syndrome. Incomplete fissure and hyperplastic or calcified lymph nodes, adherent to segmented arteries and the middle lobe bronchus, made it a formidable procedure, generally requiring proximal control of the right pulmonary artery.

Most often, middle lobectomy is performed in association with either upper or lower lobectomy for tumors that cross fissures. Combined middle and lower lobectomy was often required for the treatment of bronchiectasis.

If upper and middle lobes are resected, the bronchi are closed separately; for middle and lower lobectomy, the bronchus intermedius is divided just distal to the right upper lobe bronchus. The major fissure is opened and the lower lobe is retracted posteriorly (Fig. 27-6A). By following the posterior edge of the middle lobe as it joins the major fissure, and dissecting deep within the fissure, lymph nodes are noted, indicating the site of the interlobar pulmonary artery. The artery is dissected proximally in the subadventitial plane and the middle lobe artery is identified (Fig. 27-6B). Generally, two middle lobe arteries exist; the first one identified arises from the interlobar artery anteriorly, more or less opposite to the superior segmental artery arising posteriorly. Further proximal dissection of the interlobar artery demonstrates a second, and rarely a third, artery to the middle lobe. Occasionally, an anomalous branch of the middle artery to the upper lobe is identified. After ligation and division of the middle lobe arteries, the table is rotated posteriorly and the anterior aspect of the hilum is dissected, isolating and ligating the middle lobe vein that enters the

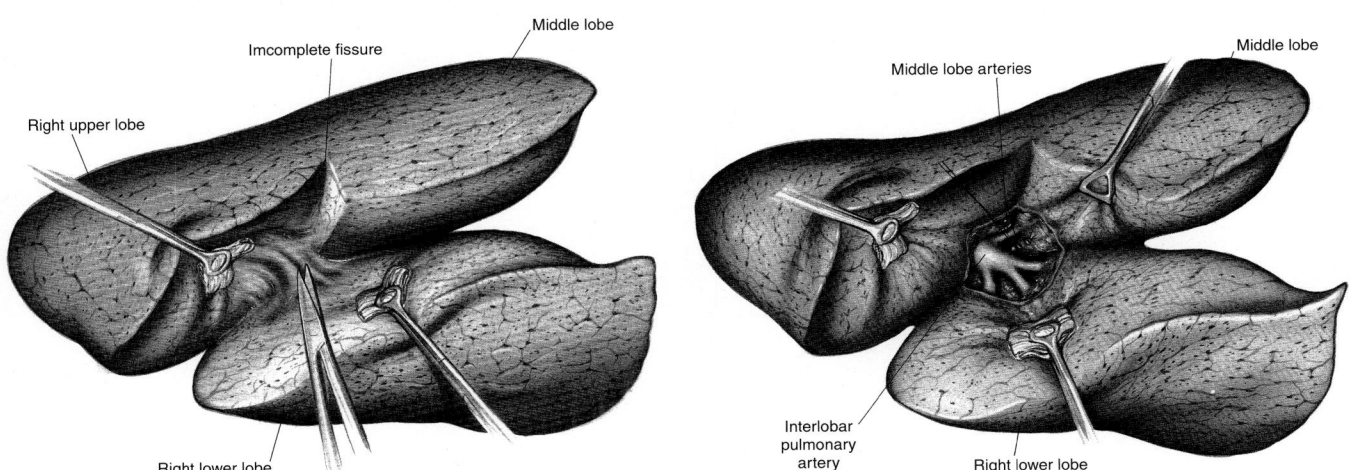

A

B

Fig. 27-6. A. and B. Dissection of the oblique fissure at its junction with the horizontal fissure demonstrates the interlobar pulmonary artery and its branches. One middle lobe artery is divided.

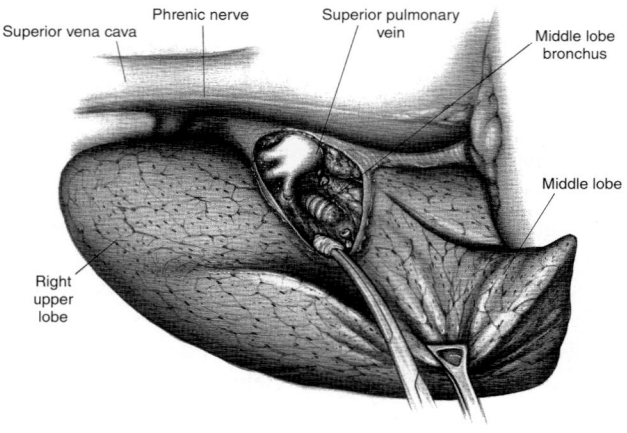

Fig. 27-7. The anterior mediastinal pleura is incised. The middle lobe vein is isolated and divided.

lower portion of the superior pulmonary vein (Fig. 27-7). After division of the middle lobe vein, the bronchus is readily accessible (Fig. 27-8A). In difficult dissections, it may be more expeditious to divide the middle lobe vein, isolate and divide the bronchus, and then ligate and divide the middle

lobe arteries. Manual suturing is generally easier than inserting a stapling device.

The closed middle lobe bronchus is deep within the parenchyma and disruption of this bronchial closure is virtually unknown. The distal portion of the transected middle lobe bronchus is grasped with a bronchus clamp. Using differential inflation and traction on the bronchus clamp, the fissure may then be completed along the lines of the intersegmental veins, by a combination of sharp and blunt dissection and stapling (Fig. 27-8B). After completion of the fissure and removal of the specimen, the raw surfaces of the upper lobe are approximated to the lower lobe by several ties to help seal air leak.

RIGHT LOWER LOBECTOMY

The oblique fissure is opened while retracting the right upper and middle lobes anteriorly and the lower lobe posteriorly. The interlobar pulmonary artery is deeply situated in the region where the oblique and horizontal fissures meet (see Fig. 27-6B). The temptation to staple and divide areas of fusion between the posterior segment of the right upper lobe and the superior segment of the lower lobe before demonstrating the

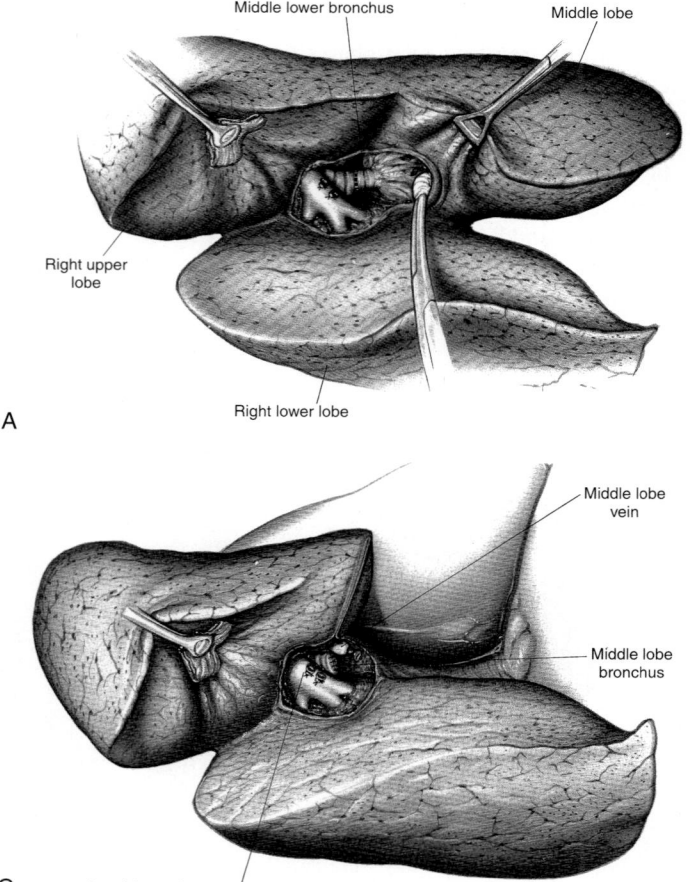

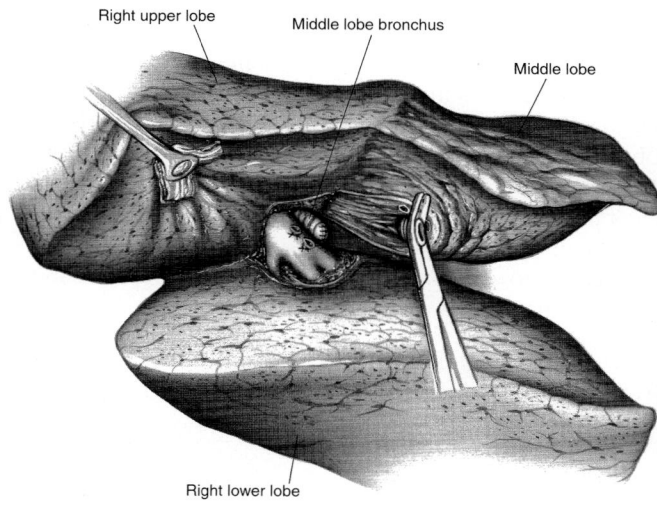

Fig. 27-8. A. The middle lobe bronchus is identified. The line of bronchial transection is illustrated. **B.** Traction on the specimen bronchus and differential inflation facilitate completion of the horizontal fissure. **C.** Hilum after middle lobectomy.

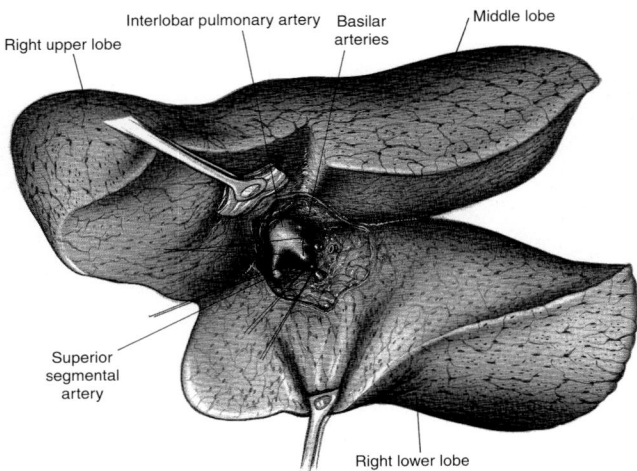

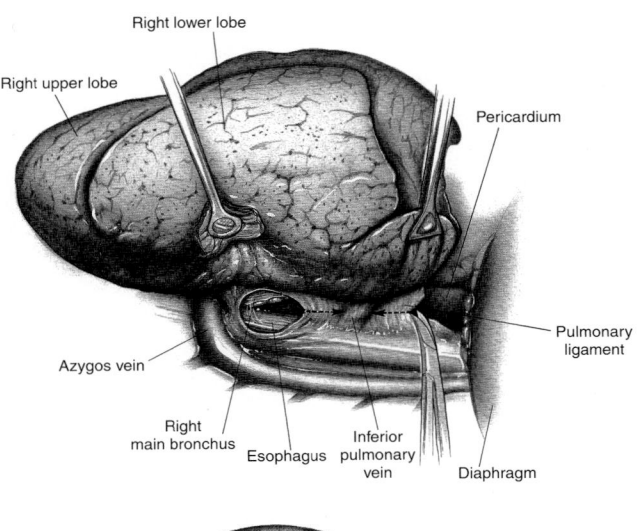

Fig. 27-9. Arterial supply of the right lower lobe. The origin of the middle lobe artery is visualized. Stapling the posterior portion of the oblique fissure facilitates the dissection of the superior segmental artery.

interlobar pulmonary artery and its branches must be avoided. The visceral pleura overlying the interlobar artery is opened and the pulmonary artery is dissected. The middle lobe artery, originating from the anteromedial surface of the interlobar artery, must be demonstrated. Directly opposite and posterolaterally lies the superior segmental artery. Rarely, the posterior ascending artery to the upper lobe originates from the superior segmental artery. Occasionally, the superior segment of the right lower lobe has two branches. Often, it is best to isolate and divide the basal arteries first, distal to the middle lobe and superior segmental arteries (Fig. 27-9). The basal arteries may have a short common trunk from which two branches originate: one supplying the anterior and medial segments and the other supplying the posterior and lateral segments. Occasionally, the four basal segmental arteries originate separately distal to the middle lobe artery, and dissection into the lung parenchyma is required to obtain adequate length for ligation and division. Attention is then directed to securing the superior segmental artery, taking care to preserve the posterior segmental artery to the right upper lobe.

The lobe is retracted anteriorly and superiorly. The inferior pulmonary ligament is divided up to the lymph node at the lower border of the inferior pulmonary vein (Fig. 27-10A). The posterior mediastinal pleura is incised over the posterior surface of the inferior pulmonary vein, which is cleared of areolar tissue, and the pleural incision is carried superiorly to above the level of the bronchus intermedius. The interval between the lower border of the bronchus and the superior pulmonary vein is dissected. The anterior surface of the inferior pulmonary vein is then cleared. With an index finger serving as a guide, the inferior pulmonary vein is then isolated, using a Semb's clamp (Fig. 27-10B). The interval between the lower lobe bronchus and the inferior vein is widened so that a vascular stapler may be inserted to occlude the cardiac end of the vein. The extrapericardial portion of the right inferior pul-

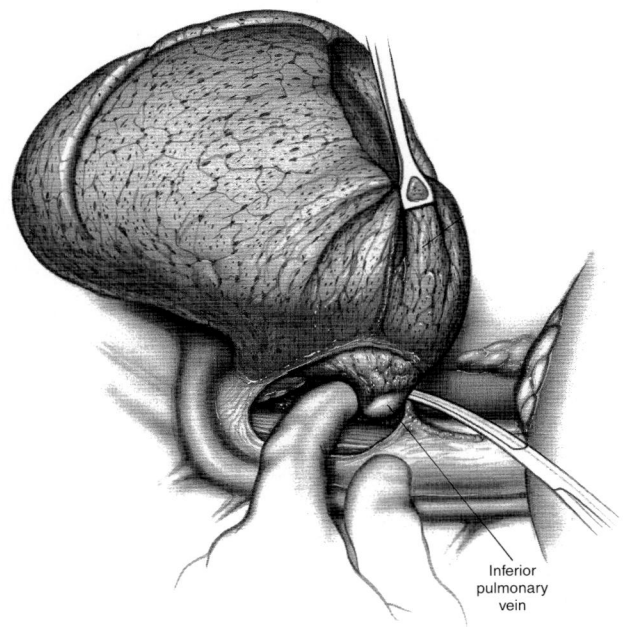

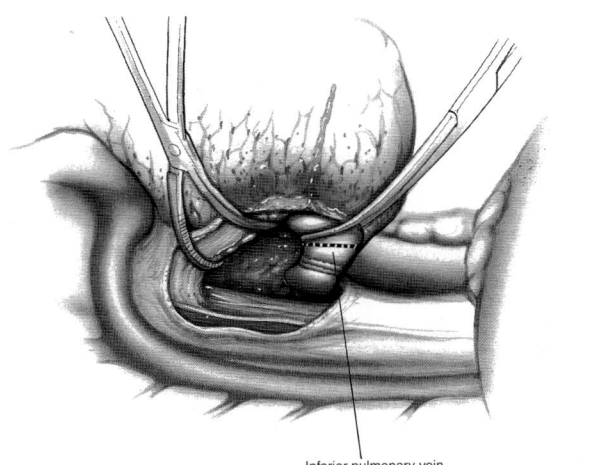

Fig. 27-10. A. The lung is retracted anteriorly. **B.** The inferior pulmonary ligament is divided. **C.** The inferior pulmonary vein is then dissected, stapled, and divided.

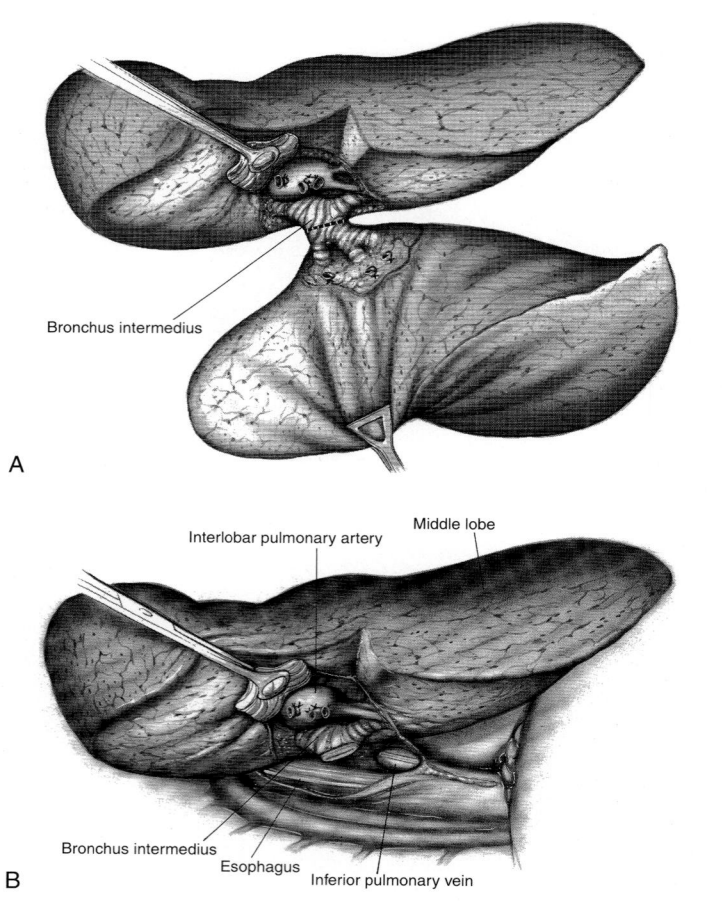

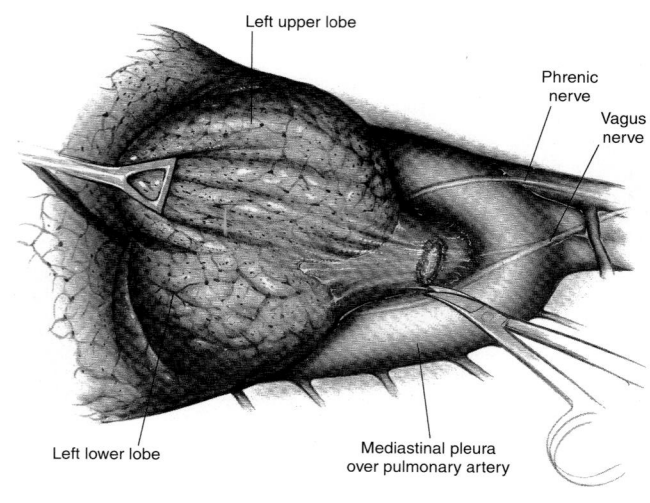

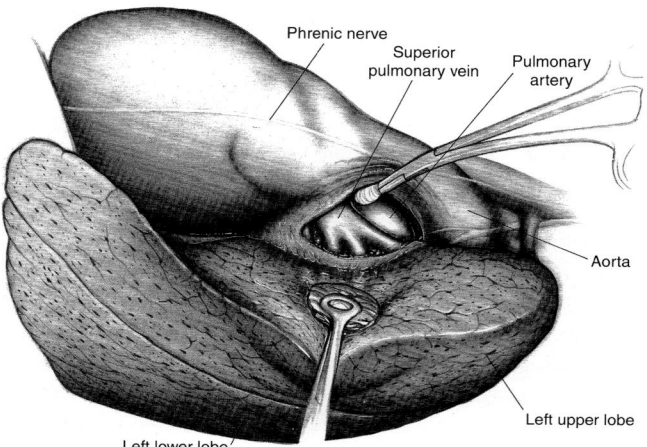

Fig. 27-11. A. and B. Oblique transection of the right lower lobe bronchus preserves patency of the middle lobe bronchus.

Fig. 27-12. A. and B. The mediastinal pleura is incised and the pulmonary artery is dissected in the subadventitial plane. The interval between the pulmonary artery and the superior pulmonary vein is defined.

monary vein is short. It is not advisable to ligate the vein because the tie may spring off the fibrous pericardium. Rather than sacrifice length, application of a Sarot's clamp to the specimen side of the vein and cutting on the clamp ensures sufficient length of the vein to be clamped and closed by a vascular suture or divided after application of a vascular stapler (Fig. 27-10C). Alternatively, the superior and basilar segmental veins are ligated individually. The lower lobe bronchus is then dissected. Because the middle lobe bronchus and the superior segmental bronchus originate from the intermediate bronchus at almost the same level, it may be necessary to close the basal segmental bronchus and the superior segmental bronchus separately to avoid obstructing the middle lobe bronchus. Usually, an oblique application of the 4.8-mm stapling device does not occlude the middle lobe bronchus (Fig. 27-11A). It is advisable to apply the stapler, close it without firing, and then re-aerate the right lung to ensure the patency of the middle lobe bronchus. Although a similar anatomic situation exists with regard to left lower lobe bronchus and the lingular bronchus, the risk of occluding the middle lobe bronchus is far greater than that of occluding the lingular bronchus. Alternatively, the lower lobe bronchus may be sutured as previously described.

LEFT UPPER LOBECTOMY

The most common anatomic variation encountered during left upper lobectomy is the number of segmental arterial branches, which vary from three to eight. The procedure is straightforward, provided the apical and anterior arteries are not injured during their isolation and division. To best accomplish this safely, proximal control of the left pulmonary artery is recommended, and these proximal branches are the last to be dissected and divided.

The left lung is retracted inferiorly, and the mediastinal pleura overlying the pulmonary artery is incised (Fig. 27-12A). After identification of the course of the phrenic nerve, the pleural incision is carried over the medial portion of the superior pulmonary vein just lateral to the pericardium (Fig. 27-12B). Posteriorly, the incision is made to a point below the level of the bronchus. The vagus nerve is visible subpleurally, marking the posterior limit of the hilar dissection (Fig. 27-

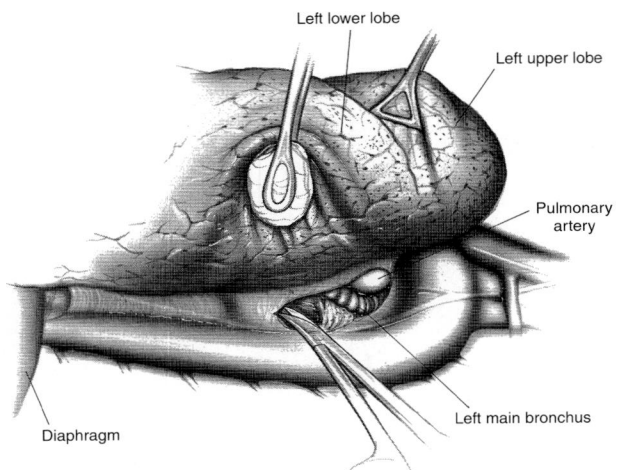

Fig. 27-13. Dissection of the posterior aspect of the left upper lobe hilum medial to the vagus nerve.

13). Areolar tissue overlying the convex surface of the pulmonary artery is cleared. The upper border of the left main bronchus is defined after division of vagal branches. A pledget dissector is used to roll the pulmonary artery away from the left main bronchus. Anteriorly, the interval between the pulmonary artery and the superior pulmonary vein is defined, and again the pulmonary artery is rolled out of its sheath, allowing an index finger to encircle the artery (Fig. 27-14). A Semb's clamp may then be used to draw a Silastic vessel loop about the artery. The ends of the loop are tied with a heavy silk suture and the loop is allowed to lie in the chest, readily accessible in the event of pulmonary artery injury.

The lung is retracted anteriorly and the pulmonary artery is dissected into the oblique fissure (Fig. 27-15A). If neces-

sary, the posterior part of the fissure is completed with clamps or a stapler with the pulmonary artery visualized. The pulmonary artery is dissected over the middle point of its presenting surface as it curves around the left upper lobe bronchus. As the fissure dissection proceeds, the posterior segmental arteries are noted opposite the superior segmental artery (Fig. 27-15B). Further distal dissection demonstrates one or two lingular arteries; the arterial dissection is complete when the basilar segmental branches are identified. With the lower lobe retracted inferiorly and the upper lobe retracted superiorly, the lingular branches are isolated and divided. The upper lobe is then rotated clockwise and the posterior segmental branches are ligated and divided. Proceeding in this fashion, from the lingular arteries proximally and rotating the lobe, makes each subsequent arterial isolation easier. The apical and anterior branches arise from the convex surface of the pulmonary artery often as a short trunk, slightly anterior to the middle point of the artery. These branches are the last to be divided (Fig. 27-16). Ligation and division of the apical segmental vein may enhance the visualization of the apical and anterior segmental arteries. The now completely mobilized pulmonary artery is rolled away from the upper lobe bronchus and is inspected for anomalous branches originating from its medial surface. This maneuver facilitates the later transection of the bronchus.

The lobe is retracted posteriorly and the anterior surface of the superior pulmonary vein is cleared of areolar tissue. The posterior surface of the pulmonary vein is freed by carrying the dissection on the anterior surface of the bronchus just external to the peribronchial connective tissue. Three or four branches enter the superior pulmonary vein and are encircled with ligatures. The extrapericardial length of pulmonary vein is often inadequate for safe ligation; therefore, it is an ideal place for the use of a vascular stapler. In the

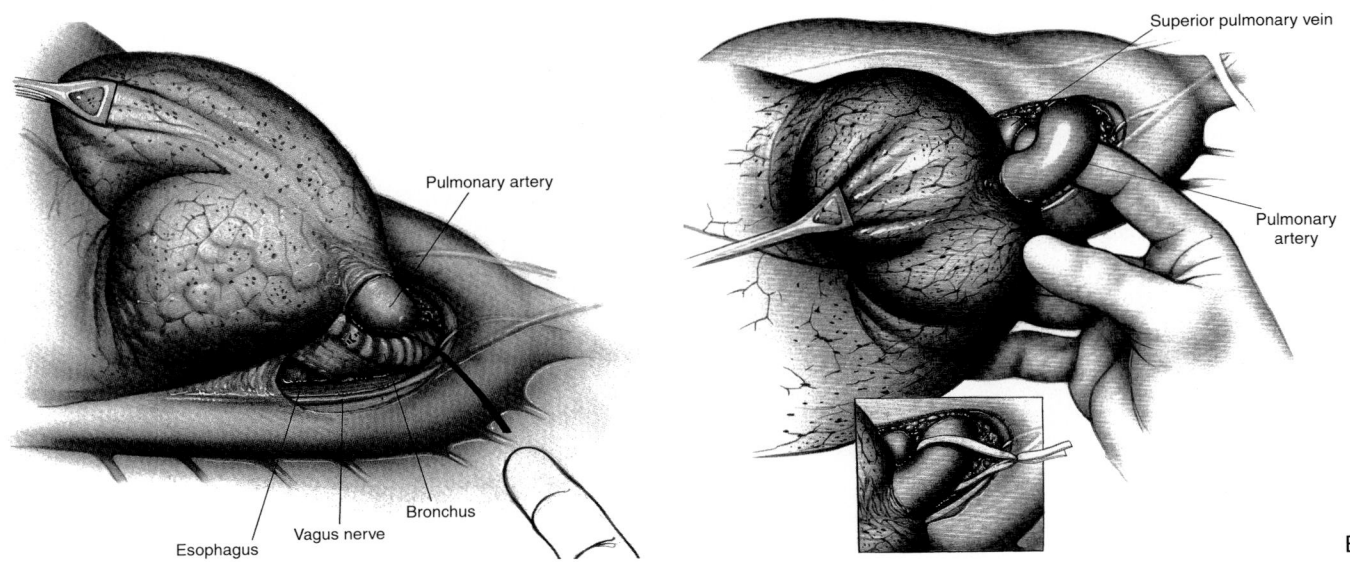

A

B

Fig. 27-14. A. and B. The left pulmonary artery is dissected from the left main bronchus and is encircled with a Silastic loop.

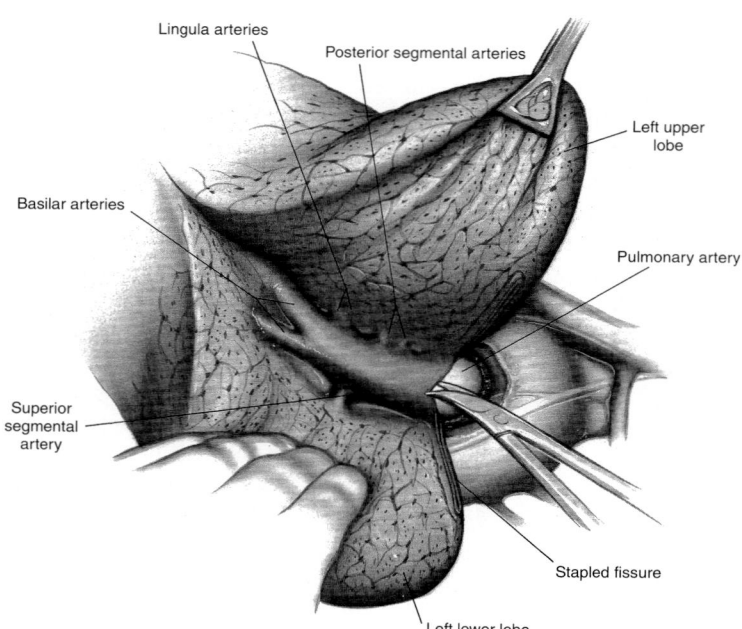

A

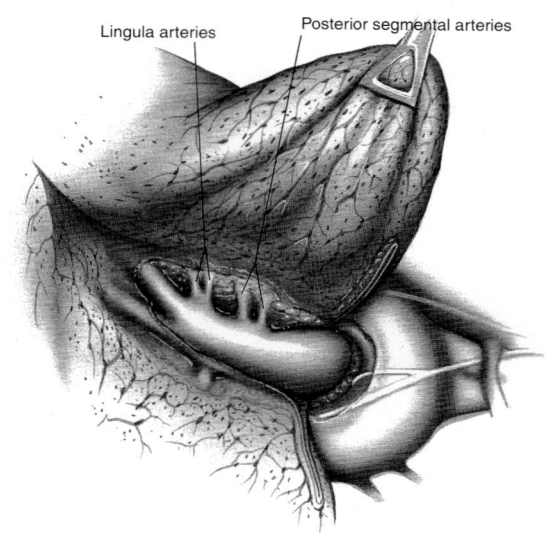

B

Fig. 27-15. A. and B. The posterior portion of the fissure is completed by stapling and the segmental arteries are demonstrated.

absence of a stapling device, the branches are tied, a vascular clamp is applied proximally, and the vein is divided and then closed with a vascular suture. It is often easier to divide the bronchus first. To divide the bronchus at the appropriate level, the interval between the lingular bronchus and the lower lobe bronchus is defined by rolling the pulmonary artery posteriorly, thus exposing the bifurcation of the left main bronchus (Fig. 27-17A). The upper lobe bronchus is occluded with a stapling device. Differential inflation ensures that the lower lobe bronchus is not

compromised; the stapler is fired and the bronchus is transected with a Semb's clamp positioned between the bronchus and the vein to protect the vein. After closure of the bronchus, the specimen end of the bronchus is grasped with a bronchus clamp. Elevation of the clamp exposes the deep surface of the superior pulmonary vein (Fig. 27-17B). The superior pulmonary vein is then managed as previously described. The inferior pulmonary ligament is divided to allow the left lower lobe to advance upward to better fill the thoracic cavity.

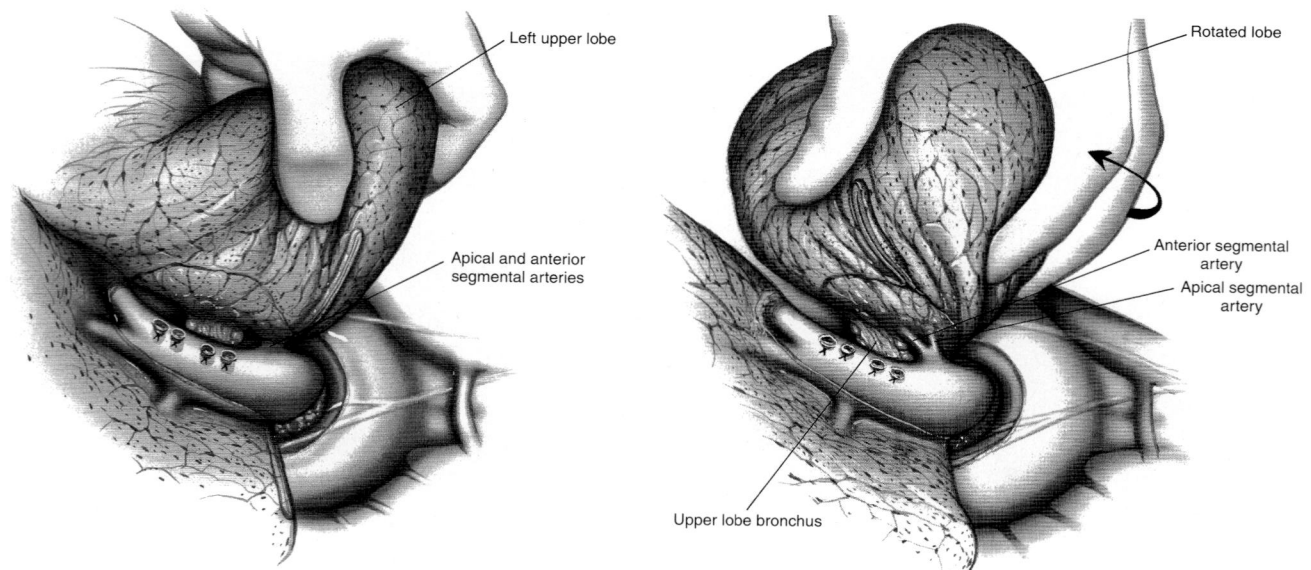

A

B

Fig. 27-16. A. and B. After division of the lingula and posterior segmental arteries, rotation of the lobe aids dissection of the apical and anterior segmental arteries.

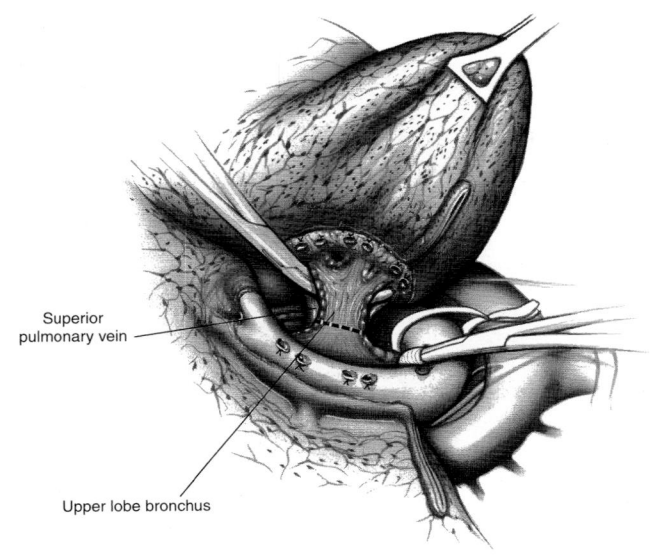

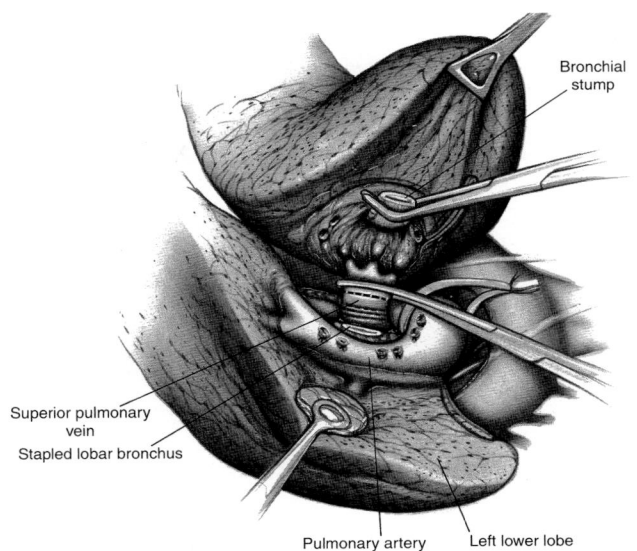

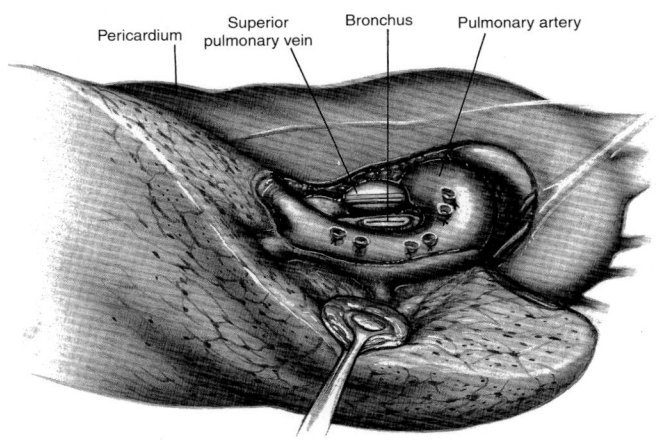

Fig. 27-17. A. The pulmonary artery is rolled away from the left upper bronchus. The site of bronchial transection is indicated. **B.** The left upper lobe bronchus is stapled and divided. The superior pulmonary vein is stapled and occluded distally by a Sarot clamp. **C.** Left upper lobe hilum after lobectomy.

LEFT LOWER LOBECTOMY

Provided that the oblique fissure is complete, left lower lobectomy is the simplest of all to perform; vascular anomalies are not commonly noted. The lung is retracted anteriorly and the posterior mediastinal pleura is incised from the level of the bronchus to the inferior pulmonary ligament, which should be divided at this time. The upper lobe is retracted anteriorly and superiorly, and the lower lobe is moved posteriorly and inferiorly, exposing the pulmonary artery in the fissure (Fig. 27-18A). It is best to commence dissection of the pulmonary artery from its sheath at the posterior aspect of the fissure. If the fissure is obliterated by adhesions, dissection of the posterior segment of the upper lobe from the superior segment of the lower lobe is accomplished by pledget dissection of the interlobar pulmonary artery from the overlying parenchyma, as well as by the creation of a tunnel so that a stapling device or clamps may be inserted to complete enough of the fissure

to allow further exposure of the interlobar artery. The anteromedial portion of the fissure is easily completed after bronchial closure. The superior segmental artery arises from the posterolateral surface of the interlobar pulmonary artery at a slightly lower level than the posterior segmental artery to the left upper lobe. Dissection of the interlobar artery along its midpoint is continued to delineate the origin of the lingular arteries, which must not be sacrificed. The basal trunk is then dissected, exposing the basal segmental branches. Occasionally, it is possible to double ligate the basal trunk distal to the lingular arteries and have one distal tie, but usually the basal branches must be ligated separately to ensure adequate length of the proximal stump (Fig. 27-18B).

The inferior pulmonary vein is then cleared of areolar tissue, demonstrating its superior segmental and basal tributaries, and the interval between the bronchus and the vein is defined (Fig. 27-19A). The extrapericardial portion of the left inferior pulmonary vein is longer than the right; double

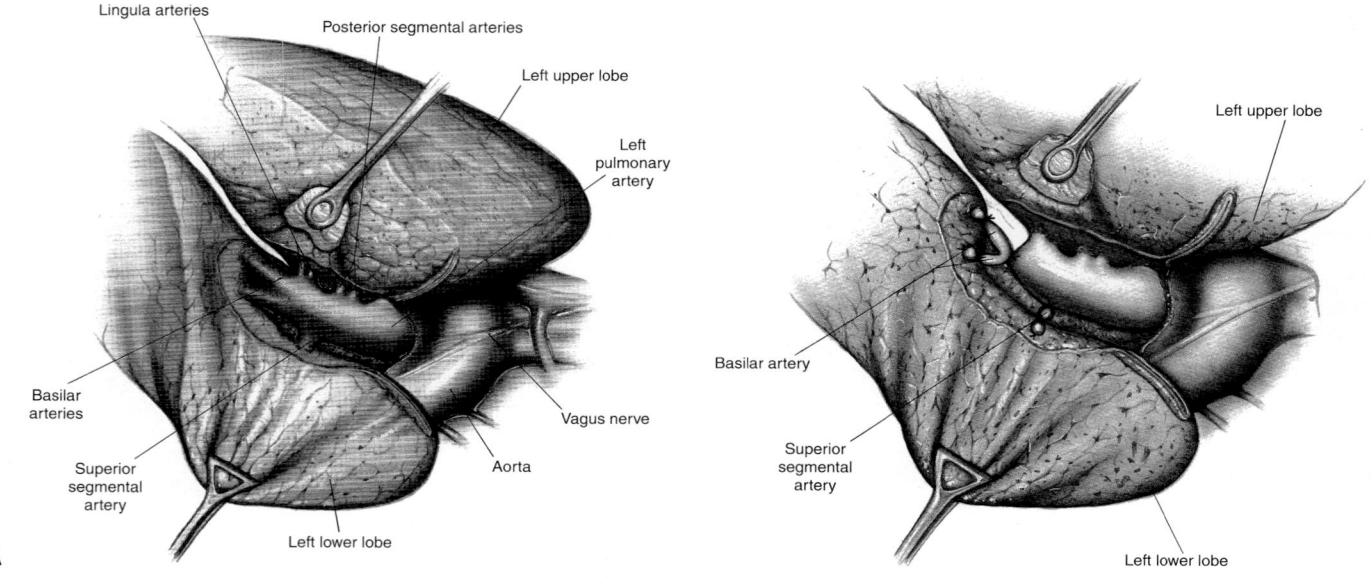

Fig. 27-18. A. Oblique fissure is completed and pulmonary artery branches are demonstrated. **B.** The superior segmental artery is ligated. Basal arteries are ligated and divided after the lingula arterial branches are demonstrated.

proximal ligation is acceptable. The preferred management, however, is stapling the cardiac end of the vein, or application of a vascular clamp and suture. Additional length may be obtained by occluding the specimen side with a Sarot's or other nonslipping clamp (Fig. 27-19B).

The bronchus is cleared of areolar tissue and the crotch below the upper lobe bronchus is dissected. The stapling device is applied just distal to the upper lobe bronchus to avoid creating a cul de sac, or the bronchus is closed manually as described previously (Fig. 27-20).

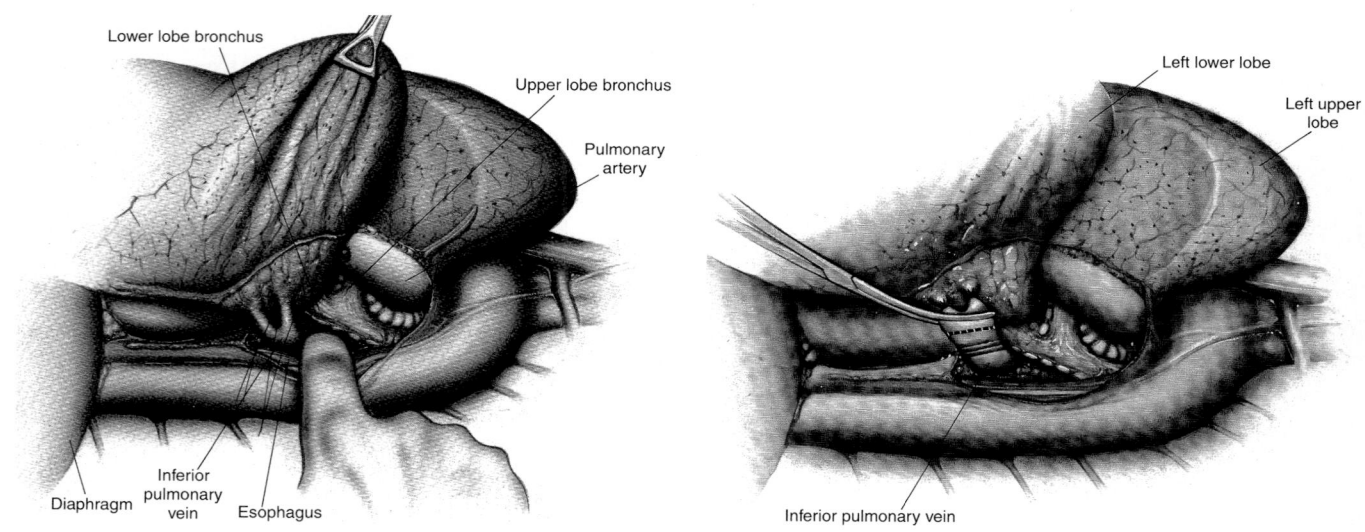

Fig. 27-19. A. The interval between the pulmonary vein and the lower lobe bronchus is defined. **B.** The inferior pulmonary vein has been stapled. A Sarot clamp is applied to the specimen side prior to transection.

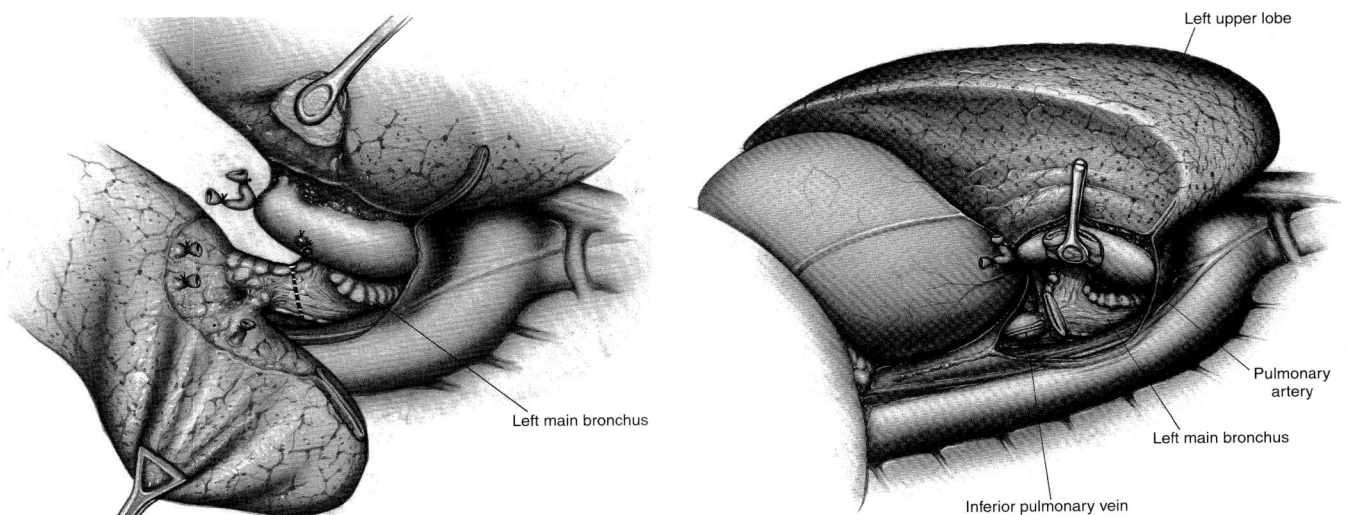

Fig. 27-20. A. Oblique transection of the bronchus prevents formation of a cul de sac. **B.** View of the hilum after left lower lobectomy.

ACKNOWLEDGMENT

The authors gratefully acknowledge the support of the Feldesman Fund for Thoracic Surgery at Montefiore Medical Center.

REFERENCES

Blades B, Kent EM: Individual ligation technique for lower lobectomy. J Thorac Surg *10*:84, 1940.
Lewis RJ, Sisler GE, Caccavale RJ: Imaged thoracic lobectomy: should it be done? Ann Thorac Surg *54*:80, 1992.

McCaughan BC, et al: Chest wall invasion in carcinoma of the lung. J Thorac Cardiovasc Surg 89:836, 1985.
Overholt RH, Langer L: The Technique of Pulmonary Resection. Springfield, IL: Charles C. Thomas, 1951.
Trastek VF, et al: En bloc (non-chest wall) resection for bronchogenic carcinoma with parietal fixation. Factors affecting survival. J Thorac Cardiovasc Surg *87*:352, 1984.

READING REFERENCES

Edmunds JH Jr, Norwood WI, Low DW: Atlas of Cardiothoracic Surgery. Philadelphia: Lea & Febiger, 1990.
Waldhausen JA, Pierce WS (eds): Johnson's Surgery of the Chest. 5th Ed. Chicago: Year Book, 1985.

CHAPTER 28

Sleeve Lobectomy

Joachim Schirren, Thomas Muley, and Ingolf Vogt-Moykopf

Bronchoplastic resection, or bronchial sleeve resection, is a well-established and valuable alternative to pneumonectomy in the treatment of benign and malignant conditions of the airway, sparing lung parenchyma by reanastomosing the healthy bronchus lying beyond the involved segment. If the section of bronchus to be resected subserves a lobe, then lobectomy must be added. Bronchoplastic resection may be combined with angioplastic procedures.

HISTORY

The first bronchoplastic operation was performed at the Brompton Hospital in London by Price Thomas in 1947. He resected the right upper lobe with a sleeve of the descending bronchus and reanastomosed the intermediate bronchus to the main bronchus, preserving the middle and lower lobes. This operation, still the most common variant, was performed for a bronchial adenoma, a frequent indication for such conservative procedures in modern practice. D'Abreau and McHale (1952) described a case in which isolated resection of the left main bronchus was performed for a bronchial adenoma, and in 1953, Gebauer used a similar technique when resecting a long tuberculous stenosis. Allison (1954) was the first to report the use of such conservative operations for bronchial carcinoma. Since then, numerous authors have reported their experiences of this surgical procedure.

Although bronchoplastic resection was originally advocated in lung cancer as a compromise in patients with insufficient reserves to tolerate pneumonectomy, it is now established as a safe and effective alternative to pneumonectomy whenever the extent of the disease permits.

Angioplasty was discussed by Allison (1954) in his original report, and Wurning (1967) described tangential resection of the pulmonary artery. A series of four successful operations, combining bronchoplastic and angioplastic resection, was reported by Pichlmaier and Spelsberg in 1971. Toomes and one of us (I.V.-M.) (1985) described the first transposition of a complete lobe. After upper bilobec-

tomy the lower lobe was transposed. Belli (1985), one of us (I.V.-M.) (1986), Read (1993) and associates, as well as Naruke (1989), subsequently have published their series.

INDICATIONS

Conservative resections such as bronchoplastic and angioplastic operations are particularly useful in elderly patients and the frail patient with limited respiratory reserve, for whom pneumonectomy would prove hazardous. In recent years, however, the value of conservative resections has been appreciated in younger, fitter patients who could withstand pneumonectomy but for whom conservative resections have less effect on exercise capacity and quality of life. Bronchoplastic resection has been used by Black and colleagues (1988) to deal with bronchial neoplasms and congenital strictures in infants and children. Although sleeve resections are technically more demanding, today no increase in perioperative risk occurs.

Bronchoplastic resection is a valid option when dealing with tumors of the bronchus, whether benign or malignant, and for bronchial stenosis after trauma or tuberculosis. The latter was described by Kato and coworkers (1993). Bronchial carcinoma is by far the most common indication for such conservative resections, salvaging lung parenchyma without compromising radicality. Bronchoplastic and angioplastic resection may be appropriate in a number of operative situations for lung cancer (Fig. 28-1A and B).

Localized, often superficial T_1 tumors of the main bronchus—more commonly the long left main bronchus—may be resected without the loss of any lung tissue. Tumors may extend from within a lobar orifice to involve the descending bronchus, making lobectomy and sleeve resection necessary. Depending on the proximity of the lobar orifice to the main carina, such tumors may be T_2 or T_3 lesions. Extrabronchial tumor extension, or metastatic hilar lymph nodes, may involve the origin of the lobar bronchus and infiltrate peribronchial tissues, the pulmonary artery, and, rarely, the vein. For such tumors pneumonectomy may be

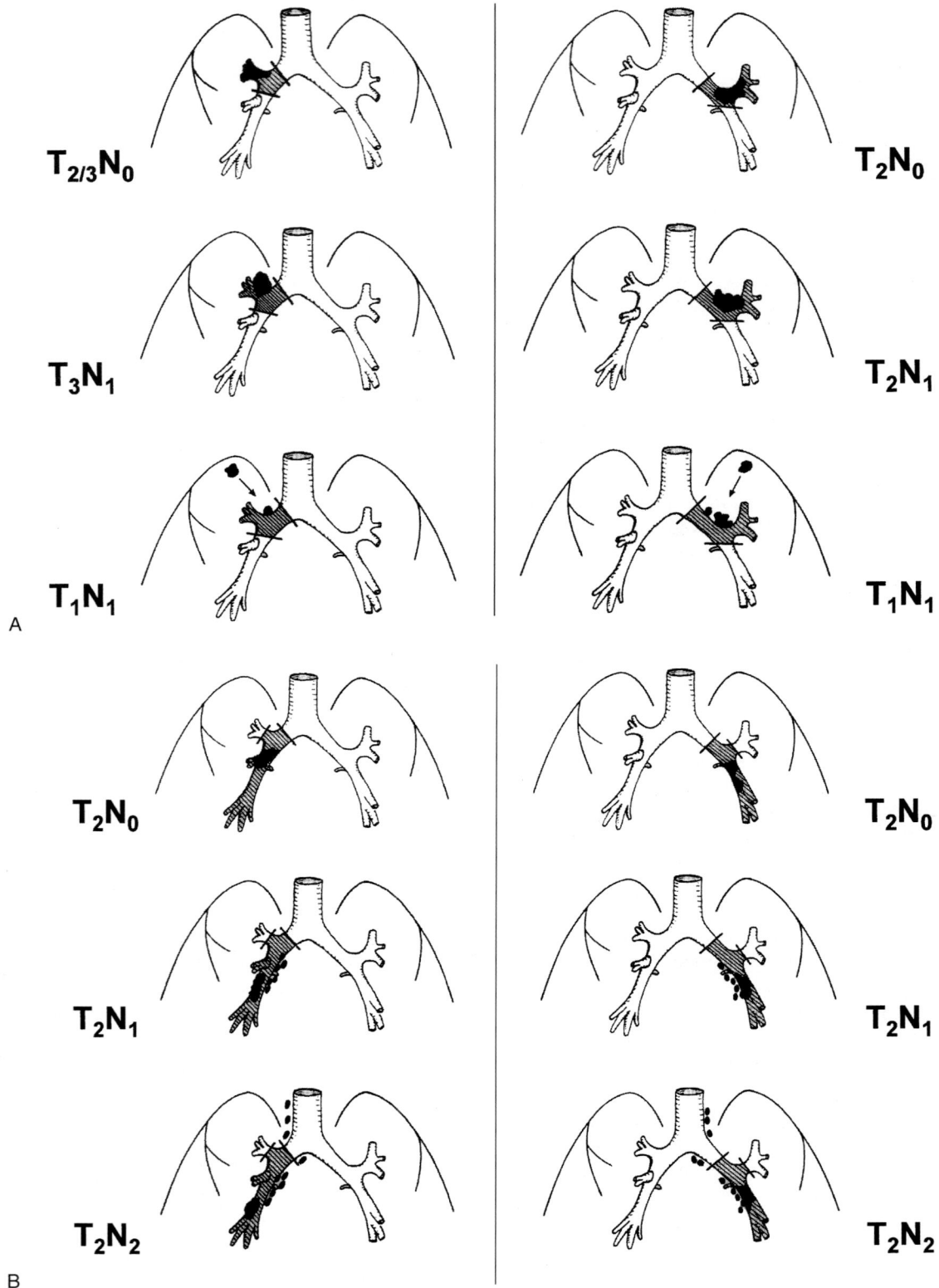

$T_{2/3}N_0$

T_2N_0

T_3N_1

T_2N_1

T_1N_1

T_1N_1

A

T_2N_0

T_2N_0

T_2N_1

T_2N_1

T_2N_2

T_2N_2

B

Fig. 28-1. Indications for sleeve resection of right- and left-sided bronchial carcinoma in relation to tumor stage. Tumor and involved lymph nodes are given in black. The extent of resection is indicated by gray. **A.** Indications for upper lobe sleeve resection of right- and left-sided tumors, respectively. **B.** Indications for lower right-sided bilobectomy and left-sided resection of the lower lobe and main bronchus (reverse or Y-sleeve resection). Arrows point to hilar or peribronchial lymph node metastases from a peripherally located tumor.

avoided by bronchoplastic resection, sometimes with an added angioplastic procedure.

Maeda and colleagues (1986) showed that lung cancer not only infiltrates microscopically from the primary tumor for a distance averaging 7.2 mm (range, 3 to 20 mm), but also that metastatic clusters of cancer cells are often found in the lymphatics, lymph nodes, bronchial arterials, and nerve sheaths present in the peribronchial and intrabronchial wall. Lung cancer may have extensive peribronchial spread, a feature that provides further rationale for the use of sleeve resections.

The role of bronchoplastic and angioplastic resection in N_1 disease and for limited N_2 disease has been debated. Early reports emphasized the poorer prognosis after such conservative resections, and many surgeons were concerned that this may be the result of compromising oncologic principles to avoid pneumonectomy. The results, however, are at least as good as for pneumonectomy when considered stage by stage, with a lower operative mortality. This was shown by the works of Rees and Paneth (1970), Bennett and Smith (1978), and Deslauriers and coworkers (1986), as well as Van Schil (1991, 1996) and Mehran (1994) and their associates.

Other, less frequent indications for bronchoplasty include bronchial carcinoid tumors and adenomas, lung metastases with endobronchial extension, and rarer tumors such as sarcomas, mucoepidermoid carcinoma, and adenoid cystic carcinoma. The results of main bronchial sleeve resection with conservation of pulmonary tissue were reported by Newton and coworkers (1991).

PREOPERATIVE ASSESSMENT

The feasibility of bronchoplastic and angioplastic resection usually can be assessed only at surgery, although the surgeon should always keep such options in mind. A careful bronchoscopic assessment should be made by the surgeon to establish a tissue diagnosis and plan surgical strategy. Routine preoperative assessment of lung function and arterial gas measurements are complemented by perfusion scintigraphy, and, in selected cases, ventilation scintigraphy, to assess the contribution each lung makes to overall function. Computed tomography is useful in determining the extent of the bronchial stenosis, assessing the extent of extrabronchial extension, and determining the state and likely recoverability of distal lung parenchyma. Kesler and coworkers (1991) have found magnetic resonance imaging of value in preoperative evaluation. When assessing patients with malignant tumors, we rely on computed tomography scanning to assess mediastinal lymph node involvement and the need for mediastinoscopy, which in our unit is principally used to exclude N_3 disease because we routinely advocate radical resection in N_2 cases. Pulmonary angiography may suggest that angioplastic surgery is required. Suri and colleagues (1997) concluded from their study that arteriographic findings may accurately show whether a sleeve lobectomy is technically possible, that only a pneumonec-

tomy is possible, or that the only safe way to ensure clearance of the pulmonary artery is to perform arterioplasty. Although the selective pulmonary arteriography may provide a detailed anatomic view, in our own experience, it does not necessarily reflect the exact intraoperative findings.

ANESTHESIA

As a routine for all major thoracic surgery, it is our practice to use continuous monitoring by pulse oximetry, central venous cannulation, and arterial cannulation to monitor blood pressure and blood gas analysis. In addition, when sleeve resection of the bronchus is contemplated, a double-lumen tube is positioned with the bronchial limb placed under bronchoscopic guidance into the contralateral main bronchus. Although several authors advocate a single-lumen endobronchial tube for such operations, this can jeopardize gas exchange until the pulmonary artery has been clamped and has proved to be a problem in patients with reduced functional reserve and in whom perfusion remains satisfactory in the lung being operated on. High-frequency jet ventilation is useful when the bronchial anastomosis is performed close to the carina, or when problems occur in positioning the bronchial tube on the right side.

SURGICAL TECHNIQUE

The most common incision used for bronchoplastic and angioplastic procedures is the standard posterolateral thoracotomy. Although a median sternotomy incision can be used, as advocated by Urschel and Razzuk (1986), we have not found this to give adequate exposure for bronchoplastic procedures on the left, and, in malignant cases, radical dissection of the mediastinal lymph nodes may be difficult in the lower mediastinum and in the paraesophageal region. Also, the additional manipulation necessary through the sternotomy approach may cause hemodynamic problems in elderly patients and those with heart disorders. We have found the posterolateral thoracotomy to be the most convenient approach, allowing thorough evaluation of the anterior and posterior hilar structures and permitting complete mediastinal node dissection with safety.

Bronchoplastic Resection

The classic operation of right upper lobectomy with sleeve resection is still the most common bronchoplastic procedure. However, right upper lobectomy with sleeve resection now includes a wide range of operations including 1) sleeve resection of the bronchus alone, preserving all lung parenchyma; 2) sleeve resection with upper lobectomy or upper and middle lobectomy, and variants in which only small volumes of lung parenchyma such as the apical segment of the lower lobe or the middle lobe are resected; and

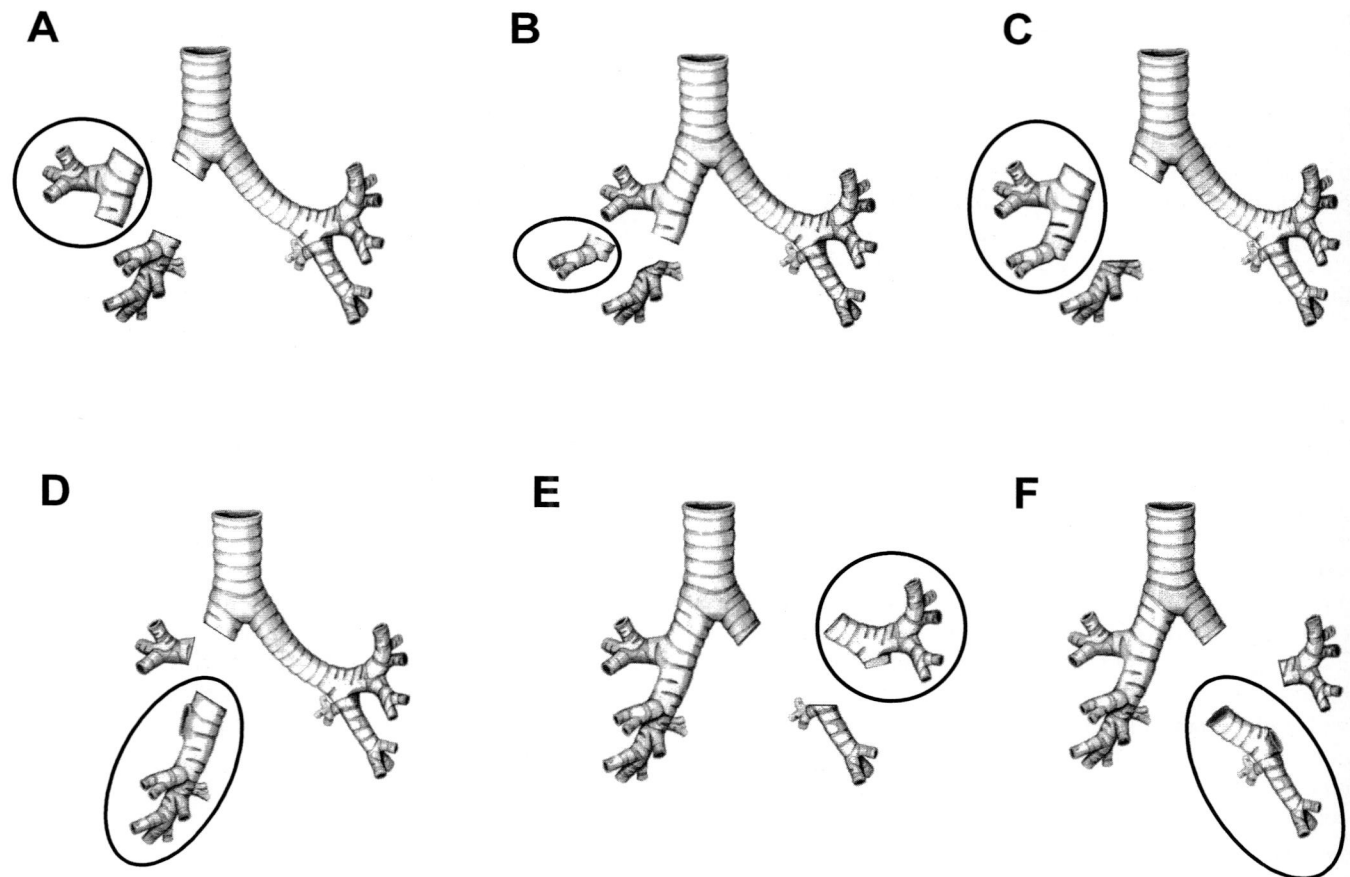

Fig. 28-2. Sleeve resection on the right and left bronchial tree including resection of corresponding lung parenchyma. Cycles indicate resected segments of the bronchial tree. **A.** Right upper lobe. **B.** Right middle lobe. **C.** Right upper bilobectomy. **D.** Right lower bilobectomy (Y-sleeve resection). **E.** Left upper lobe. **F.** Left lower lobe and main bronchus (Y-sleeve resection).

3) the reverse sleeve or Y-sleeve operation in which the upper lobe is reanastomosed to the main bronchus after resection of the descending bronchus with the lower lobe or middle and lower lobes (Figs. 28-2 and 28-3).

Other novel techniques have widened the applicability of bronchoplastic procedures in recent years. If the surgeon is anxious to conserve lung tissue in a patient with limited lung function, and yet finds it difficult to determine how much of the lung can be salvaged in situ, it is possible to remove the lung and dissect the structures at the operating table, without concerns regarding bleeding, and then reimplant the lobes or segments that can be salvaged. Occasionally, it is possible to detach the lobar vein and reimplant it into the other pulmonary vein, the so-called transposition lobectomy (Fig. 28-4). This is useful after sleeve resection of the right upper lobe and middle lobe, thus relieving tension on the bronchial and arterial anastomoses.

It is important to observe some key technical points when undertaking bronchoplasty. Great care should be exercised in preserving, as far as possible, the bronchial arterial supply to the resection margins, particularly the distal margin. The tis-

sues around the bronchus should not be removed, skeletalizing the bronchus. Nodal dissection should be performed before undertaking the anastomosis so as to avoid tension subsequently. Removing such nodes, especially if they are involved by tumor, may damage bronchial arteries, particularly those at the main carina. The resection margins should be examined by frozen section to ensure radicality. The bronchial margins should show fine petechial bleeding prior to the anastomosis. Any rough edges or projecting cartilage should be trimmed.

If the surgeon is concerned about the viability of the bronchial margins, especially when resection has been preceded by radiation therapy, other measures should be considered to provide vascularized tissue to wrap the anastomosis. A pedicle flap of the omentum can be raised through a diaphragmatic incision, taking care not to damage the pedicle during mobilization or by closing the diaphragm too tightly. The omental flap should not be too bulky. Such steps add to the length of the surgery and bring their own morbidity. Others have used intercostal muscle flaps, but these are often too bulky. A flap of pericardium or pleura is preferable. If care is taken to avoid tension on the anastomosis,

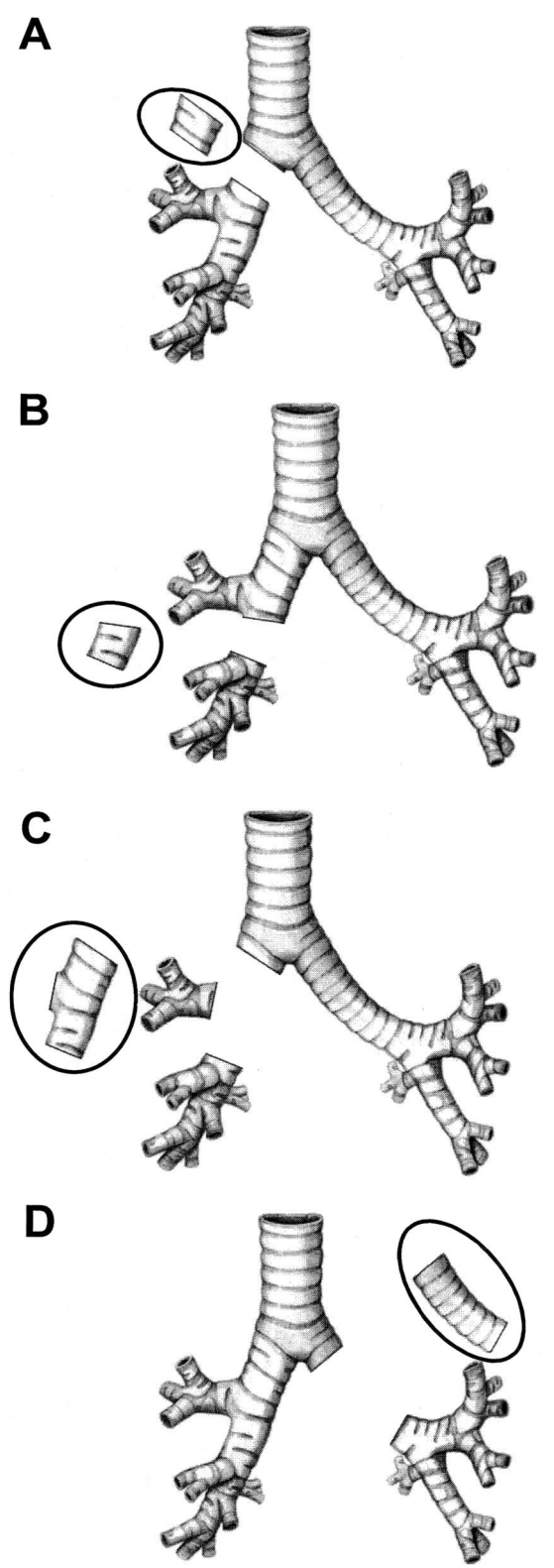

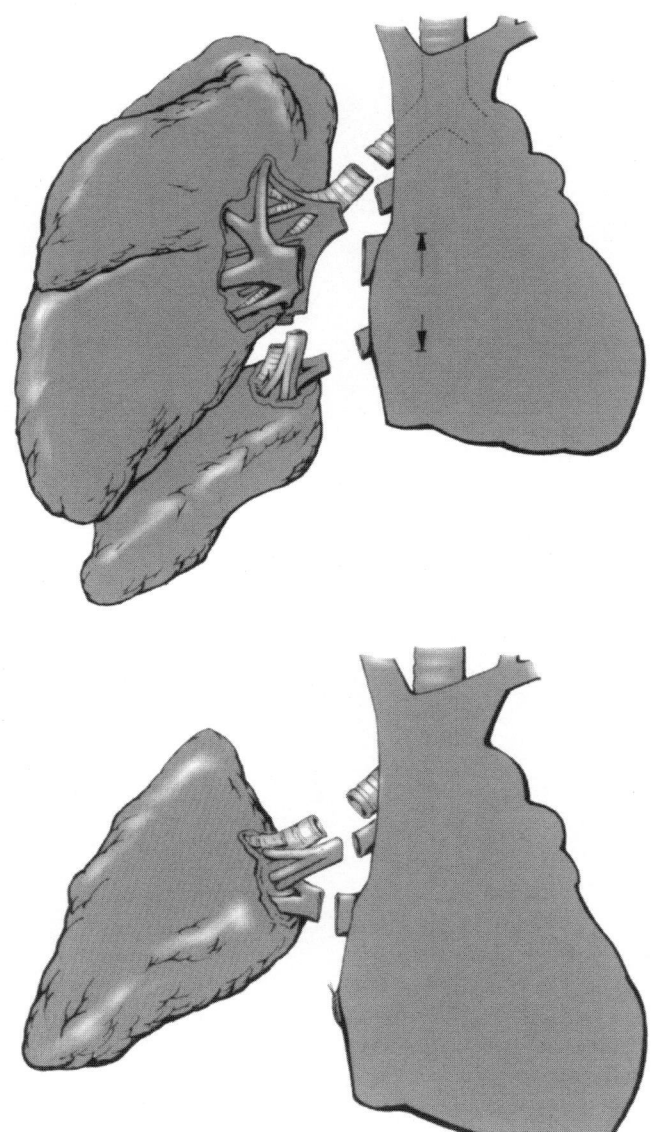

Fig. 28-4. Transposition lobectomy. Beside the double-sleeve resection of the pulmonary artery and the bronchus, the lower lobe vein is transferred to the site of the upper vein at the left vestibule. This technique can be used to achieve tension-free anastomoses in bronchial sleeves combined with segmental arterial resection in case of more extensive defects to be bridged.

Fig. 28-3. Segmental resection of bronchus without resection of lung parenchyma (e.g., resection of carcinoid tumors). **(A)** Right main bronchus, **(B)** bronchus intermedius, **(C)** right main bronchus and bronchus intermedius (triple sleeve), and **(D)** left main bronchus.

these measures are unnecessary, a point made by Deslauriers and coworkers (1986).

The anastomosis is performed edge to edge, but if great discrepancy exists between the sizes of the bronchi, the smaller distal lumen may be telescoped into the larger proximal end. If the discrepancy is slight, the anastomosis can be performed end to end, leaving the posterior wall until last, so that larger spaces can be left between sutures on the membranous portion of the larger lumen. In our experience all other methods to try to tailor the proximal lumen to match

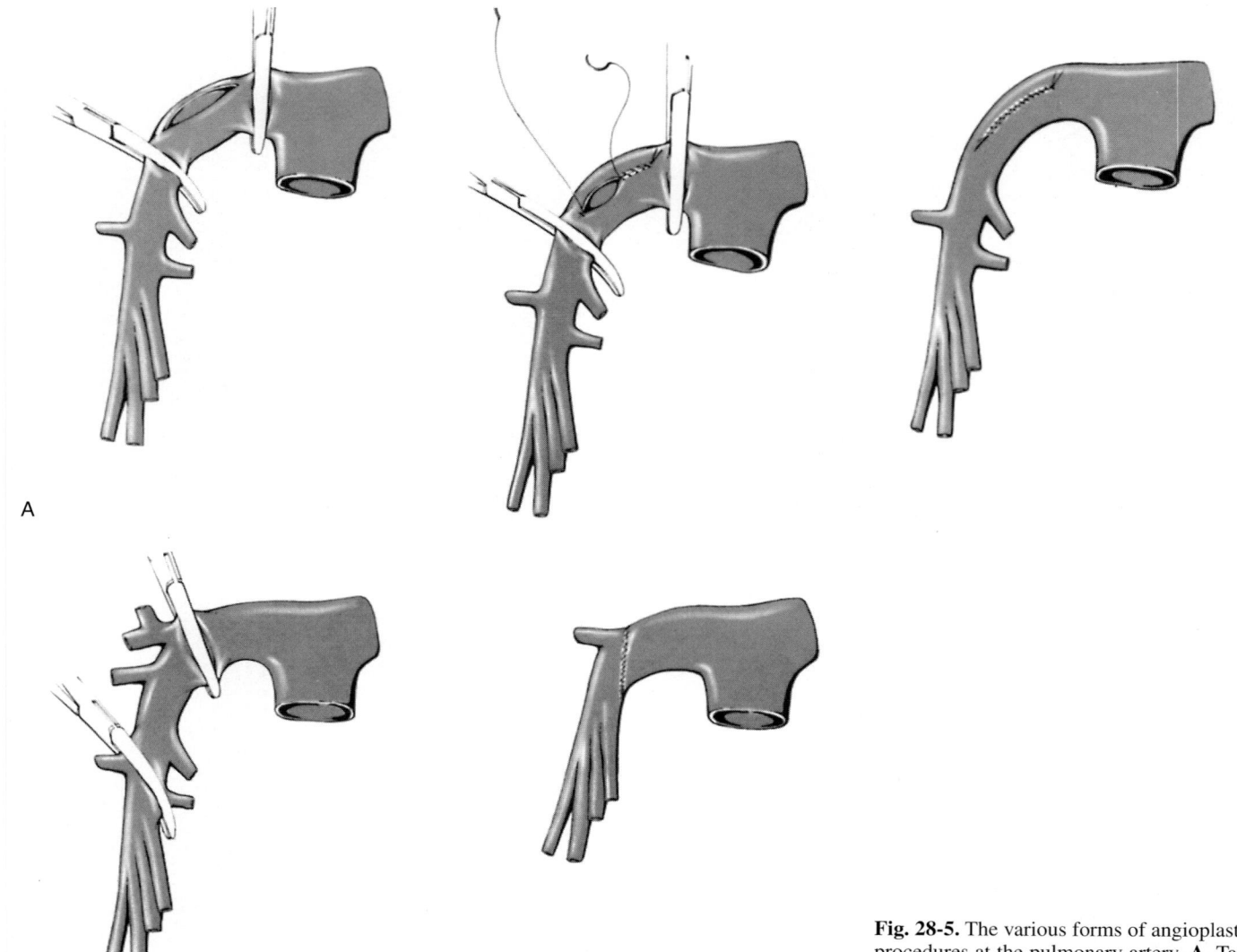

A

B

Fig. 28-5. The various forms of angioplastic procedures at the pulmonary artery. **A.** Tangential. **B.** Complete segmental resection.

the size of the distal orifice have proved unsatisfactory. The transection of the bronchus must be performed as perpendicular as possible to the axis of the bronchus. Wedge resections result in kinking at the anastomosis.

The anastomosis must be completely free of tension. It was previously held that slight tension would serve to prevent kinking, but this is not a problem if the anastomosis has been performed correctly. Mobilization of the pulmonary ligament may be sufficient to avoid tension when short segments of the bronchus have been resected, but for longer defects, up to 5 cm, other steps should be taken. These steps may include division of the azygos arch, mobilization of the aortic arch by detaching the ligament of Botalli and Marshall's fold, the performance of a circular pericardiotomy around the pulmonary vein, or transposition of the pulmonary vein.

The anastomosis is performed using a single layer of interrupted sutures of absorbable 4-0 or 5-0 monofilament material (polydioxamone). The sutures are placed around the cartilages at each end of the anastomosis, passing through the

full thickness of the bronchial wall. Trying to avoid sutures breaching the mucosa has proved impracticable in our experience, but granuloma formation is rare. It is important to retain the correct orientation of the bronchial walls and to compensate for any discrepancy by correct suture placement. The distance between sutures must be appropriate to ensure that the blood supply of the anastomosis is not impaired.

After the anastomosis has been completed, it is checked under water while the anesthetist sustains positive ventilation at 40 cm of water. Finally, before closure, flexible bronchoscopy is performed to examine the anastomosis and undertake bronchial toilet.

Angioplastic Resection

Similar ingenuity can be shown when undertaking angioplastic procedures, with tangential resection of part of the wall of the pulmonary artery (Fig. 28-5A), sleeve resection

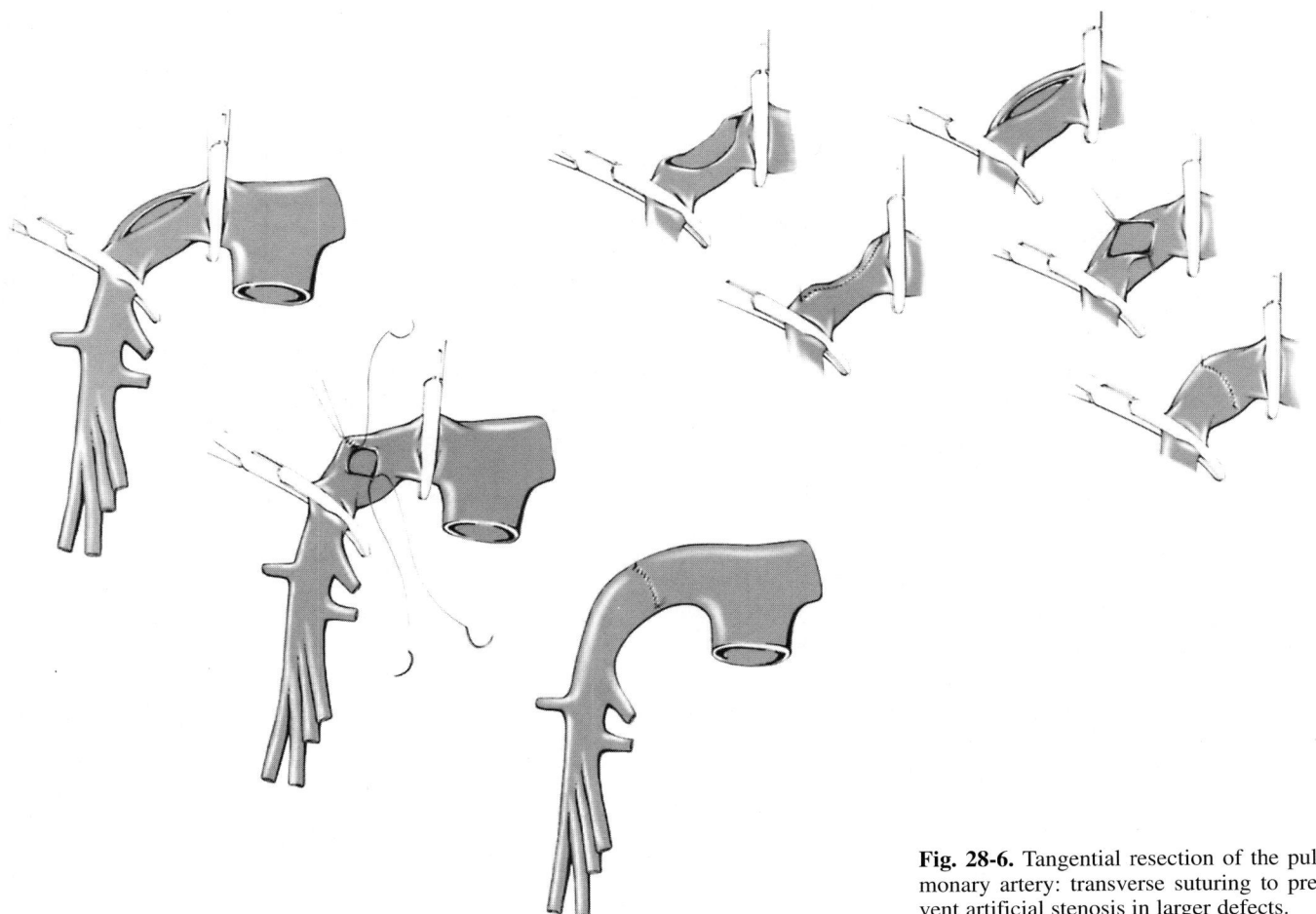

Fig. 28-6. Tangential resection of the pulmonary artery: transverse suturing to prevent artificial stenosis in larger defects.

of a length of the artery, and reanastomosis of segmental arteries (Fig. 28-5B). Angioplastic resection usually is reserved for the resection of tumors, in conjunction with bronchoplasty. Resection of the artery may be necessitated by direct tumor invasion or by involved glands. Occasionally, angioplasty is necessary when large bronchial defects result from trauma with kinking of the bronchial anastomosis. More than 90% of vascular sleeve resections are carried out in association with upper lobectomy or bilobectomy, usually combined with bronchoplasty.

At its simplest, angioplasty might entail a partial defect inside of the pulmonary artery when proximity of the tumor does not allow sufficient access to permit ligation of the segmental arteries separately. The pulmonary artery must be mobilized to its origin to accommodate an atraumatic, proximal clamp. This is facilitated by opening the pericardium, on the right by division of the azygos arch and on the left by division of the ligament of Botalli and the fold of Marshall. Back bleeding is controlled by applying a second clamp at a suitable site or by clamping the pulmonary veins. Intravascular clotting is prevented by giving 5000 to 7500 IU of heparin intravenously, depending on the patient's weight, before clamping the vessels.

The surgeon must then decide whether it is preferable to close the arterial defect longitudinally or transversely or to undertake sleeve resection of the vessel (Fig. 28-6).

The anastomosis is undertaken using a continuous suture of 5-0 or 6-0 monofilament nonabsorbable material. Any discrepancy in the size of the vessels can be accommodated by oblique division of the smaller vessel or by incising along the lumen of the distal vessel. If a gross discrepancy in size exists, interrupted sutures may be preferable.

Combined Angioplasty and Bronchoplasty

The majority of so-called double-sleeve resections are performed together with upper lobectomy (Fig. 28-7). When possible, the bronchial anastomosis is carried out first to avoid damaging the vascular anastomosis. If the surgeon has any worries about either anastomosis, the anastomosis should be wrapped with vascularized tissue such as pericardium. The omentum has proved too bulky in practice and compresses the arterial anastomosis. The avoidance of tension is of paramount importance. The aforementioned techniques should be fully used.

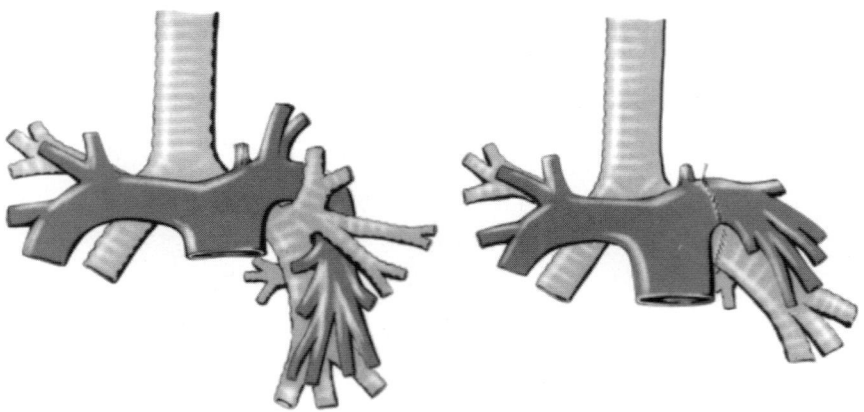

Fig. 28-7. Double-sleeve resection of the left upper lobe. The relationship between the bronchial tree and the pulmonary arteries is much closer on the left side than on the right side of the lung. To ensure radicality, sleeve resection of the left upper lobe often includes segmental resection of the pulmonary artery. In sleeve resection of the right upper lobe, with regard to the vessels, radicality can be achieved mostly by angioplastic procedures (e.g., tangential resection). Double-sleeve resection of the right upper lobe is rare.

More recently, in a patient who could not tolerate a pneumonectomy and in whom the lesion could not be resected by one of the aforementioned techniques with the lung in situ, the lung has been excised in toto and transferred to a sterile operating room table. The tumor is then removed from the excised lung—an extracorporeal resection. The tumor-free portion of the lung that can be preserved is then reimplanted into the hemithorax. Another procedure used more frequently is the transposition lobectomy. This is performed together with extensive lung resections, mostly with upper right-sided, double-sleeve bilobectomy. The procedure involves transplanting the lower lobe vein into the proximal stump of the upper lobe vein to ensure the tension-free anastomoses of both the bronchus and the artery (see Fig. 28-4). Our experience (1984 through 1994) comprises 19 patients who were treated by transposition lobectomy, extracorporeal

lung resection, or both. One patient died during the hospital stay. The postoperative follow-up is included in Long-Term Results, later in this chapter.

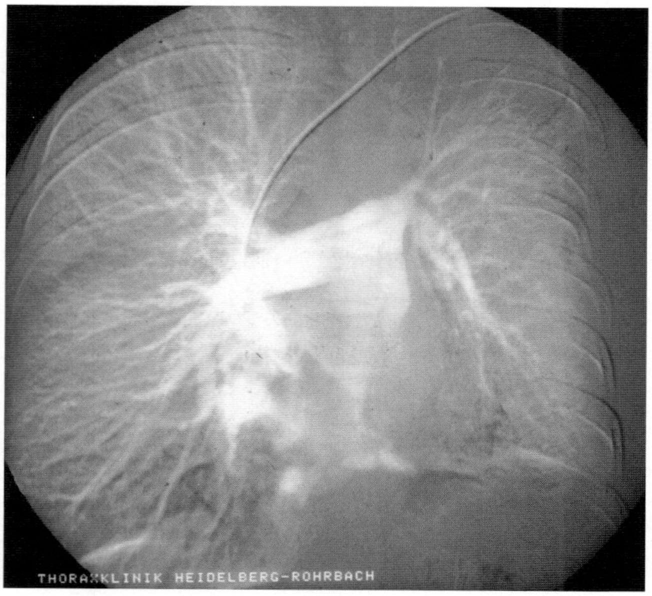

POSTOPERATIVE CARE

After bronchoplastic resection, the normal postoperative measures are supplemented by specific steps. The patient is extubated as early as possible under bronchoscopic control. The airway is cleared and any lavage sent for bacteriology. The patient is taught respiratory exercises preoperatively, and these are supplemented by mucolytics and bronchodilators, incentive spirometry, and intensive physiotherapy using percussion and postural drainage. If these measures fail to prevent sputum retention, bronchoscopy is performed and blind nasotracheal aspiration is avoided. A temporary tracheostomy is performed if persistent problems occur, thus enabling repeated bronchoscopy.

Bronchoscopy is repeated at 1 and 6 weeks. Perfusion and ventilation scintigraphy is performed before discharge. Stenosis is thus detected early and treated endoscopically by dilation, laser resection, and in severe cases, stent implantation. Pulmonary angiography (Fig. 28-8) is performed to check arterial and venous patency if concerns exist regarding vascular thrombosis. Rendina and colleagues (1992) have suggested that low-dose corticosteroids may improve bronchial healing.

COMPLICATIONS

Bronchial stricture has been reported by Firmin (1983) and Kawahara (1994) and their associates in 4 to 6% of cases after bronchoplastic resection. Impaired healing may result in superficial necrosis of the bronchial mucosa or a small fistula, but these normally heal spontaneously. In patients who require ventilation, fistulas often progress to total necrosis and complete dehiscence. This should be recognized by regular bronchoscopy. It is, however, sometimes

THORAXKLINIK HEIDELBERG-ROHRBACH

Fig. 28-8. Postoperative angiography of the pulmonary artery after double-sleeve resection of the left upper lobe. A well-perfused lower lobe artery can be demonstrated.

difficult to differentiate between superficial mucosal slough-ing and complete necrosis of the bronchial wall, and the clue is usually provided by the patient's general condition. The presence of fever, leukocytosis, persistent air leak, or an infected effusion are worrisome features. Experience is necessary in deciding whether to undertake completion pneumonectomy or to continue observation. In general, if the patient's lung function permits, completion pneumonectomy should be performed promptly once complete dehiscence is recognized. Hemoptysis is particularly worrisome and may indicate erosion of the arterial wall and impending bronchoarterial fistula. Immediate reoperation can salvage almost one-half of these patients in our experience.

Kinking of the bronchial anastomosis does not occur unless a wedge resection of the bronchus has been performed or the sleeve has been fashioned badly. The late appearance of a bronchial stricture is treated by endoscopic techniques such as the insertion of a stent, as described by Tsang and Goldstraw (1989). It is rare for such problems to lead to destruction of the remaining lobe, making completion pneumonectomy unavoidable.

Acute and chronic thrombotic occlusion may occur after angioplastic resection. Acute occlusion presents in the early postoperative period with rapid deterioration in the patient's general condition and hypoxemia. The diagnosis is confirmed by immediate angiography, and completion pneumonectomy undertaken. Chronic occlusion of the vascular anastomosis by thrombosis is insidious and usually is detected by a ventilation-perfusion mismatch on routine scintigraphy. It requires no treatment in most cases, and the lung, although functionless, can be left in place. Thrombotic occlusion of a venous anastomosis results in hemorrhagic infarction of the lung. The clinical features and management are the same as for arterial thrombosis.

Completion pneumonectomy may be necessary for the complications of conservative resection but carries a mortality of 15 to 20%, as shown in the series of Kawahara (1994) and Van Schil (1992) and their colleagues. Bronchopleural fistula has been reported to occur in 3 to 6% of cases by Kawahara and coworkers (1994), and occurred in 7.4% of our series of patients with bronchial carcinoma.

In a prospective study performed at our clinic (Thoraxklinik, Heidelberg-Rohrbach, Germany) between 1984 and 1994, 466 bronchoplastic, angioplastic, or both kinds of resections were carried out in patients with lung cancer. A total of 568 angioplastic procedures were performed (Table 28-1). Nineteen patients who were treated by extracorporeal lung resection, transposition lobectomy, or both are included.

The 30-day in-hospital mortality was related to the age of the patient and the nature of the procedure. For isolated bronchial sleeve resection the mortality was 8%, within the reported range of 0 to 9%. The mortality increased with increasing complexity of operation and varied between 7 and 17% for combined bronchoplastic and angioplastic resection. Since 1990 a steady decrease in mortality occurred, probably because of the advance in surgical tech-

Table 28-1. Bronchoplastic and Angioplastic Procedures in the Treatment of Lung Cancer

Procedure	Number
Sleeve resection left side	
Upper lobe sleeve bronchial	12
Upper lobe sleeve pulmonary artery	13
Double-sleeve resection	123
Y-sleeve resection lower lobe	45
Sleeve resection right side	
Sleeve resection upper lobe	144
Sleeve resection middle lobe	3
Sleeve resection upper bilobectomy	45
Y-sleeve resection lower bilobectomy	60
Partial bronchial sleeve	21
Angioplastic procedures	568

From Schirren J, Muley T, Schneider P, Latzke L: Chirurgische therapie des bronchial-karzinoms. *In* Drings P, Vogt-Moykopf I (eds): Thoraxtumoren–Diagnostik–Staging–gegenwärtiges Therapiekonzept. 2nd Ed. Heidelberg, Germany: Thoraxklinik Heidelberg-Rohrbach, 1998. With permission.

niques and improvements in intensive care medicine. In general, causes of death did not differ significantly from those found after standard resections.

The frequency of sleeve resection is much higher in the treatment of carcinoid tumors, compared with resection of bronchial carcinoma. Between 1984 and 1995 in Thoraxklinik Heidelberg-Rohrbach, in 132 patients with carcinoids of the lung, 61 patients underwent sleeve resection. Twenty-nine patients had classic sleeve resection of the upper lobe, nine patients had tumor resected by double-sleeve resection (bronchus and pulmonary artery), 11 patients underwent reverse or Y-sleeve resection, and in 12 patients the tumor could be resected by isolated bronchus resection without loss of parenchyma. In this group of patients the rate of severe complications was low. Bronchial fistula was seen in three patients (2.2%), with the need for secondary pneumonectomy in two patients (1.5%). The 30-day mortality was less than 1% (one patient).

LONG-TERM RESULTS

The overall 5-year survival rates after bronchoplastic resection for lung cancer vary from 30 to 46%, as shown by the reports of Bennett and Smith (1978) and Faber (1984), Watanabe (1990), and Van Schil (1996) and their associates. The survival correlates with lymph node involvement and the stage of the tumor. The 5-year survival of cases with negative node results is in the range of 50 to 67%, as described by Deslauriers (1986), Belli (1985), and Mehran (1994) and their colleagues, as well as by Naruke (1989). For N_1 cases, survival ranges from 21 to 60%, as reported in the series of Deslauriers (1986) and Van Schil (1996) and their coworkers. For stage I, II, and III cases the 5-year survival has been reported as 63 to 79%, 37 to 55%, and 21 to 30%, respec-

Table 28-2. Stage-Related Survival After Radical Bronchoplastic and Angioplastic Resections (R_0) in Patients with Bronchial Carcinoma

p-Stage (n)	I (105)	II (131)	IIIa (111)	IIIb (72)
1 yr	76%	80%	70%	53%
3 yrs	61%	52%	40%	26%
5 yrs	51%	41%	25%	nd
7 yrs	nd	38%	15%	nd
Median (mos)	73	42	24	15

nd, not determined.
From Schirren J, Muley T, Schneider P, Latzke L: Chirurgische therapie des bronchial-karzinoms. *In* Drings P, Vogt-Moykopf I (eds): Thoraxtumoren–Diagnostik–Staging–gegenwärtiges Therapiekonzept. 2nd Ed. Heidelberg, Germany: Thoraxklinik Heidelberg-Rohrbach, 1998. With permission.

tively, by Watanabe (1990) and Tedder (1992) and their associates. In our series we found 5-year survival rates between 20 and 51% depending on the tumor stage. In Table 28-2, the results in patients with complete resection by bronchoplastic, angioplastic, or both kinds of procedures are given. A clinical example is shown in Figure 28-9.

Local recurrence probably results from undetected lymphatic permeation at the hilar level and is reported to occur in 6 to 23% of cases in the series of Faber (1984), Mehran (1994), Kawahara (1994), and Van Schil (1996) and their associates. In our series local recurrence occurred in 16%. When possible, local recurrence is resected or treated by radiation therapy when resection is contraindicated.

The long-term functional recovery after bronchoplastic resection has been studied using perfusion and ventilation scintigraphy (Table 28-3). One of us (I.V.-M.) (1985) has shown significant function after bronchoplastic, angioplastic, or both kinds of resections as early as 3 weeks after surgery. Angeletti (1991), Khargi (1994), and Gaissert (1996) and their associates have shown further recovery up to 4 months. The reimplanted lobes function normally, and postoperative reduction in lung function reflects only the volume of lung parenchyma that has been resected.

In the management of lung cancer, bronchoplastic and angioplastic resection carries no higher perioperative mor-

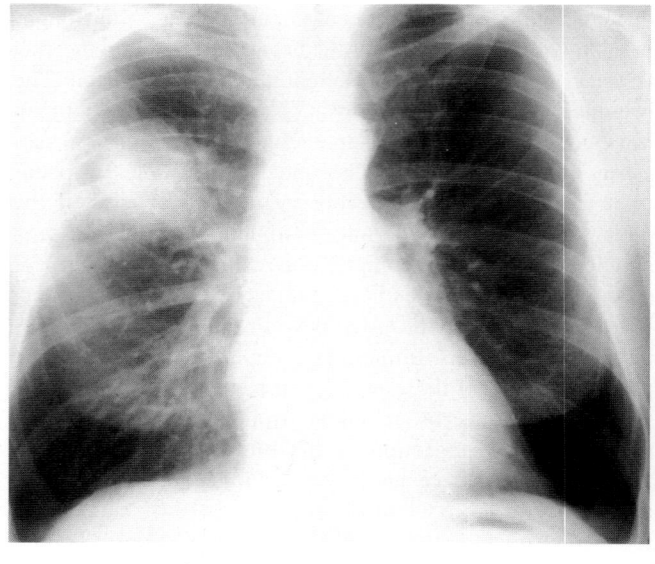

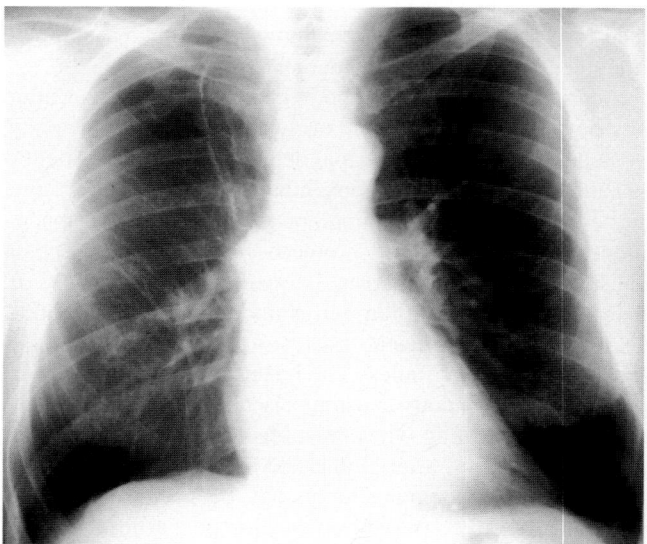

Fig. 28-9. Right upper lobe sleeve resection in a 66-year-old male patient with $pT_2pN_1pM_0$ (Union International Contra le Cancerium 1987) adenocarcinoma. **A.** Preoperative roentgenogram. **B.** Postoperative roentgenogram 7 years later.

Table 28-3. Results of Perfusion and Ventilation Scintigraphy after Double-Sleeve Resection of Left Upper Lobe in Patients with Primary or Secondary Lung Tumors (n = 38, 1994 through 1998)

	Preoperative	Postoperative Group 1 (7–27 days)		Postoperative Group 2 (44–184 days)	
	Perfusion	Perfusion	Ventilation	Perfusion	Ventilation
n^a	36	24	23	17	13
Mean ± standard deviation	40.2 ± 7.3	21.7 ± 4.0	21.0 ± 5.0	28.4 ± 5.5	27.5 ± 7.2
Range	25–63	13–29	11–30	26–41	19–40

[a]Not all patients were analyzed twice (postoperative group 1 and postoperative group 2); some were only included in postoperative group 1 or postoperative group 2, respectively.
From Dr. A. Schmäl and Dr. S. Thuengerthal, Department of Radiology, Thoraxklinik Heidelberg-Rohrbach.

tality than pneumonectomy and preserves lung function and quality of life. These techniques are valid alternatives to pneumonectomy whenever the situation permits. Nowadays, simple pneumonectomy should be the exception rather than the rule in treatment of lung cancer. In benign disease causing bronchial obstruction, bronchoplastic techniques offer a means of surgical correction that can result in improved lung function, which means preservation of quality of life.

REFERENCES

Allison PR: Course of Thoracic Surgery in Groningen, Netherlands, 1954.

Angeletti CA, et al: Functional results of bronchial sleeve lobectomy. Eur J Cardiothorac Surg 5:410, 1991.

Belli L, et al: Bronchoplastic procedures and pulmonary artery reconstruction in the treatment of bronchogenic cancer. J Thorac Cardiovasc Surg 90:167, 1985.

Bennett FW, Smith AR: A twenty-year analysis of the results of sleeve resection for primary bronchogenic carcinoma. J Thorac Cardiovasc Surg 76:840, 1978.

Black CT, Luck SR, Raffensperger JG: Bronchoplastic techniques for pediatric lung salvage. J Pediatr Surg 23:653, 1988.

D'Abreau AL, McHale SJ: Bronchial "adenoma" treated by local resection and reconstruction of the left main bronchus. Br J Surg 39:355, 1952.

Deslauriers J, et al: Long-term clinical and functional results of sleeve lobectomy for primary lung cancer. J Thorac Cardiovasc Surg 92:871, 1986.

Faber LP, Jensik RJ, Kittle CF: Results of sleeve lobectomy for bronchogenic carcinoma in 101 patients. Ann Thorac Surg 37:279, 1984.

Firmin RK, et al: Sleeve lobectomy (lobectomy and bronchoplasty) for bronchial carcinoma. Ann Thorac Surg 35:442, 1983.

Gaissert HA, et al: Survival and function after sleeve lobectomy for lung cancer. J Thorac Cardiovasc Surg 111:948, 1996.

Gebauer PW: Bronchial resection and anastomosis. J Thorac Surg 26:241, 1953.

Kato R, et al: Bronchoplastic procedures for tuberculous bronchial stenosis. J Thorac Cardiovasc Surg 106:1118, 1993.

Kawahara K, et al: Management of anastomotic complications after sleeve lobectomy for lung cancer. Ann Thorac Surg 57:1529, 1994.

Kesler KA, et al: Assessing the feasibility of bronchoplastic resection with magnetic resonance imaging. Ann Thorac Surg 52:145, 1991.

Khargi K, et al: Pulmonary function after sleeve lobectomy. Ann Thorac Surg 57:1302, 1994.

Maeda M, et al: Tracheobronchoplasty for lung cancer. Int Surg 71:221, 1986.

Mehran RJ, et al: Survival related to nodal status after sleeve resection for lung cancer. J Thorac Cardiovasc Surg 107:576, 1994.

Naruke T: Bronchoplastic and bronchovascular procedures of the tracheobronchial tree in the treatment of primary lung cancer. Chest 96:53S, 1989.

Newton JR Jr, Grillo HC, Mathisen DJ: Main bronchial sleeve resection with pulmonary conservation. Ann Thorac Surg 52:1272, 1991.

Pichlmaier H, Spelsberg F: Organerhaltende Operation des Bronchialkarzinoms. Langenbecks Arch Chir 328:221, 1971.

Price Thomas C: Conservative resection of the bronchial tree. J R Coll Surg Edinb 1:169, 1956.

Read RC, et al: Pulmonary artery sleeve resection for abutting left upper lobe lesions. Ann Thorac Surg 55:850, 1993.

Rees GM, Paneth M: Lobectomy with sleeve resection in the treatment of bronchial tumours. Thorax 25:160, 1970.

Rendina EA, Venuta F, Ricci C: Effects of low-dose steroids on bronchial healing after sleeve resection: a clinical study. J Thorac Cardiovasc Surg 104:888, 1992.

Suri RM, et al: Pulmonary arteriography for the assessment of technical feasibility of sleeve resection in lung cancer. Ann Thorac Surg 63:800, 1997.

Tedder M, et al: Current morbidity, mortality and survival after bronchoplastic procedures for malignancy. Ann Thorac Surg 54:387, 1992.

Toomes H, Vogt-Moykopf I: Conservative resection for lung cancer. In Delarue NC, Eschapasse H (eds): International Trends in General Thoracic Surgery. Vol. 1. Lung Cancer. Philadelphia: WB Saunders, 1985, p. 88.

Tsang V, Goldstraw P: Endobronchial stenting for anastomotic stenosis after sleeve resection. Ann Thorac Surg 48:568, 1989.

Urschel HC Jr, Razzuk MA: Median sternotomy as a standard approach for pulmonary resection. Ann Thorac Surg 41:130, 1986.

Van Schil PE, et al: TNM staging and long term follow up after sleeve resection for bronchogenic tumours. Ann Thorac Surg 52:1096, 1991.

Van Schil PE, et al: Long term survival after bronchial sleeve resection: univariate and multivariate analyses. Ann Thorac Surg 61:1087, 1996.

Van Schil PE, et al: Completion pneumonectomy after bronchial sleeve resection: incidence, indications and results. Ann Thorac Surg 53:1042, 1992.

Vogt-Moykopf I, et al: Bronchoplastic and angioplastic operation in bronchial carcinoma: long-term results of a retrospective analysis from 1973 to 1983. Int Surg 71:211, 1986.

Vogt-Moykopf I, et al. Manschettenresektion des Bronchus und der Pulmonlarterie. Prax Klin Pneumol 39:574, 1985.

Watanabe Y, et al: Results in 104 patients undergoing bronchoplastic procedures for bronchial lesions. Ann Thorac Surg 50:607, 1990.

Wurning P: Technische Vorteile bei der Hauptbronchusresektion rechts und links. Thoraxchir und vask Chir 15:16, 1967.

READING REFERENCES

Bjork VO, Carlens E, Craford C: The open closure of the bronchus and the resection of the carina and of the tracheal wall. J Thorac Surg 23:419, 1952.

Dortenmann I: Indikation und Technik der parenchym-erhaltenden Bronchusresektion. Thoraxchir und vask Chir 11:554, 1964.

Fujimura S, et al: Prognostic evaluation of tracheobronchial reconstruction for bronchogenic carcinoma. J Thorac Cardiovasc Surg 90:161, 1985.

Jensik RJ, et al: Sleeve lobectomy for carcinoma, a ten year experience. J Thorac Cardiovasc Surg 64:400, 1972.

Johnston JB, Jones PH: The treatment of bronchial carcinoma by lobectomy and sleeve resection of the main bronchus. Thorax 14:48, 1959.

Matthes TH: Über Möglichkeiten von Lungenteil—und Bronchusresektionen rait End-zu-End Anastomose bei ausgewählten Fällen von Bronchialkarzinomen. Thoraxchirurgie 4:106, 1956.

Naruke T: Bronchoplastic procedure for lung cancer. J Thorac Cardiovasc Surg 73:927, 1977.

Paulson DL, Shaw RR: Preservation of lung tissue by means of bronchoplastic procedures. Am J Surg 89:347, 1955.

Paulson DL, et al: Bronchoplastic procedures for bronchogenic carcinoma. J Thorac Cardiovasc Surg 59:38, 1970.

Van Den Bosch JMM, et al: Lobectomy with sleeve resection in the treatment of tumours of the bronchus. Chest 80:154, 1981.

Vogt-Moykopf I, et al: Bronchoplastic techniques for lung resection. In Baue AE, Naunheim KS (eds): Glenn's Thoracic and Cardiovascular Surgery. 5th Ed. Vol. 1. Thoracic Surgery. Norwalk: Appleton and Lange, 1990, p. 403.

Weisel RD, et al: Sleeve lobectomy for carcinoma of the lung. J Thorac Cardiovasc Surg 78:839, 1979.

Drings P, Vogt-Moykopf I (eds): Thoraxtumoren—Diagnostik—Staging—gegenwärtiges Therapiekonzept. 2nd Ed. Berlin: Springer Verlag, 1998.

CHAPTER 29

Pneumonectomy and Its Modifications

Peter Goldstraw

As necessity is the mother of invention, the increasing epidemic of lung cancer in the first half of this century, as noted by Holmes Sellors (1955) and Rigdon and Kirchoff (1958), among others, demanded the development of surgical methods for its treatment. In 1912, but reported in 1913, Morriston Davies, then at University College Hospital in London, undertook the first dissection lobectomy for lung cancer. The patient died on the eighth postoperative day, leaving Tudor Edwards at the Brompton Hospital with the credit of performing the first successful lobectomy for lung cancer in 1928, which was subsequently reported in 1932. Graham and Singer, in St. Louis, reported the first successful removal of the entire lung for cancer in 1933. As noted by Baue (1984), Graham preferred the term *pneumectomy* to describe this operation. He did not dissect the hilar structures, preferring to transfix the hilar vessels and bronchus as they emerged from the mediastinum. Important as this landmark operation was, our modern technique of pneumonectomy owes more to the dissection method first undertaken in 1930 by Churchill in Boston, as he and his associates recorded in 1950. Once more, necessity spurred progress, and when attempting pneumonectomy by mass ligation of the hilar structures, he found the tumor too close to the hilum and was forced to dissect out each structure and ligate them separately. Unfortunately, his failure to close a bronchus led to the patient's death, and it fell to Reinhoff (1936) in Baltimore to undertake the first successful dissection pneumonectomy for cancer in 1933.

Pneumonectomy then became established, as pioneers in many countries benefited from these early experiences and the scientific community witnessed parallel progress in radiology, anesthesia, and the development of blood transfusion and antibiotics. The publications of Meade (1961), Smith (1982), Burford (1958), and Churchill (1958) and their colleagues in the United Kingdom and the United States attest to this progress. Indeed, pneumonectomy became so routine that many surgeons, such as Johnson and associates (1958), considered it the only proper operation for lung cancer. Ochsner (1978) recalled the debate, quoting the strong condemnation of lesser resections by leading authorities in the 1940s. In the succeeding decades, most surgeons came to appreciate that the best operation was the least resection that removed the primary tumor and its involved lymphatics. Each more conservative resection was introduced as a compromise for the patient unable to tolerate more extensive resection, and each (i.e., lobectomy, sleeve resection, and segmentectomy) has been shown to be an adequate cancer operation, with survival as least as good as with more extensive resections, as long as the basic oncologic principle of resecting all of the primary tumor and its involved lymphatics can be achieved. Still, in many cases, however, this is only possible by pneumonectomy.

INDICATIONS FOR PNEUMONECTOMY

The majority of pneumonectomies are still performed for lung cancer. Occasionally, one may perform pneumonectomy for bronchiectasis or for a lung destroyed by chronic suppuration. Although these are common indications in the Third World, they are rare in developed countries. Pneumonectomy occasionally is performed for pulmonary metastases and rare thoracic tumors. These problems are discussed no further in favor of concentrating on pneumonectomy for lung cancer.

As the extent of resection is rarely known before surgery, all patients to undergo thoracotomy for lung cancer should be assessed for their suitability for pneumonectomy. This is essentially a cost-benefit assessment. The *cost* of operation includes many factors other than the financial cost and the time off work, but uppermost in the patient's mind is the risk of death postoperatively and the likely reduction in exercise capacity. These risks depend on the assessment of patient fitness, which is covered in Chapters 19 and 20. The *benefit* offered by pneumonectomy is the possibility of cure or extended survival, which depend on preoperative staging, discussed in Chapter 98. I have come to appreciate that no matter how carefully the preoperative staging is undertaken,

411

intraoperative staging is essential to review the situation before proceeding with resection, as Gaer and I (1990), Fry (1984), Gephardt and Rice (1990), Albertucci (1992), and Izbicki (1992) and their colleagues have stated. I (1991) think of thoracotomy as the final investigation before undertaking treatment by resection. Fernando and I (1990) showed that preoperative staging of lung cancer underestimates the extent of disease in almost one-half of the patients coming to thoracotomy. Although resection is still reasonable in 95% of patients, in some groups, who can only be identified by intrathoracic staging, complete resection is not possible or resection is not likely to offer survival advantages. In these cases, it is preferable to withdraw, causing as little damage as possible, rather than to compound the error by futile resection.

If the tumor is found at thoracotomy to be resectable only by pneumonectomy, the surgeon must weigh this added risk against the reduced prospects of cure for the tumor now known to have a more advanced stage. Although in most cases the decision is to proceed with resection, situations arise in which resection by lobectomy would have been reasonable, yet pneumonectomy is undesirable. One can reliably assess that pneumonectomy, once begun, can be accomplished, as all the hilar structures can be identified and confirmed to be free of tumor before commencing resection. Unfortunately, this does not apply to lesser resections, and one can only be sure of being able to complete lobectomy, or other conservative resections, after dividing segmental vessels and moving on to inspect the underlying lymph nodes around the bronchus. It is best to avoid this resection cascade, especially if the surgical options are restricted by physiologic considerations.

Bronchoscopy is an important component of preoperative staging, as Spiro and I noted (1984). Increasingly, the diagnosis is established by one's medical colleagues with fiberbronchoscopy. The surgeon should, however, repeat the bronchoscopy immediately before thoracotomy. Anatomic features, of little import to the physician, may affect decisions at thoracotomy. A tumor may lie in the intermediate bronchus, but the surgeon knows that if the origin of this bronchus is invaded, only pneumonectomy will suffice, whereas if the tumor lies at the termination of the same bronchus, middle and lower lobectomy may be adequate. Similarly, some abnormalities of bronchial anatomy, particularly with the right upper lobe, as noted by Le Roux (1962) and discussed in Chapter 5, may create difficulties if lobectomy is attempted. The wise anesthetist looks for distortion of the bronchial tree to aid placement of double-lumen tubes.

Although pulmonary resection is possible through a wide variety of incisions, the lateral thoracotomy approach allows a fuller assessment of the tumor and the mediastinum than the anterior, posterior, or median sternotomy incisions. It has therefore become my standard approach. It matters less whether one has been trained to use a thoracotomy through the interspace or through the bed of a rib, and the fifth or sixth rib allows adequate access for pneumonectomy. The details of these incisions are covered in Chapter 25.

At thoracotomy, the surgeon should commence with a careful intraoperative evaluation to provide answers to four key questions:

1) *What is the diagnosis?* It may seem facile to pose this question, but many legal cases hinge on the basis for the diagnosis. Surgeons often urge patients to proceed with thoracotomy on the basis of highly suspicious chest radiography results, perhaps supported by suspicious cytologic findings. Although it is right that we recommend this procedure, we have a responsibility to obtain a firm histologic diagnosis before resecting lung tissue. Rapid section histology must be on hand, and the surgeon must carefully select the tissue to biopsy. This sampling is often straightforward, but surrounding inflammatory changes occasionally obscure the underlying malignant process. It may not prove possible to get accurate biopsy samples without risk of damage to segmental bronchi or vessels. At the final analysis, the surgeon must proceed on the basis of all available evidence: the biopsy findings, radiographic appearances, and clinical features. One may have to perform lobectomy on the suspicion that an underlying malignancy cannot be excluded. Usually, this is proved to be the case when the resection specimen is subsequently sectioned. In any event, for this to be necessary, the lobe is sufficiently damaged by such an extensive inflammatory process as to have little function. Rarely, during the course of lobectomy, tumor is encountered. The surgeon then can obtain histologic confirmation at this point, and proceed with pneumonectomy if necessary. It has never proved necessary in the author's experience to perform pneumonectomy without a diagnosis justifying such an extensive resection.

2) *Can the proven malignancy now be resected by pneumonectomy?* To answer this question, the surgeon must carefully and systematically circumnavigate the hilum, checking that each structure to be divided can be controlled at a point free of tumor. The details of this step are discussed subsequently. If the hilar structures have to be exposed intrapericardially, the pericardiotomy should be limited at this stage to preserve the phrenic nerve. One is always able to confirm that complete resection is possible before dividing any vital structures, and if resection is not possible, the minimum amount of damage has been inflicted.

3) *Does the intrathoracic staging indicate that the consequences of pneumonectomy are justified by the prospects for cure?* By now, the local extent of the tumor, its T stage, has been more fully defined. Pleural metastases have been excluded, and invasion into the chest wall, diaphragm, or mediastinum has been confirmed or refuted. Critically, by now the mediastinal lymph nodes have been dissected and examined, as is described in detail in Right Pneumonectomy (later in this chapter) and a more accurate N stage has been determined.

4) *Can this proven malignancy be resected by more conservative resection without compromising prospects for cure?* It is at this point that attention is focused on the hilum, and the prospects for lobectomy, sleeve resection, or segmentectomy are evaluated. I prefer to proceed in this order because, as already mentioned, one may not be able to complete the lesser resection if tumor is encountered after dividing segmental structures; one is committed to resection, and it is better to make the decision regarding resection on the cost-to-benefit assumption of pneumonectomy.

TECHNIQUE

Let us assume that the patient comes to surgery with a firm histologic diagnosis or that we have, with rapid section analysis, answered the question of whether the proven malignancy now can be resected by pneumonectomy. Let us follow the routine steps to evaluate the hilum, dissect the mediastinal lymph nodes, decide whether staging indicates pneumonectomy or a more conservative procedure, and undertake pneumonectomy if required. The detailed steps for right pneumonectomy through a right lateral thoracotomy incision are described subsequently. All lymph node station references relate to the nodal chart of Naruke and associates (1978).

Right Pneumonectomy

Once intrapleural dissection has freed any adhesions, the operative lung can be collapsed using the double-lumen endobronchial tube. The lung is retracted posteriorly and inferiorly to gain access to the area of the pulmonary artery, superior pulmonary vein, and azygos arch (Fig. 29-1). The sheath of the pulmonary artery is opened on its superior aspect, as the upper lobe branches are arising. The nodes in this position (station 10 on the Naruke chart) are reflected upward, off the superior surface of the right main bronchus, to the undersurface of the azygos arch. As for all other nodal groups cleared while encircling the hilum, these are put on one side on a swab for more detailed evaluation before resection. It is convenient at this point to continue the dissection of the right paratracheal nodes (stations 2, 3, and 4). This maneuver is described in more detail in Chapter 100, but it is my practice to conserve the azygos vein, dissecting the nodes from beneath it, and completing the dissection of the higher nodes through a small incision in the mediastinal pleura above the arch.

The lung is then retracted anteriorly. Dissection continues posteriorly along the undersurface of the azygos arch, mobilizing the superior margin of the main bronchus. By dividing the vagal branches and bronchial arteries that lie on the posterior wall of the right main bronchus, the esophagus can be retracted (Fig. 29-2) to provide access to the main carinal

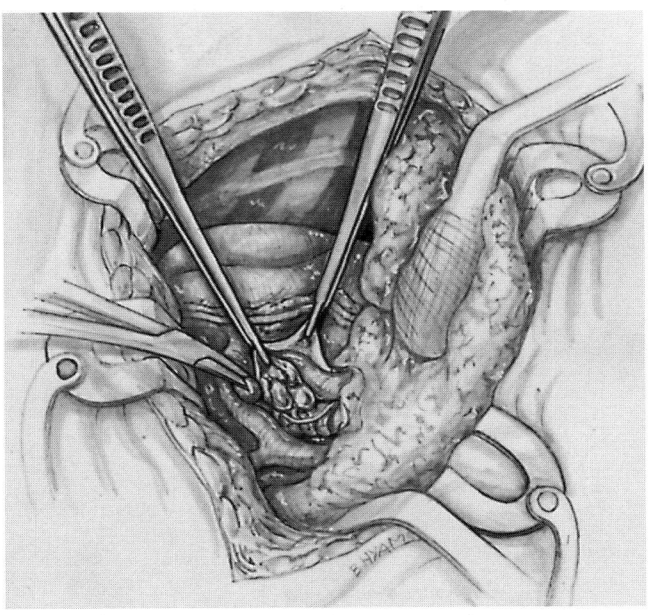

Fig. 29-1. The lung is retracted posteriorly and inferiorly to access the pulmonary artery, superior pulmonary vein, and azygos arch. The superior aspect of the pulmonary artery is opened as the upper lobe branches arise. Station 10 nodes are reflected upward, off the superior surface of the right main bronchus to the undersurface of the azygos arch.

nodes (station 7). The fascia enveloping these nodes is incised, and the nodes are removed to clear the inferior aspect of the carina. The surgeon should now be able to pass a finger around the main bronchus, ensuring resectability at this point.

Dissection can continue inferiorly along the anterior aspect of the esophagus, removing nodes in station 8, freeing the inferior pulmonary ligament with its small nodes (station 9), and identifying the inferior pulmonary vein (Fig. 29-3). Dissection should clear this vein so that a finger can be passed around it. Small vessels bleeding on the esophagus require cautery, and one must exercise great care to avoid injury to the esophagus with resultant fistula. It may be preferable to see what natural hemostasis can achieve while the operation continues.

The dissection continues around the undersurface of the inferior pulmonary vein, moving onto the anterior aspect of the hilum and moving the retractor to depress the lung posteriorly. The superior pulmonary vein is mobilized and its middle and upper lobe tributaries are identified. Anomalies of pulmonary venous anatomy occur. A pericardial reflection extends anteriorly as a ligament between the superior pulmonary vein and the pulmonary artery. This structure is incised to clear the superior margin of the superior vein and the anterior and inferior aspects of the pulmonary artery (Fig. 29-4). The surgeon should be able to encircle both these structures with a finger, confirming resectability at this point.

The surgeon has now completed the circumnavigation of the hilum. All the structures that have to be divided to per-

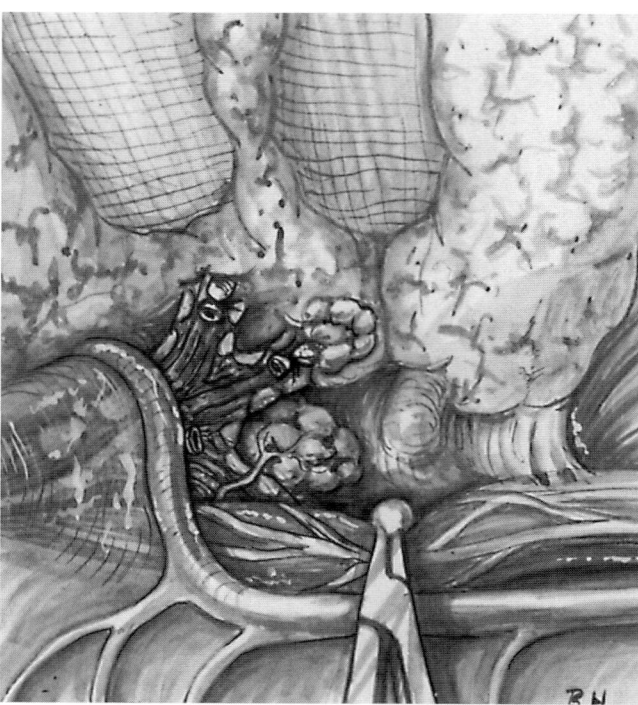

Fig. 29-2. Retraction of the esophagus gives access to the main carinal nodes.

mit pneumonectomy have been identified at a point free of tumor. If detailed examination of the resected mediastinal lymph nodes confirms that pneumonectomy could offer survival advantages to compensate for the loss of the lung parenchyma, and if lesser resection has been considered but pronounced oncologically inadequate, the surgeon proceeds with pneumonectomy.

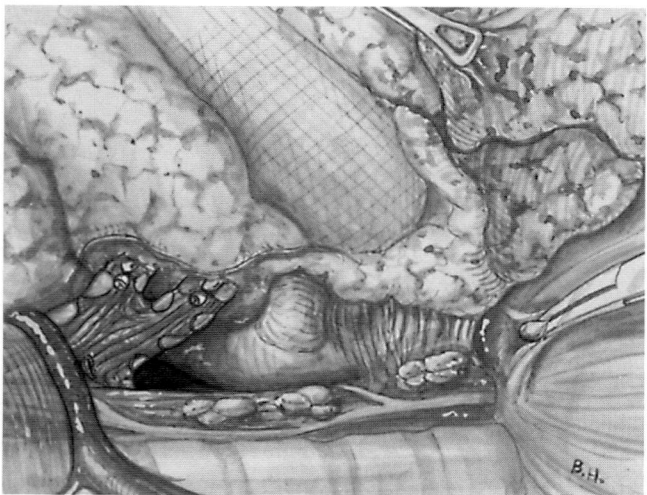

Fig. 29-3. Dissection along the anterior aspect of the esophagus allows removal of station 8 nodes, freeing of the inferior pulmonary ligament, and identification of the inferior pulmonary vein.

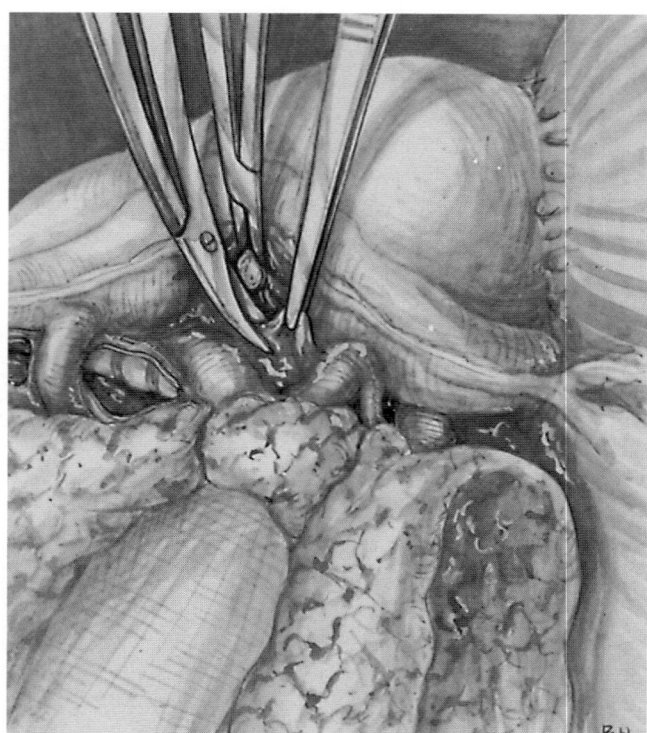

Fig. 29-4. Dissection around the undersurface of the inferior pulmonary vein, moving onto the anterior aspect of the hilum and moving the retractor to depress the lung.

The hilar structures may be divided in any order; I divide them in order of ease and convenience. I begin with the pulmonary artery. The index finger is looped around the vessel (Fig. 29-5A) to devolve it from the mediastinum, separate it from adjacent structures, and guide the passage of a crushing clamp. A Ronald Edwards clamp, which looks like a right-angled Roberts clamp, is ideal. Two clamps are applied at least 1 cm apart and the vessel is divided (Fig. 29-5B), taking care to leave a generous flange distal to the proximal clamp. Each end is transfixed with a braided 2-0 suture. It is important to transfix each margin of the vessel close to the edge (Fig. 29-5C). Only a single throw of the knot is performed at this stage. The suture then encircles the vessel, and the suture is tied, on the other side of the vessel (Fig. 29-5D). This transfixion suture is tied tight as the clamp is released, and the knot is then completed. Further reinforcing throws are used over the proximal stump (Fig. 29-5E).

The pulmonary veins are dealt with similarly. The inferior vein is best controlled by retracting the lung superiorly (Fig. 29-6).

At this stage, only the bronchus is left. Many surgeons have been trained to staple the bronchus, but it is my practice to suture the bronchial stump. The method includes a crushing clamp, but if length does not permit, the same suture technique can be used in an open method. The technique is thus applicable in all situations. al–Kattan and associates (1995) reviewed the results of this technique in 471 consecutive

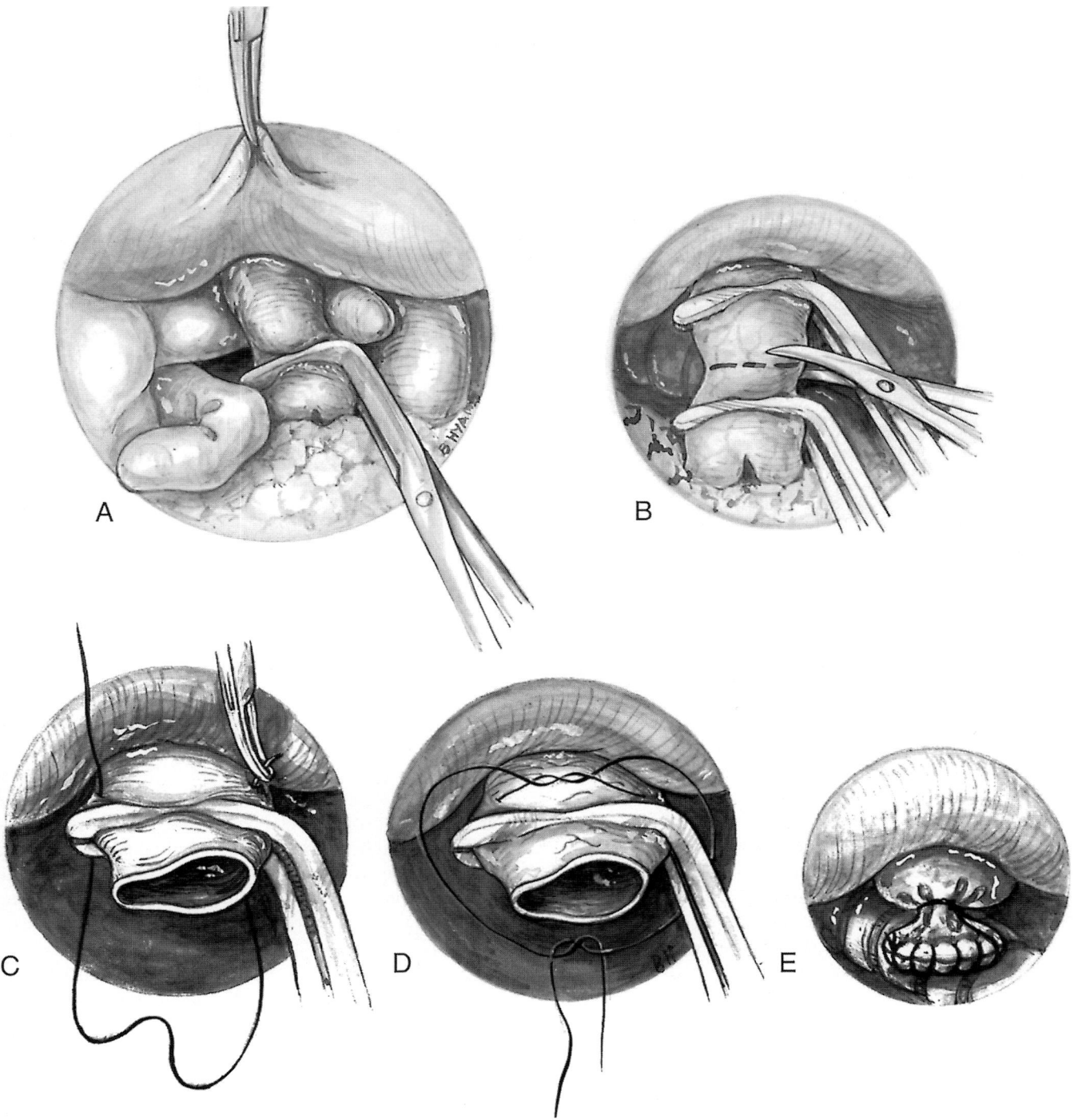

Fig. 29-5. Dividing hilar structures. **A.** The index finger devolves the pulmonary artery from the mediastinum and guides the passage of a crushing clamp. **B.** Two clamps are applied and the vessel is divided. **C.** Margins are transfixed with a braided suture. **D.** The suture circles the vessel and is tied on the other side. **E.** Reinforcing throws are used over the proximal stump.

pneumonectomies, of which 23 (4.8%) were for benign conditions such as tuberculosis, and 27 (5.7%) were completion pneumonectomies. Working in a postgraduate institution, this method has been taught to many surgeons in training with safe results. The overall fistula rate for these pneumonectomy cases is 1.5%. In the 359 pneumonectomies performed by the author, only two bronchopleural fistulae were noted, for an incidence of 0.55%. When pneumonectomy was performed by a surgeon in training, the risk of fistula increased to 4.3%, but many trainees had no failures. No evidence exists that sta-

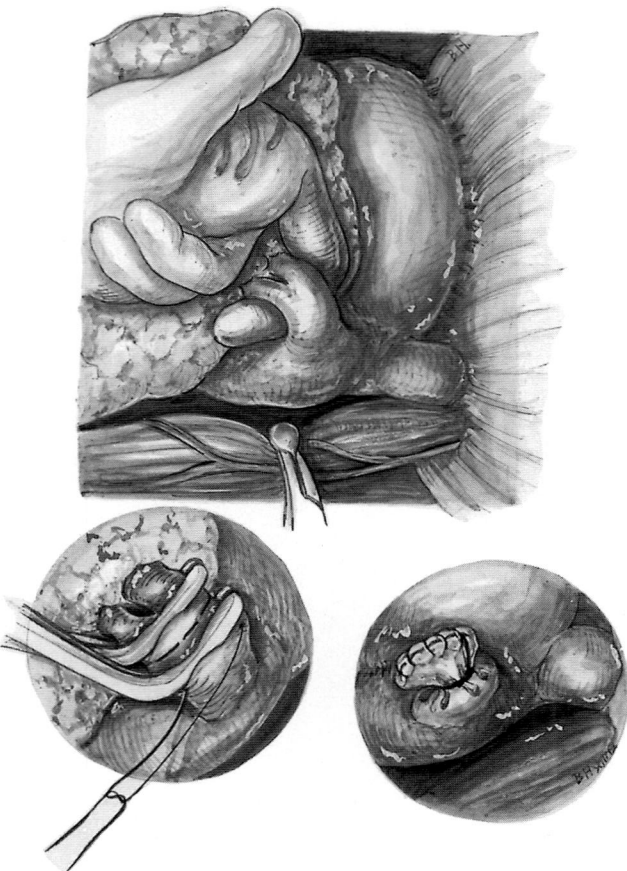

Fig. 29-6. Division of the pulmonary veins, as described in Figure 29-5. The lung is retracted superiorly to control the inferior vein.

pling is safer, even in the restricted situations in which it is applicable. Each surgeon, however, uses the technique that he or she was taught and that is safe and effective.

The lung is lifted to expose the carina (Fig. 29-7A). A crushing clamp is applied flush with the exterior landmark of the carina. If length permits, and especially if infected secretions are dammed within the lung, a second, distal clamp is applied. The bronchus is divided, leaving a flange of 2 to 3 mm distal to the proximal clamp, and the lung is removed. The stump is sutured with a 2-0 monofilament suture; I prefer using nonabsorbable material. A continuous, horizontal mattress suture runs the length of the stump, immediately proximal to the clamp, around the edge of the bronchus, and back to the standing end of the suture (Fig. 29-7B). The flange of the bronchus is then excised along the distal edge of the clamp (Fig. 29-7C) and sent for histologic evaluation. The clamp is released as the suture is tied, usually causing the stump to corrugate slightly. Closure is completed with a second suture running over and over the crushed flange distal to the previous suture (Fig. 29-7D).

The pleural space is irrigated and the bronchial stump is tested as airtight by the anesthetist, with inflation to 40 cm

of water pressure while the stump is immersed. Hemostasis is checked.

The bronchial stump is buried by apposing mediastinal tissues over it (Fig. 29-8). A continuous suture repairs the incision in the mediastinal pleura above the azygos arch, and runs across the azygos vein to pull it over the stump. The azygos vein is occluded, but its sacrifice provides a good pledget of tissue to cover the bronchial stump. This suture continues inferiorly, drawing the esophagus to the posterior aspect of the sheath of the pulmonary artery and the pericardium, to the lower limit of the mediastinal dissection at the inferior pulmonary vein.

The thoracotomy is closed without drainage. A drain is only necessary if continued bleeding is a concern, which may be the case after extensive chest wall resection or with pleuropneumonectomy. The patient is turned supine and excess air is aspirated from the pneumonectomy space (Fig. 29-9) to bring the mediastinum to the side of surgery. Usually, 1.5 to 2.0 L of air are removed. The final assessment of the mediastinal position is made by judging the tracheal position once the endobronchial tube has been removed and on postoperative chest radiography.

Left Pneumonectomy

The dissection for left pneumonectomy differs only in the area of the aortic arch (Fig. 29-10). The lung is retracted inferiorly and the vagus and phrenic nerves are identified as they lie beneath the mediastinal pleura over the aortic arch. The former lies deep to the superior intercostal vein, a useful landmark in difficult dissections. Nodes anterior to the vagus nerve (station 5) and over the anterior aspect of the arch beneath the phrenic nerve (station 6) are removed to expose the pulmonary artery. The recurrent laryngeal branch of the vagus must be identified clearly and preserved before removing the glands at station 4 lying on the upper aspect of the main bronchus beneath the aorta.

As on the right side, dissection continues over the superior and posterior aspects of the main bronchus to gain access to the nodes at the main carina (Fig. 29-11). All hilar structures are encircled as nodes are resected to complete the intrathoracic staging and to confirm resectability. The transection and closure of these structures is as described for right pneumonectomy.

The bronchial stump is buried (Fig. 29-12) by approximating the esophagus to the posterior aspect of the sheath of the pulmonary artery and pericardium, taking care not to damage the recurrent laryngeal nerve.

Intrapericardial Ligation of the Pulmonary Vessels

More advanced tumors may require the intrapericardial division of the pulmonary vessels to achieve complete clear-

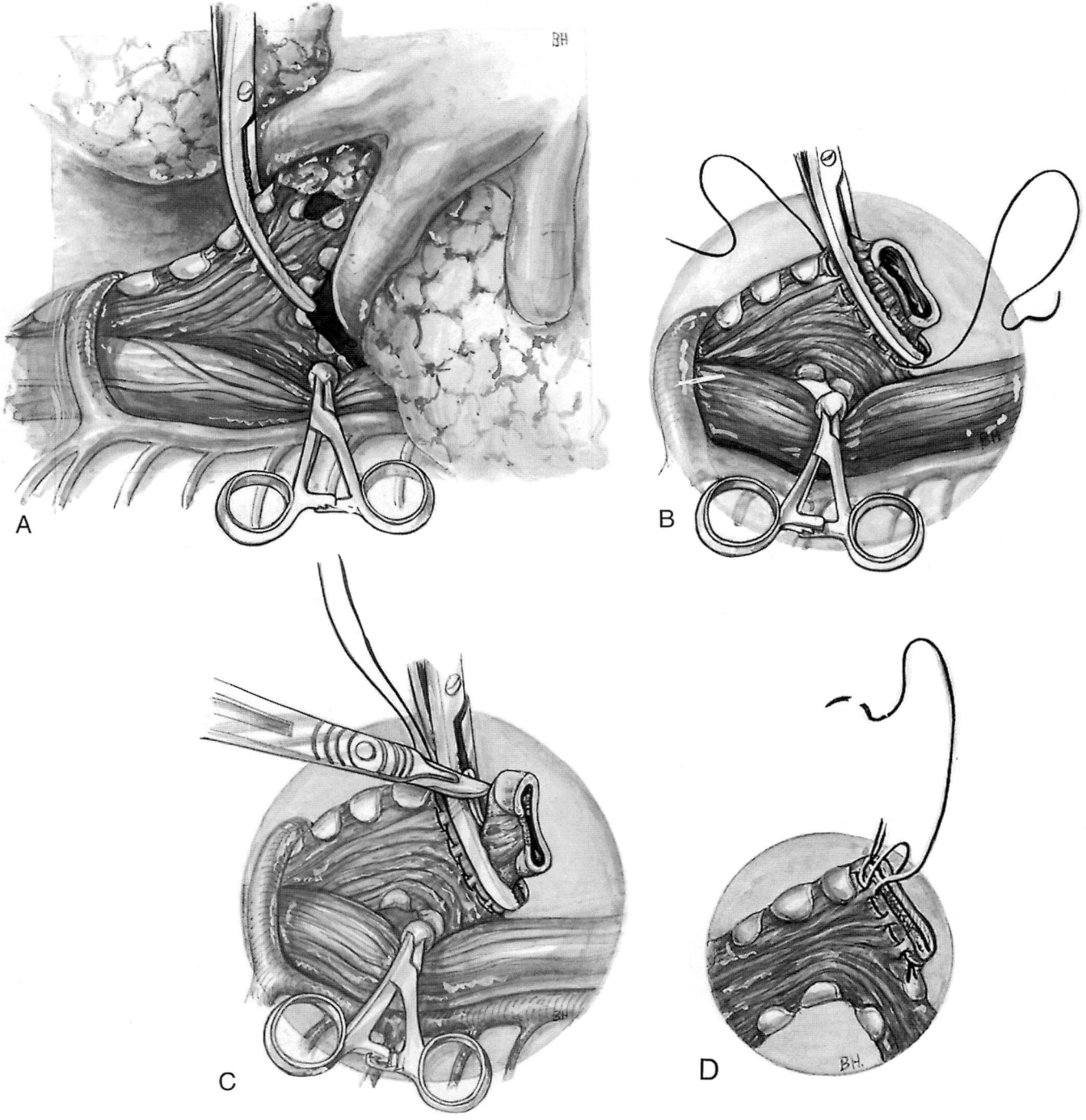

Fig. 29-7. A. The carina is exposed. **B.** Suture pattern on the bronchus stump. **C.** The flange of the bronchus is excised. **D.** Closure is completed with sutures over the crushed flange distal to the previous suture.

ance. Again, one should limit damage until complete resection is assured and until intrathoracic staging has shown pneumonectomy is desirable. The pericardium is therefore opened at a point clear of the phrenic nerve. This area may be immediately adjacent to the entry of the vessels, or if invasion of the pericardium is more widespread, anterior to the phrenic nerve. If resection proceeds, the steps are as described previously.

On the right side, the pulmonary artery is seen superiorly and the pericardial reflection usually passes obliquely across

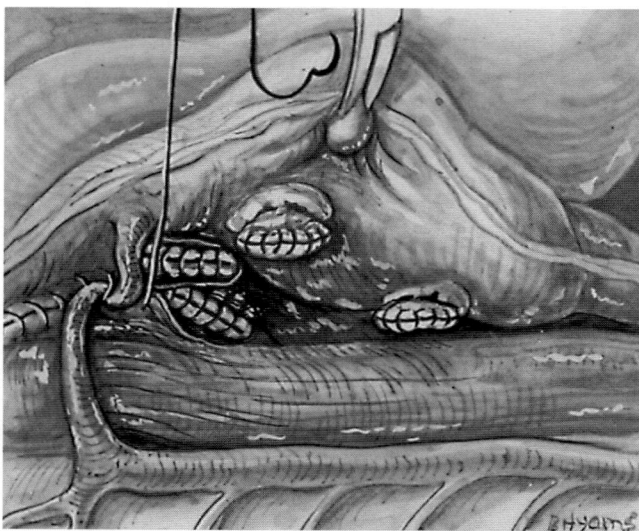

Fig. 29-8. The bronchial stump is buried by apposing mediastinal tissues.

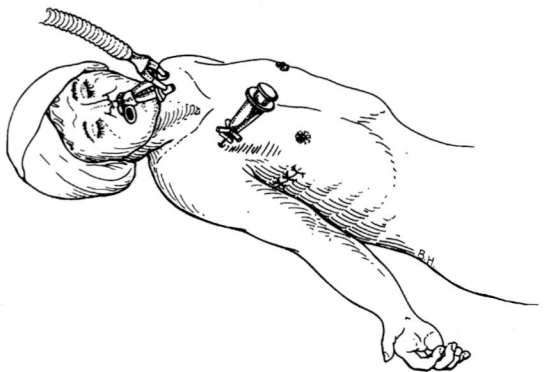

Fig. 29-9. Patient positioning after thoracotomy.

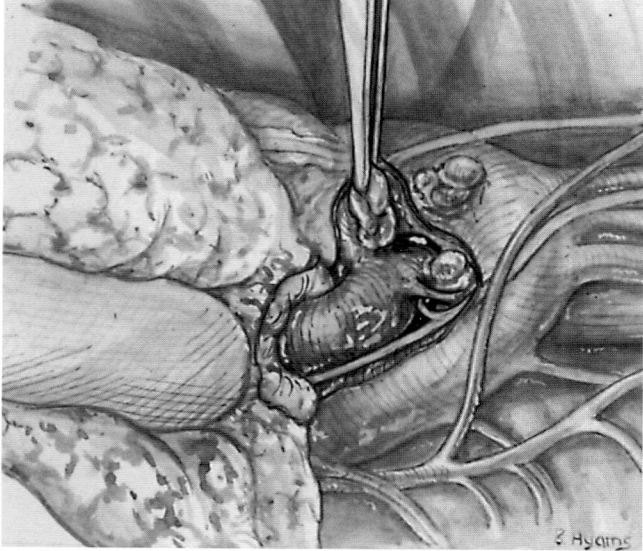

Fig. 29-10. Dissection for left pneumonectomy.

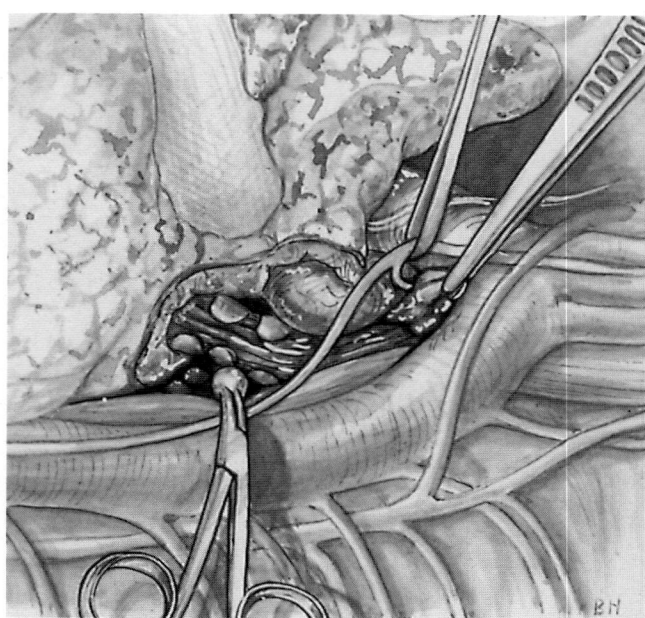

Fig. 29-11. Dissection over the superior and posterior aspects of the main bronchus allows access to the nodes at the main carina.

the artery. The vessel may be readily encircled just proximal to this point. On occasion, the pericardial reflection is more medial and the artery must then be exposed medial to the superior vena cava between this latter vessel and the aorta. The superior and inferior pulmonary veins are usually covered with the serous pericardium for approximately three-fourths of their circumference. Therefore, it is necessary to open this pericardial serous layer above and below each vessel to pass a finger about the vessel.

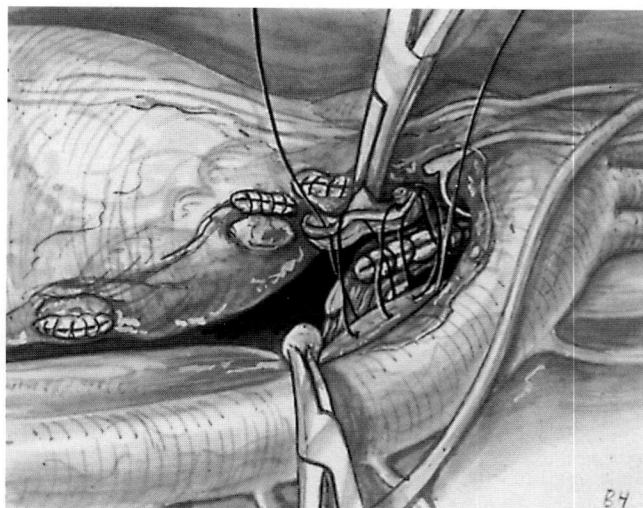

Fig. 29-12. The bronchial stump is buried by approximating the esophagus to the posterior aspect of the sheath of the pulmonary artery and the pericardium.

On the left side, the pulmonary artery is prominent and the fold of Marshall is a readily recognized landmark. Relative to the veins, approximately 75% of the superior pulmonary vein is covered with serous pericardium as it is on the right side; however, the inferior vein is almost completely covered, so only a small part of its wall is not free within the pericardial sac.

On occasion, a clamp is applied to the left atrium and both pulmonary veins are divided simultaneously. The tumor may be too close to the point of division of artery or veins to allow a second, distal clamp. The security of the proximal clamp must not be endangered by trying to insert the distal clamp or by transection of the vessel too close to leave a safe flange distal to this clamp. If this happens, the tissues may squeeze from between the clamp, with resultant severe hemorrhage. It is preferable in these circumstances to deal with the other hilar structures first, and then divide the final vessel without a distal clamp. In my experience, bleeding from the distal lumen is usually minimal because the tumor has occluded the vessel, but it is easy to suture the distal stump if any sequestrated blood threatens to obscure the operative field.

Any pericardial defect after pneumonectomy deserves attention. The options, however, differ on the right and left sides, as the consequences of cardiac herniation differ in these circumstances. After right pneumonectomy, cardiac herniation is associated with torsion and rotation on the vena cavae, which lead to venous inflow occlusion with rapid and dramatic fatality. All pericardial defects after right pneumonectomy therefore must be closed. After left pneumonectomy, however, the heart may freely prolapse into the pneumonectomy space without any physiologic upset, unless constriction occurs. After left pneumonectomy, therefore, the surgeon may close the defect in the pericardium or enlarge it sufficiently to allow free herniation. Small pericardial defects, on either side, may be closed by suturing the stumps of the pulmonary veins to the anterior margins of the defect (Fig. 29-13). The left atrium is adherent to the posterior pericardium, and rotation and herniation cannot occur posteriorly because the heart is fixed by the contralateral pulmonary veins.

Large pericardial defects on the right side usually are associated with resection of the phrenic nerve. One can use a pedicled vascular patch of the diaphragm to repair the pericardial defect and at the same time plicate the diaphragm (Fig. 29-14). The diaphragmatic patch is mobilized from the periphery of this structure, close to the costal attachment. If this step is not possible through the original thoracotomy incision, a second intercostal incision can be made three ribs lower. Once mobilization begins, the patch is reflected superiorly to visualize the inferior phrenic vessels. The diaphragmatic closure proceeds as one develops the patch (Fig. 29-15). One should be bold; a large patch is needed and the diaphragm always comes together. The patch is hinged upward on a narrow pedicle near the inferior vena cava that contains the inferior phrenic vessels. The diaphragmatic

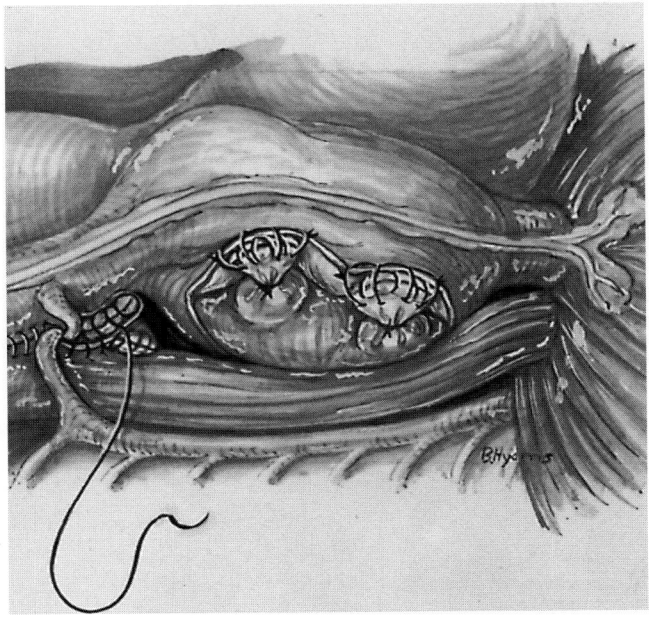

Fig. 29-13. The anterior margins of small pericardial defects are sutured to the stumps of the pulmonary veins.

defect is closed completely except for a tiny foramen around these vessels, near the inferior vena cava. The patch is then turned over and sutured to the margins of the pericardial defect with the peritoneal aspect facing outward (Fig. 29-16). It is preferable to leave a gap in this closure over the superior vena cava to avoid compression of this vessel, but small enough to prevent herniation. The bronchial stump may then be buried by suturing the esophagus to the posterior margin of the pericardial defect or to the patch (Fig. 29-17). Although this method is preferred by the author, the pericardial defect may be closed by using other adjacent tissue flaps or a prosthetic soft tissue patch, as noted in Chapter 26.

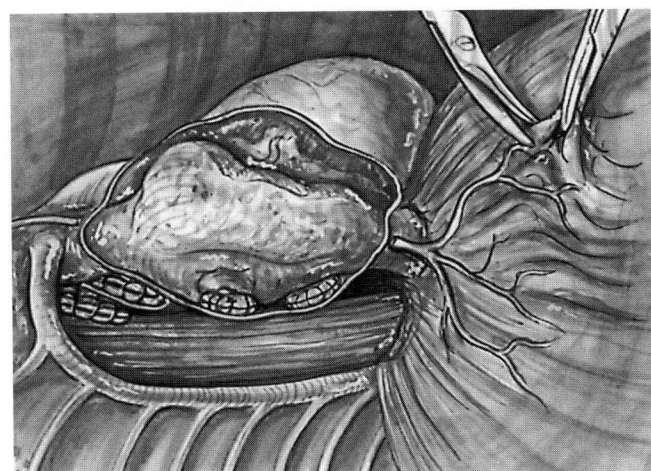

Fig. 29-14. A pedicled vascular patch of the diaphragm is used to repair a large pericardial defect.

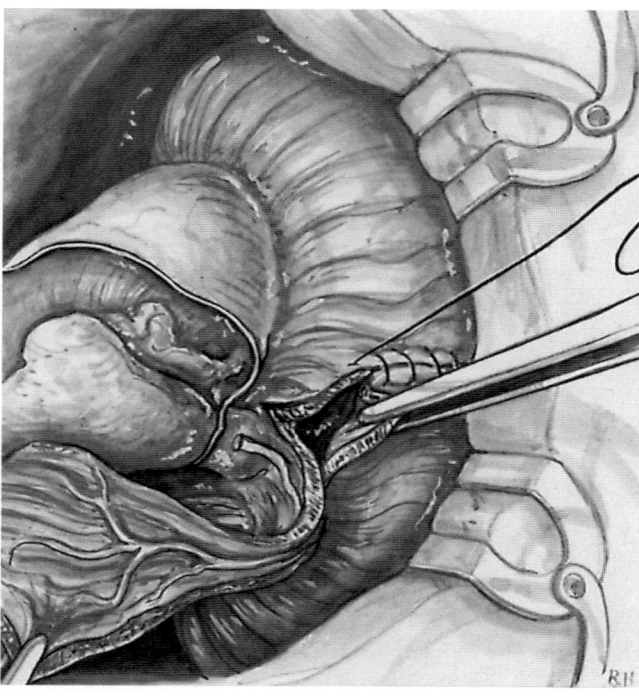

Fig. 29-15. Diaphragmatic closure proceeds as the patch is developed.

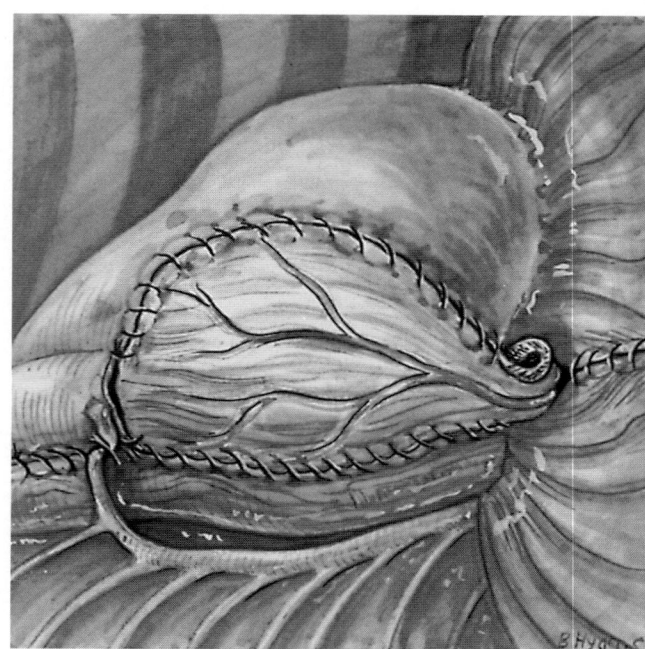

Fig. 29-17. The bronchial stump is buried by suturing the esophagus to the posterior margin of the pericardial defect or the patch.

After left pneumonectomy, small pericardial defects may be closed, but large ones are enlarged down to the diaphragm, preserving the phrenic nerve (Fig. 29-18). If the phrenic nerve has been sacrificed, the diaphragm should be plicated, through a second intercostal incision if necessary.

Other Modifications

Other modifications of pneumonectomy are rare. Pleuropneumonectomy is undertaken for chronic suppuration and involves only the extrapleural mobilization of the chronically inflamed cortex adherent to the lung. This procedure is bloody, but dissection around the hilum proceeds as described. The surgeon may encounter difficulty if adherent and calcified nodes hinder access to the vessels. The supra-aortic pneu-

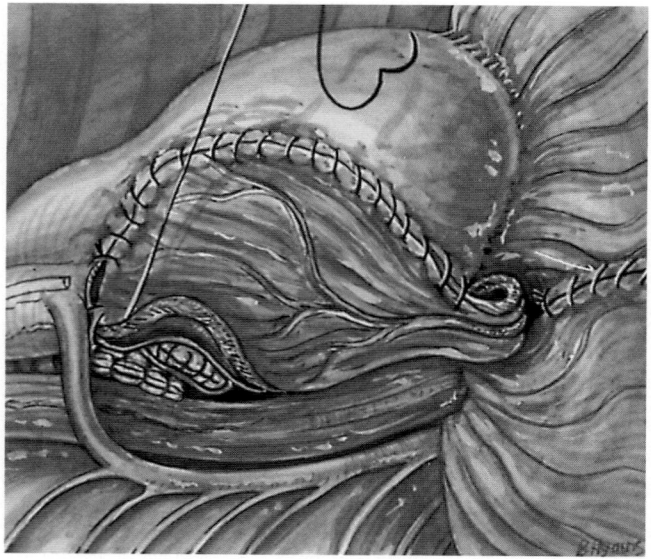

Fig. 29-16. The patch is turned over and sutured to the margins of the pericardial defect with the peritoneal aspect facing outward.

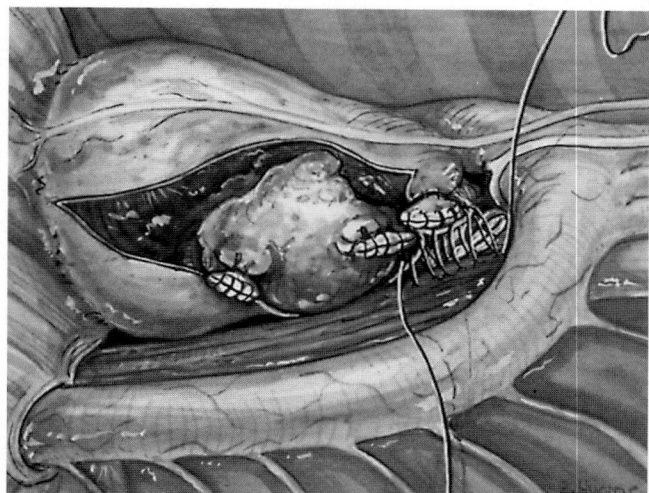

Fig. 29-18. Large pericardial defect is repaired while preserving the phrenic nerve.

monectomy described by Smith and Nigam (1979) has been abandoned by most surgeons. Sleeve pneumonectomy, resecting the carina and lower trachea with the lung, is rarely indicated in lung cancer. It is described in detail in Chapter 30.

REFERENCES

Albertucci M, et al: Surgery and the management of peripheral lung tumors adherent to the parietal pleura. J Thorac Cardiovasc Surg 103:8, 1992.

al–Kattan K, Cattelani L, Goldstraw P: Bronchopleural fistula after pneumonectomy for lung cancer. Eur J Cardiothorac Surg 9:479, 1995.

Baue AE: Evarts A Graham and the first pneumonectomy. JAMA 251:257, 1984.

Burford TH, et al: Results in the treatment of bronchogenic carcinoma: an analysis of 1008 cases. J Thorac Surg 36:316, 1958.

Churchill, ED, et al: Further studies in the surgical management of carcinoma of the lung: a further study of the cases treated at the Massachusetts General Hospital from 1950 to 1957. J Thorac Surg 36:301, 1958.

Churchill ED, et al: The surgical management of carcinoma of the lung. J Thorac Surg 20:349, 1950.

Davies HM: Recent advances in surgery of the lung and pleura. Br J Surg 1:228, 1913.

Edwards AT: The surgical treatment of intrathoracic new growths. Br Med 1:827, 1932.

Fernando HC, Goldstraw P: The accuracy of clinical evaluative intrathoracic staging in lung cancer as assessed by postsurgical pathologic staging. Cancer 65:2503, 1990.

Fry WA: Decision making at the time of exploratory thoracotomy [editorial]. Ann Thorac Surg 38:310, 1984.

Gaer JA, Goldstraw P: Intraoperative assessment of nodal staging at thoracotomy for carcinoma of the bronchus. Eur J Cardiothorac Surg 4:207, 1990.

Gephardt GN, Rice TW: Utility of frozen-section evaluation of lymph nodes in the staging of bronchogenic carcinoma at mediastinoscopy and thoracotomy. J Thorac Cardiovasc Surg 100:853, 1990.

Goldstraw P: Consensus report of the IASLC working party on pretreatment minimal staging. Lung Cancer 7:7, 1991.

Graham EA, Singer JJ: Successful removal of an entire lung for carcinoma of the bronchus. JAMA 101:1371, 1933.

Holmes Sellors T: Results of surgical treatment of carcinoma of the lung. Br Med J 1:445, 1955.

Izbicki JR, et al: Accuracy of computed tomographic scan and surgical assessment for staging of bronchial carcinoma: a prospective study. J Thorac Cardiovasc Surg 104:413, 1992.

Johnson J, Kirby CK, Blakemore WS: Should we insist on "radical pneumonectomy" as a routine procedure in the treatment of carcinoma of the lung? J Thorac Surg 36:309, 1958.

Le Roux BT: Anatomical abnormalities of the right upper bronchus. J Thorac Cardiovasc Surg 44:225, 1962.

Meade RH: The evolution of pulmonary surgery. In Meade RH (ed): A History of Thoracic Surgery. Springfield, IL: Charles C Thomas, 1961, pp. 28–97.

Naruke T, Suemasu K, Ishikawa S: Lymph node mapping and curability at various levels of metastasis in resected lung cancer. J Thorac Cardiovasc Surg 76:832, 1978.

Ochsner A: The development of pulmonary surgery, with special emphasis on carcinoma and bronchiectasis. Am J Surg 135:732, 1978.

Reinhoff WF: The surgical technique of total pneumonectomy. Arch Surg 32:218, 1936.

Rigdon RH, Kirchoff H: Cancer of the lung from 1900 to 1930. Int Abstracts Surg 107:105, 1958.

Smith RA: Development of lung surgery in the United Kingdom. Thorax 37:161, 1982.

Smith RA, Nigam BK: Resection of proximal left main bronchus carcinoma. Thorax 34:616, 1979.

Spiro SG, Goldstraw P: The staging of lung cancer (editorial). Thorax 39:401, 1984.

READING REFERENCES

Berend N, Woodcock AJ, Marlin GE: Effects of lobectomy on lung function. Thorax 35:145, 1980.

Bignall JR, Martin M, Smither DW: Survival in 6086 cases of bronchial carcinoma. Lancet 1:1067, 1967.

Firmin RK, et al: Sleeve lobectomy (lobectomy and bronchoplasty) for bronchial carcinoma. Ann Thorac Surg 35:442, 1983.

Ginsberg RJ, et al: Modern thirty-day operative mortality for surgical resections in lung cancer. J Thorac Cardiovasc Surg 86:654, 1983.

Jensik RJ, Faber LP, Kittle CF: Segmental resection for bronchogenic carcinoma. Ann Thorac Surg 28:475, 1979.

Jensik RJ, et al: Sleeve lobectomy for carcinoma; a ten-year experience. J Thorac Cardiovasc Surg 64:400, 1972.

Kirsh MM, et al: Carcinoma of the lung: results of treatment over ten years. Ann Thorac Surg 21:371, 1976a.

Kirsh MM, et al: Major pulmonary resection for bronchogenic carcinoma in the elderly. Ann Thorac Surg 22:369, 1976b.

Roxburgh JC, Thompson JC, Goldstraw P: Hospital mortality and long-term survival after pulmonary resection in the elderly. Ann Thorac Surg 51:800, 1991.

Van Mieghem W, Demedts M: Cardiopulmonary function after lobectomy or pneumonectomy for pulmonary neoplasm. Respir Med 83:199, 1989.

Wilkins EW, Scannell JG, Craver JG: Four decades of experience with resections for bronchogenic carcinoma at the Massachusetts General Hospital. J Thorac Cardiovasc Surg 76:364, 1978.

Williams DE, et al: Survival of patients surgically treated for stage 1 lung cancer. J Thorac Cardiovasc Surg 82:70, 1981.

CHAPTER 30

Tracheal Sleeve Pneumonectomy

Yoh Watanabe

Tracheal sleeve pneumonectomy is an aggressive procedure for resection of bronchial carcinoma involving the tracheobronchial angle, carina, or lower trachea and lung. The airway is reconstructed by anastomosis of the opposite main stem bronchus to the lower trachea. This procedure is a type of *extended resection*, a term suggested by Chamberlain and associates (1959).

In 1950, Abbott and associates first reported experience with the surgical resection of the carina, tracheal wall, and contralateral bronchial wall in patients undergoing right pneumonectomy. He also detailed the technical difficulties encountered in that procedure. In 1959, Gibbon also described a patient who underwent resection of the distal trachea during right pneumonectomy and anastomosis of the left bronchus to the residual trachea and survived for 6 months. After that, however, only a few reports of tracheal sleeve pneumonectomy were published for some years. Mathey and colleagues (1966) reported two patients with epidermoid carcinoma who had undergone right tracheal sleeve pneumonectomy and survived for 1.5 and 4.5 years, respectively, and Thompson (1966) reported a patient undergoing right tracheal sleeve pneumonectomy.

In 1972, Jensik and associates reported 17 cases of tracheal sleeve pneumonectomy. Since then, the results of tracheal sleeve pneumonectomy in a moderate number of patients have been reported subsequently by Jensik (1982) and Deslauriers (1979, 1985, 1989) and their associates. However, operative mortality in these reports was 27 to 31%, and the 5-year survival rate was only 13 to 23%. On the other hand, Dartevelle and colleagues (1988, 1995, 1996) reported improved survival rates with lower operative mortality.

In addition to these reports, the results of tracheal sleeve pneumonectomy were reported by Perelman and Koroleva (1980) and Grillo (1982b), as well as by Fujimura (1985), Tsuchiya (1990), Watanabe (1990a), Mathisen (1991), Muscolino (1992), Maeda (1993), Roviaro (1994), and Sharpe (1996) and their associates. These series had fewer patients, but reported a lower operative mortality. The results with respect to long-term survival, however, remained unsatisfactory.

Grillo (1982a, 1982b), who has done a large number of carinal resections for tracheal tumor, suggested that, in applying the procedure for bronchial carcinoma with carinal involvement, the patients should be restricted to those who are potentially curable on the basis of preoperative mediastinoscopy (i.e., absence of extranodal metastases, contralateral node metastasis, upper mediastinal, or extensive node metastases) and the exclusion of distant metastases.

SELECTION OF PATIENTS

Tracheal sleeve pneumonectomy may be considered in a patient in whom bronchial carcinoma is centrally located at the hilus of the lung with extension to involve the orifice of the main stem bronchus or the lateral aspect of the lower trachea. The most favorable histologic type is squamous cell carcinoma, and the best results are achieved in patients with this type of lesion.

The initial step in identifying a possible candidate for this procedure is bronchoscopy. Faber (1987) reported that a large central tumor on the right side frequently caused thickening and erythema of the mucosa at the tracheobronchial angle and indicated the possibility that standard pneumonectomy would not be technically possible. Random samples for biopsy must be taken proximally to determine the possible line of dissection in the tracheobronchial tree. According to Deslauriers and colleagues (1989, 1996), tissue should be taken from any doubtful area and also in the trachea at 3 cm above the carina. Local invasion up to that level indicated that a tension-free and tumor-free reconstruction was unlikely. Dartevelle and colleagues (1988, 1996) concluded that invasion of the trachea beyond the lower 2 cm and contralateral main bronchus beyond 1.5 cm would produce excess anastomotic tension, so that the safe limit is 4 cm between the lower trachea and the contralateral main bronchus. Roviaro and associates (1994) have shown that the operation should not be done if the tumor extends higher than three cartilage rings on the distal tracheal wall.

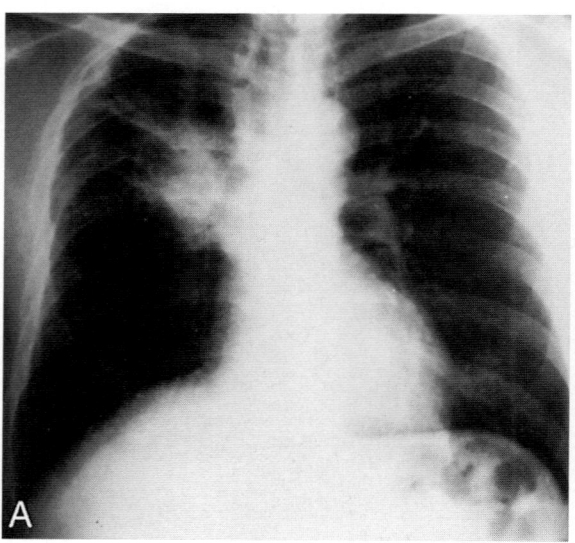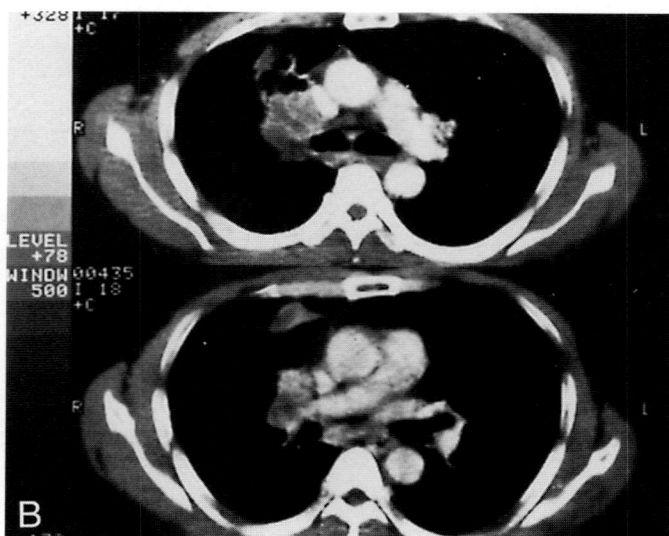

Fig. 30-1. A. Preoperative chest radiograph. **B.** Computed tomography scan of a 49-year-old man who underwent right tracheal sleeve pneumonectomy.

Tomography, computed tomography, and magnetic resonance imaging are also helpful in defining the extra-bronchial extent of the lesions (Fig. 30-1). With the aid of these examinations, precise delineation of the pulmonary artery, superior vena cava, and main bronchial involvement can be obtained along with detection of enlarged mediastinal lymph nodes. Local invasion of the superior vena cava is not a contraindication to sleeve pneumonectomy if tangential excision is possible. In the series of the author (1990a), Tsuchiya (1990), and Dartevelle (1988, 1996) and their colleagues, some patients underwent concomitant resection of the superior vena cava. Correlation of the bronchoscopic and computed tomographic findings is important in determining the appropriate type of resection.

Deslauriers (1985) and colleagues (1979, 1989, 1995) recommended mediastinoscopy as part of the preoperative staging, because neoplastic involvement of the superior mediastinal nodes (N_2 disease) generally represents an absolute contraindication to tracheal sleeve pneumonectomy. Faber (1987) also recommended mediastinoscopy when the mediastinal lymph nodes were greater than 1 cm in diameter. Both these authors believe that contraindications to resection were positive superior mediastinal nodes and positive contralateral tracheal nodes. Dartevelle and coworkers (1988, 1995, 1996) also recommended mediastinoscopy for histologic verification, if the mediastinal lymph nodes were greater than 1.5 cm in diameter. They concluded that subcarinal lymph node involvement should not be regarded as a contraindication because such tumors were resectable en bloc with the carina, and long-term results were encouraging. But N_3 disease and ipsilateral paratracheal lymph node involvement was a surgical contraindication, because there were no 2-year survivors.

Carinal resection in patients with tumor recurrence in the bronchial stump after prior pneumonectomy is another possible surgical indication for tracheal sleeve resection. In these patients, either the right or left main stem bronchus is anastomosed to the trachea after resection of the carina. We have performed such an operation in only one patient, but the carinal resection series reported by Grillo (1982a), Jensik (1972, 1982), Mathisen (1991), Faber (1987), Deslauriers (1979, 1985, 1989, 1996), and Dartevelle (1996) and their colleagues include a few cases of carinal resection after previous pneumonectomy.

PREOPERATIVE ADJUVANT THERAPY IN PATIENTS WITH BRONCHIAL CARCINOMA

As preoperative adjuvant therapy, radiation therapy, bronchial arterial infusion therapy, and induction therapy are applicable. Jensik and colleagues (1972, 1982) recommended preoperative radiation therapy for sterilization of the mediastinal lymph nodes and the primary lesion. Twenty-five of the 30 patients in their group received radiation therapy administered from either a cobalt or linear accelerator source. The dose varied from 3200 to 5000 rads, but most individuals received 4000 rads administered over a 4-week period. They experienced eight perioperative deaths, most of them related to the development of bronchial fistulas. It was difficult, they claimed, to incriminate preoperative irradiation as a causative factor for fistula. They also stated that the benefits resulting from reduction in tumor volume and the improvement of the lesion on bronchoscopic examination justify its use. Roviaro and associates (1994) recommended low-dosage preoperative radiation therapy to reduce tumor size to facilitate the anastomotic procedure.

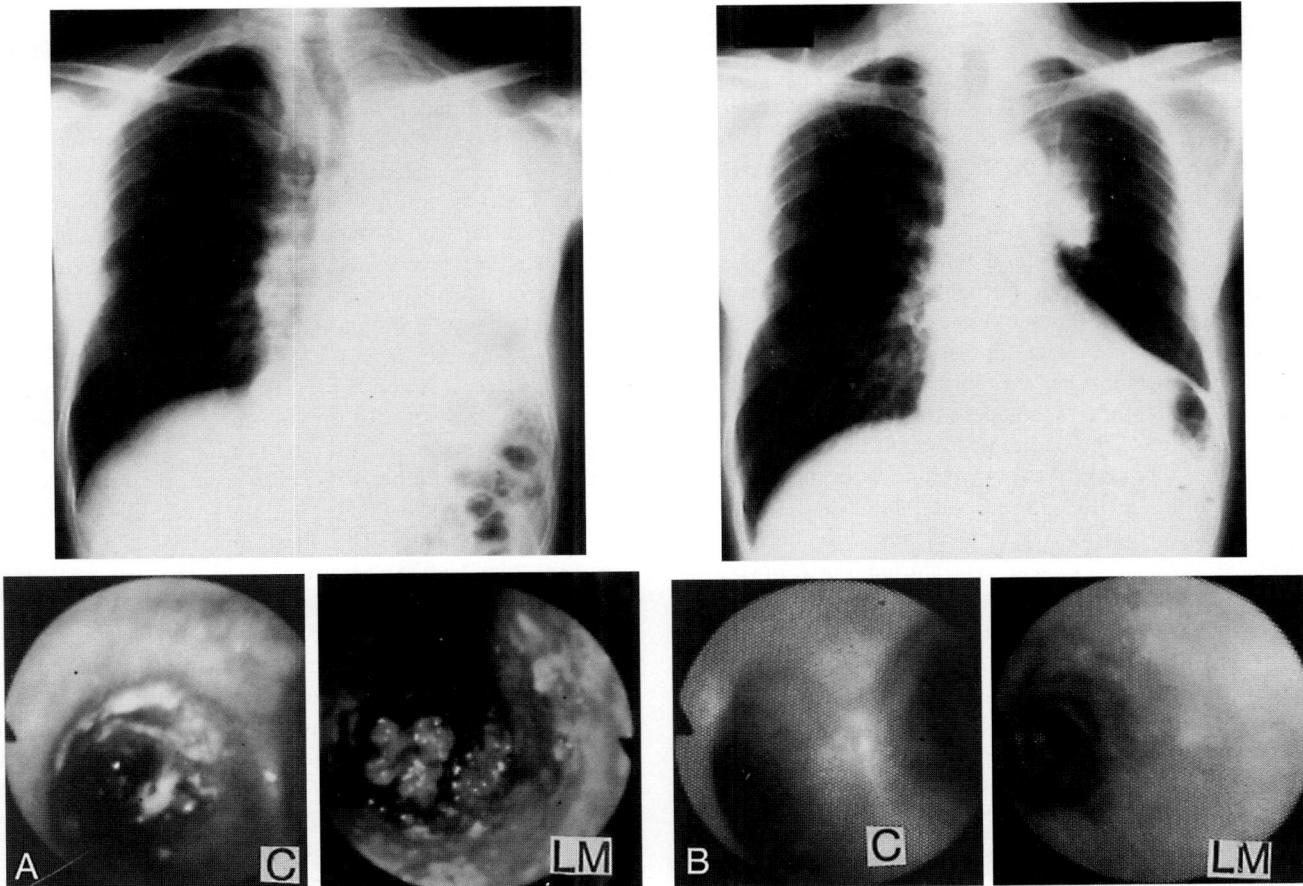

Fig. 30-2. Effect of bronchial arterial infusion (BAI) as preoperative adjuvant therapy. **A.** Chest radiograph and bronchoscopic findings in a 66-year-old man with epidermoid carcinoma of the left hilum that caused complete atelectasis of the left lung. **B.** Chest radiograph and bronchoscopic view taken 11 days after the second course of BAI therapy. The patient underwent left tracheal sleeve pneumonectomy 20 days after the second course of BAI therapy. C, carina; LM, left main bronchus.

On the other hand, Dartevelle (1988), Deslauriers (1979), and their associates emphasized that preoperative irradiation increases the risk of bronchopleural fistula.

In our series (1990b) of 18 patients, no one underwent preoperative irradiation, although five patients underwent bronchial arterial infusion therapy as a preoperative adjuvant treatment. These patients received mitomycin C (8 mg), Esquinone (carbazilquinone, 6 mg), and ACNU (nimustine, 50 mg). Figure 30-2 shows the disappearance of atelectasis related to tumor shrinkage after two courses of bronchial arterial infusion therapy. The patient subsequently underwent left tracheal sleeve pneumonectomy.

The effects of induction therapy for advanced lung cancer are still under evaluation. To date, Dartevelle (1995, 1996), Macchiarini (1994), and Roviaro (1994) and their associates have applied induction therapy in patients who were candidates for sleeve pneumonectomy. As Dartevelle's group experienced a few cases of operative deaths in patients receiving induction therapy, they concluded that the potential benefits of induction therapy should be regarded cau-

tiously because it lowers the surgical security of an already technically demanding procedure.

SURGICAL APPROACH

For right tracheal sleeve pneumonectomy, I have always used a right posterolateral thoracotomy and believe it is the best approach. Muscolino and associates (1992), however, performed right tracheal sleeve pneumonectomy by an anterior thoracotomy through the fourth intercostal space in seven patients without any surgical mortality. They concluded that anterior thoracotomy might improve the surgical management of these patients. Pearson and colleagues (1984) preferred to use median sternotomy in patients requiring carinal resection. They point out that this technique has several advantages over a right posterolateral thoracotomy in selected cases, because any type of pulmonary resection is possible through a median sternotomy. In addition, this incision also provides adequate exposure for an intrapericardial mobilization of the right pulmonary hilum, which also may be necessary to minimize tension on a tracheobronchial anastomosis.

With regard to left tracheal sleeve pneumonectomy, controversy exists regarding the best surgical approach, and it is also controversial whether this should be a one-stage or two-stage operation.

In the one-stage operation for left tracheal sleeve pneumonectomy, left posterolateral thoracotomy, median sternotomy (with or without left anterior thoracotomy), or bilateral anterolateral thoracotomy (clamshell incision) can be used. Abbott and colleagues (1950), Grillo (1982a), and Salzer and coworkers (1987) reported a one-stage operation using a left posterolateral thoracotomy, but by this approach, proper exposure of the carina underneath the aortic arch is difficult, and this lack of exposure hinders performance of the anastomosis. Grillo (1982a) and Mathisen (1996) recommend that, with flexion of the neck and with tapes placed around the lower trachea and the right main bronchus, it is possible to draw the airway up beneath the aortic arch and place appropriate traction sutures, excise the carina, and anastomose the trachea to the right main bronchus. Maeda and associates (1993) used left thoracotomy and compared two methods—that is, drawing-down approach and drawing-up approach—which was reported by Bjork (1955). They concluded that the drawing-down route was preferable to obtain a larger operative field without dividing branches of intercostal arteries.

Deslauriers (1989, 1995) and Gilbert (1984) and their associates recommend a two-stage procedure. In the first stage, left proximal pneumonectomy is carried out, and the carina is resected from the right side 3 to 5 weeks later. They emphasize caution, however, in using this operative method. Because of the local inflammatory reaction and mediastinal shift that follow pneumonectomy, mobilization of the left main stem bronchus stump is potentially dangerous and one must be aware of the proximity of the left pulmonary artery stump and left recurrent laryngeal nerve.

I have done one-stage operations by median sternotomy combined with a left anterolateral thoracotomy in one patient undergoing left tracheal sleeve pneumonectomy and one undergoing a carinal resection after prior left pneumonectomy. This approach provides excellent exposure and access for lung resection as well as reconstruction procedures, which ultimately facilitates performance of the operation. Thus, I suggest and strongly recommend the median sternotomy approach combined with a left anterolateral thoracotomy for the performance of left tracheal sleeve pneumonectomy.

MAINTENANCE OF VENTILATION

Maintenance of adequate ventilation and oxygenation is of crucial importance in tracheobronchial surgery. In general, provision of ventilation is incompatible with an unobstructed operative field; a bulky endotracheal tube permits adequate ventilation but impedes access to the operative field for anastomosis.

A tube ventilation system coming from above or across the operative field is the most conventional method. Abbott and coworkers (1950) described the use of a long tube directed into the left main stem bronchus to maintain ventilation with left endobronchial anesthesia during the operative procedure. Jensik and associates (1972, 1985) used this method in the majority of their patients, although it was modified in some instances with a supplementary sterile tube and connector, which is placed into the left main stem bronchus after it is divided. The other end of the connecting tube is directed outward through the incision and over the anesthetic screen. After the first portion of the anastomosis is completed, the tube is withdrawn and the original endobronchial tube is directed beyond the suture line into the left main stem bronchus. The anastomosis is then completed over the tube. Geffin and associates (1969) showed that this method can be adapted to all types of carinal reconstructions. This system has the disadvantage, however, of requiring repeated tube manipulations with frequent interruption of airway suturing. If the tube runs across the operative field—for example, an armored tube into the left main stem bronchus—it further restricts surgical access to the carina. Roviaro and coworkers (1994) recommend a long (45 cm) thin caliber (5.0 to 6.5 mm) tube with self-inflating polyurethane cuff, which greatly facilitates all maneuvers.

Frumin (1959) and Heller (1964) and their colleagues described the technique of prolonged apneic oxygenation for carinal reconstruction. After hyperventilating the patient with 100% oxygen, 10 to 12 minutes of total apnea can often be tolerated. Deslauriers and associates (1979) used this technique in a few cases of tracheal sleeve pneumonectomy, but they commonly noted arrhythmias, acidosis, and hypercapnia for 15 minutes after the initiation of the prolonged apneic oxygenation. Thus, this technique is used rarely because the duration of safe apnea and the cardiovascular response are unpredictable in any individual patient.

McClish and colleagues (1985) described the value of the high-flow catheter technique after using it in 18 patients undergoing tracheobronchial reconstruction. This method has specific advantages with regard to the simplicity of the equipment and anesthetic technique. It involves positive pressure ventilation with a high flow of gas and without air entrainment. Oxygen is applied from a high-pressure source capable of delivering it at a pressure of 50 psi and a flow of 100 L/min. Depending on the airway resistance and lung compliance, the inflation flow can be adjusted through a reducing valve to generate an airway pressure of 25 to 40 cm H_2O. Deslauriers and associates (1985, 1989) now use this method preferentially.

High-frequency jet ventilation (HFJV) also can be used to provide good ventilation and oxygenation. Our group (Watanabe et al. 1988) uses this ventilatory method in all our patients undergoing tracheobronchial reconstructive surgery

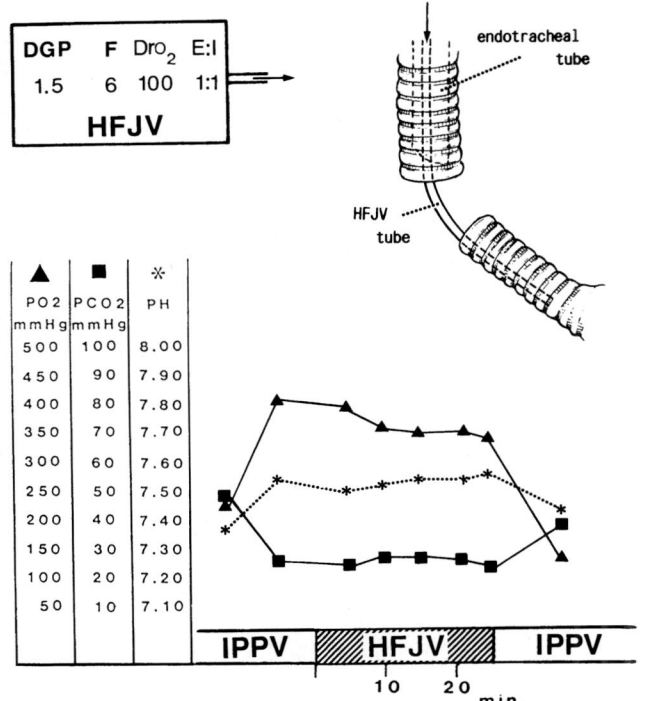

Fig. 30-3. The ventilatory method and blood gas analyses in a patient (75-year-old man) who underwent right tracheal sleeve pneumonectomy. DGP, driving gas pressure; DrO₂, O₂ content of driving gas; E:I, expiratory to inspiratory ratio; F, frequency; HFJV, high-frequency jet ventilation; IPPV, intermittent positive-pressure ventilation.

(Fig. 30-3). El-Baz and colleagues (1981) first reported the use of HFJV in six patients undergoing tracheobronchoplastic surgery. I and my colleagues (Watanabe et al. 1988) analyzed arterial blood gas values during HFJV in 21 patients receiving major airway reconstructive surgery, including nine who underwent tracheal sleeve pneumonectomy. I emphasize the advantages of HFJV over classic intermittent positive-pressure ventilation using an endotracheal tube. In tracheal sleeve pneumonectomy, a relatively high driving gas pressure (1.5 to 2.5 kg/cm²) at 360 to 480 cycles per minute provides optimal ventilation and oxygenation. This method permits greater accuracy in placing and tying sutures and eliminates the need for intermittent withdrawal and reinsertion of the endotracheal tube into the contralateral main bronchus. Use of HFJV delivered through a small-bore catheter can facilitate performance of the anastomosis and thus directly contribute to the elimination of complications along the suture line and ultimately to improving the surgical outcome. In the series of Muscolino and coworkers (1992), HFJV was used. Dartevelle and colleagues (1988, 1995, 1996) once used Grillo's ventilation method, but they have switched to HFJV since 1982 because it improves surgical exposure, avoids endotracheal manipulations, and provides satisfactory gas exchanges.

Perelman and Koroleva (1980) reported the use of hyperbaric oxygenation. They performed the first four operations

on the trachea that were ever done in a hyperbaric chamber. Compression was begun 10 to 15 minutes before entering the tracheobronchial tree. The air pressure in the operating room was raised to 2.5 to 3.0 atm, and it was possible to discontinue lung ventilation intermittently for 8 to 10 minutes.

OPERATIVE PROCEDURE

Right Tracheal Sleeve Pneumonectomy

The patient is placed in the left lateral position, and a right posterolateral thoracotomy is the approach. The thoracic cavity is entered through the fifth intercostal space. At thoracotomy, the posterior mediastinal pleura is longitudinally incised along the trachea, the right main stem bronchus, and the esophagus from the apex to the base of the right hemithorax to expose the tracheobronchial tree. It is mandatory to ligate the azygos vein and to mobilize the trachea; the pericardium may be opened at this time. After careful observation from outside the tracheobronchial tree to detect tumor extension, the feasibility of tracheal sleeve pneumonectomy is finally determined in combination with the findings obtained by preoperative endoscopic examination. Once the decision to perform a tracheal sleeve pneumonectomy is made, the pericardium is opened along the phrenic nerve to expose the right main pulmonary artery and veins. These vessels are interrupted intrapericardially. The carina is then fully mobilized from its mediastinal bed, and tapes are passed around the lower trachea and the left and right main stem bronchi.

Both trachea and left main stem bronchus are transected at the intercartilaginous ligament (Fig. 30-4A). The trachea is transected 1 cm proximal to the tumor, usually at the first or second distal tracheal ring, but sometimes transection must extend as high as 3 cm above the carina. The left main stem bronchus is divided also at a level free of tumor, but it is seldom necessary to make the division more than one ring below the carina. Frozen sections are examined to confirm that the site of transection is free of tumor.

Before starting the reconstruction procedure, mobilization of the trachea and left main stem bronchus is accomplished to lessen the tension at the anastomosis. The left main stem bronchus is relatively fixed by the aortic arch. Gentle blunt dissection of this bronchus from the aortic arch and surrounding tissue is done, excluding the posterior, membranous portion. This maneuver is continued down to the left upper lobe bronchus. The trachea is pulled down in the same way, and maximal flexion of the neck fully reduces the tension at the anastomosis.

The suture material used in all patients is absorbable 3-0 Vicryl. The anastomosis is commenced at the farthest point from the operator (Fig. 30-4B). Cartilage-to-cartilage apposition of the left lateral wall of the trachea to the lateral wall of the left main stem bronchus with the placement and tying of two sutures forms the basis of the anastomosis, and more sutures are then added to the cartilaginous part of the

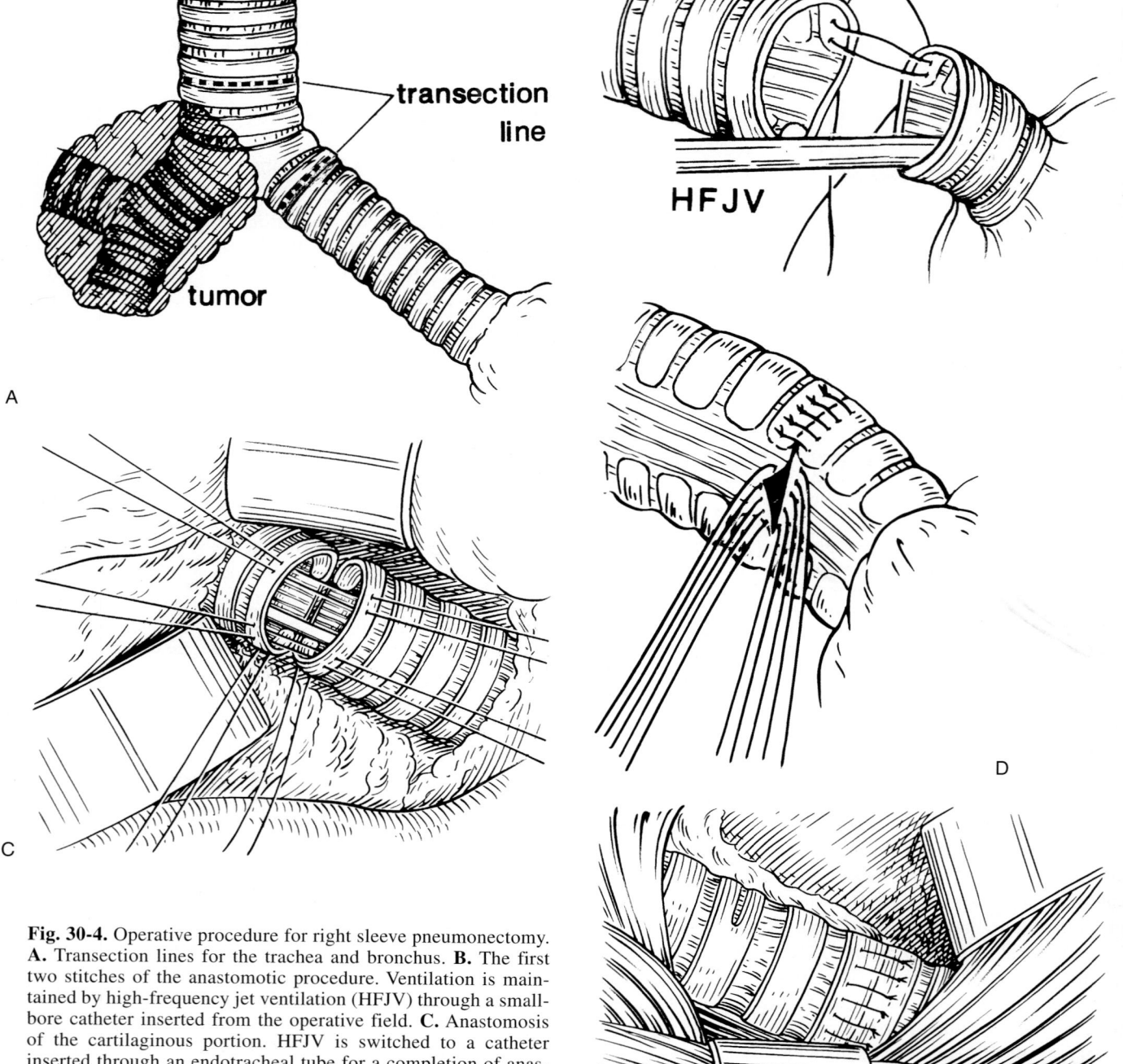

Fig. 30-4. Operative procedure for right sleeve pneumonectomy. **A.** Transection lines for the trachea and bronchus. **B.** The first two stitches of the anastomotic procedure. Ventilation is maintained by high-frequency jet ventilation (HFJV) through a smallbore catheter inserted from the operative field. **C.** Anastomosis of the cartilaginous portion. HFJV is switched to a catheter inserted through an endotracheal tube for a completion of anastomosis at the anterior part of the cartilaginous and membranous portion. **D.** Equalization of luminal disparity by crimping the membranous part. **E.** Completion of the anastomosis. The suture line is covered circumferentially by pedicled parietal pleural flap.

bronchus. Sutures are placed through the full thickness of the trachea and bronchus, making certain that the knots are tied outside of the lumen (Fig. 30-4C). The membranous part of the bronchus is anastomosed as the last part of the procedure. Luminal disparity is equalized by expanding the

membranous portion of the smaller bronchus and crimping that of the larger trachea (Fig. 30-4D). Once the anastomotic procedures are completed, the suture line should be checked for air leaks and the endotracheal tube should be located at sufficient distance above the suture line.

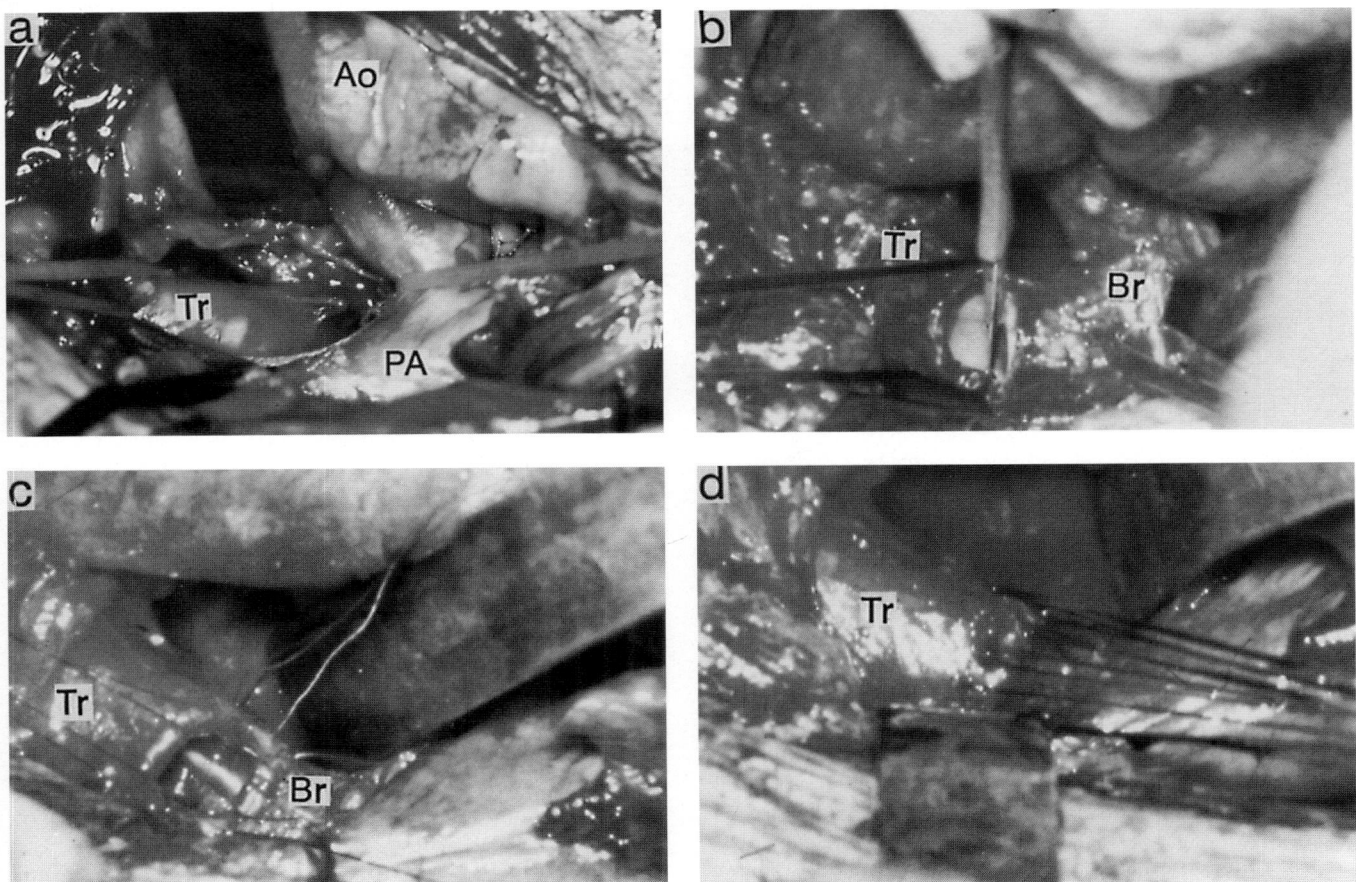

Fig. 30-5. Intraoperative view of left tracheal sleeve pneumonectomy through median stenotomy. **a.** Exposure of the trachea (Tr) and bronchus (Br) via pericardium. **b.** Transection of the distal trachea. **c.** Anastomotic procedure of the cartilaginous part. **d.** Completion of the anastomosis. Ao, aorta; PA, pulmonary artery.

The anastomotic site is covered routinely by a circumferential pleural flap to prevent suture leaks or dehiscence (Fig. 30-4E). In a tracheal sleeve pneumonectomy for bronchial carcinoma, lymph node dissection of the hilar and mediastinal nodes is also performed as in routine lobectomy or pneumonectomy for malignant lung tumors.

Left Tracheal Sleeve Pneumonectomy

Left tracheal sleeve pneumonectomy is a relatively rare procedure in every series reported. As mentioned previously, controversy still exists regarding the best surgical approach and whether a one- or two-stage operation should be performed. Our group uses a one-stage operation involving median sternotomy combined with left anterolateral thoracotomy. The operation starts with median sternotomy. Exposure of the carina and main bronchus requires a transpericardial approach. The anterior pericardium is opened vertically from the level of the innominate vein to the bottom of the pericardium to permit circumferential mobilization of the ascending aortic arch, which is then retracted leftward. The posterior

pericardium is incised vertically. The superior vena cava is displaced laterally and to the right. The right main pulmonary artery is exposed and displaced inferiorly. By these maneuvers, the entire mediastinal trachea and carina are clearly exposed (Fig. 30-5). Then, anterolateral thoracotomy at the fourth intercostal space is added to allow lung resection. By this approach, transection of the trachea and left main stem bronchus for pneumonectomy and anastomosis of the trachea and right main stem bronchus can be done easily in the same fashion as already described for right tracheal sleeve pneumonectomy. Division of the trachea at a point 1.5 cm above its bifurcation is sufficient for most tumors, but it is also possible to resect an additional length of distal trachea and elevate the right main stem bronchus for primary anastomosis, if necessary.

PERIOPERATIVE AND POSTOPERATIVE MANAGEMENT

As soon as the anastomosis is completed, intraoperative bronchoscopy is performed through an adapter while venti-

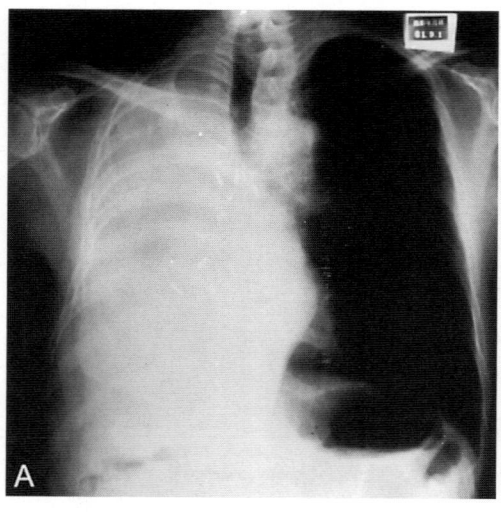
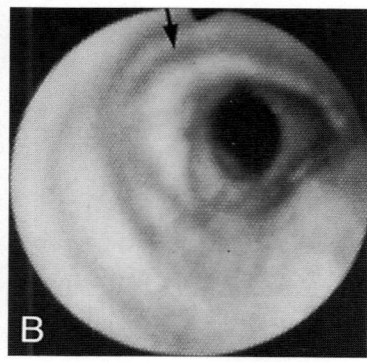

Fig. 30-6. A. Chest radiograph taken 19 months after right tracheal sleeve pneumonectomy in a 54-year-old man shows the normal caliber of the airway at the anastomotic site. **B.** Bronchoscopic view of the anastomotic site 2 years after left sleeve pneumonectomy in a 66-year-old man shows a clear anastomotic line (*arrow*).

lation is maintained. The anastomotic site is observed and blood clots or mucus is aspirated from the distal bronchus. Most patients are extubated within 4 to 5 hours after the operation. In my experience, almost all patients suffer from transient bronchorrhea, which is probably related to denervation, the interruption of lymphatics, and damage to the ciliary epithelium. It is recommended that patients are placed in the lateral decubitus position, resected side down, for postural drainage of bronchial secretions. Pernasal bronchoscopy is performed at the bedside on the first postoperative day to remove any secretions at the anastomosis and for infusion of antibiotics into the reconstructed lung. This procedure is repeated for several days, if necessary. Neck flexion is recommended for 7 days after the operation. During that time, oral intake is totally avoided and nutrition is maintained by intravenous hyperalimentation. Figure 30-6 shows a chest radiograph and bronchoscopic findings after tracheal sleeve pneumonectomy.

MORTALITY AND PROGNOSIS

In Table 30-1, the number of patients undergoing tracheal sleeve pneumonectomy, surgical mortality, long-term survivors, and 5-year survival rates are shown. Various reports have been done on tracheal sleeve pneumonectomy. However, most of them were results of a small number of patients with short-term follow-up. Three major reports have a moderate number of patients for evaluation of operative mortality and long-term survival rate in tracheal sleeve pneumonectomy. In 1982, Jensik and associates reported survival in 34 patients (30 right and four stump recurrences after prior pneumonectomy) undergoing tracheal sleeve pneumonectomy. The perioperative mortality was 29%, and the 5-year survival rate of the entire group was 15%. In 1991, Faber reported final results of 40 patients in their group (36 tracheal sleeve pneumonec-

tomies and four stump recurrences). Their overall operative mortality was 28%, and the 5-year survival rate was 20%, showing that the operative mortality was higher than the survival rate. Deslauriers and associates (1989) reported their results in 38 patients (33 right, three left, and two stump recurrences). The operative mortality was 29% and the 5-year survival rate was 13%.

On the other hand, Dartevelle and colleagues (1988, 1995, 1996) reported more favorable outcomes. In 1988, they reported 55 tracheal sleeve pneumonectomies (53 right and two left). The overall operative mortality was 11% and actuarial 5-year survival rate, excluding six operative deaths, was 23%. In the report published in 1995, their operative mortality was reduced to 7% and the 5-year survival rate including postoperative deaths was increased to 40%. In their report of 60 patients in 1996 (56 right and four left), the operative mortality was 3%, and the 5-year survival rate was 43.3%, showing encouraging results of tracheal sleeve pneumonectomy. Roviaro and associates (1994) reported 28 cases of tracheal sleeve pneumonectomy. Their operative mortality was 4%, and seven patients survived longer than 4 years, which projects to a 20% 5-year survival rate.

As shown in Table 30-1, it is true that only a few patients can survive for long among the group in which a curative operation is accomplished. Some controversy exists as to whether tracheal sleeve pneumonectomy is an appropriate procedure for bronchial carcinoma, because the mortality is similar to the long-term survival rate. According to Mathisen and Grillo (1991), carinal resection of bronchial carcinoma has a justifiable role, if one can achieve operative mortality under 10% and 5-year survival rates of 20 to 25%. Faber (1987), whose mortality and 5-year survival rate were 27% and 16%, respectively, reported that they had not performed tracheal sleeve pneumonectomy in the past 3 years, probably because they have undertaken a more aggressive preoperative treatment program consisting of combination chemotherapy and radiation therapy.

Table 30-1. Results of Tracheal Sleeve Pneumonectomy

Authors	No. of Patients	Operative Mortality (%)	Long-Term Survivors	5-Year Survival Rate (%)
Mathey et al (1966)	2	0	1 (>4 yrs)	—
Jensik et al (1972)	17	12	2 (>2 yrs)	—
Jensik et al (1982)	34	29	2 (>5 yrs)	15
Faber (1987)	37	27	6 (>5 yrs)	16
Faber (1991)	40	28	8 (>5 yrs)	20
Deslauriers et al (1979)	16	31	1 (>7 yrs)	—
Deslauriers et al (1985)	27	27	3 (>5 yrs)	23
Deslauriers et al (1989)	38	29	4 (>5 yrs)	13
Dartevelle et al (1988)	55	11	7 (>5 yrs)	23[a]
Dartevelle et al (1995)	55	7	9 (>5 yrs)	40
Dartevelle et al (1996)	60	3	12 (>2 yrs)	43
Fujimura et al (1985)	6	0	1 (>2 yrs)	—
Watanabe et al (1990)	12	17	1 (>4 yrs)	—
Tsuchiya et al (1990)	15	20	1 (>2 yrs)	—
Matheisen and Grillo (1991)	17	8[b]	—	—
Muscolino et al (1992)	7	0	2 (>4 yrs)	—
Roviaro et al (1994)	28	4	7 (>4 yrs)	20
Sharpe and Moghissi (1996)	17	0	—	—

[a]Excluding six operative deaths.
[b]Including other procedures of carinal resection.

On the contrary, the results of Dartevelle and associates (1995, 1996) are encouraging and advocate performing tracheal sleeve pneumonectomy. From the results of their series, they concluded that tracheal sleeve pneumonectomy provides a fair survival rate in selected patients. The prognosis depends mainly on lymph node involvement; the tumors most commonly amenable are squamous cell carcinoma with N_0 or N_1 disease; spread to superior mediastinal nodes is a contraindication to operation.

REFERENCES

Abbott OA, et al: Experiences with the surgical resection of the human carina, tracheal wall and contralateral bronchial wall in cases of the right total pneumonectomy. J Thorac Surg 19:906, 1950.

Bjork VO: Left-sided bronchotracheal anastomosis. J Thorac Surg 30:492, 1955.

Chamberlain JM, et al: Bronchogenic carcinoma. An aggressive surgical attitude. J Thorac Cardiovasc Surg 38:727, 1959.

Dartevelle PG, et al: Tracheal sleeve pneumonectomy for bronchogenic carcinoma: report of 55 cases. Ann Thorac Surg 46:68, 1988.

Dartevelle PG, et al: Update in 1995. Ann Thorac Surg 60:1854, 1995.

Dartevelle P, Macchiarini P: Carinal resection for bronchogenic carcinoma. Semin Thorac Cardiovasc Surg 8:414, 1996.

Deslauriers J, et al: Sleeve pneumonectomy for bronchogenic carcinoma. Ann Thorac Surg 28:465, 1979.

Deslauriers J: Involvement of the main carina. In Delarue NC, Eschapasse H (eds): International Trends in General Thoracic Surgery. Vol. 1. Philadelphia: WB Saunders, 1985, p. 139.

Deslauriers J, Beaulieu M, McClish A: Tracheal-sleeve pneumonectomy. In Shields TW (ed): General Thoracic Surgery. 3rd Ed. Philadelphia: Lea & Febiger, 1989, pp. 382.

Deslauriers J, Jacques J: Sleeve pneumonectomy. Chest Surg Clin North Am 5:297, 1995.

El-Baz NM, et al: One-lung high frequency positive-pressure ventilation for sleeve pneumonectomy. An alternative technique. Anesth Analg 60:683, 1981.

Faber LP, et al: Results of surgical treatment of stage III lung carcinoma with carinal proximity. Surg Clin North Am 67:1001, 1987.

Faber LP: Discussion of Mathisen and Grillo: carinal resection for bronchogenic carcinoma. J Thorac Cardiovasc Surg 102:16, 1991.

Frumin JM, Epstein RM, Cohen C: Apneic oxygenation in man. Anesthesiology 20:789, 1959.

Fujimura S, et al: Prognostic evaluation of tracheobronchial reconstruction for bronchogenic carcinoma. J Thorac Cardiovasc Surg 90:161, 1985.

Geffin B, et al: Anesthetic management of tracheal resection and reconstruction. Anesth Analg 48:884, 1969.

Gibbon JH, in discussion to Chamberlain M, et al: Bronchogenic carcinoma. An aggressive surgical attitude. J Thorac Cardiovasc Surg 38:727, 1959.

Gilbert A, et al: Tracheal sleeve pneumonectomy for carcinoma of the proximal left main bronchus. Can J Surg 27:583, 1984.

Grillo HC: Carinal reconstruction. Ann Thorac Surg 34:356, 1982a.

Grillo HC: Carcinoma of the lung. What can be done if the carina is involved? Am J Surg 143:694, 1982b.

Heller ML, Watson TR, Imredy DS: Apneic oxygenation in man. Polarographic arterial oxygen tension study. Anesthesiology 25:25, 1964.

Jensik RJ, et al: Tracheal sleeve pneumonectomy for advanced carcinoma of the lung. Surg Gynecol Obstet 134:231, 1972.

Jensik RJ, et al: Survival in patients undergoing tracheal sleeve pneumonectomy for bronchogenic carcinoma. J Thorac Cardiovasc Surg 84:489, 1982.

Macchiarini P, et al: Extended operations after induction therapy for stage IIIb (T4) non-small cell lung cancer. Ann Thorac Surg 57:966, 1994.

Maeda M, et al: Operative approach for left-sided carinoplasty. Ann Thorac Surg 56:441, 1993.

Mathey J, et al: Tracheal and tracheobronchial resections. Technique and results in 20 cases. J Thorac Cardiovasc Surg 51:1, 1966.

Mathisen DJ: Carinal reconstruction: techniques and problems. Semin Thorac Cardiovasc Surg 8:403, 1996.

Mathisen DJ, Grillo HC: Carinal resection for bronchogenic carcinoma. J Thorac Cardiovasc Surg 102:16, 1991.

McClish A, et al: High-flow catheter ventilation during major tracheobronchial reconstruction. J Thorac Cardiovasc Surg 89:508, 1985.

Muscolino G, et al: Anterior thoracotomy for right pneumonectomy and carinal reconstruction in lung cancer. Eur J Cardiothorac Surg 6:11, 1992.

Pearson FG, Todd LC, Cooper JD: Experience with primary neoplasms of the trachea and carina. J Thorac Cardiovasc Surg 88:511, 1984.

Perelman M, Koroleva N: Surgery of the trachea. World J Surg 4:583, 1980.

Roviaro GC, et al: Tracheal sleeve pneumonectomy for bronchogenic carcinoma. J Thorac Cardiovasc Surg 107:13, 1994.

Salzer GM, Muller LC, Kroesen G: Resection of the tracheal bifurcation through a left thoracotomy. Eur J Cardiothorac Surg *1*:125, 1987.

Sharpe DAC, Moghissi K: Tracheal resection and reconstruction: a review of 82 patients. Eur J Cardiothorac Surg *10*:1040, 1996.

Thompson DT: Tracheal resection with left lung anastomosis following right pneumonectomy. Thorax *21*:560, 1966.

Tsuchiya R, et al: Resection of tracheal carina for lung cancer. J Thorac Cardiovasc Surg *99*:779, 1990.

Watanabe Y, et al: The clinical value of high-frequency jet ventilation in major airway reconstructive surgery. Scand J Thorac Cardiovasc Surg *22*:227, 1988.

Watanabe Y, et al: Results in 104 patients undergoing bronchoplastic procedures for bronchial lesions. Ann Thorac Surg *50*:607, 1990a.

Watanabe Y, et al: Reappraisal of bronchial arterial infusion therapy for advanced lung cancer. Jpn J Surg *20*:27, 1990b.

CHAPTER 31

Segmentectomy and Lesser Pulmonary Resections

Joseph LoCicero III

Parenchyma-sparing pulmonary resections are important procedures for many patients. Although lobectomy and pneumonectomy remain standard operations for patients with primary lung cancer who can tolerate it, many authors advocate less than lobectomy as an alternative operation, particularly in patients with limited pulmonary reserve. In cases in which resection of pulmonary metastases may provide prolonged survival, a lesser parenchymal resection is an ideal procedure. These techniques are also applied for diagnosis of the indeterminate pulmonary nodule.

SEGMENTECTOMY

This form of resection, popularized in the mid-twentieth century, is an anatomic operation because it removes the segmental bronchus back to its primary branch, along with all the lung parenchyma and lymph node groupings drained by the bronchus and its associated segmental pulmonary artery. This technique was used in the treatment of pulmonary tuberculosis, bronchiectasis, and other suppurative pulmonary lesions. After development of effective antituberculous chemotherapy and broad-spectrum antibiotics for suppurative diseases, the operation became less common. Many authors since the 1970s, such as Jensik and associates (1973, 1979, 1987), Shields and Higgins (1974), and Crabbe and colleagues (1989, 1991), suggested its use in early lung cancer. Segmentectomy is an anatomic operation that obeys the principles of cancer surgery by removing the associated lymph nodes. Studies by Read and coworkers (1990) and Warren and Faber (1994) show that excellent results can be achieved in patients with early (T_1N_0) cancers. For those patients with poor pulmonary function, Kodama (1997) and Cerfolio (1996) and their associates note that segmentectomy can lead to long-term survival. Only one randomized trial on this subject exists and comes from the Lung Cancer Study Group and was reported by Ginsberg and Rubenstein (1995). However, the report combines both segmentectomy and wedge resection. Together they have a worse outcome when compared with lobectomy. Thus, controversy over the use of segmentectomy for primary lung cancer remains.

With the resurgence of *Mycobacterium tuberculosis* in urban areas and the development of drug-resistant atypical strains, this technique remains vitally important to the eradication of suppurative disease while maximally preserving a normally functioning lung. Agasthian (1996) and Ashour (1996) and their associates reported control of bronchiectasis by segmentectomy alone in 13 to 16% of patients. Segmentectomy has been used in patients with severe *Aspergillus* and pulmonary mycosis infections. However, Massard (1993) and Temeck (1994) and their colleagues noted that significant complications develop in both conditions regardless of the magnitude of the resection.

Even congenital lesions can be managed with segmental resections. Nuchtern and Harberg (1994) used segmentectomy for intralobar lung cysts. Sapin and associates (1997) were able to use segmentectomy in one-third of the patients they treated for congenital adenomatoid disease of the lung.

Technique

Standard lateral thoracotomy position using double-lumen endotracheal tube anesthesia is the most popular approach at present. A posterior approach in the prone position may be used, particularly when one expects copious secretions from a suppurative process. This approach has limited application today and should be undertaken only by those familiar with the special positioning required to avoid brachial plexus injury.

The initial steps in segmentectomy are the same as for any standard resection of the lung. The hilar structures are identified and the major fissure is opened. The surgeon must be familiar with intraparenchymal anatomy of the bronchus and pulmonary artery to accomplish a segmentectomy successfully.

On the right side, the bronchus is the most posterior hilar structure. The upper lobe branches of the pulmonary artery are the most superior hilar structures in the chest (Fig. 31-1). In the major fissure, the pulmonary artery can be exposed,

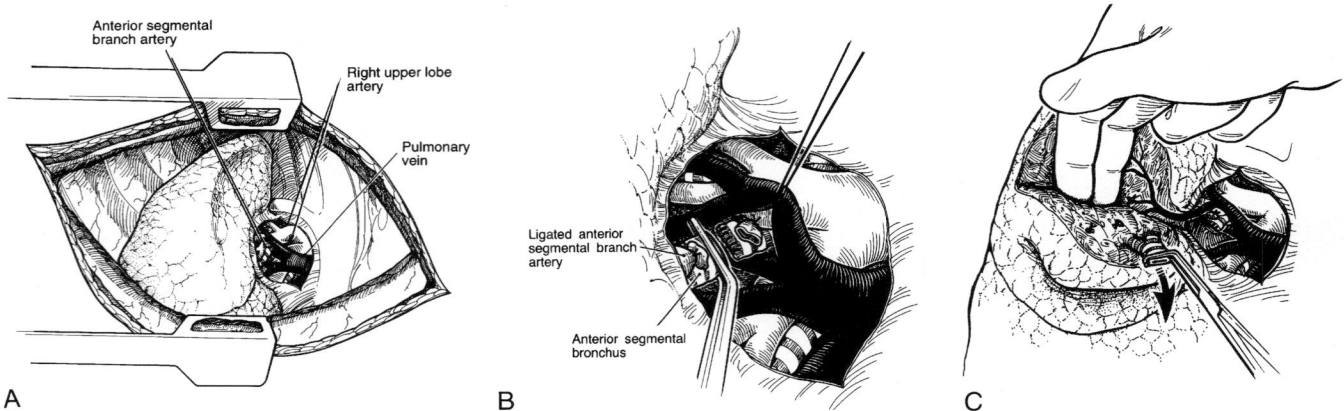

Fig. 31-1. A right anterior segmentectomy. **A.** Isolation of the right upper lobe artery and ligation of the anterior segmental branch. **B.** Division of the anterior segmental bronchus. **C.** Traction and finger fracture of the pulmonary parenchyma visualizing the pulmonary vein in the intersegmental plane.

demonstrating the continuation of the main pulmonary artery into the lower lobe. Anterior and posterior branches originate opposite one another and go, respectively, to the middle lobe and the superior segment of the lower lobe, forming a cross. Often, a posterior ascending branch arises from the posterior segmental artery and supplies part of the posterior segment of the upper lobe (Fig. 31-2).

On the left side, the pulmonary artery crosses superiorly above the left main stem bronchus to become the most posterior structure in the hilus. The apical-posterior and anterior and segmental branches are located anteriorly and superiorly. A separate posterior segmental branch is often found posteriorly on the main pulmonary artery, just at or above the major fissure (Fig. 31-3). In the major fissure, the lingular branches anteriorly and the superior segment branch posteriorly form a cross on the continuation of the pulmonary artery (Fig. 31-4).

The surgeon must be mindful of the high degree of variability of the branches of the pulmonary artery and carefully identify each branch before ligation (see Chapter 5).

The artery and bronchus are ligated and divided. When performing a segmentectomy for suppurative lung disease, it may be best to divide the bronchus first to prevent contamination of the normal lung. Controversy over whether to divide the bronchus or artery first raged through the 1930s and 1940s and has been carefully traced by Grismer and Read (1995). However, in the United States today, the order of division depends on the segment to be removed. For the apical and anterior segment of the upper lobe on the right side, the artery is ligated first and elevated to locate the segmental bronchus. For the posterior right upper lobe segment, it may be easier to divide the bronchus first and then the artery, which may be deep in the parenchyma and not easily

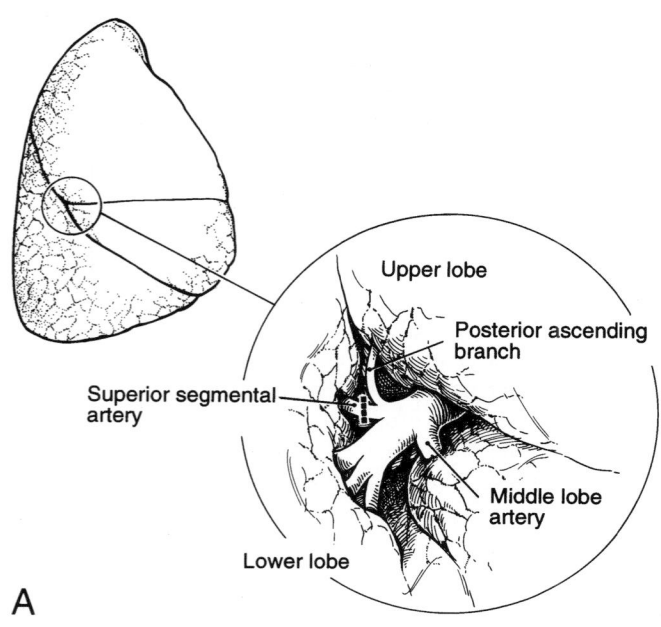

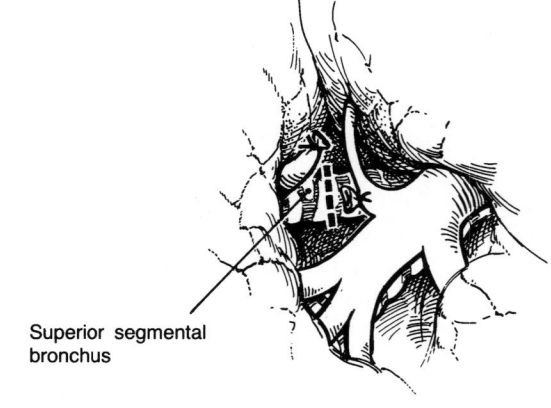

Fig. 31-2. A right superior segmentectomy. **A.** Exposure of the pulmonary artery in the fissure demonstrating the middle lobe artery and the superior segmental artery opposite one other with identification and preservation of the posterior ascending arterial branch. **B.** Division of the superior segmental bronchus.

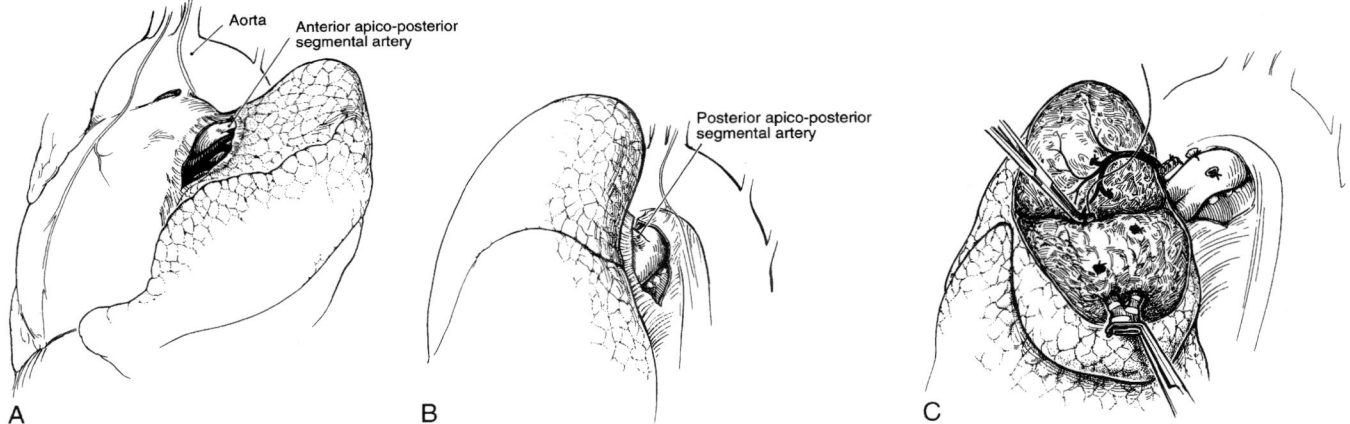

Fig. 31-3. A left apicoposterior segmentectomy. **A.** Identification and ligation of the anterior artery. **B.** Identification and ligation of the posterior artery. **C.** Parenchymal dissection of the segment exposing the vein in the intersegmental plane.

isolated anteriorly because of the other segmental branches. On the left side, the arterial branches are more easily isolated first because the bronchus is the middle structure on that side.

Before dividing the bronchus, the segment to be removed should be differentially deflated and inflated to help delineate the intersegmental planes, keeping in mind that filling of the deflated segment may occur from adjacent segments by means of collateral ventilation. With the advent of the double-lumen tube, it is often easier to inflate the entire lung, clamp the bronchus, and allow the rest of the lung to deflate. The segment remains inflated for a longer period, even with some loss from collateral ventilation. Once the appropriate segmental bronchus is identified, it is divided. The proximal stump may be closed either with a mechanical

stapler or with interrupted fine absorbable sutures. Additional coverage of the stump is usually not necessary.

After the bronchus and artery are ligated, traction is placed on the bronchus and the segment is removed in a retrograde manner. The plane is developed using digital blunt dissection with division of the pleura by scissors or cautery. The pulmonary veins course through the intersegmental planes and provide an excellent anatomic guide. Individual branches of the vein emanating from the segment into the fissure are sequentially divided.

After removal of the specimen, the raw surfaces of the adjacent segments are inspected and any significant bleeding is controlled. A sponge is applied to the expanded lung. After 5 to 10 minutes, the sponge is removed and the lung

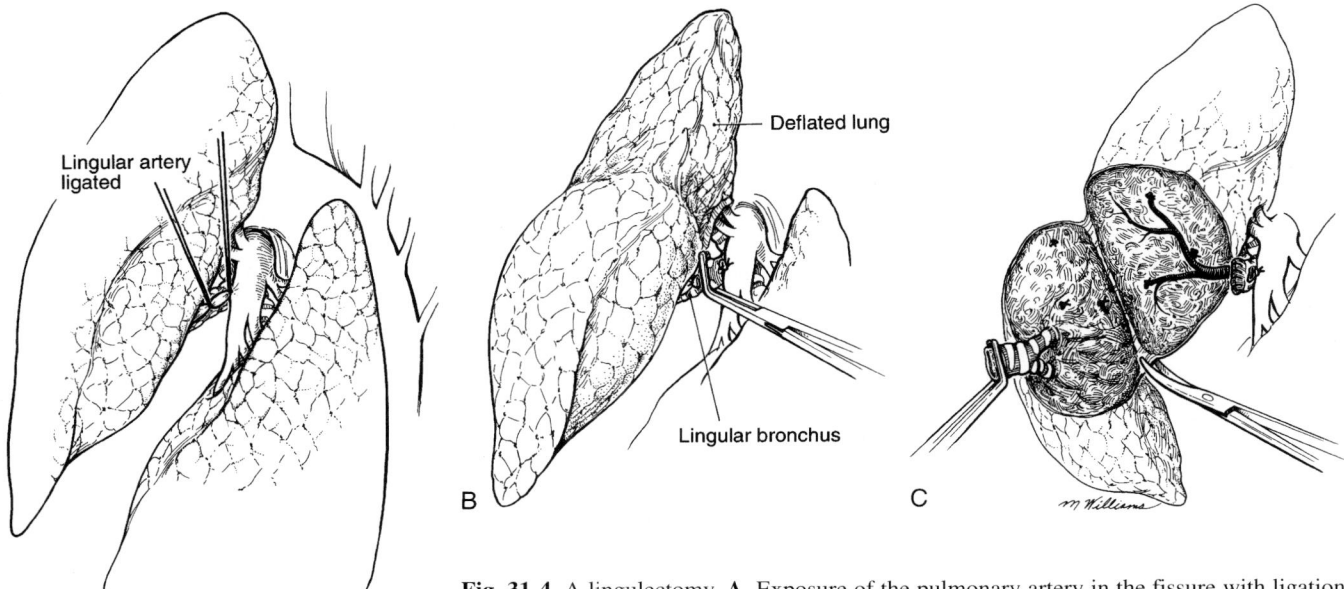

Fig. 31-4. A lingulectomy. **A.** Exposure of the pulmonary artery in the fissure with ligation of the lingular artery exposing the lingular bronchus. **B.** Identification of the intersegmental plane after deflation of the lung. **C.** Division of the pleura by sharp dissection.

surface is again inspected. If the dissection of the intersegmental plan has been done carefully, only a few alveolar air leaks will be present. These tend to seal over promptly with reexpansion of the lung during the postoperative period. Any leaking from small bronchi, however, must be recognized and controlled; this type of leak may cause persistent problems and predispose to postoperative space problems and infections. Jensik (1986) advocated covering the raw surfaces with pleural flaps or reconstituting the lung by bringing the adjacent segments together. Such a step generally is unnecessary when anatomic planes are respected and may lead to increased postoperative problems.

Management of the Pleural Space

Two thoracostomy tubes are placed into the space before the wound is closed, one anteriorly and one posteriorly. These tubes are connected to an underwater drainage system. The amount and timing of the suction to be used is at the discretion of the surgeon. Subsequent management of the pleural tubes is the same as that described for lobectomy.

Physiologic Effects

The physiologic changes after segmentectomy are the same as those noted after a lobectomy. The patient reacts in the same way as after a lobectomy because of the significant dysfunction after handling of the lobe during the operation. Late functional results are related to the number of segments removed. Over the next several months, the patient regains function of the remaining segments, although functional gain by the preservation of a segment of a lobe is generally less than expected from its volume.

Morbidity and Mortality

The nonfatal complications are similar to those occurring after a lobectomy. The major ones are prolonged air leak, either peripheral alveolar pleural fistula or a true bronchopleural fistula; empyema; and persistent pleural air space. All are interrelated and the incidence of any one alone or in combination varies most directly with the disease process and the difficulty experienced in the dissection of the intersegmental planes.

The incidence of persistent pleural air space is as high as 33% in patients with pulmonary tuberculosis. Compared with pleural air spaces occurring after lobectomy, however, only a small percentage of those noted after segmentectomy produce symptoms. When serious complications develop as a result of the space, they are most likely to be septic. The empyema with or without bronchopleural fistula must be treated in the usual manner.

Segmentectomy is essentially a benign procedure and the mortality should approximate 1%. It may, however, be as high as 4 to 6% in patients with poor pulmonary function or in those with previous pulmonary resection, as reported by Jensik (1986).

NONANATOMIC PARENCHYMA-SPARING RESECTIONS

Patients with metastatic lesions from sites such as the gastrointestinal tract, head and neck, breast, and genitourinary tract are ideal candidates for metastasectomy using nonanatomic resections. These patients may have multiple lesions or may present with additional lesions on subsequent occasions. Anatomic resections may remove a considerable amount of unaffected normal functioning lung, which might render these individuals pulmonary cripples and severely affect their quality of life. Mountain and colleagues (1984) reported an overall survival rate of 35% in large collected series of patients. McAfee and coworkers (1992) found a 5-year survival rate of 35% for colon carcinoma. Lanza and associates (1992) reported a 35% 5-year survival for breast carcinoma. Progrebniak and colleagues (1992) were able to extend median survivals of patients with renal cell carcinoma to 43 months. Patients who may also benefit from such an approach are those with marginal function who have an early stage I or stage II lung cancer. In a small series of collected patients with marginal lung function and early cancers, Miller and Hatcher (1987) showed a 5-year survival rate of 35%. Errett and associates (1985), Peters (1982), and Lewis and colleagues (1992) advocated similar approaches for the patient with marginal lung function. Currently, a National Cancer Institute Intergroup study is collecting data on combining video-assisted wedge resection with radiation for primary lung cancer in patients with marginal pulmonary function.

Several methods are available for performing nonanatomic resections of the lung, including open or video-assisted stapling, electrocautery, and laser. The techniques for each of these are similar.

Technique

Patients undergoing limited lung resection using any one of the variety of the aforementioned methods may have one of a variety of incisions ranging from a standard posterolateral incision or sternotomy for bilateral disease to the minimally invasive video-assisted thoracic surgical techniques. Most patients are placed in the lateral thoracotomy position with double-lumen tube anesthesia. After entry into the chest, thorough inspection is made to ensure that all areas of disease are identified. If the patient has multiple metastatic lesions, each should be addressed separately.

Several open and endoscopic in-line stapling devices made by a variety of companies are available to perform a nonanatomic wedge resection.

The wedge is best performed by using a U-type rather than a V-type resection. This ensures an adequate margin around the lesion. Two methods can be used. Two parallel lines are

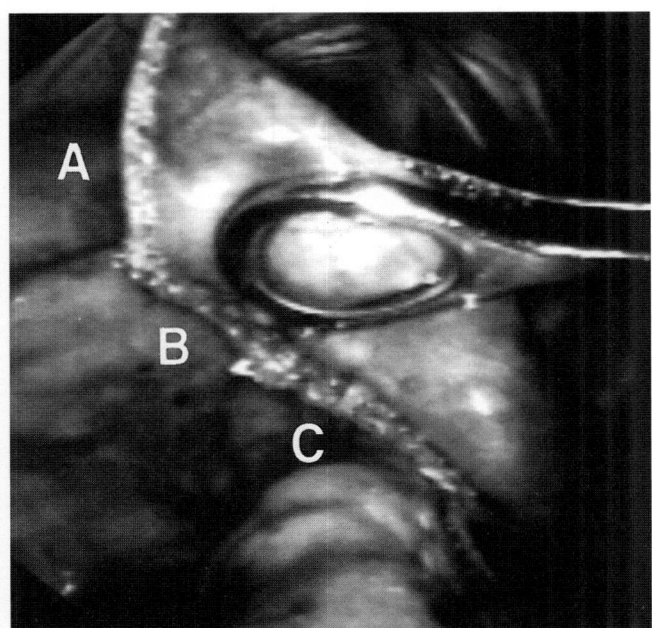

Fig. 31-5. A wedge resection. The first staple line begins resection (A). The second staple line provides a generous margin under the lesion (held in forceps) (B). The third staple line completes the margin around the lesion (C). A fourth staple line completes the resection.

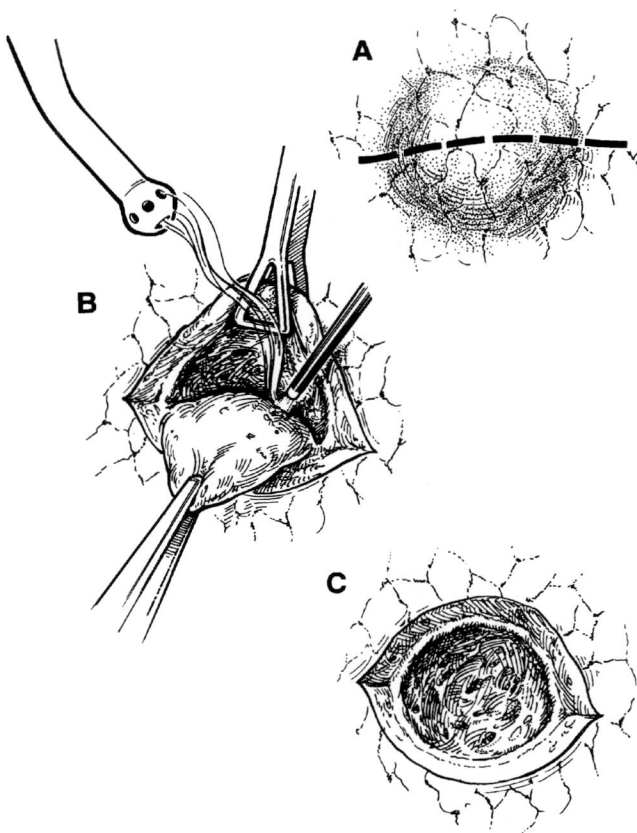

Fig. 31-6. A laser resection of a pulmonary nodule. **A.** Parenchymal incision down to the lesion. **B.** Lasering of the parenchyma using traction and countertraction. **C.** Open crater after laser excision.

placed into the lungs, several centimeters separated from the lesion. The lesion is then elevated and one or two additional staple lines are placed at the proximal margin. Alternatively, the staple line is begun near the lesion and the edge of the specimen to be removed is elevated and additional staple lines are fired until the lesion and the surrounding margin are resected. The last firing is usually performed from a different angle (Fig. 31-5). When done thoracoscopically, the latter technique is used. Such a maneuver may require three to five staple applications but it creates a contoured cut with an adequate margin around the lesion. The use of a video-assisted resection has largely supplanted the subsequent techniques, but they are included for completeness.

Electrocautery may be used to remove a lesion. This device can cut and coagulate simultaneously; the technique for its use was described by Urschel (1986). A linear incision is made over the lesion in the parenchyma and the lesion is exposed. By using traction and countertraction and applying cautery just beneath the lesion, it can be excised, leaving essentially all normal lung tissue. To accomplish this excision, a setting of at least 70 W must be applied to coagulate the tissue. At this power, resection proceeds with adequate coagulation of small and medium blood vessels. The major disadvantage is that the hot cautery blade may stick to the parenchyma.

An alternative to this approach was described by Cooper and colleagues (1986). They described the use of a bipolar cautery. When traction and countertraction are applied, small amounts of tissue are grabbed with the bipolar forceps and coagulated. All larger vessels and bronchi are ligated

individually. This technique produces good results with minimal air leak or injury to the remaining parenchyma. It is laborious and time consuming, however, and any vessel larger than 1 mm must be ligated individually.

Another tool for resection is the neodymium:yttrium-aluminum-garnet laser, an excellent cutting and coagulating tool for the surgeon. One major advantage of the yttrium-aluminum-garnet laser is that it does not have to touch the tissue, and thus no sticking occurs. At a power setting of 80 W, it can coagulate vessels up to 2 mm in diameter and seal air leaks from bronchi up to 1 mm in diameter. It produces a considerable smoke plume, which must be evacuated through filtered suction. The technique for removing a lesion was described by me and my colleagues (1989) (Fig. 31-6). Traction and countertraction are applied and the laser is used to excise the entire lesion. Because the laser produces considerable shrinkage of tissue, one must aim approximately 1 to 2 cm from the lesion. Larger blood vessels not coagulated by the laser should be individually ligated. One theoretic advantage of the laser is that because of its depth of penetration, it may be destroying additional small micrometastasis up to 4 mm away from the lesion.

Management of the Pleural Space

Thoracostomy tubes are placed into the space before the wound is closed. These tubes are connected to an underwater drainage system. Air leak with staple lines is usually minimal. But for coagulation or laser resection, when negative suction is applied to the tubes, significant air leak may result, particularly on positive-pressure ventilation. It may be best to withhold suction until the patient is in the postanesthesia care unit. When a patient is breathing spontaneously, suction may be applied cautiously. Once the lung is reexpanded, suction may be necessary to maintain this expansion. Subsequent management of the pleural tubes is the same as that described for lobectomy.

Postoperative care is similar to that of lobectomy and segmentectomy. During the early postoperative period, chest radiography frequently shows a halo around the site where the laser or cautery is used. This area eventually collapses and disappears, a process that occurs over several months. Such a scar may be difficult to evaluate radiographically, and the follow-up of malignant lesions, even by computed tomographic scans, is difficult. It is necessary to obtain a scan in the early postoperative period so that this area may be evaluated in comparison with later postoperative studies.

Physiologic Effects

The physiologic changes subsequent to a wedge resection in the absence of postoperative pleural complications are minimal. Those seen are related more directly to the thoracotomy incision than to the removal of a small portion of lung. Early in the postoperative period, the lung volume is restricted. Inspiratory capacity and expiratory reserve volume are decreased. Alveolar hypoventilation, with carbon dioxide retention and some degree of respiratory acidosis, sometimes occurs. Again, because of pain, compliance may be reduced and the chest wall may be stiff, resulting in an increased work of breathing. This situation is usually noted within the first few hours of operation, but returns gradually to normal within 1 to 2 weeks after operation.

Morbidity and Mortality

The morbidity after a wedge resection is minimal. When present, complications are most often the result of either retention of secretions or pleural problems. Persistent air spaces occur in up to 10% of cases. Most of these spaces produce no symptoms and require no treatment.

The mortality for wedge resection is near zero for patients with benign inflammatory disease and no more than 0.5% for those with malignant disease or pulmonary tuberculosis.

Reports by Saltman and me (1997) and Tovar and associates (1998) on the video-assisted methods show that such procedures can be performed even as outpatient procedures.

REFERENCES

Agasthian T, et al: Surgical management of bronchiectasis. Ann Thorac Surg 62:976, 1996.
Ashour M, et al: Surgery for unilateral bronchiectasis: results and prognostic factors. Tuber Lung Dis 77:168, 1996.
Cerfolio RJ, et al: Lung resection in patients with compromised pulmonary function. Ann Thorac Surg 62:348, 1996.
Cooper JD, et al: Precision cautery excision of pulmonary lesions. Ann Thorac Surg 41:51, 1986.
Crabbe MM, Patrisi GA, Fontenelle LJ: Minimal resection for bronchogenic carcinoma: should this be standard therapy? Chest 95:968, 1989.
Crabbe MM, Patrisi GA, Fontenelle LJ: Minimal resection for bronchogenic carcinoma: an update. Chest 99:1421, 1991.
Errett LE, et al: Wedge resection as an alternative procedure for peripheral bronchogenic carcinoma in poor risk patients. J Thorac Cardiothorac Surg 90:656, 1985.
Ginsberg RJ, Rubinstein LV: Randomized trial of lobectomy versus limited resection for T1 N0 non-small cell lung cancer. Ann Thorac Surg 60:615, 1995.
Grismer JT, Read RC: Evolution of pulmonary resection techniques and review of bronchus first method. Ann Thorac Surg 60:1133, 1995.
Jensik RJ: The extent of resection for localized lung cancer: segmental resection. In Kittle CF (ed): Current Controversies in Thoracic Surgery. Philadelphia: WB Saunders, 1986.
Jensik RJ: Mini resection of small peripheral carcinomas of the lung. Surg Clin North Am 66:951, 1987.
Jensik RJ, Faber LP, Kittle CF: Segmental resection for bronchogenic carcinoma. Ann Thorac Surg 28:475, 1979.
Jensik RJ, et al: Segmental resection for a lung cancer: A fifteen year experience. J Thorac Cardiothorac Surg 66:563, 1973.
Kodama K, et al: Intentional limited resection for selected patients with T1 N0 M0 non-small-cell lung cancer: a single-institution study. J Thorac Cardiovasc Surg 114:347, 1997.
Lanza LA, et al: Long-term survival after resection of pulmonary metastasis of the breast. Ann Thorac Surg 54:244, 1992.
Lewis R, et al: Video-assisted thoracic surgery resection of malignant lung tumors. J Thorac Cardiothorac Surg 104:1679, 1992.
LoCicero J, et al: Laser-assisted parenchyma-sparing resection. J Thorac Cardiothorac Surg 97:732, 1989.
Massard G, et al: Surgical treatment of pulmonary and bronchial aspergilloma. Ann Chir 47:147, 1993.
McAfee MK, et al: Colorectal lung metastasis: results of surgical excision. Ann Thorac Surg 53:780, 1992.
Miller JI, Hatcher CR: Limited resection of bronchogenic carcinoma in the patient with marked impairment of pulmonary function. Ann Thorac Surg 44:340, 1987.
Mountain CF, McMutery MJ, Hermes KE: Surgery for pulmonary metastasis: a twenty year experience. Ann Thorac Surg 38:323, 1984.
Nuchtern JG, Harberg FJ: Congenital lung cysts. Semin Pediatr Surg 3:233, 1994.
Peters RM: The role of limited resection in carcinoma of the lung. Am J Surg 143:706, 1982.
Progrebniak HW, et al: Renal cell carcinoma: resection of solitary and multiple metastasis. Ann Thorac Surg 54:33, 1992.
Read RC, Yoder G, Schaeffer RC: Survival after conservative resection for T1 N0 M0 non-small cell lung cancer. Ann Thorac Surg 499:391, 1990.
Saltman AE, LoCicero J: Short stay thoracic surgery. J Resp Crit Care Med 155:A482, 1997.
Sapin E, et al: Congenital adenomatoid disease of the lung: prenatal and perinatal management. Pediatr Surg Int 12:126, 1997.
Shields TW, Higgins GA: Minimal pulmonary resection in treatment of carcinoma of the lung. Arch Surg 108:420, 1974.
Temeck BK, et al: Thoracotomy for pulmonary mycoses in non-HIV-immunosuppressed patients. Ann Thorac Surg 58:333, 1994.
Tovar EA, et al: One day admission for lobectomy: an incidental result of a clinical pathway. Ann Thorac Surg 65:803, 1998.
Urschel HC, in discussion of Cooper, et al: Precision cautery excision of pulmonary lesions. Ann Thorac Surg 41:53, 1986.
Warren WH, Faber LP: Segmentectomy vs. lobectomy in patients with stage I pulmonary carcinoma: five-year survival and patterns of intrathoracic recurrence. J Thorac Cardiovasc Surg 107:1087, 1994.

CHAPTER 32

Instruments and Techniques of Video-Assisted Thoracic Surgery

Jeffrey C. Lin and Rodney J. Landreneau

BACKGROUND TO VIDEO-ASSISTED THORACIC SURGERY

Advances in videoendoscopic instrumentation and the evolution of endosurgical techniques have promoted a rapid expansion in video-assisted operative approaches in nearly every surgical discipline, including thoracic surgery. An exponential increase has occurred in the number and variety of operations performed by video-assisted thoracic surgery (VATS) techniques. VATS has pervaded the practice of general thoracic surgery just as laparoscopic approaches now dominate many aspects of general surgery.

VATS evolved from the simple pleural diagnostic procedure thoracoscopy. As Braimbridge (1993) noted in his review, the first thoracoscopic procedure reported was performed by the Swedish physician Hans Christian Jacobeus (1910). He used a primitive rigid cystoscope to explore the pleural space and to facilitate collapse therapy for pulmonary tuberculosis popular in that era. In 1921, Jacobeus presented his experience with this technique at the Society of Radiotherapy and Electrocauterization. There, he described a "two-stick" approach to directly examine the pleural cavity and to provide electrocautery access to lyse the pleural adhesions that were preventing collapse of the lung in the treatment of pulmonary tuberculosis. Jacobeus (1922, 1925) continued to use minimally invasive approaches throughout his career.

Thoracoscopy was a popular intervention in the management of pulmonary tuberculosis for the next three decades. Large European clinical experiences were summarized in reports by Fourestier and Duret (1943) and Coulaud and DesChamps (1947), detailing the technique and the effectiveness of thoracoscopic intervention for pleural-based pathology. In spite of this enthusiastic support for thoracoscopy in Europe, influential thoracic surgeons in the United States did much to forestall thoracoscopic intervention in North America. This criticism was led by John

Alexander, a pioneer in surgical treatment for pulmonary tuberculosis and a prominent figure in American academic thoracic surgery. Alexander (1937) expressed his concern over accounts of thoracoscopic disasters occurring in the tuberculosis sanatoria of his day. These sanatoria were primarily staffed by physicians who had neither a surgical background nor the technical support to handle the potentially life-threatening complications that could occur during these early thoracoscopic procedures.

The development of effective antibiotic therapy for tuberculosis in the 1950s rendered invasive treatment modalities, such as induced pneumothorax and thoracoplasty, obsolete. As a result, the practice of thoracoscopy was greatly curtailed in North America and Europe. Nonetheless, European investigators, including Brandt (1978), Swierenga and associates (1974), and Bergquist and Nordenstam (1966), continued to use thoracoscopy for the diagnosis and management of selected pleural and pulmonary processes. After a period of near abandonment over the ensuing 25 years, the development of videoendoscopic technology and effective endoscopic stapling devices renewed interest in thoracoscopy, or more accurately, VATS. Improved image resolution and the ability to televise the magnified view of the surgical field allowed others in the operating room to actively assist the surgeon. Concurrently, the development of endoscopic surgical instruments and techniques further accelerated the evolution of thoracoscopy from a diagnostic to a therapeutic modality. Since 1991, minimally invasive VATS has evolved to the preferred approach to many common thoracic surgery problems.

The goal of VATS is to reduce postoperative pain and other postthoracotomy morbidity without compromising the therapeutic efficacy of open thoracic surgery, as stressed by one of us (R.J.L.) and associates (1992b). Successful implementation of this goal has made VATS the preferred approach to the diagnosis and treatment of many thoracic disease processes (Tables 32-1 and 32-2). Clinical investiga-

Table 32-1. Potential Indications of Video-Assisted Thoracic Surgery

Diagnostic
  Indeterminate pleural effusion (benign versus malignant)
  Tissue diagnosis
    Pleural-based masses (metastatic adenocarcinoma versus mesothelioma)
    Diffuse interstitial lung disease
    Indeterminate peripheral pulmonary nodule
    Mediastinal lymph node biopsy
    Mediastinal mass biopsy
Therapeutic
  Pleuropulmonary
    Pleural effusion/empyema
    Pleurodesis (thermal/mechanical/chemical/talc)
    Bullous disease ablation/resection
    Wedge resection for early stage lung cancer in selected high-risk patients
    Anatomic resection for lung cancer
  Esophageal
    Resection of leiomyomata
    Resection of enteric cysts
    Esophagomyotomy
    Antireflex surgery for intractable gastroesophageal reflux disease
    Video-assisted esophagectomy
  Mediastinal
    Thymectomy for myasthenia gravis
    Thymectomy for stage I thymoma
    Resection of benign mediastinal tumors (teratoma)
    Resection of posterior mediastinal (neurogenic) masses
    Excision of bronchogenic, enteric, or pericardial cysts
    Drainage of pericardial effusion
    Pericardiectomy
Miscellaneous
  Dorsal sympathectomy or splanchnicectomy
  Drainage of paravertebral abscess
  Orthopedic diskectomy
  Internal mammary artery harvest for coronary artery bypass grafting

Table 32-2. Relative Contraindications for Video-Assisted Thoracic Surgery

Dense pleural symphysis
Ventilator dependency
Noncompliant lung
Severe emphysema
Pulmonary hilar lesions
Pulmonary lesions abutting the upper mediastinum or posterior paravertebral gutter
Small (<1 cm), deeply located pulmonary nodules
Large pulmonary nodules (>3 cm)
Chest wall involvement by tumor
Small thoracic cavity or significant anatomic restrictions (i.e., severe scoliosis)
Inability to achieve or tolerate single lung ventilation
Inability to achieve ipsilateral pulmonary atelectasis
Hemodynamic instability
Severe thoracic trauma or intrathoracic hemorrhage
Coagulopathy
Inadequate visualization or instrumentation to perform procedure

tions reported by one of us (R.J.L.) (1993b,c, 1994), Hazelrigg (1991, 1993a,b), and Kirby (1995) and associates have demonstrated that VATS has similar efficacy to open thoracotomy while providing the benefits of decreased pain-related morbidity, functional disability, length of hospital stay, and postoperative cardiac arrhythmias.

This chapter reviews the instrumentation, general operative setup, and basic VATS approach strategies required for optimal results. The role of VATS in the management of certain pleural and pulmonary diseases is briefly reviewed. Specific applications of VATS as a diagnostic tool and as a therapeutic modality in pulmonary and esophageal surgery, mediastinal lesions, thymectomy, and sympathectomy are discussed in detail in Chapters 18, 33, 43, 130, 158, and 173.

INSTRUMENTATION FOR IMAGING: THORACOSCOPES AND VIDEO IMAGING SYSTEMS

A 10-mm, zero-degree, rigid "operating" thoracoscope (Karl Storz Endoscopy-America, Inc., Culver City, CA) with a 5-mm biopsy channel is preferable to the "view only" thoracoscopes and laparoscopes for most VATS procedures (Figs. 32-1 and 32-2). This operative thoracoscope allows for single intercostal access for the management and biopsy of many pleural-related problems and also potentially allows for the performance of more complex VATS interventions with one less intercostal access site, as previously noted by one of us (R.J.L.) and colleagues (1992a,b, 1993a). Furthermore, when use of the neodymium:yttrium-aluminum-garnet (Nd:YAG) laser is considered, the biopsy channel of the operating thoracoscope allows for direct end-on viewing of the laser's effect on the target pathology. For similar reasons, the

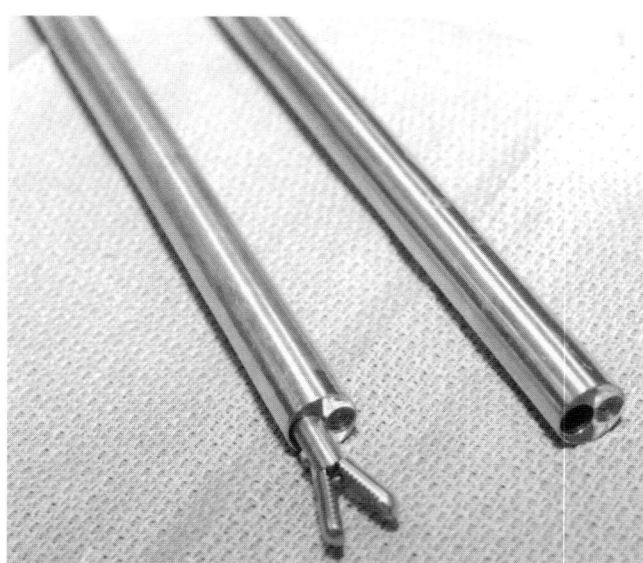

Fig. 32-1. Storz operating thoracoscope. Note the 5-mm grasper in the biopsy channel of the thoracoscope (left).

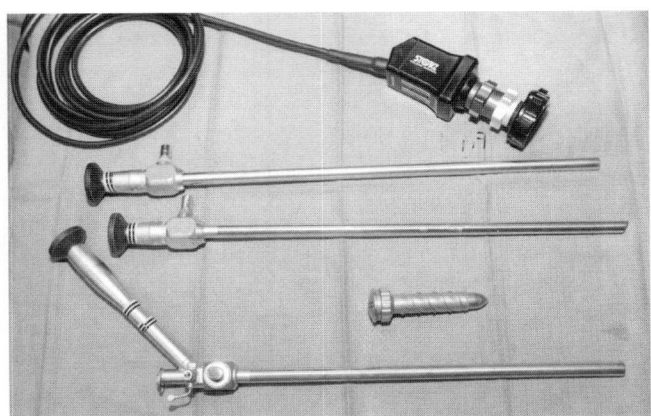

Fig. 32-2. From top to bottom: Storz Endovision Camera, zero-degree standard laparoscope, 30-degree laparoscope, reusable blunt tip thoracoscopic port, and Storz thoracoscope with biopsy channel.

zero-degree thoracoscope is preferred for the majority of VATS procedures. An angled thoracoscope is rarely needed with proper planning of the trocar sites, but may be helpful in selected instances. Flexible and semiflexible thoracoscopes are available, but maintenance of spatial orientation is more difficult with these instruments than with the rigid devices.

A three-chip digital video camera and high-resolution video monitors are paramount to accurately depict the operative field. Our practice currently uses the Karl Storz Endovision system (Karl Storz Endoscopy-America, Inc., Culver City, CA), consisting of the Tricam SL camera (see Fig. 32-2) and image-processing module (Fig. 32-3). Similar high-quality three-chip digital cameras are available (Stryker, Olympus, and so forth), but the Storz system offers a built-in zoom capability and digital image enhancement features. The camera system is also compatible with other endoscopes used in our operating room, including the 5- and 10-mm laparoscope, fiberoptic bronchoscope, and fiberoptic esophagogastroscope. A photographic printer, videotape recorder, and dual high-resolution monitors (Sony Electronics, Tokyo) complete the video equipment used by our thoracic surgical team (see Fig. 32-3).

The use of three-dimensional imaging for VATS has been explored. Given the present technological limitations of three-dimensional systems, however, we have found little need for this technology. Headsets, visors, and other devices typically used by these systems are unwieldy and uncomfortable. Furthermore, the focal distance at which most endoscopic systems provide three-dimensional or binocular vision is beyond the usual distance at which dissection and tissue manipulation are accomplished. Attempts at a closer view by advancing the thoracoscope result in loss of binocular accommodation and a blurred image. The limitations of monocular vision inherent in current systems can usually be overcome by the surgeon as experience with VATS increases. The surgeon can establish the necessary spatial perspective between the target pathology and the instruments by zooming out or withdrawing the tho-

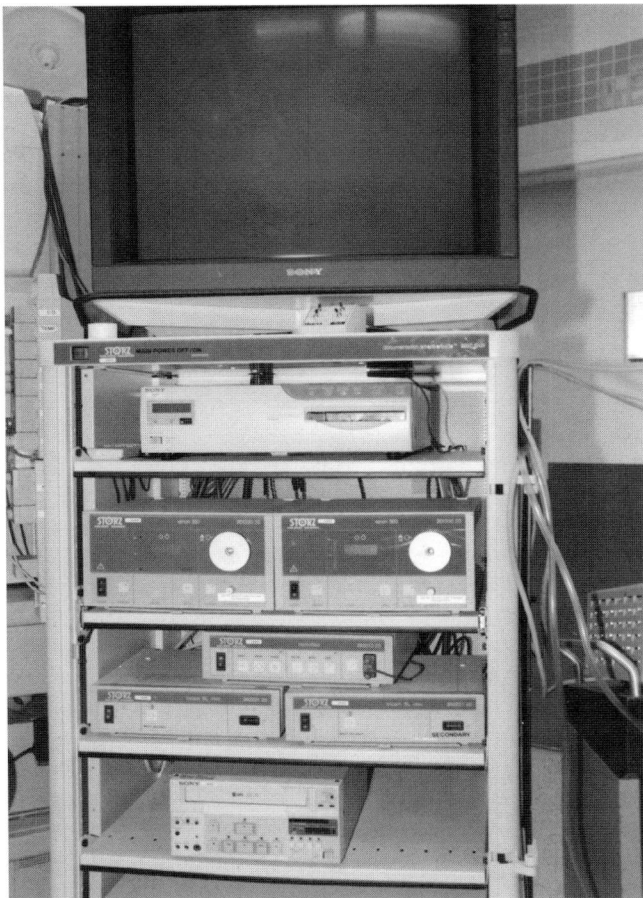

Fig. 32-3. Video endoscopic equipment, top to bottom: high-resolution video monitor, video image printer, xenon light sources (×2), video processing units (×2), and videotape recorder.

racoscope to gain a panoramic view of the operative field, or by zooming in or advancing the thoracoscope to gain a near perspective of the surgical field. Appropriate placement of the instrument ports and the thoracoscope in relation to the target also aids in maintaining spatial orientation.

Modalities for Tissue Coagulation: Electrocautery, Ultrasound, and Laser

Monopolar electrocautery (Valleylab, Inc., Boulder, CO) is used for simple dissection and coagulation during VATS in similar fashion to open surgery. Bipolar electrocautery is seldom necessary in VATS. Bipolar electrocautery is indicated when VATS is chosen for paraspinous pathology (e.g., thoracic intervertebral disc disease, neurogenic tumors, to avoid neurologic injury). At present, the argon beam coagulator (ABC; Birtcher Medical Systems, Irvine, CA), is uncommonly used in VATS, although it has been advocated by some for thermal pleurodesis. The ABC differs from standard electrocautery in that it uses a stream of inert argon

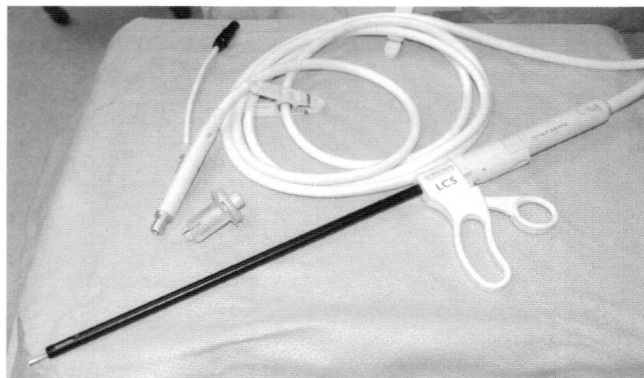

Fig. 32-4. Ten-millimeter Harmonic Scalpel/LCS Shears (Ethicon Endo-Surgery, Inc., Cincinnati, OH).

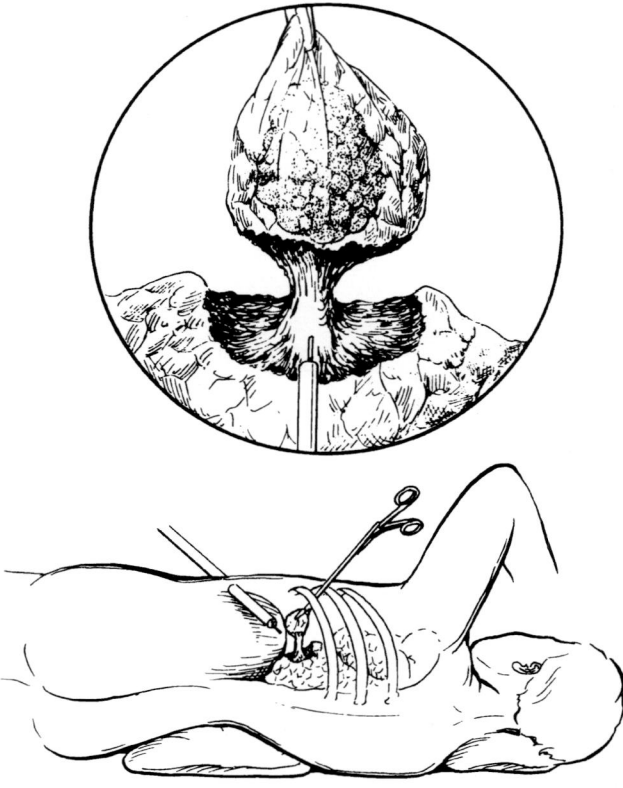

Fig. 32-5. Video-assisted thoracic surgery approach for neodymium:yttrium-aluminum-garnet laser resection of a peripheral lung nodule. From Landreneau RJ, et al: Thoracoscopic Nd:YAG laser assisted pulmonary resection. Ann Thorac Surg 52:1176, 1991b. With permission.

gas that blows away fluids and conducts the electrocautery current into a broader beam. These effects have made the ABC a useful tool in coagulating broad surfaces and solid organ parenchyma. Applications of the ABC in VATS include pleural symphysis for pneumothorax and pleural effusion and lung volume reduction through superficial cauterization and shrinkage of subpleural bullous emphysema. Results with the ABC in these settings have been good but not outstanding, because of the high incidence of prolonged air leaks, as reported by Lewis and colleagues (1993). In a study by Sawabata and associates (1996), the ABC was found to induce a significant amount of destructive coagulation on the pleural surface, leading to subsequent air leaks.

The ultrasonic dissector/coagulator (Harmonic Scalpel/UltraCision LCS Shears, Ethicon Endo-Surgery, Inc., Cincinnati, OH) (Fig. 32-4) performs on a different principle than electrocautery. Instead of applying a current of high-frequency AC electricity, the Harmonic Scalpel uses 50-kHz oscillations that are physically transmitted to the tissues in the grasp of the shears or the tip of the scalpel. This creates the intracellular and extracellular vibrations that result in heat and coagulation of the tissue. One important advantage of the Harmonic Scalpel is that little threat of injury exists to adjacent tissue outside the grasp of the forceps's jaws or the tip of the scalpel. Hemostasis is reliable, even when dividing blood vessels 3 or 4 mm in diameter. Coagulation is effective in sealing the vessels with a minimal incidence of delayed bleeding. By obviating the need for individually clipping and dividing small vessels, the operation may be expedited.

The primary role of electrocautery and the Harmonic Scalpel in VATS pulmonary surgery is division of simple adhesions and dissection of the hilar structures. Electrocautery alone is inefficient and potentially inappropriate for division of lung parenchyma or larger parenchymal blood vessels. The 1064-nm Nd:YAG laser has been well described as a tool for resection of selected pulmonary lesions by Dowling (1992a,b,c), LoCicero (1989), and one of us (R.J.L.)

(1991a,b, 1992a, 1993d) and colleagues. Indeed, until the advent of the endoscopic stapling devices, Nd:YAG laser lung resection was a common modality used for parenchymal sparing excision of pulmonary nodules. The Nd:YAG laser can function as a primary or adjunctive resective and coagulative tool for pulmonary resection (Fig. 32-5) and is the most versatile laser available for VATS applications presently available. It has been found to have superior hemostatic and pneumostatic coagulation properties compared with CO_2 lasers in reports by LoCicero (1985, 1989) and one of us (R.J.L.) (1991a,b, 1992a, 1993d) and associates.

A 30- to 40-W continuous laser mode is used as the noncontact fiberoptic laser probe is positioned 1 to 2 cm from the lung to produce a broader application of the laser beam. This maneuver enhances thermal coagulation of lung parenchyma while a more focused application of the laser energy by positioning the laser probe closer enhances cutting properties. As larger vessels are encountered (larger than 2 mm), the laser is defocused further to achieve adequate coagulation before vessel division. In addition, these larger vessels are secured by hemoclips. In essence, the pulmonary nodule and a margin of lung tissue are cored away from the surrounding lung as the laser resection proceeds

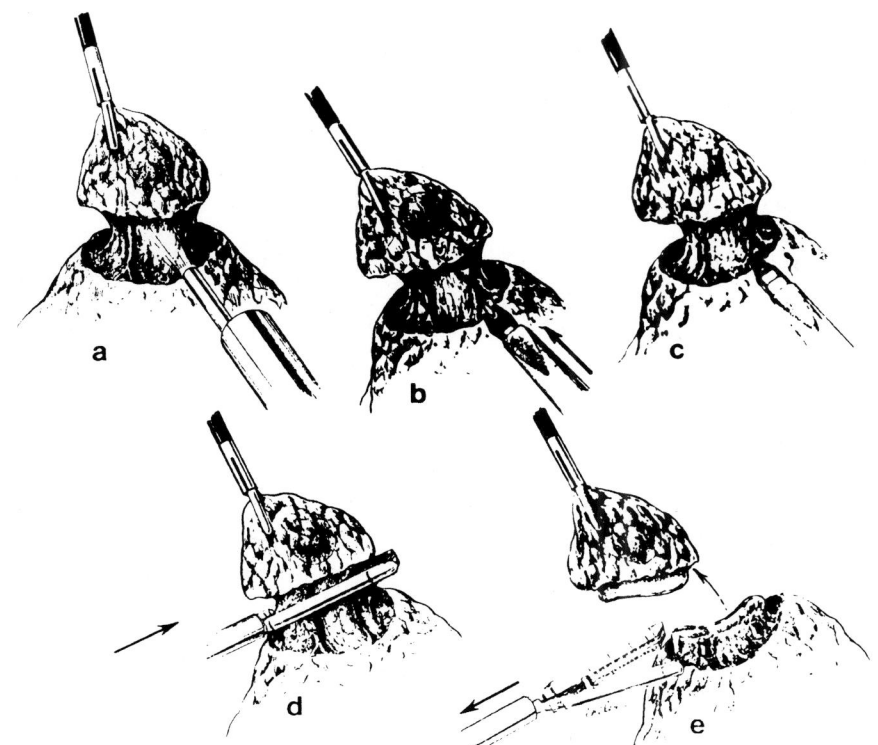

Fig. 32-6. Technique of combining application of the neodymium:yttrium-aluminum-garnet laser (**a**), surgical clips (**b**), cautery (**c**), and endoscopic stapler (**d and e**) for pulmonary wedge resection. From Landreneau RJ, et al: Thoracoscopic resection of 85 pulmonary lesions. Ann Thorac Surg *54*:415, 1992a. With permission from The Society of Thoracic Surgeons.

(see Fig. 32-5). The laser-coagulated lung surface generally exhibits good hemostasis and pneumostasis.

This technique of lung resection with the Nd:YAG laser is effective but is slow and tedious. Moreover, a significant learning curve is required for proficiency in VATS laser pulmonary resection. Hence, most thoracic surgeons have lacked enthusiasm for this approach. As a result, the general experience with VATS lung resections was limited until the introduction of effective endostapling devices. Presently, the role of the Nd:YAG laser in pulmonary resection is limited, but is perhaps most useful in patients with poor pulmonary reserve when maximal parenchymal sparing is desired. As noted by LoCicero (1989) and one of us (R.J.L.) (1993d) and coworkers, the adjuvant use of the Nd:YAG laser to stapled techniques (Fig. 32-6) may facilitate resection from difficult locations, such as the flat sur-

face of the lower lobe, or when the nodule is deep within the lung parenchyma.

Stapling Devices

Development of effective and reliable endoscopic stapling devices revolutionized and accelerated the application of VATS for pulmonary diseases, as outlined by Acuff and associates (1993). The endoscopic stapling devices are generally easy to use and reliably divide pulmonary parenchyma and vessels while maintaining excellent hemostasis and pneumostasis. Commonly available models include the EVC/ELC staplers from Ethicon (Cincinnati, OH) and the EndoGIA from United States Surgical Corporation (Norwalk, CT). A variety of staple sizes and stapler lengths are presently available (Table 32-3).

Table 32-3. Specifications of Commonly Used Thoracoscopic Staplers

Product	Staple Line (mm)	Cut Line (mm)	Rows/No. of Staples	Crown (mm)	Open Height (mm)	Closed Height (mm)
EVC 35	37	33	6/54	3.0	2.5^a/3.5	1.0^a/1.5
EndoGIA 30	32.5	27.5	6/48	3.0	2.5^a/3.5	1.0^a/1.5
EndoTA 30	32.5	N/A	3/24	3.0	2.5^a/3.5	1.0^a/1.5
ENDOCUTTER	63	60	4/64	3.0	3.85/4.5	1.5/2.0
EndoGIA 60	60	57	6/90	3.0	2.5^a/3.5/4.8	1.0^a/1.5/2.0
Ethicon 4 row	60	63	N/A 4/64	3.0	3.85/4.5	1.5/2.0
EndoTA 60	60	N/A	3/45	3.0	2.5^a/3.5/4.8	1.0^a/1.5/2.0

NA, not applicable.
^{a}Vascular.
EVC, ENDOCUTTER, Ethicon, Cincinnati, OH; EndoGIA, EndoTA, United States Surgical Corporation, Norwalk, CT.

The one grip design, such as the Ethicon EZ-45, allows the apposition of the stapler jaws and the application of the staples without the need to change the grip. Reticulating staplers are now available from US Surgical, Ethicon, and Richard Allen, and are of benefit in certain instances. We generally use the 30- or 45-mm stapler loads in pulmonary surgery. Although 60-mm stapler loads are available, Worsey and one of us (R.J.L.) (1998) noted that the jaws of the device open only slightly wider, thus making these instruments more difficult to use than the 30- or 45-mm devices.

Hand-Held Instruments and Instrument Design

The explosion in endoscopic or minimally invasive surgery in North America and Europe has fueled the industry to invest in development of both disposable and reusable hand-held instruments and accessory operative instrumentation. Although a vast array of plastic disposable instruments and trocars is available, reusable models of thoracoscopy ports and other instruments, such as retractors, graspers, and clamps, can be used. Most surgeons acquire reusable endoscopic surgical instruments when their VATS case volume justifies the cost of acquiring reusable instruments. Presently available reusable endoscopic scissors are frequently subject to rapid dulling of the blades or loosening of the hinge mechanism. This results in deterioration of the scissoring action, rendering the instrument ineffective. Some companies have developed endo-scissors with replaceable ends that incorporate a new set of scissor blades and hinge. This concept can overcome the limitations of the endo-scissors mentioned at a reduced additional cost (Snowden Pencer, Atlanta, GA) and may be preferable to the plastic disposable endoscopic scissors.

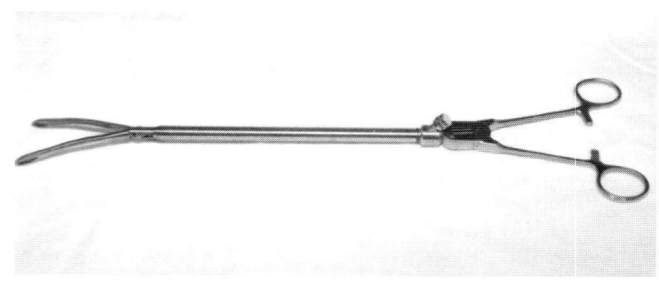

Fig. 32-8. Example of coaxial designed thoracoscopic grasper (Starr Medical Instruments, New York, NY).

A central problem facing the surgeon performing VATS relates to the inadequate design inherent in the pistol grip endosurgical instruments. Although the pistol grip design works well for some applications, such as endostaplers, it is awkward for detailed manipulation and dissection (Fig. 32-7). As a result, some surgeons use standard instruments via a utility or limited thoracotomy access incision. Coaxial endosurgical instruments that allow for unimpeded access through the intercostal port (Fig. 32-8) have been developed by Starr Medical Instruments (New York, NY, formerly Produktion Chirougischen Instrumente, Tuttingen, Germany) and Scanlan (St. Paul, MN) for true port access VATS. These instruments retain the feel of standard open surgical instruments and replicate many of the familiar standard graspers and forceps while requiring a minimal intercostal access incision (Fig. 32-9).

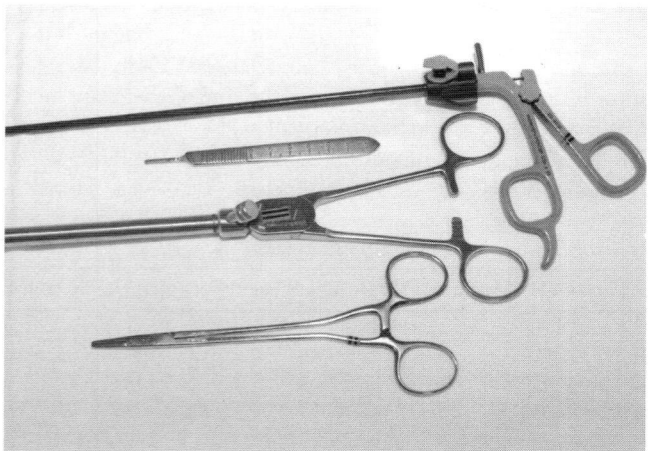

Fig. 32-7. Thoracoscopic instrument design: Pistol grip versus coaxial. Top to bottom: pistol grip, coaxial, standard open instrument for comparison.

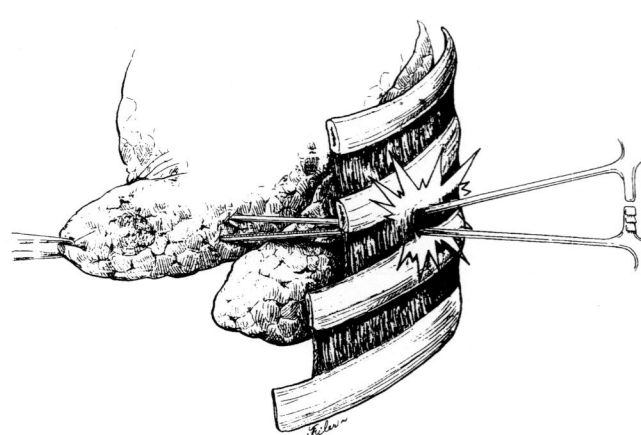

A

Fig. 32-9. A. Narrow intercostal space prevents use of standard open instruments.

BASIC VIDEO-ASSISTED THORACIC SURGERY OPERATIVE STRATEGIES

The first maneuver is proper patient selection for the operation. As with any major operative procedure, a careful assessment of the patient's physiologic reserve is mandatory, as stressed by Wernly and DeMeester (1989) and outlined by Melendez and Fischer (1997) and Teplick (1997). Another major preoperative concern facing thoracic surgeons beginning VATS is determining the adequacy of anesthesia team support available in their hospital. It is vital that anesthesia personnel be experienced in open thoracic procedures and the principles and applications of selective ventilation during the operation, as described by Benumof (1983). VATS procedures cannot be accomplished without sufficient unilateral pulmonary atelectasis. Therefore, it is crucial that the anesthesia team is well acquainted with double-lumen endotracheal intubation, bronchial blockers, and other techniques as reviewed by Wilson (1997) to achieve single lung ventilation, as well as the physiologic support required during single lung ventilation.

Intraoperative bronchoscopy is important to rule out endobronchial pathology. After placement of the double-lumen tube is confirmed, the patient is positioned in a full lateral decubitus position with appropriate padding and with the operating table extended to maximize the intercostal distances on the operative side (Fig. 32-10). The patient should be secured to the table to allow for any table position changes needed. The thorax is prepared and draped for open thoracotomy should this necessity arise. It is vital that the surgical team preparing for VATS interventions be personally familiar with standard thoracic surgical procedures. Many VATS procedures share the same potential intraoperative complications as their open counterparts. Accordingly, VATS procedures should be performed in an operating room where facilities for immediate conversion to thoracotomy are available.

A careful preoperative review of the chest roentgenogram and computed tomographic (CT) scan is vital to formulate

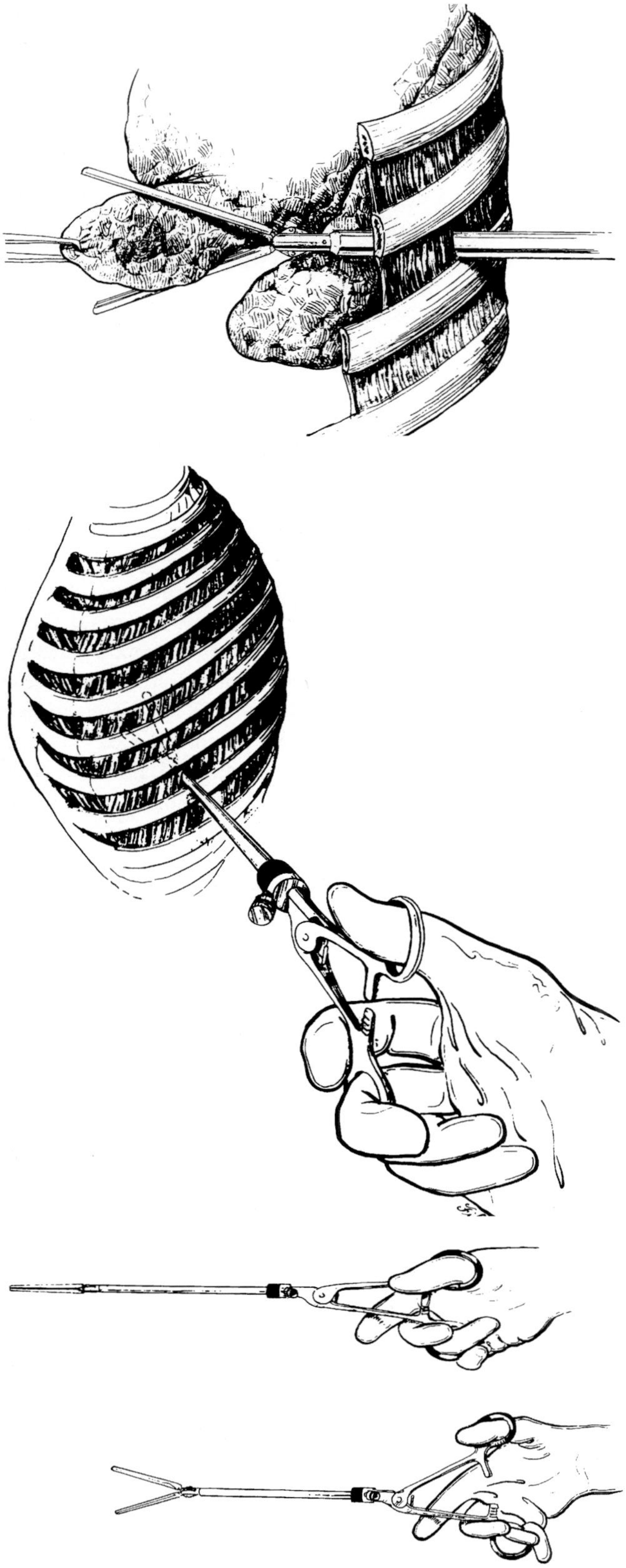

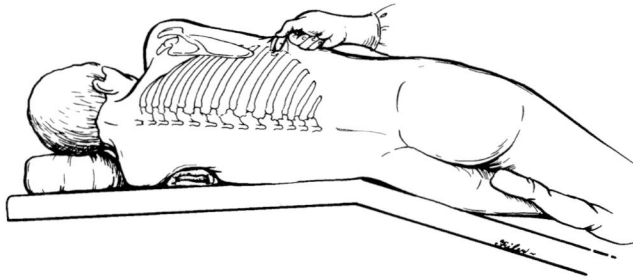

Fig. 32-10. Patient in the left lateral decubitus position with digital exploration of the proposed initial trocar site to confirm that a free pleural space is present. From Landreneau RJ, et al: Video-assisted surgery: basic technical concepts and intercostal approach strategies. Ann Thorac Surg *54*:800, 1992b. With permission.

Fig. 32-9. *Continued.* **B–D.** Coaxial thoracoscopic instruments allow use of small port incisions while retaining instrument feel of standard open instruments.

the plan for the initial and subsequent intercostal access for the thoracoscopic and surgical instruments. Furthermore, as one of us (R.J.L.) and colleagues (1992b, 1993a) have outlined, the patient's specific anatomy is an important consideration. For example, for a VATS-directed wedge biopsy of the lung for diffuse interstitial disease, a right-sided approach is preferred. Because of the trilobar anatomy of the right lung, more edges exist from which to obtain wedge biopsies. On the other hand, a left-sided approach is advised for bilateral diffuse nodular disease. This is because of the more reliable and complete collapse that can be achieved on the left side, an important factor for identifying the nodules. The left-sided approach for lung biopsy is also preferred in smaller patients, in whom double-lumen intubation may not be possible and bronchial blockers are used.

Similarly, because of anatomic considerations, we have altered our approach for VATS thymectomy (see Chapter 173). A left-sided approach was initially described by the senior author (R.J.L.) and associates (1992c) for better pulmonary collapse and visualization of the aortopulmonary window lymph nodes. With further experience, however, it was found that troublesome bleeding could arise at the region near the superior vena cava and innominate vein that is difficult to address from the left. A right-sided approach clearly visualizes this region during dissection and is now our preferred approach to VATS thymectomy unless the predominant thymic pathology is localized on the left.

The operation is begun by choosing an appropriate intercostal site of access for exploratory thoracoscopy. The skin incision is made directly over the intercostal space to be entered, as opposed to the tunnel sometimes made for simple tube thoracostomy. This allows for increased mobility of the port and reduces the incidence of postoperative intercostal neuritis secondary to excessive torquing of the thoracoscope against the rib cage and intercostal neurovascular bundle, as previously outlined by one of us (R.J.L.) and colleagues (1992b, 1993a). Careful introduction of a small curved clamp (e.g., Kelly or Crile) through the intercostal muscles and pleura is made along the superior border of the lower rib of the intercostal access site to minimize injury to the intercostal vessels and nerve. The clamp is opened to widen the intercostal space. Direct digital exploration, rather than blind trocar placement into the chest, is used to identify any local pleural adhesions and avoid injury to the underlying lung (see Fig. 32-10). Pleural adhesions to the lung can impede the introduction of instruments and potentially result in parenchymal injury. Flimsy local adhesions can be divided with blunt finger dissection. More extensive pleural symphysis in the location of the initial access site may require alternative intercostal access. Hemostasis of the port site should be meticulous, as even small amounts of bleeding dribble down the trocar and onto the thoracoscope lens.

In general, the sixth or seventh intercostal space in the midaxillary line is ideal for trocar protected thoracoscope access to the pleural cavity. This initial thoracoscope location usually provides a clear view of the mediastinum, all

pleural surfaces, and the pulmonary parenchyma. The intercostal access trocar tube is important to prevent soiling the thoracoscope lens surface during the introduction and variable positioning of the thoracoscope during the operation. Agents such as FRED (Dexide, Inc., Fort Worth, TX) can be applied to the lens to reduce lens fogging. Prewarming of the thoracoscope in a warm water bath (Circon Co., Santa Barbara, CA) further reduces lens fogging from condensation by reducing the temperature differential between the warm moist air within the pleural cavity and the cooler thoracoscope. Carbon dioxide insufflation is rarely needed to conduct VATS. Occasionally, this is used at the beginning of the procedure to facilitate a more complete and expeditious collapse of the lung. If carbon dioxide insufflation is used, the intrapleural pressure is kept below 10 mm Hg to avoid mediastinal tension and hemodynamic compromise. Exploratory thoracoscopy is then performed.

The visibility of the entire thoracic cavity obtained through the VATS approach contrasts favorably with the confined direct view of the intrathoracic structures obtained through a limited axillary, inframammary, or lateral thoracotomy as noted by one of us (R.J.L.) and coworkers (1992b, 1993a). After the initial thoracoscopic exploration is concluded, further intercostal access for VATS instrumentation is achieved under direct thoracoscopic vision (Fig. 32-11).

The specific locations of the additional port sites are determined by the site of the primary pathology (Table 32-4). In general, the ports are strategically placed about the thorax to allow for some working room between the port and the lesion. The endoscopic instruments and the thoracoscopic camera should be oriented so that they all are facing the target pathology from the same direction (Fig. 32-12). Otherwise, difficulties in instrument manipulation occur because of mirror imaging when the instruments are directed toward the thoracoscopic camera. It is paramount to conceptualize

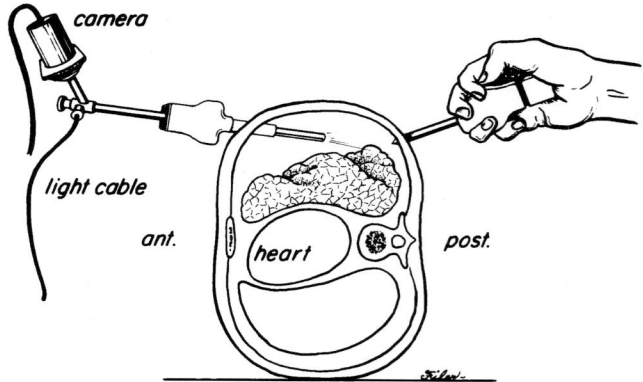

Fig. 32-11. All subsequent instruments and trocars are introduced under direct thoracoscopic visualization to ensure proper location and to avoid trauma to the intercostal neurovascular bundle or intrathoracic structures. From Landreneau RJ, et al: Video-assisted thoracic surgery: basic technical concepts and intercostal approach strategies. Ann Thorac Surg *54*;800, 1992b. With permission.

Table 32-4. Strategic Approach to Intrathoracic Pathology at Specific Locations

Area of Interest	Thoracoscope	Retractor/Grasper	Dissector/Stapler	Additional Instrument
Apices	6 mid	4 anterior	4/5 posterior	—
Anterior mediastinum	5 mid/posterior	2/3 mid	5/6 posterior	7 mid
Posterior mediastinum	5 mid	4/6 anterior	2 Ant.	3/4 anterior
Interlobar fissure				
Two port	6/7 mid/posterior	—	—	5 anterior
Three port	7/9 mid/posterior	6/7 mid/posterior	—	5 anterior
Midesophagus/aortopulmonary window	5/6 posterior	5 auscultatory triangle	4 anterior	7 mid
Distal esophagus	7 mid	4 anterior	6/8 posterior	7 anterior
Pericardium (left)	7 posterior	9 mid	5 posterior	—

Note: Instruments are often used interchangeably at more than one access site.
Anterior, mid, and posterior, anterior, mid, and posterior axillary lines; 5, fifth intercostal space; 6, sixth intercostal space, and so forth.

the three-dimensional location of the target lesion within the thorax, then place the port access sites to triangulate on the lesion. With adequate distance between the ports, fencing of the instruments can be avoided and enhancement of the surgeon's spatial perception of the operative field is achieved. In addition to the thoracoscope, trocar ports are required to protect endostaplers during their insertion into the thorax. On the other hand, other instruments such as graspers and suction devices do not require a trocar port, and increased instrument mobility can be gained by omitting the port. Strategic positioning of the thoracoscopic camera and the

endoscopic instruments is vital to the success and efficiency of the procedure (Table 32-5).

Excessive torque should be avoided when manipulating the instruments in VATS to avoid damaging the instruments as well as the complications of postoperative intercostal neuritis (Fig. 32-13). For simple biopsy procedures, a two-stick approach using a grasper through the operating thoracoscope often suffices (Fig. 32-14). This technique often requires alternating the positions of the thoracoscope and the stapler to facilitate the wedge resection (Fig. 32-15). If the view is inadequate or if the angle of the instrument is

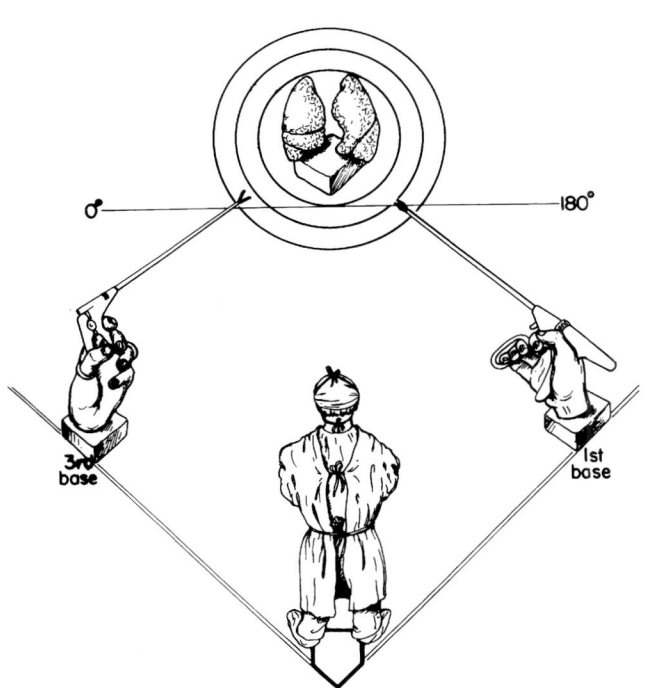

Fig. 32-12. Baseball diamond concept for triangulation of the instruments and thoracoscope for strategic visibility and manipulation of the target pathology. From Landreneau RJ: Video-assisted surgery: basic technical concepts and approach strategies. Ann Thorac Surg *54*:800, 1992b. With permission.

Table 32-5. Basic Video-Assisted Thoracic Surgery Operative Concepts

Conceptualize the three-dimensional location of the lesion from the computed tomographic scans to triangulate the trocars.

Ensure sufficient atelectasis of the operative hemithorax.

Thoracoscopy ports and thoracoscope are placed a distance across the chest cavity from the lesion to achieve a panoramic view of the operative field and to achieve room to manipulate the instruments.

Place the trocar sites in the chest wall sufficiently apart to avoid instrument crowding and fencing during manipulation of the instruments.

Thoracoscopy ports are inserted under thoracoscopic visualization, as are subsequent insertion of operating instruments, to avoid injury to lung or other intrathoracic structures.

Maintain the operative instruments and the thoracoscope in the same 180-degree arc to keep the same video-endoscopic perspective and avoid mirror-imaging.

The surgeon should use both hands to manipulate the instruments.

Manipulation and movement of the instruments should be conducted in an orderly and systematic fashion.

The instruments should be manipulated one by one, in a serial fashion, while avoiding random movements of multiple instruments.

Avoid excessive torque on the instruments or thoracoscope.

Become familiar with the operation and function of the required equipment (e.g., thoracoscope, video system, stapling devices) before surgery.

Conversion to thoracotomy is an appropriate option when the performance of VATS is limited by availability of necessary equipment, technical assistance, or clinical condition of the patient.

Use a retrieval device routinely (i.e., endobag) for extraction of suspected or potential neoplastic specimens.

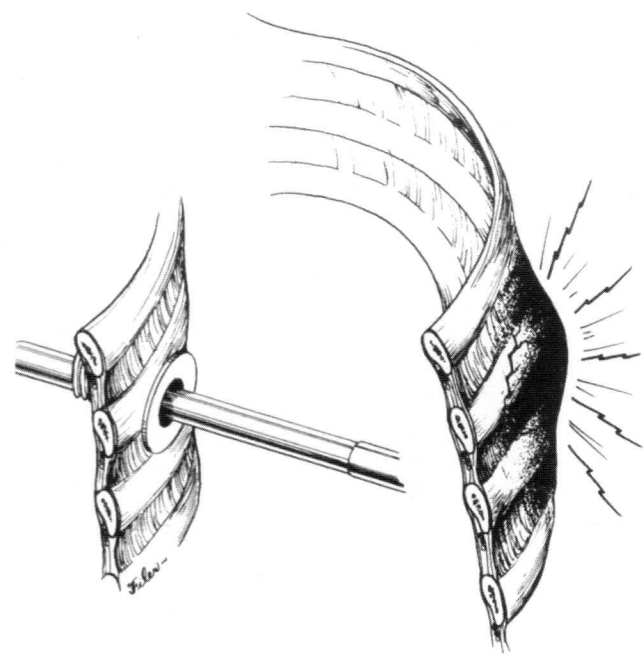

Fig. 32-13. The trocar-protected intercostal access site for thoracoscopic introduction, illustrated as a potential site of intercostal neuronal injury and rib fracture caused by excessive torquing of the instrumentation at the interspace. From Landreneau RJ, et al: Prevalence of chronic pain following pulmonary resection by thoracotomy or video-assisted thoracic surgery. J Thorac Surg *107*:1079, 1994. With permission.

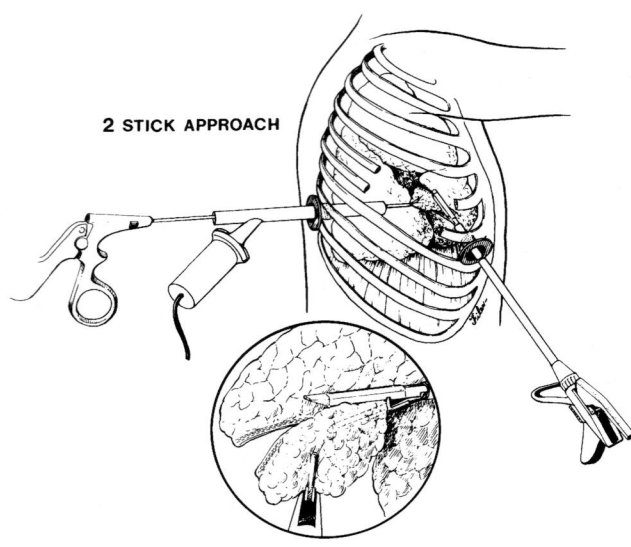

Fig. 32-14. Two-stick thoracoscopic lung biopsy approach. Insert depicts videoscopic view of the grasping instrument as it appears through the biopsy channel of the operating thoracoscope and the endoscopic stapling device crossing beneath the grasped lung tissue. From Ferson PF, et al: Thoracoscopic vs. "open" lung biopsy for the diagnosis of infiltrate lung disease. J Thorac Cardiovasc Surg *106*:194, 1993. With permission.

inappropriate for the desired manipulation, options include alternating the port sites or establishing a more favorable site of intercostal access for a three-stick approach (Fig. 32-16). Sometimes, by changing or alternating the location of the instruments and thoracoscope, a different perspective can be gained to achieve the task at hand. Last, conversion to a limited utility thoracotomy or standard open thora-

cotomy is wise if compromise of the diagnostic or therapeutic intent is otherwise jeopardized.

Manipulation of the operative table is also important in the course of a VATS procedure. For most cases, the table is rotated posteriorly to expose more of the anterior thorax. For cases involving an anterior lesion, a more posterior approach is achieved by rotating the table anteriorly and placing the ports more posteriorly. The use of Trendelenburg's and reverse Trendelenburg's positions is also helpful to allow gravity to keep the lung out of the operative field. To minimize muscular tension and fatigue in the surgeon's arms and

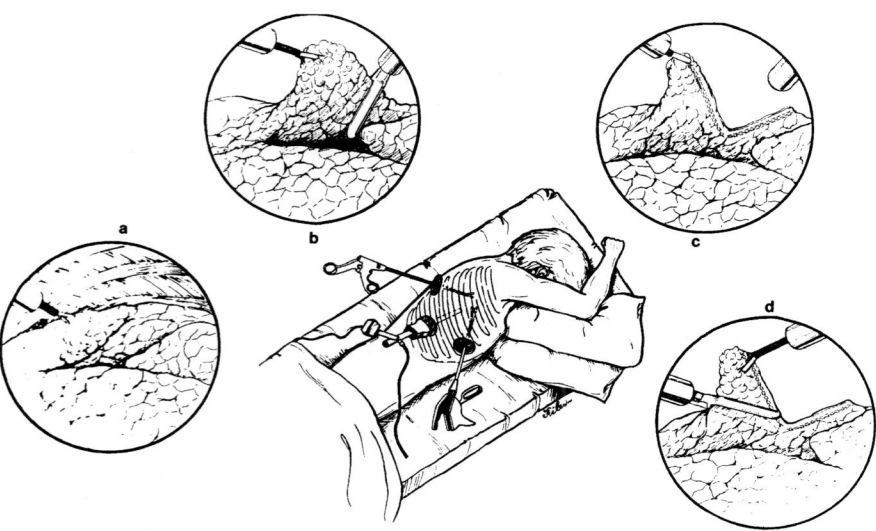

Fig. 32-15. a–d. Serial application of the endostapling device to accomplish a standard V wedge resection of the lung with a three-stick technique. Note that the intercostal access position of the stapling device and the grasping instruments are reversed to complete the stapled wedge resection expeditiously. From Dowling RD, et al: Thoracoscopic wedge resection of the lung. Surg Rounds *16*:341, 1993. With permission.

3 STICK APPROACH

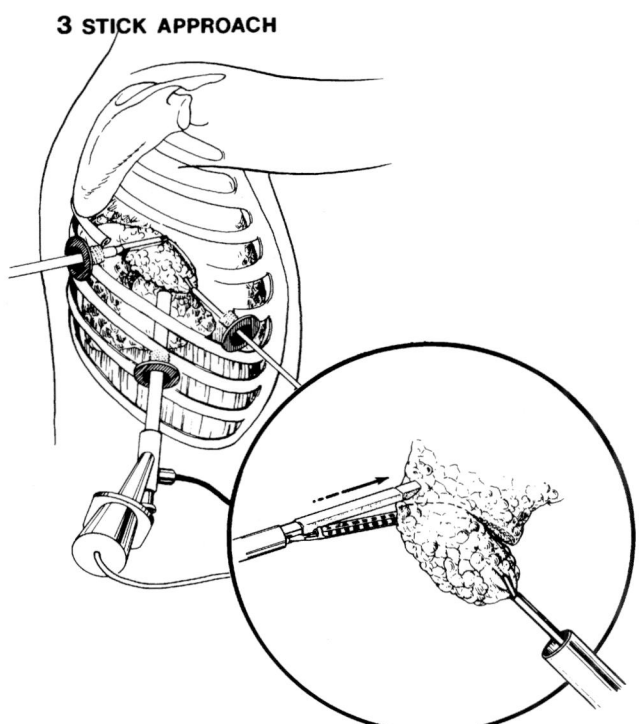

Fig. 32-16. Drawing of intercostal access typically used for a three-stick intercostal access approach for video-assisted thoracic surgical wedge resection of the lung using the endoscopic stapling device. From Ferson PF, et al: Thoracoscopic vs. "open" lung biopsy for the diagnosis of infiltrate lung disease. J Thorac Cardiovasc Surg *106*:194, 1993. With permission.

hands, the operating table should be lowered so that the handles of the instruments are at the level of the surgeon's elbow or slightly lower, thereby keeping the surgeon's wrists in neutral position and the elbows in slight extension (elbows held slightly beyond 90 degrees).

SPECIFIC PROBLEMS

Lung Nodules

Several procedures and techniques greatly facilitate VATS when used for excision of lung nodules, as Mack (1993) and one of us (R.J.L.) (1993a) and colleagues have detailed. An appreciation of the three-dimensional location of the lesion within the hemithorax by review of the radiographs is paramount. Again, complete ipsilateral pulmonary atelectasis is crucial. Pleural adhesions hindering pulmonary parenchymal collapse should be lysed by sharp dissection or electrocautery as necessary. With adequate collapse, most pleural and subpleural-based nodules 1 cm or larger are evident. Smaller nodules or nodules situated deeper in the lung may be seen as a subtle puckering of the visceral pleural surface. A sweeping motion over the surface of the lung parenchyma

with a blunt instrument where the lesion is suspected may reveal the mass as a slight irregularity in the texture of the lung. Lastly, if these maneuvers are unsuccessful, the lung can be elevated toward the chest wall for direct digital palpation. When difficulty in locating the lesion is anticipated beforehand, Mack (1993) and Schwartz (1994) and their coworkers have suggested that a preoperative CT-guided needle localization or subpleural dye injection may be a useful adjunct.

Complex Empyema and Clotted Hemothorax

The successful application of VATS to débride and drain loculated empyemas and clotted hemothoraces has been described by Hutter and associates (1985), Ridley and Braimbridge (1991), and one of us (R.J.L.) and colleagues (1996). Review of appropriate radiographs, including plain films and CT scans, is conducted to determine the site of the major pocket or loculation of the empyema. This location is confirmed intraoperatively by needle aspiration. A 10-mm port is introduced from a dependent direction into the loculation (Fig. 32-17). Specimens are sent for Gram's stain, acid-fast stain, routine and anaerobic cultures, as well as cultures for mycobacterium and fungus. Evacuation of the empyema pocket is facilitated by the use of a large-bore

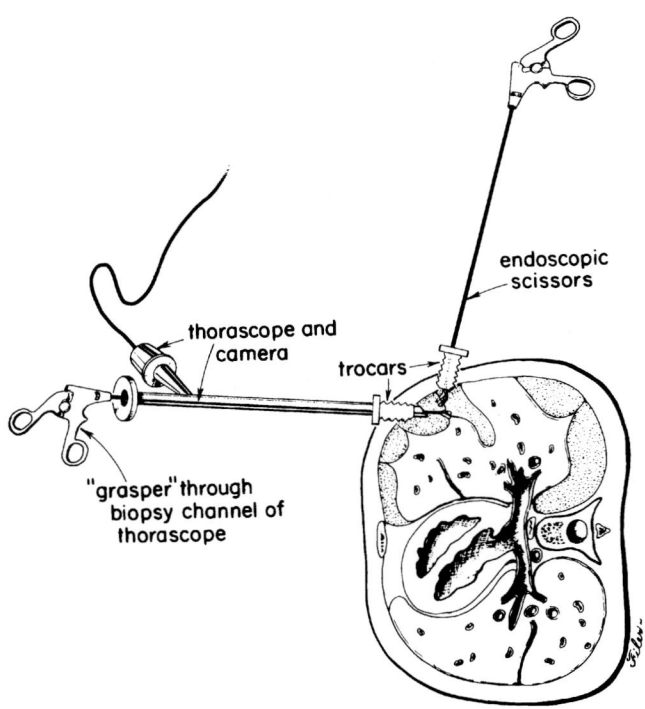

Fig. 32-17. Illustration depicting the importance of accurate intercostal access for video-assisted thoracic surgical intervention on loculated pleural effusions. From Landreneau RJ, et al: Thoracoscopy for empyema and hemothorax. Chest *109*:18, 1995. With permission.

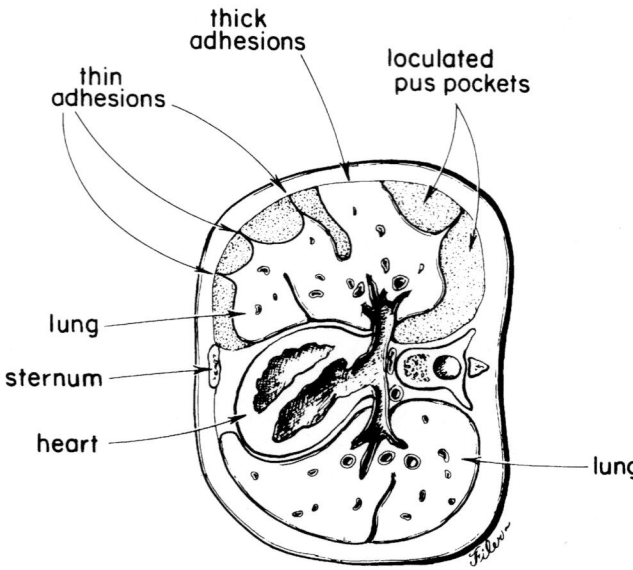

Fig. 32-18. Illustration of the pathologic processes resulting in loculated pleural processes requiring video-assisted thoracic surgical intervention. From Landreneau RJ, et al: Thoracoscopy for empyema and hemothorax. Chest *109*:18, 1996. With permission.

(No. 36 to 40F) sucker (Snowden Pencer, Inc., Tucker, GA) to remove the pus and fibrinous debris. Once the pocket is drained, additional access sites can be established under thoracoscopic guidance and additional instruments introduced. Minor loculations and adhesions are taken down, but areas of thick adhesions between the lung and the chest wall are generally left alone (Fig. 32-18). A significant risk of injury to the lung exists when mobilizing dense adhesions, with resultant bleeding or air leak, whereas it is unusual for these broad adhesions to be primarily responsible for limiting proper lung reexpansion. When the cause of the pleural process is in question, pleural biopsy is performed to evaluate for infectious (e.g., tuberculosis) or malignant etiologies.

As outlined by one of us (R.J.L.) and associates (1996), VATS can be used with a high degree of success in properly selected patients for débridement and drainage of empyema. Early empyemas and hemothoraces are excellent candidates for VATS, whereas chronic empyemas should be initially approached by VATS with a low threshold to convert to thoracotomy. Early empyemas in the exudative and fibrinopurulent phases generally were found to have thin fibrinous septae between loculations and a soft fibrinous pleural peel that was successfully débrided by VATS in 98% of cases. Similarly, we had excellent results with VATS drainage of clotted hemothoraces (100%) that had failed tube thoracostomy drainage. Associated multiorgan trauma and coagulopathy are treated before evaluation by VATS. In contrast to early empyema and clotted hemothoraces, chronic empyema is marked by the subacute nature of the inflammatory process, often with a resultant thick and fibrotic pleural peel causing varying degrees of lung entrapment. This fibrotic

process is variable. As we discovered in 54% of the chronic empyemas approached by VATS, the peel had not yet progressed to the dense fibrotic stage, and they were successfully decorticated and drained thoracoscopically. The other 46% of chronic empyemas were found to have a dense peel that required thoracotomy for adequate decortication. Experience and clinical judgment dictate when a case should be converted to thoracotomy.

In summary, we advocate VATS techniques for complex or loculated empyemas in the acute phase. Empyemas in the subacute phase (approximately 3 weeks) may still be successfully addressed by VATS in one-half the cases. Empyemas that are demonstrated, either on CT scan or intraoperative evaluation, to have a thick and fibrotic peel with lung entrapment should be decorticated by open techniques. Once issues of acute trauma and coagulopathy have been addressed, VATS should be used early in the management of the patient with a clotted hemothorax to avoid the sequelae of late fibrothorax or secondary infection of the intrathoracic clot as Mancini (1993) and one of us (R.J.L.) and coworkers (1996) have outlined.

Chest Tubes

At the conclusion of the VATS operation, one or more of the intercostal access sites is used for chest tubes in most patients. Proper placement is confirmed by thoracoscopy before removal of the thoracoscope. The remaining intercostal access sites are closed in layers, ensuring an air-tight closure. In the extremely thin patient, however, the chest tubes may have to be placed through separate incisions using an oblique subcutaneous tunnel to avoid air entry when the chest tube is removed. Administration of a long-acting local anesthetic (e.g., 0.25% bupivacaine) at the intercostal sites is helpful with postoperative pain management. Russo and associates (1998) reported on the safety and efficacy of early removal of chest tubes in the immediate perioperative period after elective VATS stapled wedge biopsy. Thirty-one of 33 patients met criteria (full lung expansion on chest radiography and no air leak) and had their chest tubes removed within 90 minutes after surgery. Five patients developed a small pneumothorax that was followed expectantly, and no patient required a repeat tube thoracostomy.

Extraction of Tissue Specimens

Removal of pathologic tissues from the thoracic cavity can be a problem encountered with VATS. Technically, extraction of a specimen is facilitated by placing it in a sterile glove or a commercially available plastic sleeved bag such as the Pleatman sac (Cabot Medical, Langhorn, PA), or EndoCatch (United States Surgical Corporation, Norwalk, CT) for retrieval through one of the intercostal access sites. Routine use of a retrieval bag avoids placing undue tension

Table 32-6. Incidence of Common Postoperative Complications after Video-Assisted Thoracic Surgery and Thoracotomy

Author	Year	No.	Persistent Air Leak >7 days	Respiratory Failure Requiring Prolonged Mechanical Ventilation	Postoperative Bleeding Requiring 1 U Transfusion or Reexploration	Superficial Sound Infections	Empyema	Deep Venous Thrombosis	Death
Yim and Liu	1996	1337	21 (1.6%)	4 (0.3%)	6 (0.4%)	13	2	1	1
Jancovici et al.	1996	937	63 (6.7%)	1 (0.01%)	18 (1.9%)		3	5	5
Inderbitzi and Grillet	1996	5280	93 (1.8%)	2 (0.04%)	23 (0.4%)			2	16
Krasna et al.	1996	348	3 (0.9%)	1 (0.3%)	3 (0.9%)		2		0
Kaiser and Bavaria	1993	266	10 (3.8%)		5 (1.9%)	5			
Hazlerigg et al.	1993a	1820	43 (3.2%)	13 (1.0)	21 (1.6%)	21	8		0
Nagasaki et al.	1982	961	16 (1.7%)			17		8	

on the specimen when it is withdrawn from the chest, risking morselization of the specimen and increasing the risk of tumor deposition. For larger specimens, a sterile plastic endoscopic video camera sleeve works well as a retrieval device. When retrieving larger specimens, the intercostal access incision can be slightly lengthened and slight rib spreading used to accommodate the size of the specimen.

COMPLICATIONS OF VIDEO-ASSISTED THORACIC SURGERY

Surgical complications after large series of VATS procedures have been reviewed by Hazlerigg and associates (1993b), Yim and Liu (1996), Jancovici and associates (1996), Inderbitzi and Grillet (1996), Krasna and coworkers (1996), and Kaiser and Bavaria (1993). These large series include the full spectrum of operations performed with VATS techniques, and common postoperative complications included prolonged air leaks, bleeding, and infection. However, the reported rates of common complications after VATS interventions were similar or less than a historical series of open thoracotomy as reported by Nagasaki and associates (1982) (Table 32-6).

However, several procedural-related complications are specific to VATS. These include complications related to the insertion of thoracoscopy ports, postoperative intercostal neuritis, stapling device failure, and port site deposition of tumor. As one of us (R.J.L.) and colleagues (1998) have reviewed, thoracoscopy port-related complications can be minimized by always inserting the port under thoracoscopic visualization, using blunt-tipped trocars designed for thoracoscopy, and avoiding the use of sharply pointed laparoscopy ports. The port should be inserted without undue force and always under control, otherwise the port may pop into the chest blindly with resultant injury to intrathoracic structures (Fig. 32-19). Intercostal neuritis is commonly caused by excessive pressure to the intercostal nerve. This is avoided by placing the skin incision for the port directly over the proposed intercostal space, instead of the more traditional oblique subcutaneous tunnel. This allows for a full 360-degree mobility of the port, reducing the amount of torque on the instruments and the intercostal nerves.

Furthermore, excessive spreading of the intercostal soft tissues and the passage of sharp or awkwardly shaped instruments should be minimized or avoided. Modern endoscopic stapling techniques are quite reliable, although instances of stapler failure have been described. However, the likelihood of stapler failure is increased if the stapler reload is not properly seated or if tissue, staples, or other debris are left on the anvil or hinge mechanism of the stapler. Thus, close attention during the reloading process to ensure that the stapler is properly assembled and the anvil is clean can avoid a potential catastrophe.

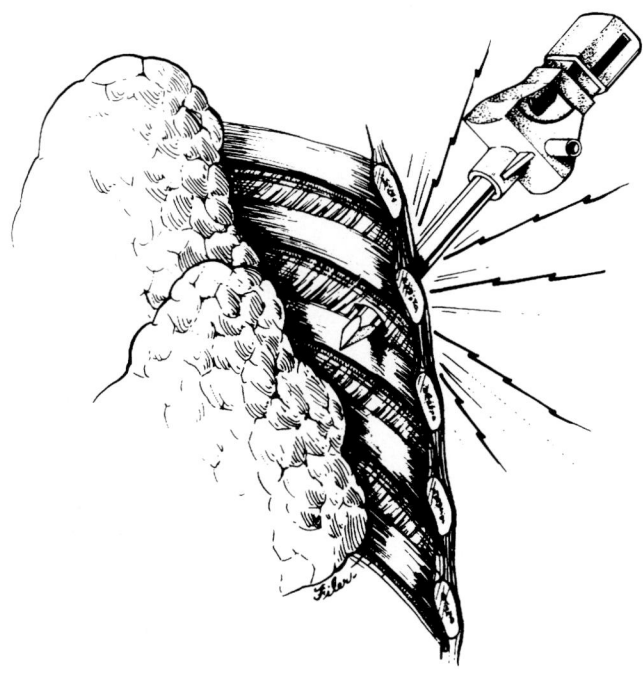

Fig. 32-19. Direct intercostal neurovascular injury related to trocar or endosurgical access during the video-assisted thoracic surgery procedure. Also note the sharply pointed laparoscopy trocar depicted that should be avoided in video-assisted thoracic surgery. From Landreneau RJ, et al: Prevalence of chronic pain following pulmonary resection by thoracotomy or video-assisted thoracic surgery. J Thorac Cardiovasc Surg *107*:1079, 1994. With permission.

Deposition and dissemination of tumor cells during VATS with subsequent tumor recurrence has been described as a potential complication after VATS biopsy of suspected lymph nodes or pulmonary wedge resections. This phenomenon is hardly unique, as access site recurrences have been reported after laparoscopic operations and after VATS for a wide variety of neoplasms, as noted by Downey and associates (1996, 1998). Many of these reports are anecdotal, involving a wide degree of pathology and surgical techniques. In a review by Collard and Reymond (1996), increased risk of parietal seeding and early local recurrence after VATS for cancer was associated with pulling the neoplastic tissue through a stab incision. Collard and Reymond (1996), Yim and Liu (1996), and Jancovici and associates (1996) all noted an increased risk of local recurrence at the thoracoscopy port sites when a retrieval device (i.e., a glove or bag) was not used. They, along with Krasna and colleagues (1996), further noted that recurrence was more likely in operations when mesothelioma, metastatic sarcoma or melanoma, or malignant pleural effusion were present.

On the other hand, these series have illustrated that many postoperative complications related to thoracic surgery, such as atelectasis, pneumonia, cardiac arrhythmias, or deep venous thrombosis, are found less commonly after VATS than open thoracotomy. This is likely a benefit of the decreased pain-related morbidity of the operation. Certainly, a central appeal of VATS has been the documented decreased postoperative pain and decreased operative morbidity to the chest, back, and shoulder muscles resulting in decreased requirements for narcotic analgesics, improved pulmonary toilet, and a more expedient return to preoperative level of activities as compared with open techniques.

REFERENCES

Acuff TE, et al: Role of mechanical stapling devices in thoracoscopic pulmonary resection. Ann Thorac Surg 56:749, 1993.

Alexander J: The Collapse Therapy of Pulmonary Tuberculosis. Springfield, IL: Charles C Thomas, 1937, pp. 313–316.

Benumof JL: Physiology of the open chest and one-lung ventilation. In Kaplan JA (ed): Thoracic Anesthesia. New York: Churchill Livingstone, 1983, pp. 287–316.

Bergquist S, Nordenstam H: Thoracoscopy and pleural biopsy in the diagnosis of pleurisy. Scand J Respir Dis 47:64, 1966.

Braimbridge MV: The history of thoracoscopic surgery. Ann Thorac Surg 56:610, 1993.

Brandt HJ: Indikation und Technik der Diagnostischen Thorakoskopie. Atemwegs Lungenkrankh 3:150, 1978.

Collard JM, Reymond MA: Video-assisted thoracic surgery (VATS) for cancer–risk of parietal seeding and of early local recurrence. Int Surg 81:343, 1996.

Coulaud E, DesChamps P: Decouverte pleuroscopique d'une importante perforation pulmonaire asymptomatique. Guerison Rapide Spontanee. Rev Tuberculose 11:825, 1947.

Dowling RD, et al: Thoracoscopic Nd:YAG laser resection of a solitary pulmonary nodule. Chest 102:1903, 1992c.

Dowling RD, Ferson PF, Landreneau RJ: Thoracoscopic resection of pulmonary metastasis. Chest 102:1450, 1992b.

Dowling RD, Wachs ME, Ferson PF: Thoracoscopic Nd:YAG laser resection of a pulmonary metastasis. Cancer 70:1873, 1992a.

Downey RJ: Complications after video-assisted thoracic surgery. In McKenna RJ (ed): Chest Surgery Clinics of North America, Philadelphia: WB Saunders, 1998, pp. 907–918.

Downey RJ, McCormack P, LoCicero J: Dissemination of malignant tumors after video-assisted thoracic surgery. J Thorac Cardiovasc Surg 111:954, 1996.

Ferson PF, et al: Thoracoscopic vs. "open" lung biopsy for the diagnosis of infiltrate lung disease. J Thorac Cardiovasc Surg 106:194, 1993.

Fourestier M, Duret M: Nécessité de la biopsie pleurale pour le diagnostic de l'endotheliome de la plevre. Presse Med 32:467, 1943.

Hazelrigg SR, et al: Cost analysis for thoracoscopy: thoracoscopic wedge resection. Ann Thorac Surg 56:633, 1993b.

Hazelrigg SR, et al: The effect of muscle sparing versus standard posterolateral thoracotomy on pulmonary function, muscle strength, and postoperative pain. J Thorac Cardiovasc Surg 101:394, 1991.

Hazelrigg SR, et al: Video assisted thoracic surgery study group. Ann Thorac Surg 56:1039, 1993a.

Hutter JA, Harari D, Baimbridge MV: The management of empyema thoracis by thoracoscopy and irrigation. Ann Thorac Surg 39:517, 1985.

Inderbitzi RG, Grillet MP: Risk and hazards of video-thoracoscopic surgery: a collective review. Eur J Cardiothorac Surg 10:483, 1996.

Jacobeus HC: The practical importance of thoracoscopy in surgery of the chest. Surg Gynecol Obstet 34:289, 1922.

Jacobeus HC: Possibility of the use of cystoscope for the investigation of the serous cavities. Munch Med Wochenschr 57:2090, 1910.

Jacobeus HC: Die Thorakoskopie und ihre praktische Bedeutung. Ergebn Ges Med 7:112, 1925.

Jancovici R, et al: Complications of video-assisted thoracic surgery: a five year experience. Ann Thorac Surg 61:533, 1996.

Kaiser LR, Bavaria JE: Complications of thoracoscopy. Ann Thorac Surg 56:796, 1993.

Kirby TJ, et al: Video-assisted thoracic surgery versus muscle-sparing thoracotomy. A randomized trial. J Thorac Cardiovasc Surg 109:997, 1995.

Krasna MJ, Deshmukh S, McLaughlin JS: Complications of thoracoscopy. Ann Thorac Surg 61:1066, 1996.

Landreneau RJ, et al: Differences in postoperative pain, shoulder function, and morbidity between video-assisted thoracic surgery and muscle sparing "open" thoracotomies. Ann Thorac Surg 56:1285, 1993b.

Landreneau RJ, et al: Effect of minimally invasive approaches on acute and chronic postoperative pain. In McKenna RJ (ed): Chest Surgery Clinics of North America. Philadelphia: WB Saunders, 1998, pp. 891–906.

Landreneau RJ, et al: Nd:YAG laser assisted pulmonary resections. Ann Thorac Surg 51:973, 1991a.

Landreneau RJ, et al: Postoperative pain-related morbidity: video-assisted thoracic surgery versus thoracotomy. Ann Thorac Surg 56:1285, 1993c.

Landreneau RJ, et al: Prevalence of chronic pain after pulmonary resection by thoracotomy or video-assisted thoracic surgery. J Thorac Cardiovasc Surg 107:1079, 1994.

Landreneau RJ, et al: Strategic planning for video-assisted thoracic surgery "VATS." Ann Thorac Surg 56:615, 1993a.

Landreneau RJ, et al: Thoracoscopy for empyema and hemothorax. Chest 109:18, 1996.

Landreneau RJ, et al: Thoracoscopic Nd:YAG laser assisted pulmonary resection. Ann Thorac Surg 52:1176, 1991b.

Landreneau RJ, et al: Thoracoscopic resection of an anterior mediastinal tumor. Ann Thorac Surg 54:142, 1992c.

Landreneau RJ, et al: Thoracoscopic resection of 85 pulmonary lesions. Ann Thorac Surg 54:415, 1992a.

Landreneau RJ, et al: VATS wedge resection of the lung using the neodymium:yttrium-aluminum garnet laser. Ann Thorac Surg 56:758, 1993d.

Landreneau RJ, et al: Video-assisted thoracic surgery: basic technical concepts and intercostal approach strategies. Ann Thorac Surg 54:800, 1992b.

Lewis RJ, Caccavale RJ, Sisler GE: Surgical treatment of diffuse end-stage bilateral bullous disease of the lung using video-assisted thoracic surgery and the argon beam coagulator. Ann Thorac Surg 55:1394, 1993.

LoCicero J III, et al: Experimental air leak in lung sealed by low-energy carbon dioxide laser irradiation. Chest 87:820, 1985.

LoCicero J III, et al: Laser-assisted parenchymal sparing pulmonary resection. J Thorac Cardiovasc Surg 97:732, 1989.

Mack MJ, et al: Techniques for localization of pulmonary nodules for thoracoscopic resection. J Thorac Cardiovasc Surg 106:550, 1993.

Mancini M, et al: Early evacuation of clotted blood in hemothorax using thoracoscopy. J Trauma 34:144, 1993.

Melendez JA, Fischer ME: Preoperative pulmonary evaluation of the thoracic surgical patient. In Wilson RS (ed): Chest Surgery Clinics of North America. Philadelphia: WB Saunders, Philadelphia, 1997, pp. 641–654.

Nagasaki F, Flehinger BJ, Martini N: Complications of surgery in the treatment of carcinoma of the lung. Chest 82:25, 1982.

Ridley PD, Braimbridge MV: Thoracoscopic debridement and pleural irrigation in the management of empyema thoracis. Ann Thorac Surg 51:461, 1991.

Russo L, et al: Early chest tube removal after video-assisted thoracoscopic wedge resection of the lung. Ann Thorac Surg 66:1751, 1998.

Sawabata N, et al: In vitro comparison between argon beam coagulation and Nd:YAG laser in lung contraction therapy. Ann Thorac Surg 62:1485, 1996.

Schwartz RE, et al: Needle localization thoracoscopic resection (NLTR) of indeterminate pulmonary nodules: impact on management of patients with malignant disease. Ann Surg Oncol 2:49, 1994.

Swierenga J, Wagenaar JP, Bergstein PG: The value of thoracoscopy in the diagnosis and treatment of diseases affecting the pleura and the lung. Pneumologie 151:11, 1974.

Teplick R: Preoperative cardiac assessment of the thoracic surgical patient. In Wilson RS (ed): Chest Surgery Clinics of North America. Philadelphia: WB Saunders, 1997, pp. 655–696.

Wernly JA, DeMeester TR: Preoperative assessment of patients undergoing lung resection for cancer. In Roth JA, Ruckedeschel JC, Weisenburger TH (eds): Thoracic Oncology. Philadelphia: WB Saunders, 1989, pp. 156–176.

Wilson RS. Lung isolation, tube design, and technical approaches. In Wilson RS (ed): Chest Surgery Clinics of North America. Philadelphia: WB Saunders, 1997, pp. 735–752.

Worsey J, Landreneau RJ: Approach strategies and special instrumentation for thoracic surgery. In Manncke K, Rosin RD (eds): Minimal Access Thoracic Surgery. Philadelphia: Chapman and Hall Medical, Lippincott–Raven, 1998, pp. 39–52.

Yim APC, Liu HP: Complications and failures of video-assisted thoracic surgery: experience from two centers in Asia. Ann Thorac Surg 61:538, 1996.

CHAPTER 33

Video-Assisted Thoracic Surgery for Wedge Resection, Lobectomy, and Pneumonectomy

Robert J. McKenna, Jr.

The expectation for minimally invasive thoracic procedures has been that they would reduce morbidity, mortality, and hospital stay and allow quicker return to regular activities for patients after procedures that formerly required major incisions. This expectation has yet to be conclusively proven, although some of the early results are encouraging. The techniques for lung resection—wedge, lobectomy, and pneumonectomy—with video-assisted thoracic surgery (VATS) are evolving, but this chapter presents details about the current approaches.

VIDEO-ASSISTED THORACIC SURGICAL RESECTION OF LUNG NODULES

Currently, lung nodules are more commonly resected with VATS than with thoracotomy. Hazelrigg and associates (1993) showed that, compared with an open procedure, VATS has a shorter hospital length of stay, although the cost savings from a shorter length of stay are equal to the additional cost of the extra equipment for the VATS procedure, so no overall cost savings exist. The VATS resections in this study were performed with disposable equipment, so a cost savings may be realized if the procedure is performed with reusable instruments.

A centrally located mass may be difficult to resect with VATS, and a small mass (smaller than 5 mm) may be difficult to locate with VATS. Video-assisted thoracic surgical wedge resection is usually undertaken for a peripherally located mass between 1 and 5 cm in size.

Operative Technique for Wedge Resection

Under one-lung general anesthesia, the patient is placed in a full lateral decubitus position, as for a posterolateral thoracotomy. A trocar and thoracoscope are placed through the eighth intercostal space to obtain the optimal panoramic view of the thoracic cavity. Usually, two additional incisions are made for an instrument to hold the lung and for the endoscopic stapler. The exact location of the incisions depends on the location of the lung nodule so the VATS incision can be extended for whatever incision is required if further lung resection is performed. Generally, a 1- to 2-cm incision is placed in the midaxillary line for palpation of the lung with a finger and a 1- to 2-cm incision in the midclavicular line in the sixth interspace for a stapler.

Localization of Lung Nodules by Video-Assisted Thoracic Surgery

Because the small incisions used for VATS limit the surgeon's ability to palpate the lung, a key to successful performance of resection of a lung mass via VATS is the ability to find the lesion. It is, therefore, important for the surgeon to correlate the location of a mass on computed tomographic scan with the patient's anatomy. An experienced thoracic surgeon can almost always find a lung mass in this fashion.

Rarely, preoperative localization of a lung nodule is helpful when a lung mass is small (usually smaller than 5 mm) or deeper (3 cm) below the pleura. Under computed tomographic guidance, the radiologist places a hooked wire in the nodule. The wire should be cut off at skin level because it does not matter if it retracts into the chest. In contrast, if the wire has been taped to the chest without being cut, the wire may become dislodged from the mass if the patient develops a pneumothorax. When the wire has been positioned, the patient is then transferred to the operating room for resection of the area of the lung with the wire. The mass can usually be palpated in the specimen without the need for a specimen radiograph to confirm that the mass has been resected. As Mack and colleagues (1993) noted, this technique is associated with minimal complications (e.g., rare dislodgment of the wire or pneumothorax). Wire localization was used more often in the early days of VATS before surgeons realized that it was rarely necessary.

Wedge Resection

The use of endoscopic staples is the most common method for wedge resections of a lung nodule. Ring forceps through two incisions position the mass for the stapler. Often, the stapler is fired through different incisions to complete the resection.

Alternatively, electrocautery or laser can resect the mass and the lung parenchyma is sutured. A fourth incision is often made for another instrument to provide good traction and countertraction on the lung for optimal function of the electrocautery. Smoke from the electrocautery can be problematic. Suction in the thoracic cavity causes the lung to reexpand unless air can flow into the thoracic cavity through at least one of the incisions. Many thoracic surgeons find endoscopic suturing difficult, so this approach is less common than wedge resection with staples.

Cancer has recurred in thoracoscopy incisions after biopsy as noted by Downey and associates (1996) in a review of 21 cases. If the lung mass could be a malignancy, it should be placed in a bag for removal to protect the incision. Several endoscopic bags are available for removal of the usual wedge resection.

GENERAL FEATURES OF A VIDEO-ASSISTED THORACIC SURGICAL LOBECTOMY

A VATS lobectomy should be the same procedure that is performed with an open operation. This includes the individual ligation of vessels and bronchus for the lobectomy and a lymph node dissection or sampling as recommended by the author and colleagues (1995). The indications and contraindications for the procedure (Tables 33-1 and 33-2) are similar to the indications for lobectomy via thoracotomy. The tumor must be small enough for removal through the VATS incisions. The author and Fischel also have demonstrated in 1994 that a lobectomy by VATS may be easier for older patients than a thoracotomy. The author and associates (1996) have found that the combination of VATS lung volume reduction surgery and VATS lobectomy allows a complete cancer operation for some patients who otherwise would not be candidates for an operation because of poor pulmonary function. Centrally located tumors require a thoracotomy to determine whether sleeve resection or a pneumonectomy is appropriate. The dissection around the vessels and in the mediastinum is more difficult after chemotherapy or radiation, so a thoracotomy is usually necessary. This section first describes the techniques that are common to all VATS lobectomies and then some features that are unique to resection of specific lobes.

One-Lung Ventilation

After induction of general anesthesia with one-lung ventilation, the patient is placed in a full lateral decubitus position. To allow the maximal time possible for the lung to collapse, one-lung ventilation is instituted while the patient is positioned and the surgeon goes to scrub his or her hands. If the lung has not collapsed enough when the procedure begins, the bronchoscope is passed into the ipsilateral main stem bronchus for suctioning to encourage further atelectasis.

Incisions

Proper placement of incisions is critical (Fig. 33-1; see Color Fig. 33-1). The trocar and thoracoscope are placed in the eighth intercostal space in the midaxillary line on the right or posterior axillary line on the left to avoid obstruction of vision by the pericardial fat pad. This provides the best panoramic view of the thoracic cavity. The 30-degree lens allows the surgeon to see around structures in the hilum better than the 0-degree lens. The camera incision is usually placed over a rib and angled superiorly to the interspace to reduce irritation of the intercostal nerve when the trocar is rotated. All other incisions are made directly over an interspace.

Through a 1- to 2-cm incision in the auscultatory triangle, a curved ring forceps manipulates the lung for inspection of the pleura and exposure of the hilum to determine the proper position for the other incisions. Lower placement of this posterior incision improves the angle of the stapler for the superior pulmonary vein and assistance with a lower lobectomy. Slightly higher placement of the incision helps with paratracheal node dissection, but makes the angle for the stapler on the pulmonary vein more difficult.

Table 33-2. Contraindications for Video-Assisted Thoracic Surgical Lobectomy

Nodal disease (benign or malignant)
Chest wall or mediastinal invasion (T_3 or T_4 tumor)
Endobronchial tumor seen at bronchoscopy
Neoadjuvant chemotherapy
Neoadjuvant radiation therapy
Positive mediastinoscopy

Table 33-1. Indications for Video-Assisted Thoracic Surgical Lobectomy

Clinical stage I lung cancer
Tumor size <5 cm
Benign disease (giant bulla, bronchiectasis, and so forth)
Physiologic operability

Position of the Surgeon

The surgeon usually stands on the front side of the patient and the dissection begins in the hilus. This is the approach used for lung resection through an anterolateral, muscle-sparing thoracotomy. This makes the procedure much easier than trying to perform the procedure with the approach for a posterolateral thoracotomy (see Right Upper Lobectomy, later in this chapter).

Hilar Dissection

Vessels in the hilus are dissected sharply through the utility thoracotomy incision with standard thoracotomy instruments, such as Metzenbaum scissors and DeBakey pickups. Hilar lymph nodes are removed as separate specimens to facilitate pathologic staging and to facilitate passage of the nonarticulating endoscopic stapler (EZ 35, Ethicon or Endo-GIA, US Surgical, Norwalk, CT) across the pulmonary vessels. Vascular isolation requires more dissection for a VATS procedure than is customary for a thoracotomy.

Stapling Devices

The fissure, bronchus, and pulmonary vessels larger than 5 mm are transected with surgical, usually endoscopic, staples (Figs. 33-2 through 33-4; see Color Fig.s 33-2 through 33-4). The vascular (20-mm) staples are used for the vessels, and the green cartridge (48-mm) staples are used on the fissure and the bronchus. Elevating the vessel with a tie aids placement of the stapler across the vessels. Articulation of the stapling devices is not necessary if the correct angle for

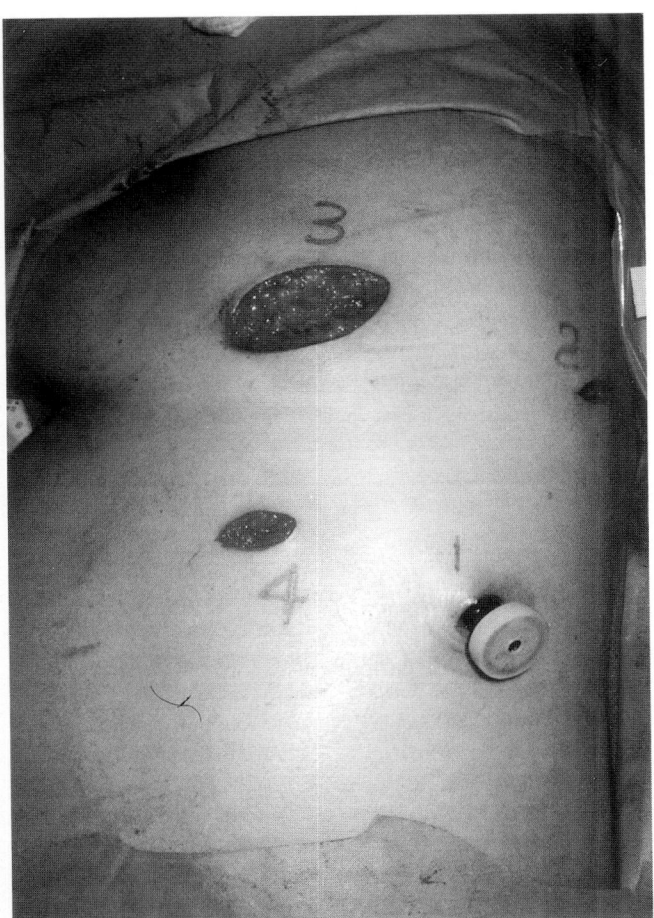

Fig. 33-1. The incisions for our approach to video-assisted thoracic surgical lobectomy including the following: (1) an incision for the trocar and the thoracoscope, (2) an incision in the auscultatory triangle for an assistant's instrument, (3) the utility thoracotomy incision, and (4) an incision in the midclavicular line for the stapler. (See Color Fig. 33-1.)

The utility thoracotomy incision is a 4- to 6-cm incision from the anterior edge of the latissimus dorsi muscle to the anterior axillary line. It is directly lateral to the superior pulmonary vein for an upper lobectomy or one interspace lower for a middle or lower lobectomy. The ribs are not spread, but a Weitlander retractor may be used to hold the soft tissues of the chest wall open for easier passage of instruments and to prevent the lung from expanding when suctioning in the chest. The hilar structures are easily accessible for dissection through this incision. Hilar vessels can be tied just as with an open procedure because a finger can usually reach through this incision to the vessels.

A 2-cm incision is made in the midclavicular line in the largest interspace close to the costal margin. A ring forceps through this incision can depress the diaphragm for visualization of the inferior pulmonary ligament or retract the middle lobe out of the visual field after the minor fissure has been completed during an upper lobectomy.

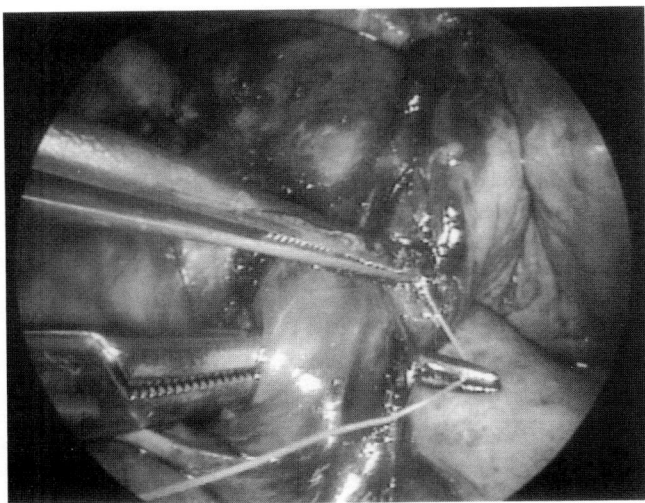

Fig. 33-2. A right-angle clamp pulls a tie around the middle lobe bronchus. (See Color Fig. 33-2.)

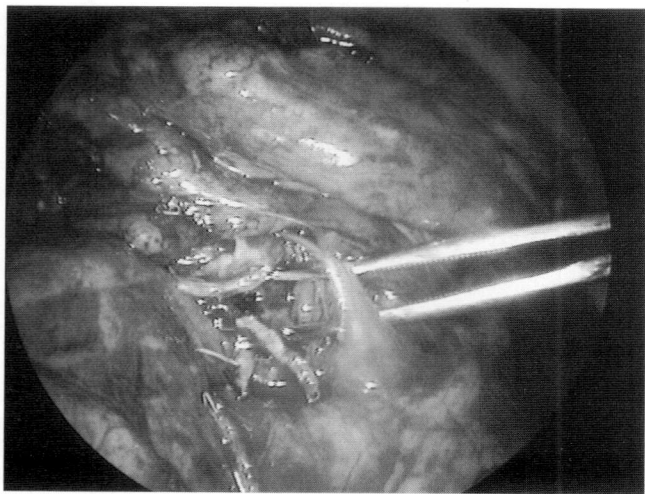

Fig. 33-3. A right-angle clamp mobilizes the right middle lobe artery. (See Color Fig. 33-3.)

the stapler is chosen. The incision that offers the best angle for stapling these structures is presented in Table 33-3.

Completeness of the Fissure

The fissure is usually completed after the vessels and bronchus are transected. The completeness of the fissure is, therefore, not a factor in determining the feasibility of performing a VATS lobectomy through an anterior approach.

Specimen Removal

To minimize the risk of contaminating the incision with the tumor, the lung specimen is placed in a bag for

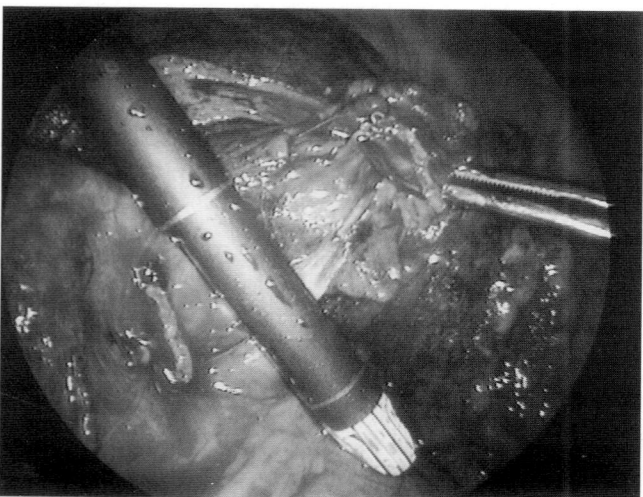

Fig. 33-4. The endoscopic stapler is across the right middle lobe artery. (See Color Fig. 33-4.)

Table 33-3. The Incision through which the Stapler Is Usually Passed for Transection of the Arteries, Veins, Bronchi, and Fissures

Incision	Tissue to Be Stapled
Posterior incision	Superior pulmonary vein
	Anterior trunk of upper lobe artery
	Middle lobe artery and vein
	Left upper lobe bronchus
Utility thoracotomy incision	Minor fissure
	Right upper lobe bronchus
	Inferior pulmonary vein
Midclavicular incision	Inferior pulmonary vein
	Anterior trunk of upper lobe artery
	Major fissure
	Additional left upper lobe arteries
	Lower lobe arteries
	Lower lobe bronchus

removal through the utility thoracotomy incision. An endocatch is large enough for a middle lobe. Removal of the other lobes or the entire lung requires the LapSac (Cook Urological, Bloomington, IN) because it is a larger bag. Some specimens are difficult to remove through the small utility thoracotomy incision. The lobes usually have a pyramidal shape. Removal of the lobe is easier if the narrow part of the lobe is removed first. The ribs may be spread for larger tumors or lobes.

Lymph Node Dissection

Either mediastinal node sampling or a complete lymph node dissection can be performed by VATS (Fig. 33-5; see Color Fig. 33-5). Paratracheal node dissection is easier if the azygos vein is transected, but that is usually not necessary. From posteriorly, a ring forceps lifts the azygos vein for exposure of the tracheobronchial angle node and pretracheal nodes. After the pleura is incised to mobilize the azygos vein, the vein is retracted inferiorly. The posterior ring forceps lifts the pleura and the paratracheal nodes as the surgeon dissects in the planes along the superior vena cava, trachea, and pericardium over the ascending aorta, from the azygos vein to the innominate artery. This exposure is easiest after a right upper lobectomy. After a middle or lower lobectomy, a ring forceps through the midclavicular incision should retract the upper lobe out of the visual field.

Anterior retraction of the lung through the utility thoracotomy incision provides exposure for subcarinal node dissection. This begins at the inferior pulmonary vein and proceeds superiorly. A ring forceps from posteriorly lifts the pleura over the nodes so the pleura can be incised along the intermediate bronchus and pericardium. Clips are applied to any tissue that does not easily separate when spreading along the bronchus and pericardium. The vagus nerve and esophagus are identified and preserved.

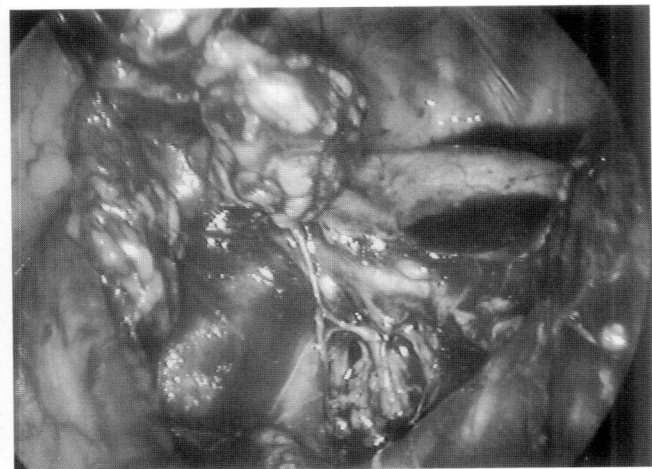

Fig. 33-5. The aortic-pulmonary window lymph nodes are elevated. This exposes the aorta, vagus nerve, and recurrent laryngeal nerve. (See Color Fig. 33-5.)

Aortopulmonary window lymph nodes usually are resected before left upper lobectomy because it makes mobilization of the arterial branches easier. Standard thoracotomy instruments perform this dissection through the utility thoracotomy incision. The pleura is cut parallel to the phrenic nerve and along the superior margin of the superior pulmonary vein from the pericardium and laterally along the apical vein as it crosses the anterior trunk. The nodes and pleura are then lifted to mobilize the tissue from the pulmonary artery. The pleura is incised along the vagus nerve. The recurrent laryngeal nerve is identified and preserved. The lymph node tissue is then dissected off the aorta.

Simultaneous Stapling Lobectomy

Lewis and Caccavale (1998) have reported thoracoscopic lobectomy with simultaneous stapling of the vessels and bronchus, rather than individual ligation, as described. This procedure has created considerable controversy because some surgeons view this as a large wedge resection. With this technique, the lobe is mobilized by partially completing the fissure. A TA stapler, used for open procedures, is fired across the remaining fissure, vessels, and bronchus.

TECHNIQUES FOR SPECIFIC LOBECTOMIES

Right Upper Lobectomy

Both an anterior and a posterior approach are possible for a right upper lobectomy. An anterior approach begins in the hilus. Removal of hilar nodes defines the middle lobe vein and the upper lobe vein. The minor fissure then can be completed with a stapler through the utility thoracotomy incision. The mobilization of the vein helps determine the proper placement of the stapler. Completion of the minor fissure provides access for a vascular stapler from the posterior incision to transect the vein. Removal of lobar nodes along the artery provides exposure of the arterial branches to the upper lobe. The best angle for the stapler to reach the anterior trunk is provided by the inferior incision in the midclavicular line. Additional, smaller branches are tied or clipped. Some thoracic surgeons may be unaccustomed to locating the posterior ascending artery anteriorly as it courses between the upper and intermediate bronchi. Through the utility thoracotomy incision, the bronchus is mobilized and stapled. The final maneuver is completion of the remaining fissure with the stapler through the midclavicular incision.

For the posterior approach, dissection of the posterior ascending artery is performed in the fissure. This approach is more limited than the anterior technique because an incomplete fissure is a contraindication to this approach. After transection of the posterior ascending artery, the fissure between the superior segment of the lower lobe and the posterior segment of the upper lobe is completed. The bronchus is mobilized and stapled from posteriorly. This provides exposure for the arteries.

Middle Lobectomy

Middle lobectomy begins with hilar dissection to remove hilar lymph nodes and mobilize the middle lobe vein. The vascular staple through the posterior incision transects the vein. This may be easier if the middle lobe is first mobilized by partially completing the fissure between the middle lobe and the lower lobe from inferiorly.

After transection of the vein, further completion of the fissure with the stapler through the anterior midclavicular incision exposes the bronchus. The posterior incision provides the best angle for stapling the middle lobe bronchus. This exposes the middle lobe artery that is usually small, so it can be tied or clipped. The final maneuver is stapling the minor fissure through the utility thoracotomy incision. Occasionally, the middle lobe has two arteries, so the surgeon should look for a second artery that is inferior to the bronchus.

Lower Lobectomy

The approach for a lower lobectomy depends on the completeness of the fissure. The operation is simpler when the fissure is well developed. The artery is mobilized in the fissure and transected with a stapler through the midclavicular incision. Through the same incision, a stapler completes the major fissure inferiorly to the level of the transected artery.

The pulmonary ligament is taken down and level 9 nodes harvested. The stapler for the inferior pulmonary vein goes through either the utility thoracotomy incision or the midclavicular incision. The bronchus is then well exposed for a stapler through the midclavicular incision. Finally, the remainder of the fissure is completed from inferiorly.

The operation for a lower lobectomy is different when the fissure is poorly developed. First, the pulmonary ligament is taken down, and the inferior pulmonary vein is transected. The bronchus and the artery can then be identified inferiorly by opening the inferior portion of the major fissure. Inferiorly, dissection along the anterior and lateral surfaces of the artery elevates the incomplete fissure off the artery. Completion of this part of the fissure provides good exposure for dissection of the artery. The artery and the bronchus can then be individually stapled. Finally, the fissure by the superior segment is completed with the stapler through the midclavicular incision.

Left Upper Lobectomy

The technique for a left upper lobectomy is similar to that for a right upper lobectomy. The approach begins anteriorly with hilar dissection and stapling of the superior pulmonary vein and anterior trunk of the artery. A stapler through the midclavicular incision is fired on the major fissure to expose the lingular artery that can be tied anteriorly or stapled posteriorly. The bronchus is thus exposed. The most dangerous part of a left upper lobectomy is mobilization of the bronchus because a right angle must be passed between the bronchus and the artery. After mobilization, the bronchus is stapled posteriorly. The remaining branches of the artery can then be seen. Dissection through the utility thoracotomy incision mobilizes these arteries to tie or clip them. Finally, the fissure is completed with multiple firings of the stapler through the midclavicular incision.

Left Lower Lobectomy

A left lower lobectomy is performed with the same technique as is used for a right lower lobectomy.

PNEUMONECTOMY

A pneumonectomy on either side is simpler than a lobectomy. The superior pulmonary vein is mobilized through the utility thoracotomy incision and stapled through the midclavicular incision. This exposes the artery. Because reports exist of endoscopic staples cutting without stapling the vessel, it is advisable to either use an endoscopic stapler with the knife removed or the TA stapler. The inferior pulmonary vein is stapled from anteriorly. Removal of subcarinal nodes provides access to the main stem bronchus at the level of the carina. Through the utility thoracotomy incision, a 30-mm TA stapler is then fired on the bronchus. An entire lung can usually be removed through the same-size incision as a lobe if the apex of the lung is passed first through the incision.

RESULTS OF VIDEO-ASSISTED THORACIC SURGICAL LOBECTOMY

Results of the larger published series of VATS lobectomy and pneumonectomy compare favorably with results expected with a thoracotomy (Table 33-4). Seven (0.6%) deaths in 1120 patients were caused by venous mesenteric infarct, myocardial infarction, respiratory failure, or unknown reasons.

In these series, complications occurred in 10.0 to 21.9% of the patients after VATS lobectomy. These included prolonged air leak (5 to 10%), arrhythmias, pneumonia, and respiratory failure. Transfusions were necessary in 0 to 3% of patients. Bronchial stump leak requiring surgical repair occurred in four cases (0.36%).

Conversion to Thoracotomy

Conversion from VATS to thoracotomy was necessary in 0 to 19.5% of patients in these series. Overall, 119 of 1120 operations were converted to thoracotomy (11.6%).

Most commonly, oncologic reasons, such as centrally located tumors requiring vascular control, a sleeve resection, or unsuspected T$_3$ tumors, attached to the chest wall,

Table 33-4. Major Published Series of Video-Assisted Thoracic Surgical Lobectomy and Pneumonectomy

Reference	No.	Cancer	Mortality	Length of Stay
Lewis and Caccavale (1998)	200	171	0	3.07
Yim et al. (1998)	214	168	1 (0.4%)	6.8
Kasada et al. (1998)	145	103	1 (0.8%)	NA
Hermansson et al. (1998)	30	15	0	4.4
Walker et al. (1996)	150	123	3 (2%)	7.2
Roviaro et al. (1998)	169	142	1 (0.5%)	NA
McKenna et al. (1998)	212	212	1 (0.5%)	4.6
Total	**1120**	**934**	**7 (0.6%)**	**5.28**

diaphragm, or superior vena cava, prompted the conversion. If a sleeve lobectomy may be required, conversion to thoracotomy is needed to evaluate the relationship of the tumor to the artery. Abnormal hilar nodes with granulomatous or metastatic disease adherent to the superior pulmonary vein are better evaluated and more safely resected with thoracotomy. Approximately 30% of the conversions to thoracotomy were for nononcologic reasons, such as pleural symphysis.

Intraoperative Hemorrhage

Bleeding from a pulmonary vessel during a VATS procedure can be troublesome and dangerous because access is limited. However, this occurs infrequently when an experienced surgeon performs the procedure. A sponge stick should be available to immediately apply pressure for controlling hemorrhage if bleeding occurs. With the bleeding thus controlled, a decision is made as to whether a thoracotomy is needed.

In these series, bleeding led to the conversion to a thoracotomy in 10 cases (0.9%). No deaths resulted from the bleeding episodes, and not all patients required transfusion. The incidence and the morbidity of this complication, therefore, is small for surgeons experienced with VATS lobectomy. A multi-institutional survey of 1560 VATS lobectomies reported by Mackinlay (1997) found that the only intraoperative death was related to an intraoperative myocardial infarction, not bleeding.

Postoperative Pain

Patients generally appear to have less pain after a VATS lobectomy than after a lobectomy by thoracotomy. Walker and associates (1996) compared the requirement for narcotic pain medicine in 83 VATS resections versus 110 patients who underwent thoracotomy during the same time period. The VATS group averaged less morphine than the thoracotomy group (57 vs. 83 mg of morphine, $P < .001$). In a randomized, prospective trial of lobectomy in 67 patients (47 by VATS and 23 by muscle-sparing thoracotomies), Giudicelli and colleagues (1994) reported that postoperative pain was significantly less ($P < .02$) after a VATS procedure. The incidence of postthoracotomy pain syndrome after VATS lobectomy (2.2%) reported by the author (1995) is lower than expected after thoracotomy.

Landreneau and associates (1994) prospectively evaluated daily narcotic requirements, hospital stay, and a visual analogue pain scale in 165 patients after muscle-sparing thoracotomy with 178 patients after VATS. The VATS group experienced less pain and greater shoulder strength in the first 6 months postoperatively, but there was no difference after 1 year.

Tumor Seeding of the Incision

Seeding of the VATS incisions occurred in 3 of 934 (0.35%) lobectomies performed for cancer. The risk of tumor recurrence in a VATS incision, therefore, appears to be low and can perhaps be even lower with the use of proper bags to protect the incisions during removal of specimens.

Adequacy of Cancer Operation

In an international survey of 1560 VATS lobectomies by 23 surgeons who had performed at least 20 VATS lobectomies, Mackinlay (1997) showed that the mediastinal nodes were biopsied with mediastinoscopy alone (22.7%), mediastinoscopy and lymph node sampling (32%), or lymph node dissection (45.5%). Kaseda and associates (1998) reported that lymph node dissection with VATS lobectomy yielded an average of 23 lymph nodes (range, 10 to 51).

Long-term disease-free survival is the ultimate measure for the adequacy of any cancer operation. Kaseda and colleagues (1998) reported a 94% 4-year survival for stage I lung cancer resected with VATS lobectomy. Lewis and Caccavale (1998) found a 94% 3-year survival for stage I, 57% for stage II, and 25% for stage III. The cure rate for lung cancer does not seem to be compromised when a complete cancer operation is performed by VATS.

REFERENCES

Downey RJ, et al: Dissemination of malignant tumors after video-assisted thoracic surgery: a report of twenty-one cases. J Thorac Cardiovasc Surg 111:954, 1996.

Giudicelli R, et al: Video-assisted minithoracotomy versus muscle-sparing thoracotomy for performing lobectomy. Ann Thorac Surg 58:712, 1994.

Hazelrigg SR, et al: Cost analysis for thoracoscopy: thoracoscopic wedge resection. Ann Thorac Surg 56:633, 1993.

Hermansson U, Konstantinov IE, Aren C: Video-assisted thoracic surgery (VATS) lobectomy: the initial Swedish experience. Semin Thorac Cardiovasc Surg 10:285, 1998.

Kaseda S, Aoki T, Hangai N: Video-assisted thoracic surgery (VATS) lobectomy: the Japanese experience. Semin Thorac Cardiovasc Surg 10:300, 1998.

Landreneau RJ, et al: Prevalence of chronic pain following pulmonary resection by thoracotomy or video-assisted thoracic surgery. J Thorac Cardiovasc Surg 107:1079, 1994.

Lewis RJ, Caccavale RJ: Video-assisted thoracic surgical non-rib spreading simultaneously stapled lobectomy (VATS(n)SSL). Semin Thorac Cardiovasc Surg 10:332, 1998.

Mack MJ, et al: Techniques for localization of pulmonary nodules for thoracoscopic resection. J Thorac Cardiovasc Surg 106;550, 1993.

Mackinlay TA: VATS Lobectomy: an international survey. Presented at the IVth International Symposium on Thoracoscopy and Video-Assisted Thoracic Surgery, Sao-Paulo, Brazil, May, 1997.

McKenna RJ Jr: VATS lobectomy with mediastinal lymph node sampling or dissection. Chest Surg Clin N Am 4:223, 1995.

McKenna RJ Jr, Fischel RJ: VATS lobectomy and lymph node dissection or sampling in eighty-year-old patients. Chest 106:1902, 1994.

McKenna RJ Jr, et al: Combined operations for lung cancer and lung volume reduction surgery. Chest 110:885, 1996.

McKenna RJ Jr, et al: VATS lobectomy: the Los Angeles experience. Semin Thorac Cardiovasc Surg 10:321, 1998.

Roviaro G, et al: Video-assisted thoracoscopic surgery (VATS) major pulmonary resections: the Italian experience. Semin Thorac Cardiovasc Surg *10*:313, 1998.

Walker WS: Video-assisted thoracic surgery (VATS) lobectomy: the Edinburgh experience. Semin Thorac Cardiovasc Surg *10*:291, 1998.

Walker WS, et al: Continued experience with thoracoscopic major pulmonary resection. Int Surg *81*:255, 1996.

Yim APC, et al: Thoracoscopic major lung resections: an Asian perspective. Semin Thorac Cardiovasc Surg *10*:326, 1998.

READING REFERENCES

Kirby TJ, et al: Lobectomy-video-assisted surgery versus muscle sparing thoracotomy. A randomized trial. J Thorac Cardiovasc Surg *109*:997, 1995.

Leaver HA, et al: Phagocyte activation after minimally invasive and conventional pulmonary lobectomy. Eur J Clin Invest *26*(Suppl 1):210, 1996.

Roviaro G, et al: Videothoracoscopic staging and treatment of lung cancer. Ann Thorac Surg *59*:971, 1995.

CHAPTER 34

Median Sternotomy and Parasternal Approaches to the Lower Trachea and Main Stem Bronchi

Aart Brutel de la Rivière

Median sternotomy as an approach to the main stem bronchi is mainly indicated in the surgical treatment of bronchopleural fistula after pneumonectomy. Other indications include main stem bronchial tumors, which require only sleeve resection of the bronchus. In patients with more extensive resection of the carina, the disadvantage of not being able to mobilize the left main bronchus precludes this approach. On the right side, however, pericardial release and full mobilization of the hilum can be accomplished safely. Rare indications include patients who require complex completion pneumonectomy in which, as a first step, transsternal ligation of the main vessels and bronchial closure permit safe removal of the remaining lung through a second lateral incision.

Median sternotomy allows preparation of the major omentum by slightly extending the incision into the abdomen. The omentum, brought up into the chest via the pericardial sac, can easily reach the main carina and plays a major role in supportive surgical techniques to promote healing of bronchial suture lines.

Median sternotomy as a means of access to the pulmonary hilum was first described by Padhi and Lynn (1960), who reported the anterolateral approach. Abruzzini (1961) described the transsternal route to the main bronchi without opening the pericardium, and Perelman (1998) subsequently popularized the technique, incorporating Bogush's advice to go through the pericardium. Azorin and coworkers (1996) reported video-assisted surgical closure of a postpneumonectomy bronchopleural fistula, approaching the main carina as in cervical mediastinoscopy.

In this chapter, I describe the median sternotomy and parasternal approaches for the management of persistent main stem bronchopleural fistula after pneumonectomy. For more conservative strategies, see the publications of Pairolero (1990) and Puskas (1995) and their associates.

TECHNIQUE OF TRANSPERICARDIAL APPROACHES

The patient lies supine on the operating table. Selective ventilation to prevent flooding of the remaining lung should be achieved either by selective bronchial intubation using a long endotracheal tube or by the use of a double-lumen tube. Selective intubation with a long tube allows the tube to be pulled back far above the main carina at the time of actually closing the bronchus, thereby diminishing tension on the suture line by removing the internal stent (i.e., the tube).

Intravenous vasodilators lower blood pressure and thus allow safe manipulation of the ascending aorta. A large-bore nasogastric tube facilitates esophageal identification during dissection. Single-shot antibiotic prophylaxis is used.

After complete median sternotomy (in redo cases, this is performed with an oscillating saw), care should be taken to avoid entering the pleural space. In patients with long-standing fistulas, the combination of severe hyperinflation and retraction of the mediastinal structures toward the operated side may cause serious displacement of the heart and great vessels. For left-sided fistulas, this may be an indication to use the parasternal route.

The pleural fold is dissected and the pericardium is opened longitudinally; stay sutures facilitate exposure. The tracheal bifurcation is reached between the superior vena cava and the ascending aorta at the lateral sides and between the innominate vein and the pulmonary artery at

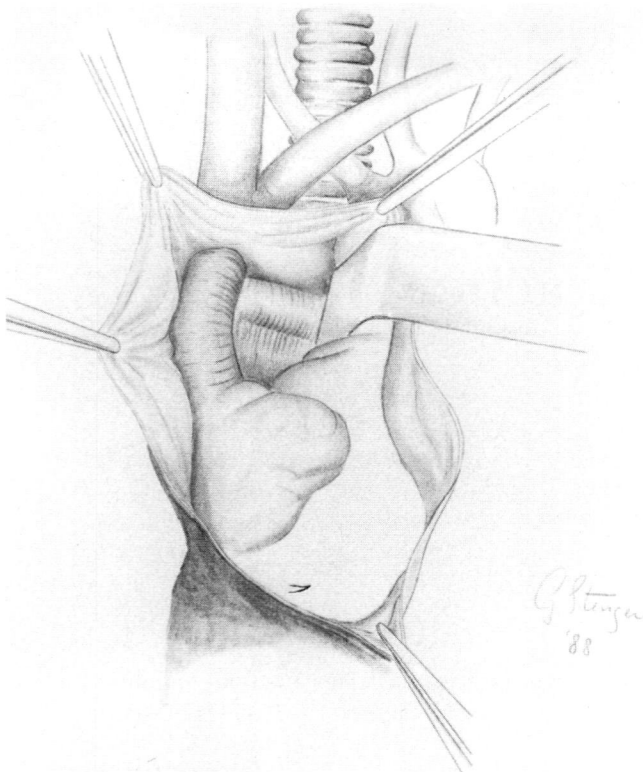

Fig. 34-1. The ascending aorta is retracted to the left with a retractor. The right pulmonary artery is visualized between the superior vena cava to the right and the retractor to the left.

the craniocaudal borders. This approach also allows lymph node sampling of the main carina and its surroundings (e.g., Naruke stations 7 and 3). A hand-held retractor should gently keep the aorta away to the left; a stay suture on the right atrial appendage brings it to a more caudal, stable position in the operative field (Fig. 34-1). Access to the main carina is obtained by opening the dorsal pericardium (Fig. 34-2A).

Right Main Bronchus

First, the residual right pulmonary artery is reamputated behind the ascending aorta, immediately at its take-off from the main pulmonary artery (Fig. 34-2B). Only the proximal end is closed (Prolene 5.0, running suture). If retraction of the great vessels to the right is extreme, the main carina can also be approached to the left of the ascending aorta.

During mobilization, care should be taken to avoid injury to the left recurrent laryngeal nerve, esophagus, and azygous vein. The right bronchus is dissected and encircled. If the bronchial stump is too short to allow safe (i.e., tension-free) closure, a carinal resection should be done (see Chapter 30).

Dissection should be limited to avoid interruption of blood supply, but a tension-free suture line is essential. Encircling the distal trachea or left main bronchus (or both) is optional (Fig. 34-3). If dense adhesions preclude going around the bronchus, it is transected stepwise in a ventrodorsal direction. The bronchus is closed with resorbable suture material: 3.0 Vicryl or 3.0 polydioxanone suture. Although automatic stapling devices are used to close the airway, their introduction and manipulation in the operative field require considerable additional space, which is usually not available in this type of operation.

Before tying the sutures, the endobronchial tube is pulled back high above the carina. The distal bronchial stump should be resected, or destroyed by electrocautery, because it may cause mucous discharge into the surrounding tissue.

Adequate coverage of the proximal stump is important: A pericardial fat pad, thymic remnants, or the omentum can be used. If the pericardium is to be closed (standard in our hands), an intrapericardial drain is left, as is a substernal drain. The patient is extubated on the table.

Left Main Bronchus

On the left, the residual bronchus (i.e., the stump) is usually longer, and the need for more extensive surgery is rare.

Transsternal Approach

After opening the dorsal pericardium between the aorta and the vena cava, the main carina is reached. The left main bronchus is dissected, paying attention to the recurrent laryngeal nerve. If dense adhesions do not permit encircling the bronchus, it should be transected gradually. Closure and handling of the distal stump are the same as those for the right distal stump.

Parasternal Approach

In patients with a left-sided fistula and severe retraction of the mediastinum to the left, transpericardial access can also be obtained by an anterolateral thoracotomy (second or third interspace) or a parasternal approach, which consists of a vertical skin incision followed by subpericostal resection of the second and third cartilages.

The thickened pleural reflection is dissected, and the pericardium is opened longitudinally, anterior to the phrenic nerve. Transsection of the left pulmonary artery and closing the main pulmonary artery with 5.0 Prolene, thereby severing Botallo's ligament, facilitates exposure of the left main bronchus. If additional mobilization is required, intrapericardial transsection of the pulmonary veins is useful.

Primary vascular control is the key to a safe operation. Closing the bronchus is as indicated; identification of the bronchial stump may be facilitated by transillumination, using a fiberoptic bronchoscope.

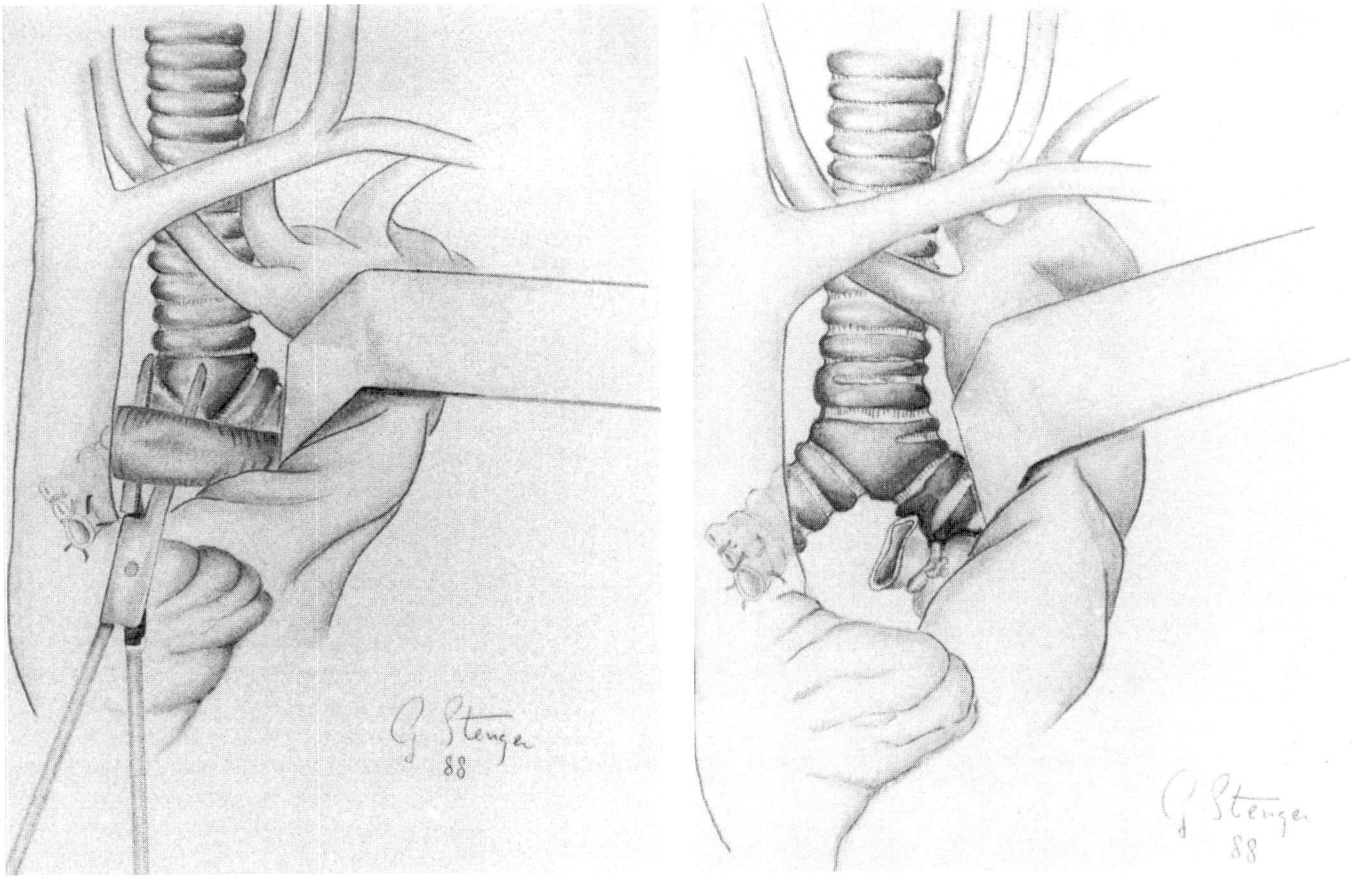

Fig. 34-2. A. The dorsal pericardium is opened, and the right pulmonary artery is encircled. **B.** After reamputation of the right pulmonary artery, behind the ascending aorta, the bronchus is dissected.

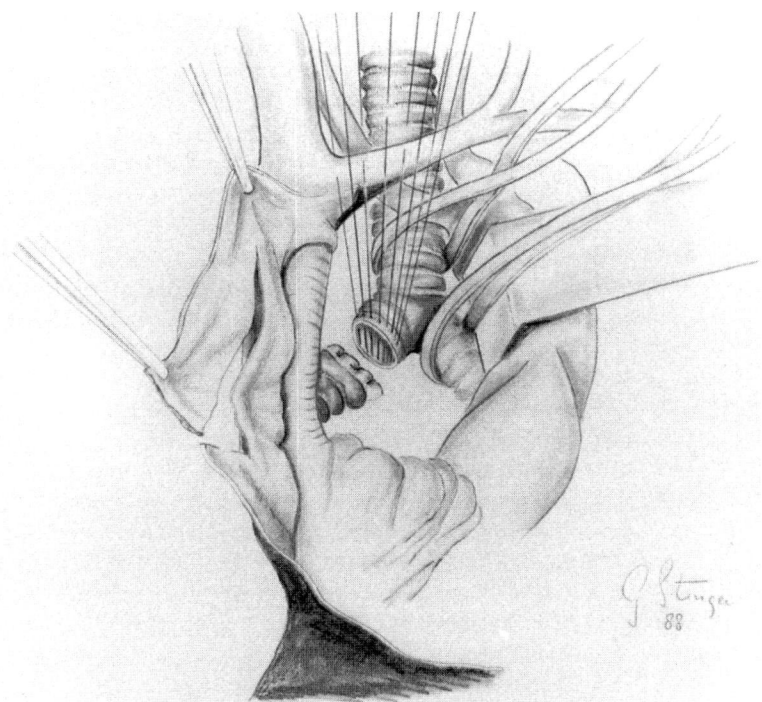

Fig. 34-3. The distal trachea and the left main bronchus are encircled, and the right main bronchus is transected and resutured. Note the pericardial flap prepared ventral to the superior vena cava to cover the newly created stump.

PERIOPERATIVE MANAGEMENT

Space infections in patients with active empyema should be properly controlled before operating on the airway. The best drainage is obtained by a large, open thoracostomy window. The pleural space is packed twice daily with gauze soaked in a 0.02% chlorhexidine solution.

The time needed to get the pleural space at least "clean" can be used to improve the patients' nutritional status using a nasogastric feeding tube. Pretreatment usually requires about 6 weeks. The thoracostomy can be closed 2 weeks after midsternal closure.

MORBIDITY AND MORTALITY

Intraoperatively, hemorrhage is the most serious complication, occurring in 2 to 5%. Postoperative complications are mostly determined by the preoperative, general condition of the patient. Apart from respiratory insufficiency, the most dreaded complication is recurrent fistula. Small recurrent fistulas can be treated conservatively; large fistulas should be attacked surgically, if the patient can tolerate the procedure.

Thirty-day mortality of the operation is reported as 0 to 5.4%. Overall hospital mortality is much higher, reaching 24%. After discharge, no recurrences have been reported.

Long-term prognosis is determined by the original pathology: For cancer patients, survival is related to the extent of their disease; for patients with benign disease, the results are excellent.

PRESENT STATUS OF PARASTERNAL APPROACH

The parasternal approach in itself is simple and effective. In the treatment of postpneumonectomy bronchopleural fistula; however, its place should be carefully defined.

Early fistulas (within 2 weeks of resection) without empyema can be resutured through the ipsilateral hemithorax, buttressing the new stump with a vascularized pedicle or the omentum.

Small, chronic fistulas can usually be obliterated without direct bronchial surgery (e.g., using biological glue) or by the use of a thoracostomy window with repeated packing for a period of 4 to 6 weeks.

Large fistulas with concomitant empyema should be treated surgically, either through the ipsilateral chest with liberal use of muscle flaps or omentum or by the transpericardial approach. The transpericardial approach is most useful when there are contraindications to an ipsilateral approach or when a carinal resection is required.

The technique has the advantage of operating in an aseptic, undisturbed field with well-defined anatomy; however, one should be highly selective using this procedure.

REFERENCES

Abruzzini P: Trattamento chirurgico delle fistole del bronco principale consecutive a pneumonectomia per tubercolosi. Chirur Torac *14*:165, 1961.
Azorin JF, et al: Closure of a postpneumonectomy main bronchus fistula using video-assisted mediastinal surgery. Chest *109*:1097, 1996.
Padhi RK Lynn RB: The management of bronchopleural fistulas. J Thorac Cardiovasc Surg *39*:385, 1960.
Pairolero PC, et al: Postpneumonectomy empyema. J Thorac Cardiovasc Surg *99*:958, 1990.
Perelman MI: Surgery for chronic bronchial fistulas after pneumonectomy. J Cardiovasc Surg *39*:137, 1998.
Puskas JD, et al: Treatment strategies for bronchopleural fistula after pneumonectomy. J Thorac Cardiovasc Surg *109*:989, 1995.

READING REFERENCES

Brutel de la Riviere A, et al: Transsternal closure of bronchopleural fistula after pneumonectomy. Ann Thorac Surg *64*:954, 1997.
Ginsberg RJ, et al: Closure of chronic postpneumonectomy bronchopleural fistula using the transsternal transpericardial approach. Ann Thorac Surg *47*:231, 1989.
Stamatis G, et al: Transsternal transpericardial operations in the treatment of bronchopleural fistulas after pneumonectomy. Eur J Cardiothorac Surg *10*:83, 1996.

CHAPTER 35

Extended Resection of Bronchial Carcinoma in the Superior Pulmonary Sulcus

Kamal A. Mansour and Fady S. Wanna

In 1924, Henry K. Pancoast, then Chairman of Radiology at the University of Pennsylvania, reported four cases of "superior sulcus tumors" and stressed the importance of careful radiographic evaluation of apical chest tumors. It is probable that his 1932 paper is the one that established the syndrome. The tumors occur at a definite location at the thoracic inlet and are characterized clinically "by pain around the shoulder and down the arm, Horner's syndrome and atrophy of the muscles of the hands and present radiographic evidence of a small, homogeneous shadow at the extreme apex, always more or less local rib destruction and often vertebral infiltration."

The definition of the superior pulmonary sulcus is obscure. Teixeira (1983) reported that, as defined by Kubik, the pulmonary sulcus is "nothing but the costovertebral gutter whose superior limit is the first rib arch and whose inferior limit is the insertion of the diaphragm in the thoracic cage." Anatomically defined, Pancoast's tumor therefore is a painful apicocostovertebral syndrome and as such should be differentiated from other bronchial carcinomas arising in the upper lobes and invading the chest wall, vena cava, and recurrent laryngeal or phrenic nerves. Paulson (1973) stressed that Pancoast's tumors are bronchial carcinomas developing in the extreme periphery of the lung and typically involve, by direct extension, structures in the thoracic inlet including the lower trunk of the brachial plexus, intercostal nerves, sympathetic trunk and stellate ganglion, subclavian vessels, adjacent ribs, and vertebrae producing severe, steady, and unrelenting pain in the eighth cervical (ulnar surface of forearm and little and ring fingers) and first thoracic nerve root distribution (ulnar aspect of arm to the elbow) and often causing Horner's syndrome (Fig. 35-1).

As is true of bronchial carcinoma in any location, the extent of the tumor and stage of nodal invasion are the dominant factors in prognosis. By definition, carcinomas in the superior pulmonary sulcus are at least T_3 lesions. Once mediastinal or vertebral column invasion occurs, these tumors become T_4 lesions. According to Mountain (1997), the most recent revision in the international system for staging lung cancer $T_3N_0M_0$ disease corresponds to a stage IIB. N_1 or N_2 nodal involvement associated with T_3 lesions advances these carcinomas to stage IIIA. Patients with stage IIB and IIIA disease can usually be resected. However, a T_4 lesion irrespective of nodal involvement places these carcinomas at a stage IIIB and these are not truly resectable.

DIAGNOSIS AND PREOPERATIVE EVALUATION

Superior pulmonary sulcus tumors account for less than 5% of all lung cancers. Histologically, these carcinomas are squamous cell in 50% of the cases, with adenocarcinoma and large cell types accounting for the remainder. Small cell cancer is rare. Nevertheless, tissue diagnosis is necessary to rule out other lesions occurring in the superior pulmonary sulcus such as acute or chronic infections, usually fungal in origin, that may mimic Pancoast's syndrome. Stanley and Lusk (1985) reported a case of actinomycosis, and Simpson (1986) and Ziomek (1992) and their associates reported cases that were caused by invasive aspergillosis and cryptococcosis, respectively. Gallagher and colleagues (1992) reported a case that was caused by a *Staphylococcus aureus* infection.

In the early stages, chest radiography may show a crescentic shadow at the apex of the lung resembling "an apical pleural cap." Regardless of its appearance in the frontal view, an apical lordotic view shows the tumor as a mass with a convex lower border indenting the lung. Destruction of the upper ribs or dorsal vertebrae, together with a unilateral apical lesion is specific for a Pancoast's tumor. Bucky films may be required for adequate visualization of the bony structures. Planigraphy and bone scanning are used to delineate the location of the tumor and the extent of involvement of the ribs, paraspinal region, and vertebrae.

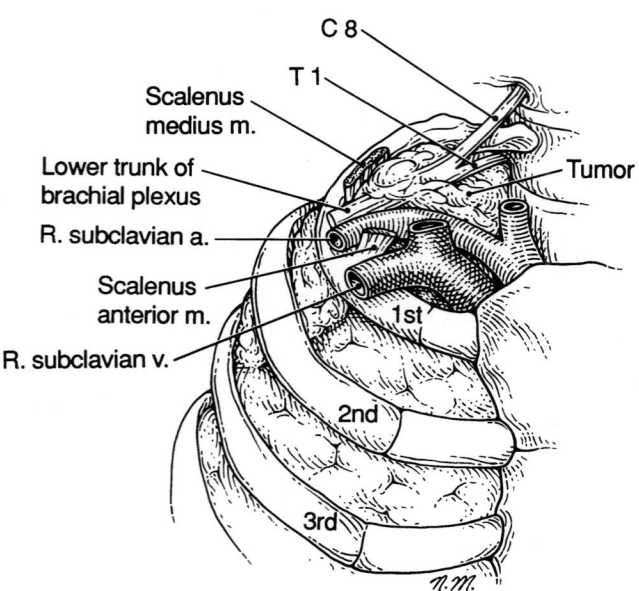

Fig. 35-1. Pancoast's tumor located in the superior section of the costovertebral gutter, invading the lower trunk of the brachial plexus, and posterior aspects of the upper ribs.

Thoracoabdominal computed tomography (CT) scan and magnetic resonance (MR) imaging are used for staging purposes and also to determine the soft tissue extent of the tumor invasion. MR imaging offers the ability to obtain coronal or sagittal planes that give a better delineation of the most superior or inferior extent of the lesion. In addition, Heelan and associates (1989) noted that sagittal and coronal MR imaging allow better appreciation of the relationship of blood vessels and nerves to the lung apex. These images also allow better assessment of invasion of these latter structures by tumor. Both CT and MR imaging can help if the vasculature is involved; however, venous angiography and subclavian arteriography may be resorted to if the MR imaging is not diagnostic. CT and MR imaging are also important in evaluating spinal disease. Noninvasive MR imaging demonstrates tumor replacement of bone marrow and the extent of epidural soft tissue disease. Although CT scans show bone fragments within the canal from pathologic compression fractures, the soft tissue detail is poor.

CT myelography is invasive but demonstrates both bony detail and cord compression. Enzmann and DeLaPaz (1990) believe it is indicated for patients who are unsuitable for MR imaging—for example, those with pacemakers, who do not have access to emergency MR facilities, or who are considered for surgical decompression and stabilization.

Cytohistologic diagnosis has been obtained in a small percentage of cases by sputum examination, bronchoscopic aspirates, brush biopsy, and a transbronchial biopsy. Tissue diagnosis can be obtained by percutaneous needle biopsy. If the tumor is large, it can be biopsied under fluoroscopy using either an anterior or posterior approach. Smaller lesions that are in difficult areas, surrounded by bony or vascular struc-

tures, or both, are usually biopsied under CT guidance. Either fluoroscopy or CT-guided biopsies should have a high degree of accuracy with a low incidence of pneumothorax. This is because the lung parenchyma is rarely entered.

Transcervical supraclavicular technique described by McGoon (1964) or the supraclavicular thoracotomy described by Dart and colleagues (1977) for removal of specimen from a superior sulcus tumor may be resorted to on rare occasions.

Scalene node biopsy for palpable nodes and mediastinoscopy or limited anterior mediastinotomy, if CT shows mediastinal node enlargement, should be performed as a staging procedure. Preoperative evaluation of these patients should also address systemic disease, and appropriate workup including scans should be obtained to rule out distant metastases to the brain, bones, and abdomen.

PREOPERATIVE IRRADIATION AND EXTENDED RESECTION

In the 1950s, tumors in the superior pulmonary sulcus were widely believed to be resistant to radiation and inaccessible to complete and curative resection. The average survival time of untreated patients after diagnosis was 10 to 14 months. Radiation therapy alone or after resection left few survivors after 1 year. Since the 1960s, results have been improving. Irradiation used alone has been reported to relieve pain, prolong survival, and in some instances effect a cure. The reports of irradiation combined with incomplete resection have been encouraging, although the results are not always comparable, because less extensive apical chest tumors are frequently confused with typical superior pulmonary sulcus tumors. Surgical resection remains the mainstay modality in the treatment of superior sulcus tumor. However, improved survival and decreased morbidity have been documented with the use of preoperative irradiation combined with extended resection. Preoperative irradiation combined with extended resection, as reported by Shaw and associates (1961), has improved survival dramatically. The reports of many investigators, including Hilaris and colleagues(1974), and Komaki and colleagues (1990), support this approach (see Chapter 103).

The purpose of preoperative irradiation is to modify the extent of the lesion and sterilize the periphery of the disease at the chest wall level. Using megavoltage equipment, a tumor dose of 4000 to 4500 rads, given in 10 fractions, is delivered over the tumor in the superior sulcus, chest wall, and superior mediastinum beyond the midline. Two to 3 weeks after the completion of irradiation, an extended en bloc resection of the carcinoma and chest wall is done, usually including the upper two or three ribs with the intercostal muscles and nerves, the posterior portions of the appropriate thoracic vertebrae, the lower trunk of the brachial plexus, a portion of the stellate ganglion, and the dorsal sympathetic chain. The involved lung is resected by means of either lobectomy or segmental resection depending on the extent of the parenchymal disease.

The pathologic effects of irradiation of the tumor are related to the length of survival after extended resection. Those patients without nodal involvement who had no residual viable carcinoma in the chest wall or margins of resection did well and were long-term survivors. Those patients who had viable tumor in the chest wall, margins of the resection, perineural lymphatics, or nerve roots at the intervertebral foramen, however, did poorly and died in less than 2 years, mainly from distant metastases, but also with local recurrence of carcinoma, regardless of postoperative external beam irradiation therapy.

Clinical and experimental observations suggest that preoperative irradiation in doses not sufficient to cause gross regression of tumor decreases local recurrence, prevents growth of disseminated tumor cells, and increases survival when compared with irradiation or operation alone.

The theoretical advantages of preoperative over postoperative irradiation depend on the treatment administered before surgical interference and its attendant risks of dissemination, implantation, or inflammation, together with violation of the vascular bed of the tumor, resulting in reduced oxygen tension and consequent diminished irradiation sensitivity. Use of additional postoperative irradiation in patients who have had preoperative irradiation and resection raises the risk of radiation fibrosis and nerve entrapment of the brachial plexus caused by the increased cumulative dose exceeding the tolerance of normal tissues. However, some evidence supports the use of postoperative irradiation in patients in whom the nodes or the margins of resection are found to be positive at the time of operation as shown by The Lung Cancer group (1986). In this select group of patients postoperative irradiation appears to decrease the incidence of local recurrence.

CHEMOTHERAPY

Although local control can be achieved with resection with or without irradiation therapy in a large number of these patients, distant relapse more frequently to a distant site remains a common cause of morbidity and mortality. Therefore, a systemic form of therapy is appealing in the management of these patients.

Both the Southwest Oncology Group trial reported in 1993 and a larger follow-up to that trial reported by Albain and associates (1995) prospectively established the trimodality approach consisting of chemotherapy, irradiation, and subsequent surgery in the treatment of stage IIIA and IIIB non–small cell lung cancer as having encouraging results in terms of improving survival rates compared with historical control. Martini and colleagues (1993), investigating the role of chemotherapy in the treatment of stage IIIA lung cancer, found increased survival in patients receiving chemotherapy followed by surgery.

Nevertheless, until 1995 there was not a prospective randomized study that addressed the role of chemotherapy in the treatment of superior pulmonary sulcus tumor. However,

in June 1995 an Eastern Cooperative Oncology Group S9416 trial started enrolling patients diagnosed as having a superior pulmonary sulcus tumor in various treatment arms. This study compares a regimen of chemotherapy with cisplatin and etoposide given concurrently with irradiation followed by surgery and additional chemotherapy, to the same regimen without surgical intervention in patients who are not surgical candidates.

CONTRAINDICATIONS FOR SURGICAL RESECTION

Contraindications to surgical intervention are extensive involvement of the brachial plexus, the paraspinal region, particularly the intervertebral foramina, and the bodies or laminae of the vertebrae; mediastinal perinodal involvement; soft tissue involvement at the base of the neck; and distant metastases, in addition to the usual cardiopulmonary limitations. Venous obstruction, although not typical of a carcinoma in the superior pulmonary sulcus, is another contraindication to the operation. In some instances, patients with ipsilateral involved mediastinal nodes have undergone resection for palliation of pain, but survival has been limited to 2 years. Similarly, resection of an extensively involved subclavian artery may rarely be necessary with grafting, although these patients usually do not survive more than 1 year.

SURGICAL TECHNIQUE

Classic Posterior Approach (Paulson Operation)

The patient is placed on his or her side with the arm over the head, exposing the axilla and scapular region. A long parascapular incision is made starting just above the level of the spine of the scapula and carried two finger breadths beyond the tip of the scapula and ending in the anterior axillary line (Fig. 35-2). The trapezius and latissimus dorsi muscles are divided, exposing the serratus anterior muscle and rhomboideus major muscle. The serratus anterior muscular attachments to the upper ribs, particularly the second, and the rhomboideus major muscle are divided, thus elevating the scapula and shoulder and exposing the apex of the chest cage. The serratus posterior superior muscle is divided at its insertion on ribs two to five, lateral to their angles, and preserved for later use.

The pleural cavity is entered through the space below the planned limit of rib resection. For example, if the third rib is involved, then the incision should be made along the top of the fourth rib, and if the first two ribs are to be removed, then the pleural space should be entered on top of the third rib. The rib spreader is then placed between the undersurface of the scapula and the third or fourth ribs, depending on the situation. Dissection is divided into anterior, superior, and posterior phases. Anterior dissection is started first

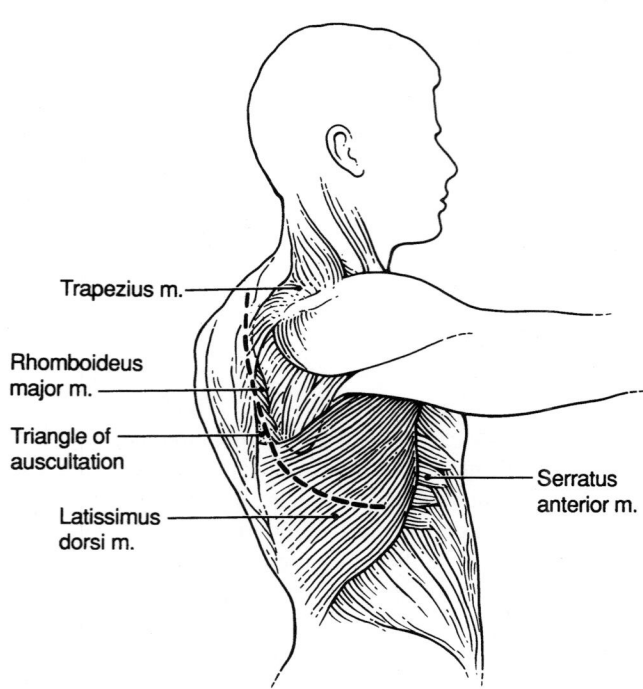

Fig. 35-2. The classic posterolateral thoracotomy incision.

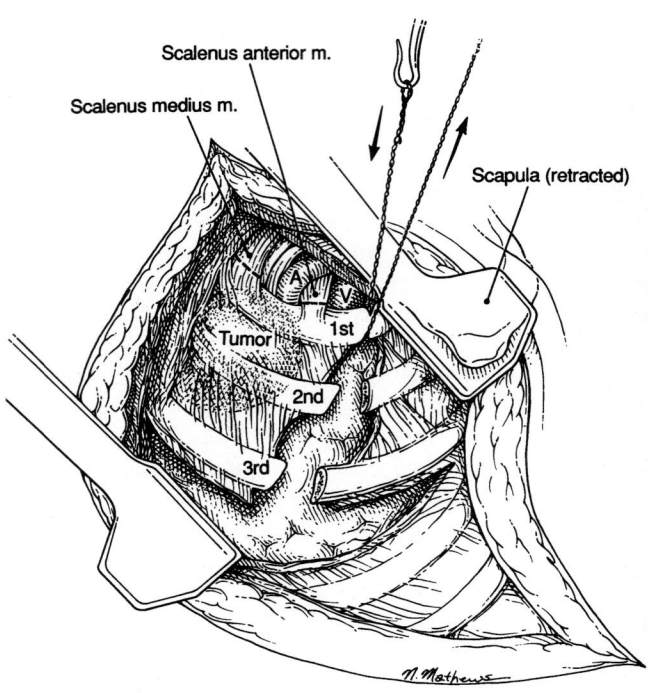

Fig. 35-3. Anterior and superior phases of dissection (division of upper ribs, scalenus anticus and medius muscles) and identification of the subclavian artery and vein by retracting the first rib inferiorly.

(Fig. 35-3). The third and second ribs and intercostal muscles, nerves, and vessels are divided approximately 2 inches anterior to the growth and involved lung. The subclavian vein is identified, and dissection is carried medially to divide the first rib anteriorly using a first rib cutter or a Gigli saw.

Superior dissection continues by grasping the first rib using a bone-holding forceps and retracting it downward to expose the attachment of the scalenus anticus to the scalene tubercle of the first rib between the subclavian vein in front and the subclavian artery behind. The scalenus anticus muscle is then divided, and dissection is carried posteriorly beyond the brachial plexus. At this time the scalenus medius muscle is divided at its attachment into the upper surface of the first rib between the tubercle of the rib and the groove for the subclavian artery.

The posterior phase of the dissection starts by dividing the first rib beyond the extent of the tumor (Fig. 35-4A). With the hand inside the chest, the first rib is cut either at its neck or beyond the attachment of its tubercle to the transverse process of the vertebral body. At this point, the lower trunk of the brachial plexus is identified, as the first rib is retracted downward and divided after the extent of its involvement by the tumor has been determined (Fig. 35-4B). The posterior phase of the dissection continues inferiorly by dividing the second and third ribs. The sacrospinalis muscle is retracted outward, and the transverse processes are divided flush with the tubercles of the ribs or more posteriorly depending on the extent of the tumor. Conversely, the posterior phase of the dissection may start from below upward, dividing the third,

second, and first ribs in that order. Using a chisel and hammer technique, the transverse processes may be divided and a section of the vertebral body may be resected depending on the degree of the tumor invasion. The intercostal nerves and vessels are clipped before division, but if uncontrolled bleeding or spinal fluid leak occurs at the intervertebral foramen, a muscle graft using a small section of an intercostal muscle is sewn over the leak. Bone wax may be used; however, it is not advisable to use oxidized regenerated cellulose (Surgicel, Johnson & Johnson, Somerville, NJ) or absorbable gelatin sponge (Gelfoam, The Upjohn Company, Kalamazoo, MI) because migration or swelling and cord compression are liable to occur with hazardous consequences as has been reported by Tashiro and associates (1987) and Short (1990). It is also not advisable to use the electrocautery in close proximity to the spinal cord because neural injury may result. The dorsal sympathetic chain is divided posteriorly, and the internal mammary artery is divided as it crosses the apex of the chest to reach the undersurface of the sternum.

The extended resection of the carcinoma is then completed by the usual technique of upper lobectomy or segmental resection depending on the extent of the disease.

Adequate pleural drainage is established by means of an upper anterior chest tube and a lower posterior tube placed in the ninth interspace so as to lie in the paravertebral gutter. The remaining lung is expanded, and hemostasis is carefully controlled. The chest is closed usually by suturing the serratus posterior superior muscle to the intrinsic dorsal muscu-

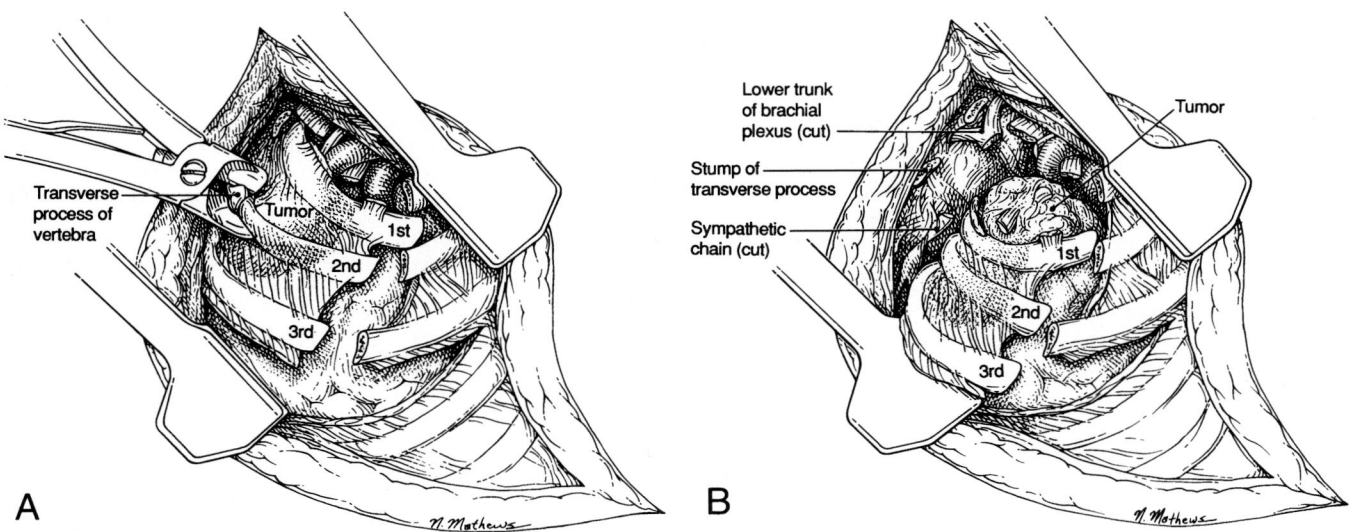

Fig. 35-4. A. Posterior approach to resection of the tumor by division of transverse processes of the vertebrae and elevation of the heads of the ribs. **B.** Division of the lower trunk of brachial plexus as the first rib is retracted inferiorly.

lature. No synthetic materials are used because the scapula furnishes the posterior support. However, if portions of more than three ribs have been removed, the use of Prolene mesh or a soft tissue patch sutured to the margins of the defect under tension is helpful in minimizing paradoxic motion.

Tumor with Mediastinal Node Invasion

The case for mediastinal node resection remains controversial. However, I perform a systematic node dissection for non–small cell carcinoma of the lung even when no perinodal involvement is obvious; this is followed by a course of irradiation therapy to the mediastinum if any nodes prove to be involved by tumor.

Tumor Involvement of the Subclavian Artery

Dissection of the growth away from the subclavian artery may be difficult, but it usually can be accomplished through the adventitial plane. If the artery is invaded, resection of the involved segment with end-to-end anastomosis or interposition graft may be considered. For the latter, a No. 6 or 8 ringed polytetrafluoroethylene graft may be used. Branches of the subclavian artery, including the internal mammary, the thyrocervical, and occasionally the vertebral, may have to be sacrificed.

Tumor Involvement of the Vertebral Bodies

Elevating the tumor in the plane of its pseudocapsule is usually preferable; however, bony attachments suggestive of tumor involvement are chiseled away carefully. As much as one-fourth of the involved vertebral body can be removed without disturbing the spinal support. If CT and preoperative myelography demonstrate destruction of the vertebral body with epidural extensions (stage IIIb), the disease is usually unresectable. Nevertheless, in selected patients, if the disease is localized to one vertebral body, aggressive treatment is important in delaying or preventing direct compression of the spinal cord. Some reports exist of giving preoperative external irradiation of a total dose to the tumor of 4000 rads in 20 fractions. The involved vertebral body is then drilled out with a high-speed drill, and portions of the body above and below are resected. All epidural tumor is resected down to the dura. Nori and associates (1982) suggest that stability of the spine be accomplished by using a bone graft supplemented with methyl methacrylate, after loading catheters are placed along the resected margins for postoperative irradiation with iridium-192 from the second through the fifth postoperative day.

SURGICAL MORBIDITY AND MORTALITY

In addition to the expected postoperative development of atelectasis caused by pain and interruption of the chest wall, unique complications consist of persistence of spinal fluid leaks and pleural drainage, both of which eventually subside, as do parenchymal air leaks. In the event of a pneumothorax and spinal fluid leak, air may pass into the spinal canal, resulting in meningitis.

Permanent neurologic deficits involving the ulnar nerve, resulting from resection of the lower trunk of the brachial plexus, are not incapacitating. If the extent of the tumor permits preservation of the eighth cervical nerve, the defect secondary to resection of the first and second thoracic nerve roots is not severe. Horner's syndrome, if not present preoperatively, develops postoperatively secondary to resection of the dorsal sympathetic chain and at least a portion of the stellate ganglion. None of these defects is disabling, and all patients surviving over 3 years are relieved of their original pain. No complications of irradiation after the doses recommended are reported.

Operative mortality has been no more than 3%. The stage of nodal involvement, the local extent of the carcinoma, and the pathologic effects of radiation at the chest wall level are the important factors in prognosis. Paulson (1979) and Miller and associates (1979) of our group report that with the combined preoperative irradiation and extended resection, a 35% survival rate at 5 years is achieved for all patients and 44% for patients without nodal involvement. It remains to be seen whether these statistics can be improved with the use of a trimodality approach for the treatment of this disease. Almost all series reporting on the value of various modalities in the treatment of superior pulmonary sulcus carcinomas are retrospective. Therefore, by definition, selection bias may account for some if not all of the findings reported in these series.

REFERENCES

Albain KS, et al: Concurrent cisplatin/etoposide plus chest radiotherapy followed by surgery for stages IIIA (N2) and IIIB non–small cell lung cancer: mature results of Southwest Oncology Group phase II study 8805. J Clin Oncol 13:1880, 1995.

Dart CH, Braitman HE, Lalarb S: Supraclavicular thoracotomy for diagnosis of apical lung and superior mediastinal lesions. Ann Thorac Surg 28:91, 1977.

Enzmann DR, DeLaPaz RL: Tumor. In Enzmann DR, DeLaPaz RL, Rubin JB (eds): Magnetic Resonance of the Spine. Baltimore: CV Mosby, 1990.

Gallagher KJ, et al: Pancoast syndrome: an unusual complication of pulmonary infection by Staphylococcus aureus. Ann Thorac Surg 53: 903, 1992.

Heelen RT, et al: Superior sulcus tumors: CT and MR imaging. Radiology 170:637, 1989.

Hilaris BS, et al: The value of preoperative radiation therapy in apical cancer of the lung. Surg Clin North Am 54:831, 1974.

Komaki R, et al: Superior sulcus tumor: treatment selection and results for 85 patients without metastasis (MO) at presentation. Int J Radiat Oncol Biol Phys 19:31, 190.

Martini N, et al: Preoperative chemotherapy for stage IIIA (N2) lung cancer: the Sloan-Kettering experience with 136 patents. Ann Thorac Surg 55:1365, 1993.

McGoon DC: Transcervical technic for removal of specimen from superior sulcus tumor for pathologic study. Ann Surg 159:407, 1964.

Miller JI, Mansour KA, Hatcher CR Jr: Carcinoma of the superior pulmonary sulcus. Ann Thorac Surg 28:44, 1979.

Mountain CF: Revisions in the international system for staging lung cancer. Chest 111:1710, 1997.

Nori D, et al: Bronchogenic carcinoma with invasion of the spine. JAMA 248:2491, 1982.

Pancoast HK: Importance of careful roentgen ray investigations of apical chest tumors. JAMA 83:1407, 1924.

Pancoast HK: Superior pulmonary sulcus tumor: tumor characterized by pain, Horner's syndrome, destruction of bone and atrophy of hand muscles. JAMA 99:1391, 1932.

Paulson DL: The importance of defining location and staging of superior pulmonary sulcus tumors [editorial]. Ann Thorac Surg 15:549, 1973.

Paulson DL: Carcinoma in the superior pulmonary sulcus [editorial]. Ann Thorac Surg 28:3, 1979.

Short HD: Paraplegia associated with the use of oxidized cellulose in posterolateral thoracotomy incisions. Ann Thorac Surg 50:178, 1990.

Simpson FG, Morgan M, Cooke NJ: Pancoast's syndrome associated with invasive aspergillosis. Thorax 41:156, 1986.

Stanley SL Jr, Lusk RH: Thoracic actinomycosis presenting as a brachial plexus syndrome. Thorax 40:74, 1985.

Tashiro C, et al: Postoperative paraplegia associated with epidural narcotic administration. Can J Anaesth 34:190, 1987.

Teixeira JP: Concerning the Pancoast tumor: what is the superior pulmonary sulcus? Ann Thorac Surg 35:577, 1983.

The Lung Cancer Group: Effects of postoperative mediastinal radiation on completely resected stage II, and III epidermoid cancer of the lung. N Engl J Med 315:1377, 1986.

Ziomek S, et al: Primary pulmonary cryptococcosis presenting as a superior sulcus tumor. Ann Thorac Surg 53:892, 1992.

CHAPTER 36

Anterior Approach to Superior Sulcus Lesions

Philippe G. Dartevelle and Paolo Macchiarini

Superior sulcus lesions include a constellation of benign or malignant tumors extending to the superior thoracic inlet. They cause steady, severe, and unrelenting shoulder and arm pain along the distribution of the eighth cervical nerve trunk and first and second thoracic nerve trunks. They also cause Horner's syndrome (i.e., ptosis, miosis, and anhidrosis) and weakness and atrophy of the intrinsic muscles of the hand, a clinical entity known as Pancoast's (1924) syndrome. Bronchial carcinoma represents the most frequent cause of superior sulcus lesions, and we refer to this cause throughout. However, Macchiarini and colleagues (1993) reported that a wide variety of other conditions can result in Pancoast's syndrome (Table 36-1); thus, a histologic diagnosis is required when the syndrome is encountered.

PRESENTATION

Superior sulcus lesions of non–small cell histology account for less than 5% of all bronchial carcinomas, as reported by Ginsberg and associates (1994). These tumors may arise from either upper lobe and tend to invade the parietal pleura, endothoracic fascia, subclavian vessels, brachial plexus, vertebral bodies, and first ribs. However, their clinical features are influenced by their location. Tumors located anterior to the anterior scalene muscle may invade the platysma and sternocleidomastoid muscles, external and anterior jugular veins, inferior belly of the omohyoid muscle, subclavian and internal jugular veins and their major branches, and the scalene fat pad (Fig. 36-1). They invade the first intercostal nerve and first rib more frequently than the phrenic nerve or superior vena cava, and patients usually complain of pain distributed to the upper anterior chest wall.

Tumors located between the anterior and middle scalene muscles may invade the anterior scalene muscle with the phrenic nerve lying on its anterior aspect; the subclavian

artery with its primary branches, except the posterior scapular artery; and the trunks of the brachial plexus and middle scalene muscle (Fig. 36-2). These tumors present with signs and symptoms related to the compression or infiltration of the middle and lower trunks of the brachial plexus (e.g., pain and paresthesia radiating to the shoulder and upper limb).

Tumors lying posterior to the middle scalene muscles are usually located in the costovertebral groove and invade the nerve roots of T1, the posterior aspect of the subclavian and vertebral arteries, paravertebral sympathetic chain, inferior cervical (stellate) ganglion, and prevertebral muscles (Fig. 36-3). Because of the peripheral location of these lesions, pulmonary symptoms, such as cough, hemoptysis, and dyspnea, are uncommon in the initial stages of the disease. Abnormal sensation and pain in the axilla and medial aspect of the upper arm in the distribution of the intercostobrachial (T2) nerve are more frequently observed in the early stage of the disease process. With further tumor growth, patients may present with full-blown Pancoast's syndrome.

PREOPERATIVE STUDIES

Any patient presenting with signs and symptoms that suggest the involvement of the thoracic inlet should undergo a careful and detailed preoperative evaluation to establish the diagnosis of bronchial carcinoma and assess operability. These patients usually present with small apical tumors that are hidden behind the clavicle and the first rib on routine chest radiographs. The diagnosis is established by history and physical examination, biochemical profile, chest radiographs, bronchoscopy and sputum cytology, fine-needle transthoracic or transcutaneous biopsy and aspiration, and computed tomography of the chest. A video-assisted thoracoscopy occasionally might be indicated to obtain tissue proof when the other investigations are negative and to eliminate the possibility of pleural

Table 36-1. Causes of Pancoast's Syndrome

Neoplasms: primary bronchial carcinomas
Other primary thoracic neoplasms
    Adenoid cystic carcinoma
    Hemangiopericytoma
    Mesothelioma
Metastatic neoplasms: carcinoma of the larynx, cervix, urinary
    bladder, and thyroid gland
Hematologic neoplasms: plasmacytoma, lymphomatoid granuloma-
    tosis, lymphoma
Infectious processes
    Bacterial: staphylococcal and pseudomonal pneumonia, thoracic
      actinomycosis
    Fungal: aspergillosis, allescheriasis, cryptococcosis
    Tuberculosis
    Parasitic hydatid cyst
Miscellaneous causes: cervical rib syndrome, pulmonary
    amyloidoma

Adapted from Arcasoy SM, Jett JR: Superior pulmonary sulcus tumors and Pancoast's syndrome. N Engl J Med *337*:1370, 1997.

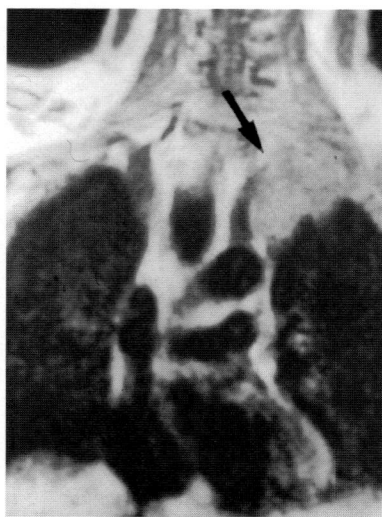

Fig. 36-2. Magnetic resonance image showing a left superior sulcus bronchial carcinoma invading the middle thoracic inlet, including the subclavian artery (*arrow*).

metastatic disease. If there is evidence of mediastinal adenopathy on chest radiographs or computed tomographic scanning, histologic proof is mandatory because patients with clinical N_2 disease are not suitable for operation. Neurologic examination and electromyography delineate the tumor's extension to the brachial plexus, phrenic nerve, and epidural space. Vascular invasion is evaluated by venous angiography, subclavian arteriography, Doppler ultrasonography (cerebrovascular disorders contraindicate sacrifice of the vertebral artery), and magnetic resonance imaging (Fig. 36-4). Magnetic resonance imaging should be performed routinely when tumors approach the intervertebral foramina to rule out invasion of the extradural space (Fig. 36-5).

The initial evaluation also includes all preoperative cardiopulmonary functional tests routinely performed before any major lung resection and investigative procedures to identify the presence of any metastatic disease.

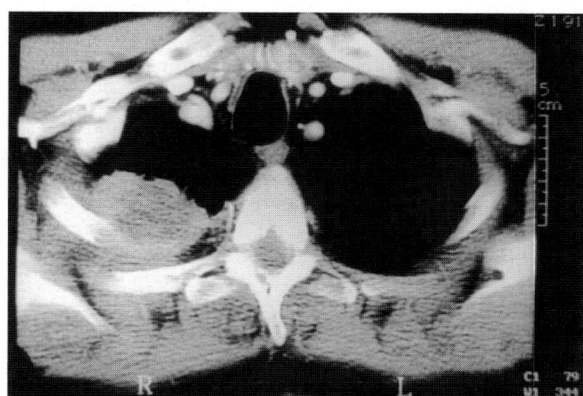

Fig. 36-3. Computed tomography showing a right superior sulcus bronchial carcinoma invading the posterior arch of the first rib. This tumor is usually approached by the posterolateral thoracotomy, as described by Shaw and colleagues (1961).

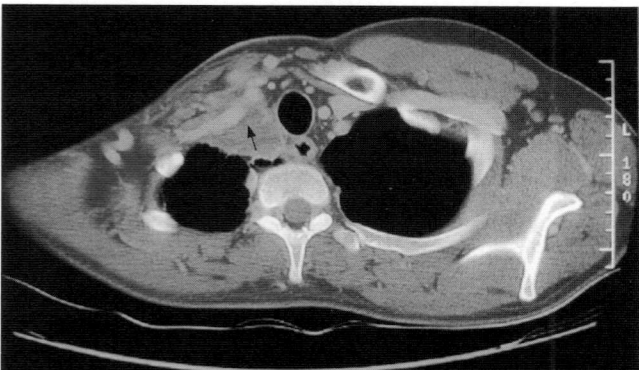

Fig. 36-1. Computed tomography showing a right superior sulcus bronchial carcinoma invading the anterior thoracic inlet, including the subclavian vein (*arrow*).

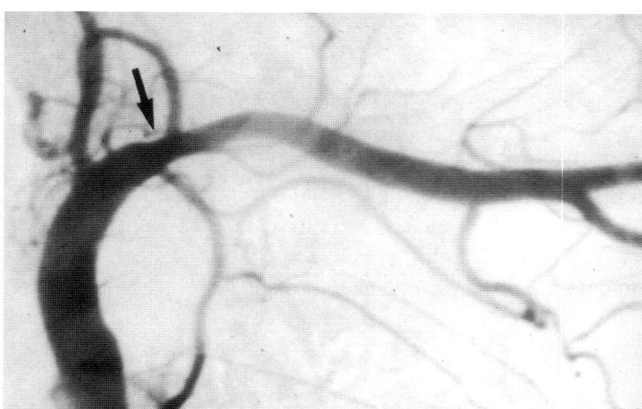

Fig. 36-4. Angiography illustrating a massive tumoral invasion of the intrascalenic left subclavian artery (*arrow*).

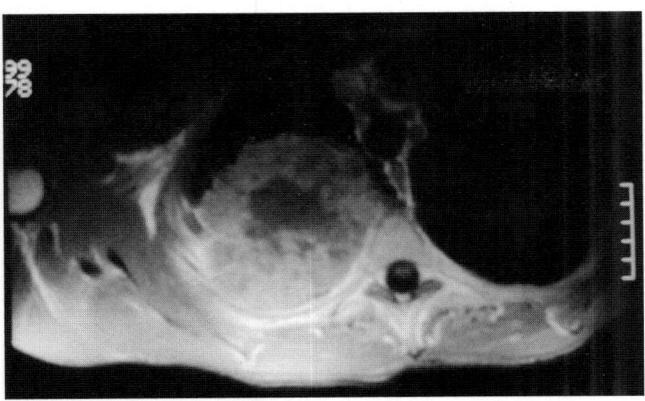

Fig. 36-5. Magnetic resonance image that rules out invasion of the intervertebral foramina by the tumor.

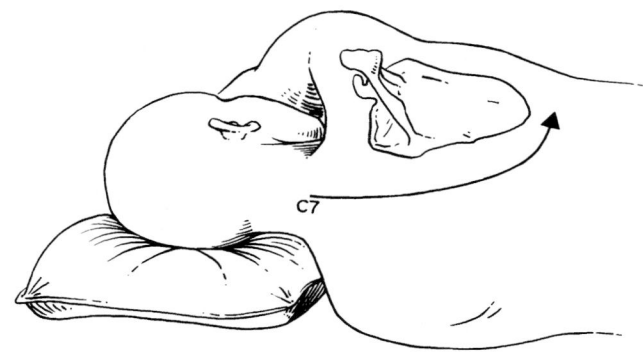

Fig. 36-6. The classic posterolateral thoracotomy incision, as described by Shaw and colleagues (1961), for superior sulcus tumors having no extension to the thoracic inlet.

TREATMENT

Despite their small size and general lack of extrathoracic metastasis at presentation, one of the most perplexing characteristics of superior sulcus tumors has been their almost universal and rapid mortality. For many years, it was believed that these tumors were not amenable to surgery until Chardack and MacCallum (1953) successfully performed a lobectomy and chest wall excision followed by radiation therapy. Five years later, Shaw and colleagues (1961) approached superior sulcus tumors with preoperative radiation therapy (30 to 45 Gy in 4 weeks, including the primary tumor, mediastinum, and supraclavicular region) followed by surgical resection. This radiosurgical approach shortly became the standard treatment, yielding better disease control and survival than other treatments. More recently, Ginsberg and colleagues (1994) provided evidence that en bloc resection of the chest wall and the involved adjacent structures as well as lobectomy must be considered the standard surgical approach for superior sulcus tumors combined with external radiation (preoperative, postoperative, or both). The goal of the operation is the complete and en bloc resection of the upper lobe in continuity with the invaded ribs, transverse processes, subclavian vessels, T1 nerve root, upper dorsal sympathetic chain, and prevertebral muscles.

We (1998) reviewed surgical approaches for the treatment of superior sulcus lesions. All of them must be known because the ultimate hope for cure depends on whether a complete resection is performed. As a general rule, superior sulcus tumors not invading the thoracic inlet are completely resectable through the classic posterior approach of Shaw and associates (1961) alone (Fig. 36-6). Because the posterior approach does not allow direct and safe visualization, manipulation, and complete oncologic clearance of all anatomic structures that compose the thoracic inlet, superior sulcus lesions extending to the thoracic inlet should be resected by the anterior transcervical approach as described by Dartevelle and colleagues (1993). This operative procedure is increasingly accepted as a standard approach for all benign and malignant lesions of the thoracic inlet structures, other than bronchial cancers (e.g., osteosarcomas of the first rib and tumors of the brachial plexus), and for exposing the anterolateral aspects of the upper thoracic vertebrae.

Contraindications to this approach include extrathoracic metastasis, invasion of the brachial plexus above the T1 nerve root, invasion of the vertebral canal and sheath of the medulla, massive invasion of the scalene muscles and extrathoracic muscles, mediastinal lymph node metastasis, and significant cardiopulmonary disease.

ANTERIOR TRANSCERVICAL TECHNIQUE

One-lung anesthesia with measurements of urine output and body temperature are necessary, as is an arterial line opposite to the primary lesion and at least two venous lines for volume expansion as necessary. The patient is supine with the neck hyperextended and the head turned away from the involved side. A bolster behind the shoulder elevates the operative field. The skin preparation extends from the mastoid downward to the xiphoid process and from the midaxillary line laterally to the contralateral midclavicular line medially.

An L-shaped cervicotomy incision is made, including a vertical presternocleidomastoid incision carried horizontally below the clavicle up to the deltopectoral groove (Fig. 36-7). The incision is then deepened with cautery. The sternal attachment of the sternocleidomastoid muscle is divided. The cleidomastoid muscle, along with the upper digitations of the ipsilateral pectoralis major muscle, is scraped from the clavicle. A myocutaneous flap is then folded back, providing full exposure of the neck and cervicothoracic junction.

Once the inferior belly of the omohyoid muscle is divided, the scalene fat pad is dissected and pathologically examined to exclude scalene lymph node metastasis. Inspection of the ipsilateral superior mediastinum after division of

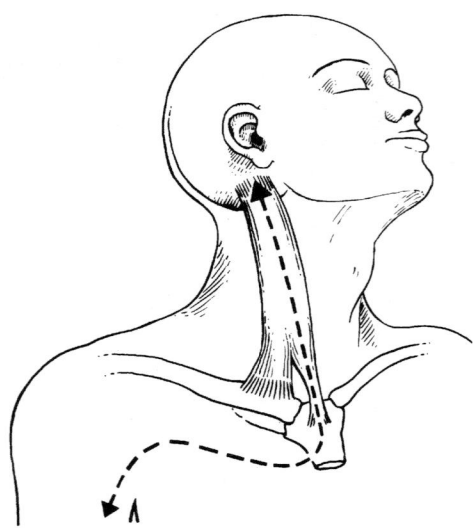

Fig. 36-7. Anterior transcervical approach, as described by one of us (P.D.) and colleagues (1993).

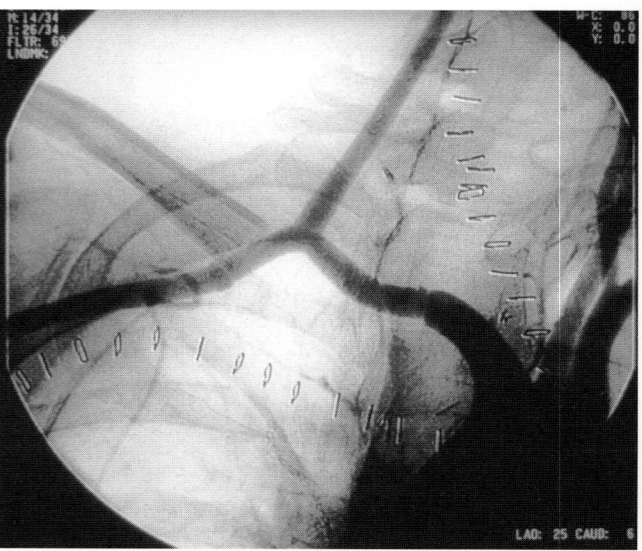

Fig. 36-8. Postoperative angiogram after resection through the anterior transcervical approach of a superior sulcus tumor invading the intrascalenic subclavian artery and vein, and origin of the right common artery (per Fig. 36-1). Revascularization was accomplished by an end-to-end anastomosis between the postscalenic right subclavian and the brachiocephalic artery and end-to-side anastomosis between the right common carotid and postscalenic arteries.

the sternothyroid and sternohyoid muscles is then made by the operator's finger along the tracheoesophageal groove. The tumor's extension to the thoracic inlet is then carefully assessed. We recommend resection of the medial half of the clavicle only if the tumor is deemed resectable.

The jugular veins are dissected first, so that branches to the subclavian vein can eventually be divided. On the left side, ligation of the thoracic duct is usually required. Division of the distal part of the internal, external, and anterior jugular veins facilitates visualization of the venous confluence at the origin of the innominate vein; do not hesitate to suture-ligate the internal jugular vein to increase exposure of the subclavian vein. If the subclavian vein is involved, it can be easily resected after proximal and distal control has been achieved. Direct extension of the tumor to the innominate vein does not preclude resection.

Next, the anterior scalene muscle is divided with cautery either at its insertion on the scalene tubercle of the first rib or in a tumor-free margin. If the tumor has invaded the upper part of this muscle, it needs to be divided at its insertions on the anterior tubercles of the transverse processes of C3–C6. Before dealing with the anterior scalene muscle, the status of the phrenic nerve is carefully assessed because its unnecessary division has a deleterious influence on the postoperative course. It should be preserved whenever possible.

The subclavian artery is then dissected. To improve its mobilization, its branches are divided; the vertebral artery is resected only if invaded and if no significant extracranial occlusive disease was detected on preoperative Doppler ultrasound. If the tumor rests against the wall of the subclavian artery, the artery can be freed following a subadventitial plane. If there is invasion of the arterial wall, resection of the artery to obtain tumor-free margins is necessary. After proximal and distal control is obtained, the

artery is divided on either side of the tumor. Revascularization is performed at the end of the procedure either with a polytetrafluoroethylene graft (6 or 8 mm) or, more often, with an end-to-end anastomosis after freeing the jugulocarotid and subclavian arteries (Fig. 36-8). During these maneuvers, the pleural space is usually opened by dividing Sibson's fascia.

The middle scalene muscle is divided above its insertion on the first rib or higher, as indicated by the extension of the tumor. This might require division of its insertions on the posterior tubercles of the transverse processes of vertebrae C2–C7, especially for apical tumors invading the middle compartment of the thoracic inlet. The nerve roots of C8 and T1 are then easily identified and dissected free from outside to inside up to where they join to form the lower trunk of the brachial plexus. Thereafter, the ipsilateral prevertebral muscles are resected, along with the paravertebral sympathetic chain and stellate ganglion, from the anterior surface of the vertebral bodies of C7 and T1. This permits oncologic clearance of the major lymphatic vessel draining the thoracic inlet and the visualization of the intervertebral foramina as well. The T1 nerve root is usually divided proximally beyond visible tumor, just lateral to the T1 intervertebral foramen. Although the tumor's spread to the brachial plexus may be high, neurolysis is usually achieved without division of the nerve roots above T1. Injury of the lateral and long thoracic nerves should be avoided because it may result in a winged scapula.

Before the upper lobectomy, the chest wall resection is completed. The anterolateral arch of the first rib is divided

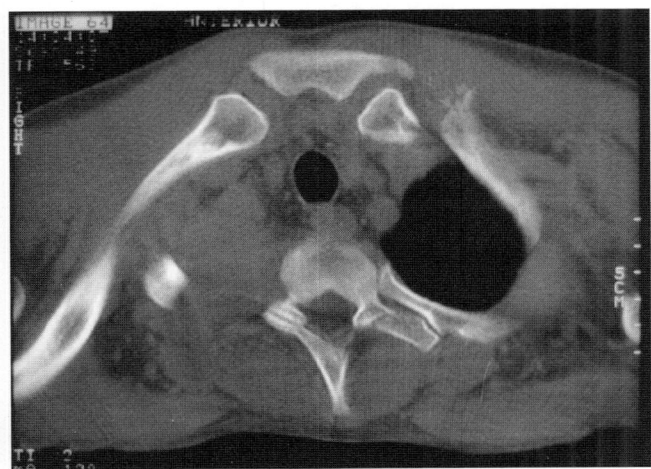

Fig. 36-9. Computed tomography of a right superior sulcus bronchial carcinoma extending into the intervertebral foramen without intraspinal extension.

at the costochondral junction. The second rib is divided at the level of its middle arch, and the third rib is scraped on the superior border toward the costovertebral angle. The specimen is then progressively freed. The divided ribs are disarticulated from the transverse processes of the first two or three thoracic vertebrae. It is through this cavity that an upper lobectomy can be performed to complete the operation, although it is technically demanding. In effect, unlike the original description by Dartevelle and colleagues (1993), it has become evident that an additional posterior thoracotomy is usually not required. The upper lobectomy and chest wall resection of the first four ribs can be performed through the transcervical approach only, without resorting to a posterolateral thoracotomy. The cervical incision is closed in two layers after the sternal insertion of the sternocleidomastoid muscle is sutured, and conventional postlobectomy drainage of the ipsilateral chest cavity is carried out.

There is increasing concern about the functional and esthetic benefit of preserving the clavicle. We believe that the indications for preserving and reconstructing the clavicle are limited to the combined resection of the serratus anterior muscle and the long thoracic nerve because this causes the scapula to rotate and draw forward. This entity (*scapula alata*), combined with the resection of the internal half of the clavicle, pushes the shoulder anteriorly and medially and leads to severe cosmetic and functional discomfort. If this circumstance is anticipated, we recommend an oblique section of the manubrium that fully preserves the sternoclavicular articulation, its intra-articular disc, and the costoclavicular ligaments rather than the simple sternoclavicular disarticulation. Clavicular osteosynthesis can then be accomplished by placing metallic wires across the lateral clavicular edges and across the divided manubrium.

One of us (P.D.) (1997) developed a technique for resecting posteriorly located superior sulcus tumors extending into the intervertebral foramen without intraspinal extension

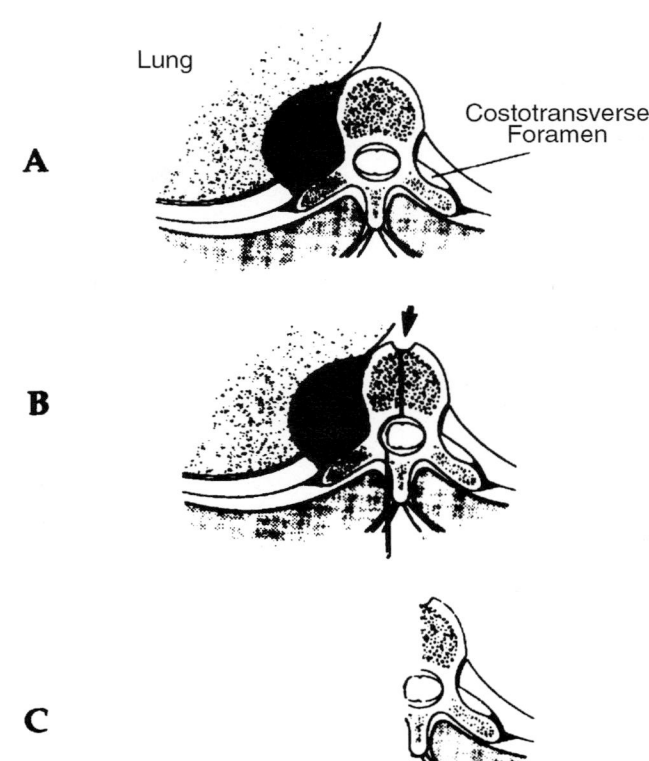

Fig. 36-10. A. Right tumor invading the first thoracic intervertebral foramen. **B.** The lesion is usually approached through transcervical (anterior) and middle (posterior) incisions for apical malignant tumors invading the first two thoracic intervertebral foramina. During the cervical step, the anterolateral aspects of the vertebral bodies of C7–T2 are safely and perfectly exposed. A median slice (*arrow*) on the prevertebral planes can greatly facilitate the section of the invaded vertebral bodies during the posterior step. Usually, tumors invade two intervertebral foramina, necessitating resection of at least hemivertebrectomy (line of transection) above and below the invaded foramen. **C.** The hemivertebrae must be fixed thereafter. From Dartevelle P: Extended operations for lung cancer. Ann Thorac Surg *63*:12, 1997. With permission.

(Fig. 36-9). The underlying principle is that one can perform a radical procedure by resecting the intervertebral foramen and dividing the nerve roots inside the spinal canal by a combined anterior transcervical and posterior midline approach. The first step of the operation includes the transcervical approach, during which resectability is assessed and all tumor-bearing areas are freed in tumor-free margins, as described. On completion, the patient is placed in a ventral position, and a median vertical incision is extended from spinal processes C7–T4. After a unilateral laminectomy on three levels, the nerve roots are divided inside the spinal canal at their emergence from the external sheath covering the spinal cord. After division of the ipsilateral hemivertebral bodies, the specimen is resected en bloc with the lung, ribs, and vessels through the posterior incision (Fig. 36-10).

VII. PULMONARY RESECTIONS

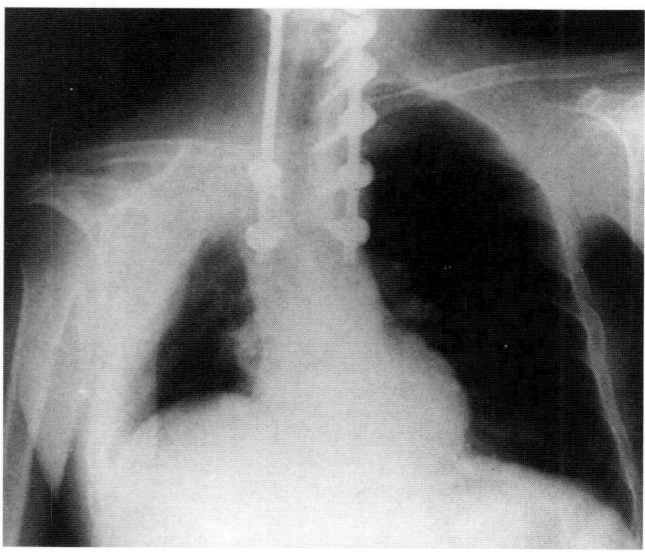

Fig. 36-11. Chest radiograph showing bilateral spinal fixation with metal rods interposed. From Dartevelle P: Extended operations for lung cancer. Ann Thorac Surg *63:12*, 1997. With permission.

On the side of the tumor, spinal fixation is performed from the pedicle above to the pedicle below the resected hemivertebrae; on the contralateral side, a screw is placed in each pedicle (Fig. 36-11). However, the presence of an anterior spinal artery penetrating the spinal canal through an invaded intervertebral foramen contraindicates surgery.

SURGICAL MORBIDITY AND MORTALITY

Surgical complications are many.

1) *Spinal fluid leakage.* The risks of air embolism into the subarachnoid space, ventricles, and central canal of the brain and spinal cord justify reoperation, for which a cerebral ventricular-venous shunt may be required.

2) *Horner's syndrome and nerve deficits.* Although division of the T1 nerve root does not induce significant muscular palsy in the nerve's distribution, resection of the lower trunk of the brachial plexus may result in atrophic paralysis of the forearm and small muscles of the hand, with paralysis of the cervical sympathetic system (Klumpke-Déjérine syndrome). This should be discussed with the patient preoperatively. Relief of the preoperative pain and cure are worth the nerve sacrifice, however, and adaptation is usually reasonable.

3) *Hemothorax* may result from extensive pleural adhesion, chest wall resection, or blood spillage from veins around the intervertebral foramina.

4) *Chylothorax* should be prevented intraoperatively by detailed and extensive ligation of the cervical and intrathoracic lymphatic vessels. Whenever this occurs, contin-

ued chest tube drainage, lung expansion, or reoperation may be necessary (see Chapter 63).

5) *Prolonged ventilatory support.* Because of chest wall dyskinesia and phrenic nerve resection—or even temporary paresis from the dissection—patients having a combined transcervical and midline approach are more likely than others to develop postoperative atelectasis and perfusion-ventilation mismatch. Thus, they are unable to breathe spontaneously in the early postoperative course.

The postoperative course is usually characterized by atelectasis because of the extended chest wall resection, with or without phrenic nerve sacrifice. Treatment involves measures to achieve complete lung expansion by ensuring the following:

- Adequate ventilation, using mechanical support if necessary
- Satisfactory chest tube function
- Prevention of retained secretions by mobilization; coughing; chest physiotherapy; nasotracheal, orotracheal, or bronchoscopic suctioning; or a temporary tracheostomy
- Adequate analgesia
- Increase of the transpulmonary pressure with incentive spirometry or continuous positive airway pressure mask

Fluid overload should be avoided and diuretics used judiciously to avoid adult respiratory distress syndrome. Chest tubes remain in place until all air leaks have stopped and there is complete lung expansion and almost no fluid drainage. Incomplete lung expansion with persistent intrapleural air space should be ignored because ultimately it will be filled with serous fluid.

Resection of the subclavian vein should be accompanied by elevation of the ipsilateral forearm to facilitate venous drainage and generation of a collateral venous pathway within 1 to 2 months. One should closely follow the radial pulse to control the patency of the revascularized subclavian artery; after a preoperative loading dose of intravenous heparin, anticoagulant treatment should be switched to oral doses for a 6-month postoperative period only.

RESULTS AND PROGNOSIS

The overall 5-year survival rates after combined radiosurgical (posterior approach) treatment of superior sulcus tumors due to bronchial carcinoma range from 18 to 56% (Table 36-2). The best prognosis is found in patients without nodal involvement who have had a complete resection, as noted by Arcasoy and Jett (1997) and Ginsberg and colleagues (1994). We (1998) reported a complete resection rate of 100% with no postoperative mortality or major complications. The 5-year and median survival rates were approximately 35% and 18 months, respectively. The local recurrence rate was less than 1.8% using our approach. Among the adverse prognostic factors, the nodal status is the only predictor of disease-free survival (Table 36-3).

Table 36-2. Results of Patients Treated Surgically for Superior Sulcus Tumors

Author (Year)[a]	No. of Cases	5-Year Survival (%)	Mortality (%)
Miller et al. (1979)	36	31	NS
Paulson (1985)	79	35	3
Anderson et al. (1986)	28	34	7
Devine et al. (1986)	40	10	8
Wright et al. (1987)	21	27	—
Shahian et al. (1987)	18	56	—
McKneally et al. (1987)	25	51	NS
Komaki et al. (1990)	25	40	NS
Sartori et al. (1992)	42	25	2.3
Maggi et al. (1994)	60	17.4	5
Ginsberg et al. (1994)	100	26	4
Okubo et al. (1995)	18	38.5	5.6
Dartevelle (1998)	70	34	—
Total	**562**	**33 ± 12[b]**	**3.5 ± 3[b]**

NS, not stated.

[a]Listed in Reading References.

[b]Values are number ± standard deviation.

Adapted from Dartevelle P, Macchiarini P: Optimal management of tumors in the superior sulcus. *In* Franco KL, Putman J Jr (eds): Advanced Therapy in Thoracic Surgery. Hamilton, Ontario: BC Decker, 1998. With permission.

Table 36-3. Factors Influencing Survival and Disease-Free Survival in Completely Resected Patients whose Superior Sulcus Tumors Invaded the Thoracic Inlet and Were Surgically Resected through the Anterior Approach[a]

Adverse prognostic factors
  Female gender
  Positive bronchoscopy
  Abnormal serum carcinoembryonic antigen
  Full-blown Pancoast's syndrome
  Positive lymph nodes (N_{1-3})
Factors without prognostic influence
  Side and site of the tumor
  Type of surgery (wedge or lobectomy)
  Subclavian vessel invasion (absent or present)
  Invasion of the intervertebral foramen

[a]By multivariate analysis, only the nodal status adversely affected disease-free survival.

Adapted from Macchiarini P, Dartevelle P: Extended resections for lung cancer. *In* Roth JA, Hong WK, Cox JD (eds): Lung Cancer. 2nd Ed. Cambridge, MA: Blackwell Scientific Publications, 1998. With permission.

REFERENCES

Arcasoy SM, Jett JR: Superior pulmonary sulcus tumors and Pancoast's syndrome. N Engl J Med *337*:1370, 1997.

Chardack WM, MacCallum JD: Pancoast syndrome due to bronchogenic carcinoma: successful surgical removal and postoperative irradiation: a case report. J Thorac Surg *54*:831, 1953.

Dartevelle P: Extended operations for lung cancer. Ann Thorac Surg *63*:12, 1997.

Dartevelle P, et al: Anterior transcervical-thoracic approach for radical resection of lung tumors invading the thoracic inlet. J Thorac Cardiovasc Surg *105*:1025, 1993.

Dartevelle P, Macchiarini P: Optimal management of tumors in the superior sulcus. *In* Franco KL, Putman J Jr (eds): Advanced Therapy in Thoracic Surgery. Hamilton, ON: BC Decker, 1998.

Ginsberg RJ, et al: Influence of surgical resection and brachytherapy in the management of superior sulcus tumor. Ann Thorac Surg *57*:1440, 1994.

Macchiarini P, et al. Technique for resecting primary or metastatic non-bronchial carcinomas of the thoracic outlet. Ann Thorac Surg *55*:6, 1993.

Macchiarini P, Dartevelle P: Extended resections for lung cancer. *In* Roth JA, Hong WK, Cox JD (eds): Lung Cancer. 2nd Ed. Cambridge, UK: Blackwell Scientific Publications, 1998.

Pancoast HK: Importance of careful roentgen-ray investigations of apical chest tumors. JAMA *83*:1407, 1924.

Shaw RR, Paulson DL, Kee JLJ: Treatment of the superior sulcus tumor by irradiation followed by resection. Ann Surg *154*:29, 1961.

READING REFERENCES

Anderson TM, Moy PM, Holmes EC: Factors affecting survival in superior sulcus tumors. J Clin Oncol *4*:1598, 1986.

Devine JW, et al: Carcinoma of the superior pulmonary sulcus treated with surgery and/or radiation therapy. Cancer *57*:941, 1986.

Ginsberg RJ, et al: Influence of surgical resection and brachytherapy in the management of superior sulcus tumors. Ann Thorac Surg *57*:1440, 1994.

Komaki R, et al: Superior sulcus tumors: treatment selection and results for 85 patients without metastasis (M0) at presentation. Int J Radiat Oncol Biol Phys *19*:31, 1990.

Maggi G, et al: Combined radiosurgical treatment of Pancoast tumor. Ann Thorac Surg *57*:198, 1994.

McKneally M: Discussion of Shahian DM, Neptune WB, Ellis FH Jr: Pancoast tumors: improved survival with preoperative and postoperative radiotherapy. Ann Thorac Surg *43*:32, 1987.

Miller JI, Mansour KA, Hatcher CR Jr: Carcinoma of the superior pulmonary sulcus. Ann Thorac Surg *28*:44, 1979.

Okubo K, et al: Treatment of Pancoast tumors. Combined irradiation and radical resection. Thorac Cardiovasc Surg *43*:84, 1995.

Paulson DL: Technical considerations in stage T3 disease: the superior sulcus lesion. *In* Delarue NC, Eschapasse H (eds): International Trends in Thoracic Surgery. Vol. 1. Philadelphia: WB Saunders, 1985, p. 121.

Sartori F, et al: Carcinoma of the superior pulmonary sulcus. Results of irradiation and radical resection. J Thorac Cardiovasc Surg *104*:679, 1992.

Shahian DM, Neptune WB, Ellis FH Jr: Pancoast tumors: improved survival with preoperative and postoperative radiotherapy. Ann Thorac Surg *43*:32, 1987.

Wright CD, et al: Superior sulcus lung tumors. Results of combined treatment (irradiation and radical resection). J Thorac Cardiovasc Surg *94*:69, 1987.

CHAPTER 37

Complications of Pulmonary Resection

Thomas W. Shields and Ronald B. Ponn

Operations for lung resection vary widely, from a small pneumonotomy for enucleation of a peripheral hamartoma to pneumonectomy. Although most procedures are unilateral, synchronous bilateral resections are not uncommon and occasionally may entail removal of a large total volume of lung tissue. In addition, the procedures may be extended to include removal of portions of the chest wall, diaphragm, pericardium, and, less commonly, other adjacent structures. Large airways and pulmonary arteries may be reconstructed to preserve lung parenchyma by avoiding pneumonectomy. Another variable is the method of exposure, which includes various types of thoracotomy and video-assisted thoracic surgery. The technical aspects and some of the problems associated with specific operations and incisions are discussed in Chapters 25 through 36.

INTRAOPERATIVE COMPLICATIONS

The three major life-threatening complications during the operation, other than those associated with the anesthetic management of the patient (Chapters 22 to 24), are injury to a major vessel with massive hemorrhage, cardiac arrhythmias and myocardial ischemia, and the development of a contralateral pneumothorax. Intraoperative complications that do not present an immediate threat to life, but often cause significant morbidity and sometimes mortality postoperatively, include injuries to an intrathoracic nerve, the thoracic duct, the esophagus, the spinal cord, or the dura. Because the consequences of these injuries are usually not detected during the operation, they are discussed as early postoperative complications. Similarly, tumor embolization is a rare occurrence that may be potentially lethal during the resection of a lung tumor but is more often diagnosed postoperatively.

Injury to a Major Pulmonary Vessel

Avoidance and management of an injury to a major pulmonary vessel are discussed in Chapter 26. It should be noted that at times, to obtain proximal control, vessels must be exposed intrapericardially.

Intraoperative Cardiac Complications

Intraoperative cardiac arrhythmias and myocardial ischemia occur most often in patients with underlying cardiac disease but may also be caused by temporary physiologic derangements in patients without clinical heart disease. The former problem is best avoided by the preoperative identification of high-risk cases and, when indicated, the use of a Swan-Ganz catheter and appropriate prophylactic preoperative and intraoperative medications to minimize ischemia. In all cases, factors that may produce cardiac dysfunction (usually hypoxemia, hypokalemia, hypervolemia or hypovolemia, tachycardia, and acidosis) must be rapidly identified and corrected. Excessive manipulation of the heart can cause arrhythmias (usually ventricular) and myocardial ischemia due to direct effects and hypotension. If retraction or compression of the heart cannot be avoided, manipulation should be limited to short intervals, with predetermined hemodynamic end points and ample time for recovery between attempts.

Although the appropriate preoperative medical treatment of coronary artery disease reduces the risk of myocardial ischemia during operation, the use of prophylactic digitalization has no effect on reducing the occurrence of intraoperative arrhythmias as noted by Ritchie and coworker (1990). The efficacy of prophylactic calcium channel blockers, such as diltiazem, as suggested by Amar and colleagues (1997), in reducing the incidence of postoperative supraventricular arrhythmias is unknown.

Contralateral Pneumothorax

The incidence of the development of a contralateral pneumothorax is low. Vogt-Moykopf (1990) reported an incidence of 0.8%. It is thought to be a greater threat in patients undergoing operation for bullous or bleb disease of the lung, but it may occur during any thoracotomy. Vogt-Moykopf (1990) stated that it may occur during an ultraradical lymph node dissection with perforation of the mediastinal pleura, but the few we have seen were the result of the spontaneous rupture of an unsuspected contralateral bleb. As a result of positive-pressure ventilation, air accumulates in the contralateral pleural space, the lung on the affected side becomes increasingly difficult to ventilate, and the effects of insufficient gas exchange become evident. With recognition of this complication, prompt evacuation of the air from the contralateral pleural space is mandatory. This is accomplished by opening the mediastinal pleura from the operative side and placing a thoracostomy tube via the mediastinum or a transcutaneous route.

POSTOPERATIVE COMPLICATIONS: MORBIDITY AND MORTALITY AFTER PULMONARY RESECTION

Multiple factors influence the incidence and types of complications, both fatal and nonfatal, after pulmonary resection. These include the age and physical status of the patient (i.e., cardiorespiratory functional status, nature of the pathologic process, type and extent of the procedure, and use of various neoadjuvant or postoperative adjuvant therapeutic modalities).

Both nonfatal and fatal complications may be classified as unique to, or directly related to, the procedure (e.g., technical, pleural, pulmonary, cardiac, hemorrhagic, or septic) and those related to the performance of any major operative procedure (e.g., cardiovascular, gastrointestinal, genitourinary, peripheral vascular, neurologic, and thromboembolic). Of the complications related to the procedure per se, more than one etiologic factor (i.e., technical, septic, or failure in healing) may play a role in the development of a complication.

Major improvements in patient selection and appropriate preoperative preparation, as well as current operative and anesthetic techniques and more effective control of postoperative pain, have reduced the rates of postoperative morbidity and mortality.

The reports of Cerfolio (1996), Ferguson (1995), Kearney (1994), Lewis (1994), Miller (1993), and Morice (1992) and Putnam (1990) and their associates emphasize exacting preoperative functional evaluation to reduce the incidence of complications. The predictive values of various studies to determine postoperative values of forced vital capacity, forced expiratory volume in 1 second (FEV_1), diffusing capacity of the lung for carbon monoxide (D_{LCO}), and maximum oxygen consumption ($\dot{V}O_2max$) in poor-risk patients are less than exact in relationship to the occurrence of nonfatal complications but somewhat more reliable regarding mortality. Ferguson and associates (1995) believe that the determination of D_{LCO} is the most valuable single study, whereas Bolliger and colleagues (1995) believe that exercise testing with determination of $\dot{V}O_2max$ expressed as a percentage of the predicted value is the single best predictor of postoperative complications. Rather than relying on a single study to predict the possibility of a postoperative complication or death, Pierce and colleagues (1994) and Melendez and Barrera (1998) have reported the usefulness of composite indices of the various lung function studies and other factors to predict the patient's outcome. The former authors developed the "predicted postoperative product" index, and the latter authors constructed the "predictive respiratory complication quotient." Each appears to be superior to any single factor in predicting postoperative mortality and morbidity, but further studies to confirm their usefulness are needed, and the ultimate answer is yet to be established. In the studies of Mitsudomi and colleagues (1996) of patients who underwent pneumonectomy, the results by univariate analysis suggest that an elevated serum lactate dehydrogenase level or a low predicted forced vital capacity or FEV_1 were significantly associated with postoperative complications. On multivariate analysis of their data, a high lactate dehydrogenase level and a low predicted FEV_1 remained independent prognostic factors. To make matters even more confusing, Duque and coworkers (1997) reported that the presence of insulin-dependent diabetes mellitus or peripheral vascular disease increased the incidence of postoperative complications, and the latter was significantly related to postoperative mortality.

In the face of the somewhat bewildering mass of data, a number of surgical groups, after what they believe to be adequate selection of the candidates for pulmonary resection, have developed postoperative management strategies in an effort to further reduce the morbidity and mortality rates after pulmonary resection. Knott-Craig and associates (1997) have suggested a regimen of postoperative digitalization, subcutaneous heparin, and the use of vaso-occlusive stockings until the patient is fully mobile. In their series of 173 pulmonary resections, the hospital mortality rate was 1.6% and the morbidity rate was only 15%. In their high-risk patients, these rates were less than 5% and 20%, respectively. However, the role of each element in achieving these salutary results remains unknown.

After pneumonectomy, the incidence of nonfatal complications varies from as low as 15% to as high as 60%. The majority of the complications are cardiac dysrhythmias, pulmonary infection, respiratory insufficiency, empyema, bronchopleural fistula, and hemothorax.

In patients who have undergone a lobectomy, the morbidity rate is frequently higher, and it may vary with the underlying disease process: inflammatory or carcinoma. In most series, complications are seen in men more often than in women. The number of complications increases in the elderly and in patients undergoing extended resections, extensive lymph node dissections, or bronchoplasty procedures. In a series of 369 lobectomies reported by Keagy and associates (1985), 41% had nonfatal complications; 224 complications occurred in 151 patients. The respiratory system was involved in one-third: 50 patients required prolonged ventilation and

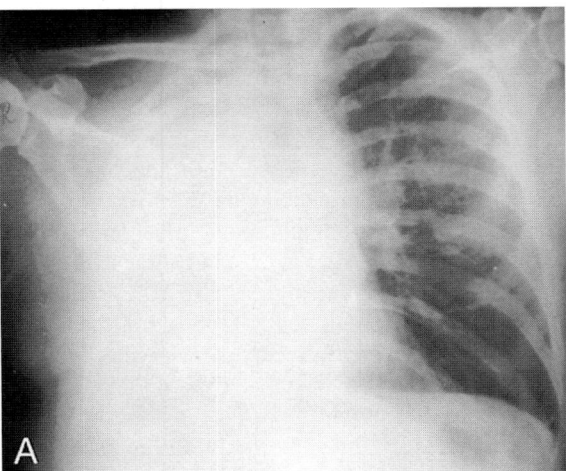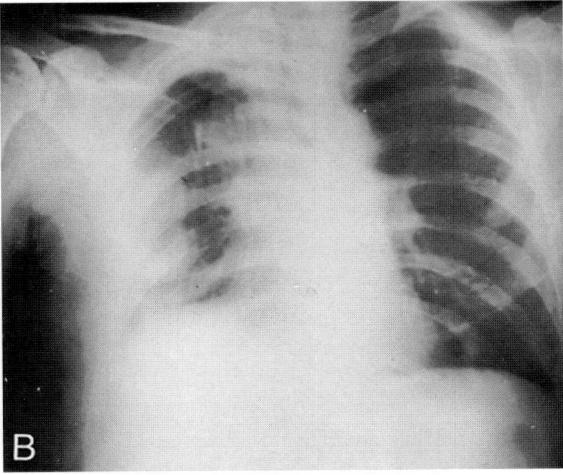

Fig. 37-1. A. Chest radiograph reveals massive atelectasis of remaining right lung 24 hours after right upper lobectomy. **B.** Reexpansion of remaining right lung after bronchoscopy.

27 had atelectasis or excessive secretions. The incidence of pneumonia per se was not documented. Cardiac complications also occurred in one-third, arrhythmias being the most common. In the remaining one-third, air leaks, pleural effusions, pneumothoraces, empyema (2.4%), postoperative hemorrhage, bronchial stump leaks (1.3%), pulmonary emboli, wound infections, and one instance of lung gangrene occurred. Postoperative massive atelectasis (Fig. 37-1), persistent residual air space (Fig. 37-2), and prolonged air leaks present problems not seen after a pneumonectomy.

After a segmentectomy, the nonfatal complications are similar to those occurring after a lobectomy. The major

complications are prolonged air leak; peripheral fistula or, rarely, true bronchopleural fistula; empyema; and persistent pleural air space. All are interrelated, and the incidence of any one alone, or in combination, varies directly with the disease process and the difficulty experienced in the dissection of the intersegmental planes.

The morbidity rate after a wedge resection is minimal. When present, the complication is most often the result of either retention of secretions or pleural problems. Persistent air spaces occur but with an incidence less than 10%. Most of these spaces produce no symptoms and require no treatment.

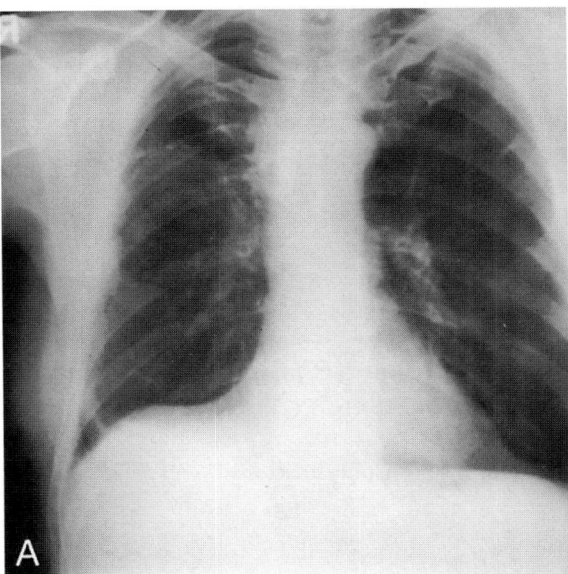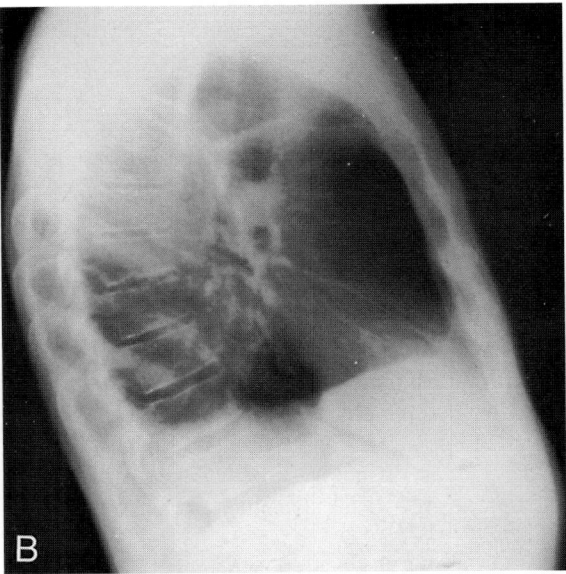

Fig. 37-2. Posteroanterior **(A)** and lateral **(B)** radiographs of the chest show an asymptomatic residual air space 4 weeks after a right upper lobectomy for carcinoma of the lung.

The complications occurring after lung volume reduction procedures, bronchoplasty and tracheoplasty operations, and video-assisted thoracoscopic pulmonary resections are discussed in Chapters 83, 28, 30, and 33, respectively.

Mortality rates after pulmonary resection, to be meaningful, must include all deaths occurring within 30 days of operation and all in-hospital deaths, regardless of the length of stay. After pneumonectomy, the mortality rates vary from as low as 1.5% to as high as 30%. The majority of deaths occur after a right pneumonectomy, as noted by Nagasaki (1982) and Cybulsky (1992) and their associates. In patients with carcinoma of the lung, the rates vary but are in the range of 5 to 15%. Ginsberg and associates (1983) in the North American Lung Cancer Study Group reported an overall 30-day postoperative mortality rate of only 6%, as did Nagasaki and colleagues (1982) from the Sloan-Kettering Cancer Center. In a review of 586 pneumonectomies for resection of lung cancer in 1 year in Japan, the incidence of postoperative mortality was reported by Wada and associates (1998) to be only 3.2%. It must be noted, however, that this study is limited by reporting only 30-day mortality, without mention of in-hospital deaths occurring after 30 days. In patients 70 years of age or older, the mortality rate may be as high as 30%. With proper preoperative selection and meticulous postoperative care, however, the mortality rate in patients older than age 70 years may be kept as low as 6%, as reported by Ginsberg and associates (1983). Wahi (1989) and Patel (1992) and coworkers reported a mortality rate of 13% in this older group, whereas Ishida and associates (1990) recorded no deaths after pneumonectomy in 11 patients in this age group. Roxburgh and associates (1991) noted a higher mortality rate after pneumonectomy in the elderly, but the difference was not significant. Patients undergoing a completion pneumonectomy for a second lung cancer have a similar rate; however, as pointed out by McGovern and colleagues (1988), when the procedure is carried out for removal of a persistent or superimposed inflammatory process, the mortality rate may be three times as high. Muysoms and associates (1998) reported a mortality rate of 37.5% in patients who underwent a completion pneumonectomy for the attempted correction of early complications of the primary operation, especially for control of a bronchopleural fistula. Terzi and colleagues (1995) experienced even higher mortality (57%) if the procedure was done for an early complication of a sleeve resection. The mortality rates for extrapleural pneumonectomy for diffuse malignant mesothelioma vary between 5 and 9%, as reported by Sugarbaker (1992) and Da Valle (1986) and their associates. Brown and Pomerantz (1995) achieved an enviable rate of only 1.6% in 62 pleuropneumonectomies, including a few completion pneumonectomies, for multiple drug–resistant tuberculosis. Dartevelle (1988), Mathisen and Grillo (1991), and Roviaro (1994) and Tsuchiya (1990) and their colleagues have recorded operative mortality rates after sleeve pneumonectomy of 10.9%, 15%, 8%, and 4%, respectively.

The major causes of death after a pneumonectomy are respiratory insufficiency; septic complications, such as postoperative pneumonia or an empyema that may or may not be associated with a bronchopleural fistula; postpneumonec-tomy pulmonary edema (PPE); myocardial infarction; and pulmonary embolus. Renal failure may be a major factor in older patients, as reported by Patel and associates (1992), as well as other concomitant medical disease.

The mortality rates are lower after lobectomy than after pneumonectomy. Patient selection and disease process are the major factors influencing the occurrence of postoperative death. In patients with pulmonary tuberculosis, the mortality rate is in the range of 1 to 2%; in patients with carcinoma of the lung, it may be as high as 8 to 10%, but as reported by Ginsberg (1983) and Keagy (1985) and their colleagues, it should be no greater than 3%. In the review by Wada and colleagues (1998), the postoperative mortality rate was 1.2% after 5609 lobectomies carried out for resection of a lung cancer, but only 30-day mortality was included. In contrast to the common experience that pneumonectomy (especially right-sided) is associated with a high mortality in elderly patients, the risk of lobectomy should be low. Our group, as reported by Pagni and associates (1997, 1998) noted a mortality of 2.4% for 293 lobectomies in patients aged 70 and older, as contrasted with 12.5% for 24 pneumonectomies during the same period, and a 4.2% mortality rate in octogenarians undergoing standard or extended lobectomy for lung cancer. In a series of 500 pulmonary resections for lung cancer in patients older than 70 years of age, Thomas and colleagues (1998) reported mortality rates of 8%, 11.8%, 7.6%, and 0%, for pneumonectomy, bilobectomy, lobectomy, and lesser resections, respectively. In this study, increasing age, male gender, low FEV_1, hypertension, and extended procedures correlated with greater risk.

The major causes of death after lobectomy are septic complications and cardiopulmonary insufficiency. Fatal pulmonary embolism occurs infrequently. Fatal cardiac and other nonpulmonary complications, such as upper gastrointestinal hemorrhage, occur occasionally.

Segmentectomy is essentially a benign procedure, and mortality rates of approximately 1% are reported when the procedure is done electively in patients with satisfactory pulmonary function. Jensik (1986) and Martini and associates (1986) reported that the mortality rate may, however, be as high as 4 to 6% in patients with poor pulmonary function, when more extensive tumor is present, or in patients with a previous pulmonary resection. Wada and colleagues (1998) reported a 30-day mortality rate of 0.8% for lesser resection in 904 patients with lung cancer.

EARLY COMPLICATIONS AFTER PULMONARY RESECTION

Hemorrhagic Complications

Postoperative Hemorrhage

Major hemorrhage after thoracotomy and resection is most commonly the result of inadequate hemostasis of a bronchial artery or a systemic vessel in the chest wall. Infrequently, the slipping of a ligature from a major pulmonary vessel or an unrecognized injury to a systemic vein (e.g., vena cava, azygos) is the cause. Bleeding related to a coagulation abnormality is rare and, when present, is often associated with the use of a large number of units of stored blood transfusions (usually more than 10) during the operative procedure. When a coagulopathy is suspected, coagulation studies are indicated, and the appropriate therapy (fresh frozen plasma, cryoprecipitate, or platelet transfusion) is given as indicated.

When chest tubes are in place, an output of blood of more than 200 mL per hour for 4 to 6 hours indicates massive bleeding, but lesser output may occur because of clot formation in the pleural space or in the drainage system. Complete reliance on the amount of drainage to determine blood loss can be misleading. When massive bleeding is the suspected cause of the patient's hypotension, radiographs of the chest to determine the degree of opacification of the ipsilateral hemithorax are indicated. Any one of the following— failure to respond to presumed adequate blood replacement, a large amount of blood in the hemithorax, or continued, excessive bleeding from the chest tubes—is an indication for reexploration.

In a series of 1428 resections, Peterffy and Henze (1983) reported 113 hemorrhagic episodes: 30% occurred after a pneumonectomy, 66% after a lobectomy, and 4% after a segmentectomy. Emergency thoracotomy was required in 37 patients (an incidence of 2.6%). Six of the patients died: four as the result of hemorrhage and two because of a subsequent bronchopleural fistula. In another three patients, massive bleeding (two from the pulmonary artery and one from a systemic vessel) was found to be the cause of death at autopsy. Thus, the overall incidence of mortality related to uncontrolled bleeding was less than 0.1%.

Sudden Massive Hemorrhage

On rare occasions, the ligature on the stump of the pulmonary artery slips off, as noted by Peterffy and Henze (1983). Less commonly, a ligature slips from a pulmonary vein closure, especially when the pericardial reflection is included in the ligature. Massive blood loss occurs rapidly into the ipsilateral hemithorax. If the patient is still unconscious, sudden inability to obtain a pulse or a blood pressure reading is the only indication of its occurrence. If the patient is awake, sudden syncope with accompanying loss of pulse and blood pressure occurs. Massive fluid infusion and ventilation with 100% oxygen may restore some degree of cardiac output and oxygenation of the vital tissues of the body. Further bleeding from the vessel may temporarily cease owing to a low or near-absent cardiac output as well as the result of the tamponading effect of the large amount of blood (which clots rapidly) in the hemithorax. If time permits, an electrocardiogram should rule out a myocardial infarction. The patient should be returned to the operating room as expeditiously as possible and the incision reopened, the clotted blood removed (bleeding from the vessel may

recur at this time), and the vessel identified and controlled. Secure closure of the vessel is best obtained by suture of the stump or by the use of a vascular stapler. A successful outcome may be anticipated if the bleeding has been recognized promptly, the fluid replacement is adequate, and the vessel is controlled without further major loss of blood volume. Use of a suture ligature placed sufficiently distal to the simple ligature or of a vascular stapler for primary closure should eliminate this complication.

Bronchovascular Fistula

The occurrence of a bronchovascular fistula with fatal hemorrhage is a rare event after a standard pulmonary resection, but it may develop in approximately 3% of patients who have undergone a bronchoplastic procedure, according to the review of Tedder and associates (1992). In most instances, the fistula is the result of a small, clinically asymptomatic abscess from a minor leak of the bronchial suture line that erodes into an adjacent ligated pulmonary artery or one of its branches or through the suture line of an adjacent angioplastic repair. It is best avoided by interposition of a viable tissue flap between the bronchial and vascular suture lines at the time of operation.

Cardiac Complications

Cardiac Herniation

When a defect in the pericardium is not repaired and remains open, herniation of the heart may occur. This rare complication usually follows pneumonectomy but has been reported after lobectomy. The incidence is equal on the right or left side. Opening of the pericardial sac on the left down to the diaphragm prevents left-sided herniation, but opening the pericardium completely on the right does not do so. Cardiac herniation usually occurs in the immediate postoperative period and is usually brought about by a change in the position of the patient. The herniation results in a varying degree of obstruction of both the inflow and outflow of the heart. On the right, cardiac rotation causes torsion of the inferior and superior venae cavae with resultant cessation of inflow to the heart. Increased venous pressure is observed, associated with peripheral hypotension, tachycardia, displaced cardiac impulse, and cardiovascular collapse. The displacement of the heart through a right-sided defect is readily identified on a standard posteroanterior or anteroposterior radiograph of the chest. The displacement on the left side cannot be identified by either of these views but can be appreciated on a lateral radiograph. Left-sided herniation through a defect in the pericardium is a true strangulation hernia, resulting in impairment of left ventricular filling and ejection as well as myocardial blood flow. Electrocardiogram changes may mimic myocardial infarction. In all cases, prompt surgical repair, involving reduction of the herniation and repair (usually with a patch of synthetic material) of the pericardial defect is essential because it may rapidly evolve into a fatal complication. A mortality rate of 50% has occurred in the 30 or more recorded cases.

Cardiac Tamponade

When the pericardium has been opened and subsequently closed to prevent the occurrence of a cardiac herniation, there is the rare possibility, as noted by Harvey and associates (1995), that undetected bleeding may occur from the pericardial incision into the pericardial space. The amount of blood that accumulates may be sufficient to result in a degree of tamponade. Hypotension, increased central venous pressure, a paradoxical pulse, and slowly developing cardiac failure may be seen. Diagnosis is established by determination of right-sided and wedge pressures, radiography, and ultrasonography. The treatment is prompt, adequate drainage of the accumulated blood by a transthoracic or subxiphoid incision or a percutaneous catheter approach.

Hypotension in the Absence of Bleeding

Hypotension associated with an elevated central venous pressure may occur with cardiac tamponade, cardiac herniation, myocardial infarction, and cardiac failure. The first two complications have been discussed, and the third is discussed under Myocardial Ischemia and Myocardial Infarction.

Heart failure caused by underlying cardiac disease is suggested by the patient's preoperative cardiac status and is managed medically with inotropic agents, afterload reduction, diuretics, and other modalities as necessary.

Cardiac Dysrhythmias

Cardiac tachydysrhythmias occur in 18% of patients undergoing noncardiac surgery, according to Amar and associates (1995). Mitsudomi and colleagues (1996) reported the incidence to be as high as 34%, and it was the most common complication after pneumonectomy for lung cancer. The dysrhythmias occur most often in patients aged 60 years or older. Rarely are they seen in anyone younger than the age of 50 years, as noted by one of us (T.W.S.) and Ujiki (1968). Generally, the incidence after pneumonectomy in the older age group is between 20% and 30%; after lobectomy the incidence is lower, in the range of 15 to 20%. Tachydysrhythmias are seen only infrequently after lesser resections. Of all the arrhythmias that occur, atrial fibrillation is the most common. Sinus tachycardia, atrial flutter, runs of premature ventricular contractions, nodal rhythm, and even bradyarrhythmias or bigeminy may occur. Infrequently occurring dysrhythmias include paroxysmal atrial tachycardia with block, multifocal atrial tachycardia, ventricular tachycardia, the sick sinus syndrome, and torsades de pointes (atypical ventricular tachycardia).

Abnormal rhythms usually arise during the first postoperative week. Ritchie and associates (1990) showed that with continuous monitoring initiated at the induction of anesthesia, more than one-half of the arrhythmias are recognized within the first 24 hours of the beginning of the operative procedure (the perioperative and early postoperative period). In their experience, this was more often the case after pneumonectomy than after lobectomy. In the majority of reports, however, the complication is recognized on the second or third day postoperatively.

The duration is variable, and, at times, the heart may revert spontaneously to a normal rhythm. This occurs most often in patients who develop atrial fibrillation, but most patients require medical therapy. Those with other supraventricular tachycardias (SVTs) and bradyarrhythmias also usually require treatment. All potentially lethal arrhythmias require urgent therapy.

The cause of the abnormal rhythms is unknown, although mediastinal shift, hypoxia, and abnormal pH of the blood, as well as other factors, have been implicated but unproved. The effect of vagal nerve irritation on the role of increased right ventricular preload and afterload, as suggested by Nakamura and colleagues (1997), is yet to be determined. What is known is that the occurrence of an arrhythmia is more common with advanced age, coronary artery disease, and a more extensive operative procedure, the incidence being highest after intrapericardial ligation of the pulmonary vessels. Krowka and colleagues (1987) also noted that arrhythmia occurred frequently in the postpneumonectomy patient who develops interstitial pulmonary edema or perihilar edema. Previous cardiac arrhythmia, frequent premature atrial or ventricular contractions preoperatively, and a complete or incomplete right bundle branch block on preoperative electrocardiogram also have been associated with increased incidence of this complication. Von Knorring and associates (1992) also recorded that an abnormal response to exercise and intraoperative hypotension were strong predictors of postoperative cardiac arrhythmias. Asamura and colleagues (1993), in a retrospective study of 267 resections, found an incidence of 23.6% of cardiac dysrhythmias and noted that extensive mediastinal lymph node dissection, the presence of lung cancer, and an age of 70 or older also appeared to be contributing factors.

Most studies have found that the occurrence of postoperative SVTs, particularly if persistent or recurrent, correlates not only with prolongation of hospitalization, but also with an increase in operative mortality. Amar and coworkers (1996) reported that patients who developed tachydysrhythmias after lung cancer surgery had a lower late survival at 1.5 years, independent of other factors such as age, tumor stage, and extent of resection. As a result of the high incidence and potential seriousness of postoperative arrhythmias, many clinicians use prophylactic digitalization in the older patient undergoing pneumonectomy or, less commonly, lobectomy. The potential danger of toxicity must be considered, but the advantages of its prophylactic use in reducing the incidence of arrhythmias, as shown by Wheat and Burford (1961) as well as by one of us (T.W.S.) and

Ujiki (1968), seem to outweigh this possible danger. These clinical trials, however, were retrospective and uncontrolled. Many surgeons, therefore, question the prophylactic use of digitalis, and numerous randomized trials have not supported its use. Krowka and associates (1987) from the Mayo Clinic are opposed to its use, but one must cite the high incidence of arrhythmias their patients experienced as well as the 25% incidence of mortality associated with these complications. In a nonrandomized study, Patel and colleagues (1992) also found the use of prophylactic digitalization to be of no benefit in the reduction of postpneumonectomy arrhythmias. These authors reported a 26% mortality rate with this complication. It is of interest, however, that neither Asamura (1993) nor Mitsudomi (1996) and their associates noted any association of mortality with the development of a dysrhythmia postoperatively.

Although many groups, including Knott-Craig and associates (1997), continue to use prophylactic digoxin, sufficient numbers of prospective randomized trials show that its use confers no protection from the development of an arrhythmia compared to the control groups who received no prophylactic antiarrhythmic therapy. Among these studies are those of Borgeat (1989, 1991), Ritchie (1990, 1992), and Amar (1997) and their associates. Prophylactic agents that appear to be efficacious include flecainide, amiodarone, verapamil, and diltiazem. Borgeat and associates (1991) used a continuous infusion of flecainide (a class Ic antiarrhythmic agent) starting at admission to the postoperative unit and continuing for 72 hours. A significant reduction in the incidence of arrhythmias was observed in the flecainide-treated group (7%) compared to untreated patients or those receiving digoxin (47%). The disadvantages of this regimen include the use of a continuous infusion, the need to measure serum drug levels, and the potential ventricular proarrhythmic effect of flecainide. Van Mieghem and colleagues (1994) used amiodarone to prevent SVT but stopped their trial owing to pulmonary toxicity caused by this drug. Similarly, β-blockers may be effective, but they are generally avoided in pulmonary patients because of the potential induction of bronchospasm or congestive heart failure. Bayliff and associates (1998), in a double-blind study, found that propranolol used as a prophylactic measure did not significantly reduce the incidence of a postoperative arrhythmia but did result in a high incidence of hypotension (49%) and bradycardia (25%). Prophylactic calcium channel blockers appear to decrease the incidence of SVT. Van Mieghem and associates (1996) noted a 50% decrease in atrial fibrillation when a constant infusion of verapamil was begun postoperatively and continued for 72 hours. However, a significant incidence of bradycardia and hypotension existed. Diltiazem, in contrast, appears to be an effective agent, without the side effects of verapamil. In a prospective, randomized study of 70 patients undergoing standard or extrapleural pneumonectomy, Amar and colleagues (1997) found a 28% incidence of supraventricular arrhythmia in the control-placebo group, 31% in the group of patients who received digoxin, and 14% in the diltiazem group. The regimen consists of an initial loading dose of 20 mg intravenously immediately postoperatively, followed by 10 mg intravenously every 4 hours for 24 to 36 hours. On day 2, 180 to 240 mg is given as a single daily oral dose and continued for 30 days. In the diltiazem group, all the dysrhythmias occurred in patients who had undergone an extrapleural pneumonectomy; none was observed in patients who had undergone a standard pneumonectomy. Of interest was the observation that the incidence of dysrhythmias after extrapleural pneumonectomy was essentially the same in the control, the digoxin, and the diltiazem groups (30 to 38%).

When an atrial tachycardia occurs postoperatively that does not revert spontaneously to a normal rhythm, intravenous administration of digoxin is begun and repeated at 4-hour intervals up to a loading dose of 1 mg. If the rhythm fails to convert to normal (typically, 80% of patients respond to this regimen) titrated small boluses of verapamil may be given. An infusion of diltiazem may be equally effective and better tolerated. It is also appropriate to use either of these calcium channel blockers as first-line therapy, in place of digoxin. β-Blockers may be administered for rate control but require careful monitoring for the induction of bronchospasm or congestive heart failure. Pairolero and Payne (1983) suggested the use of oral quinidine sulfate (200 mg three times per day) to control the dysrhythmia. Electrical cardioversion rarely is necessary but should not be delayed when drug therapy fails and the tachycardia is causing clinical deterioration. Harpole and associates (1996) suggest that after rate control has been achieved, procainamide or diltiazem should be given to patients with impaired pulmonary status. Refractory cases benefit from the input of electrophysiology specialists and possibly the use of second-line agents, such as sotalol, amiodarone, or propafenone. In all cases of postoperative SVT, inciting factors, such as inadequate respiratory status, acid–base derangement, electrolyte abnormality, and drugs (e.g., theophylline), should be rapidly identified and corrected. Although often pursued at great monetary cost, myocardial ischemia and infarction are not common etiologies of postoperative SVT.

Persistence or early frequent recurrence of SVT in the postoperative patient always raises the issue of anticoagulation to prevent thromboembolism. No exact guidelines to decide this risk-benefit question (i.e., is the risk of embolism higher than the risk of bleeding in the postsurgical patient, and when in the postoperative period does the ratio change?) exist. If bleeding has complicated the operation, anticoagulation is generally not used early. In many cases, a "low-dose" approach is used initially, either with heparin followed by warfarin (Coumadin) or by starting with warfarin alone. Aspirin may be adequate and less prone to cause hemorrhagic problems. The ideal approach in the specific setting of noncardiac thoracic surgery must await clinical trials.

When an immediate inciting factor is eliminated, in contrast to atrial arrhythmias, ventricular dysrhythmias, especially when not present preoperatively, may reflect myocardial ischemia or damage. Appropriate testing should be instituted quickly. Ventricular tachycardia should be treated promptly with an intravenous bolus of lidocaine hydrochloride, 50 to 100 mg. Once controlled, a lidocaine infusion should be continued at a rate of 1 to 3 mg per minute. Persistent problems require cardiology consultation and, possibly, electrophysiologic testing.

Bradyarrhythmia is managed by the use of atropine or intravenous isoproterenol. Cardiac pacing may be required when a third-degree atrioventricular block or a sick sinus syndrome is present.

Myocardial Ischemia and Myocardial Infarction

Transient myocardial ischemia is uncommon, but Von Knorring and associates (1992) reported this finding in 3.8% of 598 patients undergoing resection for lung cancer. Patients with coronary artery disease and previous myocardial infarction are more prone to develop this complication. Silent ischemia may be identified by postoperative monitoring and usually is seen on the second to fourth postoperative day. Khan (1993) suggested that such patients receive enteric-coated aspirin, 160 to 325 mg daily, as well as an appropriate β-blocker to protect the patient from infarction and death, although this therapy has not been proven in clinical trials.

Myocardial infarction was recorded in 1.2% of patients reported by the aforementioned authors. More significant is that the event is fatal in 50 to 75% of the patients in whom it occurs. The presence of known coronary artery disease is a predictor of a postoperative myocardial infarction, but the significance of preoperative S-T segment and T-wave changes on the electrocardiogram as predictors of a postoperative myocardial infarct is controversial. The appropriate cardiac evaluation of a prospective thoracic surgical patient is discussed in Chapter 20.

Platypnea and Orthodeoxia: Right-to-Left Shunt

Rarely, a patient develops platypnea and orthodeoxia after a pneumonectomy and even less frequently after a lobectomy, usually a right upper lobectomy or a right upper-middle bilobectomy. The patient may or may not be dyspneic in the supine position but becomes so, or the degree of dyspnea worsens, when the patient assumes an upright sitting position. Oxygen saturation is found to be less than normal in the supine position but is rapidly corrected by oxygen administration. The desaturation is exaggerated when the patient sits up or stands. The cause of this unusual event is the presence of a right-to-left interatrial shunt through a patent foramen ovale despite a normal right atrial pressure, as noted by Smeenk and Postmus (1993). Hypovolemia may exacerbate the shunt. It is postulated that the shunt occurs as a result of change in position of the heart after a right pneumonectomy that causes direct streaming of the blood flow from the inferior vena cava to the site of the foramen ovale. Mercho and colleagues (1994) demonstrated this phenome-

non in two patients after a right pneumonectomy with patent foramen ovale and normal atrial pressures by dynamic magnetic resonance (MR) imaging. At least 24 cases have been described in the literature since the original report of Schnabel and coworkers (1956). Bakris and associates (1997) recorded four patients (1997), and Zueger and colleagues (1997) reported one patient with a true septum secundum defect. The diagnosis is confirmed by echocardiography with a "bubble" study, dynamic MR imaging, shunt measurements by catheterization, or cardiac angiography. Closure of the defect is curative. This has been done most often by direct repair, but Godart and coworkers (1997) successfully used a modified button device described by Rao and colleagues (1994) to close secundum defects by a percutaneous route.

Pulmonary Complications

Postpneumonectomy Pulmonary Edema

PPE occurs in 2 to 5% of cases of pneumonectomy. PPE is lethal when unrecognized and carries a high mortality rate, even with early diagnosis. Although PPE is essentially adult respiratory distress syndrome (ARDS, noncardiogenic pulmonary edema), its devastating consequences in the postpneumonectomy patient, refractoriness to standard therapies, and the likelihood that some of the etiologic factors for PPE are unique make it reasonable to view PPE as a specific syndrome. Peters (1987) reported that it usually follows a right pneumonectomy in a patient whose preoperative pulmonary function was good and whose first 12 to 24 hours postoperatively were uneventful. Progressive dyspnea and apprehension appear first. Hypoxemia develops, and when the condition is unrecognized and untreated, death occurs. Peters postulated from clinical observations and studies in the laboratory by Zeldin and associates (1984) that perioperative excessive fluid is the etiologic factor. The single remaining lung must remove a large fluid load, and the fluid filtered in the lung exceeds the capacity of lymphatics. Fluid accumulates in the peribronchial spaces initially, which makes the lung stiffer, increasing the work of breathing. When the peribronchial space is filled, the alveoli fill rapidly with fluid, hypoxemia occurs, and death ensues.

Verheijen-Breemhaar and associates (1988) reported 11 cases of severe PPE in 243 patients (4.5%); the majority (8 of 113 patients, or 7%) were observed after a right pneumonectomy and only three after a left pneumonectomy (2%). Overhydration was the common denominator, and edema was found in three of seven patients who required reoperation for control of postoperative hemorrhage. Patel and associates (1992) recorded 30 cases of varying magnitude of PPE in 197 patients. Thirteen of these 30 patients died (a mortality rate of 43%). PPE also occurs as one of the major fatal complications after a tracheal sleeve pneumonectomy. The pulmonary edema can develop even when strict attention is paid to the amount of perioperative fluid

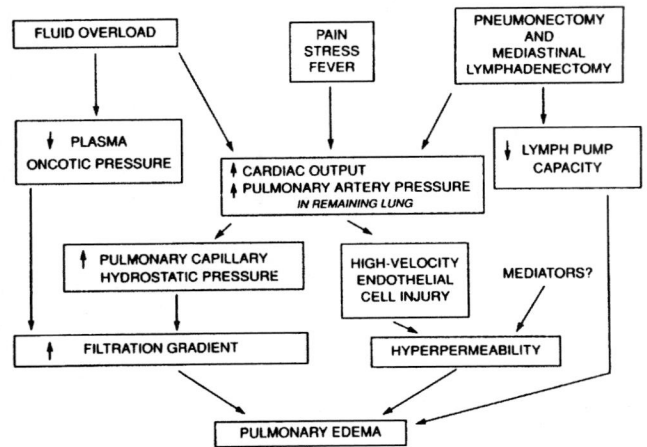

Fig. 37-3. Pathophysiology of postpneumonectomy pulmonary edema. From Shapira OM, Shahian DM: Postpneumonectomy pulmonary edema. Ann Thorac Surg 56:190, 1993. With permission.

used. Mathisen and Grillo (1991), as well as Deslauriers (personal communication, 1992), suggest that the extensive interruption of the major lymphatic channels to the remaining lung as the result of the operative procedure may play a major role in the occurrence of the edema, but this theory remains unproved.

Turnage and Lunn (1993) showed that the histologic changes seen in PPE are those of ARDS (i.e., diffuse alveolar damage). Shapira and Shahian (1993) suggest that the chain of events leading to PPE (Fig. 37-3) results from a combination of increased filtration gradient across the pulmonary microcirculation acting in concert with hyperpermeability. Abnormal capillary permeability in the patient with pulmonary edema was noted by Mathru and associates (1990). Waller and colleagues (1996) suggested that increased pulmonary endothelial permeability may be the result of increased microvascular flow rate because the linear velocity of the blood in the microcirculation increases when a reduced vascular bed is subjected to a constant cardiac output. The increase in flow may result in injury to the endothelium. In addition, Rocker and coworkers (1988) have noted a possible role of neutrophil-related enzymes in producing endothelial injury, with resultant increase in endothelial permeability. Furthermore, van der Werf and associates (1997) noted that multiple transfusions of fresh frozen plasma were associated with PPE, possibly caused by an immunologic reaction to these blood products. Deslauriers and coworkers (1998) found a 4.5% incidence of PPE and 80% mortality rate in 291 pneumonectomies. Like Waller and colleagues (1993) and Turnage and Lunn (1993), these authors did not find a correlation between PPE and fluid balance. In this series, PPE was associated with increasing extent and duration of operation and with the use of an underwater seal drainage system rather than a balanced system. Thus, PPE likely has a multifactorial etiology. It should be noted that PPE may

occur after either a left or right pneumonectomy, as well as after a right upper lobectomy.

Nonetheless, whatever the cause, excessive fluid replacement should be avoided during the operative procedure, as should the use of fresh frozen plasma. It also has been suggested that prolonged high-pressure ventilation be minimized during the operation. When the process is unrecognized (usually within the first 24 to 48 hours) until it is in a full-blown state, the accompanying ventilatory dysfunction progresses relentlessly, despite aggressive therapeutic intervention to reverse the process, and often results in the death of the patient. When the possibility of PPE is suspected, other causes of hypoxemia and radiographic infiltrates (e.g., cardiogenic pulmonary edema, bronchopleural fistula, aspiration, infection, pulmonary embolus, and other pathologic states) must be rapidly sought and in some cases empirically treated until reliably ruled out. When early therapy is instituted, consisting of restriction of fluid intake, morphine, diuretics, and mechanical ventilatory support with positive end-expiratory pressure, the mortality rate associated with this complication may be reduced.

It has been further suggested by Mathisen and associates (1998) that inhaled nitric oxide at a concentration of 10 to 20 parts per million, in addition to measures to improve the management of the patient's secretions, ventilation-perfusion matching, and antibiotics should be added to this regimen. With the institution of inhaled nitric oxide, a statistically significant improvement in oxygenation occurred in all patients so treated, and a significant decrease in postoperative mortality was observed compared to that in patients before the use of nitric oxide. The addition of intravenous steroid therapy revealed no statistically significant benefit in their patients.

Respiratory Insufficiency

Respiratory insufficiency after a pneumonectomy may manifest clinically as dyspnea, tachypnea, rapid pulse, anxiety, and mental confusion. The latter, particularly in elderly persons, may be a prominent and early sign of hypoxia. Results of blood gas studies reveal an early fall in both Po_2 and Pco_2 values, although as respiratory failure progresses, Pco_2 levels become elevated. A shift in the mediastinum toward the remaining lung, elevation of the left leaf of the diaphragm caused by gastric distention after a right pneumonectomy, retention of secretions with areas of atelectasis in the remaining lung, and restriction of chest wall movement because of severe postoperative pain are the major mechanical factors that initiate the problem. They should be corrected by appropriate therapeutic intervention. In a patient who has undergone a lobectomy or a lesser procedure, shallow breathing, reflex splinting of the chest wall, and impaired cough lead to retention of secretions in the ipsilateral lung. If the airway is not kept clear, partial or complete atelectasis of the remaining lobe or lobes on the ipsilateral side may occur. Physical findings and, if necessary, radiographic examination of the chest confirm the diagnosis. Prompt tracheobronchial suction, which may include bronchoscopic aspiration of retained secretions, is indicated. If retention of secretions continues to be troublesome, a tracheostomy may be necessary.

Pulmonary edema or pneumonia also may be a cause of, or contribute to, the magnitude of the pulmonary insufficiency. The physiologic, functional status of the cardiorespiratory system may be the underlying element in the causation of respiratory insufficiency. The remaining capacity may be inadequate for sufficient gas exchange and transportation of adequate oxygen to the tissues of the body. Impaired ventilatory function preoperatively or predicted marginal functional capacity after a proposed resection by standard lung function tests, ventilation-perfusion scans, determination of the diffusion capacity, and oxygen uptake on exercise, as discussed previously, should alert the surgeon to the possible occurrence of pulmonary insufficiency postoperatively. Reduced functional capacity may be exacerbated by the presence of retained secretions, patchy areas of atelectasis, and pulmonary edema, with resultant functional arteriovenous shunting that further contributes to the underlying difficulty. Oxygen therapy, appropriate tracheobronchial toilet, or reintubation with assisted or controlled mechanical ventilation may be indicated to sustain the patient during the acute phase. Respiratory failure is discussed in detail in Chapter 39.

Massive Atelectasis

Severe or massive atelectasis after lobectomy was reported to have an incidence of 7.8% and comprised just under 25% of the complications after lobectomy in 218 patients by Korst and Humphrey (1997). Severe atelectasis was more common after a right upper or a right upper-middle bilobectomy than after a right lower or either left lobectomies. The difference (15.5% versus 6%) was statistically significant. These authors also found no different predisposing factors in those in whom the complication developed compared to those in whom it did not occur.

Clinically, when massive atelectasis does develop, the patient becomes acutely short of breath, and a variable degree of cyanosis ensues. Associated with the tachypnea, a rapid pulse and sharp temperature elevation are observed. The physical findings and radiographic examination are diagnostic. Treatment is prompt and effective tracheobronchial toilet.

Lobar Torsion and Gangrene

A 180-degree rotation of a lobe on its bronchovascular pedicle is occasionally seen intraoperatively with excessive traction and manipulation of the lung during a pulmonary resection. It also may occur spontaneously postoperatively. Rotation is seen most commonly with a freely mobile (i.e., complete major and minor fissures) right middle lobe, as

recorded in a survey by Wong and Goldstraw (1992), but it may occur with either the upper or lower lobe of the left lung as well. If unrecognized and not corrected, vascular occlusion with resultant infarction and gangrene of the involved lobe occurs.

Obviously, the remaining lung after a lobectomy should be inspected to ensure its proper position and lack of torsion before closure of the chest incision. Also, a freely mobile middle lobe after an upper lobectomy (usually associated with torsion of the middle lobe) or lower lobectomy should be stabilized by several interrupted sutures or by stapling to the other remaining lobe to prevent torsion. Such fixation or stabilization is rarely if ever warranted on the left side despite reports of a few isolated cases by Kelly (1977), Linaudais (1980), and Kucich (1989) and their associates.

When this rare event does occur postoperatively, incomplete expansion and opacification of the lobe—often in an unusual anatomic position—can be observed on the postoperative radiographs. Lack of expansion after the usual tracheobronchial suction requires prompt bronchoscopy. Piccione and Faber (1991) report that bronchoscopy reveals a compressed bronchus with a fishmouth appearance. Although the scope may be passed through the obstruction, the involved bronchus collapses as the scope is withdrawn. Although the features of torsion on radionuclide perfusion scan, pulmonary angiography, and computed tomography (CT) have been well described, these studies are generally not required for diagnosis.

When torsion of the lobe is suggested by radiographic and bronchoscopic findings, immediate reoperation is indicated to release the torsion and to stabilize the involved lobe, if viable, in the correct anatomic position. If the lobe is not viable, a lobectomy of the involved middle lobe on the right or a completion pneumonectomy on the left side becomes necessary.

When the torsion remains unrecognized, infarction and gangrene of the involved lobe occur, with the resultant local thoracic and systemic findings of infection. Gangrene of a lobe also may occur in the absence of torsion, as noted by Piccione and Faber (1991). The underlying cause of the gangrene is an unrecognized ligation or other compromise of either the venous outflow or, less commonly, the pulmonary arterial supply of the lobe. In either instance, reoperation and resection of the involved lobe are mandatory. The rarity of lobar gangrene is supported by the data reported by Keagy and associates (1985), in which only one instance of this complication was noted in 224 complications (0.4%) in 369 patients (0.27%) who had undergone a lobectomy.

Pulmonary Infarction After Angioplasty

After pulmonary artery angioplasty accompanying a lobectomy or a bronchoplastic procedure, thrombosis may occur secondary either to kinking of the vessel or stenosis at the site of the repair. With rare exception, this leads to infarction of the supplied pulmonary parenchyma. A low-grade fever and opacification of the lung are present in the absence of a bronchial obstruction. According to Warren (1995), initially the bronchial mucosa may appear normal on bronchoscopy but soon becomes cyanotic, edematous, and hemorrhagic. The diagnosis is confirmed by a pulmonary angiogram or a perfusion scan. Once the diagnosis is made, a completion pneumonectomy is indicated.

Postoperative Pneumonia

In some patients, infection may be superimposed on unresolved atelectatic areas or may result from unrecognized episodes of aspiration. The true incidence of postoperative pneumonia is difficult to establish; in most reviews, this complication is considered together with atelectasis and major problems associated with retention of secretions. Keagy and associates (1985) noted this conglomerate group of complications in 7% of 369 patients who had undergone lobectomy, and Wahi and colleagues (1989) reported an incidence of 6.6% in 197 patients who had undergone a pneumonectomy. Although the overall incidence of pneumonia was not recorded, Von Knorring and associates (1992) reported it was the cause of death in 1.3% of 598 patients undergoing resection for lung cancer. Tedder and associates (1992), in a review of bronchoplastic procedures, noted that postoperative pneumonia per se occurred in 6.6% of the reported patients and was responsible for 15.4% of the postoperative deaths observed. Hollaus and colleagues (1997) reported that aspiration pneumonia is common in patients with a bronchopleural fistula. In these patients, the aspiration often is associated with the development of ARDS. Approximately 40% of patients die as the result of the development of this complication.

Although data are sparse, it is likely that postoperative pneumonia is seen most often in patients who require prolonged ventilatory support or who have continued inordinate difficulty in clearing their tracheobronchial secretions. Aerobic, anaerobic, and mixed infections occur, and proper collection (e.g., bronchoscopic aspiration, protected brush) and cultural procedures for identification of the offending organisms are mandatory (see Chapter 14). Although most postresection pneumonias are caused by bacteria, the possibility of viral, fungal, *Legionella*, and *Mycoplasma* pneumonia should always be kept in mind, especially in patients immunosuppressed by cancer and its treatment and those with complicated postoperative courses. Camazine and associates (1995) stress the need for a high index of suspicion of atypical infections in debilitated patients after finding that three of six patients with pneumonia and respiratory failure in a series of 54 consecutive thoracotomies for cancer had herpes simplex virus pneumonia. All three patients responded to acyclovir.

In all cases, appropriate antibiotics, nutritional support, and good tracheobronchial toilet are essential for recovery. *Pseudomonas* and *Serratia* infections, as in other clinical settings, are the most difficult.

Prolonged Air Leak

After pulmonary resections of lesser magnitude than a pneumonectomy, an air leak from a residual raw parenchymal surface is a common occurrence. With complete reexpansion of the lung and obliteration of the pleural space, the leak usually stops in 2 to 3 days. The persistence of a leak beyond 7 days is considered abnormal and is generally used to define a "prolonged" air leak. Various maneuvers—increasing or decreasing the suction applied to the water seal system, conversion to water seal drainage only, or placement of additional chest tubes—may be tried empirically. In most instances, the air leak stops even if the space persists.

Prolonged air leaks are a very frequent problem in volume reduction surgery for emphysema, occurring in 30 to 50% of cases. The various methods suggested to reduce the incidence of persistent air leak from stapled excision lines through emphysematous parenchyma are discussed in Chapter 26 and its management in Chapter 83. Rice and Kirby (1992) reported peripheral air leaks lasting more than 7 days in 35 (15.2%) of 197 patients undergoing pulmonary resection. Only three leaks (1.5%), however, persisted beyond 2 weeks. Although there were no complications directly related to the leaks, the mean postoperative length of stay was 5.6 days longer in this group.

No single correct way exists to manage a persistent air leak. The ingenuity and experience of the surgeon greatly affect the approach in the individual patient in whom infection of any accompanying air space is absent. The identification and occlusion by vascular embolization coils and fibrin glue of the subsegmental bronchi supplying the leaking site, as described by one of us (R.B.P.) and associates (1993), may be successful. Application of fibrin glue to the leaking parenchymal surface by a thoracoscopic approach has also been described. Some recommend that the presence of a prolonged air leak in patients without evidence of a pneumothorax be managed by the instillation of talc slurry. Because complications of peripheral air leaks are uncommon, reoperation is rarely warranted. As shown by McKenna (1996) and one of us (R.B.P.) (1997) and associates, most cases can be managed on an outpatient basis with Heimlich valves. If sepsis develops, however, the presence of a frank bronchopleural fistula must be assumed, and appropriate management to resolve the issue is warranted.

Bronchopleural Fistula

A bronchopleural fistula is observed in 1 to 4% of patients after a pneumonectomy or a lobectomy and less often after a segmentectomy or lesser procedure. Vester and associates (1991) reported an incidence of 3.9% after 503 pneumonectomies, 3.7% after stapled closure of the bronchus, 12.5% after suture closure, 1.1% after 1083 lobectomies, and 0.3% after 650 segmentectomies. Asamura and associates (1992) reported an incidence of 2.1% after 2359 pulmonary resections for lung cancer. al–Kattan and colleagues (1994) reported an incidence of fistula of only 1.3% in 530 consecutive pneumonectomies. The bronchial stump was closed manually with nonabsorbable monofilament 2-0 Prolene sutures. Of interest is the report of Sarsam and Moussali (1989). They recorded no fistulas after the use of a bronchoplastic method of closure using a membranous flap from the posterior bronchial wall (originally described by Jack [1965]) in a series of 332 pneumonectomies, despite the use of chromic catgut as the suture material.

A bronchopleural fistula is more common after resections for inflammatory disease of the lung, especially in patients with active tuberculosis and positive sputum. Pomerantz and colleagues (1991) noted a 10.5% incidence after resection in 85 patients with resistant mycobacterial infections. Almost all occurred after a right pneumonectomy in patients with multiple drug–resistant *Mycobacterium avium-intracellulare* infections, despite a transposed muscle flap to cover the bronchial stump. In a contrasting report, Brown and Pomerantz (1995) reported only one fistula in 62 pneumonectomies in patients with multidrug-resistant *M. tuberculosis* infections; the vast majority were extrapleural pneumonectomies and a few were completion pneumonectomies. In patients who received a full course of preoperative mediastinal and hilar irradiation, Yashar and associates (1992) reported an incidence of 9.6%. In a multivariate analysis of 1360 recent lung cancer resections, Asamura and associates (1992) noted that the significant risk factors for a bronchopleural fistula were pneumonectomy, residual tumor at the bronchial stump, preoperative irradiation, and diabetes. These authors also noted that most bronchopleural fistulas occur after resections of the right lung, particularly a right pneumonectomy (Table 37-1).

Early after a resection (1 to 2 days, even up to 7 days), a bronchopleural fistula may occur because of a technically poor closure of the bronchial stump. After pneumonectomy, an early bronchopleural fistula manifests by a massive air leak with the development of a progressive increase in clinically evident subcutaneous emphysema. A small amount of subcutaneous emphysema is normally seen because some of the air in the postpneumonectomy space at the time of clo-

Table 37-1. Prevalence of Bronchopleural Fistula According to Side of Resection

Resection	% of Operations Performed	
	Right Side	Left Side
Segmentectomy	0	0
Lobectomy	1.7	0.3
Pneumonectomy	8.6	2.3
Bronchoplasty	6.9	0
Pleuropneumonectomy	25.0	0
All resections	3.0	0.9

From Asamura H, et al: Bronchopleural fistulas associated with lung cancer operations. Univariate and multivariate analysis of risk factors, management and outcome. J Thorac Cardiovasc Surg *104*:1456, 1992. With permission.

sure is expelled into the tissue of the chest wall with coughing or is forced out with a rapid accumulation of fluid within the space. Along with the development of massive subcutaneous emphysema, the patient may exhibit varying degrees of respiratory insufficiency because the fistula physiologically represents a modified open pneumothorax. Ventilatory support, often best accomplished by the use of selective bronchial intubation or jet ventilation, may be necessary at this stage in severe cases.

When the bronchial leak occurs later in the postoperative course, it may be caused by failure of healing resulting from inadequate viable tissue coverage of the stump or infection of the fluid within the space and rupture of the empyema through the bronchial stump. At this stage, the patient expectorates variable quantities of serosanguineous, frothy fluid. Danger of flooding of the remaining lung is present. The patient should be placed with the operated side down and the head elevated. Prompt drainage of the affected pleural space is indicated.

When a bronchopleural fistula occurs later than 2 weeks after pneumonectomy, it is most likely the result of rupture of an empyema through the bronchial stump, although at times lack of healing of the bronchial stump may be the underlying cause. Clinically, the patient is most likely febrile and has a cough productive of purulent sputum. Hemoptysis may occur.

An occult bronchopleural fistula without expectoration of pleural fluid occasionally occurs (Fig. 37-4). A fall in the fluid level on a chest radiograph should arouse suspicion. It is unclear whether the fluid escapes through the bronchus and is swallowed, unnoticed, by the patient or is lost by absorption through the parietal pleura as the result of increased intrapleural pressure, which becomes potentially greater than atmospheric pressure. Nonetheless, confirmation of the diagnosis can be sought by instillation of methylene blue into the pneumonectomy space and watching for its appearance in the sputum, by bronchoscopy to examine the stump, or by radionuclide inhalation.

Management of an occult bronchopleural fistula poses a vexing clinical problem. When the patient remains asymptomatic and no signs of clinical infection are present, expectant treatment with systemic antibiotics and close observation is acceptable, as suggested by O'Meara and Slade (1974). More often than not, there is no further difficulty. If any finding of clinical infection occurs, however, prompt drainage of the pleural space is mandatory.

Management of a clinically evident bronchopleural fistula depends on the time of its development postoperatively and its underlying cause. Early in the postoperative period (up to 7 or even 14 days, according to Brutel de la Riviere (1997), reoperation and repair of the bronchial stump may be indicated. With operative repair, coverage of the new bronchial suture line is mandatory. A transposed muscle flap, the pericardial fat pad, or an omental pedicle flap may be used (see Chapter 59). Otherwise, evacuation of the fluid in the affected pleural space and institution of proper drainage are

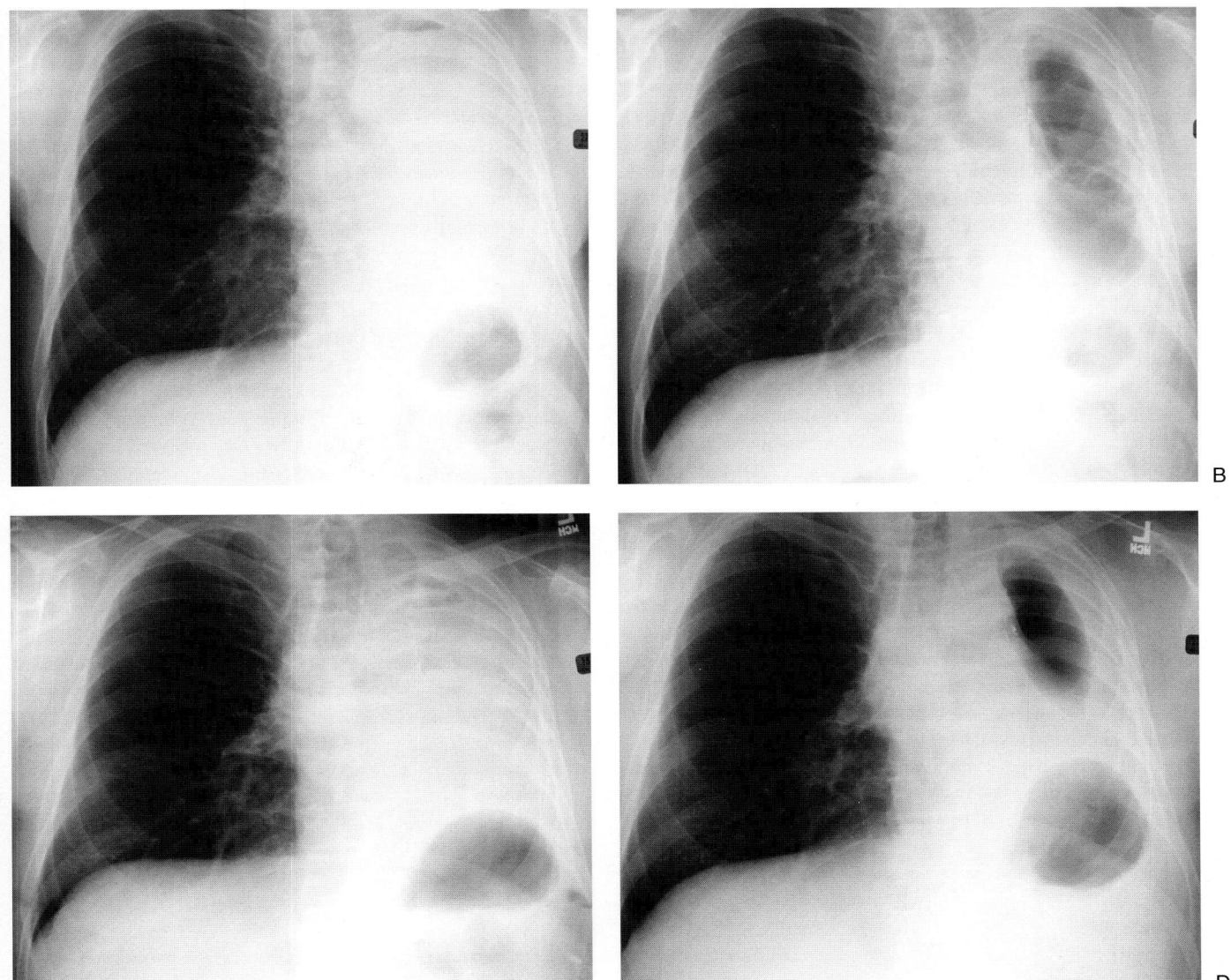

Fig. 37-4. Occult postpneumonectomy bronchopleural fistula. **A.** Chest radiograph 1 month after left pneumonectomy shows space almost completely filled with fluid. **B.** Film 2 months later at routine follow-up shows a large volume of air in the hemithorax. The patient was entirely well and had not noted cough, sputum, or symptoms of infection. Bronchoscopy at this time was negative. **C.** Fourteen months later, the hemithorax is filled with fluid and a few air pockets (1.5 years postpneumonectomy and 6 months after the hemithorax was filled with antibiotic-saline solution at the time of thoracoscopy and repeat bronchoscopy, both of which did not demonstrate a fistula or recurrent tumor). **D.** Six months afterward (2 years after pneumonectomy) a large volume of air is again seen in the pleural space. The patient remains asymptomatic and without evidence of recurrent cancer 2.5 years after diagnosis of an occult bronchopleural fistula.

indicated. Jensen and Sharma (1985) suggested using fibrin glue to occlude the opening when the fistula is small. Moritz (personal communication, 1986) had success with this method for closing small bronchopleural fistulas that developed from a technical failure with the use of a mechanical stapling device. Glover and associates (1987) also reported successful use of fibrin glue for the closure of small fistulas. Hollaus and coworkers (1998) reported that the endoscopic application of fibrin glue was most successful in the treat-

ment of fistulas less than 3 mm; endoscopic techniques alone were less satisfactory in patients with larger fistulas.

In most situations, when a major bronchopleural fistula is present, more aggressive measures to achieve closure of the fistula and to control the associated empyema are necessary. Puskas and colleagues (1995) at the Massachusetts General Hospital recommend initial drainage and the subsequent direct closure of the bronchus by a manual suture technique and support of the suture line with an omental flap. Eventual obliteration of the pleural space may be necessary. At the Mayo Clinic, Pairolero and colleagues (1990) advocate that after stabilization of the patient, open drainage be accomplished by establishing an Eloesser flap or reopening a portion of the original thoracotomy. Trastek (1997) reiterated their experience. After cleansing of the pleural space, the bronchial stump is reclosed and reinforced with vascularized tissue in the form of a transposed muscle or omental flap. Subsequent sterilization of the pleural space is accomplished by the Clagett maneuver. Gharagozloo and associates (1998) reported success with 22 early postpneumonectomy fistulas by reoperation for débridement and bronchial stump closure, continuous pleural irrigation with 0.1% povidone-iodine (40 mL per hour for 7 days) followed by saline irrigation for 24 hours. If a Gram stain of the pleural effluent was negative at that point, the hemithorax was filled with 2 L of a solution containing gentamicin, neomycin, and polymyxin B. If the Gram stain was positive, povidone-iodine irrigation was resumed and the cycle repeated. There were no recurrent fistulas or empyemas, and the mean hospitalization after repair was only 13 days. The use of muscle flaps to close bronchopleural fistulas and to obliterate the pleural space, as described by Miller (1984), is discussed in detail in Chapter 59.

Transsternal transpericardial exposure and division of a long bronchial stump associated with a bronchopleural fistula have become popular. When the distal stump cannot be removed, a tissue flap, preferably muscle, should be transposed between the divided ends. Simple stapling of the stump proximal to the leak is ineffective: Refistulization inevitably occurs. Abruzzini (1961) was one of the first to report the importance of division of the stump to control a fistula.

Maassen (1975), Bruni (1987), Perelman (1987), and Perelman and Ambatiello (1970) also recorded the use of this procedure in Europe. In the United States, Baldwin and Mark (1985) and Cosgrove (1985), and in Canada, Ginsberg and associates (1989), also have reported its use. The technique and indications for transsternal closure of a bronchopleural fistula are presented in Chapter 34. Perelman and associates (1987) also described a right posterior approach to the left main bronchial stump (Fig. 37-5) that was accomplished in 25 patients, with good results in 20. Four late deaths occurred, two related to bronchial recanalization and two related to progressive empyema. Brutel de la Riviere and associates (1997), in addition to their experience with the transsternal transpericardial closure of a long stump, reported the use of a carinal resection to eradicate a fistula in patients with a short bronchial stump. However, a high failure rate occurred with this approach. Azorin and colleagues (1996) reported a transcervical mediastinal video-assisted thoracoscopic approach to staple the left main stem bronchial stump for control of a postpneumonectomy bronchopleural fistula. The pleural space was then cleaned and drained through a thoracic approach. Although this technique appeared to be successful, the stump was not divided, and late recanalization remains a possibility.

Bronchopleural fistula rarely occurs after a lobectomy. Management of the open bronchial stump and the usually associated empyema space is like that after a pneumonectomy except that the presence of pulmonary tissue in the hemithorax modifies the management to a variable extent (see Chapter 59). Occasionally, it is advisable to perform a completion pneumonectomy, although, as noted by McGovern and colleagues (1988), the complication rate is high

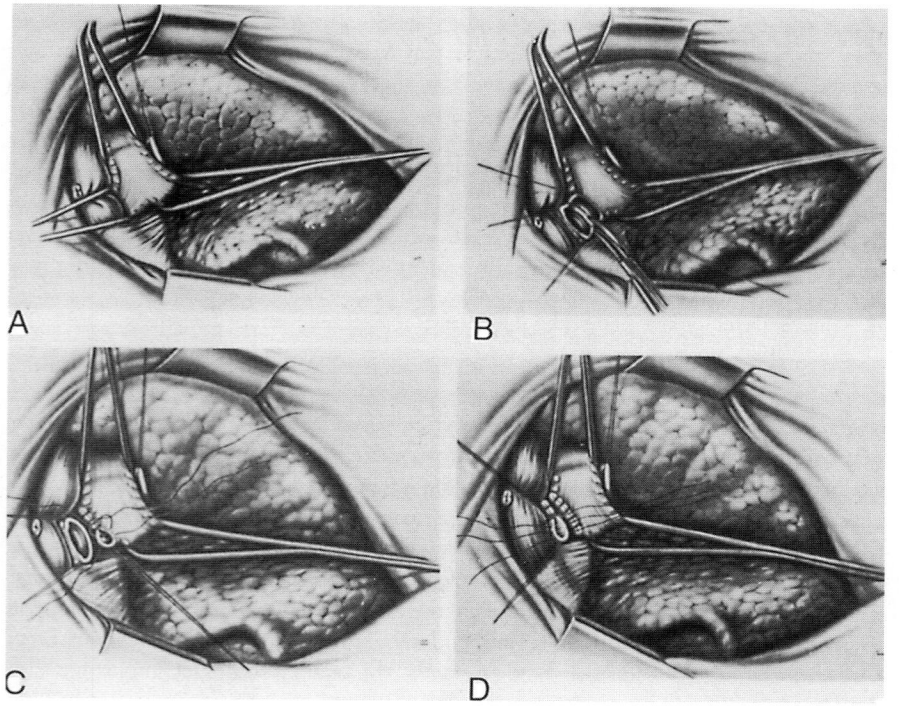

A

B

C

D

Fig. 37-5. Right posterior approach to the left main stem bronchus. **A.** The trachea and both main stem bronchi have been isolated and tapes placed around them. **B.** The left main stem bronchial stump is dissected off the trachea. **C.** The trachea is closed with interrupted sutures. **D.** The remaining distal stump is closed in a similar manner. From Perelman MI, Rymko LP, Ambatiello GP: Bronchopleural fistula: surgery after pneumonectomy. *In* Eschapasse H, Grillo H (eds): International Trends in General Thoracic Surgery. Major Challenges. Vol. 2. Philadelphia: WB Saunders, 1987. With permission.

(>50%). Deslauriers (1988) emphasized the hazard of previous irradiation when a completion pneumonectomy is contemplated. He also noted that when bronchial dehiscence is the indication for completion pneumonectomy accompanying a "benign" inflammatory process, other therapeutic options deserve serious consideration before resorting to this procedure. Bronchial dehiscence and fistula formation also occur after broncho- or tracheoplastic procedures. In a survey of 1562 such procedures performed in Japan, Maeda and associates (1989) reported this complication in 5.6% of cases, with death in 47.7% of those in whom it occurred, for an overall mortality rate of 2.7%. This complication is discussed in more detail in the specific chapters related to these procedures (see Chapters 28 and 30).

The reported mortality rate after the development of a bronchopleural fistula is variable. Rates as low as 16% to as high as 72% have been recorded. Most deaths are caused by sepsis, respiratory insufficiency, and malnutrition. Rarely, inflammatory erosion of the pulmonary artery stump occurs, with resulting fatal hemorrhage. Khargi and associates (1993) recorded a 4% incidence of this event with a 50% mortality rate. Most of the series reported have not comprised comparable patients, disease states, or operations, so that it is impossible to state categorically which patients are most likely to succumb as a result of a bronchopleural fistula. However, those who have undergone an extensive peribronchial dissection or a right-sided pneumonectomy or who received preoperative irradiation are at greatest risk. Others at high risk are those who have undergone a tracheo- or bronchoplastic procedure, have borderline pulmonary function, have a serious comorbid disease, or are elderly.

Pleural Complications

Persistent Residual Air Space

A persistent residual air space frequently occurs after a lobectomy. It is more common in older persons and in those who have undergone resection for pulmonary granulomatous diseases than in other lobectomy patients. When resection was common for the management of persistent negative cavitary *M. tuberculosis*, one of us (T.W.S.) and colleagues (1959) reported an incidence of persistent residual air space as high as 21%. Presently, most residual air spaces are seen after lobectomy for carcinoma. The space may be located superiorly in the apex (more common) or inferiorly, just above the diaphragm. The majority of spaces do not cause symptoms, and the clinical course of the patient is unaffected by their presence. An asymptomatic space gradually disappears over a period of months, by absorption of the gases within the space and further expansion of the remaining lung or by the deposition of a pleural peel in the area. A small number of the air spaces, however, do cause symptoms and require surgical intervention of varying magnitude for their eventual control. The symptoms may consist of pain, dyspnea, hemoptysis, fever, or signs of continued air leak. The persistent air leak may be caused by seepage from the alveoli (a small peripheral fistula) or from a frank bronchopleural fistula. With alveolar seepage, the composition of the gas in the space is the same as that of the gas in the alveolar spaces rather than the gas in the venous blood. Although it is impossible to maintain a negative pressure within the space because of this seepage, the space may remain sterile. In the presence of a frank bronchopleural fistula, however, not only is a major air leak present, but also an empyema ultimately develops. Such a space is controlled by drainage and obliteration of the space, as discussed in Chapter 59.

The incidence of persistent pleural air space after a segmentectomy is as high as 33% in patients with pulmonary tuberculosis (Fig. 37-6), but it is less after one for the removal of a lung tumor. Compared with the pleural air spaces occurring after a lobectomy, however, a smaller percentage of those occurring after segmentectomy become symptomatic. When serious complications develop as a result of the space, they are most likely septic.

Persistent air spaces after a wedge resection occur infrequently. The incidence is less than 10%. Almost all are benign and resolve without treatment. Space problems are common after lung volume-reduction operations (see Chapter 83). Creation of an apical pleural tent to convert the potential space to an extrapleural location has been repopularized in this group of patients and applied to other instances in which space problems may be anticipated.

Pleural Effusion

A small collection of pleural effusion at the base of the hemithorax is common after lobectomy or a lesser resection, but major collections are uncommon if satisfactory pleural drainage has been maintained. When a significant amount of fluid persists, more efficient drainage should be established. Although, in most instances, the fluid that remains is reabsorbed or becomes organized, the danger of infection persists. Pulmonary function may be affected adversely by the persistence of the fluid collection.

Empyema

Empyema occurs less frequently than in the early years of thoracic surgery but is still seen in 1 to 3% of patients who undergo a pneumonectomy. It may or may not be associated with a bronchopleural fistula. The use of prophylactic intrapleural and systemic antibiotics remains controversial. If gross contamination occurs at operation or if reoperation is necessary for control of postoperative hemorrhage or an early bronchial leak, the risk of developing an empyema increases. Gaud (1987) noted that postoperative mechanical ventilation also increased the risk.

When an empyema occurs, the patient shows a greater or lesser degree of systemic toxicity, the white blood cell count

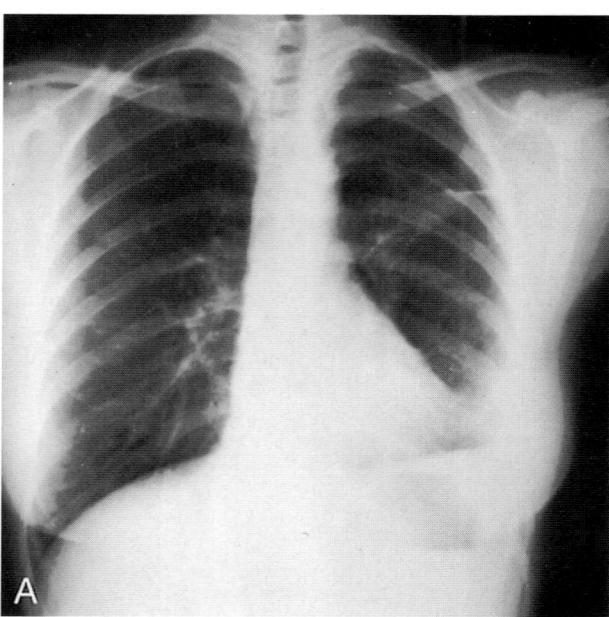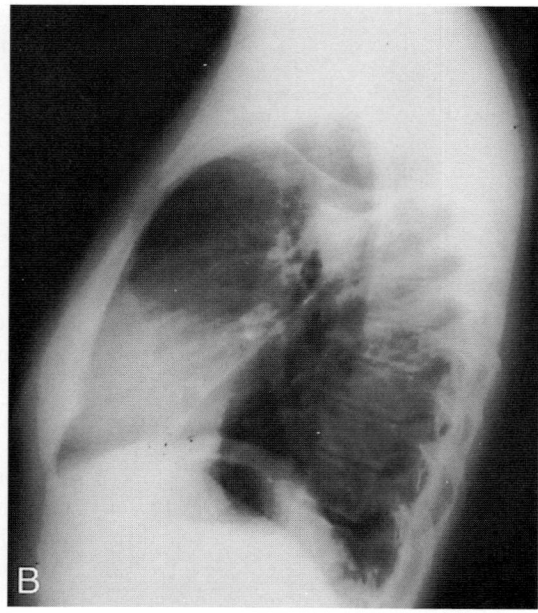

Fig. 37-6. Posteroanterior (**A**) and lateral (**B**) radiographs reveal an asymptomatic air space 6 weeks after a left apical posterior segmentectomy was performed for treatment of pulmonary tuberculosis.

is elevated with a shift to the left, the appetite is poor, and general deterioration occurs. At times, it is difficult to establish a definitive diagnosis of the presence of a frank empyema. In such situations, Icard and colleagues (1994) have stressed the use of measuring blood levels of C-reactive protein. This protein is one of the better indicators of the acute phase response to trauma, infection, and inflammation. In the presence of a smoldering empyema, the patient has persistently high C-reactive protein values or exhibits a secondary rise in the levels above 100 mg/L. Once the diagnosis is established, drainage of the space is indicated. Bacterial cultures and sensitivity studies of the exudate are obtained, and definitive management of the empyema is carried out as discussed in Chapter 59.

An empyema is also a major complication after a lobectomy. It occurs more commonly after resections for inflammatory disease than after those for the removal of a malignant or benign lung tumor. Significantly, a residual basal space seems to be associated more commonly with subsequent infection than is the more frequent apical residual space. The initial treatment consists of adequate drainage and systemic antibiotics. The space may ultimately need to be obliterated by one of the techniques described in Chapter 59. It should be noted that the ipsilateral pulmonary function is reduced by the occurrence and the treatment of an empyema.

Postresection Chylothorax

Injury to the thoracic duct with subsequent chylothorax is rare after pulmonary resection. Simpson (1990) stated

that the incidence of such injury was less than 0.05%. However, Brie (1990), Sarsam (1994), and Terzi (1994) and their associates report rates of 0.3%, 0.5%, and 0.74%, respectively. From 1950 to 1970, most injuries followed resections for benign diseases (e.g., pulmonary tuberculosis) but at present, they are more common after resections for the management of carcinoma of the lung, particularly during aggressive resection of the local tumor or mediastinal lymph nodes involved by extensive metastatic disease. Injury to the duct may occur anywhere along its course or at one of the small lymphatic channels from the lung, or may be due to injury of a channel from a mediastinal lymph node that enters directly into the thoracic duct, which were demonstrated by the anatomic study of Riquet and associates (1989). Such injuries have occurred after upper and lower lobectomies or after pneumonectomies on either side. The injury generally is not recognized until the patient resumes oral alimentation. In the postlobectomy patient, the chylothorax is manifested by the change in the character of the drainage to a milky fluid and an increase in the amount of drainage. In nine postpneumonectomy patients, Sarsam and colleagues (1994) noted a rapid accumulation of fluid in the pleural space without the onset of any ominous symptomatology in five of the nine patients, but the other four patients developed major mediastinal shift to the contralateral side with subsequent hemodynamic and respiratory embarrassment. The development of a tension chylothorax also was noted by Karwande (1986) and Brie (1990) and their colleagues in a number of their patients. Emergency thoracentesis reveals the characteristic milky fluid, and immediate closed-tube thoracostomy is indicated.

Ngan (1988) and Vallieres (1993) and their colleagues suggested that lymphangiography be performed soon after the diagnosis is made. Standard lipoidal lymphangiography, despite the risk of an occasional pulmonary complication, may demonstrate the site of the leak or the lack of one, at best. Nuclear lymphangiography, although used by Rice and associates (1987), may not be successful in this regard. Lipoidal lymphangiography is both diagnostic and prognostic. When no major leak is seen and the contrast material appears at the terminus of the thoracic duct, certain investigators believe that conservative management is more likely to be successful.

Definitive therapy in either situation (postlobectomy or postpneumonectomy) consists of an initial trial period of expectant therapy with continued drainage and total parenteral nutrition or low-fat diet and medium-chain triglycerides for 7 to 14 days. With reexpansion of the remaining lung in the postlobectomy patient, the leak frequently seals (approximately 50% or more of patients), but spontaneous closure is less likely in the postpneumonectomy patient. In a postpneumonectomy patient, a continued leak of more than 300 mL per day is an indication for surgical intervention with ligation of the thoracic duct, as described in Chapter 63. In the series reported by Brie and associates (1990), this step was necessary in all four patients who had undergone a pneumonectomy. In the postlobectomy patient, a persistent leak of 500 mL per day is an indication of failure of conservative management. Operative intervention (i.e., ligation of either the leak or the proximal thoracic duct) is then required. Stenzl (1983) and Akaogi (1989) and their associates reported successful closure of the leak with the use of fibrin glue applied through tube thoracostomies. Morita (1990) and Landreneau (1992) and their colleagues have used a video-assisted thoracoscopic surgical approach to control the chylous leak.

Esophageal Injury

Injury to the esophagus may occur during a difficult dissection in the course of a pneumonectomy performed for either inflammatory or extensive neoplastic disease. Shama and Odell (1985) reported an incidence of 0.5% in a series of 869 pneumonectomies for inflammatory disease. Van den Bosch and associates (1980) noted that most (92%) occurred on the right and, in two-thirds of all cases, after resection of inflammatory disease. Benjamin and colleagues (1969) reported its occurrence during resection for carcinoma. Massard and colleagues (1994) recorded seven esophageal injuries that occurred during lung resections: six during the removal of a carcinoma and only one during treatment of an inflammatory disease process.

In contrast to Evans' (1972) belief that most esophageal fistulas result from erosion of a peribronchial abscess into the esophagus, most surgeons now believe that the injury to the esophagus occurs at the time of surgery and that only the manifestation of the resultant empyema is recognized late.

When a difficult mediastinal dissection is encountered intraoperatively, peroral placement of a large bougie may aid in identifying the esophagus. If an injury is suspected, injection of air or methylene blue may locate the site. When recognized at operation, immediate repair usually is successful, but if the injury is overlooked, mediastinitis and empyema occur. Recognition of the source of the infection may be elusive until oral feedings are observed in the thoracic drainage. The injury may be confirmed by a barium swallow. Treatment is use of one of the many options for any late-recognized esophageal injury, as described in Chapter 132. The overall results, as noted by Massard and coworkers (1994), are poor, with prolonged morbidity and a high incidence of eventual mortality.

Wound Complications

Wound Infections

Infection of a thoracotomy or sternotomy incision after a pulmonary resection is rare. When present, the usual signs and symptoms of infection are present. Open drainage and antibiotics are indicated in its management.

Wound Dehiscence

Complete breakdown of a thoracic incision after a pulmonary resection is even less common than a wound infection. Early dehiscence requires prompt reclosure, but late dehiscence, most often the result of wound infection, may be managed initially by local débridement and pleural drainage, with subsequent reclosure when the infection has been controlled.

Subcutaneous Emphysema

Air trapped in the pleural space after a pneumonectomy, or air from a leak that is not being removed effectively by the chest tube drainage system after a lobectomy or lesser resection, may be forced out through the intercostal incision into the soft tissues of the chest wall on change of position or coughing. This subcutaneous air may be localized only to the wound area, but when excessive amounts of air are forced into the adjacent tissue planes, it may extend up into the face and down to the groin and into the scrotum. No specific therapy is required other than improving and ensuring patency of the drainage system. On occasion, a sudden massive air leak may indicate the occurrence of a bronchopleural fistula, but in most instances, subcutaneous emphysema is a benign, self-limiting situation. Upper airway obstruction as the result of the emphysema is a rare complication, and the use of cervical incisions to decompress the area is not indicated. If airway obstruction is suggested clinically, endotracheal intubation should be done.

Thoracic Neurologic Complications

Injury to Intrathoracic Nerves

Phrenic Nerve

Unsuspected injury to the phrenic nerve rarely occurs during pulmonary resection. Unintentional injury is most often due to mechanical or electrocautery attempts to control bleeding from the vein that accompanies the nerve or if dense mediastinal adhesions must be divided for hilar exposure. More often, the nerve is knowingly sacrificed in the removal of a tumor invading the mediastinum or in the excision of metastatic nodes anterior to the superior pulmonary vein. Although most patients clinically tolerate unilateral loss of diaphragmatic function, paralysis does lessen ventilatory capacity, even when present on the side of a pneumonectomy. The consequences to people with marginal pulmonary function may be significant. Purposeful injury or division of the nerve to paralyze the hemidiaphragm to reduce the volume of the ipsilateral hemithorax ("phrenic crush") is to be avoided, except in unusual circumstances.

Recurrent Laryngeal Nerve

Recurrent nerve injury occurs far more often on the left and results from mechanical or cautery dissection of mediastinal lymph nodes or invasive tumor in the aortopulmonary window at the ligamentum arteriosum. Exposure of the nerve at this time may help to avoid its injury. Right-sided injury is rare in cases of pulmonary resection, being seen only with extensive high node dissections. Unilateral damage results in hoarseness and can also cause serious problems with aspiration. In a series of complete mediastinal lymph node dissections in patients with lung cancer, Bollen and associates (1993) observed unintentional injury in 3 of 62 patients. The number of left-sided dissections was not recorded, so the actual incidence of this injury remains unknown. It should be noted that the many advocates of systematic lymph node dissection in lung cancer patients usually do not record this injury. In patients who have received neoadjuvant therapy for locally advanced lesions, injury to or the necessary removal of either the vagal or phrenic nerve because of the extent of the disease process, as noted by Yashar and colleagues (1992), may increase the number of these injuries.

Spinal Cord Injury

Injury to the spinal cord with resultant paraplegia usually results from attempts to control persistent bleeding from an intercostal vessel or to stop continued oozing at the posterior angle of the intercostal incision or at the site of removal of a portion of a vertebra. Thrombosis of the anterior spinal artery is an infrequent cause.

Use of unipolar cautery is to be avoided in these areas, as is packing of the area with hemostatic substances, such as oxidized cellulose. Either continued bleeding with egress of blood into the spinal canal or migration and swelling of the hemostatic material within the canal, as reported by Short (1990), may compromise the space and result in pressure on the spinal cord. Compression of the spinal cord is poorly tolerated, and paraplegia readily develops.

Attar and colleagues (1995) reported five instances of paraplegia from their own institution and reviewed 35 cases reported in the literature. They confirm that the major intraoperative factors contributing to this devastating complication were bleeding at the costovertebral angle and the use of oxidized cellulose to control this bleeding, with subsequent migration and swelling of the material in the spinal canal. Thrombosis of the anterior spinal artery, epidural hematoma, epidural narcotic, metastatic carcinoma, and intraoperative hypotension were infrequent causes. If bleeding in the costovertebral angle appears significant and persistent, the thoracic surgeon should seek neurosurgical assistance for widening of the foramen, bipolar cautery control, and other specialized techniques. Walker (1990) and Benfield (1990) discussed the avoidance, prophylactic management, and early recognition of this complication during the operative procedure. However, even early postoperative diagnosis and prompt neurosurgical decompression of the spinal cord frequently do not reverse the process.

Dural Laceration: Subarachnoid-Pleural Fistula

Laceration of the dura without damage to the spinal cord may occur during pulmonary resection and result in a subarachnoid pleural fistula, commonly called *a cerebrospinal fluid (CSF) leak*. Most often, this complication occurs during resection of lung neoplasms that invade the posterior chest wall in the region of the costovertebral angle. However, nerve root avulsion and CSF leak can result from rib retraction during any thoracotomy, as reported by Frantz and Battaglini (1980) and Da Silva and associates (1987), among others. If the diagnosis is made intraoperatively, usually by the identification of clear CSF draining into the operative field from the posterior aspect of the intercostal incision, closure should usually be carried out at that time. Although pleural and muscle flaps placed into the foramen have been successful, it is generally prudent to seek intraoperative neurosurgical consultation for consideration of foraminal widening, direct dural suture or patching, or a planned immediate or staged approach to the problem by posterior laminectomy.

Because of small volumes of drainage and mixing with blood during the operation, a CSF leak is more often recognized in the postoperative period. With decreasing proportions of blood, the chest tube output becomes clear and persists in higher volumes than expected. A clinical diagnosis of CSF leak can be made by this finding after an operation requiring dissection in the costovertebral region. Plain radiographs of the skull or cranial CT may show pneumocephalus in some cases. Pneumocephalus results from the entry of pleural air via sufficiently large fistulas into the subarachnoid space during the positive-pressure phases of mechanical or spontaneous ventilation. If the diagnosis remains in doubt, radionuclide myelography, as reported by Pollack and coworkers (1990) may demonstrate the fistula. Many patients are asymptomatic, but others develop headache, seizures, mental status changes, focal neurologic findings, or signs of meningeal irritation. Death has been reported. Although often discussed, frank bacterial meningitis is rare. Although some fistulas close spontaneously, early neurosurgical consultation is prudent. Closure can be performed by the aforementioned techniques. A posterior hemilaminectomy approach is generally preferable to reopening the thoracotomy.

Peripheral Tumor Emboli

A tumor embolus may be dislodged from an involved pulmonary vein during the isolation and ligation of the vessel during the operative procedure. Taber (1961) and Senderoff and Kirschner (1962) were among the first authors to report the occurrence of a massive tumor embolism during a pulmonary resection for lung carcinoma, although, in 1947, Till and Fairburn reported a spontaneous massive embolism in a patient with a far-advanced lung tumor. Whyte and associates (1992) reported two cases and reviewed another 18 cases of embolization in patients with bronchial carcinoma; an additional five patients had a sarcomatous lesion. Spencer and colleagues (1993) reported a patient with multiple tumor emboli occurring during a pneumonectomy. In 1995, Gomez and colleagues reported an additional case and noted that a total of 31 cases had been reported in the literature. Eighty-four percent of these occurred during a pulmonary resection; the remainder were spontaneous. In the review of Whyte and associates (1992), the site of embolization was the aortic bifurcation or femoral vessels in 50% of patients. Other sites included vessels of the upper extremities, cerebral circulation, and the mesenteric arteries. Fifty percent of the patients died as a result of the embolic episode. Removal of the embolus is indicated when possible. Those who survive such an episode, according to Heitmiller (1992), die as a result of the metastatic spread of the original tumor and not of the effects of the embolic episode per se. Prevention of embolization when a major pulmonary vein is involved is primarily by proximal intrapericardial ligation of the vessel, including excision of a portion of the adjacent atrium, if necessary. Use of cardiopulmonary bypass, as suggested by Mansour and colleagues (1988) to remove tumor from the atrium, except in patients with a low-grade sarcoma, would

appear to be an inappropriate procedure in patients with lung cancer.

Complications Not Unique to Pulmonary Resection

Pulmonary Embolism

Pulmonary embolism may occur in 1% to as high as 5% of individuals undergoing a pulmonary resection. Ziomek and colleagues (1993) recorded this high percentage in a prospective evaluation of 77 patients for the occurrence of a postoperative embolism. The embolus originated in the lower extremities. Occasionally, the site may be in the veins of the pelvis. Sudden death may occur, but most patients survive long enough to permit diagnosis and treatment. Nonetheless, in the postresection patient, the overall mortality rate is 50%, according to Nagasaki and associates (1982).

An unusual site of origin of the embolus in postpneumonectomy patients is a thrombus in the pulmonary arterial stump. Chuang and colleagues (1966) reported that thrombosis occurred in 1% of postpneumonectomy patients. It is said to occur twice as often after a right than after a left pneumonectomy. This may be the result of the longer length of the right arterial stump. Takahashi and associates (1993) noted that the right pulmonary artery stump is 42 to 43 mm long, whereas the left stump can be 0 to 10 mm long. The thrombosis may be result from lack of effective flow in the stump or, theoretically, could develop owing to puckering and infolding of the vessel by the ligature, which could increase the likelihood of thrombosis within the vessel. A vascular suture closure or stapling of the vessel may lessen the minimal risk of this complication.

Deep Venous Thrombosis

In the aforementioned prospective study of Ziomek and colleagues (1993), 4 of the 77 patients had evidence of deep venous thrombosis preoperatively, and 11 more cases developed postoperatively, for an overall incidence of 19%. As noted, four pulmonary emboli occurred in the 77 patients. Of interest was the observation that none of these complications occurred in 17 patients who were taking aspirin or ibuprofen preoperatively; a controlled study certainly is indicated. Ziomek and associates noted that the thromboembolic events occurred more commonly in patients who had adenocarcinoma, a large tumor, a major resection, and a higher tumor, node, metastasis stage.

Renal Failure

In most series, renal failure is a relatively rare complication. However, Patel and associates (1992) documented this event in 15% of 197 patients undergoing a pneumonectomy. The renal failure occurred most often in patients older than

70 years. These authors also found renal failure to be an important factor for in-hospital mortality.

Cerebrovascular Accident

Data relative to the frequency of this complication are lacking, but an occasional "stroke" is observed postoperatively. In cancer patients, it is imperative that a true cerebrovascular event be differentiated from the postoperative manifestation of a previously occult cerebral metastasis. The use of computed tomography and MR imaging may promptly resolve the issue.

Massive Gastrointestinal Hemorrhage

Massive gastrointestinal hemorrhage is an uncommon complication. It is rarely seen as a single event but more often in association with other life-threatening complications (e.g., severe pulmonary insufficiency and sepsis) and is often the terminal event.

LATE COMPLICATIONS

Postpneumonectomy Syndrome

In infants, children, and, infrequently, young or middle-aged adults, excessive mediastinal shift after a pneumonectomy occurs gradually. The resultant compression of the remaining contralateral bronchus leads to severe respiratory compromise. Development of the syndrome is most common after a right pneumonectomy, is infrequently seen after a left pneumonectomy in patients with a right-sided aortic arch, and is observed rarely after a left pneumonectomy in patients with a normal position of the aortic arch in the left hemithorax.

Right Postpneumonectomy Syndrome

After a right pneumonectomy, excessive displacement of the heart with a counterclockwise rotation of the great vessels and trachea leads to a stretching and narrowing of the left main stem bronchus between the aorta and the pulmonary artery, as well as compression of the left pulmonary vessels. Narrowing of the bronchus results in severe respiratory insufficiency. Adams (1972), Szarnicki (1978), and Wasserman (1979) and their associates were among the first to describe this syndrome, although Maier and Gould (1953) were the first to describe the pathophysiology resulting in the syndrome in a patient with agenesis of the right lung. Bronchoscopic examination and the findings on CT examination of the chest, as described by Shephard and colleagues (1986) are diagnostic (Fig. 37-7). The most successful treatment has been the placement of prosthetic devices in the ipsilateral hemithorax to restore the heart and lung to a more normal position and thus relieve the obstruction of the

bronchus. Such procedures have been described by Wasserman (1979), Powell (1979), Riveron (1990), Rasch (1990), Grillo (1992), Jansen (1992), and Audy (1993) and their associates. Direct approaches to correct the left main stem bronchial narrowing by use of Silastic implants and various supports of the elongated posterior wall reported by Nissen (1954), Herzog (1987), and Moser (1994) and their colleagues have been used with varying results. Direct attempts to correct severely malacic airways are difficult, and Grillo and associates (1992) have reported two deaths in three patients in whom this has been attempted. Boiselle and colleagues (1997) note that inspiratory and expiratory CT may be useful for identifying tracheomalacia in postpneumonectomy syndrome.

Left Postpneumonectomy Syndrome

Quillin and Shackelford (1991), as well as Shephard (1986) and Grillo (1992) and their associates, described the occurrence of the same obstructive syndrome after a left pneumonectomy in patients who had a right-sided aortic arch. It was believed that the syndrome could not occur with a normally situated left aortic arch. However, Shamji and colleagues (1996) described four patients with a normally located aortic arch in whom the syndrome developed after left pneumonectomy. The bronchial obstruction was believed to be caused by a clockwise rotation of the pulmonary vessels and trachea, with compression of the right main bronchus between the right pulmonary artery and the spine (Fig. 37-8). Three of the four were successfully treated with placement of a saline-filled prosthesis into the left pleural space to reposition the heart and right lung in a more normal anatomic position. The fourth patient was managed by removal of a portion of the offending thoracic vertebra.

Superimposed Late Infection

Late Empyema

Pyogenic Empyema

Empyema may occur in a residual pleural space as a result of hematogenous spread of an organism from another site in the body or from the late occurrence of an occult bronchopleural fistula, often the result of recurrent tumor. The course is often indolent and may become manifest only by the occurrence of empyema necessitatis. Drainage and subsequent management are the same as any other empyema.

Hemorrhagic Empyema

Shimada and colleagues (1991) reported the rare occurrence of a chronic expanding hematoma in the postpneu-

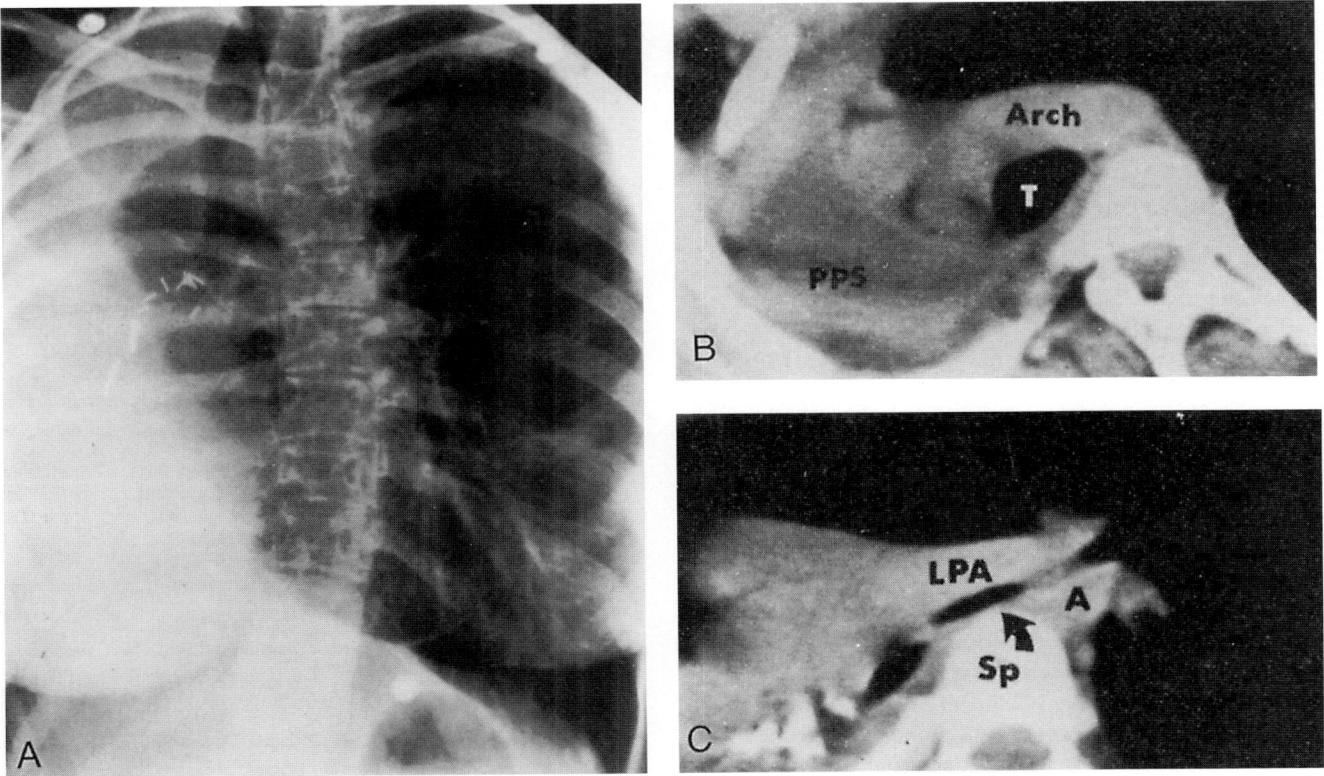

Fig. 37-7. The right postpneumonectomy syndrome. **A.** Posteroanterior chest radiograph with shift of the left lung into the right hemithorax. Computed tomographic scans reveal compression of the left main stem bronchus by the adjacent vessels. Soft tissue windows at the level of the aortic arch **(B)** and the left pulmonary artery **(C)** demonstrate a small postpneumonectomy space (PPS). The aortic arch (Arch) and pulmonary artery are rotated counterclockwise. The trachea (T) is to the right of the spine (Sp), and the left main bronchus (*arrow*) crosses anterior to the thoracic spine and posterior to the left pulmonary artery (LPA). From Grillo HC, et al: Postpneumonectomy syndrome: diagnosis, management and results. Ann Thorac Surg *54*:638, 1992. With permission.

monectomy space many years after the original procedure. Bleeding originated from granulation tissue in the space. Clinical symptomatology was the result of pressure and distortion of the mediastinal structures and the remaining contralateral lung. Surgical evacuation of the chronic hematoma was successful. The term *hemorrhagic empyema* was applied to this very uncommon late complication.

Fungal Empyema

The most commonly reported fungal infection that becomes clinically apparent late after a pulmonary resection is the result of *Aspergillus fumigatus*. Massard and associates (1992) reported 10 cases of aspergillosis that developed in a persistent pleural space after a lobectomy; the initial lobectomy was performed for the treatment of lung cancer in six, pulmonary tuberculosis in three, and aspergilloma in one. The most effective treatment was a thoracoplasty. Open drainage, as suggested by Shirakusa and colleagues (1989), is not advocated by Massard and associates (1992) because

it requires a second procedure, either a muscle transfer or an eventual thoracoplasty.

Retained Foreign Body

On rare occasions, a foreign body, usually a surgical sponge, is left in the pleural space after a primary resection. Patel and colleagues (1994) have coined the term *gossypiboma* to describe retained cotton material (sponge) in a body cavity. These authors removed by a lobectomy a retained sponge that had caused a severe pulmonary infection after a cardiac procedure. Originally, the infection was thought to be caused by an echinococcal cyst. Nomori and associates (1996) reported one case that occurred after a pulmonary resection and reviewed four additional cases in the Japanese literature. In their case, the retained sponge in the pleural space resulted in the development of a foreign body granuloma that years later eroded into a bronchus, with subsequent episodes of hemoptysis. Radiologic examination,

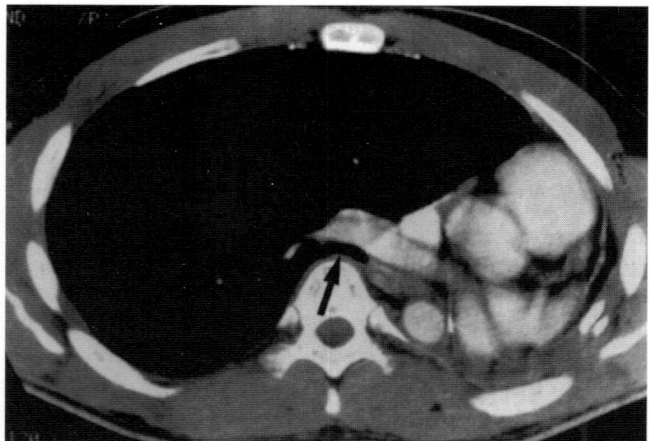

Fig. 37-8. Contrast-enhanced computed tomographic scan at the level of the right pulmonary artery and bronchus intermedius demonstrates narrowing of the airway caused by compression between the right pulmonary artery and spine (*arrow*). Marked mediastinal shift and clockwise rotation exist. From Shamji FM, et al: Postpneumonectomy syndrome with ipsilateral aortic arch after left pneumonectomy. Ann Thorac Surg 62:1627, 1996. With permission.

including MR imaging, revealed a cavitary lesion containing a mass lesion and an air crescent that resembled an aspergilloma. Resection was successfully carried out and revealed the offending foreign body.

REFERENCES

Abruzzini P: Trattenento chirurgico della fistule del broncho principale consecutive a pneumonectomia per tubercolosi. Chir Torac 14:165, 1961.

Adams HP, et al: Severe airway obstruction caused by mediastinal displacement after right pneumonectomy in a child. A case report. J Thorac Cardiovasc Surg 63:534, 1972.

Akaogi E, et al: Treatment of postoperative chylothorax with intrapleural fibrin glue. Ann Thorac Surg 48:116, 1989.

al–Kattan K, Cattalani L, Goldstraw P: Bronchopleural fistula after pneumonectomy with a hand suture technique. Ann Thorac Surg 58:1433, 1994.

Amar D, et al: Clinical and echocardiographic correlates of symptomatic tachydysrhythmias and cardiac function after pneumonectomy. Chest 108:349, 1995.

Amar D, et al: Relationship of early postoperative dysrhythmias and long-term outcome after resection of non-small cell lung cancer. Chest 110:437, 1996.

Amar D, et al: Effects of diltiazem versus digoxin on dysrhythmias and cardiac function after pneumonectomy. Ann Thorac Surg 63:1374, 1997.

Asamura H, et al: Bronchopleural fistulas associated with lung cancer operations. Univariate and multivariate analysis of risk factors, management and outcome. J Thorac Cardiovasc Surg 104:1456, 1992.

Asamura H, et al: What are the risk factors for arrhythmias after thoracic operations? A retrospective multivariate analysis of 267 consecutive thoracic operations. J Thorac Cardiovasc Surg 106:1104, 1993.

Attar S, et al: Paraplegia after thoracotomy: report of 5 cases and review of the literature. Ann Thorac Surg 59:1410, 1995.

Audy G, et al: Expandable prosthesis in right postpneumonectomy syndrome in children and adolescents. Ann Thorac Surg 56:323, 1993.

Azorin JF, et al: Closure of a postpneumonectomy main bronchus fistula using video-assisted mediastinal surgery. Chest 109:1097, 1996.

Bakris NC, et al: Right to left shunt after pneumonectomy. Ann Thorac Surg 63:198, 1997.

Baldwin JC, Mark JBD: Treatment of bronchopleural fistula after pneumonectomy. J Thorac Cardiovasc Surg 90:813, 1985.

Bayliff CD, et al: Propranolol in the prevention of postoperative arrhythmias in patients undergoing thoracic surgery. Presented at the 34th Annual Meeting of the Society of Thoracic Surgeons. New Orleans, January 26, 1998. Abstract 59, p. 172.

Benfield JR: Invited commentary of Short HD: Paraplegia associated with the use of oxidized cellulose in posterolateral thoracotomy incisions. Ann Thorac Surg 50:290, 1990.

Benjamin I, Olsen AM, Ellis FH Jr: Esophagopleural fistula: a rare postpneumonectomy complication. Ann Thorac Surg 7:139, 1969.

Boiselle PM, et al: Postpneumonectomy syndrome: another twist. J Thorac Imaging 12:209, 1997.

Bolliger CT, et al: Lung scanning and exercise testing for prediction of postoperative performance in lung resection candidates at increased risk for complications. Chest 108:341, 1995.

Bollen ECM, et al: Mediastinal lymph node dissection in resected lung cancer. Morbidity and accuracy of staging. Ann Thorac Surg 55:961, 1993.

Borgeat A, et al: Prevention of arrhythmias by flecainide after noncardiac thoracic surgery. Ann Thorac Surg 48:232, 1989.

Borgeat A, et al: Prevention of arrhythmias after noncardiac thoracic surgery: flecainide versus digoxin. Ann Thorac Surg 51:964, 1991.

Brie M, et al: Chylothorax complicating pulmonary resection. In Deslauriers J, Lacquet LK (eds): Thoracic Surgery: Surgical Management of Pleural Diseases. St. Louis: CV Mosby, 1990.

Brown J, Pomerantz M: Extrapleural pneumonectomy for tuberculosis. Chest Surg Clin N Am 5:289, 1995.

Bruni F: Bronchopleural fistula: treatment of long stump after pneumonectomy. In Eschapasse H, Grillo H (eds): International Trends in General Thoracic Surgery. Vol. 2. Philadelphia: WB Saunders, 1987.

Brutel de la Riviere, et al: Transsternal closure of bronchopleural fistula after pneumonectomy. Ann Thorac Surg 64:954, 1997.

Camazine B, et al: Herpes simplex viral pneumonia in the post-thoracotomy patient. Chest 108:876, 1995.

Cerfolio RJ, et al: Lung resection in patients with compromised pulmonary function. Ann Thorac Surg 62:348, 1996.

Chuang TH, et al: Pulmonary embolization from vascular stump thrombosis following pneumonectomy. Ann Thorac Surg 2:290, 1966.

Cosgrove DM III: Closure of postpneumonectomy bronchopleural fistula. Presented at the Clinical Congress, American College of Surgeons. Thoracic Surgery Postgraduate Course. Chicago, October 15, 1985.

Cybulsky IJ, et al: Prognostic significance of computed tomography in resected N_2 lung cancer. Ann Thorac Surg 54:533, 1992.

Dartevelle PG, et al: Tracheal and sleeve pneumonectomy for bronchogenic carcinoma: report of 55 cases. Ann Thorac Surg 46:68, 1988.

Da Silva VF, et al: Subarachnoid-pleural fistula complicating thoracotomy: case report and review of the literature. Neurosurgery 20:806, 1987.

Da Valle MJ, et al: Extrapleural pneumonectomy for diffuse malignant mesothelioma. Ann Thorac Surg 42:612, 1986.

Deslauriers J: Indications for completion pneumonectomy. Ann Thorac Surg 46:133, 1988.

Deslauriers J, Aucoin A, Gregoire J: Postpneumonectomy pulmonary edema. Chest Surg Clin N Am 8:611, 1998.

Duque JL, et al: Early complications in the surgical treatment of lung cancer: a prospective, multicenter study. Ann Thorac Surg 63:944, 1997.

Evans JP: Post-pneumonectomy oesophageal fistula. Thorax 27:674, 1972.

Ferguson MK, Reeder LB, Mick R: Optimizing selection of patients for major lung resection. J Thorac Cardiovasc Surg 109:275, 1995.

Frantz PT, Battaglini JW: Subarachnoid-pleural fistula: unusual complication of thoracotomy. J Thorac Cardiovasc Surg 79:873, 1980.

Gaud C: Role of mechanical ventilation in the genesis of empyema and bronchopleural fistula. In Grillo HC, Eschapasse H (eds): International Trends in General Thoracic Surgery. Vol. 2. Philadelphia: WB Saunders, 1987, p. 447.

Gharagozloo F, et al: Pleural space irrigation and modified Clagett procedure for the treatment of early postpneumonectomy empyema. J Thorac Cardiovasc Surg 116:943, 1998.

Ginsberg RJ, et al: Modern thirty-day operative mortality for surgical resections in lung cancer. J Thorac Cardiovasc Surg 86:654, 1983.

Ginsberg RJ, et al: Closure of chronic postpneumonectomy bronchopleural fistula using the transsternal transpericardial approach. Ann Thorac Surg 47:231, 1989.

Glover W, et al: Fibrin glue applications through the fiberoptic bronchoscope: closure of bronchopleural fistulas. J Thorac Cardiovasc Surg 93:470, 1987.

Godart F, et al: Postpneumonectomy interatrial right-to-left shunt: successful percutaneous treatment. Ann Thorac Surg 64:834, 1997.

Gomez JR, et al: Tumor embolism after pneumonectomy for primary pulmonary neoplasia. Ann Vasc Surg 9:199, 1995.

Grillo HC, et al: Postpneumonectomy syndrome: diagnosis, management and results. Ann Thorac Surg 54:638, 1992.

Harpole DH Jr, et al: Prospective analysis of pneumonectomy: risk factors for major morbidity and cardiac dysrhythmias. Ann Thorac Surg 61:977, 1996.

Harvey JC, Erdman C, Beattie EJ: Pneumonectomy. Chest Surg Clin N Am 5:253, 1995.

Heitmiller RF: Prognostic significance of massive bronchogenic tumor embolus. Ann Thorac Surg 53:153, 1992.

Herzog H, et al: Surgical therapy for expiratory collapse of the trachea and large bronchi. In Grillo HC, Eschapasse H (eds): International Trends in General Thoracic Surgery. Vol. 2. Philadelphia: WB Saunders, 1987, p. 74.

Hollaus PH, et al: Natural history of bronchopleural fistula after pneumonectomy: a review of 96 cases. Ann Thorac Surg 63:1391, 1997.

Hollaus PH, et al: Endoscopic treatment of postoperative bronchopleural fistula: experience with 45 cases. Ann Thorac Surg 66:923, 1998.

Icard P, et al: Utility of C-reactive protein measurements for empyema diagnosis after pneumonectomy. Ann Thorac Surg 57:933, 1994.

Ishida T, et al: Long-term results of operation for non-small cell lung cancer in the elderly. Ann Thorac Surg 50:919, 1990.

Jack GD: Bronchial closure. Thorax 20:8, 1965.

Jansen JP, et al: Postpneumonectomy syndrome in adulthood. Surgical correction using an expandable prosthesis. Chest 101:1167, 1992.

Jensen C, Sharma P: Use of fibrin glue in thoracic surgery. Ann Thorac Surg 39:521, 1985.

Jensik RJ: The extent of resection for localized lung cancer: segmental resection. In Kittle CF (ed): Current Controversies in Thoracic Surgery. Philadelphia: WB Saunders, 1986.

Karwande SV, Wolcott MW, Gay WA: Postpneumonectomy tension chylothorax. Ann Thorac Surg 42:585, 1986.

Keagy BA, et al: Elective pulmonary lobectomy: factors associated with morbidity and operative mortality. Ann Thorac Surg 40:349, 1985.

Kearney DJ, et al: Assessment of operative risk in patients undergoing lung resection. Importance of predicted pulmonary function. Chest 105:753, 1994.

Kelly MV, Kygere R, Miller WC: Postoperative lobar torsion and gangrene. Thorax 32:501, 1977.

Khan MG: Angina. In Khan MG, Lynch JP III (eds): Cardiac and Pulmonary Management. Philadelphia: Lea & Febiger, 1993, p. 57.

Khargi K, et al: Hemorrhage due to inflammatory erosion of the pulmonary artery stump in postpneumonectomy bronchopleural fistula. Ann Thorac Surg 56:357, 1993.

Knott-Craig F, et al: Improved results in the surgical management of surgical candidates with lung cancer. Ann Thorac Surg 63:1405, 1997.

Korst RJ, Humphrey CB: Complete lobar collapse following pulmonary lobectomy. Its incidence, predisposing factors and clinical ramifications. Chest 111:1285, 1997.

Krowka MJ, et al: Cardiac dysrhythmia following pneumonectomy. Chest 91:490, 1987.

Kucich VA, Villarreal JR, Schwartz DB: Left upper lobe torsion following lower lobe resection. Early recognition of a rare complication. Chest 95:1146, 1989.

Landreneau RJ, et al: Video-assisted thoracoscopic surgery: basic technical concepts and intercostal approach strategies. Ann Thorac Surg 54:800, 1992.

Lewis JW, et al: Right heart function and prediction of respiratory morbidity in patients undergoing pneumonectomy with moderately severe cardiopulmonary dysfunction. J Thorac Cardiovasc Surg 108:169, 1994.

Linaudais W, Cavanaugh DG, Greer TM: Rapid postoperative thoracotomy for torsion of the left lower lobe: case report. Mil Med 145:698, 1980.

Maassen W: The transsternal and transpericardial approach for surgical treatment of fistulas of the main bronchus after pneumonectomy. Thoraxchirurgie 23:257, 1975.

Maeda M, et al: Statistical survey of tracheobronchoplasty in Japan. J Thorac Cardiovasc Surg 97:402, 1989.

Maier HC, Gould WI: Agenesis of the lung with vascular compression of the tracheobronchial tree. J Pediatr 43:38, 1953.

Mansour KA, Malone CE, Craver JM: Left atrial tumor embolization during pulmonary resection: review of the literature and report of two cases. Ann Thorac Surg 46:455, 1988.

Martini N, et al: The extent of resection for localized lung cancer: lobectomy. In CF Kittle (ed): Current Controversies in Thoracic Surgery. Philadelphia: WB Saunders, 1986.

Massard G, et al: Pleuropulmonary aspergilloma: clinical spectrum and results of surgical treatment. Ann Thorac Surg 54:1159, 1992.

Massard G, et al: Esophagopleural fistula: an early and long-term complication after pneumonectomy. Ann Thorac Surg 58:1437, 1994.

Mathisen DJ, Grillo HC: Carinal resection for lung cancer. J Thorac Cardiovasc Surg 102:16, 1991.

Mathisen DJ, et al: Inhaled nitric oxide for adult respiratory distress syndrome following pulmonary resection. Ann Thorac Surg 66:1894, 1998.

Mathru M, et al: Permeability pulmonary edema following lung resection. Chest 98:1216, 1990.

McGovern EM, et al: Completion pneumonectomy: indications, complications, and results. Ann Thorac Surg 46:141, 1988.

McKenna RJ, et al: Use of the Heimlich valve to shorten hospital stay after lung reduction surgery for emphysema. Ann Thorac Surg 61:1115, 1996.

Melendez JA, Barrera R: Predictive respiratory complication quotient predicts pulmonary complications in thoracic surgical patients. Ann Thorac Surg 66:220, 1998.

Mercho N, et al: Right-to-left interatrial shunt causing platypnea after pneumonectomy. Chest 105:931, 1994.

Miller JI: Single-stage complete muscle flap closure of the postpneumonectomy empyema space: a new method and possible solution to a disturbing complication. Ann Thorac Surg 38:227, 1984.

Miller JI Jr: Physiologic evaluation of pulmonary function in candidates for lung resection. J Thorac Cardiovasc Surg 105:347, 1993.

Mitsudomi T, et al: Postoperative complications after pneumonectomy for treatment of lung cancer: multivariate analysis. J Surg Oncol 61:218, 1996.

Morice RC, et al: Exercise testing in the evaluation of patients at high risk for complications from lung resection. Chest 101:358, 1992.

Morita R, et al: A case of postoperative chylothorax successfully treated by thoracoscopic fibrin gluing. Nippon Kyobu Geka Gakkai Zasshi 38:2465, 1990.

Moser NJ, et al: Management of postpneumonectomy syndrome with a bronchoscopically placed endobronchial stent. South Med J 87:1156, 1994.

Muysoms FE, et al: Completion pneumonectomy: analysis of operative mortality and survival. Ann Thorac Surg 66:1165, 1998.

Nagasaki F, Flehinger BJ, Martini N: Complications of surgery in the treatment of carcinoma of the lung. Chest 82:25, 1982.

Nakamura T, et al: Cardiac arrhythmias following lobectomy in elderly patients. J Jpn Assoc Chest Surg 11:500, 1997.

Ngan H, Fok M, Wong J: The role of lymphangiography in chylothorax following thoracic surgery. Br J Radiol 61:1032, 1988.

Nissen R: Tracheoplastie zur Beseitigung der Erschlaffung des membranosen Teils der Intrathorakalen. Luftrohre Schweiz Med Wochenschr 84:219, 1954.

Nomori H, et al: Retained sponge after thoracotomy that mimicked aspergilloma. Ann Thorac Surg 61:1535, 1996.

O'Meara JB, Slade PR: Disappearance of fluid from the postpneumonectomy space. J Thorac Cardiovasc Surg 67:621, 1974.

Pagni S, Federico JA, Ponn RB: Pulmonary resection for lung cancer in octogenarians. Ann Thorac Surg 63:785, 1997.

Pagni S, et al: Pulmonary resection for malignancy in the elderly: is age still a risk factor? Eur J Cardiothorac Surg 14:40, 1998.

Pairolero PC, et al: Postpneumonectomy empyema: the role of intrathoracic muscle transposition. J Thorac Cardiovasc Surg 99:958, 1990.

Pairolero PC, Payne WS: Postoperative care and complications in the thoracic surgical patient. In Glenn WWL, et al (eds): Thoracic and Cardiovascular Surgery. 4th Ed. Norwalk, CT: Appleton-Century-Crofts, 1983, p. 338.

Patel AM, Trastek VF, Coles DT: Gossypibomas mimicking echinococcal cyst disease of the lung. Chest 105:284, 1994.

Patel RL, Townsend ER, Fountain SW: Elective pneumonectomy: factors associated with morbidity and operative mortality. Ann Thorac Surg 54:84, 1992.

Perelman MI: Late treatment of chronic bronchopleural fistula with long stump after pneumonectomy. In Eschapasse H, Grillo H (eds): International Trends in General Thoracic Surgery. Vol. 2. Philadelphia: WB Saunders, 1987.

Perelman MI, Ambatiello GP: Transpleuraler, transsternaler und kontralateraler Zugang bei Operationen wegen Bronchial fistel nach Pneumonectomie. Thorax Chir Vaskul Chir *18*:45, 1970.

Perelman MI, Rymko LP, Ambatiello GP: Bronchopleural fistula: surgery after pneumonectomy. *In* Eschapasse H, Grillo H (eds): International Trends in General Thoracic Surgery. Vol. 2. Philadelphia: WB Saunders, 1987.

Peterffy A, Henze A: Haemorrhagic complications during pulmonary resection. A retrospective review of 1428 resections with 113 haemorrhagic episodes. Scand J Thorac Cardiovasc Surg *17*:283, 1983.

Peters RM: Postpneumonectomy pulmonary edema. *In* Eschapasse H, Grillo H (eds): International Trends in General Thoracic Surgery. Vol. 2. Philadelphia: WB Saunders, 1987.

Piccione W Jr, Faber LP: Management of complications related to pulmonary resection. *In* Waldhausen JA, Orringer MB (eds): Complications in Cardiothoracic Surgery. St. Louis: Mosby–Year Book, 1991, p. 336.

Pierce RJ, et al: Preoperative risk evaluation for lung cancer resection: predicted postoperative product as a predictor of surgical mortality. Am J Respir Crit Care Med *150*:947, 1994.

Pollack IF, Pang P, Hall WA: Subarachnoid-pleural fistula and subarachnoid-mediastinal fistula. Neurosurgery *26*:519, 1990.

Pomerantz M, et al: Surgical management of resistant mycobacterial tuberculosis and other mycobacterial pulmonary infections. Ann Thorac Surg *52*:1108, 1991.

Ponn RB, et al: Treatment of peripheral bronchopleural fistulas with endobronchial occlusion coils. Ann Thorac Surg *56*:1343, 1993.

Ponn RB, Silverman HJ, Federico JA: Outpatient chest tube management. Ann Thorac Surg *64*:1437, 1997.

Powell RW, Luck SR, Raffensperger JG: Pneumonectomy in infants and children: the use of a prosthesis to prevent mediastinal shift and its complications. J Pediatr Surg *14*:231, 1979.

Puskas JD, et al: Treatment strategies for bronchopleural fistula. J Thorac Cardiovasc Surg *109*:989, 1995.

Putnam JB Jr, et al: Predicted pulmonary function and survival after pneumonectomy for primary lung carcinoma. Ann Thorac Surg *49*:909, 1990.

Quillin SP, Shackelford GD: Postpneumonectomy syndrome after left lung resection. Radiology *179*:100, 1991.

Rao S, et al: International experience with secundum atrial septal defect occlusion by the buttoned device. Am Heart J *128*:1022, 1994.

Rasch DK, et al: Right pneumonectomy syndrome in infancy treated with an expandable prosthesis. Ann Thorac Surg *50*:127, 1990.

Rice TW, et al: Simultaneous occurrence of chylothorax and subarachnoid pleural fistula after thoracotomy. Can J Surg *30*:256, 1987.

Rice TW, Kirby TTJ: Prolonged air leak. Chest Surg Clin N Am *2*:803, 1992.

Riquet M, Hidden G, Debesse B: Les collaterales dur canal thoracique d'origine ganglio-pulmonaire étude anatomique et chylothorax après chirurgie pulmonaire. Ann Chir Thorac Cardiovasc *43*:646, 1989.

Ritchie AJ, Bowe P, Gibbons JRP: Prophylactic digitalization for thoracotomy: a reassessment. Ann Thorac Surg *50*:86, 1990.

Ritchie AJ, Gibbons JRP: Prophylactic digitalization in pulmonary surgery. Thorax *47*:41, 1992.

Riveron FA, et al: Silastic prosthesis plombage for right postpneumonectomy syndrome. Ann Thorac Surg *50*:465, 1990.

Rocker GM, et al: Neutrophil degranulation and increased pulmonary capillary permeability following oesophagectomy: a model of early lung injury in man. Br J Surg *75*:883, 1988.

Roviaro GC, et al: Tracheal sleeve pneumonectomy for bronchogenic carcinoma. J Thorac Cardiovasc Surg *107*:14, 1994.

Roxburgh JC, Thompson J, Goldstraw P: Hospital mortality and long-term survival after pulmonary resection in the elderly. Ann Thorac Surg *51*:800, 1991.

Sarsam MA, Moussali H: Technique of bronchial closure after pneumonectomy. J Thorac Cardiovasc Surg *98*:220, 1989.

Sarsam MA, Rahman AN, Deiraniya AK: Postpneumonectomy chylothorax. Ann Thorac Surg *57*:689, 1994.

Schnabel TG et al: Postural cyanosis and angina pectoris following pneumonectomy: relief by closure of an interatrial septal defect. J Thorac Surg *32*:246, 1956.

Senderoff E, Kirschner A: Massive tumor embolism during pulmonary surgery. J Thorac Cardiovasc Surg *44*:528, 1962.

Shama DM, Odell JA: Esophageal fistula after pneumonectomy for inflammatory disease. J Thorac Cardiovasc Surg *89*:77, 1985.

Shamji FM, et al: Postpneumonectomy syndrome with ipsilateral aortic arch after left pneumonectomy. Ann Thorac Surg *62*:1627, 1996.

Shapira OM, Shahian DM: Postpneumonectomy pulmonary edema. Ann Thorac Surg *56*:190, 1993.

Shephard JO, et al: Right-pneumonectomy syndrome: radiographic findings, and CT correlation. Radiology *161*:661, 1986.

Shields TW, Ujiki G: Digitalization for the prevention of cardiac arrhythmia following pulmonary surgery. Surg Gynecol Obstet *126*:743, 1968.

Shields TW, et al: Persistent pleural air space following resection for pulmonary tuberculosis. J Thorac Cardiovasc Surg *38*:523, 1959.

Shimada J, et al: Chronic hemorrhagic empyema developing thirty-three years after right pneumonectomy. A case report. J Jpn Assoc Thorac Surg *39*:1204, 1991.

Shirakusa T, et al: Surgical treatment of pulmonary aspergilloma and Aspergillus empyema. Ann Thorac Surg *48*:779, 1989.

Short HD: Paraplegia associated with the use of oxidized cellulose in posterolateral thoracotomy incisions. Ann Thorac Surg *50*:288, 1990.

Simpson L: Chylothorax in adults: pathophysiology and management. *In* Deslauriers J, Lacquet LK (eds): Thoracic Surgery: Surgical Management of Pleural Diseases. St. Louis: CV Mosby, 1990.

Smeenk FW, Postmus PE: Interatrial right to left shunting developing after pulmonary resection in the absence of elevated right sided heart pressures. Review of the literature [Review]. Chest *103*:528, 1993.

Spencer DD, de la Garza LJ, Walker WA: Multiple tumor emboli after pneumonectomy. Ann Thorac Surg *55*:169, 1993.

Stenzl W, et al: Treatment of postsurgical chylothorax with fibrin glue. Thorac Cardiovasc Surg *31*:35, 1983.

Sugarbaker DJ, Mentzer SJ, Strauss G: Extrapleural pneumonectomy in the treatment of malignant pleural mesothelioma. Ann Thorac Surg *54*:941, 1992.

Szarnicki R, et al: Tracheal compression by the aortic arch following right pneumonectomy in infancy. Ann Thorac Surg *25*:231, 1978.

Taber RE: Massive systemic tumor embolization during pneumonectomy: a case report with comments on routine primary pulmonary vein ligation. Ann Surg *154*:263, 1961.

Takahashi T, et al: Clot in the pulmonary artery after pneumonectomy [letter]. AJR Am J Roentgenol *161*:1110, 1993.

Tedder M, et al: Current morbidity, mortality, and survival after bronchoplastic procedures for malignancy. Ann Thorac Surg *54*:387, 1992.

Terzi A, et al: Chylothorax after pleuro-pulmonary surgery: a rare but unavoidable complication. Thorac Cardiovasc Surgeon *42*:81, 1994.

Terzi A, et al: Completion pneumonectomy: experience with 47 cases. Thorac Cardiovasc Surg *43*:52, 1995.

Thomas P, et al: Clinical patterns and trends of outcome of elderly patients with bronchogenic carcinoma. Eur J Cardiothorac Surg *13*:266, 1998.

Till AS, Fairburn EA: Massive neoplastic embolism. Br J Surg *35*:86, 1947.

Trastek VF: Invited commentary of Hollaus PH, et al: Natural history of bronchopleural fistula after pneumonectomy: a review of 96 cases. Ann Thorac Surg *63*:1391, 1997.

Tsuchiya R, et al: Resection of tracheal carina for lung cancer: procedure, complications, and mortality. J Thorac Cardiovasc Surg *99*:779, 1990.

Turnage WS, Lunn JJ: Postpneumonectomy pulmonary edema. A retrospective analysis of associated variables. Chest *103*:1646, 1993.

Vallieres E, Shamji FM, Todd TR: Postpneumonectomy chylothorax. Ann Thorac Surg *55*:1006, 1993.

van den Bosch JM, et al: Postpneumonectomy oesophagopleural fistula. Thorax *35*:865, 1980.

van der Werf YD, et al: Postpneumonectomy pulmonary edema. A retrospective analysis of incidence and possible risk factors. Chest *111*:1278, 1997.

Van Mieghem W, et al: Amiodarone and the development of ARDS after lung surgery. Chest *105*:1642, 1994.

Van Mieghem W, et al: Verapamil as prophylactic treatment of atrial fibrillation after lung operations. Ann Thorac Surg *61*:1083, 1996.

Verheijen-Breemhaar L, et al: Postpneumonectomy pulmonary oedema. Thorax *45*:323, 1988.

Vester SR, et al: Bronchopleural fistula after stapled closure of the bronchus. Ann Thorac Surg *52*:1253, 1991.

Vogt-Moykopf I: Contralateral pneumothorax occurring after pulmonary surgery. *In* Deslauriers J, Lacquet LK (eds): Thoracic Surgery: Surgical Management of Pleural Diseases. St. Louis: CV Mosby, 1990, p. 158.

Von Knorring J, et al: Cardiac arrhythmias and myocardial ischemia after thoracotomy for lung cancer. Ann Thorac Surg *53*:642, 1992.

Wada H, et al: Thirty-day operative mortality for thoracotomy in lung cancer. J Thorac Cardiovasc Surg *115*:70, 1998.

Wahi R, et al: Determinants of perioperative morbidity and mortality after pneumonectomy. Ann Thorac Surg *48*:33, 1989.

Walker WE: Paraplegia associated with thoracotomy. Ann Thorac Surg *50*:178, 1990.

Waller DA, et al: Noncardiogenic pulmonary edema complicating lung resection. Ann Thorac Surg *55*:140, 1993.

Waller DA, et al: Pulmonary endothelial permeability changes after major lung resections. Ann Thorac Surg *61*:1435, 1996.

Warren WH: Surgical techniques in the dissection and reconstruction of the pulmonary artery. Chest Surg Clin N Am *5*:333, 1995.

Wasserman K, et al: Postpneumonectomy syndrome: surgical correction using silastic implants. Chest *75*:78, 1979.

Wheat MW Jr, Burford TH: Digitalis in surgery. J Thorac Cardiovasc Surg *41*:162, 1961.

Whyte RI, Starkey TD, Orringer MB: Tumor emboli from lung neoplasms involving the pulmonary vein. J Thorac Cardiovasc Surg *104*:421, 1992.

Wong PS, Goldstraw P: Pulmonary torsion: a questionnaire survey and a survey of the literature. Ann Thorac Surg *54*:286, 1992.

Yashar J, et al: Preoperative chemotherapy and radiation therapy for stage IIIa carcinoma of the lung. Ann Thorac Surg *53*:445, 1992.

Zeldin RA, et al: Postpneumonectomy pulmonary edema. J Thorac Cardiovasc Surg *87*:359, 1984.

Ziomek S, et al: Thromboembolism in patients undergoing thoracotomy. Ann Thorac Surg *56*:223, 1993.

Zueger O, et al: Dyspnea after pneumonectomy: the result of an atrial septal defect. Ann Thorac Surg *63*:1451, 1997.

Postoperative Management of the General Thoracic Surgical Patient

CHAPTER 38

General Principles of Postoperative Care

Robert J. Cerfolio

The postoperative care of the general thoracic surgical patient is challenging. Excellent results are achieved by blending the complex management of cardiopulmonary physiology with the simple, but labor intensive custodial care of pulmonary hygiene. Thoracic care also entails the unique management of the pleural space.

Despite advances in anesthesia, epidural catheters, and pulmonary preservation techniques, the mortality of elective pulmonary and esophageal resection remains two to four times higher than that of elective coronary artery bypass surgery, as reported by Ginsberg (1983) and by Deslauriers (1989) and their colleagues. Morbidity in most large series is also higher, and ranges from 10 to 70%, depending on the criteria applied, with most reports showing major or minor complications in 30 to 40% of cases, as described by Olsen (1991) and Wahi (1989) and their associates. Chapter 37 presents a complete review of the mortality and morbidity of pulmonary resection. The clinical challenge of postoperative care is increasing with the development of new technologies and the increasing numbers of operations performed in the elderly, in patients previously treated with radiation and chemotherapy, and in immunocompromised patients. The current emphasis on cost containment and managed care adds to the challenge. Outcome must not only be optimal as judged by traditional clinical end points, but good results must be achieved with shorter lengths of stay and lower expenditure.

Although postoperative morbidity is best prevented by preoperative and intraoperative management, some complications are unavoidable. General postoperative principles include preoperative preparatory techniques such as smoking cessation, incentive spirometry teaching, pulmonary rehabilitation, and nutritional supplementation. Intraoperative and postoperative considerations include meticulous hemostasis and surgical technique; minimal intravenous fluids during and after pulmonary resection; adequate pain control; appropriate cardiac and oxygen saturation monitoring; chest physiotherapy; nasotracheal suctioning, minitracheostomy, or both; bronchodilators; and early and frequent ambulation. Even with optimal management in these areas, postoperative complications occur.

This chapter presents a brief overview of the preventive techniques listed previously. The specifics of these techniques, along with the incidence, diagnosis, and management of some of the complications that can occur are discussed. More specific postoperative complications and their management, as well as the management of the unstable ventilated patient, are discussed in Chapters 37 and 39.

PREOPERATIVE PREPARATION

Most patients who come to thoracotomy with pulmonary or esophageal disease have a history of smoking. Cessation of smoking, often aided by oral or transdermal nicotine preparations or antidepressants, and pulmonary rehabilitation before surgery decrease respiratory complications. It is unrealistic to expect patients who are dealing with the stress of upcoming surgery and the fear of cancer to significantly improve their nutritional, respiratory, and cardiopulmonary status within 1 to 2 weeks before thoracotomy. Nonetheless, efforts should be made toward this goal. At a minimum, the patient should stop smoking. Smoking cessation, even for only a few days preoperatively, can positively affect morbidity. In only 3 to 5 days, smoking cessation improves ciliary clearance and decreases secretions. Furthermore, preoperative chest physiotherapy, as shown by Stein and Cassara (1970), reduces pulmonary complications, especially in the high-risk patient. Preoperative incentive spirometry and flutter valve teaching allow patients to learn how best to use these instruments before having to deal with the pain of thoracotomy and the inconvenience of being connected to many medical devices.

Another important preoperative technique is intravenous antibiotics before skin incision. Sterile surgical technique as well as preoperative antibiotics prevent wound infection. Wound infections are rare in thoracotomy patients. However, bothersome tape burns are common. At the Pain Service at

509

the University of Alabama at Birmingham, we currently place only antibiotic ointment on the incision and chest tube sites. The patient leaves the operating room with no surgical dressing or tape of any kind. This avoids tape burns on the skin around the incision, and we have had no wound infections with this technique. Tape, which is used on the chest tube site after tube removal, is applied sparingly.

A final preoperative principle that should be mentioned is deep venous thrombosis prophylaxis. Pulsatile stockings or subcutaneous heparin should be instituted before incision. We prefer the former prophylactic approach, because it avoids the minor morbidity of a needle stick; the cost of injections, needles, and syringes; and the potential for heparin-induced thrombocytopenia.

EPIDURAL ANALGESIA

Adequate control of pain is the key element for allowing a smooth, complication-free early course after thoracotomy. This area has been reviewed by Kruger and McRae (1999).

The limitations of intermittently administered systemic narcotics are well known and include inconstant tissue levels, with troughs that may be insufficient and peaks that may result in somnolence and respiratory depression. Patient-controlled analgesia solves this problem, but requires that the patient be able to understand the concept and system. Intra-operative intercostal nerve blocks provide only temporary relief, and frequent injections postoperatively risk bleeding and pneumothorax. Continuous block can be achieved by placement of indwelling catheters, but the technique is cumbersome. Intercostal block by cryoanalgesia or phenol injection results in a high incidence of permanent neuralgia.

Although careful attention to pain control using a variety of approaches can provide excellent recovery, epidural analgesia is now the preferred method, when feasible, and represents a major advance in general thoracic surgical care. Popularized by El-Baz and Ivankovich (1986), it significantly reduces respiratory complications by allowing patients to breathe more deeply, walk sooner, and mobilize secretions more effectively. These advantageous effects, moreover, have enabled safe operations on older, sicker, and weaker patients, with less cardiopulmonary reserve, thus raising the bar to such heights that there are now few, if any, patients that cannot tolerate thoracotomy. Selected patients with postoperative predicted diffusing capacity of carbon monoxide (D_{LCO}) and postoperative predicted forced expiratory volumes of 1 second (FEV_1) of even less than 25% can now undergo limited pulmonary resections mainly because of epidural analgesia. In fact, the unanswered question now may be, is there an absolute lowest limit of predicted postoperative pulmonary function that precludes resection?

The epidural space begins at the foramen magnum and is an extension of the meningeal and endosteal layers of the cerebral dura mater. The posterior thoracic epidural space is approximately 3 mm in depth. The interspinous space between the

thoracic vertebral bodies is smaller than that between the lumbar bodies. Moreover, the angulation of the thoracic spinal processes has a much steeper pitch than that of the lumbar spinal processes. It is for this reason that the paramedian approach is usually used for thoracic epidural placement instead of a median approach as is used for cervical and lumbar epidural catheter placement. A final, clinically relevant, anatomic feature is that the spinal cord lies directly anterior to the thoracic epidural space, as opposed to the cauda equina, which lies just anterior to the lumbar epidural space. Inadvertent puncture of the cord can have significant consequences, as opposed to puncture of the cauda equina, which has no real sequelae. For this reason, thoracic epidurals should be positioned with the patient awake just before surgery.

The main advantage of a thoracic epidural over a lumbar epidural is that the analgesic effect is delivered directly at the dermatomal epicenter of the incision (Fig. 38-1). Therefore, a local anesthetic such as bupivacaine can be used, and narcotics such as fentanyl or morphine can be minimized. This allows one to avoid the respiratory depressive effect of narcotics by maximizing the local analgesic effects of local anesthetics. The disadvantages of the thoracic epidural versus the lumbar epidural are based on the anatomic facts just described. Catheter placement is more difficult because of the angle of the spinal processes and the smaller space. The potential also exists of injuring the cord. The reported incidence of spinal cord injury, however, is less than 1%. In

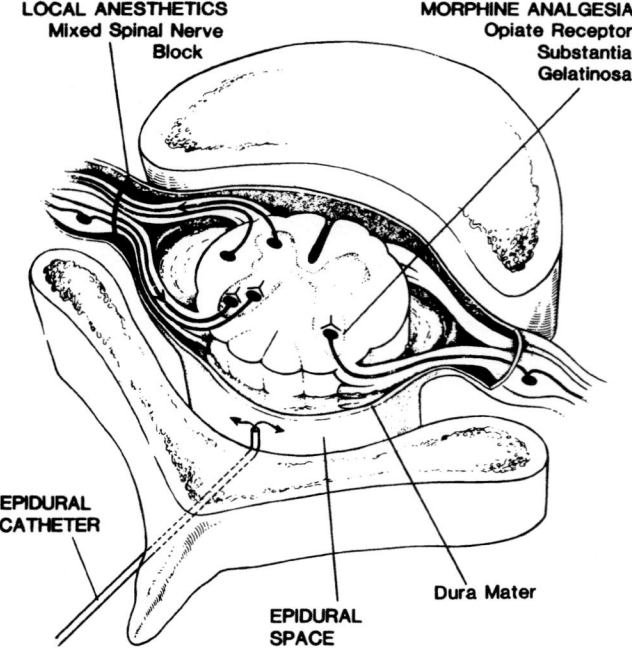

Fig. 38-1. Anatomic basis for narcotic analgesia and local anesthetic action. From El-Baz N, Ivankovich AD: Management of postoperative thoracotomy pain: continuous epidural infusion of morphine. *In* Kittle CF (ed): Current Controversies in Thoracic Surgery. Philadelphia: Saunders, 1986. With permission.

experienced hands, thoracic epidural analgesia can be offered with a minimal incidence of complications.

Several different agents can be delivered through an epidural catheter. In general, they are divided into local anesthetics and narcotics or opioids. The most commonly used local agent, bupivacaine, is less fat soluble than the most commonly used narcotic, fentanyl. The more lipophilic fentanyl, once delivered into the epidural space, traverses the space more quickly. It is this fact that allows lumbar epidurals to offer thoracic analgesia. The obvious disadvantage of this characteristic is that greater concentrations of opioids can reach the brainstem faster with thoracic epidural versus lumbar epidurals. This increases the risk of respiratory depression when narcotics are used.

The main disadvantage of local anesthetics delivered via a thoracic epidural catheter is the potential cardiovascular side effects. A chemical sympathectomy may cause decreased peripheral vascular resistance and hypotension. The problem may be compounded by a decrease in inotropy and in circulating levels of catecholamines. These latter effects result from impaired sympathetic stimulation of the adrenal medulla. Every effort should be made to avoid treating this problem with excessive intravenous administration of crystalloid fluids.

A third decision to be made concerning epidural analgesia is dosing. The ideal basal rate is one that offers sufficient analgesia that the patient never has to supplement with injections. However, because of the wide range of pain tolerance, this is often impossible. Therefore, we choose a relatively low basal rate.

The Pain Service at the University of Alabama at Birmingham uses thoracic epidurals almost exclusively for the patient who undergoes thoracotomy. We give 2 to 3 mL of 0.25% bupivacaine in the operating room near the end of the procedure. Postoperatively, the patient receives 4 mL/hour of 0.10% bupivacaine and 10 mg/mL of fentanyl. Ketorolac (Toradol), a nonsteroidal anti-inflammatory agent, is usually added to this regimen to provide multimodal analgesia. Although some surgeons are concerned about renal insufficiency induced by this agent, especially because pulmonary resection patients are often kept relatively hypovolemic, we have not experienced this problem. The new cyclooxygenase II inhibitors may eliminate this potential complication.

Complications from epidural analgesia include accidental entry into the subarachnoid space, hematoma, urinary retention, itching, nausea, and respiratory depression. A wet tap can occur when either the needle or the subsequently introduced catheter inadvertently enters the subarachnoid space. The first problem should be recognized immediately. Catheter misplacement in the subarachnoid space should be recognized when the test dose of local anesthetic agent, which should always be given after insertion, results in numbness in the chest area.

The best way to avoid most of these complications entails experienced personnel on the pain service and adequate monitoring of all patients who have epidural catheters. All patients should have a urinary catheter, and the catheter should be left in place for approximately 6 hours after the epidural is removed. We generally remove the epidural catheter after 2 days, and use the next 1 or 2 days before discharge for titration of oral pain medicines to meet each patient's specific analgesic needs.

PREVENTION OF PULMONARY INSUFFICIENCY

The incidence of respiratory insufficiency after pulmonary resection continues to decrease, despite operating on higher risk patients. Before surgery, all patients should undergo full pulmonary function testing, with special emphasis on the levels of the FEV_1, D_{LCO}, maximum voluntary ventilation, and an arterial blood gas obtained while breathing ambient air. The postoperative predicted FEV_1 and D_{LCO} should be calculated. These values can be determined by multiplying the preoperative value by the expected amount of lung that should remain after the planned pulmonary resection. If the ventilation is evenly distributed, one can easily calculate this figure based on the number of segments in each lobe. The number of remaining segments can be used to provide a reasonable estimate of postoperative function. For example, if a patient is to undergo a right lower lobectomy, the predicted postoperative FEV_1 is $14/19$ of the preoperative value, because right lower lobectomy entails removal of five segments. This approach assumes equal ventilation to the affected lung. In the patient with unequal ventilation, a quantitative ventilation-perfusion scan should be used to assess differential function, as discussed by Mjorner (1968) and Wernly and associates (1980). For example, if a patient is to undergo pneumonectomy and the affected lung has only 30% perfusion, the postoperative predicted D_{LCO} is 70% of the measured preoperative D_{LCO}. Other methods of calculation divide the lung into subsegments and factor into the calculations any totally obstructed units that are to be resected, because they do not contribute to the measured baseline parameter. I and my colleagues (1996) and Ferguson and associates (1988, 1995), among others, have shown that a predicted postoperative D_{LCO} or FEV_1 that is less than 40% of the expected value correlates with increased morbidity. Even when both predicted values are less than 40%, however, selected patients without significant comorbidities can safely undergo limited pulmonary resection if the arterial blood gas does not reveal hypercapnia. Hypercapnia is a sign of poor pulmonary reserve, and a P_{CO_2} greater than 45 mm Hg should be viewed as a marker of surgically significant pulmonary dysfunction. We perform pulmonary resections in selected patients with a P_{CO_2} greater than 55, but usually limit the extent of resection to segmentectomy or wedge excision.

Despite careful assessment of preoperative function and the use of pulmonary preserving techniques when indicated, pulmonary insufficiency can still occur after pulmonary resection. The inability to extubate a patient immediately after the operation is a poor prognostic sign, especially in the absence of an obvious anesthetic or surgical cause for this uncommon event, because the underlying problem may be inadequate remaining pulmonary function. Less ominous, and more common, is the appearance of respiratory difficulty later in the postoperative period. The difficulty usually arises on postoperative day 2 or 3, because of pneumonia, poor cough, or pulmonary edema. The patient often begins to develop signs of respiratory distress before the appearance of an infiltrate on chest film. Sputum cultures should be obtained, and broad-spectrum antibiotics should be started and tailored to the cultures and sensitivities reported later. To prevent progression of the problem, all basic aspects of pulmonary support must be maximized, including limitation of intravenous fluids, chest physiotherapy, frequent respiratory treatments with bronchodilators, incentive spirometry, ambulation with physical therapy, control of secretions, and nutritional support. If voluntary and assisted clearance of secretions is inadequate, nasotracheal suctioning should be used. If suctioning is needed repeatedly, a nasal trumpet should be inserted to facilitate easy access. If these techniques fail, minitracheostomy can be performed to allow direct suctioning. Induced diuresis is often helpful. If respiratory insufficiency and radiographic infiltrate(s) persist, and the results of standard cultures are not helpful, bronchoscopy should be considered for bronchoalveolar lavage, with protected brush sampling and transbronchial biopsy to search for unusual causes of postoperative respiratory failure.

Chest Physiotherapy, Incentive Spirometry, and Ambulation

Prevention of respiratory complications starts not only preoperatively but also in the operating room. Careful induction of anesthesia avoids aspiration. Most patients who are going to have a thoracotomy should have an epidural catheter. This, coupled with chest physiotherapy, frequent ambulation, bronchodilators, and other measures of pulmonary hygiene, help minimize complications.

Pneumonia remains a significant problem. It is the main complication that occurs from the failure to properly execute the preventive measures mentioned in this section. I and my associates (1998) and others have reported that the incidence is low (2 to 3%); postoperative pneumonia is associated with significant morbidity. Larger series, such as those of Deslauriers (1994) and Duque (1997) and their associates have reported incidences ranging up to 6%. Risk factors include prolonged preoperative hospitalization, pneumonectomy, poor pulmonary reserve, and smoking.

Atelectasis, a risk factor for the development of pneumonia, is another common complication after pulmonary and esophageal surgery. Most atelectasis is platelike, discoid, or linear and is subsegmental. These types have little clinical consequence in the patient with adequate pul-

monary reserve. However, atelectasis that is segmental or greater may cause clinical compromise and often requires bronchoscopy. Risk factors for significant atelectasis include poor cough, impaired pulmonary function, diaphragmatic dysfunction, chest wall instability, or sleeve resection, as noted by Massard and Wilhm (1998). The clinical sequelae of this type of significant atelectasis is ventilation-perfusion mismatch, leading to hypoxemia and impaired alveolar macrophage function. This combination may lead to pneumonia.

Chest physiotherapy with vibratory percussion, ambulation at least three to four times daily, and secretion control are the mainstays of prevention. Ambulation not only decreases the risk of deep venous thrombosis, but it helps rehabilitate the patient. It improves the distribution of pulmonary blood flow and minimizes areas of ventilation-perfusion mismatch. It is probably the single most important maneuver that a patient can do to help prevent many different types of complications.

Respiratory treatments are another important adjunct to achieve pulmonary hygiene. These include mist inhalation to loosen secretions, inhaled nebulized bronchodilators, and chest percussion with postural drainage, as summarized by Deschamps and colleagues (1992). Even with optimal respiratory treatment, some patients are not able to sufficiently mobilize their secretions. In this situation, nasotracheal suction via a nasal trumpet or a minitracheostomy may be required to clear the airways and avoid atelectasis and pneumonia.

Despite appropriate application of all of these techniques and the provision of adequate pain control, some patients develop a pulmonary infiltrate. Although Tobin and Grenvik (1984) showed that up to 30% of new infiltrates in the intensive care unit prove not to be pneumonia, a missed pneumonia in a postoperative patient is associated with a high rate of morbidity. In some cases, the patient develops a productive cough, fever, and elevated white blood cell count in the absence of radiographic evidence of an infiltrate. Because clinical pneumonia may precede radiologic pneumonia, especially in a dehydrated patient, broad-spectrum antibiotics should be started immediately and should often include fungal prophylaxis. If all the culture results ultimately are negative, antibiotics can be stopped.

Aspiration

Aspiration can be a dramatic or insidious but often devastating complication after pulmonary or esophageal surgery. Although it usually occurs in the early postoperative period, it may occur in a patient doing well and preparing to go home and result in multiorgan system failure and sepsis. Therefore, aspiration should be aggressively avoided. Patients should be allowed to eat or drink only when wide awake and when sitting upright in bed or in a chair. Family members should be discouraged from well-meaning attempts to help feed the patient, especially if the patient is drowsy.

MONITORING

Most significant complications after general thoracic procedures are cardiopulmonary and occur within the first 72 hours after surgery. For this reason, immediate and continuous postoperative cardiac and pulmonary monitoring is necessary. Early care in an intensive care unit has been the standard approach for thoracotomy patients. At our center, the majority of patients are sent directly to the floor. In a series of 400 consecutive thoracotomies, of which 55% had a history of cardiac or significant respiratory disease, or both, only 20% of patients were initially managed in an intensive care unit setting. Operative mortality was only 2.9%, and major morbidity was 14%. Ninety-seven percent of patients had epidural catheters. Arterial lines are rarely used postoperatively, but continuous cardiac monitoring and pulse oximetry are used early in all cases. These parameters are monitored at the nursing station by a central system equipped with alarms for low oxygen saturations or cardiac arrhythmias.

Routine blood tests are not necessary after most pulmonary resections. If the oxygen saturation is consistently acceptable and if no clinical signs of respiratory difficulty exist, serial arterial blood gases are not needed and even a baseline blood gas may be superfluous. Similarly, if the chest tube output is minimal, urinary volume is adequate (0.5 mL/kg per hour), and the blood pressure and cardiac rhythm are normal, serial hemograms and electrolyte levels are not required. Especially unwarranted is the occasional practice of obtaining electrocardiograms and cardiac enzymatic studies on all general thoracic surgical patients.

INTRAVENOUS FLUID MANAGEMENT

It is often difficult for the surgeon to convince the anesthesiologists, nurses, residents, and fellows that pulmonary surgical patients do not require and should not be given the traditional amount of fluids needed by most other postsurgical patients. Pulmonary surgery does not cause large fluid shifts, as does intraperitoneal surgery. Moreover, expansion and deflation of the lung during selective lung ventilation, intraoperative barotrauma and volutrauma to the alveoli, and surgical manipulation all lead to the potential for pulmonary edema.

Patients who undergo an uncomplicated pneumonectomy should receive no more than 500 to 800 mL of crystalloid from the time of hospital admission until they enter the recovery room. The tendency to give patients large volumes of fluids after epidural placement because of hypotension from a sympathectomy effect must be avoided. This is a difficult task and is only accomplished by continued communication between the surgical service and the pain, anesthesia,

nursing, and resident services. We prefer the use of α-agonist agents such as phenylephrine if mean arterial blood pressure decreases after epidural dosing in pulmonary surgical patients. For esophageal resections, in contrast, α-agonists should be avoided to prevent ischemia of the mobilized conduit via vasoconstriction. Fluid replacement in these cases cannot be as restricted as in patients undergoing pulmonary operations. We usually use a baseline rate of 40 mL/hour of 5% dextrose in lactated Ringer's solution (D5LR) in a 70-kg man after lobectomy and 125 mL/hour of D5LR after esophagogastrectomy. In all cases, adjustments are made on the basis of clinical assessment.

When pulmonary edema develops despite appropriate fluid management, diuretics are the mainstay of treatment. It is important to ensure that the cause is not cardiac insufficiency. If the patient continues to deteriorate, echocardiography should be performed to assess both right and left ventricular function. Blood cultures and appropriate scans should be performed to search for infection. If aggressive diuresis is not successful, and no apparent septic or cardiogenic etiology for the pulmonary edema exists, the patient may have adult respiratory distress syndrome. Diagnosis and management of this complication are discussed in Chapters 37 and 39.

POSTOPERATIVE HEMORRHAGE

The incidence of postoperative hemorrhage after elective general thoracic surgical procedures should be extremely small. In our last 2000 operations, only one patient has had to return to the operating room for control of hemorrhage. Four patients had a coagulopathy that required multiple transfusions. When excessive bleeding occurs via the chest tube(s), standard coagulation studies are performed. A thromboelastogram or bleeding time also can be performed if needed. If possible, all measured abnormalities should be corrected before reoperation.

MANAGEMENT OF CHEST TUBES AND AIR LEAKS

Although persistent air leak after pulmonary resection is a common complication, few reports exist in the literature on optimal treatment. Any patient who has had entry into the thoracic cavity has the potential to develop an air leak and a pleural space problem. The incidence ranges from 15 to 50%, depending on the definition. I and my colleagues (1998) found an incidence of air leak after elective pulmonary resection of 20 to 30% on the first postoperative day.

Intraoperative prevention requires identification of parenchymal leaks by careful inspection, and, in some cases, control by suturing, stapling, or the application of topical sealants. Prophylactic measures include the use of staple-line buttressing with bovine pericardial or polytetrafluoroethylene. Chest tube placement is critical because it helps achieve pleural apposition. Although some surgeons use only one

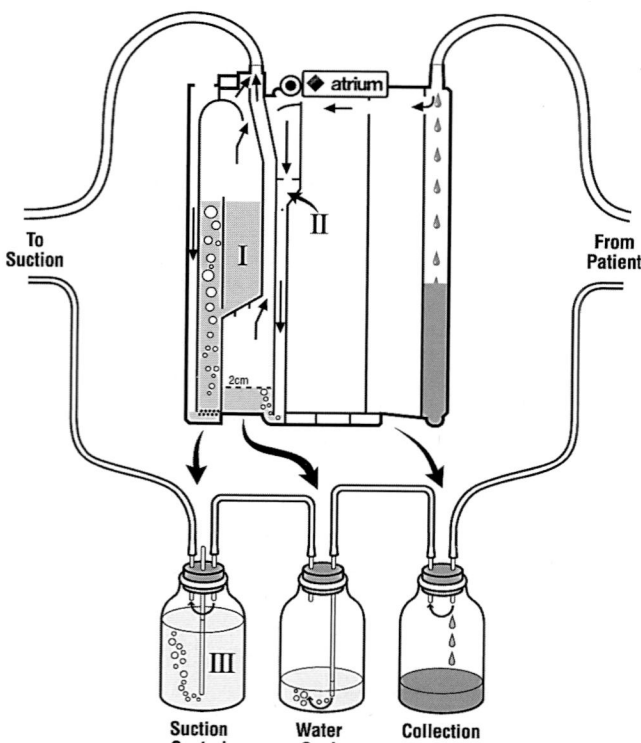

Fig. 38-2. A commercially available compartmentalized three-bottle suction apparatus. It can be used without suction as a simple water-seal device. The height of the column in the suction control chamber determines the amount of negative pressure applied to the pleural space (I). An additional feature is the ability to measure the amount of negative pressure developed by the patient (II and III).

tube after lobectomy, we prefer two tubes. We believe that the advantage of preventing a residual space problem by yielding parietal and visceral pleural apposition offsets the added cost and morbidity of an extra chest tube. The length of hospital stay is not affected, because both chest test tubes can be removed on the same day. We position two No. 28F soft chest tubes after upper lobectomy in the anterior and posterior apex. After lower lobectomy, we prefer a right-angle chest tube along the diaphragm and a straight anterior tube in the apex. We use induced pneumoperitoneum after bilobectomy to decrease the residual space and the duration of air leaks. In a current prospective study, this technique has shortened the postresection length of stay.

After surgery is completed, and the pleural space and air leaks have been controlled as well as possible, most thoracotomy tubes can be managed on water seal, at least during transfer. Even with large leaks, tension does not develop. A widely used, commercially available system for draining the pleural space is the Pleur-evac, a compact, nonbreakable, three-bottle chest drainage apparatus (Fig. 38-2). It can be used as a simple underwater seal system or attached to a vacuum line. The amount of suction is limited by the height

of the column of water in the vacuum control chamber. The third component of the unit is a compartmentalized collection chamber.

When a postoperative air leak is noted, the first step is to ensure that the air leak is from the lung and not from a problem in the drainage system. Also, if the patient has had an anatomic pulmonary resection, and the leak is large or continuous, one must exclude a bronchopleural fistula from the bronchial closure. My colleagues and I (1998) described a classification system for peripheral air leaks, based on the timing of their occurrence during the respiratory cycle and on the magnitude of the air leak. Using a commercially available air leak meter, we label air leaks as expiratory only, inspiratory only, continuous, or forced expiratory, meaning they occur only with cough. We found this classification system to be reproducible among different observers, inexpensive, and an excellent predictor of the natural history of different types of air leaks.

Our study showed that most air leaks after pulmonary resection are expiratory or forced expiratory. Continuous air leaks are rare and occur more often in patients with spontaneous rupture of an emphysematous bleb than in postoperative cases. When a continuous leak is noted after pulmonary resection, the source is usually a defect at the bronchial closure site, rather than a parenchymal fistula. Inspiratory air leaks are seen almost exclusively in mechanically ventilated patients, because of continuous positive airway pressure. Quantifying air leaks with the air leak meter enables one to treat large leaks sooner and save hospital days. Increasing magnitude of the leak as measured by the meter ranges from 1 to 7. We found that air leaks rated as 3 or less have a good chance of prompt cessation on water seal.

Although most surgeons currently use suction routinely for patients with or without air leaks, our randomized, prospective study indicates that water seal is superior to suction for earlier cessation of expiratory and forced expiratory air leaks. However, patients with large air leaks (rated as greater than 4 on the leak meter) may develop a pneumothorax when converted to water seal. A pneumothorax impedes sealing of the air leak because of the absence of visceral and parietal pleural apposition.

Most leaks immediately decrease on water seal. If pleural apposition is maintained, there is a good chance that the air leak will stop within 24 to 48 hours. Early air leaks rated as greater than 4/7, or smaller leaks that are still present by the fifth postoperative day, are managed by placement of a Heimlich valve or by bedside chemical pleurodesis. In the rare instances of late ongoing air leak, a trial of chest tube clamping, as described by Kirschner (1992), often demonstrates clinical stability and preserved lung expansion, because of adhesion formation. In such cases, the chest tube can be removed, despite the presence of an air leak. The persistent space does not become infected and resolves over time. Unless massive and associated with respiratory compromise or septic residual space problems, persistent alveolar air leaks can be managed rapidly and without the need for prolonged hospitalization, as discussed in Chapter 37.

REFERENCES

Cerfolio RJ, et al: Lung resection in patients with compromised pulmonary function. Ann Thorac Surg *62*:348, 1996.

Cerfolio RJ, et al: A prospective algorithm of the management of air leaks after pulmonary resection. Ann Thorac Surg *66*:1726, 1998.

Deschamps C, et al: Postoperative management. Chest *102*:713, 1992.

Deslauriers J, et al: Current operative morbidity associated with elective surgical resection for lung cancer. Can J Surg *32*:335, 1989.

Deslauriers J, et al: Prospective assessment of 30-day operative morbidity of surgical resections in lung cancer. Chest *106*:329S, 1994.

Duque JL, et al: Early complications in surgical treatment of lung cancer: a prospective, multicenter study. Ann Thorac Surg *63*:944, 1997.

El-Baz N, Ivankovich AD: Managment of postoperative thoracotomy pain: continuous epidural infusion of morphine. *In* Kittle CF (ed): Current Controversies in Thoracic Surgery. Philadelphia: WB Saunders, 1986.

Ferguson MK, et al: Diffusing capacity predicts morbidity and mortality after pulmonary resection. J Thorac Cardiovasc Surg *96*:894, 1988.

Ferguson MK, Reeder LB, Mick R: Optimizing selection of patients for major lung resection. J Thorac Cardiovasc Surg *109*:275, 1995.

Ginsberg RJ, et al: Modern 30 day operative mortality for surgical resections in lung cancer. J Thorac Cardiovasc Surg *86*:654, 1983.

Kirschner PA: Provocative clamping and removal of chest tubes despite persistent air leak [Letter]. Ann Thorac Surg *53*:740, 1992.

Kruger M, McRae K: Pain management in cardiothoracic practice. Surg Clin North Am *79*:387, 1999.

Massard G, Wihlm JM: Postoperative atelectasis. Chest *113*:503, 1998.

Mjorner G: ^{133}Xe radiospirometry: a clinical method for studying regional lung function. Scand J Respir Dis *64S*:5, 1968.

Olsen GN, et al: Stair climbing as an exercise test predicts the postoperative complications of lung resection—2 years experience. Chest *99*:587, 1991.

Stein M, Cassara EL: Preoperative pulmonary evaluation and therapy for surgery patients. *JAMA* 211:787, 1970.

Tobin MJ, Grenvik A: Nosocomial lung infection and its diagnosis. Crit Care Med *12*:191, 1984.

Wahi R, et al: Determinants of perioperative morbidity and mortality after pneumonectomy. Ann Thorac Surg *48*:333, 1989

Wernly JA, et al: Clinical value of quantitative ventilation-perfusion lung scans in the surgical management of bronchogenic carcinoma. J Thorac Cardiovasc Surg *80*:535, 1980.

CHAPTER 39

Ventilatory Support of Postoperative Surgical Patients

Joseph LoCicero III and Joseph B. Zwischenberger

POSTOPERATIVE PULMONARY PATHOPHYSIOLOGY

All patients who undergo major thoracic surgical procedures require careful attention to ventilatory function. Pulmonary function and resultant gas exchange deteriorate after any major surgical procedure, particularly after pulmonary resections. Minute ventilation is well preserved, but its separate components are considerably altered. Churchill and McNeil (1927) reported that vital capacity (VC) is reduced by 50 to 75% in the first 24 hours. On average, tidal volume is diminished by 20% and functional residual capacity (FRC) by 35% in thoracic and upper abdominal procedures. Normally, a return to preoperative levels is observed in 7 to 14 days. Despite the fall in tidal volume, minute ventilation is maintained by compensatory increases in respiratory rate.

Latimer and associates (1971) found that the highest rates of postoperative pulmonary complications occurred with thoracic and upper abdominal procedures. Atelectasis occurs when the closing volume of the airways exceeds the expiratory reserve volume in the early postoperative period. At special risk are the elderly and smokers, whose closing volume is already elevated. Obese patients already have a diminished expiratory reserve volume. Patients with chronic obstructive lung disease exhibit problems with expiratory reserve volume and closing volume.

Several other mechanisms contribute to a decrease in lung volume and compliance. A major increase in extravascular lung water may result not only in decreased compliance of the lung but also in hypoxemia. Such may occur even in the absence of the characteristic radiographic changes of pulmonary edema. Prys-Roberts and colleagues (1967) noted that alveolar-arterial oxygen gradients might increase without any abnormalities becoming apparent on standard chest radiographs. The increases in lung water may result from fluid overload, left ventricular failure, or impairment of the permeability characteristics of the pulmonary capillary membrane

(so-called low-pressure pulmonary edema). Low-pressure pulmonary edema has often been referred to as adult respiratory distress syndrome (ARDS) and may occur after shock, sepsis, aspiration, and multiple blood transfusions, all of which may be associated with major surgical procedures. After pulmonary surgery, these abnormalities may be exaggerated by two factors. First, the ipsilateral lung may have undergone operative trauma and contusion. In addition, its intraoperative collapse and reexpansion may result in fluid extravasation from the pulmonary capillary bed. Second, pulmonary artery pressure may increase transiently after resection of pulmonary tissue, particularly after pneumonectomy. Capillary pressure (P_c) is largely determined by both left atrial pressure (P_{la}) and pulmonary artery pressure (P_{pa}), as shown in the equation $P_c = P_{la} + 0.4(P_{pa} - P_{la})$. Therefore, any increase in pulmonary artery pressure—particularly if complicated by excessive fluid administration—results in additional fluid movement into the alveolar and interstitial spaces.

This accumulation of extravascular lung water may affect regional ventilation not only by subsequent alveolar flooding but also by augmenting airway closure via peribronchial cuffing. Atelectasis and decreased compliance alter regional ventilation and, in the end, adversely affect ventilation-perfusion ($\dot{V}/\dot{Q}$) matching. Hypoxemia results.

Although hypoxemia is seen early, hypercarbia is usually a late-appearing abnormality, often signifying that the patient is tiring and may soon require mechanical assistance. Indeed, unless pain is particularly severe or the patient is oversedated, hypocarbia is typical after surgery because the respiratory rate often increases as a function of anxiety, pain, and hypoxemia.

Several postoperative cardiovascular changes may further alter $\dot{V}/\dot{Q}$ matching. For example, a decrease in cardiac output resulting from hypovolemia, sepsis, or an increase in left ventricular afterload may affect the degree of regional pulmonary artery perfusion and further aggravate impaired $\dot{V}/\dot{Q}$ matching. Increases in right ventricular filling pressure caused by pulmonary hypertension (which may result from excision of lung tissue) may further impair left ventricular function by shifting the intraventricular septum and adversely affecting left ventricular filling.

POSTOPERATIVE INDICATIONS FOR SUPPORT

Despite the pathophysiologic alterations in pulmonary function, only a few patients eventually require mechanical ventilatory support. The decision to initiate or continue mechanical ventilation is usually based on an assessment of gas exchange, impending respiratory failure, and the patient's ability to protect the airway. The postoperative period should then be characterized by respiratory monitoring as well as a careful clinical evaluation of the patient.

Many patients have indwelling arterial lines placed by the anesthesia staff to facilitate management of one-lung anesthesia techniques. Arterial blood can and should be sampled early to assess both Pao_2 and $Paco_2$. Oxygenation can, however, be adequately assessed noninvasively through pulse oximetry as long as peripheral perfusion is satisfactory. Oxygenation should be undertaken routinely in the recovery room and in the early postoperative period.

Although respiratory fatigue, once established, should be reflected in abnormal arterial blood gas values, it is important to recognize the clinical signs of impending respiratory muscle fatigue to initiate corrective measures. Such recognition requires an assessment of the patient rather than laboratory data. Mental acuity and awareness in the face of obvious freedom from pain are encouraging. The patient who is able to converse in sentences is likely to generate an adequate tidal volume. Respiratory muscle paradox is an early and reliable sign of established muscle fatigue and is an indication for mechanical ventilatory support. It is easily assessed by placing a hand on the chest and the abdomen during inspiration and expiration. Normally, the chest and abdomen expand together when the patient inhales because diaphragmatic descent displaces abdominal viscera. In established fatigue, the diaphragm moves paradoxically upward during inspiration, resulting in the abdominal hand moving inward while the chest expands.

In the early postoperative period, the patient's level of consciousness may be impaired from inadequate reversal of anesthesia or other complications, such as postoperative cerebral vascular accident and narcotic overdosage, which may also result in central nervous system (CNS) depression sufficient to cause an inability to protect the airway. At such times, micro- or macro-aspiration may occur. Unless rapid reversal with naloxone hydrochloride (Narcan) is achieved, early intubation is advisable.

Postoperative respiratory failure can occur in one of three situations, as noted in Table 39-1. Most problems in the immediate postoperative period are related to pure ventilatory failure or a mixed picture. It is at this time that problems associated with inadequate reversal of anesthesia, narcotic

Table 39-1. Classification of Respiratory Failure

Type	Pathophysiology	Measurement
Hypoxemic	$\dot{V}/\dot{Q}$ mismatch	Pao_2, Sao_2
Ventilatory	$-V_D/V_T$, inadequate ventilation	$Paco_2$, pH
Mixed	$\dot{V}/\dot{Q}$ mismatch and $-V_D/V_T$	Pao_2, Sao_2, $Paco_2$

overdosage, perioperative aspiration, or airway obstruction secondary to laryngeal edema becomes evident. Shapiro and associates (1977) defined acute ventilatory failure as a $Paco_2$ determination greater than 50 mm Hg and a pH of less than 7.30. Table 39-2 lists other parameters. Early and temporary intubation is all that is required, unless the patient has developed a $\dot{V}/\dot{Q}$ abnormality as well from complicating aspiration, fluid overload, inadequate pulmonary reserve, or major atelectasis. Once reintubation has been accomplished, radiographic examination of the chest is necessary to ensure that none of these complications has developed.

For the patient who does well in the initial postoperative period, continued monitoring of oxygen saturation is important as long as he or she requires supplemental oxygen. This monitoring need not be continuous in the nonventilated patient, unless the fraction of inspired oxygen (Fio_2) is high or the saturation is marginally acceptable. The need for continued blood gas analysis depends on the following: 1) a preoperative elevation of $Paco_2$, 2) a postoperative elevation of $Paco_2$, and 3) unreliable or inconsistent oximetric saturation readings.

The mixed form of respiratory failure is seen in some well-defined clinical scenarios. First, it can occur when there is preexisting carbon dioxide retention. Under such circumstances, excessive oxygen administration may remove the hypoxic drive for breathing that has become a compensatory mechanism in patients with chronic hypercarbia. Too often, the goals of oxygen administration are poorly defined, and physicians assume that a high Pao_2 value provides a margin of safety. A saturation of more than 95% may actually depress respiratory effort in these patients, leading to an exacerbation of CO_2 retention and the onset of an acute respiratory acidosis wherein hypoxemia is a late feature. Second, in cases of mental obtundation, arterial oxygen desaturation may result in an inability to respond with an increased respiratory effort, and CO_2 retention complicates the hypoxia. Third, when respiratory muscle fatigue comes on quickly

Table 39-2. Variables Defining Ventilatory Failure Requiring Intubation

Respiratory rate	<4 or >35
$Paco_2$	>50 mm Hg
$V_D/\dot{V}_T$	>0.6
Vital capacity	<15 mL/kg
Negative inspiratory force	<20 cm H_2O

because of malnutrition or associated chronic disease, both depression of oxygenation and elevation of CO_2 levels occurs, particularly in the patient recovering from prolonged ventilatory support after severe lung injury. Finally, the development of a pulmonary embolus in a patient receiving mechanical ventilatory assistance is a classic example of the mixed picture. The pathophysiology of pulmonary embolism involves an increase in dead space because the vascular supply to well-ventilated alveoli is obstructed. In the spontaneously ventilated patient, reflex hyperventilation usually leads to hypocarbia. In the ventilated-controlled patient, however, such a reflex increase in minute ventilation does not occur, depending on the ventilator mode and the presence or absence of paralysis, and therefore hypercarbia develops.

NONVENTILATOR STRATEGIES

When a patient shows signs of ventilatory impairment, steps can be taken to improve function. Incentive spirometry and chest physiotherapy have been the backbone of therapy for all postoperative patients. Arguments pro and con have been presented for these time-honored methods, but the attention to the patient and the patient's own efforts have been very successful in improving ventilatory function. Hillberg and Johnson (1997) discussed noninvasive ventilation as a method of treating a V̇/Q̇ mismatch. In addition to oxygen therapy, patients may be offered continuous positive airway pressure (CPAP) oxygen with a nasal mask. These systems were developed for severe chronic obstructive pulmonary disease (COPD) but are beneficial for patients with moderately acute ventilatory failure. These masks can be applied before or after surgery to improve oxygen delivery. The devices are well tolerated, even by patients with CO_2 retention, and require little training to use properly.

VENTILATOR MANAGEMENT STRATEGIES

Many varieties of ventilatory support are available. Table 39-3 presents a rational approach to ventilator modes.

Control Mode of Ventilation

The control mode of ventilation is often used in patients with ARDS due to the high peak pressures needed to achieve adequate chest expansion. The major disadvantage with this mode is that the patient cannot cycle the ventilator; thus, the minute ventilation must be set appropriately. In the assist-control mode of ventilation, in which every breath is supported by the ventilator, a backup control rate is set, but the patient may choose any rate above the set rate. Using this mode of ventilation, the tidal volume, inspiratory flow rate, flow waveform, sensitivity, and control rate are set. Advantages are that assist-control ventilation combines the security of controlled ventilation with the possibility of synchronizing the breathing pattern of the patient and ventilator. It also ensures ventilatory support during each breath. Marini and colleagues reported in 1985 and 1986 on the disadvantages, which include the following:

- Excessive patient work occurs during inadequate peak flow or sensitivity settings, especially, as Ward and associates (1988) note, if the ventilatory drive of the patient is increased.
- It is sometimes poorly tolerated in awake, nonsedated subjects and can require sedation to ensure synchrony of patient and machine.
- Respiratory alkalosis can occur.
- It may worsen air trapping with patients who have chronic obstructive lung disease, according to Slutsky (1993).

Synchronized Intermittent Mandatory Ventilation

As described by Downs (1973) and Weisman and colleagues (1983), synchronized intermittent mandatory ventilation (SIMV) combines a preset number of ventilator-delivered mandatory breaths of preset tidal volume with the facility for intermittent patient-generated spontaneous breaths. An advantage of this technique is that the patient can perform a variable amount of respiratory work and yet have the security of a preset mandatory level of ventilation. Also,

Table 39-3. Conventional and Unconventional Forms of Ventilatory Support

	Ventilation	Lung	Medications	Other
Standard	Volume ventilation, positive end-expiratory pressure	Pulmonary toilet	Antibiotics, broncho-dilators	Nutrition support (enteral preferred)
Advanced	Pressure-limited ventilation, permissive hypercapnia, inverse ratio ventilation, tracheostomy	Prone positioning, bronchoscopy	Steroids, diuretics	Increased O_2 delivery (hematocrit, cardiac output)
Extraordinary	Nitric oxide, high-frequency ventilation or high-frequency oscillatory ventilation, intratracheal pulmonary ventilation, partial liquid ventilation	Hemofiltration, surfactant replacement	Ketoconazole, prostaglandin E_1, antioxidants	ECMO, $ECCO_2R$, IVOX, $AVCO_2R$

$AVCO_2R$, arteriovenous carbon dioxide removal; $ECCO_2R$, extracorporeal carbon dioxide removal; ECMO, extracorporeal membrane oxygenation; IVOX, intravenous oxygenation.

SIMV allows for a variation in level of support, from near total ventilatory support to spontaneous breathing, and it can be used as a weaning tool. Disadvantages include hyperventilation, respiratory alkalosis, and excessive work of breathing because of the presence of a poorly responsive demand valve, suboptimal ventilatory circuits, or inappropriate flow delivery. In each case, extra work is imposed on the patient during spontaneous breaths.

Pressure Support Ventilation

Pressure support ventilation (PSV) is a pressure-targeted, flow-cycled mode of ventilation in which the patient must trigger each breath. PSV is designed to assist spontaneous breathing; therefore, the patient must have an intact respiratory drive. Its advantages are that it is regarded as a comfortable mode of ventilation for most patients, it reduces the work of breathing, and it can be used to overcome the airway resistance caused by the endotracheal tube. In addition, PSV may be useful in patients who are difficult to wean. Disadvantages of PSV are that tidal volume is not controlled and depends on respiratory mechanics, cycling frequency, and synchrony between the patient and ventilator. Also, PSV may be poorly tolerated in some patients with high airway resistances because of the preset high initial flow rates.

In severe cases of ARDS, Gattinoni and associates (1987) showed that only a small part of the lung parenchyma remains accessible to gas delivered by mechanical ventilation. Hickling (1990) noted that tidal volumes of 10 mL/kg or more may overexpand and injure the remaining normally aerated lung parenchyma and could worsen the prognosis of severe acute respiratory failure (ARF) by extending nonspecific alveolar damage. High airway pressures may result in overdistention and local hyperventilation of more compliant parts of the diseased lung. Kolobow and coworkers (1987) found that overdistention of lungs in animals produced diffuse alveolar damage.

Volume-Cycled Ventilation

In volume-cycled ventilation, a machine-delivered tidal volume is set to be consistent with adequate gas exchange and patient comfort. The tidal volume selected for burned patients normally varies between 10 and 15 mL/kg of body weight. Kacmarek and Vengas (1987) argued that numerous factors, such as lung or thorax compliance, system resistance, compressible volume loss, oxygenation, ventilation, and barotrauma, are considered when setting volumes and rates. It is critically important to avoid overdistention, and this can generally be accomplished by ensuring that peak airway and alveolar pressures do not exceed a maximum target. Hickling and associates (1990) and Marini (1992) agree that a peak airway pressure greater than 35 cm H_2O in adults

raises concern about the development of barotrauma and that ventilator-induced lung injury increases.

Technical Aspects of Ventilator Management

Setting of the mandatory ventilator respiratory rate depends on the mode of ventilation selected, the delivered tidal volume, the ratio of dead space to tidal volume, metabolic rate, targeted Pco_2 levels, and level of spontaneous ventilation. With adults, Kacmarek and Vengas (1987) found that the set mandatory rate normally varies between 4 and 20 breaths per minute (bpm), with most clinically stable patients requiring mandatory rates in the range of 8 to 12 bpm. In patients with inhalation injury, mandatory rates exceeding 20 bpm may be necessary, depending on the desired expired volume and targeted Pco_2. Along with the Pco_2, pH, and patient comfort, the primary variables controlling the selection of the respiratory rate are the development of air trapping and automatic positive end-expiratory pressure (auto-PEEP), according to Pepe and Marini (1982).

The respiratory rates of children and infants must be set substantially higher than those of adults. For pediatric patients, the respiratory rate can be set at from 14 to 35, depending on the disease state and the desired level of targeted Pco_2. Slower respiratory rates are useful in the patient with obstructed airways because slower rates allow more time for exhalation and emptying of hyperinflated areas.

The selection of the peak inspiratory flow rate during volume ventilation is determined primarily by the level of spontaneous inspiratory effort. Peak inspiratory flows ideally should match patient peak inspiratory demands. In the 1993 American College of Chest Physicians' Consensus Conference report, Slutsky noted that this normally requires peak flows to be set at 40 to 100 L/min, depending on expired volume and inspiratory demand. As a starting point and until the level of hypoxemia is determined, a patient placed on a ventilator should receive an oxygen concentration of 100%. The concentration should be systematically lowered as soon as arterial blood gases dictate. In patients who are difficult to oxygenate, Stroller and Kacmarek (1990) showed that oxygen concentrations can be minimized by optimizing PEEP and mean airway pressures (MAPs) and by selecting a minimally acceptable oxygen saturation. PEEP is applied to recruit lung volumes, elevate MAP, and improve oxygenation. The level of PEEP used varies with the disease process. PEEP levels should start at 5 cm H_2O and be increased in 2.5-cm increments. Increasing levels of PEEP in conjunction with a prolonged inspiratory time aids in oxygenation and allows for the safe level of oxygen to be used. Optimal PEEP, defined by Suter and associates (1975), is the level of end-expiratory pressure that results in the lowering of intrapulmonary shunting, significant improvement in arterial oxygenation, and only a small change in cardiac output, arteriovenous oxygen content differences, or mixed venous oxygen tension.

Standard extubation criteria defined by Sahn and Lakshminarayan (1973) and Tahvanainen and colleagues (1983) are the following:

- Pa_{O_2} to FI_{O_2} ratio greater than 250
- Maximum inspiratory pressure greater than 60 cm H_2O
- VC of at least 15 to 20 mL/kg
- Tidal volume of at least 5 to 7 mL/kg
- Maximum voluntary ventilation of at least twice the minute volume

In general, these indices evaluate the patient's ability to sustain spontaneous ventilation. They do not assess a patient's ability to protect the upper airway. For this reason, traditional indices often do not reflect the true clinical picture of a patient with an inhalation injury.

MODES OF VENTILATORY SUPPORT

Gentle Ventilation with Permissive Hypercapnia

Perhaps the most significant ventilator management strategy aimed directly at reducing airway pressures during ARDS to avoid exacerbating barotrauma or volume trauma is the use of low-pressure, low-volume ventilation. The American College of Chest Physicians' Consensus Conference, reported by Slutsky (1993), recommended that under conditions of lung overdistention, airway pressures should be limited by reducing tidal volumes and accepting the attendant increase in arterial P_{CO_2} levels. Bidani and colleagues (1994) used permissive hypercapnia as the method of allowing blood P_{CO_2} levels to rise, with or without control of arterial blood pH. Hickling and associates (1994) described lower tidal volumes (5 to 8 mL/kg) used to prevent excessive alveolar distention and low levels of PEEP and supplemental oxygen to improve hypoxemia. Thus, even in the diseased lung, $\dot{V}/\dot{Q}$ match and arterial oxygenation can be improved, independent of the reduced level of ventilation required to excrete CO_2 during hypercapnia.

Hickling and coworkers (1990) first published retrospective data on 50 patients with severe ARDS managed with permissive hypercapnia. Peak inspiratory pressure (PIP) was limited to less than 40 cm H_2O at all times and to less than 30 cm H_2O when possible, using volume-cycled ventilation, tidal volumes as low as 5 mL/kg, and SIMV mode to allow spontaneous respirations, while the P_{CO_2} was "permitted" to increase. All patients had a lung injury score of 2.5 and a mean Pa_{O_2} to FI_{O_2} ratio of 94. The mean maximum P_{CO_2} was 62 mm Hg, and the highest was 129 mm Hg. No specific treatment was used to treat the respiratory acidosis, and the pH was allowed to fall to as low as 7.02. The mean time from initiation of ventilation to the maximum P_{CO_2} was 5.2 days; the mean duration of ventilation was 8.1 days for survivors and 9.0 days for nonsurvivors. Mortality was significantly lower than that predicted by APACHE II (i.e., 16% vs. 39.6%). Hickling and associates (1994) later evaluated the

outcome in 53 patients with severe ARDS. They were managed with spontaneous breathing using SIMV limitation of PIP to 30 to 40 cm H_2O, low tidal volumes (4 to 7 mL/kg from the start of ventilation), and permissive hypercapnia without the use of bicarbonate to buffer acidosis. The hospital mortality rate was significantly lower than that predicted by the APACHE II scores (26.4% vs. 53.3%, $P = .004$), even after correcting the latter for the effect of hypercapnic acidosis (26.4% vs. 51.1%, $P = .008$). The mean maximum P_{CO_2} was 66.5 mm Hg (range 38 to 158 mm Hg), and the mean arterial pH at the same time was 7.23 (range 6.79 to 7.45). No pneumothoraces developed during mechanical ventilation.

In 1998, Amato and colleagues compared "protective" ventilation at 6 mL/kg tidal volume with "conventional" ventilation at 12 mL/kg tidal volume in patients with ARDS. They found that protective ventilation allowed 66% of patients to be weaned from ventilators compared to 29% with conventional ventilation. Clinical barotrauma was 7% with protective ventilation and 42% with conventional; hospital mortality was 38% and 71%, respectively. In the protective ventilation group, arterial P_{CO_2} was initially 80 mm Hg, and sodium bicarbonate was given when pH fell below 7.2. Stewart and coworkers (1998), however, did not find any difference in survival between patients in whom peak airway pressure was limited to less than 30 cm H_2O and those in whom peak airway pressure was allowed to increase up to 50 cm H_2O. In their study, the tidal volume (7.2 ± 0.8 vs. 10.8 ± 1.0 mL/kg) and peak airway pressure (23.6 ± 5.8 vs. 34.0 ± 11.0 cm H_2O) were statistically different but not clinically significant. Tidal volume in the pressure-limited ventilation group was not as low as reported previously, and arterial P_{CO_2} was only in the range of 50 mm Hg. A peak airway pressure between 30 and 40 cm H_2O in the control group may not have been severe enough to exacerbate lung injury because pressure-limited ventilation did not show benefits in terms of improving survival and minimizing barotrauma.

The possible benefits of pressure limitation and the resultant hypercapnia in ARF must be balanced against any potential physiologic costs arising from alterations of CO_2 homeostasis. Carbon dioxide affects cellular function through direct molecular CO_2 effects, through "indirect" effects mediated via neurological or humoral control pathways, and by its contribution to maintenance of tissue pH. Both Bidani (1994) and Cardenas (1996) and their associates note that accumulation of CO_2 may lead to tissue acidosis, catecholamine release, and changes in hemodynamics and organ blood flow. Siesjo and colleagues (1972) note that there is a depressant effect of CO_2, presumably resulting from a combination of inert gas narcotic effect, direct inhibition of synaptic transmission, and depression of cellular function mediated by the reduction in intracellular pH.

Significant hypercapnia and respiratory acidosis may be tolerated if tissue anoxia and ischemia are prevented. Moderate degrees of chronic respiratory acidosis are well tolerated in patients with COPD and are not associated with demonstrable abnormalities in CNS, renal, or cardiovascular function. Graded decrements in minute ventilation over several hours allow time for pH compensatory mechanisms (cellular buffers, renal compensation) to adjust to the progressive hypercapnic state. Alternatively, as Cardenas and colleagues (1996) have done, bicarbonate could be administered to temporarily ameliorate the respiratory acidosis.

Increased Inspiratory Time (Inverse Ratio Ventilation)

The time allowed for the inspiratory and expiratory phases of mechanical ventilation is commonly referred to as the inspiratory to expiratory (I:E) ratio. The inspiratory part of the ratio includes the time to deliver the tidal volume before the exhalation valve opens and exhalation begins. The expiratory part of the ratio includes the time necessary for the tidal volume to exit through the exhalation valve before the next inspiration begins. The inspiratory time should be long enough to deliver the tidal volume at flow rates that do not result in turbulence and high peak airway pressures. In severe lung disease, it is acceptable to prolong the inspiratory time to allow for better distribution of gas and to exchange oxygen diffusion. Prolonged inspiratory time creates a more laminar flow, which helps to keep peak pressures lower. Fast inspiratory times are tolerated in patients with severe airway obstruction. The fast inspiratory time allows for a longer expiratory phase, which may help to decrease the amount of overinflation. Standard mechanical ventilation attempts to simulate normal physiology whereby inspiration is considerably shorter than expiration, with an I:E ratio of approximately 1:2 or 1:3. During the inspiratory phase of mechanical ventilation, positive pressure is used to overcome the impedance of the breathing circuit and conducting airways, as well as inflating the terminal alveoli. To prevent unstable alveoli with reduced compliance from collapsing during the expiratory phase, PEEP maintains persistent distending pressures in the airway, thereby promoting alveolar recruitment, increasing end-expiratory lung volume, and improving oxygenation. The combination of inspiratory pressure (PIP), expiratory pressure (PEEP), I:E ratio, and gas flow rate determines MAP, which represents overall airway pressures averaged over time during the respiratory cycle.

Prolongation of the inspiratory time has been advocated to overcome regional inhomogeneities in oxygenation to improve arterial oxygenation. Increasing inspiratory time when the I:E ratio exceeds 1:1 (e.g., 2:1, 3:1) is termed *inverse ratio ventilation* (IRV). In this scenario, the alveoli are maintained at a higher volume for a greater portion of the respiratory cycle. The theoretical benefits are improved $\dot{V}/\dot{Q}$ ratios in patent alveolar units and more effective alveolar recruitment than the transient increases normally seen with conventional settings. Recruitment of atelectatic alveoli produces two beneficial effects. First, it decreases the intrapulmonary shunt and may allow a reduction in the FIO_2 as more alveoli participate in gas exchange. Second, by reducing the repetitive opening and closing of unstable lung

units, a reduction in the shear forces applied to the parenchyma may minimize ventilator-induced injury.

One problem with IRV is the reduction of expiratory time, so there may be insufficient time for removal of the inspired tidal volume. This causes trapping of gas in the terminal air units, resulting in the phenomenon termed *auto-PEEP*. Some investigators think that auto-PEEP is a necessary component in recruiting unstable alveoli, whereas others propose that it results in regional overdistention with resultant barotrauma and possible pneumothorax. Similarly, the increase in MAP can result in marked elevations in intrathoracic pressure, impaired venous return, and reduced cardiac output, with resultant hemodynamic compromise in an already critically ill patient.

Most experience with IRV in the treatment of severe respiratory failure, as described by Rappaport and associates (1994), is limited to the pressure control mode (PC-IRV). Lessard and coworkers (1994) showed that most studies demonstrate that PIP can be reduced without a reduction in alveolar ventilation; however, no improvement in mortality was demonstrated by switching to PC-IRV. Unfortunately, the majority of patients were initiated on a volume-controlled ventilator algorithm with high PIP and FIO_2 for prolonged periods before the change to PC-IRV. A prospective, randomized trial of PC-IRV on patients with a similar illness severity who are enrolled early enough in the course of treatment is necessary to reveal any potential improvement in survival.

High-Frequency Ventilation

High-frequency ventilation (HFV) involves the delivery of respiratory tidal volumes averaging significantly less than anatomic dead space at a high frequency. Typical tidal volumes are in the range of 1 to 3 mL/kg, with a respiratory rate between 150 and 300 bpm. Compared to conventional ventilation, Arnold and associates (1994) found that PIPs during HFV are less because of the reduced tidal volumes, and, theoretically, a reduction in iatrogenic barotrauma is expected. HFV with maintenance of adequate MAPs for gas exchange without elevated peak pressures has been shown to be beneficial in infants with respiratory distress syndrome (RDS).

High-Frequency Oscillatory Ventilation

High-frequency oscillatory ventilation (HFOV) has shown some promise in the ventilation of patients with inhalation injury. In a baboon model of moderate smoke inhalation injury, Cioffi and associates (1993) showed that the barotrauma index (rate-pressure product) increased significantly during conventional ventilation compared to high-frequency flow interruption ventilation, but both attained adequate ventilation and oxygenation. In the group treated with conventional ventilation, significantly more parenchymal injury was seen than in the high-frequency flow interruption group. Retrospective studies by Cioffi (1993) and Rue (1993) and their coworkers indicate that better ventilation and survival in adults may be attained with high-frequency flow interruption ventilation in comparison to conventional (volume-limited) ventilation. Significant decreases in the incidence of pneumonia and mortality in patients with inhalation injury have been noted when high-frequency percussive ventilation was used rather than conventional ventilation. With this mode of ventilation, subtidal volumes are delivered in a progressive stepwise fashion until a preset oscillatory equilibrium is reached and exhalation is passive. HFOV uses a reciprocating piston, diaphragm, or bellows to generate a sinusoidal respiratory waveform during the breathing cycle. Characteristically, both the inspiratory and expiratory phases are active, with gas driven into and withdrawn from the lungs by the pump stroke. The frequency of oscillation ranges over a wide spectrum (1 to 50 cycles per second), and pumps with variable I:E ratios are available.

Results from randomized studies by the Hi-Fi Study Group (1989) and Clark and associates (1994) using HFOV have demonstrated a decreased incidence of barotrauma and bronchopulmonary dysplasia, as well as a reduction in the number of term infants who actually progress (i.e., deteriorate) to require extracorporeal membrane oxygenation (ECMO) therapy. The use of HFOV allows improved control of Pco_2, especially for management of persistent pulmonary hypertension in the neonate, in which intentional respiratory alkalosis can reverse a right-to-left ductal shunt or persistent fetal circulation. The improvements in oxygenation can be attributed to static inflation (up to 30 cm H_2O) with intermittent increases to assist in alveolar recruitment and reexpansion of atelectatic segments. However, the most conclusive study, the Hi-Fi study (1989), demonstrated that HFOV resulted in a significantly higher incidence of interventricular hemorrhage and other long-term sequelae without clear benefit over controls. This mode of therapy has been used mainly as a last alternative before initiation of ECMO, or as a rescue technique when infants did not respond to either conventional ventilation or an alternative advanced technique. Isolated spectacular responses in individual patients continue to stimulate further investigations of HFOV (Table 39-4).

High-Frequency Jet Ventilation

High-frequency jet ventilation (HFJV) consists of intermittent delivery of gas through a small-bore cannula positioned in the airway that delivers fresh gas in short bursts. A cycling mechanism is used to regulate rate, inspiratory time, and driving pressure. Rates are commonly 100 to 200 bpm, and the expiratory phase of the cycle is entirely passive, dependent on chest wall and lung compliance. The primary use is as a rescue therapy in adults with ARF-related hypoxemia in the face of high PEEP or a significant air leak. The use of smaller tidal volumes with increases in MAP, but not PIP, is purported to help avoid worsening barotrauma. Carlo and coworkers (1989) reported on a group of neonates with severe RDS and showed that HFJV produced a significant reduction in MAP and Pco_2 but no variation in mortality, incidents of air leak, or length of assisted ventilation compared to conventional ventilation. Complications associated with HFJV include the risk of tracheal obstruction and inflammatory tracheal injuries. Successful application has been achieved by Baumgart and associates (1992) in neonates with RDS from meconium aspiration or congenital posterolateral diaphragmatic hernias. Most responders to HFJV show the greatest improvement within the first few hours of treatment (see Table 39-4).

Intratracheal Pulmonary Ventilation

Muller and colleagues (1993) developed intratracheal pulmonary ventilation (ITPV) using a specially designed

Table 39-4. Clinical Trials in High-Frequency Ventilation

Treatment	Author	No. of Patients	Survival
HFOV	Eyal et al. (1984) (HFPPV)	25	72%
	Hi-Fi Study Group (1989)	327	82%
	Cioffi et al. (1989)	8	100%
	Cioffi et al. (1991)	54	81.5%
	Clark et al. (1992)	30	83% (30 days); 77% (to D/C)
	Rosenberg et al. (1993)	12	58%
	Hi-Fi Study Group (1993)	86	79%
	Rue et al. (1993)	61	83.6%
	Gerstmann et al. (1996)	125 (64 HFOV, 61 CV)	70%
	Fort et al. (1997)	17	47% (30 days)
	Rettwitz-Volk et al. (1998)	46	89%
HFJV	Berner et al. (1991)	6	67%
	Smith et al. (1993)	29	69%

CV, control ventilation; D/C, discharge; HFJV, high-frequency jet ventilation; HFOV, high-frequency oscillatory ventilation; HFPPV, high-frequency positive-pressure ventilation.

endotracheal tube with a conventional ventilator, which operates with continuous oxygen flow delivered at the level of the carina. The design is such that the Venturi effect produces efficient CO_2 clearance with a tidal volume that is but a fraction of conventional volumes, thus maintaining a very low airway pressure. The ventilator is used only for the expiratory phase because the ITPV catheter delivers fresh gas. Makhoul and colleagues (1995) has studied the system extensively in animals, and normal levels of CO_2 have been sustained over prolonged periods. Raszynski and associates (1993) reported the case of a girl with sickle cell chest syndrome, who was treated with intratracheal gas insufflation, weaned from ECMO, and ultimately discharged. Measurements of end-expiratory pressures demonstrated no inadvertent PEEP. ITPV remains experimental and must be studied in a clinical trial but holds promise.

Adjunctive Strategies to Mechanical Ventilation

Ventilation in the Prone Position

When ventilating a patient in the supine position, the dependent lung regions are preferentially perfused because of the effects of gravity, the mechanical distention of capillaries, and transudation of fluid in the dependent (or basal) portions of the pulmonary parenchyma. Studies by Pappert (1994) and Lamm (1994) and their colleagues demonstrated a significant improvement in oxygenation and $\dot{V}/\dot{Q}$ inequality during ventilation in the prone position. Mechanisms for this improvement are an increase in FRC, change in diaphragm motion, and redistribution of blood flow to less affected lung regions, which result in increased recruitment of previously atelectatic but uninjured lung units. The gravitational distribution of pleural pressure is much more uniform in the prone position. Ventilating a patient in the prone position presents unique nursing and resuscitative challenges and may not always be well tolerated by a patient with marginal hemodynamics. Clinical studies seem to suggest a benefit from prone ventilation in correcting ARDS-related hypoxemia in some cases (Table 39-5); it remains to be determined if this significantly affects morbidity or mortality.

Surfactant Replacement Therapy

Surfactant is inactivated during ARDS, probably related to a protein leak into the alveolus. Surfactant is known to decrease alveolar surface tension and alveolar edema and exhibits some anticytokine effects. Weg and associates (1994) demonstrated the safety of aerosolized surfactant, but the results of several trials are mixed (see Table 39-5). The use of surfactant in neonates with lung inflammation has reduced both morbidity and mortality. In contrast, Anzueto and coworkers (1996) demonstrated no improvement in 30-day survival, length of stay in the intensive care unit, duration of mechanical ventilation, or physiologic function with surfactant use in sepsis-related ARDS in adults. Routes of administration, natural versus artificial surfactants, and dosing remain controversial. Although there may be some benefit to replacement of surfactant in some patients with ARDS, further studies are warranted.

Inhaled Nitric Oxide

Reflex pulmonary vasoconstriction in response to hypoxemia during ARDS increases intrapulmonary resistance and potentially overloads the right heart in a critically ill patient. Early work with intravenous pulmonary vasodilators was largely unsatisfactory because of the unwanted side effect of systemic hypotension combined with the resultant increase in blood flow to regions in the lung, which were either collapsed or filled with fluid, thereby increasing the $\dot{V}/\dot{Q}$ mis-

Table 39-5. Clinical Trials in Strategies Adjunctive to Mechanical Ventilation

Treatment	Author	No. of Patients	Survival
Prone position ventilation	Walz and Muhr (1992)	16	68.8%
	Pape et al. (1993)	22	Pao_2 to Fio_2 ratio increased from day 0 (140 ± 45) to day 5 (237 ± 40)
	Pappert et al. (1994)	12	67% responders[a]
	Stocker et al. (1997)	25	88%
Surfactant	Perez-Benavides et al. (1995)	7	86.8%
	Pallua et al. (1998)	4	100%
Nitric oxide	Rossaint et al. (1993)	10	80%
	Abman et al. (1994)	10	50%
	Neonatal Inhaled Nitric Oxide Study Group (1997)	114	86% (120 days)
	Dellinger et al. (1998)	120	71%
Partial liquid ventilation	Gauger et al. (1996)	6	100%
	Hirschl et al. (1996)	10	50%
	Leach et al. (1996)	10	80%

[a]Improvement in Pao_2 >10 mm Hg after 30 minutes in prone position.

match and ultimately worsening hypoxia. In the late 1980s, nitric oxide (NO) was reported to be a potent pulmonary-selective vasodilator. This stemmed from work showing that the vascular endothelium played a vital role in the generation of vascular relaxing factors and was responsible for regulation of both arterial and venous smooth muscle tone. When administered via inhalation, NO is distributed to regions of the lung that contain patent alveoli and therefore are able to transfer NO to the bloodstream. By diffusion of NO to the surrounding vasculature, blood flow is increased to areas of the parenchyma that are capable of gas exchange and diverted away from poorly ventilated areas. This manifests as an increase in arterial oxygenation and a reduction in $\dot{V}/\dot{Q}$ mismatch. NO has an affinity for hemoglobin on the order of 1500 times that of carbon monoxide. On combining with hemoglobin, NO is immediately inactivated; therefore, systemic effects are rarely seen.

Some of the most extensive work has been done in the setting of the transitional period of adaptation from fetal and newborn circulation and its relation to persistent pulmonary hypertension. Kinsella and Abman (1995) used NO as a rescue therapy in newborns with severe hypoxia secondary to severe respiratory failure in an attempt to prevent the need for ECMO. NO has also been used to treat the transient, severe pulmonary hypertension seen after lung transplantation. Currently, inhaled NO is part of ongoing studies as an adjunct in the treatment of adult ARDS. Despite transient reductions in peak airway pressures and inspired oxygen levels, NO therapy may or may not have an effect on overall mortality in the ARDS population, who frequently have concomitant illnesses or injuries, each with its own attendant morbidity (see Table 39-5). Dellinger and associates (1996) reported preliminary results of the only randomized, controlled, blinded trial in nonseptic ARDS patients [NO dose: 0, 1.25, 5.0, 20, 40, and 80 parts per million (ppm)]: Different doses showed no difference in outcomes.

Potential toxicities of NO therapy are related to the formation of NO_2 and methemoglobin. Approximately 80 to 90% of inhaled NO is absorbed within the bloodstream and combines to form methemoglobin. The factors affecting the rate of conversion are related primarily to the dose of NO in ppm, hemoglobin level, and oxygen saturation. Doses in the range of 0 to 80 ppm have been investigated, and minimal toxicity from methemoglobinemia has been shown. Also, under conditions of antioxidant depletion, NO can induce free radical formation and subsequent inflammation.

Partial Liquid Ventilation

Perfluorocarbons (PFCs) have unique gas solubility properties and low vapor pressure, relatively high density, and low surface tension. They are biologically inactive, physiologically inert, insoluble in lipids and water, and have limited potential for systemic absorption. PFCs have several proposed modes of action that may affect ARDS, but their significance has yet to be rigorously determined. When instilled into the airway, PFCs distribute primarily to the dependent regions by virtue of their greater density than water. Here, they displace the inflammatory exudate, acting as a lavage, while possibly improving lung compliance via surfactantlike properties. Additionally, PFCs may help to redistribute pulmonary perfusion from the dependent, collapsed alveoli to better-ventilated, nondependent regions. PFCs are bacteriostatic and may also have anti-inflammatory activity. Overbeck and colleagues (1996) demonstrated in animal models of ARDS the efficacy of PFCs in improving gas exchange and pulmonary function. Gas exchange improved with reductions in physiologic shunt and improvements in compliance.

Gauger and colleagues (1996) initiated human studies in pediatric RDS populations, with PFC instillation to the predicted FRC of 30 mL/kg in combination with standard gas ventilation (partial liquid ventilation, or PLV). PLV was able to support gas exchange and allow some improvement in lung compliance. A subsequent trial conducted by Leach and coworkers (1996) in infants with ARF who did not respond to conventional therapy showed that all patients demonstrated some improvement in oxygenation without serious adverse events. Preliminary phase I and II studies in adults with ARDS have also demonstrated safety of PLV; however, the effects on gas exchange and outcome have been inconsistent. Again, isolated spectacular responses in individual patients have been reported. PLV may be a viable alternative for infants with RDS, but the role in pediatric and adult ARDS awaits the results of further investigations (see Table 39-5).

EXTRAPULMONARY GAS EXCHANGE TO PROVIDE LUNG REST

The hypothesis proposed by Kolobow and associates (1977a) that "lung rest" can be accomplished using an artificial lung device with extracorporeal circulation derived from animal experiments using a spiral coil membrane lung designed for CO_2 removal in chronic lung disease. During testing of these carbon dioxide membrane lungs (CDML) in spontaneously breathing animals, Kolobow and coworkers (1977b) noted that spontaneous ventilation decreased proportionally to CO_2 removal by CDML. By removal of 100% of metabolic CO_2 production by CDML, Kolobow and colleagues (1978) showed that the animals apparently could be kept completely apneic while an amount of oxygen equal to the animal's oxygen consumption was provided without ventilation (apneic ventilation). Thus, the normal physiologic reaction to a reduced need for CO_2 removal was a reduction in tidal volume and minute ventilation, resulting in a reduced excretion of CO_2 through the native lung while arterial blood P_{CO_2} remained at the normal level. Furthermore, Kolobow and colleagues (1977b) demonstrated that any increase or decrease in extracorporeal CO_2 within a few seconds was reflected in the animals by an increase or decrease in breathing and, more specifically, an increase or decrease in alveolar ventilation. The use of oxygenator technology to accomplish partial or total gas exchange (O_2 or CO_2, with or without cardiac support) is based on the premise that lung rest facilitates repair and avoids the barotrauma or volume trauma of ventilator management. The basic technique involves a permeable membrane gas exchanger, either extracorporeal or intracorporeal, with or without use of a pump. Large vessel cannulation is typically needed in patients with extracorporeal support. Depending on the design and application of the technology, the circuit orientation can be venovenous, venoarterial, as with ECMO, or arteriovenous, as with arteriovenous CO_2 removal ($AVCO_2R$). Techniques reported by Alpard and associates (1998a) have used percutaneous access to simplify $AVCO_2R$, with significant reductions in ventilator settings. Intracorporeal devices are limited by the surface area of the oxygenator within the vena cava.

Extracorporeal Membrane Oxygenation

ECMO, a modification of cardiopulmonary bypass, decreases the mortality of neonatal RDS and is capable of total gas exchange. According to the Extracorporeal Life Support Registry reported by Bartlett (1997), infants with a predicted mortality of 90% have been treated with ECMO, and a nationwide experience of more than 15,000 patients shows survival greater than 80%. Adult ECMO has also improved survival compared to historic controls; however, one recent study comparing ECMO with conventional support shows no superiority of either technique. Bartlett and colleagues (1976) began clinical trials in 1972 and reported the first successful use of ECMO in newborn respiratory failure in 1976. During the initial experience, ECMO had an overall survival rate of 75 to 95%; these results helped to establish the therapeutic effectiveness of ECMO in infants having a predicted 80 to 100% mortality. The Extracorporeal Life Support Organization database on all adults with severe respiratory failure, as reported by Tracy and colleagues (1995), demonstrates a cumulative short-term survival rate of 47%. Recent appreciation of the neonatal and pediatric populations with ARF has also yielded new therapeutic strategies that may affect the adult population (Table 39-6).

Pierre (1998) and Lessin (1996) and their coworkers have shown that ECMO can also be used as rescue therapy in pediatric burn patients with rapidly progressive ARF. Mortality in pediatric burn patients with pulmonary complications has been reported as high as 84 to 89%. Ombrellaro and associates (1994) reported the first case of a child with thermal injury and ARDS who underwent ECMO for the treatment of respiratory failure. O'Rourke and coworkers (1993) reported the Extracorporeal Life Support Organization experience: The survival rate was 71% in 14 pediatric burn patients with respiratory failure supported by ECMO.

Table 39-6. Recent Clinical Trials in Extracorporeal Membrane Oxygenation

Author	No. of Patients	Survival (%)
Bartlett et al. (1986)	100	72
Ryan and Doody (1992)	5	100
Moler et al. (1993)	220	46
Cornish et al. (1993)	17	88
Ombrellaro et al. (1994)[a]	1	100[b]
Goretsky et al. (1995)[a]	5	60
Green et al. (1996)	38	68.4
Lessin et al. (1996)[a]	2	100
Kolla et al. (1997)	100[c]	54
Pranikoff et al. (1997)	36	50[d]
Pierre et al. (1998)[a]	5	60

[a]Reports focusing on severe respiratory failure after burn injury.
[b]First reported survival of pediatric patient with thermal injury and adult respiratory distress syndrome (ARDS) using extracorporeal membrane oxygenation.
[c]A mortality rate of 50% was associated with >5 days mechanical ventilation.
[d]Forty-five patients with ARDS had a 51% survival rate.

Extracorporeal Carbon Dioxide Removal

Gattinoni (1986) introduced the use of extracorporeal carbon dioxide removal ($ECCO_2R$) in both animals and humans, in which the focus was CO_2 extraction to facilitate a reduction in ventilatory support. Carbon dioxide removal is facilitated via extracorporeal circulation through the membrane lung while oxygenation is maintained by simple diffusion across patent alveoli. Kolobow and colleagues (1978) demonstrated the validity of this *apneic oxygenation*. O_2 was supplied via constant flow to alveoli maintained with PEEP, and no deterioration in oxygenation was observed. Gattinoni and associates (1978, 1986) demonstrated a decrease in mortality in patients managed with $ECCO_2R$ and low-frequency, pressure-limited ventilation, using ECMO survival reported by Zapol and coworkers (1979) as the historic control. This improvement in survival has been duplicated at various centers using ECMO criteria as historic controls, with an overall rate of 46%. Morris and colleagues (1994), however, compared conventional ventilation ("old therapy") with pressure-controlled IRV with or without $ECCO_2R$ ("new therapy") in 40 ARDS patients. No significant difference in survival was found between the two groups, who had rates of 42% (old therapy) and 33% (new therapy) and an overall rate of 38%. Of note, the majority of patients were hypercapnic on randomization, and although mean peak airway pressures were significantly lower in the new therapy group, they remained elevated (57.8 vs. 49.5 cm H_2O). Lewandowski and associates (1992) reported on the management of 38 patients with severe ARDS, using an integrated approach that included permissive hypercapnia, pressure-controlled ventilation, frequent body position changes, and inhaled NO in 7 patients. Eighteen patients were treated with $ECCO_2R$, with bypass used initially, if they fulfilled fast ECMO criteria, or subsequently, if they worsened on the standard therapy. The overall survival rate was 84 to 100% in the patients who did not require $ECCO_2R$ and 66% in the $ECCO_2R$ group.

Intracorporeal Gas Exchange

Mortensen (1987) and Mortensen and Berry (1989) pioneered the concept of intra–vena caval oxygenation (IVOX) and CO_2 removal. IVOX is a miniature membrane lung that consists of multiple hollow fibers placed in the vena cava to oxygenate blood and remove CO_2 without the need for extracorporeal circulation or blood transfusion (Table 39-7). Cox and colleagues (1991) and one of us (J.B.Z.) and Cox (1991) showed that the amount of CO_2 removal represented approximately 30% of the CO_2 production of an adult sheep (150 to 180 mL/min). Later clinical studies (Zwischenberger and colleagues, 1992; Cox and colleagues, 1993) demonstrated 40 to 70 mL/min O_2 and CO_2 exchange (approximately 25 to 30% of metabolic demand). Conrad and coworkers (1994) found that use of IVOX allowed some reduction in ventilator settings: FIO_2, PEEP, mean or peak airway pressure, and minute ventilation were decreased by more than 10% in more than 60% of patients and by more than 25% in more than 40% of patients.

IVOX is a membrane oxygenator whose CO_2 removal capacity depends on the transmembrane PCO_2 gradient. With permissive hypercapnia and intentional gradual increase in blood PCO_2 levels, the CO_2 pressure gradient across the IVOX membrane can be increased and thus CO_2 removal can be enhanced. In addition, application of IVOX with permissive hypercapnia allowed a further reduction in ventilatory settings that could help minimize barotrauma inflicted with conventional ventilatory treatment. The clinical results of one of us (J.B.Z.) and colleagues (1994) show that as arterial PCO_2 is allowed to increase into the 60- to 80-mm Hg range, IVOX efficiency can as much as double to further reduce the required ventilator support. Tao and coworkers (1995) noted that permissive hypercapnia and active blood mixing are also effective strategies to reduce surface area requirements. Federspiel and associates (1997) at the University of Pittsburgh used these concepts in the design of other intracorporeal devices, such as the intravenous membrane oxygenator.

Arteriovenous Carbon Dioxide Removal

$AVCO_2R$ was developed as a simplified form of ECMO. The use of a simple arteriovenous shunt eliminates a substantial portion of tubing and ECMO-related components, reducing the foreign surface area, priming fluid, and blood transfusion volume. During $AVCO_2R$, CO_2 removal and O_2 transfer are uncoupled. As Kolobow and colleagues (1978) found, CO_2 is secreted through the membrane gas exchanger, whereas O_2 diffuses through the native lungs (apneic oxygenation).

Brunston and coworkers (1997) determined that long-term, high-flow $AVCO_2R$ can be tolerated by adult sheep with severe respiratory failure without sequelae. To evaluate the effect of $AVCO_2R$ on ventilator support requirements during ARDS, Tao and associates (1997) produced smoke inhalation injury in adult sheep followed by mechanical ventilation to maintain normal blood gases. The sheep were treated with full-flow $AVCO_2R$ 24 hours later. Minute ventilation was reduced from 10.3 ± 1.4 L/min at baseline to 0.5 ± 0.0 L/min at 6 hours on $AVCO_2R$, while maintaining normocapnia. Similarly, PIP decreased from 40.8 cm H_2O to 19.7 ± 7.5 cm H_2O. PaO_2 was maintained above 100 mm Hg at maximally reduced ventilator support. These data indicate that extracorporeal CO_2 removal using a low-resistance gas exchanger in an arteriovenous shunt proves to be a simple and effective treatment to avoid ventilator-induced barotrauma during severe respiratory failure. Brunston (1996) and Alpard (1998b) and their colleagues applied percutaneous $AVCO_2R$ in a recently developed model of smoke inhalation and 40% total body surface area burn injury. All animals met clinical entry criteria for ARDS within 48 hours. Percutaneous $AVCO_2R$ allowed significant reductions in minute ventilation (13 to 6 L/min), tidal volume (450 to 270 mL per breath), PIP (25 to 14 cm H_2O), respiratory rate (25 to 16 bpm), and FIO_2 (0.86 to 0.34) while normocapnia was maintained. Initial clinical trials using

Table 39-7. Clinical Trials on Intra- and Extracorporeal Gas Exchange

Treatment	Author	No. of Patients	Survival (%)
Extracorporeal CO_2 removal	Gattinoni et al. (1986)	43	48.8
	Wagner et al. (1990)	76	50
	Brunet et al. (1993)	23	50
	Cornish et al. (1993)	17	88
	Green et al. (1996)	38	68.4
Intravenous oxygenation	High et al. (1992)	5	20
	Jurmann et al. (1992)	3	33
	Gentilello et al. (1993)	8	20
	Conrad et al. (1994)	160	60[a]

[a]Mechanical support 25% in 50% of patients.

AVco$_2$R for respiratory failure have demonstrated safety and feasibility of the technique.

WEANING AND EXTUBATION

Weaning after Respiratory Failure

Most patients requiring mechanical assistance for respiratory failure present a different challenge from ARDS: Varying degrees of continued parenchymal disease, increased bronchial reactivity, respiratory muscle debility, and cardiovascular compromise demand a cautious approach to weaning. The initial problem is to identify that weaning is possible; this is usually signaled by an FIO$_2$ less than 50%, PEEP less than or equal to 7 cm H$_2$O, and a clearing of infiltrates on chest radiography. Further support for the initiation of the weaning effort can be obtained in the conscious patient by the ability to generate a forced VC of at least 7 mL/kg body weight and a minimal negative inspiratory force of 15 cm H$_2$O. Of the several methods of weaning, the focus of this section is on the classic method, intermittent mandatory ventilation (IMV), and pressure support.

Although weaning via an open airway (T piece method) has often been quoted as a variant of a classic wean, it possesses no distinct advantage. On the contrary, potential disadvantages are that the removal of end-expiratory pressure eventually results in a progressive fall in FRC and the increased probability of $\dot{V}/\dot{Q}$ mismatching. Annest (1980) and Quan (1981) and their colleagues showed that this leads to increased work of breathing.

The CPAP, or classic, method places the entire responsibility for ventilation on the patient. It provides for intermittent stresses with periods of complete rest at levels of assisted ventilation. Theoretically, this maximal stress followed by rest should provide beneficial respiratory muscle exercise. When using the classic technique, it is important to recognize that patients initially tolerate CPAP for only a short time. Extending the interval should proceed slowly: Patients should not be stressed to the point of impending failure. Cohen and associates (1982) described the clinical signs of respiratory muscle fatigue. Increased respiratory rate is followed by an alteration between rib cage and abdominal breathing, which they termed *respiratory alternans* (paradoxic abdominal and chest wall motion), and, finally, decreased Pao$_2$ accompanied by a fall in minute ventilation and hypercarbia. Electromyographic recordings from their patients revealed high- and low-frequency discharges from the intercostal muscles. A fall in the ratio of high- to low-frequency power indicated fatiguing muscle and preceded the clinical signs of failure. Clinically, a simple guide to a patient's tolerance of the weaning process can be obtained by measuring VC and negative inspiratory force at the beginning and end of the CPAP wean. The wean period should not be extended unless the beginning and ending values are comparable.

During the IMV technique, a patient must work constantly and may fail the weaning process if he or she is not able to sustain the effort. As noted, failure occurs when fatigue results in diminishing tidal volumes, which in turn reduces FRC. Gas exchange becomes increasingly impaired. In addition, the ventilator may itself impose an increased burden on the work of breathing. Marini and associates (1986) demonstrated higher workloads during patient-triggered ventilatory breaths than during spontaneous breathing. Part of the explanation for this phenomenon lies in the resistance threshold in the ventilator itself. The resistance within the internal circuitry of respirators varies greatly. For this reason, when using CPAP, it is wise to use external circuits.

PSV and the use of pressure support during weaning has become popular. During weaning, the amount of pressure support is gradually decreased until it is eliminated or until 10 cm H$_2$O has been achieved. It is a well-tolerated form of weaning. As with the classic method, however, adequate rest with maximal pressure support is a prerequisite between weaning intervals.

The Spanish weaning trials have tried to make some sense out of the controversy. Esteban and colleagues (1997) cooperated in a multicenter trial. Patients were randomly assigned to undergo a 2-hour trial of spontaneous breathing in one of two ways: with a T-tube system or with PSV of 7 cm H$_2$O. If a patient had signs of poor tolerance at any time during the trial, mechanical ventilation was reinstituted. Patients without these features at the end of the trial were extubated. Of the 246 patients assigned to the T-tube group, 192 successfully completed the trial and were extubated; 36 of them required reintubation. Of the 238 patients in the group receiving PSV, 205 were extubated and 38 of them required reintubation. The percentage of patients who remained extubated after 48 hours was not different between the two groups (63% T tube, 70% PSV; $P = .14$). The percentage of patients failing the trial was significantly higher when the T tube was used (22% vs. 14%; $P = .03$). Esteban and colleagues (1995) also performed another trial with slightly different results: 130 patients had respiratory distress during a 2-hour trial of spontaneous breathing. These patients were randomly assigned to undergo one of four weaning techniques:

1) IMV, in which the ventilator rate was initially set at a mean ± SD of 10.0 ± 2.2 bpm and then decreased, if possible, at least twice a day, usually by 2 to 4 bpm (29 patients)
2) PSV, in which pressure support was initially set at 18.0 ± 6.1 cm H$_2$O and then reduced, if possible, by 2 to 4 cm H$_2$O at least twice a day (37 patients)
3) Intermittent trials of spontaneous breathing, conducted two or more times a day if possible (33 patients)
4) Once-daily trail of spontaneous breathing (31 patients)

Standardized protocols were followed for each technique. The median duration of weaning was 5 days for IMV. Weaning lasted 4 days for the PSV group, 3 days for intermittent—

multiple—trials of spontaneous breathing, and 3 days for a once daily trial of spontaneous breathing. After adjustment for other covariates, the rate of successful weaning was higher with a once-daily trial of spontaneous breathing than with IMV (rate ratio, 2.83; 95% confidence interval, 1.36 to 5.89; $P < .006$) or PSV. There was no significant difference in the rate of success between once-daily trials and multiple trials of spontaneous breathing.

Nutrition

To wean successfully, a patient must be able to assume an ever-increasing workload of breathing as assisted ventilation is reduced. Significantly, the work of breathing must be efficient and coordinated or else fatigue develops and reintubation is required. As Roussos (1985) pointed out, respiratory muscles normally are continuously active, and when put to rest, they atrophy quickly. These muscles must be rebuilt during weaning. For this reason, adequate nutritional support is crucial to supply protein for muscle development. If necessary, total parenteral nutrition should be instituted to provide sufficient calories.

Most thoracic surgical patients can tolerate enteral feeds within 24 to 48 hours, so protein depletion is not usually a problem. Esophagectomy patients often have a jejunostomy feeding tube placed intraoperatively, and alimentation can begin. Total parenteral nutrition, however, should be instituted within 48 hours if attempts at enteral feeding fail. Nutrition requirements must be actively determined, as Dark and coworkers (1985) showed. Otherwise, increased carbohydrate calories lead to increased carbon dioxide production, which can precipitate hypercapnic respiratory failure. Unless the patient is severely catabolic, 2000 to 2500 calories are given, 50% in the form of lipids. In addition, 1 g of protein per kg body weight per day should be supplied. Requirements in septic patients may be 30 to 50% higher. Fluid balance may be a problem in the thoracic surgical patient and in those with renal insufficiency. For these patients, monitoring of daily weight is a sensitive measurement of fluid accumulation, allowing judicious use of diuretics or dialysis to maintain fluid balance. Hypophosphatemia is a well-described cause of respiratory muscle fatigue that should be corrected.

Decision to Extubate

Patients are ready for extubation when the criteria outlined in Table 39-8 are met and the patients are maintaining acceptable gas levels. Additionally, patients should be normotensive and should not have demonstrated dysrhythmia or tachycardia during the final weaning stages. Morganroth and colleagues (1984) quantitated these factors into ventilator and adverse factor scores. Not achieving the aforementioned criteria predicted an unsuccessful wean in their long-term ventilated patients. These criteria are conservative

Table 39-8. Criteria for Extubation

F_{IO_2}	<50%
CPAP/PEEP	<7.5 cm H_2O
Respiratory rate	8–25 breaths/min
Rapid shallow breathing index	<80 breaths/min
Vital capacity	10–15 mL/kg
Negative inspiratory force	>20 cm H_2O

CPAP, continuous positive airway pressure; PEEP, positive end-expiratory pressure.

and, as DeHaven and associates (1985) pointed out, may underestimate the ability of some patients to tolerate extubation. DeHaven and colleagues advocated extubation only for patients with an intrapulmonary shunt of less than 15% or PaO_2 to F_{IO_2} ratios greater than 300 with room air. Using these measures, 94% of patients were extubated successfully, even though 48% did not meet the traditional standards. Many patients in this study, however, had not undergone prolonged ventilation. In the final analysis, the ability of the patient to sustain adequate ventilation and oxygenation with spontaneous ventilation over a fixed period warrants a trial of extubation. No technique is fail-safe, however, nor does any system assess the ability to clear secretions after removal of an endotracheal tube. Nonetheless, trials of extubation are appropriate when patients can maintain their own support over several hours and reintubation is not known to be difficult.

Technique of Extubation

Before extubation, it is imperative to ensure that the patient can protect the airway (gag reflex and cough) and that significant upper airway obstruction, especially glottic edema, is not present. To ensure that the airway is adequate, the cuff of the endotracheal tube is deflated and the patient is instructed to inspire. The endotracheal tube is then occluded while the patient forcibly exhales. If the patient can exhale around the tube, glottic and subglottic edema are not critical. In the absence of such a leak, the glottis and the upper airway should be examined using a flexible bronchoscope inserted transnasally. The ability to pass the bronchoscope between the vocal cords anteriorly suggests that extubation may be attempted with caution. Postextubation stridor attributed to residual glottic edema usually responds to a helium-oxygen mixture (30% oxygen, 70% helium) and racemic epinephrine therapy. Failure to insert the bronchoscope between the vocal cords and the tube should delay extubation for 24 to 48 hours so that edema might clear.

Tracheostomy

The timing of tracheostomy remains controversial. In many centers, endotracheal intubation—particularly transnasal—is allowed to continue indefinitely. In North America, tracheostomy is traditionally undertaken after 2 weeks. Little evidence supports this arbitrary time period, although a study by Stauffer and colleagues (1981) indicated a higher incidence of tracheal stenosis and laryngotracheal ulceration in patients undergoing tracheostomy more than 14 days after endotracheal intubation. The corollary was that no advantage was found to suggest that tracheostomy was better than prolonged endotracheal intubation. Of the many reasons given for performing tracheostomies, such as difficulty in suctioning, patient discomfort, laryngotracheal lesions, oral hygiene, and glottic edema, only the last two justify this approach. Stauffer and colleagues (1981) clearly showed that difficulty in suctioning and patient discomfort were minor problems and that tracheostomy may have a higher incidence of laryngotracheal complications. Difficulty in maintaining oral hygiene is a common occurrence, however, and leads to oropharyngeal infections, sialadenitis, and mucosal ulceration. As mentioned previously, extubation is contraindicated in the presence of glottic edema, and tracheostomy maintains the airway and allows the edema to resolve. For these reasons, tracheostomy should be considered for patients intubated for 10 to 14 days and in whom it is expected that mechanical ventilatory support will be required for some time. It should be undertaken earlier when endotracheal reintubation is indicated because secretions cannot be cleared.

Percutaneous tracheostomy at the bedside has recently gained acceptance. Hazard and colleagues (1991) have demonstrated that the technique can be performed effectively and safely. It does, however, require the ability to use a flexible bronchoscope.

REFERENCES

Abman SH, et al: Acute effects of inhaled nitric oxide in children with severe hypoxemic respiratory failure. J Pediatr 124:881, 1994.

Alpard SK, et al: Severe respiratory failure secondary to smoke inhalation and cutaneous flame burn injury: initial experience with percutaneous arteriovenous CO_2 removal. J Burn Care Rehabil 19:S193, 1998a.

Alpard SK, et al: Dose dependent development of severe respiratory failure in an ovine model of smoke inhalation and cutaneous flame burn injury. Crit Care Med 26:A111, 1998b.

Amato MBP, et al: Effect of a protective-ventilation strategy on mortality in the acute respiratory distress syndrome. N Engl J Med 338:347, 1998.

Annest SJ, et al: Detrimental effects of removing end-expiratory pressure prior to extubation. Ann Surg 191:539, 1980.

Anonymous: Randomized study of high-frequency oscillatory ventilation in infants with severe respiratory distress syndrome. Hi-Fi Study Group. J Pediatr 122:609, 1993.

Anzueto A, et al: Aerosolized surfactant in adults with sepsis-induced acute respiratory distress syndrome. Exosurf Acute Respiratory Distress Syndrome Sepsis Study Group. N Engl J Med 334:1417, 1996.

Arnold JH, et al: Prospective, randomized comparison of high-frequency oscillatory ventilation and conventional mechanical ventilation in pediatric respiratory failure. Crit Care Med 22:1530, 1994.

Bartlett RH, et al: Extracorporeal membrane oxygenation (ECMO) cardiopulmonary support in infancy. Trans Am Soc Artif Intern Organs 22:80, 1976.

Bartlett RH, et al: Extracorporeal membrane oxygenation (ECMO) in neonatal respiratory failure. 100 cases. Ann Surg 204:236, 1986.

Bartlett RH: Extracorporeal life support registry report 1995. ASAIO J 43:104, 1997.

Baumgart S, et al: Diagnosis-related criteria in the consideration of extracorporeal membrane oxygenation in neonates previously treated with high-frequency jet ventilation. Pediatrics 89:491, 1992.

Berner ME, Rouge JC, Suter PM: Combined high-frequency ventilation in children with severe adult respiratory distress syndrome. Intensive Care Med 17:209, 1991.

Bidani A, et al: Permissive hypercapnia in acute respiratory failure. JAMA 272:957, 1994.

Brunet F, et al: Extracorporeal carbon dioxide removal and low-frequency positive-pressure ventilation. Improvement in arterial oxygenation with reduction of risk of pulmonary barotrauma in patients with adult respiratory distress syndrome. Chest 104:889, 1993.

Brunston RL Jr, et al: Determination of low blood flow limits for arteriovenous carbon dioxide removal (AVCO$_2$R). ASAIO J 42:M845, 1996.

Brunston RL Jr, et al: Prolonged hemodynamic stability during arteriovenous carbon dioxide removal (AVCO$_2$R) for severe respiratory failure. J Thorac Cardiovasc Surg 114:1107, 1997.

Cardenas VJ Jr, et al: Correction of blood pH attenuates changes in hemodynamics and organ blood flow during permissive hypercapnia. Crit Care Med 24:827, 1996.

Carlo WA, et al: High-frequency jet ventilation in neonatal pulmonary hypertension. Am J Dis Child 143:233, 1989.

Churchill ED, McNeil D: The reduction in vital capacity following operation. Surg Gynecol Obstet 44:483, 1927.

Cioffi WG Jr, et al: High-frequency percussive ventilation in patients with inhalation injury. J Trauma 29:350, 1989.

Cioffi WG Jr, et al: Prophylactic use of high-frequency percussive ventilation in patients with inhalation injury. Ann Surg 213:575, 1991.

Cioffi WG, et al: Decreased pulmonary damage in primates with inhalation injury treated with high-frequency ventilation. Ann Surg 218:328, 1993.

Clark RH, et al: Prospective randomized comparison of high-frequency oscillatory and conventional ventilation in respiratory distress syndrome. Pediatrics 89:5, 1992.

Clark RH, Yoder BA, Sell MS: Prospective, randomized comparison of high-frequency oscillation and conventional ventilation in candidates for extracorporeal membrane oxygenation. J Pediatr 124:447, 1994.

Cohen CA, et al: Clinical manifestations of inspiratory muscle fatigue. Am J Med 73:308, 1982.

Conrad SA, et al: Major findings from the clinical trials of the intravascular oxygenator. Artif Organs 18:846, 1994.

Cornish JD, et al: Efficacy of venovenous extracorporeal membrane oxygenation for neonates with respiratory and circulatory compromise. J Pediatr 122:105, 1993.

Cox CS Jr, et al: Use of an intravascular oxygenator/carbon dioxide removal device in an ovine smoke inhalation injury model. ASAIO Trans 37:M411, 1991.

Cox CS Jr, et al: Intracorporeal CO_2 removal and permissive hypercapnia to reduce airway pressure in acute respiratory failure. The theoretical basis for permissive hypercapnia with IVOX. ASAIO J 39:97, 1993.

Dark DS, Pingleton SK, Kerby GR: Hypercapnia during weaning. A complication of nutritional support. Chest 88:141, 1985.

DeHaven CB, Hurst JM, Branson RD: Postextubation hypoxemia treated with a continuous positive airway pressure mask. Crit Care Med 13:46, 1985.

Dellinger RP, et al: Inhaled nitric oxide in ARDS: preliminary results of a multicenter clinical trial. Crit Care Med 24:A29, 1996.

Dellinger RP, et al: Effects of inhaled nitric oxide in patients with acute respiratory distress syndrome: results of a randomized phase II trial. Inhaled nitric oxide in ARDS study group. Crit Care Med 26:15, 1998.

Downs JB, et al: Intermittent mandatory ventilation: a new approach to weaning patients. Chest 64:331, 1973.

Esteban A, et al: A comparison of four methods of weaning patients from mechanical ventilation. Spanish Lung Failure Collaborative Group. N Engl J Med 332:345, 1995.

Esteban A, et al: Extubation outcome after spontaneous breathing trials with T-tube or pressure support ventilation. The Spanish Lung Failure Collaborative Group. Am J Respir Crit Care Med 56:459, 1997.

Eyal FG, et al: High-frequency positive-pressure ventilation in neonates. Crit Care Med 12:793, 1984.

Federspiel WJ, et al: Development of a low flow resistance intravenous oxygenators. ASAIO J *43*:M725, 1997.

Fort P, et al: High-frequency oscillatory ventilation for adult respiratory distress syndrome—a pilot study. Crit Care Med 25:937, 1997.

Gattinoni L, et al: Low-frequency positive pressure ventilation with extracorporeal carbon dioxide removal (LFPPVECCO$_2$R): an experimental study. Anesth Analg 57:470, 1978.

Gattinoni L, et al: Low-frequency positive-pressure ventilation with extracorporeal CO_2 removal in severe acute respiratory failure. JAMA 256:881, 1986.

Gattinoni L, et al: Pressure-volume curve of total respiratory system in acute respiratory failure. Computed tomographic scan study. Am Rev Respir Dis *136*:730, 1987.

Gauger PG, et al: Initial experience with partial liquid ventilation in pediatric patients with the acute respiratory distress syndrome. Crit Care Med 24:16, 1996.

Gentilello LM, et al: The intravascular oxygenator (IVOX): preliminary results of a new means of performing extrapulmonary gas exchange. J Trauma 35:399, 1993.

Gerstmann DR, et al: The Provo multicenter early high-frequency oscillatory ventilation trial: improved pulmonary and clinical outcome in respiratory distress syndrome. Pediatrics 98:1044, 1996.

Goretsky MJ, et al: The use of extracorporeal life support in pediatric burn patients with respiratory failure. J Pediatr Surg 30:620, 1995.

Green TP, et al: The impact of extracorporeal membrane oxygenation on survival in pediatric patients with acute respiratory failure. Pediatric Critical Care Study Group. Crit Care Med 24:323, 1996.

Hazard P, Jones C, Benitone J: Comparative clinical trial of standard operative tracheostomy with percutaneous tracheostomy. Crit Care Med 19:1018, 1991.

Hickling KG. Ventilatory management of ARDS: can it affect the outcome? Intensive Care Med 16:219, 1990.

Hickling KG, Henderson SJ, Jackson R: Low mortality associated with low volume pressure limited ventilation with permissive hypercapnia in severe adult respiratory distress syndrome. Intensive Care Med 16:372, 1990.

Hickling KG, et al: Low mortality rate in adult respiratory distress syndrome using low-volume, pressure-limited ventilation with permissive hypercapnia: a prospective study. Crit Care Med 22:1568, 1994.

Hi-Fi Study Group: High-frequency oscillatory ventilation compared with conventional mechanical ventilation in the treatment of respiratory failure in preterm infants. N Engl J Med 88:320, 1989.

High KM, et al: Clinical trials of an intravenous oxygenator in patients with adult respiratory distress syndrome. Anesthesiology 77:856, 1992.

Hillberg RE, Johnson DC: Noninvasive ventilation. New Engl J Med *337*:1746, 1997.

Hirschl RB, et al: Initial experience with partial liquid ventilation in adult patients with the acute respiratory distress syndrome. JAMA 275:383, 1996.

Jurmann MJ, et al: Intravascular oxygenation for advanced respiratory failure. ASAIO J 38:120, 1992.

Kacmarek RM, Vengas J: Mechanical ventilatory rates and tidal volumes. Respir Care 32:466, 1987.

Kinsella JP, Abman SH: Recent developments in the pathophysiology and treatment of persistent pulmonary hypertension of the newborn. J Pediatr *126*:853, 1995.

Kolla S, et al: Extracorporeal life support for 100 adult patients with severe respiratory failure. Ann Surg 226:544, 1997.

Kolobow T, et al: The carbon dioxide membrane lung (CDML): a new concept. Trans Am Soc Artif Intern Organs 23:17, 1977a.

Kolobow T, et al: Control of breathing using an extracorporeal membrane lung. Anesthesiology 46:138, 1977b.

Kolobow T, et al: An alternative to breathing. J Thorac Cardiovasc Surg 75:261, 1978.

Kolobow T, et al: Severe impairment in lung function induced by high peak airway pressure during mechanical ventilation. An experimental study. Am Rev Respir Dis *135*:312, 1987.

Lamm WJ, Graham MM, Albert RK: Mechanism by which the prone position improves oxygenation in acute lung injury. Am J Respir Crit Care Med *150*:184, 1994.

Latimer RG, et al: Ventilatory patterns and pulmonary complications after upper abdominal surgery determined by preoperative and postoperative computerized spirometry and blood gas analysis. Am J Surg *122*:622, 1971.

Leach CL, et al: Partial liquid ventilation with perflubron in premature infants with severe respiratory distress syndrome. The LiquiVent Study Group. N Engl J Med 335:761, 1996.

Lessard MR, et al: Effects of pressure-controlled with different I:E ratios versus volume-controlled ventilation on respiratory mechanics, gas exchange, and hemodynamics in patients with adult respiratory distress syndrome. Anesthesiology 80:983, 1994.

Lessin MS, et al: Extracorporeal membrane oxygenation in pediatric respiratory failure secondary to smoke inhalation injury. J Pediatr Surg 31:1285, 1996.

Lewandowski K, Slama K, Falke K: Approaches to improve survival in severe ARDS. In Vincent JL (ed): Update of Intensive Care and Emergency Medicine. Berlin: Springer-Verlag, 1992, pp. 372–383.

Makhoul IR, et al: Intratracheal pulmonary ventilation versus conventional mechanical ventilation in a rabbit model of surfactant deficiency. Pediatr Res 38:878, 1995.

Marini JJ: New approaches to the ventilatory management of the adult respiratory distress syndrome. J Crit Care 87:256, 1992.

Marini JJ, Capps JS, Culver BH: The inspiratory work of breathing during assisted mechanical ventilation. Chest 87:612, 1985.

Marini JJ, Rodriguez RM, Lamb V: The inspiratory workload of patient initiated mechanical ventilation. Am Rev Respir Dis *134*:902, 1986.

Moler FW, Palmisano J, Custer JR: Extracorporeal life support for pediatric respiratory failure: predictors of survival from 220 patients. Crit Care Med *21*:1604, 1993.

Morganroth MJ, et al: Criteria for weaning from prolonged mechanical ventilation. Arch Intern Med *144*:1012, 1984.

Morris AH, et al: Randomized clinical trial of pressure-controlled inverse ratio ventilation and extracorporeal CO_2 removal for adult respiratory distress syndrome. Am J Respir Crit Care Med *149*:295, 1994.

Mortensen JD: An intravenacaval blood gas exchange (IVCBGE) device. A preliminary report. ASAIO Trans 33:570, 1987.

Mortensen JD, Berry G: Conceptual and design features of a practical, clinically effective intravenous mechanical blood oxygen/carbon dioxide exchange device (IVOX). Int J Artif Organs *12*:384, 1989.

Muller EE, et al: How to ventilate lungs as small as 12.5% of normal: the new technique of intratracheal pulmonary ventilation. Pediatr Res *34*:606, 1993.

Neonatal Inhaled Nitric Oxide Study Group: Inhaled nitric oxide in full-term and nearly full-term infants with hypoxic respiratory failure. N Engl J Med 336:597, 1997.

Ombrellaro M, et al: Extracorporeal life support for the treatment of adult respiratory distress syndrome after burn injury. Surgery 115:523, 1994.

O'Rourke PP, et al: Extracorporeal membrane oxygenation: support for overwhelming pulmonary failure in the pediatric population. Collective experience from the extracorporeal life support organization. J Pediatr Surg 28:523, 1993.

Overbeck MC, et al: Efficacy of perfluorocarbon partial liquid ventilation in a large animal model of acute respiratory failure. Crit Care Med 24:1208, 1996.

Pallua N, et al: Intrabronchial surfactant application in cases of inhalation injury: first results from patients with severe burns and ARDS. Burns 24:197, 1998.

Pape HC, et al: Effect of continuous change in axial position in treatment of posttraumatic lung failure (ARDS). A clinical study. Unfallchirurgie 19:329, 1993.

Pappert D, et al: Influence of positioning on ventilation-perfusion relationships in severe adult respiratory distress syndrome. Chest *106*:1511, 1994.

Pepe PE, Marini JJ: Occult positive pressure in mechanically ventilated patients with airflow obstruction. Am Rev Respir Dis *126*:166, 1982.

Perez-Benavides F, Riff E, Franks C: Adult respiratory distress syndrome and artificial surfactant replacement in the pediatric patient. Pediatr Emerg Care *11*:153, 1995.

Pierre EJ, et al: Extracorporeal membrane oxygenation in the treatment of respiratory failure in pediatric patients with burns. J Burn Care Rehabil *19*:131, 1998.

Pranikoff T, et al: Mortality is directly related to the duration of mechanical ventilation before the initiation of extracorporeal life support for severe respiratory failure. Crit Care Med 25:28, 1997.

Prys-Roberts C, et al: Radiographically undetectable pulmonary collapse in the supine position. Lancet 2:399, 1967.

Quan SF, Falltrick RT, Schlobohm RM: Extubation from ambient or expiratory positive airway pressure in adults. Anesthesiology 55:53, 1981.

Rappaport SH, et al: Randomized, prospective trial of pressure-limited versus volume-controlled ventilation in severe respiratory failure. Crit Care Med 22:22, 1994.

Raszynski A, et al: Rescue from pediatric ECMO with prolonged hybrid intratracheal pulmonary ventilation. A technique for reducing dead space ventilation and preventing ventilator induced lung injury. ASAIO J 39:M681, 1993.

Rettwitz-Volk W, et al: A prospective, randomized, multicenter trial of high-frequency oscillatory ventilation compared with conventional ventilation in preterm infants with respiratory distress syndrome receiving surfactant. J Pediatr 132:249, 1998.

Rosenberg RB, et al: High-frequency ventilation for acute pediatric respiratory failure. Chest 104:1216, 1993.

Rossaint R, et al: Inhaled nitric oxide for the adult respiratory distress syndrome. N Engl J Med 328:399, 1993.

Roussos C: Function and fatigue of respiratory muscles. Chest 88:142S, 1985.

Rue LW, et al: Improved survival of burned patients with inhalation injury. Arch Surg 128:772, 1993.

Ryan DP, Doody DP: Treatment of acute pulmonary failure with extracorporeal support: 100% survival in a pediatric population. J Pediatr Surg 27:1111, 1992.

Sahn SA, Lakshminarayan S: Bedside criteria for discontinuation of mechanical ventilation. Chest 63:1002, 1973.

Shapiro BA, Harrison RA, Walton JR: Clinical Application of Blood Gases. 2nd Ed. Chicago: Year Book, 1977.

Siesjo BK, Folbergrova J, MacMillan V: The effect of hypercapnia upon intracellular pH in the brain, evaluated by the bicarbonate-carbonic acid method and from the creatine phosphokinase equilibrium. J Neurochem 19:2483, 1972.

Slutsky AS: Mechanical ventilation. American College of Chest Physicians' Consensus Conference [published erratum appears in Chest 106:656, 1994]. Chest 104:1833, 1993.

Smith DW, et al: High-frequency jet ventilation in children with the adult respiratory distress syndrome complicated by pulmonary barotrauma. Pediatr Pulmonol 15:279, 1993.

Stauffer JL, Olson DE, Petty TL: Complications and consequences of endotracheal intubation and tracheostomy: a prospective study of 150 critically ill adult patients. Am J Med 70:65, 1981.

Stewart TE, et al: Evaluation of a ventilation strategy to prevent barotrauma in patients at high risk for acute respiratory distress syndrome. Pressure and Volume-Limited Ventilation Strategy Group. N Engl J Med 338:355, 1998.

Stocker R, et al: Prone positioning and low-volume pressure-limited ventilation improve survival in patients with severe ARDS. Chest 111:1008, 1997.

Stroller JK, Kacmarek RM: Ventilatory strategies in the management of the adult respiratory distress syndrome. Clin Chest Med 11:755, 1990.

Suter PM, Fairley HB, Isenberg MD: Optimum end-expiratory airway pressure in patients with acute respiratory failure. N Engl J Med 292:284, 1975.

Tahvanainen J, Salmenpera M, Nikki P: Extubation criteria after weaning from IMV and CPAP. Crit Care Med 11:702, 1983.

Tao W, et al: Strategies to reduce surface area requirements for carbon dioxide removal for an intravenacaval gas exchange device. ASAIO J 41:M567, 1995.

Tao W, et al: Significant reduction in minute ventilation and peak inspiratory pressures with arteriovenous carbon dioxide removal during severe respiratory failure. Crit Care Med 25:689, 1997.

Tracy TF Jr, Delosh T, Stolar CJH: The registry of the Extracorporeal Life Support Organization. In Zwischenberger JB, Bartlett RH (eds): ECMO. Extracorporeal Cardiopulmonary Support in Critical Care. Ann Arbor, MI: Extracorporeal Life Support Organization, 1995, pp. 251–260.

Wagner PK, et al: Extracorporeal gas exchange in adult respiratory distress syndrome: associated morbidity and its surgical treatment. Br J Surg 77:1395, 1990.

Walz M, Muhr G: Continuously alternating prone and supine position in acute lung failure. Chirurg 63;931, 1992.

Ward ME, et al: Optimization of respiratory muscle relaxation during mechanical ventilation. Anesthesiology 69:29, 1988.

Weg JG, et al: Safety and potential efficacy of an aerosolized surfactant in human sepsis-induced adult respiratory distress syndrome. JAMA 272:1433, 1994.

Weisman IH, et al: Intermittent mandatory ventilation. Am Rev Respir Dis 127:641, 1983.

Zapol WM, et al: Extracorporeal membrane oxygenation in severe acute respiratory failure. A randomized prospective study. JAMA 242:2193, 1979.

Zwischenberger JB, Cox CS Jr: A new intravascular membrane oxygenator to augment blood gas transfer in patients with acute respiratory failure. Tex Med 87:60, 1991.

Zwischenberger JB, et al: Intravascular membrane oxygenation and carbon dioxide removal—a new application for permissive hypercapnia? Thorac Cardiovasc Surg 40:115, 1992.

Zwischenberger JB, et al: IVOX with gradual permissive hypercapnia: a new management technique for respiratory failure. J Surg Res 57:99, 1994.

READING REFERENCE

Zwischenberger JB, Bartlett RH (eds): ECMO. Extracorporeal Cardiopulmonary Support in Critical Care. Ann Arbor, MI: Extracorporeal Life Support Organization, 1995, pp. 251–260.

SECTION IX

The Chest Wall

CHAPTER 40

Chest Wall Deformities

Robert C. Shamberger

A broad spectrum of congenital chest wall deformities exists. The severe life-threatening deformities, ectopia cordis and asphyxiating thoracic dystrophy, are rare in comparison with the more frequent and milder pectus excavatum and carinatum. Congenital anterior thoracic deformities can be conveniently considered in five categories: 1) pectus excavatum; 2) pectus carinatum; 3) Poland's syndrome; 4) sternal defects, including ectopia cordis; and 5) miscellaneous conditions, including vertebral and rib anomalies, asphyxiating thoracic dystrophy (Jeune's disease), and rib dysplasia.

Congenital heart disease has been identified by Shamberger and associates (1988b) in 1.5% of infants and children undergoing chest wall correction at the Children's Hospital in Boston (Table 40-1). The frequency of chest wall deformities among all patients with congenital heart disease evaluated at this institution was only 0.17%.

PECTUS EXCAVATUM

Posterior depression of the sternum and costal cartilages produces the characteristic findings of pectus excavatum: funnel chest, or *trichterbrust*. The first and second ribs and the manubrium are usually in their normal position (Fig. 40-1), but the lower costal cartilages and the body of the sternum are depressed. In older adolescents and adults, the most anterior portion of the osseous ribs may also be curved posteriorly. The extent of sternal and cartilaginous deformity is quite variable. Numerous methods of grading and defining these deformities have been proposed by Hümmer and Willital (1984), Oelsnitz (1981), Welch (1980), and Haller and associates (1987), as well as others, but none has been universally accepted. Asymmetry of the depression is present frequently. Often the right side is more depressed than the left, and the sternum may be rotated as well. Many children with pectus excavatum have a characteristic physique with a broad thin chest, dorsal lordosis, "hook shoulder" deformity, costal flaring, and poor posture.

Pectus excavatum is present at birth or within the first year of life in the majority of affected children (86%), as shown in Figure 40-2. Although the deformity rarely resolves, it may worsen during the period of rapid adolescent growth. Waters and associates (1989) identified scoliosis in 26% of 508 patients with pectus excavatum. Hence, all patients with pectus deformities should be evaluated clinically for scoliosis. Asymmetric pectus excavatum with a deep right gutter and sternal rotation often is accompanied by more serious scoliosis. Correction of the associated pectus excavatum may stabilize the curve in conjunction with exercises or bracing, thereby avoiding spinal fusion.

Asthma may be identified in patients with pectus excavatum and carinatum. In a review of 694 consecutive cases, Shamberger and Welch (1988b) found a subgroup of 35 patients were identified with asthma (5.2%), which is comparable to the occurrence of asthma in the general pediatric population.

Etiology and Incidence

Ravitch (1977) reported that pectus excavatum may occur as frequently as 1 in 300 to 400 live births and that it is rare in blacks. It occurs more frequently in boys than girls, by almost a 4:1 ratio. Although the sternal depression appears to be caused by overgrowth of costal cartilages, the etiology of pectus deformities is unknown. Early investigators, such as Lester (1957), attributed its development to an abnormality of the diaphragm. Little evidence has supported this theory other than the occurrence reported by Greig and Azmy (1990) of pectus excavatum in children after repair of agenesis of the diaphragm. Hecker and associates (1981) described histopathologic changes in the costal cartilages similar to those seen in scoliosis, aseptic osteonecrosis, and inflammatory processes, but the etiology of these findings and their significance are unknown.

An increased familial incidence exists. In a review by Shamberger and colleagues (1988c), 37% of 704 patients had a family history of chest wall deformity. Three of four siblings were involved in one family. Scherer and colleagues (1988) reported a high incidence of chest wall deformities in

Table 40-1. Congenital Heart Disease Associated with Pectus Excavatum and Carinatum (No. of Cases)

Aortic ring	1
Aortic regurgitation	1
Atrial septal defect primum	2
Atrial septal defect secundum	3
Complete atrioventricular canal	3
Dextrocardia	3
Ebstein's malformation	1
Idiopathic hypertrophic subaortic stenosis	2
Patent ductus arteriosus	1
Pulmonic stenosis	1
Total anomalous pulmonary venous return	1
Transposition of great arteries	6
Tetralogy of Fallot	3
Tricuspid atresia	1
Truncus arteriosus	1
Ventricular septal defect	6

From Shamberger RC, et al: Anterior chest wall deformities and congenital heart disease. J Thorac Cardiovasc Surg 96:427, 1988. With permission.

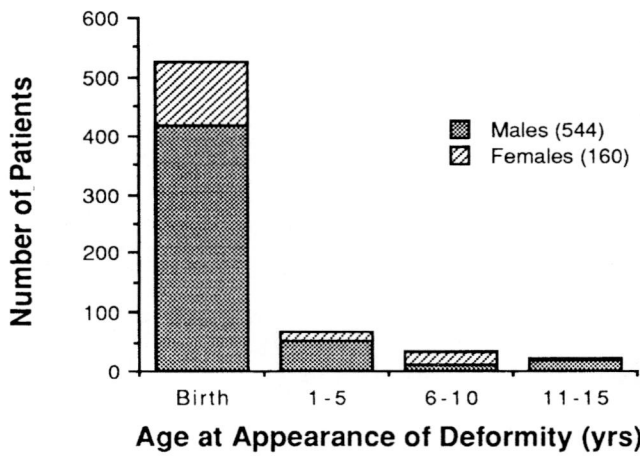

Fig. 40-2. Age at appearance of pectus excavatum deformity in 704 infants and children. Note the large proportion identified at birth or within the first year of life and the predominance of males with the deformity. From Shamberger RC, Welch KJ: Surgical repair of pectus excavatum. J Pediatr Surg 23:615, 1988. With permission.

children with Marfan's syndrome that are often severe and usually accompanied by scoliosis. Patients with abdominal musculature deficiency syndrome (prune-belly syndrome) commonly have pectus excavatum [8 of 43 patients in the experience of Welch and Kearney (1974)]. Pectus excavatum also occurs with other myopathies and chromosomal defects, such as Turner's syndrome. A summary of the associated musculoskeletal abnormalities is shown in Table 40-2.

Symptoms

Pectus excavatum is well tolerated in infancy and childhood. The anterior depression in an infant with a flexible chest may be magnified by upper airway obstruction from tonsillar and adenoidal hypertrophy, but they do not primarily produce the pectus deformity. Older children may complain of pain in the area of the deformed cartilages or of precordial pain after sustained exercise. A few patients have palpitations, presumably due to transient atrial arrhythmias. These patients may have mitral valve prolapse and associated atrial arrhythmias.

Pathophysiology

Some authors, including Haller and associates (1970), contend that no cardiovascular or pulmonary impairment results from pectus excavatum. This contrasts, however, with the clinical impression that many patients have increased stamina after surgical repair. These findings date back to the surgical repair performed by Sauerbruch in 1913 (1920). The patient was an 18-year-old boy who developed dyspnea and palpitations with very limited exercise. Three years after his operation, he could work 12 to 14 hours a day without tiring and without palpitations. Anecdotal reports during the next three decades confirmed this observation. Since then, investigators have sought to identify the physiologic abnormality or combination of abnormalities that could explain this symptomatic improvement after surgery. Early physiologic measurements of cardiac and

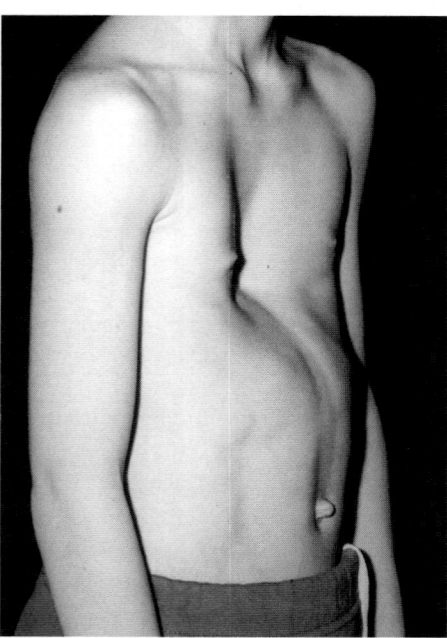

Fig. 40-1. An 8-year-old boy with a symmetric pectus excavatum deformity. Note that the depression extends to the sternal notch.

Table 40-2. Musculoskeletal Abnormalities Identified in 130 of 704 Cases of Pectus Excavatum

Scoliosis	107
Kyphosis	4
Myopathy	3
Marfan's syndrome	2
Pierre Robin syndrome	2
Prune-belly syndrome	2
Neurofibromatosis	3
Cerebral palsy	4
Tuberous sclerosis	1
Congenital diaphragmatic hernia	2

From Shamberger RC, Welch KJ: Surgical repair of pectus excavatum. J Pediatr Surg 23:615, 1988. With permission.

pulmonary function were crude and did not yield convincing evidence of a cardiopulmonary deficit. In many early studies, summarized by Shamberger and Welch (1988a), the results fell within the broad range of normal values, if often at the lower limit.

A systolic ejection murmur is frequently identified in patients with pectus excavatum and is magnified by a short interval of exercise. It is attributed to the close proximity between the sternum and the pulmonary artery, which results in transmission of a flow murmur.

Electrocardiographic abnormalities are common and Schaub and Wegmann (1954) attributed them to the abnormal configuration of the chest wall and the displacement and rotation of the heart into the left thoracic cavity. Preoperative electrocardiographic findings reported by Welch (1980) in 32 patients with pectus excavatum are shown in Table 40-3. Most significant are the cases of conduction blocks or arrhythmias. Patients with a history of palpitations should have a 24-hour electrocardiogram as well as an echocardiogram to evaluate for mitral valve prolapse. Resolution of these supraventricular arrhythmias has been anecdotally reported after correction of a pectus excavatum deformity.

Deformity of the chest wall led many authors to attribute the symptomatic improvement in patients after surgery to

Table 40-3. Electrocardiographic Findings in a Group of 32 Patients with Pectus Excavatum

Abnormality	Number of Patients
Right axis deviation	15
Depressed ST-T segments (2,3,aVF)	11
Tall P waves	7
Right bundle branch block	5
Combined block	3
Left ventricular hypertrophy	4
Left atrial hypertrophy	1
Paroxysmal atrial tachycardia	1

From Welch KJ: Chest wall deformities. In Holder TM, Ashcraft KW, eds. Pediatric Surgery. Philadelphia: WB Saunders, 1980. With permission.

initial impairment in pulmonary function. This was difficult to prove, however, with the wide range of pulmonary function that exists from individual to individual and its dependence on physical training and body habitus.

Pulmonary Function Studies

As early as 1951, Brown and Cook performed respiratory studies on patients before and after surgical repair. They demonstrated that although vital capacity (VC) was normal, the maximum breathing capacity diminished (50% or more) in nine of 11 cases and increased an average of 31% after surgical repair. Weg and associates (1967) evaluated 25 Air Force recruits with pectus excavatum and compared them with 50 unselected basic trainees. Although the lung compartments of both groups were equal, as were the vital capacities, the maximum voluntary ventilation was significantly lower in those with pectus excavatum than in the control population. Castile and coworkers (1982) evaluated seven patients with pectus excavatum, five of whom were symptomatic with exercise. The mean total lung capacity of the group was 79% of predicted. Flow volume configurations were normal, excluding airway obstruction. Workload tests demonstrated normal response to exercise in the dead space to tidal volume ratio and alveolar-arterial oxygen difference. The measured oxygen uptake, however, increasingly exceeded predicted values as workload approached maximum in the four "symptomatic" subjects with pectus excavatum. This pattern of oxygen consumption was different from that in normal subjects and in the three asymptomatic subjects with pectus excavatum, in whom a linear response was seen. The mean oxygen uptake in the symptomatic subjects at maximal effort exceeded the predicted values by 25.4%. The three asymptomatic subjects, on the other hand, demonstrated normal linear oxygen uptake during exercise. Increased oxygen uptake suggests increased work of breathing in these symptomatic individuals despite the normal or mildly reduced vital capacities. Increases in tidal volume with exercise were uniformly depressed in those with pectus excavatum.

Cahill and coworkers (1984) performed pre- and postoperative studies in five children and adolescents with pectus carinatum and in 14 with pectus excavatum. No abnormalities were demonstrated in the pectus carinatum group. The low normal vital capacities in excavatum patients were unchanged by operation, but a small improvement in the total lung capacity and a significant improvement in the maximal voluntary ventilation were seen. Exercise tolerance improved in those with pectus excavatum after operation, as determined both by total exercise time and maximal oxygen consumption. In addition, at any given workload, those with pectus excavatum demonstrated a lower heart rate, stable oxygen consumption, and higher minute ventilation after repair. Mead and associates (1985) studied rib cage mobility by assessing intra-abdominal pressure. Normal abdominal pressure tracings in pectus excavatum suggested normal rib cage mobility.

Blickman and colleagues (1985) assessed pulmonary function in 17 children with pectus excavatum by xenon perfusion and ventilation scintigraphy before and after surgery. Ventilation studies were abnormal in 12 children before surgery and improved in seven after repair. Perfusion scans were abnormal in ten children before surgery and improved after operation in 6 children. The ventilation-perfusion ratios were abnormal in ten of the 17 children preoperatively and normalized after repair in six children.

Derveaux and colleagues (1989) evaluated 88 patients with pectus excavatum and carinatum by pulmonary function tests before and 1 to 20 years after repair (mean was 8 years). The surgical technique used a fairly extensive chest wall dissection. Preoperative studies were within the normal range (>80% of predicted) except in subjects with both scoliosis and pectus excavatum. The postoperative values for forced expiratory volume in 1 second and VC were decreased in all groups when expressed as percent of predicted, although the absolute values at follow-up may have been greater than at preoperative evaluation. Radiologic evaluation of these individuals confirmed improved chest wall configuration, so the relative deterioration in pulmonary function was not the result of recurrence of the pectus deformity. An inverse relationship was found between preoperative and postoperative function. Those with less than 75% of predicted function had improved function after surgery, but results were worse after repair if the preoperative values were greater than 75% of predicted. Almost identical results were found in a study by Morshuis and associates (1994a), who evaluated 152 subjects before and a mean of 8 years after surgery for pectus excavatum. These physiologic results were in contrast to the subjective improvement in symptoms from the subjects and the improved chest wall configuration. The decline in pulmonary function in the postoperative studies was attributed to the operation because the preoperative defect appeared to be stable regardless of the age at initial repair. Both studies were marred by the obvious lack of an age and severity-matched control group without surgery.

Derveaux and colleagues (1988) evaluated transpulmonary and transdiaphragmatic pressures at total lung capacity in 17 individuals with pectus excavatum. Preoperative and long-term follow-up evaluations were performed a mean of 12 years apart. Reduced transpulmonary and transdiaphragmatic pressures suggested that the increased restrictive defect was produced by extrapulmonary rather than pulmonary factors, or that surgery produced increased rigidity of the chest wall.

Wynn and colleagues (1990) assessed 12 children with pectus excavatum by pulmonary function tests and exercise testing. Eight children had repair and were evaluated pre- and postoperatively. Four children had two sets of evaluation but no operation. A decline in total lung capacity was identified in the repaired children compared with stable values in the control group. Cardiac output and stroke volume increased appropriately with exercise before and after operation in both groups, and the operation was believed to have produced no physiologically significant effect on the response to exercise.

Kaguraoka and associates (1992) evaluated pulmonary function in 138 individuals preceding and after repair of pectus excavatum. A decrease in VC occurred during the first 2 months after surgery, with recovery to preoperative levels by one year after operation. At 42 months, the values were maintained at baseline, despite a significant improvement in the chest wall configuration. Tanaka and coworkers (1993) found similar results in individuals who had the more extensive sternal turnover technique; in fact, they demonstrated a more significant and long-term decrease in VC. Morshuis and coworkers (1994b) evaluated 35 subjects who had had pectus excavatum repaired as teenagers or young adults; ages were 17.9 ± 5.6 years. Preoperative evaluations were performed and repeated 1 year after surgery. Preoperative total lung capacity ($86.0 \pm 14.4\%$ of predicted) and VC ($79.7 \pm 16.2\%$) were significantly decreased from predicted valves and decreased further after surgery ($-9.2 \pm 9.2\%$ and $-6.6 \pm 10.7\%$, respectively). The efficiency of breathing at maximal exercise improved significantly after operation. Ventilatory limitation of exercise occurred in 43% of the subjects before repair, and there was a tendency toward improvement after operation. However, the group with no ventilatory limitation initially demonstrated a limitation after operation with a significant increase in oxygen consumption.

Quigley and colleagues (1996) evaluated 36 adolescents with pectus excavatum and ten age-matched healthy controls at baseline and then an average of 8 months after surgery in 15 subjects and 9 months in controls. Adolescents with pectus excavatum had a decrease in VC compared with controls, although the mean values remained in the normal range. The mean total lung capacity was normal. There was no difference in workload between subjects with pectus excavatum and the controls, with both groups achieving a similar duration and level of exercise. No significant change in follow-up pulmonary function tests was seen in either group. The duration of exercise as well as the level of work increased significantly in those who had surgery but not in the controls. The absence of adverse effects on pulmonary function after surgery was attributed to a less extensive surgical procedure than was used in the studies reported by Derveaux (1988) and Morshuis (1994a, 1994b) and their colleagues.

In composite, these studies of pulmonary function over the last four decades have failed to document consistent improvement in pulmonary function resulting from surgical repair. In fact, studies have demonstrated deterioration in pulmonary function at long-term evaluation that was attributable to increased chest wall rigidity after surgical repair. Despite this finding, workload studies have shown improvement in exercise tolerance after repair.

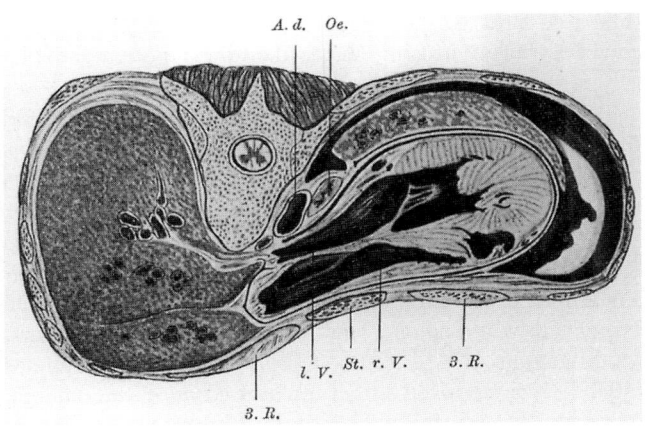

Fig. 40-3. Anatomic drawing from an autopsy of a male with pectus excavatum reported in 1912 demonstrates compression of the heart, particularly the right ventricle by the sternum. From Bien G: Zur Anatomie und Åtiologie der Trichterbrust. Beitr Pathol Anat Allg Pathol *52*:567, 1912. With permission.

Cardiovascular Studies

Posterior displacement of the sternum can produce a deformity of the heart, particularly anterior indentation of the right ventricle. Early pathologic studies demonstrated this finding (Fig. 40-3). Garusi and D'Ettorre (1964) showed by angiography displacement of the heart to the left, often with a sternal imprint on the anterior wall of the right ventricle. Howard (1959) demonstrated by angiography its resolution by surgical repair. Elevated right heart pressures have been reported by some authors, as have pressure curves similar to those seen in constrictive pericarditis. In 1962, Bevegård studied 16 individuals with pectus excavatum by right heart catheterization and exercise testing. The physical work capacity in pectus excavatum at a given heart rate was significantly lower in the sitting than the supine position. Those with 20% or greater decline in physical work capacity from the supine to the sitting position had shorter sternovertebral distances than did those with less decrease in their physical work capacity. The measured stroke volume at rest decreased from supine to sitting positions a mean of 40.3%, similar to normal subjects. In the supine position, stroke volume increased with exercise 13.2%. In the sitting position, the increase in stroke volume from rest to exercise was 18.5% for the pectus excavatum group, significantly lower ($P < .001$) than the 51% increase seen in normal subjects. Thus, in the pectus excavatum group, an increased cardiac output could be achieved primarily by increased heart rate because limited enhancement of the stroke volume could occur. Intracardiac pressures measured at rest and with exercise were normal in all subjects despite this apparent limitation of ventricular volume. Gattiker and Bühlmann (1967) confirmed this limitation of the stroke volume in a study of 19 subjects. In the upright position at a heart rate of 170 beats per minute, the physical work capacity was lower

than in the supine position (mean 18% decrease) because of the decrease in stroke volume. Beiser and associates (1972) performed cardiac catheterization in six adolescents and young adults with moderate degrees of pectus excavatum. Normal pressure and cardiac index were obtained at rest in the supine position. The cardiac index during moderate exercise was normal, but the response to upright exercise was below that predicted in two patients and at the lower limit of normal in three patients. The cardiac index was 6.8 ± 0.8 L/min/m^2 compared with 8.9 ± 0.3 L/min/m^2 in a group of 16 normal controls ($P < .01$). The difference in cardiac performance again appeared to be produced primarily by a smaller stroke volume in the group with pectus excavatum in an upright position. Stroke volume was 31% lower and cardiac output 28% lower during upright as compared with supine exercise. Postoperative studies were performed in three individuals: Two of them achieved a higher level of exercise tolerance after surgery. The cardiac index increased an average of 38%. Because heart rate at maximal exercise was not higher after repair, an enhanced stroke-volume response was responsible for this increase.

Peterson and associates (1985) performed radionuclide angiography and exercise studies in 13 children with pectus excavatum. Ten of 13 were able to reach the target heart rate before surgical repair, four without symptoms. After operation, all but one child reached the target heart rate during the exercise protocol, and nine of 13 reached the target without becoming symptomatic. The left and right ventricular end-diastolic volumes were consistently increased after repair at rest, and the mean stroke volume was increased 19% after repair. These findings substantiated the ventricular volume changes previously demonstrated by cardiac catheterization, although an increase in the cardiac index was not demonstrated.

Additional studies are needed to further define the relationship between pectus excavatum and cardiopulmonary function. Recent dynamic or exercise studies have been most promising in this area. Methods to more effectively evaluate preoperative cardiopulmonary function are needed to identify which children may achieve symptomatic and physiologic improvement from surgical repair.

Echocardiographic Studies

Bon Tempo (1975), Salomon (1975), and Schutte (1981) and their associates reported mitral valve prolapse in patients with narrow anterior-posterior chest diameters, anterior chest wall deformities, and scoliosis. Echocardiographic prospective studies of adults with pectus excavatum demonstrated mitral valve prolapse in six of 33 (18%) subjects studied by Udoshi and associates (1979) and in 11 of 17 subjects (65%) of Saint-Mezard and colleagues (1986). Anterior compression of the heart by the depressed sternum may deform the mitral annulus or the ventricular chamber and produce mitral valve prolapse in these patients. Preoperative evaluation by echocardiogram of children with pectus excavatum by the author and associates (1987) identified 23 children with mitral valve prolapse. Postoperative studies did not demonstrate mitral valve prolapse in 10 (43%) of these children, suggesting resolution after correction of the chest wall deformity.

Surgical Repair

The first surgical corrections of pectus excavatum were reported by Meyer in 1911 and Sauerbruch in 1920. In 1939, Ochsner and DeBakey summarized early experience with various techniques. In 1949, Ravitch reported a technique that included excision of all deformed costal cartilages with the perichondrium, division of the xiphoid from the sternum, division of the intercostal bundles from the sternum, and a transverse sternal osteotomy securing the sternum anteriorly in an overcorrected position. He used Kirschner wire fixation in the first two patients and silk suture fixation in later patients.

Baronofsky (1957) and Welch (1958) reported a technique for the correction of pectus excavatum that emphasized total preservation of the perichondrial sheaths as well as the attachment of the upper sheaths and intercostal bundles to the sternum. Anterior fixation of the sternum was achieved with silk sutures. The technique I use today remains unchanged from these methods except for the use of strut fixation in older children, in those with severe deformities in whom complete correction is difficult to achieve by suture fixation alone, and in all patients with Marfan's syndrome. Haller and associates (1970) later developed a technique labeled *tripod fixation*, in which subperichondrial resection of the abnormal cartilages is performed followed by a posterior sternal osteotomy. The most cephalad normal cartilages are then divided obliquely in a posterolateral direction. When the sternum is elevated, the sternal ends of the cartilage rest on the costal ends, providing further anterior support of the sternum.

Several authors have promoted supporting the sternum by metallic struts after mobilization of the costal cartilages. Rehbein and Wernicke (1957) developed struts that could be placed into the marrow cavity of the ribs at the costochondral junction. An arch was then formed by the struts anterior to the sternum, and the sternum was secured to this arch. Paltia and associates (1958) placed a transverse strut through the caudal end of the sternum, firmly fixing its location. The two ends of the strut are supported by the ribs laterally. Adkins and Blades (1961) and Jensen and associates (1970) used retrosternal elevation by a metallic strut. Willital (1981) employed a similar retrosternal strut after creating multiple chondrotomies in the costal cartilages to provide flexibility. Recent innovations in these methods include bioabsorbable struts, Marlex mesh, or a Dacron vascular graft as a strut, but there is no evidence these methods are preferable to traditional methods. No randomized studies have compared the recurrence or complication rates between

suture or strut fixation. Oelsnitz (1981) and Hecker and coworkers (1981), using suture fixation, reported satisfactory repairs in their large series in 90 to 95%.

The *sternal turnover* was first proposed by Judet and Judet (1954) and Jung (1956) in the French literature. In this method, the sternum is mobilized and the costal cartilages are divided, allowing the sternum to be rotated 180 degrees. Wada and colleagues (1970) have reported a very large series from Japan using this technique, which is essentially a free graft of sternum. It is a radical approach and has been associated with major complications if infection occurs. Modifications of this technique by Taguchi and associates (1975) have involved either preservation of the internal mammary vessels by wide dissection or reimplantation of the internal mammary artery. These methods were developed because of the reported incidence of osteonecrosis and fistula formation, which occurred in up to 46% of patients older than 15 years.

A method described by Allen and Douglas (1979) is that of implantation of Silastic molds into the subcutaneous space to fill the deformity. Although this approach may improve the external contour of the chest, extrusion of the molds has occurred, and this method does nothing to increase the volume of the thoracic cavity. A method of elevation of the sternum with a retrosternal bar without resection or division of the costal cartilages has been reported by Nuss and colleagues (1998), but confirmation of the safety and efficacy of this method await its replication by other centers.

Surgical Technique

The surgical technique for correction of pectus excavatum is depicted in Figure 40-4. In girls, particular attention is taken to place the incision within the projected inframammary crease, thus avoiding the complications of breast deformity and development described by Hougaard and Arendrup (1983). Skin flaps are mobilized by electrocautery to the angle of Louis superiorly and to the xiphoid inferiorly. Pectoral muscle flaps are elevated off the sternum and costal cartilages, thus preserving the entire pectoralis major and portions of the pectoralis minor and serratus anterior muscles in the flap (see Fig. 40-4A). Ellis and associates (1997) have described elevating the skin and muscle together in a single flap, which is a reasonable alternative method.

Perioperative antibiotics are used, giving one dose of cefazolin immediately before operation and three postoperative doses. The Hemovac drain is removed when the drainage is less than 15 mL for an 8-hour period. All patients are warned to avoid aspirin-containing compounds for 2 weeks before surgery.

I currently use the retrosternal bar (Baxter Healthcare Co., Deerfield, IL) for internal fixation to secure the sternum firmly in an anterior position and to avoid the need to skeletonize the sternum to achieve adequate mobility for suture

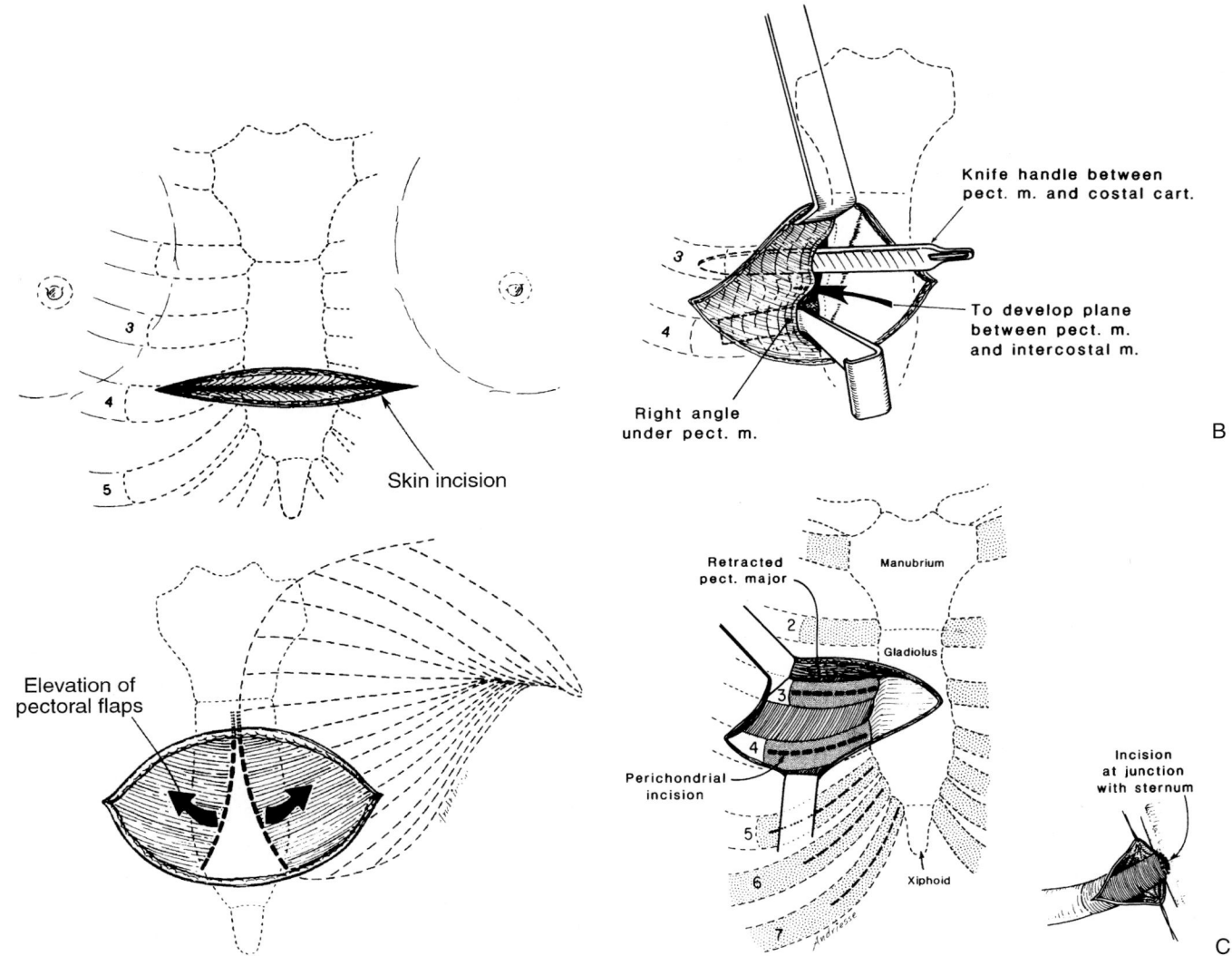

Fig. 40-4. Surgical technique for repair of pectus excavatum. **A.** A transverse incision is placed below and well within the nipple lines and, in females, at the site of the future inframammary crease. The pectoralis major muscle is elevated from the sternum along with portions of the pectoralis minor and serratus anterior bundles. **B.** The correct plane of dissection of the pectoral muscle flap is defined by passing an empty knife handle directly anterior to a costal cartilage after the medial aspect of the muscle is elevated with electrocautery. The knife handle is then replaced with a right-angle retractor, which is pulled anteriorly. The process is then repeated anterior to an adjoining costal cartilage. Anterior distraction of the muscles during the dissection facilitates identification of the avascular areolar plane and avoids entry into the intercostal muscle bundles. Muscle elevation is extended bilaterally to the costochondral junctions of the third to fifth ribs. **C.** Subperichondral resection of the costal cartilages is achieved by incising the perichondrium anteriorly. It is then dissected away from the costal cartilages in the bloodless plane between perichondrium and costal cartilage. Cutting back the perichondrium 90 degrees in each direction at its junction with the sternum (*inset*) facilitates visualization of the back wall of the costal cartilage. (*Continued*)

fixation. Although correction of pectus excavatum is technically most easily performed in a young child, I have become increasingly concerned about long-term recurrence in these children as well as impairment in growth of the chest wall. I currently delay surgery until the children are well into their pubertal growth. At this age, the chest has less remaining growth and opportunity for recurrence of the pectus excavatum (Fig. 40-5). In contrast, Humphreys and Jaretzki (1980) and Backer and associates (1961) have found no correlation between the age at repair and frequency of recurrence.

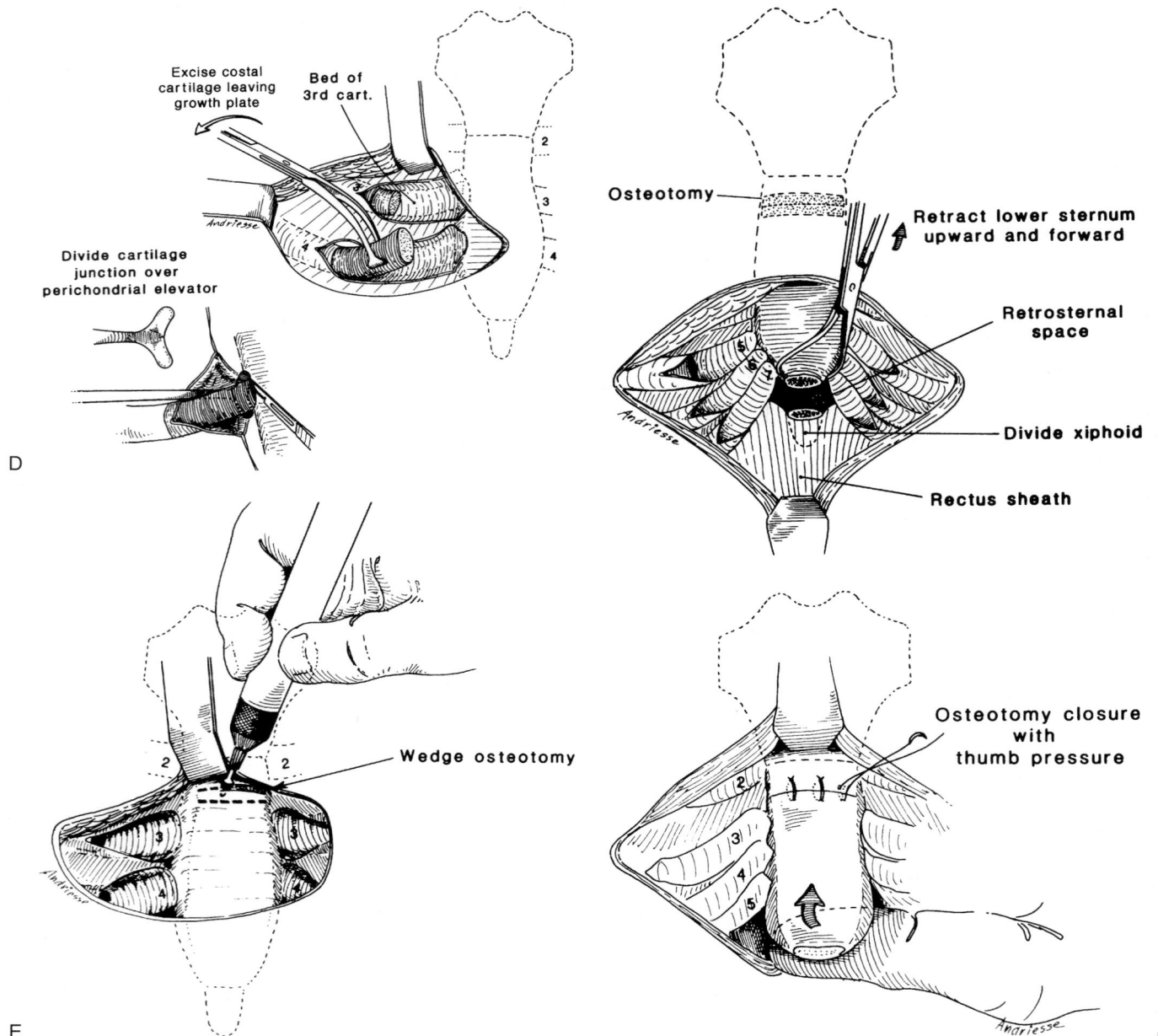

Fig. 40-4. (*Continued*) **D.** The cartilages are divided at their junction with the sternum with a knife having a Welch perichondrial elevator held posteriorly to elevate the cartilage and protect the mediastinum (*inset*). The divided cartilage can then be held with an Allis clamp and elevated. The costochondral junction is preserved with a segment of costal cartilage on the osseous ribs by incising the cartilage with a scalpel. Costal cartilages three through seven are generally resected, but occasionally the second costal cartilages must be removed if posterior displacement or funneling of the sternum extends to this level, as may be seen in older patients (see Fig. 40-1). Segments of the sixth and seventh costal cartilages are resected to the point where they flatten to join the costal arch. Familiarity with the cross-sectional shape of the medial ends of the costal cartilages facilitates their removal. The second and third cartilages are broad and flat, the fourth and fifth are circular, and the sixth and seventh are narrow and deep. **E.** The sternal osteotomy is created above the level of the last deformed cartilage and the posterior angulation of the sternum, generally the third cartilage but occasionally the second. Two transverse sternal osteotomies are created through the anterior cortex with a Hall air drill (Zimmer USA, Inc., Warsaw, IN) 2 to 4 mm apart. **F.** The base of the sternum and the rectus muscle flap are elevated with two towel clips, and the posterior plate of the sternum is fractured. The xiphoid can be divided from the sternum with electrocautery, allowing entry into the retrosternal space. This step is not necessary with the use of a retrosternal strut. Preservation of the attachment of the perichondrial sheaths and xiphoid avoids an unsightly depression that can occur below the sternum. **G.** When a strut is not used, the osteotomy is closed with several heavy silk sutures as the sternum is elevated by the assistant. (*Continued*)

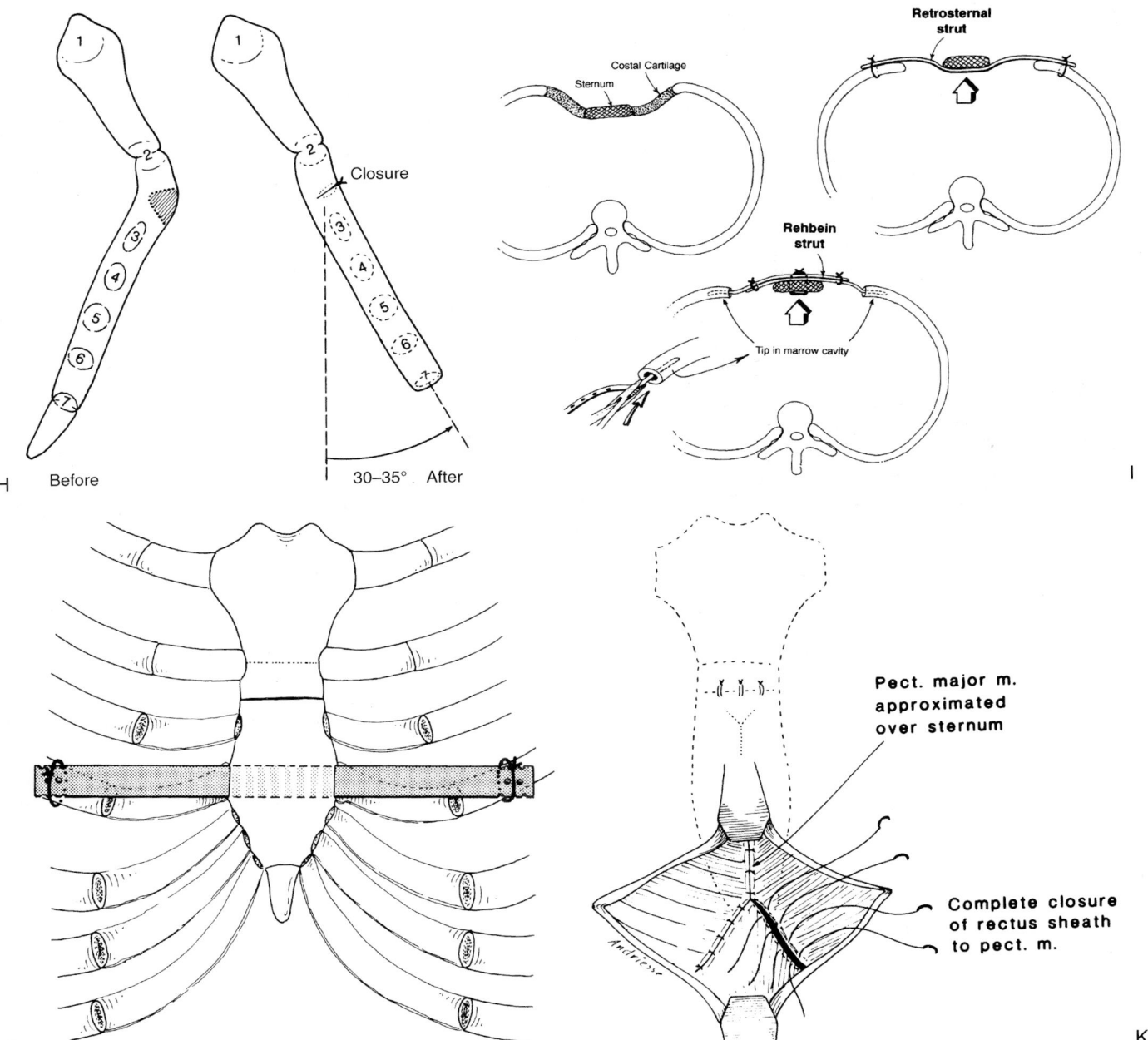

Fig. 40-4. (*Continued*) **H.** Correction of the abnormal position of the sternum is achieved by creation of a wedge-shaped osteotomy, which is then closed, bringing the sternum anteriorly into an overcorrected position. **I.** This figure demonstrates the use of both retrosternal struts and Rehbein struts. Rehbein struts are inserted into the marrow cavity (*insert*) of the third or fourth rib, and the struts are then joined medially to create an arch anterior to the sternum. The sternum is sewn to the arch to secure it in its new anterior position. The retrosternal strut is placed behind the sternum and is secured to the rib ends laterally to prevent migration. **J.** Anterior depiction of the retrosternal struts. The perichondrial sheath to either the third or fourth rib is divided from its junction with the sternum, and the retrosternal space is bluntly dissected to allow passage of the strut behind the sternum. It is secured with two pericostal sutures laterally to prevent migration. The wound is then flooded with warm saline and cefazolin solution to remove clots and inspect for a pleural entry. A single-limb medium Hemovac drain (Snyder Laboratories, Inc., New Philadelphia, OH) is brought through the inferior skin flap to the left of the sternum and placed in a parasternal position to the level of the highest resected costal cartilage. **K.** The pectoral muscle flaps are secured to the midline of the sternum, advancing the flaps to obtain coverage of the entire sternum. The rectus muscle is then joined to the pectoral muscle flaps, closing the mediastinum. A–H and K from Shamberger RC, Welch KJ: Surgical repair of pectus excavatum. J Pediatr Surg 23:615, 1988. With permission. D and F adapted from original figure.

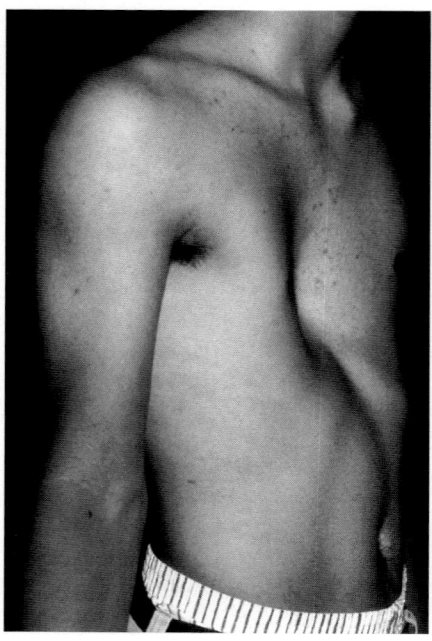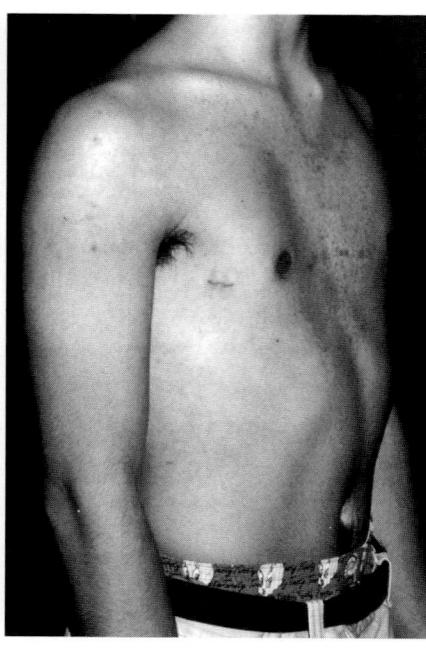

A,B

Fig. 40-5. Pectus excavatum repair. **A.** Preoperative. **B.** Seven months postoperative photograph of a 14-year-old boy repaired using retrosternal struts.

Complications

Complications of pectus excavatum repair that Shamberger and Welch (1988b) reported in 704 patients (Table 40-4) are few and relatively unimportant, except for major recurrence in 17 patients. In 2% of patients, a limited pneumothorax required aspiration or was simply observed. Tube thoracostomy has not been required in the past decade and was used in only four patients in the entire series. Wound infection is rare with use of perioperative antibiotic coverage.

The most distressing complication after surgical correction of pectus excavatum is major recurrence of the deformity. It is difficult to predict which patients will have a major recurrence, but it appears to occur with increased frequency in children with poor muscular development and an asthenic or "marfanoid" habitus. All children with Marfan's syndrome should be repaired with strut fixation because of

Table 40-4. Complications of Pectus Excavatum Repair: 70 Cases in 704 Patients

Pneumothorax[a]	11
Wound infection	5
Wound hematoma	3
Wound dehiscence	5
Pneumonia	3
Seroma	1
Hemoptysis	1
Hemopericardium	1
Major recurrence	17
Mild recurrence	23

From Shamberger RC, Welch KJ: Surgical repair of pectus excavatum. J Pediatr Surg *23*:615, 1988. With permission.
[a]Four patients required chest tube placement.

the high risk of recurrence reported without struts. Scherer and associates (1988) reported a low recurrence rate (one of 8 cases) using a retrosternal strut.

Although recurrences appear symmetric, they are in fact frequently right sided, with a deep right parasternal gutter and sternal obliquity. The third, fourth, and fifth rib ends migrate medially, with apparent "foreshortening" of the costal cartilages. Correction of recurrent pectus excavatum is generally a formidable task. Sanger and associates (1968) reported their experience in secondary correction. They resected the regenerated fibrocartilage plate, repeated the osteotomy, and closed the pectoral muscles behind the sternum. Ten patients had an early good result. In the Boston Children's Hospital experience, 12 children and adolescents underwent secondary repair. Resection of the segments of the third to fifth costal cartilages was necessary to correct the deformity. After clearing the tip of the sternum, resection of the left fibrocartilage plate to the level of the third or second perichondrial sheath allowed the sternum to be brought forward and rotated to an acceptable position. Ten of 12 repeat operations were accomplished without pleural entry. Follow-up of patients with secondary correction ranged from 10 to 17 years. Eight have acceptable thoracic contour; two have a broad shallow depression; and two have frank recurrence. I recommend use of strut fixation on all patients with secondary repair because cartilage regeneration will be slower and less adequate than that after primary operation.

In 1990, Martinez and associates first described a deficiency in thoracic growth in children after repair of pectus excavatum that was most noticeable in children repaired early during the preschool years. In 1995, Haller reported three boys who had presented in their teens with apparent limited growth of the ribs after resection of the costal cartilages at an early age, pro-

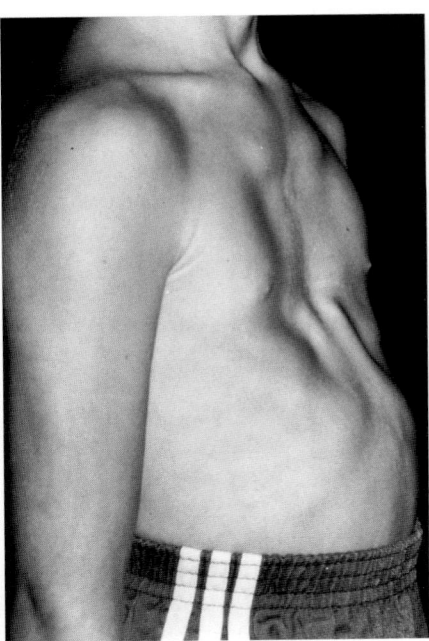
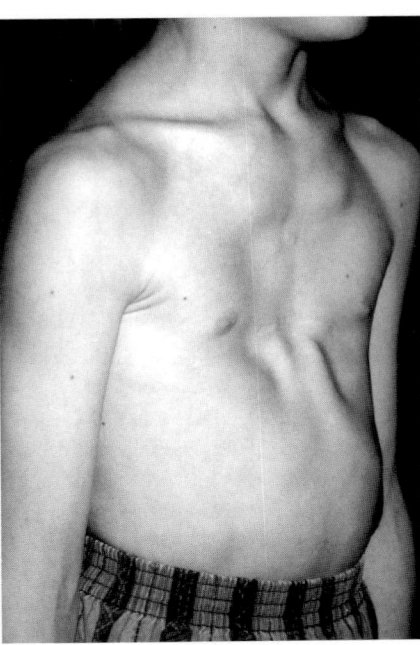
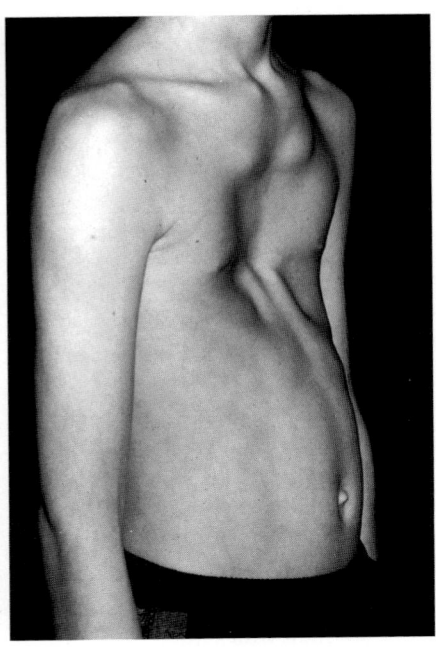

A–C

Fig. 40-6. Sequence of figures demonstrating deterioration in the quality of a repair that can occur with time. This boy had an initial excellent result from a Welch repair with suture fixation of the sternum at age 4 years 3 months. The follow-up photographs at 7 years 6 months (**A**), 9 years 3 months (**B**), and 12 years 9 months (**C**) demonstrate progressive depression of the sternum and costal cartilages and relative "overgrowth" of the upper chest.

ducing a bandlike narrowing of the mid chest (*acquired Jeune's disease*) (Fig. 40-6). In some cases, the first and second ribs in which the costal cartilages have not been resected have apparent relative overgrowth, producing anterior protrusion of the upper sternum (Fig. 40-7). Haller (1995) attributed this occurrence to injury during surgical repair of the costochondral junctions, which are the longitudinal growth centers for the ribs, and to decreased growth of the sternum resulting from injury to its growth centers or vascular supply.

Martinez and associates (1990) demonstrated experimentally in 6-week-old rabbits that resection of the costal cartilages produced a marked impairment in chest growth, particularly the anterior-posterior diameter, during a 5.5-month period of observation. Less severe impairment occurred if only the medial three-fourths of the costal cartilage was resected, preserving the growth centers at the costochondral junction. This impairment was attributed to fibrosis and scarring within the perichondrial sheaths. Perichondrial sheaths, bone, or other prosthetic tissues that cannot grow also should not be joined posterior to the sternum because they will form a bandlike stricture across the chest. This complication of delayed thoracic growth was described primarily in children repaired in early childhood and can be avoided by delaying surgery until the children are older. Preservation of the costochondral junction leaving a segment of the cartilage on the osseous portion of the rib may partially minimize growth impairment. Patients are followed after surgery to full growth: age 16 for girls and 19 for boys. Use

of clinical and Moiré photography, as reported by Shochat and associates (1981), for initial evaluation and follow-up studies leads to improved clinical assessment of results and obviates the need for multiple radiographic examinations.

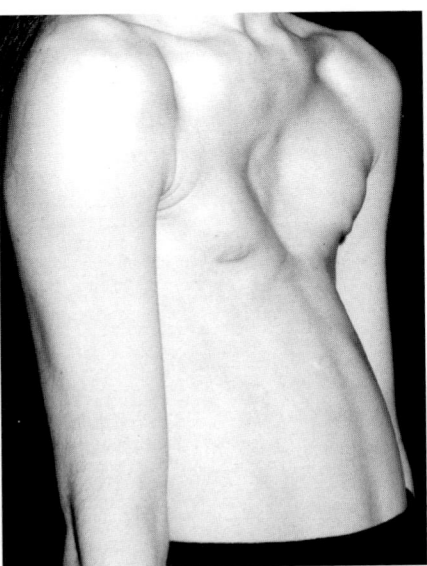

Fig. 40-7. A 10-year-old girl 7 years after repair of pectus excavatum. She demonstrates relative "overgrowth" of the upper costal cartilages, which were not resected during her repair, and a bandlike narrowing of her chest below that level.

Table 40-5. Frequency of Pectus Carinatum Deformities

Chondrogladiolar	
Symmetric	89
Asymmetric	49
Mixed carinatum and excavatum	14
Chondromanubrial	3
Total number of cases	155

From Shamberger RC, Welch KJ: Surgical correction of pectus carinatum. J Pediatr Surg 22:48, 1987. With permission.

PECTUS CARINATUM

Pectus carinatum, or anterior protrusion of the sternum, is much less frequent than pectus excavatum: 16.7% of all chest wall deformities in the Boston Children's Hospital experience. The anterior protrusion occurs in a spectrum of configurations often divided into four categories (Table 40-5). The most frequent form, termed *chondrogladiolar* by Brodkin (1949), consists of anterior protrusion of the body of the sternum with symmetric protrusion of the lower costal cartilages. Howard (1958) described it as appearing as if a giant hand had pinched the chest from the front, forcing the sternum and medial portion of the costal cartilages forward and the lateral costal cartilages and ribs inward (Fig. 40-8). Asymmetric deformities with anterior displacement of the costal cartilages on one side and normal cartilages on the contralateral side are less common (Fig. 40-9). Mixed lesions have a carinate deformity on one side and a depression or excavatum deformity on the contralateral side, often with sternal rotation. Some authors classify these as a variant of the excavatum deformities. The most infrequent deformity is the upper chondromanubrial or "pouter pigeon" deformity. It consists of protrusion of the manubrium and

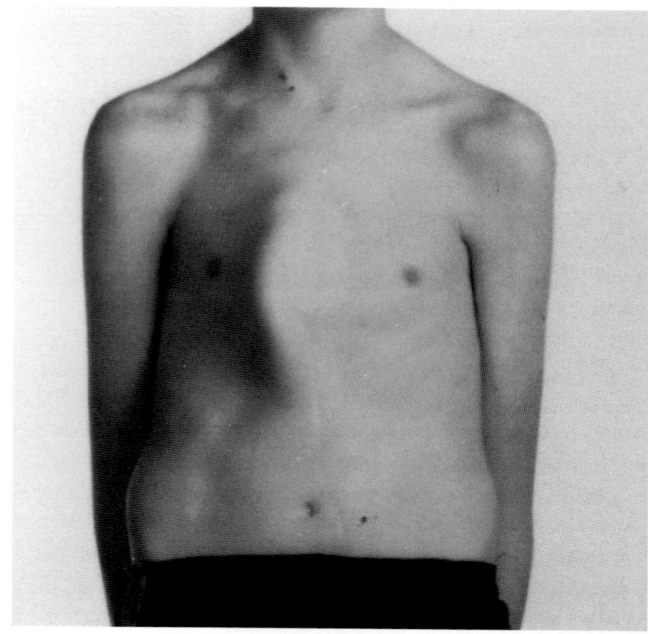

Fig. 40-9. A 12-year-old boy with marked asymmetric pectus carinatum demonstrates protrusion of the costal cartilages limited to the right side.

second and third costal cartilages with relative depression of the body of the sternum (Fig. 40-10).

Etiology

The etiology of pectus carinatum is no better understood than that of pectus excavatum. It appears as an overgrowth

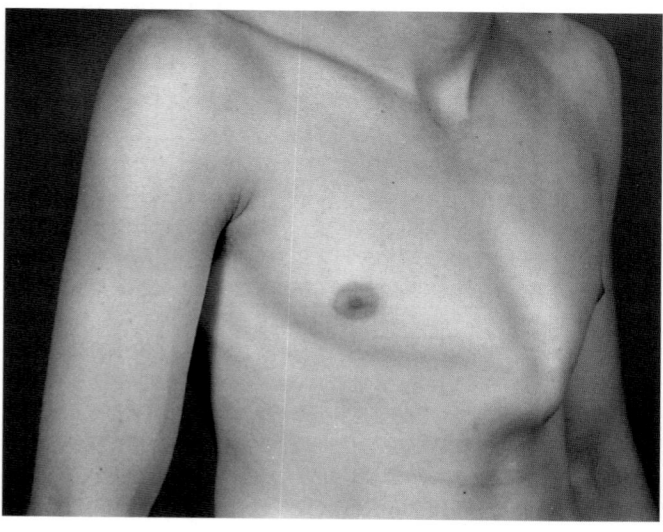

A

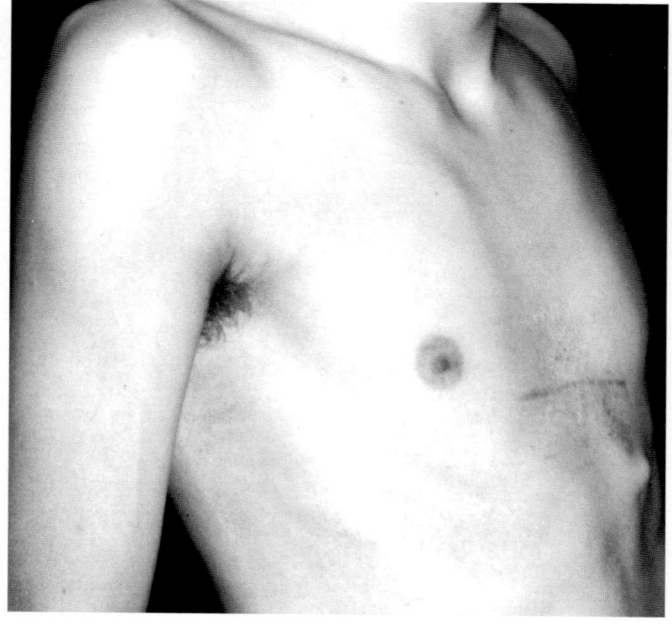

B

Fig. 40-8. A. Symmetric chondrogladiolar pectus carinatum in a 19-year-old man. **B.** Postoperative photograph shows correction of the protruding sternum and costal cartilages.

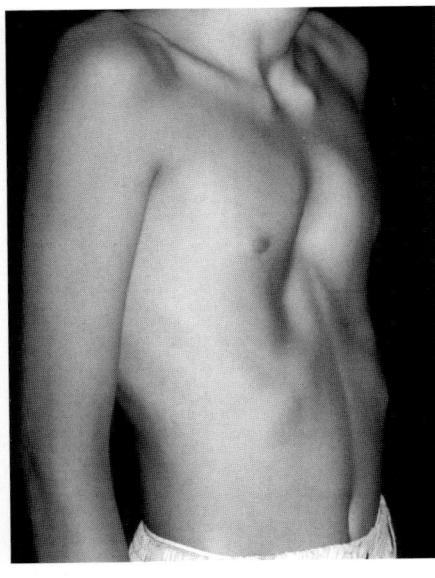
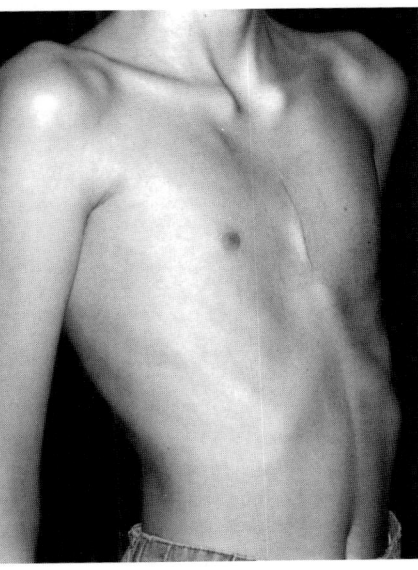

B

Fig. 40-10. **A.** A 15-year-old boy with the chondromanubrial deformity. Note the posterior depression of the lower sternum, accentuated by the anterior bowing of the second and third costal cartilages. **B.** After repair, the sternal contour is improved and costal cartilages are reformed in a more appropriate fashion. From Shamberger RC, Welch KJ: Surgical correction of chondromanubrial deformity. J Pediatr Surg 23:319, 1988. With permission.

of the costal cartilages with forward buckling and anterior displacement of the sternum. Again, there is a clear-cut increased family incidence, which suggests a genetic basis. In a review by the author and colleagues (1987) of 152 patients, 26% had a family history of chest wall deformity. A family history of scoliosis was obtained in 12% of the patients. It is much more frequent in boys (119, or 78%) than in girls (33, or 22%). Scoliosis and other deformities of the spine are the most common associated musculoskeletal anomalies (Table 40-6).

Pectus carinatum usually appears in childhood, and in almost one-half of patients, the deformity was not identified until after the eleventh birthday (Fig. 40-11). The deformity may appear in mild form at birth but often progresses during early childhood, particularly in the period of rapid growth at puberty. The chondromanubrial deformity, in contrast with the chondrogladiolar form, is often noted at birth and is associated with a truncated, comma-shaped sternum with absent sternal segmentation or premature obliteration of the sternal sutures (Fig. 40-12). Currarino and Silverman (1958) described its association with an increased risk of congenital heart disease. Lees and Caldicott (1975) reviewed 1915 radiographs and identified 135 children with sternal fusion

anomalies. Eighteen percent of these children had documented congenital heart disease.

Surgical Repair

Correction of carinate deformities has had a colorful history, beginning with the first repair by Ravitch (1952) of a chondromanubrial deformity. He resected multiple costal cartilages and performed a double sternal osteotomy. In 1953, Lester reported two methods of repair for chondrogladiolar deformity. The first approach, resection of the anterior portion of the sternum, was abandoned because of excessive blood loss and unsatisfactory results. The second method, subpe-

Table 40-6. Musculoskeletal Abnormalities Identified in 30 of 152 Cases of Pectus Carinatum

Scoliosis	23
Neurofibromatosis	2
Morquio's disease	2
Vertebral anomalies	1
Hyperlordosis	1
Kyphosis	1

From Shamberger RC, Welch KJ: Surgical correction of pectus carinatum. J Pediatr Surg 22:48, 1987. With permission.

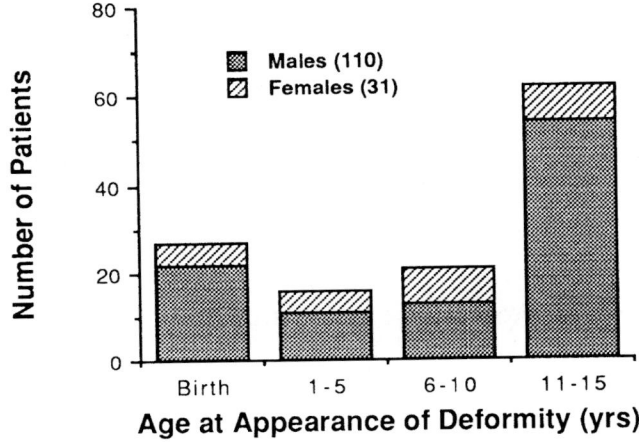

Fig. 40-11. Age at appearance of the pectus carinatum deformity in 141 infants and children. Note the appearance of protrusion in almost one-half of the children at puberty. From Shamberger RC, Welch KJ: Surgical correction of pectus carinatum. J Pediatr Surg 22:48, 1987. With permission.

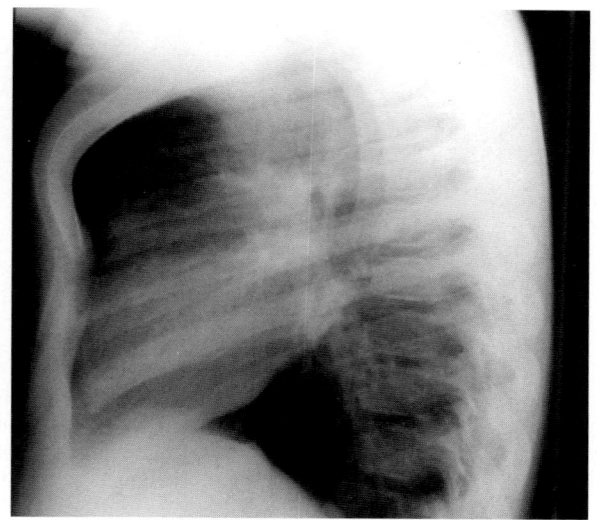

Fig. 40-12. Lateral chest radiograph in a boy with chondromanubrial pectus carinatum. The short, comma-shaped sternum lacking segmentation is apparent.

riosteal resection of the entire sternum was a no less radical technique. Chin (1957), and later Brodkin (1958), advanced the transected xiphoid and attached the rectus muscles to a higher site on the sternum, the xiphosternopexy. This produced posterior displacement of the sternum in younger patients with a flexible chest wall. Howard (1958) combined this method with subperichondrial costal cartilage resection and a sternal osteotomy. Ravitch (1960) reported repair of the chondrogladiolar deformity by resection of costal cartilage in a one- or two-stage procedure, with placement of "reefing" sutures to shorten and posteriorly displace the perichondrium. A sternal osteotomy was used in one of three cases. Robicsek and associates (1963) described repair by subperichondrial resection of costal cartilages, transverse sternal osteotomy, and resection of the protruding lower portion of the sternum. The xiphoid and rectus muscles were reattached to the new lower margin of the sternum, pulling it posteriorly. In 1973, Welch and Vos reported an approach to these deformities that I continue to use today. Recent attempts at treating children with pectus carinatum by orthotic bracing (Haje and Bowen

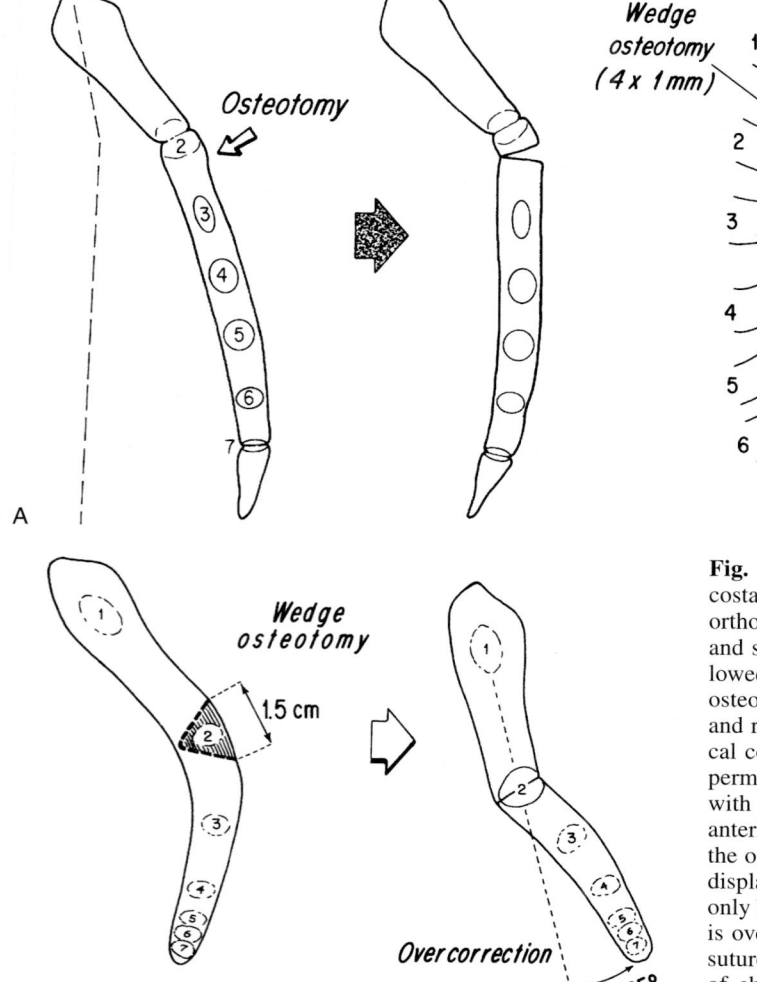

Fig. 40-13. A. A single or double osteotomy after resection of the costal cartilages allows posterior displacement of the sternum to an orthotopic position. **B.** The mixed pectus deformity is corrected by full and symmetric resection of the third to seventh costal cartilages, followed by transverse offset (0- to 10-degree wedge-shaped sternal osteotomy). Closure of this defect achieves both anterior displacement and rotation of the sternum. From Shamberger RC, Welch KJ: Surgical correction of pectus carinatum. J Pediatr Surg 22:48, 1987. With permission. **C.** The chondromanubrial type of deformity is depicted with a broad, wedge-shaped sternal osteotomy placed through the anterior cortex at the obliterated sternomanubrial junction. Closure of the osteotomy after fracture of the posterior cortex achieves posterior displacement of the superior portion of the sternum, which is secured only by its attachment to the first rib. The lower portion of the sternum is overcorrected 20 to 35 degrees and secured in position by strut or suture fixation. From Shamberger RC, Welch KJ: Surgical correction of chondromanubrial deformity. J Pediatr Surg 23:319, 1988. With permission.

Table 40-7. Complications of Pectus Carinatum Repair: 7 Cases in 152 Patients

Pneumothorax[a]	4
Atelectasis	1
Wound infection	1
Local tissue necrosis	1

[a]Two patients required chest tube placement.

[1992]; Mielke and Winter [1993]) have been reported, and success has been achieved in younger children.

Surgical Technique

The placement of the skin incision, mobilization of the pectoral muscle flaps and subperichondrial resection of the costal cartilage are identical to the method described for pectus excavatum. Management of the sternum is shown in Figure 40-13 for the various deformities. In the chondromanubrial deformity, the costal cartilages must be resected from the second cartilage inferiorly, as described by Welch and I (1988). A single-limb medium Hemovac drain (Snyder Laboratories, Inc., New Philadelphia, OH) is brought through the inferior skin flap, as for excavatum patients, with the suction ports in a parasternal position to the level of the highest resected costal cartilage. The pectoralis muscle flaps and skin flaps are closed. Perioperative antibiotics are used as in pectus excavatum.

Operative Results

Results are overwhelmingly successful in these patients. In a review of 152 cases by Welch and I (1987), postoperative recovery was generally uneventful. Blood transfusions are rarely required, and none has been given in the last 10 years. There is a 3.9% complication rate (Table 40-7). Only three patients have required revision, each having additional lower costal cartilages resected for persistent unilateral malformation of the costal arch.

POLAND'S SYNDROME

In 1841, Poland described congenital absence of the pectoralis major and minor muscles associated with syndactyly. Despite prior report of this entity by Froriep (1839), the label *Poland's syndrome* has been used since 1962, when Clarkson first applied it to a group of similar patients. Subsequent reports have described other components of the syndrome, including absence of ribs, chest wall depression, and abnormalities of the breasts. Each component of the syndrome may occur with variable severity. The extent of thoracic involvement may range from hypoplasia of the sternal head of the pectoralis major and minor muscles with normal underlying ribs to complete absence of the anterior portions of the second to fifth ribs and costal cartilages (Fig. 40-14). Breast involvement is frequent, ranging from mild hypopla-

sia to complete absence of the breast (amastia) and nipple (athelia) (see Fig. 40-14C). Minimal subcutaneous fat and an absence of axillary hair are components. Hand deformities may include hypoplasia (brachydactyly) and fused fingers (syndactyly), primarily involving the central three digits. The most severe expression of the anomaly, mitten or claw deformity (ectromelia) is rare, as noted by Clarkson (1962) and Walker and associates (1969). Poland's syndrome may also occur in combination with Sprengel's deformity, in which there is decreased size, elevation, and winging of the scapula.

Poland's syndrome is present from birth and has an estimated incidence of 1 in 30,000 to 1 in 32,000, as reported by Freire-Maia and colleagues (1973) and McGillivray and Lowry (1977). Abnormalities in the breast can be defined at birth by absence of the underlying breast bud and the hypoplastic nipple, which is often superiorly displaced. The etiology of Poland's syndrome is unknown. Bouvet and associates (1978) have proposed hypoplasia of the ipsilateral subclavian artery as the origin of this malformation, but, as noted by David (1979), decreased blood flow to the extremity may be the consequence rather than the cause of decreased muscle mass of the hypoplastic limb. Although some forms of syndactyly have been described as autosomal dominant traits, a similar pattern has not been demonstrated in patients with Poland's syndrome, which is generally sporadic. Multiple cases within a family are rare, as described by Sujansky and coworkers (1977), David (1982), and Cobben and associates (1989). Poland's syndrome is associated with a second rare syndrome, the Möbius syndrome: bilateral or unilateral facial palsy and abducens oculi palsy. Nineteen such cases have been identified by Fontaine and Ovlaque (1984), but a unifying etiology is lacking. Boaz and colleagues (1971) have reported an unusual association between Poland's syndrome and childhood leukemia.

The Boston Children's Hospital experience with Poland's syndrome from 1970 to 1987, reported by myself and associates (1989), included 41 children and adolescents, of whom 21 were males. The lesion was right sided in 23 patients, left sided in 17 patients, and bilateral in 1 patient. Hand anomalies were noted in 23 (56%) and breast anomalies in 25 (61%). In 10 children, the underlying thoracic abnormality required reconstruction, and in three children, rib or cartilage grafts were needed for complete repair.

Surgical Repair

Assessment of the extent of involvement of the various musculoskeletal components is critical for optimal thoracic reconstruction. If the extent of the deformity is limited to the sternal component of the pectoralis major and minor muscles, there is little functional deficit and repair is not necessary, except to facilitate breast augmentation in females (Fig. 40-15). If the underlying costal cartilages are depressed or absent, repair must be considered to minimize the concavity, to eliminate the

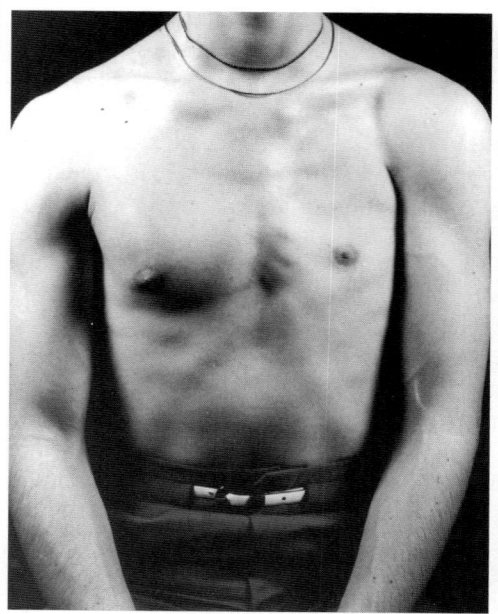
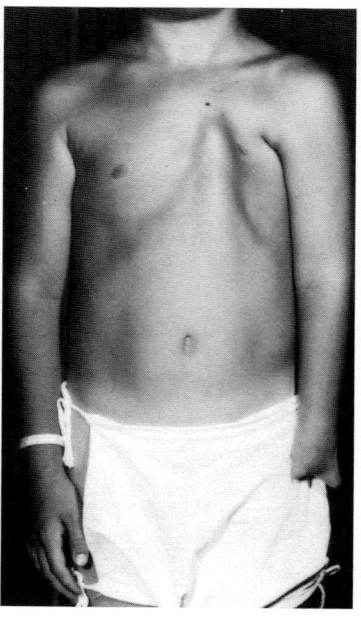
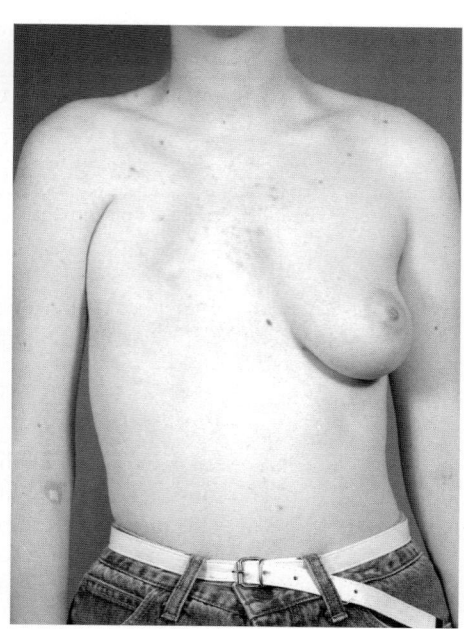

A–C

Fig. 40-14. A. Muscular 15-year-old boy with Poland's syndrome with loss of the left axillary fold owing to absence of the pectoralis major muscle. He has an orthotopic sternum and normal cartilages. He compensates adequately for loss of the pectoralis major and minor muscles. Surgery is not indicated in males with these findings. **B.** Eight-year-old boy with Poland's syndrome and more extensive thoracic involvement. The pectoralis major and minor muscles and the serratus to the level of the fifth rib are absent. There is sternal obliquity, and the third to fifth ribs are aplastic, ending at the level of the nipple. The corresponding cartilages are absent. The endothoracic fascia lies beneath a thin layer of subcutaneous tissue. Note the hypoplastic nipple and ectromelia of the ipsilateral hand, the most severe malformation of the hand associated with Poland's syndrome. **C.** Fourteen-year-old girl with Poland's syndrome. Note the high position of the right nipple, amastia, sternal rotation, and depressed right chest. The anterior second to fourth ribs and cartilages were missing. Breast augmentation will be required after the ipsilateral breast achieves full growth.

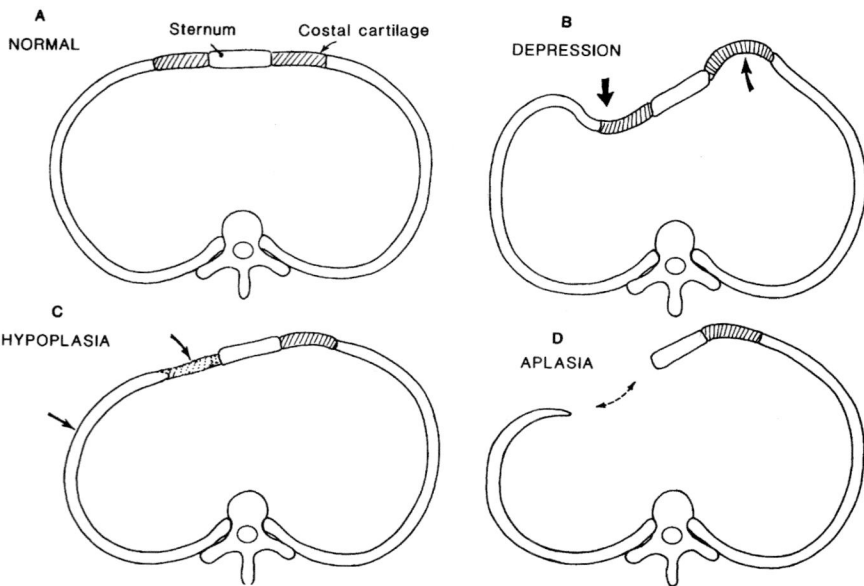

Fig. 40-15. A. The spectrum of thoracic abnormality seen in Poland's syndrome. Most frequently, an entirely normal thorax is present, and only pectoral muscles are absent. **B.** Depression of the involved side of the chest wall, with rotation and often depression of the sternum. A carinate protrusion of the contralateral side is frequently present. **C.** Hypoplasia of ribs on the involved side but without significant depression may be seen. It usually does not require surgical correction. **D.** Aplasia of one or more ribs is usually associated with depression of adjacent ribs on the involved side and rotation of the sternum. From Shamberger RC, Welch KJ, Upton J III: Surgical treatment of thoracic deformity in Poland's syndrome. J Pediatr Surg 24:760, 1989. With permission.

Table 40-8. Sternal Defects Reported in 109 Cases of Cleft Sternum

Upper cleft	46
Upper cleft to xiphoid	33
Complete cleft	23
Lower defect with manubrium or midsegment intact	5
Central defect with manubrium and xiphoid intact (skin ulceration noted in only three cases)	2

From Shamberger RC, Welch KJ: Sternal defects. Pediatr Surg Int 5:156, 1990. With permission.

num and cervicofacial hemangiomas, which were reported in 14 cases since the first description of this association by Fischer in 1879.

Surgical Repair

Maier and Bortone accomplished the first primary repair of cleft sternum in 1949 in a 6-week-old infant. The flexibility of the newborn chest allows approximation of the sternum without cardiac compression (Fig. 40-17). A summary of the reported repairs for cleft sternum in 69 cases is shown in Table 40-9.

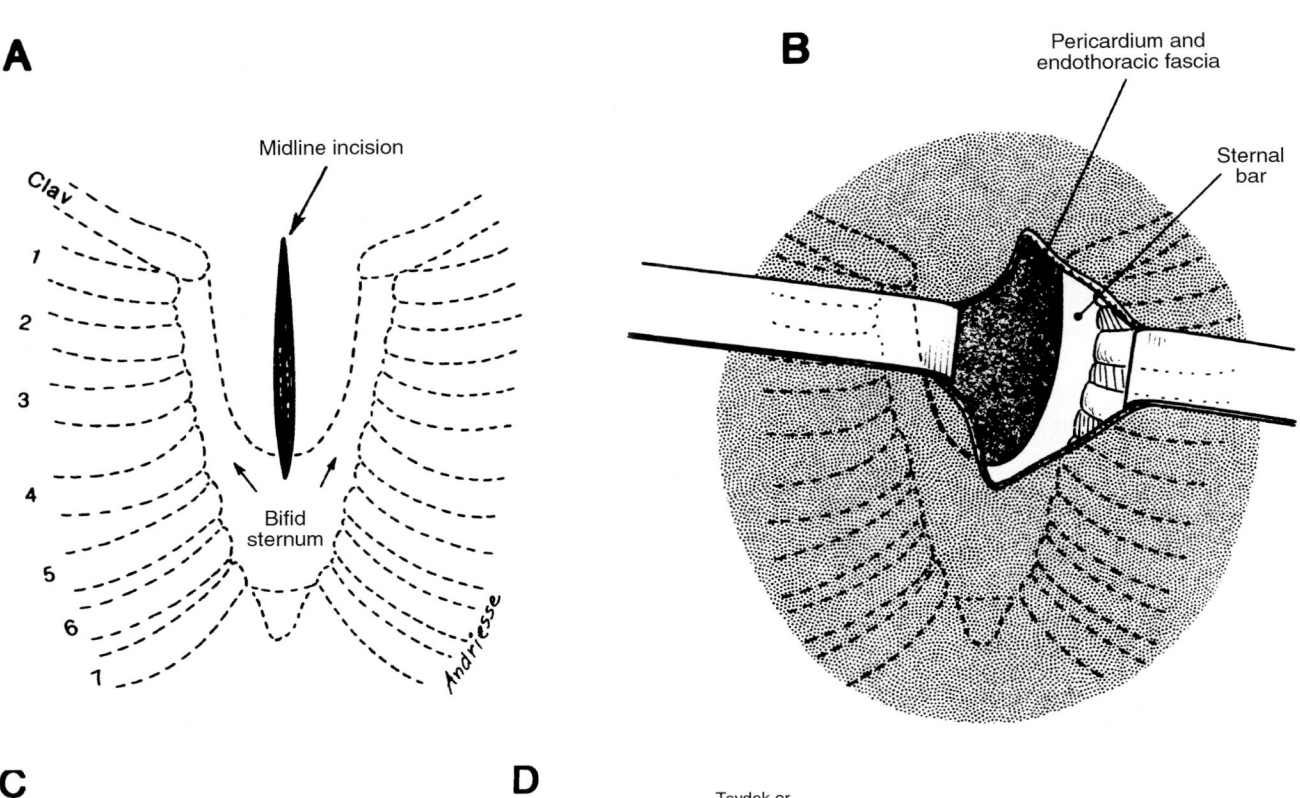

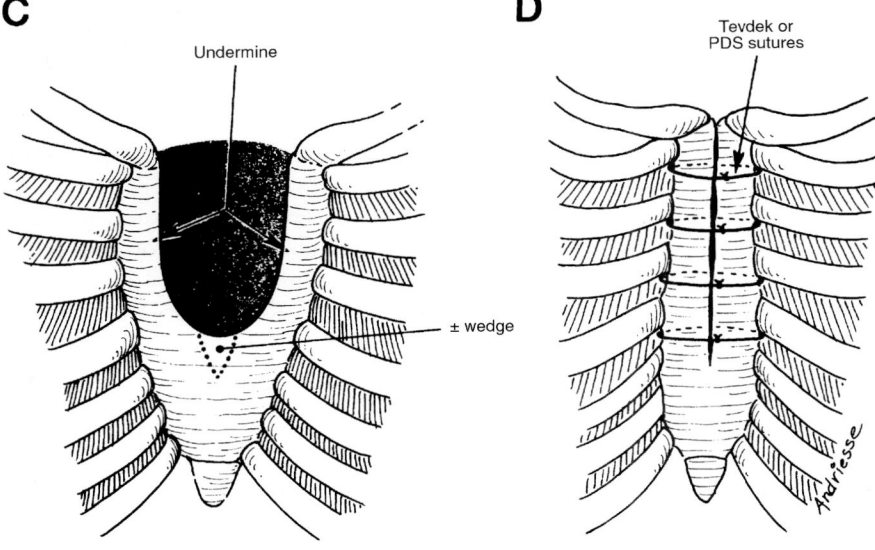

Fig. 40-17. **A.** Repair of bifid sternum is best performed through a longitudinal incision extending the length of the defect. **B.** Directly beneath the subcutaneous tissues the sternal bars are encountered, with pectoral muscles present lateral to the bars. The endothoracic fascia and pericardium are just below these structures. **C.** The endothoracic fascia is mobilized off the sternal bars posteriorly with blunt dissection to allow safe placement of the sutures. Approximation of the sternal bars may be facilitated by excising a wedge of cartilage inferiorly. **D.** Closure of the defect is achieved with 2-0 Tevdek or PDS (Ethicon, Inc., Sommerville, NJ) sutures. From Shamberger RC, Welch KJ: Sternal defects. Pediatr Surg Int 5:156, 1990. With permission.

Table 40-9. Methods of Repair of Cleft Sternum in 69 Cases

Primary approximation and repair	25
Primary repair with sliding chondrotomies (Sabiston)	19
Primary repair with rotating chondrotomies (Meissner)	3
Primary repair with other chondrotomy	4
Bone or cartilage graft	8
Prosthetic mesh graft	4
Sternocleidomastoid muscle transposition	3
Transposition of local soft tissues	2
Skin closure with excision of ulcer	1

From Shamberger RC, Welch KJ: Sternal defects. Pediatr Surg Int 5:156, 1990. With permission.

Sabiston reported reconstruction of cleft sternum using multiple oblique chondrotomies (1958). The chondrotomies increase the chest wall dimensions and flexibility. The technique is useful in older infants and children with a less flexible chest and a wide defect. Meissner (1964) described a variation of repair in which the cartilages are divided laterally and swung medially to cover the defect. Autologous grafts of costal cartilage, split ribs, and segments of the costal arch have been used since Burton (1947) first repaired this defect with a portion of the costal arch. Repairs with prosthetic material are far less satisfactory because of the risks of infection and the inability of these tissues to grow with the child. Most authors now recommend treatment of cleft sternum in the newborn period, when simple direct closure is possible without the use of prosthetic materials or grafts.

Ectopia Cordis

Although treatment of isolated cleft sternum is routinely successful, surgical repair of ectopia cordis has a high mortality, particularly thoracic ectopia cordis. The lethal factor in thoracic ectopia cordis and cervical ectopia cordis is the extrathoracic location of the heart, which makes tissue coverage difficult. In thoracoabdominal ectopia cordis [the Cantrell pentalogy (1958)], the major impediment to survival is the high incidence of intrinsic congenital heart disease.

Etiology

The etiology of thoracic ectopia cordis and thoracoabdominal ectopia cordis is much debated. Higginbottom (1979), Opitz (1985), Hersh (1985), and Kaplan (1985) and their colleagues consider these anomalies to be the result of disruption of the amnion and possibly disruption of the chorionic layer or yolk sac as well. This disruption occurs during the third or fourth week of gestation at a time when cardiac chamber formation is occurring rapidly. This timing may account for the high incidence of abnormal cardiac development. VonPraagh (personal communication, 1987) has the intriguing notion, based on embryology studies by Patten (1946) and Bremer (1939), that acute hyperflexion of the craniocervical segment of the embryo pins the heart down in

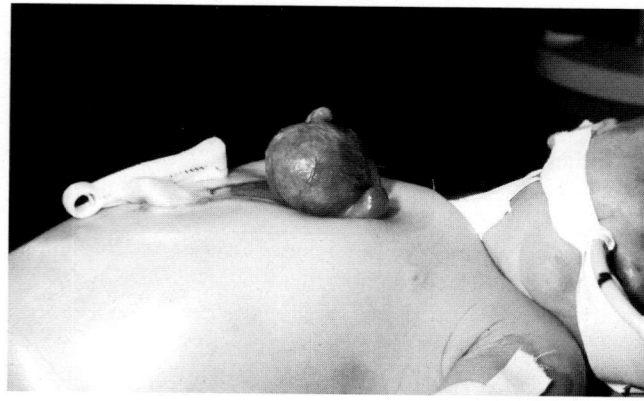

Fig. 40-18. An infant with thoracic ectopia cordis without a significant abdominal wall defect. The cardiac apex is cephalad. Any movement of the heart resulted in bradycardia and arrest. The patient had severe aortic overriding and complex tetralogy of Fallot.

the extrathoracic position with the submental cardiac apex. The abnormal fetal configuration produced by oligohydramnios may persist to delivery and oppose traction by the gubernaculum cordis, which normally pulls the cardiac apex into caudal alignment. Chromosome abnormalities have been reported by Say and Wilsey (1978), King (1980), and Stoll and associates (1987), who also commented on the supraumbilical raphe and gubernaculum cordis.

Thoracic Ectopia Cordis

Thoracic ectopia cordis is one of the most dramatic occurrences in the delivery room (Fig. 40-18). The naked beating heart is external to the thorax. Clearly visible are the atrial appendages, coronary vasculature, and cephalic orientation of the cardiac apex. The gubernaculum cordis initially extends to the supraumbilical raphe. Thoracic ectopia cordis was first reported by Stensen (1671). Stensen's report was later translated by Willius (1948). Stensen identified the four components of the tetralogy of Fallot in this patient with thoracic ectopia cordis (such is the fate of eponyms). Cardiac anomalies are unusually frequent in thoracic ectopia cordis. Table 40-10 lists the cardiac anomalies reported up to 1990. Only four of 75 cases had no intrinsic cardiac anomalies.

Infants with thoracic ectopia cordis are severely deficient in the midline somatic tissues that normally cover the heart. Many attempts at primary closure fail because of the inability to mobilize adequate tissues for coverage. An abdominal defect is often present as well. Recent computed tomogram evaluation by Haynor and associates (1984) also shows reduced intrathoracic volume in these infants. Most allegedly successful repairs have been not of true thoracic ectopia cordis but, rather, thoracoabdominal ectopia cordis. Cutler and Wilens first attempted repair in 1925 by skin flap coverage but failed because of cessation of cardiac function,

Table 40-10. Intrinsic Cardiac Lesions Reported: 75 Cases of Thoracic Ectopia Cordis

Tetralogy of Fallot	16
Pulmonary artery stenosis	6
Transposition of great arteries and pulmonary artery stenosis or atresia	8
Patent ductus arteriosus (PDA)	2
Tricuspid and pulmonary atresia	3
Ventricular septal defect (VSD) and atrial septal defect (ASD)	6
VSD	5
ASD and PDA	4
ASD	1
Truncus arteriosus	3
Coarctation, ASD, and PDA	1
Coarctation	1
Aortic hypoplasia	1
Double-outlet left ventricle	2
Double-outlet right ventricle	2
Aortic stenosis, ASD, and PDA	1
Single atrium, single ventricle	3
Double atrium, single ventricle	3
Cor triatriatum	1
Aberrant right subclavian artery	1
Bilateral superior vena cava[a]	1
Normal	4

[a]Also present in association with many of the listed anomalies.
From Shamberger RC, Welch KJ: Sternal defects. Pediatr Surg Int 5:156, 1990. With permission.

presumably from compression of the heart. Only three reported survivors of more than 29 attempts have been recorded (Table 40-11).

The first successful repair of ectopia cordis was achieved by Koop in 1975 and was reported by Saxena (1976). An infant with a normal heart had skin flap coverage at 5 hours of age, with inferior mobilization of the anterior attachments of the diaphragm. The sternal bars were 2 inches apart and could not be approximated primarily without cardiac compression and compromise. At 7 months of age, an acrylic resin of Dacron and Marlex mesh was inserted to close the sternal cleft, followed by primary skin closure. Necrosis of the skin flaps complicated the postoperative course with infection of the prosthetic material, which was later removed. This child survives to age 20 years and is reported to be entirely well.

Successful closure in two other infants is reported. Dobell and associates (1982) also achieved closure in two stages. Skin flap coverage was provided for the newborn. Rib strut grafts were placed over the sternal defect at 19 months of age and covered with pectoral muscle flaps. The pericardium was divided from its anterior attachments to the chest wall, allowing the heart to fall back partially into the thoracic cavity. Only Amato and colleagues (1988) achieved complete coverage of the heart in one stage. The unifying theme of successfully managed cases is mobilization of adequate soft tissue to cover the heart in its extrathoracic location and avoiding attempts to return the heart to an orthotopic location. Of note, in the successful cases, intrinsic cardiac lesions and associated abdominal defects were absent. These are the characteristics that most distinguish the successes from the failures, rather than any differences in surgical techniques. Coverage of the heart with autologous tissues, whether by flap rotation or bipedicle flaps, generally produces excessive compression on the heart, which limits cardiac output either by kinking outflow vessels or impeding cardiac filling. In most instances, attempts are abandoned in the operating room because of severe cardiac impairment. In patients who are repaired with autologous tissue grafts (bone or cartilage) or synthetic materials, infection and extrusion of the graft invariably occurs. Ultimate success with this lesion will be achieved only by accomplishing tissue coverage of the heart that avoids posterior displacement into an already limited thoracic space. This will require use of tissues from sites distant from the chest wall. Severe intracardiac defects associated with thoracic ectopia cordis in most cases also limit survival. The only recent advancement in management of this lesion has been early ultrasonographic diagnosis, as described by Kragt (1985) and Mercer (1983) and their colleagues, including definition of the intracardiac lesion and termination of the pregnancy, if acceptable to the parents.

Abdominal wall defects are also frequent in these patients, including an upper abdominal omphalocele or diastasis recti and, rarely, eventration of the abdominal viscera (Fig. 40-19). Associated abdominal defects are summarized in Table 40-12. The presence of abdominal defects should not, however, lead to classification of these lesions as thora-

Table 40-11. Reported Survivors of Thoracic Ectopia Cordis and Their Repair

Author	Year	Cardiac Lesion	Method of Sternal Closure
Koop and Saxena	1975	None	Skin flap closure at 5 hours. Acrylic resin applied to sternal cleft at 7 months.
Dobell	1982	None	Perinatal skin closure in one stage. Second-stage repair with rib grafts.
Amato, Cotroneo, and Gladieri	1988	None	Skin flaps mobilized, diaphragm moved inferiorly, Gore-Tex[a] membrane used to close defect with skin flaps over it. Child survived but died of aspiration at 11 months of age.

From Shamberger RC, Welch KJ: Sternal defects. Pediatr Surg Int 5:156, 1990. With permission.
[a]Gore-Tex: WL Gore & Associates, Inc., Flagstaff, AZ.

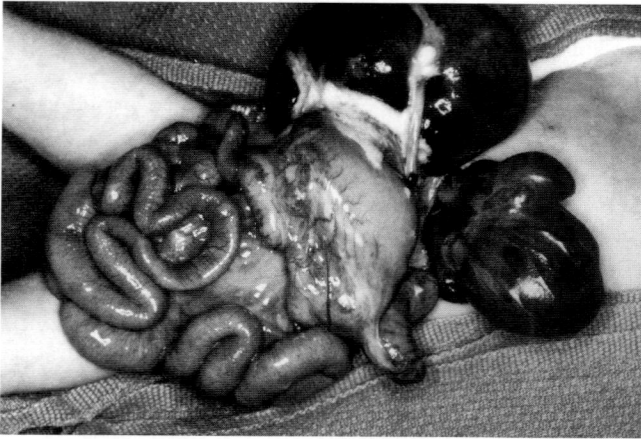

Fig. 40-19. Infant with thoracic ectopia cordis and eventration of the abdominal viscera.

coabdominal ectopia cordis, which should be reserved for those infants in whom the heart is covered at birth.

Thoracoabdominal Ectopia Cordis (Cantrell's Pentalogy)

In thoracoabdominal ectopia cordis, the heart is covered by an omphalocele-like membrane or thin skin, which is often pigmented in a child with thoracoabdominal ectopia cordis. The sternum is cleft inferiorly, and the heart lacks the severe anterior rotation present in thoracic ectopia cordis. An early report of this lesion by Wilson in 1798 clearly defined the associated somatic defects of the abdominal wall, diaphragm, and pericardium (Fig. 40-20) as well as the intrinsic cardiac anomalies. This entity was subsequently reviewed by Major (1953) and Cantrell and associates (1958). It is now frequently called Cantrell's pentalogy, although it was described long before Cantrell's relatively recent review. The five essential features of thoracoabdominal ectopia cordis are a cleft lower sternum, a half moon–shaped anterior diaphragmatic defect resulting from lack of development of the septum transversum, absence of the parietal pericardium at the diaphragmatic defect, omphalocele (Table 40-13), and in most patients, an intrinsic cardiac anomaly (Table 40-14; Fig. 40-21). A left ventricular diverticulum occurs with surprising frequency in this anomaly. In many cases, the diverticulum protrudes through the diaphragmatic and pericardial defects into the abdominal cavity.

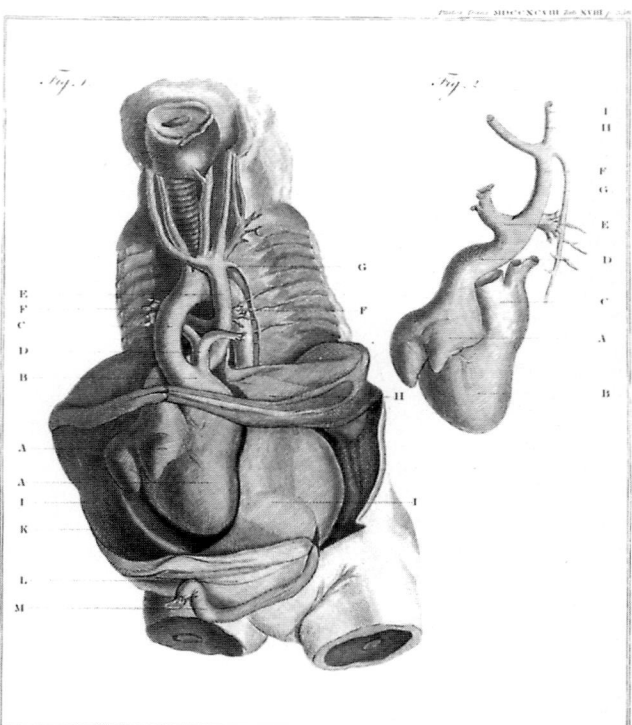

Fig. 40-20. Earliest drawing of thoracoabdominal ectopia cordis. It clearly demonstrates the anterior semilunar diaphragmatic and pericardial defects, allowing abdominal displacement of the heart. The cardiac defect was a single atrium and single ventricle (cor biloculare with truncus arteriosus). An omphalocele was found as well but is not shown. From Wilson J: A description of a very unusual formation of the human heart. Philos Trans R Soc Lond *11*:346, 1798. With permission.

Successful repair and long-term survival are more frequent in thoracoabdominal ectopia cordis than in thoracic ectopia cordis. Arndt attempted the first repair in 1896, but return of the heart to the thoracic cavity resulted in death. Wieting performed the first successful surgical repair in 1912. He achieved primary closure of the diaphragm and abdominal wall fascia but ignored the ventricular diverticulum. Initial surgical intervention must address the skin defects overlying the heart and abdominal cavity. Primary excision of the omphalocele with skin closure avoids infection and mediastinitis, although several cases have been successfully managed by local application of topical astringents, thus allowing

Table 40-12. Abdominal Wall Defects Reported in 75 Cases of Thoracic Ectopia Cordis

Omphalocele	36
Diastasis recti (or ventral hernia)[a]	6
Eventration	4

From Shamberger RC, Welch KJ: Sternal defects. Pediatr Surg Int 5:156, 1990. With permission.
[a]Often covered by thin, pigmented dermis.

Table 40-13. Abdominal Wall Defects Reported in Patients with Thoracoabdominal Ectopia Cordis

Omphalocele	64
Diastasis recti (or ventral hernia)	40
Diaphragmatic defect	71
Pericardial defect	46

From Shamberger RC, Welch KJ: Sternal defects. Pediatr Surg Int 5:156, 1990. With permission.

Table 40-14. Intrinsic Cardiac Lesions Reported in Patients with Thoracoabdominal Ectopia Cordis

Tetralogy of Fallot	13
Tetralogy of Fallot and diverticulum of left ventricle	1
Diverticulum of left ventricle	16
Diverticulum of left ventricle and VSD	9
Diverticulum of left ventricle, pulmonary stenosis, and VSD	1
Diverticulum of left ventricle and ASD	1
Diverticulum of left ventricle, ASD, and VSD	1
Diverticulum of left ventricle, VSD, and mitral stenosis	1
Diverticulum left ventricle, hypoplastic left ventricle, and VSD	1
VSD	8
VSD and ASD	2
VSD and single atrium	1
ASD	3
ASD, VSD, and total anomalous pulmonary venous connection	1
Truncus arteriosus	5
Single atrium and single ventricle	5
Pulmonary atresia and single ventricle	2
Pulmonary atresia, VSD, and PDA	1
Pulmonary stenosis and VSD	3
Tricuspid atresia	4
Double-outlet left ventricle	2
Double-outlet right ventricle	2
Transposition of the great arteries, mitral atresia, and pulmonary artery hypoplasia	1
Transposition of the great arteries and pulmonary artery stenosis	2
Transposition great arteries and VSD	1
Aortic stenosis, ASD, and VSD	1
Bilateral superior vena cava[a]	1
Normal	5

From Shamberger RC, Welch KJ: Sternal defects. Pediatr Surg Int 5:156, 1990. With permission.
ASD, atrial septal defect; PDA, patent ductus arteriosus; VSD, ventricular septal defect.
[a]Also present in association with many of the listed anomalies.

Table 40-15. Reported Methods of Repair of Thoracoabdominal Ectopia Cordis

Primary closure of diaphragm and abdominal wall defect	8
Primary closure of skin only and excision of omphalocele	7
Primary closure of diaphragm	4
Primary closure of abdominal wall defect	2
Coverage of abdominal defect with Silastic pouch and secondary epithelialization	3
Resection of lower ribs and sternum to increase room in chest with inferior attachment of diaphragm and primary skin coverage	1
Staged repair with initial skin closure with secondary prosthetic mesh closure of the abdominal and thoracic defect	1
Staged repair with initial skin closure with secondary closure of abdominal wall and diaphragm	1

From Shamberger RC, Welch KJ: Sternal defects. Pediatr Surg Int 5:156, 1990. With permission.

secondary epithelialization to occur. Several early cases, as in that of Cullerier (1806), document the long-term viability of individuals with thoracoabdominal ectopia cordis with intact skin coverage despite the abnormal location of the heart.

Advances in cardiac surgery now allow correction of the intrinsic cardiac lesions, which were previously fatal. An aggressive approach to repair in infants with thoracoabdominal ectopia cordis is appropriate. Repair of the abdominal wall defect or diastasis has been achieved by primary closure or prosthetic mesh (Table 40-15). Primary closure of the thoracoabdominal defect may be difficult to achieve because of the wide separation of the rectus muscles and their superior attachment to the costal arches. Complete repair of the intracardiac defect is best performed before placement of prosthetic mesh overlying the heart. Repair of the abdomen and chest wall is important primarily for mechanical protection of the heart and abdominal viscera. Early diagnosis by prenatal ultrasound has not altered the surgical approach or overall mortality of this lesion. Three cases in the Boston Children's Hospital series had severe pulmonary hypoplasia, which was lethal in two reported by Shamberger and Welch (1990), a previously unreported association.

THORACIC DEFORMITIES IN DIFFUSE SKELETAL DISORDERS

Asphyxiating Thoracic Dystrophy (Jeune's Disease)

In 1954, Jeune and colleagues described a newborn with a narrow rigid chest and multiple cartilage anomalies. The patient died of respiratory insufficiency early in the perinatal period. Subsequent authors have further characterized this form of osteochondrodystrophy, which has variable degrees of skeletal involvement. It is inherited in an autosomal recessive pattern and is not associated with chromosomal abnormalities. Its most prominent feature is a narrow, bell-shaped thorax and protuberant abdomen. The thorax is narrow in both the transverse and sagittal axis and has little respiratory

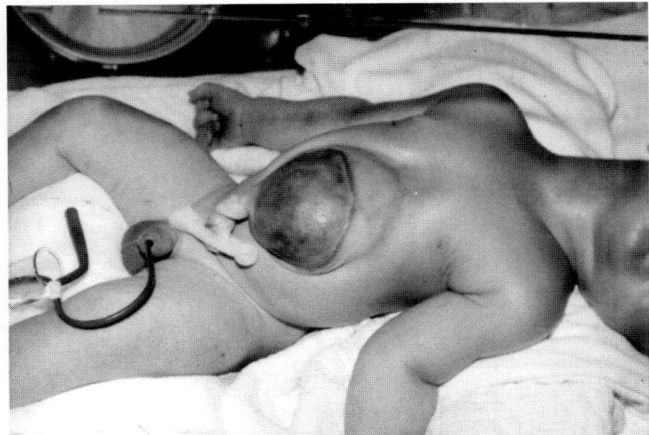

Fig. 40-21. Newborn male with thoracoabdominal ectopia cordis. Note flaring of the lower sternal area merging with a large epigastric omphalocele. The septum transversum and the inferior portion of the pericardium were absent. Tetralogy of Fallot was present.

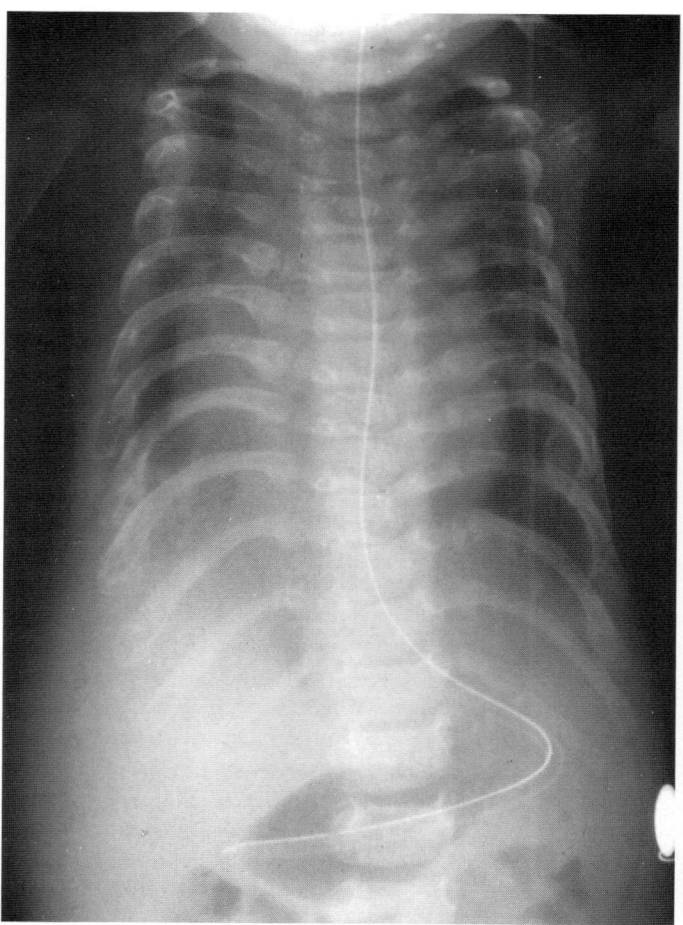

A

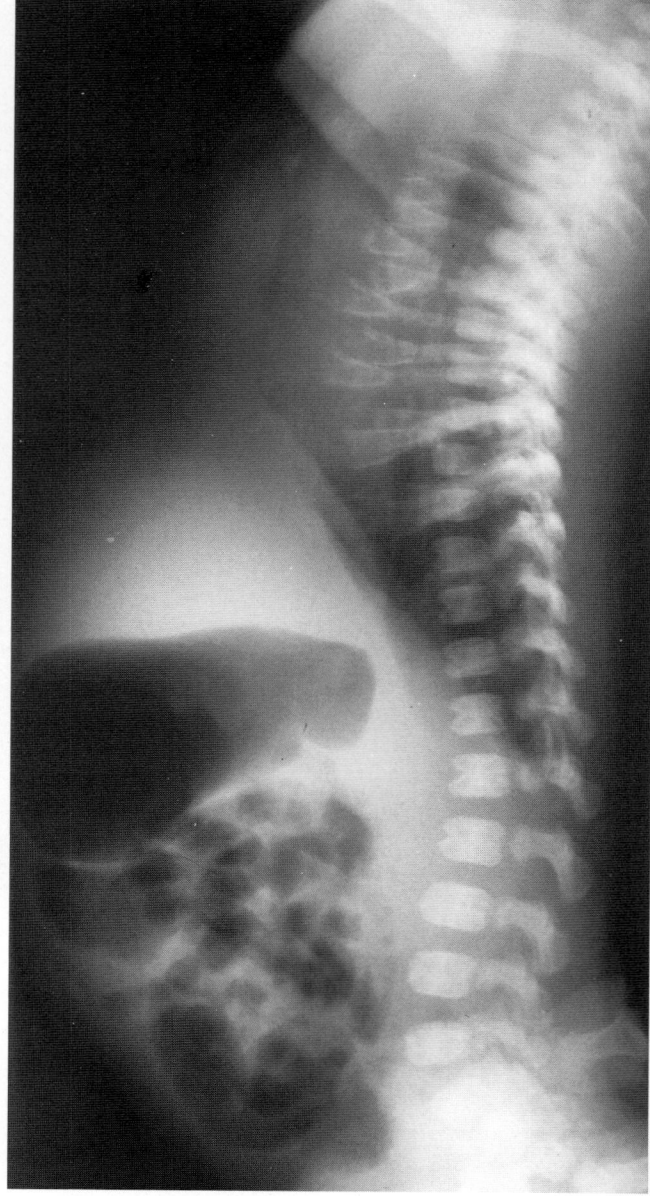

B

Fig. 40-22. Jeune's disease (asphyxiating thoracic dystrophy). **A.** Anteroposterior radiograph shows short horizontal ribs and narrow chest. **B.** Lateral radiograph demonstrates that the short ribs end at the midaxillary line. Abnormal flaring at the costochondral junctions is also present. The patient died of progressive respiratory insufficiency at 1 month of age. There was no surgical intervention. Postmortem examination revealed alveolar hypoplasia.

motion due to the horizontal direction of the ribs (Fig. 40-22). The ribs are short and wide, and the splayed costochondral junctions barely reach the anterior axillary line. The costal cartilage is abundant and irregular, like a rachitic rosary. Microscopic examination of the costochondral junction demonstrates disordered and poorly progressing endochondral ossification, resulting in decreased rib length.

Skeletal abnormalities associated with this syndrome include short stubby extremities with relatively short and wide bones. The clavicles are in a fixed and elevated position, and the pelvis is small and hypoplastic, with square iliac bones.

The syndrome has a variable extent of pulmonary impairment. Although the initial cases reported resulted in neonatal deaths, subsequent reports by Kozlowski and Masel (1976) and others have documented a wide range of survival of children with this syndrome. The pathological findings in autopsy cases reveal a range of abnormal pulmonary development. In most cases, the bronchial development is normal and there are fewer alveolar divisions, as described by Williams and associates (1984).

Spondylothoracic Dysplasia (Jarcho-Levin Syndrome)

Spondylothoracic dysplasia is an autosomal recessive deformity with multiple vertebral and rib malformations, described by Jarcho and Levin in 1938. Infants and children

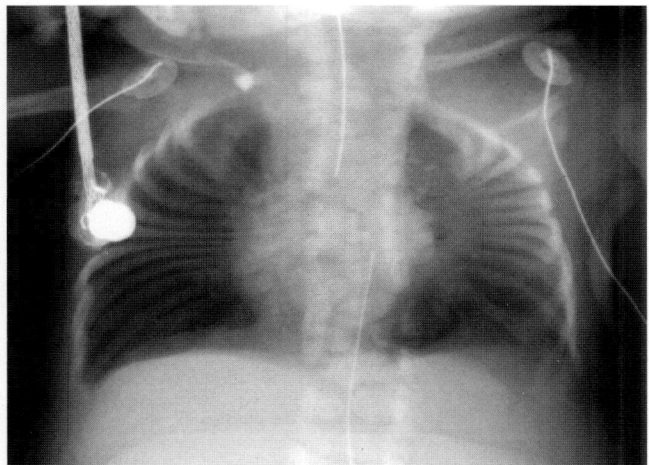

Fig. 40-23. Chest radiograph of an infant with spondylothoracic dysplasia. Severe abnormality of the spine is apparent, with multiple alternating hemivertebrae and "crablike" ribs.

with this syndrome have multiple alternating hemivertebrae in most, if not all, of the thoracic and lumbar spine. The vertebral ossification centers rarely cross the midline, although bone formation is normal. Multiple posterior fusions of the ribs and remarkable shortening of the thoracic spine result in a "crablike" radiographic appearance of the chest (Fig. 40-23).

The thoracic deformity is secondary to the spine anomaly, which results in close posterior approximation of the origin of the ribs. Although most infants with the entity succumb before 15 months of age, as reviewed by Roberts and colleagues (1988), no surgical efforts have been proposed or attempted. One-third of patients with this syndrome have associated malformations, including congenital heart disease and renal anomalies. Heilbronner and Renshaw (1984) have reported its occurrence primarily in Puerto Rican families (15 of 18 cases).

REFERENCES

Pectus Excavatum

Adkins PC, Blades B: A stainless steel strut for correction of pectus excavatum. Surg Gynecol Obstet 113:111, 1961.

Allen RG, Douglas M: Cosmetic improvement of thoracic wall defects using a rapid setting silastic mold: a special technique. J Pediatr Surg 14:745, 1979.

Backer OG, Brünner S, Larsen V: The surgical treatment of funnel chest: initial and follow-up results. Acta Chir Scand 121:253, 1961.

Baronofsky ID: Technique for the correction of pectus excavatum. Surgery 42:884, 1957.

Beiser GD, et al: Impairment of cardiac function in patients with pectus excavatum, with improvement after operative correction. N Engl J Med. 287:267, 1972.

Bevegård S: Postural circulatory changes at rest and during exercise in patients with funnel chest, with special reference to factors affecting the stroke volume. Acta Med Scand 171:695, 1962.

Blickman JG, et al: Pectus excavatum in children: pulmonary scintigraphy before and after corrective surgery. Radiology 156:781, 1985.

Bon Tempo CP, et al: Radiographic appearance of the thorax in systolic click-late systolic murmur syndrome. Am J Cardiol 236:27, 1975.

Brown AL, Cook O: Cardio-respiratory studies in pre and post operative funnel chest (Pectus excavatum). Dis Chest 20:378, 1951.

Cahill JL, Lees GM, Robertson HT: A summary of preoperative and postoperative cardiorespiratory performance in patients undergoing pectus excavatum and carinatum repair. J Pediatr Surg 19:430, 1984.

Castile RG, Staats BA, Westbrook PR: Symptomatic pectus deformities of the chest. Am Rev Respir Dis 126:564, 1982.

Derveaux L, et al: Mechanism of pulmonary function changes after surgical correction for funnel chest. Eur Respir J 1:823, 1988.

Derveaux L, et al: Preoperative and postoperative abnormalities in chest x-ray indices and in lung function in pectus deformities. Chest 95:850, 1989.

Ellis DG, Snyder CL, Mann CM: The "re-do" chest wall deformity correction. J Pediatr Surg 32:1267, 1997.

Garusi GF, D'Ettorre A: Angiocardiographic patterns in funnel-chest. Cardiologia 45:312, 1964.

Gattiker H, Bühlmann A: Cardiopulmonary function and exercise tolerance in supine and sitting position in patients with pectus excavatum. Helv Med Acta 33:122, 1967.

Greig JD, Azmy AF: Thoracic cage deformity: a late complication following repair of an agenesis of diaphragm. J Pediatr Surg 25:1234, 1990.

Haller JA. Severe chest wall constriction from growth retardation after too extensive and too early (<4 years) pectus excavatum repair: an alert. Ann Thorac Surg 60:1857, 1995.

Haller JA, et al: Pectus excavatum: a 20 year surgical experience. J Thorac Cardiovasc Surg 60:375, 1970.

Haller JA, et al: Use of CT scans in selection of patients for pectus excavatum surgery: a preliminary report. J Pediatr Surg 22:904, 1987.

Hecker WC, Procher G, Dietz HG: Results of operative correction of pigeon and funnel chest following a modified procedure of Ravitch and Haller. Z Kinderchir 34:220, 1981.

Hougaard K, Arendrup H: Deformities of the female breasts after surgery for funnel chest. Scand J Thorac Cardiovasc Surg 17:171, 1983.

Howard R: Funnel Chest: its effect on cardiac function. Arch Dis Child 32:5, 1959.

Hümmer HP, Willital GH: Morphologic findings of chest deformities in children corresponding to the Willital-Hümmer classification. J Pediatr Surg 19:562, 1984.

Humphreys GH II, Jaretzki A III: Pectus excavatum: late results with and without operation. J Thorac Cardiovasc Surg 80:686, 1980.

Jensen NK, et al: Pectus excavatum and carinatum: the how, when and why of surgical correction. J Pediatr Surg 5:4, 1970.

Judet J, Judet R: Thorax en entonnoir. Un procédé opératoire. Rev Orthop 40:248, 1954.

Jung A: Le traitement du thorax en entonnoir par le "retournement pédiculé" de la cuvette sterno-chondrale. Mém Acad Chir 82:242, 1956.

Kaguraoka H, et al: Degree of severity of pectus excavatum and pulmonary function in preoperative and postoperative periods. J Thorac Cardiovasc Surg 104:1483, 1992.

Lester CW: The etiology and pathogenesis of funnel chest, pigeon breast, and related deformities of the anterior chest wall. J Thorac Surg 34:1, 1957.

Martinez D, et al: The effect of costal cartilage resection on chest wall development. Pediatr Surg Int 5:170, 1990.

Mead J, et al: Rib cage mobility in pectus excavatum. Am Rev Respir Dis 132:1223, 1985.

Meyer L: Zur chirurgischen behandlung der angeborenen trichterbrust. Verh Berliner Med Gesellschaft 42:364, 1911.

Morshuis W, et al: Pulmonary function before surgery for pectus excavatum and at long-term follow-up. Chest 105:1646, 1994a.

Morshuis WJ, et al: Exercise cardiorespiratory function before and one year after operation for pectus excavatum. J Thorac Cardiovasc Surg 107:1403, 1994b.

Nuss D, Kelly RE, Croitoru DP: A 10 year review of a minimally invasive technique for the correction of pectus excavatum. J Pediatr Surg 33:545, 1998.

Ochsner A, DeBakey M: Chone-chondrosternon: report of a case and review of the literature. J Thorac Surg 8:469, 1939.

Oelsnitz G: Fehlbildungen des brustkorbes. Z Kinderchir 33:229, 1981.

Paltia V, et al: Operative technique in funnel chest: experience in 81 cases. Acta Chir Scand 116:90, 1958.

Peterson RJ, et al: Noninvasive assessment of exercise cardiac function before and after pectus excavatum repair. J Thorac Cardiovasc Surg 90:251, 1985.

Quigley PM, et al: Cardiorespiratory function before and after corrective surgery in pectus excavatum. J Pediatr 128:638, 1996.

Ravitch MM: The operative treatment of pectus excavatum. Ann Surg 129:429, 1949.

Ravitch MM: Congenital deformities of the chest wall and their operative correction. Philadelphia: WB Saunders, 1977.

Rehbein F, Wernicke HH: The operative treatment of the funnel chest. Arch Dis Child 32:5, 1957.

Saint-Mezard G, et al: Prolapsus valvulaire mitral et pectus excavatum: association fortuite ou groupement syndromique? La Presse Médicale 15:439, 1986.

Salomon J, Shah PM, Heinle RA: Thoracic skeletal abnormalities in idiopathic mitral valve prolapse. Am J Cardiol 36:32, 1975.

Sanger PW, Robicsek F, Daugherty HK: The repair of recurrent pectus excavatum. J Thorac Cardiovasc Surg 56:141, 1968.

Sauerbruch F: Die Chirurgie der Brustorgane. Berlin: Springer, 1920, p. 437.

Schaub VF, Wegmann T: Elektrokardiographische veränderungen bei trichterbrust. Cardiologia 24:39, 1954.

Scherer LR, et al: Surgical management of children and young adults with Marfan syndrome and pectus excavatum. J Pediatr Surg 23:1169, 1988.

Schutte J, et al: Distinctive anthropometric characteristics of women with mitral valve prolapse. Am J Med 71:533, 1981.

Shamberger RC, Welch KJ: Cardiopulmonary function in pectus excavatum. Surg Gynecol Obstet 166:383, 1988a.

Shamberger RC, Welch KJ: Surgical repair of pectus excavatum. J Pediatr Surg 23:615, 1988b.

Shamberger RC, et al: Anterior chest wall deformities and congenital heart disease. J Thorac Cardiovasc Surg 96:427, 1988c.

Shamberger RC, Welch KJ, Sanders S: Mitral valve prolapse associated with pectus excavatum. J Pediatr Surg 111:404, 1987.

Shochat SJ, et al: Moiré phototopography in the evaluation of anterior chest wall deformities. J Pediatr Surg 16:353, 1981.

Taguchi K, et al: A new plastic operation for pectus excavatum: sternal turnover surgical procedure with preserved internal mammary vessels. Chest 67:606, 1975.

Tanaka F, et al: Postoperative lung function in patients with funnel chest. J Jpn Assoc Thorac Surg 41:2161, 1993.

Udoshi M, et al: Incidence of mitral valve prolapse in subjects with thoracic skeletal abnormalities—A prospective study. Am Heart J 97:303, 1979.

Wada J, et al: Results of 271 funnel chest operations. Ann Thorac Surg 10:526, 1970.

Waters PM, et al: Scoliosis in children with pectus excavatum and pectus carinatum. J Pediatr Orthop 9:551, 1989.

Weg JG, Krumholz RA, Harkleroad LE: Pulmonary dysfunction in pectus excavatum. Am Rev Respir Dis 96:936, 1967.

Welch KJ: Satisfactory surgical correction of pectus excavatum deformity in childhood: a limited opportunity. J Thorac Surg 36:697, 1958.

Welch KJ, Kearney GP: Abdominal musculature deficiency syndrome: prune belly. J Urol 111:693, 1974.

Welch KJ: Chest wall deformities. In Pediatric Surgery, Holder TM, Ashcraft KW (eds). Philadelphia: WB Saunders, 1980.

Willital GH: Operationsindikation-Operationstechnik bei Brustkorbdeformierungen. Z Kinderchir 33:244, 1981.

Wynn SR, et al: Exercise cardiorespiratory function in adolescents with pectus excavatum. J Thorac Cardiovasc Surg 99:41, 1990.

Pectus Carinatum

Brodkin HA: Congenital chondrosternal prominence (Pigeon breast) a new interpretation. Pediatrics 3:286, 1949.

Brodkin HA: Pigeon breast—Congenital chondrosternal prominence. Arch Surg 77:261, 1958.

Chin EF: Surgery of funnel chest and congenital sternal prominence. Br J Surg 44:360, 1957.

Currarino G, Silverman FN: Premature obliteration of the sternal sutures and pigeon-breast deformity. Radiology 70:532, 1958.

Haje SA, Bowen JR. Preliminary results of orthotic treatment of pectus deformities in children and adolescents. J Pediatr Orthop 12:795, 1992.

Howard R: Pigeon chest (protrusion deformity of the sternum). Med J Aust 2:664, 1958.

Lees RF, Caldicott WJH: Sternal anomalies and congenital heart disease. AJR Am J Roentgenol 124:423, 1975.

Lester CW: Pigeon breast (pectus carinatum) and other protrusion deformities of the chest of developmental origin. Ann Surg 137:482, 1953.

Mielke CH, Winter RB. Pectus carinatum successfully treated with bracing: a case report. Int Orthop 17:350, 1993.

Ravitch MM: Unusual sternal deformity with cardiac symptoms-operative correction. J Thorac Surg 23:138, 1952.

Ravitch, MM: The operative correction of pectus carinatum (pigeon breast). Ann Surg 151:705, 1960.

Robicsek F, et al: The surgical treatment of chondrosternal prominence (pectus carinatum). J Thorac Cardiovasc Surg 45:691, 1963.

Shamberger RC, Welch KJ: Surgical correction of pectus carinatum. J Pediatr Surg 22:48, 1987.

Shamberger RC, Welch KJ: Surgical correction of chondromanubrial deformity (Currarino Silverman Syndrome). J Pediatr Surg 23:319, 1988.

Welch KJ, Vos A: Surgical correction of pectus carinatum (pigeon breast). J Pediatr Surg 8:659, 1973.

Poland's Syndrome

Boaz D, Mace JW, Gotlin RW: Poland's syndrome and leukemia. Lancet 1:349, 1971.

Bouvet JP, et al: Vascular origin of Poland syndrome? A comparative rheographic study of the vascularisation of the arms in eight patients. Eur J Pediatr 128:17, 1978.

Clarkson P: Poland's syndactyly. Guy Hosp Rep 111:335, 1962.

Cobben JM, et al: Poland anomaly in mother and daughter. Am J Med Genet 33:519, 1989.

David TJ: Vascular origin of Poland syndrome? Eur J Pediatr 130:299, 1979.

David TJ: Familial Poland anomaly. J Med Genet 19:293, 1982.

Fontaine G, Ovlaque S: Le syndrome de Poland-Möbius. Arch Fr Pediatr 41:351, 1984.

Freire-Maia N, et al: The Poland Syndrome—Clinical and genealogical data, dermatoglyphic analysis, and incidence. Hum Hered 23:97, 1973.

Froriep R: Beobachtung eines Falles Von Mangel der Brustdrüse. Notizen aus dem Gebiete der Naturund Heilkunde 10:9, 1839.

Haller J, et al: Early reconstruction of Poland's syndrome using autologous rib grafts combined with a latissimus muscle flap. J Pediatr Surg 19:423, 1984.

McGillivray BC, Lowry RB: Poland syndrome in British Columbia: incidence and reproductive experience of affected persons. Am J Med Genet 1:65, 1977.

Ohmori K, Takada H: Correction of Poland's pectoralis major muscle anomaly with latissimus dorsi musculocutaneous flaps. Plast Reconstr Surg 65:400, 1980.

Poland A: Deficiency of the pectoralis muscles. Guy Hosp Rep 6:191, 1841.

Ravitch MM: Atypical deformities of the chest wall—Absence and deformities of the ribs and costal cartilages. Surgery 59:438, 1966.

Shamberger RC, Welch KW, Upton J III: Surgical treatment of thoracic deformity in Poland's syndrome. J Pediatr Surg 24:760, 1989.

Sujansky E, Riccardi VM, Matthew AL: The familial occurrence of Poland syndrome. Birth Defects 13:117, 1977.

Walker JC, Meijer R, Aranda D: Syndactylism with deformity of the pectoralis muscle-Poland's syndrome. J Pediatr Surg 4:569, 1969.

Sternal Clefts

Burton JF: Method of correction of ectopia cordis. Arch Surg 54:79, 1947.

Fischer H: Fissura sterni congenita mit partieller Bauchspalte. Dtsch Z Chir 12:367, 1879.

Maier HC, Bortone F: Complete failure of sternal fusion with herniation of pericardium. J Thorac Surg 18:851, 1949.

Meissner F: Fissura sterni congenita. Zentralbl Chir 89:1832, 1964.

Sabiston DC Jr: The surgical management of congenital bifid sternum with partial ectopia cordis. J Thorac Surg 35:118, 1958.

Shamberger RC, Welch KJ: Sternal defects. Pediatr Surg Int 5:156, 1990.

Thoracic Ectopia Cordis

Amato JT, Cotroneo JV, Gladieri RJ: Repair of complete ectopia cordis [Film]. Presented at the American College of Surgeons Clinical Congress, Chicago, October 23–28, 1988.

Bremer L: Textbook of Embryology. Philadelphia: WB Saunders, 1939.

Cantrell JR, Haller JA, Ravitch MM: A syndrome of congenital defects involving the abdominal wall, sternum, diaphragm, pericardium, and heart. Surg Gynecol Obstet 107:602, 1958.

Cutler GD, Wilens G: Ectopia cordis: report of a case. Am J Dis Child *30*:76, 1925.

Dobell ARC, Williams HB, Long R: Staged repair of ectopia cordis. J Pediatr Surg *17*:353, 1982.

Haynor DR, et al: Imaging of fetal ectopia cordis: roles of sonography and computed tomography. J Ultrasound Med *3*:25, 1984.

Hersh JH, et al: Sternal malformation/vascular dysplasia association. Am J Med Genet *21*:177, 1985.

Higginbottom MC: The amniotic band disruption complex: timing of amniotic rupture and variable spectra of consequent defects. Pediatrics 95:544, 1979.

Kaplan LC, et al: Ectopia cordis and cleft sternum: evidence for mechanical teratogenesis following rupture of the chorion or yolk sac. Am J Med Genet *21*:187, 1985.

King CR: Ectopia cordis and chromosomal errors. Pediatrics *66*:328, 1980.

Kragt H, et al: Case report: prenatal ultrasonic diagnosis and management of ectopia cordis. Eur J Obstet Gynecol Reprod Biol *20*:177, 1985.

Mercer LJ, Petres RE, Smeltzer JS: Ultrasound diagnosis of ectopia cordis. Obstet Gynecol *61*:523, 1983.

Opitz JM: Editorial comment following paper by Hersh et al and Kaplan et al on sternal cleft. Am J Med Genet *21*:201, 1985.

Patten BM: Human Embryology. Toronto: Blakiston, 1946.

Saxena N: Ectopia cordis child surviving; prosthesis fails. Pediatr News *10*:3, 1976.

Say B, Wilsey CE: Chromosome aberration in ectopia cordis (46,XX,17q⁺). Am Heart J *95*:274, 1978.

Stensen N: An unusually early description of the so-called tetralogy of Fallot. *In* Acta Medica et Philosophica Hafnienca, Vol. 1. Edited by T Bartholin, 1671–1672, p. 202. Translated into English by FA Willius Proc Staff Meet Mayo Clin 23:316, 1948.

Stoll SC, Vivier M, Renaud R: A supraumbilical midline raphe with sternal cleft in a 47,XXX woman. Am J Med Genet *27*:229, 1987.

Willius FA: An unusually early description of the so-called tetralogy of Fallot. Proc Staff Meet Mayo Clin *23*:316, 1948.

Thoracoabdominal Ectopia Cordis and Cantrell's Pentalogy

Arndt C: Nabelschnurbruch mit Herzhernie. Operation durch Laparotomie mit tödlichem Ausgang. Centralbl Gynäkol 20;632, 1896.

Cantrell JR, Haller JA, Ravitch MM: A syndrome of congenital defects involving the abdominal wall, sternum, diaphragm, pericardium, and heart. Surg Gynecol Obstet *107*:602, 1958.

Cullerier M: Observation sur un déplacement remarquable du coeur; par M. Deschamps, médecin à Laval. J Général Méd Chir Pharmacie *26*:275, 1806.

Major JW: Thoracoabdominal ectopia cordis. J Thorac Surg *26*:309, 1953.

Wieting: Eine operative behandelte Herzmissbildung. Dtsch Z Chir *114*:293, 1912.

Wilson J: A description of a very unusual formation of the human heart. Philos Trans R Soc Lond Biol Sci 2:346, 1798.

Miscellaneous Conditions

Heilbronner DM, Renshaw TS: Spondylothoracic dysplasia. J Bone Joint Surg *66A*:302, 1984.

Jarcho S, Levin PM: Hereditary malformation of the vertebral bodies. Bull Johns Hopkins Hosp *62*:216, 1938.

Jeune M, et al: Polychondrodystrophie avec blocage thoracique d'evolution fatale. Pediatrie *9*:390, 1954.

Kozlowski K, Masel J: Asphyxiating thoracic dystrophy without respiratory disease: report of two cases of the latent form. Pediatr Radiol *5*:30, 1976.

Roberts AP, et al: Spondylothoracic and spondylocostal dysostosis: hereditary forms of spinal deformity. J Bone Joint Surg *70B*:123, 1988.

Williams AJ, Vawter G, Reid LM: Lung structure in asphyxiating thoracic dystrophy. Arch Pathol Lab Med *108*:658, 1984.

CHAPTER 41

Infections of the Chest Wall

Joseph LoCicero III

Chest wall infections can be categorized either as primary problems arising spontaneously or as secondary infections caused by previous procedures or preexisting disease states. The result is the same, with equally devastating potential complications. Management of such infections may be as simple as administering routine antibiotic therapy or may require multiple and prolonged drainage procedures and complex reconstructive operations. Prompt intervention is essential to minimize serious morbidity.

SKIN AND SOFT TISSUE INFECTIONS

The thorax accounts for one-fifth of the total body surface area and thus can be afflicted with many common, nonspecific soft tissue infections. Furuncles and boils common to any hair-bearing surface frequently occur. Superficial infections often develop in minor injuries and burns of the chest, as they do elsewhere in the body.

Abscesses

Soft tissue abscesses may occur anywhere on the chest wall. They are characterized by the usual signs and symptoms of an abscess anywhere on the body and are rarely associated with an abnormal chest radiograph. Two potentially serious infections specific to the chest wall and involving large potential spaces are subpectoral and subscapular abscesses. These occasionally present as primary infections but more often are secondary to a chronically infected thoracotomy incision. They are characterized by local pain, with or without swelling, combined with fever and leukocytosis. Computed tomography (CT) easily identifies and localizes the problem. Prompt drainage and appropriate antibiotic therapy usually lead to successful resolution. Suction catheters are rarely required because these spaces are obliterated once drained. Occasionally when the abscess is

large, several counterincisions are made to débride and pack the space more completely.

With the worldwide rise in tuberculosis and immigration of people from the Third World to North America, pulmonary tuberculosis may be seen in any thoracic surgical practice. Like scrofula, mycobacteria can cause a soft tissue infection of the chest wall. Hsu and colleagues reviewed its management in 1995. Patients present with a slowly enlarging painless mass on the chest wall. A CT scan is helpful to rule out the possibility of pulmonary involvement. Diagnosis can be made with a diagnostic aspiration of the abscess. Treatment should be combination antituberculous therapy for 6 to 9 months. Surgical débridement is reserved for failures. If the diagnosis is not made before débridement, a broad-spectrum antibiotic should be added. Fungal infections of the chest wall should also receive long-term antibiotic therapy, but radical débridement is a mandatory part of the therapy.

Gangrene

Necrotizing soft tissue infections may occur as a complication of empyema or trauma. These infections frequently begin when the pleural material is drained through the soft tissues either by chest tube or thoracotomy. Pingleton and Jeter (1983) reported extensive synergistic gangrene of the chest wall with *Bacteroides melaninogenicus* and *Streptococcus viridans* after tube thoracostomy for empyema. Delay in recognition led to the patient's demise. LoCicero and Vanecko (1985) reported destruction of the pectoralis major and serratus muscles that was caused by clostridial myonecrosis at the site of a tube thoracostomy in a patient with Boerhaave's syndrome. Radical débridement and daily dressing changes under general anesthesia eventually led to a successful outcome. Viste and colleagues (1997) reported a case of necrotizing infection caused by gastric herniation after laparoscopic fundoplication. Urschel and associates

(1997) reviewed the world literature and found a 90% mortality rate for this devastating problem.

Infections of the head and neck as well as dental manipulation have been identified as sources of necrotizing fasciitis of the chest. Steel (1987) described a case of necrotizing ulceration of the chest wall after dental manipulation; it was successfully treated by surgical débridement and chemotherapy. He noted that the primary suspect organisms were *Streptococcus milleri* and *Bacteroides* species. Nallathambi and colleagues (1987) reviewed the current literature and discovered 28 chest wall and mediastinal infections related to dental manipulation or pharyngeal abscesses. These rapidly progressive, mixed aerobic and anaerobic infections have been associated with a 32% mortality rate. Antibiotic prophylaxis for deep dental manipulations and careful follow-up for any early signs of sepsis are essential.

Early recognition, radical débridement of all involved necrotic tissue, high-dose antibiotic therapy, prolonged ventilatory support, and delayed closure with biologic tissue represent the only salvation for these patients. The antibiotic of choice used to be single-drug treatment with high-dose penicillin, but many organisms of the normal flora above the diaphragm have become resistant to penicillin. Therapy should begin presumptively with a combination that includes penicillin or ampicillin, an aminoglycoside, and clindamycin or metronidazole. Once cultures and susceptibilities are available, the antibiotic regimen should be tailored accordingly.

INFECTIOUS CHEST WALL INVASION

With drug resistance and superinfection during antibiotic therapy, virulent organisms occasionally cause pneumonia that has the capability of direct chest wall invasion. Suchyta and associates (1987) reported a community-acquired chronic *Acinetobacter calcoaceticus* pneumonia with direct chest wall involvement discovered only at autopsy. Yuan and associates (1992) successfully treated a patient with pneumonia and extensive chest wall involvement attributed to *Actinobacillus actinomycetemcomitans*. This patient required high-dose penicillin therapy for 3 months. However, as Hseih and colleagues (1993) point out, *Actinomyces* species (i.e., *israelii, naeslundii,* and *odontolyticus*) infections usually respond to antibiotic (penicillin) therapy, and surgical intervention may not be necessary if pretherapeutic diagnosis can be made.

EMPYEMA NECESSITATIS

Infrequently seen today, the soft tissue infection called empyema necessitatis is caused by an undrained underlying pleural infection. An untreated empyema may eventually burrow through the chest wall and into the subcutaneous tissue of the chest. Suspicion of this entity should be raised by the patient's history and confirmed by physical and radiographic examination of the chest. The soft tissue component may require separate drainage but often resolves with appropriate drainage of the empyema.

MONDOR'S DISEASE

Mondor's disease is a benign condition consisting of localized thrombophlebitis occurring in the superficial veins of the breast and anterior chest wall. The true incidence of this entity is unknown. Reports have been infrequent. Because the condition produces few symptoms and signs, most examples are probably not referred to informed examiners for study.

The earliest description was by Fagge (1869). Williams (1931) attributed the disease to thrombophlebitis, as did Mondor (1939), for whom the condition is named. Most cases occur in women, and frequently no antecedent cause can be found. Radical mastectomy may predispose to the development of this disease, as Herrman (1966) proposed, whereas benign conditions, such as fibrocystic disease, have no association with this entity. In a few instances in which a biopsy was performed, Farrow (1955) described a sclerosing endophlebitis with complete or partial obliteration of the lumen.

Clinically, the disease presents as a cordlike structure in the subcutaneous tissue of the axilla, chest, or abdomen. Its greatest significance may be the possible confusion with inflammatory carcinoma of the breast. It does not tend to recur or lead to thromboembolism. In most subjects, no specific therapy is indicated because it regresses spontaneously.

MISCELLANEOUS INFECTIONS

Several other conditions may manifest as infections of the chest wall. Golladay and associates (1985) noted three benign conditions in 24 children who presented with chest wall masses. These included trichinosis, nodular fasciitis, and myositis ossificans, all confirmed by excisional biopsy. The latter two were almost certainly secondary to localized trauma.

Cartilage and Bony Structures

Tietze's Syndrome

Painful, nonsuppurative swelling of the costal cartilages without abnormal histologic change is referred to as Tietze's syndrome. This condition, which is not a disease, was described in two patients by Tietze (1921), who attributed the changes to tuberculosis. This has never been confirmed. Since his publication, case reports have been sporadic. Kayser (1956), who reviewed the world literature, could find only 156 cases.

The true frequency of this condition is not known, but the symptom complex appears to be common. Peyton (1983) described 76 women in his office practice and 156 men and women visiting an emergency room who complained of this syndrome. Symptoms include chest pain and swelling of the costochondral junction. The junction, usually the second, is usually prominent and is tender to deep palpation. He noted that emotional tension is frequently associated with this symptom complex. In a study by Disla and colleagues (1994), of 122 consecutive patients with chest wall complaints presenting to the emergency room, 30% met criteria for diagnosis of costochondritis and 8% met the American College of Rheumatology criteria for fibromyalgia. After 1 year, 55% of the patients with costochondritis still had symptoms.

Rarely are further tests necessary to confirm this diagnosis, but Edelstein and colleagues (1985) pointed out that CT scan of the chest is helpful to exclude chest wall masses in these patients.

As might be expected for a condition as vague as this, several invasive treatments have been advocated, from hydrocortisone infiltration to surgical removal of the involved area. The latter hardly seems justified. In most patients, reassurance and symptomatic treatment with compounds containing ibuprofen are sufficient.

Costochondritis

Infections of the costal cartilage cause great debility. They are chronic beyond all expectation and thus demoralizing to the patient and the surgeon alike. When recognized and treated properly, response is rapid, but the required treatment is exceedingly radical for what appears to be such a minor problem. This often leads to delay in appropriate management. Recognizing the basic problem, Moschowitz (1918) pointed out that chronicity resulted less from the type of infecting organism than from the avascular nature of the cartilage. He correctly urged removal of the cartilage for cure.

Before 1940, most chondritis was spontaneous, usually caused by tuberculosis. Some cases were caused by typhoid or paratyphoid fever. Today most infections are surgical complications. Most follow median sternotomy performed for cardiac procedures; some follow thoracotomy, tube thoracostomy, or chest wall trauma. Occasionally, fungal infections may burrow through the chest wall to cause chondritis.

Because the fifth to ninth costal cartilages are contiguous or fused, infections involving any one of these segments dictate a major resection for cure. The xiphoid is partially a cartilaginous structure and thus may promote bilateral spread of the infection. This avascular hyaline cartilage behaves like a foreign body, once infected. When free of perichondrium, it begins to take on a moth-eaten appearance in the depths of a draining wound. The disintegration of the cartilage occurs slowly, but the cartilage is never completely reabsorbed. Sequestra that are characteristic of chronic osteomyelitis do not classically form in chondritis. The car-

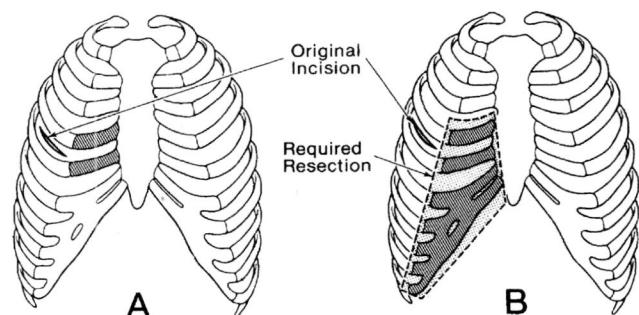

Fig. 41-1. Cartilage resection necessary for proper treatment of costochondritis. **A.** Initial incision and costal involvement. **B.** Delay may lead to secondary costal arch involvement, necessitating arch removal.

tilage remains exposed and unmoved in the depths of the narrow, granulating wound.

Many organisms have been cultured from costochondritis. The primary infecting organisms include *Escherichia coli, Streptococcus pneumoniae, Pseudomonas aeruginosa, Mycobacterium tuberculosis*, staphylococci, streptococci, and *Nocardia*. Once the wound is opened and drained, subsequent cultures may grow a variety of organisms, depending on the environment and the antibiotic regimen the patient is receiving.

Usually, the disease manifests as a draining sinus in the region of the cartilages. Local pain and tenderness are present. As with any other chronic infection, general debility and, perhaps, low-grade fever accompany an elevated white cell count. In most patients, the diagnosis is confirmed by tenderness over the cartilages and infection in the vicinity.

The preferred therapy is radical excision, as Murphy (1916) and Moschowitz (1918) advocated. Any involved cartilage should be removed completely (Fig. 41-1). If the lower ribs are involved, all fused segments must be excised. No bare cartilage should remain in the infected wound. The more conservative approach is to pack the wound and reconstruct it later, as Lewis (1967) and Talucci and Webb (1983) advocated. Others, such as Hines and Lee (1983) and Arnold and Pairolero (1984), have shown that the defect may be closed in one stage with minimal morbidity. Techniques of reconstruction are discussed later in the chapter.

Osteomyelitis

Sternal Osteomyelitis

Although spontaneously appearing osteomyelitis of the sternum or ribs did occur when tuberculosis was prevalent, it is rare today. Even when tuberculosis was more common, osteomyelitis of the sternum was uncommon. In a series of more than 1000 patients with bone and joint tuberculosis reported by Wassersug (1941), the sternum was involved in only 1.1%. Today, primary sternal osteomyelitis occurs in heroin addicts. More often, secondary infections, usually

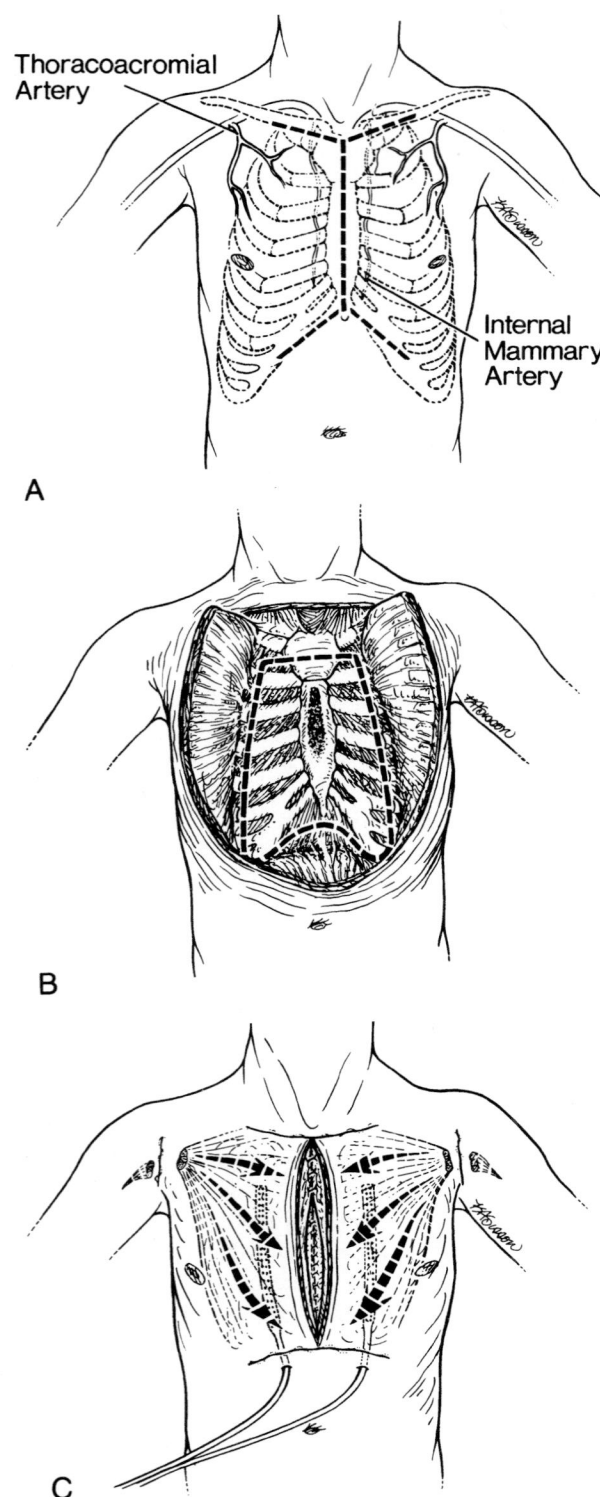

Fig. 41-2. Depiction of one-stage operation for chronic sternal osteomyelitis. **A.** The H-shaped incision used to expose the sternum and costal cartilages. **B.** Bilateral pectoralis major myocutaneous flaps have been raised. The extent of the planned resection is shown. **C.** Humeral detachment of the pectoralis muscles with advancement and closure over suction drains. From Johnson P, et al: Management of chronic sternal osteomyelitis. Ann Thorac Surg *40*:69, 1985. With permission.

after cardiac surgical procedures, are the etiologic factors. Ochsner and associates (1972) noted a 1.5% infection rate with an overall 10% mortality. Rates today are similar.

The factors implicated in the development of postoperative sternal infections, enumerated by Talamonti and associates (1987), include diabetes, low cardiac output, use of bilateral internal thoracic artery grafts, and, most significantly, reoperation for excessive postoperative bleeding.

Manifestations of this condition are similar to those of chondritis. When osteomyelitis involves the sternum, an associated chondritis may occur, which can be mistaken for the principal cause of chronicity. The first sign of postoperative sternal osteomyelitis may be an unstable sternum or serosanguineous discharge.

In chronic sternal osteomyelitis, the most successful results have been achieved by extensive sternal and chondral removal followed by myocutaneous reconstruction. The most commonly used reconstruction is bilateral pectoralis major flap advancement, as described by Johnson and associates (1985). A modified H incision is used to mobilize the pectoralis major muscles, with the blood supply based on the thoracoacromial artery (Fig. 41-2A). This also allows adequate exposure of the sternum, which is then excised (Fig. 41-2B). If possible, the upper manubrium with the clavicular attachments is left intact. This prevents skeletal problems as the shoulders rotate anteriorly and inferiorly. Next, the humeral heads of the pectoralis major muscles are transected, and the flaps are advanced over drains to close the defect (Fig. 41-2C). This gives a good cosmetic result with preservation of pulmonary function.

Rib Osteomyelitis

Diagnosis of osteomyelitis of the ribs is usually made because of local inflammatory signs and symptoms or because of a persistently draining sinus. When the infection is secondary to open drainage of an empyema, it can be one cause of a slowly healing wound. Sequestration from ribs affected by osteomyelitis has been reported. The sequestrum may even pass into the lungs, as Roe and Benioff (1955) noted.

Confirmation is usually made by chest radiography. Although CT scanning of the chest is usually not necessary for confirmation of the diagnosis, it may help in evaluating possible underlying associated intrathoracic pathology, as suggested by Wechsler and Steiner (1989).

Excision of all diseased bone usually provides adequate treatment for osteomyelitis of the ribs. To prevent the problem after empyema drainage, Churchill (1929) recommended a clean division of the ribs, leaving no rib exposed or unprotected by periosteum. Occasionally, extensive excision may be required. In patients in whom the infection is overwhelming and an extensive excision is required, mechanical ventilation may be necessary until the infection is obliterated and reconstruction can be safely attempted.

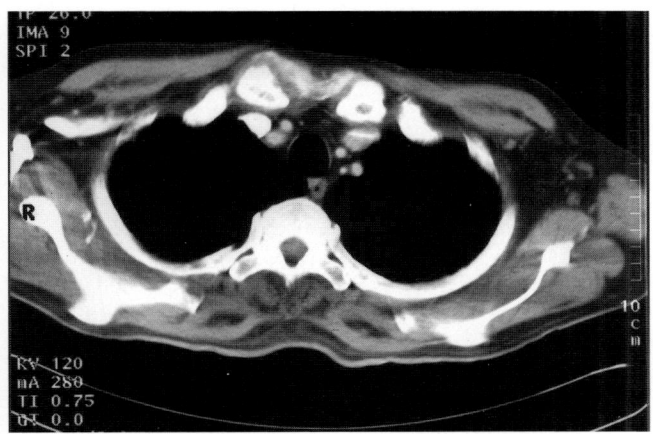

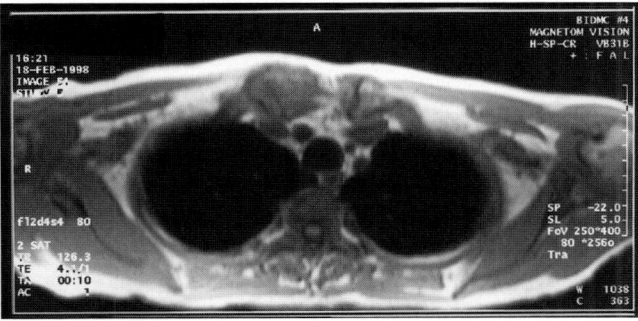

Fig. 41-3. Computed tomographic (CT) and magnetic resonance (MR) imaging scans of a patient with sternoclavicular osteomyelitis. The changes on CT scan are subtler than the changes seen on MR imaging. **A.** The CT scan shows the right sternoclavicular joint with some minimal swelling around it and bony erosion that looks nearly the same as the opposite side. **B.** The MR imaging is more striking, with obliteration of the cartilage of the clavicular head with striking soft tissue involvement.

Sternoclavicular Osteomyelitis

Sternoclavicular osteomyelitis is a relatively new problem that occurs not only in addicts but also in individuals who have had subclavian catheters, as well as in patients with no known antecedent interventions. However, the latter group is usually ill, either with a chronic debilitating illness such as diabetes mellitus or liver failure or an overwhelming acute illness such as sepsis from a remote site.

The inciting organisms vary widely, depending on the etiology. In my experience, both gram-positive organisms, such as *Staphylococcus* and group B streptococcus, and gram-negative organisms cause these infections. Buescher and colleagues (1994) recorded a case of aspergillus infection in a patient undergoing chemotherapy for acute myelogenous leukemia. An interesting report by Berrocal and associates (1993) from Peru found seven cases of brucellar sternoclavicular arthritis among 1729 cases of primary brucellosis.

These patients present with fever and severe unremitting pain in the joint. Some patients even demonstrate instability of the joint and have difficulty lifting objects and even writing in severe cases. Routine radiographs are not helpful.

Even CT scans may be of little help. These scans may not show much bony destruction because the damage begins in the joint (Fig. 41-3A). The condition must be inferred from the surrounding soft tissue involvement. Magnetic resonance imaging is a much more sensitive tool than CT for detecting joint disease and therefore presents a more dramatic image (Fig. 41-3B). The joint as well as the soft tissue swelling is more clearly defined.

Treatment requires the same radical débridement as other cases reported here. To remove the joint completely and any possibility of recurrence, one must bear in mind that the sternoclavicular joint is contiguous with the clavicle, sternum, and first rib. This area should be removed en bloc. To create the best closure, I have found that removal of a portion of the second rib is helpful, whether it is involved or not. A trapdoor incision is made beginning above the clavicle, extending to the midline, down the midline, and across the anterior chest below the disease, usually the third rib. A flap is made, including the pectoralis muscle. Sometimes, it is involved in the infection and a portion must be sacrificed, but every effort should be made to salvage as much of it as possible. The internal thoracic artery and vein are ligated above the third rib. The platysma and scalene muscles are divided above and the sternum is bisected to the third rib. The second and third ribs are divided beyond the infection, and the clavicle is cut in half or more. The first rib is cleared at this point and divided. The specimen is removed and cultures taken before sending the specimen to the pathology laboratory. Closed suction drains are placed, and the flap is advanced into place with interrupted sutures. Foreign material or mesh should be avoided. The long-term result is excellent for both infection control and chest wall function (Fig. 41-4).

Osteoradionecrosis

One of the most difficult problems encountered by the thoracic surgeon is a large necrotic ulcer of the chest wall after radiation therapy for carcinoma of the breast or other condition. Often, more infection and necrosis exist than are visible externally. Prosthetic materials usually cannot be used in the infected field. With radiation becoming a standard in the minimal surgical techniques of breast cancer, and despite all the precautions taken by radiation therapists, these problems are on the rise. Treatment requires close cooperation between the thoracic surgeon and the plastic and reconstructive surgeon.

The foremost principle in the treatment of a radionecrotic ulcer is wide surgical excision and primary coverage of the defect, as Arnold and Pairolero (1984, 1989) described. Tissue of the affected area should be sent for pathologic analysis when radiation was performed for a local malignancy to ensure that no residual tumor is present.

Provisions for covering the expected defect with viable tissue must be carefully considered before the surgical procedure. Understanding and use of myocutaneous flaps have advanced. Jurkiewicz and colleagues (1980) described a variety of flaps, including pectoralis major, rectus abdo-

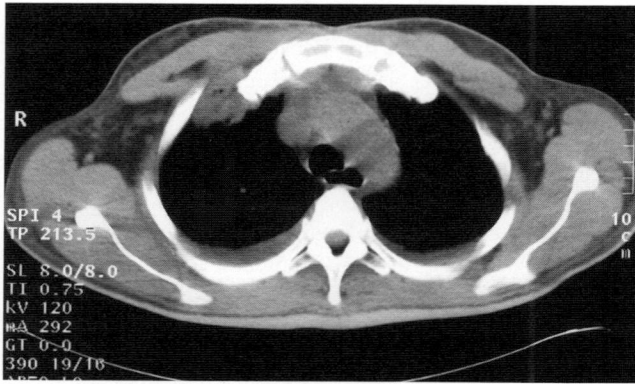

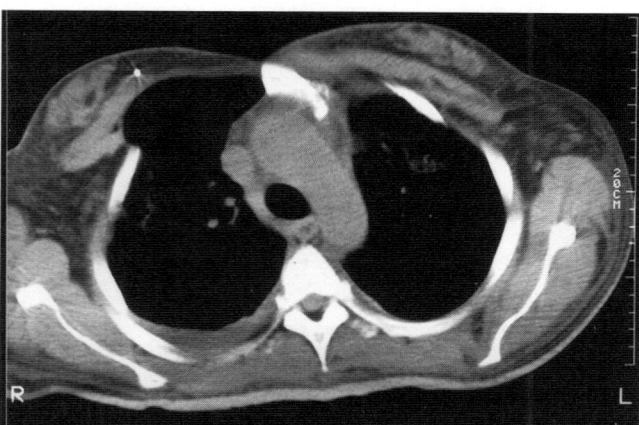

Fig. 41-4. Before and after computed tomographic scans of a patient with sternoclavicular osteomyelitis. **A.** Subtle bony changes are associated with soft tissue fluid collection. **B.** Two years after resection and primary closure, the hemisternum is healed, and the pectoralis muscle covers the defect to the midline.

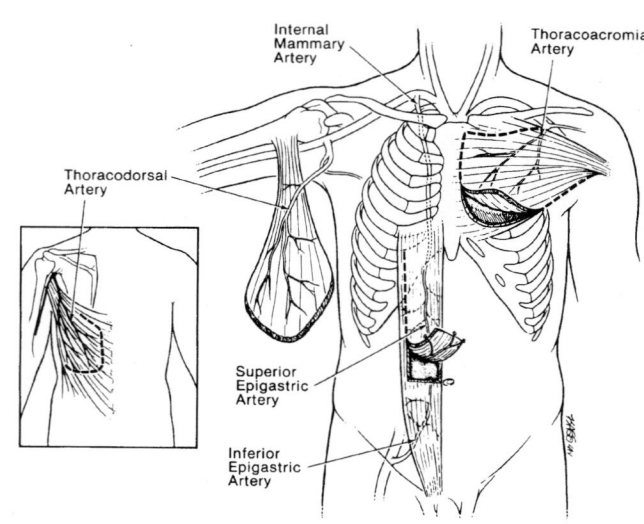

Fig. 41-5. Representation of the most common myocutaneous muscle flaps with their individual blood supply used for chest wall reconstruction.

minis, and latissimus dorsi flaps (Fig. 41-5). Other innovative flaps include segmentally split pectoral girdle flaps [proposed by Tobin (1990)] and free extended forearm flaps [suggested by Schmidt and colleagues (1987)].

The latissimus flap was first described by Tansini (1906) but was rediscovered by McCraw and colleagues (1978). Hines and Lee (1983) used this flap in five patients and noted that even if the primary blood supply—the thoracodorsal artery—was cut at the time of initial mastectomy, collateral blood supply appeared adequate. They also pointed out that the muscle, albeit smaller and thinner when the thoracodorsal nerve has been resected, remains usable. Within the past few years, plastic and reconstructive surgeons have applied microvascular techniques to this flap. Free flaps have been used with great success, with and without the associated skin as well as inside the chest, as reported by Hammond and associates (1993) and outside the chest as described by Hidalgo and colleagues (1993).

In most instances, foreign material should be avoided when infection is present. Usually, the resulting paradoxical movement of the chest wall in these patients is minimally debilitat-

ing and not worth the risk of secondary infection. Myocutaneous flaps have been beneficial when a large portion of the chest wall or sternum must be removed (see Chapter 46).

IMMUNOCOMPROMISED PATIENTS

Patients who are immunocompromised because of malignancy, malnutrition, or human immunodeficiency virus infection present special problems. In granulocytopenic patients, findings of severe chest wall infections may be subtle. Aranha and coworkers (1988) recommend antibiotic therapy and surgical débridement with the early findings of erythema, localized tenderness, and temperature elevation. Golladay and Baker (1987) note that in immunocompromised children, invasive aspergillosis is the offending infection one-third of the time, with high mortality rates even with early aggressive intervention.

In patients infected with human immunodeficiency virus, common organisms often cause serious chest wall infection. Martos and colleagues (1989) reported two cases of tuberculosis of the chest wall. Rodriguez-Barradas and associates (1992) found chest wall infections related to pneumococcal pneumonia. Despite the uniformly fatal nature of the underlying disease, standard surgical principles of aggressive débridement and antibiotic therapy result in gratifyingly good long-term results.

REFERENCES

Arnold PG, Pairolero PC: Intrathoracic muscle flaps: a 10-year experience in the management of life threatening infections. Plast Reconstruct Surg *84*:92, 1989.

Aranha GV, et al: Soft tissue infections in the compromised host. Am Surg *54*:463, 1988.

Berrocal A, et al: Sternoclavicular brucellar arthritis: a report of 7 cases and a review of the literature. J Rheumatol 20:1184, 1993.

Buescher TM, et al: Resection of the chest wall and central veins for invasive cutaneous aspergillus infection in an immunocompromised patient. Chest 105:1283, 1994.

Churchill E: The technic of rib resection and osteomyelitis of the rib ends. JAMA 92:644, 1929.

Disla E, et al. Costochondritis. A prospective analysis in an emergency department setting. Arch Intern Med 154:2466, 1994.

Edelstein G, et al: CT observation of rib abnormalities: spectrum of findings. J Comput Assist Tomogr 9:65, 1985.

Fagge CH: Remarks on certain cutaneous affections: with cases. Guy Hosp Rep 15:259, 1869.

Farrow JH: Thrombophlebitis of the superficial veins of the breast and anterior chest wall (Mondor's disease). Surg Gynecol Obstet 101:63, 1955.

Golladay ES, Baker SB: Invasive aspergillosis in children. J Pediatr Surg 22:504, 1987.

Golladay ES, et al: Chest wall masses in children. South Med J 78:292, 1985.

Hammond DC, et al: Intrathoracic free flaps. Plast Reconstr Surg 91:1259, 1993.

Herrman JB: Thrombophlebitis of breast and contiguous thoracoabdominal wall (Mondor's disease). NY State J Med 66:3146, 1966.

Hidalgo DA, et al: Free flap chest wall reconstruction for recurrent breast cancer and radiation ulcers. Ann Plast Surg 30:375, 1993.

Hines GL, Lee G: Osteoradionecrosis of the chest wall: management of post resection defects using Marlex mesh and a rotated latissimus dorsi: myocutaneous flap. Am Surg 49:608, 1983.

Hseih MJ, et al: Thoracic actinomycosis. Chest 104:366, 1993.

Hsu HS, et al: Management of primary chest wall tuberculosis. Scand J Thorac Cardiovasc Surg 29:119, 1995.

Johnson P, et al: Management of chronic sternal osteomyelitis. Ann Thorac Surg 40:69, 1985.

Jurkiewicz MJ, et al: Infected median sternotomy wound: successful treatment by muscle flaps. Ann Surg 191:738, 1980.

Kayser HL: Tietze's syndrome: a review of the literature. Am J Med 21:982, 1956.

Lewis FJ: Chondritis as a postoperative complication. Lancet 87:247, 1967.

LoCicero J, Vanecko RM: Clostridial myonecrosis of the chest wall complicating spontaneous esophageal rupture. Ann Thorac Surg 40:396, 1985.

Martos JA, et al: Chondrocostal and chondrosternal tuberculosis in two heroin addicts infected with human immunodeficiency virus. Med Clin (Barc) 93:467, 1989.

McCraw JB, Penix JO, Baker JW: Repair of major defects of chest wall and spine with a latissimus dorsi myocutaneous flap. Plast Reconstr Surg 62:197, 1978.

Mondor MH: Tronculite soucutane subaigue de la paroi thoracique anteolaterale. Mem Acad Chir 65:1271, 1939.

Moschowitz A: The treatment of diseases of the costal cartilages. Ann Surg 68:168, 1918.

Murphy JB: Bone and joint diseases in relation to typhoid fever. Surg Gynecol Obstet 23:119, 1916.

Nallathambi MN, et al: Craniocervical necrotizing fasciitis: critical factors in management. Can J Surg 30:61, 1987.

Ochsner JL, Mills NL, Woolverton WC: Disruption and infection of the median sternotomy incision. J Cardiovasc Surg 13:394, 1972.

Peyton FW: Unexpected frequency of idiopathic costochondral pain. Obstet Gynecol 62:605, 1983.

Pingleton SK, Jeter J: Necrotizing fasciitis as a complication of tube thoracostomy. Chest 83:925, 1983.

Rodriguez-Barradas MC, et al: Unusual manifestations of pneumococcal infection in human immunodeficiency virus-infected individuals: past revisited. Clin Infect Dis 14:192, 1992.

Roe BB, Benioff MA: Late hemoptysis from rib sequestrum thirty-four years following empyema drainage. Surgery 38:764, 1955.

Schmidt RG, et al: Chest wall reconstruction with a free extended forearm flap: a case report. J Reconstr Microsurg 3:189, 1987.

Steel A: An unusual case of necrotizing fasciitis. Br J Oral Maxillofac Surg 25:328, 1987.

Suchyta MR, et al: Chronic Acinetobacter calcoaceticus var anitratus pneumonia. Am J Med Sci 294:117, 1987.

Talamonti MS, et al: Early re-exploration for excessive postoperative hemorrhage lowers wound complication rates in open heart surgery. Am J Surg 53:102, 1987.

Talucci RC, Webb WR: Costal chondritis of the costal arch. Ann Thorac Surg 35:318, 1983.

Tansini I: Sopra il mio nuovo processo di amputazione dell mammella. Riforma Medica (Palermo) 12:757, 1906.

Tietze A: Ueber eine eigenartige Haufung von Fallen mit Dystrophie der Rippenknorpel. Berl Klin Wochenschr 58:829, 1921.

Tobin GR: Segmentally split pectoral girdle muscle flaps for chest wall and intrathoracic reconstruction. Clin Plast Surg 17:683, 1990.

Urschel JD, et al: Necrotizing soft tissue infection of the chest wall. Ann Thorac Surg 64:276, 1997.

Viste A, et al: Herniation of the stomach and necrotizing chest wall infection following laparoscopic Nissen fundoplication. Surg Endosc 11:1029, 1997.

Wassersug JD: Tuberculosis of the sternum. N Engl J Med 225:445, 1941.

Wechsler RJ, Steiner RM: Cross sectional imaging of the chest wall. J Thorac Imaging 4:29, 1989.

Williams GA: Thoraco-epigastric phlebitis producing dyspnea. JAMA 96:2196, 1931.

Yuan A, et al: Actinobacillus actinomycetemcomitans pneumonia with chest wall involvement and rib destruction. Chest 101:1450, 1992.

READING REFERENCES

Arnold PG, Pairolero PC: Chest wall reconstruction: experience with 100 consecutive patients. Ann Surg 199:725, 1984.

Culliford AT, et al: Sternal and costochondral infections following open heart surgery. J Thorac Cardiovasc Surg 72:714, 1976.

CHAPTER 42

Thoracic Outlet Syndrome

Harold C. Urschel, Jr.

Thoracic outlet syndrome consists of compression of the subclavian vessels and brachial plexus at the superior aperture of the thorax. It was designated previously according to presumed etiologies, such as scalenus anticus, costoclavicular, hyperabduction, cervical rib, and first rib syndromes. The various syndromes are similar, and the specific compression mechanism is often difficult to identify; however, the first rib seems to be a common denominator against which most compressive factors operate.

The symptoms are neurologic, vascular, or mixed, depending on which component is compressed. Occasionally, the pain is atypical in distribution and severity and is experienced predominantly in the chest wall and parascapular area, simulating angina pectoris.

Diagnosis of the nerve compression group can be objectively substantiated by determining the ulnar nerve conduction velocity. In the vascular compression group, diagnosis is usually established clinically, rarely requiring the use of angiography.

The ulnar nerve conduction velocity test (UNCV), as described by Jebson (1967) and Caldwell and associates (1971) has widened the clinical recognition of this syndrome and has improved diagnosis, selection of treatment, and assessment of therapeutic results.

Physiotherapy to improve posture, strengthen shoulder girdle muscles, and stretch neck muscles is used initially in most cases of thoracic outlet syndrome and is often successful in cases of mild compression. Surgical treatment involves extirpation of the first rib, usually through the transaxillary approach, and is for cases of severe compression that have not responded to medical therapy.

ANATOMIC CONSIDERATIONS

The subclavian vessels and brachial plexus traverse the cervicoaxillary canal to reach the upper extremity. The outer border of the first rib divides this canal into a proximal division triangle. This proximal division is composed of the sca-

lene triangle and the space bounded by the clavicle and the first rib (the costoclavicular space). The distal division comprises the axilla. The proximal division is the most critical for neurovascular compression. It is bounded superiorly by the clavicle and the subclavius muscle; inferiorly by the first rib; anteromedially by the border of the sternum, the clavipectoral fascia, and the costocoracoid ligament; and posterolaterally by the scalenus medius muscle and the long thoracic nerve. The scalenus anticus, inserting on the scalene tubercle of the first rib, divides the costoclavicular space into two compartments: an anterior compartment, containing the subclavian vein, and a posterior compartment, containing the subclavian artery and brachial plexus. The axilla, which is the outer division of the cervicoaxillary canal, with its underlying structures, including the pectoralis minor muscle, the coracoid process, and the head of the humerus, is also an area of potential compression.

Compression Factors

Many factors can cause compression of the neurovascular bundle at the thoracic outlet. The basic factor, which was pointed out by Rosati and Lord (1961), is deranged anatomy, to which congenital, traumatic, and atherosclerotic factors may contribute (Table 42-1).

Bony abnormalities are present in approximately 30% of patients, either as a cervical rib, a bifid first rib, fusion of first and second ribs, clavicular deformities, or previous thoracoplasty.

Pathologic changes in the configuration of the cervicoaxillary canal alter the normal functional dynamics and serve as the basis of the clinical maneuvers used in the diagnosis of thoracic outlet syndrome.

Adson or Scalene Test

The Adson or scalene test, described by Adson in 1951, tightens the anterior and middle scalene muscles, thus

Table 42-1. Etiologic Factors in Thoracic Outlet Syndrome

Anatomic
   Potential sites of neurovascular compression
      Interscalene triangle
      Costoclavicular space
      Subcoracoid area
   Congenital
      Cervical rib and its fascial remnants
      Rudimentary first thoracic rib
      Scalenus muscles
         Anterior
         Middle
         Minimus
   Adventitious fibrous bands
      Bifid clavicle
      Exostosis of first thoracic rib
      Enlarged transverse process of C7
      Omohyoid muscle
      Anomalous course of transverse cervical artery
      Brachial plexus posterior fixation
      Flat clavicle
   Traumatic
      Fracture of clavicle
      Dislocation of head of humerus
      Crushing injury to upper thorax
      Sudden, unaccustomed muscular efforts involving shoulder girdle muscles
      Cervical spondylosis and injuries to cervical spine
Atherosclerosis

decreasing the interscalene space and magnifying any preexisting compression of the subclavian artery and brachial plexus. The patient is instructed to 1) take and hold a deep breath, 2) extend his or her neck fully, and 3) turn his or her face toward the side. Obliteration or diminution in the radial pulse suggests compression.

Costoclavicular Test: Military Position

In the costoclavicular test, the shoulders are drawn downward and backward. This maneuver narrows the costoclavicular space by approximating the clavicle to the first rib, thus tending to compress the neurovascular bundle. Changes in the radial pulse with production of symptoms indicate compression.

Hyperabduction Test

When the arm is hyperabducted to 180 degrees, the components of the neurovascular bundle are pulled around the pectoralis minor tendon, coracoid process, and the head of the humerus. If the radial pulse decreases, compression should be suspected.

Arm Claudication Test

In the arm claudication test, the shoulders are drawn upward and backward. The arms are raised to the horizontal position with the elbows flexed 90 degrees. With exercises

of the hands, numbness or pain is experienced in the hands and forearms if compression is present.

SIGNS AND SYMPTOMS

The symptoms of thoracic outlet syndrome depend on whether the nerves or blood vessels, or both, are compressed at the thoracic outlet.

My associates and I (1971 and 1972) observed that symptoms of nerve compression occur most frequently, pain and paresthesia being present in about 95% of patients and motor weakness in approximately 10%. Pain and paresthesia are segmental in 75% of cases, with 90% occurring in the ulnar nerve distribution. Pain is usually insidious in onset and commonly involves the neck, shoulder, arm, and hand. In some patients, the pain is atypical, involving the anterior chest wall or the parascapular area, and is termed *pseudoangina* because it simulates angina pectoris. As my associates and I (1973) reported, these patients have normal coronary arteriograms and decreased ulnar nerve conduction velocities, strongly suggesting the diagnosis of thoracic outlet syndrome. The usual shoulder, arm, and hand symptoms that might have provided the clue for the diagnosis of thoracic outlet syndrome are initially either absent or minimal compared to the severity of the chest pain. Without a high index of suspicion, the diagnosis of thoracic outlet syndrome is frequently overlooked, and many of these patients become "cardiac cripples" without an appropriate diagnosis or develop severe psychological depression when told that their coronary arteries are normal and that they have no significant cause for their pain.

The two distinct groups of patients with pseudoangina are as follows. Group I patients have symptoms and clinical findings that suggest angina pectoris but have normal coronary arteriograms and significant depression of ulnar nerve conduction velocity. Group II patients have both significant coronary artery disease, as evidenced by 75% or greater stenosis in one or more of the major coronary arteries on coronary arteriography, and thoracic outlet syndrome, as evidenced by depression of ulnar nerve conduction velocity. A high index of suspicion of thoracic outlet disease in such individuals must be maintained so that the appropriate methods of diagnosis and management can be exercised. Objective laboratory tests that are important for differentiating these two groups of patients include electrocardiogram, exercise stress tests, coronary arteriogram, electromyography, UNCV, cine esophagram, and radiographs of the chest.

To understand the symptomatic overlap between coronary artery disease and this atypical manifestation of the thoracic outlet syndrome (i.e., pseudoangina), it is necessary to review the neuroanatomy, innervation, and pain pathways of the arm, chest wall, and heart.

At least two types of pain pathways are present in the arm. These are the commonly acknowledged C5–T1 cutaneous "more superficial" fibers and the T2–T5 afferent spinal fibers, which travel with the sympathetic nerves and transmit "deeper" painful stimuli from the ulnar median and parascapular distribution, as reported by Kuntz (1951). The cell bodies of the two types of afferent neurons are situated in the dorsal root ganglia of the corresponding spinal segments. They synapse in the dorsal gray matter of the spinal cord and the axons of the second-order neurons, cross the midline, and ascend in the spinothalamic tract to the brain.

Compression of the "superficial" C8–T1 cutaneous afferent fibers elicits stimuli that are transmitted to the brain and recognized as integumentary pain or paresthesias in the ulnar nerve distribution. In contrast, compression of the predominantly "deeper" sensory fibers elicits impulses that are interpreted by the brain as deep pain originating in the arm or referred to the chest wall.

The pseudoangina experienced in thoracic outlet compression shares with angina pectoris the same dermatomal distribution, in that the heart, arm, and chest wall have afferent fibers convergent on T2–T5 spinal cord segments and cell bodies that are located in the corresponding dorsal root ganglia. Referred pain to the chest wall is a component of both pseudoangina and angina pectoris. Because somatic pain is more common than visceral pain, the brain interprets activity arriving in a given pathway as a pain stimulus in a particular somatic area.

Two theories attempt to explain the mechanism of referred pain from the heart or arm stimuli to chest wall. The convergence theory holds that somatic and visceral afferents converge on the same spinothalamic neurons; when the same pathway is stimulated by activity in visceral afferents, the signal reaching the brain is the same and the pain is projected to the somatic area. The facilitation effort theory holds that because of subliminal fringe effects, incoming impulses from visceral structures (e.g., heart) lower the threshold of spinothalamic neurons receiving afferents from somatic areas. Thus, minor activity in the pain pathways from the somatic areas (activity that would normally die out in the spinal cord) passes on to the brain and is interpreted as somatic pain rather than pain in the viscera, where the stimulus was initiated.

Symptoms of vascular compression in thoracic outlet syndrome, much less common than those of neurologic compression, include coldness, weakness, easy fatigability of the arm and hand, and pain that is usually more diffuse in distribution. Raynaud's phenomenon is occasionally noted. Venous compression is recognized by edema, venous distention, and discoloration of the arm and hand. Thrombosis of the subclavian vein ("effort thrombosis" or Paget-Schroetter syndrome) is infrequently noted but was described by Lang in 1962.

Objective physical findings, in contrast, are more common in patients with primarily vascular rather than neural compression. Loss or diminution of radial pulse and reproduction of symptoms can be elicited with Adson's test, costoclavicular (military) position, and hyperabduction maneuvers in most patients with vascular compression. Other possible findings are venous distention and edema, trophic changes, Raynaud's phenomenon, temperature changes, subclavian vein thrombosis, and even arterial occlusion and claudication. In cases of neural compression, the objective neurologic findings, which

occur less frequently, consist of hypoesthesia, anesthesia, and occasional muscular weakness or atrophy.

DIAGNOSIS

The basic diagnostic considerations for thoracic outlet syndrome include the history and physical examination, radiographs of the chest and cervical spine, neurologic consultation, electromyography, and UNCV. On occasion, a cervical myelogram, coronary angiogram, and venograms may be necessary to elicit the diagnosis.

Cardinal for the establishment of the thoracic outlet diagnosis in pseudoangina is the elimination of the possibility of significant coronary artery disease by submaximal exercise stress testing and coronary arteriography when indicated. Subsequently, after excluding pulmonary, esophageal, and chest wall causes, the diagnosis of thoracic outlet syndrome must be entertained and established by the appropriate clinical evaluation and the slowing of the ulnar nerve conduction velocity.

Nerve Conduction Velocity

Motor conduction velocities of the ulnar, median, radial, and musculocutaneous nerves can be reliably measured, as described by Jebson (1967). Caldwell and associates (1971) improved and adapted to clinical use the technique of measuring UNCV in evaluating patients with thoracic outlet compression. Conduction velocities over proximal and distal segments of the ulnar nerve are determined by recording the action potentials generated in the hypothenar or first dorsal interosseous muscles. The points of stimulation are the supraclavicular fossa, mid-upper arm, area below the elbow, and wrist. The Meditron 201-AD or the TECA B-3 electromyogram, including the coaxial cable with three-needle or surface electrodes, can be used for this examination. The normal average UNCV values are 72 m/second across the thoracic outlet, 55 m/second around the elbow, 59 m/second in the forearm, and 2.5 to 3.5 m/second at the wrist. In patients with thoracic outlet syndrome, I and my colleagues (1971) found that the average UNCV value is reduced to 53 m/second across the outlet, with a range of 32 to 65 m/second.

Angiography

Simple clinical observations usually suffice to determine the degree of vascular impairment in the upper extremity and, as Lang (1962) noted, peripheral angiography is rarely needed. Bruits in the supra- or infraclavicular spaces suggest stenoses, and absence of pulse denotes total obstruction. In these instances, retrograde or antegrade arteriograms of the subclavian and brachial arterial systems are indicated to demonstrate localized pathologic changes. Using arteriography or phlebog-

Table 42-2. Differential Diagnosis of Nerve Compression

Cervical spine
    Ruptured intervertebral disc
    Degenerative disease
    Osteoarthritis
    Spinal cord tumors
Brachial plexus
    Superior sulcus tumors
    Trauma (postural palsy)
Peripheral nerves
    Entrapment neuropathy
    Carpal tunnel (median nerve)
    Ulnar nerve (elbow)
    Radial nerve
    Suprascapular nerve
Medical neuropathies
Trauma
Tumor

raphy routinely for demonstrating temporary occlusion of the vessels in different arm positions would seem redundant to an adequate clinical examination in most patients and is associated with some morbidity—unnecessary although minimal. The UNCV is usually depressed in patients with vascular compression as well as nerve compression. It serves to satisfy the physician and patient about objective testing; moreover, it is less expensive and safer. In instances of venous stenosis or obstruction, as in Paget-Schroetter syndrome, phlebography is indicated to discern the extent of thrombosis to determine the status of collateral venous circulation.

Differential Diagnosis

Thoracic outlet syndrome should be differentiated from a variety of neurologic, vascular, pulmonary, and esophageal lesions. It is necessary to differentiate it from lesion of the cervical spine, brachial plexus, and peripheral nerves (Table 42-2).

Several arterial and venous phenomena (Table 42-3) can be confused with thoracic outlet syndrome; however, the differentiation can often be made clinically.

Table 42-3. Differential Diagnosis of Vascular Compression

Arterial
    Arteriosclerosis
    Aneurysm
    Occlusive disease
    Thromboangiitis obliterans
    Embolism
    Functional
    Raynaud's disease
Reflex vasomotor dystrophy
Causalgia: Vasculitis, collagen disease, panniculitis
Venous thrombophlebitis
    Mediastinal venous obstruction
    Malignant
    Benign

In patients with atypical presentations, such as chest pain, a high index of suspicion of thoracic outlet syndrome in addition to angina pectoris must be maintained.

THERAPY

Patients with thoracic outlet syndrome usually should receive physiotherapy before operative intervention. Such therapy must be properly performed because many of these patients receive the same treatment as do people with cervical syndrome, which often exaggerates the symptoms of thoracic outlet compression. Proper physiotherapy for thoracic outlet compression includes heat massages, active neck exercises, scalenus anticus muscle stretching, strengthening of the upper trapezius muscle, and posture instruction. Because sagging of the shoulder girdle, common among middle-aged people, is a major etiologic factor in this syndrome, many patients with less severe disease benefit from strengthening the shoulder girdle and improving posture. More than one-half of patients seen in consultation required no surgical procedure but improved significantly with conservative management.

Most patients with a UNCV above 60 m/second improve with conservative management. Most patients with a UNCV below 60 m/second require surgical resection of the first rib and correction of other bony abnormalities.

As Roos (1966) and Roos and Owens (1966) suggested, resection of the first rib, and a cervical rib when present, is best performed through the transaxillary approach for complete removal, with decompression of the seventh and eighth cervical and first thoracic nerve roots. It can be accomplished without major muscle division, as in the posterior approach advocated by Clagett (1962) or retraction of the brachial plexus, as in the anterior supraclavicular approach suggested by Falconer and Li (1962). The infraclavicular approach does not allow complete removal of the first rib. The transaxillary approach shortens the postoperative disability and provides better cosmetic results compared to both anterior and posterior approaches. The latter is especially important because 80% of patients are women.

Technique of Transaxillary Resection of First Rib

The patient is placed in the lateral position with the involved extremity abducted to 90 degrees by traction straps wrapped carefully around the forearm and attached to an overhead pulley. An appropriate amount of weight, usually 1 to 2 pounds, depending on the patient's build, is used to maintain this position without undue traction. For additional exposure, traction can be increased intermittently by the anesthesiologist. The axilla and forearm are prepared and draped. A transverse incision is made below the hairline between the pectoralis major and the latissimus dorsi muscles and deepened to the external intercostal fascia. Care should be taken to prevent injury to the intercostobrachial cutaneous nerve, which passes from the chest wall to the subcutaneous tissue in the center of the operative field. The dissection is extended cephalad next to the external intercostal fascia up to the first rib. With gentle dissection, the neurovascular bundle is identified and its relation to the first rib and both scalene muscles is clearly outlined to avoid injury to the neurovascular bundle. The insertion of the scalenus anticus muscle on the first rib is dissected and the muscle is divided. The first rib is dissected subperiosteally with a periosteal elevator and carefully separated from the underlying pleura to avoid pneumothorax. The rib is then divided at its middle portion. With use of an alligator forceps, the anterior portion of the rib is pulled away from the vein, the costoclavicular ligament is cut, and the rib is divided at its sternal attachment. The anterior venous compartment is thus decompressed. The posterior segment of the rib is then grasped with alligator forceps and retracted away from its bed to facilitate its dissection and separation from the subclavian artery and brachial plexus posteriorly. The scalenus medius muscle should not be cut from the rib but rather stripped with a periosteal elevator to avoid injuring the long thoracic nerve that lies on its posterior margin. The dissection of this rib segment is carried to its articulation with the transverse process of the vertebra and divided. If the dissection is kept in the subperiosteal plane, no damage occurs to the first thoracic nerve root, which lies immediately under the rib. Complete removal of the neck and head of the first rib is achieved by a long, special double-action pituitary rongeur. The eighth cervical and first thoracic nerve roots can be visualized clearly at this point. If a cervical rib is present, it is removed at this time, and the seventh cervical nerve root can be observed. Only the subcutaneous tissues and skin require closure because no large muscles have been divided. Only occasional, intermittent firm traction is required for exposure, and no evidence of brachial plexus stretching or neuritis has been observed when this technique is used. The patient is encouraged to use the arm normally and can be discharged from the hospital between 2 and 3 days after the surgical procedure.

It is preferable to remove the entire first rib, including its head and neck, to avoid future irritation of the plexus because a residual portion, particularly if it is long, may cause recurrence of symptoms. The periosteum should be fragmented and destroyed to prevent callus formation and "regeneration" of the rib.

Removal of incompletely resected or regenerated rib and lysis of adhesions of the brachial plexus in symptomatic patients with decreased ulnar nerve conduction velocity can best be accomplished through the posterior approach. The anterior supraclavicular approach is used for arterial bypass and reconstructive procedures.

Results

The clinical results of first rib resections in properly selected patients are good in 85%, fair in 10%, and poor in 5%. A good result is indicated by complete relief of symptoms, a fair result by improvement with some residual or recurrent mild symptoms, and a poor result by no change from the preoperative status.

Uniform improvement of symptoms is usually obtained in patients with primarily vascular compression.

In patients with predominantly nerve compression, however, two groups with different rates of improvement are observed. The first group includes patients with the classic manifestations of ulnar neuralgia and elicitation of pulse diminution, in whom an average preoperative UNCV is reduced to 53 m/second. Ninety-five percent of patients in this group are improved by first rib resection. In the second group are patients with atypical pain distribution who may or may not have shown pulse changes by compression tests and in whom the average preoperative ulnar nerve conduction velocity was only reduced to 60 m/second. Surgical intervention is carried out in such patients as a therapeutic trial after prolonged conservative therapy has failed. Although many patients in the second group are improved, the fair and poor results mostly occur in these patients, as the author and Razzuk (1972) have noted.

The UNCV and clinical status are highly correlated. Patients with good postoperative results have a preoperative average UNCV of 51 m/second and show return to a normal average of 72 m/second after operation. In those who have fair results, the preoperative UNCV averages 60 m/second and increases to an average of only 63 m/second after operation. In the poor-result group, no appreciable change occurs in the postoperative from the preoperative values; in fact, the average conduction time was only 58 m/second.

No hospital mortality has been directly related to this procedure. Postoperative morbidity after the transaxillary approach includes clinically inconsequential pneumothorax in 15%, hematoma in 1%, and infection in 1%.

PAGET-SCHROETTER SYNDROME

"Effort" thrombosis of the axillary-subclavian vein, or Paget-Schroetter syndrome, usually occurs as a result of unusual or excessive use of the arm in addition to the presence of one or more compressive elements in the thoracic outlet, as the author and Razzuk (1991) have recorded.

Sir James Paget in 1875 in London and von Schroetter in 1884 in Vienna described this syndrome of thrombosis of the axillary-subclavian vein, which bears their names. The word *effort* was added to thrombosis because of the frequent association with exertion producing either direct or indirect compression of the vein. The thrombosis results from trauma or unusual occupations requiring repetitive muscular activity, as has been observed in professional athletes, Linotype operators, painters, and beauticians. Cold and traumatic factors, such as carrying skis over the shoulder, tend to increase the proclivity for thrombosis. Elements of increased thrombogenicity also increase the incidence of this problem and exacerbate its symptoms on a long-term basis.

For years, patients with effort thrombosis were treated with anticoagulants and conservative exercises; if recurrent symptoms developed when they returned to work, they were considered candidates for first rib resection. Use of thrombolytic agents with early surgical decompression of the neurovascular compression has reduced morbidity, such as a postphlebitic syndrome, and the necessity for thrombectomy. A review of 67 patients seen by the author and Razzuk (1991) over 25 years showed that 34 were initially treated with heparin sodium and then crystalline warfarin sodium (Coumadin). Recurrent symptoms developed in 21 of these patients after they returned to work, necessitating transaxillary first rib resection to relieve symptoms; eight also underwent thrombectomy. In 1993, Machleder described 43 patients initially treated with thrombolytic agents and heparin, followed promptly by early first rib resection. The evaluation and efficacy of this therapy have been established by frequent and repetitive venograms and careful follow-up of patients. Most patients showed improvement with thrombolytic therapy. Remaining stenoses that suggested intravascular thrombosis were usually related to external compression of the vein by the clavicle, costoclavicular ligament, rib, or scalenus anterior muscle. Venous thrombectomy was necessary in only four patients, in whom the clot was not controlled by thrombolytic therapy and operative release of compression. No deaths were reported in this series.

Adams and DeWeese (1971) reported long-term results in patients treated conservatively with elevation and warfarin. They noted a 12% incidence of pulmonary embolism. Development of occasional venous distention occurred in 18%, and late residual arm symptoms of swelling, pain, and superficial thrombophlebitis were noted in 68% of patients (i.e., deep venous thrombosis with postphlebitic syndrome). One patient had phlegmasia cerulea dolens. These findings substantiate observations made by myself and Razzuk (1991) that a more aggressive operative approach after thrombolytic therapy is indicated, particularly for younger patients engaged in precipitating occupations.

One advantage of urokinase over streptokinase is the direct action of urokinase on the thrombosis distal to the catheter, which produces a local thrombolytic effect. Streptokinase produces a systemic effect involving the alteration of serum plasminogen and increasing potential complications. Heparin is given postoperatively until the catheter is removed. A decrease in the need for thrombectomy after use of the thrombolytic agent followed by aggressive surgical intervention is another advantage because some of the long-term disability is related to morbidity from thrombectomy as well as recurrent thrombosis.

The natural history of Paget-Schroetter syndrome suggests moderate morbidity with conservative treatment alone. Bypass with vein or other conduits has limited application. Causes other than thoracic outlet syndrome must be treated individually. Intermittent obstruction of the subclavian vein can lead to thrombosis, and decompression should be used prophylactically.

RECURRENT THORACIC OUTLET SYNDROME

Extirpation of the first rib offers relief of symptoms in patients with thoracic outlet syndrome that is not improved by physiotherapy. Ten percent of surgically treated patients develop variable degrees of shoulder, arm, and hand pain and paresthesias; these are usually mild and short lasting and usually respond well to a brief course of physiotherapy and muscle relaxants. In 1.6% of patients, however, symptoms persist, become progressively more severe, and often involve a wider area of distribution because of entrapment of the intermediate trunk in addition to the lower trunk and C8 and T1 nerve roots. Symptoms may recur from 1 month to 10 years after initial rib resection. However, as my colleagues and I noted (1976), in most instances, recurrence is within the first 3 months. Symptoms consist of aching or burning pain, often associated with paresthesia, involving the neck, shoulder, parascapular area, anterior chest wall, arm, and hand. Vascular lesions are uncommon and consist of causalgia minor and infected false aneurysms.

Two distinct groups of patients required reoperation. Pseudorecurrences happen in patients who never had relief of symptoms after the initial operation. Cases can be separated etiologically as follows: 1) the second rib was mistakenly resected instead of the first; 2) the first rib was resected, leaving a cervical rib; 3) a cervical rib was resected, leaving an abnormal first rib; or 4) a second rib was resected, leaving a rudimentary first rib. The second group, in whom true recurrence takes place (Urschel and Razzuk 1986), includes a group of patients whose symptoms were relieved after the initial operation but who developed recurrence because a significant piece of the first rib was left in place at the initial operation. A second group had complete resection of the first rib but demonstrated excessive scar formation involving the brachial plexus.

Physiotherapy should be instituted in all patients with symptoms of neurovascular compression after first rib resection. If symptoms persist and conduction velocity remains below normal, reoperation is indicated.

Reoperation for recurrent thoracic outlet syndrome is always performed through the posterior thoracoplasty approach to provide better exposure of the nerve roots and brachial plexus, thereby reducing the danger of injury to these structures as well as providing adequate exposure of the subclavian artery and vein. It also provides a wider field for easy resection of any bony abnormalities or fibrous bands and allows extensive neurolysis of the nerve roots and brachial plexus, which are not always accessible through the limited exposure of the transaxillary approach. The anterior or supraclavicular approach is inadequate for reoperation.

The basic elements of reoperation include 1) resection of persistent or recurrent bony remnants of either a cervical or the first rib, 2) neurolysis of the brachial plexus and nerve roots, and 3) dorsal sympathectomy. Sympathectomy removes the T1, T2, and T3 thoracic ganglia. The surgeon should avoid damaging the C8 ganglion (upper aspect of the stellate ganglion), which produces Horner's syndrome. The sympathectomy provides relief of major and minor causalgia and alleviates the paresthesias in the supraclavicular and interclavicular areas. The incidence of postsympathetic syndrome has been negligible in this group of patients. The use of a nerve stimulator to differentiate scar from nerve root is cardinal in avoiding damage in reoperation.

The technique of the operation includes a high thoracoplasty incision, extending from 3 cm above the angle of the scapula, halfway between the angle of the scapula and the spinous processes, and caudad 5 cm from the angle of the scapula. The trapezius and rhomboid muscles are divided the length of the incision. The scapula is retracted from the chest wall by incising the latissimus dorsi over the fourth rib. The posterior superior serratus muscle is divided, and the sacrospinalis muscle is retracted medially. The first rib remnant and cervical rib remnant, if present, are located and removed subperiosteally. After the rib remnants have been resected, the regenerated periosteum is extirpated. In my experience, most regenerated ribs occur from the end of an unresected segment of rib rather than from periosteum, although the latter is possible. At the initial operation, therefore, it is important to remove the first rib totally to reduce the incidence of bony regeneration in all patients with primarily nerve compression and pain symptoms.

If excessive scar is present after removal of any bony rib remnant, it may be prudent to perform the sympathectomy initially. This involves resection of a 1-in. (2.5 cm) segment of the second rib posteriorly to locate the sympathetic ganglion. In that way, the first thoracic nerve may be easier to locate beneath rather than through the scar.

Neurolysis of the nerve root and brachial plexus is performed using a nerve stimulator. Neurolysis is carried down to but not into the nerve sheath. It is extended peripherally over the brachial plexus as far as any scar persists. Excessive neurolysis is not indicated, and opening of the nerve sheath produces more scar than it relieves. To minimize excessive scar, efforts in the initial operation for thoracic outlet syndrome should include complete extirpation of the first rib; avoidance of hematomas by adequate drainage, either by catheter or by opening the pleura; and avoidance of infection.

The subclavian artery and vein are released if symptoms mediate. The scalenus medius muscle is débrided. The dorsal sympathectomy is completed via extrapleural dissection. Meticulous hemostasis is effected, and a large, round Jackson-Pratt catheter drain is placed in the area of the brachial plexus, although not touching it. This drain is brought out through the subscapular space through a stab wound into the axilla. Methylprednisolone acetate (Depo-Medrol), 80 mg, is left in the area of the nerve plexus, although the patient is not given systemic steroids unless keloid formation has previously occurred. The wound is closed in layers with interrupted heavy Vicryl sutures to provide adequate strength, and the arm is kept in a sling to be used gently for the first 3 months. Range-of-motion exercises are prescribed to prevent shoulder limitation; however, overactivity is contraindicated because it may result in excessive scar formation. The use of hyaluronic acid may also decrease adhesions.

When the problem is vascular, involving false or mycotic aneurysms, special techniques for reoperation are used. A bypass graft is interposed from the innominate or carotid artery proximally, through a separate tunnel distally, to the brachial artery. Usually, the saphenous vein is used, although other conduits may be selected. The arteries feeding and leaving the infected aneurysm are ligated. At a subsequent stage, the aneurysm is resected through a transaxillary approach with no fear of bleeding or ischemia of the arm.

Special instruments have been devised to provide adequate resection through the transaxillary or posterior route. These include a modified strengthened pituitary rongeur and a modified Leksell double-action rongeur for first rib removal without danger to the nerve root.

The sympathectomy relieves chest wall pain that mimics angina pectoris, esophageal disease, or even a lung tumor by denervating the deep fibers that travel with the arteries and bone.

Results of reoperation have been excellent if an accurate diagnosis was established and the proper procedure was executed. Follow-up of more than 1000 patients has ranged from 6 months to 15 years. All patients improved initially after reoperation; in 79%, improvement was maintained for more than 5 years. Fourteen percent of patients developed symptoms that were easily managed with physiotherapy. Seven percent of patients required a second reoperation, in every instance because of rescarring. No deaths occurred, and only one case of significant infection requiring drainage was recorded.

REFERENCES

Adams JT, DeWeese JA: Effort thrombosis of the axillary and subclavian veins. J Trauma 11:923, 1971.

Adson AW: Cervical ribs: symptoms, differential diagnosis for section of the scalenus anticus muscle. J Int Coll Surg 16:546, 1951.

Caldwell JW, Crane CR, Krusen EM: Nerve conduction studies: an aid in the diagnosis of the thoracic outlet syndrome. South Med J 64:210, 1971.

Clagett OT: Presidential address: research and prosearch. J Thorac Cardiovasc Surg 44:153, 1962.

Falconer MA, Li FWP: Resection of the first rib in costoclavicular compression of the brachial plexus. Lancet 1:59, 1962.

Jebson RH: Motor conduction velocities in the median and ulnar nerves. Arch Phys Med 48:185, 1967.

Kuntz A: Afferent innervation of peripheral blood vessels through sympathetic trunks. South Med J 44:673, 1951.

Lang EK: Roentgenographic diagnosis of the neurovascular compression syndromes. Radiology 79:58, 1962.

Machleder HI: Evaluation of a new treatment strategy for Paget-Schroetter syndrome: spontaneous thrombosis of the axillary-subclavian vein. J Vasc Surg 17:305, 1993.

Paget J: Clinical Lectures and Essays. London: Longmans Green, 1875.

Roos DB: Transaxillary approach for first rib resection to relieve thoracic outlet syndrome. Ann Surg 163:354, 1966.

Roos DB, Owens JC: Thoracic outlet syndrome. Arch Surg 93:71, 1966.

Rosati LM, Lord JW: Neurovascular compression syndromes of the shoulder girdle. In Modern Surgical Monographs. New York: Grune and Stratton, 1961, p. 168.

Urschel HC Jr: Thoracic outlet syndrome: reoperation. In Grillo HC, Eschapasse H (eds): International Trends in General Thoracic Surgery: Major Challenges. Vol. 2. Philadelphia: WB Saunders, 1987, p. 374.

Urschel HC Jr, Razzuk MA: Current concepts: management of the thoracic outlet syndrome. N Engl J Med 286:1140, 1972.

Urschel HC Jr, Razzuk MA: Improved management of the Paget-Schroetter syndrome secondary to thoracic outlet compression. Ann Thorac Surg 52:1271, 1991.

Urschel HC Jr, Razzuk MA: The failed operation for thoracic outlet syndrome: the difficulty of diagnosis and management. Ann Thorac Surg 42:523, 1986.

Urschel HC Jr, et al: Objective diagnosis (ulnar nerve conduction velocity) and current therapy of the thoracic outlet syndrome. Ann Thorac Surg 12:608, 1971.

Urschel HC Jr, et al: Thoracic outlet syndrome masquerading as coronary artery disease. Ann Thorac Surg 16:239, 1973.

Urschel HC Jr, et al: Reoperation for recurrent thoracic outlet syndrome. Ann Thorac Surg 21:19, 1976.

Von Schroetter L: Erkrankungen der Gefässe. In Nathnogel R (ed): Handuch der Pathologie und Therapie. Vienna: Holder, 1884.

READING REFERENCES

Adson AW, Coffey IR: Cervical rig: a method of anterior approach for relief of symptoms by division of the scalenus anticus. Ann Surg 85:839, 1927.

Aziz S, Straehley CJ, Whelan TJ: Effort-related axillosubclavian vein thrombosis. Am J Surg 152:57, 1986.

Molina JE: Surgery for effort thrombosis of the subclavian vein. J Thorac Cardiovasc Surg 103:341, 1992.

Rob CG, Standover A: Arterial occlusion complicating thoracic outlet compression syndrome. BMJ 2:709, 1958.

Roos DB: Experience with first rib resection for thoracic outlet syndrome. Ann Surg 173:429, 1971.

Telford ED, Mottershead S: Pressure at the cervicobrachial junction. J Bone Joint Surg Am 30:249, 1948.

Urschel Jr HC, Paulson DL, McNamara JJ: Thoracic outlet syndrome. Ann Thorac Surg 61:1, 1968.

CHAPTER 43

Thoracic Thoracoscopic Sympathectomy

William Scott Arnold and Thomas M. Daniel

Greenwood (1967) and Brown (1926) noted that surgical sympathectomy was first used clinically in the late nineteenth century by Jaboulay and later by Jonnesco. Adson et al. (1935) were among the first in the United States to describe a sympathectomy for vasomotor disorders and hyperhidrosis. Since then, there has been an evolution in surgical approaches to the thoracic sympathetic chain and in the extent of resection of the rami and ganglia (Table 43-1). This evolution culminated in the modern thoracoscopic sympathectomy, which provides an effective, minimally invasive, anatomically exact, and cosmetically appealing therapy with a low complication rate for specific pseudomotor, vasomotor, or sweat gland disorders. The most commonly used technique is one of thoracoscopic T2 and T3 en bloc ganglionectomy with preservation of the T1 stellate ganglion and division of Kuntz's nerve, as described under Technique. Gossot (1997) has reintroduced selective sympathectomy, or ramisectomy.

ANATOMY

The descending autonomic fibers project to cell bodies that lie in the intermediolateral or intermediomedial gray columns of the spinal cord. Sympathetic fibers then emanate from T1 to L2 or L3 and travel out from the thoracolumbar cord in the ventral roots, then via white rami into the sympathetic chain. There, the fibers may synapse and exit at the same level, synapse and travel up the chain to exit at another level, travel and then synapse, or pass through the chain to synapse more peripherally. The postganglionic fibers exit via nonmyelinated gray rami at all spinal cord segments (Fig. 43-1).

As reviewed by Harati (1993), the preganglionic sympathetic fibers to the upper extremity originate from the intermediolateral cell columns of T2 through T6; ascend, synapse in, or pass through the stellate ganglion; and enter the lower trunk of the brachial plexus, mainly the medial cord. They travel to the upper extremity primarily via the median and ulnar nerves. The T2 and T3 roots contain most of the vasoconstrictor fibers to the upper extremity. As noted by Lemmens (1982), the T2 outflow is the most important sympathetic innervation for both vasomotor and pseudomotor nerves of the hand. Axillary sympathetic innervation derives from T4 and T5. Significantly, as best described by Cross (1993), the sympathetic outflow to the ciliary muscle of accommodation and the pupillary constrictor of the eye arises from T1, ascends through the stellate ganglion without synapsing, and travels to the superior cervical ganglion. There, the fibers synapse and pass along with branches of the carotid to the eye (see Fig. 43-1). This knowledge is important in preventing the complication of Horner's syndrome, which is ipsilateral ptosis, miosis, and facial anhidrosis. Finally, there are alternate pathways of sympathetic innervation to the upper extremity. The best described is the nerve of Kuntz (Kuntz et al. 1937), a variable intrathoracic nerve that arises from approximately T2 and bypasses the sympathetic chain by parallel vertical fibers to flow directly to the lower brachial plexus (Fig. 43-2). A basic knowledge of this anatomy allows one to understand the importance of preservation of the T1 rami and stellate ganglion in preventing Horner's syndrome. It also becomes clear why an en bloc T2–T3 ganglionectomy with ablation of Kuntz's nerve can provide a nearly complete autonomic innervation of the upper extremity: It removes T2 and T3 outflow directly and removes ascending fibers from the lower thoracic segments of T4 and T5. A selective sympathectomy, or ramisectomy, as reviewed by Gossot (1997), involves division of the rami only and theoretically could allow selective T2–T3 denervation and possibly less compensatory hyperhidrosis.

INDICATIONS

The main indications for thoracic sympathectomy are primary hyperhidrosis of the upper extremity and reflex sympathetic dystrophy in its early phases.

Table 43-1. Approaches to Thoracic Sympathectomy

Open
    Posterior: Adson (1935), Smithwick (1936), Cloward (1969)
    Supraclavicular: Telford (1935)
    Transthoracic: Goetz and Marr (1944)
    Transaxillary: Atkins (1954), Roos (1971)
Minimally invasive
    Percutaneous radiofrequency ablation: Wilkinson (1984)
    Thoracoscopic: Kux (1954, 1978)

Data taken from studies cited in the chapter and the following studies: Atkins MJB: Sympathectomy by the axillary approach. Lancet *1*:538, 1954; Cloward RB: Hyperhidrosis. J Neurosurg *30*:545, 1969; Goetz RH, Marr JAS: The importance of the second thoracic ganglion for the sympathetic supply of the upper extremities: with description of two new approaches for its removal in cases of vascular disease: preliminary report. Clin Proc *3*:102, 1944; Kux M: Thorakoskopische Engriffe an Nervensystem. Stuttgart: George Thieme Verlag, 1954; Kux M: Thoracic endoscopic sympathectomy in palmar and axillary hyperhidrosis. Arch Surg *113*:264, 1978; Smithwick RH: Modified dorsal sympathectomy for vascular spasm of the upper extremities. Am Surg *104*:339, 1936; Telford ED: Technique of sympathectomy. Br J Surg *23*:448, 1935; and Wilkinson HA: Radiofrequency percutaneous upper thoracic sympathectomy: technique and review of indications. N Engl J Med *311*:34, 1984.

Primary hyperhidrosis is a disorder of excessive sweat production of the palms and often axillae and soles. The triggers are primarily emotional but may also relate to heat or exercise. The sweating is profuse and palpable to the patient and visible to others. It is socially debilitating and can cause maceration of the skin. Employment is often jeopardized. Hyperhidrosis has a slight female predominance and an increased incidence in Asians and Sephardic Jews. There is often a familial predisposition. Medical treatment, as reviewed by White (1986), consists of therapy with topical aluminum chloride, iontophoresis, systemic or topical anticholinergic therapy, or biofeedback. Excision of axillary sweat glands has also been performed. Surgical sympathectomy is highly effective and safe and should be considered for all patients with significant primary hyperhidrosis. As reported by Edmondson (1992) and Gossot (1997), thoracoscopic sympathectomy has a 90% success rate for hyperhidrosis.

Schwartzman et al. (1997) reported a high success rate with thoracoscopic sympathectomy in the treatment of carefully selected patients with early-phase reflex sympathetic dystrophy. In this study, 100% of patients with symptom duration of 12 months or less had long-term relief, whereas only 44% had relief if symptoms had been present longer than 24 months.

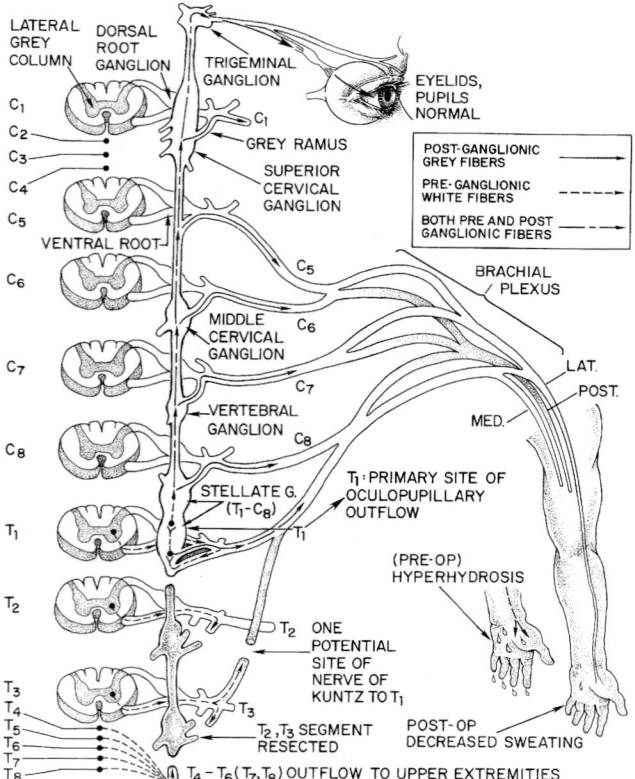

Fig. 43-1. Schematic representation of the sympathetic pathway to the upper extremity and face. Note T1 outflow to eye.

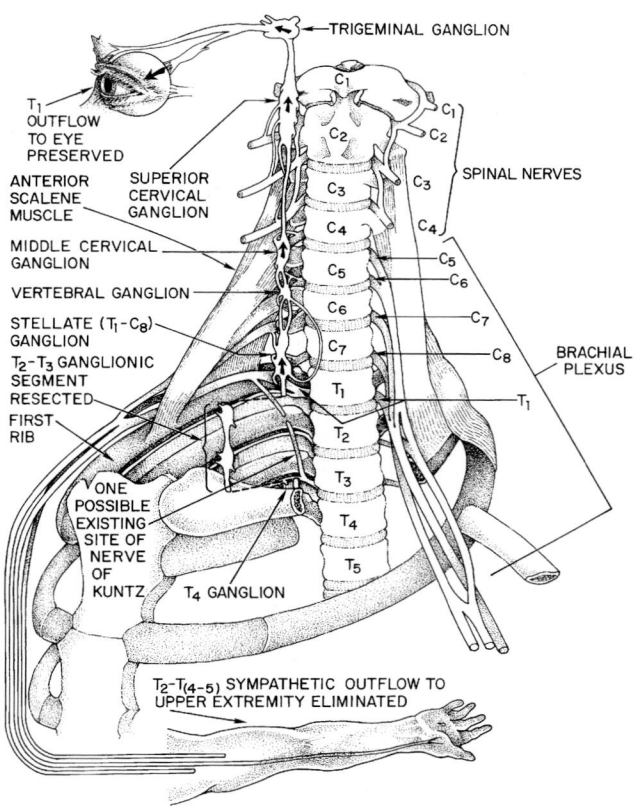

Fig. 43-2. Anatomy of the cervicothoracic region, with emphasis on landmarks for sympathectomy.

Sympathectomy is rarely used for Raynaud's syndrome or Berger's disease. These disorders respond variably to surgery, generally have a benign course, or are best treated with smoking cessation, withdrawal of β-blockers, avoidance of cold temperatures, and pharmacotherapy with calcium channel blockers or α-antagonists. Sympathectomy has other rare indications, including sympatholysis after nonrevascularizable upper extremity arterial embolization to the palmar arch, refractory angina, and long QT syndrome.

TECHNIQUE

We use dual-lumen anesthesia and position the patient in a modified decubitus position with the patient slightly forward, approximately 15 degrees beyond perpendicular. This allows the ipsilateral lung to fall away from the posteriorly located sympathetic chain. A 30-degree thoracoscope is inserted in the fifth intercostal space at the midaxillary line, and the lung is allowed to passively deflate with the head of the bed elevated to allow the apex to fall away from the chest wall (Fig. 43-3). We then use two 5-mm working trocars in the third intercostal space, one anteriorly and one posteriorly.

The first rib is often difficult to visualize via thoracoscope. It is often covered by an area of bright yellow fat at its costovertebral junction, which serves as a useful landmark. The surgeon should thoracoscopically "palpate" the soft tissue above the apparent first rib to be sure there is no further cephalad rib. Once the first rib is localized, the pleura is opened and the second rib identified. Dissection is not carried out above the upper border of the second rib to preserve the stellate ganglion. This also decreases the chances

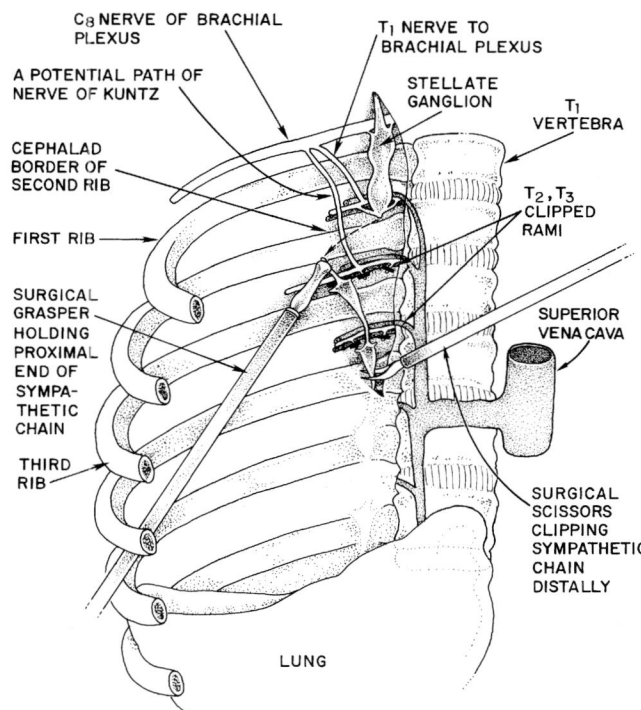

Fig. 43-4. Depiction of thoracoscopic T2–T3 ganglionectomy. The second rib is identified, and the rami and main trunk are clipped and cut.

of injury to the T1 outflow to the lower cord of the brachial plexus (see Fig. 43-2). The sympathetic chain is grasped, elevated, and bluntly dissected. The rami from T2 and T3 are hemoclipped and divided, and the chain is hemoclipped proximally and distally and dissected out, removing T2 and T3 en bloc (Fig. 43-4).

A selective sympathectomy or ramisectomy, in which only the rami are divided from T2 to T5, may also be used. This procedure, as reported by Gossot (1997), has a somewhat higher recurrence rate but a decreased severity of compensatory hyperhidrosis. Here the rami are clipped and divided from T2 to T5. T5 is easily identified because it is just at or below the azygous vein.

Finally, the bodies of the second and third ribs are scored horizontally with cautery from the costovertebral angle laterally for 3 to 4 cm. This divides any accessory fibers, such as the nerves of Kuntz. Use of cautery is otherwise minimized, particularly near the rami to prevent intercostal neuralgias. No indwelling chest tube is required if hemostasis is adequate.

COMPLICATIONS

Specific complications include compensatory hyperhidrosis, which occurs in 60 to 70% of patients. It consists of excessive sweating in nondenervated areas, such as the back and groin. It is often tolerable but can be severe. Its

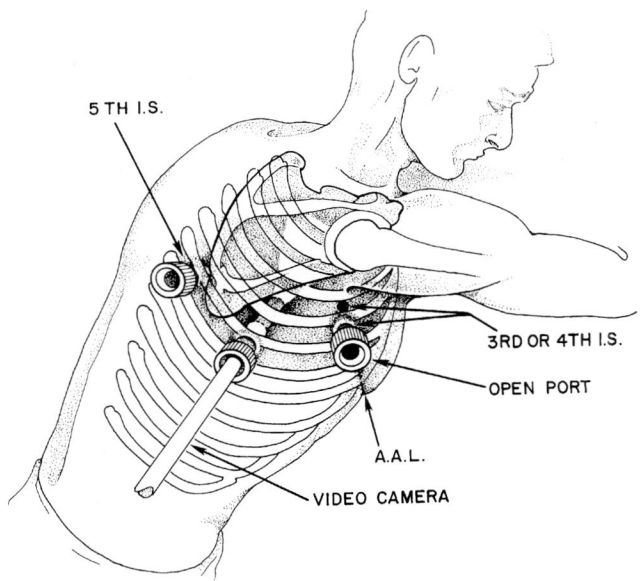

Fig. 43-3. Patient positioning and trocar placement. The patient is slightly forward (approximately 15 degrees past perpendicular), with the head of the bed slightly elevated. A.A.L., anterior axillary line; I.S., intercostal space.

etiology is unclear but may well represent a normal thermoregulatory compensation.

Edmondson et al. (1992) reported a 48% incidence of gustatory sweating (i.e., facial sweating with salivary stimuli).

Horner's syndrome is rare with preservation of T1. It may occur in 5 to 10% of patients, however, because of anatomic variability in the formation of the stellate ganglion. Other specific complications include recurrence, intercostal neuralgias, pneumothorax, and injury to the subclavian vessels or the esophagus.

REFERENCES

Adson AW, Craig WM, Brown GE: Essential hyperhidrosis cured by sympathetic ganglionectomy and trunk resection. Arch Surg 31:794, 1935.

Atkins MJB: Sympathectomy by the axillary approach. Lancet 1:538, 1954.

Brown GE: The treatment of peripheral vasomotor disturbances of the extremities. JAMA 87:379, 1926.

Cloward RB: Hyperhidrosis. J Neurosurg 30:545, 1969.

Cross FA: Autonomic innervation of the eye. In Low PA (ed): Clinical Autonomic Disorders. New York: Little, Brown, 1993.

Edmondson RA, Banerjee AK, Rennie JA: Endoscopic thoracic sympathectomy in the treatment of hyperhidrosis. Ann Surg 215:289, 1992.

Goetz RH, Marr JAS: The importance of the second thoracic ganglion for the sympathetic supply of the upper extremities: with description of two new approaches for its removal in cases of vascular disease: preliminary report. Clin Proc 3:102, 1944.

Gossot D, et al: Thoracoscopic sympathectomy for upper limb hyperhidrosis: looking for the right operation. Ann Thorac Surg 64:975, 1997.

Greenwood B: The origins of sympathectomy. Med Hist 11:165, 1967.

Harati Y: Anatomy of the spinal and peripheral autonomic nervous system. In Low PA (ed): Clinical Autonomic Disorders. New York: Little, Brown, 1993.

Kuntz A, Alexander F, Furcolo L: Role of pre-ganglionic fibers of the first thoracic nerve in sympathetic innervation of the upper extremity. Proc Soc Exp Biol Med 37:282, 1937.

Kux M: Thorakoskopische Engriffe an Nervensystem. Stuttgart: George Thieme Verlag, 1954.

Kux M: Thoracic endoscopic sympathectomy in palmar and axillary hyperhidrosis. Arch Surg 113:264, 1978.

Lemmens HAJ: Importance of the second thoracic segment for the sympathic denervation of the hand. Vasc Surg 16:23, 1982.

Roos DB: Experience with first rib resection for thoracic outlet syndrome. Ann Surg 173:429, 1971.

Schwartzman RJ, et al: Long term outcomes following sympathectomy for complex regional pain syndrome type I (RSD). J Neurol Sci 150:149, 1997.

Smithwick RH: Modified dorsal sympathectomy for vascular spasm of the upper extremities. Am Surg 104:339, 1936.

Telford ED: Technique of sympathectomy. Br J Surg 23:448, 1935.

White JW: Treatment of primary hyperhidrosis. Mayo Clin Proc 61:951, 1986.

Wilkinson HA: Radiofrequency percutaneous upper thoracic sympathectomy: technique and review of indications. N Engl J Med 311:34, 1984.

CHAPTER 44

Anterior Transthoracic Approaches to the Spine

Robert M. Vanecko and Thomas W. Shields

During the last third of the twentieth century, the anterior transthoracic approaches to the spinal column have become the preferred techniques to manage most problems involving the lower cervical, thoracic, and upper lumbar portions of the spine in children and adults. Hodgson and Stock (1956) and Hodgson and coworkers (1960) in Hong Kong were the first to suggest the transthoracic approach in the management of Pott's disease (tuberculosis of the spine) and its complication, Pott's paraplegia. The reports of Cauchoix and Binet (1957) suggested the use of median sternotomy to expose the vertebral bodies from C7 to T4. Perot and Munro (1969), Dwyer and colleagues (1969), and Harrington (1981) recorded the transthoracic approach for the removal of a midline thoracic disc protrusion, the management of scoliosis, and the management of fracture-dislocations of the spine due to metastatic malignant disease, respectively. Cook (1971) was also among the initial surgeons to bring to the attention of American surgeons the anterior thoracic approach to the spine. In addition to these early reports, a large number of publications on this subject appeared in orthopedic and neurosurgical, as well as general thoracic, literature over the past 30 years.

INDICATIONS FOR THE TRANSTHORACIC APPROACH TO THE SPINE

Indications for the use of a transthoracic approach (i.e., posterolateral thoracotomy, median sternotomy, or thoracoabdominal incision) to expose the spine are the presence of a destructive process of one or more vertebral bodies or intervertebral discs, fractures of the thoracic or lumbar spine, and major spinal deformities (Table 44-1). The incidence of the various lesions managed by these anterior approaches varies in children and adults. Spinal deformities are much more common in children and adolescents, whereas degenerative disorders, both infectious and malignant, are more common in adults. In children and adolescents, Burrington (1976) and Janik (1997) and their

colleagues at Children's Hospital in Denver listed scoliosis (366 patients) and kyphosis (132 patients) as the major primary diagnoses. These conditions were the result of idiopathic disease, neuromuscular disorders, hemivertebra-fracture pseudoarthrosis, Scheuermann's disease, and tumors—primarily neurofibromatosis—as well as some other uncommon causes. In adults, Anderson and colleagues (1993) found the indications for these approaches to be the presence of a herniated nucleus pulposus (30%), metastatic disease to the spine (27%), infection (22%), spinal deformities (12%), fracture (6%), and primary tumor involving the spine (3%). In regard to metastatic tumors and primary tumors of the spine or an adjacent structure (lung or mesenchymal or neurogenic tumor) involving the spine, McAfee and Zdeblick (1989) and Walsh and coworkers (1997) found that metastatic disease was by far the most common cause of destruction of a vertebral body. The common primary tumors were of the lung, kidney, breast, melanoma, multiple myeloma, pancreas, and thyroid. The indications for operation in these patients were severe pain or impending paraplegia. Lesions from the lung (primarily Pancoast tumors), neurogenic tumors (neuroblastoma or ganglioneuroblastomas), as well as the benign neurofibroma, Wilms' tumor, and mesenchymal tumors (liposarcomas, chondrosarcomas, and chordomas), are among the tumors that may secondarily involve or deform a vertebral body. Primary tumors of the vertebral body are uncommon and include osteosarcoma, plasmacytoma, and chondrosarcoma. Operation may be for cure or at times only for palliation. Rarely, an astrocytoma may require a spinal decompression as noted by Naunheim and associates (1994), or a destructive aneurysmal bone cyst as recorded by Janik and colleagues (1997) may require vertebrectomy and spinal stabilization. Traumatic injury with fracture and impending or present neurological complications has been a major indication for transthoracic exposure of the thoracic, thoracolumbar, or lower cervical spine, as recorded in the series of McElvein (1988) and Naunheim (1994) and their associates, 40% and 36%, respectively.

Table 44-1. Etiology of Spinal Disorders That Indicate Anterior Thoracic Approaches

Destructive disorders of vertebral body or disc
  Infection
    Tuberculosis
    Pyogenic infection
    Parasitic infestation
  Malignancy
    Metastatic disease
    Involvement by adjacent primary tumors
    Primary tumor of vertebral body
  Degenerative disc disease: herniated nucleus pulposus
  Trauma
    Fracture-dislocation
    Compression fracture
  Spinal deformities
    Scoliosis
    Kyphosis
    Lordosis

OPERATIVE APPROACHES

In general, the spine can be divided into four levels: 1) C7–T2, 2) T2–T6, 3) T6–T12, and 4) T12–L3. According to Thurer and Herskowitz (1996), exposure of vertebral bodies C7–T2 may be obtained via a low cervical incision, a transaxillary thoracotomy, or a vertical cervical incision along the anterior border of the sternocleidomastoid muscle combined with an upper median sternotomy (Fig. 44-1).

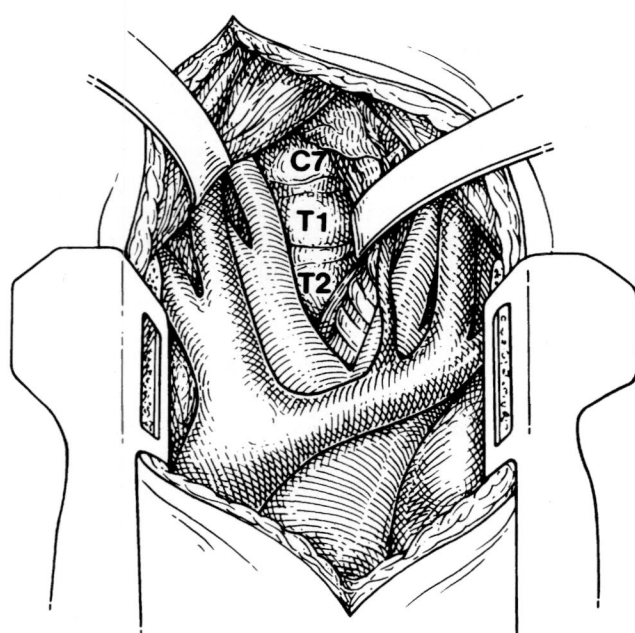

Fig. 44-1. Surgical exposure of C7–T2 through combined oblique neck and upper sternotomy incision. From Anderson TM, Mansour KA, Miller JI Jr: Thoracic approaches to anterior spinal operations: anterior thoracic approaches. Ann Thorac Surg 55:1447, 1994. Reprinted with permission from the Society of Thoracic Surgeons.

With the latter approach, Walsh and colleagues (1997) suggest that a left-sided neck incision be used unless contraindicated by the laterality of the disease process because there is less likelihood of injury to the contralateral recurrent laryngeal nerve by retraction of the trachea and esophagus to obtain the appropriate exposure. Furthermore, these authors note that good exposure may be obtained from C4 to T3 by this approach.

Both of the aforementioned authors and associates, as well as Anderson and coworkers (1993), among others, recommend a right posterolateral thoracotomy approach to lesions of T2–T6 vertebral bodies or discs. A left-sided approach may be used if the disease process extends primarily to the left side of the spine, if there is involvement of the left lung or other left-sided structure, or if a previous operation has been done on the right side.

For exposure of T6–T12, either a left or a right lateral thoracotomy may be used. It should be noted that the intercostal incision or rib resection should be at least one or more, often two, levels above the uppermost vertebral involvement. In patients with scoliosis, the laterality of the incision is determined by the direction in which the apex of the curvature points.

Exposure of vertebral bodies T12–L3 is varied. A right thoracotomy with retroperitoneal exposure by posterior division of the hemidiaphragmatic leaf for lesions of T12 or L1 may be used. For greater exposure of T8–L2, a left thoracotomy with an additional circumferential incision of the hemidiaphragmatic leaf from the chest wall may be carried out. In this situation or when even more exposure is necessary, a thoracoabdominal incision affords the best access. Either a right or left incision may be used. Some prefer the left-sided approach because they believe it is easier to retract the spleen than it is the liver on the right and also because of the presence of the inferior vena cava on the right. Others, such as McElvein and colleagues (1988), believe these anatomical relationships to be of no great concern.

PREOPERATIVE AND OPERATIVE TECHNIQUES

Preoperative Embolization

Some patients with metastatic disease involving a vertebra (e.g., renal cell carcinoma and thyroid carcinoma) may have excessive vascularity of the metastatic lesion. Walsh and associates (1997) suggest preoperative embolization to reduce the excessive blood supply. This procedure was done in eight of their patients, but in three patients, a major complication occurred: an asymptomatic aortic dissection, DeBakey type III; transient Brown-Séquard's syndrome, which improved significantly; and a spinal artery syndrome, which resulted in motor paraplegia that did not improve with time. Thus, it would appear that embolization should be resorted to only if absolutely necessary.

Anesthesia

A single-lumen endotracheal tube is satisfactory for the general anesthesia given to patients in whom a cervical incision, a cervical-median sternotomy, or a thoracoabdominal incision is to be used. When a thoracotomy alone is to be carried out, a double-lumen endotracheal tube is preferred so that one-lung anesthesia with deflation of the ipsilateral lung may be accomplished during the exposure for management of the spinal disease and subsequent stabilization of the spine.

Position of the Patient

The patient in whom a cervical incision or cervical-median sternotomy is to be carried out is placed in a supine position. The neurosurgeon or orthopedic surgeon of the team determines placement and position of the head and upper body. When a standard axillary or lateral thoracotomy is to be done, the patient is placed in a lateral decubitus position. When a thoracoabdominal incision is to be made, the patient is placed in a 45-degree angle so that easy exposure of the abdomen is obtained.

Surgical Incisions

The low cervical, transaxillary thoracotomy, cervical-median sternotomy, and standard posterolateral thoracotomy incisions have been described in detail elsewhere in the text. The thoracoabdominal approach to this area that one of us (R.M.V.), who has collaborated with orthopedic surgeons in the management of many patients with scoliosis, prefers is a thoracoabdominal incision carried out as follows: An oblique incision is made over the tenth or rarely the eleventh rib and extended onto the abdomen for several inches. The thoracic muscles are incised to expose the rib, which is then removed subperiostially. The chest is then entered, and any adhesions of the lung to the lower chest wall or diaphragm are freed. After the external oblique muscle of the abdomen is incised, the costal cartilage of the previously removed rib is identified. The cartilage is cut in half, exposing an area that is devoid of any structure other than properitoneal fat and peritoneum. This provides safe, easy access to the retrodiaphragmatic area, the inner aspect of the abdominal musculature, and the retroperitoneal area. The peritoneum can then be freed from these structures by blunt dissection, using both index fingers working in opposite directions against the muscle. Folded sponges on a ring forceps or cottonoid dissectors may also be helpful. As the dissection progresses posteriorly, the iliopsoas muscle is identified and the peritoneum is freed from the iliopsoas toward the midline. The intact peritoneum with the contained abdominal contents can be displaced medially. The diaphragm can now be detached in a circumferential fashion from the tip of the cartilage to the area where the vertebral bodies pass beneath the diaphragm. A convenient way to accomplish this is to make a series of cuts with curved Mayo scissors. The full length of the cutting edge of the scissors is inserted along the diaphragm, aligning it approximately 0.75 to 1 inch from the attachment of the diaphragm to the chest wall. The cut is then made, leaving an adequate cuff or diaphragm on the chest wall, useful for the eventual reattachment of the diaphragm. Two sutures are placed opposite one another at the end of the incision. These are quite helpful in realigning the diaphragm at the time of closure.

The diaphragm is progressively detached by repeating the maneuver of making a curvilinear cut in the diaphragm and then placing marking sutures until the midline and vertebral bodies and the right crus of the diaphragm are reached. The pleura over the vertebral bodies of the lower thoracic spine can be incised and mobilized if exposure of these vertebrae is essential to the orthopedic procedure. A rib spreader is inserted. Further exposure in the abdominal portion of the incision may be needed. It can be accomplished by stripping the peritoneum from the inside of the abdominal musculature and then incising the internal oblique muscle and the transversalis muscle. Depending on the level of the rib that is removed and the extent of the abdominal muscle incised, the vertebrae from T9 to L4 can be exposed.

Exposure of the Spine and Management of Its Vascular Supply

Exposure of the Spine

After the lung has been collapsed, the parietal pleura is incised vertically to expose the spinal area involved or the abdominal peritoneum, and its contents are retracted to expose the vertebral bodies without injury to the ureters or other retroperitoneal structures. Injury to either the arterial supply to the vertebra or to any adjacent venous channels, especially in the lumbar area, must be guarded against. The use of Bovie unipolar cautery or packing near a neuroforamen is to be avoided because of potential infarction of the anterior spinal artery or compression of the spinal cord (see Chapter 37).

Vascular Supply

The lower cervical region is supplied by radicular branches of the vertebral, thyrocervical, and costocervical arteries. The thoracic and lumbar areas receive their blood supply from the aorta. The vascular supply to the spine is segmental and paired at each vertebral level. These vessels arise from the aorta and supply the vertebral body and the intraspinal structures (Fig. 44-2). Approximately 75% of the blood supply to the anterior spinal artery comes from these vessels. In the lower thoracic spine, blood supply to the anterior spinal artery is supplemented by that from the artery of Adamkiewicz; in fact, it may be the major blood supply

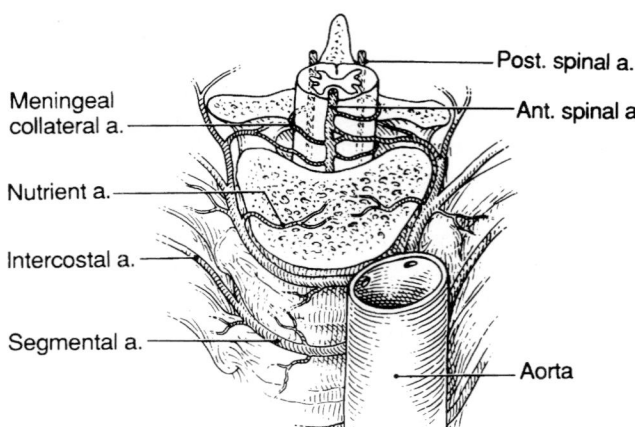

Fig. 44-2. Anatomy of segmental arteries in relation to aorta and intercostal arteries. a., artery; Ant., anterior; Post., posterior. From Anderson TM, Mansour KA, Miller JI Jr: Thoracic approaches to anterior spinal operations: anterior thoracic approaches. Ann Thorac Surg 55:1447, 1994. Reprinted with permission from the Society of Thoracic Surgeons.

to the lower half of the spinal cord. This artery arises from an intercostal vessel anywhere from the level of T7–L2 but generally arises at T8–T10. In 75 to 80% of patients, it arises on the left side; in 20 to 25%, it arises from the right side (Fig. 44-3). There is controversy as to whether this vessel must be visualized by preoperative angiography before operation on the lower thoracic spine, but many, including McElvein (1993), believe it is unnecessary. The segmental arterial branches on the ipsilateral side are divided over the body of the vertebra close to the aorta, including one segmental branch above and below the extent of the pathologic process. Evoked potentials are obtained to ensure that injury to the spinal cord does not occur.

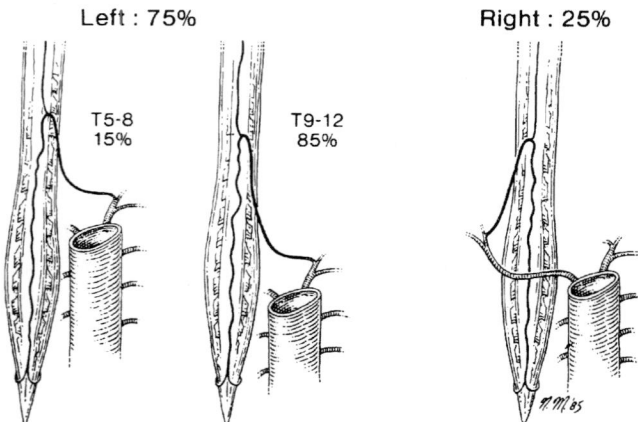

Fig. 44-3. Variation in the origin of the artery of Adamkiewicz from the intercostal vessels of the thoracic arch. From Shields TW, Reynolds M: Neurogenic tumors of the thorax. Surg Clin North Am 68:645, 1988. With permission.

Management of the Diseased Vertebra or Intervertebral Disc

The management of the vertebra and intervertebral disc generally is carried out by the neurosurgeon or orthopedic surgeon and depends on the disease process present. In Pott's disease or other infectious processes, a paraspinal abscess is evacuated and precise curettage of the diseased vertebra is carried out. In patients with malignant involvement, Walsh and associates (1997) remove the vertebral body and perform a discectomy above and below the involved vertebra. The tumor is removed down to the posterior longitudinal ligament, which is incised and retracted to expose the dural sac to decompress the sac. The nerve roots must be visualized as well as the bony end plates of the vertebrae above and below the resected discs. These structures must be free of gross tumor. In patients with a complex kyphoscoliotic deformity, extensive exposure is necessary to manage both upper and lower ends of the spinal curvature as noted by Janik and associates (1997).

Reconstruction and Fixation

Reconstruction may be carried out by bone grafts; autogenous bone is preferred. Most of these are not vascularized, but McElvein and colleagues (1988) suggest the use of a vascularized rib segment. A methylmethacrylate strut may be fashioned and used instead of a bone graft. Walsh and associates (1997) have presented their technique with this material.

Fixation, when indicated, is carried out anteriorly by using locking plate and screw constructs whenever possible. When this cannot be done, posterior constructs are placed via a separate posterior incision, either during the same operative procedure or several days later. The former is preferred over the latter approach whenever possible. In patients with scoliosis, special instrumentation (e.g., Dwyer internal fixation apparatus, Harrington rods) is required, as is also the case with fracture-dislocations of C7–T1.

MORTALITY AND MORBIDITY

The mortality rate after anterior exposure of the spine varies from zero to as high as 8.2% (Table 44-2). These rates depend primarily on the disease process present, patient selection, and the age group operated on. Cancer patients appear to have the highest incidence of postoperative mortality; although Naunheim and colleagues (1994), by multivariate analysis of their data, showed that the only significant independent predictor of a postoperative fatality was the presence of osteomyelitis, and this was associated with a mortality of 25%.

Postoperative morbidity rates vary from 7.8% to as high as 29.5% (see Table 44-2). The major complications are res-

Table 44-2. Mortality and Morbidity Rates after Anterior Spinal Operations

Author	Date	Mortality Rate (%)	Morbidity Rate (%)
Richardson et al.	1976	4.5	NR
McAfee and Zdeblick	1989	0	17.0
McElvein et al.	1988	0	17.7
Anderson et al.	1993	2.7	22.0
Naunheim et al.	1994	3.2	NR
Janik et al.	1997	0	9.8
Walsh et al.	1997	8.2	29.5

NR, not recorded.

piratory: pulmonary dysfunction, retained secretions, atelectasis, pulmonary edema, adult respiratory distress syndrome, effusion, and pneumothorax from air leaks. Cardiac complications comprise the second largest number and consist of dysrhythmias, myocardial infarction, and congestive failure. Urinary tract infection, cerebrovascular accident, gastrointestinal complications, and wound infection and dehiscence are recorded in a varying number of patients.

RESULTS

The results of these various anterior spinal procedures can be considered very satisfactory to excellent in most patients, depending on the underlying disease process. In patients with Pott's disease, Richardson and coworkers (1976) reported that 77.2% of their patients were completely rehabilitated, and those who had a major neurologic deficit—paraplegia—evidenced a 100% recovery. McAfee and Zdeblick (1989) and Walsh and associates (1997) noted substantial pain relief in 93% and 90% of their surviving patients, respectively. Neurologic defects were ameliorated in almost all patients, and ambulation was regained in 85% and 75%, respectively, in the two aforementioned series in patients who were unable to walk preoperatively. In the report by Naunheim and colleagues, existing neurologic defects were lessened in 97%. These results contrast with those reported by Siegal and Siegal (1985), who used posterior laminectomies plus stabilization to relieve spinal cord compression by malignant epidural tumors. They reported neurologic improvement in only 44% of patients. Moreover, their operations were accompanied by wound complications and infection in 28% of cases. Bohlman and Zdeblick (1988) used a transthoracic approach in eight patients with herniated thoracic discs. They reported an excellent result (full recovery) in 62.4% and a good result (mild muscular weakness or mild pain) in 37.4%. More spe-

cific details of results in patients with fracture-dislocations or major spinal deformities (e.g., scoliosis or kyphosis) are found in the reading references. Overall, the results after operations carried out by the anterior route appear to amply justify this approach.

REFERENCES

Anderson TM, Mansour KA, Miller JI Jr: Thoracic approaches to anterior spinal operations: anterior thoracic approaches. Ann Thorac Surg 55:1447, 1993.

Bohlman HH, Zdeblick TA: Anterior excision of herniated thoracic discs. J Bone Joint Surg 70:1038, 1988.

Burrington JD, et al: Anterior approach to the thoracolumbar spine: technical considerations. Arch Surg 111:456, 1976.

Cauchoix J, Binet J: Anterior surgical approaches to the spine. Ann R Coll Surg Engl 27:237, 1957.

Cook WA: Transthoracic vertebral surgery. Ann Thorac Surg 12:54, 1971.

Dwyer AF, Newton NC, Sherwood AA: An anterior approach to scoliosis. A preliminary report. Clin Orthop 62:192, 1969.

Harrington KD: The use of methylmethacrylate for vertebral-body replacement and anterior stabilization of pathological fracture-dislocations of the spine due to metastatic malignant disease. J Bone Joint Surg Am 63:36, 1981.

Hodgson AR, Stock FE: Anterior spinal fusion: a preliminary communication on radical treatment of Pott's disease and Pott's paraplegia. Br J Surg 44:266, 1956.

Hodgson AR, et al: Anterior spinal fusion: the operative approach and pathologic findings in 412 patients with Pott's disease of the spine. Br J Surg 48:172, 1960.

Janik JS, et al: Anterior exposure of spinal deformities and tumors: a 20-year experience. J Pediatr Surg 32:852, 1997.

McAfee PC, Zdeblick TA: Tumors of the thoracic and lumbar spine: surgical treatment via the anterior approach. J Spinal Disord 2:145, 1989.

McElvein RB: In discussion of Anderson TM, Mansour KA, Miller JI Jr: Thoracic approaches to anterior spinal operations: anterior thoracic approaches. Ann Thorac Surg 55:1447, 1993.

McElvein RB, et al: Transthoracic exposure for anterior spinal surgery. Ann Thorac Surg 45:278, 1988.

Naunheim KS, et al: Anterior exposure of the thoracic spine. Ann Thorac Surg 57:1436, 1994.

Perot PL Jr, Munro DD: Transthoracic removal of midline thoracic disc protrusions causing spinal cord compression. Neurosurgery 31:452, 1969.

Richardson JD, et al: Transthoracic approach for Pott's disease. Ann Thorac Surg 21:552, 1976.

Siegal T, Siegal T: Surgical decompression of anterior and posterior malignant epidural tumors compressing the spinal cord: a prospective study. Neurosurgery 17:424, 1985.

Thurer RJ, Herskowitz K: Open approaches to posterior mediastinal tumors and the spine. Chest Surg Clin N Am 6:117, 1996.

Walsh GL, et al: Anterior approaches to the thoracic spine in patients with cancer: indications and results. Ann Thorac Surg 64:1611, 1997.

READING REFERENCES

Bridwell K, Dewald R: Spinal Surgery. Philadelphia: JB Lippincott, 1996.

Hoppenfeld S, deBoer P: Surgical Exposure in Orthopedics. Philadelphia: JB Lippincott, 1991.

Watkins R: Surgical Approach to the Spine. New York: Springer-Verlag, 1983.

CHAPTER 45

Chest Wall Tumors

Peter C. Pairolero

Chest wall tumors encompass a kaleidoscopic panorama of bone and soft tissue disease. Included among these tumors are benign and malignant primary neoplasms of the bony skeleton; chest wall metastases; neoplasms that invade the chest wall from the lung, pleura, mediastinum, muscle, and breast; and benign nonneoplastic conditions (Table 45-1). Nearly all of these disorders have at one time or another been irradiated either as the treatment of choice or in combination with chest wall resection, and patients commonly present with a postradiation necrotic chest wall tumor. The thoracic surgeon is frequently asked to evaluate all of these patients, most often to establish a diagnosis. The thoracic surgeon is also sometimes called on to treat the condition until it is cured and occasionally is asked to manage necrotic, foul-smelling chest wall ulcers. All are diagnostic and therapeutic challenges. Surgical extirpation in many of these patients is frequently the only remaining modality of treatment; this may be compromised by incorrect diagnosis or an inability to reconstruct large chest wall defects. From a practical standpoint, however, treatment for cure is most often limited to resection of primary chest wall tumors.

INCIDENCE

Primary tumors of the chest wall are uncommon, and few series have been reported. Most reports such as those by Pascuzzi and colleagues (1957), Groff and Adkins (1967), and Stelzer and Gay (1980), excluded patients with soft tissue tumors and included only patients with primary bone tumors. When combined, however, the soft tissues become a major source of chest wall tumors, as noted by Graeber and colleagues (1982), the author and Arnold (1985), and King (1986), Ryan (1989), Eng (1990), Evans (1990) and their associates, as well as Farley and Seyfer (1991). Indeed, soft tissues are the most common source of primary chest wall malignancy, accounting for nearly 50% of these tumors treated surgically in adults. More recently, Andrassy and associates (1998) reported that soft tissue sarcomas were also

the most common chest wall tumors in children. Altogether, primary tumors of the chest wall, including bony and soft tissue tumor, account for approximately 2% of all primary tumors found in the body. The reported incidence of malignancy in these tumors varies from approximately 50 to 80%, with the higher malignancy rate found in those series including soft tissue tumors. Malignant fibrous histiocytoma, chondrosarcoma, and rhabdomyosarcoma are the most common primary malignant neoplasms that the thoracic surgeon is asked to manage, and cartilaginous tumors, desmoids, and fibrous dysplasias are the most common primary benign tumors (Table 45-2). Radiation-associated malignant tumors of the chest wall are also increasing. Schwarz and Burt (1996) reported that osteosarcoma is the most common tumor seen after radiation.

BASIC PRINCIPLES

Signs and Symptoms

Chest wall tumors generally present as slowly enlarging masses. Most are initially asymptomatic, but with continued growth, pain invariably occurs. At first the pain is frequently generalized, and the patient is often treated for a neuritis or musculoskeletal complaint. Nearly all malignant tumors are likely to become painful, as compared to only two-thirds of benign tumors. In some instances of rib tumors, a mass may not be apparent on physical examination but instead is detected on radiograph of the chest. On occasion, fever, leukocytosis, and eosinophilia accompany some of these tumors.

Diagnosis

The diagnostic evaluation of patients with suspected chest wall tumors should include a careful history and physical and laboratory examination followed by conventional plain and

Table 45-1. Classification of Chest Wall Tumors

Primary neoplasms of chest wall
    Malignant
    Benign
Metastatic neoplasms to chest wall
    Sarcoma
    Carcinoma
Adjacent neoplasms with local invasion
    Lung
    Breast
    Pleura
Nonneoplastic disease
    Cyst
    Inflammation

tomographic chest radiography. Previous radiographs of the chest are important in determining growth rate. In general, magnetic resonance (MR) imaging is the preferred method of imaging chest wall tumors, as pointed out by Fortier and associates (1992, 1994), Siegel and Luken (1996), and Wyttenbach and associates (1998). Not only does MR imaging distinguish the tumor from nerves and blood vessels, but it also allows visualization in different planes, such as coronal or sagittal. MR imaging, however, does not accurately assess pulmonary nodules or the extent of calcification within the lung. Thus, if the lung parenchyma needs evaluation for metastatic disease, computed tomography is preferable.

Chest wall tumors that are clinically suspected of being primary neoplasms, either benign or malignant, require tissue diagnosis by histologic examination. Because most malignant primary tumors have a benign counterpart, adequate tissue sampling is mandatory, and an open biopsy provides more thorough sampling than needle aspiration. The biopsy, however, should not interfere with subsequent treatment. An improperly placed biopsy site, extensive soft tissue

Table 45-2. Primary Chest Wall Tumor

Malignant
    Myeloma
    Malignant fibrous histiocytoma
    Chondrosarcoma
    Rhabdomyosarcoma
    Ewing's sarcoma
    Liposarcoma
    Neurofibrosarcoma
    Osteogenic sarcoma
    Hemangiosarcoma
    Leiomyosarcoma
    Lymphoma
Benign
    Osteochondroma
    Chondroma
    Desmoid
    Fibrous dysplasia
    Lipoma
    Fibroma
    Neurilemoma

dissection, and wound infection can all complicate subsequent treatment by delaying definitive resection, radiation therapy, or chemotherapy.

Most pathologists are reluctant to diagnose chest wall tumors on frozen section examination, preferring instead to obtain special stains and multiple tissue sections and to confer with their colleagues. Consequently, definitive diagnosis is frequently not available until several days after the biopsy is obtained.

Small primary neoplasms (3 to 5 cm) should be diagnosed by excisional biopsy with minimal margins (1 cm). Chest wall closure for these small lesions is usually straightforward and does not require skeletal reconstruction. If the lesion eventually proves to be benign or is a malignancy better treated with irradiation, chemotherapy, or both (as discussed later), no further operative intervention is indicated. If malignant and wide radical excision is required, however, the patient should be returned to the operating room, where the biopsy site is completely excised and a 4-cm margin of chest wall is obtained. Primary chest wall tumors bigger than 5 cm should be diagnosed by incisional biopsy. The skin incision should be positioned in such a location that wound healing is not compromised, thereby preventing ulceration and infection. To prevent cancer dissemination, skin flaps should not be elevated and the pleural space should not be entered. After pathologic examination is complete, treatment can proceed as indicated. Needle aspiration should be reserved only for those patients with a known primary tumor elsewhere and who are clinically suspected of having a metastasis; if nondiagnostic, however, open biopsy is indicated.

Treatment

Wide resection of primary malignant chest wall neoplasm is essential to successful management. The extent of resection should not be compromised because of an inability to close the chest wall defect. Consequently, the mandatory ingredients for successful management of these neoplasms are wide resection and dependable reconstruction, as I and Arnold (1985, 1986) and Arnold and I (1979, 1984, 1996) pointed out.

Opinions about what constitutes wide resection differ. King and associates (1986) analyzed the effect of extent of resection on long-term survival in patients with primary malignant chest wall neoplasm. The percentage of patients with a 4-cm or more margin of resection remaining free from cancer at 5 years was 56%, compared to only 29% for patients with a 2-cm margin (Fig. 45-1). Many surgeons consider a margin of resection free of tumor of several centimeters to be adequate. Although this may be adequate for chest wall metastases, benign tumor, and certain low-grade malignant primary bone neoplasms (such as chondrosarcoma), a 2-cm resection margin is inadequate for more malignant neoplasms, such as malignant fibrous histiocy-

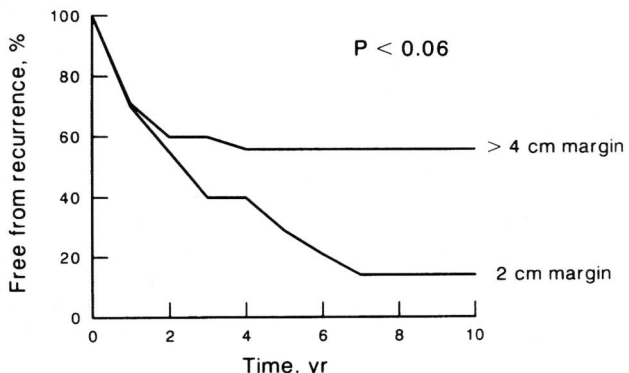

Fig. 45-1. Percentage of patients with malignant chest wall neoplasms remaining free from recurrent cancer by extent of resection margin. Zero time on abscissa represents day of chest wall resection. From King RM, et al: Primary chest wall tumors: factors affecting survival. Ann Thorac Surg *41*:597, 1986. With permission.

toma and osteogenic sarcoma, that can spread within the marrow cavity or along such tissue planes as the periosteum or parietal pleura. Consequently, all primary malignant neoplasms initially diagnosed by excisional biopsy should have further resection to include at least a 4-cm margin of normal tissue on all sides. High-grade malignancies should also have the entire involved bone resected. For neoplasms of the rib cage, this includes removal of the involved ribs, the corresponding anterior costal arches if the tumor is located anteriorly, and several partial ribs above and below the neoplasm. For tumors of the sternum and manubrium, resection of the entire involved bone and corresponding costal arches bilaterally is indicated. Any attached structures, such as lung, thymus, pericardium, or chest wall muscles, should also be excised.

The role of resection for chest wall metastases and recurrent breast cancer is controversial. Nonetheless, most thoracic surgeons would agree that tumor ulceration is an indication for excision. For these patients, wound hygiene is crucial, and surgical excision is frequently the only treatment option available. The goal in treating patients with necrotic tumor should be a healed wound after local excision. Although the length of survival is not increased after resection, the quality of life is certainly improved.

SPECIFIC TUMORS

Primary Bone Tumors

Primary chest wall tumors historically have included neoplasms and nonneoplastic conditions, such as cysts, infections, and fibromatosis. Although these tumors represent an array of different causes, combining them is still prudent because most present similarly, and many have common radiographic features. Primary bone neoplasms constitute the majority of these tumors.

Primary bone neoplasms involving the chest wall are uncommon. In the Mayo Clinic's series of 6034 bone tumors reported by Dahlin and Unni (1986), 355 (5.9%) occurred in either the ribs (85%) or the sternum (15%). Overall, 89% were malignant and only 11% were benign. Sternal tumors were slightly more likely to be malignant (96% versus 88%). The most common benign bone neoplasms were cartilaginous in origin—osteochondroma and chondroma. The most common malignant neoplasms were myeloma, chondrosarcoma, malignant lymphoma, and Ewing's sarcoma.

Benign Rib Tumors

Osteochondroma

Osteochondroma is the most common benign bone neoplasm, constituting nearly 50% of all benign rib tumors. The incidence, however, may actually be higher, because most patients are asymptomatic, and the tumors are often not removed. Men are affected three times more frequently than women. The neoplasm begins in childhood and continues to grow until skeletal maturity is reached. The onset of pain in a previously asymptomatic tumor may indicate malignant degeneration.

Osteochondromas arise from the metaphyseal region of the rib and present as a stalked bony protuberance with a cartilaginous cap. A rim of calcification may be present at the periphery of the tumor, and stippled calcification is often present within the tumor (Fig. 45-2). Microscopically, bony proliferation occurs to varying degrees; the thickness of the cartilaginous cap also varies.

All osteochondromas occurring in children after puberty or in adults should be resected. Asymptomatic osteochondromas may occur before puberty, but if pain or increase in size occurs, the tumor should be resected. Rarely, an osteochondroma may cause injury to either the diaphragm, as reported by Fujiu and associates (1996), or to the pleura with the occurrence of a hemothorax. Fujiu and associates collected 12 such cases in the literature, including those reported by Tomares (1994) and Harrison (1994) and their colleagues. Repair of injury and excision of the offending rib lesion are indicated.

Chondroma

Chondromas constitute 15% of all benign neoplasms of the rib cage. Most occur anteriorly at the costochondral junction. Both sexes are affected equally, and the tumor can occur at any age. These neoplasms usually present as a slowly enlarging mass that may be nontender or slightly painful. Radiographically, chondroma is an expansile lesion causing thinning of the cortex. The differentiation between a chondroma and a chondrosarcoma is impossible on clinical

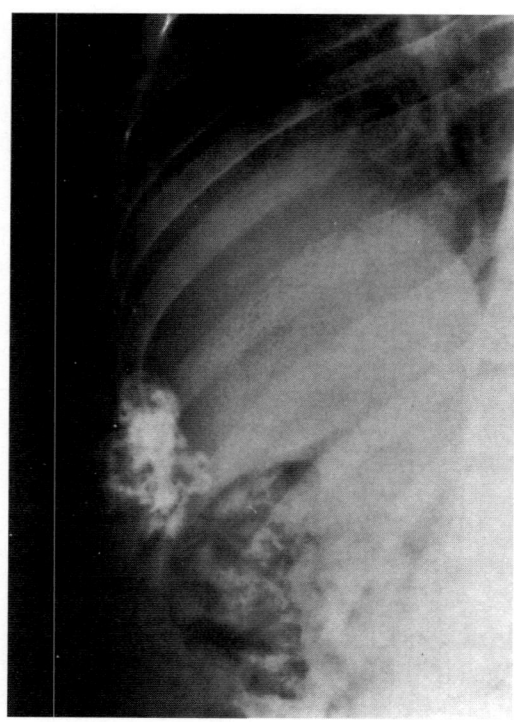

Fig. 45-2. A 52-year-old man with osteochondroma arising in the anterior right ninth rib. Note intact cortex and stippled calcification within the tumor.

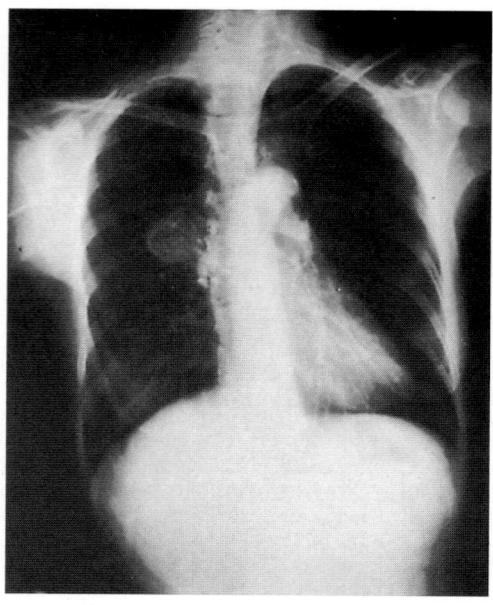

Fig. 45-3. Fibrous dysplasia involving the posterior ribs. Resection necessitated excision of the lateral portion of the adjacent vertebral body.

and radiographic examination. Grossly, chondroma presents as a lobulated mass. Microscopically, the tumor is characterized by lobules of hyaline cartilage. The microscopic differentiation between a chondroma and a low-grade chondrosarcoma can be extremely difficult. All chondromas must be considered malignant and should be treated by wide excision. Although this resection may seem extensive for what may turn out to be a benign tumor, modern reconstructive techniques make the risk negligible, and long-term results are excellent.

Fibrous Dysplasia

Fibrous dysplasia is a cystic, nonneoplastic lesion and is probably a developmental abnormality characterized by fibrous replacement of the medullary cavity of the rib. Most cases present as solitary lesions; when multiple lesions are encountered, Albright's syndrome (multiple bone cysts, skin pigmentation, and precocious sexual maturity in girls) should be suspected.

Fibrous dysplasia is usually manifested by a slowly enlarging, nonpainful mass in the posterolateral rib cage. Both sexes are affected equally. The disease begins in childhood, often in infancy, but is not detected until routine screening chest radiography in young adulthood. Radiographically, its appearance is characteristic, consisting of expansion and thinning of the bony cortex with a central ground-glass appearance (Fig. 45-3). Microscopically, some

degree of calcification with bony trabeculation and fibrous formation appears. Treatment should be conservative. Many lesions stop growing at puberty. Local excision is indicated for painful, enlarging lesions.

Histiocytosis X

Histiocytosis X is not a neoplasm but is a part of the spectrum of disease involving the reticuloendothelial system, including eosinophilic granuloma, Letterer-Siwe disease, and Hand-Schüller-Christian disease. Microscopically, all three components are similar and consist of a mixed inflammatory infiltrate of eosinophils and histiocytes.

Eosinophilic granuloma is limited to only bone involvement, whereas Hand-Schüller-Christian disease and Letterer-Siwe disease may have systemic signs and symptoms such as fever, malaise, weight loss, lymphadenopathy, and splenomegaly; leukocytosis, eosinophilia, and anemia are also often present with these two diseases. Most patients with eosinophilic granuloma present with pain limited to the area of skeletal involvement. Histiocytosis X occurs in persons younger than 50 years. Letterer-Siwe disease typically occurs in infants, Hand-Schüller-Christian disease in children, and eosinophilic granuloma in young to middle-aged adults.

Bone lesions occur in all three clinical variants of histiocytosis X. The skull is most commonly involved, but 10 to 20% of patients have rib lesions. The radiographic appearance is similar for all three forms of the disease. The lesion presents as an expansile lesion in the ribs, with periosteal new bone formation and uneven destruction of the cortex producing endosteal scalloping. Confusion with osteomyelitis may occur because of accompanying fever, malaise, and elevated white blood cell count.

Because of the expansile nature of histiocytosis X, excisional biopsy is required to establish the diagnosis. In patients with eosinophilic granuloma, excision alone should result in cure if the lesion is solitary. For patients with multiple lesions of eosinophilic granuloma, low-dose radiation therapy (300 to 600 rads) to each lesion has been helpful. Characteristically, the other two variants of the disease run a chronic course requiring corticosteroids and chemotherapy.

Malignant Rib Tumors

Myeloma

Myeloma is the most common primary malignant rib neoplasm, accounting for one-third of all tumors in the Mayo Clinic series reported by Dahlin and Unni (1986). Most myelomas involving the chest wall occur as a manifestation of systemic multiple myeloma, and a patient with a myeloma of the rib cage almost inevitably develops the manifestations of the systemic disease. Solitary myeloma involving the rib is secondary only to solitary vertebral involvement. Myeloma is most common in the fifth through seventh decades of life and is rare in people younger than 30 years. Two-thirds of the patients are men. Pain is the most common symptom and often occurs without a palpable mass. Most patients are anemic, with an increase in the erythrocyte sedimentation rate. Abnormal protein electrophoresis is present in 85% of patients, and up to 50% have hypercalcemia and Bence Jones protein in their urine.

Radiographically, myeloma presents as a punched-out osteolytic lesion with cortical thinning. Pathologic fracture is common. Grossly, the tumor is typically gray and friable. Microscopically, sheets of closely packed cells with abundant cytoplasm is observed. Mitosis is rare, but hyperchromatism and multinuclear cells are present.

Whether the rib changes are solitary or multiple, local excision is done to confirm the diagnosis, and radiation therapy is the treatment of choice for solitary and both irradiation and chemotherapy for multiple lesions. Five-year survival is approximately 20%.

Chondrosarcoma

Accounting for nearly 30% of all primary malignant bone neoplasms, chondrosarcoma is most frequently a neoplasm of the anterior chest wall, with 75% arising in either the costochondral arches or the sternum. The tumor most commonly occurs in the third and fourth decades of life and is relatively uncommon in persons younger than 20 years. Chondrosarcoma is more frequent in men. Nearly all patients present with a slowly enlarging mass that has usually been painful for many months. Grossly, chondrosarcoma is a lobulated neoplasm that may grow to massive proportions and consequently may extend internally into the pleural space or outwardly into the muscle and adipose tissue of the chest wall (Fig. 45-4). Microscopically, the findings range from normal cartilage to obvious malignant changes. Lichtenstein and Jaffe (1943) described the characteristic findings of plump, atypical, and multiple nuclei, which may be more apparent in the peripheral areas of a growing tumor (Fig. 45-5). Differentiation from chondroma may be extremely difficult. From a practical standpoint, all tumors arising in the costal cartilages should be considered to be malignant and should be treated by wide resection.

The cause of chondrosarcoma is unknown. Although malignant degeneration of benign cartilaginous tumors (secondary chondrosarcoma) has been reported, most chondrosarcomas arise de nova. Lichtenstein (1977) was the first to suggest an association between trauma and chondrosarcoma. McAfee and associates (1985) subsequently reported that 12.5% of their patients had sustained severe crushing injury to the ipsilateral chest wall.

Radiographically, chondrosarcoma has a characteristic appearance. The tumor appears as a lobulated mass arising in the medullary portion of the bone (Fig. 45-6). The cortex is often destroyed, and the margins of the tumor are poorly defined (Fig. 45-7). Mineralization of the tumor matrix is common, producing a mottled type of calcification. Pathologic fracture is uncommon. Computed tomography can be helpful in determining the extent of the neoplasms (Fig. 45-8).

Definitive diagnosis of chondrosarcoma can only be made pathologically. Histologic confirmation, however, is sometimes difficult, because most chondrosarcomas are well differentiated. This tendency to be well differentiated may result in misdiagnosis of chondroma and subsequent undertreatment, leading to local recurrences. Generous sampling in the pathology laboratory of different areas within the tumor may facilitate histologic diagnosis. For this reason, excisional biopsy rather than incisional or needle biopsy of all chest wall masses suspected of being chondrosarcoma is indicated.

Chest wall chondrosarcoma typically grows slowly and recurs locally. If it is left untreated, metastases occur late. Prompt, complete control of the primary neoplasm is the main determinant of survival; the objective of the first operation should be resection wide enough to prevent local recurrence. This involves resection of a 4-cm margin of normal tissue on all sides. Wide resection results in cure in nearly all patients (Fig. 45-9), with 10-year survival approaching 97%, as reported by McAfee and associates (1985).

Ewing's Sarcoma

Ewing's sarcoma involving the rib cage accounts for 12% of all primary malignant neoplasms of the bony thorax. Two-thirds of all cases of Ewing's sarcoma occur in persons younger than 20 years, but young infants rarely develop this tumor. Boys are affected twice as often as girls. Signs and symptoms are common. A painful, enlarging mass is common. Fever, malaise, anemia, leukocytosis, and

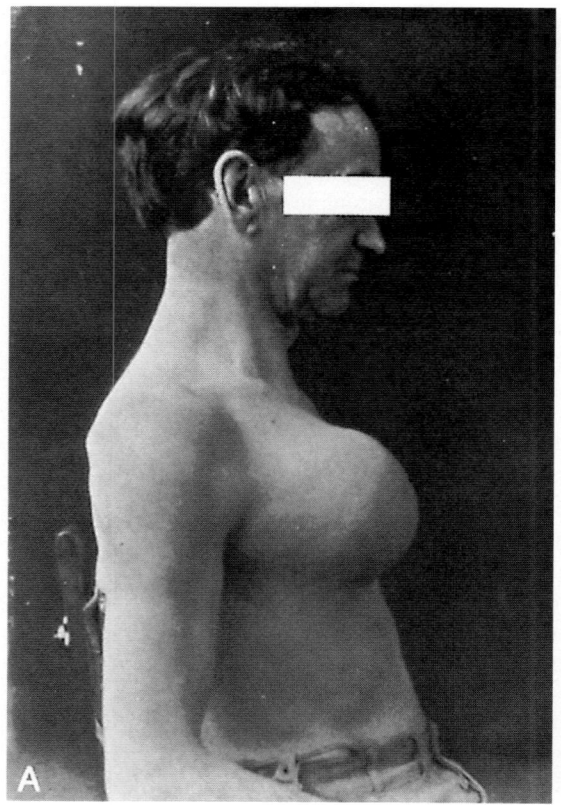

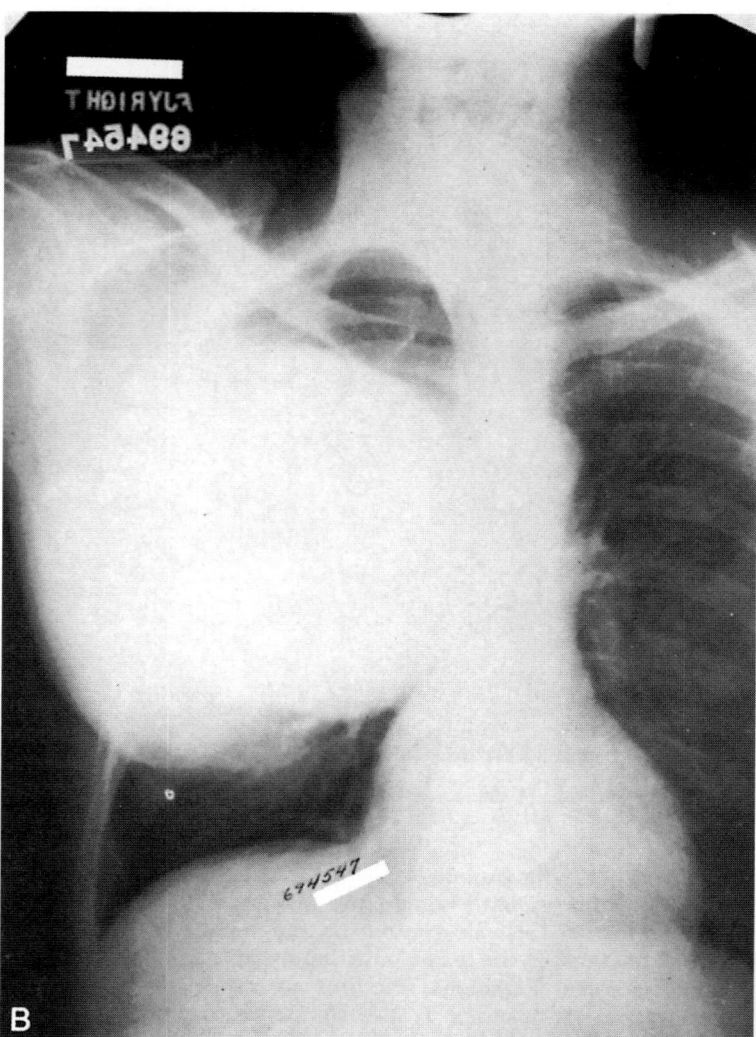

Fig. 45-4. A. A 56-year-old man with a huge chondrosarcoma arising from the right anterior third costochondral arch. **B.** Chest radiograph of the same patient.

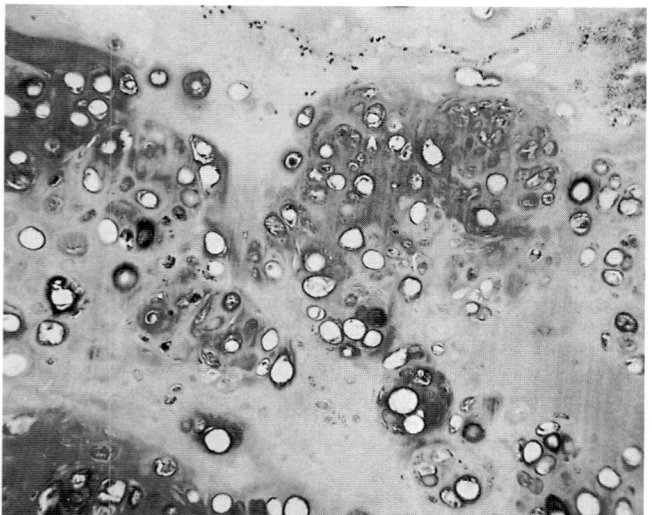

Fig. 45-5. Photomicrograph demonstrating typical cellular changes of chondrosarcoma.

an increased sedimentation rate may be present. Radiographically, mottled destruction containing lytic and blastic areas appears. An onion-skin appearance of the surface of the bone, caused by elevation of the periosteum and multiple layers of subperiosteal new bone formation, may be seen, but this feature is not pathognomonic because it may be found in other bone tumors, both benign and malignant. Radiating spicules may also be present on the surface of the bone, which makes the lesion indistinguishable from osteogenic sarcoma. Pathologic fractures are rare. The radiographic appearance is also similar to that of osteomyelitis. This similarity, combined with fever, leukocytosis, and an increase in sedimentation rate, may lead to the erroneous diagnosis of osteomyelitis.

Ewing's sarcoma tends to be whitish-gray and is soft and not encapsulated. Histologically, the tumor is cellular, and distinguishing Ewing's sarcoma from lymphoma may be difficult. Early spread to the lungs and to other bones is common and occurs in 30 to 75% of patients.

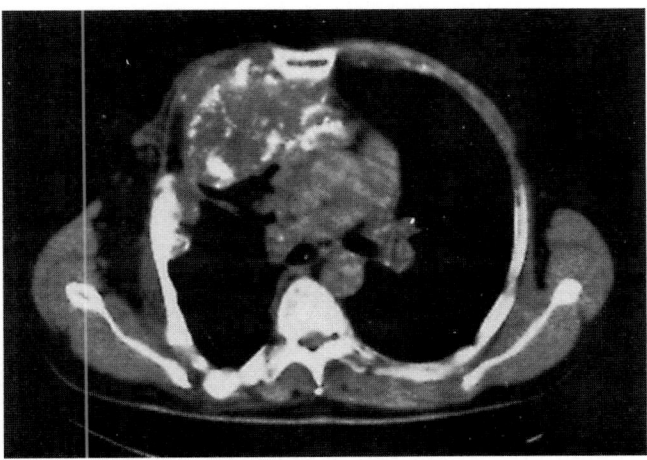

Fig. 45-8. Computed tomographic scan of a 59-year-old man with chondrosarcoma arising in the right anterior chest wall. Note destruction of cortex and stippling within the neoplasm.

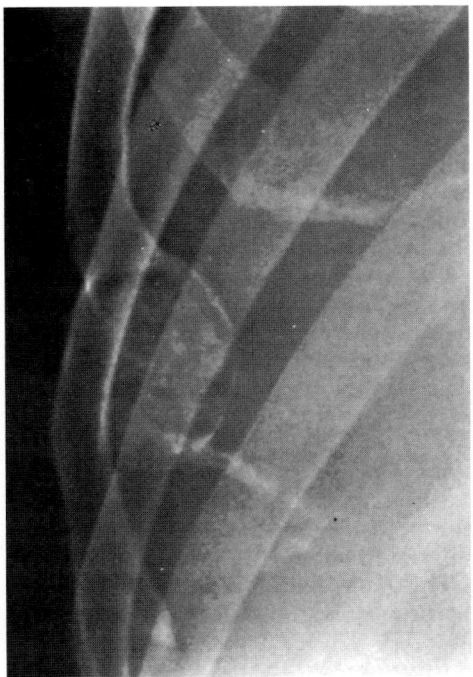

Fig. 45-6. A 53-year-old man with chondrosarcoma of the right anterior sixth rib. Mass had been present 18 months without pain. From McAfee MK, et al: Chondrosarcoma of the chest wall: factors affecting survival. Ann Thorac Surg *40*:535, 1985. With permission.

Adequate biopsy is necessary for correct diagnosis. Ewing's sarcoma is radiosensitive; thus, irradiation is the treatment of choice. Adjuvant chemotherapy is also used. Five-year survival is 40 to 50%.

Osteogenic Sarcoma

Osteosarcoma of the bony thorax is less common than chondrosarcoma and constitutes 6% of all primary malignant bone neoplasms. Unfortunately, it is more malignant and, hence, carries a much less favorable prognosis. Osteogenic sarcoma generally occurs in teenagers and young adults and commonly affects more young men than women. Most patients present with a rapidly enlarging tumor that is often painful. Serum alkaline phosphatase lev-

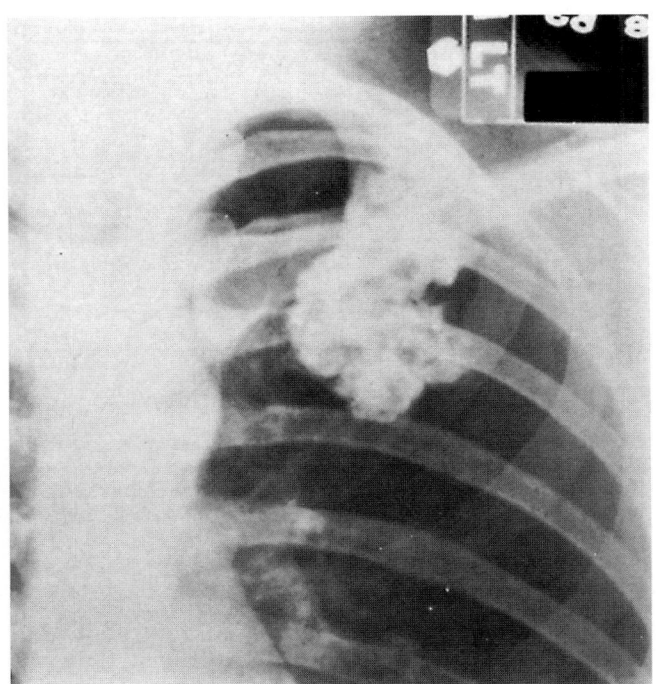

Fig. 45-7. A 32-year-old woman with chondrosarcoma of the left anterior first rib. Both supraclavicular pain and a mass had been present for 2 months. From McAfee MK, et al: Chondrosarcoma of the chest wall: factors affecting survival. Ann Thorac Surg *40*:535, 1985. With permission.

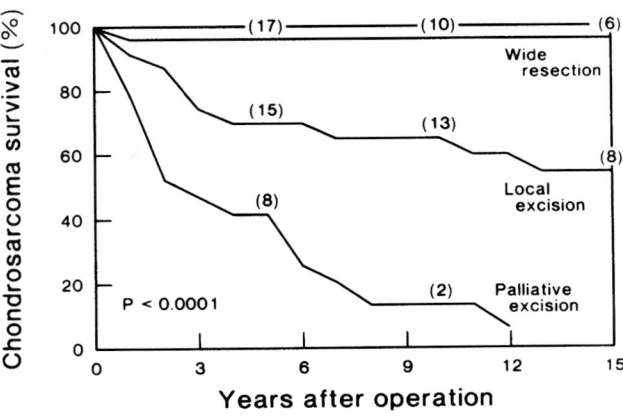

Fig. 45-9. Survival of patients with chest wall chondrosarcoma by extent of operation. Zero time on abscissa represents day of operation. From McAfee MK, et al: Chondrosarcoma of the chest wall: factors affecting survival. Ann Thorac Surg *40*:535, 1985. With permission.

els are frequently elevated. Radiographically, bone destruction with indistinct borders that gradually merge into adjacent normal bone appears. Calcification characteristically occurs at right angles to the cortex, producing a sunburst appearance. Pathologic fractures are rare. Grossly, the tumor is large and lobulated, with extension through cortical bone and into adjacent soft tissue. Microscopically, the predominant component may be bony, cartilaginous, or fibrous.

The treatment of osteogenic sarcoma consists of wide resection of the tumor, including the entire involved bone (rib or sternum) and adjacent soft tissues (lung or muscle). Radiation therapy has not been valuable in managing this neoplasm, and the role of chemotherapy remains controversial. In general, the prognosis is poor: the 5-year survival rate is 20%.

Radiation-Associated Malignant Tumors

Malignant postirradiation tumors of the chest wall are uncommon, but the frequency appears to be increasing. Schwarz and Burt (1996) reported on 361 patients with primary chest wall tumors, 21 (6%) of whom previously had received irradiation in the area of the tumor. Indication for the initial radiation therapy most commonly was either lymphoma or breast cancer. Osteosarcoma and soft tissue sarcoma were the most common postirradiation tumors observed. Survival after wide resection was similar to survival following resection for tumors arising de novo. Because the outcome following resection appears to be similar, these patients should be offered identical treatment to those patients whose tumor arises de novo.

Tumors of the Manubrium, Sternum, Scapula, and Clavicle

Dahlin and Unni (1986) reported that primary neoplasms of the manubrium and sternum constitute 15% of all primary chest wall bone tumors. Nearly all (96%) are malignant. The majority are chondrosarcomas, myeloma, malignant lymphoma, and osteogenic sarcomas. In addition, the sternum is a frequent site of metastatic neoplasms, such as carcinomas originating in the breast, thyroid gland, or kidney; the last two often present as pulsating tumors. Benign tumors, such as chondromas, hemangiomas, and bone cysts, have been reported.

The scapula, as Dahlin and Unni (1986) noted, is a common site for primary bone neoplasms, having an incidence of 2.8%, which is approximately half those of the ribs and sternum combined (5.9%). Although it is an infrequent site for metastatic tumors, the same kinds of primary bone neoplasms occur in the scapula as in the rib cage. The malignant tumors include myeloma, Ewing's sarcoma, chondrosarcoma, osteogenic sarcoma, and lymphoma.

Primary neoplasms of the clavicle are uncommon, accounting for less than 1% of all primary bone tumors. Ninety percent are malignant. Over two-thirds of the malignant tumors are radiosensitive, being either myelomas (43%) or Ewing's sarcoma (22%). The clavicle is more likely to be a site of metastatic disease than of primary tumors.

Arnold and I (1978) emphasized that primary malignant neoplasms of the manubrium, sternum, scapula, and clavicle should be treated by wide resection, including all of the involved bone and a 4-cm margin.

Primary Soft Tissue Tumors

Primary soft tissue tumors may arise from any component of the thoracic cage, and a variety have been reported, based on a histologic diagnosis of the predominant cell type. Preoperative differentiation between these neoplasms is difficult. Pain often is present. Progressive enlargement is usually apparent by both physical and radiographic examination. Wide resection of the tumor and adjacent structures is the treatment of choice.

Benign Soft Tissue Tumors

Various benign tumors involving all chest wall structures have been reported. Predominant among these are fibromas; lipomas; giant cell tumors; neurogenic tumors; vascular tumors, such as hemangiomas with or without arteriovenous fistulas; and, less commonly, benign tumors of connective tissue. Malignant degeneration is uncommon, and all should be treated by local excision.

Desmoid

Desmoid tumor deserves special consideration. Forty percent of all desmoids occur in the shoulder and chest wall. Encapsulation of the brachial plexus and the vessels of the arm and neck is common. The tumor often extends into the pleural cavity, markedly displacing mediastinal structures (Fig. 45-10). Initially, the tumor presents as a poorly circumscribed mass with little or no pain. Paresthesias, hyperesthesia, and motor weakness occur later, after neural encasement. Veins or arteries are rarely occluded. Desmoid tumor occurs most commonly between puberty and 40 years of age and is rarely observed in infants or the very old. Men and women are affected equally.

Grossly, the tumor originates in muscle and fascia and frequently extends along tissue planes. Microscopically, a monotonous pattern of elongated spindle-shaped cells infiltrating the surrounding tissue is invariably seen. Most pathologists consider desmoids to be a form of benign fibromatosis, as do Goellner and Soule (1980) and Hayry and associates (1982). Because these tumors invade adjacent structures, however, and because Soule and Scanlon (1962) reported malignant degeneration, some, including Hajdu (1979), consider it to be a low-grade fibrosarcoma. Whatever the cause, the tumor tends to be recurrent if inadequately excised and should be treated with wide resection, like primary malignant chest wall neoplasms. Encapsulation of thoracic outlet structures presents a special

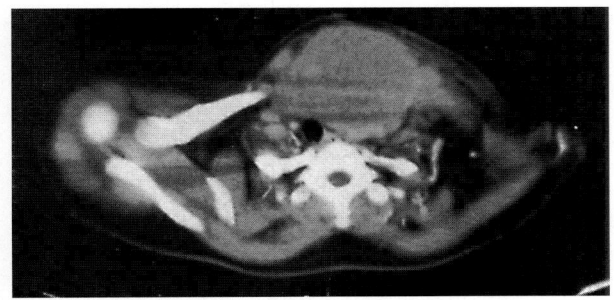

Fig. 45-10. Computed tomographic scan of a 35-year-old woman with desmoid tumor arising in the left axilla. Note the intrathoracic component displacing the trachea and brachiocephalic vessels to the right.

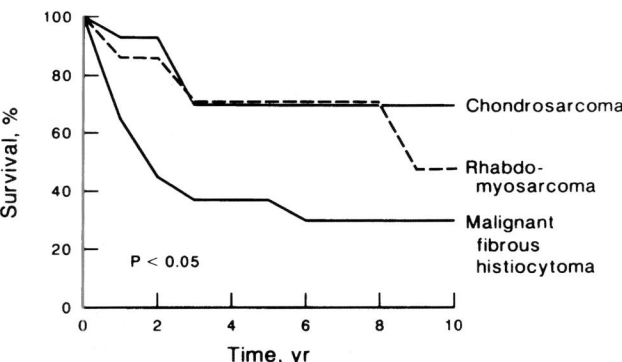

Fig. 45-11. Overall survival of patients with chest wall malignant neoplasms after resection. Zero time on abscissa represents day of chest wall resection. From King RM, et al: Primary chest wall tumors: factors affecting survival. Ann Thorac Surg *41*:597, 1986. With permission.

problem in management. Enucleation of the tumor from these structures followed by radiation therapy is current practice.

Malignant Soft Tissue Tumors

Malignant Fibrous Histiocytoma

As I and Arnold (1985) and King and associates (1986) pointed out, malignant fibrous histiocytoma is the most common primary chest wall neoplasm the thoracic surgeon is asked to evaluate. The tumor characteristically occurs in late adult life, with the majority of cases occurring between the ages of 50 and 70 years. These neoplasms are rare in childhood, and approximately two-thirds occur in men. Malignant fibrous histiocytoma often presents as a painless, slowly enlarging mass. Pregnancy, however, may accelerate the growth rate, resulting in pain. Weiss and Enzinger (1978) reported that fever and leukocytosis with neutropenia or eosinophilia are occasionally present. Excellent circumstantial evidence suggests that some chest wall malignant fibrous histiocytomas are radiation-induced; Weiss and Enzinger (1978) reported the development of this tumor within the irradiated area following therapy for breast cancer, Hodgkin's lymphoma, and myeloma.

Grossly malignant fibrous histiocytoma tends to be lobulated and spread for considerable distances along fascial planes or between muscle fibers, which accounts for its high recurrence rate after resection. Histologically, the tumor has a highly variable morphologic pattern, ranging from well-differentiated, elongated spindle cells to highly anaplastic pleomorphic histiocyte–like cells. The neoplasm is unresponsive to both irradiation and chemotherapy and should be treated by wide resection. Five-year survival is approximately 38% (Fig. 45-11).

Rhabdomyosarcoma

Rhabdomyosarcoma is the second most common chest wall soft tissue malignant neoplasm and occurs most frequently in children and young adults. These tumors are rare after the age

of 45 years, and men are affected only slightly more often than women. Rhabdomyosarcomas present as a rapidly enlarging mass that is usually deep-seated and is intimately associated with striated muscle tissue. Generally, the tumor is neither painful nor tender, despite evidence of rapid growth. Grossly and microscopically, it has few neoplastic characteristics. As with most rapidly growing tumors, the overall appearance reflects the degree of cellularity and the extent of secondary changes, such as hemorrhage and necrosis.

Modern therapy has profoundly altered the clinical course of this disease. Wide resection followed by irradiation and multidrug chemotherapy has resulted in 5-year survivals of 70% (see Fig. 45-11). Inadequately treated, the tumor rapidly recurs both locally and metastatically.

Liposarcoma

Liposarcoma is primarily a neoplasm of adult life, with the peak incidence between the ages of 40 and 60 years. It rarely occurs in infants and small children. Most patients are men. Malignant degeneration of a preexisting lipoma is rare. Association with antecedent trauma has been reported.

Grossly, liposarcomas are well encapsulated and lobulated. Microscopically, abundant anaplastic lipoblasts are common. Treatment is with wide excision. Five-year survival is approximately 60%, and recurrence is usually local, reflecting incomplete excision. Radiation therapy and chemotherapy have little to offer.

Neurofibrosarcoma

Chest wall neurofibrosarcoma frequently occurs along the intercostal nerve and is typically a disease of adult life, occurring in persons between 20 and 50 years of age. Three-fourths of these neoplasms occur in men, and approximately half are associated with von Recklinghausen's disease. Grossly, the tumor is encapsulated. Microscopically, a monotonous pattern of elongated spindle-like cells spread for considerable distances along the nerve sheath. Treatment is by wide excision.

Leiomyosarcoma

Leiomyosarcomas are primarily neoplasms of adult life but occur less frequently than malignant fibrous histiocytoma and liposarcoma. Approximately two-thirds of patients are women. Children rarely develop these tumors. Most neoplasms present as a slowly enlarging mass that may be painful.

Grossly, leiomyosarcomas are whitish gray and lobulated, with foci of hemorrhage and necrosis. Cyst formation is often present. Microscopically, the tumor appears as swirling, elongated, spindle-like cells. Treatment is with wide excision. Recurrence is local and metastatic.

CLINICAL EXPERIENCE

Since the 1970s, Arnold and I (1996) have resected chest wall tumors in 275 patients; 115 were primary neoplasms. Nearly two-thirds of these neoplasms were malignant. Malignant fibrous histiocytoma and chondrosarcoma were the most common malignant neoplasm, and desmoid tumor was the most common benign tumor. The patients' ages ranged from 6 to 80 years, with a median of 44 years. An average of 3.6 ribs were resected. Total or partial sternectomies were performed in 18 patients. Skeletal defects were closed with prosthetic material in 44 patients and with autogenous ribs in 5. Ninety-four patients underwent 141 muscle transpositions, including 79 pectoralis major, 33 latissimus dorsi, seven serratus anterior, five external oblique, three rectus abdominis, three trapezius, and 11 other muscles. The omentum was transposed in 10 patients. Patients were generally extubated the evening of the operation or the next day. Three patients required tracheostomy. Most other patients had only minor changes in pulmonary function. Median hospitalization was 8 days. No 30-day postoperative deaths occurred.

Long-term survival of patients with malignant primary chest wall tumors depends on cell type and extent of resection. In the Mayo Clinic series, overall 5-year survival was 57%. Wide resection for chondrosarcoma resulted in a 5-year survival of 96% compared to only 70% for patients who had local excision (see Fig. 45-9). Five-year survival for patients with either chondrosarcoma or rhabdomyosarcoma was 70%, in contrast to only 38% for patients with malignant fibrous histiocytoma (see Fig. 45-11). Recurrent neoplasm, however, was an ominous sign; only 17% of patients in whom recurrence developed survived 5 years.

CONCLUSION

The key to successful treatment of all chest wall tumors is still early diagnosis with aggressive surgical resection and adequate chest wall reconstruction. This procedure can generally be performed in one operation, with minimal respiratory insufficiency and with low operative mortality. Most important, these techniques allow potential long-term survival for all patients with primary chest wall tumor.

REFERENCES

Andrassy RJ, et al: Thoracic sarcomas in children. Ann Surg 227:170, 1998.

Arnold PG, Pairolero PC: Chondrosarcoma of the manubrium. Resection and reconstruction with pectoralis major muscle. Mayo Clin Proc 53:54, 1978.

Arnold PG, Pairolero PC: Use of pectoralis major muscle flaps to repair defects of anterior chest wall. Plast Reconstr Surg 63:205, 1979.

Arnold PG, Pairolero PC: Chest wall reconstruction: experience with 100 consecutive patients. Ann Surg 199:725, 1984.

Arnold PG, Pairolero PC: Chest wall reconstruction: an account of 500 consecutive patients. Plast Reconstr Surg 98:804, 1996.

Dahlin DC, Unni KK: Bone Tumors: General Aspects and Data on 8,542 Cases. Springfield, IL: Charles C. Thomas, 1986.

Eng J, et al: Primary bony chest wall tumours. J R Coll Surg Edinb 35:44, 1990.

Evans KG, et al: Chest wall tumours. Can J Surg 33:229, 1990.

Farley JH, Seyfer AE: Chest wall tumors: experience with 58 patients. Mil Med 156:413, 1991.

Fortier MV, et al: Chest wall lesions: findings on MR images in 41 cases [abstract]. Radiology 185:356, 1992.

Fortier M, et al: MR imaging of chest wall lesions. Radiographics 14:597, 1994.

Fujiu K, et al: Hemothorax in a patient with multiple osteochondroma: a case report. J Jpn Assoc Chest Surg 10:838, 1996.

Goellner JR, Soule EH: Desmoid tumors: an ultrastructural study of eight cases. Hum Pathol 11:43, 1980.

Graeber GM, et al: Initial and long-term results in the management of primary chest wall neoplasms. Ann Thorac Surg 34:664, 1982.

Groff DB, Adkins PC: Chest wall tumors. Ann Thorac Surg 4:260, 1967.

Hajdu SI: Pathology of soft tissue tumors. Philadelphia: Lea & Febiger, 1979, p. 122.

Harrison NK, et al: Osteochondroma of the rib: an unusual cause of hemothorax. Thorax 49:618, 1994.

Hayry P, et al: The desmoid tumor. II. Analysis of factors possibly contributing to the etiology and growth behavior. Am J Clin Pathol 77:674, 1982.

King RM, et al: Primary chest wall tumors: factors affecting survival. Ann Thorac Surg 41:597, 1986.

Lichtenstein L: Bone Tumors. 5th Ed. St. Louis: CV Mosby, 1977, p. 186.

Lichtenstein L, Jaffe HL: Chondrosarcoma of bone. Am J Pathol 19:553, 1943.

McAfee MK, et al: Chondrosarcoma of the chest wall: factors affecting survival. Ann Thorac Surg 40:535, 1985.

Pairolero PC, Arnold PG: Chest wall tumors: experience with 100 consecutive patients. J Thorac Cardiovasc Surg 90:367, 1985.

Pairolero PC, Arnold PG: Thoracic wall defects: surgical management of 205 consecutive patients. Mayo Clin Proc 61:557, 1986.

Pascuzzi CA, Dahlin DC, Clagett OT: Primary tumors of the ribs and sternum. Surg Gynecol Obstet 104:390, 1957.

Ryan MB, McMurtrey MJ, Roth JA: Current management of chest-wall tumors. Surg Clin North Am 69:1061, 1989.

Schwarz RE, Burt M: Radiation-associated malignant tumors of the chest wall. Ann Surg Oncol 3:387, 1996.

Siegel MJ, Luker GD: Pediatric chest MR imaging: noncardiac clinical uses. Magn Reson Imaging Clin N Am 4:559, 1996.

Soule EG, Scanlon PW: Fibrosarcoma arising in an extraabdominal desmoid tumor: report of a case. Mayo Clin Proc 37:443, 1962.

Stelzer P, Gay WA Jr: Tumors of the chest wall. Surg Clin North Am 60:779, 1980.

Tomares SM, et al: Hemothorax in a child as a result of costal exostosis. Pediatrics 93:523, 1994.

Weiss SW, Enzinger FM: Malignant fibrous histiocytoma: an analysis of 200 cases. Cancer 41:2250, 1978.

Wyttenbach R, Vock P, Tschappeler H: Cross-sectional imaging with CT and/or MRI of pediatric chest tumors. Eur Radiol 8:1040, 1998.

CHAPTER 46

Chest Wall Reconstruction

Peter C. Pairolero

For over a century, chest wall reconstruction has been a challenge that surgeons have confronted with varying levels of fear and trepidation, as evidenced by Parham's (1898) description of the surgically created pneumothorax:

> . . . one of the most startling clinical pictures that the surgeon can ever be called upon to witness. At such a sight the stoutest heart will quaver. No wonder the older surgeons discountenanced such operations. . . . So sudden in my case was the pneumothorax and so striking were the manifestations of profound shock, threatening almost instant dissolution before our eyes, that I resolved to acquaint myself more thoroughly with the dangers of thoracic surgery.

Surgeons have subsequently worked diligently at "acquainting" themselves with the various dangers and have dealt with them in various and fascinating ways. O'Dwyer (1887) and Fell (1891) described positive-pressure airway ventilation and the importance of upper airway control. They introduced tracheal intubation and provided a large experience with this technique. Lund (1913), Hedblom (1921), Harrington (1927), and Zinninger (1930) classified tumors of the chest wall. In the early 1930s, Graham and Singer (1933) performed the first successful pneumonectomy for carcinoma of the lung. In addition, the risk of pulmonary and chest wall resections was dramatically improved by combining endotracheal ventilation with closed chest drainage and later with antibiotics.

The 1940s brought further contributions in the form on reconstruction techniques. Watson and James (1947) discussed the use of fascia lata grafts for closure of chest wall defects. Maier (1947) treated large anterior defects due to cancer and radiation therapy with cutaneous flaps that commonly included the remaining breast. Bisgard and Swenson (1948) used rib grafts as horizontal struts to reconstruct the resected sternum. Pickrell and associates (1948) advanced surgical treatment of recurrent breast carcinoma by resecting a portion of chest wall.

The latissimus dorsi musculocutaneous flap was originally described by Tansini (1906) for coverage of the anterior chest wall after radical mastectomy. Hutchins (1939) used the latissimus dorsi muscle to close radical mastectomy defects. The latissimus dorsi flap was again presented to the surgical world by Campbell (1950) when he reconstructed a full-thickness defect in the anterior thorax and covered the muscle immediately with a split-thickness skin graft. Regrettably, this method of reconstruction went unnoticed for nearly 20 years, until interest in muscle transposition was revived and the technique was rediscovered and refined. Graham and colleagues (1960), Le Roux (1964), Rees and Converse (1965), and Starzynski (1969) and Martini (1969) and their associates all made further refinement of chest wall reconstructive techniques in the 1960s. Many of these procedures were and continue to be multistaged. Kiricuta (1963), of Rumania, described transposition of the greater omentum for reconstruction of chest wall defects due to excision of malignancies of the chest.

Since 1970, numerous authors have made significant contributions to reconstruction of the thorax. Muscle and musculocutaneous flaps of the latissimus dorsi, pectoralis major, serratus anterior, rectus abdominis, and external oblique muscles have been used most frequently. The clarification of the functional anatomy and blood supply of these muscles has resulted in more aggressive resections in the treatment of chest wall tumors and in the surgical amelioration of the ravages of radiation therapy. Reports by McCormack (1981), Larson (1982) and Arnold (1984) and their colleagues, as well as by the author and Arnold (1985, 1986a, 1986b) confirmed that aggressive resection of the chest wall with immediate, dependable reconstruction is reasonable for managing these problems.

ETIOLOGY

Defects of the chest wall occur almost always as a result of neoplasm, irradiation, or infection (Table 46-1). The chest wall defect produced by resection of most neoplasms involves loss of the skeleton and frequently the overlying soft

Table 46-1. Etiology of Chest Wall Defects

Neoplasm
    Primary chest wall
    Metastatic chest wall
    Contiguous lung cancer
    Contiguous breast cancer
Infection
    Median sternotomy wound
    Lateral thoracotomy wound
    Osteomyelitis
    Costochondritis
Radiation necrosis
Trauma

Table 46-2. Considerations for Reconstruction of Chest Wall Defects

Location
Size
Depth
    Partial thickness
    Full thickness
Duration
Condition of local tissue
    Irradiation
    Infection
    Residual tumor
    Scarring
General condition of patient
    Chemotherapy
    Corticosteroid
    Chronic infection
Lifestyle and type of work
Prognosis

tissues. Infection, radiation necrosis, and trauma produce partial or full-thickness defects, depending on their severity.

PREOPERATIVE EVALUATION

Chest wall resection and reconstruction are major undertakings and have the full potential for life-threatening complications. As discussed by Azarow and associates (1989), accurate preoperative assessment is critical because it will allow the detection and treatment of correctable problems. The patient at high risk for developing postoperative complications can often be identified by history and by physical, radiographic, and routine laboratory examinations. The importance of a careful respiratory history cannot be overemphasized. The patient's smoking habits, occupational exposure, and other possible exposure to pulmonary irritants should also be obtained. The presence of dyspnea, cough, sputum, and wheeze should be thoroughly evaluated. The extent of any underlying lung disease should be documented. Routine pulmonary function testing, such as spirometry, should be obtained in all patients. Nonpulmonary risk factors, such as cardiovascular and renal risks, are equally important. Age itself, however, is relatively unimportant if the patient is otherwise in good health.

CONSIDERATION FOR RECONSTRUCTION

The ability to close large chest wall defects is the main consideration in the surgical treatment of most chest wall afflictions. Excision should not be undertaken if the surgeon does not have the confidence and ability to close the defect. The critical questions of whether the reconstructed thorax will support respiration and protect the underlying organs must be answered when the extent of resection and the method of reconstruction are considered. This is true whether the thorax is involved with a neoplasm, an infection, or radiation necrosis. Adequate resection and dependable reconstruction are the mandatory ingredients for successful treatment. These two important items are accom-

plished most safely, as Arnold and I (1984) noted, by the joint efforts of a thoracic surgeon and a plastic surgeon.

Reconstruction of chest wall defects involves consideration of many factors (Table 46-2). The location and size are of utmost importance, but the medical history and local conditions of the wound may drastically alter a reconstructive choice. Primary closure remains the best option available when possible. If the defect is partial thickness and will accept and support a skin graft, reconstruction in this manner is quite reasonable. If a partial thickness defect will not reliably accept a skin graft, a situation that frequently occurs with radiation necrosis, omental transposition with skin grafting is used. If full-thickness reconstruction is required, the structural stability of the thorax and soft tissue coverage must be considered.

SPECIAL CONSIDERATIONS

Radiation Injury

Radiation therapy has undoubtedly saved many lives and benefited countless other patients. In Arnold's and my experience (1986, 1989), however, the reconstructive surgeon is rarely, if ever, asked to see a recipient of such therapy who has had absolutely no problems. Rather, most patients have impending or actual chest wall ulceration, complicated by the ever-present possibility of recurrent cancer. Certainly, situations arise when resection and reconstruction are reasonable alternatives in spite of the possible presence of metastatic disease. In many of these patients, the quality of life can be vastly improved with such a procedure. It is also important to understand the extent of radiation injury in adjacent tissues. Computed tomography and magnetic resonance imaging are helpful because they more accurately delineate the condition of the underlying lung and mediastinum. Such information may, in fact, be more important

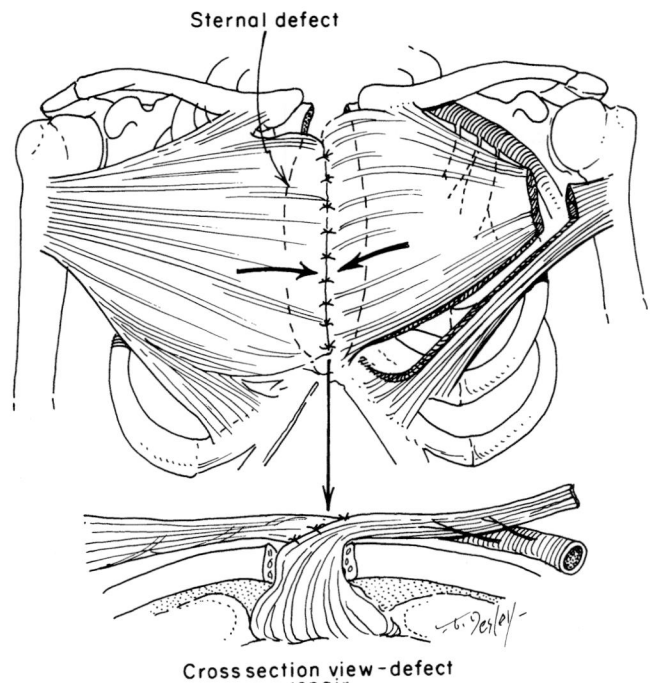

Sternal defect

Cross section view–defect repair

Fig. 46-1. Use of pectoralis major muscle for infected median sternotomy. The left (nondominant) pectoralis major muscle is separated from its humeral attachment. The lateral aspect of the muscle is left intact to maintain an anterior axillary fold. The left muscle is transposed into the mediastinum to obliterate dead space and is sutured to the right (dominant) pectoralis major muscle, which is advanced to the midline (*inset*). From Pairolero PC, Arnold PG: Management of recalcitrant median sternotomy wounds. J Thorac Cardiovasc Surg 88:357, 1984. With permission.

than the presence or absence of distant metastases. Knowledge of the presence of a mediastinal abscess or destroyed lung is critical for successful chest wall resection and reconstruction. If a history of chest wall bleeding is present, consideration should be given to angiography if any suspicion of involvement of the heart or great vessels exists. Similarly, parasternal ulceration deserves careful evaluation because of potential erosion into the internal mammary vessel, with severe hemorrhage as its sequela.

Infected Median Sternotomy Wounds

Infected median sternotomy wounds are life-threatening complications. Left untreated, these infections can extend to cardiac and aortic suture lines, prosthetic grafts, and intracardiac prostheses. I and Arnold (1984) and with my associates (1991) believe that these wounds should be inspected under general anesthesia in the operating room, where the subcutaneous space and sternum are opened and all foreign material is removed. All recesses of the previously dissected mediastinum must be thoroughly explored. However, every

effort should be made to avoid entering the pleural spaces if no clinical or radiographic evidence of empyema is present.

After debridement, the sternotomy wound is dressed with gauze moistened with saline solution. The wound dressing is changed every 4 to 6 hours. If at any time evidence of new or persistent necrotic tissue is present, the patient is returned to the operating room for further debridement. Secondary closure is performed when the wound is clean.

I and Arnold (1984) prefer to obliterate the mediastinum with pectoralis major muscle flaps (Fig. 46-1), reserving rectus abdominis muscle transposition as a backup procedure. Usually, both pectoralis major muscles are mobilized. The humeral attachments are divided as needed to permit the degree of rotation and advancement required. The overlying skin and subcutaneous tissues are closed either directly or later. Miller and Nahai (1989), however, prefer to leave the medial edge of the pectoralis muscle attached to the chest wall and obliterate the mediastinum by a turnover of the muscle.

SKELETAL RECONSTRUCTION

Reconstruction of the bony thorax is controversial. Differences of opinion exist about who should be reconstructed and what type of reconstruction should be done. In general, all full-thickness skeletal defects that have the potential for chest wall paradox should be reconstructed. The decision not to reconstruct the skeleton depends on the size and location of the defect. Defects less than 5 cm in greatest diameter anywhere on the thorax are usually not reconstructed. Posterior defects less than 10 cm likewise do not require reconstruction because the overlying scapula provides support. Larger defects, however, should be reconstructed, and autogenous tissue such as fascia lata or ribs and prosthetic material such as the various meshes, metals, or methyl methacrylate have been used.

Stabilization of the bony thorax is best accomplished with prosthetic material such as Prolene mesh (Ethicon, Inc., Somerville, NJ) or 2-mm polytetrafluoroethylene (Gore-Tex) soft tissue patch (W. L. Gore and Associates, Flagstaff, AZ). Placing either of these materials under tension improves the rigidity of the prosthesis in all directions. The soft tissue patch is superior because it prevents movement of fluid and air across the reconstructed chest wall. Marlex mesh (Daval, Inc., Providence, RI) is used less frequently because when placed under tension, it is rigid in one direction only. Although I and Arnold (1985, 1986a) believe that reconstruction with rigid materials such as methyl methacrylate–impregnated meshes is not necessary, McCormack (1989) has been a strong advocate of this procedure.

Full-thickness skeletal defects resulting from excision of tumors of both the sternum and lateral chest wall should be reconstructed if the wound is not contaminated. If the wound is contaminated from previous radiation necrosis or necrotic neoplasm, reconstruction with prosthetic material is not advised, as the prosthesis may subsequently become infected,

Table 46-3. Autogenous Tissue Available for Chest Wall Reconstruction

Muscle
  Latissimus dorsi
  Pectoralis major
  Rectus abdominis
  Serratus anterior
  External oblique
  Trapezius
Omentum

resulting in obligatory removal. In this situation, reconstruction with a musculocutaneous flap alone is preferred. Similarly, resection of the bony thorax in a patient who has been previously irradiated may not require skeletal reconstruction as the lung frequently adheres to the underlying parietal pleura and paradox does not occur. Covering radiation skin necrosis with soft tissue is frequently adequate.

SOFT TISSUE RECONSTRUCTION

Muscle and omental transposition can be used to reconstruct soft tissue chest wall defects (Table 46-3). Muscle is the tissue of choice for soft tissue coverage of full-thickness defects for which skeletal reconstruction is not required. Muscle can be transposed as muscle alone or as a musculocutaneous flap. The omentum should be reserved for partial-thickness reconstruction or as a backup procedure for muscle transposition that has failed in full-thickness defects.

Muscle Transposition

Latissimus Dorsi

The latissimus dorsi muscle is the largest flat muscle of the thorax. Its dominant thoracodorsal neurovascular leash has an arc of rotation that allows coverage of the lateral and central back as well as the anterolateral and central front of the thorax, as Campbell (1950) and Bostwick and associates (1979) pointed out. Its dependable musculocutaneous vascular connections also make it a reliable musculocutaneous flap. This muscle flap can cover huge chest wall defects because virtually one-half of the back can be elevated on the blood supply of a single latissimus dorsi muscle in the uninjured, nonirradiated patient (Fig. 46-2). The donor site may need skin grafts when large musculocutaneous flaps are elevated, but this represents a small disadvantage when considering that large, robust flaps can be transposed to either the anterior or posterior chest for full-thickness reconstruction. If the dominant blood supply has been compromised from previous trauma or surgery, Fisher and colleagues (1983) showed the muscle can still dependably be transposed on the branch of the adjacent serratus anterior muscle.

Pectoralis Major

The pectoralis major muscle is the second largest flat muscle on the chest wall and in many respects is the mirror image of the latissimus dorsi muscle. As Arnold and I (1979) reported, its dominant thoracoacromial neurovascular leash, which enters posteriorly about midclavicle, allows elevation of the muscle, either as a muscle or musculocutaneous flap, and rotation centrally for chest wall reconstruction. The pectoralis major muscle is equally as reliable as the latissimus dorsi flap. I and Arnold (1984, 1986b) showed that it is beneficial in reconstructing anterior chest wall defects such as those resulting from sternal tumor excisions and infected median sternotomy wounds (Fig. 46-3). Generally, only the muscle is transposed, and the skin can be closed primarily, thereby avoiding the distortion created by centralizing the breast. Reconstruction in this manner is more symmetric and aesthetically acceptable. If central skin must be excised, symmetry of the breast can still be maintained, because the transposed muscle readily accepts and supports an overlying skin graft. If necessary, the muscle can also be transposed on its secondary blood supply through the perforators from the internal mammary vessels.

Rectus Abdominis

Use of the rectus abdominis muscle for chest wall reconstruction is based on the internal mammary neurovascular leash. The inferior epigastric vessels must be divided to allow rotation to the chest wall. This muscle can be mobilized and moved either as a muscle or as a musculocutaneous flap (Fig. 46-4) with the skin component oriented horizontally, vertically, or both. The vertical skin flap, however, is more reliable because it is oriented along the long axis of the muscle and thus maintains more musculocutaneous perforators. The donor site is usually closed primarily.

I and Arnold (1985) believe the rectus abdominis muscle is most useful in reconstruction of lower sternal wounds. Either muscle can be used, as their arcs of rotation are identical. The muscle that has patent and uninjured internal mammary vessels must be chosen. Angiographic demonstration of vessel patency may help determine which musculocutaneous unit is most reliable, particularly in previously irradiated patients or in patients with infected sternotomy wounds. Also, in many infected sternotomy wounds, the internal mammary artery may have previously been used for coronary artery bypass.

Serratus Anterior

The serratus anterior muscle is a small, flat muscle located in the midaxillary line between the latissimus dorsi and pectoralis major muscles. Its blood supply comes from the serratus branch of the thoracodorsal vessels and from the long thoracic artery and vein. This muscle can be used alone or as an adjunctive muscle with the pectoralis major or the latissimus dorsi muscles. As Arnold and colleagues (1984)

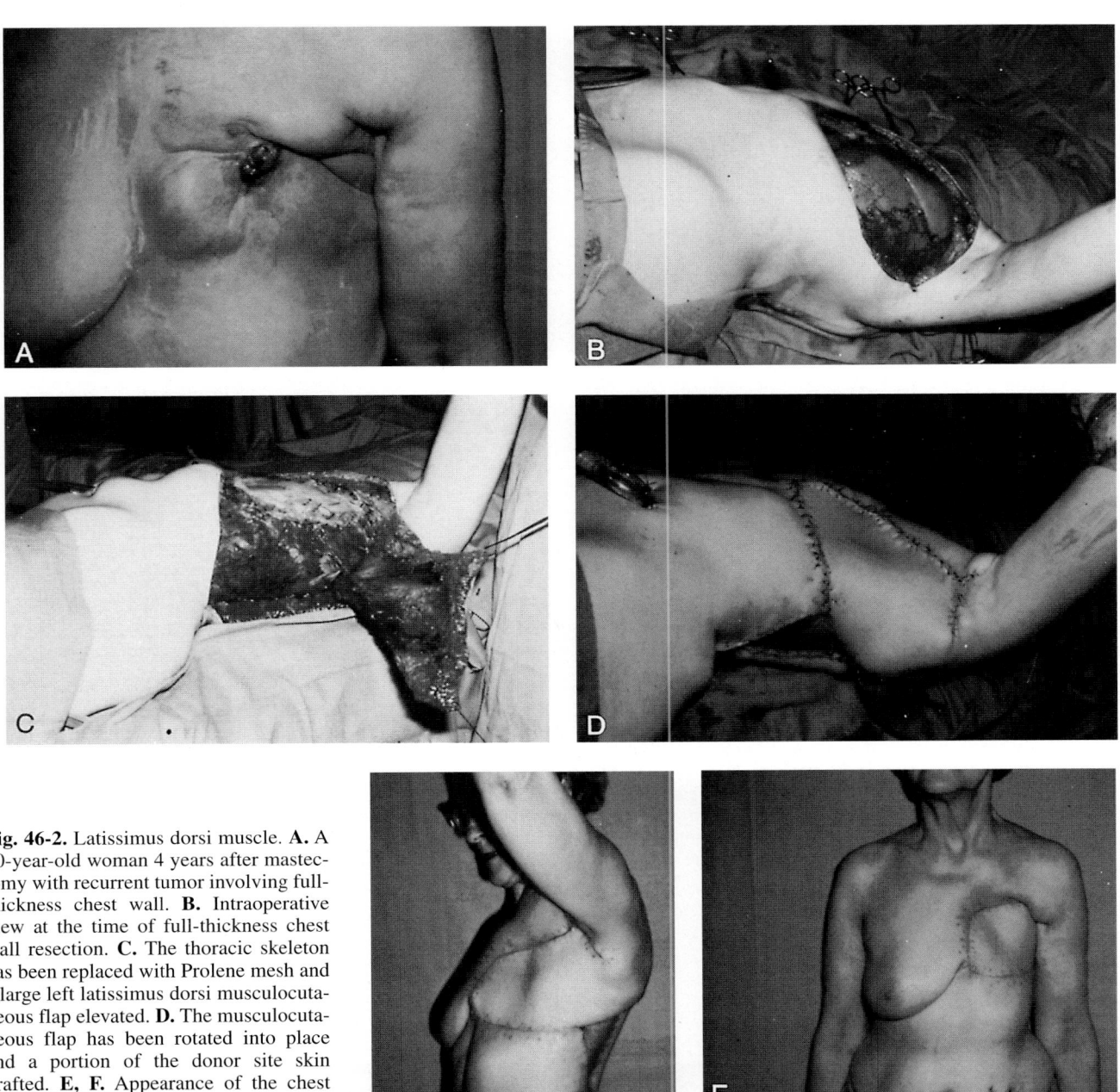

Fig. 46-2. Latissimus dorsi muscle. **A.** A 60-year-old woman 4 years after mastectomy with recurrent tumor involving full-thickness chest wall. **B.** Intraoperative view at the time of full-thickness chest wall resection. **C.** The thoracic skeleton has been replaced with Prolene mesh and a large left latissimus dorsi musculocutaneous flap elevated. **D.** The musculocutaneous flap has been rotated into place and a portion of the donor site skin grafted. **E, F.** Appearance of the chest wall 3 months following resection. From Arnold PG, Pairolero PC: Chest wall reconstruction: experience with 100 consecutive patients. Ann Surg *199*:725, 1984. With permission.

pointed out, the muscle also augments the skin-carrying ability of either adjacent muscle. The author and colleagues (1983) found that this muscle is particularly useful as an intrathoracic muscle flap.

External Oblique

The external oblique muscle can also be transposed as a muscle or musculocutaneous flap (Fig. 46-5) and is most useful in closing defects of the upper abdomen and lower thorax. It reaches the inframammary fold without tension but, as Hodgkinson and Arnold (1980) noted, does not readily extend higher. The primary blood supply is from the lower thoracic intercostal vessels, as Lund (1913), Hedblom (1921), Harrington (1927), Zinninger (1930), Maier (1947), Watson and James (1947), and Bisgard and Swensen (1948) demonstrated. With this muscle, lower chest wall defects can be closed without distorting the breast.

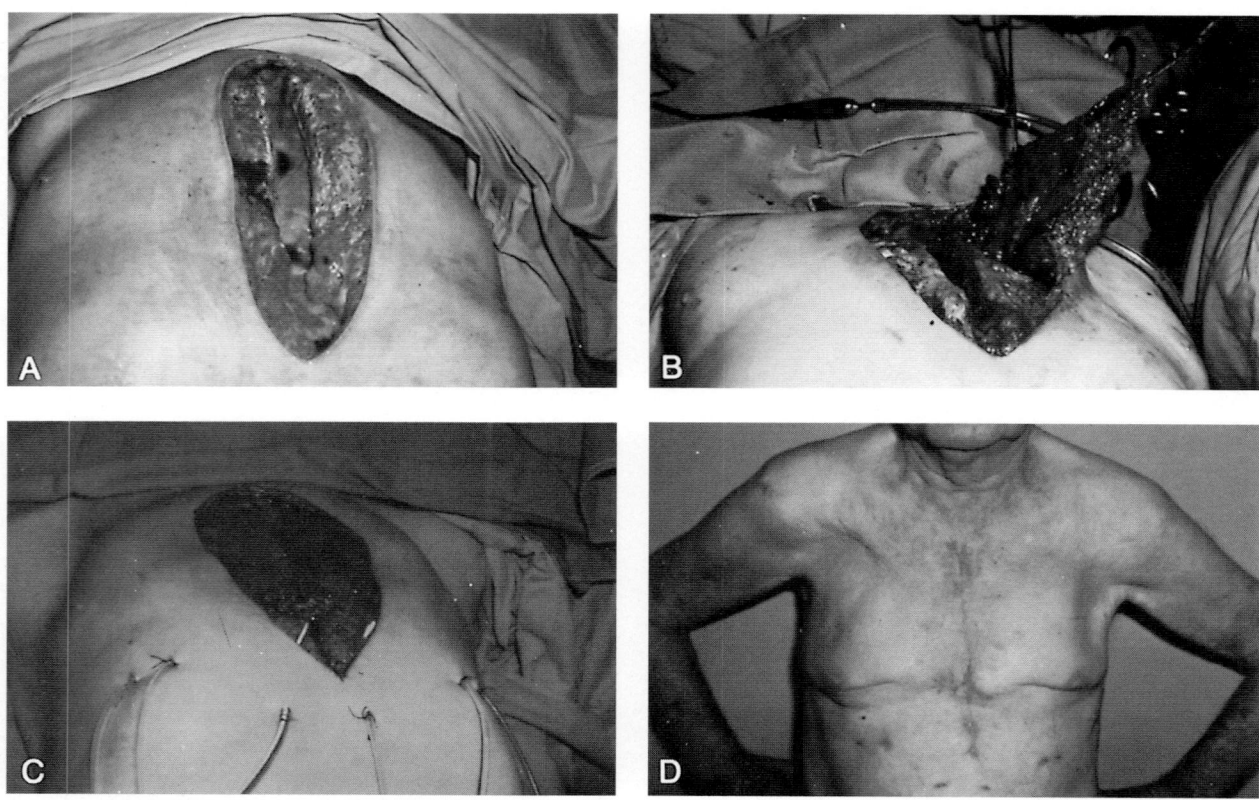

Fig. 46-3. Pectoralis major muscle. A 72-year-old man had median sternotomy for coronary artery bypass graft for coronary artery disease. **A.** Approximately 3 months later, after multiple débridements that removed essentially the central portion of the sternum. **B.** At the time of closure the left pectoralis major muscle is totally mobilized and separated from the humeral attachment. The right pectoralis major muscle is mobilized over the midaxillary line but not separated from its humeral attachment. **C.** The two muscles are sutured together in the midline, and a large portion of the left pectoralis major muscle is draped into the defect in the central sternal area. **D.** Appearance approximately 3 months after closure. From Arnold PG, Pairolero PC: Chest wall reconstruction: experience with 100 consecutive patients. Ann Surg *199*:725, 1984. With permission.

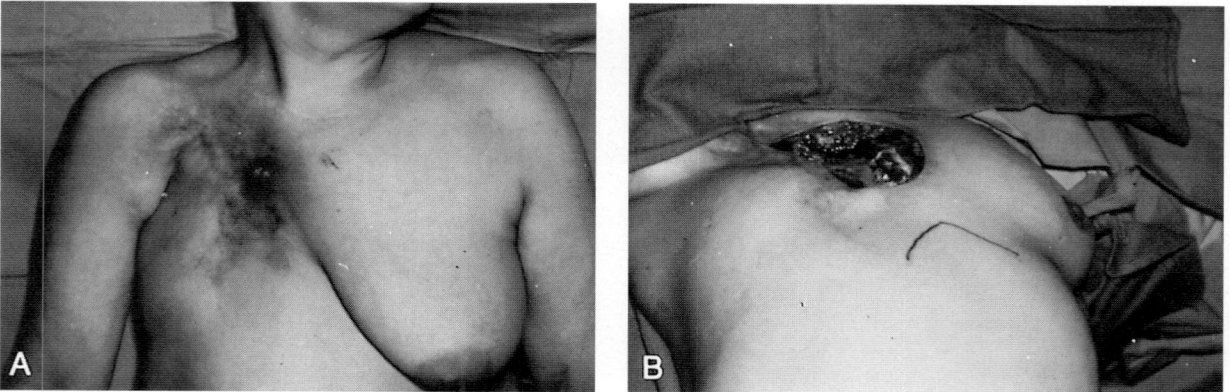

Fig. 46-4. Rectus abdominis muscle. **A.** A 49-year-old woman 5 years after mastectomy and radiation therapy with radionecrotic area on the right chest. **B.** The wound is excised, including a portion of the right sternum and the right anterior chest wall. (*Continued*)

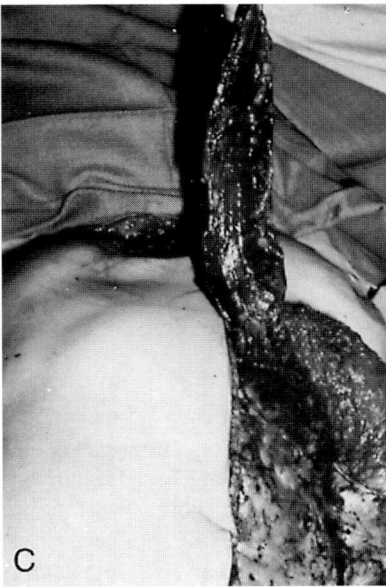

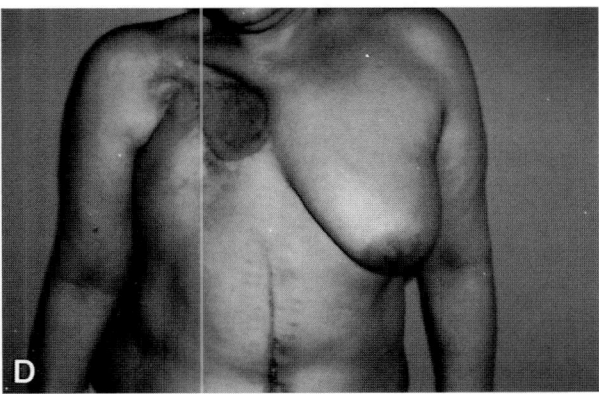

Fig. 46-4. (*Continued*) **C.** Contralateral (left) rectus abdominis muscle is elevated for transposition into the defect. **D.** Four months after closure with split-thickness skin graft over the transposed rectus abdominis muscle. From Arnold PG, Pairolero PC: Chest wall reconstruction: experience with 100 consecutive patients. Ann Surg *199*:725, 1984. With permission.

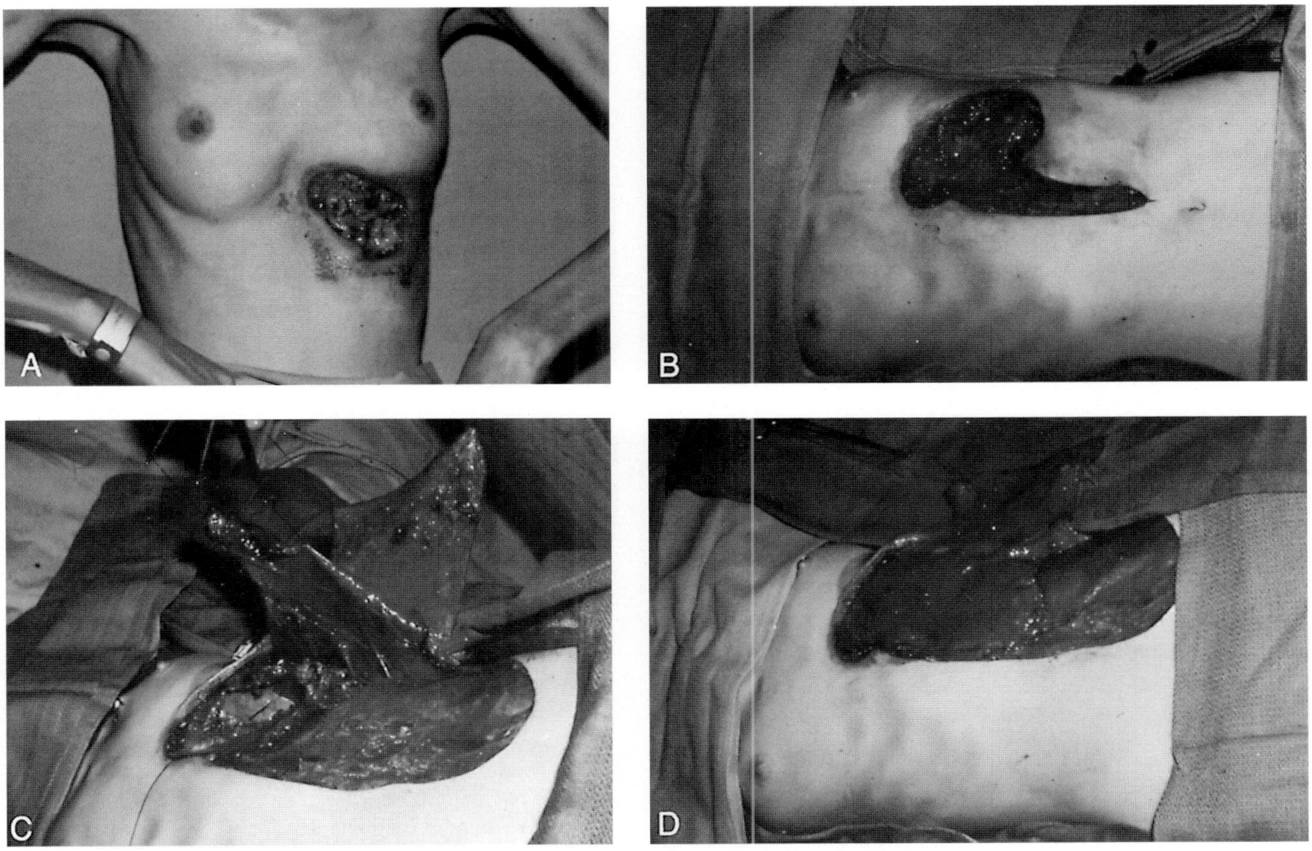

Fig. 46-5. External oblique muscle. **A.** A 31-year-old woman with radiation ulcer of the chest after therapy for Hodgkin's disease. Ulcer present for 18 months. **B.** The chest wall defect after excision of distal sternum, xiphoid cartilage, costal cartilage, and ribs 5 through 9. **C.** External oblique muscle elevated as a separate flap to close thoracic defect. The overlying skin-fascia flap was also advanced to close the cutaneous defect, which was smaller. **D.** Muscle flap sutured into position to close the chest wall defect. (*Continued*)

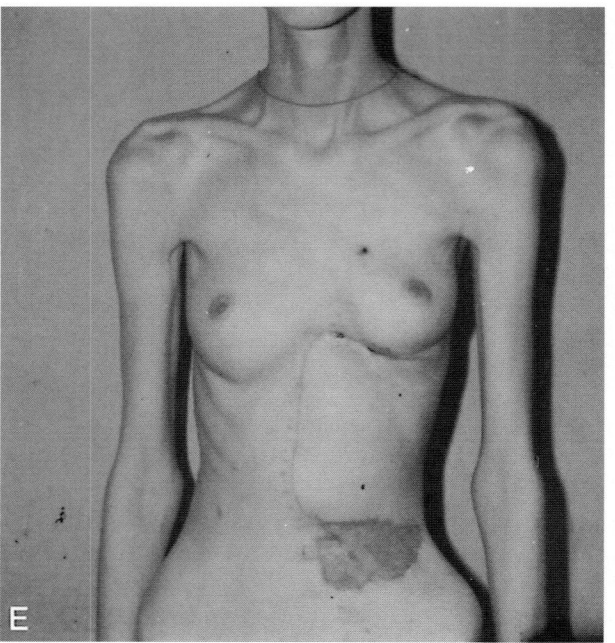

Fig. 46-5. *(Continued)* E. Four months postoperatively. From Hodgkinson DJ, Arnold PG: Chest wall reconstruction using the external oblique muscle. Br J Plast Surg *33*:216, 1980. With permission.

Trapezius Muscle

The trapezius muscle has been useful to close defects at the base of the neck or the thoracic outlet but is not consistently useful for other chest wall reconstructions. Its primary blood supply is the dorsal scapular vessels.

Omental Transposition

Omental transposition, as Jurkiewicz and Arnold (1977) noted, has been most useful in reconstructing partial-thickness chest wall defects, particularly in radiation necrosis that does not involve tumor (Fig. 46-6).

In this situation, the skin and soft tissue are débrided down to what remains of the thoracic skeleton, which may be either bone or cartilage but frequently is only irradiated ischemic scar. The transposed omentum with its excellent blood supply from the gastroepiploic vessels adheres to the irradiated wound and readily accepts and supports an overlying skin graft. Because the omentum has no structural stability of its own, it is not particularly useful in full-thickness defects because additional support, such as fascia lata, bone, or prosthetic material, is necessary.

Omental transposition is helpful when planned muscle flaps have failed with partial necrosis. Generally, this results

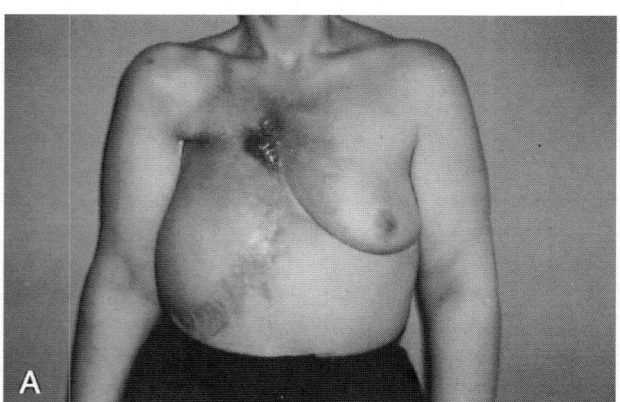

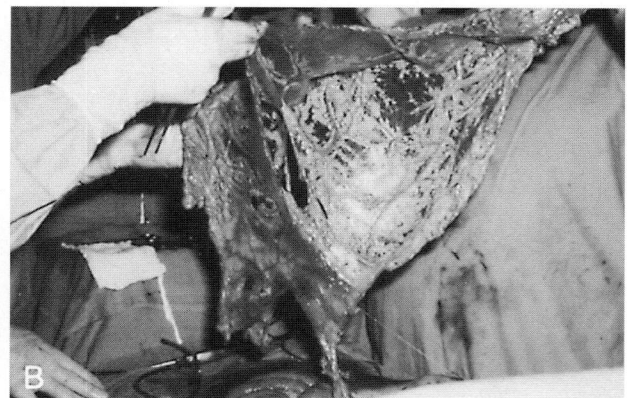

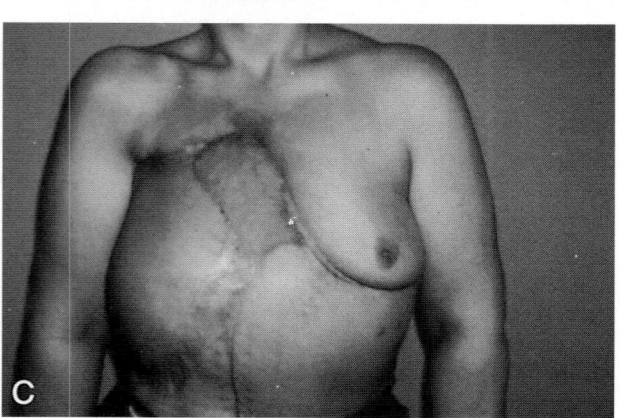

Fig. 46-6. Omentum. A 44-year-old woman had a modified mastectomy with radiation therapy. Radiation necrosis was treated by rotation of a large cutaneous flap based on the right. **A.** Wound breakdown developed, requiring excision of skin and soft tissue only; no evidence of recurrent tumor was present. **B.** Greater omentum was mobilized on right gastroepiploic vessels in preparation for transposition into the defect. **C.** Appearance of chest 6 months after closure, with a stable split-thickness skin graft. From Arnold PG, Pairolero PC: Chest wall reconstruction: experience with 100 consecutive patients. Ann Surg *199*:725, 1984.

in only a soft tissue defect, and pleural seal with respiratory stability is not required, thus allowing a most threatening situation to be salvaged.

Although infections of the lower sternum are best treated with a rectus abdominis muscle flap, the blood supply, based on the distal aspect of the internal mammary artery, may have been interrupted previously either by use of this artery for coronary revascularization or by ligation with sternal resection. If the internal mammary artery is not intact or if the wound is large, omental transposition is performed, followed by split-thickness skin grafting 48 hours later.

CLINICAL EXPERIENCE

Arnold and I (1996) reported 500 chest wall reconstructions at the Mayo Clinic. This experience represents the combined efforts of a single plastic surgeon and a single general thoracic surgeon and does not represent the entire experience at our institution. Two-hundred seventy-five patients had chest wall tumors, 142 had infected median sternotomy wounds, 119 had radiation necrosis, and 121 had a combination of these. The patients ranged in age from 1 day to 85 years (average 55 years). Skeleton resection of the chest wall was done in 443 patients. An average of 3.9 ribs were resected in 241 patients. Total or partial sternectomies were performed in 231 patients. Skeletal defects were closed with prosthetic material in 184 patients; 116 with 2-mm expanded polytetrafluoroethylene (Gore-Tex soft tissue patch), 55 with polypropylene mesh (Prolene mesh), and 13 with autogenous rib. Four hundred seven patients underwent 611 muscle transpositions including 355 pectoralis major, 141 latissimus dorsi, 30 external oblique, 27 serratus anterior, 18 rectus abdominis, six trapezius, and 34 others. The omentum was transposed in 51 patients.

The 500 patients underwent an average of 2.3 operations. Most of the multiple operations were debridements in patients with infected wounds. Hospitalization averaged 21 days. Fifteen perioperative deaths occurred. Twenty-three patients required tracheostomy. Most other patients, as Meadows and associates (1985) reported, had only minor changes in pulmonary function.

Follow-up averaged 57 months. Two-hundred twenty-nine late deaths occurred. The cause of death was cancerous in 147 patients, cardiac in 49, pulmonary in seven, and other in 26. No late deaths occurred related to either resection or reconstruction of the chest wall. At the time of last follow-up, 403 of the 485 patients (83.1%) who were alive 30 days after operation had excellent results with a healed, asymptomatic chest wound.

REFERENCES

Arnold PG, Pairolero PC: Use of pectoralis major muscle flaps to repair defects of the anterior chest wall. Plast Reconstr Surg 63:205, 1979.

Arnold PG, Pairolero PC: Chest wall reconstruction: experience with 100 consecutive patients. Ann Surg 199:725, 1984.

Arnold PG, Pairolero PC: Surgical management of the radiated chest wall. Plast Reconstr Surg 77:605, 1986.

Arnold PG, Pairolero PC: Reconstruction of the radiation-damaged chest wall. Surg Clin North Am 69:1081, 1989.

Arnold PG, Pairolero PC: Chest wall reconstruction: an account of 500 consecutive patients. Plast Reconstr Surg 98:804, 1996.

Arnold PG, Pairolero PC, Waldorf JC: The serratus anterior muscle: intrathoracic and extrathoracic utilization. Plast Reconstr Surg 73:240, 1984.

Azarow KS, et al: Preoperative evaluation and general preparation for chest-wall operations. Surg Clin North Am 69:899, 1989.

Bisgard JD, Swenson SA Jr: Tumors of the sternum: report of a case with special operative technic. Arch Surg 56:570, 1948.

Bostwick J III, et al: Sixty latissimus dorsi flaps. Plast Reconstr Surg 63:31, 1979.

Campbell DA: Reconstruction of the anterior thoracic wall. J Thorac Surg 19:456, 1950.

Fell GE: Forced respirations. JAMA 16:325, 1891.

Fisher J, Bostwick J, Powell RW: Latissimus dorsi blood supply after thoracodorsal vessel division: the serratus collateral. Plast Reconstr Surg 72:502, 1983.

Graham EA, Singer JJ: Successful removal of an entire lung for carcinoma of the bronchus. JAMA 101:1371, 1933.

Graham J, et al: Marlex mesh as a prosthesis in the repair of thoracic wall defects. Ann Surg 151:469, 1960.

Harrington SW: Surgical treatment of intrathoracic tumors and tumors of the chest wall. Arch Surg 14:406, 1927.

Hedblom CA: Tumors of the bony chest wall. Arch Surg 3:56, 1921.

Hodgkinson DJ, Arnold PG: Chest-wall reconstruction using the external oblique muscle. Br J Plast Surg 33:216, 1980.

Hutchins EH: A method for the prevention of elephantiasis chirurgica. Surg Gynecol Obstet 69:795, 1939.

Jurkiewicz MJ, Arnold PG: The omentum: an account of its use in the reconstruction of the chest wall. Ann Surg 185:548, 1977.

Kiricuta I: L'emploi du grand epiploon dans la chirugie du sein cancéreux. Presse Med 71:15, 1963.

Larson DL, et al: Major chest wall reconstruction after chest wall irradiation. Cancer 49:1286, 1982.

Le Roux BT: Maintenance of chest wall stability. Thorax 19:397; 1964.

Lund FB: Sarcoma of the chest wall. Ann Surg 58:206, 1913.

Maier HC: Surgical management of large defects of the thoracic wall. Surgery 22:169, 1947.

Martini N, Starzynski TE, Beattie EJ Jr: Problems in chest wall resection. Surg Clin North Am 49:313, 1969.

McCormack P, et al: New trends in skeletal reconstruction after resection of chest wall tumors. Ann Thorac Surg 31:45, 1981.

McCormack P: Use of prosthetic materials in chest-wall reconstruction: assets and liabilities. Surg Clin North Am 69:965, 1989.

Meadows JA III et al: Effect of resection of the sternum and manubrium in conjunction with muscle transposition on pulmonary function. Mayo Clin Proc 60:604, 1985.

Miller JI, Nahai F: Repair of the dehisced median sternotomy incision. Surg Clin North Am 69:1091, 1989.

O'Dwyer J: Fifty cases of croup in private practice treated by intubation of the larynx, with a description of the method and of the dangers incident thereto. Med Rec 32:557, 1887.

Pairolero PC, Arnold PG: Management of recalcitrant median sternotomy wounds. J Thorax Cardiovasc Surg 88:357, 1984.

Pairolero PC, Arnold PG: Chest wall tumors: experience with 100 consecutive patients. J Thorac Cardiovasc Surg 90:367, 1985.

Pairolero PC, Arnold PG: Thoracic wall defects: surgical management of 205 consecutive patients. Mayo Clin Proc 61:557, 1986a.

Pairolero PC, Arnold PG: Primary tumors of the anterior chest wall. Surgical Rounds 9:19, 1986b.

Pairolero PC, Arnold PG, Harris JB: Long-term results of pectoralis major muscle transposition for infected sternotomy wounds. Ann Surg 213:583, 1991.

Pairolero PC, Arnold PG, Piehler JM: Intrathoracic transposition of extrathoracic skeletal muscle. J Thorac Cardiovasc Surg 86:809, 1983.

Parham FW: Thoracic resection of tumor growing from the bony wall of the chest. Trans South Surg Gynecol Assoc 11:223, 1898.

Pickrell KL, Kelley JW, Marzoni FA: The surgical treatment of recurrent carcinoma of the breast and chest wall. Plast Reconstr Surg *3*:156, 1948.

Rees TD, Converse JM: Surgical reconstruction of defects of the thoracic wall. Surg Gynecol Obstet *121*:1066, 1965.

Starzynski TE, Snyderman RK, Beattie EJ Jr: Problems of major chest wall reconstruction. Plast Reconstr Surg *44*:525, 1969.

Tansini I: Sopra il mio nuovo processo di amputazione della mammella. Gazz Med Ital Torino *57*:141, 1906.

Watson WL, James AG: Fascia lata grafts for chest wall defects. J Thorac Surg *16*:399, 1947.

Zinninger MM: Tumors of the wall of the thorax. Ann Surg *92*:1043, 1930.

READING REFERENCES

Blades B, Paul JS: Chest wall tumors. Ann Surg *131*:976, 1950.

Boyd AD, et al: Immediate reconstruction of full-thickness chest wall defects. Ann Thorac Surg *32*:337, 1981.

Brown RG, Fleming WH, Jurkiewicz MJ: An island flap of the pectoralis major muscle. Br J Plast Surg *30*:161, 1977.

Burnard RJ, Martini N, Beattie EJ Jr: The value of resection in tumors involving the chest wall. J Thorac Cardiovasc Surg *68*:530, 1974.

Irons GB, et al: Use of the omental free flap for soft-tissue reconstruction. Ann Plast Surg *11*:501, 1983.

Jurkiewicz MJ, et al: Infected median sternotomy wound: successful treatment by muscle flaps. Ann Surg *191*:738, 1980.

McGraw JB, Penix JO, Baker JW: Repair of major defects of the chest wall and spine with the latissimus dorsi myocutaneous flap. Plast Reconstr Surg *62*:197, 1978.

Myre TT, Kirklin JW: Resection of tumors of the sternum. Ann Surg *144*:1023, 1956.

Ramming KP, et al: Surgical management and reconstruction of extensive chest wall malignancies. Am J Surg *144*:146, 1982.

SECTION X

The Diaphragm

CHAPTER 47

Embryology and Anatomy of the Diaphragm

Thomas W. Shields

The diaphragm serves as the anatomic division between the thoracic and the abdominal cavities and, as such, is a muscular structure that is dealt with by both abdominal and thoracic surgeons. The surgical correction of acquired and congenital abnormalities of the diaphragm may be made from either abdominal or thoracic approaches, depending on the nature of the lesion, the location of the lesion, other abnormalities of the chest or abdomen, and the particular training and experience of the involved surgeon. The diaphragm exists as an anatomic barrier but is not a surgical barrier; a competent surgeon should be able to handle any surgical problem involving the diaphragm and therefore should be versatile enough to approach diaphragmatic lesions from either above or below.

EMBRYOLOGY

The diaphragm originates from an unpaired ventral portion (septum transversum), from paired dorsal lateral portions (pleuroperitoneal folds), and from an irregular medial dorsal portion (dorsal mesentery) (Fig. 47-1). The septum transversum, formed during the third week of gestation, separates the pericardial region from the rest of the body cavity. This part of the diaphragm grows dorsad from the ventral body wall and moves caudad with the other contributors to the diaphragm to reach the normal position of the diaphragm at approximately 8 weeks. The pleuroperitoneal folds arise on the lateral body walls, at the level where the cardinal veins swing around to enter the sinus venosus of the heart. These folds extend medially and somewhat caudad to join with the septum transversum and the dorsal mesentery to complete the development of the diaphragm at about the seventh week; the right pleuroperitoneal canal closes somewhat earlier than the left. Muscle fibers migrate from the third, fourth, and fifth cervical myotomes, carrying along their innervation, and grow between the two membranes to complete the structures of the diaphragm. During the tenth week, the intestines return from the yolk sac to the abdomi-

nal cavity and, at approximately 12 weeks, rotation and fixation of the intestines occur.

A delay or variation in the described timetable may result in a variety of congenital hernias with or without a hernial sac, or may even result in a congenital eventration of a hemidiaphragm. Early return of the intestines to the abdomen before closure of the pleuroperitoneal membrane results in a hernia through this opening (a so-called foramen of Bochdalek hernia). A sac usually is not present, but if it is, the return of the intestines may have occurred after the closure of the pleuroperitoneal membrane but before the migration of the cervical myotomes between the membranes. Foramen of Morgagni hernias occur anteriorly, almost always have a sac, and therefore probably result from lack of ingrowth of the cervical myotomes. A congenital short esophagus is related to late closure of the diaphragm and early return of the intestine to the abdomen. Congenital eventration may be a total error of ingrowth of cervical myotomes in one or both hemidiaphragms and therefore is actually a large congenital diaphragmatic hernia and not an eventration. An absent diaphragm probably represents an error of growth of the septum transversum and other embryologic elements. Duplication of a hemidiaphragm can occur. The fusion and formation timetable variations also may involve defects in the diaphragm in association with certain vascular anomalies of the lungs and heart.

ANATOMY

Gross Features

The diaphragm is a dome-shaped structure of muscular fibers radiating out from either side of an irregularly shaped central tendon; it consists of the right and the left hemidiaphragms. In structure and function, the diaphragm differs from any other muscle in the body. It is a muscular septum between the abdominal and thoracic cavities, serving as the

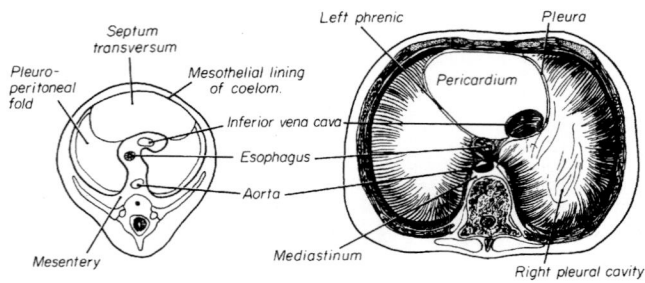

Fig. 47-1. Embryologic components of the diaphragm. Redrawn from Shields TW: The diaphragm. *In* Nora P, ed: Operative Surgery: Principles and Techniques. Philadelphia: Lea & Febiger, 1972.

major muscle of respiration. Its domelike shape allows important abdominal structures, such as the liver and the spleen, to have the protection of the lower ribs and the chest wall. The dome of the right hemidiaphragmatic leaf is normally at a higher level than is that of the left. It has been generally thought that this is the result of the liver mass beneath the right leaf. However, this view has been brought into question by the studies of Reddy and colleagues (1994). Their observations support the concept that the cardiac mass is responsible for the lower portion of the left hemidiaphragm rather than the former hypothesis.

Voluntary muscular fibers originate from the xiphisternum, from the lateral lower six ribs on each side, and from the external and internal arcuate ligaments that arise from the upper three lumbar vertebrae. Bilaterally, the muscle fibers insert into the central tendon of the diaphragm. The muscle mass of the diaphragm is considered by De Troyer and associates (1982) and Rochester (1985) as comprising two distinct parts: a thin costal muscle mass and a thicker crural portion. Although both muscle masses are innervated by the phrenic nerves, their activity on stimulation is different. The differences that result in diaphragmatic and lower chest wall movement are discussed in Chapter 48. Suffice to mention that the movement of the crural portion has the lesser effect on ventilatory exchange.

The central tendon is a thin aponeurosis of closely interwoven fascial fibers in the form of a three-leaf clover. The two lateral leaves form the dome of the diaphragm and the third (anterior) leaf is fused with the diaphragmatic surface of the pericardium.

Major interest in the muscular portion of the diaphragm centers about the two crura, which play varying roles in the formation of the esophageal hiatus. The right crus arises from the bodies of the first and second lumbar vertebrae, and the fibers divide as they pass to the left, normally overlapping in front and behind to form the entire esophageal hiatus. Collis and associates (1954), however, found this arrangement in only a little more than half of their subjects. In the others, the left crus contributed to a varying degree to the makeup of the hiatus, and in approximately 2%, the left crus made up the major portion of the esophageal hiatus.

The hiatal opening is situated at the level of the tenth thoracic vertebra just to the left of the midline and just ventral to where the aorta passes into the abdomen. The inferior vena cava passes through the tendinous portion of the right side of the diaphragm between the anterior leaf and the right lateral leaf at the level of the eighth thoracic vertebra. The other normal openings are the parasternal foramina (i.e., the foramina of Morgagni) through which the internal mammary arteries pass into the abdomen to become the superior epigastric arteries. Evidence suggests that in some subjects a variable number of fenestrations or pores are present, or are potentially so, in either hemidiaphragmatic leaf. These are more commonly observed on the right than on the left and are located posteriorly when present. These fenestrations are of no importance normally but may become the route of fluid or air to traverse from the peritoneal cavity into the pleural space, as demonstrated by the studies of Park and Pham (1995) and Urhahn and Gunther (1993) (see Addendum, Significance of Pores in the Diaphragm, later in this chapter).

The thoracic side of the diaphragm is covered with the parietal pleura, and the abdominal surface with peritoneum, except at the naturally occurring openings, and the bare area occupied by a portion of the liver.

Blood Supply

The principal blood supply of the diaphragm is derived directly from the aorta or from its most superior abdominal branches (Fig. 47-2), and its venous drainage empties into the inferior vena cava. Both the arterial supply and the venous drainage (the right and left inferior phrenic veins) are found on the undersurface of the diaphragm (Fig. 47-3). The inferior phrenic artery usually bifurcates posteriorly near the dome of the diaphragm and the branches course along the margins of the central tendon. The smaller posterior division courses laterally above the dorsal and lumbocostal origin of the diaphragm, where it has collateral anastomoses with the lower five intercostal arteries. The larger anterior division runs anterosuperiorly to the edge of the central tendon, where it anastomoses freely with the pericardiacophrenic artery. The venous pattern is similar except that the veins generally course along the posterior aspect of the central tendon to join the inferior vena cava. Veins on the inferior surface of the diaphragm communicate with the hepatic veins through the left triangular and coronary ligaments of the liver.

Nerve Distribution

The right and left phrenic nerves arise from their respective third, fourth, and fifth cervical nerve roots and constitute the total nerve supply for the ipsilateral hemidiaphragm. The distribution of each nerve is important in reference to

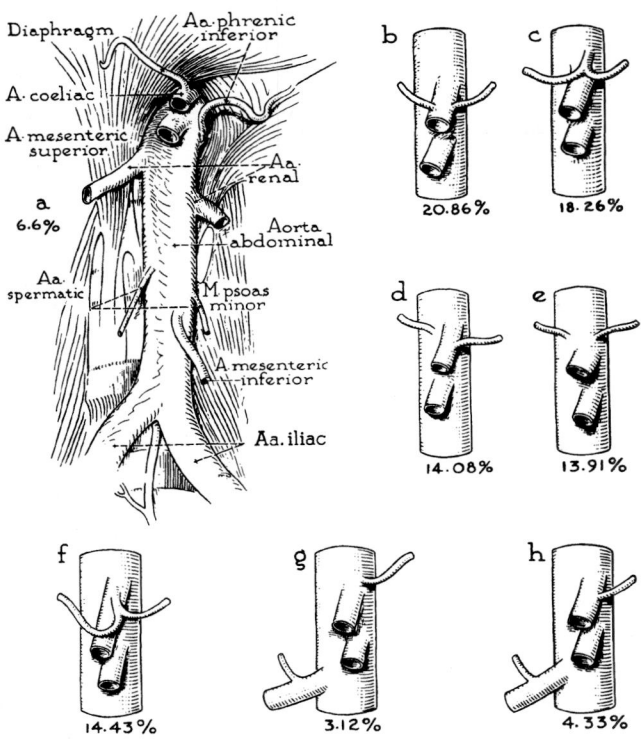

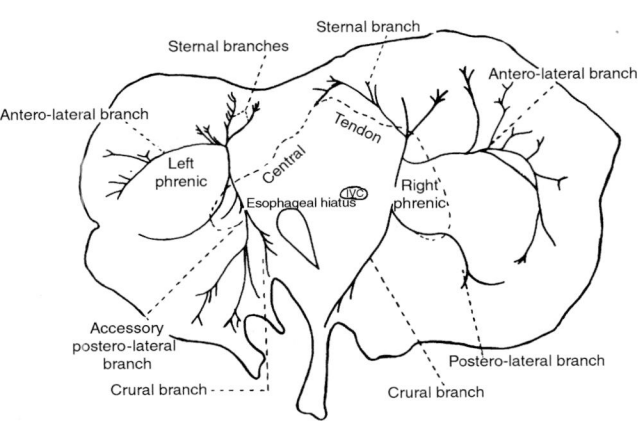

Fig. 47-4. Distribution of the phrenic nerves as seen from above. Redrawn from Merendino KA, et al: The intradiaphragmatic distribution of the phrenic nerve with particular reference to the placement of diaphragmatic incisions and controlled segmental paralysis. Surgery *39*:189, 1956.

Fig. 47-2. The arterial supply of the diaphragm from the abdominal aorta with variations in the origin of the inferior phrenic arteries. Redrawn from Anson BJ, McVay C: Surgical Anatomy. 5th Ed. Philadelphia: WB Saunders, 1971.

incisions into the diaphragm. The course of each has been described by Merendino and colleagues (1956). The right phrenic nerve reaches the diaphragm just lateral to the inferior vena cava, and the left just lateral to the left border of the heart. Generally, the nerves divide, either just above or at the level of the diaphragm, into several terminal branches. Some are distributed to the pleural and peri-

toneal surfaces, but the great bulk of each nerve passes into, or through, the diaphragm and most often divides into four major rami to supply the various muscular portions. Usually, two of the rami share a common trunk for a varying distance so that three muscular branches arise from each phrenic nerve: one anteromedially, one laterally, and the remaining one posteriorly (Fig. 47-4). Injury to any of these branches causes paralysis of the supplied portion of the hemidiaphragm.

Surgical Incisions

Incisions into the diaphragm must be made to avoid injury to the major branches of the phrenic nerves. Incision through the central tendon rarely causes diaphragmatic paralysis (Fig. 47-5A, B), but this approach provides only minimal exposure of the adjacent compartment. A more satisfactory access is provided by a circumferential incision at the periphery of the diaphragm, which permits excellent exposure of the upper abdominal contents from the thorax and vice versa with little or no possibility of injury to any major branch of the ipsilateral phrenic nerve (Fig. 47-5C). On the left, the incision may be started at the esophageal hiatus and carried from behind forward circumferentially 2.5 to 3.0 cm away from the attachment of the diaphragm to the chest wall. The crural or posterior branch of the phrenic nerve is divided, but this division is of little consequence. The main branch of the left inferior phrenic artery is usually encountered with this incision and requires division and ligation. Alternatively, the incision may be started anteriorly just lateral to the pericardium and extended circumferentially as far posteriorly as necessary. The ipsilateral hemidiaphragm may then be raised as a trapdoor and retracted medially for exposure. Closure of the incision is accom-

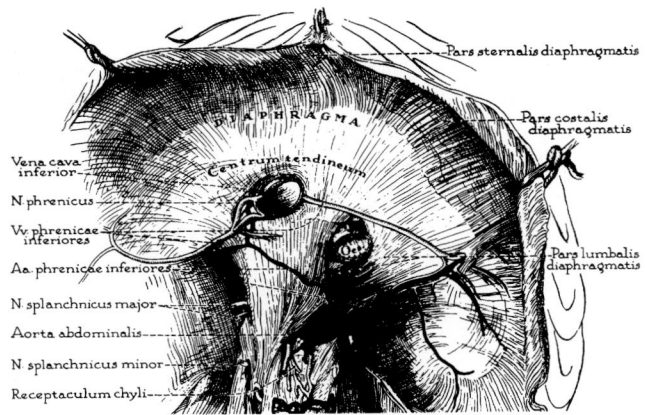

Fig. 47-3. The arterial and venous distribution on the undersurface of the diaphragm. Redrawn from Anson BJ, McVay C: Surgical Anatomy. 5th Ed. Philadelphia: WB Saunders, 1971.

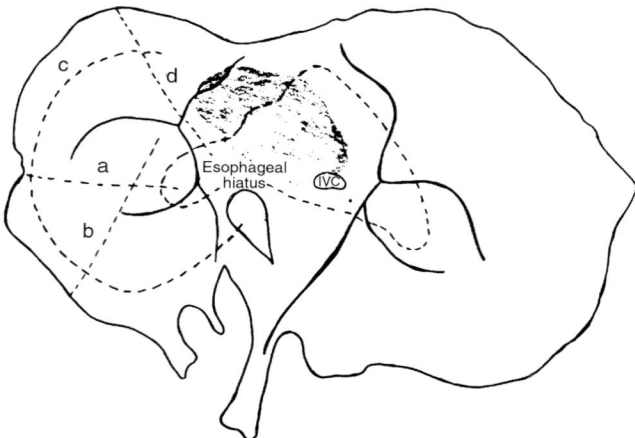

Fig. 47-5. Safe areas for incision into the diaphragm. Redrawn from Merendino KA, et al: The intradiaphragmatic distribution of the phrenic nerve with particular reference to the placement of diaphragmatic incisions and controlled segmental paralysis. Surgery *39*:189, 1956.

plished readily by approximating the cut edges of the hemidiaphragm with multiple interrupted simple or mattress sutures of 0 or 2-0 nonabsorbable material of the surgeon's choice. A similar incision may also be carried out on the right.

When a combined abdominothoracic approach is used, the incision in the diaphragm may be extended medially between the pericardial attachment to the diaphragm and the entrance of the phrenic nerve into the diaphragm, with severance of only the small sternal division of the nerve (Fig. 47-5D). The incision is then carried to the apex of the esophageal hiatus. To ensure adequate exposure, the phrenic nerve and pericardiacophrenic vessels must be freed from the pericardium proximally and retracted laterally. Care must be exercised to prevent injury to these structures during this retraction. This incision is closed the same as a circumferential incision. Sicular (1992) reported the use of this latter incision with the use of the 90 GIA stapling instrument in more than 50 patients with no compromise of exposure. Moreover, he reported no clinical evidence of phrenic nerve injury postoperatively. Incisions in the diaphragm other than a circumferential or a very medial one must be avoided because the anterolateral and posterolateral branches of the nerve are likely to be divided.

ADDENDUM

Significance of Pores in the Diaphragm

Kirschner (1998) has globally categorized the clinical occurrence of peritoneopleural transphrenic passage of fluids or gases via either congenital or acquired pores in the diaphragm as *porous diaphragm syndromes*. The numerous clinical entities are listed in Table 47-1. Kirschner (1998)

Table 47-1. Porous Diaphragm Syndromes According to Substance Traversing the Diaphragm

Fluids
  Spontaneous ascites
    Cirrhosis of the liver[a]
    Meigs' syndrome
    Pancreatic ascites[a]
    Chylous ascites[a]
  Iatrogenic ascites
    Peritoneal dialysis[a]
  Hemoperitoneum
    Abdominal/tubal pregnancy
    Ruptured spleen
    Ruptured aortic aneurysm
    Operative hemorrhage
    Endometriosis[a]
Gases
  Pneumoperitoneum
    Catamenial pneumothorax[a]
    Therapeutic pneumoperitoneum[a]
    Spontaneous pneumoperitoneum[a]
    Laparoscopic pneumoperitoneum[a]
    Diagnostic pneumoperitoneum[a]
Tissue
  Endometriosis
    Catamenial pneumothorax[a]
    Pleural endometriosis[a]
Exudates/secretion
  Subphrenic abscess[a]
  Liver abscess[a]
  Pancreatic pseudocyst[a]
  Bilothorax[a]
Intestinal contents
  Perforated peptic ulcer[a]

[a]Defect observed.
From Kirschner PA: Porous diaphragm syndromes. Chest Surg Clin North Am *8*:449, 1998. With permission.

has described these in detail, but only a few of the more important ones are discussed briefly in this addendum. The diaphragmatic pores permit the egress of ascitic fluid from the abdomen in some cirrhotic patients into the ipsilateral hemithorax pleural space, resulting in a cirrhotic hydrothorax. When identified, closure of the pore is curative, as reported by Lieberman and Peters (1970), and Mouroux (1996) and Temes (1997) and their colleagues, among others. Hydrothorax also may occur during peritoneal dialysis when these pores are present, and Nomoto and associates (1989) reported an incidence of 1.6% of this complication. The role of diaphragmatic pores in the etiology of catamenial pneumothorax is questioned by many, but these pores have been found in over one-third of the cases; in some reports, such as that of Stern and colleagues (1980), all explored patients were found to have these pores, whereas Lillington and associates (1972) only identified 3 of 18 patients as having these diaphragmatic fenestrations. One of the arguments against their role in the development of catamenial pneumothorax has been the failure to identify air in the abdomen. However, Downey and colleagues (1990) reported the presence of a pneumoperitoneum associated with a catamenial pneumothorax in a patient on three separate occasions, a finding that tends to refute the aforementioned argument. Last, the occurrence of a tension pneumothorax during the course of laparoscopy is to be noted. This event may be life-threatening and has been reported by Heddle and Platt (1984), Whiston and associates, (1991), and Childers and Caplinger (1995). This complication must be differentiated from other anesthetic complications presenting with similar clinical features.

REFERENCES

Childers JM, Caplinger P: Spontaneous pneumothorax during operative laparoscopy secondary to congenital diaphragmatic defects: a case report. J Reprod Med 40:151, 1995.

Collis JL, Kelly TD, Wiley AM: Anatomy of the crura of the diaphragm and the surgery of hiatus hernia. Thorax 9:175, 1954.

De Troyer A, et al: Action of costal and crural parts of the diaphragm on the rib cage in dogs. J Appl Physiol 53:30, 1982.

Downey DB, et al: Pneumoperitoneum with catamenial pneumothorax. AJR Am J Roentgenol 155:29, 1990.

Heddle RM, Platt AJ: Tension pneumothorax during laparoscopic cholecystectomy. Br J Surg 79:374, 1984.

Kirschner PA: Porous diaphragm syndromes. Chest Surg Clin North Am 8:449, 1998.

Lieberman FL, Peters RL: Cirrhotic hydrothorax. Further evidence that an acquired diaphragmatic defect is at fault. Arch Intern Med 125:114, 1970.

Lillington GA, Mitchell SP, Wood GA: Catamenial pneumothorax. JAMA 219:1328, 1972.

Merendino KA, et al: The intradiaphragmatic distribution of the phrenic nerve with particular reference to the placement of diaphragmatic incisions and controlled segmental paralysis. Surgery 39:189, 1956.

Mouroux J, et al: Management of pleural effusion of cirrhotic origin. Chest 109:1093, 1996.

Nomoto Y, et al: Acute hydrothorax in continuous ambulatory peritoneal dialysis: a collaborative study of 161 centers. Am J Nephrol 9;363, 1989.

Park CH, Pham CD: Hepatic hydrothorax. Scintigraphic confirmation. Clin Nucl Med 20:278, 1995.

Reddy V, Sharma S, Cobanoglu A: What dictates the position of the diaphragm—the heart or the liver? A review of sixty-five cases. J Thorac Cardiovasc Surg 108:687, 1994.

Rochester DF: The diaphragm: Contractile properties and fatigue. J Clin Invest 75:1397, 1985.

Sicular A: Direct septum transversum incision to replace circumferential diaphragmatic in operations on the cardia. Am J Surg 164:167, 1992.

Stern H, Toole AL, Merino M: Catamenial pneumothorax. Chest 78:480, 1980.

Temes RT, et al: Videothoracoscopic treatment of hepatic hydrothorax. Ann Surg 64:1468, 1997.

Urhahn R, Gunther RW: Transdiaphragmatic leakage of ascites in cirrhotic patients: evaluation with ultrafast gradient echo MR imaging and intraperitoneal enhancement. Magn Reson Imaging 11:1067, 1993.

Whiston RJ, et al: Tension pneumothorax during laparoscopic cholecystectomy. Br J Surg 78:1325, 1991.

READING REFERENCES

Anson BJ: Atlas of Human Anatomy. Philadelphia: WB Saunders, 1950.

Anson BJ, McVay C: Surgical Anatomy. 5th Ed. Philadelphia: WB Saunders, 1971.

Patten B: Human Embryology. 3rd Ed. New York: McGraw-Hill, 1968, p. 406.

Shields TW: The diaphragm. In Nora P: Operative Surgery: Principles and Techniques. Philadelphia: Lea & Febiger, 1972.

CHAPTER 48

Diaphragmatic Function, Diaphragmatic Paralysis, and Eventration of the Diaphragm

Thomas W. Shields

Although the major anatomic function of the diaphragm is the separation of the thoracic and abdominal cavities, its major physiologic function is its role in ventilation. The movement of this musculotendinous structure is responsible for the largest fraction of air moved during inspiration. With quiet breathing, this accounts for approximately 75 to 80% of the total amount of air brought into the lungs. In the supine position, it contributes 60% of the minute volume.

Primarily, the diaphragm is a muscle of inspiration, and the downward descent of the central tendon results from a coordinated contraction of all its muscle fibers. The resultant vertical movement is approximately 1 to 2 cm during quiet breathing but may be as much as 6 to 7 cm with deep, forced breathing. Each centimeter of vertical movement is estimated to contribute an intake of approximately 300 to 400 ml of air during normal breathing.

As noted by De Troyer and associates (1982) and Rochester (1985), however, the muscle mass of the diaphragm is considered to comprise two functionally distinct parts: costal and crural portions. The fiber composition of each is different: The costal muscle is thin, and the crural portion is thicker. Both groups of fibers are innervated by the phrenic nerves, but stimulation by phrenic activity results in two different actions on the chest wall. Contraction of the costal portion causes the diaphragm to flatten and the lower ribs to lift; both activities enlarge the thoracic cavity. The crural portion only causes some downward displacement of the diaphragm and is thus less effective in overall ventilatory activity of the structure.

Some muscular activity of the diaphragm occurs during exhalation. Contraction of the diaphragmatic muscle fibers does not cease abruptly at the onset of expiration but gradually declines during the initial portion of expiration and reaches zero at about the midpoint of expiration. Persistent diaphragmatic activity during the early phase of expiration provides precise regulation of the shift in air flow from inspiration to expiration. During vigorous breathing efforts, activity of the diaphragm also occurs toward the end of max-

imum expiratory efforts. The muscular activity at this time, as Agostoni and Torri (1962) reported, limits the degree to which the lungs collapse.

PARALYSIS OF THE DIAPHRAGM

Either the right or left hemidiaphragm may be paralyzed without significant respiratory embarrassment in the adult. Although ventilation on the paralyzed side is maintained by transmission of the cyclic pressure changes produced by the functioning hemidiaphragm across the mediastinum, a 20 to 30% reduction initially occurs in the vital capacity and the total lung capacity. Fackler and colleagues (1967) reported the return of these lung volumes to normal after 6 months. Clinically, in an adult, respiratory distress is minimal, although the patient may complain of chest pain and a nonproductive cough. The patient may spontaneously sleep in a semirecumbent position or in the lateral decubitus position with the side of the paralyzed hemidiaphragm down. Bilateral diaphragmatic paralysis may be tolerated by normal adults, but as McCredie and associates (1962) noted, a marked reduction of vital capacity and expiratory flow rates results, particularly while the individual is supine. In a patient with bilateral paralysis, excessive movement of the accessory muscles of respiration may be seen. Rochester (1985) has noted that such individuals are prone to chronic respiratory failure.

In infants and young children, unilateral paralysis may cause severe respiratory embarrassment, and mechanical ventilation is necessary. Bilateral paralysis is even more life threatening and is fatal unless the infant or child receives prompt ventilatory support.

In the infant or child, the lower rib cage, as noted by Hagan and colleagues (1977), may move paradoxically, even with quiet respiration. When the infant is in the lateral decubitus position, Robotham (1979) has reported that, with the paralyzed diaphragmatic leaf up, the inward paradoxic motion of the subcostal area of the upper abdomen can be seen readily. In the adult, paradoxic movement of the lower chest wall or abdomen is not evident.

Paralysis of the hemidiaphragm may be suggested by elevation of that leaf of the diaphragm on a standard chest radiograph, and evidence of some basilar atelectasis on the involved side may also be present. Paralysis may be positively identified only by the fluoroscopic observation of paradoxic movement of the paralyzed hemidiaphragm on sudden inspiration. This is best demonstrated by the classic "sniff" test. The sudden inspiratory movement causes the normal hemidiaphragm to descend, whereas the paralyzed hemidiaphragm moves in the opposite direction. In critically ill patients requiring mechanical ventilation, electrophysiologic evaluation of the phrenic nerves has been suggested by Moorthy and associates (1985). This appears to be a reliable and satisfactory method for determining the presence of paralysis of a diaphragmatic leaf under adverse clinical conditions.

Etiology of Diaphragmatic Paralysis

In infants the most common cause of unilateral hemidiaphragmatic paralysis is injury of one of the phrenic nerves during a cardiac procedure. Stone and associates (1987) reported an incidence of only 0.3%, but Watanabe and colleagues (1987) noted one of 1.6%. The incidence was slightly higher for open heart procedures and somewhat lower for closed heart operations (1.9% versus 1.3%). The Mustard procedure and the Glenn anastomosis had the highest incidences in each respective group. Procedures after previous operations had almost twice the incidence of an initial procedure. Most of the injuries were temporary (84%) but initially were associated with considerable morbidity. Before modern management, Shoemaker and colleagues (1981) recorded an overall mortality of 20 to 25%; the high rate was due mainly to underlying cardiac conditions. Birth trauma is also an occasional cause of phrenic nerve injury, as is the removal of a mediastinal tumor in an infant or young child. In pubescent girls, Helps and associates (1993) reported that a high incidence of right phrenic nerve injury occurred when a low submammary incision was used as the access for a right thoracotomy in the repair of secundum atrial defect as compared to a low rate of injury with the use of a midline sternal approach. It is suggested that the former approach be abandoned in this group of patients.

In adults, posttraumatic injury after a cardiac procedure, particularly with the use of topical hypothermia with ice slush, is the most common cause. Scannell and associates (1963) initially reported two deaths in four patients with cold injury to the phrenic nerves. Subsequently, Dajee and colleagues (1983) reported an incidence of topically hypothermic-induced injury of 9.6% but with no resulting mortality. Usually, the left phrenic nerve is the involved nerve, but right or bilateral nerve injury does occur. Some degree of paresis probably occurred in even a much higher percentage in the early experience with topical hypothermia.

Wheeler and associates (1985) reported the use of a cardiac insulation pad to reduce the incidence of injury. Hypothermic injury, however, is now less of a problem with the avoidance of opening of the pleural space, and if this does occur, inflation of the lung to protect the nerve from contact with the ice slush has reduced the incidence to less than 2% in most centers. When injury does occur, it is generally only temporary but can be permanent in 15 to 25% of patients.

Other traumatic causes of phrenic nerve damage are involvement by tumor (e.g., primary carcinoma of the lung, invasive thymoma, malignant germ cell tumors, and non-Hodgkin's lymphoma). Surgical injury likewise may occur and has been noted after mediastinotomy, surgical resections in the thorax and neck, and even placement of a subclavian or jugular vein catheter or electrode. High cervical spinal cord injuries may also result in diaphragmatic paralysis.

Idiopathic diaphragmatic paralysis is not uncommon in adults. It frequently is the result of a subclinical viral infection. The paralysis is most often unilateral, but patients with bilateral involvement have been reported by Spitzer (1973), Camfferman (1985), and Celli (1987) and their associates. Piehler and colleagues (1982) reviewed the records of 142 patients with unexplained diaphragmatic paralysis. Less than half were symptomatic. Subsequent improvement was better in those who had pain or cough than in those with dyspnea. The diaphragm returned to a normal position in less than 10%. Only 3.5% had an underlying malignancy and only one patient (0.7%) had progressive atrophy.

Management of Diaphragmatic Paralysis

In infants and young children, initial therapy is mechanical ventilation, including continuous positive airway pressure. Proper positioning with the involved side down appears helpful. If continued support is required beyond 2 weeks, Watanabe and colleagues (1987) advise operative plication of the involved diaphragmatic leaf, as suggested by Shoemaker and associates (1981), for example. The technique of plication (i.e., central pleating, as described by Schwartz and Filler [1978]), which does not require muscle resection and minimizes the possibility of injury to the phrenic nerve branches of the hemidiaphragm, is suggested as the method of choice. A different approach has been suggested by Jaklitsch and colleagues (1997). They reported the successful use of radial diaphragmatic plication in infants with moderate to severe respiratory distress. In their technique via a lateral thoracotomy, multiple sutures reinforced with Teflon pledgets are placed circumferentially in the periphery of the hemidiaphragm that avoid the central tendon. This minimizes the possibility of further injury to the phrenic nerve or injury to the blood supply of the central tendon. Moores (personal communication, 1997) suggests a somewhat similar approach to hemidiaphragmatic plication that uses only four sutures that are radially placed into the central tendon and then brought out at the peripheral margin of the hemidiaphragm and encircles the adjacent rib. This latter procedure can be accomplished readily by a video-assisted thoracoscopic surgical approach. The effect of plication of the paralyzed leaf of the diaphragm is the immobilization of the leaf in the flat position to maximally reduce its paradoxic movement with the associated shift of the mobile mediastinum to the contralateral side on inspiration. Ventilatory exchange becomes more efficient, and the infant may be more readily weaned from ventilatory support. The value of early plication has been supported further by the long-term study reported by Stone and colleagues (1987), who showed that plication did not prevent return of diaphragmatic function.

At times, direct repair of a severed nerve may be attempted. Brouillette and associates (1986) reported the successful repair of one transected phrenic nerve but failure of an interposed nerve graft in the other in a patient with bilateral nerve transections during the operative removal of a mediastinal lesion.

In adults and children older than 2 years, conservative therapy is most often indicated. Surgical intervention and plication of the involved diaphragmatic leaf has been done with good success, however, by Wright and colleagues (1985) in patients with continuing disability. Graham and associates (1990) reported the use of plication in 17 adult patients who had persistent dyspnea and orthopnea that were due to paralysis of a hemidiaphragm with a reduction in the forced vital capacity and lung volume. All showed subjective and objective improvement. In a 5- to 12-year follow-up in six patients, objective improvement in the lung functions were maintained. In patients with idiopathic bilateral paralysis, Celli and associates (1987) have reported salutary results by the use of intermittent external negative-positive ventilation.

Therapeutic Use of Phrenic Nerve Paralysis

Therapeutic temporary paralysis of a phrenic nerve has been used in the past for treatment of pulmonary tuberculosis. This procedure can be used to elevate the hemidiaphragm to help obliterate the pleural space after the removal of a portion of the lung when there is insufficient residual lung tissue to fill the pleural space. Temporary paralysis can be obtained postoperatively by percutaneous infiltration about the nerve trunk in the neck with local anesthetic. At times, direct exposure of the nerve in the neck is required. Additional elevation of the paralyzed diaphragm can be obtained by the induction of a temporary pneumoperitoneum.

EVENTRATION OF THE DIAPHRAGM

Eventration of the diaphragm is a rare anomaly, the cause of which remains to be understood completely. In general, congenital eventration of the diaphragm or the eventration occurring in newborn infants is probably a true congenital defect acquired during the fetal period. Severe cardiorespiratory symptoms in the newborn or neonate with a large unilateral eventration may be present because of secondary hypoplasia of the lung on the involved side. The appropriate resuscitative measures are required to correct acid–base balance, ventilatory insufficiency, and poor systemic perfusions, as in the neonate with a symptomatic congenital posterolateral diaphragmatic hernia (see Chapter 50). After the newborn's condition is stabilized, surgical correction of the eventration is indicated.

The repair of the defect is an emergency procedure in newborns or neonates with respiratory distress. It usually is accomplished through a thoracic approach. An incision is made in the circumference of the diaphragm, a few centimeters from the costal margin. The thinned-out diaphragm then is put on a stretch and reattached to the costal margin.

Eventration that occurs in older children and adults is thought to be caused by an acquired complete or incomplete paralysis of the diaphragmatic leaf. More often than not, localized eventration, which usually occurs on the right, with protrusion of liver through the defect, does not require surgical treatment. With a major hernia or a complete eventration, the patient may have cardiorespiratory symptoms, gastrointestinal symptoms, or both secondary to the elevation of the diaphragmatic leaf. Operative repair is indicated for older patients who have symptoms. Peters (1994) succinctly defines the value of plication of the diaphragm, but he emphasizes that it only should be done when evidence exists of ventilatory compromise leading to ventilatory insufficiency because of the paradoxic movement of the involved hemidiaphragmatic leaf:

> Plication of the diaphragm substitutes a fixed for a paradoxical diaphragm. The patient wastes less energy if the position of the diaphragm at end-expiration results in an adequate preload on the remaining inspiratory muscles. If the paralyzed diaphragm is made very tight to assume the position of maximum inspiration, this should decrease the ventilatory work by eliminating the paradoxical motion and at the same time result in a better preload on the inspiratory muscles by providing a more subatmospheric pleural pressure at end-expiration. Plication of the paralyzed diaphragm increases both end-expiratory and end-inspiratory lung volumes by preventing the abdominal contents from displacing the lung during both inspiration and expiration. In a patient with chronic obstructive lung disease who has poor elastic recoil of the lungs and chronic hyperexpansion of the lungs, fixing the paradoxical diaphragm in the inspiratory position provides more room for the large lungs and results in a more subatmospheric end-expiratory pressure, which exerts greater force to pull in the chest and elevate the innervated diaphragm to provide a better preload to the inspiratory muscles.

A transthoracic approach is preferred. Entry into the pleural space is made through the bed of the eighth rib or the eighth intercostal space. After any adhesions that may be present are freed, the thinned-out diaphragmatic leaf is repaired by plication (Fig. 48-1). A second method is by incision of the leaf, and the repair then is carried out by imbricating one

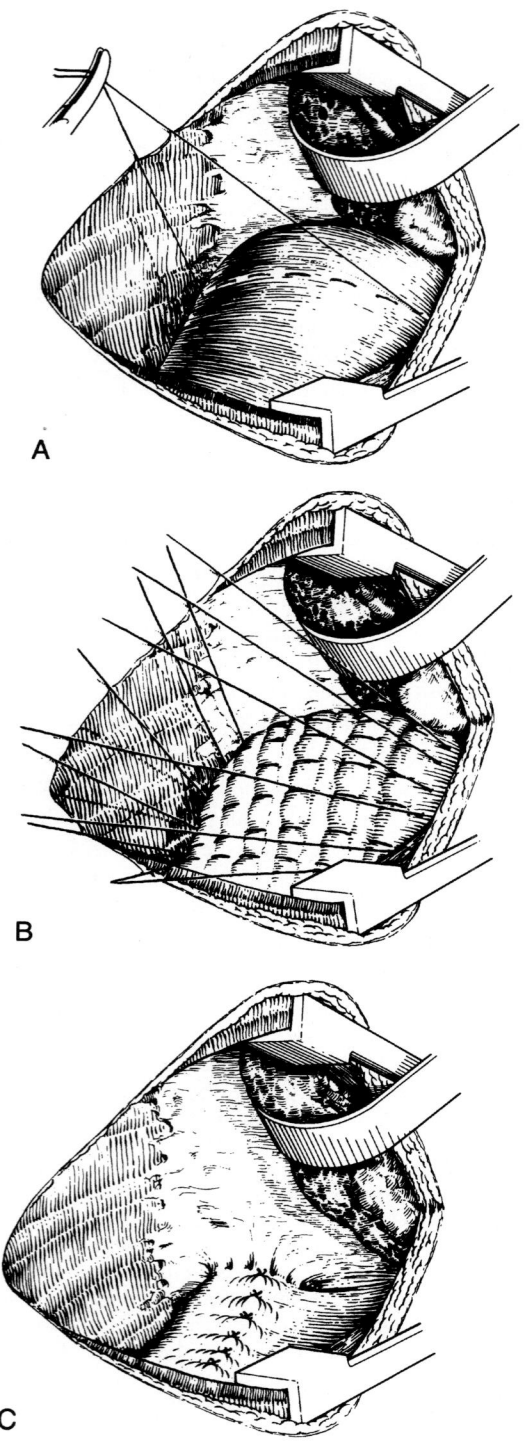

A

B

C

Fig. 48-1. Technique of plication of an eventration of the diaphragm. **A.** Four to six rows of 00 or 000 nonabsorbable sutures are inserted into the hemidiaphragm in an anterolateral to a posterolateral direction. Each row consists of five to six pleats. The branches of the phrenic nerve are avoided when the nerve is still functional. **B.** The sutures are left untied until all rows are in place. **C.** Sutures are tied to plicate and shorten the nonfunctioning leaf. From Spitz L: *In* Jackson JW, Cooper DKC (eds): Rob and Smith's Operative Surgery: Thoracic Surgery. 4th Ed. London: Butterworths, 1986, p. 7. With permission.

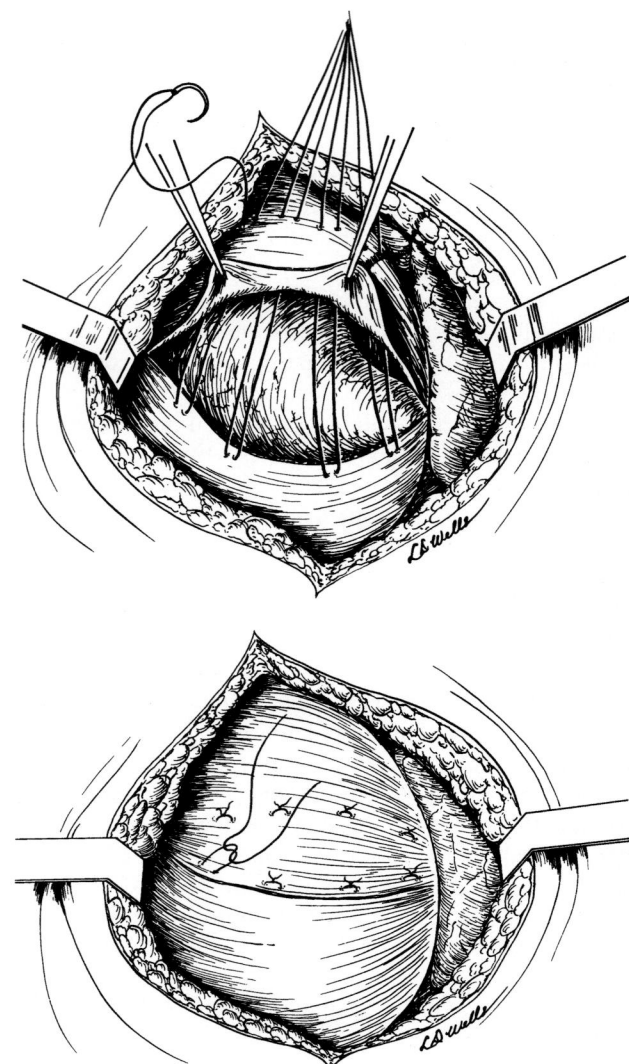

Fig. 48-2. Technique of repair of symptomatic eventration of the diaphragm. From Shields TW: The diaphragm. *In* Nora P (ed): Operative Surgery: Principles and Techniques. Philadelphia: Lea & Febiger, 1972. With permission.

layer over the other with interrupted sutures of No. 00 or No. 0 silk or other nonabsorbable suture material (Fig. 48-2). Either repair is usually attended with low mortality and morbidity rates; however, plication of the diaphragmatic leaf is the preferred method. Mouroux and colleagues (1996) have suggested that the repair of an eventration be carried out by a video-assisted thoracoscopic approach rather than by a standard thoracotomy. The diaphragmatic leaf is invaginated and held in place by two rows of continuous sutures (Fig. 48-3). Wright (1985) and Graham (1990) and their associates achieved excellent relief of exertional dyspnea and orthopnea after transthoracic diaphragmatic plication of unilateral, nonmalignant diaphragmatic paralysis. A significant increase occurred in arterial oxygen tension and all lung volumes except residual volume in the patients.

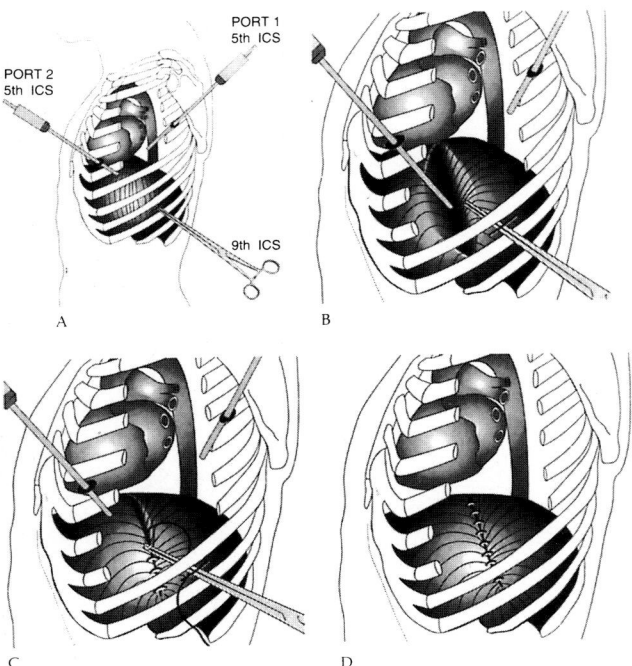

Fig. 48-3. A. Position of the two thoracoscopic ports: PORT 1 for the thoracoscope and PORT 2 for site of insertion of the forceps used to group the apex of the eventration. A minithoracotomy is made over the ninth intercostal space (ICS) for the suturing of the diaphragm. **B.** With the use of a Duval forceps, the apex of the eventration is pushed down toward the abdomen. **C.** The created transverse fold of the diaphragm is sutured with nonabsorbable material. **D.** Completed operation. From Mouroux J, et al: Technique for the repair of diaphragmatic eventration. Ann Thorac Surg 62:205, 1996. With permission.

Agenesis of the diaphragm and the presence of an accessory diaphragm have been reported by Nazarian (1971) and Geisler (1977) and their colleagues. A syndrome described by Spitz and associates (1975) consists of multiple supraumbilical abdominal wall defects, defects of the lower sternum, deficiency of the anterior diaphragm and diaphragmatic pericardium, and congenital cardiac defects (i.e., Cantrell's pentalogy) (see Chapter 40).

REFERENCES

Agostoni E, Torri G: Diaphragm contraction as a limit to maximum expiration. J Appl Physiol 17:427, 1962.

Brouillette RT, et al: Successful reinnervation of the diaphragm after phrenic nerve transection. J Pediatr Surg 21:63, 1986.

Camfferman F, et al: Idiopathic bilateral diaphragmatic paralysis. Eur J Respir Dis 66:65, 1985.

Celli BR, Rassulo J, Corral R: Ventilatory muscle dysfunction in patients with bilateral idiopathic diaphragmatic paralysis: reversal by intermittent external negative pressure ventilation. Am Rev Respir Dis 136:1276, 1987.

Dajee A, et al: Phrenic nerve palsy after topical cardiac hypothermia. Int Surg 68:345, 1983.

DeTroyer A, et al: Action of costal and crural parts of the diaphragm on the rib cage in dogs. J Appl Physiol 53:30, 1982.

Fackler CD, Perret GE, Bedell GN: Effect of unilateral phrenic nerve section on lung function. J Appl Physiol 23:923, 1967.

Geisler F, Gottlieb A, Fried D: Agenesis of the right diaphragm repaired with Marlex. J Pediatr Surg 12:587, 1977.

Graham DR, et al: Diaphragmatic plication for unilateral diaphragmatic paralysis: a 10 year experience. Ann Thorac Surg 49:248, 1990.

Hagan R, et al: Neonatal chest wall afferents and regulation of respiration. J Appl Physiol 42:362, 1977.

Helps B-A, et al: Phrenic nerve damage via a right thoracotomy in older children with secundum ASD. Ann Thorac Surg 53:328, 1993.

Jaklitsch MT, et al: Twenty-year experience with peripheral radial plication of the diaphragm. Presented at the 33rd Annual Meeting of the Society of Thoracic Surgery. February 3, 1997, San Diego, CA.

McCredie M, Lovejoy FW Jr, Kalfrieder NL: Pulmonary function in diaphragmatic paralysis. Thorax 17:213, 1962.

Moorthy SS, et al: Electrophysiologic evaluation of phrenic nerves in severe respiratory insufficiency requiring mechanical ventilation. Chest 88:211, 1985.

Mouroux J, et al: Technique for the repair of diaphragmatic eventration. Ann Thorac Surg 62:905, 1996.

Nazarian M, et al: Accessory diaphragm: report of a case with complete physiological evaluation and surgical correction. J Thorac Cardiovasc Surg 61:293, 1971.

Peters RM: Invited commentary of Takeda S, et al: Plication of the hemidiaphragm after sleeve pneumonectomy, p. 1755, and Glassman LR, et al: Successful plication for postoperative diaphragmatic paralysis in an adult, p. 1754. Ann Thorac Surg 58:1757, 1994.

Piehler JM, et al: Unexplained diaphragmatic paralysis: a harbinger of malignant disease? J Thorac Cardiovasc Surg 84:861, 1982.

Robotham JL: A physiological approach to hemidiaphragm paralysis. Crit Care Med 7:563, 1979.

Rochester DF: The diaphragm: contractile properties and fatigue. J Clin Invest 75:1397, 1985.

Scannell SC: Results of open heart operation for acquired aortic valve disease. J Thorac Cardiovasc Surg 45:47, 1963.

Schwartz MZ, Filler RM: Plication of the diaphragm for symptomatic phrenic nerve paralysis. J Pediatr Surg 13:259, 1978.

Shoemaker R, et al: Aggressive treatment of required phrenic nerve paralysis in infants and small children. Ann Thorac Surg 32:250, 1981.

Spitz L, et al: Combined anterior abdominal wall, sternal, diaphragmatic, pericardial and intracardiac defects: a report of five cases and their management. J Pediatr Surg 10:491, 1975.

Spitzer SA, Korczym AD, Kalaci J: Transient bilateral diaphragmatic paralysis. Chest 64:355, 1973.

Stone KS, et al: Long-term fate of the diaphragm surgically plicated during infancy and early childhood. Ann Thorac Surg 44:62, 1987.

Watanabe T, et al: Phrenic nerve paralysis after pediatric cardiac surgery. Retrospective study of 125 cases. J Thorac Cardiovasc Surg 94:383, 1987.

Wheeler WE, et al: Etiology and prevention of topical cardiac hypothermia-induced phrenic nerve injury and left lower lobe atelectasis during cardiac surgery. Chest 88:680, 1985.

Wright CD, et al: Results of diaphragmatic plication for unilateral diaphragmatic paralysis. J Thorac Cardiovasc Surg 90:195, 1985.

READING REFERENCES

Campbell EJM: The Respiratory Muscles and the Mechanics of Breathing. London: Lloyd-Luke, 1958.

Easton PA, et al: Respiratory function after paralysis of the right hemidiaphragm. Am Rev Respir Dis 127:125, 1983.

Haller JA Jr, et al: Management of diaphragmatic paralysis in infants with special emphasis on selection of patients for operative plication. J Pediatr Surg 14:779, 1979.

Keltz H, Kaplan S, Stone DJ: Effect of quadriplegia and hemidiaphragmatic paralysis on the thoraco-abdominal pressure during respiration. Am J Phys Med 48:109, 1969.

Koontz AR, Levin MB: Agenesis of the right half of the diaphragm. Am Surg 34:657, 1968.

McNamara JJ, et al: Eventration of the diaphragm. Surgery 64:1013, 1968.

Ribet M, Linder JL: Plication of the diaphragm for unilateral eventration or paralysis. Eur J Cardiothorac Surg 6:357, 1992.

Thomas TV: Congenital eventration of the diaphragm. Ann Thorac Surg 10:180, 1970.

CHAPTER 49

Pacing of the Diaphragm

John A. Elefteriades and Jacquelyn A. Quin

The concept of using electricity to stimulate artificial respiration that was noted by Beard and Rockwell in 1875 dates back to a suggestion by Cavallo of using electrical stimulation of the phrenic nerve as a technique for cardiopulmonary resuscitation in his 1777 treatise on the uses of electricity for human ailments. Several years later, Hufeland (1783), in his doctoral dissertation, entitled "The Use of Electricity in Asphyxia," recommended stimulation of the phrenic nerve to induce contraction of the diaphragm. In 1818, Ure (1819) demonstrated the feasibility of electrical stimulation of the phrenic nerve in a "freshly hung criminal." "The success of it was truly wonderful. Full . . . breathing instantly commenced. The chest heaved and fell; the belly was protruded and again collapsed, with the relaxing and retiring diaphragm" (Fig. 49-1). Electrical stimulation of the phrenic nerve was popularized subsequently by Duchenne de Boulogne during a cholera epidemic in 1849 as a technique for cardiopulmonary resuscitation as a treatment for asphyxia, as noted by Erdmann in 1858. In a subsequent monograph on the use of phrenic nerve stimulation, Duchenne (1872) reported, "It is apparent from all my experiments on men and on animals, alive and dead, that stimulation of the phrenic nerve by electrical current can produce contraction of the diaphragm." In 1927, Isreal reported on the use of transcutaneous stimulation of the phrenic nerves for ventilation of six apneic newborns, all of whom survived. In the 1950s, Sarnoff and associates (1950) used electrophrenic respiration extensively to treat victims of the polio epidemic.

Long-term, continuous pacing of the conditioned diaphragm as it exists today became possible through the efforts of Glenn and associates (1964, 1972, 1976, 1984, 1986). Applying their experience with radiofrequency cardiac pacemakers, they reported first on continuous radiofrequency stimulation of the phrenic nerve for several days in an animal model in 1964, and first applied to a patient with chronic ventilatory insufficiency in 1966, as reported by Judson and Glenn in 1968. Complete ventilatory support of a quadriplegic patient was achieved in 1972. In 1980, continuous bilateral, low-frequency stimulation of the conditioned diaphragm for complete respiratory support was advocated by Glenn (1980) and colleagues (1984), who recognized that bilateral high-frequency ventilation induced excessive fatigue.

A number of organized programs for diaphragm pacing have been established in the United States and abroad. Presently, an estimated 1000 pacemakers have been implanted; a majority of patients derive benefit from placement of the pacemaker.

Advances and improvements in electrophrenic respiration continue as experimental developments in pacing technique are applied to clinical practice. One such example is intercostal muscle recruitment, in which ventilation is conducted by stimulation of the upper thoracic nerve roots using spinal cord epidural electrodes, as reported in the studies of DiMarco and associates (1987, 1989, 1994). Intercostal muscle recruitment has been shown to maintain ventilation independently for brief periods of time; when used in combination with phrenic nerve stimulation, Supinski (1991) reported that a synergistic effect on ventilation may be seen.

INDICATIONS

Pacing of the diaphragm has become an established mode of ventilatory support in two clinical settings: central alveolar hypoventilation and high cervical spinal cord injury. These two indications account for the vast majority of clinical cases of diaphragm pacing.

The use of diaphragm pacing has been studied in two additional conditions: intractable hiccups and end-stage chronic obstructive pulmonary disease. Diaphragm pacing was found by Glenn and the senior author (1991) to be effective in treating patients with intractable hiccups; however, the number of patients with truly intractable hiccups who require such surgical control are few. As previously suggested by Glenn and colleagues (1978), diaphragm pacing also has been used in patients with end-stage chronic obstructive pulmonary disease in whom ventilatory drive is based on hypoxia rather than hypercarbia. The administra-

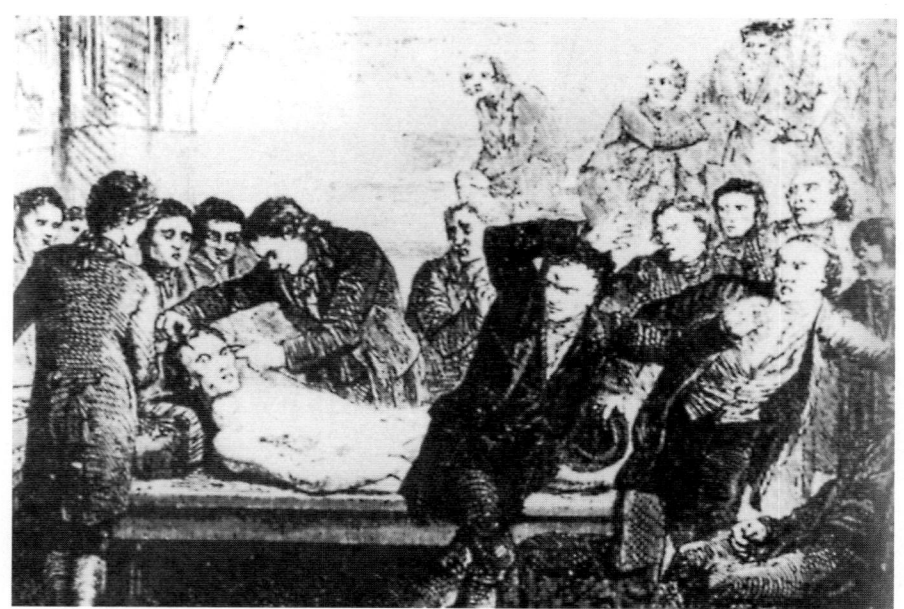

Fig. 49-1. Ure's induction of artificial respiration (Glasgow, 1818) by galvanic stimulation of the left phrenic nerve in a "freshly hung criminal." From Ure A: An account of some experiments made on the body of a criminal immediately after execution, with physiological and practical observations. J Sci Arts (Lond) 6:283, 1819.

tion of as little as 24% oxygen may cause episodic respiratory failure in these patients, as the hypoxic drive becomes increasingly diminished. Diaphragm pacing can provide oxygen-protected ventilation (continued adequacy of ventilation despite loss of hypoxic drive). As with hiccups, the number of patients with such severe progression of chronic obstructive pulmonary disease is limited.

Central Alveolar Hypoventilation

The various sleep apnea syndromes and terminology should be distinguished, because treatment modalities differ. Shneerson (1988) has provided a comprehensive review. The most basic distinction is between *obstructive* and *central* sleep apnea. In obstructive sleep apnea, upper airway obstruction during inspiration prevents adequate ventilation; however, the respiratory drive is normal, and respiratory muscle activity is preserved. The dilemma for these patients is anatomic, as the brain tells the muscles to breathe, but closure of the upper airway prevents exchange of air. Causes of obstructive apnea include pharyngeal tumors, dysmorphology of the pharynx, obesity, or exaggerated relaxation of the pharyngeal musculature during sleep. Obstructive sleep apnea is not treated with phrenic nerve pacing but rather through correction of the underlying mechanical obstruction. Intermittent positive-pressure breathing, or nasal bilevel positive airway pressure, may be used to support ventilation in these circumstances. The positive pressure overcomes the mechanical airway obstruction. The apparatus usually is applied at night when needed and removed during the day.

Distinct from obstructive sleep apnea is central sleep apnea (central hypoventilation), in which a failure of the respiratory

drive itself exists, rather than an anatomic obstruction to ventilation. The brain fails to direct ventilation. This disease process stems from malfunction of the respiratory control center of the medulla. Such may occur when the medulla becomes involved in a number of disease processes including infection (e.g., encephalitis), stroke, or trauma including iatrogenic injury. Some cases, which are thought to be idiopathic, probably represent dysfunction of the medullary chemoreceptors that normally detect hypoxia and hypercarbia.

It is increasingly recognized that the blunted nocturnal response to hypoxia and hypercapnia that characterizes central sleep apnea also prevails during the day in many, if not most, afflicted patients; however, ventilation may be augmented to a certain extent in the awake individual by conscious effort. For this reason, *central alveolar hypoventilation* is a preferred descriptor over *sleep apnea*. The term *Ondine's curse* also has been used extensively in the literature to describe this condition. The term originates from the Latin word *unda*, or *wave*. Undines were water spirits. In 1811 and translated into English in 1839, German baron Friedrich Heinrich Karl de la Motte Fouque published *Undine*, the fictional story of a water nymph who placed a curse on her mortal husband for unfaithfulness. From these original works evolved *Ondine*, from French playwright Giraudoux (1946), which told the story of a mortal who was cursed to stop breathing whenever he fell asleep, for having married a water nymph.

Patients with central alveolar hypoventilation often, but not always, have a characteristic pickwickian habitus. The chronic hypoxia and hypercapnia, as well as the fragmented sleep pattern itself, lead to daytime somnolence. Over time, pulmonary vasoconstriction, secondary to chronic hypoxia, may lead to fixed pulmonary hypertension, which may ultimately result in right-sided heart failure.

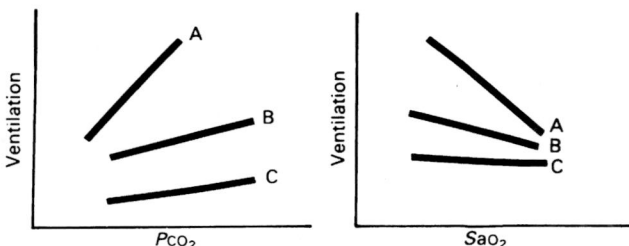

Fig. 49-2. The ventilatory response to hypercapnia and hypoxia. Normal individuals (A). Patients with chest wall disorders (B). Patients with central hypoventilation (C).

The adequacy of the respiratory drive is assessed by ventilatory response to hypercapnia and hypoxia (Fig. 49-2). Ventilation normally increases linearly with increasing P_{CO_2}. Ventilation should increase linearly with decreasing O_2 saturation, and increase exponentially as the partial pressure of oxygen (P_{O_2}) decreases. An impaired response to each of these parameters is seen in patients with central alveolar hypoventilation. Intermediate responses can be seen in individuals with primary weakness of the muscles of respiration, which can mimic central hypoventilation; however, standard spirometric tests of pulmonary function can usually readily distinguish between the two conditions. In diagnosing central alveolar hypoventilation, the senior author routinely performs a 24-hour respiratory control study, with hourly assessment of asleep-awake status, end-tidal CO_2, and O_2 saturation. Patients with central hypoventilation demonstrate a characteristic pattern of severe nocturnal hypoventilation and hypercarbia, with milder daytime hypercarbia.

Central alveolar hypoventilation is an appropriate indication for diaphragm pacing. The artificially induced ventilation satisfactorily compensates for the lack of respiratory drive.

Quadriplegia

The other common affliction that may be treated by diaphragm pacing is cervical spinal cord injury. With increased public awareness of cardiopulmonary resuscitation techniques, improved emergency care delivery systems, widespread availability of positive-pressure ventilation, and improved long-term respiratory care, more patients are surviving the accident that causes quadriplegia and being sustained for longer periods than in earlier eras. Spinal cord injuries, which may be as high as 56.1 per 1 million population in some countries, occur most often from motor vehicle crashes. Burney and colleagues (1993) have observed that the cervical region of the spinal cord is most commonly involved; over one-half of these injuries have been reported to result in quadriplegia or some degree of quadriparesis. In the adolescent population, Noguchi (1994), as well as others, has pointed out that sporting event accidents are also a common cause of cervical injury. Spivak and associates

(1994) note that cervical injuries in the elderly population often occur secondary to an accidental fall. Iatrogenic injuries may be seen as well. In addition to traumatic etiologies, infections, developmental and vascular abnormalities, and infarctions also can produce quadriplegia.

The lower motor neurons of the phrenic nerve are located in the spinal cord at the levels of C3–5. Spinal cord disruption below these levels causes quadriplegia but does not disrupt respiration by virtue of an intact phrenic nerve with upper motor neuron communication. Spinal cord injury, which involves the C3–5 levels, where the cell bodies of the phrenic nerve are located, may cause a partially injured phrenic nerve. The patient may retain a limited ability to ventilate. However, ventilation may not be improved with the addition of diaphragm pacing, because the phrenic nerve is compromised from degeneration. The decision to pace under these circumstances requires careful consideration, because the benefit from doing so may be limited.

High cervical quadriplegia (at the C2–3 levels or higher) eliminates spontaneous ventilation by disrupting the tracts that lead from the medullary respiratory control center to the spinal cord (Fig. 49-3). However, the integrity of the phrenic

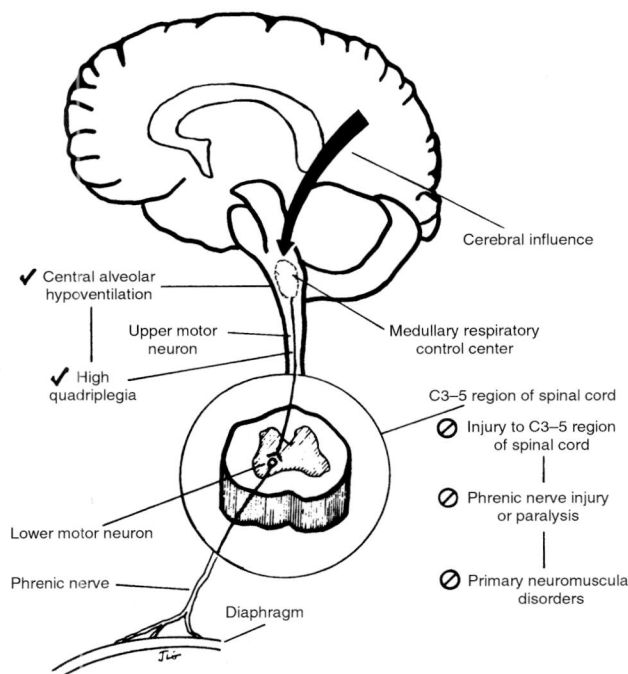

Fig. 49-3. Respiratory control system as regards disorders appropriate or inappropriate for diaphragm pacing. The involuntary medullary respiratory control center is subject to a degree of cerebral voluntary influence. The upper motor neurons of the phrenic system have their cell bodies in the medullary respiratory control center. The axons of the upper motor neurons synapse in the spinal cord with the lower motor neurons, at the level of C3–5. The phrenic nerve proper is composed of the axons of those lower motor neurons. Check marks indicate appropriate indications for diaphragm pacing. International *verboten* symbols identify inappropriate indications.

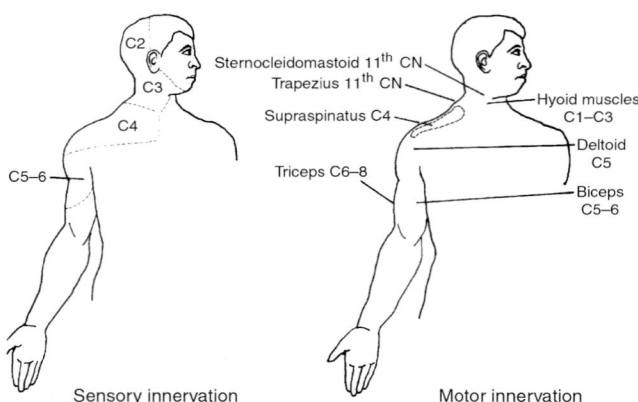

Fig. 49-4. Sensory and motor findings that allow discrimination of *high* quadriplegia. Quadriplegia at C2–3 or higher is well treated by diaphragm pacing. CN, cranial nerve.

nerve is maintained, because the cell bodies of the phrenic nerve are spared from injury.

High cervical spinal cord lesions also denervate the intercostal (T1–T12), abdominal (T7–L1), and pelvic (L1–S2) accessory muscles of respiration. Only the sternocleidomastoid and trapezius muscles, which are innervated by the spinal accessory nerve (cranial nerve XI), remain functional with quadriplegia at or above the C2–3 level. The neurologic findings that distinguish high quadriplegia (C2–3 or higher) are shown in Figure 49-4. In general, patients with high quadriplegia demonstrate intact sensation only to the clavicles; motor function is disrupted from the deltoid muscle and below.

The respiratory paralysis from high quadriplegia is directly correctable by diaphragm pacing. When a patient with high quadriplegia manifests respiratory paralysis and the phrenic nerve is found to be intact, diaphragm pacing is indicated if the patient's overall status permits.

PACING PREREQUISITES

Purposeful diaphragm pacing requires at least an intact phrenic nerve and a functional diaphragm. Phrenic nerve stimulation is not indicated for patients in whom the nerve is injured or dysfunctional. Examples include direct nerve injury from trauma, as a complication of cardiac surgery, as pointed out by Dimopoulou (1998) and Luc Diehl (1994) and their associates, or via involvement from malignancy or infection. Figure 49-3 illustrates schematically the levels of neurologic insult that represent appropriate and inappropriate circumstances for diaphragm pacing.

It is also critical that the diaphragm muscle be inherently sound in order to tolerate pacing. In general, a diaphragm affected by a primary muscular disorder such as myasthenia gravis or muscular dystrophy is not appropriate for pacing. Patients with central hypoventilation should demonstrate at least a 5-cm maximal excursion of the diaphragm with spontaneous breathing before embarking on diaphragm pacing; 8 to 10 cm is average. Quadriplegic patients are not required

to exhibit the same degree of excursion with phrenic nerve stimulation as spontaneously ventilating patients. The diaphragm is expected to atrophy with disuse from quadriplegia and can be corrected with gradual conditioning. However, some brisk downward deflection of the diaphragm with percutaneous stimulation of the phrenic nerve should be observed even in quadriplegia.

Diaphragm pacing requires that the ability of the lungs to oxygenate and ventilate be preserved. In most cases, pulmonary function test results should be normal or minimally compromised, because pacing cannot compensate for severe restrictive or obstructive lung disease. For similar reasons, major deformities of the chest wall contraindicate diaphragm pacing by virtue of their mechanical interference with ventilatory function.

Equally imperative for successful diaphragm pacing is a knowledgeable and cooperative patient. Patients who have suffered permanent cognitive impairment are not appropriate candidates for pacing. Aside from important issues of health care allocation, a brain-damaged status prevents appreciation of many of the benefits of diaphragm pacing. Paramount to the success of an individual patient is a supportive network of family members and friends, and a professional team of health care providers who are familiar with pacing techniques and the long-term aftercare.

Phrenic Nerve Function

Because an intact phrenic nerve is essential for pacing, accurate assessment of nerve function assumes paramount importance. Sarnoff (1951) and Shaw (1980) and their colleagues have described the technique for transcutaneous testing of phrenic nerve conduction (Fig. 49-5). The overall technique is similar to that for any electromyelography or nerve conduction test. A thimble electrode facilitates testing of the phrenic nerve. The *motor point* of the nerve is located medial to the lateral edge of the clavicular head of the sternocleidomastoid muscle. With the sternocleidomastoid muscle retracted medially, stimulation is applied by the thimble electrode; the current is directed posteriorly. We look for a brisk ipsilateral hemidiaphragmatic contraction, which is visible and grossly palpable on physical examination. Additionally, the muscle action potential of the diaphragm and the phrenic nerve conduction time may be measured with the use of surface electrodes. Two electrodes are placed at approximately the level of the eighth intercostal space, one in the anterior axillary line and the other in the posterior axillary line. A ground electrode is placed at the xiphoid. The phrenic nerve conduction time is measured as the elapsed time from phrenic nerve stimulation at the neck until a diaphragmatic action potential is recorded by an oscilloscope. The phrenic nerve conduction time for the adult is normally 7.5 to 10.0 ms. A prolonged conduction time (greater than 11 ms) is considered abnormal; however, slightly prolonged times (11 to 14 ms) do not necessarily preclude pacing.

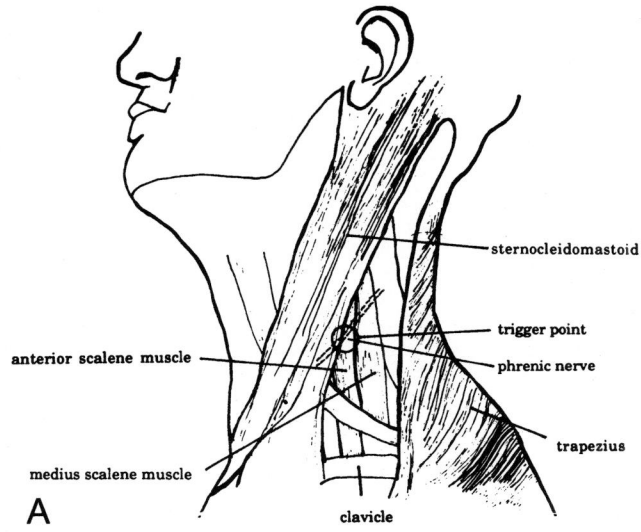

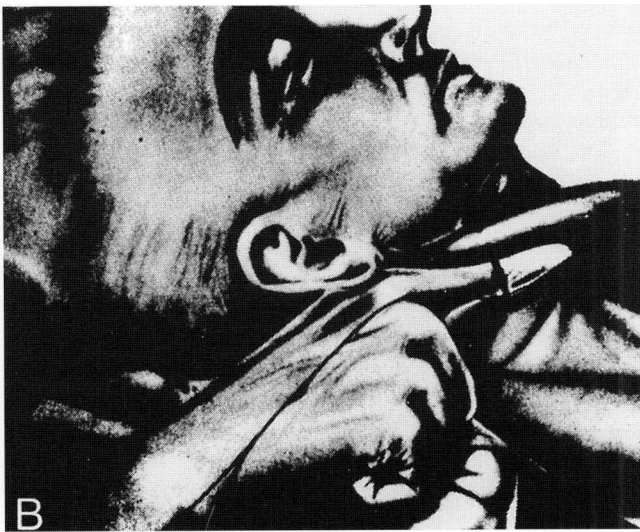

Fig. 49-5. Testing for viability of the phrenic nerve by percutaneous electrical stimulation. **A.** The trigger point at the border of the clavicular head of the sternocleidomastoid where the phrenic nerve is accessible to stimulation as it crosses on the scalene muscles. **B.** Application of the thimble electrode.

Phrenic nerve conduction time also may be assessed using cervical magnetic stimulation. A magnetic coil placed on the neck causes depolarization of the intraforaminal segments of cervical nerve roots C3–5. Bilateral, simultaneous stimulation of the nerve roots is usually performed; however, Mills and coworkers (1995) have shown that unilateral stimulation is possible. Because depolarization is applied to the intraforaminal segments of the roots that make up the phrenic nerve rather than the nerve per se, *cross-stimulation* of additional muscles that may be partially or completely supplied by the same intraforaminal segments may occur. Careful interpretation of results with cervical magnetic stimulation is necessary, because the results cannot be directly compared with those of percutaneous electromagnetic stimulation in which the phrenic nerve is directly and specifically stimu-

lated. Although Similowski and associates (1996, 1997) have reported on the usefulness of cervical magnetic stimulation for the selection of phrenic pacing candidates when used in combination with cortical magnetic stimulation, the number of patients evaluated is small, and application of this device for phrenic nerve assessment is not standard.

The clinical response of the diaphragm to nerve stimulation is paramount. Intact conduction produces a dramatic and easily recognized contraction of the hemidiaphragm. Simple clinical inspection is often adequate; however, fluoroscopy can be used to quantify the amount of hemidiaphragm contraction. Failure to elicit a strong contraction almost invariably indicates a nonviable phrenic nerve. In rare instances, nerve viability cannot be ascertained by noninvasive methods. Under these circumstances, if pacing is deemed critical, operative exploration and direct stimulation of the nerve should ensue.

Patients with spinal cord injury may have delayed recovery of respiratory function such that an initially ventilator-dependent patient may recover spontaneous respiratory function. Therefore, an interim period of at least 3 months after injury is best undertaken before the final decision for diaphragm pacing is made. This waiting period allows many issues related to the acute injury to resolve. Patients find time to establish rehabilitation regimens, including those related to altered bowel and bladder function and the prevention of decubitus ulcers. The quadriparetic patient also may require a time period of psychological adjustment to the neurologic injury itself. In the event pacing is eventually determined necessary, proper attention to these related issues is essential to its overall success.

TECHNIQUES

Pulse Train Stimulation

Unlike cardiac muscle, which is able to propagate a single electrical impulse to allow contraction, the diaphragm is not an electrical syncytium. Thus, a single stimulus, such as that delivered by a cardiac pacemaker, is insufficient to effect contraction of the diaphragm. Rather, a series of multiple stimuli is required to produce a mechanically effective diaphragm contraction. A series of such repeated stimuli is termed a *pulse train*, and several electrical parameters are defined in pulse train stimulation (Fig. 49-6). The rate determines the overall number of pulse trains delivered by diaphragm pacing per minute; this corresponds to the respiratory rate. The pulse train duration determines the length of time of the pulse train, which, in turn, determines the duration of inspiration. The pulse width determines the length of time for any one individual impulse, and the number of impulses within a pulse train is called the *frequency*. Frequency also can be expressed by its inverse, the pulse interval, which determines the length of time between individual impulses within a pulse train. Specifically, frequency (Hz) = 1000 ms/pulse interval. The amplitude determines the voltage of each stimulus within the

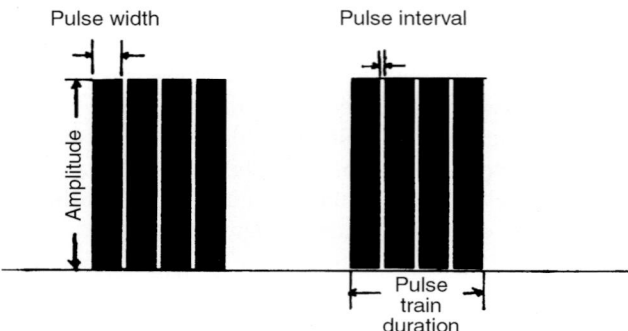

Fig. 49-6. Pulse train stimulation. Characteristics (and unit measurements) describing pulse train stimulation: rate (breaths per minute, bpm), overall number of pulse trains delivered per minute; amplitude (v), voltage of each stimulus in a pulse train series; pulse width (ms), duration of an individual pulse; pulse interval (ms), duration between pulses in a train; frequency (Hz), timing of stimuli within a pulse train (frequency [Hz] = 1000/pulse interval); pulse train duration (ms), overall duration of one train of pulses, corresponding to inspiratory duration.

pulse train; this determines the strength of the diaphragm contraction and the resulting tidal volume.

Electrode stimulation of the phrenic nerve may be performed in either monophasic or biphasic fashion. Biphasic stimulation, in which alternating positive and negative currents are used, requires less electrical energy and may reduce nerve injury. Likewise, stimulation may be done in unipolar or bipolar mode, depending on the number of electrodes in contact with the nerve.

It cannot be overemphasized that diaphragm pacing requires an intact and functional phrenic nerve. Although experimental studies of direct intramuscular stimulation of the phrenic nerve have been performed by Peterson and associates (1994a, 1994b), these techniques have found limited clinical application. Intramuscular stimulation of the diaphragm probably occurs through the branches of the phrenic nerve as the nerve divides in the central portion of the diaphragm. Unfortunately, atrophy of the denervated muscle in cases of phrenic nerve injury would probably diminish the strength of the diaphragmatic contraction even in the event direct diaphragm stimulation was realized. Although successful phrenic nerve repair has been reported by Merav and colleagues (1983), and grafting by Baldissera (1993) and Krieger (1994) and their associates, the long-term merit of such endeavors remains unproved in terms of primary nerve function and ability to pace.

Pacing Equipment

Unlike cardiac pacemakers, which are totally implantable, diaphragm pacemakers have an extracorporeal generator, approximately the size of a clock radio, in addition to the surgically implanted nerve electrode and receiver. Output

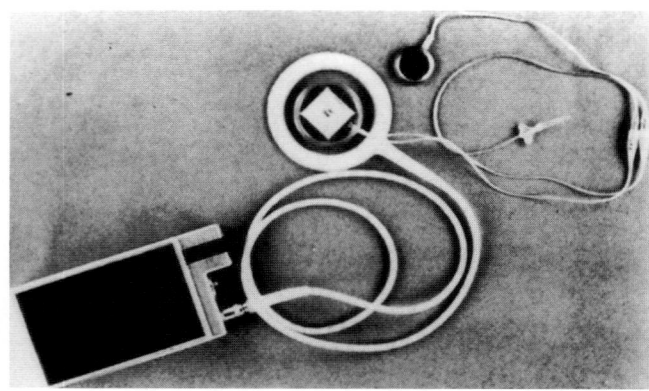

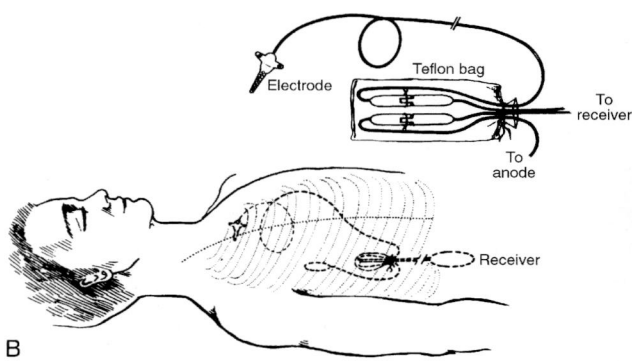

Fig. 49-7. The apparatus for diaphragm pacing. **A.** The hardware. The transmitter, external antenna, implantable receiver, and phrenic nerve electrode are shown. The transmitter remains outside the body, as does the antenna, which is taped securely to the skin over the implanted receiver. **B.** Equipment in place in patient. Note placement of phrenic nerve electrode at the level of the upper thorax. The implanted receiver is situated over a flat portion of the lower chest wall.

from the generator is carried through an antenna, the coil of which is taped securely to the patient's skin over the receiver site. The antenna transmits a radiofrequency signal to the implanted receiver, which resembles a pocket watch in size and shape. Through inductive coupling, a stimulating signal is conducted to the receiver and across the electrode to stimulate the phrenic nerve (Fig. 49-7). Despite the external position of the generator and the inductive coupling arrangement for transmission of the signal to the body, the system is reliable and relatively simple to teach. A portable generator also exists for ambulatory patients, which is approximately the size of a compact disc player. Designed by Glenn and colleagues (1972), the system remains the prototype for the three commercial pacing systems currently in use.

Although the goal of a totally implanted pacemaker has been long since achieved in an animal model by Hogan and coworkers (1976, 1989), a commercially available implant for clinical use has not been realized. The relatively low volume of diaphragm pacemakers implanted annually and the need for a battery adequate to power pulse train stimulation have contributed to the slow progress. Lanmüller and associ-

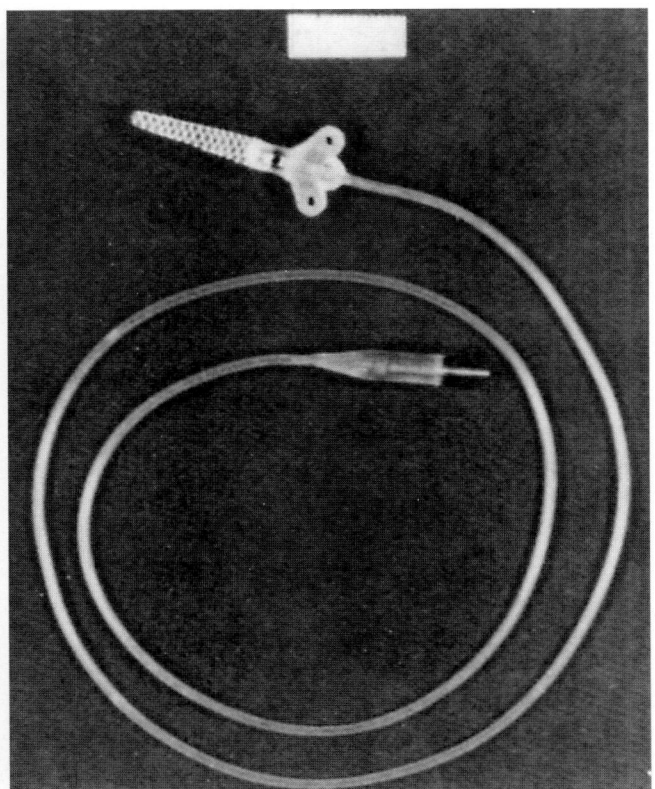

Fig. 49-8. Detailed view of the 180-degree half-cuff phrenic nerve electrode.

ates (1997) have reported their progress with an implantable pacemaker. The anticipated battery life is 3 to 5 years, depending on the electrode type. The development of a rate-responsive diaphragm pacemaker, a feature already available in cardiac pacemakers, remains to be accomplished.

Commercial Devices

Currently, three pacing systems are in clinical use; each varies slightly with respect to design. The Avery system (Avery Laboratories, Glen Cove, NY) uses the half-cuff or 180-degree unipolar electrode as originally developed at Yale (Fig. 49-8). The system is also used for skeletal muscle stimulation in other clinical applications. The electrode is placed preferentially in 180-degree contact to avoid the potential nerve entrapment and injury from scar tissue that may occur with a 360-degree or full-cuff contact. Letsou and associates (1992) found experimentally that pacing with either the half-cuff or full-cuff configurations were comparable. The Avery system is the only commercially manufactured device in the United States; however, technical difficulties with receiver function and longevity have prompted the group at Yale to reconsider its use.

Currently, the Jukka Astrostim model (Atrotech OY, Tampere, Finland) is used at Yale and elsewhere with favorable results. This model differs from the Avery device by virtue of a quadripolar electrode. Two strips of Teflon, each carrying two electrode contacts, are opposed to the nerve, one behind and one in front. Any of the four electrode contacts may serve as the cathode with its opposite contact serving as the anode. Stimulation of the phrenic nerve occurs through only one of the electrode contacts at any given time, permitting incomplete stimulation of the nerve fascicles and associated muscle bundles. Such selective stimulation is thought to resemble more closely natural respiration, in which incomplete recruitment of nerve fascicles allows some muscle bundles to do the work of breathing while others recover. At regular intervals, an increased tidal volume is effected using an increased stimulation current. These "sighs" allow additional conditioning of the diaphragm in the event recruitment of muscle mass is needed for increased ventilation requirements. An adapter is available to connect the Avery electrode with the Astrostim receiver for patients who have undergone previous placement of the former.

Similar to the Astrostim model, the Vienna phrenic pacemaker, designed by Medimplant, Inc. (Vienna, Austria) stimulates the nerve using multiple electrode contacts with incomplete stimulation of the nerve. The electrode is also a quadripolar unit of carousel design (Fig. 49-9). Both phrenic nerves are activated through one receiver.

Device Implantation

In implanting the system, extreme caution is taken in placing the electrode to the phrenic nerve, because damage to the nerve during implantation would essentially preclude pacing. The operation is done through a limited anterior thoracotomy in the second or third intercostal space (Fig. 49-10). The pectoral muscle is divided in the direction of its fibers. The internal mammary artery and vein are divided deliberately to avoid accidental disruption while transecting the intercostal muscles. On entering the thorax, the phrenic nerve is identified on the mediastinal surface, anterior to pulmonary hilum. A location is chosen superior to the heart where the phrenic nerve is accessible and where the electrode can be placed so as to lie perfectly flat beneath the nerve. The mediastinal pleura is incised parallel to the nerve, both anteriorly and posteriorly, and several millimeters away from the neurovascular bundle itself. The electrode is slipped atraumatically behind the mobilized phrenic structures, such that the phrenic bundle rests inside the half-cuff platinum contact of the electrode in the case of the unipolar electrode. The Silastic portions of the electrode are secured by suture to the mediastinal pleura. Perfect lie of the electrode must be obtained such that no distortion or traction on the nerve results; delayed injury or dysfunction of the nerve may result otherwise. Bleeding from the artery or vein accompanying the nerve is not treated if minor. This usually stops spontaneously; application of cautery could well injure the delicate nerve. With

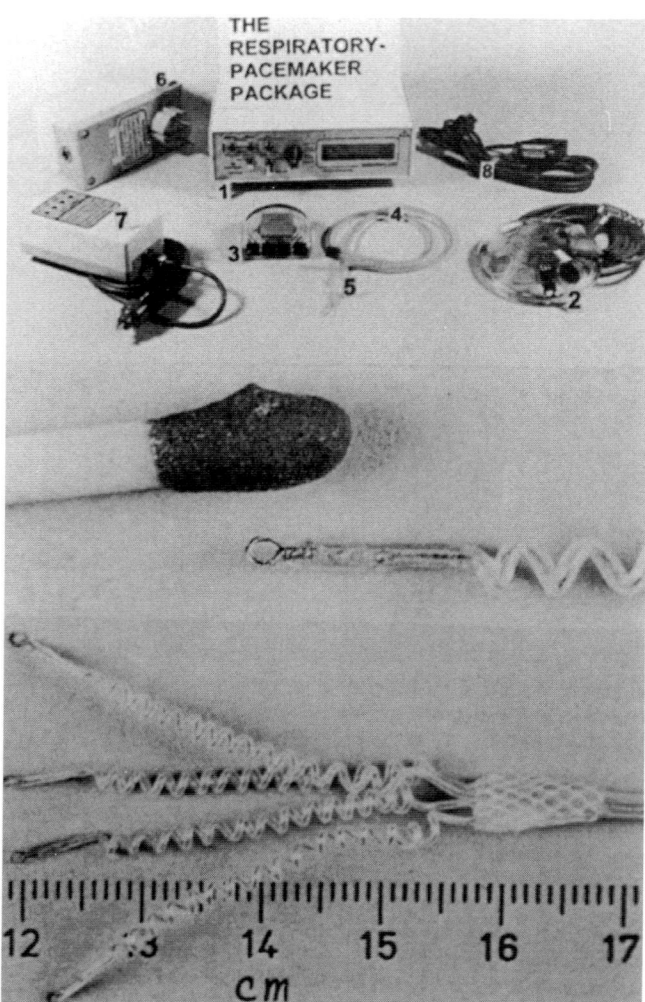

Fig. 49-9. Vienna phrenic pacemaker by Medimplant (Vienna, Austria). **(Top)** the complete respiratory package including (1) battery-powered control, (2) radiofrequency transmission coil (external), (3) eight-channel implanted nerve stimulator, (4) electrode leads, (5) electrode contacts (see bottom frame), (6) power transformer for household current, (7) car battery power transformer, and (8) trigger unit for respirator (used during training). **(Middle)** Epineural electrode. Match head placed for size comparison. **(Bottom)** Actual four-prong quadripolar electrode. From Creasey G, et al: Electrical stimulation to restore respiration. J Rehab Res Dev *33*:123, 1996. With permission.

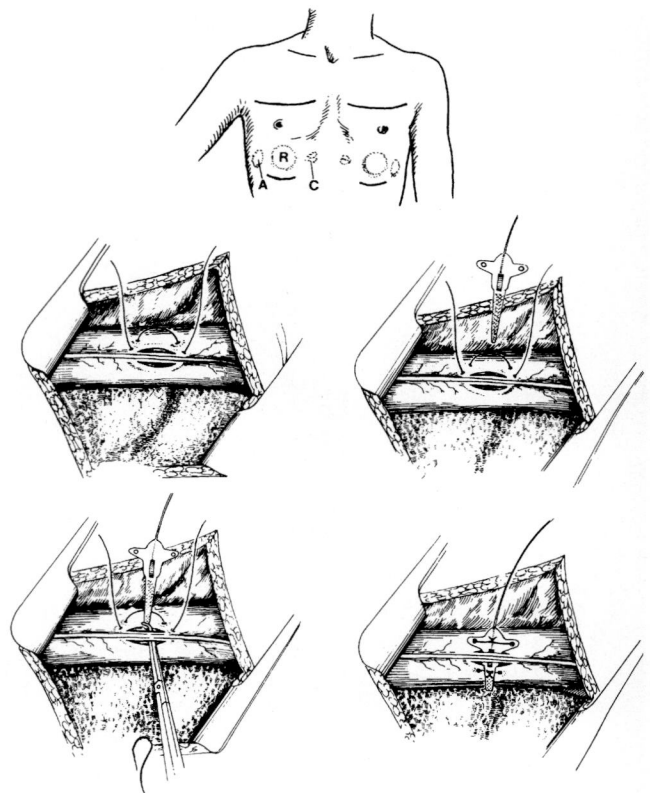

Fig. 49-10. Transthoracic approach to the phrenic nerves for diaphragm pacing. **(Top)** Incisions in the second interspace for nerve access. Incisions at the costal margin for implantation of receiver (R), anode plate (A), and connectors (C). **(Middle and bottom)** Sequential steps in implantation of 180-degree electrode behind the phrenic nerve. Modified from Glenn WWL: The diaphragm. *In* Glenn WWL (ed): Thoracic and Cardiovascular Surgery. 4th Ed. East Norwalk, CT: Appleton-Century-Crofts, 1983, p. 363.

careful attention to atraumatic technique, injury to the phrenic nerve should be avoidable.

The other end of the electrode is passed carefully through the chest wall using a chest tube to avoid trauma during its passage. Redundant wire is left within the thorax, on the surface of the lung, to avoid tension on the electrode with lung excursion. The excess wire is placed into a Teflon bag to facilitate future access. A precise subcutaneous pocket is created over a flat portion of the lower anterolateral rib cage to house only the receiver, with precise closure of the pocket to prevent receiver migration. As with any device implanta-

tion, the incision is closed away from the underlying receiver, to avoid any undue pressure, which can result in improper healing, dehiscence, or both.

Implantation of a cervical electrode is somewhat controversial. Advocates of this approach cite technical ease of electrode placement in the neck, compared with that via the thoracic approach, especially in the patient with a mildly deformed thorax or with an element of pulmonary parenchymal disease. Bilateral concurrent implantation of the nerves may be performed. However, the cervical approach is discouraged for several reasons, the most important of which is the existence of accessory phrenic nerve radicals that originate below the C3–5 level that do not join the phrenic nerve until a mediastinal location (Fig. 49-11), as pointed out by Kelly (1950) as well as by Glenn and Sairenji (1985). A cervically placed electrode would not stimulate these radicals. Other anatomic variations also exist within the neck. The nerve may be adjacent to the brachial plexus, intramuscular in the scalenus anticus muscle, or bifurcated; under these circumstances, electrode placement may prove awkward.

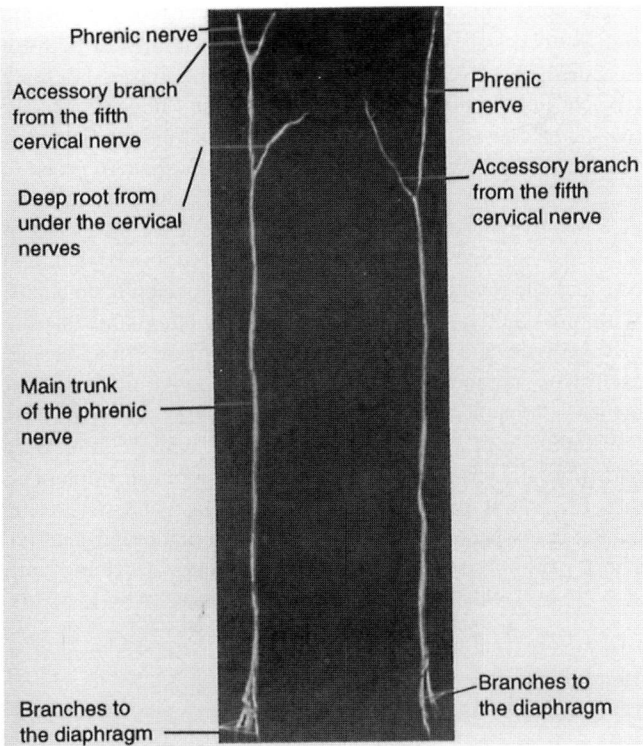

Fig. 49-11. Phrenic nerves removed by the operation of exeresis, a treatment in the early twentieth century for apical tuberculosis. To effect diaphragm paralysis, surgeons removed the phrenic nerve and associated branches by avulsion in the neck. *Nebenphrenicus*, probably the branch of the fifth cervical, the so-called accessory branch, is presumed to join the nerve trunk at the cervical level on the right. On the left side, the branch joins the nerve trunk at a lower level and would probably not be stimulated by an electrode in the cervical location. From Glenn WWL, Sairenji H: Diaphragm pacing in the treatment of chronic ventilatory insufficiency. *In* Roussos C, Macklem PT (eds): The Thorax, Part B. New York: Marcel Dekker, 1985, p. 1434. With permission.

In the event cervical placement is chosen, patients should be temporarily intubated if a tracheostomy is not already present. When a tracheostomy is present, the site is covered with an occlusive dressing to decrease the risk of contamination during electrode placement. An incision of approximately 5 cm is made above and parallel to the midportion of the clavicle. The lateral border of the sternocleidomastoid muscle is identified and retracted medially with the internal jugular vein. At this level, the nerve is almost always found overlying the scalenus anticus muscle, just deep to the scalene fascia, as it crosses from the lateral to medial aspect of the muscle. A stimulation probe is positioned and 2 to 10 mA of current applied. Diaphragm contraction confirms correct identification of the nerve. Nerve dissection and placement of the permanent nerve electrode and radiofrequency receiver proceed in a fashion similar to that used in the chest. The subcutaneous pocket is created in the infraclavicular region by blunt dissection through the existing cervical incision.

Placement of the Medimplant device is usually performed through a median sternotomy, as both electrodes are stimulated from a single receiver. The prongs of the electrode are carefully sutured using microsurgical technique to the epineural tissue using fine (8-0) polypropylene suture.

The system is tested in the operating room to confirm function before the patient is undraped. Testing is performed with a sterile antenna passed off the operating field, to the extracorporeal generator. Excellent contraction of the diaphragm with pacing should occur in a threshold range of 1.0 to 2.0 mA. Pacing that requires high-threshold values, or failure to pace at all, requires reevaluation of the lead for improper placement or displacement, injury to the lead, or injury to the phrenic nerve itself. Infection is avoided via the use of meticulous technique and prophylactic antibiotics. Implantation of the right and left pacemaker systems are usually performed approximately 2 weeks apart.

Device Settings

Fluoroscopy, performed at the initial evaluation of the diaphragm and at pacemaker implantation, is used to determine proper threshold current settings. A fluoroscopically visible ruler is placed beneath the diaphragm with numeral 1 visible at the dome of the diaphragm. The anteroposterior distance of the x-ray tube is kept constant at 30 cm for all diaphragm evaluations. Maximal voluntary descent is determined for patients with central hypoventilation. The threshold current, the amount needed to produce a contraction of the diaphragm that is just discernible, is measured. The amount of current needed for maximal contraction of the diaphragm is measured, and the degree of descent associated with this current is measured. For clinical pacing, the current is set just above that needed for maximal excursion. Reassessment of the diaphragm with respect to current settings is performed at intervals thereafter.

The respiratory rate is individualized for each patient. In adult patients undergoing bilateral pacing, 6 to 10 breaths per minute usually suffice. Adults who are paced unilaterally and children require a faster rate. Pacemaker default settings for inspiratory duration and pulse width are usually preset by the manufacturer. For adults, the inspiratory duration is usually 1.3 seconds, and pulse width is 150 ms. Inspiration duration for children is adjusted to 0.9 seconds. Frequency and pulse interval settings are discussed subsequently in the context of diaphragm conditioning.

Conduct of Pacing

Pacing is not begun until 2 weeks after device implantation is complete; it has been noted that earlier initiation led to the development of bloody pleural effusions. This may represent disruption of immature adhesions by the strong diaphragm contraction elicited by pacing.

Several modes of pacing are possible: unilateral, pacing on alternating sides (usually at 12-hour intervals), or simultaneous bilaterally pacing. Unilateral pacing may suffice in selected circumstances, such as in patients with central alveolar hypoventilation; however, the preference of the Yale group is to condition the diaphragm for low-frequency, continuous bilateral stimulation.

No skeletal muscle, including the diaphragm, is able to perform maximal continuous work. Although the diaphragm contracts incessantly to provide respiration, activation of the individual nerve fascicles and muscle bundles is staggered such that during any given breath, a percentage of dormant motor units is allowed metabolic recovery from previous activation. Because pulse train stimulation of the phrenic nerve activates most, if not all, of the nerve's fascicles and muscle bundles, individual motor units are not allowed to rest and the unconditioned diaphragm tires easily.

Because of these issues, a program of gradual conditioning is used to allow the diaphragm to acclimate to pulse train electrical stimulation and, in the case of quadriplegia, restore the diaphragm, which has atrophied from disuse. The pacing schedule usually begins with 15 minutes of pacing per hour, in the supine position, for several hours a day. The number of minutes per hour and the number of hours per day are gradually increased in a systematic fashion until full-time pacing is achieved. Increases in the pacing regimen are made approximately every 7 to 14 days as tolerated by the patient. The adaptive process may require weeks to months, depending on the condition of the diaphragm at the inception of pacing. Quadriplegic patients require longer conditioning times than patients with central hypoventilation. Along with progressive increases in the pacing period, the frequency of stimuli in the pulse train is decreased progressively, usually to approximately 7.1 Hz, corresponding to a pulse interval of 140 ms, to minimize diaphragm fatigue and allow longer pacing periods. Also to minimize fatigue, the number of breaths per minute is progressively decreased to the lowest number that provides adequate ventilation. When the patient is sitting, the ventilatory rate is increased by one breath per minute to maintain adequate ventilation. A snug abdominal binder is placed in sitting quadriplegic patients.

Tidal volume, minute volume, end-tidal partial pressure of carbon dioxide, and oxygen saturation are monitored at the beginning and end of each pacing period as well as at regular intervals during pacing. Measurements are usually done hourly until the patient is well advanced on the pacing protocol. Noninvasive monitoring, using oxygen saturation and end-tidal carbon dioxide monitors, are correlated periodically with arterial blood gases.

A decrease in the tidal volume or increase in end-tidal partial pressure of carbon dioxide, in the absence of specific correctable pulmonary problems, is considered to be evidence of diaphragm fatigue. The patient is rested temporarily on mechanical ventilation, and pacing is resumed with a shorter pacing period.

The fully conditioned diaphragm demonstrates histologic and biochemical changes that underlie its ability to perform sustained work. Normally, the diaphragm is composed of three types of muscle fibers. The majority of type I fibers (55%) are oxidative, slow-twitch fibers that easily resist fatigue. Type IIB fibers (24%) are glycolytic, fast-twitch fibers that are prone to fatigue. Type IIA (21%) fibers have intermediate characteristics: fast-twitch, fatigue-resistant, and oxidative. This ratio of different fiber types allows the normally functioning diaphragm considerable flexibility in meeting various metabolic demands. With prolonged periods of pulse train stimulation, this mixture of glycolytic and oxidate fibers is transformed into a state exclusively composed of slow-twitch, oxidative fibers, allowing for continuous sustained mechanical work.

Patients with central hypoventilation who require only part-time, nocturnal, pacing of 8 to 12 hours can implement their full pacing plan immediately; the period of time that the patient is not paced is adequate to prevent diaphragm fatigue. These patients usually undergo high-frequency pacing with 20 to 25 Hz, with corresponding pulse interval of 40 to 50 ms.

Tracheostomy

Once full-time ventilation is achieved, a Teflon tracheal button can be substituted in place of the conventional tracheostomy tube (Fig. 49-12). This tracheal device maintains the airway similarly to a tracheostomy; however, the button is more cosmetically appealing by virtue of being barely visible when in place. In addition, patients have more normal speech and reduced tracheal irritation and injury. The inner plug of the button is removed during sleep to ensure an unobstructed airway.

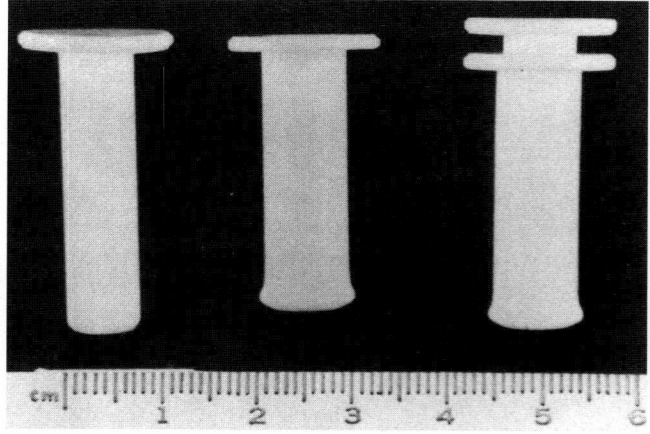

Fig. 49-12. The *tracheal button* used to replace the tracheostomy tube in conditioned, full-time pacing patients. The inner plug is shown on the left, the open tube in the middle, and the two assembled components on the right. The flange of the button sits flush with the skin when the button is in place in the stoma, maintaining patency indefinitely, while maintaining cosmesis. From Glenn WWL, et al: Long-term ventilatory support by diaphragm pacing in quadriplegia. Ann Surg *183*:566, 1976. With permission.

Ideally, even patients who have achieved full-time, continuous pacing should retain a permanent tracheostomy. It is known that pacing can produce extremely vigorous diaphragm contractions that, when combined with a lack of muscle coordination in the upper airway, can cause upper airway obstruction. All patients are instructed to leave the stoma open during sleep. In addition, a maintained tracheostomy provides secure airway access in the event malfunction of the pacemaker system occurs, necessitating immediate positive-pressure ventilation.

Complications

Unlike cardiac pacemakers, which require minimal associated care, diaphragm pacemakers mandate a thorough understanding of the device and its limitations and the principles of pacing technique to produce successful pacing. Potential complications of the pacemaker include receiver and electrode failure. Weese-Mayer and colleagues (1996) conducted a study of component failure in 33 patients who underwent phrenic pacing. The most common complication was receiver failure, occurring, on average, at 56.3 months. Failure may occur as the epoxy capsule of the receiver breaks down over time; an ingress of fluid results, causing an electrical short of the internal components of the receiver. In patients with cardiac pacemakers, one must also be cognizant of the potential complication of cross-talk between the two devices.

Other complications, not necessarily involving the pacing device itself, include acute and chronic phrenic nerve injury, diaphragm fatigue, and infection. Temporary and chronic stresses, especially as occur in quadriplegic patients, include bladder and pulmonary infections, pressure ulcers, and orthopedic deformities, especially scoliosis. These situations often increase the pacing requirements of the patient. Unfortunately, the pacing system does not automatically adjust to increased ventilatory demand; careful assessment of the patient's condition and readjustment of the pacemaker is required to avoid the disastrous situation in which a pacing patient is returned to and maintained unnecessarily on mechanical ventilation.

RESULTS

The review of Glenn and colleagues (1988) of the worldwide experience with 477 patients who had undergone diaphragmatic pacemaker insertion demonstrated the feasibility of diaphragm pacing. Of the 165 patients in this series with detailed follow-up, pacing was completely successful in meeting the ventilation needs in 47%, partially successful in 35%, and unsuccessful in 17%. Twenty-seven percent of patients in this series paced full time and 61% of patients paced part time. Although no recent study of similar magnitude with which to compare the current status of phrenic pacing has been done, several smaller studies have examined long-term outcome.

Long-term follow-up for quadriplegic patients who were conditioned at Yale, when last reported by the senior author and associates (1992), revealed that of 14 patients, 7 continued to pace full time. At present, six of the original patients continue to pace full time; all have done so for over 10 years. Two patients have died. Six patients who failed pacing, or pace only sporadically, do so for various reasons including insufficient nursing and supportive care, progressive disability from quadriplegia, insufficient funds to continue pacing, and patient noncompliance.

Similarly, Fodstad's series (1995) of 42 patients who underwent diaphragm pacemaker placement (33 bilateral and nine unilateral) over a 13-year period revealed that 19 patients continued to pace full time at a mean follow-up of 62 months. Seven patients died after pacing for periods that ranged from 4 months to 11 years. Five patients pace intermittently, and eight patients have stopped pacing for reasons including phrenic nerve root (C3–5) injury in six patients and voluntary cessation in two patients. Three patients died before pacing was achieved.

Weese-Mayer and associates (1996) reviewed the results of 64 patients, including 35 children, who underwent quadripolar electrode pacing. At a mean follow-up of 2 years for children, pacing was successful in 94%. Successful pacing without complications, however, was substantially lower in adults (60%). At a mean follow-up of 2.2 years for the adults, the success rate and complication-free success rates were 86% and 52%, respectively. Electrode dysfunction was the most common complication overall (19%); infection occurred in 2.9% and phrenic nerve damage developed in 3.8%.

Results of the Medimplant device were reviewed in children and adults. Mayr and associates (1993) reported on 15 patients with high cervical injury (C3 and above) who underwent pacemaker placement. Eleven patients achieved conditioned diaphragm pacing and paced for a mean of 43.3 months. Four patients died after pacing for 60, 58, 31, and 7 months. Causes of death were pulmonary embolism, pneumonia, and sepsis in three patients. The reason for one death was unclear. Girsch and colleagues (1996) reported eight children, whose ages ranged from 2 to 13 years, who underwent placement of the Vienna pacemaker. One child was diagnosed with central alveolar hypoventilation; the other seven children suffered high cervical or brain stem damage from tumor or trauma. Full-time pacing was achieved in four patients with a mean conditioning time of 13 months. These children have paced for 10, 28, 38, and 48 months. One child continues to undergo conditioning. Pacing was intermittent in two children. One child refused to pace secondary to social difficulties despite the physical ability to do so.

Hunt (1978) and Brouillette (1988) and their associates have clarified certain characteristics specific to pacing of infants and young children. Their experience in 32 patients with predominantly congenital central hypoventilation demonstrated that pacing can be effective; 25 of 32 patients survived and the vast majority were rehabilitated adequately to allow return home. Both Hunt (1978) and Brouillette (1988) and their colleagues have established that pacing of one diaphragm is poorly tolerated because of excess mediastinal motion; that shorter inspiration duration (0.9 seconds) is more efficient; and that full-time bilateral pacing of the infant or young child is not well tolerated. Motoyama (1977) attributes this intolerance of children to continuous pacing to the immaturity of the pediatric musculoskeletal system. By the age of 8 to 10 years, these issues have largely resolved and pacing tolerance and technique more closely approximate those for the adult.

At present, no prospective trial has been performed to compare diaphragm pacing with mechanical ventilation or other modes of ventilatory support, nor is one foreseen. The number of patients who require or qualify for pacing is limited and the population of patients is heterogeneous. Whether diaphragm pacing imparts improved survival in either patients with quadriplegia or central hypoventilation remains unclear. However, it has been the experience of the group at Yale that, at least in patients with central alveolar hypoventilation, progressive respiratory deterioration is common and death from hypoventilation is possible in the untreated individual. Moreover, the sequelae of prolonged hypoventilation and hypoxia include cor pulmonale from chronic hypoxic vasoconstriction and permanent cerebral dysfunction. In this regard, diaphragm pacing is thought to retard the decline in overall function that would otherwise result from untreated hypoxia.

Similarly, although no comparative trials have established the superiority of pacing over mechanical ventilation in patients with quadriplegia, some inferences may be drawn from accumulated clinical data. Carter and associates (1987a, 1987b) at the Texas Institute for Rehabilitation and Research compared their experience over 17 years in treating ventilator-dependent patients with spinal cord injury with mechanical ventilation (19 patients) versus diaphragm pacing (18 patients). The survival rates of diaphragm-paced patients and ventilated patients were 39% and 32%, respectively. Although pacing survival was slightly greater, no statistically significant difference was seen. However, as the specific mode of pacing was not mentioned and the study somewhat dated, it is proposed that a more favorable result in the paced population of patients might be seen if all had been paced with continuous, bilateral, low-frequency stimulation.

ADVANTAGES AND CAVEATS OF DIAPHRAGM PACING

Diaphragm pacing offers a number of advantages over positive-pressure ventilation. Most important to quadriplegic patients is the increased geographic independence afforded by paced ventilation. Patients who successfully complete a pacing program readily attest to the increased ease with which they are able to travel, whether for work, study, or pleasure. In this regard, the development of a totally implanted pacemaker for clinical use would represent an even greater advance; its arrival is eagerly anticipated.

In addition to increased freedom, paced patients have more natural phonation and speech. The advent of the tracheal button decreases their risk for tracheal complications associated with prolonged ventilation, such as tracheal stenosis, erosion, and tracheoesophageal fistula. Pacing patients are not exposed to the potential complications of mechanical ventilation such as accidental disconnection from the ventilator and tracheostomy occlusion from excessive airway secretions.

Patients who undergo diaphragm pacing also may find reduced health care costs as many are able to reside at home or outside of an institutionalized setting. After the initial cost of the pacing equipment and conditioning period, a maintained pacing system is relatively inexpensive.

Nonetheless, it must be emphasized that successful pacing requires critical patient selection including a thorough assessment of the patient's phrenic nerve and diaphragm function, underlying pulmonary function, and cognitive ability. The social environment in which the patient is expected to pace is equally important. Patients who fail to meet the prerequisites for pacing, or have questionable indications for pacing, often do not pace successfully, despite a considerable emotional, physical, and financial investment. Conversely, patients with the proper indications and adequate medical, psychological, and social support enjoy the benefits of successful pacing, which are readily apparent in terms of quality of life, medical condition, and financial savings.

REFERENCES

Baldissera F, et al: Diaphragm reinnervation by laryngeal motoneurons. J Appl Physiol 75:639, 1993.

Beard GM, Rockwell AD: Practical Treatise on the Medical and Surgical Uses of Electricity. 2nd Ed. London: Lewis, 1875, pp. 214–318.

Brouillette RT, et al: Stimulus parameters for phrenic nerve pacing in infants and children. Pediatr Pulmonol 4:33, 1988.

Burney RE, et al. Incidence, characteristics, and outcome of spinal cord injury at trauma centers in North America. Arch Surg 238:596, 1993.

Carter RE: Comparative study of electrophrenic nerve stimulation and mechanical ventilation in traumatic spinal cord injury. Paraplegia 25:86, 1987a.

Carter RE: Respiratory aspects of spinal cord injury management. Paraplegia 25:262, 1987b.

de La Motte Fouque FHK: Undine. A Miniature Romance. Translated by Rev Thomas Tracy. Standard Library. London: W. Smith, 1839, pp. 1–32.

DiMarco AF, Budzinska K, Supinski GS: Artificial ventilation by means of electrical activation of the intercostal accessory muscles alone in anesthetized dogs. Am Rev Respir Dis 139:961, 1989.

DiMarco AF, et al: Activation of the inspiratory intercostal muscles by electrical stimulation of the spinal cord. Am Rev Respir Dis 136:1385, 1987.

DiMarco AF, et al: Evaluation of intercostal pacing to provide artificial ventilation in quadriplegics. Am J Respir Crit Care Med 150:934, 1994.

Dimopoulou I, et al: Phrenic nerve dysfunction after cardiac operations: electrophysiologic evaluation of risk factors. Chest 113:8, 1998.

Duchenne GBA: De l'ectrisation localisée et de son application a la pathologie et a le therapeutique par courant induits et par courants galvaniques interrompus et continus par le Dr. Duchenne. Paris: Bailliere, 1872.

Elefteriades JA, et al: Long-term follow-up of bilateral pacing of the diaphragm in quadriplegia. N Engl J Med 326:1433, 1992.

Erdmann, BA. Die ortliche Anwendung der Elektricitat in der Physiologie, Pathologie und Therapie. 2nd Ed. Leipzig, Germany: Berlag von Joh. Ambr. Barth, 1858, p. 240.

Fodstad H: Phrenicodiaphragmatic pacing. In Roussos C (ed): The Thorax. 2nd Ed. Paris: Marcel Dekker, 1995, p. 2597.

Giraudoux JH: Ondine, Ides et Calendes. Paris: Neuchatel & Paris, 1946, pp. 162–267.

Girsch W, et al: Vienna phrenic pacemaker—experience with diaphragm pacing in children. Eur J Pediatr Surg 6:140, 1996.

Glenn WWL: The treatment of respiratory paralysis by diaphragm pacing. Ann Thorac Surg 30:106, 1980.

Glenn WWL: The diaphragm. In Glenn WWL (ed): Thoracic and Cardiovascular Surgery. 4th Ed. East Norwalk, CT: Appleton-Century-Crofts, 1983, p. 363.

Glenn WWL, Elefteriades JA. The diaphragm: dysfunction and induced pacing. In Baue AE, et al (eds): Glenn's Thoracic and Cardiovascular Surgery. 5th Ed. Norwalk, CT: Appleton-Century-Crofts, 1991.

Glenn WWL, Gee BL, Schachter EN: Diaphragm pacing: application to a patient with chronic obstructive pulmonary disease. J Thorac Cardiovasc Surg 75:273, 1978.

Glenn WWL, Sairenji H: Diaphragm pacing in the treatment of chronic ventilatory insufficiency. In Roussos C, Macklem PT (eds): The Thorax. New York: Marcel Dekker, 1985, p. 1407.

Glenn WWL, et al: Electrical stimulation of excitable tissue by radio-frequency transmission. Ann Surg 160:338, 1964.

Glenn WWL, et al: Total ventilatory support in a quadriplegic patient with radiofrequency electrophrenic respiration. N Engl J Med 286:513, 1972.

Glenn WWL, et al: Long-term ventilatory support by diaphragm pacing in quadriplegia. Ann Surg 183:566, 1976.

Glenn WWL, et al: Ventilatory support for pacing of the conditioned diaphragm in quadriplegia. N Engl J Med 310:1150, 1984.

Glenn WWL, et al: Twenty years of experience in phrenic nerve stimulation to pace the diaphragm. PACE 9:780, 1986.

Glenn WWL, et al: Fundamental considerations in pacing of the diaphragm for chronic ventilatory insufficiency: a multi-center study. PACE 11:2121, 1988.

Hogan JF, Holcomb WG, Glenn WWL: A programmable, totally implantable, battery-powered diaphragm pacemaker: design characteristics. In Saha S (ed): Proceedings of the Fourth New England Bioengineering Conference. Elmsford, NY: Pergamon, 1976, p. 221.

Hogan JF, Koda H, Glenn WWL: Electrical techniques for stimulation of the phrenic nerve to pace the diaphragm: inductive coupling and battery powered total implant in asynchronous and demand modes. PACE 12:847, 1989.

Hufeland CW: Usum uis electriciae in asphyxia experimentis illustratum. Göttingen, Germany: Dissertatio Inauguralis Medica, 1783.

Hunt CE, et al: Central hypoventilation syndrome: experience with bilateral phrenic nerve pacing in 3 neonates. Am Rev Respir Dis 118:23, 1978.

Isreal F: Uber die Wiederbelebung scheintoter Neugeborener mit Hilfe des elektrischen Stroms. Z Geburtshilfe Gynakol 91:602, 1927.

Judson JP, Glenn WWL: Radiofrequency electrophrenic respiration: Long-term application to a patient with primary hypoventilation JAMA 203:1033, 1968.

Kelly WD: Phrenic nerve paralysis: special consideration of the accessory nerve. J Thorac Surg 19:923, 1950.

Krieger AJ, Gropper MR, Adler RJ: Electrophrenic respiration after intercostal to phrenic nerve anastomosis in a patient with anterior spinal artery syndrome: a technical case report. Neurosurgery 35:760, 1994.

Lanmüller H, et al: Useful applications and limits of battery powered implants in functional electrical stimulations. Artif Organs 21:210, 1997.

Letsou GV, et al: Comparison of 180-degree and 360-degree skeletal muscle nerve cuff electrodes. Ann Thorac Surg 54:925, 1992.

Luc Diehl J, Lofaso F, Deleuze P: Clinically relevant diaphragmatic dysfunction after cardiac operations. J Thorac Cardiovasc Surg 107:487, 1994.

Mayr W, et al: Multichannel stimulation of phrenic nerves by epineural electrodes: clinical experience and future developments. ASAIO J 39:M729, 1993.

Merav AD, Attai LA, Condit DD: Successful repair of the transected phrenic nerve with restoration of diaphragmatic function. Chest 84:642, 1983.

Mills GH, et al: Unilateral magnetic stimulation of the phrenic nerve. Thorax 50:1162, 1995.

Motoyama EK: Pulmonary mechanics during early postnatal years. Pediatr Res 11:220, 1977.

Noguchi T: A survey of spinal cord injuries resulting from sport. Paraplegia 32:170, 1994.

Peterson DK, et al. Long-term intramuscular electrical activation of the phrenic nerve: safety and reliability. IEEE Trans Biomed Eng 41:1115, 1994a.

Peterson DK, et al. Long-term intramuscular electrical activation of the phrenic nerve: efficacy as a ventilatory prosthesis. IEEE Trans Biomed Eng 41:1127, 1994b.

Sarnoff SJ, et al: Electrophrenic respiration in acute bulbar poliomyelitis. AMA 143:1383, 1950.

Sarnoff SJ, et al: Electrophrenic respiration. VII. The motor point of the phrenic nerve in relation to external stimulation. Surg Gynecol Obstet 93:90, 1951.

Shaw RK, et al: Electrophysiological evaluation of phrenic nerve function in candidates for diaphragm pacing. J Neurosurg 53:345, 1980.

Shneerson J: Disorders of Ventilation. Oxford, England: Blackwell Scientific, 1988.

Similowski T, et al: Assessment of the motor pathway to the diaphragm using cortical and cervical magnetic stimulation in the decision-making process of phrenic pacing. Chest 110:1551, 1996.

Similowski T, et al: Comparison of magnetic and electrical phrenic nerve stimulation in assessment of phrenic nerve conduction time. J Appl Physiol 82:1190, 1997.

Spivak JM. et al: Cervical spine injuries in patients 65 and older. Spine 19:2303, 1994.

Supinski GS: Effect of synchronizing intercostal muscle and diaphragm contraction on inspired volume production [abstract]. Am Rev Respir Dis 143:A566, 1991.

Ure A: An account of some experiments made on the body of a criminal immediately after execution, with physiological and practical observations. J Sci Arts (Lond) 6:283, 1819.

Weese-Mayer DE, et al: Diaphragm pacing with a quadripolar phrenic nerve electrode: an international study. PACE Pacing Clin Electrophysiol 19:1311, 1996.

READING REFERENCES

Agostoni E, et al: Static feature of the passive rib cage and abdomen-diaphragm. J Appl Physiol 20:1187, 1965.

Alander DH, Andreychik DA, Stauffer ES: Early outcome in cervical spinal cord injured patients older than 50 years of age. Spine 19:2299, 1994.

Chervin, RD, Guilleminault C: Diaphragm pacing: review and reassessment. Sleep 17:176, 1994.

Elefteriades JA: Discussion of Miller JI, et al: Phrenic nerve pacing in quadriplegia. J Thorac Cardiovasc Surg 99:35, 1990

Lan C, et al: Traumatic spinal cord injuries in rural region of Taiwan: an epidemiological study in Hualien county 1986–90. Paraplegia 31:398, 1993.

MacLean IC, Mattioni TA: Phrenic nerve conduction studies: a new technique and its application in quadriplegic patients. Arch Phys Med Rehabil 62:70, 1981.

Markland ON, et al: Electrophysiologic evaluation of diaphragm by transcutaneous phrenic nerve stimulation. Neurology 34:604, 1984.

McCreery DB, Agnew WF: Mechanisms of stimulation-induced neural damage and their relation to guidelines for safe stimulation. In Agnew WF, McCreery DB (eds): Neural Prostheses: Fundamental Studies. Englewood Cliffs, NJ: Prentice-Hall, 1990.

McGory BJ, et al: Acute fractures and dislocations of the cervical spine in children and adolescents. J Bone Joint Surg Am 75:988, 1993.

Mellins RB, et al: Failure of automatic control of ventilation (Ondine's curse): report on an infant born with this syndrome and review of the literature. Medicine (Baltimore) 49:487, 1970.

Mills KR, et al: The optimal current direction for excitation of human cervical motor roots with a double coil magnetic stimulator. Electroencephalogr Clin Neurophysin 89:138, 1933.

Oda T, et al: Evaluation of electrical parameters for diaphragm pacing: an experimental study. J Surg Res 30:142, 1981.

Price C, et al. Epidemiology of traumatic spinal cord injury and acute hospitalization and rehabilitation charges for spinal cord injuries in Oklahoma, 1988–90. Am J Epidemiol 139:37, 1994.

Serif NS: Central alveolar hypoventilation syndrome. Trans Am Neurol Assoc 89:252, 1964.

Severinghaus JW, Mitchel RA: Ondine's curse. Failure of respiratory center automaticity while awake. Clin Res 10:122, 1962.

Shingu H, et al: Spinal cord injuries in Japan: a nationwide epidemiological survey in 1990. Paraplegia 32:3, 1994.

Whiteneck GG, et al: A collaborative study of high quadriplegia. Grant Report, US Department of Education, Rehabilitation Research and Demonstrations—Field Initiated Research. 1985.

CHAPTER 50

Congenital Posterolateral Diaphragmatic Hernias and Other Less Common Hernias of the Diaphragm in Infants and Children

Marleta Reynolds

CONGENITAL POSTEROLATERAL DIAPHRAGMATIC HERNIAS

The diagnosis of congenital diaphragmatic hernia can be made in utero with a great deal of accuracy. Early diagnosis allows time for parents to receive genetic and pediatric surgical consultation. Perinatal management can be altered to facilitate optimal care. The combination of early diagnosis and advances in prenatal and postnatal therapies have improved the outcome for babies born with congenital diaphragmatic hernia. A plethora of research related to congenital diaphragmatic hernia has provided insight into the pathophysiology of this complex anomaly. Infants and older children who are found to have a congenital diaphragmatic hernia are not as severely affected as the neonate and should have 100% predicted survival.

Embryology

The classic congenital diaphragmatic hernia of Bochdalek is a posterolateral defect in the diaphragm thought to be caused by failure of the pleuroperitoneal canal to close at 8 weeks' gestation (Fig. 50-1). Kluth and associates (1996), studying an animal model of congenital diaphragmatic hernia, believe the hernia results from defective formation of the posthepatic mesenchymal plate portion of the developing diaphragm. The defect occurs on the left side 80% of the time and is occasionally bilateral. The hole can range in size from a 1- to 2-cm round defect to total absence of the hemidiaphragm.

When the intestines return to the abdomen from the yolk sac at 10 weeks' gestation the intestines and other abdominal viscera may herniate into the chest. The mediastinum is pushed toward and into the contralateral hemithorax. Autopsy studies by the author and colleagues (1984) and Geggel and associates (1985) demonstrate pulmonary hypoplasia of both lungs. The ipsilateral lung's weight may be 20 to 50% below normal. Geggel and colleagues (1985) found the contralateral lung's volume to be 12 to 42% below normal. The pulmonary hypoplasia consists of a decrease in the number of bronchioles, arterioles, and in the number and size of the alveoli. Excessive muscularization of the pulmonary arterioles also occurs. Kluth and associates (1996) suggest that the pulmonary hypoplasia results from a reduction in spatial proportions of the ipsilateral lung. Miyazaki and colleagues (1998) have found strong insulin-like growth factor I in the hypoplastic lungs of affected babies and proposed that the lung hypoplasia results from a failure to progress in the developing lung.

Bollmann and associates (1995) reported that in 72% of fetuses diagnosed prenatally with congenital posterolateral diaphragmatic hernia, one or more extradiaphragmatic malformations were present. Eighteen percent of the fetuses studied in their group had chromosomal anomalies. Only 36.3% of the babies diagnosed postnatally had associated malformations. Congenital heart disease; neural tube defects; genitourinary, skeletal, and craniofacial anomalies; and abdominal wall defects can be found. Anomalies of intestinal rotation and fixation are always present.

Attempts to identify prognostic factors based on prenatal ultrasound findings have been problematic. Prenatal diagnosis alone was once considered a bad prognostic factor, but as the numbers of routine ultrasounds increased, the significance of this factor decreased. At present, observation of the liver in the chest is still considered a bad prognostic factor. Teixeira and colleagues (1997) have found that fetal abdominal circumference below the fifth percentile is a poor prognostic

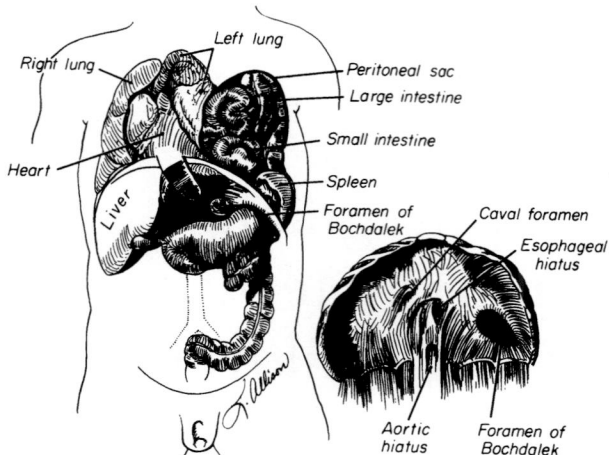

Fig. 50-1. Congenital diaphragmatic hernia of Bochdalek. From Shields TW: The diaphragm. *In* Nora P, ed: Operative Surgery: Principles and Techniques. Philadelphia: Lea & Febiger, 1972. With permission.

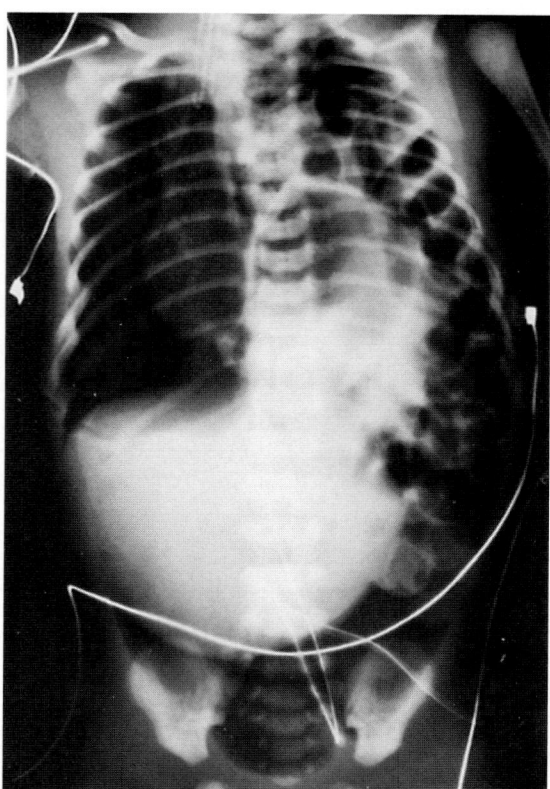

Fig. 50-2. This "babygram" demonstrates multiple loops of intestine on the left side of the chest and a few loops in the abdomen. The mediastinum is shifted to the contralateral side.

sign. Metkus and associates (1996) also found that the size of the contralateral lung measured as a ratio of lung area to head circumference was the only absolute predictor of survival.

Presentation

A congenital posterolateral diaphragmatic hernia may cause life-threatening respiratory distress in the first hours or days of life. The defect can cause respiratory distress or feeding intolerance in later infancy or childhood or may be identified on a radiograph obtained for unrelated reasons in an asymptomatic patient. The morbidity and mortality associated with a congenital diaphragmatic hernia is directly related to the age of the patient at presentation (Table 50-1).

Some babies with congenital posterolateral diaphragmatic hernia become symptomatic in the delivery room. The diagnosis is suspected if the abdomen is scaphoid and heart sounds are heard in the right chest. Radiography of the baby demonstrates gas-filled loops of intestines in the chest (Fig. 50-2). An oral-gastric tube placed into the stomach to decompress the intestines may appear in the chest, and a paucity of gas exists in the abdomen (Fig. 50-3).

Table 50-1. Infants with Congenital Posterolateral Diaphragmatic Hernia, 1962 through 1983

Onset and Severity of Symptoms	No.	Mortality (%)
<6 hours, critical	44	33–83
<6 hours, noncritical	53	6–11
6–24 hours	15	0
24 hours	32	0
Total	**144**	

Any baby with respiratory distress at birth who is suspected of having a posterolateral diaphragmatic hernia should be quickly intubated and ventilated. Mask bagging only increases the distention of the herniated stomach and intestines and further compromises ventilation.

Mechanical ventilation with 100% FIO_2 and low airway pressures (less than 25 cm H_2O with 5 cm of positive end-expiratory pressure) should be used. Vascular access using an umbilical artery catheter is adequate for arterial blood gas sampling and fluid and drug administration. The baby should be rapidly transported to a center with a surgeon, a neonatal intensive care unit equipped to care for such an infant, and extracorporeal membrane oxygenation (ECMO) capabilities. Profound respiratory acidosis is typically found with the first arterial blood gas. Ventilation is individualized to prevent or treat hypercarbia and hypoxemia. Prolonged hypoxemia, acidosis, and hypercarbia produce pulmonary vasoconstriction and persistent fetal circulation. Myocardial dysfunction may necessitate support with dobutamine and renal perfusion with low-dose dopamine. Because dopamine in higher doses may constrict the pulmonary vasculature, it is used only in low doses. Five percent albumin can be used to treat systemic hypotension in boluses of 10 to 15 mL.

A congenital posterolateral diaphragmatic hernia may be found incidentally in an older infant or child. Newman and colleagues (1986) found that the older infant or child with a

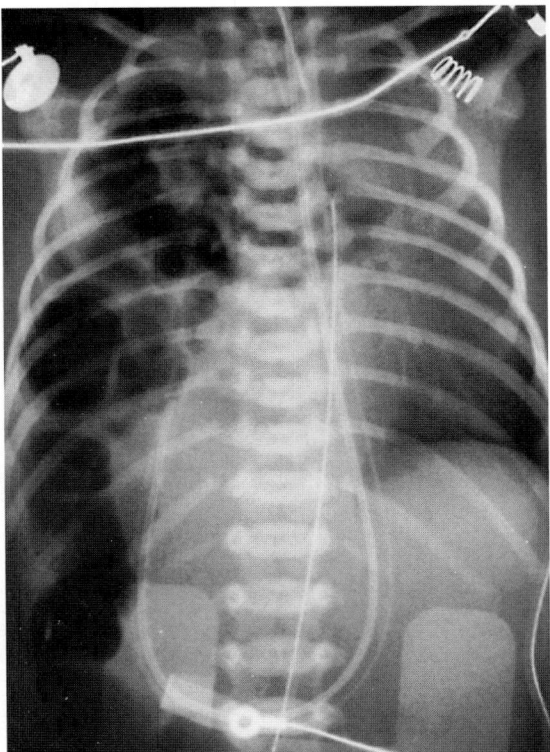

Fig. 50-3. Radiograph demonstrates a right-sided diaphragmatic hernia. The orogastric tube is seen in the right side of the chest, identifying the location of the stomach.

Table 50-2. Management Strategy in Newborns with Congenital Posterolateral Diaphragmatic Hernia

Nasal intubation
No muscle relaxants
No hyperventilation or alkalosis
Permissive hypercapnia, attempting to maintain $PaCO_2$ <60 mm Hg
Attempt to maintain preductal SaO_2 >90%
Provide adequate chest wall movement
Administer dobutamine, dopamine as needed
Use a time-cycled, pressure-limited, continuous-flow infant ventilator

Conventional mode →
30–40 breaths/min
20–30 cm H_2O peak inspiratory pressure
3–5 cm H_2O positive end-expiratory pressure
6–8 L/min gas flow

If during conventional mode:
   Preductal SaO_2 is <85%
   Preductal $PaCO_2$ is >65–70 mm Hg
   Spontaneous breathing is labored and ineffective
         Then switch to unconventional mode
               ↓
     100 breaths/min
     20–22 cm H_2O peak inspiratory pressure
     0 cm H_2O positive end-expiratory pressure
     12–15 L/min gas flow

Modified from Hirschl RB: Innovative therapies in the management of newborns with congenital diaphragmatic hernia. Semin Pediatr Surg 5:256, 1996.

posterolateral diaphragmatic hernia also may present with respiratory or gastrointestinal symptoms. Diagnosis is made with chest radiography or barium studies of the gastrointestinal tract. The hernia should be repaired at the time of diagnosis. The lungs of these children are not hypoplastic, and the operative mortality should be 0%.

Management

Once the newborn with a congenital posterolateral diaphragmatic hernia is transferred to a center with ECMO capabilities, an effort is made to stabilize the baby for at least 72 hours before considering operative repair. In the past, hyperventilation and alkalosis were used to control pulmonary hypertension and persistent fetal circulation. Wung and associates (1995) proposed permissive hypercapnia with spontaneous ventilation in an effort to minimize ventilator-induced lung injury. Although slow to gain acceptance, their strategy is being applied by many centers (Table 50-2).

Inhaled nitric oxide is a selective pulmonary vasodilator that has been successfully used to treat pulmonary hypertension in newborns. Once believed to be the answer for babies with congenital posterolateral diaphragmatic hernia, results of its use were disappointing. It is certainly worth trying as an adjunctive therapy before, during, or after ECMO.

The newest therapy under study is partial liquid ventilation. Hirschl (1996) describes the technique of instilling perfluorocarbon into the trachea and lungs. Standard mechanical ventilation is performed through the liquid. Because perfluorocarbon can carry more oxygen and carbon dioxide, it can enhance gas exchange.

If these strategies are not successful in reversing persistent fetal circulation, ECMO is considered for newborns who meet institutional criteria (Fig. 50-4).

Operative Correction

In the past, repair of a congenital posterolateral diaphragmatic hernia was considered a surgical emergency. Babies were operated on in the delivery room or were taken directly

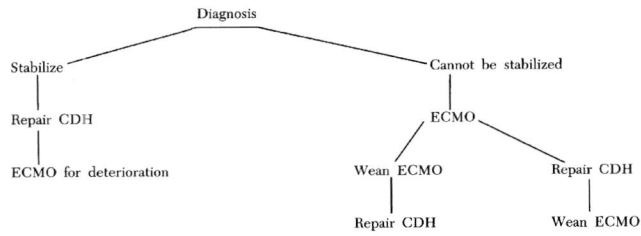

Fig. 50-4. Algorithm for a symptomatic baby with congenital diaphragmatic hernia.

from the transport ambulance to the operating suite. Retrospective analysis of this treatment plan has shown little advantage or improvement in survival. In fact, Sakai and associates (1987) have demonstrated that early surgery causes deterioration in pulmonary mechanics. Nakayama and associates (1991) have shown that preoperative stabilization results in an improvement in pulmonary compliance in a group of babies with delayed repair of the hernia. Glick (1992) and Suen (1993) and their associates have demonstrated that the lungs of fetuses with congenital Bochdalek's diaphragmatic hernias are biochemically premature, and some babies have been shown to benefit from surfactant replacement therapy during this stabilization period, as reported by Bos and colleagues (1990, 1991). In light of these studies, most centers attempt to stabilize these babies before repair of the diaphragmatic hernia.

Once stable, the neonatal ventilator is moved from the neonatal intensive care unit to the operating room for use during the operation, or the surgery is performed in the intensive care unit. Any sudden deterioration of vital signs during transport, in the operating room, or during the postoperative period usually indicates a pneumothorax on the contralateral side. Gibson and Fonkalsrud (1983) and Srouji and associates (1981) reported that a contralateral pneumothorax or a pneumomediastinum is associated with an increase in mortality and should be prevented with the use of low airway pressures. A tube thoracostomy with a No. 10F chest tube should be rapidly placed if a pneumothorax is suspected.

The correction of a congenital posterolateral diaphragmatic hernia is performed through a paramedian incision. The abdominal viscera are returned to the abdomen from the chest, and the hernia sac, if present, is excised. Extralobar pulmonary sequestrations, often an associated malformation in infants with congenital diaphragmatic hernia, are resected at the time of hernia repair. A small diaphragmatic defect is closed with permanent suture and Teflon pledgets. Larger defects can be closed with polytetrafluoroethylene membrane. When the hemidiaphragm is completely absent, a polytetrafluoroethylene membrane can be sutured to the ribs, both anteriorly and posterolaterally. The medial portion of the membrane can be sutured to the contralateral diaphragmatic leaf and the adventitia overlying the aorta and esophagus. A chest tube is placed in the ipsilateral thorax and attached to a three-way stopcock and closed. Topical thrombin and cryoprecipitate are applied to the surgical field to prevent postoperative bleeding if ECMO becomes necessary (Fig. 50-5).

Controversy continues regarding the best method of thoracic drainage. Suggestions have included no chest tube, bilateral prophylactic chest tubes, underwater seal, and tubes exposed to atmospheric pressure. Tyson and associates (1985) recommended "balanced thoracic drainage" to maintain normal intrathoracic pressure. The ipsilateral chest tube attached to a three-way stopcock allows removal of air or fluid, depending on the clinical picture and the finding on radiography of the chest. The author prefers this latter method.

Associated intra-abdominal anomalies should be corrected at the time of hernia repair if the baby's condition is stable. If fascial closure causes compromise of respiratory

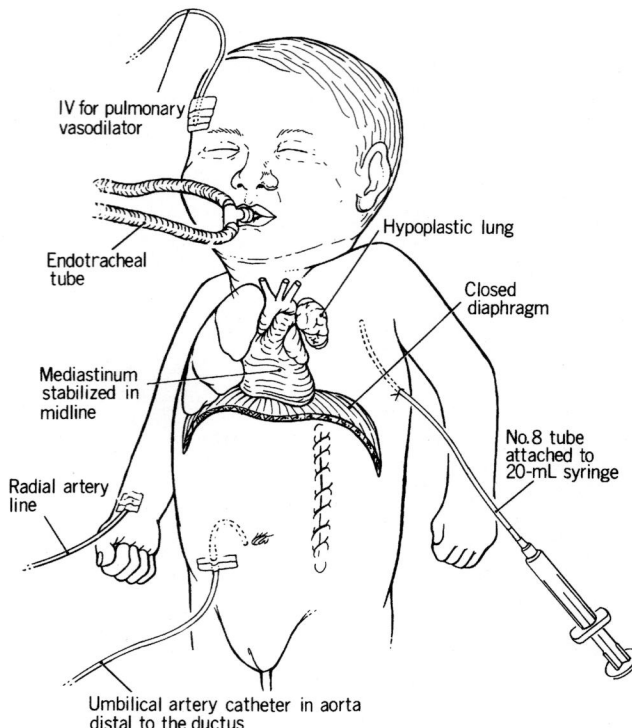

Fig. 50-5. Total postoperative management of a poor-risk infant. The mediastinum is stabilized with the pleural catheter, blood gases are monitored above and below the ductus arteriosus, and the intravenous lines are used for the administration of vasodilator drugs. From Ramenofsky MD, Luck SR: Diaphragmatic anomalies. *In* Raffensperger JC, ed: Swenson's Pediatric Surgery. 4th Ed. East Norwalk, CT: Appleton-Century-Crofts, 1980, p. 675. With permission.

excursion, a ventral hernia can be created by closing the skin only. Occasionally, even the skin cannot be closed, and a *silo* of Silastic sheeting can be used to temporarily contain the abdominal viscera.

Extracorporeal Membrane Oxygenation

ECMO has been successfully used in more than 100 centers in the United States to treat reversible respiratory failure in newborn infants. Hardesty (1981), Bartlett (1986), Weber (1987), Redmond (1987), and Langham (1987) and their colleagues reported survival rates among infants with congenital diaphragmatic hernia treated with ECMO ranging from 38 to 77%. This wide range in survival rates probably reflects differences in selection criteria and the experience of the particular center. Standard criteria have not been established, but in general include alveolar-arterial oxygen gradient ($A aDO_2$) less than 600 for 12 hours; oxygen index greater than 40; acute deterioration (pH less than 7.15 or Pao_2 less than 55 mm Hg) for 2 consecutive hours; failure of conventional management; and progressive barotrauma.

Contraindications to the use of ECMO, as described by Bartlett and associates (1986), include preexisting intraventricular hemorrhage, weight less than 2000 g, and congenital or neurologic abnormalities incompatible with normal life.

Reickert and associates (1998) reported the outcome of babies with congenital Bochdalek's diaphragmatic hernia treated at 16 different institutions that used multimodal therapies. Overall survival in 411 patients was 69%. Survival for babies placed on ECMO was 55% and 81% for those who did not need ECMO. Currently, ECMO is reserved for those babies who cannot be stabilized or deteriorate after hernia repair. If ECMO is needed before hernia repair, the hernia can be repaired after ECMO is no longer needed or in a final effort to wean a baby from ECMO.

Factors in Survival

Several methods have been used to predict survival in infants with congenital posterolateral diaphragmatic hernia. Boix-Ochoa and colleagues (1977) reported that an arterial blood pH less than 7.0 with a Pco_2 greater than 100 is an early predictor for a poor outcome. Touloukian and Markowitz (1984) devised a scoring system based on preoperative radiographic findings. The radiographic findings include the side of the diaphragmatic hernia, location of the stomach, presence of pneumothorax, and relative volume of aerated ipsilateral and contralateral lung. A total score can be derived for each patient and identifies the high-risk patient.

$Aado_2$ is used more frequently to predict survival. Harrington (1982) and Manthei (1983) and their associates reported that preoperative and postoperative $Aado_2$ greater than 500 mm Hg correlated with little chance of survival. Manthei and colleagues (1983) also noted that initial postoperative improvement, as evidenced by a transient decrease in $Aado_2$, was followed by a sudden increase in $Aado_2$. Expecting this deterioration allows prompt institution of aggressive measures to prevent and treat the decline in oxygenation.

Bohn and associates (1987) used ventilatory parameters to predict survival by plotting Pco_2 versus ventilation index (ventilation index = ventilation rate multiplied by mean airway pressure) in the pre-ECMO era. Wilson and associates (1991) have shown that the best postductal Pco_2 and the oxygenative-ventilation index (Pco_2/mean airway pressure multiplied by respiratory rate multiplied by 100) were predictors of mortality. Infants who did not respond to conventional mechanical ventilation (best postductal Po_2 less than 100; best postductal Pco_2 greater than 40, with ventilation index greater than 1000) did not benefit from ECMO.

Future Prospects

Because the degree of pulmonary hypoplasia determines survival in infants with congenital posterolateral diaphragmatic hernia, investigations of in utero correction began. Harrison (1980a) and Adzick (1985) and their associates developed a model for congenital posterolateral diaphragmatic hernia in the fetal lamb and observed that changes identical to those found in humans occurred in the fetal lamb. Harrison and colleagues (1980b) reported that the in utero correction of the defect in fetal lambs allowed sufficient lung growth for survival. The optimal time predicted for in utero intervention in humans is between 22 and 28 weeks' gestation. As Harrison and coworkers (1985) pointed out, ultrasound diagnosis of other anomalies and chromosomal analysis are prerequisites for maternal intervention. Although technically feasible, the results of clinical trials, such as those by Harrison and colleagues (1993), did not show improved outcome and in utero repair was abandoned.

Lipsett and associates (1998) have shown that antenatal tracheal occlusion can reverse the lung hypoplasia in a lamb model of congenital diaphragmatic hernia using morphometric analysis. Attempts to apply the technique to the human fetus have been difficult and since 1995 several investigators have been studying the feasibility of tracheal occlusion as a means of reversing pulmonary hypoplasia in a congenital diaphragmatic hernia experimental model. Problems with open hysterotomy have led to attempts to apply endoscopic techniques to accomplish the same goal. Vander Wall and associates (1996) described the use of a fetal endoscopic tracheal clip, and Benachi and associates (1997) used endoscopic placement of a tracheal balloon. Benachi and colleagues (1998) reported that although tracheal occlusion of the fetus with congenital Bochdalek's diaphragmatic hernia was feasible and could reverse hypoplasia, a significant reduction in the number of type II pneumocytes and surfactant production in experimental animals was seen. Harrison and colleagues (1998) reported a series of fetuses treated with open and endoscopic tracheal clip application. Survival was better for those treated with the endoscopic technique (75% vs. 15%). Whether in utero treatment with tracheal occlusion will prove to be beneficial in a large series of fetuses with congenital diaphragmatic hernia remains to be seen.

Long-Term Follow-Up

Several short- and long-term studies, such as that by Ijsselstijn and associates (1997), have identified the long-term morbidity associated with the diagnosis of congenital Bochdalek's diaphragmatic hernia. Jeandot and colleagues (1989) evaluated survivors after 1 to 2 years and found a persistent reduction in perfusion but improved ventilation of the ipsilateral lung based on lung ventilation and perfusion scintigraphy. Chest radiography confirmed continuing changes (Fig. 50-6). Vanamo (1996) and Zaccara (1996) and their associates studied older survivors and found no clinical impairment but identified some reduced exercise tolerance and minor ventilatory impairment. Other sequelae documented by Nobuhara and colleagues (1996) included anterior chest wall deformities in 21%, scoliosis in 10.5%, and gastroesophageal reflux in more than 50%. Naik and associates (1996) found that morbidity could be correlated with

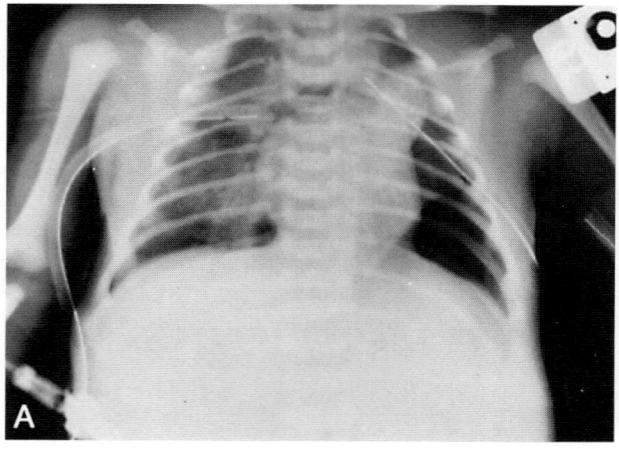

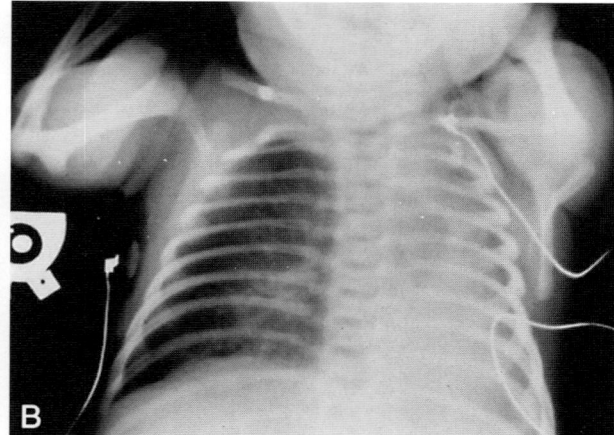

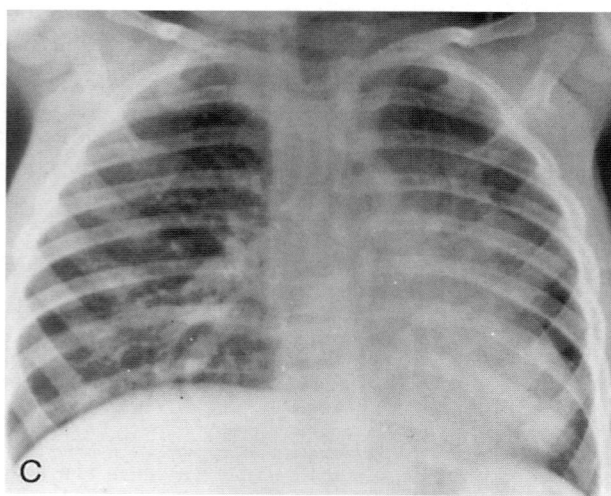

Fig. 50-6. A. Early postoperative radiograph shows a small left lung. B. One month later, hyperinflation of the contralateral lung is seen, and the mediastinum has shifted into the ipsilateral chest. C. Even 2 years after repair of the diaphragmatic hernia, the contralateral lung and mediastinum are still in the ipsilateral chest. The child was asymptomatic at the time.

the length of time the infant required ventilatory support or supplemental oxygen. Of those babies requiring ECMO, Stolar and associates (1995) found cognitive outcome to be worse when compared with babies treated with ECMO for other reasons. Sensorineural hearing loss was reported by Nobuhara and colleagues (1996) to develop in 18% of their survivors. The author has found a similar incidence in her institution. Recurrent posterolateral diaphragmatic hernia can develop, especially in those babies that require patch repair. Small bowel obstruction can also plague these children at any time.

MISCELLANEOUS CONGENITAL DIAPHRAGMATIC HERNIAS

Hernias through the Central Tendon of the Diaphragm

Hernias may occur through the central portion of the diaphragm. Partial or localized eventration of the diaphragm with marked thinning of the tissues to form a ring and a hernial sac may occur also. When such a hernia occurs on the

right side, a mushroomlike projection of liver that has grown through the opening in the right diaphragmatic leaf may be found. On radiography of the chest, this projection is occasionally misinterpreted as a diaphragmatic tumor. Differentiation may be made by instituting a pneumoperitoneum, after which, air appears to surround the liver protrusion. Repair of this type of hernia is unnecessary if clear identification can be made by the pneumoperitoneum. If not, exploration is required to rule out the possibility of a primary tumor of the diaphragm.

If the hernia is on the left side, the stomach is occasionally herniated through the central portion of the diaphragm; it usually is identified as an air-containing cyst on the top of the diaphragm. The hernia may be associated with a partial absence of the pericardium, and the stomach and small intestine may herniate into the pericardial sac and cause cardiac symptoms. In general, when such a defect occurs through the central portion of the left hemidiaphragm or into the pericardial sac, the hernia should be repaired as soon as it is discovered. In infants and children, the repair usually is accomplished through an abdominal approach, similar to that described for the repair of the foramen of Bochdalek hernia. In contrast, in the older child and adult, repair is accomplished through a thoracic approach.

Paraesophageal Hernia in Infants and Children

A paraesophageal hernia diagnosed in infancy or childhood may be congenital or acquired. The acquired variety usually occurs as a complication of the surgical treatment of gastroesophageal reflux. A congenital paraesophageal hernia first may be suggested by the findings on chest radiography (Fig. 50-7A). An upper gastrointestinal series demonstrates the herniated stomach and other abdominal contents in the chest (Fig. 50-7B). In some children, anemia may develop from gastritis, or esophagitis and vomiting from obstruction or incarceration. The symptoms depend on the size of the defect, the position of the stomach, the amount of obstruction at the gastroesophageal junction or pylorus, and the presence of other viscera within the hernia sac.

Surgery is indicated in all cases and should include reduction of the intestinal contents, excision of the sac, reapproximation of the diaphragmatic crura, and, in some cases, as suggested by Jawad and associates (1998), an antireflux procedure or gastropexy should be carried out (see Chapter 136).

Foramen of Morgagni Hernia

Anatomy

On each side of the sternum is a potential space, known as the *foramen of Morgagni*, or the *space of Larrey*, through which passes the internal mammary artery to become the superior epigastric artery. This triangular space is between the muscular fibers originating from the xiphisternum and the costal margin that insert on the central tendon of the diaphragm. The left space is less likely to develop a hernia because it is protected by the pericardial sac. The ligamentum teres defines the medial border of the hernia through either space.

Most often in infants and children, a foramen of Morgagni hernia contains only a piece of omentum that is caught up in the defect that may enlarge over a period of time. Rarely, a portion of one of the abdominal viscera, often the stomach, is contained in the hernia (Fig. 50-8). A portion of the liver, as reported by Newman and Davis (1989) may be present in the hernia sac.

Incidence

Hernias through the foramen of Morgagni are uncommon at any age but are even rarer in the child than in the adult. Berman and associates (1989) reported only 15 infants and children with Morgagni hernias collected over a 20-year period at the Hospital for Sick Children in Toronto. Pokorny and associates (1984) reported only five hernias of this type in infants in a 6-year period at the Texas Children's Hospital.

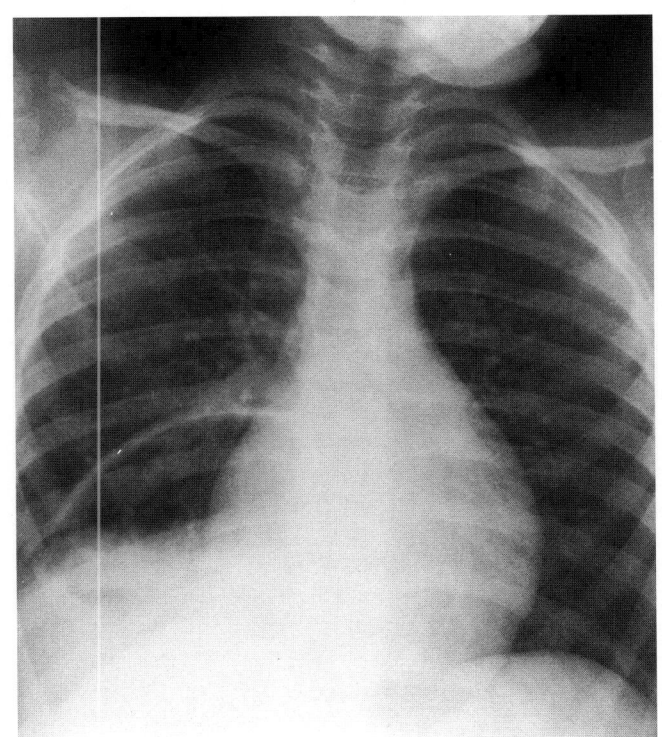

A

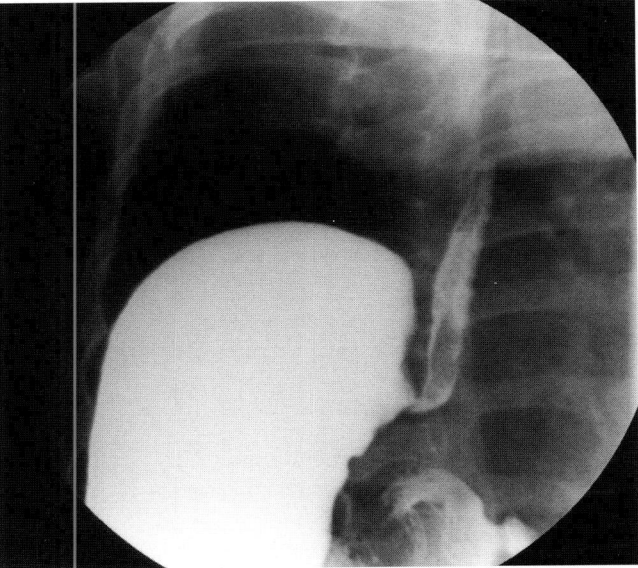

B

Fig. 50-7. A. Chest radiograph illustrating the presence of a large cystic air space located behind the right side of the cardiac shadow. B. The barium swallow revealed the stomach to be present in a large paraesophageal hiatus hernia.

The unusual occurrence of foramen of Morgagni hernias in identical twins was recorded by Harris and associates (1993).

Symptoms

A small foramen of Morgagni hernia usually is unrecognized and asymptomatic in infants and young children.

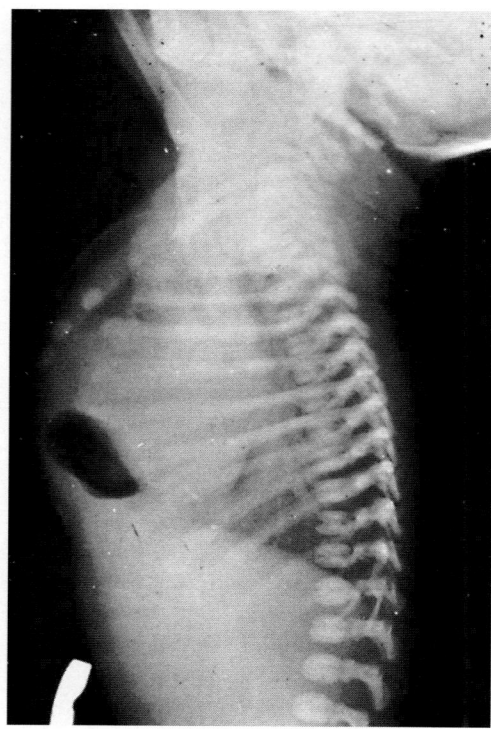

Fig. 50-8. Lateral chest radiograph of the chest in an infant with a congenital foramen of Morgagni hernia that was found to contain most of the stomach at the time of repair.

Larger ones, often because of the presence of an abdominal viscus in the hernia, may produce respiratory symptoms. Neonates with large hernias can present with severe respiratory distress similar to the dramatic clinical picture associated with the more common posterolateral Bochdalek's hernia. In addition, neonates and infants with foramen of Morgagni hernia may have associated congenital anomalies, such as Down, Turner's, or Noonan's syndrome, pentalogy of Cantrell, pectus deformities, bowel malrotation, and genitourinary malformations.

A foramen of Morgagni hernia, however, is more often symptomatic in older children and adolescents. Exercise and other athletic activity, as noted by Valases and Sills (1988), may precipitate the occurrence of symptoms. The older child or adolescent with a foramen of Morgagni hernia may complain of dull pain in the right subcostal area. Rarely, intermittent, partial intestinal obstruction may occur, including gastric volvulus, but complete obstruction is uncommon. Dyspnea is observed only occasionally in patients past early childhood.

Diagnosis

Radiographic studies of the chest reveal a density, either solid or containing air, adjacent to the right or left side of the heart. A computed tomographic examination of an anterior cardiophrenic mass may reveal the presence of bowel, thus

confirming the diagnosis. Sonographic and magnetic resonance imaging may at times be valuable, as noted in the report of Newman and Davis (1989). Contrast studies of the large intestine and often of the upper gastrointestinal tract may be indicated in the evaluation of some patients.

Surgical Repair

Surgical repair is recommended for all hernias because of the lifetime risk of intestinal obstruction. In infants and young children an open repair is indicated. The abdominal approach for surgical repair of this hernia is chosen if the diagnosis is known preoperatively. A subcostal incision or a right epigastric paramedian incision may be used. With the latter incision, the rectus muscle is retracted laterally to expose the posterior rectus and transversalis fascia. After the abdomen has been opened, the contents of the hernia are reduced into the peritoneal cavity and the margins of the hernial sac are identified. As noted, the ligamentum teres defines the medial border of the hernia. The hernia sac is removed when possible. The repair of the muscular defect is made with interrupted mattress sutures, and usually it is necessary to pull the diaphragm up to the posterior part of the sternum and to the posterior rectus sheath. After repair, the abdomen is closed. In most patients, it is not necessary to enter into the chest or to drain the pleural space. In the older child or adolescent, one could consider laparoscopic repair, as has been carried out by Hussong (1997) and Orita (1997) and their colleagues in older adults.

Rarely, in children, a foramen of Morgagni hernia is encountered while the anterior mediastinum is being explored for an undiagnosed mediastinal mass in either of the anterior cardiophrenic angles. As soon as the mass has been identified as a foramen of Morgagni hernia, the sac is opened and explored, and the contents are reduced into the peritoneal cavity. The repair is then accomplished in a manner similar to that just described. In this instance, it is also best to suture the diaphragm to the posterior part of the sternum and the rectus sheath. On occasion, because of the size of the defect and a deficiency of available tissue, it is necessary to sew in a small piece of plastic mesh or a soft tissue Gore-Tex patch. A recurrence of a foramen of Morgagni hernia is rare.

Peritoneal Pericardial Hernia

A rare diaphragmatic defect between the peritoneal cavity and pericardial sac also has been reported. Ake and colleagues (1991) reported the prenatal diagnosis of a fetus with such a hernia. The infant was asymptomatic at birth, and the hernia was repaired through the abdomen on the fifth day of life. Milne and associates (1990) reported two patients with an identical defect associated with a giant omphalocele. The author has treated an infant with this defect who presented at birth with severe respiratory distress, hypotension, and persistent fetal circulation (Fig. 50-9). Urgent repair was done; at operation the stomach was found inside the pericardium.

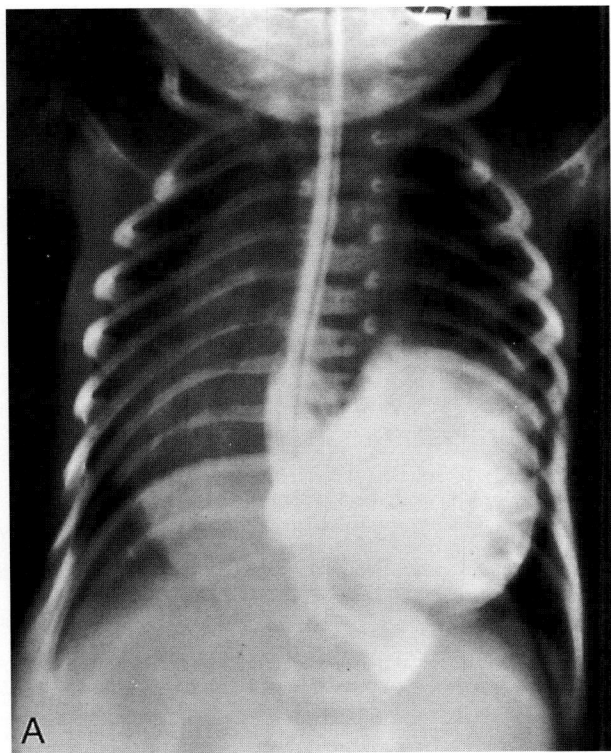

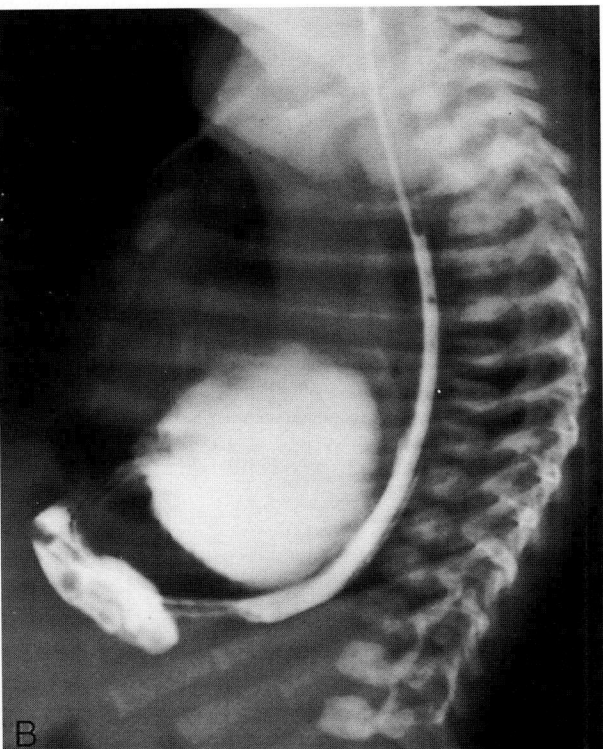

Fig. 50-9. Anteroposterior **(A)** and lateral radiographic **(B)** views of a barium swallow in an infant with a peritoneal pericardial hernia.

Reduction of the stomach immediately improved cardiac function. The defect was closed with interrupted Ticron pledget sutures. The patient had no further difficulty postoperatively. Milne and associates (1990) suggested that this defect is secondary to failure of fusion of the pars sternalis portion of the septum transversum in the development of the diaphragm. Repair may be performed through the abdomen or chest. The abdominal approach is preferred.

REFERENCES

Adzick NS, et al: Correction of congenital diaphragmatic hernia in utero. IV. An early gestation fetal lamb model for pulmonary vascular morphometric analysis. J Pediatr Surg 20:673, 1985.

Ake E, et al: Short communication: in utero sonographic diagnosis of diaphragmatic hernia with hepatic protrusion into the pericardium mimicking an intrapericardial tumour. Prenat Diagn 11:719, 1991.

Bartlett RH, et al: Extracorporeal membrane oxygenation (ECMO) in neonatal respiratory failure. 100 cases. Ann Surg 204:236, 1986.

Benachi A, et al: Tracheal obstruction in experimental diaphragmatic hernia: an endoscopic approach in the fetal lamb. Prenat Diagn 17:629, 1997.

Benachi A, et al: Lung growth and maturation after tracheal occlusion in diaphragmatic hernia. Am J Respir Crit Care Med 157:921, 1998.

Berman L, et al: The late-presenting pediatric Morgagni hernia: a benign condition. J Pediatr Surg 24:970, 1989.

Boix-Ochoa J, et al: The important influence of arterial blood gases on the prognosis of congenital diaphragmatic hernia. World J Surg 1:783, 1977.

Bohn DJ, et al: Ventilatory predictors of pulmonary hypoplasia in congenital diaphragmatic hernia confirmed by morphologic assessment. J Pediatr 111:423, 1987.

Bollmann R, et al: Associated malformations and chromosomal defects in congenital diaphragmatic hernia. Fetal Diagn Ther 10:52, 1995.

Bos AP, et al: Congenital diaphragmatic hernia: impact of prostanoids in the perioperative period. Arch Dis Child 65:994, 1990.

Bos AP, et al: Surfactant replacement therapy in high-risk congenital diaphragmatic hernia. Lancet 338:1279, 1991.

Geggel RL et al: Congenital diaphragmatic hernia: arterial structural changes and persistent pulmonary hypertension after surgical repair. J Pediatr 107:457, 1985.

Gibson C, Fonkalsrud EW: Iatrogenic pneumothorax and mortality in congenital diaphragmatic hernia. J Pediatr Surg 18:555, 1983.

Glick PL, et al: Pathophysiology of congenital diaphragmatic hernia. II: The fetal lamb CDH model is surfactant deficient. J Pediatr Surg 27:382, 1992.

Hardesty RL, et al: Extracorporeal membrane oxygenation. Successful treatment of persistent fetal circulation following repair of congenital diaphragmatic hernia. J Thorac Cardiovasc Surg 81:556, 1981.

Harrington J, Raphaely RC, Downes JJ: Relationship of alveolar-arterial oxygen tension difference in diaphragmatic hernia of the newborn. Anesthesiology 56:473, 1982.

Harris GJ, Soper RT, Kimura KK: Foramen of Morgagni hernia in identical twins: is this an inheritable defect? J Pediatr Surg 28:177, 1993.

Harrison MR, Jester JA, Ross NA: Correction of congenital diaphragmatic hernia in utero. I. The model: intrathoracic balloon produces fatal pulmonary hypoplasia. Surgery 88:174, 1980a.

Harrison MR, et al: Correction of congenital diaphragmatic hernia in utero. II. Simulated correction permits fetal lung growth with survival at birth. Surgery 88:260, 1980b.

Harrison MR, et al: Fetal diaphragmatic hernia: fetal but fixable. Semin Perinatol 9:103, 1985.

Harrison MR, et al: Correction of congenital diaphragmatic hernia in utero: VI. Hard-earned lessons. J Pediatr Surg 28:1411, 1993.

Harrison MR, et al: Correction of congenital diaphragmatic hernia in utero: IX: fetuses with poor prognosis (liver herniation and low lung-to-head ratio) can be saved by fetoscopic temporary tracheal occlusion. J Pediatr Surg 33:1017, 1998.

Hirschl RB: Innovative therapies in the management of newborns with congenital diaphragmatic hernia. Semin Pediatr Surg 5:256, 1996.

Hussong RL Jr, Landreneau RJ, Cole FH Jr: Diagnosis and repair of a Morgagni hernia with video-assisted thoracic surgery. Ann Thorac Surg 63:1474, 1997.

Ijsselstijn H, et al: Long-term pulmonary sequelae in children with congenital diaphragmatic hernia. Am J Respir Crit Care Med 155:174, 1997.

Jawad AJ, et al: Congenital para-oesophageal hiatal hernia in infancy. Pediatr Surg Int 13:91, 1998.

Jeandot R, et al: Lung ventilation and perfusion scintigraphy in the follow-up of repaired congenital diaphragmatic hernia. Eur J Nucl Med 15:591, 1989.

Kluth D, et al: Embryology of congenital diaphragmatic hernia. Semin Pediatr Surg 5:224, 1996.

Langham MR Jr, et al: Extracorporeal membrane oxygenation following repair of congenital diaphragmatic hernias. Ann Thorac Surg 44:247, 1987.

Lipsett J, et al: Effect of antenatal tracheal occlusion on lung development in the sheep model of congenital diaphragmatic hernia: a morphometric analysis of pulmonary structure and maturity. Pediatr Pulmonol 25:257, 1998.

Manthei U, Vaucher Y, Crowe CP Jr: Congenital diaphragmatic hernia: immediate preoperative and postoperative oxygen gradients identify patients requiring prolonged respiratory support. Surgery 93:83, 1983.

Metkus AP, et al: Sonographic predictors of survival in fetal diaphragmatic hernia. J Pediatr Surg 31:148, 1996.

Milne LW, et al: Pars sternalis diaphragmatic hernia with omphalocele: a report of two cases. J Pediatr Surg 25:726, 1990.

Miyazaki E, et al: Altered insulin-like growth factor I mRNA expression in human hypoplastic lung in congenital diaphragmatic hernia. J Pediatr Surg 33:1476, 1998.

Naik S, et al: Prediction of morbidity during infancy after repair of congenital diaphragmatic hernia. J Pediatr Surg 31:1651, 1996.

Nakayama DK, Motoyama EK, Tagge EM: Effect of preoperative stabilization on respiratory system compliance and outcome in newborn infants with congenital diaphragmatic hernia. J Pediatr 118:793, 1991.

Newman B, Davis PL: Sonographic and magnetic resonance imaging of an anterior diaphragmatic hernia. Pediatr Radiol 20:110, 1989.

Newman BM, et al: Presentation of congenital diaphragmatic hernia past the neonatal period. Arch Surg 121:813, 1986.

Nobuhara KK, et al: Long-term outlook for survivors of congenital diaphragmatic hernia. Clin Perinatol 23:873, 1996.

Orita M, et al: Laparoscopic repair of a diaphragmatic hernia through the foramen of Morgagni. Surg Endosc 11:668, 1997.

Pokorny WJ, McGill CW, Harberg FJ: Morgagni hernias during infancy. Presentation and associated anomalies. J Pediatr Surg 19:394, 1984.

Redmond CR, et al: Extracorporeal membrane oxygenation for respiratory and cardiac failure in infants and children. J Thorac Cardiovasc Surg 93:199, 1987.

Reickert CA, et al: Congenital diaphragmatic hernia survival and use of extracorporeal life support at selected level III nurseries with multimodality support. Surgery 123:305, 1998.

Reynolds M, Luck SR, Lappen R: The "critical" neonate with diaphragmatic hernia: a 21-year perspective. J Pediatr Surg 19:364, 1984.

Sakai H, et al: Effect of surgical repair on respiratory mechanics in congenital diaphragmatic hernia. J Pediatr 111:432, 1987.

Srouji MN, Buck B, Downes JJ: Congenital diaphragmatic hernia: deleterious effects of pulmonary interstitial emphysema and tension extrapulmonary air. J Pediatr Surg 16:45, 1981.

Stolar CJJ, Crisafi MA, Driscoll YT: Neurocognitive outcome for neonates treated with extracorporeal membrane oxygenation: are infants with congenital diaphragmatic hernia different? J Pediatr Surg 30:366, 1995.

Suen HC, et al: Biochemical immaturity of lungs in congenital diaphragmatic hernia. J Pediatr Surg 28:471, 1993.

Teixeira J et al: Abdominal circumference in fetuses with congenital diaphragmatic hernia: correlation with hernia content and pregnancy outcome. J Ultrasound Med 16:407, 1997.

Touloukian RJ, Markowitz RI: A preoperative x-ray scoring system for risk assessment of newborns with congenital diaphragmatic hernia. J Pediatr Surg 19:252, 1984.

Tyson KR, Schwartz MZ, Marr CC: "Balanced" thoracic drainage is the method of choice to control intrathoracic pressure following repair of diaphragmatic hernia. J Pediatr Surg 20:415, 1985.

Valases C, Sills C: Anterior diaphragmatic hernia (hernia of Morgagni). Case report. NJ Med 85:603, 1988.

Vanamo K, et al: Long-term pulmonary sequelae in survivors of congenital diaphragmatic defects. J Pediatr Surg 31:1096, 1996.

Vander Wall KJ, et al: Fetal endoscopic ("Fetendo") tracheal clip. J Pediatr Surg 31:1101, 1996.

Weber TR, et al: Neonatal diaphragmatic hernia. An improving outlook with extracorporeal membrane oxygenation. Arch Surg 122:615, 1987.

Wilson JM, et al: Congenital diaphragmatic hernia: predictors of severity in the ECMO era. J Pediatr Surg 26:1028, 1991.

Wung JT, et al: Congenital diaphragmatic hernia: survival treated with very delayed surgery, spontaneous respiration, and no chest tube. J Pediatr Surg 30:406, 1995.

Zaccara A, et al: Maximal oxygen consumption and stress performance in children operated on for congenital diaphragmatic hernia. J Pediatr Surg 31:1092, 1996.

READING REFERENCES

Baran EM, Houston HE, Lynn HB: Foramen of Morgagni hernias in children. Surgery 62:1076, 1967.

Bently G, Lister J: Retrosternal hernia. Surgery 57:567, 1965.

Breaux CW, et al: Improvement in survival of patients with congenital diaphragmatic hernia utilizing a strategy of delayed repair after medical and/or extracorporeal membrane oxygenation stabilization. J Pediatr Surg 26:333, 1991.

Weber TR, et al: Congenital diaphragmatic hernia beyond infancy. Am J Surg 162:643, 1991.

CHAPTER 51

Foramen of Morgagni Hernia

John A. Federico and Ronald B. Ponn

In 1769, Morgagni first described the rare anterior, retrosternal diaphragmatic defect that now bears his name. He noted this condition in the autopsy of an Italian stonecutter who died from gangrenous colon herniated through an opening beneath the sternocostal junction. Because Napoleon's surgeon, Larrey, described a surgical approach to the pericardial sac through an anterior retrosternal diaphragmatic defect, this area has also been termed the *space of Larrey*.

ANATOMY

The embryology of the diaphragm is discussed in Chapter 47. Lack of fusion or muscularization of the pleuroperitoneal membrane anteriorly leads to a defect in the costosternal trigones known as a Morgagni foramen. This triangular space is located between the muscle fibers from the xiphisternum and the costal margin fibers that insert on the central tendon (Fig. 51-1). The internal mammary artery traverses this space to enter the rectus sheath and become the superior epigastric artery. Because the peritoneum is intact, there is usually a true hernia sac. In most cases, the hernia contains only omentum, but the colon is involved occasionally, and the small bowel or stomach rarely. A left-sided defect is less likely to result in herniation because it is protected by the pericardium. The ligamentum teres defines the medial border of the hernia on either side.

INCIDENCE

Clinically evident hernias through the foramen of Morgagni are uncommon at any age. Despite their congenital etiology, they are detected less often in children than in adults. Comer and Clagett (1966) reported 50 patients (7%) with foramen of Morgagni hernia of a total of 750 patients with diaphragmatic hernias of all kinds found over 32 years. Harrington (1948) listed only seven foramen of Morgagni hernias (1.5%) in a series of 430 patients who were

operated on for diaphragmatic hernia. Overall, the incidence of Morgagni hernia among all diaphragmatic defects in adults and children is 3 to 4%. For the anatomic reason noted above, about 90% of the hernias occur on the right, 8% are bilateral, and only 2% are limited to the left. Morgagni hernias are detected more often in women than in men and in obese people more often than in those of average or below-average weight.

SYMPTOMS

In a literature review of 132 adult and pediatric cases, Berardi and associates (1997) reported that approximately one-third of patients are asymptomatic. Those with symptoms most frequently describe chronic gastrointestinal complaints, such as crampy pain or constipation from partial intermittent colonic obstruction. Symptoms due to intermittent gastric volvulus or small bowel obstruction are less frequent. Patients often complain only of vague epigastric or substernal fullness or a dull right subcostal discomfort. Complete obstruction, incarceration, or strangulation with necrosis of a hollow viscus contained in a Morgagni hernia is rare, and is associated with an acute or subacute presentation. In the aforementioned series, 12 patients had complete bowel obstruction and one had gangrenous intestine.

Cardiorespiratory symptoms (mainly dyspnea and palpitations) are less common overall than gastrointestinal complaints. Although children are more often asymptomatic than are adolescents and adults, they have an approximately equal incidence of respiratory and gastrointestinal symptoms.

As with other hernias, conditions that produce prolonged or sudden severe increased intra-abdominal pressure can precipitate the onset of or exacerbate existing symptoms due to a Morgagni hernia. Valases and Sills (1988) reported that exercise and athletic activity may cause the occurrence of symptoms. Ellyson and Parks (1986) reported that trauma could initiate symptoms. Lin and Maginot (1999) described a patient who became symptomatic during pregnancy.

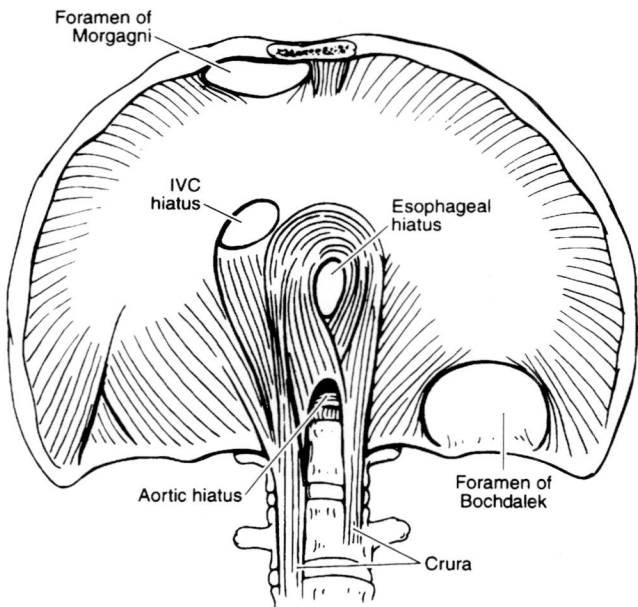

Fig. 51-1. Illustration of posterolateral (Bochdalek) and anterior (Morgagni) diaphragmatic hernia. Note location of the latter between muscle fibers from the xiphisternum and from the costal arch that insert on the central tendon. From Naunheim KS: Adult presentation of unusual diaphragmatic hernias. Chest Surg Clin North Am 8:359, 1998. With permission.

DIAGNOSIS

The diagnosis of a foramen of Morgagni hernia is made by radiography, prompted either by symptoms or performed for

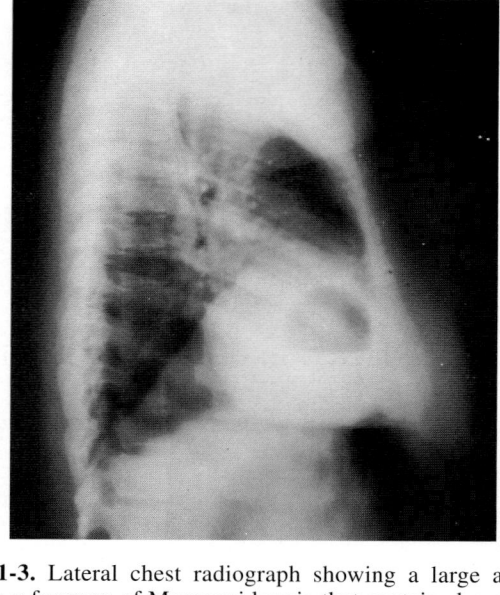

Fig. 51-3. Lateral chest radiograph showing a large air-fluid level in a foramen of Morgagni hernia that contained part of the stomach.

unrelated reasons. In very small hernias, Lanuza (1971) described "the sign of the cane": a curvilinear accumulation of fat continuous with the properitoneal fat line of the anterior abdominal wall. This sign suggests that a small anterior cardiophrenic mass may be a Morgagni hernia. More commonly, the standard chest radiograph shows obvious right, left, or bilateral pericardiophrenic abnormalities that are solid or contain air. The usual finding is a rounded opacity at the right cardiophrenic angle. The lateral chest film localizes

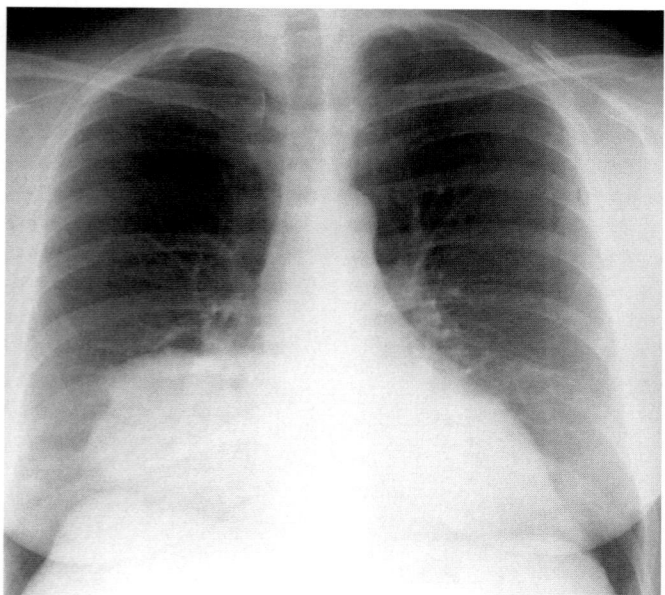

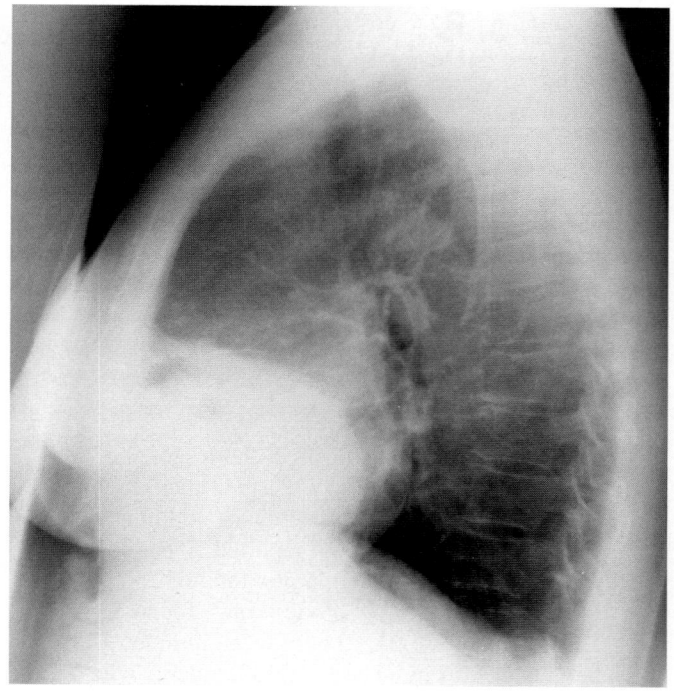

Fig. 51-2. A. Posteroanterior radiograph shows a round right pericardiophrenic density. **B.** Lateral film localizes the opacity to the retrosternal area.

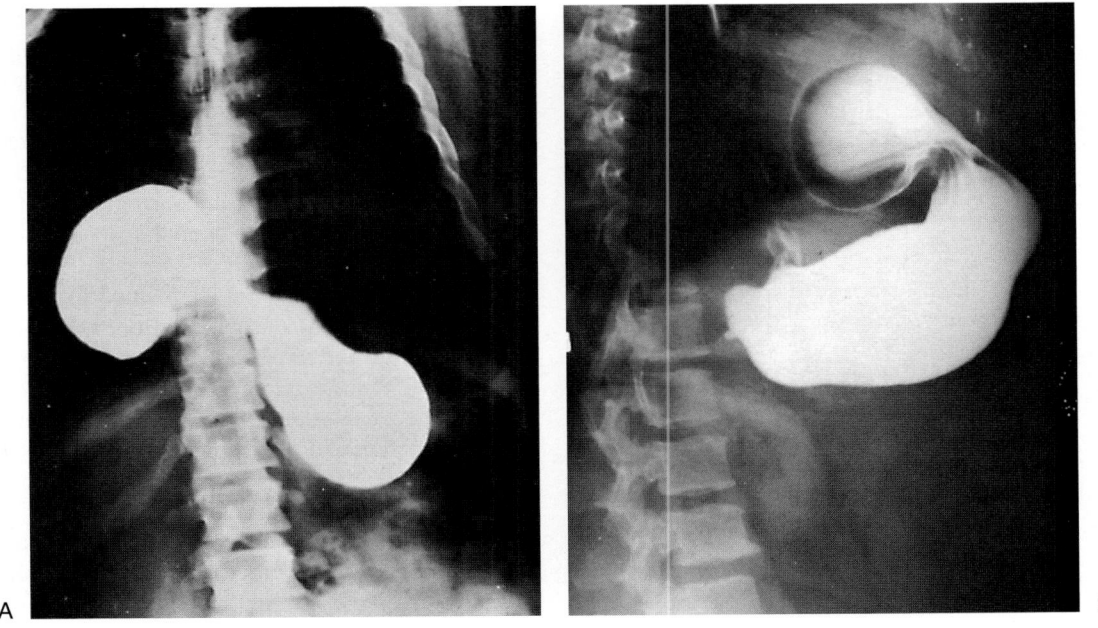

Fig. 51-4. Posteroanterior film (**A**) and lateral view (**B**) of a barium-filled stomach partially herniated into the chest through a right-sided foramen of Morgagni hernia.

this density to the anterior retrosternal space (Fig. 51-2). The opacification is generally due to omentum rising through the hernia defect. When the transverse colon, small bowel, or stomach herniates through the defect, an air-fluid level may be seen on chest film (Fig. 51-3). In adults, pericardial cyst, prominent fat pad, loculated pneumothorax, bronchial carcinoma in the cardiophrenic region, and atypical mediastinal tumor may mimic the radiographic features of herniation through the foramen of Morgagni.

Contrast studies of the colon or upper gastrointestinal tract can confirm the diagnosis in patients with visceral herniation (Fig. 51-4). Computed tomographic scan is diagnostic in cases with or without visceral herniation because it demonstrates the presence of fat, a hollow viscus, or both, without the need for gastrointestinal contrast. The usual computed tomographic finding is a retrosternal mass of fat density representing herniated omentum (Fig. 51-5) or a combination of omentum and an air-containing viscus (Fig. 51-6). Magnetic resonance imaging can provide similar information but is usually not required. Although radiographs after induced pneumoperitoneum have been used to outline the hernia sac for definitive diagnosis, this approach is rarely needed.

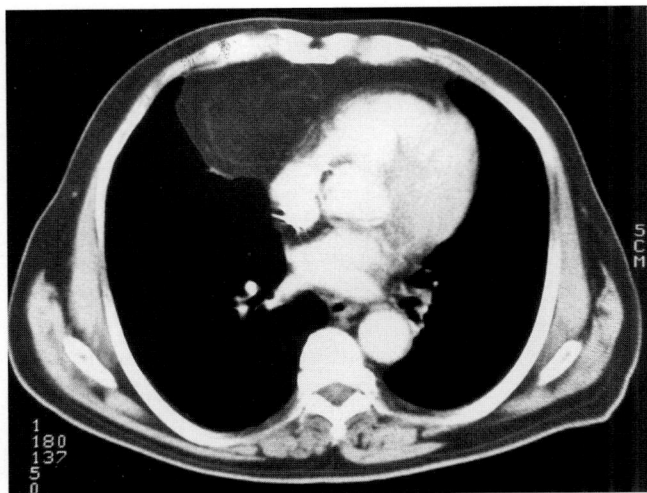

Fig. 51-5. Computed tomographic scan showing a right retrosternal mass consisting entirely of fat in herniated omentum.

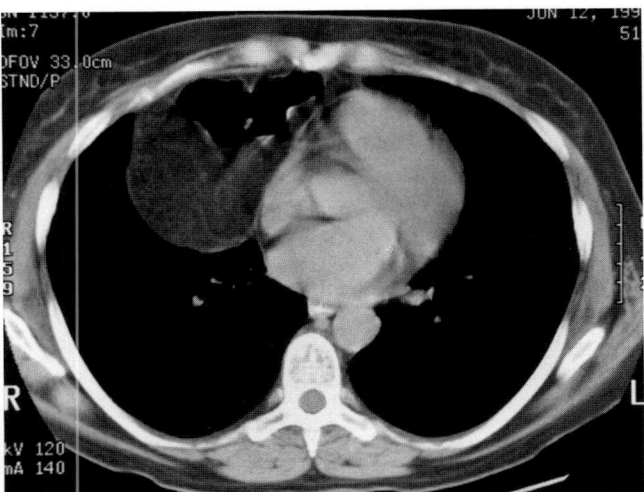

Fig. 51-6. Computed tomographic scan showing a right retrosternal hernia containing both omentum and transverse colon.

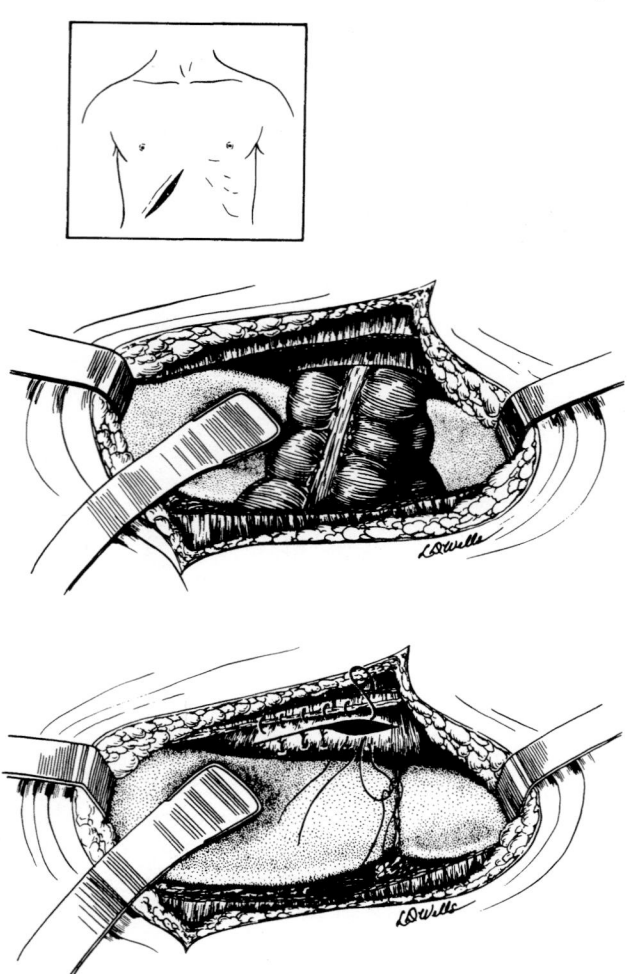

Fig. 51-7. Technique of closure of a foramen of Morgagni hernia by an open transabdominal approach. From Shields TW: The diaphragm. *In* Nora P (ed): Operative Surgery: Principles and Techniques. Philadelphia: Lea & Febiger, 1972.

SURGICAL REPAIR

The treatment of a Morgagni hernia is surgical. All symptomatic adults should undergo repair. We agree with most recent reports in also recommending repair in most asymptomatic adults because hernias may enlarge over time and there is a low but definite risk of progression to incarceration and strangulation. Thus, a safe elective operation can become a potentially high-risk procedure. In some asymptomatic cases, however, it is reasonable to follow the patient without repair. This group includes people with only herniated omentum who have comorbidities that increase the risk of operation.

Repair is generally performed transabdominally through an upper midline, subcostal, or paramedian incision. A midline approach allows easy access to both sides in the event that bilateral hernias are encountered. Adhesions are taken down, and the contents of the hernia are reduced into the peritoneal cavity. The margins of the hernia sac are identified, and the sac is generally resected. As in all types of hernia surgery, a

tension-free closure is required to prevent recurrence. For small defects that can be closed primarily, repair of the muscular defect is performed with heavy (0-gauge) interrupted nonabsorbable mattress sutures. It is usually necessary to pull the diaphragm up to the posterior part of the sternum and to the posterior rectus sheath (Fig. 51-7). Prosthetic patches are used to close larger defects. In many patients, it is not necessary to enter the chest or to drain the pleural space.

Occasionally, a foramen of Morgagni hernia is encountered during a thoracotomy performed for an undiagnosed mediastinal mass or other indication. Once identified, the sac is opened and explored, and the contents are reduced into the peritoneal cavity. Primary or prosthetic patch repair of the defect can often be performed in a manner similar to the transabdominal technique. In some cases, adequate repair requires passing the sutures around a rib anteriorly or through the sternal periosteum.

Experience is increasing with minimally invasive approaches to the treatment of foramen of Morgagni hernias. Laparoscopy is used most commonly, as reported by Kuster (1992) and Orita (1997) and their colleagues, as well as Fernandez-Cebrian and De Oteyza (1996), among others. Hussong and associates (1997) reported success with a thoracoscopic approach.

The results of surgical repair of Morgagni hernias are excellent. Operative mortality and morbidity are low, especially for elective repair. There were five deaths (3.8%), involving one child and four adults, in the series of 132 patients reviewed by Berardi and coworkers (1997). Of paramount importance is that all five deaths occurred in patients with strangulated bowel. Although there are no reliable data on recurrence rates, individual reports of recurrences are rare. Follow-up is limited, but the results of endoscopic repair so far appear to be excellent.

REFERENCES

Berardi RS, et al: An update on the surgical aspects of Morgagni's hernia. Surgical Rounds, Sept. 1997, pp. 370–376.

Comer TP, Clagett OT: Surgical treatment of hernia of the foramen of Morgagni. J Thorac Cardiovasc Surg 52:461, 1966.

Ellyson JH, Parks SN: Hernia of Morgagni in trauma patients. J Trauma 26:569, 1986.

Fernandez-Cebrian JM, De Oteyza JP: Laparoscopic repair of hernia of foramen of Morgagni. J Laparoendosc Surg 6:61, 1996.

Harrington SW: Various types of diaphragmatic hernia treated surgically. Surg Gynecol Obstet 86:735, 1948.

Hussong RL, Landreneau RJ, Cole FH: Diagnosis and repair of a Morgagni hernia with video-assisted thoracic surgery. Ann Thorac Surg 63:1474, 1997.

Kuster GGR, Kline LE, Garzo G: Diaphragmatic hernia through the foramen of Morgagni: laparoscopic repair. J Laparosc Surg 2:93, 1992.

Lanuza A: The sign of the cane: a new radiological sign for the diagnosis of small Morgagni hernias. Radiology 101:293, 1981.

Lin JC, Maginot AE: Postpartum incarcerated Morgagni's hernia: an unusual presentation of Morgagni's hernia. Surgical Rounds, Feb. 1999, pp. 70–72.

Orita M, et al: Laparoscopic repair of a diaphragmatic hernia through the foramen of Morgagni. Surg Endosc 11:668, 1997.

Valases C, Sills C: Case report: anterior diaphragmatic hernia (hernia of Morgagni). NJ Med 85:603, 1988.

CHAPTER 52

Paraesophageal Hiatal Hernia

Keith S. Naunheim and Lawrence L. Creswell

The esophageal hiatus is formed by muscle fibers of the right crus of the diaphragm with little or no contribution from the left crus. These fibers overlap inferiorly, where they attach over and along the right side of the median arcuate ligament, which is attached to the lateral aspects of the vertebral bodies. The orifice is therefore teardrop shaped, with the point to the right of the aorta and the rounded portion in the midline close to the connecting portion of the central tendon of the diaphragm. The crural fibers form a tunnel that encloses the esophagus. The phrenoesophageal ligament is formed by fusion of the endothoracic and endoabdominal fascia at the diaphragmatic hiatus. This ligament holds the distal esophagus in place. The lower esophagus normally resides within the abdomen.

Herniation of abdominal contents through the esophageal hiatus into the thoracic cavity has been recognized for several centuries. Bowditch (1853) reported such a case but credited Ambrose Paré with a description of a patient with herniation of the stomach through the esophageal hiatus in 1610. One of the first successful repairs was accomplished by Potempski in 1884 and reported by him in 1889.

CLASSIFICATION

Hiatal hernias are generally classified into four types, the most common of which is the sliding, or type I hiatal hernia.

Type I Hiatal Hernia

In the sliding type of hiatal hernia, the gastroesophageal junction moves through the esophageal hiatus into the visceral mediastinum so that it occupies an intrathoracic position cephalad to the stomach, which follows it. This process occurs because of circumferential weakening of the phrenoesophageal ligament. Factors that may contribute to the development of this hernia include increased abdominal pressure (e.g., with pregnancy, obesity, or vomiting) and

vigorous esophageal contraction, which may pull the gastroesophageal junction up into the mediastinum. This type of hiatal hernia is frequently accompanied by loss of tone and competence of the lower esophageal sphincter (LES), which may result in gastroesophageal reflux and esophagitis. The LES effects may be related to the loss of mechanical advantage at the gastroesophageal junction when it is displaced into the chest. Many sliding hiatal hernias do not produce symptoms. A peculiar abnormality is incompetence of the gastric cardia or the LES without radiologic evidence of a hiatal hernia, which Hiebert and Belsey (1961) called a "patulous cardia." The diagnosis and treatment of reflux esophagitis and type I hiatal hernia are reviewed in Chapter 139.

Type II Hiatal Hernia

The paraesophageal, or type II, hiatal hernia is an uncommon disorder that is distinct from the sliding hiatal hernia. In a paraesophageal hiatal hernia, the phrenoesophageal membrane is not weakened diffusely but rather is weakened focally, anterior and lateral to the esophagus. The gastric cardia and lower esophagus remain below the diaphragm. The gastric fundus protrudes or rolls through the defect into the mediastinum (Fig. 52-1). Paraesophageal hiatal hernia is by far less common than the sliding hiatal hernia. Hill and Tobias (1968), Ozdemir and colleagues (1973), and Sanderud (1967) reported that this condition accounted for only 3 to 6% of all patients undergoing surgical repair of hiatal hernias. Because most patients with hiatal hernia do not undergo operative repair, probably only 1 to 2% of all hiatal hernias are type II defects. Allen and colleagues (1993) found only 147 patients (0.32%) with paraesophageal hiatal hernias, with 75% or more of the stomach in the chest among 46,236 patients with hiatal hernia at the Mayo Clinic from 1980 to 1990. In 124 of their patients who underwent operation, 51 patients (41%) had a type II hiatal hernia, 52 patients had a type III (mixed sliding and parae-

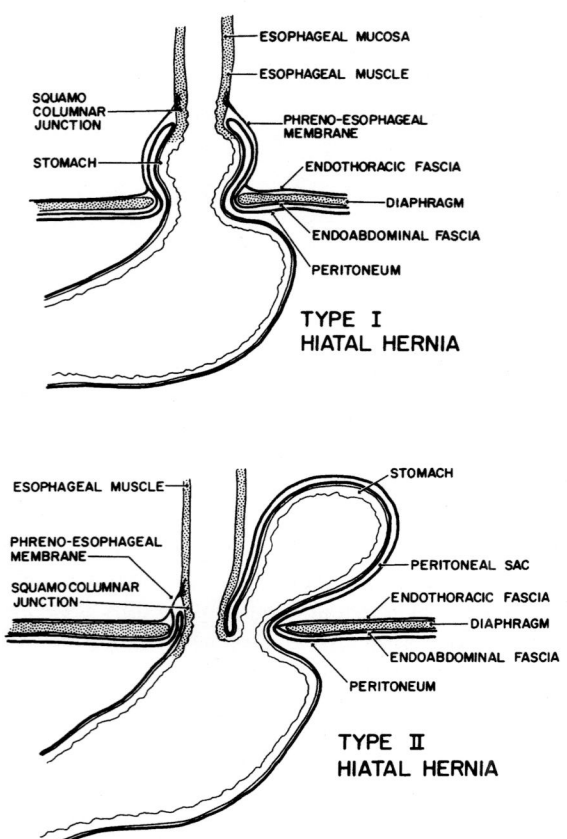

ESOPHAGEAL MUCOSA
ESOPHAGEAL MUSCLE
SQUAMO COLUMNAR JUNCTION
PHRENO-ESOPHAGEAL MEMBRANE
STOMACH
ENDOTHORACIC FASCIA
DIAPHRAGM
ENDOABDOMINAL FASCIA
PERITONEUM
TYPE I HIATAL HERNIA

ESOPHAGEAL MUSCLE
STOMACH
PHRENO-ESOPHAGEAL MEMBRANE
SQUAMO COLUMNAR JUNCTION
PERITONEAL SAC
ENDOTHORACIC FASCIA
DIAPHRAGM
ENDOABDOMINAL FASCIA
PERITONEUM
TYPE II HIATAL HERNIA

Fig. 52-1. Two types of hiatal hernia. Type I hiatal hernia is not a true hernia in that the endoabdominal fascial lining of the abdomen remains intact. In type II hiatal hernia, a defect in the fascia allows a peritoneal sac to pass through the opening in the esophageal hiatus and enter the pleural cavity.

sophageal) hiatal hernia (43%), and 21 patients (17%) had a type IV hiatal hernia (i.e., with herniation of other organs in addition to the stomach).

The term *parahiatal hernia* has been used in the past, but this type of defect may not actually exist. We have never encountered a defect in the diaphragm alongside the esophageal hiatus with protrusion of stomach into the chest and identifiable crural or diaphragmatic fibers between the hernia orifice and the esophageal hiatus.

Type III Hiatal Hernia

The type III, or mixed, hiatal hernia is a combination of types I and II: a sliding *and* rolling hernia.

If a type I hiatal hernia enlarges, the attenuated phrenoesophageal membrane may also weaken focally anteriorly, allowing protrusion of the gastric fundus. Rotation of the stomach may result in the body or fundus obtaining a higher position within the chest than the cardia, a situation usually found only in type II hiatal hernias. Pearson and colleagues

(1983) stated that true type II hiatal hernias are rare and suggested that most are, in fact, misdiagnosed type III defects with a supradiaphragmatic LES. Little support exists for this controversial viewpoint, however. How often a type II paraesophageal hiatal hernia becomes a type III hiatal hernia is not known. Frequently, however, when a patient has a large paraesophageal hiatal hernia with rotation of the body and fundus of the stomach into the chest, the gastroesophageal junction is in a location superior to the esophageal hiatus of the diaphragm. In such circumstances, however, the gastroesophageal junction is in the posterior aspect of the hiatus, and the patient does not usually have symptoms of an attenuated intrinsic sphincter with reflux esophagitis. A type III defect is frequently present when a type II hiatal hernia has been present for many years, presumably due to gradual enlargement of the esophageal hiatus so that the gastroesophageal junction no longer lies within or below the hiatus. Attachments of the gastroesophageal junction remain intact posteriorly. Evidence increasingly suggests that a type I hiatal hernia is caused by esophageal contraction abnormalities with a pull on the gastroesophageal junction. Patients with severe esophagitis rarely have a paraesophageal herniation, and patients with a large paraesophageal hiatal hernia seldom have significant esophagitis despite a supradiaphragmatic gastroesophageal junction.

Type IV Hiatal Hernia

Progressive enlargement of the diaphragmatic opening eventually can lead to herniation of organs other than the stomach. The transverse colon and omentum are most commonly involved, but the spleen and small bowel also may herniate into the chest.

ANATOMY AND PHYSIOLOGY

In a true paraesophageal hiatal hernia, the lower esophagus and cardia remain fixed below the diaphragm in the posterior aspect of the diaphragmatic hiatus. A focal weakening of the phrenoesophageal membrane occurs anterior or lateral to the esophagus, and the combination of negative intrathoracic and positive intra-abdominal pressure pushes the abdominal viscera through the defect. The protruding organs are covered circumferentially by a layer of peritoneum that forms a true hernia sac, unlike the type I hiatal hernia, in which the stomach forms the posterior wall of the hernia sac. The intrathoracic migration of the stomach evolves by so-called organoaxial rotation (Fig. 52-2). The lesser curve of the stomach is anchored in the abdomen by the posterior attachments of the lower esophagus, the left gastric artery, and the retroperitoneal fixation of the pylorus and duodenum. These three points define the long axis of the stomach, and they remain relatively fixed in the abdomen in a type II hiatal hernia. The greater curve of the stomach, however, is relatively mobile and rotates about the "long axis" by mov-

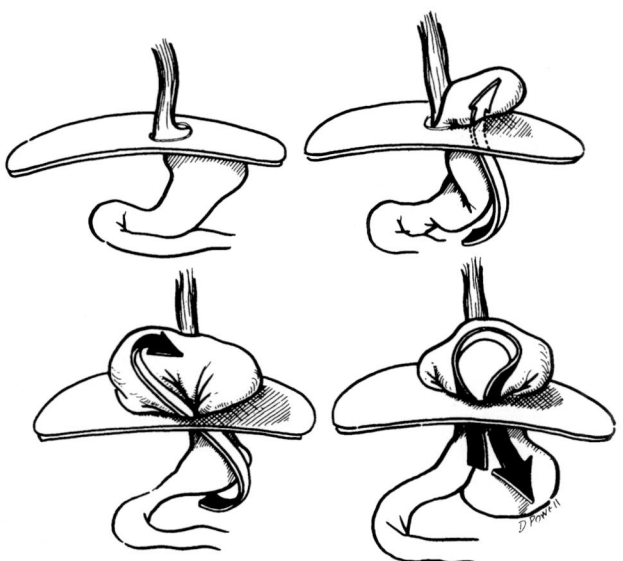

Fig. 52-2. Mechanics of incarceration and strangulation with paraesophageal hiatal hernia. Note that the fundus may prolapse back into the abdomen. From Postlethwait RW (ed): Surgery of the Esophagus. 2nd Ed. East Norwalk, CT: Appleton-Century-Crofts, 1986. With permission.

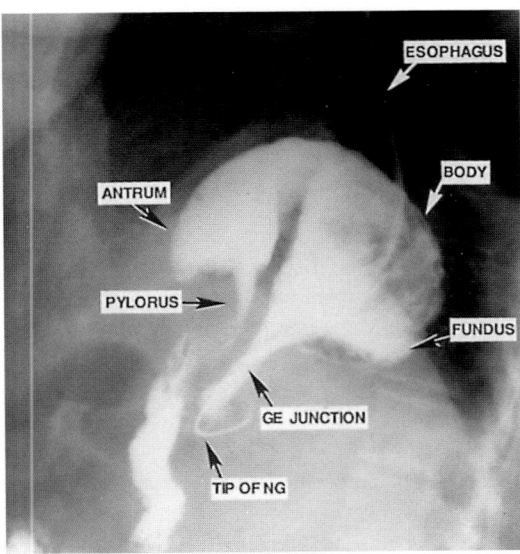

Fig. 52-3. Barium study of the stomach that demonstrates the "upside-down" appearance of the stomach in the thoracic cavity. Note the nasogastric (NG) tube extending through the length of the esophagus with the tip at the gastroesophageal (GE) junction below the esophageal hiatus. The fundus, body, and antrum of the stomach are above the diaphragm.

ing first anteriorly and then upward, as the hernia evolves. The fundus is the first part of the stomach to protrude upward through the anterior hernia sac. As the hiatal defect enlarges, the body and antrum continue the axial rotation and migrate into the thorax, leaving the cardia and pylorus in the abdomen. The stomach then resides "upside down" in the chest, with the greater curve pointing cephalad and the cardia remaining below the diaphragm (Fig. 52-3). The stomach initially may occupy a retrocardiac position, but as the hernia enlarges, rotation occurs into the right chest. With huge hernias, most of the stomach lies within the right hemithorax, with the greater curve of the stomach pointing toward the right shoulder. This rotation places an upward tension on the omentum and may facilitate herniation of the transverse colon into the sac. The organoaxial rotation of the stomach is most commonly upward into the chest and to the right. This is the path of least resistance because of the aorta to the left and the heart anterior and to the left. Occasionally, however, the stomach may rotate superiorly but not to the right, so that the greater curve lies transversely behind the heart.

As with any true anatomic hernia, the potential complications include bleeding, incarceration, volvulus, obstruction, strangulation, and perforation. Gastritis and ulceration have been visualized endoscopically in as many as 30% of the patients who have type II hiatal hernias. Wichterman and colleagues (1979) suggested that these ulcers are the result of poor gastric emptying and torsion of the gastric wall, particularly after repeat incarcerations, which may impair the blood supply and lymphatic drainage. Although brisk bleeding can occur, these ulcers more frequently cause a slow, chronic blood loss and anemia.

The most serious complication of the type II hiatal hernia is gastric volvulus associated with incarceration and strangulation. Hill and Tobias (1968) and Ozdemir (1973) and Wichterman (1979) and their colleagues reported that approximately 30% of patients with paraesophageal hernias present with gastric volvulus, but this complication may not be so common today. Perdikis and colleagues (1997) reported this complication in only 6% of patients with type II hiatal hernias, and some series have reported *no* patients with this complication. After a meal, the fundus may prolapse down from the hernia sac and back into the abdomen (see Fig. 52-2). This twists and angulates the stomach in its midportion just proximal to the antrum, resulting in partial or complete obstruction. Distention of the intrathoracic stomach and further rotation of the fundus can result in obstruction at the gastroesophageal junction. Still further twisting may lead to pyloric obstruction, which results in an incarcerated gastric segment and closed-loop obstruction. If unchecked, this process ultimately leads to strangulation, necrosis, and perforation. Unless this process is recognized and corrected, the resulting mediastinitis and shock are fatal.

Allen and colleagues (1993) reported five patients who required emergency operations for suspected strangulation. Three of these patients had gastric necrosis and one died. Borchardt's triad (1904) of chest pain, retching with an inability to vomit, and inability to pass a nasogastric tube indicates volvulus of the stomach and was present in three of Allen and colleagues' patients (1993). Twenty-three of their patients were followed without surgery. Four of these patients developed progressive symptoms, and one died of aspiration.

A type III defect is frequently present when a type II hiatal hernia has been present for many years. This may be due to gradual enlargement of the hiatus so that the gastroesophageal junction no longer lies within or below the hiatus. The attachment of the gastroesophageal junction remains intact posteriorly. Most of these hernias are very large when the diagnosis is made. It may be that the symptoms are so mild or nonspecific when the hernia is small that the patients do not seek medical attention. It may also be that once this type of hernia begins to develop, it progresses rapidly to a large size because of negative intrathoracic and positive intra-abdominal pressures.

SYMPTOMS

Many type II hiatal hernias cause few or no symptoms and remain undiagnosed for years until recognized on a routine chest radiograph. Chronic bleeding from gastritis or ulceration of the intrathoracic gastric segment may lead to iron-deficiency anemia, resulting in fatigue and exertional dyspnea. Most patients, however, present with complaints of postprandial discomfort, caused by an intrathoracic gastric segment that becomes dilated by food and swallowed air. Frequently, these complaints have been present for many years. Patients usually describe sensations of substernal fullness or pressure, and this is often mistaken for angina. This discomfort is frequently accompanied by nausea and is somewhat relieved by belching or regurgitation. Although Pearson and colleagues (1983) reported that most of their patients had severe symptoms, it is probably because of the high percentage of mixed (type III) hiatal hernias in their patient population. Ellis and colleagues (1986) noted that symptoms of gastroesophageal reflux were very uncommon in their patients with type II hiatal hernias. Fuller and colleagues (1996) reported that reflux-related symptoms (e.g., heartburn, regurgitation) were predominant in only 27% of patients and that hernia-related symptoms (e.g., dysphagia, distention, anemia, or bleeding) were predominant in 73% of patients. True dysphagia is uncommon. Finally, a large type III or IV hiatal hernia may occupy a portion of the thoracic cavity and result in postprandial respiratory symptoms of breathlessness with a sense of suffocation. Symptoms may be mild despite a huge hernia. Many patients become accustomed to and tolerate these gas-bloat symptoms well.

When gastric volvulus and obstruction occur, patients present in extreme distress. Most such patients give a long history of complaints but have never sought medical advice. The chief complaints at the time of presentation are severe pain and pressure in the chest or the epigastric region. The discomfort is usually accompanied by nausea and may be misdiagnosed as an acute myocardial infarction. Vomiting may occur, but more frequently the patient complains of retching and an inability to regurgitate. The patient may also complain of the inability to swallow saliva. If the volvulus is allowed to progress, strangulation of the intrathoracic portion of stomach occurs, resulting in a toxic clinical picture including fever, "third-spacing" of fluid, and hypovolemic shock. The

mortality rate in this situation approaches 50%. Kafka (1994) and Oliver (1990) and their colleagues reported acute hemorrhagic pancreatitis in association with paraesophageal hernia, either because of herniation of the pancreatic head or distortion of the pancreatic duct with impaired drainage.

DIAGNOSIS

The diagnosis of paraesophageal hiatal hernia is usually first suspected because of an abnormal chest radiograph. The most frequent finding is a retrocardiac air bubble with or without an air-fluid level (Fig. 52-4). In a giant paraesophageal hernia, the hernia sac and its contents occasionally protrude into the right thoracic cavity. The differential diagnosis includes mediastinal cyst or abscess and dilated obstructed esophagus, as in end-stage achalasia. A barium study of the upper gastrointestinal tract is the diagnostic study of choice. The pathognomonic finding is an upside-down stomach in the chest (see Fig. 52-3). The radiologist must pay careful attention to the position of the cardia. This not only confirms the diagnosis of a type II defect but may be important in deciding whether an antireflux procedure should be performed at the same time as the anatomic hernia repair. A barium enema may help determine if any portion of colon is involved.

After the presence of the paraesophageal hiatal hernia has been established radiographically, one must determine whether it has a functional effect on the competence of the LES. This is best accomplished by endoscopy and esophageal function testing.

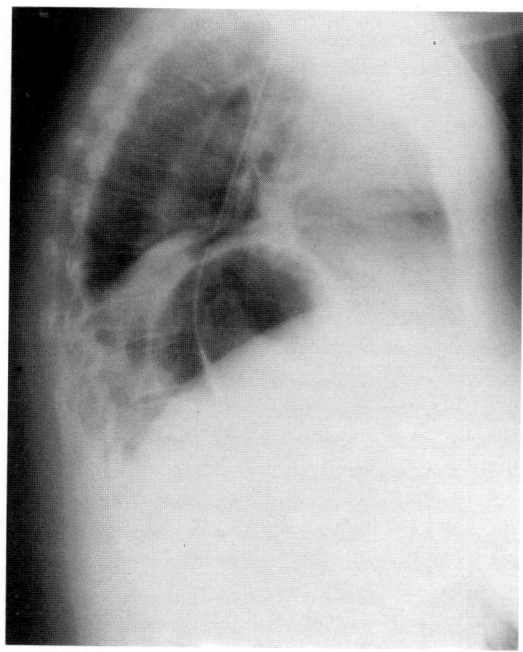

Fig. 52-4. Retrocardiac air bubble and type II hiatal hernia. Note the wedge of atelectatic lung compressed by a large hernia sac.

Although symptoms of gastroesophageal reflux may be uncommon in patients with a pure type II hiatal hernia, they are occasionally present and may indicate pathologic peptic esophagitis. Preoperative esophageal testing may help confirm or refute this suspicion. Esophageal manometry is useful for determining the location of the LES, which marks the gastroesophageal junction, an area that can be difficult to locate on barium study. An LES at a supradiaphragmatic level suggests a huge paraesophageal hiatal hernia or a type III (mixed paraesophageal and sliding hiatal) hernia, which is more likely to have a component of reflux and esophagitis. Ambulatory 24-hour esophageal pH testing can help to identify gastroesophageal reflux, which is best treated by a fundoplication procedure at the time of surgical correction (Chapter 139). Walther and colleagues (1984) found pH evidence for pathologic reflux in 9 of 15 patients (60%) with type II hiatal hernias. Fuller and colleagues (1996) found similar evidence in 69% of their patients.

The role of esophagoscopy in the evaluation of patients with type II hiatal hernias remains unclear. Pearson and colleagues (1983) performed endoscopy on all 51 patients with primary incarcerated giant hiatal hernias. They found that 30% had grade 1 esophagitis, and another 30% had grade 2 to 4 esophagitis, but virtually all these patients had type III hiatal hernias. Ellis and colleagues (1986) reported a series that included 39 patients with primary type II defects and found only 5 patients (13%) with endoscopic evidence of mild-to-moderate esophagitis, an incidence similar to that reported by Walther and colleagues (1984). Most recently, Fuller and colleagues (1996) found esophagitis in 5 of 15 patients (33%) with type II hiatal hernias, including three with grade 2 esophagitis, one with grade 3 esophagitis, and one with stricture. Significantly, these investigators also reported that endoscopy did not identify pathologic reflux in 58% of their patients who had gastroesophageal reflux demonstrated by pH monitoring.

Apparently, pure type II hiatal hernias are not frequently associated with an incompetent LES or significant gastroesophageal reflux, which probably occurs more frequently in patients with type III defects. Preoperative endoscopy and esophageal motility studies can help to establish the location of the gastroesophageal junction and LES with relation to the diaphragm. The combination of esophageal pH testing and endoscopy may determine whether significant gastroesophageal reflux or pathologic esophagitis is present. These tests should be used before elective operation for any patient with a type II hiatal hernia and symptoms of gastroesophageal reflux. They should also be used routinely for any patient with known or suspected type III hernia with a supradiaphragmatic LES.

THERAPY

There is no acceptable medical treatment regimen for patients with paraesophageal hiatal hernia. Patients followed expectantly are at great risk, as noted by Skinner and Belsey (1967), who found a 29% mortality rate in 21 patients treated without operation. Because of the serious and life-threatening nature of the complications of this disorder, the presence of the hernia is, in itself, a surgical indication.

When a patient with a type II hiatal hernia presents with gastric volvulus and obstruction, decompression with a nasogastric tube must be performed promptly. In the absence of signs of toxicity, an operation can then be scheduled at the earliest convenience. The inability to decompress a gastric volvulus in this situation constitutes a surgical emergency and mandates immediate operative intervention, whether or not signs of toxicity are present.

Operative Approaches

Although the necessity for operation is universally recognized, there is still controversy about which operation should be performed and by which operative approach. The repair can be performed easily through either an abdominal or thoracic approach and can be performed laparoscopically as well. Each of these approaches has strong proponents. Regardless of the approach, however, the operative principles for hernia repair apply: reduction of the hernia, resection of the sac, and closure of the defect.

Advocates of the thoracic approach emphasize the ease of intrathoracic dissection of the hernia contents and sac. In patients with type III defects, the thoracic approach allows a thorough dissection of the esophagus in cases of moderate-to-severe esophageal shortening. This approach may allow reduction of a fundoplication beneath the esophageal hiatus without the need for an esophageal lengthening procedure. The proponents of a transthoracic repair, however, usually neglect to note the increased morbidity and discomfort associated with the thoracotomy approach. In addition, a transthoracic repair may allow the stomach to rotate organoaxially after it is pushed back into the peritoneal cavity. This then produces a volvulus of the body of the stomach in which the greater curve of the stomach adheres to the liver. Wichterman and colleagues (1979) reported two patients in whom this occurred; these patients required a laparotomy postoperatively to correct the volvulus.

Those who suggest an abdominal approach point out that the procedure is easily performed through the abdomen and that additional abdominal procedures can be undertaken simultaneously. In addition, this approach allows placement of a gastrostomy tube, which obviates the need for a postoperative nasogastric tube and may also decrease the risk of recurrent volvulus. The only patient in whom this approach might prove difficult is one with a proven type III hiatal hernia with known gastroesophageal reflux and a foreshortened esophagus. In this case, the thoracic approach may be a better alternative. Familiarity with the dissection of the esophagus (as for transhiatal esophagectomy), however, allows mobilization of most of the esophagus through an enlarged esophageal hiatus.

Advocates of the laparoscopic procedure emphasize the less invasive nature of this approach. Particularly for elderly patients who may have comorbid conditions, the laparoscopic hernia repair may offer a safe, less traumatic alternative to a conventional operation and may result in a quicker recovery. Although many primary care physicians may be reluctant to refer asymptomatic or mildly symptomatic patients with type II hiatal hernias for conventional surgery, they might be more willing to refer patients for laparoscopic procedures. Even the strongest proponents of this approach, however, recognize that the laparoscopic operation is technically difficult, particularly regarding excision of the hernia sac. Critics of the laparoscopic approach point out that even in experienced hands, the laparoscopic approach may be associated with greater morbidity (e.g., operative complications or conversion to an "open" procedure) and lead to more postoperative difficulties that require treatment (e.g., second operation, esophageal dilatation for dysphagia, gastroesophageal reflux).

Should an Antireflux Procedure Be Included?

The indications for an antireflux procedure at the time of correction of the anatomic hernia remain controversial. Many authors, including Pearson (1983) and Ozdemir (1973) and their colleagues have written that they routinely perform an antireflux procedure in all patients, regardless of the presence or absence of gastroesophageal reflux symptoms. Allen and associates (1993) reported that nearly 95% of their patients with intrathoracic stomach underwent a transthoracic repair with the addition of an uncut Collis-Nissen fundoplication, Belsey Mark IV fundoplication, or Nissen fundoplication. The remainder of their patients underwent an abdominal repair with an antireflux procedure. Thus, they routinely performed an antireflux procedure despite the fact that only 15% of their patients had esophagitis. They reported excellent results for all types of repair. At the other extreme, Hill and Tobias (1968) espoused simple anatomic repair alone and reported excellent results with no recurrences and no postoperative gastroesophageal reflux in 19 patients.

Other authors have reported a selective approach for the inclusion of an antireflux procedure. Ellis and colleagues (1986) suggested that patients with type II hiatal hernia should undergo preoperative endoscopy, esophageal manometry, and pH testing. This group also suggested that only patients with symptoms or objective evidence of gastroesophageal reflux should be considered for an antireflux repair, usually a Belsey Mark IV fundoplication or a loose Nissen fundoplication. Williamson and colleagues (1993) reviewed 117 patients with paraesophageal hiatal hernias. The most common presenting symptom was epigastric or substernal pain in 76% of patients. Only 17 patients underwent antireflux procedures in addition to anatomic repair of the hernia. The antireflux procedures were performed for esophagitis determined by symptoms and by esophagoscopy, with a hypotensive LES (<10 mm Hg) or positive 24-hour pH monitoring. Postoperatively, however, two of their patients (1.7%) developed severe gastroesophageal reflux symptoms and findings, and 17 others (14.5%) developed mild and controllable symptoms. They reported the development of a recurrent hernia in 10 of 117 patients, with good to excellent results in 86% of patients. Fuller and colleagues (1996) considered the role of fundoplication in 15 patients with type II hiatal hernia. These authors concluded that with careful preoperative assessment via endoscopy and pH monitoring, objective evidence of gastroesophageal reflux was present in the majority of patients and that an antireflux procedure was indicated for most, if not all, patients.

Operative Technique: Conventional Abdominal Approach

We prefer and recommend the abdominal approach through an upper midline incision. The left lobe of the liver is mobilized and retracted to the right. The contents of the hernia sac are reduced back into the peritoneal cavity by gentle traction. If resistance is encountered while the hernia contents are being reduced, a small rubber catheter inserted in the hernia sac allows entry of air as downward tension is placed on the contents of the sac. This decreases the suction effect that holds the viscera in the chest. Occasionally, in cases of a tight incarceration, the hiatal ring itself may have to be incised to allow return of the organs to the abdominal cavity. This can be performed safely on the left side of the crus posteriorly along the side of the aorta.

The hernia sac is dissected free from the thoracic cavity and resected. Once this has been accomplished, the dead space in the mediastinum disappears as the lungs expand. No drainage of this space is necessary. The large diaphragmatic defect is located anterior to the lower esophagus. In type II hiatal hernias, the gastroesophageal junction usually remains within the abdomen, bound posteriorly by fibrous attachments. Care is taken during the ensuing dissection not to take down this posterior attachment, which maintains the LES in an intra-abdominal position. A circumferential dissection is performed on the lower 4 to 8 cm of esophagus through the enlarged esophageal hiatus. With anterior traction on the lower esophagus, the crural repair can begin at the level of the aorta and continue anteriorly until the esophagus is returned to its normal anatomic position at the anterior rim of the esophageal hiatus. This repair is usually performed with simple, interrupted nonabsorbable 0 sutures placed at 1-cm intervals. These sutures must be placed well back from the apparent crural edge due to the attenuated nature of the crura.

If the patient has objective evidence of significant reflux esophagitis preoperatively, an antireflux procedure is now performed. If the posterior attachments of the lower esophagus are taken down during dissection, it is likely that the LES has been disturbed and will be incompetent postopera-

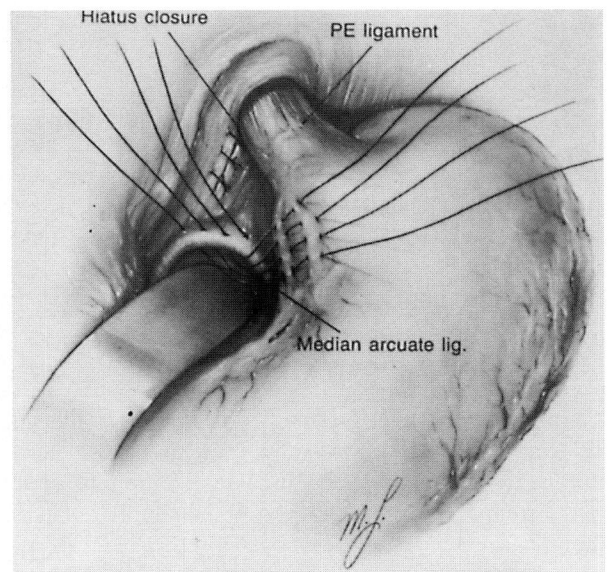

Fig. 52-5. Hill suture plication after reduction of the paraesophageal (PE) hernia and repair of the hiatal defect to maintain the position of the gastroesophageal junction within the abdominal cavity. From Postlethwait RW (ed): Surgery of the Esophagus. 2nd Ed. East Norwalk, CT: Appleton-Century-Crofts, 1986, p. 245. With permission.

tively. In these patients, we also perform an antireflux procedure at this time, and our procedure of choice is a loose Nissen fundoplication. If there is doubt about whether the gastroesophageal junction is below the esophageal hiatus, it is best to mobilize the junction and the lower esophagus. Sufficient mobilization allows the junction to be brought 4 to 5 cm below the esophageal hiatus. The esophageal hiatus can then be narrowed or repaired by approximating the crura, beginning posteriorly over the aorta and behind the esophagus. This displaces the esophagus anteriorly into its normal position as it passes through the esophageal hiatus.

If no fundoplication is to be performed, the stomach is fixed within the peritoneal cavity by two methods. The first is a modified Hill suture plication, in which three interrupted nonabsorbable sutures are placed between the lesser curve of the stomach and the preaortic fascia (Fig. 52-5). These sutures hold the gastroesophageal junction within the abdominal cavity and prevent the development of a type I (sliding) hiatal hernia postoperatively. If the esophagus has been mobilized during the repair, these sutures can be attached to the crural repair posteriorly. The second technique is a Stamm gastrostomy, which serves two functions. First, it eliminates the need for a nasogastric tube. Many patients with incarcerated type II hiatal hernias have a prolonged period of postoperative gastric stasis, and a gastrostomy allows continued drainage without the discomfort or complications of an indwelling nasogastric tube. Second, the gastrostomy fixes the stomach to the anterior abdominal wall, thereby maintaining its position within the abdominal cavity and preventing an intra-

abdominal gastric volvulus, a reported complication of transthoracic repairs. The gastrostomy tube can be removed 8 to 12 days after the operation.

If gangrene or perforation is found at the time of operation, all devascularized tissue must be resected and all infected tissue must be débrided. Broad-spectrum antibiotics that include anaerobic coverage are strongly advised in this setting because of the possibility of perforation and mediastinal contamination.

Operative Technique: Laparoscopic Approach

Laparoscopic repair of paraesophageal hiatal hernia was first described by Congreve (1992). Larger series have recently been reported by Perdikis (1997) and Willekes (1997) and their colleagues. The operation is usually performed supine, in steep Trendelenburg's position (Fig. 52-6). In one approach, five 10- to 12-mm ports are used:

1) 12 cm caudad from the xiphoid
2) Just left of the midline, 2 to 3 cm beneath the costal margin in the left upper quadrant
3) Just lateral to the rectus muscle, 4 to 5 cm beneath the costal margin in the left upper quadrant
4) At the level of the umbilicus in the left anterior axillary line
5) In the right anterior axillary line at the level of the umbilicus

The surgeon works through the two ports in the left upper quadrant.

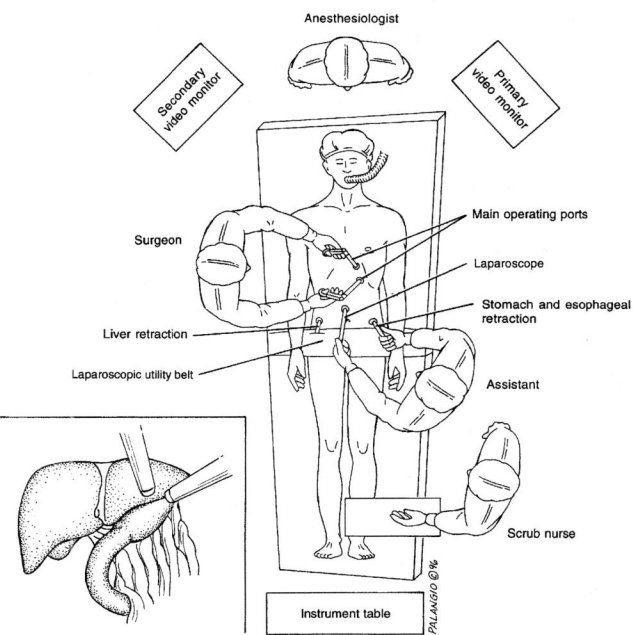

Fig. 52-6. Operative setup for laparoscopic repair of paraesophageal hernia. From Willekes CL, et al: Laparoscopic repair of paraesophageal hernia. Ann Surg 225:31, 1997. With permission.

Table 52-1. Operative Mortality for Paraesophageal Hernia Repair[a]

Author	Elective (%)	Emergency[b] (%)
Beardsley and Thompson (1964)	—	3/10 (30)
Sanderud (1967)	0/14 (0)	1/7 (14)
Hill & Tobias (1968)	0/19 (0)	2/10 (20)
Ozdemir et al. (1973)	0/19 (0)	2/12 (16)
Wichterman et al. (1979)	0/16 (0)	1/6 (16)
Carter et al. (1980)	—	1/14 (7)
Pearson et al. (1983)	0/47 (0)	1/4 (25)
Walther et al. (1984)	0/15 (0)	—
Ellis et al. (1986)	1/39 (2)	—
Landreneau et al. (1992)	0/12 (0)	0/5 (0)
Allen et al. (1993)	0/119 (0)	1/5 (20)
Williamson et al. (1993)[c]	1/112 (0.9)	1/7 (14)
Perdikis et al. (1997)[c]	0/65 (0)	—
Willekes et al. (1997)[c]	0/30 (0)	—
Total	1/507 (0.2)	13/90 (14)

[a]Operative mortality is reported as number of deaths divided by number of operated patients.
[b]*Emergency* is defined as gastric volvulus.
[c]Using laparoscopic approach.

Just like the conventional "open" procedure, the operation is performed in four major stages: reduction of the hernia, excision of the hernia sac, crural repair, and fundoplication, if necessary. Reduction of the hernia sac into the abdominal cavity and excision of the sac can be very difficult and it may not be necessary to remove the hernia sac from the anterior surface of the gastroesophageal junction. The crural repair is usually accomplished with interrupted, nonabsorbable sutures, but the use of prosthetic materials [e.g., Gore-Tex (W.L. Gore, Flagstaff, AZ)] has also been described. If warranted, a laparoscopic fundoplication can be performed. Laparoscopic gastrostomy can be used to fix the stomach to the anterior abdominal wall and provide an alternative to a nasogastric tube.

Operative Morbidity and Mortality

Elective surgical repair of paraesophageal hernias is safe. A collective review of 300 patients (Table 52-1) reveals that the operative mortality rate was less than 0.5%, a figure similar to that quoted for repair of sliding hiatal hernias. Emergency procedures in cases of gastric volvulus, however, carry a much higher mortality rate of approximately 14% (see Table 52-1). This marked increase in operative risk underscores the need for elective repair at the time of the initial diagnosis.

The postoperative complications are the same as those for antireflux procedures, with two additions. First, in patients with gastric volvulus and obstruction, pulmonary complications apparently increase, probably because of episodes of regurgitation and aspiration. Second, prolonged gastric stasis may persist for a period of 7 to 10 days after operative repair because of lingering inflammation and edema in the released gastric segment.

For patients undergoing laparoscopic repair, Willekes (1997) and Perdikis (1997) and their colleagues reported conversion to an "open" procedure in 0% and 3% of patients, respectively. There were no operative deaths. Complications occurred in approximately one-third of patients and included gastric perforation, gastric bleeding, slipped Nissen fundoplication, small-bowel obstruction, and atelectasis.

RESULTS

The long-term results, as noted by Martin and colleagues (1997), are generally excellent, regardless of whether an antireflux procedure is performed in addition to simple repair. Hill and Tobias (1968) performed simple repair and had no recurrence or gastroesophageal reflux in 22 patients over a 15-year follow-up period. Wichterman and colleagues (1979), who routinely performed concomitant antireflux procedures, noted identical results. Recurrent type I hernias with gastroesophageal reflux, however, have been reported in 10% by Ozdemir and colleagues (1973), in 8% by Pearson and colleagues (1983), and in 8% by Sanderud and colleagues (1967) despite fundoplication at the time of initial repair. Simultaneous fundoplication is therefore apparently ineffective prophylaxis against recurrent herniation with resultant gastroesophageal reflux. More appropriately, fundoplication might be used selectively in patients with documented gastroesophageal reflux.

Allen and colleagues (1993) report excellent results in 60% of their patients, good results in 33%, fair results in 5.2%, and poor results in 1.7%. In Williamson and colleagues' (1993) report, the results were considered excellent in 53.9%, good in 29.5%, fair in 4.3%, and poor in 12.1%. The poor results in this series resulted mainly from symptomatic recurrence of the paraesophageal hiatal hernia in 10% and the infrequent development of severe gastroesophageal reflux in 2% of the patients who did not have a concomitant antireflux procedure at the time of hernia repair.

Although there are acceptable early results after laparoscopic repair of paraesophageal hiatal hernias, the long-term results after operation by this approach remain unknown. As such, the laparoscopic approach cannot be recommended routinely to patients with paraesophageal hiatal hernia.

REFERENCES

Allen MS, et al: Intrathoracic stomach: presentation and results of operation. J Thorac Cardiovasc Surg *105*:253, 1993.

Beardsley JM, Thompson WR: Acutely obstructed hiatal hernia. Ann Surg *159*:49, 1964.

Borchardt M: Zur Pathogie und Therapie des Magen Volvulus. Arch Klin Chir *74*:243, 1904.

Bowditch HI: Peculiar case of diaphragmatic hernia. Buffalo Med J Month Rev *9*:1, 1853.

Carter R, Brewer LA, Hinshaw DB: Acute gastric volvulus: a study of 25 cases. Am J Surg *140*:99, 1980.

Congreve DP: Laparoscopic paraesophageal hernia repair. J Laparoendosc Surg *2*:45, 1992.

Ellis FH, Crozier RE, Shea JA: Paraesophageal hiatus hernia. Arch Surg *121*:416, 1986.

Fuller CB, et al: The role of fundoplication in the treatment of type II paraesophageal hernia. J Thorac Cardiovasc Surg *111*:655, 1996.

Hiebert CA, Belsey R: Incompetency of the gastric cardia without radiologic evidence of hiatal hernia. J Thorac Cardiovasc Surg *42*:352, 1961.

Hill LD, Tobias JA: Paraesophageal hernia. Arch Surg *96*:735, 1968.

Kafka NJ, et al: Acute pancreatitis secondary to incarcerated paraesophageal hernia. Surgery *115*:653, 1994.

Landreneau RJ, et al: Clinical spectrum of paraesophageal herniation. Dig Dis Sci *37*:537, 1992.

Martin TR, Ferguson MK, Naunheim KS: Management of giant paraesophageal hernia. Dis Esophagus *10*:47, 1997.

Oliver MJ, et al: Acute pancreatitis and gastric volvulus occurring in a congenital diaphragmatic hernia. J Pediatr Surg *25*:1240, 1990.

Ozdemir IA, Burke WA, Ikins PM: Paraesophageal hernia: a life-threatening disease. Ann Thorac Surg *16*:547, 1973.

Pearson FG, et al: Massive hiatal hernia with incarceration: a report of 53 cases. Ann Thorac Surg *35*:45, 1983.

Perdikis G, et al: Laparoscopic paraesophageal hernia repair. Arch Surg *132*:586, 1997.

Potempski P: Nuovo processo operativo per lar riduzione cruenta della ernie diaframmatiche de trauma e per la sutura delle ferite del diaframma. Bul Reale Accad Med Roma *15*:191, 1889.

Sanderud A: Surgical treatment for the complications of hiatal hernia. Acta Chir Scand *133*:223, 1967.

Skinner DB, Belsey RHR: Surgical management of esophageal reflux and hiatus hernia: long-term results with 1030 patients. J Thorac Cardiovasc Surg *53*:33, 1967.

Walther B, et al: Effect of paraesophageal hernia on sphincter function and its implication on surgical therapy. Am J Surg *147*:111, 1984.

Wichterman K, et al: Giant paraesophageal hiatal hernia with intrathoracic stomach and colon: the case for early repair. Surgery *86*:497, 1979.

Willekes CL, et al: Laparoscopic repair of paraesophageal hernia. Ann Surg *225*:31, 1997.

Williamson WA, et al: Paraesophageal hiatal hernia: is an anti-reflux procedure necessary? Ann Thorac Surg *56*:447, 1993.

CHAPTER 53

Tumors of the Diaphragm

Robert J. Downey

The diaphragm is commonly involved with neoplasms, such as malignant pleural disease, both primary and metastatic, or malignant peritoneal disease. Only rarely, however, is the diaphragm the source of either benign or malignant processes. In this chapter, the presentation, evaluation, and treatment of benign and malignant primary tumors of the diaphragm are discussed.

HISTORIC BACKGROUND

Little has been written on the subject of primary neoplasms of the diaphragm, which reflects the rarity of these tumors. Grancher (1868) is commonly credited with providing the first description of a primary diaphragmatic tumor, a benign fibroma, unsuspected until discovered at autopsy. Other authors give primacy to Clark (1886) for a report of a primary lipoma of the diaphragm. Isolated case reports have predominated subsequent reports; these were summarized in three major reports published by Nicholson and Whitehead (1956), Wiener and Chou (1965), and Olafsson and associates (1971). The last report found a total of only 71 case reports in the world literature up to that time.

PRESENTATION AND EVALUATION

A review of the case reports available in the literature suggests that diaphragmatic tumors are not associated with any characteristic symptoms. Approximately 50% were asymptomatic and were discovered either incidentally on radiographs or at the time of surgical exploration performed for unrelated reasons. If any symptom is characteristic, it is that of a sense of lower chest discomfort or heaviness, with possible referred pain to the top of the shoulder. Larger masses may give rise to compression of adjacent structures, such as the lung, which causes cough, dyspnea, and hemoptysis, or the heart, with lower extremity edema found if venous return is compromised. Other physical findings appear to be rare,

although some authors have noted masses palpable in the upper abdomen or bulging through rib interspaces.

Evaluation before surgery is almost exclusively radiographic. Older reports, such as that of Ackerman in 1942, suggested fluoroscopy in conjunction with the performance of diagnostic pneumoperitoneum and pneumothorax; subsequent reports suggested the use of angiography. These measures are rarely used today, having been replaced by ultrasound, computed tomography (CT), and magnetic resonance (MR) imaging, as discussed by Yeh (1990), Brink (1994), and Kanematsu (1995) and their associates, respectively.

Given the rarity of diaphragmatic lesions, it is reasonable to suggest that evaluation should be directed toward consideration of the possible presence of more common benign or malignant lesions arising in proximity to, but not from, the diaphragm. The presence of normal diaphragmatic anatomical variants that may be confused with neoplasms should also be considered. These distinctions can be very difficult. The differential diagnosis can be summarized as follows: The diaphragm may be involved by nonneoplastic processes, such as infections (including *Mycobacterium tuberculosis*), hematomas, congenital abnormalities, and hernias, or it may be secondarily involved by neoplasms metastatic to the diaphragm. Organs in the region of the diaphragm may be involved by processes that may be confused with primary diaphragmatic processes, particularly infectious processes. Primary or secondary neoplastic diseases of the liver, lung, pericardium, thymus (particularly thymolipoma), stomach, or spleen also should be kept in mind.

If the initial test suggesting the presence of a lower thoracic cavity density is a chest radiograph, decubitus films may suggest the presence of a free-flowing effusion. Further evaluation usually consists of some combination of CT scans, MR imaging, and ultrasound. Structural abnormalities of the diaphragm, such as lobulations, localized eventrations, slips, and hypertrophic crus, may simulate neoplastic masses. However, such structural abnormalities can usually be distinguished from neoplastic processes by their appearance. For example, Ferguson and Westcott (1976) and Yeh and colleagues (1990) discuss the fact that lobulations are usually multiple, and eventrations generally conform to or retain the overall shape of the diaphragm. Distinguishing a mass that apparently arises from the diaphragm from one originating in the lung parenchyma may be facilitated by reconstructions of CT images if a low-attenuation plane can be seen between the mass and the diaphragm. The radiology literature suggests that further support for localizing a mass in the lung may be offered by the suggestion of irregular margins with the nearby lung, the presence of acute angles between the diaphragm and the mass, and focal volume loss in the lung, with pulmonary vessels and bronchi appearing to curve into the lesion. A pleural origin for a mass is suggested by the presence of obtuse angles between the lesion and the diaphragm. Imaging of herniated hollow viscera through the diaphragm may be enhanced by the use of orally or intravenously administered contrast. Ultrasound or MR imaging of the liver may help to localize a mass in the liver parenchyma. The choice among the wide range of currently available diagnostic imaging modes depends largely on the suspected diagnosis, but to some extent, extensive radiographic investigations may be replaced by video-assisted thoracic surgical techniques, or laparoscopy, or both, because they offer the possibilities of diagnosis and of treatment.

PRIMARY BENIGN NEOPLASTIC LESIONS

The most commonly reported benign neoplasm of the diaphragm is the lipoma. Other reported benign diaphragmatic lesions include fibroma and congenital cysts. Case reports of chondroma, angioma, lymphangioma, hemangioendothelioma, rhabdomyofibroma, and neurofibroma also have been published (Table 53-1).

Table 53-1. Primary Tumors of the Diaphragm

Benign	Malignant
Mesothelial origin	
Angiofibroma	Chondrosarcoma
Chondroma	Fibroangioendothelioma
Fibroma	Fibromyosarcoma
Fibrolymphangioma	Fibrosarcoma
Fibromyoma	Hemangioendothelioma
Hamartoma	Hemangiopericytoma
Lymphangioma	Leiomyosarcoma
Leiomyoma	Mesothelioma
Lipoma	Myosarcoma
Rhabdomyofibroma	Rhabdomyosarcoma
	Sarcoma, various cell types
	Synovioma
Neurogenic origin	
Neurilemmoma	Neurogenic sarcoma
Neurofibroma	
Others	
Adenoma	
Cysts	

Historic Background

As noted previously, the first reported case of a primary lipoma dates to Clark in 1886, and approximately 23 cases were subsequently reported. More than one-half of these cases were previously unsuspected findings at autopsy; the symptoms attributed to these lesions in the remaining patients were largely those of vague lower chest wall discomfort. No cases have been reported in pediatric patients, but given that the majority came to light either at autopsy or as asymptomatic radiographic findings, it is possible that they are present but undiagnosed in the pediatric population.

Description

Kalen (1970), Gallia (1968), Ferguson and Westcott (1976), and Tihansky and Lopez (1988) have described the radiologic appearance of lipomas, suggesting that by and large, they appear as sharp-bordered, smooth, possibly lobulated masses. The reported lipomas are usually described pathologically as encapsulated, ranging from 1 to 10 cm, and having the same gross appearance of lipomatous tissue found elsewhere throughout the body. Because they appear to arise from the substance of the diaphragm, the reported cases often have an "hourglass" or "dumbbell" shape due to protrusions into thoracic and abdominal cavities, extending through centimeter-sized defects in the diaphragm, with residual diaphragmatic muscle fibers interdigitated with the fatty tissue. Wiener and Chou (1965) summarize reported cases, finding that they arise predominantly from the left and posterolateral areas of the diaphragm, although essentially every portion of the diaphragm has been involved. The diagnosis may be suggested by the findings of fat-density material on CT scan. Treatment is excision with removal of as little of the normal diaphragm as necessary, with surgery being performed largely to provide a definitive diagnosis. Sampson and colleagues (1960) reported a lipoma apparently undergoing degeneration into a liposarcoma; however, because I have been unable to find any other reported case of a liposarcoma of the diaphragm, this may reasonably be held to be an exceedingly rare event.

The other two groups of benign lesions predominating in collected series are cystic formations, such as bronchial, mesothelial, or teratoid cysts, which Olafsson and colleagues (1971) found to comprise up to 35% of benign series, and neurogenic tumors (neurilemmoma and neurofibroma), as discussed by McClenathan and Okada (1989). These lesions are too varied to summarize meaningfully other than to say that approximately 50% came to attention because of symptoms, with the remainder diagnosed incidentally by radiographs performed for apparently unrelated reasons. It is interesting to note, however, that numerous investigators, including Trivedi (1958), Wiener and Chou (1965), and McClenathan and Okada (1989) recorded that one-half of the reported neurogenic tumors of the diaphragm were associated with hyper-

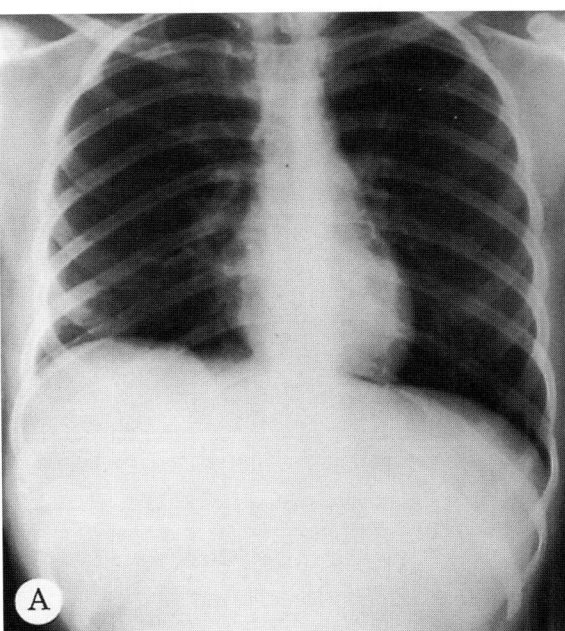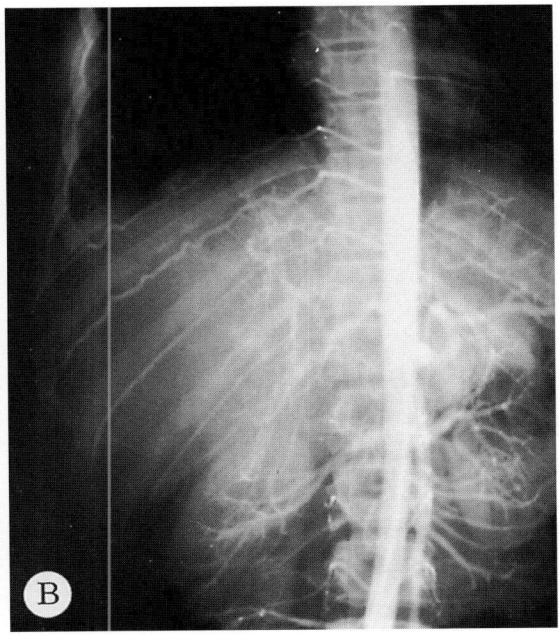

Fig. 53-1. A. Posteroanterior radiograph of the chest revealing an elevated right hemidiaphragm. Suggestion of a mass occupying the lateral three-fourths of the right hemidiaphragmatic leaf is noted. **B.** Aortogram of the same patient demonstrates displacement of the normal vascular structures in the liver by a large neurofibroma of the diaphragm. Hypertrophy of the intercostal muscle is visualized clearly on this aortogram.

trophic pulmonary osteoarthropathy or clubbing of the fingers, or both. These are rare findings with other diaphragmatic tumors: Only one patient with clubbing of the fingers was recorded in 63 non-neural tumors of the diaphragm collected by Wiener and Chou (1965). McClenathan and Okada (1989) found that most neural lesions—symptomatic or not—are benign (77%) (Fig. 53-1). Various other benign lesions have been reported, as noted previously (see Table 53-1).

Treatment

Once suspected, surgical resection of all benign lesions is definitive treatment and offers a uniform excellent prognosis. Resection is likely to be considered for any benign mass, either to confirm the diagnosis or to relieve symptoms, if present.

PRIMARY MALIGNANT NEOPLASTIC LESIONS OF THE DIAPHRAGM

The majority of the reported cases of malignant tumors have been of mesenchymal origin, which is not surprising, given the cell structure of the diaphragm. Histology varies, including reports of such rare tumors as leiomyosarcoma by Parker (1985), malignant fibrous histiocytoma by Tanaka and coworkers (1982), and fibrosarcomas by Sbokos and associates (1977). Almost unique cases, such as epithelioid

hemangioendothelioma, were reported by Bevelaqua and colleagues (1988), and hemangiopericytoma by Seaton (1974) (Fig. 53-2). The presentation of these tumors resembles that of the benign lesions, with the exception that symptoms of locoregional spread may be present.

In reported cases, surgical resection with or without chemotherapy or radiation therapy was often performed in an attempt to cure. The tumor and adjacent involved areas are removed en bloc, when possible, with a wide margin of normal diaphragm. Primary closure of the diaphragm is usually not possible, but on occasion, the remaining diaphragmatic tissue may be advanced up the chest for reattachment to the rib cage. More often than not, closure of the defect necessitates the use of a prosthetic soft tissue patch of Gore-Tex or other similar suitable material. Interrupted sutures are used to secure the prosthetic material to the cut edges of the diaphragm or to the chest wall as necessary. Morbidity and mortality rates after excision of these tumors should be low. As expected, ventilatory loss on the side of the resection is noted, but the magnitude of such losses has not been documented. The effectiveness of surgical resection is hard to evaluate because many cases were reported for their radiologic interest, without long-term outcomes. However, for the small number of cases reported with outcome data, the prognosis appears grim, even after apparently curative resection. Because the majority of patients with primary diaphragmatic malignancies come to medical attention owing to symptoms that usually indicate locoregionally advanced disease, long-term survival was only

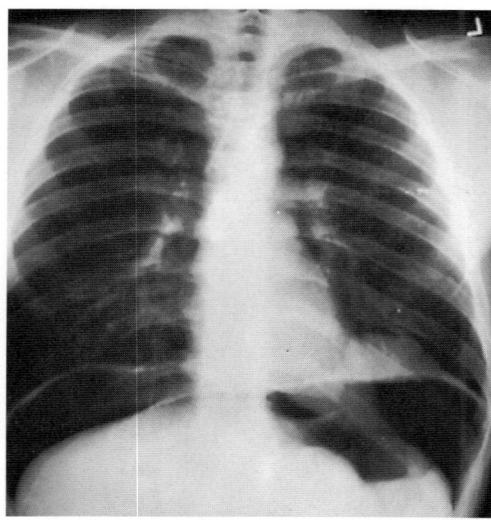

Fig. 53-2. The diagnosis of a diaphragmatic tumor was easily confirmed by a pneumoperitoneum. This tumor was excised and found to be a fibrosarcoma.

rarely achieved, with the majority of patients having either local or distant metastatic recurrences.

REFERENCES

Ackerman AJ: Primary tumors of the diaphragm roentgenologically considered. AJR Am J Roentgenol 47:711, 1942.

Bevelaqua RA, Valensi Q, Hulnick D: Epithelioid hemangioendothelioma; a rare tumor with variable prognosis presenting as a pleural effusion. Chest 93:665, 1988.

Brink JA, et al: Abnormalities of the diaphragm and adjacent structures: findings on multiplanar spiral CT scans. AJR Am J Roentgenol 163: 307, 1994.

Clark FW: Subpleural lipoma of diaphragm. Trans Pathol Soc Lond 38:324, 1886.

Ferguson DD, Westcott JL: Lipoma of the diaphragm: report of a case. Radiology 118:527, 1976.

Gallia FJ: Nodular lesion of the diaphragm. JAMA 203:725, 1968.

Grancher M: Tumeur vegetante du centre phrenique du diaphragme. Bull Soc Anat Paris 43:85, 1868.

Kalen NA. Lipoma of the diaphragm. Scand J Respir Dis 51:28, 1970.

Kanematsu M, et al: Dynamic MRI of the diaphragm. J Comput Assist Tomogr 19:67, 1995.

McClenathan JH, Okada F: Primary neurilemmoma of the diaphragm. Ann Thorac Surg 48:126, 1989.

Nicholson F, Whitehead R. Tumors of the diaphragm. Br J Surg 43:633, 1956.

Olafsson G, Rausing A, Holen O: Primary tumors of the diaphragm. Chest 59:568, 1971.

Parker MC: Leiomyosarcoma of the diaphragm—a case report. Eur J Surg Oncol 11:171, 1985.

Sampson CC, et al: Liposarcoma developing in a lipoma. Arch Pathol 69:506, 1960.

Sbokos CG, et al: Primary fibrosarcoma of the diaphragm. Br J Dis Chest 71:49, 1977.

Seaton D: Primary diaphragmatic haemangiopericytoma. Thorax 29:595, 1974.

Tihansky DP, Lopez GM: Bilateral lipomas of the diaphragm. N Y State J Med 88:151, 1988.

Tanaka F, et al: Prosthetic replacement of the entire left hemidiaphragm in malignant fibrous histiocytoma of the diaphragm. J Thorac Cardiovasc Surg 83:278, 1982.

Trivedi SA: Neurolemmoma of the diaphragm causing severe hypertrophic pulmonary osteoarthropathy. Br J Tuberc 52:214, 1958.

Wiener MF, Chou WH. Primary tumor of the diaphragm. Arch Surg 90:143, 1965.

Yeh HC, Halton KP, Gray CE: Anatomic variations and abnormalities in the diaphragm seen with US. Radiographics 10:1019, 1990.

SECTION XI
The Pleura

CHAPTER 54

Anatomy of the Pleura

Thomas W. Shields

EMBRYOLOGY

The paired pleural cavities are derivatives of the intraembryonic portion of the primitive coelom. The primitive coelom arises by splitting of the lateral mesoderm on either side of the embryo into splanchnic and somatic layers. These paired cavities are later separated by three partitions into three subdivisions: the pericardial cavity, the pleural cavities, and the peritoneal cavity. The partitions are the unpaired septum transversum, the paired pleuropericardial folds, and the paired pleuroperitoneal folds. The right and left coelomic chambers dorsal to the septum transversum remain relatively unexpanded for a period as the so-called pleural canals; these lie on either side of the mediastinal region. The development of the pleuroperitoneal folds completes the separation of the pleural canals from the other two body cavities: the pericardial cavity and the peritoneal cavity. At the fourth week of development, the laryngotracheal outgrowth from the floor of the pharynx is noted, and in the fifth week, the two lung buds begin to enlarge into the respective pleural canals. According to Patten (1968), the pleural spaces open up in advance of lung growth, and the lungs move (bulge) into the space prepared to receive them. With growth, the lungs and the pleuropericardial membranes come to lie on either side of the heart, and the pleuroperitoneal folds become part of the diaphragm. In this process of expansion of the lungs into the pleural canals, the splanchnic mesoderm is pushed out as a covering over the mesenchyma-packed bronchial trees (Fig. 54-1). The splanchnic mesoderm becomes thinned to form the mesothelial layer of the pleura, and the mesenchymal tissue immediately beneath this layer becomes the connective tissue of the pleura. The splanchnic mesoderm is thus the origin of the visceral pleura, and the somatic mesoderm is the origin of most of the parietal pleura.

HISTOLOGY

The two pleural layers have similar histologic features, with the exception of the presence of stomata in the parietal pleura and their absence in the visceral pleura. According to Antony and colleagues (1992), each layer consists of 1) an innermost mesothelial cell layer, 2) a submesothelial interstitial connective tissue layer, 3) an inner thin elastic fiber layer, 4) an outer interstitial connective tissue layer, and 5) a thick elastic fiber layer. In addition, according to Hammer (1995), a fatty layer separates the parietal pleura and the muscles of the chest wall. The mesothelial cells in both visceral and parietal pleura, according to Wang (1982, 1985), vary in thickness from less than 1 µm to more than 4 µm and from 16.4 ± 6.8 to 41.9 ± 9.5 µm in diameter. Their shape may vary according to their location in the pleural membrane.

Ultrastructurally, the mesothelial cells demonstrate microvilli. Tight apical junctions are present, but gap junctions, desmosomes, or half desmosomes occur infrequently on the basal part of the cell membrane.

Immunohistochemically, the mesothelial cells, as reported by Dervan (1986) and Bolen (1986) and their associates, express both low- and high-molecular-weight cytokeratin. The normal mesothelial cells are negative for reaction to vimentin, epithelial membrane antigen, carcinoembryonic antigen, and factor VIII–related antigen.

Beneath the basal membrane of the mesothelial layer is a collection of loose connective tissue. This submesothelial layer contains collagen tissue, elastic fibers, small blood vessels, lymphatic networks, and nerve fibers. The mesenchymal cells in this layer, according to Keating (1978), Said (1984), and England (1989) and their coworkers, have the characteristics of fibroblasts. The cells are negative for cytokeratin, carcinoembryonic antigen, and factor VIII–related antigen.

The visceral and parietal pleural layers are approximately the same thickness, averaging 30 to 40 µm, according to Staub and colleagues (1985). Large dehiscences, or stomata, have been documented in the parietal pleura. Chretien and Huchon (1990) state that these stomata, ranging from 2 µm to more than 6 µm in diameter, connect the pleural cavity with the subpleural lymphatic network and permit egress of material into the lymphatics from the pleural space. Wang (1985) has described focal accumulations of macrophages,

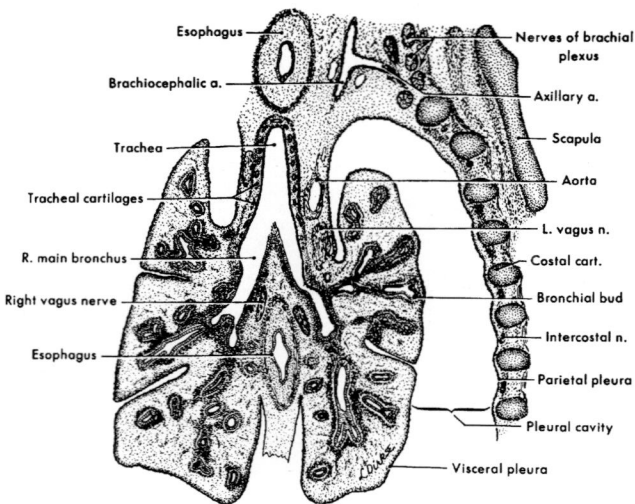

Esophagus

Brachiocephalic a.

Trachea

Tracheal cartilages

R. main bronchus

Right vagus nerve

Esophagus

Nerves of brachial plexus

Axillary a.

Scapula

Aorta

L. vagus n.

Costal cart.

Bronchial bud

Intercostal n.

Parietal pleura

Pleural cavity

Visceral pleura

Fig. 54-1. Frontal section through the developing lungs in an 8-week-old embryo. Projection drawing (original magnification ×25) from University of Michigan Collection, EH 352, CR 25 mm. From Patten BM: Human Embryology. 3rd Ed. New York: McGraw-Hill, 1968. With permission.

along with pluripotential mesenchymal, lymphoid, and plasma cells (called Kampmeier's foci) in the caudal portions of the mediastinal pleura that may be functionally related to the stomata.

GROSS ANATOMIC FEATURES

The visceral pleura is closely applied to the lung surfaces from the hila outward. It lines the major and minor fissures to the extent that each is developed; the minor fissure on the right may be incomplete to absent in 50% of humans. It also may delineate the various accessory fissures (see Chapter 5) when present. The pulmonary ligament, which extends caudad from each hilus to near the diaphragm, consists of two apposed layers of visceral (splanchnic) pleura and becomes continuous with the parietal pleura.

The visceral pleura adheres to the lung parenchyma. A naturally occurring cleavage plane is absent. When the visceral pleura is stripped from the lung parenchyma, a raw surface with innumerable air leaks, and at times small bleeding vessels, is left behind.

The parietal pleura lines the chest wall (the costal pleura), the mediastinum, and the diaphragm and forms the cupula or plural dome at the thoracic inlet bilaterally. The mediastinal pleura extends from the sternum ventrally to the thoracic spine dorsally and covers the mediastinal structures and the pericardium. The diaphragmatic pleura adheres tightly to the diaphragmatic tissues, and a cleavage plane between the two is basically nonexistent. Similarly, the mediastinal pleura is densely adherent to the pericardium. In contrast, the remainder of the mediastinal pleura, the pleura of the cupula, and the costal pleura can be readily dissected from the underly-

ing tissues. The plane of cleavage from the chest wall lies between the loose connective and fatty tissue layer and the endothoracic fascia attached to the underlying osseous, muscular, and vascular structures of the chest wall.

Topographically, the borders of the pleura are formed by continuity of the outer surface of costal, mediastinal, and diaphragmatic pleurae. A sharp anterior border of the pleura is defined along the line at which costal and mediastinal pleurae meet, subjacent to the sternum. The inferior border of the pleura is formed by the line of union between costal and diaphragmatic pleurae. The posterior border is outlined by the meeting of costal pleura with the posterior margin of mediastinal pleura near the thoracic vertebrae. The anterior reflection of mediastinal and costal pleurae forms a thin, sharp costomediastinal recess within the pleural sac. A similar recess, the costodiaphragmatic recess, formed at the base of the pleural sac by reflections of costal and diaphragmatic pleurae, may be related to overlying structures of the thoracic cage. The topographic localization of the anterior, inferior, and posterior borders of the pleura vary somewhat. The anterior pleural borders of the pulmonary cupulae are separated by visceral structures at the base of the neck. As they descend medially behind the sternum, they appose one another at the sternal angle and form the anterior mediastinal line seen on the chest radiograph in Figure 54-2. The right anterior border continues downward close to the midline. At the lower limits of the body of the sternum, it diverges laterally along the sixth or seventh costal cartilage to become the inferior pleural border. The left anterior pleural border may follow a similar course, but more commonly, it diverges laterally at the fourth costal cartilage, lies at the lateral sternal margin at the fifth, courses still further laterally at the sixth cartilage, and then diverges laterally with increasing severity at the seventh costal cartilage. The lateral displacement of the left anterior pleural border between the fourth and sixth costal cartilages forms the cardiac notch, or cardiac incisura. Radiographically, a lateral view demonstrates this area as a soft tissue shadow bounded by an interface between lung and the heart and adjacent fat. The interface has been termed the *retrosternal line* by Whalen and associates (1973).

The inferior borders of both pleural sacs diverge laterally along the seventh costal cartilage and then cross ribs eight, nine, and ten. They reach their lowest level at about the middle of the eleventh rib in the midaxillary line. From this point, they follow an almost horizontal course, cutting across the twelfth rib to meet the posterior pleural border at the twelfth thoracic vertebra. If the twelfth rib is short, the posterior pleural border may lie below it. In some individuals, as noted by Melnikoff (1923), the inferior border may be sufficiently high that it does not cross the twelfth rib at all, instead, it meets the posterior borders of the pleura at the eleventh thoracic vertebra.

The posterior pleural borders ascend alongside or in front of the bodies of thoracic vertebrae until they diverge superiorly near the pulmonary cupulae. They are rounded, in con-

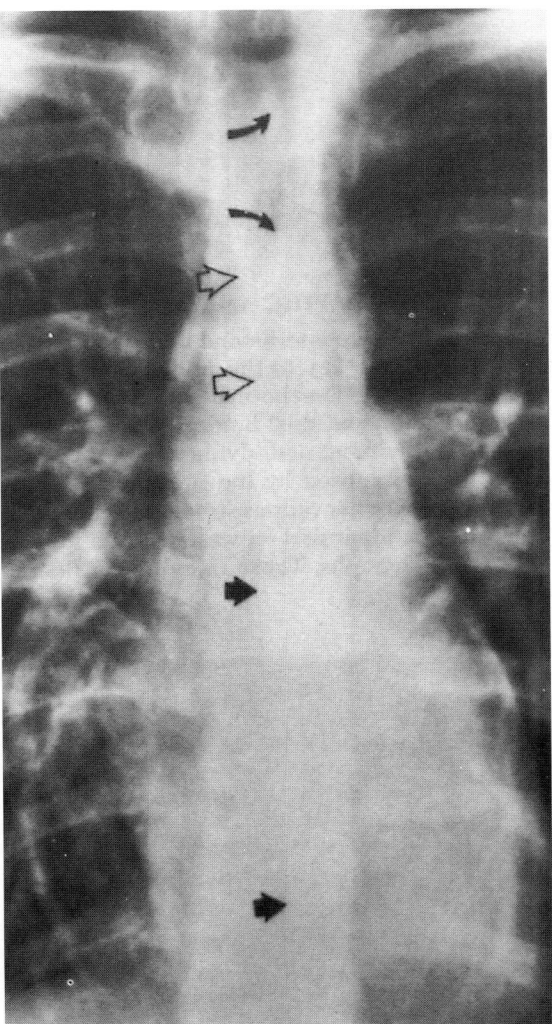

Fig. 54-2. Posteroanterior chest radiograph reveals the azygoesophageal recess, superior esophageal recess, and anterior mediastinal line. A slightly curved shadow convex to the right (*solid arrows*) projected in front of the thoracic spine from below the right main bronchus and extending down to just above the diaphragm is the azygoesophageal recess. Superiorly, a second curved linear shadow convex to the left (*curved arrows*) projected over the tracheal air column represents the superior esophagopleural recess. Between the two is a third linear shadow projected over the lower half of the tracheal air column (*open arrows*), representing the anterior mediastinal line. From Fraser RG, Pare JAP: Diagnosis of Diseases of the Chest. 2nd Ed. Philadelphia: WB Saunders, 1983. With permission.

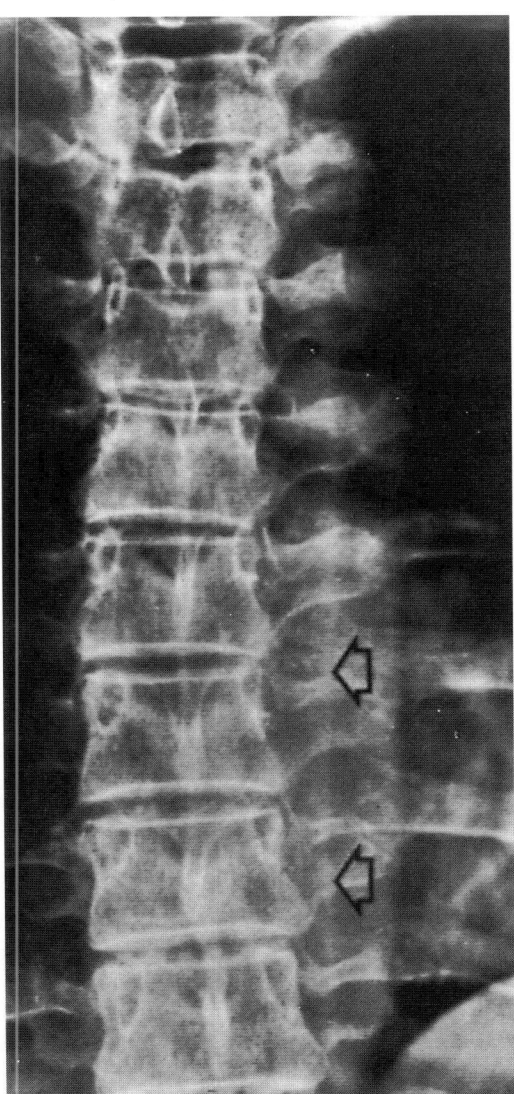

Fig. 54-3. Radiograph of the mediastinum (anteroposterior, with patient supine) reveals the longitudinal shadow (*arrows*) extending from the arch of the aorta to the diaphragm, representing the paraspinal line. From Fraser RG, Pare JAP: Diagnosis of Diseases of the Chest. 2nd Ed. Philadelphia: WB Saunders, 1983. With permission.

sophageal recess and the *superior esophageal recess* (see Fig. 54-2). The left paraspinal line, which also is frequently seen, is related to the reflection of the parietal pleura from the vertebral bodies over the descending aorta (Fig. 54-3). Fraser and colleagues (1989) discuss in detail the explanations for these lines as seen on radiographs of the chest.

BLOOD SUPPLY

The visceral pleura was believed to be supplied by both the bronchial and pulmonary arterial systems. The investigations of Albertine and associates (1982) in sheep, how-

trast to either anterior or inferior borders. Right and left posterior borders may be in close apposition in front of the vertebral bodies. Where this situation occurs, thin retroesophageal recesses are formed behind the esophagus and in front of the aorta and the hemiazygos and azygos veins.

As a result of these recesses, lines, usually two, are visible within the mediastinal contour on a well-exposed frontal chest radiograph. These lines have been termed the *azygoe-*

ever, revealed that the visceral pleural blood supply was entirely from the bronchial arterial system. There is no reason to believe it is otherwise in the human. Venous drainage is by way of the pulmonary veins. The blood supply to the parietal pleura is from the various systemic arterial vessels supplying the chest wall, diaphragm, and mediastinum and from vessels to the cupula from the subclavian arteries in the neck. Venous drainage is to the corresponding veins and, at times, directly into the superior vena cava.

LYMPHATIC DRAINAGE

The subpleural space of the visceral pleura has a large network of lymphatic channels, but only rarely is a subpleural lymph node identified. Trapnell (1964) reported the incidence of intrapulmonary lymph nodes to be 18%, but no nodes were found in a subpleural location. Greenberg (1961), however, described a lymph node in this location that was removed surgically because it had been identified radiographically as a coin lesion.

The lymphatic drainage of the visceral pleura is primarily to the deep pulmonary plexus located in the interlobar and peribronchial spaces. Riquet and associates (1989), however, described direct subpleural lymphatic connections to the mediastinal nodes in approximately 22 to 25% of lung segments studied. These subpleural connections were present more often in the upper lobes than in the lower lobes.

The lymphatic drainage of the parietal pleura is into the parietal pleural lymphatic channels. The aforementioned stomata and Kampmeier's foci play important roles in this process. The lymphatic networks of the chest wall drain into the internal mammary chain anteriorly and the intercostal chain posteriorly. The drainage of the diaphragmatic pleura is to the retrosternal and mediastinal lymph nodes as well as to the celiac lymph nodes in the abdomen.

NERVE SUPPLY

The parietal pleura is innervated by both somatic and sympathetic and parasympathetic fibers via the intercostal nerves. The diaphragmatic pleura is supplied by the phrenic nerves. The visceral pleura is devoid of somatic innervation.

REFERENCES

Albertine KH, et al: Structure, blood supply, and lymphatic vessels of the sheep's visceral pleura. Am J Anat *165*:277, 1982.

Antony VB, et al: Pleural cell biology in health and disease. Am Rev Respir Dis *145*:1236, 1992.

Bolen JW, Hammer SP, McNutt MA: Reactive and neoplastic serosal tissue. A light microscopic, ultrastructural, and immunocytochemical study. Am J Surg Pathol *10*:34, 1986.

Chretien J, Huchon GJ: New contributions to the understanding of pleural space structure and junction. *In* Deslauriers J, Lacquet LK (eds): Thoracic Surgery: Surgical Management of Pleural Diseases. International Trends in General Thoracic Surgery. Vol 6. St. Louis: CV Mosby, 1990.

Dervan PA, Tobin B, O'Connor M: Solitary (localized) fibrous mesothelioma: evidence against mesothelial cell origin. Histopathology *10*:867, 1986.

England DM, Hochholzer L, McCarthy MJ: Localized benign and malignant fibrous tumors of the pleura. A clinicopathologic review of 223 cases. Am J Surg Pathol *13*:640, 1989.

Fraser RG, et al: Diagnosis of Diseases of the Chest. 3rd Ed. Philadelphia: WB Saunders, 1989.

Greenberg HB: Benign subpleural lymph node appearing as a pulmonary "coin" lesion. Radiology *77*:97, 1961.

Hammer SP: Pleural diseases. *In* Dail DH, Hammer SP, Colby TV (eds): Pulmonary Pathology—Tumors. New York: Springer-Verlag, 1995, p. 405.

Keating S, et al: Solitary fibrous tumor of the pleura: An ultrastructural and immunohistochemical study. Thorax *42*:976, 1978.

Melnikoff A: Die chirurgische Anatomie des Sinus costodiaphragmaticus. Arch Klin Chir Berl *123*:133, 1923.

Patten BM: Human Embryology. New York: McGraw-Hill, 1968, pp. 87, 406.

Riquet M, Hidden G, Debesse B: Direct lymphatic drainage of lung segments to the mediastinal nodes. An anatomic study on 260 adults. J Thorac Cardiovasc Surg *97*:623, 1989.

Said JW, et al: Localized fibrous mesothelioma: an immunohistochemical and electron microscopic study. Hum Pathol *15*:440, 1984.

Staub NC, Wiener-Kronish JP, Albertine KM: Transport through the pleura: Physiology of normal liquid and solute exchange in the pleural space. *In* Chretien J, Bignon J, Hirsch A (eds): The Pleura in Health and Disease. New York: Marcel Dekker, 1985, pp. 169–193.

Trapnell DH: Recognition and incidence of intrapulmonary lymph nodes. Thorax *19*:44, 1964.

Wang NS: Morphological data of the pleura: Normal conditions. *In* Chretien J, Hirsch A (eds): Diseases of the Pleura. Paris: Masson, 1982, pp. 10–24.

Wang NS: Mesothelial cells in situ. *In* Chretien J, Bignon J, Hirsch J (eds): The Pleura in Health and Disease. New York: Marcel Dekker, 1985, pp. 23-24.

Whalen JP, et al: The retrosternal line: A new sign of an anterior mediastinal mass. AJR Am J Roentgenol *117*:861, 1973.

CHAPTER 55

Resorption of Gases from the Pleural Space

Yvon Cormier

Under normal circumstances, there are no free gases in the pleural space. A variety of conditions, however, can lead to the accumulation of gases in this cavity. Because the virtual space between the parietal and visceral pleura is under negative pressure, any communication with the surrounding structures (bronchi, alveoli, extrathoracic communication through the chest wall) immediately causes gases to enter the pleural space (i.e., produce a pneumothorax). The pressure in the pleural space is negative in relation to the atmosphere because of the elastic properties of the lungs, which tend to collapse, and that of the chest wall, which, at volumes below 75% of the total lung capacity, tends to expand. In normal individuals, at functional residual capacity when respiratory muscles of the thoracic wall are in the relaxed state, this pressure is approximately 5 cm/H_2O lower than that of the surrounding atmosphere. This pressure further decreases during inspiration, especially in the presence of airway obstruction. During a Müller maneuver (i.e., maximal inspiratory efforts against a closed glottis) pleural pressure can transiently become negative, to lower than 100 cm/H_2O.

When gases enter the pleural space, pressure gradients and the physical laws of gases favor their eventual resorption.

FACTORS DETERMINING GAS RESORPTION

Gas resorption from the pleural space is achieved by a simple diffusion from the pleural space into the venous blood. This diffusion, which can occur in both directions, is possible because the pleura and capillary walls are permeable to gases and because the partial pressures of gases in the pleural space and those in the venous blood can differ. For example, a positive pressure gradient between the gases in the pneumothorax and those dissolved in the venous blood would favor the passage of those gases from the pneumothorax into the venous blood. No active transport mechanisms for gas resorption exist; the only driving forces that determine gas resorption are pressure gradients.

The rate of gas resorption depends on four variables: 1) diffusion properties of the gases present in the pleural space; 2) the pressure gradients for the gases in the pleural space in relation to the venous blood; 3) the area of contact between the pleural gas and the pleura; and 4) permeability of the pleural surface (e.g., a thickened fibrotic pleura absorbs less than a normal pleura).

Because the solubility and diffusion properties of different gases vary considerably, the speed of resorption depends on the type of gas involved. For example, oxygen is resorbed 62 times faster than nitrogen (N_2). Water vapor (H_2O) and carbon dioxide (CO_2) equilibrate almost instantaneously, CO_2 being 23 times more soluble than O_2.

Depending on the clinical situation, a pneumothorax can initially contain room air (i.e., a leak from the outside) or alveolar air (i.e., a leak through the lungs). The alveolar air contains different proportions of CO_2, O_2, or N_2, depending on the ventilation of the patient and the presence of supplemental O_2 given to the patient at the time of the leak into the pleural space. If a patient is receiving 100% O_2, the pleural gases will be composed mostly of this gas and contain no N_2, the slowest gas to be resorbed. Initial gas compositions in a pneumothorax when the air entry is room air or alveolar air with the patient breathing room air or 100% O_2 are presented in Figure 55-1.

PARTIAL PRESSURE OF GASES IN VENOUS BLOOD

Because pressure gradients that favor gas resorption are those between the pneumothorax and those in the venous blood, it is also important to consider the venous blood partial gas pressures. Under normal circumstances, the total gas pressure in a pneumothorax is within a few millimeters of mercury of that of the atmosphere (760 mm Hg), whereas that in the venous blood is 702 mm Hg, 58 mm Hg lower. This positive pressure gradient between the pneumothorax

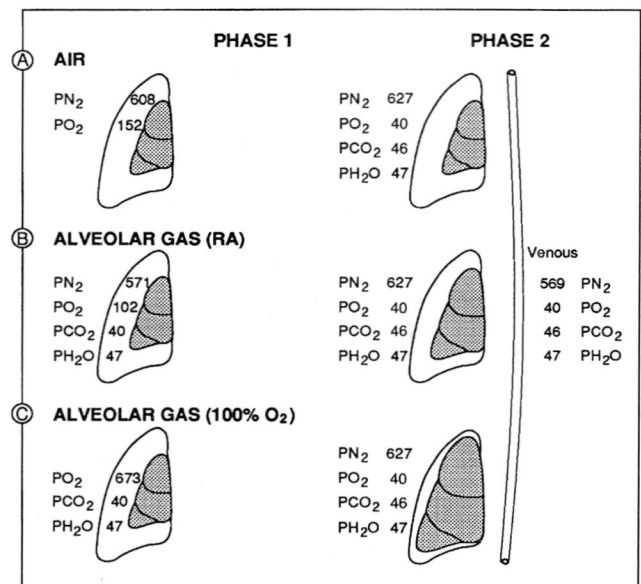

Fig. 55-1. Gas partial pressures initially present in a pneumothorax when air entry comes from room air (**A**); alveoli, subject breathing room air (RA) (**B**); and alveoli, subject breathing 100% O_2 (**C**). After equilibration (phase 1) the resulting gas partial pressures become identical regardless of the initial gas composition. Note that the volume change of the pneumothorax during phase 1 is least when the pneumothorax was initially constituted with room air; intermediate when with alveolar air, patient breathing room air; and much greater when the patient was breathing 100% O_2.

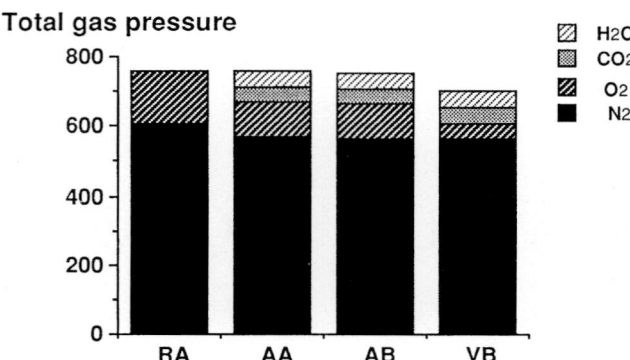

Fig. 55-2. The total and partial gas pressures in room air (RA), alveolar air (AA), arterial blood (AB), and in venous blood (VB). The total pressure for RA and AA is the same, whereas a small total pressure decrease occurs between AA and AB (7 mm Hg) and a further, more significant decrease is seen between AB and VB (51 mm Hg). The difference between RA and VB therefore equals 58 mm Hg.

and the venous blood constitutes the driving force responsible for gas resorption from a pneumothorax.

MECHANISMS OF THE GAS PRESSURE GRADIENTS BETWEEN THE PNEUMOTHORAX AND THE VENOUS BLOOD

A schematic approach is used here to explain the gas composition in venous blood. Dry room air contains, for all practical purposes, 80% N_2 and 20% O_2. Other gases (e.g., CO_2, argon, and so forth) are of minute quantities. The normal atmospheric pressure is 760 mm Hg (1031 cm/H_2O); therefore, the partial pressure of N_2 in dry room air is 608 mm Hg, whereas that of O_2 is 152 mm Hg. When room air enters the alveoli, it gains H_2O vapor and CO_2 and loses O_2; the resulting gas composition is now N_2 = 571 mm Hg, O_2 = 102 mm Hg, H_2O = 47 mm Hg, and CO_2 = 40 mm Hg. The alveoli being in close communication with the atmosphere, the total gas pressure at this level must equal 760 mm Hg. This alveolar gas composition is in contact with the blood at the alveolar capillary level, and gas exchange occurs. The resulting normal arterial gas composition is PaO_2 = 97 mm Hg, $PaCO_2$ = 40 mm Hg, and PaN_2 = 569 mm Hg, water vapor remains constant at 47 mm Hg;

the total arterial gas pressure is 753 mm Hg. Note that a 7-mm Hg pressure gradient exists between the alveolar gas pressure and that of the arterial blood. Our cells consume O_2 and produce CO_2, consuming 300 mL of O_2 for 240 mL of CO_2 produced, a respiratory quotient of 0.8. Despite this small difference between the quantity of O_2 consumed compared with that of CO_2 produced, the metabolic changes increase the $PaCO_2$ by 6 mm Hg and decrease that of oxygen by 57 mm Hg in its passage through the capillaries from the arterial to the venous system. This large difference in the changes in O_2 and CO_2 partial pressures is caused by the difference in the solubility and transport capacity of the blood for these two gases. N_2 is not metabolized and therefore remains unchanged between the arterial and venous blood. Water vapor also remains constant at 47 mm Hg. The resulting venous gas pressure is therefore $P\bar{v}O_2$ = 40 mm Hg, $P\bar{v}CO_2$ = 46 mm Hg, $P\bar{v}N_2$ = 569 mm Hg, $P\bar{v}H_2O$ = 47 mm Hg, for a total gas pressure of 702 mm Hg (i.e., 51 mm Hg less than that in the arterial blood and 58 mm Hg less than that of alveolar or room air total gas pressures). A schematic summary of gas pressures from room air to the venous blood is given in Figure 55-2. A pneumothorax results because of a communication between the pleural cavity and the atmosphere, either via the thoracic wall or the lung. Because of this communication, the initial gas pressure in a pneumothorax equals that of the atmosphere at 760 mm Hg, thus creating a 58-mm Hg gradient between the two.

PHASES OF GAS RESORPTION

There are two phases in the gas resorption from the pleural space: phase 1, equilibration of gases partial pressures, and phase 2, constant resorption.

Phase 1: Equilibration

The first phase represents the equilibration of gases initially placed into the pleural cavity with that of venous blood. Its duration and the amount of gas resorbed during this phase depends on the composition of the initial gases in the pneumothorax. The second phase is the constant resorption rate that follows once the equilibration has occurred.

Regardless of the quality of gases initially in the pneumothorax, the first phase results in an equilibrating period, after which the composition of the remaining gases in the pneumothorax are all similar in all situations. It follows, therefore, that gases can enter or leave the pleural cavity as this equilibration takes place. If the initial pneumothorax contained 100% O_2, the N_2 partial pressure would be greater in the venous blood than in the pleural cavity; in this condition the N_2 gradient favors N_2 to leave the venous blood and enter the pleural space. However, because O_2 is more soluble, more O_2 leaves the pleural cavity than N_2 will enter. Therefore, the total quantity of gases in the pleural cavity decreases, despite ingoing N_2. If one filled a pleural cavity with 100% N_2, the initial phase of equilibration would produce an increase in the quantity of gases in the pneumothorax because more O_2 and CO_2 would enter the cavity than N_2 would leave. The gas composition at equilibrium is determined by the partial pressures of gases in the venous blood. At this time, the gas composition in the remaining pneumothorax is the same, regardless of the composition of the initial gas. The following can be different: the volume resorbed during the equilibrating phase (see Fig. 55-1), the greater the quantity of the more soluble gases and the greater the gradient between the pleural space and the venous blood, the faster the resorption. The high solubility and resorption rate of CO_2 is the reason this gas is infused into the abdominal cavity for laparoscopy.

If a patient receives supplemental O_2 for more than 2 or 3 minutes, the P_{N_2} in the alveoli and in the blood decrease proportionally. For example, if a subject received 50% O_2, the partial pressure of N_2 would decrease in the alveolar air, and subsequently in the venous blood, from 569 to approximately 350 mm Hg. Because the $P\bar{v}_{O_2}$ does not increase significantly with an increase of inspired O_2, the pressure gradient between a pneumothorax would be greatly increased in such a situation, from 58 to 277 mm Hg in this case.

Phase 2: Constant Resorption

If all gases in the pleural space were at equilibrium with the venous gas pressure, the intrapleural total gas pressure would be $O_2 + CO_2 + H_2O + N_2 = 702$ mm Hg, or 58 mm Hg less than atmosphere. Such a negative pleural pressure (58 mm Hg) is impossible on a long-term basis.

CLINICAL SITUATIONS OF PNEUMOTHORACES

Three potential situations of pneumothoraces result in different behavior of gas resorption from the pleural cavity. The pneumothorax can behave as 1) a closed rigid cavity, 2) a closed collapsible cavity, and 3) an open cavity. Clinical conditions and mechanisms of gas resorption under these three conditions are discussed separately.

Closed Rigid Cavity

In theory, a closed rigid pneumothorax (e.g., non–reexpandable lung) could remain air filled. As gases are resorbed along each gas partial pressure as previously described, the pressure inside the pleural space would progressively decrease until it stabilizes at a pressure of 58 mm Hg lower than the atmosphere. At this negative pressure, no pressure gradient remains to ensure continued resorption. Although such a negative pleural pressure is possible on a short-term basis, if this negative pressure is maintained, fluid eventually seeps into the pleural cavity and gradually fills it with liquid, which subsequently solidifies and fibroses. Permanent residual pneumothorax equals a persistent opening as, for example, a bronchopleural fistula.

Closed Collapsible Cavity

This situation is by far the most frequent form of pneumothorax. This condition occurs when gases enter the pleural space, the opening responsible for the pneumothorax becomes occluded, and the lungs are freely reexpandable. As gases are resorbed, no new gases enter the pleural space, and the reexpansion of the lungs compensates for the volume of resorbed gases, therefore preventing the appearance of negative intrapleural pressure. All gases eventually are resorbed, and the lungs take their normal place, leaving no physical pleural cavity.

As the intrapleural gas pressure tends to decrease as a result of gas resorption, the lung reexpands, and the amount of air in the pleural cavity progressively decreases until it is all resorbed. At the so-called equilibrium, therefore, O_2, CO_2, and H_2O partial pressures are similar in the venous blood and in the pleural cavity. The slower N_2, however, is 58 mm Hg higher in the pleural cavity, which is at or close to atmospheric pressure, than that in the venous blood, which is 58 mm Hg subatmospheric. The decreasing volume of the pneumothorax prevents large intrapleural negative pressures and ensures the persistence of this positive partial pressure gradient between gases in the pleural cavity and the venous blood. The intrapleural pressure is not allowed to decrease to −58 mm Hg, as in a closed rigid cavity, where such a gradient would no longer exist and all gas resorption would cease. The time required to absorb all gases in a pneumothorax is quite variable and depends on previously described characteristics. It has been estimated that 6% of a pneumothorax is absorbed in 24 hours.

Open Cavity

As long as the communication between the pleural cavity and the lung or through the thoracic wall persists, the lung does not reexpand because all absorbed gases are replenished from the outside. In this condition, gases in the pleural space are resorbed as for the closed cavity; however, the gases resorbed are determined by what is returned into the pleural cavity. Because the composition of pleural gases remains constant, what comes in is what is resorbed. For example, if the pleural cavity is opened to the outside, O_2 and N_2 are resorbed at a proportion of 20:80, corresponding to the gas composition of dry room air.

EFFECTS OF BAROMETRIC PRESSURE ON PLEURAL GASES

People living at different altitudes live in different barometric pressures (e.g., the barometric pressure at 11,000 feet above sea level is 500 mm Hg compared with 760 mm Hg at sea level). However, the gas fractions in the atmosphere always remain the same, regardless of the altitude. For an atmospheric pressure of 500 mm Hg, the P_{N_2} in the atmosphere would be 400 mm Hg and the P_{O_2} would be 100 mm Hg, dry air. Changes in these gas pressures from room air to the venous blood would follow the same principle as when the atmospheric pressure is 760 mm Hg. At 11,000 feet, the arterial pressure of O_2 would be approximately 60 mm Hg and that of venous blood not significantly different from that at sea level (40 mm Hg), giving an arterial to venous oxygen pressure decrease of only 20 mm Hg compared with 51 mm Hg at sea level. Because the O_2 decrease between arterial and venous blood is the major cause of the lower total gas pressure in the venous blood and the eventual N_2 gradient between the venous blood and gases in a pneumothorax at equilibrium, this N_2 gradient would therefore be much smaller at this high altitude. Such differences in pressure gradients would decrease the rate of N_2 resorption.

Although the proportions of different gases do not change with changing barometric pressures, the volume occupied by a given quantity of gases does. For example, a pneumothorax of 1-L volume would increase by 33% if the patient was transported in an airplane pressurized at 8000 feet, which is common practice. If a pneumothorax developed in a deep sea diver at 30 feet below the surface, the volume of the pneumothorax would double as the diver resurfaces, and this when no new gases enter the pleural space.

THERAPEUTIC CONSIDERATIONS

The dynamics of gas resorption from the pleural space can be used clinically. A potential application is to give 100% O_2 to a patient during a maneuver that is at risk of creating a pneumothorax. A typical example for which this is useful is transthoracic lung biopsy. When 100% O_2 is given during the procedure, any resulting pneumothorax resorbs much faster for two reasons: 1) The pneumothorax is filled with the more soluble O_2; and 2) the pressure gradient between the pneumothorax and the venous blood is larger, because giving 100% O_2 washes out N_2 from the alveoli and eventually the venous blood. Giving 100% O_2 to a patient when the pneumothorax is already in place also increases the rate of gas resorption by decreasing $P\bar{v}_{N_2}$ and therefore increasing the pressure gradient for this gas between the pneumothorax and the venous blood. This beneficial effect, however, is relatively small and probably not clinically useful.

READING REFERENCES

Cormier Y, Laviolette M, Tardif A: Prevention of pneumothorax in needle lung biopsy by breathing 100% oxygen. Thorax 35:37, 1980.
Dale WA, Rahn H: Rate of gas absorption during atelectasis. Am J Physiol 170:606, 1952.
Kircher LT, Swartzel RL: Spontaneous pneumothorax and its treatment. JAMA 155:24, 1954.
Loring SH, Butler JP: Gas exchange in body cavities. In Fishman AP, Farhi LE, Tenney MR (eds): Handbook of Physiology. Section 3. The Respiratory System. Washington, DC: American Physiological Society, 1987, p. 238.
Piiper J: Physiological equilibria of gas cavities in the body. In Fenn NO, Rahn H (eds): Handbook of Physiology. Vol. 2. Respiration. Washington, DC: American Physiological Society, 1965, p. 1205.

CHAPTER 56

Pneumothorax

Willard A. Fry and Kerry Paape

Pneumothorax or air in the chest is a phenomenon that has been appreciated since ancient time and has been well discussed by Seremetis (1970), Lindskog and Halasz (1957), Killen and Gobbel (1968), Gobbel and associates (1963), and Kittle (1986). Hippocrates and Galen were aware of disease processes involving the pleural space. Adams (1960) notes that Vesalius, in the sixteenth century, was aware of the necessity for positive-pressure inflation of the trachea to keep the lungs expanded once the pressure seal of the pleural space had been broken. It was not until the nineteenth century, however, that physicians began to appreciate the various subtleties of disease in the pleural space. The development of the stethoscope by Laënnec and the development of radiology by Roentgen brought great advances in the diagnosis of intrathoracic disease. By 1898, John B. Murphy, in Chicago, stimulated by his European colleagues, wrote about the use of artificial pneumothorax in the treatment of pulmonary tuberculosis. The designation of tuberculosis as the primary etiologic agent for spontaneous pneumothorax was finally put to rest by Kjaergaard in 1932.

The thoracic surgeon is called to treat pneumothorax on a regular basis, and the most common presentations are primary spontaneous and secondary after medical procedures. In some areas, pneumothorax associated with *Pneumocystis carinii* pneumonia is unusually common. Controversy continues over the best method to treat pneumothorax. The explosive development of thoracoscopy in the 1990s and the availability of purified talc have fueled the controversies. Some of the most heated debates in current medical literature involve treatment programs for spontaneous pneumothorax. In this chapter, we describe the means that we find the most practical and useful and list alternatives that we consider appropriate.

ETIOLOGY

The most common cause of primary spontaneous pneumothorax is the rupture of an apical subpleural bleb (Fig.

56-1). The etiology of such blebs is obscure. Some authors have postulated a difference in alveolar pressure in the upright human between the base and the apex of the lung. In the absence of an associated disorder, spontaneous pneumothorax is rarely seen before puberty. It is more common in men than in women by a ratio of 6:1, and it is more common in smokers than in nonsmokers, as described by Lindskog and Halasz (1957) and Bense (1987) and Sadikot (1997) and their associates. The typical patient with a spontaneous pneumothorax is a young, tall, thin man in late adolescence or early adulthood who experiences the sudden onset of chest pain and shortness of breath and who has not been engaging in any unusual or strenuous activity. This clinical picture is in contrast to that of the rarer condition of spontaneous pneumomediastinum, which is invariably associated with strenuous exertion, such as bench-press weight lifting. Children who present with spontaneous pneumothorax often have an underlying condition, such as cystic fibrosis, as described by Wilcox and colleagues (1995).

The causes of pneumothorax are listed in Table 56-1. Special mention must be made of secondary spontaneous pneumothorax associated with acquired immunodeficiency syndrome (AIDS) because it is prevalent in certain centers, as described by Beers and colleagues (1990). Sepkowitz (1991), Coker (1993), Shanley (1991), and Renzi (1992) and their associates have raised the question of its precipitation by pentamidine aerosol. Wait and Dal Nogare (1994), Metersky (1995), and Pastores (1996) and their associates emphasize the gravity of spontaneous pneumothorax in AIDS patients with *Pneumocystis* pneumonia.

The most common sarcomas contributing to pneumothorax are osteosarcoma and synovial sarcomas, as described by Dines and coworkers in 1973. Special mention is made of spontaneous rupture of the esophagus, for if it presents as pneumothorax without gastrointestinal symptoms, and if the diagnosis is not suspected, an unfavorable outcome is virtually certain. The physician should be alerted by the nature of the accompanying pleural fluid. In the instances of pneu-

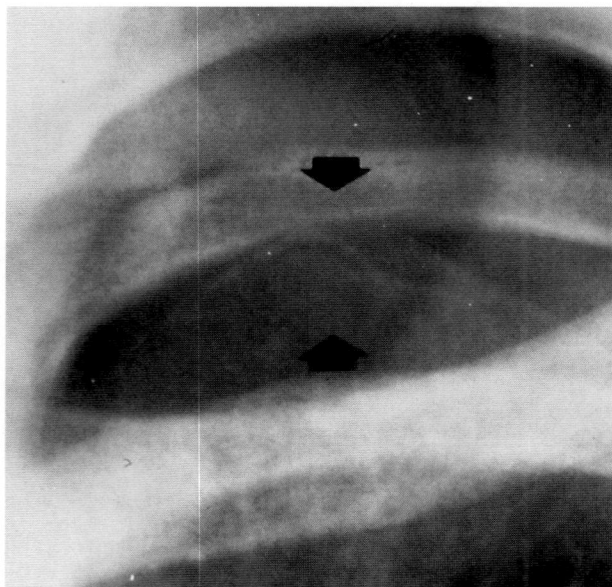

Fig. 56-1. Apical subpleural blebs (*arrows*) in a male adolescent with a recurrent spontaneous pneumothorax.

Table 56-1. Classification of Pneumothorax

Spontaneous
  Primary
    Subpleural bleb rupture
  Secondary
    Bullous disease, including chronic obstructive pulmonary
      disease
    Cystic fibrosis
    Spontaneous rupture of the esophagus
    Marfan's syndrome
    Eosinophilic granuloma
    Pneumocystis carinii, especially in patients with acquired
      immunodeficiency disease
    Metastatic cancer, especially sarcoma
    Pneumonia with lung abscess
    Catamenial
    Asthma, secondary to mucous plugging
    Lung cancer
    Lymphangioleiomyomatosis
  Neonatal
Acquired
  Iatrogenic
    Subclavian (percutaneous) catheterization
      Central lines
      Pacemaker insertion
    Transthoracic needle biopsy
    Transbronchial lung biopsy
    Thoracocentesis
    Chest tube malfunction
    After laparoscopic surgery
  Barotrauma
  Traumatic
    Blunt trauma
      Motor vehicle accidents
      Falls
      Sports-related
    Penetrating trauma
      Gunshot wounds
      Stab wounds

mothorax associated with asthma and mucus plugs, the postulated mechanism is obstructive atelectasis of one lobe or segment with hyperinflation of other portions of the lung and resultant parenchymal disruption (Fig. 56-2).

Spontaneous pneumothorax occurring in patients with established chronic obstructive pulmonary disease (COPD), especially with bulla formation, is troublesome. These patients tolerate even small degrees of collapse poorly, and they should be treated aggressively rather than by observation, as described by Dines and colleagues in 1970. This group of patients is discussed in detail in Chapter 83. Spontaneous pneumothorax complicating cystic fibrosis is treated differently because of the development of effective bipulmonary lung transplantation, described by Pasque and associates (1990). Whereas in years past, obliteration of the pleural space in cystic fibrosis patients prone to spontaneous pneumothorax was a high priority, less aggressive therapy is now being recommended to facilitate an easier operative field for the lung transplant surgeon.

Shearin (1974), Maurer (1968), and Lillington (1972) and their colleagues have described catamenial pneumothorax, or pneumothorax that occurs—and recurs—during the first 3 days of menses. Fleisher and associates (1990) have reviewed the possible causes of this problem. In the classic descriptions, nonovulatory states, such as pregnancy and oral contraceptive use, were not associated with pneumothorax. We have encountered primary spontaneous pneumothorax complicating pregnancy more often than catamenial pneumothorax. This has also been described by Dhalla and Teskey (1985) and Van Winter (1996).

Spontaneous pneumothorax may occur as a rare manifestation of lung cancer. Steinhauslin and Cuttat (1985) described the possible mechanisms. They also noted that lung cancer is estimated to cause only 0.03 to 0.05% of cases of spontaneous pneumothorax. Another rare cause of spontaneous pneumothorax is lymphangioleiomyomatosis, which is seen in young women (see Chapter 111).

Pneumothorax in the neonatal period tends to be treated by the neonatologist and is listed only for completeness. Colombani and Haller (1990) presented a review of this subject.

Acquired pneumothorax is most often iatrogenic, except in institutions with a high incidence of civilian trauma. The placement of central lines and pacemakers by percutaneous subclavian vein catheterization, transthoracic needle biopsy, thoracocentesis, and transbronchoscopic lung biopsy are all frequent causes of pneumothorax. Many are directly related to physician experience, but the risk of inducing pneumothorax from such procedures is always present. Breathing high concentrations of oxygen before

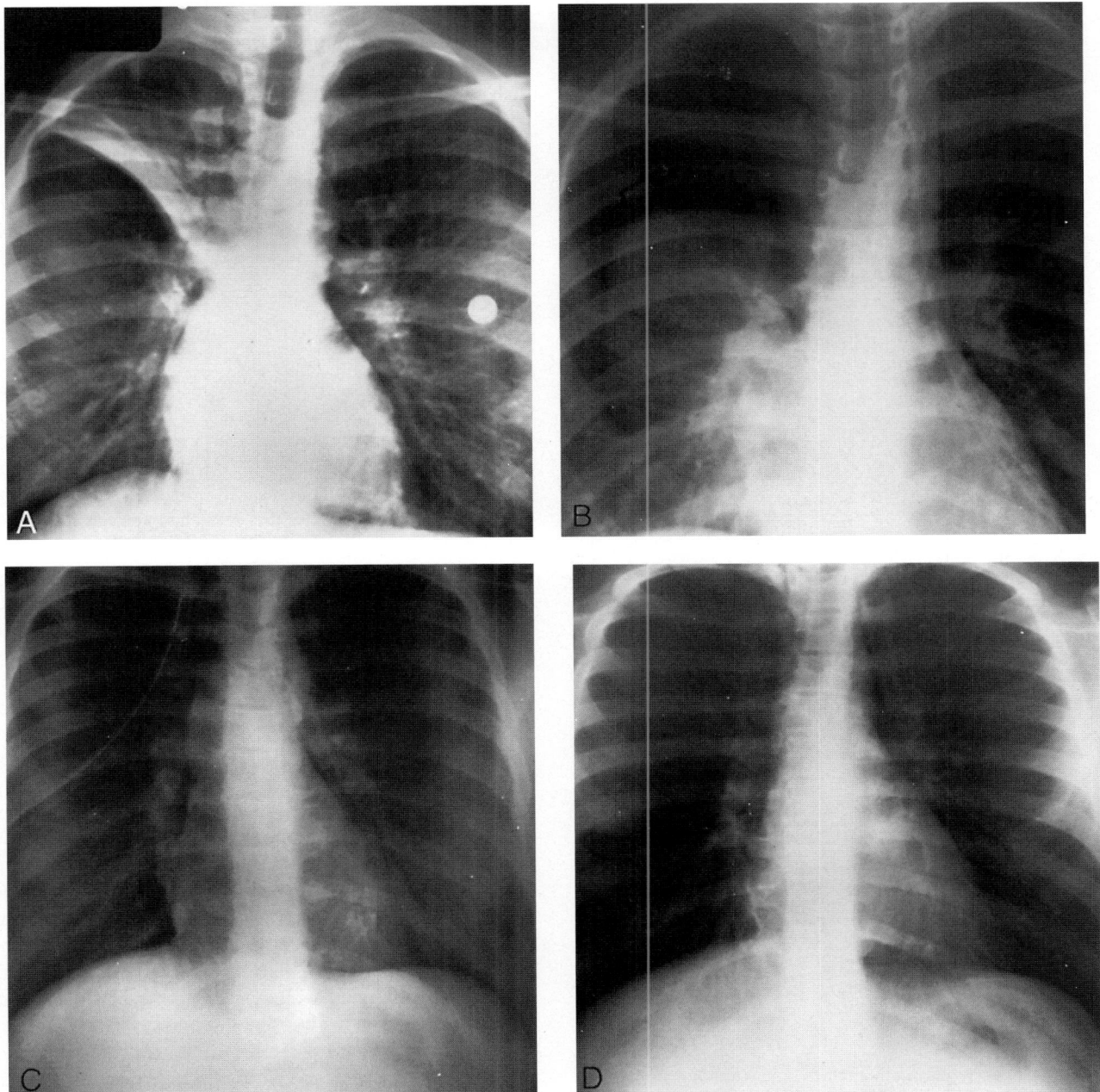

Fig. 56-2. Pneumothorax complicating asthma in a 12-year-old girl. **A.** Right upper lobe atelectasis (*arrow*) attributed to mucous plugs. **B.** Pneumothorax attributed to overdistention of nonatelectatic lung. **C.** Reexpansion of the lung by tube thoracostomy with clearing of the atelectasis. **D.** Continued reexpansion of the lung after chest tube removal.

transthoracic needle procedures has been recommended (see Chapter 55). Farn and associates (1993) described pneumothorax during laparoscopic surgery as a sequela of previous transdiaphragmatic surgical intervention. Another cause of pneumothorax that is often overlooked is chest tube dysfunction attributable to inadequately sophisticated medical personnel. Such situations include not refilling a water seal bottle with the appropriate amount of water, not filling the U-manometer in the Pleur-evac type of chest

drainage systems, and not adequately securing a chest tube to the chest drainage system tubing, thereby permitting the occasional disconnection, with resulting potential for an open pneumothorax.

Barotrauma pneumothorax is defined as that occurring in a patient receiving positive-pressure ventilation. It is always treated by intervention rather than observation because patients relying on mechanical ventilation are already in a compromised state and the positive airway pressure result-

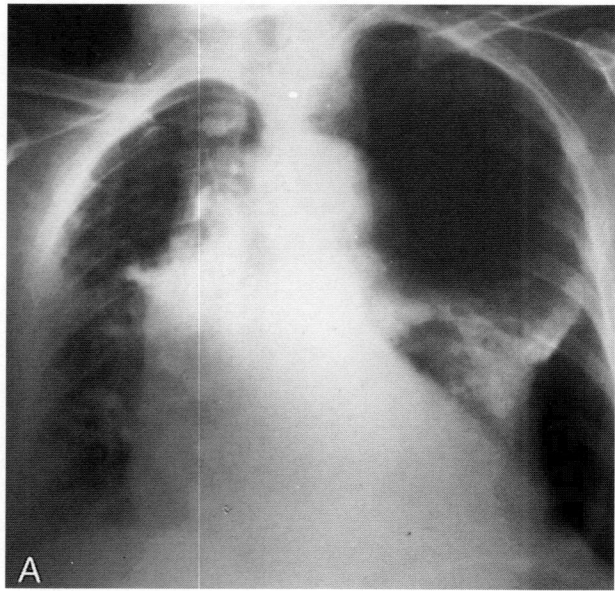

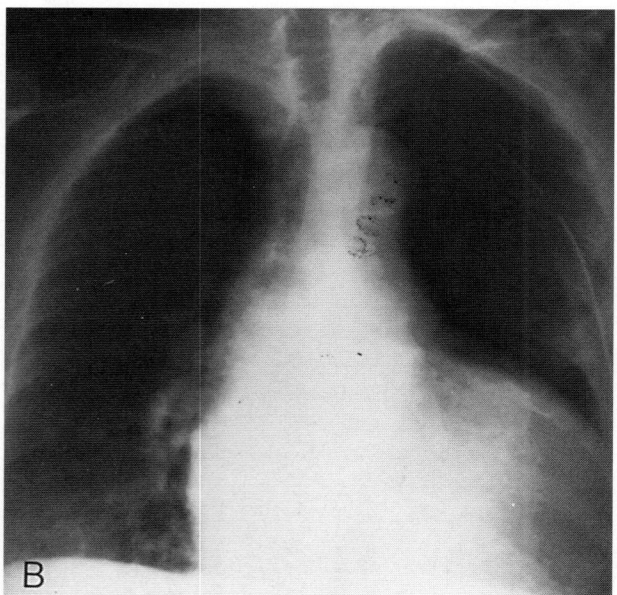

Fig. 56-3. Tension pneumothorax in a 72-year-old woman. It resulted from a focal bulla and eventually required surgical treatment. **A.** Shift of the mediastinum to the right side. A single adhesion kept part of the lung fixed to the chest wall. **B.** Prompt resolution of the pneumothorax with tube thoracostomy. Note return of the mediastinum to its normal position.

ing from the mechanical ventilation is a "setup" for tension pneumothorax. Barotrauma pneumothorax is often attributed to areas of the lung that become overdistended during mechanical ventilation as other areas are consolidated and poorly ventilated. As a general rule, any barotrauma pneumothorax is an indication for tube thoracostomy, as discussed by Kirby and Ginsberg (1992). This topic is discussed in more detail in Chapter 71.

Traumatic pneumothorax resulting from either blunt or penetrative chest trauma is dealt with in Chapter 70. We urge the placement of a chest tube for traumatic pneumothorax of whatever size whenever there is any other associated injury because the prompt reexpansion of the collapsed lung immediately eliminates a treatment variable for that patient. Contact sports, such as football and hockey, occasionally produce a sports-related pneumothorax, as reported by Partridge and associates (1997), in the absence of a detectable rib fracture.

PRESENTATION

The symptoms of spontaneous pneumothorax are the sudden onset of chest pain, shortness of breath, and cough. They can be mild or severe. True tension pneumothorax is relatively uncommon, but it is accompanied by tachycardia, sweating, hypotension, and a pallor that are striking and that result from mediastinal shift, reduced preload, and intense stimulation of the sympathetic nervous system (Fig. 56-3). As previously mentioned, the usual primary spontaneous pneumothorax occurs without warning or precipitating activity. As the lung collapses, the leak is usually obliterated, thereby limiting the amount of collapse and the progression to tension pneumothorax.

The physical findings of a pneumothorax usually vary with the amount of collapse. If the collapse is significant, findings include diminished tactile fremitus, hyperresonance to percussion, and decreased breath sounds on the affected side. In instances of mild collapse, physical findings can be misleadingly normal, so that if the history suggests pneumothorax and yet the physical examination is normal, a chest radiograph should be obtained. In instances of tension pneumothorax, the aforementioned classic physical findings are accentuated and accompanied by a tracheal shift, on palpation of the trachea in the suprasternal notch, to the uninvolved side. A clinical diagnosis of tension pneumothorax made on the basis of appropriate history and physical findings is adequate to allow for the emergency placement of a chest tube without preliminary confirmatory chest radiography, if the clinical situation so demands, and we so instruct our students and house staff.

DIAGNOSIS

The chest radiograph is the standard procedure in making the diagnosis of a pneumothorax. It should be upright and preferably in the posteroanterior projection. It is possible to miss a pneumothorax in a semisupine portable anteroposterior view. If the patient cannot be upright, a lateral decubitus view with the suspect side positioned up may be helpful. Radiographs obtained in exhalation may accentuate the pneumothorax, but we have not found this technique useful enough in most clinical situations to warrant the double radi-

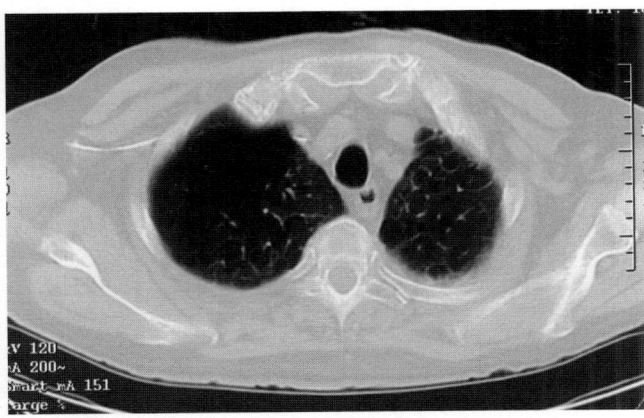

Fig. 56-4. Computed tomographic scan of the lungs of a 72-year-old man with extensive bullous disease who presented with a spontaneous pneumothorax.

Table 56-2. Treatment Options for Pneumothorax

Observation
Needle aspiration
Percutaneous catheter to drainage
    Water-seal or Pleur-evac type
    Heimlich valve
Tube thoracostomy
    Water-seal or Pleur-evac
    Heimlich valve
Tube thoracostomy with instillation of pleural irritant
Video-assisted thoracic surgery
Thoracotomy

ographic exposure (see Fig. 56-7B). Rhea and colleagues (1982) presented a nomogram for estimating the percentage of pneumothorax. In general, the percentage of collapse is underestimated. Skin folds are occasionally misread as pneumothorax. The skin fold artifact, however, has a denser shadow just under the "line," which is the opposite of a pneumothorax, in which the lung is more dense in its central portion. Computed tomography of the lungs gives an excellent evaluation of pneumothorax, as described by Warner (1991) and Lesur (1990) and their associates, but the cost effectiveness of such a procedure must be questioned (Fig. 56-4). Small fluid collections are frequently encountered if the pneumothorax lasts longer than 24 hours. The fluid is usually clear, and it is not necessary to analyze it. Large effusions often are bloody and suggest a torn vascular adhesion. Some patients may require immediate operation to control the hemorrhage from a vascular chest wall adhesion that has been torn because such adhesions have a systemic arterial blood supply.

It is important to exclude a giant bulla in the differential diagnosis because tube drainage of such bullae is unrewarding.

The physiologic consequences of a pneumothorax range from little, such as 10% spontaneous pneumothorax in a college student, to life threatening, such as a tension pneumothorax in an older patient with already compromised cardiopulmonary function aggravated by mediastinal shift and compression of the contralateral lung. Gustman and coauthors (1983) described a laboratory model of tension pneumothorax resulting in respiratory failure. The consequences of airline travel and its attendant pressure abnormalities are discussed in Chapter 55. In general, patients with a known pneumothorax should not be encouraged to travel by air.

TREATMENT

Treatment options are listed in Table 56-2. A small spontaneous pneumothorax in an otherwise healthy patient can be observed and followed to its resorption (Fig. 56-5),

although, as discussed by Carr (1963) and Lippert (1991) and their colleagues, the results of observational therapy have been under question. Baumann and Strange (1997) present a comprehensive review of treatment from the pulmonologist's point of view. As discussed in Chapter 55, supplying extra oxygen to such patients theoretically hastens the resolution of the pneumothorax, but the true cost-effectiveness of such treatment must be questioned. Kircher and Swartzel (1954) estimated that 1.5% of the air is reabsorbed over each 24-hour period.

Needle or small-catheter aspiration of a mild-to-moderate spontaneous pneumothorax may hasten the resolution, as noted by Delius and associates (1989), if a persistent leak is absent. A plastic needle of the Medicut or Angiocath variety is recommended. Numerous manufacturers have available products. We tend to use that supplied in a disposable thoracocentesis tray, which has a 14-gauge pliable Teflon catheter that can be advanced over a 17-gauge 6-inch needle. The needle can be fitted to an automated two-way valve for easy aspiration. Needle aspiration has some particularly devoted advocates in the United Kingdom. The British Thoracic Society, as reported by Harvey and Prescott (1994), recommends it as a primary treatment option for primary spontaneous pneumothorax. Miller (1998) presents a strong argument in favor of considering aspiration as initial therapy. We find that simple aspiration is particularly useful in a smaller pneumothorax with a delayed diagnosis, when the passage of time suggests that the process will be self-limited (Fig. 56-6).

A tube thoracostomy should be carried out for pneumothoraces over 30% to hasten recovery, or for lesser degrees of collapse in patients with symptoms of associated disorders, such as heart disease or COPD. We prefer to use a 24 to 28F catheter directed toward the apex. If the tube is placed in the anterior to midaxillary line, less muscle tissue has to be traversed. An anterior tube placed through the second interspace does, on the other hand, provide excellent apical air clearance. Anterior tubes are to be avoided in women of almost all ages for cosmetic and esthetic reasons. Foley catheters have been placed in the past, but we no longer recommend their use. It has been suggested that rubber tubes are more irritating than plastic tubes and that rubber tubes are

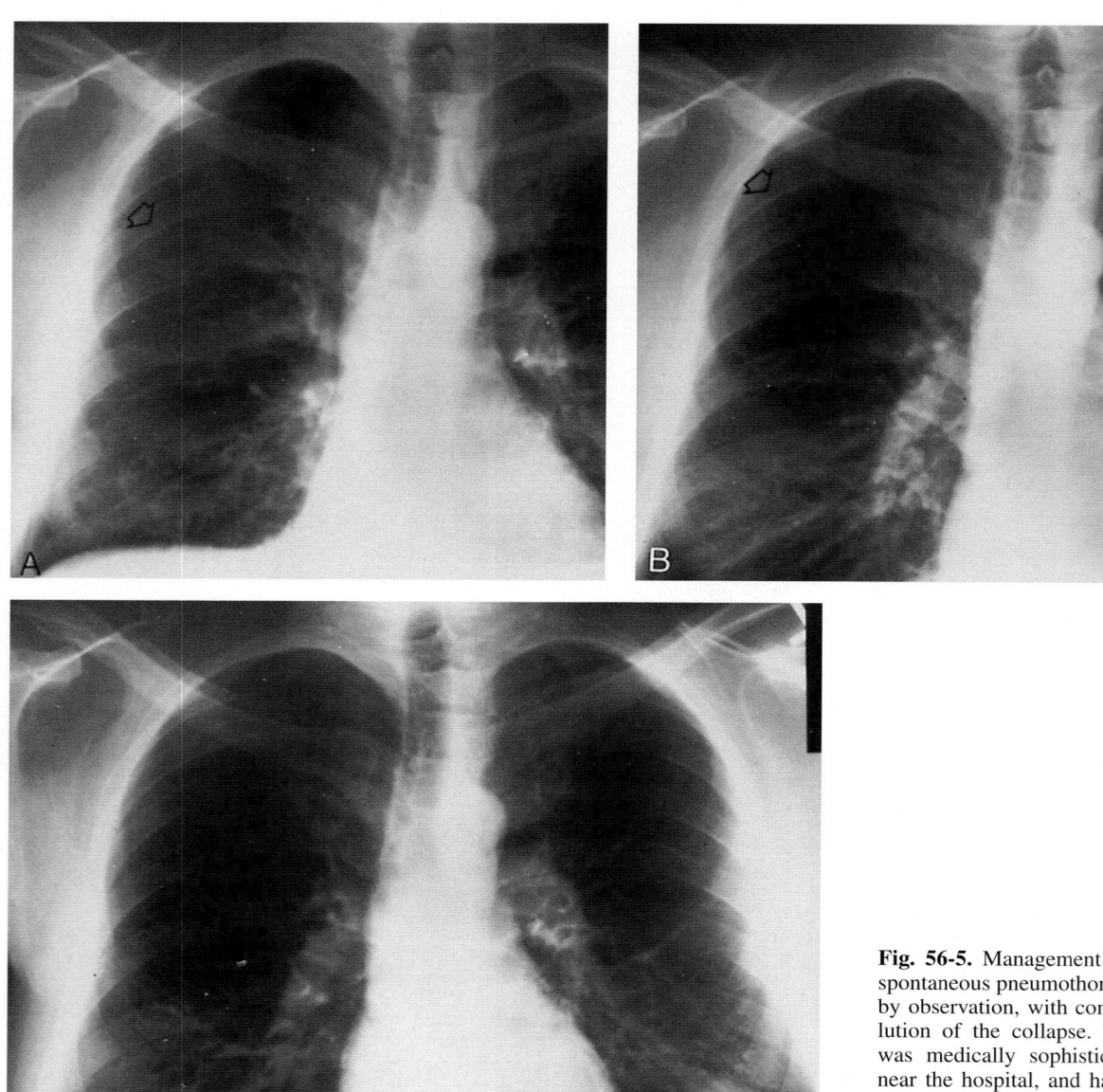

Fig. 56-5. Management of primary spontaneous pneumothorax (*arrows*) by observation, with complete resolution of the collapse. The patient was medically sophisticated, lived near the hospital, and had an occupation that was not physically demanding. **A**, **B**, and **C** were taken at weekly intervals.

preferable in patients with primary spontaneous pneumothorax because they promote focal pleural symphysis. We are unaware of any randomized clinical trial that has addressed this issue. Whether the tube is placed by clamp or by trocar is at the discretion of the thoracic surgeon. We tend to prefer the trocar technique for its speed and convenience (Fig. 56-7). Small-to-medium pneumothoraces can be treated successfully on an outpatient basis, as described by Peters and Kubitschek (1984), as well as by Mercier (1976), Obeid (1985), and Cannon (1981) and their associates, by smaller polyvinyl catheters passed percutaneously; several commercial sets are available. Whether to use a water seal or Pleurevac drainage system or a Heimlich valve is left to the discretion of the surgeon. We prefer a Pleur-evac drainage system set to water seal alone, and gentle suction of about 20 cm H_2O is used only if the lung is not completely reexpanded. We tend to eschew routine suction so as to avoid reexpansion pulmonary edema, as described by Matsuura and colleagues (1991) and Light (1990) (Fig. 56-8).

Indications for operative intervention are listed in Table 56-3. Surgical treatment of a pneumothorax is recommended for a persistent air leak over 5 to 7 days, for a second recurrence in the typical patient, and for the first episode in a patient with only one lung (Fig. 56-9). Certain occupations (e.g., divers and airplane pilots) suggest that an operation should be performed after the first episode. The chance of recurrence is estimated at 20 to 50% by Seremetis (1970) and Lindskog and Halasz (1957).

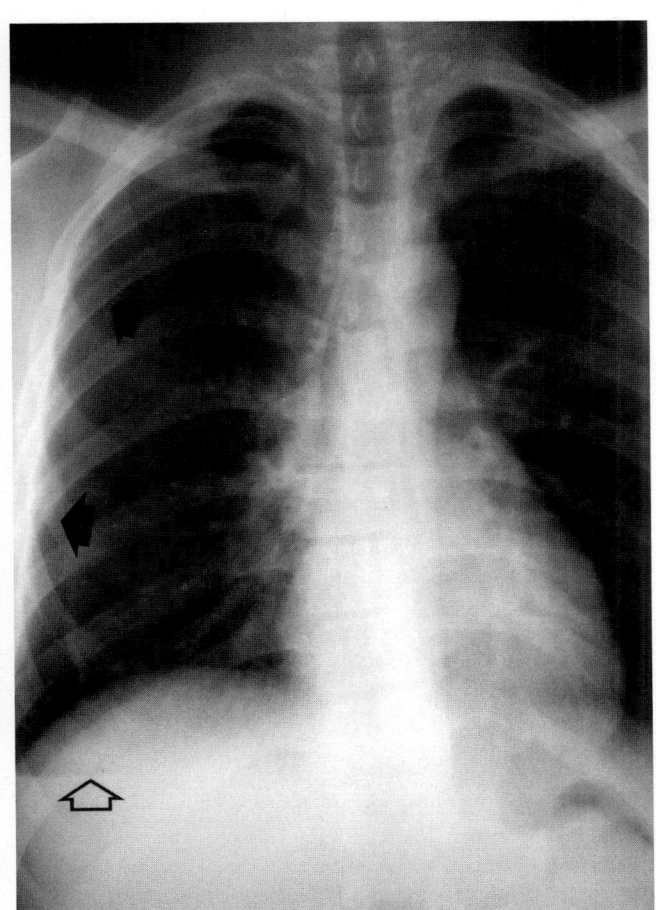

Fig. 56-6. Small pneumothorax (*solid arrows*) successfully treated by aspiration. This is also an example of a sports-related pneumothorax. The patient is a 20-year-old football player who was hit in the right chest by an opponent's helmet 2 days before this film. Note the air-fluid level at the base (*open arrow*), which suggests a degree of chronicity. A single-needle aspiration immediately reexpanded the lung. There was no air leak.

The various surgical options are listed in Table 56-4. The preferred form of surgical treatment is much debated. Various agents have been placed in the pleural space to induce pleural symphysis. The list is long, but it includes silver nitrate, talc, hypertonic glucose, urea, oil, nitrogen mustard, and various antibiotics. A clinical trial described by Light and colleagues in 1990 suggested that intrapleural tetracycline instillation could reduce the incidence of recurrence. We believe, however, that the reduction in recurrence was not overwhelming, considering the short follow-up period. Tetracycline has become difficult to obtain in the United States, and most tetracycline enthusiasts have switched to doxycycline. Talc has been recommended by Weissberg (1990), van de Brekel (1993), and Almind (1989) and their associates, but talc therapy, whether by tube and slurry or by thoracoscopy with insufflation, should, in the opinion of many surgeons, be reserved for malignant effusions, not benign pneumothorax.

However, Milanez (1994) and Tschopp (1997) and their coworkers report favorable experience with talc for spontaneous pneumothorax. Neither series gives long-term results, which is a matter of concern when dealing with benign disease. Deslauriers (1980), Thomas (1993), and Murray (1993) and their colleagues, as well as Weeden and Smith (1983), reported series of open operations by limited lateral or axillary incision with bleb excision and pleural abrasion or limited apical pleurectomy with excellent results, low recurrence rates, and no mortality. Dumont and colleagues (1995) reported an excellent series of 400 such operations using a muscle-sparing incision with only one recurrence (0.25%). Our experience with such minithoracotomies has also been favorable. Such results should be kept in mind when reviewing video-assisted thoracic surgery (VATS) series. Complete parietal pleurectomy, popularized by Gaensler (1956), should be reserved for open treatment failures, for postpneumonectomy patients with a first pneumothorax, and for older patients, usually with COPD, with pneumothorax associated with bullous disease. Mills and Baisch (1965) and Clagett (1968) have raised serious objections to using parietal pleurectomy on a routine basis. Patients with known bilateral pneumothoraces—concurrent or separate—can be considered for bilateral treatment via median sternotomy. Bilateral VATS procedures at a single sitting could also be considered.

The goal of surgical treatment is to find the offending bleb, remove it, and do some manipulation to encourage adhesion formation—but not too dense an adhesion. It is hoped that such adhesions would keep the lung "up" should another bleb develop and leak in subsequent years. If no bleb is found, the apex of the upper lobe should be stapled off. In such instances, many surgeons recommend a limited apical pleurectomy. We generally abrade the parietal pleura over the upper half of the chest wall with dry gauze. Marlex mesh and cautery cleaning pads are also used.

The role of thoracoscopy and VATS in the surgical treatment of pneumothorax is evolving. Preliminary reports by Melvin (1992), Nathanson (1991), Inderbitzi (1993) and their associates, as well as by LoCicero (1992), have been encouraging. Subsequent reports by Waller (1994), Naunheim (1995), Bertrand (1996), Mouroux (1996), and Passlick (1998) and their colleagues reinforce the earlier recommendations to consider VATS as the primary mode of surgical intervention. Most series do report a recurrence rate with VATS that is slightly higher than that with minithoracotomy. Our results using the VATS approach in the surgical treatment of pneumothorax have been similar. The offending bleb can often be identified and stapled with an endo-GIA through the thoracoscope or with a TA-type stapler through an accessory incision, as described by Lewis and coworkers (1992). Using single-lung anesthesia and a double-lumen endotracheal tube, the anesthesiologist can apply gentle positive pressure to the operated lung to assist in locating the air leak. Pleural abrasion and pleurectomy can also be performed using VATS techniques. At present, our preference is to recommend treatment of the

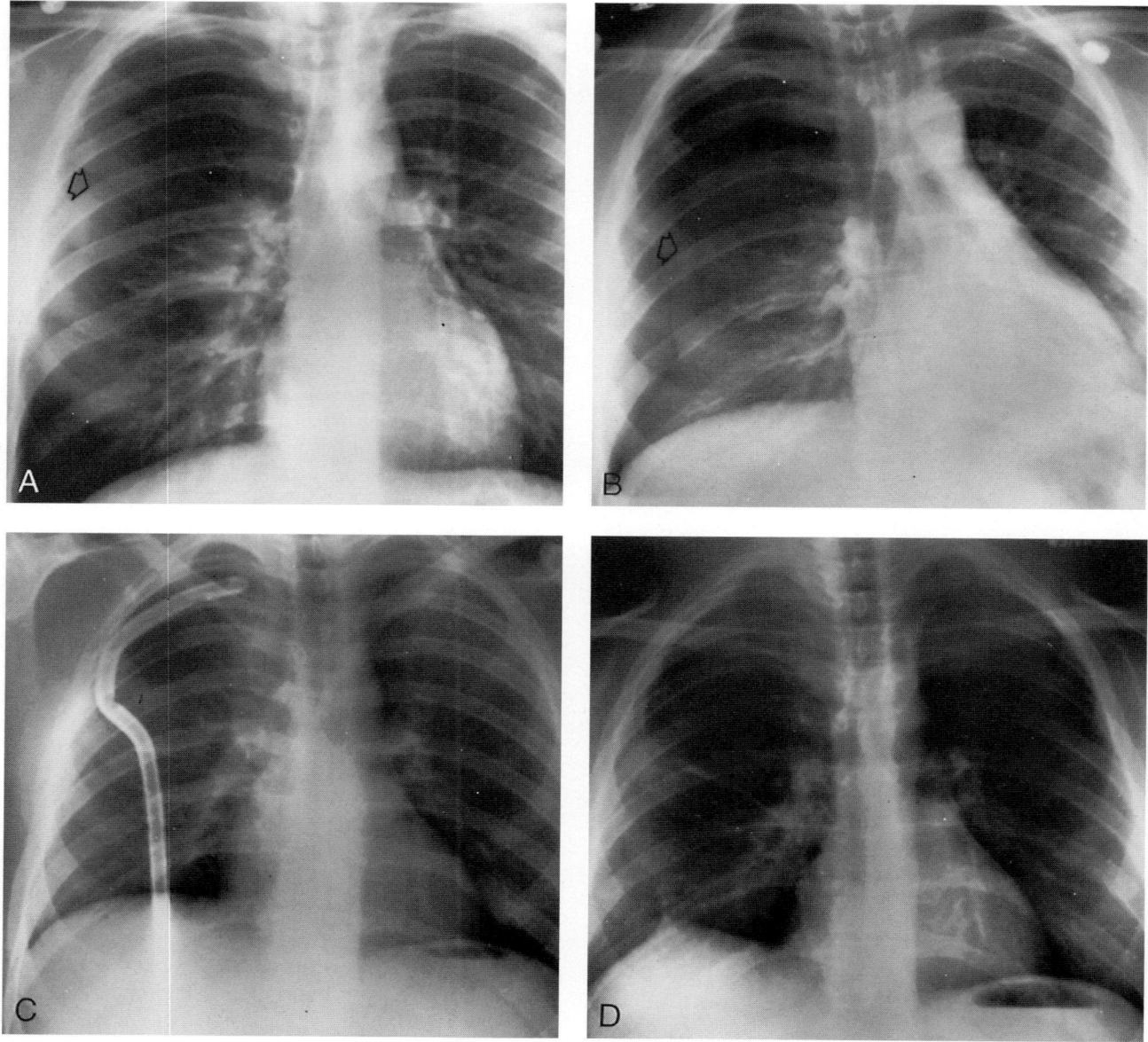

Fig. 56-7. Treatment of primary spontaneous pneumothorax by tube thoracostomy. **A.** On inspiration, there is significant collapse (*arrow*), estimated at 30% in a 22-year-old man. **B.** On exhalation, note accentuation of the pneumothorax (*arrow*) because the pleural air remains constant, but the thoracic volume is smaller. Note a slight shift of the mediastinum to the uninvolved side. **C.** Tube thoracostomy with a rubber tube directed to the apex. **D.** Follow-up chest radiograph demonstrated continued reexpansion of the lung.

uncomplicated pneumothorax that nonetheless qualifies for surgical treatment by the VATS approach with stapling of the bleb, if found, or of the ever-present apical abnormality if no bleb as such is found. Pleural abrasion is done with dry gauze that has been passed into the chest through the accessory incision or one of the ports. We place two or three rubber chest tubes through the ports to encourage pleural irritation, and they usually are removed on the third postoperative day (Fig. 56-10). It is our impression that more

surgeons use plastic drain tubes. We have already explained our preference for rubber drains. We prefer the more open surgical approach by axillary thoracotomy if we expect to encounter significant bullous disease or unusual adhesion formation, if there has been a previous surgical failure, or if a complete parietal pleurectomy is planned. Massard and associates (1998) present an excellent review of the recent and pertinent literature on VATS for pneumothorax. Cole (1995) and Kim (1996) and their colleagues express doubt

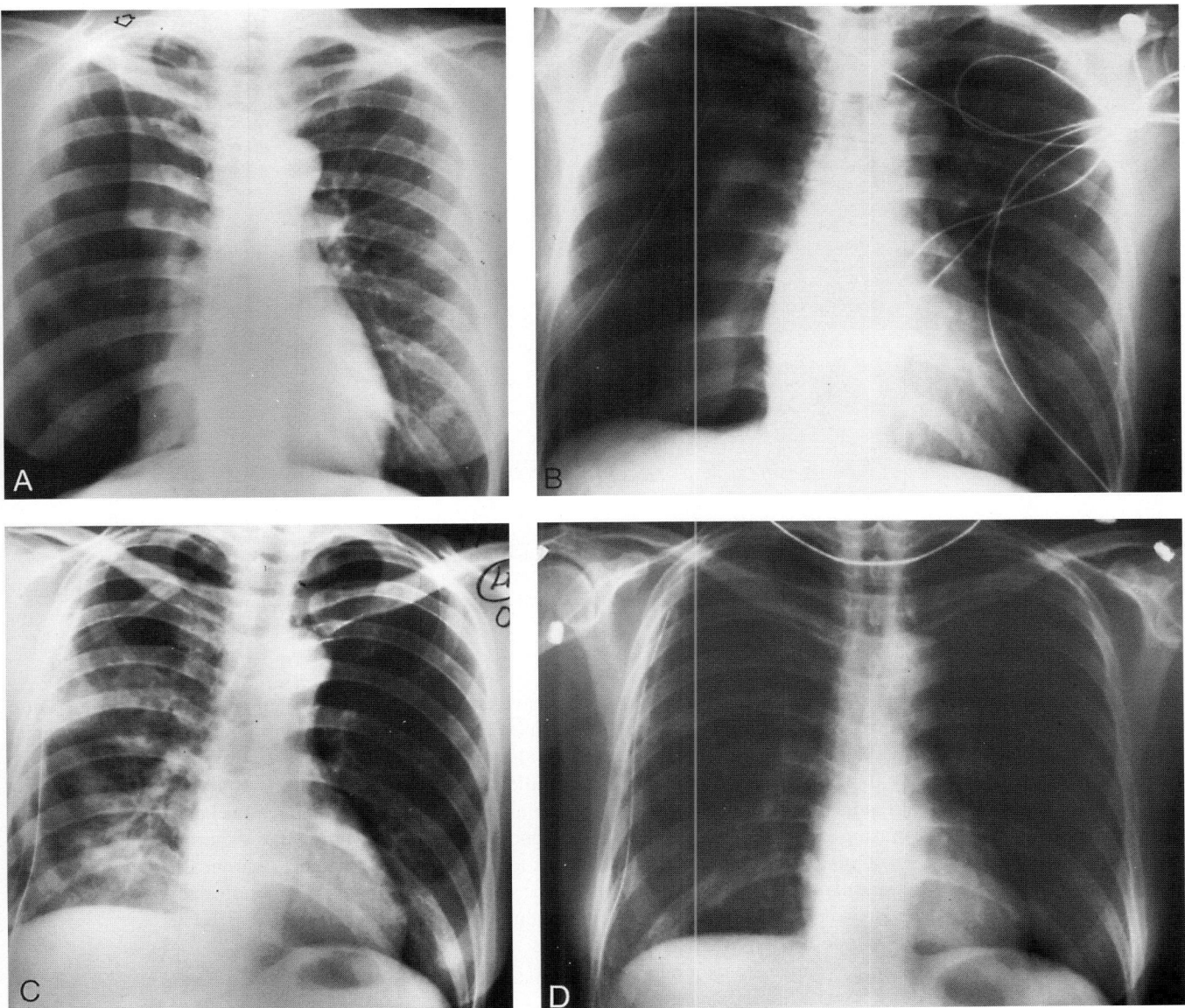

Fig. 56-8. Effect of suction and appearance of reexpansion pulmonary edema in a 52-year-old woman who was a smoker. **A.** Near total collapse from primary spontaneous pneumothorax. An apical adhesion is noted (*arrow*). **B.** On water seal alone, reexpansion is only minimal. **C.** After application of suction of −20 cm H_2O, the lung is completely reexpanded. Note the reexpansion pulmonary edema, which was asymptomatic in this case. **D.** Twenty-four hours later, the edema has disappeared.

about the effectiveness of the VATS approach. Another series of patients reported by Dumont and coworkers (1997) also raises the issue of whether the recurrence rate is higher after VATS than after minithoracotomy.

The selection of surgical treatment in AIDS patients is more difficult, as described by Gerein (1991) and Crawford (1992) and their associates, as well as by Wait and Estrera (1992), because persistent air leak in spite of standard treat-

Table 56-3. Indications for Operative Intervention for Pneumothorax

Persistent air leak
Recurrent pneumothorax
First episode in a patient with prior pneumonectomy
First episode with occupational hazard
    Airplane pilot
    Diver

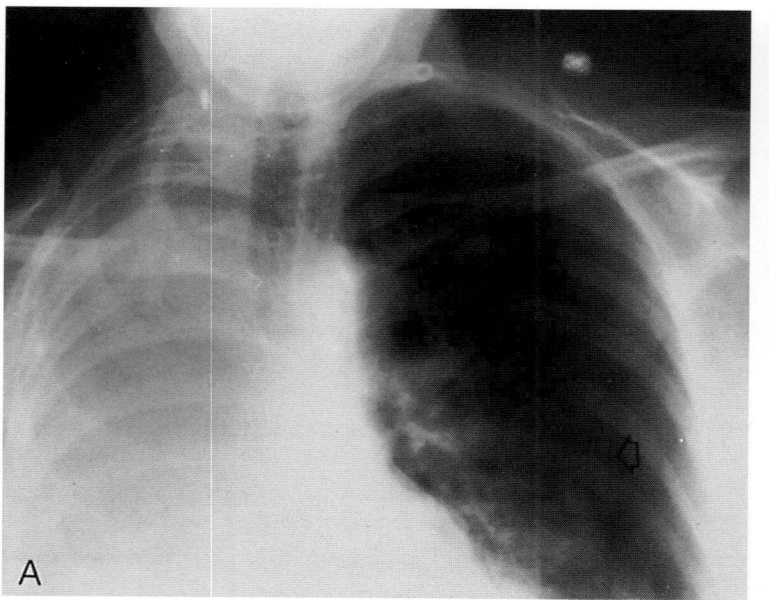
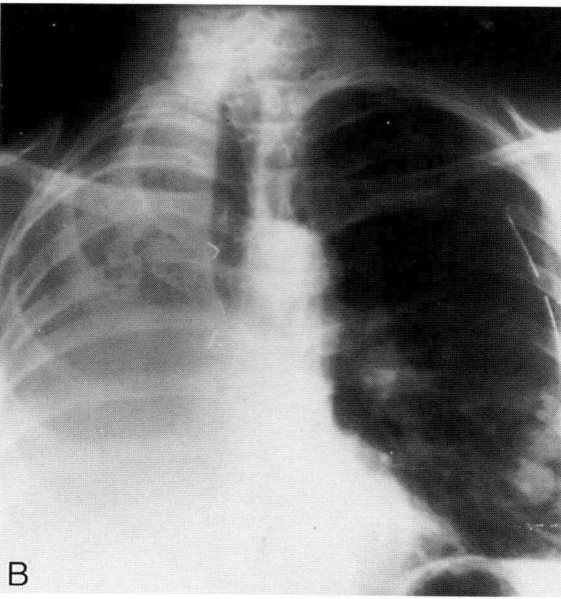

Fig. 56-9. Secondary spontaneous pneumothorax in a 50-year-old woman with only one lung. **A.** Significant, symptomatic collapse secondary to metastatic adenocarcinoma of the lung (*arrows*). **B.** Immediate reexpansion by tube thoracostomy. This woman's performance status was good; therefore, she underwent immediate parietal pleurectomy through a small axillary incision.

ment implies a poor prognosis. Hauck and associates (1991) described a thoracoscopic approach using a fibrin glue derivative. Torre and Belloni (1989) described use of an yttrium-aluminum-garnet laser thoracoscopically. Patients in poor medical condition that renders them inoperable can also be effectively handled by using Heimlich valves, thus permitting hospital discharge in some instances.

Some maneuvers in the treatment of pneumothorax deserve mention. A persistent air leak in a patient with a properly placed chest tube who is a poor operative risk can sometimes be encouraged to close by using pneumoperitoneum, as described by Brooks (1973). Sometimes, high-volume suction can "get the lung out" in patients with COPD who are poor operative candidates. The usual Pleur-evac type drainage systems do not provide this type of suction, but the old-fashioned water-seal bottles attached to a high-force suction source, such as the Emerson apparatus, accomplishes the task.

The training background of the physician treating pneumothorax by VATS is pertinent. Waller (1997) makes a per-

suasive argument that it be a thoracic surgeon. The culture of medical practice varies from community to community. We strongly believe that the thoracoscopist should be able to handle all surgical complications of a VATS procedure.

Finally, we plead for patience on behalf of the thoracic surgeon. Sometimes, waiting a few more days allows an air leak to seal. On the other hand, if surgical treatment is going to be necessary, the sooner it is performed, the sooner that patient can resume a routine lifestyle.

Table 56-4. Surgical Procedures for Pneumothorax

Pleural abrasion
Parietal pleurectomy
Apical
Complete
Talcage
By slurry
By insufflation

Note: All include excision or obliteration of the offending bleb or bulla.

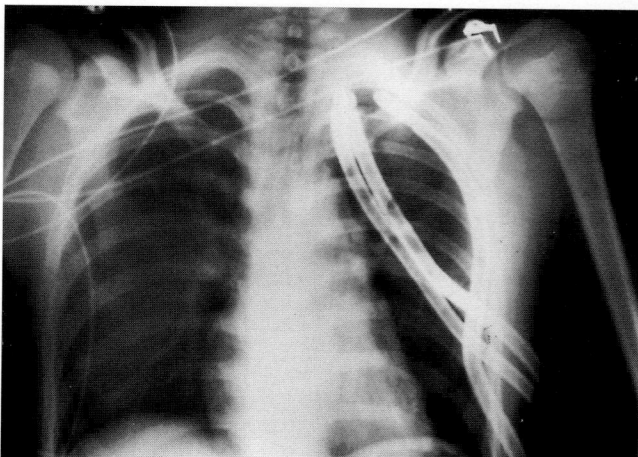

Fig. 56-10. Chest radiograph after video-assisted bleb excision and pleural abrasion in a 14-year-old boy (same patient as in Fig. 56-1). Three rubber tubes were placed through the three ports. He has had no recurrence.

REFERENCES

Adams WE: Pulmonary reserve and its influence on the development of lung surgery. J Thorac Cardiovasc Surg *40*:141, 1960.

Almind M, Lange P, Viskum K: Spontaneous pneumothorax: comparison of simple drainage, talc pleurodesis, and tetracycline pleurodesis. Thorax *44*:627, 1989.

Baumann MH, Strange C: Treatment of spontaneous pneumothorax: a more aggressive approach? Chest *112*:789, 1997.

Beers MF, Sohn M, Swartz M: Recurrent pneumothorax in AIDS patients with *Pneumocystis* pneumonia. A clinicopathologic report of three cases and review of the literature. Chest 98:266, 1990.

Bense L, Eklund G, Wiman LG: Smoking and the increased risk of contracting spontaneous pneumothorax. Chest *92*:1009, 1987.

Bertrand PC, et al. Immediate and long-term results after surgical treatment of primary spontaneous pneumothorax by VATS. Ann Thorac Surg *61*:1641, 1996.

Brooks JW: Open thoracotomy in the management of spontaneous pneumothorax. Ann Surg *177*:798, 1973.

Cannon WB, Mark JBD, Jamplis RW: Pneumothorax: a therapeutic update. Am J Surg *142*:26, 1981.

Carr DT, Silver AW, Ellis FH Jr: Management of spontaneous pneumothorax: with special reference to prognosis after various kinds of therapy. Mayo Clin Proc *38*:103, 1963.

Clagett OT: The management of spontaneous pneumothorax. J Thorac Cardiovasc Surg *55*:761, 1968.

Coker RJ, et al: Pneumothorax in patients with AIDS. Respir Med *87*:43, 1993.

Cole FH Jr, et al: Video-assisted thoracic surgery: primary therapy for spontaneous pneumothorax? Ann Thorac Surg *60*:931, 1995.

Colombani PM, Haller JA: Neonatal pneumothorax. *In* Deslauriers J, Lacquet LK (eds): Thoracic Surgery: Surgical Management of Pleural Diseases. St. Louis: CV Mosby, 1990, p. 149.

Crawford BK, et al: Treatment of AIDS-related bronchopleural fistula by pleurectomy. Ann Thorac Surg *54*:212, 1992.

Delius RE, et al: Catheter aspiration for simple pneumothorax. Experience with 114 patients. Arch Surg *124*:833, 1989.

Deslauriers J, et al: Transaxillary pleurectomy for treatment of spontaneous pneumothorax. Ann Thorac Surg *30*:569, 1980.

Dhalla S, Teskey JM: Surgical management of recurrent spontaneous pneumothorax during pregnancy. Chest *88*:301, 1985.

Dines DE, Clagett OT, Payne WS: Spontaneous pneumothorax in emphysema. Mayo Clin Proc *45*:481, 1970.

Dines DE, et al: Malignant pulmonary neoplasms predisposing to spontaneous pneumothorax. Mayo Clin Proc *48*:541, 1973.

Dumont P, et al: Surgical treatment of pneumothorax. Study of a series of 400 cases. Ann Chir *49*:235, 1995.

Dumont P, et al: Does a thoracoscopic approach for surgical treatment of spontaneous pneumothorax represent progress? Eur J Cardiothorac Surg *11*:27, 1997.

Farn J, Hammerman AM, Brunt LM: Intraoperative pneumothorax during laparoscopic cholecystectomy: a complication of prior transdiaphragmatic surgery. Surg Laparosc Endosc *3*:219, 1993.

Fleisher AG, Clement PB, Nelems B: Catamenial pneumothorax: pathophysiology and management. *In* Deslauriers J, Lacquet LK (eds): Thoracic Surgery: Surgical Management of Pleural Diseases. St. Louis: CV Mosby, 1990, p. 132.

Gaensler EA: Parietal pleurectomy for recurrent spontaneous pneumothorax. Surg Gynecol Obstet *102*:293, 1956.

Gerein AN, et al: Surgical management of pneumothorax in patients with acquired immunodeficiency syndrome. Arch Surg *126*:1272, 1991.

Gobbel WG Jr, et al: Spontaneous pneumothorax. J Thorac Cardiovasc Surg *46*:331, 1963.

Gustman P, Yerger L, Wanner A: Immediate cardiovascular effects of tension pneumothorax. Am Rev Respir Dis *127*:171, 1983.

Hauck H, Bull PG, Pridun N: Complicated pneumothorax: short- and long-term results of endoscopic fibrin pleurodesis. World J Surg *15*:146, 1991.

Harvey J, Prescott RJ: Simple aspiration versus intercostal tube drainage for spontaneous pneumothorax in patients with normal lungs. BMJ *309*:1338, 1994.

Inderbitzi RG, et al: Thoracoscopic pleurectomy for treatment of complicated spontaneous pneumothorax. J Thorac Cardiovasc Surg *105*:84, 1993.

Killen DA, Gobbel WG Jr: Spontaneous Pneumothorax. Boston: Little, Brown, 1968, pp. 1–35.

Kim KH, et al: Transaxillary minithoracotomy versus video-assisted thoracic surgery for spontaneous pneumothorax. Ann Thorac Surg *61*:1510, 1996.

Kirby TJ, Ginsberg RJ: Management of the pneumothorax and barotrauma. Clin Chest Med *13*:97, 1992.

Kircher LT Jr, Swartzel RL: Spontaneous pneumothorax and its treatment. JAMA *155*:24, 1954.

Kittle CF: The surgical management of recurrent or persistent pneumothorax. *In* Current Controversies in Thoracic Surgery. Philadelphia: WB Saunders, 1986, pp. 41–42.

Kjaergaard H: Spontaneous pneumothorax in the apparently healthy. Acta Med Scand *43*(Suppl):159, 1932.

Lesur O, et al: Computed tomography in the etiologic assessment of idiopathic spontaneous pneumothorax. Chest *98*:341, 1990.

Lewis RJ, et al: One hundred consecutive patients undergoing video-assisted thoracic operations. Ann Thorac Surg *54*:421, 1992.

Light RW: Reexpansion Pulmonary Edema in Pleural Diseases. 2nd Ed. Philadelphia: Lea & Febiger, 1990, pp. 256–257.

Light RW, et al: Intrapleural tetracycline for the prevention of recurrent spontaneous pneumothorax. JAMA *264*:2224, 1990.

Lillington GA, Mitchell SP, Wood GA: Catamenial pneumothorax. JAMA *219*:1328, 1972.

Lindskog GE, Halasz NA: Spontaneous pneumothorax. Arch Surg *75*:693, 1957.

Lippert HL, et al: Independent risk factors for cumulative recurrence rate after first spontaneous pneumothorax. Eur Respir J *4*:324, 1991.

LoCicero J: Minimally invasive thoracic surgery, video-assisted thoracic surgery and thoracoscopy. Chest *102*:330, 1992.

Massard G, Thomas P, Wilhm J-M: Minimally invasive management for first and recurrent pneumothorax. Current review. Ann Thorac Surg *66*:592, 1998.

Matsuura Y, et al: Clinical analysis of reexpansion pulmonary edema. Chest *100*:1562, 1991.

Maurer ER, Schaal JA, Mendez FL Jr: Chronic recurrence of spontaneous pneumothorax due to endometriosis of the diaphragm. JAMA *168*:2013, 1968.

Mercier C, et al: Outpatient management of intercostal tube drainage in spontaneous pneumothorax. Ann Thorac Surg *22*:163, 1976.

Melvin WS, Krasna MJ, McLaughlin JS: Thoracoscopic management of spontaneous pneumothorax. Chest *102*:1877, 1992.

Metersky ML, et al: AIDS-related spontaneous pneumothorax. Risk factors and treatment. Chest *108*:946, 1995.

Milanez JR, et al: Intrapleural talc for the prevention of recurrent pneumothorax. Chest *106*:1162, 1994.

Miller AC: Treatment of spontaneous pneumothorax: the clinician's perspective on pneumothorax management. Communication to the editor. Chest *113*:1423, 1998.

Mills M, Baisch BF: Spontaneous pneumothorax. Ann Thorac Surg *1*:286, 1965.

Mouroux J, et al: Video-assisted thoracoscopic treatment of spontaneous pneumothorax: technique and results of one hundred cases. J Thorac Cardiovasc Surg *112*:385, 1996.

Murphy JB: Surgery of the lung. JAMA *31*:151, 208, 281, 341, 1898.

Murray KD, et al: A limited axillary thoracotomy as primary treatment for recurrent spontaneous pneumothorax. Chest *103*:137, 1993.

Nathanson LK, et al: Videothoracoscopic ligation of bulla and pleurectomy for spontaneous pneumothorax. Ann Thorac Surg *52*:316, 1991.

Naunheim KS, et al: Safety and efficacy of video-assisted thoracic surgical techniques for the treatment of spontaneous pneumothorax. J Thorac Cardiovasc Surg *109*:1198, 1995.

Obeid FN, et al: Catheter aspiration for simple pneumothorax (CASP) in the outpatient management of simple traumatic pneumothorax. J Trauma *25*:882, 1985.

Partridge RA, et al: Sports-related pneumothorax. Ann Emerg Med *30*:539, 1997.

Pasque MK, et al: Improved technique for bilateral lung transplantation: rationale and initial clinical experience. Ann Thorac Surg *49*:785, 1990.

Passlick B, et al: Efficiency of video-assisted thoracic surgery for primary and secondary spontaneous pneumothorax. Ann Thorac Surg *65*:324, 1998.

Pastores SM, et al: Review: pneumothorax in patients with AIDS-related pneumocystis carinii pneumonia. Am J Med Sci *312*:229, 1996.

Peters J, Kubitschek KR: Clinical evaluation of a percutaneous pneumothorax catheter. Chest *86*:714, 1984.

Renzi PM, et al: Bilateral pneumothoraces hasten mortality in AIDS patients receiving secondary prophylaxis with aerosolized pentamidine. Chest *102*:491, 1992.

Rhea JT, DeLuca SA, Greene RE: Determining the size of pneumothorax in the upright patient. Radiology *144*:733, 1982.

Sadikot RT, et al: Recurrence of primary spontaneous pneumothorax. Thorax *52*:805, 1997.

Sepkowitz KA, et al: Pneumothorax in AIDS. Ann Intern Med *114*:455, 1991.

Seremetis MG: The management of spontaneous pneumothorax. Chest *57*:65, 1970.

Shanley DJ, et al: Spontaneous pneumothorax in AIDS patients with recurrent *Pneumocystis carinii* pneumonia despite aerosolized pentamidine prophylaxis. Chest *99*:502, 1991.

Shearin RPN, Hepper NGG, Payne WS: Recurrent spontaneous pneumothorax concurrent with menses. Mayo Clin Proc *49*:98, 1974.

Steinhauslin CA, Cuttat JF: Spontaneous pneumothorax: a complication of lung cancer? Chest *88*:709, 1985.

Thomas P, et al: Résultats du traitement chirurgical des pneumothorax persistants ou récidivants. Ann Chir *47*:136, 1993.

Torre M, Belloni P: Nd:YAG laser pleurodesis through thoracoscopy: new curative therapy in spontaneous pneumothorax. Ann Thorac Surg *47*:887, 1989.

Tschopp JM, Brutsche M, Frey JG: Treatment of complicated spontaneous pneumothorax by simple talc pleurodesis under thoracoscopy and local anesthesia. Thorax *52*:329, 1997.

van de Brekel JA, Duurkens VAM, Vanderschueren RGJ: Pneumothorax. Results of thoracoscopy and pleurodesis with talc poudrage and thoracotomy. Chest *103*:345, 1993.

Van Winter JT et al: Management of spontaneous pneumothorax during pregnancy: case report and review of the literature. Mayo Clin Proc *71*:249, 1996.

Wait MA, Dal Nogare AR: Treatment of AIDS-related spontaneous pneumothorax: a decade of experience. Chest *106*:693, 1994.

Wait MA, Estrera A: Changing clinical spectrum of spontaneous pneumothorax. Am J Surg *164*:528, 1992.

Waller DA: Video-assisted thoracoscopic surgery (VATS) in the management of spontaneous pneumothorax. Thorax *52*:307, 1997.

Waller DA, Forty J, Morritt GN: Video-assisted thoracoscopic surgery versus thoracotomy for spontaneous pneumothorax. Ann Thorac Surg *58*:372, 1994.

Warner BW, Bailey WW, Shipley RT: Value of computed tomography of the lung in the management of primary spontaneous pneumothorax. Am J Surg *162*:39, 1991.

Weeden D, Smith GH: Surgical experience in the management of spontaneous pneumothorax, 1972–82. Thorax *38*:737, 1983.

Weissberg D: Role of chemical methods to induce adhesive pleuritis. *In* Deslauriers J, Lacquet LK (eds): Thoracic Surgery: Surgical Management of Pleural Diseases. St. Louis: CV Mosby, 1990, p. 130.

Wilcox DT, et al: Spontaneous pneumothorax: a single-institution, 12-year experience in patients under 16 years of age. J Pediatric Surg *30*:1452, 1995.

CHAPTER 57

Physiology of Pleural Fluid Production and Benign Pleural Effusion

Richard W. Light

The author (1995) has estimated that more than 1 million cases of pleural effusions occur annually in the United States. The possibility of a pleural effusion should be considered whenever a patient with an abnormal chest radiograph result is evaluated. Increased densities on chest radiography are frequently attributed to parenchymal infiltrates when they actually represent pleural fluid. Free pleural fluid is best demonstrated with lateral decubitus chest radiography, ultrasonography, or computed tomographic (CT) scans. If, on lateral decubitus chest radiography, the distance between the inside of the chest wall and the outside of the lung is greater than 10 mm, a diagnostic thoracentesis usually is indicated. If this distance is less than 10 mm, the pleural effusion is probably not clinically significant and a thoracentesis is not indicated. The presence of loculated pleural fluid is best demonstrated with ultrasonography.

FORMATION AND RESORPTION OF PLEURAL FLUID

Pleural fluid has several possible origins. It can originate in the capillaries in the parietal or visceral pleura. It can come from the interstitial spaces of the lung, or it can come from the peritoneal cavity through small holes in the diaphragm. Wiener-Kronish and coworkers (1984) have reported that the rate of entry of fluid into the pleural space in normal individuals is approximately 0.01 mL/kg per hour.

Capillary Origin

The movement of fluid across the pleural membranes is believed to be governed by Starling's law of transcapillary exchange. When this law is applied to the pleura:

$$Q_f = L_p \times A[(P_{cap} - P_{pl}) - \sigma_d (\pi_{cap} - \pi_{pl})]$$

where Q_f is the liquid movement; L_p is the filtration coefficient per unit area or the hydraulic water conductivity of the membrane; A is the surface area of the membrane; P and π are the hydrostatic and oncotic pressures, respectively, of the capillary (cap) and pleural (pl) space; and σ_d is the solute reflection coefficient for protein, a measure of the membrane's ability to restrict the passage of large molecules. Kinasewitz and colleagues (1984) have estimated that σ_d is approximately 0.80 in humans.

Estimates for the magnitude of the pressures affecting fluid movement in and out of the pleural space are shown in Figure 57-1. When the parietal pleura is considered, a gradient for fluid filtration is normally present. The hydrostatic pressure in the parietal pleura is approximately 30 cm H_2O, whereas the pleural pressure is approximately –5 cm H_2O. The net hydrostatic pressure gradient is therefore 30 – (–5) = 35 cm H_2O and favors the movement of fluid from the capillaries in the parietal pleura to the pleural space. Opposing this hydrostatic pressure gradient is the oncotic pressure gradient. The oncotic pressure in the plasma is approximately 34 cm H_2O. Because the oncotic pressure of the small amount of pleural fluid is approximately 5 cm H_2O, the net oncotic gradient is 34 – 5 = 29 cm H_2O. Thus, the net gradient is 35 – 29 = 6 cm H_2O, favoring the movement of fluid from the capillaries in the parietal pleura to the pleural space.

Albertine and coworkers (1984) have shown that the blood supply to the visceral pleura in humans is from the bronchial artery rather than the pulmonary artery. The net gradient for fluid movement across the visceral pleura in humans is probably close to zero. The pressure in the visceral pleural capillaries is approximately 6 cm H_2O less than that in the parietal pleural capillaries because the former drain into the pulmonary veins. Because this is the only pressure that differs from those affecting fluid movement across the parietal pleura and because the net gradient for the parietal pleura is 6 cm H_2O, it follows that the net gradient for fluid movement across the visceral pleura is approximately zero. It is also

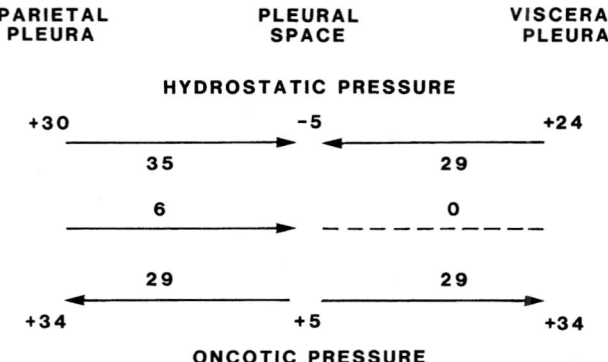

Fig. 57-1. Diagram of the various pressures that influence the movement of fluid in and out of the pleural space in humans. From Light RW: Pleural Diseases. 3rd Ed. Baltimore: Williams & Wilkins, 1995, p. 9. With permission.

quite likely that the filtration coefficient (L_p) for the visceral pleura is substantially less than that for the parietal pleura because Albertine and coworkers (1982) have shown that the capillaries in the visceral pleura are much farther from the pleural space than are those in the parietal pleura.

Interstitial Origin

Convincing evidence has been presented that the origin of a substantial percentage of pleural fluid is the interstitial spaces of the lung. Broaddus and coworkers (1990) have demonstrated that when sheep, a species with pleurae similar to that in humans, were volume overloaded by administration of 20% of their body weight as Ringer's lactate, transudative liquid flowed across the visceral pleura of the isolated, in situ lungs. The pleural fluid contained the same protein concentration as did the lung lymph and the interstitial edema liquid in the lung. The volume of pleural fluid constituted approximately 25% of all edema formed in the lung. In other experiments, Allen and colleagues (1989) have shown that with high-pressure pulmonary edema in sheep, pleural fluid accumulates only after pulmonary edema develops. In the clinical situation, Wiener-Kronish and coworkers (1985) have shown that in patients with congestive heart failure, the presence of pleural effusions on ultrasound correlates more closely with the pulmonary venous pressure than with the systemic venous pressure and that the likelihood of pleural effusions increases as the severity of the pulmonary edema on chest radiography increases.

Exudates found in association with increased permeability pulmonary edema probably also originate from the lung interstitium. When Wiener-Kronish and associates (1988) induced increased permeability edema in sheep by the infusion of oleic acid, pleural fluid accumulated only after pulmonary edema developed. In this report, no detectable injury to the visceral pleura was seen by morphologic studies. They found that approximately 20% of the excess lung liquid that formed after oleic acid-induced lung injury was cleared from the lung

through the pleural space. Other researchers have come to similar conclusions. Amouzadeh and colleagues (1991) concluded that the high-protein pleural effusion that developed in rats after the administration of xylazine had its origin in the parenchymal interstitial spaces of the lung. Bernaudin and associates (1986) made similar conclusions about the exudative pleural effusions induced by hypoxia in rats.

Peritoneal Origin

Fluid that is free in the peritoneal cavity can move directly into the pleural space if the diaphragm has holes in it. This mechanism is responsible for the pleural effusions that occur in conjunction with cirrhosis and ascites, pancreatic ascites, Meigs' syndrome, and peritoneal dialysis.

Lymphatic Clearance

Figure 57-1 might lead one to conclude that pleural fluid should continuously accumulate because Starling's equation favors fluid formation through the parietal pleura and no gradient exists for fluid absorption through the visceral pleura. Fluid clearance via the pleural lymphatics is thought to explain the lack of fluid accumulation normally. Wang (1975) demonstrated that, at least in rabbits, the pleural space is in communication with the lymphatic vessels by means of stomas located within the parietal pleura. No such stomas are present in the visceral pleura. Gaudio and coworkers (1988) were unable to demonstrate these stomas in parietal pleura from humans. Stewart (1963) demonstrated that proteins, cells, and all other particulate matter are removed from the pleural space by these lymphatics in the parietal pleura.

Most fluid that enters the pleural space is removed via the lymphatics. Broaddus and coworkers (1988) produced artificial hydrothoraces in awake sheep by injecting an autologous protein solution at a volume of 10 mL/kg with a protein level of 1.0 g/dL. They found that the hydrothorax was removed almost completely by the lymphatics in a linear fashion at a rate of 0.28 mL/kg per hour. This linearity suggests that the lymphatics operate at maximum capacity once the pleural liquid exceeds a certain threshold volume. Note that the capacity for lymphatic clearance is 28 times as high as the normal rate of pleural fluid formation.

In the experiments of Broaddus and colleagues (1988) previously referred to, the fluid that was introduced into the pleural space had an oncotic pressure of approximately 5 cm H_2O. From Figure 57-1 one might speculate that if fluids with oncotic pressures other than 5 cm H_2O were introduced, the equilibrium would have been altered such that fluid would enter the pleural space from visceral pleura in animals with high pleural fluid oncotic pressures and would leave the pleural space through the visceral pleura in animals with low pleural fluid oncotic pressures. This does not appear to be the case. Aiba and coworkers (1984) produced artificial pleural effusions in dogs with protein levels ranging from 0.1 to 9.0 g/dL. Even when the induced pleural effusion had an oncotic pressure of 0.1 g/dL, no increase in the concentration of protein occurred with time, indicating that the low oncotic pressure did not induce a rapid efflux of fluid out of the pleural space. When the protein concentration of the induced effusions was greater than 4 g/dL, the concentration of protein in the pleural fluid did decrease with time, indicating a net transfer of protein-free fluid into the pleural space. However, the net amount of fluid entering the pleural space, even with a protein level of 9.0 g/dL, was only 0.22 mL/kg per hour. This degree of fluid flux is similar to the lymphatic clearance of 0.22 mL/kg per hour reported in the same studies. These observations explain why protein levels and hematocrits remain relatively stable in individuals with hemothoraces.

The amount of fluid that can be cleared through these lymphatics is substantial. Stewart (1963) found that the mean lymphatic flow from one pleural space in seven patients was 0.40 mL/kg per hour, whereas Leckie and Tothill (1965) found that the mean lymphatic flow was 0.22 mL/kg per hour in seven patients with congestive heart failure. In both these studies, marked variability was noted from one patient to another. If these results from patients with congestive heart failure can be extrapolated to the normal person, a 60-kg individual should have the capacity to absorb approximately 20 mL/hour or 500 mL/day from each pleural space through the lymphatics.

In summary, if the experimental results in sheep can be extrapolated to humans, it appears that a small amount (0.01 mL/kg per hour) of fluid constantly enters the pleural space from the capillaries in the parietal pleura. Almost all of this fluid is removed by the lymphatics in the parietal pleura, which can remove approximately 0.20 mL/kg per hour. Little net fluid movement occurs across the visceral pleura. A pleural effusion develops when the amount of fluid that enters the pleural space exceeds the amount that can be removed via the lymphatics. Accordingly, pleural effusions can develop and are caused by increased pleural fluid formation, decreased lymphatic clearance from the pleural space, or a combination of these two factors. The three primary origins of pleural fluid are the pleural capillaries, pulmonary interstitial spaces, and peritoneal cavity.

DIFFERENTIAL DIAGNOSIS

Pleural effusions can occur as complications of many different diseases and therapeutic procedures (Table 57-1). The initial step in evaluation of the patient is the differentiation between exudative and transudative effusions.

Separation of Exudates from Transudates

When it is found that a patient has a pleural effusion that measures more than 10 mm on decubitus radiography, a diagnostic thoracentesis should usually be performed. If the

Table 57-1. Differential Diagnoses of Pleural Effusions

I. Transudative pleural effusions
  A. Congestive heart failure
  B. Pericardial disease
  C. Cirrhosis
  D. Nephrotic syndrome
  E. Peritoneal dialysis
  F. Superior vena cava obstruction
  G. Myxedema
  H. Pulmonary emboli
  I. Sarcoidosis
  J. Urinothorax
II. Exudative pleural effusions
  A. Neoplastic diseases
    1. Metastatic disease
    2. Mesothelioma
  B. Infectious diseases
    1. Bacterial infections
    2. Tuberculosis
    3. Fungal infections
    4. Viral infections
    5. Parasitic infections
  C. Pulmonary embolization
  D. Gastrointestinal disease
    1. Esophageal perforation
    2. Pancreatic disease
    3. Intra-abdominal abscesses
    4. Diaphragmatic hernia
  E. Collagen vascular diseases
    1. Rheumatoid pleuritis
    2. Systemic lupus erythematosus
    3. Drug-induced lupus
    4. Immunoblastic lymphadenopathy
    5. Sjögren's syndrome
    6. Wegener's granulomatosis
    7. Churg-Strauss syndrome
  F. After surgical procedures
    1. Postcardiac injury syndrome
    2. Post–coronary artery bypass surgery
    3. Post–lung transplantation
    4. Post–liver transplantation
    5. Postabdominal surgery
    6. Post–endoscopic variceal sclerotherapy
  G. Asbestos exposure
  H. Sarcoidosis
  I. Uremia
  J. Meigs' syndrome
  K. Yellow nail syndrome
  L. Drug-induced pleural disease
    1. Nitrofurantoin
    2. Dantrolene
    3. Methysergide
    4. Bromocriptine
    5. Procarbazine
    6. Amiodarone
  M. Trapped lung
  N. Radiation therapy
  O. Electrical burns
  P. Urinary tract obstruction
  Q. Iatrogenic injury
  R. Ovarian hyperstimulation syndrome
  S. Chylothorax
  T. Hemothorax

patient has obvious congestive heart failure, consideration can be given to postponing the thoracentesis until the heart failure is treated. If such a patient, however, is febrile or has pleuritic chest pain or if the effusions are not of comparable size on both sides, a thoracentesis should be performed without delay. Shinto and I (1990) have shown that the characteristics of pleural fluid associated with heart failure change little with diuresis over several days.

The first question to be answered with a diagnostic thoracentesis is whether the patient has a transudative or an exudative pleural effusion. Broaddus and I (1992) have modified the classic definitions of the transudates and exudates to take into account the newer theories concerning the formation and resorption of pleural fluid. By this new definition, transudative effusions arise from increased hydrostatic pressures or decreased oncotic pressure, whereas exudative effusions result from increased permeability. This differentiation can be made by simultaneous analysis of the protein and lactic acid dehydrogenase (LDH) levels in the pleural fluid and in the serum. Exudative pleural effusions meet at least one of the following criteria, whereas transudative pleural effusions meet none, according to the classic definitions of the author and colleagues (1972): 1) pleural fluid protein to serum protein greater than 0.5, 2) pleural fluid LDH to serum LDH greater than 0.6, and 3) pleural fluid LDH greater than two-thirds upper normal limit for serum. If none of these criteria are met, the patient has a transudative pleural effusion and the pleural surfaces and the lung can be ignored while the congestive heart failure, cirrhosis, or nephrosis is treated. Remember, however, that a transudative pleural effusion can result from pulmonary embolization.

The previously mentioned criteria occasionally misidentify a transudative effusion as an exudative effusion. If a patient appears to have a transudative effusion clinically, but the pleural fluid meets exudative criteria, the difference between the serum and pleural fluid albumin levels should be assessed. Burgess and coworkers (1995) have shown that if this difference exceeds 1.2 g/dL, the patient in all probability has a transudative effusion.

Differentiating Exudative Pleural Effusions

Once it has been determined that a patient has an exudative pleural effusion, one should attempt to determine which of the diseases listed in Table 57-1 is responsible, remembering that pneumonia, malignancy, and pulmonary embolization account for the great majority of all exudative pleural effusions. It is recommended that the following tests be obtained on the pleural fluid from a patient with an undiagnosed exudative pleural effusion: glucose level, amylase level, LDH level, differential cell count, microbiological studies, and cytology. In selected patients, other tests on the pleural fluid, such as the pH, adenosine deaminase (ADA) level, interferon-γ level, polymerase chain reaction (PCR) for tuberculous DNA, and lipid analysis may be of value.

Appearance of Pleural Fluid

The gross appearance of the pleural fluid should always be described and its odor noted. If the pleural fluid smells putrid, the patient has a bacterial infection, probably anaerobic, of the pleural space. If the pleural fluid smells like urine, the patient probably has a urinothorax caused by obstruction of the ureters. If the pleural fluid is bloody, a pleural fluid hematocrit should be obtained. If the pleural fluid hematocrit is greater than 50% that of the peripheral blood, the patient has a hemothorax, and one should consider inserting chest tubes. If the pleural fluid is turbid, milky, or bloody, the supernatant should be examined after centrifugation. If the supernatant is clear, then the turbidity was caused by cells or debris in the pleural fluid. If the turbidity persists, then the patient probably has a chylothorax or a pseudochylothorax.

Pleural Fluid White Blood Cell Count and Differential

The absolute pleural fluid white blood cell count is of limited usefulness. Counts greater than 10,000 per μL are most common with parapneumonic effusions but also are seen with pancreatitis, pulmonary embolism, collagen vascular disease, malignancy, and tuberculosis. The differential cell count on the pleural fluid is of more usefulness than is the absolute cell count. If the pleural fluid contains predominantly polymorphonuclear leukocytes, then it is caused by an acute disease process such as pneumonia, pulmonary embolization, pancreatitis, intra-abdominal abscess, or early tuberculosis. If the pleural fluid contains predominantly mononuclear cells, then malignancy, tuberculosis, or a resolving acute process is probably responsible for the effusion. The majority of patients with pleural fluid eosinophilia have either blood or air in their pleural space. If neither air nor blood is present in the pleural space, several unusual diagnoses should be considered. Benign asbestos pleural effusions are frequently eosinophilic. Patients with pleural effusions secondary to drug reactions (e.g., nitrofurantoin, bromocriptine, or dantrolene) typically have pleural fluid eosinophilia. The pleural fluid of patients with pleural paragonimiasis is typically eosinophilic with a low glucose, low pH, and a high LDH level. No diagnosis is ever determined for approximately 20% of exudative pleural effusions, and pleural fluid eosinophilia is found in approximately 40% of these effusions. The demonstration that more than 50% of the white blood cells in an exudative pleural effusion are small lymphocytes indicates that the patient probably has a malignant or a tuberculous pleural effusion.

Pleural Fluid Glucose

The presence of a reduced pleural fluid glucose level (less than 60 mg/dL) narrows the diagnostic possibilities to seven: parapneumonic effusion—empyema, malignant effusion, tuberculous effusion, rheumatoid effusion, hemothorax, or paragonimiasis or the Churg-Strauss syndrome. If a patient with a parapneumonic effusion has a pleural fluid glucose level less than 40 mg/dL, tube thoracostomy should be performed. Most patients with rheumatoid pleural effusions have a pleural fluid glucose level below 30 mg/dL.

Pleural Fluid Amylase

An elevated (i.e., above the upper normal limit of serum) pleural fluid amylase indicates that the patient has esophageal perforation, pancreatic disease, or malignant disease. The best screening test for a ruptured esophagus is probably the pleural fluid amylase. The origin of the amylase in this instance is the salivary glands. It is important to establish this diagnosis expeditiously, because the mortality exceeds 50% if the mediastinum is not explored within 24 hours of the perforation. Approximately 10% of patients with acute pancreatitis have an accompanying pleural effusion, and in an occasional patient, the chest symptoms dominate the clinical picture and the elevated pleural fluid amylase is the first clue that the primary problem is pancreatic rather than pulmonary. Patients with chronic pancreatic disease may develop a sinus tract between the pancreas and the pleural space, which leads to a chronic illness dominated by a large pleural effusion. Unless the pleural fluid amylase level is measured, one may wrongly ascribe the chronic illness and the large pleural effusion to malignancy. The pleural fluid amylase level is elevated in approximately 10% of malignant pleural effusions. Analysis of the amylase isoenzymes permits differentiation of pancreatic disease from malignant disease because Kramer and associates (1989) have shown that the amylase associated with malignancy is of the salivary subtype.

Pleural Fluid Lactic Acid Dehydrogenase

The pleural fluid LDH level should be measured every time a diagnostic thoracentesis is performed because the level of LDH in the pleural fluid is a good indicator of the degree of inflammation in the pleural space. If the pleural fluid LDH level increases with serial thoracentesis, the degree of inflammation is worsening, and one should be more aggressive in pursuing a diagnosis. Alternatively, a decreasing pleural fluid LDH level indicates that the pleural inflammation is improving.

Pleural Fluid Cytology

Pleural fluid cytology is quite useful in establishing the diagnosis of malignant pleural effusion because the diagno-

sis can be established in 40 to 90% of patients, depending on the tumor type, the amount of fluid submitted, and the skill of the cytologist. Prakash and coworkers (1985) have shown that the cytology result is usually positive if the primary tumor is an adenocarcinoma whereas it is usually not positive if the primary tumor is a squamous cell carcinoma, lymphoma, or mesothelioma. Lee and coworkers (1996), among others, have shown that the use of immunohistochemical tests using monoclonal antibodies facilitates the differentiation of adenocarcinoma cells, benign mesothelial cells, and malignant mesothelial cells.

Culture and Bacteriologic Stains

Pleural fluid from patients with undiagnosed exudative pleural effusions should be cultured for bacteria, both aerobically and anaerobically, mycobacteria, and fungi. A Gram's stain of the fluid should be obtained also.

Pleural Fluid pH and P_{CO_2}

The pleural fluid pH is most useful in determining whether chest tubes should be inserted in patients with parapneumonic effusions. If the pleural fluid pH is less than 7, the patient invariably has a complicated parapneumonic effusion, and tube thoracostomy should be instituted. If the pleural fluid pH is greater than 7.20, the patient probably does not require tube thoracostomy. The pleural fluid pH can be reduced to less than 7.20 with eight other conditions: systemic acidosis, esophageal rupture, rheumatoid pleuritis, tuberculous pleuritis, malignant pleural disease, hemothorax, paragonimiasis, or the Churg-Strauss syndrome. When the pleural fluid pH is used as a diagnostic test, it must be measured with the same care as arterial pH. The fluid should be collected anaerobically in a heparinized syringe and placed in ice for transfer to the laboratory to avoid spontaneous acid generation by the fluid. The pleural fluid pH must be measured with a blood gas machine. Cheng and coworkers (1998) have shown that pleural fluid pH measured with either a pH meter or pH indicator strips is not sufficiently accurate for clinical decision making.

Pleural Fluid Tests for the Diagnosis of Tuberculous Pleuritis

Three tests, namely the pleural fluid ADA level, the pleural fluid interferon-γ level, and the PCR for tuberculous DNA have been shown to be useful in the diagnosis of tuberculous pleuritis. In a study reported from Spain by Valdes and coworkers (1998), 253 of 254 patients (99.6%) with tuberculous pleuritis had a pleural fluid ADA level above 47 U/L. Burgess and associates (1996) have shown that the specificity of the pleural fluid ADA level for tuberculosis can be increased if it is combined with a pleural fluid lymphocyte to neutrophil ratio of greater than 0.75. In their series, the specificity of the pleural fluid ADA level increased from 81 to 95% if the diagnosis of tuberculosis was based on an ADA level above 50 U/L and a lymphocyte neutrophil ratio of 0.75 or higher. However, I know of no commercial laboratories that perform this test in the United States at the present time.

Patients with tuberculous pleuritis tend to have a high pleural fluid interferon-γ level. In a study of 345 patients with exudative pleural effusions, Villena and coworkers (1996) reported that the sensitivity of a pleural fluid interferon-γ with a cutoff level of 3.7 U/mL was 0.99 whereas the specificity was 0.98. The PCR for tuberculous DNA on pleural fluid also appears to be useful in the diagnosis of tuberculous pleuritis. Querol and associates (1995) reported that the sensitivity and specificity of PCR and ADA were comparable for the diagnosis of tuberculous pleuritis. It is likely that the results with PCR will improve as its technology is refined.

Other Diagnostic Tests on Pleural Fluid

If the supernatant of the pleural fluid is cloudy, levels of cholesterol and triglycerides in the pleural fluid should be obtained to differentiate chylothorax from pseudochylothorax. With chylothorax, the pleural fluid triglyceride levels are usually elevated above 110 mg/dL. With pseudochylothorax, the pleural fluid cholesterol level is elevated.

Numerous reports have advocated the use of tumor markers in the pleural fluid for diagnosing malignant pleural effusion. However, the use of tumor markers for the diagnosis of pleural malignancy is not recommended because no tumor marker has yet been found that is 100% specific and one does not want to falsely establish the diagnosis of malignant pleural effusions.

Various reports have advocated measuring other enzymes and proteins in the pleural fluid including antinuclear antibody levels, rheumatoid factor, lysozyme, and alkaline and acid phosphatase. However, none have proven to be useful in the differential diagnosis or management of patients with pleural effusions.

INVASIVE TESTS FOR UNDIAGNOSED EXUDATIVE PLEURAL EFFUSIONS

In the majority of patients, the cause of the pleural effusion is apparent after the initial clinical assessment and a diagnostic thoracentesis. If the diagnosis is not apparent, the following invasive tests might be considered: needle biopsy of the pleura, thoracoscopy, bronchoscopy, and open biopsy of the pleura. It is important to remember that no diagnosis is established for approximately 20% of exudative pleural effusions and these resolve spontaneously leaving no residua. Three factors should influence the vigor with which one pursues the diagnosis in patients with undiagnosed exudative effusions.

1) The symptoms and clinical course of the patient: If the symptoms are minimal or if they are improving, a less aggressive approach is indicated.
2) The trend of the pleural fluid LDH level: If the pleural fluid LDH tends to increase with serial thoracenteses, a more aggressive approach is indicated because the process is getting worse.
3) The attitude of the patient: If the patient is desperate to know why he or she has developed a pleural effusion, an aggressive approach should be taken.

Needle Biopsy of the Pleura

With special needles, small specimens of the parietal pleura can be obtained relatively noninvasively. Since the 1930s, the diagnosis of tuberculous pleuritis has been established primarily via needle biopsy of the pleura. However, as outlined previously under Differential Diagnosis, noninvasive tests for establishing the diagnosis of tuberculous pleuritis have been developed and hence needle biopsy of the pleura is usually not necessary to establish this diagnosis. The other main diagnosis that is established with needle biopsy of the pleura is malignant pleural disease. Prakash and associates (1985) have demonstrated that needle biopsy results of the pleura are usually negative in patients who have negative cytology results. If the diagnosis of malignancy is strongly suspected and the cytology result on the fluid is negative, it is preferable to proceed to thoracoscopy rather than needle biopsy of the pleura.

Thoracoscopy

With this procedure, discussed in more detail in Chapter 18, the pleural surfaces can be directly visualized through a scope introduced through a small incision in the chest wall. The instrumentation for video-assisted thoracic surgery has improved dramatically, and video-thoracoscopy has become the primary means of diagnosing pleural malignancy in patients who have negative cytology results.

Thoracoscopy is excellent at establishing the diagnosis of malignancy. As shown by Loddenkemper (1998), thoracoscopy establishes the diagnosis of malignant pleural disease in 95% of patients with pleural malignancy. When one does a diagnostic thoracoscopy, one should be prepared to insufflate talc at the time of the procedure because this is the most effective way to prevent recurrence of the pleural effusion. Although the diagnosis of tuberculous pleuritis also can be made with thoracoscopy, other benign etiologies for pleural effusions are rarely established with thoracoscopy. If a thoracoscopy is nondiagnostic, one can say with reasonable certainty, however, that the patient has neither pleural malignancy nor pleural tuberculosis.

Bronchoscopy

Bronchoscopy is sometimes useful in the evaluation of patients with an undiagnosed exudative pleural effusion. Not all patients with an undiagnosed pleural effusion should undergo bronchoscopy. Chang and Perng (1989) demonstrated that bronchoscopy was useful only if the patient had a parenchymal abnormality or hemoptysis. Patients with an undiagnosed pleural effusion should undergo CT of the chest. Then bronchoscopy is performed only if the CT scan demonstrates parenchymal abnormalities or if the patient has hemoptysis. At the time of bronchoscopy, special attention is paid to those portions of the lung in which the parenchymal abnormalities were demonstrated.

Bronchoscopy is probably not indicated for the patient with a pleural effusion and no parenchymal abnormality, hemoptysis, and less than a massive effusion. Poe and associates (1994) reported that bronchoscopy was diagnostic in only 1 of 48 (2%) such patients. Similarly bronchoscopy is rarely diagnostic in the patient with a cytologically positive pleural effusion and no parenchymal abnormality. Feinsilver and coworkers (1986) reported that bronchoscopy was diagnostic in 2 of 17 (12%) such patients.

Open Biopsy of the Pleura

Thoracotomy with direct biopsy of the pleura provides the best biopsy specimens. However, it has been replaced by video-thoracoscopy in centers in which this procedure is available. It should be emphasized that open pleural biopsy does not always provide a diagnosis in patients with pleural effusions. Ryan and coworkers (1981) reported that between 1962 and 1972, 51 patients with pleural effusion at the Mayo Clinic had no diagnosis after an open pleural biopsy. In 31 of these patients, there was no recurrence of the pleural effusion and no cause ever became apparent. However, 13 of the patients were eventually proven to have malignant disease.

BENIGN CONDITIONS CAUSING PLEURAL EFFUSION

The remainder of this chapter deals with specific conditions that cause pleural effusion. The reader is referred to the following chapters for a discussion of other diseases of the pleura: Chapter 58 for parapneumonic effusion, Chapter 60 for tuberculous and fungal pleural infections, Chapter 63 for chylothorax, Chapter 65 for mesothelioma, and Chapter 68 for malignant pleural effusions.

TRANSUDATIVE PLEURAL EFFUSIONS

Transudative pleural effusions occur because of increased hydrostatic or decreased oncotic pressures.

Congestive Heart Failure

Congestive heart failure is responsible for more pleural effusions than any other disease process. The pleural effusions that occur with congestive heart failure tend to be bilateral and of approximately the same size on each side. Almost all patients with pleural effusions secondary to congestive heart failure have left ventricular or biventricular failure. Patients with congestive heart failure and pleural effusion should undergo diagnostic thoracentesis if the effusions are not bilateral and comparable in size, if the patients are febrile, or if they have pleuritic chest pain to verify that the fluid is transudative. Otherwise, the effusion can be observed while the heart failure is treated, and it usually resolves.

Rarely, a patient with congestive heart failure has a persistent pleural effusion despite intensive therapy. If such patients are dyspneic and if their dyspnea is relieved by a therapeutic thoracentesis, consideration can be given to attempting a pleurodesis with a sclerosing agent such as a doxycycline or talc slurry.

Hepatic Hydrothorax

Pleural effusions occur in approximately 5% of patients with cirrhosis and ascites. The predominant mechanism responsible for the pleural effusion is the direct movement of peritoneal fluid through small holes in the diaphragm into the pleural space. The effusions are usually right sided and frequently are large enough to produce severe dyspnea. If medical management of the cirrhosis and ascites does not control the pleural effusion, several options exist.

The ideal treatment is to reverse the liver disease. This is best done with a liver transplant, but not all patients with a hepatic hydrothorax are candidates for transplantation. The next best treatment is probably implantation of a transjugular intrahepatic portal systemic shunt. Strauss and associates (1994) performed this procedure in five patients and reported that the requirement for thoracenteses was eliminated in four and was greatly reduced in the fifth patient.

If liver transplantation or transjugular intrahepatic portal systemic shunt is not feasible, then the best treatment is probably videothoracoscopy with closure of the diaphragmatic defects and talc insufflation. Mouroux and coworkers (1996) performed this procedure on eight patients. They found diaphragmatic defects that could be closed in six of the eight patients, and none of these six patients developed recurrent pleural effusions. The remaining two patients did develop recurrent effusions but they only occupied approximately one-third of the hemithorax. Pleurodesis also can be attempted with an agent such as doxycycline or talc slurry after tube thoracostomy, but Runyon and coworkers (1986) believe that this procedure is contraindicated in these patients because of the danger of hypovolemia and even death.

An alternative treatment is the insertion of a peritoneo-jugular shunt. As demonstrated by Park and coworkers (1997), these shunts can sometimes control the effusion. However, they frequently do not control the effusion because fluid preferentially moves to the pleural space where the hydrostatic pressure is less than it is in the central veins.

One possibility that must be kept in mind when managing a patient with a hepatic hydrothorax is a spontaneous bacterial empyema. Spontaneous bacterial empyema is the infection of a preexisting hepatic hydrothorax in which a parapneumonic infection has been excluded. In a prospective study at a university-based referral hospital, Xiol and associates (1996) reported that 16 of 120 patients (13%) admitted with a diagnosis of hepatic hydrothorax had a spontaneous bacterial empyema. The criteria for the diagnosis of a spontaneous empyema are a positive pleural fluid culture result and a pleural fluid neutrophil count greater than 250 cells/mL with the exclusion of a pneumonic process. Culture-negative spontaneous bacterial empyema is diagnosed in patients with a negative pleural fluid culture result, but with a compatible clinical course and a neutrophil count greater than 500 per mL. Xiol and coworkers reported that 10 of 24 episodes (43%) were not associated with bacterial peritonitis. Treatment of spontaneous empyema requires tube thoracostomy.

Nephrotic Syndrome

Pleural effusions that are caused by decreased plasma oncotic pressure occur in approximately 20% of patients with the nephrotic syndrome. The possibility of pulmonary emboli should always be considered in patients with this syndrome, and a lung scan, pulmonary arteriography, or both should be obtained to exclude this diagnosis. Optimally, treatment of the nephrotic syndrome results in an increased level of protein in the serum and resolution of the pleural effusion.

Peritoneal Dialysis

Large pleural effusions occasionally complicate peritoneal dialysis. The mechanism appears to be a diaphragmatic defect as it is for the hydrothorax seen with cirrhosis and ascites. Frequently, one wants to continue the dialysis in these patients. Such cases are best managed, as recommended by Chow and associates (1988), by chemical pleurodesis induced by a tetracycline derivative combined with a short period of small-volume, intermittent peritoneal dialysis.

EXUDATIVE PLEURAL EFFUSIONS

Pleural Effusions That Are Caused by Pulmonary Embolization

The diagnosis most commonly overlooked in the differential diagnosis of a patient with an undiagnosed pleural effusion is pulmonary embolization. The symptoms of patients with pleural effusions accompanying pulmonary embolization are no different from those in patients with emboli but without pleural effusion. Dyspnea is reported by more than 80% of the patients and is usually greater than one would expect from a similar-sized effusion with a different etiology.

The pleural effusion associated with pulmonary embolization usually occupies less than one-third of the hemithorax. Coche and associates (1998) reported that 13 of 26 patients (50%) with pulmonary emboli had pleural effusions. The pleural effusions were bilateral in 6 of the 13 and were not necessarily related to the side of the effusion. Nothing is characteristic about the pleural fluid associated with pulmonary embolization. It may be a transudate or an exudate; may be bloody or clear; and may contain mostly neutrophils, lymphocytes, or other mononuclear cells.

Any patient with an undiagnosed pleural effusion should undergo perfusion lung scanning or contrast-enhanced spiral CT. If doubt persists, pulmonary arteriography should be performed. The treatment of the patient with a pleural effusion secondary to pulmonary embolism is the same as for any patient with pulmonary emboli. If the pleural effusion increases in size with treatment, the patient probably has recurrent emboli or another complication such as a hemothorax or a pleural infection.

Pleural Effusions Secondary to Diseases of the Gastrointestinal Tract

Esophageal Perforation

The possibility of esophageal rupture should be considered in acutely ill patients with pleural effusion, because the mortality from this condition approaches 100% if it is not appropriately diagnosed and treated within 48 hours. Esophageal rupture occurs spontaneously in patients who have vomited or iatrogenically after endoscopy or insertion of a Blakemore tube. Patients with esophageal rupture are acutely ill with chest pain and dyspnea caused by the mediastinal and pleural infection. Subcutaneous emphysema in the suprasternal notch is suggestive of the diagnosis. The best screening test for esophageal rupture is the measurement of the level of amylase in the pleural fluid. With esophageal rupture, the pleural fluid amylase level is elevated because of the high amylase level in the saliva that enters the pleural space. The diagnosis is confirmed with the demonstration of esophageal disruption via contrast studies.

The treatment of choice for esophageal perforation is exploration of the mediastinum with primary repair of the esophageal tear and drainage of the pleural space and mediastinum. Large doses of parenteral antibiotics should be given to treat the mediastinitis and the pleural infection. If exploration of the mediastinum is delayed more than 48 hours after rupture, primary repair is usually not possible because of the damaged tissue. Such patients may be managed with T-tube intubation of the esophageal defect, as suggested by Bufkin and associates (1996) (see Chapter 132 for a detailed discussion of this problem).

Acute Pancreatitis

A high prevalence of pleural effusions occurs in patients with acute pancreatitis. In a study of 133 patients with acute pancreatitis with contrast-enhanced CT scans, Lankisch and coworkers (1994) found that the prevalence of pleural effusions with acute pancreatitis is approximately 50%. Fifty-one of the effusions were bilateral, 10 were unilateral left-sided, and five were unilateral right-sided. At times, with acute pancreatitis, respiratory symptoms consisting of pleuritic chest pain and dyspnea may dominate the clinical picture. The prevalence of pancreatic pseudocyst is much higher in patients with pleural effusion than in those without pleural effusion. If the pleural effusion does not resolve within 2 weeks of starting appropriate therapy for the pancreatitis, the possibility of a pancreatic abscess or a pancreatic pseudocyst should be considered.

Chronic Pancreatic Disease

Patients with chronic pancreatic disease on occasion develop a sinus tract from their pancreas through the diaphragm into the mediastinum and then into the pleural space. The clinical picture of patients with chronic pancreatic disease and pleural effusion is usually dominated by chest symptoms such as dyspnea, cough, and chest pain. Rockey and Cello (1990) found that most patients do not have abdominal symptoms, because the pancreaticopleural fistula decompresses the pseudocyst. The pleural effusion is usually massive and recurs rapidly after thoracentesis. The effusion is most commonly left sided but may be right sided or bilateral.

The diagnosis is suggested by a high pleural fluid amylase level and is confirmed by abdominal CT scan or ultrasound. Endoscopic retrograde cholangiopancreatography usually documents the fistulous tract or other pathology in the pancreas.

Patients with chronic pancreatic pleural effusions should be given a trial of conservative therapy for 2 to 3 weeks. Rockey and Cello (1990) recommended that this therapy

consist of nasogastric suction, no oral intake, suppression of pancreatic secretion with atropine, and repeated therapeutic thoracenteses. Pederzoli and associates (1986) reported that the administration of a continuous infusion of somatostatin may decrease the secretions through the fistula and facilitate closure. If conservative treatment fails, which Parekh and Segal (1992) reported is much more common when the patient has severe pancreatitis, a laparotomy should be performed. The anatomy of the pancreatic ductal system should be assessed preoperatively with endoscopic retrograde cholangiopancreatography or at the time of operation with an operative pancreatogram. If a sinus tract is found, it should be ligated or excised. The pancreas should be partially resected, drained with a Roux-en-Y loop, or both. Faling and colleagues (1984) suggested an alternate approach whereby the pancreatic pseudocyst was drained by percutaneous catheter drainage. Decortication of the pleura may be necessary for some patients.

Intra-abdominal Abscess

Pleural effusions frequently accompany intra-abdominal abscesses, including subphrenic (80%), pancreatic (40%), intrasplenic (35%), and intrahepatic (20%). The pleural fluid is a sterile exudate with predominantly neutrophils. The possibility of an intra-abdominal abscess should be considered seriously in a patient with a persistent neutrophilic pleural effusion and no parenchymal infiltrates. The diagnosis is best established by abdominal CT scan, and treatment consists of antibiotics plus drainage.

Pleural Effusions after Surgical Procedures

After Cardiac Injury Syndrome

The postcardiac injury syndrome, also called the postpericardiectomy or postmyocardial infarction (Dressler's) syndrome, is characterized by pericarditis, pleuritis, or pneumonitis, or a combination of these, that occurs after injury to the myocardium or pericardium. The syndrome typically develops approximately 3 weeks after the injury but can occur anytime between 3 days and 1 year. The pleural fluid is an exudate that is frequently serosanguineous or bloody. The treatment of choice is the use of anti-inflammatory agents such as aspirin or indomethacin. Patients with this syndrome after coronary artery bypass procedures should be treated with corticosteroids because the pericarditis may cause graft occlusion.

After Coronary Artery Bypass Surgery

A high prevalence of small pleural effusions occurs after coronary artery bypass surgery. Peng and coworkers (1992) and Hurlbut and associates (1990) have reported that the incidence of pleural effusion after coronary artery bypass surgery exceeds 40%. The incidence is comparable whether saphenous vein graphs or internal mammary artery grafts are used. The pathogenesis of the effusions is unknown, but Peng and coworkers (1992) have speculated that they are caused by pericardial inflammation. The effusions are predominantly small and on the left side. In almost all cases, the effusions resolve spontaneously without treatment over several weeks.

A few patients develop larger symptomatic pleural effusions after coronary artery bypass surgery. In a prospective study, Rodriguez and colleagues (1998) reported that 29 of 320 patients had effusions that occupied more than 25% of the hemithorax 28 days postoperatively. Although chylothorax, pleural infection, the postcardiac injury syndrome, pulmonary embolism, and congestive heart failure can all cause pleural effusions after coronary artery bypass surgery, most of these larger effusions have no clear-cut etiology. These unexplained exudative effusions can be divided into two categories: bloody and nonbloody. The bloody effusions tend to reach their maximal size within 30 days of surgery, frequently are associated with peripheral eosinophilia, have a high pleural fluid LDH, and respond to one or two therapeutic thoracenteses. In contrast, the nonbloody exudative pleural effusions tend to reach their maximal size more than 30 days postoperatively, have more than 50% small lymphocytes, and have a relatively low pleural fluid LDH. These nonbloody pleural effusions are more difficult to manage, frequently requiring pleurodesis with a sclerosing agent. The bloody pleural effusions are probably related to blood in the pleural space secondary to surgery. No known etiology for the nonbloody pleural effusions exists.

After Fontan Procedure

With this procedure, the right ventricle is bypassed by an anastomosis between the superior vena cava, the right atrium, or the inferior vena cava and the pulmonary artery. This surgery is usually performed for tricuspid atresia or univentricular heart. As reported by Laks and coworkers (1984), a transudative pleural effusion occurs postoperatively in nearly every patient and is a significant problem postoperatively in many patients. Spicer and associates (1996) have demonstrated that effusions are more likely to occur in patients who have significant aortopulmonary collateral vessels preoperatively. They recommend embolization of these vessels at preoperative angiography. The treatment of choice for this condition is probably the insertion of a pleuroperitoneal shunt, as suggested by Sade and Wiles (1990). An alternative treatment is creation of a late fenestration as suggested by Rychik and coworkers (1997).

After Abdominal Surgery

The author and George (1976) reported that the incidence of pleural effusion in the 2 to 3 days after abdominal surgery is approximately 50%. The incidence of postoperative pleural effusion is greater in patients undergoing upper abdominal surgery, in patients with postoperative atelectasis, and in those patients with free abdominal fluid at surgery. The pleural effusion in the postoperative period is probably caused either by diaphragmatic irritation or the transdiaphragmatic movement of intra-abdominal fluid. If a patient develops a significant amount of fluid postoperatively, a diagnostic thoracentesis should be performed to rule out pleural infection as a cause of the effusion. The possibility of pulmonary embolization also should be considered. If the effusion develops more than 72 hours postoperatively, it is probably not related to the surgical procedure itself, and alternate explanations must be found such as pulmonary embolization, intra-abdominal abscess, or hypervolemia.

After Endoscopic Variceal Sclerotherapy

Endoscopic variceal sclerotherapy has become one of the principal forms of therapy for patients who have bled from ruptured esophageal varices. Edling and Bacon (1991) have reported that small pleural effusions complicate this procedure approximately 50% of the time. The pleural effusion is thought to result from the extravasation of the sclerosant into the esophageal mucosa, which results in an intense inflammatory reaction in the mediastinum and pleura. The effusions can be right sided, left sided, or bilateral, and the fluid is exudative. If the effusion persists for more than 24 to 48 hours and is accompanied by fever or if the effusion occupies more than 25% of the hemithorax, a thoracentesis should be done to rule out an infection or an esophagopleural fistula. The latter diagnosis is suggested by a high pleural fluid amylase level.

After Liver Transplantation

Almost all patients who undergo an orthotopic liver transplantation develop a pleural effusion postoperatively. Spizarny and associates (1993) prospectively evaluated 42 liver transplant recipients and reported that 40 of 42 patients (95%) developed a right-sided pleural effusion within 72 hours of transplantation. The effusions may be large. Bilik and coworkers (1992) reported that 23 of 48 children (48%) receiving transplants developed effusions large enough to cause respiratory compromise and that tube thoracostomy was necessary in 15 patients (31%). The pathogenesis of the pleural effusion after liver transplantation is not definitely known, but it has been suggested that the effusion is caused by injury or irritation of the right hemidiaphragm caused by the extensive right upper quadrant dissection and retraction. Uetsuji and associates (1994) have shown that the pleural effusions can be largely prevented if a fibrin sealant is sprayed on the undersurface of the diaphragm around the insertion of the liver ligaments. The natural history of these effusions is that they increase in size over the first 3 postoperative days and then gradually resolve over a period ranging from several weeks to several months. If the effusion increases in size after the first 3 days, subdiaphragmatic pathology such as a hematoma, abscess, or biloma should be suspected.

After Lung Transplantation

With lung transplantation, the lymphatics that normally drain the lung are severed. Accordingly, fluid that normally leaves the lung via these lymphatics exits via the pleural space. Nevertheless, pleural effusions are usually not evident in the few days after lung transplantation because chest tubes are in place. Judson and associates (1996) reported that the mean daily pleural fluid drainage via chest tube dropped from 400 mL on the first postoperative day to 200 mL on the fourth postoperative day. The pleural fluid drainage reached almost 1000 mL in a patient who developed the postreimplantation response.

As might be expected, patients who develop pleural complications post–lung transplantation are likely to develop pleural effusions. Judson and Sahn (1996) reported that pleural effusions occurred with 14 of 19 (74%) episodes of acute rejection, seven of eight (88%) instances of chronic rejection, 6 of 11 (55%) episodes of infection, and three of four (75%) instances of lymphoproliferative disease.

Pleural Effusions That Are Caused by Miscellaneous Diseases

Acquired Immunodeficiency Syndrome and Pleural Effusion

Pleural effusions are relatively uncommon in patients with acquired immunodeficiency syndrome (AIDS). As reported by Strazzella and Safirstein (1991) parapneumonic effusions are the most common cause of pleural effusion in patients with AIDS, and these parapneumonic effusions are more likely to be complicated in patients with AIDS than in immunocompetent patients. Other common causes of pleural effusions in patients with AIDS include Kaposi's sarcoma, tuberculosis, cryptococcosis, lymphoma, and, rarely, *Pneumocystis carinii* infection.

Rheumatoid Pleuritis

Approximately 5% of patients with rheumatoid arthritis have a pleural effusion sometime during their life. Most effusions occur in the older man with subcutaneous nodules. The pleural fluid with rheumatoid pleuritis is distinctive, characterized by a glucose level less than 30 mg/dL, a high LDH level (700 IU/L), and a low pH (less than 7.20). The pleural effusion usually resolves spontaneously within 3 months. No controlled study has documented the efficacy of any treatment.

Lupus Erythematosus

Approximately 40% of patients with systemic lupus erythematosus or drug-induced systemic lupus erythematosus develop a pleural effusion during the course of their disease. The pleuritis may be the first manifestation of the underlying disease. Most patients with lupus pleuritis have pleuritic chest pain and are febrile. The diagnosis is made primarily via the clinical picture and serologic test results on the serum. Khare and coworkers (1994) have shown that an elevated pleural fluid antinuclear antibody titer is not diagnostic of lupus pleuritis. Patients with lupus pleuritis should be treated with prednisone, 80 mg every other day, with rapid tapering once the symptoms are controlled.

Asbestos Exposure

Pleural effusions develop in approximately 3% of individuals who have had moderate to heavy asbestos exposure. The resulting exudative pleural effusion usually develops between 5 and 20 years of the initial exposure. Patients with pleural effusion are usually asymptomatic. The diagnosis of benign asbestos effusion is one of exclusion and requires the following: asbestos exposure, exclusion of other causes (e.g., infection, pulmonary embolism, malignancy), and a follow-up of at least 2 years to verify that it is benign.

Drug Reactions

Administration of nitrofurantoin, dantrolene, methysergide, and bromocriptine at times is associated with a syndrome characterized by fever, dyspnea, chest pain, and peripheral blood and pleural eosinophilia, which develop weeks to months after initiation of therapy. Discontinuation of the offending medication results in resolution of the syndrome.

Uremia

Uremia may be complicated by a fibrinous pleuritis and pleural effusion. Approximately 3% of uremics have an exudative pleural effusion, and no close relationship exists between the degree of uremia and the occurrence of a pleural effusion. After dialysis is initiated, the effusion gradually disappears within 4 to 6 weeks in the majority of patients.

REFERENCES

Aiba M, Inatomi K, Homma H: Lymphatic system or hydro-oncotic forces. Which is more significant in drainage of pleural fluid? Jpn J Med 23:27, 1984.

Albertine KH, et al: Structure, blood supply, and lymphatic vessels of the sheep's visceral pleura. Am J Anat 165:277, 1982.

Albertine KH, Wiener-Kronish JP, Staub NC: The structure of the parietal pleura and its relationship to pleural liquid dynamics in sheep. Anat Rec 208:401, 1984.

Allen S, Gabel J, Drake R: Left atrial hypertension causes pleural effusion formation in unanesthetized sheep. Am J Physiol 257(2 Pt 2):H690, 1989.

Amouzadeh HR, et al: Xylazine-induced pulmonary edema in rats. Toxicol Appl Pharmacol 108:417, 1991.

Bernaudin JF, et al: Protein transfer in hyperoxic induced pleural effusion in the rat. Exp Lung Res 210:23, 1986.

Bilik R, Yellen M, Superina RA: Surgical complications in children after liver transplantation. J Pediatr Surg 27:1371, 1992.

Broaddus VC, et al: Removal of pleural liquid and protein by lymphatics in awake sheep. J Appl Physiol 64:384, 1988.

Broaddus VC, Light RW: What is the origin of pleural transudates and exudates? (Editorial). Chest 102:658, 1992.

Broaddus VC, Wiener-Kronish JP, Staub ND: Clearance of lung edema into the pleural space of volume-loaded anesthetized sheep. J Appl Physiol 68:2623, 1990.

Bufkin BL, Miller JI Jr, Mansour KA: Esophageal perforation: emphasis on management. Ann Thorac Surg 61:1447, 1996.

Burgess LJ, Maritz FJ, Taljaard JJ: Comparative analysis of the biochemical parameters used to distinguish between pleural transudates and exudates. Chest 107:1604, 1995.

Burgess LJ, et al: Combined use of pleural adenosine deaminase with lymphocyte/neutrophil ratio. Increased specificity for the diagnosis of tuberculous pleuritis. Chest 109:414, 1996.

Chang S-C, Perng RP: The role of fiberoptic bronchoscopy in evaluating the causes of pleural effusions. Arch Intern Med 149:855, 1989.

Cheng D-S, et al: Comparison of pleural fluid pH values obtained using blood gas machine, pH meter and pH indicator strip. Chest 1998 (in press).

Chow CC, et al: Massive hydrothorax in continuous ambulatory peritoneal dialysis: diagnosis, management and review of the literature. NZ Med J 27:475, 1988.

Coche EE, et al: Acute pulmonary embolism: ancillary findings at spiral CT. Radiology 207:753, 1998.

Edling JE, Bacon BR: Pleuropulmonary complications of endoscopic variceal sclerotherapy. Chest 99:1252, 1991.

Faling LJ, et al: Treatment of chronic pancreatic pleural effusion by percutaneous catheter drainage of abdominal pseudocyst. Am J Med 76:329, 1984.

Feinsilver SH, Barrows AA, Braman SS: Fiberoptic bronchoscopy and pleural effusion of unknown origin. Chest 90:514, 1986.

Gaudio E, et al: Surface morphology of the human pleura. A scanning electron microscopic study. Chest 92:149, 1988.

Hurlbut D, et al: Pleuropulmonary morbidity: internal thoracic artery versus saphenous vein graft. Ann Thorac Surg 50:959, 1990.

Judson MA, Handy JR, Sahn SA: Pleural effusions following lung transplantation. Time course, characteristics, and clinical implications. Chest 109:1190, 1996.

Judson MA, Sahn SA: The pleural space and organ transplantation. Am J Respir Crit Care Med 153:1153, 1996.

Khare V, et al: Antinuclear antibodies in pleural fluid. Chest 106:866, 1994.

Kinasewitz GT, et al: Role of pulmonary lymphatics and interstitium in visceral pleural fluid exchange. J Appl Physiol 56:355, 1984.

Kramer MR, Cepero RJ, Pitchenik AE: High amylase in neoplasm-related pleural effusion. Ann Intern Med 110:567, 1989.

Laks H, et al: Experience with the Fontan procedure. J Thorac Cardiovasc Surg 88:939, 1984.

Lankisch PG, Groge M, Becher R: Pleural effusions: a new negative prognostic parameter for acute pancreatitis. Am J Gastroenterol 89:1849, 1994.

Leckie WJH, Tothill P: Albumin turnover in pleural effusions. Clin Sci 29:339, 1965.

Lee JS, et al: Immunohistochemical panel for distinguishing between carcinoma and reactive mesothelial cells in serious effusions. Acta Cytol 40:631, 1996.

Light RW: Pleural Diseases. 3rd Ed. Baltimore: Williams and Wilkins, 1995.

Light RW, et al: Pleural effusions: the diagnostic separation of transudates and exudates. Ann Intern Med 77:507, 1972.

Light RW, George RB: Incidence and significance of pleural effusion after abdominal surgery. Chest 69:621, 1976.

Light RW, et al: Large pleural effusions occurring after coronary artery bypass surgery (CABG). Am J Respir Crit Care Med 157:A65, 1998.

Loddenkemper R. Thoracoscopy—state of the art. Eur Respir J 11:213, 1998.

Mouroux J, et al: Management of pleural effusion of cirrhotic origin. Chest 109:1093, 1996.

Parekh D, Segal I: Pancreatic ascites and effusion. Risk factors for failure of conservative therapy and the role of octreotide. Arch Surg 127:707, 1992.

Park SZ, et al: Treatment of refractory, nonmalignant hydrothorax with a pleurovenous shunt. Ann Thorac Surg 63:1777, 1997.

Pederzoli P, et al: Conservative treatment of external pancreatic fistulas with parenteral nutrition alone or in combination with continuous intravenous infusion of somatostatin, glucagon or calcitonin. Surg Gynecol Obstet 163:428, 1986.

Peng M-J, et al: Postoperative pleural changes after coronary revascularization. Comparison between saphenous vein and internal mammary artery grafting. Chest 101:327, 1992.

Poe RH, et al: Sensitivity, specificity, and predictive values of closed pleural biopsy. Arch Intern Med 144:325, 1984.

Poe RH, et al: Use of fiberoptic bronchoscopy in the diagnosis of bronchogenic carcinoma. A study in patients with idiopathic pleural effusions. Chest 105:1663, 1994.

Prakash URS, Reiman HM: Comparison of needle biopsy with cytologic analysis for the evaluation of pleural effusion: analysis of 414 cases. Mayo Clin Proc 60:158, 1985.

Querol JM, et al: Rapid diagnosis of pleural tuberculosis by polymerase chain reaction. Am J Respir Crit Care Med 152:1977, 1995.

Rockey DC, Cello JP: Pancreaticopleural fistula. Report of 7 cases and review of the literature. Medicine 69:332, 1990.

Rodriguez RM, et al: Incidence of pleural effusions 30 days post coronary artery bypass surgery. Chest 114:1998 (in press).

Runyon BA, Greenblatt M, Ming RHC: Hepatic hydrothorax is a relative contraindication to chest tube insertion. Am J Gastroenterol 81:566, 1986.

Ryan CJ, et al: The outcome of patients with pleural effusion of indeterminate cause at thoracotomy. Mayo Clin Proc 56:145, 1981.

Rychik J, Rome JJ, Jacobs ML: Late surgical fenestration for complications after the Fontan operation. Circulation 96:33, 1997.

Sade RM, Wiles HB: Pleuroperitoneal shunt for persistent pleural drainage after Fontan procedure. J Thorac Cardiovasc Surg 100:621, 1990.

Shinto RA, Light RW: The effects of diuresis upon the characteristics of pleural fluid in patients with congestive heart failure. Am J Med 88:230, 1990.

Spicer RL, et al: Aortopulmonary collateral vessels and prolonged pleural effusions after modified Fontan procedures. Am Heart J 131:1164, 1996.

Spizarny DL, Gross BH, McLoud T: Enlarging pleural effusion after liver transplantation. J Thorac Imaging 8:85, 1993.

Stewart PB: The rate of formation and lymphatic removal of fluid in pleural effusions. J Clin Invest 42:258, 1963.

Strauss RM, et al: Transjugular intrahepatic portal systemic shunt for the management of symptomatic cirrhotic hydrothorax. Am J Gastroenterol 89:1520, 1994.

Strazzella WD, Safirstein BH: Pleural effusions in AIDS. NJ Med 88:39, 1991.

Uetsuji S, et al: Prevention of pleural effusion after hepatectomy using fibrin sealant. Int Surg 79:135, 1994.

Valdes L, et al: Tuberculous pleurisy: a study of 254 cases. Arch Intern Med 1998 (in press).

Villena V, et al: Interferongamma in 388 immunocompromised and immunocompetent patients for diagnosing pleural tuberculosis. Eur Respir J 9:2635, 1996.

Wang NS: The preformed stomas connecting the pleural cavity and the lymphatics in the parietal pleura. Am Rev Respir Dis 111:12, 1975.

Wiener-Kronish JP, et al: Protein egress and entry rates in pleural fluid and plasma in sheep. J Appl Physiol 56:459, 1984.

Wiener-Kronish JP, et al: Relationship of pleural effusions to pulmonary hemodynamics in patients with congestive heart failure. Am Rev Respir Dis 132:1253, 1985.

Wiener-Kronish JP, et al: Relationship of pleural effusions to increased permeability pulmonary edema in anesthetized sheep. J Clin Invest 82:1422, 1988.

Xiol X, et al. Spontaneous bacterial empyema in cirrhotic patients: a prospective study. Hepatology 23:719, 1996.

CHAPTER 58

Parapneumonic Empyema

Joseph S. McLaughlin and Mark J. Krasna

Pleural effusion is a common accompaniment of the inflammation of bacterial pneumonia. These "uncomplicated effusions" are nonpurulent, have a negative Gram's stain result for bacteria, have negative results by culture, and are generally free flowing. Light (1985, 1991) and associates (1980), using biochemical parameters, noted a pH greater than 7.30, a normal glucose level, and a lactic acid dehydrogenase (LDH) concentration less than 1000 IU/L. Most parapneumonic effusions resolve with appropriate antibiotic treatment and resolution of the pulmonary infection.

Thoracic empyema occurs when bacteria invade the normally sterile pleural space. The process was described by Andrews and colleagues, reporting for the American Thoracic Society in 1962, as a continuum of three stages (Table 58-1).

Stage 1 is characterized by the presence of an exudative effusion from increased permeability of the inflamed and swollen pleural surfaces. This stage corresponds to the uncomplicated parapneumonic effusion of Light and colleagues (1980) and is initially sterile. Fibrin is deposited and polymorphonuclear leukocytes are present in small numbers. With bacterial invasion, the process blends into the fibropurulent stage 2, true empyema or Light's "complicated" pleural effusion. Initially, the fluid is still relatively clear and yellow, but the white blood cell count is greater than 500 cells per µL, the specific gravity is greater than 1.018, and the protein level is greater than 2.5 g/dL. The pH is less than 7.2 and the LDH levels reach 1000 IU/L. Although fibrin deposits and early angioblastic and fibroblastic proliferation are seen in later phases of the exudative stage, these processes accelerate, and heavy fibrin deposition takes place on both pleural surfaces, particularly the parietal pleura. The effusion becomes purulent, with a white cell count above 15,000 cells per µL. Biochemically, the pH decreases to levels below 7.0, the glucose decreases to less than 50 mg/dL, and the LDH increases to greater than 1000 IU/L. Stage 3 begins as early as 1 week after infection with collagen organization and deposition on both pleural surfaces and entrapment of the underlying lung. This process is mature in 3 to 4 weeks, and the organized collagen on the pleural surface is termed a *peel*. The effusion at this point is grossly purulent and at least 75% of the volume is sediment on standing. Chronicity is characterized by dense fibrosis, contraction and trapping of the lung, atelectasis and prolonged pulmonary infection, and reduction of the size of the hemithorax. Fibrothorax with invasion of the chest wall and narrowing of the intercostal spaces may be thought of as the end stage of this process.

Complications of the empyema process may take place early or late. Necrosis of the visceral pleural surface, as noted by Hankins and associates (1978), may result in bronchopleural fistula heralded by sudden expectoration of, at times, copious amounts of purulent sputum. Marks and Eickhoff (1970) described that the necrosis of the parietal pleura and the chest wall and skin results in empyema necessitatis. These conditions are usually seen in patients treated with antibiotics for pneumonia who have unrecognized empyema. Often, these patients have persistent low-grade fever until the empyema drains through the chest wall or into the lung. Rarely, osteomyelitis of the ribs or spine may occur. Invasion of the mediastinum with pulmonary esophageal fistula and pericarditis have been reported also. Metastatic spread is unusual, but Scheld (1998) has suggested that up to 12% of brain abscesses are from pleuropulmonary disease including empyema.

BACTERIOLOGY

The bacterial etiology of empyema has changed over the years. Before the development of antibiotics, 10% of patients who survived pneumonia developed empyema. According to Ehler (1941), *Streptococcus* and *Pneumococcus* were the most frequent organisms. After the introduction of antibiotics, the incidence of empyema from these organisms was markedly reduced as was the mortality. *Staphylococcus* became much more prevalent and, in the 1950s and 1960s, Ravitch and Fein (1961) found that this organism produced 90% of empyema in children under age 2 years. In more recent times, as pointed out by Varkey and associates (1981) and Bergeron (1990), penicillin-resistant *Staphylo-*

Table 58-1. American Thoracic Society Classification of Empyema

Stage 1	Exudative with swelling of the pleural membranes
Stage 2	Fibrinopurulent with heavy fibrin deposits
Stage 3	Organization with ingrowth of fibroblasts and deposition of collagen

From Andrews NC, et al: Management of nontuberculous empyema: a statement of the subcommittee on surgery. Am Rev Respir Dis 85:935, 1962. With permission.

coccus, gram-negative bacteria, and anaerobic organisms have been the predominant microbes. Bartlett and colleagues (1974a) reported that 76% of empyema patients had positive culture results for either anaerobes exclusively (35%) or anaerobes in combination with aerobes (41%). Anaerobic bacteria are normal flora of the mouth, intestine, and female genital tract. They are difficult to culture, being extremely oxygen sensitive. Multiple organisms are frequently cultured (50 in the series of Sullivan and colleagues [1973]), but the most common is *Peptostreptococcus*. Similar findings were recorded by Ali and Unrah (1990).

Brook and Frazier (1993) independently studied 197 patients with culture-positive empyema from two military hospitals. Aerobic organisms were isolated in 127 patients (64%), mixed aerobic and anaerobic organisms in 45 patients (23%), and anaerobic organisms in 25 patients (13%). The predominant aerobic or facultative bacterial isolates were *Streptococcus pneumoniae* (70), *Staphylococcus aureus* (58), *Escherichia coli* (17), *Klebsiella pneumoniae* (16), and *Haemophilus influenzae* (12). The predominant anaerobes were anaerobic cocci (36), pigmented *Prevotella* and *Porphyromonas* (24), *Bacteroides fragilis* (22), and *Fusobacterium* spp. (20). Most patients from whom *S. pneumoniae* and *H. influenzae* were cultured had pneumonia. Most patients from whom *S. aureus* were recovered had pneumonia, aspiration pneumonia, or lung abscesses. Recovery of anaerobic bacteria was associated with the diagnosis of aspiration pneumonia and lung, dental, and oropharyngeal abscesses.

In children, the clinical and bacteriologic scenario has changed as well. Empyema is more often seen in older children as opposed to infants and is most commonly caused by *Pneumococcus*. In a study by Hardie and coworkers (1996) of community-acquired pneumonia complicated by empyema in children reported in 1996, 40% of empyemas were caused by *S. pneumoniae*, 15% of which were penicillin-resistant, and 44% had negative culture results. None of the empyemas were associated with *S. aureus* or *H. influenzae*, and only one was caused by group A *Streptococcus*. Miller (1990) suggests that the culture-negative status of these children is now a common finding because of pretreatment with antibiotics in the community setting.

The propensity for developing empyema varies considerably with the type of bacteria producing the primary pneu-

Table 58-2. Etiology of Pneumonia

Agent	Incidence (%)[a]
Community-acquired pneumonia	
Streptococcus pneumoniae	60–75
Hemophilus influenzae[b]	5–10
Staphylococcus aureus	<5
Mycoplasma pneumoniae	1–10
Legionella pneumophila	1–5
Chlamydia pneumoniae	1–5
Streptococcus pyogenes[c]	<1
Unknown	35%
Hospital-acquired pneumonia	
Aerobic gram negative	45+
Klebsiella pneumoniae	
Escherichia coli	
Pseudomonas aeruginosa[d]	
S. aureus	<10

[a]Incidence varies with series.
[b]Empyema complicates 10% of *H. influenzae* pneumonias in children, but is rare in adults.
[c]Empyema in 30% or greater. Incidence may be much higher in children.
[d]Most common cause of pneumonia in intensive care unit, with significant potential for empyema.

monia, the setting in which the infection is acquired, and the alteration in these produced by antibiotic therapy administered for primary pneumonia or for concurrent conditions. For example, as reported by Bartlett and colleagues (1974a), Fang and colleagues (1990), Light (1990), and Johnson and Finegold (1994), *S. pneumoniae* is responsible for 60 to 75% of community-acquired pneumonias, but only 2% of patients with pneumococcal pneumonia develop empyema (Tables 58-2 through 58-4). *S. pneumoniae* accounts for 1 to 2% of community-acquired pneumonias, but up to 10% of adults and 50% of children develop empyema. In hospital settings, *Staphylococcus* and aerobic, gram-negative bacteria are the most common agents producing pneumonia. Both have significant potential to produce empyema.

Table 58-3. Incidence of Empyema According to Bacteria-Causing Pneumonia

Organism	Effusion (%)	Incidence of Empyema (%)
Aerobic		
Gram positive		
Streptococcus pneumoniae	50	<5
Staphylococcus aureus (children)	70	80
S. aureus (adults)	40	20
Gram negative		
Escherichia coli	50	90
Pseudomonas	50	90
Anaerobic	35	90

Table 58-4. Frequency of Causative Organisms of Parapneumonic Empyemas

Organism	n (%)
Peptostreptococcus	5 (12)
Staphylococcus epidermidis	5
Streptococcus viridans	4 (10)
Peptococcus	3 (7)
Diphtheroids	3
Staphylococcus aureus	3
Streptococcus pyogenes	2 (5)
Haemophilus influenzae	2
Fusobacterium nucleatum	2
Acinetobacter	2
Bacteroides (*Prevotella*)	2
Enterobacter aerogenes	1 (2)
Klebsiella pneumoniae	1
Pseudomonas	1
Microaerophilic streptococci	1
Micrococcus spp.	1
Streptococcus pneumoniae	1
Clostridium spp.	1
Anaerobic gram-positive cocci	1
Anaerobic gram-positive bacilli	1
Total	**42**

From Ali I, Unruh H: Management of empyema thoracis. Ann Thorac Surg *50*:335, 1990. With permission.

CLINICAL FEATURES

Empyema may be heralded by an exacerbation or recurrence of the septic course of pneumonia, or it may present as a continuation of symptoms and manifestations of the primary pneumonic process. Antibiotics have blunted and changed the clinical picture so that progression from the symptoms and signs of pneumonia to those of empyema may be subtle. The most common presenting symptoms of empyema according to Varkey and colleagues (1981) are shortness of breath (82%), fever (81%), cough (70%), and chest pain (67%). All of these are common to pneumonia as well. The presence of these symptoms in a patient with febrile respiratory illness or the accentuation or prolongation of these symptoms in a patient with pneumonia should alert the clinician to the possibility of empyema. The clinician should be aware that the incidence of pleuritic chest pain and leukocytosis is similar whether or not pleural effusion is present.

Empyema from aerobic bacterial pneumonia usually presents as an acute febrile illness with chest pain, sputum production, and leukocytosis. Anaerobic pleural infection is more indolent and, in Bartlett and colleagues' series (1974a), averaged 10 days before presentation. The majority of these patients have a history of alcoholism or unconsciousness, have lost weight, and have mild anemia, although hospital-acquired infection and immunosuppression may alter this course.

Physical examination reveals a toxic, anxious patient with tachycardia and tachypnea. Restricted and guarded chest wall excursion may be present. Percussion of the chest wall may elicit pain and dullness over the empyema area. With chronicity, the patient may develop clubbing of the fingers, contraction of the chest wall, inanition, and other signs of chronic illness.

DIAGNOSIS

Chest Radiography

The presence of a significant pleural effusion in association with a lower respiratory illness is typical, but this clinical picture may be seen also with pulmonary embolism, acute pancreatitis, Dressler's syndrome, tuberculosis, and other conditions. Light and associates (1980) have suggested that bilateral decubitus chest radiography be performed. With the involved side down, the distance between the inside of the chest wall and the outside of the lung normally should not exceed 10 mm. If this distance exceeds 10 mm, thoracocentesis should be done immediately. If no fluid is free flowing, one must assume that loculation has taken place.

A number of techniques for localizing empyema collections are now available. Because the posterior lateral

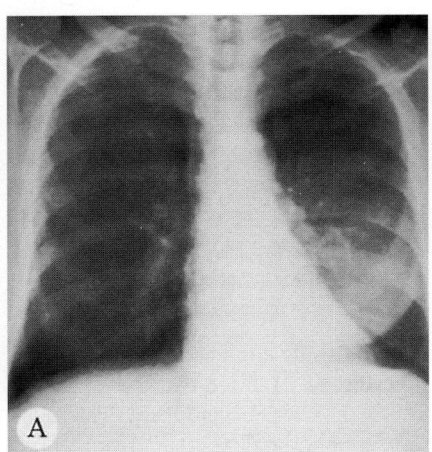 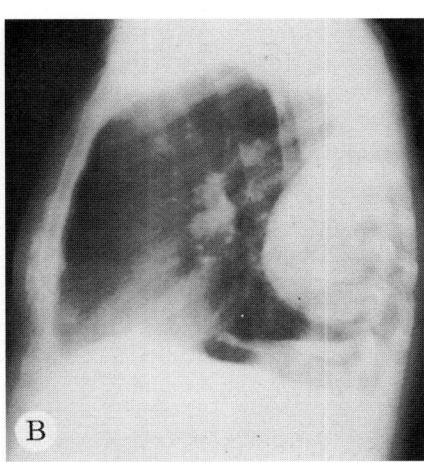

Fig. 58-1. A. Posteroanterior radiograph of patient with encapsulated pleural effusion. **B.** *Inverted D* or *pregnant lady sign* on lateral view is classic, if not typical, of encapsulated empyema.

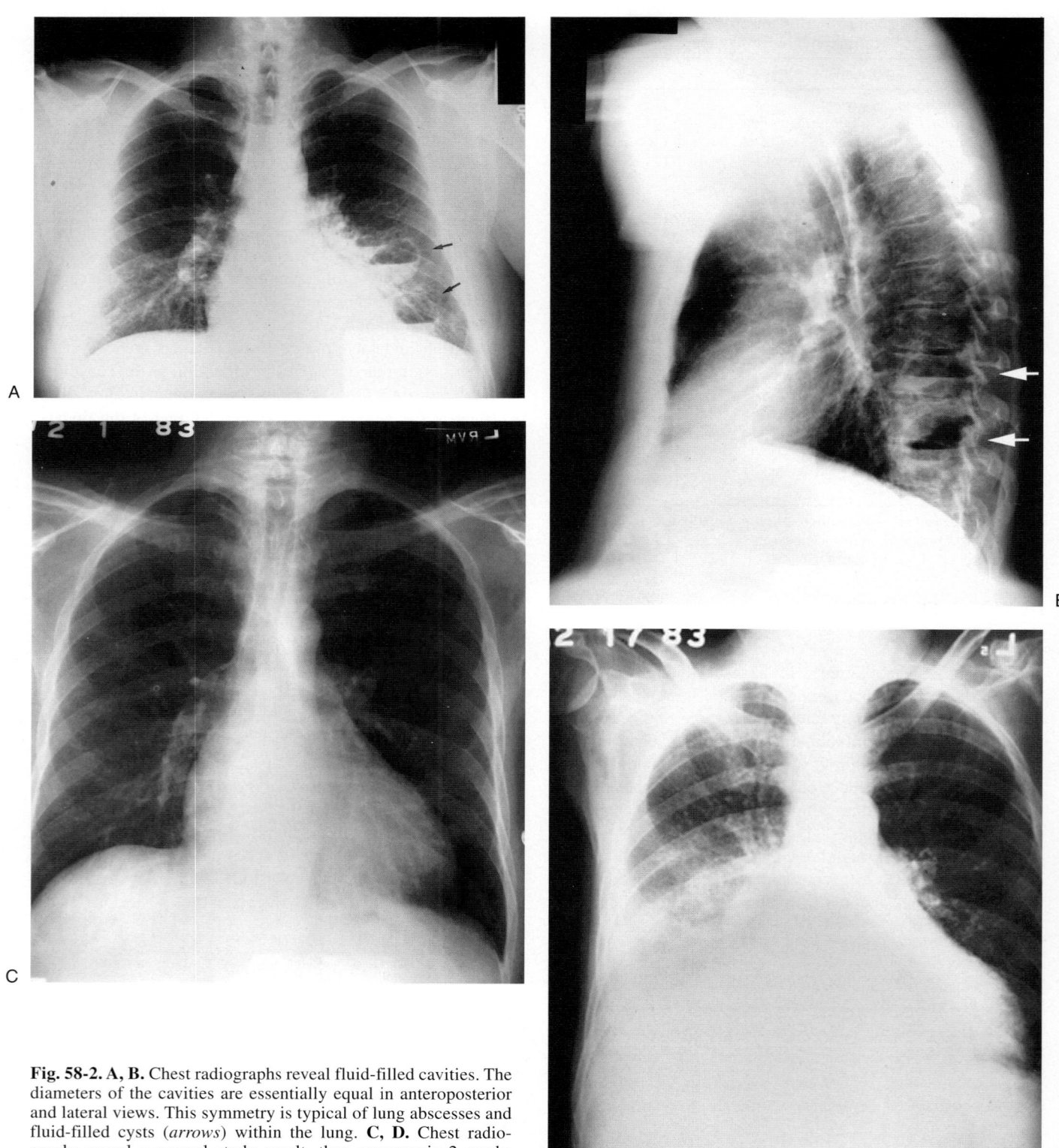

Fig. 58-2. A, B. Chest radiographs reveal fluid-filled cavities. The diameters of the cavities are essentially equal in anteroposterior and lateral views. This symmetry is typical of lung abscesses and fluid-filled cysts (*arrows*) within the lung. **C, D.** Chest radiographs reveal a normal study result, then pneumonia 2 weeks later. (*Continued*)

diaphragmatic angle is the most dependent position of the thorax, most empyemas are found in this area. The *inverted D* or *pregnant lady sign*, as coined by LeRoux and Dodds (1964), on the lateral view is classic (Fig. 58-1). The differentiation of lung abscess with effusion from empyema and bronchopleural fistula may also be suggested by plain chest radiographic examination (Fig. 58-2). Friedman and Hellekani (1977) have noted that lung abscess air-fluid levels are usually the same dimensions in both the posteroanterior and lateral views, whereas empyema air-fluid levels are rarely the

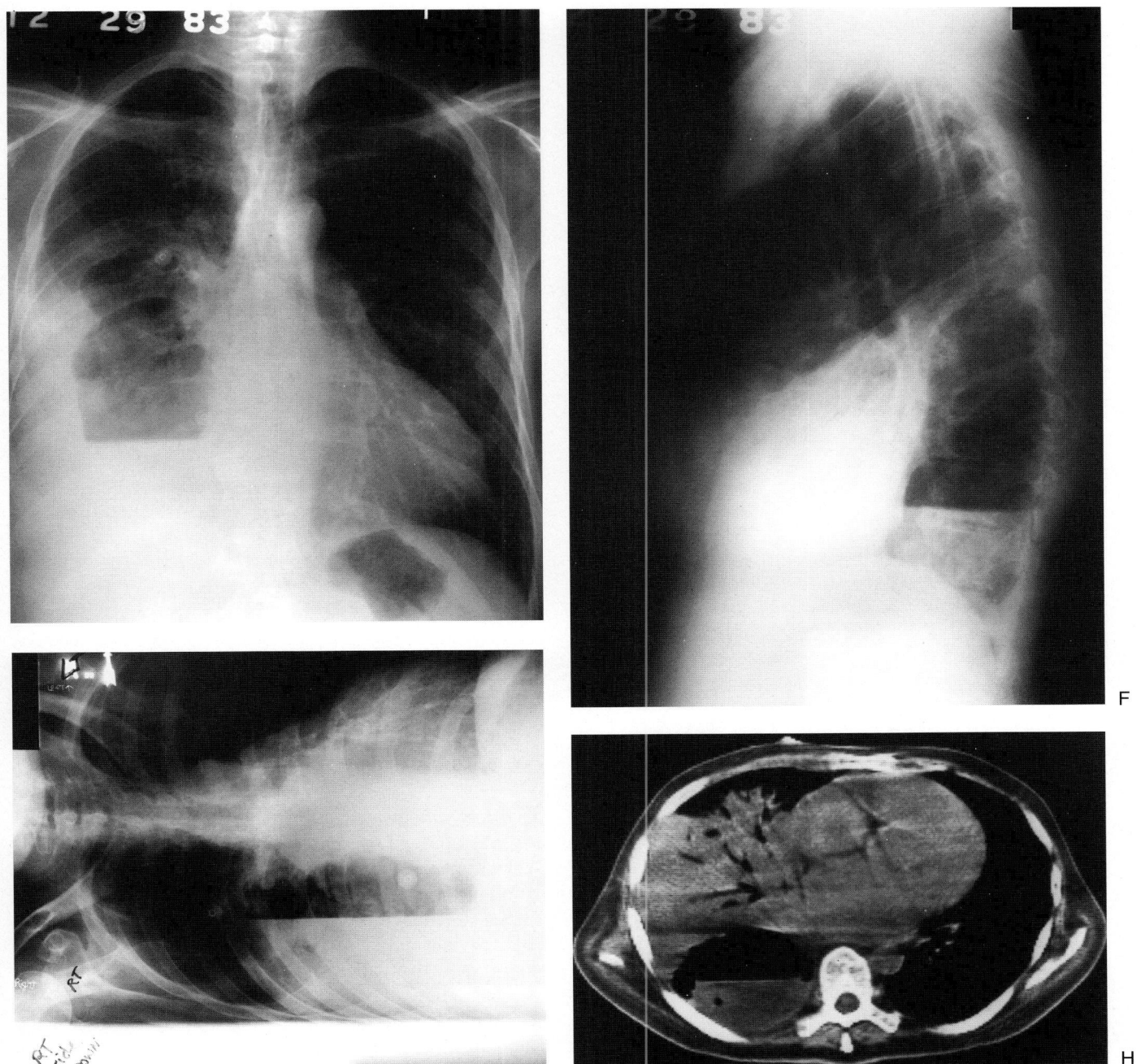

Fig. 58-2. (*Continued*) **E, F.** This study reveals an asymmetric air-fluid space typical of bronchopleural fistula and empyema. **G, H.** A decubitus study confirms the large empyema and the computed tomography scan confirms the large air- and fluid-filled space outside the lung.

same in these views, and these findings are helpful in differentiating the two conditions.

Computed Tomography

Computed tomographic (CT) scanning is useful in localizing collections, identifying underlying parenchymal disease, and distinguishing empyema from lung abscess (Fig. 58-3). Fluid density and the presence of loculations can be determined, the latter being an important factor in treatment planning. CT-guided thoracocentesis is a highly accurate and safe technique that is used routinely.

Sonography

Alternately, sonography of the chest may be used. Sonography can demonstrate pleural fluid collections, loculations, and parenchyma involvement and may be used to

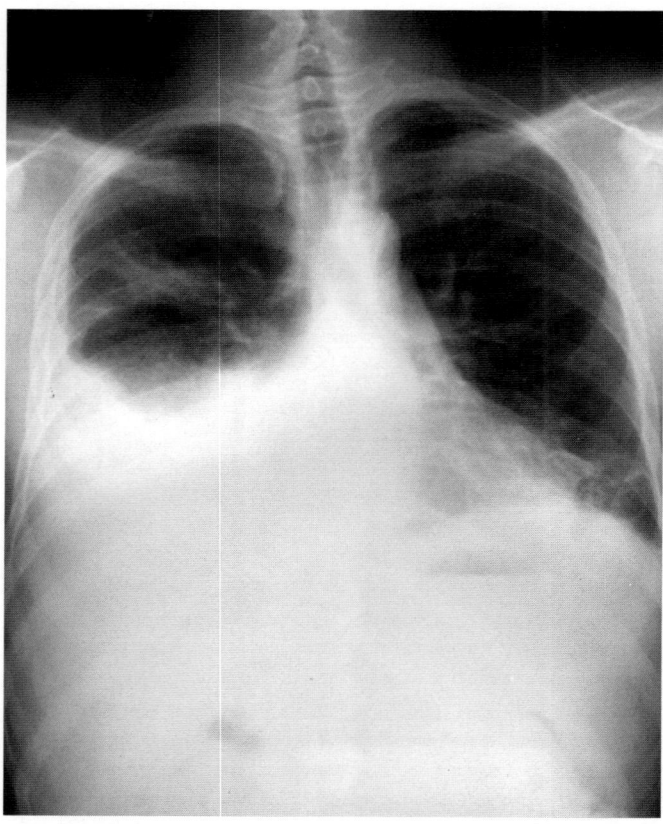

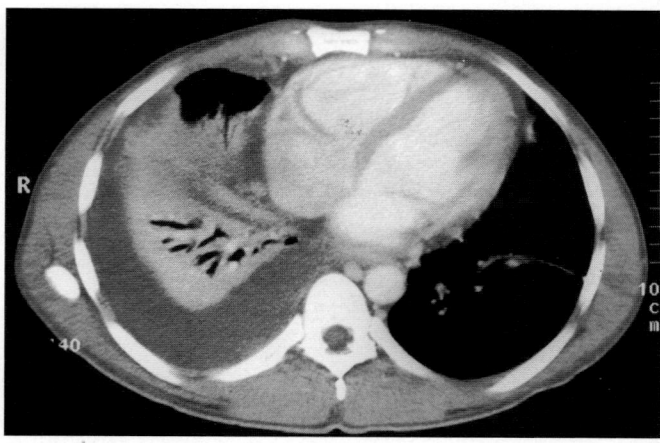

Fig. 58-3. Patient with acute lower respiratory illness. **A.** Patient upright radiograph reveals density in right lower lung field. **B.** Computed tomography scan reveals large empyema collection with atelectatic lobe and consolidation.

guide thoracocentesis. The choice of this technique is institutionally dependent.

Thoracentesis

The appearance of the fluid provides a first and major source of information concerning diagnosis and treatment. Straw-colored, clear, or slightly cloudy fluid is found in sterile *parapneumonic* effusions. This condition corresponds to early stage 1 of the American Thoracic Society classification, the "uncomplicated" effusion of Light (1985), the "benign" effusion of Potts and associates (1976), and the "low pH" pleural effusion of Van Way and colleagues (1988). Twenty percent to 70% of these clear with appropriate treatment of the primary pneumonia. The problem and dilemma is that benign-appearing fluid may herald an impending frank empyema. Therefore, the fluid must be examined by Gram's stain, cultured for aerobic and anaerobic bacteria, and tested for antibiotic sensitivity. Biochemical changes (i.e., low pH, low glucose, and high LDH) indicate and precede culture positivity and, according to Light (1991) and others, can serve as a guide to therapy. Cloudy or frankly purulent fluid is diagnostic. Aerobic pus has little or no offensive odor. Anaerobic pus is usually foul smelling.

MANAGEMENT

Effective management of empyema requires 1) control of infection and sepsis by appropriate antibiotic therapy, 2) evacuation of pus from the pleural space, and 3) obliteration of the empyema cavity. Once the diagnosis is established, treatment must proceed with all possible haste. In Bartlett and associates' (1974b) series of 43 anaerobic empyemas, five patients (12%) died. All five deaths were attributed to a delay in appropriate drainage. In Ashbaugh's (1991) series, delay in instituting drainage increased the mortality from 3.4 to 16%.

Antibiotic Therapy

Appropriate intravenous antibiotics should be administered promptly. Many patients, when first seen by the surgeon, have already been treated with antibiotics and their culture results may be negative. Despite this, cultures of the blood and empyema fluid should be obtained. According to Bergeron (1990) and Hughes and Van Scoy (1991), Gram's staining of the empyema fluid and empyema history are excellent guides to initial antibiotic therapy. For community-acquired pneumonia and empyema, a third-generation cephalosporin or clindamycin are good initial choices, par-

Table 58-5. Choice of Antibiotics against Pathogens in Empyema

Organism	Antibiotic
Community-acquired infections	
Gram-positive bacteria	
Streptococcus pneumoniae[a]	Third-generation cephalosporin (ceftriaxone)
	Extended-spectrum quinolone (levofloxacin)
Haemophilus influenzae	Third-generation cephalosporin
Staphylococcus aureus	Oxacillin, nafcillin
Streptococcus pyogenes[b]	High-dose penicillin
Gram-negative bacteria	
Klebsiella pneumoniae	Third-generation cephalosporin
Suspected anaerobes[c]	Clindamycin
	Amoxicillin/clavulanate
Hospital-acquired infections	
Gram-positive bacteria	
S. aureus	Oxacillin, nafcillin
	Vancomycin
Gram-negative bacteria	
Pseudomonas aeruginosa	Ciprofloxacin and gentamicin
	Imipenem and gentamicin
Klebsiella pneumoniae	Third-generation cephalosporin
	Piperacillin/tazobactam
Anaerobes	Clindamycin
	Amoxicillin/clavulanate

[a]Fifteen percent or more resistant to penicillin.
[b]Resistant to erythromycin.
[c]Pneumonia and empyema associated with indolent course, a history of aspiration, periodontal disease, lung abscess, and foul-smelling sputum.

ticularly if the Gram's stain reveals gram-positive cocci. For gram-negative empyemas or if anaerobes are suspected, a third-generation cephalosporin and clindamycin are usually effective (Table 58-5). For hospital-acquired pneumonia and empyema, antibiotic therapy should be guided by culture and sensitivity studies.

Thoracocentesis

Needle aspiration of the fluid should be carried out with an 18-gauge needle under local anesthesia. If the fluid appears benign, is not loculated, and can be removed totally or nearly so, thoracocentesis may be all that is necessary to control the disease process. Leukocyte count, Gram's stain, cultures, and glucose and LDH levels of the fluid should be carried out. If negative, resolution usually occurs. Chest radiographic examination should be repeated in 24 hours to ascertain the status of the effusion. If the volume has increased, repeat thoracocentesis is indicated. Light and colleagues (1980) have advised that if the fluid is positive by biochemical evaluation, staining, or culture, closed tube thoracostomy drainage is required.

Chest Tube Drainage

Closed chest tube drainage is usually the first step in the treatment of acute empyema. It is highly effective in treating uncomplicated parapneumonic effusions and classic empyema without loculation. A No. 36F or larger tube is placed in the most dependent area of the empyema cavity as determined by previous thoracocentesis and radiographic examination. Underwater seal drainage with moderate suction (-20 cm H_2O) is then applied to drain the purulent fluid and to obliterate the space.

When this approach is successful, clinical improvement is generally noted within 48 to 72 hours. Chest radiography reveals evacuation of the fluid and reexpansion of the lung. Drainage should progressively decrease and the fluid should clear. When the drainage has decreased to 50 mL within a 24-hour period and the lung has re-expanded, the chest tube can be removed. This usually occurs within 5 to 10 days. Antibiotics should be continued for 6 weeks.

Success of closed chest drainage depends primarily on the state of the empyema when treated. Van Way and associates (1988) published a classification of empyema that is useful in predicting success of closed chest tube drainage in complicated parapneumonic effusions: 1) class I, low pH pleural effusion, with pleural fluid with a pH less than 7.20 and negative pleural fluid culture; 2) class II, classic empyema, with positive pleural fluid cultures and no loculations; and 3) class III, complicated empyema, with multiple loculations on chest radiography, initially or subsequently, or trapped lung.

These authors reported that 10 of 12 patients (83%) in class I were managed successfully with a single chest tube and with no deaths. There were 28 patients in class II. All of their effusions were successfully managed with chest tubes, but there were two deaths. There were 40 patients in class III. Eight of these (20%) were managed successfully with multiple chest tubes, but 32 (80%) required thoracotomy.

Intrapleural Fibrinolytic Agents

Loculation of empyema cavities is produced by membranes composed of fibrin. The use of fibrinolytic agents to dissolve these membranes was reported by Tillett and Sherry in 1949. These authors instilled streptokinase and streptodornase into empyema pockets and found that these agents broke up loculations and aided in the drainage of thick pus. Significant systemic reaction was associated with the use of these enzymes and, because results in most institutions were unsatisfactory, their use fell into disfavor.

More recently, streptokinase has been purified and it, along with urokinase, which is not as allergenic, have been the subject of a number of reports. These reports indicate that streptokinase and urokinase are efficient debriding agents. Mitchell (1989), Willsie-Ediger (1990), Aye (1991), Rosen (1993) and their associates reported success rates of up to 80% with the use of streptokinase in patients with loculated empyema despite the fact that, in most series, only small catheters were used for chest drainage. Success rates of 90% were reported by Moulton (1989) and Lee (1991) and their colleagues with the use of urokinase.

The enzyme is inserted into the empyema cavity through the chest tube while the patient is in the decubitus position, empyema side up. Streptokinase (250,000 U) or urokinase (100,000 U) mixed in 100 mL of normal saline is injected, via syringe and 21-gauge needle, through the tube, which is then clamped for 6 to 8 hours. This procedure is repeated daily and is generally followed by increased chest tube drainage and radiographic evidence of loculation dissolution and cavity shrinkage.

Bouros and associates (1997) compared streptokinase and urokinase in a double-blind study of 50 consecutive patients with either complicated pleural effusion or frank empyema who had inadequate drainage through the chest tube (less than 70 mL/24 hours). Clinical and radiologic improvement was noted in all but two patients (8%) in each group who required surgical intervention. The mean volume of drainage was significantly increased (urokinase, 420 mL/24 hours; streptokinase, 380 mL/24 hours). The mean number of installations was six in both groups, and the mean lengths of stay were approximately 11 days. Two patients in the streptokinase group suffered high fever. The total cost for drug therapy was approximately twice as much in the urokinase group. The authors concluded that fibrinolytic therapy is a valuable adjunct to chest tube drainage and that, despite the cost, urokinase may be desirable because of local systemic reactions to streptokinase. These reactions included fever, chills, and chest pain. In Laisaar and colleagues' (1996) series, enzymatic treatment was effective in 72% of patients, but 28% required further treatment such as decortication or lung resection. Chin and Lim (1997), in a controlled study of 52 patients (29 treated with drainage only and 23 treated with drainage plus streptokinase daily), noted increased drainage in the streptokinase group, but no difference in hospital stay duration, mortality, or need for decortication.

Open Drainage

In cases in which closed tube drainage is not successful, prolonged drainage may be achieved by an open method although Graham and Bell, reporting for the Empyema Commission in 1918, demonstrated that open drainage must not be carried out in the acute phase of the disease. If performed, an open pneumothorax is created with reduced ventilation, hypoxia, and death. Once the lung has fixed to the chest wall, however, ventilation is ensured and open drainage is safe. In the past, these conditions were heralded by increased sediment in fluid drained by thoracocentesis from the empyema cavity. When sediment reached 75%, open drainage was said to be safe.

Open drainage may be achieved by cutting off the chest tube a few centimeters from the skin and anchoring it in place with a safety pin and tape. This may be safely accomplished in 2 to 3 weeks when the space is obliterated, no gross up and down movements occur in the water column, and pneumothorax does not occur when the tube is open to atmospheric pressure. The tube may be withdrawn a few centimeters each week as granulation tissue fills the tract and drainage decreases.

Open drainage also may be achieved through rib resection and use of a modified Eloesser's flap (1935) technique, as reported by Symbas and coworkers (1971). In this modification, the original U-shaped flap is converted to an inverted U-shaped flap to maintain the patency of the tract. Ali and associates (1996) suggest that this is a useful procedure in instances in which a large space exists and prolonged drainage is anticipated.

Video-Assisted Thoracoscopy

Video-assisted thoracoscopy (VATS) has become the primary modality for treating complicated empyema after initial therapy, with or without chest tube drainage, in many institutions, including our own, as recorded by Angelillo Mackinlay (1996) and Landreneau (1996) and their associates, as well as by one of us (M.J.K.) and colleagues (1996, 1998). VATS allows adhesiolysis and débridement with better exposure than minithoracotomy. Decortication for lung expansion before fibrosis can be accomplished with equal facility. Although chest tube drainage combined with enzymatic débridement is effective, VATS therapy results in a higher success rate (90%), shorter hospital stay, and less cost. Wait and associates (1997) point out that it can routinely salvage patients in whom chest tube drainage with enzymatic débridement is not successful.

The VATS procedure is described in Chapter 18. A dual-lumen endotracheal tube is inserted for single-lung ventilation. Its position is confirmed by bronchoscopy. Blood pressure, central venous pressure, SaO_2, and end tidal CO_2 are monitored continuously. The patient is placed in the lateral decubitus position. A three-port triangle approach is used with the ports later serving as chest tube drainage sites. The empyema cavity is entered, loculations broken up, adhesions lysed with endoscopic scissors and cauterized, fibrin and purulent material removed mechanically and by suction, and chest cavity irrigated with copious amounts of saline. The lung surface is wiped clean and the lung re-expanded. Morbidity is low, and the chest tubes usually can be removed sequentially beginning in 3 to 4 days, depending on the virulence of the infection, the presence of a bronchopleural fistula, and the state of the patient. If complete reexpansion is not achieved, the remaining, dependent chest tube can be cut off and converted to an open empyema drainage tube.

Thoracotomy, Minithoracotomy, and Decortication

Although VATS has the advantages of better exposure and patient tolerance, open thoracotomy with débridement and decortication is an effective means of dealing with empyema. Most studies of this technique predate the widespread use of VATS. Van Way and associates (1988) reported on 22 patients in whom débridement and decortication were carried out and in whom drainage was established through a limited thoracotomy. The process resolved completely in all, and no deaths occurred in this series. Miller (1990) described 52 patients treated with open thoracotomy. Good results were obtained in 50 of these patients, and no operative deaths occurred.

Empyemectomy

Empyemectomy is rarely performed. It requires an extrapleural dissection of the parietal pleural surface and tedious dissection of the sac from the lung. Just as in decortication of a chronically collapsed and trapped lung, lung damage requiring undesirable and unnecessary resection is often the result.

CHRONIC EMPYEMA

Chronicity refers to a state of continued infection associated with both fibrosis and a pleural space that is often associated with bronchopleural fistula. Fortunately, this is an uncommon occurrence after appropriate treatment. In the past, such spaces were treated by some form of thoracoplasty. This generally took the form of a modified Shede procedure. Ribs were resected over the cavity, the parietal pleura was removed, and the muscle bundles were allowed to fall against the visceral pleura. The procedure was effective, but mutilating. Presently, as noted by Hankins and colleagues (1978), muscle translocation into the cavity with occasional rib resection is the more desirable and effective procedure.

TREATMENT OF EMPYEMA IN CHILDREN

Empyema in infants and children is usually associated with pneumonia. Its incidence has diminished greatly in response to the successful treatment of pneumonia with antibiotics. In addition, its bacterial etiology has changed concomitantly with the evolution of microbial resistance. According to Foglia and Randolph (1987), during the past decade, the most frequent causes of empyema were *H.*

influenzae, β-hemolytic streptococci, *S. pneumoniae*, and anaerobes. Hardie and associates (1996), however, noted that *S. pneumoniae*, often resistant to penicillin and erythromycin, is the most common organism. Gustafson and colleagues (1990) have stressed the observation that anaerobic bacteria produce effusions that loculate quickly and are difficult to drain, whereas staphylococcal effusions are most commonly unilocular and relatively easier to drain.

Fever is the most common presenting symptom in childhood empyema. Fever, cough, and dyspnea are present in 75% of children on admission. Decreased breath sounds, tactile and vocal fremitus, and tachypnea and tachycardia are often present, as reported by Middlekamp (1969) and McLaughlin (1984) and their colleagues, as well as by Chonmaitree and Powell (1983). Other symptoms are grunting respiration, intercostal retraction, and lethargy. The polymorphic leukocyte count is virtually always elevated. Chonmaitree and Powell (1983) noted pulmonary lobar infiltrate in 52% of patients with empyema, segmental infiltrate in 33%, and bilateral patchy infiltrate in 14%. Foglia and Randolph (1987) note that CT scanning is extremely useful in clarifying the extent of parenchymal lung and pleural involvement.

The treatment of empyema in children remains controversial, but the goals of therapy have been clearly outlined by Mayo and associates (1982) (Table 58-6).

The possibility of empyema in children as heralded by clinical signs and symptoms and radiographic evidence of pleural involvement or infusion requires prompt attention. A CT scan should be carried out if the presence of fluid is in question and thoracocentesis should be performed for visual, biochemical, and cultural evidence of infection.

Antibiotics administered intravenously, according to Gram's stain, culture, and sensitivity studies, and pleural drainage are the mainstays of treatment. Foglia and Randolph (1987) demonstrated that most children treated with appropriate antibiotics and chest tube drainage recover. This course depends on the disease stage, type of bacteria, and degree of lung trapping. If rapid recovery does not occur, additional intervention is indicated. Various authors, such as Raffensperger and colleagues (1982), have recommended minithoracotomy or full thoracotomy. Gustafson

Table 58-6. Goals of Therapy in Empyema in Children

Save life
Eliminate the empyema
Reexpand the trapped lung
Restore mobility of the chest wall and diaphragm
Return respiratory function to normal
Eliminate complications or chronicity
Reduce the duration of hospital stay

From Mayo P, Saha SP, McElvein RB: Acute empyema in children treated by open thoracotomy and decortication. Ann Thorac Surg 34:401, 1982. With permission.

and colleagues (1990) noted that aggressive care, including early thoracotomy, led to early recovery and excellent long-term results. In older children, VATS delocation, decortication, if necessary, and drainage were used. Open drainage is never indicated in children because of late skeletal deformities. We do not believe that the use of enzymatic débridement is indicated in children. Rosen and associates (1993), however, have reported some success with adjuvant use of enzymatic débridement.

REFERENCES

Ali SM, Siddiqui AA, McLaughlin JS: Open drainage of massive tuberculous empyema with progressive reexpansion of the lung: an old concept revisited. Ann Thorac Surg 62:218, 1996.

Ali I, Unruh H: Management of empyema thoracis. Ann Thorac Surg 50:355, 1990.

Andrews NC, et al: Management of nontuberculous empyema: a statement of the subcommittee on surgery. Am Rev Respir Dis 85:935, 1962.

Angelillo Mackinlay TA, et al: VATS debridement versus thoracotomy in the treatment of loculated postpneumonia empyema. Ann Thorac Surg 61:1626, 1996.

Ashbaugh DG: Empyema thoracis. Factors influencing morbidity and mortality. Chest 99:1162, 1991.

Aye RW, Forese DP, Hill LD: Use of purified streptokinase in empyema and hemothorax. Am J Surg 161:560, 1991.

Bartlett JG, Finegold SM: Anaerobic infections of the lung and pleural space. Am Rev Respir Dis 110:56, 1974.

Bartlett JG, et al: Bacteriology of empyema. Lancet 1:338, 1974.

Bergeron MG: The changing bacterial spectrum and antibiotic choice. In Deslauriers J, Lacquet LK (eds): International Trends in General Thoracic Surgery. Vol. 6. St. Louis: CV Mosby, 1990.

Bouros D, et al: Intrapleural streptokinase versus urokinase in the treatment of complicated parapneumonic effusions: a prospective, double-blind study. Am J Respir Crit Care Med 155:291, 1997.

Brook I, Frazier EH: Aerobic and anaerobic microbiology of empyema. A retrospective review in two military hospitals. Chest 103:1502, 1993.

Chin NK, Lim TK: Controlled trial of intrapleural streptokinase in the treatment of pleural empyema and complicated parapneumonic effusions. Chest 111:275, 1997.

Chonmaitree T, Powell KR: Parapneumonic pleural effusion and empyema in children. Review of a 19-year experience, 1962–1980. Clin Pediatr 22:414, 1983.

Ehler AA: Non-tuberculous thoracic empyema: a collective review of the literature from 1934 to 1939. Int Abstr Surg 72:17, 1941.

Eloesser L: An operation for tuberculous empyema. Surg Gynecol Obstet 60:1096, 1935.

Fang GD, et al: New and emerging etiologies for community-acquired pneumonia with implications for therapy. A prospective multicenter study of 359 cases. Medicine 69:307, 1990.

Foglia RP, Randolph J: Current indications for decortication in the treatment of empyema in children. J Pediatr Surg 22:28, 1987.

Friedman PJ, Hellekani CAG: Radiologic recognition of bronchopleural fistula. Radiology 124:289, 1977.

Graham EA, Bell RD: Open pneumothorax: its relation to the treatment of acute empyema. Am J Med Sci 156:839, 1918.

Gustafson RA, et al: Role of lung decortication in symptomatic empyemas in children. Ann Thorac Surg 49:940, 1990.

Hankins JR, et al: Bronchopleural fistula. Thirteen-year experience with 77 cases. J Thorac Cardiovasc Surg 76:755, 1978.

Hardie W, et al: Pneumococcal pleural empyemas in children. Clin Infect Dis 22:1057, 1996.

Hughes CE, Van Scoy RE: Antibiotic therapy in pleural empyema. Semin Respir Infect 6:94, 1991.

Johnson CC, Finegold SM: Pyogenic bacterial pneumonia, lung abscess and empyema. In Murray JF, Nadel JA (eds): Textbook of Respiratory Medicine. Vol. 1. 2nd Ed. Philadelphia: WB Saunders, 1994.

Krasna MJ: Thoracoscopic decortication. Surg Laparosc Endosc 8:283, 1998.

Krasna MJ, Deshmukh S, McLaughlin JS: Complications of thoracoscopy. Ann Thorac Surg 61:1066, 1996.

Laisaar T, Puttsepp E, Laisaar V: Early administration of intrapleural streptokinase in the treatment of multiloculated pleural effusions and pleural empyemas. Thorac Cardiovasc Surg 44:252, 1996.

Landreneau RJ, et al: Thoracoscopy for empyema and hemothorax. Chest 109:18, 1996.

Lee KS, et al: Treatment of thoracic multiloculated empyemas with intracavitary urokinase: a prospective study. Radiology 179:771, 1991.

LeRoux BT, Dodds TC: A Portfolio of Chest Radiographs. Edinburgh: E and S Livingston, 1964.

Light RW: Parapneumonic effusions and empyema. Clin Chest Med 6:55, 1985.

Light RW: Parapneumonic effusions and infections of the pleural space. In Light RW (ed): Pleural Diseases. 2nd Ed. Philadelphia: Lea & Febiger, 1990.

Light RW: Management of parapneumonic effusions. Chest 100:892, 1991.

Light RW, et al: Parapneumonic effusions. Am J Med 69:507, 1980.

Marks MI, Eickhoff TC: Empyema necessitatis. Am Rev Respir Dis 101:759, 1970.

Mayo P, Saha SP, McElvein RB: Acute empyema in children treated by open thoracotomy and decortication. Ann Thorac Surg 34:401, 1982.

McLaughlin FJ, et al: Empyema in children: clinical course and long-term follow-up. Pediatrics 73:587, 1984.

Middlekamp JN, Purkerson ML, Burford TH: The changing pattern of empyema thoracis in pediatrics. J Thorac Cardiovasc Surg 47:165, 1964.

Miller JI: Empyema thoracis. Ann Thorac Surg 50:343, 1990.

Mitchell ME, et al: Intrapleural streptokinase in management of parapneumonic effusions: report of series and review of literature. J Fla Med Assoc 76:1019, 1989.

Moulton JS, Moore PT, Mencini RA: Treatment of loculated pleural effusions with transcatheter intracavitary urokinase. AJR Am J Roentgenol 153:941, 1989.

Potts DE, Levin DC, Sahn SA: Pleural fluid pH in parapneumonic effusions. Chest 70:328, 1976.

Raffensperger JG, et al: Mini-thoracotomy and chest tube insertion for children with empyema. J Thorac Cardiovasc Surg 84:477, 1982.

Ravitch M, Fein R: The changing picture of pneumonia and empyema in infants and children: a review of the experience at the Harriett Lane Home from 1934 through 1958. JAMA 175:1039, 1961.

Rosen H, et al: Intrapleural streptokinase as adjunctive treatment for persistent empyema in pediatric patients. Chest 103:1190, 1993.

Scheld WM: Bacterial meningitis, brain abscess and other suppurative intracranial infections. In Harrison's Principles of Internal Medicine. 14th Ed. New York: McGraw-Hill, 1998.

Sullivan KM, et al: Anaerobic empyema thoracis. The role of anaerobes in 226 cases of culture-proven empyemas. Arch Intern Med 131:521, 1973.

Symbas PN, et al: Nontuberculous pleural empyema in adults. The role of a modified Eloesser procedure in its management. Ann Thorac Surg 12:69, 1971.

Tillett WS, Sherry S: The effect in patients of streptococcal fibrinolysin (streptokinase) and streptococcal desoxyribonuclease on fibrinous, purulent and sanguinous pleural effusions. J Clin Invest 28:173, 1949.

Van Way C III, Narrod J, Hopeman A: The role of early limited thoracotomy in the treatment of empyema. J Thorac Cardiovasc Surg 96:436, 1988.

Varkey B, et al: Empyema thoracis during a ten-year period. Analysis of 72 cases and comparison to a previous study (1952 to 1967). Arch Intern Med 141:1771, 1981.

Wait MA, et al: A randomized trial of empyema therapy. Chest 111:1548, 1997.

Willsie-Ediger SK, et al: Use of intrapleural streptokinase in the treatment of thoracic empyema. Am J Med Sci 300:296, 1990.

CHAPTER 59

Postsurgical Empyema

Joseph I. Miller, Jr.

The second most frequent cause of empyema is the postsurgical development of infection in the pleural space after surgery of the esophagus, lungs, or mediastinum (Table 59-1). Postsurgical empyema accounts for 20% of all cases of empyema. It most frequently follows pneumonectomy, occurring in 2 to 12% of patients. It may occur in 1 to 3% of patients after lobectomy. LeRoux and associates (1986) report that in 8 to 11% of patients, the preceding lesion causing an empyema thoracis is an unrecognized subphrenic abscess in the patient who has undergone an abdominal, urologic, or pelvic operation. Empyema may occur secondary to a spontaneous pneumothorax with a persistent bronchopleural fistula; it may occur after parasitic infection or secondary to retained foreign bodies in the bronchial tree, or it may have a number of miscellaneous causes. The etiology of empyema in 215 patients is given in Table 59-2.

Factors that may promote the development of a postsurgical empyema are listed in Table 59-3.

NONRESECTIONAL POSTSURGICAL EMPYEMA

The development of nonresectional thoracic surgical empyema is related to the predisposing cause. It may follow esophageal surgery with resultant leak into the pleural space; it may develop after subdiaphragmatic surgery on the stomach, pancreas, or spleen with the accumulation of fluid in the subdiaphragmatic space. It may occur after rupture of an infected pleural bleb or secondary to lung abscess.

Infection in the pleural space unrelated to a pulmonary resection generally can be treated in the same manner as a nonsurgical empyema, with correction of the underlying cause, appropriate antibiotics, and drainage with closed chest tube thoracostomy.

EMPYEMA AFTER RESECTION

Empyema that complicates pulmonary resection must be considered separately from empyema that occurs sponta-
neously or after trauma. When empyema complicates a pulmonary resection that is less than a pneumonectomy, the ability of the remaining lung to fill the pleural space after management of the empyema by drainage or decortication, and thereby to obliterate the pleural space, depends on the state of the remaining lung and its location, apical or basal. Empyema after upper lobectomy nearly always requires more than simple drainage, which nearly always suffices after lower lobectomy. After pneumonectomy, the empyema space is inevitably large and nearly always permanent. In these circumstances, alternative methods of treatment include sterilization, permanent drainage, thoracoplasty, and obliteration of the space by muscle flap transposition.

The incidence of empyema after pulmonary resection varies with the indications for the resection (inflammatory or neoplastic disease), with or without preoperative radiation. With resection for pulmonary tuberculosis, sputum conversion having been achieved, the incidence of bronchopleural fistula with empyema in the series Lynn (1958) reported was 6.7% after lobectomy. When sputum results were still positive for acid-fast organisms, Teixera (1968) reported it was 10%.

With pneumonectomy, as opposed to lesser resections, LeRoux and associates (1986) reported that the incidence of empyema varies from 2 to 13%. When pneumonectomy is completed through an empyema, the incidence of continued pleural infection is 45%.

Although empyema may occur at any time postoperatively, even years later, most empyemas develop in the early postoperative period. The pleural space may be contaminated at the time of pulmonary resection with the development of a bronchopleural or esophagopleural fistula, or from blood-borne sources. After pulmonary resection that is less than a pneumonectomy, empyema occurs more often when the pleural space is incompletely filled by expansion of the remaining lung, mediastinal shift, and elevation of the diaphragm. Symptoms and signs vary, and if resection was performed for neoplastic disease, they may be difficult to distinguish from those caused by dissemination of tumor. The possibility of empyema must be considered in any

Table 59-1. Etiology of Surgical Empyema

I. Postresectional
    A. Post–open lung biopsy or wedge resection
    B. Postsegmentectomy
    C. Postlobectomy
    D. Postpneumonectomy
II. Infection secondary to general or thoracic surgical procedures or intra-abdominal complications
    A. Gastric or pancreatic
    B. Esophageal
    C. Cardiac
    D. Pulmonary
    E. Others
        1. Perforated intra-abdominal viscus
            a. Duodenal ulcer
            b. Diverticulum of the colon
            c. Appendiceal abscess
        2. Other causes of peritonitis

patient with clinical features of infection after pulmonary resection. Expectoration of serosanguineous liquid and purulent discharge from the wound or the drain sites is almost diagnostic. On radiography of the chest, usually a pleural opacity is seen, with or without a fluid level, when resection has been less than a pneumonectomy. After pneumonectomy, a decrease in the fluid level early postoperatively, or the appearance of a new fluid level when the pneumonectomy site was uniformly opaque, strongly suggests an infected pleural space with bronchopleural fistula. The timing of surgical intervention and the type of operative procedure undertaken are tailored to the individual patient. An algorithm for the management of postresectional empyema is given in Figure 59-1.

General Principles of Treatment

When the diagnosis of postresectional empyema, with or without a bronchopleural fistula, is made, surgical drainage by closed chest tube thoracostomy and institution of appro-

Table 59-2. Etiology of Empyema in 215 Patients

Event or State	Number	Percent
Pulmonary infection	122	57
After surgical procedures	42	20
After trauma	13	6
Spontaneous pneumothorax	7	3
Esophageal perforation	5	2
After thoracentesis	4	2
Subdiaphragmatic infection	4	2
Undetermined	18	8
Total	**215**	**100**

Compiled from Snider GL, Saleb SS: Empyema of thorax in adults: review of 105 cases. Chest *54*:12, 1968; and Hall DP, Elkin RG: Empyema thoracis: a review of 110 cases. Am Rev Respir Dis *88*:785, 1963.

Table 59-3. Factors That Promote Development of Postsurgical Empyema

Delay in diagnosis
Improper choice of antibiotics
Loculation or encapsulation by a dense inflammatory reaction
Presence of a bronchopleural fistula
Foreign body in the pleural space
Chronic infection
Entrapment of lung by thick visceral peel
Inadequate previous drainage or premature removal of a tube

priate antibiotic therapy are crucial. Once adequate drainage has been established and the patient is stabilized, usually in 10 to 14 days, the course of management can be determined. If a bronchopleural fistula is present, the fistula should be closed by a myoplasty or omentoplasty, followed by single-stage muscle flap closure of the remaining space. If the patient is medically unstable, the closed chest tube thoracostomy can be converted to open drainage by Eloesser's procedure.

If the patient has only an empyema space without a bronchopleural fistula, the cavity is sterilized by irrigation with the appropriate antibiotic solution, as determined by the antibiotic sensitivities of the chest tube drainage, and a single-stage muscle flap closure of the remaining cavity is performed. A complete discussion of muscle flap closure is given later in this chapter. If the patient is medically unstable, closed chest tube thoracostomy can be converted to an open Eloesser's flap.

Postpneumonectomy Empyema

Postpneumonectomy empyema remains a problem. It is associated with a bronchopleural fistula in approximately 40% of patients, and in only 20% of patients does the bronchopleural fistula close spontaneously. One of the most important advances in the treatment of this complication was the report by Clagett and Geraci (1963) in which they described rib resection with antibiotic irrigation and closure of the space in 6 to 8 weeks. Stafford and Clagett (1972) reported a success rate of 75 to 88% in using this method in sterilization of the empyema and permanent closure. My experience with this method has not achieved that success rate. When the offending organism is *Staphylococcus aureus*, a fair chance of success exists, but when multiple bacterial organisms are present, the rate of success is only approximately 20%.

Figure 59-2 presents an algorithm for treatment of the postpneumonectomy empyema space. Once the diagnosis of postpneumonectomy empyema, with or without bronchopleural fistula, has been established, prompt pleural drainage by closed chest tube thoracostomy is mandatory. Chest tube thoracostomy is continued until the mediastinum becomes stabilized, generally requiring approximately 2

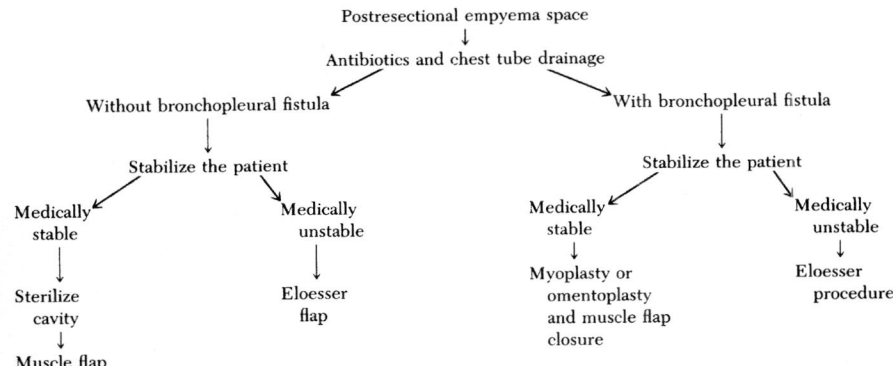

Fig. 59-1. Management of postresectional empyema.

weeks. Thereafter, open drainage or another modality of therapy for the empyema space can be undertaken safely without shift of the mediastinum. Once the patient is medically stable and has entered into the chronic phase at 3 to 4 weeks, if no bronchopleural fistula is present, a modified Clagett's procedure is performed. A second small chest tube is inserted into the second intercostal space, and a continuous inflow-outflow irrigation system is established through the pleural cavity. The irrigant is based on antibiotic sensitivities to the pleural drainage. This is generally 2 g of cephalosporin in 500 mL of 5% dextrose in water, running at a rate of 50 mL/hour through the inflow catheter, with continuous drainage through the outflow catheter. Occasionally, if gram-negative organisms are present, I use 0.25% neomycin as the irrigant. This method achieves sterilization of the space in approximately 50% of patients. If the method is successful and the return irrigant is negative on 3 consecutive days after 2 weeks of irrigation, the chest tubes can be removed, and pleural fluid is allowed to reaccumulate to fill the remaining space. If the modified Clagett's technique fails, a complete muscle flap closure of the pneumonectomy space can be performed.

If a patient with a postpneumonectomy empyema has a bronchopleural fistula, it is likewise treated during the acute phase with closed chest tube thoracostomy, with conversion to open drainage at the appropriate time when mediastinal stabilization has occurred. If the fistula closes, one can attempt the aforementioned modified Clagett's sterilization of the cavity. In the patient in whom the bronchopleural fistula persists, the fistula and space are then managed by transposition of muscle flaps into the empyema space, as the author and associates (1984) reported.

Muscle Flap Closure of the Postpneumonectomy Empyema Space

I believe that the best way to treat a postpneumonectomy space is single-stage muscle flap closure, completely obliterating the pneumonectomy space by the transposition of the thoracic skeletal muscles.

Abrashanoff (1911) reported extrathoracic muscle transposition for closure of a bronchopleural fistula. Since then, muscle flaps have been used to obliterate spaces, close a

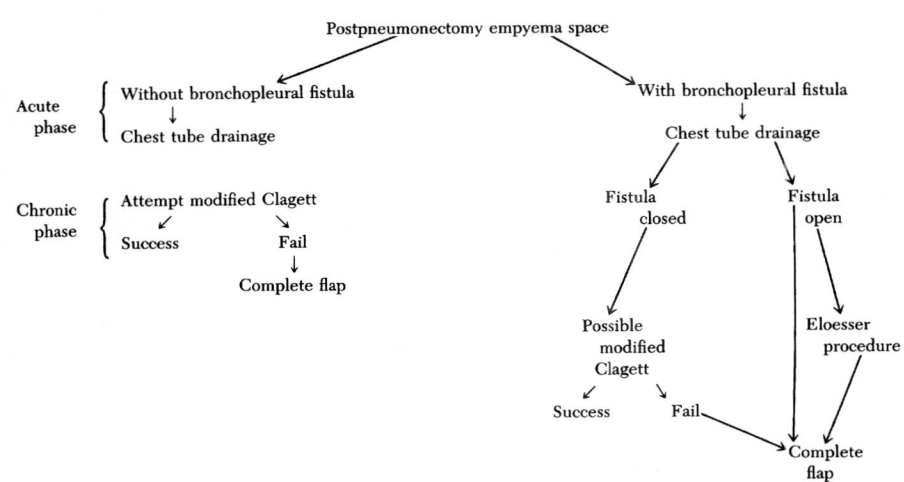

Fig. 59-2. Treatment of postpneumonectomy empyema space.

bronchopleural fistula, and reinforce tracheobronchial and esophageal anastomosis. In the late 1970s, our group used extrathoracic muscle flaps to close bronchopleural fistula and postlobectomy empyema cavities, but not until 1980 did we attempt to fill an entire pneumonectomy space with muscle flaps.

Because of their excellent blood supply and ability by pedicle flap to reach almost any location in the pleural space, muscle flaps are ideal tissue to fill a contaminated space. The extrathoracic muscle flaps used in various combinations in our patients (1984) in order of frequency are the latissimus dorsi, serratus anterior, pectoralis major, omentum, and rectus abdominis. The percentage of flap coverage of normal pneumonectomy space in the adult by each flap is latissimus dorsi (30 to 40%), serratus anterior (10 to 15%), pectoralis major (20 to 30%), pectoralis minor (0 to 2%), omentum (5 to 15%), and the rectus abdominis (5 to 15%). These figures are based on clinical estimation of coverage at the time of operation and cadaver studies.

Extrathoracic muscle flaps require a route of entry when transposed into the thoracic cavity. Segments of rib, determined by the blood supply of the muscles (Fig. 59-3), are resected to prevent kinking, constriction, and consequent

swelling and ischemia of the muscle when the muscle is transposed into the pleural space.

Specific Muscle Flaps and Omentum

Omentum

The omentum can be brought into the pleural space as a flap or a free graft. It is the flap of choice to cover an open bronchial stump because of the excellent vascular supply. Neovascularization is evident in the stump within 48 hours after placement of an omental flap around a closed stump. The omental flap is usually brought up through a separate anterior opening in the diaphragm and is laid over the bronchial stump; tacking sutures are placed around the flap (Fig. 59-4). Normally, I do not use this flap unless an open bronchial stump is present or not enough muscle is available to fill the space.

Pectoralis Major

The pectoralis major flap is one of the two most commonly used extrathoracic muscle flaps. It has a dual blood

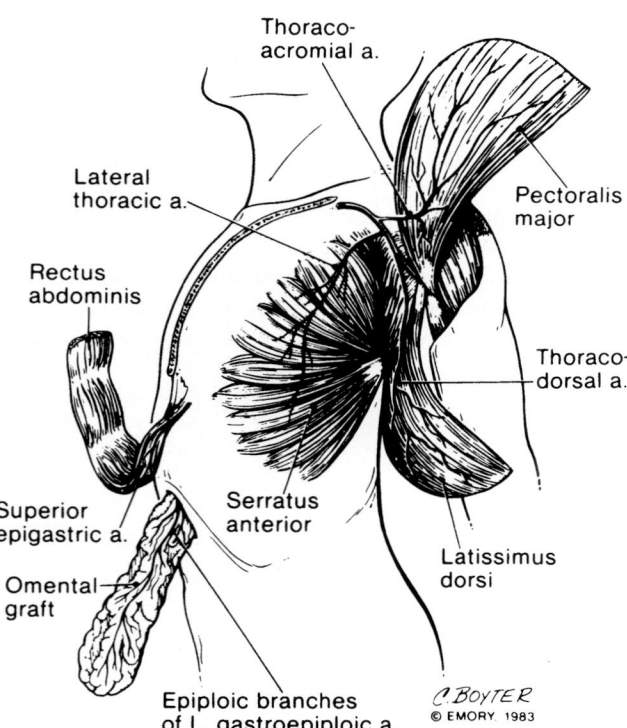

Fig. 59-3. Extrathoracic muscle flaps that can be used in closure of a postpneumonectomy empyema cavity. a, artery. From Miller JI, et al: Single-stage complete muscle flap closure of the postpneumonectomy empyema space: a new method and possible solution to a disturbing complication. Ann Thorac Surg 38:227, 1984. With permission.

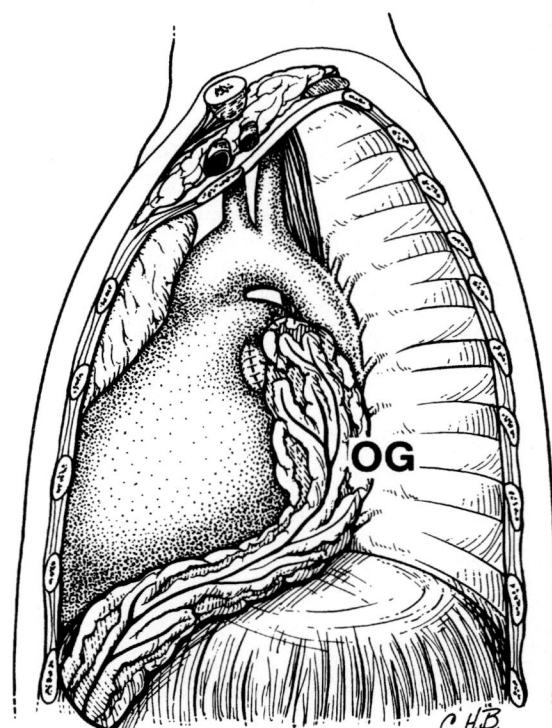

Fig. 59-4. The omental flap is brought through an anterior opening in the diaphragm and placed over the bronchial stump. OG, omental graft. From Miller JI, et al: Single-stage complete muscle flap closure of the postpneumonectomy empyema space: a new method and possible solution to a disturbing complication. Ann Thorac Surg 38:227, 1984. With permission.

supply from the predominant thoracoacromial artery to the major pedicle, and from the internal mammary to the major pedicle and secondary pedicles. It can be used as a reverse turnover flap or placed directly into the wound. It requires a 5-cm rib resection for entry into the chest. It is the flap of choice for sternal infections and ranks after the latissimus dorsi and serratus anterior for the pleural space.

Latissimus Dorsi

The latissimus dorsi flap is the most commonly used flap for thoracic defects. Its predominant blood supply is from the thoracodorsal artery. It can be used as a turnover flap or placed directly into the wound. It may be brought through the incision or through a separate small rib resection.

Serratus Anterior

The serratus anterior is my second choice of flap for filling a pneumonectomy space and is particularly good for filling a small space. The entrance into the chest is through the primary chest incision.

Rectus Abdominis

In general, the rectus abdominis is used for closure of the lowest one-third of sternal defects. It is held in reserve for problems involving the pleural space in case a residual space remains. It is generally the last flap applied.

Surgical Technique of Single-Stage Complete Muscle Flap Closure

Single-stage muscle flap closure is performed for a persistent postpneumonectomy empyema space at approximately 3 months for benign disease and 6 months to 1 year for malignant disease. The six basic steps for complete flap closure are 1) appropriate antibiotics are given, based on the sensitivities of the pleural drainage; 2) the original incision is reopened; 3) the cavity is débrided widely so that good granulation tissue is present; 4) a bronchopleural fistula is identified, and if present, the edges are freshened, and the fistula is closed, if technically possible; an omental flap is brought up through the anterior diaphragmatic incision (see Fig. 59-4) and tacked around the fistula with 3-0 Prolene sutures; 5) appropriate muscle flaps are then swung to fill the pleural space; and 6) the procedure is begun with a latissimus dorsi flap and followed with any necessary flaps to fill the entire space, depending on the anatomic location and size of the space. The filling of the entire pleural space is shown in Figure 59-5. Mathes and Nahai (1982) discussed in detail the technique of flap mobilization in their excellent work on muscle and musculocutaneous flaps.

All extrathoracic muscle flaps require a route of entry into the chest. The location of the opening is usually deter-

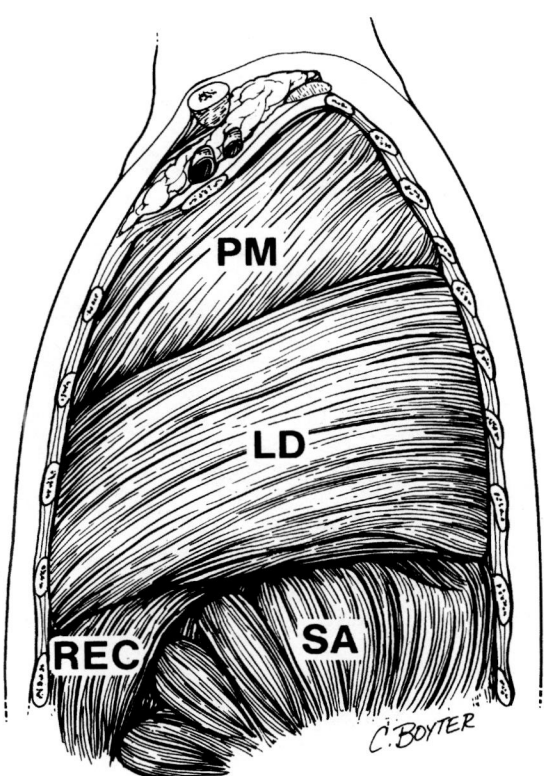

Fig. 59-5. An entire pleural space filled with muscle flaps and their usual anatomic location. LD, latissimus dorsi; PM, pectoralis major; REC, rectus abdominis; SA, serratus anterior. From Miller JI, et al: Single-stage complete muscle flap closure of the postpneumonectomy empyema space: a new method and possible solution to a disturbing complication. Ann Thorac Surg *38*:227, 1984. With permission.

mined by the blood supply of the muscle and should be placed so that the blood supply is under no tension after transposition. Generally, 4 to 5 cm of the appropriate rib is all that must be resected to allow for flap entry. Figure 59-6 shows the typical site of entry for the pectoralis major and latissimus dorsi flaps. The sine qua non for success with single-stage complete muscle flap closure is that the entire space must be filled. If a space is left, it is usually just beneath the fifth or sixth rib in the midaxillary line and can be closed by a short resection of the ribs over it without cosmetic deformity. Following transposition of the muscle flaps, the wound is closed primarily, and chest tubes are connected to Pleur-evac suction for 7 to 10 days. Appropriate antibiotics are given.

The two predominant points in this surgical technique are that no residual space can be left and that a sufficient number of flaps must be available so that any intrathoracic space can be filled. To date, I have used this technique in over 35 patients, with only 6 failures (17.2%).

An alternative method of dealing with the infected postpneumonectomy space has been popularized by Pairelero and his colleagues at the Mayo Clinic. This is a two-stage pro-

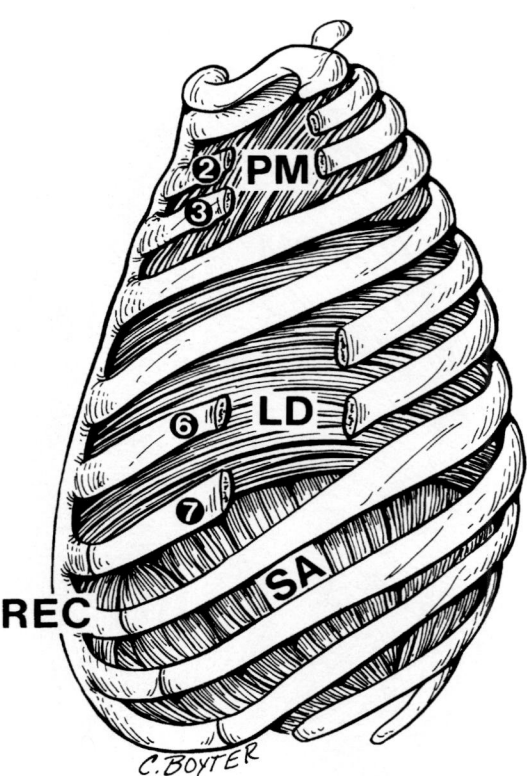

Fig. 59-6. Usual sites of rib resection for entrance of the pectoralis major (PM) and latissimus dorsi (LD) flaps into the pleural spaces. REC, rectus abdominis; SA, serratus anterior. From Miller JI, et al: Single-stage complete muscle flap closure of the postpneumonectomy empyema space: a new method and possible solution to a disturbing complication. Ann Thorac Surg 38:227, 1984. With permission.

wound is then left open and packed daily for 6 weeks to 3 months. The second stage is obliteration of the pleural space by filling it with an antibiotic solution and then closing the wound in layers.

Pairelero (personal communication, 1998) reported on 62 patients treated in this manner. The age range was from 29 to 77 years, with a mean age of 60. Hospitalization ranged from 4 to 137 days, with a median of 34. Thirty-eight patients had a bronchopleural fistula and 24 did not. There were eight postoperative deaths (13%). Of the 38 patients with a bronchopleural fistula, 33 (87%) healed well and 5 (13%) failed to heal. In the total of 62 patients, 44 patients had their chest totally closed at a second stage. In this group, 34 patients healed completely but nine failed to heal and one was lost to follow-up.

In the total group of 62 who underwent the procedure, 17 never had the second stage performed and the chest was left open. Reasons for this were as follows: carcinoma (five), respiratory failure (five), recurrent bronchopleural fistula (three), cardiac hemorrhage (two), infarction (one), and refusal (one). This technique is a highly effective procedure but is associated with prolonged hospitalization and a significant mortality; however, it has been popularized by Pairelero and his colleagues.

In summary, the principles of dealing with a pneumonectomy space are the same regardless of the technique used. The infected space must be drained and sterilized. A bronchopleural fistula, if present, must be closed and covered with autologous material. The space must then be obliterated with muscle or antibiotic solution.

Postresectional Lobectomy Empyema

Our group's algorithm for the treatment of the postresectional empyema space after lobectomy is given in Figure 59-7. The basic principles that apply to the pneumonectomy space apply to the management of the empyema space after resectional lobectomy. In general, a persistent lower lobec-

cedure. The first stage consists of reopening the thoracotomy wound and leaving it open. If the cavity is markedly purulent, it is left alone until it starts to clear up, which generally requires 5 to 7 days. If the cavity is not too purulent and a bronchopleural fistula is present, the fistula is closed primarily and covered with a serratus anterior muscle. The

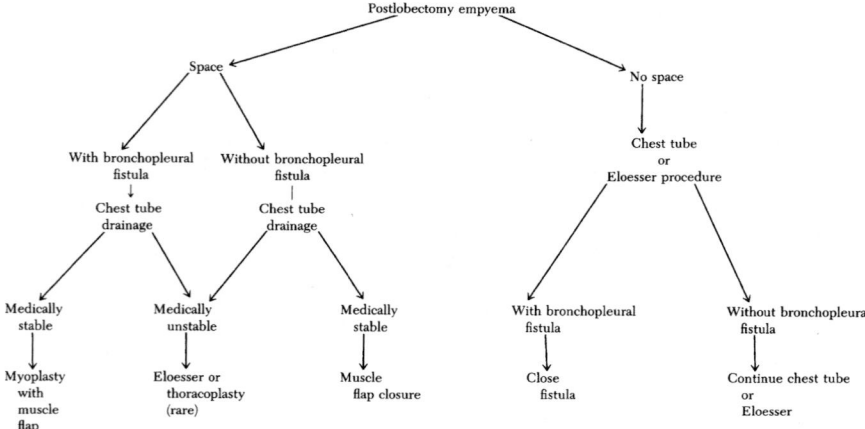

Fig. 59-7. Treatment of postlobectomy empyema.

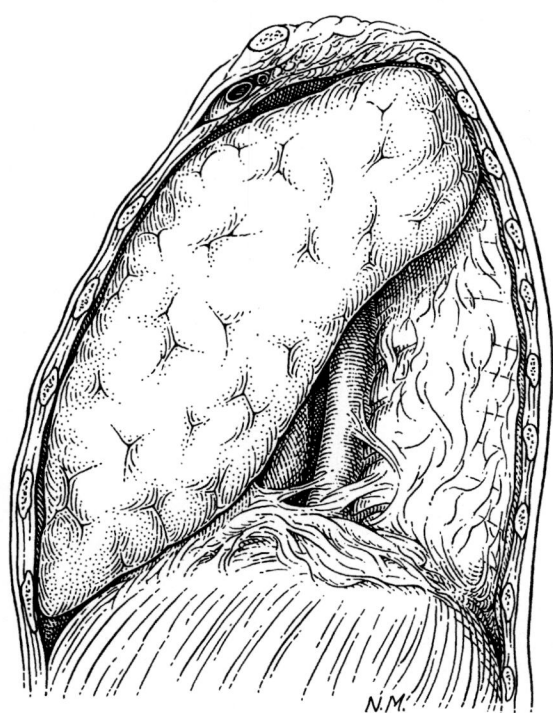

Fig. 59-8. A residual empyema cavity after a lower lobectomy.

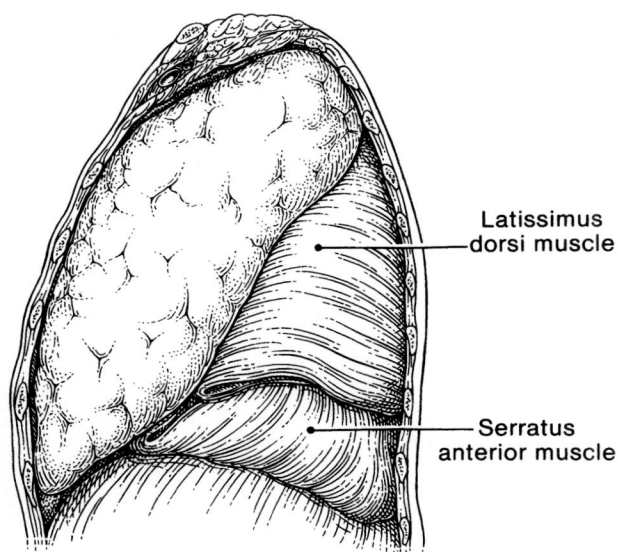

Fig. 59-9. Flap closure of a lower lobectomy empyema cavity with the latissimus dorsi and serratus anterior muscles.

tomy space (Fig. 59-8) can be easily closed and filled by application of the serratus anterior and latissimus dorsi flap. This is illustrated in Figure 59-9. If a bronchopleural fistula is present, it is closed by myoplasty, using a pedicled intercostal muscle flap, followed by obliteration of the space with the latissimus dorsi and serratus anterior muscles. If an upper lobe space persists following lobectomy, with or without bronchopleural fistula, the fistula is closed with a pedicle intercostal muscle flap, followed by a reverse pectoralis major turnover flap into the superior space through the second intercostal space.

REFERENCES

Abrashanoff: Plastische Methode der Schliessung von Fistelgangen, welche von inneren Organen kommen. Zentralbl Cir 38:186, 1911.

Clagett OT, Geraci JE: A procedure for the management of postpneumonectomy empyema. J Thorac Cardiovasc Surg 45:141, 1963.

LeRoux BT, et al: Suppurative diseases of the lung and pleural space. Part 1. Empyema thoracis and lung abscess. Curr Probl Surg 23:6, 1986.

Lynn RB: The bronchial stump. J Thorac Surg 36:70, 1958.

Mathes SJ, Nahai F: Clinical Applications for Muscle and Musculocutaneous Flaps. St Louis: CV Mosby, 1982.

Miller JI, et al: Single-stage complete muscle flap closure of the postpneumonectomy empyema space: a new method and possible solution to a disturbing complication. Ann Thorac Surg 38:227, 1984.

Stafford EG, Clagett OT: Postpneumonectomy empyema: neomycin instillation and definitive closure. J Thorac Cardiovasc Surg 63:771, 1972.

Teixera J: The present status of thoracic surgery in tuberculosis. Dis Chest 53:19, 1968.

READING REFERENCES

Beck C: Thoracoplasty in America and visceral pleurectomy with report of a case. JAMA 28:58, 1897.

Bowditch HI: Paracentesis thoracis: an analysis of 25 cases of pleuritic effusion. Am Med Monthly 3, 1853.

Eggers C: Radical operation for chronic empyema. Ann Surg 77:327, 1923.

Fowler GR: A case of thoracoplasty for the removal of a large cicatricial fibrous growth from the interior of the chest, the result of an old empyema. Med Record 44:938, 1893.

Graham EA, Bell RD: Open pneumothorax: its relation to the treatment of acute empyema. Am J Med Sci 156:939, 1918.

Hewitt C: Drainage for empyema. Br Med J 1:317, 1876.

Hippocrates: Major Classic Descriptions of Disease. Springfield, IL: Charles C Thomas, 1965.

Hood RM: History of empyema management. In Hood RM (ed): Surgical Diseases of the Pleura and Chest. Philadelphia: WB Saunders, 1986.

Lawrence GH: Empyema. In Lawrence GH (ed): Problems of the Pleural Space. Philadelphia: WB Saunders, 1983.

Trousseau A: Lectures on clinical medicine delivered at the Hotel-Dieu, Paris. McCormick JR (trans). London: The New Sydenham Society 3:198, 1870.

CHAPTER 60

Tuberculous and Fungal Infections of the Pleura

Gilbert Massard and Jean-Marie Wihlm

Mycobacterial and fungal infections of the pleural space are uncommon disorders in the Western world. Pleural tuberculosis (TB) is most often a side phenomenon of primary infection and seldom requires operative intervention except for diagnostic purposes. Empyema caused by reactivation of TB rarely occurs in patients who received adequate medical treatment but represents a real challenge to the thoracic surgeon. In a series of 380 empyema patients reported by Weissberg and Refaely (1996), no case of fungal infection was mentioned. Fungal empyema typically occurs in residual pleural spaces after previous resection or radiation therapy; these cases are particularly difficult, marked by chronic illness and consumption. Although expertise from a large number of cases is obviously lacking, the general guidelines used for treatment of any empyema also apply to the latter categories. A first step is to clean gross contamination, either with tube thoracostomy or open window thoracostomy. Once the pleural space has been cleaned, a complete and definitive obliteration of the space must be achieved to prevent further relapse of the infection. The procedure of choice is decortication, which requires an expandable underlying lung. Open window thoracostomy may be a life-saving procedure in acutely ill patients but jeopardizes the possibility of subsequent decortication; permanent loss of function must be expected when the lung remains trapped below an armor of fibrotic scar tissue. The common feature of chronic mycobacterial and fungal infections is that often the underlying lung cannot be reexpanded to fill the pleural space, either because of previous partial resection or because of diffuse fibrosis. In the latter patients, the goal of treatment may be achieved either with thoracoplasty or with various pedicled flaps developed from the chest wall muscles or the greater omentum. Extrapleural pneumonectomy for destroyed lung complicated with empyema is a high-risk procedure and cannot be recommended as standard practice.

In this discussion, we describe separately tuberculous empyema, *Aspergillus* empyema, and finally miscellaneous conditions, because the patients differ considerably. We do not detail the technical aspects of procedures such as decor-

tication, thoracoplasty, and muscle transfers; these procedures are presented in Chapters 61, 62, and 59, respectively.

PLEURAL TUBERCULOSIS

Tuberculous infection of the pleura appears as a disease of the past when one refers to the paucity of recent publications. Indeed, most of the principles defined during the 1950s and 1960s are still valuable today. Langston and colleagues (1967) stated that TB of the pleura may manifest itself clinically and pathologically in a variety of ways. The gamut runs from the thin idiopathic effusion that may yield acid-fast bacilli with difficulty, if at all, to the thick purulent exudates that have positive results on direct smears. All gradations and combinations of extent as well as character of pleural involvement or bacteriologic content are seen, as noted by Langston and associates (1967). Nevertheless, for clarification, we artificially subdivide the subsequent discussion into three groups defined by the natural history of disease:

1) During primary TB, pleural effusions appear in approximately 8% of patients. The fluid is usually serofibrinous, and this condition should be called *tuberculous pleuritis*.
2) During reactivation of TB, pleural infection turns to a true empyema, characterized by an opaque and purulent effusion. Such tuberculous empyemas may be either pure or mixed: In the case of bronchopleural fistula, other micro-organisms can infect the pleura together with *Mycobacterium tuberculosis*.
3) The particular setting of late complications of collapse therapy for TB, which are infrequently encountered nowadays, present varying complex problems.

Tuberculous Pleuritis

According to Jereb and colleagues (1991), the pleural space is the second most common site of extrapulmonary

TB, the first being the lymphatic system. Pleural infection, as noted by Weir and Thornton (1985), is supposed to originate from subpleural pulmonary lesions. The clinical presentation is well known. General signs include low-grade fever, weakness, weight loss, and night sweats. Revealing respiratory symptoms are nonproductive cough, pleuritic chest pain, and dyspnea correlated to the extent of effusion. In the elderly, silent disease is not uncommon. Chest radiography shows a pleural effusion; concomitant parenchymal disease is observed in approximately one-third of cases. At the early stage of disease, the tuberculin skin test result is positive in 75% of patients, but, according to Berger and Mejia (1973), it should be positive in virtually all patients by 2 months, except in patients with acquired immunodeficiency syndrome (AIDS). Positive diagnosis relies on direct sampling of the pleural fluid and on pleural biopsies. Gross analysis of pleural fluid reveals an exudative fluid with a protein level in excess of 40 g/L and a white cell count of 1 to 6 g/L with predominant lymphocytes. Absence of desquamated mesothelial cells suggests TB, as reported by Weir and Thornton (1985). Glucose level determination is not really useful; cultures take 3 to 6 weeks, and the results are inconsistently positive. Only 30% become positive in Berger and Mejia's (1973) experience. In the study of Caminero and colleagues (1993), determination of IgG antibody levels to mycobacterial antigen 60 with a cut-off value of 150 U/mL had a sensitivity of 50% and a specificity of 100%. The sophisticated determination of adenosine deaminase has been found by Berenguer and associates (1992) to have a poor sensitivity and specificity. Falk (1965) noted that cultures from sputum or gastric content are expected to be negative unless radiologic evidence exists for parenchymal disease. Therefore, the most reliable investigation is pleural biopsy. Bates (1979) and Berger and Mejia (1973) reported that pleural biopsy with the Abrams needle or similar devices yields a positive result in 60 to 80% of patients. According to Yim (1996), video-assisted thoracic surgery achieves a high level of specificity because multiple biopsies increase the diagnostic threshold. Regarding the remarkably low operative risk, it seems reasonable to proceed with thoracoscopy when direct examination of bacteriologic samples is negative, rather than waiting several weeks for the result of cultures. Histologic evidence of caseating epithelioid granulomas is indicative of TB; Levine and colleagues (1970) recommended that immediate antituberculous therapy should be commenced, although only identification of acid-fast bacilli is completely diagnostic.

In summary, the diagnostic criteria defined by Langston and associates (1967) are still valuable today. Tuberculous pleuritis may be assumed for one or more of the following specific findings: 1) positive tuberculin skin test result; 2) secretions positive for *M. tuberculosis*, sputum, or gastric content; 3) pleural fluid positive for *M. tuberculosis*; and 4) pleural disease consistent with tuberculous granuloma on histologic study of biopsy or resected tissue.

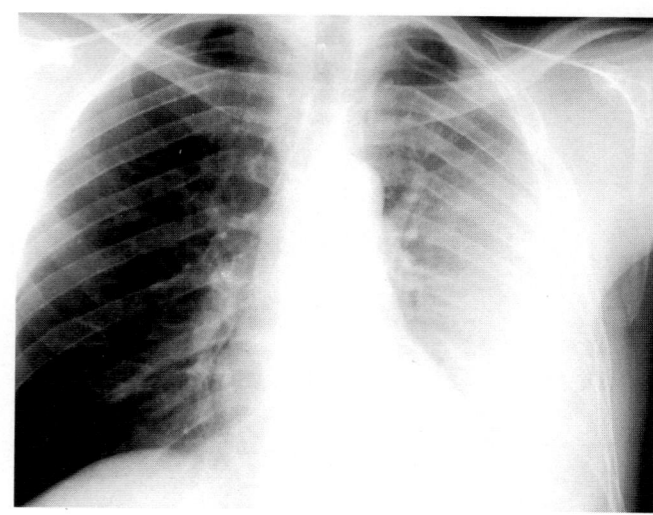

Fig. 60-1. Posteroanterior chest radiograph showing a large left pleural effusion. Needle biopsy disclosed tuberculous granuloma initially. The effusion failed to resolve after 4 months of adequate treatment.

The natural history of tuberculous pleuritis is usually benign, with spontaneous resorption even if untreated. Usual management includes antituberculous treatment, repeated thoracentesis as required, and close observation. Most often, patients respond favorably. However, depending on the individual patient's immunologic status, excessive production of exudative material may start a diffuse thickening of the visceral pleura, leading to an entrapment of the lung, regardless of whether adequate antituberculous treatment is used (Fig. 60-1). Such residual pleural disease is a threat for reactivation of TB or further development of a bronchopleural fistula, and therefore decortication should be considered.

Indications for decortication rely on careful examination of medical imaging. Previously, the indication for decortication was confirmed with lateral chest radiography. It was assumed that pleural disease seen on a posteroanterior projection but not visible on lateral films, is diffuse around the pleural sac, and that a minor thickness of the pleural peel occurs; such cases were expected to clear progressively, with return of normal motion of the chest wall. On the other hand, an effusion visible on both anteroposterior and lateral views corresponds to a large posterior pocket with a relatively thick pleural peel, by virtue of dependent accumulation. Such encapsulated pleural processes are not likely to resolve completely unless small at the onset, and in the cases with a thick pleural peel, decortication was recommended by Langston and colleagues (1967). Computed tomography (CT) scan has confirmed this approach and also has replaced bronchography for assessment of the underlying lung (Fig. 60-2).

Determination of the appropriate timing of surgical intervention was clearly defined in 1967, and no obvious reason exists to change anything in Langston and associates' (1967) criteria: 1) decortication is indicated when thoracentesis fails

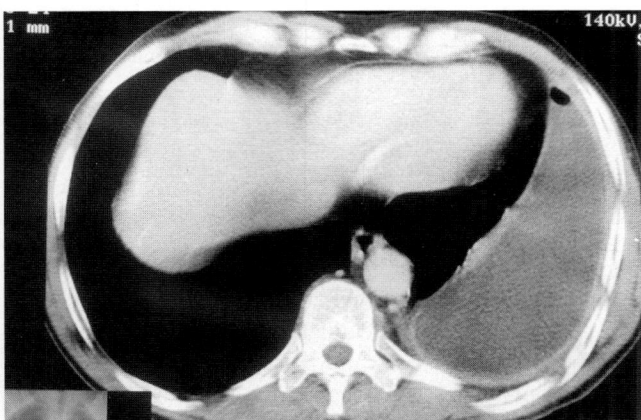

Fig. 60-2. Same patient as seen in Figure 60-1. Computed tomographic scan demonstrated a thickened visceral pleural peel entrapping the lung and requiring decortication for reexpansion.

Table 60-1. Treatment Plan for Chronic Mycobacterial or Fungal Empyema

I. Decortication
  A. Lung expandable
    No extensive circumferential calcifications
    No cavitations or cystic bronchiectasis
  B. Previous resection
    Add thoracoplasty
  C. When is additional resection necessary?
    Multidrug resistance present
    Hemoptysis
    Aspergilloma
    Cystic bronchiectases/infected
    Avoid pneumonectomy whenever possible
  D. When is additional resection not indicated?
    Reactivated tuberculosis, converted sputum, asymptomatic destroyed lung
  E. What to do when poor expansion of lung is present during decortication
    Consider immediate thoracoplasty
    May elect prolonged drainage plus pneumoperitoneum
  F. What to do when there is poor expansion postoperatively
    Consider deferred thoracoplasty
II. Open window thoracostomy
  A. Lung not expandable
    Circumferential calcification
  B. Poor-risk patient
  C. Previous resection complicating IIA or IIB
    Consider isolated thoracoplasty for apical space

to yield fluid or fails to alter radiographic appearance, 2) the extent of pleural involvement should be equivalent to one-third or one-fourth of the hemithorax and cast a clearly discernible shadow in the posterior basal gutter, and 3) decortication should be made as early as is consistent with good judgment (i.e., after 2 to 4 months of drug therapy).

Technical aspects of decortication are discussed in Chapter 61. In our opinion, a generous thoracotomy is still required. It remains preferable to proceed with the lung inflated for precise peeling of the visceral pleura and thus to achieve optimal reexpansion. At present, this seems not to be easily reproducible with minimally invasive alternatives to a standard thoracotomy, although Yim (1996) and others have reported that isolated cases have been managed successfully by video-assisted thoracic surgery techniques.

Tuberculous Empyema

Pleural reactivation of TB has been a threat in patients who did not receive major antituberculous drug therapy. Moreover, chronic empyema was frequently complicated by bronchopleural fistula, leading to a so-called mixed empyema characterized by a contamination with both *M. tuberculosis* and common pyogens. Chronic empyema following TB adequately treated with antituberculous antibiotics is seldom associated with reactivation of TB in the pleural space. For example, none of the 22 patients treated by Garcia-Yuste and coworkers (1998) had any evidence for ongoing mycobacterial infection.

Diagnosis is easy in patients with known sequelae of TB. Low-grade fever, constitutional complaints, and increasing dyspnea with or without chest pain are the major symptoms. Abundant sputum suggests bronchopleural fistula. On chest radiography, the obvious finding is an increase of the extent of the pleural involvement; the appearance of an air-

fluid level heralds a bronchopleural fistula. Thoracentesis yields purulent fluid, which should be sent routinely for both bacterial and fungal cultures. Thoracentesis may be difficult in patients with a calcified pleura and requires an experienced operator. As soon as empyema is confirmed, adequate drainage should be instituted. Our preference is the tube thoracostomy, whereas others prefer immediate open thoracostomy. We limit open thoracostomy to the severely ill patient with a poor operative risk, because it may jeopardize subsequent decortication. In patients with documented reactivation of TB, the classic principle—to convert sputum cultures with medical treatment before resection—should still be applied as recommended by Treasure and Seaworth (1995).

The next step is to plan for definitive treatment, which implicates major thoracic surgery with often complicated outcome (Table 60-1). Unfortunately, video-assisted thoracic surgery has no place, though otherwise it should be particularly useful for those patients who are debilitated, thus making them poor candidates for conventional open surgery.

The first question is to determine whether the underlying lung is re-expandable. Ideally, one should prefer the most conservative approach, which consists of reexpanding the lung with decortication. The CT scan is most helpful in the evaluation of the entrapped lung; bronchography is no longer required. Areas with cavitations or large cystic bronchiectases obviously will not reexpand. Conversely, Mouroux and associates (1996), as well as Treasure and

Seaworth (1995), have found that a patent bronchopleural fistula does not preclude decortication.

The second question is to determine whether parenchymal resection is required. Metatuberculous lungs are relatively stiff, and loss of volume leads to residual pleural space, which represents a factor for persistent empyema postoperatively. Therefore, combined parenchymal resections should strictly adhere to the classic indications for resection as reported by Pomerantz (1991) and Mouroux (1996) and their colleagues as well as by Treasure and Seaworth (1995): 1) multiple drug-resistant disease, 2) threat of hemoptysis, and 3) infectious complications such as bronchiectasis or aspergilloma. Current criteria for drug resistance are 1) clinical or radiologic evidence of progressive disease and 2) persistent mycobacteria on sputum examination after 3 months of a four-drug treatment; at an earlier stage, bacillar casts may be visible on direct examination of smears, but fail to grow in culture. When the remaining lung is extensively destroyed, extrapleural pneumonectomy is to be considered. We would, however, raise some admonitions against a difficult and potentially dangerous procedure. Publications by Halezeroglu (1997) and Conlan (1995) and their associates as well as by Odell and Henderson (1985) conclude that both previous TB and coexistent empyema are significant risk factors for procedure-related morbidity and mortality.

As we and our colleagues (1995b) pointed out, the postoperative course after decortication with or without additional parenchymal resection may be complicated mainly by pleural space disease. Prolonged air leaks ultimately seal with prolonged drainage, provided that the lung is completely expanded. Persisting pleural spaces after decortication may be managed either with muscle plombage or with thoracoplasty. Thoracoplasty has an unwarranted bad name and should be rehabilitated in patients with marked malnutrition; a four-rib thoracoplasty with a stable and retracted mediastinum may be expeditiously carried out, as noted by Hopkins and associates (1985), compared with the preparation and transfer of two or three muscle flaps. Rather than performing an immediate thoracoplasty as in former years, we prefer to test the expansion potential of the remaining lung and to proceed with second-stage thoracoplasty only when it proves to be necessary.

Creating an open window thoracostomy initially is an important decision, because decortication cannot be performed in a second stage. However, Garcia-Yuste and colleagues (1998) suggest that a two-stage management with thoracostomy and subsequent muscle plombage of the cleaned residual space is a reasonable alternative in cases unsuitable for decortication. Poor general health status and extensive calcifications precluding decortication are indications for this type of management. In the case of a largely destroyed but asymptomatic lung, two-stage myoplasty may help avoid the temptation to proceed with extrapleural pneumonectomy.

Regardless of the type of surgical management decided on, adjuvant antituberculous treatment is mandatory in cases of documented reactivation of TB.

Late Pleural and Extrapleural Complications of Collapse Therapy

Until the early 1960s, when major antituberculous drugs became available and began the end of a long-standing plague, the only active treatment for TB was the so-called collapse procedures. The common objective of these procedures was to collapse cavitated lung tissue and to obtain progressively scarring of the tuberculous area. Most physicians used to these treatments have retired, and few patients still survive. Thoracic surgeons of the younger generation have had virtually no exposure to such patients.

The first stage of collapse therapy was creation of an artificial intrapleural pneumothorax; because of the spontaneous resorption of the intrapleural air, reinjections of air were required at 2-week intervals. The first indication for thoracoscopic surgery was apical adhesiolysis to promote apical collapse by Dumarest and coworkers in 1945. When extensive apical adhesions precluded adequate collapse with intrapleural pneumothorax, extrapleural pneumolysis was the preferred procedure. Similarly, as carried out by Roberts (1948), the collapse space was maintained by periodic injections of air. After 2 to 3 years of treatment, the injections of air were discontinued, and the space progressively filled with serous fluid and retracted to a small and permanent residual space. The considerable burden of pneumothorax, and the infectious risk depending on repeated thoracenteses as well, led to the conception of extramusculoperiosteal plombage, also called the *birdcage operation*, which was most popular between 1948 and 1955 as reported by Wilson and coworkers (1956) and Shepherd (1985). In the latter operation, the periosteum and intercostal muscles were stripped off the ribs, similar to thoracoplasty, and pushed inside the chest cavity to collapse the underlying cavity. The collapse was maintained with methyl methacrylate balls packed between the denuded ribs and the surface of pneumolysis; initially, extraperiosteal pneumolysis was believed to avoid thoracoplasty. However, the many infectious complications, as well as the frequently reported migrations of material, necessitated that the plombage be removed several months later and thoracoplasty be performed to obliterate the extraperiosteal space. In Chicago and some areas of the Pacific Northwest of the United States, the use of paraffin as the plombage material became common during the same time period. Lees (1951) and Fox (1962) and their associates reviewed their extensive experience with this material. Infectious complications were rare, but migration of the wax plomb occurred in more than 25% of the patients as early as 5 to 6 months to as late as 10 years or more. A thoracoplasty was rarely necessary after the removal of the

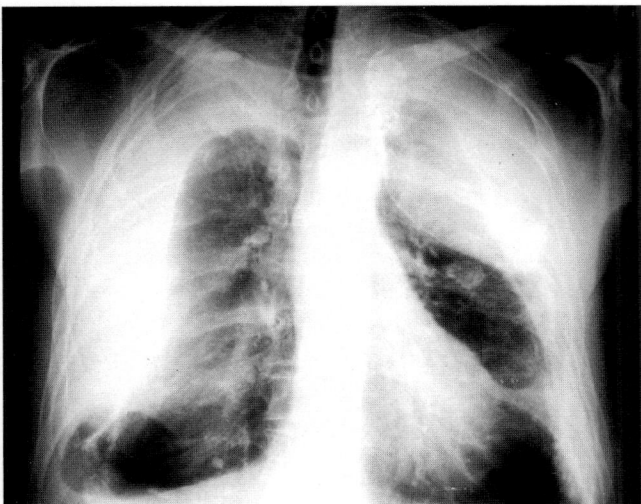

Fig. 60-3. Bilateral tension effusion at the site of a right-sided intrapleural and a left-sided extrapleural pneumothorax.

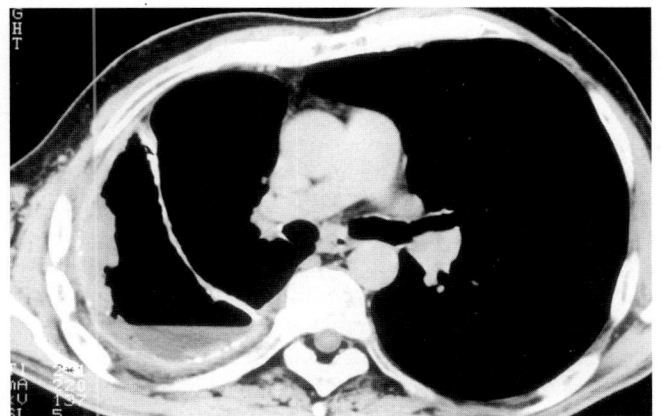

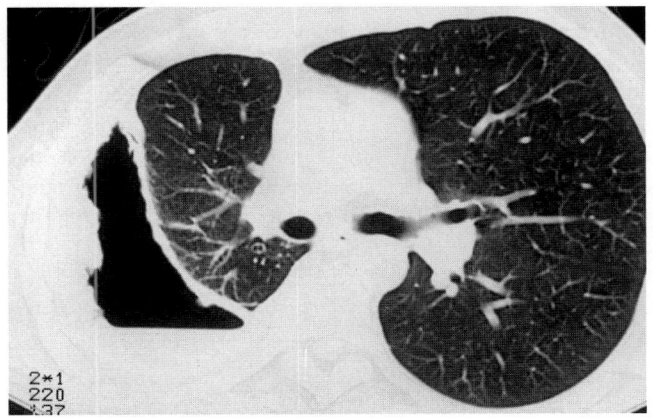

Fig. 60-4. Patient with tuberculous empyema complicating a previous intrapleural pneumothorax. **A.** Mediastinal window. A broad pleural peel is clearly outlined. **B.** Parenchymal window obviates relatively normal underlying lung tissue prone to reexpansion after decortication.

migrated plomb in contrast to the Lucite plombage. All these procedures rapidly vanished with the advent of antituberculous chemotherapy.

Late infectious complications at the site of previous intrapleural or extrapleural pneumothorax present as either progressively acquired swelling of the residual pocket (Fig. 60-3) or appearance of an air-fluid level because of a bronchopleural fistula. One-half of the patients only are symptomatic and complain of fever, increasing dyspnea, pain, or hemoptysis; productive cough usually indicates bronchopleural fistula. The diagnosis is made, as pointed out by us and our associates (1995a), when comparing consecutive surveillance chest films in asymptomatic patients. Surprisingly, the pleural fluid is sterile on culture in more than one-half the patients. Furthermore, the incidence of proven tuberculous empyema is relatively low. In our experience (1995a), 13 patients out of 28 had positive microbiology results, and four only had proved pleural TB. Similarly, Schmid and De Haller (1986) observed a single case of reactivated TB in a series of 15 patients. These observations are consistent with earlier data reported by Neff and Buchanan (1975), which showed that tuberculous empyema was a rather usual early complication of collapse therapy but did not contribute significantly to the late morbidity.

The preferred mode of treatment of late empyema is decortication. The underlying lung is expected to re-expand because no previous parenchymal resection has been performed. Simple open window drainage is not satisfactory per se but is a fair treatment for debilitated and otherwise inoperable patients. On the other extreme, the risk of extrapleural pneumonectomy is certainly prohibitive in this particular setting. Both sequelae of TB and coexisting empyema are significant risk factors as noted by Halezeroglu (1997) and the authors (1996) and associates. Furthermore, these patients are in their seventh decade of life and frequently present with

significant respiratory or cardiovascular comorbidity. Thoracoplasty should be restricted to either space problems following decortication or diffuse and heavy calcifications obliterating the extrapleural dissection plane.

Decortication is well-tolerated, although it is complicated by prolonged air leaks in most patients. We and our colleagues (1995b) found that the average drainage time was 16 days; however, drainage time was increased to a mean of 20 days in symptomatic patients and in patients with positive microbiology results. The reexpansion potential of such chronically entrapped lungs is surprising but may be anticipated from careful inspection of CT of the underlying lung (Fig. 60-4). Technical details do not diverge from those of any decortication. Briefly, double-lumen tube intubation is mandatory to prevent flooding of the opposite lung. A generous posterolateral thoracotomy is necessary for adequate exposure. Resection of the fifth or sixth rib is usually necessary because of the considerable retraction of the rib cage; the extrapleural plane is entered through the posterior periosteum. The parietal pleura is freed up to the mediastinal reflections, which requires considerable strength in case of extensive calcifications. Overenthusiastic dissection along the paraspinal gutter may lead to avulsion of the azygos vein on the right side or of intercostal vessels on the left side. The lung is identified ideally at the anterior mediastinal recess. However, when this adequate cleavage plane is not easily found, the pleural pocket should be entered and the visceral pleura incised directly over the lung; the thickened pleura is progressively freed and excised from the center to the periphery. One should refrain from resecting any lung, because the previous tuberculous areas have scarred over the years. We recommend triple drainage connected to strong suction (100 to 150 mm Hg), because air leaks stop only when the apposition of pleural surfaces is restored. Because compliance of such lungs is decreased, strong suction is required to shift the mediastinum and elevate the diaphragm. Antituberculous therapy is mandatory and should be guided by sensitivity studies. The functional recovery after such procedures is debated. We do not anticipate any restoration of lung function. In our opinion, the aim of the operation is to use the lung as a natural prothesis to fill the pleural space and to resolve the empyema and, of course, avoid extrapleural pneumonectomy.

Late complications occurring in extraperiosteal plombage cavities were more frequently frank infections; in 1997 we reported eight proved infections in a total of 10 exudates; four of them were tuberculous empyemas. When infection occurs, the usual finding is recent onset of swelling along the thoracoplasty incision or in the subclavicular area; infection facilitates erosion of the devitalized ribs and migration of the plombage material, which can be palpated beneath the skin. The procedure of choice is removal of the plombage and immediate thoracoplasty (Figs. 60-5 and 60-6). The approach is made through the previous thoracoplasty incision. Ablation of the devitalized, sometimes partly eroded ribs, is usually simple. We emphasize that the first rib should

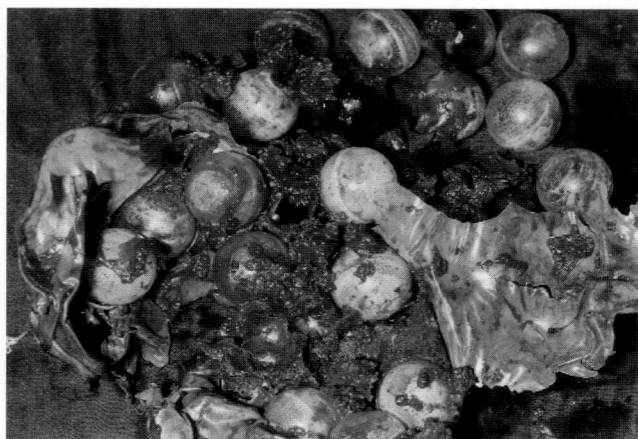

Fig. 60-6. Same patient as seen in Figure 60-5. Freshly removed plombage material.

be resected to prevent any residual space, which could be the bed for relapse of infection; this technical step is in agreement with Hopkins and associates (1985). Intraoperative fluoroscopy is mandatory to check for complete removal of any foreign material; Lucite balls may be embedded into calcified tissues at the floor of the collapse space and be hidden from the surgeon's eye or fingers. Calcifications of the floor of the collapse space usually determine a peripheral rim, which must be trimmed away to provide adequate collapse. Double drainage for irrigation is placed before standard closure in layers. Naturally, adjuvant antituberculous therapy is mandatory.

ASPERGILLUS EMPYEMA

Pleural infection with *Aspergillus fumigatus* is a rather infrequent disease; Kearon and colleagues (1987) listed only 30 cases in an exhaustive review of the literature. Even in the immunodeficient setting of lung transplantation, *Aspergillus* empyema remains rare. In a series of 31 graft recipients with positive *Aspergillus* culture results reported by Westney and colleagues (1996), only one patient developed *Aspergillus* empyema. Contamination of the pleural space with *Aspergillus* sporae or hyphae results either from direct intrapleural seeding during surgery or by aspiration of aerosolized particles through a bronchopleural fistula. Fungal growth requires a persistent pleural space, which provides excellent atmospheric conditions with an ambient temperature of 37°C, a moisture of 100%, and abundant proteins readily available to digestion by fungal catalase or chymotrypsin. Pleural aspergillosis presents in two clinical pictures that differ considerably. Acute *Aspergillus* empyema develops usually during the immediate postoperative course after an intrapleural thoracic procedure and presents with similar findings as any postoperative pleural infection. Late *Aspergillus* empyema presents similarly to

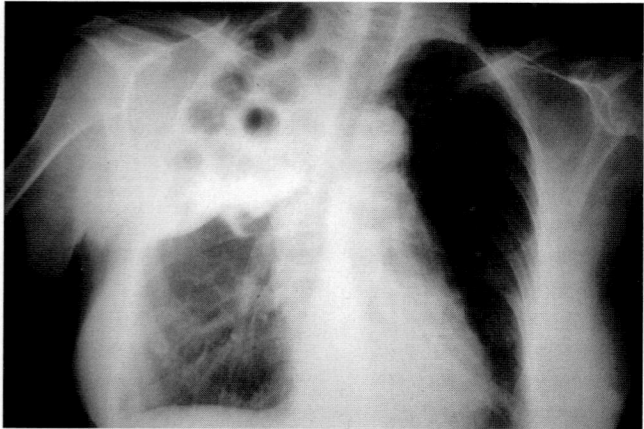

Fig. 60-5. Extraperiosteal plombage with methyl methacrylate balls. Late infectious complication with exudative distention of the collapse space.

pulmonary aspergilloma as a chronic process of the saprophytic type. The following section refers mainly to our personal data, originally published in 1992(a).

Acute *Aspergillus* Empyema

As noted by Herring and Pecora (1976), acute *Aspergillus* empyema most often occurs after a surgical procedure undertaken to treat an aspergilloma. We have reported seven cases of acute pleural infection (1992a). Five of them resulted from gross intraoperative contamination, with four patients being operated on for a known aspergilloma. A fifth patient was operated on for spontaneous hemopneumothorax and underwent resection of an apical bulla; retrospectively, a small mycetoma was identified by review of the preoperative CT scan.

The most common operation preceding acute *Aspergillus* empyema is partial lung resection such as lobectomy or segmentectomy. One of our personal cases (1992a) occurred after diagnostic thoracoscopy for a metastatic pleural effusion; this procedure was complicated with multiple parenchymal fistulae. Another case reported by Purcell and Corris (1995) describes a patient with bronchopulmonary aspergillosis, who developed *Aspergillus fumigatus* empyema subsequent to a spontaneous pneumothorax. Nakanishi and colleagues (1996) noted that percutaneous instillation of antifungal agents into a parenchymal cavity hosting a mycetoma is also known to foster pleural seeding.

A threat of pneumonectomy exists in patients with aspergilloma. These operations are characterized by major intraoperative difficulties because of the usually dense and highly vascular adhesions. Virtually all patients operated on by our group (1996) had excessive intraoperative bleeding, and six of eight developed postpneumonectomy empyema. However, only a single case had the pleural space contaminated with *Aspergillus*. After this experience, we recommend removal of the fungus ball and a thoracoplasty to obliterate the parenchymal cavity when feasible, as described in 1992(a), rather than proceeding with an extrapleural pneumonectomy.

The most common clinical finding after partial lung resection is prolonged air leak and persistent drainage of fluid; in addition, fever and weight loss are usual. The residual pleural space hosting the infection is not always apparent on standard chest radiography. More particularly, anterior spaces most often require CT studies to be identified. After pneumonectomy, the signs of empyema are well known to all thoracic surgeons: General malaise, fever, and pallor identify the patient at risk. Infection is confirmed by elevated white blood cell count and persisting high C-reactive protein levels that were reported by Icard and associates (1994). Chest radiography shows a rapid increase of the pleural air-fluid level because of increased exudation of pleural fluid; the mediastinum is occasionally shifted toward the contralateral lung.

Diagnosis of *Aspergillus* empyema is easily confirmed by appropriate analysis of pleural fluid samples. Serodiagnosis is less reliable, because it may be negative at the early stages of the disease.

Cure of acute *Aspergillus* empyema requires sterilization and complete and definitive obliteration of the pleural space. Various strategies such as pleural lavage through a chest tube, surgical débridement, and open window thoracostomy achieve a satisfactory gross cleaning of the pleural space. But the final decision as to how to obliterate the space depends on the reexpansion potential of the remaining lung. After resections less than lobectomy, expansion is clearly possible as soon as air leaks have sealed. In such patients, conservative management with antifungal treatment has a fair chance for success. According to Chatzimichalis and coworkers (1998), because of the hyperemia of the acutely infected pleura, the tissue penetration of itraconazole is satisfactory and sufficiently high local concentrations are easily obtained similar to invasive pulmonary aspergillosis. A lone case of success of treatment with aerosolized liposomal amphotericin B has been reported by Purcell and Corris (1995); high local tissue concentrations are expected in the presence of a bronchopleural fistula. The problem is different in patients who have undergone a lobectomy. Clearly, intraoperative seeding results from parenchymal tears because of a difficult dissection. This means that such patients had complex aspergilloma as pointed out by Daly and colleagues (1986) and that the remaining lung is expectedly sclerotic with reduced reexpansion potential. In favorable cases, institution of a pneumoperitoneum sufficiently increases the diaphragm to obtain contact of the pleural surfaces. In the event of larger pleural spaces, aggressive management is mandatory to shorten the spontaneous evolution. In our opinion, apical spaces are best dealt with by thoracoplasty. Muscle flaps are often disappointingly thin in emaciated patients marked by chronic illness; further, the largest flap (i.e., the latissimus dorsi) usually has been sacrificed during the initial thoracotomy. None of the six patients we treated with thoracoplasty developed recurrent disease (1992a).

Management of *Aspergillus* empyema after pneumonectomy does not differ from management of postpneumonectomy empyema in general. Once the diagnosis is established, the pleural space must be drained. Aggressive management is mandatory to obtain quick cleaning of gross purulent material. Most authors proceed with an open window thoracostomy as described by Clagett and Geraci (1963). In our current practice, we prefer surgical débridement followed by irrigations through a chest tube. It is questionable whether a tedious cleaning by video-assisted thoracic surgery techniques offers any advantage over a short thoracotomy in this situation. To obliterate the cleaned pleural space, the debate is between the proponents of muscle plombage procedures, such as Shirakusa (1989, 1990) and Pairolero (1990) and their colleagues, as well as Ali and Unruh (1990), and the partisans of thoracoplasty including Horrigan and Snow (1990) as well as Grégoire (1987) and Hopkins (1985) and their associates.

Chronic *Aspergillus* Empyema

Chronic *Aspergillus* empyema is fostered by a residual pleural space communicating with the bronchial tree. The cavity is penetrated by aerosolized fungal material similarly to parenchymal cavities. Further development of the fungus is favored by progressive erosion of the surrounding structures by its proteolytic enzymes. As we have shown (1992a), the most frequent setting is previous partial lung resection for TB or lung cancer. Adjuvant or neoadjuvant radiation therapy has been retrospectively identified in four of our six patients operated for lung cancer (1992a) and, as suggested by Utley (1993), might be a contributing factor. In addition, occasional *Aspergillus* empyemas are encountered in patients with sequelae of previous collapse therapy, as previously noted. The common problem in these patients is that medical therapy with itraconazole is likely to fail. The first reason is that tissue penetration in chronic lesions surrounded by fibrotic scar tissue, as pointed out by Chatzimichalis and associates (1998) is expected to be low, similar in this aspect to an aspergilloma. The second reason is that the possibility of infection persists as long as a residual pleural space exists. The obligate operative management is one of the most challenging situations in general thoracic surgery. The precarious health status of patients with *Aspergillus* empyema is best described by Krakowka and colleagues (1970), who reported five deaths during treatment in a series of 10 patients.

Two clinical presentations are to be discussed, corresponding to postresectional empyema and empyema in previous collapse spaces. Chronic postresectional empyema may be detected on routine chest radiography but is usually symptomatic. The symptoms are similar to those of pulmonary aspergilloma: hemoptysis, bronchorrhea, dyspnea, and chest pain. Chest radiography shows either a partial hydropneumothorax indicating a bronchopleural fistula or a progressive thickening of known pleural sequelae that was noted by Libshitz and associates (1974). True intrapleural megamycetomas are uncommon. Empyema in previous intrapleural or extrapleural collapse spaces or residual pockets after tuberculous pleurisy may be silent and appear as an enlargement of the pleural thickening on sequential surveillance chest radiography. Otherwise, fever and chest pain are the usual symptoms. Cough and increased sputum indicate bronchopleural fistula, which is characterized by an air-fluid level on chest films (Figs. 60-7 and 60-8).

A positive diagnosis relies on direct identification of *Aspergillus* species or serodiagnosis. Sampling of pleural fluid is easy in patients with hydropneumothorax only. Fortunately, serodiagnosis is most reliable because it is nearly always positive in patients with chronic infection. Our current criteria for *Aspergillus* infection are the following:

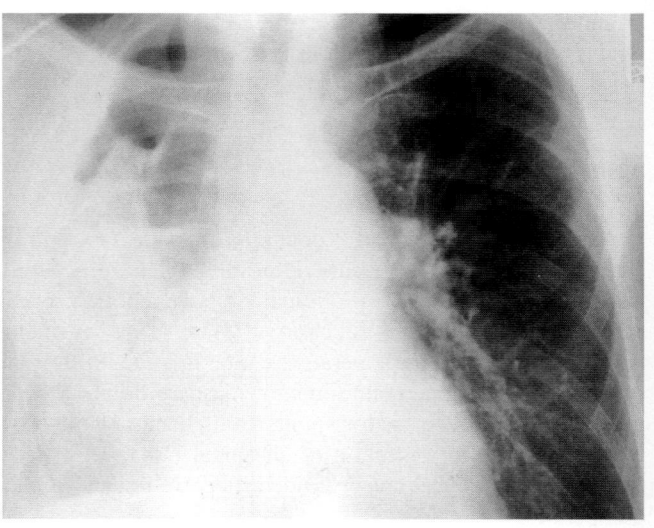

Fig. 60-7. *Aspergillus* empyema caused by bronchopleural fistula complicating an intrapleural pneumothorax. Note the apical pneumothorax and basal effusion, determining a midthoracic air-fluid level. Extensive pleural calcifications; translucent trapped lung packed against the hilum.

either at least two precipitations on immunoelectrophoresis, or a single precipitation with positive catalase activity. In our previous series (1992a), the average number of precipitations was 7.2 (range, 2 to 15); all but one patient had a positive result for catalase activity.

Treatment options differ between postresectional and postcollapse empyema. In any event, the underlying lung should be left in place when feasible, because a significantly increased risk for mortality and major morbidity exists after pneumonectomy in patients with preoperative empyema; this has been estimated to be close to 40% by Halezeroglu (1997) and Conlan (1995) and their associates, as well as by Odell and Henderson (1985). Furthermore, according to McGovern and colleagues (1988), the risk of completion pneumonectomy in this situation is prohibitive. The operative mortality of 9.4% after completion pneumonectomy for cancer was increased to 27.6% after completion pneumonectomy for benign disease in the Mayo Clinic experience. Similarly, the prevalence of empyema was 20.7% and 9.3%, and the prevalence of bronchopleural fistula was 17.2% and 3.1%, respectively, for benign and malignant disease. Therefore, further resection is only legitimized when persisting infectious lesions such as lung abscess or bronchiectases would otherwise jeopardize the outcome. In extreme situations, completion pneumonectomy and immediate thoracoplasty have been advocated by Utley (1993).

In postresectional empyema, the remaining lobe is usually fibrosed because of previous TB or radiation therapy. Therefore, decortication is likely to fail. Muscle transfers are less than optimal in these malnourished patients with marked chronic illness; besides, as previously noted, the latissimus dorsi muscle has usually been sacrificed during the initial thoracotomy. Although some successes have been obtained

leagues (1985) and Horrigan and Snow (1990). Incomplete apical collapse is a concern when the first rib is left in place. Of course, such operations are risky because of the disabled status of these patients. In our experience, mortality of thoracoplasty has been 7%, caused by respiratory infection. More than one-half the patients in our series (1992a) experienced major perioperative bleeding (>1500 mL) because of the usual hypervascularization of aspergillized cavities; preoperative embolization as suggested by Hughes and associates (1986) usually fails to reduce intraoperative bleeding because the perilesional vascular network is supplied by multiple pedicles as pointed out by Chen and colleagues (1997). We suggest generous rib resection, because more than 40% of our patients had persistent space problems after thoracoplasty. The postoperative course is usually prolonged, with an average hospital stay of 49 days in our experience; this is the result of the disease rather than of the procedure used. However, long-term results show no evidence for recurrent infection at a mean follow-up of 7 years. Thoracoplasty offers the possibility for a one-stage cure. Management with open window thoracostomy followed by muscle flap transfer or omentoplasty to fill the residual space seems less aggressive than thoracoplasty, but duration of the complete treatment plan takes at best 6 months as reported by Shirakusa and colleagues (1989).

Treatment of long-term complications of residual collapse spaces is initiated with tube thoracostomy and irrigations. CT scan reveals some expandable underlying parenchyma in most cases, although perfusion scan shows a dramatic decrease of perfusion (see Fig. 60-8). Knowing the risk of pneumonectomy through an empyema (1995a), we advocate decortication in the latter cases. Inexperienced surgeons might be frightened by the sight of the residual lung with multiple parenchymal leaks, as it presents at the conclusion of the operation. Triple drainage put to strong suction, and a good deal of patience, lead finally to sealing of the leaks and cure of the patient. One should remember that postoperative drainage is significantly prolonged, as we have noted (1995b), in symptomatic patients and patients with positive microbiology findings.

MISCELLANEOUS CONDITIONS

Several other fungal diseases, such as blastomycosis, histoplasmosis, cryptococcosis, and sporotrichosis, may occasionally involve the pleura during acute pulmonary infection with pleural perforation. Patients with AIDS are particularly prone to such infections. The main problem in these patients is appropriate microbiological diagnosis. With adequate antifungal treatment, the infection should resolve without any need for surgical management except for drainage of large effusions.

Two agents, *Coccidioides immitis* and *Candida albicans*, are of particular interest. Coccidioidomycosis may cause diffuse lung destruction similar to TB and may result in similar

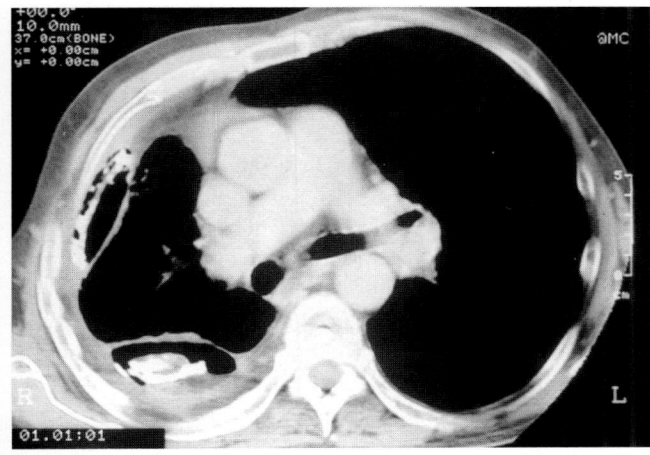
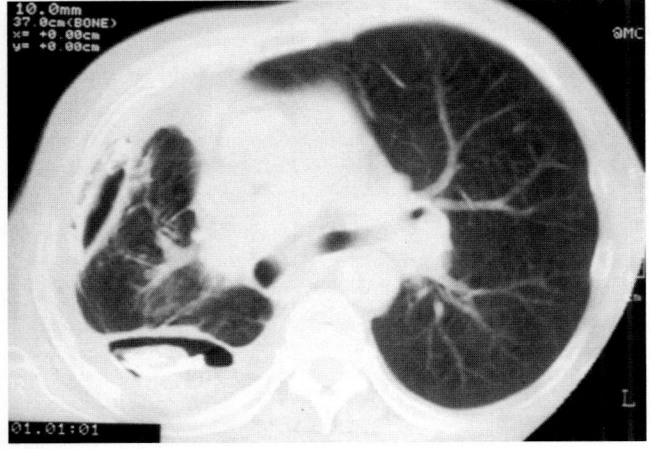

Fig. 60-8. *Aspergillus* empyema caused by bronchopleural fistula complicating an intrapleural pneumothorax. Same patient as seen in Figure 60-7. **A.** Mediastinal window: thickened parietal and visceral pleura with extensive calcifications. **B.** Parenchymal window: the trapped lung tissue is nearly normal and did reexpand after decortication.

with omental transfer, as reported by Shirakusa and associates (1990), we would add some caveats to this technique. In malnourished patients, the tissue volume is spare. Harvest of the omentum exposes the patient to the additional risk of laparotomy. When the omentum is used, one should avoid a direct passage through the diaphragm to prevent herniation of abdominal viscera as we noted (1992b). It is mandatory to use indirect tunneling, either through Morgagni's hiatus or through the phrenohepatic ligaments as suggested by Jurkiewicz and Arnold (1977). The most appropriate management should include careful curettage of all fungal material, followed by a retailoring of the chest wall with thoracoplasty. Many authors such as Grégoire and colleagues (1987) recommend leaving the first rib in place to avoid scoliosis. However, others including Loynes (1972) believe that scoliosis is determined by extensive rib resections and resection of the transverse processes of the vertebra. We stress the need to routinely resect the first rib, as do Hopkins and col-

surgical problems. The presence of yeast cells within a pleural effusion suggests the presence of an esophagopleural fistula.

Coccidioidomycosis

Pleural infection with *C. immitis* seldom has been referred to in the literature. A review published by Drutz and Catanzaro (1978a, 1978b) describes two situations depending on the natural history of disease. An acute infection appears in 40% of infected patients and mimics an influenza-like acute respiratory infection. The pleural effusion that may appear simultaneously to the pulmonary infiltrate is usually sterile. Approximately 5% of patients develop irreversible pulmonary lesions such as cavitations or bronchiectases. Rupture of a cavitation into the pleural space leads to a coccidioidal or mixed empyema. Amphotericin B is the basis of treatment; surgical indications are carried out along identical guide lines as for pleural TB.

The difficulties of chronic pulmonary coccidioidomycosis with empyema are perfectly illustrated by a case reported by Utley (1993). This patient presented with bronchopleural fistula and simultaneous granulomatous infection of the lung and pleural space 10 years after left lower lobectomy for coccidioidomycosis. Operative intervention was prompted by major hemoptysis. Completion pneumonectomy was required because of cavitations in the remaining lobe. A mass closure of hilar vessels and bronchus with transfixing mattress sutures was used because of inability to individually close the vessels and bronchus because of fibrous scarring of the hilum, and the pleural space was obliterated by an immediate thoracoplasty.

Candida albicans

Though usually seen in immunocompromised individuals, such as patients with AIDS or transplant recipients, as noted by Emery and associates (1991), empyema with yeast cells should suggest an esophageal fistula. Typically, microbiology reveals combined infection together with saprophytic oropharyngeal bacteria or gram-negative bacilli. Jones and Ginsberg (1992) noted that diagnosis of an esophagopleural fistula is usually simple in case of spontaneous or iatrogenic disruption.

Sehti and Takaro (1978) reported that an esophagopleural fistula complicates approximately 0.5% of pneumonectomies. This complication is relatively unknown, although Takaro and colleagues reported its occurrence in their collective review in 1960. Intraoperative injury causing a direct tear, or devascularization with subsequent necrosis, leads to an early fistula that becomes apparent during the postoperative recovery period. The empyema is managed by insertion of a chest tube, and the diagnosis is often established by simple observation of draining saliva or food particles. Recurrent cancer or inflammatory changes are the cause of late esophagopleural fistulae and are revealed by the occurrence of an empyema. We and our associates (1994) observed the presence of tiny and sinuous tracts that are sometimes tedious to close and require careful barium swallow studies in various positions, especially lateral decubitus with the pneumonectomy space in the dependent position. Curative treatment may be offered to any patient without recurrent cancer and requires two steps: 1) closure of the esophageal defect by direct repair reinforced with a myoplasty or omentoplasty, and 2) eradication of the empyema by definitive obliteration of the pneumonectomy space; this is achieved with either thoracoplasty or muscle flap transfers as we (1994) and Engelman (1970) and colleagues have suggested.

REFERENCES

Ali I, Unruh H: Management of empyema thoracic. Ann Thorac Surg 50:355, 1990.

Bates JH: Diagnosis of tuberculosis. Chest 76:757, 1979.

Berenguer J, et al: Tuberculous meningitis in patients infected with the human immunodeficiency virus. N Engl J Med 326:668, 1992.

Berger HW, Mejia E: Tuberculous pleurisy. Chest 63:88, 1973.

Caminero JA, et al: Diagnosis of pleural tuberculosis by detection of specific IgG anti-antigen 60 in serum and pleural fluid. Respiration 60:58, 1993.

Chatzimichalis A, et al: Surgery for aspergilloma: a reappraisal. Ann Thorac Surg 65:927, 1998.

Chen JC, et al: Surgical management for pulmonary aspergilloma: a 28 year experience. Thorax 52:810, 1997.

Clagett OT, Geraci J: A procedure for the management of post-pneumonectomy empyema. J Thorac Cardiovasc Surg 45:141, 1963.

Conlan AA, et al: Elective pneumonectomy for benign lung disease: modern-day mortality and morbidity. J Thorac Cardiovasc Surg 110:1118, 1995.

Daly RC, et al: Pulmonary aspergilloma. Results of surgical treatment. J Thorac Cardiovasc Surg 92:981, 1986.

Drutz DJ, Catanzaro A: Coccidioidomycosis. Part I. Am Rev Respir Dis 117:559, 1978a.

Drutz DJ, Catanzaro A: Coccidioidomycosis. Part II. Am Rev Respir Dis 117:727, 1978b.

Dumarest J, et al: La Pratique du Pneumothorax Thérapeutique. Paris: Masson, 1945.

Emery RW, et al: Treatment of end-stage chronic obstructive pulmonary disease with double lung transplantation. Chest 99:533, 1991.

Engelman RM, Spencer FC, Berg P: Postpneumonectomy esophageal fistula. Successful one-stage repair. J Thorac Cardiovasc Surg 59:871, 1970.

Falk A: Tuberculosis pleurisy with effusion. Diagnosis and results of chemotherapy. Postgrad Med 38:631, 1965.

Fox RT, et al: Extraperiosteal plomb thoracoplasty. J Thorac Cardiovasc Surg 44:371, 1962.

Garcia-Yuste M, et al: Open-window thoracostomy and thoracomyoplasty to manage chronic pleural empyema. Ann Thorac Surg 65:818, 1998.

Grégoire J, et al: Thoracoplasty: its forgotten use in the management of non-tuberculous post-pneumonectomy empyema. Can J Surg 30:343, 1987.

Halezeroglu S, et al: Factors affecting postoperative morbidity and mortality in destroyed lung. Ann Thorac Surg 64:1635, 1997.

Herring M, Pecora D: Pleural aspergillosis: a case report. Am Surg 42:300, 1976.

Hopkins RA, et al: The modern use of thoracoplasty. Ann Thorac Surg 40:181, 1985.

Horrigan TP, Snow NJ: Thoracoplasty: current application to the infected pleural space. Ann Thorac Surg 50:695, 1990.

Hughes CF, Waugh R, Lindsay D: Surgery for pulmonary aspergilloma: preoperative embolization of the bronchial circulation. Thorax 41:324, 1986.

Icard P, et al: Utility of C-reactive protein measurements for empyema diagnosis after pneumonectomy. Ann Thorac Surg 57:933, 1994.

Jereb JA, et al: Tuberculosis morbidity in the United States: final data, 1990, in CDC surveillance summaries. MMWR Morb Mortal Wkly Rpt 40:23, 1991.

Jones WG, Ginsberg RJ: Esophageal perforation: a continuing challenge. Ann Thorac Surg 53:534, 1992.

Jurkiewicz MJ, Arnold PG: The omentum: an account on its use in the reconstruction of the chest wall. Ann Surg 185:548, 1977.

Kearon MC, et al: Pleural aspergillosis in a 14 year old boy. Thorax 42:477, 1987.

Krakowka P, Rowinska E, Halweg H: Infection of the pleura by Aspergillus fumigatus. Thorax 25:245, 1970.

Langston HT, Barker WL, Graham AA: Pleural tuberculosis. J Thorac Cardiovasc Surg 54:511, 1967.

Lees WM, et al: Results in 278 patients who had the modern type of thoracoplasty for tuberculosis. J Thorac Surg 22:329, 1951.

Levine H, et al: Diagnosis of tuberculous pleurisy by culture of pleural biopsy specimen. Arch Intern Med 126:269, 1970.

Libshitz HI, Atkinson GW, Israel HL: Pleural thickening as a manifestation of Aspergillus superinfection. AJR Am J Roentgenol 120:883, 1974.

Loynes RD: Scoliosis after thoracoplasty. J Bone Joint Surg 54:484, 1972.

Massard G, et al: Pleuropulmonary aspergilloma: clinical spectrum and results of surgical treatment. Ann Thorac Surg 54:1149, 1992a.

Massard G, et al: Eventration diaphragmatique compliquant l'épiplooplastie après résection pariétale thoracique. Ann Chir Plast Esthét 37:329, 1992b.

Massard G, et al: Esophagopleural fistula: an early and long term complication after pneumonectomy. Ann Thorac Surg 58:1437, 1994.

Massard G, et al: Early and long term results after completion pneumonectomy. Ann Thorac Surg 59:196, 1995a.

Massard G, et al: Decortication is a valuable option for late empyema after collapse therapy. Ann Thorac Surg 60:888, 1995.

Massard G, et al: Pneumonectomy for chronic infection is a high risk procedure. Ann Thorac Surg 62:1033, 1996.

Massard G, et al: Long-term complications of extraperiosteal plombage. Ann Thorac Surg 64:220, 1997.

McGovern EM, et al: Completion pneumonectomy: indications, complications and results. Ann Thorac Surg 46:141, 1988.

Mouroux J, et al: Surgical management of pleuropulmonary tuberculosis. J Thorac Cardiovasc Surg 111:662, 1996.

Nakanishi Y, et al: Empyema following the percutaneous instillation of antifungal agents in patients with aspergillosis. Intern Med 35:657, 1996.

Neff TA, Buchanan BD: Tension pleural effusion: a delayed complication of pneumothorax therapy in tuberculosis. Am Rev Respir Dis 111:543, 1975.

Odell JA, Henderson BJ: Pneumonectomy through empyema. J Thorac Cardiovasc Surg 89:423, 1985.

Pairolero PC, et al: Postpneumonectomy empyema. The role of intrathoracic muscle transposition. J Thorac Cardiovasc Surg 99:958, 1990.

Pomerantz M, et al: Surgical management of resistant mycobacterial tuberculosis and other mycobacterial pulmonary infections. Ann Thorac Surg 52:1108, 1991.

Purcell IF, Corris PA: Use of nebulized liposomal amphotericin B in the treatment of Aspergillus fumigatus empyema. Thorax 50:1321, 1995.

Roberts ATM: Extrapleural pneumolysis: a review of 128 cases. Thorax 3:166, 1948.

Schmid FG, De Haller R: Late exudative complications of collapse therapy for pulmonary tuberculosis. Chest 89:822, 1986.

Sehti GK, Takaro T: Esophagopleural fistula following pulmonary resection. Ann Thorac Surg 25:74, 1978.

Shepherd MP: Plombage in the 1980s. Thorax 40:328, 1985.

Shirakusa T, et al: Surgical treatment of aspergilloma and Aspergillus empyema. Ann Thorac Surg 48:779, 1989.

Shirakusa T, et al: Use of pedicled omental flap in treatment of empyema. Ann Thorac Surg 50:420, 1990.

Takaro T, Walkup HE, Okano T: Esophagopleural fistula as a complication of thoracic surgery. J Thorac Cardiovasc Surg 40:179, 1960.

Treasure RL, Seaworth BJ: Current role of surgery in mycobacterium tuberculosis. Ann Thorac Surg 59:1405, 1995.

Utley JR: Completion pneumonectomy and thoracoplasty for bronchopleural fistula and fungal empyema. Ann Thorac Surg 55:672, 1993.

Weir MR, Thornton GF: Extrapulmonary tuberculosis: experience of a community hospital and review of the literature. Am J Med 79:467, 1985.

Weissberg D, Refaely Y: Pleural empyema: 24-year experience. Ann Thorac Surg 62:1026, 1996.

Westney GE, et al: Aspergillus infection in single and double lung transplant recipients. Transplantation 61:915, 1996.

Wilson NJ, et al: Extraperiosteal plombage thoracoplasty: operative technique and results with 161 cases with unilateral surgical problems. J Thorac Surg 32:797, 1956.

Yim AP: The role of video-assisted thoracoscopic surgery in the management of pulmonary tuberculosis. Chest 110:829, 1996.

CHAPTER 61

Fibrothorax and Decortication of the Lung

Thomas W. Rice

Decortication of the lung is the process of peeling or stripping a constricting membrane from the pleural surfaces. Fowler (1893) and Delorme (1894) were the first physicians to describe how to free an entrapped lung and in 1896 Delorme first used the term *decortication*. Decortication departed from the classic approach of aspiration, open drainage, and thoracoplasty for the treatment of chronic empyema and fibrothorax. Further refinements of the initial procedure by Lloyd (1908), Lund (1911), Mayo and Beckman (1914), Lilenthal (1915), Ware (1917), and Eggers (1923) included intercostal incision, wide exploration of the pleural cavity, full mobilization of the lung, removal of the fibrous peel, but not the visceral pleura, and suction drainage of the complicated pleural space.

Despite individual surgical successes with decortication for chronic empyema, scant enthusiasm developed for this procedure. Milfeld and colleagues (1978) opined that before World War II this was primarily because of the inadequacies of anesthesia, antimicrobial agents, blood transfusion, and technical expertise. The lack of therapy for organizing hemothorax complicating penetrating thoracic trauma, however, reactivated interest in decortication during World War II, as documented by the publications of Price Thomas and Cleland (1945), Samson and Burford (1947), Burford (1945), Samson (1946), and Tuttle (1946) and their associates. This experience, coupled with the development of effective antituberculous medication, encouraged many surgeons including Ackman and Madore (1951), Mulvihill and Klopstock (1948), Gurd (1947), Himmelstein (1948), Gordon (1949), O'Rourke (1949), Weinberg (1948 and 1949), and Waterman and Domm (1951) and their coworkers to explore the use of decortication in the treatment of fibrothorax and iatrogenic pneumothorax complicating pulmonary tuberculosis. More than 50 years from its inception, decortication of the lung in the treatment of fibrothorax was finally established. This surgical evolution was the result of one world war and three disease processes.

Today, an established fibrothorax is optimally managed by thoracotomy and decortication of the lung. In patients with empyema and hemothorax, videothoracoscopy and video-assisted thoracoscopic surgery, as noted by Angelillo Mackinlay (1996), and Davidoff (1996), Hutter (1985), Landreneau (1996), and Sendt (1995) and their associates, as well as by Ridley and Baimbridge (1991) and Silen and Weber (1995), facilitate early irrigation, débridement, and drainage of the pleural space. Despite earlier diagnosis and minimally invasive abilities to drain the pleural space and prevent fibrothorax, entrapment of the lung still occurs.

PATHOPHYSIOLOGY

Samsom (1955) pointed out that if pleural fluid is left undrained, regardless of its nature (Table 61-1), an inflammatory response deposits fibrin on the visceral and parietal pleura. As inflammation proceeds, a thin layer of immature blood vessels and loose collagen forms over the pleural surfaces (Fig. 61-1; see Color Fig. 61-1). Organization produces a dense, avascular collagen matrix that walls off the insulting fluid but does not affect the underlying pleura. In this fibrous cavity, between the visceral and parietal pleura, the fluid decomposes (Fig. 61-2; see Color Fig. 61-2). The extent of inflammatory reaction is determined by the nature of the fluid and varies from the microscopically thin glistening membrane in transudative pleural effusions to the thick fibrous peel of empyema and hemothorax.

Fluid in the pleural space also results in pulmonary compression and, if sufficient quantity, atelectasis. The compressed atelectatic lung is trapped by inflammatory tissue coating the visceral pleura. The underlying lung is usually unaffected unless the pleural fluid production began as a destructive parenchymal process (e.g., tuberculosis, necrotizing pneumonia, or penetrating trauma). The chest wall and diaphragm are similarly coated by the fibrous process, which is typically thicker and more exuberant over the parietal pleura than over the visceral pleura. Entrapment of the lung and encasement of the thoracic cage produces a restrictive ventilatory defect and, as described by Liu and colleagues (1991), is characterized by reduction of lung

Table 61-1. Causes of Fibrothorax

Common
    Empyema
    Hemothorax
    Pleural effusion
    Pneumothorax
    Tuberculosis
Uncommon
    Asbestosis (Sterling and Herbert 1990)
    Cholelithiasis (Willekes and Widman 1996)
    Chylothorax (Fairfax et al. 1986)
    Liver abscess (Morton et al. 1970)
    Pancreatitis (Shapiro et al. 1970)
    Paragonimiasis (Dietrick et al. 1981)
    Silicon (Rice et al. 1995)
    Ventriculopleural shunt (Yellin et al. 1992)

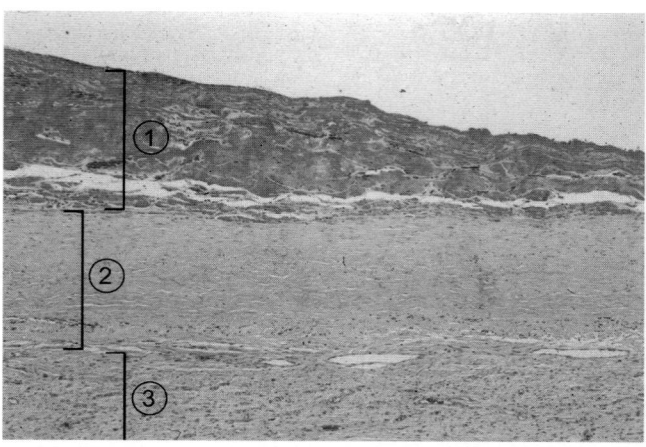

Fig. 61-2. Photomicrograph of a mature pleural peel consists of (1) debris, (2) mature collagen, and (3) a loose vascular matrix overlying the visceral pleura. (Hematoxylin and eosin, original magnification ×40.) (See Color Fig. 61-2.)

volumes (forced vital capacity; total lung capacity; vital capacity; forced expiratory volume in 1 second, decreased diffusing capacity of the lungs for carbon monoxide), Kco (carbon monoxide transfer coefficient), and an increase of the residual volume to total lung capacity ratio. The diffusing capacity of the lungs for carbon monoxide corrected for these reduced volumes is normal, indicative of extrapulmonary restriction with normal underlying lung. The bronchospirometric study of Autio (1959) showed that the alterations of pulmonary function in tuberculous pleural disease generally exceed those of tuberculous parenchymal disease.

Pulmonary vasoconstriction results in a significant reduction of perfusion of the entrapped lung. Perfusion abnormality usually exceeds the reduction of ventilation of the involved lung. This mechanism prevents hypoxia if contralateral lung function is preserved. Generally, normal oxy-

gen saturation occurs at rest, but moderate reduction occurs with exercise, as shown by the cardiac catheterization studies carried out by Muller in 1959. In severe or bilateral disease, Robin and associates (1966) noted that hypoxia, hypercarbia, pulmonary hypertension, and cor pulmonale may result.

DIAGNOSIS AND EVALUATION

Although a history of penetrating thoracic trauma, pneumonia, or tuberculosis may be elicited, according to Deslauriers and Perrault (1995) no inciting cause is found in 50% of patients. The most common complaint is progressive dyspnea on exertion. Occasionally, patients may experience chest discomfort ranging from tightness to frank pain, dry nonproductive cough, fatigue or malaise, or both. Ghoshal and colleagues (1997) have emphasized that cough with expectoration, hemoptysis, or fever should alert the examining physician of underlying pulmonary parenchymal disease. Physical examination demonstrates unilateral fixation of the chest wall with reduced excursion of the ipsilateral hemidiaphragm. The chest is dull to percussion with impaired transmission of breath sounds on auscultation.

Findings on chest radiography are uniform. Maffessanti and associates (1996) describe these features as dependent radiodensities that involve the diaphragmatic surface and lower lateral chest wall with obliteration of the costophrenic sulcus. This may progress superiorly and, in extreme cases, can obliterate the pleural space (Fig. 61-3). Chest wall findings include narrowed intercostal spaces and diminished size of the hemithorax with retraction of the mediastinum toward the fibrothorax. Pleural calcifications may occur on the inner aspect of the peel, providing an accurate measurement of the thickness of the rind (Figs.

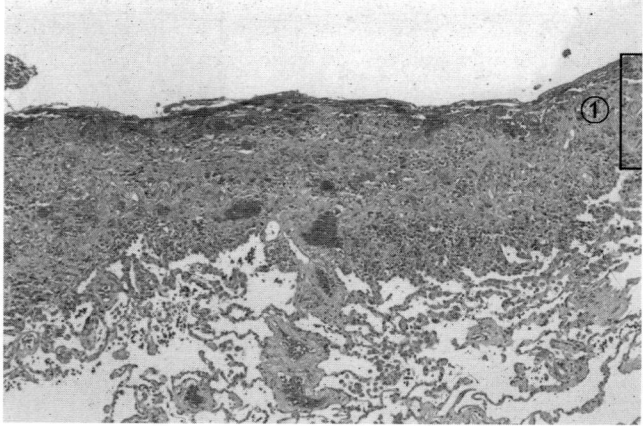

Fig. 61-1. Photomicrograph shows that a distinct boundary between early pleuritis (1) and the visceral pleura does not yet exist. Decortication before maturation of the pleural peel develops a plane between the visceral pleura and pulmonary parenchyma. (Hematoxylin and eosin, original magnification ×100.) (See Color Fig. 61-1.)

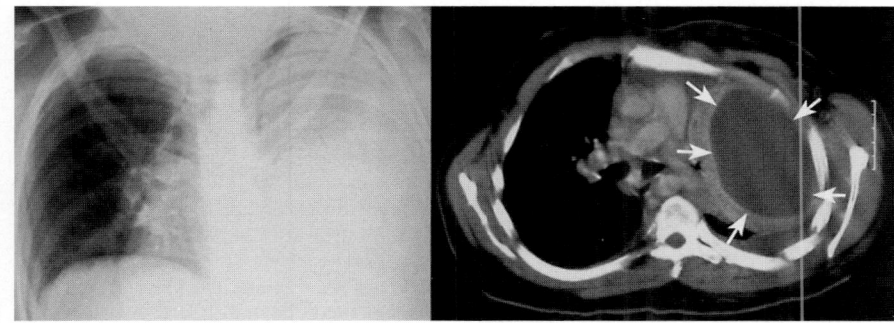

Fig. 61-3. Empyema. **A.** Nearly complete opacification of the left hemithorax in a patient with cerebral palsy who is recovering from *Staphylococcus* pneumonia. **B.** A midthoracic computed tomographic section demonstrates a homogeneous pleural fluid collection with enhancing margins [split pleura sign (*arrows*)].

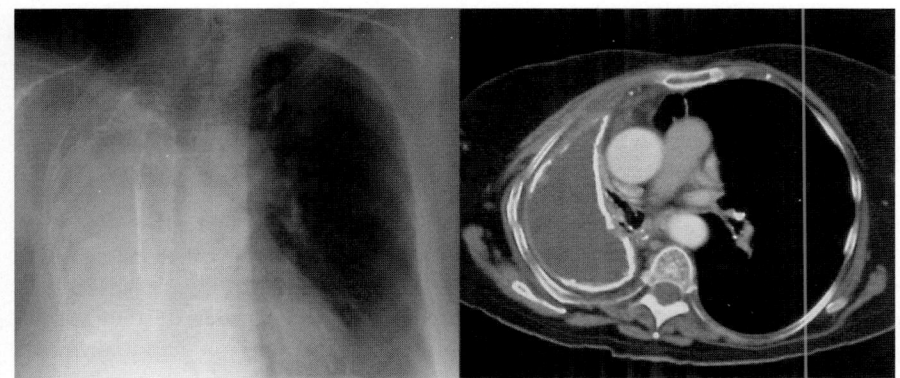

Fig. 61-4. Tuberculous empyema. **A.** A chronic tuberculous empyema filling the right hemithorax. **B.** A computed tomographic section at the pulmonary hilum demonstrates a calcified tuberculous empyema cavity. The right main bronchus is visualized, but destruction of the right lung has occurred.

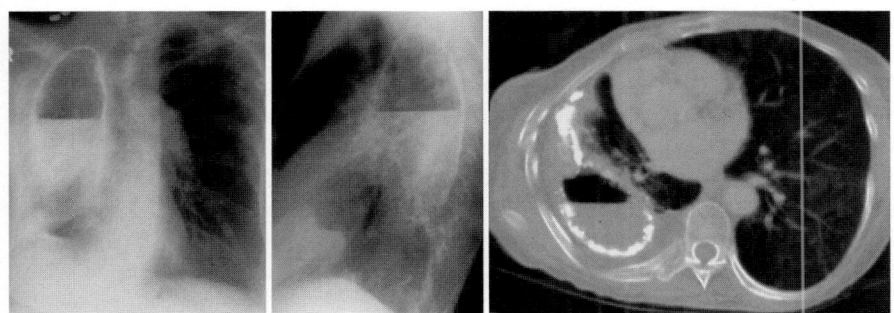

Fig. 61-5. Tuberculous empyema with bronchopleural fistula. **A, B.** Posteroanterior and lateral chest roentgenograms of a tuberculous empyema with calcified margins and an air-fluid level. Aerated pulmonary parenchyma is visualized inferior to the empyema cavity. **C.** A midthoracic computed tomographic section demonstrates the calcified empyema cavity with an air-fluid level. Although significant volume loss has occurred, a compressed aerated right lung without parenchymal destruction is seen.

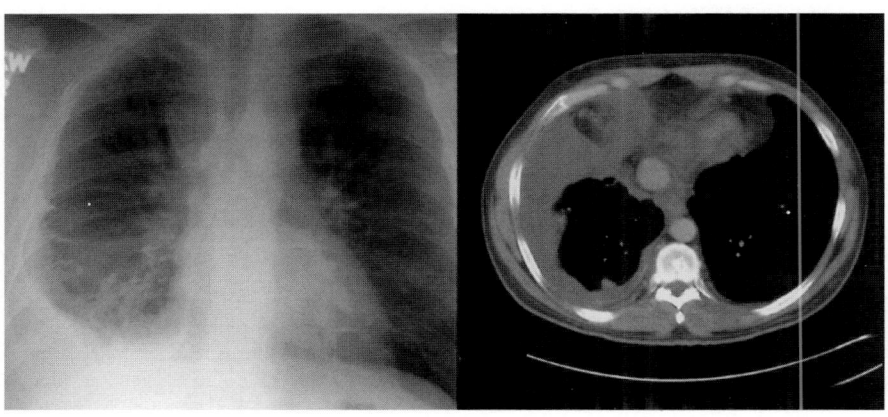

Fig. 61-6. Neglected pleural effusion. **A.** An idiopathic chronic right pleural effusion. **B.** A computed tomographic section of the lower chest demonstrates a homogeneous low-density fluid collection. At thoracoscopy, a constricting pleural peel was found that required decortication.

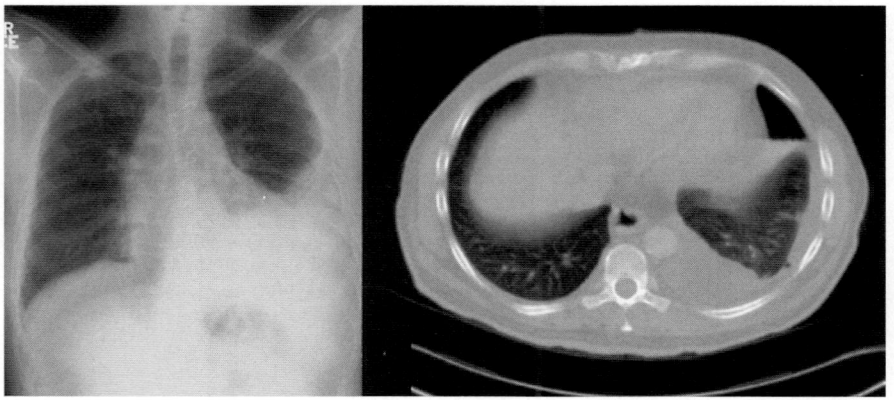

A,B

Fig. 61-7. Neglected pleural effusion. **A.** A chronic left pleural effusion complicating coronary artery bypass surgery. **B.** A lower thoracic computed tomographic section demonstrates a hydropneumothorax after thoracentesis. A constricting pleural peel is suggested because of the inability of thoracentesis to evacuate the pleural collection and expand the lung. The evacuation of fluid by thoracentesis from this rigid cavity required replacement with an equal volume of air.

61-4 and 61-5). The extent of the fibrothorax is best appreciated by computed tomographic (CT) scan, which images the pleural peel as a smooth, symmetric, tissue density extrapulmonary mass (Fig. 61-6 and 61-7). Fibrothorax complicating hemothorax has a heterogeneous character on computed tomographic scan (Fig. 61-8). A nodular appearance is suspicious for mesothelioma or pleural metastases; Im and colleagues (1991) note that a fat component is seen in tuberculous fibrothorax or with chronic corticosteroid administration. More important, CT scans enable surgeons to assess the underlying pulmonary parenchyma for tuberculosis, bronchiectasis, and mass lesions. Rounded atelectasis may masquerade as a carcinoma, but as Cohen and associates (1993) demonstrated, it is caused by pleural entrapment of the lung and is a parenchymal finding of fibrothorax.

Preoperative physiologic evaluation includes conventional pulmonary function testing with spirometry, diffusion studies (diffusing capacity of the lungs for carbon monoxide), arterial blood gas analysis, and exercise testing. These evaluations are useful to quantify the degree of respiratory impairment and also may be used for comparisons in postoperative follow-up. A quantitative perfusion scan confirms the unilateral reduction of pulmonary perfusion.

TREATMENT

Indications and Contraindications for Decortication

Decortication of the lung is indicated for patients with symptomatic extraparenchymal restrictive disease secondary to fibrothorax. Surgery is considered if thoracentesis, tube drainage, or thoracoscopy have failed to drain the pleural space and expand the lung and if malignant pleural disease has been excluded. Precise timing of the operation depends on the underlying disease process. In patients with hemothorax, decortication is performed more than 6 weeks after the injury. This allows maturation of the pleural peel and establishes a plane of dissection. Samson and coworkers (1946) recommended that if after conventional therapy the lung is not completely expanded, especially if more than 50% compression exists, the apex is collapsed, or both, then decortication is indicated. When pleural drainage fails to resolve an empyema, decortication re-expands the lung, controls the pleural space, and eliminates infection. Decortication is indicated in patients with tuberculosis if pleural disease persists after chronic antituberculous therapy. If thoracentesis fails to yield fluid or if no changes are seen on chest radiography, decortication

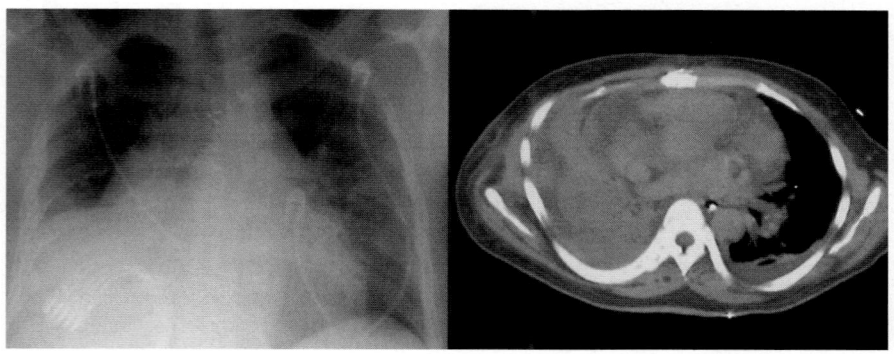

A,B

Fig. 61-8. Traumatic hemothorax. **A.** A right hemothorax complicates a gunshot wound to the upper abdomen that caused liver injury. Tube thoracostomy ineffectively treated this traumatic hemothorax. **B.** Computed tomography demonstrates a heterogeneous pleural collection typical of hemothorax.

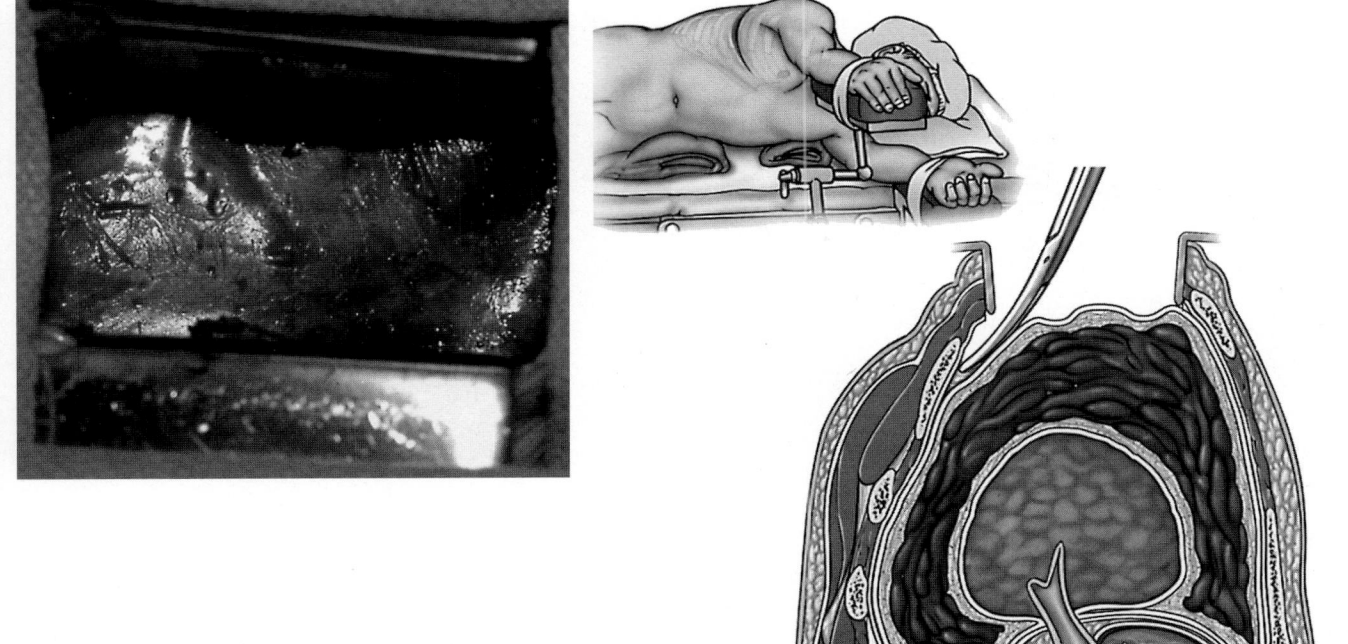

Fig. 61-9. The parietal pleura is bluntly dissected from the chest wall in the area of the incision, before the rib retractor is inserted.

should be considered. There should be considerable opacification on the lateral projection and opacification of at least one-quarter to one-third of the posteroanterior radiograph. Decortication is indicated also for complications after collapse therapy or plombage.

Surgery is contraindicated in patients with major bronchial obstruction, pulmonary destruction, uncontrolled sepsis, contralateral disease, chronic debilitation, or prohibitive concomitant organ system dysfunction. Fibrothorax must be differentiated from mesothelioma and malignancies metastatic to the pleural space. Thoracentesis, percutaneous biopsy, or thoracoscopy should precede thoracotomy if the diagnosis of fibrothorax is in question.

Technique of Decortication

Bronchoscopy is performed initially to exclude endobronchial processes that prohibit expansion of the entrapped lung. A double-lumen endotracheal tube (versus a single-lumen tube with or without a bronchial blocker) allows variations in ventilation that may facilitate decortication (i.e., positive pressure ventilation, pressurization of the lung without ventilation, clamped endotracheal lumen at the end of positive pressure expansion of the lung, or no ventilation). The preferred operative approach is in the lateral decubitus position with posterior lateral thoracotomy. The early

reports of Rudström and Thoren (1955) and Samson (1955) advocated resection of one or two ribs for improved exposure. This may be necessary when the intercostal spaces are so severely contracted that the ribs touch or overlap. However, rib resection is generally not required if the parietal pleura is bluntly dissected from the chest wall in the area of the incision, before the rib retractor is inserted, as described by Waterman and Domm (1951) (Fig. 61-9). Entry into the thorax at the sixth or seventh interspace according to Williams (1950) provides better exposure of the lower lobe and the hemidiaphragmatic leaf where the fibrothorax may be more dense. Savage and Fleming (1955) suggest that a second, superior intercostal incision in the fourth or fifth interspace may improve exposure of the upper thorax with this low intercostal approach.

According to Wright and associates (1949), the need for parietal pleurectomy and freeing of the chest wall, diaphragm, and mediastinum spurred great debate. Parietal pleurectomy was discouraged by Samson and Burford (1947) and Tuttle and colleagues (1947) because of increased operative time and the potential for excessive blood loss. However, many physicians, including Ackman and Madore (1951) and Waterman and Domm (1957), as well as some of the aforementioned European surgeons, recognized that freeing these structures allowed the movement necessary for ventilation. Today, most surgeons would add at least a partial or, if possible, complete decortication of the

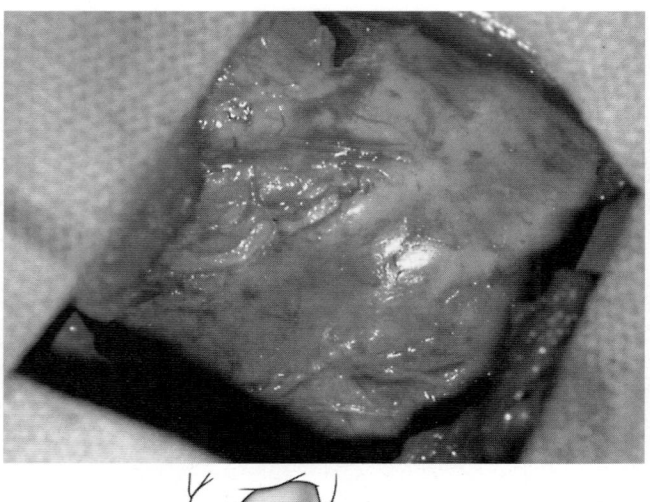

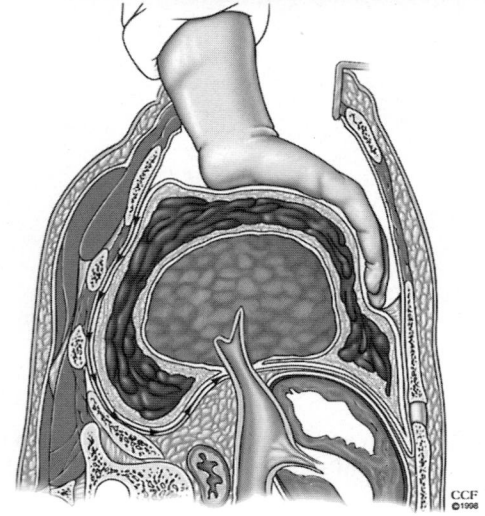

Fig. 61-10. Blunt dissection of the parietal peel occurs in the plane between the endothoracic fascia and the parietal pleura.

parietal pleura. The surgeon proceeds with blunt dissection of the parietal peel (Fig. 61-10). The plane of dissection is between the endothoracic fascia and the parietal pleura. The dissection may be carried beyond the chest wall to include the diaphragm and mediastinal pleura. Decortication of the hemidiaphragm and mediastinum may be facilitated by delaying this portion of the parietal dissection until the lung has been decorticated. These two surfaces may then be freed retrograde from the pulmonary hilum and antegrade from the chest wall. Caution must be taken to prevent injury to the diaphragmatic leaf or phrenic nerve as noted by Waterman and Domm (1951) and Mayo and associates (1982). In areas of dense fibrosis with obliteration of the plane of dissection, patches of fibrous tissue may be left on these structures. No advantage is gained if aggressive freeing of the diaphragm or mediastinum near the phrenic nerve results in diaphragmatic dysfunction.

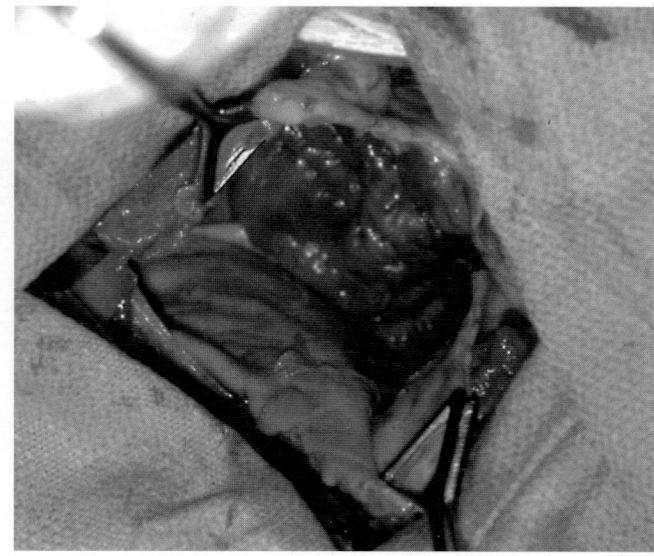

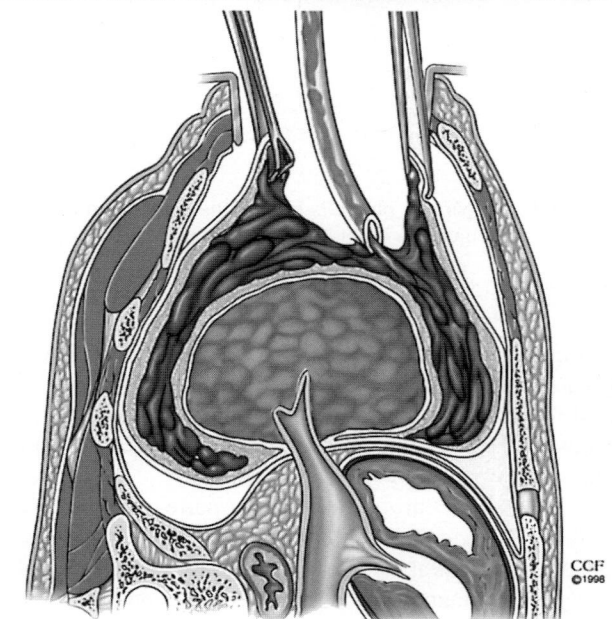

Fig. 61-11. The thickened parietal peel is incised and the pleural cavity evacuated of fluid and debris.

The thickened parietal peel is incised and the pleural cavity entered (Fig. 61-11). An empyectomy with preservation of the integrity of the cavity was recommended by Samson (1955) for tuberculous empyema. In nontuberculous empyema, entrance into the cavity causes temporary contamination of the operative field and is generally unavoidable. Perioperative antibiotics and complete expansion of the lung with obliteration of any potential pleural space minimizes postoperative empyema. The pleural cavity is entered and evacuated of fluid and debris. This material is cultured. Pulmonary decortication

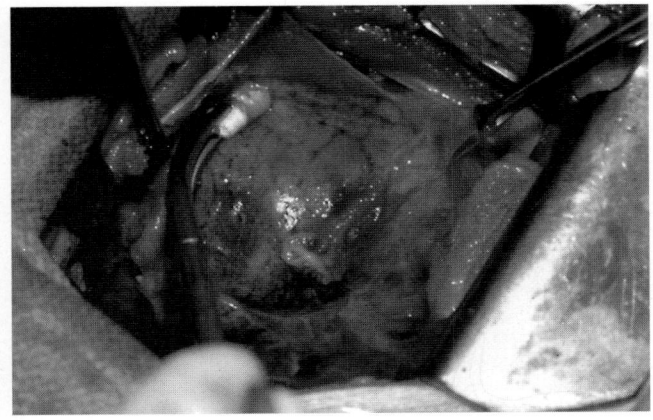

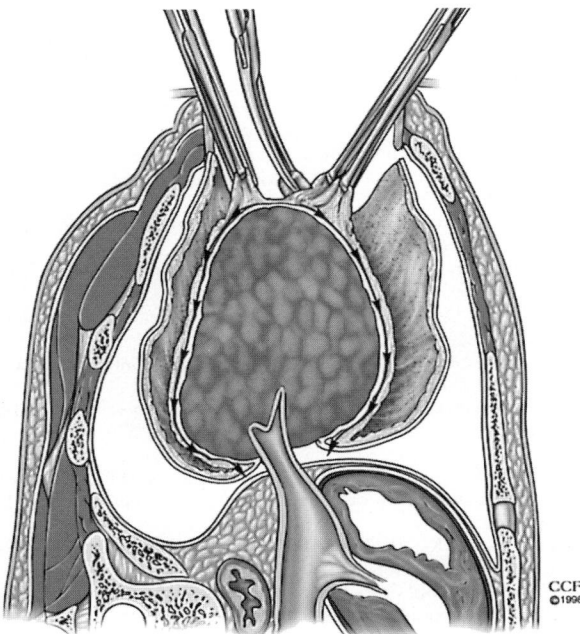

Fig. 61-12. Unlike parietal decortication, the plane of visceral decortication lies between the visceral pleura and the fibrous peel. The plane of dissection is initiated with a blunt spatula-type instrument. The peel is firmly grasped and gentle traction applied. Blunt dissection is done with Kittner's dissectors or a gauze-covered finger.

begins with incision of the fibrous peel overlying the visceral pleura. Many layers in the fibrous peel may be divided before the glistening gray visceral pleura is encountered (Fig. 6-12). Gentle reexpansion of the lung may facilitate this process, but pulmonary collapse may expedite the freeing of the entrapped lung without visceral pleural damage. Decortication may not be possible in areas of underlying parenchymal disease or when pulmonary injury resulted from penetrating trauma. In these cases, the pleural peel may be left on the pulmonary surface or the underlying lung may be resected if it is

destroyed by the underlying disease process. If the correct plane is not identified, decortication includes the visceral pleura and pulmonary parenchyma. Excessive bleeding and large air leaks from deep parenchymal injury must be controlled. Fortunately, the injury is usually limited to the subpleural parenchyma and is controlled with reexpansion of the lung.

The pleural space is drained with two or three chest tubes. They are positioned low in the thoracic cavity and pass posteriorly into the costovertebral sulcus to the apex of the thorax, anteriorly into the hilum to the apex of the thorax, and inferiorly along the diaphragm into the posterior costophrenic sulcus. On completion of the operation, the patient should be reintubated with a large, single-lumen endotracheal tube and bronchoscopy performed to free the airway of secretions. A short period of positive pressure ventilation may facilitate pulmonary expansion. Chest tube suction should be sufficient to evacuate the pleural space of blood and air. Excessive suction fostering air leaks is not a major concern in the early postoperative period.

Mortality and Morbidity

Mayo (1985) reported that operative mortality ranges from 0 to 8% and depends on the severity of illness and general state of health. Morbidity is the result of underlying disease processes or operative complications. Sepsis, wound infection, empyema, hemorrhage, prolonged air leak, and bronchopleural fistula are the most common complications. These postoperative problems are minimized by meticulous surgical techniques that control air leaks and bleeding and ensure complete re-expansion of the lung with obliteration of the pleural space.

RESULTS

Patton (1952), Siebens (1956), and Barker (1965) and their associates have found that absence of underlying parenchymal disease is the best predictor of improved pulmonary function after decortication. Operative complications such as phrenic nerve injury or empyema may diminish the benefits of decortication as noted by Siebens and colleagues (1956). The postoperative physiologic studies of Morton and coworkers (1970) have shown that improvement after decortication may be less in patients with tuberculosis than in patients with pyogenic infection or trauma. Both Carroll (1951) and Patton (1952) and their colleagues reported that a shorter duration of pleural disease is associated with better results. However, restoration of pulmonary function has been reported more than 50 years after onset of pleural tuberculosis by Hughes (1975). Petty (1961) and Massard (1995) and their coworkers also reported favorable results after durations of 20 to over 30 years of the disease process. Ultimate gain in pulmonary function may be limited by the presence of pleural infection as observed by Patton and associates (1952). On the other hand, continued postoperative improvement in pulmonary function has been reported for up to 3 years by these latter authors. A report by Ilic (1996) of early decortication for traumatic hemothorax showed stable postoperative pulmonary function immediately after chest tube removal and at 6 months postoperatively. Normalization of pulmonary function seen on chest radiography, as pointed out by Barker and associates (1965), correlates with functional improvement.

Failure to obtain improvement in pulmonary function after decortication may be the result of inappropriate patient selection, operative difficulties, or postoperative complications. Expansion of a severely damaged lung or the inability to expand a fibrotic lung prohibits improved pulmonary function that is expected with decortication. Persistent restriction may result from the inability to free the chest wall or diaphragm. Damage of the phrenic nerve or diaphragm impairs ventilation and may worsen pulmonary function. Decortication in the parenchymal plane deep to the visceral pleura causes increased bleeding and air leak and may result in postoperative bronchopleural fistula and recurrence of hemothorax and empyema.

REFERENCES

Ackman FD, Madore P: Decortication preceding thoracoplasty for the elimination of long-standing tuberculous empyema. J Thorac Surg 22:358, 1951.

Angelillo Mackinlay TA, et al: VATS debridement versus thoracotomy in the treatment of loculated postpneumonia empyema. Ann Thorac Surg 61:1626, 1996.

Autio V: The reduction of respiratory function by parenchymal and pleural lesions. A bronchospirometric study of patients with unilateral involvement. Acta Tuberc Scand 37:112, 1959.

Barker WL, Neuhaus H, Langston HT: Ventilatory improvement following decortication in pulmonary tuberculosis. Ann Thorac Surg 1:532, 1965.

Burford TH, Parker EF, Samson PC: Early pulmonary decortication in the treatment of posttraumatic empyema. Ann Surg 122:163, 1945.

Carroll D, et al: Pulmonary function following decortication of the lung. Am Rev Tuberc 63:231, 1951.

Cohen AM, et al: Rounded atelectasis and fibrotic pleural disease: the pathologic continuum. J Thorac Imaging 8:309, 1993.

Davidoff AM, et al: Thoracoscopic management of empyema in children. J Laparoendosc Surg 6:S-51, 1996.

Delorme E: Nouveau traitment des empyèmes chroniques. Gaz Hop 67:94, 1894.

Delorme E: Du traitment des empyèmes chronique par la decortication du poumon. Dixième Congrès Francis de Chirugie 379, 1896.

Deslauriers J, Perrault LP: Fibrothorax and decortication. In Pearson FG, et al (eds): Thoracic Surgery. New York: Churchill Livingstone, 1995, p. 1107.

Dietrick RB, Sade RM, Pak JS: Results of decortication in chronic empyema with special reference to paragonimiasis. J Thorac Cardiovasc Surg 82:58, 1981.

Eggers C: Radical operation for chronic empyema. Ann Surg 77:327, 1923.

Fairfax AJ, McNabb WR, Spiro SG: Chylothorax: a review of 18 cases. Thorax 41:880, 1986.

Fowler GR: A case of thoracoplasty for removal of a large fibrous growth from the interior of the chest, the result of an old empyema. Med Record 44:838, 1893.

Ghoshal AG, et al: Fibrothorax—problem, profile and prevention. J Indian Med Assoc 95:610, 1997.

Gordon J, Brook R, Welles ES: Decortication in pulmonary tuberculosis including studies of respiratory physiology. J Thorac Surg 18:337, 1949.

Gurd FB: Decortication in chronic empyema of tuberculous origin. J Thorac Surg 16:587, 1947.

Himmelstein A, Miscall L, Kirschner PA: Decortication in tuberculosis. Surg Clin North Am 28:1601, 1948.

Hughes RL, et al: Evaluation of unilateral decortication. A patient successfully treated 44 years after onset of tuberculosis. Ann Thorac Surg 19:704, 1975.

Hutter JA, Harari D, Braimbridge MV: The management of empyema thoracic by thoracoscopy and irrigation. Ann Thorac Surg 39:517, 1985.

Ilic N: Functional effects of decortication after penetrating war injuries to the chest. J Thorac Cardiovasc Surg 111:967, 1996.

Im JG, et al: Apical opacity associated with pleural tuberculosis: high-resolution CT findings. Radiology 178:727, 1991.

Landreneau RJ, et al: Thoracoscopy for empyema and hemothorax. Chest 109:18, 1996.

Lilenthal H: Empyema. Exploration of the thorax with primary mobilization of the lung. Ann Surg 62:309, 1915.

Liu CT, et al: Pulmonary function in patients with pleural effusions of varying magnitude and fibrothorax. Panminerva Med 33:86, 1991.

Lloyd S: The surgical treatment of "unresolved pneumonia." NY Post-Grad M Sch Hosp 177, 1908.

Lund FB: The advantage of the so-called decortication of the lung in empyema. JAMA 57:693, 1911.

Maffessanti M, Bortolotto P, Grotto M: Imaging of pleural disease. Monaldi Arch Chest Dis 51:138, 1996.

Massard G, et al: Decortication is a valuable option for late empyema after collapse therapy. Ann Thorac Surg 60:888, 1995.

Mayo CH, Beckman EH: Visceral pleurectomy for chronic empyema. Am Surg 59:884, 1914.

Mayo P: Early thoracotomy and decortication for nontuberculous empyema in adults with and without underlying disease. A twenty-five year review. Am Surg 51:230, 1985.

Mayo P, Saha SP, McEelvein RB: Diaphragmatic avulsion following decortication. A case review of acute nontuberculous empyema. Ala J Med Sci 19:81, 1982.

Milfeld DJ, Mattox KL, Beall AC Jr: Early evacuation of clotted hemothorax. Am J Surg 136:686, 1978.

Morton JR, Boushy SF, Guinn GA: Physiological evaluation of results of pulmonary decortication Ann Thorac Surg 9:321, 1970.

Muller C. Cardiopulmonary hemodynamics in chronic lung disease with special reference to pulmonary tuberculosis, cardiac catheterization studies at rest and on exercise. Scand J Clin Lab Invest 11(Suppl 44):1, 1959.

Mulvihill DA, Klopstock R: Decortication of the nonexpandable postpneumothorax tuberculous lung. J Thorac Surg 17:723, 1948.

O'Rourke P, O'Brien EJ, Tuttle WL: Decortication of the lung in patients with pulmonary tuberculosis. Am Rev Rep Dis 59:30, 1949.

Patton WE, Watson TR, Gaensler EA: Pulmonary function before and at intervals after surgical decortication of the lung. Surg Gynecol Obstet 95:477, 1952.

Petty TL, Filley GF, Mitchell RS: Objective functional improvement by decortication after twenty years of artificial pneumothorax for pulmonary tuberculosis. Am Rev Respir Dis 84:572, 1961.

Price Thomas C, Cleland WP: Decortication in clotted and infected haemothoraces. Lancet 1:327, 1945.

Rice DC, et al: Silicone thorax: a complication of tube thoracostomy in the presence of mammary implants. Ann Thorac Surg 60:1417, 1995.

Ridley PD, Baimbridge MV: Thoracoscopic debridement and pleural irrigation in the management of empyema thoracis. Ann Thorac Surg 51:461, 1991.

Robin ED, et al: Pulmonary hypertension and unilateral pleural constriction with speculation on pulmonary vasoconstrictive substance. Arch Intern Med 118:391, 1966.

Rudström P, Thoren L: Decortication of the lung. Acta Chir Scand 110:437, 1955.

Samson PC: Some surgical considerations in pulmonary decortication. Am J Surg 89:364, 1955.

Samson PC, Burford TH: Total pulmonary decortication. Its evolution and present concepts of indications and operative technique. J Thorac Surg 16:127, 1947.

Samson PC, et al: The management of war wounds of the chest in a base center. The role of early pulmonary decortication. J Thorac Surg 15:1, 1946.

Savage T, Fleming HA: Decortication of the lung in tuberculous disease. A study of 43 cases. Thorax 10:293, 1955.

Sendt W, Förster E, Hau T: Early thoracoscopic debridement and drainage as definite treatment for pleural empyema. Eur J Surg 161:73, 1995.

Shapiro DH, Anagnostopoulos CE, Dineen JP. Decortication and pleurectomy for the pleuropulmonary complications of pancreatitis. Ann Thorac Surg 9:76, 1970.

Siebens AA, et al: The physiologic effects of fibrothorax and the functional results of surgical treatment. J Thorac Surg 32:53, 1956.

Silen ML, Weber TR: Thoracoscopic debridement of loculated empyema thoracis in children. Ann Thorac Surg 59:1166, 1995.

Sterling GM, Herbert A: Lung en cuirasse: restrictive pleurisy associated with asbestos exposure. Thorax 35:715, 1990.

Tuttle WM, Langston HT, Crowley RT: The treatment of organizing hemothorax by pulmonary decortication. J Thorac Surg 16:117, 1947.

Ware MW: The trend of surgery in empyema of the thorax. Ann Surg 65:320, 1917.

Waterman DH, Domm SE: Decortication of the unexpandable pneumothorax lung. Dis Chest 19:1, 1951.

Weinberg J, Davis JD: Pleural decortication in pulmonary tuberculosis. Am Rev Tuberc 60:288, 1949.

Weinberg J, Horner JC, Davis JD: Decortication of the unexpanded tuberculous lung following induced pneumothorax. Surg Clin North Am 28:1591, 1948.

Willekes CL, Widman WD: Empyema from lost gallstones: a thoracic complication of laparoscopic cholecystectomy. J Laparoendosc Surg 6:123, 1996.

Williams MK: The technique of pulmonary decortication and pleurolysis. J Thorac Surg 20:652, 1950.

Wright GW, et al: Physiologic observations concerning decortication of the lung. J Thorac Surg 18:372, 1949.

Yellin A, et al: Fibrothorax associated with a ventriculopleural shunt in a hydrocephalic child. J Pediatr Surg 27:1525, 1992.

CHAPTER 62

Thoracoplasty

Thomas W. Shields

The operative removal of the skeletal support of a portion of the chest is called a *thoracoplasty*. This procedure is accomplished by the subperiosteal removal of a varying number of rib segments. The removal of the rib segments permits the unsupported portion of the chest wall to sink in toward the mediastinum and thus reduces the size of the hemithorax. Although a great variety of thoracoplasty procedures have been described, the extraperiosteal paravertebral thoracoplasty described by Alexander (1937) is the standard operation.

At present, a thoracoplasty is used primarily in the treatment of chronic thoracic empyema in cases in which either insufficient or no remaining pulmonary tissue exists to obliterate the pleural space. The more recent experiences with the approach have been chronicled by Grégoire (1987), Young and Ungerleider (1990), Stamatis (1992), Peppas (1993), Puchetti (1994) and their associates, as well as by McMillan (1987) and Barker (1994). Nonetheless, a conventional thoracoplasty is carried out less often than it once was, and many surgeons use thoracoplasty only as a procedure of last resort.

It is rarely used in patients with pulmonary tuberculosis, except for pleural and occasionally extensive combined pleuropulmonary disease. Massard and colleagues (1992) believe this to be the recommended approach to the management of late-recurring *Aspergillus fumigatus* infection of a persistent pleural space after a pulmonary resection. A limited preresection *tailoring* thoracoplasty and the plombage type of thoracoplasty may be used on rare occasions in a patient with extensive parenchymal disease and markedly reduced pulmonary function, but again is seldom used.

In the tailoring thoracoplasty, a limited number of ribs of the upper portion of the chest are removed a week or so before thoracotomy, when it is expected that the proposed resection would result in an insufficient amount of remaining lung tissue to fill the normal sized thoracic cage. In a plombage thoracotomy, an inert, foreign substance is placed in a space created beneath the rib cage by extraperiosteal stripping of the ribs of the upper portion of the chest. How-

ever, using a foreign substance to obtain collapse in the presence of underlying pleural infection is contraindicated.

When the desired collapse cannot be obtained by a conventional thoracoplasty or the space cannot be obliterated by a muscle flap transposition, and a persistent infected space remains, a Schede thoracoplasty or one of its many modifications may be necessary.

OPERATIVE TECHNIQUE

Conventional Thoracoplasty

The standard procedure is that outlined by Alexander (1937). Now that the operation is used to control a chronic thoracic empyema, the procedure is accomplished in one stage. When it was used to treat pulmonary tuberculosis, it was done in two or more stages to circumvent adverse physiologic changes of paradoxic chest wall motion occurring in the postoperative period. The magnitude of the collapse procedure depends on the size of the empyema cavity. Ordinarily, seven ribs are resected, which allows the scapula and attached extracostal musculature to drop into the space and helps to maintain the collapse. Should fewer ribs be resected, the lower portion of the scapula may have to be excised, so that it does not impinge on the remaining ribs. This would prevent it from falling into the created space to help obtain optimal collapse. Special attention postoperatively must be paid to ensure proper functioning of the ipsilateral shoulder girdle when an extensive thoracoplasty has been done.

With the patient in the lateral decubitus position, a parascapular incision is begun at the level of the spine of the scapula and extended inferiorly and laterally to the midaxillary line. The subjacent extracostal muscles (trapezius, rhomboids, and latissimus dorsi) are incised to expose the rib cage and to allow the scapula to be retracted anteriorly and superiorly (Fig. 62-1). Posteriorly, the attachments of the serratus posterior and erector spinae muscle groups are

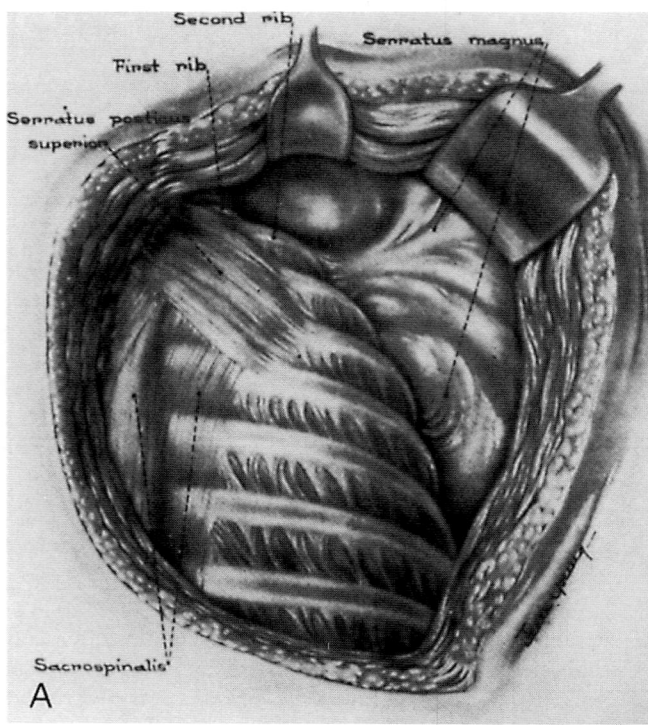

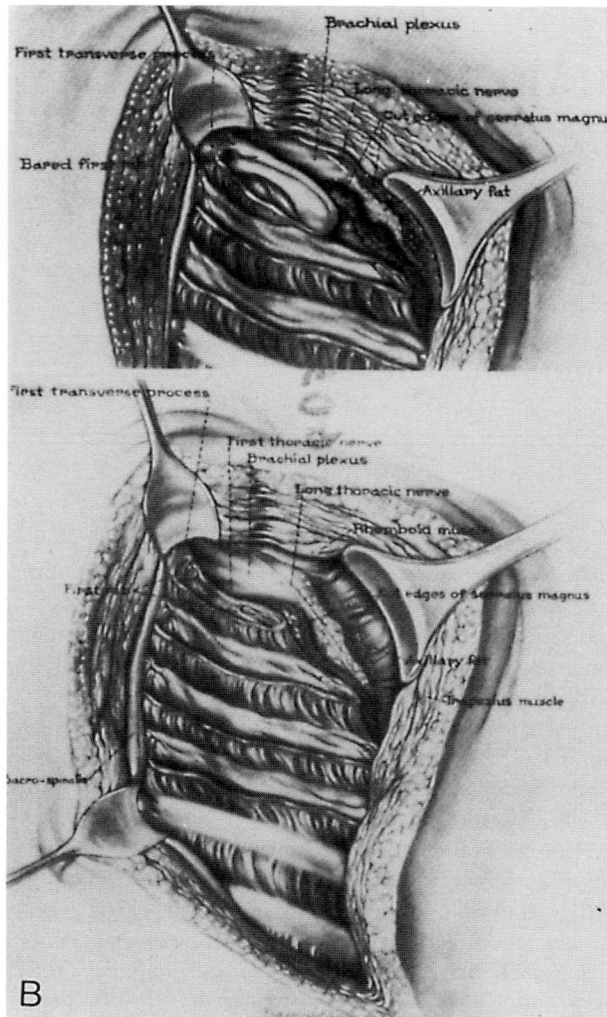

Fig. 62-1. Alexander-type thoracoplasty. **A.** Elevation of scapula to expose chest wall. **B.** Ribs resected as described in text. From Alexander J: The Collapse Therapy of Pulmonary Tuberculosis. Springfield, IL: Charles C Thomas, 1937. With permission.

separated from the ribs of the upper half of the chest. Similarly, the insertions of the serratus anterior muscle are separated from the upper three or four ribs.

After exposure of the rib cage, the posterior half of the third rib is resected after incising and stripping off its periosteal investment. In patients with an empyema, the transverse process of the vertebral body generally need not be excised, but this can be done if necessary to achieve maximal collapse. This excision is facilitated by division of the costotransverse ligaments (Fig. 62-2). The transverse process is best removed by the use of a rongeur after retraction of the sacrospinalis muscles medially. The rib is then resected further posteriorly to the level of the base of the transverse process. Some surgeons also prefer to excise the head of the rib as well, avulsing it from its articulation with the vertebral body. Next, the second rib is resected subperiosteally from the costochondral junction to the vertebral body; the second transverse process also may be removed. It is essential that no residual space remain in the costovertebral sulcus.

The first rib is removed if a limited thoracoplasty is done for obliteration of an apical empyema space that has occurred after a lobectomy. If the procedure is done for the collapse of a chronic postpneumonectomy empyema space, however, the first rib may not have to be removed and, in fact, Deslauriers (personal communication, 1987) believes it should always be left in place to preserve the structural integrity of the neck, shoulder girdle, and upper thorax. If any doubt exists of any apical residual space remaining, however, the first rib should be removed, as suggested by McMillan (1987). When this is indicated, the first rib is exposed and the periosteum incised on its lower edge. This usually is accomplished by scraping the edge with a periosteal elevator. The flat inferior surface is stripped of its periosteum. Starting far posteriorly, the outer or superior surface is stripped of its periosteum; care must be taken to protect the brachial plexus and subclavian vessels at this time. This is best accomplished by inserting a finger to retract the neurovascular structures away from the rib. Extreme caution is necessary at the scalene tubercle. The rib

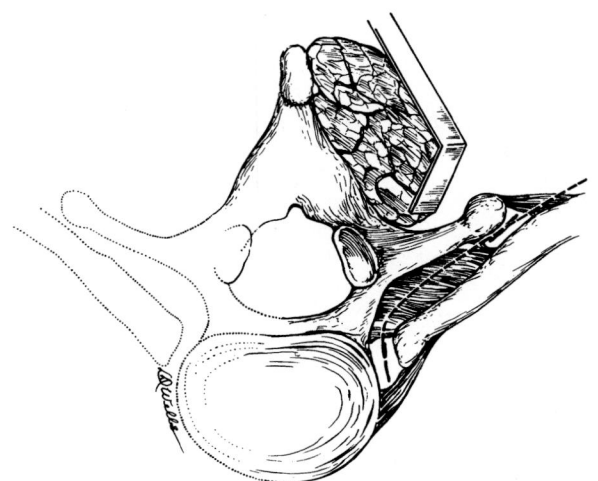

Fig. 62-2. Site of division of the costotransverse ligaments to facilitate removal of the head of the rib and the transverse process.

then is divided at the level of the tip of the transverse process and avulsed from its costochondral junction anteriorly. The head of the first rib and the first transverse process are not resected. A portion of the remaining third rib and segments of the lower ribs are then resected subperiosteally to ensure complete obliteration of the empyema space.

Bjork (1954) and others have suggested the use of an osteoplastic technique of thoracoplasty. Initially, the first rib was divided as well as the second through the fifth ribs; however, now, as described by Conlan (1990), the first rib is left intact, and only a subperiosteal resection of the posterior portions of the second through fifth ribs is carried out. The apex is then freed by extrapleural mobilization and permitted to drop, thus preserving the first rib. The residual lengths of the second to fifth ribs and underlying chest wall are sutured down to the sixth rib. This gives the chest wall stability, but this step would appear to be unnecessary when the collapse is done to obliterate an empyema cavity.

Axillary Thoracoplasty

Pomerantz (personal communication, 1998) has performed a small number of apical thoracoplasties with a transaxillary approach. The skin incision is made as in the operation for the removal of the first rib in patients with a thoracic outlet syndrome. The first rib is removed by essentially the same technique as described in these patients (see Chapter 42). Once the first rib has been removed, varying lengths of the posterior portions of the second, third, and fourth ribs are removed subperiosteally to obtain the desired degree of collapse to obliterate the residual apical space. This procedure is obviously less traumatic than the standard conventional thoracoplasty and thus should be better toler-

ated by the ill patients who require such intervention. The success of this more limited approach to a thoracoplasty is yet to be documented, but it may become a new technique in our surgical armamentarium.

Thoracomyopleuroplasty

Rather than carry out an Alexander extraperiosteal paravertebral thoracoplasty, Dupon (1990) has suggested the use of thoracomyopleuroplasty (i.e., thoracomediastinal plication) originally described by Andrews (1961) (Fig. 62-3). In this technique, only the ribs overlying the empyema space are resected. The remainder of the chest wall, including the apex, is freed as necessary by mobilizing the musculoperiosteal wall from the remaining overlying portions of the rib cage. The empyema space is then entered, and débridement of parietal and visceral surfaces of the space is carried out. The cavity is then obliterated by suturing (mattressing) the pleuromusculoperiosteal wall to the mediastinal or visceral pleura. The thoracotomy incision is then reapproximated down to the space and closed without drainage. The stated advantages are that this procedure is much smaller than the standard thoracoplasty, is less mutilating, is well tolerated by the poor-risk patient, and obtains similar results.

Grow (1946) and Kergin (1953) reported earlier similar modifications of the thoracoplasty procedure, as that suggested by Andrews (1961). All ribs are resected over the empyema space, but the intercostal bundles are left intact. By incisions through one or more of the exposed periosteal beds, a parietal decortication is accomplished. Superficial curettage of the underlying visceral pleural peel is executed. The intercostal muscle bundles, with their vascular supply intact, are allowed to fall across the visceral surface of the cavity. A bronchopleural fistula, if present, may be excised and closed by suturing a pedicled muscle graft over the opening. The incision is closed loosely over drains lying superficial to the muscle bundles. External pressure dressings are used to ensure apposition of the tissues.

Plombage Thoracoplasty

The plombage thoracoplasty modification of the conventional thoracoplasty was developed to overcome the adverse effects of decostalization of a portion of the chest wall. A foreign substance (e.g., paraffin, Lucite spheres in a polyethylene bag, or fiberglass) was inserted in a space created between the ribs and the thoracic fascia and freed periosteal and intercostal musculature to maintain optimal collapse. The technique of this procedure was described by Fox and the author (1972) in the first edition of this text. Talamonti and associates (1989) have reported the use of an inflatable tissue expander to obtain the degree of collapse desired. However, as noted previously, the use of a foreign body

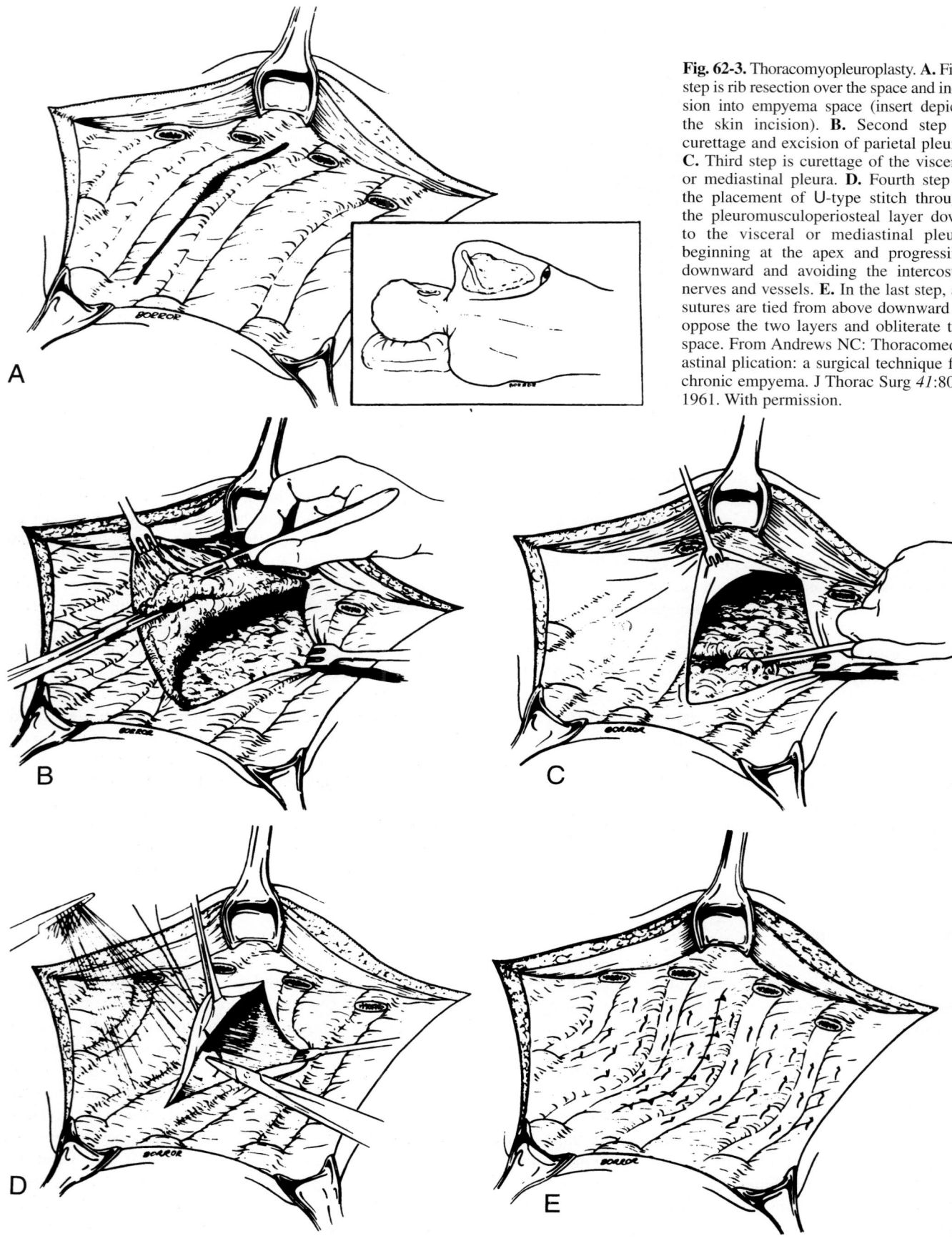

Fig. 62-3. Thoracomyopleuroplasty. **A.** First step is rib resection over the space and incision into empyema space (insert depicts the skin incision). **B.** Second step is curettage and excision of parietal pleura. **C.** Third step is curettage of the visceral or mediastinal pleura. **D.** Fourth step is the placement of U-type stitch through the pleuromusculoperiosteal layer down to the visceral or mediastinal pleura beginning at the apex and progressing downward and avoiding the intercostal nerves and vessels. **E.** In the last step, all sutures are tied from above downward to oppose the two layers and obliterate the space. From Andrews NC: Thoracomediastinal plication: a surgical technique for chronic empyema. J Thorac Surg *41*:809, 1961. With permission.

plomb is contraindicated in the management of a chronic empyema. Consequently, these procedures have been discarded, except in the rare patient with otherwise uncontrollable mycobacterial infection. Talamonti and associates (1989) reported the use of a modified plombage thoracoplasty to control a progressive *Mycobacterium avium* complex infection, and Jouveshomme and colleagues (1998) have reported its use in selected patients with extensive disease caused by multidrug-resistant mycobacteria.

Schede Thoracoplasty

The operation described by Schede (1890) for obliteration of a chronic empyema space is rarely if ever performed at present but has been widely modified by many surgeons. The Schede operation consists of radical unroofing of an empyema space by resecting the overlying ribs, intercostal bundles, and subjacent parietal pleural peel. The extracostal muscles and skin are partially closed over gauze packing. The wound is repacked at intervals. The desired effect is that freshly granulating tissue sets up an obliterative healing process and eventually closes the space.

PHYSIOLOGIC CHANGES AFTER THORACOPLASTY

The immediate physiologic sequelae of a standard extraperiosteal paravertebral thoracoplasty noted previously, when performed to manage parenchymal tuberculosis, were related to the development of an area of paradoxic motion of the chest wall. The effort of breathing increased as the result of the abnormal volume displacement and greater pleural pressure changes necessary to move air in and out of the lungs. If the mediastinum was mobile, mediastinal flutter occurred. *Pendelluft* (i.e., air flow from one lung to the other during the ventilatory cycle) may theoretically occur. Maloney and associates (1961), however, reported that, in the presence of a closed chest, the lung on the side of the paradoxic chest wall motion actually expands on the inspiration. Also, Gaensler (1965) showed, by using a pneumotachographic screen at the carina, that no air moves from one lung to the other after a thoracoplasty, as long as the proximal airway is patent.

Retained secretions, however, caused partial airway obstruction. The cough mechanism was reduced in effectiveness as a result of the inability to generate a high positive pressure in the pleural space because of the unsupported portion of the chest wall. The postoperative problems attendant to these changes were directly proportional to the number and length of the segments of rib resected. However, when a thoracoplasty is performed to obliterate a chronic empyema cavity, the rigidity of the underlying visceral and parietal peels prevents paradoxic motion. The early physiologic changes enumerated do not occur, and the procedure can be tolerated by most patients except the very poor-risk patient.

The late physiologic changes after the operation are related not only to the extent of the rib resections and underlying lung collapse but also to the late skeletal deformity that occurs. A greater or lesser degree of rotoscoliosis develops subsequent to the removal of the ribs and the transverse processes. This results in a diminution of function of the contralateral lung. Gaensler and Strieder (1951) found that when a thoracoplasty was done over a nonfunctioning lung, a permanent loss of approximately 27% of the preoperative vital capacity and 21% of maximal voluntary ventilation of the contralateral lung followed. In late survivors, Bredin (1989) observed an average reduction of 50% in both the vital capacity and maximum voluntary ventilation, a 60% decrease in the forced expiratory volume in 1 second, and a 40% reduction in the total lung capacity in 15 patients who were evaluated 30 years after a thoracoplasty. Some obstructive disease as well as a reduction of exercise performance also was noted.

The physiologic changes after a Schede thoracoplasty are related to the unstable chest wall and the degree of paradoxic motion that develops. In addition, sacrifice of the intercostal nerves results in paresis of the ipsilateral abdominal wall.

MORBIDITY

Postoperative morbidity after thoracoplasty is related not only to the type of procedure used but also to the disease process present. The complications directly related to a conventional thoracoplasty are those caused by injury of the vessels or nerves during removal of the first rib or injury to the thoracic duct with resultant chylous effusion, retention of secretions with atelectasis, and septic complications.

Wound infection is uncommon, but infection of the apical or subscapular space may occur when the operation is performed to treat a chronic empyema. However, even if the empyema space is entered during the procedure, this occurrence is unusual.

MORTALITY

Death after a thoracoplasty is most often related to the underlying chronic disease process rather than to the operation per se. Hopkins and coworkers (1985) reported a 13% mortality in their entire series but noted a decline in this figure in the second half of their experience. Young and Ungerleider (1990) reported a mortality of 10% and Dupon (1990) a rate of 5.4%. Grégoire and colleagues (1987) reported no deaths in their series of 17 patients. In a series of 37 thoracoplasties to control septic complications after a previous resection, or less often for the management of an uncontrolled parapneumonic empyema, Peppas and associates

(1993) reported a mortality of 10.8%. Of interest was the observation that the mortality was twice as high in those patients in whom the original resection had been done for the removal of a lung cancer.

RESULTS

The overall success rate of a thoracoplasty in eliminating intrathoracic space problems has improved over the years. Hopkins and coworkers (1985) reported a failure rate of 33% before 1976 but only 17% since then. Grégoire (1987), from Deslauriers' group, reported an early failure rate of only 12% in 17 patients with chronic postpneumonectomy empyema. In a similar group of patients, Dupon (1990) reported a complete recovery in 84% of cases, and in 2 to 15 years after the procedure, 75% of the patients had returned to normal activity. Peppas and associates (1993) also noted that the quality of life was improved in the majority of the survivors in their series.

LATE COMPLICATIONS

Over the years, a number of late complications in long-term survivors of a thoracoplasty have been reported. Serious complications account for only a small number of the complications when one considers the total number of either conventional or plombage procedures that have been done in the past.

Complications after Plombage Thoracoplasty

Migration of a paraffin plomb is a common event. This late complication was recorded in as many as 25% of the patients by Fox and associates (1962). Simple removal, except in the rare secondarily infected space, was generally all that was necessary to resolve the problem. However, Tanaka and colleagues (1996) reported four cases of an expanding paraffin plombage space causing dyspnea and pain as a result of a hematoma developing from granulomatous tissue associated with the occurrence of a capillary hemangioma. A fatal hemorrhage into a large, symptomatic cyst (recurrent nerve paralysis and superior vena cava syndrome) associated Polystan pack plombage performed 38 years earlier was reported by Skinner and Sinclair (1992).

In patients in whom Lucite spheres have been used for the plombage, infection, either with pyogenic or mycobacterial organisms, may occur within months of their placement. However, in some patients this event does not occur until years later. In this situation, migration of one or more spheres is common. The sphere may migrate into the lung, a vascular structure, or chest wall, as noted by Horowitz (1992) and Massard (1997) and their colleagues. In one patient reported by Horowitz and associates (1992), a sphere

eroded into the esophagus and subsequently resulted in a small-bowel obstruction.

Complications after a Standard Thoracoplasty

Hanagiri and coworkers (1997) reported one case of an expanding hematoma in a post-thoracoplasty space 42 years after the procedure had been done. The source of the hemorrhage was a vessel in the fibrous tissue of the wall. Surgical evacuation was successful.

Association of the Late Occurrence of Malignancy

In three patients with extraperiosteal Lucite sphere plombage, a malignant lesion has been reported to have occurred in various tissues adjacent to the plombage space 30 to 40 years after the operation. Harland and colleagues (1993) noted the development of a squamous cell carcinoma in the adjacent lung; Roggli and associates (1982) reported the occurrence of a malignant mesothelioma, and Thompson and Entin (1969) recorded the development of an extraskeletal chondrosarcoma. The exact relationship between the occurrence of these tumors and the Lucite sphere plombage remains unknown. Rather than being an etiologic factor, a more likely explanation is that the association is only coincidental.

REFERENCES

Alexander J: Collapse Therapy of Pulmonary Tuberculosis. Springfield, IL: Charles C Thomas, 1937, p. 402.
Andrews NC: Thoraco-mediastinal plication: a surgical technique for chronic empyema. J Thorac Surg 41:809, 1961.
Barker WL: Thoracoplasty. Chest Surg Clin North Am 4:593, 1994.
Bjork VD: Thoracoplasty: a new osteoplastic technique. J Thorac Surg 28:194, 1954.
Bredin CP: Pulmonary function in long-term survivors of thoracoplasty. Chest 95:18, 1989.
Conlan AA: Prophylaxis and management of postlobectomy infected spaces. In Deslauriers J, Lacquet LK (eds): Thoracic Surgery: Surgical Management of Pleural Diseases. St. Louis: CV Mosby, 1990, p. 279.
Dupon H: Andrews technique of thoracomyopleuroplasty. In Deslauriers J, Lacquet LK (eds): Thoracic Surgery: Surgical Management of Pleural Diseases. St. Louis: CV Mosby, 1990, p. 255.
Fox RT, et al: Extraperiosteal plombage thoracoplasty. J Thorac Cardiovasc Surg 44:371, 1962.
Fox RT, Shields TW: Thoracoplasty. In Shields TW (ed): General Thoracic Surgery. Philadelphia: Lea & Febiger, 1972, p. 351.
Gaensler EA: Lung displacement: abdominal enlargement, pleural space disorders, deformities of the thoracic cage. In Fenn WO, Rahan H, (eds): Handbook of Physiology. Baltimore: Williams & Wilkins, 1965.
Gaensler EA, Strieder JW: Progressive changes in pulmonary function after pneumonectomy: the influence of thoracoplasty, pneumothorax, oleothorax, plastic sponge plombage on the side of pneumonectomy. J Thorac Surg 22:1, 1951.
Gregoire R, et al: Thoracoplasty: its forgotten role in the management of nontuberculous postpneumonectomy empyema. Can J Surg 30:343, 1987.
Grow JB: Chronic pleural empyema. Dis Child 12:26, 1946.
Hanagiri T, et al: Chronic expanding hematoma in the chest. Ann Thorac Surg 64:559, 1997.

Harland RW, Sharma M, Rosenzweig DY: Lung carcinoma in a patient with Lucite sphere plombage thoracoplasty. Chest *103*:1295, 1993.

Hopkins RA, et al: The modern use of thoracoplasty. Ann Thorac Surg *40*:181, 1985.

Horowitz MD, et al: Late complications of plombage. Ann Thorac Surg *53*:803, 1992.

Jouveshomme S, et al: Preliminary results of collapse therapy with plombage pulmonary disease caused by multidrug-resistant mycobacteria. Am J Respir Crit Care Med *157*:1609, 1998.

Kergin FG: An operation for chronic pleural empyema. J Thorac Surg *26*:430, 1953.

Maloney JV Jr, Schmutzer KJ, Raschke E: Paradoxical respiration and "pendelluft." J Thorac Cardiovasc Surg *41*:291, 1961.

Massard G, et al: Pleuropulmonary aspergilloma: clinical spectrum and results of surgical treatments. Ann Thorac Surg *54*;1159, 1992.

Massard G, et al: Long-term complications of experiosteal plombage. Ann Thorac Surg *64*:220, 1997.

McMillan IKR: Bronchopleural fistula: treatment by space reduction. *In* Grillo HC, Eschapasse H (eds): International Trends in General Thoracic Surgery, Vol 2. A Major Challenge. Philadelphia: WB Saunders, 1987, p. 440.

Peppas G, et al: Thoracoplasty in the context of current surgical practice. Ann Thorac Surg *56*:903, 1993.

Puchetti V, et al: La toracoplastica oggi. Rivisitazione di una tecnica del passato. Chir Ital *46*:57, 1994.

Roggli VI, et al: Pumonary asbestos body counts and electron probe analysis of asbestos body cores in patients with mesothelioma: a study of 25 cases. Cancer *50*:2423, 1982.

Schede M: Die Behandlung der Empyeme. Verh Cong Innere Med Wiesb *9*:41, 1890.

Skinner JS, Sinclair DJ: Fatal mediastinal compression as a late complication of surgical plombage. Thorax *47*:321, 1992.

Stamatis G, et al: Die heutige Rolle der Thorakoplastik zur Behandlung des chronischen Pleuraempyems. Pneumoligie *46*:564, 1992.

Talamonti MS, et al: A new method of extraperiosteal plombage for atypical pulmonary tuberculosis. Chest *96*:237S, 1989.

Tanaka H, et al: Expanding plombage space developing as a late complication of extraperiosteal paraffin plombage in four cases. J Jpn Assoc Chest Surg *10*:685, 1996.

Thompson JR, Entin SD: Primary extraskeletal chondrosarcoma. Report of a case arising in conjunction with extrapleural Lucite ball plombage. Cancer *23*:936, 1969.

Young WG, Ungerleider RM: Surgical approach to the chronic empyema: thoracoplasty. *In* DesLauriers J, Lacquet LK (eds): Thoracic Surgery: Surgical Management of Pleural Diseases. St. Louis: CV Mosby, 1990, p. 247.

CHAPTER 63

Anatomy of the Thoracic Duct and Chylothorax

Joseph I. Miller, Jr.

Embryologically, the thoracic duct is a bilateral structure and has the potential of having many varied anatomic patterns. The pattern and anatomy of the thoracic duct is considered standard, as reported by Davis (1915), in only 65% of humans. Many anatomic variations occur in lymphatic and lymphaticovenous anastomosis (Fig. 63-1).

TYPICAL PATTERN OF THE THORACIC DUCT

The usual anatomic pattern of the thoracic duct is shown in Figure 63-2. The thoracic duct is the main collecting vessel of the lymphatic system and is far larger than the right terminal lymphatic duct. Most commonly, the thoracic duct originates from the cisterna chyli in the midline at the level of the second lumbar vertebra. The cisterna chyli is 3 to 4 cm long and 2 to 3 cm in diameter. It is generally found along the vertebral column at the level of L2, but may be found anywhere between T10 and L3, generally to the right side of the aorta.

From the cisterna chyli, the thoracic duct ascends to enter the chest through the aortic hiatus at the level of T10–T12, just to the right of the aorta. Above the diaphragm, the duct lies on the anterior surface of the vertebral column behind the esophagus and between the aorta and the azygos vein. The duct usually lies in front of the right intercostal arteries with the nerves close by. The duct continues upward on the right side of the vertebral column to approximately the level of the fifth or sixth thoracic vertebra, where it crosses behind the aorta and aortic arch into the left posterior portion of the visceral compartment of the mediastinum. From there, it passes superiorly in close approximation to the left side of the esophagus and the pleural reflection into the neck. Before exiting the mediastinum, the duct receives tributaries from the bronchomediastinal trunk of the right lymphatic duct. Once the duct enters the neck, it arches 2 to 3 cm above the clavicle and swings laterally anterior to the subclavian artery and thyrocervical arteries. It continues deeper into the neck in front of the phrenic nerve and the scalenus anticus muscle. At this point, it passes behind the left carotid sheath and jugular vein before anastomosing with the left subclavian jugular junction (Fig. 63-3). The anatomic manner in which the thoracic duct ends varies. It may enter the jugular vein as a single trunk or as multiple trunks. It most commonly enters at the junction of the left internal jugular and subclavian veins.

MAJOR VARIATIONS OF THE THORACIC DUCT

The only thing constant about the anatomy of the thoracic duct is the numerous anatomic variations. Davis (1915) reported nine major variations, and Anson (1950) listed 12 different anatomic variations of the lower portion of the thoracic duct (Fig. 63-4).

Major variations of the thoracic duct itself include doubling, left-sidedness, and right or bilateral termination, as well as the rare azygos vein termination. The embryologic basis for these variations is the plexiform nature of the trunks from which the duct arises. Doubling was reported in 4.7% of patients by Adachi (1953) and in 39% in a larger series by Van Pernis (1949); the lower figure is probably correct for extensive duplication. In a few instances, the abdominal components of the trunk may pass upward to both sides or only to the left of the aorta. Rarely, as noted by Adachi (1953) as well as Davis (1915), the duct may be left-sided throughout its course. Adachi also reported that only the upper part of the duct may be double so that it terminates in both the right and left sides of the neck (1.8%) or the right side alone (1.6%). At its termination, the duct may enter into a short plexus with its tributary trunks so that in approximately 20% of people it enters the vein by two or more branches. Termination of the duct in the azygos system is rare. Edwards (1972) reported, in an autopsy subject, that he had observed the duct to enter the hemiazygos vein. In its cervical course, Adachi (1953) noted that the duct may run posterior rather than anterior to the vertebral or the subclavian artery.

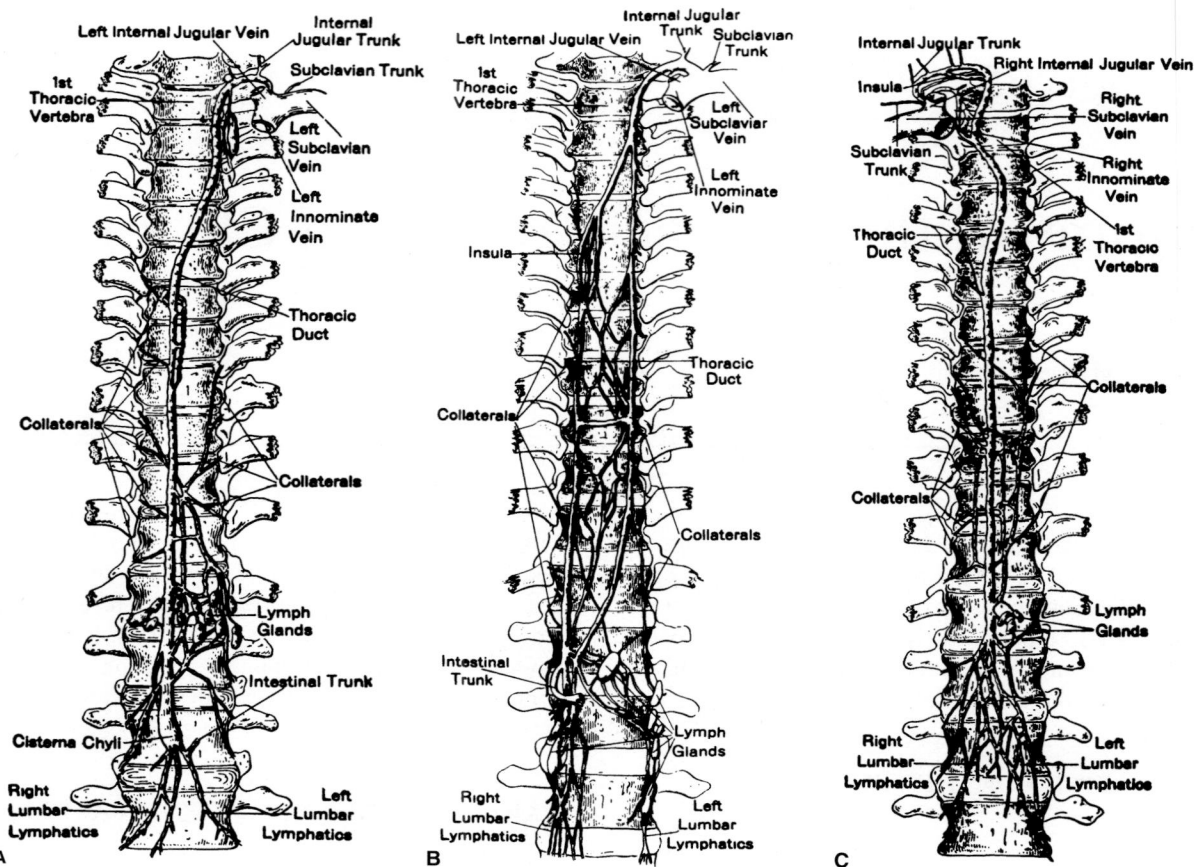

Fig. 63-1. Variations of the thoracic duct. **A.** A duct conforming to the usual description. **B.** Absence of a cisterna chyli and duplication of much of the course of the duct. **C.** Absence of a cisterna and right-sided termination. From Edwards EA, Malone PD, Collins JJ Jr: Operative Anatomy of the Thorax. Philadelphia: Lea & Febiger, 1972. With permission.

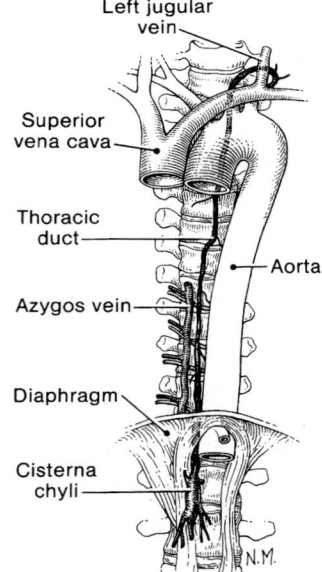

Fig. 63-2. Usual anatomic pattern of the thoracic duct. From Miller JI: Chylothorax and anatomy of the thoracic duct. *In* Shields TW (ed): General Thoracic Surgery. 3rd Ed. Philadelphia: Lea & Febiger, 1989. With permission.

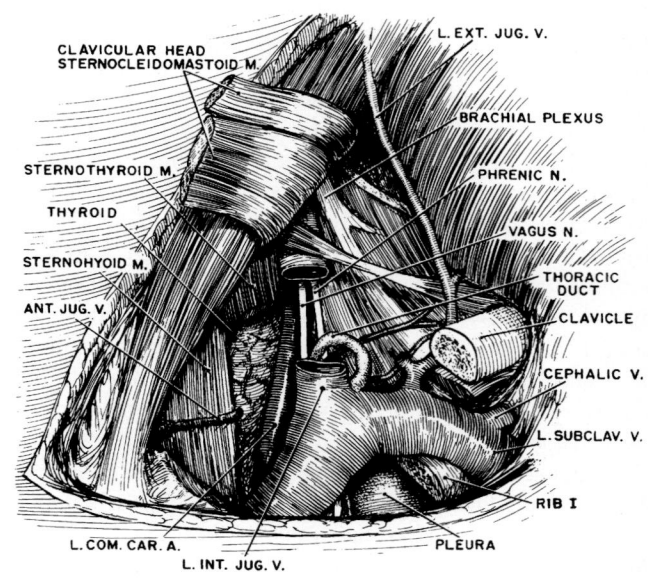

Fig. 63-3. Termination of the thoracic duct. A., aorta; M., muscle; V., vein. From Edwards EA, Malone PD, Collins JJ Jr: Operative Anatomy of the Thorax. Philadelphia: Lea & Febiger, 1972. With permission.

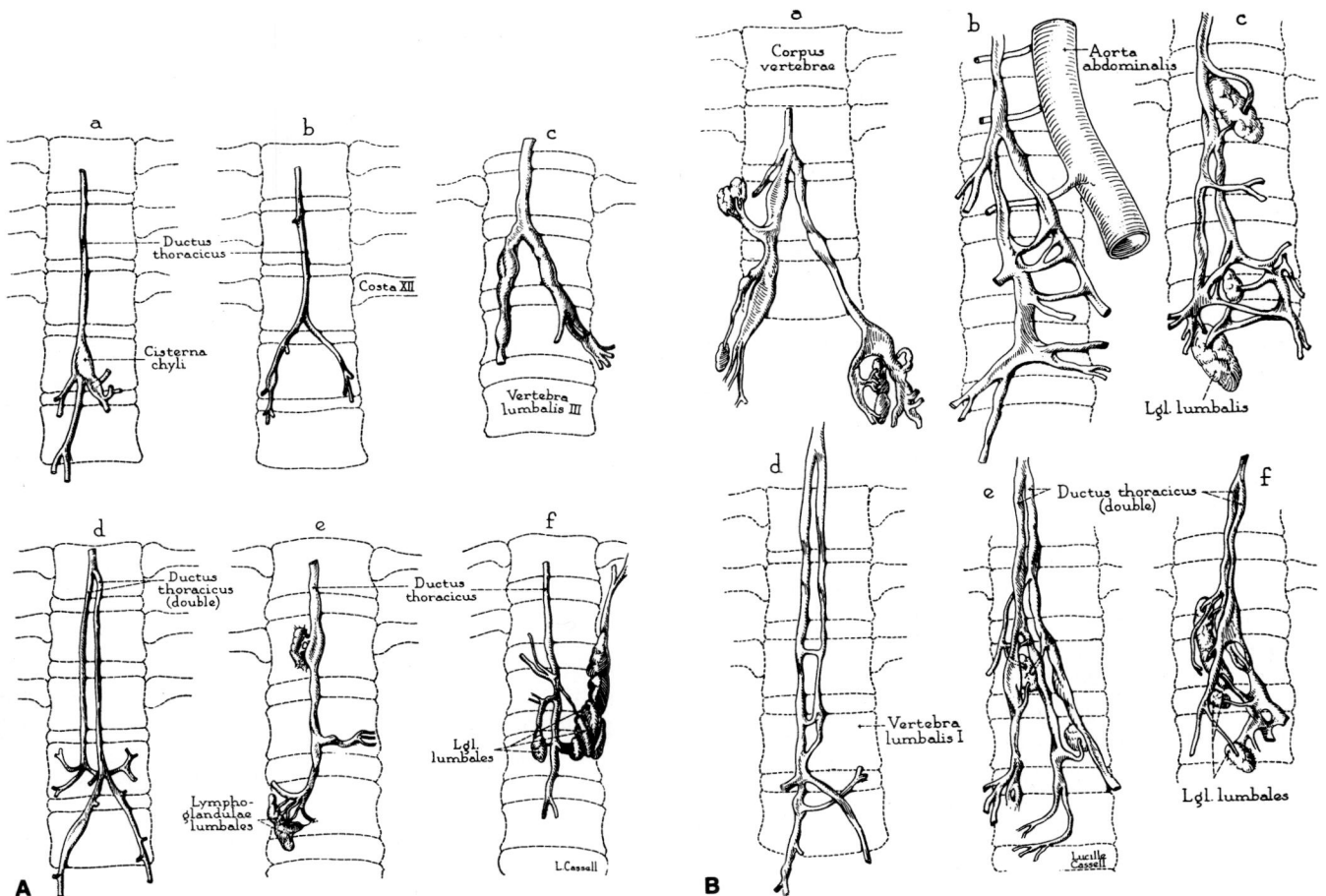

Fig. 63-4. Thoracic duct. Variations and vertebral relations. **A.** a and c, ducts possessing sacculations of considerable size; b and d, ducts of slender form; e and f, ducts of elongated form. **B.** a, duct of common, Y-shaped form; b through d, ducts possessing numerous anastomoses between the bilateral tributaries; e and f, trifid ducts. From Anson BJ: An Atlas of Human Anatomy. Philadelphia: Saunders, 1963. With permission.

In 1922, Lee reported a detailed study of the collateral circulation of the lymphatic system in the mediastinum. He identified various connections between the thoracic duct and the azygos vein, as well as other connections between intercostal veins and the thoracic duct within the chest. The thoracic duct contains valves in various locations throughout its entire course.

Lymph from the right side of the head, neck, and chest wall, as well as from the right lung and the lower half of the left lung, through the bronchomediastinal trunk, drain into the right lymphatic duct. This duct also carries lymph from the heart and the dome of the liver and from the right diaphragm. Bessone and colleagues (1971) pointed out that the right lymphatic duct is small and is rarely visualized.

COMPOSITION OF CHYLE

The term *chyle* comes from the Latin *chylus*, meaning *juice*. It is the lymph that originates in the intestine. The fat contained in the intestinal lymph gives chyle its characteristic appearance. Thoracic duct lymph is not pure chyle, but a mixture of lymphatic fluid originating in the intestine, liver, abdominal wall, and lower extremities. Ninety-five percent of the volume of the thoracic duct lymph originates in the liver and the intestinal tract. Under normal circumstances, the amount of lymph originating in the extremities is negligible.

The primary function of the thoracic duct is the transport of digestive fat to the venous system. Munk and Rosenstein (1891) observed a thoracic duct fistula and recognized that the thoracic duct lymph was clear during fasting but became milky after a fatty meal. Approximately 60 to 70% of the ingested fat is absorbed by the intestinal lymphatic system and conveyed to the bloodstream by the thoracic duct. The composition of chyle is listed in Table 63-1. The main component of chyle is fat.

Thoracic duct lymph contains from 0.4 to 5.0 g of fat per 100 mL and 50 to 70% of absorbed fat is conveyed to the bloodstream by way of the thoracic duct. This is made up of neutral fat, free fatty acids, sphingomyelin, phospholipids, cholesterol, and cholesterol esters. The total amount of cholesterol ranges from 65 to 220 mg/100 mL.

Table 63-1. Composition of Chyle

Component	Amount (per 100 mL)
Total fat	0.4–5.0 g
Total cholesterol	65–220 mg
Total protein	2.21–5.9 g
Albumin	1.2–4.1 g
Globulin	1.1–3.6 g
Fibrinogen	16–24 g
Sugar	48–200 g
Electrolytes	Similar to plasma
Cellular elements	
Lymphocytes	400–6800 per μL
Erythrocytes	50–600 per μL
Antithrombin globulin	25% plasma concentrate
Prothrombin	25% plasma concentrate
Fibrinogen	25% plasma concentrate

Those fatty acids with less than 10 carbon atoms in the chain are absorbed directly by the portal venous system. This particular fact forms the basis for the use of medium-chain triglycerides as an oral diet in the conservative management of chylothorax. Neutral fat, as Ross (1961) noted, is found in the lymph in the form of minute globules that are smaller than 0.5 mm in diameter. Ingested fat passes from the intestine to the systemic circulation in approximately 1.5 hours, with a peak absorption at 6 hours after ingestion.

Ross (1961) and Roy and associates (1967) reported that the total protein content of thoracic duct lymph ranges from 2.2 to 5.9 g/100 mL, approximately one-half of that found in the plasma. Thoracic duct lymph contains as much as 4% protein, consisting of albumin, globulin, fibrinogen, and prothrombin, with an albumin ratio of 3:1. Sugar concentration in thoracic duct lymph ranges from 40 to 200 g/100 mL. The electrolyte composition is similar to that found in plasma, with sodium, potassium, chloride, calcium, and inorganic phosphorus being the predominant electrolyte components.

Antithrombin globulin, prothrombin, and fibrinogen are all present in human thoracic duct lymph in concentrations greater than 25% of plasma levels. Stuttman and associates (1965) reported that factors V and VIII are present in concentrations of approximately 8.9% and 4.5%, respectively, in thoracic lymph.

The main cellular elements of thoracic duct lymph are lymphocytes. They range from 400 to 6800 cells per μL. As Hyde and colleagues (1974) noted, most of these lymphocytes are T lymphocytes. Thoracic duct lymphocytes differ qualitatively and quantitatively from peripheral blood lymphocytes in their reactivity to antigenic stimulation.

In clear lymph, approximately 50 red cells per μL exist, whereas in the postabsorptive states, as Shafiroff and Kau (1959) reported, the number may increase to 600 red cells per μL of thoracic duct lymph. In addition, fat-soluble vitamins, antibodies, enzymes (including pancreatic lipase, alkaline phosphatase, serum glutamic-oxaloacetic transaminase, and serum glutamic-pyruvic transaminase), and urea nitrogen also are present in thoracic duct lymph. Because of the numerous constituents of thoracic duct lymph, it is readily apparent why the persistent loss of this fluid can interfere with nutrition and immunity.

PHYSIOLOGY OF THE THORACIC DUCT

The function of the thoracic duct is the transport of ingested fat to the venous system. Volume and weight of flow of lymph have been estimated to be 1.38 mL/kg of body weight per hour. Crandall and associates (1943) found that the rate of flow increases after ingestion of food and water, and also during abdominal massage, with a maximum flow of 3.9 mL/minute and a minimum flow of 0.38 mL/minute. Hepatic lymph increases by 150% after meals, whereas intestinal lymph increases to up to 10 times the basal flow after fatty meals. Starvation and complete rest decrease the flow of thoracic duct lymph.

The forward flow of chyle from the cisterna chyli to the entrance into the left subclavian-internal jugular vein junction is influenced by several factors:

1) The inflow of chyle into the lacteal system creates a vis a tergo, which is in turn produced by the intake of food and liquid into the intestine and is augmented by intestinal movement.
2) Negative intrathoracic pressure on inspiration and the resultant gradient between this negative pressure and positive intra-abdominal pressure helps the upward flow of chyle.
3) Muscular contractions of the thoracic duct wall are probably the most important factor. Contractions of the duct wall occur every 10 to 15 seconds independent of respiratory movements. The intraductal pressure ranges from 10 to 25 cm H_2O, and with obstruction, as Shafiroff and Kau (1959) observed, it may increase to 50 cm H_2O. These rhythmic contractions cause the duct to empty into the subclavian vein. The thoracic duct valves, located throughout its course but mostly in the upper portion, permit only upward unidirectional flow.

The flow of chyle varies greatly with the content of the meal and is particularly increased when the fat content of the food is high. Volumes up to 2500 mL of chyle in 24 hours have been collected from the cannulated human thoracic duct. Most of the body's lymphocytes are transported through the thoracic duct system back to the venous system.

The lymph circulation performs the vital function of collecting and transporting excess tissue fluid, extravasated plasma protein, absorbed lipids, and other large molecules from the interstitial spaces back to the bloodstream.

ETIOLOGY OF CHYLOTHORAX

Chylothorax is the presence of lymphatic fluid in the pleural space resulting from a leak of the thoracic duct or one of its major divisions. This condition is being recog-

Table 63-2. Etiology of Chylothorax

Congenital
    Atresia of thoracic duct
    Thoracic duct, pleural fistula space
    Birth trauma
Traumatic
    Blunt
    Penetrating
    Surgical
        Cervical
            Excision of lymph nodes
            Radical neck dissection
        Thoracic
            Ligation of patent ductus arteriosus
            Excision of coarctation
            Esophagectomy
            Resection of thoracic aortic aneurysm
            Resection of mediastinal tumor
            Left pneumonectomy
        Abdominal
            Sympathectomy
            Radical lymph node dissection
Diagnostic procedures
    Lumbar arteriography
    Subclavian vein catheterization
Neoplasms
Miscellaneous

nized more frequently, after both cardiac and general thoracic surgery. Increased understanding of the physiology, pathogenesis, diagnosis, and management of chylothorax has decreased the initial 50% mortality to a mortality of 10% in major medical centers.

Numerous classifications of chylothorax have been suggested. Most have been based on information obtained at postmortem examination. In 1971, Bessone and colleagues suggested classifying chylothorax into 1) congenital chylothorax, 2) postoperative traumatic chylothorax, 3) nonsurgical traumatic chylothorax, and 4) nontraumatic chylothorax. DeMeester (1983), however, has published a more thorough classification (Table 63-2).

Congenital Chylothorax

Chylothorax in the neonate, although rare, is the leading cause of pleural effusion in this age group. In most cases, the exact cause cannot be ascertained. Birth trauma or congenital defects in the duct wall, or both, may be precipitating factors. Increased venous pressure in birth trauma, causing thoracic duct rupture, has been suggested as a possible cause. In rare instances, malformations of the lymphatic system, particularly in the thoracic duct itself, have been shown to be the cause of congenital chylothorax. The thoracic duct may be absent or atretic, and, in occasional instances, multiple, dilated lymphatic channels with abnormal communications have been noted, as well as multiple fistulae between the thoracic duct and pleural space.

Traumatic Chylothorax

The second major cause of chylothorax is traumatic chylothorax, which may occur with either blunt or penetrating trauma or after a surgical procedure. The most common form of nonpenetrating injury to the thoracic duct is produced by a sudden hyperextension of the spine with rupture of the duct just above the diaphragm. Sudden stretching over the vertebral bodies may be enough in itself to tear the duct, but usually the duct has been fixed as a result of prior disease or malignancy. This may be secondary to a blast or blunt trauma. Episodes of vomiting or a violent bout of coughing also can result in tearing of the thoracic duct. Biet and Connolly (1951) believe this is generally caused by a shearing of the thoracic duct by the right crus of the diaphragm. These are the most commonly mentioned causes of chylothorax resulting from nonpenetrating injuries to the chest. Penetrating injury from a gunshot or a stab wound to the thoracic duct is unusual and is apt to be overshadowed by damage to other structures of more immediate importance.

Operative Injuries

Injury at operation is fairly common. Chylothorax has been reported after almost every known thoracic surgical procedure, including operations on the aorta, esophagus, heart, lungs, and sympathetic nervous system. Injury also has been reported after surgery in the neck, after such operations as radical neck resection and scalene node biopsy. It has been reported also after abdominal operations of sympathectomy and radical lymph node dissection. In addition, it has been reported with translumbar aortography and subclavian venous catheterization. An occasional instance has been reported after an attempt to introduce a cannula into the left internal jugular vein.

Often, a latent interval of 2 to 10 days passes between the time of injury and the development of a chylothorax that becomes clinically evident. This is because of the accumulation of lymph in the posterior mediastinum until the mediastinal pleura ruptures, usually on the right side at the base of the pulmonary ligament. Once established, the thoracic duct pleural fistula does not tend to close, in contrast to the dictum that in the absence of obstruction a fistula closes. Spontaneous sealing of a fistula after a closed injury may be expected in only approximately 50% of patients, and death generally ensues in the remaining patients unless the fistula is surgically closed.

Intraoperatively, the duct is most vulnerable to damage in the upper part of the left chest, particularly, as Higgins and Molder (1971) noted, with procedures involving mobilization of the aortic arch, the left subclavian artery, or the esophagus. The classically described course of the duct explains why damage to it below the level of the fifth or sixth thoracic vertebra usually results in a right-sided chylous effusion, and why damage above this level usually results in effusion on the left side.

Neoplastic Chylothorax

Ross (1961) stated that the thoracic duct can be involved in both benign and malignant disease by direct lymphatic permeation in continuity with the primary growth, by direct invasion of the duct by the primary growth, or by tumor embolus in the main duct. The chylothorax may be either unilateral or bilateral. DeMeester (1983) reported that the predominant mechanism of the leak is by rupture of distended tributaries because of back pressure from the neoplastic obstruction or actual erosion of the duct itself. It has been most frequently reported after lymphosarcoma, retroperitoneal lymphoma, or primary carcinoma of the lung. Rarely, malignant chylous leaks may fill the pericardial sac with chyle and produce signs and symptoms of cardiac tamponade.

Miscellaneous Causes

Infections, filariasis, pancreatic pseudocysts, thrombosis of the jugular and subclavian veins, cirrhosis of the liver, and tuberculosis can all cause chylothorax.

Benign lymphangiomas arising in the thoracic duct also may produce single or multiple cystlike spaces filled with chyle.

Pulmonary lymphangioleiomyomatosis, reported by Cunn (1973) and Silverstein (1974) and their associates, is a rare cause of chylothorax. This condition is seen in women of reproductive age who have shortness of breath as the major complaint. Pneumothorax and hemoptysis can be seen in addition to chylothorax, and these women usually die of pulmonary insufficiency within 10 years of presentation.

PATHOLOGIC PHYSIOLOGY

Chylothorax can cause cardiopulmonary abnormalities, as well as serious metabolic and immunologic deficiencies. The accumulation of chyle in the chest can result in compression of the underlying lung, with a reduction of vital capacity and mediastinal shift, resulting in shortness of breath, and, occasionally, symptoms of marked respiratory distress. In general, the development is insidious, and symptoms occur gradually. In contrast, with rapid accumulation, shock, tachypnea, tachycardia, and hypotension can occur. Chyle is thought to be bacteriostatic because of its lecithin and fatty acid content and therefore is usually sterile. Because it is nonirritating, chyle does not tend to form a peel that can result in a trapped lung.

The loss of protein, fat-soluble vitamins, and fat contained in chyle can lead to serious metabolic defects and death in patients with chylothorax. Shafiroff and Kau (1959)

emphasized that the loss of lymphocytes and antibodies can interfere also with the immunologic status of a patient with chylothorax.

DIAGNOSIS

Diagnosis of a chylothorax is suggested by the presence of a nonclotting, milky fluid, which is obtained from the pleural space at thoracentesis or chest tube insertion. The diagnosis is confirmed by the finding of free microscopic fat and fat content of the fluid higher than that of the plasma. In traumatic chylothorax, the chyle may initially appear bloodstained, and this may be misleading. On microscopic examination, the presence of fat globules that clear with alkali and ether, or stain with Sudan-3, is diagnostic. Lymphocytes are the predominant cells found in chyle, whereas in traumatic chylus effusion, red blood cells are at least initially present. Chylous effusions must be distinguished from pseudochyle and cholesterol pleural effusions. Boyd (1986) noted that pseudochyle occurs with malignant tumors or infection and is milky in appearance because of the presence of lecithin-globulin complex. Pseudochyle contains only a trace of fat, and fat globules cannot be seen with Sudan-3 stain smears. Milky pleural effusions also can be seen secondary to tuberculosis, and Bower (1968) reported milky pleural effusions to occur in rheumatoid arthritis.

Cholesterol pleural effusions that are seen in these two disease entities acquire their milky appearance from a high concentration of cholesterol crystals. If it is still difficult to distinguish chyle from pseudochyle or cholesterol pleural fluid, a test consisting of feeding a patient a fat stained with green No. 6 dye, which stains the chylous effusion approximately 1 hour after ingestion of the dye, is a helpful diagnostic test. Obtaining cholesterol and triglyceride levels of the fluid can help because most chylous effusions have a cholesterol to triglyceride ratio of less than 1, whereas nonchylous effusions have a ratio greater than 1. In addition, if the fluid has a triglyceride level of more than 110 mg/100 mL, a 99% chance exists that the fluid is chyle. If the triglyceride level is less than 50 mg/100 mL, Staats and colleagues (1980) noted that only a 5% chance exists that the fluid is chyle.

Another helpful index in determining if a leak is related to a chylous leak is the rate of fluid accumulation in the chest. The rate of accumulation in the chest from a chylous fistula exceeds 400 to 500 mL/day and averages approximately 700 to 1200 mL/day in a 70-kg adult. The flow rate is obviously proportionately less in infants and children, depending on the body surface area. A detailed analysis of the effusion should produce values similar to those listed in Table 63-1 if the effusion is indeed a chylous effusion. Once a chylothorax is diagnosed, a complete history and physical examination should be performed to discern the etiology. Chylothorax in a postoperative period generally develops 7 to 14 days postoperatively. Surgery in the region of the aorta, esophagus, or posterior mediastinum should suggest the presence or the possibility of a chylothorax. Blunt trauma 2 to 6 weeks earlier also should suggest the presence of a potential chylothorax.

In nontraumatic chylothorax, an extensive search for the cause of the pleural effusion must be undertaken. Computed tomography and lymphangiography are diagnostic techniques that are helpful in the study of chylothorax. Occasionally, lymphangiography details the exact site of leakage and also the anatomic abnormalities of the thoracic duct. A computed tomography examination of the chest is a good way to demonstrate the presence of mediastinal disease that could cause a chylothorax. A mediastinal mass or enlarged mediastinal nodes, as well as primary lung cancer, could easily be demonstrated by this technique.

MANAGEMENT

The ideal management of the patient with chylothorax is unknown. The disease occurs in various situations, and opinion about which types of chylothorax should be treated operatively is diverse: the postsurgical or post-traumatic types only, or the nontraumatic types as well. Whether young children should undergo surgery is also controversial. The development of a lymphatic leak in the thorax certainly necessitates decisive management if considerable morbidity and mortality are to be avoided. Well-standardized guidelines have emerged that have enhanced the understanding and treatment of this difficult clinical problem.

Table 63-3 lists the various modalities used in the treatment of chylothorax. They can be divided into conservative therapy, operative therapy, and radiation therapy.

Current treatment of chylothorax is thoracic duct ligation, introduced by Lampson and associates (1948). They showed that the mortality from chylothorax decreased from 50 to 15%. Before this report of successful control of traumatic chylothorax by direct ligation of the thoracic duct, the mortality for this condition was 45%; nontraumatic chylothorax had a mortality of 100%. Treatment of the condition before 1948 consisted of thoracentesis or closed chest tube thoracostomy and a low-fat diet. Today, the crucial decision in the management of these patients is when to advocate surgical intervention. No unanimous opinion exists on whether to operate or, if surgery is not undertaken initially, on how long conservative management should be used before resorting to surgical intervention.

Conservative therapy consists of maintaining effective thoracostomy tube drainage with good expansion of the lung. The most important aspect is to maintain adequate nutrition, as loss of chylous fluid causes electrolyte imbalance and increases nutritional needs. Central hyperalimentation is routinely used while giving the patient nothing by mouth. Any oral feedings increase output through the fistula. No standard exists of how long conservative therapy should

Table 63-3. Modalities Used in Treatment of Chylothorax

Conservative
　Nothing by mouth
　Medium-chain triglycerides
　Central hyperalimentation
　Drainage of pleural space
　　Thoracentesis
　　Closed chest tube thoracostomy
　Complete expansion of lung
Operative
　Direct ligation of thoracic duct
　Mass ligation of thoracic duct tissue
　Pleuroperitoneal shunting
　Pleurectomy
　Fibrin glue
Radiation therapy

be tried before considering operative intervention. Williams and Burford (1964) as well as Selle and associates (1971) recommended that 14 days is a maximum limit for conservative therapy before surgical intervention. In approximately 50% of patients, the thoracic duct leak closes spontaneously, and the other 50% require surgical intervention. When chest tube drainage is consistently greater than 500 mL/day for 2 weeks, surgical intervention is definitely indicated, except for those patients for whom thoracotomy is contraindicated, such as those with vertebral fractures or with nonresectable tumors. If a lung is entrapped and pleural synthesis cannot be achieved with reexpansion by closed chest tube thoracostomy, then early surgical intervention is indicated. If chylous drainage is still present after a period of carefully supervised nonoperative conservative therapy, patients with congenital, traumatic, or postoperative chylothorax should undergo surgical treatment.

OPERATIVE THERAPY OF A CHYLOUS FISTULA

Several techniques may be used to control a chylous fistula, singly or in a combination: direct ligation of the thoracic duct, mass ligation of the thoracic duct, pleuroperitoneal shunting, and pleurectomy. Occasionally, decortication may be required when the lung is entrapped. Stenzel and colleagues (1983) suggested that fibrin glue be applied in some instances.

In unilateral chylothorax, the chest should be opened on the side of the effusion. When the effusion is bilateral, it is more prudent to explore the right side first, with ligation of the duct low in the right chest. Exploration of the left side is done later, if necessary. Ross (1961) stated that the easiest way to find the duct and the leakage point is to give the patient 100 to 200 mL of olive oil through a nasogastric tube 2 to 3 hours before the operation; what remains in the stomach at the time of anesthetic induction can be removed by the same nasogastric tube. This causes filling of the duct with milky chyle, which is readily recognized throughout the course of the operation. An alternative method is to inject a 1% aqueous solution of Evans blue dye into the leg. This causes staining of the thoracic duct within 5 minutes that lasts up to 12 minutes. The disadvantage of the dye is that the adjacent tissues are also stained when free escape of chyle occurs.

Ligation of the thoracic duct just above the diaphragm through the right chest is currently favored by most authors, including Selle (1971), Patterson (1981), and Milson (1985) and their associates, regardless of the site of the chylous leak. As noted, the thoracic duct is a single structure from T12–T8 in more than 75% of all patients.

The three techniques used to control the leak of chyle are direct closure of the fistula, suture of the leaking mediastinal pleura, and supradiaphragmatic ligation of the duct. The best method is to find the actual point of leakage and to close it with nonabsorbable sutures with the use of Teflon pledgets, compressing the leakage point in the adjacent tissue between the two pledgets, and, if possible, allowing the main portion of the duct to remain patent. Either of the first two techniques, and particularly the second, should be combined with supradiaphragmatic ligation of the duct. This alone is entirely effective in instances in which no attempt has been made to directly close the fistula. The most favorable site for elective ligation is low in the right chest just above the right crus of the diaphragm where the duct lies on the vertebral column between the aorta and the azygos vein (Fig. 63-5).

If a definite source of leak cannot be identified when the right side of the chest is explored, despite use of the previously described ingestion of fat (milk or cream) or olive oil before surgery, then supradiaphragmatic ligation of the duct should be performed. This method was originally described by Murphy and Piper (1977) and subsequently championed by Patterson and colleagues (1981).

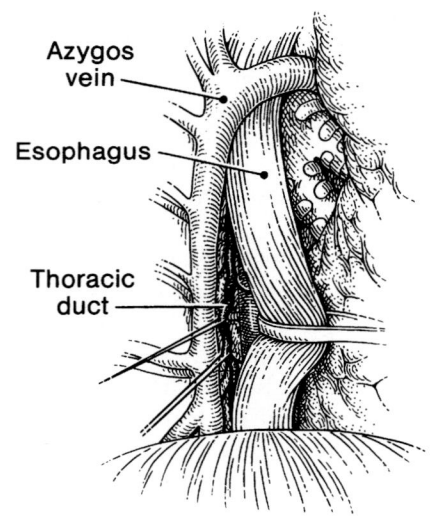

Fig. 63-5. Surgical anatomy of the thoracic duct in the right suprahepatic location.

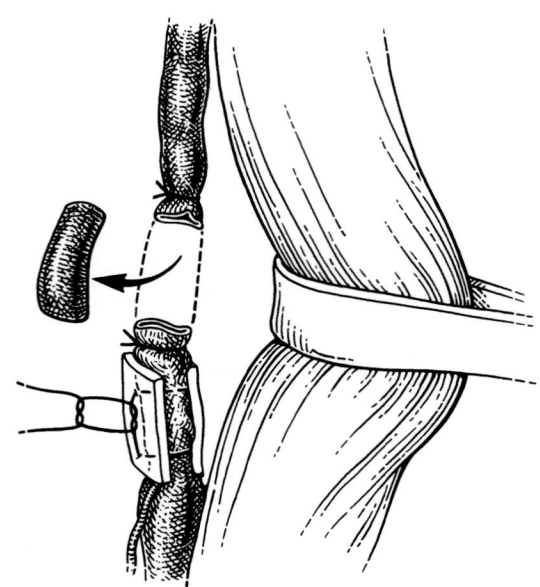

Fig. 63-6. Mass ligation of the thoracic duct using Teflon pledgets with nonabsorbable suture.

Supradiaphragmatic Ligation of the Thoracic Duct

A standard posterolateral thoracotomy incision is made, going through the bed of the resected right sixth rib. Generally, the pleura has a shaggy appearance because of fibrin deposits. After these deposits are cleaned off, the pulmonary ligament is divided between clamps and the pulmonary ligament swept upward to the level of the inferior pulmonary vein. The retropleural area is often thickened up to 1 to 2 cm and should be biopsied, if this is the case. It is best to ligate the duct en masse by going around the duct, taking a generous bite of tissue around the duct, and going close to the vertebral bodies, but avoiding the esophagus, aorta, and azygos vein. This suture should be tied with large pledgeted sutures on either end, as shown in Figure 63-6. This effects a mass ligature in the area between the azygos vein and the aorta just above the diaphragm. One must take care not to enter the wall of the esophagus. In effect, all tissue between the azygos vein and the aorta is ligated in the mass ligature.

A parietal pleurectomy is performed to achieve pleural synthesis. At the same time, if the underlying lung is trapped, it is decorticated. Two chest tube catheters are placed into the thoracic cavity and the chest closed in the usual fashion. In general, the chest tubes can be removed in 5 to 7 days, and recovery is rapid.

Other Techniques to Control Chylothorax

Milson and associates (1985) and Weese and Schouten (1984) reported the successful use of pleuroperitoneal shunt-

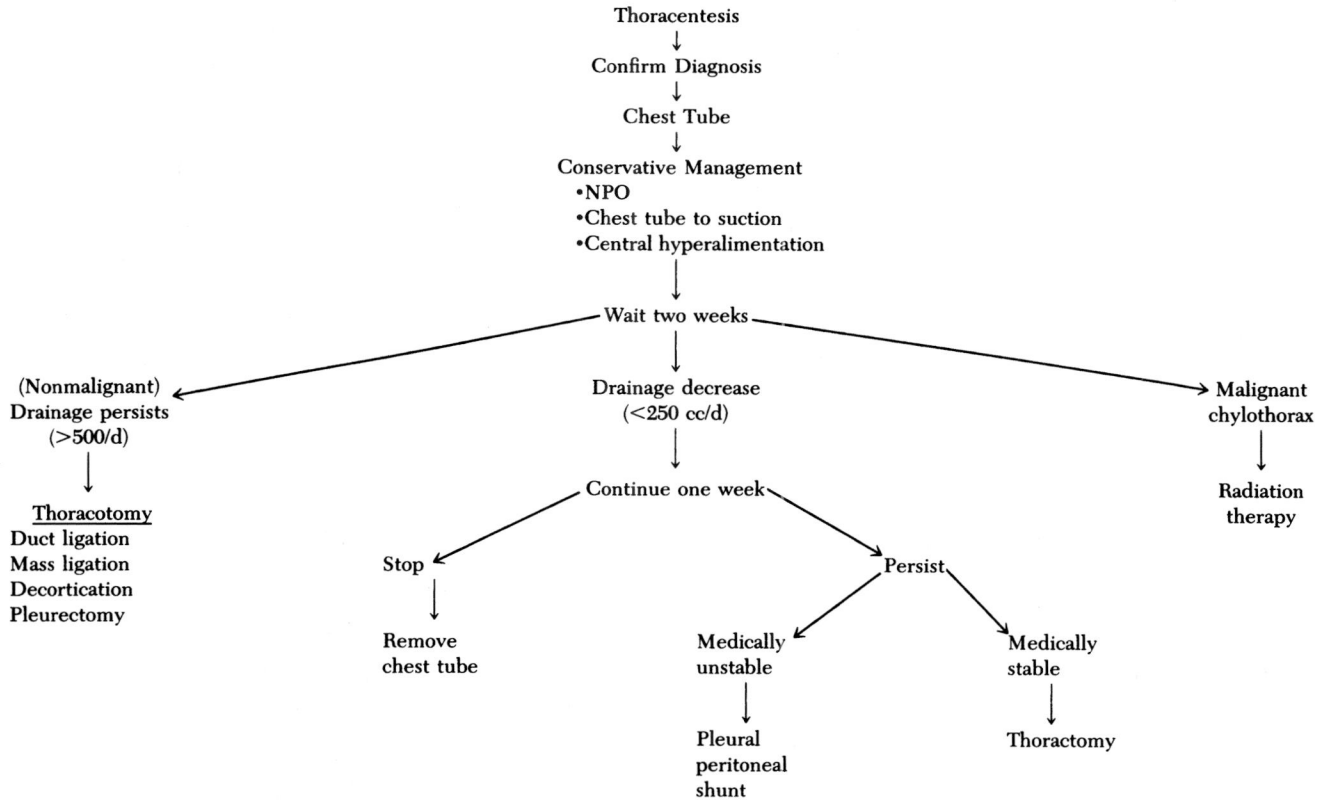

Fig. 63-7. Management of chylothorax.

ing with the double-valve Denver peritoneal shunt in the treatment of chylothorax. I have used this method with success.

Stenzel and colleagues (1983) reported the successful use of fibrin glue in one case of postsurgical chylothorax after an extrapleural ligation of the patent ductus arteriosus.

In nontraumatic chylothorax, the cause must be determined, and if neoplasm or infection is the cause, it must be treated specifically with radiation therapy, chemotherapy, or antibiotic therapy. If chylous drainage persists in these situations, pleural synthesis by catheter drainage of the pleura with instillation of nitrogen mustard or other irritants can be tried. In some cases, even though not desirable, thoracic duct ligation or pleurectomy may be needed to control the chylothorax. Radiation therapy has been successful in managing chylothorax in patients with mediastinal lymphoma and carcinoma. Irradiation of the pleural lymphatics to 2000 rads causes closure of the thoracic duct leak in most cases. I have observed four patients with nontraumatic chylothorax in whom no malignancy could be found and who received radiation therapy to the pleural lymphatics to 2000 rads with success in all cases.

GUIDELINES FOR MANAGEMENT

In an excellent review of the indications for surgery, Selle and colleagues (1971) established the following guidelines:

1) Idiopathic cases in the neonate usually respond well to thoracentesis.
2) Nontraumatic chylothorax, exclusive of the neonatal group, usually suggests a widespread fatal illness, and operative intervention is usually ineffective and should, therefore, be avoided.
3) In cases resulting from trauma, an initial trial of nonoperative therapy is indicated. Transthoracic ligation of the duct is indicated when the average daily chyle loss has exceeded 1500 mL/day in adults for more than 5 days.
4) If the chyle flow has not diminished within 14 days or if nutritional complications appear imminent, surgery is indicated.

Figure 63-7 lists my approach in the management of chylothorax. Thoracentesis is performed to confirm the diagnosis. Once the diagnosis of chylothorax has been established, a chest tube is inserted by closed thoracostomy. The patient is given nothing by mouth, and nutritional replacement is begun, using central hyperalimentation. Rarely is the patient allowed to drink, and if so, a medium-chain triglyceride diet is used. This method is continued for 2 weeks. If drainage greater than 500 mL/day persists, and the underlying cause is nonmalignant, the patient is taken to the operating room for surgical control of the leak in the aforementioned manner. A success rate of greater than 90%

may be expected with surgical intervention. Moreover, the mortality should be zero.

If the drainage is less than 250 mL/day and appears to be decreasing, I may continue to try conservative therapy for 1 more week. If the leakage stops, the chest tube is removed. If this is to be done, one should give a trial of a high-fat diet before removing the chest tube. If leakage persists at this time, pleuroperitoneal shunting could be performed if the patient is a medically compromised candidate, or thoracotomy and the previously mentioned procedures can be performed. If conservative therapy fails to control the chylothorax after 2 weeks, and the underlying condition is a malignancy, then irradiation is administered. Generally, radiation therapy to the amount of 2000 rads controls most cases of this variety of chylothoraces.

REFERENCES

Adachi B: Der Ductus Thoracicus des Japaner. Tokyo: Kenkyursha, 1953.
Anson BJ: An Atlas of Anatomy. Philadelphia: WB Saunders, 1950, pp. 336–337.
Bessone LN, Ferguson TB, Burford TH: Chylothorax: a collective review. Ann Thorac Surg 12:527, 1971.
Biet AB, Connolly NK: Traumatic chylothorax: a report of a case and a survey of the literature. Br J Surg 39:564, 1951.
Bower BC: Chyliform pleural effusion in rheumatoid arthritis. Am Rev Respir Dis 47:4515, 1968.
Boyd A: Chylothorax. In RM Hood, et al (eds): Surgical Disease of the Pleura and Chest Wall. Philadelphia: WB Saunders, 1986.
Crandall L Jr, Barker SB, Graham DC: A study of the lymph from a patient with thoracic duct fistula. Gastroenterology 1:1040, 1943.
Cunn B, Liebow AA, Friedman PJ: Pulmonary lymphangiomatosis: a review. Am J Pathol 79:398, 1973.
Davis MK: A statistical study of the thoracic duct in man. Am J Anat 171:212, 1915.
DeMeester TR: The pleura. In Sabiston DC, Spencer EC (eds): Surgery of the Chest. 4th Ed. Philadelphia: WB Saunders, 1983.
Edwards AE: The thoracic duct. In Edwards EA, Malone PD, Collins JJ Jr: Operative Anatomy of Thorax. Philadelphia: Lea & Febiger, 1972, p. 227.
Higgins CB, Molder DG: Chylothorax after surgery for congenital heart disease. J Thorac Cardiovasc Surg 61:411, 1971.
Hyde PV, Jerky J, Gishen P: Traumatic chylothorax. S Afr J Surg 12:57, 1974.
Lampson RS, et al: Traumatic chylothorax: a review of the literature and report of a case treated by mediastinal ligation of the thoracic duct. J Thorac Surg 17:778, 1948.
Lee FC: The establishment of collateral circulation following ligation of the thoracic duct. Johns Hopkins Hosp Bull 33:21, 1922.
Milson JW, et al: Chylothorax: an assessment of current surgical management. J Thorac Cardiovasc Surg 89:221, 1985.
Munk I, Rosenstein A: Zur Lehre von der Resporption in Darm nach Untersuchungen an einer Lymph (chylus) fistel beim Menschen. Virchuis Arch Pathol Anat 123:484, 1891.
Murphy TO, Piper CA: Surgical management of chylothorax. Ann Surg 43:719, 1977.
Patterson GA, et al: Supradiaphragmatic ligation of the thoracic duct in intractable chylous fistula. Ann Thorac Surg 32:44, 1981.
Ross JK: A review of surgery of the thoracic duct. Thorax 16:12, 1961.
Roy PH, Carr DT, Payne WS: The problem of chylothorax. Mayo Clin Proc 42:457, 1967.
Selle JG, Synder WA, Schreiber JT: Chylothorax. Ann Surg 177:245, 1971.
Shafiroff GP, Kau QY: Cannulation of the human thoracic lymph duct. Surgery 45:814, 1959.
Silverstein EF, et al: Pulmonary lymphangiomyomatosis. Am J Roentgenol Radium Ther Nucl Med 120:832, 1974.
Staats RA, et al: The lipoprotein profile of chylous and unchylous pleural effusion. Mayo Clin Proc 55:700, 1980.
Stenzel W, et al: Treatment of post surgical chylothorax with fibrin glue. J Thorac Cardiovasc Surg 31:35, 1983.
Stuttman LJ, Dumont AE, Shinowara G: Coagulation factors in human lymph and plasma. Am J Med Sci 250:292, 1965.
Van Pernis PA: Variations of the thoracic duct. Surgery 26:806, 1949.
Weese JL, Schouten JT: Internal drainage of intractable malignant pleural effusions. Wis Med J 83:21, 1984.
Williams KR, Burford TH: The management of chylothorax. Ann Surg 160:131, 1964.

READING REFERENCES

Blalock A, Cunningham RS, Robinson CS: Experimental production of chylothorax by occlusions of the superior vena cava. Ann Surg 104:359, 1936.
Donini I, Batteggati M: The Lymphatic System. London: Piccin Medical Books, 1972, pp. 11–26.
Goorwitch J: Traumatic chylothorax and thoracic duct ligation. J Thoracic Surg 29:467, 1955.
Klepser RG, Berny JF: The diagnosis and surgical management of chylothorax with the aid of lipophilic dyes. Dis Chest 25:409, 1954.

CHAPTER 64

Localized Fibrous Tumors of the Pleura

Thomas W. Shields and Anjana V. Yeldandi

Localized fibrous tumors of the pleura have previously been most often classified as localized mesotheliomas of the pleura, either benign or malignant. The malignant variety also has been classified by some investigators, including Martini and associates (1987), as fibrosarcomas. Scharifker and Kaneko (1979), among others, have suggested that the cell origin of these tumors is a noncommitted mesenchymal cell present in the areolar tissue subjacent to the mesothelial lining of the pleura and is not from the mesothelial cells of the pleura, as the earlier name implies. The most appropriate term for the malignant variety is a *localized malignant fibrous tumor of the pleura.*

The studies of Dalton (1979), Said (1984), Dervan (1986), Keating (1987), and England (1989) and their associates, as well as the studies of Witkin and Rosai (1989) and El-Naggar (1989) and Steinetz (1990) and their colleagues, have supported this concept of the mesenchymal origin of both the benign and malignant localized fibrous tumors of the pleura. Additional, but oblique, support of this concept is the observation that a history of asbestos exposure is lacking in the patients with these tumors; although a single case reported by Metintas and colleagues (1997) shows an association of malignant fibrous tumor in a person exposed to tremolite asbestos. Because no immunohistochemical studies were done in this case, one could speculate whether this case represented a localized malignant mesothelioma, which is in marked contrast to those patients with diffuse malignant mesothelioma in whom asbestos exposure is recorded in more than 60%.

BENIGN LOCALIZED FIBROUS TUMORS OF THE PLEURA

Pathologic Characteristics

Gross Features

Most benign localized fibrous tumors arise from the visceral pleura on a stalk and project into the pleural space in a pedunculated manner. Sessile attachment to the pleura occurs, and inward growth into the lung parenchyma may be seen infrequently. Yousem and Flynn (1988) reported three intraparenchymal localized fibrous tumors, only one of which was attached to the visceral pleura. They theorized that the other two may have arisen from mesenchymal cells in the interlobular septa or even de nova in the lung tissue. Localized fibrous tumors may also occasionally develop within a fissure. The benign tumors also may arise from the mediastinal, diaphragmatic, or costal portions of the parietal pleura. Tumors in these locations, however, including those arising within a fissure or growing into the lung, often prove to be malignant. Grossly, the benign tumors may have vascular adhesion between the tumor and the adjacent visceral or parietal pleura. They are almost always solitary and are ovoid or round. The external surface may be smooth or bosselated. According to England and associates (1989), a thin, membranous capsule is present in approximately one-half of the cases. The size may vary greatly from a small nodule to a huge mass that may completely fill the hemithorax. On cut section, the mass is composed of dense, whorled fibrous tissue that may contain cystlike structures filled with a clear viscid fluid in 10 to 15% of cases. Calcifications may be present within the tumor.

Histologic Features

Microscopically, one or more histologic patterns can be seen. The most common pattern seen is the patternless pattern described by Stout (1971). Fibroblastlike cells and connective tissue are observed in varying proportions and are arranged in a disorderly or random pattern (Fig. 64-1). The tumor cells are spindle or plump ovoid cells with round to oval nuclei and small nucleoli. Collagen and elastin bundles are readily identified. Pleomorphism and mitosis are seen infrequently. The second most common pattern is described as hemangiopericytomalike and is often combined with the patternless pattern. In this variety, closely packed tumor cells are arranged around open or collapsed, irregular branching capillaries. Other uncommon patterns, always mixed with

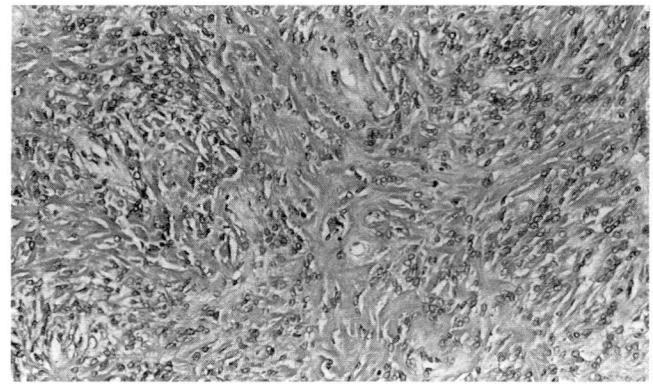

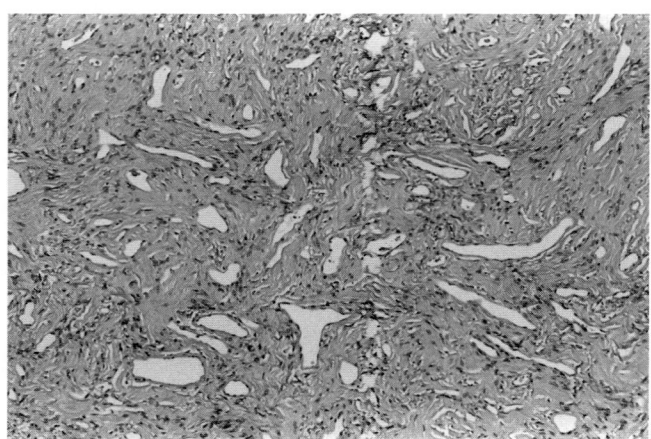

Fig. 64-1. A. Localized benign fibrous tumor of pleura with dense, wirelike strands of collagen sprinkled with plump fibroblastlike cells forming a patternless pattern. **B.** Photomicrograph of a hemangiopericytic pattern from a benign localized fibrous tumor of the pleura.

Table 64-1. Differentiation of Localized Fibrous Tumor and Diffuse Mesothelioma of the Pleura: Immunoreactivity

	Localized Fibrous Tumor	Mesothelioma
CD34 (reactivity in hemato-poietic stem cells)	+	–
Vimentin	+	++
Epithelial membrane antigen	–	(+)
Actin	(+)	–
Cytokeratin	–	++
Carcinoembryonic antigen	–	–

+, positive; –, negative; (+), variably or weakly positive; ++, strongly positive.

antigen, carcinoembryonic antigen, factor VIII–related antigen, neurofilament, or S-100 protein. The cells, however, have positive results with vimentin and weakly to variably positive results for muscle-specific actin. Westra (1994), Van de Rijn (1994), Flint and Weiss (1995), and Hanan (1995) and their coworkers reported consistent positivity of these tumors to CD34 monoclonal antibodies. CD34 reactivity is characteristically described as present in hematopoietic stem cells, endothelium, vascular tumors, and smooth muscle tumors. The lack of keratin reactivity and positive CD34 antigen differentiates these fibrous tumors of the pleura from a desmoplastic mesothelioma (Table 64-1). Suster and colleagues (1998) in their study of *bcl*-2 in spindle cell tumors showed strong positivity with this proto-oncogene in fibrous tumors of the pleura.

Flow-Cytometric DNA Studies

El-Naggar and colleagues (1989) described a diploid DNA pattern in all 12 nonrecurrent benign fibrous tumors in their study. The S-phase was low in all 12 as well.

Clinical Features

Benign localized fibrous tumors of the pleura occur with equal frequency in both sexes, although Milano (1990) reported a greater incidence in women. The tumor may occur in any age group but is more common in the fifth to eighth decades of life. More than one-half of the tumors are asymptomatic. Previously, Briselli and associates (1981), in a review of 368 patients with these tumors recorded in the literature, including eight of their own cases, noted that 64% were reported to have had symptomatic lesions. However, this included many patients diagnosed late, and in addition, 12% of these patients had malignant lesions. Okike (1978) and England (1989) and their colleagues reported that chronic cough, chest pain, and dyspnea were the most common complaints (Table 64-2). Chest pain is most often manifested when the lesion arises from the parietal pleura. Occasionally, in a patient with a large tumor, symptoms of bronchial compression

one of the aforementioned patterns, are described as storiform, herringbone, leiomyomalike, or neurofibromalike. Moran and associates (1992) have discussed the histologic growth patterns in both the benign and the malignant solitary fibrous pleural tumors.

Ultrastructural Features

Ultrastructurally, single to clusters of fusiform to round cells are found interspaced between focal or abundant collagen. The cells, according to Said and colleagues (1984), most closely resemble mesenchymal cells of fibroblastic type. Keating and coworkers (1987) noted that no basal lamina, intracellular junctions, or microvilli are seen. The observations of El-Naggar (1989) and Steinetz (1990) and their associates support the fibroblastic nature of these cells.

Immunohistologic Features

Immunohistochemically, the spindle cells that make up these tumors do not express low- or high-molecular-weight keratin reactivity; nor do they express epithelial membrane

Table 64-2. Symptoms of Benign Localized Fibrous Tumors of the Pleura

Symptom	Okike et al. (1978) 52 Patients	England et al. (1989) 138 Patients
Asymptomatic	28	92
Chronic cough	17	16
Chest pain	12	26
Dyspnea	10	15
Fever	9	1
Hypertrophic pulmonary osteo-arthropathy with or without clubbing	10	—
Pleurisy	3	—
Weight loss	3	3
Hemoptysis	1	0
Pneumonitis	1	—

and atelectasis may occur. Okike and colleagues (1978) recorded the occurrence of hypertrophic pulmonary osteoarthropathy in 20% of their patients. Briselli and associates (1981), in their collective review, reported an incidence of 22%. Frequently, the tumor is of large size (larger than 7 cm) when this is observed.

Hypertrophic Pulmonary Osteoarthropathy

This symptom complex occurs in association with many intrathoracic disease processes. Clagett and colleagues (1952) at the Mayo Clinic reported that hypertrophic pulmonary osteoarthropathy occurred in 66% of cases of localized fibrous tumor of the pleura, although their later data presented by Okike and associates (1978) noted this association in only 20% of instances. Nonetheless, this pattern contrasts markedly with the overall 5% incidence of hypertrophic pulmonary osteoarthropathy in bronchial carcinoma, as reported in one of the lead articles in the *Lancet* (Lead Article, 1959). We have observed the incidence to be only 2 to 3% in this latter disease.

Osteoarthropathy describes a rheumatoidlike disease of the bones and joints. It is frequently associated with clubbing of the fingers, but it may be present without clubbing. Gynecomastia is similarly seen with hypertrophic pulmonary osteoarthropathy yet also occurs as a solitary extrathoracic manifestation of an intrathoracic neoplasm.

The classic findings in hypertrophic pulmonary osteoarthropathy include stiffness of the joints, edema over the ankles and occasionally of the hands, arthralgia, and pain along the surfaces of the long bones, especially the tibia. At times, the joint and bone pain is severe.

The joint and bone involvement is usually bilateral. The distal ends of the ulna and radius are most frequently involved, and radiographic evidence of the periosteal thickening is most commonly seen here. The bones of the hands, ankles, knees, elbows, and shoulders are involved in that approximate order.

Finger pressure on the anterior surface of the distal tibia often elicits pain in advance of any radiologic changes.

Clinical symptoms vary from minimally detectable stiffness of the wrists to systemic toxicity. Some of the systemic manifestations seem to be related to one or more endocrine, collagen, or immunologic mechanisms of the body that are not directly related to the osteoarthropathy. Chills and spiking temperature, markedly elevated sedimentation rate, and malaise with obvious systemic toxicity may be present.

Hypertrophic pulmonary osteoarthropathy may be associated with clubbing of the fingers and toes, although many investigators believe the latter is not actually part of the syndrome. Martinez-Lavin (1987), as well as Shneerson (1981), however, have suggested that the two processes are related and arise from the same underlying cause, most likely the overproduction or lack of metabolism by the lung of a growthlike hormone.

Clubbing

Clubbing is the enlargement of the distal phalanges, usually of both the hands and feet. Diner (1962) described periosteal new growth with lymphocytic and plasma cell infiltration of connective tissue around the nail beds, resulting in increased fibrous tissue between the nail bed and phalanx. Van Hazel (1940) reported the digital arteries to be enlarged and elongated 10 to 15 times normal. Also, Cudkowicz and Armstrong (1953) noted the presence of arteriovenous anastomosis in the distal finger segments near the junction of the dermis and the subcutaneous tissue.

Clinically, the distal phalanx is enlarged, especially widened, with a loss of the obtuse angle that the nail bed normally forms with the plane of the proximal skin surface. A spongy sensation on depression of the proximal nail bed is characteristic.

According to Martinez-Lavin (1987), a common denominator appears to be present in the various processes associated with clubbing. These processes can be broadly classified into pulmonary, cardiac, and extrathoracic. Only the first category is discussed.

Neoplastic lesions of the lung causing clubbing are generally associated with hypertrophic pulmonary osteoarthropathy, whereas the congenital structural and inflammatory pulmonary lesions associated with clubbing rarely show signs of arthropathy. Nonneoplastic pulmonary disorders seen with clubbing include pulmonary arteriovenous fistula, lung abscess, bronchiectasis, empyema, pulmonary infarction, emphysema, chronic bronchitis, chronic inflammation of the lung, sarcoidosis, idiopathic pulmonary fibrosis, diffuse interstitial fibrosis, primary pulmonary hypertension, pneumoconiosis, and atelectasis.

Etiology

The etiology of hypertrophic pulmonary osteoarthropathy and clubbing remains an enigma. A single cause for these two frequently associated yet distinct phenomena seems unlikely. Flavell (1956) reported relief from the pain of hypertrophic osteoarthropathy after division of the vagus nerve at the hilus of the lung in patients with inoperable pulmonary neoplasms. Diner (1962) described dramatic relief of symptoms after cervical or thoracic vagotomy. Ginsburg (1958) found that blood flows in the hand and foot were similar in a control group and in patients with hypertrophic pulmonary osteoarthropathy. Lovell (1950), however, demonstrated increased blood flow in patients with clubbing secondary to congenital cyanotic heart disease. These patients had dilatated venous plexuses in the skin of the nail bed area, accompanied by increased caliber in the digital arteries and abnormal arteriovenous communications.

Although the cause of these conditions remains unknown, several observations may be made. First, clubbing of the fingers has some connection with arteriovenous shunting. Whether these abnormal arteriovenous communications permit a substance that is normally altered or detoxified in the lung to appear in the systemic circulation or whether small emboli that are usually filtered out by the lung are allowed to appear there is unanswered, but certainly the latter is highly debatable. Cudkowicz and Armstrong (1953) demonstrated precapillary bronchopulmonary anastomosis in patients with clubbing. Desaturation of the blood per se seems an unlikely explanation because the incidence of clubbing in severely emphysematous patients is so low. Second, circumstantial evidence exists in the relationship of hypertrophic pulmonary osteoarthropathy and involvement of the pleura. This aspect is borne out by the occurrence of the syndrome in some patients with localized fibrous tumors of the pleura, as well as in patients with peripheral bronchial carcinomas. A neoplastic process involving the pleura, the embryologic origin of which is pluripotential, may elaborate a substance that elicits osseous articular responses. This same neoplastic process also might create an arteriovenous fistula, producing clubbing. It has been suggested by Steiner (1968) and Gosney (1990) and their colleagues that ectopic production of a growth hormone–like substance by a tumor may result in the development of clubbing, as well as in pulmonary osteoarthropathy.

The clinical significance of hypertrophic pulmonary osteoarthropathy is greater in its diagnostic than its therapeutic implications. Removal of the pulmonary lesion for the most part gives dramatic remission of the arthralgia and peripheral edema. In the series reported by Okike and associates (1978), 8 of 10 patients with localized fibrous tumors experienced complete relief of the symptom complex after operative removal of the tumor. Osseous radiographic changes regress much more slowly. Recurrence of a localized fibrous tumor is usually heralded by a return of the symptoms present with the original osteoarthropathy.

Hypoglycemia

A large benign localized fibrous tumor of the pleura may be associated with a severe hypoglycemia. An incidence of 3 to 4% has been stated. In addition, a number of diverse mesenchymal tumors also have been reported to have an infrequent association with this condition. In 1968, Devroede and Tirol reported that 58 examples of hypoglycemia secondary to a mesenchymal tumor had been recorded in the literature up to that time. According to Silverstein and associates (1964), most of those were fibrosarcomas, although examples of neurofibroma, rhabdomyosarcoma, liposarcoma, leiomyosarcoma, hemangiopericytoma, and mesothelioma were also noted.

As in the instances of hypoglycemia from other causes, the patient can present with varying symptoms of central nervous system deprivation of glucose. Convulsions, syncope, and even coma may occur. Death may result if the severe hypoglycemia is not corrected promptly.

Nelson and coworkers (1975) reviewed the numerous theories to explain the mechanism of hypoglycemia. Among these are 1) increased glucose consumption by the tumor; 2) a defect in glucose regulators (i.e., adrenocorticotropic hormone, growth hormone, or glucagon); 3) ectopic secretion of insulin by the tumor, the presence of a stimulator of insulin release, or a potentiator of circulating insulin; 4) the inhibition of glycogenolysis; 5) the inhibition of lipolysis and hepatic gluconeogenesis; and 6) the presence of nonsuppressible insulinlike activity and insulin growth factors I and II. Most of these theories have been disproved, and Nelson and associates (1975) suggested that increased glucose use by the tumor was probably a partial explanation. Bunn and Ridgway (1989), however, reported that tumor use of glucose to a degree that causes hypoglycemia has not yet been substantiated. Currently, these latter authors believe the most likely, although far from established, mechanism is tumor production of nonsuppressible insulinlike active substances, called *somatomedins*, and insulinlike growth factors. Somatomedins are reported by Van Wyk and associates (1974) to be a family of peptide hormones produced by the liver under growth hormone regulation. Zaph (1981), Gordon (1981), and Li (1983) and their colleagues have reported these substances in various examples of extrapancreatic tumor hypoglycemia. Cole (1990) and Strøm (1991) and their associates have demonstrated insulinlike growth factors in one patient each who had associated hypoglycemia with a benign fibrous pleural tumor. The hypoglycemia was relieved in each with removal of the tumor. The relief of the hypoglycemia associated with a benign fibrous tumor is typical after complete removal of the tumor.

Galactorrhea

Galactorrhea is a rare finding in patients with fibrous tumors of the pleura. It has been reported, however, by Briselli (1981) and McCaughey (1985) and their associates.

Radiographic Features

The appearance of a localized fibrous tumor of the pleura is for the most part indistinguishable from that of other nod-

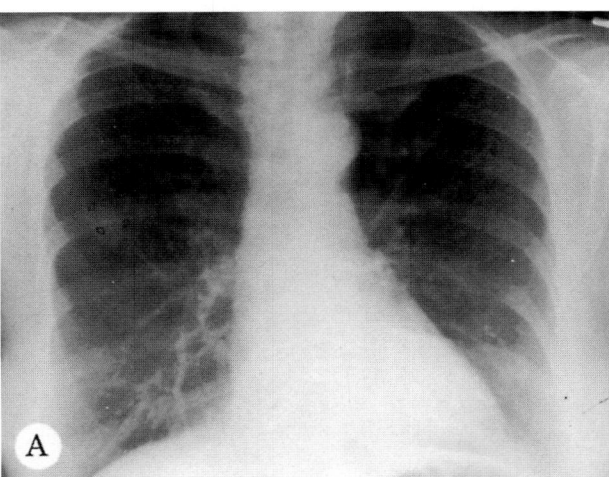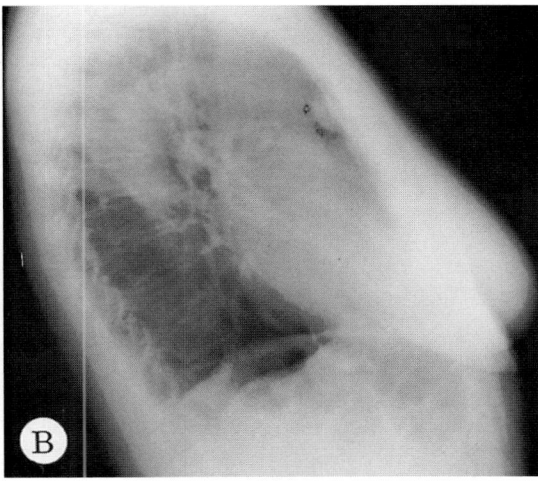

Fig. 64-2. Posteroanterior (**A**) and lateral (**B**) radiographs of the chest of a 68-year-old woman revealing a small peripheral mass in the anterior aspect of right upper lobe. At thoracotomy the mass was found to be a pedunculated fibrous tumor attached to the visceral pleura of the right upper lobe.

ules of the lung (Fig. 64-2). A circumscribed mass of varying size usually is located in the lung periphery or in the projection of an interlobar fissure. The larger neoplasms may have irregular shapes, although the margins are usually sharply defined. These tumors arise, more often from a pedicle from the visceral pleura. Desser and Stark (1998) have reviewed the radiologic findings. Occasionally, movement of the mass may be demonstrated with changes in position, as recorded by Lewis and associates (1985), when the tumor is on a stalk. Zirinsky and Hsu (1982) also demonstrated this change in location by computed tomography. However, computed tomographic examination per se has little to add to the standard radiographic examination of these lesions. Mendelson and colleagues (1991) have reviewed the computed tomographic findings relative to this tumor. Infrequently, a pleural effusion may be present. In the collective review of England and associates (1989), 8% of 138 patients had a pleural effusion as the initial clinical finding.

Diagnosis

Fine-needle aspiration biopsy appears to be a valuable tool in establishing a diagnosis in these peripherally located tumors. Milano (1990) has suggested that it may occasionally be diagnostic. Dusenbery (1991), Apple (1997) and Weynand (1998) and their colleagues reported cytologic features of solitary fibrous tumors of the pleura. Their studies are based on fine-needle aspiration of these peripherally located tumors, preparation of cell blocks from the aspirations, and immunohistochemistry performed on the cell block. Immunohistochemically, the spindle cells of the tumor have negative results to keratin and positive results to CD34 antibodies. In association with cytologic features,

immunohistochemistry, and characteristic radiologic findings, a precise diagnosis can be made preoperatively.

Treatment

Localized fibrous tumors of the pleura are usually amenable to surgical resection (Fig. 64-3). Tumors that are considered benign on the basis of being localized, however, may be malignant both histologically and clinically, so adequate removal of the original lesion must be ensured. Nothing in our experience suggests that lobectomy is preferable to local resection of a pedunculated lesion arising from the visceral pleura. If the lesion is within the lung parenchyma, however, resection of the lobe is advisable. A segmentectomy is occasionally sufficient, but even a bilobectomy may be necessary when the lesion is located within a fissure. Localized fibrous tumors of the mediastinal, diaphragmatic, and parietal pleura should be excised as widely as can be accomplished satisfactorily because these locations are more often associated with a malignant lesion.

Prognosis

Almost all patients with benign localized fibrous tumors of the pleura are cured by adequate excision of the lesion. Nomori and associates (1997) describe a benign fibrous tumor arising from the diaphragm with subsequent recurrence of the tumor to the parietal pleura within an area of contact from the primary tumor. England and associates (1989) noted only two recurrences in 98 patients (2%) and in both patients a second curative resection was possible. Any recurrences, however, must be viewed with suspicion.

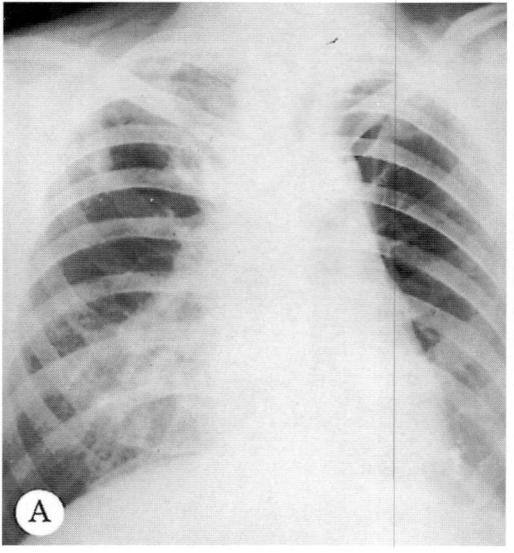 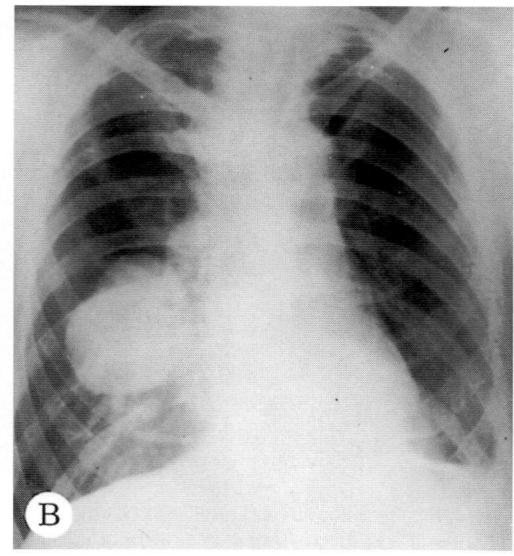

Fig. 64-3. A. Radiograph of chest revealing a 3-cm solitary nodule at the level of the fifth interspace anteriorly in the right lung. **B.** Radiograph of the same patient 10 years later, revealing marked enlargement of the mass. At thoracotomy a benign fibrous tumor was readily removed.

MALIGNANT LOCALIZED FIBROUS TUMORS OF THE PLEURA

Incidence

The relative incidence of malignant localized fibrous tumors as compared with that of the benign lesions is unknown. Thirty-six percent of the fibrous pleural tumors reviewed by England and associates (1989) were malignant, but all of the 223 cases had been referred to the Armed Forces Institute of Pathology for study and represent a biased database. In the review of 360 cases by Briselli and colleagues (1981), the incidence of malignant tumors was 12%. In the report from the Mayo Clinic by Okike and coworkers (1978), the incidence was 13%; these latter figures may represent a more appropriate incidence of malignancy.

Pathologic Characteristics

Gross Features

The malignant variety of fibrous tumor, as compared with benign tumors, tends to be large, to be more often located atypically (from the parietal pleura, intralobar in location, or to exhibit inverted growth into the pulmonary parenchyma), and to show areas of necrosis and hemorrhage (Table 64-3 and Fig. 64-4).

Microscopic Features

Malignant fibrous tumors of the pleura, in contrast to benign tumors, show an increased cellularity, cellular pleo-

morphism, and an increased number of mitotic figures (Fig. 64-5; see Table 64-3). El-Naggar and associates (1989) observed higher mitotic counts than in the benign tumors. Extensive areas of myxomatous change, hemorrhage, and necrosis also are seen commonly.

Other Features

Immunohistochemically, no differences exist between benign and malignant tumors. The ultrastructural findings are not truly distinguishable from those tumors of the

Table 64-3. Pathologic Features That Distinguish Benign and Malignant Localized Fibrous Tumor of Pleura

Feature	Benign (n = 141)		Malignant[a] (n = 82)	
	n	%	n	%
Gross				
Pedunculated	73	52	21	26
Atypical location[b]	67	48	55	67
Size (>10 cm)	34	24	45	55
Necrosis and hemorrhage	21	15	53	65
Microscopic				
Increased cellularity	18	13	62	76
Pleomorphism[c]	14	10	69	84
Mitosis (>4 mf/10 hpf)	2	1	63	77

[a]For all features, the differences between benign and malignant tumors are statistically significant by the Chi-square test (P <.05).
[b]Tumor attached to parietal pleura, fissure, or mediastinum or inverted into peripheral lung.
[c]Pleomorphism expressed as increased nuclear grades.
From England DM, Hochholzer L, McCarthy MJ: Localized benign and malignant fibrous tumors of the pleura. A clinicopathologic review of 223 cases. Am J Surg Pathol *13*:640, 1989. With permission.

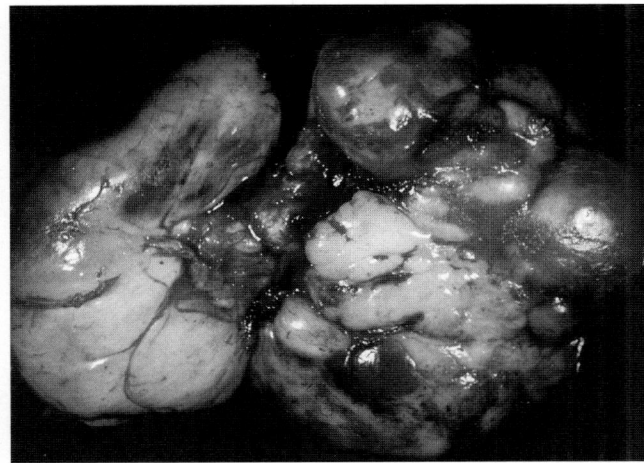

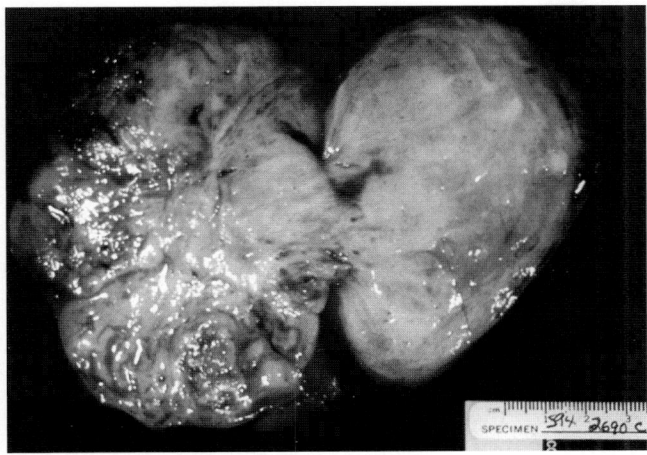

Fig. 64-4. Gross morphology of a malignant fibrous tumor in a 77-year-old man. **A.** The lobulated mass weighed 624 g and measured 15 × 11 × 5 cm. **B.** Cut section of the tumor shows a firm tumor with areas of necrosis and hemorrhage. The tumor recurred in 8 months and the patient died after 17 months.

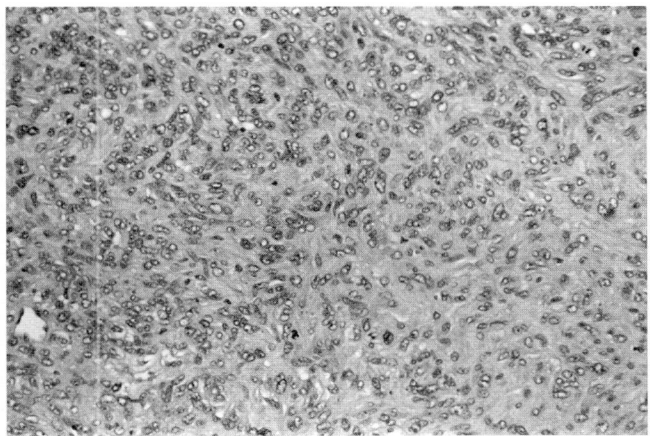

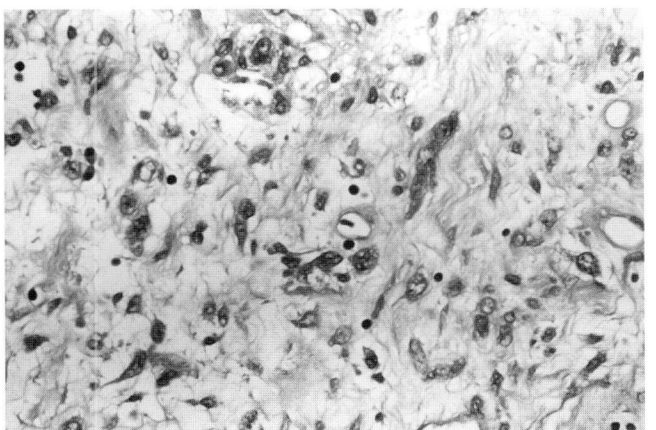

Fig. 64-5. Microscopic section of a malignant fibrous tumor of the pleura. **A.** Histology demonstrates increased cellularity and increased number of mitotic figures. **B.** High power shows cellular pleomorphism.

benign variety. Flow cytometric DNA studies showed an elevated S-phase in contrast to a low S-phase in benign lesions according to the study of El-Naggar and associates (1989). Uzoaru and associates (1994) described a single case of malignant fibrous tumor occurring in a 15-year-old girl; flow cytometric analysis revealed an aneuploid population of tumor cells.

Clinical Features

Most of these patients, approximately three-quarters, in contrast to those with localized benign mesotheliomas, have symptoms. Chest pain, cough, dyspnea, and fever are the most common symptoms. Osteoarthropathy rarely, if ever, occurs with the localized malignant lesion. Hypoglycemia, however, is more commonly seen in patients with the malignant than the benign fibrous tumors of the pleura. An inci-

dence of 11% as compared with 3%, respectively, is found according to the data of England and associates (1989).

Radiographic Features

The radiographic findings in patients with malignant fibrous tumors of the pleura are similar to those seen in patients with the benign variety, except the lesions tend to be larger and pleural effusion is seen more often. An incidence of associated pleural effusion of 32% was recorded by England and associates (1989). Occasionally, rib erosion may occur as the result of invasion of the chest wall.

Diagnosis

In most instances, the diagnosis is not apparent until histologic examination of the resected specimen. Invasion of the chest wall or other adjacent structures within the chest grossly establishes the malignant nature of the lesion.

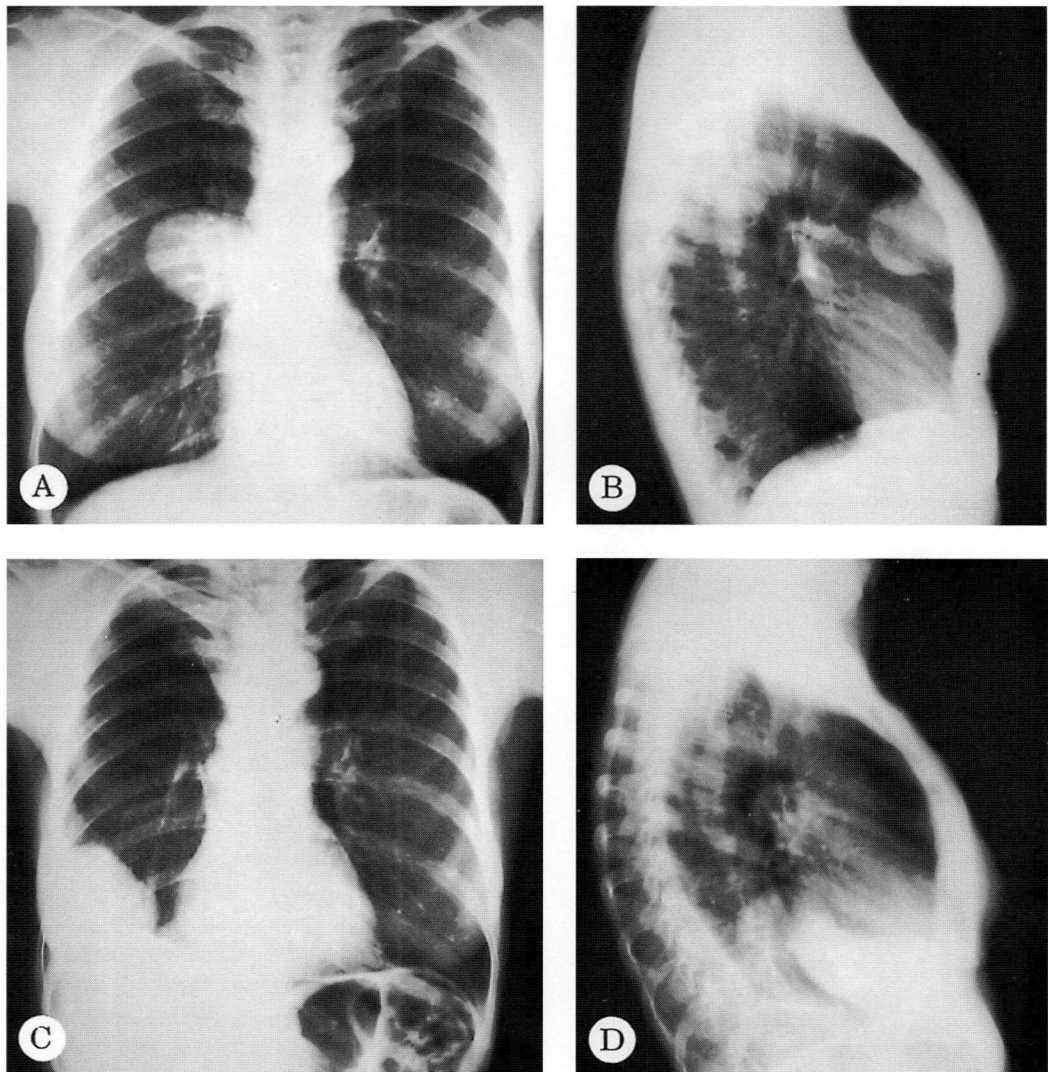

Fig. 64-6. A and B. Posteroanterior and lateral radiographs of the chest revealing a large solitary mass, which was diagnosed as a benign fibrous tumor on its removal by a right upper lobectomy. **C and D.** Posteroanterior and lateral radiographs of the chest 6 months after removal of the tumor, revealing rapid recurrence of the tumor, which required a pneumonectomy for its complete removal. The mass was frankly malignant on histologic examination. The patient succumbed to recurrent malignant fibrous tumor of the pleura.

Recurrence of a lesion originally thought to be benign must be regarded as suggesting the true malignant nature of the lesion (Fig. 64-6).

Treatment

Wide local excision, including pulmonary and pleural resections, is carried out as indicated. Resection of a lesion arising from the parietal pleura should include the adjacent chest wall. When complete resection is possible, postoperative adjuvant therapy (irradiation or chemotherapy) is not indicated. When the resection is incomplete, Martini and

associates (1987) suggest that radiation therapy, both internal (brachytherapy) and external, should be used. Localized recurrence of a solitary malignant fibrous tumor should be evaluated for possible resection.

Prognosis

Okike and colleagues (1978) reported only a 12% long-term survival in patients with localized malignant tumors. England and associates (1989), however, reported a survival of 45% among 71 patients they considered to have had malignant lesions; most of the survivors had either pedun-

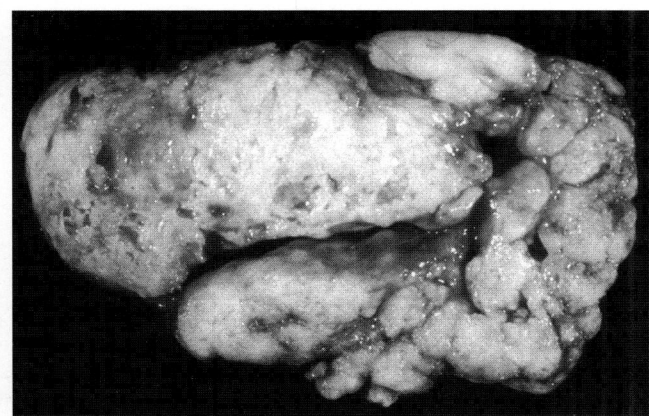

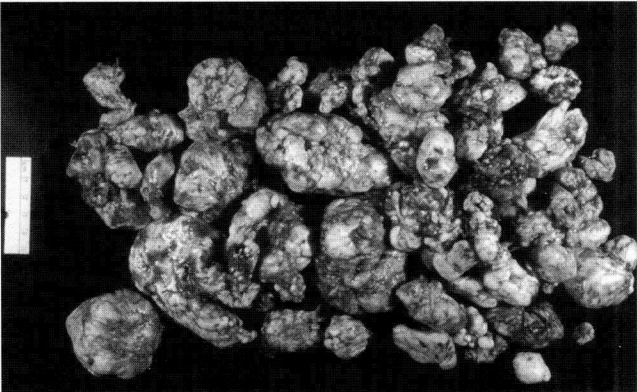

Fig. 64-7. Gross morphology of a recurrent malignant fibrous tumor from a 60-year-old woman. **A and B.** Multiple nodules of various sizes are seen.

culated or well-circumscribed tumors. Chest wall or pericardial invasion does not preclude long-term survival if a complete excision can be carried out. Pleural effusion is a poor prognostic feature in the patients with a malignant fibrous tumor of the pleura.

Martini and colleagues (1987) reported 10 patients with long-term survival after complete resection of the tumor. England and associates (1989) concur that the most important indicator of clinical outcome is whether the tumor can be totally excised initially. Patients with incomplete excision all die from their disease.

Recurrences of even completely excised lesions do occur. Initially, these are almost always local at the site of excision. However, spread to other sites within the thorax or into the abdomen occurs (Fig. 64-7). Lymph node metastases are seen, as are blood-borne metastases, in patients with persistent or recurrent disease. The sites of metastases recorded, in order of decreasing frequency, are the liver, central nervous system, spleen, peritoneum, adrenal gland, gastrointestinal tract, kidney, intra-abdominal lymph nodes, and bone. Most patients with recurrent disease survive less than 5 years.

REFERENCES

Apple SK, Nieberg RK, Hirschowitz SL: Fine needle aspiration biopsy of solitary fibrous tumor of the pleura. A report of two cases with discussion of diagnostic pitfalls. Acta Cytol *42*:1528, 1997.

Briselli M, Mark EJ, Dickersin R: Solitary fibrous tumors of the pleura: eight new cases and review of 360 cases in the literature. Cancer *47*:2678, 1981.

Bunn PA Jr, Ridgway EC: Paraneoplastic syndromes. *In* DeVita VT Jr, Hellman S, Rosenberg SA (eds): Cancer: Principles and Practice of Oncology. 3rd Ed. Philadelphia: JB Lippincott, 1989, p. 1896.

Clagett OT, McDonald JR, Schmidt HW: Localized fibrous mesothelioma of the pleura. J Thorac Surg *24*:213, 1952.

Cole FH, et al: Benign fibrous pleural tumor with elevation of insulin-like growth factor and hypoglycemia. South Med J *83*:690, 1990.

Cudkowicz L, Armstrong JB: Finger clubbing and changes in the bronchial circulation. Br J Tuberc Dis Chest *47*:277, 1953.

Dalton WR, et al: Localized primary tumors of the pleura: an analysis of 40 cases. Cancer *44*:1465, 1979.

Dervan PA, Tobin B, O'Connor M: Solitary localized fibrous mesothelioma: evidence against mesothelial cell origin. Histopathology *10*:867, 1986.

Desser TS, Stark P: Pictorial essay: solitary tumor of the pleura. J Thorac Imaging *13*:27, 1998.

Devroede J, Tirol AF: Grant pleural mesothelioma associated with hypoglycemia and hyperthyroidism. Am J Surg *116*:130, 1968.

Diner WC: Hypertrophic osteoarthropathy. JAMA *181*:555, 1962.

Dusenbery D, Grimes MM, Frable WJ: Fine needle aspiration cytology of localized fibrous tumor of pleura. Diagn Cytopathol *8*:444, 1992.

El-Naggar AK, et al: Localized fibrous tumor of the serosal cavities: immunohistochemical, electron-microscopic and flow-cytometric DNA study. Am J Clin Pathol *92*:561, 1989.

England DM, Hochholzer L, McCarthy MJ: Localized benign and malignant fibrous tumors of the pleura: a clinicopathologic review of 223 cases. Am J Surg Pathol *13*:640, 1989.

Flavell G: Reversal of pulmonary hypertrophic osteoarthropathy by vagotomy. Lancet *1*:260, 1956.

Flint A, Weiss SW: CD-34 and keratin expression distinguishes solitary fibrous tumor (fibrous mesothelioma) of pleura from desmoplastic mesothelioma. Human Pathol *26*:428, 1995.

Ginsburg J: Observations on the peripheral circulation in hypertrophic pulmonary osteoarthropathy. Q J Med *27*:335, 1958.

Gordon P, et al: Hypoglycemia associated with non-let cell tumors and insulin like growth factors. N Engl J Med *305*:1452, 1981.

Gosney MA, Gosney JR, Lye M: Plasma growth hormone and digital clubbing in carcinoma of the bronchus. Thorax *45*:545, 1990.

Hanan CA, Mietinen M: Solitary fibrous tumor: histological and immunohistochemical spectrum of benign and malignant variants presenting at different sites. Hum Pathol *26*:440, 1995.

Keating S, et al: Solitary fibrous tumor of the pleura: an ultrastructural and immunohistochemical study. Thorax *42*:976, 1987.

Lead article: Lancet *2*:389, 1959.

Lewis MI, et al: The case of the moving intrathoracic mass. Chest *88*:897, 1985.

Li TCM, et al: Surgical cure of hypoglycemia associated with cystosarcoma phylloides and elevated NSILP. Am J Med *74*:1080, 1983.

Lovell RRH: Observations on the structure of clubbed fingers. Clin Sci *9*:299, 1950.

Martinez-Lavin M: Digital clubbing and hypertrophic osteoarthropathy: a unifying hypothesis. J Rheumatol *14*:6, 1987.

Martini N, et al: Pleural mesothelioma: current review. Ann Thorac Surg *43*:113, 1987.

McCaughey WTE, Kannerstein M, Churg J (eds): Tumors of submesothelial origin. *In* Tumors and Pseudotumors of the Serous Membranes. Bethesda, MD: Armed Forces Institute of Pathology, 1980, p. 81.

Mendelson DS, et al: Localized fibrous pleural mesothelioma: CT findings. Clin Imaging *15*:105, 1991.

Metintas M, et al: Malignant localized fibrous tumor of the pleura occurring in a person environmentally exposed to tremolite asbestos. Respiration *64*:236, 1997.

Milano MJ: Benign mesothelioma. *In* Deslauriers J, Lacquet LK (eds): Thoracic Surgery: Surgical Management of Pleural Disease. St. Louis: CV Mosby, 1990.

Moran CA, Suster S, Koss MN: The spectrum of histologic growth patterns in benign and malignant fibrous tumors of the pleura. Semin Diagn Pathol 9:169, 1992.

Nelson R, et al: Hypoglycemic coma associated with benign pleural mesothelioma. J Thorac Cardiovasc Surg 69:306, 1975.

Nomori H, et al: Contacting metastasis of a fibrous tumor of the pleura. Eur J Cardiothorac Surg 12:928, 1997.

Okike N, Bernatz PE, Woolner LB: Localized mesothelioma of the pleura. Benign and malignant variants. J Thorac Cardiovasc Surg 75:363, 1978.

Said JW, et al: Localized fibrous mesothelioma: an immunohistochemical and electron microscopic study. Hum Pathol 15:440, 1984.

Scharifker D, Kaneko M: Localized fibrous "mesothelioma" of pleura (submesothelial) fibroma: a clinicopathologic study of 18 cases. Cancer 43:627, 1979.

Shneerson JM: Digital clubbing and hypertrophic osteoarthropathy: the underlying mechanisms. Br J Dis Chest 75:113, 1981.

Silverstein MN, Wakin KE, Bahn RC: Hypoglycemia associated with neoplasia. Am J Med 36:415, 1964.

Steiner H, Dahlback O, Waldenstrom J: Ectopic growth hormone production and osteoarthropathy in carcinoma of the bronchus. Lancet 1:783, 1968.

Steinetz C, et al: Localized fibrous tumors of the pleura: correlation of histopathological, immunohistochemical and ultrastructural features. Pathol Res Pract 186:344, 1990.

Stout AP: Tumors of the pleura. Harlem Hosp Bull 5:54, 1971.

Strøm EH, et al: Solitary fibrous tumor of the pleura. An immunohistochemical, electron-microscopic and tissue culture of a tumor producing insulin-like growth factor I in a patient with hypoglycemia. Pathol Res Pract 187:109, 1991.

Suster S, Fisher C, Moran CA: Expression of bcl-2 oncoprotein in benign and malignant spindle cell tumors of soft tissue, skin, serosal surfaces, and gastrointestinal tract. Am J Surg Pathol 22:863, 1998.

Uzoaru I, Chou P, Reyes-Mugica M: Malignant solitary fibrous tumor of the pleura. Pediatr Pathol 14:11, 1994.

Van de Rijn M, Lombard CM, Rouse RV: Expression of CD34 by solitary fibrous tumors of the pleura, mediastinum, and lung. Am J Surg Pathol 18:814, 1994.

Van Hazel W: Joint manifestations associated with intrathoracic tumors. J Thorac Surg 9:495, 1940.

Van Wyk JJ, et al: The somatomedans: a family of insulin-like hormones under growth hormone control. Recent Prog Horm Res 30:259, 1974.

Westra WH, Gerald WL, Rosai J: Solitary fibrous tumor. Consistent CD34 immunoreactivity and occurrence in the orbit. Am J Surg Pathol 18:992, 1994.

Weynand B, Collard P, Galant C: Cytopathological features of solitary fibrous tumor of the pleura: a study of 5 cases. Diagn Cytopathol 18:118,1998.

Witkin FB, Rosai J: Solitary fibrous tumor of the mediastinum, a report of 14 cases. Am J Surg Pathol 13:547, 1989.

Yousem SA, Flynn DS: Intrapulmonary localized fibrous tumor: intraparenchymal so-called localized fibrous mesothelioma. Am J Clin Pathol 89:365, 1988.

Zaph J, Walter H, Froesch ER: Radioimmunological determination of insulin-like growth factors I and II in normal subjects and in patients with growth disorders and extrapancreatic tumor hypoglycemia. J Clin Invest 68:1321, 1981.

Zirinsky K, Hsu JT: Flopping mass in an asymptomatic woman. Chest 81:733, 1982.

READING REFERENCES

Arkless D, Goranow I, Krastinow G: Hypoglycemia in an intrathoracic fibroma. Med Bull Vet Admin 19:225, 1942.

Arrigoni MC, et al: Benign tumors of the lung: a ten-year surgical experience. J Thorac Cardiovasc Surg 60:589, 1970.

Aufiero TX, et al: Intrapulmonary benign fibrous tumor of the pleura. J Thorac Cardiovasc Surg 110:549, 1995.

Barclay N, Ogbeide M, Grillo A: Gross hypertrophic pulmonary osteoarthropathy in a 7-year-old child. Thorax 25:484, 1970.

Barrett NR: The pleura. Thorax 25:515, 1970.

Berne AS, Heitzman ER: The roentgenologic signs of pedunculated pleural tumors. AJR Am J Roentgenol 87:892, 1962.

Cudkowicz L, Wraith DC: A method of study of the pulmonary circulation in finger clubbing. Thorax 12:313, 1957.

Hernandez FJ, Fernandez BB: Localized fibrous tumors of pleura: a light and electron microscopic study. Cancer 34:1667, 1974.

Maier HC, Barr D: Intrathoracic tumors associated with hypoglycemia. J Thorac Cardiovasc Surg 44:321, 1962.

Marie P: De l'ostéoarthropathie hypertrophiante pneumonique. Rev Med Paris 10:1, 1890.

Sanguinetti CM, et al: Localized fibrous pleural tumour of the interlobular pleura. Eur Respir J 9:1094, 1996.

Spry CI, Williamson DH, James ML: Pleuromesothelioma and hypoglycemia. Proc R Soc Med 61:1105, 1968.

Sternon I, Paramentier G, Rutsaert J: Comas hypoglycemiques et mesotheliome pleural benin. Acta Clin Belg 26:44, 1971.

Von Bamberger E: Ueber Knochenveranderungen bei chronischen Lungen- und Herzkrankheiten. Z Klin Med 18:193, 1890.

Wierman H, Clagett OT, McDonald JR: Articular manifestations in pulmonary diseases. JAMA 155:1459, 1954.

CHAPTER 65

Diffuse Malignant Mesothelioma

Valerie W. Rusch

Diffuse malignant pleural mesothelioma is an uncommon and lethal cancer for which there is currently no standard treatment. The first report of a primary pleural tumor, presumably a mesothelioma, is attributed to Lieutaud in 1767, but there was no precise pathologic description until Klemperer and Rabin (1937) classified mesotheliomas as either localized or diffuse. Cell culture experiments by Stout and Murray (1942) examined the histological origin of these tumors. However, mesothelioma was largely regarded as a medical curiosity until 1960, when Wagner and coworkers reported 33 cases of diffuse malignant pleural mesothelioma in asbestos mine workers from the Northwestern Cape Province of South Africa. Subsequent studies, especially work by Selikoff and associates (1965) and Whitwell and Rawcliffe (1971) in the United States, confirmed that asbestos exposure was the major risk factor for malignant mesothelioma. The epidemiology of diffuse malignant mesothelioma is now well understood, but its biological behavior remains an enigma, and the treatment of this cancer is still controversial.

The incidence of malignant mesothelioma is increasing because of the large number of individuals who were exposed to asbestos during the 1930s to 1960s in asbestos mines and asbestos-related industries, before the causal relationship between asbestos and mesothelioma was recognized. An estimated 2000 to 3000 cases occur annually in the United States. It is important for thoracic surgeons to be knowledgeable about mesothelioma because they are often called on to make the diagnosis and to recommend treatment.

EPIDEMIOLOGY AND INCIDENCE

A relationship between asbestos exposure and interstitial lung disease was first recognized in 1906, when deaths among asbestos textile workers from pneumoconiosis were reported in England and France by Murray (1907) and Auribault (1906). Scattered case reports by Wedler (1943a,b), Cartier and Smith (1952), and Van der Schoot (1958) suggested a link between asbestos exposure and diffuse malignant mesothelioma, but this was not clearly established until Wagner's reports (1960, 1986). Wagner was appointed Asbestosis Research Fellow at the South Africa Pneumoconiosis Research Unit in 1954 and was charged with determining if all types of asbestos caused the same diseases. An increasing frequency of a fatal pleural tumor in patients hospitalized at the Tuberculosis Hospital in the asbestos mining region of South Africa led Wagner and associates to study pleural biopsies on these patients. The surprise finding of mesothelioma in these biopsies prompted a careful epidemiologic study. Asbestos exposure was the single factor common to all these cases. Subsequently, Wagner went to Great Britain to study this problem further, and he again demonstrated an epidemiologic relationship between asbestos exposure and mesothelioma among asbestos workers and insulators.

The second direct demonstration of the link between asbestos exposure and mesothelioma, described by Layman (1992) and Musk and colleagues (1989), occurred in Western Australia where, from 1943 to 1966, approximately 7000 individuals at the Wittenoom asbestos mines had extensive exposure to asbestos. The first case of mesothelioma was diagnosed in 1960. By the end of 1986, 94 cases of mesothelioma, 141 cases of lung cancer, and 356 successful compensation claims for asbestosis were recorded among former miners and their family members. An additional 692 cases of mesothelioma are expected to occur in this cohort between 1987 and 2020. The Wittenoom asbestos industry is considered the worst industrial disaster in Australian history.

As reported by de Klerk and Armstrong (1992), the type of asbestos fiber plays a critical role in the risk of developing mesothelioma. Asbestos belongs to the family of silicate fibers and includes two mineralogical groups: amphibole and serpentine fibers. Chrysotile asbestos is the only member of the serpentine group, whereas crocidolite, amosite, tremolite, anthrophyllite, and actinolite asbestos belong to the amphibole group. Pooley (1987) reports that these minerals differ considerably in their structure and composition. Serpentine fibers are large, curly shaped fibers that do not travel beyond the major airways, whereas amphibole fibers are narrow and straight fibers that migrate through the lymphatics of the pulmonary parenchyma and accumulate in the interstitial spaces and the subpleural region. It is the amphibole fibers, especially crocidolite asbestos ("blue asbestos") that are most clearly associated with malignant mesothelioma. Chrysotile is more closely associated with the development of lung cancer.

Crocidolite asbestos is found only in South Africa and Western Australia but has been exported all over the world for various industrial uses. Chrysotile ("white asbestos") accounts for 97% of worldwide asbestos production and is mined principally in the Ural Mountains in Russia, Quebec Province in Canada, Zimbabwe and Swaziland in South Africa, the Italian Alps, and Cyprus. Churg and DePaoli (1988) and McDonald and coworkers (1989) report that chrysotile itself is not thought to cause mesothelioma but is often contaminated with amphibole fibers, such as tremolite or amosite ("brown asbestos").

Individuals can be exposed to asbestos in many situations because it has a thousand uses, as reported by Huncharek (1992). However, as discussed by Andersson and Olsen (1985), Malker and associates (1985), and McDonald and McDonald (1980), the areas of the world that have a high incidence of mesothelioma are those with asbestos mines and countries that have shipyards, insulation, construction, and automobile industries that use large amounts of asbestos. In North America, the highest incidence areas include the provinces of Quebec and British Columbia in Canada, which have asbestos mines, and Seattle, Hawaii, San Francisco–Oakland, New York–New Jersey, New Orleans, and Norfolk, Virginia, which have large shipyards or asbestos industries. It is difficult to document a relationship between the duration or intensity of asbestos exposure and the risk of developing mesothelioma, but Levine (1981) has reported that patients with peritoneal mesothelioma usually have a history of heavier exposure than do patients with pleural disease.

Mesothelioma is also caused by other naturally occurring and manufactured silicate fibers that share the physical properties of amphibole asbestos fibers. These properties are a diameter of smaller than 0.25 μm and a length greater than 5.0 μm. The most notable example is erionite, a zeolite fiber found in volcanic deposits in central Turkey, where it is the major material for building homes. Baris (1987) found that in Karain, Turkey, a village of 604 persons, malignant mesothelioma was the single most common cause of death, with 62 cases recorded from 1970 to 1981. In this village, mesothelioma frequently occurs in individuals who are in their 20s or 30s because they have been exposed to erionite from birth.

Less common causes of malignant mesothelioma exist. Lerman and associates (1991) record that radiation exposure at periods ranging from 10 to 31 years before the development of mesothelioma is the most clearly documented of these causes (e.g., individuals who received mantle radiation

Table 65-1. Nonasbestos Causes of Mesothelioma

Agent	Species Tumor Observed in or Induced in[a]
Naturally occurring mineral fibers	
Zeolites (eronite)	Human, rat
Minerals	
Nickel	Rat
Silica powder	Rat
Beryllium	Rat, ?human
Radiation	Human, rat
Organic chemicals	
Polyurethane, polysilicone	Rat
Sterigmatocystin (aflatoxin B1-related compound)	Rat
Ethylene oxide	Rat
N-Methyl-N-nitrosourea	Guinea pig
N-Methyl-N-nitrosourethane	Mouse
3-Methylcholanthrene	Mouse
Methyl nitrosamine	Rat
1-Nitroso-5, 6-dihydrouracil	Rat
Diethylstilbestrol	Monkey
Stilboestrol	Dog
3, 4, 5-Trimetholxycinnamaldehyde	Rat
Mineral oil	Human
Liquid paraffin	Human
Viruses	
MC 29 avian leukosis virus	Chicken
SV 40	Hamster
Chronic inflammation	
Recurrent lung infections	Human
Tuberculous pleuritis	Human
Recurrent diverticulitis	Human
Familial Mediterranean fever	Human
Nonspecific industrial exposure	
Shoe industry workers	Human
Petrochemical–oil industry workers	Human
Stone cutters	Human
Leather factory or textile workers	Human
Occupations involving exposure to copper, nickel, fiberglass, rubber or glass dust	Human
Cocarcinogens	
3-Methylcholanthrene-asbestos	Rat
Radiation-asbestos	Rat
N-Methyl-N-nitrosourea-asbestos	Rat
Hereditary predisposition	Human

[a]Note: In some instances the tumors induced in animals by various agents may represent sarcomas rather than mesotheliomas.
From Hammar SP, Bolen JW: Pleural neoplasms. In Dail DH, Hammar SP (eds): Pulmonary Pathology. New York: Springer, 1988, p. 979. With permission.

for Hodgkin's disease as young adults). Extravasation of radioactive thorium dioxide (Thorotrast, a contrast agent previously used for radiologic procedures) and exposure to isoniazid in utero are anecdotally reported by Antman (1983, 1984) and Anderson (1985) and their coworkers to cause mesothelioma. A variety of other substances, summarized by Peterson and associates (1984) and Hammar and Bolen (1988) in Table 65-1, are thought to be possible risk factors for malignant mesothelioma, based on epidemiologic or experimental animal studies. However, in contrast to lung cancer, for which asbestos and smoking act as synergistic carcinogens, smoking is not a risk factor for malignant mesothelioma.

The peak age for the development of malignant mesothelioma is the sixth decade of life. Because most patients develop mesothelioma as a result of occupational exposure to asbestos, the increased incidence of this disease has occurred in men. In the United States, the incidence in women remains at the baseline level of 3 cases/million population, whereas in men it has risen to 15 cases/million people per year. Malignant mesothelioma is predominantly a disease of older adults because of the long latency period (at least 20 years) between exposure to causative agents and the development of cancer, but Fraire and colleagues (1988) report that it can occur in childhood. In that setting, it is usually idiopathic. Malignant mesothelioma sometimes develops in young adults because of exposure to risk factors during childhood, as reported by Kane and colleagues (1990).

PATHOLOGY AND MOLECULAR BIOLOGY

Mesotheliomas arise from multipotential mesothelial or subserosal cells that can develop into either an epithelial or a sarcomatoid neoplasm. In contrast to localized fibrous tumors of the pleura described by Scharifker and Kenko (1979), diffuse mesotheliomas always have an epithelial component. However, they exhibit a wide array of histologic patterns (Table 65-2) and, often, a mixture of epithelial and sarcomatoid features (Figs. 65-1 and 65-2). In a review of 819 cases, Hillerdal (1983) reported that 50% were of epithelial type, 34% were of mixed type, and 16% were of the sarcomatoid type. The histologic appearance of mesotheliomas is easily confused with that of other neoplasms, and there is often disagreement among pathologists when light microscopy is used as the sole method of diagnosis. The rate at which tumors originally diagnosed as mesotheliomas are reclassified ranges

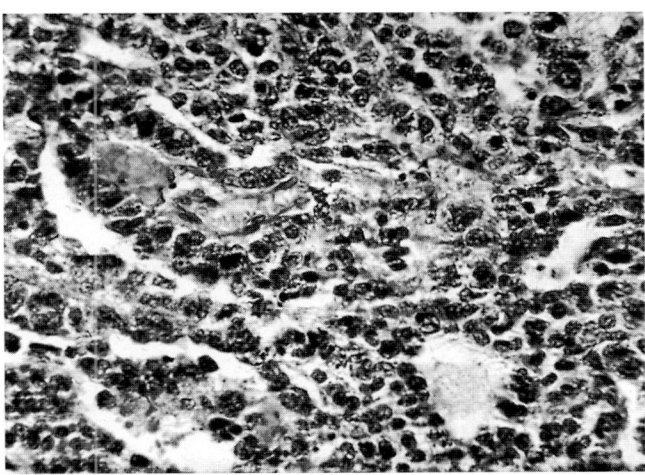

Fig. 65-1. Photomicrograph of epithelial type of malignant mesothelioma.

from 30 to 84% when these specimens are reviewed by panels of reference pathologists. The usual challenge for the pathologist is to distinguish epithelial mesotheliomas from metastatic adenocarcinoma. However, as Cantin and associates (1982) report, very early mesotheliomas can be difficult to distinguish from benign mesothelial hyperplasia, and the rare desmoplastic form of mesothelioma often resembles benign fibrosis because of its predominantly fibroblastic cell type and sparsely cellular appearance.

Several histochemical stains help to distinguish malignant mesothelioma from other tumors. Pulmonary adenocarcinomas usually stain positively with mucicarmine, whereas mesothelioma does not. Approximately 20% of epithelial mesotheliomas produce an acidic mucosubstance, hyaluronic acid, which can be seen either within or between cells with an Alcian blue or colloidal iron stain. However, immunohistochemistry and electron microscopy are now routinely used to establish a definitive pathologic diagnosis. Battifora and Kopinski (1985) and Wirth (1991) and Mezger (1990) and their colleagues report that useful immunohistochemical stains include antibodies to high- and low-molecular-weight cytokeratins, to vimentin, to human milk fat globule, to carcinoembryonic antigen, and to Leu-M1. Mesotheliomas stain positively for low-molecular-weight cytokeratins, a feature that distinguishes them from sarcomas. They almost never stain for carcinoembryonic antigen, a feature that distinguishes them from adenocarcinomas. If immunohistochemical stains yield equivocal results, electron microscopy usually provides a definitive diagnosis. Burns and associates (1985) have emphasized that the most prominent feature of mesotheliomas is that they have numerous, long, sinuous microvilli, whereas adenocarcinomas have short, straight microvilli that are covered by a fuzzy glycocalyx.

As summarized by Pass and Mew (1996), relatively little is understood about the biology of diffuse malignant mesothelioma. Burmer and coworkers (1989) reported that

Table 65-2. Histologic Classification of Mesothelioma

Epithelial
  Tubulopapillary
  Epithelioid
  Glandular
  Large cell (giant cell)
  Small cell
  Adenoid-cystic
  Signet ring
Sarcomatoid (fibrous, sarcomatous, mesenchymal)
Mixed epithelial-sarcomatoid (biphasic)
Transitional
Desmoplastic
Localized fibrous mesothelioma

From Hammar SP, Bolen JW: Pleural neoplasms. *In* Dail DH, Hammar SP (eds): Pulmonary Pathology. New York: Springer, 1988, p. 979. With permission.

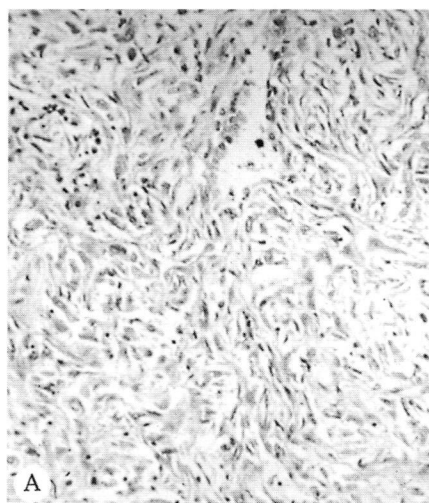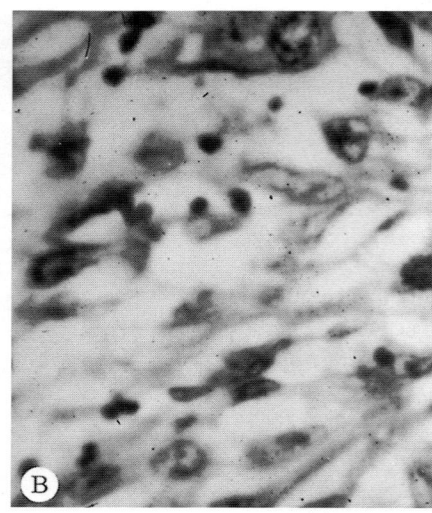

Fig. 65-2. Photomicrograph of a malignant mesothelioma of the sarcomatous variety. **A.** Low-power magnification. **B.** High-power magnification.

approximately 65% of malignant mesotheliomas were diploid on flow cytometry and had surprisingly low proliferative rates. However, a study by Tammilehto (1992) has shown that low S-phase fraction is an independent prognostic factor. Molecular biological information has frequently derived from mesothelioma cell lines, although chromosomal abnormalities are increasingly studied in primary tumor specimens. These abnormalities include alterations, usually deletions, on chromosomes 1, 3, 4, 9, 11, 14, and 22, as reported by Popescu (1988), Hagemeijer (1990), Taguchi (1993), and Lee (1996) and their associates. Xiao and colleagues (1995) also reported that deletion of both the *p15* and *p16* inhibitor genes within the chromosome band 9p21 occurred in 72% of 50 primary mesotheliomas studied. Additional copies of the short arm of chromosome 7 have also been seen by Tiainen and colleagues (1989) and may be an indicator of poor prognosis. Overexpression of the platelet-derived growth factors (PDGFs) and of their receptors has been a consistent finding by Gerwin and associates (1987) in human mesothelioma cell lines compared to normal cell lines. Versnel and coworkers (1988) have noted the expression of C-*sis* (PDGF B-chain) and PDGF A-chain genes in some cell lines. Abnormalities of the tumor suppressor gene, *p53*, have also been reported by Cote and coinvestigators (1991). However, other investigators, including Mor and associates (1997), have found that *p53* mutations are rare in primary mesothelioma, in contrast to most solid tumors. Transfection experiments conducted by Reddel and colleagues (1989) using the activated C-Ha-*ras* (HRAS1) oncogene EJ-*ras* in a human mesothelial cell line suggest that activation of this oncogene could play a critical role in the malignant transformation of mesothelial cells. Even stronger evidence of a viral etiology exists. Simian virus 40 (SV40) DNA sequences have been shown by Carbone (1994) and Testa (1998) and their colleagues to be present in primary mesotheliomas. Because asbestos is also found in most of the specimens containing SV40 DNA, it is thought that these two agents may function as cocarcinogens. How these preliminary pieces of information fit together in the overall sequence of carcinogenesis in mesothelioma remains to be seen.

CLINICAL AND RADIOLOGIC PRESENTATION

The clinical presentation of diffuse malignant mesothelioma is insidious and nonspecific. Mesothelioma has traditionally been portrayed as a diffuse, massive tumor that causes excruciating chest pain. In fact, these signs and symptoms are seen only when mesothelioma reaches a locally advanced stage. In the early stages of disease, dyspnea is the predominant symptom and is related to the presence of an effusion. When the effusion is drained, patients are asymptomatic. As the tumor grows, patients develop ill-defined, mild, but continuous chest discomfort. Dyspnea may actually improve during this phase of the disease because, with tumor growth, the pleural surfaces fuse, and the effusion resolves. Only when the disease becomes locally advanced does the patient develop severe chest pain, which is related to tumor infiltration of the chest wall and intercostal nerves. This is accompanied by a sense of chest tightness and dyspnea caused by entrapment of the lung by tumor. In the final stages of disease, dyspnea and chest pain become severe and unremitting. These symptoms are related to encasement of the chest wall, lung, and mediastinum, sometimes associated with mediastinal shift and compression of the contralateral lung. The tumor may extend directly though the pericardium, causing a pericardial effusion or myocardial metastases. The symptoms of locally advanced pleural disease can also be compounded by the development of ascites from direct extension of the tumor through the diaphragm or a contralateral pleural effusion from metastatic disease. Elmes and Simpson (1976) and Ruffie and associates (1989) report a variety of other symptoms, such as bone pain, which can occur in terminal patients who develop extrathoracic metastases.

Thus, dyspnea and chest pain are the most common presenting symptoms, occurring in 90% of patients. Weight loss occurs in approximately 30% of patients but is seen only in the advanced stages of the disease. Uncommon symptoms include cough, weakness, anorexia, fever, hemoptysis, hoarseness, dysphagia, and Horner's syndrome. A few cases presenting with a spontaneous pneumothorax have been reported by Sheard and colleagues (1991).

In the early stages of disease, the findings on physical examination are nonspecific. Dullness to percussion and decreased breath sounds may be noted because of the presence of a pleural effusion, but the chest examination is otherwise normal. In the late stages of disease when tumor encases the hemithorax, the excursion of the chest with respiration diminishes, and the chest wall is noticeably contracted. Diffuse dullness to percussion and decreased breath sounds are present over the entire hemithorax. There is a subtle fullness of the intercostal spaces. Palpable soft tissue masses may be found in the chest wall if the tumor has grown through the intercostal spaces or has implanted in the site of a previous thoracentesis or thoracotomy incision. Palpable supraclavicular or axillary nodes or an obvious ascites may be present if the tumor has metastasized to these areas, as described by Law and colleagues (1982a).

Paraneoplastic syndromes are uncommon, but autoimmune hemolytic anemia, hypercalcemia, hypoglycemia, the syndrome of inappropriate secretion of antidiuretic hormone, and hypercoagulability not related to thrombocytosis have been reported by Ruffie and associates (1989). Olesen and Thorshauge (1988) found that thrombocytosis, defined as a platelet count of 400,000/mL or greater. occurs in approximately 30 to 40% of patients, is sometimes associated with a leukemoid reaction, but does not seem to increase the risk of thromboembolic episodes.

Mesothelioma patients often have abnormal electrocardiographic (ECG) and echocardiographic findings. In a review of 64 patients, Wadler and coworkers (1986) found that 55 patients (89%) had an abnormal ECG. Sinus tachycardia was seen in 42% of patients, non–life-threatening ventricular or atrial arrhythmias occurred in 17% of patients, and more than one-third of patients had some form of bundle branch block. Although pericardial invasion or myocardial involvement was a common finding at autopsy in these patients, most ECG abnormalities occurred more than 6 months before death, which suggests that they are not solely related to the presence of advanced disease. Echocardiography was somewhat insensitive but highly specific for involvement of the pericardium or myocardium by tumor: Three patients who had pericardial effusions by echocardiogram had pericardial and myocardial involvement at

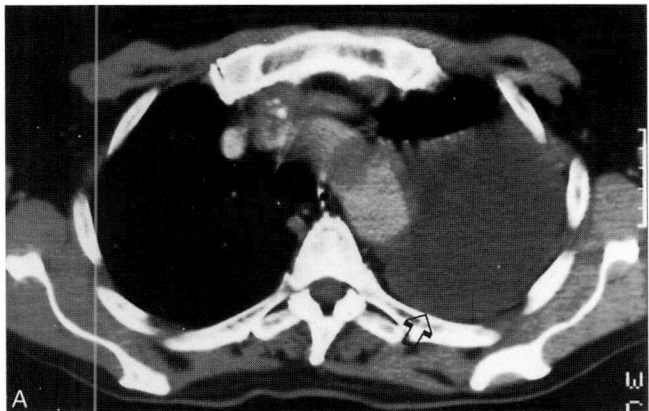
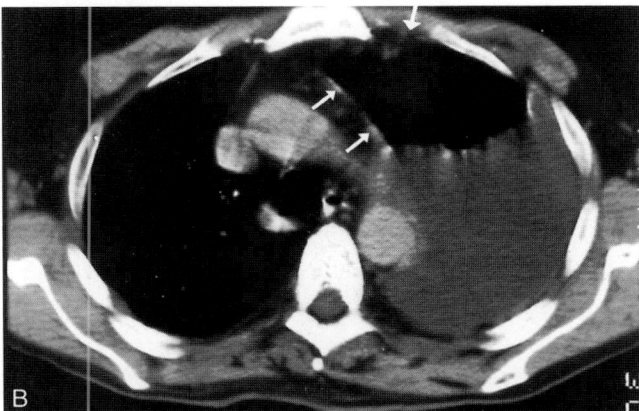

Fig. 65-3. Computed tomographic (CT) scans of an early-stage diffuse mesothelioma. **A.** The CT scan at the level of the aortic arch shows a large left pleural effusion (*arrow*) with no evidence of pleural disease. **B.** The second CT scan at the level of the aortopulmonary window shows mild pleural thickening and irregularity (*arrows*) in addition to the effusion. At thoracotomy, there was diffuse studding of the pleura with tumor nodules that were 1 to 2 mm.

autopsy, whereas five patients who had pericardial tumor at autopsy had had a normal echocardiogram.

No tumor markers are routinely used for malignant mesothelioma. Serum hyaluronan may be elevated in some patients, which is not surprising given the positive staining for hyaluronic acid seen in many epithelial mesotheliomas. In one study of 37 patients, Dahl and colleagues (1989) found that a rise in serum hyaluronan had a sensitivity of 65% and a specificity of 85% as a predictor of progressive disease. Hyaluronan can be measured using a commercial kit, but the kit is not readily available in most hospitals. CA-125 was reported by Rusch and colleagues (1994) to be elevated in approximately 20% of patients, and its use as a serum marker is therefore limited.

The radiographic appearance of malignant mesothelioma is variable and is related to the stage of the tumor at diagnosis. In early-stage mesothelioma, a large pleural effusion is often the only sign of disease (Fig. 65-3). Sub-

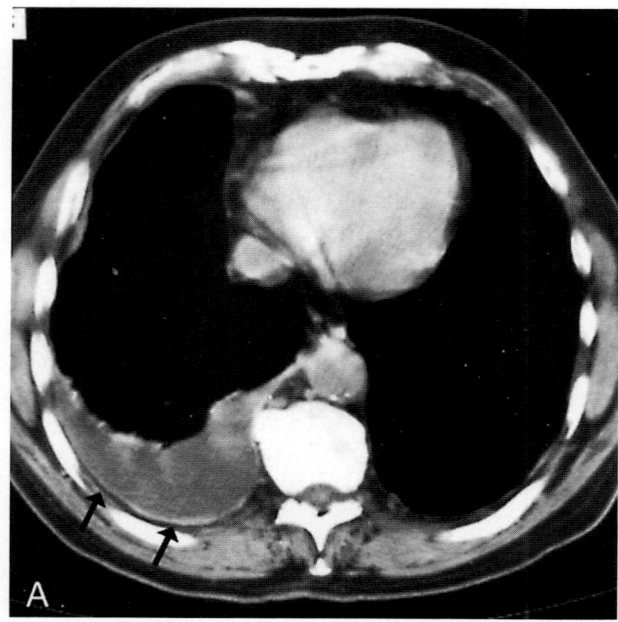

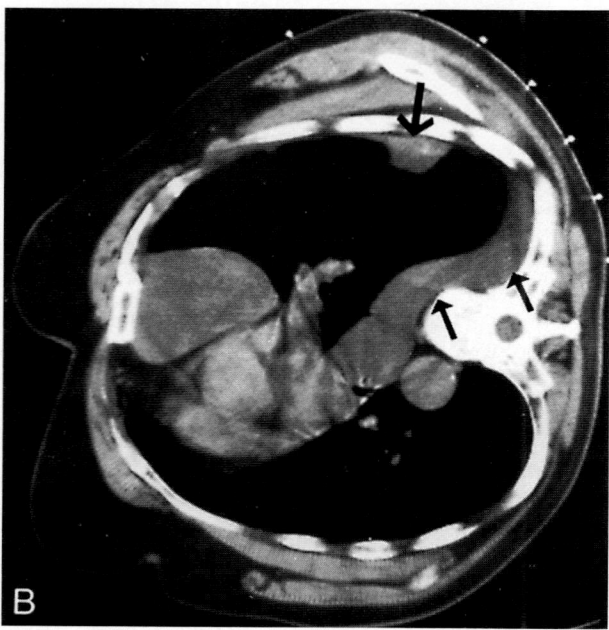

Fig. 65-4. Computed tomographic (CT) scans of an early-stage mesothelioma. **A.** There is a large pleural effusion with diffuse mild pleural thickening and irregularity (*arrows*). **B.** A CT scan obtained with the patient in the lateral position shows a dominant chest wall mass (*large arrow*) and a freely flowing effusion (*small arrow*).

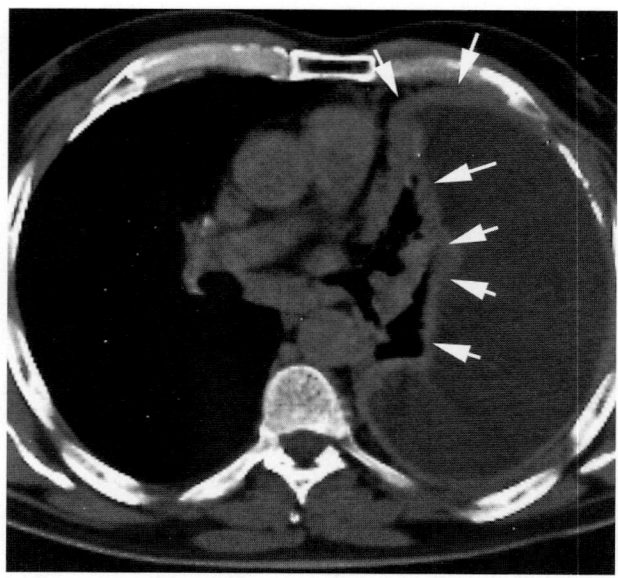

Fig. 65-5. Computed tomographic scan of a locally advanced mesothelioma. There is a thick confluent pleural peel along the chest wall (*large arrows*), encasing the collapsed lung and extending into the fissure (*small arrows*).

tle pleural thickening or small, discrete, pleural-based masses may be seen on computed tomography (CT) (Fig. 65-4). Subsequently, larger pleura-based masses become evident and are often intermixed with multiloculated effusions. Gotfried and colleagues (1983) note that rarely, a dominant pleural-based mass may be the initial presenta-

tion, but ultimately the involvement of the pleura is always diffuse. Eventually, a thick confluent pleural rind develops, with encasement of the lung and obliteration of the pleural space (Fig. 65-5). Mediastinal adenopathy, direct extension of the tumor into the mediastinum, involvement of the pericardium with pericardial effusion, and extension into the chest wall or through the diaphragm are seen with locally advanced disease (Fig. 65-6). Rabinowitz (1982), Mirvis (1983), Law (1982a), and Alexander (1981) and their colleagues report that CT permits a far better assessment of the extent of the disease than does standard radiography, which cannot demonstrate many of these abnormalities. CT is currently the most accurate noninvasive way to stage patients, to assess response to treatment, and to detect recurrent disease postoperatively, but, as reported by Rusch and associates (1988), it is often inaccurate in diagnosing chest wall involvement or extension through the diaphragm. It was hoped that magnetic resonance imaging (MR scan) would prove more accurate in this regard. However, in a recent study comparing CT and MR imaging for preoperative staging, Heelan and associates (1998) have shown that MR imaging is not significantly better than CT in defining the local extent of tumor. Therefore, CT remains the standard imaging study.

The role of positron emission tomography (PET) scanning is currently being investigated. Bénard and associates (1998) report that PET correctly identified the presence of malignant mesothelioma in all 26 patients studied. It is unclear whether PET will be useful as a staging study.

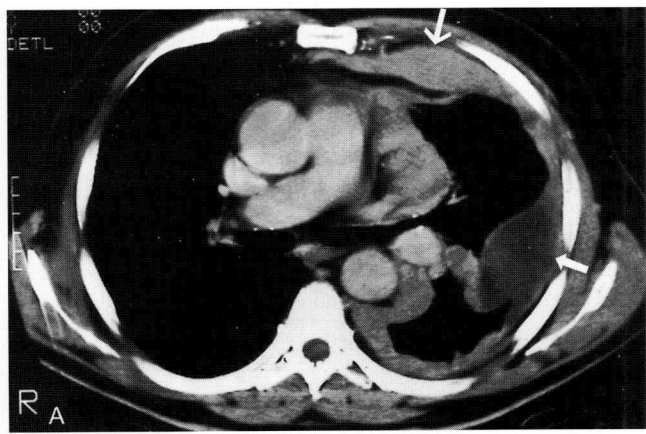

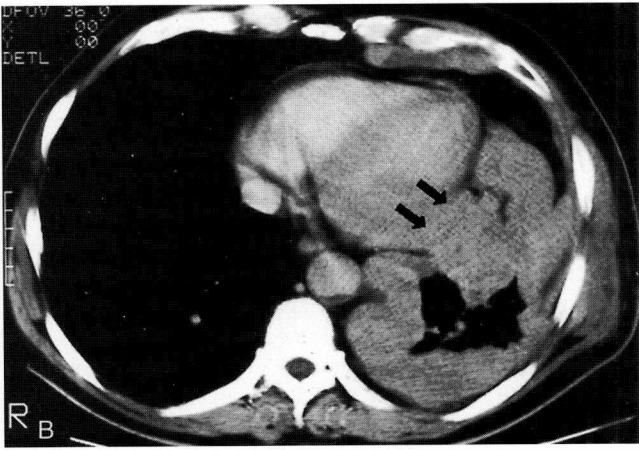

Fig. 65-6. Computed tomographic (CT) scan of a locally advanced mesothelioma. **A.** The CT scan at the level of the pulmonary artery shows a thick, irregular, confluent pleural peel (*large arrow*) with a loculated pleural effusion (*small arrow*). **B.** The CT scan at the level of the midheart shows massive tumor encasing and collapsing the lung and suggests invasion of the pericardium (*arrows*).

DIAGNOSIS

A thoracentesis is usually the initial diagnostic procedure because most patients present with a pleural effusion. Pleural fluid cytology is positive for malignancy in only 30 to 50% of patients. Percutaneous pleural biopsy yields a diagnosis of malignancy in up to one-third of cases. As emphasized by Battifora and Kopinski (1985) and Wirth (1991) and Mezger (1990) and their colleagues, it usually does not provide a large enough specimen for the immunohistochemical or electron microscopic studies that are critical for a definitive diagnosis. As described by Boutin and associates (1991b, 1993a,) thoracoscopy is the optimal diagnostic procedure because it yields a diagnosis in at least 80% of patients without committing the patient to a major surgical procedure. The appearance of the pleural space is variable and depends on the extent of disease and the cell type. In the earliest stage of

mesothelioma, involvement of the pleura is microscopic, and the only visible finding is a large pleural effusion. As the disease progresses, the thoracoscopic appearance evolves from tumor studding of the parietal pleura with a free pleural space and a large pleural effusion to studding of both parietal and visceral pleurae. The next stage is larger but still discrete masses with multiloculated pleural effusions and finally, a confluent irregular sheet of tumor with obliteration of the pleural space. The tumor ranges from soft, friable, and hypervascular to densely fibrotic, depending on the mixture of cell types. No clinical findings are pathognomonic of malignant mesothelioma.

When thoracoscopy is not technically feasible because the pleural space is obliterated by locally advanced tumor, the small incision made for thoracoscopy is extended to a length of 6 cm and used for open pleural biopsy by resection of a short segment of the overlying rib. Because mesothelioma has a notorious propensity to implant in the chest wall, this incision should be placed in line with a possible subsequent thoracotomy incision, so that it can be excised at the time of the definitive operation. Exploratory thoracotomy should be avoided because it exposes patients who have metastatic adenocarcinoma to the unnecessary morbidity of a major operation and complicates definitive surgical resection in patients with mesothelioma. Most important, pleural biopsies should be submitted fresh to the pathologist so that they can be placed in the appropriate fixative for electron microscopy.

No additional studies or procedures beyond thoracoscopy and CT scans of the chest and abdomen are routinely necessary to diagnose and stage patients with malignant mesothelioma. Bronchoscopy is done only to exclude the possibility of a primary lung cancer with endobronchial tumor. It is uniformly normal in patients with mesothelioma, as noted by Lewis and coworkers (1981). Mediastinoscopy may demonstrate involved mediastinal nodes, but the role of mediastinoscopy in selecting patients for treatment has not been carefully assessed. Additional imaging studies, such as bone scans, are indicated only to evaluate specific symptoms (i.e., localized bone pain or laboratory abnormalities, such as an elevated alkaline phosphatase). As a general rule, distant metastases are seen only in patients who have very locally advanced tumor.

NATURAL HISTORY AND STAGING

The successful treatment of any cancer is based on an understanding of its natural history. However, our understanding of the natural history and prognostic factors in malignant mesothelioma is still limited. Until recently, there was not even an accurate, universally accepted staging system. The staging system used most frequently in the past was the one proposed by Butchart and colleagues (1976) (Table 65-3), which had imprecise descriptors for the primary tumor

Table 65-3. Staging Proposed by Butchart and Colleagues

Stage I
    Tumor confined within the "capsule" of the parietal pleura
       (i.e., involving only ipsilateral pleura, lung, pericardium, and
       diaphragm)
Stage II
    Tumor invading chest wall or involving mediastinal structures
       (e.g., esophagus, heart, opposite pleura)
    Lymph node involvement in the chest
Stage III
    Tumor penetrating diaphragm to involve peritoneum; involve-
       ment of opposite pleura
    Lymph node involvement outside the chest
Stage IV
    Distant blood-borne metastases

From Butchart EG, et al: Pleuropneumonectomy in the management of diffuse malignant mesothelioma of the pleura: experience with 29 patients. Thorax *31*:15, 1976. With permission.

and for the lymph node involvement. A stage I tumor, for instance, could include patients who had minimal pleural studding, a free pleural space, and pleural effusion as well as patients who had a thick, confluent sheet of tumor with obliteration of the pleural space but without invasion of the mediastinum or opposite pleura. Yet clinical experience indicates that the latter is more locally advanced tumor with a poorer prognosis. In addition, the exact sites, incidence, and prognostic implications of lymph node involvement are still controversial. The inclusion of "lymph node involvement in the chest" in stage II and "lymph node involvement outside the chest" in stage III is empiric. Allen and coworkers (1994) did not find any association between lymph node metastases and survival in 96 patients who underwent surgical resection. However, reports from Sugarbaker and associates (1993, 1996) and Rusch and Venkatraman (1996) indicate that patients who have positive mediastinal nodes have a poorer prognosis. These data must be confirmed in larger numbers of patients subjected to systematic lymph node dissection.

Dimitrov and McMahon (1987) describe several other proposed staging systems, including a tumor, node, metastasis (TNM)-based system by Chahinian (1983). This system is more precise than the Butchart system but does not fully reflect the usual findings at thoracotomy. For instance, the T1 descriptor (involvement of the parietal and visceral pleural surfaces with sparing of the diaphragm) does not reflect what we now know is the pattern of disease progression: tumor studding of all parietal pleural surfaces followed by involvement of the visceral pleura. The greatest tumor burden is almost always in the lower half of the hemithorax and on the diaphragm. In an effort to improve and unify the staging system for malignant mesothelioma, the Union Internationale Contre le Cancer proposed another TNM-based system. The T-status descriptors are more detailed than in previous systems, and the descriptors for nodal involvement in this system are borrowed directly from the

current international staging system for non–small cell lung cancer. However, this system was developed without clinicopathologic correlation.

More recently, the author (1995) reported for the International Mesothelioma Interest Group a new TNM-based staging system that updates and reconciles all previous systems (Table 65-4). This staging system is based on current data about patterns of disease progression and the correlation between T and N status and survival. The development of this system facilitates outcome analyses and the design of clinical trials.

Another issue that confounds the interpretation of the published literature is that most reports do not stage patients by CT scan but assess them only by symptoms, physical examination, and chest radiographs. The inaccuracy of such a clinical assessment leads to a heterogeneous patient population that makes it hard to decipher the results of treatment for mesothelioma. Many series also record outcome in small numbers of patients seen over long periods and treated in a highly individualized manner. Little wonder that reported survival rates vary widely. Law and coworkers (1984) reported a median survival of 18 months for 64 patients treated with supportive care, with no differences in survival according to cell type. Twelve of the 64 patients survived longer than 5 years, but the diagnosis of mesothelioma in this study was based on histology alone, and less than one-third of all patients were staged by CT scan. Hulks and colleagues (1989) reported a median survival of 30 weeks for 68 patients treated with supportive care. They based their pathologic diagnosis on immunohistochemistry as well as histology. No CT scanning was performed, and patients were classified principally according to their symptoms. Patients who presented with dyspnea lived significantly longer than did patients who presented with pain, for a median survival of 44 versus 22 weeks, probably reflecting the extent of disease at diagnosis. Cell type did not appear to influence survival.

Other authors, notably Tammilehto (1992), Ruffie (1989), Adams (1986), and Antman (1988) and their colleagues, have tried to identify prognostic factors in malignant mesothelioma but have done this mainly in the setting of retrospective reviews of patients with different stages of disease, treated with widely varying regimens. Contrary to the data reported by Law (1982b) and Hulks (1989) and their associates, epithelial histology has generally been a favorable prognostic factor. Absence of chest pain and good performance status are also thought to be favorable prognostic factors but probably reflect only an early stage of the disease. Other factors, including female gender and age younger than 50 years, have incidentally been cited as favorable prognostic factors. In several series, thrombocytosis (defined as a platelet count >400,000/mL), appears to have a negative impact on survival.

Malignant mesothelioma was long thought to be a tumor that remained localized to the chest, as described by Nauta

Table 65-4. New International Staging System for Diffuse Malignant Pleural Mesothelioma

T_1	T_{1a}	Tumor limited to the ipsilateral parietal ± mediastinal ± diaphragmatic pleura
		No involvement of the visceral pleura
	T_{1b}	Tumor involving the ipsilateral parietal ± mediastinal ± diaphragmatic pleura
		Tumor also involving the visceral pleura
T_2		Tumor involving each of the ipsilateral pleural surfaces (parietal, mediastinal, diaphragmatic, and visceral pleura) with at least one of the following features:
		Involvement of diaphragmatic muscle
		Extension of tumor from visceral pleura into the underlying pulmonary parenchyma
T_3		Locally advanced but potentially resectable tumor
		Tumor involving all the ipsilateral pleural surfaces (parietal, mediastinal, diaphragmatic, and visceral pleura) with at least one of the following features:
		Involvement of the endothoracic fascia
		Extension into the mediastinal fat
		Solitary, completely resectable focus of tumor extending into the soft tissues of the chest wall
		Nontransmural involvement of the pericardium
T_4		Locally advanced technically unresectable tumor
		Tumor involving all the ipsilateral pleural surfaces (parietal, mediastinal, diaphragmatic, and visceral pleura) with at least one of the following features:
		Diffuse extension or multifocal masses of tumor in the chest wall, with or without associated rib destruction
		Direct transdiaphragmatic extension of tumor to the peritoneum
		Direct extension of tumor to the contralateral pleura
		Direct extension of tumor to mediastinal organs
		Direct extension of tumor into the spine
		Tumor extending through to the internal surface of the pericardium with or without a pericardial effusion; or tumor involving the myocardium

N (lymph nodes)

N_X	Regional lymph nodes cannot be assessed
N_0	No regional lymph node metastases
N_1	Metastases in the ipsilateral bronchopulmonary or hilar lymph nodes
N_2	Metastases in the subcarinal or the ipsilateral mediastinal lymph nodes, including the ipsilateral internal mammary nodes
N_3	Metastases in the contralateral mediastinal, contralateral internal mammary, ipsilateral or contralateral supraclavicular lymph nodes

M (metastases)

M_X	Presence of distant metastases cannot be assessed
M_0	No distant metastasis
M_1	Distant metastasis present

Stage I			
Ia	T_{1a}	N_0	M_0
Ib	T_{1b}	N_0	M_0
Stage II	T_2	N_0	M_0
Stage III	Any T_3	Any N_1	M_0
		Any N_2	
Stage IV	Any T_4	Any N_3	Any M_1

From Rusch VW: A proposed new international TNM staging system for malignant pleural mesothelioma. From the International Mesothelioma Interest Group. Chest *108*:1122, 1995. With permission.

and colleagues (1982). Several autopsy series have now disproved this. Ruffie and coinvestigators (1989) found that 45 of 92 (49%) patients had distant metastases at autopsy. The liver was the most common site and the contralateral lung the second most common site of distant disease, but metastases were also found in sites as widely disseminated as the prostate, brain, and thyroid. Elmes and Simpson (1976) found distant metastases in 48 of 148 patients (33%) patients at autopsy. The metastases were widely disseminated, but the liver and the contralateral lung were once again the most common sites of disease. Similar findings have been reported by Roberts (1976) and by Whitwell and Rawcliffe (1971). The uncommon but definite occurrence of brain and spine metastases has been emphasized in several reports, notably those of Walters and Martinez (1975), as well as those of Kaye (1986) and Ruffie (1989) and their associates. Virtually all patients have advanced local or regional disease at death. As pointed out by Nauta and colleagues (1982), however, the symptoms related to locoregional tumor are usually the most difficult to palliate and therefore the most obvious clinically. Patients with malignant mesothelioma face a dual problem: control of the locoregional tumor throughout the course of their disease and prevention of distant metastases as a late manifestation of their cancer.

TREATMENT

As for any other cancer, the treatment options for malignant mesothelioma include surgery, radiation, chemotherapy, immunotherapy, supportive care, or some combination of these modalities. However, the choice of treatment is influenced by factors that do not apply to some other malignancies: the location and extent of the tumor, and the general medical condition of these patients who are usually older and have significant medical comorbidities. The assessment of treatment regimens for malignant mesothelioma is hampered by a lack of large prospective clinical trials. Most patients have been treated in a highly individualized manner. Reported series are often small and retrospective.

Radiation Therapy

It is difficult to evaluate the success of radiation therapy as the only treatment because it is usually given in conjunction with surgical resection or chemotherapy. Radiation therapy as the sole treatment is generally used to palliate an area of symptomatic tumor in the chest wall or mediastinum.

According to Brady (1981), Ball and Cruickshank (1990), and Gordon and coworkers (1982), the use of radiation is limited by the volume of the primary tumor that involves the entire hemithorax and by proximity of the tumor to many vital structures that are intolerant of high doses of radiation.

For the most part, radiation doses to the affected hemithorax have been kept at 4500 cGy or less to prevent toxicity to the heart, esophagus, lung, and spinal cord. Maasilta (1991) documented the severe pulmonary toxicity caused by higher-dose hemithoracic irradiation. The radiographic changes and the deterioration in pulmonary function and oxygenation that develop over the year after radiation therapy are compatible with a total loss of lung function on the irradiated side. Sinoff and associates (1982) have shown that the toxicity of irradiation may also be potentiated by the administration of chemotherapy, including drugs such as doxorubicin.

One way to circumvent these problems is to administer radiation therapy as adjuvant treatment after surgical resection of gross tumor. A variety of techniques can be used to minimize the radiation dose to the lung. The largest and most consistent experience with this approach was reported by Hilaris (1984) and Kutcher (1987) and their colleagues at the Memorial Sloan-Kettering Cancer Center. After subtotal resection of gross tumor by pleurectomy-decortication, any residual tumor was implanted intraoperatively with ^{125}I or ^{192}Ir implants. Patients then received external beam irradiation to the entire hemithorax using a mixed photon-electron beam technique to a total dose of 4500 cGy, attempting to spare the underlying lung. In an updated report by Mychalczak and coworkers (1989), 105 patients treated in this manner from 1976 to 1988 at Memorial Sloan-Kettering Cancer Center experienced a median survival of 12.6 months with 1- and 2-year actuarial survivals of 52 and 23%, respectively. However, the 27 patients who had pure epithelial histology and minimal gross residual disease requiring only external beam irradiation without brachytherapy had a median survival of 15 months, and 1- and 2-year survivals of 68 and 35%, respectively. There were 19 complications, including 12 cases of radiation pneumonitis and eight patients with pericarditis and tamponade. The most common site of relapse was local. Ipsilateral recurrent pleural tumor was seen in 64 of the 105 patients (63%). Both this experience and some experimental work by Soubra and associates (1990) indicate that a low-dose mixed photon-electron beam, although theoretically attractive, does not spare the pulmonary parenchyma or provide long-term local control for most patients.

External beam radiation therapy has also been administered after extrapleural pneumonectomy. At the Dana Farber Cancer Institute and Joint Center for Radiation Therapy, Baldini and associates (1997) gave adjuvant cyclophosphamide, Adriamycin (doxorubicin), and cisplatin (CAP) chemotherapy and hemithoracic irradiation to 49 patients who had undergone extrapleural pneumonectomy. After a median radiation dose of 30.6 Gy (range, 20 to 41.4 Gy), 16 patients (35%) developed a local recurrence. This high rate of recurrent disease in the ipsilateral hemithorax emphasizes that low- to moderate-dose radiation therapy does not provide adequate local control.

The use of high-dose (54-Gy) hemithoracic irradiation as adjuvant therapy after extrapleural pneumonectomy is being evaluated in a prospective trial at Memorial Sloan-Kettering Cancer Center. The successful use of fast neutron therapy to control local bulky disease has been described in a case report by Blake and coworkers (1985), but this has not yet been confirmed in larger series. Small-series studies have been reported on the intrapleural use of radioactive colloidal compounds, including radioactive gold (^{198}Au) and chromic phosphate (^{32}P), but as described by Brady (1981), these seem ineffective in treating any substantial tumor bulk in the pleural cavity.

The most successful use of irradiation is as an adjuvant therapy to prevent tumor implantation in the chest wall after thoracoscopy. Boutin and associates (1995) reported that in a small randomized trial, 8 of 20 (40%) patients who did not receive radiation therapy to the chest wall after thoracoscopy developed tumor implantation compared to none of the 20 patients who did receive radiation. Because the radiation regimen was a short course (700 cGy daily for 3 days), this treatment is worth considering in patients for whom further surgical intervention is planned. Low and colleagues (1995) confirmed the experience, using this radiation regimen in 20 patients and found no evidence of local recurrence in irradiated sites.

Overall, the contribution of radiation therapy to the local control of malignant mesothelioma has been disappointing. It is generally agreed that hemithoracic radiation therapy is not a feasible primary treatment for malignant mesothelioma because the doses of radiation therapy that might be effective in controlling the tumor are not tolerated by the underlying lung or surrounding mediastinal structures. It is not even clear that radiation therapy palliates the pain caused by locally advanced tumor involving the chest wall. Radiation therapy may be effective in adjuvant treatment, particularly after extrapleural pneumonectomy, when it becomes possible to deliver higher-dose irradiation to the hemithorax. Adjuvant short-course radiation therapy to the chest wall after thoracoscopy seems to prevent the development of chest wall tumor implants after thoracoscopy.

Chemotherapy

Numerous phase II studies of chemotherapeutic agents have been performed in malignant mesothelioma testing virtually all the currently available drugs. These have been well summarized by Antman and associates (1988) and more recently reviewed in detail by Krarup-Hansen and Hansen (1991) and Ong and Vogelzang (1996) (Table 65-5). Response rates as high as 30 to 40% have been reported in small single-institution studies, but in pooled data from multiple studies, response rates are generally in the 20% range. The results of these studies are influenced by the inclusion of patients with varying stages of disease and different mesothelioma cell types and by the lack of use of CT scanning to assess response. Dimitrov (1982), Chahinian (1978), Dabouis (1981), Raghavan (1990), and

Table 65-5. Series of ≥15 Patients with Malignant Mesothelioma Treated with Single-Agent Chemotherapy

Agent	First Author/Year[a]	No. of Patients	Responders No.	%	95% Confidence Interval (%)
Doxorubicin	Lerner/1983	51	7	14	7–26
Doxorubicin	Sorenson/1985	15	0	0	0–20
Detorubicin	Colbert/1985	35	9	26	14–42
Pirarubicin	Kaukel/1987	35	8	22	11–38
Epirubicin	Magri/1991	21	1	5	1–23
Epirubicin	Mattson/1992	48	7	15	6–28
Mitoxantrone	Eisenhauer/1986	28	2	7	2–22
Mitoxantrone	van Breukelen/1991	34	1	3	0–27
Cisplatin	Mintzer/1985	24	3	13	4–31
Cisplatin	Zidar/1988	35	5	14	6–29
Carboplatin	Mbidde/1986	17	2	12	0–27
Carboplatin	Raghavan/1990	31	5	16	5–34
Carboplatin	Vogelzang/1990	40	3	7	2–21
Vindesine	Kelsen/1983	17	1	6	0–17
Vindesine	Boutin/1987	21	0	0	0–15
Vincristine	Martensson/1989	23	0	0	0–14
Vinblastine	Cowan/1988	20	0	0	0–16
Paclitaxel	Vogelzang/1994	15	2	13	4–38
Cyclophosphamide	Sorenson/1985	16	0	0	0–19
Ifosfamide	Alberts/1988	17	4	24	10–48
Ifosfamide	Zidar/1992	26	2	8	1–25
Ifosfamide	Falkson/1992	40	1	3	1–14
Mitomycin	Bajorin/1987	19	4	21	8–43
Methotrexate	Solheim/1992	60	22	37	26–50
Trimetrexate	Vogelzang/1994	51	6	12	2–33
Edatrexate	Belani/1994	20	5	25	9–49
Edatrexate + leucovorin	Belani/1994	17	3	18	6–41
CB3717	Cantwell/1986	18	1	6	0–27
5-FU	Harvey/1984	20	1	5	1–24
Dihydro-5-azacytidine	Harmon/1991	42	7	17	9–31
Amsacrine	Falkson/1980	19	1	5	1–24
Diaziquone	Eagan/1986	20	0	0	0–17
Bacille Calmette-Guérin	Webster/1982	30	NA	NA	NA
Acivicin	Alberts/1988	19	0	0	0–17
Interferon-α-2a	Christmas/1993	25	3	12	4–30
Interleukin-2	Eggermont/1991	17	4	24	10–48
Interferon-γ	Boutin/1991	22	5	23	10–44

NA, not available.

[a]See original article for list of references.

From Ong ST, Vogelzang NJ: Chemotherapy in malignant pleural mesothelioma: a review. J Clin Oncol *14*:1007, 1996. With permission.

Umsawasdi (1991) and their associates have shown that active agents include doxorubicin, detorubicin, ifosfamide, cisplatin, carboplatin, mitomycin, methotrexate, edatrexate, 5-azacitidine, and 5-fluorouracil. Combination treatment has not proved clearly superior to a single agent (Table 65-6). Overall, the response rates for currently available chemotherapy drugs in malignant mesothelioma remain disappointing.

Immunotherapy

Interferons are known to have a direct antiproliferative effect on mesothelioma cell lines. Studies by Sklarin and coworkers (1988) on mesothelioma xenografts in nude mice have shown the efficacy of recombinant human interferon-α-2a combined with mitomycin C. These experimental data prompted the development of clinical trials using interferon, either alone or in combination with chemotherapy. However, these trials (see Table 65-6) have not demonstrated response rates that are superior to single-agent cisplatin alone.

The use of interferon-γ as an intrapleural treatment in patients with early-stage disease has recently been reported by Boutin and associates (1991a). Twenty-two patients were treated with a solution of interferon-γ (40 × 106 U) infused into the pleural space twice weekly for 2 months. Response was assessed by serial CT scans and repeat thoracoscopy. A 56% overall response rate was observed. These promising initial results will undoubtedly stimulate additional clinical trials. Intrapleural immunotherapy, however, requires a free

Table 65-6. Series of ≥15 Patients with Malignant Mesothelioma Treated with Combination Chemotherapy

Agent	First Author/Year[a]	No. of Patients	Responders		
			No.	%	95% Confidence Interval (%)
Doxorubicin + cyclo-phosphamide	Samson/1987	36	4	11	6–21
Doxorubicin + DTIC + cyclophosphamide	Samson/1987	40	5	13	6–21
Doxorubicin + cyclo-phosphamide + DTIC	Dhingra/1983	20	5	25	11–47
Doxorubicin + ifosfamide	Carmichael/1989	16	2	12.5	1–38
Doxorubicin + cisplatin	Ardizzoni/1991	24	6	25	10–47
Doxorubicin + cisplatin	Chahinian/1993	35	5	14	5–30
Mitomycin + cisplatin	Chahinian/1983	35	9	26	12–43
Doxorubicin + cisplatin + cyclophosphamide	Shin/1993	23	6	26	12–46
Epirubicin + ifosfamide	Magri/1992	17	1	6	1–27
Rubidazone + DTIC	Zidar/1983	23	0	0	0–14
DHAC + cisplatin	Samuels/1994	30	4	13	5–29
Mitomycin + bleomycin + cisplatin + doxorubicin	Breau/1991	25	11	44	27–63
Cisplatin + etoposide	Eisenhauer/1988	26	3	12	4–30
Pirarubicin + cisplatin	Koschel/1991	39	6	15	7–29
Doxorubicin + 5-azacyti-dine	Chahinian/1982	36	8	22	12–38
Doxorubicin + interferon-α	Upham/1993	25	4	16	6–35
Mitomycin + cisplatin + interferon-α	Tansan/1994	20	2	11	3–30
Cisplatin + interferon-α	Trandafir/1994				
Low-dose interferon		22	8	36	19–57
High-dose interferon		15	3 + 1CR	27	11–52

[a]See original article for list of references
CR, conditioned response; DHAC, dihydro-5-azacytidine; DTIC, (dimethyltriazeno)imidazole carboxamide (dacarbazine).
From Ong ST, Vogelzang NJ: Chemotherapy in malignant pleural mesothelioma: a review. *J Clin Oncol* *14*:1007, 1996. With permission.

pleural space to be effective and therefore can be administered only to patients with early-stage disease who have a free-flowing effusion and minimal tumor involving the pleural surfaces.

Goey and colleagues (1995) studied intrapleural interleukin 2 (IL-2) in a phase I trial in patients with stage I or II mesothelioma. IL-2 was administered as a continuous infusion using a dose-escalation schedule ranging from 3×10^4 to 36×10^6 IU daily. A partial response was seen in 4 of 21 evaluable patients. There were no complete responses, and the median overall survival was 15.6 months. IL-2 appears to have antitumor activity in mesothelioma but has not been studied further.

Surgery

Because of the limitations of radiation therapy and chemotherapy, surgical resection is still the mainstay of treatment for malignant mesothelioma. Three operations have been performed: extrapleural pneumonectomy (also termed *pleuropneumonectomy*), pleurectomy-decortication, and a palliative limited pleurectomy.

Extrapleural pneumonectomy is an en bloc resection of the pleura, lung, ipsilateral hemidiaphragm, and pericardium. As described by the author and coinvestigators (1991), pleurectomy-decortication is an attempt to remove all gross pleural disease without removing the underlying lung. The hemidiaphragm and pericardium are also removed and reconstructed if necessary. A palliative pleurectomy involves limited resection of the parietal pleura to control a pleural effusion by creating a durable pleurodesis. The details of the surgical technique for these operations are described in other chapters and are not reviewed here (see Chapters 61 and 66).

Another operation performed for strictly palliative purposes is thoracoscopy and talc poudrage. As reported by Ruffie (1989) and Boutin (1991b) and their colleagues, this is highly effective in controlling effusions and provides excellent palliation for patients whose general medical condition precludes more aggressive treatment.

Role of Surgical Resection

Complete resection of all gross tumor seems to convey a modest but definite improvement in survival in several large series. However, the value of extrapleural pneumonectomy relative to pleurectomy-decortication remains controversial. Extrapleural pneumonectomy has the esthetic appeal of removing the tumor en bloc, but either operation, if performed well in properly selected patients, allows the removal of all gross tumor. On the other hand, resection of the tumor with wide, microscopically negative margins, as can be achieved with a lung, breast, or colon cancer, is simply not feasible in malignant mesothelioma because the margins of resection are vital structures, such as the aorta, cavae, and esophagus.

In an initial report by Butchart and associates (1976), extrapleural pneumonectomy carried an operative mortality of 30%. More recent data show a substantial reduction in this mortality, probably reflecting better patient selection and improved perioperative care. Preoperative CT scanning, careful pulmonary function testing, ventilation-perfusion lung scanning, and improved methods of evaluating cardiac function noninvasively now allow selection of patients who have completely resectable tumors and have the cardiopulmonary reserve to tolerate the operation safely. Intraoperative monitoring and anesthetic management are much better than they were in the 1970s. In one prospective multi-institutional study reported by the author and coinvestigators (1991), the mortality rate was 15%. However, as reported by DeLaria (1978), Sugarbaker (1991, 1996), DeValle (1986), and Allen (1994) and their associates and by the author and Venkatraman (1996), mortality rates as low as 6% have been achieved in single-institution retrospective studies in which patients have been carefully selected and operated on by experienced surgeons.

By contrast, McCormack and associates (1982) at Memorial Sloan-Kettering reported an operative mortality of 1.8% for pleurectomy-decortication. These results are similar to what is seen with pulmonary resections for lung cancer, namely, that operative mortality is directly linked to the extent of resection and is 5 to 10% for a standard pneumonectomy. Both pleurectomy-decortication and particularly extrapleural pneumonectomy are technically complex and are not frequently performed by most surgeons. Therefore, patients may benefit by referral to centers dedicated to the treatment of malignant mesothelioma.

Controversy exists with regard to surgical treatment centers on the relative value of an extrapleural pneumonectomy versus a pleurectomy-decortication: Is the higher operative mortality of extrapleural pneumonectomy justified by a better overall survival? One problem is that extrapleural pneumonectomy cannot be performed in some patients because they have underlying cardiopulmonary disease that does not permit resection of an entire lung. However, pneumonectomy facilitates some forms of adjuvant treatment, especially postoperative irradiation, which can be administered to a much higher total dose after pneumonectomy than after pleurectomy-decortication.

In addition, some patients do not have a tumor that is technically resectable by pleurectomy-decortication. A con-

fluent sheet of tumor encasing the lung with obliteration of the pleural space is resectable only by extrapleural pneumonectomy. This situation can usually be identified by the preoperative CT scan (see Figs. 65-3 and 65-4). It is not known whether a patient who has early-stage disease that is technically completely resectable by either extrapleural pneumonectomy or by pleurectomy-decortication is better served by one operation versus the other. The issue is unresolved, but ultimately, the long-term outcome of such a patient after complete resection of all gross tumor may be determined not by the operation but by the type and effectiveness of the adjuvant treatment.

Combined Modality Treatment

Both extrapleural pneumonectomy and pleurectomy-decortication permit only the removal of gross tumor without wide surgical margins. The author and coinvestigators (1991) have shown that patients treated with surgical resection alone relapse rapidly. Therefore, most treatment regimens have focused on multimodality treatment. It is difficult, however, to evaluate the results of combined modality treatment because most series, including Achatzy (1989), Chahinian (1982), and Alberts (1988) and their associates, report small numbers of patients treated in a highly individualized manner over long periods. In addition to the Memorial Sloan-Kettering experience with pleurectomy-decortication and radiation therapy described previously, another large and relatively uniform experience with combined modality treatment has been reported by the Dana Farber Cancer Center. From 1980 to 1995, Sugarbaker and colleagues (1996) performed an extrapleural pneumonectomy in 120 patients, followed by CAP chemotherapy and subsequent hemithoracic irradiation. The overall survival rates were 45% at 2 years and 22% at 5 years. The 2- and 5-year survival rates were 65% and 27%, respectively, for patients with epithelial cell type and 2% and 0% for patients with sarcomatous or mixed histology tumors. Nodal metastases were a significant adverse prognostic factor. It is difficult to assess how much the irradiation or chemotherapy each contribute to these survival rates because these have not been tested individually as adjuvant treatment. A prospective trial of adjuvant high-dose (54-Gy) radiation therapy without chemotherapy has been completed at Memorial Sloan-Kettering Cancer Center, but the results of this study are not yet reported.

Several novel treatment strategies have been investigated. At the National Cancer Institute, Pass and coworkers (1994) performed a phase I trial evaluating the use of photodynamic therapy (PDT) immediately after pleurectomy-decortication or extrapleural pneumonectomy. PDT seeks to improve local control by eliminating microscopic residual disease immediately after surgical resection. This approach is based on experimental data with mesothelioma cell lines, reported by Keller and coworkers (1990) and a previous small clinical trial reported by Ris and colleagues (1991), which suggested the feasibility of this approach. Pass and associates (1994) reported that 42 patients received PDT after maximal surgical tumor debulking using escalating light doses of 15 to 35 J/cm². There was one mortality and three serious complications. Overall, this trial demonstrated the feasibility and safety of combined surgical resection and PDT.

I and my colleagues (1994) tested another approach in a phase II trial at Memorial Sloan-Kettering Cancer Center. Patients received a single dose of intrapleural cisplatin (75 mg/m²) and mitomycin (8 mg/m²) after complete resection of all gross tumor by pleurectomy-decortication. Additional chemotherapy was administered systemically starting 1 month postoperatively using two cycles of cisplatin 50 mg/m² per week × 4 and mitomycin 8 mg/m² × 1. This approach of surgical resection and short, intensive chemotherapy tried to address the problems of both local control and potential distant metastases. It was based on the established use of intraperitoneal chemotherapy in ovarian cancer and on a smaller but successful experience with intracavitary chemotherapy in both pleural and peritoneal mesothelioma, reported by Lederman (1987), Markman (1986), and Mintzer (1985) and their associates.

I and my coinvestigators (1994) also found that 23 patients treated with pleurectomy-decortication and adjuvant chemotherapy tolerated the treatment but had a high risk of local recurrence (16 of 20 patients). Although overall survival was favorable (40% at 2 years) the high rate of local relapse after intensive chemotherapy was believed not to warrant further trials of incorporating this approach into treatment.

More recently, Sterman and colleagues (1998) have explored the feasibility of treating early-stage malignant mesothelioma with intrapleural gene therapy. Using human mesothelioma tumors growing in the peritoneal cavities of severe combined immunodeficient mice, Hwang and colleagues (1995) reported that the herpes simplex virus thymidine kinase (*HSVtk*) gene could be successfully transferred to tumor via an adenovirus. Administration of the antiviral drug ganciclovir then led to selective tumor cell death. This treatment approach is currently being evaluated in phase I and II human clinical trials.

REFERENCES

Achatzy R, et al: The diagnosis, therapy and prognosis of diffuse malignant mesothelioma. Eur J Cardiothorac Surg *3*:445, 1989.

Adams VI, et al: Diffuse malignant mesothelioma of pleura. Diagnosis and survival in 92 cases. Cancer *58*:1540, 1986.

Alberts AS, et al: Malignant pleural mesothelioma: a disease unaffected by current therapeutic maneuvers. J Clin Oncol *6*:527, 1988.

Alexander E, et al: CT of malignant pleural mesothelioma. Am J Roentgenol *137*:287, 1981.

Allen KB, Faber LP, Warren WH: Malignant pleural mesothelioma. Extrapleural pneumonectomy and pleurectomy. Chest Surg Clin N Am *4*:113, 1994.

American Joint Committee on Cancer: Manual for Staging of Cancer. 4th Ed. Philadelphia: JB Lippincott, 1992.

Anderson KA, et al: Malignant pleural mesothelioma following radiotherapy in a 16-year-old boy. Cancer *56*:273, 1985.

Andersson M, Olsen JH: Trend and distribution of mesothelioma in Denmark. Br J Cancer *51*:699, 1985.

Antman KH, et al: Multimodality therapy for malignant mesothelioma based on a study of natural history. Am J Med *68*:356, 1980.

Antman KH, et al: Malignant mesothelioma following radiation exposure. J Clin Oncol *1*:695, 1983.

Antman KH, et al: Mesothelioma following Wilms' tumor in childhood. Cancer *54*:367, 1984.

Antman KH, et al: Malignant mesothelioma: prognostic variables in a registry of 180 patients, the Dana-Farber Cancer Institute and Brigham and Women's Hospital experience over two decades, 1965–1985. J Clin Oncol *6*:147, 1988.

Auribault M: Bulletin de l'Inspection du Travail, 1906, p. 126.

Baldini EH, et al: Patterns of failure after trimodality therapy for malignant pleural mesothelioma. Ann Thorac Surg *63*:334, 1997.

Ball DL, Cruickshank DG: The treatment of malignant mesothelioma of the pleura: review of a 5-year experience, with special reference to radiotherapy. Am J Clin Oncol *13*:4, 1990.

Baris YI: Asbestos and Erionite Related Chest Diseases. Ankara, Turkey: Semik Ofset Matbaacilik, 1987.

Battifora H, Kopinski MI: Distinction of mesothelioma from adenocarcinoma. An immunohistochemical approach. Cancer *55*:1679, 1985.

Bénard F, et al: Metabolic imaging of malignant pleural mesothelioma with fluorodeoxyglucose positron emission tomography. Chest *114*:713, 1998.

Blake PR, Catterall M, Errington RD: Treatment of malignant melanoma by fast neutrons. Br J Surg *72*:517, 1985.

Boutin C, Rey F: Thoracoscopy in pleural malignant mesothelioma: a prospective study of 188 consecutive patients. Part 1: Diagnosis. Cancer *72*:389, 1993a.

Boutin C, et al: Thoracoscopy in pleural malignant mesothelioma: a prospective study of 188 consecutive patients. Part 2: Prognosis and staging. Cancer *72*:394, 1993b.

Boutin C, Rey F, Viallat J-R: Prevention of malignant seeding after invasive diagnostic procedures in patients with pleural mesothelioma. A randomized trial of local radiotherapy. Chest *108*:754, 1995.

Boutin C, et al: Activity of intrapleural recombinant gamma-interferon in malignant mesothelioma. Cancer *67*:2033, 1991a.

Boutin C, Viallat JR, Aelony Y: Practical Thoracoscopy. Berlin: Springer-Verlag, 1991b.

Brady LW: Mesothelioma—the role for radiation therapy. Semin Oncol *8*:329, 1981.

Burmer GC, et al: Flow cytometric analysis of malignant pleural mesotheliomas. Hum Pathol *20*:777, 1989.

Burns TR, et al: Ultrastructural diagnosis of epithelial malignant mesothelioma. Cancer *56*:2036, 1985.

Butchart EG, et al: Pleuropneumonectomy in the management of diffuse malignant mesothelioma of the pleura. Experience with 29 patients. Thorax *31*:15, 1976.

Cantin R, Al-Jabi M, McCaughey WTE: Desmoplastic diffuse mesothelioma. Am J Surg Pathol *6*:215, 1982.

Carbone M, et al: Simian virus 40-like DNA sequences in human pleural mesothelioma. Oncogene *9*:1781, 1994.

Cartier P, Smith WE: Survey of some current British and European studies of occupational tumor problems. Arch Indust Hygiene Occup Med *5*:242, 1952.

Chahinian AP: Therapeutic modalities in malignant pleural mesothelioma. *In* Chretien J, Hirsch A (eds): Diseases of the Pleura. New York: Masson, 1983.

Chahinian AP, et al: Cisplatin with adriamycin or mitomycin for malignant mesothelioma: a randomized phase II trial. Proc ASCO *6*:183, 1987 (abst).

Chahinian AP, et al: Diffuse malignant mesothelioma. Prospective evaluation of 69 patients. Ann Intern Med *96*:746, 1982.

Chahinian AP, et al: Diffuse pulmonary malignant mesothelioma. Response to doxorubicin and 5-azacytidine. Cancer *42*:1687, 1978.

Churg A, DePaoli L: Environmental pleural plaques in residents of a Quebec chrysotile mining town. Chest *94*:58, 1988.

Cote RJ, et al: Genetic alterations of the p53 gene are a feature of malignant mesotheliomas. Cancer Res *51*:5410, 1991.

Dabouis G, Le Mevel B, Corroller J: Treatment of diffuse pleural malignant mesothelioma by cis dichloro diammine platinum (C.D.D.P.) in nine patients. Cancer Chemother Pharmacol *5*:209, 1981.

Dahl IMS, et al: A longitudinal study of the hyaluronan level in the serum of patients with malignant mesothelioma under treatment. Hyaluronan as an indicator of progressive disease. Cancer 64:68, 1989.

de Klerk NH, Armstrong BK: The epidemiology of asbestos and mesothelioma. In Henderson DW, et al (eds): Malignant Mesothelioma. New York: Hemisphere, 1992.

DeLaria GA, et al: Surgical management of malignant mesothelioma. Ann Thorac Surg 26:375, 1978.

DeValle MJ, et al: Extrapleural pneumonectomy for diffuse, malignant mesothelioma. Ann Thorac Surg 42:612, 1986.

Dimitrov NV, et al: High-dose methotrexate with citrovorum factor and vincristine in the treatment of malignant mesothelioma. Cancer 50:1 245,1982.

Dimitrov NV, McMahon S: Presentation, diagnostic methods, staging, and natural history of malignant mesothelioma. In Antman K, Aisner J (eds): Asbestos-Related Malignancy. Orlando: Grune & Stratton, 1987.

Elmes PC, Simpson MJC: The clinical aspects of mesothelioma. QJM New Series 45:427, 1976.

Fraire AE, et al: Mesothelioma of childhood. Cancer 62:838, 1988.

Gerwin BI, et al: Comparison of production of transforming growth factor-beta and platelet-derived growth factor by normal human mesothelial cells and mesothelioma cell lines. Cancer Res 47:6180, 1987.

Goey SH, et al: Intrapleural administration of interleukin 2 in pleural mesothelioma: a phase I-II study. Br J Cancer 72:1283, 1995.

Gordon W Jr, et al: Radiation therapy in the management of patients with mesothelioma. Int J Radiat Oncol Biol Phys 8:19, 1982.

Gotfried MH, Quan SF, Sobonya RE: Diffuse epithelial pleural mesothelioma presenting as a solitary lung mass. Chest 84:99, 1983.

Hagemeijer A, et al: Cytogenetic analysis of malignant mesothelioma. Cancer Genet Cytogenet 47:1, 1990.

Hammar SP, Bolen JW: Pleural neoplasms. In Dail DH, Hammar SP (eds): Pulmonary Pathology. New York: Springer-Verlag, 1988.

Heelan RT, et al: Malignant pleural mesothelioma: comparison of CT and MR imaging for staging. Am J Radiol 1998 (in press).

Hilaris BS, et al: Pleurectomy and intraoperative brachytherapy and post-operative radiation in the treatment of malignant pleural mesothelioma. Int J Radiat Oncol Biol Phys 10:325, 1984.

Hillerdal G: Malignant mesothelioma 1982: review of 4710 published cases. Br J Dis Chest 77:321, 1983.

Hulks G, Thomas JS, Waclawski E: Malignant pleural mesothelioma in western Glasgow 1980–6. Thorax 44:496, 1989.

Huncharek M: Changing risk groups for malignant mesothelioma. Cancer 69:2704, 1992.

Hwang HC, et al: Gene therapy using adenovirus carrying the herpes simplex-thymidine kinase gene to treat in vivo models of human malignant mesothelioma and lung cancer. Am J Respir Cell Mol Biol 13:7, 1995.

Kane MJ, Chahinian AP, Holland JF: Malignant mesothelioma in young adults. Cancer 65:1449, 1990.

Kaye JA, et al: Malignant mesothelioma with brain metastases. Am J Med 80:95, 1986.

Keller SM, Taylor DD, Weese JL: In vitro killing of human malignant mesothelioma by photodynamic therapy. J Surg Res 48:337, 1990.

Klemperer P, Rabin CB: Primary neoplasms of the pleura. A report of five cases. Arch Pathol 11:385, 1937.

Krarup-Hansen A, Hansen HH: Chemotherapy in malignant mesothelioma: a review. Cancer Chemother Pharmacol 28:319, 1991.

Kutcher GJ, et al: Technique for external beam treatment for mesothelioma. Int J Radiat Oncol Biol Phys 13:1747, 1987.

Law MR, et al: Malignant mesothelioma of the pleura: a study of 52 treated and 64 untreated patients. Thorax 39:255, 1984.

Law MR, et al: Computed tomography in the assessment of malignant mesothelioma of the pleura. Clin Radiol 33:67, 1982a.

Law MR, Hodson ME, Heard BE: Malignant mesothelioma of the pleura: relation between histological type and clinical behaviour. Thorax 37:810, 1982b.

Layman L: The blue asbestos industry at Wittenoom in Western Australia: a short history. In Henderson DW, et al (eds): Malignant mesothelioma. New York: Hemisphere, 1992.

Le Roux BT: Pleural tumors. Thorax 17:111, 1962.

Lederman GS, et al: Long-term survival in peritoneal mesothelioma. The role of radiotherapy and combined modality treatment. Cancer 59:1882, 1987.

Lee W-C, et al: Loss of heterozygosity analysis defines a critical region in chromosome 1p22 commonly deleted in human malignant mesothelioma. Cancer Res 56:4297, 1996.

Lerman Y, et al: Radiation associated malignant pleural mesothelioma. Thorax 46:463, 1991.

Levine RL: Asbestos: An Information Resource (NIH Publication No. 81-1681). Bethesda, MD: National Institutes of Health, 1981.

Lewis RJ, et al: Diffuse, mixed malignant pleural mesothelioma. Ann Thorac Surg 31:53, 1981.

Low EM, et al: Prevention of tumour seeding following thoracoscopy in mesothelioma by prophylactic radiotherapy. Clin Oncol 7:317, 1995.

Maasilta P: Deterioration in lung function following hemithorax irradiation for pleural mesothelioma. Int J Radiat Oncol Biol Phys 20:433, 1991.

Malker HSR, et al: Occupational risks for pleural mesothelioma in Sweden, 1961–79. J Natl Cancer Inst 74:61, 1985.

Markman M, et al: Cisplatin administered by the intracavitary route as treatment for malignant mesothelioma. Cancer 58:18, 1986.

McCormack PM, et al: Surgical treatment of pleural mesothelioma. J Thorac Cardiovasc Surg 84:834, 1982.

McDonald AD, McDonald JC: Malignant mesothelioma in North America. Cancer 46:1650, 1980.

McDonald JC, et al: Mesothelioma and asbestos fiber type. Evidence from lung tissue analyses. Cancer 63:1544, 1989.

Mezger J, Lamerz R, Permanetter W: Diagnostic significance of carcinoembryonic antigen in the differential diagnosis of malignant mesothelioma. J Thorac Cardiovasc Surg 100:860, 1990.

Mintzer DM, et al: Phase II trial of high-dose cisplatin in patients with malignant mesothelioma. Cancer Treat Rep 69:711, 1985.

Mirvis S, et al: CT of malignant pleural mesothelioma. AJR Am J Roentgenol 140:655, 1983.

Mor O, et al: Absence of p53 mutations in malignant mesotheliomas. Am J Respir Cell Mol Biol 16:9, 1997.

Murray M: Report of the Departmental Committee on Compensation for Industrial Diseases. London: HMSO, 1907.

Musk AW, et al: The incidence of malignant mesothelioma in Australia, 1947–1980. Med J Aust 150:242, 1989.

Mychalczak BR, et al: Results of treatment of malignant pleural mesothelioma with surgery, brachytherapy, and external beam irradiation [Abstract]. Endocurie Hypertherm Oncol 5:245, 1989.

Nauta RJ, et al: Clinical staging and the tendency of malignant pleural mesotheliomas to remain localized. Ann Thorac Surg 34:66, 1982.

Olesen LL, Thorshauge H: Thrombocytosis in patients with malignant pleural mesothelioma. Cancer 62:1194, 1988.

Ong ST, Vogelzang NJ: Chemotherapy in malignant pleural mesothelioma: a review. J Clin Oncol 14:1007, 1996.

Pass HI, et al: Intrapleural photodynamic therapy: results of a phase I trial. Ann Surg Oncol 1:28, 1994.

Pass HI, Mew DJY: In vitro and in vivo studies of mesothelioma. J Cell Biochem Suppl 24:142, 1996.

Peterson JT, Greenberg SD, Buffler PA: Non-asbestos-related malignant mesothelioma. A review. Cancer 54:951, 1984.

Pooley FD: Asbestos mineralogy. In Antman K, Aisner J (eds): Asbestos-Related Malignancy. Orlando, FL: Grune & Stratton, 1987.

Popescu NC, Chahinian AP, DiPaolo JA: Nonrandom chromosome alterations in human malignant mesothelioma. Cancer Res 48:142, 1988.

Rabinowitz JG, et al: A comparative study of mesothelioma and asbestosis using computed tomography and conventional chest radiography. Radiology 144:453, 1982.

Raghavan D, et al: Phase II trial of carboplatin in the management of malignant mesothelioma. J Clin Oncol 8:151, 1990.

Reddel RR, et al: Tumorigenicity of human mesothelial cell line transfected with EJ-ras oncogene. J Natl Cancer Inst 81:945, 1989.

Ris H-B, et al: Photodynamic therapy with chlorins for diffuse malignant mesothelioma: initial clinical results. Br J Cancer 64:1116, 1991.

Roberts GH: Distant visceral metastases in pleural mesothelioma. Br J Dis Chest 70:246, 1976.

Ruffie R, et al: Diffuse malignant mesothelioma of the pleura in Ontario and Quebec: a retrospective study of 332 patients. J Clin Oncol 7:1157, 1989.

Rusch VW: Pleurectomy/decortication and adjuvant therapy for malignant mesothelioma. Chest 103:382S, 1993.

Rusch VW, Godwin JD, Shuman WP: The role of computed tomography scanning in the initial assessment and the follow-up of malignant pleural mesothelioma. J Thorac Cardiovasc Surg 96:171, 1988.

Rusch VW, Piantadosi S, Holmes EC: The role of extrapleural pneumonectomy in malignant pleural mesothelioma. J Thorac Cardiovasc Surg *102*:1, 1991.

Rusch VW, The International Mesothelioma Interest Group: A proposed new international TNM staging system for malignant pleural mesothelioma. Chest *108*:1122, 1995.

Rusch VW, Venkatraman E: The importance of surgical staging in the treatment of malignant pleural mesothelioma. J Thorac Cardiovasc Surg *111*:815, 1996.

Rusch VW, et al: A phase II trial of pleurectomy/decortication followed by intrapleural and systemic chemotherapy for malignant pleural mesothelioma. J Clin Oncol *12*:1156, 1994.

Scharifker D, Kenko M: Localized fibrous "mesothelioma" of pleura (submesothelial fibroma). A clinicopathologic study of 18 cases. Cancer *43*:627, 1979.

Selikoff IJ, Churg J, Hammond EC: Relation between exposure to asbestos and mesothelioma. N Engl J Med *272*:560, 1965.

Sheard JDH, et al: Pneumothorax and malignant mesothelioma in patients over the age of 40. Thorax *46*:584, 1991.

Sinoff C, et al: Combined doxorubicin and radiation therapy in malignant pleural mesothelioma. Cancer Treat Rep *66*:1605, 1982.

Sklarin NT, et al: Augmentation of activity of cis-diamminedichloroplatinum (II) and mitomycin c by interferon in human malignant mesothelioma xenografts in nude mice. Cancer Res *48*:64, 1988.

Smythe WR, et al: Use of recombinant adenovirus to transfer the herpes simplex virus thymidine kinase (*HSVtk*) gene to thoracic neoplasms: an effective in vitro drug sensitization system. Cancer Res *54*:2055, 1994.

Soubra M, et al: Physical aspects of external beam radiotherapy for the treatment of malignant pleural mesothelioma. Int J Radiat Oncol Biol Phys *18*:1521, 1990.

Stanton MF, Wrench C: Mechanisms of mesothelioma induction with asbestos and fibrous glass. J Natl Cancer Inst *48*:797, 1972.

Sterman DH, Kaiser LR, Albelda SM: Gene therapy for malignant pleural mesothelioma. Hematol Oncol Clin North Am *12*:553, 1998.

Stout AP, Murray MR: Localized pleural mesothelioma. Arch Pathol *34*:951, 1942.

Sugarbaker DJ, et al: Extrapleural pneumonectomy, chemotherapy, and radiotherapy in the treatment of diffuse malignant pleural mesothelioma. J Thorac Cardiovasc Surg *102*:10, 1991.

Sugarbaker DJ, et al: Trimodality therapy of malignant pleural mesothelioma. J Clin Oncol *11*:295, 1992.

Sugarbaker DJ, et al: Node status has prognostic significance in the multimodality therapy of diffuse, malignant mesothelioma. J Clin Oncol *11*:1172, 1993.

Sugarbaker DJ, et al: Extrapleural pneumonectomy in the multimodality therapy of malignant pleural mesothelioma. Results in 120 consecutive patients. Ann Surg *224*:288, 1996.

Taguchi T, et al: Recurrent deletions of specific chromosomal sites in 1p, 3p, 6q, and 9p in human malignant mesothelioma. Cancer Res *53*:4349, 1993.

Tammilehto L: Malignant mesothelioma: prognostic factors in a prospective study of 98 patients. Lung Cancer *8*:175, 1992.

Testa JR, et al: A multi-institutional study confirms the presence and expression of simian virus 40 in human malignant mesotheliomas. Cancer Res *58*:4505, 1998.

Tiainen M, et al: Chromosomal abnormalities and their correlations with asbestos exposure and survival in patients with mesothelioma. Br J Cancer *60*:618, 1989.

Umsawasdi T, et al: A case report of malignant pleural mesothelioma with long-term disease control after chemotherapy. Cancer *67*:48, 1991.

Van der Schoot HC: Asbestosis en pleuragezwellen. Ned Tijdschr Geneeskd *102*:1125, 1958.

Versnel MA, et al: Expression of c-*sis* (PDGF B-chain) and PDGF A-chain genes in ten human malignant mesothelioma cell lines derived from primary metastatic tumor. Oncogene *2*:601, 1988.

Vokes EE, Weichselbaum RR: Concomitant chemoradiotherapy: rationale and clinical experience in patients with solid tumors. J Clin Oncol *8*:911, 1990.

Wadler S, et al: Cardiac abnormalities in patients with diffuse malignant pleural mesothelioma. Cancer *58*:2744, 1986.

Wagner JC: Mesothelioma and mineral fibers. Cancer *57*:1905, 1986.

Wagner JC, Slegg CA, Marchand P: Diffuse pleural mesotheliomas and asbestos exposure in Northwestern Cape Province. Br J Ind Med *17*:260, 1960.

Walters KL, Martinez AJ: Malignant fibrous mesothelioma. Metastatic to brain and liver. Acta Neuropathol (Berl) *33*:173, 1975.

Wedler HW: Uber den Lungenkrebs bei Asbestose. Dtsch Arch Klin Med *191*:189, 1943a.

Wedler HW: Asbestose und Lungenkrebs. Dtsch med Wschr *69*:575, 1943b.

Whitwell F, Rawcliffe RM: Diffuse malignant pleural mesothelioma and asbestos exposure. Thorax *26*:6, 1971.

Wirth PR, Legier J, Wright Jr GL: Immunohistochemical evaluation of seven monoclonal antibodies for differentiation of pleural mesothelioma from lung adenocarcinoma. Cancer *67*:655, 1991.

Xiao S, et al: Codeletion of *p15* and *p16* in primary malignant mesothelioma. Oncogene *11*:511, 1995.

CHAPTER 66

Technique of Pleural Pneumonectomy in Diffuse Mesothelioma

Scott J. Swanson, Sean C. Grondin, and David J. Sugarbaker

The technique of extrapleural pneumonectomy has been described since the late 1940s, initially by Sarot (1949) for the treatment of tuberculous empyema and in the 1980s and 1990s for other noninfectious pleural diseases, such as malignant pleural mesothelioma (i.e., diffuse mesothelioma). Worn (1974), Faber (1986), and Butchart (1976), DeLaria (1978), DaValle (1986), Rusch (1991), and Allen (1994) and their colleagues have described the surgical approach and the pathophysiologic and histologic consequences of extrapleural pneumonectomy for malignant pleural mesothelioma. Most authors, however, have reported a high perioperative mortality and morbidity when compared with that of nonextrapleural pneumonectomy (Table 66-1). One of us (D.J.S.) and colleagues (1999), however, have reported on a series of 183 patients who underwent extrapleural pneumonectomy followed by adjuvant chemotherapy and radiation therapy for malignant mesothelioma. This large cohort had an operative mortality of 3.8%, which is a significant improvement over previous reports. Improvement in operative mortality since the 1970s is multifactorial, but is due largely to improvements in patient selection and preoperative preparation, intraoperative management, and postoperative care of patients with this extremely complex disease.

This chapter describes our approach to staging and patient selection for surgical resection, specifically extrapleural pneumonectomy. The surgical technique for right-sided extrapleural pneumonectomy is explained in detail, with a supplement on the variations required for the left-sided approach. The clinical results from our 10-year experience at the Brigham and Women's Hospital Thoracic Surgery Division and Dana-Farber Surgical Services are also described.

STAGING

At present, no consensus exists among clinicians regarding which staging system for malignant pleural mesothelioma should be used universally. In 1976, a staging scheme was proposed by Butchart and associates (1976) that has been used worldwide (see Table 65-3). In the years following, a number of classifications have been proposed, including a new tumor, node, metastasis system by the International Mesothelioma Interest Group in 1995, reported by Rusch (1995) (see Table 65-4). The weakness of these systems is that they fail to adequately stratify patient survival by stage.

Using the Butchart staging system, surgical resection is only appropriate for stage I disease. Extension of tumor into the mediastinum or through the diaphragm (Butchart stages II, III) or the presence of metastatic disease (stage IV) prohibits resection because survival beyond 1 year is extremely low.

With increasing evidence published by Rusch and Venkatraman (1996) to support the importance of concise surgical staging in the treatment of malignant mesothelioma, one of us (D.J.S.) and colleagues (1999) of the Oncology Program at the Division of Thoracic Surgery, Brigham and Women's Hospital and Dana-Farber Cancer Institute, proposed a staging system based on the prognostic indicators of resectability, nodal status, and tumor histology (Table 66-2). The importance of these indicators has been demonstrated in the analysis of 183 patients by one of us (D.J.S.) and associates (1999). The classification defines patients who have Brigham stage I or II disease as potentially resectable.

Patients with either of these two stages of disease are technically resectable. They could be further assessed for treatment by determining the preresectional lymph node status of their disease. For this reason, preresectional staging of nodes by using minimally invasive surgical techniques, such as thoracoscopy, mediastinoscopy, and laparoscopy, are important not only in the selection of appropriate patients for specific types of operative management but also in assessing stage-specific adjuvant trials. In the near future, radiologic imaging using positron

Table 66-1. Reported Mortality with Extrapleural Pneumonectomy

Author (year)	No. of Patients	Epithelial Cell Type	Operative Mortality (%)	2-Year Survival (%)	5-Year Survival (%)
Worn (1974)	62	—	—	37	10
Butchart et al. (1976)	29	11	31	10	3
DeLaria et al. (1978)	11	9	0	27	—
DaValle et al. (1986)	33	20	9	24	6
Rusch et al. (1991)	20	—	15	33	—
Allen et al. (1994)[a]	40	26	7.5	22.5	10
Sugarbaker et al. (1999)[b]	183	103	3.8	37	14

[a]Extrapleural pneumonectomy followed by chemotherapy [cyclophosphamide, Adriamycin (doxorubicin), and prednisone (cisplatin) (CAP)].
[b]Extrapleural pneumonectomy followed by adjuvant radiation therapy (40.5 Gy ±14.4 Gy boost dose to areas of residual disease, localized lymph nodes and/or localized positive resection margins) and chemotherapy [doxorubicin (nine patients), CAP (80 patients) and carboplatin/paclitaxel (94 patients)]. The 2- and 5-year survival for 176 patients who survived surgery were 38% and 15%, respectively.

emission tomography scanning may also prove to be a helpful staging tool.

Trimodality Therapy

Attempts to improve survival using surgical therapy were unsuccessful until treatment plans involving a trimodality approach were introduced by one of us (D.J.S.) and coworkers (1991, 1993, 1996, 1997). The approach is derived from a traditional treatment strategy that achieves local control by using pleuropneumonectomy followed by radiation therapy and control of systemic disease with chemotherapy.

Careful preoperative assessment and selection are required if the appropriate patients with malignant pleural

Table 66-2. Revised Staging System for Malignant Pleural Mesothelioma

Stage	Description
I	Disease completely resected within the capsule of the parietal pleura without adenopathy: ipsilateral pleura, lung, pericardium, diaphragm, or chest-wall disease limited to previous biopsy sites
II	All of stage I with positive resection margins and/or intrapleural adenopathy
III	Local extension of disease into chest wall or mediastinum; heart or through diaphragm or peritoneum; or with extrapleural lymph node involvement
IV	Distant metastatic disease

Note: Butchart stage II and III patients (Butchart et al. 1976) are combined into stage III. Stage I represents resectable patients with negative nodes. Stage II represents resectable patients that have positive nodal status.
Modified from Sugarbaker DJ, et al: Resection margins, extrapleural nodal status, and cell type determine postoperative long-term survival in trimodality therapy of malignant pleural mesothelioma: results in 183 patients. J Thorac Cardiovasc Surg *117*:54, 1999. With permission.

mesothelioma are to be selected for these aggressive treatment regimens that include extrapleural pneumonectomy.

PATIENT SELECTION

To be considered initially for extrapleural pneumonectomy, a patient is required to have a Karnofsky performance status higher than 70, normal liver and renal function tests, a room air arterial Pco_2 less than 45 mm Hg, and a room air arterial Po_2 more than 65 mm Hg.

As a result of the obliterative nature of the pleural disease, preoperative pulmonary function tests, notably forced expiratory volume in 1 second (FEV_1) and forced vital capacity (FVC), may not fully predict a patient's postoperative pulmonary function. Patients with malignant pleural mesothelioma may behave as though the diseased lung is functionally absent before surgery. For patients in whom lung function is borderline (i.e., predicted postoperative FEV_1 less than 1 L), the use of quantitative ventilation-perfusion scanning, when combined with knowledge of FEV_1 and FVC, results in a reliable prediction of the postoperative lung function after surgery. Echocardiography to measure left and right ventricular function is helpful in assessing preexisting alterations in ventricular function and providing a baseline for monitoring cardiac toxicity during postoperative chemotherapy.

Preoperative chest magnetic resonance (MR) imaging and computed tomography (CT) are essential in determining the extent of intrathoracic and extrathoracic disease preoperatively. Determining the presence of transdiaphragmatic extension or mediastinal invasion, especially of the vena cava, trachea, esophagus, or aorta and in invasion of the paravertebral sulcus, is required to determine the extent of tumor in these patients. The presence of mediastinal invasion or abdominal disease precludes surgical resection, because no long-term survivors have been reported in this setting. Chest MR imaging has been shown by Patz and associates (1992) to be of value in addition to CT scanning in making these determinations.

TECHNIQUE OF PLEUROPNEUMONECTOMY IN DIFFUSE MESOTHELIOMA

Right Pleuropneumonectomy

After induction of anesthesia and placement of a left-sided double-lumen tube, the patient is positioned in a left lateral decubitus position in preparation for an extended right posterolateral thoracotomy. A nasogastric tube should be placed to facilitate palpation of the esophagus during the dissection and to maintain a decompressed stomach postoperatively, particularly in the setting of a neodiaphragm.

These patients are monitored with arterial lines, continuous oximetry, and a central venous line. Thoracic epidural catheters are placed preoperatively and may be used for intraoperative management and postoperative pain control.

Before making the thoracotomy incision, a limited subcostal incision is made to explore for possible transdiaphragmatic involvement if suggested by the preoperative MR imaging. Laparoscopic exploration may be preferred by surgeons with experience in this technique. If peritoneal involvement is discovered, the procedure should be terminated and no attempt at thoracic resection made. The diaphragm may be distended with the tumor, but frank invasion into the peritoneal space should be documented with biopsy before abandoning the procedure.

An incision is made along the bed of the sixth rib, as suggested by Garcia and associates (1997) (Fig. 66-1). The incision is taken from 2 cm lateral to the costovertebral junction following the bed of the sixth rib to the costochondral junction. After periosteal stripping, the sixth rib is excised in its entirety to provide adequate exposure. The posterior periosteum, in the bed of the excised sixth rib, is then incised, and a widely based extrapleural dissection is advanced superiorly toward the apex of the thorax using both sharp and blunt dissection. The anterior component of the dissection is completed first, both superiorly and inferiorly toward the diaphragm. The posterior dissection is carried out after adequate exposure has been obtained anteriorly. This provides a safe view of the mediastinal structures in the posterior portion of the visceral compartment. After adequate initial dissection has been achieved to allow room for self-retaining retractors, two chest retractors are positioned anteriorly and posteriorly within the chest. Combined sharp and blunt dissection continues toward the apex of the hemithorax. The brachial triangle is exposed carefully to avoid avulsion of the subclavian artery and vein. In general, the parietal pleura thins out in this region, and special attention to the plane of dissection should be maintained.

On the anterior border, the internal mammary artery and vein, as noted by Garcia and colleagues (1997), must be protected from injury, because they can be easily avulsed from the superior vena cava and the subclavian artery (Fig. 66-2). Posterosuperiorly, the dissection is carried from the apex of the hemithorax down to the azygos vein (Fig. 66-3). The dissection is extrapleural until the right main stem bronchus and upper lobe are visualized. The extrapleural tissues are then dissected from the superior vena cava and azygos vein. At this point, the surgeon must rule out any disease extension that precludes an extrapleural pneumonectomy. The pericardium is opened and the pericardial space is palpated

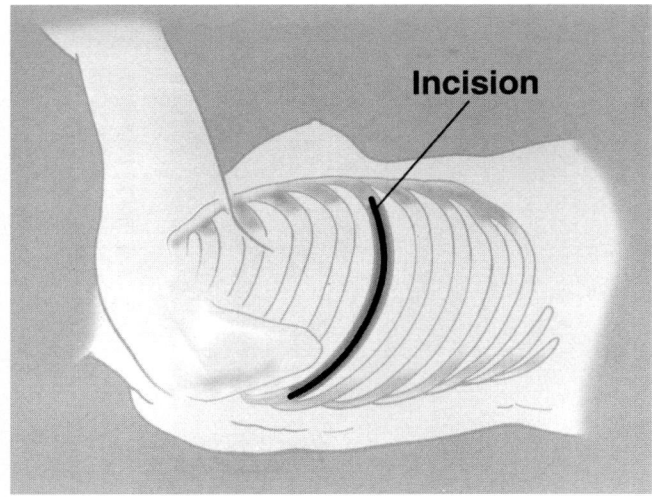

Fig. 66-1. The extended right thoracotomy incision. From Garcia JP, Richards WG, Sugarbaker DJ: Surgical treatment of malignant mesothelioma. *In* Kaiser LR, Kron IL, Spray TL (eds): *Mastery of Cardiothoracic Surgery.* Philadelphia: Lippincott–Raven, 1998. With permission.

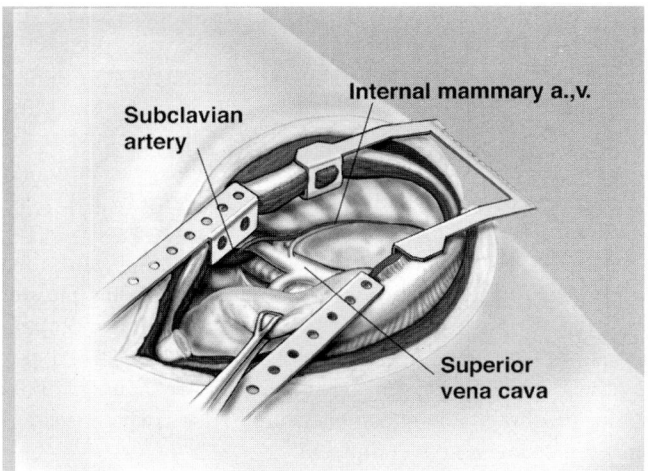

Fig. 66-2. Internal mammary artery (a.) and vein (v.) originating from subclavian artery and superior vena cava, respectively. From Garcia JP, Richards WG, Sugarbaker DJ: Surgical treatment of malignant mesothelioma. *In* Kaiser LR, Kron IL, Spray TL (eds): *Mastery of Cardiothoracic Surgery.* Philadelphia: Lippincott–Raven, 1998. With permission.

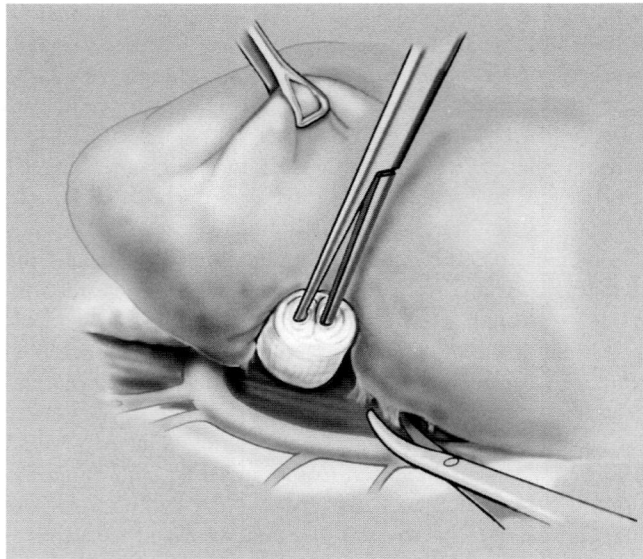

Fig. 66-3. Right lung dissected medially away from azygous vein. From Garcia JP, Richards WG, Sugarbaker DJ: Surgical treatment of malignant mesothelioma. *In* Kaiser LR, Kron IL, Spray TL (eds): Mastery of Cardiothoracic Surgery. Philadelphia: Lippincott–Raven, 1998. With permission.

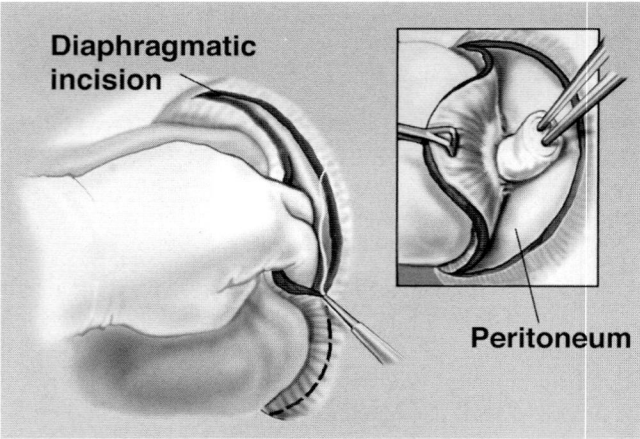

Fig. 66-4. Dissection of the pleural envelope off the diaphragm. From Garcia JP, Richards WG, Sugarbaker DJ: Surgical treatment of malignant mesothelioma. *In* Kaiser LR, Kron IL, Spray TL (eds): Mastery of Cardiothoracic Surgery. Philadelphia: Lippincott–Raven, 1998. With permission.

to rule out invasion. Posteriorly, palpation is carried out to confirm the absence of aortic or esophageal invasion. Without signs of unresectable disease, attention is turned to the diaphragmatic resection.

The anterior dissection at the base of the lung is completed when the circumferential diaphragmatic margin is dissected. The diaphragm is incised at its lateral margin in a circumferential fashion as far as the anterior border of the pericardium. Garcia and coworkers (1997) stress that care should be taken to maintain continuity of the pleural envelope, which typically requires dissection of the envelope off the edge of the diaphragm before the division of the diaphragm (Fig. 66-4). The diaphragm is dissected off the peritoneum by blunt dissection using a sponge stick (see Fig. 66-4, inset). After the diaphragm has been divided anteriorly to the pericardium, it is incised along the caval-esophageal hiatuses. The pericardium is incised to view the inferior vena cava fully during division of the diaphragm. Palpation of the nasogastric tube during the posterior portion of the dissection helps prevent inadvertent injury to the esophagus and facilitates mobilization of the specimen from the aorta and esophagus. Then, just lateral to the inferior vena cava and the esophagus, the posterior diaphragmatic attachments are divided. The diaphragmatic incision is now completed.

Completion of the pericardial incision is performed anteromedially to the phrenic nerve and hilar vessels, as described by Garcia and coworkers (1997) (Fig. 66-5). The main pulmonary artery is then dissected, isolating it from the superior vena cava and superior pulmonary vein. A soft, flanged catheter is passed around the pulmonary artery to

guide subsequent safe passage of an endovascular stapler in a technique described previously by one of us (D.J.S.) and associates (1997). One jaw of the endovascular stapler is placed in the flange of the endoleader catheter. This catheter delivers the stapler safely around the vessel. The pulmonary artery is divided intrapericardially. The superior and inferior pulmonary veins are each stapled between two lines of vascular staples using the endoleader maneuver (Fig. 66-6).

The pericardial resection is completed by dividing the pericardium posterior to the hilum. The surgical specimen is then brought forward anteriorly. Now dissection is advanced posteriorly to the pericardium and lateral to the esophagus.

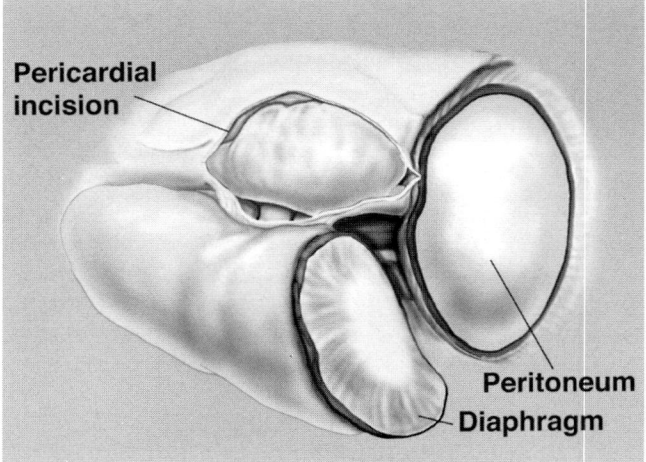

Fig. 66-5. Pericardium is opened anteromedially to the phrenic nerve and hilar vessels. From Garcia JP, Richards WG, Sugarbaker DJ: Surgical treatment of malignant mesothelioma. *In* Kaiser LR, Kron IL, Spray TL (eds): Mastery of Cardiothoracic Surgery. Philadelphia: Lippincott–Raven, 1998. With permission.

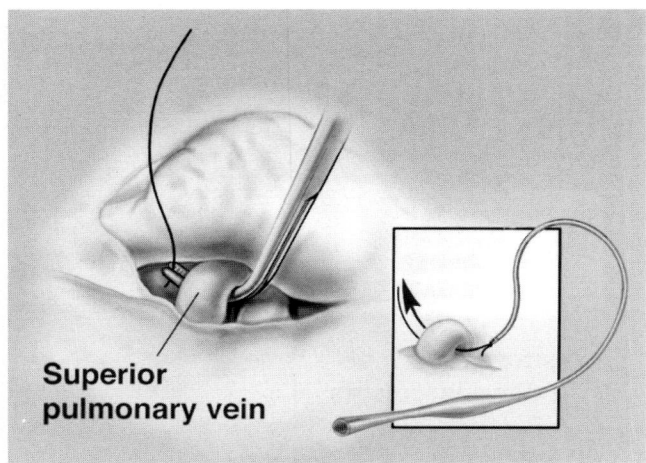

Fig. 66-6. The superior pulmonary vein is dissected within the pericardium. Inset: illustration of a safe technique for dissection of the hilar vessels using a pliable, plastic, self-dilating guidance catheter. One jaw of the endoscopic stapler fits into the end of this catheter, thus allowing safe placement of the stapler. From Garcia JP, Richards WG, Sugarbaker DJ: Surgical treatment of malignant mesothelioma. *In* Kaiser LR, Kron IL, Spray TL (eds): Mastery of Cardiothoracic Surgery. Philadelphia: Lippincott–Raven, 1998. With permission.

At this point, we perform a subcarinal node dissection. The right main bronchus is dissected as far as the carina and stapled with a heavy gauge wire bronchial stapler (TA-30, Ethicon Endo-Surgery, Johnson & Johnson, Cincinnati, OH) using the endoleader technique (Fig. 66-7); subsequently, the surgical specimen is removed for pathologic assessment.

At the time of surgery, the specimen is examined grossly and microscopically by the pathologist for the status of the resection margins. Approximately 20 sections are taken through each specimen to identify positive microscopic margins remaining along the chest wall, the bronchus, the pericardium, and diaphragm. Paratracheal, hilar, paraesophageal, inferior pulmonary ligament, peridiaphragmatic, and subcarinal nodes are also sampled to facilitate staging. Sampling of aortopulmonary nodes is added for a left-sided resection.

A pericardial fat pad based on a superior vascular pedicle is raised and rotated over the bronchial stump. It is secured circumferentially around the stump using self-absorbing 3-0 sutures (polyglactin, Vicryl, Ethicon, Somerville, NJ). The pericardium on the right side is always reconstructed with a prosthetic patch to prevent cardiac herniation. A 0.1-mm synthetic membrane (Gore-Tex, WL Gore and Associates, Inc., Flagstaff, AZ) is secured to the posterior, inferior and anterior pericardial margins with running 3-0 polypropylene sutures (Prolene, Ethicon, Somerville, NJ). It is also tacked superiorly in several places to prevent superior displacement of the heart. The diaphragm is also reconstructed using a prosthetic impermeable patch (2-mm Gore-Tex) that is sewn with a running monofilament (polypropylene, Prolene, Ethicon, Somerville, NJ) 0 suture (Fig. 66-8). The diaphragmatic patch is secured posteriorly to the diaphragmatic remnant, medially to hiatal musculature, and anteriorly to the chest wall. Use of permeable patches in this situation can result in peritoneal fluid filling the right pneumonectomy space, which may result in a severe mediastinal shift or cardiac tamponade. The pericardial patch should be fenestrated to prevent tamponade physiology caused by fluid accumulating postoperatively in a closed pericardial space (Fig. 66-9).

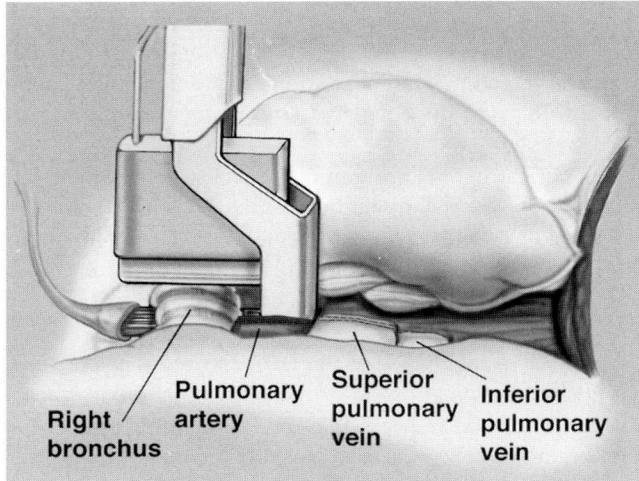

Fig. 66-7. The right main stem bronchus is transected with a heavy gauge stapler near the carina after the pulmonary artery and veins have been divided. Note the guidance catheter (full view in Fig. 66-6) is also used to place the bronchial stapler. From Garcia JP, Richards WG, Sugarbaker DJ: Surgical treatment of malignant mesothelioma. *In* Kaiser LR, Kron IL, Spray TL (eds): Mastery of Cardiothoracic Surgery. Philadelphia: Lippincott–Raven, 1998. With permission.

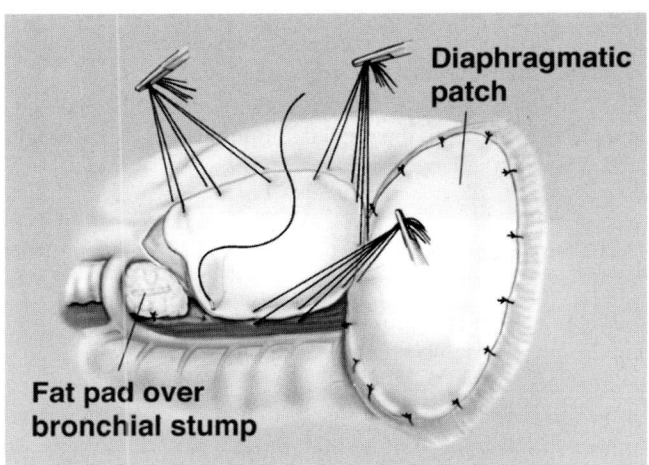

Fig. 66-8. The pericardium and diaphragm are reconstructed and a fat pad placed over the bronchial stump. From Garcia JP, Richards WG, Sugarbaker DJ: Surgical treatment of malignant mesothelioma. *In* Kaiser LR, Kron IL, Spray TL (eds): Mastery of Cardiothoracic Surgery. Philadelphia: Lippincott–Raven, 1998. With permission.

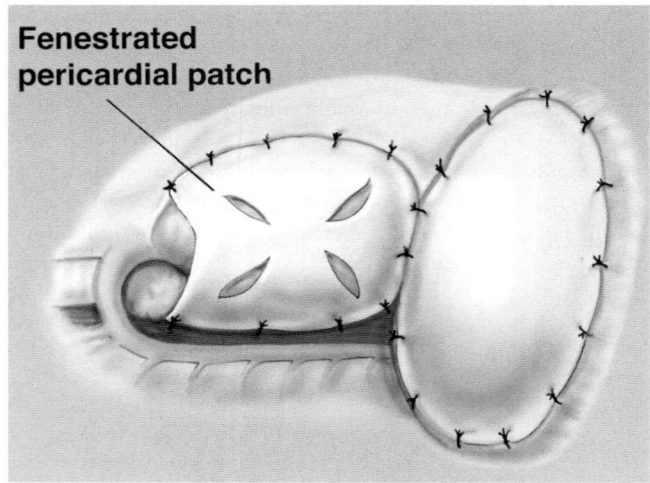

Fig. 66-9. Fenestrations in the pericardial patch are made to prevent tamponade. From Garcia JP, Richards WG, Sugarbaker DJ: Surgical treatment of malignant mesothelioma. *In* Kaiser LR, Kron IL, Spray TL (eds): Mastery of Cardiothoracic Surgery. Philadelphia: Lippincott–Raven, 1998. With permission.

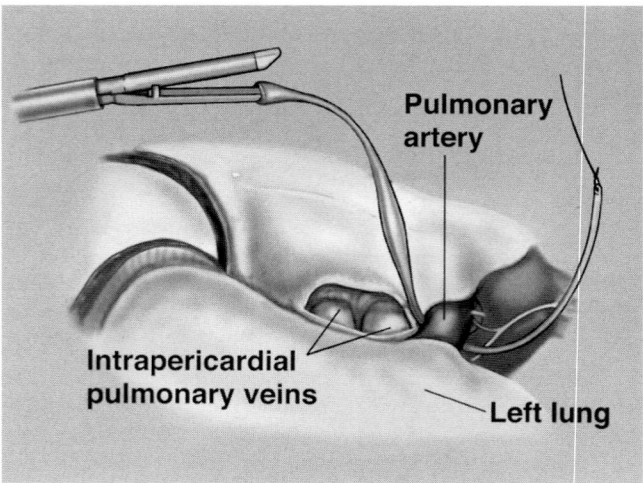

Fig. 66-10. The left pulmonary artery is divided as it leaves the pericardium and enters the left chest. From Garcia JP, Richards WG, Sugarbaker DJ: Surgical treatment of malignant mesothelioma. *In* Kaiser LR, Kron IL, Spray TL (eds): Mastery of Cardiothoracic Surgery. Philadelphia: Lippincott–Raven, 1998. With permission.

If an area of gross disease cannot be resected after pneumonectomy, it is delineated using radiopaque clips, which facilitate targeting for postoperative radiation therapy. The chest is then closed in the usual fashion to ensure an airtight closure. A small (e.g., No. 12F) red rubber catheter is placed in the residual pleural space to allow mediastinal positioning. Postoperatively, before extubation, the pneumonectomy space is reduced in size by removal of 750 cc of air in women and 1000 cc in men with the use of a 50-cc syringe attached to the red rubber catheter with a three-way stopcock. In the recovery room, a radiograph of the chest is obtained to check for midline position of the heart and mediastinal structures. If these are not midline on the chest radiograph, the mediastinum can be balanced by introducing or removing air; subsequently, the catheter can be removed. If a hemothorax is present, then a standard chest tube is placed and put to water-seal. It is used to monitor drainage overnight and removed the next day.

Left Pleuropneumonectomy

Placing either an endobronchial blocker or a right double-lumen tube for lung isolation is appropriate in left pleuropneumonectomy. The dissection for a diffuse mesothelioma of the left hemithorax is similar to that on the right, but some important differences should be noted.

Technically, the dissection on this side is less difficult because of the position of the caval, aortic and esophageal hiatuses. During dissection of the posteromedial aspect of the specimen, entering the correct plane in the preaortic region to prevent avulsion of the intercostal vessels is important. These intercostal vessels or the aorta itself may also be injured during the dissection of the aortodiaphragmatic hiatus. The assessment of the aorta is the critical step on the left side in determining tumor resectability because aortic involvement may preclude resection. The esophagus in its location anterior to the aorta should be identified and protected, particularly during dissection at the base of the diaphragm posteriorly.

Garcia and associates (1997) have recommended that the left main pulmonary artery, being much shorter than the right main pulmonary artery, be dissected and divided in an extrapleural, extrapericardial plane to prevent encroachment on the right pulmonary artery (Fig. 66-10). The pulmonary veins may be dissected intrapericardially, and the pericardial resection is completed posteriorly. The left main stem bronchus must be dissected up to the carina to ensure a short bronchial stump.

The pericardium is not routinely reconstructed on the left side, because the risk of cardiac herniation is low. The heart is tethered by the cavae and projected into the left hemithorax. Therefore, although the heart can rotate or herniate into an empty right hemithorax, it will not herniate into an empty left hemithorax. If a small pericardial resection is carried out, risk of strangulation of the left ventricular apex exists, but given the typical extent of mesothelioma, this is generally not a relevant issue. Because of the reduced size of the left hemithorax, less air is removed at the end of the procedure: 500 cc in women, 750 cc in men.

Hemostasis

Routine blood loss during this procedure is 750 mL for a right pneumonectomy and 500 mL for a left pneumonectomy. During the mobilization of the specimen, surgical hemostasis is best accomplished using electrocautery and by rapidly packing bleeding areas resulting from pleural dissection. Once the specimen has been removed, liberal use of the argon beam coagulator and electrocautery is needed to coagulate the numerous small vessels in the extrapleural plane bleeding on the chest wall surface. It is important to devote extra attention to hemostasis because bleeding from the chest wall can be the source of significant postoperative morbidity.

POSTOPERATIVE MANAGEMENT

The goals of postoperative management are not dissimilar from those with patients undergoing other standard pneumonectomy procedures. These are to control pain and minimize intravascular volume changes. Postoperatively, we routinely use thoracic epidural catheters for the first 3 to 5 days. Pain control is vital to minimize postoperative atelectasis and its resulting pulmonary dysfunction. Patients are monitored in a thoracic stepdown unit with arterial lines, central venous lines, continuous oximetry, and respiratory rate monitors. Nursing is on a one-to-two basis with regular chest physiotherapy. Deep vein thrombosis prophylaxis is done with pneumatic boots and subcutaneous heparin. Patients are placed on bedrest for 48 hours postoperatively to facilitate mediastinal stability. After 48 hours, ambulation and chest physiotherapy are routine.

Patients are routinely placed on a 1-L, 24-hour fluid restriction for 3 to 5 days postoperatively. This is owing to the tendency of these patients to retain fluid and to have mild episodes of capillary leak in the remaining lung, which can lead to desaturation. Desaturation of oxygen levels is usually treated with diuresis and chest physiotherapy. If this is not effective, bronchoscopy is carried out. Daily chest radiographs are closely evaluated for mediastinal shift that might lead to tamponade or in-flow obstruction. Contralateral infiltrates are treated aggressively in this patient population. Because the nasogastric tube can impede effective cough, the tube is removed on postoperative day 1 if clinical parameters are acceptable. The patient, however, should avoid any oral intake until evidence exists of return of gastric function, because aspiration is a highly morbid event in this group of patients.

CLINICAL RESULTS AND DISCUSSION

In 1999, one of us (D.J.S.) and associates reported a series of 183 patients who underwent pleuropneumonectomy with a consistent postoperative mortality rate (3.8%) comparable to that of standard pneumonectomy, as reported by Ginsberg and associates (1983) (see Table 66-1). Clearly, patient selection is an important factor in this lowered mortality, as are advances in preoperative preparation, intraoperative management, and postoperative care.

Cell type, adequate surgical resection margins and node status, when combined with postoperative chemotherapy (cisplatin/paclitaxel) and radiation therapy (40.5 Gy ±14.4 Gy boost dose to areas of residual disease, localized lymph nodes, and/or localized positive resection margins) have been shown to demonstrate prognostic importance. Patients with epithelial cell pleural mesothelioma enjoyed a survival advantage over patients with mixed or pure sarcomatous cell type treated with surgery, chemotherapy, and radiation therapy. As one of us (D.J.S.) and colleagues (1999) have noted, the inability to obtain negative resection margins or the presence of nodal involvement at the time of surgical resection were predictors of poorer survival. Overall, 2- and 5-year survival of 38% and 15%, respectively, were noted in the 176 patients who survived pleuropneumonectomy and were treated with trimodality therapy. However, the 31 patients who had all three predictors of improved survival (epithelial histology, negative lymph nodes, and resection margins) had a 2- and 5-year survival of 68% and 46%, respectively. These data also support the survival stratification using the Brigham modified staging system (see Table 66-2).

Innovative therapeutic agents and delivery systems are being investigated that would allow the direct application of these agents into the chest. Kaiser (1997) has reported that novel therapies, such as photodynamic therapy, cytokines, and gene therapy, are being targeted as potential treatment strategies.

REFERENCES

Allen KB, Faber LP, Warren WH: Malignant pleural mesothelioma. Extrapleural pneumonectomy and pleurectomy. Chest Surg Clin North Am 4:113, 1994.
Butchart EG, et al: Pleuropneumonectomy in the management of diffuse malignant mesothelioma of the pleura. Experience with 29 patients. Thorax 31:15, 1976.
DaValle MJ, et al: Extrapleural pneumonectomy for diffuse, malignant mesothelioma. Ann Thorac Surg 42:612, 1986.
DeLaria GA, et al: Surgical management of malignant mesothelioma. Ann Thorac Surg 26:375, 1978.
Faber LP: Malignant pleural mesothelioma: operative treatment by extrapleural pneumonectomy. In Kittle CF (ed): Current Controversies in Thoracic Surgery. Philadelphia: WB Saunders, 1986, p. 80.
Garcia JP, Richards WG, Sugarbaker DJ: Surgical treatment of malignant mesothelioma. In Kaiser LR, Kron IL, Spray TL (eds): Mastery of Cardiothoracic Surgery. Philadelphia: Lippincott–Raven, 1998.
Ginsberg RJ, et al: Modern thirty-day operative mortality for surgical resections in lung cancer. J Thorac Cardiovasc Surg 86:654, 1983.
Kaiser LR: New therapies in the treatment of malignant pleural mesothelioma. Semin Thorac Cardiovasc Surg 9:383, 1997.
Patz EF Jr, et al: Malignant pleural mesothelioma: value of CT and MR imaging in predicting resectability. AJR Am J Roentgenol 159:961, 1992.
Rusch VW, Piantadosi S, Holmes EC: The role of extrapleural pneumonectomy in malignant pleural mesothelioma. A Lung Cancer Study Group trial. J Thorac Cardiovasc Surg 102:1, 1991.
Rusch VW, The International Mesothelioma Interest Group: A proposed new international TNM staging system for malignant pleural mesothelioma. Chest 108:1122, 1995.
Rusch VW, Venkatraman E: The importance of surgical staging in the treatment of malignant pleural mesothelioma. J Thorac Cardiovasc Surg 111:815, 1996.
Sarot IA: Extrapleural pneumonectomy and pleurectomy in pulmonary tuberculosis. Thorax 4:173, 1949.

Sugarbaker DJ, Norberto JJ, Swanson SJ: Extrapleural pneumonectomy in the setting of multimodality therapy for diffuse malignant pleural mesothelioma. Semin Thorac Cardiovasc Surg 9:373, 1997.

Sugarbaker DJ, et al: Extrapleural pneumonectomy, chemotherapy, and radiotherapy in the treatment of diffuse malignant pleural mesothelioma [see comments]. J Thorac Cardiovasc Surg 102:10, 1991.

Sugarbaker DJ, et al: Node status has prognostic significance in the multimodality therapy of diffuse, malignant mesothelioma. J Clin Oncol 11:1172, 1993.

Sugarbaker DJ, et al: Extrapleural pneumonectomy in the multimodality therapy of malignant pleural mesothelioma. Results in 120 consecutive patients. Ann Surg 224:288, 1996.

Sugarbaker DJ, et al: Resection margins, extrapleural nodal status, and cell type determine postoperative long-term survival in trimodality therapy of malignant pleural mesothelioma: results in 183 patients. J Thorac Cardiovasc Surg 117:54, 1999.

Worn H: Moglichkeiten und Ergebnisse der chirurgischen Behandlung des malignen Pleuramesotheliomas. Thoraxchir Vask Chir 22:391, 1974.

CHAPTER 67

Uncommon Tumors of the Pleura

Thomas W. Shields and Anjana V. Yeldandi

RARE PRIMARY BENIGN TUMORS OF THE PLEURA

Calcifying Fibrous Pseudotumor of the Pleura

Pinkard and associates (1996) described the occurrence of a benign, pleural-based tumor in three young adults. The pleural lesions were identified on standard chest radiography and did not reveal any calcification. Computed tomography, however, revealed calcification within the masses; Erasmus and colleagues (1996) published the significant radiographic and computed tomographic features in these three patients. On resection, the masses were found to be unencapsulated and were seen to arise from either the parietal or visceral pleural surface. In two of the patients, the lesions were solitary, whereas in the other, multiple lesions were seen. Histologically, the tumors were composed of hyalinized collagenous fibrotic tissue interspersed with lymphoplasmacytic infiltrates and calcification; many of these had psammomatous features. No evidence of malignancy existed in these tumors. Surgical resection appears to be curative.

RARE PRIMARY MALIGNANT TUMORS OF THE PLEURA

Except for a few rare primary malignant tumors of the pleura, most malignant lesions involving the pleura are either diffuse malignant mesotheliomas, metastatic lesions involving the pleural surface, or direct invasion of adjacent tumors from the lung or chest wall. Many of the metastatic and invasive lesions mimic a diffuse malignant mesothelioma in both their pathologic features and clinical course. The metastatic lesions include adenocarcinomas from various sites, primarily the lung, including the so-called pseudomesotheliomatous adenocarcinoma of the lung, which was initially described by Harwood and colleagues (1976) and further defined by Dessy and Pietra (1991) and Koss (1992) and Freidman (1993) and their associates, melanomas, thymomas, and metastatic epithelioid sarcomas, as well as tumors from other sites of origin. These secondary tumors must be differentiated from true diffuse mesotheliomas by ultrastructural and immunohistochemical features, the discussion of which is not germane to this chapter. However, the few rare primary malignant pleural lesions deserve further comment.

Biphasic Synovial Sarcoma of the Pleura

Battifora (1994) reported one case and Gaertner and associates (1996) reported five cases of biphasic tumors that were interpreted as synovial sarcomas arising in the pleural cavity. These tumors resembled the synovial (biphasic) tumors of the mediastinum reported by Witkin and colleagues (1989) (see Chapter 185). The pleural tumors occurred in young adults and appeared to be pseudoencapsulated, but had a rapidly fatal course. Differentiation by light microscopy, electron microscopy, and immunohistochemistry, as noted by Henderson and associates (1997), is necessary to separate this tumor from a primary malignant mesothelioma.

Epithelioid Hemangioendothelioma Involving the Pleura

Dail (1988) and Battifora (1993) reported the occurrence of an epithelioid hemangioendothelioma involving the pleura. Lin and associates (1996) reported seven similar cases. These tumors markedly resemble malignant mesotheliomas but can be differentiated by labeling the tumor with antibodies to von Willebrand's factor (factor VIII) and to other monoclonal antibodies from endothelial-derived cells (CD34, UEA-I, QBEND10, and CD31). Furthermore, these tumors are negative to or have low reactivity to low-molecular-weight cytokeratin. The clinical outlook of these patients is grave; the tumor responds poorly to treatment and early death is the result of disseminated disease.

Angiosarcoma of the Pleura

A few cases of angiosarcoma of the pleura have been recorded. McCaughey and colleagues (1983) reported one case, and Hammer (1995) noted the observation of one case. Although this tumor, when it occurs in the pleura, may resemble a diffuse malignant mesothelioma, its true nature may be suggested by the presence of vascular-appearing spaces by light microscopy. The presence of Weibel-Palade bodies and the tumor's positive reaction to vimentin and factor VIII–related antigen plus its negative reaction to cytokeratin antigens establishes the vascular origin of the tumor. The clinical course of the patient is poor.

Primary Smooth Muscle Tumors of the Pleura

Moran and colleagues (1995) described five cases of primary smooth muscle tumors of the pleura. These tumors are extremely rare and should be distinguished from other spindle cell neoplasms. These tumors test positive for muscle markers, such as smooth muscle action and desmin, by immunohistochemistry. It should be noted that Gibbs (1995) is not convinced that these tumors represent a true entity.

Primary Pleural Liposarcoma

Liposarcomas of the pleura are exceedingly rare. Only nine cases of primary pleural liposarcomas have been reported. Wong and associates (1994), in their report of a single case, also review eight other cases reported in the literature. Histologically, three were myxoid liposarcomas, one a well-differentiated liposarcoma, and four liposarcomas were not subtyped. Patients were symptomatic only when the tumors reached a large size. The most common symptom was dyspnea. Treatment consisted of surgical excision and adjuvant radiation therapy.

Primary Extraskeletal Myxoid Chondrosarcoma of the Pleura

Goetz and associates (1992) reported a single case of chondrosarcoma of the pleura that clinically mimicked a malignant mesothelioma. This tumor was seen in a patient with a 15-year history of exposure to asbestos. The tumor encased the lung and grossly was nodular with a gelatinous texture. Histologically, the tumor had typical features of myxoid chondrosarcoma. Immunochemically, only vimentin was expressed. Many ferruginous bodies also were seen in histologic sections. A metastatic sarcoma from a distant primary site was excluded clinically. A sarcomatoid mesothelioma was excluded by lack of keratin expression and by the presence of microtubular aggregates with rough endoplasmic reticulum by ultrastructural examination.

Primary Pleural Thymomas

Most cases reported in the literature as pleural thymomas have been shown, as noted by Moran and coworkers (1992), to be an extension to the pleural surfaces of an underlying malignant thymoma originating in the thymus gland in the mediastinum. Such was the case in the report of Fukayama and colleagues (1998). However, some cases of thymomas have involved the pleura but in which no evidence of involvement of the thymus gland could be found, and these have been regarded as primary pleural lesions. Moran and associates (1992) described eight cases of thymomas presenting as pleural tumors. Histologically, six cases were indistinguishable from mediastinal thymomas: The tumors had lobular architecture with lymphocytic and epithelial components. Radiologically, four cases had diffuse pleural thickening mimicking mesothelioma. Whether these tumors represent thymomas arising from ectopic thymic tissue or invasive thymomas from an occult mediastinal primary is unclear.

Localized Malignant Mesothelioma

Crotty and associates (1994) described six cases of localized malignant mesotheliomas of the pleura. In four patients, the tumors presented as sessile broad-based pleural tumors and two were pedunculated. Histologically, three were purely epithelioid and three were biphasic. Immunohistochemically and ultrastructurally, these tumors had a malignant mesothelioma phenotype. Three patients had recurrences and died of their disease, and three were free of disease after surgical resection.

Primary Squamous Cell Carcinoma of the Pleura

Willen and associates (1976) reported the occurrence of a squamous cell carcinoma arising from the pleural surface in six patients who had been treated over long periods by a pneumothorax to maintain an extrapleural pneumolysis for the management of pulmonary tuberculosis. In four other patients treated in the same manner, they identified areas of squamous metaplasia of the pleural surface. They suggested that such areas of metaplasia could become the site of origin of squamous cell carcinomas they identified. Ruttner and Heinzl (1977) described a similar case and noted an earlier case reported by Ender (1966). Treatment is complete resection, if possible. The role of irradiation is unknown. Other squamous cell carcinomas have been described that have originated in pleurocutaneous fistulas, but these are not true pleural lesions. The occurrence of squamous cell carcinoma in chronic sinus and fistulous tracts is a well-known entity.

Adenosquamous Cell Carcinoma of the Pleura

Hammer (1995) mentions one patient who had a squamous cell carcinoma of the pleura. Some of the cells in this tumor stained for the presence of mucicarmine, thus suggesting the diagnosis of adenosquamous cell carcinoma. Kwee and colleagues (1981) reported the presence of an "adenosquamous" mesothelioma of the pleura. Again, whether this is a rare primary pleural tumor or only a variant of a diffuse mesothelioma remains conjecture.

Primary Melanoma of the Pleura

According to Dail (1995), only one case of probable primary pleural melanoma has been reported. This case was presented by Smith and Opipari (1978), and no evidence of a reported primary site of a melanoma was uncovered by the history or autopsy carried out 3 weeks after biopsy of a large pleural-based melanoma. Their major criteria for a primary lung melanoma were met, equally applicable to primary pleural melanoma as espoused by Jensen and Egedorf (1967): 1) no previously removed skin tumor, 2) no ocular tumor, 3) a solitary specimen, and 4) autopsy proof of no other organ involvement.

Malignant Peripheral Nerve Sheath Tumor

Ordóñez and Tornos (1997) described a single case of primary malignant peripheral nerve sheath tumor of the pleura in a 57-year-old man that clinically mimicked a malignant mesothelioma. Histologically, the tumor had features of epithelioid malignant peripheral nerve sheath tumor. In this case, rhabdomyoblasts were seen in addition to spindle and epithelioid cells. The immunohistochemical features of this tumor were as follows: the spindle and epithelioid cells expressed S-100 protein; the epithelioid cells had local reaction to heavy keratins; and the rhabdomyoblasts were positive for desmin and myoglobin and negative for S-100 protein. No reactivity occurred for muscle actin, synaptophysin, chromogranin, or anti-melanoma monoclonal antibody (HMB45). The patient had a fatal course and died from the disease.

Other Primary Malignant Tumors

Malignant solitary localized fibrous tumors of the pleura are generally readily differentiated from other malignant tumors involving the pleura. As noted previously in Chapter 64, these tumors do not express cytokeratin, whereas they label positive for CD34.

Other malignant sarcomas, because of their site of origin and lack of expression for cytokeratin reactivity, are usually not confused as being diffuse malignant mesotheliomas. In rare instances, diagnostic (as a rule purely academic) dilemmas do occur.

REFERENCES

Battifora H: Case six biphasic synovial sarcoma invading the pleura. *In* Short Course of Tumors and Tumor-Like Lesions of Serosal Membranes. XX International Congress of the International Academy of Pathology. Hong Kong, 1994.

Battifora H: Epithelioid hemangioendothelioma imitating mesothelioma. Appl Immunohistochem *1*:220, 1993.

Crotty TB, et al: Localized malignant mesothelioma: a clinicopathologic and flow cytometric study. Am J Surg Pathol *18*:357, 1994.

Dail DH: Uncommon tumors. *In* Dail DH, Hammar SP (eds): Pulmonary Pathology. New York: Springer-Verlag, 1988, p. 847.

Dail DH: Uncommon tumors. *In* Dail DH, Hammar SP, Colby TV (eds): Pulmonary Pathology—Tumors. New York: Springer-Verlag, 1995, p. 157.

Dessy E, Pietra GG: Pseudomesotheliomatous carcinoma of the lung. An immunohistochemical and ultrastructural study of three cases. Cancer *68*:1747, 1991.

Ender A: Ein Beitrag zum primaren pflasterzellkarzinom der Pleura nach extrapleuralem Pneumothoraax. Juris-Verlag, Thesis, University of Zurich, 1966.

Erasmus JJ, et al: Calcifying fibrous pseudotumor of pleura: radiographic features in three cases. J Comput Assist Tomogr *20*:763, 1996.

Freidman HD, Litovsky SH, Abraham JL: Mucin-positive epithelial mesothelioma and pseudomesotheliomatous adenocarcinoma. Arch Pathol Lab Med *117*:967, 1993.

Fukayama M, et al: Pulmonary and pleural thymoma. Diagnostic application of lymphocyte markers to the thymoma of unusual site. Am J Clin Pathol *89*:617, 1988.

Gaertner E, et al: Biphasic synovial sarcomas arising in the pleural cavity: a clinicopathologic study of five cases. Am J Surg Pathol *20*:36, 1996.

Gibbs AR: Smooth muscle tumors of the pleura. Histopathology *27*:295, 1995.

Goetz SP, Robinson RA, Landas SK: Extraskeletal myxoid chondrosarcoma of the pleura: report of a case clinically simulating mesothelioma. Am J Clin Pathol *97*:498, 1992.

Hammar SP: Pleural diseases. *In* Dail DH, Hammar SP, Colby TV (eds): Pulmonary Pathology—Tumors. New York: Springer-Verlag, 1995, p. 405.

Harwood TR, Gracey DR, Yokoo H: Pseudomesotheliomatous carcinoma of the lung: a variant of peripheral lung cancer. Am J Clin Pathol *65*:159, 1976.

Henderson DW, et al: Malignant mesothelioma of the pleura: current surgical pathology. *In* Corrin B (ed): Pathology of Lung Tumors. New York: Churchill Livingstone, 1997, p. 241.

Jensen QA, Egedorf J: Primary melanoma of the lung. Scand J Respir Dis *48*:127, 1967.

Koss M, et al : Pseudomesotheliomatous adenocarcinoma: a reappraisal. Semin Diagn Pathol *9*:117, 1992.

Kwee WS, et al: Primary "adenosquamous" mesothelioma of the pleura. Virchows Arch [A] *393*:353, 1981.

Lin BT, et al : Malignant vascular tumors of the serous membranes mimicking mesothelioma. A report of 14 cases. Am J Surg Pathol *20*:1431, 1996.

McCaughey WTE, Dardick I, Barr JR: Angiosarcoma of serous membranes. Arch Pathol Lab Med *107*:304, 1983.

Moran CA, et al: Thymomas presenting as pleural tumors. Report of eight cases. Am J Surg Pathol *16*:138, 1992.

Moran CA, Suster S, Koss MN: Smooth muscle tumours presenting as pleural neoplasms. Histopathology *27*:227, 1995.

Ordóñez NG, Tornos C. Malignant peripheral nerve sheath tumor of the pleura with epithelial and rhabdomyoblastic differentiation: report of a case clinically simulating mesothelioma. Am J Surg Pathol *20*:1515, 1997.

Pinkard NB, et al: Calcifying fibrous pseudotumor of pleura. A report of three cases of a newly described entity involving the pleura. Am J Clin Pathol *105*:189, 1996.

Ruttner JR, Heinzl S: Squamous-cell carcinoma of the pleura. Thorax *32*:497, 1977.

Smith S, Opipari MI: Primary pleural melanoma. A first reported case and literature review. J Thorac Cardiovasc Surg *75*:827, 1978.

Willen R, et al: Squamous epithelial cancer in metaplastic pleura following extrapleural pneumothorax for pulmonary tuberculosis. Virchows Arch [A] *370*:225, 1976.

Witkin GB, Miettinen M, Rosai J: A biphasic tumor of the mediastinum with features of synovial sarcoma. A report of four cases. Am J Surg Pathol *13*:490, 1989.

Wong WW, et al: Liposarcoma of the pleura. Mayo Clin Proc *69*:882, 1994.

CHAPTER 68

Malignant Pleural Effusions

Steven A. Sahn

DEFINITION AND INCIDENCE

Malignant pleural effusions are diagnosed by finding malignant cells in the pleural fluid or pleural tissue by closed needle biopsy, by biopsy through thoracoscopy or thoracotomy, or at autopsy. In some cases of established malignancy with an associated pleural effusion, malignant cells cannot be demonstrated in either pleural fluid or pleural tissue and probably are not present at the time of the diagnostic procedure. I (1985) have termed these effusions "paramalignant" because they are associated with and caused by the malignancy but do not result from pleural invasion. Paramalignant effusions can be caused by a direct local effect of the tumor, by systemic manifestations of the malignancy, or as a consequence of therapy (Table 68-1). Impaired pleural space lymphatic drainage is an important mechanism responsible for the formation of both paramalignant and malignant pleural effusions.

Virtually all cancers metastasize to the pleura. Lung cancer is the most common to involve the pleura because of its proximity to the pleural surface and, as Meyer (1966) suggested, its propensity to invade the pulmonary arteries and embolize to the visceral pleura. Breast cancer also frequently metastasizes to the pleura, causing approximately 25% of malignant pleural effusions. Ovarian carcinoma and gastric cancer are next in frequency, and each represents less than 5% of malignant pleural effusions. I (1998) found that approximately 7% of patients with malignant pleural effusions, however, have an unknown primary site at the time of the initial diagnosis of the malignant effusion.

I (1998) have noted that lymphomas account for approximately 10% of all malignant pleural effusions and, according to Valentine and Raffin (1992), are the most common cause of chylothorax. Both Hodgkin's disease and non-Hodgkin's lymphoma have been associated with pleural effusions with variable incidences and usually through different mechanisms. Pleural effusions result more commonly from impaired lymphatic drainage of the pleural space in Hodgkin's disease, whereas direct pleural involvement tends

to be more common in non-Hodgkin's lymphoma. These observations were recorded by Weick (1973), Jenkins (1981), and Xaubet (1985) and their associates.

Diffuse malignant mesothelioma arises from mesothelial cells or possibly from a precursor cell that is situated in the submesothelial connective tissue. The association of asbestos exposure and malignant mesothelioma was established in 1960 by the report of Wagner and colleagues (1960). McDonald and coworkers (1970) recorded that the incidence of malignant mesothelioma is approximately one per million per year in the general population that is not exposed to asbestos. Emont and associates (1970) reported that the incidence can rise 20-fold in certain populations and is even higher in shipyard communities.

PATHOGENESIS

Impaired lymphatic drainage of the pleural space is probably the most important mechanism responsible for accumulation of large volumes of pleural fluid in malignancy. The lymphatic system can be blocked at any point from the stoma of the parietal pleura to the mediastinal and parasternal (internal mammary) lymph nodes. The autopsy studies by Meyer (1966) and Chernow and myself (1977) have demonstrated the association of mediastinal lymph node involvement and the presence of substantial pleural fluid. Conversely, these studies showed evidence of pleural involvement with tumor in the absence of pleural effusions, lending support to this mechanism. Furthermore, as Meyer (1966) noted, pleural effusions usually do not occur when the pleura is involved by sarcoma because of the absence of lymphatic metastasis. Weick and associates (1973) noted that Hodgkin's disease tends to cause pleural effusions by lymphatic obstruction, and Xaubet and associates (1985) noted that non-Hodgkin's lymphoma tends to produce effusions by both lymphatic obstruction and direct pleural invasion.

The inflammatory response to pleural tumor invasion results in increased microvascular permeability and pro-

Table 68-1. Causes of Paramalignant Pleural Effusions

Cause	Comment
Local effects of tumor	
Lymphatic obstruction	Important mechanism for pleural fluid accumulation
Bronchial obstruction with pneumonia	Parapneumonic effusion; does not exclude operability in lung cancer
Bronchial obstruction with atelectasis	Transudate; does not exclude operability in lung cancer
Trapped lung	Owing to extensive tumor involvement of visceral pleura
Chylothorax	Disruption of thoracic duct; non-Hodgkin's lymphoma most common cause
Superior vena cava syndrome	Transudate; caused by increased systemic venous pressure
Systemic effects of tumor	
Pulmonary embolism	Hypercoagulable state
Hypoalbuminemia	Serum albumin less than 1.5 g/dL; associated with anasarca
Complications of therapy	
Radiation therapy	
Early	Pleuritis 6 weeks to 6 months after radiation completed
Late	Fibrosis of mediastinum; constrictive pericarditis; superior vena caval obstruction
Chemotherapy	
Methotrexate	Pleuritis or effusion; ± blood eosinophilia
Procarbazine	Fever and chills; blood eosinophilia
Cyclophosphamide	Pleuropericarditis
Mitomycin	Associated with interstitial disease
Bleomycin	Associated with interstitial disease

Modified from Sahn SA: Malignant pleural effusions. Clin Chest Med 6:114, 1985.

duces small volumes of pleural effusion. Chretien and Jaubert (1985) suggested that oxygen radicals, arachidonic acid metabolites, proteases, lymphocytes, and immune complexes are probably causative.

Pleural effusion is an early manifestation of a malignant mesothelioma and probably results from a combination of increased capillary permeability from direct pleural invasion and impaired lymphatic drainage of the pleural space. As the tumor progresses and the visceral and parietal pleura fuse, the fluid diminishes or disappears.

Autopsy series have shown that in patients with carcinoma of the lung, pleural metastasis is almost always found on both the visceral and parietal pleural surfaces. Meyer (1966) noted that rarely is only the visceral pleural surface involved, and isolated parietal pleural metastases were never identified. Visceral pleural metastasis in lung cancer appears to result from contiguous spread or through pulmonary arterial invasion and embolization. Once seeded with tumor, these malignant cells migrate from the visceral to parietal pleural surface along either preformed or tumor-induced

pleural adhesions. Alternatively, free tumor cells exfoliated from the visceral pleural surface can adhere to the parietal pleura and multiply. Chernow and I (1977) reported that adenocarcinoma of the lung is the most common cell type to involve the pleura, presumably owing to its peripheral location. When bilateral pleural metastases occur in lung cancer, hepatic spread and parenchymal invasion in the contralateral lung usually is causative. Once contralateral lung metastasis occurs, pulmonary artery invasion and embolization follow, as in the ipsilateral lesion. The data concerning the laterality of the pleural effusion in relation to the primary lesion support this mechanism.

Chernow and I (1977) pointed out that in lung cancer, pleural effusions occur either ipsilaterally or bilaterally and virtually never occur solely in the contralateral pleural space. With other cancers, pleural involvement is usually from tertiary spread from established liver metastases with no predilection for side. Fentiman and associates (1981) summarized the conflicting data in breast carcinoma, with some studies showing a high incidence of ipsilateral pleural effusion and others no predilection for side. Probably two mechanisms are operative: chest wall lymphatic invasion resulting in ipsilateral effusion, and hepatic spread with bilateral or contralateral hematogenous spread.

CLINICAL PRESENTATION

The most common presenting symptom of patients with carcinoma or lymphoma of the pleura and a large pleural effusion is dyspnea on exertion. In diffuse pleural mesothelioma, patients generally present with the insidious onset of either dyspnea or chest pain. Taryle and colleagues (1976) noted that almost all patients with a malignant mesothelioma present with some symptoms whereas Chernow and I (1977) and Weick and associates (1973) reported that up to 25% of patients with carcinoma or lymphoma of the pleura, respectively, may be relatively asymptomatic when the pleural effusion is initially discovered on a routine chest radiograph.

Because malignant involvement of the pleura signals advanced disease, these patients frequently have weight loss and appear chronically ill. Chernow and I (1977) found that pleural effusion provided the initial diagnosis of cancer in almost 50% of these patients.

Patients with carcinoma of the pleura may have chest pain caused by involvement of the parietal pleura, ribs, or chest wall. Elmes and Simpson (1976) emphasized, however, that the chest pain associated with malignant mesothelioma is more common and impressive but is nonpleuritic and frequently referred to the upper abdomen or shoulder.

Chernow and I (1977) noted that signs of a pleural effusion are typically found on physical examination and cachexia and lymphadenopathy may be seen in cancer; but the examination may be unremarkable in malignant mesothelioma, except for the findings of a moderate to large pleural effusion.

RADIOGRAPHS OF THE CHEST

The pleural effusion associated with lung cancer is ipsilateral to the primary lesion. This may be because of direct pleural involvement, mediastinal lymph node infiltration, or an endobronchial lesion with pneumonia or atelectasis. With other primary sites, with the possible exception of breast cancer, there appears to be no ipsilateral predilection and bilateral effusions are common. As Chernow and I (1977) have pointed out, these effusions usually are the result of mediastinal lymph node metastasis.

Patients with carcinomatous pleurisy usually present with a moderate to large effusion (500 to 2000 mL; 10% have effusions less than 500 mL and a similar number have massive pleural effusion with complete opacification of the hemithorax). Malignancy is the most common cause of a massive pleural effusion; in a series by Maher and Berger (1972), 67% of 46 massive pleural effusions were caused by malignancy (Fig. 68-1). The radiographic finding of bilateral effusions with a normal heart size suggests malignancy, most commonly carcinoma, which Rabin and Blackman (1957) noted (Fig. 68-2). Benign effusions associated with this radiographic finding include lupus pleuritis, esophageal rupture, hepatic hydrothorax, nephrotic syndrome, and constrictive pericarditis.

When an apparently large pleural effusion is present (1500 mL) with an absence of contralateral mediastinal shift, malignancy is almost always the cause, and the patient has a poor prognosis. The following diagnoses should be considered in this context: 1) carcinoma of the ipsilateral main stem bronchus causing atelectasis, 2) a fixed mediastinum caused by malignant lymph nodes, 3) malignant mesothelioma (the density represents mostly tumor with a small effusion), and 4) extensive tumor infiltration of the ipsilateral lung radiographically mimicking a large effusion.

As Whitcomb and associates (1972) and MacDonald (1977) described, in Hodgkin's disease, patients with pleural effusions usually have associated lymphadenopathy and parenchymal infiltrates. In contrast, Jenkins and colleagues (1981) reported that in non-Hodgkin's lymphoma, intrathoracic lymphadenopathy occurs in few of the cases associated with either pulmonary disease or pleural effusions.

Heller and colleagues (1970) noted that in malignant mesothelioma the initial chest radiograph usually shows a moderate to large unilateral pleural effusion. After therapeutic thoracentesis, the pleura may show thickening or nodularity. Evidence of asbestos exposure, such as interstitial lung disease or pleural plaques, may be identified in the contralateral lung and pleura. Radiographic clues suggesting that the large effusion may be caused by mesothelioma rather than carcinoma are pleural nodularity, absence of con-

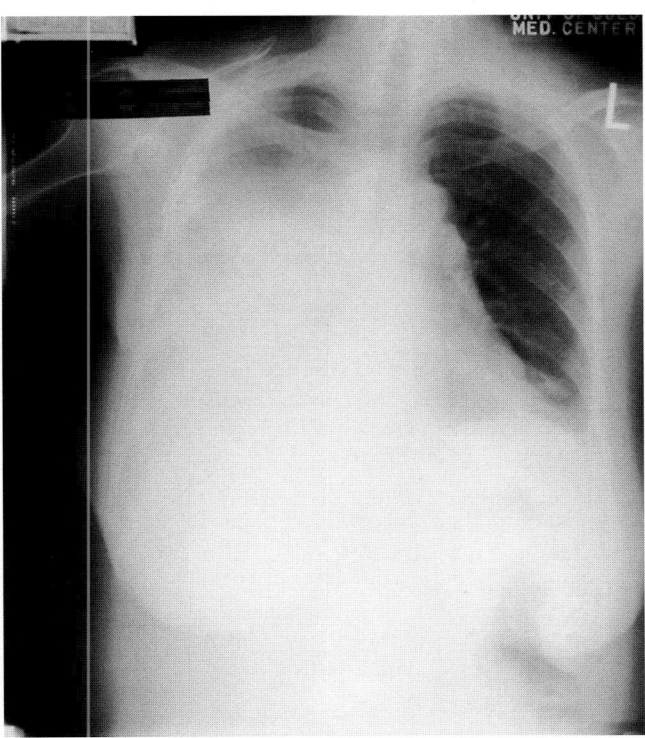

Fig. 68-1. A 60-year-old woman with adenocarcinoma of the lung with a massive right pleural effusion. Note the contralateral mediastinal shift.

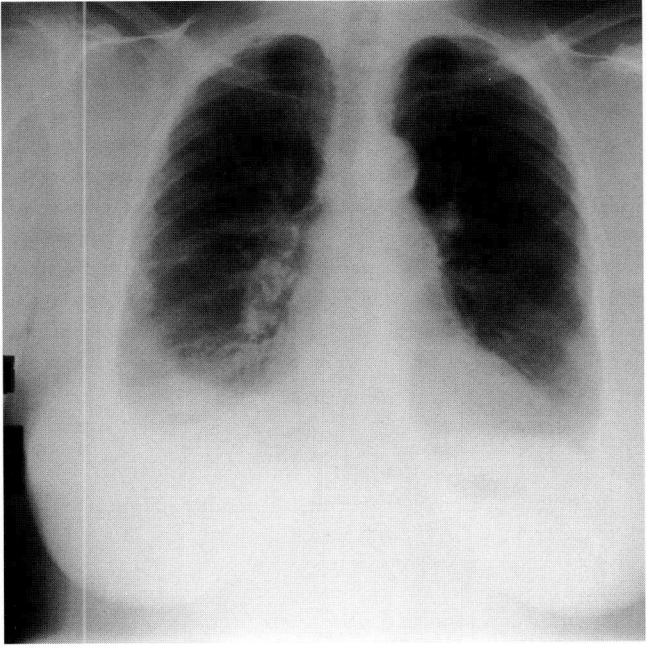

Fig. 68-2. A 64-year-old woman who presented with progressive dyspnea on exertion. She had a salivary amylase-rich pleural effusion. Note the bilateral pleural effusions, a cardiac silhouette at the upper limits of normal, and no evidence of congestive heart failure.

tralateral mediastinal shift with an apparent large effusion, and a tendency for loculation.

PLEURAL FLUID CHARACTERISTICS

Malignant pleural effusions may be serous, serosanguineous, or grossly bloody. A grossly bloody effusion suggests direct pleural involvement, whereas a serous effusion results from either lymphatic obstruction or an endobronchial lesion with atelectasis. Light and coworkers (1973) suggested that when the red blood cell count in the pleural fluid is greater than 100,000/μL in the absence of trauma, malignancy is the most likely diagnosis. Most of the nucleated cells (2500 to 4000/μL) in pleural fluid, as Yam (1967) noted, are lymphocytes, macrophages, and mesothelial cells; more than 50% of the cellular population are lymphocytes in approximately one-half of the cases. The percentage of polymorphonuclears (PMNs) usually is less than 25% of the cell population but on rare occasions, when there is intense pleural inflammation, the PMN may predominate. In a prospective study, Rubins and Rubins (1996) reported that pleural fluid eosinophilia occurred in 7.8% (10 of 128) of patients with malignant effusions and that malignancy is as prevalent among eosinophilic as well as noneosinophilic effusions.

Carcinomatous pleural effusions typically are exudates, with a protein concentration of approximately 4 g/dL; Chernow and I (1977) and Light and associates (1972), however, reported protein concentrations from 1.5 to 8.0 g/dL. Approximately 5 to 10% of malignant pleural effusions are transudates. These transudative malignant effusions are caused by early stages of lymphatic obstruction, atelectasis from bronchial obstruction, or concomitant congestive heart failure. When an effusion meets exudative criteria by lactate dehydrogenase (LDH) but not protein, Light and associates (1972) emphasized that malignancy should be suspected. I and my colleague Good (1988) found that approximately one-third of patients with malignant pleural effusions have a low pleural fluid pH (less than 7.30, range of 6.95 to 7.29) and a low glucose concentration (less than 60 mg/dL or pleural fluid to serum ratio of less than 0.5) at presentation. These effusions usually have been present for several months and are associated with a large tumor burden and fibrosis of the pleural surface. Good and colleagues (1985) suggested that the abnormal pleural membrane reduces glucose entry into the pleural space and impairs glucose end-product efflux, resulting in a local acidosis. Furthermore, I and my colleague Good (1988) noted that low pH-low glucose malignant effusions are associated with short survival, ease of diagnosis by cytology and pleural biopsy, and a poor response to intrapleural sclerosing agents.

Pleural effusions caused by lymphoma have characteristics similar to those of carcinoma of the pleura. These effusions, however, tend to be less hemorrhagic and less likely to result in pleural fluid acidosis and low glucose concentrations. Both

myself (1985) and Gottehrer and colleagues (1990) have pointed out that a pleural effusion in malignant mesothelioma is more likely to have a low pH and low glucose content and greater protein and LDH concentrations than effusions from carcinoma of the pleura. Because of an overlap of values, however, these data are not helpful in separating carcinoma from mesothelioma in an individual patient.

DIAGNOSIS

From my (1998) compilation of several large series totaling more than 500 cases of malignancy, pleural fluid cytology had a diagnostic yield of 66%, and percutaneous pleural biopsy had a diagnostic yield of 46%. When both procedures were performed, a positive diagnosis was obtained in 73% of cases.

With a standardized approach and an experienced cytopathologist, diagnostic yields in cases of proven malignancy approximate 90% on the initial pleural fluid examination with an additional 2 to 4% yield with a second sample as recorded by Johnston (1985), Hsu (1987), and Star and Sherman (1991). Several observations can be made from these data: 1) the diagnostic yield is dependent on the extent of disease and primary malignancy; 2) pleural fluid cytology is more sensitive than pleural biopsy; 3) the tests are complementary, but pleural biopsy adds little to cytologic examination; 4) the lower yield from pleural biopsy is the result of the pattern of pleural metastasis, sampling error and operator technique; and 5) the wide range of incidence of positive results with both tests probably relates to imprecise handling of specimens, expertise of the cytopathologist, and the possibility that the pleural effusion was paramalignant at the time of the procedure. From the thoracoscopy data of Canto (1983), the yield of percutaneous pleural biopsy probably could be increased by performing the procedure as close to the diaphragm and midline as possible because pleural metastases tend to originate near the diaphragm and spread cephalad toward the costal pleura.

Some patients with exudative pleural effusions remain without a diagnosis after a repeat cytologic examination with or without repeat pleural biopsy. Options at this time include observation, thoracoscopy, or open pleural biopsy. Recommending an invasive procedure is easier psychologically for the physician but creates morbidity and economic burden for the patient. However, with experienced operators, thoracoscopy is a highly effective diagnostic procedure with minimal morbidity and essentially no mortality. Boutin and coworkers (1981) diagnosed 131 of 150 (87%) malignant pleural effusions, both carcinoma and mesothelioma, while pleural fluid cytology and percutaneous needle biopsy performed the day before thoracoscopy provided the diagnosis in only 41% of patients. During the 10 years of study, the diagnostic yield for malignancy rose from 78 to 97% with better instrumentation. Loddenkemper and Boutin (1993) reported a prospective study comparing the diagnostic yield of pleural fluid cytology, percutaneous needle biopsy and medical thoracoscopy in 208 patients. Cytology had a 62% sensitivity and needle biopsy a 44% sensitivity, with a combined sensitivity of 74%, compared to 95% sensitivity with thoracoscopy. Open pleural biopsy requires a thoracotomy with associated morbidity, a low mortality rate, and economic burden. Treatable causes of exudative effusions, such as tuberculous pleurisy and pulmonary embolism, should be excluded before invasive procedures are undertaken. Approximately 5 to 14% of patients with tuberculous pleural effusions are not diagnosed by pleural fluid and tissue culture and pleural histologic examination; and if tuberculous pleurisy is not treated, 65% of patients develop active tuberculosis within 5 years. Therefore, patients with a positive tuberculin skin test and an undiagnosed lymphocyte-predominant exudate should be treated with antituberculous drugs. Bronchoscopy should be done before thoracoscopy or open pleural biopsy if there is absence of contralateral shift with a large effusion, evidence of ipsilateral volume loss, a pulmonary lesion in addition to the pleural effusion, or the presence of hemoptysis. According to Feinsilver and associates (1986), the value of bronchoscopy in an undiagnosed pleural effusion without the aforementioned factors is limited.

An alternate approach is observation with repeat cytology and pleural biopsy at a later time if the effusion has not regressed. Malignant pleural effusions almost never resolve spontaneously; an increase in the size of the pleural effusion heightens the suspicion of malignancy. Furthermore, if the clinician does not diagnose a malignant pleural effusion for several weeks, rarely has a disservice been done to the patient who has widespread, incurable disease. Diagnosis of a malignancy that characteristically is responsive to therapy, such as breast, prostate, thyroid, small cell lung cancer, and germ cell cancer and lymphoma, however, should be pursued more aggressively in the appropriate clinical settings.

Measurements of carcinoembryonic antigen, hyaluronic acid, and LDH isoenzymes have no diagnostic value. Chromosomal analysis of pleural fluid is expensive and not available in all laboratories but may be helpful in the diagnosis of lymphoma and leukemia.

The antemortem diagnosis of malignant mesothelioma requires both clinical and histologic observations. Diagnosis from exfoliative cytology is difficult, and Whitaker (1978) questions its value. Even when malignancy is diagnosed, it may be impossible to differentiate metastatic adenocarcinoma from a malignant mesothelioma. Percutaneous needle biopsy, because of the small amount of tissue, does not consistently yield a definitive diagnosis and frequently prompts a misleading diagnosis of adenocarcinoma. High levels of hyaluronic acid have been thought to be helpful in establishing the diagnosis of mesothelioma; however, Rasmussen and Faber (1967) observed that most patients with mesothelioma have intermediate levels, frequently seen in metastatic carcinoma and other inflammatory diseases. Experienced thoracoscopists, such as Boutin and Rey (1993), report a 98% (185 of 188 patients) diagnostic yield in malignant mesothe-

lioma compared to 26% and 21% for cytology and percutaneous needle biopsy, respectively. Mesotheliomas, as Edge and Choudhury (1978) noted, tend to invade surgical sites. Prophylactic irradiation should be given postoperatively. On occasion, even after adequate tissue has been examined from thoracoscopy or thoracotomy, diagnosis remains uncertain. The subsequent course or biopsy from a tumor implant at the surgical site often provides the diagnosis.

Most pathologists can confidently diagnose a sarcomatous or mixed histologic variant but have difficulty in differentiating the epithelial form of mesothelioma from the more common metastatic adenocarcinoma. Special tissue stains, newer immunologic techniques, and electron microscopy aid in the antemortem diagnosis of patients with the epithelial variety of mesothelioma (see Chapter 65).

PROGNOSIS

I and my colleague Good (1988) noted that the diagnosis of a malignant pleural effusion portends a poor prognosis. Patients with carcinoma of the lung, stomach, and ovary generally survive only a few months from the time of diagnosis of the malignant effusion, whereas patients with breast cancer may survive several months to years, depending on the response to chemotherapy. Patients with lymphomatous pleural effusions tend to have a survival intermediate between breast cancer and other carcinomas.

I and my colleague Good (1988) observed that patients with low pH (less than 7.30) and low glucose (less than 60 mg/dL) malignant effusions survive only a few months, whereas those with a normal pH and glucose malignant effusion survive for approximately 1 year. Thus, the biochemical findings in the pleural fluid provide the clinician with information that is helpful in deciding on a rational plan of palliative treatment.

Although a pleural effusion is an ominous sign in lung cancer, usually excluding operability, Decker and colleagues (1978) reported that approximately 5% of these patients have a paramalignant effusion or effusion from another cause and may be operative candidates. The burden falls to the clinician to diagnose the cause of the pleural effusion before making a decision about possible curative surgery. Circumstances suggesting that the pleural effusion in lung cancer is paramalignant and that the patient may still be cured by resection are squamous cell type, radiographic volume loss, serous effusion, transudate, and parapneumonic effusion. If the cause of the effusion cannot be established clinically, thoracoscopy should be done to investigate the cause.

TREATMENT

When the pleural effusion has been documented to be malignant or paramalignant and the patient is not a surgical candidate, the clinician must make a decision concerning palliation. Factors that must be considered in this decision are the patient's general condition, symptoms, and expected survival. Management options range from observation in the asymptomatic patient to thoracotomy with pleurectomy. Most asymptomatic patients eventually develop progressive pleural effusions, producing dyspnea that requires therapy, while the minority probably reach a new steady state of pleural fluid formation and absorption and do not progress to a symptomatic stage requiring therapy. In the debilitated patient with a short expected survival, based on the extent of disease, general status, and the biochemical characteristics of the fluid, it is more prudent to perform a therapeutic thoracentesis periodically on an outpatient basis than to recommend hospitalization and tube thoracostomy or thoracoscopy with pleurodesis, with their associated morbidity and cost.

Pleurectomy with pleural abrasion is virtually always effective in obliterating the pleural space and controlling recurrence of the effusion. Pleural abrasion with or without talc poudrage or pleurectomy should be carried out in most patients who undergo thoracotomy for an undiagnosed pleural effusion and are found to have malignancy because this prevents the subsequent development of a symptomatic pleural effusion. Pleurectomy, however, even when indicated, as Martini and colleagues (1975) and Fry and Khandekar (1995) discussed, is a major surgical procedure associated with substantial morbidity and mortality. Thus, this procedure should be reserved for patients with an expected survival of at least 6 months, who are in relatively good condition, who have a trapped lung, or who have failed pleurodesis.

TECHNIQUE OF PLEURECTOMY*

Beattie (1963) has provided an excellent description of pleurectomy. The thorax is entered by a posterolateral incision, with entrance into the pleural space, preferably by an intercostal incision in the fifth or sixth interspace. The extrapleural dissection is begun in the plane between the parietal pleura and the extrathoracic fascia at the margins of the intercostal incision before the rib spreader is inserted. The parietal pleura is then stripped circumferentially to the mediastinum; more tumor tends to be present at the diaphragmatic costopleural junction than at the apical pleura, and it is recommended that the upper half of the pleural dissection be completed first. Care must be taken in continuing the pleural dissection over the mediastinal surface to avoid injury to the phrenic, recurrent laryngeal, or sympathetic nerves or stellate ganglion. Damage to the vascular structures of the mediastinum likewise must be avoided. Dissection is continued down from the apex to the pulmonary hilus, which completes the initial phase of the procedure. The inferior portion of the parietal pleura is then dissected free. Care must be taken at the costophrenic sulcus

---

*Addendum by the Senior Editor, TW Shields.

not to remove the diaphragmatic attachment to the chest wall. It is unnecessary, as well as often impossible, to remove the diaphragmatic pleura, but the reflection of the pleura posteriorly on the lower mediastinal surface in association with the pulmonary ligament should be freed to the inferior border of the hilus. Dissection of the mediastinal pleura from pericardium is difficult and should not even be attempted in the region of the phrenic nerve. If the lung is free and ventilates well, no visceral pleural dissection is indicated. If, on the other hand, the lung is bound down with fibrin, a standard decortication is necessary. After hemostasis is obtained satisfactorily, pleural drainage and closure are completed in the standard manner.

The procedure is applicable only to a highly selected group of patients in good general condition whose malignant pleural effusion has failed to respond to local therapy. Best results are obtained when the primary lesion is a carcinoma of the breast or, occasionally, a melanoma. Results vary but are more often poor in patients with carcinoma of the lung. Complications are frequent, as high as 23%, and mortality rates are significant, 10 to 18%. When decortication of the lung is necessary in conjunction with the pleurectomy, the mortality rate is significantly increased.

CHEMOTHERAPY OR IRRADIATION

In general, systemic chemotherapy is disappointing for the control of malignant pleural effusions. Nonetheless, patients with lymphoma [according to Weick (1973) and Xaubet (1985) and their associates], patients with breast cancer [from the reports of Fentiman (1981) and Jones (1975) and their colleagues], or small cell carcinoma of the lung [as Livingston and coworkers (1982) noted] may respond well to chemotherapy. Information about steroid receptors obtained from malignant pleural fluid in patients with breast cancer can provide a source for determining potential response to hormonal manipulation. In general, radiation therapy is of limited value in controlling carcinomatous malignant pleural effusions. Roy and associates (1967) suggested, however, that when there is predominantly mediastinal node involvement, irradiation may be valuable for patients with lymphoma or small cell carcinoma of the lung or when the effusion is a chylothorax.

PLEURODESIS

For most patients, the most cost-effective and least morbid method for controlling a symptomatic, malignant pleural effusion is chest tube drainage with instillation of a sclerosing agent. Tetracycline hydrochloride was most commonly used, but in 1991 Lederle Laboratories, the only manufacturer of intravenous and intramuscular tetracycline hydrochloride, ceased production of this drug as a result of the unavailability of the sterile tetracycline salt, which was now required by the U.S. Food and Drug Administration. Walker-Renard and associates (1993) reported that other tetracyclines (minocycline, 300 mg, and doxycycline, 500 mg) have produced complete response rates of 86% (six of seven patients) and 72% (43 of 60 patients), respectively. Many patients treated with intrapleural doxycycline have required more than one instillation compared to only a single dose of minocycline. The most common adverse effects of the tetracycline drugs have been chest pain and fever. The effectiveness of the tetracyclines depends primarily on their fibrogenicity rather than antineoplastic activity. Dryzer and colleagues (1993b) have shown in a rabbit model that both tetracycline and minocycline produce a marked inflammatory response and extensive pleural fibrosis and symphysis in a dose-dependent manner as I and my colleague Good (1981) have previously pointed out.

Walker-Renard and colleagues (1993) reported that talc, mainly poudrage but also slurry, resulted in a complete success rate of 93% (153 of 165 patients) in the treatment of malignant pleural effusions. The complete success rate of talc in control of malignant effusions was found superior to the complete success rate of all other chemical agents, including bleomycin at 54% (108 of 199 patients) and the tetracycline drugs at 68% (290 of 427 patients). The complete success rate with all non-antineoplastic agents was 75% (577 of 770 patients) compared to a complete success rate of only 44% (175 of 398 patients) for all antineoplastic agents. The most commonly reported adverse effects were pain (265 of 1440 patients, 23%) and fever (220 of 1144 patients, 19%) with variability depending on the chemical agent used.

Kennedy and I (1994) reviewed all published series of talc pleurodesis for the treatment of pleural effusions, the majority being malignant. In this review, success was based on clinical criteria and radiographic findings and both complete and partial success were considered; partial success was defined as some recurrence of pleural fluid but not requiring further pleural space drainage. When analyzed by method of administration, both talc poudrage (418 of 461 patients) and slurry (168 of 185 patients) resulted in similar success rates (complete and partial) of 91% for treatment of pleural effusions. Talc received from chemical suppliers is asbestos-free with a particle size generally smaller than 50 μm. While talc is not packaged sterilely by the manufacturer, limitation on the number of microorganisms is a part of specification and total bacterial count cannot exceed 500 organisms per gram of talc. Bacillus species can be routinely cultured from unsterilized talc. Currently, there is no standard method of sterilization; however, dry heat, gamma irradiation, and ethylene oxide gas have all been shown to be effective methods of sterilization by Kennedy and colleagues (1995). Once the packets of talc are sterilized, they remain culture negative for at least 1 year.

The degree of pain associated with talc has been reported from nonexistent to severe; however, in most patients, pain is not a major adverse effect with talc. Fever after talc poudrage or slurry has been reported to occur in 16 to 69% of patients. Fever generally occurs 4 to 12 hours after talc instillation and may last for 72 hours. Despite the efficacy of talc pleurodesis, there are concerns about its short-term safety. There have been a number of reports of respiratory failure after both talc poudrage and talc slurry by Factor (1975), and Rinaldo (1983) and Campos (1997) and their associates. Some of the patients did not survive the episode of respiratory failure. Doses used have been 2 to 14 g. Talc crystals have been found in the bronchoalveolar lavage fluid of some of these patients and, at autopsy, talc crystals have been detected in the lungs and other organs. However, it is uncertain, as noted by Campos and colleagues (1997) and by Kennedy and I (1994), whether talc dissemination from the pleural space is related to the acute respiratory failure. It is doubtful that the method of administration plays a major role in the development of respiratory failure, although the dose and particle size may be important.

If the clinician has documented that therapeutic thoracentesis results in relief of dyspnea and the rate of recurrence and the return of symptoms is rapid, instillation of talc, minocycline, or doxycycline through a chest tube or talc poudrage via thoracoscopy should be considered. If the expected survival is several months, the patient is not debilitated, and the pleural fluid pH is greater than 7.20 or 7.30, the patient is a good candidate for pleurodesis. Attempting pleurodesis is useless if the lungs cannot be expanded fully; this would occur in main stem bronchial obstruction with atelectasis or a trapped lung. I and Good (1988), as well as Sanchez-Armengol and Rodriguez-Panadero (1993), have reported that the documentation of a low pleural fluid pH (less than 7.30 or less than 7.20, respectively) not only suggests a limited survival but a poor response to tetracycline pleurodesis and talc poudrage, respectively. The large tumor bulk and fibrosis involving the pleural surfaces in the low-pH effusions diminishes the effectiveness in producing pleural symphysis, which may be caused by trapped lung, the inability of the pleurodesis agent to injure the mesothelial cell, or the blockage of fibroblast migration into the pleural space.

The technique for chemical pleurodesis is critical for a successful result in the properly selected patient (Table 68-2). The pleural surfaces must be juxtaposed at the time inflammation is induced and remain in close contact over the ensuing 48 to 72 hours; this is best accomplished with chest tube drainage of the pleural space. If the effusion is large, the fluid probably should be drained slowly over the first several hours with intermittent clamping of the tube to decrease the risk of unilateral pulmonary edema. Pulmonary edema is most likely to occur when there is an endobronchial obstruction or trapped lung that does not allow the lung to expand to the chest wall with removal of fluid, resulting in a precipitous drop in pleural pressure. Furthermore, pleurodesis should not be attempted in the aforementioned situations because it will not be successful. Minocycline, 300 mg; doxycycline, 500 mg; or talc slurry, 2

Table 68-2. Procedure for Pleurodesis

1. Place chest tube in midaxillary line directed toward diaphragm.
2. Remove fluid in controlled manner under water seal.
3. Assess tube position on radiograph to position patient for optimal drainage.
4. Connect chest tube to suction (–20 cm H_2O).
5. Demonstrate minimal tube drainage at bedside and lung expansion and small or absent effusion on radiograph.
6. Give intravenous narcotic and midazolam.
7. Instill minocycline, 300 mg, or doxycycline, 500 mg, in 50 mL of saline or talc in 2–5 g in 100 mL of saline through chest tube and clamp 1 hour.
8. Rotate patient given talc slurry.
9. Connect chest tube to suction (–20 cm H_2O).
10. Remove chest tube when drainage is less than 100 mL per day.

to 5 g, should be instilled into the pleural space when the pleural effusion is absent or minimal and the lung is expanded fully. Lorch and colleagues (1988), working in my laboratory, have radiolabeled tetracycline and demonstrated that after intrapleural instillation, tetracycline is distributed completely throughout the pleural space within seconds and that the distribution is not enhanced by patient rotation. This study suggested that the patient need not be rotated through various positions after tetracycline instillation to ensure adequate distribution of the pleurodesis agent. In a follow-up clinical study from our group, Dryzer and colleagues (1993a) showed no difference in success rate with both tetracycline and minocycline in those patients not rotated compared to those who were rotated through various positions after drug instillation. Thus, my recommendation is that patients receiving doxycycline or minocycline pleurodesis need not be rotated through various positions after instillation, thus avoiding discomfort for the patient and additional personnel time. However, I currently rotate patients receiving talc slurry owing to the possibility that the suspension may not be evenly distributed. No studies have evaluated the optimum dwell time; a 1-hour dwell time for the pleurodesis agent should be adequate as experimental studies have shown immediate mesothelial injury. The chest tube should be removed when pleural space drainage is minimal—approximately less than 100 mL/day. With appropriate patient selection and the use of proper technique, the malignant effusion should be controlled in 80 to 95% of patients. Success need not be defined as the production of complete pleural symphysis but as diminishing the reaccumulation of pleural fluid so that dyspnea is relieved and repeat therapeutic thoracentesis is not required. Wooten and associates (1988) noted that both tetracycline and lidocaine, the latter used by some clinicians in an attempt to ameliorate chest pain, are absorbed systematically and reach therapeutic levels by 30 to 60 minutes; a history of allergic reactions to either drug is a contraindication to its use. The dose of lidocaine should not exceed 150 mg or 3 mg/kg, whichever

is less. Strange and associates (1993), in my laboratory, have found similar rapid systemic absorption of minocycline from the rabbit pleural space.

The average wholesale price of talc is less than $1. Minocycline, 300 mg, and doxycycline, 500 mg, cost approximately $80 each. In contrast, the usual 1 U/kg-dose of bleomycin costs $1100. Thus, cost consideration must be kept in mind in the management of the malignant effusion.

The management of malignant mesothelioma is discussed in Chapter 65. Judgment in the management of these patients is the keynote of appropriate care.

REFERENCES

Beattie EJ Jr: The treatment of malignant pleural effusions by partial pleurectomy. Surg Clin North Am 43:99, 1963.
Boutin C, Cargnino P, Viallat JR: Thoracoscopy in malignant effusion. Am Rev Respir Dis 124:588, 1981.
Boutin C, Rey F: Thoracoscopy in pleural malignant mesothelioma: a prospective study of 188 consecutive patients. Part 1. Diagnosis. Cancer 72:389, 1993.
Campos JRM, et al: Respiratory failure due to insufflated talc. Lancet 349:351, 1997.
Canto A, et al: Points to consider when choosing a biopsy method in cases of pleurisy of unknown origin. Chest 84:176, 1983.
Chernow B, Sahn SA: Carcinomatous involvement of the pleura: an analysis of 96 patients. Am J Med 63:695, 1977.
Chretien J, Jaubert F: Pleural responses in malignant metastatic tumors. In Chretien J, Bignon J, Hirsch A (eds): The Pleura in Health and Disease. New York: Marcel Dekker, 1985, p. 489.
Decker DA, et al: The significance of a cytologically negative pleural effusion in bronchogenic carcinoma. Chest 74:640, 1978.
Dryzer SR, et al: A comparison of rotation and nonrotation in tetracycline pleurodesis. Chest 104:1763, 1993a.
Dryzer SR, et al: Early inflammatory response of minocycline and tetracycline on the rabbit pleura. Chest 104:1585, 1993b.
Edge JR, Choudhury SL: Malignant mesothelioma of the pleura in Barrow-in-Furness. Thorax 33:26, 1978.
Elmes PC, Simpson MJC: The clinical aspects of mesothelioma. QJM 45:427, 1976.
Emont et al: Epidemiology of primary malignant mesothelial tumors in Canada. Cancer 26:914, 1970.
Factor SM: Granulomatous pneumonitis. A result of intrapleural instillation of quinacrine and talcum powder. Arch Pathol 99:499, 1975.
Feinsilver SH, Barrows AA, Braman SB: Fiberoptic bronchoscopy and pleural effusion of unknown origin. Chest 90:516, 1986.
Fentiman IS, et al: Pleural effusion in breast cancer: a review of 105 cases. Cancer 47:2087, 1981.
Fry WA, Khandekar JD: Parietal pleurectomy for malignant pleural effusion. Ann Surg Oncol 2:160, 1995.
Good JT Jr, Taryle DA, Sahn SA: The pathogenesis of low glucose, low pH malignant effusions. Am Rev Respir Dis 131:737, 1985.
Gottehrer A, et al: Hypothyroidism and pleural effusions. Chest 98:1130, 1990.
Heller RM, Janower ML, Weber AL: The radiological manifestations of malignant pleural mesothelioma. AJR Am J Roentgenol 108:53, 1970.
Hsu C: Cytologic detection of malignancy in pleural effusion: a review of 5,255 samples from 3,811 patients. Diagn Cytopathol 3:8, 1987.
Jenkins PF, et al: Non-Hodgkin's lymphoma, chronic lymphatic leukemia, and the lung. Br J Dis Chest 75:22, 1981.
Johnston WW: The malignant pleural effusion. A review of cytopathological diagnoses of 584 specimens from 472 consecutive patients. Cancer 56:905, 1985.
Jones SE, Durie BGM, Salmon SE: Combination chemotherapy with adriamycin and cyclophosphamide for advanced breast cancer. Cancer 36:90, 1975.
Kennedy L, Sahn SA: Talc pleurodesis for the treatment of pneumothorax and pleural effusion. Chest 106:1215, 1994.

Kennedy L, et al: Sterilization of talc for pleurodesis: available techniques, efficacy and cost analysis. Chest *107*:1032, 1995.

Light RW, Erozan YS, Ball WC: Cells in pleural fluid: their value in differential diagnosis. Arch Intern Med *132*:854, 1973.

Light RW, et al: Pleural effusions: the diagnostic separation of transudates and exudates. Ann Intern Med 77:507, 1972.

Livingston RB, et al: Isolated pleural effusion in small cell lung carcinoma: favorable prognosis. Chest *81*:208, 1982.

Loddenkemper R, Boutin C: Thoracoscopy: diagnostic and therapeutic indications. Eur Respir J *6*:1544, 1993.

Lorch DG, et al: The effect of patient positioning on the distribution of tetracycline in the pleural space during pleurodesis. Chest *93*:527, 1988.

MacDonald JB: Lung involvement in Hodgkin's disease. Thorax *32*:664, 1977.

McDonald JB, et al: Epidemiology of primary malignant mesothelial tumors in Canada. Cancer *26*:914, 1970.

Maher GG, Berger HW: Massive pleural effusions: malignant and non-malignant causes in 46 patients. Am Rev Respir Dis *105*:458, 1972.

Martini N, Bains MS, Beattie EJ, Jr: Indications for pleurectomy in malignant effusion. Cancer *35*:734, 1975.

Meyer PC: Metastatic carcinoma of the pleura. Thorax *21*:437, 1966.

Rabin CB, Blackman NS: Bilateral pleural effusion. Its significance in association with a heart of normal size. J Mt Sinai Hosp *24*:45, 1957.

Rasmussen KN, Faber V: Hyaluronic acid in 247 pleural fluids. Scand J Respir Dis *48*:366, 1967.

Rinaldo JE, Owens GR, Rogers RM: Adult respiratory distress syndrome following intrapleural instillation of talc. J Thorac Cardiovasc Surg *85*:523, 1983.

Roy PH, Carr DT, Payne WS: The problem of chylothorax. Mayo Clin Proc *42*:457, 1967.

Rubins JB, Rubins HB: Etiology and prognostic significance of eosinophilic pleural effusions. Chest *110*:1271, 1996.

Sahn SA: Malignant pleural effusions. Clin Chest Med *6*:113, 1985.

Sahn SA: Malignant pleural effusions. *In* Fishman AP, Elias JA, Fishman JA, Grippi MA, Kaiser LR, Senior RM (eds): Pulmonary Diseases and Disorders, 3rd Ed. New York: McGraw-Hill, 1998.

Sahn SA, Good JT Jr: The effect of common sclerosing agents on the rabbit pleural space. Am Rev Respir Dis *124*:65, 1981.

Sahn SA, Good JT Jr: Pleural fluid pH in malignant effusion: diagnostic, prognostic and therapeutic implications. Ann Intern Med *108*:345, 1988.

Sanchez-Armengol A, Rodriguez-Panadero F: Survival and talc pleurodesis in metastatic pleural carcinoma, revisited. Report of 125 cases. Chest *104*:1482, 1993.

Starr RL, Sherman ME: The value of multiple preparations in the diagnosis of malignant pleural effusions. Acta Cytol *35*:533, 1991.

Strange C, et al: Minocycline and tetracycline are rapidly absorbed through the rabbit pleural space. Am Rev Respir Dis *147*:A795, 1993.

Taryle DA, Lakshminarayan S, Sahn SA: Pleural mesotheliomas. An analysis of 18 cases and review of the literature. Medicine (Baltimore) *55*:153, 1976.

Valentine VG, Raffin TA: The management of chylothorax. Chest *102*:586, 1992.

Wagner JC, Sleggs CA, Marchand P: Diffuse pleural mesothelioma and asbestos exposure in the North Western Cape Province. Br J Ind Med *17*:260, 1960.

Walker-Renard PB, Vaughan LM, Sahn SA: Chemical pleurodesis for the treatment of malignant pleural effusions: Review of the world's literature. (Submitted) Ann Intern Med 1993.

Weick JK, et al: Pleural effusion in lymphoma. Cancer *31*:848, 1973.

Whitaker D: The cytology of malignant mesothelioma in Western Australia. Acta Cytol *22*:67, 1978.

Whitcomb ME, et al: Hodgkin's disease of the lung. Am Rev Respir Dis *106*:79, 1972.

Wooten SA, et al: Systemic absorption of tetracycline and lidocaine following intrapleural instillation. Chest *94*:960, 1988.

Xaubet A, et al: Characteristics and prognostic value of pleural effusions in non-Hodgkin's lymphomas. Eur J Respir Dis *66*:135, 1985.

Yam LT: Diagnostic significance of lymphocytes in pleural effusions. Ann Intern Med *66*:972, 1967.

READING REFERENCES

Antman KH: Multimodality treatment for malignant mesothelioma based on a study of natural history. Am J Med *68*:356, 1980.

Hillerdal G: Malignant mesothelioma 1982: review of 4710 published cases. Br J Dis Chest *77*:321, 1983.

Schienger M, et al: Mesotheliomes pleuraux malins. Bull Cancer (Paris) *56*:265, 1969.

CHAPTER 69

Malignant Pericardial Effusions

Darroch W. O. Moores and Juan A. Cordero, Jr.

Malignant pericardial effusions remain a challenging clinical problem. Patients with malignant pericardial effusions may be asymptomatic or have myriad clinical symptoms. Press and Livingston (1987) noted that one-half of all patients with malignant effusions present with cardiac tamponade. Approximately 50% of pericardial effusions in patients with known malignancy are benign, in that no evidence exists of malignant cells within the pericardium or pericardial fluid. For this reason, proof of pericardial involvement is paramount in planning therapy. A significant difference in survival occurs between patients with malignant effusion and those with underlying cancer who do not have pericardial involvement (Fig. 69-1). As noted by one of us (D.W.O.M.) and associates (1995), as well as by Mills and colleagues (1995), lung and breast carcinoma account for the majority of malignant pericardial effusions (Table 69-1). Among patients with malignant pericardial effusion, those with breast cancer appear to have significantly better survival rates after drainage than patients with either lung or other types of cancer (*P* <.01; Fig. 69-2). This differentiation is important in planning long-term care of these patients. The treatment of malignant pericardial effusions is controversial, and each modality has its strong proponents.

ETIOLOGY AND PATHOPHYSIOLOGY

Obstruction of lymphatic flow is the primary mechanism involved in the development of pericardial effusions. Hancock (1990) has noted that malignancy spreads to the pericardium primarily through the lymphatics. Although lymphatic networks are present throughout the pericardium, Fraser and associates (1980), Roberts and Spray (1976), and Miller (1971) and Fraser (1980) and their colleagues have emphasized the importance of the cardiac lymphatic networks in the pathogenesis of pericardial effusions. Cardiac metastases with retrograde involvement of the pericardium can lead to pericardial effusions. Mediasti-

nal lymphatic obstruction by lung, breast, and hematologic malignancies is a second mechanism in the development of pericardial effusions as noted by Thurber and colleagues (1962). Metastatic deposits in the serosa of the pericardium can lead to exudation of fluid into the pericardial space as well as obstruction of the venous and lymphatic drainage of the pericardium, leading to cardiac tamponade. Cardiac tamponade is a common presenting symptom of malignant pericardial effusions. As noted by Spodick (1983), tamponade is a mechanical compromise of cardiac filling that defeats compensatory mechanisms. The rate of pericardial fluid accumulation is the most important factor in the compromise of cardiac function. Large pericardial effusions that develop slowly may remain asymptomatic, whereas small effusions that accumulate rapidly can lead to hemodynamic instability.

CLINICAL PRESENTATION

The presentation of patients with malignant pericardial effusions may range from asymptomatic to cardiac tamponade with hemodynamic compromise. Fraser (1980) and Lopez (1983) and their associates have found that the most common presentation of patients with a malignant pericardial effusion is cardiac tamponade. Increasing dyspnea can also be a common presenting symptom in these patients as noted by Fincher (1993). The most important factor in the development of symptoms is the rate of pericardial fluid accumulation. The pericardium is quite distensible, and large effusions that have accumulated slowly may remain asymptomatic. Mild compression of the heart by fluid may produce only elevated central venous pressures with a normal systolic blood pressure. Acute cardiac tamponade results when pericardial fluid accumulates rapidly, compromising ventricular filling during diastole. This results in decreased cardiac output and dyspnea. Cardiac decompensation and death can quickly ensue in these patients.

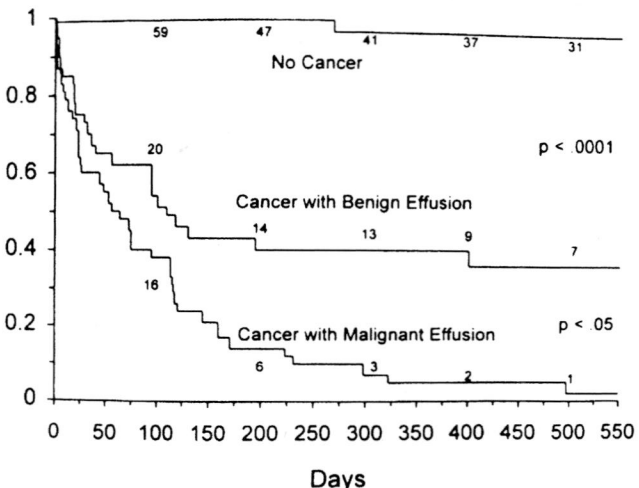

Fig. 69-1. Patients with cancer and benign effusion had significantly longer median survival rates than patients with malignant pericardial effusion. From Moores DWO, et al: Subxiphoid pericardial drainage for pericardial tamponade. J Thorac Cardiovasc Surg *109*:546, 1995. With permission.

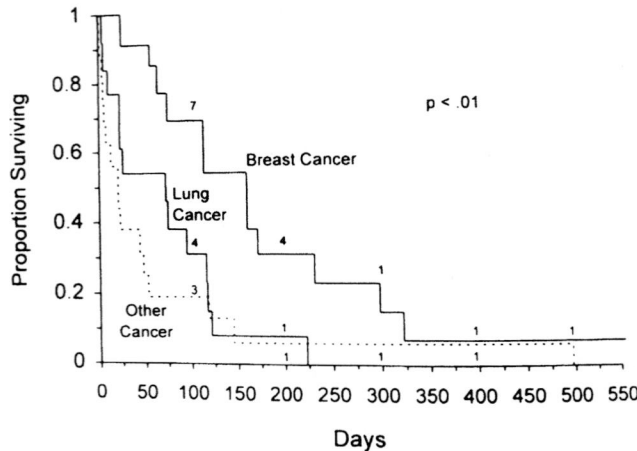

Fig. 69-2. Survival for patients with malignant pericardial effusion. Patients with breast cancer had significantly longer median survival than patients with lung or other types of cancer. From Moores DWO, et al: Subxiphoid pericardial drainage for pericardial tamponade. J Thorac Cardiovasc Surg *109*:546, 1995. With permission.

DIAGNOSIS

The diagnosis of malignant pericardial effusion is based on finding malignant cells within the pericardial fluid or pericardial tissue. Patients usually present with distended neck veins, dyspnea, and pulsus paradoxus. Electrocardiographic changes consist of diminished QRS complexes. In asymptomatic patients the diagnosis is usually made on the basis of an enlarged cardiac silhouette on plain chest radiography, whereas subacute tamponade usually manifests as progressive dyspnea. Patients suspected of having pericardial effusion based on signs, symptoms, and plain radiography require further diagnostic evaluation.

Echocardiography is the most helpful adjunct in the diagnosis of pericardial effusions (Fig. 69-3). Echocardiography can quantify the volume and location of a pericardial effu-

sion as well as the presence of loculations or adhesions. Furthermore, echocardiography can provide physiologic evidence of tamponade such as right ventricular collapse during end-diastole, paradoxical septal motion, and systolic collapse with inward movement of the right atrial and ventricular walls during early systole. Computed tomography and magnetic resonance imaging have both been used to evaluate malignant pericardial disease. Both of these studies provide excellent anatomic evidence of pericardial effusive

Table 69-1. Tumor Types in Patients with Cancer

Type	No. of Cases	%
Primary tumors		
Lung	30	40.0
Breast	23	30.6
Lymphoma	7	9.3
Mesothelioma	5	6.6
Other primary tumors	7	9.3
Gastric	(2)	(2.6)
Sarcoma	(3)	(4.0)
Thymoma	(2)	(2.6)
Unknown primary tumor	3	4.0
Total	**75**	

From Moores DWO, et al: Subxiphoid pericardial drainage for pericardial tamponade. J Thorac Cardiovasc Surg *109*:546, 1995.

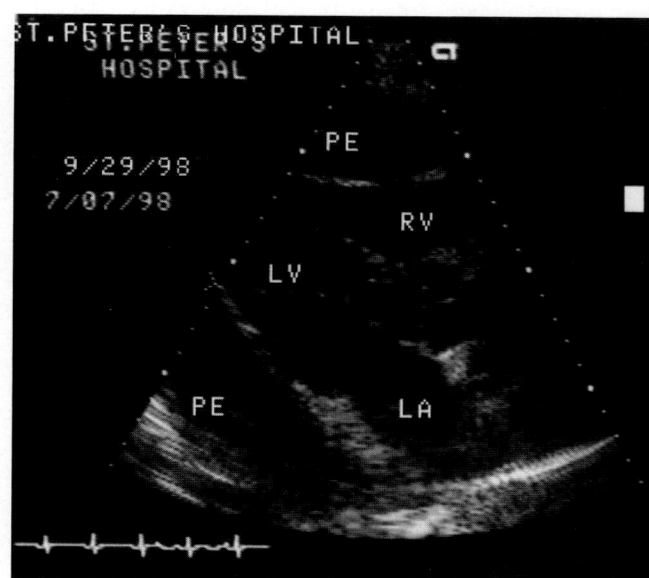

Fig. 69-3. Echocardiogram demonstrating a large pericardial effusion. LA, left atrium; LV, left ventricle; PE, pericardial effusion; RV, right ventricle.

disease but are unable to provide any physiologic evidence of tamponade.

TREATMENT

Malignant pericardial effusions require drainage to confirm the pathologic diagnosis and prevent cardiac tamponade and hemodynamic compromise. The optimal drainage procedure may vary from patient to patient, and selection should be made by considering the particular circumstances of each patient and the experience of the surgeon. Relevant factors include the need for diagnosis, prevention of recurrence, immediate treatment of tamponade, coexistence of pericardial constriction, and patient tolerance of anesthetics. In patients with cancer, proof of pericardial involvement is necessary for planning therapy, because survival is significantly decreased in patients with malignant effusions (see Fig. 69-1). If pericardiocentesis fails to yield malignant cells, an open procedure with biopsy of the pericardium may be necessary. Options in the treatment of pericardial effusions include needle or catheter pericardiocentesis, pericardiocentesis and intrapericardial sclerosis, systemic chemotherapy and radiation therapy, percutaneous balloon pericardiotomy, pericardioperitoneal shunt, pericardiectomy performed by an open thoracotomy, pericardial window performed through a left anterolateral thoracotomy, video-assisted thoracic surgery (VATS), pericardiectomy, and subxiphoid tube pericardiostomy. The most effective method of drainage to prevent recurrence is subject to controversy.

Pericardiocentesis

In use since 1840, needle pericardiocentesis, or aspiration of fluid from the pericardial cavity, can provide dramatic and lifesaving results in patients with pericardial tamponade. Traditionally, the needle is inserted at the right side of the xiphisternum and angled 30 to 45 degrees cephalad toward the posterior aspect of the left shoulder, while aspirating with a syringe. Once fluid is encountered, the needle can be changed over a wire to a Silastic catheter (Fig. 69-4). Pericardiocentesis seems relatively noninvasive because no incision is made and little anesthesia is administered, but the risk of complications is between 5 and 50% as noted by Wong and associates (1979). The most feared complication is cardiac laceration, which can be fatal. The risks are high with small or loculated effusions, with failure to use echocardiography, and in patients with thrombocytopenia. Conversely, pericardiocentesis is safest when echocardiography demonstrates a large free anterior effusion. Wong and associates (1979) have advocated that pericardiocentesis be done with electrocardiographic monitoring, fluoroscopy, and right-sided heart catheterization to minimize complications.

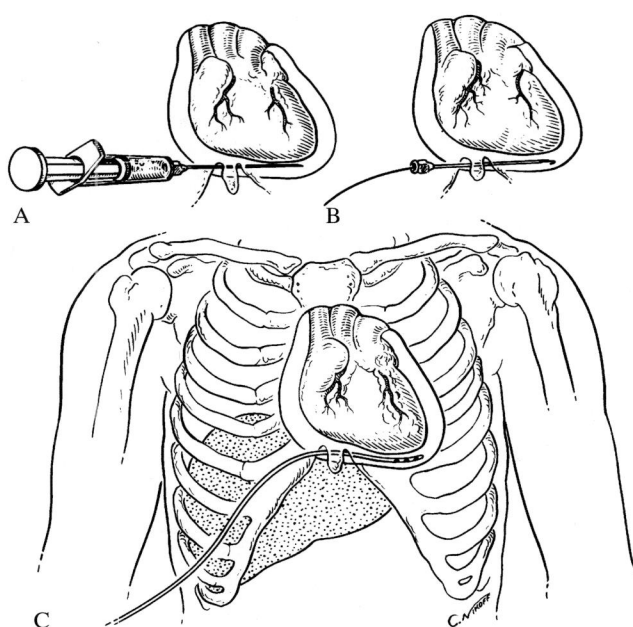

Fig. 69-4. A. Needle pericardiocentesis by the subxiphoid approach. **B.** Guidewire introduced through needle into the pericardial space. **C.** Percutaneous catheter drainage of the pericardial space. From Moores DWO, Dziuban SW Jr: Pericardial drainage procedures. Chest Surg Clin North Am 5:359, 1995. With permission.

Several series of patients undergoing subxiphoid pericardiocentesis attest to its initial effectiveness. Clarke and Cosgrove (1987) and Celermajer and colleagues (1991) have reported on 24 and 36 patients, respectively, who underwent subxiphoid pericardiocentesis for malignant effusions. Their initial success in removing fluid and alleviating symptoms ranged from 94.4 to 100.0%. One patient in this collective series died secondary to a cardiac laceration. Vaitkus and colleagues (1994) have noted that even when pericardiocentesis is initially effective, recurrence of effusion and tamponade occurs in greater than 50% of patients. Wong and associates (1979) reported a series of 52 patients with pericardial tamponade who were treated with pericardiocentesis. Seventeen of the 52 patients (32%) had unproductive or unsuccessful pericardiocentesis, and 8 of the 52 patients (15%) had serious complications. These complications included one death, one cardiac arrest, one subdiaphragmatic abscess, and five ventricular punctures without adverse sequelae.

A variation of needle pericardiocentesis involves the placement of a Silastic catheter for indwelling pericardial drainage. As noted by Vaitkus and colleagues (1994), a slightly higher efficacy than with pericardiocentesis can be obtained with this procedure, but catheter occlusion can occur and the risks and limitations of pericardiocentesis apply as well. Indwelling pericardial catheters tend to be used in conjunction with systemic chemotherapy. One inherent limitation of pericardiocentesis is the inability to obtain tissue for diagnosis. When a suspicion of malignancy exists, positive fluid cytology results are diagnostic but negative cytology results are indeterminate. Therefore, it is reasonable to forego pericardiocentesis and instead perform an open surgical drainage with pericardial biopsy, especially in patients who do not have tamponade, because their risk from anesthesia and surgery is low. Because of its limitations and complications, pericardiocentesis alone is being used less frequently in favor of other techniques such as open surgical drainage.

Intrapericardial Sclerosis

Many sclerosing agents have been instilled into the pericardium in an effort to prevent the recurrence of pericardial effusions. Most agents are intended to induce an inflammatory response and obliterate the pericardial space. All patients in these series underwent an initial pericardiocentesis to gain access to the pericardial space. Shepherd and associates (1987) reported a series of 58 patients with malignant pericardial effusions treated with intrapericardial tetracycline hydrochloride. Forty-three patients (74%) had control of their effusions for longer than 30 days. Eight patients (14%) did not achieve control and two had catheter-related complications. There were five patients who developed atrial arrhythmia and one cardiac arrest. Three patients had reaccumulation of fluid after catheter removal. Davis and colleagues (1984) achieved slightly better results with intrapericardial tetracycline sclerosis in 33 cases. In their series, 30 patients had control of the effusions and resolution of cardiac tamponade. The three failures were related to catheter complications. Girardi and associates (1997) reported their experience with intrapericardial sclerotherapy with thiotepa. In their series, 37 patients underwent sclerotherapy, with a 13% recurrence rate based on three failures and two catheter obstructions. Maher and associates (1996) reported on 93 patients treated with intrapericardial sclerosis using tetracycline or doxycycline. These authors achieved control of the effusion in 68 patients (73%). Eight of their patients could not undergo sclerosis because of technical failure. Two patients had cardiac arrest before sclerosis could be attempted. Complications included atrial arrhythmia in eight patients and infection in one patient. Variable results have been reported in the literature with the use of sclerosing agents in the treatment of malignant pericardial effusions. Pericardiocentesis in combination with the instillation of a sclerosing agent appears safe and may be effective in controlling malignant pericardial effusions. However, the results obtained with these modalities are inferior in terms of effectiveness and recurrence to open surgical procedures.

Systemic Chemotherapy and Radiation Therapy

Systemic chemotherapy and radiation therapy have been used with variable success in the treatment of malignant pericardial effusions. Most patients who receive systemic therapy undergo an initial therapeutic pericardiocentesis. Primrose and colleagues (1983) have reported complete resolution of a malignant pericardial effusion in a patient with bronchial carcinoma treated with vinblastine. Similarly, Reynolds and associates (1977) had a series of three patients with breast carcinoma treated with combination chemotherapy who had complete resolution of their effusions. Vaitkus and coworkers (1994) describe success in 67% of patients treated with systemic chemotherapy. Prevention of recurrence was unrelated to concurrent pericardiocentesis. The majority of the patients in this review had breast carcinoma. Variable results also have been reported with the use of radiation therapy in the treatment of malignant pericardial effusions. Cham and colleagues (1975) reported a series of 38 patients with malignant pericardial effusions treated with 2500 to 3500 rads over 3 to 4 weeks. They recorded improvement in 60% of the patients with a duration of 12 to 36 months. A significant proportion of the patients in this series had breast cancer. Patients with tumors that are sensitive to these modalities may benefit from such adjunctive therapy after initial pericardiocentesis.

Balloon Pericardiotomy

The use of a percutaneous balloon to create a pericardial window was initially described in 1991 by Palacios and associates. Percutaneous balloon pericardiotomy involves the use of a balloon-dilating catheter to create a nonsurgical pericardial window (Fig. 69-5). Palacios and associates (1991) performed percutaneous balloon pericardial window in eight patients with malignant pericardial effusion and tamponade. A left or bilateral pleural effusion occurred in all patients after treatment. There were no recurrences at a mean follow-up of 6 months. Similarly, Ziskind and colleagues (1993) reported a multicenter trial that involved 50 patients with malignant effusions treated with percutaneous balloon pericardiotomy. They obtained a successful result in 46 of 50 patients with a mean follow-up of 3.6 months. Two patients required an early operation for complications of the procedure, and two patients required a late operation for recurrence of tamponade. In addition, eight patients required either thoracentesis or tube thoracostomy. Long-term follow-up with a larger number of patients is needed to further assess the exact role of this modality in the treatment of malignant pericardial effusions.

Pericardial to Peritoneal Drainage

Pericardial to peritoneal drainage in the treatment of malignant pericardial effusions was described by Wang and associates (1994). If the peritoneum is opened, the subxiphoid approach can be used to create a communication between the pericardium and the abdominal cavity. It is not clear why fluid

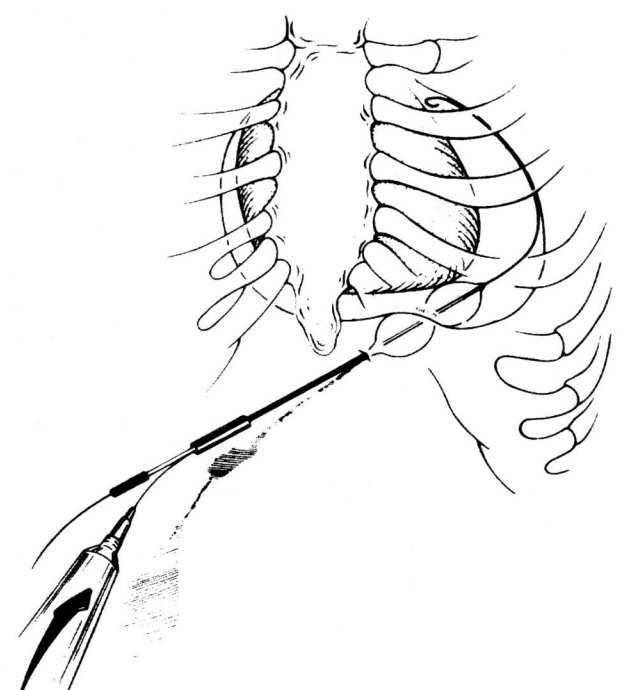

Fig. 69-5. Balloon pericardiotomy technique. The dilating balloon is advanced over a guidewire to straddle the pericardial margin. It is then manually inflated to create the pericardial window. From the American College of Cardiology, Ziskind AA, et al: Percutaneous balloon pericardiotomy for the treatment of cardiac tamponade and large pericardial effusions: description of technique and report of the first 50 cases. J Am Coll Cardiol 21:1, 1993. With permission.

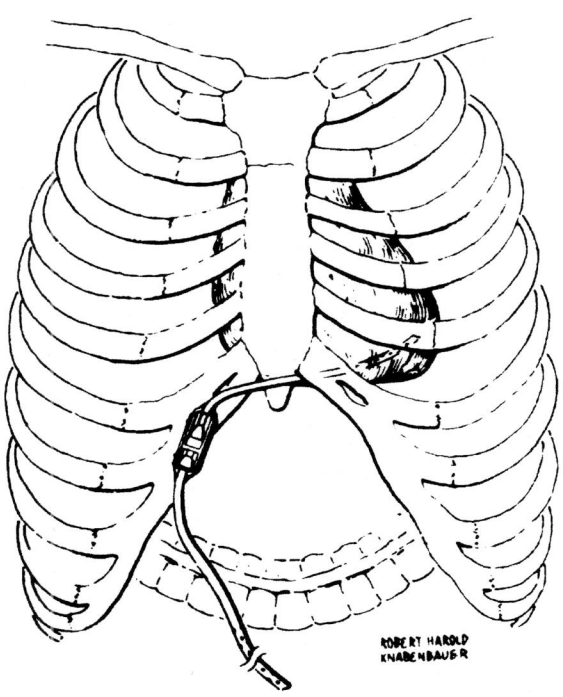

Fig. 69-6. Pericardioperitoneal shunt. From Wang N, et al: Pericardioperitoneal shunt: an alternative treatment for malignant pericardial effusion. Ann Thorac Surg 57:289, 1994. With permission from The Society of Thoracic Surgeons.

should drain in only one direction from the negative pressure thoracic cavity to the positive pressure abdominal cavity. This type of window probably closes relatively quickly with adhesions to the liver and omentum. Similarly, the subxiphoid approach can be used to implant a Denver shunt from the pericardial cavity to the peritoneal cavity (Fig. 69-6). Wang and colleagues (1994) reported on four patients with malignant pericardial effusions that were treated with Denver pericardioperitoneal shunts. Three of the patients died of the disease process without evidence of recurrence. The efficacy of this technique requires further study.

Pericardiectomy

Pericardiectomy can provide definitive therapy for patients with malignant pericardial effusive disease. The procedure involves resection of the parietal pericardium through either a median sternotomy (Fig. 69-7) or left anterior thoracotomy. Piehler and associates (1985) reviewed their experience with pericardiectomy in the treatment of malignant pericardial effusions in 72 patients. These patients were treated by either partial or complete pericardiectomy. In their experience, the incidence of recurrence

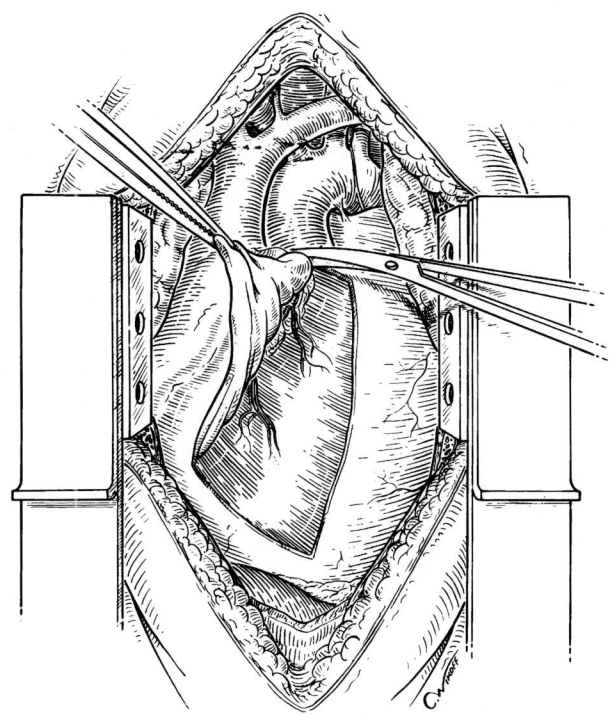

Fig. 69-7. Pericardial resection initiated through median sternotomy. From Moores DWO, Dziuban SW Jr: Pericardial drainage procedures. Chest Surg Clin North Am 5:359, 1995. With permission.

necessitating reoperation was more prevalent in patients who had undergone partial pericardiectomy. The authors suggested a direct relationship between the extent of pericardial resection and the incidence of recurrent effusion and advocated complete pericardiectomy. Within this series, however, only 13 patients underwent subxiphoid drainage and only 1 of the 13 required reoperation (7.7%). Five of 24 patients in this series who underwent transthoracic pericardiectomy required reoperation (20.8%). Naunheim and colleagues (1991) reported no significant difference in survival or recurrence in patients treated by subxiphoid or transthoracic drainage. In their series, postoperative respiratory complications were more prevalent in patients treated by transthoracic drainage than in patients treated by subxiphoid drainage. Vaitkus and colleagues (1994) reported a success rate of 83.3% and a mortality of 13.3% for transthoracic pericardiectomy in the treatment of malignant effusions. The disadvantages of this procedure are the requirement for general anesthesia and a thoracotomy. Transthoracic pericardiectomy with its attendant morbidity and mortality appears disadvantageous over less invasive procedures in the treatment of these gravely ill patients.

Video-Assisted Thoracoscopic Pericardiectomy

Pericardial drainage can be accomplished via VATS in patients with malignant pericardial effusive disease. The procedure requires general anesthesia and a double-lumen endotracheal tube for single-lung ventilation. Patients with cardiac tamponade must undergo initial pericardiocentesis before VATS pericardiectomy. The patient is positioned in the lateral decubitus position and three trocars are used (Fig. 69-8). Division of adhesions between lung and pericardium may be required. One or two chest tubes can be left after

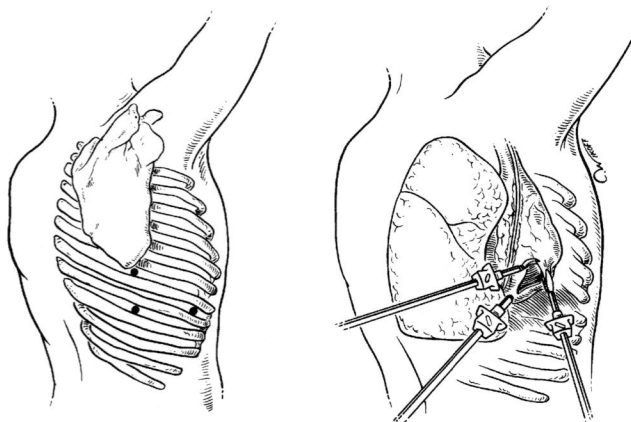

Fig. 69-8. Video-thoracoscopic approach to pericardial window showing three trocars introduced from the right side. Left side approach is also feasible. From Moores DWO, Dziuban SW Jr: Pericardial drainage procedures. Chest Surg Clin North Am 5:359, 1995. With permission.

completion of the procedure. Hazelrigg and associates (1993) reported their experience with thoracoscopic pericardiectomy in patients with pericardial effusive disease. Eighteen patients in this series had malignant pericardial effusions. They reported no recurrences and four complications that included two cases of dysrhythmia and two cases of pneumonia. Similarly, Mack and associates (1993) treated nine patients with malignant pericardial effusions via VATS pericardiectomy. Drainage of the pericardial space and control of symptoms was obtained in all patients in their series. They reported no major complications. Thoracoscopic pericardial drainage offers relatively little advantage over subxiphoid pericardial drainage as an initial procedure. It is more time consuming, requires double-lumen endotracheal intubation, and is more expensive than subxiphoid pericardiostomy. Thoracoscopic pericardiectomy is a viable alternative to anterior thoracotomy in patients who fail initial subxiphoid drainage.

Subxiphoid Tube Pericardiostomy

Larrey (1829) was the first to describe pericardial drainage via the subxiphoid approach in the early 1800s. This procedure is expeditious, has low morbidity, and can be performed under local anesthesia. We believe that this is the procedure of choice for the majority of patients with malignant pericardial effusive disease. In a 5-year series, one of us (D.W.O.M.) and associates (1995) reported on 82 patients with malignant pericardial effusions treated via subxiphoid tube pericardiostomy. Recurrent pericardial tamponade necessitating further surgical intervention occurred in two patients (2.4%). No mortality was attributable to the surgical procedure, and postoperative survival was determined by the underlying disease process. Vaitkus and colleagues (1994) in a collective review found the subxiphoid approach to be successful in controlling malignant pericardial effusions in 91.5% of patients with low rates of complications. Allen and associates (1999) compared subxiphoid pericardiostomy versus percutaneous catheter drainage in patients with cardiac tamponade. In their study, subxiphoid pericardiostomy was associated with no operative deaths and a complication rate of 1.1%, whereas percutaneous drainage had a mortality of 4% and a complication rate of 17%. Effusions recurred in 1.1% of patients following subxiphoid pericardiostomy compared with 30.4% with percutaneous drainage. Patients were preselected in that percutaneous drainage was used for patients with hemodynamic instability, precluding subxiphoid pericardiostomy.

Surgical drainage affords the opportunity for digital exploration and pericardial biopsies to obtain histology. The procedure is performed through a vertical incision from the xiphisternal junction down to the tip of the xiphoid process (Fig. 69-9). The upper linea alba is opened and the xiphoid is split or resected. Blunt dissection is then used to define the retrosternal plane. The pericardium can then be approached through the peritoneal cavity or extraperi-

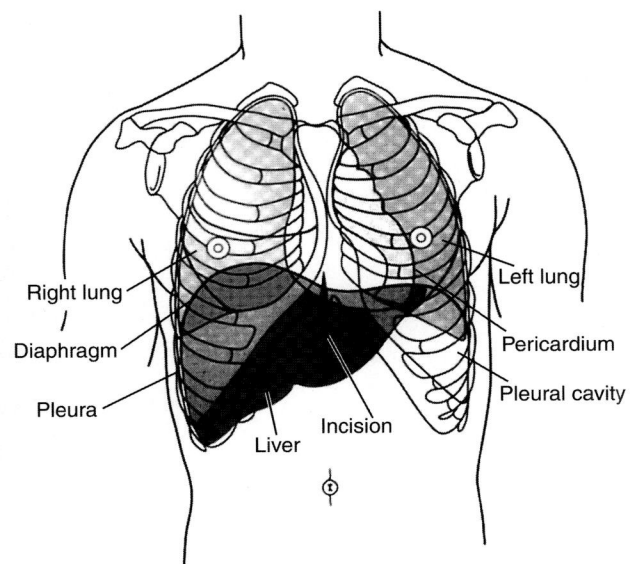

Fig. 69-9. Location of subxiphoid incision and its relation to surface and underlying anatomy. From Moores DWO, Dziuban SW Jr: Pericardial drainage procedures. Chest Surg Clin North Am 5:359, 1995. With permission.

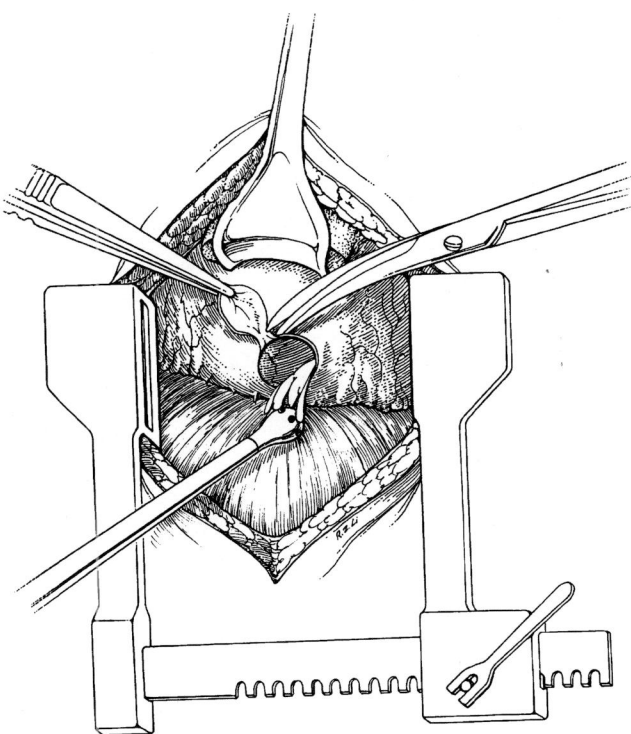

Fig. 69-10. Pericardial segment removed via the subxiphoid approach. From Moores DWO, et al: Subxiphoid pericardial drainage for pericardial tamponade. J Thorac Cardiovasc Surg 109:546, 1995. With permission.

toneally. A scalpel is used to open the pericardium, taking care to avoid any myocardial adhesions. Fluid is then collected for cytology and microbiology and the pericardial space is explored by digital palpation. A pericardial biopsy can then be obtained for histology and microbiology studies (Fig. 69-10). A No. 28F thoracostomy tube is then placed into the pericardial space from a separate lateral or inferior incision (Fig. 69-11). The chest tube is maintained on negative suction for approximately 4 days. We believe that postoperative tube suction drainage allows adhesions to form between the pericardium and epicardium, thus obliterating the pericardial space and preventing reaccumulation of fluid. In the aforementioned series (D.W.O.M. 1995) all eight of the patients who subsequently underwent autopsy were found to have obliteration of the pericardial space by dense adhesions.

The subxiphoid approach can be performed under local or general anesthesia. Local anesthesia reduces the risk of cardiovascular collapse at the expense of a more technically difficult procedure. Agitated or symptomatic patients may not tolerate the supine position under local anesthesia. We generally prefer general anesthesia with intubation because it offers more control, muscular relaxation, and technical accuracy. Patients with minimal echocardiographic evidence of right-sided heart compression tolerate general anesthesia well.

Our experience leads us to believe that subxiphoid tube pericardiostomy provides expeditious, effective, and durable treatment in patients with malignant pericardial effusive disease with low morbidity. It is the method we use in the majority of patients.

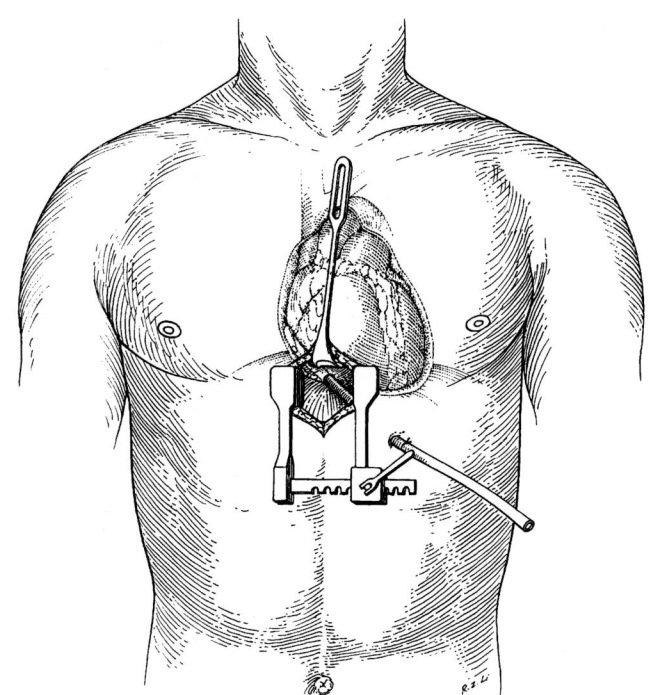

Fig. 69-11. Subxiphoid pericardial drainage tube brought out through a separate stab incision. From Moores DWO, et al: Subxiphoid pericardial drainage for pericardial tamponade. J Thorac Cardiovasc Surg 109:546, 1995. With permission.

REFERENCES

Allen KB, et al: Pericardial effusion: subxiphoid pericardiostomy versus percutaneous catheter drainage. Ann Thorac Surg (in press).

Celermajer DS, et al: Pericardiocentesis for symptomatic malignant pericardial effusion: a study of 36 patients. Med J Aust 154:19, 1991.

Cham WC, et al: Radiation therapy of cardiac and pericardial metastases. Radiology 114:701, 1975.

Clarke DP, Cosgrove DO: Real-time ultrasound scanning in the planning and guidance of pericardiocentesis. Clin Radiol 38:119, 1987.

Davis S, Rambotti P, Grignani F: Intrapericardial tetracycline sclerosis in the treatment of malignant pericardial effusion: an analysis of 33 cases. J Clin Oncol 2:631, 1984.

Fincher RME: Case report: malignant pericardial effusion as the initial manifestation of malignancy. Am J Med Sci 305:106, 1993.

Fraser RS, Viloria JB, Wang NS: Cardiac tamponade as a presentation of extracardiac malignancy. Cancer 45:1697, 1980.

Girardi LN, Ginsberg RJ, Burt ME: Pericardiocentesis and intrapericardial sclerosis: effective therapy for malignant pericardial effusions. Ann Thorac Surg 64:1422, 1997.

Hancock EW: Neoplastic pericardial disease. Cardiol Clin 8:673, 1990.

Hazelrigg SR, et al: Thoracoscopic pericardiectomy for effusive pericardial disease. Ann Thorac Surg 56:792, 1993.

Larrey DJ: New surgical procedure to open the pericardium in case of fluid in its cavity. Clin Chir 2:303, 1829.

Lopez JM, et al: Massive pericardial effusion produced by extracardiac malignant neoplasms. Arch Intern Med 143:1815, 1983.

Mack MJ, et al: Video thoracoscopic management of benign and malignant pericardial effusions. Chest 103:390S, 1993.

Maher EA, Shepherd FA, Todd TJR: Pericardial sclerosis as the primary management of malignant pericardial effusion and cardiac tamponade. J Thorac Cardiovasc Surg 112:637, 1996.

Miller AJ, Jain S, Levin B: Radiographic visualization of the lymphatic drainage of the heart muscle and pericardial sac in the dog. Chest 59:271, 1971.

Mills SA, Graeber GM, Nelson MG: Malignant tumors involving the heart and pericardium. In Roth JA, Ruckdeschel JC, Weisenburger TH (eds): Thoracic Oncology. Philadelphia: WB Saunders, 1995, pp. 492–513.

Moores DWO, et al: Subxiphoid pericardial drainage for pericardial tamponade. J Thorac Cardiovasc Surg 109:546, 1995.

Naunheim KS, et al: Pericardial drainage: subxiphoid vs transthoracic approach. Eur J Cardiothorac Surg 5:99, 1991.

Palacios IF, et al: Percutaneous balloon pericardial window for patients with malignant pericardial effusion and tamponade. Cathet Cardiovasc Diagn 22:244, 1991.

Piehler JM, et al: Surgical management of effusive pericardial disease. Influence of extent of pericardial resection on clinical course. J Thorac Cardiovasc Surg 90:506, 1985.

Press OW, Livingston R: Management of malignant pericardial effusion and tamponade. JAMA 257:1088, 1987.

Primrose WR, Clee MD, Johnston RN: Malignant pericardial effusion managed with Vinblastine. Clin Oncol 9:67, 1983.

Reynolds PM, Byrne MJ. The treatment of malignant pericardial effusion in carcinoma of the breast. Aust NZ J Med 7:169, 1977.

Roberts WC, Spray TL: Pericardial heart disease: a study of its causes, consequences and morphologic features. Cardiovasc Clin 7:11, 1976.

Shepherd FA, et al: Medical management of malignant pericardial effusion by tetracycline sclerosis. Am J Cardiol 60:1161, 1987.

Spodick DH: Pericardial windows are suboptimal [letter]. Am J Cardiol 51:607, 1983.

Thurber DL, Edwards JE, Anchor RWP: Secondary malignant tumors of the pericardium. Circulation 26:228, 1962.

Vaitkus PT, Herrmann HC, LeWinter MM: Treatment of malignant pericardial effusion. JAMA 272:59, 1994.

Wang N, et al: Pericardioperitoneal shunt: an alternative treatment for malignant pericardial effusion. Ann Thorac Surg 57:289, 1994.

Wong B, et al: The risk of pericardiocentesis. Am J Cardiol 44:1110, 1979.

Ziskind AA, et al: Percutaneous balloon pericardiotomy for the treatment of cardiac tamponade and large pericardial effusions: description of technique and report of the first 50 cases. J Am Coll Cardiol 21:1, 1993.

SECTION XII
Thoracic Trauma

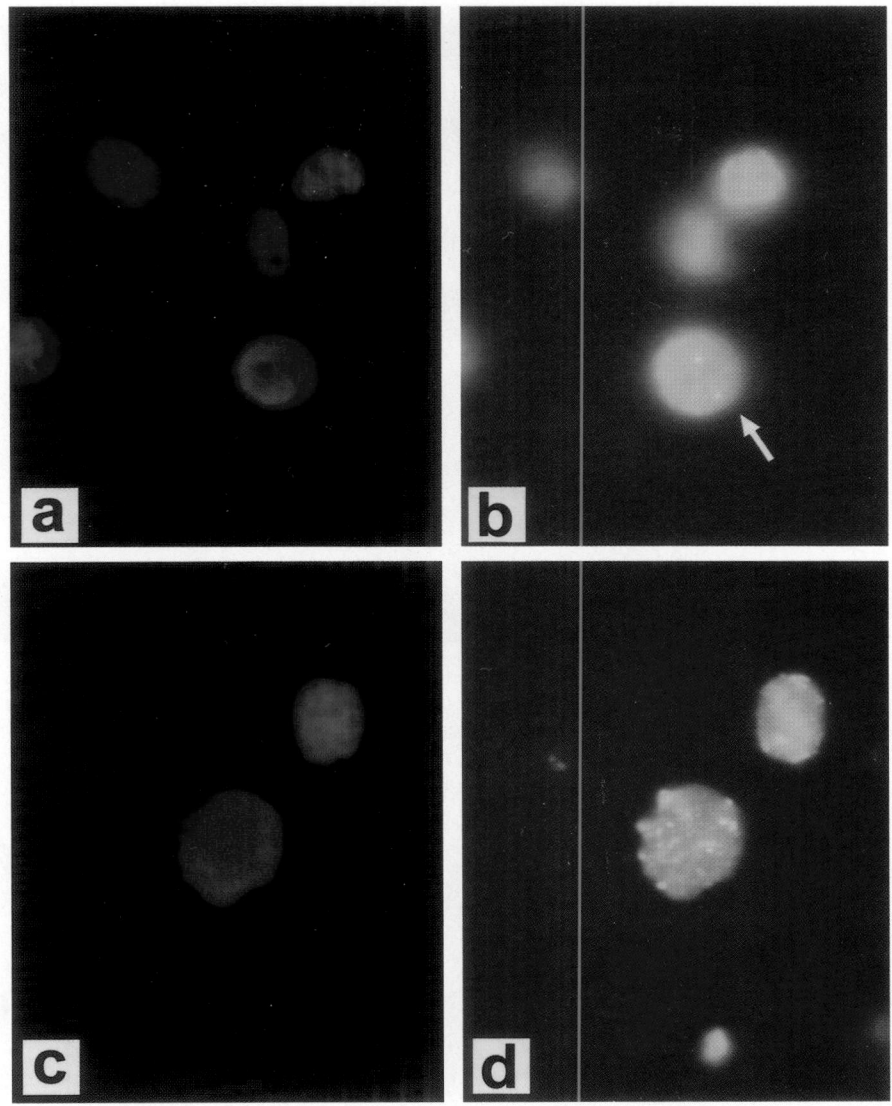

Color Fig. 15-1. Fluorescent in situ hybridization (FISH) demonstrating diploid complement of c-*erb*-b2/*HER*2/*neu* in normal cells. **a.** DAPI staining of cells. **b.** FISH (*arrow* designates diploid signal) and cancer cell line with amplification of c-*erb*-b2/*HER*2/*neu*. **c.** DAPI staining of cells. **d.** FISH. Courtesy of Dr. Paula Capodieci.

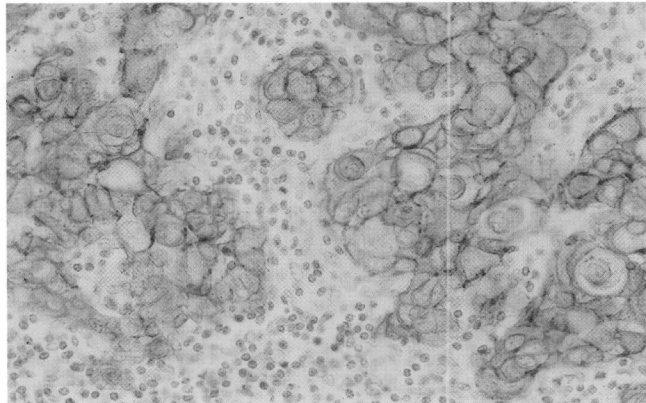

Color Fig. 15-2. Metastatic squamous cell carcinoma to a lymph node with positive staining of c-*erb*-b2/*HER2*/*neu*/*p185^{neu}* by immunohistochemistry.

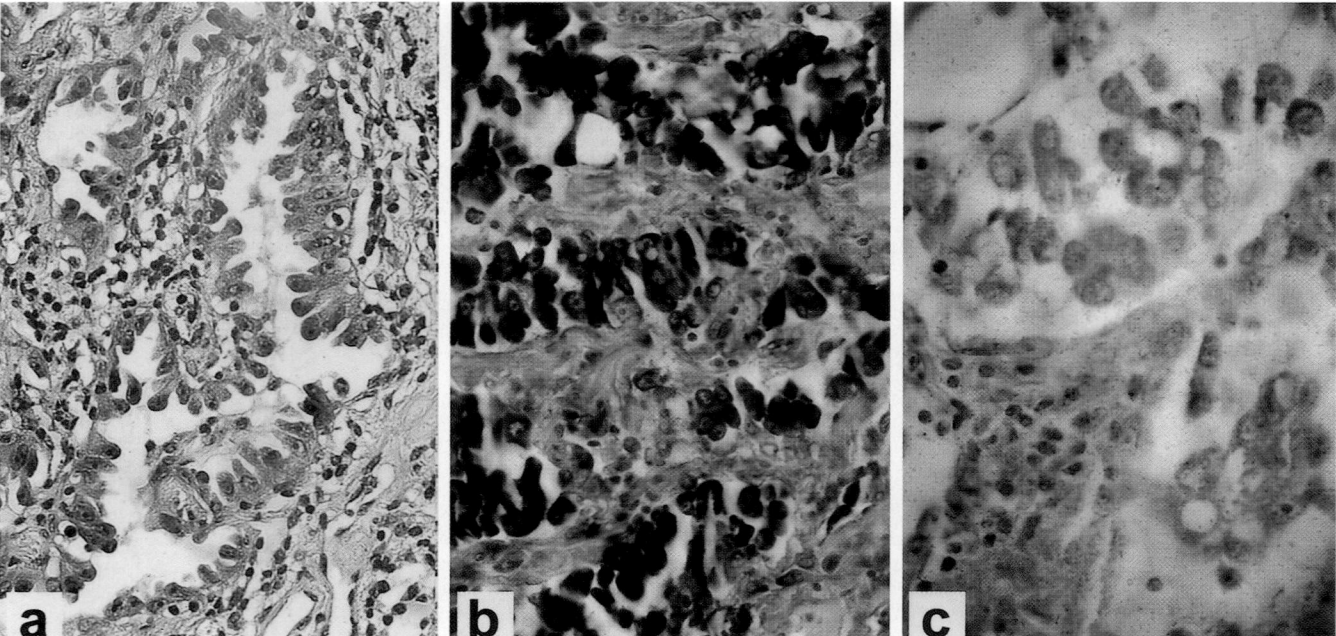

Color Fig. 15-3. a. Bronchioalveolar carcinoma stained by hematoxylin and eosin. **b.** In situ hybridization with antisense probe for mitogen-activated protein kinase phosphatase-1 demonstrating positive signal in the tumor cells. **c.** Control sense probe with absent signal in the tumor cells.

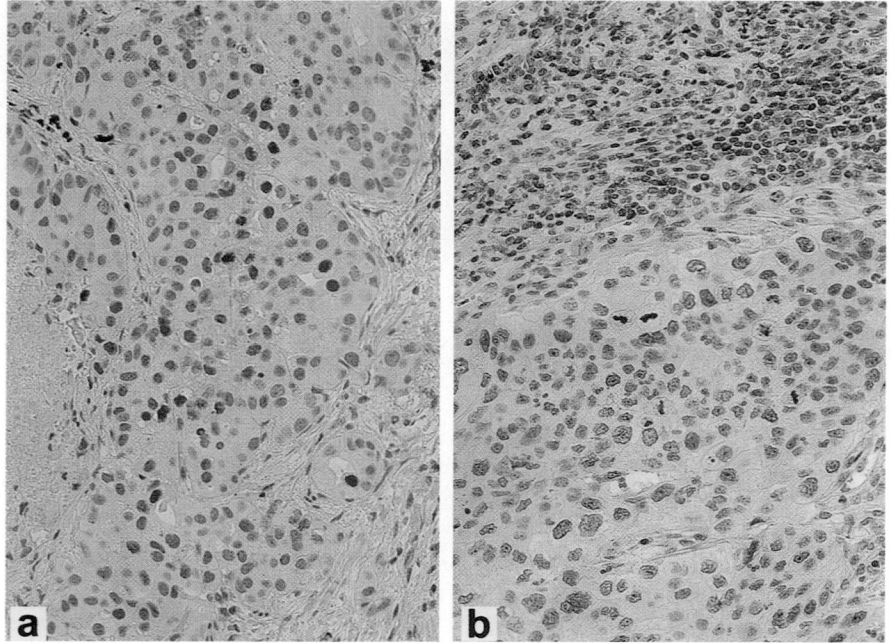

Color Fig. 15-4. *p27* expression by immunohistochemistry in non–small cell lung carcinoma. **a.** High expression of *p27* in tumor cells. **b.** Low expression of *p27* in tumor cells with lymphocytes serving as positive internal control. Courtesy of Dr. Michael Murphy.

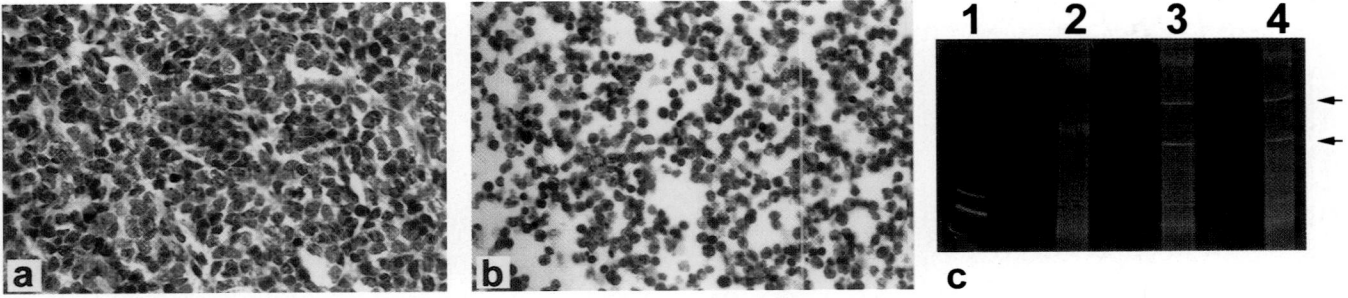

Color Fig. 15-5. T-lymphoblastic lymphoma in a lymph node **(a)** and subsequent pleural effusion with atypical lymphoid population **(b)**, producing identical monoclonal banded patterns by polymerase chain reaction single-strand conformational polymorphism–based TCR- gene rearrangement analysis **(c**; lanes 3 and 4, *arrows*). Courtesy of Dr. Michael Murphy.

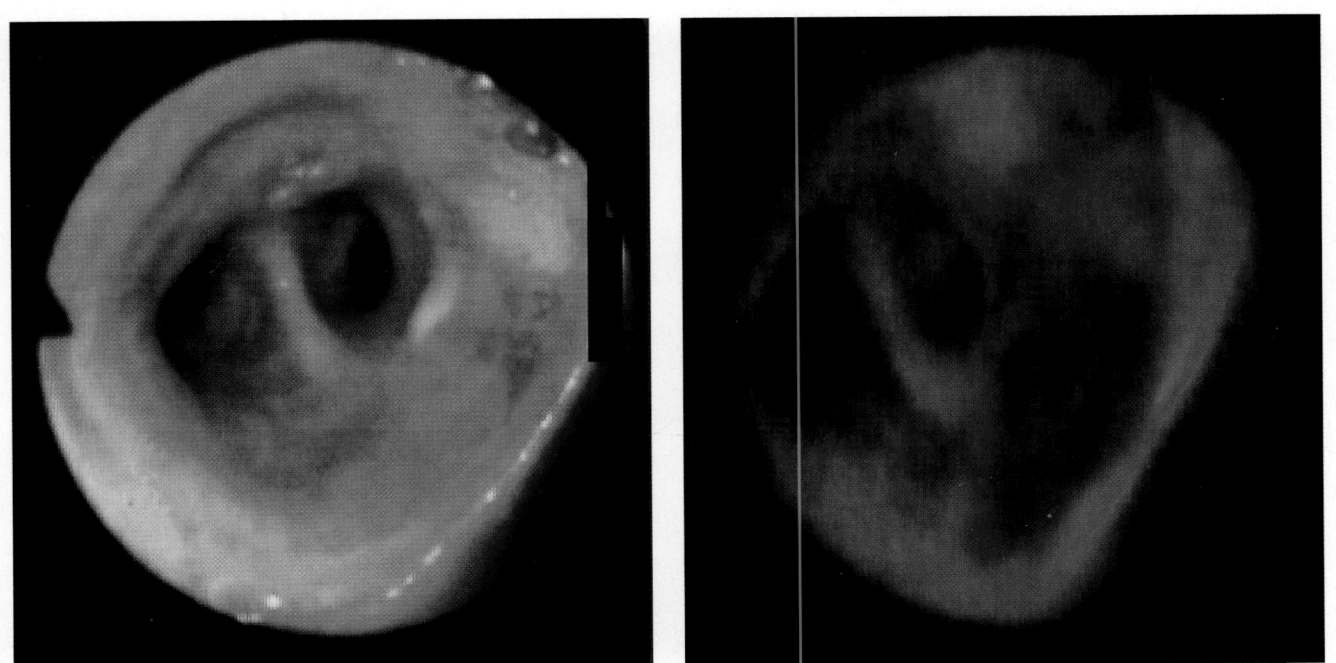

Color Fig. 16-7. A. Photograph of a normal-appearing bronchial mucosa using a white light source. **B.** Photograph of the same bronchial mucosa using a helium-cadmium laser light source to induce autofluorescence.

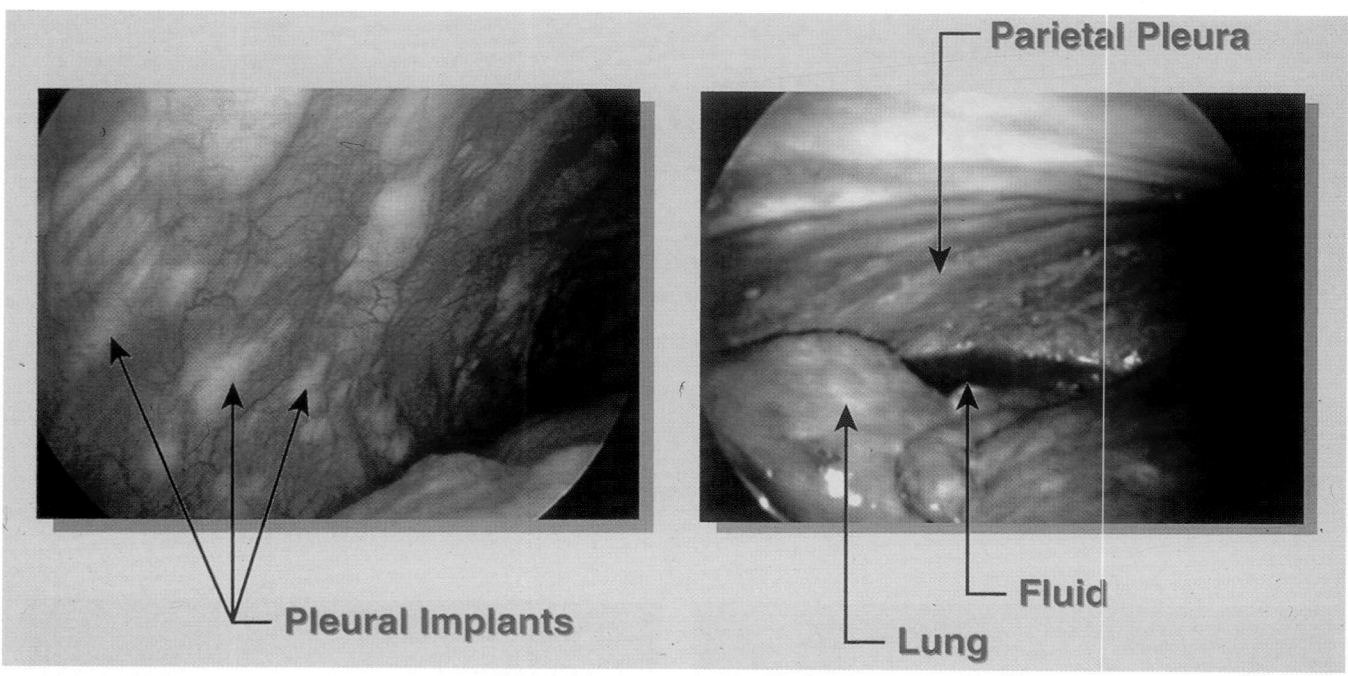

Color Fig. 18-4. Malignant pleural disease.

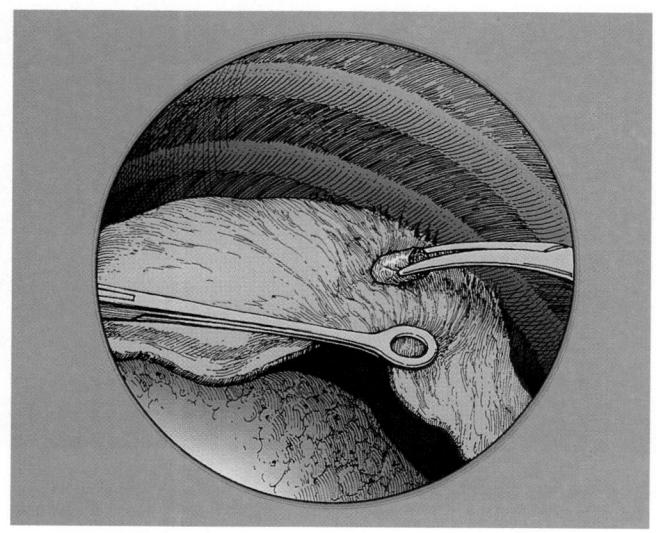

Color Fig. 18-5. Elevating pleura from chest wall.

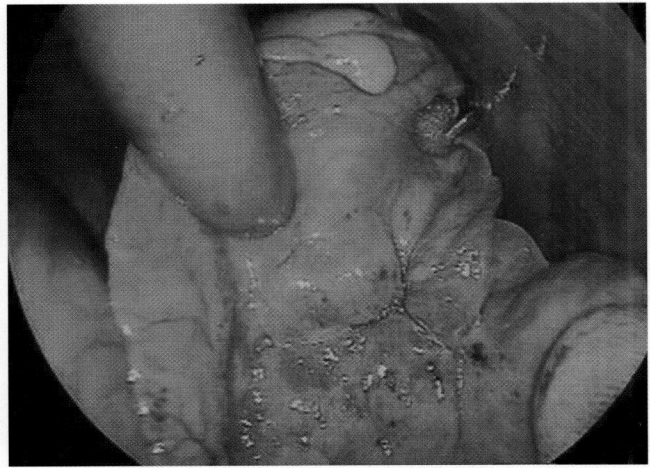

Color Fig. 18-6. Finger palpation of lung nodule.

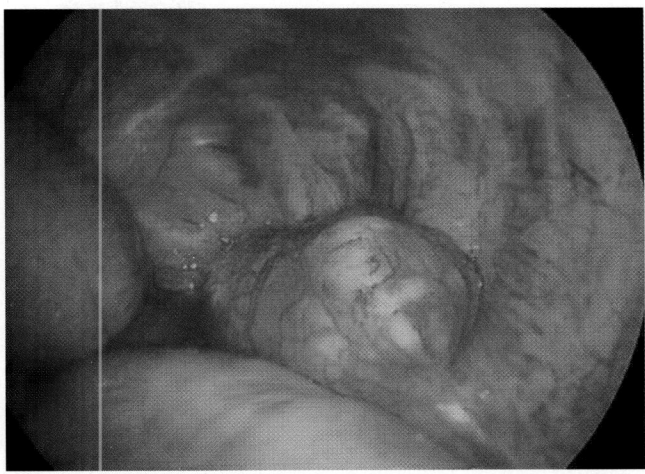

Color Fig. 18-10. Appearance of mediastinal mass as seen from right thorax.

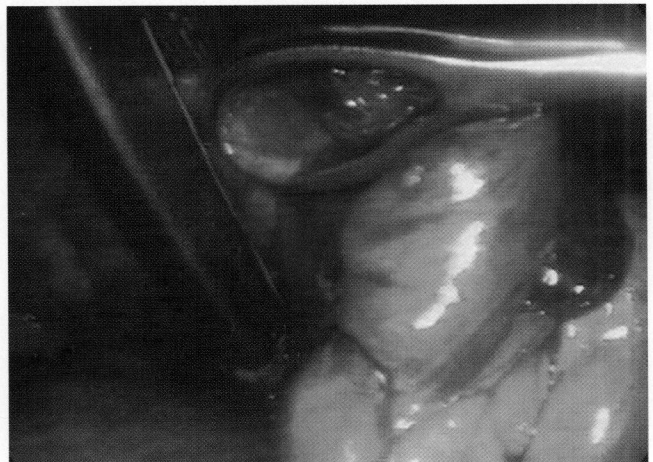

Color Fig. 18-8. Nodule within ring forceps with linear stapler in position.

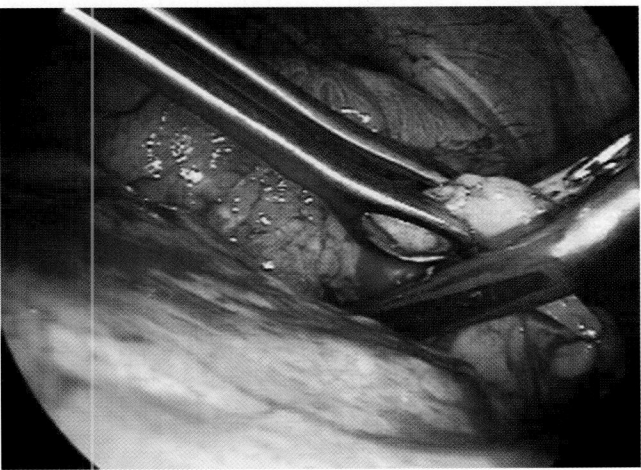

Color Fig. 18-11. Biopsy being performed using linear stapler for hemostasis (pathology: nodular sclerosing Hodgkin's lymphoma).

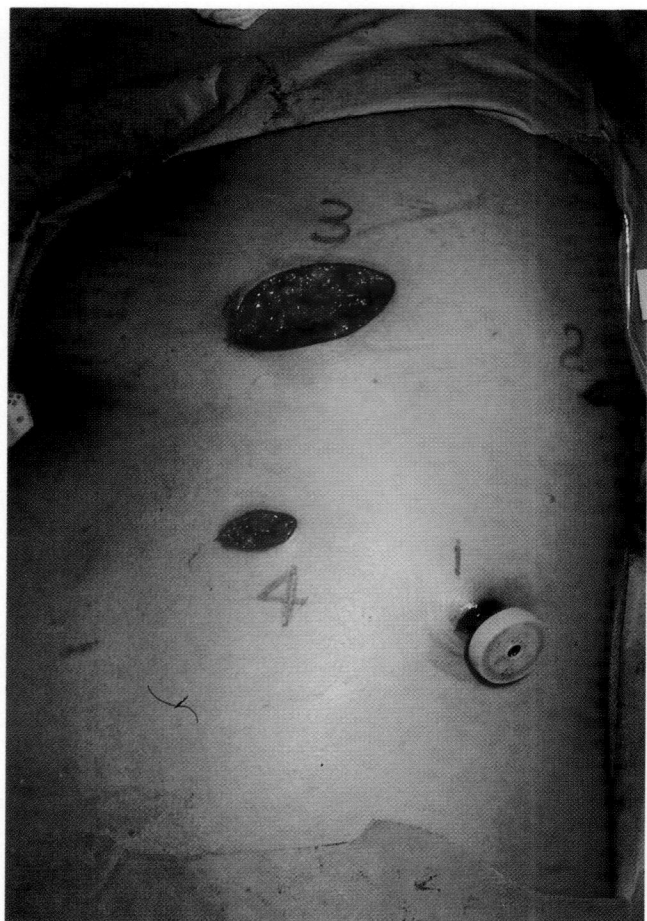

Color Fig. 33-1. The incisions for our approach to video-assisted thoracic surgical lobectomy including the following: (1) an incision for the trocar and the thoracoscope, (2) an incision in the auscultatory triangle for an assistant's instrument, (3) the utility thoracotomy incision, and (4) an incision in the midclavicular line for the stapler.

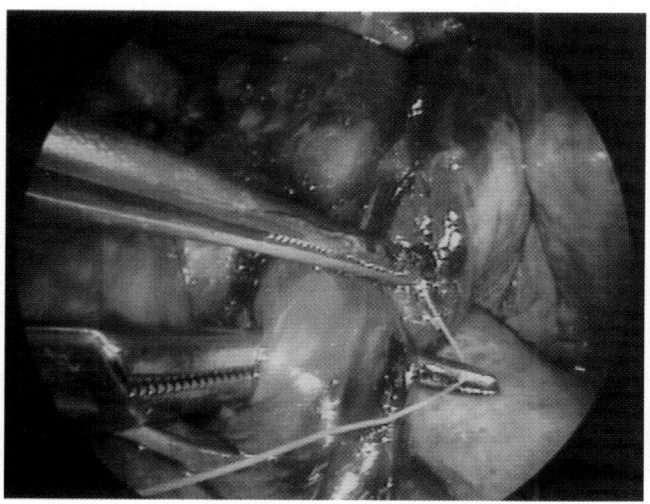

Color Fig. 33-2. A right-angle clamp pulls a tie around the middle lobe bronchus.

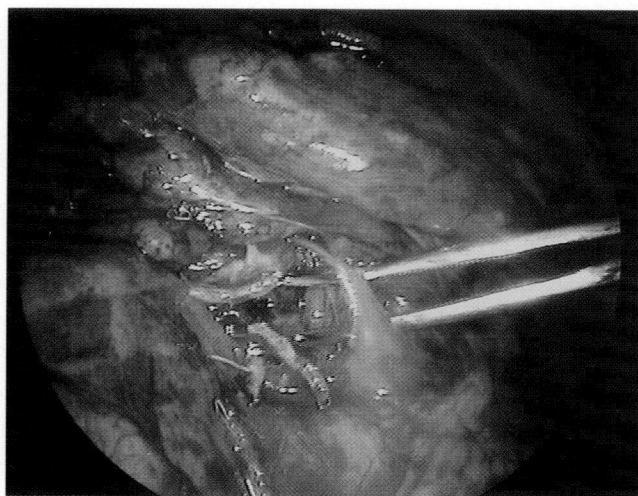

Color Fig. 33-3. A right-angle clamp mobilizes the right middle lobe artery.

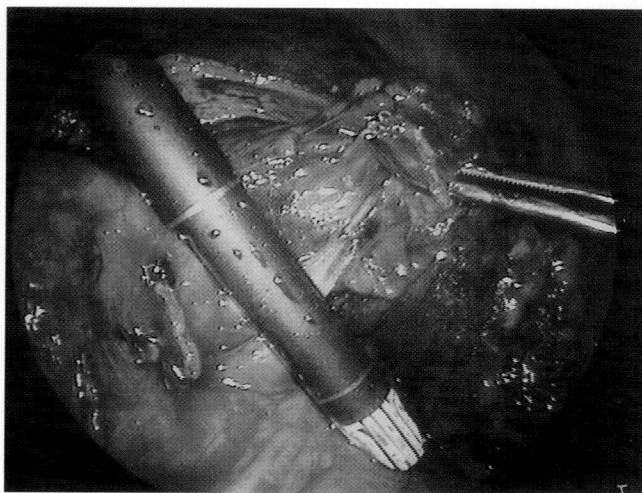

Color Fig. 33-4. The endoscopic stapler is across the right middle lobe artery.

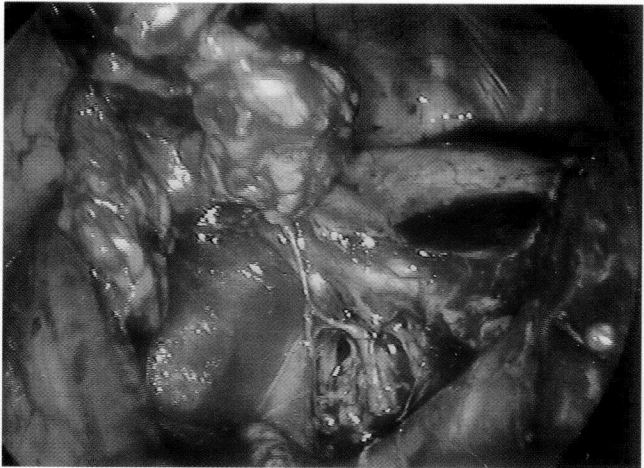

Color Fig. 33-5. The aortic-pulmonary window lymph nodes are elevated. This exposes the aorta, vagus nerve, and recurrent laryngeal nerve.

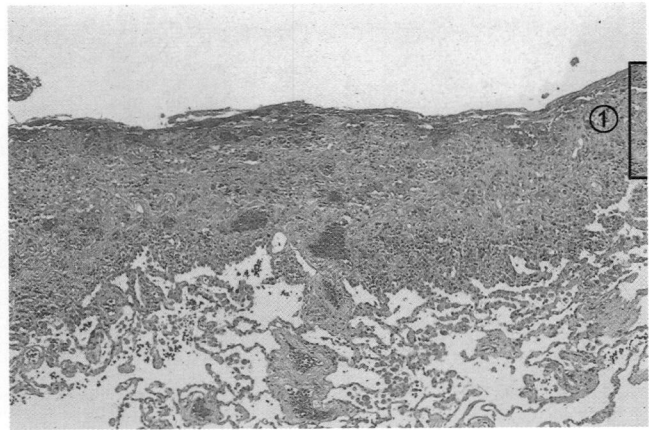

Color Fig. 61-1. Photomicrograph shows that a distinct boundary between early pleuritis (1) and the visceral pleura does not yet exist. Decortication before maturation of the pleural peel develops a plane between the visceral pleura and pulmonary parenchyma. (Hematoxylin and eosin, original magnification 100.)

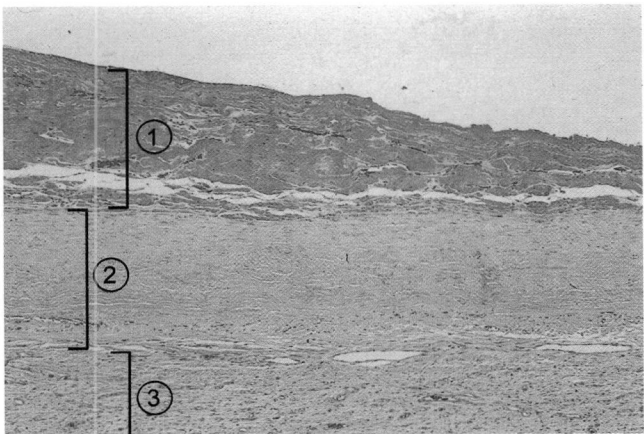

Color Fig. 61-2. Photomicrograph of a mature pleural peel consists of (1) debris, (2) mature collagen, and (3) a loose vascular matrix overlying the visceral pleura. (Hematoxylin and eosin, original magnification 40.)

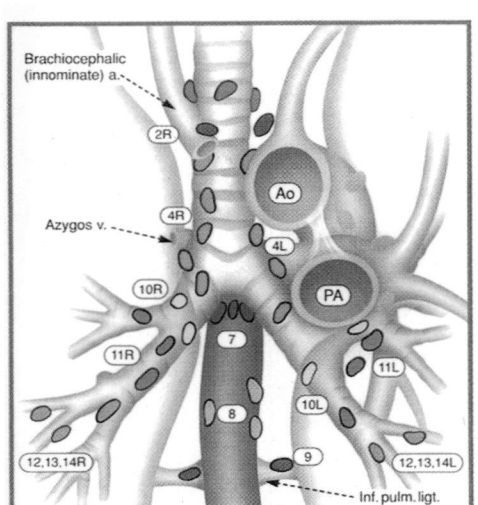

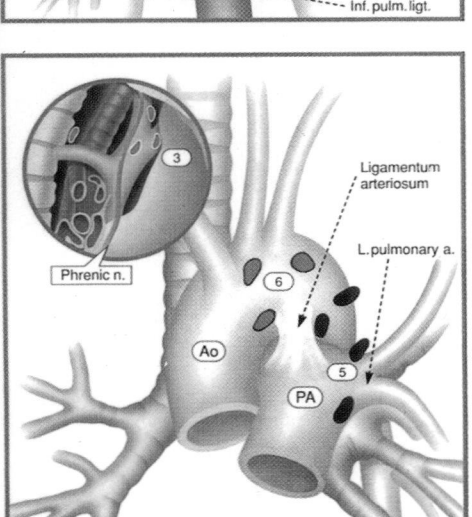

Superior Mediastinal Nodes

● 1 Highest Mediastinal

● 2 Upper Paratracheal

● 3 Pre-vascular and Retrotracheal

● 4 Lower Paratracheal
   (including Azygos Nodes)

N_2 = single digit, ipsilateral
N_3 = single digit, contralateral or supraclavicular

Aortic Nodes

● 5 Subaortic (A-P window)

● 6 Para-aortic (ascending
   aorta or phrenic)

Inferior Mediastinal Nodes

● 7 Subcarinal

● 8 Paraesophageal
   (below carina)

● 9 Pulmonary Ligament

N_1 Nodes

○ 10 Hilar

● 11 Interlobar

○ 12 Lobar

○ 13 Segmental

○ 14 Subsegmental

Color Fig. 98-1. Regional lymph node stations. Ao, aorta; PA, pulmonary artery.

CHAPTER 70

Blunt and Penetrating Injuries of the Chest Wall, Pleura, and Lungs

Felix D. Battistella and John R. Benfield

Thoracic trauma has challenged physicians since earliest recorded medical history. The Edwin Smith Papyrus of approximately 3000 BC described three cases involving chest injuries. Hippocrates and Galen proposed treatments for blunt and penetrating thoracic injuries that persisted for centuries. For example, Galen's recommendation of open packing of penetrating chest injuries with a poultice was followed until the thirteenth century when Theodoric advised débriding and closing chest wounds. In the sixteenth century, Ambroise Paré advocated delayed closure of chest wounds when there had been significant bleeding. During the seventeenth century, numerous irrigating cannulas were developed and used for the treatment of empyema. Johannes Scultetus (1674) described these in *The Surgeon's Storehouse*. During this time, physicians used professional "wound suckers" to drain intrathoracic collections. Not until 1707 did Anel adapt a syringe to the instruments used in sucking wounds, thus eliminating the need for human wound suckers.

A major step forward in the nineteenth century occurred with the development of closed drainage of the chest. The use of cannulas eventually led to the development of chest tubes. Although the underwater seal method was first described by Playfair in 1875, the use of closed chest drainage systems did not become popular until World War II.

Perhaps the most famous chest wound was reported by William Beaumont in 1825. His patient, after treatment of a close range gunshot wound to the lower chest, developed a chronic gastric fistula, allowing Beaumont to develop his classic observations on gastric physiology.

The discovery of x-rays by Roentgen in 1895 ushered in a new era in the diagnosis of thoracic pathology. The twentieth century brought the development of endotracheal intubation and the introduction of mechanical ventilators in the 1950s. Control of thoracic pain was achieved with the introduction of intercostal nerve blocks by Latteri; more recently, the use of epidural analgesia has become widespread.

Overall mortality from chest wounds has decreased from 62% during the Civil War to 4 to 7% in recent civilian experience. Among other developments, this improved survival rate was associated with the description of "wet lungs" by Burford and Burbank in 1945. The term *traumatic respiratory insufficiency* was subsequently used to describe the entity that is currently referred to as *acute respiratory distress syndrome* (ARDS). To this day, ARDS and multisystem organ dysfunction are the major barriers in the quest for improved survival of multiple-trauma victims.

EPIDEMIOLOGY

Although trauma is known to be the leading cause of death in the first four decades of life, statistics regarding the true incidence of chest trauma are scant. LoCicero and Mattox (1989) have estimated that 20 to 25% of trauma deaths—approximately 16,000 deaths per year—are attributable to thoracic injuries. According to Shorr and associates (1987), blunt trauma from motor vehicle accidents has accounted for 70 to 80% of thoracic injuries. Besson and Saegesser (1983) have noted that up to one-third of patients hospitalized after automobile accidents have evidence of major chest trauma.

When blunt thoracic trauma is considered, the victim's age is a critical variable. Children's elastic and flexible chest walls simultaneously protect them from rib and sternal fractures and enhance their exposure to force on the thoracic viscera. Thus, Nakayama and colleagues (1989) stress that children are at high risk for major intrathoracic injuries. Elderly patients have brittle chest walls that are subject to major injury secondary to low-energy trauma while affording poor protection for the underlying viscera. Hence, as noted by Shackford (1986) and Shorr and associates (1989), older people have a high mortality rate, even from minor chest wall injuries.

Penetrating thoracic injuries are rare in children and in old people but are increasingly common in young adults. Most civilian gunshot wounds are from low-velocity handguns. These do not transfer a large amount of energy to the surrounding tissues. In military situations, and occasionally in civilian settings, high-velocity gunshot wounds and close-range shotgun wounds dissipate large amounts of lateral shock wave energy that result in considerable amounts of devitalized tissue that require débridement.

Although most chest trauma can be managed without thoracotomy, Shackford (1986) and Kish and coworkers (1976) emphasize that thoracic injuries require prompt evaluation and treatment to avoid preventable mortality. This chapter addresses only injuries of the chest wall, pleura, tracheobronchial tree, and lungs. Diaphragmatic and esophageal injuries are discussed in Chapters 74 and 132, respectively.

EVALUATION AND MANAGEMENT

General Considerations

The priority for evaluation and management of any trauma victim is to assess the airway and to establish adequate ventilation. Arterial blood gas determinations are useful when circumstances allow; however, decisions about airway management should be based on rather simple clinical observations. A respiratory rate higher than 30 breaths per minute or labored respirations should trigger evaluation for easily correctable causes of respiratory distress. Immediate intubation and mechanical ventilation are required for patients with a respiratory rate higher than 35 breaths per minute or for patients with labored respirations, profound shock, or severe head injuries. Circulation should be assessed and supported with the necessary resuscitative measures almost simultaneous to airway management. In hypotensive patients, evaluation of the thorax for reversible causes of shock is critical (Table 70-1).

The circumstances surrounding the accident should be ascertained, because they may help in providing a correct diagnosis. For example, patients requiring extrication from behind steering wheels, or crushed by automobiles, are likely to have life-threatening intrathoracic injuries. Rapid deceleration accidents increase the index of suspicion for shearing injuries of the thoracic aorta or main stem bronchi. In hypotensive

Table 70-1. Etiology of Shock after Thoracic Trauma

Tension pneumothorax
Hemothorax
Cardiac tamponade
Myocardial dysfunction due to contusion
Air emboli
Injury to the great vessels
Large pulmonary contusion
Ruptured diaphragm

Table 70-2. Injuries Associated with Blunt Thoracic Trauma

Type of Injury	Percentage
Cranial injury	44
Abdominal injury	21
Extremity fractures	54
Pelvic fractures	12
Spinal fractures	6

Compiled from Galan G, et al: Blunt chest injuries in 1696 patients. Eur J Cardiothorac Surg 6:284, 1992; Glinz W: Symposium paper: priorities in diagnosis and treatment of blunt chest injuries. Injury 17:318, 1986; and Kulshrestha P, et al: Chest injuries: a clinical and autopsy profile. J Trauma 28:844, 1988.

patients, evaluation of the chest begins with examination of the neck veins. Distention of these veins differentiates cardiac compressive shock that is due to tension pneumothorax or cardiac tamponade from hypovolemic shock, which is usually associated with collapsed veins. Inspection of the chest wall during spontaneous respirations may reveal paradoxical motion associated with a flail chest. Palpation may reveal less conspicuous instability of the chest wall, or it may demonstrate crepitus that is due to subcutaneous emphysema associated with pneumothorax. Point tenderness can be elicited over rib, sternal, or clavicular fractures.

Isolated thoracic injury after blunt thoracic trauma is uncommon (Table 70-2). Associated extrathoracic injuries have been reported by Shorr and colleagues (1987), Besson and Saegesser (1983), Glinz (1991), and others in more than 75% of thoracic trauma patients. Among 200 patients with systolic blood pressures less than 100 mm Hg, more than one-half had major intra-abdominal injuries fully or in part responsible for their hemodynamic instability.

The location of penetrating wounds should be noted, but they should not be probed. If the wound is located below the fifth rib, evaluation of the abdomen is necessary because the possibility of diaphragmatic penetration and intra-abdominal injury must be excluded. Visualization of the diaphragm to exclude injury can be accomplished by a variety of means, including video-assisted thoracotomy—thoracoscopy, laparoscopy, laparotomy, or thoracotomy. In patients with multiple injuries that involve the chest and abdomen who have been hemodynamically unstable, we recommend laparotomy as the first avenue of intervention. This approach allows control of abdominal bleeding, which is often easily corrected, before proceeding with further evaluation and perhaps operative intervention for complex intrathoracic injuries.

All critically injured patients, except those who require resuscitative thoracotomy in the emergency department or patients with clinical evidence of a tension pneumothorax, should have an immediate radiograph of the chest. In addition to looking for the common post-traumatic abnormalities, particular attention should be paid to possible findings that may be easily overlooked (Table 70-3). Up to 35% of patients with ruptured diaphragms may initially have normal

Table 70-3. Frequently Overlooked Chest Radiograph Findings in Polytrauma Victims

Soft tissue injuries
Skeletal injuries
Ruptured diaphragm
Widened mediastinum
Foreign bodies
Mediastinal air

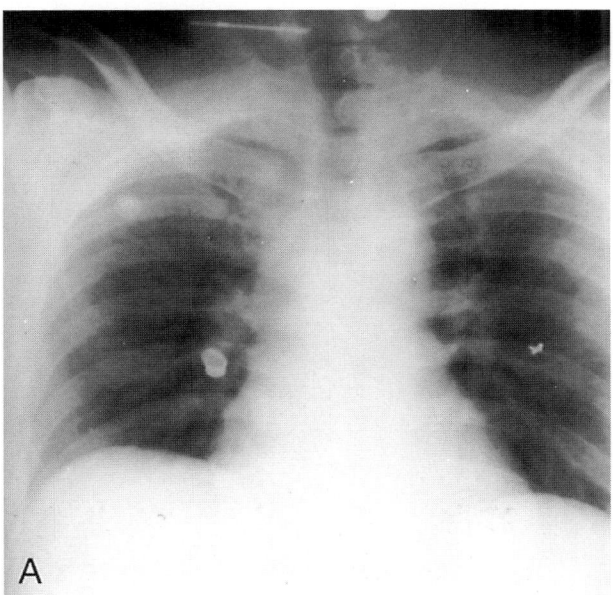

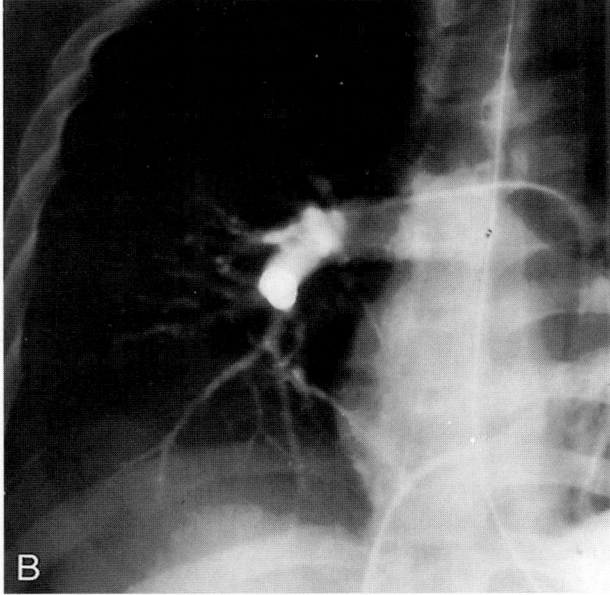

Fig. 70-1. Foreign body embolization. **A.** This chest radiograph depicts two foreign bodies lodged in the pulmonary arteries after a gunshot wound to the abdomen that injured the iliac vein. **B.** Pulmonary angiogram confirms the foreign body's location within the pulmonary artery.

or minimally abnormal chest radiographs. Penetrating wounds should be identified with radiopaque markers before radiographs are obtained. The initial location of bullets is noteworthy, because they may embolize (Fig. 70-1).

Stab wounds and low-velocity gunshot wounds lead to minimal chest wall trauma unless associated with injury to an intercostal or internal mammary artery. Penetrating injuries of the chest wall are typically managed expectantly unless continued bleeding occurs. Persistent hemorrhage from the aforementioned arteries is an indication for thoracotomy and ligation of the offending vessel. High-velocity gunshot wounds or close-range shotgun wounds, conversely, lead to devastating chest wall injuries and major injuries to the underlying structures. Management of such injuries almost always requires operation.

Trauma to the lower chest wall raises concern about possible intra-abdominal injuries. Penetrating injuries below the fifth rib may be associated with diaphragmatic hernias and injuries to intra-abdominal organs in 42% of patients, as reported by Murray and colleagues (1997). In hemodynamically stable patients, laparoscopy can be used to assess the integrity of the diaphragm; if the diaphragm has been violated, laparotomy should be performed to inspect the abdominal contents. Hemodynamically unstable patients with penetrating lower chest wall injury should undergo urgent laparotomy. Blunt trauma to the lower thorax is also associated with injuries to the underlying abdominal organs.

Chest wall injuries are most commonly the result of a motor vehicle accident and are often associated with injuries to the underlying structures, as pointed out by Campbell (1992), and to other areas of the body (see Table 70-2). In one series reported by Glintz (1991), more than three-fourths of patients hospitalized with thoracic trauma had other associated injuries. These associated injuries take precedence over chest wall injuries. On completion of the initial evaluation and treatment of life-threatening injuries, attention should be directed to pain control and pulmonary physiotherapy. Inadequate pain management and poor pulmonary hygiene lead to ventilatory compromise and various pulmonary complications.

Mediastinal and Subcutaneous Emphysema

Injuries to the tracheobronchial tree, esophagus, and lungs can all lead to mediastinal emphysema. Although rupture of the lung substance due to a penetrating injury typically leads to a pneumothorax, blunt rupture can involve part of the lung facing the hilar vessels or the bronchi. Air then dissects back along the bronchi and vessels to the mediastinum. If the leak is large, air migrates into the subcutaneous space of the neck, from where it can extend to the face and torso down to the inguinal ligament and occasionally to the external genitalia. Tracheobronchial injury should be suspected when a large amount of mediastinal air is present, especially if the pneumomediastinum seems to increase with

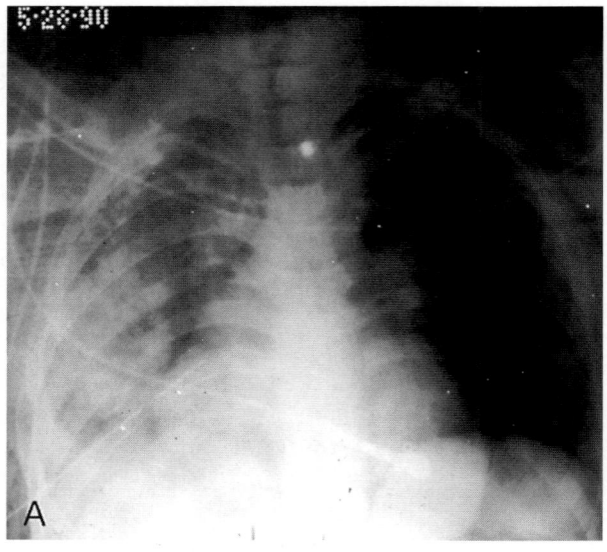

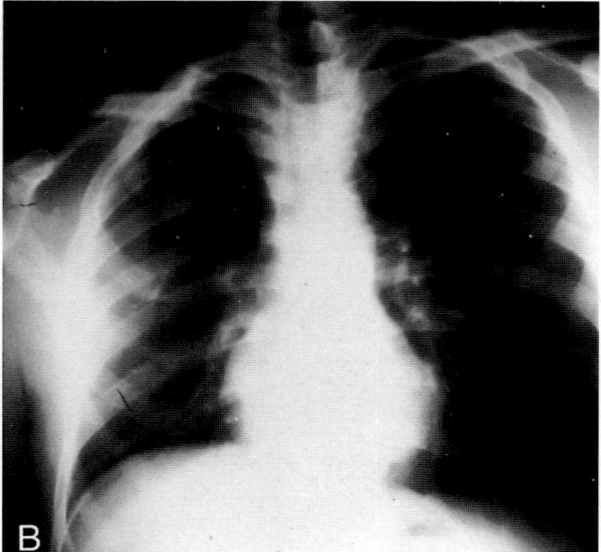

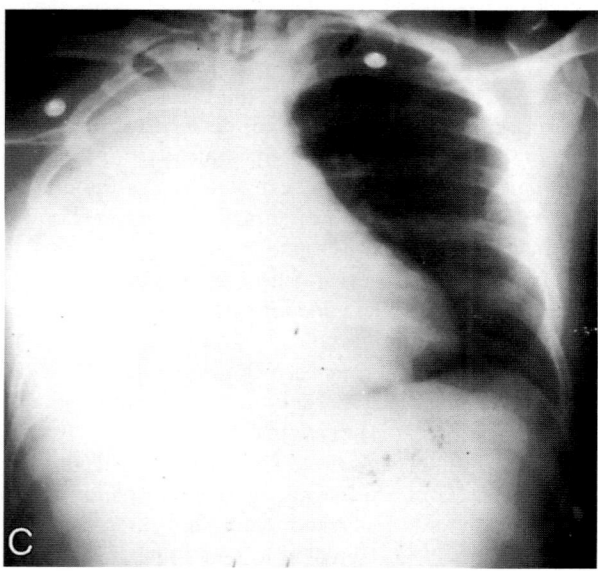

Fig. 70-2. Delayed recognition of bronchial rupture. Chest radiographs. **A.** Large amount of subcutaneous emphysema and mediastinal air after a crushing injury of the chest. **B.** Partial aeration after the chest tube removal approximately 2 weeks later; the patient was discharged from the hospital, doing well. **C.** Total collapse of the right lung 3 days later, when a stenotic obstruction of the right main stem bronchus from a torn bronchus was recognized.

mechanical ventilation (Fig. 70-2). The tracheobronchial tree and the esophagus should be assessed in a victim with penetrating injury to the mediastinum. Treatment and management should address the etiology of the mediastinal or subcutaneous emphysema. Decompression incisions in the skin are rarely, if ever, indicated.

INJURIES OF THE CHEST WALL, PLEURA, AND LUNGS

Rib Fractures

Rib fractures have been reported by Kemmerer and colleagues (1961) and Conn and colleagues (1963) in 35 to 40% of thoracic trauma victims, making these fractures the most common major thoracic injury. The diagnosis is based primarily on clinical findings. Post-traumatic pleuritic chest pain is usually diagnostic of rib fractures; these fractures can be localized by palpation. We consider the added expense of films made for the purpose of showing rib detail unnecessary. It is nonetheless important to quantitate the severity of rib fractures for prognosis and to map which ribs are fractured to assist in making a judgment as to possible types of associated injuries. Chest radiographs are largely used to identify associated intrathoracic injuries.

Fractures of the first and second ribs indicate the possible existence of additional serious intrathoracic injury. Although routine aortography has been advocated for patients with upper rib fractures, we agree with Poole (1989) that it is not needed unless other signs of injury to the thoracic aorta or great vessels are present. However, as noted by Richardson and colleagues (1975), fractures of the upper ribs and scapula have been associated with a mortality rate up to 36% and are hallmarks of severe trauma. According to the aforementioned authors, concomitant injuries to the head (53%), abdomen (33%), and thorax (64%) are often found in these patients.

Management of upper rib fractures is directed at identifying associated injuries and at controlling the associated pain that leads to splinting of the chest wall and hypoventilation. Decreased excursions of the chest wall and poor pulmonary hygiene may lead to atelectasis, pneumonia, and respiratory failure. Our experience, like that of Wisner (1990), has shown that the prompt use of epidural analgesia results in a lower morbidity and mortality than parenteral narcotics, particularly in elderly patients. Early mobilization, deep inspiratory efforts, and frequent coughing should be encouraged. Pulmonary physiotherapy, nasotracheal suctioning, and prompt bronchoscopy should be instituted in patients unable to clear secretions. Although young patients with single rib fractures might be managed with oral narcotics, more severe injuries may require parenteral narcotics. In general, young patients with multiple rib fractures or the older patient with less than three fractured ribs obtain adequate relief of discomfort with patient-controlled intravenous analgesia using the narcotic of choice. Old patients with three or more rib fractures or patients with pre-existing compromised pulmonary status are best managed with epidural analgesia. In the experiences of Worthley (1985), Mackersie and colleagues (1987), and Wisner and colleagues (1990), continuous administration of epidural analgesia is universally useful in patients with severe chest wall injuries such as multiple bilateral rib fractures, flail chests, or a combined thoracoabdominal injury.

Alternative methods for controlling pain due to thoracic injury include intercostal nerve blocks, intrapleural catheter analgesia, or transcutaneous electric nerve stimulation. Each of these modalities has disadvantages. Intercostal nerve blocks require repeated administration, and each injection exposes patients to the risk of pneumothorax. Intrapleural regional analgesia with a catheter in the pleural cavity achieves adequate pain control without sedation or respiratory depression. However, catheter placement carries the risk of pneumothorax and, based on the report by Luchette and colleagues (1994), appears to be less effective than epidural analgesia. Transcutaneous electric nerve stimulation is of no benefit immediately after trauma; this method should be limited to controlling pain in the chronic setting.

Wilson and colleagues (1977) and Garcia and colleagues (1990) have documented that the outcome of treatment and therefore the prognosis for rib fractures is related to the number of ribs injured, the patient's age, and the patient's underlying pulmonary status. Conn and associates (1963) and Worthley (1985) have noted that the mortality rate from isolated rib fractures in the elderly has been as high as 10 to 20%. Rib fractures in children as recorded by Nakayama and coworkers (1987) have been associated with a mortality rate of 5%. Thus, the full significance of rib fractures has too often been inadequately recognized. Morbidity and mortality from rib fractures can be minimized if associated injuries are identified and treated promptly and adequate pain control is achieved. These principles are especially important in the care of elderly patients.

Flail Chest

Instability of the chest wall from unilateral or bilateral multiple rib fractures, or from disruptions of the costochondral junctions, results in an estimated 5% of patients with thoracic trauma according to the data of LoCicero and Mattox (1989). The force needed to create a flail chest depends on the compliance of the ribs; old people may suffer an unstable chest wall after low energy impacts, whereas, as noted by Nakayama and associates (1989), flail chest occurs in less than 1% of children after severe thoracic trauma.

Paradoxical chest wall motion leads to a reduction in vital capacity and to ineffective ventilation that, along with associated pulmonary contusion, can lead to ARDS. Early documentation of respiratory compromise and frequent monitoring of respiratory rate, oxygen saturation, and arterial blood gasses is crucial. The clinical appearance of patients with flail chest may be misleading. Objective information obtained from arterial blood gas determinations should be the supervening guide to therapy. Unless there is evidence of rapid improvement after brief observation and aggressive pain management, we recommend endotracheal intubation and ventilator assistance for patients whose respiratory rate is more than 30 breaths per minute, whose Pao_2 is less than 60 torr, or whose $Paco_2$ is more than 45 torr.

Treatment of the unstable chest wall remains somewhat controversial. Previous attempts at external stabilization of the involved segment including the use of sand bags and towel clips are now considered anachronistic. Internal stabilization using positive pressure ventilation was introduced by Avery and associates in 1956; this method became the routine until it was superseded by the current recommendations. We now use the same therapeutic guidelines for flail chest as for simple rib fractures—that is, prompt and aggressive pain control, vigorous pulmonary hygiene, and selective endotracheal intubation with mechanical ventilation in patients with respiratory decompensation. The reports of other surgeons, including those of Trinkle and colleagues (1975), Shackford and colleagues (1976), Freedland and colleagues (1990), and Clark and colleagues (1988), and our experience have taught us that prophylaxis and early intervention must be the guiding principles. Endotracheal intubation and mechanical ventilation are instituted early, based primarily on physiologic evidence of ventilatory insufficiency, respiratory fatigue, or deterioration. Mechanical ventilation is instituted for treatment of respiratory insufficiency rather than for its ability to splint chest wall instability, and it is maintained until pain control permits the patient to perform adequate pulmonary hygiene. Patients are given aggressive pulmonary physiotherapy with incentive spirometry, encouraged to cough deeply, and are treated with suctioning, humidification of air, and chest percussion with postural drainage. Bronchoscopy is used liberally to remove retained secretions promptly and to expand areas of collapsed lung.

Operative fixation of flail segments has not gained widespread acceptance, although several techniques have been developed by Haasler (1990), Paris and colleagues (1991), and Landreneau and colleagues (1991). We use operative fixation of flail chest wall segments when thoracotomy is being done for other indications. In addition, we rarely use internal fixation for patients with isolated extensive flail segment associated with poorly controlled pain.

Survival after flail chest injuries has improved with selective ventilatory support and improved pain management. The mortality rate of flail chest of approximately 30 to 40% reported by Shackford and colleagues (1976) and Thomas and colleagues (1978) in the mid-1970s fell to 11 to 16% in the late 1980s, as recorded by Freedland (1990) and Clark (1988) and their colleagues. Associated injuries such as underlying pulmonary contusion, as pointed out by Clark and associates (1988), continue to contribute significantly to the persistently high mortality rate, perhaps causing it to be twice as high in patients with associated injuries as in individuals with isolated chest wall trauma. Other commonly associated injuries such as central nervous system injuries and intra-abdominal trauma contribute to mortality and increase the likelihood that mechanical ventilation will be needed.

Landercasper and coworkers (1984) noted that flail chest injuries may have long-term consequences. Impaired pulmonary function has been documented in long-term survivors; 63% of patients reported dyspnea, and 49% of patients reported persistent pain as subjective abnormalities. Objective evidence of chronic disability revealed 57% of patients had abnormal spirometry and 70% had abnormal treadmill tests. The etiology of these persistent pulmonary abnormalities is unclear, and whether internal stabilization of the chest wall would reduce their incidence is unknown.

Traumatic Asphyxia

Traumatic asphyxia results from a severe crush injury of the thorax. It manifests itself with facial and upper chest petechiae, subconjunctival hemorrhages, cervical cyanosis, and occasionally neurologic symptoms. Temporary impairment or loss of vision, presumed to be due to retinal edema, may be present rarely. Factors implicated in the development of these striking physical characteristics include thoracoabdominal compression after deep inspiration against a closed glottis, which results in venous hypertension in the valveless cervicofacial venous system. Williams and colleagues (1968) and M. C. Lee and colleagues (1991) recommend that treatment is primarily supportive; concurrent injuries, however, should be excluded.

Sternal Fractures

Sternal fractures, according to Otremski and colleagues (1990), occur in approximately 4% of patients involved in major motor vehicle accidents. Older patients and front-seat vehicle occupants involved in frontal collisions are at greatest risk. The fracture is typically transverse and is located in

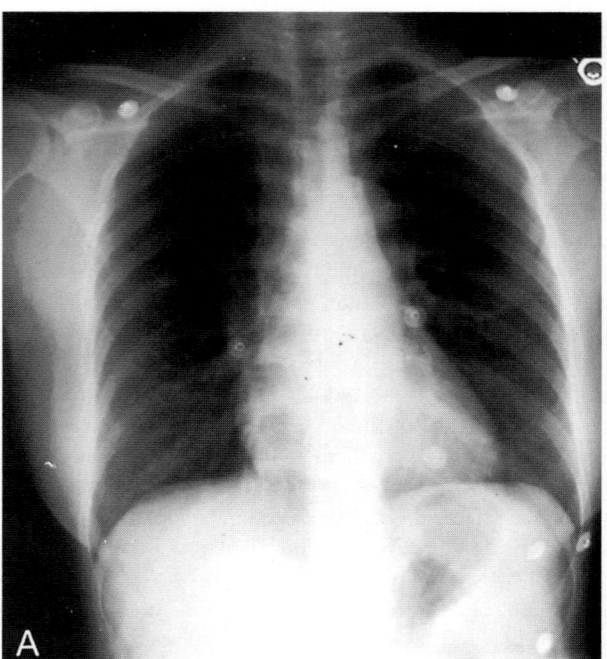

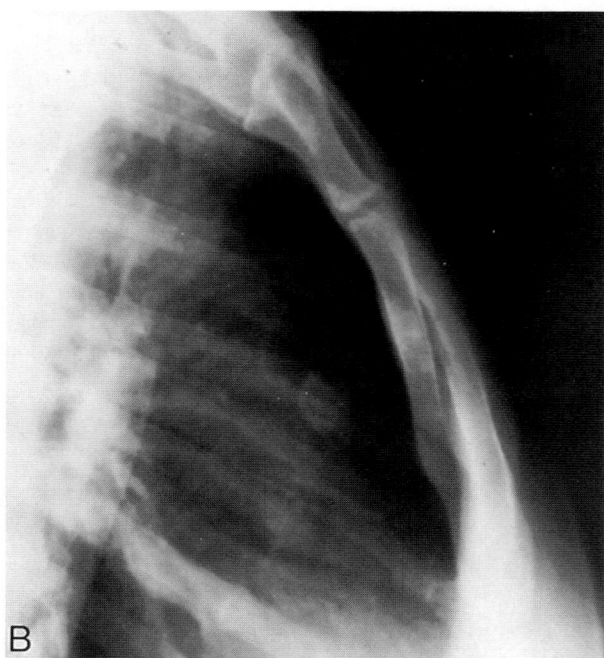

Fig. 70-3. Sternal fracture. **A.** Posteroanterior chest radiograph fails to reveal the fracture sustained after a head-on motor vehicle accident. **B.** Lateral projection shows the fracture with the two overriding fragments.

the upper and midportions of the body of the sternum. Diagnosis can be made on physical examination with the identification of localized tenderness, swelling, and deformity. Radiographic confirmation of these fractures requires a lateral view because they are rarely apparent on the anteroposterior chest film (Fig. 70-3).

Sternal fractures, like other chest wall injuries, as noted by Buckman and coworkers (1987), are frequently associated with other significant intra- and extrathoracic injuries. Injury to the underlying myocardium has been variably reported depending on the diagnostic test used to identify its presence. Although the clinical significance of abnormal test results in hemodynamically stable patients has been challenged by the studies of Wisner and associates (1990), myocardial injury should be considered in the hemodynamically unstable patient with evidence of anterior chest wall injury.

Treatment of sternal fractures is similar to that for rib fractures; it consists primarily of pain control and pulmonary hygiene. If the fracture is severely displaced, open reduction through a midline incision with internal fixation using cross wires is indicated. In the rare patient with a flail sternum that is due to disruption of the costochondral junctions, internal fixation as recommended by Shackford and colleagues (1976) or external fixation as recommended by Henley and colleagues (1991) has been advocated to minimize the need for positive pressure ventilation.

Scapular and Clavicular Fractures

Fractures of the scapula are uncommon, and they are due to a severe force of impact. This results in an 80 to 90% incidence of associated injuries, according to MaGahan and colleagues (1980) and Thompson and colleagues (1985); Armstrong and Van der Spuy (1984) report a 10% mortality rate. Because of the high incidence of concurrent brachial plexus injuries, a careful neurovascular examination should be documented. Treatment consists of shoulder immobilization with subsequent early range of motion exercises. Guttentag and Rechtine (1988) have pointed out that surgical repair may be indicated when glenohumeral joint function is impaired.

Clavicular fractures, on the other hand, are common and often isolated. Isolated clavicular fractures rarely, if ever, compromise ventilation, and treatment by immobilization of the shoulder with a sling and analgesia is effective and usually without complications. Only rarely is operative repair necessary for severely displaced fractures. Damage to the underlying subclavian vessels or the brachial plexus is rare, but this possibility should be considered.

Penetrating Chest Wall Wounds

Wounds from stabbings or low-velocity gunshot wounds are quite different from large chest wall defects associated with penetration from high-velocity missiles or shotgun wounds. Sucking chest wounds present life-threatening emergencies, and they are often associated with devastating intrathoracic injuries. The equilibration of intrathoracic pressure with atmospheric pressure associated with an open pneumothorax leads to decreased alveolar ventilation. A patient's inability to ventilate can be temporarily corrected in part by covering the defect. In the field, this can be accomplished by covering the wound with a plastic sheet that is taped on three sides, leaving one side free to act as a one-way valve. In the emergency department, the wound can be covered with an impermeable dressing, and a chest tube can be placed to reexpand the lung. Management of large open wounds requires operative débridement with removal of devitalized tissue, foreign bodies such as shotgun wadding materials and bone fragments, and formal chest wall closure. Often this can be accomplished by mobilizing the surrounding tissues; however, large soft tissue defects require rotational or free myocutaneous flaps. The pectoralis muscle, latissimus dorsi, or rectus abdominis flaps can be used (Fig. 70-4). The use of synthetic materials such as Marlex, Gore-Tex, or methylmethacrylate may be appropriate for elective chest wall reconstruction, but we do not recommend their use after acute trauma because of the risk of infection from the contamination associated with the injury.

Most low-velocity handgun and stab wounds can be managed nonoperatively, usually with only tube thoracostomy. Although the appearance of gunshot wounds should be described in detail, it is best to avoid describing wounds as entrance or exit wounds, because appearance can be deceiving. We prefer to leave this determination to the discretion of the forensic pathologist, because often it is of great medical-legal importance.

High-velocity missiles from military weapons or rifles are associated with surprisingly large lateral shock waves that cause extensive tissue injury and temporary cavities that often are not externally apparent. Therefore, these injuries require enhanced suspicion of significant internal viscus injury, débridement of surface wounds, and liberal use of exploratory thoracotomies when the indications for operation are marginal. We have experienced instances of delays in proceeding with thoracotomy after high-velocity bullet wounds with subsequent adverse consequences. However, we cannot recall an instance of regret for having proceeded with early operation in such a case.

Asymptomatic penetrating chest wall wounds of the type usually seen in civilian practice without evidence of intrathoracic injury can be observed in the emergency department with a repeat chest radiograph obtained 6 hours after the initial chest film. If re-evaluation shows no evidence of deterioration, patients may not need to be admitted to the hospital, and appropriate follow-up can be accomplished with outpatient visits, as documented by the data of Ordog and colleagues (1983), Karanfilian and colleagues (1981), Weigelt and colleagues (1982), and Ammons and colleagues (1986). Delayed evidence of hemothorax or pneumothorax under such circumstances can be expected in about 7 to 9% of patients.

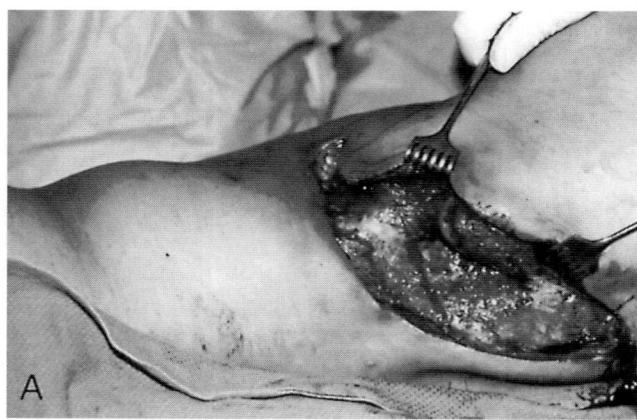

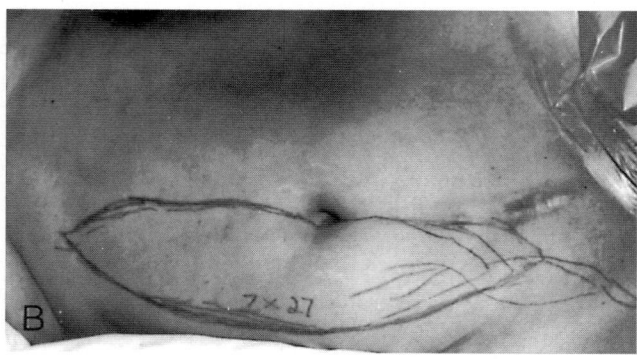

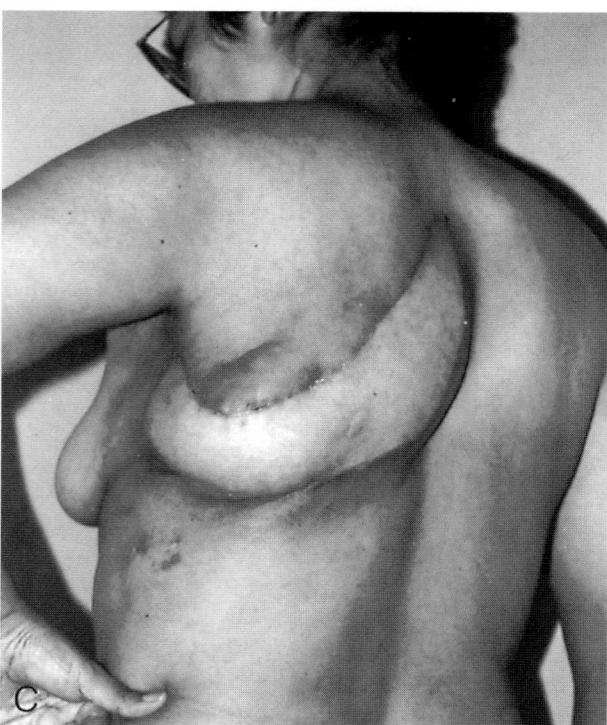

Fig. 70-4. Myocutaneous flap. **A.** Post-traumatic chest wall defect. **B.** Rectus abdominis flap. **C.** Postoperative result.

Pneumothorax

Simple Pneumothorax

Post-traumatic pneumothoraces may not always come to attention during the initial assessment of critically injured victims because of the noisy environment of the resuscitation room. Therefore, the chest radiograph should be obtained early in the evaluation and inspected carefully for the presence of lung markings extending to the periphery. We recommend chest tube drainage of post-traumatic pneumothoraces, even for small collections of air, especially in patients who require positive-pressure ventilation. When a large air leak is present or reexpansion of the lung is difficult, a tracheobronchial injury should be suspected and bronchoscopy should be performed.

Tension Pneumothorax

Physical examination in patients with a tension pneumothorax usually reveals severe respiratory distress, distended neck veins, a deviated trachea, and absent breath sounds on the affected side. In such cases, placement of a thoracostomy tube before obtaining a chest radiograph helps restore the patient's blood pressure, because decompression with a chest tube is an immediately effective treatment. Tension pneumothorax should be suspected in any patient with chest wall trauma receiving general anesthesia when a sud-

den cardiopulmonary deterioration associated with a marked increase in ventilatory pressures is present. Some surgeons routinely insert thoracotomy tubes in patients with rib fractures even though no evidence is present of underlying pulmonary injury or a pneumothorax to prevent the possible occurrence of an intraoperative tension pneumothorax if the injured patient is to undergo a general anesthetic. We recommend monitoring these patients carefully and have a low threshold for inserting a tube thoracostomy if the patient's cardiopulmonary status deteriorates.

Hemothorax

Massive intrathoracic hemorrhage that is recognized during emergency department resuscitative thoracotomy requires rapid assessment of the bleeding source. Temporary placement of a large vascular clamp on the hilum of the lung may prove lifesaving while the patient is transported to the operating room.

Bedside ultrasound, which is used to detect hemoperitoneum in the initial evaluation of the blunt trauma victim, can also be used to detect traumatic pleural effusions. As reported by Sisley and colleagues (1998), ultrasound can be rapidly performed by the surgeon performing the initial evaluation of the injured patient. More commonly, recognition of a hemothorax relies on the chest radiographic findings. Because initial radiographs are obtained with the patient in the supine position and pleural fluid lies posteriorly, detecting a small hemothorax may be difficult. In patients with moderate-sized collections, the chest film may reveal a slight opacification of the affected hemithorax. Treatment is directed at correcting the hypovolemia and evacuating the blood from the pleural cavity. Initial drainage of the pleural space should be established with a chest tube. If the chest cavity is adequately drained with a No. 36F chest tube and bleeding has stopped, this should be ample treatment. However, thoracotomy is indicated if the initial chest tube output is more than 1,500 mL (>20 mL/kg) or if the hourly output continues without abatement at more than 200 mL/hour (>2 mL/kg/h) for 2 to 4 hours. If opacification of the chest radiograph persists, this indicates an inadequately drained hemothorax. The clotted hemothorax should be evacuated to prevent the formation of a fibrous peel and to reduce the risk of empyema. We recommend using video-assisted thoracic surgery (VATS) techniques to evacuate large retained clotted hemothoraces. Evacuation of the clotted hemothorax is not an emergency if bleeding has stopped. VATS drainage of the pleural cavity is best performed 1 to 3 days postinjury to reduce the risk of rebleeding from the injured lung.

Sources for intrathoracic bleeding include intercostal vessels, pulmonary parenchymal injuries, major pulmonary vessels, and injury to the heart or great vessels. Most pulmonary parenchymal injuries can be managed with a tube thoracostomy simply by evacuating the hemothorax and allowing the lung to reexpand. The pulmonary distention associated with reexpansion of the lung tamponades parenchymal bleeding after most injuries. If a thoracotomy is needed because of injury to the intercostal vessels or the internal mammary artery, management requires adequate exposure. Often, the exposure can be enhanced by cutting a rib or two posteriorly. In patients who are exsanguinating, a large rib shear can be used to fracture ribs without skeletonizing them. In patients with large chest wall injuries whose bleeding is diffuse and difficult to localize, ligation of the intercostal vessels near their origins may be a lifesaving maneuver. If bleeding from intercostal vessels occurs at the level of the intervertebral foramen, control may require laminectomy; packing of the foramen should be avoided because it may place patients at risk for spinal cord injury and subsequent paraplegia.

If inflation of the lung fails to control pulmonary parenchymal bleeding, the patient may require pulmonary resection. Lobar or segmental resections are rarely necessary. Frequently a tractotomy can be performed along the course of a penetrating injury using a stapling device as described by Asensio and colleagues (1997) and Wall and colleagues (1998). Hemorrhage can then be controlled rapidly by selective vascular ligation. In the patient with large pulmonary lacerations, contusion, and major hemorrhage, bleeding can be controlled with standard anatomic lobar resection. Thompson and colleagues (1988), Bowling and colleagues (1985), and Baumgartner and colleagues

(1996) report that pneumonectomy in the trauma victim carries a mortality rate approaching 100% and should be considered only as a last resort. Gunshot wounds in the periphery of the lung may be amenable to wedge resections. Central penetrating injuries with massive pulmonary hemorrhage may require intrapericardial control of the pulmonary artery and the pulmonary veins. On rare occasions in moribund patients, rapid control of pulmonary bleeding can be achieved by using stapling devices across the pulmonary hilum to rapidly control hemorrhage from multiple lobes or from a central pulmonary injury.

If a major air leak is present, the source should be identified. Small air leaks from the lung periphery usually resolve without need for repair. Lacerations of the trachea or major bronchi require repair with 4-0 or 3-0 absorbable sutures. It is usually best to begin by gaining control of the pulmonary vasculature so that the airway can be exposed with relative leisure and under the best possible conditions.

Air Embolism

Thomas and Roe (1973) and Yee and colleagues (1983) reported that air embolism often follows penetrating and blunt chest injury. In the experience of Swanson and Trunkey (1989), it occurred in 4% of all major thoracic trauma cases. Sixty-five percent of cases resulted from penetrating injuries to the chest, and 35% of cases from blunt chest trauma, almost invariably because of lacerations of the lung secondary to rib fractures.

The key to diagnosis of air embolism is to have a high index of suspicion. The pathophysiology is a fistula between a bronchus and a pulmonary vein. In those patients who are breathing spontaneously, the pressure differential is from the pulmonary vein to the bronchus so that air is not aspirated into the vascular system; hemoptysis may occur in approximately one-fourth of such patients. When the patient is intubated with positive pressure, however, the pressure differential is from the bronchus to the pulmonary vein, resulting in air being carried to the left side of the heart and being ejected into the aorta, causing systemic air embolism. These patients present in one of three ways: 1) with focal or lateralizing neurologic signs, 2) sudden cardiovascular collapse, or 3) froth when the initial arterial blood specimen is obtained. Any patient with focal or lateralizing neurologic findings who has a chest injury but no head injury could have air embolism as an explanation for the neurologic deficit. Confirmation may be obtained by funduscopic examination showing air in the retinal vessels. When a patient comes into the emergency department in extremis and an emergency thoracotomy is carried out, air should always be looked for in the coronary vessels. If it is found, the hilum of the offending lung should be immediately clamped to stop the ingress of air into the left side of the heart.

The treatment of air embolism is immediate thoracotomy, preferably in the operating room, although many of these patients have thoracotomies in the emergency department. The hilum of the affected lacerated lung is cross-clamped, the patient is placed in the head-down (Trendelenburg's) position, and the left ventricle is vented to remove any residual contained air. Other resuscitative measures in patients who have had cardiac arrest from air embolism include internal cardiac massage to re-establish perfusion and to clear the coronary vessels of any contained air. One milliliter of 1:1,000 epinephrine can be injected intravenously or into the endotracheal tube to provide an alpha-adrenergic effect, driving air out of the systemic microcirculation. Definitive treatment is to oversew the lacerations of the lung, and in some instances a lobectomy and rarely a pneumonectomy may be required. Using aggressive diagnosis and treatment, Swanson and Trunkey (1989) achieved a 55% salvage rate in patients with air embolism secondary to penetrating trauma and a 20% salvage rate in patients with air embolism from blunt trauma.

Pulmonary Contusion

Pulmonary contusion, which usually results from blunt trauma, consists of hemorrhage into the alveolar and interstitial spaces. Contusions can result from penetrating injury, especially high-velocity missile wounds (Fig. 70-5). Although Nakayama and coworkers (1989) have reported that pulmonary contusions can occur as isolated injuries in children, in adults they are typically associated with other injuries and have an overall mortality rate of 22 to 30%, as has been recorded by Besson and Saegesser (1983) and Stellin (1991). Many contusions are small and contribute little to patients' morbidity, but large contusions lead to hypoxia and the need for mechanical ventilation. The increased use of computed tomographic (CT) scanning in the evaluation of acute chest trauma, as described by Wagner and Jamieson (1989) and Trupka and colleagues (1997), has improved the sensitivity and makes the diagnosis easier than using plain roentgenographs.

Pulmonary contusion should be suspected in any patient with major chest wall injury; it can be confirmed by radiologic evaluation. Most clinically significant contusions appear on the initial chest radiographs and may be difficult to differentiate from aspirations. Several characteristics aid in distinguishing between the two entities. Pulmonary contusions are usually present on the initial film. The first post-trauma chest radiograph of patients suffering from aspiration may be normal, with the development of an infiltrate occurring during the next several hours. Infiltrates that are due to aspiration may be confined by anatomic pulmonary segments; those associated with pulmonary contusions outline the area of impact that may or may not correspond to the lobar or segmental anatomy of the lung. Among the most helpful features that permit distinction between contusion and aspiration pneumonia is the nature of the tracheobronchial secretions: aspiration is associated with copious secretions that usually contain particulate matter, whereas contusions may be associ-

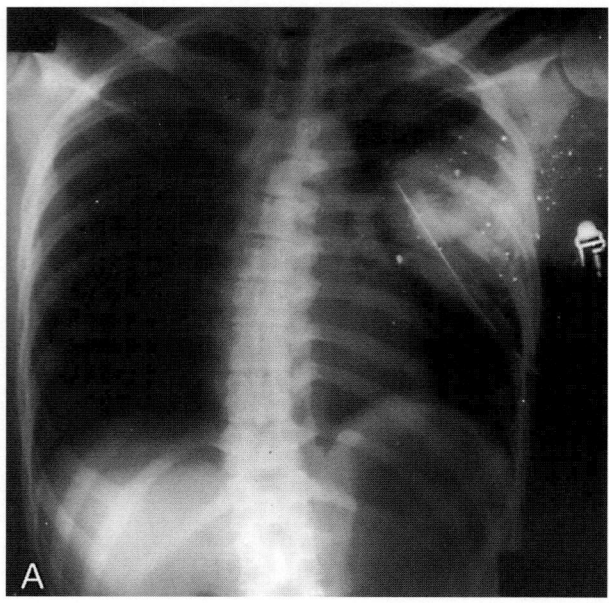
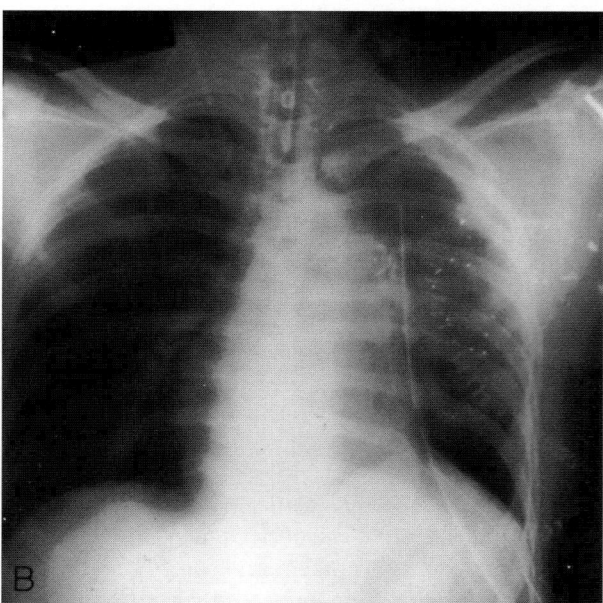

Fig. 70-5. High-velocity missile wounds. **A.** Chest radiograph shows an injury from a high-power rifle wound sustained through a bulletproof vest. **B.** Postoperative chest radiograph. The contusion and pulmonary parenchymal bleeding was confined to the upper lobe that was resected.

ated with bloody secretions. Initial care for both conditions is supportive and is based on serial physiologic measurements and sequential radiographs. Patients with aspiration, however, often benefit from early bronchoscopy.

Pulmonary hematoma is another condition that may be difficult to differentiate from pulmonary contusion because of the surrounding intraparenchymal hemorrhage. However, 24 to 48 hours after the injury, a hematoma typically develops into a discrete mass with distinct margins. CT scans can be helpful in distinguishing between contusion and hematoma. In most cases, the hematoma itself does not interfere with gas exchange and with time is resorbed spontaneously. Only rarely can these hematomas become secondarily infected and present as an abscess requiring drainage.

CT evaluation of the chest after blunt trauma has been advocated by Toombs (1981) and Wagner (1988) and their colleagues as a more sensitive and accurate means of diagnosing pulmonary contusions. Additionally, CT has led to the finding that pulmonary lacerations are frequently associated with pulmonary contusions. A classification system has been proposed to quantitate injury and thus allow comparison of various treatment modalities. However, present treatment recommendations for pulmonary contusion do not depend on CT findings. Thus, neither the risk involved in transport for patients who are unstable and require intensive support nor the expense of CT studies is warranted.

Our current recommendations for treatment of patients with pulmonary contusions include ventilatory support, as needed, based on clinical and laboratory findings. Associated injuries to the chest wall, pleura, and lungs should be identified and treated. Fluid administration should be adequate to resuscitate shock; oxygen delivery and consumption should be made optimal. Because of increases in capillary endothelial permeability associated with pulmonary contusion, some authors have encouraged fluid restriction. Judicious administration of fluids with cardiovascular monitoring is appropriate, particularly in elderly patients; however, fluid restriction and the administration of diuretics in the treatment of pulmonary contusion is appropriate only in patients with evidence of fluid overload. Filling pressures should be returned to normal, using either blood products or crystalloid or colloid solutions, to maintain adequate oxygen delivery. Massive pulmonary contusions associated with large shunt fractions and hypoxemia with differential lung compliances between the affected and unaffected lungs can be managed with dual lung ventilation or, rarely, with resection of the affected lung.

Occasionally pulmonary injuries require lung resections to control massive intrathoracic hemorrhage, particularly with high-velocity missile injuries, as documented by wartime experiences recorded by Fischer and associates (1974). Contusions surrounding low-velocity gunshot wounds seen in the civilian experience can usually be managed without the need for operation. In all cases, the extent of resection should be as conservative as possible and according to anatomic boundaries, if feasible.

TRACHEOBRONCHIAL TRAUMA

Mechanisms

The self-healing potential of the large airways was first described by Winslow in 1874 when he reported evidence of a remote bronchial injury that had healed in a canvasback duck that subsequently had been killed by a hunter. Since that time, progress has been made in the recognition and treatment of airway injuries, and an increased incidence of this injury has been reported, which is in part due to improvements in prehospital care. In spite of improved recognition, bronchial injury remains rare, with less than a 1% incidence in major trauma victims. Injuries to the tracheobronchial tree occur due to both blunt and penetrating injuries, with the latter predominating. Both blunt and penetrating injuries to the cervical tracheal are more common than those to the intrathoracic portion of the tracheobronchial tree.

Injuries to the large airways due to penetrating trauma are usually associated with other major injuries, especially vascular injuries that require early operative intervention. This often leads to the diagnosis of the tracheobronchial injury at the time of exploration. Partial tears of the airway after blunt trauma are often missed on initial evaluation; they can present months to years later with a stenosis of the airway and collapse, infection, or both, of the distal portion of the lung.

Blunt injuries to the intrathoracic airway usually occur within 2 cm of the carina. Penetrating injuries can occur along any portion of the airway. Although direct trauma to the airway is responsible for penetrating and blunt injuries to the cervical trachea, several mechanisms are postulated in the genesis of blunt intrathoracic injuries. These include 1) linear rupture of the membranous portion of the trachea due to an abrupt increase in large airway pressure caused by thoracic compression in a patient with a closed glottis, 2) disruption of the trachea at points of fixation (the carina and the cricoid) that is due to the shearing forces seen with rapid deceleration, and 3) laceration or transection of the trachea near the carina that is due to lateral traction on the lungs caused by crushing chest injuries that acutely decrease the anterior-posterior diameter of the thoracic cavity.

Diagnosis

The degree of challenge in diagnosing tracheobronchial trauma depends on the location of the injury. Injuries to the cervical trachea can readily be identified on the basis of history and physical findings. Symptoms associated with injury to the cervical trachea can include subcutaneous emphysema, dyspnea, dysphonia, and hemoptysis. Patients with penetrating injuries and these findings should be explored after an adequate airway has been established. Blunt injuries to the cervical trachea can be evaluated with bronchoscopy and CT of the neck.

Timely diagnosis of injuries to the intrathoracic tracheobronchial tree requires a high index of suspicion. Injuries to the intrathoracic tracheobronchial tree may manifest with persistent, massive air leaks. The findings, however, may be much more subtle and, because of this, partial tears of a main stem bronchus are often missed at the time of initial presentation. For example, subcutaneous emphysema, pneumomediastinum, air outlining a bronchus, deviation of an endotracheal tube, or the "fallen lung sign" (collapse of the lung toward the lateral chest wall), as described by Unger and colleagues (1989), can be clues to the presence of a tracheobronchial injury. Inability to reexpand the lung with tube thoracostomy or a persistent air leak in the postinjury period may also indicate a tracheobronchial injury. Patients with tracheobronchial tears that are not recognized progress to develop either a suppurative lung infection or a complete collapse of the affected lung. Management of delayed presentations of bronchial injuries is discussed in the section on complications of thoracic trauma.

Patients with suspected tracheobronchial injuries should undergo immediate bronchoscopy to evaluate the airways. Either rigid or flexible bronchoscopy can be used, and the examination is best performed in the operating room by an experienced endoscopist. Any blood or clots found in the airway should be cleared because it can interfere with detection of an injury and can impede ventilation. Not only is bronchoscopy a sensitive diagnostic tool for the detection of tracheobronchial injuries, but it also can often aid in establishing a secure airway. Bronchoscopy is nearly always diagnostic for major trauma to the tracheobronchial tree, as noted by Hara and Prakash (1989) and Velly and associates (1991).

Treatment

Although surgical intervention is indicated in most patients with documented injuries to the large airways, small tracheobronchial tears involving less than one-third of the circumference can be managed nonoperatively if the lung is fully reexpanded after tube thoracostomy and if the patient does not require high pressure mechanical ventilation. These patients should be watched closely for signs of respiratory insufficiency and for evidence of infection, especially mediastinitis.

Injuries to the cervical trachea can usually be managed through a collar incision. The development of skin flaps below the platysma allows exposure of the entire cervical trachea, and with some dissection, the proximal retrosternal trachea can be mobilized into the field for repair. Injuries should be débrided and repairs should be made with fine interrupted absorbable suture. Major tracheal injury with tissue loss may require conversion into a tracheostomy. Injuries near the thyroid cartilage should be examined for possible laryngeal injury and should be managed with a tracheostomy. When performed, the tracheostomy should be brought out through a separate incision, if possible, to avoid contaminating the entire wound. Injuries to the cervical trachea, away from the larynx, can be repaired primarily with interrupted absorbable suture. The repair can be stented for short periods of time with an endotracheal tube.

Combined injuries to the trachea and esophagus should have viable tissue such as a strip of sternocleidomastoid muscle interposed between the repairs. Should the injury

extend down into the mediastinum, further exposure can be obtained by performing a median sternotomy or a partial sternotomy with a trap door to expose the proximal intrathoracic trachea. The entire chest should be prepared for inclusion in the operative field.

Exposure of the mediastinal trachea, the carina, and the right main stem bronchus is best achieved through a right posterior-lateral thoracotomy through the fourth intercostal space. The proximal left main stem bronchus can be dealt with through a right thoracotomy; however, complete transection of the left main stem bronchus is best exposed through a standard left thoracotomy.

The first priority on identifying the injury should be to establish an adequate airway so that the repair can be accomplished safely. Establishing an adequate airway is best achieved by selectively cannulating and ventilating the uninjured lung. If the area of injury involves the carina or the trachea, the repair can be performed over the endotracheal tube. Although some surgeons have advocated the use of cardiopulmonary bypass for the repair of tracheobronchial injuries, we disagree with this recommendation. The systemic anticoagulation required for cardiopulmonary bypass is best avoided, if possible, in polytrauma victims. Adequate ventilation and oxygenation can be achieved with either single or double selective endobronchial intubation or with a jet ventilator.

After the area of injury is identified, the proximal and distal airway is dissected free enough so that a repair can be performed using well-vascularized tissues without tension. Care should be taken not to dissect any more than is necessary, especially in the lateral peritracheal planes, because it avoids recurrent laryngeal nerve injuries and minimizes devascularization of the trachea. Devitalized tissue should be débrided and the mucosa should be approximated with 3-0 or 4-0 interrupted absorbable sutures. We rarely, if ever, find it advisable to encircle the cartilaginous rings above and below an area of injury. When large amounts of tissue require débridement, repair of the tracheobronchial tree can be facilitated by dissecting and mobilizing the hilum and incising the inferior pulmonary ligament. Methods to enhance mobilization of the trachea and bronchi, which are sometimes needed for the management of acute injuries, are described in detail in Chapter 75. After completion of a repair, a strip of pleura, an intercostal muscle pedicle, or an omental pedicle should be used to buttress the suture line. It is best to avoid using any periosteum from the ribs when mobilizing the intercostal muscle pedicle, because this can recalcify and lead to stenosis of the airway. Interposing a strip of viable tissue between the trachea and esophagus is especially important when both structures are injured. As pointed out by Flynn and colleagues (1989), this decreases the incidence of postoperative leak and of tracheoesophageal fistula formation. Injuries to the large airways distal to the lobar divisions are best treated by lobectomy because these injuries are rarely isolated. Typically they are associated with major vascular injuries that can be controlled simultaneously with pulmonary resection.

Most victims with major airway injuries die shortly after their accident due to asphyxia; however, overall morbidity and mortality for patients with tracheobronchial trauma who survive to reach the emergency department depend on their associated injuries. Of victims evaluated and treated, the best prognosis is associated with isolated airway injuries, injuries to the cervical trachea, and penetrating injuries. Long-term functional results after tracheobronchial repair are good.

PROCEDURES FOR THE MANAGEMENT OF THORACIC TRAUMA

The surgical techniques used are standard for thoracic surgery; therefore, the following comments are intended only to give our references and recommendations.

Tube Thoracostomy

For most cases, we recommend insertion at the fourth or fifth intercostal space (i.e., nipple line) between the anterior and midaxillary lines. In hemodynamically stable patients, a short subcutaneous tunnel is made before penetrating the pleural cavity; in critically injured patients, however, no subcutaneous tract is formed because it may delay insertion of the tube. In adult patients, we recommend a No. 36F tube. Insertion of chest tubes with a trocar should be avoided in trauma patients. If, according to immediate follow-up radiograph, evacuation of a hemothorax or pneumothorax is incomplete, remedial action appropriate for the underlying injury should be pursued immediately.

Thoracotomy

Baker and colleagues (1998) recommend resuscitative thoracotomy in the emergency department for victims of penetrating thoracic injuries who suffer cardiopulmonary arrest within 5 minutes of presentation to the emergency department. The use of resuscitative emergency department thoracotomy in blunt trauma victims is arguable because survival for blunt trauma victims suffering cardiac arrest is dismal, as emphasized by Bodai and associates (1983). Therefore we rarely use emergency department thoracotomy in blunt trauma victims with cardiac arrest. Cardiac arrest resulting from penetrating trauma, especially due to stab wounds to the heart, is associated with a higher survival rate, averaging approximately 30% in several series reviewed by Ivatury and Rohman (1987). An aggressive approach to the victim with penetrating thoracic trauma with cardiac arrest is therefore recommended.

Urgent thoracotomy is indicated in patients with large or persistent hemothorax or with air leaks that preclude adequate ventilation. When an air leak is the major indication for urgent

operation and circumstances permit, preoperative bronchoscopy is done. Its role, however, remains to be determined.

Techniques of Pulmonary Resection

Standard lung resections according to anatomic divisions are infrequently required for the management of trauma. If they are needed, segmental resections should be used in preference to lobectomies, and pneumonectomies should be avoided whenever possible because of the high mortality associated with pneumonectomy, even after adequate hemostasis and resuscitation have been achieved. Damaged pulmonary parenchyma has a remarkable ability to recover, and pleural surfaces with troublesome oozing of blood or air leaks can be effectively treated in some instances with use of the Argon beam coagulator or fibrin glue or expectantly with adequate drainage of the chest cavity. We believe reoperating promptly is better, if necessary, than sacrificing potentially functioning lung tissue. Hemostasis can be rapidly achieved in patients with a penetrating lung injury with major hemorrhage by opening the tract and selectively ligating bleeding vessels. The tractotomy can be performed rapidly using a device that staples and cuts simultaneously.

Bronchoscopy

Both flexible and rigid instruments should be available for a bronchoscopy. We use rigid instruments when massive bleeding is present in the airways or to establish an airway. Large foreign bodies such as broken teeth that have been aspirated and are obstructing a bronchus are also best removed endoscopically with a rigid bronchoscope. For diagnostic examinations or clearing secretions, we prefer to use flexible instruments.

Methods of Tracheobronchial Reconstruction

Tracheobronchial repair of major airways has been discussed previously. The technical principles that apply are as follows: 1) prompt repair of an acute injury is better than delayed repair; 2) débridement of nonviable tissue and approximation of viable edges without tension is needed; 3) tissue conservation is an important goal, even in young, healthy patients; and 4) the use of fine absorbable suture materials is recommended, though monofilament suture materials with knots tied outside the airway lumen are acceptable alternatives.

COMPLICATIONS OF THORACIC TRAUMA

Empyema

The incidence of empyema after thoracic trauma is approximately 3 to 4% in the experience of Helling and col-

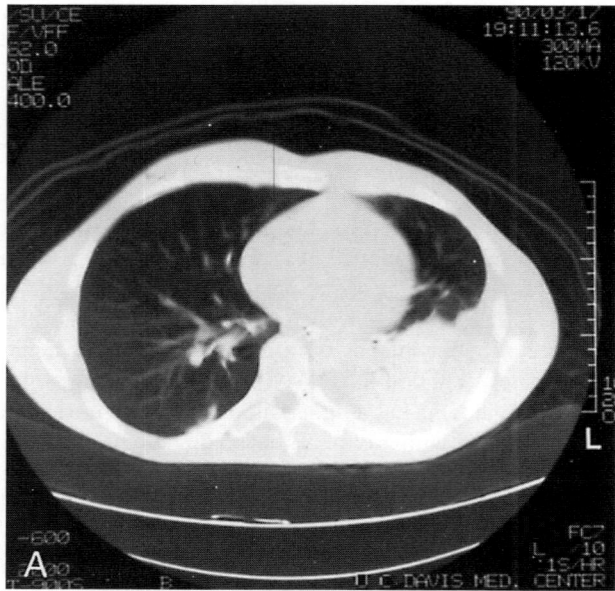

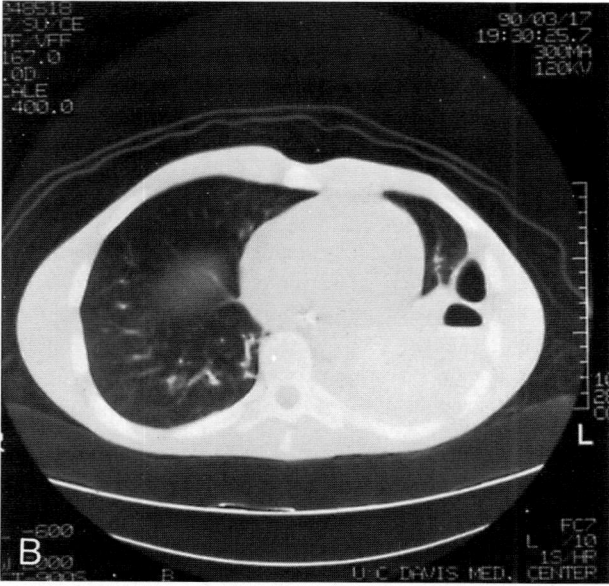

Fig. 70-6. Post-traumatic empyema. Computed tomographic scan. **(A)** Well-localized fluid collection, separated from adjacent pulmonary parenchyma, and persistent despite chest tube placement. **B.** Air-fluid level consistent with bronchopleural fistula and empyema.

leagues (1989), LeRoux and colleagues (1986), and Aguilar and colleagues (1997). This incidence can be minimized by using meticulously sterile technique while inserting thoracostomy tubes and by ensuring good apposition of the pleural surfaces so that no space remains for the accumulation of fluid or blood. The risk of empyema increases in patients with persistent bronchopleural fistula, pulmonary contusions, and residual clotted hemothoraces.

Empyema rarely manifests itself with overt septic shock; it mostly presents as an indolent infectious process. CT scans aid in defining the size and location of loculated collections (Fig. 70-6). A visceral pleural peel can be identified by the characteristic "split pleura sign" described by Hanna and colleagues (1991) and Waite and colleagues (1990), which represents intravenous contrast enhancement of the parietal and visceral pleurae.

Thoracentesis and appropriate culture of the fluid obtained often identifies the offending organisms and assists with antibiotic selection. The most common organisms are skin flora such as staphylococcus or streptococcus. Gram-negative enteric organisms should be suspected when the initial trauma involved combined thoracic and abdominal injuries. Although initial antibiotic coverage should be broad, it should be promptly focused based on the results of culture and sensitivity studies. This avoids the development of resistant organisms or opportunistic fungal infections.

The treatment of empyema depends on the clinical stage of its development (see Chapters 58 and 59). The initial phase is an exudative state that is often amenable to drainage with thoracostomy tube and intravenous antibiotic administration. During this time, the pleural space has relatively few adhesions, and the likelihood that the collections are loculated is low. At this stage, VATS can be very helpful in establishing adequate drainage of the infected pleural fluid. However, the diagnosis is more commonly established beyond the early exudative phase, in the fibrinopurulent phase. This transitional phase is characterized by loculated collections of gelatinous material and the early development of a pleural peel. In our experience as reported by Scherer and colleagues (1998), VATS can frequently be used to successfully drain post-traumatic empyemas in this transitional phase. Therefore, we recommend that VATS should be the initial operative approach to patients with suspected post-traumatic empyema. The surgical team should be prepared to convert to open thoracotomy if adequate decortication cannot be achieved through the smaller incisions used with VATS or if the lung cannot be adequately collapsed to permit visualization. The later chronic or organizing phase of empyema is characterized by the development of a thick, fibrotic pleural rind that entraps the lung. This stage typically requires open surgical intervention to adequately decorticate the thick pleural peel.

Alternative treatment modalities that have been proposed in the management of post-traumatic empyema but have not been well studied include the use of intracavitary fibrinolytic agents that have been suggested by K. S. Lee and colleagues (1991) and Moulton and colleagues (1989). We are skeptical that fibrinolytic therapy will be anything more than an adjunct to surgical drainage and decortication.

Clotted Hemothorax

Incomplete evacuation of a hemothorax after thoracic trauma is best prevented with early, effective tube thoracostomy drainage. As reported by Kish and colleagues (1976) and Helling and colleagues (1989), incomplete drainage has been reported in approximately 15% of cases. Patients with significant volume loss due to residual hemothorax should undergo operative drainage. If performed within 2 weeks of the original trauma, VATS can be useful in draining a clotted hemothorax and avoiding rib-spreading thoracotomy. Meyer and colleagues (1997) found significant advantages when VATS was used to evacuate clotted hemothoraces compared with a second tube thoracostomy. Our favorable experience and that reported by Heniford and coworkers (1997) support the use of VATS to drain retained post-traumatic pleural collections early postinjury. Effective and complete drainage longer than 2 weeks after the injury almost certainly requires a standard, open thoracotomy because of adhesions between the visceral and parietal pleurae and a tenacious inflammatory peel that envelops the lung.

Bronchopleural Fistula

Persistent air leak is an unusual complication after thoracic trauma. When a persistent bronchopleural fistula is present, injury to the proximal airways should be suspected and surgically repaired if present. Rarely, a thoracostomy tube may be lodged within the pulmonary parenchyma. If this is suspected, the tube should be removed and a new one placed. Care should be taken to avoid injury to the lung when replacing the tube by slowly dissecting into the pleural space and probing the cavity with a finger to ensure that the lung is free of the chest wall where the tube will be placed.

Bronchopleural fistulas also occur in the intensive care unit as a result of the barotrauma of mechanical ventilation. In such cases treatment should be limited to draining any pneumothorax present (most of which are loculated) and to supporting the patient's ventilatory status. Most of these air leaks improve as the patient's pulmonary compliance improves. Care should be taken in placing thoracostomy tubes in such patients because numerous adhesions are usually present in the thoracic cavity and the lung can be quite firm and vulnerable to injury because of changes in the consistency of the lung induced by the inflammatory process. Patients with stiff lungs and massive air leaks may require intubation of each lung and independent lung ventilation with two ventilators to optimize their pulmonary status. Dual lung ventilation improves pulmonary function by improving ventilation to both the affected and unaffected lungs. In our experience, patients with massive air leaks requiring dual lung ventilation have a poor prognosis due to the severity of their underlying ARDS.

Treatment of a persistent bronchopleural air leak, other than from a major airway injury, rarely requires operative intervention. Occasionally we discharge patients with chronic bronchopleural fistulas from the hospital with chest tubes and Heimlich valves. Usually, the air leaks stop by the time of the patient's first return visit, which is in 1 week. Rarely, the thoracostomy tube is placed to open drainage, and it is then advanced along its fibrous tract slowly over days until it is out. Even more rarely, if the bronchopleural fistula persists in spite of the aforementioned treatment, a pulmonary resection or an Eloesser flap may be required.

Bronchial Stenosis

Tracheobronchial injuries may present with minimal findings; Velly and colleagues (1991) reported that 17% of bronchial tears are diagnosed on a delayed basis. In such cases the partial tear will permit ventilation and reexpansion of the lung after the acute injury; however, as the bronchus heals, a stricture forms, leading to distal collapse of the lung (Fig. 70-7). If the distal lung is not infected, the atelectatic lung may not give rise to any symptoms and will remain undiagnosed until a subsequent chest radiograph is obtained. Distal infection presents with findings consistent with a pneumonia or pulmonary abscess. Bronchoscopy is diagnostic and should be performed whenever evidence exists of lobar collapse in the post-traumatic patient. CT scanning of the chest may be helpful in determining whether distal infection is present.

The decision to repair the bronchus or to resect the involved lung should be based on whether distal infection is present. An atelectatic lung can certainly be aerated even after long periods of time with excellent functional results (see Fig. 70-7), as one of us (J.R.B., 1958), and Eastridge and associates (1970) have reported. This requires resection of the bronchial stenosis with primary repair using fine absorbable sutures in an interrupted fashion, as previously described. A suppurative infection of the distal lung, however, precludes repair because of the acute morbidity associated with advanced infection. This infection often spills over into the normal lung after continuity between the injured bronchus and the tracheobronchial tree has been re-established. In addition, the infected lung distal to the stenosis is usually severely damaged, as manifested by bronchiectasis. This poses a risk for chronic recurrent infections in the affected lung segment. Therefore, grossly infected lung distal to a bronchial stricture should be resected, with bronchial repair being reserved for patients with atelectatic lung.

Chylothorax

The accumulation of chyle in the thorax, caused by injury to the thoracic duct, is a rare complication that can occur after blunt trauma, as recorded by Dulchavsky and colleagues (1988). More commonly, it occurs due to a penetrating injury. Findings on presentation include large and persistent chest tube drainage (500–2000 mL/day) that is milky in character when the patient has an oral diet. This finding may not be present early in the post-traumatic period, which is due to the reduced lymph flow and the clear appearance of the chyle in the fasting state. Analysis of the fluid reveals a high triglyceride level and stains positive with

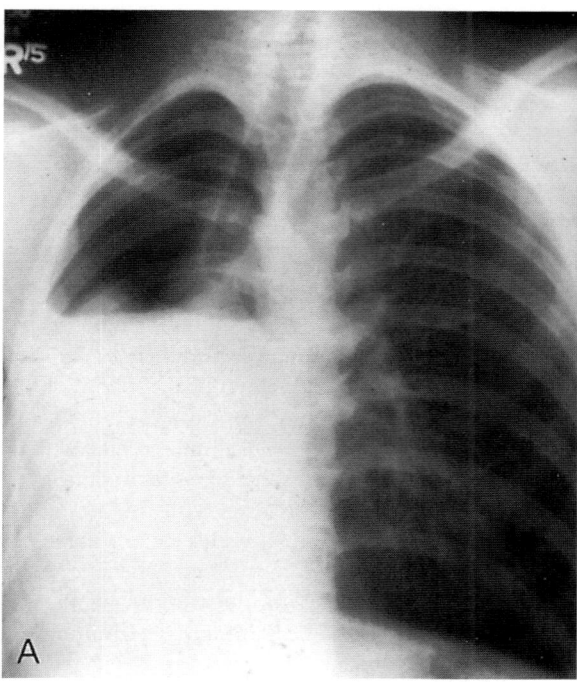 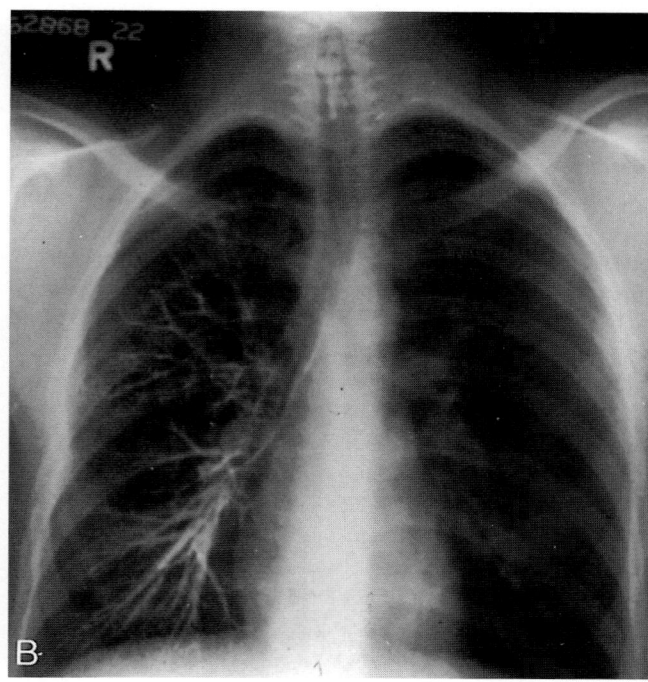

Fig. 70-7. Ruptured bronchus. Chest roentgenograph. **A.** Hemopneumothorax associated with complete main stem bronchial disruption. **B.** Bronchogram after repair of a transected bronchus reveals excellent long-term results.

the fat stain Sudan III. Infection is rare because of the bacteriostatic nature of chyle.

After the diagnosis of chylothorax is established, initial treatment should consist of adequate drainage of the chest, bowel rest, and total parenteral nutrition for nutritional support. If significant drainage persists beyond 2 weeks of observation, operative management should be pursued. Milson and associates (1985) have reviewed the current surgical management strategies used in patients who have failed nonoperative management; insertion of a pleuroperitoneal shunt or transthoracic ligation of the thoracic duct at the diaphragmatic hiatus will, as a rule, successfully treat this difficult clinical problem. As a result of the infrequent occurrence of this problem, the ideal treatment is not well established (see Chapter 63).

REFERENCES

Aguilar MM, et al: Posttraumatic empyema. Risk factor analysis. Arch Surg *132*:647, 1997.

Ammons MA, Moore EE, Rosen P: Role of the observation unit in the management of thoracic trauma. J Emerg Med *4*:279, 1986.

Anel D. L'Art de Succet les Plaies. Amsterdam: Francois Ander Plaats, 1707, p 13.

Armstrong CP, Van der Spuy J: The fractured scapula: importance and management based on a series of 62 patients. Injury *15*:324, 1984.

Asensio JA, et al: Stapled pulmonary tractotomy: a rapid way to control hemorrhage in penetrating pulmonary injuries. J Am Coll Surg *185*:486, 1997.

Avery EE, Mörch ET, Benson DW: Critically crushed chests. J Thorac Surg *32*:291, 1956.

Baker JM, et al: Use of cardiopulmonary bypass to salvage patients with multiple-chamber heart wounds. Arch Surg *133*:855, 1998.

Baumgartner F, et al: Survival after trauma pneumonectomy: the pathophysiologic balance of shock resuscitation with right heart failure. Am Surg *62*:967, 1996.

Benfield JR, et al: The reversibility of chronic atelectasis. Surg Forum *8*:473, 1958.

Besson A, Saegesser F: Color Atlas of Chest Trauma and Associated Injuries. Vol. 1. Oradell, NJ: Medical Economics, 1983, p. 9.

Bodai BI, et al: Emergency thoracotomy in the management of trauma: a review. JAMA *249*:1891, 1983.

Bowling R, et al: Emergency pneumonectomy for penetrating and blunt trauma. Am Surg *51*:136, 1985.

Buckman R, et al: The significance of stable patients with sternal fractures. Surg Gynecol Obstet *164*:261, 1987.

Burford TH, Burbank B: Traumatic wet lung. J Thorac Surg *14*:415, 1945.

Campbell DB: Trauma to the chest wall, lung, and major airways. Semin Thorac Cardiovasc Surg *4*:234, 1992.

Clark GC, Schecter WP, Trunkey DD: Variables affecting outcome in blunt chest trauma: flail chest vs. pulmonary contusion. J Trauma *28*:298, 1988.

Conn JH, et al: Thoracic trauma: analysis of 1022 cases. J Trauma *3*:22, 1963.

Dulchavsky SA, Ledgerwood AM, Lucas CE: Management of chylothorax after blunt chest trauma. J Trauma *28*:1400, 1988.

Eastridge CE, et al: Tracheobronchial injury caused by blunt trauma. Ann Rev Respir Dis *101*:230, 1970.

Fischer RP, Geiger JP, Guernsey JM: Pulmonary resections for severe pulmonary contusions secondary to high-velocity missile wounds. J Trauma *14*:293, 1974.

Flynn AE, Thomas AN, Schecter WP: Acute tracheobronchial injury. J Trauma *29*:1326, 1989.

Freedland M, et al: The management of flail chest injury: factors affecting outcome. J Trauma *30*:1460, 1990.

Galan G, et al: Blunt chest injuries in 1696 patients. Eur J Cardiothorac Surg *6*:284, 1992.

Garcia VF, et al: Rib fractures in children: a marker of severe trauma. J Trauma *30*:695, 1990.

Glinz W: Symposium paper: priorities in diagnosis and treatment of blunt chest injuries. Injury *17*:318, 1986.

Glinz W: Causes of early death in thoracic trauma. *In* Webb WR, Besson A (eds): Thoracic Surgery: Surgical Management of Chest Injuries. Vol. 7. St. Louis: Mosby–Year Book, 1991.

Guttentag IJ, Rechtine GR: Fractures of the scapula: a review of the literature. Orthop Rev *17*:147, 1988.

Haasler GB: Open fixation of flail chest after blunt trauma. Ann Thorac Surg *49*:993, 1990.

Hanna JW, Reed JC, Choplin RH: Pleural infections: a clinical-radiologic review. J Thorac Imaging *6*:68, 1991.

Hara KS, Prakash UBS: Fiberoptic bronchoscopy in the evaluation of acute chest and upper airway trauma. Chest *96*:627, 1989.

Helling TS, et al: Complications following blunt and penetrating injuries in 216 victims of chest trauma requiring tube thoracostomy. J Trauma *29*:1367, 1989.

Heniford BT, et al: The role of thoracoscopy in the management of retained thoracic collections after trauma. Ann Thorac Surg *63*:940, 1997.

Henley MB, et al: External fixation of the sternum for thoracic trauma. J Orthop Trauma *5*:493, 1991.

Ivatury RR, Rohman M: Emergency department thoracotomy for trauma: a collective review. Resuscitation *15*:23, 1987.

Karanfilian R, Machiedo GW, Bolanowski PJ: Management of nonpenetrating stab and gunshot wounds of the chest. Surg Gynecol Obstet *153*:395, 1981.

Kemmerer WT, et al: Patterns of thoracic injuries in fatal traffic accidents. J Trauma *1*:595, 1961.

Kish G, et al: Indications for early thoracotomy in the management of chest trauma. Ann Thorac Surg *22*:23, 1976.

Kulshrestha P, et al: Chest injuries: a clinical and autopsy profile. J Trauma *28*:844, 1988.

Landercasper J, Cogbill TH, Lindesmith LA: Long-term disability after flail chest injury. J Trauma *24*:410, 1984.

Landreneau RJ, Hinson JM, Hazelrigg SR: Strut fixation of an extensive flail chest. Ann Thorac Surg *51*:473, 1991.

Lee KS, et al: Treatment of thoracic multiloculated empyemas with intracavitary urokinase: a prospective study. Radiology *179*:771, 1991.

Lee MC, et al: Traumatic asphyxia. Ann Thorac Surg *51*:86, 1991.

LeRoux BT, et al: Suppurative diseases of the lung and pleural space. Part I: Empyema thoracis and lung abscess. Curr Probl Surg *23*:1, 1986.

LoCicero J, Mattox KL: Epidemiology of chest trauma. Surg Clin North Am *69*:5, 1989.

Luchette FA, et al: Prospective evaluation of epidural versus intrapleural catheters for analgesia in chest wall trauma. J Trauma *36*:865, 1994.

Mackersie RC, et al: Continuous epidural fentanyl analgesia: ventilatory function improvement with routine use in treatment of blunt chest injury. J Trauma *27*:1207, 1987.

MaGahan JP, Rab GT, Dublin A: Fractures of the scapula. J Trauma *20*:880, 1980.

Meyer DM, et al: Early evacuation of traumatic retained hemothoraces using thoracoscopy: a prospective, randomized trial. Ann Thorac Surg *64*:1396, 1997.

Milson JW, et al: Chylothorax: an assessment of current surgical management. J Thorac Cardiovasc Surg *89*:221, 1985.

Moulton JS, Moore PT, Mencini RA: Treatment of loculated pleural effusions with transcatheter intracavitary urokinase. Am J Roentgenol *153*:941, 1989.

Murray JA, et al: Penetrating left thoracoabdominal trauma: the incidence and clinical presentation of diaphragm injuries. J Trauma *43*:624, 1997.

Nakayama DK, Ramenofsky ML, Rowe MI: Chest injuries in childhood. Ann Surg *210*:770, 1989.

Ordog GJ, Balasubramanium S, Wasserberger J: Outpatient management of 3757 gunshot wounds to the chest. J Trauma *23*:832, 1983.

Otremski I, et al: Fracture of the sternum in motor vehicle accidents and its association with mediastinal injury. Injury *21*:81, 1990.

Paris F, Tarrazona V, Garcia-Zarza A: Controversial aspects of surgical fixation for traumatic flail chest. *In* Webb WR, Besson A (eds): Thoracic Surgery: Surgical Management of Chest Injuries. Vol. 7. St Louis: Mosby–Year Book, 1991.

Playfair: Case of empyema treated by repeated aspiration and subsequently by drainage: recovery. Br Med J *1*:45, 1875.

Poole GV: Fracture of the upper ribs and injury to the great vessels. Surg Gynecol Obstet *169*:275, 1989.

Richardson JD, McElvein RB, Trinkle JK: First rib fracture: a hallmark of severe trauma. Ann Surg *181*:251, 1975.

Scherer LA, et al: Video-assisted thoracic surgery in the treatment of posttraumatic empyema. Arch Surg *133*:637, 1998.

Scultetus J: The Surgeon's Storehouse. London: Starkey, 1674, p. 159.

Shackford SR: Blunt chest trauma: the intensivists's perspective. Intensive Care Med *1*:125, 1986.

Shackford SR, et al: The management of flail chest: a comparison of ventilatory and nonventilatory treatment. Am J Surg *132*:759, 1976.

Shorr RM, et al: Blunt thoracic trauma: analysis of 515 patients. Ann Surg *206*:200, 1987.

Shorr RM, et al: Blunt chest trauma in elderly. J Trauma *29*:234, 1989.

Sisley AC, et al: Rapid detection of traumatic effusion using surgeon-performed ultrasonography. J Trauma *44*:291, 1998.

Stellin G: Survival in trauma victims with pulmonary contusion. Am Surg *57*:780, 1991.

Swanson J, Trunkey DD: Trauma to the chest wall, pleura and thoracic viscera. *In* Shields TW (ed): General Thoracic Surgery. 3rd Ed. Philadelphia: Lea & Febiger, 1989.

Thomas AH, Roe BB: Air embolism following penetrating lung injuries. J Thorac Cardiovasc Surg *66*:533, 1973.

Thomas AN, et al: Operative stabilization for flail chest after blunt trauma. J Thorac Cardiovasc Surg *75*:793, 1978.

Thompson DA, et al: Urgent thoracotomy for pulmonary or tracheobronchial injury. J Trauma *28*:276, 1988.

Thompson DA, Flynn TC, Miller PW: The significance of scapular fractures. J Trauma *25*:974, 1985.

Toombs BD, Sandler CM, Lester RG: Computed tomography of chest trauma. Radiology *140*:733, 1981.

Trinkle JK, et al: Management of flail chest without mechanical ventilation. J Thorac Surg *19*:355, 1975.

Trupka A, et al: Value of thoracic computed tomography in the first assessment of severely injured patients with blunt chest trauma: results of a prospective study. J Trauma *43*:405, 1997.

Unger JM, Schuchmann GG, Grossman JE: Tears of the trachea and main bronchi caused by blunt trauma: radiologic findings. Am J Roentgenol *153*:1175, 1989.

Velly JF, et al: Post traumatic tracheobronchial lesions: a follow-up study of 47 cases. Eur J Cardiothorac Surg *5*:352, 1991.

Wagner RB, Crawford WO, Schimpf PP: Classification of parenchymal injuries of the lung. Radiology *167*:77, 1988.

Wagner RB, Jamieson PM: Pulmonary contusion: evaluation and classification by computed tomography. Surg Clin North Am *69*:31, 1989.

Waite RJ, et al: Parietal pleural changes in empyema: appearances at CT. Radiology *175*:145, 1990.

Wall, MJ, et al: Pulmonary tractotomy as an abbreviated thoracotomy technique. J Trauma *45*:1015, 1998.

Weigelt JA, et al: Management of asymptomatic patients following stab wounds to the chest. J Trauma *22*:291, 1982.

Williams JS, Minken SL, Adams JT: Traumatic asphyxia — reappraised. Ann Surg *167*:384, 1968.

Wilson RF, Murray C, Antonenko DR: Nonpenetrating thoracic injuries. Surg Clin North Am *57*:17, 1977.

Winslow WH: Rupture of bronchus from wild duck. Philadelphia Med Times, April 15, 1874, p. 22.

Wisner DH: A stepwise logistic regression analysis of factors affecting morbidity and mortality after thoracic trauma: effect of epidural analgesia. J Trauma *30*:799, 1990.

Wisner DH, Reed WH, Riddick RS: Suspected myocardial contusion. Ann Surg *212*:82, 1990.

Worthley LIG: Thoracic epidural in the management of chest trauma: a study of 161 cases. Intensive Care Med *11*:312, 1985.

Yee FS, Thomas AN, Wilson R: Management of air embolism in blunt and penetrating thoracic trauma. J Thorac Cardiovasc Surg *85*:661, 1983.

READING REFERENCES

Beaumont W: Experiments and Observations on the Gastric Juice and the Physiology of Digestion. New York: Dover Publications, 1959. (Original work published 1825.)

Breadsted JH: The Edwin Smith Surgical Papyrus. Vol. 1. Chicago: University of Chicago Press, 1930, p. 391.

Johnston JR, McCaughey W: Epidural morphine: a method of management of multiple fractured ribs. Anesthesia *35*:155, 1980.

Meade RH: A History of Thoracic Surgery. Springfield, IL: Bannerston House, 1961, p. 3.

Rovenstine EA, Byrd ML: The use of nerve block during treatment for fractured ribs. Am J Surg *46*:303, 1939.

Theodoric: Surgery (AD 1267). Vol. 1. Campbell E, Colton J (trans). Norwalk, CT: Appleton-Century-Crofts, 1955.

CHAPTER 71

Barotrauma and Inhalation Injuries

Joseph B. Zwischenberger, Weike Tao, Scott K. Alpard, Akhil Bidani, and Joseph LoCicero III

Occasionally, the thoracic surgeon is called on to assist in the management of patients with complex pulmonary problems in the intensive care unit. Two of the more common are barotrauma and inhalation injuries. To adequately manage these conditions, it is important to understand the underlying mechanisms of injury. Support and specific therapies then can be administered properly.

BAROTRAUMA

Cullen and Caldera (1979) noted that the incidence of pneumothorax in ventilated patients in the intensive care unit ranges between 0.5 and 15%. Macklin and Macklin (1944) described the most common mechanism of injury. A small airway or alveolus ruptures and the air dissects through the bronchovascular connective tissue proximally into the mediastinum, ultimately rupturing into the pleural space.

Etiology

Although it is obvious that an air sack must rupture to produce a pneumothorax, the mechanism of that rupture is a subject of debate (Table 71-1). Most theories are based on overdistention or pressurization of the alveolus. Traditional supportive management for severe respiratory failure has used volume-controlled mechanical ventilation using tidal volumes of 10 to 15 mL/kg because Bendixen and associates (1963) noted that high lung volumes minimize atelectasis and prevent deterioration in oxygenation in patients undergoing anesthesia. This strategy often requires high airway pressures (>35 cm H_2O) to deliver these volumes to maintain normocapnia in patients with severe lung injury. In fact, the original description of adult respiratory distress syndrome (ARDS) by Ashbaugh and colleagues (1967) included high inspiratory ventilator pressures as part of the definition.

Webb and Tierney (1974) first recognized ventilator-induced parenchymal lung injury as separate from the previously recognized forms of barotrauma. Rats ventilated at high airway pressures (45 cm H_2O) developed alveolar edema, hypoxemia, and decreased lung compliance, with death occurring within 1 hour. They proposed that interstitial edema may be caused by pulmonary interdependence and that the alveolar edema may be from depletion or inactivation of surfactant. Peevy and associates (1990) studied isolated perfused rabbit lungs, examining various methods of ventilation. They ventilated four sets of lungs with either a low or high gas flow rate while holding the peak inspiratory pressure (PIP) either low (27 cm H_2O) or high (50 cm H_2O). They found that the high PIP group produced significant microvascular injuries. Injury occurred in the higher flow rate and low-pressure group but not to the same extent as the high-pressure low-flow rate group. They concluded that the peak airway pressure was the most important mechanism of injury.

Conversely, Marini and Ravenscraft (1992) used geometric and mathematic modeling to evaluate mean airway pressure. They found that under conditions of passive inflation, mean arterial pressure correlated with arterial oxygenation, hemodynamic performance, and barotrauma.

Alveolar distensibility, a measure of alveolar energetics, is a precursor to barotrauma. Tsuno and colleagues (1990) studied regional pressure-related overdistention of healthy alveoli, termed *barotrauma* or *volutrauma*, that can result in a pattern of diffuse alveolar damage that is histologically indistinguishable from other causes of ARDS. Dreyfuss and coworkers (1988) demonstrated increases in capillary permeability edema and inactivation of surfactant during intermittent positive-pressure hyperventilation with high inflation pressures. Brown (1986) and Macklin and Macklin (1984) have reported that pulmonary barotrauma occurs with an incidence ranging from 0.5 to 64.0% in patients who require mechanical ventilation. Mannino and colleagues (1976) found that the average is 5 to 15%. Mathru (1983)

Table 71-1. Potential Causes of Barotrauma

High peak airway pressures
High mean airway pressures
Alveolar overdistension, increased volume
Positive end-expiratory pressure

and Moylan (1978) and their associates noted that barotrauma is an immediate cause of death in 13 to 35% of occurrences. Elevated PIP, high mandatory respiratory rate, oxygen toxicity, and alveolar overdistension may explain the occurrence of barotrauma. Diakun (1991) reasoned that PIP requirements remain the single best predictor of barotrauma because of the higher pressures necessary to deliver an adequate minute volume when the lungs sustain a severe injury that decreases pulmonary compliance. Peterson and Baier (1983) reported a 43% incidence of barotrauma when the PIP exceeded 70 cm H_2O. If PIP was 50 to 70 cm H_2O, the incidence of barotrauma decreased to 8%, and when the PIP was less than 50 cm H_2O, the incidence of barotrauma was 0% in 157 patients.

PIP was initially considered safe if it was less than 50 cm H_2O, but even this level may be too high if an underlying pulmonary pathologic condition exists that predisposes the patient to barotrauma. Overdistension of alveoli and distal airways, regardless of the pressure involved, also has been proposed by Hillman and Barber (1980), as well as by Hurd (1984) and Alpan (1984) and their associates as a cause of barotrauma. It occurs either through selection of a tidal volume that is too large or nonuniform lung disease. Nonuniform lung disease causes preferential ventilation of normal alveoli, which leads to overdistension of these normal alveoli as they try to accommodate most of the tidal volume. Animal studies have suggested that alveolar overdistension, whether produced by positive or negative pressure, is responsible for the initiation, propagation, or both of the injury. Tsuno and colleagues (1991) analyzed the histopathologic changes in lungs of baby pigs after mechanical ventilation at a PIP of 40 cm H_2O for 22 ± 11 hours. Alveolar hemorrhage, alveolar neutrophil infiltration, alveolar macrophage and type II pneumocyte proliferation, interstitial congestion and thickening, interstitial lymphocyte infiltration, emphysematous change, and hyaline membrane formation were all consistent with the early stages of ARDS. Animals ventilated with conventional ventilatory parameters (tidal volume 15 mL/kg; Pco_2 at 40 mm Hg) for an additional 3 to 6 days showed the aforementioned findings coupled with prominent organized alveolar exudate, which resemble the changes seen in the late stages of ARDS. A control group ventilated at a PIP of 18 cm H_2O showed no histopathologic changes in the lung. Dreyfuss and coworkers (1985) likewise showed that application of high inflation pressure ventilation in rats resulted in pulmonary edema after only 20 minutes, with histologic findings similar to those seen in human ARDS.

Adkins and colleagues (1991) varied PIP while ventilating young and old rabbits. They found that the young rabbits were more susceptible to pneumothorax and concluded that for the same inspiratory pressure, higher volumes would be presented in the young lungs and that overdistension was the etiologic factor. In an intriguing report, Colebatch and Ng (1991) studied 14 men who developed pneumothoraces during shallow water diving and compared their pulmonary mechanics with 34 healthy nonsmokers and 10 age-matched healthy male divers. They found that those who had developed pneumothoraces had stiffer airways and smaller air spaces. They concluded that such a situation would magnify the elastic stresses in the peribronchial alveolar tissue, which would increase the likelihood of interstitial gas dissection. It is known that patients with ARDS have markedly decreased compliance associated with smaller thickened alveoli, and this clinical situation might be analogous to the observed findings in the divers who developed pneumothoraces.

Ranieri and associates (1991) studied the effects of positive end-expiratory pressure (PEEP) on alveolar recruitment in patients with respiratory distress syndrome. Observing the pressure-volume loops on zero end-expiratory pressure and PEEP, they found two populations of patients. Some patients showed evidence of alveolar recruitment as evidenced by an upward concavity of the pressure-volume curve during zero end-expiratory pressure ventilation, which increased with PEEP. Other patients demonstrated an upward convexity, noting volume displacement without alveolar recruitment. This was aggravated with PEEP. They believed that this subpopulation of patients would be susceptible to barotrauma.

Patients at risk for barotrauma range from infants receiving physiologic continuous positive airway pressure (5 cm H_2O), as reported by Alpan and associates (1984), to adults requiring controlled mechanical ventilation and high levels of PEEP, as reported by Mathru and associates (1983) and Kohn and Bellamy (1982). Mathru and coworkers (1983) and Reines (1981) noted that patients who are treated with volume-cycled or controlled mechanical ventilation have a higher incidence of barotrauma when compared to patients who are treated with pressure-limited or intermittent mandatory ventilation. As pointed out by Carlon (1983) and Parker (1993) and their associates, this is probably because of the higher airway pressures that are generated by volume-cycled ventilators compared with pressure-limited ventilators. Also, the controlled mechanical ventilators usually are associated with a higher respiratory rate and more asynchronous breathing than intermittent mandatory ventilation-type ventilators. Gattinoni and colleagues (1987) observed that ARDS is a heterogeneous, not diffuse, lung injury, with areas of relatively normal lung interspersed with areas of alveolar and interstitial edema. The term *baby lungs* has been used to describe the smaller physiologic lung volume. Exposure of relatively normal alveoli with near normal compliance characteristics to high distending pressures results in a larger delivered volume per lung unit, marked overdistention, and the possible increased risk of further lung injury. This scenario occurs regardless of which mode of ventilation generates the high inspiratory pressures.

The exact mechanism of barotrauma or volutrauma remains unclear. Kawano and coworkers (1987) used a saline lung lavage followed by controlled mechanical ventilation (tidal volume of 12 mL/kg) on three groups of rabbits: a normal group, a group rendered neutropenic by pretreatment with nitrogen mustard, and a nitrogen mustard group that was retransfused with granulocytes before the study was begun. The first and third groups developed a high permeability pulmonary edema with hyaline membrane formation, whereas the neutropenic group showed none of these changes. These experimental findings suggest a prominent role for inflammatory cells in the development of the lung injury and argue against an injury that is entirely mechanical.

Presentation

One of the earliest radiographic signs of barotrauma is mediastinal air. Although this finding is often a precursor of pneumothorax, not all patients with pneumomediastinum develop a pneumothorax. In addition, pneumomediastinum usually does not give a clue as to the site of origin. Once pneumomediastinum develops, vigilance is important to discover early signs of pneumothorax.

Often, the first sign of barotrauma is not seen on routine chest radiography but presents as an acute change in hemodynamics or oxygenation. Any patient with poor compliance on positive-pressure ventilation and PEEP who becomes acutely hypotensive or hypoxemic may have a pneumothorax. In patients who have severe respiratory distress syndrome, the pneumothorax may not be large. The loss of even a small amount of lung volume may be sufficient to alter the steady state. Auscultation of the chest in pneumothorax may demonstrate disparate breath sounds, which may be confirmed by chest radiography.

Management

In a patient who has acutely developed barotrauma and is hemodynamically unstable, a needle catheter thoracostomy may be diagnostic as well as life-saving. A sterile needle placed through the second or third intercostal space lateral to the midclavicular line allows the air to escape and should stabilize the patient until a more definitive catheter or tube can be placed. A large tube, preferably a No. 28F or 32F, should be placed in the fifth or sixth intercostal space at the anterior axillary line. The large tube is used to remove any high-volume leak produced. Because many of these severely ill patients also have associated effusions, the tube should be directed posteriorly.

Sometimes the surgeon is notified of a critically ill ventilated patient when the patient develops a pneumomedi-

astinum. Because the side of origin cannot be determined in such a case, the choice is observation or bilateral tube thoracostomy. Our preference is to assemble in the room the equipment necessary for both a needle and a tube thoracostomy but to await the development of a pneumothorax and treat only that side.

Because of the underlying disease, the lungs are stiff and may not completely reexpand. However, positive-pressure ventilation is being used on these patients. Because of these two facts, negative suction on the drainage system is unnecessary. Air from the air leak escapes through the water seal. Tubes should be left in place until the compliance significantly improves and the PEEP levels are consistently below 10 cm H_2O.

Prevention

Adjustment of ventilation to prevent barotrauma is as varied as the theories concerning its etiology. Because the major pulmonary mechanical changes in respiratory distress syndrome are decreased compliance and defect in diffusion, ventilation must be adjusted to optimize these values. Both pressure and volume determine alveolar distention and compliance. Theories show that peak airway pressure and PEEP are the major contributors to barotrauma. Optimal management is accomplished by delivering the tidal volume (10 to 15 mL/kg) at a rate sufficient to maintain a normal Pco_2 at the lowest flow rates possible, which decreases the peak airway pressure and mean airway pressures, yet delivers relatively normal lung volumes, thus optimizing compliance. The slower breath delivered by lower flow rates may also allow accommodation of the alveolar wall, thus decreasing local wall tension. As suggested by Shapiro and colleagues (1984), PEEP should be adjusted to the lowest levels necessary, as measured by the best improvement in shunt fraction and oxygen delivery with the lowest dead space ventilation and inspired oxygen concentration.

INHALATION INJURIES

The most common pulmonary injury associated with burns is smoke inhalation. According to Ryan and associates (1998), inhalation injury remains a major factor responsible for the mortality of the thermally injured. Burn mortality from associated inhalation injury ranges from 20 to 84%. Herndon and coworkers (1987) found the incidence of inhalation injury to be as high as 33% of all major burns. Demling (1989) stated these injuries account for at least 50% of the burn deaths at the accident scene. Death occurs by lethal chemical inhalation. Over the past decade, the synergy of the inhalation injury, concurrent with ventilator-induced barotrauma, has forced investigators to readdress the pathophysiology of smoke inhalation injury. Smoke inhalation not only directly affects the respiratory tract and lung, but also inflammatory mediators affect other major organ systems as well. In addition, treatment of smoke inhalation with positive-pressure mechanical ventilation may further exacerbate the lung injury.

Two major types of pulmonary injuries occur in burn victims: inhalation injury at the time of acute trauma and pulmonary injury secondary to the management of cutaneous burns. The latter includes a wide variety of injuries from pulmonary edema secondary to massive crystalloid fluid resuscitation to acute lung injury and respiratory distress from sepsis and multiple organ failure. These injuries are no different from any other critically ill patient. Management of these conditions is covered in Chapter 72.

Etiology of Inhalation Injury

The term *pulmonary burn* is a misnomer. The lungs are rarely burned secondary to inhalation injury. The oropharynx, nasopharynx, and upper airway sufficiently cool the gases that are inhaled so that thermal injury is minimal in the lungs. When a burn does occur, it is almost always fatal. Two circumstances in which this occurs are steam injuries in a closed space and overheated gases in ventilated patients. One of us (J.L.) has managed a patient who received superheated (45°C) ventilator gases for 8 hours from a faulty heating unit. This patient exhibited severe bronchorrhea and acute lung injury resistant to ventilator therapy and succumbed within 48 hours.

Pathophysiology

Birky and Clarke (1991) reported that approximately 80% of fire-related deaths result not from burn injury but from inhalation of the toxic compounds of combustion. Inhalation injury may occur independently from cutaneous burn injury, although they usually occur together. The injury is notable both for its inhomogeneous distribution within a patient and its variable severity between patients. The physicochemical properties of the causative agent, amount of smoke inhaled, and pre-existing diseases that might decrease the resistance of the recipient to injury determine the site and degree of injury.

Common household items produce a variety of toxic chemicals (Table 71-2). Davies (1986) identified more than 50 chemicals in the blood of inhalation victims who died at the scene of fires. Carbon monoxide (CO), a colorless gas, binds avidly to hemoglobin with over 200 times the affinity of oxygen. It causes severe tissue hypoxia. Hydrogen cyanide is a product of incomplete combustion of plastics and blocks oxidative metabolism. Its effects are not seen for up to 40 minutes after exposure and are dose dependent. Ammonia combines with water on contact with mucosa to form ammonium hydroxide, a strong alkali that produces liquefaction necrosis. Aldehydes, produced by combustion

Table 71-2. Toxic Elements in Common Fire Smoke

Source	Toxin	Effect
Any organic matter	Carbon monoxide	Tissue hypoxia
	Carbon dioxide	Narcosis
	Nitrogen dioxide	Pulmonary edema and bronchial irritation
Wood, wallpaper	Aldehydes	Mucosal damage
Nylon	Ammonia	Mucosal irritation
Petroleum plastics	Benzene	Mucosal irritation
	Hydrogen chloride	Mucosal irritation
Polyvinyl chloride	Carbonyl chloride	Mucosal irritation

of wood, initiate severe pulmonary edema. Exposure to greater than 30 parts per million can produce death in 10 minutes. Hydrogen chloride released in the combustion of plastics produces glottic and pulmonary edema. Nitrogen dioxide produced from combustion of cellulose usually causes no immediate problems. However, within a few hours, it can cause severe respiratory epithelial damage and pulmonary edema. It can react also with the blood to produce methemoglobin. Carbonyl-chloride (Phosgene), produced in the combustion of polyvinyl chloride, causes necrosis of epithelium and pulmonary edema. Because of its low concentration in fires, it usually produces only chest tightness and mucosal irritation.

The magnitude of the chemical problem is illustrated by the studies of the deadly fire that occurred in the Stardust Nightclub in Dublin in 1981. Woolley (1984) reported on a re-enactment. A portion of the nightclub was re-created and monitored during a controlled fire. Within minutes of starting the fire, smoke production exceeded 1000 m³/minute and visibility dropped to less than 1 m. Near the fire, the oxygen concentration was only 2%, with a 3% CO level. Other toxic chemicals in lethal concentrations were hydrogen cyanide and hydrogen chloride. Near the exit, the oxygen concentration averaged 13%, whereas other toxic chemicals remained in lethal concentrations.

The pathophysiology of smoke inhalation can be categorized into two aspects: direct injury to the airway and progressive injury secondary to the inflammatory response. The upper airway of the respiratory tract normally thermoregulates and humidifies inspired air. Because of the relatively low heat content and the intrinsic ability of the upper airway to dissipate heat, Zikria (1975) and Dowell (1971) and their coworkers, as well as Traber and Herndon (1990), have reiterated that the airway and lungs are initially damaged from incomplete products of combustion, most importantly aldehydes and oxides of sulfur and nitrogen. CO exposure is ubiquitous during smoke inhalation and may contribute to severe hypoxia immediately following the injury. Many of these compounds may act together to increase mortality, especially for CO and hydrogen cyanide as reported by Prien and Traber (1988). Moore and colleagues (1991) found that a CO synergism exists that exacerbates tissue hypoxia and acidosis. This synergism may also decrease cerebral oxygen consumption and metabolism as reported by Pitt and associates (1979). The extent of inhalation damage produced depends on ignition source, temperature, concentration, and solubility of the toxic gases generated. The more caustic materials, such as acrolein and other aldehydes, damage the airway and set off reactions that are inflammatory to the bronchi and parenchyma. On the other hand, CO and cyanide rarely damage the airway but do affect gas exchange. CO toxicity remains one of the most frequent immediate causes of death after smoke-induced inhalation injury. Inhalation of a 0.1% CO mixture may result in generation of a carboxyhemoglobin level as high as 50%. A low or normal CO level does not rule out the presence of inhalation injury. Patients should receive 100% oxygen until their CO level is 0%. In fact, CO has an affinity for hemoglobin that is 200 to 250 times that of oxygen. Prien and Traber (1988) showed that the oxygen-hemoglobin dissociation curve loses its sigmoid shape and is shifted to the left, thus further impairing tissue oxygen availability. Goldbaum and associates (1976) demonstrated that competitive inhibition with cytochrome oxidase enzyme systems, most notably cytochromes a and P450, results in an ability of cellular systems to use oxygen. Toxic symptoms manifest at levels greater than 20%, and death may occur at levels greater than 60%.

Herndon and colleagues (1988) chronicled the pathophysiology of the tracheobronchial tree after smoke inhalation. Isago (1991) and Kramer (1989) and their coworkers noted increased capillary permeability and edema. Hinder (1997) and Abdi (1991) and their associates found a marked increase in tracheobronchial blood flow. Ahn and colleagues (1990) described epithelial shedding, congestion, regional emphysema, and progressive separation of the epithelium with formation of pseudomembranous casts with resultant partial or complete airway obstruction. Traber and Herndon (1990) described the copious exudate in the airway containing β-glucuronidase and thromboxane caused by smoke. Abdi and associates (1995) found that the cyclo-oxygenase inhibitor ibuprofen attenuates changes in vascular resistance, and Kimura and colleagues (1988) noted a parallel decrease in the lung lymph flow seen after smoke inhalation injury.

Traber and associates (1985) and later Linares and coworkers (1989) implicated leukocytes and the production of oxygen radicals and proteolytic enzymes in the pathogenesis of lung injury after smoke inhalation. Prien and colleagues (1988) noted that pulmonary damage and changes in pulmonary arterial resistance and lymph flow were significantly attenuated in sheep depleted of leukocytes by nitrogen mustard. Basadre and associates (1988) found that the production of oxygen radicals, as indicated by plasma-conjugated dienes, and the consumption of antiprotease, as measured by α_2-macroglobulin levels in lung lymph, were not changed in these animals, whereas both of these vari-

ables were elevated in the smoked group. Ahn and associates (1990) postulated that pretreatment with xanthine oxidase inhibitor also attenuated many of these changes, indicating an ischemia-reperfusion phenomenon.

Several forms of pulmonary dysfunction may result from the complex pathophysiologic reactions to inhalation injury. Hypoxia, ventilation-perfusion mismatching, increased airway resistance, decreased pulmonary compliance, and increased pulmonary vascular resistance may result from the initial release of vasoactive substances from the damaged epithelium. Sloughed necrotic epithelium, serous exudate, blood cells, and mucus form casts that may cause atelectasis and exacerbate ventilation-perfusion mismatching and hypoxia. In studying percussive ventilation, Cioffi and colleagues (1989) described air trapping that occurs distal to obstruction caused by casts, resulting in barotrauma; alternatively, total occlusion of the airways by casts produces atelectasis and increases the risk of pneumonia. Decreased compliance and increased airway resistance may lead to elevated airway pressures and barotrauma. Mean airway pressures exceeding the mucosal capillary perfusion pressure may result in ischemia of the already damaged tracheobronchial mucosa, compounding the initial epithelial insult. Increasing amounts of mucosal slough, interstitial edema, and decreasing compliance lead to further elevation in ventilatory pressures and worsening barotrauma, as well as increased likelihood of the development of pneumonia. Hyperemia, edema, superficial mucosal sloughing, and ulceration of the tracheal mucosa are often present before arterial blood gas abnormalities; deteriorating pulmonary function test results or respiratory failure signal the presence of inhalation injury.

Diagnosis

Many times, patients present with carbonaceous material around the nose and mouth or inside the oropharynx, making the diagnosis of smoke inhalation easy. Other times manifestations may be subtle, and only a high index of suspicion and laboratory testing lead to the diagnosis.

Clark and Nieman (1988) describe a variety of situations. Patients with severe cases die at the scene. Some patients may respond initially to resuscitation, only to die of severe hypoxia. Patients with less severe cases may enter the hospital in respiratory distress that is caused by airway edema and bronchorrhea. These patients may have stridor, wheezing, and decreased breath sounds. The mildest group may appear relatively comfortable but deteriorate within the first 24 hours, developing severe respiratory compromise.

A high index of suspicion for inhalation injury is essential to avoid missed injuries. Clark and colleagues (1989) noted a majority (56%) of patients with inhalation injury present with some combination—three or more—of history and physical findings indicating inhalation injury including the signs and symptoms listed in Table 71-3. Fiberoptic bron-

Table 71-3. Signs and Symptoms Suggesting Possible Inhalation Injury

Signs
Conjunctivitis
Carbonaceous sputum
Facial burns
Singed nasal vibrissae
Stridor
Bronchorrhea
Dyspnea
Disorientation
Obtundation
Coma
Symptoms
Lacrimation
Severe brassy cough
Hoarseness
Shortness of breath
Anxiety
Wheezing

choscopy and intravenous xenon 133 ventilation scanning, which identifies regions of complete or incomplete small airway obstruction secondary to inhalation injury, can be used to establish the diagnosis. To confirm injury, particularly in mild cases, one must rely on laboratory evaluation and bronchoscopy. Arterial blood gases are usually diagnostic. Although the Pco_2 may be normal, carboxyhemoglobin and cyanmethemoglobin levels are elevated. Mildly elevated carboxyhemoglobin may not be diagnostic, because it may be elevated in smokers. Elevated cyanmethemoglobin levels, however, are diagnostic. Fitzpatrick and Cioffi (1995) found that the combination of bronchoscopy and xenon 133 scanning is 93% accurate in the diagnosis of smoke inhalation injury. Fiberoptic bronchoscopy also allows immediate institution of therapy when severe inhalation injury or airway obstruction is diagnosed.

Treatment

According to Clark (1992), patients surviving the acute accident scene with isolated smoke inhalation injury usually experience illness for only several days and then begin to improve, allowing cautious withdrawal of support. Long-term sequelae directly from smoke inhalation are uncommon.

In the management of inhalation injury, one must constantly reassess the patency of the airway and the adequacy of ventilation. Even at the scene of the accident, intubation may be required. Haponik and Summer (1987) noted that as many as 50% of surviving inhalation victims may require intubation. Bronchoscopy is rarely required to determine the need for intubation.

Oxygen is an important component of early therapy. Because of the mucosal edema that is present, high inspired concentrations may help to improve arterial oxygenation.

Because CO has such a great affinity for hemoglobin, a high Po_2 is required to displace it.

Conservative approaches to the management of inhalation injury stress the use of measures to avoid intubation and positive-pressure ventilation, and if ventilatory support is necessary, permissive hypercapnia and borderline adequacy of oxygenation are preferable to attaining arbitrarily normal blood gases at the cost of inflicting barotrauma and volutrauma. The endpoints of resuscitation are not changed by the presence of an inhalation injury; a urine output of 30 to 50 mL/hour in adults or 0.5 to 1.0 mL/kg per hour in children weighing 30 kg or less is the best indication that appropriate fluid resuscitation is being administered to the patient. Several retrospective clinical reviews by Scheulen and Munster (1982), Navar (1985), Hughes (1989), and Herndon (1988) and their associates have shown that coexisting inhalation injury increases the fluid resuscitation requirements of patients with cutaneous thermal injury, particularly in the first 24 hours, by 40 to 75% (range, 13.5 to 110.0%) in comparison with patients without inhalation injury. A prospective animal study by Herndon and colleagues (1986) demonstrated that inadequate fluid resuscitation after smoke inhalation injury was detrimental. Limiting fluid resuscitation "to protect the lung" may actually lead to increased extravascular lung water, hypoxia, and decrements in lung function, along with the risks of inadequate tissue perfusion, renal failure, and possible death from hypovolemic shock.

Therapeutic coughing, chest physiotherapy, early ambulation, airway suctioning, and pharmacologic agents, all of which are effective in mobilizing and removing retained secretions, are essential to respiratory management of patients with smoke inhalation injury. Tracheobronchial suctioning is important for the removal of debris that cannot be cleared by patients with an incapacitated mucociliary apparatus and ineffective cough. Adequate humidification of inspired gas is essential to help limit inspissation of mucus in the injured airways. Despite adequate humidification, inspissation of secretions still occurs in many patients with severe inhalation injury. In experimental ovine models of inhalation injury, heparin, administered either systemically as demonstrated by Cox and colleagues (1993) or by nebulizer as demonstrated by Brown and associates (1988), prevented or decreased the formation of tracheobronchial casts. In two separate prospective clinical trials conducted by Levine and coworkers and Moylan and Alexander, both reported in 1978, corticosteroids have not been beneficial in altering morbidity or mortality after inhalation injury and may be associated with a higher rate of infection-related complications; therefore, they should be avoided unless the patient was corticosteroid dependent before injury or has persistent bronchospasm unresponsive to other therapy. Fiberoptic bronchoscopy, although labor intensive and expensive, has proved effective when all other therapies fail to remove secretions. Treatment algorithms for pathophysiologic events resulting from mild and moderate inhalation injury are listed in Table 71-4.

Table 71-4. Treatment Algorithms for Mild and Moderate Inhalation Injury

Problem	Seen in	Diagnostic/Treatment
Hypoxia	All injuries	Supplemental oxygen
Reactive bronchorrhea, copious secretions	All injuries	Incentive spirometry; chest physiotherapy, nasotracheal suctioning
Inspissated secretions	Moderate and severe injuries	Humidification, nasotracheal suctioning
Wheezing	Moderate and severe injuries	Diagnostic bronchoscopy to distinguish endobronchial obstruction (plugging) from bronchospasm and edema
Plugging (inspissated mucus or mucosal slough)	Moderate and severe injuries	Humidification; therapeutic bronchoscopy (as needed); aerosolized heparin
Bronchospasm	Moderate and severe injuries	Nebulized β_2-agonists; if effective, then intravenous aminophylline

Florid respiratory failure is present in some victims. Patients with marginal oxygenation who fail to improve rapidly are treated vigorously because alveolar volume loss and total atelectasis is such a prominent feature in this illness. It is easier to prevent collapse than it is to restore alveolar volume.

REFERENCES

Abdi S, et al: Lung edema formation following inhalation injury: role of the bronchial blood flow. J Appl Physiol 71:727, 1991.

Abdi S, et al: Effects of ibuprofen on airway vascular response to cotton smoke injury. Eur J Pharmacol 293:475, 1995.

Adkins WK et al: Age affects susceptibility to pulmonary barotrauma in rabbits. Crit Care Med 19:390, 1991.

Ahn SY, et al: Effects of allopurinol on smoke inhalation in the ovine model. J Appl Physiol 68:228, 1990.

Alpan G, Goder K, Glick B: Pneumopericardium during continuous positive airway pressure in respiratory distress syndrome. Crit Care Med 12:1080, 1984.

Ashbaugh DG, et al: Acute respiratory distress in adults. Lancet 2:319, 1967.

Basadre JO, et al: The effect of leukocyte depletion on smoke inhalation injury in sheep. Surgery 104:208, 1988.

Bendixen HH, Hedley-Whyte J, Laver MB: Impaired oxygenation in surgical patients during general anesthesia with controlled ventilation: a concept of atelectasis. N Engl J Med 269:991, 1963.

Birky MM, Clarke FB: Inhalation of toxic products from fires. Bull NY Acad Med 57:997, 1991.

Brown DL: Pulmonary barotrauma. In Kirby RR, Taylor RW (eds): Respiratory Failure. Chicago: Year Book, 1986, p. 602.

Brown M, et al: Dimethylsulfoxide with heparin in the treatment of smoke inhalation injury. J Burn Care Rehabil 9:22, 1988.

Carlon GC, Howland WS, Ray C: High frequency jet ventilation: a prospective randomized evaluation. Chest 84:551, 1983.

Cioffi WG Jr, et al: High-frequency percussive ventilation in patients with inhalation injury. J Trauma 29:350, 1989.

Clark WR Jr: Smoke inhalation: diagnosis and treatment. World J Surg 16:24, 1992.

Clark WR, Bonaventura M, Myers W: Smoke inhalation and airway management at a regional burn unit: 1974–1983. Part I: Diagnosis and consequences of smoke inhalation. J Burn Care Rehab 10:52, 1989.

Clark WR Jr, Nieman GF: Smoke inhalation. Burns Incl Thermal Inj 14:473, 1988.

Colebatch HJ, Ng CK: Decreased pulmonary distensibility and pulmonary barotrauma in divers. Respir Phys 96:293, 1991.

Cox CS Jr, et al: Heparin improves oxygenation and minimizes barotrauma after severe smoke inhalation in an ovine model. Surg Gynecol Obstet 176:339, 1993.

Cullen DJ, Caldera DL: The incidence of ventilation-induced pulmonary barotrauma in critically ill patients. Anaesthesia 50:185, 1979.

Davies JWL: Toxic chemicals versus lung tissue—an aspect of inhalation injury revisited. J Burn Care Rehab 7:213, 1986.

Demling RH: Management of the burn patient. In Schumaker HB, et al. (eds): Textbook of Critical Care. 2nd Ed. Philadelphia: WB Saunders, 1989.

Diakun TA: Carbon dioxide embolism: successful resuscitation with cardiopulmonary bypass. Anesthesiology 74:1151, 1991.

Dowell AR, Kilburn KH, Pratt PC: Short-term exposure to nitrogen dioxide. Effects on pulmonary ultrastructure, compliance, and the surfactant system. Arch Intern Med 128:74, 1971.

Dreyfuss D, et al: Intermittent positive-pressure hyperventilation with high inflation pressures produces pulmonary microvascular injury in rats. Am Rev Respir Dis 132:880, 1985.

Dreyfuss D, et al: High inflation pressure pulmonary edema. Respective effects of high airway pressure, high tidal volume, and positive end-expiratory pressure. Am Rev Respir Dis 137:1159, 1988.

Fitzpatrick JC, Cioffi WG Jr: Diagnosis and treatment of inhalation injury. In Herndon DN (ed): Total Burn Care. Philadelphia: WB Saunders, 1995, pp. 184–192.

Gattinoni L, et al: Pressure-volume curve of total respiratory system in acute respiratory failure. Computed tomographic scan study. Am Rev Respir Dis 136:730, 1987.

Goldbaum LR, Orellano T, Dergal E: Mechanism of the toxic action of carbon monoxide. Ann Clin Lab Sci 6:372, 1976.

Haponik ER, Summer WR: Respiratory complications in burn patients: diagnosis and management of inhalation injury. J Crit Care 2:121, 1987.

Herndon DN, Traber DL, Traber LD: The effect of resuscitation on inhalation injury. Surgery 100:248, 1986.

Herndon DN, et al: Pulmonary injury in burned patients. Surg Clin North Am 67:31, 1987.

Herndon DN, et al: Inhalation injury in burned patients: effects and treatment. Burns Incl Therm Inj 14:349, 1988.

Hillman KM, Barber JD: Asynchronous independent lung ventilation (AILV). Crit Care Med 8:390, 1980.

Hinder F, et al: Inhalation injury increases the anastomotic bronchial blood flow in the pouch model of the left ovine lung. Shock 8:131, 1997.

Hughes KR, et al: Fluid requirements of patients with burns and inhalation injuries in an intensive care unit. Intensive Care Med 15:464, 1989.

Hurd TE, Novak R, Gallagher TJ: Tension pneumopericardium: a complication of mechanical ventilation. Crit Care Med 12:200, 1984.

Isago T, et al: Analysis of pulmonary microvascular permeability after smoke inhalation. J Appl Physiol 71:1403, 1991.

Kawano T, et al: Effect of granulocyte depletion in a ventilated surfactant-depleted lung. J Appl Physiol 62:27, 1987.

Kimura R, et al: Ibuprofen reduces the lung lymph flow changes associated with inhalation injury. Circ Shock 24:183, 1988.

Kohn S, Bellamy P: Pulmonary barotrauma in patients with adult respiratory distress syndrome (ARDS) during continuous positive pressure ventilation (CPPV). Am Rev Respir Dis 125:129A, 1982.

Kramer GC, et al: Effects of inhalation injury on airway blood flow and edema formation. J Burn Care Rehabil 10:45, 1989.

Levine BA, Petroff PA, Slade CL: Prospective trials of dexamethasone and aerosolized gentamicin in the treatment of inhalation in the burned patient. J Trauma 18:188, 1978.

Linares HA, Herndon DN, Traber DL: Sequence of morphological events in experimental smoke inhalation. J Burn Care Rehabil 10:27, 1989.

Macklin MT, Macklin CC: Malignant interstitial emphysema of the lungs and mediastinum. Medicine 23:281, 1944.

Macklin MT, Macklin CC: Malignant interstitial emphysema of the lungs and mediastinum as an important occult complication in many respiratory diseases and other conditions: an interpretation of the clinical deterioration in light of the laboratory experiment. Medicine 23:281, 1984.

Mannino FL, Feldman BH, Heldt GP: Early mechanical ventilation in RDS with prolonged inspiration. Pediatr Res *10*:464, 1976.

Marini JJ, Ravenscraft SA. Mean airway pressure: physiologic determinants and clinical importance. Part II. Clinical implications. Crit Care Med *20*:1604, 1992.

Mathru M, Rao TLK, Venus B: Ventilator-induced barotrauma in controlled mechanical ventilation versus intermittent mandatory ventilation. Crit Care Med *11*:359, 1983.

Moore SJ, Ho IK, Hume AS: Severe hypoxia produced by concomitant intoxication with sublethal doses of carbon monoxide and cyanide. Toxicol Appl Pharmacol *109*:412, 1991.

Moylan FMB, Walker AM, Kramer S: The relationship of bronchopulmonary dysplasia to the occurrence of alveolar rupture during positive pressure ventilation. Crit Care Med *6*:140, 1978.

Moylan JA, Alexander LG Jr: Diagnosis and treatment of inhalation injury. World J Surg *2*:185, 1978.

Navar PD, Saffle JR, Warden GD: Effect of inhalation injury on fluid resuscitation requirements after thermal burn. Am J Surg *150*:716, 1985.

Parker JC, Hernandez LA, Peevy KJ: Mechanisms of ventilator-induced lung injury. Crit Care Med *21*:131, 1993.

Peevy KG, et al: Barotrauma and microvascular injury in lungs of non-adult rabbits: effect of ventilation pattern. Crit Care Med *18*:634, 1990.

Peterson GW, Baier H: Incidence of pulmonary barotrauma in a medical ICU. Crit Care Med *11*:67, 1983.

Pitt BR, et al: Interaction of carbon monoxide and cyanide on cerebral circulation and metabolism. Arch Environ Health *34*:345, 1979.

Prien T, Traber DL: Toxic smoke compounds and inhalation injury—a review. Burns Incl Therm Inj *14*:451, 1988.

Prien T, et al: Lack of hematogenous mediated pulmonary injury with smoke inhalation. J Burn Care Rehabil *9*:462, 1988.

Ranieri VM, et al: The effects of positive inexpiratory pressure on alveolar recruitment and gas exchange in patients with adult respiratory distress syndrome. Am Rev Respir Dis *144*:544, 1991.

Reines HD: Manifestations of barotrauma in acute respiratory failure. Am Surg *47*:421, 1981.

Ryan CM, et al: Objective estimates of the probability of death from burn injuries [see comments]. N Engl J Med *338*:362, 1998.

Scheulen JJ, Munster AM: The Parkland formula in patients with burns and inhalation injury. J Trauma *22*:869, 1982.

Shapiro BA, Kane RD, Harrison RA: Positive end expiratory therapy in adults with special reference to acute lung injury: review of the literature and suggested clinical correlation. Crit Care Med *12*:127, 1984.

Traber DL, et al: Pulmonary edema and compliance changes following smoke inhalation. J Burn Care Rehabil *6*:490, 1985.

Traber DL, Herndon DN: Pathophysiology of smoke inhalation. *In* Haponik EF, Münster AM (eds): Respiratory Sequelae of Burns. New York: McGraw-Hill, 1990, pp. 61–71.

Tsuno K, Prato P, Kolobow T: Acute lung injury from mechanical ventilation at moderately high airway pressures. J Appl Physiol *69*:956, 1990.

Tsuno K, et al: Histopathologic pulmonary changes from mechanical ventilation at high peak airway pressures. Am Rev Respir Dis *143*:1115, 1991.

Webb HH, Tierney DF: Experimental pulmonary edema due to intermittent positive pressure ventilation with high inflation pressures. Protection by positive end-expiratory pressure. Am Rev Respir Dis *110*:556, 1974.

Woolley WB: The Stardust Disco fire: Dublin 1981: studies of combustion products during simulation experiments. Fire Safe J *7*:267, 1984.

Zikria BA, et al: What is clinical smoke poisoning? Ann Surg *181*:151, 1975.

CHAPTER 72

Acute Respiratory Distress Syndrome

John G. Williams and C. James Carrico

Acute respiratory distress syndrome (ARDS), previously known as the adult respiratory distress syndrome, is a syndrome of noncardiogenic pulmonary dysfunction characterized by refractory hypoxemia, decreased pulmonary compliance, and diffuse interstitial infiltrates on chest radiography. Although many definitions of ARDS have been proposed since Ashbaugh and colleagues' initial description in 1967, the American-European Consensus Conference (AECC) on ARDS' recommended definition, reported by Bernard and associates (1994a, 1994b), has been widely accepted since 1994. Early definitions of ARDS had focused on patients with severe pulmonary dysfunction, often using a PaO_2/FiO_2 of 150 mm Hg as the primary criterion of impaired gas exchange. The AECC accommodated a broader spectrum of pulmonary dysfunction by defining two clinical entities: acute lung injury and ARDS (Table 72-1).

Acute lung injury is defined by 1) acute onset, 2) PaO_2/FiO_2 less than 300 mm Hg regardless of the level of positive end-expiratory pressure (PEEP), 3) bilateral infiltrates on frontal chest radiography, and 4) pulmonary artery occlusion pressure less than 18 mm Hg when measured or no evidence of left atrial hypertension. ARDS is defined by 1) acute onset, 2) PaO_2/FiO_2 less than 200 mm Hg regardless of the level of PEEP, 3) bilateral infiltrates on frontal chest radiography, and 4) pulmonary artery occlusion pressure less than 18 mm Hg when measured or no evidence of left atrial hypertension. With the adoption of these definitions, a uniform standard is now present to characterize the natural history, pathogenesis, and management outcomes of ARDS. A prospective comparison by Moss and colleagues (1995a) of the definition proposed by the AECC and two alternative definitions, the Lung Injury Score and the Modified Lung Injury Score, found that similar patients were identified by all three definitions.

Although ARDS is a relatively common clinical entity, its prevalence is not well established. The published recommendations of the AECC emphasize the need for definitive studies to determine the true incidences of acute lung injury and ARDS. It has been estimated by Bernard and associates (1994a, b) that 100,000 to 150,000 patients develop ARDS

in the United States per year. The reported incidence of ARDS, as noted by Murray (1977) and Webster (1988) and their colleagues, ranges from 5 to 50 cases per 100,000.

ARDS mortality is 40 to 60%. The mortality was virtually unchanged over the 20 years from 1967, when Ashbaugh and colleagues reported a 58% mortality, to 1987, when Artigas and coworkers (1991) of the European Collaborative Study reported a 59% mortality. Large series in the 1990s have shown similar mortality, but several studies of Hudson (1995), Suchyta (1992), and Milberg (1995) and their associates suggest a reduction in ARDS mortality to approximately 40%. Montgomery (1985), Bell (1983), and Gee (1990) and their colleagues note that mortality is influenced by a variety of factors including the underlying cause of ARDS, preexisting medical conditions, and patient age. Deaths that occur within 72 hours of developing ARDS, according to Montgomery and associates (1985) are typically caused by the primary disease process, whereas late deaths are from sepsis and multiple organ failure. Irreversible respiratory failure is infrequently the primary cause of death, with only 16% of deaths attributable to fulminant respiratory failure. ARDS is a relatively frequent manifestation of severe inflammatory insults that produce organ dysfunction, but it is the combined failure of other organ systems that is responsible for the high mortality of ARDS.

BRIEF HISTORY

Although references to an ARDS-like pulmonary dysfunction were made as early as World War I, it was not until 1967 that Ashbaugh and associates definitively described an ARDS in adults that Petty and Ashbaugh (1971) later named the *adult respiratory distress syndrome*. In the 1960s and early 1970s, significant advances in resuscitation and ventilatory support led to a greater recognition of respiratory failure in patients with sepsis, shock, aspiration pneumonia, pancreatitis, and severe traumatic injuries. A number of terms including *shock lung*, *wet lung*, *Da Nang lung*, *post-*

Table 72-1. Acute Lung Injury and Acute Respiratory Distress Syndrome

	Timing of Onset	Oxygenation Pao_2/Fio_2	Chest Radiography	Evaluation of Cardiogenic Causation
Acute lung injury	Acute	<300 mm Hg regardless of positive end-expiratory pressure	Bilateral infiltrates	PAOP <18 mm Hg or absence of clinical evidence of elevated left atrial pressure
Acute respiratory distress syndrome	Acute	<200 mm Hg regardless of positive end-expiratory pressure	Bilateral infiltrates	PAOP <18 mm Hg or absence of clinical evidence of elevated left atrial pressure

PAOP, pulmonary artery occlusion pressure.
Adapted from Bernard GR, et al: The American-European Consensus Conference on ARDS. Am J Respir Crit Care Med *149*:818, 1994.

perfusion lung, and *traumatic wet lung* were used to describe the pulmonary dysfunction that developed in these patients.

ARDS, however, is not a new entity. In 1925, Osler observed that "uncontrolled septicemia leads to a frothy pulmonary edema that resembles serum, not the sanguinous transudative edema fluid seen in dropsy or congestive heart failure." Early observations of the association between pulmonary dysfunction and trauma were made by Burford and Burbank in 1945 when they reported acute respiratory failure ("traumatic wet lung") after thoracic injury and noted its association with increased interstitial and intra-alveolar fluid. Mallory and colleagues (1950) subsequently described some of the classic features of pulmonary pathology in necropsy cases of traumatic shock from World War II. In 1950, Jenkins and associates used the term *congestive atelectasis* to refer to the respiratory failure seen in patients with sepsis, trauma, and peritonitis.

Ashbaugh and coworkers provided the first detailed clinical and histopathologic description of ARDS in 1967. They reported findings in 12 patients with respiratory insufficiency after trauma, severe viral infection, acute pancreatitis, and shock. Histopathologic features of this syndrome included hemorrhagic interstitial and intra-alveolar edema, atelectasis, hyaline membrane formation, and the presence of numerous alveolar macrophages. They further noted that the characteristics of the syndrome described resembled those of fat embolism syndrome, respiratory distress syndrome in infants, congestive atelectasis, and postperfusion lung. These seminal observations indicated that the respiratory dysfunction seen in ARDS was associated with an acute inflammatory response in the lung. It has since become apparent, as noted by Montgomery (1985) and one of us (C.J.C.) (1986) and associates, that uncontrolled systemic inflammation, whether elicited by sterile or infectious insult, is capable of producing acute dysfunction in other organ systems.

RISK FACTORS AND BIOCHEMICAL MARKERS

Clinical risk factors, physiologic responses, and biochemical markers have been used to identify patients at risk for developing ARDS. It has long been recognized that both direct and indirect causes of pulmonary injury are associated with the development of ARDS (Table 72-2). The studies of Bernard (1994a, 1994b), Hudson (1995), Fowler (1983), and Pepe (1982) and their colleagues have noted that the most common causes of ARDS caused by direct lung injury are pulmonary contusion, gastric aspiration, and pulmonary infection, whereas ARDS caused by indirect lung injury most commonly results from sepsis, severe trauma, and prolonged shock. Webster (1988) and Fowler (1983) and their associates have noted that nearly 80% of patients who develop ARDS have one or more of these risk factors. Moreover, Fowler (1983) and Pepe (1982) and their associates have pointed out that the risk of developing ARDS ranges from 2 to 40% in patients with a single risk factor. These same authors, as well as Hudson and colleagues (1995), note that patients with uncontrolled sepsis, pulmonary contusion, aspiration pneumonia, prolonged shock, and severe polytrauma are at greatest risk for ARDS. Fowler (1983) and Pepe (1982) and their colleagues reported that the probability of developing ARDS is disproportionately increased when more than one risk factor is present. The latter authors also recorded that the percentage of patients who develop ARDS is increased 2.3-fold when two risk factors are present and 4.7-fold with three risk factors.

ARDS risk also depends on the magnitude of the physiologic insult, as indicated by correlation with the systemic

Table 72-2. Clinical Risk Factors

Direct injury
    Pulmonary contusion
    Aspiration
    Toxic inhalation
    Pulmonary infection
    Near drowning
Indirect injury
    Sepsis syndrome
    Severe extrathoracic trauma
    Hypertransfusion for emergency resuscitation
    Cardiopulmonary bypass

Adapted from Bernard GR, et al: The American-European Consensus Conference on ARDS. Am J Respir Crit Care Med *149*:818, 1994.

Table 72-3. Acute Respiratory Distress Syndrome Risk

	Percent of Patients with Acute Respiratory Distress Syndrome
Systemic inflammatory response syndrome: number of criteria met	
2	2
3	3
4	6
Apache II score, first 24 hours	
0–9	13
10–19	21
20–24	41
25–29	39
>29	44
Injury severity score	
1–9	0
10–19	20
20–29	26
30–39	26
40–49	35
>49	50

Adapted from Rangel-Frausto MS, et al: The natural history of the systemic inflammatory response syndrome (SIRS). JAMA *273*:117, 1995; and Hudson LD, et al: Clinical risk for development of the acute respiratory distress syndrome. Am J Respir Crit Care Med *151*:293, 1995.

inflammatory response syndrome, the injury severity score (ISS), and the acute physiology and chronic health evaluation (APACHE) score (Table 72-3). The systemic inflammatory response syndrome, an early nonspecific index of systemic inflammation according to Rangel-Frausto and associates (1995), is associated with a modest increased risk of ARDS. This risk increases with the number of systemic inflammatory response syndrome criteria met, but only 2 to 6% of patients with systemic inflammatory response syndrome develop ARDS. Similarly, ARDS risk increases with increasing ISS and APACHE II scores. Webster and coworkers (1988) have observed that 50% of patients with an ISS greater that 49 and 44% of patients with an APACHE II score greater than 29 develop ARDS.

Early changes in oxygenation have been shown by Weigelt (1981), Pepe (1983), and T. J. Donnelly (1994) and their colleagues to predict ARDS. Weigelt and associates (1981) reported a 95% probability of developing ARDS in patients with a PaO_2 less than 100 mm Hg on 40% O_2 or a PaO_2 less than 350 mm Hg on 100% O_2. T. J. Donnelly and coworkers (1994) found significant differences in the PaO_2/FIO_2 ratios of patients who developed ARDS as early as 4 hours postinjury. Pepe and associates (1983) have used these differences in the initial PaO_2/FIO_2 ratio, combined with clinical risk factors and ISS, to create a scoring system that estimates ARDS risk.

A number of biochemical markers have been examined as potential indicators of the cellular or humoral events that precede clinically apparent lung injury. Miller and colleagues (1992, 1996) have found that interleukin 8 (IL-8), an impor-

tant neutrophil chemoattractant implicated in lung injury, is elevated in the lung lavage of patients with ARDS and has been correlated with clinical outcomes. Retrospective analysis of lung lavage IL-8 by Donnelly and associates (1993) and Reid and Donnelly (1996) showed a positive predictive index of 80%. Soluble forms of intracellular adhesion molecule-1 (ICAM-1) and the endothelial adhesion molecules E- and P-selectin have not been shown to predict ARDS by Sakamaki (1995), Sessler (1995), and Boldt (1995) and their colleagues, but do correlate with outcomes and may therefore have prognostic value. Another marker of endothelial injury, von Willebrand's factor antigen, has been shown to be elevated in patients with acute respiratory failure but has a positive predictive value of only 65% in patients with nonpulmonary sepsis syndrome and no predictive value in patient populations with more diverse risk factors in the studies of Carvalho (1982), Rubin (1990), and Moss (1995b) and their associates. Abnormalities in surfactant and surfactant-associated proteins have been detected by Hallman (1982) and Pison (1992) and their coworkers in patients with respiratory failure. Additional studies will be necessary to determine whether these alterations can be used to accurately predict the development of ARDS. A variety of neutrophil products have been examined as potential predictors of ARDS. Elastase, soluble L-selectin, and CD11b/CD18 are increased in patients with ARDS, as reported in the studies of S. C. Donnelly (1994, 1995) and Laurent (1994) and their associates, as well as by Simms and D'Amico (1991), but have not yet been studied prospectively to establish their predictive value. Although complement activation is an important humoral component of systemic inflammatory responses, the presence of activated complement proteins such as C3a and C5a does not reliably predict ARDS according to Duchateau (1984) and Tennenberg (1987) and their colleagues. To date, biochemical markers of ARDS have relatively low predictive value for any given individual but may be useful in characterizing patient populations at risk.

PATHOGENESIS

Studies of the pathogenesis of ARDS have had to accommodate three simple, yet challenging observations: 1) The characteristics of ARDS are remarkably consistent despite its diverse clinical causes, 2) inflammatory stimuli presenting on either side of the alveolar-capillary membrane produce the same syndrome of pulmonary dysfunction, and 3) identical insults do not produce lung injury in all individuals. The earliest accounts of ARDS highlighted the similarity of lung injuries produced by such diverse insults as sepsis, shock, fat embolism, gastric aspiration, and pulmonary contusion. This suggested the presence of a final common pathway(s) of lung injury that could be elicited by a heterogeneous group of primary stimuli. In addition, because both direct and indirect insults produce ARDS, the final common pathway(s) involved in lung injury must be elicited by either intravascular or intra-alveolar stimuli. The third and most challenging observation (that the same stimulus does not induce lung injury in all individuals) requires that hypotheses involving the pathogenesis of ARDS provide an explanation for the heterogeneity of individual responses to a given stimulus.

Initial clinical and histologic investigations by Ashbaugh (1967) and Jenkins (1950) and their colleagues suggested that the refractory hypoxemia characteristic of ARDS was directly related to increased pulmonary capillary permeability and extravascular lung fluid. Intra-alveolar and interstitial edema are consistent early features of ARDS and, as noted by Mitchell and associates (1992), extravascular lung water is increased from three to eight times normal. A second important characteristic of ARDS [the presence of leukocyte and platelet microthrombi, according to Bachofen and Weibel (1977)] indicates that ARDS is associated with an acute intravascular inflammatory process. Observations suggesting that an acute inflammatory process alters the integrity of the alveolar-capillary membrane have provided the basis for more than three decades of research into the cellular and molecular mechanisms of acute lung injury. A number of critical proinflammatory events associated with the development of ARDS, including macrophage activation, neutrophil recruitment and activation, endothelial injury, platelet aggregation and degranulation, the activation of plasma proteins, and alveolar epithelial injury, have been identified in the studies of Weiland (1986), Groeneveld (1997), and Heffner (1987) and their colleagues, as well as Tate and Repine (1983) (Table 72-4).

Macrophage Activation

Pulmonary interstitial and alveolar macrophages are key signaling and effector cells in acute lung injury. These resident leukocytes of the lung are ideally positioned to initiate local inflammatory responses. They do so by elaborating a variety of secreted and membrane-associated mediators including cytokines, reactive oxygen intermediates, eicosanoids, tissue factor, and HLA-DR antigen. Macrophage activation promotes neutrophil recruitment, antigen presentation, phagocytosis, and sequestration at the inflammatory site. In addition to providing these beneficial actions, a number of macrophage products including reactive oxygen intermediates, tumor necrosis factor (TNF), and IL-1 have been implicated in acute lung injury by Brackett and McCay (1994), Simpson and Casey (1989), and Koy and associates (1996). Meduri and colleagues (1995) have reported that TNF, IL-1, and IL-8 are elevated in bronchoalveolar lavage fluid from patients with ARDS and correlate with mortality. Studies by Molloy and coworkers (1993) examining altered macrophage function in acute lung injury suggest that a failure of counterregulatory mechanisms that normally limit inflammatory responses may result in the pathologic release of proinflammatory substances that contribute to lung injury.

Neutrophil Recruitment and Activation

Neutrophil participation in ARDS has been established by the studies of Harlan (1987), Idell and Cohen (1985), and Weiland (1986) and Hinson (1983) and their associates, demonstrating the presence of activated neutrophils in the lungs of patients with ARDS, the ability of neutrophil-derived mediators to induce lung injury, and the attenuation of lung injury following neutrophil depletion or blocking experiments. Simms and D'Amico (1991) have reported that neutrophil margination and transendothelial migration are mediated by chemoattractants and the upregulation of neutrophil-endothelial binding. Donnelly (1993), Hammerschmidt (1980), and Garcia (1988) and their colleagues have observed that neutrophil chemoattractants IL-8, LTB4, and C5a are increased in acute lung injury. IL-8 concentrations have been shown by Goodman and coworkers (1996) to correlate with the number of neutrophils present in the bronchoalveolar lavage fluid of patients with ARDS. Expression of neutrophil and endothelial adhesion molecules is also increased in acute lung injury. Simms and D'Amico (1991), as well as O'Leary (1996) and Wang (1997) and their associates, reported that proinflammatory mediators including TNF, IL-1, and endotoxin released during conditions that predispose to ARDS upregulate neutrophil expression of a number of adhesion molecules including CD11b/CD18, ICAM-1, and L-selectin. In addition to their role in neutrophil margination, Shappell and colleagues (1990) have suggested that integrins may further contribute to lung injury by inducing the release of reactive oxygen species. Blockade of CD11/CD18 on neutrophils or ICAM-1 on endothelial cells with monoclonal antibodies, as noted by Horgan and associates (1990, 1992) attenuates pulmonary

Table 72-4. Pathogenesis of Acute Respiratory Distress Syndrome

Cellular mechanisms
  Macrophage activation
  Neutrophil recruitment and activation
  Endothelial injury
  Platelet aggregation and degranulation
  Plasma protein activation
  Alveolar epithelial injury
Tissue responses
  Increased pulmonary microvascular permeability
  Microvascular thrombosis
  Intra-alveolar and interstitial edema
  Intra-alveolar fibrin deposition
  Altered pulmonary vasomotor tone
Pathophysiology
  Hypoxemia
  Decreased pulmonary compliance
  Increased shunt fraction
  Decreased functional residual capacity
  Increased work of breathing

neutrophil sequestration and lung injury. Janoff (1985) and Weiland and coworkers (1986), as well as Anderson and associates (1991), have observed that activated neutrophils produce reactive oxygen intermediates, elastase, gelatinases, and collagenase; all capable of producing lung injury. Despite evidence that neutrophils play an important role in the pathogenesis of ARDS, neutrophil-independent mechanisms also appear to be involved in lung injury. Acute lung injury has been demonstrated in severely neutropenic patients by Ognibene and colleagues (1986) and in animal models with impaired neutrophil adherence or attenuated neutrophil function by Carraway and associates (1998).

Endothelial Injury

Pulmonary capillary injury is a hallmark of ARDS. Ashbaugh and colleagues (1967) initially stated that the early evidence of this injury included hemorrhagic interstitial and intra-alveolar edema, microvascular occlusion with platelet and neutrophil aggregates, and the loss of normal endothelial histocytologic architecture; these features were confirmed by Hasleton (1983). More recently, biochemical markers of endothelial cell activation and injury (e.g., von Willebrand's factor antigen and tissue factor pathway inhibitor) have been shown by Sabharwarl and associates (1995) to be elevated in patients with ARDS. Grau and coworkers (1996) have reported that expression of TNF receptor p75 and adhesion molecules ICAM-1 and vascular cell adhesion molecule-1 (VCAM-1) is also increased in pulmonary microvascular endothelial cells from patients with ARDS. It is hypothesized that neutrophil adherence and the creation of a protected microenvironment between the neutrophil and endothelial cell are prerequisites for neutrophil-mediated injury to endothelium. Inflammatory mediators released in response to injury or infection induce the expression of endothelial adhesion molecules. Chuluyan and colleagues (1995) have noted that IL-1 upregulates E-selectin, ICAM-1, and VCAM-1 expression. TNF and IL-1 have been shown by Shalaby and associates (1987) to enhance endothelial injury by neutrophils and reactive oxygen intermediates. Minamiya and colleagues (1995) have observed that bacterial lipopolysaccharides also promote neutrophil-endothelial adherence and release of hydrogen peroxide into the pulmonary microcirculation. Endothelial injury associated with neutrophil adherence and activation is accompanied by a loss of endothelial integrity that is characterized by cytoskeletal changes, increased permeability, and proteolytic injury to endothelial surface elements. Recovery of a number of endothelial membrane-associated proteins from extracellular fluids is increased. In patients with ARDS, these include thrombomodulin and soluble E-selectin as noted by MacGregor (1997) and Ruchaud-Sparagano (1998) and their associates. The latter investigators also have noted that release of soluble E-selectin may further exacerbate endothelial injury by decreasing neutrophil chemotaxis and

increasing the production of reactive oxygen intermediates and integrin-mediated adhesion.

Platelet Aggregation and Degranulation

Platelet aggregation and microvascular thrombosis normally act to sequester and limit inflammatory responses. In contrast, disseminated platelet activation contributes to pulmonary dysfunction by redistributing microvascular blood flow, increasing capillary permeability, and activating leukocytes. In the mid-1970s, thrombocytopenia and pulmonary platelet sequestration were noted in patients with ARDS by Bone (1976) and Hill (1976) and their associates. These findings were associated with extensive microvascular thrombosis, pulmonary hypertension, and pulmonary edema. According to the studies of Heffner and coworkers (1987), platelet activation is initiated by bacterial lipopolysaccharides, platelet-activating factor, thromboxane, and thrombin. These authors also reported that degranulation further amplifies the local inflammatory response, producing vasoconstriction and neutrophil recruitment by the release of platelet-activating factor, thromboxane, serotonin, and platelet-derived growth factor.

Activation of Plasma Protein Systems

A number of important plasma protein systems are activated in ARDS. Craddock (1977) and Hammerschmidt (1980) and their colleagues observed that complement activation is a common feature of ARDS and has been used experimentally to produce lung injury. Complement fragments, as described by Duchateau and associates (1984), are potent activators of neutrophils, stimulating aggregation, chemokinesis, and adhesion to endothelium. However, both Flick (1986) and Dehring (1987) and their colleagues have shown that depletion of complement does not prevent septic lung injury, indicating that other mechanisms contribute. A second plasma protein system commonly activated in ARDS is the coagulation cascade as reported by Bone and coworkers (1976). Dorinsky and Gadek (1989) have recorded that clinically evident coagulopathy is present in 26% of patients with ARDS. Intravascular and intra-alveolar fibrin deposition are also frequent findings according to Idell and associates (1987). Coagulation is promoted by the upregulation of endothelial and monocyte and macrophage tissue factor. In a study by Johnson and colleagues (1983), the infusion of thrombin in animals results in increased microvascular permeability and lung injury, suggesting that rather than being a consequence of lung injury, coagulation is involved in the pathogenesis of lung injury. Saldeen (1983) reported that the inhibition of fibrinolysis contributes to the hypercoagulation seen in ARDS. The inhibition of intra-alveolar fibrinolytic activity is caused in part by increased plasminogen-activator inhibitor type 1 release according to the investigations of Bertozzi and coworkers (1990).

Alveolar Epithelial Injury

Although alveolar epithelial injury is evident in histopathologic and ultrastructural studies of patients with ARDS, biochemical assessment and quantification of epithelial injury has been lacking because of the absence of markers of epithelial injury. The identification of an alveolar epithelial type I cell specific protein has been used as a marker of epithelial cell injury by McElroy and associates (1995) in an animal model of pneumonia. A second potential marker of epithelial injury, epithelial cell-derived neutrophil activator-78, has been shown by Goodman and colleagues (1996) to be elevated in the bronchoalveolar fluid of patients with ARDS. Evidence of functional injury has previously been demonstrated by Hallman and associates (1982) and more recently by Lewis and Jobe (1993) by abnormalities in epithelial surfactant. Gunther and colleagues (1996) have shown that lung lavages of patients with ARDS contain decreased total phospholipids, decreased large surfactant aggregates, and decreased surfactant protein A and have increased surface tension. Abnormalities in surfactant may not directly reflect injury to the type II epithelial cell. Plasma proteins with access to the alveolus because of capillary injury are known to influence surfactant activity and may be responsible for some alterations in surfactant activity as Seeger and coworkers (1985) have observed. It is also true, however, that epithelial cells are subject to injury by many of the same macrophage- and neutrophil-derived mediators implicated in endothelial cell injury as shown by Sulkowska (1997). Bacteria and bacterial products (e.g., exoenzyme S and phospholipase A) can injure alveolar epithelium as demonstrated by the studies of Wiener-Kronish and associates (1991, 1993).

The initial sequence of cellular events that precede ARDS depends on the nature and site of the insult. Well-recognized differences in the nature of insults (e.g., sterile versus infectious) activate distinct inflammatory pathways. Recognition of the importance of the site of the primary insult in determining early inflammatory responses has increased. For example, indirect pulmonary insults (e.g., sepsis, shock, pancreatitis) involve systemic mediators that upregulate adhesion molecule expression, neutrophil adherence and activation, and the activation of plasma protein systems as early events. In contrast, insults presented via the tracheobronchial tree (e.g., gastric aspiration, pneumonia, inhalation burn) first produce a local inflammatory response mediated in large part by alveolar macrophages. Subsequent diffuse lung injury appears to depend on a failure of regulatory mechanisms to contain or localize the inflammatory response. In this setting the participation of intravascular components of the inflammatory response including neutrophil recruitment and activation occur as secondary events. The failure of initial attempts to treat ARDS by modifying inflammatory responses is in large part because of an incomplete understanding of the complexity of the factors that dictate host responses to injury and infection.

The primary pathophysiologic correlates of the cellular events enumerated early by Iliff and colleagues (1972) that result in ARDS are an increase in transcapillary fluid flux, interstitial edema, decreased pulmonary compliance, impaired oxygenation, and increased work of breathing. Zapol and Snider (1977) also noted that the release of vasoactive substances from platelets, neutrophils, and macrophages is accompanied by a period of pulmonary hypertension. Initial injury to the alveolar-capillary membrane is compounded by diminished surfactant activity. The redistribution of intrapulmonary blood flow because of microvascular thrombosis and altered vasomotor responses, in conjunction with the loss of alveolar gas exchange units because of collapse and intra-alveolar fluid accumulation, leads to ventilation-perfusion mismatching, an increase in the shunt fraction Qs/Qt, and decreased functional residual capacity.

DIAGNOSIS

The diagnoses of acute lung injury and ARDS are made using the criteria established by the AECC (see Table 72-1). A number of scoring systems have been developed to further stratify the severity of lung injury. These systems are particularly useful in studies that seek to quantify the progression of pulmonary dysfunction and are commonly used in natural history studies and clinical efficacy trials. The most widely accepted scoring system is the Lung Injury Score developed by Murray and associates (1988) (Table 72-5).

Table 72-5. Lung Injury Score

Chest Radiographic Score		Compliance (mL/cm H_2O)	
No alveolar consolidation	0	≥80	0
Consolidation in 1 quadrant	1	60–79	1
Consolidation in 2 quadrants	2	40–59	2
Consolidation in 3 quadrants	3	20–39	3
Consolidation in 4 quadrants	4	≤19	4
Oxygenation (Pao_2/Fio_2)		PEEP (cm H_2O)	
≥300	0	≤5	0
225–299	1	6–8	1
175–224	2	9–11	2
100–174	3	12–14	3
≤100	4	≥15	4
Sum of values divided by number of components used			
No injury	0		
Mild to moderate injury	0.1–2.5		
Severe injury (acute respiratory distress syndrome)	>2.5		

Adapted from Murray JF, et al: An expanded definition of the adult respiratory distress syndrome. Am Rev Respir Dis *138*:720, 1988.

Table 72-6. Adult Respiratory Distress Syndrome Management

Objectives
    Identify and treat reversible causes of lung injury
    Achieve adequate oxygenation
    Maintain tissue perfusion
    Prevent iatrogenic pulmonary injury
Ventilatory support
    Conventional
        Supplemental oxygen
        Pressure-limited positive-pressure ventilation
        Positive end-expiratory pressure
        Hemodynamic monitoring to identify and correct cardiac
            dysfunction
    Alternative
        Permissive hypercapnea
        Inverse ratio ventilation
        High-frequency ventilation

MANAGEMENT

Traditional management of ARDS consists of the identification and treatment of the primary cause(s) of respiratory failure and supportive ventilatory care (Table 72-6). A number of different strategies have been used in an attempt to provide adequate ventilatory support while preventing iatrogenic lung injury. However, proven therapies, pharmacologic or mechanical, that directly affect the outcomes of ARDS by attenuating or reversing acute inflammatory lung injury have not been identified. It is essential therefore to identify and treat primary causes of ARDS. Because sepsis is the most common cause of ARDS, septic foci must be sought out and treated. Both Fry (1980) and Montgomery (1985) and their colleagues, among others, have pointed out that intra-abdominal infection is the most frequent source of infection in surgical patients with sepsis-related ARDS.

Conventional Ventilatory Management

All patients with acute respiratory insufficiency require attention to pulmonary toilet to minimize the risks of atelectasis, endobronchial mucus plugging, and pneumonia. However, it has not been possible to prevent or reverse ARDS with early ventilatory support. It has become progressively clearer that the objective of ventilatory management is to maintain adequate oxygenation and ventilation while preventing ventilator-induced lung injury and maintaining adequate tissue perfusion (see Table 72-6). This usually has been accomplished with supplemental oxygen, pressure-limited positive-pressure ventilation, and PEEP. Patients with ARDS should be placed on a ventilatory mode that minimizes the work of breathing. This can be accomplished with either volume- or pressure-cycled, assist control modes. Controversy regarding the use of pressure-cycled versus volume-cycled ventilatory modes is based largely on differences in

the rate at which positive pressure and gas flow develop in these two modes. Older volume-cycled ventilators produced rapid, sustained flows that stopped abruptly (*square wave* flow pattern) that may be detrimental by increasing maldistribution of ventilation and producing barotrauma. Davis and associates (1996) have noted that the newer ventilators allow the regulation of flow rates in volume-cycled ventilatory modes and have largely eliminated this concern. Small tidal volumes of 6 to 10 mL/kg and limited peak airway pressures less than 40 to 45 cm H_2O as suggested by Gammon and coworkers (1992), as well as by Dreyfuss and Saumon (1992), are used to minimize the risk of iatrogenic lung injury. PEEP is applied to minimize the need for supplement oxygen to an FIO_2 of 0.6 or less. By attenuating progressive atelectasis and increasing functional residual capacity, PEEP partially corrects ventilation-perfusion mismatching in the lung and thus improves oxygenation. Valta and associates (1993) have noted that alveolar recruitment by PEEP, previously cited as a cause of improved oxygenation, is minimal.

Ventilator and fluid management are closely linked in patients with ARDS. In contrast to normal negative-pressure ventilation, which augments cardiac venous return, increased mean airway pressures that accompany the application of PEEP result in increased intrathoracic pressure and may decrease venous return. Thus, positive-pressure ventilation can decrease left ventricular end-diastolic volume, increase pulmonary vascular resistance, and significantly impair cardiac performance. Appropriate fluid management depends on the recognition that adequate filling pressures must be maintained to ensure optimal cardiac performance and tissue perfusion. Excessive fluid administration exacerbates hypoxemia in these patients with pulmonary capillary injury and increased permeability. The pulmonary artery catheter provides valuable information in this setting and should be used as soon as it is apparent that the severity of respiratory dysfunction requires increasing PEEP and mean airway pressures in order to maintain oxygenation.

Permissive Hypercapnea

Permissive hypercapnea, or pressure-targeted ventilation, is a lung-protective strategy suggested by Hickling and colleagues (1990) in which hypoventilation and hypercapnea are accepted to avoid peak airway pressures above 40 to 45 cm H_2O. The pathophysiologic consequences of hypercapnea (e.g., central nervous system dysfunction, neuromuscular weakness, and intracranial hypertension) are primarily related to the magnitude and the rate of change of intracellular pH. Arterial partial pressures of CO_2 in the range of 80 to 100 mm Hg and even respiratory acidosis with pH in the range of 7.05 to 7.15 that develop over several hours are remarkably well tolerated if oxygenation is preserved. An increase of 10 to 20 mm Hg per hour in the PCO_2 allows compensatory mechanisms to maintain intracellular pH. Sodium bicarbonate is commonly administered for an acidosis of less than 7.2. Although permissive hypercapnea is regarded by many as an experimental approach, in practice it is relatively common to accept hypercapnea when minute ventilation becomes rate-limited because of low lung volumes and high airway pressures. However, given the effect of hypercapnea on cerebral vessels, the use of permissive hypercapnea in patients with head injuries should be avoided until its use in this group of patients has been thoroughly examined.

Inverse Ratio Ventilation

Inverse ratio ventilation (IRV) is a labor-intensive ventilatory technique that improves oxygenation by increasing the fraction of inspiratory time in the respiratory cycle. Normal inspiratory-expiratory ratios of 1:3 are increased to 2:1, 3:1, or 4:1. Indications for its use are high peak airway pressures and persistent hypoxemia despite maximal conventional ventilatory support. Gurevitch and colleagues (1986) have reported that improved oxygenation is achieved by prolonging the period of inhalation and thus the interval of positive airway pressure. This maintains alveolar gas exchange units at lower levels of PEEP and lower peak airway pressures than can be achieved with conventional techniques but increases mean airway pressure. It also has been suggested by Marcy and Marini (1991) that increasing the inspiratory-expiratory ratio promotes alveolar recruitment, decreases dead-space ventilation, and improves gas mixing. Patients ventilated using IRV should be sedated and pharmacologically paralyzed. IRV can be initiated with either pressure- or volume-controlled ventilatory modes. Volume-cycled IRV is achieved by decreasing the inspiratory flow rate or adding a pause after inspiration. An important practical point to remember when using IRV is that as the ventilatory rate increases, the amount of time allowed for exhalation decreases and effective ventilation decreases. At high inspiratory-expiratory ratios and ventilatory rates, PCO_2 increases dramatically as ventilatory rate increases.

High-Frequency Ventilation

High-frequency ventilation is being investigated as an alternative ventilatory technique in patients with ARDS. This technique uses ventilatory rates from 60 to 3600 cycles per minute combined with continuous positive airway pressures. The high ventilatory frequency promotes rapid gas mixing throughout the lung despite low tidal volumes. This technique appears to be most applicable to patients with large thoracostomy tube air leaks and possibly to patients with severe ARDS who fail conventional techniques and IRV. A preliminary study of patients with ARDS caused by sepsis, trauma, and gastric aspiration by Fort and coworkers

(1997) demonstrated improvement in oxygenation with high-frequency ventilation while mean airway pressures were maintained in the low 30 cm H_2O. Concerns that the increased mean airway pressures used in high-frequency ventilation would impair cardiac function were not borne out in this study. No significant changes in cardiac function were observed, although many patients had an early, transient increase in pulmonary artery pressure.

Surfactant

Surfactant is a type II alveolar epithelial cell-derived phospholipid that decreases alveolar surface tension and opening pressure. Neonatal respiratory distress syndrome has been treated successfully with surfactant. The role of replacement surfactant therapy in ARDS is unclear. Human and animal studies by Lewis and Jobe (1993) and by Pison (1989) and Gregory (1991) and their colleagues have shown that surfactant activity is impaired in acute lung injury and that these abnormalities correlate with the severity of respiratory dysfunction. But although preliminary studies using bovine or synthetic surfactant showed promising results, subsequent trials have had mixed results, according to the studies of Walmrath (1996) and Anzueto (1996) and their associates. This is in part because of differences in the formulations of surfactant that have been used. The activity of surfactant depends on its association with apoproteins; surfactant proteins A, B, and C. One of the experimental agents, Exosurf, used in early studies evaluating the efficacy of surfactant replacement therapy in patients with ARDS contained only the phospholipid component. Although the results of these early studies have left many people skeptical about its efficacy, additional work is needed to determine whether a biologically active form of surfactant can improve pulmonary function.

Inhalational Nitric Oxide

Nitric oxide is a locally active vasodilator that can be delivered directly to ventilated areas of the lung to improve perfusion. Frostell and colleagues (1993) have reported that inhaled nitric oxide at concentrations of 5 to 80 ppm results in selective pulmonary vasodilation without systemic hypotension. In addition to its direct effects on vasomotor tone, Gries and associates (1998) have suggested that nitric oxide may decrease lung inflammation by inhibiting platelet aggregation. The studies of Rossaint (1993), Gerlach (1993), and McIntyre (1995) and their coworkers show that nitric oxide reduces the pulmonary hypertension associated with early acute lung injury but its effects on oxygenation are less consistent. Improved oxygenation and decreased shunt are observed in 60 to 65% of patients, but no survival benefit has been shown in the experience of Rossaint and associates (1995). The efficacy of nitric oxide in patients with ARDS is currently being evaluated in prospective, randomized clinical trials.

Extracorporeal Membrane Oxygenation and Partial Liquid Lung Ventilation

Extracorporeal membrane oxygenation and extracorporeal CO_2 removal were evaluated as salvage techniques in patients with severe refractory hypoxemia as early as 1979 by Zapol and colleagues and more recently by Morris and associates (1994). Early experiences with extracorporeal membrane oxygenation showed prohibitive complication rates and mortality, but technical improvements such as those reported by Gattinoni and coworkers (1986) have resulted in fewer complications and improved survival. A 47% survival was reported in a subset of patients enrolled in a phase 1 trial of extracorporeal membrane oxygenation by Anderson and colleagues (1993). Neither technique has shown survival benefit in prospective randomized studies.

Partial liquid lung ventilation exploits the unique ability of perfluorocarbons to dissolve large quantities of respiratory gases and their low surface tension. Perfluorocarbons have been studied in animal models of severe lung injury and show modest improvement in pulmonary compliance and oxygenation. Partial liquid ventilation uses conventional ventilatory modes with a volume of perfluorocarbon equivalent to the functional residual capacity. Preliminary work by Hirschl (1996) and Gauger (1996) and their colleagues indicates improvements in oxygenation, compliance, and shunt. Additional studies are needed to establish the role of partial liquid lung ventilation as a salvage technique in patients with severe lung injury unresponsive to conventional management.

Anti-Inflammatory Agents

Numerous anti-inflammatory agents have been investigated in acute lung injury and sepsis. Antioxidant therapy using allopurinol, superoxide dismutase, catalase, vitamin E, and N-acetylcysteine have shown mixed results in animal and human studies conducted by Warner (1986) and Kunimoto (1987) and their associates, as well as by Bernard (1991). Antibody and receptor antagonist therapies directed at blocking the biological activities of endotoxin, TNF, IL-1, and cell adhesion molecules have been examined primarily in sepsis, the major cause of ARDS. An early report of decreased respiratory failure in patients with gram-negative sepsis treated with endotoxin antibody has not been supported by subsequent studies reported by Greenman (1991), Ziegler (1991), and McCloskey (1994) and their colleagues. Anticytokine therapies have produced mixed results. Although animal studies often indicate significant survival benefits, controlled clinical studies fail to confirm these findings. The IL-1 receptor antagonist study reported by Fisher and associates

(1994a), for example, failed to show improved survival in septic patients, but a posthoc subset analysis (1994b) showed benefit. Inhibitors of eicosanoid synthesis and phosphodiesterase inhibitors have shown beneficial anti-inflammatory actions in animal models but do not have clinically proven benefit as shown by Haupt (1991) and Ardizzoia (1993) and their colleagues in preventing or treating sepsis or ARDS. Similarly, Bone and associates (1989) have shown that prostaglandin E_1 treatment has failed to improve survival in patients with ARDS.

Corticosteroids have potent anti-inflammatory effects that have been shown to decrease pulmonary capillary injury when administered before lung injury in experimental models, as noted in the review of Metz and Sibbald (1991) but have not been shown to improve clinical outcomes when administered during the early phase of ARDS in the studies of Bernard (1987), Bone (1987), and Luce (1988) and their colleagues. Corticosteroids may have applications in the later phases of acute lung injury. Several studies reported by Ashbaugh and Maier (1985), Hooper and Kearl (1990), and Meduri and associates (1991, 1998) indicate a benefit of corticosteroids administered during the fibroproliferative phase of ARDS when infection is absent. Despite intensive efforts to identify anti-inflammatory agents effective in the prevention or treatment of ARDS, to date no prospective randomized trial has demonstrated benefit from any of the agents studied. Intensive investigation continues in this area.

REFERENCES

Anderson BO, Brown JM, Harken AH: Mechanisms of neutrophil-mediated tissue injury. J Surg Res 51:170, 1991.

Anderson H 3rd, et al: Extracorporeal life support for adult cardiorespiratory failure. Surgery 114:161, 1993.

Anzueto A, et al: Aerosolized surfactant in adults with sepsis-induced acute respiratory distress syndrome. Exosurf Acute Respiratory Distress Syndrome Sepsis Study Group. N Engl J Med 334:1417, 1996.

Ardizzoia A, et al: Respiratory distress syndrome in patients with advanced cancer treated with pentoxifylline: a randomized study. Support Care Cancer 1:331, 1993.

Artigas A, et al: Clinical presentation, prognostic factors, and outcome of ARDS in the European Collaborative Study (1985–1987). In Zapol WM, Lemaire F (eds): Adult Respiratory Distress Syndrome. New York: Marcel Dekker Inc, 1991, p. 37.

Ashbaugh DG, et al: Acute respiratory distress in adults. Lancet 2:319, 1967.

Ashbaugh DG, Maier RV: Idiopathic pulmonary fibrosis in adult respiratory distress syndrome. Arch Surg 120:530, 1985.

Bachofen M, Weibel ER: Alterations of the gas exchange apparatus in adult respiratory insufficiency associated with septicemia. Am Rev Respir Dis 116:589, 1977.

Bell RC, et al: Multiple organ system failure and infection in adult respiratory distress syndrome. Ann Intern Med 99:293, 1983.

Bernard GR: N-acetylcysteine in experimental and clinical acute lung injury. Am J Med 91:(suppl 3c):54, 1991.

Bernard GR, et al: High-dose corticosteroids in patients with the adult respiratory distress syndrome. N Engl J Med 317:1565, 1987.

Bernard GR, et al: The American-European consensus conference on ARDS. Am J Respir Crit Care Med 149:818, 1994a.

Bernard GR, et al: Report of the American-European consensus conference on acute respiratory distress syndrome. J Crit Care 9:72, 1994b.

Bertozzi P, et al: Depressed bronchoalveolar urokinase activity in patients with adult respiratory distress syndrome. N Engl J Med 322:890, 1990.

Boldt J, et al: Do plasma levels of circulating soluble adhesion molecules differ between surviving and non surviving critically ill patients? Chest 107:787, 1995.

Bone RC, Francis PB, Pierce AK: Intravascular coagulation associated with the adult respiratory distress syndrome. Am J Med 61:585, 1976.

Bone RC, et al: Early methylprednisolone treatment for septic syndrome and the adult respiratory distress syndrome. Chest 92:1032, 1987.

Bone RC, et al: Randomized double-blind, multicenter study of prostaglandin E₁ in patients with the adult respiratory distress syndrome. Chest 96:114, 1989.

Brackett DJ, McCay PB: Free radicals in the pathophysiology of pulmonary injury and disease. Adv Exp Med Biol 366:147, 1994.

Burford TH, Burbank B: Traumatic wet lung. J Thorac Cardiovasc Surg 14:415, 1945.

Carraway MS, et al: Antibody to E- and L-selectin does not prevent lung injury or mortality in septic baboons. Am J Respir Crit Care Med 157:938, 1998.

Carrico CJ, et al: Multiple organ failure syndrome. Arch Surg 121:196, 1986.

Carvalho ACA, et al: Altered factor VIII in acute respiratory failure. N Engl J Med 307:1113, 1982.

Chuluyan HE, et al: IL-1 activation of endothelium supports VLA-4 (CD49d/CD29)-mediated monocyte transendothelial migration to C5a, MIP-1a, RANTES, and PAF but inhibits migration to MCP-1: a regulatory role for endothelium-derived MCP-1. J Leukoc Biol 58:71, 1995.

Craddock PR, et al: Complement and leukocyte-mediated pulmonary dysfunction in hemodialysis. N Engl J Med 296:769, 1977.

Davis K Jr, et al: Comparison of volume control and pressure control ventilation: is flow waveform the difference? J Trauma 41:808, 1996.

Dehring DJ, et al: Complement depletion in a porcine model of septic acute respiratory disease. J Trauma 27:615, 1987.

Donnelly SC, et al: Interleukin-8 and development of adult respiratory distress syndrome in at-risk patient groups. Lancet 341:643, 1993.

Donnelly SC, et al: Role of selectins in development of adult respiratory distress syndrome. Lancet 344:215, 1994.

Donnelly SC, et al: Plasma elastase levels and the development of the adult respiratory distress syndrome. Am J Respir Crit Care Med 151:1428, 1995.

Donnelly TJ, et al: Cytokine, complement, and endotoxin profiles associated with the development of the adult respiratory distress syndrome after severe injury. Crit Care Med 22:768, 1994.

Dorinsky PM, Gadek JE: Mechanisms of multiple nonpulmonary organ failure in ARDS. Chest 96:885, 1989.

Dreyfuss D, Saumon G: Barotrauma is volutrauma, but which volume is the one responsible? Intensive Care Med 18:139, 1992.

Duchateau J, et al: Complement activation in patients at risk of developing the adult respiratory distress syndrome. Am Rev Respir Crit Care Med 130:1058, 1984.

Fisher CJ Jr, et al: Initial evaluation of human recombinant interleukin-1 receptor antagonist in the treatment of sepsis syndrome: a randomized, open-label, placebo-controlled multicenter trial. The IL-IRA Sepsis Syndrome Study Group. Crit Care Med 22:12, 1994a.

Fisher CJ Jr, et al: Recombinant human interleukin-1 receptor antagonist in the treatment of patients with sepsis syndrome. Results from a randomized, double-blind, placebo-controlled trial. Phase III rhIL-Ira Sepsis Syndrome Study Group. JAMA 271:1836, 1994b.

Flick MR, et al: Reduction of total hemolytic complement activity with Naja haje cobra venom factor does not prevent endotoxin-induced lung injury in sheep. Am Rev Respir Dis 133:62, 1986.

Fort P, et al: High-frequency oscillatory ventilation for adult respiratory distress syndrome—a pilot study. Crit Care Med 25:937, 1997.

Fowler AA, et al: Adult respiratory distress syndrome: risk with common predispositions. Ann Intern Med 98:593, 1983.

Frostell CG, et al: Inhaled nitric oxide selectively reverses human hypoxic pulmonary vasoconstriction without causing systemic vasodilation. Anesthesiology 78:427, 1993.

Fry DE, et al: Multiple system organ failure: the role of uncontrolled infection. Arch Surg 115:136, 1980.

Gammon RB, Shin MS, Buchalter SE: Pulmonary barotrauma in mechanical ventilation: patterns and risk factors. Chest 102:568, 1992.

Garcia JGN, et al: Inflammatory events after fibrin microembolization alterations in alveolar macrophage and neutrophil function. Am Rev Respir Dis 137:630, 1988.

Gattinoni L, et al: Low frequency positive pressure ventilation with extracorporeal CO₂ removal in severe acute respiratory failure. JAMA 256:881, 1986.

Gauger PG, et al: Initial experience with partial liquid ventilation in pediatric patients with the acute respiratory distress syndrome. Crit Care Med 24:16, 1996.

Gee MH, et al: Physiology of aging related to outcome in the adult respiratory distress syndrome. J Appl Physiol 69:822, 1990.

Gerlach H, et al: Time-course and dose-response of nitric oxide inhalation for systemic oxygenation and pulmonary hypertension in patients with adult respiratory distress syndrome. Eur J Clin Invest 23:499, 1993.

Goodman RB, et al: Inflammatory cytokines in patients with persistence of the acute respiratory distress syndrome. Am J Respir Crit Care Med 154:602, 1996.

Grau GE, et al: Phenotypic and functional analysis of pulmonary microvascular endothelial cells from patients with acute respiratory distress syndrome. Lab Invest 74:761, 1996.

Greenman RL, et al: A controlled clinical trial of E5 murine monoclonal IgM antibody to endotoxin in the treatment of gram-negative sepsis. JAMA 266:1097, 1991.

Gregory TJ, et al: Surfactant chemical composition and biophysical activity in acute respiratory distress syndrome. J Clin Invest 88:1976, 1991.

Gries A, et al: Inhaled nitric oxide inhibits human platelet aggregation p-selectin expression, and fibrinogen binding in vitro and in vivo. Circulation 97:1481, 1998.

Groeneveld ABJ, et al: Systemic coagulation and fibrinolysis in patients with or at risk for the adult respiratory distress syndrome. Thromb Haemost 78:1444, 1997.

Gunther A, et al: Surfactant alterations in severe pneumonia, acute respiratory distress syndrome, and cardiogenic lung edema. Am J Respir Crit Care Med 153:176, 1996.

Gurevitch MJ, et al: Improved oxygenation and lower peak airway pressure in severe adult respiratory distress syndrome. Treatment with inverse ratio ventilation. Chest 89:211, 1986.

Hallman M, et al: Evidence of lung surfactant in respiratory failure study of bronchoalveolar lavage phospholipids, surface activity, phospholipase activity, and plasma myoinositol. J Clin Invest 70:673, 1982.

Hammerschmidt DE, et al: Association of complement activation and elevated plasma-C5a with adult respiratory distress syndrome. Lancet 1:947, 1980.

Harlan JM: Neutrophil-mediated vascular injury. Acta Med Scand Suppl 715:123, 1987.

Hasleton PS: Adult respiratory distress syndrome—a review. Histopathology 7:307, 1983.

Haupt MT, et al: Effect of ibuprofen in patients with severe sepsis: a randomized, double-blind, multicenter study. Crit Care Med 19:1339, 1991.

Heffner JE, Sahn SA, Repine JE: The role of platelets in the adult respiratory distress syndrome. Culprits or bystanders. Am Rev Respir Dis 135:482, 1987.

Hickling KG, Henderson SJ, Jackson R: Low mortality associated with low volume pressure limited ventilation with permissive hypercapnia in severe adult respiratory distress syndrome. Intensive Care Med 16:372, 1990.

Hill JD, et al: Pulmonary pathology in acute respiratory insufficiency: lung biopsy as a diagnostic tool. J Thorac Cardiovasc Surg 71:64, 1976.

Hinson JM, et al: Effect of granulocyte depletion on altered lung mechanics after endotoxemia in sheep. J Appl Physiol 55:92, 1983.

Hirschl RB, et al: Evaluation of gas exchange, pulmonary compliance, and lung injury during total and partial liquid ventilation in the acute respiratory distress syndrome. Crit Care Med 24:1001, 1996.

Hooper RG, Kearl RA: Established ARDS treated with a sustained course of adrenocortical steroids. Chest 97:138, 1990.

Horgan MJ, Wright SD, Malik AB: Antibody against leukocyte integrin (CD18) prevents reperfusion-induced lung vascular injury. Am J Physiol 259:L315, 1990.

Horgan MJ, et al: Role of ICAM-1 in neutrophil-mediated lung and vascular injury after occlusion and reperfusion. Am J Physiol 261:H1578, 1992.

Hudson LD, et al: Clinical risk for development of the acute respiratory distress syndrome. Am J Respir Crit Care Med 151:293, 1995.

Idell S, Cohen AB: Bronchoalveolar lavage in patients with the adult respiratory distress syndrome. Clin Chest Med 6:459, 1985.

Idell S, et al: Procoagulant activity in bronchoalveolar lavage in the adult respiratory distress syndrome: contribution of tissue factor associated with factor VII. Am Rev Respir Dis 136:1466, 1987.

Iliff LD, Greene RE, Hughes JMB: Effect of interstitial edema on distribution of ventilation and perfusion in isolated lung. J Appl Physiol 33:462, 1972.

Janoff A: Elastase in tissue injury. Annu Rev Med 36:207, 1985.

Jenkins MT, et al: Congestive atelectasis—a complication of the intravenous infusion of fluids. Ann Surg 132:327, 1950.

Johnson A, Tahamont MV, Malik AB: Thrombin-induced lung vascular injury. Am Rev Respir Dis 128:38, 1983.

Koy Y, et al: Tumor necrosis factor induced lung leak in rats: less than with interleukin-1. Inflammation 20:461, 1996.

Kunimoto F, et al: Inhibition of lipid peroxidation improves survival rate of endotoxic rats. Circ Shock 21:15, 1987.

Laurent T, et al: CD11B/CD18 expression, adherence, and chemotaxis of granulocytes in adult respiratory distress syndrome. Am J Respir Crit Care Med 149:1534, 1994.

Lewis JF, Jobe AH: Surfactant and the adult respiratory distress syndrome. Am Rev Respir Dis 147:218, 1993.

Luce JM, et al: Ineffectiveness of high-dose methylprednisolone in preventing parenchymal lung injury and improving mortality in patients with septic shock. Am Rev Respir Dis 138:62, 1988.

MacGregor IR, et al: Modulation of human endothelial thrombomodulin by neutrophils and their release products. Am J Respir Crit Care Med 155:47, 1997.

Mallory TB, et al: The general pathology of traumatic shock. Surgery 27:629, 1950.

Marcy TW, Marini JJ: Inverse ratio ventilation in ARDS: rationale and implementation. Chest 100:494, 1991.

McCloskey RV, et al: Treatment of septic shock with human monoclonal antibody HA-1A: a randomized, double-blind, placebo-controlled trial. Ann Intern Med 121:1, 1994.

McElroy MC, et al: A type I cell-specific protein is a biochemical marker of epithelial injury in a rat model of pneumonia. Am J Physiol 268:L181, 1995.

McIntyre RC, et al: Inhaled nitric oxide variably improves oxygenation and pulmonary hypertension in patients with acute respiratory distress syndrome. J Trauma 39:418, 1995.

Meduri GU, et al: Fibroproliferative phase of ARDS: clinical findings and effects of corticosteroids. Chest 100:943, 1991.

Meduri GU, et al: Inflammatory cytokines in the BAL of patients with ARDS. Chest 108:1303, 1995.

Meduri GU, et al: Effect of prolonged methylprednisolone therapy in unresolving acute respiratory distress syndrome. A randomized controlled trial. JAMA 280:159, 1998.

Metz C, Sibbald WJ: Anti-inflammatory therapy for acute lung injury. A review of animal and clinical studies. Chest 100:1110, 1991.

Milberg JA, et al: Improved survival of patients with acute respiratory distress syndrome (ARDS): 1983–1993. JAMA 273:306, 1995.

Miller EJ, Cohen AB, Matthay MA: Increased interleukin-8 concentrations in the pulmonary edema fluid of patients with acute respiratory distress syndrome from sepsis. Crit Care Med 24:1448, 1996.

Miller EJ, et al: Elevated levels of NAP-1/interleukin-8 are present in the airspaces of patients with the adult respiratory distress syndrome and are associated with increased mortality. Am Rev Respir Dis 146:427, 1992.

Minamiya Y, et al: Endotoxin-induced hydrogen peroxide production in intact pulmonary circulation of rat. Am J Respir Crit Care Med 152:348, 1995.

Mitchell JP, et al: Improved outcome based on fluid management in critically ill patients requiring pulmonary artery catheterization. Am Rev Respir Dis 145:990, 1992.

Molloy RG, et al: Mechanism of increased tumor necrosis factor production after thermal injury. Altered sensitivity to PGE2 and immunomodulation with indomethacin. J Immunol 151:2142, 1993.

Montgomery AB, et al: Causes of mortality in patients with the adult respiratory distress syndrome. Am Rev Respir Dis 132:485, 1985.

Morris AH, et al: Randomized clinical trial of pressure-controlled inverse ratio ventilation and extracorporeal CO_2 removal for adult respiratory distress syndrome. Am J Respir Crit Care Med 149:295, 1994.

Moss M, et al: Establishing the relative accuracy of three new definitions of the adult respiratory distress syndrome. Crit Care Med 23:1629, 1995a.

Moss M, et al: Von Willebrand factor antigen levels are not predictive for the adult respiratory distress syndrome. Am J Respir Crit Care Med 151:15, 1995b.

Murray JF, and the staff of the Division of Lung Diseases, National Heart, Lung and Blood Institute: Mechanisms of acute respiratory failure. Am Rev Respir Dis 115:1071, 1977.

Murray JF, et al: An expanded definition of the adult respiratory distress syndrome. Am Rev Respir Dis 138:720, 1988.

Ognibene FP, et al: Adult respiratory distress syndrome in patients with severe neutropenia. N Engl J Med 315:547, 1986.

O'Leary EC, Marder P, Zuckerman SH: Glucocorticoid effects in an endotoxin-induced rat pulmonary inflammation model: differential effects on neutrophil influx, integrin expression, and inflammatory mediators. Am J Respir Cell Molec Biol 15:97, 1996.

Osler W. The principles and practice of medicine, designed for the use of practitioners and students of medicine. 10th Ed. thoroughly revised by Thomas McCrae. New York: Appleton, 1925. Cited in: Wiedemann HP, Tai DY: Adult respiratory distress syndrome: current management, future directions. Cleve Clin J Med 64:365, 1997.

Pepe PE, et al: Clinical predictors of the adult respiratory distress syndrome. Am J Surg 144:124, 1982.

Pepe PE, et al: Early prediction of the adult respiratory distress syndrome by a simple scoring method. Ann Emerg Med 12:749, 1983.

Petty TL, Ashbaugh DG: The adult respiratory distress syndrome: clinical features, factors influencing prognosis and principles of management. Chest 60:233, 1971.

Pison U, et al: Surfactant abnormalities in patients with respiratory failure after multiple trauma. Am Rev Respir Dis 140:1033, 1989.

Pison U, et al: Surfactant protein a (A-SP-A) is decreased in acute parenchymal lung injury associated with polytrauma. Eur J Clin Invest 22:712, 1992.

Rangel-Frausto MS, et al: The natural history of the systemic inflammatory response syndrome (SIRS). JAMA 273:117, 1995.

Reid PT, Donnelly SC: Predicting acute respiratory distress syndrome and intrapulmonary inflammation. Br J Hosp Med 55:499, 1996.

Rossaint R, et al: Inhaled nitric oxide for the adult respiratory distress syndrome. N Engl J Med 328:399, 1993.

Rossaint R, et al: Efficacy of inhaled nitric oxide in patients with severe ARDS. Chest 107:1107, 1995.

Rubin DB, et al: Elevated von Willebrand factor antigen is an early plasma predictor of acute lung injury in nonpulmonary sepsis syndrome. J Clin Invest 86:474, 1990.

Ruchaud-Sparagano MH, et al: Potential pro-inflammatory effects of soluble E-selectin upon neutrophil function. Eur J Immunol 28:80, 1998.

Sabharwarl AK, et al: Tissue factor pathway inhibitor and von Willebrand factor antigen levels in adult respiratory distress syndrome and in a primate model of sepsis. Am J Respir Crit Care Med 151:758, 1995.

Sakamaki F, et al: Soluble form of p-selectin in plasma is elevated in acute lung injury. J Respir Crit Care Med 151:1821, 1995.

Saldeen T: Clotting microembolism, and inhibition of fibrinolysis in adult respiratory distress. Surg Clin N Am 63:285, 1983.

Seeger W, et al: Alteration of surfactant function due to protein leakage: special interaction with fibrin monomer. J Appl Physiol 58:326, 1985.

Sessler CN, et al: Circulating ICAM-1 is increased in septic shock. Am J Respir Crit Care Med 151:1420, 1995.

Shalaby MR, et al: Receptor binding and activation of polymorphonuclear neutrophils by tumor necrosis factor-alpha. J Leukoc Biol 41:196, 1987.

Shappell SB, et al: Mac-1 (CD11b/CD18) mediates adherence-dependent hydrogen peroxide production by human and canine neutrophils. J Immunol 144:2702, 1990.

Simms HH, D'Amico R: Increased PMN CD11b/CD18 expression following post-traumatic ARDS. J Surg Res 50:362, 1991.

Simpson SQ, Casey LC: Role of tumor necrosis factor in sepsis and acute lung injury. Crit Care Clin 5:27, 1989.

Suchyta MR, et al: The adult respiratory distress syndrome: a report of survival and modifying factors. Chest 101:1074, 1992.

Sulkowska M: Effect of human recombinant tumor necrosis factor-alpha and pentoxifylline on the ultrastructure of type II alveolar epithelial cells in pregnant and non pregnant rabbits. J Comp Pathol 117:227, 1997.

Tate RM, Repine JE: Neutrophils and the adult respiratory distress syndrome. Am Rev Respir Dis 128:552, 1983.

Tennenberg SD, Jacobs MP, Solomkin JS: Complement-mediated neutrophil activation in sepsis- and trauma-related adult respiratory distress syndrome. Clarification with radioaerosol lung scans. Arch Surg 122:26, 1987.

Valta P, et al: Does alveolar recruitment occur with positive end expiratory pressure in adult respiratory distress syndrome patients? J Crit Care 8:34, 1993.

Walmrath D, et al: Bronchoscopic surfactant administration in patients with severe adult respiratory distress syndrome and sepsis. Am J Respir Crit Care Med *154*:57, 1996.

Wang JH, et al: Intercellular adhesion molecule-1 (ICAM-1) is expressed on human neutrophils and is essential for neutrophil adherence and aggregation. Shock *8*:357, 1997.

Warner BW, Hasselgren P-O, Fischer JE: Effect of allopurinol and superoxide dismutase on survival rate in rats with sepsis. Curr Surg *43*:292,1986.

Webster NR, Cohen AT, Nunn JF: Adult respiratory distress syndrome—how many cases in the UK? Anaesthesia *43*:923, 1988.

Weigelt JA, Snyder WH, Mitchell RA: Early identification of patients prone to develop adult respiratory distress syndrome. Am J Surg *142*:687, 1981.

Weiland JK, et al: Lung neutrophils in the adult respiratory distress syndrome: clinical and pathophysiologic science. Am Rev Respir Dis *133*:218, 1986.

Wiener-Kronish JP, Albertine KH, Matthay MA: Differential responses of the endothelial and epithelial barriers of the lung in sheep to *Escherichia coli* endotoxin. J Clin Invest *88*:864, 1991.

Wiener-Kronish JP, et al: Alveolar epithelial injury and pleural empyema in acute *P. aeruginosa* pneumonia in anesthetized rabbits. J Appl Physiol *75*:1661, 1993.

Zapol WM, Snider MT: Pulmonary hypertension in severe acute respiratory failure. N Engl J Med *296*:476, 1977.

Zapol WM, et al: Extracorporeal membrane oxygenation in severe acute respiratory failure. JAMA *242*:2193, 1979.

Ziegler EJ, et al: Treatment of gram-negative bacteremia and septic shock with HA-1A human monoclonal antibody against endotoxin. N Engl J Med *324*:429, 1991.

CHAPTER 73

Management of Foreign Bodies of the Airway

Jeffrey P. Ludemann, C. Anthony Hughes, and Lauren D. Holinger

On March 27, 1897, whilst eating some soup, [J.W.] aspirated a bone. This accident was followed by attacks of violent cough and dyspnoea, which, however, became gradually less . . . . On direct laryngeal examination by means of Kirstein's spatula, the patient being seated with his head strongly deflected to the left, I saw in the right principal bronchus a white mass. On the following day I introduced, under cocaine anaesthesia, a straight tube of 9 millimetres diameter and 25 centimetres length through the larynx and the trachea until I came near the foreign body. The curvature of the trachea was thus removed, and the foreign body could be seen distinctly. I had great difficulty in catching hold of the foreign body, using a pair of slender forceps which had specially and quickly been made. The difficulties were great, as at that time . . . I was still without the necessary practice which enables one to look easily, and even more to operate, through long tubes. Eventually I succeeded in catching the bone and in extracting it. The patient was able to return home on the following day.

Gustav Killian (1902)

Foreign body aspiration is a serious and potentially fatal occurrence. Through advances in prevention, first aid, and endoscopic technology, a nearly 20% decrease in deaths from foreign body aspiration within the United States has occurred over the last decade. Nevertheless, in 1996, the National Safety Council reported an average of more than eight deaths per day from foreign body aspiration in the United States. Generally, the longer a foreign body has been lodged within the tracheobronchial tree, the greater the morbidity. Thus, an early diagnosis remains a key to successful and uncomplicated management of these accidents.

The first extraction of an airway foreign body was performed by Gustav Killian near the end of the nineteenth century; and the basic principles of extraction were meticulously developed by Chevalier Jackson during the first half of the twentieth century. Jackson's concepts of the various mechanical problems and demonstrations of their solutions remain valid today. At any given institution, airway foreign body problems should be managed by the individuals with the best training and most experience, regardless of their particular subspecialty. As Jackson (1938) stated and Hughes and colleagues (1996) reiterated, the techniques of foreign body extraction should be mastered through practice on lung models and then on anesthetized laboratory animals before they are attempted in human beings.

EPIDEMIOLOGY AND ETIOLOGY

Older infants and toddlers constitute the vast majority of patients with foreign body aspiration. Darrow and Holinger (1995) reviewed multiple case series and found that children younger than 5 years of age account for approximately 84% of cases and children younger than 3 years of age account for 73%. The high incidence in this age group reflects the tendency of children to explore the world using their mouths. In addition, these children have not developed a full posterior dentition and may have immature neuromuscular mechanisms for swallowing and airway protection. Moreover, many youngsters are allowed to talk, run, or play with food or other objects in their mouths. For uncertain reasons, boys aspirate foreign bodies more frequently than girls by the ratio of approximately 2:1. In adults, other factors such as neurologic dysfunction or dental trauma may play a role in foreign body aspiration.

Although adults most commonly aspirate bones from fish, birds, or small mammals, children usually aspirate vegetable matter. Darrow and Holinger (1995) found that nuts, particularly peanuts, account for approximately 34% of cases of foreign bodies found in the pediatric airway. Even nut fragments found in crunchy peanut butter have been aspirated. Other commonly aspirated types of vegetable matter include pieces of raw carrot, apple, dried beans, popcorn, and sunflower, watermelon, or pumpkin seeds.

The spectrum of airway foreign bodies varies from country to country, depending on the diet and customs of the population. For example, Mu and colleagues (1990) reported that in mainland China, nearly 95% of aspirated foreign bodies in children were organic. In contrast, more industrialized countries have a greater incidence of aspiration of plastic foreign bodies, because plastic parts are used frequently by the toy industry. Other reported examples of the cultural influence on these accidents include aspiration of Mardi Gras beads, pieces of crab shell, holiday decorations and gifts, and straight pins by Middle Eastern women and girls, who hold the pins between their lips while securing their facial scarves. Fortunately, ingestion of safety pins has become rare, since the advent of disposable diapers. Rarely, medical therapy itself may be responsible. Aspiration of pills, a thermometer fragment, and an object within a metered-dose inhaler has been reported.

HISTORY

Three stages of symptoms result from the aspiration of an object into the airway:

Initial event: Violent paroxysms of coughing, choking, gagging, and possibly airway obstruction occur immediately after a foreign body is aspirated. An esophageal foreign body large enough to cause posterior tracheal compression may cause similar symptoms. Such a history can be elicited in most cases, but unfortunately many parents tend to downplay the significance of such an event or do not recall the incident until after the foreign body has been extracted. Some parents engage in wishful thinking and minimize the symptoms, hoping that nothing is wrong and that no surgical intervention will be required. Older children often are reluctant to admit to such an episode for fear of being punished.

Asymptomatic interval: During the second stage, the foreign body becomes lodged, reflexes fatigue, and the immediate irritating symptoms subside. This stage is the most treacherous and accounts for a large percentage of delayed diagnoses and overlooked foreign bodies. It is during this second stage that the physician is inclined to minimize the possibility of a foreign body accident, being reassured by the absence of signs and symptoms.

Complications: In this third stage, obstruction, erosion, or infection develop and again direct attention to the presence of a foreign body. Signs include fever, cough, and hemoptysis. Complications include formation of bronchial granulation tissue, atelectasis, pneumonia, lung abscess, and, eventually, bronchocutaneous fistula. Such complications occur more rapidly after aspiration of vegetable matter and sharp objects compared with plastics and other biologically inert materials.

The current medical practice of treating an asthmatic or "croupy" child with antibiotics or corticosteroids may obscure signs and symptoms that normally would be expected with a retained foreign object. Clearing of symptoms with these agents cannot always be assumed to be diagnostic of a specific disease process. The fact that a wheeze disappears or a pneumonic process temporarily clears may merely mean that the patient's reaction to a foreign body has been controlled temporarily. The recurrence of "asthma" after tapering of therapy should heighten a physician's suspicion of an aspirated foreign body.

A positive history must never be ignored. A negative history may be misleading. Choking or coughing episodes accompanied by wheezing are highly suggestive of foreign body aspiration. The literature reveals that diagnosis is delayed more than 24 hours in 50% of cases as noted by Wiseman (1984); and more than 1 week in 15% of cases as reported by Reilly and colleagues (1997). Disregarding a child's story because of age or lack of symptoms may cause a delay in diagnosis, which may make removal more difficult and complicated. As Wetmore (1994) stated, once an aspirated foreign body is suspected, the burden of proof is on the bronchoscopist. Furthermore, Mantor and colleagues (1989) suggested that "some negative bronchoscopies are necessary in order to prevent the morbidity that occurs from a missed foreign body aspiration."

PHYSICAL EXAMINATION

Laryngeal Foreign Bodies

Large globular foreign bodies that become lodged between the vocal cords usually cause complete obstruction and asphyxiation unless promptly expelled. Flat, thin, and sharp objects, such as eggshell and bone, may become lodged between the vocal cords in the sagittal plane. Dysphonia, croupy cough, stridor, and varying degrees of dyspnea ensue, all of which increase as edema and inflammation progress. Odynophagia may occur also.

Tracheal Foreign Bodies

Jackson and Jackson (1936) described three features of tracheal foreign bodies. The *audible slap* and the *palpatory thud* result from the impact of a mobile foreign body against the tracheal wall on deep inspiration or coughing. The *asthmatoid wheeze* results from partial bronchial obstruction from the foreign body and the inflammatory reaction. Biphasic stridor also may occur if the foreign body is within the extrathoracic trachea.

Bronchial Foreign Bodies

Wiseman (1984) noted that the classic triad of wheezing, coughing, and decreased air entry to the obstructed side was present in only 31% of children examined within 24 hours of bronchial foreign body aspiration and only 47% of children examined after 24 hours. Moreover, physical signs may change rapidly with migration of the foreign body and with the development of edema and infection. If the foreign body eventually lodges within one bronchus, the physical examination may stabilize.

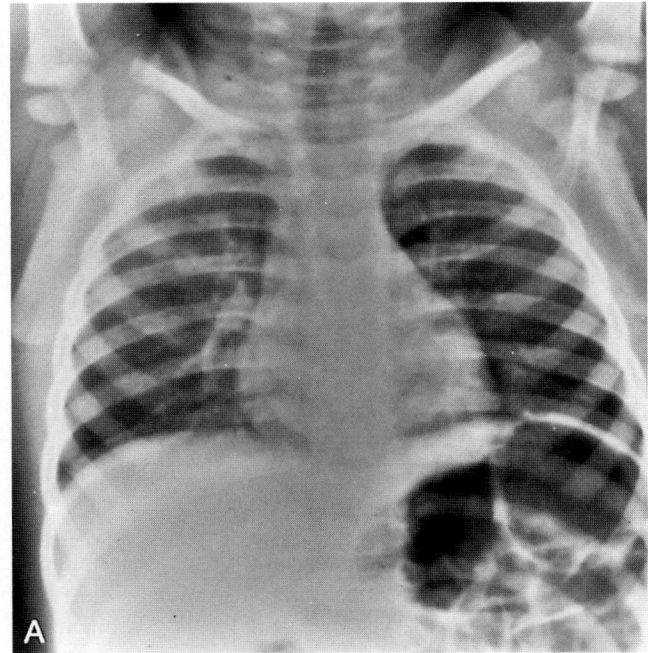

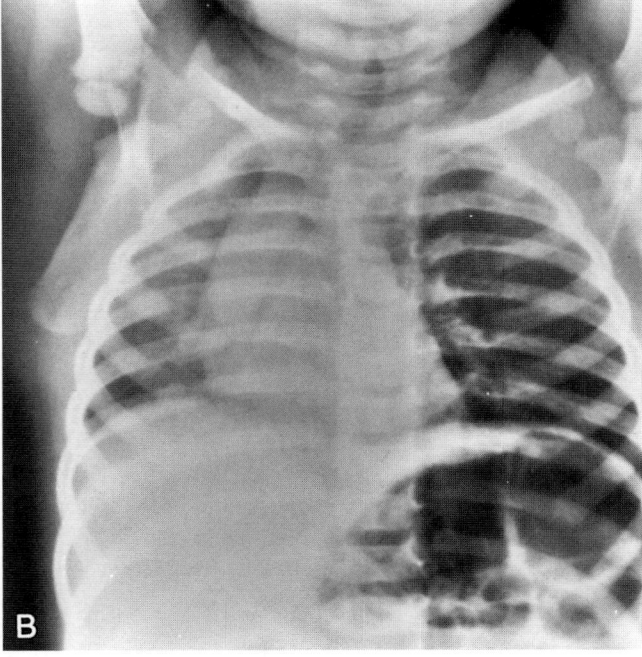

Fig. 73-1. A. Anteroposterior radiograph of the chest during inspiration. **B.** Anteroposterior radiograph of the chest during expiration. Note the trapping of air in the left lung field caused by a peanut in the left main stem bronchus.

RADIOLOGIC EVALUATION

Inspiratory and expiratory posteroanterior and lateral chest radiography is standard when foreign body aspiration is suspected. If the foreign body is radiopaque, a film is taken in the greatest diameter of the object for accurate localization before endoscopy. More than 90% of foreign bodies, however, are radiolucent, as reported by Vane and colleagues (1988). This percentage is likely to increase as more polyethylenes are used to make toys.

Jackson and Jackson (1950) described the pathophysiology behind the radiographic diagnosis of radiolucent bronchial foreign bodies. Initially, the object creates a bypass valve, which still allows ingress and egress of air. At this stage, radiography results are normal. As edema of the surrounding bronchial wall develops, a check valve is created. On inspiration, the bronchus dilates and permits ingress of air. However, on expiration, the bronchus constricts, and contact of the edematous bronchus with the foreign body blocks the egress of air. Thus, air trapping (obstructive emphysema) results. Radiographically, when a check valve is created, the inspiratory film is normal, whereas the expiratory film shows hyperinflation of the affected lung and shift of the mediastinum to the opposite side (Fig. 73-1). If inspiratory and expiratory films are not possible because a child is tachypneic or uncooperative, lateral decubitus chest films or fluoroscopy may also identify air trapping.

Eventually, when enough edema develops to block both ingress and egress of air, a stop valve is created. Obstructive atelectasis is seen radiographically. This late complication usually takes days or weeks to develop.

Although reports vary, Black and colleagues (1994) found that inspiratory and expiratory chest radiography was diagnostic in 83% of 440 children with tracheobronchial foreign bodies. In cases of suspected tracheal foreign bodies, posteroanterior and lateral soft tissue neck films (high kilovoltage airway films) are the radiographic test of choice. As Esclamado and Richardson (1987) reported, airway films are abnormal in 92% of children with tracheal foreign bodies, whereas chest radiography is abnormal in only 58%. Pneumomediastinum is a rare but highly diagnostic finding. It was reported by Burton and colleagues (1989) in 7% of patients with tracheobronchial foreign bodies.

In rare cases, when a radiolucent foreign object is lodged too far in the lung periphery for endoscopic management, it may be precisely localized by bronchography, computed tomography, or in certain cases, magnetic resonance imaging. Imaizumi and colleagues (1994) noted that, because of their high lipid content, peanut fragments appear as high-intensity signals on T1-weighted images. Such information would confirm the diagnosis and would assist in localization if thoracotomy and segmentectomy were to become necessary.

TREATMENT

An airway foreign body usually does not constitute an acute emergency. In general, the treatment of choice is reasonably prompt endoscopic removal under conditions of maximum safety and minimum trauma. Too often, foreign bodies are considered emergencies, leading to hasty, inadequate preoperative planning and poorly prepared, improper attempts at removal. Most patients with foreign bodies who have come to the endoscopic surgeon have already passed the acute phase. When no urgent danger to the patient's life exists, the problem is approached with complete and thoughtful consideration of the physiologic and mechanical factors involved.

The endoscopic removal can be scheduled once trained personnel are available, instruments have been checked, and techniques have been tested. However, untoward delay of bronchoscopic removal is potentially harmful because the foreign body may become dislodged from the bronchus and impacted in the larynx, causing asphyxiation. Therefore, endoscopy is deferred only until preoperative studies have been obtained and the patient has been prepared for surgery by adequate hydration and emptying of the stomach. Foreign bodies in the larynx or tracheobronchial tree are usually removed on the same day the diagnosis is considered.

Two situations exist, however, in which an airway foreign body does constitute an acute emergency.

Actual or Potential Airway Obstruction

Of Things that endanger stopping of the breath in swallowing, some are Sharp, and some Blunt. . . . I have heard of a Child in Woodstreet strangled with a Grape.

Stephen Bradwell (1633)

The most serious complication of foreign body aspiration is complete obstruction of the airway. Globular food objects, such as hot dogs, grapes, nuts, and candies, are the most frequent offenders, whereas rubber balloons and other toys are common among nonfood objects. Large or multiple esophageal foreign bodies also can cause airway obstruction, by posterior compression.

Although the yearly death toll from foreign body aspiration in the United States remains at approximately 3000, the incidence of asphyxiation in the pediatric population has demonstrated a progressive decline. Among children between birth and 4 years of age, 650 died of foreign body ingestion in 1968. By 1990, this number had decreased to 261. As Ryan and colleagues (1990) reported, this trend probably is the result of improved public awareness and prevention, the development of rapid response paramedic teams, and the introduction of and public education about the Heimlich maneuver.

Hot dogs rarely are seen as foreign bodies by the endoscopist. Toddlers who choke on hot dogs usually asphyxiate on the spot unless the incident is recognized and treated at the scene. Recognition of complete airway obstruction is critical to the success of first aid efforts. Coughing, gagging, and throat clearing are reflexes that protect the airway and are indications that the obstruction is not complete. First aid delivered to such a patient is unnecessary and potentially dangerous. Probing the hypopharynx with a finger may drive a loose foreign body into the larynx, transforming a partial obstruction into a complete obstruction. The foreign body also may be forced into the esophagus, where compression of the trachea against the upper sternum may cause

an obstruction that cannot be relieved even by tracheotomy. Similarly, back blows with the victim inverted also are ill-advised in the incompletely obstructed child. Such treatment may cause a bronchial foreign body to lodge in the glottis from below, precipitating complete obstruction.

Complete airway obstruction may be recognized in the conscious child as sudden respiratory distress with an inability to speak or cough. An older child or adult might use the choking distress signal, which is the gesture of clutching the neck between the thumb and index finger. In the completely obstructed patient, attempts at rescue breathing are unsuccessful, resulting in no chest expansion.

The best management of the child with complete airway obstruction caused by foreign body aspiration is controversial and evolving. In 1986, the Committee on Accident and Poisoning prevention of the American Academy of Pediatrics revised its policy statement on first aid for the choking child to advocate back blows followed by chest thrusts as primary therapy for infants. Because of the risk of rupture of abdominal viscera, abdominal thrusts are not recommended for children less than 1 year of age. For all others, abdominal thrusts as described by Heimlich (1975) are recommended. If laryngeal obstruction persists despite these efforts, cardiopulmonary resuscitation continues until skilled medical personnel and appropriate equipment are available to secure the airway via laryngoscopy and foreign body extraction, cricothyroidotomy, or tracheostomy. These recommendations conform with those of the American Heart Association and the American Red Cross.

Dried Beans or Peas

When a main bronchus is obstructed by a dried bean or pea for more than 24 hours, absorbed moisture may cause the capsule to burst (Fig. 73-2). As the bean rapidly swells,

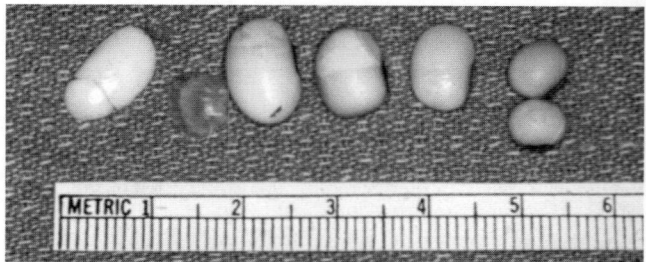

Fig. 73-2. When 8-year-old J. B. fell into a huge trailer filled with soybeans, he essentially drowned, aspirating multiple soybeans, four of which are seen on the left. The two soybeans on the right were brought in by his father for comparison. They contained approximately 13% moisture when harvested from the field and are about one-half the size of the moisture-swollen beans that were extracted from the tracheobronchial tree. Despite preoperative cyanosis, the patient recovered without sequelae. From Holinger LD: Foreign bodies of the airway and esophagus. *In* Holinger LD, Lusk RP, Green CG (eds): Pediatric Laryngology and Bronchoesphagology. Philadelphia: Lippincott–Raven, 1997, p. 236. With permission.

the airway becomes increasingly obstructed. If the patient does not asphyxiate, the swelling at least obliterates forceps spaces, making the technical aspects of bronchial foreign body extraction extremely difficult. Most children raised on farms are taught from a young age not to play near large containers of dried beans or peas, to prevent drowning and asphyxiation.

Similarly, a sucralfate tablet can also cause rapid airway obstruction, even in adults. Overdahl and Wewers (1994) hypothesized that obstruction occurs because an aspirated sucralfate tablet not only expands rapidly but also binds to mucosa. The sooner such a patient undergoes bronchoscopy, the greater the probability of a successful endoscopic retrieval.

Disc Battery Ingestion and Esophageal Perforation

The bronchoesophagologist may encounter two other foreign body situations that mandate urgent intervention: disc battery ingestion with esophageal lodging and esophageal perforation. Maves and colleagues (1984) demonstrated that disc batteries cause esophageal mucosal damage after 1 hour, erosion into the muscular layers within 2 to 4 hours, and esophageal perforation within 8 to 12 hours. Thus, a disc battery that is lodged in the esophagus must be removed urgently. Similarly, any patient exhibiting signs and symptoms of esophageal perforation should undergo prompt confirmatory diagnostic studies followed by retrieval of the foreign body and appropriate medical and surgical therapy. Discussion of esophageal foreign bodies is presented in Chapter 131.

Preoperative Preparation

When foreign body aspiration is not an acute emergency, the endoscopist gathers as much information as possible and prepares equipment before the patient enters the operating room. If the parents know what the foreign body might be, they are asked to return home to obtain a duplicate. If this is not possible, they are asked to draw the object as accurately as possible. They are questioned carefully about the object's size, color, and texture. When a duplicate object can be obtained, it is tested to determine which bronchoscope and forceps are best suited for extraction. When the object has multiple contours, a method of disimpaction, disentanglement, or version and seizure should be worked out for each possible presentation. As Holinger (1962) pointed out, "if two hours are spent in such preparation, the safe endoscopic removal of the foreign body may take only two minutes. But if only two minutes are taken for preparation, the endoscopist may find himself attempting makeshift ineffective procedures for the next frustrating two hours."

Because the patient's family may be distraught, the preoperative discussion with them is an essential part of the preparation for endoscopy. The risks of the procedure, including complete airway obstruction, the need for tempo-

rary tracheotomy, possible rupture of the trachea or bronchi, and failed extraction are discussed, but in such a way that the patient or parents do not delay the procedure unnecessarily. A thorough medical history is taken and careful assessment of the child's general medical condition is carried out. This may include additional laboratory studies and control of medical problems such as dehydration or asthma. Patients with sharp and potentially contaminated foreign bodies are also given tetanus prophylaxis.

Instrumentation

Rigid bronchoscopes are the instruments of choice for foreign body extraction, especially within the pediatric airway. The major drawback of flexible instruments is that they lack control of the foreign body and provide inadequate control of the airway. The rigid bronchoscopes are available in a greater range of size, allow the use of a greater variety of forceps, provide better exposure of the foreign body, and permit sheathing of sharp points within the tube during extraction. The flexible bronchoscope may be of some help in a patient who is unable to extend the head and neck or in the occasional adult patient with a foreign body lodged far in the lung periphery.

For pediatric airway foreign body extraction, the size 3.75 × 30.0 cm Doesel-Huzly rigid bronchoscope with rod-lens telescope is most commonly used. In general, the shortest, widest bronchoscope that atraumatically reaches the foreign body is chosen. Two laryngoscopes and two bronchoscopes are lighted and available; should a light fail or a forceps become jammed in the scope, a back-up is immediately available.

Passive action forceps offer a wide range of blades for the various type of mechanical problems. Four types exist: forward grasping, rotation, ball-bearing (globular object), and hollow object forceps. At least 60 variations of these four basic types have been designed. Positive action forceps have the advantage of a narrower shaft and have the capacity to dilate a bronchus. This may be critical when a round object is wedged in a distal bronchus and forceps spaces are not apparent. The blades of the positive action forceps can be used to dilate the bronchial wall to advance past the equator of the object.

The standard forward grasping forceps has a powerful grip that pulls the object proximally. It is useful for dense foreign bodies that require a firm grasp to prevent stripping off. For more delicate manipulation, and particularly for friable foreign bodies, a lighter forceps such as a fenestrated peanut forceps or a positive action forceps with delicate curved blades is best. A magnified view may be obtained with a rod-lens telescope or the optical forceps. Finally, a relatively large duck-billed forceps is also selected in case the foreign body becomes lodged within the larynx or hypopharynx.

A complete instrumentation is essential. Failure to remove a foreign body or loss of a patient can never be excused or justified by the lack of proper equipment. Many of the complications and failures of attempted foreign body removal arise because the endoscopist lacks the instruments specifically designed for the problem. This is not a valid excuse, but merely a regrettable explanation of the failure. If a full range of rigid scopes and foreign body forceps is not available, the procedure should not be attempted.

The equipment must be in perfect repair and working order. The forceps are adjusted and lubricated so they are smooth in operation and so the blades close completely when the handles are closed. At least two forceps are selected before surgery because unexpected circumstances arising during the procedure may require an alternative. Ideally, all instruments should be sterile and stored in a cabinet with glass doors so they are readily available in an emergency. Potential problems may arise if instruments are wrapped in sterile packages and kept in storage areas outside the endoscopy suite.

Surgical Team

Adequate training and experience are important for the anesthesiologist, nursing personnel, and endoscopist. The importance of cooperation, communication, and a team approach to foreign body extraction cannot be overemphasized. The anesthesiologist, scrub nurse, circulating nurse, and endoscopist all must have experience with the extraction of foreign bodies. If such a team cannot be assembled promptly, consideration is given to delaying the procedure until they are available. A plan for orderly removal of the object is discussed with each member of the team and his or her role in that plan is delineated clearly. The procedure is not begun until all members of the team are prepared and positioned appropriately.

Anesthesia

General anesthesia is used for endoscopic extraction of foreign bodies. Preoperative sedation is generally avoided. Instead, the parents, anesthesiologist, and nursing staff help keep the child calm before induction to avoid dislodgment of the foreign body because of crying. Electrocardiography, pulse, oxygen saturation, and end-tidal carbon dioxide are routinely monitored. A large-bore intravenous catheter is placed.

Spontaneous respiration during the procedure is preferred because it is somewhat safer than apneic techniques in which the patient is completely paralyzed and therefore cannot move any air if the airway is temporarily lost. Positive-pressure ventilation (bagging) is avoided because this tends to drive the foreign body further peripherally. As anesthesia lightens, an occasional cough actually may help propel the foreign body toward the bronchoscope.

An inhalation anesthetic, typically halothane, is delivered through the closed system of a rigid bronchoscope. The larynx and trachea are sprayed with topical 4% lidocaine before the bronchoscope is introduced. Once the bronchoscope is in place, lidocaine also can be administered to the

bronchi. During the actual attempts at extraction, 100% oxygen is given through the bronchoscope.

Basic Technique

Prepared by practice with a duplicate of the foreign body and review of the radiographs, the surgeon introduces the bronchoscope. Once the bronchoscope has been advanced into the trachea, ventilation is established and confirmed by the endoscopist. The tracheobronchial tree is inspected completely because multiple foreign bodies are present in up to 9% of cases, as emphasized by Hughes and colleagues (1996). Inspection begins with the normal bronchus. All secretions are aspirated to ensure optimal respiratory function when the involved side is inspected. The location of the foreign body is approached slowly and carefully to avoid overriding or displacement. Care is taken to avoid driving the foreign body further down. Suction is used to remove secretions from around the foreign body, but it is not used in the attempt at extraction.

The endoscopist must resist the impulse to seize the foreign body as soon as it is discovered. Before any attempt at extraction, a careful study is made to determine the size, shape, position, probable location of unseen parts, and relation to surrounding structures. As determined by the appearance of the presenting part, combined with the knowledge obtained from the radiographic studies, the endoscopist may suspect that sharp points are buried deep within the mucosa or outside the wall in the mediastinum. The presentation of the foreign body may be modified with the tip of the scope, a technique that is especially helpful when establishing forceps spaces between the object and the lumen walls. When the most favorable point in position for grasping has been ascertained, the closed forceps is inserted through the scope (Fig. 73-3).

All manipulation is gentle and delicate. The forceps is advanced until it lightly touches the foreign body, and the endoscope is withdrawn a short distance to permit the forceps blades to be opened. The forceps blades are advanced until the tips pass the equator of the object; then the forceps blades are closed. The tip of the scope is advanced against the foreign body, which is held against the tube mouth. The grasp of the forceps is maintained firmly by the fingers of the right hand while all traction for withdrawal is made by the left hand. The thumb of the left hand firmly clamps the forceps to lock the relationship between the forceps and the scope during extraction so that the three units are extracted as one. The bronchoscope keeps the vocal cords apart until the foreign body has exited the glottis. Just before exiting the glottis, the foreign body is rotated to the sagittal plane, which is the largest diameter of the laryngeal lumen.

After removal of a foreign body from the tracheobronchial tree, the laryngoscope is reinserted and a second pass is made with the bronchoscope. Retained secretions are aspirated and the entire tracheobronchial tree is rechecked to be certain that no fragments or other objects remain. Granulation tissue is resected as necessary and bleeding can be controlled with a

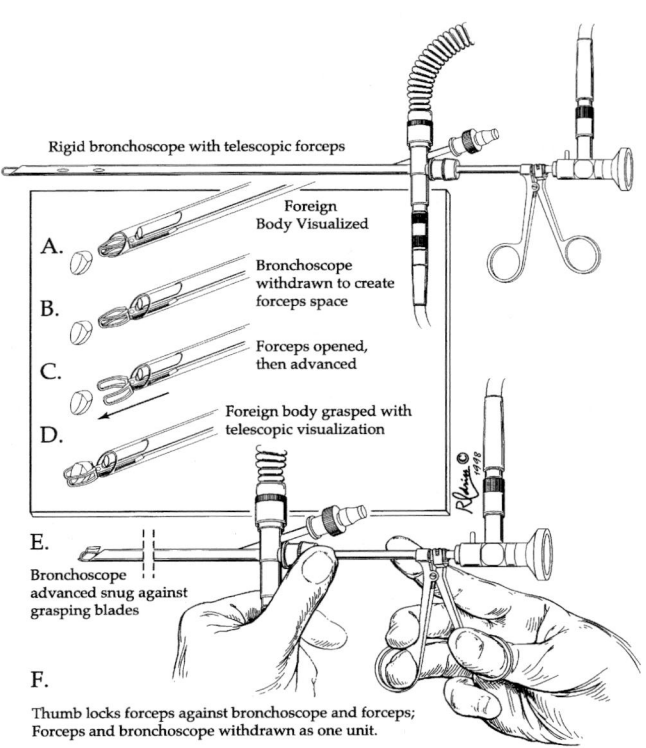

Fig. 73-3. Basic technique of airway foreign body extraction. Modified from Jackson C, Jackson CL: Diseases of the Air and Food Passages of Foreign Body Origin. Philadelphia: WB Saunders, 1936.

topical vasoconstrictive agent. Oxymetazoline probably has the greatest therapeutic index for the respiratory mucosa, as demonstrated by Riegle and colleagues (1992).

Special Techniques

In the rare circumstance that a spherical foreign body cannot be removed, a Fogarty catheter may be lubricated and passed through the bronchoscope, distal to the object. The balloon is then inflated and withdrawn in order to dislodge the object proximally and allow its extraction. Good and Deutsch (1998) suggest a Fogarty catheter may be especially useful in the case of a hollow spherical object, such as a hair bead.

Special techniques have been developed for the extraction of pointed objects (Fig. 73-4). The endoscopist must resist being pressured into hasty action without thorough preparation. The first priority during the extraction procedure is to localize the point. The point is released and sheathed within the scope. It often is necessary to accomplish this by first moving the object distally to disengage the point, then advancing the scope over the object, rather than pulling the object into the tube.

Long, pointed objects typically lodge with the point facing upward. This occurs even if the object enters point first. The point becomes engaged by the mucosa and the object

tumbles, then proceeds with the point trailing. Pins, needles, and similar long, pointed objects fall into two categories: breakable needles and pins and bendable pins. A pin-bending forceps may be useful in extracting these objects.

Special techniques for long, pointed objects include aligning the bronchus to approach the object by its long axis. Biplane fluoroscopy may be of assistance in this situation. Magnets have been used also. Tacks, nails, and large-headed foreign bodies in the tracheobronchial tree are released, sheathed, and removed with an inward rotation method that is used for pins and needles with imbedded points. A side-grasping forceps captures the pin at the point. A corkscrew motion is used to push the pin distally while rotating it clockwise, freeing the point and aligning the shaft with the long axis of the forceps. The scope is then advanced over the point to sheath it for extraction.

Double-pointed objects sometimes can be bent to convert them to a single point for extraction. A broad-tack forceps or wide-staple forceps may be used to protect both points simultaneously during extraction.

When a point cannot be sheathed, the foreign body may be withdrawn with the point trailing. A rotation forceps allows a point to rotate and trail.

For a sharp bone that could not be safely dislodged, Boelcskei and colleagues (1995) described the use of the neodymium:yttrium-aluminum-garnet laser to cut the bone into smaller fragments to facilitate extraction.

Fluoroscopic assistance is used for radiopaque upper lobe foreign bodies, pins in the lung periphery, and sharp or irregular foreign bodies, such as dental bridge work. For accurate localization, simultaneous biplane fluoroscopy is required; it may be available only in a special procedures room within the radiology department. The technique is deceptively simple but extremely hazardous because the fluoroscope does not visualize the tissues that lie between the forceps blades and the foreign body.

Stripping Off

As a foreign body is brought out through the larynx, the lateral pressure of the vocal folds may strip it from the forceps grasp. Because complete airway obstruction ensues, a prompt, efficient response is required. The airway is reestablished immediately by removing the object or by pushing it down into the bronchus in which it had been lodged, allowing ventilation of the good lung. The faulty technique is corrected and the object is relocated and extracted.

A foreign body lost in the trachea usually is carried into the normal bronchus. This occurs because the previously obstructed lung or lobe moves little air and is edematous or narrowed by granulation tissue. This creates an immediate and critical emergency because the child's only functional lung is completely obstructed. The object must be removed immediately or relocated into the other bronchus. If the foreign body cannot be visualized readily, it may be found next

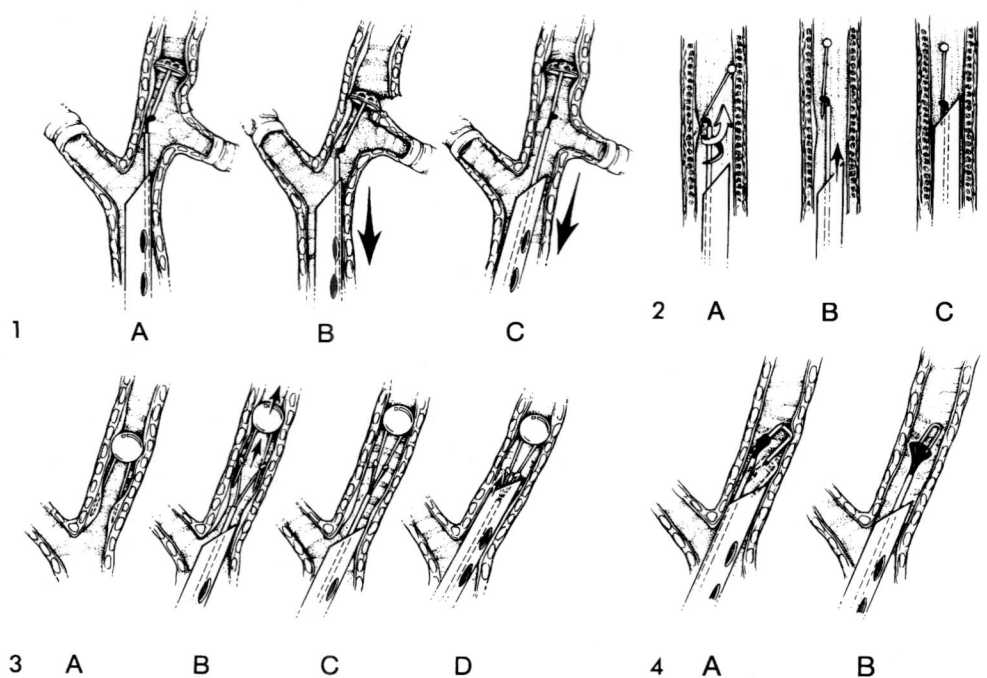

Fig. 73-4. Techniques of endoscopic removal. **1.** Long axis traction is particularly important for pointed objects with large heads. The point may be easily located (**A**), but greater hazard lies in risk of tearing the bronchial wall with the head of the tack (**B**). Positioning the patient's head toward the opposite side straightens the axis of airway, permitting relatively safe, slow, and steady withdrawal of the object (**C**). **2.** Inward rotation method is used for pins or needles with imbedded point. Side-grasping forceps capture pin near point (**A**). Corkscrew motion is used to push the pin distally while rotating it clockwise, freeing the point and aligning the shaft with the long axis of the forceps (**B**). The scope is advanced over the point to sheathe (**C**) for extraction. **3.** Technique of managing bendable double-pointed objects. Points buried in the mucosal wall (**A**) are released by moving them distally (**B**). Points are approximated (**C**), then sheathed for extraction by advancing the rigid scope (**D**). **4.** Tucker staple forceps (**A**) is angled to permit sheathing of both points within the beveled tip of the bronchoscope. Jackson broad-staple forceps (**B**) grasps and protects both points during advancement of the bronchoscope to sheathe them. From Holinger LD: Management of sharp and penetrating foreign bodies of the upper aerodigestive tract. Ann Otol Rhinol Laryngol 99:684, 1990. With permission.

to the scope, below the vocal folds, or in the mouth, hypopharynx, or nasopharynx.

"Stripping off" may result from factors related to the forceps or the foreign body itself. Forceps factors include faulty application of the forceps, use of the wrong forceps for the problem, mechanically imperfect forceps, and poorly adjusted or poorly constructed forceps. Three foreign body factors can lead to stripping off: poor orientation of the foreign body (solution: rotate 90 degrees at the vocal folds); insecure grasp of the foreign body (solution: sheath the foreign body with the end of the bronchoscope and lock the forceps against the bronchoscope with the left thumb); and a foreign body is too large for the laryngeal lumen (solution: fragment the foreign body or remove it through a tracheotomy).

Postoperative Treatment

After endoscopic foreign body extraction, the patient is usually admitted to the hospital for overnight observation. Antibiotics are prescribed only if there was a preoperative diagnosis of pneumonia. In cases of pneumonia or purulent bronchitis, chest physical therapy is indicated. On the day after the procedure, if the patient is afebrile and the lungs are clear to auscultation, the patient is discharged home. However, if the patient remains febrile or has persistent pulmonary signs or symptoms, chest radiography is performed and appropriate therapeutic measures are taken.

COMPLICATIONS

Immediate complications of endoscopic extraction or attempted extraction include pneumomediastinum, laryngeal impaction and complete obstruction, and failure to recover the object, which necessitates thoracotomy. In the recovery room, laryngeal edema or bronchospasm may compromise the airway. Late complications include pneumonia, atelectasis, and granuloma or stricture formation, with their resulting problems.

Traumatic laryngitis and laryngeal edema are treated with elevation of the head of the bed, humidity, racemic epinephrine, and high-dose corticosteroids (1 mg/kg of dexamethasone, up to 20 mg, intravenously as a bolus). When laryngeal edema is anticipated, corticosteroid therapy should be initiated in the operating room. Laryngeal edema is proportional to the time the bronchoscope is in the larynx, the trauma of the procedure, and the size of the bronchoscope in relation to the size of the larynx. To prevent laryngeal edema, smaller bronchoscopes that pass easily through the larynx are preferred, although there may be a slight leak if positive pressure is required.

Repetition of any endoscopic procedure after an unsuccessful attempt at removal is avoided until laryngeal symptoms resolve. Three to 7 days usually is adequate. It is wise to use this waiting period in patients who have had previous attempts at endoscopic extraction elsewhere. The presence of severe respiratory obstruction is an obvious exception to these guidelines.

If the initial attempt at endoscopic extraction is unsuccessful because of abundant, bleeding granulation tissue and purulent bronchitis, the patient should be treated for approximately 3 days with intravenous and nebulized dexamethasone and intravenous antibiotics. Such treatment has resulted in dramatic resolution of the granulation tissue before endoscopic extraction has been reattempted.

The aspirated foreign body that is most likely to result in failed endoscopic extraction is the flowering head of grasses such as timothy. Jackson (1952) noted that by means of its long, stiff bristles, the grasshead propels itself through tissues with each breath, until it emerges days to months later via a bronchocutaneous fistula. At bronchoscopy, usually only granulation tissue and purulent secretions are seen. Thus, thoracotomy and segmentectomy are almost always indicated.

Complications of Nonendoscopic Means of Foreign Body Extraction

Postural drainage (chest physical therapy) and bronchodilators were suggested by Burrington and Cotton (1972) as an alternative to bronchoscopic removal of airway foreign bodies. This ill-advised and poorly conceived technique has led to at least four cases of respiratory arrest, one of which also involved transient cortical blindness. This throwback to the nineteenth century does no more than serve as a makeshift alternative for those who are unskilled in modern bronchoscopic techniques. Although Campbell and Cotton (1982) retracted this recommendation for the treatment of foreign bodies in the main bronchi, they continue to advocate its use for peripheral foreign bodies. In a subsequent series of 28 such cases, only 18 were treated successfully with this therapy. Endoscopic extractions salvaged 8 of the 10 failures.

PREVENTION

Potentially all cases of foreign body aspiration are preventable. In 1923, Jackson initiated the first public awareness campaign, directed chiefly at parents, teachers, and nurses. Continued public education is of paramount importance. A reasonable goal would be to instruct every caregiver about foreign body aspiration prevention strategies and first aid techniques at their first visit with a pediatrician. An informative pamphlet entitled "Choking Prevention and First Aid for Infants and Children, Guidelines for Parents" is available from the American Academy of Pediatrics.

Continued vigilance by the Consumers Products Safety Commission is also necessary. In 1979, the Consumers Products Safety Commission issued federal regulations to ban certain toys from children under 3 years of age. Hazardous toys are identified by their ability to pass through a "small parts" cylinder. However, as Reilly (1990) noted, many spherical objects that have caused childhood asphyxiation actually pass this test. Therefore, tighter standards in toy testing are indicated.

Foods could also be made safer. In 1984, Harris and colleagues suggested that the United States government adopt labeling regulations for dangerous food products, as is done in Sweden. For example, package labels should instruct parents not to feed nuts or crunchy peanut butter to children under 4 years of age. Additionally, labels should instruct parents not to feed hot dogs or grapes to toddlers until these foods are cut into small quarter sections.

Despite such measures, it is unlikely that all cases of foreign body aspiration can be prevented. Therefore, prevention of unnecessary complications should be considered. As stated initially, a key to preventing complications is an early diagnosis. Schimpl and colleagues (1991) found that the complication rate of pediatric foreign body aspiration is increased 17 times when bronchoscopy is delayed more than 12 hours. To facilitate early diagnosis, a radiopaque material should be placed within all plastic toys. Furthermore, to educate our colleagues, the fundamentals of diagnosis of foreign body aspiration should be taught routinely within medical school and pediatric residency curricula.

REFERENCES

American Academy of Pediatrics: Choking prevention and first aid for infants and children, guidelines for parents. Elk Grove Village, IL: American Academy of Pediatrics, 1990.
Black RE, Johnson DG, Matlak ME: Bronchoscopic removal of foreign bodies in children. J Pediatr Surg 29:682, 1994.
Boelcskei PL, Wagner M, Lessnau KL: Laser-assisted removal of a foreign body in the bronchial system of an infant. Laser Surg Med 17:375, 1995.
Bradwell S: Helps for sudden accidents endangering life. London: Thomas Purfoot, 1633.
Burrington JD, Cotton EK: Removal of foreign bodies from the tracheobronchial tree. J Pediatr Surg 7:119, 1972.
Burton EM, et al: Pneumomediastinum caused by foreign body aspiration in children. Pediatr Radiol 20:45, 1989.
Campbell DM, Cotton EK, Lilly JR: A dual approach to tracheobronchial foreign bodies in children. Surgery 91:178, 1982.
Darrow DH, Holinger LD: Foreign bodies of the larynx, trachea, and bronchi. In Bluestone CD, Stool S, Kenna MA (eds): Pediatric Otolaryngology. 3rd Ed. Philadelphia: WB Saunders, 1995.
Esclamado RN, Richardson MA: Laryngotracheal foreign bodies in children. Am J Dis Child 141:259, 1987.

Good GA, Deutsch ES: Method for removing endobronchial beads. Ann Otol Rhinol Laryngol 107:291, 1998.

Harris CS, et al: Childhood asphyxiation by food. A national analysis and overview. JAMA 251:2231, 1984.

Heimlich HJ: A life-saving maneuver to prevent food-choking. JAMA 234:398, 1975.

Holinger LD: Management of sharp and penetrating foreign bodies of the upper aerodigestive tract. Ann Otol Rhinol Laryngol 99:684, 1990.

Holinger LD: Foreign bodies of the airway and esophagus. In Holinger LD, Lusk RP, Green CG (eds): Pediatric Laryngology and Broncho-esophagology. Philadelphia: Lippincott–Raven, 1997.

Holinger PH: Foreign bodies in the air and food passages. Trans Am Acad Ophthalmol Otolaryngol 66:193, 1962.

Hughes CA, Baroody FM, Marsh BR: Pediatric tracheobronchial foreign bodies: historical review from the Johns Hopkins Hospital. Ann Otol Rhinol Laryngol 105:555, 1996.

Imaizumi H, et al: Definitive diagnosis and location of peanuts in the airways using magnetic resonance imaging techniques. Ann Emerg Med 23:1379, 1994.

Jackson C: The Life of Chevalier Jackson. New York: Macmillan, 1938.

Jackson C, Jackson CL: Diseases of the air and food passages of foreign body origin. Philadelphia: WB Saunders, 1936.

Jackson C, Jackson CL: Bronchoesophagology. Philadelphia: WB Saunders, 1950.

Jackson CL: Grasses as foreign bodies in the bronchus and lungs. Laryngoscope 62:897, 1952.

Killian G: Direct endoscopy of the upper air-passages and oesophagus: its diagnosis and therapeutic value in the search for and removal of foreign bodies. J Laryngol Rhinol Otol 17:461, 1902.

Mantor PC, Tuggle DW, Tunell WP: An appropriate negative bronchoscopy rate in suspected foreign body aspiration. Am J Surg 158:622, 1989.

Maves MD, Carithers JS, Birck HG: Esophageal burns secondary to disc battery ingestion. Ann Otol Rhinol Laryngol 93:364, 1984.

Mu LC, Sun DQ, He P: Radiologic diagnosis of aspirated foreign bodies in children: review of 343 cases. J Laryngol Otol 104:778, 1990.

National Safety Council: Accident Facts. 1997 Ed. Chicago: National Safety Council, 1997.

Overdahl MC, Wewers MD: Acute occlusion of a mainstem bronchus by a rapidly expanding foreign body. Chest 105:1600, 1994.

Reilly JS: Prevention of aspiration in infants and young children: federal regulations. Ann Otol Rhinol Laryngol 99:273, 1990.

Reilly JS, et al: Pediatric aerodigestive foreign body injuries are complications related to timeliness of diagnosis. Laryngoscope 107:17, 1997.

Riegle EV, et al: Comparison of vasoconstrictors for functional endoscopic sinus surgery in children. Laryngoscope 102:820, 1992.

Ryan CA, et al: Childhood deaths from toy balloons. Am J Dis Child 144:1221, 1990.

Schimpl G, et al: [Foreign body aspiration in children. The advantages of emergency endoscopy and foreign body removal.] [German] Anaesthesist 40:479, 1991.

Vane DW, et al: Bronchoscopy for aspirated foreign bodies in children. Experience in 131 cases. Arch Surg 123:885, 1988.

Wetmore RF: Foreign bodies of the aerodigestive tract. In Gates GA (ed): Current Therapy in Otolaryngology-Head and Neck Surgery. 5th ed. St. Louis: Mosby–Year Book, 1994.

Wiseman NE: The diagnosis of foreign body aspiration in childhood. J Pediatr Surg 19:531, 1984.

CHAPTER 74

Diaphragmatic Injuries

Panagiotis N. Symbas

Diaphragmatic lacerations may result from penetrating or blunt trauma to this musculotendinous structure that separates the thoracic and abdominal cavities. If the laceration is unrecognized and not promptly repaired, one or more of the abdominal viscera will herniate into the thoracic cavity, with resulting early or late compromise of ventilatory or gastrointestinal function. Immediate herniation is most often associated with a large tear in one of the diaphragmatic leaves, but the symptoms of the herniation usually are obscured by the symptoms of other associated injured organs or structures. Small rents such as those caused by stab wounds rarely are symptomatic early, but if they are unrepaired, progressive abdominal visceral herniation occurs because of the pressure gradient between the thoracic and peritoneal cavities. As the herniation of abdominal viscera progresses, the likelihood of ventilatory compromise or of mechanical obstruction, with or without strangulation, of a portion of the contained gastrointestinal tract increases.

Diaphragmatic injuries usually are caused by penetrating or blunt trauma, and rarely they may be due to iatrogenic injury, to spontaneous rupture during pregnancy, or to unexplained spontaneous rupture. They can be separated into two categories: those recognized at the time of initial hospitalization for the evaluation of an episode of trauma and those missed initially and recognized at some time remote from the first hospitalization.

RECOGNITION DURING INITIAL HOSPITALIZATION

The mechanism, symptoms, and other features of blunt and penetrating injuries are dissimilar. Therefore, the initial recognition and management of these two types of injury are best discussed separately.

Blunt Diaphragmatic Trauma

Rupture of a portion of the diaphragm usually results from decelerating injuries suffered in motor vehicle accidents or from falls from great heights. Other crushing injuries to the lower chest or upper abdomen also may result in laceration of the diaphragm. Beal and McKennan (1988) reported an incidence of 3% of ruptured diaphragm in those patients experiencing severe blunt trauma who survived long enough to be admitted to the hospital.

The rupture most commonly occurs in the left leaf. Contrary to common belief, the right hemidiaphragm is not immune from injury. The ratio of rupture of the left versus the right hemidiaphragm in my experience (1986) was 5:1; Estrera and colleagues (1985) reported a 34% incidence of right-sided rupture; and Shah and colleagues (1995), in a collective review of the literature, found rupture of the left diaphragm in 68.5%, the right in 24.2%, bilateral in 1.5%, pericardial in 0.9%, and unclassified in 4.9%. Injuries on the right side are usually posterolateral to the central tendon. The pericardial or central portion of the diaphragm also may be ruptured, and avulsion of the diaphragm from the rib cage infrequently occurs.

Pathology

On the left side, the organs most commonly herniated into the chest are the stomach, spleen, large bowel, liver, small intestine, and omentum. On the right, when herniation occurs, the liver is always present and the colon is occasionally herniated, as Brown and Richardson (1985) reported. Vascular injuries (tears of the juxtahepatic vena cava and hepatic vein injuries) as well as lacerations of the liver frequently are associated with rupture of the right hemidiaphragm.

Symptomatology

Symptoms and signs of diaphragmatic rupture (e.g., respiratory distress, cardiac disturbances, deviated trachea, and bowel sounds in the chest) are present in the minority of patients initially seen after the blunt injury; most symptoms present are related to other organ system injuries or to the presence of hypovolemic shock.

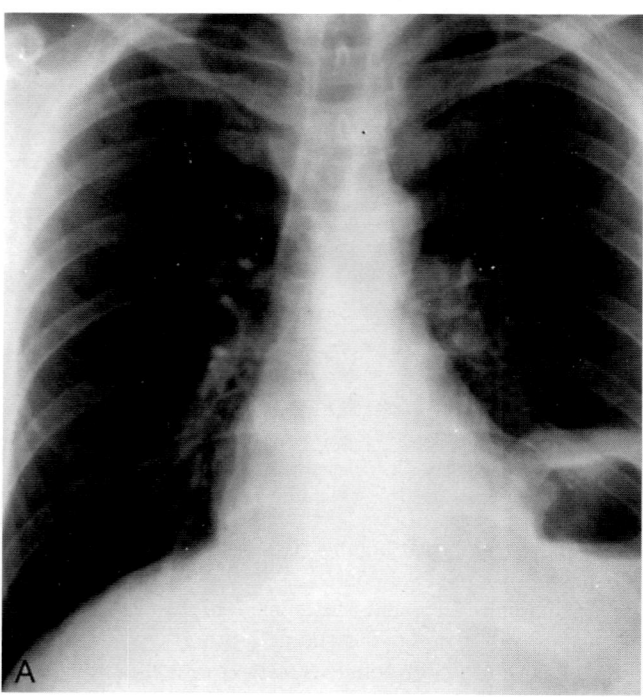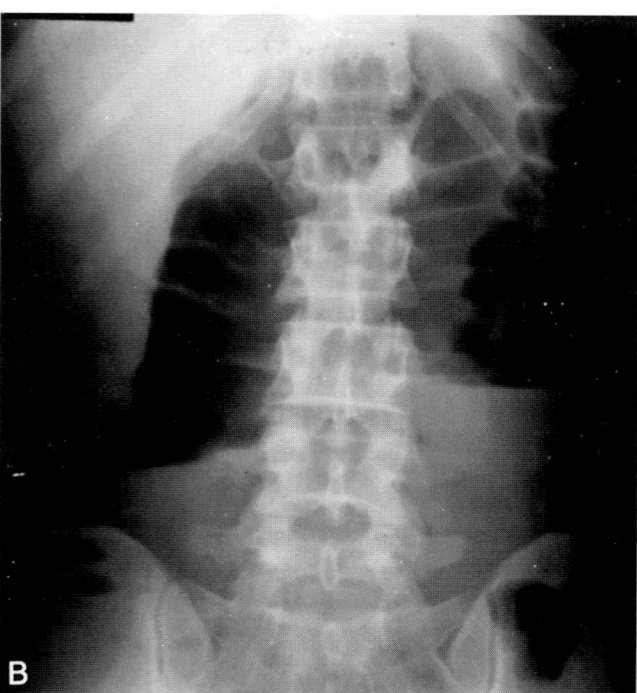

Fig. 74-1. Radiographs of a 30-year-old man after a vehicular accident. **A.** Frontal view of the chest shows abnormal diaphragmatic silhouette. **B.** Plain radiograph of the abdomen reveals upward displacement of the transverse colon. From Symbas PN, Vlasis SE, Hatcher C Jr: Blunt and penetrating diaphragmatic injuries with or without herniation of organs into the chest. Ann Thorac Surg *42*:158, 1986. With permission.

Radiographic Examinations

Routine radiography of the chest is the most efficient study when the patient is stable enough to have the procedure done. It is abnormal in almost all and is diagnostic of rupture in over one-half of the patients. Abnormal radiography results of the chest show an elevated, obscured, or irregular diaphragmatic dome on the side of the visceral herniation. The costophrenic angle is almost always blunted because of contained fluid. With lacerations on the left, one or more air-fluid levels and radiolucency in the lower lung field, with or without shifting of the mediastinum away from the side of the hernia, appear (Fig. 74-1). Occasionally, the nasogastric tube can be seen to turn upward into the chest (Fig. 74-2). With right-sided injuries, the right leaf is markedly elevated with or without an associated fluid collection; air-fluid levels are less frequently observed. Occasionally, a rounded shadow protruding above the leaf appears on the lateral film, which is highly diagnostic for right-sided rupture (Fig. 74-3). Nondiagnostic findings of a pneumothorax, hydrothorax (hemothorax), or both, are also frequently present.

Diagnosis

Radiography of the chest may be diagnostic, as noted. In those patients too ill to be moved, Ammann and colleagues (1983) suggested using bedside real-time sonographic examination. In patients not requiring emergency operation, the diagnosis may be confirmed with barium contrast studies of either the upper or lower gastrointestinal tract. Computed tomography, as Heiberg (1980) and Toombs (1981) and their associates reported, can likewise be used to demonstrate the herniation. When right-sided injury is suspected and conditions permit, fluoroscopic examination and radionuclide liver scan, as well as ultrasonography and computed tomography, can be done to delineate the herniated portion of the liver. The use of diagnostic pneumoperitoneum is rarely indicated. In patients requiring emergency operation for control of bleeding or correction of other life-threatening injuries, the diagnosis must be made at operation. Both leaves of the diaphragm, therefore, must be adequately inspected in all patients who are operated on with severe blunt chest and upper abdominal injuries.

On rare occasions when the diagnosis cannot be established by the previously mentioned tests and the patient is stable, magnetic resonance imaging, as reported by Carter and associates (1996), or video-assisted thoracoscopy, as recorded by Spann (1995) and Lindsey (1997) and their colleagues, establishes the diagnosis.

Treatment

Because of the danger of development of respiratory and even circulatory embarrassment or visceral obstruction, with

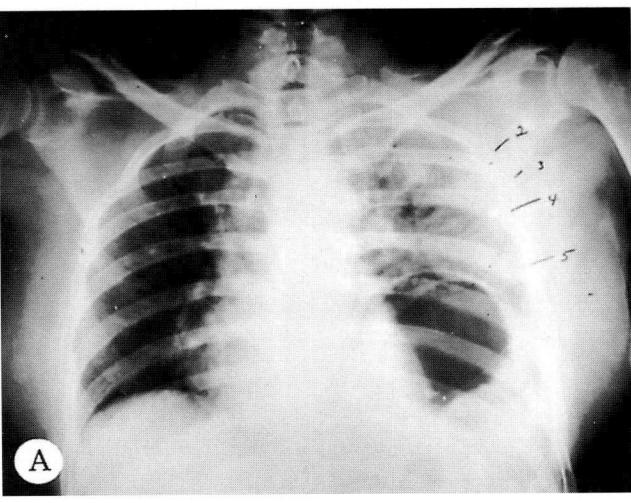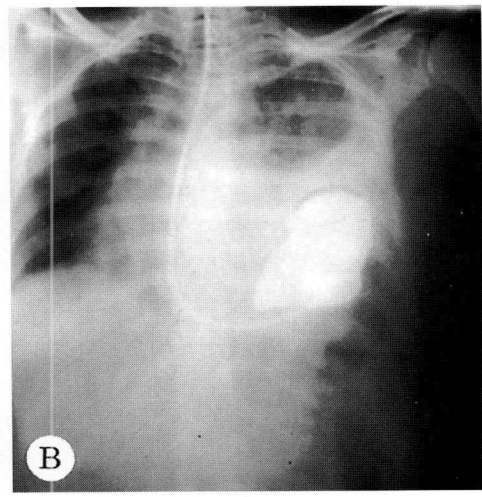

Fig. 74-2. A. Radiograph of chest made 12 hours after severe trauma, showing multiple rib fractures and a large gas bubble in the lower portion of the left side of the chest. B. Barium study revealed the large gas shadow to be the stomach, which had herniated through the ruptured diaphragm.

incarceration or strangulation of the involved portion of the gastrointestinal tract, diaphragmatic injury should be repaired surgically as soon as possible after the diagnosis is established and when the patient's clinical condition permits. Although a diaphragmatic leaf may be best exposed through the chest, the approach chosen should be based on the clinical findings in each patient. Because the major source of massive bleeding is usually a lacerated abdominal viscus, Beal and McKennan (1988) prefer the abdominal approach. During the acute postinjury period, the diaphragmatic injury should be repaired through the incision required for the emergency repair of other organ injuries. In all the patients who were operated on by the author and associates (1986) shortly after the injury, laparotomy was the incision used.

Tears of the left hemidiaphragm are most often repaired through the abdomen because of frequently associated injuries to intra-abdominal organs, although in the absence of any symptoms suggesting such injury, a left thoracotomy is adequate. Tears of the right hemidiaphragm, when recognized preoperatively, are best repaired through a right thoracotomy, as Estrera and associates described in 1979. In 1985, however, these authors recommended that the approach be individualized, depending primarily on which cavity (thorax or abdomen) shows continued evidence of bleeding. When injury to the retrohepatic vena cava or hepatic veins is encountered during an abdominal approach, Estrera and associates (1985) extend the incision by a median sternotomy to place a temporary vena cava shunt to control the bleeding.

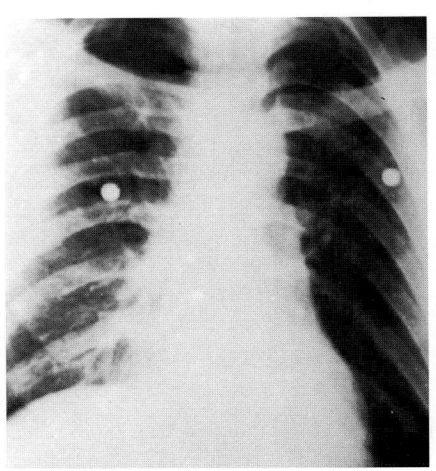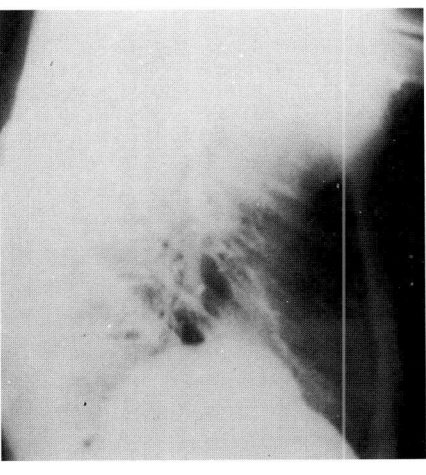

,B

Fig. 74-3. Chest radiographs of a patient with ruptured right hemidiaphragm and partial herniation of the liver. A. Posteroanterior view suggested only minimal elevation of the right hemidiaphragm. B. Lateral view was fairly impressive. From Estrera A, et al: Blunt traumatic rupture of the right hemidiaphragm: experience in 12 patients. Ann Thorac Surg 39:525, 1985. With permission.

After control and repair of other associated visceral injuries, the diaphragmatic tear is closed with interrupted figure-of-eight No. 0 nonabsorbable sutures. Prosthetic material is rarely needed in acute blunt trauma injuries. Disruption of the repaired diaphragmatic leaf is rare.

Mortality

The mortality may be high in these patients, not as the result of the diaphragmatic injury per se but as the consequence of other severe visceral trauma. The author and associates (1986) reported a 22% mortality in this group of patients. Brooks (1978) and Brown and Richardson (1985) reported rates of 14% and 17%, respectively. Beal and McKennan (1988) reported a mortality of 40.5%. Ninety-seven percent of their patients had associated injuries, and 87% of those who died were in severe hypovolemic shock when admitted to the hospital.

Penetrating Diaphragmatic Injuries

Penetrating diaphragmatic injuries usually result from stab wounds or gunshot wounds of the lower chest (e.g., below the nipples), the upper abdomen (e.g., epigastrium), the flanks, or the back; one-half of the patients treated by me and my associates (1986) had a wound of the chest below the nipples, but injuries of all other sites of the trunk were associated with a diaphragmatic wound. Injury to either diaphragmatic leaf occurs with almost equal frequency.

Pathology

The diaphragmatic injury is generally small, and herniation of the abdominal viscera into the chest is usually absent early. Only if the injury is missed does late herniation occur because of the different pressures in the two cavities.

Symptomatology

The history and physical examination per se do not indicate diaphragmatic injury. The presence of abdominal complaints or findings in a patient who has sustained a chest wound, however, are strongly suggestive of diaphragmatic injury, as is the presence of chest findings when the site of entrance of the wound is the abdomen or flank. Many patients, however, only have findings associated with the cavity of entrance, and the diaphragmatic injury remains unsuspected until the time of exploration or, unfortunately, is occasionally missed entirely when exploration of either the chest or abdomen was thought not to be indicated. This latter event most often occurs with stab wounds, because patients with gunshot wounds of the trunk usually undergo either emergency abdominal or thoracic exploration.

Radiographic Findings

In 93 instances of penetrating injuries of the diaphragm, Miller and associates (1984) reported the radiograph of the chest to have been normal in 43% and abnormal in 57%. The abnormalities were a hemothorax, pneumothorax, or both in 96% and herniated abdominal contents or pneumoperitoneum in 2% each. The author and associates (1986) found the radiograph results to be normal in one-third of 185 patients with this type of injury.

Diagnosis

A high index of suspicion of the presence of a diaphragmatic injury must be present in all penetrating injuries of the trunk and particularly in those with wounds from the nipple line to the umbilicus. Miller and associates (1984), among others, have suggested that all such penetrating injuries, symptomatic or not, should be explored and complete inspection of both leaves of the diaphragm be carried out. In their series, 13% of the patients had no associated injuries. The author concurs with this policy for any gunshot wound, but at times a more conservative approach can be used in the management of stab wounds, most of which are explored because of associated symptomatology. In the absence of any findings or suggestion of injury to the diaphragm or any visceral injury, however, exploration may not be mandatory. A few stab wound injuries to the diaphragm will undoubtedly be missed with this approach, possibly as high as 13%, according to Miller and associates' (1984) report. Pneumoperitoneum and abdominal paracentesis generally are of no aid in identifying these missed injuries early, and ultrasonography and computed tomographic examinations are of limited value. When the diagnosis cannot be established with these tests and chest radiography shows an otherwise unexplained, persistent abnormality of the diaphragm or the lower lung field or both, laparoscopy, as reported by Ivatury and coworkers (1992), or video-assisted thoracoscopy, as recorded by Spann and associates (1995), reliably diagnoses or rules out diaphragmatic injury. Elective barium studies should be recommended in a 4- to 6-week period after the patient's discharge when routine exploration or thoracoscopy has not been done.

Treatment

In the absence of intrathoracic organ injury or major intrapleural bleeding, the abdominal approach is always preferred because it permits detection and treatment of nonevident intra-abdominal injury and enables the surgeon to examine both diaphragmatic leaflets, which is not possible through a transthoracic approach. Any injury to the diaphragm can be repaired readily with No. 0 nonabsorbable interrupted sutures.

Mortality

Diaphragmatic injury should not cause death. Associated organ injury, however, results in a variable number of

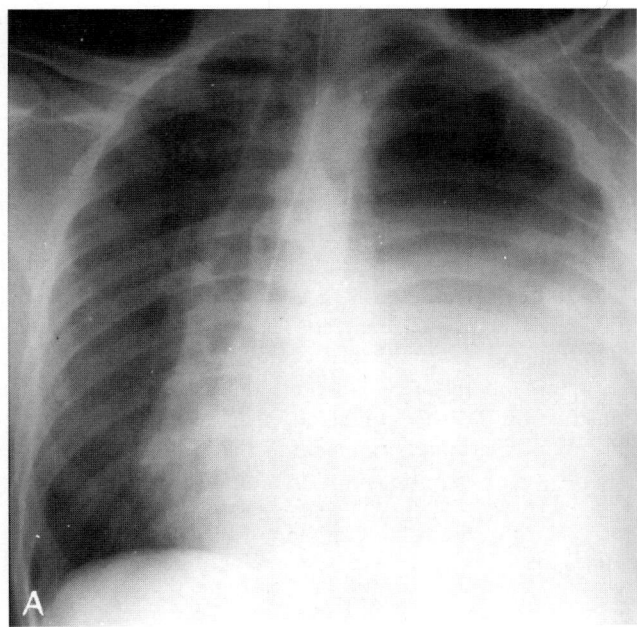

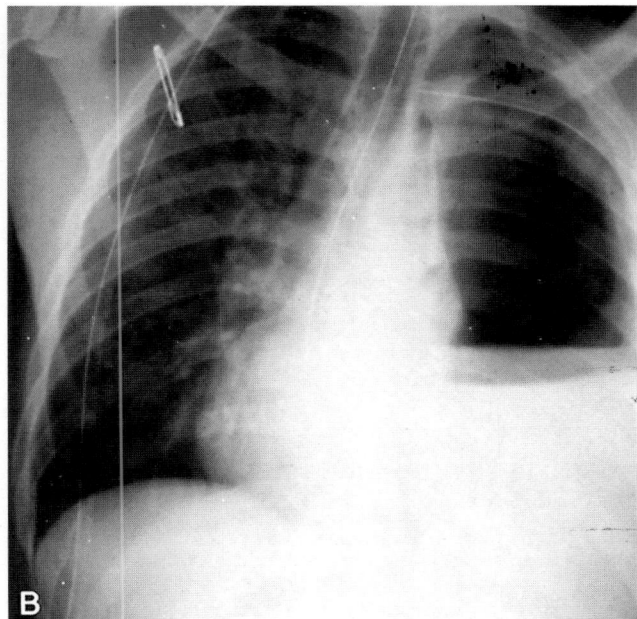

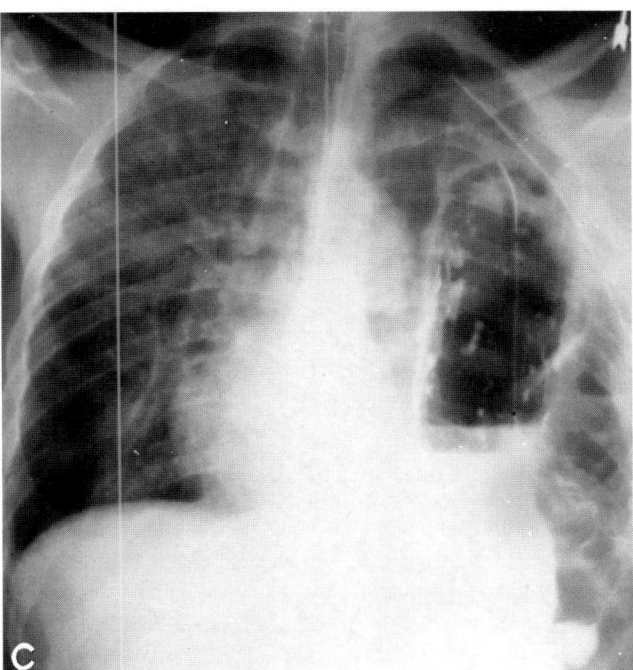

Fig. 74-4. Chest radiographs of a 46-year-old man who was involved in a car accident 6 years earlier. **A.** Supine chest radiograph shows radiodensity of the lower left lung field and radiolucency of the upper left field with displacement of the mediastinum. **B.** Erect frontal view shows two air-fluid levels. **C.** Upper gastrointestinal series and barium enema demonstrate both the stomach and large bowels in the left chest. From Symbas PN, Vlasis SE, Hatcher C Jr: Blunt and penetrating diaphragmatic injuries with or without herniation of organs into the chest. Ann Thorac Surg *42*:158, 1986. With permission.

deaths. In my series of 185 penetrating injuries, four deaths occurred—a mortality of 2.2%.

LATE RECOGNITION

The initial injury to the diaphragm, from either blunt or penetrating trauma, may be undetected during the patient's first hospitalization and may only become manifest because of symptoms or signs related to a hernia of one or more abdominal viscera into the chest. Although no large body of data is available, it is most likely that more late diaphragmatic hernias result from missed stab wound injuries than from blunt trauma. In a small series reported by Hegarty and colleagues (1978), 22 of 25 late hernias were from previous stab wounds. Nonetheless, many examples of herniation caused by blunt injuries have been observed (Figs. 74-4 and 74-5).

These hernias may be recognized any time from a few weeks to over three or four decades after the original injury. The hernias resulting from blunt trauma tend to be larger,

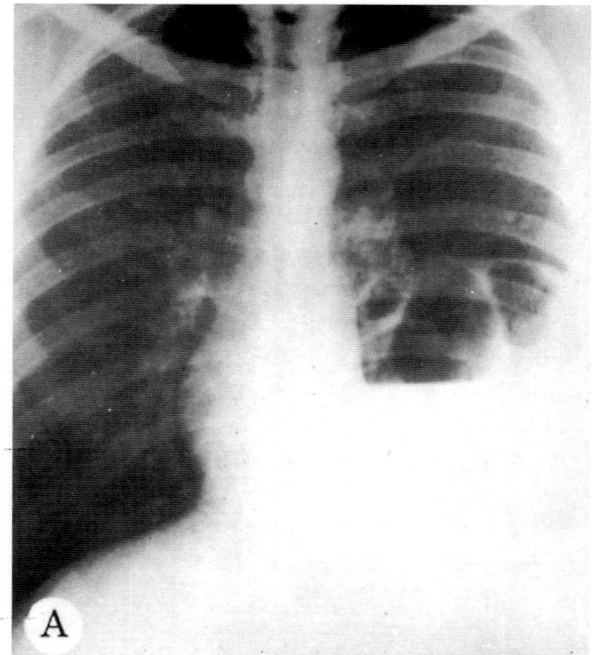

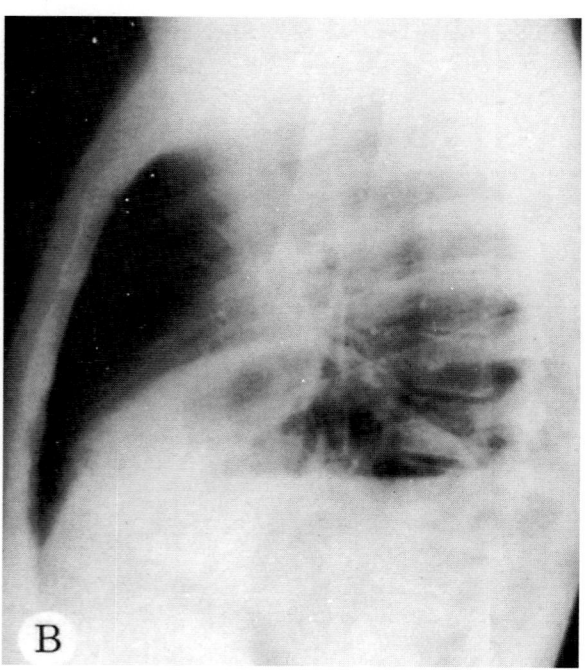

Fig. 74-5. Traumatic diaphragmatic hernia through the left paracardiac portion of the left hemidiaphragm discovered 15 years after the initial injury. **A.** Posteroanterior radiograph of chest showing multiple air-fluid spaces in the lower one-half of the left chest. **B.** Lateral radiograph made with the patient in the upright position.

especially those involving the left hemidiaphragm, and to contain multiple abdominal viscera. In order of frequency, as the author and associates (1986) have noted, the stomach, colon, small bowel, omentum, and spleen herniate through a left diaphragmatic traumatic defect, whereas the colon and liver are the most commonly herniating organs through a

right defect. Those from penetrating trauma tend to contain only colon or a portion of the stomach, or both.

Symptomatology

The larger hernias are more likely to produce ventilatory signs and symptoms caused by the reduction of the lung volume on the side of the hernia. Gastrointestinal problems caused by interference of the normal functioning of the contained viscera may occur also. The smaller hernias that contain only a loop of large bowel or stomach become symptomatic because of partial, and at times of complete, obstruction of the contained segment. When complete obstruction occurs, strangulation of the herniated visceral segment may develop and is an ominous complication.

Diagnosis

The diagnosis of traumatic diaphragmatic hernia should be suspected in any patient who has sustained blunt or penetrating trauma of the trunk, particularly of the chest or epigastrium, and in whom chest radiography shows an abnormal diaphragmatic silhouette or lower lung field. The abnormality may include only an obscured or abnormal diaphragmatic shadow, a radiodensity, a radiolucency, or one or more air-fluid levels in the lung fields with or without mediastinal shift. The radiographic examination of the chest, however, does not differentiate diaphragmatic hernia from various other conditions that can cause these abnormalities, unless a nasogastric tube has been inserted and is seen in the chest cavity, which indicates the stomach is herniated in the thorax.

The most important studies for the diagnosis are either barium by mouth or a barium enema, as Felson (1973) pointed out. He noted that whichever of the organs is herniated, stomach or colon, the point of entry and exit through the torn diaphragmatic leaf is most often through a small single defect. Moreover, the edges of the defect are closely applied to the herniated viscus. Thus, the points of entry and exit are closely applied and constricted. This results in a side-by-side, beaklike narrowing of the barium column (Figs. 74-6 and 74-7). Carter and associates (1951) reported that if the herniated bowel becomes obstructed, the number of beaks is reduced to one, and dilatation proximal to the site of constriction is observed (Fig. 74-8). The obstruction within the hernia is often of the closed loop type, so distention of the loop within the hernia may be great. These authors also noted that the combination of a high left hemidiaphragm and the presence of splenic flexure obstruction is almost diagnostic of a traumatic diaphragmatic hernia.

Other diagnostic studies such as pneumoperitoneum, pneumothorax, and angiography are less rewarding than the barium studies. Ultrasonography and computed tomographic studies may be helpful at times but probably less so than in the evaluation of patients thought to have acute injury of the diaphragm.

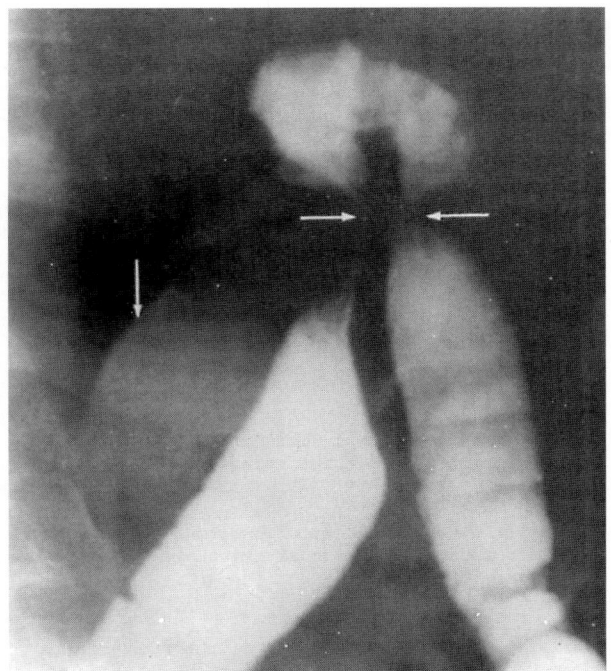

Fig. 74-6. Counter-incision breakdown after hiatal hernia repair. Nonobstructive hernia. The medial portion of the diaphragm is visible (*vertical arrow*). The "lovebird sign" is well shown (*horizontal arrows*). From Felson B: Chest Roentgenology. Philadelphia: WB Saunders, 1973, p. 421. With permission.

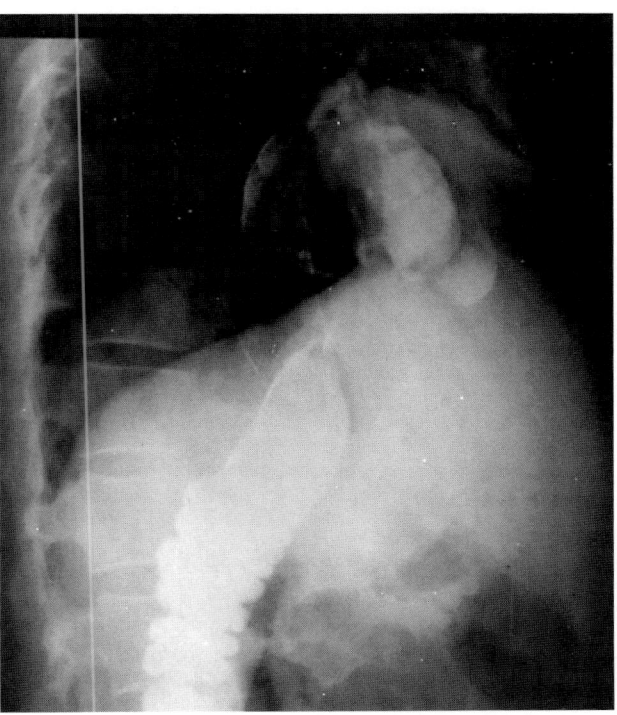

Fig. 74-7. Barium enema showing apposition of loops of large bowel herniating into the thorax through a previous stab wound of the diaphragm. From Symbas PN, Vlasis SE, Hatcher C Jr: Blunt and penetrating diaphragmatic injuries with or without herniation of organs into the chest. Ann Thorac Surg *42*:158, 1986. With permission.

Treatment

Once the hernia is recognized, reduction of the hernia and repair of the diaphragmatic defect through the transthoracic route is indicated. The frequent presence of marked adhesions between the herniated viscus and thoracic contents necessitates this route. In the presence of obstruction, with or without strangulation of the contained viscus, the incarcerated diaphragmatic hernia must be approached by the transthoracic route. After mobilization of the obstructed or strangulated viscus, the abdomen may need to be entered through an abdominal incision to complete the necessary operative repair or resection and diversion of the involved viscus. The repair of the diaphragmatic defect is accomplished by direct suture repair in almost all instances. Only rarely in the presence of large tears from original blunt trauma is a prosthetic graft necessary.

Morbidity and Mortality

The morbidity after repair of a diaphragmatic hernia that was recognized late is that seen after any major thoracotomy. The mortality, however, may vary greatly, depending on the status of the hernia at the time of its repair. When the procedure is done electively, the mortality should approach zero. In marked contrast, however, is the excessive

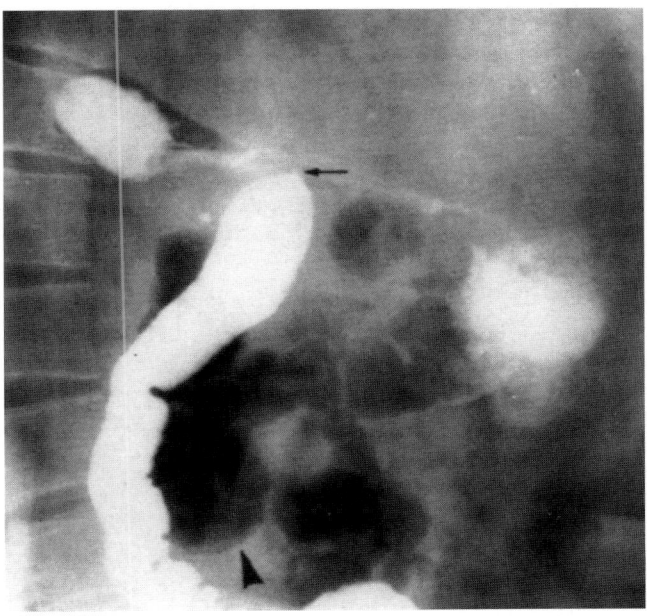

Fig. 74-8. Obstruction of the distal segment, lateral view. Note the single beak (*arrow*). The stomach, outlined with barium, is not herniated. The proximal colon shows moderate gaseous distention (*arrowhead*). From Felson B: Chest Roentgenology. Philadelphia: WB Saunders, 1973, p. 421. With permission.

mortality experienced in those patients who present with a strangulated, gangrenous viscus in the hernia. In such instances, the mortality may be as high as 80%, as Hegarty and associates (1978) reported. These missed hernias, therefore, must be recognized and repaired before obstruction and gangrene of the contained visceral segment occur.

REFERENCES

Ammann AM, et al: Traumatic rupture of the diaphragm: real time sonographic diagnosis. AJR Am J Roentgenol 140:915, 1983.

Beal SL, McKennan M: Blunt diaphragm rupture: a morbid injury. Arch Surg 123:828, 1988.

Brooks JW: Blunt traumatic rupture of the diaphragm. Ann Thorac Surg 26:199, 1978.

Brown GL, Richardson JD: Traumatic diaphragmatic hernia: a continuing challenge. Ann Thorac Surg 39:170, 1985.

Carter BN, Giuseffi J, Felson B: Traumatic diaphragmatic hernia. AJR Am J Roentgenol 65:56, 1951.

Carter EA, et al: Case report: Cine MRI in the diagnosis of a ruptured right hemidiaphragm. Clin Radiol 51:137, 1996.

Estrera AS, Platt MR, Mills LJ: Traumatic injuries of the diaphragm. Chest 75:306, 1979.

Estrera AS, Landay MJ, McClelland RN: Blunt traumatic rupture of the right hemidiaphragm: experience in 12 patients. Ann Thorac Surg 39:525, 1985.

Felson B: Chest Roentgenology. Philadelphia: WB Saunders, 1973, p. 437.

Hegarty MM, et al: Delayed presentation of traumatic diaphragmatic hernia. Ann Surg 188:229, 1978.

Heiberg E, et al: CT recognition of traumatic rupture of the diaphragm. AJR Am J Roentgenol 135:369, 1980.

Ivatury RR, et al: Laparoscopy in the evaluation of the intrathoracic abdomen after penetrating injury. J Trauma 33:101, 1992.

Lindsey I, et al: Laparoscopic management of blunt diaphragmatic injury. Aust N Z J Surg 67:619, 1997.

Miller LW, et al: Management of penetrating and blunt diaphragmatic injury. J Trauma 24:403, 1984.

Shah R, et al: Traumatic rupture of diaphragm. Ann Thorac Surg 60:1444, 1995.

Spann JC, et al: Evaluation of video-assisted thoracoscopic surgery in the diagnosis of diaphragmatic injuries. Am J Surg 170:628, 1995.

Symbas PN, Vlasis SE, Hatcher CR Jr: Blunt and penetrating diaphragmatic injuries with or without herniation of organs into the chest. Ann Thorac Surg 42:158, 1986.

Toombs BD, Sandler CM, Lester RG: Computed tomography of chest trauma. Radiology 140:733, 1981.

READING REFERENCES

Clay RC, Hanlon CR: Pneumoperitoneum in the differential diagnosis of diaphragmatic hernia. J Thorac Cardiovasc Surg 21:57, 1951.

Ebert PA, Gaertner RA, Zuidema GD: Traumatic diaphragmatic hernia. Surg Gynecol Obstet 125:59, 1967.

Fagan CJ, et al: Traumatic diaphragmatic hernia into the pericardium: verification of diagnosis by computed tomography. J Comput Assist Tomogr 3:405, 1979.

Hood RM: Traumatic diaphragmatic hernia [collective review]. Ann Thorac Surg 12:311, 1971.

Lucido JL, Wall CA: Rupture of the diaphragm due to blunt trauma. Arch Surg 86:989, 1963.

Mansour KA, et al: Diaphragmatic hernia caused by trauma: experience with 35 cases. Am Surg 41:97, 1975.

Nelson JB Jr, et al: Diaphragmatic injuries and posttraumatic hernia. J Trauma 2:36, 1960.

Sutton JP, Carlisle RB, Stephenson SE Jr: Traumatic diaphragmatic hernia: a review of 25 cases. Ann Thorac Surg 3:136, 1967.

Symbas PN: Blunt traumatic rupture of the diaphragm. Ann Thorac Surg 26:193, 1978.

SECTION XIII

The Trachea

CHAPTER 75

Surgical Anatomy of the Trachea and Techniques of Resection

Hermes C. Grillo

ANATOMY

Functionally, the trachea serves principally as a conduit for ventilation. Viewed in this way, it would seem to be an ideal structure for replacement or reconstruction when involved by surgical disease. Anatomically, however, it presents several unique features that partially account for the difficulty in its surgical management. These features are its unpaired nature, unique structural rigidity, short length, relative lack of longitudinal elasticity, proximity to major cardiovascular structures, and blood supply.

My colleagues and I (1964) reported that the adult human trachea averages 11.8 cm in length (range, 10 to 13 cm) from the infracricoid level to the top of the carinal spur. Usually from 18 to 22 cartilaginous rings occur within this length, approximately two rings per centimeter. Occasionally, rings are incomplete or bifid. In an adult man, the internal diameter of the trachea measures approximately 2.3 cm laterally and 1.8 cm anteroposteriorly. These measurements vary roughly in proportion to the size of the individual and are usually smaller in women. The cross-sectional shape in the adult is approximately elliptic. In infants and children, it is more nearly circular. The configuration may change with disease. Thus, the lower two-thirds may be flattened in tracheomalacia or rigidly narrowed from side to side to produce *saber-sheath trachea*.

The surgeon usually visualizes the trachea as he or she learned to see it in the thyroidectomy position, with the neck extended, as a structure that is one-half cervical and one-half thoracic. Mulliken and the author (1968) pointed out that the trachea becomes almost entirely mediastinal when the neck is flexed, for the cricoid cartilage drops to the level of the thoracic inlet. This may be the permanent position in the aged because of cervical kyphosis. These simple observations contributed to the development of surgical reconstructive techniques that obviate the requirement for prostheses.

The trachea, when viewed laterally in the upright individual, courses backward and downward at an angle from a nearly subcutaneous position at the infracricoid level to rest against the esophagus and vertebral column at the carina. The larynx and the origin of the esophagus are intimately related anatomically at the cricopharyngeal level. Below this point, the posterior membranous wall of the trachea maintains a close spatial relationship to the esophagus. A distinct, easily separable plane is present below the cricoid level, but a common blood supply is shared. Anteriorly, the thyroid isthmus passes over the trachea in the region of the second ring. The lateral lobes of the thyroid are closely applied to the trachea, and a common blood supply is obtained from the branches of the inferior thyroid artery. Lying in the groove between trachea and esophagus are the recurrent nerves, coursing from beneath the arch of the aorta on the left side and therefore having a longer course in proximity to the trachea there than on the right side, where the nerve has looped around the subclavian artery and then approached the groove. A nonrecurrent nerve rarely is present on the right in conjunction with an anomalous subclavian artery. These nerves enter the larynx between the cricoid and thyroid cartilages just anterior to the inferior cornua of the thyroid cartilage.

The anterior pretracheal plane may be developed easily in the cervical region. Fibrofatty tissue, lymph nodes, and fine branches of the anterior jugular vein are present in front of this plane. The innominate vein lies anteriorly, away from the trachea. The innominate artery, however, crosses over the midtrachea obliquely from its point of origin from the aortic arch to the right side of the neck. In children, the innominate artery is higher and is encountered in the lower part of the neck. In some adults, the artery is unusually high and crosses the trachea at the base of the neck when slight extension is present. Occasionally, a tiny branch of this artery may be encountered in the segment of the artery that crosses the trachea. At the level of the carina, the left main bronchus passes beneath the aortic arch and the right beneath the azygos vein. The pulmonary artery lies just in front of the carina. On either side of the trachea lies fibrofatty tissue containing lymph node chains; a large packet of nodes lies just beneath the carina (see Chapter 6).

The course of the trachea from the anterior cervical position to the posterior mediastinal position with close relationships to major vascular structures makes access to the entire trachea through a single incision difficult. I (1969) emphasized that these anatomic facts demand precise definition of the extent and nature of the tracheal lesions in planning surgical procedures.

The cartilaginous rings give the human trachea its lateral rigidity. The rings extend approximately two-thirds of the circumference. The posterior wall is membranous. The trachea is lined with respiratory mucosa, which is tightly applied to the inner surface of the cartilages grossly. The normal epithelium is columnar and ciliated. The cilia clear particulate matter and secretions. Mucous glands are liberally present. In chronic smokers and in persons with other chronic irritation, squamous metaplasia frequently occurs; in extreme instances, few ciliated cells remain. Such individuals must clear secretions by coughing vigorously. This observation, plus the demonstrated feasibility of cutaneous reconstructions and occasional successes with prosthetic interpositions, makes it clear that ciliated epithelium, although highly desirable, is not essential for tracheal reconstruction. Between the cartilaginous rings and in the membranous wall, the submucosa is fibromuscular.

Considerable contraction of the muscular membranous wall can occur with coughing and with spasm, the tips of the cartilages being drawn inward. Such transient narrowing of the airway may be observed fluoroscopically and during bronchoscopy in normal individuals. Some longitudinal flexibility exists; a degree of elasticity is present that

appears to be greater in youth and to decrease with age. Calcification of the rings is seen most often with advancing age, although to lesser degree than in the cricoid cartilage. Local trauma or operation may lead to calcification. The normal trachea slides easily in its layer of fibrofatty areolar tissue from neck to mediastinum.

The blood supply of the human trachea is segmental, largely shared with the esophagus and derived principally from multiple branches of the inferior thyroid artery above and the bronchial arteries below. The arteries approach laterally and fine branches pass anteriorly to the trachea and posteriorly to the esophagus. Miura and I (1966) noted that the inferior thyroid artery nourishes the upper trachea, usually through a pattern of three principal branches with fine subdivisions and extremely fine collateral vessels, but with many variations, as noted by Salassa and colleagues (1977). The bronchial vessels nourish the lower trachea. Sometimes, the internal mammary artery contributes (Fig. 75-1). Excessive circumferential dissection with division of the lateral pedicles during an operative procedure can easily devascularize the trachea.

METHODS OF RECONSTRUCTION OF THE TRACHEA

The surgical approach to the trachea developed more slowly than other areas of thoracic surgery, because of the rarity of tracheal tumors, the anatomic complexities of reconstruction, and the biological incompatibilities that met efforts at prosthetic reconstruction. Earlier hesitations because of problems of physiologic management during reconstruction proved to be less formidable. The growth in frequency of postintubation benign lesions, as a result of the success of modern respiratory therapy, increased the urgency of developmental work.

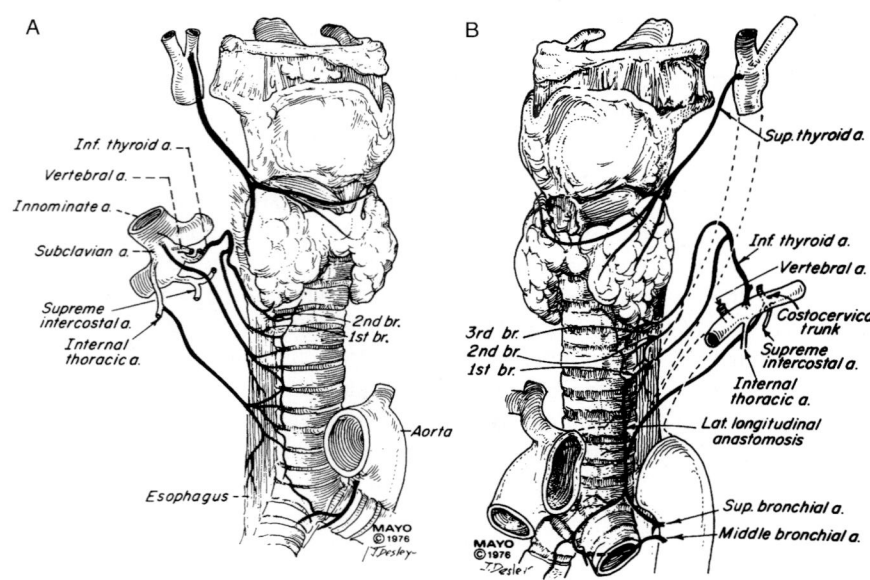

Fig. 75-1. Blood supply of the trachea. A. Right anterior view. B. Left anterior view. The right side varies in some respects. From Salassa JR, Pearson BW, Payne WS: Gross and microscopical blood supply of the trachea. Ann Thorac Surg 24:100, 1977. With permission.

The concept of direct end-to-end anastomosis of trachea to trachea was generally accepted as the ideal method of tracheal repair after reconstruction. It was long believed, however, as stated by Belsey (1950), that no more than 2 cm (approximately four tracheal rings) could be removed and anastomosis consistently made. As a result, lateral resection was done when possible, with attempts made to patch the defect in various ways, using fascia, skin, pericardium, other tissues, and foreign materials. When such a technique was applied to malignant neoplasms, inadequate removal of tumor resulted, with early recurrence. Such patches also failed to heal. Partial cicatrization was an additional factor. Attention was directed early to the development of an artificial trachea.

Prosthetic Replacement

Many materials have been used for prosthetic replacement of the trachea. Most work has been done in animals, but a scattered experience in humans has been reported. Replacements have consisted of tubes made of glass or metal; stainless steel mesh in either tubes or coils and tantalum mesh; Lucite, polyethylene, and other plastic cylinders; tubes of Ivalon or Marlex mesh; Teflon with combinations of Ivalon or Dacron; and, more recently, polytetrafluoroethylene and Silastic tubes, often with stainless steel wire or plastic rings to supply rigidity. Early prostheses were usually solid tubes that bridged defects between the two ends of the trachea. Their failure led to use of rigid mesh cylinders that were intended to allow incorporation into the surrounding connective tissue. More recently, flexible meshwork has been supported by splinting plastic rings. These meshwork prostheses were based on the theory that they would be incorporated by connective tissue and that epithelium would then grow down over this bed of new connective tissue; the rigid rings would maintain an open airway. In most experiments, only short prosthetic bridges have been incorporated to any extent. Some of the longer prostheses maintain an open airway, but firm healing with full tissue encasement and epithelialization has not occurred. This basically unhealed state might be acceptable as an airway, but these longer prostheses have been subject, in a high percentage of instances, to occlusion by formation of granulation tissue at the nonhealing ends, strictures at these ends, sepsis causing rejection of the prosthesis, or erosion of major vessels with fatal hemorrhage. An occasional long-term success has occurred, largely as an exception rather than as the rule. The problem is the biological instability caused by placing a foreign body in a bed of connective tissue adjacent to an epithelium that necessarily is contaminated with bacteria. With a foreign body in place, a chronic abscess is presented to the mediastinum, with the described results. Borrie and Redshaw (1970) attempted to solve these problems by accepting a foreign tube as a permanent airway, but making it with cuffs that could be sutured that they hoped would be incorporated by connective tissue.

Neville and associates (1990) reported successes with a similar prosthesis. Vogt-Moykopf and Mickisch (1987) noted the many complications that occur.

Chemically fixed tracheal tissue grafts are essentially bioprostheses, subject sooner or later to resorption and cicatricial replacement. Allografts require augmentation of blood supply, such as an omental pedicle, to safeguard viability. The usual immunologic problems are present, and a major concern is that the principal need for tracheal replacement today is for extensive malignant tumors, usually a contraindication to transplantation.

Anatomic Mobilization

Perhaps most crucial to the evolution of mobilization techniques for tracheal reconstruction was recognition that the cervical trachea, as seen in the hyperextended surgical *thyroid* position, may be delivered into the mediastinum by cervical flexion. A few reports of clinical resections greater than 2 cm appeared, but few systematic studies of the anatomic potential are recorded. Michelson and associates (1961) noted that careful mobilization of the entire trachea in eight cadavers allowed for anastomosis with 1 lb of tension, after resection of 4 to 6 cm, with an additional 2.5 to 5.0 cm obtained by division of the left main bronchus.

Our detailed anatomic studies in cadavers attempted to answer the surgical questions of how much trachea could be resected and primary anastomosis made when the trachea was approached in progressive fashion from either a cervical or a transthoracic approach, depending on the location of the lesion. In one study, Mulliken and I (1968) mobilized the trachea through a cervicomediastinal approach, carefully preserving the lateral tissue that bears the blood supply. Using a standard tension of 1000 to 1200 g for approximation, it was possible, with the neck in 15 to 35 degrees of flexion, to resect an average length of 4.5 cm (approximately seven rings) and to increase this by 1.4 cm by entering the pleural space and mobilizing the right hilus (Fig. 75-2A). With greater degrees of cervical flexion, even longer resections are possible. Suprahyoid laryngeal release, described by Montgomery (1974), adds 1.0 to 1.5 cm while minimizing the difficulties in swallowing that attended earlier techniques for release. Alternating lateral division of the intercartilaginous ligaments of the trachea to obtain extension has been proposed experimentally but not applied clinically to any extent. This technique has the disadvantages of probable interference with tracheal blood supply and the need for extensive tracheal exposure to obtain a rather limited extension of length.

In approaching the lower half of the trachea, my colleagues and I (1964) accomplished mobilization progressively by first freeing the hilus of the right lung and dividing the pulmonary ligament; second, freeing the pulmonary vessels from their pericardial attachments; and third, transplanting the left main bronchus, which is held in place by

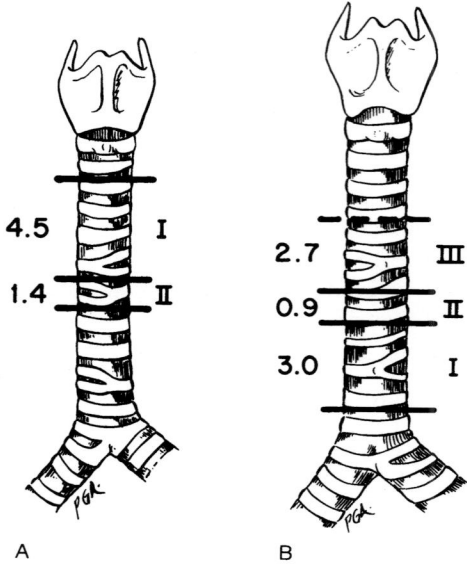

Fig. 75-2. The amounts of trachea that can be removed and yet permit primary anastomosis. **A.** Cervicomediastinal mobilization permitted removal of 4.5 cm under 1000-g tension, with cervical flexion. Intrathoracic dissection permitted removal of an additional 1.4 cm. **B.** Transthoracic hilar dissection and division of the pulmonary ligament, with the cervical spine in the neutral position, permitted removal of 3 cm, intrapericardial dissection an additional 0.9 cm, and division of the left main bronchus with reimplantation in the bronchus intermedius an additional 2.7 cm. The use of cervical flexion has demonstrated that the area designated I may be significantly greater than 3 cm. From Grillo HC: Surgical approaches to the trachea. Surg Gynecol Obstet *129*:347, 1969. With permission.

the arch of the aorta, to the bronchus intermedius. In these earlier studies, we did not use cervical flexion but instead held the neck in the neutral position. At tensions under 1000 g, the first maneuver allowed for resection of 3 cm and the second for 0.9 cm additionally; the radical measure of bronchial implantation permitted an additional 2.7 cm (Fig. 75-2B). It has since become clear that cervical flexion combined with hilar and pericardial mobilization plus division of the pulmonary ligament allows lengths of 5 to 6 cm to be removed by the transthoracic approach. These figures represent only guidelines. The length of trachea that may be resected safely in an individual varies widely with age, posture, bodily habitus, extent of disease, and prior tracheal surgery. Bronchial implantation has been reserved for carinal excision or similar complex maneuvers to avoid adding another unnecessary risk to operation. Reimplantation of the left main bronchus into the bronchus intermedius was first used clinically by Barclay and associates (1957).

The limits of safety with varying anastomotic tensions have not been established in humans. Cantrell and Folse (1961) found in dogs that tensions below 1700 g permitted safety from disruption after anastomosis. In anatomic studies in the cadaver, we found that an average tension of 675 g only was required for approximation (maximum, 1000 g) after a 7-cm resection. Such clinical measurements as we

have made show tensions of approximately 600 g in resections of 4 to 5 cm in length.

Anatomic and clinical observations show that great attention must be paid to the lateral blood supply in tracheal mobilization. This fine segmental supply cannot be disrupted safely, particularly for anastomosis of a long distal segment to a short proximal segment; the distal segment must not be freed circumferentially.

Another peculiarity of tracheal reconstruction depends on the relative rigidity of the anterolateral walls. Transverse wedging of the anterior wall of the trachea may buckle the posterior wall into a partially obstructing valve. Circumferential resection, which may, however, be beveled, is most often preferable.

SURGERY OF THE TRACHEA

Anesthesia

The airway must be under full control at all times during reconstructive surgery of the trachea, so that hasty maneuvers are unnecessary and hypoxia does not occur. The patient should breathe spontaneously during the operation and at its conclusion so that ventilatory support is not necessary. Cardiopulmonary bypass has been used for tracheal surgery, but it is not necessary for relatively simple resection and, as noted by Geffin and colleagues (1969), presents real hazards for more complex procedures requiring extensive manipulation of the lung. Procedures are explained carefully to the patients before the operation. Induction is carried out slowly and gently, especially in a patient with a highly obstructed trachea. If a benign stenosis presents an airway diameter of less than 5 mm, dilatation is performed and an endotracheal tube is passed beyond the lesion, to prevent arrhythmia caused by CO_2 buildup during the early stages of operation. Occasionally, a nearly obstructing tumor has required prompt bronchoscopy with a ventilating bronchoscope shortly after induction, with subsequent intubation. Obstructing tumor may be cored out with the rigid bronchoscope aided by biopsy forceps. Frequent monitoring of blood gases and electrocardiography are essential. Bronchoscopic examination should be done by both the surgeon and the anesthetist, who must deal with this airway until surgical access distal to the lesion has been obtained. If tracheostomy is already present, induction is simplified. Initial dissection is always done carefully to avoid increasing the degree of obstruction by roughness or pressure. The area below the obstruction is isolated first, so that a transection of the trachea can be performed at any point and an airway can be introduced across the operative field, should the degree of obstruction increase. Sterile anesthesia tubing, connectors, and endotracheal tubes are available in the operative field. I have not found it necessary to make distal incisions in the tracheobronchial tree for insertion of ventilatory catheters but, rather, have proceeded as described. If transthoracic resection is performed close to the carina, the endotracheal tube is passed into the left main bronchus and that lung alone is ventilated; if the Po$_2$ decreases toward unsatisfactory levels, a previously isolated right pulmonary artery is temporarily clamped to eliminate the shunt through the right lung. This is rarely required. Slow increase in shunting may occur during prolonged operation because of low tidal ventilation, increasing atelectasis, and aspiration of secretions and must be guarded against, as noted by Wilson (1987). High-frequency ventilation is a useful adjunct, especially in complex carinal reconstruction, as reported by El-Baz and associates (1982).

Surgical Approaches

Lesions in the upper half of the trachea that are known to be benign are best approached cervically (Fig. 75-3A). If a malignant lesion is present, be prepared for the cervicomediastinal and, possibly, thoracic approach. Placement of the cervical incision depends on the pathologic state, the presence of existing stomas, and the possible need for sternotomy. If a postoperative temporary tracheostomy stoma may be required after a difficult laryngotracheal anastomosis, then the incision must be planned so that a stoma can be made away from the incision. If the initial dissection through the neck indicates need for further exposure, the upper sternum is split to a point just beyond the angle of Louis; horizontal division of the sternum into an intercostal space is not necessary. Because the great vessels present anteriorly, division of more than the upper sternum is not helpful; division simply allows room to maneuver in managing the more distal trachea (Fig. 75-4B). Innominate vein division also adds nothing.

Rarely, this incision must be extended through the fourth intercostal space on the right to permit additional mobilization of the intrathoracic trachea by freeing the hilus of the right lung. Such an incision permits wide exposure of the entire trachea from cricoid to carina. This is almost never necessary in benign stenosis. If extirpative surgery and terminal tracheostomy are expected, the incision should avoid a vertical limb even if sternal division is needed. A large bipedicled flap is prepared through two horizontal incisions, as I suggested in 1966. A long-segment cutaneous tracheal replacement also may be so fashioned. Such circumstances are unusual but should be kept in mind in planning extensive procedures.

Neoplastic lesions of the lower half of the trachea are most easily approached directly through a high right thoracotomy incision (Fig. 75-3B). It is possible to excise even low benign lesions from the anterior approach described. Cervical flexion devolves sufficient trachea into the mediastinum so that lower tracheal tumors are usually approachable completely through the right side of the chest without a sternal component. The fourth intercostal space or fourth rib resection is used. Median sternotomy with dissection between the superior vena cava and aorta, and anterior and posterior pericardial division, provides access to the lower trachea and carina, but the exposure is poor for extensive dissection or complex reconstruction.

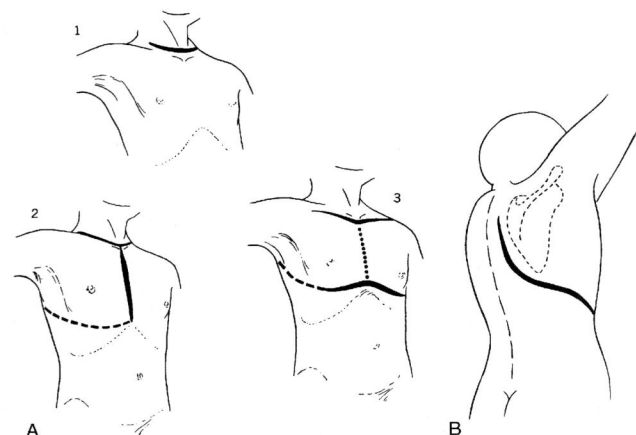

Fig. 75-3. A. Incisions for approach to the upper portion of the trachea. (1) Cervical incision allows access to upper trachea and to the mediastinum with somewhat limited exposure. (2) Median sternotomy, usually carried only through the upper one-third of the sternum, allows more extended dissection into the mediastinum. Extension of the incision to the right fourth intercostal space (*dotted line*) allows exposure of the entire trachea from cricoid to carina and permits mobilization of the hilus. (3) Cervicomediastinal approach is here carried out beneath a bipedicled anterior skin flap. The flap is kept intact in case it is necessary to fashion a mediastinal tracheostomy. Such an incision is rarely needed. **B.** Incision for approach to the lower trachea and carina. The thorax is entered through the fourth intercostal space or the bed of the resected fourth rib. The high incision shown permits the scapula to be drawn out of the way. From Grillo HC: Surgical approaches to the trachea. Surg Gynecol Obstet *129*:347, 1969. With permission.

Reconstruction of the Upper Trachea

The upper flap is raised with or without circumcising an existing tracheostomy incision or including it in the original incision; individualization is required in each patient. Many existing tracheostomy stomas, even if they are to be allowed to close spontaneously later, usually have to be remade in another opening in the skin because of changed postoperative relationships between trachea and overlying skin. If the lesion is high, benign, and short, only a limited field is required. Dissection is confined chiefly to the midline, the upper flap being raised to the level of the cricoid and the lower to the sternal notch to allow dissection in the pretracheal plane as needed. Dense scar is often present in association with benign stenosis and dissection is done close to the trachea to avoid damage to the recurrent nerves, especially near the cricoid. Isolation of the nerves is avoided because this would increase the danger of injury. Freeing the trachea below the lesion early allows easy establishment of airway control and expe-

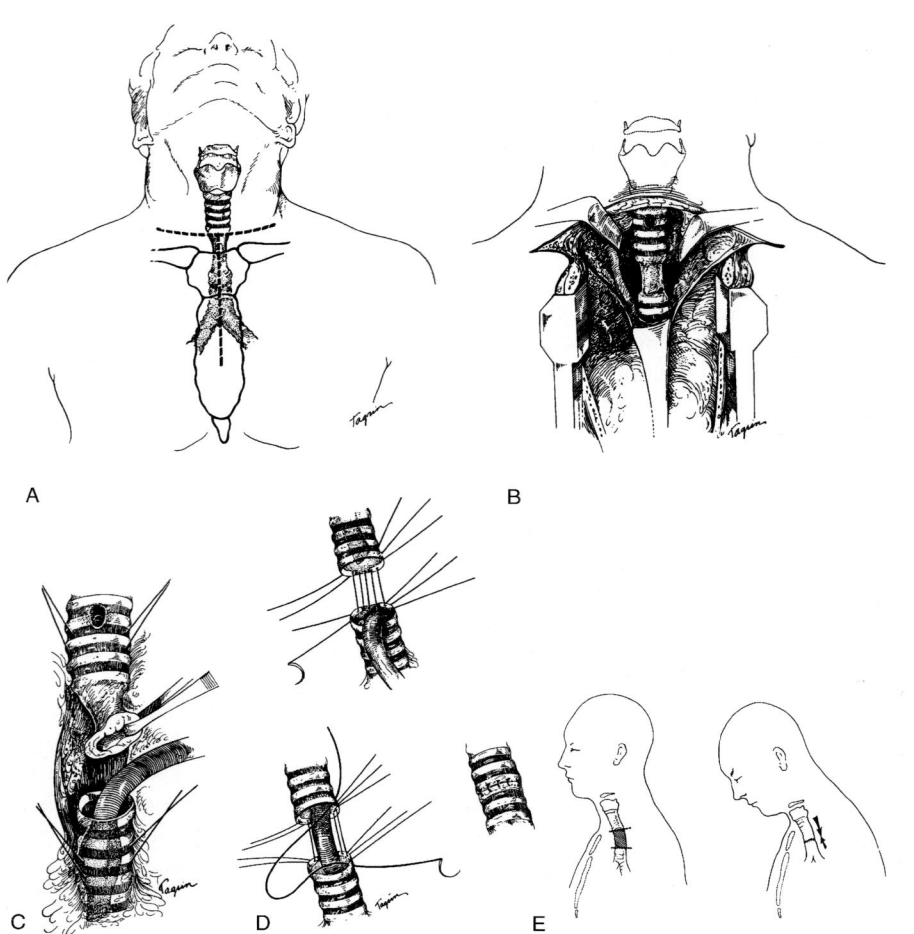

Fig. 75-4. Reconstruction of the upper trachea. **A.** The collar incision is often adequate for benign lesions in the upper and midtrachea. Partial division of the sternum allows access to the mediastinum over the great vessels. **B.** The innominate vein is retracted but not divided because greater exposure is not so obtained because of the posterior position of the lower trachea. The pleura is intact. **C.** Direct intubation has been performed after division of the trachea below an adherent stenotic lesion. Dissection is now simplified. Traction sutures are shown and also the scar of the prior tracheostomy. **D.** Details of placement of sutures. Interrupted sutures passing through the cartilage and membranous wall are used. Knots are tied on the outside. **E.** Diagram to indicate that the majority of mobilization in the approach to the upper trachea is obtained by cervical flexion with downward devolution of the trachea and a lesser amount by upward movement of the distal trachea. A–D, From Grillo HC: Surgery of the trachea. Curr Probl Surg 7:3, 1970. With permission.

dites dissection of a cicatrized segment from the esophagus. Mobilization is made as required before and behind the trachea both proximally and distally. Tentative approximation with traction sutures, while the neck is flexed by the anesthetist, demonstrates whether approximation may be accomplished or whether further dissection is needed. A single layer of anastomotic sutures is placed in interrupted fashion so that the knots are tied on the outside. Fine No. 4-0 absorbable polymeric sutures are preferred. I prefer Vicryl. In many instances, the sutures become inaccessible to direct vision during tying and must not break (Fig. 75-4). The anterior approach also may be used for tumor, but in this situation, sternotomy is often required for adequate removal of paratracheal tissue. In this instance, the recurrent nerves are usually identified and preserved, if they are not involved by tumor.

When benign stenosis of the upper trachea also involves the subglottic larynx, one-stage reconstruction is possible. As I (1982a) reported, the technique is complex. The anterior subglottic larynx is resected and, in cases in which the stenosis is circumferential, the posterior cricoid lamina is bared but preserved in order to protect the recurrent laryngeal nerves (Fig. 75-5). The distal tailored trachea is advanced to replace the anterior subglottic laryngeal wall with cartilages and to resurface the posterior cricoid plate with membranous tracheal wall.

I and Mathisen (1992) have had generally good results. Stenting of the anastomosis is not necessary if the repair is precise.

Reconstruction of the Lower Trachea

After confirmation of the extent of a tumor, anatomic mobilization is usually accomplished before severing the trachea. If obstruction appears to be imminent during mobilization, the trachea is transected and distally intubated. If the line of transection is supracarinal, the left main bronchus is intubated. Access to the subcarinal lymph nodes and lower paratracheal nodes is excellent. The recurrent nerves reach a point adjacent to the trachea promptly and should be sacrificed deliberately only if required. Cervical flexion by the anesthetist devolves a fair segment of trachea into the chest even in the lateral position, and this, in combination with the mobilization maneuvers earlier noted, permits end-to-end anastomosis (Fig. 75-6). Complex maneuvers may be necessary for excision and reconstruction of carinal lesions or lesions involving the right main stem bronchus or upper lobe bronchus (Fig. 75-7). In general, my principle is to excise the tumor with a satisfactory margin and then use a suitable reconstruction for the specific situation. As I have described (1965, 1970, 1982b), a second-

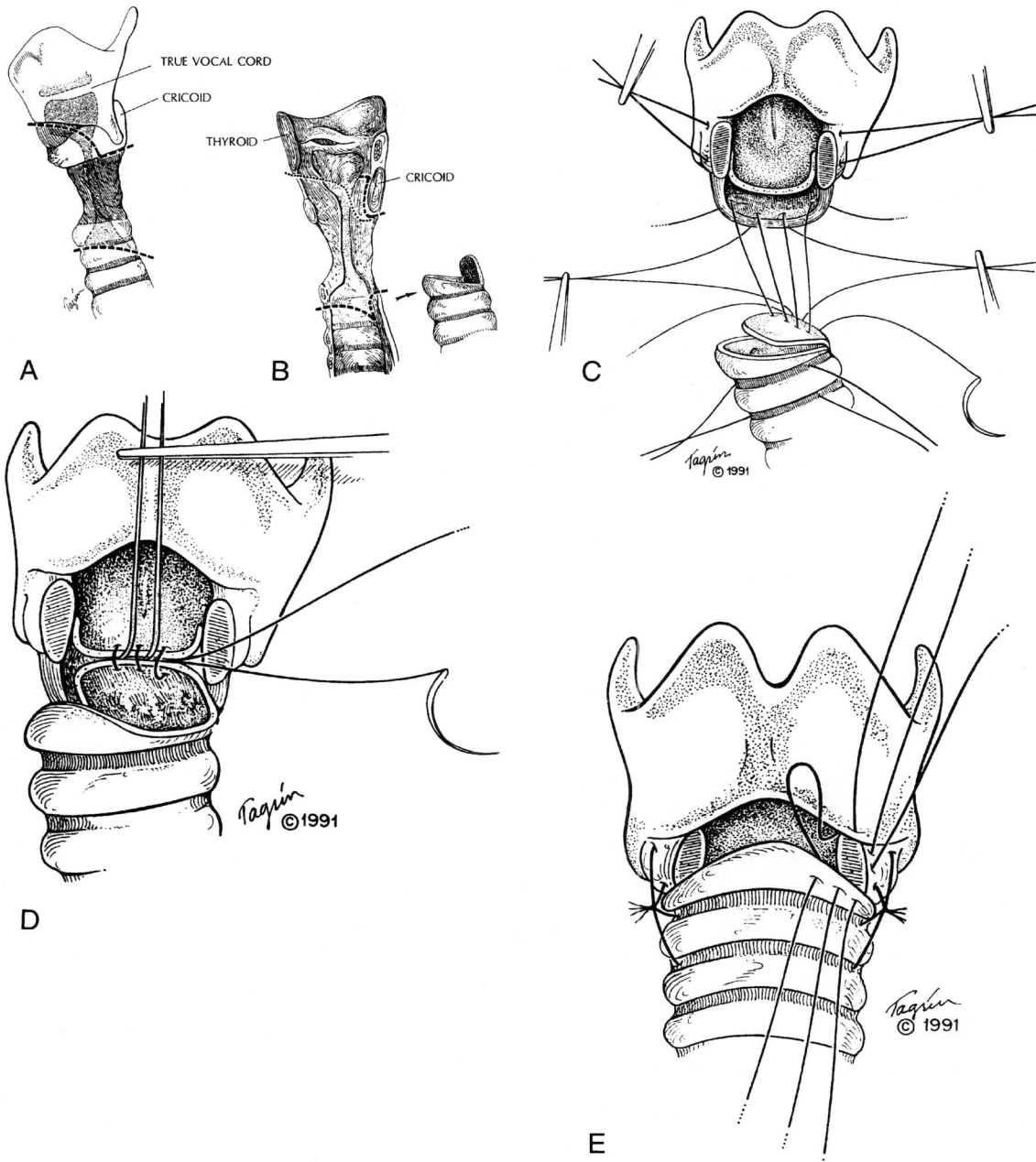

Fig. 75-5. Technique of laryngotracheal resection and reconstruction. **A.** External lines of division of the larynx and trachea are indicated by dashed lines. The anterior cricoid arch is removed. **B.** When the subglottic intralaryngeal stenosis is circumferential, scar is removed from the front of the posterior cricoid lamina, baring the cartilage. The residual posterior cricoid lamina protects the recurrent laryngeal nerves. Distally, the trachea is beveled over the length of one cartilage to fit the anterolateral subglottic defect that has been created. A broad-based flap of membranous tracheal wall is fashioned to resurface the bared cricoid plate. **C.** The posterior flap is fixed to the lower margin of the cricoid plate with four extraluminal sutures (4-0 Tevdek). The lateral traction sutures (2-0 Vicryl) are shown also in the larynx proximally and in the trachea distally. **D.** Posterior mucosal anastomotic sutures (4-0 Vicryl) are placed with knots to lie behind the mucosa. Traction sutures are omitted in this diagram for simplicity. **E.** After placement of all the posterior and posterolateral anastomotic sutures as far anteriorly as the lateral stay sutures, the patient's neck is flexed, the stay sutures are tied, the sternal fixing Tevdek sutures are tied, and then the posterior mucosal sutures are tied. The anterior and anterolateral anastomotic sutures are then placed and finally tied serially. A and B, From Grillo HC: Primary reconstruction of airway after resection of subglottic laryngeal and upper tracheal stenosis. Ann Thorac Surg *33*:3, 1982. With permission. C–E, From Grillo HC, Mathisen DJ, Wain JC: Laryngotracheal resection and reconstruction for subglottic stenosis. Ann Thorac Surg *53*:54, 1992. With permission.

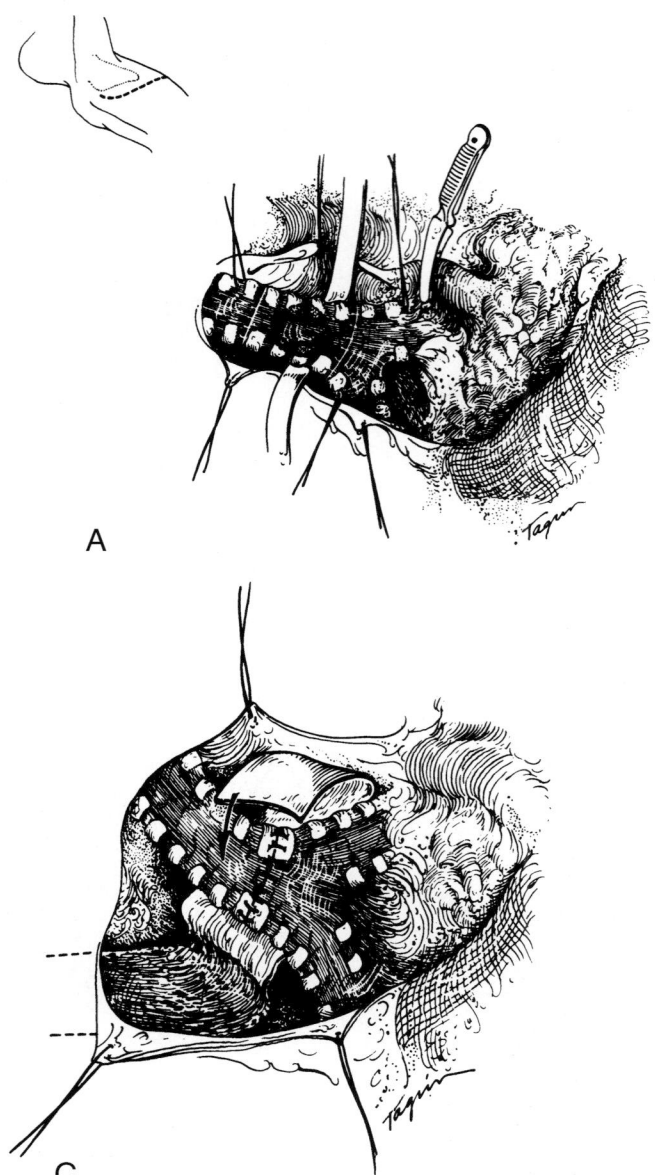

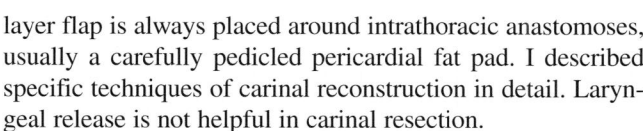

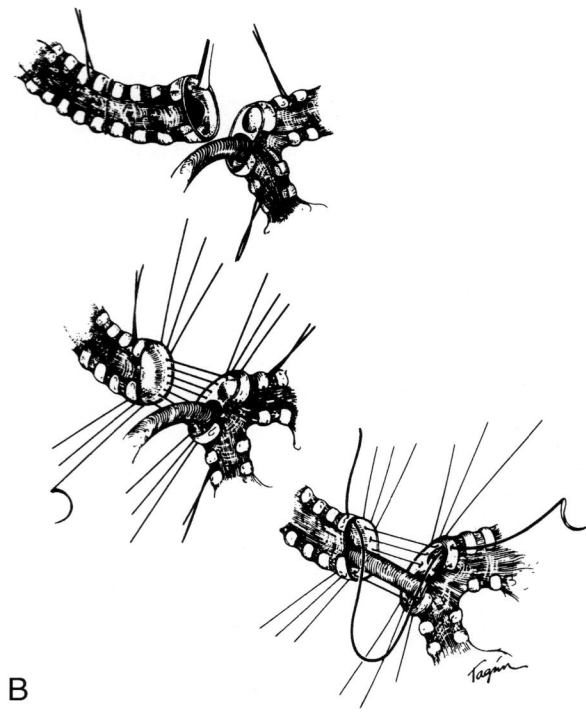

Fig. 75-6. Reconstruction of the lower trachea. **A.** Exposure through a thoracotomy. Hilar mobilization has been accomplished and also circumferential dissection of the trachea. When a tumor is present, paratracheal nodal tissue is excised with the specimen. Traction sutures have been placed proximally and distally. The lines of resection are shown. A clamp may be placed on the pulmonary artery later if the patient fails to maintain adequate oxygenation on intubation of the left main bronchus alone. This step has been necessary in lesions close to the carina as well as in carinal resections. **B.** Details of management of resection and suturing. Intubation has been carried out across the operative field and the specimen is then removed. After placement of sutures on the anterior and lateral walls of the trachea, an elongated endotracheal tube is passed from above into the left main bronchus and the balance of the posterior sutures are placed before their being tied. **C.** After completion of the anastomosis, which is facilitated by flexion of the patient's neck, a second layer of pedicled pleural flap is placed about the anastomosis. From Grillo HC: Surgery of the trachea. Curr Probl Surg 7:3, 1970. With permission.

layer flap is always placed around intrathoracic anastomoses, usually a carefully pedicled pericardial fat pad. I described specific techniques of carinal reconstruction in detail. Laryngeal release is not helpful in carinal resection.

Tracheostomy is avoided after tracheal reconstruction to avoid drying of secretions or injury to the anastomosis. On rare occasions, it may be necessary, temporarily, after laryngotracheal anastomosis.

Complex Methods

One sees few benign lesions or potentially curable malignant lesions that require resection of lengths of trachea and still leave a functional larynx, in which end-to-end reconstruction may not be done by present methods. In a rare instance, I (1965)

applied an extension of an earlier method developed experimentally and clinically for replacement of cervical trachea by fashioning an invaginated, horizontally bipedicled tube of full-thickness skin supported by fully buried polypropylene rings. Results have been no more dependable than the use of prostheses. At present, I believe both should be avoided. The alternatives are T-tubes for benign lesions and irradiation for malignant lesions nonresectable because of length.

Mediastinal Tracheostomy

Rarely, when a lesion involves a large portion of trachea and larynx but seems to be within possible bounds of cure, resection of both larynx and trachea may be indicated, either for palliation of severe airway obstruction or for potential

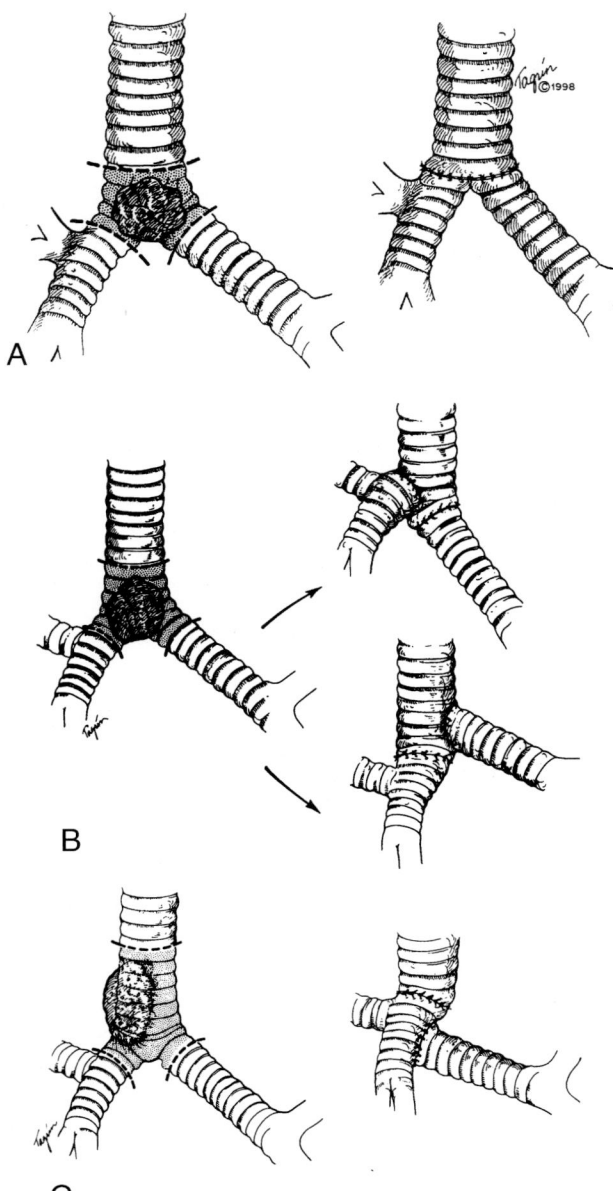

Fig. 75-7. Tracheal reconstruction after carinal resection. **A.** When the lesion is of limited extent, a neocarina may be fashioned. **B.** Following carinal resection without removal of a long segment of trachea, reconstruction is most frequently performed by implanting the left main bronchus into the stump of the devolved lower trachea. The right main bronchus is then implanted preferentially in a side opening fashioned in the lower portion of the trachea. **C.** When a longer segment of trachea has been resected, it frequently is necessary to mobilize the right lung and elevate the right main bronchus to reach the trachea, which also has been devolved as far distally as it will go. In such cases, the left main bronchus may have to be anastomosed to the bronchus intermedius. Preservation of some blood supply for all of these segments of airway is essential for the repair to heal successfully. From Grillo HC: Tracheal tumors: surgical management. Ann Thorac Surg 26:112, 1978. With permission.

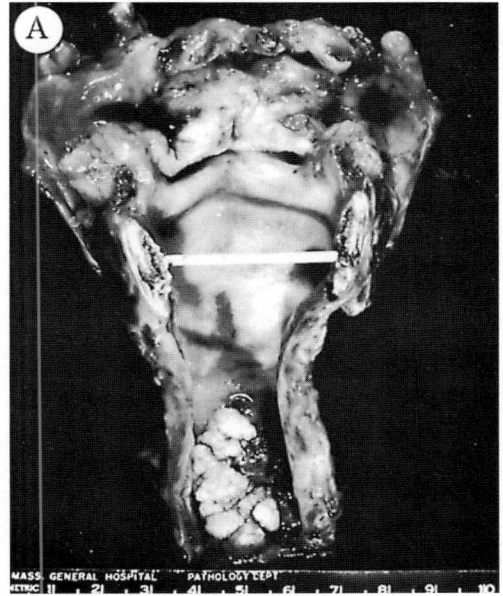

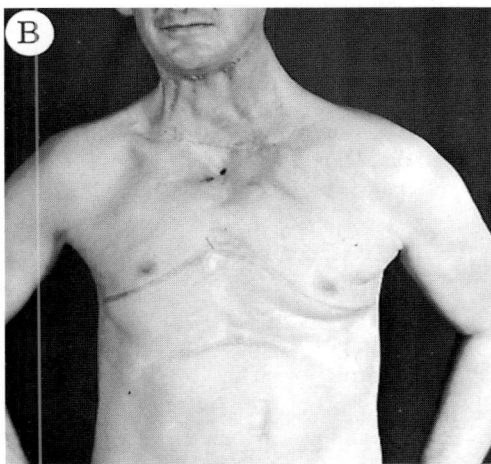

Fig. 75-8. Mediastinal tracheostomy. **A.** Laryngotracheal specimen to remove two obstructing lesions, mucoepidermoid carcinoma of the larynx and squamous cell carcinoma of the trachea, concurrently. Regional node dissections were done later. From Grillo HC: Surgery of the trachea. Curr Probl Surg 7:3, 1970. **B.** Photograph of a patient 18 months after initial resection shows the anatomic features of a low mediastinal tracheostomy. The procedure was carried out between two horizontal incisions, one across the base of the neck and the other beneath the nipples. The upper chest wall defect is the result of the removal of the upper sternum and medial ends of clavicles and upper two ribs. The stoma sits just above the aortic arch. The short horizontal incision just below the stoma was necessary for control of bleeding in the innominate artery postoperatively. The horizontal incision below the xiphoid was initially placed as a relaxing incision to allow advancement of flaps upward.

cure. The cervical esophagus may also have to be removed en bloc. Attempts to pull the deeply situated distal tracheal stump to the surface place excess tension on the suture line; attempts to carry complex skin tubes down to the trachea led to separation at the suture lines, sepsis, and osteomyelitis of the sternum. Massive hemorrhages from the innominate artery and aortic arch have been frequent complications of such methods. Muscle flaps have not fully protected these vessels. A technique that I devised (1966) attempted to eliminate these problems by bringing the anterior skin down to the stump of the trachea by removing the heads of the clavicles, the upper portion of sternum, and the medial ends of the first two ribs (Fig. 75-8). This procedure is done extrapleurally. Excellent blood supply is present in the flap, and the anastomosis is made to a circular opening in the middle point of the flap so that the suture line is simple. If a large amount of skin has to be excised with the lesion, alternative myocutaneous flaps are designed. Hazards of bleeding do attend such procedures, however, if primary healing is not obtained. Elective division of the innominate artery, with appropriate preoperative angiography and intraoperative electroencephalographic monitoring, plus advancement of pedicled omental flaps to the upper mediastinum, as recorded by the author and Mathisen (1990), have avoided such incidents. Waddell and Cannon (1959) and Orringer (1992) recommended transposition of the tracheostome to the right of the innominate artery.

TRACHEOSTOMY AND ITS PROBLEMS

Immediate complications of tracheostomy, such as intraoperative and early postoperative hemorrhage, incorrect placement, injury to adjacent structures, and hypoxia during the procedure, essentially have been eliminated by the deliberate performance of tracheostomy over an emergency airway established by endotracheal intubation or rigid bronchoscopy. Later complications, such as plugging of the tube, valvelike obstruction at the tip caused by dry secretions, slippage of cuffs or of the tube, and local sepsis, have been reduced in incidence by meticulous care of the tracheostomy, and their consequences have been minimized by early recognition and correction. In addition to the late obstructive complications to be discussed in Chapter 69, erosion of the innominate artery and tracheoesophageal fistula must be remembered, as pointed out by Mulder and Rubush (1969) as well as others. I and my colleagues (1976) described a single-stage method for repair of postintubation tracheoesophageal fistula, which has given excellent results.

I prefer to perform a tracheostomy through a short horizontal incision approximately 1 cm below the cricoid and to identify the cricoid precisely so that the correct level of second and third rings may be selected. The thyroid isthmus usually must be divided. A vertical incision in the trachea is used. Extreme care should be exercised to avoid injuring the first ring, because subsequent erosion may damage the cricoid and produce a subglottic stricture that is extremely difficult to repair. If necessary, the tracheal opening should include the fourth ring also. A tube with an inner cannula is preferable. Initially, it is held not only by tapes but also by skin sutures passed through the flanges and tied.

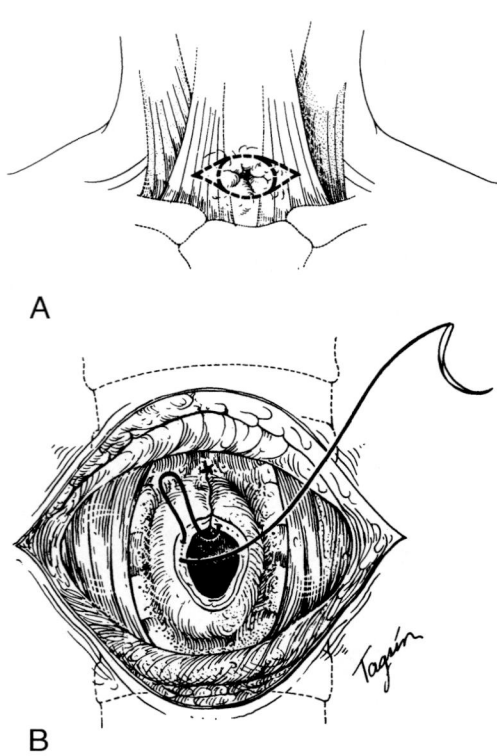

Fig. 75-9. Technique for closure of persistent tracheal stoma. **A.** The skin around the margin of the stoma is elevated with a circumferential incision. The lateral extensions create an ellipse to provide access and permit plastic closure. **B.** After dissection of the skin and platysma above and below, and mobilization of the strap muscles laterally, the central circular flap is created, with great care not to destroy its basal blood supply. It is now closed with a subcuticular suture. The epithelial surface faces the lumen. The strap muscles are next approximated and the skin and platysma are closed above in a horizontal layer. From Lawson DW, Grillo HC: Closure of a persistent tracheal stoma. Surg Gynecol Obstet *130*:995, 1970. With permission.

Another rare complication of tracheostomy is a persistent stoma that does not close even after many months. This situation usually results from a long, persistent tracheostomy, a large stoma caused by the operative procedure or sepsis, healing of skin to tracheal epithelium, and debilitating systemic states that depressed the healing response. Lawson and I (1970) devised a technique for closure that circumscribes the stoma, using the healed skin as a first-stage circular flap (Fig. 75-9). When this skin is inverted with a subcuticular suture, a healed epithelial surface is presented to the tracheal lumen. The strap muscles are approximated and the skin and platysma are closed horizontally over this area. Results of repair by this method have been excellent.

REFERENCES

Barclay RS, McSwan N, Welsh TM: Tracheal reconstruction without the use of grafts. Thorax *12*:177, 1957.
Belsey R: Resection and reconstruction of the intrathoracic trachea. Br J Surg *38*:200, 1950.

Borrie J, Redshaw NR: Cervical tracheal reconstruction in sheep, using silastic prostheses with subterminal suture cuffs. Proc Univ Otago Med School 48:32, 1970.

Cantrell JR, Folse JR: The repair of circumferential defects of the trachea by direct anastomosis: experimental evaluation. J Thorac Cardiovasc Surg 42:589, 1961.

El-Baz N, et al: One-lung high-frequency ventilation for tracheoplasty and bronchoplasty. Ann Thorac Surg 34:564, 1982.

Geffin B, Bland J, Grillo HC: Anesthetic management of tracheal resection and reconstruction. Anesth Analg 48:884, 1969.

Grillo HC: Circumferential resection and reconstruction of mediastinal and cervical trachea. Ann Surg 162:374, 1965.

Grillo HC: Terminal or mural tracheostomy in the anterior mediastinum. J Thorac Cardiovasc Surg 51:422, 1966.

Grillo HC: Surgical approaches to the trachea. Surg Gynecol Obstet 129:374, 1969.

Grillo HC: Surgery of the trachea. Curr Probl Surg 7:3, 1970.

Grillo HC: Primary reconstruction of airway resection of subglottic laryngeal and upper tracheal stenosis. Ann Thorac Surg 33:3, 1982a.

Grillo HC: Carinal reconstruction. Ann Thorac Surg 34:356, 1982b.

Grillo HC, Mathisen DJ: Cervical exenteration. Ann Thorac Surg 49:401, 1990.

Grillo HC, Dignan EF, Miura T: Extensive resection and reconstruction of mediastinal trachea without prosthesis or graft: an anatomical study in man. J Thorac Cardiovasc Surg 48:741, 1964.

Grillo HC, Mathisen DJ, Wain JC: Laryngotracheal resection and reconstruction for subglottic stenosis. Ann Thorac Surg 53:54, 1992.

Grillo HC, Moncure AC, McEnany MT: Repair of inflammatory tracheoesophageal fistula. Ann Thorac Surg 22:112, 1976.

Lawson DW, Grillo HC: Closure of a persistent tracheal stoma. Surg Gynecol Obstet 130:995, 1970.

Michelson E, et al: Experiments in tracheal reconstruction. J Thorac Cardiovasc Surg 41:784, 1961.

Miura T, Grillo HC: The contribution of the inferior thyroid artery to the blood supply of the human trachea. Surg Gynecol Obstet 123:99, 1966.

Montgomery WW: Suprahyoid release for tracheal anastomosis. Arch Otolaryngol 99:255, 1974.

Mulder DS, Rubush JL: Complications of tracheostomy: Relationship to long-term ventilatory assistance. J Trauma 9:389, 1969.

Mulliken J, Grillo HC: The limits of tracheal resection with primary anastomosis. Further anatomical studies in man. J Thorac Cardiovasc Surg 55:418, 1968.

Neville WE, Bolandowski PJ, Kotia GG: Clinical experience with silicone tracheal prosthesis. J Thorac Cardiovasc Surg 99:604, 1990.

Orringer M: Anterior mediastinal tracheostomy with and without cervical exenteration. Ann Thorac Surg 54:628, 1992.

Salassa JR, Pearson B, Payne WS: Growth and microscopic blood supply of the trachea. Ann Thorac Surg 23:100, 1977.

Vogt-Moykopf I, Mickisch GH: Prosthetic replacement of the trachea: Discussion. In Grillo HC, Eschapasse H (eds): International Trends in General Thoracic Surgery. Vol. 2. Philadelphia: WB Saunders, 1987, p. 147.

Waddell W, Cannon B: A technique for subtotal excision of the trachea and establishment of a sternal tracheostomy. Ann Surg 149:1, 1959.

Wilson RS: Anesthetic management for tracheal reconstruction. In Grillo HC, Eschapasse H (eds): International Trends in General Thoracic Surgery. Vol. 2. Philadelphia: WB Saunders, 1987, p. 3.

CHAPTER 76

Management of Nonneoplastic Diseases of the Trachea

Hermes C. Grillo

A wide spectrum of benign conditions that affect the trachea are described under the general headings of lesions that are caused by infection; posttraumatic lesions, including iatrogenic injuries; extrinsic lesions compressing the trachea; and miscellaneous, including a variety of lesions largely of unknown origin. Additional topics that are dealt with in other chapters are congenital lesions of the trachea (see Chapter 77) and acute traumatic injury (see Chapter 70).

INFECTION

Tuberculosis

Tuberculosis of the upper airway appears principally to involve the lower trachea, main bronchi, or both. Acute ulcerative tuberculous tracheitis is treated medically. As the acute process heals, stenosis may evolve. Typically, the stenosis shows a pattern of submucosal fibrosis laid down in circumferential manner with marked narrowing or occlusion of the airway. The tracheal cartilages appear to be grossly intact, although peribronchial or peritracheal fibrosis is seen. The lesions may be quite lengthy and thus present a marked or insuperable surgical challenge. Active tuberculosis should be arrested and controlled before surgical resection and reconstruction is performed. In one patient in whom surgery was forced because of acute disease obstructing both the distal trachea and the carina, healing was unsatisfactory, and fatal disruption occurred. In three patients who required carinal resection and reconstruction for excision of mature stenoses, two had excision of the right upper lobe as well with reimplantation of the bronchus intermedius. Complete stenosis of the left main bronchus has been managed by total excision of that bronchus and advancement and reimplantation of the bifurcation of

the left upper and lower lobes to the carina, as described by Newton and associates (1991).

Histoplasmosis

Histoplasmosis may affect the airways in several ways. It may produce massive mediastinal fibrosis with involvement of distal trachea, carina, and main bronchi, or it may involve principally the right bronchial tree in relation to the masses of lymph nodes in the right paratracheal and pretracheal area and in the middle lobe sump. The fibrosing process may extend centrally to involve the right pulmonary artery up to its point of origin even within the pericardium. The lesions may be a composite of airway compression plus intrinsic fibrotic involvement. Massive histoplasmoma at the carina may compress the airway. In such lesions there may be central caseation with a fibrotic capsule that actually involves one or both main bronchial walls intimately. Another presentation is with densely fibrotic and calcified subcarinal and precarinal lymph nodes, which may invade and erode through the wall of the trachea, carina, or bronchi. Broncholiths also occur peripherally in the lobar bronchi. Secondary infection and hemorrhage may follow. More recently, broncholithiasis in general has been associated with histoplasmosis rather than with tuberculosis, as it was in an earlier era. These clinical manifestations have been described by Mathisen and myself (1992). The organism *Histoplasma capsulatum* is more often identified by special stains in pathologic material removed at surgery rather than on cultures. Organisms have been identified in fewer than 50% of patients who are presumed to have disease originating from this source. It has been theorized that the continuing fibrotic process is a reaction to products of the infection rather than to viable organisms. Thus, diagnosis is often presumptive, based on pathologic and radiologic findings as well as on a history of exposure and clinical evolution of the disease.

Other Inflammatory Disease Processes

A small number of patients have been seen who have suffered from diphtheria in childhood and presented many years later with tracheal stenosis or laryngotracheal stenosis. Because most of these patients had tracheostomies in infancy or early childhood for treatment of the acute disease, it is difficult to differentiate whether the late stenoses were caused by the disease or the treatment. Reconstruction may be possible.

Scleroma is a rare disease that may involve the airways as well as the nasopharynx. It is found in Mexico and Central America. A rare case of necrosing mucormycosis involving the trachea or carina as well as the lungs may be seen in diabetic patients or in people who are immunosuppressed or undergoing chemotherapy, particularly for lymphomas. Prompt and radical surgical excision with the protection of vigorous and prolonged treatment with amphotericin may save some of these patients, as noted by Tedder and associates (1994).

POST-TRAUMATIC LESIONS

Blunt Trauma

Ruptures of the trachea, carina, or main bronchi that are caused by blunt trauma may go unrecognized. Such patients almost always have a history of pneumothorax treated by tube drainage, often bilateral in the case of tracheal rupture. They present with shortness of breath or wheezing. The trachea or bronchus may be reduced to only a tiny opening when the diagnosis is made at last. Treatment consists of prompt excision of stenosis and surgical repair. When the bronchus is injured, every effort is made to salvage the distal lung. This is usually possible unless severe infection has ensued. Deslauriers and associates (1982) have demonstrated adequate function of reimplanted lungs. Functional return appears to be roughly inversely proportional to the length of time that the lung was compromised.

In patients who have suffered tracheal separation caused by blunt injury in the neck and who have been treated by tracheostomy only, total stenosis of the area of separation follows. Both recurrent laryngeal nerves are usually at least temporarily paralyzed and often permanently. Such patients must be evaluated carefully some months after their injury when the local inflammation has subsided. Laryngeal reconstruction, when necessary, with stabilization of the glottic aperture, is generally accomplished first. The larynx is then reconnected to the trachea, as described by Mathisen and myself (1987). An effective although unmodulated voice is

obtained. Pharyngoesophageal separation that was not repaired initially is reconstructed at the same time.

Inhalation Burns

Inhalation burns of the larynx, trachea, and bronchi are particularly difficult injuries to manage. The agent may have been chemical, thermal, or a combination of both. These patients often show little damage to the pharynx or supraglottic larynx once the immediate injury has subsided. Persistent damage often commences in the subglottis just below the vocal cords and extends down the airway in a gradually diminishing intensity of injury. The depth of injury as well as the length of airway injured probably relate to the dose received as well as to the actual injury potential of the agent. Gaissert and I and our colleagues (1993) found that in 18 patients treated for tracheal stenosis that was caused by inhalation injury, 14 had subglottic strictures as well and two had main bronchial stenosis. Although it is sometimes difficult to differentiate later injuries from the intubation with which the patients were treated acutely, three of our patients had laryngotracheal strictures without any history of intubation.

In most cases, the tracheal rings were not destroyed and the injuries were confined to various depths of mucosal and submucosal damage. Attempts at resection of injuries, especially in the early phase, should not be made. First, involvement often commences immediately below the cords and involves the entire subglottic larynx, making repair almost impossible. Second, the burned airway responds poorly to early surgery, even where the lesion appears to be limited, much in the way that burned skin elsewhere in the body does (i.e., by the reformation of massive scarring). With appropriately placed splinting, silicone T-tubes, and a great deal of patience, a stable and open airway may usually be obtained in most of these patients in time.

Posttherapeutic Stenosis

Stenosis of the trachea after tracheal reconstruction in most cases is caused by excessive tension on the anastomosis, and this is related to overzealous resection of too great a length of trachea. Dangerous tensions in tracheal resection may be reached at approximately the 50% level of length of resection in the adult and at the 30 to 40% level in the child. Carinal resections are particularly at risk because of their complex nature. Patients chronically on high doses of prednisone are especially at risk if extensive tracheal resection is performed. Unnecessary disturbance of the blood supply to the trachea by extensive circumferential dissection also leads to stenosis or separation. Profuse, hypertrophic granulations at the anastomosis, which were seen when nonabsorbable sutures were used for tracheal repair, have vanished since the introduction of Vicryl sutures.

Stenoses also may result from radiation therapy and laser injury. Brachytherapy has also contributed a number of main bronchial stenoses. The contribution of lasering to tracheal damage is more difficult to assess because the lasering is often applied for attempted treatment of pre-existing lesions and in conjunction with a tracheostomy performed to safeguard the airway. Whereas laser injury may often be dealt with by subsequent resectional surgery, irradiation injuries may either be surgically uncorrectable when first seen or correctable only with considerable risk.

The special problem of obtaining healing after reconstruction in a previously irradiated trachea (when the dosage has exceeded 4000 cGy approximately 1 year or more earlier) has been largely successfully met by advancement of an omental buttress, as described by Muehrcke and me (1995).

Postintubation Damage

Intubation either with oral or nasal endotracheal tubes or with tracheostomy tubes is most commonly used to deliver mechanical ventilatory support in respiratory failure. Assistance supplied through cuffed tubes has thus far proved to be the only practicable method of management for adults with poor pulmonary or chest wall compliance. High-flow respirators with uncuffed tubes, electrophrenic respirators, and negative pressure tank respirators have not been satisfactory for managing these severe problems. High-frequency ventilation for long-term use remains developmental. A whole spectrum of tracheal lesions resulting from such treatment was discerned by Andrews and Pearson (1971) and by me (1969, 1970) (Fig. 76-1). The most common lesions, and those most amenable to definitive treatment, are those responsible for airway obstruction. Because a single patient may have more than one lesion and because the treatment of these lesions differs, precise definition of the pathologic state is essential in planning treatment. Lindholm (1970) showed that endotracheal tubes may cause injury at the laryngeal level even after only 48 hours of intubation: glottic edema; vocal cord granulomas; erosions, particularly over the arytenoids; formation of granulation tissue; polypoid obstructions; and actual stenosis, particularly at the subglottic intralaryngeal level. Subglottic injury is produced also by cricothyroidotomy and by cricoid erosion caused by high tracheostomy in the presence of kyphosis. Montgomery (1968) noted that subglottic stenosis may be difficult to correct. Sometimes it is impossible.

At the tracheostomy site, granulomas that can obstruct the airway may form during healing. If the tracheostomy stoma has been made too large by turning a large flap or excising a large window in the initial tracheostomy, or if erosion is caused by sepsis and heavy prying equipment, cicatricial healing may produce an anterior A-shaped stenosis that can severely compromise the airway. The posterior wall of the trachea may be relatively intact in these patients. At the level of the inflatable cuff, whether placed on a tracheostomy tube or

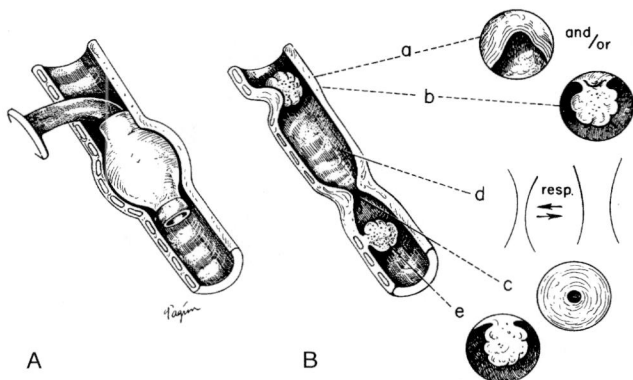

Fig. 76-1. Diagram of inflammatory lesions related to cuffed tracheostomy tubes. **A.** Location of the stoma and the distorting effect of a conventional cuff. **B.** Lesions developing at corresponding sites of injury. At the stoma, an anterior stricture (a) or a granuloma (b), or a combination may occur. At the cuff site (c), circumferential stricture occurs. Between the stoma and such a stricture, varying degrees of tracheal malacia may result, with functional occlusion (d). At the site of erosion by the tip of the tube (e), a granuloma may occur. Innominate erosion and a tracheoesophageal fistula are seen at both cuff level and tip level.

an endotracheal tube, circumferential erosion of the tracheal wall may occur. If this erosion is deep enough, all the anatomic layers of the trachea may be destroyed, so that cicatricial repair results in a tight circumferential stenosis (Fig. 76-2). Malacia may result also. Below this level at the point where the tip of the tube may pry against the tracheal wall, additional erosion may occur with formation of granuloma, especially in children, for whom uncuffed tubes are used. In the segment between the stomal and cuff level, varying degrees of chondromalacia with resulting tracheomalacia may occur. Here, the cartilages are not totally destroyed but only thinned. Bacterial infection in this segment of the trachea during the period of ventilatory support probably contributes to this process.

The etiologic basis of the cuff stenosis has been variously attributed to pressure necrosis by the cuff, irritating quality

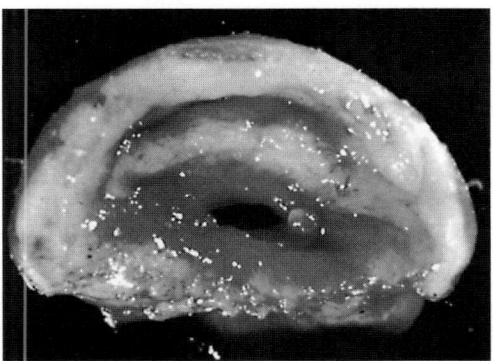

Fig. 76-2. Circumferential stenosis at cuff level. This surgical specimen shows the narrow size to which the lumen may be reduced before recognition of symptoms.

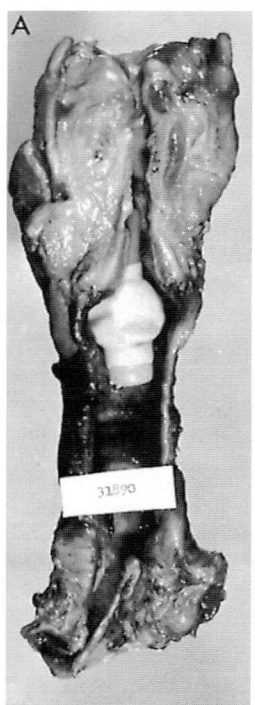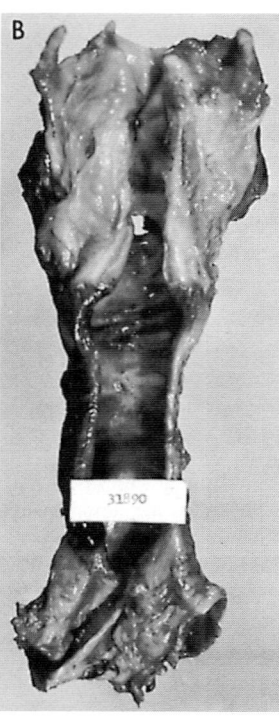

Fig. 76-3. Autopsy specimen of larynx and trachea reveals tracheal injury caused by cuffed tracheostomy tube. **A.** Portex tracheostomy tube had been in place for 19 days. Note the dilatation of the trachea where the cuff had been inflated. **B.** Inflammatory erosive changes have bared multiple cartilages. Note also a distal erosion caused by the tip of the tube. Similar injuries occur with metal or rubber tubes. From Grillo HC: Surgery of the trachea. Curr Probl Surg 7:3, 1970. With permission.

of materials in rubber and plastic cuffs and tubes, irritant materials produced by gas sterilization, hypotension, and bacterial infection. Studies by Cooper and me (1969a), as well as by Florange and colleagues (1965), of autopsy specimens of patients who had been on ventilators with inflated cuffs (Fig. 76-3), prospective studies of similar patients by Andrews and Pearson (1971), and analysis of surgically removed lesions caused by cuffs and experimental reproduction of these lesions under controlled conditions by Cooper and the author (1969a, 1969b) point to pressure necrosis as the principal etiologic agent. As my associates and I (1971) showed, if standard Rusch cuffs are inflated to just provide a seal at ventilatory pressures of approximately 25 cm H_2O, intracuff pressures increase to 180 to 250 mm Hg. Carroll and associates (1969) noted that, although these pressures are not exactly those exerted on the tracheal mucous membrane, high pressures are indeed exerted. The trachea has an elliptic form, so it becomes deformed at the point where a seal is obtained. If perfusion pressures in the patient are lower than normal, necrosis can occur even more easily. The mucosa overlying the cartilage is initially destroyed. The bared cartilages become necrotic and ultimately slough. Attempts at repair after full-thickness damage to the tracheal wall lead only to scar formation. Because

the erosion is circumferential, the resultant strictures are also. Even further erosive damage can lead to tracheoesophageal fistula posteriorly or to perforation of the innominate artery anteriorly.

Patients with stenosis and malacia develop symptoms and signs of airway obstruction consisting of dyspnea on exertion, stridor, cough, and obstructive episodes. Hemoptysis does not occur. In a few patients, pneumonia, sometimes bilateral, has been noted. On occasion, a patient, while still intubated, begins to develop obstruction from formation of granulations around the tip of the tube. In most instances, the obstruction appears only after extubation, because the tube splints a cuff stenosis or potential stomal stenosis as long as it remains in place. Any patient who develops symptoms of airway obstruction who has been intubated for over 24 hours or more within the previous 2 years must be considered to have organic obstruction until proved otherwise. Many such patients have been treated for varying lengths of time with the incorrect diagnosis of asthma. Such errors resulted from lack of awareness of these lesions and the fact that in most patients routine radiography of the chest shows normal lung fields.

Symptoms occurred in a few patients within 2 days of extubation; most demonstrated symptoms between 10 and 42 days after extubation, and a few at greater intervals, usually within a few months. If a patient remains sedentary while recovering from the original disease, the airway may shrink to a critical diameter of 4 to 5 mm before symptoms become obvious. At this aperture, fatal obstruction may occur at any time.

Although general improvement has occurred with design of large-volume cuffs, most of these cuffs can still produce tracheal injury if slightly overinflated beyond their resting maximal volume, because of their relatively inextensible materials. Stomal injuries continue to occur for the reasons described. Cricothyroidotomy may lead to severe or irreparable subglottic injury.

Three additional and particularly severe injuries to the airway may occur from intubation. These are tracheoesophageal fistula, tracheoinnominate artery fistula, and subglottic laryngeal or laryngotracheal stenosis. Tracheoesophageal fistula occurs most commonly in patients who have a ventilating cuff in the trachea for a long period of time along with a feeding tube in the esophagus. The two foreign bodies pincer the "party wall" between trachea and esophagus, leading first to inflammation, which seals one against the other, and then perforation, which may enlarge to include the entire membranous wall of the trachea. Concomitant circumferential injury to the trachea is usually present as well because this is basically a cuff lesion.

Anterior erosion of the trachea may lead to a fistula into the innominate artery. A small number of anterior erosions were seen in the past, which were caused by angulation of a tube tip or a high-pressure cuff itself directly eroding through into the artery. More common, although still rare, are erosions of the artery, which occur at the inferior margin of a low-placed tracheostomy stoma, which is in immediate contiguity with the artery. The inner curve of the tube erodes its way through the arterial wall. It is seen most often in children and young adults in whom tracheostomy is placed too low, because on hyperextension more than one-half of the trachea rises up into the neck. If the stoma is placed with respect to the sternal notch rather than to the cricoid cartilage, the tracheostomy then resides just above the elevated innominate artery. Deslauriers and colleagues (1975) called attention to this complication.

Stenosis of the upper trachea may be associated with a severe subglottic stenosis as well. Stenosis of the subglottic larynx arises from three causes. The principal one is from erosion, which is caused by an endotracheal tube that has been left in place for some time. The principal factor at fault may be use of a tube that has a bore too large for the patient. One of the narrowest parts of the upper airway is at the level of the cricoid cartilage. The second most common cause is erosion by a tracheostomy tube upward through the cricoid cartilage to affect the lower anterior larynx. It occurs most commonly in older patients who are kyphotic and in whom the cricoid cartilage is close to the sternal notch. A third cause of subglottic stenosis is the deliberate use of cricothyroidostomy for ventilation. If damage occurs at the stomal level, it is by surgical selection within the larynx. Lesions that involve the subglottic larynx as well as the upper trachea are much more difficult to repair surgically, although single-staged techniques have been devised by myself (1982), Pearson (1975), and Couraud (1979) and their associates.

Tracheoesophageal fistula becomes manifest by a sudden increase in tracheal secretions and the appearance of any ingested material in the trachea. If the patient is on a respirator, gastric distention may appear. Tracheoinnominate arterial fistulas are rare but may be announced by premonitory hemorrhage or by massive initial hemorrhage. In treating bleeding from a tracheostomy, it is important to differentiate between erosion of tracheal granulations or mucosa and arterial fistula. Sometimes angiography demonstrates a false aneurysm that soon bleeds massively.

EXTRINSIC LESIONS

Goiter

Large goiters, either cervical or mediastinal, may gradually compress the airway sufficiently to cause symptoms. The slow growth of the goiter may deform cartilaginous rings without destroying them. When the goiter is removed, the trachea may remain distorted in shape and narrowed, but clinically significant airway obstruction is rarely present. Quite frequently, removal of the goiter leads to immediate improvement in respiratory symptoms. If, however, sufficient softening of the cartilages has occurred that is caused by the prolonged compression, removing the supporting

mass of thyroid tissue actually allows the trachea to collapse with respiratory effort. This is determined by intraoperative bronchoscopy, local examination and palpation in the operative field, and, finally, by observation of the patient in the operating room after extubation. Several methods of managing this problem have evolved, including intubation with an uncuffed tube followed by tracheostomy, preferably with insertion of a silicone T-tube several days later when the wound is sealed, immediate buttressing of the trachea with specially made polypropylene plastic rings, or in Europe, by using traction sutures from the tracheal wall tied over either internal or external buttons.

An anterior substernal goiter usually does not exert pressure on the trachea because of its position in front of the great vessels. Katlic and colleagues (1985) reported that the trachea was more likely to be compressed by posterior descending goiters that enter the thoracic strait lateral to the esophagus and trachea.

Vascular Compression

Symptoms of tracheal compression may be produced by congenital vascular rings or by aneurysms of the innominate artery or of an anomalous subclavian artery that passes behind the trachea and esophagus. In children, compression may be produced by the innominate artery itself (see Chapter 78).

Patients with a right aortic arch that rises high, turns down sharply in a hairpin configuration, and descends on the right (accompanied by a left anomalous subclavian artery, often a diverticulum of Kummerell, a ligamentum arteriosum, and also with a narrow anteroposterior chest with or without a degree of pectus excavatum) may suffer tracheal compression that becomes severely symptomatic. Excision of the diverticulum and transplantation of the anomalous subclavian may not relieve the obstruction. Aortopexy of the arch or even arch division after aortic bypass may be required.

Mediastinal Masses

Most mediastinal masses that compress the trachea are malignant neoplasms. On rare occasions, however, my colleagues and I have seen a large bronchogenic cyst located at the carina actually compress the airway and also have seen an infant trachea compressed by a large thymic cyst.

Postpneumonectomy Syndrome

After right pneumonectomy, the mediastinum may move completely over to the right axilla and posteriorly, and in so doing, the aortic arch becomes rotated horizontally. This may lead to angulation and compression of the remaining tracheobronchial tree with obstruction either at the carina or in the proximal left main bronchus. The bronchus is actually compressed between the pulmonary artery, which is stretched in front of it, and either the aorta or the vertebral bodies posteriorly. It cannot be predicted which patient will suffer this distortion after pneumonectomy. It was formerly thought that this was principally a syndrome seen in children, but my colleagues and I (1992b) described a number of patients in whom the problem appeared after pneumonectomy in adulthood. The reverse situation may be seen after left pneumonectomy in the presence of a right aortic arch. The patient's symptoms may be rapidly progressive and lead to total disability (see Chapter 37). Rarely, the syndrome may follow left pneumonectomy with a normal aortic arch.

MISCELLANEOUS LESIONS

Relapsing Polychondritis

Relapsing polychondritis is a disease of unknown origin and uncertain course. Cartilaginous structures in the body may be affected, most prominently the nasal and ear cartilages and those of the tracheobronchial tree. The airway changes may precede the more diagnostic changes in the nose and ears, sometimes by years. When the lower trachea and bronchi are affected first, the disease manifests itself by progressive airway obstruction with difficulty in clearing secretions and ultimately pulmonary infections. The disease may extend into the segmental bronchi. Relapsing polychondritis also may affect the larynx and uppermost trachea. Here, the cartilages become inflamed and thickened, and constrictive narrowing of the subglottic and subcricoid airways occurs. The disease may then progress distally, but without predictability. Surgical therapy is usually not applicable. Sometimes it is necessary to provide an airway with a tracheostomy tube, and at times stenting with a silicone T-tube or T-Y tube may provide palliation for a time. The disease is unrelenting.

Wegener's Granulomatosis

Wegener's granulomatosis may affect the larynx and trachea with inflammatory lesions that lead to airway obstruction. The rate and extent of involvement are highly unpredictable. With response to medical treatment, an apparently stable stenosis may result.

Sarcoidosis

Sarcoidosis may produce airway obstruction through the mechanism of massive enlargement of mediastinal lymph nodes compressing the airway and distorting it and, also, by intrinsic fibrotic changes in the wall of the trachea and bronchi. A circumferential stenosis results that usually involves a long segment of trachea and main bronchi. Indeed, it may involve bronchi more distally also. These lesions are not amenable to surgical treatment because of diffuseness and extent, but periodic dilatation is effective for some time.

Amyloid

Amyloid disease on rare occasions involves the trachea and main bronchi in an extensive process leading to narrowing throughout the tracheobronchial tree. The lesion most often is too extensive to permit surgical resection and reconstruction.

Tracheopathia Osteoplastica

Tracheopathia osteoplastica manifests itself pathologically by the formation of calcified nodules beneath the mucosa, adjacent to but not actually originating from the cartilages, as described by Young and associates (1980). The involvement may commence in the subglottic larynx and extend throughout the trachea and more distally into the bronchial tree. It appears in adults, progressing insidiously. Patients have difficulty in raising their tenacious secretions as the disease progresses. Ultimately, severe obstructive symptoms may ensue. In some patients, however, the disease remains a curiosity and does not seriously impair them. Some reported cases have been discovered incidentally on autopsy. I have seen three patients who have required surgical relief.

Tracheobronchiomegaly

Tracheobronchiomegaly (Mounier-Kuhn syndrome) is probably of congenital origin, although it usually becomes clinically manifest in adulthood. The symptoms are progressive dyspnea on exertion and difficulty in raising secretions. The trachea may be hugely widened on radiographic examination, with both unusually elongated cartilages, which are markedly deformed, and a redundant membranous wall. The cartilages tend gradually to assume a reverse curve, which brings the redundant membranous wall up against the cartilages, causing obstruction. The main bronchi are also involved.

Saber-Sheath Trachea

Saber-sheath trachea is a deformity seen usually as an incidental finding in patients with varying degrees of chronic obstructive pulmonary disease later in their life, usually in their 50s and 60s. The radiologic presentation was detailed by Greene and Lechner (1975). The lower two-thirds of the trachea, the intrathoracic trachea, gradually assume a configuration in which the side-to-side diameter diminishes progressively and the anteroposterior diameter increases. The cartilages are not malacic. The configuration of the airway changes. In early stages it causes no difficulty, but as it become more and more marked, the posterior part of the cartilages approximate with attempts to cough and breathe deeply, and the patient finds that he or she cannot clear secretions. The proximal cervical portion of the trachea usually appears quite normal.

Idiopathic Tracheal Stenosis

Idiopathic stenosis presents over a wide spectrum of age, almost exclusively in women, with progressive dyspnea on exertion and wheezing. Patients with idiopathic tracheal stenosis are usually found to have a short stenosis (approximately 2 to 3 cm) involving the uppermost trachea, and in many cases, the subglottic larynx as well. Distally, the trachea appears quite normal. The patients have no history of trauma, infection, inhalation injury, intubation for ventilation, or any other tracheal or airway disease. In a series of 49 patients that my colleagues and I described (1993), only three had any systemic symptoms. Two had mild arthralgias, and one had poorly defined arteritis. Many who had been followed for as long as 15 years had never developed any other systemic symptoms. The stricture itself is roughly circumferential and pathologically shows only chronic inflammation with marked submucosal fibrosis. The cartilages are uninvolved. The pathology is distinct from polychondritis, Wegener's granulomatosis, or any of the aforementioned conditions. The patients do not have mediastinal fibrosis or pathologic processes involving mediastinal lymph nodes. Of the patients in whom an antinuclear cytoplasmic antibody test was done, only the patient with polyarteritis had a positive antinuclear cytoplasmic antibody result. Interestingly, only one patient showed progression of stenosis after surgical resection.

In addition to this quite well-defined lesion, I have seen a small number of patients with stenosis involving a large part of the trachea and others in which the carina or main bronchi, or both, were involved in an undefined inflammatory fibrotic process. In this small group of patients, no other incriminating signs, symptoms, or laboratory findings occurred to implicate any known disease or syndrome. The process tends to progress in these patients.

Tracheal Malacia

Tracheal and tracheobronchial malacia remain poorly defined for the most part. A segmental area of malacia may result from postintubation injury either at the level of a cuff lesion or in the segment between the stoma and the cuff lesion. With chronic obstructive pulmonary disease, including emphysema and chronic bronchitis, malacia may develop in the lower trachea, main bronchi, and sometimes the more distal bronchi. In this situation the tracheal rings take on the shape of an archer's bow with elongation of the membranous wall. When the patient attempts to expire forcefully or to cough, the membranous wall approximates to the anterior softened and flattened cartilage, causing nearly total obstruction. Herzog and associates (1987) have carefully defined this entity. It is entirely different from the characteristics of saber-sheath trachea. A smaller number of patients have been seen who have malacia involving a large portion or even the entire trachea wherein the rings are thinned to a point at which they no longer support the airway. The airway almost takes on the appearance of the esophagus. In these patients, the malacia is total in contrast with the picture just described of anteroposterior collapse. The limited malacia that may result from compression by a goiter or thyroid adenoma has been previously mentioned.

DIAGNOSTIC STUDIES

Tracheal lesions often are recognized late despite a prolonged period of symptoms. As physicians become aware of the possibility of tracheal lesions, they are increasingly suspicious of a diagnosis of adult-onset asthma. Appropriate radiographic examinations are used to rule out the possibility of a tracheal lesion in any patient who has obstructive airway symptoms with radiographic demonstration of normal lung fields. Rarely, even specialized techniques fail to reveal an unusual lesion, and bronchoscopic examination is required.

Radiographic Examination of the Trachea

Radiographic studies of the trachea are used not only to rule in or out the presence of a tracheal lesion but also to define the location, extent, and sometimes the character of the lesion (Fig. 76-4). Furthermore, these studies demonstrate the involvement of paratracheal structures by neoplastic lesions. I (1970) have found the following radiographs to be helpful.

Lateral films of the neck with the chin raised demonstrate most lesions of the upper half of the trachea. Careful technique shows the cartilaginous structures of the larynx as well as the trachea and the relationship of the trachea to the vertebral column posteriorly. If the patient has an existing tracheostomy stoma or has a tracheostomy scar, a radiopaque marker placed on the skin at this level helps to identify its relationship to inflammatory post-tracheostomy lesions.

Anteroposterior views of the airway from larynx to carina, using a copper filter, provide useful overall assessment. Oblique views throw the tracheal air column into relief. Fluoroscopy demonstrates malacia and clarifies vocal cord function.

Tracheal laminography helps give precise measurement of the extent of lesions and their relative distances from landmarks such as the vocal cords and the carina. A magnifying effect occurs in the radiographs, but at the same time

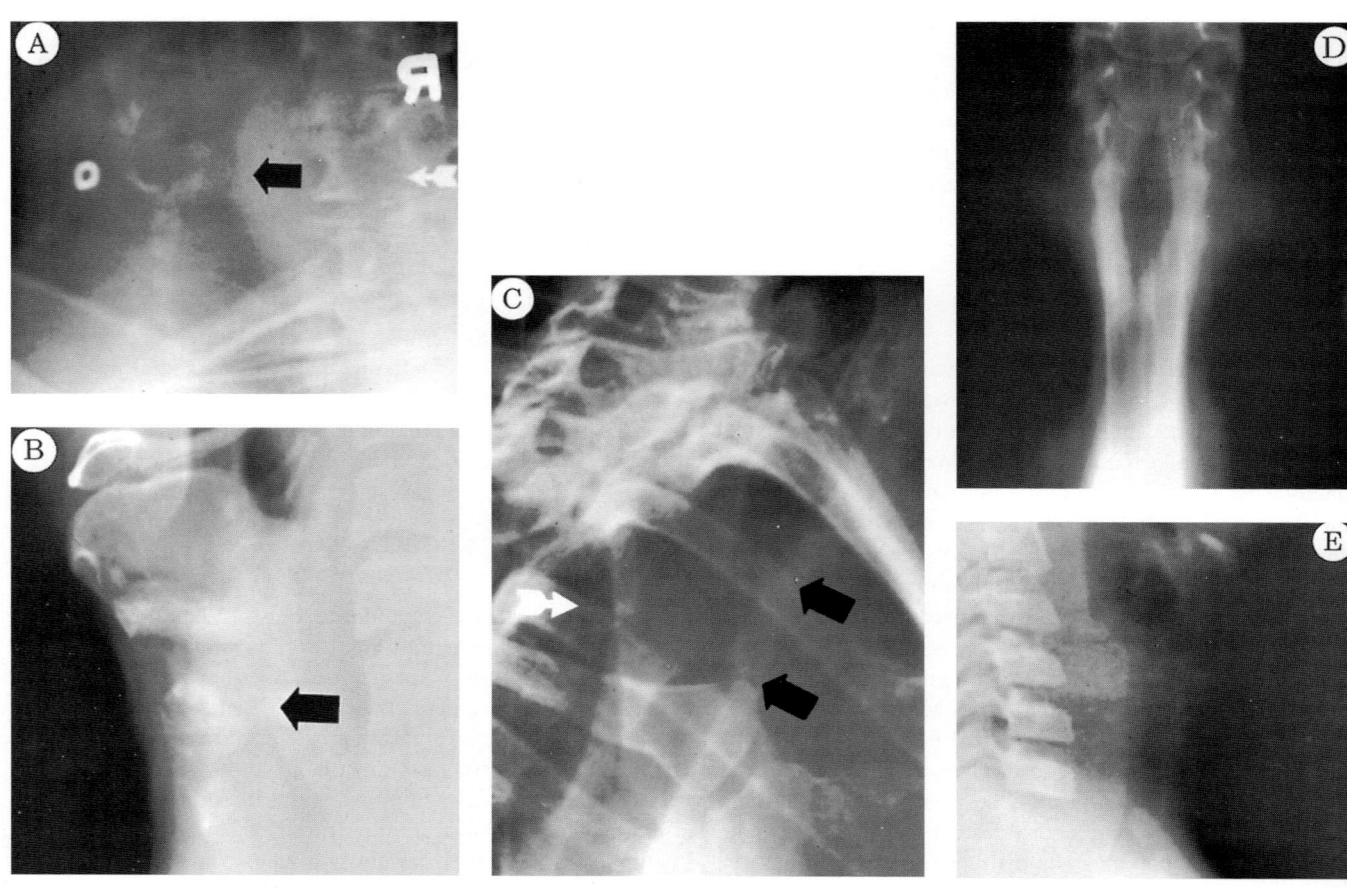

Fig. 76-4. Radiographs showing various injuries from tracheostomy tubes. **A.** Lateral view of the neck. The circular opaque marker is on the skin at the tracheostomy site. The black arrow points to a large inflammatory granuloma occluding the tracheal lumen. Some narrowing of the trachea is seen at this level. Endoscopic removal alone was required. **B.** Similar view showing an anterior stomal stricture. A deep indentation of the anterior trachea is seen at the level marked by the arrow. Resection and reconstruction were necessary. From Grillo HC: Surgery of the trachea. Curr Probl Surg 7:3, 1970. With permission. **C.** Detail of left anterior oblique view of the chest showing a lengthy midtracheal stenosis marked by the two black arrows. From Grillo HC: Surgery of the trachea. Curr Probl Surg 7:3, 1970. With permission. **D.** Laminogram showing the stenosis in **C**. The upper narrowing is at the laryngeal level and is normal. **E.** Lateral neck view with hyperextension to demonstrate granuloma in a child's trachea at the level of the tube's tip. Ventilatory support without a cuff had been given after a cardiac operation in this child.

the trachea is somewhat foreshortened because of its oblique passage through the chest. When viewing all radiographs, as well as during bronchoscopy, it should be noted that the level of the vocal cords is not that of the lowermost portion of the larynx. Approximately 1.5 to 2.0 cm of larynx occur between the vocal cords and the inferior border of the cricoid cartilage. Planning for operative procedures must take this into account.

Contrast studies of the trachea add little information, except with a tracheoesophageal fistula, and this is better shown by barium esophagography.

Computed tomography is valuable only in showing the mediastinal extent of a tumor. It is of little use in assessing benign stenosis except in special cases such as goiter, vascular lesions, or histoplasmosis. Inspiratory and expiratory computed tomography scans help to clarify dynamic states such as tracheobronchomalacia and postpneumonectomy syndrome.

If a patient with tracheal stenosis still has a tracheostomy tube in place, it should be removed during radiographic examination to obtain useful information. Even if a tube has been in place for many months, it should be removed cautiously, with provision made for immediate reinsertion. Emergency equipment including suctioning devices and a range of replacement tubes should be available. The physician must be competent to perform such intubation under slight difficulty. The airway often becomes nearly totally obstructed within 20 to 40 minutes after removal of such a tube. Occasionally, considerable force is required for reinsertion of an airway. Weber and I

(1978) described the radiographic findings in tracheal tumors and stenosis.

Bronchoscopy

Bronchoscopic examination is required, sooner or later, in all of these patients. When a lesion is known to be present, whether it is neoplastic or inflammatory, and when all else points to its surgical correctability, bronchoscopy is best deferred until preparations have been made for definitive treatment of the lesion. The trauma of bronchoscopy in a patient who is subtotally obstructed may precipitate complete obstruction. Little is lost by delaying the bronchoscopy until the time of definitive operation. Frozen sections may be obtained for histologic diagnosis. In the presence of most obstructive lesions, the requirements for resection are clear at the outset. The bronchoscopy is done with the patient under general anesthesia, permitting unhurried, atraumatic examination and manipulation. Bronchoscopic examination and removal are all that is required in patients with polypoid granulomas at the stomal site or at the site of the tube tip. Esophagoscopy is performed also when neoplasms are examined. Rigid bronchoscopy, under general inhalation anesthesia, using pediatric bronchoscopes serially, is used to dilate severe stenosis for emergency relief. Urgent operation is almost never required. Obstructing tumors may similarly be relieved in an emergency situation or if time is needed to assess a patient, by coring out tumor tissue with the tip of the bronchoscope assisted with biopsy forceps. In 30 years, I have never encountered dangerous bleeding or obstruction. The use of laser has been unnecessary for either benign or malignant lesions.

Other Diagnostic Studies

Pulmonary function studies in patients with obstructing lesions of the trachea confirm a high degree of airway obstruction. Measurements are sometimes useful in clarifying the presence of parenchymal disease and may alter the extent of the operative approach. Obstructing lesions generally require surgical relief. Function studies provide a useful basis for measurement of results, especially forced expiratory volume in 1 second, peak expiratory flow rate, and flow-volume loops.

Bacteriologic cultures are made of tracheal secretions and of tracheostomy wounds. Antibiotic sensitivities guide the prophylactic program for perioperative protection.

OPERATIVE VERSUS NONOPERATIVE TREATMENT

The preferred treatment of benign obstruction of the trachea is resection and reconstruction when the patient can tolerate it. With careful evaluation, planning, and execution, most patients with lesions such as postintubation tracheal stenosis can be successfully treated operatively when they have recovered from the primary disease that led to the stenosis. A properly conducted anesthesia and operative repair from the anterior approach do not have a great physiologic effect on the patient. Nonoperative methods of temporizing are, however, available. When the disease is not malignant, undue risks must not be taken. Rarely, the medical condition may not permit even the relatively benign procedure required. If the patient has serious neurologic or psychiatric deficits that prevent cooperation in the postoperative phase, reconstruction is best deferred. The patient and anesthesia must be selected to avoid the need for ventilatory support postoperatively. If ventilatory support is needed postoperatively in a shortened trachea, the cuff may rest against the anastomosis and may lead to dehiscence.

The temporizing methods available are repetitive bronchoscopic dilation of a stenosis or reinstitution of a tracheostomy, dilation of the stricture, and passage of a tracheostomy tube or a silicone T-tube through the lesion to splint the airway. Lesions in the immediate supracarinal position are not easily managed in this way. A tube long enough to remain seated often causes episodes of obstruction when it is near the carina, and a T-Y tube may lead to bronchial granulations. Generally, however, it is wiser to use a T-tube for a permanent airway than to undertake a hazardous reconstruction that has a high risk for failure. Gaissert and I (1993) and Cooper (1989) and colleagues have detailed the uses and results of T-tube management of complex airway problems.

Repeated dilation and splinting have been proposed as definitive methods for treating tracheal stenosis. In most severe lesions in which the whole thickness of the tracheal wall has been converted to scar tissue, even prolonged stenting for many years does not lead to permanent recovery. Numerous patients have been treated this way. Despite repeated trials, it has been impossible, with only rare exceptions, to remove the splinting tube. When lesser degrees of damage have occurred, either in the completeness of a stricture of the circumference of the trachea or in the depth of the tracheal wall, a period of prolonged splinting, on occasion, may result in an adequate airway after removal of the splint. Such a result has been reported in children. Toty and colleagues (1987) pointed out that laser treatment can lead to cure only in granuloma, also easily removed by bronchoscopy, and thin, weblike stenosis. Such stenoses are rare. The principal effect of the laser in these lesions has been to delay definitive treatment and, sometimes, to worsen the lesion. Particularly to be deplored is reestablishment of tracheostomy to permit laser treatment, which is usually ineffective.

Few, if any, patients with postintubation tracheal stenosis cannot be repaired successfully when first identified. Successive failed or inappropriate therapies make such patients' stenoses unreconstructible.

Prevention of Postintubation Tracheal Stenosis

The incidence of stenosis at the stomal level can be reduced by careful placement of the stoma, avoidance of large apertures, elimination of heavy and prying ventilatory connecting equipment, and meticulous care of the tracheostomy.

Many proposals have been made to reduce the formerly inevitable occurrence of some stenoses at the cuff level. These methods included use of double-cuff tubes, changes in materials and sterilization techniques, attempts to avoid cuffs altogether, use of disk and sponge seals instead of cuffs, use of spacers to relocate the cuff level periodically, and pre-stretching of plastic cuffs. The only promising methods, accepting the present need for cuffs in management of adult patients in severe respiratory failure, have been intermittent inflation of cuffs cycled to the respirator, described by Arens and colleagues (1969), and, more simply, the development of large-volume, low-pressure cuffs that conform to the shape of the trachea rather than deforming it, described by Cooper and me (1969b) and by me and my coworkers (1971) (Fig. 76-5). Such a cuff provided a seal at intracuff pressures of 33 mm Hg compared with 270 mm Hg in a comparative Rusch standard cuff. Thus, in a series of 45 patients in whom such a cuff was compared, on a randomized basis, with standard cuffs, 25 patients with the soft cuff showed one-half as much damage, scaled on the basis of endoscopic observations at the time of deflation of the cuff, as 20 patients with standard cuffs. All severe damage was in the standard group. The inci-dence of cuff stenosis has decreased markedly as equipment has improved, but low-pressure cuffs must be inflated care-fully to avoid converting them to high-pressure cuffs. Failure to do so has continued to produce a steady flow of stenoses requiring reconstruction.

Cricothyroidostomy should be avoided. Although laryn-geal injury is rare, it may not be correctable when it occurs. Tracheal injuries, also rare, are reparable when they first occur. Inappropriate treatment has served to make some incorrectable.

This section on operative versus nonoperative treatment and on prevention of lesions has been confined to the most frequent lesion (postintubation stenosis). Space does not permit consideration of each of the other varied benign lesions described earlier in this chapter.

RESULTS OF TREATMENT

I and my colleagues (1995) reported 503 patients who underwent reconstruction for postintubation tracheal injury between 1965 and early 1992. One hundred four of the referred patients had undergone prior reconstructive attempts or other major tracheal procedures. Two hundred fifty-one had postintubation stenoses at the site of an inflat-able cuff. There were 178 stomal stenoses and 38 stomal and cuff stenoses, and in 36 the origin was uncertain. Sixty-two had involvement of the subglottic larynx. Twenty patients

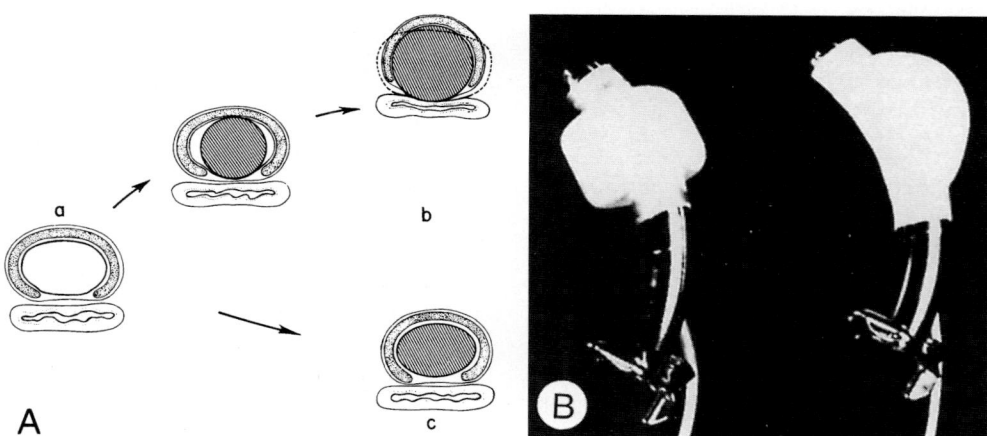

Fig. 76-5. A. Diagram of the mechanism of pressure necrosis by a tracheostomy cuff and its avoidance. (a) Nor-mal elliptic shape of the trachea. When a conventional cuff is inflated, it may expand in circular fashion in its widest diameter but at this point fails to occlude the basically irregularly elliptic shape of the trachea. (b) Further distention has been required to effect a seal. At this point the trachea is deformed by the cuff, and much of the considerable intracuff tension is transmitted to the tracheal wall. (c) A large-volume low-pressure cuff has been inflated with a minimal amount of air. The cuff conforms to the irregular shape of the lumen and provides a seal at low intracuff pressures. Correspondingly low pressures are transmitted to the tracheal wall. **B.** Comparison of a standard cuff and a large-volume, low-pressure cuff. On the left, the large-volume cuff is shown spontaneously filled with air. No stretch has been placed on the rubber of the cuff wall at this point. The volume is sufficient to occlude most adult tracheas. On the right, a Rusch cuff has been distended with 8 mL of air. It is tense and eccen-tric. The stretching of the rubber has created a hard structure that exerts considerable pressure on the trachea, which it must deform to provide a seal. From Grillo HC, et al: A low pressure cuff for tracheostomy tubes to min-imize tracheal injury: a comparative clinical trial. J Thorac Cardiovasc Surg 62:898, 1971. With permission.

with tracheoesophageal fistula were corrected by the technique I reported with my colleagues (1976). One presented with a tracheoinnominate arterial cuff fistula. Corrective reconstructive surgery was effected through the cervical route alone in 350 of these patients, with the addition of an upper sternotomy in 145, through the transthoracic route in 6, and a skin tube replacement was constructed in one patient for a total of 521 operations in 503 patients (see Chapter 75).

In 440 patients, the results were good or excellent. An *excellent* result denotes an anatomically and functionally normal airway. The patient suffers no limitation whatsoever because of the airway, and on either radiographic or bronchoscopic examination, or both, essentially no narrowing is demonstrated at the anastomotic site. Patients classified as having a *good* result have no functional difficulty whatsoever but may have a minimal anatomic narrowing that is definable on either radiographic study or bronchoscopic examination.

The results in 31 patients were classified as *satisfactory*. These patients are able to carry out all of their normal daily activities but have enough narrowing of the airway to limit major physical effort.

Twenty patients had treatments listed as failures. Causes of failure included inadequate appreciation of existing neurologic dysphagia, cardiac decompensation requiring postoperative ventilation, unappreciated severe laryngeal dysfunction, and restenosis. Five deaths occurred. In four of the patients who died, the patients were sent to us on respirators and hence reconstruction was contraindicated but undertaken because no therapeutic alternative existed. The other developed bilateral pneumonia and could not be weaned from postoperative respiratory support. My colleagues and I (1986) described the complications of tracheal surgery for both benign stenosis and neoplasms in detail. Donahue and I and our colleagues (1997) were surprised to find that the outcome was good or satisfactory in 92% of 75 patients operated after unsuccessful initial repairs.

Pearson and Andrews (1971) reported 60 patients with tracheal stenosis. In 34 the stenosis was at the stomal and in 26 at the cuff level. Thirty-seven segmental resections were performed. In 33 of the patients, the results were good, and in one the result was fair. There was one failure and two operative deaths. Six of the patients developed significant restenosis, and re-resection was performed with good results in all but one of the group. Laryngeal release was used as an adjunctive procedure in five of these patients.

The management of acquired benign tracheoesophageal fistula depends on whether the adjacent segment of trachea is circumferentially damaged, as it almost always is in postintubation lesions, or whether the posterior wall fistula is the sole tracheal pathology, as it usually is in fistulas that are caused by foreign bodies. In the first case, concomitant tracheal resection is done with lateral excision of the fistula in the esophageal wall. In the latter, tracheal resection is unnecessary, and both membranous tracheal wall and esophageal wall are precisely repaired after division of the fistulae. Healthy tissue, such as strap muscles from the anterior approach or intercostal transthoracically, is always interposed between the two suture lines to prevent recurrence. Mathisen and associates (1991) noted excellent results after repair of 27 postintubation fistulas, with one death after anastomotic separation consequent to an extensive tracheal resection. Three deaths also occurred after transthoracic repair of distal posttraumatic fistulas in the presence of established mediastinal sepsis. All three required postoperative ventilation. Prompt recognition and repair following the initial injury would likely have been successful.

I reported the results, with my colleagues (1992a), of single-stage laryngotracheal resection and repair of postintubation subglottic stenosis involving larynx and upper trachea in 50 patients. An additional 30 patients had stenoses in the same location from other causes: trauma, seven; idiopathic, 19; and miscellaneous, four. Long-term results were excellent in 18 patients, good in 51, satisfactory in eight, and failed in two. One died of acute myocardial infarction. Maddaus (1992) and Couraud (1979) and their colleagues have produced similar encouraging results.

Mathisen and I (1987) found that 16 of 17 patients treated for laryngotracheal stenosis resulting from trauma had good airways and voices, despite the initial presence of vocal cord paralysis in 14. Four also had esophageal injury requiring repair. Eight needed intralaryngeal procedures before laryngotracheal repair.

Gaissert and coworkers (1993) found that complex laryngotracheal strictures caused by burns responded well in many cases to prolonged stenting (mean, 28 months) with recovery of a functional airway and voice in most patients. In a few, resection of subglottic stenosis was necessary. Early tracheal resection was best avoided. Of 16 patients treated, nine required no airway support, four have permanent tracheal tubes, two died (one from respiratory failure and one from an unrelated cause), and one was lost to follow-up.

After a failed attempt at tracheal reconstruction with postoperative stenosis, it is best to wait for a prolonged period to permit resolution of the scar and inflammation in the operative field. A minimum of 4 months and preferably 6 months should be allowed. In the meanwhile, it may be necessary to insert a tracheal T-tube or tracheostomy tube to maintain the airway. Reoperation is often extremely difficult. It is surprising, however, to find in some situations in which there appeared to be tension at the original anastomosis that re-resection of a limited stricture may be done with the finding that no apparent tension exists at the time of the second repair. This, however, is not universally true. The greatest enemy of secondary resection is the possibility of anastomotic tension, which may have led to the first failure. Much, therefore, depends on the individual history of the patient.

Histoplasmosis can present nearly insuperable problems in airway management. In the description of the manifestations of mediastinal fibrosis and histoplasmosis, Mathisen and I (1992) listed nine patients who had undergone tracheobronchoplastic procedures: right carinal pneumonectomy in four, carinal reconstruction in one, sleeve lobectomy in three, and main bronchial sleeve resection in one. Three died postoperatively, one from anastomotic separation after extended resection, and two from postpneumonectomy respiratory distress syndrome.

With my colleagues, I (1992b) presented the results of surgical attempts to treat severe postpneumonectomy syndrome in 11 adults. Ten underwent mediastinal repositioning. Five who had not also developed tracheobronchomalacia did well. Another died from presumed pulmonary embolism. Four suffered malacic obstruction unrelieved by repositioning. Aortic division with bypass to relieve compression and resection of malacic airway in these desperately ill patients produced only one success. Clearly, correction must be done early, before malacia develops.

Extrinsic compression caused by substernal or intrathoracic goiter is generally relieved, without the need for tracheal procedures, by thyroidectomy, as shown by Katlic and colleagues (1985) in a series of 80 patients. Dyspnea was present preoperatively in 28% and stridor in 16%; 79% had tracheal deviation. Flow-volume loops showed tracheal obstruction. No deaths occurred. The procedure is well tolerated even by frail and aged patients: Only a few required tracheal splinting. No effective medical treatment exists.

I and my associates (1993) defined the clinical and pathologic characteristics of idiopathic laryngotracheal stenosis and reported results of surgical treatment in 35 patients. Twenty-nine underwent single-stage laryngotracheal resection and reconstruction, and six underwent cricotracheal segmental resection and reconstruction. Thirty-two achieved good or excellent results in voice and airway, two needed annual dilatations, and one has a permanent tracheostomy.

In three patients who presented with severely obstructive tracheopathia osteoplastica, I performed a tracheal fissure from the cricoid to the carina and inserted a Tor T-Y (Hood, Inc., Pembroke, MA) tube for splinting. Once the trachea has been divided anteriorly, because the membranous wall is not involved by the disease process, it is possible to hinge the two anterolateral walls on either side outward so that a wide lumen is created by the T-tube. The tracheal wall can then be sutured together again. The T-tube is allowed to remain in place for 4 to 6 months to allow firm healing of the trachea in an open position. The tube is removed, having established an adequate airway. Prior attempts have been made to use the laser but failed. One patient required a permanent T-tube.

An attempt at splinting and shortening the posterior membranous wall combined with an attempt to reshape the reverse curve of the cartilages failed in one patient with Mounier-Kuhn disease in whom it was attempted. It was necessary to insert an in-lying permanent tracheal T-tube. Two other patients have been treated in similar fashion since that time, and all have achieved satisfactory palliative results.

In two patients with such extreme saber-sheath trachea that they were unable to clear secretions, the trachea was splinted with external special polypropylene ring splints.

The tracheal wall was sutured to the splints, pulling it outward. The sternohyoid muscles were turned down to embed the rings against the tracheal wall to maintain correction after nonabsorbable sutures ultimately pull through. The procedure permitted the patients to clear secretions, which they had not been able to do before.

In patients with tracheobronchial malacia affecting the lower two-thirds of the trachea and main bronchi, who have softened, splayed out cartilages in an archer's bow configuration, and redundant membranous tracheal wall, reshaping the trachea was proposed and described by Herzog and colleagues (1987). A strip of splinting material is placed along the membranous wall of the trachea in a width corresponding to estimated normal. The corners of the cartilages on either side are sutured to the splint, and the membranous wall is quilted to the splint as well. Pulling the two ends of the cartilages together posteriorly causes the cartilages to arch forward, re-creating a more nearly normal cross-sectional configuration. The redundant membranous wall is fixed to the splint posteriorly so that it cannot pout forward to obstruct the lumen. Herzog originally used fascia lata and eventually moved to use of Gore-Tex. Other materials that have been used include lyophilized bone and perforated plastic splints.

Gore-Tex, in my experience, gave an initially excellent result. In one patient, however, after some months, fluid accumulated between the Gore-Tex and the membranous wall where sutures had pulled through, because Gore-Tex does not become enmeshed in scar tissue. Strips of pericardium harvested within the operative field may be satisfactory. Marlex mesh, which has pores large enough to permit ingrowth of connective tissue to fuse it to the membranous wall, works equally well. Although this procedure does not correct the underlying obstructive pulmonary disease from which most of these patients suffer, it does improve the delivery of gases through the major airways and provide more effective cough. It is possible from the right thoracotomy approach to splint not only the lower two-thirds of the trachea but also the right main bronchus and bronchus intermedius and the left main bronchus to its bifurcation.

REFERENCES

Andrews MJ, Pearson FG: The incidence and pathogenesis of tracheal injury following cuffed tube tracheostomy with assisted ventilation: an analysis of a two year prospective study. Ann Surg 173:249, 1971.

Arens JF, Oschner JL, Gee C: Volume-limited intermittent cuff inflation for long-term respiratory assistance. J Thorac Cardiovasc Surg 58:837, 1969.

Carroll R, Hedden M, Safar P: Intratracheal cuffs: performance characteristics. Anesthesia 31:275, 1969.

Cooper JD, Grillo HC: The evolution of tracheal injury due to ventilatory assistance through cuffed tubes: a pathologic study. Ann Surg 169:334, 1969a.

Cooper JD, Grillo HC: Experimental production and prevention of injury due to cuffed tracheal tubes. Surg Gynecol Obstet 129:1235, 1969b.

Cooper JD, et al: Use of silicone stents in the management of airway problems. Ann Thorac Surg 47:371, 1989.

Couraud L, et al: Intérêt de la résection cricoidienne dans le traitement des sténoses cricotrachéales après intubation. Ann Chir Thorac Cardiovasc 33:242, 1979.

Couraud L, et al: Posttraumatic disruption of the laryngo-tracheal junction. Eur J Cardio Thorac Surg 3:441, 1989.

Deslauriers J, et al: Innominate artery rupture: a major complication of tracheal surgery. Ann Thorac Surg 20:671, 1975.

Deslauriers J, et al: Diagnosis and long-term follow-up of major bronchial disruptions due to nonpenetrating trauma. Ann Thorac Surg 33:32, 1982.

Donahue DM, et al: Reoperative tracheal rejection and reconstruction for unsuccessful repair of postintubation stenosis. J Thorac Cardiovasc Surg 114:934, 1997.

Florange W, Muller J, Forster E: Morphologie de la nécrose trachéale après trachéotomie et l'utilisation d'une prosthèse respiratoire. Anesth Analg 22:693, 1965.

Gaissert HA, Lofgren RH, Grillo HC: Upper airway compromise after inhalation injury. Complex strictures of larynx and trachea and their management. Ann Surg 218:672, 1993.

Greene RE, Lechner GL: "Saber-sheath" trachea: a clinical and functional study of marked coronal narrowing of the intrathoracic trachea. Radiology 115:265, 1975.

Grillo HC: The management of tracheal stenosis following assisted respiration. J Thorac Cardiovasc Surg 57:52, 1969.

Grillo HC: Surgery of the trachea. Curr Probl Surg 7:3, 1970.

Grillo HC: Primary reconstruction of airway after resection of subglottic laryngeal and upper tracheal stenosis. Ann Thorac Surg 33:3, 1982.

Grillo HC, et al: A low pressure cuff for tracheostomy tubes to minimize tracheal injury: a comparative clinical trial. J Thorac Cardiovasc Surg 62:898, 1971.

Grillo HC, et al: Postintubation tracheal stenosis: treatment and results. J Thorac Cardiovasc Surg 109:486, 1995.

Grillo HC, et al: Idiopathic laryngotracheal stenosis: the entity and its management. Ann Thorac Surg 56:80, 1993.

Grillo HC, Mathisen DJ, Wain JC: Laryngotracheal resection and reconstruction for subglottic stenosis. Ann Thorac Surg 53:54, 1992.

Grillo HC, Moncure AC, McEnany MT: Repair of inflammatory tracheoesophageal fistula. Ann Thorac Surg 22:112, 1976.

Grillo HC, et al: Postpneumonectomy syndrome: diagnosis, management and results. Ann Thorac Surg 54:638, 1992.

Grillo HC, Zannini P, Michelassi F: Complications of tracheal reconstruction. J Thorac Cardiovasc Surg 91:322, 1986.

Herzog H, et al: Surgical therapy for expiratory collapse of the trachea and large bronchi. In Grillo HC, Eschapasse (eds): International Trends in General Thoracic Surgery: Major Challenges. Philadelphia: WB Saunders, 1987, p. 74.

Katlic MR, Grillo HC, Wang CA: Substernal goiter: analysis of 80 Massachusetts General Hospital cases. Am J Surg 149:283, 1985.

Lindholm CE: Prolonged endotracheal intubation. Acta Anaesth Scand 33(Suppl):1, 1970.

Maddaus MA, et al: Subglottic tracheal resection and synchronous laryngeal reconstruction. J Thorac Cardiovasc Surg 104:1443, 1992.

Mathisen DJ, Grillo HC: Laryngotracheal trauma. Ann Thorac Surg 43:254, 1987.

Mathisen DJ, Grillo HC: Clinical manifestations of mediastinal fibrosis and histoplasmosis. Ann Thorac Surg 54:1053, 1992.

Mathisen DJ, et al: Management of acquired nonmalignant tracheoesophageal fistula. Ann Thorac Surg 52:759, 1991.

Montgomery WW: The surgical management of supraglottic and subglottic stenosis. Ann Otol 77:534, 1968.

Muehrcke DD, Grillo HC, Mathisen DJ: Reconstructive airway surgery after irradiation. Ann Thorac Surg 59:14, 1995.

Newton JR, Grillo HC, Mathisen DJ: Main bronchial sleeve resection with pulmonary conservation. Ann Thorac Surg 52:1272, 1991.

Pearson FG, Andrews MJ: Detection and management of tracheal stenosis following cuffed tube tracheostomy. Ann Thorac Surg 12:359, 1971.

Pearson FG, et al: Primary tracheal anastomosis after resection of the cricoid cartilage with preservation of recurrent laryngeal nerves. J Thorac Cardiovasc Surg 70:806, 1975.

Tedder M, et al: Pulmonary mucormycosis: results of medical and surgical therapy. J Thorac Cardiovasc Surg 57:1044, 1994.

Toty L, et al: Laser treatment of postintubation lesions. In Grillo HC, Eschapasse H (eds): International Trends in General Thoracic Surgery. Vol. 2. Philadelphia: WB Saunders, 1987, p. 31.

Weber AL, Grillo HC: Tracheal stenosis: an analysis of 151 cases. Radiol Clin North Am 16:291, 1978.

Young RH, Sandstrom RE, Mark EJ: Tracheopathia osteoplastica: clinical, radiologic, pathologic and histogenetic features. J Thorac Cardiovasc Surg 79:537, 1980.

CHAPTER 77

Benign and Malignant Tumors of the Trachea

L. Penfield Faber and William H. Warren

Tumors of the trachea are rare, despite their histologic similarity to tumors of the main stem bronchus and lung. They are approximately 100 times less common than bronchial tumors and constitute only 2% of all upper respiratory tract tumors, as reported by Perelman and Koroleva (1987). Tracheal cancer is responsible for less than 0.1% of all cancer deaths, as noted by Pearson and Gulane (1995). Malignant tumors of the trachea are more common than benign tumors. Houston and associates (1969) reviewed 30 years of experience at the Mayo Clinic, and 53 of 90 tracheal tumors were malignant. Hajdu and colleagues (1970) reported a series of 41 primary malignancies of the trachea that were treated over a period of 33 years at a major cancer hospital. This number represents slightly more than one malignant tracheal tumor per year seen at a major referral center, which emphasizes the relative rarity of these tumors. In a center study of 208 patients with primary tracheal tumors reported by Regnard and associates (1996), 181 were malignant and 27 were benign. The most common malignant tumors are squamous cell carcinoma and adenoid cystic carcinoma. In a review of 43 tracheal tumors occurring in infants and children, Gilbert and associates (1953) noted that 93% were benign. Desai and associates (1998) reviewed 36 reported tracheal tumors in infants and children from 1965 to 1995: 23 were benign and 13 were malignant. Malignant fibrous tumors and mucoepidermoid carcinoma were the more common malignant variants in children. The predominant benign tumors in children are hemangiomas, fibromas, and papillomas.

Secondary tumors also involve the trachea. Direct extension into the trachea occurs from cancers of the thyroid, larynx, lung, and esophagus. Mediastinal tumors may directly invade the trachea; the most common is lymphoma. Metastasis to the trachea is uncommon, but breast cancer, melanoma, and sarcomas have all been found in the trachea.

SYMPTOMS AND FINDINGS

Dyspnea and shortness of breath on exertion are the most common presenting symptoms and, according to Perelman

and Koroleva (1987), occur when the tracheal lumen has been reduced to one-third of its normal cross-sectional area. Perelman and coworkers (1996) noted inspiratory dyspnea in 80% of patients. Regnard and associates (1996) reported that 42% of 208 patients had a presenting complaint of dyspnea. Cough is a common symptom associated with tracheal neoplasms, but no particular salient features are associated with a cough to indicate that it is caused by a tracheal tumor. As the airway narrows, the classic symptom of wheezing becomes apparent. Stridor is a more prominent form of wheezing and indicates significant compromise of the airway. Often, a patient with a tracheal tumor is treated for asthma for a prolonged period.

Hemoptysis occurs in approximately 20% of patients with tracheal neoplasms and is most commonly seen in patients with squamous cell carcinoma. People with benign tumors rarely, if ever, present with hemoptysis. A change in voice quality can be related to paralysis of the vocal cord resulting from invasion of the recurrent laryngeal nerve or by direct extension of an upper tracheal tumor into the larynx. Recurrent pneumonitis, either unilateral or bilateral, can occur from obstruction of a main bronchus. Perelman and Koreleva (1987) reported that the interval between the onset of early symptoms and diagnosis was approximately 25 months for benign tumors and 8 months for malignant tumors. Regnard and associates (1996) noted that the mean duration of symptoms for patients with adenoid cystic carcinoma was 12 months and 4 months for tracheal cancers. The long duration of symptoms is emphasized by the finding of Perelman and colleagues (1996) that 23% of patients with tracheal tumor arrived at the Center for Surgery with life-threatening asphyxia. Regnard and associates (1996) also noted acute respiratory failure in 29% of patients.

Dysphagia is an uncommon symptom that indicates esophageal compression by a large bulky neoplasm. Auscultation of the chest reveals a coarse wheeze that is enhanced by rapid and deep inspiration. The wheeze is more prominent on inspiration than on expiration and is different from the wheezing commonly associated with bronchial asthma.

Obstruction from a tracheal tumor can be heard if the examiner places an ear close to the patient's open mouth during deep and forceful breathing. This is a simple but major finding associated with laryngeal or tracheal obstruction. The neck and supraclavicular fossae should be examined carefully for evidence of enlarged lymph nodes, which may indicate spread of a malignant tumor. Location of tumors in the trachea, as reported by Perelman and associates (1996), was the thoracic trachea in 77, the cervical trachea in 26, and the carinal region in 41 patients.

DIAGNOSIS

Radiographic Features

Careful inspection of tracheal air column on posteroanterior and lateral chest radiographs sometimes reveals a tracheal tumor (Fig. 77-1). Oblique views of the trachea and lateral neck radiographs and hyperextension reveal the presence of the tumor but do not provide specific information necessary for a planned resection and reconstruction. Linear tomography, as described by Weber and Grillo (1992), provides excellent visualization of the extent of the tumor (Fig. 77-2). Tracheal tomograms, however, are not effective for determining extraluminal extension of the tumor or lymph node invasion. Computed tomography (CT) has generally replaced linear tomography as the primary method of radiologic evaluation of a tracheal tumor. Mediastinal extension, esophageal compression, and tracheal lumen size are all seen clearly on the CT scan (Fig. 77-3). Using thin-cut CT sections and knowing the distance between the cuts can permit a moderately accurate measurement of the length of trachea that is involved by the tumor. Gross pathologic characteristics of the tumor are also identified on CT scan. Benign lesions are frequently round and smooth and approximately 2 cm in diameter. The tumor is generally inside the lumen of the trachea, and the well-circumscribed nature of the tumor is clearly evident. Calcification is a characteristic of benign lesions and is seen in tumors, such as chondromas and hamartomas (Fig. 77-4). Calcification is also present, however, in a chondrosarcoma. Malignant tumors extend up and down the trachea for several centimeters, and the surface of the tumor is irregular and possibly ulcerated. The tracheal wall is obviously invaded by the tumor at its base, and extraluminal growth may be present (Fig. 77-5). Enlarged lymph nodes usually indicate metastatic spread. The CT scan should always be done with infusion to delineate clearly the relationship of the tumor to the superior vena cava and other vascular structures in the mediastinum. No specific radiologic findings that differentiate malignant tumors of the trachea exist.

Magnetic resonance (MR) imaging can offer some advantages in the assessment of tracheal neoplasms. Coronal, oblique, and sagittal views can be obtained that demonstrate long lengths of the trachea and delineate a more precise length of tracheal involvement by the tumor. T_1-weighted

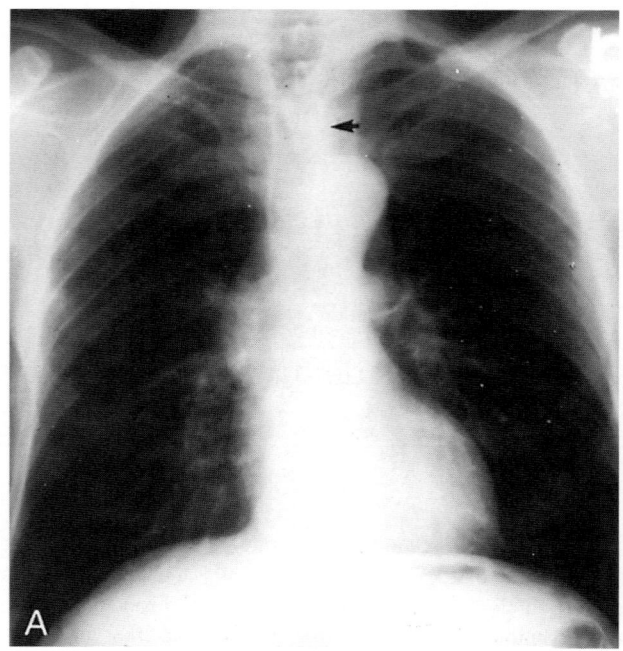

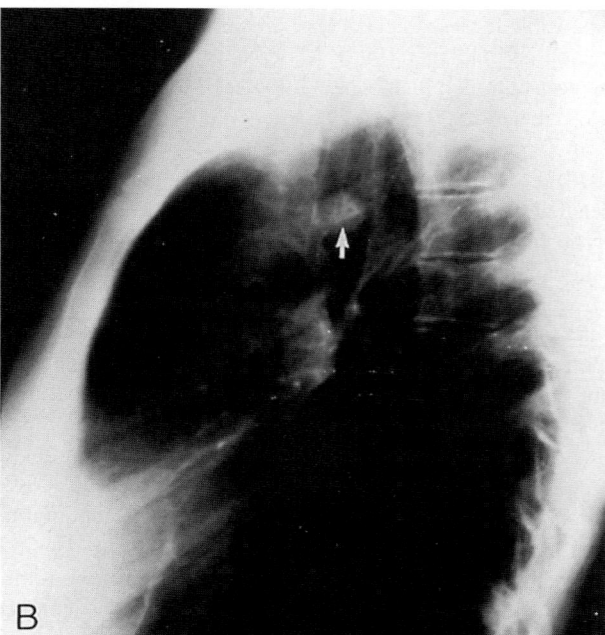

Fig. 77-1. A. A chondroma can be seen on this frontal chest radiograph (*arrow*). **B.** Tracheal hamartoma is clearly identified on this lateral chest radiograph (*arrow*).

images characterize the anatomy of the trachea and adjacent soft tissues quite well. MR imaging also clearly depicts adjacent vascular structures and permits assessment of possible invasion of these structures. MR angiography can be used in place of conventional angiography when vena caval obstruction is evaluated.

Three-dimensional helical CT of the central airway can provide precise anatomic information for the planning of

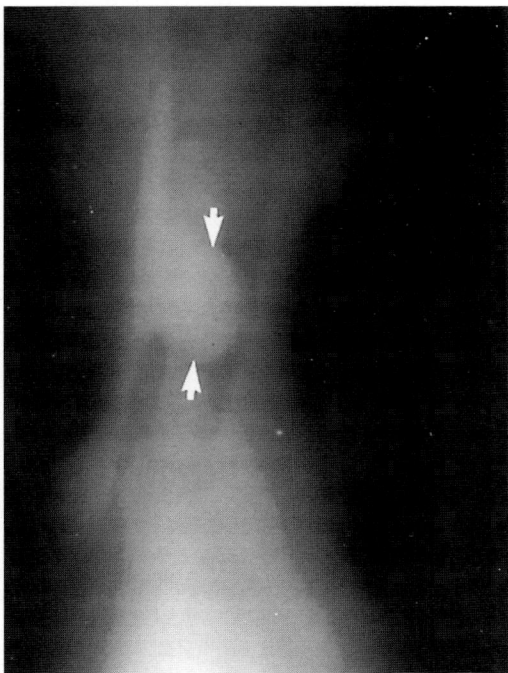

Fig. 77-2. Linear tomogram clearly depicts the length of involvement of a carcinoid tumor of the trachea (*arrows*).

endobronchial and surgical procedures. Kauczor and associates (1996) evaluated 36 patients with proven airway obstruction. The majority had bronchial carcinoma or mediastinal or hilar lymphadenopathy. Bronchoscopic correlation was completed in all patients. Anatomy of the lesions

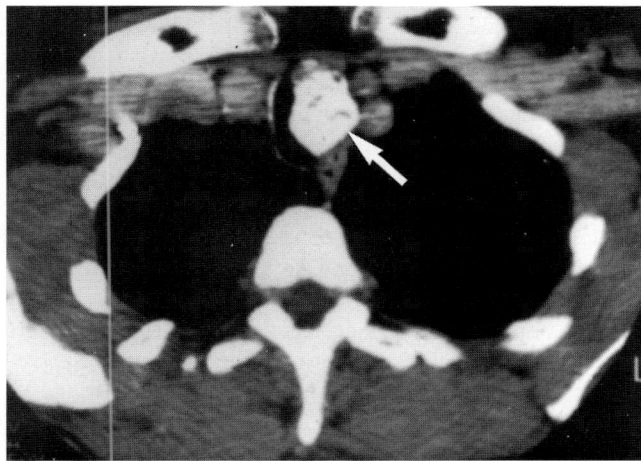

Fig. 77-4. The computed tomogram demonstrates almost total calcification of a tracheal chondroma (*arrow*).

was clearly depicted and closely correlated to the bronchoscopic findings. Three-dimensional helical CT provided added information in assessing the distal airway when the bronchoscope could not be passed through the obstructing lesion. This radiologic technique will become most valuable in planning tracheal resections or in monitoring palliative efforts for tracheal neoplasms.

If the patient complains of dysphagia, a barium examination of the esophagus can demonstrate compression or possibly invasion. This study may also further define the extraluminal extent and size of the tracheal neoplasm.

Pulmonary function studies reveal airway obstruction characterized by a reduced volume of air expired in one second, a significantly decreased peak flow rate, and a flattened expiratory flow volume loop. Maximum voluntary ventilation is diminished. Pulmonary function tests may also delineate the presence or absence of parenchymal lung disease.

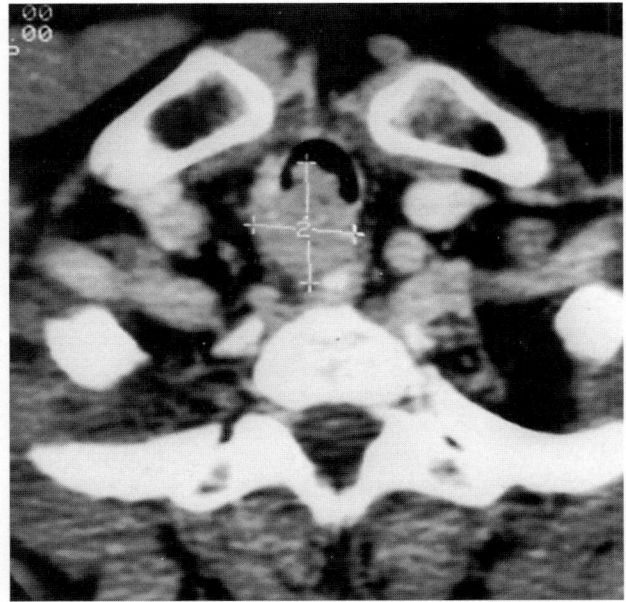

Fig. 77-3. Computed tomogram identifies posterior mediastinal extension of an adenoid cystic carcinoma.

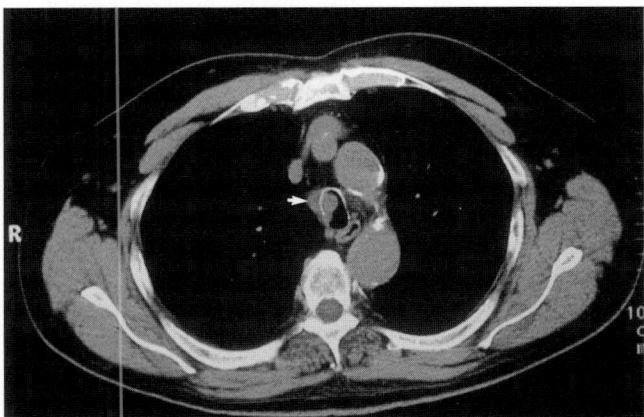

Fig. 77-5. Computed tomographic scan shows adenoid cystic carcinoma extending through the tracheal cartilage (*arrow*).

Bronchoscopy

Bronchoscopy is a necessary step in the diagnosis and clinical evaluation of a patient with a tracheal tumor. Biopsy and manipulation of a tracheal tumor is potentially hazardous, however, because bleeding can cause complete tracheal obstruction. A sedated or anesthetized patient may be unable to maintain adequate ventilation, and the passage of an endotracheal tube may not be possible because of the obstructing tumor. The bronchoscopic examination should be carried out by an experienced endoscopist, who can insert an open-tube bronchoscope through the tumor to establish an airway and manage any complications of hemorrhage.

A bronchoscopic examination is always conducted in the operating room, where ventilating bronchoscopes and biopsy forceps are available and a trained anesthesiologist is close at hand. Grillo (1989) believes that when the indications for primary tracheal resection are clear-cut, bronchoscopy can be deferred until the time of the operative procedure and frozen sections are used to determine histology. With the flexible fiberoptic bronchoscope, however, a careful examination and biopsy can be accomplished in the awake patient. A preresection bronchoscopy offers several advantages:

1) Vocal cord function is evaluated and the entire larynx and cricoid cartilage are seen clearly. This visualization is particularly important for upper tracheal lesions in which a partial resection of the cricoid or laryngectomy may be required.
2) The gross characteristics of the tumor are noted, and an impression can be gained whether the tumor is benign or malignant.
3) The size of the tracheal lumen is clearly noted. this assessment is extremely helpful in planning anesthetic management of the airway during the initial phase of tracheal resection.
4) A biopsy sample can be obtained with the small biopsy forceps through the flexible instrument, and knowing the histology is of benefit in planning the treatment program.
5) Frequently, the small flexible fiberoptic bronchoscope can be inserted past the neoplasm and the distal airway can be carefully examined. The length of the tumor can be carefully measured and correlated with the radiologic measurements.

These findings are extremely helpful in planning the surgical approach and resection.

The bronchoscopy is performed with the flexible fiberscope passed through a topically anesthetized nasopharynx to a position above the larynx. Supplemental oxygen is provided through the mouth. Several aliquots of 4% lidocaine (Xylocaine) are instilled on and through the vocal cords until satisfactory topical anesthesia is achieved. The vocal cords and larynx are examined carefully, and the bronchoscope is then passed into the trachea to visualize the tumor. Decision for biopsy depends on the vascularity of the tumor and the size of the tracheal lumen. The decision for biopsy requires careful judgment, and the biopsy should not be done if there is any possibility of airway compromise (Fig. 77-6). Houston

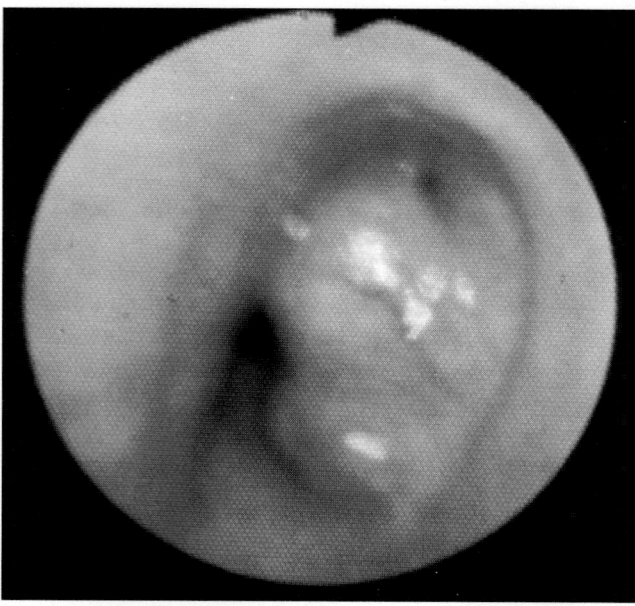

Fig. 77-6. Adenoid cystic carcinoma partially obstructs the tracheal lumen. The flexible bronchoscope passed easily and biopsy was done with evaluation of the distal trachea.

and colleagues (1969) reported that, of 53 primary cancers of the trachea, the diagnosis was established by bronchoscopic biopsy without complication in 47 patients (Fig. 77-7).

When life-threatening airway obstruction occurs from a tracheal tumor or bleeding from a biopsy obstructs the airway, an adequate tracheal lumen can be established by coring out the tumor with the rigid bronchoscope and biopsy forceps, as described by Mathisen and Grillo (1989). Regnard and associ-

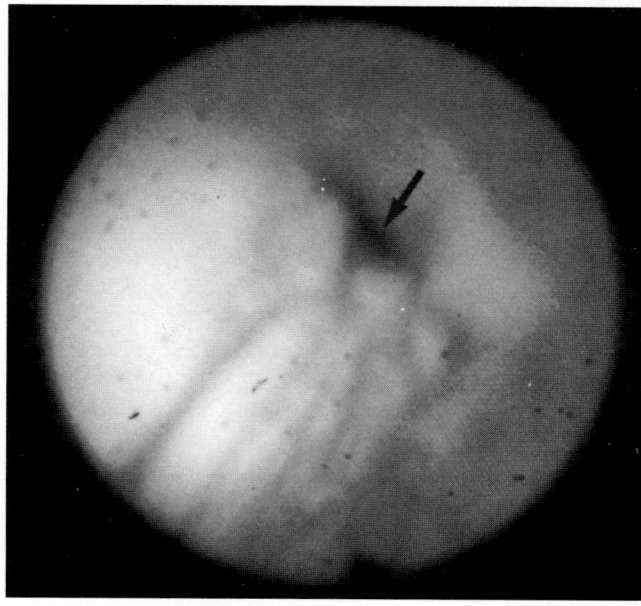

Fig. 77-7. A trachea almost totally occluded by adenoid cystic carcinoma (*arrow*). Bleeding from biopsy or manipulation could be life threatening.

ates (1996) recommend the relief of tracheal obstruction to better define location and size of the tumor and to provide a more adequate airway. In their series of 208 tracheal tumors, airway obstruction in 62 of 71 patients was relieved by laser treatment, by bronchoscopic débridement in five, and by cryotherapy in two. Tracheostomy was done to provide an adequate airway in two patients. Daddi and associates (1998) describe several advantages associated with the endoscopic treatment of airway obstruction before attempted curative resection. They included the improvement of respiratory function, a better assessment of the exact location of the tumor by endoscopic means, more reliable CT scanning of the airway, and improvement of the patient's performance status with associated pulmonary therapy and antibiotics. Endoscopic débridement was accomplished with ventilating rigid bronchoscopes and the neodymium:yttrium-aluminum-garnet (Nd:YAG) laser.

BENIGN TUMORS

Gilbert and associates (1953) reported that the common benign tumors of the trachea are chondroma, papilloma, fibroma, and hemangioma. Benign tumors most often occur in the upper one-third of the trachea in children and are more common in the lower one-third in adults, frequently arising from the membranous portion of the trachea (Table 77-1).

Chondroma

According to Mark (1983), the most common benign mesenchymal tumor of the trachea is a chondroma (Fig. 77-8).

Table 77-1. Benign Tracheal Tumors

Tumor Type	No. [Perelman and Koroleva (1987)]	No. [Grillo and Mathisen (1990)]
Squamous papillomata	9	5
Multiple	—	4
Solitary	—	1
Pleomorphic adenoma	4	2
Granular cell tumor	—	2
Fibrous histiocytoma	—	1
Leiomyoma	1	2
Chondroma	—	2
Chondroblastoma	—	1
Nerve sheath tumor	6	2
Paraganglioma	—	2
Vascular tumor	4	1
Vascular malformation	—	2
Myoblastoma	1	—
Lipoma	1	—
Xanthoma	1	—
Pseudosarcoma	—	1
Total	**27**	**23**

Note: Some of the tumors listed have been reclassified from the original source.
From Gilbert JG, et al: Primary tracheal tumors in the infant and adult. Arch Otolaryngol Head Neck Surg 58:1, 1953. With permission.

These tumors histologically duplicate normal cartilage and can exhibit vascular invasion. Endoscopically, a chondroma appears as a firm, white nodule projecting into the lumen of the trachea. The tumor occurs in a 4:1 preponderance in men, and it is more common in adults than in children. No definite

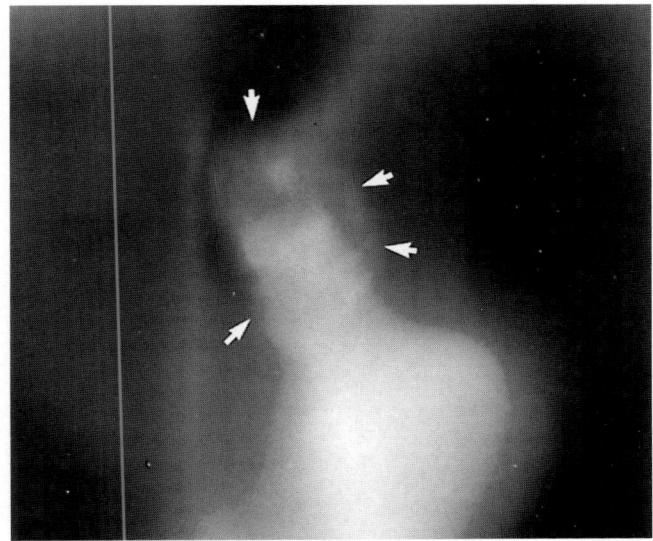

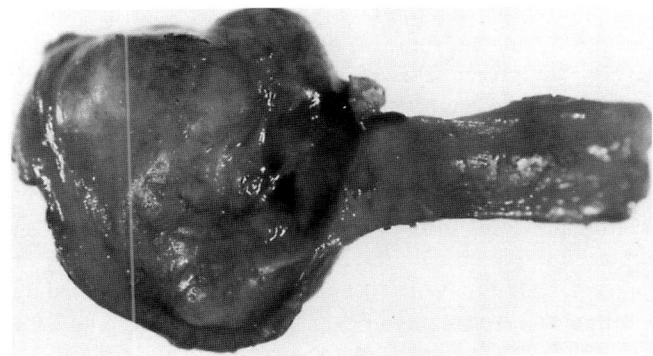

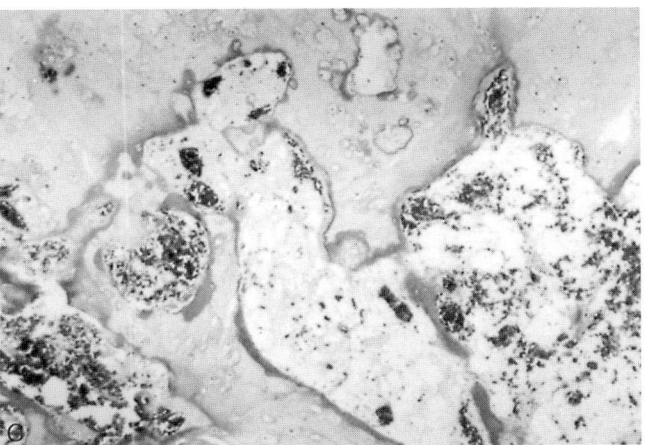

Fig. 77-8. A. Linear tomogram depicts a calcified chondroma (*arrows*). B. The benign chondroma is removed by segmental tracheal resection. C. Microscopic examination reveals areas of ossification in a largely cartilaginous tumor.

etiology for this lesion has been described. A chondroma occurs more frequently in the larynx than in the trachea. Biopsy of the lesion can be difficult because of its firm consistency, and this characteristic can indicate the diagnosis. Vascularity is minimal, and the lesion can be removed easily through the bronchoscope. Recurrence after endoscopic removal has been observed, however, and Salminen and colleagues (1990) reported malignant transformation to chondrosarcoma. Recommended treatment is segmental tracheal resection.

Papilloma

A solitary papilloma of the trachea is rare, but this lesion does occur in adults. A solitary benign papilloma is easily removed through the bronchoscope and the base of the tumor can be ablated with the Nd:YAG laser. Periodic endoscopic surveillance is indicated, and recurrence can be treated with laser ablation.

Juvenile laryngotracheal papillomatosis is common in children and is seen more frequently than is solitary papilloma of the trachea. It accounts for 60% of benign tracheal tumors in children, according to Beattie and associates (1992). It has been linked with the human papilloma virus of types 6 and 11. Papillomatosis more commonly involves the larynx, but it is found in the tracheobronchial tree in 20% of patients. It follows a relatively benign course, requiring repeated endoscopic removal, with recurrence rates as high as 90%. Complications include chronic cavitary respiratory papillomatosis resulting from proliferation of the virus in the distal bronchial tree, as noted by Karley and colleagues (1989). Malignant transformation of papillomatosis has been reported in patients with a history of radiation therapy or smoking, but it may also occur in nonsmokers, as noted by Guillou and associates (1991). The types of therapy for the more invasive form of the disease include photodynamic therapy with sensitization of the papilloma cells using hematoporphyrin diacetate, as described by Kavuru (1990) and Basheda (1991) and their colleagues. Leventhal and associates (1991) reported successful treatment with the use of lymphoblastoid interferon-α-N1.

Fibroma

Fibroma accounts for approximately 20% of all benign tumors in adults, according to Beattie and colleagues (1992). Mark (1983) reported that fibroma is more common than fibrosarcoma and can be difficult to distinguish from a fibrous histiocytoma. A benign fibroma is easily removed through the bronchoscope, followed by careful laser ablation of the base of the tumor. Local recurrence would be unusual, but if it does occur, segmental tracheal resection would then be indicated.

Hemangioma

Mark (1983) noted that hemangioma of the trachea is similar to hemangioma of the skin in infants, with an increase in size at 1 month of age followed by a spontaneous decrease in size at 1 year. It may arise in the trachea or extend into the tracheal lumen from a hemangioma located in the mediastinum. Treatment may require tracheostomy to provide an adequate airway, followed by repeated small doses of radiation therapy to shrink the tumor. Weber and coworkers (1990) used steroids to cause regression. Many lesions require no treatment, and natural regression frequently occurs. Larger hemangiomas of the lower trachea may require direct surgical intervention. In this instance, a careful plan must be developed for airway control during excision of the tumor. Franks and Rothera (1990) used cardiopulmonary bypass to resect a low-lying tracheal hemangioma.

Other Benign Tumors

Granular Cell Tumor

The granular cell tumor occurs less frequently in the trachea than it does in the tongue, neck, or larynx. Burton and associates (1992) summarized the reported experience with this tumor in the trachea and identified 24 cases. The tumor is thought to be of neurogenic origin and derives from Schwann cells. Malignant transformation of the granular cell tumor does occur in other sites, but it has never been reported in the trachea. Both endoscopic and partial tracheal resection have been successful as treatment of this lesion. Burton and associates (1992), however, described a case of local recurrence after endoscopic resection that then required partial tracheal resection. Daniel and colleagues (1980) recommended removal of tumors larger than 1 cm by a segmental tracheal resection because of the increased risk for full-thickness wall involvement with tumors of this size. Smaller lesions (<1 cm) are easily ablated by endoscopic Nd:YAG laser therapy. Cunningham and coworkers (1989) recommend the use of bipolar cautery. Endoscopic therapy would certainly be applicable to large tumors as well, with resection reserved for local recurrence, because malignant transformation of this tumor in the trachea has yet to be reported.

Fibrous Histiocytoma

Fibrous histiocytoma is a histologically benign tumor in the trachea, but it can be locally infiltrative (Fig. 77-9). An associated prominent inflammatory component can cause the tumor to be termed an *inflammatory pseudotumor*. The behavior of this tumor in the trachea appears to be benign, but because of its local infiltration, segmental resection is the treatment of choice. Resection of a malignant fibrous histiocytoma of the trachea was reported by Randleman and associates (1990) with identification of one other case in the literature.

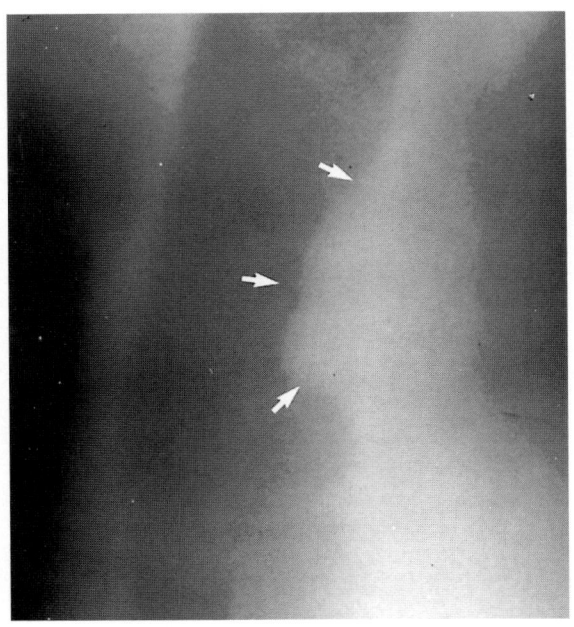

Fig. 77-9. A broad-based fibrous histiocytoma (*arrows*) removed by segmental tracheal resection.

Glomus Tumor

Glomus tumor is a benign neoplasm arising from specialized cells surrounding arterial venous anastomoses. Garcia-Prats and colleagues (1991) reviewed the literature and found six cases of tracheal origin. All tumors were treated by segmental tracheal resection.

Lipoma

Tracheal lipoma is a rare lesion, with five cases reported (Fig. 77-10). Chen (1990) described a patient with a tracheal lipoma requiring major tracheal resection for complete removal. Other authors describe endoscopic removal. It is only logical to approach this tumor with endoscopic removal because it is a completely benign tumor, and any local recurrence can be treated successfully with laser therapy.

Leiomyoma

A leiomyoma may occur as a primary tracheal tumor and, according to Mark (1983), it usually occurs in the distal

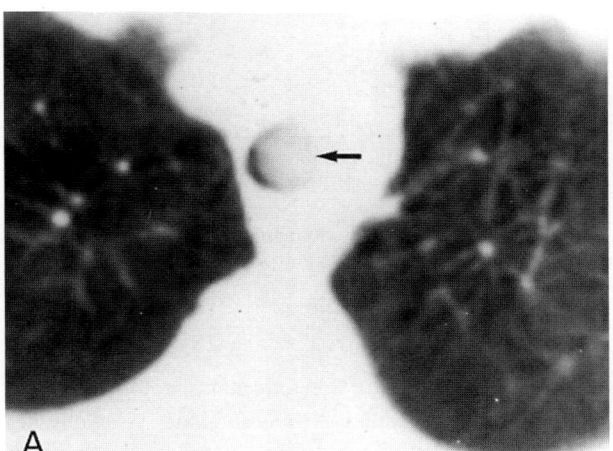

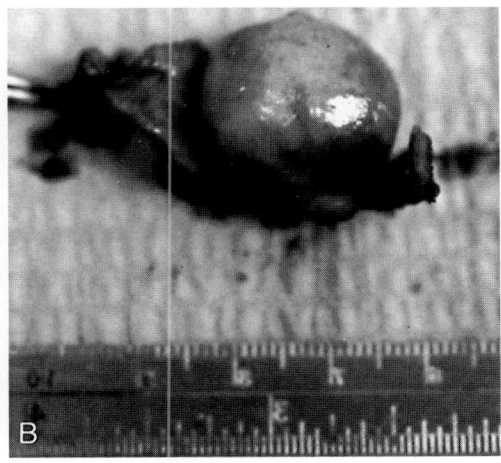

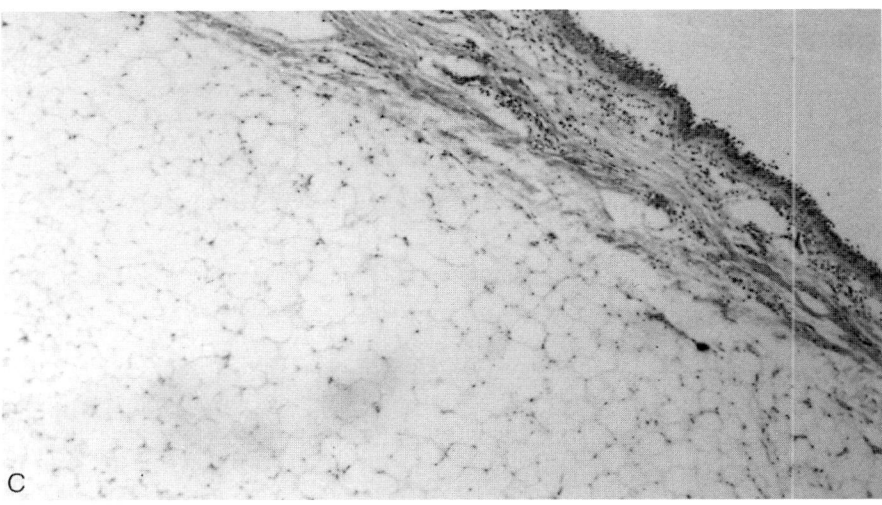

Fig. 77-10. A. Computed tomogram shows almost total tracheal obstruction by a lipoma (*arrow*). **B.** Tracheal resection was required for the removal of the broad-based lesion. **C.** On microscopic examination, the fatty tumor is seen in the submucosa of the trachea.

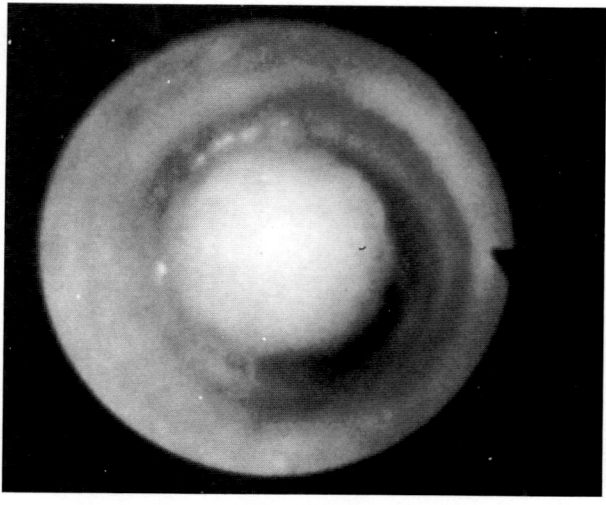
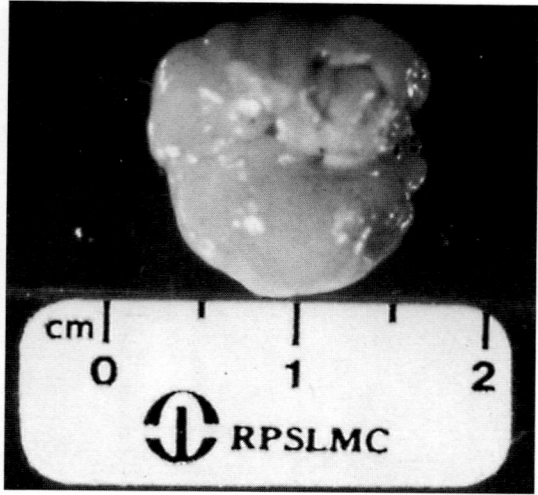

A,B

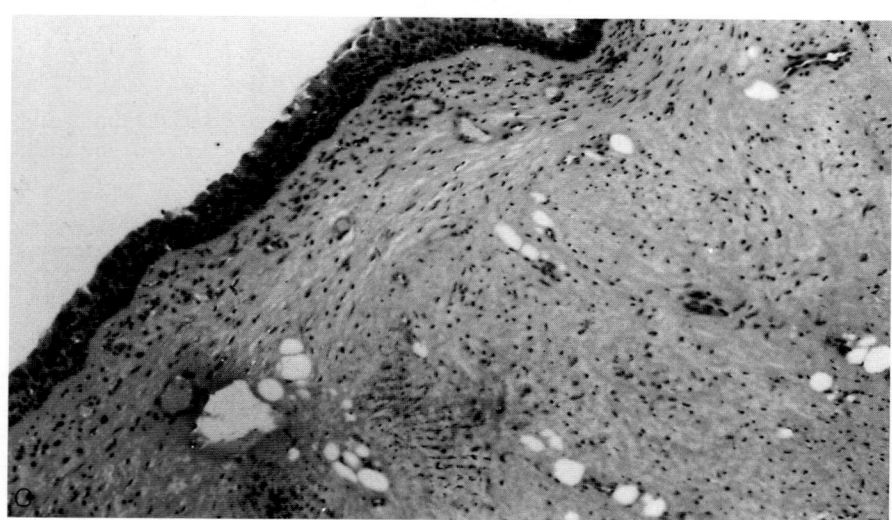

C

Fig. 77-11. A. Bronchoscopic appearance of a tracheal hamartoma. **B.** Resection was accomplished through a rigid, open bronchoscope. **C.** Fibrous hamartoma. Microscopic examination reveals dense connective tissue, fat, and smooth muscle in tracheal submucosa.

one-third of the trachea. Both tracheal resection and endoscopic removal have been described in rare case reports.

Neurofibroma

The neurofibroma can occur in the trachea as a primary tumor, but it is not associated with generalized neurofibromatosis. This tumor can invade the wall of the trachea, and segmental resection would be the treatment of choice.

Pang (1989) presented two cases of primary neurilemoma (schwannoma) of the trachea. His review identified 14 other reported cases. These tumors derive from the Schwann cell and are typically slow growing. The tumor usually has a broad base, and complete removal by bronchoscopy would be difficult. These tumors can recur with malignant potential, and segmental tracheal resection is the treatment of choice.

Hamartoma

Hamartoma is a benign tumor composed of tissues normally found in that organ or structure, but the normal-

appearing tissues are not in their normal histologic pattern. Most hamartomas are found in the pulmonary parenchyma, but 10% are located in the main bronchus or trachea. They are polypoid in appearance and can cause symptoms of respiratory obstruction. The CT scan can be diagnostic in detecting fat and calcification in a smooth and rounded lesion. They do not become malignant, and endoscopic resection is the treatment of choice (Fig. 77-11).

MALIGNANT PRIMARY TRACHEAL TUMORS

The most frequent malignant primary tracheal tumors in the adult are squamous cell carcinoma and adenoid cystic carcinoma. Manninen and associates (1991) reported a national registry study in Finland of tracheal carcinoma that demonstrated the overall rarity of this malignancy. They noted that primary carcinoma of the trachea accounted for 0.03% of all detected malignancies registered in Finland between the years 1967 and 1985. Tracheal malignancy accounted for less than 0.2% of all malignancies of the res-

Table 77-2. Malignant Tumors of the Trachea (Number of Patients)

Tumor Type	Eschapasse (1987)	Grillo and Mathisen (1990)	Gelder and Hetzel (1993)	Perelman et al. (1996)	Regnard et al. (1996)
Adenoid cystic carcinoma	4	80	34	66	65
Squamous cell carcinoma	16	70	174	21	94
Carcinoid tumors	—	11	1	20	9
Typical	—	10	—	14	—
Atypical	—	1	—	6	—
Mucoepidermoid tumor	—	4	—	1	5
Hemangiopericytoma	—	—	1	2	—
Adenocarcinoma	2	1	13	1	4
Small cell carcinoma	—	1	16	3	—
Fibrosarcoma	—	—	1	1	—
Melanoma	—	1	—	—	1
Chondrosarcoma	—	1	—	—	1
Spindle cell carcinoma	—	2	2	—	—
Rhabdomyosarcoma	—	1	—	—	—
Adenosquamous cell carcinoma	—	1	—	—	—
Plasmacytoma	—	—	4	3	2
Others	5	—	26	3	—
Total	**27**	**173**	**272**	**121**	**181**

piratory tract over the same period, and squamous cell carcinoma was the most common tumor. In a review of 198 patients with tracheal tumors, Grillo and Mathisen (1990) reported 80 patients with adenoid cystic carcinoma and 70 with squamous cell carcinoma. In a series of 144 patients who underwent surgery for primary tumors of the trachea, Perelman and associates (1996) recorded 66 adenoid cystic carcinomas and 21 squamous cell carcinomas. Squamous cell carcinomas seem to be more prominent in Europe. Regnard and associates (1996) reported 94 squamous cell carcinomas and 65 adenoid cystic carcinomas in 181 malignant tumors of the trachea, and Gelder and Hetzel (1993) recorded 174 squamous cell carcinomas and 34 adenoid cystic carcinomas in 272 reported cases (Table 77-2).

Squamous Cell Carcinoma

Squamous cell carcinoma of the trachea occurs most commonly in the distal one-third of the trachea and originates frequently along the posterior wall (Fig. 77-12). It affects men approximately four times more frequently than women, spreads to regional lymph nodes, and invades adjacent mediastinal structures. It accounts for approximately 50% of all primary tracheal malignancies, and most patients are heavy smokers. It is not unusual for these patients to develop or have had a secondary primary cancer of the larynx or lung. At the time of diagnosis, Mark (1983) states that invasion into the tracheal wall has occurred in 50% of patients, extension into the mediastinum in 33%, and metastasis to cervical lymph nodes in 33%. Grillo and associates (1992a) noted that, in approximately two-thirds of patients with squamous cell carcinoma, the lesion is resectable at the time of presentation. Limitations to resectability include an excessive linear extent of the tumor, leaving insufficient trachea for reconstruction, invasion of critical mediastinal

structures, and distant metastasis. In patients with squamous cell carcinoma, the status of lymph nodes in the mediastinum at the time of resection and the presence of tumor at the margin of surgical resection serve as major determinants of prognosis.

Adenoid Cystic Carcinoma

Adenoid cystic carcinoma more commonly arises in the upper one-third of the trachea in contrast to squamous cell carcinoma (Fig. 77-13). In many series, it is the most common tracheal malignancy. According to Mark (1983), it is proportionately more prevalent in the trachea than in the main stem bronchus. This tumor is frequently referred to as a cylindroma, but this terminology should be abandoned because it implies that the tumor is benign. The adenoid cystic carcinoma is a slow-growing neoplasm, and patients frequently have experienced symptoms for longer than 1 year before diagnosis is made. This tumor arises from bronchial glands and is histologically identical to those that arise in the salivary glands. Tobacco exposure is not a risk factor. It classically infiltrates the submucosa of the trachea for a distance greater than is grossly apparent. This pathologic feature accounts for an increased likelihood of a positive microscopic surgical margin at the time of tracheal resection (Fig. 77-14). The tumor grows through the tracheal cartilaginous rings and infiltrates the sheath of nerves adjacent to the trachea. It frequently pushes adjacent mediastinal structures aside rather than directly invading them. The adenoid cystic carcinoma less commonly spreads to regional lymph nodes but does metastasize to the lung or other distant organs. Local recurrence after resectional therapy can occur many years later, and these patients should be followed for the rest of their lives. Because of the relatively slow growth of these tumors, sig-

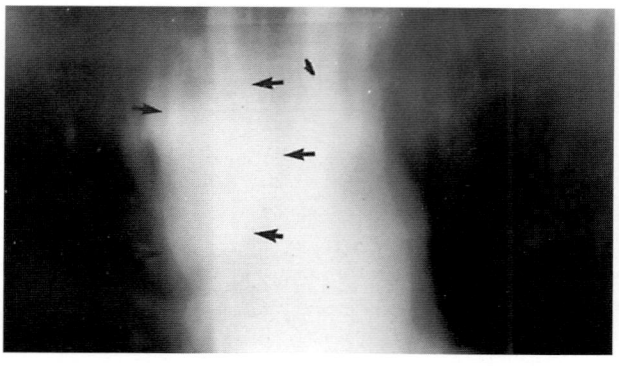
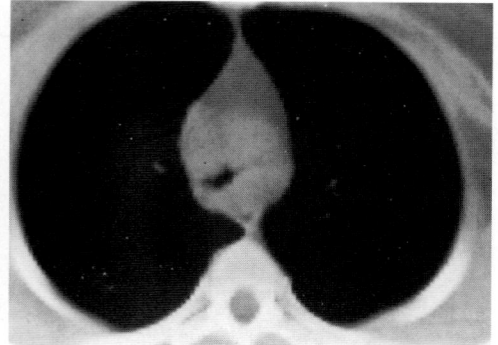

A,B

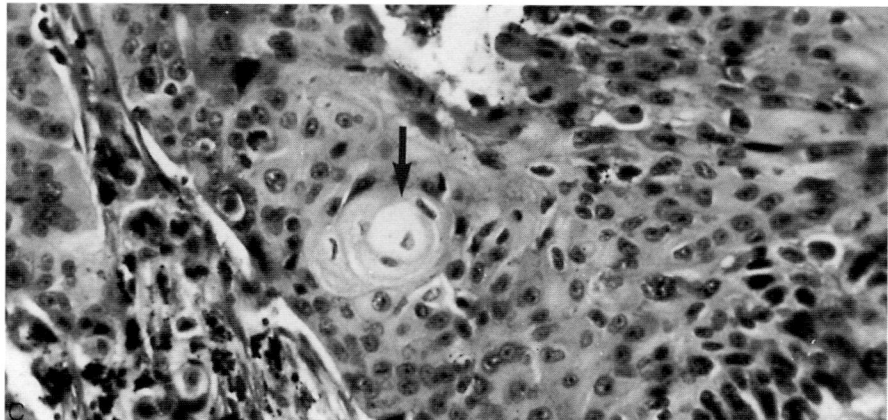

C

Fig. 77-12. A. Extensive tracheal squamous cell carcinoma (*arrows*) is seen on the radiograph of the chest. **B.** Computed tomogram reveals significant involvement of the tracheal lumen. **C.** Biopsy revealed a squamous carcinoma. A keratin pearl is seen (*arrow*) in the center of the microscopic section.

nificant palliation can be achieved by resections that are associated with a positive margin. Postoperative radiation therapy is a determinant in achieving long-term control. Grillo and Mathisen (1990) reported that prognosis did not appear to depend on a positive resection margin or the presence of positive lymph nodes.

In a review of 38 patients with adenoid cystic carcinoma of the upper airway, Maziak and associates (1996) noted that lymphatic metastases were relatively uncommon, and subsequent hematogenous metastasis occurred in 17 of the 38 patients. Pulmonary metastasis occurred in 13 patients.

Carcinoid Tumors

Carcinoid tumors are the third most common malignant tumors of the trachea. Briselli and colleagues (1978) published a review of the occurrence of this tumor in the trachea. Tracheal carcinoids may be of the typical or atypical histologic types. The typical carcinoids behave in a "benign" fashion; only minimal margins beyond the tumor are required at the time of resection. The atypical carcinoids are of greater malignant potential and may invade tissues beyond the trachea. Lymph node metastases may be present. In such cases, more aggressive resection is required.

Other Primary Malignant Tumors

Tracheal Adenocarcinoma

Tracheal adenocarcinoma accounts for approximately 10% of all primary tracheal malignancies, as reported by Mark (1983) (Fig. 77-15); this does not include adenocarcinomas arising from a main stem bronchus that extend to the lower trachea or carina. Adenocarcinoma carries a poor long-term prognosis because of its propensity to spread directly into the mediastinum and to metastasize to regional lymph nodes. Therapy is primary resection, if technically feasible.

Small Cell Carcinoma

Small cell carcinoma of the trachea is rare compared to its more common bronchial presentation. Prognosis is extremely poor, and its natural history parallels that of small cell carcinoma of the lung. Primary treatment is chemotherapy and local radiation therapy.

Other Uncommon Malignant Tumors

Other malignant tumors include mucoepidermoid tumor, which was reported by Heitmiller and associates (1989), mixed tumor, and various mesenchymal tumors, including

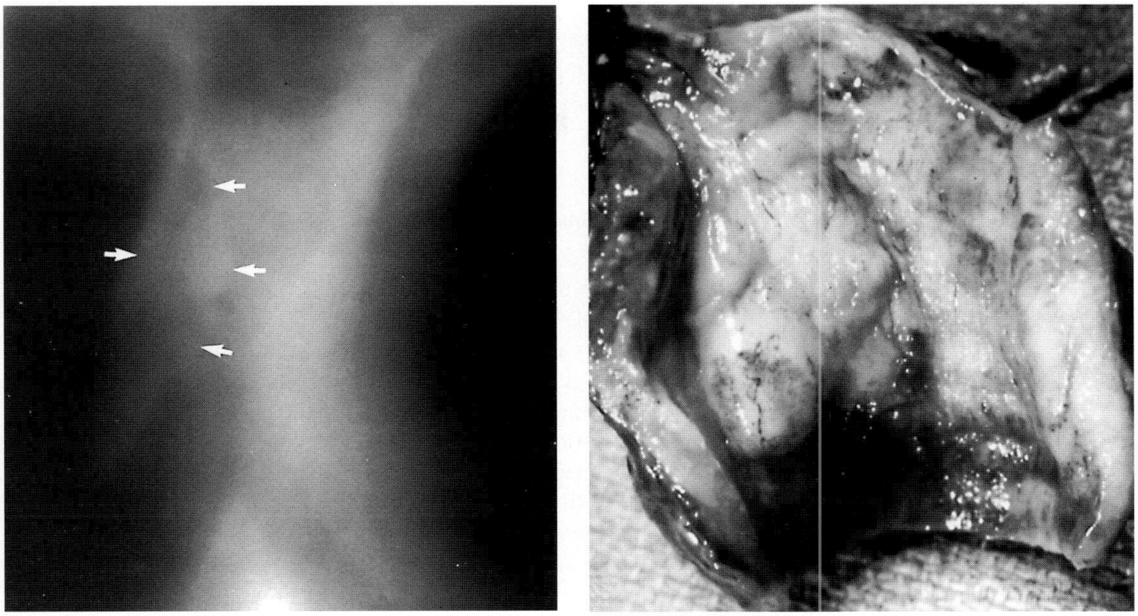

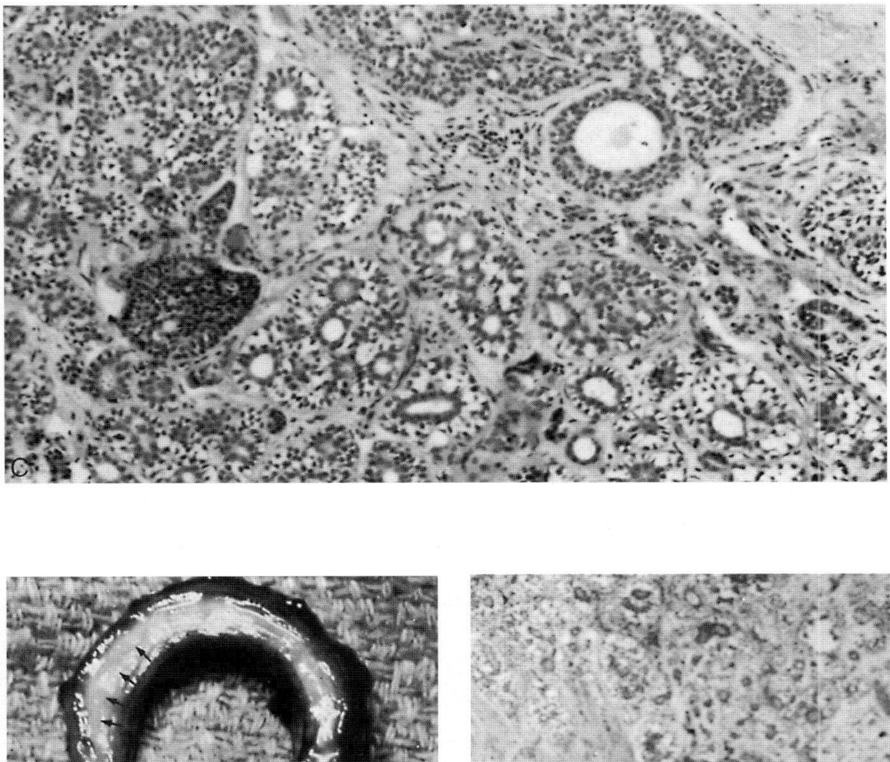

Fig. 77-13. A. Adenoid cystic carcinoma is seen on a linear tomogram (*arrows*). **B.** Six centimeters of trachea were resected for the adenoid cystic carcinoma seen in **A**. **C.** Adenoid cystic carcinoma. Microscopic examination reveals a cribriform pattern within nests of tumor cells separated by a hyalinized stroma.

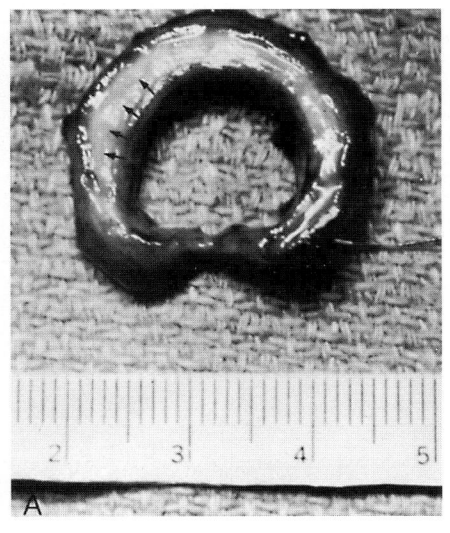
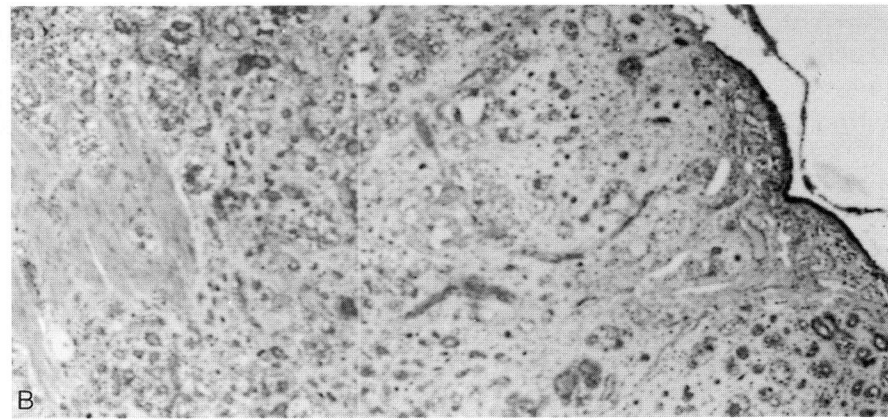

Fig. 77-14. A. Gross examination reveals submucosal extension of adenoid cystic carcinoma at the distal margin of resection. **B.** Microscopic examination reveals submucosal infiltration of the tumor at the margin of resection.

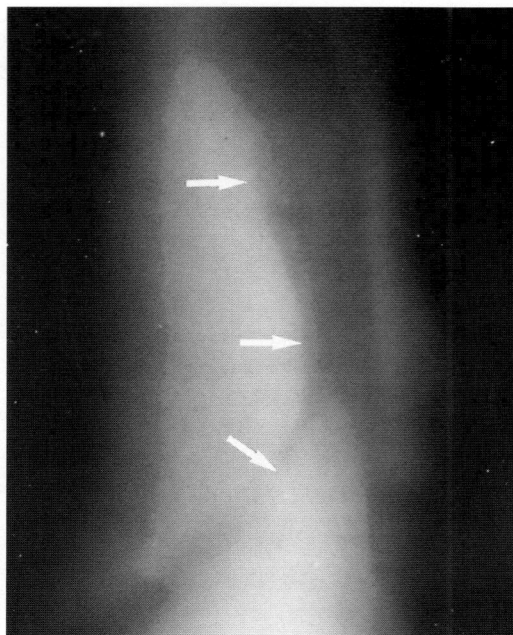

Fig. 77-15. Tracheal adenocarcinoma (*arrows*) involving the main stem bronchus and carina.

chondrosarcoma and fibrosarcoma. Thedinger and coworkers (1991) reported a patient with a tracheal leiomyosarcoma. Kaplan and associates (1992) described primary lymphoma of the trachea. Treatment of lymphoma depends on stage of the disease, as well as histologic subtype. A localized lymphoma responds to primary radiation therapy. Plasma cell tumor of the trachea has been reported, and when the diagnosis is established, therapy is initial endoscopic removal and subsequent radiation therapy. The patient should be monitored closely for the late development of multiple myeloma.

SECONDARY MALIGNANT TRACHEAL TUMORS

The trachea is subject to invasion by adjacent malignancies, including laryngeal, thyroid, lung, and esophageal cancer. Metastasis from distant primary tumors is also possible, including melanoma and tumors of the breast, kidney, and stomach.

Laryngeal Carcinoma

Extension of laryngeal carcinoma into the upper portion of the trachea is a common phenomenon; it is treated by surgical excision during the course of laryngectomy with end tracheostomy formation. Recurrence of the cancer at the stoma is rarely resectable for cure and is best treated with palliative radiation therapy, chemotherapy, or both. Sisson (1975) and Krespi (1985) and their colleagues used an aggressive surgical approach in the treatment of tracheal stomal recurrences.

The morbidity and mortality rates, however, are high. Ujiki and associates (1987) recorded the major and frequent problems that accompany the associated reconstruction of gastrointestinal continuity, with transposition of the stomach and a pharyngogastric anastomosis in a previously irradiated field.

Thyroid Carcinoma

In a review of thyroid cancer invading the trachea, Zannini and Melloni (1996) noted that the incidence of this occurrence varied from 0.5 to 21%. The variation of incidence was attributed to the criteria used to define airway invasion and the number of cases of undifferentiated thyroid cancer included in the various series. Shin and associates (1993) defined a staging system for differentiated thyroid cancer invading the trachea. In stage I, the cancer abuts the external perichondrium, and in stage IV, there is invasion into the tracheal mucosa. Ozaki and associates (1995) examined the spread of tracheal cancer into the tracheal wall and found that circumferential spread on the mucosal side of the trachea was greater than the extent of thyroid cancer on the adventitial side. Thyroid cancer invading the airway is frequently asymptomatic because the tumor has not protruded into the tracheal lumen. Symptoms include wheezing, stridor, hemoptysis, and dyspnea on exertion. Recommended diagnostic evaluation includes high-resolution and spiral CT scans to define the upper airway and search for metastatic pulmonary disease, endoscopic examination of the larynx and trachea to assess vocal cord mobility and possible tracheal invasion, and assessment for bony metastatic disease. The most frequent well-differentiated thyroid carcinomas are the papillary and follicular types, and there is no difference in their tendency to invade the trachea or larynx. Undifferentiated and antiplastic tumors have a greater tendency to invade the trachea. Frequently, invasion of the trachea by thyroid cancer is an intraoperative finding. The decision on the extent of resection must be based on expected morbidity, extent of tracheal invasion, and ability to achieve airway reconstruction. The shave technique of resection has been advocated by McCarty and associates (1997). Nishida and associates (1997) also noted that well-differentiated thyroid carcinomas with limited tracheal invasion could be treated successfully by nonresectional management of the trachea. Postoperative adjuvant irradiation is recommended for these patients. Patients with deep invasion of the trachea or intraluminal extension require segmental tracheal resection.

Patients with locally recurrent thyroid cancer after a previous resection are usually symptomatic (Fig. 77-16). In a review by Grillo and associates (1992b), the most common presentation was that of a patient with previous thyroid surgery in whom the cancerous gland had to be "shaved" off the underlying trachea. This group of patients was often treated with radioactive iodine or external radiation therapy postoperatively. Recurrence at the site of prior resection is particularly troublesome, with recurrent airway bleeding and eventual suffocation from tumor progression. Therefore, as emphasized by Grillo and associates

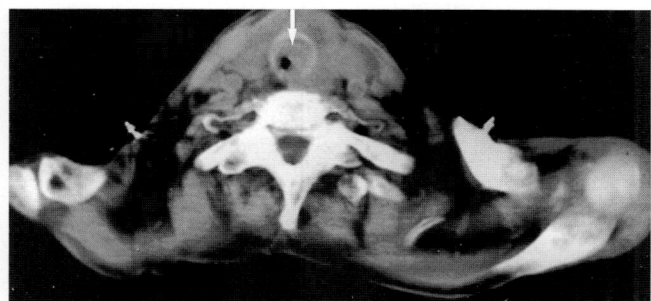

Fig. 77-16. Recurrent thyroid carcinoma (*arrow*) invading the trachea. Clinical signs were hemoptysis and severe stridor.

(1992b), palliation and, in some instances cure, can be achieved by segmental tracheal resection or by laryngotracheal resection and reconstruction at the site of recurrence.

Carcinoma of the Lung

Carcinoma of the lung involves the trachea and tracheal carina by proximal extension from tumors arising from a main stem bronchus or extrinsic compression and invasion from disease in the paratracheal or subcarinal lymph nodes. Most, if not all, patients with local invasion from metastatic disease in mediastinal lymph nodes are not candidates for resection. Electrocautery or laser ablation and brachytherapy, however, may be palliative in the management of intraluminal obstructive growth. The role of neoadjuvant multimodality therapy followed by excision must be evaluated. Direct involvement of the tracheal carina by proximal extension of a main stem bronchial tumor without mediastinal lymph node involvement may be considered for possible resection (tracheal sleeve pneumonectomy), especially if the postoperative mortality can be kept in the range of 10% (see Chapter 30).

Esophageal Cancer

Invasion of esophageal malignancy into the trachea often results in esophagorespiratory fistula. Burt and coworkers (1991) reviewed the extensive experience with this problem at Memorial Hospital in New York. The approach to this problem has varied, with many people advocating esophageal stents or gastrostomy for feeding purposes. Esophageal exclusion with gastric or colon bypass is a major operative procedure that is associated with a high operative mortality and, most often, only brief postoperative survival.

Other Malignancies

Metastasis to the trachea from distant sites is usually treated with endoscopic resection and Nd:YAG laser abla-

tion to debulk the lesion. Systemic chemotherapy or radiation therapy is used as indicated.

PRINCIPLES AND RESULTS OF SURGICAL TREATMENT

History

Belsey (1950) reported experience with tracheal resection and listed 2 cm as the maximal length of trachea that could be circumferentially resected. Rob and Bateman (1949) reported resection of part of the tracheal wall with reconstruction by autologous or synthetic material. These procedures frequently were complicated by fistula, mediastinal infection, and stenosis. In subsequent years, some authors described successful resection of longer lengths of trachea. The door was opened to extended and aggressive tracheal surgery by Grillo and associates (1964) when they thoroughly and systematically described the amount of trachea that could be removed from thoracic and cervical mediastinal approaches. The landmark conclusion was that approximately one-half of the trachea could be removed and reapproximated. Many reports by Grillo and colleagues (1964, 1983, 1989, 1990, 1992) on techniques and results of resection of tracheal tumors and stenosis paved the way for modern techniques of tracheal resection. Pearson and associates (1975) were among the first to describe resection techniques for high tracheal lesions that involved the cricoid. In 1995, Pearson and Gullane updated their experience with these techniques.

Prosthetic Replacement of the Trachea

A significant number of animal experiments have been carried out in an attempt to develop a prosthesis that could replace a long segment of the trachea. Tube grafts of stainless steel, plastic, and glass have all met with failure. This failure is related to granulation tissue that obstructs or results in strictures at the anastomosis and to migration of the prosthesis, leading to erosion of mediastinal vessels. Neville and associates (1990) reported 19 years of experience with the use of a silicone tube to reestablish airway continuity in cases of malignant and benign tracheal obstruction. In some patients, the silicone tube was used as a stent and in others, resection of the trachea with primary anastomosis of the tube to the proximal and distal trachea was accomplished. Successful use of this prosthesis has not been duplicated in other centers, and its use is not recommended.

Selection of Surgical Procedure

Tracheal resection and end-to-end anastomosis using various release techniques to minimize tension is the primary form of therapy for tracheal neoplasms. The standard techniques are discussed in Chapter 75.

Benign tumors must be approached with a full knowledge of the pathology of the tumor to be treated. Benign tumors that are broad based and have a likelihood of local recurrence are best managed by tracheal resection. These tumors usually involve the trachea for a distance of 1 or 2 cm, and the resection and anastomosis is accomplished without difficulty. Benign tumors, such as lipoma, solitary papilloma, and hamartoma, can be removed through the rigid bronchoscope. The Nd:YAG laser has facilitated the total ablation of these tumors, and after endoscopic removal, the base of the tumor is ablated with the laser. Endoscopic surveillance is indicated to be certain that local recurrence does not occur.

Malignant primary tumors of the trachea should be treated by primary resection when the clinical findings indicate that the tumor most likely can be removed and tracheal reconstruction can be accomplished safely. Grillo and Mathisen (1990) reported 147 resections in 198 tracheal tumors seen from 1962 to 1989. These resections included laryngotracheal resection, staged reconstruction, and carinal resection. There were 82 "pure" tracheal resections, and of these, 32 were for squamous carcinoma and 22 for adenoid cystic carcinoma. The operative mortality in the tracheal reconstructions was 1% (1 in 82).

Perelman and associates (1996) reported 48 sleeve resections of the trachea with anastomosis for malignant tumors. Operative mortality was 4.2% (2 in 48 patients). A silicone prosthesis was used in five patients when the length of trachea resected was too long to permit an anastomosis. Mortality in this group was 40% (2 in 5 patients). Regnard and associates (1996) noted that postoperative mortality was three times greater for tracheal cancers than for adenoid cystic carcinoma and other tumors. In their series, the best prognostic factor for tracheal cancers was the completeness of resection. Postoperative complications and mortality was not affected by the age of the patient, positive margins at resection, or lymph node involvement. Maziak and associates (1996) reported a mortality rate of 6.3% in 32 tracheal resections for adenoid cystic carcinoma. However, four of these patients had reconstruction with a Marlex mesh prosthesis.

Squamous Cell Carcinoma

Grillo and associates (1992a) evaluated 70 patients with squamous cell carcinoma of the trachea. Fifty patients were deemed suitable for attempted resection. The tumor was excised in 44 patients, and sleeve resections of the trachea were done in 32, carinal resection in nine, and other types of procedures in three. In 98 resected tracheal cancers reported by Regnard and associates (1996), the resection margin was positive in 26%. Grillo and Mathisen (1990) noted a 23% positive resection margin in resected tracheal cancers. These findings confirm the necessity of performing frozen-section analysis on resected margins during the operative procedure as well as the difficulty of achieving a complete resection in patients with tracheal cancers. Because resection margins are frequently limited and preservation of residual tracheal blood supply negates the ability to carry out a wide en bloc dissection, Grillo and Mathisen (1990) and Regnard (1996) recommend postoperative radiation therapy for all patients undergoing tracheal resection for squamous cell carcinoma.

Adenoid Cystic Carcinoma

Prognosis does not depend on a positive resection margin or the finding of positive lymph nodes. This factor is important to keep in mind at the time of the surgical resection because patients who have grossly negative resection margins but a positive frozen-section margin do not require more aggressive resection, with its attendant higher risk of anastomotic separation. Additional tracheal tissue should be resected if the microscopic margin is positive on frozen section and a satisfactory anastomosis can still be safely accomplished. The best long-term results are achieved in patients who have had a complete resection (Fig. 77-17). Maziak and associates (1996) reported excellent long-term results after both complete and incomplete resections for adenoid cystic carcinoma of the trachea. Grillo and Mathisen (1990) and Maziak (1996) recommend postoperative irradiation for all patients with adenoid cystic carcinoma, whether or not the margins are positive.

Other Malignant Tumors

All other types of primary tracheal malignant tumors should be resected, if it is technically feasible. The decision for postoperative radiation therapy is based on the completeness of the surgical resection and the histologic type of tumor. Atypical carcinoid tumor with negative margins at resection is not a candidate for adjuvant radiation.

Prognosis

Squamous Cell Carcinoma

Grillo and Mathisen (1990) reported that 49% (20 of 41) of patients with squamous cell cancer are alive without evidence of tumor after resection. These results included patients who also had a carinal resection. Negative factors that affected long-term survival in patients with squamous cell carcinoma were positive nodes and microscopic tumor at the resection margin. Grillo and Mathisen (1990) state that "resection combined with irradiation provides a tripled survival time for squamous cell carcinoma" compared to radiation alone. Median survival of resected squamous cell carcinoma with postoperative irradiation was 34 months. Perelman and Koroleva (1987) reported a survival for resected tracheal squamous cell carcinoma of 27% at 3 years and 13% at 5 and 10 years. Pearson and coworkers (1984) identified four of nine patients with tracheal squamous cell carcinoma who were alive from 6 to 56 months after resection.

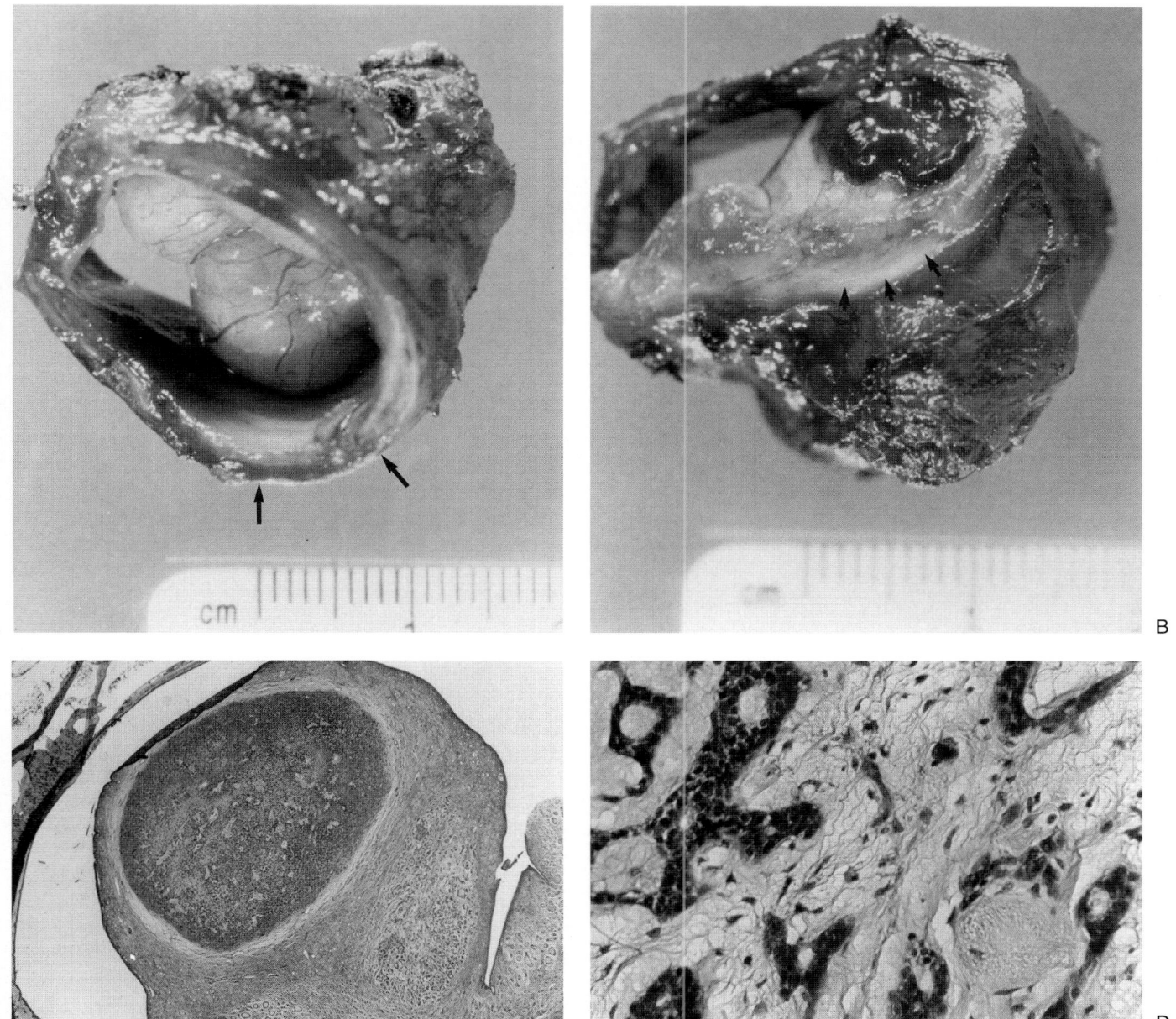

Fig. 77-17. A. Polypoid adenoid cystic carcinoma. Arrows depict distal resection margin. **B.** Positive margin at proximal resection site. A portion of the trachea was used for frozen-section analysis. Additional tracheal resection achieved a tumor-free margin. Central portion of polypoid tumor mass has pattern of a mixed salivary gland tumor. **C.** The majority of tumor is typical pattern of adenoid cystic carcinoma. **D.** Cells are arranged in ribbons and cords.

Regnard and associates (1996) reported 5- and 10-year survival rates of 47% and 36%, respectively, for resected tracheal cancers in their multicenter retrospective analysis. Their data revealed that postoperative radiation therapy did not improve survival in patients with completely resected tracheal cancers. Postoperative irradiation did significantly improve survival in patient with an incomplete resection. An interesting finding in their study was that lymph node involvement in resected tracheal cancers did not affect long-term survival. However, 80% of these patients did receive postoperative radiation therapy when lymph nodes were positive.

Adenoid Cystic Carcinoma

Adenoid cystic carcinoma is a malignant tumor of the trachea that can recur many years after resection. Therefore, reporting accurate final results is somewhat difficult given the possibility of local recurrence at 10 or 15 years postoperatively. Despite an increased incidence of tumor at the resection margin, however, Grillo and Mathisen (1990) reported that 75% (39 of 52) of patients were alive and free of disease, with a median survival of 118 months. Perelman and Koroleva (1987) reported an overall survival for resected adenoid cystic carcinoma of the trachea of 71% at 3 years, 66% at 5 years, and 56% at 10 and 15 years. Maziak and associates (1996) reported 32 resections for adenoid cystic carcinoma, of whom 16 were complete and potentially curative. There were two operative deaths in this group, and mean survival in the 14 remaining patients was 9.8 years. The median mean survival in 15 surviving patients undergoing an incomplete resection was 7.5 years. Calculated actuarial survival was 51% at 10 years in the 32 patients treated by primary resection. Metastatic tumor was found in regional lymph nodes in five patients. Regnard and associates (1996) reported 5- and 10-year survivals of 73% and 57%, respectively, for resected adenoid cystic carcinomas of the trachea. There was not a significant difference in survival in patients with a complete resection than in those with an incomplete resection. It also was noted that postoperative irradiation did not improve survival in either complete or incomplete resections. Synchronous metastatic pulmonary disease decreases median survival time and also occurs late in the course of the disease. Long-term prognosis for patients with adenoid cystic carcinoma is obviously better than that for those with squamous cell carcinoma.

RADIATION THERAPY

In patients with a primary malignant tumor of the trachea that does not meet the criteria for resection, radiation therapy can be an alternative form of therapy, although it does not appear to be as effective as primary resection for providing long-term control. Rostom and Morgan (1978) reported radiation therapy for 39 patients with primary malignant tumors of the trachea, of which 28 were squamous cell carcinomas and three were adenoid cystic carcinomas. In these 31 patients, five were reported to be free of disease at 4 to 11 years after treatment, six died of unrelated causes, and the remainder expired from local recurrence or metastatic cancer. Radiation dose varied from 5000 to 7000 cGy. Patients with disease limited to the trachea had a better prognosis, and 58% (11 of 19) with tumors confined to the trachea were controlled locally at the time of death or at the last follow-up evaluation (3 to 16 years). Fields and colleagues (1989) reported on 24 patients with primary malignant tumors of the trachea who received radiation therapy as all or part of their treatment. This group included 13 with squamous cell carcinomas and 4 with adenoid cystic carcinomas. The median actuarial survival was 10 months, with 5-year and 10-year survival rates of 25 and 13%, respectively. For patients treated with radiation therapy alone, response was related to dose, and a dose of more than 6000 cGy was statistically significant in achieving a complete response. Five patients developed serious complications,

however, including innominate artery rupture, tracheoesophageal fistula, and esophageal structure. In this series, it appeared that radiation therapy had no survival advantage over surgery for localized lesions and that primary tumor control was infrequent with the more advanced lesions. Survival was significantly better for patients with adenoid cystic carcinoma than for those with squamous carcinoma. Median survivals were 126 months and 6.5 months, respectively. Grillo and Mathisen (1990) compared their patients who underwent resection and postoperative radiation therapy with those that underwent irradiation alone. Significantly better results were achieved with resection and postoperative irradiation. Maziak and associates (1996) reported six patients with adenoid cystic carcinoma of the trachea who had irradiation as primary therapy. Mean survival was 6.2 years, with two patients developing airway obstruction as a result of local recurrence 7 and 8 years after radiation. Grillo and Mathisen (1990) reported on 12 patients with adenoid cystic carcinoma treated with radiation alone. Only three patients were alive without evidence of disease. However, these tumors were extensive at the time of initial diagnosis.

Treatment planning by CT and neutron therapy with modern techniques of deliverance may enhance the radiation treatment of primary tracheal malignancies. At present, however, irradiation is to be considered only as a primary form of therapy when the tumor cannot be technically resected or the patient is medically unfit for surgery.

ENDOSCOPIC MANAGEMENT

Palliation of obstructing or bleeding tracheal malignancies can be achieved with current endoscopic procedures. Modern intravenous anesthetic techniques permit spontaneous ventilation during open tube bronchoscopy, which provides safety for the compromised airway. Dumon and colleagues (1982) described the use of a specially designed bronchoscope through which the Nd:YAG laser fiber is passed, along with débridement forceps. Nd:YAG laser resection is particularly valuable in establishing an open airway in a patient with an obstructing tracheal neoplasm. The laser controls hemorrhage after tumor débridement with biopsy forceps or the end of the open-tube bronchoscope. Gelb and colleagues (1988) described 13 patients who underwent palliative Nd:YAG laser treatment for relief of malignant tracheal obstruction. Tracheal diameter was significantly increased after single or multiple laser treatments with improvement of inspiratory flow rates. Symptomatic relief occurred for 4 to 48 months.

The Nd:YAG laser can penetrate deeply into tumor tissue, with resultant photocoagulation of superficial and deep blood vessels with thermal necrosis. Tumor shrinkage, reduction in blood supply, and vaporization occurs. Careful use of this energy source is necessary to avoid bronchial or pulmonary artery rupture. It is practical to use the Nd:YAG laser for revascularization and tumor shrinkage, with subsequent debulking of the tumor through the rigid bronchoscope with the use of biopsy forceps. Cavaliere and associates reported on 2610 Nd:YAG laser resections in 1838 patients with obstructing lung cancer. There were 10 deaths, and the median time to regrowth and stenosis was approximately 3 months.

Cryotherapy uses a probe passed through an open-tube bronchoscope that freezes the tissue for the purpose of destroying it. Necrosis of the tumor and thrombosis of vessels do occur, but the basic architecture of the bronchus is maintained. A second open-tube bronchoscopic procedure is necessary to remove sloughed necrotic material. Its use does not appear to have significant advantages over Nd:YAG laser resection or endoscopic débridement.

Photodynamic therapy involves the use of a porphyrin-based photosensitizing agent (hematoporphyrin derivative) that, when exposed to a light of proper wavelength, forms toxic oxygen radicals and destroys the tumor. It has been used primarily for the treatment of patients with early-stage lung cancer limited to the mucosa or submucosal areas. However, it is also used for large obstructing cancers of the trachea and main stem bronchi. Newer photosensitizing agents with fewer side effects are being developed, and photodynamic therapy may prove to be efficient in débriding obstructing neoplasms of the airway.

Brachytherapy is effective in providing high-dose radiation in a localized radiation field, as described by Spratling and Speiser (1996). The high-activity isotope iridium 192 is placed into a catheter that is appropriately positioned in the lumen of the tumor after endoscopic débridement. Specific after-loading radiation machines are also available for this type of therapy. Hetzel and Smith (1991) reported that brachytherapy is complementary to laser resection, and effective palliation of the airway can be achieved. Fritz and associates (1991) described a new applicator to position the after-loading catheter centrally to minimize irregular dose distribution.

After endoscopic ablation of an intraluminal tumor, an endobronchial stent can be used to maintain an adequate airway, as suggested by Cooper and coworkers (1989). Tojo and associates reported on 25 patients with life-threatening tracheobronchial stenosis in whom expandable metal stents or silicone stents were placed. Tumor ingrowth occurred through the uncovered metal stents, and the authors' conclusion was that expandable metal stents are effective for external compression of the trachea or major bronchus, but covered metal stents or silicone stents are preferable for intraluminal tumors. Silicone stents can be positioned properly through the open-tube bronchoscope. They are easily removed and prevent tumor ingrowth. However, recurrent cancer can grow over the end of the stent, necessitating tumor débridement and repositioning of the stent. Silicone-covered metal stents can now be inserted through a small commercially available catheter, with insertion adjacent to the fiberoptic bronchoscope. The uncovered stainless steel stents have been used for maintenance of a major airway,

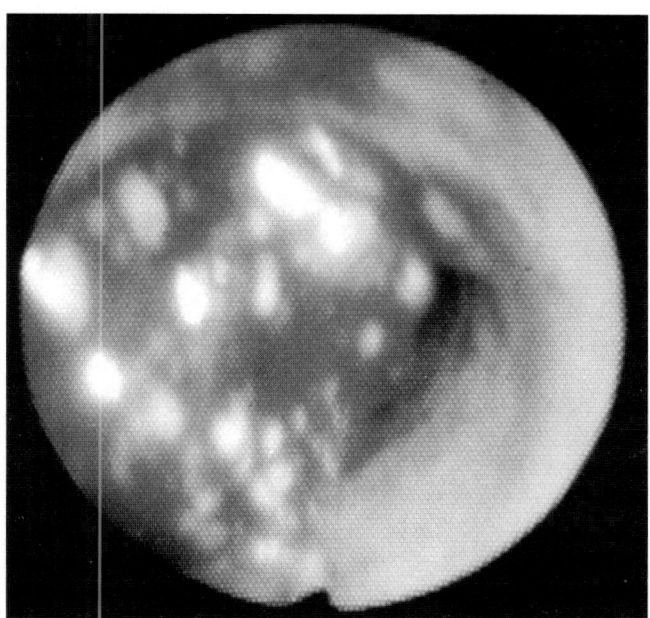

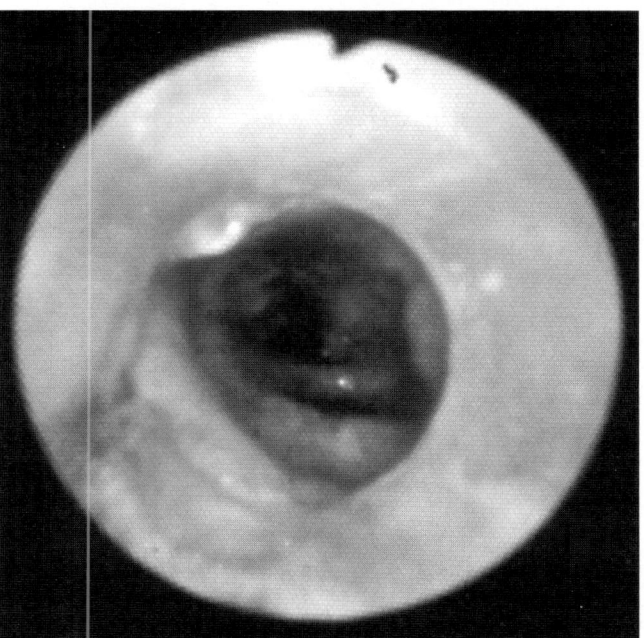

Fig. 77-18. A. Obstructing squamous carcinoma of trachea. B. Silicone stent placement after neodymium:yttrium-aluminum-garnet resection of the tumor.

but placement and repositioning are particularly difficult, and the tumor can grow through the interstices of the stent. The stainless steel stent is difficult to remove once it has been expanded into position. Wasserman (1996) reported that 10 patients with severe malignant obstruction of the trachea benefited significantly from placement of a silicone prosthesis. Median survival from stent insertion was 8 months, with stent replacement necessary in five patients (Fig. 77-18).

MANAGEMENT OF SECONDARY TUMORS INVOLVING THE TRACHEA

Grillo and associates (1992b) evaluated 52 patients with thyroid cancer invading the upper airway between 1964 and 1991. There were 34 patients in whom resection could be accomplished: 27 patients had resection and reconstruction, and seven underwent cervical exenteration. In the patients who had reconstruction, there were 16 papillary cancers, five follicular cancers, four of mixed histology, and two poorly differentiated thyroid cancers. In the reconstruction group, 17 patients had undergone prior resection, and nine patients were identified as having tracheal involvement before primary resection of the thyroid cancer. One patient had been treated only with iodine 131. Thirteen patients were referred because of recurrence, and it was specifically noted in this group of patients that the tumor had been shaved off the trachea at the time of the original resection. There were 10 tracheal sleeve resections, and the remainder had complex laryngotracheal resection and reconstruction. Mortality was 7.4% (2 of 27). Thirteen of 25 patients survived, and their long-term survival averaged 5 years and 9 months. Twelve patients were free of disease, and one patient had pulmonary metastasis. Eleven patients died of their cancer, with an average duration of survival of 3 years and 7 months. It is important to note that only two patients in this group had local recurrence, which attests to the value of radical resection for thyroid cancer invading the airway. Seven patients in the reconstruction group had metastatic disease, and the average survival for this entire group was 4.2 years, which illustrates the slow progression of pulmonary metastasis. This finding does not negate resection of recurrent thyroid cancer, if technically feasible. Grillo and associates (1992b) stressed that complete resection of local disease, including the trachea, provides the best long-term therapy. It is their opinion that the shave procedure followed by radiation therapy does not provide satisfactory long-term management. Successful long-term palliation can also be achieved when microscopic margins remain positive.

In contrast, McCarty and associates (1997) reported on 35 patients with superficial invasion of thyroid cancer who underwent the shave procedure followed by adjuvant radiation therapy. They reported that 25 patients were alive and free of recurrent disease at a mean follow-up of 81 months. Six patients developed local regional recurrence, and they underwent a second surgical procedure or repeat radiation therapy. All these patients remained free of disease at a mean follow-up of 5 years. Five patients in this series had intraluminal invasion of thyroid cancer, and all underwent laryngotracheal reconstruction. Four patients in this group were free of disease at a mean follow-up of 5 years. Nishida and coworkers (1997) reported on 13 patients who had superficial invasion of the trachea by thyroid cancer in whom nonresectional management was carried out (the shave procedure). In these patients, the carcinoma was histologically present on the tracheal side of the resected thyroid gland, but gross disease was not left behind. At a mean follow-up of 7.2 years, 9 of 13 patients were alive without evidence of recurrence. Three patients died of their cancer, and there was one operative death. These results were compared to a group of 40 patients who underwent tracheal resection for a deep tracheal invasion: There was no statistical difference identified in local, regional, or distant recurrence. Nishida and colleagues concluded that superficial invasion of thyroid cancer into the trachea can be treated by nonresectional management. They also concluded that deep invasion was best treated by tracheal resection. Antiplastic thyroid cancer invading the trachea has to be considered as a separate issue because these patients frequently expire from metastatic disease soon after an extensive resection. Ishihara and colleagues (1991) described 60 patients with advanced thyroid cancer in whom the tumor was resected along with a portion of the trachea. A complete resection was achieved in 34 patients, and 5-year actuarial survival in this group was 78%. In the patients undergoing incomplete resection, the 5-year actuarial survival was 44%.

Resection of a portion of the trachea or larynx, or both, in patients with invading thyroid carcinoma can offer significant palliation from bleeding and obstruction and, possibly, cure.

In a rare instance, tracheal involvement is the only extramural spread of the esophageal malignancy, and partial tracheal resection with musculocutaneous flap reconstruction of the trachea has been accomplished. This operation, as reported by Sodeyama and associates (1990), is often done in association with total laryngoesophagectomy, in which the reconstruction is part of a cervical or mediastinal tracheostomy construction.

REFERENCES

Basheda SG, et al: Endobronchial and parenchymal juvenile laryngotracheobronchial papillomatosis. Effect of photodynamic therapy. Chest 100:1458, 1991.

Beattie EJ, Bloom ND, Harvey JC: Trachea. In Beattie EJ, Bloom ND, Harvey JC (eds): Thoracic Surgical Oncology. New York: Churchill Livingstone, 1992, pp. 273–281.

Belsey R: Resection and reconstruction of the intrathoracic trachea. Br J Surg 38:200, 1950.

Briselli M, Mark GJ, Grillo HC: Tracheal carcinoids. Cancer 42:2870, 1978.

Burt M, et al: Malignant esophagorespiratory fistula: management options and survival. Ann Thorac Surg 52:1222, 1991.

Burton DM, Heffner DK, Paptow CA: Granular cell tumors of the trachea. Laryngoscope 102:807, 1992.

Cavaliere S, et al: Endoscopic treatment of malignant airway obstructions in 2,008 patients. Chest 110:1536, 1996.

Chen TF, et al: Obstructing tracheal lipoma: management of a rare tumor. Ann Thorac Surg 49:137, 1990.

Cooper JD, et al: Use of silicone stents in the management of airway problems. Ann Thorac Surg 47:371, 1989.

Cunningham L, et al: Treatment of tracheobronchial granular cell myoblastomas with endoscopic bipolar cautery. Chest 96:427, 1989.

Daddi G, et al: Resection with curative intent after endoscopic treatment of airway obstruction. Ann Thorac Surg 65:203, 1998.

Daniel TM, et al: Transbronchoscopic versus surgical resection of tracheobronchial granular cell myoblastomas. J Thorac Cardiovasc Surg 80:898, 1980.

Desai DP, Holinger LD, Gonzalez-Crussi F: Tracheal neoplasms in children. Ann Otol Rhinol Laryngol 107:790, 1998.

Dumon JF, et al: Treatment of tracheo-bronchial lesions by laser photo-resection. Chest 81:278, 1982.

Eschapasse H: Primary tumors of the trachea. In Grillo HC, Eschapasse H (eds): International Trends in General Thoracic Surgery. Vol. 2. Philadelphia: WB Saunders, 1987, p. 107.

Fields JN, Rigaud G, Emami BN: Primary tumors of the trachea. Results of radiation therapy. Cancer 63:2429, 1989.

Franks R, Rothera M: Cardiopulmonary bypass for resection of low tracheal hemangioma. Arch Dis Child 65:630, 1990.

Fritz P, et al: A new applicator, positionable to the center of tracheo-bronchial lumen for HDR-1R-192-afterloading of tracheobronchial tumors. Int J Radiat Oncol Biol Phys 20:1061, 1991.

Garcia-Prats MD, et al: Glomus tumour of the trachea; report of a case with microscopic, ultrastructural and immunohistochemical examination and review of the literature. Histopathology 19:459, 1991.

Gelb AF, et al: Diagnosis and Nd-YAG laser treatment of unsuspected malignant tracheal obstruction. Chest 94:767, 1988.

Gelder CM, Hetzel MR: Primary tracheal tumours: a national survey. Thorax 48:688, 1993.

Gilbert JG, Mazzarella LA, Geit LJ: Primary tracheal tumors in the infant and adult. Arch Otolaryngol Head Neck Surg 58:1, 1953.

Grillo HC: Tracheal tumors: diagnosis and management. In Choi NC, Grillo HC (eds): Thoracic Oncology. New York: Raven Press, 1983, pp. 271–278.

Grillo HC: Benign and malignant disease of the trachea. In Shields TW (ed): General Thoracic Surgery. 3rd Ed. Philadelphia: Lea & Febiger, 1989.

Grillo HC, Dignan EF, Mirua T: Extensive resection and reconstruction of mediastinal trachea without prosthesis or graft: an anatomical study in man. J Thorac Cardiovasc Surg 48:471, 1964.

Grillo HC, Mathisen DJ: Primary tracheal tumors: treatment and results. Ann Thorac Surg 49:69, 1990.

Grillo HC, Mathisen DJ, Wain JC: Management of tumors of the trachea. Oncology 6:61, 1992a.

Grillo HC, et al: Resectional management of thyroid carcinoma invading the airway. Ann Thorac Surg 54:3, 1992b.

Guillou L, et al: Squamous cell carcinoma of the lung in a nonsmoking, nonirradiated patient with juvenile laryngotracheal papillomatosis. Am J Surg Pathol 15:891, 1991.

Hajdu SI, et al: Carcinoma of the trachea. Clinicopathologic study of 41 cases. Cancer 25:1448, 1970.

Heitmiller RF, et al: Mucoepidermoid lung tumors. Ann Thorac Surg 47:394, 1989.

Hetzel MR, Smith SGT: Endoscopic palliation of tracheobronchial malignancies. Thorax 46:325, 1991.

Houston HE, et al: Primary cancers of the trachea. Arch Surg 99:132, 1969.

Ishihara T, et al: Surgical treatment of advanced thyroid carcinoma invading the trachea. J Thorac Cardiovasc Surg 102:717, 1991.

Kaplan MA, et al: Primary lymphoma of the trachea with morphologic and immunophenotypic characteristics of low-grade B-cell lymphoma of mucosa-associated lymphoid tissue. Am J Surg Pathol 16:71, 1992.

Karley SW, et al: Chronic cavitary respiratory papillomatosis. Arch Pathol Lab Med 113:1166, 1989.

Kauczor HU, et al: Three-dimensional helical CT of the tracheobronchial tree: evaluation of imaging protocols and assessment of suspected stenoses with bronchoscopic correlation. AJR Am J Roentgenol 167:419, 1996.

Kavuru MS, Mehta AC, Eliachar I: Effect of photodynamic therapy and external beam radiation therapy on juvenile laryngotracheobronchial papillomatosis. Am Rev Respir Dis 141:509, 1990.

Krespi YP, Wurster CF, Sisson GA: Immediate reconstruction after total laryngopharyngoesophagectomy and mediastinal dissection. Laryngoscope 95:156, 1985.

Leventhal BG, et al: Long-term response of recurrent respiratory papillomatosis to treatment with lymphoblastoid interferon (-N1. N Engl J Med 325:613, 1991.

Manninen MO, et al: Occurrence of tracheal carcinoma in Finland. Acta Otolaryngol (Stockh) 111:1162, 1991.

Mark E: Pathology of tracheal neoplasms. In Choi NC, Grillo HC (eds): Thoracic Oncology. New York: Raven Press, 1983, pp. 256–269.

Mathisen DJ, Grillo HC: Endoscopic relief of malignant airway obstruction. Ann Thorac Surg 48:469, 1989.

Maziak DE, et al: Adenoid cystic carcinoma of the airway: thirty-two-year experience. J Thorac Cardiovasc Surg 112:1522, 1996.

McCarty TM, et al: Surgical management of thyroid cancer invading the airway. Ann Surg Oncol 4:403, 1997.

Neville WE, Bolanowski PJ, Kotia GG: Clinical experience with the silicone tracheal prosthesis. J Thorac Cardiovasc Surg 99:604, 1990.

Nishida T. Kazuyasu N. Masayasu H: Differential thyroid carcinoma with airway invasion: indication for tracheal resection based on the extent of cancer invasion. J Thorac Cardiovasc Surg 114:84, 1997.

Ozaki O, et al: Surgery for patients with thyroid carcinoma invading the trachea: circumferential sleeve resection followed by end-to-end anastomosis. Surgery 117:268, 1995.

Pang LC: Primary neurilemmoma of the trachea. South Med J 82:785, 1989.

Pearson FG, Gullane P: Subglottic resection with primary tracheal anastomosis including synchronous laryngotracheal reconstruction. Acta Otorhinolaryngol Belg 49:389, 1995.

Pearson FG, Todd TRJ, Cooper JD: Experience with primary neoplasms of the trachea and carina. J Thorac Cardiovasc Surg 88:511, 1984.

Pearson FG, et al: Primary tracheal anastomosis after resection of the cricoid cartilage with preservation of recurrent laryngeal nerves. J Thorac Cardiovasc Surg 70:806, 1975.

Perelman MI, Koroleva NS: Primary tumors of the trachea. In Grillo HC, Eschapasse H (eds): International Trends in General Thoracic Surgery. Philadelphia: WB Saunders, 1987, pp. 91–110.

Perelman MI, et al: Primary tracheal tumors. Semin Thorac Cardiovasc Surg 8:400, 1996.

Randleman CD, Unger ER, Mansour KA: Malignant fibrous histiocytoma of the trachea. Ann Thorac Surg 50:458, 1990.

Regnard JF, Fourquier P, Levasseur P: Results and prognostic factors in resections of primary tracheal tumors: a multicenter retrospective study. The French Society of Cardiovascular Surgery. J Thorac Cardiovasc Surg 111:808, 1996.

Rob CG, Bateman GH: Reconstruction of the trachea and cervical esophagus. Br J Surg 36:202, 1949.

Rostom AY, Morgan RL: Results of treating primary tumors of the trachea by irradiation. Thorax 33:387, 1978.

Salminen U, et al: Recurrence and malignant transformation of endotracheal chondroma. Ann Thorac Surg 49:830, 1990.

Shin DH, et al: Pathologic staging of papillary carcinoma of the thyroid with airway invasion based on the anatomic manner of extension to the trachea: a clinicopathologic study based on 22 patients who underwent thyroidectomy and airway resection. Hum Pathol 24:866, 1993.

Sisson GA, Bytelle E, Edison BD: Transsternal radical neck dissection for control of stomal recurrence—end results. Laryngoscope 85:1504, 1975.

Sodeyama H, et al: Platysma musculocutaneous flap for reconstruction of trachea in esophageal cancer. Ann Thorac Surg 50:485, 1990.

Spratling L, Speiser BL: Endoscopic brachytherapy. Chest Surg Clin N Am 6:293, 1996.

Thedinger BA, et al: Leiomyosarcoma of the trachea. Ann Otol Rhinol Laryngol 100:337, 1991.

Tojo T, et al: Management of malignant tracheobronchial stenosis with metal stents and Dumon stents. Ann Thorac Surg 61:1074, 1996.

Ujiki GT, et al: Mortality and morbidity of gastric pull-up for replacement of the pharyngoesophagus. Arch Surg 122:644, 1987.

Wasserman K. Emergency stenting of malignant obstruction of the upper airways: long term follow up with two types of silicone prostheses. J Thorac Cardiovasc Surg 112:859, 1996.

Weber AL, Grillo HC: Tracheal lesions—assessment by conventional films, computed tomography and magnetic resonance imaging. Israel J Med Sci 28:233, 1992.

Weber TR, et al: Complex hemangiomas of infants and children. Arch Surg 125:1017, 1990.

Zannini P, Melloni G: Surgical management of thyroid cancer invading the trachea. Chest Surg Clin N Am 6:777, 1996.

CHAPTER 78

Compression of the Trachea by Vascular Rings

Carl L. Backer

Vascular ring refers to a group of congenital vascular anomalies of the aortic arch complex that form an anatomic ring that constricts and compresses the trachea or the esophagus, or both. In 1737, Hommel, cited by Turner (1962) described the first vascular ring, a double aortic arch. Almost all clinically significant vascular rings become symptomatic in infants or young children and initially present with airway obstruction from tracheal compression. Esophageal compression and obstruction usually becomes apparent later when solid foods are started. The classification of vascular rings that has been used at Children's Memorial Hospital in Chicago is based on specific anatomic features, particularly the location of the aortic arch (Table 78-1). The table also indicates the relative frequency of anomalies as they have presented for surgical intervention since the 1940s. As indicated, some of these anomalies are anatomically complete rings, or true vascular rings; others are anatomically incomplete, or partial vascular rings, but are grouped with true vascular rings because they present with similar pathophysiology and, hence, clinical symptoms. I have included complete tracheal rings because of their close association with pulmonary artery sling and their similar respiratory symptoms. Gross (1945) reported the first successful operation for a vascular ring when he divided a double aortic arch that was causing tracheal obstruction in a 1-year-old infant. Gross (1948) also reported the first successful suspension of the innominate artery to the sternum for innominate artery compression syndrome in a 4-month-old infant with wheezing and respiratory distress.

Potts and colleagues (1954) coined the term *pulmonary artery sling* in their report of successful repair of that anomaly in a 5 month old with intermittent attacks of dyspnea and cyanosis. Idriss and colleagues (1984) first reported the successful use of pericardium as a tracheoplasty technique in a 7 month old with complete tracheal rings.

EMBRYOLOGY

Congdon (1922) reported an extensive study of the embryonic development of the human aortic arch system, showing that six pairs of aortic arches connect the two primitive ventral and dorsal aortae (Fig. 78-1). Most portions of the first, second, and fifth arches regress. The third arches become the carotid arteries. A branch from the ventral bud of the sixth arch meets the lung bud to form the pulmonary artery. On the right side, the dorsal contribution to the sixth arch disappears; on the left, it persists as the ductus arteriosus. The formation of a vascular ring depends on preservation or deletion of specific segments of the embryonic aortic arch complex. To help visualize this, Edwards (1948) proposed a schematic model with a double aortic arch system and bilateral ductus arteriosus. By convention, the "location" of the aortic arch is determined by its relationship to the trachea. In the normal arch formation, the right fourth arch regresses, leaving a left aortic arch system (i.e., apex of aortic arch to left of trachea). If both fourth arches persist, a double aortic arch is formed. If the left fourth arch regresses, a right aortic arch system is created (apex of aortic arch to right of trachea). This is schematically demonstrated in Figure 78-2.

CLINICAL FEATURES, DIAGNOSES, AND SURGICAL TREATMENT

Double Aortic Arch

Anatomy and Clinical Features

The double aortic arch is the most common complete vascular ring that causes tracheoesophageal compression. Potts and associates (1948) noted that patients typically present in the first months of life with symptoms of stridor, respiratory distress, and a cough that sounds like a seal's bark. A simple "cold" may precipitate severe respiratory difficulty. The ascending aorta divides into two arches that pass around the trachea and esophagus and join posteriorly to form the descending aorta (see Fig. 78-2). I and my associates (1989) showed that in two-thirds of these infants, the right-sided (posterior) arch is dominant, and in one-third, the left-sided (anterior) arch is dominant. Rarely, the arches are of equal

Table 78-1. Classification of Vascular Rings and Children's Memorial Hospital Experience, 1947–1998

Vascular Rings	No. of Patients
Complete	
Double aortic arch	92
Right aortic arch with left ligamentum	81
Incomplete	
Innominate artery compression	82
Pulmonary artery sling	23
Complete tracheal rings	26
Total	**304**

size (balanced arches). The carotid and subclavian arteries originate symmetrically and separately from each arch. The tight, constricting ring thus formed compresses the trachea and esophagus.

Diagnosis

The diagnosis can be suspected on examination of the chest radiograph because the location of the aortic arch in relation to the trachea is indeterminate. In addition, the tracheal air column often shows compression, which is more prominent on the side of the dominant arch. Ideally, the next study is a barium esophagogram, which Arciniegas (1979) and Stark (1985) and their colleagues have shown to be the most reli-

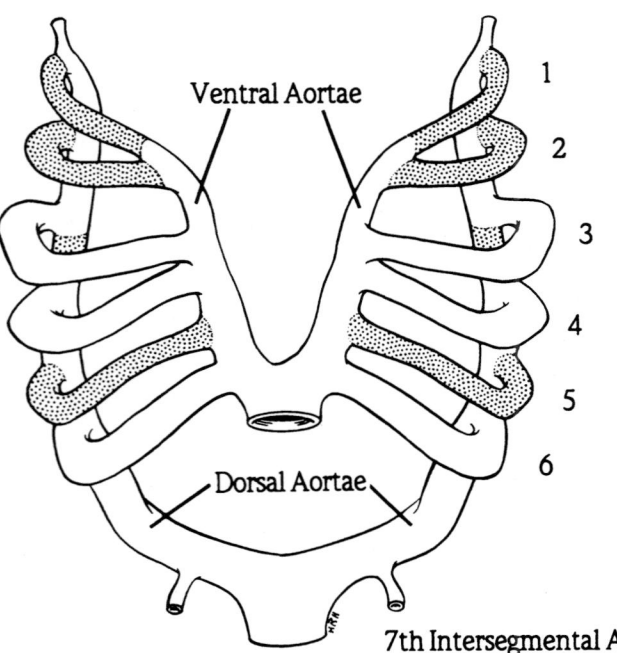

Fig. 78-1. The embryonic aortic arches. Six pairs of aortic arches develop between the dorsal and ventral aortae. Areas that are shaded regress. The seventh intersegmental arteries migrate cephalad to form the subclavian arteries. From Lowe GM, Donaldson JS, Backer CL: Vascular rings: 10-year review of imaging. Radio-Graphics *11*:637, 1991. With permission.

able study for diagnosis of vascular rings. It is also very cost effective in the current era of managed care and capitation. The double aortic arch on an anteroposterior esophagram appears as bilateral indentations of unequal size that persist in location (Fig. 78-3). At the Children's Memorial Hospital of Chicago, it is believed that a barium esophagogram provides sufficient information to plan for surgical intervention; however, many clinicians also obtain a computed tomogram (CT) or magnetic resonance (MR) image before surgical referral. McLoughlin and coworkers (1981) have shown that CT scanning is very accurate in the identification of vascular anomalies of the aortic arch and great vessels. A double aortic arch is diagnosed with certainty when both limbs are patent and are enhanced with the administration of contrast material (Fig. 78-4). As described by Lowe and associates (1991), one clue to an arch anomaly (specifically, a double aortic arch or a right aortic arch with retroesophageal subclavian artery and a ligamentum arteriosum) is the four artery sign. This is seen on sections cephalad to the aortic arch and consists of two dorsal subclavian arteries and two ventral carotid arteries spaced evenly around the trachea. The sign is present when the two dorsal subclavian arteries arise directly from the aorta rather than from a brachiocephalic artery (Fig. 78-5). Cardiac catheterization is recommended only for infants with associated congenital cardiac anomalies. Sometimes, bronchoscopy obtained as the initial study because of severe stridor shows external compression of the trachea.

Treatment

All infants with double aortic arch should be operated on; a narrowed trachea, when further compromised by mucosal edema from even a mild upper respiratory infection, can cause hypoxic or apneic episodes. As Midulla and associates (1994) reported, these children are also at risk for aortic dissection. In addition, as Heck (1993) and Othersen (1996) and their colleagues have reported, improper management of respiratory obstruction with prolonged intubation and nasogastric tube irrigation may lead to catastrophic erosion of an arch into the esophagus.

Surgical approach is through a left thoracotomy, except in cases of associated intracardiac lesions, in which case simultaneous repair can be effected through a median sternotomy. The left thoracotomy can be performed with a muscle-sparing technique, elevating the serratus anterior and the latissimus dorsi, and entering the thorax through the fourth intercostal space. The vascular ring caused by the double aortic arch is released by dividing the lesser of the two arches, usually where it inserts into the descending aorta (Fig. 78-6). In 30 to 40% of the patients, this portion of the arch is atretic. After applying the vascular clamps, the anesthesiologist carefully checks the carotid and radial pulses on both sides to ensure that blood flow is not interrupted. The arch is then divided between the vascular clamps, and the stumps are oversewn with Prolene sutures; simple ligation should not be done. The ligamentum arteriosum is also divided. Careful dissection is

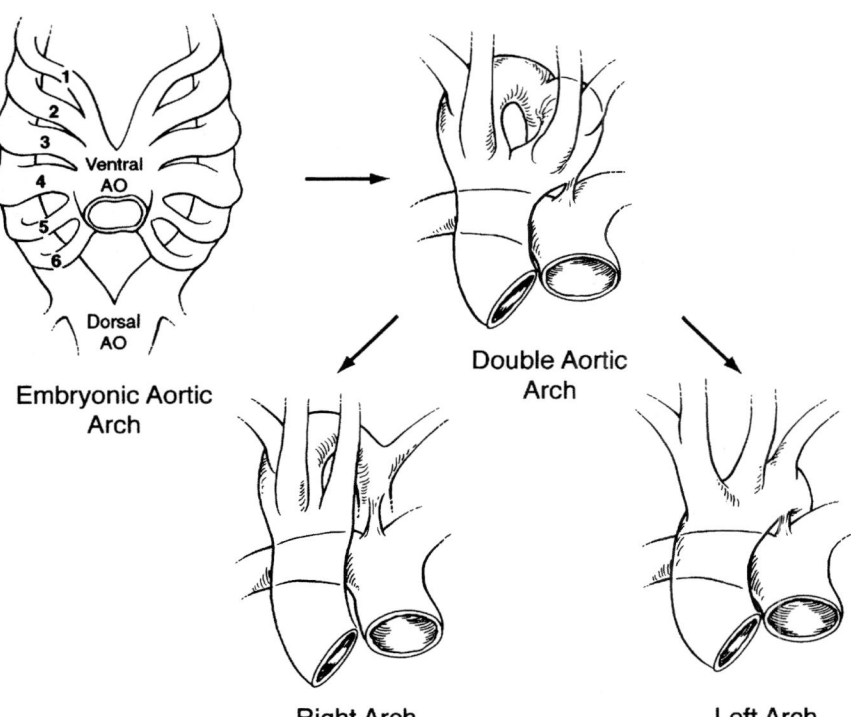

Fig. 78-2. Aortic arch development. Beginning with the embryonic aortic arch, the first, second, and fifth arches involute to form Edward's classic double aortic arch. If development stops at this point, the child has a double aortic arch. If the right fourth arch involutes, a normal left arch is formed. If the left fourth arch involutes, a right aortic arch is formed. AO, aorta. From Backer CL, Mavroudis C: Surgical approach to vascular rings. *In* Karp R, et al. (eds): Advances in Cardiac Surgery. Vol. 9. St. Louis: Mosby–Year Book, 1997, p. 31. With permission.

then performed around the trachea and esophagus to lyse any residual adhesive bands. The recurrent laryngeal and phrenic nerves are identified and protected throughout the procedure. The mediastinal pleura is not sutured closed because this could contribute to scar formation that might re-create the problems caused by the original vascular ring. For many years, my institution has routinely not placed a chest tube but

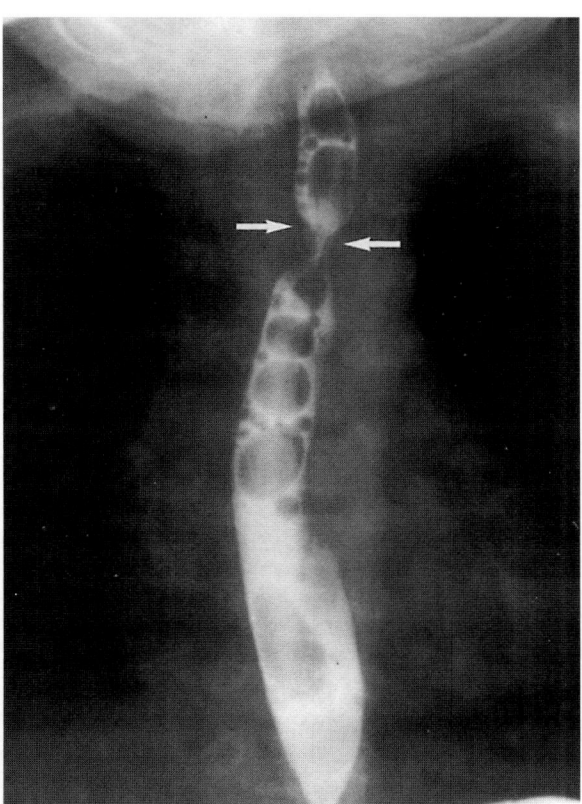

Fig. 78-3. Anteroposterior esophagogram of a 4-month-old boy who presented with stridor and was found to have a double aortic arch (*arrows*). From Backer CL, Ilbawi MN, et al: Vascular anomalies causing tracheoesophageal compression. Review of experience in children. J Thorac Cardiovasc Surg *97*:725, 1989. With permission.

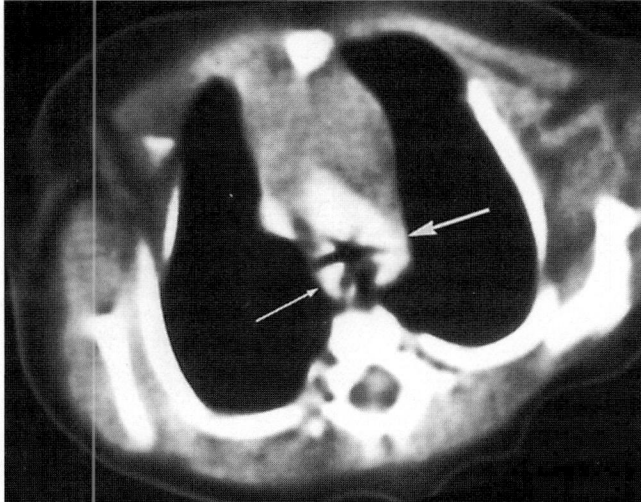

Fig. 78-4. Contrast-enhanced computed tomographic scan of a 3-week-old girl presenting with severe stridor shows a double aortic arch, left arch dominant. The right arch was successfully divided through a left thoracotomy. The large arrow points to the dominant left (anterior) arch. The small arrow points to the smaller right (posterior) arch.

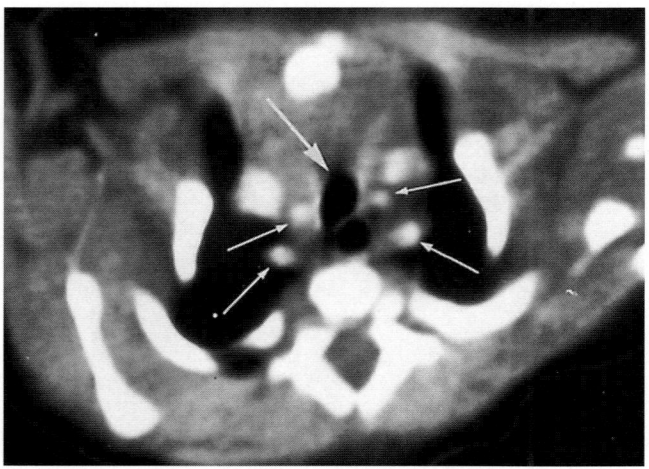

Fig. 78-5. Same infant as in Figure 78-4. The small arrows point to the four brachiocephalic vessels; large arrow points to trachea.

simply used a plastic suction catheter to evacuate pleural air, pulling it out as the skin is closed. One technical factor that the surgeon should be aware of is that when the clamps are placed on the vascular ring before ring division, the ring is temporarily tightened by inserting the clamps into the area between the ring and the trachea and esophagus. Patients may have a drop in oxygen saturation, requiring increased ventilatory pressures to provide adequate ventilation while the clamps are on the vascular ring. The postoperative care includes high humidity to loosen secretions; oxygen therapy, when needed, as monitored by pulse oximetry; vigorous chest physiotherapy; and nasopharyngeal suctioning.

Results

Results of surgical intervention are excellent. At Children's Memorial Hospital, no surgical mortality has resulted

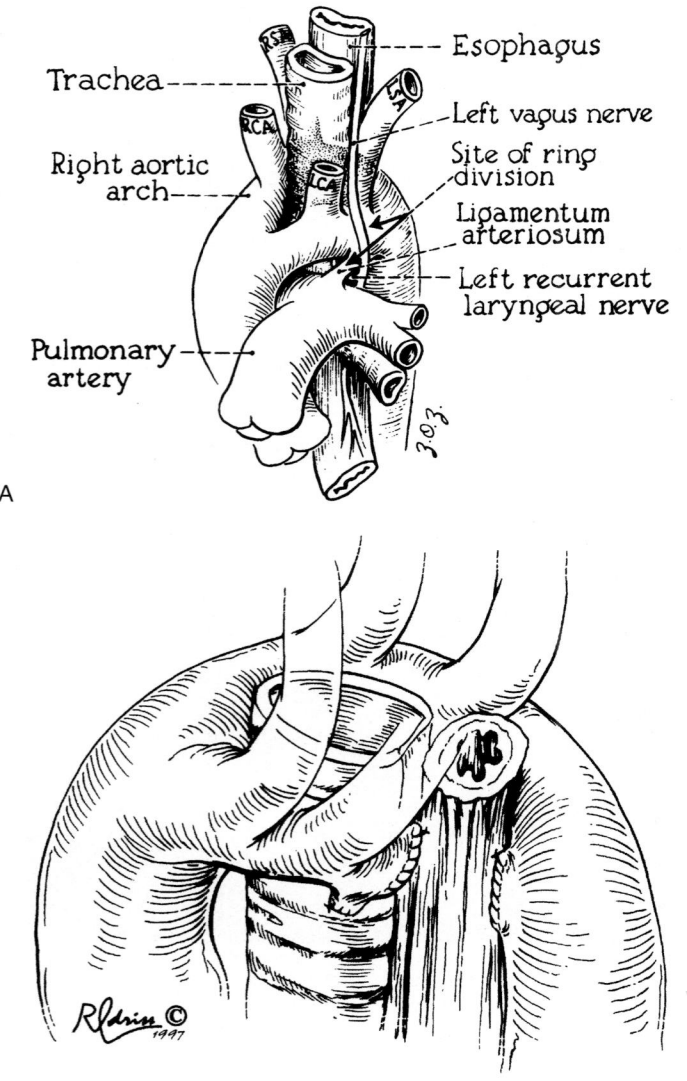

Fig. 78-6. A. Double aortic arch with right arch dominant. The vascular ring is divided at the sites shown by the arrows. LCA, left carotid artery; LSA, left subclavian artery; RCA, right carotid artery, RSA, right subclavian artery. From Backer CL, Idriss FS: Tracheoesophageal compressive syndromes of vascular origin: rings and slings. *In* Baue AE, et al. (eds): Glenn's Thoracic and Cardiovascular Surgery. 5th Ed. Norwalk, CT: Appleton-Century Crofts, 1991. With permission. **B.** Division of double aortic arch via left thoracotomy. A patent left aortic arch is being divided. A Potts ductus clamp is on the proximal portion of the arch, and a Castaneda clamp is on the distal arch adjacent to the descending thoracic aorta. The vascular ring has been partially transected and a single polypropylene suture placed on the distal portion of the divided arch. The ligamentum has already been divided and oversewn. **C.** Completed repair with clamps removed. The stumps of the vascular rings have now separated nicely and the esophagus is clearly visible. From Backer CL, Mavroudis C: Surgical approach to vascular rings. *In* Karp R, et al. (eds): Advances in Cardiac Surgery. Vol. 9. St. Louis: Mosby–Year Book, 1997, p. 41. With permission.

from a double aortic arch procedure since 1952. Most patients are discharged within 24 hours of the operation. As Nikaidoh and associates (1972) reported, some children have residual noisy breathing for 6 months to 2 years, but in nearly all instances, it gradually resolves.

Right Aortic Arch

Anatomy and Clinical Features

Right aortic arch with a left ligamentum arteriosum completing the vascular ring is almost as common as a double aortic arch. The ring is usually not as tight, however, and children typically present somewhat later in life (6 to 12 months of age). Symptoms are similar to those in infants with double aortic arch, including stridor, barklike cough,

and respiratory distress. In older children, dysphagia may be present. Some of these children eat very slowly and tend to be the last child to leave the table because they have to chew their food carefully as a learned procedure to prevent choking. Embryologically, depending on the exact site or sites of interruption of the left fourth arch and the branching pattern to the left subclavian artery, left carotid artery, and ductus arteriosus, different configurations of right aortic arch are possible. Felson and Palayew (1963) showed that two common variations are retroesophageal left subclavian artery (65%) and mirror-image branching (35%) (Fig. 78-7A and B). In either case, the left ligamentum arteriosum between the descending aorta and the left pulmonary artery completes the ring. Although D'Cruz and colleagues (1966) reported that one-third of patients with tetralogy of Fallot and truncus arteriosus have a right aortic arch, my group did not find a reverse association with a specific cardiac defect

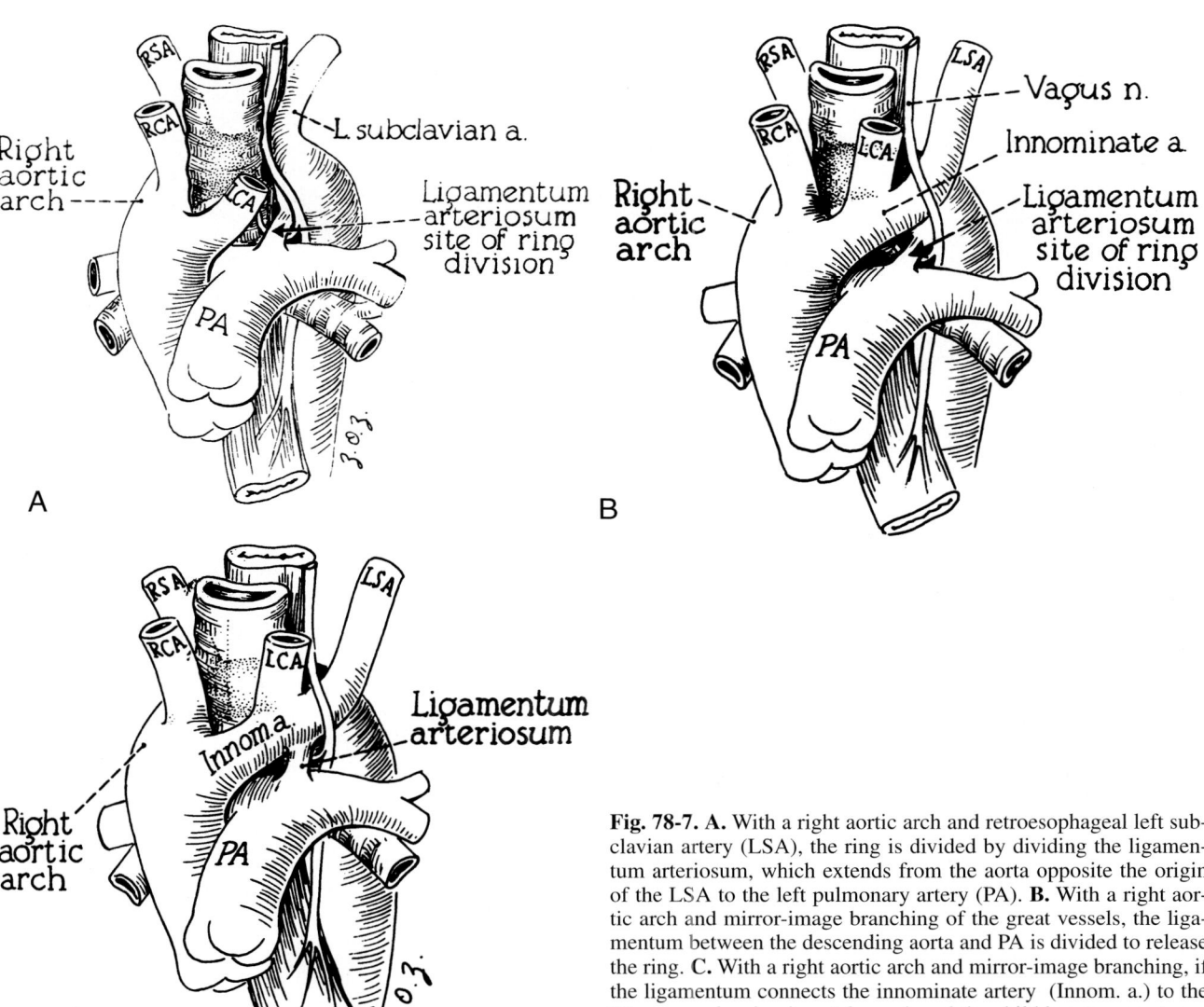

Fig. 78-7. A. With a right aortic arch and retroesophageal left subclavian artery (LSA), the ring is divided by dividing the ligamentum arteriosum, which extends from the aorta opposite the origin of the LSA to the left pulmonary artery (PA). B. With a right aortic arch and mirror-image branching of the great vessels, the ligamentum between the descending aorta and PA is divided to release the ring. C. With a right aortic arch and mirror-image branching, if the ligamentum connects the innominate artery (Innom. a.) to the PA, a vascular ring is not formed, and the child has no symptoms. LCA, left carotid artery; RCA, right carotid artery; RSA, right subclavian artery.

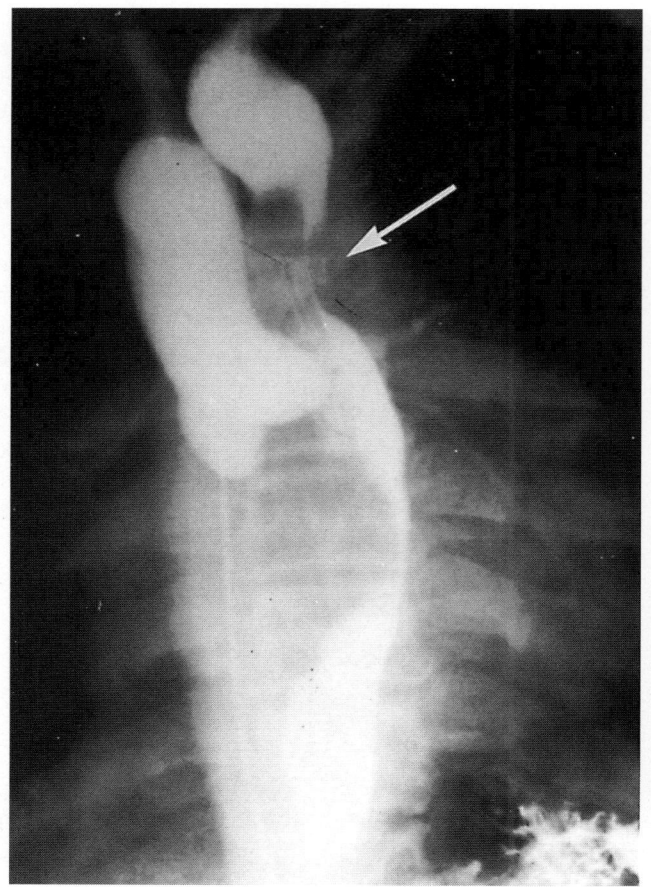
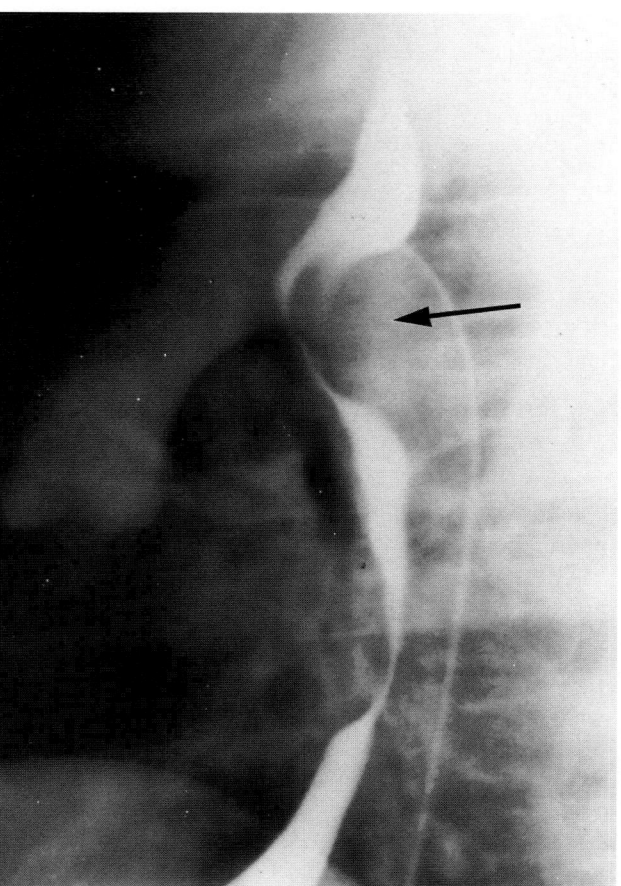

Fig. 78-8. Anteroposterior (**A**) and lateral (**B**) views of simultaneous esophagogram and aortogram in a patient with a right aortic arch and left ligamentum. The origin of the left subclavian artery is aneurysmal, forming a Kommerell's diverticulum. The combination of the tight ligamentum and the diverticulum (*arrows*) severely compresses the esophagus. In particular, the lateral film shows a classic deep posterior indentation from the large right arch.

when a vascular ring is formed by a right arch. In most infants with a cardiac defect and a right aortic arch, there is mirror-image branching with the ligamentum from the innominate artery to the pulmonary artery, so a vascular ring is not formed (Fig. 78-7C).

Diagnosis

The diagnosis is suggested by the chest radiograph, which shows an aortic arch to the right of the tracheal air column. In children who have a ligamentum completing the ring, compression of the trachea by the aorta is often quite impressive. The single most effective diagnostic examination, again, is the barium esophagram (Fig. 78-8). However, the referring clinician often obtains a CT or MR image before referring the patient for surgery. Bisset and associates (1987) have shown that MR imaging, like CT, is useful for identification of vascular rings. Axial images provide the same information as CT without ionizing radiation or intravenously administered contrast material. In addition, coronal and sagittal sections or images can be helpful in confusing

cases. A disadvantage to MR imaging is the length of time required for the study, which necessitates sedation. Figure 78-9 shows an MR image in a patient with a right aortic arch, left ligamentum, and retroesophageal left subclavian artery.

Treatment

The surgical approach is through a left thoracotomy (median sternotomy is reserved for patients with associated intracardiac lesions). After careful dissection and identification of the configuration of the aortic arch, the ligamentum arteriosum is identified as compressing the esophagus. The ring is released by dividing the ligamentum between vascular clamps and oversewing the stumps. Any adhesive bands are lysed. Chun and associates (1992) have emphasized the importance of an associated Kommerell's (1936) diverticulum. Embryologically, this diverticulum is a remnant of the left fourth aortic arch that did not undergo complete involution. The diverticulum may independently compress the esophagus or trachea, even with the ring divided. This aneurysmal dilatation should either be resected or, if small,

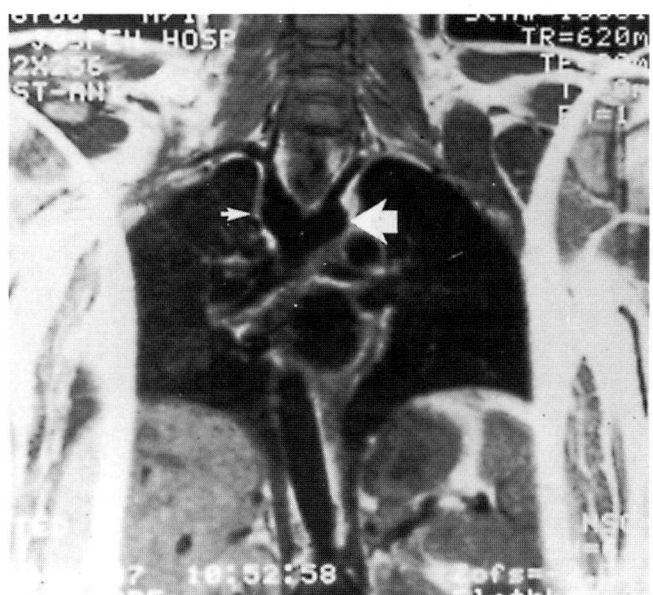

Fig. 78-9. A 17-year-old patient with dysphagia. Magnetic resonance image of a right aortic arch (*small arrow*) and a Kommerell's diverticulum (*large arrow*) at the origin of the left subclavian artery. From Backer CL, et al: Vascular anomalies causing tracheoesophageal compression. Review of experience in children. J Thorac Cardiovasc Surg 97:725, 1989. With permission.

fixed to the chest wall or vertebral bodies to prevent this complication.

I have reoperated on two children who had had their vascular ring (ligamentum) divided without addressing the associated Kommerell's diverticulum. Both were severely symptomatic, with a barklike cough, particularly with exercise. Both responded to reoperation with resection of the diverticulum and had complete resolution of airway symptoms. In one patient, the left subclavian artery was transected and reimplanted into the left carotid to relieve a taut arch compressing the trachea.

A very rare group of children with a right aortic arch and left ligamentum have a left-sided descending thoracic aorta, the so-called circumflex aorta. Robotin and colleagues (1996) have described an aortic "uncrossing" operation for these rare patients (3 of 468 patients in their series of patients with vascular rings). This procedure is performed through a median sternotomy with cardiopulmonary bypass and hypothermic circulatory arrest. The aortic arch is mobilized, divided, and brought in front of the tracheobronchial tree, then reanastomosed end-to-side to the lateral aspect of the ascending aorta. All three patients described by Robotin and coworkers (1996) had prior ligamentum division via left thoracotomy.

Results

The results of surgical intervention for this anomaly are very good. At Children's Memorial Hospital, there has been no mortality after surgery for an isolated right aortic arch since 1959. Like patients with a double aortic arch, it may take 6 to 12 months for airway symptoms to resolve.

Innominate Artery Compression Syndrome

Anatomy and Clinical Features

Innominate artery compression syndrome results from anterior compression of the trachea by the innominate artery. A "normal" left aortic arch exists, but the innominate artery appears to originate somewhat more posteriorly and leftward on the aortic arch than usual. Ardito and associates (1980) have described how, as the artery courses to the right, upward, and posterior to reach the thoracic outlet, it compresses the trachea anteriorly. These infants present with stridor, respiratory distress, cyanosis, and apnea with feeding. The infant may hold his or her head hyperextended to splint the trachea and improve breathing. Apnea or cyanosis may be precipitated by swallowing a bolus of food that presses on the soft posterior trachea with the innominate artery compressing the anterior trachea.

Diagnosis

Enthusiasm for the diagnosis of innominate artery compression syndrome increased in the late 1970s, when bronchoesophagologists switched from local to general anesthesia for bronchoscopy. As experience with these patients increased, however, the selection criteria for surgery became more stringent. The diagnosis is made with rigid bronchoscopy, which should demonstrate a pulsatile anterior compression of the trachea extending from left to right, with at least a 70% obstruction of the tracheal lumen. Anterior compression of the tracheal wall by the bronchoscope may compress the innominate artery and temporarily obliterate the right radial pulse. CT scan confirms the diagnosis, which demonstrates flattening and obliteration of the tracheal lumen by the contrast-filled innominate artery (Fig. 78-10). Radionuclide studies for gastroesophageal reflux, sleep studies, and neurologic evaluation, including CT of the brain and electroencephalograms, should be performed to rule out other causes of apnea. Barium esophagram is normal in these infants.

Treatment

When indicated, classic management of compression of the trachea by the innominate artery has been suspension of the innominate artery to the posterior aspect of the sternum, as originally described by Gross and Neuhauser (1948). At Children's Memorial Hospital, we have preferred a small right submammary thoracotomy. The right lobe of the thymus is excised, taking care not to injure the right phrenic nerve. The innominate artery is secured with pledget-supported

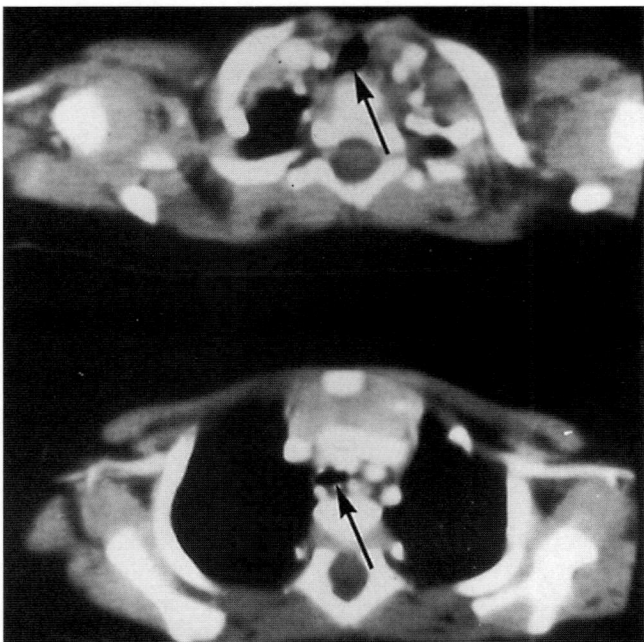

Fig. 78-10. Computed tomographic scan with contrast of an infant with innominate artery compression syndrome. The superior cut shows a normal-size trachea (*arrow*). The inferior cut shows the trachea (*arrow*) compressed by the innominate artery.

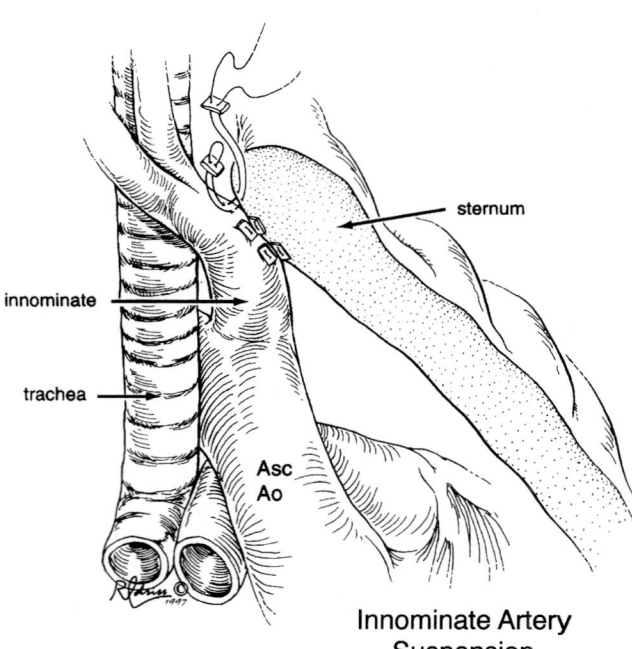

Innominate Artery
Suspension

Fig. 78-11. Innominate artery suspension. Exposure is through a right submammary thoracotomy. Fixing the adventitia of the innominate artery to the posterior table of the sternum with pledgeted sutures pulls the innominate artery anteriorly and actively pulls the tracheal wall forward and opens it. Asc Ao, ascending aorta. From Backer CL, Mavroudis C: Surgical approach to vascular rings. *In* Karp R, et al. (eds): Advances in Cardiac Surgery. Vol. 9. St. Louis: Mosby–Year Book, 1997, p. 49. With permission.

sutures to the posterior periosteum of the sternum to lift the innominate artery away from the trachea, simultaneously pulling the anterior tracheal wall open (Fig. 78-11). Hawkins and colleagues (1992) have described using a median sternotomy with division of the innominate artery and reimplantation into the ascending aorta at a site more to the right and anterior to the original site. This technique seems to sacrifice the active suspending mechanism on the tracheal wall provided by the classic technique and to pose some risk of cerebrovascular accident.

Results

At Children's Memorial Hospital, the author and colleagues (1992b) reported suspension for 76 (now 82) children, with 2 to 3% undergoing reoperation, 71 to 93% relieved of symptoms, and no deaths related to the actual procedure. Innominate artery compression of the trachea historically has been well managed by innominate artery suspension through a right anterolateral thoracotomy, and I continue to recommend this approach. Jones and coworkers (1994) have also reported good results with standard innominate artery suspension.

Pulmonary Artery Sling

Anatomy and Clinical Features

A pulmonary artery sling is a rare vascular anomaly in which the left pulmonary artery originates from the right pulmonary artery and encircles the right main stem bronchus and distal trachea before coursing anterior to the esophagus and descending aorta to enter the hilum of the left lung (Fig. 78-12). Glaevecke and Doehle (1897) were the first to report this anomaly as a postmortem finding in a 7-month-old infant with severe respiratory distress. Sade and associates (1975) reported that, embryologically, a pulmonary artery sling occurs when the developing left lung captures its arterial supply from derivatives of the right sixth aortic arch through capillaries caudad rather than cephalad to the developing tracheobronchial tree. The sling compresses and compromises the distal trachea and right main stem bronchus. Cosentino and coworkers (1991) have shown that many of these infants also have complete tracheal rings, which Berdon and colleagues (1984) have appropriately referred to as the "ring-sling" complex. Nearly all infants with pulmonary artery sling present within the first months of life with respiratory distress, particularly if there are associated complete tracheal rings.

Diagnosis

A chest radiograph may show unilateral hyperaeration of the right lung field. A barium esophagogram shows anterior compression of the esophagus on the lateral views (Fig. 78-13). Diagnosis is also obtained by cardiac echocardiogram, CT, or MR imaging; angiography is no

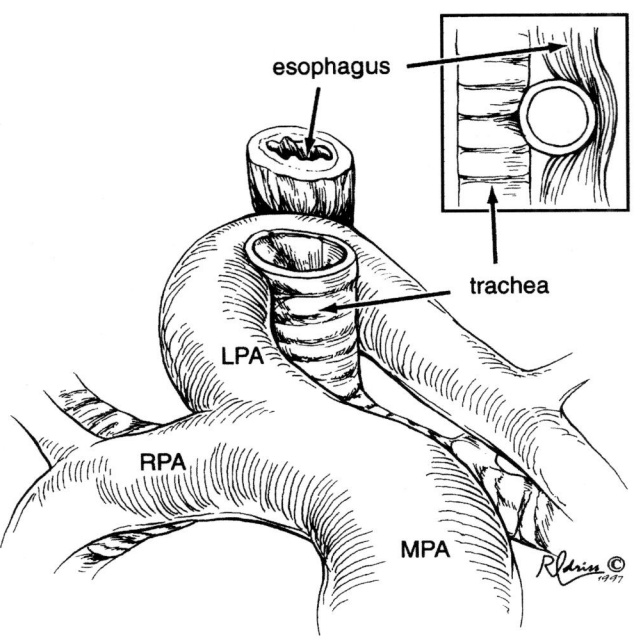

Pulmonary Artery Sling

Fig. 78-12. Pulmonary artery sling. The left pulmonary artery (LPA) originates from the right pulmonary artery (RPA) and courses between the esophagus and trachea to reach the left lung. Inset shows lateral relationship of LPA to esophagus; this view can be diagnostic on a barium swallow. MPA, main pulmonary artery. From Backer CL, Mavroudis C: Surgical approach to vascular rings. *In* Karp R, et al. (eds): Advances in Cardiac Surgery. Vol. 9. St. Louis: Mosby–Year Book, 1997, p. 52. With permission.

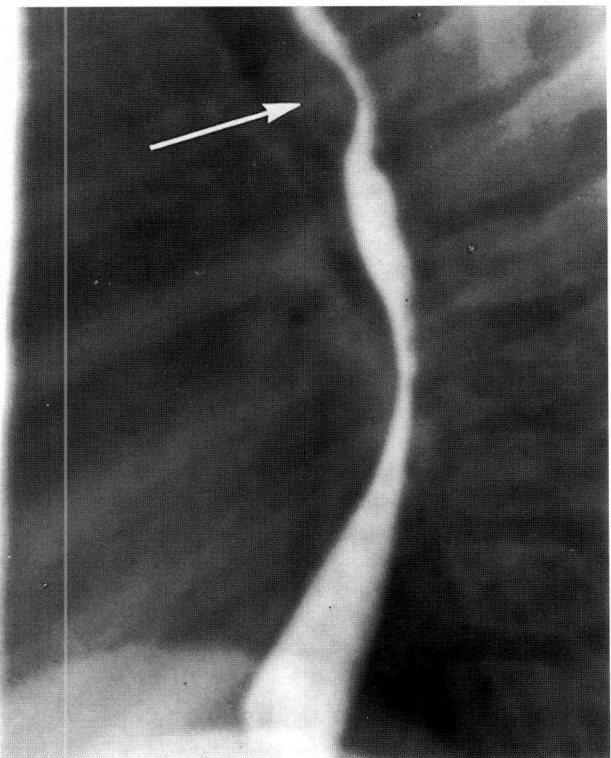

Fig. 78-13. Lateral esophagogram of an 18 month old with chronic upper respiratory tract infections. Arrow points to the anomalous left pulmonary artery compressing the esophagus anteriorly.

longer recommended unless an associated congenital cardiac anomaly is suspected. Both CT and MR imaging show clearly the left pulmonary artery originating from the right pulmonary artery, encircling the trachea, and coursing to the hilum of the left lung (Fig. 78-14). Currently, however, echocardiography is our diagnostic procedure of choice for pulmonary artery sling. Alboliras and associates (1996) reviewed our results using two-dimensional and color flow Doppler to make this diagnosis, and noted that the correct diagnosis was made in seven of seven patients. Many of these infants have a tenuous respiratory status, and it is much safer to do an echocardiogram at the bedside than to move them to the scanner. Bronchoscopy should be performed in all these infants to check for associated complete tracheal rings. In our experience, these were found in 50% of patients with pulmonary artery sling. Tracheograms are indicated only in select cases and must be done with extreme caution to avoid further ventilatory compromise.

Treatment

Surgical intervention should be undertaken as soon as the diagnosis is made because of the usual tenuous respiratory status. Potts and coworkers (1954) performed the first suc-

cessful operation for pulmonary artery sling at Children's Memorial Hospital, through a right thoracotomy. Potts operated on a 5-month-old infant who did not have an exact preoperative diagnosis but was believed to have vascular compression of the lower trachea and right bronchus by a

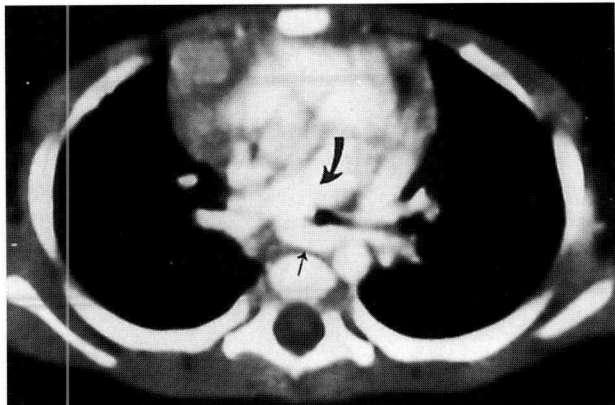

Fig. 78-14. Computed tomographic scan with contrast from a 14-month-old girl with pulmonary artery sling and complete tracheal rings from the fourth tracheal ring to the carina. Curved arrow points to main pulmonary artery. Small arrow points to left pulmonary artery, which wraps around the trachea from right to left. Note that the tracheal lumen is small from complete tracheal rings.

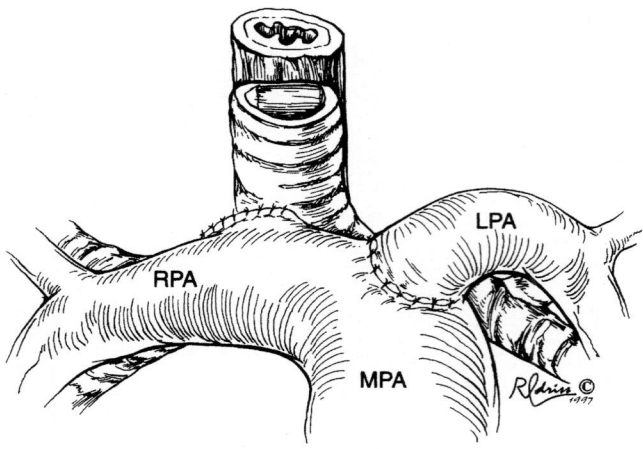

Repaired Pulmonary Artery Sling

Fig. 78-15. Operative technique. Repair is performed by transecting the left pulmonary artery (LPA) at its origin from right pulmonary artery (RPA) and anastomosing the LPA to the main pulmonary artery (MPA) anterior to the trachea at a site that approximates the usual anatomic configuration. From Backer CL, Mavroudis C: Surgical approach to vascular rings. *In* Karp R, et al. (eds): Advances in Cardiac Surgery. Vol. 9. St. Louis: Mosby–Year Book, 1997, p. 54. With permission.

vascular structure of some sort. He made the correct intraoperative diagnosis and considered several surgical alternatives, including right pneumonectomy, before deciding to transect the left pulmonary artery and reanastomosing it to the main pulmonary artery anterior to the trachea. That particular child survived the surgery and is still alive; however, as Campbell and colleagues (1980) reported, the left pulmonary artery is occluded. The next several patients operated on at Children's Memorial Hospital were reported by Koopot and associates (1975), with the approach through a left thoracotomy and using the technique described by Potts. This approach was reported by Pawade and colleagues (1992) to have good results (18 patients, one death), except in infants with associated tracheal stenosis.

My associates and I (1992a) advocate an approach with median sternotomy and the use of extracorporeal circulation. This allows accurate ligation and division of the left pulmonary artery with implantation into the main pulmonary artery anterior to the trachea (Fig. 78-15). The operation can be performed without respiratory compromise, and enough time and care can be taken to ensure patency of the left pulmonary artery. Because nearly 50% of patients with pulmonary artery sling have associated complete tracheal rings (the ring-sling complex), the median sternotomy approach allows simultaneous tracheoplasty. Since 1954, 23 patients with pulmonary artery sling have been repaired at Children's Memorial Hospital. From 1985 to 1998, 15 infants had repair using a median sternotomy approach and cardiopulmonary bypass. Thirteen of these 23 children (56%) had associated complete tracheal rings. There has

been no operative mortality and only two late deaths, both in patients having pericardial tracheoplasty for complete tracheal rings, with death occurring at 7 months and 2.5 years postoperatively. All left pulmonary arteries repaired on cardiopulmonary bypass are patent, and the mean percentage blood flow to the left lung by nuclear scan is 44%.

Complete Tracheal Rings

Anatomy and Clinical Features

As illustrated in Figure 78-16, when the child has complete tracheal rings, there is congenital absence of the membranous trachea causing the cartilage to be circumferential. This causes tracheal stenosis, which often leads to severe

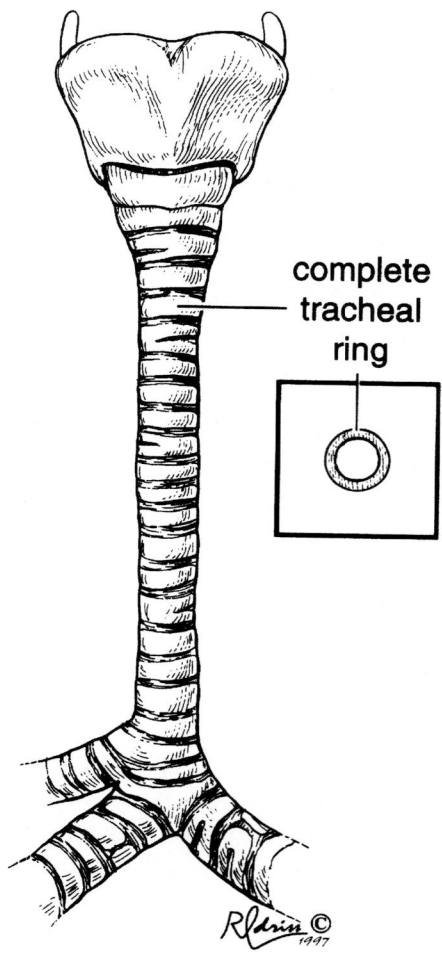

complete tracheal ring

Fig. 78-16. Complete tracheal rings causing long-segment congenital tracheal stenosis from the third tracheal ring to the carina. The membranous portion of the trachea is absent, and the cartilages are circumferential. This patient has an associated tracheal right upper lobe bronchus. From Backer CL, Mavroudis C: Surgical approach to vascular rings. *In* Karp R, et al. (eds): Advances in Cardiac Surgery. Vol. 9. St. Louis: Mosby–Year Book, 1997, p. 56. With permission.

respiratory distress in infancy. Benjamin and associates (1981) reported that medical management of this lesion is associated with a 43% mortality rate. Cantrell and Guild (1964) classified these patients into three categories: 1) segmental stenosis, 2) funnellike stenosis, and 3) generalized hypoplasia. Although the number of rings and extent of the stenosis can be variable, most of our patients have had complete tracheal rings from one or two rings below the cricoid extending to the carina.

Diagnosis

This diagnosis and the extent of involvement is established by rigid bronchoscopy. Often the bronchoscope itself cannot pass through the stenosis, but the fine telescope can pass.

Treatment

Surgical options for the management of children with long-segment congenital tracheal stenosis from complete tracheal rings include 1) pericardial patch tracheoplasty, 2) cartilage tracheoplasty, 3) slide tracheoplasty, 4) tracheal homograft, and 5) tracheal autograft. At Children's Memorial Hospital from 1982 to 1998, 28 patients had pericardial tracheoplasty, two underwent slide tracheoplasty, two had resection of short segments of complete rings, and six had repair using a free tracheal autograft. Twelve of these patients (32%) had simultaneous pulmonary artery sling repair. Six patients (16%) had simultaneous intracardiac repair of complete atrioventricular canal; two patients had double-outlet right ventricle, tetralogy of Fallot, ventricular septal defect, and pulmonary atresia. Our current approach is to use the tracheal autograft, supplemented with pericardium if necessary.

Pericardial Tracheoplasty

The technique of pericardial tracheoplasty was first described by Idriss and associates (1984). The approach is through a median sternotomy, and cardiopulmonary bypass is used for respiratory support. Bronchoscopy is used to guide an anterior incision in the trachea, which is extended proximal and distal to the complete tracheal rings. The trachea is patched open with an autologous pericardial patch anchored with interrupted 6-0 Vicryl sutures (Fig. 78-17). The patch is usually 1.5 to 2.0 cm wide and extends the length of the stenosis. The patch is stented open with an endotracheal tube for 7 to 10 days. Cosentino and coworkers (1991) reported our intermediate results, and Dunham and associates (1994) discussed the role of postoperative bronchoscopy to remove secretions and granulation tissue and perform dilation as needed. Cheng and colleagues (1997) reported complete re-epithelization of the graft site with ciliated pseudostratified columnar epithelium, thereby suggesting the likelihood of normal mucociliary flow. We have used the pericardial patch technique in 28 patients, with two early and four late deaths. One early death resulted

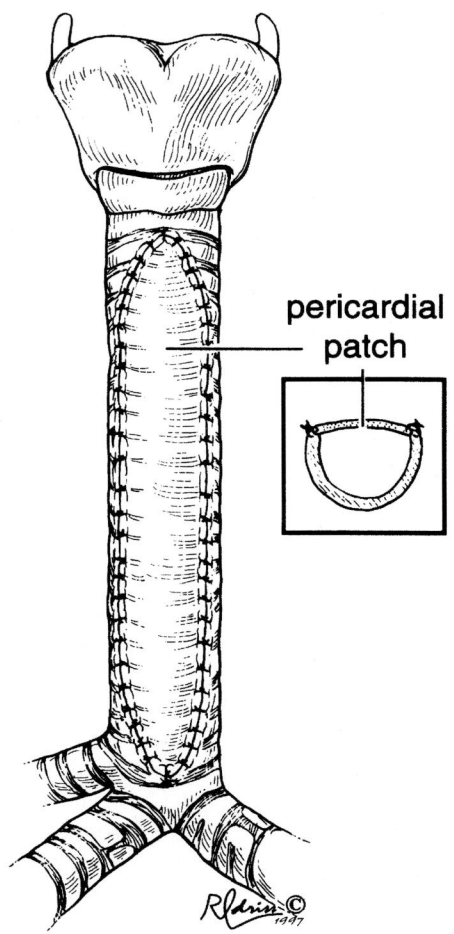

Fig. 78-17. Completed pericardial patch tracheoplasty augments the trachea anteriorly, opening the tracheal lumen significantly, as shown in the inset. From Backer CL, Mavroudis C: Surgical approach to vascular rings. *In* Karp R, et al. (eds): Advances in Cardiac Surgery. Vol. 9. St. Louis: Mosby–Year Book, 1997, p 57. With permission.

from patch dehiscence and mediastinitis. The other was related to complications of postoperative extracorporeal membrane oxygenation. Three late deaths were related to residual or recurrent airway stenosis, and one to pulmonary hypertension. I and my colleagues (1997) reported that six of these patients required surgical revision: four with cartilage grafts and two with pericardium. As Furman and associates (1999) reported, three of these patients have required seven Palmaz stents. These balloon-expandable metallic stents were placed in the distal trachea or proximal bronchi with a bronchoscope under fluoroscopic guidance, as originally described by Filler and coworkers (1995).

Slide Tracheoplasty

The "slide" tracheoplasty was first described by Tsang and colleagues (1989) and was modified by Grillo (1994). Although both described using direct ventilation through the

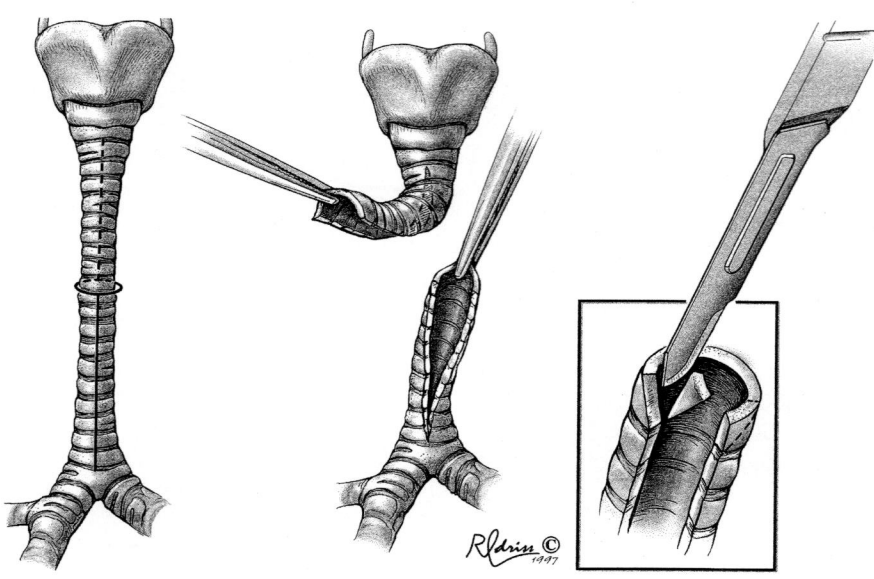

Fig. 78-18. The trachea is transected at the midpoint of the complete tracheal rings. The upper trachea is opened posteriorly; the lower trachea is opened anteriorly. The corners of the two tracheal ends are trimmed. Courtesy of Rashid Idriss, with permission.

open trachea, we have used this technique with a median sternotomy approach and cardiopulmonary bypass. The midportion of the trachea is identified bronchoscopically, and the trachea is then transected at this site. The lower trachea is opened anteriorly, the upper trachea is opened posteriorly (Fig. 78-18). The two tracheal openings then slide, one on top of the other, after the very corners of the transected trachea are trimmed. The two are anastomosed with interrupted Vicryl sutures (Fig. 78-19). This creates a trachea that is one-half as long as the original but has four times the diameter. Of course, the patient still has complete circumferential tracheal rings. Dayan and associates (1997)

reported our results using this technique in two infants. One child did very well and was discharged at 18 days; the other had considerable growth of granulation tissue and severe tracheomalacia, requiring a stent, and eventually died 4 months postoperatively.

Tracheal Autograph Technique

Because of the high reoperation rate after pericardial tracheoplasty and the aforementioned results with slide tracheoplasty, our group has tried a new technique, called *tracheal autograft technique*. We had found that, in children

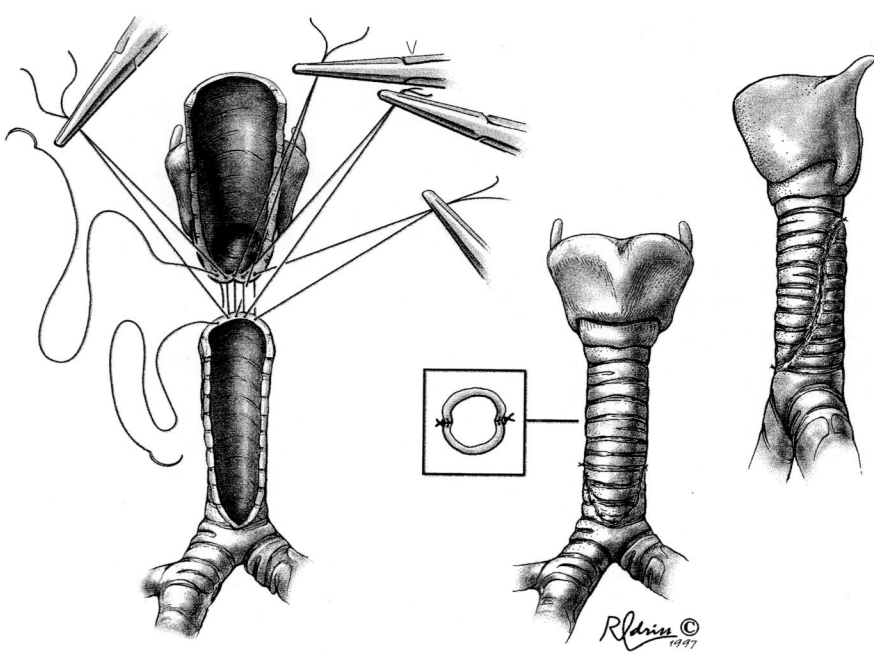

Fig. 78-19. Anastomosis between upper and lower trachea is performed with interrupted polydioxanone (PDS, Ethicon, Sommerville, NJ) or Vicryl sutures. The length of the trachea has been reduced by almost one-half; the luminal diameter has been increased by four. Courtesy of Rashid Idriss, with permission.

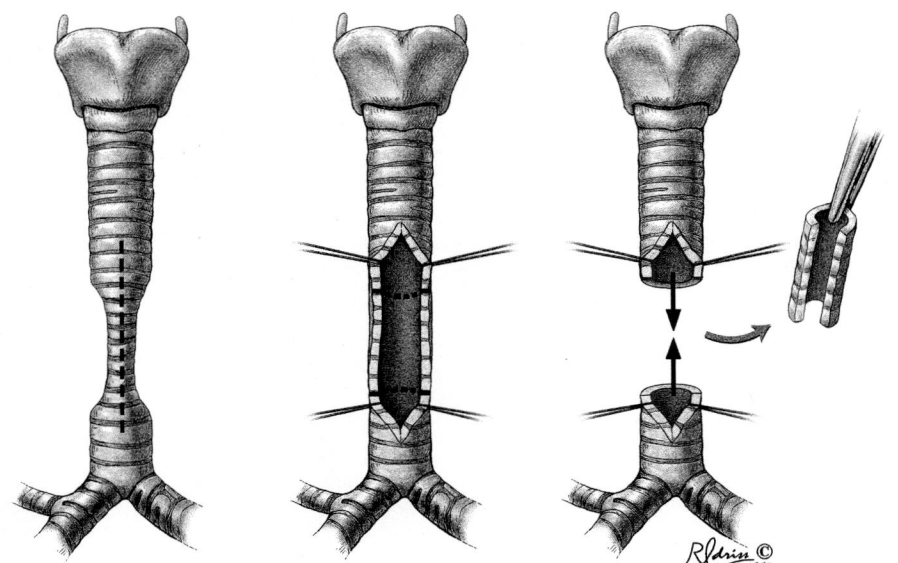

Fig. 78-20. Tracheal autograft technique. The lower trachea is incised anteriorly through 12 tracheal rings (eight complete rings). A 1.5-cm segment of trachea (essentially, the extent of the complete tracheal rings) is excised. Courtesy of Rashid Idriss, with permission.

with complete tracheal rings, the trachea is frequently longer than normal. Because of this, a pericardial tracheoplasty may result in an excessively long patch that does not have intrinsic support. In a 1995 case, I therefore excised a 1.5-cm portion of the trachea and reanastomosed the trachea posteriorly before the anterior pericardial patch was placed. Shortly thereafter, I noted in the case report by Jacobs and associates (1996a) the use of cryopreserved homograft for repair of complete tracheal rings. The portion of trachea I had excised and sent to pathology looked just like the piece of homograft Jacobs and colleagues (1996a) used for their repair. For the next child with complete tracheal rings that I operated on, I used a portion of the trachea as a free autograft.

The technique uses a median sternotomy approach and cardiopulmonary bypass for respiratory support during the tracheal repair. Under bronchoscopic guidance, the trachea is incised anteriorly though the extent of the stenosis (Fig. 78-20). A segment of trachea (1.3 to 2.2 cm) is excised, generally in the midportion of the trachea. The trachea is then reapproximated posteriorly (Fig. 78-21) with interrupted Vicryl sutures. The portion of trachea that was resected is brought in anteriorly as a free autograft. The corners of the autograft are trimmed, and it is sutured in place with additional Vicryl sutures. In a patient like the one illustrated, this completes the repair. In a child with longer stenosis, the autograft is used as a distal patch at the critical junction of the carina and left and right main stem bronchi. The remaining opening in the upper trachea is augmented with a pericardial patch 1.5 to 3.0 cm long.

Since January 1996, our group has used this technique in six infants, with a mean age of 4.9 months. Two operations were completed with the autograft alone, four required pericardial augmentations. All patients survived the procedure, were extubated at a mean of 13 days, and were discharged at

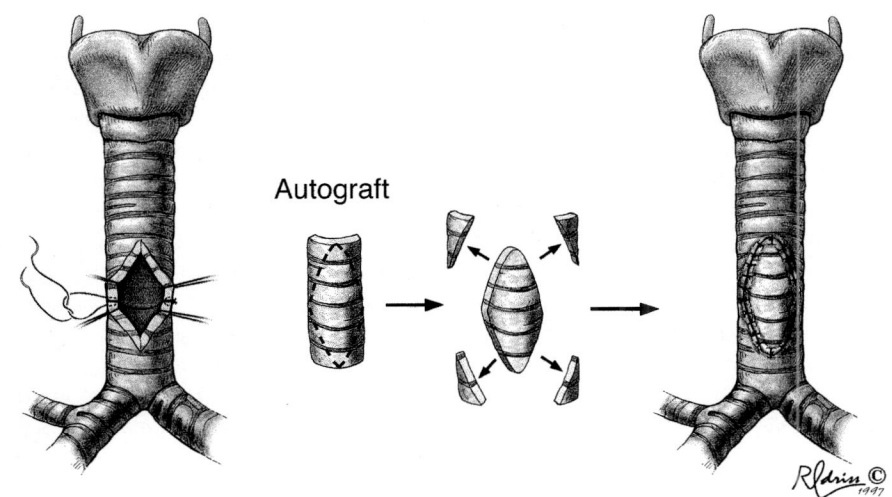

Autograft

Fig. 78-21. The two cut ends of the trachea are anastomosed posteriorly with interrupted sutures. The corners of the autograft are trimmed so that the autograft fits in the remaining anterior tracheal opening, where it is sutured in place. Courtesy of Rashid Idriss, with permission.

a mean of 23 days. One infant had recurrent tracheal stenosis related to the pericardial patch and required a stent and tracheostomy 4 months postoperatively. The mean follow-up is now 16 months, and all patients currently have widely patent tracheal lumens.

Tracheal Homografts

As mentioned earlier, European surgeons have reported using cadaveric treated homograft for congenital tracheal stenosis. Jacobs and colleagues (1996a) reported the use of cadaveric trachea, which is harvested fresh, fixed in formalin, washed in thimerosal, and stored in acetone. The stenosed trachea is patched open with the tracheal homograft and placed over a temporary silicone-rubber intraluminal stent. Jacobs and colleagues (1996b) reported on 24 children (mean age 8 years): 20 children survived, of whom 16 are free of airway symptoms. Six of these patients had long-segment congenital tracheal stenosis, had prior tracheal operation, and were approached with a median sternotomy. The homograft technique was successful in three of the six children.

Aberrant Right Subclavian Artery

A left aortic arch with aberrant origin of the right subclavian artery from the descending thoracic aorta may cause posterior indentation of the esophagus (Fig. 78-22). Gross (1946) described this as the cause of dysphagia lusoria. Abbott (1936) reported that this is the most common vascular anomaly of the aortic arch system, occurring in 0.5% of humans. As Beabout and associates (1964) confirmed, however, it is usually not a source of symptoms severe enough to cause surgical intervention, unless there is aneurysmal dilatation of the subclavian origin. Our group has not operated on a child with this diagnosis since 1973. In adults, however, the base of the aberrant right subclavian artery may become dilatated and aneurysmal, compressing the esophagus and causing symptoms of dysphagia. In that case, the right subclavian artery should be divided, the aneurysm resected, and the right subclavian artery implanted into the aorta or carotid artery. Pifarre and colleagues (1971) described this as a one-stage procedure with a left thoracotomy approach. More recently, van Son and associates (1990) have recommended a surgical approach through a right thoracotomy. Esposito and coworkers (1988) found only 26 cases of aneurysm of an aberrant subclavian artery in the world literature, and only 16 patients had been operated on. They recommended an initial approach through a right cervical incision to divide the right subclavian distal to the aneurysmal dilatation and anastomosis of the distal end to the right carotid artery to preserve blood flow to the distal distribution of the artery. The patient is then placed in a right lateral decubitus position, and the aneurysm is excised through a left thoracotomy approach. These authors believe that this approach obviates the possible complications of

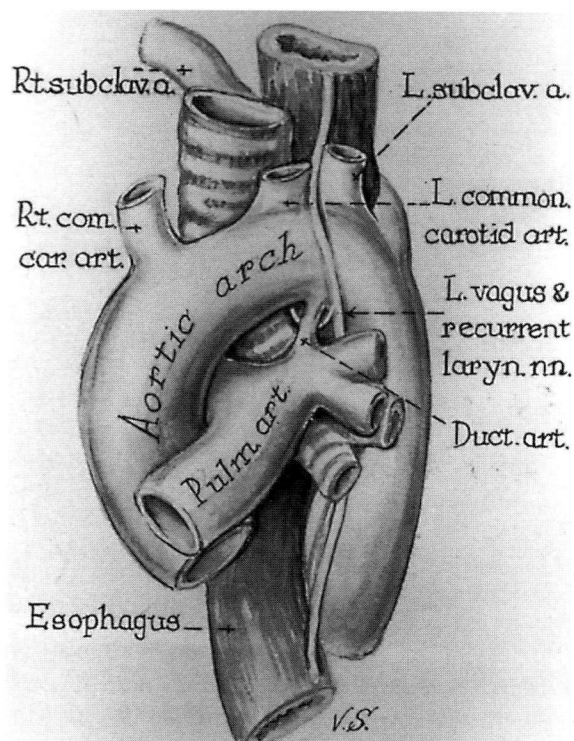

Fig. 78-22. Aberrant right subclavian artery originating as the last branch from the aortic arch. The artery courses posterior to the esophagus up to the right arm. From Idriss FS, et al: Surgery for vascular anomalies causing obstruction of the trachea and esophagus. *In* Tucker BL, Lindesmith GG (eds): Congenital Heart Disease. New York: Grune & Stratton, 1979, p. 125. With permission.

upper limb ischemia, cerebral embolization, and intraoperative hemorrhage.

Rare Vascular Rings

A cervical aortic arch may ascend into the neck and compress the trachea and esophagus. An anomalous left carotid artery may compress the trachea as it courses from right to left across the trachea. Whitman and associates (1982) reported that a left aortic arch with right-sided ligamentum and right-sided descending aorta is another unusual cause of tracheoesophageal compression. Watanabe and associates (1995) found that this anomaly has been reported approximately 19 times in the world literature. It is one of the very rare vascular rings that, as McFaul and colleagues (1981) reported, may necessitate a right thoracotomy for successful correction. These infants often have associated cardiac anomalies, such as absent left pulmonary artery, ventricular septal defect, tetralogy of Fallot, and transposition of the great arteries, as noted by Park and coworkers (1976), and the diagnosis is made by cardiac catheterization. The esophagogram also has a very distinctive appearance, with extrinsic indentation in the upper left posterior aspect of the esophagus at the level of the second thoracic vertebra. I have operated on one patient with a right aortic arch and a right ligamentum compressing the right main bronchus. This child had no left pulmonary artery. I divided the ligamentum through a median sternotomy approach because of severe hyperinflation and blebs of the right lung. Binet and colleagues (1978) described a single case report of a ductus arteriosus traversing from the right pulmonary artery to the descending aorta between the trachea and esophagus with an aberrant right subclavian artery. The ductus was compressing the trachea and right bronchus in a manner analogous to pulmonary artery sling. Ben-Shachar and associates (1985) reported a hemitruncal sling creating a vascular ring. The right pulmonary artery originated from the ascending aorta and coursed in a dorsocranial direction, wrapping around the trachea.

VIDEO-ASSISTED THORACOSCOPIC SURGERY

Video-assisted thoracoscopic surgery (VATS) has been used for the division of vascular rings. It is an extension of the use of VATS for patent ductus arteriosus ligation, as reported by Laborde and colleagues (1993). Burke and coworkers (1995) reported the use of VATS for eight patients with vascular rings. Anatomy of the rings included double aortic arch with an atretic left arch (three patients) and right aortic arch and left ligamentum arteriosum (five patients). Three patients (37.5%) required a thoracotomy to complete the procedure. The median operating time was 4 hours, and the median hospital stay was 3 days. The mean hospital stay of our vascular ring patients has been 1 day, so we have not considered the VATS technique a sufficient improvement to recommend its use. It is interesting to note that no patients in the series by Burke and colleagues (1995) had a patent arch. A real concern for the patient with a patent arch is that once the clips are applied and the ring divided, the two stumps retract because of tension on the ring. The posterior stump often retracts into the mediastinum, and if the clip should slip off, the risk of hemorrhage is great. It is not always possible to tell externally whether a segment of the ring is atretic or patent. This is another reason not to use VATS for these patients.

REFERENCES

Abbott ME: Atlas of Congenital Cardiac Disease. New York: The American Heart Association, 1936, p. 16.

Arciniegas E, et al: Surgical management of congenital vascular rings. J Thorac Cardiovasc Surg 77:721, 1979.

Alboliras ET, et al: Pulmonary artery sling: diagnostic and management strategy. Pediatrics 98:530A, 1996.

Ardito JM, et al: Innominate artery compression of the trachea in infants with reflex apnea. Ann Otol 89:401, 1980.

Backer CL, et al: Vascular anomalies causing tracheoesophageal compression. J Thorac Cardiovasc Surg 97:725, 1989.

Backer CL, et al: Pulmonary artery sling. J Thorac Cardiovasc Surg 103:683, 1992a.

Backer CL, et al: Reoperation after pericardial patch tracheoplasty. J Pediatr Surg 32:1108, 1997.

Backer CL, et al: Repair of congenital tracheal stenosis with a free tracheal autograft. J Thorac Cardiovasc Surg 115:869, 1998.

Backer CL, Holinger LD, Mavroudis C: Invited letter concerning: innominate artery compression—division and reimplantation versus suspension. J Thorac Cardiovasc Surg 103:817, 1992b.

Backer CL, Mavroudis C: Surgical approach to vascular rings. In Karp R, et al (eds): Advances in Cardiac Surgery. Vol 9. St. Louis: CV Mosby Year Book, 1997, pp. 29–64.

Beabout JW, Stewart JR, Kincaid OW: Aberrant right subclavian artery, dispute of commonly accepted concepts. AJR Am J Roentgenol 92:855, 1964.

Ben-Shachar G, et al: Hemitruncal sling: a newly recognized anomaly and its surgical correction. J Thorac Cardiovasc Surg 90:146, 1985.

Benjamin B, Pitkin J, Cohen D: Congenital tracheal stenosis. Ann Otol Rhinol Laryngol 90:364, 1981.

Berdon WE, et al: Complete cartilage-ring tracheal stenosis associated with anomalous left pulmonary artery: the ring-sling complex. Radiology 152:57, 1984.

Binet JP, et al: Ductus arteriosus sling: report of a newly recognized anomaly and its surgical correction. Thorax 33:72, 1978.

Bisset GS, et al: Vascular rings: MR imaging. AJR Am J Roentgenol 149:251, 1987.

Burke RP, et al: Video-assisted thoracoscopic surgery for congenital heart disease. J Thorac Cardiovasc Surg 109:499, 1995.

Campbell CD, et al: Aberrant left pulmonary artery (pulmonary artery sling): successful repair and 24 year follow-up report. Am J Cardiol 45:316, 1980.

Cantrell JR, Guild HG: Congenital stenosis of the trachea. Am J Surg 108:297, 1964.

Cheng ATL, et al: Histopathologic changes after pericardial patch tracheoplasty. Arch Otolaryngol Head Neck Surg 123:1069, 1997.

Chun KF, et al: Diagnosis and management of congenital vascular rings: a 22-year experience. Ann Thorac Surg 53:597, 1992.

Congdon ED: Transformation of the aortic arch system during the development of the human embryo. Contrib Embryol 14:47, 1922.

Cosentino CM, et al: Pericardial patch tracheoplasty for severe tracheal stenosis in children: intermediate results. J Pediatr Surg 26:879, 1991.

Dayan SH, et al: Slide tracheoplasty in the management of congenital tracheal stenosis. Ann Otol Rhinol Laryngol 106:914, 1997.

D'Cruz IA, et al: Right-sided aorta. Br Heart J 28:722, 1966.

Dunham ME, et al: Management of severe congenital tracheal stenosis. Ann Otol Rhinol Laryngol 103:351, 1994.

Edwards JE: Anomalies of derivatives of aortic arch system. Med Clin North Am 32:925, 1948.

Esposito RA, et al: Surgical treatment for aneurysm of aberrant subclavian artery based on a case report and review of the literature. J Thorac Cardiovasc Surg 95:888, 1988.

Felson B, Palayew MJ: The two types of right aortic arch. Radiology 81:745, 1963.

Filler RM, et al: The use of expandable metallic airway stents for tracheobronchial obstruction in children. J Pediatr Surg 30:1050, 1995.

Furman RH, et al: The use of expandable metallic stents in the treatment of pediatric tracheobronchomalacia. Arch Otolaryngol Head Neck Surg 125:203, 1999.

Glaevecke, D: Ueber eine seltene angeborene Anomalie der Pulmonalarterie. Munch Med Wochenschr 44:950, 1897.

Grillo HC: Slide tracheoplasty for long-segment congenital tracheal stenosis. Ann Thorac Surg 58:613, 1994.

Gross RE: Surgical relief for tracheal obstruction from a vascular ring. N Engl J Med 233:586, 1945.

Gross RE: Surgical treatment for dysphagia lusoria. Ann Surg 124:532, 1946.

Gross RE, Neuhauser EBD: Compression of the trachea by an anomalous innominate artery: an operation for its relief. Am J Dis Child 75:570, 1948.

Hawkins JA, Bailey WW, Clark SM: Innominate artery compression of the trachea: treatment by reimplantation of the innominate artery. J Thorac Cardiovasc Surg 103:678, 1992.

Heck HA Jr, et al: Esophageal-aortic erosion associated with double aortic arch and tracheomalacia: experience with 2 infants. Tex Heart Inst J 20:126, 1993.

Idriss FS, et al: Tracheoplasty with pericardial patch for extensive tracheal stenosis in infants and children. J Thorac Cardiovasc Surg 88:527, 1984.

Jacobs JP, et al: Successful complete tracheal resection in a three-month-old infant. Ann Thorac Surg *61*:1824, 1996a.

Jacobs JP, et al: Pediatric tracheal homograft reconstruction: a novel approach to complex tracheal stenoses in children. J Thorac Cardiovasc Surg *112*:1549, 1996b.

Jones DT, Jonas RA, Healy GB: Innominate artery compression of the trachea in infants. Ann Otol Rhinol Laryngol *103*:347, 1994.

Kommerell B: Verlagerung des Osophagus durch eine abnorm verlaufende Arteria Subclavia Dextra (Arteria Lusoria). Fortsch Geb Rontgenstr *54*:590, 1936.

Koopot R, Nikaidoh H, Idriss FS: Surgical management of anomalous left pulmonary artery causing tracheobronchial obstruction: pulmonary artery sling. J Thorac Cardiovasc Surg *69*:239, 1975.

Laborde F, et al: A new video-assisted thoracoscopic surgical technique for interruption of patent ductus arteriosus in infants and children. J Thorac Cardiovasc Surg *105*:278, 1993.

Lowe GM, Donaldson JS, Backer CL: Vascular rings: 10-year review of imaging. RadioGraphics *11*:637, 1991.

McFaul R, Millard P, Nowicki E: Vascular rings necessitating right thoracotomy. J Thorac Cardiovasc Surg *82*:306, 1981.

McLoughlin MJ, et al: Computed tomography in congenital anomalies of the aortic arch and great vessels. Radiology *138*:399, 1981.

Midulla PS, et al: Aortic dissection involving a double aortic arch with a right descending aorta. Ann Thorac Surg *58*:874, 1994.

Nikaidoh H, Riker WL, Idriss FS: Surgical management of "vascular rings." Arch Surg *105*:327, 1972.

Othersen HB Jr, et al: Aortoesophageal fistula and double aortic arch: two important points in management. J. Pediatr Surg *31*:594, 1996.

Park SC, et al: Left aortic arch with right descending aorta and right ligamentum arteriosum: a rare form of vascular ring. J Thorac Cardiovasc Surg *71*:779, 1976.

Pawade A, et al: Pulmonary artery sling. Ann Thorac Surg *54*:967, 1992.

Pifarre R, Niedballa RG, Dieter RA Jr: Definitive surgical treatment of the aberrant retroesophageal right subclavian artery in the adult. J Thorac Cardiovasc Surg *61*:154, 1971.

Potts WJ, Gibson S, Rothwell R: Double aortic arch: report of two cases. Arch Surg *57*:227, 1948.

Potts WJ, Holinger PH, Rosenblum AH: Anomalous left pulmonary artery causing obstruction to right main bronchus: report of a case. JAMA *155*:1409, 1954.

Robotin MC, et al: Unusual forms of tracheobronchial compression in infants with congenital heart disease. J Thorac Cardiovasc Surg *112*:415, 1996.

Sade RM, et al: Pulmonary artery sling. J Thorac Cardiovasc Surg *69*:333, 1975.

Stark J, et al: The diagnosis of airway obstruction in children. J Pediatr Surg *20*:113, 1985.

Tsang V, et al: Slide tracheoplasty for congenital funnel-shaped tracheal stenosis. Ann Thorac Surg *48*:632, 1989.

Turner W: On irregularities of the pulmonary artery, arch of the aorta and the primary branches of the arch with an attempt to illustrate their mode of origin by a reference to development. Br Foreign Med Chir Rev *30*:173, 1962.

van Son JAM, et al: Anatomic support of surgical approach of anomalous right subclavian artery through a right thoracotomy. J Thorac Cardiovasc Surg *99*:1115, 1990.

Watanabe M, et al: Left aortic arch with right descending aorta and right ligamentum arteriosum associated with d-TGA and large VSD: surgical treatment of a rare form of vascular ring. J Pediatr Surg *30*:1363, 1995.

Whitman G, Stephenson LW, Weinberg P: Vascular ring: left cervical aortic arch, right descending aorta, and right ligamentum arteriosum. J Thorac Cardiovasc Surg *83*:311, 1982.

SECTION XIV

Congenital, Structural, and Inflammatory Diseases of the Lung

CHAPTER 79

Congenital Lesions of the Lung

Marleta Reynolds

Most congenital lesions of the lung are recognized when respiratory symptoms develop in the newborn or infant. Some are identified in the asymptomatic child on an incidental radiograph of the chest. The remainder are diagnosed in the older child during evaluation for a respiratory infection. In an infant with severe respiratory distress, knowledge of the pathology and the ability to make a quick and accurate diagnosis based on a radiograph of the chest may be critical. In the past, arteriography and bronchography were the additional diagnostic studies of choice when time permitted, but now ultrasound and computed tomography (CT) allow greater diagnostic accuracy.

TRACHEAL AGENESIS AND ATRESIA

Tracheal agenesis or atresia leads to respiratory distress at birth and is usually fatal. Floyd and colleagues (1962) categorized the anomalies into three subtypes. Type I (10%) includes partial atresia of the trachea with a normal short segment of distal trachea arising from the anterior esophageal wall. Type II (59%) is complete tracheal agenesis with normal bronchi, bifurcation, and carina, with the carina connecting to the esophagus. Type III (31%) is complete agenesis of the trachea, with the bronchi arising from the esophagus. Affected babies may be premature, and maternal polyhydramnios is often associated. At birth, the babies turn blue and do not have an audible cry. An endotracheal tube cannot pass beyond the vocal cords, but esophageal intubation may temporarily improve ventilation. Associated anomalies are present in 84% and include other bronchopulmonary malformations, cardiac defects, vertebral anomalies, and gastrointestinal anomalies, as reported by Manschot and associates (1994). Although Kerschner and Klotch (1997) reported no long-term survivors from attempts at reconstruction, Hiyama and colleagues (1994) described a baby with tracheal atresia who was successfully managed with multiple surgical procedures. The first procedure for the type II lesion included banding of the distal

esophagus and gastrostomy. An endotracheal tube was then passed into the esophagus to just above the bronchoesophageal fistula. After 9 months of mechanical ventilation and gastrostomy feedings, a tracheostomy was created into the upper trachea. The esophagus was disconnected from the trachea and later reconstructed with a colon interposition. At the time of the report, the child was 4 years old.

BRONCHIAL ANOMALIES

Abnormal bronchial development may result in complete bronchial atresia, an aberrant origin of a main stem or segmental bronchus from the trachea, or the abnormal communication of the bronchus with another foregut derivative. Structural abnormalities of a bronchus may lead to lobar emphysema (Fig. 79-1).

Tracheal Bronchus and Diverticulum

A tracheal diverticulum may arise from the cervical or thoracic portion of the trachea and end blindly or in a rudimentary lung. The diverticulum resembles a bronchus. If the bronchial structure connects to a normal segment or lobe of lung, it is referred to as a *tracheal bronchus*. The accessory lung has normal pulmonary arterial and venous supply. Symptoms may result from stenosis of the tracheal bronchus or from other associated pulmonary anomalies. A radiograph of the chest obtained because of recurrent pneumonia, stridor, or newborn respiratory distress reveals the portion of lung involved (Fig. 79-2). At bronchoscopy, the tracheal bronchus can be seen, and an assessment of the entire tracheobronchial tree should be performed. Conventional CT and high-resolution CT can be used to demonstrate a tracheal bronchus. Wong and colleagues (1998) recommend serial coronal CT scans to better demonstrate a tracheal bronchus. Bronchography is seldom needed. Surgical resection of the tracheal bronchus and adjoining lung tissue is necessary only

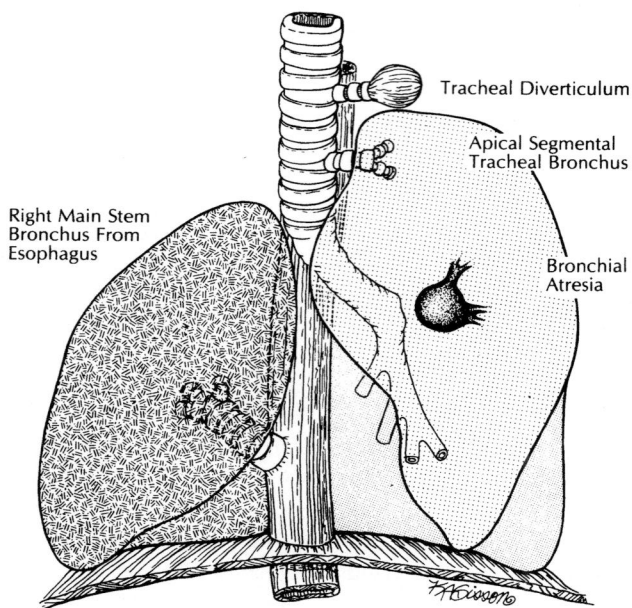

Fig. 79-1. Bronchial anomalies resulting from abnormal bronchial development. Symptoms result from bronchial obstruction and pulmonary infection. From Luck SR, et al: Congenital bronchopulmonary malformations. Curr Probl Surg 23:251, 1986. With permission.

when it is clinically indicated (Fig. 79-3). McLaughlin and colleagues (1985) recorded 18 children with tracheal bronchi who presented with recurrent pneumonia and other respiratory symptoms. Bronchography revealed bronchial stenosis and bronchiectasis of the involved lung segment in five of the children. Their symptoms were relieved by surgical resection. Vevecka and colleagues (1995) reported a 1-year-old

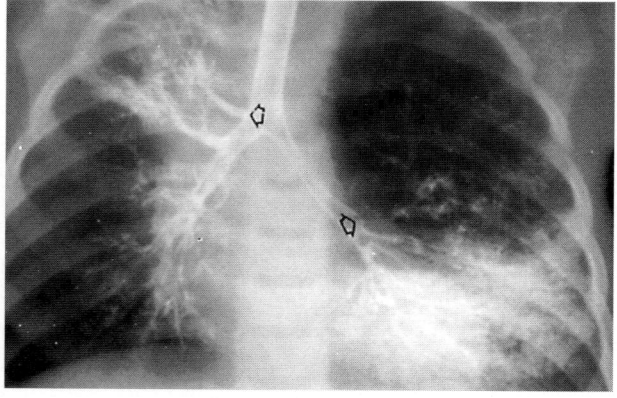

Fig. 79-2. Incidental tracheal bronchus. The patient, a 3 year old with a history of wheezing, also had an obstructed left upper lobe apical bronchus and emphysema of the left upper lobe. Left upper lobectomy was curative. From Congenital malformations of the lung. In Raffensperger JG (ed): Swenson's Pediatric Surgery, 4th Ed. Norwalk, CT: Appleton-Century-Crofts, 1980, p. 700. With permission.

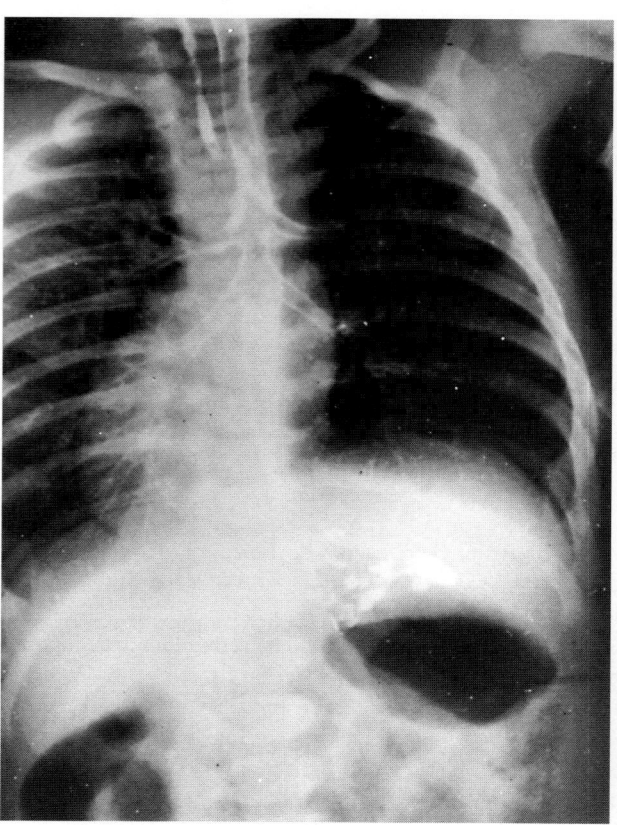

Fig. 79-3. Bilateral tracheal bronchi in a child being evaluated for chronic cough. Conservative treatment was recommended. From Holinger PH: Abnormalities of the larynx and tracheobronchial tree. In Swenson O (ed): Swenson's Pediatric Surgery, 3rd Ed. Norwalk, CT: Appleton-Century-Crofts, 1969, p. 297. With permission.

child who was found to have a cystic adenomatoid malformation connecting to a tracheal bronchus.

Bronchial Atresia

An atretic bronchus ends blindly in lung tissue. At birth, the portion of lung adjacent to the atretic bronchus is filled with fluid. The fluid is soon reabsorbed and replaced by air from the adjacent lung tissue through the pores of Kohn. Eventually, retained secretions result in a mucocele. Compression of adjacent normal bronchial structures leads to emphysematous change in the lung. Symptoms of wheezing and stridor may develop, and there is significant risk of pulmonary infection. A radiograph of the chest shows a hilar mass with radiating solid channels surrounded by hyperaerated lung. CT can differentiate the centrally placed cystic mucocele characteristic of bronchial atresia from a bronchogenic cyst or lobar emphysema. Resection is indicated to prevent pulmonary sepsis. For 9 years, Haller and colleagues (1980) observed a child with mild symptoms who had bronchial atresia and associated lobar emphysema. Progressive respiratory symptoms eventually prompted resection of the involved segment. The report documents the natural history of the lesion and further supports timely resection. Kuhn and Kuhn (1992) described the fourth reported case of an infant with bronchial atresia and bronchogenic cyst. Van Klaveren and associates (1992) reported two patients with bronchial atresia and pectus excavatum. Resection is indicated to prevent pulmonary sepsis.

Anomalous Bronchi

The most common communication between the trachea or bronchus and another foregut derivative is a tracheoesophageal fistula. Other anomalous connections are rare. Since 1950, Gans and Potts (1951) and Nikaido and Swenson (1971) have reported three infants from my institution who had an esophageal bronchus. All presented with respiratory distress and pneumonia and were found by esophagram to have a portion of lung communicating with the esophagus through a bronchial structure.

The anomalous origin of a lobar or segmental bronchus from the esophagus ("esophageal bronchus") may be right- or left-sided and may involve the upper or lower lobes. The vascular supply to the involved lobe varies; some lobes have a normal pulmonary vascular pattern and others a systemic supply. Extralobar and intralobar sequestrations (identified by the anomalous blood supply and absence of bronchial communication) occasionally communicate with the esophagus or other foregut derivatives. Confusion over terminology has prompted some authors to refer to all these anomalies as *congenital bronchopulmonary foregut malformations*.

Persistent or recurrent pneumonia in an infant or child may be caused by bronchial communication with the esophagus. An esophagogram outlines the esophageal bronchus (Fig. 79-4). Resection of the chronically infected portion of the lung is indicated. Lallemand and associates (1996) reported three cases of esophageal bronchi. In two cases, the anomalous bronchus was the main stem bronchus. These

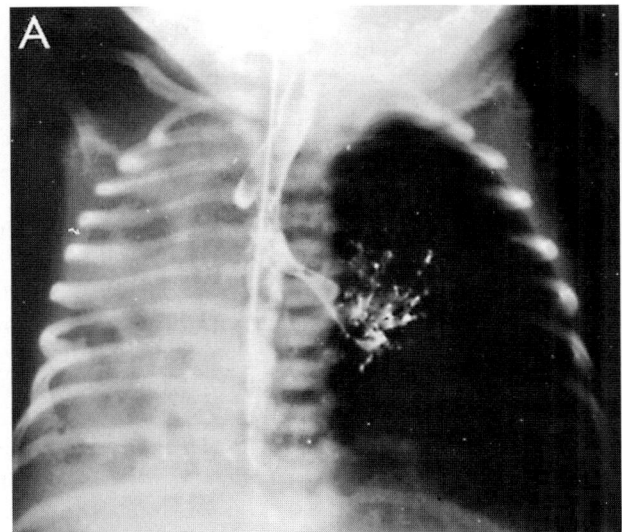
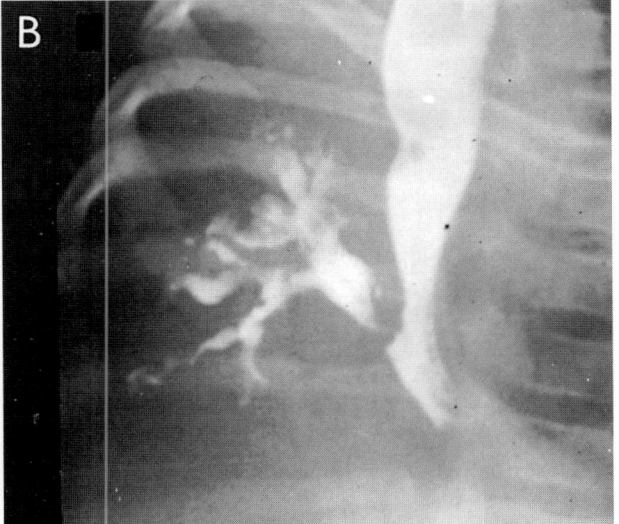
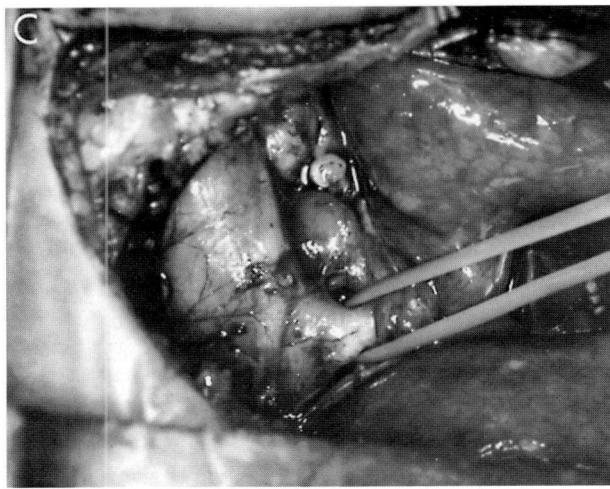

Fig. 79-4. A. Atretic right bronchus in a 1-month-old girl who presented with respiratory distress, cough, and fever. **B.** The esophagogram outlines the right bronchus and lung. **C.** At surgery, the right esophageal bronchus is identified. A right pneumonectomy was performed. She has had significant morbidity in the 4 years postoperatively. From Congenital malformations of the lung. *In* Raffensperger JG (ed): Swenson's Pediatric Surgery, 4th Ed. Norwalk, CT: Appleton-Century-Crofts, 1980, p. 700. With permission.

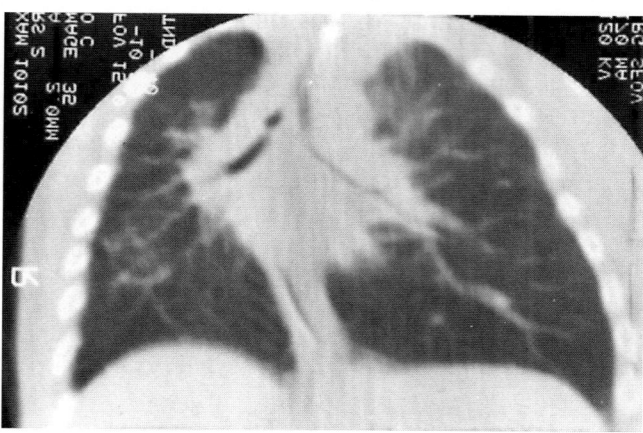

Fig. 79-5. Recurrent right upper lobe and entire right lung atelectasis in an infant with hyaline membrane disease who required prolonged intubation and ventilation. The right main stem bronchus was stenotic. Repeated dilations were palliative. This computed tomographic scan was obtained to clarify distal anatomy or identify other pathologic change. Note two areas of significant stenosis in the right main stem bronchus.

two patients were treated by implantation of the anomalous bronchus into the trachea.

Bronchial Stenosis

A true congenital bronchial stenosis is rare. Bronchial stenosis is seen most often in the right main stem bronchus secondary to inflammatory changes after improper and frequent suctioning of an infant on prolonged ventilatory support. Granulation tissue builds up at the main stem orifice. The lung distal to the obstruction becomes chronically infected or emphysematous (Fig. 79-5). Repeated bronchial dilations may be necessary to restore normal lung function and treat the infection. Jaffe (1997) reported successful balloon dilation in four of six patients with congenital and acquired tracheal and bronchial stenosis. Bronchoplastic procedures may reduce the need for pulmonary resection when the chronic infection does not resolve after attempts at bronchial dilation.

Bronchobiliary Fistula

The most uncommon bronchopulmonary malformation is the bronchobiliary fistula. Only 17 cases have been reported. Affected infants present with mild or severe respiratory distress and may have bile-stained secretions. Recurrent pneumonias may prompt a chest radiograph. Bronchography has been the diagnostic test of choice. Egrari and associates (1996) used a hepatoiminodiacetic acid scan to demonstrate the anomaly in an affected infant. The fistula usually joins the right main stem bronchus near the carina. Division of the fistula is usually curative. Ferkol and colleagues (1994)

described an infant with bronchobiliary fistula. The biliary drainage of the left lobe liver was through the fistulous tract in this patient. Division of the fistula was followed several days later by resection of the fistulous tract and the abnormal left lobe of the liver because of biliary sepsis.

CONGENITAL LOBAR EMPHYSEMA

Congenital lobar emphysema refers to the isolated hyperinflation of a lobe in the absence of an extrinsic bronchial obstruction. The left upper lobe is involved most often, followed in incidence by involvement of the right middle lobe. Boland and colleagues (1956) found hypoplastic cartilage in the bronchus of two of seven patients with lobar emphysema. Lincoln and associates (1971) described hypoplastic or absent cartilage in 22 of 28 examples reviewed. A series collected by Scarpelli and Auld (1978) reported a 25% incidence of dysplasia of the bronchial cartilage. Stovin (1959) reported abnormal orientation and distribution of the bronchial cartilage in his series of patients.

A subset of lobar emphysema is the polyalveolar lobe, first described by Hislop and Reid (1970). In an infant with classic congenital lobar emphysema, they found an increase in the number of alveoli in the affected lobe. A subsequent report by Tapper and associates (1980) reevaluated a group of infants with congenital lobar emphysema and found that 6 of 16 had the abnormal characteristics of the polyalveolar lobe.

Lobar emphysema produces symptoms in infancy. Often, a history of tachypnea, retraction of the chest wall, and wheezing since birth exists. An upper respiratory infection may complicate the condition and precipitate severe respiratory distress. Most children with lobar emphysema present before 6 months of age. Some infants develop symptoms in the first few days of life and require urgent intervention. Physical examination reveals a shift of the trachea and mediastinum to the contralateral hemithorax. Breath sounds are decreased on the affected side, with associated hyperresonance. Radiographs of the chest show hyperaeration of the affected lobe with atelectasis of the adjacent lobes and a mediastinal shift (Fig. 79-6). Careful inspection of vascular markings reduces the risk of misdiagnosis of this lesion as a tension pneumothorax.

In a newborn with severe respiratory distress, a radiograph of the chest is the only preoperative study that is indicated. In an infant with mild to moderate respiratory distress, CT can establish the diagnosis of congenital lobar emphysema by showing the hyperlucent expanded lobe and stretched, attenuated vessels. The CT can also exclude extrinsic causes of lobar emphysema, such as vascular anomalies or a mediastinal mass. In selected patients, Markowitz and colleagues (1989) recommend a radionuclide ventilation-perfusion scan to confirm the absent function of the involved lobe. Stigers (1992) and Doull (1996) and their associates recommend bronchoscopy to exclude

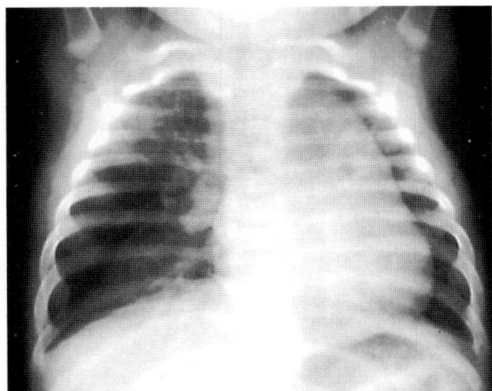

Fig. 79-6. Radiograph of a newborn with lobar emphysema involving the right middle lobe. Note the compressed right lower lobe and mediastinal shift.

intraluminal pathology and to assess the extent of bronchial collapse during ventilation.

Any infant with moderate to severe respiratory symptoms and a diagnosis of congenital lobar emphysema should be treated with lobectomy. Infants with mild symptoms may be carefully followed, although this management strategy is controversial. At operation, the chest is opened as soon as possible after induction of anesthesia. Positive-pressure ventilation causes further overinflation of the involved lobe and increases the risk of cardiovascular compromise. Gupta and associates (1998) recommend selective intubation of the contralateral lung with controlled ventilation in these infants. The abnormal lobe usually herniates through the thoracotomy incision. The lobe feels like sponge rubber, does not deflate, and bounces back into shape after it is compressed. Its edges are rounded and poorly defined. The remaining lung is atelectatic. Before resection, the mediastinum must be carefully examined for lesions that could have obstructed the bronchus. After lobectomy, the remaining lung expands to fill the chest. The emphysematous lobe characteristically does not deflate, even after it is removed from the chest.

Infants with hyaline membrane disease who require prolonged mechanical ventilation may develop acquired lobar emphysema (Fig. 79-7). The right lower lobe is most frequently affected. Suction trauma may cause squamous metaplasia of the bronchial orifice, and repeated barotrauma contributes to the ruptured alveoli and emphysematous changes. Radionuclide scans demonstrate poor perfusion of the affected lobe. Cooney and colleagues (1977) recommended lobectomy when the infant cannot be weaned from the ventilator because of the acquired emphysematous lobe.

In older infants with a history of respiratory problems, CT may help identify other causes of acquired lobar emphysema, such as extrinsic bronchial compression from enlarged lymph nodes, a bronchogenic cyst, or anomalous blood vessels. In an older child with an acute onset of symptoms, bronchoscopy is indicated to rule out an aspirated foreign body or

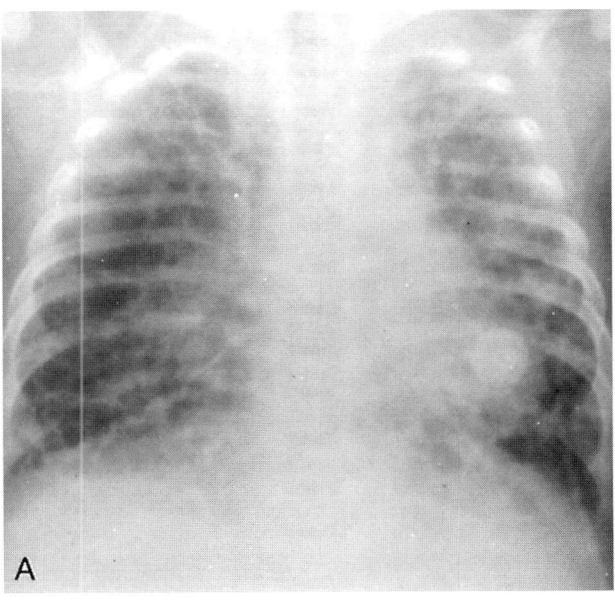

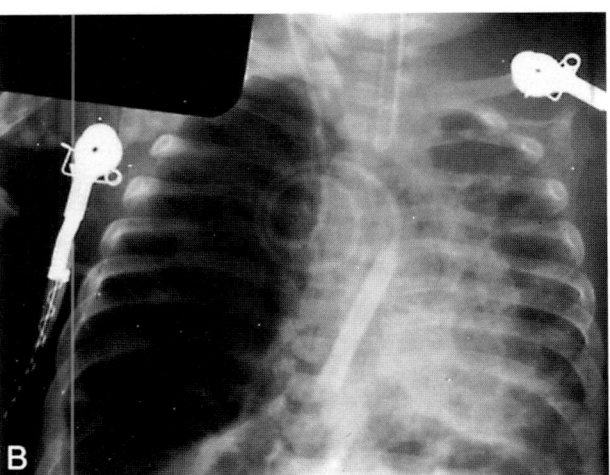

Fig. 79-7. A. Radiograph of the chest of a 2-month-old infant with bronchopulmonary dysplasia. **B.** Within 3 months, lobar emphysema developed in his right lower lobe. Further mediastinal shift and increasing ventilator requirements prompted lobectomy.

an endobronchial mass. The bronchoscopy should be planned to immediately precede thoracotomy. Oxygen, antibiotics, and humidity are administered prophylactically.

PULMONARY DYSPLASIA

Pulmonary Agenesis and Aplasia

Unilateral pulmonary agenesis results from lack of development of a single lung bud. Lung parenchyma and pulmonary vessels are lacking. Sbokos and McMillan (1977) reported a 50% incidence of associated cardiac disease, especially when the agenesis was on the right side.

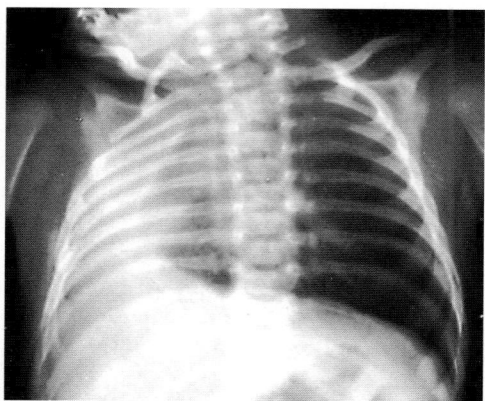

Fig. 79-8. Radiograph of the chest of a newborn with respiratory distress and agenesis of the right lung. Marked mediastinal shift to the ipsilateral side exists.

Say and associates (1980) noted that pulmonary agenesis may be associated with a chromosomal abnormality (46,XX,2p+).

A newborn with unilateral pulmonary agenesis may be asymptomatic or present with tachypnea, dyspnea, and cyanosis. Older infants or children may present with wheezing that suggests asthma or bronchitis. On physical examination, the trachea and mediastinal structures are shifted to the involved side. The overall shape of the chest is normal. Signs of airway obstruction and poor bronchial drainage may be recognizable. A radiograph of the chest reveals absence of lung markings and mediastinal shift to the ipsilateral side (Fig. 79-8). The differential diagnosis includes total lung atelectasis, total lung sequestration, or lung with an esophageal bronchus. The normal position of the diaphragm and normal intercostal spaces precludes atelectasis. An esophagogram and CT scan exclude the other possibilities. Echocardiography helps in diagnosing the associated cardiac lesions. No particular treatment exists for pulmonary agenesis, but correction of the cardiac anomaly may relieve some of the symptoms. Massumi and associates (1966) reported that 30% of infants with agenesis die in the first year of life, and 50% die within the first 5 years. The mortality was higher with right-sided agenesis. Maltz and Nadas (1968) reviewed the world literature and found 164 cases of pulmonary agenesis. Of the 36 patients reported by 1954, 24 were alive in 1968.

Bilateral pulmonary agenesis is incompatible with life, although Claireaux and Ferreira (1958) reported one infant who survived for 15 minutes. The trachea ends blindly or into primitive lung tissue. The incidence of associated anomalies is high.

Pulmonary aplasia is similar to pulmonary agenesis in that pulmonary parenchyma and vessels are absent. The blind bronchial stump may serve as a source of repeated infection in the normal contralateral lung. The stump may be identified by bronchoscopy or CT. Once recognized, the chronically infected stump should be resected (Fig. 79-9).

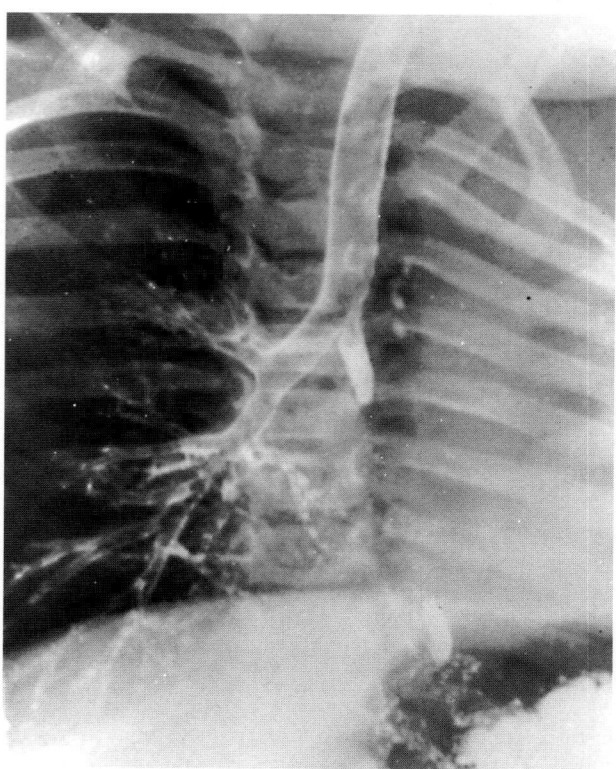

Fig. 79-9. The blind bronchial stump of pulmonary aplasia. Retained secretions in the stump led to recurrent pulmonary infections. In this setting, bronchography has been replaced by computed tomography and bronchoscopy. From Holinger PH: Abnormalities of the larynx and tracheobronchial tree. *In* Swenson O (ed): Swenson's Pediatric Surgery, 3rd Ed. Norwalk, CT: Appleton-Century-Crofts, 1969, p. 298. With permission.

Primary Pulmonary Hypoplasia

Pulmonary hypoplasia can be identified pathologically by the radial alveolar count and the ratio of lung weight to body weight. Pulmonary hypoplasia is primary if no obvious cause for the hypoplasia can be found. Swischuk and associates (1979) reported that four of eight infants with primary pulmonary hypoplasia had mean radial alveolar counts lower than normal and thickening of the pulmonary arteriolar wall. The hypertrophy of the muscular layer of the pulmonary arteriole develops in response to fetal stress. This hypertrophy is frequently found in infants with pulmonary hypoplasia and other causes of pulmonary hypertension. Haworth (1981) suggested that the normal postnatal regression of the pulmonary arteriolar muscle does not occur.

Primary pulmonary hypoplasia produces symptoms immediately after birth. An infant develops severe respiratory distress that is often unresponsive to supplemental oxygen. A radiograph of the chest demonstrates small lungs and the absence of other causes for respiratory distress. The thickened pulmonary arterioles predispose the infant to an exaggerated response to hypoxemia, acidosis, and hypercarbia. Therapy is aimed at lowering the pulmonary vascular resistance and preventing the inevitable persistent fetal circulation. Right-to-left shunting of blood occurs at three levels: across the patent foramen ovale, across the patent ductus arteriosus, and within the pulmonary capillary bed. Six of the eight infants reported by Swischuk and associates (1979) died despite aggressive management.

Secondary Pulmonary Hypoplasia

Secondary pulmonary hypoplasia is associated with various fetal and maternal abnormalities (Table 79-1). One of the most common is Potter's syndrome, in which bilateral renal agenesis results in oligohydramnios and compression of the developing fetus by the uterus. The fetus's face is distorted, and the chest is bell-shaped. Lung volume is small, with a decrease in the number of airway generations and alveoli (Fig. 79-10). The alveoli and pulmonary arterioles are smaller than normal. Other conditions that result in oligohydramnios (e.g., amniotic fluid leaks and renal dysplasias) are also associated with pulmonary hypoplasia.

Neurologic or musculoskeletal conditions that depress fetal respiratory movements are associated with hypoplastic

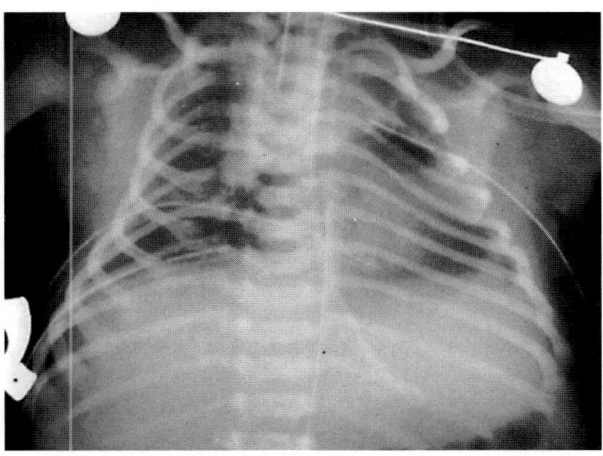

Fig. 79-10. Potter's syndrome with secondary pulmonary hypoplasia. The chest is bell shaped. Chest tubes were inserted to manage pneumothoraces resulting from barotrauma. From Luck SR, et al: Congenital bronchopulmonary malformations. Curr Probl Surg 23:251, 1986. With permission.

Table 79-1. Conditions Associated with Secondary Pulmonary Hypoplasia

Oligohydramnios
  Potter's syndrome (bilateral renal agenesis)
  Renal dysplasias
  Amniotic fluid leak
Bone dysplasias with a small or rigid chest wall
  Achondroplasia
  Chondrodystrophia fetalis calcificans
  Spondyloepiphyseal dysplasia
  Osteogenesis imperfecta
  Thanatophoric dwarfism
  Neonatal hypophosphatemia
Decreased fetal respiratory movements
  Congenital arthrogryposis multiplex congenita
  Camptodactyly and multiple ankylosis syndrome
  Congenital myotonic dystrophy
  Asphyxiating thoracic dystrophy
Diaphragmatic elevation
  Membranous diaphragm
  Abdominal mass or ascites
  Phrenic nerve agenesis
Intrathoracic space-occupying lesions
  Congenital diaphragmatic hernia
  Congenital cystic adenomatoid malformation
  Mediastinal neoplasms and cystic hygroma
  Enteric cysts (esophageal duplication)
Pulmonary vascular anomalies
  Pulmonary artery agenesis
  Scimitar syndrome
Miscellaneous
  Omphalocele
  Down syndrome
  Rhesus isoimmunization of the fetus

From Luck SR, et al: Congenital bronchopulmonary malformations. Curr Probl Surg 23:251, 1986.

lungs. Vilos and associates (1984) observed the fetus of a woman with myotonic dystrophy using ultrasound; the fetus had no respiratory movements, and the lungs were hypoplastic at birth. Wigglesworth and Desai (1979) reported that in experimental animals, the in utero transection of the spinal cord and the resulting inability of the animal to make respiratory movements result in significant pulmonary hypoplasia.

Infants who have congenital bony dysplasias may also have small and rigid chests and associated hypoplastic lungs; thanatophoric dwarfism is a good example. Most of these infants die from respiratory problems (Fig. 79-11). Jeune's syndrome, a familial chondrodystrophy, is also called *asphyxiating thoracic dystrophy*. These infants' chests are small and rigid and the lungs hypoplastic (Fig. 79-12). Futile attempts at chest reconstruction have been made, but survival has not been reported.

The developing lungs can also be affected by the abnormal development or function of the diaphragm. Phrenic nerve agenesis results in poor diaphragmatic muscle development and pulmonary hypoplasia. Infants with large abdominal masses or ascites have restricted lung development because of the elevation of the diaphragm. Hershenson and associates (1985) evaluated chest size in infants with giant omphaloceles and found them significantly decreased compared to controls. Many of the infants in their series had prolonged respiratory insufficiency, and autopsy study of one infant confirmed the presence of pulmonary hypoplasia.

The most common cause of secondary pulmonary hypoplasia is a congenital diaphragmatic hernia (see Chapter 50). The herniated viscera physically restrict lung growth on the ipsilateral side. In addition, shift of mediastinal structures results in contralateral pulmonary hypoplasia (Fig. 79-13). Kitagawa and associates (1971) reported that the lungs of infants with congenital diaphragmatic hernia had

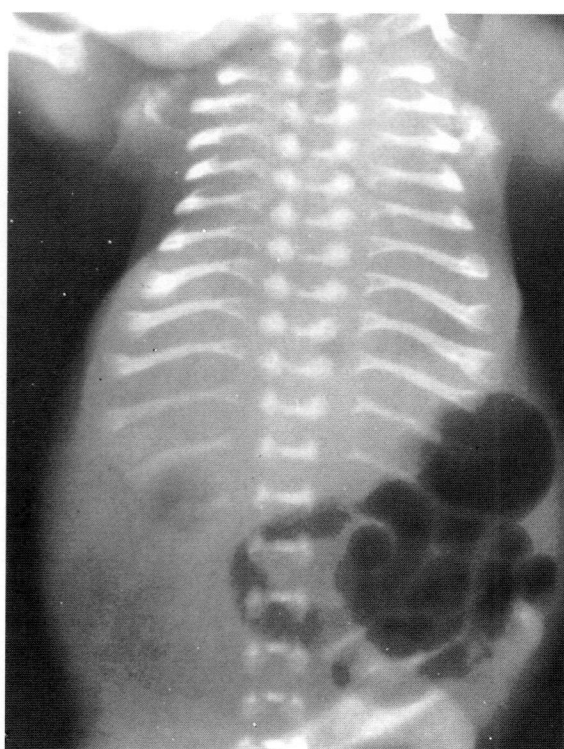

Fig. 79-11. Thanatophoric dwarf. Normal lung development is restricted by the size of the chest. From Luck SR, et al: Congenital bronchopulmonary malformations. Curr Probl Surg 23:251, 1986. With permission.

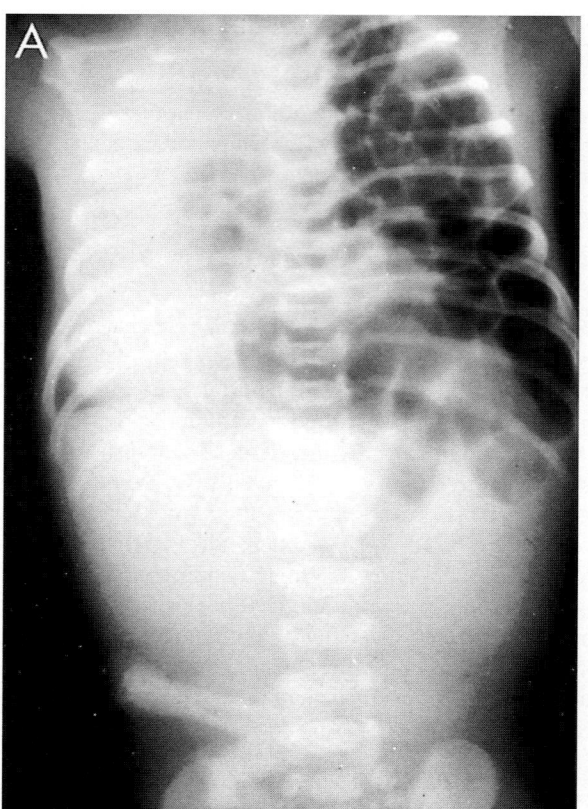

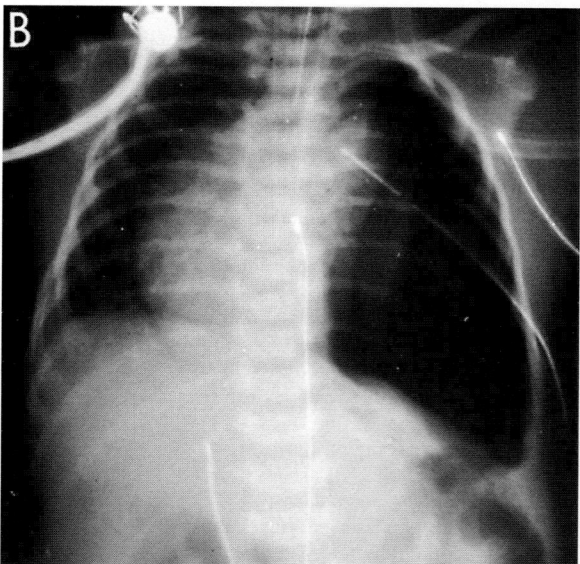

Fig. 79-13. Congenital diaphragmatic hernia. **A.** The left side of the chest is filled with intestines, and the mediastinum is shifted to the contralateral side. The abdomen lacks normal intestinal gas pattern. **B.** After surgical repair of the hernia, the severely hypoplastic ipsilateral lung is identified. The contralateral lung is also hypoplastic. From Luck SR, et al: Congenital bronchopulmonary malformations. Curr Probl Surg 23:251, 1986. With permission.

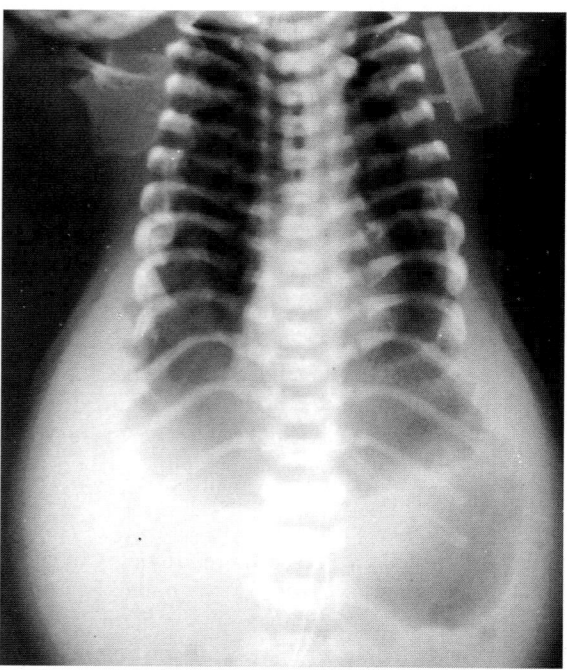

Fig. 79-12. Jeune's syndrome or asphyxiating thoracic dystrophy. The size and shape of the chest precludes normal lung development. From Luck SR, et al: Congenital bronchopulmonary malformations. Curr Probl Surg 23:251, 1986. With permission.

fewer airway generations, alveoli, and pulmonary arterioles than normal. Clinical correlation with the autopsy findings demonstrates that the most severe respiratory failure was present in infants in whom the muscularization of the pulmonary arterioles extended out from the preacinar arterioles into the interacinar arterioles. The high mortality rate associated with congenital diaphragmatic hernia is directly related to the pulmonary hypoplasia. High pulmonary vascular resistance and persistent fetal circulation are treated with high-frequency ventilation, 100% oxygen, sedation, alkalinization, and vasodilators. Extracorporeal membrane oxygenation has been used successfully to save 70% of infants with congenital diaphragmatic hernia who would otherwise have succumbed to respiratory failure.

Some cases of secondary pulmonary hypoplasia cannot be readily explained. For instance, Cooney and Thurlbeck (1982) reported that Down syndrome is associated with pulmonary hypoplasia. The autopsy study of seven children with Down syndrome revealed hypoplastic lungs in six, without evidence of congenital heart disease or other pulmonary anomalies. Chamberlain and colleagues (1977) found that infants with rhesus isoimmunization have associated pulmonary hypoplasia. Respiratory insufficiency is a frequent cause of death in these infants. The etiology and pathophysiology of the associated pulmonary hypoplasia are unknown.

SEQUESTRATION

Pulmonary sequestration describes a segment or lobe of lung tissue that has no bronchial communication with the normal tracheobronchial tree. The arterial blood supply is from a systemic vessel. The vessel often arises from the abdominal aorta, travels upward, and penetrates the diaphragm to supply the sequestration. The venous return is usually through the pulmonary veins but may be to the systemic venous system. An extralobar sequestration is separate from the normal lung and has its own visceral pleura. An intralobar sequestration is situated within normal lung parenchyma (Fig. 79-14).

A sequestration probably arises from a lung bud that is pinched off from the caudal foregut with its own blood supply. Boyden (1958) proposed this theory after reviewing data collected from embryos. Further study by Iwai and associates (1973) corroborated these findings.

Antenatal diagnosis of a sequestration can be made between 16 and 24 weeks' gestation by ultrasound. Sakala and associates (1994) reviewed the literature and reported a boy-girl ratio of 3:1. In one-half of the cases, mediastinal shift, polyhydramnios, and hydropic changes were found. All fetal deaths in this group of 11 cases occurred with hydropic changes. Four of the five survivors were noted to have regression of the lesions in utero, with resolution of the mediastinal shift. Sonographic differentiation of pulmonary sequestration and congenital cystic adenomatoid

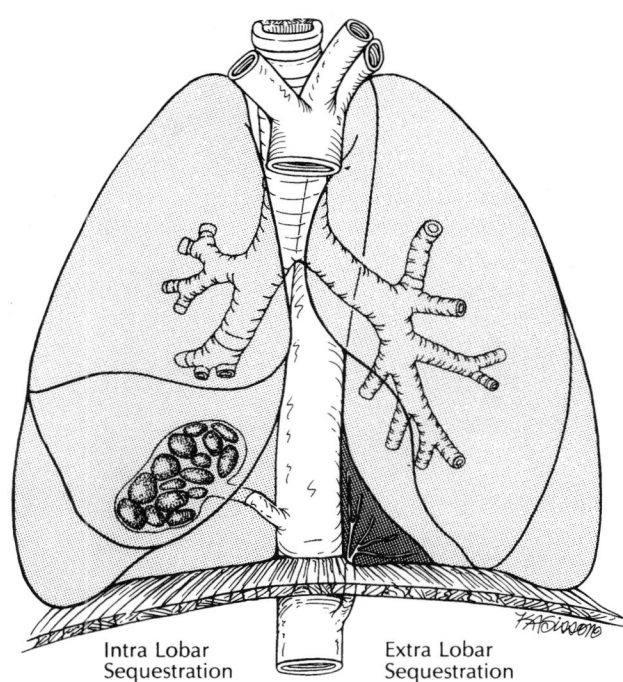

Fig. 79-14. Pulmonary sequestrations may be intralobar or extralobar. No bronchial communications exist, and the arterial supply to the segment or lobe is systemic. From Luck SR, et al: Congenital bronchopulmonary malformations. Curr Probl Surg 23:251, 1986. With permission.

malformation (CCAM) may be difficult. A sequestration appears as a solid, well-defined echogenic mass. Color flow Doppler ultrasound can be used to detect the systemic arterial supply. Careful follow-up of the fetus is warranted. Hubbard and Crombleholme (1998) and Becmeur and colleagues (1998) suggest that early delivery may be indicated if hydropic changes develop. Fetal intervention for drainage of polyhydramnios or thoracoamniotic shunting may also be considered.

Extralobar Sequestration

Twenty-five percent of sequestrations are extralobar. They are triangular, and they occur in the left chest 90% of the time. Usually found in the posterior costophrenic angle, they may also occur in the mediastinum or within or beneath the diaphragm in a periadrenal location. Some of the latter lesions may have a connection with the foregut. Diaphragmatic hernias are associated in 30%. Ultrasound and CT are useful screening examinations (Fig. 79-15). Color flow Doppler and magnetic resonance (MR) imaging are superior to CT in identifying the systemic arterial supply. Angiography is seldom necessary.

In most infants and children with extralobar sequestration, the lesion is found on an incidental radiograph of the chest. Repeated infections in the lesion may develop if a

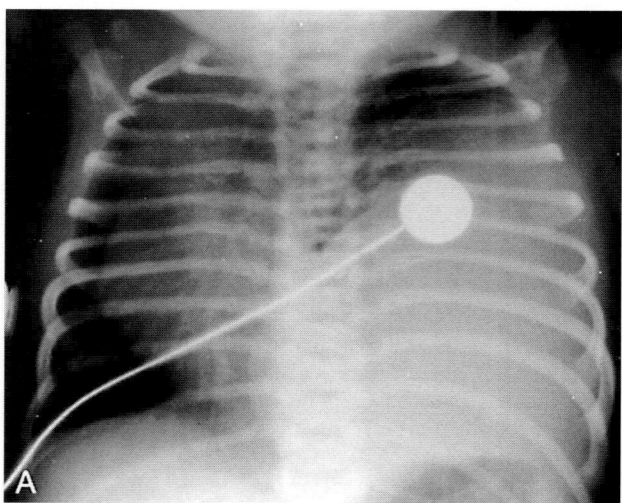

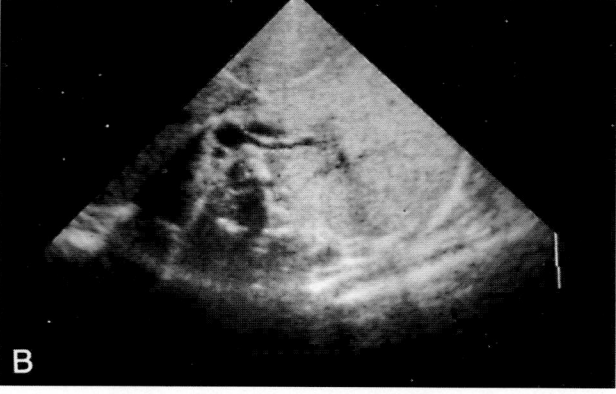

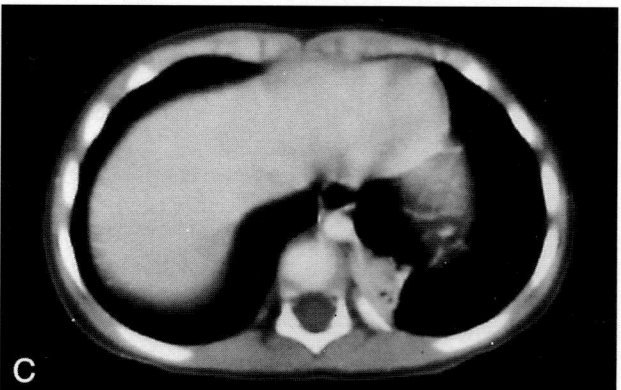

Fig. 79-15. A. Abnormal radiograph of the chest of a newborn with respiratory distress. **B.** Ultrasound identified the anomalous vessel coursing through the diaphragm and entering the sequestration. **C.** This computed tomographic scan clearly demonstrates the anomalous artery arising from the thoracic aorta and entering the sequestered lung.

communication with the foregut is present. Some are found and removed at the time of diaphragmatic hernia repair.

Intralobar Sequestration

Savic and associates (1979) reviewed a large series of sequestrations, and of 391 intralobar sequestrations, 164 were in the right lower lobe and 227 were in the left lower lobe. Only nine instances of sequestration occurred in the upper or middle lobes. In 96% of the sequestrations in this series, the venous return was to the pulmonary venous system.

Communication through the pores of Kohn may lead to chronic infection in the sequestered lobe. Children and young adults with recurrent left lower lobe pneumonia should be suspected of having an intralobar sequestration (Fig. 79-16). Infection can also lead to abscess formation and further cloud the diagnostic picture. In some children and adults, degenerative arteriosclerotic changes in the systemic artery supplying the sequestration may lead to hemoptysis. One of my patients presented with hemoptysis and an expanding lung mass. The systemic artery leading to the sequestration had become atherosclerotic and developed a false aneurysm within the sequestered lobe (Fig. 79-17). Rubin and colleagues (1994) reported fatal hemoptysis in a young adult diagnosed in infancy with an intralobar sequestration. An aneurysm of the anomalous

vessel had ruptured into the tracheobronchial tree. In the newborn, high flow through the systemic artery with normal pulmonary venous return may result in congestive heart failure.

Diagnosis in the newborn can be made with chest radiograph and color flow Doppler ultrasound. In the older child, CT can be diagnostic, although MR imaging can bet-

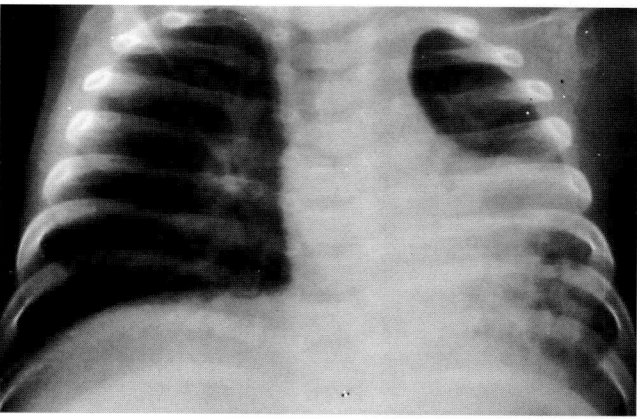

Fig. 79-16. A recurrent left lower pneumonia should suggest the possibility of an intralobar sequestration. From Luck SR, et al: Congenital bronchopulmonary malformations. Curr Probl Surg 23:251, 1986. With permission.

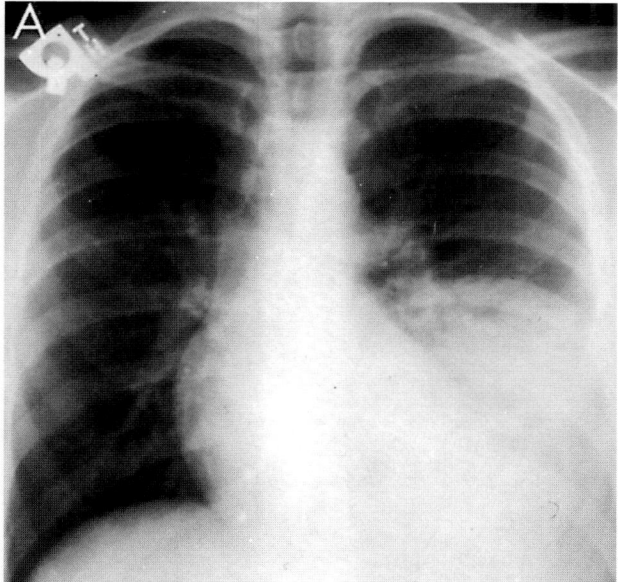

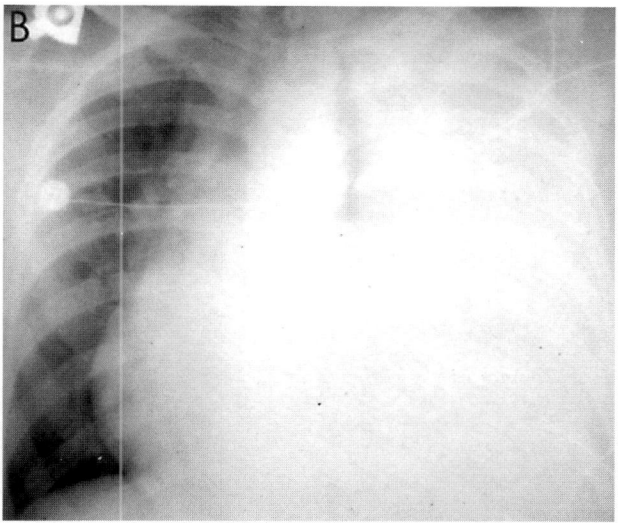

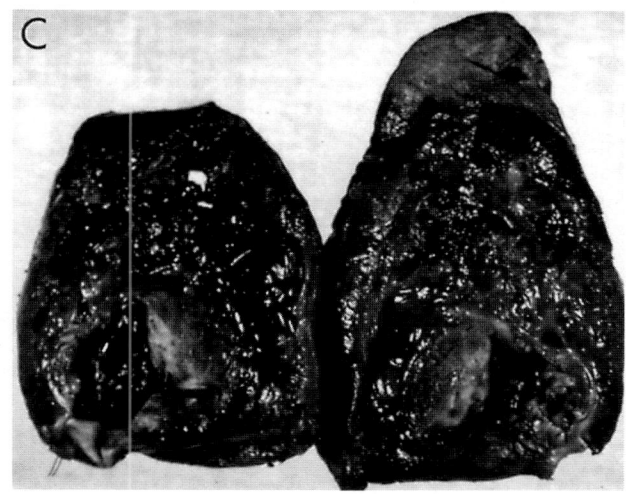

Fig. 79-17. A. This boy had had repeated right lower lobe pneumonia and presented at age 12 years with hemoptysis and a consolidated right lower lobe. **B.** Rupture of the sequestration produced a massive hemothorax and shock. Emergency left lower lobectomy was performed. **C.** The pathologic specimen reveals an aneurysm of the atherosclerotic vessel arising from the aorta. From Luck SR, et al: Congenital bronchopulmonary malformations. Curr Probl Surg *23*:251, 1986. With permission.

ter demonstrate the vascular supply. Angiogram is seldom indicated (Fig. 79-18).

Treatment consists of a segmental resection of the sequestration or, at times, a lobectomy, when inflammatory changes prevent resection of the sequestered segment alone. Careful identification of the arterial supply and suture ligation is necessary. Nuchtern and Harberg (1994) reported six patients with intralobar sequestration who all required lobectomy. There was no mortality and minimal morbidity in their group of patients. Harris and Lewis (1940) reported an attempted lobectomy in a 5 year old; it ended in exsanguinating hemorrhage when the systemic arterial supply was not recognized and was divided before control was obtained. The venous return must also be identified before resection. Thilenius (1983) and Alivizatos (1985) and their colleagues reported pulmonary infarction after inadvertent ligation of the total venous return of the right lung during resection of right lower lobe sequestration. Shermeta (personal communication, 1985) identified a similar anomaly and successfully reanastomosed the pulmonary veins of the upper and

middle lobe to the left atrium. Anomalous venous drainage of a single lobe or lobes of the right lung to the inferior vena cava below the diaphragm or to the right atrium is referred to as *scimitar syndrome*. This anomaly is discussed further in Chapter 81.

PARENCHYMAL PULMONARY LESIONS

Congenital parenchymal pulmonary lesions include isolated cystic lesions or diffuse cystic disease. Primary lymphangiectasia usually presents as diffuse cystic disease in infancy and is fatal. Other diffuse cystic disease is associated with various syndromes or diseases (e.g., Marfan's syndrome, interstitial fibrosis, histiocytosis, and Ehlers-Danlos syndrome). Surgical therapy is not indicated.

An isolated cystic lesion may be congenital or acquired, and differentiation between the two may be difficult. Careful review of all chest radiographs made since birth helps to make the differentiation. CT is excellent for differentiating

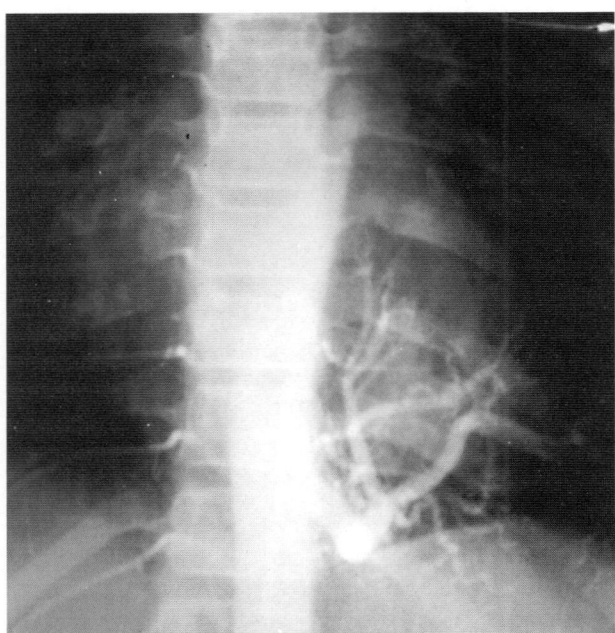

Fig. 79-18. This aortogram demonstrates the systemic arterial supply of an intralobar sequestration. Angiography is indicated if computed tomography does not accurately identify the lesion or if concomitant congenital heart disease is suspected. From Congenital malformations of the lung. *In* Raffensperger JG (ed): Swenson's Pediatric Surgery, 4th Ed. Norwalk, CT: Appleton-Century-Crofts, 1980, p. 703. With permission.

and identifying a bronchogenic cyst or CCAM from an isolated pulmonary cyst.

BRONCHOGENIC CYSTS

Bronchogenic cysts can be found in the hilum of the lung, mediastinum, posterior sulcus, and pulmonary parenchyma (Fig. 79-19), as well as in uncommon extrathoracic locations (see Chapter 187). The cysts are lined with ciliated columnar or cuboidal epithelium on a fibromuscular base. Squamous metaplasia may replace the epithelial lining, and when secondarily infected, the

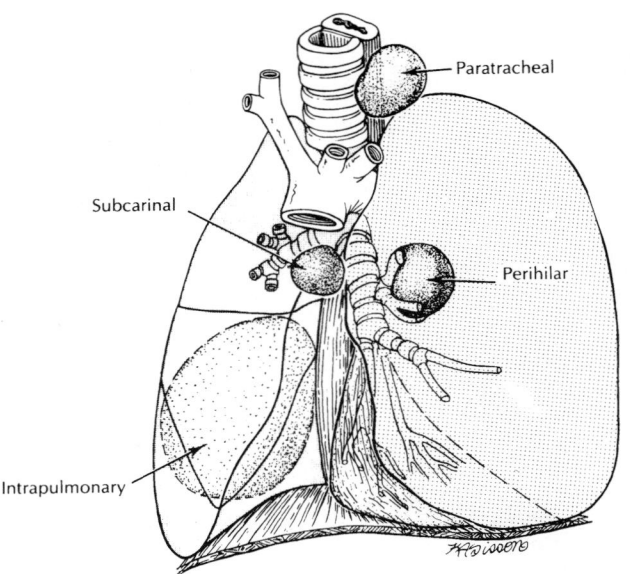

Fig. 79-19. Bronchogenic cysts are formed by abnormal budding of the respiratory tract and may be found in a variety of locations. From Luck SR, et al: Congenital bronchopulmonary malformations. Curr Probl Surg *23*:251, 1986. With permission.

epithelium may be destroyed. The cyst walls are thin and may contain cartilage and bronchial glands. The cysts are usually single but may be multilocular or multiple. The lower lobes have been reported as most commonly involved with parenchymal bronchogenic cysts. According to Ribet and colleagues (1996), however, of 21 cysts in infants and children, the right upper and left upper lobes were involved in seven cases each, the left lower lobe in six cases, and the right lower lobe in only one case. Parenchymal bronchogenic cysts frequently communicate with the tracheobronchial tree. Parenchymal cysts usually present with signs of pulmonary sepsis; however, approximately 20% of the infants and children are asymptomatic, according to Ribet and colleagues (1996). In four of their patients, the cyst was identified by antenatal ultrasonography.

An air-filled bronchogenic cyst on a chest radiograph is sharply defined and round (Fig. 79-20). The cyst can expand

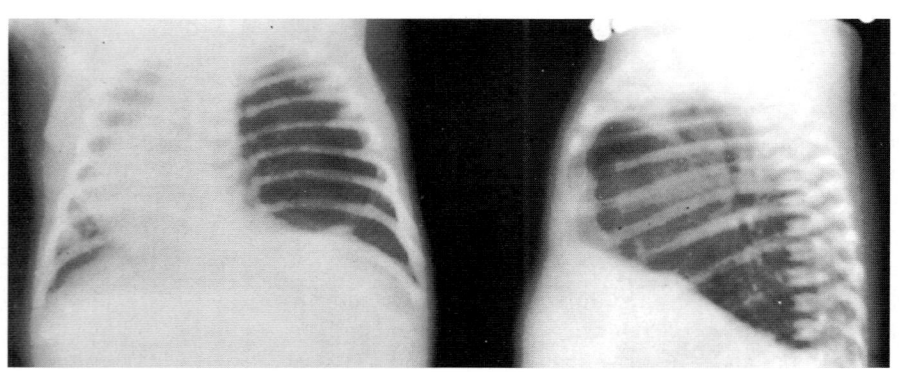

Fig. 79-20. Radiographs of the chest demonstrate a bronchogenic cyst of the left upper lobe.

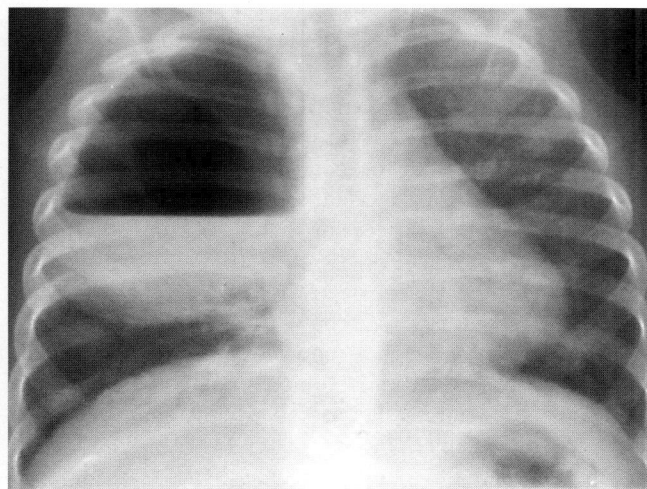

Fig. 79-21. An air-fluid level in an infected bronchogenic cyst is seen in this radiograph. This 10-month-old girl presented with a 4-day history of fever and cough. From Luck SR, et al: Congenital bronchopulmonary malformations. Curr Probl Surg *23*:251, 1986. With permission.

rapidly, and if it ruptures it may produce a tension pneumothorax. Needle aspiration may temporize, but prompt surgical resection is necessary.

A cystic lesion that communicates with the airways and contains secretions or pus has an air-fluid level on a decubitus or upright chest radiograph (Fig. 79-21). The infected cyst often has a surrounding pneumonia. Sometimes the infected cysts are difficult to differentiate from an empyema or solid pulmonary lesion (Fig. 79-22). A triangular shadow on the radiograph usually indicates an empyema. CT may differentiate a solid from a cystic lesion (Fig. 79-23). At times, a bronchogenic cyst has a high Hounsfield number on CT, which makes it difficult to differentiate the lesion from

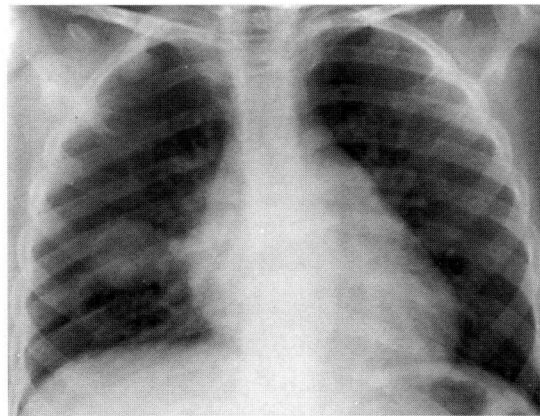

Fig. 79-22. This intrapulmonary bronchogenic cyst resembles a solid pulmonary lesion. This 4-year-old patient presented with hemoptysis. From Luck SR, et al: Congenital bronchopulmonary malformations. Curr Probl Surg *23*:251, 1986. With permission.

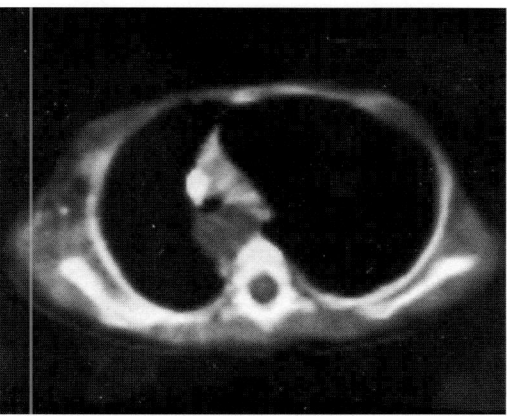

Fig. 79-23. Mediastinal bronchogenic cyst. From Snyder M, et al: Diagnostic dilemmas of mediastinal cysts. J Pediatr Surg *20*:812, 1985. With permission.

a solid mass. Nakata and associates (1993), in their study of eight mediastinal bronchogenic cysts, reported that in such instances MR imaging may help to establish the cystic nature of the lesion by the presence of relatively high signal intensities on the T_1-weighted images and very high signal intensities on T_2-weighted imaging.

Surgical resection is indicated for all bronchogenic cysts in infants and children. Parenchymal cysts require segmental or lobar resection. Morbidity and mortality should be near zero in these cases.

CONGENITAL CYSTIC ADENOMATOID MALFORMATION

A spectrum of cystic and solid lesions of the lung can be identified histologically as CCAMs. In all varieties, there is an overgrowth of terminal bronchiolar-type tubular structures and a lack of mature alveoli (Fig. 79-24). Luck and associates (1986) summarized the histologic appearance of CCAMs as follows:

1) An adenomatoid increase of terminal respiratory bronchiolelike structures lined by ciliated columnar epithelium occurs. Interspersed cysts may resemble immature alveoli. Connective tissue stroma contains disorganized elastic tissue and smooth muscle.
2) The mucosa of cysts lined with bronchial-type epithelium may show polypoid overgrowth projecting into the lumen of the cysts.
3) Bronchial mucoserous glands and cartilaginous plates are absent throughout the cystic parenchyma.
4) Occasional groups of alveolar cysts may be lined with mucus-secreting cells that resemble intestinal mucosa and do not resemble normal bronchial cells.

Stocker and associates (1977) and Bale (1979) outlined the classification of these lesions based on the clinical

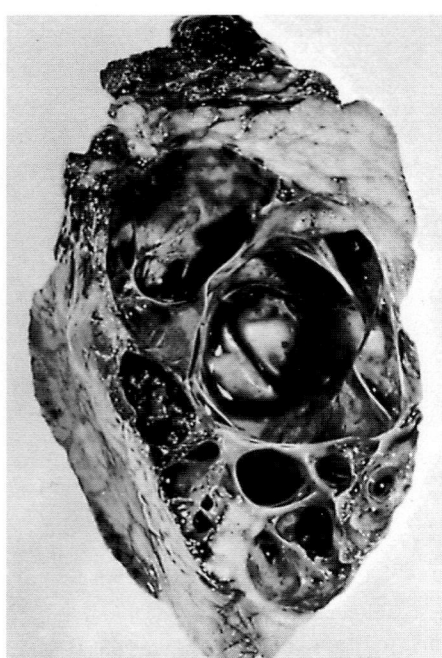

Fig. 79-24. Specimen removed from an infant with cystic adenomatoid malformation. Microscopically, there was marked proliferation of terminal bronchioles, and cartilage was lacking.

presentation and pathologic picture (Table 79-2). A predominantly solid lung mass is usually found in the stillborn or premature infant and is associated with fetal anasarca, ascites, and maternal polyhydramnios (Fig. 79-25). The combined solid-cystic lesion may produce respiratory distress in the near-term infant at birth. The primarily cystic lesion is usually found in the older infant, child, or adult because of an associated unresolving or recurrent pneumonia (Fig. 79-26).

Fetal ultrasound diagnosis of CCAM is being made with increasing frequency. Vergnes (1989) and McCullagh (1994) and their colleagues report that ultrasound is a sensitive method of identifying pulmonary pathology, but there are no specific features that can always distinguish CCAM from other congenital thoracic pathology. Prognosis and survival depend on the presence of hydrops, degree of hypoplasia of the remaining lung, histologic subtype, and timely diagnosis. Spontaneous resolution of this lesion has been reported by Mashiach and associates (1993), as well as others. Adzick and Harrison (1993) devised a useful algorithm for managing the fetus with a suspected CCAM. If or when hydrops develops, consideration for fetal intervention in the form of resection of the CCAM or shunting for hydrothorax may be beneficial.

Table 79-2. Classification of Congenital Cystic Adenomatoid Malformations

Bale[a]—Clinical Presentation	Cystic Lesion[b]	Intermediate Lesion[b]	Solid (Adenomatoid) Lesion[b]
Age	Term newborn or older	Infant	Stillborn or premature
Fetal anasarca or ascites	—	—	—
Maternal polyhydramnios	None	±	Occasional
Other anomalies	Rare	Rare	Common
Gross appearance	Cystic; sometimes solid areas	Either or both	Solid; sometimes cystic areas
Histopathology			
Bronchiolar proliferation	+	Varying degrees	+++
Alveolar appearance	Mature; separating bronchiole-type cysts	—	Immature
Mucoid epithelium or cartilage	Occasional	Occasional	Common
Prognosis	Good	Good	Poor

Stocker[c]—Clinical Presentation	Type I Lesion	Type II Lesion	Type III Lesion
Age	Term, occasional stillborn	Stillborn or premature	
Fetal anasarca or maternal polyhydramnios	Rare	Common	Common
Other anomalies	Rare	Common	Never reported
Gross appearance	Single or multiple large cysts; 2-cm diameter	Multiple, evenly spaced cysts; 1-cm diameter	Large mass, no or tiny cysts
Histopathology			
Bronchiolar proliferation	+	++	+++
Mucoid epithelium or cartilage	Mucoid cells in one-third of cases; rare cartilage; prominent bands of smooth muscle and elastic tissue	None	None
Cyst wall	—	Striated muscle in 5 of 16 cases	—
Prognosis	Good	Poor	Poor

[a]Based on 21 cases with only nine neonates; four autopsies.
[b]+ to +++ indicates increasing proportion.
[c]Based on 38 stillborn or newborn cases; 26 autopsies.
From Luck SR, et al: Congenital bronchopulmonary malformations. Curr Probl Surg 23:251, 1986. With permission.

Surgical resection is indicated to treat the presenting symptoms. The newborn with a large CCAM presents with severe respiratory distress secondary to the space-occupying mass, the compression of the contralateral lung, and the inadequate volume of functioning lung tissue at the time of presentation. The contralateral lung may also be hypoplastic. Emergency thoracotomy and lobectomy is often life saving. In the older child or adult, surgical resection is required to remove the source of recurrent pneumonia. Granata and colleagues (1998) have updated the literature pertaining to the development of malignancy in CCAM and have suggested that resection in infancy is advisable. Luck and associates (1986) summarized the reports of malignant tumors in 10 children with cystic lung disease and advocated lobectomy for the treatment of all CCAMs, symptomatic or not.

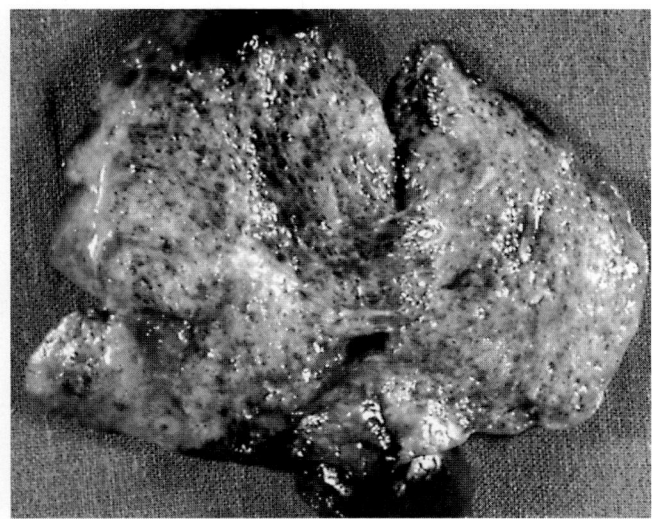

Fig. 79-25. This solid type of cystic adenomatoid malformation was found at autopsy in an infant who died shortly after birth. From Luck SR, et al: Congenital bronchopulmonary malformations. Curr Probl Surg *23*:251, 1986. With permission.

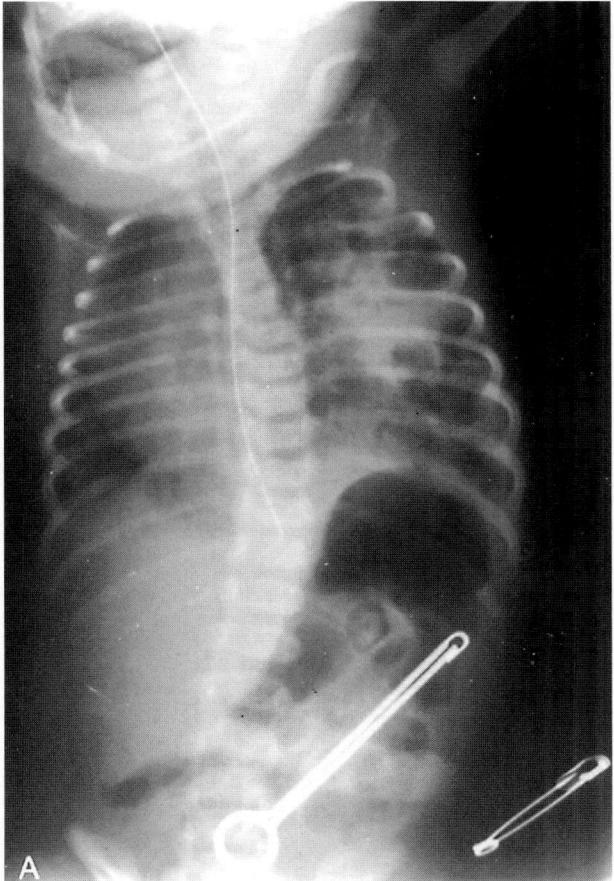

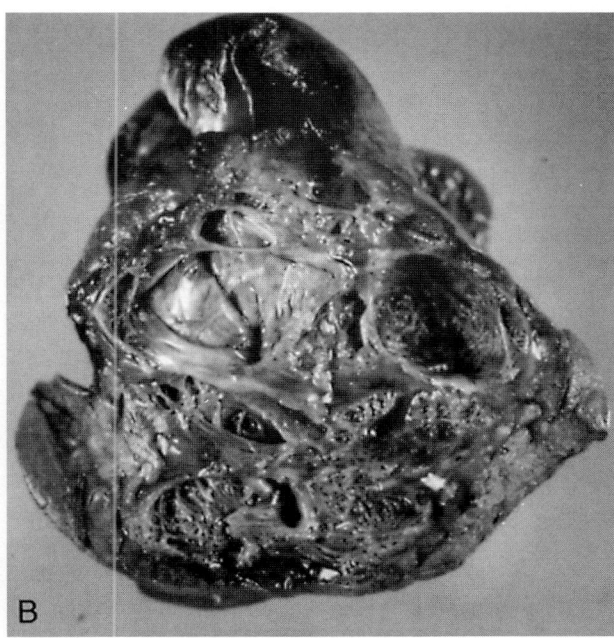

Fig. 79-26. A. This "babygram" demonstrates what appears to be multiple air-filled spaces in the left chest. The normal appearance of the gas in the abdomen suggests a cystic adenomatoid malformation in the chest rather than a congenital diaphragmatic hernia. **B.** A left upper lobectomy was performed. The specimen reveals both solid and cystic elements of the malformation. From Luck SR, et al: Congenital bronchopulmonary malformations. Curr Probl Surg *23*:251, 1986. With permission.

REFERENCES

Adzick NS, Harrison MR: Management of the fetus with a cystic adenomatoid malformation. World J Surg 17:342, 1993.

Alivizatos P, et al: Pulmonary sequestration complicated by anomalies of pulmonary venous return. J Pediatr Surg 20:76, 1985.

Bale RM: Congenital cystic malformation of the lung. A form of congenital bronchiolar ("adenomatoid") malformation. Am J Clin Pathol 71:411, 1979.

Becmeur F, et al: Pulmonary sequestrations: prenatal ultrasound diagnosis, treatment and outcome. J Pediatr Surg 33:492, 1998.

Boland RB, Schneider AF, Boggs J: Infantile lobar emphysema. Arch Pathol 61:289, 1956.

Boyden EA: Bronchogenic cysts and the theory of intralobar sequestration; new embryonic data. J Thorac Cardiovasc Surg 33:604, 1958.

Chamberlain D, et al: Pulmonary hypoplasia in babies with severe rhesus isoimmunisation: a quantitative study. J Pathol 122:43, 1977.

Claireaux A, Ferreira HP: Bilateral pulmonary agenesis. Arch Dis Child 33:364, 1958.

Cooney DR, Menke JA, Allen JE: "Acquired" lobar emphysema: a complication of respiratory distress in premature infants. J Pediatr Surg 12:897, 1977.

Cooney TP, Thurlbeck WM: Pulmonary hypoplasia in Down's syndrome. N Engl J Med 307:1170, 1982.

Doull IJM, Connett GJ, Warner JO: Bronchoscopic appearances of congenital lobar emphysema. Pediatr Pulmonol 21:195, 1996.

Egrari S, et al: Congenital bronchobiliary fistula: diagnosis and postoperative surveillance with HIDA scan. J Pediatr Surg 31:785, 1996.

Ferkol T, et al: Sinopulmonary manifestations of congenital bronchobiliary fistula. Clin Pediatr 33:181, 1994.

Floyd J, Campbell DC, Dominy DE: Agenesis of the trachea. Am Rev Respir Dis 86:557, 1962.

Gans SL, Potts WJ: Anomalous lobe of lung arising from the esophagus. J Thorac Surg 21:313, 1951.

Granata C, et al: Bronchioloalveolar carcinoma arising in congenital cystic adenomatoid malformation in a child: a case report and review on malignancies originating in congenital cystic adenomatoid malformation. Pediatr Pulmonol 25:62, 1998.

Gupta R, et al: Management of congenital lobar emphysema with endobronchial intubation and controlled ventilation. Anesth Analg 86:71, 1998.

Haller JA Jr, et al: The natural history of bronchial atresia. Serial observations of a case from birth to operative correction. J Thorac Cardiovasc Surg 79:868, 1980.

Harris HA, Lewis I: Anomalies of the lungs with special reference to the danger of abnormal vessels in lobectomy. J Thorac Cardiovasc Surg 9:666, 1940.

Haworth SG: Normal structural and functional adaptation to extrauterine life. J Pediatr 98:915, 1981.

Hershenson MB, et al: Respiratory insufficiency in newborns with abdominal wall defects. J Pediatr Surg 20:348, 1985.

Hislop A, Reid L: New pathological findings in emphysema in childhood. 1. Polyalveolar lobe with emphysema. Thorax 25:682, 1970.

Hiyama E, et al: Surgical management of tracheal agenesis. J Thorac Cardiovasc Surg 108:830, 1994.

Hubbard AM, Crombleholme TM: Anomalies and malformations affecting the fetal/neonatal chest. Semin Roentgenol 33:117, 1998.

Iwai K, et al: Intralobar pulmonary sequestration, with special reference to developmental pathology. Am Rev Respir Dis 107:911, 1973.

Jaffe RB: Balloon dilation of congenital and acquired stenosis of the trachea and bronchi. Radiology 203:405, 1997.

Kerschner J, Klotch DW: Tracheal agenesis: a case report and review of the literature. Otolaryngol Head Neck Surg 116:123, 1997.

Kitagawa M, et al: Lung hypoplasia in congenital diaphragmatic hernia. A quantitative study of airway, artery, and alveolar development. Br J Surg 58:342, 1971.

Kuhn C, Kuhn JP: Coexistence of bronchial atresia and bronchogenic cyst: diagnostic criteria and embryologic considerations. Pediatr Radiol 22:568, 1992.

Lallemand D, Quignodon JF, Courtel JV: The anomalous origin of

bronchus from the esophagus: report of three cases. Pediatr Radiol 26:179, 1996.

Lincoln JCR, et al: Congenital lobar emphysema. Ann Surg 173:55, 1971.

Luck SR, Reynolds M, Raffensperger JG: Congenital bronchopulmonary malformations. Curr Probl Surg 23:245, 1986.

Maltz DL, Nadas AS: Agenesis of the lung: presentation of eight new cases and review of the literature. Pediatrics 42:175, 1968.

Manschot HJ, Van Den Anker JN, Tibboel D: Tracheal agenesis. Anaesthesia 49:788, 1994.

Markowitz RI, et al: Congenital lobar emphysema: the roles of CT and V/Q scan. Clin Pediatr 28:19, 1989.

Mashiach R, et al: Antenatal ultrasound diagnosis of congenital cystic adenomatoid malformation of the lung: spontaneous resolution in utero. J Clin Ultrasound 21:453, 1993.

Massumi R, Taleghani M, Ellis I: Cardiorespiratory studies in congenital absence of one lung. J Thorac Cardiovasc Surg 51:561, 1966.

McCullagh M, et al: Accuracy of prenatal diagnosis of congenital cystic adenomatoid malformation. Arch Dis Child 71:F111, 1994.

McLaughlin FJ et al: Tracheal bronchus: association with respiratory morbidity in children. J Pediatr 106:751, 1985.

Nakata H, et al: MRI of bronchogenic cysts. J Comput Assist Tomogr 17:267, 1993.

Nikaido H, Swenson O: The ectopic origin of the right main bronchus from the esophagus. A case of pneumonectomy in a neonate. J Thorac Cardiovasc Surg 62:151, 1971.

Nuchtern JG, Harberg FJ: Congenital lung cysts. Semin Pediatr Surg 3:233, 1994.

Ribet MF, Copin MC, Gosselin BH: Bronchogenic cysts of the lung. Ann Thorac Surg 61:1636, 1996.

Rubin EM, et al: Fatal massive hemoptysis secondary to intralobar sequestration. Chest 106:954, 1994.

Sakala EP, Perrott WS, Grube GL: Sonographic characteristics of antenatally diagnosed extralobar pulmonary sequestration and congenital cystic adenomatoid malformation. Obstet Gynecol Surv 49:647, 1994.

Savic B, et al: Lung sequestration: report of seven cases and review of 540 published cases. Thorax 34:96, 1979.

Say B, et al: Agenesis of the lung associated with a chromosome abnormality (46,XX,2p+). J Med Genet 17:477, 1980.

Sbokos CG, McMillan IK: Agenesis of the lung. Br J Dis Chest 71:183, 1977.

Scarpelli EA, Auld P: Pulmonary Disease of the Fetus, Newborn, and Child. Philadelphia: Lea & Febiger, 1978, p. 194.

Stigers K, Woodring JH, Kanga JF: The clinical and imaging spectrum of findings in patients with congenital lobar emphysema. Pediatr Pulmonol 14:160, 1992.

Stocker JT, Madewell JE, Drake RM: Congenital cystic adenomatoid malformation of the lung. Hum Pathol 8:155, 1977.

Stovin P: Congenital lobar emphysema. Thorax 14:254, 1959.

Swischuk LE, et al: Primary pulmonary hypoplasia and the neonate. J Pediatr 95:573, 1979.

Tapper D, et al: Polyalveolar lobe: anatomic and physiologic parameters and their relationship to congenital lobar emphysema. J Pediatr Surg 15:931, 1980.

Thilenius OG, et al: Spectrum of pulmonary sequestration: association with anomalous pulmonary venous drainage in infants. Pediatr Cardiol 4:97, 1983.

Van Klaveren RJ, et al: Congenital bronchial atresia with regional emphysema associated with pectus excavatum. Thorax 47:1082, 1992.

Vergnes P, et al: Antenatal diagnosis of lung malformations. Apropos of 9 case reports. Chir Pediatr 30:185, 1989.

Vevecka E, et al: Tracheal bronchus associated with congenital cystic adenomatoid malformation. Pediatr Pulmonol 20:413, 1995.

Vilos GA, et al: Absence or impaired response of fetal breathing to intravenous glucose is associated with pulmonary hypoplasia in congenital myotonic dystrophy. Am J Obstet Gynecol 148:558, 1984.

Wigglesworth JS, Desai R: Effect on lung growth of cervical cord section in the rabbit fetus. Early Hum Dev 3:51, 1979.

Wong KS, Wang CR, Hsieh KH: Demonstration of tracheal bronchus associated with tracheal stenosis using direct coronal computed tomography. Pediatr Pulmonol 25:133, 1998.

CHAPTER 80

Pulmonary Complications of Cystic Fibrosis

Susan R. Luck

Cystic fibrosis (CF) is an inherited disease of the epithelial tissues of exocrine glands. Ductal obstruction by thick secretions results in multiple organ dysfunction. CF is the most common lethal genetic disease in the white population and is most commonly found in persons of Northern European ancestry. This autosomal recessive disease has an estimated incidence in the white population of 1 in every 2000 live births; in blacks, the incidence is 1 in every 17,000 live births. CF is virtually unknown in Asian populations. Although the frequency is approximately equal in male and female children, women and girls in the United States reportedly die at younger ages, especially after the age of 16 years. Hudson and Phelan did not find this gender-related discrepancy in their 1987 review of a large CF population in Australia. Specially dedicated CF centers throughout the world have increased patient survival and promoted research into all aspects of diagnosis and treatment. FitzSimmons (1993) summarized the data on 18,000 patients from the United States submitted to the Cystic Fibrosis Foundation registry in 1990 and compared the results with registry reports dating to 1969. The proportion of adult patients increased from 8% in 1969 to 33% in 1990. In 1990, most patients were younger than 15 years, but 33% were 18 years or older; more than 7% were 31 years or older. From 1969 to 1990, the median age of survival doubled from 14 to 28 years. The median age of survival of male patients in 1990 was 30 years, compared with 25 years for female patients.

The epithelial tissues of CF patients are impermeable to the passage of chloride ions, which normally are transported through channels in the apical cell membranes. The chloride channels are part of a complex membrane protein [CF transmembrane regulator protein (CFTR)] that is encoded by the CF gene. The structure of CFTR was first described by Riordan (1989). Tizzano and Buchwald (1992, 1993) and Collins (1992) reviewed the subsequent research on the location and function of CFTR and mutant proteins. The CFTR structure includes two areas or domains that cross the cell membrane and serve as the channels. Binding of phosphorylating nucleotides, including adenosine monophosphate, to intra-cellular domains of the protein is essential for CFTR function. Using monoclonal antibodies against the CFTR molecule, Kartner and coworkers (1992) confirmed the distribution of CFTR in the epithelial cells of pancreatic ducts, reabsorptive ducts of sweat glands, intestinal crypts, and the submucosal glands of respiratory epithelia. Quinton (1990) reviewed the research that delineated the mechanism of chloride ion transport. The absence of chloride absorption in the sweat tubules results in the retention of excessive amounts of chloride ions as well as sodium ions and water in the sweat. In the respiratory epithelia, chloride secretion is deficient, and the epithelial cells absorb more sodium than normal. Water passively follows the chloride and sodium ions into the cells with dehydration of mucus secretions. Knowles and associates (1981) showed that the cellular concentration of chloride ions results in a more negative bioelectric potential difference across CF epithelia compared to normal tissues. The resting transepithelial elective potential is elevated in individuals with CF from the normal range of 25 to 30 mV to 55 to 90 mV. Some drugs, such as amiloride, selectively inhibit the sodium pump and thus may reduce the transepithelial potential to nearly 0 mV. The chloride flux response normally increased by β-antagonists, such as isoproterenol, is absent in individuals with CF.

CLINICAL MANIFESTATIONS AND DIAGNOSIS

The levels of sodium and chloride in the eccrine sweat of patients with CF are almost always elevated to three to six times normal, usually more than 60 to 80 mEq/L. This abnormality is present from birth and persists without any relationship to the severity of pancreatic or pulmonary disease. Hyponatremic collapse can occur after heat exposure and excessive sweating. Before 1989, the diagnosis of CF was confirmed by the demonstration of an elevated sweat chloride concentration in a patient with typical chronic pulmonary disease or pancreatic insufficiency, or both. Now, genetic testing can identify patients with unusual variants of the disease who may have normal sweat chloride levels. Strong and associates (1991) described two sisters who had progressive lung disease beginning in early adulthood and repeatedly normal sweat tests. They were homozygous for an unusual CF gene mutation.

The major clinical sequelae of CF and their approximate incidence are as follows:

- Pancreatic insufficiency with malabsorption of fat and fat-soluble vitamins (85%)
- Chronic pulmonary disease with bronchiolar obstruction and recurrent infection (eventually nearly 100%)
- Azoospermia resulting from atrophy of the wolffian duct structures with absence of the vas deferens
- Meconium ileus, or neonatal bowel obstruction from inspissated meconium (15%)

Related conditions include poor weight gain, delayed sexual maturation in boys, absent or delayed menarche in girls, pancreatitis and glucose intolerance, and rectal prolapse. Women experience reduced fertility, possibly related to thick cervical mucus. Intussusception and meconium ileus equivalent, recurrent abdominal pain, and bowel obstruction are seen in older children and adults with hard, impacted stool. Biliary tract abnormalities include an increased incidence of cholelithiasis (as high as 25%), focal biliary cirrhosis, and portal hypertension (symptomatic in 5 to 10%). Severe liver disease may be unsuspected. Stern and colleagues (1980) reported that 8 of 61 patients who died with cor pulmonale had asymptomatic biliary cirrhosis. Lanng and coworkers (1991) found a steady increase in the incidence of diabetes mellitus with advancing age. Diabetes occurred in 32% of adults older than 25 years, and another 23% had an abnormal glucose tolerance test. Finkelstein and colleagues (1988) reported diabetes mellitus in 7% of adults older than 20 years of age; the onset of this complication was associated with accelerated clinical deterioration. Reisman and coworkers (1990), however, found no significant difference between diabetic and nondiabetic patients of comparable pulmonary and nutritional status. Osteoporosis is regarded as a late symptomatic complication in adult patients with CF, although low bone densities and fractures may occur in children. Aris and associates (1998) were able to obtain a history of fractures during childhood in 52.8% of 70 patients with CF, and Henderson and Specter (1994) reported an incidence of 25.1% in 143 children; both rates are well above the expected rate. Rib and vertebral compression fractures are more common. Bone densities (g/cm^2) in both men and women with CF were found to be 35% and 26% lower, respectively, by Bachrach and colleagues (1994) than in normal persons. The mechanism of this occurrence is unknown, but Ott and Aitken (1998) note that the contributing factors to the lower bone densities in patients with severe pulmonary disease are malabsorption of vitamin D, calcium, and other nutrients; hypogonadism; inactivity; respiratory acidosis; and cytokines from chronic infection. Although severe problems are found in only a minority of

CF patients, severe osteoporosis with major kyphosis and vertebral fractures may contraindicate lung transplantation. Furthermore, as pointed out by Aris and coworkers (1996), any existing osteoporosis is made more severe after lung transplantation. Hypertrophic pulmonary osteoarthropathy and inappropriate antidiuretic hormone secretion may occur in CF, as in other types of chronic pulmonary disease. Although the initial description of CF by Anderson (1938) was that of a fatal disease of infancy, the symptoms may not be recognized or even manifested until the patient is an adolescent or adult.

Most CF patients develop chronic sinusitis. The maxillary and ethmoid sinuses are opacified in 90 to 100% of children older than age 8 months; the frontal sinuses rarely develop. Most patients present with symptoms of nasal obstruction and purulent rhinorrhea between 5 and 14 years of age. Treatment is with oral antibiotics and nasal steroids. Ramsey and Richardson (1992) estimate that 20% of CF patients require surgical treatment. Nasal polyposis is commonly associated, although these may resolve by late adolescence. Lewiston and colleagues (1991) suggested that all CF patients who are candidates for lung transplantation should have operative drainage of the maxillary sinuses, because they typically are contaminated with *Pseudomonas aeruginosa* and are a source of pulmonary infection. Zuckerman and Kotloff (1998) believe intensive medical therapy is better than invasive procedures.

In 1958, Shwachman and Kulczycki introduced a scoring system (S-K score) for children with CF that quantitates the severity of clinical disease and accurately predicts the results of pulmonary function testing. Doershuk and colleagues (1964) revised this widely used system to apply to all patients. Four separate criteria of clinical status are evaluated by a detailed history and physical examination. Each is assigned an equal value of 25 points, with 100 representing a perfect score. These criteria include 1) the activity level, as compromised by respiratory symptoms; 2) physical examination and an estimate of the effort required for breathing; 3) nutritional status, with consideration of deviation from ideal body weight; and 4) chest radiographic findings. A score of 55 or less indicates severe disease.

ADULT AND ADVANCED DISEASE

Several groups, including Shwachman and associates (1977), di Sant'Agnese and Davis (1979), as well as MacLusky (1985) and Penketh (1987) and their associates, detailed the progression and treatment of this disease in adults. Huang and colleagues (1987) found that a poor S-K score, low weight percentile, and *Burkholderia (Pseudomonas cepacia)* colonization all indicated a poor prognosis. Young adults with a clinical S-K score of 65 to 75 had a median survival of 12 additional years. Pinkerton and coworkers (1985) compared the coping patterns of 200 adults with CF to those of a similar group with chronic end-stage renal failure. Even the CF patients who appeared to cope well had a high incidence of depression, self-devaluation, and body image distortion. Shepherd and associates (1990) found that, compared to healthy peers, adults with CF were less likely to be employed, had fewer years of education, and were more likely to live with parents. Neither report found a correlation between the level of physical health or pulmonary function with the degree of patient autonomy or psychosocial problems.

Long-standing hypoxia and lung infection eventually result in pulmonary vasoconstriction and fibrosis, with a chronic increase in right ventricular afterload. The physical signs of right ventricular failure are overshadowed by those of extreme pulmonary disease. Weight loss is common even after the development of peripheral edema. Hepatomegaly and a murmur of tricuspid insufficiency develop. Ascites is rare. Most of the 60 patients with cor pulmonale reviewed by Stern and colleagues (1980) were completely disabled. Their mean survival after the diagnosis of this condition was 8 months; 80% had died by 12 months. These patients may benefit from salt restriction and diuretics, with supplemental oxygen at night. Moss (1982) outlined the diagnostic criteria for cor pulmonale in CF:

- An S-K clinical score of 40 or less
- Vital capacity less than 60% of predicted normal
- The inability to raise arterial Po_2 to 300 mm Hg after breathing 100% oxygen for 10 minutes

Because the hyperinflated lungs surround the heart, cardiomegaly and right ventricular hypertrophy are absent or underestimated on the chest radiograph and electrocardiogram. Lester and coworkers (1980) correlated the echocardiographic abnormalities with the progression of cardiac decompensation and with the S-K score.

Because lung transplantation has become a treatment option for selected patients, aggressive therapy may be offered to those previously considered preterminal. Mechanical ventilation preceded lung transplantation in 10 of 54 patients with CF reported by Massard and associates (1993); four of these patients survived. The waiting period for a donor organ may be prolonged, and in the series reported by Whitehead (1991) and Shennib (1992) and their colleagues, 20% or more accepted transplant candidates expired. The complex ethical considerations in balancing a rational acceptance of terminal disease and recommendation of aggressive treatment as a prelude to possible transplantation are well outlined by Fiel (1991) and Warner (1991). They describe a negative experience for both patients and families in many cases. Recommendations for palliative and supportive care or transplant referral should be made at a reasonable time before disabling disease intervenes. Kerem and associates (1992) studied nearly 700 patients followed over 10 years and assessed factors predictive of mortality of greater than 50% in 2 years. These were a forced expiratory volume in 1 second (FEV_1) of less than 30% of predicted value; an arterial Po_2 of less than 55 mm Hg; or an arterial Pco_2 greater than 50 mm Hg. When a patient has reached this level of disease, future treatment options should be discussed realistically.

GENETICS OF CYSTIC FIBROSIS

An explosion in research and knowledge about the genetics and molecular and cellular biology of CF has occurred since 1989. Rommens (1989), Riordan (1989), and Kerem (1989) and their associates isolated and cloned the CF gene; identified and characterized CFTR, the protein product of the gene; and pinpointed the DNA sequence of the defective gene involved with most cases. The normal gene is composed of 250,000 nucleotide base pairs and is located on the long arm of chromosome 7 (7q31.3). Tsui (1992) reviewed the nearly 300 different gene mutations that have been reported to the Cystic Fibrosis Genetic Analysis Consortium. One specific mutant allele (ΔF508) is found in 67% of patients. The deletion of three nucleotides from the midportion of the gene causes the deletion of a single phenylalanine at position 508 of the protein. An affected individual has two abnormal CF genes and may be homozygous or heterozygous for the ΔF508 allele or for a non-ΔF508 allele. Carriers of only one gene usually are asymptomatic; however, Davis and Vargo (1987), among others, documented increased airway reactivity and an increased incidence of wheezing in heterozygous parents of children with CF. Anguiano and associates (1992) investigated a group of 25 infertile men with bilateral absence of the vas deferens, none of whom had pulmonary symptoms. Thirteen were carriers for ΔF508 and three had a ΔF508/non-ΔF508 genotype. Seven other mutant alleles are fairly common. The ΔF508 allele and alleles whose DNA sequencing is known can be detected by specific DNA testing, thereby allowing accurate detection of carriers and of patients who have atypical or minimally symptomatic disease. Such identification is difficult if the alleles can be identified only by their relationship to known DNA markers and with comparison to the DNA of affected family members. ΔF508 allele is the most common CF gene found in white patients of Northern European descent, especially Danish, and is found less frequently in Southern European, black, and Ashkenazi Jewish patients.

Kerem (1990a) and Kristidis (1992) and their associates have shown that different alleles appear to influence the clinical severity of disease, particularly of the pancreas. Patients who are homozygous for ΔF508 tend to have severe classic CF, and almost all have pancreatic insufficiency. As many as 10% of the non-ΔF508 alleles, however, lead to a mild form of CF in which the patient has pancreatic function sufficient for normal digestion. These alleles appear to be dominant over ΔF508. No good correlation of genotype with the degree of lung disease or liver disease exists. Neither Kerem (1989) nor Santis (1990) and their colleagues could correlate pulmonary function testing with genotype unless the patients were subdivided according to pancreatic function. Gaskin (1982) and Corey (1988) and their colleagues have shown that individuals with pancreatic sufficiency tend to have better pulmonary function, perhaps on the basis of better nutrition.

The development of a "cure" for CF must involve the alteration of the mutant CFTR or the transfer of one normal CF gene into enough respiratory epithelial cells to overcome the basic cellular defect. Further delineation of the intracellular function of normal and mutant CFTR may accelerate since the protein has been purified and reconstituted in an in vitro system by Bear and colleagues (1992). New forms of treatment can be evaluated in the mouse models produced by Snouwaert (1992) and Dorin (1992) and their colleagues in which the CFTR protein has been inactivated. Because CF is a recessive disorder determined by a lack of gene function, adding one normal gene to the nuclei of the appropriate cells should convert the cell to a carrier state and allow normal function. Only 5% of normal gene expression should be necessary. The normal CF gene has been delivered directly into respiratory epithelial cells using adenovirus and retrovirus as vectors. First, DNA material that allows the virus to replicate within the infected cell is removed; then, the foreign gene for CFTR production is inserted into the viral genome. Large quantities of the replication-deficient recombinant virus can be produced in cell culture. Rosenfeld and coworkers (1992) showed that CFTR protein is expressed within the airway epithelial cells of rats for up to 6 weeks after infection with an adenovirus vector. The adenovirus can transfer the gene into differentiated tissues that are not undergoing frequent cell division, but the effect on the respiratory cells may last only several weeks. Drumm and colleagues (1990) used recombinant retroviruses to transform cells in vitro to express normal CFTR channel function. Although the effect of retrovirus gene transmission is expected to be long lasting, only cells undergoing mitosis can be infected and the retrovirus may activate oncogenes. Zeitlin (1998) has classified the basic defect of CFTR into five categories:

Class I: Complete absence of CFTR
Class II: Defective protein folding and trafficking
Class III: Defect in regulation of CFTR function

Class IV: Chloride channel conduction defect
Class V: Reduction in synthesis affecting CFTR promoter to reduce messenger RNA transcription

Examples of gene mutation, resulting defect, and possible general therapeutic modalities are listed in Table 80-1. Some of the specific treatment regimens are now being evaluated in phase I studies.

PATHOPHYSIOLOGY OF PULMONARY DISEASE

Pulmonary infection with *P. aeruginosa* is the most significant clinical component of CF. Kerem and colleagues (1990b) documented the variable but persistent decline in pulmonary function that occurs after *P. aeruginosa* colonization of the respiratory tract. Pier (1985), Thomassen and coworkers (1987), and Berger (1991) reviewed the properties of this organism and its unique interaction with the human host. *P. aeruginosa* adheres to damaged or abnormal mucosa through specific interactions between bacterial adhesions and the cell surfaces. The mucosa may be damaged by early childhood infection with viruses, *Staphylococcus aureus*, and *Haemophilus influenzae*. Prober (1991) documented the importance of viral infection in the exacerbation of bacterial infection and decline in pulmonary function. The abnormally viscid CF secretions impede mucociliary clearance of bacteria. Mucoid strains of *P. aeruginosa* predominate in CF infection. Noninvasive colonies of mucoid organisms are protected from the action of antibiotics, immunoglobulins, and neutrophils by an extracellular polysaccharide matrix called *alginate*. Complex interactions occur between the bacteria and the large numbers of antibodies, immunoglobulins, and neutrophils that are attracted to the site of infection. Both neutrophils and *P. aeruginosa* organisms release elastase and other proteolytic enzymes that are destructive to bronchial connective tissue. The deleterious effects of neutrophil elastase include stimulation of mucosecretory differentiation of respiratory epithelium with increased mucus secretion; destruction of structural fibers of the airway; inhibition of phagocytosis; and inactivation of antipseudomonal antibod-

Table 80-1. Organization of Cystic Fibrosis Transmembrane Conductance Regular Mutations According to Defect and Therapeutic Modality

Class of Mutation	Example of Mutation	Defect	General Therapeutic Modality	Specific Clinical Examples
I	W1282X	Unstable mRNA	Aminoglycoside read-through of early termination codon	Gentamicin
II	ΔF508	Trafficking block	Chemical or molecular chaperones	Phenylbutyrate, CPX, genistein, milrinone
III	G551D	Inoperative channel	Gene or protein replacement	Gene therapy
IV	R117H	Partial conduction defect	Conduction repair or augmentation	Genistein, milrinone
V	3840 + 10 kb C → T	Normal protein levels reduced	Increased level of mRNA and protein synthesis	Gene therapy

CPX, 8-cyclopentyl-1,3-dipropylxanthine; mRNA, messenger RNA.
From Zeitlin PL: Therapies directed at the basic defect in cystic fibrosis. Clin Chest Med 19:515, 1998. With permission.

ies. The concept of actual bronchial tissue destruction is supported by the laboratory and pathologic evidence assembled by Bruce and associates (1985). Uninhibited elastase activity is indicated by the increased urinary excretion of amino acid degradation products of elastin and by the presence of fragmented elastin fibers in the CF lung at autopsy. Chronic mucosal infection, excessive production of viscid secretions, and the progressive destruction of bronchial tissue are self-perpetuated in a vicious cycle as the inflammatory and hyperimmune response from the host continues unabated. Chemical evidence of this response is hypergammaglobulinemia, increased numbers of immune complexes in sputum and serum, and increase in circulating *P. aeruginosa* antibodies found in patients with progressively severe lung disease and clinical deterioration. Chest physiotherapy and postural drainage of secretions help reduce the load of inflammatory and proteolytic products. Antibiotic therapy can temporarily ameliorate infection but also undoubtedly helps select resistant and more virulent organisms. *Burkholderia cepacia* has arisen as a virulent pathogen in the CF population since the early 1980s. The biology and multiple drug resistance of this bacterium has been detailed by Goldmann and Klinger (1986). Lewin and colleagues (1990) reviewed the course of patients colonized with this organism at several CF centers. Earlier clinical deterioration and death occurred in those who also had moderate or advanced lung disease. However, a smaller percentage of CF patients are colonized with this organism than with *P. aeruginosa*.

The gross and histopathologic findings of the CF lung reflect the effects of the cellular defect and chronic infection. Esterly and Oppenheimer (1968) noted that the earliest histologic changes appear in the tracheobronchial submucosal glands, which become obstructed and dilatated. These glands are the main site within the airway for the expression of the CF cell protein. Thereafter, thick mucus obstructs bronchioles and bronchi in a scattered fashion throughout the lungs. Bacterial colonization and mucosal infection follow. Ciliated cells are destroyed as bronchial epithelium undergoes metaplasia; the submucosa is infiltrated by inflammatory cells, with submucosal abscess formation; and adjacent lymphoid tissue proliferates. The proteolytic destruction of bronchial tissue results in fibrosis with weakening of the integrity of bronchial walls and progressive bronchiectasis. Bedrossian and coworkers (1976) showed that the incidence of bronchiectasis rises steadily after 1 year of age. Tomashefski and colleagues (1986) analyzed and quantified these bronchiectatic changes. Airway volume, as opposed to parenchymal volume, increases with progressive disease. The airway volume in the CF patient is 10 to 20% of the total lung volume, as opposed to 4% in the normal individual. This increased proportion of bronchial volume and the occurrence of cystic lesions are seen primarily in the upper lobes. Zach (1990) speculates that this difference may reflect a decrease in the clearance of secretions and their proteolytic contents from the upper lobes,

perhaps because of a smaller excursion of the upper lobes during ventilation.

PULMONARY FUNCTION STUDIES

The wide spectrum in the degree of pulmonary dysfunction among patients reflects the variable progression of airway disease. Wessel (1983) reviewed the measurements of lung volume and pulmonary mechanics that provide an objective basis for long-term follow-up and assessment of the efficacy of specific treatment. Most children can cooperate with testing by the age of 5 to 6 years, and pulmonary function studies are performed at regular intervals thereafter. The early and scattered obstruction of peripheral airways causes predictable abnormalities in arterial oxygenation, pulmonary volumes and capacities, and airflow mechanics. The uneven apportionment of inspired gases and blood flow to the alveoli results in an increase in the alveolar-arterial Po_2 gradient and arterial hypoxemia. The normally ventilated areas of lung continue to maintain a normal carbon dioxide tension. An increase in carbon dioxide tension is a preterminal finding associated with cor pulmonale. Volume displacement spirometry gives measurable evidence of increased dead-space ventilation and air trapping. Sensitive indicators of abnormal lung volumes are an increase in residual volume (RV) and in functional residual capacity. The ratio of RV to total lung capacity usually is increased and suggests air trapping. Vital capacity and total lung capacity are decreased only in patients with moderate to advanced lung involvement who have the restrictive effects of lung destruction and fibrosis. Because early disease is confined to the small airways, maximum expiratory air flows are decreased initially only at small lung volumes. Therefore, the maximum expiratory airflow after expiration of 75% of vital capacity and the average maximum expiratory flow during the middle 50% of vital capacity are more sensitive than the FEV and the FEV_1.

Zach (1990) emphasized the complexity of advancing lung disease. The walls of the central bronchi, progressively weakened by proteolytic damage to connective tissue, are unstable. These bronchi can overdistend during inspiration in response to negative intrathoracic pressure and then collapse during expiration, especially if forced. The high flow peak of expiration corresponds to the emptying of distended central bronchi (a dead-space effect). Severely compromised end-expiratory flow rates indicate peripheral airway flow in addition to any effect from now partially collapsed proximal bronchi. Patients with more severe disease may have a complex and variable combination of peripheral, partly bronchospastic airway obstruction and a central, primarily bronchiectatic, airway instability.

RADIOGRAPHIC FINDINGS

The earliest radiographic abnormalities are evidence of hyperinflation with flattening of the domes of the diaphragm and an increased anteroposterior diameter of the chest. Bron-

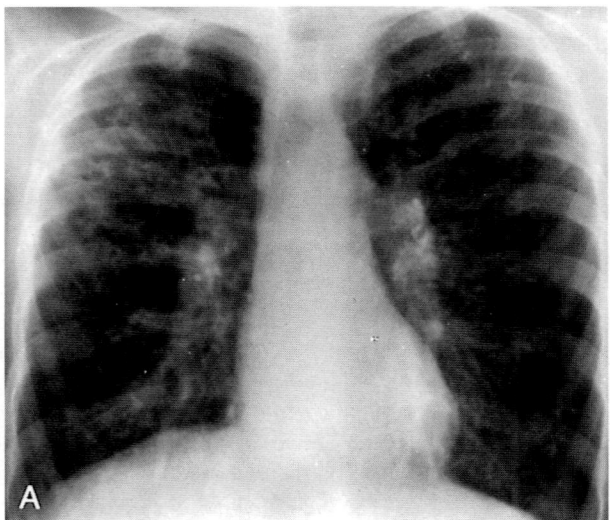

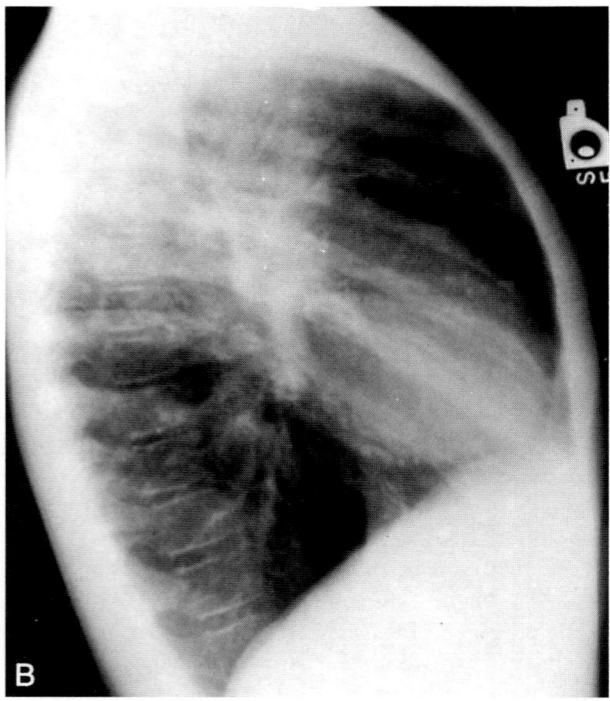

Fig. 80-1. Anteroposterior **(A)** and lateral **(B)** radiographs of a 12-year-old boy show hyperexpansion of the chest wall and depressed diaphragm from overinflated lungs. Linear and patchy densities are concentrated in a contracted right upper lobe. Note the normal heart size and the prominent pulmonary arteries. The vertebral column is osteoporotic.

chovascular markings are prominent, especially in the upper lobes. Atelectasis of the right upper lobe, right middle lobe, or left lower lobe in infants and young children should suggest the diagnosis of CF. The chest radiograph of a patient with well-established disease reveals a diffuse cystic interstitial process with maximum involvement of the upper lung fields (Fig. 80-1). Brasfield and colleagues (1980) reported that the most frequently occurring abnormalities include

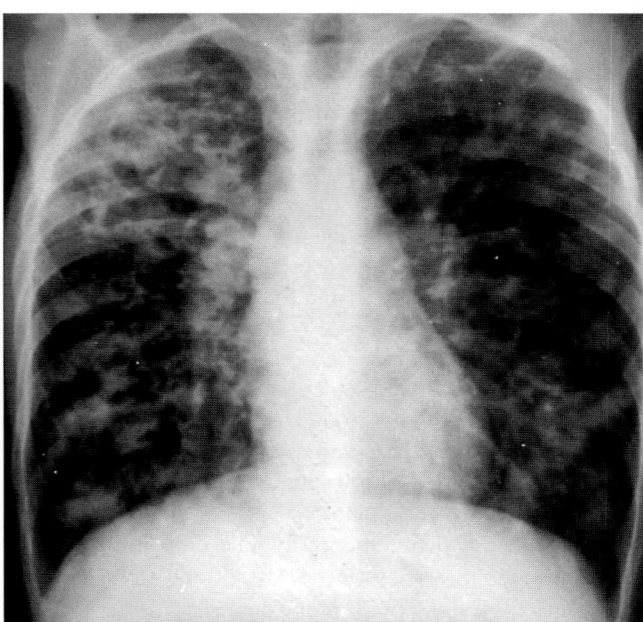

Fig. 80-2. Nodular cystic changes (bronchiectasis and scarring) and linear densities are prominent in the radiographs of a 16 year old with severe disease.

hyperinflation, usually of the upper lobes; patchy linear and nodular densities, probably representing bronchiectasis or small peribronchial abscesses; and lobar segmental atelectasis (Fig. 80-2). Fellows and associates (1979) suggested that increasingly prominent densities may represent dilatated bronchial artery collaterals. Apical blebs appear in older patients. Chest radiograph scoring can predict pulmonary function in children. Rosenberg and coworkers (1992) also have shown a strong correlation between chest radiographs of adult patients and pulmonary function, especially the FEV_1. Changes in the radiograph, however, lagged behind decreases in FEV_1 over 5 years of follow-up. Schwartz and Holsclaw (1974) suggested that the differential diagnosis in an older patient with undiagnosed interstitial disease should include CF in addition to chronic bronchitis, sarcoidosis, histiocytosis X, tuberculosis or other granulomatous infection, and connective tissue disease. The impression of microcardia, seen late in the course of the disease, is related to extensive pulmonary overinflation. A normal-sized or small heart does not rule out cor pulmonale. Computed tomography can specifically delineate radiopaque lesions, particularly the extent and severity of bronchiectasis.

COMPREHENSIVE TREATMENT

Intensive therapeutic and prophylactic regimens initiated in the late 1950s were targeted to control pulmonary secretions and avoid atelectasis, to treat and prevent pulmonary infection, and to ameliorate other medical problems affecting these patients. These measures have resulted in the current prolonged survival of many patients without halting the progressive course of the disease. Early and compulsive care can retard pulmonary damage for lengthy periods, and a better quality of life can be sustained in those with more advanced disease. Fick and Stillwell (1989), Stern (1989), and Fiel (1993) summarized the current approach to comprehensive and everyday management. Specific treatment now available or under active investigation includes regulation of transepithelial ion transport, mucolytic therapy, and amelioration of lung inflammation.

The mainstay of therapy is to encourage deep breathing and coughing, which efficiently mobilize secretions. Hofmeyer and colleagues (1986) reported that segmental postural drainage, chest percussion or vibration, breathing exercises, and active aerobic exercise, when feasible, all contribute to the mechanical removal of secretions. Active breathing exercises alone, although attractive to the older patient, do not appear to maintain pulmonary function. Reisman and colleagues (1988) have shown deterioration greater than that expected in patients who omitted routine physiotherapy in favor of breathing exercises over a 3-year period. Zach and Oberwaldner (1987) state that the mechanical clearance of mucopurulent secretions and their load of antigens and proteolytic agents is as important as antibiotic therapy and that the beneficial effects are longer lasting. Mist or nebulization therapy can help thin the thick sputum and provoke coughing. Room humidification, especially at night, is recommended. In some cases, chest physiotherapy can be more effective if preceded by aerosol inhalation of a bronchodilator, such as albuterol, in patients with demonstrable bronchial hyperreactivity. Bronchoscopy and bronchial lavage have been used to clean out accumulations of tenacious secretions in failing patients but without sustained improvement. Stern and associates (1978b) stated the technique is indicated only for persistent lobar or segmental atelectasis. Associated respiratory tract lesions (e.g., sinusitis, nasal polyps, and hypertrophied tonsils and adenoids) should be treated as indicated.

New methods to alter the tenacious adherence of the respiratory secretions are under investigation. DNA released by degenerating inflammatory cells further increases the viscosity of mucus. Human deoxyribonuclease, which can degrade the large DNA molecules into smaller strands, has been cloned and can be produced in large quantities. Hubbard and colleagues (1992) reported thinning of the sputum and improvement in pulmonary function testing in 16 patients with CF after 1 week of aerosol treatments. Knowles and associates (1990, 1991) have improved hydration of the secretions by blocking sodium absorption and stimulating chloride secretion. Application of amiloride hydrochloride, a potassium-sparing diuretic, to the respiratory epithelium blocks both sodium and water absorption. When amiloride was administered in an aerosol to adult patients, the sputum became less viscid and the expected decline in pulmonary function over 6 months was not seen. The half-life of

amiloride in the airway is only 40 minutes; the drug must be administered several times a day. The triphosphate nucleotides (adenosine triphosphate and uridine triphosphate) can stimulate a chloride channel not related to CFTR. These chloride secretogogues also improve secretions in patients but appear to work better after pretreatment with amiloride. Aerosol treatments with the mucolytic agent N-acetyl-L-cysteine have been recommended in the past, but this drug is an irritant and causes bronchospasm.

Hata and Fick (1988) and Mouton and Kerrebijn (1990) have reviewed current antibiotic therapy for pulmonary infection in CF. The prescription of "suppressive" oral antibiotics is controversial. Conventional treatment for exacerbations of infection has included carbenicillin or ticarcillin and an aminoglycoside. Piperacillin, another synthetic penicillin, has a lower sodium load. The renal clearance of aminoglycosides is increased in patients with CF, and these drugs must be administered more frequently. Ceftazidime, a third-generation cephalosporin, is bactericidal for many Gram-negative organisms, including some that are resistant to the aminoglycosides. Imipenem, a carbapenem antibiotic, has a broad spectrum of activity and is bactericidal for *P. aeruginosa*. This drug is administered with cilastatin, which inhibits degradation of the drug in the kidney and possible renal damage. Ciprofloxacin, a fluoroquinolone, is active against *S. aureus* and *H. influenzae* as well as *P. aeruginosa*. Oral, twice-daily administration is a great advantage. The hepatic clearance of theophylline and warfarin (Coumadin) is decreased by ciprofloxacin; the doses of these drugs must be carefully monitored. Ciprofloxacin is not approved for use in children. When frequent or prolonged courses are necessary, the drugs can be administered at home through a temporary peripheral catheter, a central venous catheter, or a subcutaneous port. Many of these antibiotics can be administered by aerosol, and this technique does not appear to accelerate the emergence of resistant organisms. *Pseudomonas*-specific immunoglobulin has been administered intravenously to patients by Winnie (1989) and Van Wye (1990) and their associates. In these limited clinical studies, they found significant improvement in pulmonary function during acute exacerbation of infection in patients with moderately severe lung disease.

The host inflammatory response to lung infection can be decreased with anti-inflammatory drugs. Auerbach and colleagues (1985) reduced morbidity and reported an improvement in pulmonary function in 45 patients empirically treated with alternate-day steroids (2 mg prednisone/kg) for 4 years. On the other hand, Rosenstein and Eigen (1991) found an unacceptable incidence of complications, such as cataracts, growth failure, and glucose intolerance. However, a later multicenter study of 4 years' duration reported by Eigen and colleagues (1995) used alternate-day dosing regimens of prednisone versus a placebo in 285 CF patients (aged 6 through 64 years) with mild-to-moderate lung disease. They found that a beneficial effect on lung function occurred in the prednisone-treated patients, especially in patients colonized with *P. aeruginosa*. Although the aforementioned complications were observed, it was concluded that the benefit outweighed the adverse effects when the regimen lasted less than 24 months. Konstan (1998) recommends the use of prednisone 1 mg/kg every other day for a limit of less than 2 years in patients with mild to moderate lung disease; therapy should be discontinued if no improvement in pulmonary function is noted after 6 months of treatment. Greally and coworkers (1994) suggest the use of a short course of prednisolone: 2 mg/kg every day for 2 weeks tapered to 1 mg/kg on alternate days for 10 weeks. This regimen was shown to improve functional vital capacity and FEV$_1$ and was associated with a decrease in serum immunoglobulin G and cytokine concentration compared with the use of a placebo, as an adjunct to the treatment of exacerbations of the disease. The use of the inhaled route of dosage of steroids is still under investigation. Ibuprofen inhibits the release of an inflammatory product, a leukotriene, from neutrophils; this drug was shown by Konstan and colleagues (1990) to ameliorate the inflammatory response to lung infection in a rat model. Konstan and associates (1995) reported that high-dose ibuprofen (20 to 30 mg/kg, up to 1600 mg twice a day) slowed the progression of pulmonary disease in mildly affected patients (i.e., FEV$_1$ >60% predicted), particularly in children aged 5 to 12 years. In adults, the occurrence of gastrointestinal bleeding, increased risk of hemoptysis, or renal toxicity may outweigh any benefit of the drug. Konstan (1998) further notes that there are no data to actually support the use of this drug in adults but that its use can be recommended in children with mild reduction of their pulmonary function (FEV$_1$ >60% predicted). To date, according to Oermann and colleagues (1999), both prednisone and ibuprofen are underused in the management of patients with CF. The primary natural inhibitor of neutrophil elastase in the lung is α$_1$-antitrypsin. McElvaney and associates (1991) administered this agent as an aerosol to 12 patients with CF and found that post-treatment bronchial lavage fluid had a greater bactericidal activity against *Pseudomonas*. Other anti-inflammatory therapies for CF lung disease are listed in Table 80-2. Clinical trials are under way to evaluate these agents.

Many patients with CF have positive skin tests to inhalant allergens, and some have asthmalike symptoms. An aerosolized bronchodilator, such as albuterol, should be prescribed for patients with wheezing if pulmonary function improves after a treatment. The empiric administration of steroids rests on the impression of a good clinical response. *Aspergillus fumigatus* frequently colonizes the respiratory mucosa of patients with CF, and approximately 10% of them develop evidence of hypersensitivity to the organism. Allergic bronchopulmonary aspergillosis should be suspected in patients with asthma symptoms and progressive disease or recurrent exacerbations despite otherwise adequate therapy. Brown plugs may be expectorated. Hiller (1990) reviewed the criteria for diagnosis. Eosinophilia, an increase in serum immunoglobulin E and in immunoglobulin E specific for *A. fumigatus*, and positive serum precipitins to *A. fumigatus*

Table 80-2. Anti-inflammatory Therapies for Cystic Fibrosis Lung Disease

Corticosteroids
  Prednisone
  Inhaled steroids
Nonsteroidal anti-inflammatory drugs
  Ibuprofen
  Piroxicam
Eicosanoid modulators
  Fish oil
Cytokine inhibitors
  Pentoxifylline
Antiproteases
  α$_1$-Antitrypsin
  Recombinant secretory leukoprotease inhibitor
  Beta-lactam inhibitor
  Recombinant human elastase inhibitor
Antioxidants
  Beta-carotene
  Alpha-tocopherol (vitamin E)
  Ascorbic acid (vitamin C)
  Glutathione

From Konstan MW. Therapies aimed at airway inflammation in cystic fibrosis. Clin Chest Med *19*:505, 1998. With permission.

can be demonstrated in most affected patients. Laufer and associates (1984) believed that allergic bronchopulmonary aspergillosis probably plays a role in destructive pulmonary disease that steroids could prevent. Improvement is usually seen within 2 weeks, although repeat therapy may be needed. Invasive aspergillosis rarely occurs. Antifungal drugs should be reserved for patients with significant side effects from steroids or with uncontrolled symptoms. Atypical mycobacteria should be sought in the sputum of patients who show unexpected clinical deterioration. Hjelte and associates (1990) reported six patients with positive sputum smears and cultures for these organisms, all of whom improved with antituberculous chemotherapy.

Pancreatic exocrine insufficiency prevents the normal absorption of long-chain fats and fat-soluble vitamins. Despite the administration of pancreatin-containing tablets, an increased caloric intake is indispensable for normal growth. The diet should be high in protein, with fat intake adjusted to individual tolerance. All patients should receive increased doses of multivitamins and water-soluble preparations of vitamin E. Vitamin K is given in the first year of life and thereafter for specific indications. Additional salt and fluid are advised during warm weather. Those with less pancreatic involvement exhibit better growth, less pulmonary disease, and prolonged longevity. Energy requirements increase as respiratory disease progresses. Fried and associates (1991) showed that the resting expenditure of energy is normal in patients with an FEV$_1$ greater than 85% of predicted, but it increases in a curvilinear fashion as the FEV$_1$ declines. The importance of supplemental nutrition to the maintenance and recovery of pulmonary function has received increasing attention. Corey and colleagues (1988) found a difference in the median age of survival of patients with CF treated in Boston (21 years) as opposed to Toronto (30 years), where nutritional management received priority. Both Levy (1985) and Shepherd (1986) and their colleagues reported that long-term enteral supplementation through a nasogastric tube, gastrostomy, or jejunostomy are associated with an improvement or stabilization of pulmonary function. They could not demonstrate a long-term improvement in pulmonary function in older patients.

SURGICAL EVALUATION AND INTERVENTION

Ten percent of young children followed by di Sant'Agnese (1953) in the 1940s and 1950s developed lobar atelectasis and bronchiectasis. Persistent lesions were resected. Operative intervention also was required during that period for staphylococcal pyopneumothorax, empyema, and lung abscesses, as reported by Andersen (1958), Holsclaw (1970), and Taussig and colleagues (1974). Holsclaw (1970) and Lester and colleagues (1983) noted that the rare large pulmonary abscess usually responds to prolonged antibiotic therapy and bronchoscopic aspiration (Fig. 80-3). Otherwise, pulmonary resection is indicated. Today, bronchiectasis rarely is localized and suitable for resection. The focus of thoracic surgery has shifted to adolescents and adults whose major pulmonary complications are pneumothorax, hemoptysis, and pulmonary failure. Late sequelae of a pneumothorax, of a bout of hemoptysis, or of a specific type of treatment are impossible to predict in this disease. Any complication may precipitate a further decline in precarious pulmonary reserve, culminating in death a few months later from cardiorespiratory failure. Current recommendations are based on experience with relatively small numbers of patients, often accumulated over many years, that bridges various advances in medical therapeutics. Treatment is neither randomized nor prospectively determined in any report; long-term follow-up is not always available.

Preoperative Preparation

A systematic evaluation of all involved organ systems is obtained. The results of previous pulmonary function and clinical scoring and a current echocardiogram are vital for estimation of operative risks and prognosis of long-term outcome. Appropriate studies should determine the presence of previously unsuspected portal hypertension, diabetes mellitus, gastroesophageal reflux, or cholelithiasis, which can complicate recovery. Specific preoperative measures include vigorous chest physiotherapy, systemic antibiotics based on current sputum cultures, correction of any coagulation deficits, and relief of stool impaction with enemas or oral polyethylene glycol-electrolyte solution, or both. Full and maximal caloric support should be guaranteed by peripheral or central parenteral nutrition or enteral formula supplements.

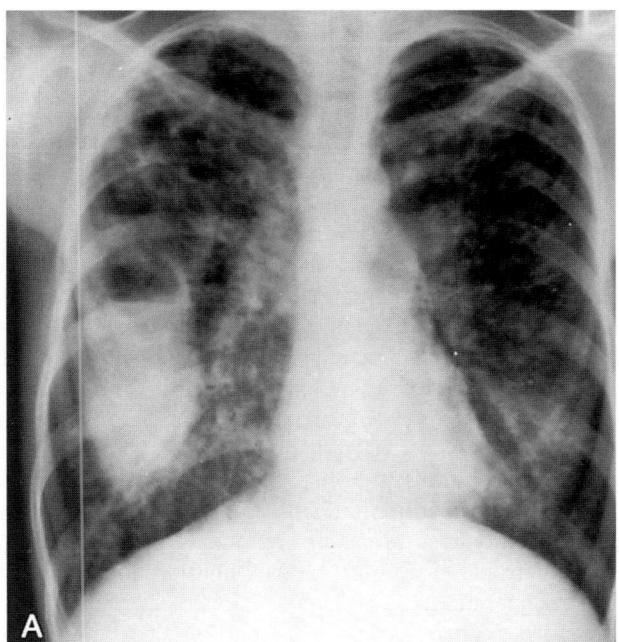

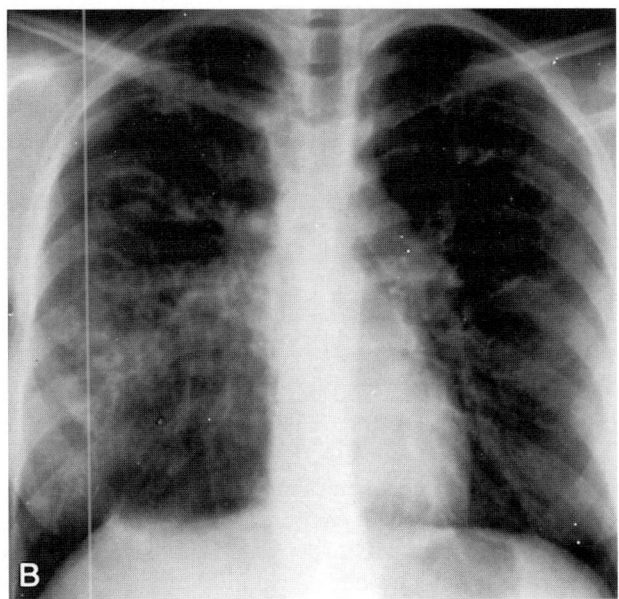

Fig. 80-3. A. A 17-year-old girl developed a multiloculated abscess after a prolonged pulmonary exacerbation of infection. **B.** The abscess had cleared with scarring 2 months after antibiotic therapy.

Anesthetic Considerations

Most postoperative complications are respiratory, and these can be limited with appropriate care. Lamberty and Rubin (1985) reviewed 77 patients who underwent general anesthesia for various procedures. The long-term decline of pulmonary function was comparable to that expected in other patients at similar ages. The pathophysiology of the disease must be considered in choosing anesthetic techniques. The ventilation-perfusion imbalance and pulmonary fibrosis lead to the slow diffusion of inhaled gases, including oxygen. Therefore, prolonged anesthetic induction and emergence time are seen with inhalant agents. Intravenous induction should be used in all cases. Spontaneous respiration may depend on a hypoxic respiratory drive, and tidal volumes decrease if spontaneous respiration is allowed under anesthesia. Assisted or controlled ventilation must be maintained through a cuffed endotracheal tube. Light nonnarcotic preoperative sedation and awaken extubation are mandatory. The postoperative respiratory drive is depressed by hyperventilation and hypocarbia. Many patients are prone to develop laryngospasm, bronchospasm, and paroxysmal attacks of coughing. Increased secretions continue to accumulate during the operation and require frequent endotracheal suctioning. Ketamine produces bronchorrhea and is contraindicated. Inspired air and gases must be well humidified during and after the operation.

A pulse oximeter, an end-tidal carbon dioxide monitor, an airway pressure monitor, and an arterial catheter provide useful data during and after the operation. Intravenous atropine is given at the time of induction. A nasotracheal tube should not be passed if the patient has extensive nasal polyps. Single-lung ventilation and fluid overload should be avoided. The use of nitrous oxide is contraindicated in the presence of a pneumothorax or large bullae. Hypoalbuminemia and aminoglycoside therapy may prolong the action of nondepolarizing muscle relaxants. At the conclusion of the procedure, all narcotics and muscle relaxants must be completely reversed. The patient should be thoroughly suctioned, awake, and coughing before extubation. Both Schuster and Fellows (1977) and Rich and associates (1978) found that prompt extubation was feasible in many cases. Robinson and Branthwaite (1984) electively ventilated all those in whom a delay in adequate spontaneous respiration was expected. Patients who are extremely ill from malnutrition or liver disease are easily oversedated and have decreased tolerance for local anesthetics. Humidified oxygen is provided postoperatively. Chest physiotherapy should be resumed immediately. Postoperative analgesia by intercostal or epidural block is helpful.

Pneumothorax

Pneumothorax is the most common surgical complication of pulmonary disease in CF. A pneumothorax follows the rupture of subpleural air cysts through pleura weakened by the effects of chronic inflammation. Tomashefski and associates (1985b) identified three different pathologic types of air cysts in older patients with CF who were dying of pulmonary disease. All cysts occur more frequently in the upper lobes. Bronchiectatic cysts are the only ones large enough to be well defined on chest radiographs, but their thick collagenous walls seem to prevent rupture. Smaller subpleural emphysematous cysts, which give the lung surface a bubbly appearance, are the likely site of pleural rupture. Interstitial air cysts located adjacent to interlobular septa may cause interstitial air dissection with pneumomediastinum. Di Sant'Agnese and Vidaurreta (1960), Lifschitz and associates (1968), and Holsclaw (1970) described pneumomediastinum and subcutaneous emphysema with and without pneumothorax in a few patients.

Tomashefski and colleagues (1985a) reported that visceral pleura obtained from CF patients during pleurectomy for pneumothorax or at autopsy shows little difference from that of patients with spontaneous pneumothorax of other cause. Pleural elastic fibers overlying air cysts are disrupted and degenerated, probably as a result of the action of neutrophil and bacterial elastase. Pneumothorax commonly occurs in adolescents and adults with advanced pulmonary disease and severe airflow obstruction. By 1970, several groups had recognized the increased frequency and the attendant morbidity and mortality of this complication (Table 80-3). As older groups of patients are followed for long periods, the incidence of pneumothorax increases from 12% of children older than 10 years of age to 20% of adults older than 20 years. McLaughlin and colleagues (1982) reported, however, that the occurrence of pneumothorax correlated better with clinical scoring and increasing pulmonary disease than with age. This complication is more common in boys and young men, perhaps because of their longer life expectancy.

Most patients cough and complain of chest pain, increased dyspnea, and, on occasion, mild hemoptysis. Chest radiographs often reveal bullous disease in the upper lobes and evidence of tension within the pleural space (Fig. 80-4). No predilection as to the side of occurrence is noted. Thirty to 50% of all affected patients eventually develop a pneumothorax on both sides. A potentially lethal tension pneumothorax may occur in up to 40% of cases. Almost every reported series describes a few patients who died with a tension or concomitant bilateral pneumothorax before treatment could be instituted. Associated mortality is high even in the patients who survive initial treatment. Thirteen percent of 72 patients with pneumothorax followed by Schuster (1983) from 1969 to 1982 died during hospitalization for management of the initial episode even though the pneumothorax was under control at the time of death. Penketh and associates (1987) reported that 25% of 61 patients followed at the Brompton Hospital, London, from 1965 to 1983, died with a pneumothorax.

Observation, needle aspiration, and closed-tube thoracostomy were the methods of treatment used initially. Disappointing results have been reported (Table 80-4). Fifty to 80% of all episodes of pneumothorax observed or aspirated

Table 80-3. Incidence of Pneumothorax in Patients with Cystic Fibrosis

Institution	No. of Patients Followed	No. of Patients with Pneumo-thorax (%)	Average or Median Age at First Pneumothorax (yrs)	No. of Episodes of Pneumothorax	No. of Patients with Bilateral Pneumothorax (%)
Babies' Hospital, New York					
Lifschitz, 1953–1967	710	20+ (3)	14	36+	6 (30)
Rainbow Babies' and Children's Hospital, Cleveland					
Stowe, 1957–1974	666	29 (4)	—	47	9 (30)
Children's Memorial Hospital, Chicago					
Luck, 1971–1976	280 total				
	144 ≥10 yrs	18 (12)	15	40	6 (33)
University of Minnesota Hospitals					
Rich, 1963–1977	440 total	28 (6)	—	—	—
	245 ≥10 yrs	27 (11)	15½	52	13 (48)
Brompton Hospital, London					
Mitchell-Hegge, 1964–1969	49	7 (14)	16	10	3 (49)
Penketh (1982), 1965–1981	243	46 (19)	17	106	—
Penketh (1987), 1965–1983	316	61 (19)	—	133	—
Children's Hospital Medical Center, Boston					
Holsclaw, 1950–1970	~2200	51 (2)	15	93	—
Schuster (1983), 1969–1982	—	72	18	180	27 (39)

either do not resolve or recur. The rate of failure or recurrence after closed-tube thoracostomy is 30 to 75%. Full pulmonary expansion may require more than one chest tube. Even the insertion of multiple tubes does not guarantee suf-

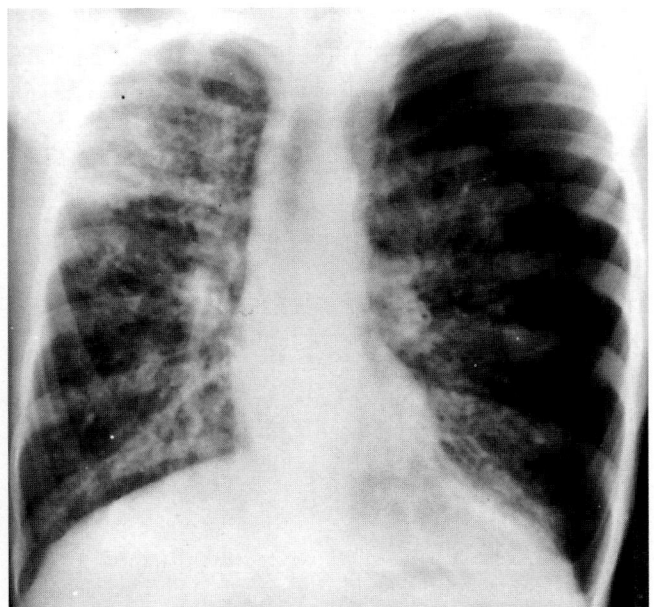

Fig. 80-4. Radiograph of the same patient as in Figure 80-1, now 14 years of age. Note a left tension pneumothorax with hyperexpansion of the left hemithorax and mediastinal shift to the right. He was treated by pleural abrasion after emergency tube thoracostomy. A right pneumothorax occurred 1 year later, and a right abrasive pleurodesis was performed.

ficient pleural reaction to prevent a subsequent tension pneumothorax (Fig. 80-5). In autopsy studies, Boat (1969), Schuster (1983), and Tomashefski (1985a) and their associates were unable to correlate the numbers of chest tubes placed with the degree of pleural symphysis. Prolonged and multiple-tube thoracostomy decompression is painful, restricts ambulation, and impedes chest physiotherapy. As resolution of the pneumothorax is delayed, the patient faces increasing anesthetic and operative risks.

Aggressive attempts to ensure the prompt formation of a pleural symphysis have been advocated in the past. If the patient might become a lung transplant candidate, however, extensive pleural adhesions should be avoided. Previous pleurodesis or pleurectomy is not an absolute contraindication to transplantation at most centers, but hemorrhage is inevitable when these lungs are mobilized. Noyes and Orenstein (1992) recommended treating recurrent pneumothorax in such patients through a limited thoracotomy or thoracoscopy with ablation of apical blebs (the most common source of pneumothorax). If transplantation does not appear indicated or possible, treatment alternatives include chemical sclerosis, pleural abrasion, and pleural stripping with or without the resection or oversewing of apical lung bullae. Chemical sclerosis with aqueous solutions of quinacrine or tetracycline has been used in a small percentage of the cases in most of the earlier series. The random instillation of variable amounts of sclerosant has produced inconsistent results, although each drug can create diffuse pleural adhesions when used in sufficient amounts. Quinacrine was used with moderate success in earlier series, but occasional severe toxicity with large doses was reported. Boat (1969), Cattaneo (1973), Kattwinkel (1973), Stowe (1975), and Schuster (1983) and

Table 80-4. Treatment of Pneumothorax by Observation, Needle Aspiration, or Tube Thoracostomy

Institution	No. of Episodes of Pneumothorax	Observation or Aspiration		Closed-Tube Thoracostomy	
		No. Treated	No. Failed or Recurred (%)	No. Treated	No. Failed or Recurred (%)
Babies' Hospital, New York					
Lifschitz, 1953–1967	35	14	7 (50)	21	7 (30)
Rainbow Babies' and Children's Hospital, Cleveland					
Stowe, 1957–1974	47	14	6 (43)	20	14 (70)
Children's Memorial Hospital, Chicago					
Luck, 1971–1976	44	18	14 (78)	25	14 (56)
University of Minnesota Hospitals					
Rich, 1963–1977	52	8	6 (75)	19	14 (74)
Brompton Hospital, London					
Penketh (1982), 1965–1981	81	31	17 (55)	43	27 (63)
Children's Hospital Medical Center, Boston					
Schuster (1983), 1969–1982	180	77	61 (80)	94	70 (74)

their colleagues, as well as Jones and Giammona (1976), reported a successful resolution in 20 of 22 patients. Although this drug is not available commercially in liquid form, a hospital pharmacy can prepare a sterile solution from tablets. Janzing and associates (1993) resurrected this drug as a preferred sclerosant. They report that patients have less chest pain than with tetracycline. Effective chemical sclerosis with tetracycline depends on the total dose of instilled drug. Sahn and Potts (1978) showed that a solution of 35 mg/kg body weight consistently produced complete obliteration of the pleural cavity in rabbits, as opposed to a solution of 7 mg/kg, which produced early fibrinous adhesions but not long-term

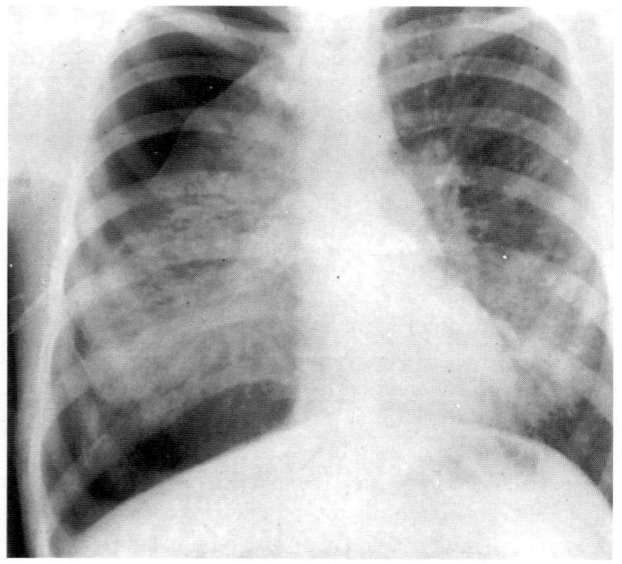

Fig. 80-5. A 15-year-old girl had recurrent right pneumothorax after the treatment of four previous episodes of pneumothorax by tube thoracostomy. Localized pleural adhesions have not prevented a tension effect with flattening of the right diaphragm.

symphysis. This dose-related response may explain the recurrence of pneumothorax in six of seven patients reported by Schuster and colleagues in 1983 because they used small doses of the drug. The clinical acceptance of tetracycline as a sclerosant is limited by immediate and severe chest pain. Tetracycline hydrochloride is now unavailable in an intravenous form. A similar effect may be produced by two semisynthetic tetracyclines that are manufactured for intravenous administration: minocycline hydrochloride (Minocin, Lederle Laboratories, Wayne, NJ) and doxycycline hyclate (Vibramycin, Roerig Division of Pfizer, Inc., New York, NY).

Daniel and associates (1990) treated nine CF patients with pneumothorax by talc (dry USP pure talc) insufflation of the pleural cavity with thoracoscopy using regional or general anesthesia. This minimally invasive procedure was uncomplicated; no recurrences were reported. After the division of all pleural adhesions, approximately 2 g of sterile talc powder is insufflated under direct vision, thoroughly coating the pleural surfaces. Spector and Stern (1989) also described the use of talc in five patients, with no recurrence in the four survivors. This technique combines a high rate of pleural symphysis with minimal risks of patient discomfort or complications.

Lifschitz and coworkers (1968) first reported thoracotomy for pleural abrasion and apical bleb resection in children with CF. Extensive experience with both pleurectomy and pleural abrasion has accumulated since 1970 (Table 80-5). Morbidity and mortality are low, considering the depressed physical status of these patients. Even staged bilateral procedures have been performed successfully by most groups. The operation should be performed after stabilization of the patient, which may include emergency placement of a chest tube. The operative approach should include a limited incision that preserves the major chest wall muscles. Abrasive pleurodesis can be accomplished through a small axillary incision using dry gauze or other sterile abrasive surface. Chest tubes are removed after the air leak has ceased and the lung is

Table 80-5. Treatment of Pneumothorax by Pleurectomy, or Abrasive Pleurodesis

Institution	No. of Patients Treated	No. of Episodes Treated	No. Failed or Recurred	Complications	Deaths
Rainbow Babies' and Children's Hospital, Cleveland					
Stowe (1957–1974)	15	17	2	2 hemorrhage, 1 deep wound infection	2 within 6 months
Olsen (1970–1985)	28	30	2	—	—
Spector and Stern (1959–1987)	57	57	9	1 phrenic nerve paralysis	1 at 1 week
University of Minnesota Hospital					
Rich, 1963–1977	20	31	1	2 hemorrhage, atelectasis	1 with severe malnutrition
Brompton Hospital, London					
Robinson, 1966–1982	18	25	5	2 hemorrhage, 3 air leak, subcutaneous emphysema, 1 atelectasis	5 within 6 months (1 at 1 week)
Children's Hospital Medical Center, Boston					
Schuster (1983), 1969–1982	20	20	0	1 empyema (*Pseudomonas*)	2 within 4 months

well expanded. Rich and colleagues (1978) believe that a stapled resection of apical blebs is contraindicated because the noncompliant lung prevents adequate closure. Immediate operative and anesthetic complications are uncommon. Pleurectomy carries a higher risk of hemorrhage than does abrasive pleurodesis. Patients with severe air-flow obstruction or with cor pulmonale may survive the procedure, but Boat and associates (1969), Mitchell-Heggs and Batten (1970), and I and my associates (1977) reported that the mortality is high at 6 months. Atelectasis and recurrent pneumothorax were particularly devastating in the series described by Penketh and associates (1987); five of six patients with these complications died within 6 months. Spector and Stern (1989) favored pleurectomy as the most successful procedure; when performed in 57 patients, however, the procedure failed in 5% and pneumothorax recurred in 11%. McLaughlin (1982), Rich (1978), Stowe (1975) and their associates and Robinson and Branthwaite (1984) reported postoperative assessment of pulmonary function in limited numbers of patients. A minimal long-term decline occurs compared to that expected on the basis of progression of the underlying lung disease. Seddon and Hodson (1988) found no significant differences in postoperative respiratory function, incidence of recurrence, or incidence of major complications in a group of 27 adults who had either an operative pleurodesis or a pleurectomy.

Ideal treatment would ensure rapid resolution of the pneumothorax, eliminate the possibility of recurrence, and incur the least morbidity and mortality. The following conclusions are warranted:

1) Pneumothorax occurs in patients with long-standing pulmonary infection and with severe and progressive air-flow obstruction.
2) Bilateral occurrence of pneumothorax is high.
3) Any form of treatment is palliative, and no improvement in baseline status can be expected, although mortality increases when definitive treatment is delayed and pulmonary function is severely depressed.
4) Closed-tube thoracostomy and chemical sclerosis are appropriate primary therapy for a patient who is not a transplant candidate. Talc poudrage and quinacrine sclerosis are both effective, and quinacrine can be instilled without a general anesthetic.
5) Lung transplantation is more difficult in the presence of diffuse adhesions, and apical bleb ablation or resection should be recommended for any possible transplant candidate.

Hemoptysis

Hemoptysis, like pneumothorax, occurs in older patients with well-established lung disease. Enlarged bronchial arteries supply multiple bronchopulmonary anastomoses in areas of bronchiectasis or abscess, usually in the upper lobes. The arrest (often immediate) of hemoptysis by bronchial artery embolization confirms this source of bleeding. Initial massive hemoptysis (>300 mL of blood loss/24 hours) is first seen at an average age of 15 years and occurs in at least 8% of patients who survive beyond the age of 15 years. Blood streaking of sputum may be observed for several years before the occurrence of massive hemoptysis. The most common precipitating event is an exacerbation in pulmonary infection, although such episodes may be difficult to distinguish from advancing pulmonary disease. Coagulopathy is uncommon. As a group, patients with massive hemoptysis do not appear to have a worse prognosis than do those with a similar degree of lung disease who never bleed. The natural history of untreated hemoptysis in patients with CF has been documented at two large centers, but with differing conclusions and therapeutic recommendations. Holsclaw and associates (1970) described 19 patients treated between 1959 and 1969. Their patients had severe pulmonary disease with an S-K score of 55 or less in 15 (79%) and an associated pneumothorax in five. In six patients, the initial attack was terminal. Five died within 1 month; two others died within 6 months. These authors concluded that this ominous complication, with a 6-month mortality of 68%, should be treated by early lung resection whenever feasible. On the other hand, all 38 patients reviewed by Stern and colleagues (1978a) stopped bleeding within 4 days and survived the acute episode; 17 (45%) had recurrence of massive hemoptysis. Only five patients required blood transfusion. Without specific intervention, 14 (37%) survived longer than 5 years, one for 20 years. The S-K score was the most accurate prognostic finding. All five patients with a score less than 35 died, whereas 15 with scores greater than 60 survived.

The dramatic onset of profuse bleeding, with the potential for asphyxiation and exsanguination, inspires a sense of urgency for definitive treatment. Levitsky and associates (1970) first reported emergency bronchial artery ligation and pulmonary resection (pneumonectomy) for hemoptysis in a patient with CF. The series of Schuster and Fellows (1977) and Porter and coworkers (1983) detailed successful operative results. Some patients with poor pulmonary function may even improve temporarily because much of the bleeding and resected lung tissue is nonfunctional and has acted as a source of continuing sepsis. Swersky and coworkers (1979) applied tamponade for bronchial bleeding with Fogarty balloons placed through a bronchoscope in four patients. Profuse hemorrhage ceased in a man treated by Bilton and colleagues (1990) after intravenous infusion of vasopressin began. This drug may allow for immediate medical stabilization, but prolonged administration causes fluid retention and bronchoconstriction.

Selective bronchial artery embolization is the preferred treatment. Remy (1977), Uflacker (1985), and Tonkin (1991) and their associates, as well as Sweezey and Fellows (1990), accomplished long-term control of bleeding with minimal risk of serious complication (Fig. 80-6). Cohen and colleagues (1990) state that this approach is appropriate for patients without severe hemoptysis but with bleeding that is chronic or slowly increasing or that interferes with daily life and chest physiotherapy. Angiography and embolization can be performed in virtually every patient through a transfemoral catheter using local anesthesia and mild sedation. The bronchial arteries may arise from the aorta at a sharp angle, inviting subintimal dissection by the catheter tip. Numerous patterns of bronchial artery anatomy are seen. Retrograde aortic flushing is minimized by the hand injection of small volumes of contrast media through a catheter tip well seated 2 to 3 cm within the bronchial arterial trunk. Contrast shunted through anastomoses with the pulmonary circulation may highlight the pulmonary veins, but the contrast medium rarely extravasates at the bleeding point. Nonionic contrast media are less toxic to the spinal cord, and the use of these agents should minimize the dangers of transverse myelitis. The visualization of spinal radicular branches is not an absolute contraindication for embolization (as the rare demonstration of the artery of Adamkiewicz certainly would be). Cohen and coworkers (1990) noted spinal arteries

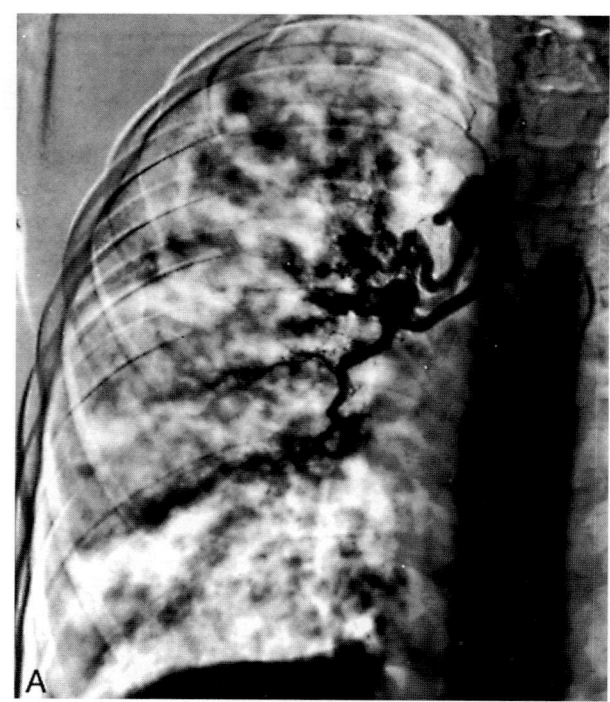

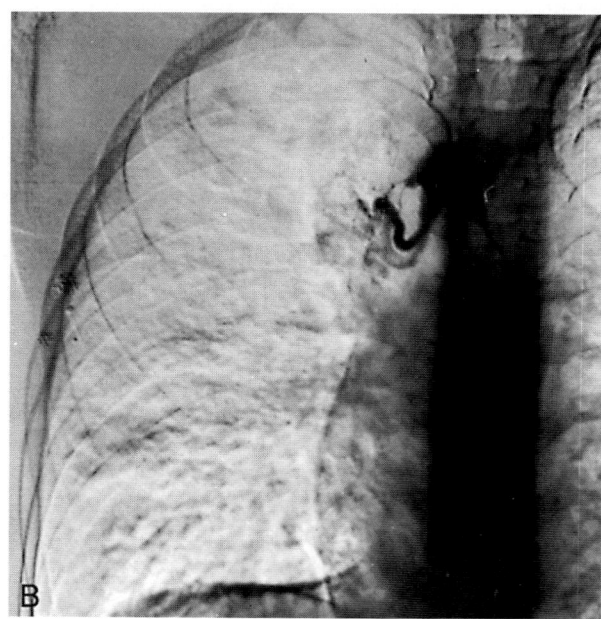

Fig. 80-6. Radiographs of the patient as in Figure 80-2, who was admitted with hemoptysis of more than 500 mL of blood and a recent history of increasing pulmonary disability. **A.** A selective injection of the right upper lobe bronchial artery shows dilatation and tortuosity of the vessel. The site of hemorrhage was not identified. **B.** After embolization of the artery with absorbable gelatin sponge (Gelfoam) a repeat bronchial injection shows near-complete occlusion of the artery. The bleeding stopped after the procedure.

branching from bronchial vessels in 11 of 20 patients. Pieces of absorbable gelatin sponge (1 to 3 mm in diameter) or beads of synthetic polyvinyl alcohol are aspirated into a tuberculin syringe and then slowly injected through the wedged catheter. The smaller emboli are injected first to occlude the most peripheral branches. Twenty to 100 fragments per artery are necessary for near-complete embolization. Blood is aspirated frequently between injections, confirming catheter position in the lumen. The embolization of each artery is concluded when approximately 90% of the peripheral runoff has been blocked. At this point, forward arterial flow is so slow that further injection may flush retrograde into the aorta. In some cases, multiple vessels must be embolized to control recurrent hemorrhage, a time-consuming procedure. Immediate side effects include transient fever and chest pain. Distal aortic embolization has caused small intestinal gangrene and transient cerebral and extremity ischemia. Dysphagia and esophagobronchial fistula have been reported. The value of preangiographic bronchoscopy to guide specific bronchial artery embolization is doubtful because 1) most patients can determine the side of hemorrhage, 2) most bleeding comes from the upper lobes and from the right more often than from the left, and 3) regardless of the actual site of bleeding, multiple vessel embolization is probably indicated whenever possible.

This technique stops acute hemorrhage in 80 to 100% of all patients. Revascularization and recannulization occur with time. Tomashefski and associates (1986) examined the lungs at autopsy of patients who underwent embolization. They found extensive transmural destruction of arterial walls with fibrous replacement and extrusion of particles of polyvinyl alcohol. Despite initial control of bleeding by embolization in 25 patients, Sweezey and Fellows (1990) reported an increase in mortality from cardiorespiratory failure during the following 3 months. With extended follow-up, severe bleeding recurred in almost 50% of the 19 patients who survived more than 3 months. Nonetheless, most were free of hemoptysis for longer than 1 year. Embolization should be repeated if hemorrhage recurs. Angiography should include the head, neck, and chest wall to search for unusual collateral supply. Cohen and colleagues (1992) reported one patient in whom collaterals of a right bronchial artery arose from the right and left thyrocervical trunks and from the right internal mammary artery.

Atelectasis and Bronchiectasis

Mearns (1972) and Schuster (1964) and their colleagues reviewed two series of children who underwent resection for bronchiectasis between 1947 and 1967. The median age was 6 years and the predominant organism was *S. aureus*. Most had localized disease in the right upper lobe (Fig. 80-7). The lower lobe and lingula were the sites involved on the left. Marmon and associates (1983) described nine older children operated on between 1969 and 1981. No operative complications or deaths were reported. The 14 patients of Smith and colleagues (1991) who underwent lobectomy (13) and pneu-

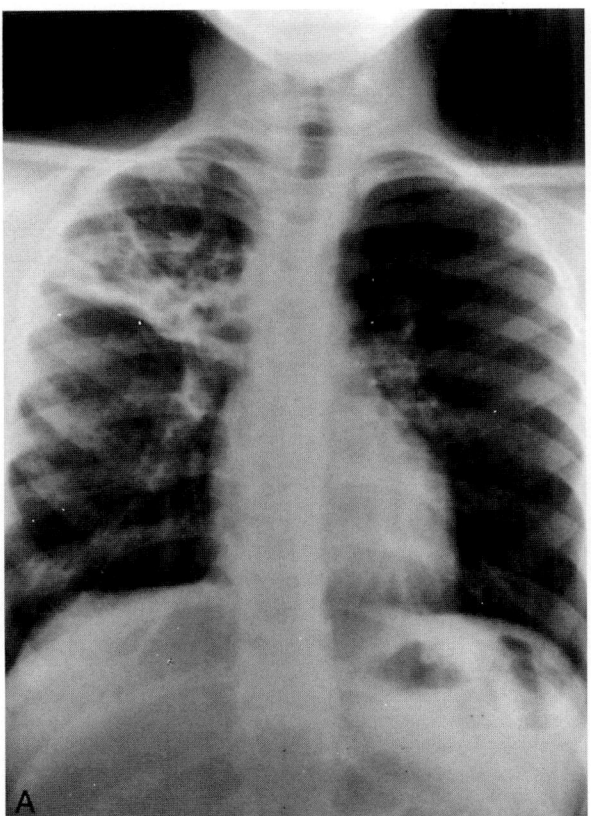
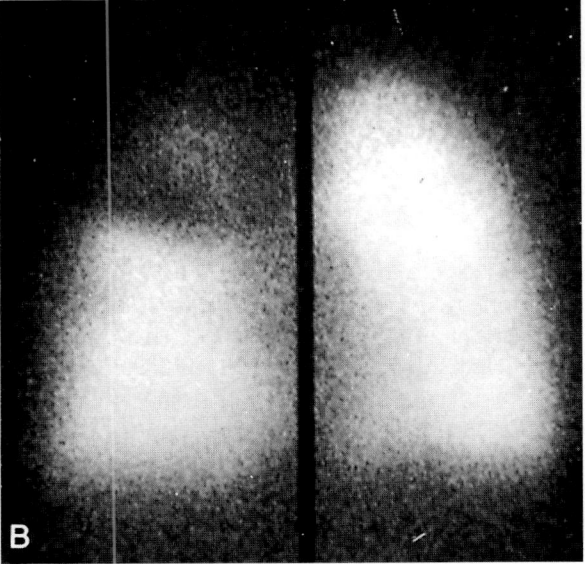

Fig. 80-7. A 9-year-old girl had a persistently productive cough despite intensive treatment. **A.** Radiograph shows that the right upper lobe remained contracted with extensive cystic changes for 4 years. Peribronchial abscesses contain air-fluid levels. **B.** An anterior projection pulmonary perfusion scintigram performed with technetium 99m albumin microspheres confirms the poorly perfused status of this bronchiectatic lobe.

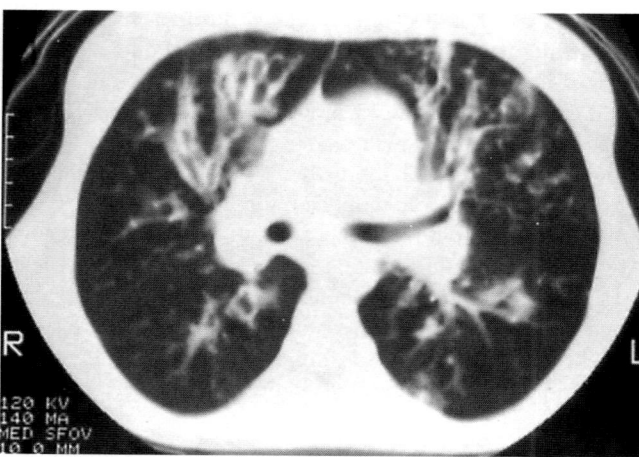

Fig. 80-8. Computed tomography demonstrates bilateral saccular bronchiectasis in multiple lung segments (worse in the lingula and right middle lobe) of a 17-year-old girl with increasing and now nocturnal cough that produced purulent secretions. The bronchi are surrounded by edema and inflammation. The hilar lymph nodes are enlarged.

Table 80-6. Standard Selection Criteria for Lung Transplantation

Age younger than 60 to 65 years
Absence of significant extrapulmonary disease
Daily steroids regimen not in excess of 20 mg prednisone or equivalent
No malignancy within the previous 5 years
Within 20% of ideal body weight
Ambulatory and capable of participating in a pretransplantation pulmonary rehabilitation program
Motivated patient who is able to understand and comply with the post-transplantation medical and rehabilitative regimen
No active cigarette smoking or drug or alcohol abuse
No major psychiatric issues
Financial resources adequate to cover the cost of transplantation, posttransplantation care, and medications

From Zuckerman JB, Kotloff RM: Lung transplantation in cystic fibrosis. Clin Chest Med 19:535, 1998. With permission.

monectomy (4) had a predominance of right-sided lesions. A significant decrease in FEV_1 was noted after operation, although subsequently, these children required fewer hospitalizations. Those with a preoperative FEV_1 of less than 30% did poorly. Symptomatic localized bronchiectasis is now seen less frequently. Lobar atelectasis is avoided or treated expeditiously in most patients. The disease seen in older adolescents and adults usually involves more than one lobe. Computed tomography provides a noninvasive technique to evaluate the entire lung field for extent and severity of disease (Fig. 80-8). If pulmonary resection is indicated, the intensive preoperative program outlined previously should be instituted.

LUNG TRANSPLANTATION

Cropp (1984), Scott (1988), and Jones (1988) and their associates reported the first cases of patients with CF who underwent heart-lung transplantation (HLT). HLT, bilateral en bloc or double transplantation (DLT), and bilateral separate or sequential transplantation (BSLT) have been successfully performed in this population with results similar to those of others undergoing transplantation (see Chapter 92). Because of the paucity of cadaveric heart and lung in bilateral lung donors, Bisson (1994) and Starnes (1996) and their associates, as well as other investigators, have used bilateral pulmonary lobar transplants from two living donors. The left lower lobe and right middle and lower lobes are the lobes of choice. Starnes and colleagues (1996) reported on 38 recipients from 76 donors with no mortality and minimal morbidity. The early results (1-year actuarial survival of 61%) compare favorably with conventional cadaveric HLT, DLT, and BSLT. According to Zuckerman and Kotloff (1998), 61 such procedures had been performed as of

November 1997. The average age at the time of transplantation in CF patients in an earlier series reported by Starnes and coworkers (1992) was 27 ± 8 years of age.

The selection criterion for transplantation in patients with CF is end-stage disease with probable death within 2 years. Women and patients younger than the age of 18 years are more often candidates than are men. As noted previously, Kerem and coinvestigators (1992) suggest that an FEV_1 less than 30% predicted, Po_2 less than 55 mm Hg, and Pco_2 more than 50 mm Hg predicts 50% mortality within 2 years.

Zuckerman and Kotloff (1998) have listed what they consider the standard selection criteria for lung transplantation in CF patients (Table 80-6). Other factors, of course, such as frequency of hospitalization, presence of pulmonary hypertension, and progressive weight loss, as well as an unacceptably poor quality of life, must also be considered.

Many of these patients have chronic colonization of the lungs with *P. aeruginosa*, which is predictive of 10% mortality within 1 year of transplantation. A smaller number of transplant candidates have superinfection with *B. cepacia* that, according to Aris and associates (1997), may result in 50% mortality within 1 year of transplantation. Griffith and colleagues (1993) found that, in the presence of resistant bacterial organisms, there was only 40% 1-year survival versus an 84% survival in the absence of such infection. Of interest is the study of Snell and coworkers (1993), who noted a subset of transplant patients in whom a *B. cepacia* infection was not recognized until after transplantation and in whom the mortality was 80% versus 30% if the infection was identified preoperatively.

The presence of *Aspergillus* is now thought not to be of great importance unless invasive aspergillosis occurs after transplantation. Paradowski (1997) and Kanj and colleagues (1997) believe that the presence of saprophytic fungal infection is no different in CF patients than in other patients undergoing lung transplantation.

In addition to parenchymal infection, the presence of sinusitis, advanced liver disease, and osteoporosis can affect eventual outcome to a greater or lesser degree. Sinusitis is

Table 80-7. Potential Contraindications to Lung Transplantation in the Cystic Fibrosis Patient

Liver disease with significant hepatocellular dysfunction or portal hypertension

Severe malnutrition (<80% of ideal body weight)

Extensive pleural scarring from prior thoracic surgery

Ventilator dependence (excluding noninvasive ventilation)

Airway colonization with *Pseudomonas Burkholderia cepacia*

Aspergilloma with extensive pleural reaction

Severe osteoporosis with history of vertebral compression fractures

Note: Policies on transplantation of patients with the above features vary among centers; none should be viewed as an absolute contraindication.
From Zuckerman JB, Kotloff RM: Lung transplantation in cystic fibrosis. Clin Chest Med *19*:535, 1998. With permission.

best treated medically rather than by invasive procedures. Severe liver disease must be treated by prior liver transplantation or by simultaneous lung-liver transplantation. Severe osteoporosis may adversely affect the outcome, and a marked degree of reduction of bone density and a history of multiple bone fractures, especially those of the spine, may preclude consideration of transplantation. Zuckerman and Kotloff (1998) have suggested the potential contraindications to lung transplantation in patients with CF (Table 80-7).

The specifics of lung transplantation and the operative techniques are presented in Chapter 92. With CF patients, both septic lungs must be removed at the time of transplantation, thus necessitating HLT or DLT. The operative technique for HLT was described originally by Reitz and colleagues (1982), and it has since been changed only slightly, as reported by Jamieson and associates (1984). Currently, HLT, as described by Yacoub and coworkers (1990), with transplantation of the CF recipient's heart to a second patient, continues to be performed in the United Kingdom, where extensive experience with these patients has accumulated. Pasque (1990) and Kaiser (1991) and their associates published early results with BSLT through bilateral anterolateral thoracotomies connected by a transverse sternotomy. This technique is increasingly popular in the United States, Canada, and France. Advantages of this method are the avoidance of cardiopulmonary bypass in most cases and excellent exposure of the pleural cavities. Apical adhesions are readily exposed, and hemorrhage is less of a problem. On the other hand, the bronchial anastomoses are more likely to become ischemic, and anastomotic stricture requiring further intervention is more common than with HLT. The use of living donors and bilateral lobar transplantation has been noted.

Postoperative immunosuppression is, in most cases, based on a three-drug protocol using cyclosporine, azathioprine, and corticosteroids. These patients, as noted by Starnes (1991) and Armitage and colleagues (1991), are subject to the usual complications of immunosuppression, including infection, hypertension, renal dysfunction, malignancy, and growth retardation. Postoperatively, rejection is

monitored with bronchoscopy and biopsies graded according to the Standard Working Formulation for Lung Rejection, reported by the International Society for Heart Transplantation (1990).

Patients with CF pose several specific postoperative problems. Because of poor absorption from the gastrointestinal tract, as pointed out by Scott and associates (1989), unusually large doses of cyclosporine (a lipid-soluble agent) must be given. Patients with CF often need two to three times as much cyclosporine as patients without CF. To improve the levels of cyclosporine, the drug is often given three times per day with exogenous pancreatic enzyme. Insulin-dependent post-transplant diabetes is part of the pancreatic insufficiency syndrome present in patients with CF. Corticosteroids exaggerate the diabetic syndrome during periods of rejection when high-dose pulsed steroids are administered. Chronic infection of the oral sinuses with resistant *Pseudomonas* or *Aspergillus* species, or both, poses a threat of infection to the transplanted lungs, particularly in view of the attendant necessity of immunosuppression. Clinicians at many centers recommend drainage of the maxillary sinuses and selective antimicrobial therapy before lung transplantation.

Infectious complications decrease with time from transplantation. As with other patients, obliterative bronchiolitis from chronic rejection is the limiting factor for long-term survival. Survival of CF patients after HLT has been similar to survival of patients with other diagnoses after HLT. Starnes and associates (1992) at Stanford University reported an actuarial survival rate of 76% at 1, 2, and 3 years after 13 HLT and two DLT for CF. Nineteen percent of patients developed obliterative bronchiolitis, and 30% of patients listed for transplant in this series died awaiting a donor. De Leval and colleagues (1991) reported 83 patients accepted for HLT for terminal CF. Twenty-six died while awaiting the operation, and 32 underwent HLT. Cumulative survival was 72% at 1 year and 56% at 3 years. No difference in survival, infection, or rejection was noted compared to results after HLT in patients with a diagnosis other than CF. Yacoub and coworkers (1990) performed HLT for CF in 27 patients between 1984 and 1988. The actuarial patient survival was 78% at 1 year and 72% at 2 years. Bacterial respiratory infections were common in the early postoperative period and necessitated vigorous medical therapy. In this series, 20 hearts were used for subsequent domino heart transplantation, and immediate heart function was satisfactory in all cases. The actuarial survival of the recipients of these domino heart transplants was 75% at 1 year. Métras and associates (1993) reported actuarial survival of 70% at 3 years for 19 children with CF who underwent DLT. In this series, no operative deaths occurred. Métras and colleagues (1993) believe that in small children, HLT may be preferable to DLT because of the size of the airway anastomosis at risk. Cooper and associates (1994) reported 20 patients undergoing bilateral lung transplantation for CF, with 85% of the group alive at 12 months. Bronchiolitis obliterans affected 25% of the survivors. Sweet and colleagues (1997) reported an 85% one-year actuarial survival, and 67% at two years can be expected. However, according to the St. Louis International Lung Transplantation Registry as of 1997, the overall actuarial survival was 72%, 55%, and 47% at 1, 3, and 5 years, respectively. Operative mortality due to technical problems and infection have declined from a high of 29%, as reported by Ramirez (1992), 16% by Shennib (1992), and 15% by Madden (1992) and their coworkers. Operative mortality has been as low as 6%, reported by Sweet (1997) and Starnes (1992) and their colleagues, and 0%, reported by Egan (1995) and Starnes (1996) and their associates. Late deaths are still most commonly caused by infection (e.g., with *B. cepacia, P. aeruginosa,* and cytomegalovirus).

CF does not recur in the transplanted lung. Wood and associates (1989) have shown normal bioelectric potential differences in the donor airway mucosa even as the upper airway continues to exhibit abnormal negative potential. Pulmonary function after HLT and lung transplantation in patients with CF is improved over the preoperative morbid state; however, some of these patients, as noted, develop obliterative bronchiolitis with subsequent deterioration of FEV_1 in the first year after transplantation. Métras and colleagues (1993) reported an increase in FEV_1 from 25.5% of predicted before transplantation to 75% of predicted at 3 months after DLT. This value increased to 95% of predicted at 6 months and then decreased slightly at 1 year because of the development of obliterative bronchiolitis. De Leval and associates (1991) reported that most patients achieved an FEV_1 of 80% or more of predicted by 3 months after transplantation. Cooper and coworkers (1994) reported the results of a 6-minute walk increasing from 348 meters pretransplant to 711 meters after transplant. The Po_2 in these patients averaged 48 before transplantation and 98 after transplantation. Although these results are encouraging, obliterative bronchiolitis continues to be a frustrating problem after lung transplantation or HLT. Concerns that immunosuppression in these patients would cause overwhelming postoperative infection have proved unfounded. Poor nutritional status is a risk factor for death while awaiting transplantation, and approximately 30% of these patients die while listed for transplantation. CF does not develop in transplanted organs. Although early and midterm results of HLT and DLT for terminal CF are encouraging, the shortage of donor organs limits the potential of lung transplantation to have a significant impact on the quality of life and on survival for the majority of people with CF.

CONCLUSIONS

Six decades of persistent medical care and investigation have expanded the horizons of each child and adult with CF. Prolonged survival is possible for many, although the emotional and financial consequences of life-long therapy are formidable. Definition of the genetic and cellular basis of the disease is beginning to allow the development of specific preventive and therapeutic measures for lung injury. At the same time, lung transplantation can offer further prolongation of life and a better quality of life to some patients with end-stage lung disease. Despite these advances, pulmonary complications continue to occur in patients who are not transplant candidates, usually when the effects of the disease are escalating. The patient is ill served by delay of definitive management. The thoracic surgeon must be prepared to recommend an appropriate and well-defined approach to operative and angiographic intervention. The goal of Mearns and colleagues (1972) for the thoracic surgeon treating CF patients continues to hold true today: The aim of surgical treatment is to slow the progression of the disease; to prolong life; and, most important, to improve the quality of that life.

REFERENCES

Anderson DH: Cystic fibrosis of the pancreas: a review. J Chronic Dis 7:58, 1958.

Anderson DH: Cystic fibrosis of the pancreas and its relation to celiac disease: a clinical pathologic study. Am J Dis Child 56:344, 1938.

Anguiano A, et al: Congenital bilateral absence of the vas deferens: a primarily genital form of cystic fibrosis. JAMA 267:1794, 1992.

Aris RM, et al: Severe osteoporosis before and after lung transplantation. Chest 109:1176, 1996.

Aris RM, et al: The effects of panresistant bacterial in cystic fibrosis patients on lung transplant outcome. Am J Respir Crit Care Med 155:1699, 1997.

Aris RM, et al: Increased rate of fractures and severe kyphosis: sequelae of living into adulthood with cystic fibrosis. Ann Intern Med 128:186, 1998.

Armitage JM, et al: Posttransplant lymphoproliferative disease in thoracic organ transplant patients: ten years of cyclosporine-based immunosuppression. J Heart Lung Transplant 10:877, 1991.

Auerbach HS, et al: Alternate-day prednisone reduces morbidity and improves pulmonary function in cystic fibrosis. Lancet 2:686, 1985.

Bachrach LK, Loutit CW, Moss RB: Osteopenia in adults with cystic fibrosis. Am J Med 96:27, 1994.

Bear CE, et al: Purification and functional reconstitution of the cystic fibrosis transmembrane regulator (CFTR). Cell 68:809, 1992.

Bedrossian CMW, et al: The lung in cystic fibrosis. A quantitative study including prevalence of pathologic findings among different age groups. Hum Pathol 7:195, 1976.

Berger M: Inflammation of the lung in cystic fibrosis. Clin Rev Allergy 9:119, 1991.

Bilton D, et al: Life threatening haemoptysis in cystic fibrosis: an alternative therapeutic approach. Thorax 45:975, 1990.

Bisson A, et al: Bilateral pulmonary lobe transplantation: left lower and right middle and lower lobes. Ann Thorac Surg 57:219, 1994.

Boat TF, et al: Pneumothorax in cystic fibrosis. JAMA 209:1498, 1969.

Brasfield D, et al: Evaluation of scoring system. AJR Am J Roentgenol 134:1195, 1980.

Bruce MC, et al: Biochemical and pathologic evidence for proteolytic destruction of lung connective tissue in cystic fibrosis. Am Rev Respir Dis 132:529, 1985.

Cattaneo SM, Sirak HD, Klassen KP: Recurrent spontaneous pneumothorax in the high-risk patient. J Cardiovasc Surg 66:467, 1973.

Cohen AM, Doershuk SF, Stern RC: Bronchial artery embolization to control hemoptysis in cystic fibrosis. Radiology 175:401, 1990.

Cohen AM, Antoun VW, Stern RC: Left thyrocervical trunk bronchial artery supplying right lung: Source of recurrent hemoptysis in cystic fibrosis. AJR Am J Roentgenol 158:1131, 1992.

Collins FS: Cystic fibrosis: Molecular biology and therapeutic implications. Science 256:774, 1992.

Cooper JD, Patterson GA, Trulock EP: Results of single and bilateral lung transplantation in 131 consecutive recipients. Washington University Lung Transplant Group. J Thorac Cardiovasc Surg 107:460, 1994.

Corey M, et al: A comparison of survival, growth, and pulmonary function in patients with cystic fibrosis in Boston and Toronto. J Clin Epidemiol 41:483, 1988.

Cropp G, et al: Heart-lung transplantation in cystic fibrosis. Cystic Fibrosis Club Abstract 25:17, 1984.

Daniel TM, Tribble CG, Rodgers BM: Thoracoscopy and talc poudrage for pneumothoraces and effusions. Ann Thorac Surg 50:186, 1990.

Davis PB, Vargo K: Pulmonary abnormalities in obligate heterozygotes for cystic fibrosis. Thorax 42:120, 1987.

de Leval MR, et al: Heart and lung transplantation for terminal cystic fibrosis: a 4½-year experience. J Thorac Cardiovasc Surg 101: 633, 1991.

di Sant'Agnese PA: Bronchial obstruction with lobar atelectasis and emphysema in cystic fibrosis of the pancreas. J Pediatr 12:178, 1953.

di Sant'Agnese PA, Davis PB: Cystic fibrosis in adults. Am J Med 66:121, 1979.

di Sant'Agnese PA, Vidaurreta AM: Cystic fibrosis of the pancreas. JAMA 172:2065, 1960.

Doershuk CF, et al: A 5-year clinical evaluation of a therapeutic program for outpatients with cystic fibrosis. J Pediatr 65:677, 1964.

Dorin J, et al: Cystic fibrosis in the mouse by targeted insertional mutagenesis. Nature 359:211, 1992.

Drumm ML, et al: Correction of the cystic fibrosis defect in vitro by retrovirus-mediated gene transfer. Cell 62:1227, 1990.

Egan TM, et al: Improved results of lung transplantation for patients with cystic fibrosis. J Thorac Cardiovasc Surg 109:224, 1995.

Eigen H, et al: A multicenter study of alternate-day prednisone therapy in patients with cystic fibrosis. Cystic Fibrosis Foundation Prednisone Trial Group. J Pediatr 126:515, 1995.

Esterly JR, Oppenheimer EH: Observations in cystic fibrosis of the pancreas. 3. Pulmonary lesions. Johns Hopkins Med Bull 122:94, 1968.

Fellows KE, et al: Selective bronchial arteriography in patients with cystic fibrosis and massive hemoptysis. Radiology 114:551, 1979.

Fick RB Jr, Stillwell PC: Controversies in the management of pulmonary disease due to cystic fibrosis. Chest 95:1319, 1989.

Fiel SB: Heart-lung transplantation for patients with cystic fibrosis. A test of clinical wisdom [commentaries]. Arch Intern Med 151:870, 1991.

Fiel SB: Clinical management of pulmonary disease in cystic fibrosis. Lancet 341:1070, 1993.

Finkelstein SM, et al: Diabetes mellitus associated with cystic fibrosis. J Pediatr 112:373, 1988.

FitzSimmons SC: The changing epidemiology of cystic fibrosis. J Pediatr 122:1, 1993.

Fried MD, et al: The cystic fibrosis gene and resting energy expenditure. J Pediatr 119:913, 1991.

Gaskin K, et al: Improved respiratory prognosis in patients with cystic fibrosis with normal fat absorption. J Pediatr 100:857, 1982.

Goldmann DA, Klinger JP: Pseudomonas cepacia: Biology, mechanisms of virulence, epidemiology. J Pediatr 108:806, 1986.

Greally P, et al: Interleukin-1 alpha, soluble interleukin-2 receptor, and IgG concentrations in cystic fibrosis treated with prednisolone. Arch Dis Child 71:35, 1994.

Griffith BP, et al: A decade of lung transplantation. Ann Surg 218:310, 1993.

Hata JS, Fick RB Jr: Pseudomonas aeruginosa and the airways disease of cystic fibrosis. Clin Chest Med 9:679, 1988.

Henderson RC, Specter BB: Kyphosis and fractures in children and young adults with cystic fibrosis. J Pediatr 125:208, 1994.

Hiller EJ: Pathogenesis and management of aspergillosis in cystic fibrosis. Arch Dis Child 65:397, 1990.

Hjelte L, et al: Prospective study of mycobacterial infections in patients with cystic fibrosis. Thorax 45:397, 1990.

Hofmeyer JL, Webber BA, Hodson ME: Evaluation of positive expiratory pressure as an adjunct to chest physiotherapy in the treatment of cystic fibrosis. Thorax 41:951, 1986.

Holsclaw DS: Common pulmonary complications of cystic fibrosis. Clin Pediatr 9:346, 1970.

Holsclaw DS, Grand RJ, Schwachman H: Massive hemoptysis in cystic fibrosis. J Pediatr 76:829, 1970.

Huang NN, et al: Clinical features, survival rate, and prognostic factors in young adults with cystic fibrosis. Am J Med 82:871, 1987.

Hubbard RC, et al: A preliminary study of aerosolized recombinant human deoxyribonuclease I in the treatment of cystic fibrosis. N Engl J Med 326:812, 1992.

Hudson I, Phelan PD: Are sex, age at diagnosis, or mode of presentation prognostic factors for cystic fibrosis. Pediatr Pulmonol 3:288, 1987.

International Society for Heart Transplantation, Yousem SA, et al: A working formulation for the standardization of nomenclature in the diagnosis of heart and lung rejection: Lung rejection study group. J Heart Transplant 9:593, 1990.

Jamieson SW, et al: Operative technique for heart-lung transplantation. J Thorac Cardiovasc Surg 87:930, 1984.

Janzing HMJ, et al: Intrapleural quinacrine instillation for recurrent pneumothorax or persistent air leak. Ann Thorac Surg 55:368, 1993.

Jones K, Higenbottam T, Wallwork J: Successful heart-lung transplantation for cystic fibrosis. Chest 93:644, 1988.

Jones RE, Giammona ST: Intrapleural quinacrine for pneumothorax in a child with cystic fibrosis. Am J Dis Child 130:777, 1976.

Kaiser LR, et al: Bilateral sequential lung transplantation: the procedure of choice for double-lung replacement. Ann Thorac Surg 52:438, 1991.

Kanj SS, et al: Infections in patients with cystic fibrosis following lung transplantation Chest 112:924, 1997.

Kartner N, et al: Mislocalization of d-F508 CFTR in cystic fibrosis sweat gland. Nat Genet 1:321, 1992.

Kattwinkel J, et al: Intrapleural instillation of quinacrine for recurrent pneumothorax. JAMA 226:557, 1973.

Kerem B-S, et al: Identification of the cystic fibrosis gene: genetic analysis. Science 245:1073, 1989.

Kerem E, et al: The relationship between genotype and phenotype in cystic fibrosis: analysis of the most common mutation (d508). N Engl J Med 323:1517, 1990a.

Kerem E, et al: Pulmonary function and clinical course in patients with CF after pulmonary colonization with Pseudomonas. J Pediatr 116:714, 1990b.

Kerem E, et al: Prediction of mortality in patients with cystic fibrosis. N Engl J Med 326:1187, 1992.

Knowles M, Gatzy J, Boucher R: Increased bioelectric potential difference across respiratory epithelia in cystic fibrosis. N Engl J Med 305:1489, 1981.

Knowles MR, Clark LL, Boucher RC: A pilot study of aerosolized amiloride for the treatment of lung disease in cystic fibrosis. N Engl J Med 322:1189, 1990.

Knowles MR, et al: Activation by extracellular nucleotides of chloride secretion in the airway epithelia of patients with cystic fibrosis. N Engl J Med 325:533, 1991.

Konstan MW: Therapies aimed at airway inflammation in cystic fibrosis. Clin Chest Med 19:505, 1998.

Konstan MW, Vargo KM, Davis PB: Ibuprofen attenuates the inflammatory response to Pseudomonas aeruginosa in a rat model of chronic pulmonary infection. Am Rev Respir Dis 141:186, 1990.

Konstan MW, et al: Effect of high-dose ibuprofen in patients with cystic fibrosis. N Engl J Med 332:848, 1995.

Kristidis P, et al: Genetic determination of exocrine pancreatic function in cystic fibrosis. Am J Hum Genet 50:1178, 1992.

Lamberty JM, Rubin BK: The management of anaesthesia for patients with cystic fibrosis. Anaesthesia 40:448, 1985.

Lanng S, et al: Glucose tolerance in cystic fibrosis. Arch Dis Child 66:612, 1991.

Laufer PO, et al: Allergic bronchopulmonary aspergillosis and cystic fibrosis. J Allergy Clin Immunol 73:44, 1984.

Lester LA, et al: Echocardiography in cystic fibrosis: A proposed scoring system. J Pediatr 97:742, 1980.

Lester LA, et al: Case report: Aspiration and lung abscess in cystic fibrosis. Am Rev Respir Dis 127:786, 1983.

Levitsky S, Lapeu A, di Sant'Agnese PA: Pulmonary resection for life-threatening hemoptysis in cystic fibrosis. JAMA 213:125, 1970.

Levy DL, et al: Effects of long-term nutritional rehabilitation on body composition and clinical status in malnourished children and adolescents with cystic fibrosis. J Pediatr 107:225, 1985.

Lewin LO, Byard PJ, Davis PB: Effect of Pseudomonas cepacia colonization on survival and pulmonary function of cystic fibrosis patients. J Clin Epidemiol 43:125, 1990.

Lewiston N, et al: Cystic fibrosis patients who have undergone heart-lung transplantation benefit from maxillary sinus antrostomy and repeated sinus lavage. Transplant Proc 23:1207, 1991.

Lifschitz MK, et al: Pneumothorax as a complication of cystic fibrosis. Am J Dis Child 116:633, 1968.

Luck SR: Management of pneumothorax in children with chronic pulmonary disease. J Thorac Cardiovasc Surg 74:834, 1977.

MacLusky J, McLaughlin FJ, Levison J: Cystic fibrosis. 1 and 2. Curr Probl Pediatr 15:1, 1985.

Madden BP, et al: Intermediate-term results of heart-lung transplantation for cystic fibrosis. Lancet 339:1583, 1992.

Marmon L, et al: Pulmonary resection for complications of cystic fibrosis. J Pediatr Surg 18:811, 1983.

Massard G, et al: Double-lung transplantation in mechanically ventilated patients with cystic fibrosis. Ann Thorac Surg 55:1087, 1993.

McElvaney NG, et al: Aerosol α-1-antitrypsin treatment for cystic fibrosis. Lancet 337:392, 1991.

McLaughlin FJ, Matthews WJ, Strieder DJ: Pneumothorax in cystic fibrosis: Management and outcome. J Pediatr 100:863, 1982.

Mearns MB, et al: Pulmonary resection in cystic fibrosis—results in 23 cases, 1957–1970. Arch Dis Child 47:499, 1972.

Métras D, et al and the Joint Marseille-Montréal Lung Transplant Program: Double-lung transplantation in children: a report of 20 cases. Ann Thorac Surg 55:352, 1993.

Mitchell-Heggs PF, Batten JC: Pleurectomy for spontaneous pneumothorax in cystic fibrosis. Thorax 25:165, 1970.

Moss AJ: The cardiovascular system in cystic fibrosis. Pediatrics 70:728, 1982.

Mouton JW, Kerrebijn KF: Antibacterial therapy in cystic fibrosis. Med Clin North Am 74:837, 1990.

Noyes BE, Orenstein DM: Treatment of pneumothorax in cystic fibrosis in the era of lung transplantation [editorial]. Chest 101:1187, 1992.

Oermann CM, Sockrider MM, Konstan MW: The use of anti-inflammatory medications in cystic fibrosis: trends and physician attitudes. Chest 115:1053, 1999.

Ott SM, Aitken ML: Osteoporosis in patients with cystic fibrosis. Clin Chest Med 19:555, 1998.

Paradowski LJ: Saprophytic fungal infections and lung transplantation—revisited. J Heart Lung Transplant 16:524, 1997.

Pasque MK, et al: Improved technique for bilateral lung transplantation: Rationale and initial clinical experience. Ann Thorac Surg 49:785, 1990.

Penketh A, et al: Management of pneumothorax in adults with cystic fibrosis. Thorax 37:850, 1982.

Penketh ARL, et al: Cystic fibrosis in adolescents and adults. Thorax 42:526, 1987.

Pier GB: Pulmonary disease associated with Pseudomonas aeruginosa in cystic fibrosis: Current status of the host-bacterium interaction. J Infect Dis 151:575, 1985.

Pinkerton D, et al: Cystic fibrosis in adult life: a study of coping patterns. Lancet 2:761, 1985.

Porter DK, Von Every MJ, Mack JW: Emergency lobectomy for massive hemoptysis in cystic fibrosis. J Thorac Cardiovasc Surg 86:409, 1983.

Prober CG: The impact of respiratory viral infections in patients with CF. Clin Rev Allergy 9:87, 1991.

Quinton PM: Cystic fibrosis: a disease in electrolyte transport. FASEB J 4:2709, 1990.

Ramirez JC, et al: Bilateral lung transplantation for cystic fibrosis. J Thorac Cardiovasc Surg 103:287, 1992.

Ramsey F, Richardson MA: Impact of sinusitis in cystic fibrosis. J Allergy Clin Immunol 90:547, 1992.

Reisman J, et al: Role of conventional physiotherapy in cystic fibrosis. J Pediatr 113:632, 1988.

Reisman J, et al: Diabetes mellitus in patients with cystic fibrosis: effect on survival. Pediatrics 86:374, 1990.

Reitz BA, et al: Heart-lung transplantation. Successful therapy for patients with pulmonary vessel disease. N Engl J Med 306:557, 1982.

Remy J, et al: Treatment of hemoptysis by embolization of bronchial arteries. Radiology 122:33, 1977.

Rich RH, Warwick WJ, Leonard AS: Open thoracotomy and pleural abrasion in the treatment of spontaneous pneumothorax in cystic fibrosis. J Pediatr Surg 13:237, 1978.

Riordan JR, et al: Identification of the cystic fibrosis gene: cloning and characterization of complementary DNA. Science 245:1066, 1989.

Robinson DA, Branthwaite MA: Pleural surgery in patients with cystic fibrosis. Anaesthesia 39:655, 1984.

Rommens JM, et al: Identification of the cystic fibrosis gene: chromosome walking and jumping. Science 245:1059, 1989.

Rosenberg SM, Howatt WF, Grum CM: Spirometry and chest roentgenographic appearance in adults with cystic fibrosis. Chest 101:961, 1992.

Rosenfeld MA, et al: In vivo transfer of the human cystic fibrosis transmembrane conductance regulator gene to the airway epithelium. Cell 68:143, 1992.

Rosenstein BJ, Eigen H: Risks of alternate-day prednisone in patients with cystic fibrosis. Pediatrics 87:9188, 1991.

Sahn SA, Potts ED: The effect of tetracycline on rabbit pleura. Am Rev Respir Dis 117:493, 1978.

St. Louis International Lung Transplantation Registry, January 1997 Report. Washington University School of Medicine, 1997.

Santis G, et al: Linked marker haplotypes and the d508 mutation in adults with mild pulmonary disease and cystic fibrosis. Lancet 335:1426, 1990.

Schuster S, et al: Pulmonary surgery for cystic fibrosis. J Thorac Cardiovasc Surg 48:750, 1964.

Schuster SR, Fellows KE: Management of major hemoptysis in patients with cystic fibrosis. J Pediatr Surg 12:889, 1977.

Schuster SR, et al: Management of pneumothorax in cystic fibrosis. J Pediatr Surg 18:492, 1983.

Schwachman H, Kulczycki LL: A report of one hundred and five patients with cystic fibrosis of the pancreas studied over a five to fourteen year period. Am J Dis Child 96:6, 1958.

Schwartz EE, Holsclaw DS: Pulmonary involvement in adults with cystic fibrosis. AJR Am J Roentgenol 122:708, 1974.

Scott J, Higenbottom T, Hutter J: Heart-lung transplantation for cystic fibrosis. Lancet 2:192, 1988.

Scott JP, et al: Cyclosporin dosing in cystic fibrosis patients following heart-lung transplantation [letter]. Transplantation 48:543, 1989.

Seddon DJ, Hodson ME: Surgical management of pneumothorax in cystic fibrosis. Thorax 43:739, 1988.

Shennib J, et al: Double-lung transplantation for cystic fibrosis. The Cystic Fibrosis Transplant Study Group. Ann Thorac Surg 54:27, 1992.

Shepherd RW, et al: Nutritional rehabilitation in cystic fibrosis: controlled studies of effects on nutritional growth retardation, body protein turnover, and course of pulmonary disease. J Pediatr 109:788, 1986.

Shepherd SL, et al: A comparative study of the psychosocial assets of adults with cystic fibrosis and their healthy peers. Chest 97:1310, 1990.

Shwachman H, Kowalski M, Khaw K-T: Cystic fibrosis: a new outlook: 70 patients above 25 years of age. Medicine 56:129, 1977.

Smith MB, et al: Predicting outcome following pulmonary resection in cystic fibrosis patients. J Pediatr Surg 26:655, 1991.

Snell GI, et al: Pseudomonas cepacia in lung transplant recipients with cystic fibrosis. Chest 103:466, 1993.

Snell GI, et al: Pseudomonas cepacia in lung transplant recipients with cystic fibrosis. Chest 103:466, 1993.

Snouwaert J, et al: An animal model for cystic fibrosis made by gene targeting. Science 257:1083, 1992.

Spector ML, Stern RC: Pneumothorax in cystic fibrosis: a 26-year experience. Ann Thorac Surg 47:204, 1989.

Starnes VA: Risks of childhood immunosuppression. J Heart Lung Transplant 10:832, 1991.

Starnes VA, et al: Cystic fibrosis. Target population for lung transplantation in North America in the 1990s. J Thorac Cardiovasc Surg 103:1008, 1992.

Starnes VA, et al: Living-donor lobar lung transplantation experience: intermediate results. J Thorac Cardiovasc Surg 112:1284, 1996.

Stern RC: The primary care physician and the patient with cystic fibrosis. J Pediatr 114:31, 1989.

Stern RC, et al: Treatment and prognosis of massive hemoptysis in cystic fibrosis. Am Rev Respir Dis 117:825, 1978a.

Stern RC, et al: Treatment and prognosis of lobar and segmental atelectasis in cystic fibrosis. Am Rev Respir Dis 118:821, 1978b.

Stern RC, et al: Treatment and prognosis of cor pulmonale with failure of the right side of the heart. Am J Dis Child 134:267, 1980.

Stowe SM, et al: Open thoracotomy for pneumothorax in cystic fibrosis. Am Rev Respir Dis 111:611, 1975.

Strong T, et al: Cystic fibrosis gene mutation in two sisters with mild disease and normal sweat chloride levels. N Engl J Med 325:1630, 1991.

Sweet SC, et al: Pediatric lung transplantation at St. Louis Children's Hospital. Am J Respir Crit Care Med 155:1027, 1997.

Sweezey NB, Fellows KE: Bronchial artery embolization for severe hemoptysis in cystic fibrosis. Chest 97:1322, 1990.

Swersky RB, et al: Endobronchial balloon tamponade of hemoptysis in patients with cystic fibrosis. Ann Thorac Surg 27:262, 1979.

Taussig LM, Belmonte MM, Beaudry PH: Staphylococcus aureus empyema in cystic fibrosis. J Pediatr 84:724, 1974.

Thomassen MJ, Demko CA, Doershuk CF: Cystic fibrosis: a review of pulmonary infections and interventions. Pediatr Pulmonol 3:334, 1987.

Tizzano EF, Buchwald M: Cystic fibrosis: beyond the gene to therapy. J Pediatr 120:337, 1992.

Tizzano EF, Buchwald M: Recent advances in cystic fibrosis research. J Pediatr 122:985, 1993.

Tomashefski JF, Cohen AM, Doershuk CF: Long-term histopathologic follow-up of bronchial arteries after therapeutic embolization with polyvinyl alcohol (Ivalon) in patients with cystic fibrosis. Hum Pathol 19:555, 1988.

Tomashefski JF, Dahms B, Bruce M: Pleura in pneumothorax. Arch Pathol Lab Med 109:910, 1985a.

Tomashefski JF, et al: Pulmonary air cysts in cystic fibrosis: Relation of pathologic features to radiographic findings and history of pneumothorax. Hum Pathol 16:253. 1985b.

Tomashefski JF, et al: Regional distribution of macroscopic lung disease in cystic fibrosis. Am Rev Respir Dis 133:535, 1986.

Tonkin IL, et al: Bronchial arteriography and embolotherapy for hemoptysis in patients with cystic fibrosis. Cardiovasc Intervent Radiol 14:241, 1991.

Tsui L-C: The spectrum of cystic fibrosis mutations. Trends Genet 8:392, 1992.

Uflacker R, et al: Bronchial artery embolization in the management of hemoptysis: technical aspects and long-term results. Radiology 157:637, 1985.

Van Wye JE, et al: Pseudomonas hyperimmune globulin passive immunotherapy for pulmonary exacerbation in cystic fibrosis. Pediatr Pulmonol 9:7, 1990.

Warner JO: Heart-lung transplantation: all the facts. Arch Dis Child 66:1013, 1991.

Wessel HU: Lung function in cystic fibrosis. In Lloyd-Still JD (ed): Textbook of Cystic Fibrosis. Boston: John Wright, PSG Inc., 1983, pp. 199–215.

Whitehead B, et al: Heart-lung transplantation for cystic fibrosis. 1. Assessment. Arch Dis Child 66:1018, 1991.

Winnie GB, Cowan RG, Wade NA: Intravenous immune globulin treatment of pulmonary exacerbation in cystic fibrosis. J Pediatr 114:309, 1989.

Wood A: Airway mucosal bioelectrical potential difference in cystic fibrosis after lung transplantation. Am Rev Respir Dis 140:1645, 1989.

Yacoub MH, et al: Heart lung transplantation for cystic fibrosis and subsequent domino heart transplantation. J Heart Transplant 9:459, 1990.

Zach MS: Lung disease in cystic fibrosis—an updated concept. Pediatr Pulmonol 8:188, 1990.

Zach MS, Oberwaldner B: Chest physiotherapy—The mechanical approach to anti-infective therapy in cystic fibrosis. Infection 5:381, 1987.

Zeitlin PL: Therapies directed at the basic defect in cystic fibrosis. Clin Chest Med 19:515, 1998.

Zuckerman JB, Kotloff RM: Lung transplantation in cystic fibrosis. Clin Chest Med 19:535, 1998.

READING REFERENCES

Davis PB (ed): Cystic Fibrosis. New York: Marcel Dekker, 1993.

Dodge JA, Brock DJH, Widdicombe JH (eds): Cystic Fibrosis—Current Topics. Chichester: John Wiley & Sons, 1993.

Marcus CL, et al: Supplemental oxygen and exercise performance in patients with cystic fibrosis with severe pulmonary disease. Chest 101:52, 1992.

Moss RB (ed): Cystic Fibrosis—Infection, Immunopathology, and Host Response. Clifton NJ: Humana Press, 1990.

Olsen MM, et al: Surgery in patients with cystic fibrosis. J Pediatr Surg 22:613, 1987.

Orenstein DA, et al: Exercise conditioning and cardiopulmonary fitness in cystic fibrosis. Chest 80:392, 1981.

CHAPTER 81

Congenital Vascular Lesions of the Lungs

Thomas W. Shields

The incidence of congenital vascular malformations of the lung is low despite the complex embryologic derivation of the pulmonary vasculature (see Chapter 2). Some of the anomalies can be associated with significant disability and still be amenable to appropriate surgical management. A classification of congenital abnormalities that affect the main branches of the pulmonary vessels and their tributaries was suggested by Ellis and associates (1964) and has been modified for completeness (Table 81-1). Although arbitrary, such a classification encourages more accurate diagnostic delineations of such defects, which may lead to eventual surgical repair in many.

AGENESIS AND STENOSIS OF THE PULMONARY ARTERY

Agenesis and stenosis of pulmonary arteries are rare but provide unusual challenges in diagnosis and management. Most affected persons with these defects die at an early age from right-sided ventricular failure and hypertension in the pulmonary artery of the unaffected side. A few patients are asymptomatic or are hampered by some dyspnea and recurrent pulmonary infections. The natural history of the anomaly is not well understood. Gregg (1941) reported that these anomalies are associated with maternal rubella.

In this abnormality, the affected lung has a small volume and decreased markings (the hyperlucent lung syndrome) (Fig. 81-1). The thoracic cage is contracted and ventilation is reduced. Ventilation-perfusion scans demonstrate vascular hypoperfusion, and decreased ventilation and obstructive bronchiolar disease can be demonstrated with bronchographic contrast material. Angiocardiography delineates the pulmonary artery anomaly. Stenosis of the pulmonary artery may occur at its origin (Fig. 81-2) or at isolated, multiple peripheral sites. In agenesis of the pulmonary artery, an anomalous artery from the aorta (Fig. 81-3) usually supplies the involved lung, but dilated bronchial arteries may be the main source of the blood that maintains some viability of the affected lung.

Surgical treatment has been reported uncommonly, and although McGoon and Kincaid (1964) reported repair of multiple peripheral areas of stenosis, most have been at the origin of either main stem artery. The success of patch arterioplasty or graft replacement of absent or stenosed pulmonary arteries depends largely on the extent of the vascular anomaly and the degree of bronchial and parenchymal lung damage secondary to infection and fibrosis. Dilatation by balloons has proved to be successful in certain cases of isolated, discrete stenosis of pulmonary arteries. Rocchini and associates (1984) reported that balloon dilation may be the procedure of choice for multiple stenotic lesions. In older patients with unilateral agenesis of the pulmonary artery, persistent respiratory infection is the most prominent complaint. Pneumonectomy is usually required, and care to identify and control any systemic artery to the lung is mandatory. Canver and colleagues (1991) reported the necessity of a pneumonectomy in a neonate with agenesis of the right pulmonary artery who developed an uncontrollable necrotizing bronchopneumonia in the involved lung. This, as these authors noted, is an unusual complication in the infant or child with this disorder.

PULMONARY ARTERIOVENOUS FISTULAS

Pulmonary arteriovenous fistulas are congenital malformations that result from errant capillary development, with incomplete formation or disintegration of the vascular septa that normally divide the primitive connections between the venous and arterial plexuses. Tobin (1966) verified that some pulmonary arteriovenous shunting exists in normal lungs. This shunting may be hemodynamically important in pathologic conditions associated with venous or arterial pulmonary hypertension, portal cirrhosis, and obstructive lung disease.

Table 81-1. Classification of Congenital Vascular Lesions of the Lung

Abnormalities of the pulmonary circulation
    Pulmonary arteries
        Agenesis of a pulmonary artery
        Stenosis of a branch or branches of the pulmonary arteries
        Pulmonary arteriovenous fistula
    Pulmonary veins
        Abnormal pulmonary venous connection
        Varicosities of the pulmonary veins
    Lymphangiectasia

Modified from Ellis FH, McGoon DC, Kincaid OW: Congenital vascular malformations of the lungs. Med Clin North Am *48*:1069, 1974.

Classification

A review of the embryology of the pulmonary vascular system indicates that pulmonary arteriovenous abnormalities may occur as isolated or combined lesions at the arterial, capillary, or venous level. Anabtawi and colleagues (1965) presented an anatomic classification based on the size and position of arteriovenous communications (Table 81-2). The classification according to the blood supply has both hemodynamic and prognostic importance because the fistulas supplied by systemic arteries have the same hemodynamic consequences as arteriovenous fistulas of the gen-

eral circulation have. Also, as Dines and associates (1974) noted, it is important to divide the entire group into those associated with Rendu-Osler-Weber disease (ROWD), also called hereditary hemorrhagic telangiectasis (HHT), and those not associated with it, because this stratification has important prognostic value. Patients with cutaneous telangiectasis (ROWD) more often have multiple pulmonary fistulas, a predictable progression of symptoms, and a higher rate of complications.

Patients with HHT have a high incidence of multiple organs involved with telangiectases: the skin, mucous membranes of the nose, lungs, brain, gastrointestinal tract, and liver. The organ involvement occurs in various combinations, and the sites of involvement appear to be governed by the underlying genetic defect. At present, at least three different phenotypes have been identified. Type I is related to a defect at chromosome 9q33-34 that relates to protein product endoglin, transforming growth factor-β (TGF-β) receptor, and mutation and is most often associated with pulmonary arteriovenous malformations. This specific phenotype has been described by Heutink and associates (1994). Type II, described by Porteous (1994) and McAllister (1994) and their coworkers, is related to chromosome 3q22, which also codes for a transforming growth factor-βII receptor and is associated, although less frequently, with pulmonary arteriovenous fistulae. Type III is related to chromosome 12q (the complete phenotype is not yet known) and was described by Vincent and colleagues (1995). This latter

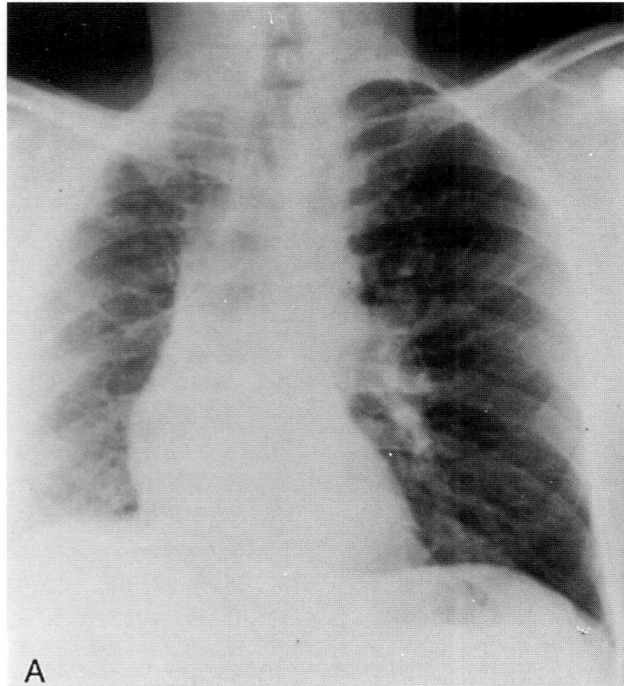
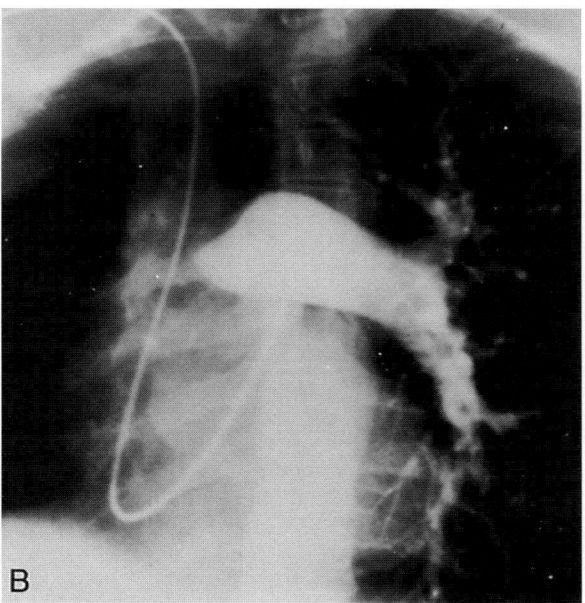

Fig. 81-1. Sawyer-James syndrome. **A.** Posteroanterior chest radiograph demonstrating small right lung with decreased vascular markings. **B.** Pulmonary angiogram in a patient with agenesis of the right pulmonary artery and minimal vascular markings (hyperlucent lung syndrome).

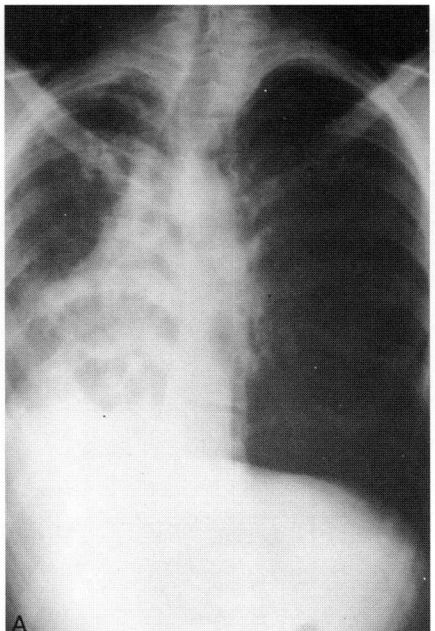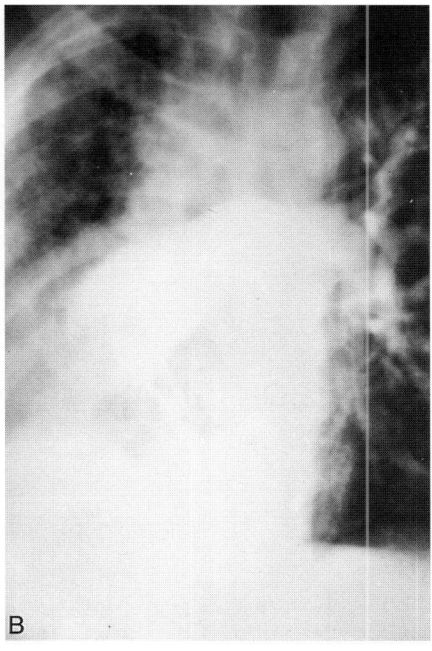

Fig. 81-2. A. Posteroanterior chest radiograph of young adult man with severe pulmonary infection in the right lung with marked shift of the mediastinum and heart into the right hemithorax. **B.** Angiogram revealing agenesis of the right pulmonary artery.

phenotype does not appear to be associated with pulmonary arteriovenous malformations.

Pulmonary Arteriovenous Fistulas with Pulmonary Arterial Supply

Clinical Aspects

Congenital pulmonary arteriovenous fistulas occur more frequently in women and are transmitted as a dominant gene with incomplete penetrance. Hodgson and Kaye (1963) reported a family that had hereditary hemorrhagic telangiectasis; 6.4% of those surveyed radiographically had pulmonary arteriovenous fistulas. Jeresaty and associates (1966) reported that symptoms began in childhood and consisted of dyspnea and easy fatigability in 25 to 50% of patients. In patients with HHT, epistaxis is an early sign and may begin in adolescence. It eventually is observed in up to 85% of the afflicted patients. Other frequent extrapulmonary symptoms and signs are headaches in 43%, transient ischemic attacks in 57%, and cerebral vascular accidents in 18%, as noted by Goodenberger (1998).

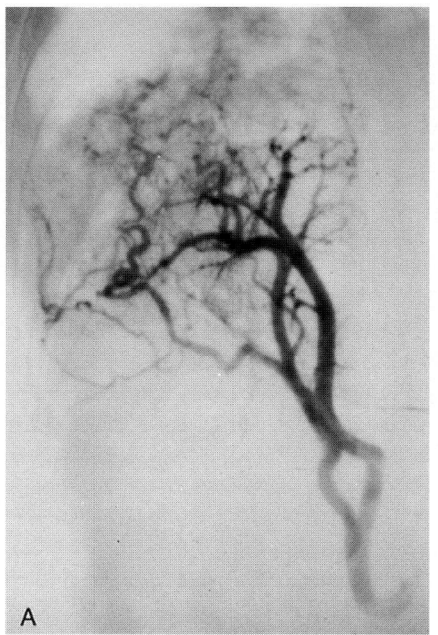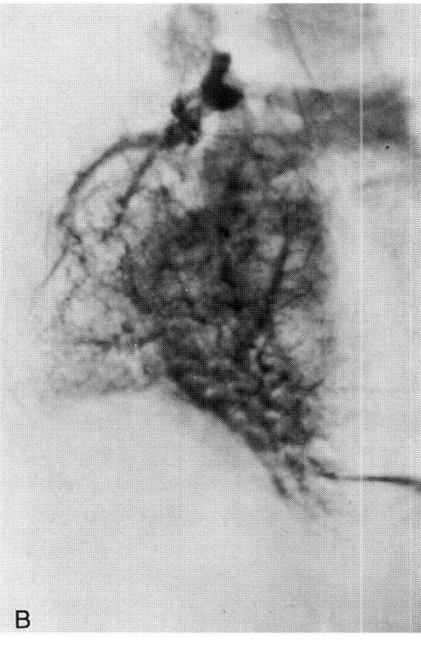

Fig. 81-3. A. This aortogram of the patient shown in Figure 81-2 demonstrates a large ectopic systemic artery that supplies the lower portion of the right lung and that arises from the subdiaphragmatic portion of the aorta. **B.** Delayed radiograph showing venous drainage through normal right pulmonary veins.

Table 81-2. Classification of Pulmonary Arteriovenous Malformations

I	Multiple small arteriovenous fistulas without aneurysm
II	Large single arteriovenous aneurysm, peripheral
IIIa	Large single arteriovenous aneurysm, central
IIIb	Large arteriovenous aneurysm with anomalous venous drainage
IIIc	Multiple small arteriovenous fistulas with anomalous venous drainage
IVa	Large single venous aneurysm with systemic artery communication
IVb	Large single venous aneurysm without fistula, varix of pulmonary vein
V	Anomalous venous drainage without fistula

Adapted from Anabtawi IN, Ellison RG, Ellison LT: Pulmonary arteriovenous aneurysms and fistulas: anatomic variations, embryology, and classification. Ann Thorac Surg *1*:277, 1965.

Exertional dyspnea, palpitations, and easy fatigability are the most frequent symptoms, usually appearing in the third or fourth decade of life and present in approximately 50% of patients. Hemoptysis is common when the fistula is associated with cutaneous telangiectasis (ROWD). A continuous bruit is present over the lesion in 75% of patients who have associated hereditary telangiectasis and in 38% of those who are without such an association. The typical bruit has a rough, humming, continuous sound that is accentuated in systole and with deep inspiration; the diastolic accentuation is more subtle. The audibility of the bruit can change with position. It may be associated with mitral valve prolapse in these patients.

The classic triad of cyanosis, polycythemia, and clubbing of the fingers or toes has been noted in approximately 20% of the patients. The presence of cyanosis indicates that at least 25 to 30% of the blood in the lesser circulation is being shunted from the right to the left side of the heart through the fistula.

Physiologic Findings

PO_2 and oxygen saturation are decreased. Intracardiac and intravascular pressure proximal to the fistula are normal; as a result, the cardiac output is usually normal, although it may be increased at times. The systemic blood pressure and the electrocardiographic findings are also normal. The heart is usually not enlarged. Blood volume study results reveal an increased red cell mass in most cases. The plasma volume remains normal.

Radiographic Features

In one-half to two-thirds of the patients, the fistulas are single. The remainder are multiple and may be bilateral in 8 to 10% of the patients. Radiographs of the chest show the fistulas as lobulated, fairly well-defined densities connected to the hilar structures by broad linear shadows because of

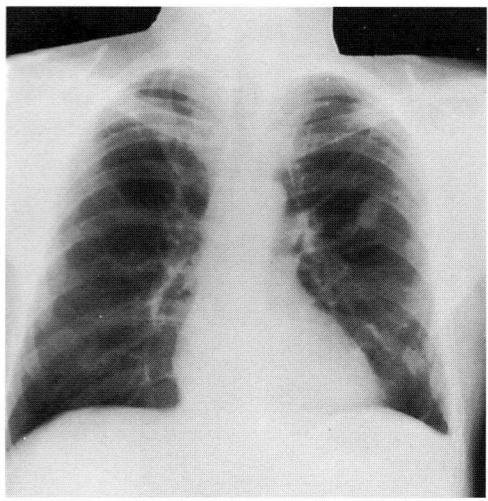

Fig. 81-4. Arteriovenous fistula in the left upper lobe with vascular connections to left hilus.

the dilated vascular connections (Fig. 81-4). Eighty percent of the lesions are subpleural or superficial. Usually, fistulas are seen more frequently in the lower than in the upper lobes. A solitary lesion initially may be interpreted as a solitary pulmonary nodule, but the characteristic lobulation (the *Mickey Mouse sign*; L Sider, personal communication, 1993) (Fig. 81-5) should alert one to the true nature of the lesion. On fluoroscopy, they may be seen to pulsate or become

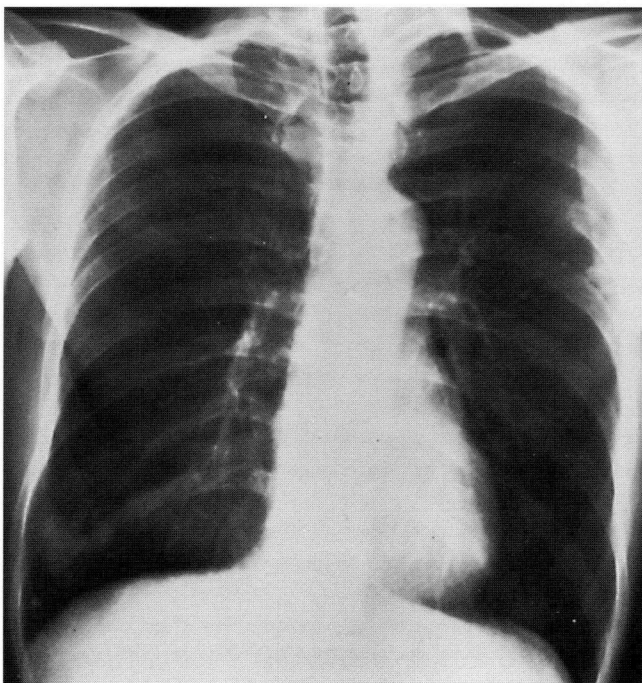

Fig. 81-5. Posteroanterior radiograph of the chest revealing a lobulated mass in the lower right lung field. The mass has a *Mickey Mouse* configuration. The arteriovenous malformation was confirmed on computed tomographic examination.

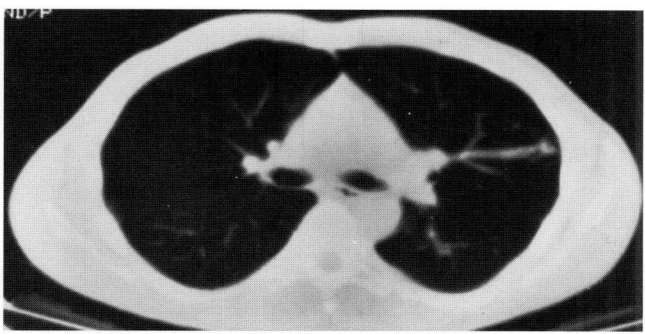

Fig. 81-6. Contrast-enhanced computed tomographic scan of the same patient as shown in Figure 81-5 showing a different level from the mass seen in the radiograph reveals several additional arteriovenous malformations in the left lung. The vascular connection to the venous system is clearly demarcated.

smaller with the Valsalva maneuver. Also on fluoroscopy, because of the increased blood flow, there may be an increased amplitude of pulsation of the hilar vessels. Computed tomography (CT) usually demonstrates the lesion sufficiently well to be diagnostic (Fig. 81-6). Remy and associates (1992) reported that CT enabled identification of 98.2% of 109 pulmonary arteriovenous fistulas in 40 patients versus only 59.6% identified by angiography (Fig. 81-7). Angiography, however, is more reliable in the analysis of the angioarchitecture and is a necessary follow-up of the CT scan in those patients who are to undergo interventional management of the fistula(s). Helical CT is also an excellent diagnostic tool and may eventually obviate the need for angiography.

Additional Diagnostic Studies

Burke and Raffin (1986) suggested the use of noninvasive studies before the use of pulmonary angiography in patients suspected of having pulmonary arteriovenous fistulas. These studies include contrast echocardiography, described by

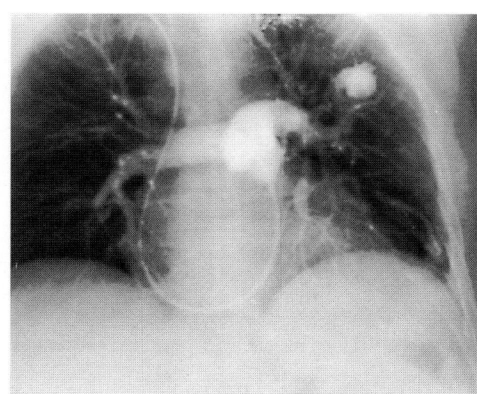

Fig. 81-7. Angiocardiogram delineating multiple arteriovenous fistulas: a large fistula in left upper lobe and an additional fistula in the left lower lobe.

Shub and associates (1976), and perfusion lung scintigraphy, reported by Lewis and colleagues (1978). A negative result excludes the presence of right-to-left shunt and thus excludes the presence of a fistula. A positive result confirms the suspected diagnosis without risk to the patient. In addition, perfusion lung scintigraphy provides a quantitative estimation of the magnitude of the shunt. With the reliability of CT scans, as noted by Remy and associates (1992), it would appear that neither of these examinations is necessary nor would they supplant the use of contrast angiography in patients who are candidates for invasive therapy.

Complications

Stringer and associates (1955) reported 30 instances of serious complications or death among 140 patients with pulmonary arteriovenous fistulas. Dalton and coworkers (1967) recorded nine instances of intrapleural rupture. Others including Iwabuchi and colleagues (1993) have noted the occurrence of this potentially fatal complication. Takenaka and associates (1996) reported the successful resection of the offending fistula in a patient who developed a massive left-sided hemothorax. In addition, these authors reviewed eight additional successful resections of ruptured fistulae reported in the Japanese literature. Massive hemoptysis is uncommon. White (1984) noted that paradoxic embolization and stroke as the result of a bland embolus to the brain may occur. Dines and associates (1974) observed a stroke to have occurred in 10% of all untreated patients followed for 4 to 10 years in whom a pulmonary arteriovenous fistula was seen on the radiograph or if there was hypoxemia on room air. Cerebral abscesses also have been reported, but none of 96 patients reported by Dines and colleagues (1983) had cerebral abscess or intrapleural rupture. The report of Puskas and colleagues (1994) noted the occurrence of a brain abscess in several of their patients who were untreated or who had a failed previous balloon occlusion of a pulmonary arteriovenous malformation. Yeung and associates (1995) have observed that neurologic manifestations, especially in those patients with ROWD, occur in 4 to 12% of the cases.

Treatment

Most patients with one or more pulmonary arteriovenous fistulas are candidates for resection or obliteration of the lesions. Only those few who have a small lesion (10 to 15 mm in diameter) and who are asymptomatic with a minimal shunt may be observed. In this subset, however, the risk of paradoxic embolization is present, as previously noted. In patients with ROWD, treatment is indicated in all patients, if at all possible, because the complication rate is highest in this group. Interventional therapy is likewise indicated in all symptomatic patients and even in those whose symptoms are minimal if the lesion can be identified on the standard chest radiographs or CT scans or if hypoxemia is present when the patient breathes room air.

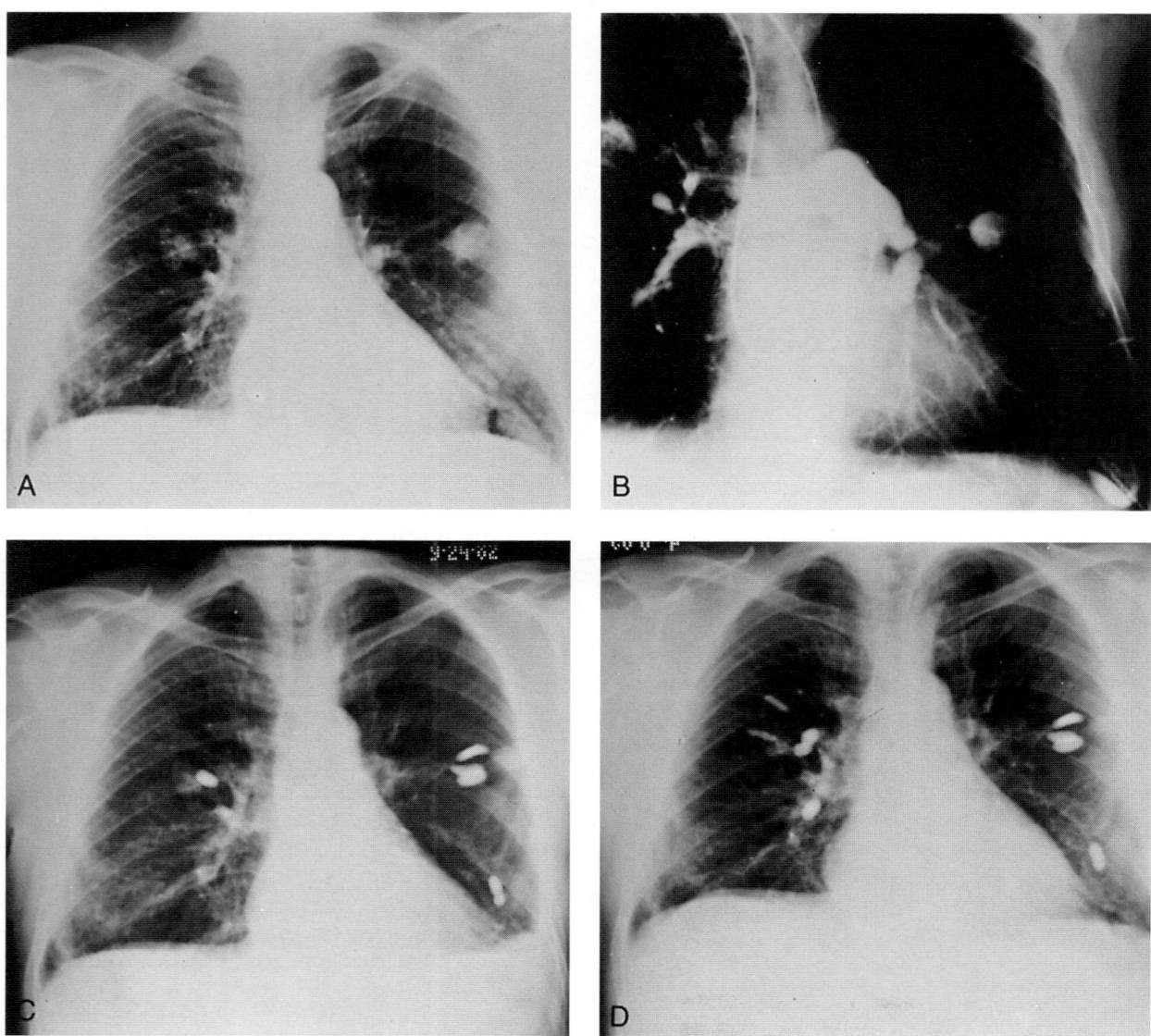

Fig. 81-8. A. Posteroanterior radiograph of a 64-year-old white man with multiple bilateral pulmonary infiltrates, frequent nosebleeds, a Po$_2$ of 52 mm Hg, and increasing shortness of breath. **B.** Pulmonary angiogram revealing multiple bilateral pulmonary arterial venous fistulas. **C.** Posteroanterior radiograph in August 1982 after balloon embolization of a number of the fistulas by R. I. White, Jr., of Johns Hopkins University, with moderate symptomatic improvement. **D.** Posteroanterior radiograph in March 1983 following balloon embolization of remaining arteriovenous fistulas, with complete relief of previous dyspnea and return of oxygen saturation and Po$_2$ levels to normal on room air. Courtesy of R. E. Otto.

Single lesions are best managed by conservative surgical excision. Some multiple lesions also may be treated by excision, but most patients with multiple or bilateral lesions are best managed by radiographically guided embolization.

Surgical Therapy

Surgical excision of an isolated, single pulmonary arteriovenous fistula is successful, with minimal mortality and morbidity and little chance of recurrence of the lesion. Surgical excision is the procedure of choice when it can be accomplished. Because most fistulas are located subpleurally, they can be removed with conservative local resections. In difficult cases in which the feeding vessel is not definitely localized preoperatively, Almeida and colleagues (1998) suggest the use of transesophageal echocardiography with agitated blood and saline contrast during the procedure in order to assist in localizing the vessel. Puskas and associates (1994) reported the successful excision of a solitary arteriovenous fistula in nine patients; one patient had staged excision of bilateral lesions. All patients were relieved of dyspnea, and no recurrences or neurologic complications occurred in the follow-up of these patients. As noted, multiple fistulas are occasionally suitable for resection. Patients with symptoms and one or more enlarging fistulas are candidates for operation. Dines and associates (1974) suggested that patients with a single fistula and HHT should be operated on because enlargement, symptoms, and complications are more frequent. Sperling and colleagues (1977) reported, however, that the combination of pulmonary hypertension and arteriovenous fistulas is a contraindication for surgical excision.

Embolic Obliteration

Selective radiographically guided embolization of multiple pulmonary arteriovenous fistulas unsuitable for surgical resection has proved to be a valuable therapeutic modality. The patients with multiple lesions are frequently severely disabled by the presence of a large right-to-left shunt, and occlusion of the multiple fistulas permits a return to a near-normal status.

Taylor and associates (1978) first reported therapeutic embolization of the fistula by pulmonary arterial catheterization and the use of small steel guidewires with 3-cm wool tails. Tadavarthy and colleagues (1975) had described the use of polyvinyl alcohol sponge (Ivalon) as an embolic agent, but its use has been infrequent in the management of pulmonary arteriovenous fistulas. The popular materials used at present are detachable silicone balloons devised by White and coworkers (1980) (Fig. 81-8) and stainless steel coils introduced by Gianturco and associates (1975).

The occluding element is placed precisely into the feeding pulmonary arterial branch beyond all of the artery's normal branches to the lung. Proper placement is guided by video monitoring, digital subtraction angiography, or both. White (1983) described his technique and pointed out that approximately 79% of the fistulas have a single feeding artery and a single draining vein, so occlusion is relatively easy to achieve; the remaining 21% have two or more feeding and draining branches, which makes the embolization process more difficult. Anderson and colleagues (1979) and Hatfield and Fried (1981) described the successful use of the Gianturco mini stainless steel coil in patients with multiple fistulas. These coils (Fig. 81-9) cause clotting and obstruction of the fistula and can be seen on the postprocedure chest film (Fig. 81-10). Hartnell and Allison (1989) have detailed the technique of coil embolization in the management of these lesions.

With proper technique and experience, the results are gratifying. With permanent occlusion of the fistulas by either of the occluding elements, the hypoxemia is corrected. White and colleagues (1988) reported persistent relief of hypoxemia and only minimal growth of small remaining arteriovenous malformations after 5 years of

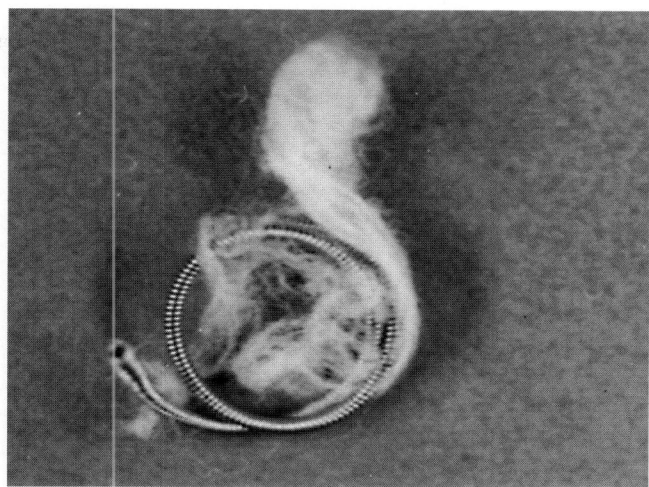

Fig. 81-9. Stainless steel coil that can be inserted via cardiac catheter to occlude and thrombose a pulmonary arteriovenous fistula.

follow-up. The low "recurrence" rates were also noted by Remy and associates (1992). Chilvers and colleagues (1990), however, pointed out that blood flow through small residual, nonoccluded malformations could account for the persistence of right-to-left shunts after occlusion of the malformations with larger feed vessels identified by angiographic study. Minimal pulmonary infarction may occur postocclusion, and chest pain may be troublesome early. Haitjema and associates (1995) reported that in a series of embolizations in 32 patients, postembolization pulmonary infarction or pleurisy occurred in 11% of the patients and occasional systemic embolism or cardiac arrhythmias were observed. More important, late recanalization occurred in 5 to 10% of the patients. Late neurologic complications have been noted by Puskas and colleagues (1994) in some patients who have undergone previous balloon occlusion. Of interest was these authors' observation of the disappearance of the occluding balloon in several patients. The fate of the previously present occluding balloon remained unknown, even in the patients in whom the arteriovenous malformation was subsequently removed surgically. Despite these criticisms raised by the aforementioned reports, Lee and associates (1997), of White's group, reiterated their strong support for the use of embolization for the management of pulmonary arteriovenous malformations; not only those with small feeding vessels but those with large ones as well. They reported that in the treatment of 221 consecutive patients with pulmonary arteriovenous malformations, 45 patients with 52 lesions resupplied by feeding arteries 8 mm in diameter or larger were managed successfully. Thirty-eight patients had 44 pulmonary arteriovenous malformations cured by the first attempt at embolization by either a balloon, a coil, or both. They agree that complications are seen: pleurisy in 31%, angina in 2%, and paradoxical embolization of a device during deployment in 4%; all of these events were self-limiting. Seven patients (11%) had persistence of the shunt because of recanalization or later

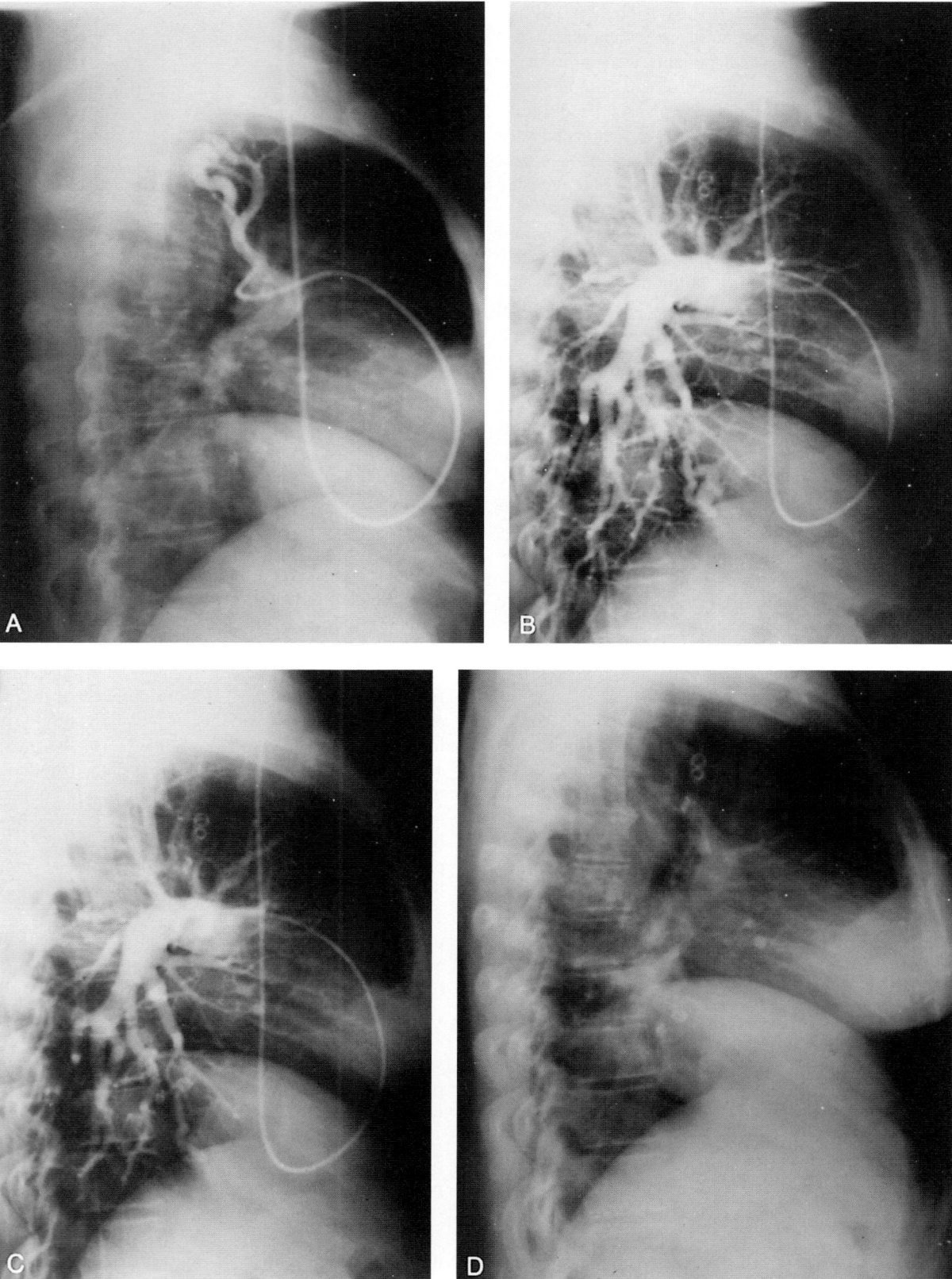

Fig. 81-10. A. Lateral view of pulmonary angiogram with selective demonstration of an upper lobe arteriovenous fistula in a patient with multiple fistulas and Rendu-Osler-Weber syndrome. **B.** The same patient with a nonselective pulmonary angiogram that demonstrates occlusion of the upper lobe fistula by the coil, which is visible on the film, and demonstration of a second fistula in the lower lobe. **C.** The same patient with both upper and lower lobe fistulas occluded by coils. **D.** The same patient's lateral chest film demonstrating multiple coils that have been used to occlude fistulas.

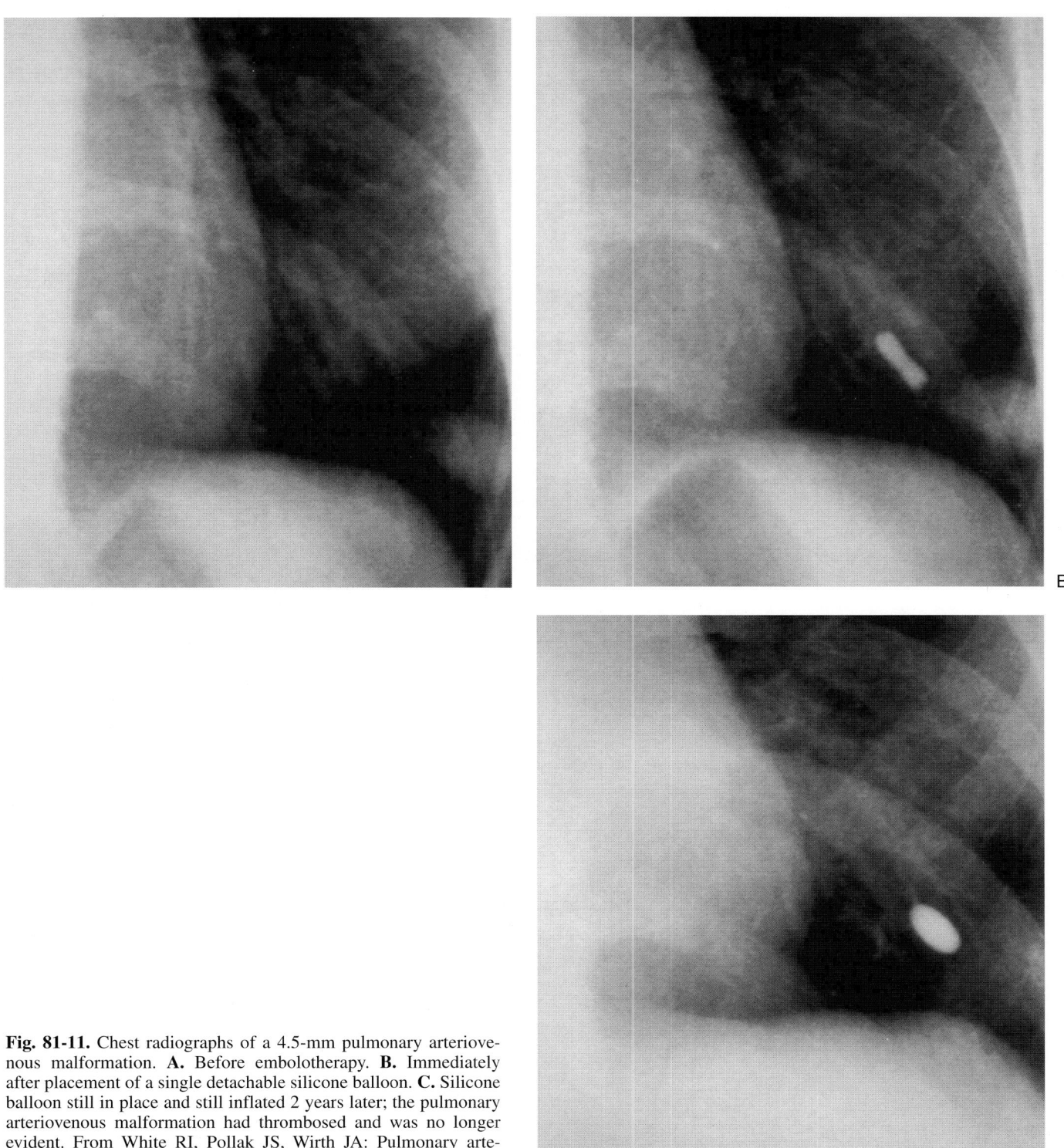

Fig. 81-11. Chest radiographs of a 4.5-mm pulmonary arteriovenous malformation. **A.** Before embolotherapy. **B.** Immediately after placement of a single detachable silicone balloon. **C.** Silicone balloon still in place and still inflated 2 years later; the pulmonary arteriovenous malformation had thrombosed and was no longer evident. From White RI, Pollak JS, Wirth JA: Pulmonary arteriovenous malformations: diagnosis and transcatheter embolotherapy. J Vasc Intervent Radiol 7:787, 1996. With permission.

ingrowth of an accessory artery; these patients were managed by a second or third procedure. They reported that a latex balloon usually deflates within a month because of slow leakage but that the deflated balloon remains in place and the fistula does not recur because thrombosis of the feeding vessel usually occurs within 20 days. However,

White (personal communication, 1998) no longer uses the latex balloon but only uses the silicone variety. When filled with iso-osmotic solution the silicone balloon remains inflated for at least 2 years and at times as long as 3 years (Fig. 81-11). White and Pollak (1994) did not observe the occurrence of a brain abscess or stroke in any of their patients.

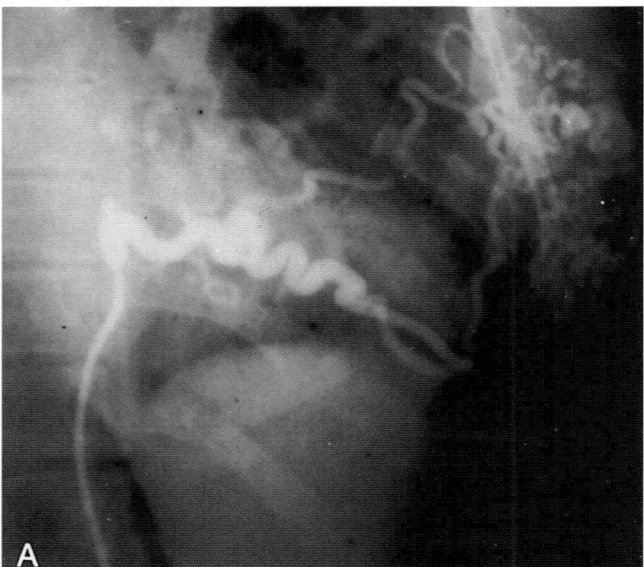

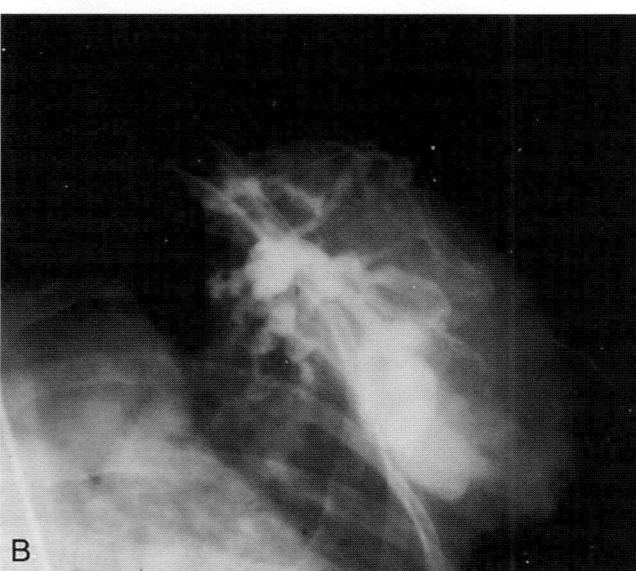

Fig. 81-12. A. Selective angiogram of an intercostal artery of a patient with a large systemic arteriovenous fistula of the chest wall. The fistula was draining into the lung. The patient had high-output congestive failure and was refractory to any occlusive therapy or surgical therapy of these multiple communications. **B.** Venous phase of the arteriovenous fistulas demonstrating drainage into the lung with rapid run-off into the pulmonary venous system.

Systemic Pulmonary Arteriovenous Fistulas

Pulmonary arteriovenous fistulas that have a systemic blood supply are rare. The bronchial arteries, internal mammary arteries, or aorta are the primary and immediate sources of the systemic arterial blood. Resection is indicated, although the extensive collateral circulation in the chest wall may provide formidable technical challenges. Involvement adjacent to the spinal column may preclude

complete resection, but partial resection of the systemic arterial sources of blood, in particular, removes the threat of serious hemorrhagic and hemodynamic complications of high-output congestive failure (Fig. 81-12).

PULMONARY ARTERY ANEURYSMS

Aneurysmal dilatation of the pulmonary artery secondary to associated congenital cardiovascular anomalies is not a rare entity, but true aneurysms of this vessel secondary to disintegration of its wall are indeed rare. Aneurysms consequent to long-standing hypertension or high pulmonary blood flow are associated most frequently with patent ductus arteriosus and by definition would be acquired and not congenital. This problem of etiology is not easily solved. Natelson and associates (1970) described aneurysms secondary to cystic medial necrosis of the pulmonary arteries that have caused striking clinicopathologic findings related to pulmonary hypertension, dissection, and rupture of the vessel. Ungaro and associates (1976) classified pulmonary artery aneurysms into specific causes (i.e., tuberculosis, syphilis, trauma) and nonspecific causes (i.e., mycotic, pulmonary hypertension, arteriosclerotic, those related to congenital defects in the vessel wall, and iatrogenic). Most so-called congenital aneurysms of the pulmonary artery, although acquired, are associated with some other congenital anomaly. Because the truly peripheral and often solitary aneurysms rupture in as many as 60% of patients, Ungaro and colleagues (1976) emphasized the necessity of definitive diagnosis and early treatment. Conservative pulmonary resection usually suffices.

Significant dilatation of both the right and the left pulmonary arteries may be present with isolated pulmonary valvular insufficiency or may be associated with the tetralogy of Fallot. This anomaly may result in the so-called Mickey Mouse heart, a sign named for its distinctive appearance on a plain chest film. This aneurysmal dilatation can cause airway problems with pressure on one or both main stem bronchi. Pierce and associates (1970) reported that an emphysematous lobe may be associated with pulmonary artery aneurysm of any etiology. Frequently, correction of the pulmonary valvular insufficiency by conduit replacement may remedy the problem, but resection of the enlarged vessels may be needed to cure the airway problems. Murphy and colleagues (1987) reported successful resection of a peripheral artery aneurysm using cardiopulmonary bypass.

PULMONARY VARIX

An isolated pulmonary varix (aneurysmal dilatation) is rare, and fewer than 50 cases have been reported. The cause of these varices is unknown, but a varix may be congenital. Steinberg (1967) reported that an enlarged variceal central portion of a pulmonary vein can be mistaken for either pulmonary or hilar

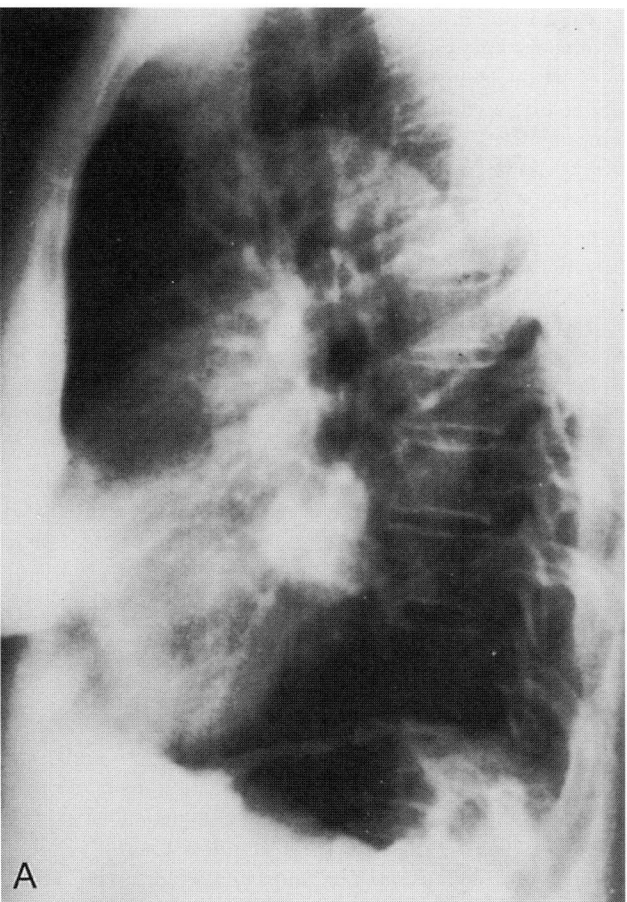 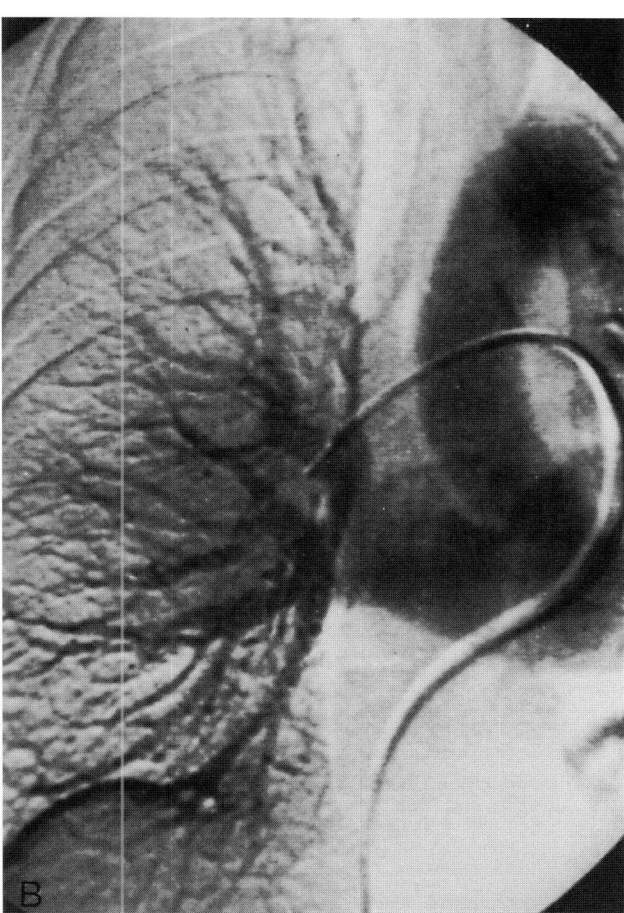

Fig. 81-13. A. Lateral radiograph of the chest of an asymptomatic 69-year-old woman with a perihilar mass. Computed tomographic scan revealed a lobulated mass in the posterior hilum. **B.** Angiogram revealed filling of large pulmonary varix in the venous phase. From Mannes GPM, van der Jagt E, Postmus PE: An asymptomatic hilar mass. Chest *101*:553, 1992. With permission.

disease on the standard chest radiographs. Batram and Strickland (1971), as well as others, have reconfirmed this impression. The patient with a pulmonary varix most often presents with an asymptomatic perihilar or hilar mass discovered on an incidental chest radiograph. Lobulation of the central mass may be present. The presence of calcification has not been reported. Rarely, complications such as systemic emboli that are caused by the release of clots from within the varix or, even more infrequently, bleeding into the bronchial tree or pleural space that is caused by rupture of the varix may occur. On the standard radiographs, an initially indeterminate perihilar or a hilar mass may be recognized (Fig. 81-13). The diagnosis, if suspected, may be supported by changes in size of the lesion on fluoroscopy when the patient performs Valsalva and Müller maneuvers. The diagnosis is confirmed by angiography, and according to Mannes and associates (1992), five characteristic features are present: 1) the arterial phase is normal without shunting, 2) the varix fills in the venous phase, 3) the varix drains directly into the left atrium, 4) emptying of the varix is delayed, and 5) the varix affects only the proximal portion of the vein. The value of CT scan or magnetic resonance imaging

in the diagnosis of this lesion has not been reported. A pulmonary varix requires no treatment. Unfortunately, the nature of the mass often is unrecognized preoperatively, and an unnecessary thoracotomy is done.

ABNORMAL PULMONARY VENOUS CONNECTION

A complete discussion of anomalous pulmonary venous connections is beyond the scope of this text.

Anomalous venous drainage of the right lung into the inferior vena cava (the scimitar syndrome), however, is often associated with bronchial anomalies, hypoplasia, and abnormal systemic arterial supply of the right lung. Although the abnormal left-to-right shunt may be the major cause of clinical problems in most patients with the syndrome, pulmonary symptoms, often of chronic severe pulmonary infection, may be the dominant clinical feature. Thus, consideration of the syndrome is important to the general thoracic surgeon.

Scimitar Syndrome

Scimitar syndrome consists of a constellation of abnormalities, the constant being total or partial anomalous pulmonary venous drainage of the right lung to the inferior vena cava. Neill and associates (1960) emphasized that the gently curved vertical shape of this vein on a chest radiograph resembles the curved Turkish sword or scimitar. Associated findings that may or may not be present are dextroposition of the heart, hypoplasia of the right lung and right pulmonary artery, malformation of the bronchial tree, and anomalous systemic arteries to the right lung from the abdominal aorta or its branches. Trell and colleagues (1971) reported that intracardiac defects are present in up to 40% of these patients.

Symptoms are related to the degree of left-to-right shunting, pulmonary hypertension, parenchymal lung disease, and associated intracardiac lesions. Kiely and coworkers (1967) documented in 70 cases that the more common symptoms were fatigue, dyspnea, decreased exercise tolerance, cough, recurrent respiratory tract infections, and failure to thrive. Chest radiography shows a small right lung, cardiac displacement to the right, and the shadow of the anomalous vein (Fig. 81-14). Electrocardiography reveals right ventricular hypertrophy. Echocardiography is useful in identifying associated intracardiac lesions and the location of the anomalous vein penetrating the diaphragm. Cardiac catheterization and angiocardiography are diagnostic.

The decision for operative intervention must be individualized depending on the degree of symptoms and the findings at cardiac catheterization. For large left-to-right shunts, physiologic correction is preferred. Kirklin and associates (1956) reported that either the anomalous vessel can be anastomosed directly to the left atrium or an intracardiac patch can be used to tunnel the flow from the anomalous vein to the left atrium through an atrial septal defect. Sanger and colleagues (1963) suggested that if inflammatory parenchymal changes are extensive, pulmonary resection or pneumonectomy should be considered. Resection eliminates the left-to-right shunt as well as the lung infection. In all instances, the systemic arterial supply to the lung is divided.

Results depend chiefly on the degree of preoperative pulmonary hypertension and associated cardiac lesions. Older patients with minimal symptoms have an excellent prognosis. Canter and associates (1986) pointed out that infants with cyanosis, failure to thrive, and severe pulmonary hypertension have a high mortality.

LYMPHANGIECTASIA

Primary pulmonary lymphangiectasia does occur or may be associated with generalized lymphangiectasia. Noonan and coworkers (1970) reported that this anomaly is associated with a syndrome that consists of pulmonary stenosis, atrial septal defect, and mental retardation. This anomaly also has been reported as a familial lesion by Scott-Emuakpor and associates (1981). Chest radiography may show a pattern similar to hyaline membrane disease or may show cystic infiltrates. The patients may develop pleural effusions or chylothorax that require drainage. The only therapy is supportive, and the disease is usually progressive and fatal.

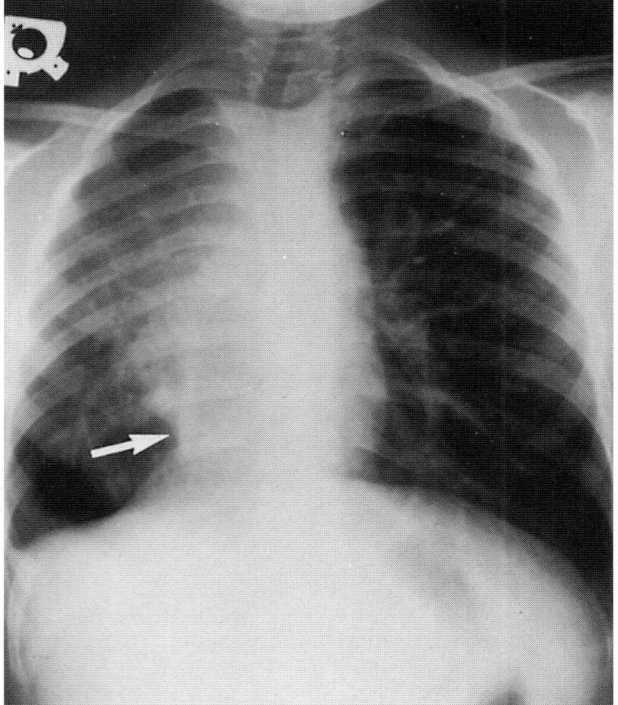

Fig. 81-14. Chest radiograph of a child with scimitar syndrome. Arrow points to the anomalous vein, which resembles a Turkish saber. Note the dextroposition of the heart and hypoplasia of the right lung.

REFERENCES

Almeida AA, et al: Transesophageal echocardiography in an operation for pulmonary arteriovenous malformations. Ann Thorac Surg 65:267, 1998.

Anabtawi IN, Ellison RG, Ellison LT: Pulmonary arteriovenous aneurysms and fistulas: anatomical variations, embryology, and classification. Ann Thorac Surg 1:277, 1965.

Anderson JH, et al: "Mini" Gianturco stainless steel coils for transcatheter vascular occlusion. Radiology 132:301, 1979.

Batram C, Strickland B: Pulmonary varices. Br J Radiol 44:927, 1971.

Burke CM, Raffin TA: Pulmonary arteriovenous malformations, aneurysms, and reflections. Chest 89:771, 1986.

Canter CE, et al: Scimitar syndrome in childhood. Am J Cardiol 58:652, 1986.

Canver CC, Pigott JD, Mentzer RM Jr: Neonatal pneumonectomy for isolated unilateral pulmonary artery agenesis. Ann Thorac Surg 52:294, 1991.

Chilvers ER, et al: Effect of percutaneous transcatheter embolization on pulmonary function, right-to-left shunt and arterial oxygenation in patients with pulmonary arteriovenous malformations. Am Rev Respir Dis 142:420, 1990.

Dalton ML Jr, et al: Intrapleural rupture of pulmonary arteriovenous aneurysm: report of a case. Chest 52:97, 1967.

Dines DE, et al: Pulmonary arteriovenous fistulas. Mayo Clin Proc 49:460, 1974.

Dines DE, et al: Pulmonary arteriovenous fistulas. Mayo Clin Proc 58:176, 1983.

Gianturco C, Anderson JH, Wallace S: Mechanical devices for arterial occlusion. Am J Roentgenol 124:428, 1975.

Goodenberger DM: Pulmonary arteriovenous malformations. In Fishman AP, et al (eds): Fishman's Pulmonary Diseases and Disorders. 3rd Ed. New York: McGraw-Hill, 1998.

Gregg NM: Congenital cataract following German measles in the mother. Trans Ophthalmol Soc Australia 3:35, 1941.

Haitjema TJ, et al: Embolisation of pulmonary arteriovenous malformations: results and follow up in 32 patients. Thorax 50:719, 1995.

Hartnell GG, Allison DJ: Coil embolization in the treatment of pulmonary arteriovenous malformations. J Thorac Imaging 4:81, 1989.

Hatfield DR, Fried AM: Therapeutic embolization of diffuse pulmonary arteriovenous malformations. Am J Roentgenol 137:861, 1981.

Heutink P, et al: Linkage of haemorrhagic telangiectasia to chromosome 9q^{34} and evidence for locus heterogeneity. J Med Genet 31:933, 1994.

Hodgson CH, Kaye RL: Pulmonary arteriovenous fistula and hereditary hemorrhagic telangiectasia: a review and report of 35 cases of fistula. Chest 43:449, 1963.

Iwabuchi S, et al: Intrapleural rupture of a pulmonary arteriovenous fistula occurring beneath the pleura: report of a case. Jpn J Surg 23:468, 1993.

Jeresaty RM, Knight HF, Hart WE: Pulmonary arteriovenous fistulas in children: report of two cases and review of literature. Am J Dis Child 111:256, 1966.

Kiely B, et al: Syndrome of anomalous venous drainage of the right lung to the inferior vena cava: a review of 67 reported cases and three new cases in children. Am J Cardiol 20:102, 1967.

Kirklin JW, Ellis FH, Wood EH: Treatment of anomalous venous connections in association with interatrial communications. Surgery 39:389, 1956.

Lee DW, et al: Embolotherapy of large pulmonary arteriovenous malformations: long term results. Ann Thorac Surg 64:930, 1997.

Lewis AB, Gates GF, Stanley P: Echocardiography and perfusion scintigraphy in the diagnosis of pulmonary arteriovenous fistula. Chest 73:675, 1978.

Mannes GP, van der Jagt EJ, Postmus PE: An asymptomatic hilar mass. Roentgenogram of the month. Chest 101:553, 1992.

McAllister KA, et al: Genetic heterogeneity in hereditary haemorrhagic telangiectasia: possible correlation with clinical phenotype. J Med Genet 31:927, 1994.

McGoon DC, Kincaid OW: Stenosis of branches of the pulmonary artery: surgical repair. Med Clin North Am 48:1083, 1964.

Murphy JP, et al: Peripheral pulmonary artery aneurysm in a patient with limited respiratory reserve: controlled resection using cardiopulmonary bypass. Ann Thorac Surg 43:323, 1987.

Natelson EA, Watts HD, Fred HL: Cystic medionecrosis of the pulmonary arteries. Chest 57:333, 1970.

Neill CA, et al: The familial occurrence of hypoplastic right lung with systemic arterial supply and venous drainage: "Scimitar" syndrome. Bull Johns Hopkins Hospital 107:1, 1960.

Noonan JA, et al: Congenital pulmonary lymphangiectasis. Am J Dis Child 120:314, 1970.

Pierce WS, et al: Concomitant congenital heart disease and lobar emphysema in infants: incidence, diagnosis, and operative management. Ann Surg 172:951, 1970.

Porteus ME, et al: Genetic heterogeneity in hereditary haemorrhagic telangiectasia. J Med Genet 31:925, 1994.

Puskas JD, et al: Pulmonary arteriovenous malformations: therapeutic options. Ann Thorac Surg 56:253, 1994.

Remy J, et al: Pulmonary arteriovenous malformations: evaluation with CT of the chest before and after treatment. Radiology 182:809, 1992.

Rocchini AP, et al: Use of balloon angioplasty to treat peripheral pulmonary stenosis. Am J Cardiol 54:1069, 1984.

Sanger PW, Taylor FH, Robicsek F: The "scimitar syndrome," diagnosis and treatment. Arch Surg 86:84, 1963.

Scott-Emuakpor AB, et al: Familial occurrence of congenital pulmonary lymphangiectasis. Genetic implications. Am J Dis Child 135:532, 1981.

Shub C, et al: Detecting intrapulmonary right-to-left shunt with contrast echocardiography: observations in a patient with diffuse pulmonary arteriovenous fistulas. Mayo Clin Proc 51:81, 1976.

Sperling DC, et al: Pulmonary arteriovenous fistulas with pulmonary hypertension. Chest 71:753, 1977.

Steinberg I: Pulmonary varices mistaken for pulmonary and hilar disease. AJR Am J Roentgenol 101:947, 1967.

Stringer CJ, et al: Pulmonary arteriovenous fistula. Am J Surg 89:1054, 1955.

Tadavarthy SM, Moller JH, Amplatz K: Polyvinyl alcohol (Ivalon)—a new embolic material. Am J Roentgenol 125:609, 1975.

Takenaka K, et al: Intrapleural rupture of pulmonary arteriovenous fistula: a case report. J Jpn Assoc Chest Surg 10:479, 1996.

Taylor BG, et al: Therapeutic embolization of the pulmonary artery in pulmonary arteriovenous fistula. Am J Med 64:360, 1978.

Tobin CE: Arteriovenous shunts in the peripheral pulmonary circulation in the human lung. Thorax 21:197, 1966.

Trell E, et al: The scimitar syndrome with particular reference to its pathogenesis. Z Kardiol 60:880, 1971.

Ungaro R, et al: Solitary peripheral pulmonary artery aneurysms: pathogenesis and surgical treatment. J Thorac Cardiovasc Surg 71:566, 1976.

Vincent P, et al: A third locus for hereditary haemorrhagic telangiectasia maps to chromosome 12q. Hum Molec Genet 4:945, 1995.

White RI Jr: Angioarchitecture of pulmonary arteriovenous malformations: an important consideration before embolotherapy. Am J Roentgenol 140:681, 1983.

White RI Jr: Embolotherapy in vascular disease. Am J Roentgenol 142:27, 1984.

White RI Jr, Pollak JS: Pulmonary arteriovenous malformations: options for management [letter to the editor]. Ann Thorac Surg 57:519, 1994.

White RI Jr, et al: Detachable silicone balloons: results of experimental study and clinical investigations in hereditary hemorrhagic telangiectasia. Ann Radiol (Paris) 23:338, 1980.

White RI Jr, et al: Pulmonary arteriovenous malformations: technique and long-term outcome of embolotherapy. Radiology 169:663, 1988.

Yeung M, et al: Transcranial Doppler ultrasonography and transesophageal echocardiography in the investigation of pulmonary arteriovenous malformation in a patient with hereditary hemorrhagic telangiectasia presenting with stroke. Stroke 26:1941, 1995.

READING REFERENCES

Bosher LH Jr, Blaki DA, Byrd BR: An analysis of the pathologic anatomy of pulmonary arteriovenous aneurysms with particular reference to the applicability of local excision. Surgery 45:91, 1959.

Good CA: Certain vascular abnormalities of lungs. Hickey Lecture. AJR Am J Roentgenol 85:1009, 1961.

Hepburn J, Dauphinee JA: Successful removal of hemangioma of the lung followed by the disappearance of polycythemia. Am J Med Sci 204:681, 1942.

Hipona FA, Jamshidi A: Observations on the natural history of varicosity of pulmonary veins. Circulation 35:471, 1967.

Kaufman SL: Intrathoracic interventional vascular techniques in congenital cardiovascular disease. J Thorac Imaging 2:1, 1987.

Kiphart RJ, et al: Systemic-pulmonary arteriovenous fistula of the chest wall and lung: a report of a case review of the literature. J Thorac Cardiovasc Surg 54:113, 1967.

Remy-Jardin M, Remy J: Comparison of vertical and oblique CT in evaluation of bronchial tree. J Comput Assist Tomogr 12:956, 1988.

Smith HL, Horton BT: Arteriovenous fistula of the lung associated with polycythemia vera: report of a case in which the diagnosis was made clinically. Am Heart J 18:589, 1939.

White RI, Pollak JS, Wirth JA: Pulmonary arteriovenous malformations: diagnosis and transcatheter embolotherapy. J Vasc Intervent Radiol 7:787, 1996.

Wolfe WG, Anderson RW, Sealy WC: Hyperlucent lung. Pathophysiology and surgical management. Ann Thorac Surg 18:172, 1974.

CHAPTER 82

Chronic Pulmonary Emboli

Renee S. Hartz

The modern era of surgery for chronic thromboembolic pulmonary hypertension (CTEPH) began in the 1980s. Until that time pulmonary thromboendarterectomy (PTE) was performed infrequently and essentially at a single medical center, the University of California at San Diego (UCSD). It posed a formidable technical challenge and was associated with both high operative mortality (more than 20%) and excessive morbidity caused by respiratory and multisystem organ failure.

Currently, PTE is performed at numerous medical centers throughout the world, largely because of the pioneering efforts of those surgeons who developed and perfected the operation at UCSD. Operative mortality has fallen and postoperative complications have become less common.

Although no longer simply an autopsy curiosity, CTEPH continues to be an underdiagnosed condition. Increased awareness and better diagnosis will lead to curative surgery in more patients worldwide.

Because most episodes are clinically silent, the true incidence of pulmonary embolism is unknown. In the United States more than a half million patients are afflicted annually and approximately 10% die within the first hour of the event. According to Dalen and Alpert (1975), accurate diagnosis is made in only one-third of the survivors so that at least 400,000 cases of pulmonary embolus are missed annually in the United States alone (Fig. 82-1). Because complete resolution of the thrombus depends on adequate anticoagulant therapy, it is likely that many patients in the subgroup with missed diagnosis go on to develop the chronic and progressively debilitating form of the disease known as CTEPH. Previously considered by many authors to represent a rare and aberrant outcome of acute pulmonary embolism, CTEPH may actually represent a logical physiologic outcome of untreated or recurrent emboli: organization of the thrombi, incorporation into the wall of the pulmonary artery, occlusion and recanalization, all occurring in repeated cycles and eventually leading to pulmonary hypertension and right-sided heart failure.

PATHOPHYSIOLOGY OF CHRONIC THROMBOEMBOLIC PULMONARY HYPERTENSION

The pulmonary hypertension observed in CTEPH is caused by chronic obstruction and subsequent medial proliferation in the central pulmonary arteries: main, lobar, and segmental. With progressive elevation of pulmonary artery pressure (PAP) and pulmonary vascular resistance (PVR), right-sided heart failure and hypoxemia occur. At this advanced stage, prognosis without surgical therapy is poor.

Microscopically, chronic emboli are fibrous, organized, and adherent to the pulmonary arterial intima. In large vessels, recanalization frequently occurs with resultant vascular bands and webs composed of dense fibrous tissue traversing some lumens. Medial hypertrophy also occurs in the larger pulmonary arteries. In the distal vessels organized lesions, resulting from ingrowth of collagen and elastin, often mimic the plexiform changes seen in primary pulmonary hypertension. These peripheral lesions are not surgically removable.

CTEPH is a dynamic process with repeated cycles of thrombosis and recanalization occurring throughout the pulmonary arterial circulation. It tends to be more pronounced in the right lung and has been found by Tartulier and associates (1984) to be present in up to 3% of autopsy series. Although etiologic factors have not been completely elucidated, it is clear that adequate anticoagulation for acute pulmonary embolism prevents its occurrence completely.

Both Wilhelmsen (1972) and Sabiston (1977) and their associates proposed that recurrent embolization was responsible for CTEPH and Sabiston and colleagues (1977) believed that inadequate thrombolysis was also involved. Riedel and coworkers (1982) subsequently stated that occult pulmonary embolism is responsible for virtually all cases of chronic pulmonary hypertension and Chitwood and associates (1984) concurred but proposed several contributing factors including embolization of previously organized thrombi into more distal arterial branches. Rich and colleagues (1988), as well as others, postulated active intravascular thrombosis after they

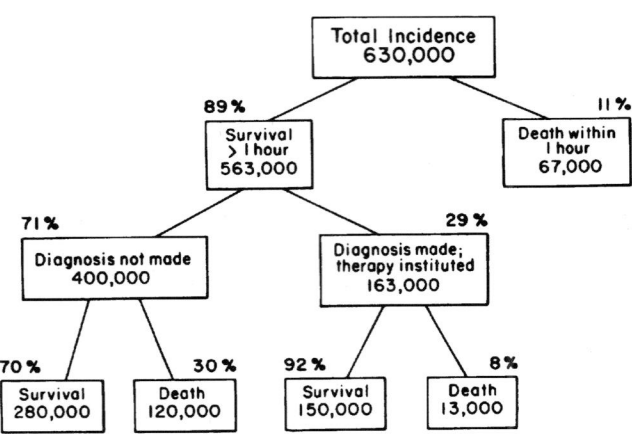

Fig. 82-1. Incidence of pulmonary embolism per year in the United States. From Dalen JE, Alpert JS: Natural history of pulmonary embolism. Prog Cardiovasc Dis *17*:257, 1975. With permission.

demonstrated increased levels of fibrinopeptide A in the sera of their patients with CTEPH. The levels decreased to normal after institution of heparin therapy.

Given these considerations it seems unnecessary to invoke an abnormality in the pulmonary endothelium as the cause for this condition. Rather, if the diagnosis of deep venous thrombosis is missed, any subsequent emboli tend to be more organized and less likely to spontaneously resolve with intrinsic fibrinolysis. When a shower of such organized thrombi occurs, or if repeated small emboli are thrown to the lungs, the stage is set for the process described by Presti and associates (1990), who performed postmortem examinations on numerous patients who died of CTEPH; the thrombi are incorporated into the arterial wall of the pulmonary arteries and endothelial proliferation occurs at the margins of the thrombi. Fresh thrombus is continually deposited when the patient is not anticoagulated appropriately. Fibrovascular organization and recanalization occur in some vessels, whereas fresh thrombosis of others occurs. The vessel wall underlying the thrombus has cleftlike spaces similar to those seen in cystic medial necrosis, the thrombi are made more adherent by varying degrees of neovascularization and fibrous attachment, and the lumens are filled with thrombus of varying age. If anticoagulation therapy is initiated at this point, the vicious cycle of thrombosis and recanalization can be stopped, but according to Presti and associates (1990), resolution of fibrous tissue and obstructive thickened intima and media cannot occur without surgical therapy.

FACTORS PREDISPOSING TO CHRONIC THROMBOEMBOLIC PULMONARY HYPERTENSION

Until recently, it was thought that most patients with CTEPH did not have a prothrombotic state and that only a small percentage of patients (0.1 to 0.2%) with pulmonary emboli went on to develop the chronic form. However, given the fact that the diagnosis of acute pulmonary embolism is missed in the majority of cases, any prothrombotic state should increase the likelihood of the development of CTEPH. The most common coagulation abnormality seen is the presence of lupuslike anticoagulant. Reported by Jamieson and coworkers (1993) to be present in only 10% of patients at UCSD, Sandoval and associates (1996) noted an incidence of 20% in a small series in Mexico, and Simonneau and colleagues (1995) noted a 30% incidence in France. These authors suggest that CTEPH should be added to the list of known vascular complications seen in the antiphospholipid syndrome. Other coagulation abnormalities described by Simonneau and associates (1995) include protein C, protein S, and antithrombin III deficiency. Therefore, even though the majority of patients with CTEPH do not have a coagulation disorder, it can no longer be stated that the incidence of such disorders in CTEPH is not higher than in the general population.

Both Woodruff (1986) and Schamroth (1987) and their colleagues described other conditions that have been associated with chronic thromboembolic disease, including malignancy, the presence of indwelling venous catheters, and atrial septal defect.

CLINICAL PRESENTATION

Progressive dyspnea on exertion is the hallmark of CTEPH. As in mitral stenosis, the course is often so insidious that patients do not remember their onset of the illness. Eventually, however, when more than 50% of the pulmonary circulation becomes obstructed, PAP increases rapidly and right-sided heart failure and hypoxemia occur. The patient's symptoms then progress to class III or IV over weeks to months. When cardiac output is extremely low, angina, indistinguishable from that seen with obstructive coronary artery disease, and syncope may occur also.

The diagnosis is missed in most patients, despite the inexorable progression of symptoms, largely because the medical community has only recently become aware that it is so common. In addition, only one-half of the patients with CTEPH have a history suggestive of phlebitis, and according to Presti and colleagues (1990), 20% have no recollection whatever of an inciting event. It also appears that a *honeymoon period* occurs, lasting months to years between the initial thromboembolic event(s) and the development of dyspnea that masks the true nature of the illness in most patients. Indeed, doctor shopping is common, and most patients with CTEPH have seen several physicians before they are diagnosed correctly. The physical examination in CTEPH is that of a patient with pulmonary hypertension and right-sided heart failure with no characteristics to distinguish it from primary pulmonary hypertension except for the occasional presence of low murmurs over the lung fields caused by partial obstruction at the pulmonary arteries as noted by Moser and associates (1992). Patients typically have a prominent right ventricular impulse, loud second heart sound, murmur of tricuspid regurgitation, engorged liver and neck veins, peripheral edema, and cyanosis. Rarely do they have stigmata of deep venous disease.

DIAGNOSIS

The diagnosis of pulmonary hypertension should be straightforward for any student of cardiopulmonary disease, but because a thromboembolic etiology is rarely considered, the diagnosis of CTEPH is often delayed or made only at autopsy.

Chest radiography may show hilar fullness, caused by enlarged central pulmonary arteries, clear or oligemic lung fields, and right ventricular enlargement. Electrocardiography usually demonstrates right ventricular hypertrophy and strain. Neither of these tests is definitive. The ventilation-perfusion lung scan is the single most important test in the differential diagnosis of primary versus obstructive pulmonary hypertension. A completely normal lung scan essentially precludes the diagnosis of CTEPH but even a single ventilation-perfusion mismatch should cause suspicion and is distinctly different than the mottled, patchy, or plexiform pattern seen in primary pulmonary hypertension. When a patchy pattern is seen, it is unnecessary to perform pulmonary arteriography to confirm the diagnosis of primary pulmonary hypertension. Any segmental or subsegmental perfusion defect, however, should lead to pulmonary arteriography. Long considered to be the standard of diagnosis in CTEPH by Moser and associates (1992), angiography is the examination that also determines technical operability. In addition, it has been demonstrated by Rich (1988) and Ryan (1988) and their colleagues that the lung scan underestimates the severity of the disease and that angiography provides a much better estimate of the obstructive process.

Auger and coworkers (1992) have demonstrated the safety of pulmonary arteriography in patients with obstructive pulmonary hypertension. In a series of 250 patients undergoing the examination, they observed no mortality, serious arrhythmia, or hemodynamic compromise using a standard approach involving a single injection of nonionic contrast into each main pulmonary artery. Based on their series, they described the typical angiographic features of CTEPH: "pouching" defects at the site of abrupt occlusions, webs or bands across lumens caused by fibrovascular organization, abrupt vascular narrowings, and complete obstructions (Fig. 82-2). Oligemia or absence of perfusion in some or all pulmonary segments was universally present distal to the obstructed vessels.

At the time of pulmonary arteriography, hemodynamic data should be obtained (i.e., cardiac output, PAP, and PVR)

because this information is needed to determine whether the patient should undergo surgery to relieve the obstructions. Generally, a patient who is severely symptomatic, who has no other life-threatening illness, and whose PVR is greater than 300 dynes/sec per cm^5 is a candidate for PTE, presuming that evidence exists of obstructive disease in the central pulmonary arteries.

Some degree of tricuspid regurgitation is universally present in this disease and may be evaluated at right-sided heart catheterization, as may be the presence or absence of a patent foramen ovale. Left-sided heart catheterization should be reserved for those patients with suspected coronary or valvular heart disease.

Echocardiography is becoming an increasingly useful screening procedure in all forms of cardiovascular disease and CTEPH is no exception. Right-sided heart dimensions, degree of tricuspid insufficiency, presence or absence of a patent foramen ovale, and an estimate of the PAP can all be readily obtained and used as a baseline for postoperative studies. Dittrich and colleagues (1988) performed preoperative and postoperative right-sided heart studies and echocardiography on 30 patients undergoing PTE and documented the marked changes noted with successful operation (Tables 82-1 and 82-2).

Computed tomographic (CT) scanning has become more important in the diagnosis of CTEPH, especially outside of the United States. At the University Hospital in Mainz, Germany, where the second largest series of PTE has been reported, Schwickert and coworkers (1994) performed both unenhanced and enhanced scans in 75 patients, 63 of whom subsequently underwent PTE. The authors described both vascular and parenchymal changes in CTEPH. Visualization of thrombus in the central pulmonary arteries, present in 53 of 75 patients, was the most important direct criterion for the diagnosis (Fig. 82-3), and vascular findings were 77% sensitive in determining technical operability in this group of patients. Lung parenchymal changes included inhomogeneous areas of hyperattenuation in underperfused areas. These areas were nodular or wedge shaped and pleural based, occurred in patients with central thrombi, and were unchanged after injection of contrast medium. Areas of *mosaic oligemia*, sharply demarcated areas of hyperattenuation and hypoattenuation, disappeared on postoperative scans in 20 of 23 patients who had serial examinations. King and associates (1994) at UCSD, however, did not find CT scans useful in the vascular evaluation of CTEPH. In a group of five patients studied, they used the scan for the parenchymal findings and axial single-photon emission CT perfusion scanning for the vascular examination. Rich and colleagues (1988), on the other hand, found the cine CT scan particularly useful in delineating central thrombus.

Finally, definitive diagnosis cannot be made in a small percentage of patients with the previously mentioned examinations. Shure and coworkers (1985) have described the use of fiberoptic angioscopy in this subset of patients.

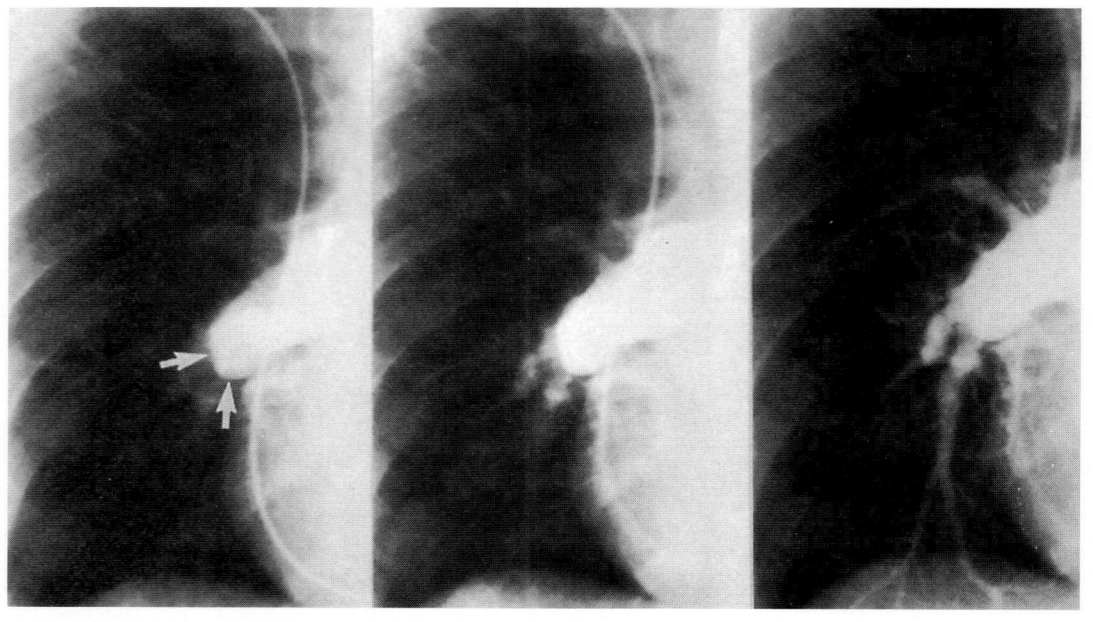

A

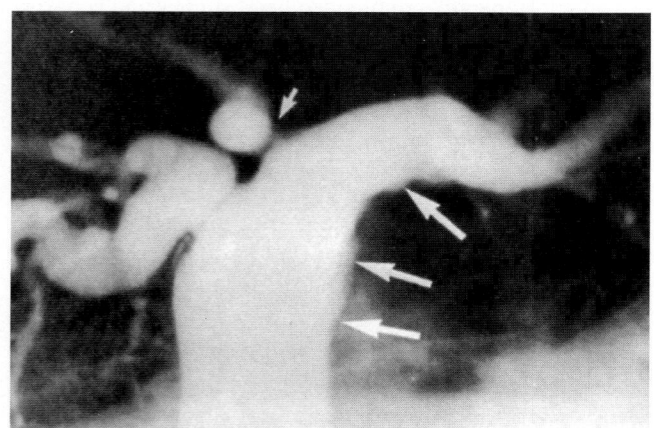

B

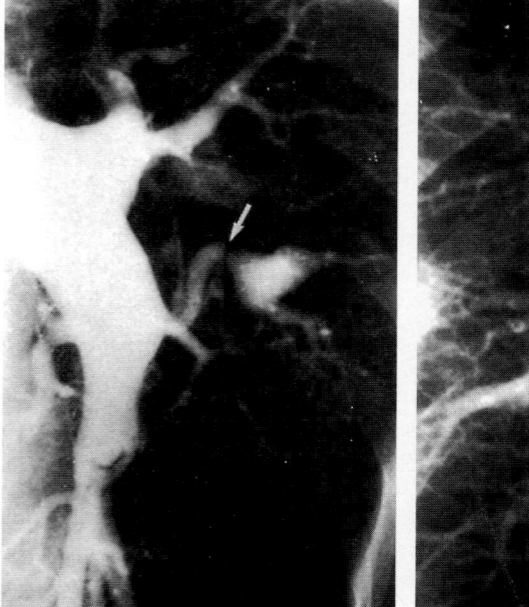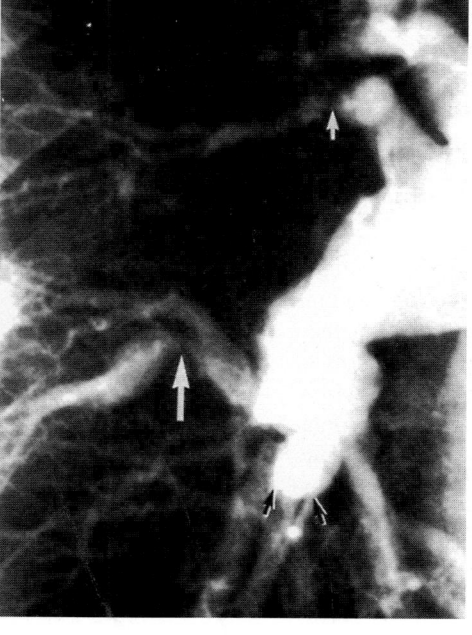

C

Fig. 82-2. Angiographic findings in chronic thromboembolic pulmonary hypertension. **A.** Pouchlike defect (*arrows*) eventually gives rise to more distal vessels. **B.** Small arrow points out a fibrous band. Large arrows depict vascular irregularity that proved to represent a large amount of thrombus at the time of surgery. **C.** Numerous vascular webs and vessel narrowings are shown at arrows. Note oligemia in lung periphery. From Auger WR, et al: Chronic major-vessel thromboembolic pulmonary artery obstruction: appearance at angiography. Radiology *182*:393, 1992. With permission.

Table 82-1. Improvements Noted Immediately Postoperatively in Hemodynamic Values in 30 Patients Who Underwent Pulmonary Thromboendarterectomy

	Preoperative	P Value	Postoperative
Right atrial mean (mm Hg)	13 ± 8	NS	11 ± 5
Right ventricular systolic (mm Hg)	76 ± 20	a	47 ± 15
PA systolic (mm Hg)	76 ± 20	a	46 ± 14
PA diastolic (mm Hg)	34 ± 11	a	18 ± 7
PA mean (mm Hg)	48 ± 12	a	28 ± 8
PA wedge (mm Hg)	9 ± 5	NS	11 ± 4
Cardiac index (L/min per m^2)	2.0 ± 0.5	a	2.9 ± 0.6
Pulmonary vascular resistance (dynes/sec per cm^5)	935 ± 620	a	278 ± 252

[a]$P < .001$. All values are expressed as mean plus or minus standard deviation.
NS, not significant; PA, pulmonary artery.
Modified from Dittrich HC, et al: Early changes of right heart geometry after pulmonary thromboendarterectomy. J Am Coll Cardiol *11*:934, 1988. With permission from the American College of Cardiology.

Table 82-2. Improvements Noted Immediately Postoperatively in Echocardiographic Values in 30 Patients Who Underwent Pulmonary Thromboendarterectomy

	Preoperative Diameter (cm)	P Value	Postoperative Diameter (cm)	Normal Subjects (n = 15)
Pulmonary artery	2.8 ± 0.3	a	2.4 ± 0.4	1.9 ± 0.4
Left atrium	3.7 ± 0.6	b	4.0 ± 0.7	3.2 ± 0.4
Inferior vena cava	2.9 ± 0.6	a	2.2 ± 0.4	1.8 ± 0.3
RA long axis	6.8 ± 1.5	a	59.0 ± 1.5	4.4 ± 0.5
RV long axis	8.7 ± 0.9	a	8.1 ± 0.9	6.9 ± 0.7
RV short axis	4.5 ± 0.8	a	3.7 ± 0.8	3.2 ± 0.6
Area (cm^2)				
RA end-systole	31 ± 12	a	24 ± 8	14 ± 4
RV end-diastole	33 ± 7	a	24 ± 8	21 ± 3
LV end-systole	14 ± 5	NS	16 ± 4	13 ± 3
LV end-diastole	24 ± 8	c	28 ± 6	31 ± 6
Eccentricity index	1.25 ± 0.20	a	0.94 ± 0.12	0.86 ± 0.08

[a]$P < .001$. All values are expressed as mean plus or minus standard deviation.
[b]$P < .05$.
[c]$P < .01$.
LV, left ventricle; RA, right atrium; RV, right ventricle.
Modified from Dittrich HC, et al: Early changes of right heart geometry after pulmonary thromboendarterectomy. J Am Coll Cardiol *11*:934, 1988. With permission from the American College of Cardiology.

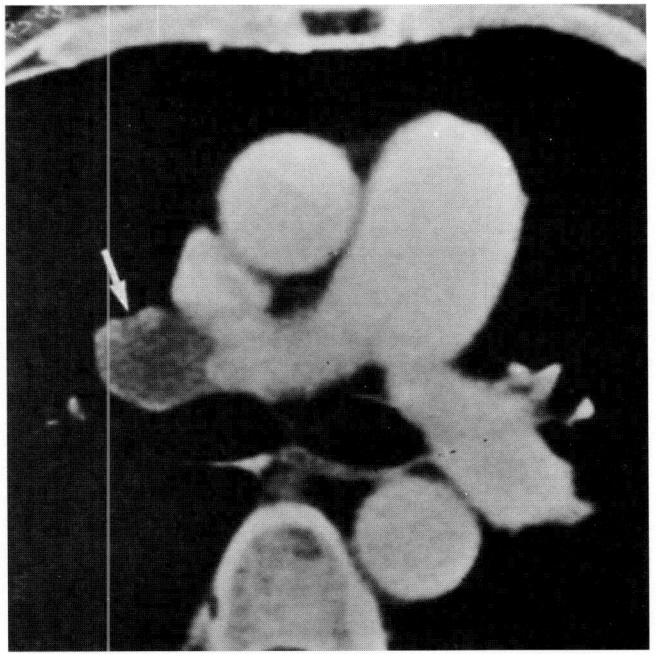

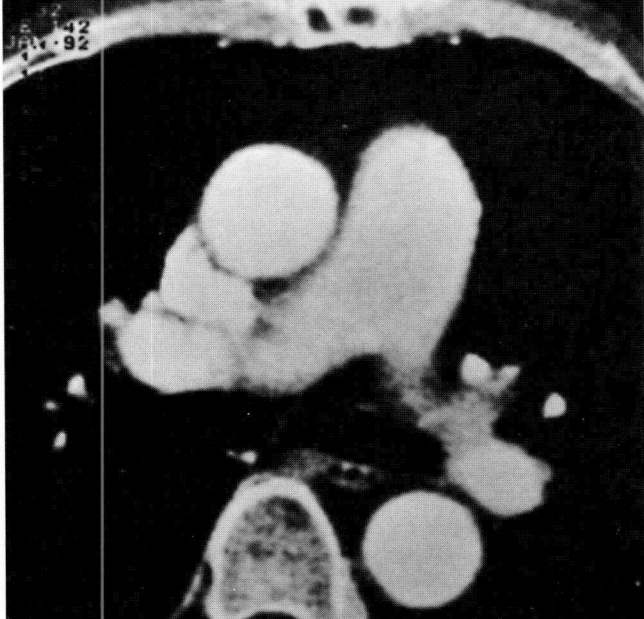

Fig. 82-3. Thrombus in the proximal right pulmonary artery on computed tomographic scan (**A**) preoperatively (*arrow*) and (**B**) absent after successful pulmonary thromboendarterectomy. From Schwickert HC, et al: Pulmonary arteries and lung parenchyma in chronic pulmonary embolism: preoperative and postoperative computed tomographic findings. Radiology *191*:351, 1994. With permission.

The ventilation-perfusion lung scan is the key examination in the differential diagnosis of thrombotic pulmonary hypertension, but either pulmonary angiography or CT scanning by an experienced radiographer should be used to verify the extent of obstruction and to determine technical operability.

TREATMENT

The natural history of pulmonary hypertension secondary to thromboembolic disease was described by Dalen and Alpert in 1975 (Fig. 82-4). When the mean PAP reaches 30

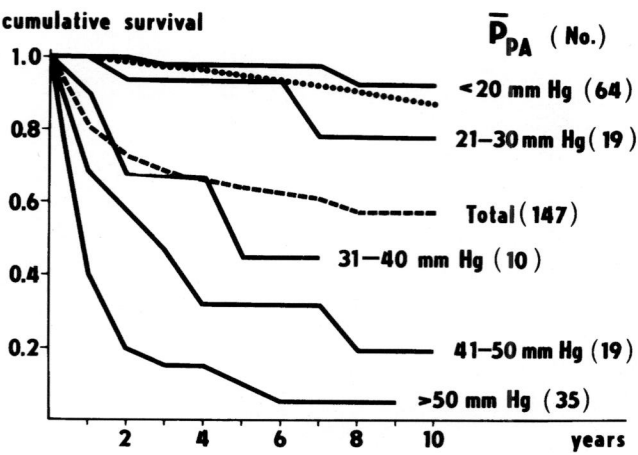

Fig. 82-4. Cumulative survival curves according to initial mean pulmonary artery pressure in pulmonary hypertension secondary to thromboembolic disease. From Riedel M, et al: Longterm follow-up of patients with pulmonary thromboembolism. Late prognosis and evolution of hemodynamic and respiratory data. Chest *81*:151, 1982. With permission.

mm Hg, survival at 5 years is 30%; and at 50 mm Hg, 5-year survival is only 10%. Both Levinson and associates (1986) and I and my colleagues (1996) found that survival was unaffected by either anticoagulant or vasodilator therapy. For these reasons Jamieson and coworkers (1993), who have performed the largest number of PTEs to date, recommends PTE for almost all patients with documented severe CTEPH; more than 90% of patients referred to UCSD for PTE undergo the procedure. Some groups prefer lung transplantation in select patients. Of 72 patients with CTEPH evaluated by Simonneau and colleagues (1995) at Antoine Beclere Hospital in France, only 11 (15%) underwent PTE and eight had lung transplantation. The authors believed that most patients referred to their institution were not candidates for PTE because of angiographic demonstration of severe distal disease. Similarly, only 45% of 75 patients with CTEPH evaluated by us at the University of Illinois Hospital underwent PTE because the remainder were thought to have inoperable distal disease.

The reported number of patients who have undergone PTE is now just under 1000 cases, almost all performed since 1984. The evolution of the procedure can be divided into three historical eras: In the introductory era (1958 to 1976), the first successful procedure was performed by Snyder and associates (1963). By 1977 a total of 18 cases had been reported by Sabiston and associates, with an overall operative mortality of 22%. In this era, the operation was not standardized, many were performed without the use of cardiopulmonary bypass or median sternotomy, and the procedure was frequently unilateral. Crucial in this era was the observation by Sabiston and associates (1977) that "good back bleeding" predicted successful outcome after PTE. The photograph of one of his operative specimens clearly estab-

lished the fact that the procedure was a thromboendarterectomy even though he referred to it as a thromboembolectomy. The operative description and the good results obtained in five of six patients operated on at Duke University ushered in the second era of PTE, the developmental era (1976 to 1984). A review article by Chitwood and colleagues (1984) stated that the number of reported procedures increased from 22 to approximately 90 during this era, but overall mortality remained in the range of 22%. Surgeons at Duke continued to use lateral thoracic incisions, avoidance of cardiopulmonary bypass, and "counterincisions" in the pulmonary arteries to ensure removal of thrombus. At UCSD, Moser and colleagues (1992) established a referral base for patients with thrombotic hypertension, allowing surgeons there to perfect techniques. In 1982 Utley and coworkers reported a series of 10 patients operated on with profound hypothermia and circulatory arrest, all with bilateral pulmonary embolectomies performed through central pulmonary arteriotomies. Although there was only one death in this series, excessive morbidity occurred. Utley and associates' (1982) series led to the modern era of treatment (1986 to the present); surgical groups at UCSD, led by Daily and colleagues (1991) and then Jamieson and associates (1993), progressively refined the operation to its present state. The number of PTEs performed at UCSD by early 1996 was 700 and the mortality had fallen to 6.6% for the last 300 patients operated on (personal communication, 1998). Several moderate-sized series were reported outside of UCSD. Table 82-3 is a list of the reported series in the modern era.

Details of Patient Selection

The indications for operation have already been described. The patient should be severely symptomatic, generally New York Heart Association class III or IV, have no other life-threatening illness, have a PVR greater than 300 dynes/sec per cm^5, and have documented disease of the central pulmonary arteries. It should be noted that Jamieson (personal communication, 1998) has liberalized criteria in younger patients and is currently operating on patients with less severe symptoms and more distal disease. Criteria for inoperability in terms of distal disease have not been established by him. Rather, it is Jamieson's opinion that any patient who manifests central disease should undergo pulmonary endarterectomy no matter how far distally the disease progresses.

Preoperative Preparation

Aside from the extensive diagnostic evaluation detailed previously, little preoperative preparation is required. All patients are on warfarin therapy at the time of diagnosis, and some physicians may prefer to admit the patient for conversion to heparin. I have found this approach unnecessary and treat patients with subcutaneous heparin at home for a few

Table 82-3. Series of Pulmonary Thromboendarterectomies Reported in the Modern Era of Pulmonary Thromboendarterectomy

Author	Year	Location	No. of Patients	Mean Pulmonary Artery Pressure (mm Hg)	Mean Pulmonary Vascular Resistance (dynes)	Operative Mortality (%)
Simmoneau et al.	1995	France	11	39	823	18
Mayer et al.	1996	Germany	119	491	1015	24
Sandoval et al.	1996	Mexico	3	NA[b]	NA	33
Alfieri et al.	1995	Italy	15	56	NA	20
Hartz et al.	1996	University of Illinois	34	54	1094	23
Daily et al.	1990	University of California, San Diego	127	46	813	12.6
Jamieson et al.[a]	1993	University of California, San Diego	150	48	937	8.7

[a]Number of cases; operative mortality in last 500 cases 6.4% (SW Jamieson, personal communication, 1993).
[b]Not available.

days before operation. The patient is admitted either the night before or morning of the planned procedure.

It is important not to treat the patient with vasodilators preoperatively. These drugs are contraindicated because the PAP cannot be lowered until the mechanical obstruction is relieved. Preoperative vasodilators may actually complicate the postoperative care of the patient. At UCSD all patients have a vena cava filter placed preoperatively unless the thrombi have come from arm veins, but the author places filters only in those patients who have documented thrombi in their leg veins at the time of the diagnostic evaluation.

Technique of Operation

Because the best published description of the operative procedure is that in Jamieson and associates' 1993 publication, this information is summarized with comments made on variations used by my group. All patients are extensively monitored; arterial line, Swan-Ganz thermodilution catheter, bladder and nasopharyngeal temperature probes, and transesophageal echocardiography are routine. We place the Swan-Ganz catheter at the beginning of the operation but remove the balloon from the tip before closing the pulmonary arteriotomies so that wedge-pressure determinations cannot be made postoperatively. Although Jamieson and colleagues (1993) recommend routine electroencephalographic monitoring, we have discontinued this practice because we try to minimize or avoid circulatory arrest.

The patients are usually polycythemic because of their prolonged hypoxia, and it is usually possible to remove two units of autologous blood after the monitoring lines are in place. This is particularly important because Daily and coworkers (1990) found that avoidance of homologous blood products decreases the morbidity of the operation.

PTE is always performed on cardiopulmonary bypass with ascending aortic and bicaval cannulation. Left ventricular venting through the right superior pulmonary vein is crucial. Jamieson and his group (1993) also prefer to vent the pulmonary artery temporarily during cooling, but we simply vent through the pulmonary arteriotomies. Gradual

cooling is begun immediately and both pulmonary arteries are extensively dissected. This can be done with electrocautery as long as care is taken to avoid the phrenic nerves. In addition, extensive mobilization of the superior vena cava is undertaken to provide better exposure of the entire proximal right pulmonary artery.

As the temperature is lowered, pump flows are appropriately decreased. At 23°C the aorta is clamped—we clamp as soon as the heart fibrillates—and a large dose of antegrade blood cardioplegia is administered. Retrograde cardioplegia does not add to right ventricular protection and is avoided if the coronary arteries are unobstructed. We prefer to repeat the antegrade dose every 20 to 30 minutes, but Jamieson and colleagues (1993) rely on systemic and topical hypothermia after the first dose. A topical cooling jacket is used for external myocardial cooling.

Since Utley and colleagues' publication in 1992, each surgical group at UCSD has stated that circulatory arrest is mandatory for the performance of this operation. Although this principle may not be inviolate, circulatory arrest is certainly desirable during the learning curve of this difficult operation.

The right pulmonary endarterectomy is usually performed first. After the caval tapes have been tightened, an arteriotomy is begun just to the right of the aorta and carried to the division of the lower lobe branches (Fig. 82-5A). Mobilization of the superior vena cava medially is recommended and is greatly facilitated by the hinged, blunt-tipped Weitlander retractor shown in Figure 82-5B. Establishing the correct endarterectomy plane is the most crucial phase of the operation, as too superficial a plane results in removal of only thrombus and too deep a plane in inadvertent perforation of the pulmonary artery. After loose thrombus is extracted, the endarterectomy plane is started directly posteriorly (Fig. 82-5C), rather than at the cut edges of the arteriotomy, although it is tempting to do so. Several reasons exist for this approach. First, it is easy to develop the wrong plane at the arteriotomy edge because the layers of the pulmonary artery tend to separate here. Second, it is desirable to leave a rim of thickened arteriotomy for subsequent closure of the pulmonary arteriotomy. Finally, when the plane is begun posteriorly and proximally, the specimen starts

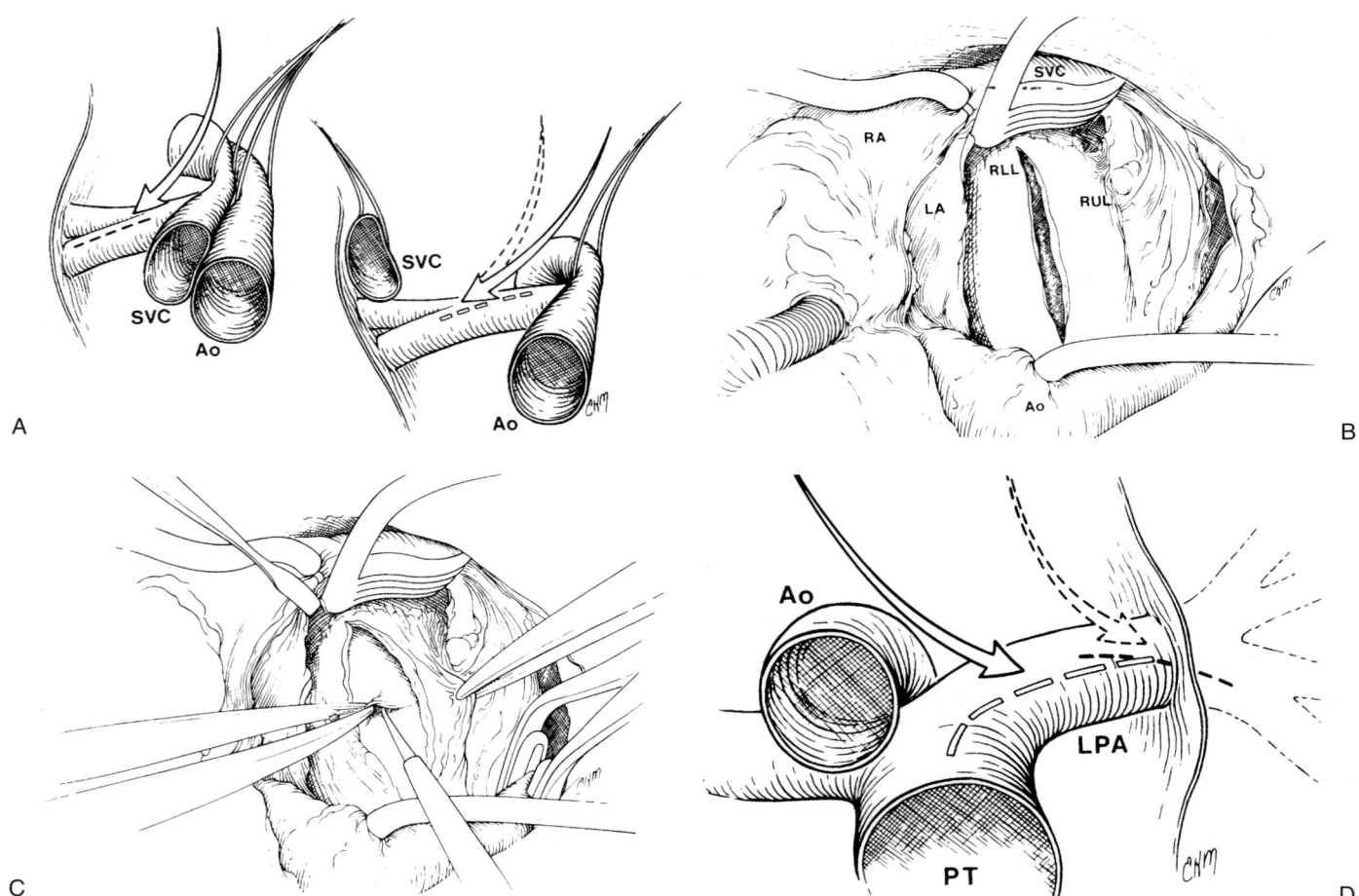

Fig. 82-5. Details of pulmonary thromboendarterectomy. **A.** Exposure of right pulmonary artery by retracting the aorta (Ao) and superior vena cava (SVC) rather than between the great vessels. **B.** Blunt-tipped retractor aids in maintaining exposure and pulmonary arteriotomy is made. **C.** Note that the endarterectomy plane is begun posteriorly rather than at the cut edges of the arteriotomy. **D.** The left pulmonary arteriotomy should also be quite proximal (*arrow*) and affords better visualization than a more distal approach (*dotted arrow*). LA, left atrium; LPA, left pulmonary artery; PT, pulmonary trunk; RA, right atrium; RLL, right lower lobe; RUL, right upper lobe. From Jamieson SW, et al: Experience and results of 150 pulmonary thromboendarterectomy operations over a 29 month period. J Thorac Cardiovasc Surg *106*:116, 1993. With permission.

out quite thin but gets thicker as the surgeon progresses further distally into the arterial branches. This automatically results in development of the correct plane while making it possible to keep the specimen intact. It is quite easy to tell when the plane is too deep because visualization of pinkish tissue indicates that the adventitia has been exposed. A new plane should be begun elsewhere.

Intense focus, good lighting, and proper instruments are mandatory for a thorough endarterectomy. An array of blunt-tipped suction dissectors have been designed at UCSD (Fig. 82-6) and described by Dailey and colleagues (1991). They are available in an assortment of lengths and angles, but it is possible to use a single straight one on every case or to do the procedure entirely with a small tonsil sucker. Because it is highly desirable that the specimen be kept intact on each side, a hand-over-hand technique is used and the assistant must be ready to repeatedly exchange the

sucker-dissector with a blunt forceps so that the surgeon need never release the specimen. In essence, the pulmonary artery is actually peeled off the specimen with a gentle motion of the dissector, rather than vice versa. The fact that the specimen is quite elastic and does not fragment as easily as arteriosclerotic plaques seen in the systemic circulation facilitates the procedure. When the subsegmental branches are reached, the feathered ends of the specimen literally pop out of the arteries. If not, excessive traction must not be placed on the specimen. Rather, it should be sharply amputated to avoid rupture of the pulmonary artery distally where repair is impossible. The entire endarterectomy can be performed through the single arteriotomy and counterincisions are unnecessary. Jamieson and associates (1993) limit circulatory arrest periods to 20 minutes and can generally perform the entire procedure on each side in that period of time. If not, reperfusion for a minimum of 10 minutes is carried

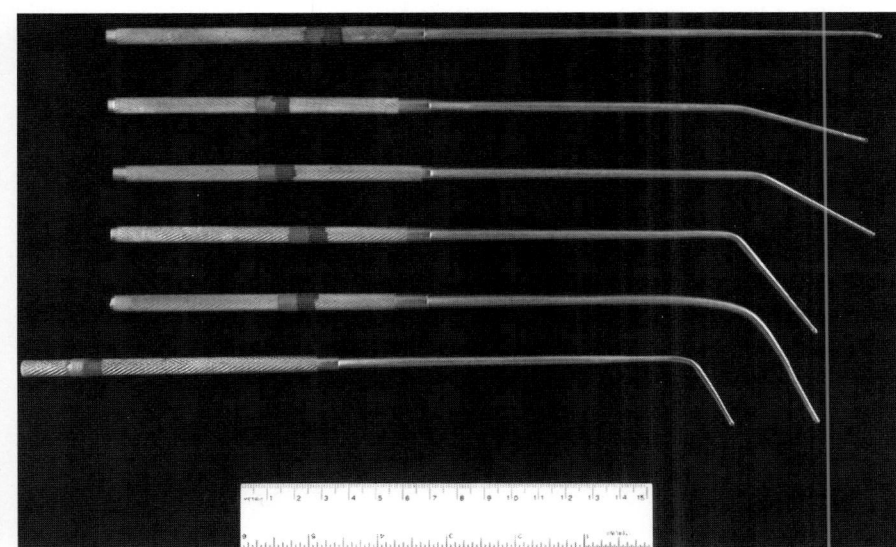

Fig. 82-6. Blunt-tipped suction-dissectors designed at the University of California, San Diego, for pulmonary thrombo-endarterectomy. From Daily PO, Dembitsky WP, Daily RP: Dissectors for pulmonary thromboendarterectomy. Ann Thorac Surg *51*:842, 1991. With permission from the Society of Thoracic Surgeons.

out before continuing. We prefer to avoid circulatory arrest and perform as much as possible of the endarterectomy at flows of 500 to 1000 mL/minute.

After completion of the right side, the pulmonary arteriotomy can be closed immediately or attention can be turned to the left side; the open right arteriotomy can be used for venting the pulmonary artery. As mentioned previously, the disease is usually less extensive on the left side. For this reason the plane may be more difficult to develop and the specimen less organized. The arteriotomy begins proximally on the left pulmonary artery and again extends to the lower lobe branch takeoff (see Fig. 82-5D). The endarterectomy then proceeds in a fashion similar to that on the right.

After completion of the endarterectomies, rewarming is immediately begun. During this time the pulmonary arteriotomies are closed with running polypropylene suture.

Jamieson and colleagues (1993) routinely inspect the interatrial septum for a patent foramen ovale at this point in the procedure. We use an intraoperative echo contrast study, performed by an experienced anesthesiologist or echocardiographer, to determine the presence or absence of an atrial shunt. Ancillary cardiac procedures also can be performed at this point, but it is not necessary to address the tricuspid regurgitation.

If desired, a dose of warm, substrate-enhanced cardioplegia can be administered over 15 to 20 minutes before removing the cross-clamp. This provides repletion of energy stores in the hypertrophied right ventricle while raising the temperature of the systemic perfusate.

During separation from cardiopulmonary bypass, nitroglycerin and prostaglandin E$_1$ should be available. Inotropes for low cardiac output also may be necessary, especially when the PAP has not been lowered to normal ranges. In general, however, the patient is dramatically improved and can be removed from bypass with no difficulty once normothermia is reached. The patient's autologous blood is then rein-

fused and the heparin reversed. If no bleeding occurs, the activated clotting time need not be completely normalized.

Postoperative Care

Postoperatively, anticoagulation with heparin is begun as soon as possible. At UCSD subcutaneous heparin is given on the night of surgery. Alternatively a low-dose heparin infusion (400 to 500 U/hour) can be initiated as soon as the patient's condition is stabilized and bleeding from the chest tubes is minimal. In any case, some form of early heparinization is imperative so that thrombosis of the freshly endarterectomized pulmonary arteries does not occur. The Swan-Ganz catheter is left in place for at least 24 hours and until it is clear that the patient is not developing severe reperfusion pulmonary edema. As during the operation, homologous blood and blood products should be avoided.

RESULTS OF SURGERY

Operative mortality has been discussed previously and is detailed in the modern era of PTE in Table 82-3. Death usually occurs from either severe right-sided heart failure when sufficient reduction in PAP is not achieved, or from pulmonary failure caused by reperfusion pulmonary edema. Virtually all patients who require right ventricular assist devices expire intraoperatively, those with reperfusion pulmonary edema within a few days, and an occasional patient with multiorgan system failure may linger for days to weeks. Thus, the course is usually characterized by rapid recovery or swift demise. The mortality has decreased from the 22% observed in the earlier era, to less than 10% at UCSD. At the University of Illinois, I and my colleagues (1996) showed that operative mortality was six times greater

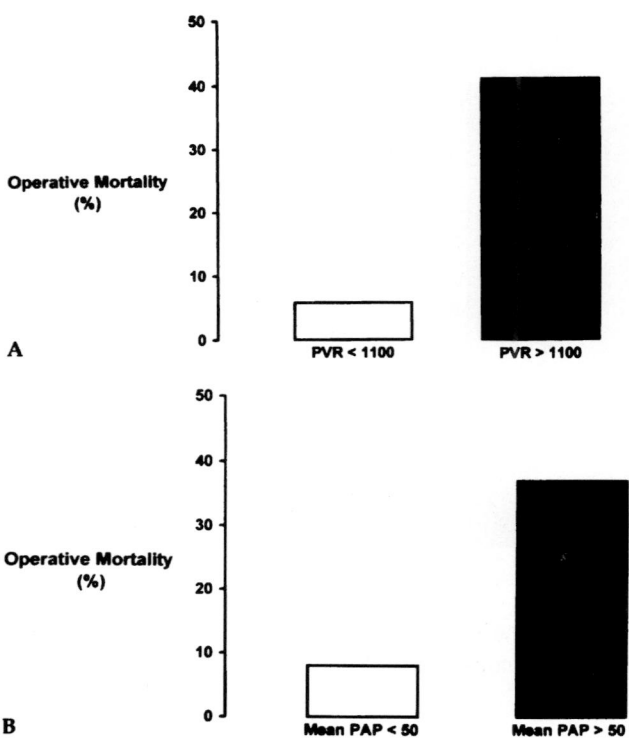

Fig. 82-7. Operative mortality for pulmonary thromboendarterectomy at the University of Illinois was six times greater in patients with pulmonary vascular resistance (PVR) greater than 1100 dynes (**A**) and five times greater in patients with mean pulmonary artery pressure (PAP) more than 50 mm Hg (**B**). From Hartz RS, et al: Predictors of mortality in pulmonary thromboendarterectomy. Ann Thorac Surg *62*:1255, 1996. With permission from the Society of Thoracic Surgeons.

in patients with preoperative PVR greater than 1100 dynes and five times greater in patients with preoperative mean PAP greater than 50 mm Hg (Fig. 82-7). Mortality in our patients with PVR less than 1100 dynes was 5.8%.

Table 82-4. Preoperative and Postoperative Hemodynamics in 150 Patients Operated by Jamieson et al. (1993)

Measurement	Preoperative	Postoperative[a]	P Value
Cardiac output (L/min)	3.8 ± 1.2	5.6 ± 1.5	<.0001
Pulmonary artery pressure, systolic (mm Hg)	78.8 ± 22.3	47.0 ± 16.9	<.0001
Pulmonary artery pressure, mean (mm Hg)	48.5 ± 13.7	28.9 ± 10.8	<.0001
Pulmonary vascular resistance (dyne/sec per cm⁻⁵)	939.9 ± 44.5	299.4 ± 16.0	<.0001

[a]The postoperative values were those recorded just before removal of the thermodilution catheter, usually on postoperative day 2 or 3. Modified from Jamieson SW, et al: Experience and results of 150 pulmonary thromboendarterectomy operations over a 29 month period. J Thorac Cardiovasc Surg *106*:116, 1993.

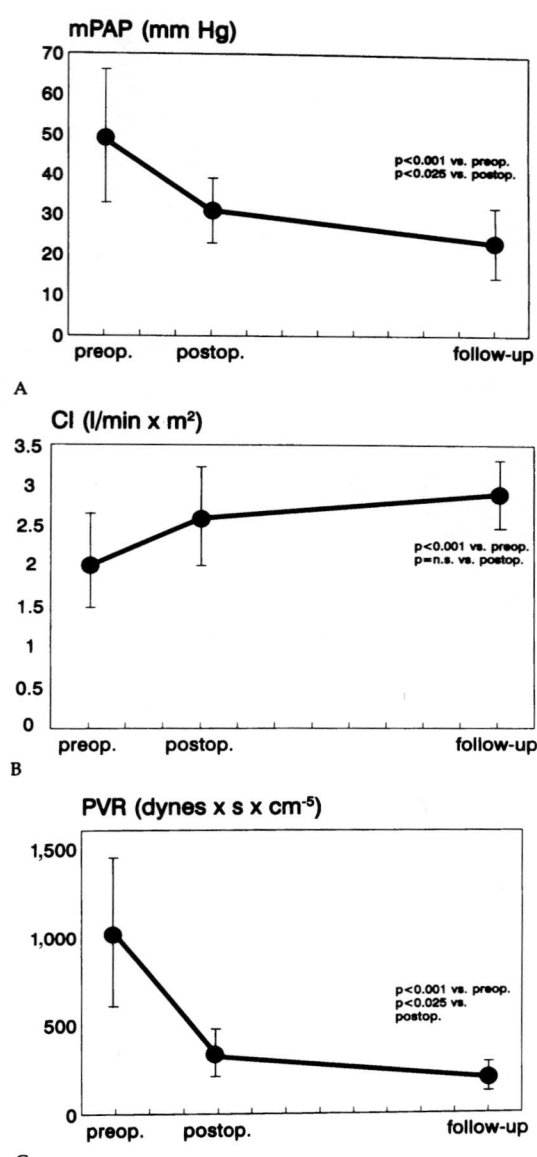

Fig. 82-8. Midterm results after pulmonary thromboendarterectomy (mean follow-up at 27 months). Note sustained improvements in mean pulmonary artery pressure (mPAP) (**A**), cardiac index (CI) (**B**), and pulmonary vascular resistance (PVR) (**C**). From Mayer E, et al: Mid-term results of pulmonary thromboendarterectomy for chronic thromboembolic pulmonary hypertension. Ann Thorac Surg *61*:1788, 1996. With permission from the Society of Thoracic Surgeons.

In addition to the usual array of complications seen after any surgery performed on cardiopulmonary bypass, two problems are particularly prominent. Reperfusion pulmonary edema occurred in all of Utley and associates' 10 patients, reported in 1982, and was present in 10% of patients in Jamieson and colleagues' 1993 series. According to Levinson and coworkers (1986), it is characterized by sustained arterial hypoxemia, radiographic infiltrates in regions distal to endarterectomized vessels, and normal left-sided filling pressures. Treatment consists of fluid restriction, use of the lowest possible inspired oxygen concentration to maintain the arterial saturation above 90%, and with mechanical ventilation and positive end-expiratory pressure when severe.

Delirium is also common after the procedure and, according to Wragg and associates (1988), is associated with deep hypothermia and circulatory arrest time. A total arrest time greater than 55 minutes was 82% sensitive and 80% specific for delirium. It occurred in 77% of patients operated on at UCSD up to 1987 and peaked 72 hours postoperatively. At the University of Illinois, where every attempt has been made to minimize or avoid circulatory arrest, we have seen only one case of severe postoperative delirium. All series report immediate and gratifying relief of symptoms in most patients. The favorable hemodynamic and echocardiographic results demonstrated immediately postoperatively by Dittrich and coworkers (1988) have been verified by most surgical groups. Jamieson and colleagues (1993) showed highly significant improvements in cardiac output, peak systolic PAP, mean PAP, and PVR (Table 82-4). In addition, Mayer and associates (1996) reported on midterm results after PTE. Sixty-five of the 119 patients who have undergone the procedure had hemodynamic evaluation 13 to 48 months after surgery (mean, 27 months). Sixty-two of the patients were in New York Heart Association class III or IV preoperatively, and 62 were in class I or II postoperatively. In addition, sustained improvements in cardiac output, PAP, and PVR were noted (Fig. 82-8).

COMMENTS

Although it is unlikely that PTE will be performed in more than a handful of centers in the United States for the foreseeable future, it is clear from a review of the world literature that CTEPH is a common illness. As increased recognition occurs, it is obvious that in any country or region where large numbers of cardiac surgical procedures are performed at least one surgical group should become familiar with the disease and its surgical treatment.

Because results of surgery clearly depend on proper patient selection, and because it is unclear what makes the patient technically inoperable, it is important that the surgeon embarking on a PTE program choose patients who are least ill early in their series (i.e., relatively young patients with only moderate elevation of PAP and PVR who have clearly demonstrated proximal thrombus angiographically or on CT scan). In this group, an operative mortality less than 10% can be readily achieved. As more experience is gained the surgeon will be able to offer the procedure to sicker patients, including those with more distal disease.

Fortunately, the serious morbidity seen in the early days of PTE has practically disappeared. Multisystem organ failure with prolonged stays in the intensive care unit are rare, and ischemic complications (e.g., neurologic impairment and prolonged pulmonary failure) have decreased as circulatory arrest times have been minimized. It is still doubtful whether the entire thromboendarterectomy can be per-

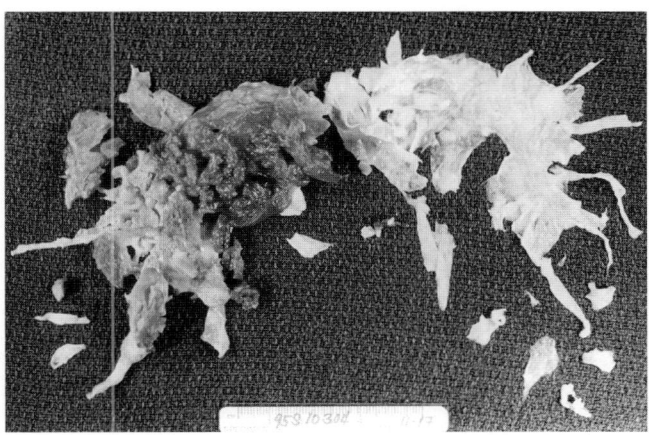

Fig. 82-9. Pulmonary embolus specimen removed at University of Illinois without circulatory arrest. From Hartz RS, et al: Predictors of mortality in pulmonary thromboendarterectomy. Ann Thorac Surg 62:1255, 1996. With permission from the Society of Thoracic Surgeons.

formed without circulatory arrest, especially when bronchial back bleeding is profuse. However, an occasional patient can be operated on without arresting the circulation. Figure 82-9 shows a specimen removed by my group with no circulatory arrest.

CTEPH is a fascinating illness that is not uncommon. Although lung transplantation is occasionally considered an option, the true cure of the disease is with surgical thromboendarterectomy followed by lifelong anticoagulation. The results of surgery are gratifying and a low operative mortality can be achieved after a relatively short learning curve.

REFERENCES

Alfieri O, et al: La tromboendoarterectomia polmonare nel trattamento chirurgico dell'ipertensione polmonare cronica tromboembolica. Prime esperienze italiane. Cardiologia 40:561, 1995.

Auger WR, et al. Chronic major-vessel thromboembolic pulmonary artery obstruction: appearance at angiography. Radiology 182:393, 1992.

Chitwood WR Jr, Sabiston DC Jr, Wechsler AS: Surgical treatment of chronic unresolved pulmonary embolism. Clin Chest Med 5:507, 1984.

Daily PO, Dembitsky WP, Daily RP: Dissectors for pulmonary thromboendarterectomy. Ann Thorac Surg 51:842, 1991.

Daily PO, et al: Risk factors for pulmonary thromboendarterectomy. J Thorac Cardiovasc Surg 99:670, 1990.

Dalen JE, Alpert JS: Natural history of pulmonary embolism. Prog Cardiovasc Dis 17:257, 1975.

Dittrich HC, et al: Early changes of right heart geometry after pulmonary thromboendarterectomy. J Am Coll Cardiol 11:937, 1988.

Hartz RS, et al: Predictors of mortality in pulmonary thromboendarterectomy. Ann Thorac Surg 62:1255. 1996.

Jamieson SW, et al: Experience and results of 150 pulmonary thromboendarterectomy operations over a 29-month period. J Thorac Cardiovasc Surg 106:116,1993.

King MA, et al: Chronic pulmonary thromboembolism: detection of regional hypoperfusion with CT. Radiology 191:359, 1994.

Levinson RM, Shure D, Moser KM: Reperfusion pulmonary edema after pulmonary artery thromboendarterectomy. Am Rev Respir Dis 134:1241, 1986.

Mayer E, et al: Mid-term results of pulmonary thromboendarterectomy for chronic thromboembolic pulmonary hypertension. Ann Thorac Surg 61:1788, 1996.

Moser KM, et al: Chronic thromboembolic pulmonary hypertension: clinical picture and surgical treatment. Eur Respir J 5:334, 1992.

Presti B, Berthrong M, Sherwin RM: Chronic thrombosis of major pulmonary arteries. Hum Pathol 21:601, 1990.

Rich S, Levitsky S, Brundage BH: Pulmonary hypertension from chronic pulmonary thromboembolism. Ann Intern Med 108:425, 1988.

Riedel M, et al: Longterm follow-up of patients with pulmonary thromboembolism. Late prognosis and evolution of hemodynamic and respiratory data. Chest 81:151, 1982.

Ryan KL, et al: Perfusion scan findings understate the severity of angiographic and hemodynamic compromise in chronic thromboembolic pulmonary hypertension. Chest 93:1180, 1988.

Sabiston DC Jr, et al: Surgical management of chronic pulmonary embolism. Ann Surg 185:699, 1977.

Sandoval J, et al: Primary antiphospholipid syndrome presenting as chronic thromboembolic pulmonary hypertension. Treatment with thromboendarterectomy. J Rheumatol 23:772, 1996.

Schamroth CL, et al: Pulmonary arterial thrombosis in secundum atrial septal defect. Am J Cardiol 60:1152, 1987.

Schwickert HC, et al: Pulmonary arteries and lung parenchyma in chronic pulmonary embolism: preoperative and postoperative CT findings. Radiology 191:351, 1994.

Shure D, Gregoratos G, Moser KM: Fiberoptic angioscopy: role in the diagnosis of pulmonary arterial obstruction. Ann Intern Med 103:844, 1985.

Simonneau G, et al: Surgical management of unresolved pulmonary embolism. A personal series of 72 patients. Chest 107:52S, 1995.

Snyder WD, Kent CD, Baisch BF: Successful endarterectomy of chronically occluded pulmonary artery. J Thorac Cardiovasc Surg 45:482, 1963.

Tartulier M, Boutarin J, Ritz B: Chronic pulmonary thromboembolism. G Ital Cardiol 14(Suppl 1):13, 1984.

Utley JR, et al: Pulmonary endarterectomy for chronic thromboembolic obstruction: recent surgical experience. Surgery 92:1096, 1982.

Wilhelmsen L, Hagman M, Werko L: Recurrent pulmonary embolism: incidence, predisposing factors and prognosis. Acta Med Scand 192:565,1972.

Woodruff WW III, et al: Chronic pulmonary embolism in children. Radiology 159:511, 1986.

Wragg RE, et al: Operative predictors of delirium after pulmonary thromboendarterectomy. A model for postcardiotomy delirium? J Thorac Cardiovasc Surg 96:524, 1988.

CHAPTER 83

Bullous and Bleb Diseases, Emphysema of the Lung, and Lung Volume Reduction Operations

Jean Deslauriers and Pierre LeBlanc

Emphysema is one of several conditions collectively referred to as *chronic obstructive pulmonary disease* (COPD). It is an insidious, progressive, and disabling condition that leads to permanent destruction of functional air spaces in the lung.

The pathology of emphysema involves permanent enlargement of the alveoli and alveolar ducts accompanied by destruction of the alveolar walls. In severe disease, damage to parenchymal tissue reduces mechanical support for the airway, leading to its eventual collapse. These obstructive changes are implicated in the extensive gas trapping occurring in the lung, which is characteristic of emphysema.

Physiologically, the effects of emphysema are compounded by decreased elastic recoil in the lung and loss of pulmonary capillary surface area in the alveoli. The loss of the mechanical support of small airways combined with inflammation reduces the expiratory airflow and causes hyperinflation of the lung. Because of the progressive increase in thoracic volume, the function of the respiratory muscles of the chest wall and diaphragm become further impaired, making it even harder to breathe. Disruption of the microcirculation around the alveoli has additional detrimental effects on respiratory function by decreasing the efficiency of gas exchange. As the disease advances, patients experience increasing dyspnea after mild exertion or even at rest and become progressively restricted in their ability to carry out normal activities. Significant mortality occurs in patients whose forced expiratory volume in 1 second (FEV_1) falls below 0.75 to 0.80 L or below 30% of predicted values.

Several forms of medical therapy are available for emphysema and these include not only drugs but also pulmonary rehabilitation, exercise programs, and the use of supplemental oxygen. Such treatments have only a limited effect on the quality of life and survival of patients, however, particularly those who are severely affected. This poor patient response to medical approaches, particularly in the advanced disease state, has encouraged efforts to explore other forms of therapy, including the use of surgical intervention.

At present, the only cure for emphysema is lung transplantation, but the option is only viable for a minority of patients because most emphysema patients are beyond the age limit for consideration as transplant recipients. Alternative surgical solutions include resection of a bulla, which may be followed by a lessening of dyspnea, and lung volume reduction surgery (LVRS), which has been shown to produce significant functional and symptomatic improvements.

This chapter on the surgical management of COPD clarifies some of the most important definitions used in the understanding of patients with the disease. It also describes some of the functional abnormalities associated with emphysema and how surgery could be of help in improving function and symptoms. Finally, this chapter gives some perspective on the results and benefits of surgery.

TERMINOLOGY AND DEFINITIONS

Emphysema

The American Thoracic Society (1962) defines emphysema as "a condition of the lung characterized by abnormal and permanent enlargement of air spaces distal to the terminal bronchiole accompanied by destruction of their walls and without obvious fibrosis." Emphysema differs from chronic bronchitis, although both disorders are characterized by obstruction of the pulmonary air flow, and, in general, patients have a combination of both. The two features in the definition of emphysema that are most important to surgeons are the permanence of enlargement and the destruction of the alveolar wall, because they indicate that the process is irreversible and that surgery should, at best, be considered palliative. Azary and coworkers (1962) have shown that, in general, emphysema is closely associated with aging.

At the close of the 19th century, Matthew Baillie (1799, 1807) was the first to describe "unnatural holes in the

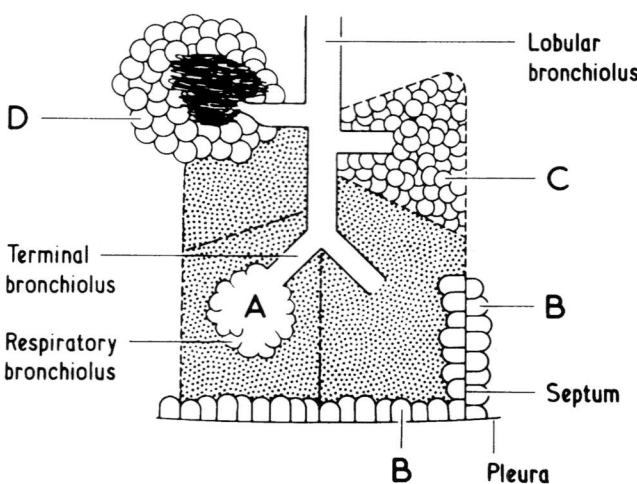

Fig. 83-1. The various forms of emphysema. Centriacinar (centrilobular) (A); (B) periacinar or paraseptal; (C) panacinar; and (D) irregular (scar). From Gaensler EA, Cagell DW, Knudson RJ, et al: Surgical management of emphysema. Clin Chest Med 4:443, 1983. With permission.

lungs." As reported by Rosenblatt (1972), he clearly defined some of the pathologic features of emphysema, such as failure of the lung to collapse when the thorax was opened, dissemination of distended vesicles on its surfaces, and the occurrence of large air spaces enclosed by their membranes of pulmonary tissue. In his volume on diseases of the chest, Laennec (1819) collected further important observations about emphysematous lungs and introduced the term *emphysema*. He recognized that air spaces were dilatated and that, in this disorder, there was partial obstruction of the smaller bronchi and bronchioles.

Gough (1952) and Gough and Wentworth (1949), as well as Leopold and Gough (1957), used sections of whole inflation-fixed lungs mounted on paper to lay the foundations for the current understanding of the anatomy of emphysema. Based on the portion of acinus predominantly involved (an acinus being a unit of bronchopulmonary tissue distal to a terminal bronchiole), three pathologic subsets of emphysema can be observed in minor to moderate disease (Fig. 83-1). As emphysema progresses, classification into specific subtypes becomes increasingly difficult, and the significance of these patterns is unknown. All three varieties of emphysema can be associated with bulla formation.

Centriacinar Emphysema (Centrilobular and Proximal)

Centriacinar emphysema develops in the proximal portion of the acinus, and is associated with destruction of the respiratory bronchioles typically caused by cigarette smoking. Snider (1983) has shown that, as the emphysematous process spreads outward from the respiratory bronchiole to adjacent respiratory structures, a microbulla is produced. Centriacinar emphysema is most common in the upper lung fields.

Panacinar Emphysema (Panlobular)

In panacinar emphysema, all portions of the acinus are similarly and uniformly destroyed; panacinar emphysema is often called *diffuse* emphysema. Progressive loss of orderly arrangement of the tissues results in progressive enlargement of the air spaces. Ultimately, little remains other than the supporting framework of vessels, septa, and bronchi. It is sometimes associated with α_1-antitrypsin deficiencies, as described by Laudell and Eriksson (1963). Panacinar emphysema is classically associated with low diffusing capacity, decreased arterial oxygen saturation on exercise, and pruning of the peripheral vasculature as seen on computed tomographic (CT) scans or pulmonary angiography.

As described by Hugh-Jones and Whimster (1978), panlobular and centrilobular emphysema are believed to be truly distinct entities, not only because of their different appearance within the lobule, but also because the lobules affected by centrilobular disease tend to be confined to the lung apices, whereas those affected by panlobular disease are more generally distributed throughout the lung.

Paraseptal Emphysema (Distal)

Paraseptal emphysema results from disruption of subpleural alveoli. Gaensler and associates (1983) noted that initial tiny disruptions tend to coalesce into larger air spaces (blebs) with possible formation of giant subpleural bullae. These blebs and bullae commonly are located along the upper borders of the lung and are responsible for most spontaneous pneumothoraces. Giant bullae associated with paraseptal emphysema are usually well demarcated and offer the best results after surgical intervention.

Cicatricial Emphysema

Air space enlargement with fibrosis is common but bears little clinical significance. It is seen with scarred tuberculosis (cicatricial emphysema) or with diffuse and chronic inflammatory disease such as sarcoidosis, granulomatosis, or pneumoconiosis (honey comb lung) (Fig. 83-2).

Blebs and Bullae

Pulmonary Blebs

Miller (W.S.) (1926) defined pulmonary blebs (Fig. 83-3) as well-circumscribed intrapleural air spaces separated from the underlying parenchyma by a thin pleural covering. They are the result of subpleural alveolar rupture, which occurs when the elastic fibers in the alveoli have been stretched beyond the breaking point. Air dissection can then proceed through the interstitial tissues and into the fibrous layer of

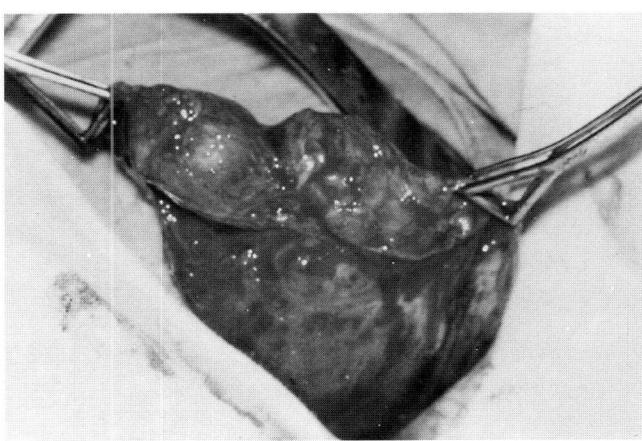

Fig. 83-3. Pulmonary blebs. Operative photograph shows well-circumscribed subpleural blebs at the apex of the lung.

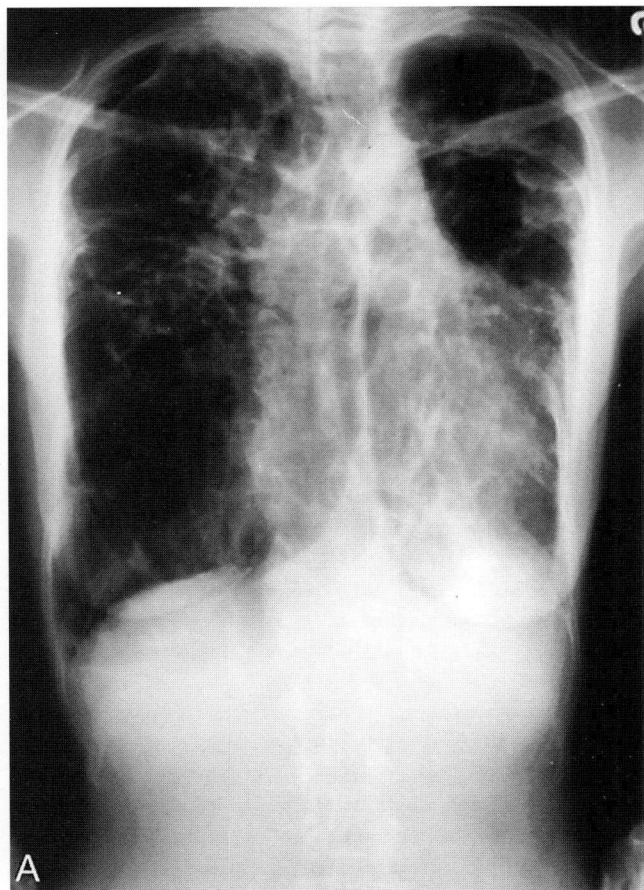

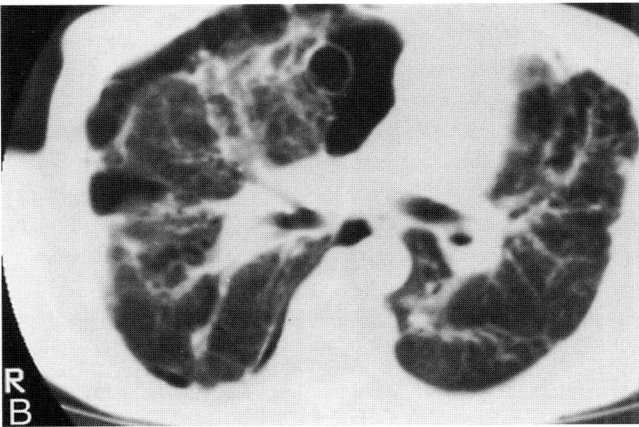

Fig. 83-2. Posteroanterior chest radiograph (**A**) and computed tomographic scan (**B**) of a 47-year-old woman with end-stage pulmonary fibrosis. Note the multiple bullae throughout both lungs.

visceral pleura. The outer wall of a bleb is made of visceral pleura and the underlying lung is normal.

Blebs are small, peripheral, and usually located at the apex of the upper lobes. They also may occur along the upper border of the superior segment of the lower lobes or scattered along the borders of any lobe. Occasionally, they coalesce to form large air spaces.

Pulmonary Bullae

Bullae were defined at the 1959 Ciba symposium as emphysematous spaces of larger than 1 cm in diameter in the inflated lung, usually but not necessarily demarcated from surrounding lung by curved hairline shadows. It was recognized that bullous disease is secondary to emphysema and that bullae can be associated with any variety of emphysema. Pathologically, bullae consist of air spaces covered by a thin membrane made of visceral pleura and connective tissue and traversed by fine blood vessels. The walls of the bulla are made of destroyed lung and the inside of the air space is crisscrossed by fibrous strands that are the remnants of the interlobular septae. Multiple small bronchial or parenchymal openings are at the base of the bulla. Davies and colleagues (1966) grouped bullae into three types. Type 1 represents a small amount of lung greatly overdistended. The bulla has a narrow neck and is well demarcated by pleura. Type 2 represents a shallow but wide layer of lung, greatly overinflated. The neck is broad and strands of tissue traverse the space and are most frequent near its base. Type 3 represents a large volume of lung that is slightly overinflated.

Most authors prefer a practical classification of bullous emphysema that is based on the presence or absence of structural changes of obstructive lung disease in the nonbullous parenchyma.

Group 1: Bullae Associated with Almost Normal Underlying Parenchyma

Group 1 bullae account for approximately 20% of all bullous lung disease. In these patients, the bullae (Fig. 83-4) are well demarcated and often are at the apex. These typically have a broad base of implantation within the parenchyma. Smaller bullae also may be visible over the remaining lung surface and, from a pathologic standpoint,

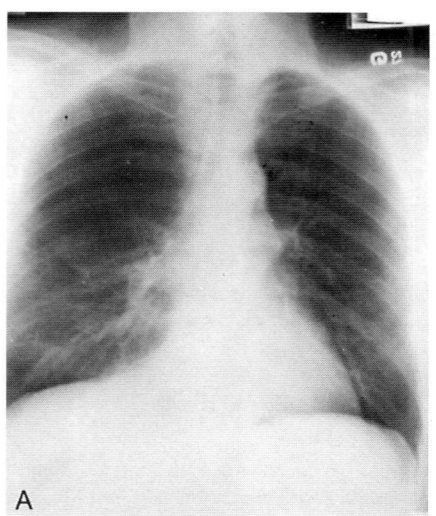

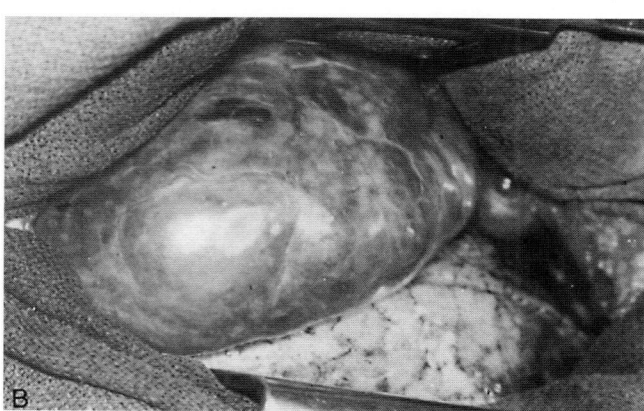

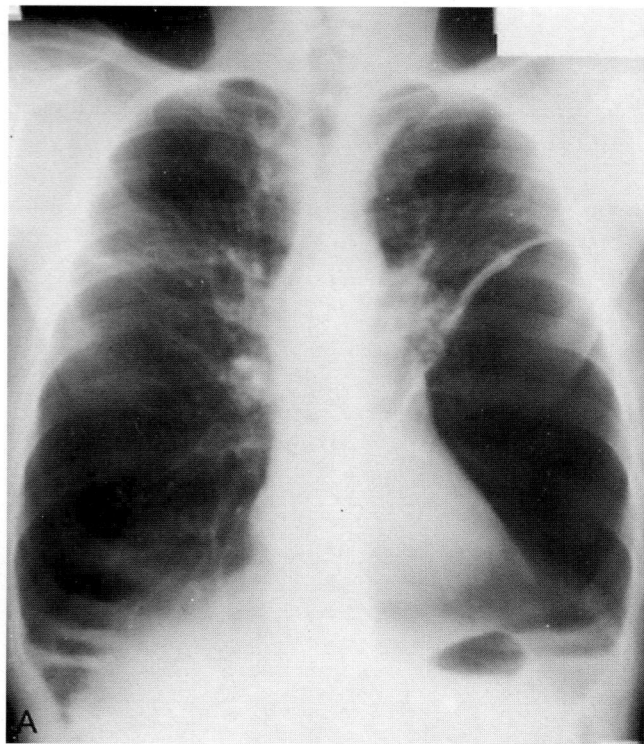

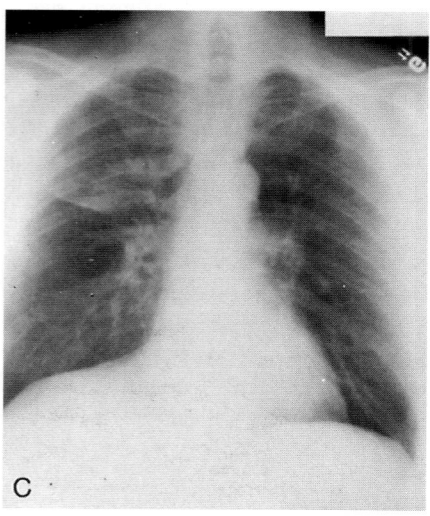

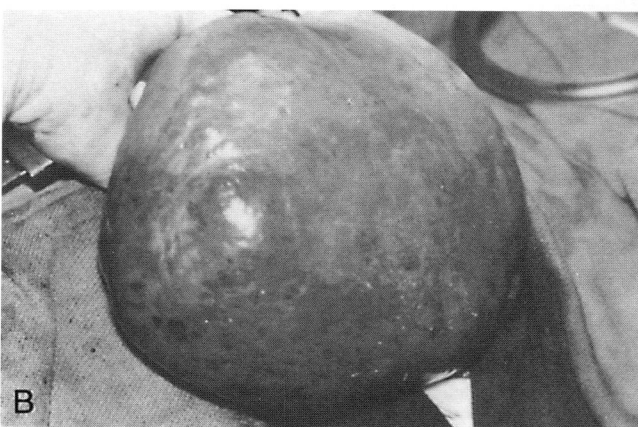

Fig. 83-5. Bulla associated with diffuse emphysema. This 47-year-old emphysematous man was admitted for worsening dyspnea. **A.** Chest radiograph shows bilateral basal bullae with flattening of the hemidiaphragms. Lung function was impaired, with a forced expiratory volume in 1 second of 0.3 L (8% of predicted) and a value for diffusing capacity of the lungs for carbon monoxide of 8.60 mL/min per mm Hg (49% of predicted). **B.** Operative photograph shows that the bulla is in fact a local exaggeration of diffuse panacinar emphysema.

Fig. 83-4. Bulla associated with almost normal underlying parenchyma. A 52-year-old man was admitted for rapidly progressive dyspnea. **A.** Chest radiograph shows decreased vascular markings in the right upper lobe area. Lung function was almost normal with a forced expiratory volume in 1 second of 2.55 L (65% of predicted) and a vital capacity of 4.94 L (95% of predicted). **B.** Operative photograph shows a large bulla herniating through the thoracotomy wound with normal underlying parenchyma. **C.** After bullectomy, the expanded lung fills the hemithorax.

bullae seen in those patients are a variant of paraseptal emphysema. When the bulla is large, it may displace adjacent lung, but the patient remains relatively free of symptoms and the pulmonary function is close to normal. By definition, a giant bulla is a bulla that fills at least one-half the hemithorax.

Group 2: Bullae Associated with Diffuse Emphysema and Vanishing Lung

Group 2 bullae represent 80% of all patients with bullous lung disease, the bullae being initially a local exaggeration of diffuse panacinar emphysema (Fig. 83-5). The bullae are usually multiple and bilateral, and they vary considerably in extent and size. Associated symptoms depend not only on the size of the bullae but also on the severity of underlying emphysema.

The vanishing lung shows complete loss of parenchyma with distended air spaces but without well-demarcated bullae. It has a broad base of implantation within the lung (Fig. 83-6).

ORIGIN AND PATHOPHYSIOLOGY OF BULLOUS LUNG DISEASE

Conventional views on the origin and behavior of bullous lung disease are based on early observations made by Baldwin and colleagues (1950) and Cooke and Blades (1952) who believed that a ball valve mechanism, present in the bronchial communication between bulla and adjacent airways, was responsible for progressive enlargement of the bulla. It was postulated that because destroyed and inflamed bronchi existed at the base of the bulla, gas was allowed to enter the air space but not allowed to leave. The bulla became progressively larger because of increased intrabullous pressure that eventually caused compression and collapse of the unsupported adjacent emphysematous lung tissue. The physiologic alterations associated with a bulla were, therefore, those of a space-occupying lesion that compressed and interfered with adjacent normal and functional lung. FitzGerald and coworkers (1973) further believed that the resulting decrease in lung volume and loss of elastic recoil caused by emphysema would lead to relaxation of peribronchial tension, narrowing of small airway diameter, and, eventually, expiratory obstruction affecting the less diseased portions of the lung.

More recently, Morgan and colleagues (1986, 1989) have shown through dynamic CT scan observations, intrabullous gas and pressure measurements, and pathologic examination that bullae are unlikely to grow and behave in the manner previously thought. According to these authors and Klingman and associates (1991), the lung surrounding a bulla is less compliant than the bulla itself and, therefore, the pressure required to inflate it exceeds the pressure necessary to inflate the bulla. In other words, when bulla and lung are exposed to the same negative intrapleural pressure, the bulla is preferentially and always completely full before the adjacent lung. Consequently, once a parenchymal weakness exceeds a certain size, it results in a space within the lung that fills preferentially. Progressively, the forces of elastic recoil produce more retraction of the adjacent lung away from the bulla, and this action tends to further enlarge the bulla.

Based on this understanding, the purpose of surgery in bullous lung disease may be more to permit the lung to regain its architecture and elasticity than to remove a space-occupying lesion.

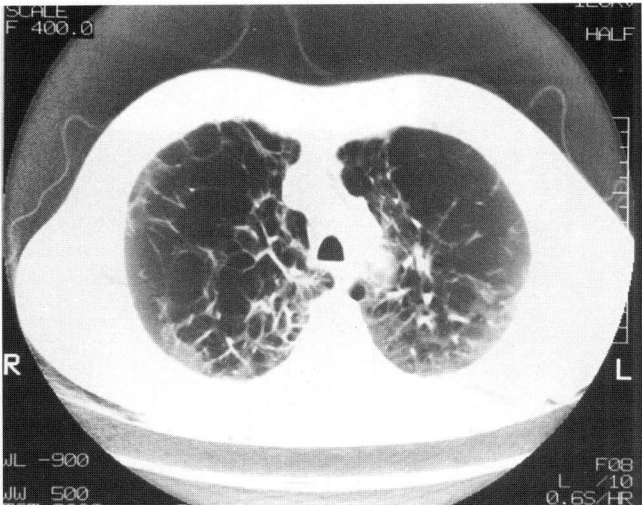

Fig. 83-6. Vanishing lung syndrome. Standard chest radiograph (**A**) and computed tomographic scan (**B**) of a 65-year-old man with vanishing lung syndrome. Note the presence of multiple small bullae disseminated throughout both lung fields.

AIRFLOW OBSTRUCTION

The major determinant of functional impairment in COPD is airflow obstruction that allows outgoing air to be trapped within the alveoli. Thurlbeck (1976, 1977) has shown that generally a good correlation exists between indices of airflow obstruction such as FEV_1 and severity of emphysema.

In 1960, Wright published the results of an autopsy study in which he compared the lungs of 20 patients with severe emphysema with those of 20 other patients with no pulmonary disease. He was able to demonstrate that cartilage atrophy in the walls of the segmental and first three orders of subsegmental bronchi in emphysematous lungs was a significant factor in the airflow obstruction seen in advanced lesions. This cartilage atrophy makes the small bronchi more vulnerable to expiratory collapse, thereby producing airflow obstruction. Linhartova (1977) and Thurlbeck (1974) and their colleagues also have documented cartilage atrophy, as well as gross irregularities in shape with tortuosity and narrowing of peripheral airways in emphysema.

Anderson and Furaker (1962) as well as Pratt and colleagues (1961) have shown that the small bronchi and bronchioles are almost entirely dependent on the radial traction forces of the surrounding expanded lung to remain open during expiration. If the elastic properties of the pulmonary tissues are altered by emphysema, these radial forces are lost and the smaller airways collapse during expiration, further contributing to airflow obstruction. Nagai and coworkers (1985a,b) have demonstrated also that airflow obstruction may be caused by cigarette-associated bronchiolar disease such as chronic bronchitis, increased airway irritability (bronchoconstriction), bronchiolar narrowing and deformities, and further narrowing of already stenotic bronchioles as seen in end-stage emphysema. According to Snider (1983), emphysematous lungs also have an increased amount of mucus in the lumens of small airways.

Many of those changes are reversible or at least can be improved by proper medical therapy, including cessation of smoking and the use of drugs. Airflow limitation resulting from a loss of elastic recoil also may be improved by the surgical resection of nonfunctional parenchyma such as is done with bullectomies or other procedures aimed at reducing lung volume.

COURSE AND PROGNOSIS OF CHRONIC OBSTRUCTIVE LUNG DISEASE

The natural history of emphysema is poorly understood because some patients may have a rapid decline, whereas others remain relatively stable for long periods. If the patient does not stop smoking, however, it is likely that the disease will progress rapidly and that annual declines in FEV_1 will be in the range of 80 to 100 mL/year as opposed to 30 mL/year if the patient stops smoking or has never smoked.

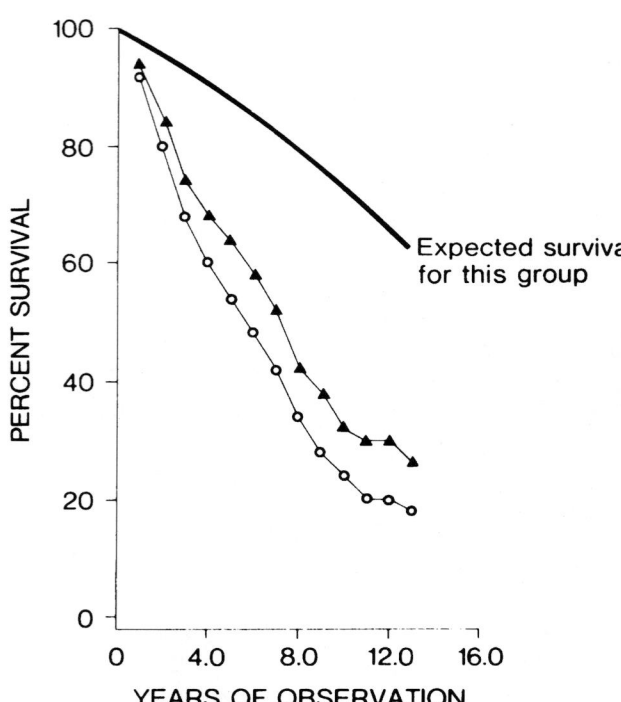

Fig. 83-7. Survival data for the entire series (200 patients). Open circle, all deaths; closed triangle, respiratory deaths. From Diener CV, Burrows B: Further observations on the course and prognosis of chronic obstructive lung disease. Am Rev Respir Dis *111*:719, 1975. With permission.

Dornhorst (1985) has also shown that patients with clinical signs of chronic bronchitis (blue bloaters), recurrent infections, or marked weight loss have a worse prognosis, and all of these criteria are considered important in the selection of patients for emphysema surgery.

In 1975, Diener and Burrows presented long-term survival data for 200 patients with chronic airway obstruction who had been enrolled in a prospective study approximately 14 years previously. All patients selected for this study had FEV_1 less than 60% of both predicted and measured vital capacities. Survival data for the entire series (Figs. 83-7 and 83-8) show the poor long-term prognosis for patients with chronic obstructive lung disease. According to Figure 83-8, the risk of death was relatively low for patients who were mildly impaired on entry into the study, whereas it approached 10% per year when the FEV_1 was mean 1.0 L. Five-year survival figures on the order of 25% were noted in patients whose FEV_1 scores were 0.75 mL or less.

LVRS or any other kind of surgery for emphysema can possibly move the patient from the lower to the upper survival curve (see Fig. 83-8) by increasing the patient's FEV_1. The improvement may be greater if the patient stops smoking and has optimal medical treatment. These expectations form the basis for the renewed interest in emphysema surgery and should remain the best standard of achievement for these procedures.

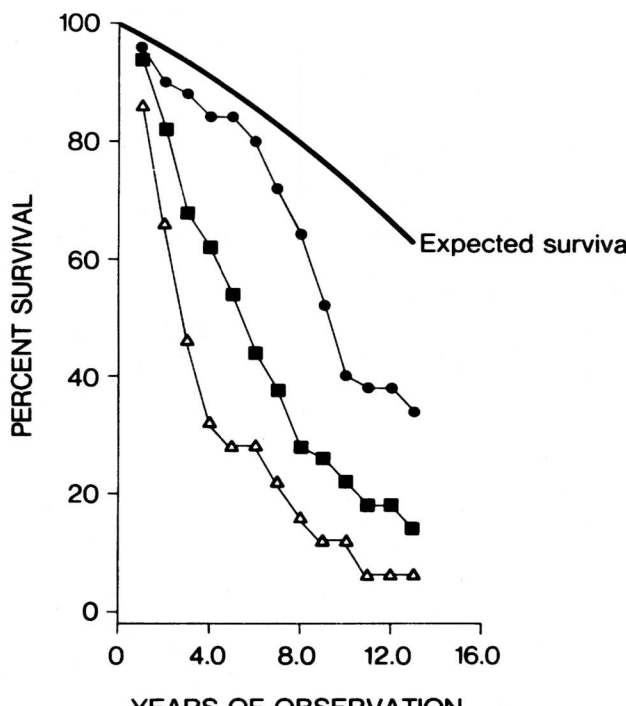

YEARS OF OBSERVATION

Fig. 83-8. Survival of groups distinguished on the basis of their forced expiratory volume in 1 second (FEV_1) at the time of enrollment in the study. Closed circle, FEV_1 >1.25 L; closed square, FEV_1 ≥0.75 L, but ≤1.25 L; δ, FEV_1 <0.75 L. From Diener CV, Burrows B: Further observations on the course and prognosis of chronic obstructive lung disease. Am Rev Respir Dis *111*:719, 1975. With permission.

HISTORY OF SURGERY FOR CHRONIC OBSTRUCTIVE LUNG DISEASE

During most of the 20th century, surgery has been used in an attempt to improve the quality of life of patients with emphysema. Knudson and Gaensler (1965) noted that these procedures included operations on the chest wall, diaphragm, pleura, nervous system and pulmonary innervation, major airways, and the lungs themselves.

Based on the observed development of a barrel chest, Freund (1906) described the operation of costochondrectomy that was conceived as a way of allowing the lungs to expand further, without constriction of the chest wall. Typically, and often under local anesthesia, four to six costal cartilages would be divided. This was frequently performed bilaterally and often in association with a transverse sternotomy, totally disrupting the integrity of the thoracic cage and so allowing further expansion of the enlarged lungs. Bircher (1918) reported the success of this procedure, claiming improvement as cure in 26 of his 30 patients. The operation did not become established, however, as it was soon recognized that it did not address the true basis of emphysema.

Attempts were then made to deal with the hyperinflation of COPD by reducing the thoracic and lung volumes. Thoracoplasty and phrenic denervation were tried and although early results seemed promising, this initial optimism proved unfounded. As Laforet (1972) explained: "Undaunted, and starting with a new set of premises, surgeons were soon advocating such procedures as thoracoplasty and phrenic nerve interruption, each calculated to reduce the volume of the overdistended lung. The alleged benefits of these maneuvers were frequently lost on patients whose worsening dyspnea left them with little energy to debate with their surgeons."

After the chest wall, the next structure to be attacked was the diaphragm. It was thought that this structure was the main cause of dyspnea in emphysema: If its flattening could be corrected, its function would be improved and patients would feel better. The first published attempts to use this approach used abdominal belts. Compression of the upper abdomen via a screw mechanism aimed to raise the diaphragm and improve respiratory function. Apart from the disadvantage of its impracticality, only patients with small abdomens could wear the device. Despite these drawbacks, Alexander and Kountz (1934) published the outcome of a study involving 25 patients treated with the belt. Nineteen reported improvement with a mean increase in forced vital capacity of 39%. A similar kind of thinking was the rationale for pneumoperitoneum. To restore the normal curvature of the diaphragm and to improve its function during normal respiration and cough, approximately 800 mL of a helium and oxygen mixture was introduced into the abdomen. As was the case with previous procedures, the early results were impressive. In a study reported by Carter and colleagues (1950), 10 of 18 patients improved, with an average increase in vital capacity (VC) of 18%, which was associated with improved diaphragmatic excursion on radiographic imaging. However, the procedure was abandoned as impractical, rather than ineffective, as gas had to be replaced every 2 weeks and such refills were associated with pain, discomfort, nausea, and the risk of infection.

The next group of anatomic structures to gain attention was the nerves of the thoracic wall and viscera. Almost every identifiable anatomic nervous structure related to the lung became "at risk" in the effort to relieve patients with COPD. The rationale behind total lung denervation was to abolish reflex bronchoconstriction and hypersecretion. These were complex procedures that did not gain widespread acceptance. Glomectomy, on the other hand, became a relatively common procedure in the 1950s. The glomus or carotid body is a small group of nerve cells located between the origin of the internal and external carotid arteries. It is a chemoreceptor, sensitive to changes in Pao_2, arterial $Paco_2$, and pH, and its removal was aimed at reducing bronchoconstriction and hypoxic drive. Nakayama (1961) published a series of almost 4000 glomectomies with improvement in 80% of patients at 6 months, decreasing to 58% by 5 years. However, controlled trials failed to confirm the value of the operation. The Albuquerque trial reported by Curran and

Graham (1971), for instance, compared glomectomy with a sham operation. Although the numbers are small, it showed that patients undergoing sham surgery did better in terms of symptoms and lung function measurement than those having glomectomy. The operation was condemned by the American Thoracic Society in a statement by the Committee on Therapy (1968) and is no longer performed.

Other interesting operations were aimed at treating airway collapse or were designed to increase blood supply to the lung by stimulating collateral circulation from the chest wall through parietal pleurectomy or talc poudrage.

The only operation that has somewhat stood the test of time is bullectomy in which distended air spaces are resected to allow the reexpansion of restricted but potentially functional adjacent lung tissue. Better preoperative workup through the use of high-resolution CT and less traumatic surgical techniques such as video thoracoscopic operations have improved the outcome of patients suitable for bullectomy. The application of similar volume reduction surgery in diffuse emphysema was first advocated by Brantigan and Mueller (1957) as a means of improving the mechanical function of the lung. In the mid-1990s, this concept was reintroduced by Cooper and associates (1995) and since then, sustained improvements in lung function parameters have been reported postoperatively.

SURGICAL MANAGEMENT OF BULLOUS DISEASE

Rationale and Indications for Surgery

Nondyspneic Patients

In patients without ventilatory symptoms (Table 83-1), surgical intervention is mostly indicated for complications such as pneumothorax, infection, or hemoptysis that are clearly attributable to the bulla. Gaensler and coworkers (1986) noted that bullous emphysema predisposes to pneumothorax and that, in such circumstances, a pneumothorax

Table 83-1. Rationale and Indications for Surgery in Patients with Complications of Their Bullae

Principal Indication	Rationale
Pneumothorax, first episode or recurrence	Further reduction of function in patients who may be compromised
	Radiologic difficulties in recognizing pneumothorax
	Prolonged air leak
True infection of bulla, pus within the bulla	Failure of response to medical treatment
Suspicion of lung cancer	Suspicion of occult carcinoma
Massive hemoptysis	Specific complications: hemoptysis, pleural rupture with pyothorax
Chest pain	Increased air trapping during hyperventilation

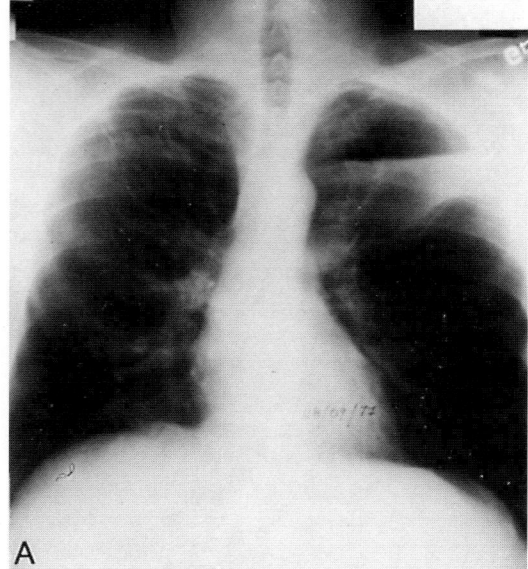

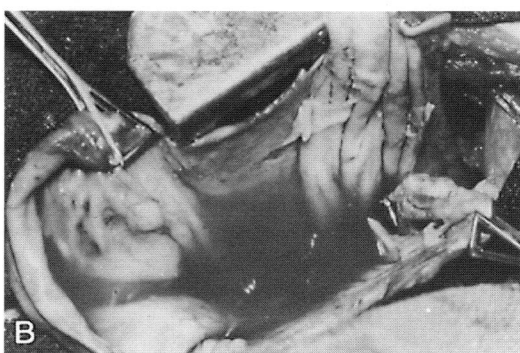

Fig. 83-9. Bulla containing an air-fluid level. **A.** This 35-year-old man with previous bullectomy on the right side has an asymptomatic loculation in the left upper lobe. **B.** At operation, he was found to have a large bulla containing serous and noninfected fluid.

can be troublesome for the following reasons: further reduction of function in already compromised patients, radiographic difficulties in diagnosing a pneumothorax when multiple bullae are present, prolonged air leak that is often less responsive to tube drainage than when associated with primary spontaneous pneumothorax, and higher risk of recurrence than for patients with primary spontaneous pneumothorax. In a series of 67 patients with secondary spontaneous pneumothoraces, Tanaka and colleagues (1993) showed that the most common underlying diseases were emphysema and tuberculosis and that the most frequent presenting symptom was dyspnea.

Infection of bullae is unusual and most bullae containing a fluid level (Fig. 83-9) are only the site of an inflammatory reaction secondary to peribullous infection. Surgery is not indicated for this problem alone, and Rubin and Buchberg (1968) showed that fluid resorption may be associated with significant shrinkage and resolution of the bulla (autobullectomy) (Fig. 83-10). In a series of 10 patients with fluid

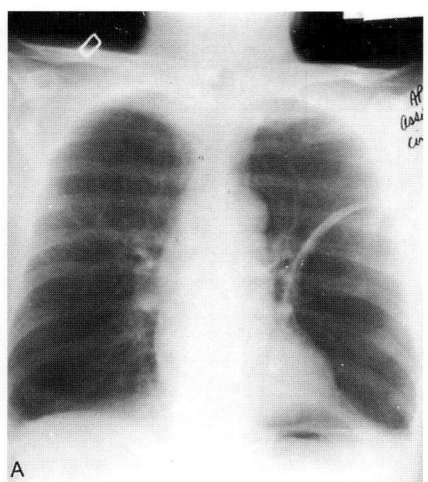 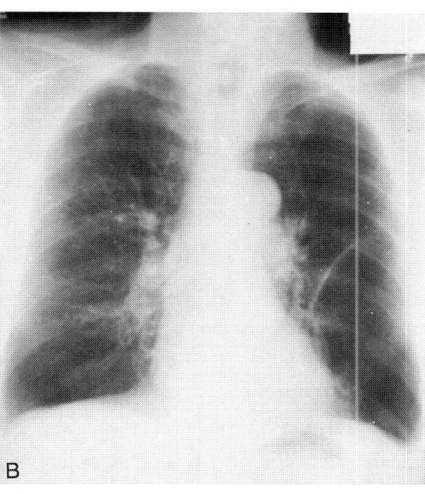

Fig. 83-10. Shrinkage of a bulla after peribullous infection. **A.** This 74-year-old man had a left basal bulla that shrank significantly. **B.** After a 3-month episode of pulmonary infection.

within a bulla reported by Mahler and colleagues (1979), the air-fluid levels disappeared in 3 days to 36 weeks (mean, 11 weeks), whereas the alveolar infiltrate generally cleared at a slower rate.

Truly infected bullae (Fig. 83-11) should be managed conservatively, even though medical treatment is often unsuccessful because of the poor communications between the infected bulla and the bronchial tree. Surgical indications for resection are the same as for primary lung abscesses: failure of response to a 6-week course of adequate medical management; suspicion of occult bronchial carcinoma; and specific complications of the abscess, such as hemoptysis or free pleural space rupture. Dean and colleagues (1987) showed that percutaneous drainage of the abscess should be considered instead of resection for high-risk patients.

Hemoptysis from an eroded artery is even more uncommon than infections. Berry and Ochsner (1972) reported one

of the few cases in which hemoptysis was thought to be secondary to rupture of thin-walled pulmonary vessels passing through the alveolar wall and fibrous septae of a bulla. Because hemoptysis is seldom associated with bullous emphysema, another lesion in a different lung zone that could account for the bleeding should always be ruled out before surgery.

Gaensler and associates (1983) and Witz and Roeslin (1980) described cases in which chest pain was the main symptom and sole indication for surgery. The pain was most often retrosternal and related to exercise, and, in some cases, it mimicked angina. This symptom was explained by overdistention of the bulla during hyperventilation with secondary mediastinal shift. All patients improved after surgical removal of their bullae.

Primary lung cancer closely associated with a large bulla was analyzed in 32 patients by Tsutsui and colleagues (1988) in an attempt to elucidate radiographic features of

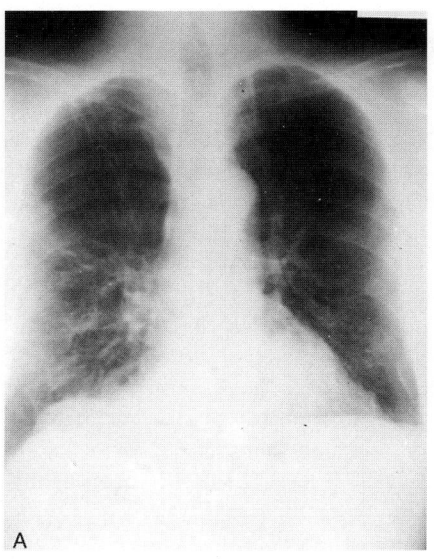 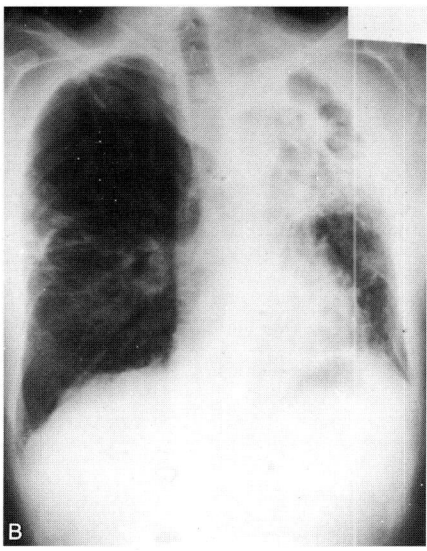

Fig. 83-11. True infection of the bulla. **A.** Initial chest radiograph of a 64-year-old man with bilateral apical bullae. **B.** This patient was readmitted 3 years later for high fever, chest pain, and hemoptysis. The radiograph shows multiple loculations within the left bulla. At surgery, he had a pyogenic infection of the bulla.

the tumor. They proposed three radiographic patterns of neoplasm development: nodular opacity within or adjacent to the bulla, partial or diffuse thickening of the bulla wall, and secondary signs of the bulla, such as changed diameter, fluid retention, and pneumothorax. Stoloff and associates (1971) investigated the population of Philadelphia between 1947 and 1967 and found that the frequency of lung cancer in men without emphysema was 0.19%, whereas in individuals with bullous emphysema, the frequency was 6.1%. Similarly Goldstein and coworkers (1967) found that in 411 patients with bullous emphysema 4.3% had lung cancer. Nickoladze (1993) proposed the following hypothesis to explain this phenomenon: 1) lung cancer occurs more frequently in lung scars that favor development of bullae, 2) dystrophic changes in lung parenchyma caused by bullous emphysema promote development of lung cancer, and 3) bullae are unventilated or poorly ventilated spaces in which carcinogens linger and predispose to the development of lung cancer.

Other unusual complications of bullous emphysema include cervical herniation of an apical bulla, such as in the case reported by Victor and colleagues (1987).

Preventive Surgery

Preventive surgery is defined as the resection of asymptomatic bullae on the premise that most of them ultimately lead to serious and irreversible complications. Its role is unclear because of the limited number of studies describing the natural history of untreated and asymptomatic bullae. Boushy and associates (1968) observed that apical bullae tend to enlarge, but this enlargement was not seen in every case and it could not be predicted. They could not document any relationship between change in bulla size and deterioration of pulmonary function. Ribet (1992) reported 23 patients in whom the bullae were first discovered on chest radiography before the appearance of any symptoms. In this group, only 4 of 23 patients were symptomless when operated on, with a delay between discovery of the bulla and the operation of 0 to 12 years, with a mean of 39 months.

Most authors agree that preventive surgery is legitimate when the bulla occupies one-half or more of the hemithorax, compresses normal lung, or has enlarged over a period of years. Spear and associates (1961) believed that any bulla occupying one-third or more of the hemithorax would ultimately be associated with impaired drainage, infection, and permanent tissue damage to the adjacent compressed lung.

Dyspneic Patients

Based on physiologic observations, the removal of bullae in emphysema and dyspneic patients can be done for the following reasons: removal of a space-occupying and possibly compressive lesion; reduction in expiratory airway resistance; and reduction of dead-space ventilation (Table 83-2).

Table 83-2. Rationale and Indications for Surgery in Dyspneic Patients with Diffuse Emphysema

Principal Indication	Rationale
Expansion of previously collapsed lung	Increase in vital capacity and forced expiratory volume in 1 second
	Improvement in gas exchange (higher ventilation-perfusion ratio and arterial Po$_2$)
Hemodynamic improvement	Increase in cardiac output; better exercise tolerance
Restoration of normal curve of diaphragm	Improvement in diaphragmatic contractility and function
Restoration of elastic recoil and reduction in airway resistance	Bullae increase the loss of elasticity in the emphysematous lung
	Loss of elastic recoil causes an extrinsic airway obstruction
Removal of an area of dead space ventilation	Reduction in volume of wasted ventilation
	Decrease in work of breathing

Removal of a Space-Occupying and Possibly Compressive Lesion

Compression of relatively healthy lung near the bullae may impair overall gas exchange, with low ventilation-perfusion ratios in the restricted lung zone. Expansion of previously restricted lung should increase the VC and arterial oxygen saturation.

High intrathoracic pressures generated by the bullae also may result in major hemodynamic dysfunction. Expiratory compression of the pulmonary arterial system and systemic venous return significantly decreases cardiac output both at rest and, more important, during exercise. Lowering intrathoracic pressures by removing large bullae may correct some of these hemodynamic parameters and decrease the degree of dyspnea.

Bullous emphysema, particularly when localized to the lower lobes, may finally have a deleterious effect on the function of the diaphragm. Restoration of the normal diaphragmatic configuration is likely to improve its contractility.

Reduction in Expiratory Airway Resistance

Ting and colleagues (1963) showed that bullae have little, if any, elastic recoil. At low volume, small variations in pressure bring important volumetric changes. At a critical level, however, compliance becomes extraordinarily low and the bulla cannot be stretched any more. Bullae can be compared with paper bags that are extremely compliant until they are full, when they become tense.

When associated with emphysema, the low compliance of the bulla significantly decreases the elastic recoil of the intervening lung and causes relaxation of the peribronchial tension. Ultimately, it creates an extrinsic airway obstruction affecting the less diseased portions of parenchyma around the bulla.

Removal of bullae may improve the elastic recoil of the previously restricted lung tissue, thus reducing the tendency of airways to collapse on exhalation.

Table 83-3. Selection of Patients for Surgery

Area of Investigation	Diagnostic Technique	Most Suitable	Least Suitable
Anatomy of the bulla			
Bullous area	Posteroanterior and lateral chest radiographs, computed tomography	Large and localized apical bulla (50%)	Multiple small bullae
		Unilateral disease	Bilateral disease
	Comparison with old radiographs	Gradual enlargement	No enlargement
Clinical appraisal			
Dyspnea index	Clinical evaluation	Rapidly progressive dyspnea	Slowly progressive dyspnea
			No dyspnea
Other clinical features		Nonsmokers	Smokers
		Pink puffers	Chronic bronchitis (blue bloaters)
		Minimal weight loss	Important weight loss
Function of the bulla	Inspiratory/expiratory radiographs	Nonventilated bulla	Ventilated bulla
	Body plethysmography		
	Angiography	Nonperfused bulla	Perfused bulla
Compression index	Posteroanterior and lateral chest radiographs	High index of compression (3/6)	Low index of compression (<3/6)
	Pulmonary angiography, computed tomography		Vanishing lung syndrome
State of compressed lung			
Overall function (extent of disease)	Chest radiograph	Localized disease	Widespread emphysema
	Inspiratory/expiratory views		
	Pulmonary function studies	Forced expiratory volume in 1 second >40%	Forced expiratory volume in 1 second <35%
		Preserved diffusing capacity of the lung for carbon monoxide and PaO_2 at rest	Reduced diffusing capacity of the lung for carbon monoxide and PaO_2 at rest
		No hypoxemia during exercise	Hypoxemia during exercise
Regional function (potential for reexpansion)			
Perfusion	Angiography	Good capillary filling in compressed lung	Poor capillary filling
	Perfusion scans		
	Chest radiography, electrocardiography	Normal cardiac function	Right-sided heart failure
	Heart catheterization		Cor pulmonale
			Pulmonary hypertension
Patient medical status		Younger age	Older age
			Severe intercurrent disease
		No respiratory failure	Frank respiratory failure
Choice of operation		Bullectomy	Lobectomy, segmentectomy

Reduction of Dead-Space Ventilation

If a bulla is well ventilated and underperfused (high ventilation-perfusion), the aim of surgery is to reduce this physiologic dead space and thereby decrease the work of breathing. Isotopic perfusion-ventilation studies have shown, however, that most bullae are neither perfused nor ventilated. The bulla was acting as a site of significant dead-space ventilation in only 1 of 14 patients studied by Pride and coworkers (1973).

Selection of Patients

Because of the emergence of modern techniques for lung imaging and functional evaluation, guidelines have been proposed to help select individuals likely to benefit from surgical intervention (Table 83-3). No single preoperative test, however, is considered an absolute predictor of improvement, and no absolute indications or contraindications exist to operation.

Because the premise for successful surgery is the presence of a symptomatic and nonfunctioning bulla adjacent to collapsed but potentially functional lung, a complete evaluation should attempt to answer the following questions: 1) Is there a localized or enlarging air space disorder, or both? 2) Is the patient dyspneic, and if so, what is the pathogenesis of the dyspnea? 3) Does the patient have associated chronic bronchitis, weight loss, or both? 4) Is the area to be resected nonfunctional? 5) Does the bulla compress adjacent lung, mediastinum, or diaphragm? 6) What is the status of the collapsed lung, and can the lung reexpand to become

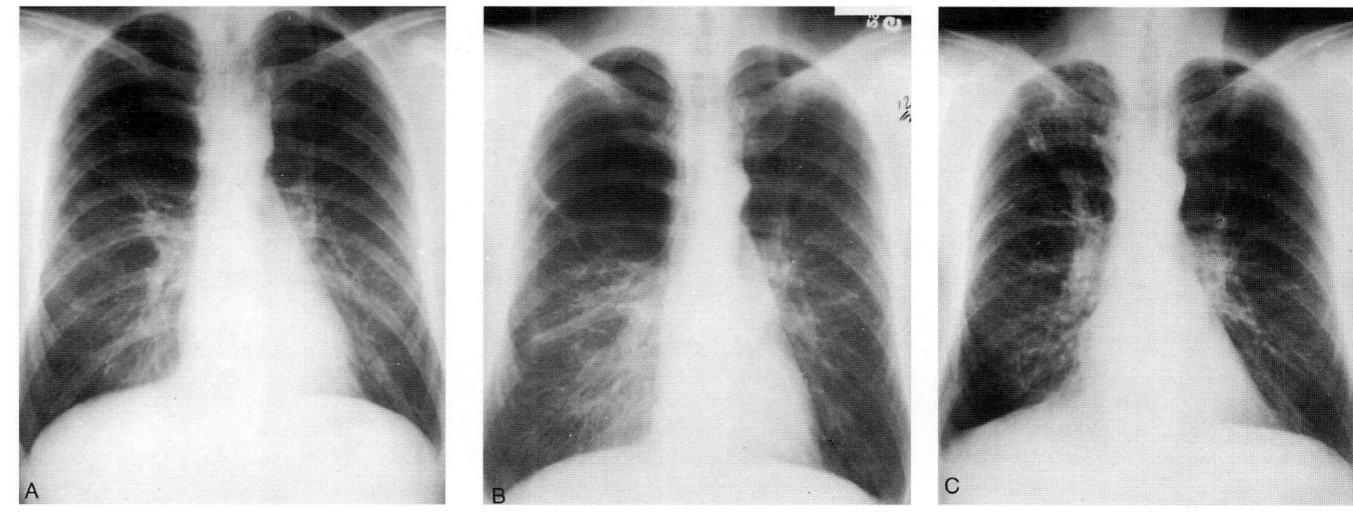

Fig. 83-12. Enlargement of a bulla. Serial radiographs demonstrate enlargement of an isolated right upper lobe bulla over 8 years. **A.** Only minimal overdistention. **B.** A well-demarcated apical bulla. **C.** After bullectomy, the underlying parenchyma reexpanded adequately.

functional? 7) What is the cardiac performance? 8) Can the patient withstand an operation?

Delineation of Bullous Area

Bullae are recognized by increased radiolucencies (avascular areas) surrounded by arcuate hairline shadows (cyst wall). Their diagnosis, number, location, and volume can be estimated from standard posteroanterior and lateral radiographs of the chest, but radiographs taken at maximum inspiration should be used to determine the true size of a given bulla. The observation that a bulla has enlarged is per-

tinent, especially if the enlargement is associated with concomitant deterioration in pulmonary reserve (Fig. 83-12).

CT is a sensitive diagnostic tool because it clearly shows the full extent of bullous disease, which is sometimes not discernible on simple posteroanterior and lateral radiographs (Fig. 83-13). For this reason, CT scanning should always be performed when evaluating patients with emphysema, whether they have obvious bullous disease or not. CT may also help in differentiating a pneumothorax from a large emphysematous bulla.

With the help of CT, Morgan and associates (1986) were able to differentiate between patients with generalized

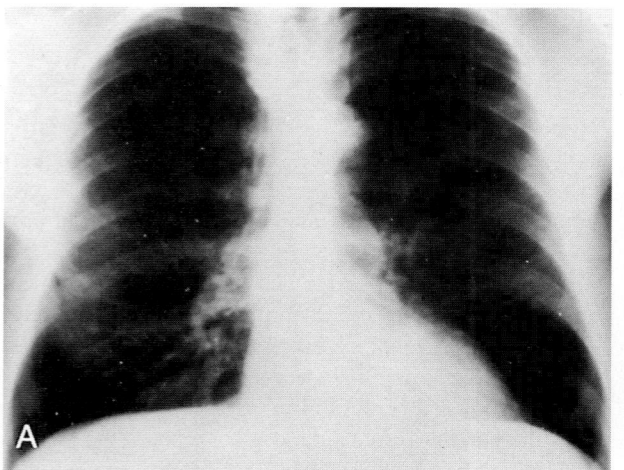
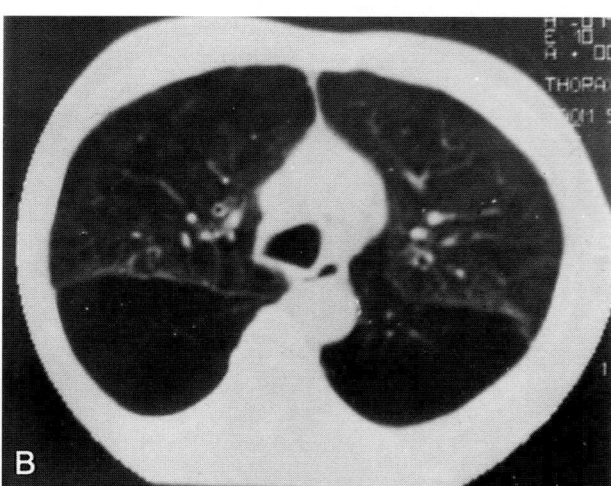

Fig. 83-13. A 53-year-old man had dyspnea. **A.** The standard posteroanterior radiograph shows almost normal parenchyma. **B.** The computed tomographic scan demonstrates well-demarcated bilateral basal bullae. Postoperatively, his forced expiratory volume in 1 second rose from 1.1 to 1.7 L and his vital capacity from 2.9 to 3.3 L. Courtesy of Dr. Marcel Dahan.

emphysema that was locally worse in the area of the suspected bulla and patients with well-defined bullae that were potentially operable. They also used CT scanning to measure the volume and ventilation of bullae, and these measurements confirmed that most true bullae do not contribute to ventilation.

Morgan and Strickland (1984) showed that CT scans obtained during expiration (dynamic CT) can offer important advantages over traditional radiology. According to these authors, the advantages of CT scanning are 1) clarification of features visible on plain radiographs, such as number, size, and position of bullae; 2) disclosure of features invisible on the plain radiographs, such as small bullae at the lung apices or in the costophrenic sinuses; 3) assessment of features often obscured by other diseases on standard radiographs, such as scoliosis; and 4) clarification and assessment of associated lung diseases.

Carr and Pride (1984) suggested that with its refinements, CT scanning has become the ultimate imaging technique for the preoperative assessment of patients with bullous emphysema.

Dyspnea Index

Because the primary objective of operation is to relieve dyspnea, selection should be based on clinical considerations. For patients with diffuse emphysema, the dyspnea must be disabling enough to limit work or everyday activities, or both, despite adequate medical treatment. Incapacitating dyspnea associated with hypoxia and hypercapnia is not considered a contraindication to operation, but surgery for patients requiring mechanical ventilation is controversial.

Clinical evaluation must also rule out any other comorbidities, such as heart disease, that may contribute to the intensity of dyspnea.

Other Clinical Features

Gaensler and associates (1986) showed that virtually all patients with bullae have a history of smoking and that smoking cessation improves the chances for a good surgical result. Hughes and colleagues (1984) also showed that among 11 patients who had received surgical treatment for bullous emphysema, all lung function variables declined at a faster rate in those who continued to smoke than in ex-smokers, the difference in rate being significant ($P < .05$) for FEV_1, and diffusing capacity of the lung for carbon monoxide (D_{LCO}).

Patients with clinical signs of chronic bronchitis, bronchospasm, recurrent infections, or dramatic weight loss generally have a higher surgical risk and a lower chance of sustained good result. Some studies have shown, however, that improved postoperative pulmonary function often results in a return to normal eating habits and significant weight gain.

Age alone is not an absolute contraindication for surgery, although emphysema is more severe and the expected oper-

ative mortality is higher in older people. Woo-Ming and associates (1963) noted that the mean age at operation of patients who had a good result was 45.4 years, whereas the mean age of patients who experienced a fair or poor result was 54.5 years.

Function of the Bulla

The distinction between communicating and noncommunicating bullae may be relevant to the understanding of the pathophysiology of a given bulla, but it is relatively unimportant in making a surgical decision. Pulmonary areas that are to be resected, however, must be areas of poor perfusion.

Most bullae are not ventilated or poorly ventilated, so the change in size in inspiration and exhalation is small. The amount of trapped air in the bulla, however, as estimated by the difference between functional residual capacity measured by the helium dilution method and by plethysmography, is large. This difference reflects the true volume occupied by the bulla. After resection of such bullae, an increase in VC and FEV_1 is expected. Morgan and associates (1986) have shown by CT scan studies of the volume of bullae and of their VC that, with few exceptions, little change in the volume of true bullae occurs between full inspiration (mean, 1454 mL) and full exhalation (mean, 1333 mL).

Bullae that communicate freely have large volume variations between inspiratory and expiratory images, but small volume difference between plethysmographic and helium dilution measurements. Little change is expected in postoperative VC, but FEV_1 improves if the space taken by the bulla is replaced by normal lung parenchyma.

Compression Index

Once it is decided that a symptomatic space-occupying bulla is present, the next step is to demonstrate that it is compressive and prevents adequate expansion of adjacent parenchyma. This is a key consideration because overstretching of nonrestricted lung may ultimately lead to some functional loss. Laros and colleagues (1986) noted that in patients with vanishing lung syndrome, the destroyed lobe had a buffer function in preventing overexpansion of the remaining lung.

Brochard and associates (1986) described a simple but effective compression index based on initial radiographic data. Patients were rated 0 to 6, according to the number of compression signs present: 1) vascular crowding in the parenchyma adjacent to the hyperinflated lung; 2) arcuate displacement of blood vessels in the periphery of the bulla; 3) displacement of the hilum; 4) mediastinal displacement during inspiration, exhalation, or both; 5) anterior mediastinal herniation of the lung; and 6) displacement of lung fissures. They were able to correlate subjective results of surgery with the severity of compression.

Most of these signs can readily be seen on standard radiography or CT scan of the chest. Pulmonary artery angiogra-

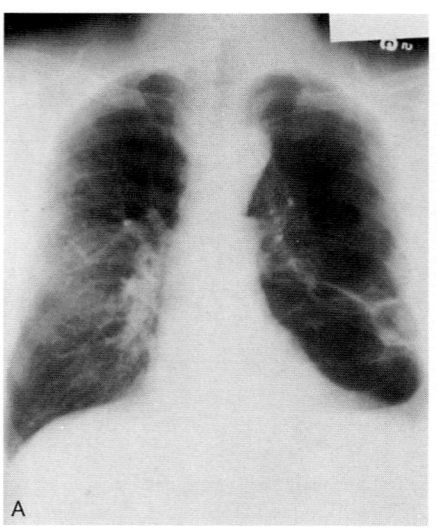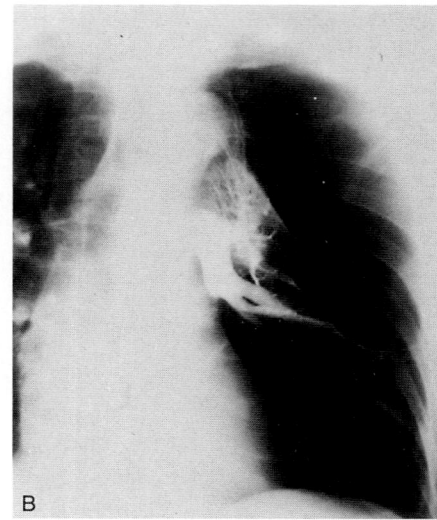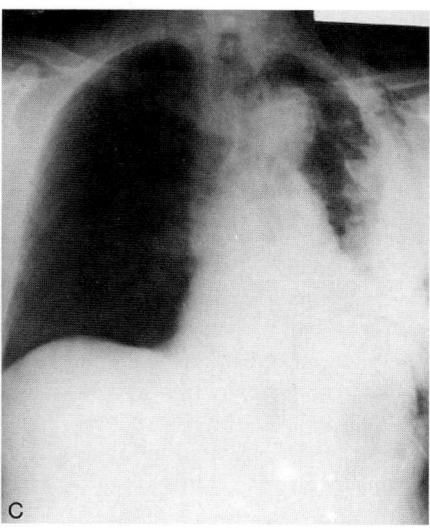

Fig. 83-14. Angiography. **A.** Chest radiograph of a 64-year-old man with previous left lower lobectomy and extensive bullous disease in the remaining upper lobe. **B.** The angiogram demonstrates a large bullous lesion with significant vascular compression. **C.** Postoperatively, the lung expands adequately.

phy may occasionally be useful not only to document vascular crowding (Fig. 83-14) but also to assess capillary filling in the periphery of adjacent parenchyma. Thinning or disruption of pulmonary capillaries (Fig. 83-15) suggests the presence of widespread emphysema and poor response to surgery.

State of Lung Adjacent to the Bulla

Because diffuse emphysema is more likely to be associated with poor outcome or at least short-lasting benefits, one

major goal of preoperative evaluation is to assess its severity. By analysis of posteroanterior and lateral radiographs of the chest, including inspiratory and expiratory images, CT, and simple pulmonary function studies, one can usually answer this question.

Pulmonary overdistention and attenuation of vascular shadows as seen on standard radiographs correlate poorly with the severity of emphysema. CT provides better information, but few data have correlated image, function, and histopathology. Gaensler and associates (1986) showed that

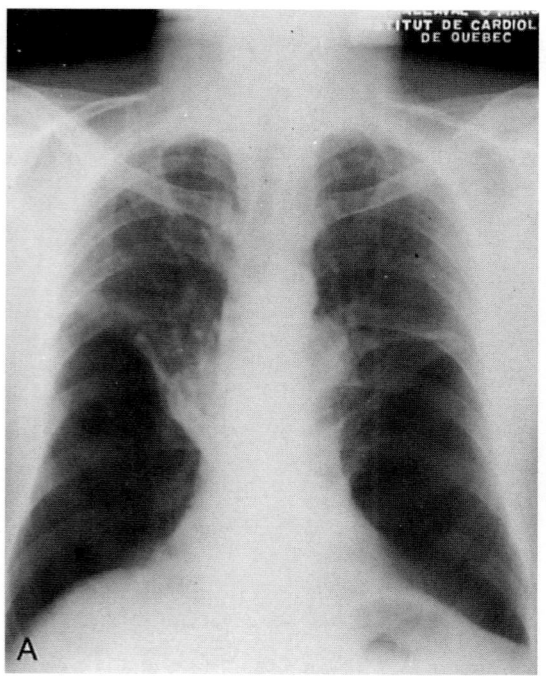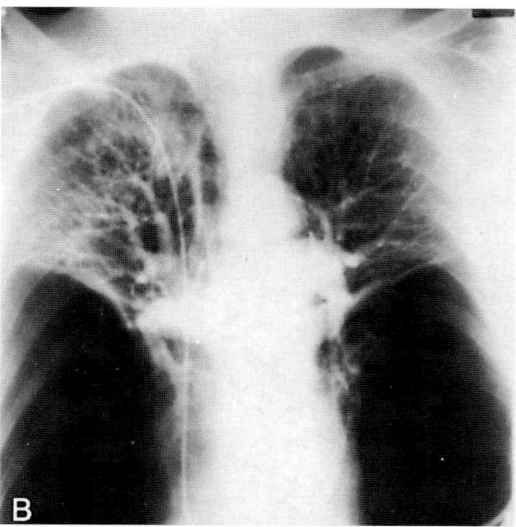

Fig. 83-15. Chest radiograph (**A**) and angiogram (**B**) of a 57-year-old man with severe chronic obstructive lung disease and large basal bullae. This patient is not an ideal surgical candidate because of a low index of compression. Peripheral capillaries in the left upper lung zone are significantly thinned.

mothorax occurring intraoperatively. In addition, the anesthetist must try to provide a quiet operative field during resection of the bulla.

Spontaneous Respiration

Because of increased peripheral airway resistance, it is best to maintain spontaneous respiration throughout most of the procedure. The active expiration of emphysematous patients contributes significantly to the maintenance of satisfactory gas exchange, especially during anesthesia. All patients are intubated under topical anesthesia, and during the procedure, they are anesthetized by inhalation of a mixture of halothane and oxygen. Continuous administration of epidural narcotics perioperatively (the catheter is inserted before induction) has decreased the need for intravenous medication or anesthetic agents. When required, spontaneous respiration can be hand-assisted with low peak inspiratory pressure.

Once the operation is completed, assisted ventilation is discontinued as soon as the patient has regained full consciousness and body temperature has returned to normal. Most patients are extubated in the operating room unless they are unable to maintain adequate blood gas values.

Intraoperative Complications

The possibility of tension pneumothorax or overdistention of the bulla precludes the use of nitrous oxide and restricts the indications for intermittent positive-pressure ventilation. What type of endotracheal tube to use is a matter of debate, but Benumof (1987) showed that a double-lumen tube is far safer than a single-lumen tube, especially if complications occur. Normandale and Feneck (1985) reported that high-frequency ventilation with low tidal volume and low airway pressure is a way to avoid pneumothorax or overdistention of the bulla.

The surgeon must be present in the operating room during induction because the pleural space may need quick decompression in the event of a pneumothorax, which may become a catastrophic event because of the impairment of venous return as well as further compromise of ventilation. At the end of the operation, the patient routinely has bronchoscopy for aspiration of blood and mucus.

Technique

Standard Technique of Bullectomy

Pedunculated bullae are dealt with easily through suture ligation of the pedicle and excision of the bulla. For patients with diffuse disease, the basic technique of plication is simple (Fig. 83-17). The development of surgical staplers has made the procedure even easier, and a modification of the Naclerio and Langer method (1947), as reported by Nelems (1980), is now used.

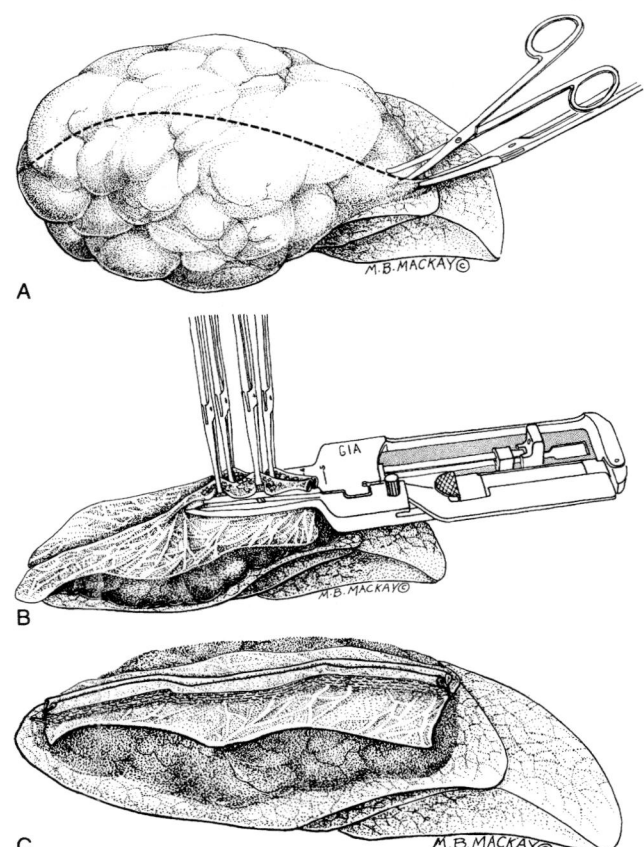

Fig. 83-17. Operative technique. **A.** Longitudinal opening of the bulla. **B.** Folding of visceral pleura over the raw surface of the lung and stapling of the entire base of the cyst. **C.** Completed bullectomy. Courtesy of Dr. J. D. Cooper.

The largest bulla is opened longitudinally and the cavity is explored from within. Strands of fibrous septae are excised (Fig. 83-18) and long Allis forceps are applied from inside so that they grasp the pleura at the reflection of relatively normal parenchyma with the cyst cavity. The visceral pleura (cyst wall) is then folded back over the remaining raw surface of lung and the GIA stapler is applied along the base of the bulla. The stapler is applied as many times as necessary until the raw surfaces of the entire base of the cyst are closed off. This double layer of pleura acts as a buttress for the staples. This reduces and may even prevent air leakage from the staple margin. Biological glues are useful to improve airtightness, but they limit pulmonary reexpansion somewhat when applied over lung surfaces. Other techniques designed to improve airtightness and minimize leakage from the suture line include the use of mechanical suture line reinforced by a polydioxianone ribbon, as described by Juettner and associates (1989), by Teflon strips, as reported by Connolly and Wilson (1989), or bovine pericardial strips (Peri-Strips, Bio-Vascular, Inc., St. Paul, MN), as described by Cooper (1994). In Parmar and colleagues' series (1987) of eight bullectomies done in seven patients, two strips of

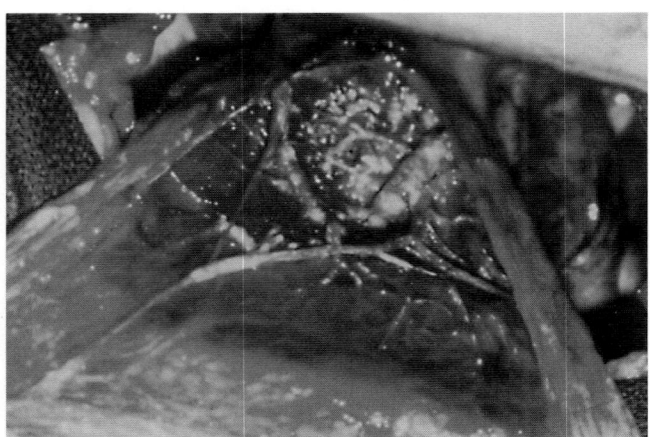

Fig. 83-18. Operative photograph shows trabeculations and fibrous septae that must be excised before stapling of the bulla.

Teflon felt approximately 1 cm wide were applied on either side of the line of resection and a continuous horizontal mattress suture of 2-0 silk was passed through all layers. All drains could be removed within 8 days with a mean interval of 4.5 days, and no patient developed a pneumothorax or atelectasis. In some cases, the parietal pleura can be cut into thin slices and wrapped around the GIA stapler before firing it as described by Whitlark and Hsu (1994).

According to Braimbridge (1989), Sir Clement Price Thomas never excised a bulla for fear of massive air leaks. He used one-lung anesthesia and allowed the lung to collapse and the bullae to become threads or tubes of thin material. He then used heavy chronic catgut, ligating the neck with three or four sutures.

The dilemma is to resect as much disease as possible while avoiding tissue reduction so extensive that it precludes lung reexpansion. In fact, the lung must be tailored to fit the hemithorax.

Some authors have stressed the importance of associating a pleurectomy or a pleural tent to the bullectomy. Eschapasse and Berthomieu (1980) advocated parietal pleurectomy, not only to prevent pneumothoraces, but also to reinforce the periphery of the lung in the hope of preventing further bulla formation. Pleural space reduction by tailoring the pleura (pleural tent), as Miscall and Duffy (1953) described, is useful when the lung does not appear to be large enough to fill the entire space. This tent is made out of parietal pleura mobilized from the apex and sutured to the lower border of the incision. Pneumoperitoneum is indicated only occasionally for patients with subpulmonic residual spaces. Because of the considerable air leak that may follow bullectomy, two properly placed drainage tubes should be left in the pleural space.

Video-Assisted Blebectomy and Bullectomy

The surgery of bullous disease by video-assisted thoracic surgery (VATS) techniques brings direct visual inspection of the lung and pleural space to minimal access surgery. It has expanded the indications for conventional bullectomy to include patients who are at high risk of operative mortality and morbidity.

Blebs and bullae can be stapled, ligated with the Endoloop (Ethicon UK Ltd., Edinburgh, Scotland), or cauterized with electrocautery, argon beam electrocoagulator, or laser. Like Landreneau and colleagues (1992), we advocate VATS staple resection of bullous disease with the Endo-GIA 30 or 60 staplers (Auto-Suture, United States Surgical Corporation, Norwalk, CT).

General endotracheal double-lumen anesthesia is always used with the patient positioned for a full posterolateral thoracotomy. Three trocars are usually necessary to perform the procedure. The first trocar, the thoracoscopic trocar, is inserted in the same location (i.e., approximately two finger breadths below the tip of the scapula, through the sixth or seventh intercostal space). A 12-mm Surgigrip is then inserted halfway between the posterior border of the scapula and the spine. If a Surgigrip cannot be inserted, which could happen in smaller or obese individuals, the skin and muscle incision should be wide enough to allow the free passage of an EndoGIA stapler without a trocar. Once the bullae are seen and their bases are well demarcated, they are suspended with an Endo dissect clamp and excised using multiple applications of the EndoGIA, usually six to eight for large bullae. A subtotal parietal pleurectomy can then be done with Endoshears. During the pleurectomy, care must be taken to remain within the endothoracic fascia to preserve the intercostal pedicle and to stay away from the costovertebral angle to avoid the sympathetic chain.

Several reports have focused on the use of VATS techniques in the management of blebs and bullae. Nathanson and associates (1991) reported on two patients with recurrent pneumothorax in whom the lung was collapsed with a CO_2 insufflator and the bullae were ligated with the Endoloop using chronic catgut and a pretied Roeder's knot. Wakabayashi (1989) also reported his experience with thoracoscopic ablation of blebs in the treatment of recurrent or persistent pneumothorax by using electrocautery. Ablation was successful in 9 of 10 patients, and the mean hospital stay of those successful cases was 2.1 days.

The use of the argon beam coagulator was evaluated by Rusch and associates (1990), and they showed that it is effective both in controlling blood loss and sealing air leaks after resection. The instrumentation is safe and it causes less tissue injury than does standard electrocautery. Lewis and colleagues (1993) reported eight patients with end-stage bullous disease, unresponsive to medical therapy, and not considered candidates for a thoracotomy, who underwent unilateral VATS ablation of bullae using the argon beam coagulator. Hospitalization averaged 13.6 days, all patients made a complete recovery, and each was subjectively improved.

Torre and Belloni (1989) reported the use of neodymium:yttrium-aluminum-garnet laser pleurodesis through thoracoscopy in 14 patients. The fiber of the laser was advanced through the operative channel of the thoracoscope, and the blebs were coagulated with low-power laser pulses. No side effects were recorded, and in 13 patients, the treatment was successful without recurrences. Wakabayashi and associates (1990) reported the use of the CO_2 laser in the treatment of patients with apical blebs and diffuse bullous emphysema. The procedure was conducted under general anesthesia with a double-lumen tube and the entire inner surfaces of the bullae were exposed to the laser. The air leaks were successfully sealed in all but one patient.

External Drainage of a Bulla

External drainage of a bulla, reported by Head and Avery (1949), is a simple, useful, and expeditious technique that can be used as a temporary or permanent measure for patients considered at poor risk for thoracotomy. The procedure can be done using local anesthesia and does not preclude later bullectomy. Because tension pneumothorax is a potentially serious complication of the technique, MacArthur and Fountain (1977) recommended removing 2.5 cm of rib over the center of the bulla and inserting a purse-string suture between parietal wall and cyst wall.

Venn and associates (1988) reported 22 intracavitary intubations performed on 20 patients for the relief of symptoms of bullous lung disease. They used the technique initially introduced by Monaldi (1938, 1947) to drain pulmonary cavities after tuberculous infection. A limited thoracotomy (5 to 7 cm) is performed to resect a portion of the underlying rib, the site of incision being determined according to the anatomy of the bulla and the disposition of adjacent compressed lung tissue. Once the pleura is opened and the bulla is incised, the interior of the bulla is inspected and the septae are perforated to allow free communication with adjacent loculae or bullae. Iodized talc is then liberally insufflated into the bullous cavity. A large Foley catheter (32F) is inserted into the cavity through a separate stab incision, and the balloon is inflated with 30 to 40 mL of air to function as a self-retaining drain. Previously inserted purse-string sutures are then tied around the catheter and an intrapleural drain is inserted at the most dependent part of the pleural space. Postoperatively, the Foley catheter remains on underwater seal drainage and is removed at 8 days, irrespective of residual air leak. After removal of the drain, the bronchocutaneous fistula spontaneously closes within 24 to 48 hours. Shah and Goldstraw (1994) reported

58 patients who underwent this procedure over a 10-year period (1983 to 1992). The operative mortality was 6.9% (four patients), and 52 patients (89.6%) noted symptomatic improvement. In all patients, improvement in symptoms was accompanied by an objective improvement in lung function.

To reduce the amount of postoperative air leakage from the bulla, Oizumi and colleagues (1990) proposed adding bronchofiberoptic occlusion of the drainage bronchus with fibrin glue to external drainage of the bulla. The fibrin glue is injected both in the base of the bulla and into the feeding segmental bronchus.

In the series of 20 patients who had external drainage of their bulla reported by Venn and associates (1988), three patients died after surgery and symptomatic improvement was reported in 16 of the remaining 17 patients; this improvement was maintained over a median follow-up of 1.6 years. Potential advantages of intracavitary drainage over standard bullectomy are that no lung tissue is removed, and both the limited incision and brief anesthesia are better tolerated by the patient.

Results

Mortality

The reported mortality varies, but in general, age at operation, patient selection, surgical approach and technique, presence or absence of cor pulmonale, and severity of diffuse emphysema are excellent predictive variables.

Witz and Roeslin (1980) reported a mortality of 1.5% for 151 patients with relatively normal underlying lung, but mortality was 11% in patients with diffuse emphysema. Most deaths resulted from respiratory failure or pleuropulmonary infection. By contrast, only two deaths (2.3%) were clearly related to surgery in the series reported by FitzGerald and associates (1974). This significant difference relates to patient selection, which was more standardized in the series of FitzGerald and associates (1974) (one institution) than in the series of Witz and Roeslin (1980) (data collected from 27 institutions in five different European countries). In three series from the 1980s (Table 83-5), no operative fatalities occurred among 66 patients who underwent bullectomy or lobectomy for bullous disease. The operative mortality for bullous emphysema should range between 1 and 5%.

Table 83-5. Operative Mortality

Authors	Years of Study	No. of Patients	No. of Operative Deaths	Percent Mortality
Witz and Roeslin (1980)	—	Group I: 151	2	1.5
		Group II: 272	25	11.0
FitzGerald et al. (1974)	1949–1972	84	2	2.3
Laros et al. (1986)	1958–1977	27	0	0.0
O'Brien et al. (1986)	1974–1981	20	0	0.0
Connolly and Wilson (1989)	1968–1988	19	0	0.0

Morbidity

Adequate postoperative care must include monitoring in an intensive care unit, prompt recognition and treatment of potential problems, early ambulation, drug treatment when needed, and above all, aggressive chest physiotherapy. This care is possible only with appropriate pain control. New techniques, such as epidural narcotic perfusion, cryoanalgesia, and patient-controlled intravenous analgesia, have been significant developments in the prophylaxis of complications.

Most problems specific to bullectomy operations relate to delayed expansion of the remaining lung, prolonged air leaks, or pleuropulmonary infections. All of these complications are troublesome, but eventually, most lungs reexpand and virtually every air leak stops. Billing and associates (1968) noted that of seven patients with persistent postoperative spaces, only one developed an empyema that required a second procedure. Air leakage is a frequent and often troublesome complication of bullectomies. It occurs because small staple or needle holes in abnormal emphysema lung tear as the lung is reexpanded, creating air leaks that can persist for many weeks postoperatively. Most air leaks can be prevented intraoperatively by the use of meticulous surgical technique. Treatment includes patience, proper suction drainage to promote full lung reexpansion, or the use of a Heimlich valve, as described by McKenna and coworkers (1996c).

Respiratory failure is uncommon if patients are well selected, and when a giant bulla is removed, the pulmonary function improves. Elective tracheotomy should be avoided, because most patients can maintain satisfactory gas exchange on spontaneous respiration. For debilitated patients, nutritive support may be required before and after surgery.

Functional Results

Assessing surgical results is difficult because most reported series are small, and as Gaensler and colleagues (1986) pointed out, bulla size, preoperative evaluation, indications for surgery, type of surgery, and quality of follow-up vary among the various series. In addition, no randomized prospective clinical trial comparing standard medical therapy with surgery has been done. From our review of more than 100 articles written since 1960, it is obvious that only general concepts can be outlined.

One of the difficulties in reporting results is the choice of parameters considered representative of good results. Certainly, decreased dyspnea and improved exercise tolerance are the primary objectives of operative intervention. Such improvement may translate into a return to useful levels of activity or even a return to full-time employment. For some patients, a decrease in the severity of chronic bronchitis also may be noted, as well as better overall quality of life. As mentioned previously, substantial weight gain can be expected after bullectomy.

Objective improvement is more difficult to quantitate, and several authors have stressed the poor correlation between relief of dyspnea and documented improvement in pulmonary function. For most patients, pulmonary function studies improve only marginally, whereas considerable relief of dyspnea is noted. In general, the degree of clinical improvement correlates reasonably well with increased air flow as measured by FEV_1, improved arterial oxygen saturations, and decreased trapped gas as measured by plethysmography. Anatomic improvement is easier to demonstrate because the expanded lung usually fills the hemithorax and isotopic studies show increased activity over previously radiolucent areas.

Early Results

With proper selection, approximately two-thirds of patients experience significant postoperative relief of dyspnea, whether they have widespread emphysema, or this improvement can be documented by pulmonary function studies. As Capel and Belcher (1957) observed, improvement is noted within 3 months of operation and is generally sustained for 2 to 3 years postoperatively.

Determining the best predictors of early good results is more difficult (Table 83-6). Bulla size is an important variable in determining clinical and physiologic outcome. Capel and Belcher (1957) reported that patients with larger cysts benefited more from operations. Gaensler and associates (1986) showed that when bullae had occupied less than one-third of the lung, no postoperative improvement was noted. With large bullae, however, postoperative increase of FEV_1 ranged from 50 to 200%. Patients likely to benefit from operation have well-documented and enlarging apical bullae occupying at least 50% of the volume of their hemithoraces. Cases of smaller bullae or multiple bullae disseminated throughout both lungs are less favorable. Laros and associates (1986) showed that patients with vanishing lungs, as recognized by prune vessels and septae within the bullous zone, should not have surgery, because soon after operation, the preoperative situation reappears in the remaining parenchyma with loss of pulmonary function.

Many authors regard the degree of compression, as documented by chest radiography, angiography, or CT scanning, as the most significant predictive variable. Gunstensen and McCormack (1973) noted that the worst results were in

Table 83-6. Best Predictors of Good Postoperative Outcome

Early results
    Bulla size and rate of enlargement
    Degree of compression
    State of underlying lung and potential for reexpansion and function
    Degree of regional asymmetry
Late results
    Severity of emphysema

patients who did not have signs of compression. Brochard and colleagues (1986) showed that when the index of compression was equal to or greater than 3, all patients had significant postoperative clinical and functional improvement. No patients with an index lower than 2 improved. Laros and associates (1986) reported that 27 patients with bullous emphysema improved after bullectomy, and their mean survival was longer than 7 years. Patients were selected for surgery based on the size of the bulla (50%) or well-documented and definite displacement of adjacent structures and on the exclusion of the presence of a vanishing lung. Connolly and Wilson (1989) and Potgieter and coworkers (1981) also showed that better results were obtained in patients with convincing evidence of compression of normal lung parenchyma.

Foreman and coworkers (1968) showed that perhaps the most useful information for selecting patients was given by the assessment of the underlying lung; it should be adequately perfused, as demonstrated by angiography, and have continued ability to wash out inhaled gas. Nakahara and associates (1983) observed that patients who did not benefit from bullectomy had disturbed ventilatory function in all lung regions, regardless of the location of the bulla. Patients with good results had relatively normal washout at the base.

By comparing initial contribution of the involved lung with postoperative increase in FEV_1, FitzGerald and colleagues (1974) noted a good correlation between regional imbalance and postoperative functional results. When the lung operated on contributed less than 10% of total function, FEV_1 always increased by more than 50% postoperatively. With a lung that initially contributed near normal perfusion, small or no increases in postoperative FEV_1 were noted.

Plication of bullae results in larger increases in FEV_1 and better clinical results than lobectomy. Rogers and colleagues (1968) investigated the effect of surgical resection on airway conductance. They observed an increase in airway conductance in all patients who underwent bullectomy. These authors attributed this increase to improved lung elastic recoil. In four of five patients who had lobectomy for carcinoma, a reduction was observed both in the airway conductance and in the functional residual capacity with relatively little change in the conductance to volume ratio. Woo-Ming and associates (1963) noted that 12 of 28 patients who had a bullectomy had a good result, whereas only 2 of 15 patients who had lobectomy could maintain a good result for any length of time. In a series reporting long-term results in 84 patients who underwent 95 procedures over 23 years, FitzGerald and associates (1974) showed that better results were obtained with giant bullae simply excised in patients with lesser degrees of chronic obstructive lung disease. Poorest results were seen in patients with smaller bullae, diffuse emphysema, and severe bronchitis who underwent lobectomy.

Other factors that may be less predictive of early good results are a large amount of trapped air in the bulla as measured by plethysmography, a severe disability before surgery, and the absence of diffuse emphysema in the remaining lung.

Late Results

Although most series have shown good to excellent initial postoperative results, dyspnea gradually returns to preoperative levels after the fifth postoperative year. The severity of emphysema seems to be the main limiting factor for sustained good results. In a series of 18 patients with bullous emphysema treated surgically, Pride and coworkers (1973) showed that increases in FEV_1 were largest in patients who preoperatively had had the least severe generalized airway obstruction. These results imply that when expiratory volumes suggest widespread emphysema, the chances of bullectomy leading to a significant and long-lasting improvement are decreased.

In the series of Witz and Roeslin (1980), patients were divided into two groups. In group I patients (151) with localized bullous disease and near normal underlying lung, 73% improved with surgery and most were able to return to work. In most cases, this improvement persisted during the years of follow-up. In group II patients (272) with more diffuse emphysema, only 50% were still improved after 5 years and 20% after 10 years. The degree of degradation paralleled the severity of emphysema.

In the series of FitzGerald and associates (1974), 47 long-term survivors with a mean follow-up time of 9 years were divided into three groups. Group I patients (16) with small and well-demarcated bullae of the paraseptal emphysema type, had sustained good results, and their long-term decline in function differed little from that of normal aging. In group II patients (16) with larger but still localized bullae, initial good results were sustained for approximately 4 to 5 years, but then function declined, only to return to preoperative levels within 7 to 10 years. In 15 patients with diffuse emphysema (group III) the average decline in FEV_1 during the follow-up period was 101 mL/year, and the functional improvement persisted for only 1 to 2 years. This annual decline is more than the expected 80 mL/year for patients with chronic obstructive lung disease and 28 mL/year for normal individuals.

Pearson and Ogilvie (1983) reviewed nine patients 5 to 10 years after surgery, and all had gradual return of their initial symptoms, with an annual decline in FEV_1 of 82 mL/year. They found no new bullae on chest radiography and no enlargement of preexisting bullae.

This clinical information suggests that surgery for bullous disease associated with diffuse emphysema is worthwhile for short-term relief, but that sustained improvement is highly unusual.

SURGICAL MANAGEMENT OF DIFFUSE EMPHYSEMA

Historical Background

In the late 1950s, Brantigan (1957) and coworkers (1957, 1959) were the first to present the concept of lung reduction for emphysema. They theorized that in the normal state, the

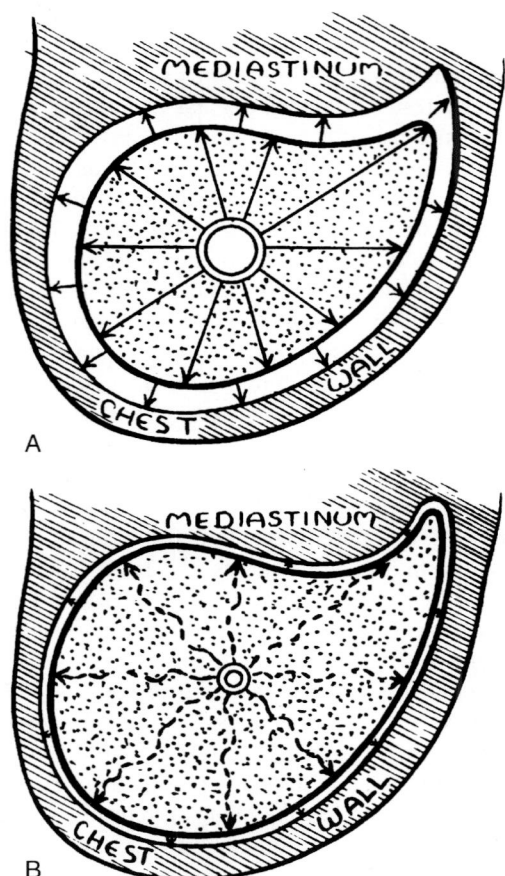

Fig. 83-19. A. The negative intrapleural pressure and the elastic fibers of the lung acting together to assert a circumferential pull on the bronchi. **B.** Loss of normal negative intrapleural pressure and the pull of the elastic fibers with no circumferential pull on bronchi to keep them open. From Brantigan OC, et al: A surgical approach to pulmonary emphysema. Am Rev Respir Dis 80:194, 1959. With permission.

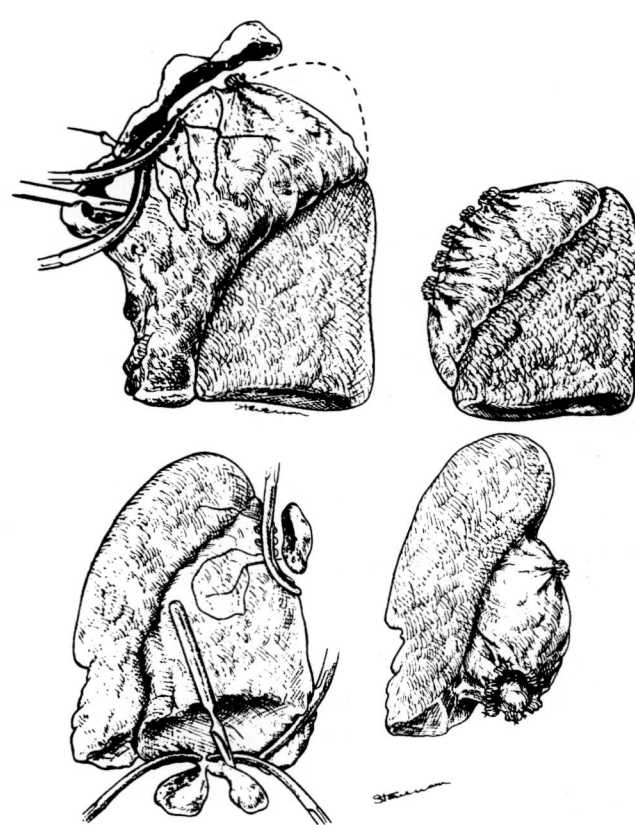

Fig. 83-20. Brantigan's method of reducing lung volume for generalized emphysema. It is done by clamp excision of the most useless areas. From Brantigan OC, et al: A surgical approach to pulmonary emphysema. Am Rev Respir Dis 80:194, 1959. With permission.

elasticity of the expanded lung is transmitted to the pliable bronchi, which are held open by a circumferential elastic pull. In emphysema, the lung has lost its elasticity and the circumferential pull holding the bronchioles open is greatly impaired, therefore accounting for a greater obstruction to airflow (Fig. 83-19). Brantigan postulated that by surgically reducing lung volume, one could restore part of this circumferential pull on the bronchioles, therefore reducing airflow obstruction and improving dyspnea (Fig. 83-20). In addition, he hoped that, by volume reduction, one could bring about a higher diaphragm with more efficient function and reduce the size of the thoracic cage, allowing for better contraction of the intercostal muscles.

Brantigan's operation consisted of reducing lung volume by the resection of the most useless areas of the lung, so that at the end, the lung would fit the volume of the pleural space on full expiration. Denervation of the lung was also added to the procedure. Among 33 patients who had this operation, there were six operative deaths (18%) and, according to Brantigan, at least two of the six deaths were caused by technical errors. All patients who survived the operation were subjectively helped, although no objective data were presented.

Soon after, Kennedy and coworkers (1960) presented a similar series of 13 patients with one operative death, one later death, and variable degree of subjective improvement among the survivors. Function measurements were inconclusive. Other procedures, such as bronchial diversion operations (D. Munro, personal communication, 1995), in which the bronchus and lung fissures were divided, were also done to achieve volume reduction.

A review of the previous work done by Georges (1966), Even (1980), and Dahan (1989) and their colleagues presented an interesting study on the use of hemodynamic data to select patients who might be candidates for volume reduction. Based on the concept of dynamic expiratory compression of both venous and pulmonary arterial flow, 10 patients were identified for disabling dyspnea, diffuse bullous emphysema, and evidence of hemodynamic impairment. Five of 10 patients who had a high compression index before surgery were improved after unilateral volume reduction.

Three years later, Crosa-Dorado and coworkers (1992) presented a detailed account of their technique involving hemostatic and pneumostatic suturing of the emphysematous lungs. The technique had been done in 76 patients between 1980 and 1991 with apparently good results in remodeling the lung for diffuse emphysema. The most recent chapter on volume reduction was written by Cooper and Patterson (1995) who presented data on 20 patients who had undergone bilateral volume reduction done through a median sternotomy incision. Preliminary results showed improvement in dyspnea, quality of life, and pulmonary function in nearly all patients who had been prepared for surgery by enrollment in a supervised rehabilitation program for a minimum of 6 weeks. A number of trials have since been carried out by various groups and have generated an increasing amount of data from which to assess the short-term effect of this procedure. An important aspect of this evaluation is the identification of selection criteria that can predict a successful outcome.

Rationale for Surgery

The rationale behind lung volume reduction procedures is the surgical excision of nonfunctional distended air spaces thought to interfere with optimal function of the surrounding more normal parenchyma. Several physiologic factors are interactive in the benefits that can be obtained after these operations.

Airflow Obstruction

In emphysema, airflow obstruction results from the loss of elastic recoil combined with an increase in airway resistance. In the normal individual, a linear relationship exists between airflow and alveolar pressure, this relationship being caused by the constant caliber of the small airways at the beginning of expiration. At the end of expiration or during forced expiration, no longer is there an increase in airflow because of dynamic compression of small airways by the surrounding lung. Hogg and coworkers (1968) have shown that because of hyperinflation, this phenomenon is increased with displacement of the airflow/alveolar pressure curve to the left, suggesting that because of the loss of elastic recoil, the lowered alveolar pressure at the beginning of expiration cannot overcome the collapse of the small airways. One of the principles of volume reduction procedures therefore involves the resection of hyperinflated but nonfunctional areas of emphysematous tissue to improve elastic recoil in the remaining lung. This in turn increases radial traction around terminal bronchioles, allowing them to remain open throughout the respiratory cycle, thus improving ventilation and relieving dyspnea.

Respiratory Muscles

Derenne and colleagues (1978) have shown that respiratory muscles such as the diaphragm, intercostals, or even the scalenes have an efficiency that is directly proportional to their shortening index and therefore to the length of their fibers during active contraction.

The anatomic modifications associated with thoracic hyperinflation place these muscles at a disadvantageous position for adequate function. Loring and Mead (1982) have shown that this phenomenon is particularly significant for the diaphragm whose lowered position limits its contractility. In addition to being at a disadvantageous position, the elevated alveolar pressures seen at end expiration add to the load that these muscles must work against. One of the objectives of the volume reduction procedure is therefore to improve contractility of the diaphragm by restoring its normal curvature.

Two additional goals can be achieved by surgery. Sweer and Zwillich (1990) have shown that in severe emphysema, patients are often in a state of denutrition with significant muscle atrophy. Correction of this status by rehabilitation programs, such as described by Cockcroft and coworkers (1981), by supplemented diets, or by surgery can significantly improve function and therefore decrease the severity of dyspnea. Bellemare and Grassino (1983) have also shown that the arterial hypoxemia seen in emphysema can place the diaphragm and other respiratory muscles in unfavorable conditions of anaerobiosis with increased fatigability. Correction of this hypoxemia by volume reduction may therefore improve muscle function.

Ventilation-Perfusion Mismatch

Cosio and Majo (1995) have shown that when distended air spaces do not have a homogeneous distribution, as is the case in most patients with emphysema, some areas of the lung have a greatly lowered elastic recoil although it is preserved in other areas. It is this heterogeneity that defines targets to be resected because these areas have poor ventilation and even poorer perfusion. In addition, compressed lung adjacent to these distended air spaces are generally well perfused but poorly ventilated, creating physiologic shunting and contributing to the arterial hypoxemia.

Cardiovascular Hemodynamics

As described in bullous emphysema, the low pressure pulmonary circulation may be the site of dynamic expiratory compression. Nakhjavan (1966) and Butler (1988) and their coworkers have shown that excessive contraction of respiratory muscles, notably during expiration, can raise intrathoracic pressures to levels high enough to generate significant decreases in systemic venous return and have a negative mechanical effect on cardiac contractility.

Pulmonary hypertension is generally seen at a late stage of emphysema. Naunheim and Ferguson (1996) have shown that elevated pulmonary vascular resistance stems from disruption in the microcirculation, which by itself is rarely sufficient to generate resting pulmonary hypertension. In a study of 21 patients who underwent LVRS, Thurnheer and colleagues (1998) found that no patient had significant pulmonary hypertension and only six had mild elevation of pulmonary artery pressure (mean, greater than or equal to 20 and less than 25 mm Hg). In that study, the pulmonary artery pressure did not change after surgery. Often, this pulmonary hypertension is secondary to arterial hypoxia, and Stark and colleagues (1973) have shown that it can be lowered by oxygen therapy.

Fixed pulmonary hypertension with secondary cor pulmonale is the result of severe destruction of the pulmonary capillary unlikely to be improved by volume reduction surgery.

Variety of Emphysema

In general terms, patients with both variations of emphysema, centriacinar and panacinar, can be candidates for volume reduction surgery. Centriacinar emphysema is commonly seen in smokers and is characterized by heterogenous patterns of disease affecting mostly the upper lobes of the lungs. In this type of emphysema, often intrinsic small-airway disease exists related to chronic inflammatory processes.

In panacinar emphysema, the disease is more uniform throughout the lung so that fewer possibilities of recruiting normal lung exist after volume reduction. In addition, less improvement in airway expiratory collapse can be expected because these small airways are intrinsically normal. One must also consider that in panacinar emphysema, reduction of lung volume may create increased inflation pressures, aggravating already existing hyperinflation.

Current Status of Lung Volume Reduction

Preoperative Assessment

LVRS is a palliative procedure that, at present, is considered appropriate treatment for a rigorously selected group of patients. Although preoperative assessment may vary between institutions, the major prerequisite is the presence of severe emphysema, as documented by CT and pulmonary function studies. The preoperative workup currently suggested can be divided into investigations trying to define the morphology of disease and those measuring pulmonary function.

Morphology

Inspiratory and expiratory chest radiography provide information regarding general thoracic configuration, hyperinflation, position of the hemidiaphragm, and severity of emphysema. Slone and Gierada (1996) have shown that chest radiography might also be useful to demonstrate associated pulmonary abnormalities such as infectious processes, interstitial diseases, or lung nodules.

CT provides a more detailed examination of the lung parenchyma. Structural changes associated with emphysema include areas of low attenuation, pruning of blood vessels, and decreased lung density gradients. Modern technologies such as high-resolution CT (thin section thickness and high-resolution reconstruction) or spiral CT allow for the calculation of the severity of emphysema as well as the three-dimensional reconstruction of the parenchyma. Combined inspiratory and expiratory CT can be used to calculate lung volume and chest wall excursion.

In an interesting study, Wisser and coworkers (1998a) defined four variables identified to quantify the severity of emphysema. These variables were 1) the degree of hyperinflation (0 to 4), 2) degree of impairment of diaphragmatic mechanics (0 to 4), 3) degree of heterogeneity (0 to 4), and 4) severity of parenchymal destruction (0 to 48). In a series of 47 consecutive patients, the authors were able to show that the degree of heterogeneity had a significant influence on functional improvement as documented by FEV_1 increase ($P = .0413$), and that the severity of parenchymal destruction was significantly associated with 30-day mortality. In a similar study, Weder and colleagues (1997) showed that the morphology of emphysema was an important predictor of outcome. In their study of 50 consecutive patients, functional improvement after LVRS was best in markedly heterogenous emphysema as defined by CT scanning. In that group, the increase in FEV_1 was $81 \pm 17\%$ as compared with $44 \pm 10\%$ for intermediately heterogenous emphysema.

Several centers finally recommend fiberoptic bronchoscopy to study endobronchial morphology in patients scheduled to have LVRS. This examination is useful to assess and grade the severity of associated malacia and to evaluate the significance of airway inflammation. Indeed, bronchoscopy is also useful to rule out occult bronchial carcinomas.

As mentioned by Naunheim and Ferguson (1996), most evaluations include a quantitative ventilation-perfusion isotope scan because this examination allows for the identification of target areas characterized by low perfusion and greatest gas retention. In addition, the amount of gas retention in various lung zones is used to predict the potential for function of the residual lung (Fig. 83-21).

Pulmonary Function

The cornerstone of pulmonary function testing is the spirometry that is used to appreciate the significance of airflow obstruction as well as its reversibility with bronchodilator drugs. Lung volumes are measured by plethysmography rather than by dilution techniques because the latter measurements tend to underestimate the degree of trapped gas and residual volume.

Other parameters of pulmonary function routinely assessed include resting arterial blood gases (arterial Po_2 and Pco_2) as well as those recorded during formal exercise testing. These are indicative of the patient's pulmonary

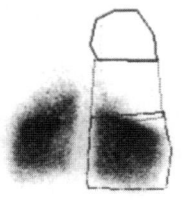
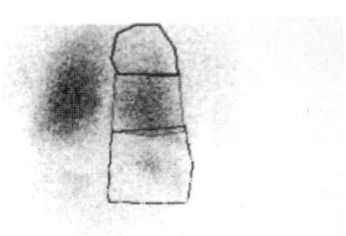

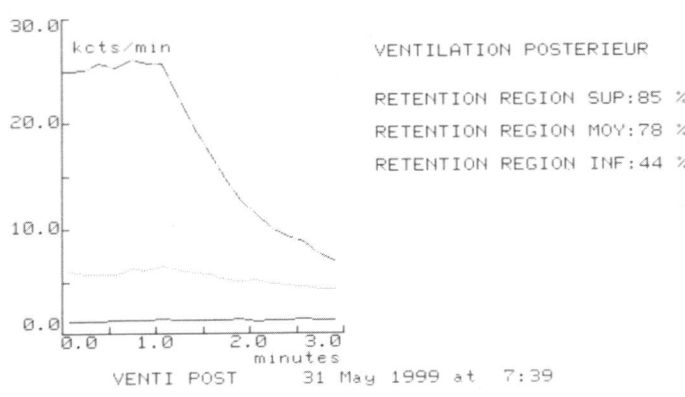

VENTILATION POSTERIEUR

RETENTION REGION SUP: 85 %

RETENTION REGION MOY: 78 %

RETENTION REGION INF: 44 %

VENTI POST   31 May 1999 at   7:39

Fig. 83-21. Ventilation-perfusion scan. Amount of xenon retained in various lung zones. Areas of low retention are likely to be functional after resection of target areas. In this figure, the lower curve represents the upper one-third of the lung with little ventilation and poor washout at 1 minute (44%). The upper curve represents the lower lung, which has good ventilation and good washout at 1 minute (85%). This is an ideal case for lung volume reduction surgery because the remaining lung (lower lung) has good potential for function based on an excellent washout.

reserve and in many ways of his or her potential for recovery after volume reduction. The diffusing capacity as measured by DLCO values is used to evaluate the severity of destruction of the pulmonary capillary bed.

Exercise Capacity

The 6-minute walk test evaluates the cardiorespiratory function quantified by the distance walked during the 6-minute exercise and by the oxygen supplement necessary to maintain oxygen saturation above 90%. More extensive evaluation of exercise capacity may be done by an ergocycle exercise test. The ventilatory response and gas exchanges may be assessed more precisely.

Cardiovascular Function

A careful evaluation of cardiac function is always done before volume reduction surgery. This evaluation includes careful taking of medical history, routine electrocardiography, and, in most cases, Doppler echocardiography to estimate ventricular function and pulmonary artery pressure. In patients with suspected coronary artery disease, a thallium-dipyridamole study should be done also.

Right-sided heart catheterization with a Swan-Ganz catheter is performed if pulmonary hypertension is suspected, not only because this finding increases the operative risk but also because it often compromises functional improvement. The test also allows for some documentation of the hemodynamic abnormalities associated with severe emphysema.

Diaphragmatic Function

Benditt (1997) and Teschler (1996) and their coworkers have shown that the evaluation of diaphragmatic function may be important if one is to understand the benefits of volume reduction surgery on the respiratory mechanics. One method commonly used is to simultaneously record abdominal and pleural pressures through catheters located in the stomach and esophagus. Because of inefficient diaphragmatic function seen in advanced emphysema, the intra-abdominal pressure becomes negative during inspiration. As shown by Dodd and associates (1984), it also becomes positive early during expiration because of the recruitment of abdominal muscles whose action is to favorably reposition the diaphragm before the next inspiration.

Some direct and indirect evidence exists to confirm improved diaphragmatic function after LVRS. Our own experience, as well as that of Slone and Gierada (1996), shows radiologic improvement in thoracic configuration, with less distention of the chest wall, as well as increased curvature and higher position of the diaphragm (Fig. 83-22).

Nutritional Status

Careful nutritional assessment must always be done because most patients with chronic obstructive lung disease are protein deficient, as shown by Donahoe and Rogers (1990). Some individuals are also overweight, a feature that may have an added detrimental effect on diaphragmatic function.

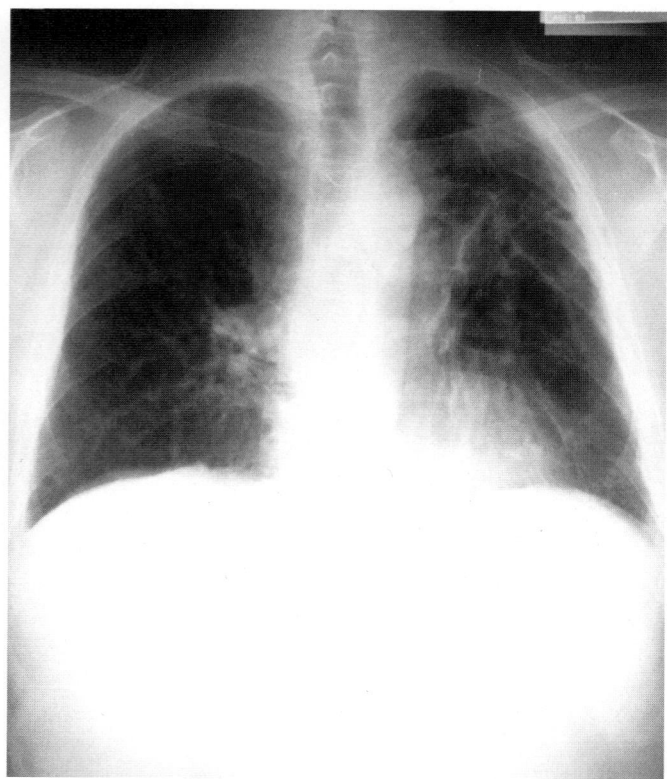

Fig. 83-22. Inspiratory posteroanterior chest radiograph of a 50-year-old male patient **(A)** before and **(B)** 6 months after bilateral lung volume reduction surgery done through median sternotomy. Improvements in diaphragmatic position are observed with higher position, increased curvature, and restored zone of apposition of the diaphragm.

Selection for Surgery

Although selection criteria may vary between institutions, important prerequisites are the presence of severe emphysema as documented by CT scanning, airflow obstruction, disabling dyspnea despite optimal medical treatment, and hyperinflated lungs by chest radiography and lung volume measurements. Other criteria include the presence of defined target areas of emphysema, smoking cessation, high personnel motivation, and ability and willingness to participate in a vigorous pulmonary rehabilitation program. Conversely, reasons to exclude patients from surgical interventions include advanced age, pulmonary hypertension, lack of suitable target areas, poor diffusing capacity, or high corticosteroid dependency, often indicative of associated chronic bronchitis or asthma.

Understanding that some patients are in a gray zone and that no preoperative test is absolutely predictive of good postoperative result, patients should be selected for surgery based on a profile determined by complete clinical, morphologic, and functional assessment. Patients with the best profiles are accepted for LVRS, whereas surgery is not offered to patients with worse profiles. As a general rule, most patients referred for surgery are not appropriate candidates and only 5 to 10% of referrals eventually have volume reduc-

tion. Indeed Miller (J.I.) and colleagues (1996) recommend that the selection process be extremely strict and selective.

Best Profile for Lung Volume Reduction Surgery

The criteria used in most institutions to select patients for surgery are outlined in Table 83-7. Like Miller (J.I.) and associates (1996), we believe that the age of 70 years should be used as a cutoff point, not only because older patients are likely to have a significantly higher postoperative morbidity or mortality, but they also have poor functional recovery. McKenna and colleagues (1997) have shown that patients aged 70 years or older experienced a 48% improvement in FEV_1 compared with an increase of 76% in younger patients. Despite these findings, and because there were no operative deaths in 17 patients older than 75 years of age, these authors, however, concluded that no absolute upper age limit could be identified.

It is essential that patients have stopped smoking for at least 6 months before operation, and random checks for nicotine are performed to ensure compliance. Patients should also be on no more than 10 mg of corticosteroids daily because higher doses may increase the risk of postoperative morbidity, especially prolonged air leaks or pulmonary infection.

Table 83-7. Best Profile for Lung Volume Reduction Surgery

Clinical guidelines
    End-stage emphysema refractory to medical treatment
    Significant dyspnea at rest or at minimal activity
    Minimal corticosteroids (<10 mg daily)
    Ability to complete rehabilitation program of 6–10 weeks
    Age <70 years and no significant comorbidity
    High motivation and acceptance of operative risk
    Abstinence of cigarette smoking for at least 6 months preoperatively
    Satisfactory nutritional status
Physiologic and morphologic guidelines
    Severe airflow limitation (forced expiratory volume in 1 second 20–35% of predicted)
    Hyperinflation (total lung capacity >130% of predicted)
    $PaCO_2$ <55 mm Hg; diffusing capacity of the lung for carbon monoxide >20% predicted
    Pulmonary artery pressure <35 mm Hg (mean)
    Heterogeneous distribution of disease
    Potential for ventilation and perfusion of residual lung

The ability to complete a preoperative rehabilitation program of 6 to 10 weeks is considered essential in most centers. As originally described by Biggar and associates (1993) and reemphasized by Miller (J.I.) and coworkers (1996), these programs include exercise arm ergometry, stationary bicycle, and exercise treadmill. Ergometry strengthens the upper extremities, whereas the stationary bike and treadmill improve overall endurance and lower extremity strength. Miller (J.I.) and colleagues (1996) even stated that pulmonary rehabilitation was undoubtedly the most important component of the entire program and that patients who could not meet the targeted rehabilitation goals of 30 consecutive minutes on the stationary bicycle and 30 consecutive minutes on the treadmill should not be operated on. As demonstrated by Debigaré and colleagues (1999), pulmonary rehabilitation programs can now be carried out entirely at home. It is also during that 6- to 10-week period that patients are better educated about their disease and eventual surgery, that their nutritional status is improved, that the amount of corticosteroids taken daily is decreased to 10 mg or less daily, and that psychological counseling and

support is provided. A summary of clinical guidelines abstracted from leading articles is given in Table 83-8.

Morphologically, the ideal candidate for LVRS is the one whose distribution of disease is heterogenous, with clearly defined targets of diseased lung. We find that ventilation-perfusion scans provide reliable information, not only about diseased areas of the lung, but also on the potential for reexpansion of the residual lung and availability of sufficient residual functional capacity. In general, patients with upper lobe disease (Fig. 83-23) are better candidates for surgery than those whose disease predominates in the lower lobes, although in lower-lobe disease, diaphragmatic function can sometimes be most compromised. Patients with α_1-antitrypsin deficiencies are not ideal candidates because the entire lung is involved by disease, and over time the residual lung also becomes hyperinflated with loss of function. In Cooper and coworkers' series (1996) of 150 consecutive bilateral lung volume reductions, 18 patients had lower lobe disease (11 with α_1-antitrypsin deficiency) and in these 18 individuals, the mean improvement in FEV_1 was 26%, the reduction in residual volume was 28%, and the increase in PaO_2 was 5 mm Hg. These values were considerably less than for the overall series, but nonetheless, Cooper and associates (1996) believed that most of these patients had experienced significant functional improvement. Ideally, the patient best suited for surgery also has radiologic signs clearly indicative of hyperinflation, with outward flaring of the lateral aspects of the thoracic cage, diaphragmatic depression and scalloping of diaphragmatic insertion, and a large anterior air space between sternum and cardiac shadow.

Physiologic parameters indicative of a good outcome after surgery include FEV_1 in the range of 20 to 35% of the predicted value and total lung capacity more than 130% of that predicted, suggesting significant pulmonary hyperinflation. Miller (J.I.) and coworkers (1996) have shown that patients who cannot reach an FEV_1 of at least 0.5 L or patients whose diffusion is less than 20% of predicted should not have LVRS and are better suited for lung transplantation or maintenance on rehabilitation programs.

Eugene and associates (1997), however, prospectively evaluated 44 patients with FEV_1 of 0.5 L or less who under-

Table 83-8. Summary of Clinical Guidelines for the Selection of Patients for Lung Volume Reduction Surgery

Criteria	Cooper et al. (1995)	Miller (J.I.) et al. (1996)	Argenziano et al. (1996)	Sciurba et al. (1996)	Miller (D.L.) et al. (1996)	McKenna et al. (1996a)
Age (yrs)	<75	<70	>75	—	<75	<80
Ambulatory	Yes	Yes	Yes	Yes	Yes	Yes
Ventilator	No	No	No	No	No	No
Prednisone requirements (mg daily)	<10	<15	<20	<20	High dose	<20
Preoperative oxygen requirement	<6 L	<6 L	—	—	—	—
Smoke free	6 mos	1 yr	6 mos	6 mos	6 mos	6 mos
Rehabilitation	Yes	Yes	Yes	No	Yes	No

Adapted from McKenna RJ, et al: Patient selection criteria for lung volume reduction surgery. J Thorac Cardiovasc Surg *114*:957, 1997.

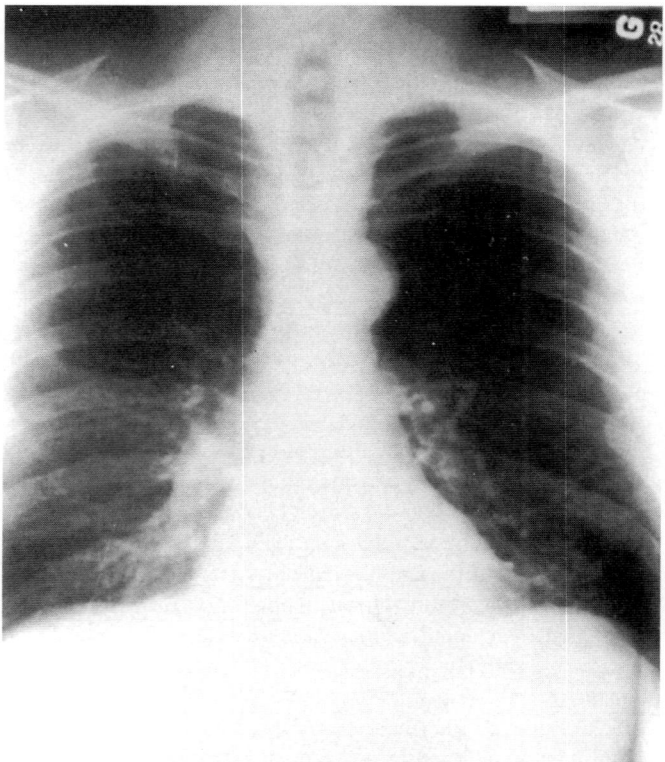

A

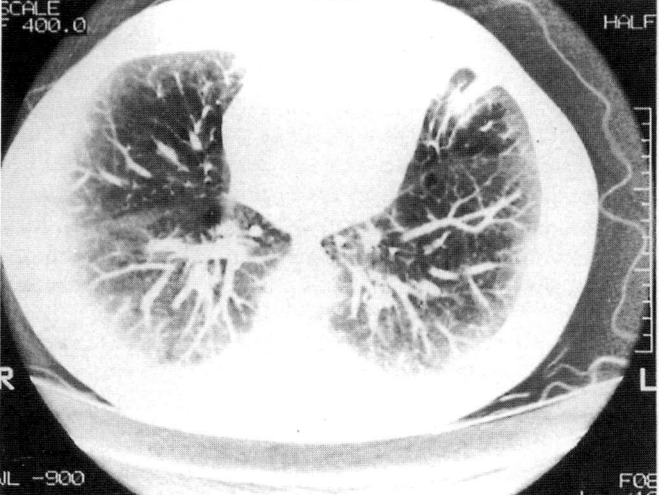

B

C

Fig. 83-23. Upper lobe disease. **A.** Chest radiograph of a suitable candidate for lung volume reduction surgery: increased lucency of the upper zones, without bullae, and relatively normal lower zones (centriacinar emphysema). **B.** Computed tomographic scan showing more severe disease in the upper lobes than **(C)** in lower lobes, therefore providing adequate target areas. This patient underwent open bilateral lung volume reduction surgery and his forced expiratory volume in 1 second improved from 1.35 to 2.19 L at 1 year postoperatively.

went volume reduction for dyspnea uncontrolled by medical management. In that series, the mean FEV_1 was 0.41 L (range, 0.23 to 0.50 L), with 80% of patients having hypercarbia and 66% pulmonary hypertension. There was one death within 30 days, and subjective improvement was noted in 89% of the cohort. FEV_1 was 0.62 L at 1 year, a 51% improvement. The authors concluded that patients with severely impaired lung function can successfully undergo operation for emphysema. In a similar study, Argenziano and colleagues (1996) concluded that profound pulmonary dysfunction characterized by FEV_1 less than 0.5 L did not preclude successful lung volume reduction and should not be regarded as absolute contraindication to surgery. Despite the results of these two studies, most investigators do not advocate surgery for patients with severe lung dysfunction.

It is generally agreed that patients with the best profile have a resting arterial Pco_2 of less that 50 mm Hg and a mean pulmonary artery pressure of less than 35 mm Hg. In

a group of four patients with hypercapnia, Miller (J.I.) and coworkers (1996) reported a 100% incidence of major complications resulting in death in two of the four patients. Wisser and associates (1998b) studied functional improvement and clinical outcome in 22 patients with chronic hypercapnia (Pco_2 greater than or equal to 45 mm Hg) who underwent LVRS, and these were compared with all other patients ($N = 58$) without hypercapnia. They concluded that hypercapnia alone was not associated with significantly higher mortality and morbidity, and therefore should not be considered an exclusion to LVRS. However, the presence of additional risk factors, such as homogeneity of disease, high degree of parenchymal destruction, or pulmonary hypertension should be considered as contraindications to the procedure.

A summary of physiologic and morphologic guidelines generally accepted for the selection of patients is given in Table 83-9.

Table 83-9. Summary of Physiologic and Morphologic Guidelines for the Selection of Patients for Lung Volume Reduction Surgery

Criteria	Reference					
	Cooper et al. (1995)	Miller (J.I.) et al. (1996)	Argenziano et al. (1996)	Sciurba et al. (1996)	Miller (D.L.) et al. (1996)	McKenna et al. (1996a)
Heterogeneous computed tomographic scan	Yes	Yes	Yes	Yes	Yes	Yes
Forced expiratory volume in 1 second	>15%	<30%	<35%	<35%	<35%	<35%
Total lung capacity	>125%		—	RV >200%	—	
P_{CO_2}	<55	<55	<50	<50	<55	<55
Diffusing capacity of the lung for carbon monoxide	—	—	—	>25%	—	—
Pulmonary artery mean pressure	<35	<35	—	—	<35	—

RV, residual volume.
Adapted from McKenna RJ, et al: Patient selection criteria for lung volume reduction surgery. J Thorac Cardiovasc Surg *114*:957, 1997.

Worst Profile for Lung Volume Reduction Surgery

The criteria used in most institutions to exclude patients for surgery are given in Table 83-10. Most of these criteria, however, do not represent absolute contraindications to surgery and none taken by itself is an absolute exclusionary criterion. It is rather the presence of several risk factors for poor outcome that is the contraindication for the procedure.

Dependence on a ventilator and a patient who is bedridden or wheelchair bound are almost absolute contraindications. In a series of 44 patients with advanced emphysema in which FEV_1 was less than 500 mL presented by Eugene and associates (1997), only six were bedridden or wheelchair bound, and none was dependent on the ventilator. Similarly, none of the 85 patients reported by Argenziano and colleagues (1996) were ventilator dependent, although 35 (41%) were unable to complete the rehabilitation program and nine (11%) had a P_{CO_2} greater than 55 mm Hg.

Severe impairment of gas exchange as documented by low D_{LCO}, low Pa_{O_2} (less than 40 mm Hg at room air), and high Pa_{CO_2} (greater than 55 mm Hg) are also considered contraindications because these values reflect the poor quality of

Table 83-10. Worse Profile for Lung Volume Reduction Surgery

Clinical guidelines
   Bronchitic symptoms or asthma
   Age >70 yrs
   Severe cachexia or obesity
   Previous pleurodesis or thoracotomy
   Severe left ventricular dysfunction or coronary artery disease
   Acquired thoracic deformity
   Alcohol dependency
Physiologic and morphologic
   Homogeneous distribution of disease
   Inability of residual lung to ventilate and perfuse
   Pa_{CO_2} >55 mm Hg
   Pulmonary hypertension (mean, >35 mm Hg)
   Diffusing capacity of the lung for carbon monoxide <20% of predicted
   Ventilator dependency

the residual lung as well as the near absence of pulmonary reserve. In a series of 154 consecutive patients who underwent bilateral thoracoscopic staple lung volume reduction reported by McKenna and coworkers (1997), 68% of patients receiving oxygen before the operation were weaned from oxygen supplementation completely after the procedure. In contrast, only 4 (22%) of the 18 patients with preoperative Pa_{O_2} less than 50 mm Hg were successfully weaned from supplementary oxygen. In the same series, 10 patients had room air Pa_{CO_2} greater than 55 mm Hg, and in this group, the postoperative room air blood gas showed a mean Pa_{CO_2} of 42.1 mm Hg. Shade and associates (1999) showed in 33 consecutive patients with a preoperative Pa_{CO_2} between 32 and 56 mm Hg that patients with higher baseline values of Pa_{CO_2} had the greatest reduction in Pa_{CO_2} post-LVRS. No substantial data exist for patients with Pa_{CO_2} at higher levels.

Signs of cor pulmonale associated with fixed pulmonary hypertension (mean greater than 35 mm Hg, systolic greater than 45 mm Hg) are poor prognostic signs and generally accepted exclusion criteria for LVRS. Similarly, anatomic airway disease, such as acquired tracheobronchomalacia, bronchitis, or bronchiectasis, are also considered indicative of a poor outcome. The problem of tracheobronchomalacia is particularly interesting and has never really been investigated in relation to volume reduction. This disorder, which is associated with advanced emphysema, is characterized by abnormalities in the elastic fibers of the membranous airways and by bronchial cartilage atrophy. Because of these features, the membranous portion of the airway becomes floppy and collapses during expiration, particularly at the level of the trachea and main bronchi where no pulmonary retraction exists capable of counteracting the collapse (soft trachea). The degree of collapse is greater during forced expiration or cough, because at that point the transmural pressure (difference between intrathoracic pressure surrounding the airways and intraluminal pressure) is greater. Several surgical methods including the use of bone chips, Gore-Tex rectus sheath, and fascia lata have been proposed to help stabilize the trachea but none has ever become popular because the results are variable and unpredictable.

Other anatomic conditions that may preclude successful surgery must be taken into account before intervention. These include pleural symphysis because of previous surgery or pleurodesis, and acquired thoracic deformities such as kyphoscoliosis or narrowing of vertebral bodies, which, because of the secondary fixation of the thoracic cage, prevent improvement even if the hyperinflation is corrected.

Miller (J.I.) and colleagues (1996) have shown that obese patients should not be operated on because their excess weight prevents them from performing early postoperative rehabilitation. In their series, four patients were considered obese and only one did well postoperatively. Similarly, they recommend against operation if a patient is receiving significant preoperative tranquilizers as the incidence of postoperative panic attacks approaches 35 to 40% in this group, such attacks being associated with a marked increase in complications. Our group also excludes from surgery patients with a low level of motivation or willingness to accept the postoperative risks, patients without strong family support, and patients with significant uncontrolled comorbidity.

Pulmonary Rehabilitation

At most institutions, pulmonary rehabilitation is the norm before performing LVRS and, in general, the goal is to achieve 30 minutes of aerobic capacity on a treadmill or bicycle with supplemented O_2 as needed. This type of program is believed to be important to improve the strength and aerobic conditioning of the patients, making surgery less traumatic and postsurgical recovery faster. Indeed, at some institutions, attainment of the exercise goals is a requirement for surgery, whereas other centers encourage patients to participate in rehabilitation programs but do not require its goals to be met before surgery.

At present, few data exist to demonstrate how useful rehabilitation is in preparing for LVRS. Although rehabilitation seldom changes the parameters of pulmonary function it improves quality of life as demonstrated by Debigaré and coworkers (1999). Postoperative rehabilitation is also essential because patients need to relearn how to breathe and use atrophied muscles.

Regardless of the time spent in formal rehabilitation, patients are expected to maintain their general fitness for the rest of their lives.

Anesthetic Considerations

Patients subjected to LVRS have friable lungs, and Triantafillou (1996) has shown that in such cases, positive-pressure ventilation may contribute to overdistention of the lungs with secondary decreases in venous return and cardiac output. It also may cause tension pneumothoraces because of the rupture of bullae or other abnormal tissues. In providing general anesthesia, the anesthetist must finally take into consideration the fact that these patients have severe underlying lung disease often associated with hypoxemia and hypercarbia.

In general, the same principles as described for the management of bullous disease are applicable to LVRS. General anesthesia is given with a double-lumen tube, and administration of long-acting narcotics or anesthetic is avoided so that extubation can be carried out immediately at the end of surgery.

Postoperative pain control is achieved through a thoracic epidural catheter located at the T3–T4 level. Miller (J.I.) and coauthors (1996) have shown that during the first 24 hours after operation, pain control should be optimized to its maximum extent using fentanyl, bupivacaine, and ketorolac tromethamine. Beginning on the third postoperative day, and subsequently thereafter, pain control is optimized with bupivacaine and tromethamine because this combination tends to minimize postoperative gastrointestinal problems seen in this particular group of patients. Subsequently, all patients are placed on a patient-controlled analgesia regimen using morphine.

Cooper and coworkers (1996) recommend that the thoracic epidural catheter be placed under fluoroscopic guidance and be used during surgery to decrease the need for narcotics or respiratory depressants and permit extubation at the end of the procedure. In their series, this goal was achieved in all ($N = 149$) but one patient who was successfully extubated the following morning.

Surgical Options

Two procedures, laser ablation and lung reduction by stapling, are currently available for the surgical treatment of diffuse emphysema amid continuing debate concerning the relative merits of these techniques. The proponents of each method claim that the lung so treated is made smaller, therefore achieving the primary goal of volume reduction.

The theoretical basis for laser action is through thermal coagulation and contraction of peripheral, emphysematous lung tissue, and Wakabayashi (1996) and colleagues (1991) have published several studies claiming success of this method. Their results are, however, open to criticism because of a lack of comprehensive follow-up and inclusion of patients with large bullae. Two papers authored by McKenna (1996b) and Hazelrigg (1996) and their associates have found laser ablation to be less satisfactory than stapling and have recommended that laser use be discontinued. In McKenna and colleagues' study (1996a) the efficacy of these two procedures was compared and patients ($N = 72$) were prospectively randomized to either neodymium:yttrium-aluminum-garnet contact laser surgery or stapled lung reduction surgery by unilateral thoracoscopy. The mean postoperative improvement in FEV_1 at 6 months was significantly greater for the patients undergoing the staple technique (32.9% versus 13.4%, $P = .01$) than for the laser treatment group, and the authors were also able to demonstrate fewer delayed air leaks in the stapler group.

Little (1997b) and coworkers (1995) also showed that improvements after laser reduction were only between 50 and 60% of those obtained with a resection technique. These authors recommend that laser be used only in areas difficult to resect, such as deep in a fissure, or in parts of the lung where resection is not planned, as an adjunctive measure to resection elsewhere. Eugene and colleagues (1995) and Wakabayashi (1996) also have presented data suggesting that the combined approach (laser and stapler) may be optimal. The report by Wakabayashi (1996) concerns 500 consecutive procedures using a combination of stapled resection and neodymium:yttrium-aluminum-garnet laser ablation of bullous disease. At follow-up, patients were found to have a statistically significant improvement in their FEV_1 of 26%, but only 203 patients out of the initial 500 were analyzed.

Further debate surrounds the relative merits of unilateral and bilateral procedures, and the use of median sternotomy versus VATS. In general, bilateral procedures have been found to give better results than unilateral reductions, with no increase in morbidity or mortality, as demonstrated by McKenna and associates (1996b). In that study, bilateral procedures (thoracoscopic stapled lung volume reduction) produced a mean improvement in the FEV_1 of 57% compared with 31% for unilateral reduction procedures ($P < .01$). In a similar study, Argenziano and coworkers (1997) showed that unilateral LVRS resulted in comparable improvements in exercise capacity and dyspnea, but that improvements in spirometric indices of pulmonary function were less in patients undergoing unilateral than bilateral LVRS.

Individual cases still exist in which a unilateral operation is more appropriate, such as when only one lung is diseased or in patients with contraindications to operation on one side such as those with prior thoracotomy or pleurodesis. In a series of 34 patients presented by Mineo and colleagues (1998), 14 selected patients had asymmetric distribution of emphysema, and they underwent unilateral volume reduction. No operative deaths occurred and at the 3-month follow-up, the mean FEV_1 increased from 0.8 to 1.2 L ($P < .001$). The authors concluded that asymmetric distribution was not an uncommon finding, and that unilateral thoracoscopic reduction pneumoplasty may represent an ideal approach in this group. Two other groups have shown good results with unilateral thoracoscopic volume reduction. Naunheim and colleagues (1996) reported their experience with the application of unilateral VATS stapled LVRS in 50 patients. Early follow-up obtained in 25 patients revealed a 30% improvement in FEV_1 and a significant improvement in Pao_2. Keenan and coworkers (1996) reported their experience with 57 patients who underwent stapled unilateral VATS LVRS. Early follow-up at 3 months revealed a 25% improvement in FEV_1.

Surgical Access and Resection of Lung

Access to the lung for volume reduction may be obtained by one of two approaches: median sternotomy and thoracoscopy. Lateral thoracotomy is no longer used, and muscle-sparing anterior thoracotomy has only been advocated by de

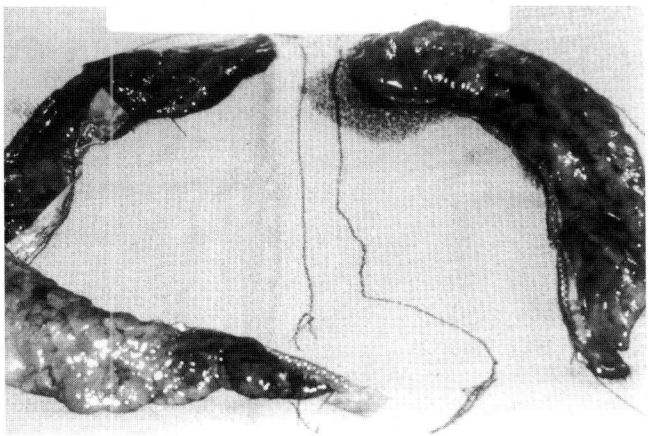

Fig. 83-24. Operative specimen showing resected lung with lung volume reduction surgery.

Perrot and coworkers (1998). In their paper, they reported that the main advantage of this approach was the excellent exposure offered to both upper and lower lobes, thus contributing to reducing the operating time and minimizing lung trauma.

In their initial paper, Cooper and associates (1995) advocated the open approach by median sternotomy. The use of this method was predicated on the desire to achieve maximum benefit at one operation with a minimum of overall morbidity. In that initial series of 20 patients, no operative mortality occurred, with an 82% increase in FEV_1, 6 mm Hg increase in oxygen tension, marked diminution in oxygen use, and significant improvement in quality of life. The follow-up paper by Cooper and colleagues (1996) and those of other authors such as Miller (J.I.) (1996), Miller (D.L.) (1996), Daniel (1996), and Date (1998) and their associates also advocate the use of median sternotomy. For all these authors, the operative technique involves staple resection of 20 to 30% of the volume of each lung (Fig. 83-24). The worse lung is done first and in upper lobe disease, a continuous staple line is used to excise the upper one-half to two-thirds of the lung (Fig. 83-25). In most cases, some destroyed lung must be left behind because, as Cooper and Patterson (1996) have pointed out, excessive removal has the potential for leaving postoperative air spaces, which promote prolonged air leaks. If such an air space is likely to be a problem, a pleural tent can be made by dissecting the parietal pleura from the chest wall. As shown by Cooper and Patterson (1996), this maneuver reduces the boundaries of the free pleural space and allows the pleural surfaces to be in apposition in the hope of sealing air leaks. With lower lobe disease, the inferior pulmonary ligament is divided and a standard U-shaped resection is carried out. As described by Cooper (1994), most authors reinforce the staple lines with bovine pericardial strips that have been shown to reduce air leakage often caused by tearing of the lung by the staples. Hazelrigg and colleagues (1997a) have also shown

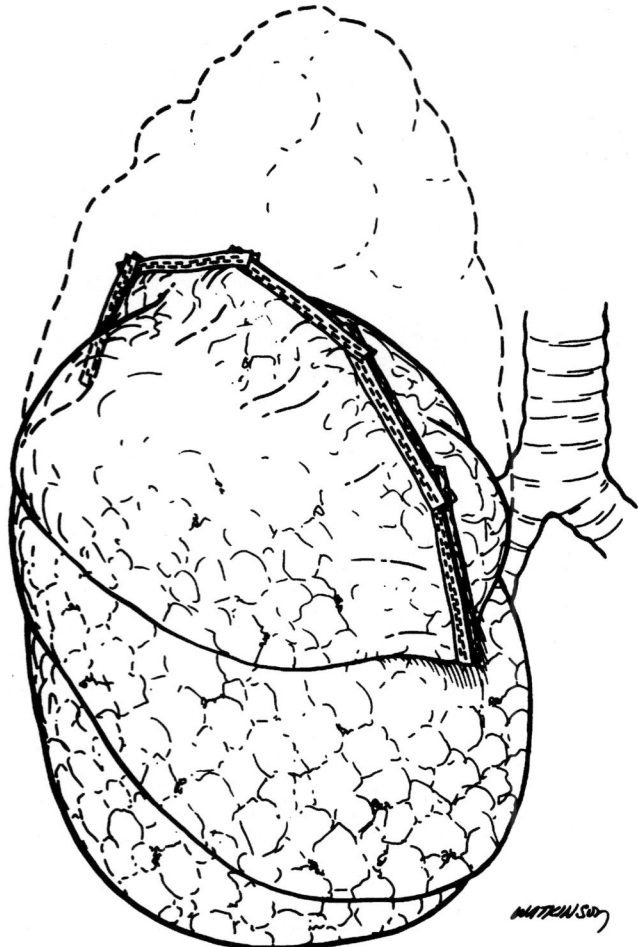

Fig. 83-25. Upper lobe lung volume reduction. A continuous staple line is used to excise the upper one-half to two-thirds of the upper lobes. The excision begins at the medial aspect of the lobe and is directed upward, over the top, and down the back side at a 45-degree angle to the sagittal pleura. From Cooper JD, Patterson GA: Lung volume reduction for severe emphysema. Chest Surg Clin N Am 5:815, 1995. With permission.

that bovine pericardial sleeves result in shorter duration of postoperative air leaks and hospital stay.

After completion of the first side, ventilation is resumed to that lung and the opposite lung is done in a similar fashion. As reported by Argenziano and coworkers (1996), a clam-shell incision can be used for the same purpose with perhaps less chance of wound dehiscence and infection. In addition, access to lower lobes may be better than through a sternotomy.

Volume reduction appears to be an ideal procedure for thoracoscopic surgery (VATS), not only because the technique is associated with lower operative morbidity, a not insignificant factor in patients with advanced emphysema, but also because the operation involves the resection of peripheral lung, which is readily accessed with thoracoscopic instrumentation. One of the inconveniences of the

VATS approach, however, is the repositioning of the patient, which is necessary if a bilateral volume reduction is to be performed in one stage. Despite this inconvenience, Little (1997a) believes that the potential benefit to these typically elderly and malnourished patients of the least stressful operative challenge is considerable. To alleviate the problem of changing position during the operation, Vigneswaran and Podbielski (1997) have described a technique in which the patient is positioned supine on the operating table with both arms extended over the head.

Kotloff and colleagues (1996) have reported similar improvements in pulmonary function and exercise tolerance after bilateral volume reduction by either median sternotomy ($N = 80$) or VATS ($N = 40$). VATS, however, was associated with a lower incidence of respiratory failure and in-hospital mortality, from which the authors concluded that this procedure may be preferable for high-risk patients. In another study reported by Roberts and associates (1998), VATS bilateral volume reduction was compared with median sternotomy with regard to postoperative complications. Significant differences were found in intensive care unit stays, days intubated, life-threatening complications, respiratory complications, requirement for tracheostomy, and death that favored VATS over sternotomy. Success also has been reported by Bingisser and coworkers (1996), who in 20 bilateral VATS volume reductions demonstrated a 38% increase in FEV_1 with a concomitant 39% increase in functional capacity as measured by a 12-minute walk test. By contrast, Wisser (1997) found that both surgical approaches resulted in similar improvement in lung function and that the incidence of air leaks, the duration of chest tube drainage, and the hospital stay were the same for both procedures.

Postoperative Management

To minimize complications and shorten hospital stay, the postoperative management of LVRS patients must be optimal. All patients are extubated immediately after completion of the procedure, if possible. This strategy is considered important by Cooper and coworkers (1996) because early extubation tends to decrease the importance and severity of air leaks.

In most institutions, patients have two chest tubes in each pleural space. These are placed with underwater seal, which tends to reduce the severity of air leaks and prevent the suctioning of a large percentage of inspired air. Occasionally, severe dryness of the airways occurs if a large air leak is present and is suctioned by active systems. If a pleural tent has been used, the tubes are placed below the tent, and if a lower lobe volume reduction has been carried out, chest tubes (straight or right angled) are left above the diaphragm. Indications for active suction drainage are the presence of a major air leak or major persistent air space. McKenna and associates (1996c) recommend the use of a Heimlich valve to facilitate earlier hospital discharge. In their series of 107 patients who underwent LVRS, 25 experienced a prolonged air leak (longer than 5 days) and were discharged from the hospital after a mean postoperative stay of 9.1 days. Chest tubes were removed an average of 7.7 days later and all apical air spaces resolved, with no deaths, empyemas, or pneumonias.

Active respiratory care must be started before the operation and compulsively carried out as soon as the patient is out of the anesthesia in the recovery room. This includes the use of physical therapies, breathing exercises, early mobilization, and bronchodilator drugs. Patients receiving systemic corticosteroids must have larger doses for 2 to 3 days postoperatively and then are reverted and maintained on the same dosage as before surgery.

Careful monitoring of the patient is important at least for the first few postoperative days. This monitoring includes blood pressure, heart rate, and urinary output as well as arterial blood gases and oxygen saturation. In these patients, it is also important to monitor breathing patterns and state of consciousness, because they occasionally retain CO_2 and become lethargic or confused.

Adequate pain control is essential for patient cooperation with bronchopulmonary hygiene and early ambulation, and this is best accomplished through the use of a thoracic epidural catheter. Other drugs routinely used during the postoperative period include broad-spectrum antibiotics and prophylactic heparin given at a dosage of 5000 U twice a day.

Results

Operative Morbidity and Mortality

Of the centers who have reported results of LVRS done between 1995 and 1997, the operative mortality varied between 5 and 10%, and most deaths were caused by pulmonary insufficiency, lung infection, or cardiac events. Little (1997b) has shown that respiratory failure is usually multifactorial and induced by lung infection, prolonged air leak, or chronic malnutrition and that cardiac complications leading to death included right-sided heart failure and myocardial ischemia. More recently, institutions have reported operative mortalities below 5%, undoubtedly the result of better patient selection and improved familiarity with the procedure. However, it is likely that the operative mortality is higher in smaller institutions with less expertise and a lower case load.

Major morbidity is encountered in an additional 15 to 20% of patients. Rigorous selection criteria and perioperative rehabilitation have kept the incidence of respiratory failure relatively low. Occasionally, however, patients need short- or long-term ventilatory assistance, which in some cases requires tracheotomy. Pneumonia is relatively uncommon because of adequate preoperative preparation, good postoperative pain control, and use of prophylactic antibiotics. If the presence of a pulmonary infiltrate is noted on chest radiography, specific antibiotics are quickly started and daily bronchoscopies may be needed to aspirate retained mucus or pus.

Prolonged air leaks (longer than 7 days) are the most frequent complications reported after LVRS, and their incidence varies from 10 to 50%. Improvement in surgical techniques, including the use of reinforced stapler lines, and avoidance of chest suction have helped lessen this problem. We have found that in cases of prolonged air leaks, the use of pneumoperitoneum to raise the diaphragm and reduce the boundaries of the pleural space is helpful. Occasionally, a patient with a significant air leak needs reexploration, especially if the importance of the air leak prevents effective ventilation. It is generally thought, although not clear from the literature, that thoracoscopic volume reduction has less morbidity than open surgery.

Miller (J.I.) and coworkers (1996) have shown that panic attacks and gastrointestinal complications are specific to volume reduction, because they are almost never seen after other types of pulmonary surgery such as lung resection for carcinoma. Panic attacks or anxiety crises are usually caused by breathing difficulties, and their incidence can be reduced or their importance minimized by proper preoperative counseling and refusal to operate on patients with psychiatric backgrounds or patients who rely on heavy doses of tranquilizers. The familiarity of the patient with all health workers involved in the postoperative care and the involvement of close relatives during that period has also helped to reduce the incidence of these problems. Another specific complication described by Miller (J.I.) and coworkers (1996) consists of marked colon distention, likely because of the slower intestinal peristalsis associated with epidural analgesia combined with the enormous swallowing of air in anxious patients. This latter factor can be partially corrected by discussing it openly with the patient and relatives before surgery.

Functional Results

The largest reported series of LVRS is that of Cooper and associates (1996) who analyzed 150 consecutive patients with only one patient lost to follow-up. In that series, clinical evaluation at 6 months showed a significant reduction in dyspnea as quantified on a dyspnea scale and index and improvement in the quality of life as documented by two questionnaires. Overall, 80% of operated patients believed that they were much better than before the surgery. Spirometry showed an improvement of FEV_1 by 51% and of forced vital capacity of 20%. Both total lung capacity (−14%) and residual volume (−28%) were significantly reduced. Gas exchange was also improved with the Pa_{O_2} being +8 mm Hg and the P_{CO_2} −4 mm Hg as compared with preoperative values. This improvement in gas exchange translated into a lower proportion of patients requiring O_2 supplements at rest (−30%) and during exercise (−48%). Although not as well documented, these results appear to be maintained at 1 and 2 years. Similar results have been reported by other groups using bilateral volume reduction whether done through an open or thoracoscopic technique. A summary of postoperative results published in the literature is given in Table 83-11.

Table 83-11. Postoperative Functional Results after Lung Volume Reduction Surgery

Series (Year)	Approach	No. of Patients	Operative Mortality (%)	Forced Expiratory Volume in 1 Second (M)	Residual Volume	6-Minute Walk Test
Naunheim et al. (1996)	Unilateral VATS	50	4.0	+ 35% (3)	−33%	+20%
Keenan et al. (1996)	Unilateral VATS	67	1.7	+ 27% (3)	−15%	+14%
Mineo et al. (1998)	Unilateral VATS	14	0	+50% (3)	−20%	+22%
McKenna et al. (1996a)	Unilateral VATS	87	2.5	+31% (3–12)	—	—
	Bilateral VATS	79	3.5	+57% (3–12)	—	—
Bingisser et al. (1996)	Bilateral VATS	20	0	+42% (3)	−23%	+39%[a]
Kotlof et al. (1996)	Bilateral VATS	40	2.5	+41% (3–6)	−23%	+35%
	Bilateral sternotomy	80	4.2	+41% (3–6)	−28%	+21%
Hazelrigg et al. (1998)	Bilateral VATS (staged)	50	0	+40% (12)	−37%	+47%
	Bilateral sternotomy	29	0	+44% (12)	−28%	+26%
Cooper et al. (1996)	Bilateral sternotomy	150	4.0	+51% (6)	−28%	+17%
Bousamra et al. (1997)	Bilateral sternotomy	37	7.0	+59% (6)	—	+30%
Date et al. (1998)	Bilateral sternotomy	39	0	+40% (3–6)	−25%	+19%

M, number of months postoperatively; VATS, video-assisted thoracic surgery.
[a] A 12-minute walk test.

Gaissert and coworkers (1996) compared the functional results after volume reduction ($N = 33$) and lung transplantation (single, $N = 39$; bilateral, $N = 27$). At 6 months, mean FEV_1 was improved by 79% (LVRS), by 231% (single lung transplant), and by 498% (bilateral lung transplant) over preoperative values. Exercise endurance as measured by the 6-minute walk distance increased by 28% (LVRS), 47% (single lung transplantation), and 79% (bilateral lung transplantation) over preoperative values. The authors concluded that LVRS was a suitable alternative in selected patients eligible for transplantation and that LVRS provided an earlier treatment option in patients who may require transplantation at some future date.

In another interesting study, Meyers and colleagues (1998) compared 22 volume reduction candidates denied operation with 65 contemporaneous and comparable volume-reduction recipients. Patients denied operation experienced a progressive worsening of their function, whereas volume reduction patients experienced sustained improvements. Absolute survival at the time of publication was 82% for the surgical group and 64% for the nonsurgical group.

A pressing concern is how long improvements are expected to last. Fessler and Wise (1999) reviewed the results of all reports providing follow-ups longer than 12 months postoperatively. The authors showed that the best FEV_1 was obtained at 6 months after operation and that thereafter the annual loss of FEV_1 was in the range of 150 to 200 mL, a rate that exceeds what is normally expected in patients with chronic obstructive lung disease. These data suggest that LVRS may accelerate the functional deterioration of the lung left behind.

Special Problems

Volume Reduction and Lung Cancer

Because lung cancer and emphysema have common etiologic patterns, it is not surprising to find that both conditions are often seen in the same individual. Indeed, Marshall and Olsen (1993) have estimated that 90% of patients with lung cancer have some degree of COPD and that at least 20% have severe disease with FEV_1 less than or equal to 1.2 L. Hazelrigg and colleagues (1997) also reported an incidence of cancer of 6.4% in a group of 281 patients who underwent a lung volume reduction operation and Pigula and associates (1996) showed that 7.8% of 128 patients who underwent LVRS had lung cancer identified during preoperative evaluation or at pathologic analysis of resected tissue. In this group, surgery is often denied because of inadequate reserve or a limited resection is carried out with higher local recurrence rates as compared with lobectomy.

Two papers have addressed the issue of combined adequate cancer resection with volume reduction. In DeMeester and coworkers' paper (1998), five patients with severe emphysema and proven or suspected lung cancer underwent lobectomy combined with volume reduction of one or more additional lobes. All five patients did well postoperatively, and each had subjective and objective improvement in respiratory function on serial postoperative studies. DeRose and colleagues (1998) also presented a series of 14 patients who underwent combined lung volume reduction and pulmonary nodule resection (11 wide wedges and three lobectomies). One operative death occurred, and at 6-month follow-up, all survivors were improved in dyspnea index, FEV_1, and 6-minute walk test. The authors concluded that simultaneous lung volume reduction and tumor resection should be considered in patients with emphysema and marginal reserve.

Volume Reduction and Lung Transplantation

The experience of institutions performing both LVRS and lung transplantation suggests that 30 to 50% of patients with advanced disease are concerned with both procedures. Cooper (1996) and Naunheim (1996) and their colleagues have suggested that LVRS can improve the quality of life of patients on a waiting list for transplant and in some cases delay transplantation. Furthermore, Zenati and associates (1995) have shown that ipsilateral LVRS does not compromise the chances of a technically successful transplantation at a later date. Kapelanski (1996) and Kroshus (1996) and their coworkers also have shown that some patients may benefit from LVRS on the native lung if it overexpands after contralateral single lung transplantation. In Kroshus and colleagues' series (1996), 3 of 66 patients who underwent single lung transplantation had development of native lung hyperexpansion and mediastinal shifting causing compression of the transplanted lung 12 to 42 months after transplantation. Unilateral LVRS was performed in all three patients, who experienced substantial relief of dyspnea and improvement in exercise tolerance after the procedure.

In general, patients with an FEV_1 of 20 to 30% of predicted and heterogeneous pattern of disease on CT should have LVRS. Patients with an FEV_1 smaller than 20% and homogeneous pattern are better suited for transplantation, whereas patients with an FEV_1 smaller than 20% of predicted but with ideal anatomic circumstances may benefit from LVRS. Zenati and associates (1998) studied 20 patients who underwent LVRS as an alternative to transplant. At follow-up of 32 ± 4 months, 19 patients were alive and 15 were off the transplant list with FEV_1 of 40 ± 18% predicted at 2 years compared with 22.7 ± 6% preoperatively. The authors concluded that LVRS has the potential to offer an effective palliation alternative to lung transplant. This is even more so in that a substantial number of emphysema patients are in fact ineligible for transplantation because of age or comorbidities.

Conclusion

Although lung volume reduction for emphysema is still a recent innovation with relatively few clinical trials that have been published, some conclusions can be drawn from the limited information available: 1) Surgery appears to offer benefits in terms of quality of life for rigorously selected subsets of patients who have exhausted other treatment options, 2) some evidence exists that bilateral LVRS offers a better result than unilateral resection and that LVRS done by thoracoscopy results in lower postoperative morbidity, 3) stapling appears to offer more consistent results than laser ablation, and in several direct comparative studies has been found to be superior, 4) pulmonary rehabilitation before surgery facilitates recovery, and 5) surgery for emphysema should be considered a palliative procedure because the remaining parenchyma must be expected to deteriorate further.

Other issues concerning LVRS are still outstanding, as highlighted in an editorial written by Rusch (1996). For instance, the most appropriate and predictable patient profiles have yet to be defined and validated. Similarly, the understanding of the role played by preoperative exercise on treatment outcomes must be improved, and methods of

objective assessment of the type, range, and frequency of tests that are necessary to monitor and evaluate postoperative progress must be developed. Some answers, such as the potential duration of benefit from LVRS, will only emerge with time. As with any new treatment, carefully controlled, prospective, randomized clinical trials are needed to generate the necessary information. Such trials are being done in Canada, as reported by Miller and coworkers (1999), and in the United States. A final consideration is the cost effectiveness of LVRS related to prolonged medical treatment. This issue has not yet been carefully addressed.

REFERENCES

Alexander HL, Kountz WB: Symptomatic relief of emphysema by an abdominal belt. Am J Med Sci 187:687, 1934.
American Thoracic Society: Chronic bronchitis, asthma, and pulmonary emphysema. A statement by the committee on diagnostic standards for non tuberculous respiratory diseases. Am Rev Respir Dis 85:762, 1962.
Anderson AE Jr, Furaker AG: Relative dimensions of bronchioles and parenchymal spaces in lungs from normal subjects and emphysematous patients. Am J Med 32:218, 1962.
Argenziano M, et al: Extended indications for lung volume reduction surgery in advanced emphysema. Ann Thorac Surg 62:1588, 1996.
Argenziano M, et al: Functional comparison of unilateral versus bilateral lung volume reduction surgery. Ann Thorac Surg 64:321, 1997.
Azary A, Anderson AE Jr, Foraker AG: The morphologic spectrum of aging and emphysematous lungs. Ann Intern Med 57:1, 1962.
Baillie M: A Series of Engraving, Accompanied with Explanations which Are Intended to Illustrate the Morbid Anatomy for Some of the Most Important Parts of the Human Body, Divided into 10 Fascicles. London: W Bulmer and Co., 1799.
Baillie M: The Morbid Anatomy of Some of the Most Important Parts of the Human Body. 3rd Ed. London: W Bulmer and Co., 1807.
Baldwin E, et al: Pulmonary insufficiency. A study of 16 cases of large pulmonary air cysts or bullae. Medicine 29:169, 1950.
Bellemare F, Grassino A: Force reserve of the diaphragm in patients with chronic obstructive pulmonary disease. J Appl Physiol 55:8, 1983.
Benditt JO, et al: Changes in breathing and ventilatory muscle recruitment patterns induced by lung volume reduction surgery. Am J Respir Crit Care Med 155:279, 1997.
Benumof JL: Sequential one-lung ventilation for bilateral bullectomy. Anesthesiology 67:268, 1987.
Berry BE, Ochsner A Jr: Massive hemoptysis associated with localized pulmonary bullae requiring emergency surgery. J Thorac Cardiovasc Surg 63:94, 1972.
Biggar DG, et al: Pulmonary rehabilitation before and after lung transplantation. In Principles and Practice of Pulmonary Rehabilitation. Philadelphia: WB Saunders, 1993.
Billing DM, Boushy BK, Kohen R: Surgical treatment of bullous emphysema. Arch Surg 97:744, 1968.
Bingisser R, et al: Bilateral volume reduction surgery for diffuse pulmonary emphysema by video-assisted thoracoscopy. J Thorac Cardiovasc Surg 112:875, 1996.
Bircher E: Die erfolge der freundschen operation beim lungen emphysem. Ditsch Med Ws Chr 44:225, 1918.
Bousamra M II, et al: Functional and oximetric assessment of patients after lung reduction surgery. J Thorac Cardiovasc Surg 113:675, 1997.
Boushy SF, et al: Bullous emphysema: clinical roentgenologic and physiologic study of 49 patients. Dis Chest 54:17, 1968.
Braimbridge MV: Discussion of Connolly JE, Wilson A: The current status of surgery for bullous emphysema. J Thorac Cardiovasc Surg 97:351, 1989.
Brantigan OC: Surgical treatment of pulmonary emphysema. Md State Med J 6:409, 1957.
Brantigan OC, Mueller E: Surgical treatment of pulmonary emphysema. Am Surg 23:789, 1957.
Brantigan OC, Muller E, Kress MB: A surgical approach to pulmonary emphysema. Am Rev Respir Dis 80:194, 1959.

Brochard L, et al: Evaluation de l'efficacité du traitement chirurgical de l'emphysème pan-lobulaire. Rev Mal Respir 4:187, 1986.

Butler J: Cause of the raised wedge pressure on exercise in chronic obstructive pulmonary disease. Am Rev Respir Dis 138:350, 1988.

Capel LH, Belcher JR: Surgical treatment of large air cysts of the lung. Lancet 1:759, 1957.

Carr DH, Pride NB: Computed tomography in preoperative assessment of bullous emphysema. Clin Radiol 35:43, 1984.

Carter MG, Gaensler EA, Kyllonen A: Pneumoperitoneum in the treatment of pulmonary emphysema. N Engl J Med 243:549, 1950.

Ciba Guest Symposium Report: Terminology, definitions and classification of chronic pulmonary emphysema and related conditions. Thorax 14:286, 1959.

Cockcroft AE, Saunders MJ, Berry G: Randomised controlled trial of rehabilitation in chronic respiratory disability. Thorax 36:200, 1981.

Committee on Therapy: Current status of the surgical treatment of pulmonary emphysema and asthma. A statement by the Committee on Therapy. Am Rev Respir Dis 97:486, 1968.

Connolly JE, Wilson A: The current status of surgery for bullous emphysema. J Thorac Cardiovasc Surg 97:351, 1989.

Cooke FN, Blades B: Cystic diseases of the lung. J Thorac Surg 23:546, 1952.

Cooper JD: Technique to reduce air leaks after resection of emphysematous lung. Ann Thorac Surg 57:1038, 1994.

Cooper JD, Patterson GA: Lung volume reduction surgery for severe emphysema. Chest Surg Clin N Am 5:815, 1995.

Cooper JD, Patterson GA: Lung volume reduction surgery for severe emphysema. Semin Thorac Cardiovasc Surg 8:52, 1996.

Cooper JD, et al: Bilateral pneumectomy (volume reduction) for chronic obstructive pulmonary disease. J Thorac Cardiovasc Surg 109:106, 1995.

Cooper JD, et al: Results of 150 consecutive bilateral lung volume reduction procedures in patients with severe emphysema. J Thorac Cardiovasc Surg 112:1319, 1996.

Cosio MG, Majo J: Overview of the pathology of emphysema in humans. Chest Surg Clin N Am 5:603, 1995.

Crosa-Dorado UL, et al: Treatment of dyspnea in emphysema: pulmonary remodeling. Hemo- and pneumostatic suturing of the emphysematous lung. Res Surg 4:152, 1992.

Curran WS, Graham WGB: Long-term effects of glomectomy: follow-up of a double-blind study. Am Rev Respir Dis 103:566, 1971.

Dahan M, et al: Intérêt de l'exploration hémodynamique dans les indications chirurgicales des emphysèmes. Ann Chir 43:669, 1989.

Daniel TM, et al: Lung volume reduction surgery: case selection, operative technique, and clinical results. Ann Surg 223:526, 1996.

Date H, et al: Bilateral lung volume reduction surgery via median sternotomy for severe pulmonary emphysema. Ann Thorac Surg 65:939, 1998.

Davies GM, Simon G, Reid L: Pre- and postoperative assessment of emphysematous bullae. Br J Dis Chest 60:120, 1966.

de Perrot M, et al: Muscle-sparing anterior thoracotomy for one-stage bilateral lung volume reduction operation. Ann Thorac Surg 66:582, 1998.

Dean NC, Stein MG, Stullbarg MS: Percutaneous drainage of an infected lung bulla in a patient receiving positive pressure ventilation. Chest 91:928, 1987.

Debigaré R, et al: Feasibility and efficacy of home exercise training in emphysema before lung volume reduction. J Cardiopulm Rehabil (in press).

DeMeester SR, et al: Lobectomy combined with volume reduction for patients with lung cancer and advanced emphysema. J Thorac Cardiovasc Surg 115:681, 1998.

Derenne JPH, et al: The respiratory muscles: mechanics, control, and pathophysiology. Am Rev Respir Dis 118:581, 1978.

DeRose, JJ, et al: Lung reduction operation and resection of pulmonary nodules in patients with severe emphysema. Ann Thorac Surg 65:3141, 1998.

Diener CV, Burrows B: Further observations on the course and prognosis of chronic obstructive lung disease. Am Rev Respir Dis 111:719, 1975.

Dodd DS, et al: Chest wall mechanics during exercise in patients with severe chronic air-flow obstruction. Am Rev Respir Dis 129:33, 1984.

Donahoe M, Rogers RM: Nutritional assessment and support in chronic obstructive pulmonary disease. Clin Chest Med 11:487, 1990.

Dornhorst AC: Respiratory insufficiency (Frederick W Pride memorial lecture). Lancet 1:1185, 1985.

Eschapasse H, Berthomieu F: La chirurgie de l'emphysème pulmonaire. Bronchopneumologie 30:173, 1980.

Eugene J, et al: Video-thoracic surgery for treatment of end-stage bullous emphysema and chronic obstructive pulmonary disease. Am Surg 61:934, 1995.

Eugene J, et al: Reduction pneumoplasty for patients with a forced expiratory volume in 1 second of 500 milliliters or less. Ann Thorac Surg 63:186, 1997.

Even P, et al: Hémodynamique des bulles d'emphysème. Un nouveau syndrome: la tamponnade cardiaque emphysémateuse. Rev Fr Mal Respir 8:117, 1980.

Fessler HE, Wise RA: Lung volume reduction surgery. Is less really more? Am J Respir Crit Med 159:1031, 1999.

FitzGerald MX, Keelan PJ, Gaensler EA: Surgery for bullous emphysema. Respiration 30:187, 1973.

FitzGerald MX, et al: Long-term results of surgery for bullous emphysema. J Thorac Cardiovasc Surg 68:566, 1974.

Foreman S, et al: Bullous disease of the lung: physiologic improvement after surgery. Ann Intern Med 69:757, 1968.

Freund WA: Zur operativen behandlung gewisser lungenkrankheiten, insbesondere des aufstarrer thorax dilatation berubenden alveolaren emphysem (mit einem operationsfalle). Z Exp Pathol Therap 3:479, 1906.

Gaensler EA, Jederlinic PJ, FitzGerald MX: Patient work-op for bullectomy. J Thorac Imaging 1:75, 1986.

Gaensler EA, et al: Surgical management of emphysema. Clin Chest Med 4:443, 1983.

Gaissert HA, et al: Comparison of early functional results after volume reduction or lung transplantation for chronic obstructive pulmonary disease. J Thorac Cardiovasc Surg 111:294, 1996.

Georges R, et al: Données hémodynamiques de l'emphysème pulmonaire diffus. J Fr Med Chir Thorac 20:373, 1966.

Goldstein MJ, et al: Bronchial carcinoma and giant bullous disease. Am Rev Respir Dis 97:1062, 1967.

Gough J: The pathological diagnosis of emphysema. Proc R Soc Med 45:576, 1952.

Gough J, Wentworth JE: The use of thin sections of entire organs and morbid anatomical studies. J R Microsc Soc 69:231, 1949.

Gunstensen J, McCormack RJM: The surgical management of bullous emphysema. J Thorac Cardiovasc Surg 65:920, 1973.

Harris J: Severe bullous emphysema. Chest 70:658, 1976.

Hazelrigg SR, et al: Thoracoscopic laser bullectomy: a prospective study with three-month results. J Thorac Cardiovasc Surg 112:319, 1996.

Hazelrigg SR, et al: Effect of bovine pericardial strips on air leak after stapled pulmonary resection. Ann Thorac Surg 63:1573, 1997a.

Hazelrigg SR, et al: Incidence of lung nodules found in patients undergoing lung volume reduction. Ann Thorac Surg 64:303, 1997b.

Hazelrigg SR, et al: Comparison of staged thoracoscopy and median sternotomy for lung volume reduction. Ann Thorac Surg 66:1134, 1998.

Head JR, Avery EE: Intra-cavitary suction (Monaldi) in the treatment of emphysematous bullae and blebs. J Thorac Surg 18:761, 1949.

Hogg JC, et al: Site and nature of airway obstruction in chronic obstructive lung disease. N Engl J Med 278:1355, 1968.

Hughes JA, et al: Long-term changes in lung function after surgical treatment of bullous emphysema in smokers and ex-smokers. Thorax 39:140, 1984.

Hugh-Jones P, Whimster W: The etiology and management of disabling emphysema. Am Rev Respir Dis 117:343, 1978.

Iwa T, Watanabe Y, Fukatani G: Simultaneous bilateral operations for bullous emphysema by median sternotomy. J Thorac Cardiovasc Surg 81:732, 1981.

Juettner FM, et al: Reinforced staple line in severely emphysematous lungs. J Thorac Cardiovasc Surg 97:362, 1989.

Kapelanski DP, et al: Volume reduction of the native lung after single-lung transplantation. J Thorac Cardiovasc Surg 111:898, 1996.

Keenan RJ, et al: Unilateral thoracoscopic surgical approach for diffuse emphysema. J Thorac Cardiovasc Surg 111:308, 1996.

Kennedy PA, et al: The surgical approach to diffuse obstructive emphysema. Preliminary report. NY State J Med 60:4002, 1960.

Klingman RR, Angelillo VA, Demeester TR: Cystic and bullous lung disease. Ann Thorac Surg 52:576, 1991.

Knudson RJ, Gaensler EA: Surgery for emphysema. Ann Thorac Surg 1:332, 1965.

Kotloff RM, et al: Bilateral lung volume reduction surgery for advanced emphysema. A comparison of median sternotomy and thoracoscopic approaches. Chest 110:1399, 1996.

Kroshus TJ, et al: Unilateral volume reduction after single-lung transplantation for emphysema. Ann Thorac Surg 62:363, 1996.

Laennec RT: De l'auscultation médiate, ou traité du diagnostic des maladies des poumons et du cœur. Paris: Brosson et Choudé, 1819.

Laforet EG: Surgical management of chronic obstructive lung disease. N Engl J Med 287:175, 1972.

Landreneau RJ, et al: Video-assisted thoracic surgery: basic technical concepts and intercostal approach strategies. Ann Thorac Surg 54:800, 1992.

Laros CD, et al: Bullectomy for giant bullae in emphysema. J Thorac Cardiovasc Surg 91:63, 1986.

Laudell CB, Eriksson S: The electrophoretic alpha-1-globulin pattern of serum in alpha-1-antitrypsin deficiency. Scand J Clin Lab Invest 15:132, 1963.

Leopold JG, Gough J: The centrilobular form of hypertrophic pulmonary emphysema and its relation to chronic bronchitis. Thorax 12:219, 1957.

Lewis RJ, Caccavale RJ, Sisler GE: VATS-argon beam coagulator treatment of diffuse end-stage bullous disease of the lung. Ann Thorac Surg 55:1394, 1993.

Lima O, et al: Median sternotomy for bilateral resection of emphysematous bullae. J Thorac Cardiovasc Surg 82:892, 1981.

Linhartova A, et al: Further observations on luminal deformity and stenosis of non respiratory bronchioles in pulmonary emphysema. Thorax 32:53, 1977.

Little AG: Pro: lung reduction surgery is of proven therapeutic benefit. J Cardiothorac Vasc Anesth 11:522, 1997a.

Little AG: Surgical treatment of emphysema. Adv Surg 30:189, 1997b.

Little AG, et al: Reduction pneumoplasty for emphysema: early results. Ann Surg 222:365, 1995.

Loring SH, Mead J: Action of the diaphragm on the rib cage inferred from a force-balance analysis. J Appl Physiol 53:756, 1982.

MacArthur AM, Fountain SW: Intracavitary suction and drainage in the treatment of emphysematous bullae. Thorax 32:668, 1977.

Mahler DA, Gertstenhaber BJ, D'Esopo ND: Air-fluid levels in lung bullae associated with pneumonitis. Am Rev Respir Dis 119(Suppl):331, 1979.

Marshall MC, Olsen GN: The physiologic evaluation of the lung resection candidate. Clin Chest Med 14:305, 1993.

McKenna RJ, et al: A randomized prospective trial of stapled lung reduction versus laser bullectomy for diffuse emphysema. J Thorac Cardiovasc Surg 111:317, 1996a.

McKenna RJ, et al: Should lung volume reduction for emphysema be unilateral or bilateral? J Thorac Cardiovasc Surg 112:1331, 1996b.

McKenna RJ, et al: Use of the Heimlich valve to shorten hospital stay after lung reduction surgery for emphysema. Ann Thorac Surg 61:1115, 1996c.

McKenna RJ, et al: Patient selection criteria for lung volume reduction surgery. J Thorac Cardiovasc Surg 114:957, 1997.

Meyers BF, et al: Outcome of Medicare patients with emphysema selected for but denied a lung volume reduction operation. Ann Thorac Surg 66:331, 1998.

Miller DL, et al: Effects of lung volume reduction surgery on lung and chest wall mechanics. Abstract and paper presented at the 32nd Annual Meeting of the Society of Thoracic Surgeons, Orlando, Florida, Jan. 29–31, 1996.

Miller JD, et al: Lung volume reduction for emphysema and the Canadian Lung Volume Reduction Surgery (CLVR) project. Can Respir J 6:26, 1999.

Miller JI Jr, Lee RB, Mansour KA: Lung volume reduction surgery: lessons learned from emphysema. Ann Thorac Surg 61:1464, 1996.

Miller WS: A study of the human pleura pulmonalis: its relation to the blebs and bullae of emphysema. AJR Am J Roentgenol 15:399, 1926.

Mineo TC, et al: Unilateral thoracoscopic reduction pneumoplasty for asymmetric emphysema. Eur J Cardiothorac Surg 14:33, 1998.

Miscall L, Duffy RW: Surgical treatment of bullous emphysema. Dis Chest 24:489, 1953.

Monaldi V: Tentativi di aspirazione endocavitaria nelle caverne tuberculari del polmone. Lotta Contro la Tuberculosi 9:910, 1938.

Monaldi V: Endocavitary aspiration: its practical applications. Tubercle 28:223, 1947.

Morgan MDL, Strickland B: Computed tomography in the assessment of bullous lung disease. Br J Dis Chest 78:10, 1984.

Morgan MDL, Denison DM, Strickland B: Value of computed tomography for selecting patients with bullous lung disease for surgery. Thorax 41:844, 1986.

Morgan MDL, et al: Origin and behaviour of emphysematous bullae. Thorax 44:533, 1989.

Naclerio E, Langer L: Pulmonary cysts: special reference to surgical treatment of emphysematous blebs and bullae. Surgery 22:516, 1947.

Nagai A, et al: The National Institutes of Health intermittent positive pressure breathing trial 1. Interrelationship between morphologic lesions. Am Rev Respir Dis 132:937, 1985a.

Nagai A, et al: The National Institutes of Health intermittent positive pressure breathing trial 1. Correlation between morphologic findings, clinical findings and evidence of expiratory airflow obstruction. Am Rev Respir Dis 132:946, 1985b.

Nakahara H, et al: Functional indications for bullectomy of giant bulla. Ann Thorac Surg 35:480, 1983.

Nakayama K: Surgical removal of the carotid body for bronchial asthma. Dis Chest 40:595, 1961.

Nakhjavan FK, et al: Influence of respiration on venous return in pulmonary emphysema. Circulation 33:8, 1966.

Nathanson LK, et al: Video thoracoscopic ligation of bulla and pleurectomy for spontaneous pneumothorax. Ann Thorac Surg 52:316, 1991.

Naunheim KS, Ferguson MK: The current status of lung volume reduction operations for emphysema. Ann Thorac Surg 62:601, 1996.

Naunheim KS, et al: Unilateral video-assisted thoracic surgical lung reduction. Ann Thorac Surg 61:1092, 1996.

Nelems JMB: A technique for controlling bullous cysts of lungs. Abstract of the Postgraduate Course in General Thoracic Surgery, University of Toronto, May 1980.

Nickoladze GD: Bullae and lung cancer. Letter to the editor. J Thorac Cardiovasc Surg 106:186, 1993.

Normandale JP, Feneck RO: Bullous cystic lung disease. Anaesthesia 40:1182, 1985.

O'Brien CJ, Hughes CF, Gianoutsos P: Surgical treatment of bullous emphysema. Aust N Z J Surg 56:241, 1986.

Oizumi H, et al: Surgery of giant bulla with tube drainage and bronchofiber optic bronchial occlusion. Ann Thorac Surg 49:824, 1990.

Parmar JM, Hubbard WG, Matthews HR: Teflon strip pneumostasis for excision of giant emphysematous bullae. Thorax 42:144, 1987.

Pearson MG, Ogilvie C: Surgical treatment of emphysematous bullae: late outcome. Thorax 38:134, 1983.

Pigula FA, et al: Unsuspected lung cancer found in work-up for lung reduction operation. Ann Thorac Surg 61:174, 1996.

Potgieter PD, et al: Surgical treatment of bullous lung disease. Thorax 36:885, 1981.

Pratt PC, Hague A, Klugh GA: Correlation of post-mortem functional structure in normal and emphysematous lungs. Am Rev Respir Dis 83:856, 1961.

Pride NB, Barter CE, Hugh-Jones P: The ventilation of bullae and the effect of their removal on thoracic gas volume and tests of pulmonary function. Am Rev Respir Dis 107:83, 1973.

Ribet ME: Cystic and bullous lung disease. Letter to the editor. Ann Thorac Surg 53:1147, 1992.

Roberts JR, et al: Comparison of open and thoracoscopic bilateral volume reduction surgery: complications analysis. Ann Thorac Surg 66:1759, 1998.

Rogers RM, Dubois AB, Blackemore WS: Effect of removal of bullae on airway conductance and conductance volume ratios. J Clin Invest 47:2569, 1968.

Rosenblatt MB: Emphysema: historical perspective. Bull N Y Acad Med 48:823, 1972.

Rubin EH, Buchberg AS: Capricious behavior of pulmonary bullae developing fluid. Dis Chest 54:60, 1968.

Rusch VW: Lung reduction surgery: a true advance? [editorial]. J Thorac Cardiovasc Surg 111:293, 1996.

Rusch VW, et al: Use of the argon beam electrocoagulator for performing pulmonary wedge resections. Ann Thorac Surg 49:287, 1990.

Sciurba FC, et al: Improvement in pulmonary function and elastic recoil after lung reduction surgery for diffuse emphysema. N Engl J Med 334:1095, 1996.

Shade D, et al: Relationship between resting hypercapnia and physiologic parameters before and after lung volume reduction surgery in severe chronic obstructive pulmonary disease. Am J Respir Crit Care Med *159*:1405, 1999.

Shah SS, Goldstraw P: Surgical treatment of bullous emphysema: experience with the Brompton technique. Ann Thorac Surg *58*:1452, 1994.

Slone RM, Gierada DS: Radiology of pulmonary emphysema and lung volume reduction surgery. Semin Thorac Cardiovasc Surg *8*:61, 1996.

Snider GL: A perspective on emphysema. Clin Chest Med *4*:329, 1983.

Spear HG, et al: The surgical management of large pulmonary blebs and bullae. Am Rev Respir Dis *87*:186, 1961.

Stark RD, et al: Long-term domiciliary oxygen in chronic bronchitis with pulmonary hypertension. BMJ *3*:467, 1973.

Stoloff IL, Karnofsky P, Mogilner L: The risk of lung cancer in males with bullous disease of the lung. Arch Environ Health *22*:163, 1971.

Sweer L, Zwillich CW: Dyspnea in the patient with chronic obstructive pulmonary disease. Clin Chest Med *11*:417, 1990.

Tanaka F, et al: Secondary spontaneous pneumothorax. Ann Thorac Surg *53*:372, 1993.

Teschler H, et al: Effect of surgical lung volume reduction on respiratory muscle function in pulmonary emphysema. Eur Respir J *9*:1779, 1996.

Thurlbeck WM: Chronic airflow obstruction in lung disease. Philadelphia: WB Saunders, 1976.

Thurlbeck WM: Aspects of chronic airflow obstruction. Chest *73*:341, 1977.

Thurlbeck WM, et al: Bronchial cartilage in chronic obstructive lung disease. Am Rev Respir Dis *109*:73, 1974.

Thurnheer R, et al: Effect of lung volume reduction surgery on pulmonary hemodynamics in severe pulmonary emphysema. Eur J Cardiothorac Surg *13*:253, 1998.

Ting EY, Klopstock R, Lyons HA: Mechanical properties of pulmonary cysts and bullae. Am Rev Respir Dis *87*:538, 1963.

Torre M, Belloni P: Nd:YAG laser pleurodesis through thoracoscopy: new curative therapy in spontaneous pneumothorax. Ann Thorac Surg *47*:887, 1989.

Triantafillou AN: Anesthetic management for bilateral volume reduction surgery. Semin Thorac Cardiovasc Surg *8*:94, 1996.

Tsutsui M, et al: Characteristic radiographic features of pulmonary carcinoma associated with large bulla. Ann Thorac Surg *46*:679, 1988.

Venn GE, Williams PR, Goldstraw P: Intracavitary drainage for bullous, emphysematous lung disease: experience with the Brompton technique. Thorax *43*:998, 1988.

Victor S, et al: Giant cervical herniation of an apical pulmonary bulla. J Thorac Cardiovasc Surg *93*:141, 1987.

Vigneswaran WT, Podbielski FJ: Single-stage bilateral, video-assisted thoracoscopic lung volume reduction operation. Ann Thorac Surg *63*:1807, 1997.

Vishnevsky AA, Nickoladze GD: One-stage operation for bilateral bullous lung disease. J Thorac Cardiovasc Surg *99*:30, 1990.

Wakabayashi A: Thoracoscopic ablation of blebs in the treatment of recurrent or persistent pneumothorax. Ann Thorac Surg *48*:651, 1989.

Wakabayashi A: Thoracoscopic laser pneumoplasty in the treatment of diffuse bullous emphysema. Ann Thorac Surg *60*:936, 1996.

Wakabayashi A, et al: Thoracoscopic treatment of spontaneous pneumothorax using carbon dioxide laser. Ann Thorac Surg *50*:786, 1990.

Wakabayashi A, et al: Thoracoscopic carbon dioxide laser treatment of bullous emphysema. Lancet *337*:881, 1991.

Weder W, et al: Radiographic emphysema morphology is associated with outcome after surgical lung volume reduction. Ann Thorac Surg *64*:313, 1997.

Whitlark JD, Hsu HK: Technique to reduce air leaks after the resection of emphysematous lung. Ann Thorac Surg *58*:1560, 1994.

Wisser W: Functional improvement after volume reduction: sternotomy versus videoendoscopic approach. Ann Thorac Surg *63*:822, 1997.

Wisser W, et al: Morphologic grading of the emphysematous lung and its relation to improvement after lung volume reduction surgery. Ann Thorac Surg *65*:793, 1998a.

Wisser W, et al: Chronic hypercapnia should not exclude patients from lung volume reduction surgery. Eur J Cardiothoracic Surg *14*:107, 1998b.

Witz JP, Roeslin N: La chirurgie de l'emphysème bulleux chez l'adulte: ses résultats éloignés. Rev Fr Mal Respir *8*:121, 1980.

Woo-Ming M, Capel LH, Belcher JR: The results of surgical treatment of large air cysts of the lung. Br J Dis Chest *57*:79, 1963.

Wright RR: Bronchial atrophy and collapse in chronic obstructive pulmonary emphysema. Am J Pathol *37*:63, 1960.

Zenati M, et al: Lung reduction as bridge to lung transplantation in pulmonary emphysema. Ann Thorac Surg *59*:1581, 1995.

Zenati M, et al: Lung volume reduction or lung transplantation for end-stage pulmonary emphysema? Eur J Cardiothorac Surg *14*:27, 1998.

READING REFERENCES

Benfield JR, et al: Current approach to the surgical management of emphysema. Arch Surg *93*:59, 1966.

Boushy SF, Billig DM, Kohen R: Changes in pulmonary function after bullectomy. Am J Med *47*:916, 1969.

Brenner M, et al: Lung volume reduction for emphysema. Chest *110*:205, 1996.

Emery RW, et al: Treatment of end-stage chronic obstructive pulmonary disease with double lung transplantation. Chest *99*:533, 1991.

Fein AM, et al: Lung volume reduction surgery. Am J Respir Crit Care Med *154*:1151, 1996.

Fitzpatrick MJ, et al: Prolonged observations of patients with cor pulmonale and bullous emphysema after surgical resection. Am Rev Tuberc *77*:387, 1958.

Hugh-Jones P, Ritchie BC, Dollery CT: Surgical treatment of emphysema. Br Med J *1*:1133, 1966.

Kuwabara M, et al: The surgical treatment of bullous emphysema: a new method for management of giant bulla. Bronchopneumologie *30*:202, 1980.

O'Donnell DE, et al: Mechanisms of relief of exertional breathlessness following unilateral bullectomy and lung volume reduction surgery in emphysema. Chest *110*:18, 1996.

Patterson GA, et al: Comparison of outcomes of double and single lung transplantation for obstructive lung disease. J Thorac Cardiovasc Surg *101*:623, 1991.

Pride NB, et al: Changes in lung function following the surgical treatment of bullous emphysema. QJM *153*:49, 1970.

Snider GL, et al: The definition of emphysema. Am Rev Respir Dis *132*:182, 1985.

Szekely LA, et al: Preoperative predictors of operative morbidity and mortality in COPD patients undergoing bilateral volume reduction surgery. Chest *111*:550, 1997.

Thurlbeck WM: Overview of the pathology of pulmonary emphysema in humans. Clin Chest Med *4*:337, 1983.

Tschernko EM, et al: The influence of lung volume reduction on ventilatory mechanisms in patients suffering from severe chronic obstructive pulmonary disease. Anesth Analg *83*:996, 1996.

Uyama T, et al: Drainage of giant bulla with bullous catheter using chemical irritant and fibrin glue. Chest *94*:1289, 1988.

Weitzenblum E: Physiopathologie de l'emphysème diffus et de l'emphysème bulleux. Rev Fr Mal Respir 8:109, 1980.

Wesley JR, Macleod WM, Mullard KS: Evaluation and surgery of bullous emphysema. J Thorac Cardiovasc Surg *63*:945, 1972.

Yusen RD, et al: Results of lung volume reduction surgery in patients with emphysema. Semin Thorac Cardiovasc Surg *8*:99, 1996.

CHAPTER 84

Bacterial Infections of the Lungs and Bronchial Compressive Disorders

Joseph I. Miller, Jr.

Suppurative diseases of the lung and certain bronchocompressive disorders formed the basis for the development of thoracic surgery as a separate surgical specialty. Despite the development of antibiotics and newer techniques in diagnosis and management, these disorders continue to form an important part of the specialty of general thoracic surgery. As noted by Hood (1994a), a number of factors contribute to the continued frequency with which these disease entities are seen. These include the emergence of antibiotic-resistant organisms, increased numbers of immunosuppressed individuals, increased drug abuse, increased aging population, and the emergence of nosocomial pulmonary infections.

The prevalence of these conditions requires that the thoracic surgeon have knowledge and surgical skills to handle these disease entities. An outline of the surgical spectrum of bacterial infections and bronchocompressive disorders of the lung is given in Table 84-1.

BRONCHIECTASIS

The term *bronchiectasis* is derived from the Greek *bronchus* and *ektasis*, meaning dilatation. In essence, as pointed out by Hodder and colleagues (1995), the term refers to the abnormal permanent dilation of subsegmental airways. The history of bronchiectasis parallels that of thoracic surgery and has been outlined previously by Lindskog (1986). The techniques of segmental resection were developed in large part because of this entity. Detailed anatomic descriptions of segmental anatomy by Boyden (1955) led to the development of individual ligation of the hilar bronchovascular structures and significantly decreased postoperative complications. With the development of antibiotics in the 1940s, this entity has not been seen as frequently, but with the emergence of drug-resistant micro-organisms and

increasing frequency of drug-resistant tuberculosis, an increased incidence of postinfectious bronchiectasis is being noted.

An outline of the etiology of bronchiectasis is given in Table 84-2. Etiologic conditions can be divided into congenital and acquired. The most frequent congenital causes are cystic fibrosis, hypogammaglobulinemia, and Kartagener's syndrome. The most frequent acquired cause is secondary to an infectious process.

Barker (1995) has emphasized that the pathophysiology of bronchiectasis requires an infectious process plus impairment of bronchial drainage, airway obstruction, or a defect in host defense. Bronchial obstruction can be caused by foreign body aspiration or enlarged lymph nodes compressing a bronchus, as seen in middle lobe syndrome. Barker (1995) noted that in immunocompromised patients, there may be ciliary dyskinesia, airway immune effector cells, neutrophilic proteases, and inflammatory cytokines. Regardless of the cause, an intense inflammation results in transmural inflammation, mucosal edema, and bronchial neovascularization.

The terms *cylindrical*, *varicose*, and *saccular* have been used to describe the pathology of bronchiectasis. A classification of bronchiectasis is given in Table 84-3. Saccular bronchiectasis follows a major pulmonary infection or results from a foreign body or bronchial stricture and is the principal type of surgical importance. Cylindrical bronchiectasis consists of bronchi that do not end blindly but communicate with lung parenchyma. This is associated frequently with tuberculosis and immune disorders. Hood (1994b) has noted a third type referred to as *varicose*, a mixture of the former two, and is distinguished by alternating areas of cylindrical and saccular disease. *Pseudobronchiectasis*, a term first reported by Blades and Dugan (1944), is a cylindrical dilatation of a bronchus after an acute pneumonic process that is temporary and disappears in several weeks or

Table 84-1. Surgical Spectrum of Bacterial Infections of the Lung and Bronchial Compressive Disease

Spectrum of surgical infectious disease
  Bronchiectasis
  Lung abscess
  Organizing pneumonia
  Pulmonary infection in granulomatous disease of childhood
  Tuberculosis and fungal disease
  Thoracic empyema
Bronchial compressive pulmonary disorders
  Right middle lobe syndrome
  Broncholithiasis
  Inflammatory lymphadenopathy
  Congenital processes
  Sclerosing mediastinitis
  Cardiovascular disease
    Congenital
      Vascular ring
      Aberrant left pulmonary artery
    Acquired aortic disease
      Aortic arch aneurysm
      Traumatic false aneurysm

months. This type has no surgical implications. In addition, certain genetic syndromes may be associated with some form of bronchiectasis. These include cystic fibrosis, α_1-antitrypsin deficiency, and immunoglobulin A (IgA) and IgG deficiency.

The distribution and frequency of bronchiectasis is given in Tables 84-4 and 84-5. The distribution to some extent is characteristic of the etiologic cause. For example, in patients with Kartagener's syndrome, hypogammaglobulinemia, and cystic fibrosis, the areas of involvement are generally diffuse and bilateral and involve multiple cystic segments of both upper and lower lobes. Tuberculosis is either unilateral or bilateral and generally involves the upper lobes or superior segment of the lower lobes.

Table 84-2. Etiology of Bronchiectasis

Congenital
  Congenital cystic bronchiectasis
  Selective immunoglobulin A deficiency
  Primary hypogammaglobulinemia
  Cystic fibrosis
  α_1-Antitrypsin deficiency
  Kartagener's syndrome
  Congenital deficiency of bronchial cartilage
  Bronchopulmonary sequestration
Acquired
  Infection
  Bronchial obstruction
    Intrinsic: tumor, foreign body
    Extrinsic: enlarged lymph nodes
  Middle lobe syndrome
  Scarring secondary to tuberculosis
  Acquired hypogammaglobulinemia

Table 84-3. Classification of Bronchiectasis

Saccular bronchiectasis
Cylindrical bronchiectasis
Pseudobronchiectasis
Posttuberculosis bronchiectasis
Genetic-related bronchiectasis

Middle lobe syndrome is caused by the involvement of lymph nodes and the middle lobe bronchus from a granulomatous process.

Clinical Diagnosis

Clinical bronchiectasis is characterized by repeated episodes of respiratory tract infection. The key symptom is cough with mucopurulent and tenacious secretions lasting months to years. This may be accompanied by intermittent hemoptysis, dyspnea, wheezing, and pleurisy. It is most frequently characterized by clinically repeated episodes.

Methods of Diagnosis

After a thorough history and physical examination, the most frequently used techniques in the diagnosis of bronchiectasis are imaging modalities, fiberoptic bronchoscopy, and bronchograms. Before the advent of computed tomography (CT), a bronchogram was the standard procedure for diagnosis (Fig. 84-1). A high-resolution CT scan has replaced this procedure in the diagnosis of bronchiectasis. The detailed images demonstrate bronchial

Table 84-4. Anatomic Distribution of Bronchiectasis in Order of Frequency

Left lower lobe
Right middle lobe, left lingula
Total left lung
Total right lung
Right upper lobe
Left upper lobe

Table 84-5. Frequency of Distribution of Bronchiectasis: Area of Involvement

Left lung more often than right lung (9:7)
Left lower lobe, most frequently involved
Right middle lobe and lingula, next most frequently involved
Total left bronchiectasis, fourth most commonly involved
Right lower and total right are less often involved
Right upper lobe is involved more often than left upper lobe (4:1)

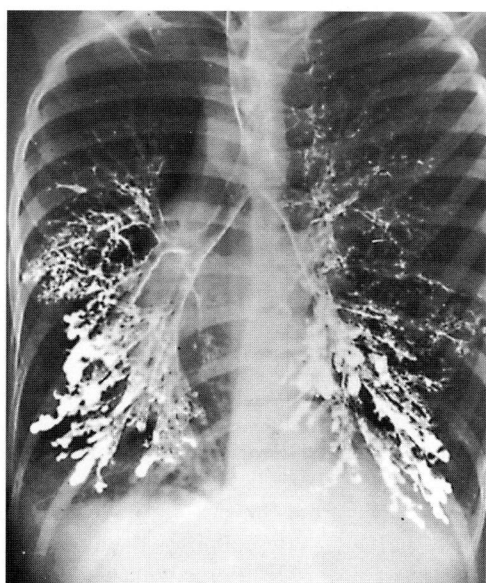

Fig. 84-1. Bilateral saccular bronchiectasis, characteristic of the preantibiotic era, involving the lower lobes, lingula, and right middle lobe. From Ferguson TB, Burford TH: The changing pattern of pulmonary suppuration: surgical implications. Dis Chest 53:396, 1968. With permission.

dilatation, peribronchial inflammation, and parenchymal disease. According to Barker (1995), the diagnosis can be made with a 2% false-negative and a 1% false-positive rate.

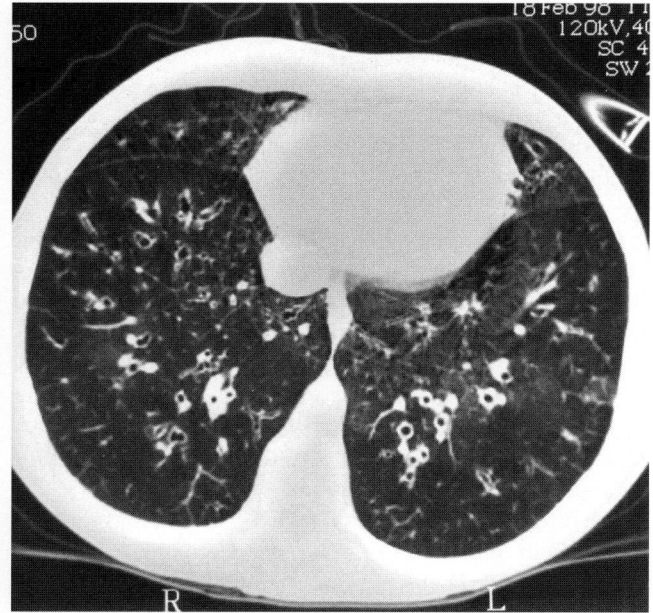

Fig. 84-2. High-resolution computed tomographic scan of bronchiectasis.

Table 84-6. Treatment of Bronchiectasis

Medical
   Prevention and control
   Antibiotics
   Postural drainage
Surgical
   Unilateral, segmental, or lobar distribution
   Persistent, recurrent symptoms when medication is discontinued
   Recurrent infection and hemoptysis
Transplantation

Figure 84-2 shows a typical high-resolution CT for lower lobe bronchiectasis.

Treatment of Bronchiectasis

An outline for the medical and surgical management of bronchiectasis is given in Table 84-6. The goals of medical management include prevention and control, appropriate antibiotic therapy, and postural drainage.

Surgical management of bronchiectasis has strict limitations and guidelines. Surgical treatment is based on three premises: 1) the disease is segmental and unilateral, 2) complete resection of all disease is possible, and 3) complete resection of all disease prevents recurrence. This does not apply to those patients with immunologic or genetic abnormalities. Specific surgical indications are listed in Table 84-6. The immediate goal of surgical resection is the removal of most, preferably all, involved segments or lobes and preservation of nonsuppurative areas. The results of surgical resection for bronchiectasis are given in Table 84-7. Hodder and associates (1995) report that the mortality varies from 0 to 8.3%.

Lung transplantation may be performed for patients with suppurative lung disease. Barker (1995) noted that of 3160 lung transplants reported by The St. Louis Lung Transplant Registry in 1994, 466 patients had transplants for cystic fibrosis and 82 for bronchiectasis. The actuarial survival at 1 year is 72% for cystic fibrosis and 57% at 3 years.

Table 84-7. Results of Surgical Resection for Bronchiectasis

Author	Patients	Mortality (%)	Morbidity (%)
Sealy et al. (1966)	140	1.4	3
Sanderson et al. (1974)	242	0.4	33
Annest et al. (1982)	24	8.3	13
Dogan (1989)	487	3.5	11

Modified from Hodder RV, Cameron R, Todd TRJ: Bacterial infections. *In* Pearson FG, et al. (eds): Thoracic Surgery. New York: Churchill Livingstone, 1995.

Table 84-8. Classification of Lung Abscess

Primary lung abscess (acute or chronic)
    Related to anaerobic aspiration
    Related to specific pneumonia
Secondary lung abscess
    With existing lung disease
    Metastatic from extrathoracic source
    Obstructing bronchial carcinoma
    Bronchoesophageal fistula
    Foreign body inhalation
    Pulmonary infarction
    Bullous emphysema

Table 84-10. Bacteriology of Lung Abscess

Anaerobic
    Bacteroides fragilis
    Fusobacterium bacilli
    Streptococcus, β-hemolytic streptococcus
Aerobic
    Klebsiella pneumoniae
    Pseudomonas aeruginosa
    Staphylococcus aureus
    Streptococcus pneumoniae
    Haemophilus influenzae

LUNG ABSCESS

Lung abscess has been recognized since the time of Hippocrates; Wiedemann and Rice (1995) quote Hippocrates:

> As time goes by, the fever becomes more severe, coughing begins and the patient cannot lie any more on the healthy side but only on the diseased side. The feet and eyes swell. When the 15th day after the rupture has occurred, prepare a warm bath, sit him upon a stool, shake him by the shoulders and listen to where the noise is heard. At that place, make an incision then it produces death more rarely.

Before the antibiotic era it was realized that unless drainage was achieved, death was inevitable. With the development of antibiotics, treatment improved and mortality decreased. With the development of increasing numbers of immunosuppressed individuals and the increased incidence of nosocomial pneumonia, lung abscess continues to be a problem for practicing thoracic surgeons.

Geppert (1994) defines a lung abscess as a subacute pulmonary infection in which the chest radiograph shows a cavity within the pulmonary parenchyma. It is a localized collection of pus that is contained within the cavity formed by the disintegration of the surrounding tissues. An abscess is defined as acute when the duration of symptoms is less than 6 weeks. In general, the abscess is solitary but occasionally may be multiple, particularly in the immunocompromised individual.

A classification of lung abscess is given in Table 84-8. Contributing factors to the development of a lung abscess are listed in Table 84-9. Anaerobic infections remain the most frequent etiologic agents. Periodontal disease and aspiration are the two most frequent causes. Fewer than

Table 84-9. Contributing Factors to Lung Abscess

Dental and periodontal disease
Anesthesia
Alcohol abuse
Seizure disorders
Immunosuppression
Neuromuscular disorders with bulbar dysfunction
Esophageal motor disorders
Bronchial obstruction

20% of patients with an anaerobic lung abscess do not have a history of one or the other of these aforementioned causes.

The typical patient has a history of an antecedent event or history of pulmonary infection or pneumonia. Patients have an intermittent febrile course with weight loss, night sweats, and cough. Later in its course, the production of purulent sputum becomes quite common. The patient may have foul breath and often appears quite ill.

The most frequent micro-organisms associated with lung abscess are listed in Table 84-10. The micro-organism is most likely related to the etiologic cause. The most frequent anaerobic cause is *Bacteroides* and the most frequent aerobic causes are *Staphylococcus aureus* and *Streptococcus pneumoniae*.

Diagnostic techniques include a complete history and physical examination with emphasis on a predisposing event such as dental work or possible aspiration. The symptoms of fever and purulent foul-smelling sputum are highly suggestive. Analysis of the sputum is necessary in the attempt to identify the causative micro-organism.

Fiberoptic bronchoscopy is indicated for two reasons. It helps in the bacteriologic assessment with the use of a sterile brush and in obtaining bacterial washings for bacterial analysis. It is also important to rule out an endobronchial tumor or obstruction and determine if the abscess is draining internally.

Radiographic imaging is generally required to determine for certainty the presence of a lung abscess. Posteroanterior and lateral chest radiography and CT scanning of the chest are the most frequent modalities used (Figs. 84-3 and 84-4). The most frequent sites of involvement are in the superior segments of the right and left lower lobes and the lateral part of the posterior segment of the right upper lobe (the axillary subsegment) (Fig. 84-5). Ninety-five percent of all lung abscesses occur in these locations.

The differential diagnosis of cavitary lung lesions revolves around four entities: 1) cavitating carcinoma, generally squamous cell; 2) tuberculous or other fungal diseases; 3) pyogenic lung abscess; and 4) empyema with bronchopleural fistula. The patient's history is important in separating the differential diagnosis. Hood (1994a) suggested that the absence of fever, lack of purulent sputum, and a nor-

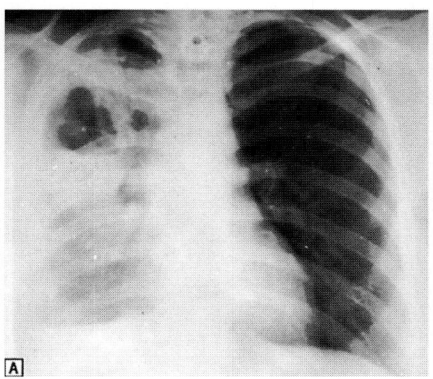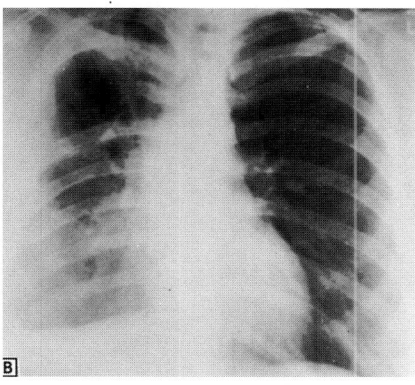

Fig. 84-3. A. Lung abscess of the preantibiotic era involving the left upper lobe. The abscess followed tonsillectomy. B. Same patient 3 weeks later showing spread to the right lung. From Ferguson TB, Burford TH: The changing pattern of pulmonary suppuration: surgical implications. Dis Chest *53*:396, 1968. With permission.

mal white blood cell count should make one highly suspicious of an underlying neoplasm.

Once the diagnosis is established, appropriate therapy must be instituted. Principles of therapy are given in Table 84-11. The etiologic organisms must be identified as quickly as possible through the techniques previously discussed. Appropriate antibiotics should be instituted based on drug sensitivity. If an aerobic micro-organism is suspected, the patient is generally started on clindamycin and gentamicin while awaiting sensitivity study results. Antibiotics are continued for a prolonged period, generally 6 to 8 weeks.

Adequate drainage must be achieved by chest physiotherapy, fiberoptic bronchoscopy, or percutaneous catheter drainage. Only when the abscess does not drain internally into the tracheobronchial tree is external drainage indicated. Wiedemann and Rice (1995) report that 80 to 90% of aerobic lung abscesses respond to medical therapy.

When the abscess does not drain internally and the patient experiences a septic course, external drainage can be achieved by closed chest tube thoracostomy, CT-directed catheter drainage, or open pneumonostomy (Fig. 84-6).

Development of percutaneous catheter drainage has significantly improved the treatment of patients with a lung abscess and decreased the need for surgical intervention. The procedure can be done with low morbidity and mortality. Occasionally, it may be used to prepare a septic patient for surgery. The results from some published series are pre-

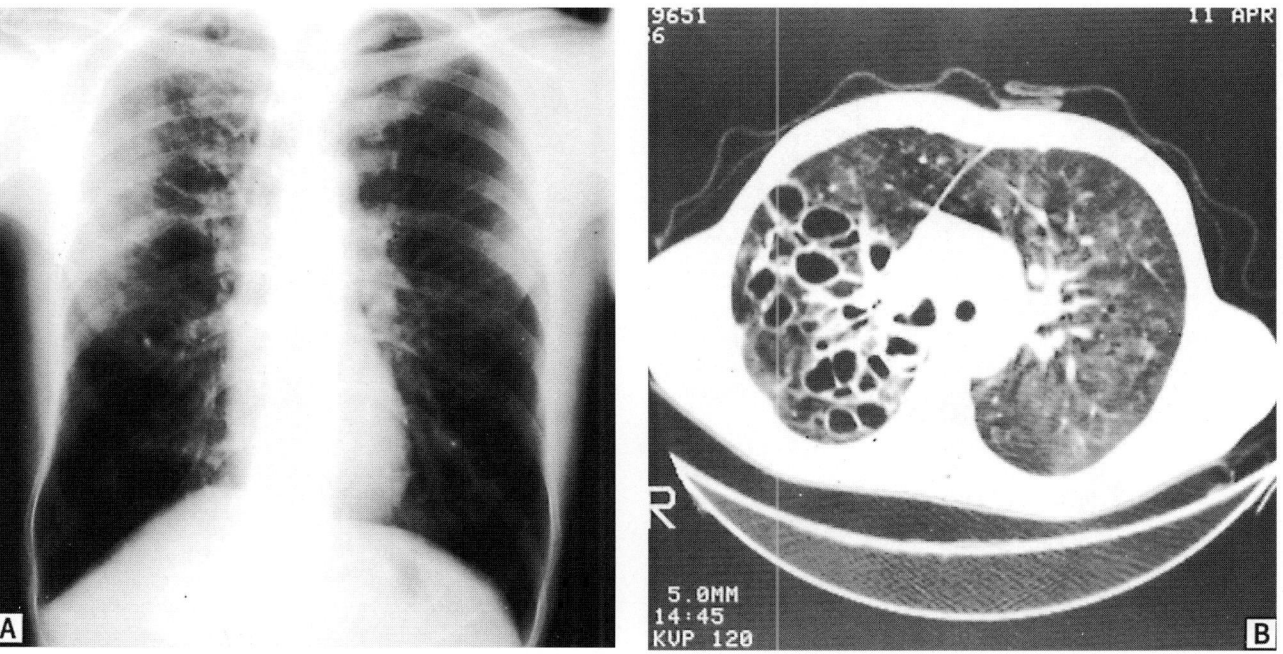

Fig. 84-4. A. Posteroanterior chest radiograph of a patient admitted with a lifelong history of pulmonary infection and hemoptysis demonstrates extensive cystic disease of the right lung. B. A computed tomographic film clearly illustrates the cystic nature of the bronchiectasis. From Hood RM: Bacterial infections of the lungs. *In* Shields TW (ed): General Thoracic Surgery. 4th Ed. Baltimore: Williams & Wilkins, 1994. With permission.

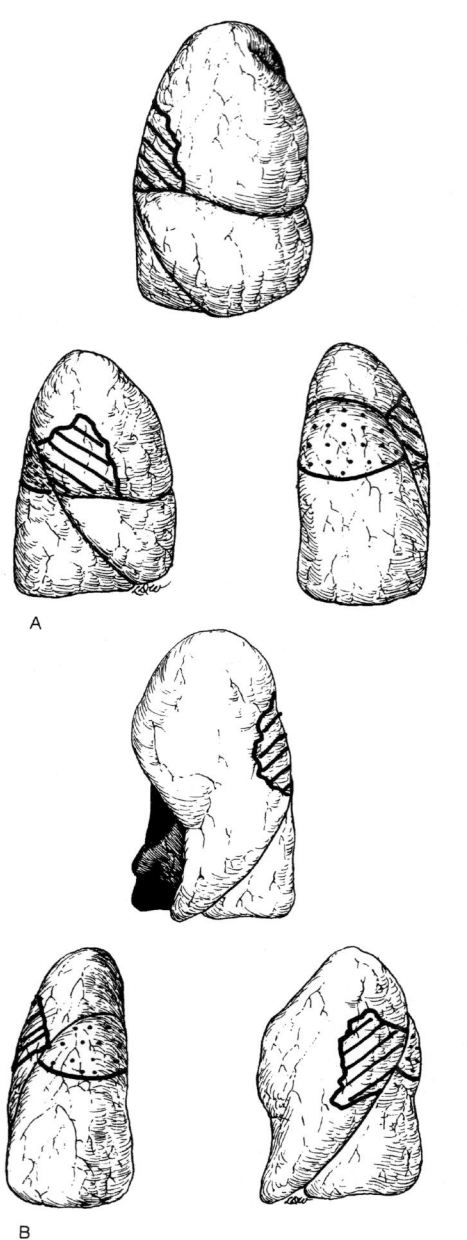

Fig. 84-5. Axillary subsegment of the posterior segment at the upper lobe and superior segment of the lower lobe. **A.** Right lung. **B.** Left lung. From Hood RM: Bacterial infections of the lungs. *In* Shields TW (ed): General Thoracic Surgery. 4th Ed. Baltimore: Williams & Wilkins, 1994. With permission.

Table 84-11. Principles of Therapy for Lung Abscess

Identification of etiologic organism
Prolonged antimicrobial therapy
Adequate drainage in acute stage
    Chest physiotherapy
    Bronchoscopy
    Percutaneous catheter drainage
Emergency surgical treatment
    Specific indication
    External drainage (only in emergent situation)

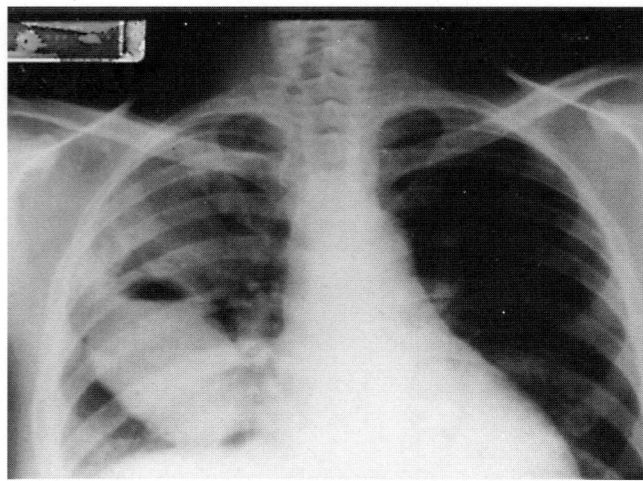

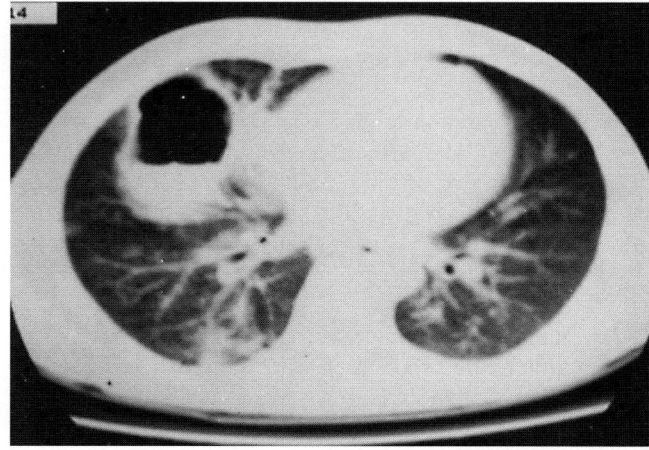

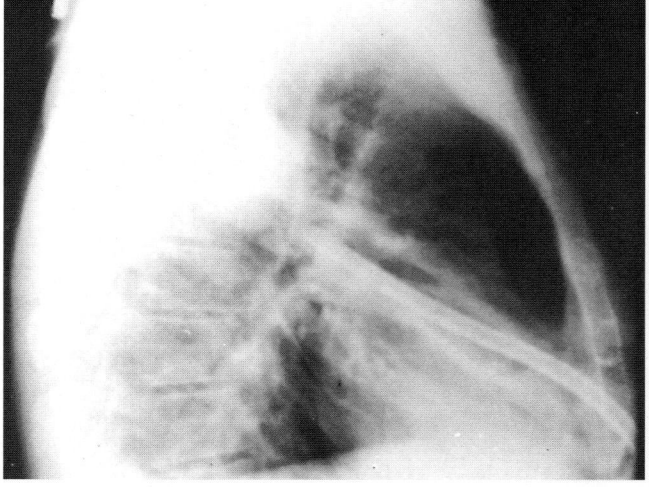

Fig. 84-6. A. Anteroposterior view of a patient with a large aspiration abscess of the middle lobe. Poor bronchial drainage exists, and the patient was toxic. **B.** Computed tomographic examination of the patient. **C.** Lateral view after Monaldi drainage. The patient recovered. This patient was unresponsive to antibiotic therapy and shows the occasional need for surgical drainage. This patient was admitted in 1984. From Hood RM: Bacterial infections of the lungs. *In* Shields TW (ed): General Thoracic Surgery. 4th Ed. Baltimore: Williams & Wilkins, 1994. With permission.

Table 84-12. Percutaneous Catheter Drainage of Lung Abscess

Author	No. of Patients	Mortality	Morbidity	Empyema	Duration, Days (mean)	Cure (%)
Weissberg (1984)	7	0	0	0	4–24 (10)	100
Crouch et al. (1987)	4	0	0	0	NS	100
Parker et al. (1987)	6	0	16.7	0	10–59 (18)	83.4
Rice et al. (1987)	11	0	18	0	NS	73
vanSonnenberg et al. (1991)	19	0	21	0	4–38	84

Modified from Wiedemann HP, Rice TW: Lung abscess and empyema. Semin Thorac Cardiovasc Surg 7:119, 1995.

sented in Table 84-12. Although generally avoidable, surgical resection may be required in up to 30% of patients undergoing percutaneous catheter drainage.

Surgical intervention is now required in only approximately 10% of patients with lung abscess. The indications for surgery in lung abscess are listed in Table 84-13. Specific indications include unsuccessful medical management over a period of 8 weeks; suspicion of cancer; complication of lung abscess, such as empyema or bronchopleural fis-

Table 84-13. Indications for Surgery in Lung Abscess

Acute stage (emergency)
    Complications
        Bronchopleural fistula
        Empyema
        Bleeding
Chronic stage (definitive)
    Persistent symptoms and signs
    Recurrent complications (empyema, bronchopleural fistula)
    Suspicion of carcinoma
    Persistence of lung abscess larger than 6 cm after 8 weeks of treatment

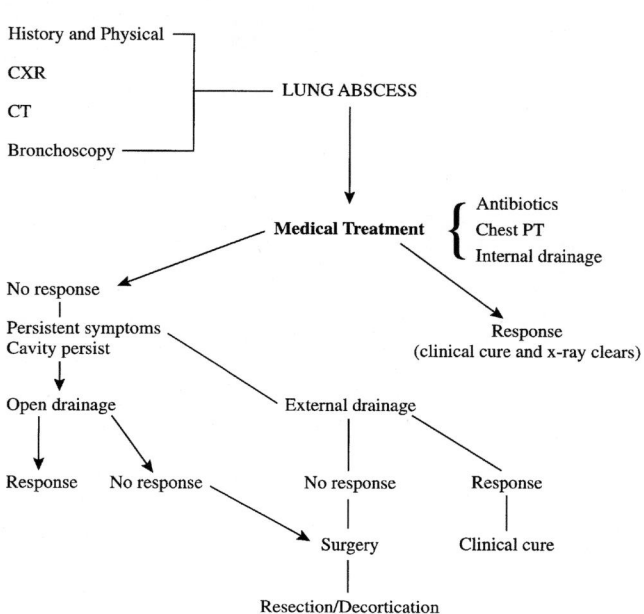

Fig. 84-7. Algorithm for management of lung abscess. CT, computed tomography; CXR, chest x-ray; PT, pneumothorax.

tula; persistence of a cavity larger than 6 cm after 8 weeks of treatment; and the presence of massive hemoptysis. An algorithm for the management of lung abscess is given in Figure 84-7.

BACTERIAL INFECTIONS OF SURGICAL IMPORTANCE IN IMMUNOSUPPRESSED PATIENTS

Bacterial infections in immunocompromised individuals continue to present problems to the general thoracic surgeon. They continue to be a major source of morbidity and mortality. These individuals are susceptible to a wide variety of organisms, but specific infections tend to occur in well-defined settings. The type of infection can be predicted based on the nature and severity of the immune defect, past patient exposures, chemotherapy given, radiographic presentation, and acuteness of illness. New treatments with oral antifungal agents and antiviral agents have improved some of the infectious complications, but in selected cases the definitive attention of the general thoracic surgeon is still needed. The general thoracic surgeon is most frequently consulted for management of pneumothoraces, need for open lung biopsy, particularly in the immunocompromised patient with bilateral infiltrates, and management of bacterial and fungal complications such as hemoptysis. The most common immunologic defects and infectious organisms are listed in Table 84-14.

Pneumothorax

The majority of pneumothoraces in immunocompromised individuals can be handled with closed chest tube thoracostomy and an experienced general thoracic surgeon competent in the management of prolonged air leaks. The majority of these pneumothoraces occur in immunocompromised individuals with human immunodeficiency virus. During the early and mid-1980s, the author operated on a significant number of immunocompromised individuals with human immunodeficiency virus. Beginning in 1990, the author began to use the Heimlich valve in the control of pneumothoraces combined with talc sclerosis. The author's group has treated more than 150 individuals since 1990, with none requiring further surgical intervention. Essentially any leak that occurs in an immunocompromised individual can be

Table 84-14. Immunologic Defects and Infectious Complication in Immunosuppressed Individuals

Defect	Common Infection
Granulocytopenia	Bacteria
	Pseudomonas
	Klebsiella
	Escherichia coli
	Staphylococcus aureus
	Staphylococcus epidermidis
	Hemolytic streptococcus
	Fungi
	Aspergillus
	Mucor
B cell (humoral)	Bacteria
	Haemophilus influenzae
T cell (cell-mediated)	Bacteria
	Legionella
	Nocardia
	Mycobacteria
	Fungi
	Cryptococcus
	Histoplasma
	Coccidioides
	Protozoa
	Pneumocystis
	Virus
	Cytomegalovirus
	Herpes simplex

Modified from White DA: Pulmonary infection in the immunocompromised patient. Semin Thorac Cardiovasc Surg 7:78, 1995.

handled by this technique. This chapter does not permit a detailed analysis of the tricks of tube management.

Open Lung Biopsy or Thoracoscopic Biopsy

The thoracic surgeon is often called to see an immunocompromised patient who is on a ventilator and in whom the pulmonologist has exhausted all interventions short of open lung biopsy to establish a diagnosis. In this situation, open lung biopsy is frequently indicated. In the emergency situation, the video-assisted thoracic surgery technique should not be used, but a 20-minute open procedure with conventional ventilation is most likely to obtain the diagnosis in the most cost-efficient manner. It should also be stated that in the author's 25 years of experience with open lung biopsy on bone marrow transplant patients, not one patient has survived nor has open lung biopsy changed the postoperative course.

Interventional Surgery

The third scenario in which the general thoracic surgeon is contacted to see an immunocompromised patient is when significant hemoptysis has developed. In this situation, the surgeon's role is to localize the site of hemoptysis through bronchoscopy and CT scanning. Once identified, bronchial embolization with gel foam or coils should be carried out. In the majority of patients, this controls the hemoptysis.

The other situation in which surgery may be readily indicated is in the patient with hemoptysis secondary to infection with aspergillosis in the fungal cavity. Another situation is the immunocompromised patient with diabetes mellitus who is infected with mucormycosis. In this case, surgical resection of the affected lung parenchyma may be the only chance of survival in these immunocompromised patients despite therapy with amphotericin B.

ORGANIZING PNEUMONIA

An occasional patient with pneumonitis, even with appropriate antibiotic therapy, does not follow the usual predictable course and develops an organized pneumonic process. This also is seen in some patients who receive little or no therapy. The course varies considerably, but the infectious process resolves into a protracted chronic course, and little or no resolution is seen on chest radiography. The volume usually slowly decreases and may even progress to complete atelectasis of the involved area. Hood (1994a) notes that the process may be either lobar or segmental in extent. Pathologically, the involved area is airless and densely fibrotic with bronchial distortion or bronchiectasis (Fig. 84-8). Microscopically, the lung structure is destroyed.

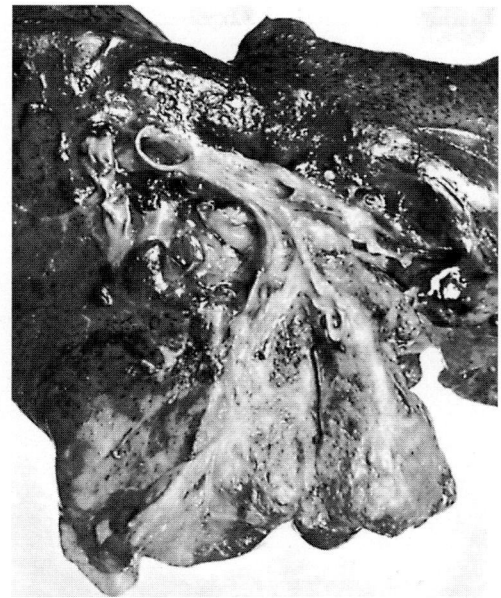

Fig. 84-8. Right lower lobe resected for organizing pneumonia shows extensive replacement of the parenchyma by scar tissue. From Hood RM: Bacterial infections of the lungs. *In* Shields TW (ed): General Thoracic Surgery. 4th Ed. Baltimore: Williams & Wilkins, 1994. With permission.

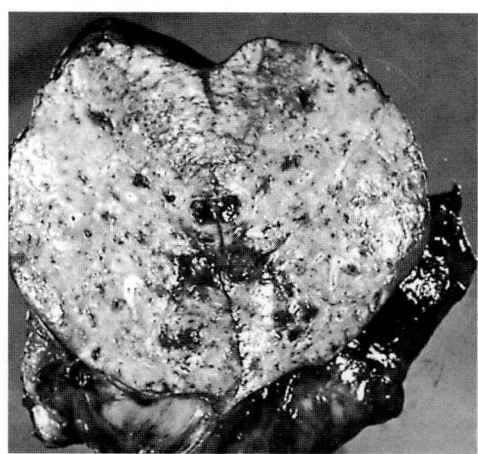

Fig. 84-9. Gross specimen of lobe removed in the treatment of lipoid pneumonia. From Hood RM: Bacterial infections of the lungs. *In* Shields TW (ed): General Thoracic Surgery. 4th Ed. Baltimore: Williams & Wilkins, 1994. With permission.

The lesion must be differentiated from an obstructing carcinoma, primary pulmonary tuberculosis, mycotic infection, foreign body aspiration, mucoid impaction, or lipoid pneumonia, among other chronic processes. Hood (1994) notes that lipoid pneumonia may be exogenous from aspiration of mineral oil or may be endogenous lipoid pneumonia resulting from some inflammatory or toxic injury to the lung (Fig. 84-9).

Regardless of its cause, the area of organized pneumonia should be resected. The outcome is satisfactory in nonimmunocompromised patients, but is poor in the immunocompromised host.

PULMONARY INFECTIONS IN CHRONIC GRANULOMATOUS DISEASE OF CHILDHOOD

Chronic granulomatous disease is a rare genetically transmitted disease in which the host's phagocytes are unable to respond to stimuli with a normal respiratory burst (i.e., production of superoxide and hydrogen peroxide by the nicotinamide adenine dinucleotide phosphate oxidase systems). The normal respiratory burst leads to the killing of ingested micro-organisms. Recurrent severe infections with common as well as with catalase-positive organisms occur. Fungal infections are frequent. The lung is the most common site of infection, and pulmonary suppuration is the cause of death in more than one-half of children with chronic granulomatous disease.

Clinical Course

Initial pulmonary infections occur in early childhood, but the diagnosis of the underlying process is usually not made until several years later. Chronic, repeated infections and, ultimately, death in the first or second decade of life were the usual course of the disease until the use of routine prophylaxis with antibiotics. The use of trimethoprim-sulfamethoxazole prophylaxis reported by Weening (1983) and Margolis (1990) and their colleagues also reduced the incidence of nonfungal infections in these patients. Margolis and associates (1990) noted that the incidence of fungal infections was not changed. Life expectancy has increased, but the incidence of acute or chronic pulmonary infection remains high. These patients present diagnostic and treatment challenges to the physician.

Radiographic Features

According to Pogrebniak and associates (1993), three radiographic patterns are noted: focal unilateral disease, focal bilateral disease, and diffuse bilateral infiltrates. Focal disease is usually confined to a pulmonary segment or lobe.

Diagnosis

The diagnosis of chronic granulomatous disease is made by the nitroblue tetrazolium test, the Western/Northern blot analyses, or both. A report from the National Institutes of Health by Abati and associates (1996) reported that cytologic specimens demonstrated a pathologic organism in only 18% of patients, but that a combination of cytology and microbiology provided a diagnosis of the infectious agent in 45%. The etiology of the lung infection, on the other hand, is often best made by an open procedure to obtain an adequate tissue specimen for cultures.

Treatment

Medical therapy is the primary approach. Surgical resection of unresolving focal disease was suggested by Roback and colleagues in 1971. Pogrebniak and associates (1993) have reported their experience with a similar aggressive surgical approach in the management of persistent focal pulmonary disease in these patients. Major resections, including segmentectomy, bisegmentectomy, lobectomy, and even pneumonectomy, were done in 12 patients. Thirteen wedge resections for diagnosis were done also. Morbidity and mortality were high from postoperative infections caused by fungal and *Pseudomonas* organisms. Temeck and colleagues (1994) reported 17 patients with chronic granulomatous disease who were proved to have *Aspergillus* as the infecting agent by open surgical procedures, most of which were wedge resections (7), and the remainder either a lobectomy (4) or a segmentectomy. Fourteen patients (82.3%) did well after operation, but three patients (17.6%) died of postoperative fungemia and multiple system organ failure.

Postoperative antibiotics and antifungal agents as indicated by the results of culture of the excised specimens are essential. The use of interferon-γ to reduce the frequency of recurrent infection has been suggested by Abramson (1990) and is now being studied by the International Chronic Granulomatous Disease Cooperative Study Group (1991). Of interest, the 14 patients in Temeck and associates' (1994) series all received white blood cell transfusions and nine also received recombinant human interferon-γ.

BRONCHOCOMPRESSIVE PULMONARY DISORDERS

Bronchocompressive disorders of the pulmonary system are an uncommon but important group of disorders of which the thoracic surgeon must be aware (see Table 84-1). The most frequent of these disorders are right middle lobe syndrome and broncholithiasis.

Right Middle Lobe Syndrome

The term *right middle lobe syndrome* was originally coined by Graham and associates (1948). These authors reported on 12 patients with right middle lobe atelectasis and bronchial compression caused by nontuberculous enlarged lymph nodes. The syndrome was characterized by episodes of hemoptysis, chronic cough, and episodes of repeated pulmonary infection. All patients were treated by lobectomy. Brock and associates (1937) described the secondary effects of tuberculous lymphadenopathy surrounding the middle lobe bronchus. They described the syndrome of bronchial compression characterized by atelectasis, bronchiectasis, and repeated pneumonic episodes. Subsequently, Paulson and Shaw (1949) reported their experience with 32 patients with disease contributed to by bronchial compression. In 1966, Culiner challenged the hypothesis of bronchial compression as the primary cause of right middle lobe syndrome. He postulated that the basic pathogenesis of the right middle lobe syndrome lay in the isolation of the right middle lobe and the loss of collateral ventilation. Lindskog and Spear (1966) reported seven cases of right middle lobe atelectasis having seven different causes.

Since 1966, the term *right middle lobe syndrome* has included all diseases of the right middle lobe. Thus, according to Wagner and Johnson (1983) the definition of the term *right middle lobe syndrome* has been modified to include all types of right middle lobe atelectasis even when bronchial compression is not present. Wagner and Johnson (1983) published a review of 933 cases reported in the literature. In their review, the following etiologic causes of right middle lobe syndrome were noted: inflammation, 47%; bronchiectasis, 15%; malignant tumors, 22%; benign tumors, 2%; tuberculosis, 9%; aspiration, 2%; and miscellaneous, 3%. It was not documented whether the atelectasis was caused by

active disease or nodal compression. Before the development of antibiotic medication, it was thought that the majority of cases of middle lobe atelectasis in childhood were caused by tuberculosis.

Pathophysiology of Middle Lobe Syndrome

Brock and associates (1937) originally proposed that the right middle lobe bronchus is a long, narrow structure surrounded by glands that lie in the inferior angle formed by its origin from the stem bronchus (Figs. 84-10 and 84-11). Later, inadequate collateral ventilation caused by lobar isolation was postulated as a second cause.

Two theories are now recognized as etiologic explanations. One view implies bronchial obstruction as the initial event. More recently, anatomic isolation of the right middle lobe with resultant loss of collateral ventilation has been indicated as the causative factor. Proponents of this view state that alveolar ventilation through the pores of Kohn is an important mechanism in preventing distal atelectasis during episodes of segmental or lobar obstruction. It is interesting to note that Hovelacque and colleagues (1937) reported that 29% of patients had complete minor fissures, 51% had partial fissures, and 20% had no fissure, and that Brock (1954) reported that 37% of patients had complete minor fissures, 53% had partial fissures, and 10% had no fissures.

Diagnosis

The hallmarks of diagnosis are based on historical findings, endoscopy, and radiographic analysis. The majority of symptomatic patients have repeated episodes of infection, intermittent hemoptysis, and persistent atelectasis of the right middle lobe. The patients may have a history of years of repeated pulmonary infections. Endoscopic findings include bronchostenosis, tumor, and abnormal but nonspecific findings. A summary of seven series of 613 patients from the world literature reported by Wagner and Johnson (1983) showed 38% with stenosis or tumor and 17% with abnormal but nonspecific changes. Forty-five percent of this group had normal findings.

Before 1985, bronchograms were the standard method by which the diagnosis was made. CT is now the preferred imaging modality. Findings include evidence of bronchostenosis, lobar collapse, inflammatory changes, and bronchiectasis.

Management of the Right Middle Lobe Syndrome

Patients who have repeated episodes of infection with lobar collapse and evidence of bronchostenosis, tumor, or obstruction from enlarged lymph nodes are best treated by surgical resection. If no endobronchial obstruction is present, the patient can generally be treated medically. Patients with diminished volume in their middle lobe who remain asymptomatic can be treated medically.

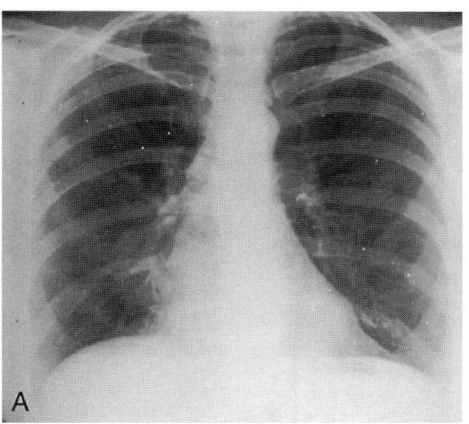
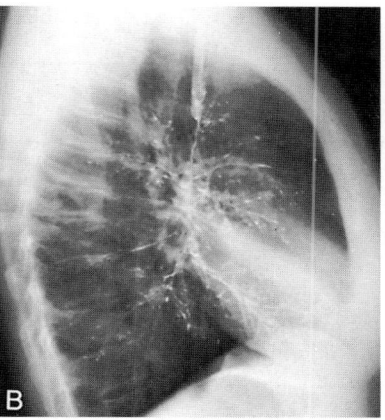
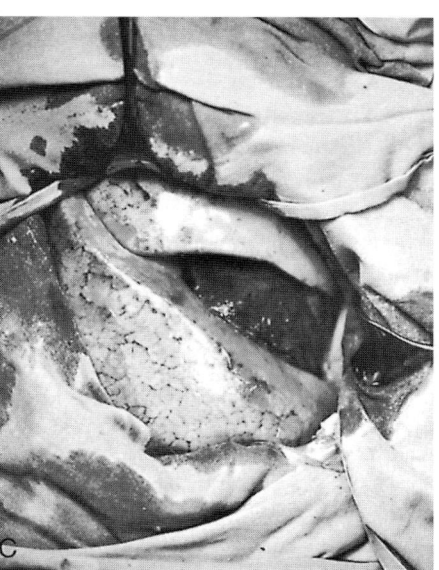

Fig. 84-10. A. and B. Radiographs of a patient with bronchial compressive disease of the right middle lobe with complete atelectasis. Note obliteration of the heart border on the right side by the inflammatory process. **C.** Appearance of the right middle lobe at the time of operation. From Hood RM: Bacterial infections of the lungs. *In* Shields TW (ed): General Thoracic Surgery. 4th Ed. Baltimore: Williams & Wilkins, 1994. With permission.

Broncholithiasis

Broncholithiasis is an uncommon pulmonary problem that may present with life-threatening complications. It is generally defined as an isolated area of bronchial compressive disease. The name implies that at least a portion of a calcified lymph node has eroded into the lumen of a bronchus. In general, as pointed out by Hood (1994a), this is considered to be a dynamic process with a spectrum of presentations.

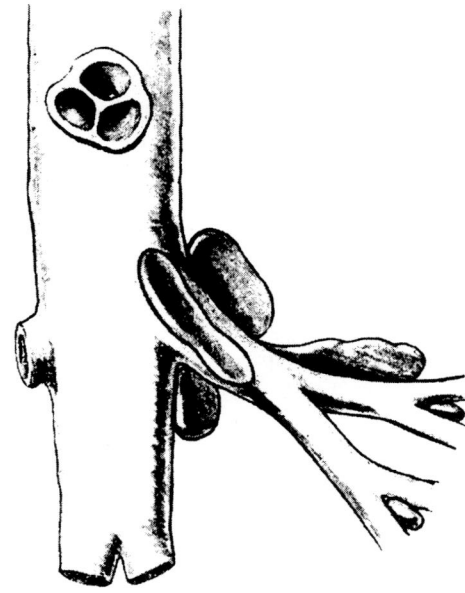

Fig. 84-11. The middle lobe bronchus and the surrounding collar of lymph nodes. From Brock RC: The Anatomy of the Bronchial Tree. 2nd Ed. London: Oxford University Press, 1954, p. 122. With permission.

According to Trastek and associates (1985), the spectrum of presentations include 1) erosion of a calcified lymph node into the lumen of a bronchus producing a broncholith, 2) distortion or partial obstruction of the tracheobronchial tree by calcified peribronchial lymph nodes, and 3) simulation of a cancer. To these must be added the occurrence of varying degrees of hemoptysis and the rare occurrence of erosion into other adjacent structures.

The pathogenesis of broncholithiasis is thought to be caused by the tissue response to a healing granulomatous inflammation as noted by Trastek and colleagues (1985). The most frequently involved diseases are histoplasmosis and tuberculosis. After spread to the central lymph nodes from the pulmonary parenchyma, calcium salts are deposited in the nodes during the healing process. Because of the dynamics of respiration, these nodes may erode into the tracheobronchial tree. They may likewise erode into adjacent organs, such as the esophagus or pulmonary vascular tree.

The majority of patients have characteristic cough with sputum production, hemoptysis, fever, and chills. Broncholithiasis may present as massive hemoptysis or as an esophagobronchial fistula. An occasional patient may cough up part of broncholithic stones.

The diagnosis should be suspected on routine chest radiography by the presence of centralized or infiltrating calcified lymph nodes or tracheobronchial distortion. CT confirms these observations.

Endoscopic findings consist of tracheobronchial distortion, inflammation, a visible broncholith, bleeding, and inflammation. An occasional patient may have endoscopic findings of a fistula in either the esophagus or the tracheobronchial tree. Trastek and associates (1985) note that a tracheoesophageal fistula can be confirmed by a meglumine diatrizoate (Gastrografin) swallow.

According to Trastek and colleagues (1985), indications for surgery include intractable cough, recurrent hemoptysis, chronic infection resulting from bronchostenosis, or a secondary esophagobronchial fistula. The presence of a calcified node alone does not warrant surgery. Goals of treatment should be removal of all offending calcification and irreversibly damaged bronchi or lung, along with conservation of as much normal pulmonary parenchyma as possible. As the tracheobronchial obstruction is frequently associated with postoperative pneumonitis, lung abscess, or bronchiectasis, resection rather than broncholithectomy is often required.

At surgery, the calcified lymph nodes and subsequent intense inflammatory response make dissection extremely difficult and potential intraoperative complications of hemorrhage and esophageal perforation possible. Proximal control of the pulmonary artery should be obtained early, before beginning dissection in the area of calcified nodes. At times, it is prudent to incise the capsule of the node and to curettage its contents to avoid injury to adjacent structures.

The extent of surgery depends on the anatomy, presence of calcified nodes, and extent of pulmonary parenchymal destruction. Ideally, an endoscopic broncholithectomy is the treatment of choice, but frequently is not possible. The author has used successfully the yttrium-aluminum-garnet laser in two patients who were poor candidates for open surgery. However, a thoracotomy is generally required with broncholithectomy and removal of all damaged pulmonary parenchyma.

Trastek and associates (1985) reported on 52 patients with broncholithiasis. Forty patients were treated with thoracotomy. In this group, broncholithectomy was achieved in all patients and 32 required pulmonary resection of various types. In the bronchoscopy group, success was achieved in eight patients with three requiring thoracotomy. Postoperative complications developed in 12.8% of the thoracotomy group and 37.5% of the bronchoscopy group. One postoperative death occurred. They concluded that broncholithectomy by way of thoracotomy is the preferred method of management. Resection should be conservative, but removal of all diseased pulmonary parenchyma should be included.

Sclerosing Mediastinitis

Sclerosing mediastinitis is an uncommon manifestation of a bronchocompressive disorder but can have devastating consequences. Although it may result from any number of etiologic causes, it most frequently follows infection with *Histoplasma capsulatum*. As the author has noted, the most frequent malignant cause is Hodgkin's disease. The other causes of granulomatous mediastinitis with fibrosis are listed in Table 84-15.

For purposes of this chapter, the discussion is limited to sclerosing mediastinitis secondary to *H. capsulatum* and mediastinal granuloma. The inability to grow the microorganism from biopsy specimens has led to the conclusion that this severe complication is not a result of active foreign proliferation but a hypersensitive reaction to a healed infec-

Table 84-15. Etiologic Factors in Granulomatous Mediastinitis with Fibrosis

Fungal infections
  Histoplasmosis
  Aspergillosis
  Mucormycosis
  Cryptococcosis
  Blastomycosis
Mycobacterial infections
  Mycobacterium tuberculosis
  Other mycobacterial infections
Bacterial infections
  Nocardiosis
  Actinomycosis
Autoimmune disease
Sarcoidosis
Rheumatic fever
Neoplasms
Trauma
Drugs
Idiopathic

Adapted from Marchevsky AM, Kaneko M: Surgical Pathology of the Mediastinum. 2nd Ed. New York: Raven, 1992.

tion. The delayed hypersensitivity results from the intense inflammation in parenchymal foci and lymph nodes, leading to caseous necrosis. Healing occurs by encapsulation and an intense fibrous process.

This extensive fibrotic process may result in severe complications. It is the most common cause of benign superior vena caval syndrome. Involvement of the tracheobronchial tree can result in stenosis at all levels of the airway. In addition, esophageal obstruction and esophagorespiratory fistulae have been reported. The most common symptoms are dyspnea, hemoptysis, postobstructive pneumonia, and superior vena caval syndrome.

Mathisen and Grillo (1992) reported on 20 patients of whom 18 underwent complex tracheobronchial procedures. They stressed the tremendous surgical challenges that this entity presented because of the intense inflammatory lung response. They had three fatalities in this group of patients. Surgeons who undertake to treat this condition should be aware of the technical challenges and the potential for high morbidity and potential mortality. Mathisen and Grillo (1992) emphasized the need for resection for large asymptomatic mediastinal granulomas before the process of sclerosing mediastinitis develops.

Inflammatory Lymphadenopathy

Enlargement of mediastinal and bronchial lymph nodes may result in a bronchocompressive disorder. This is most frequently associated with tuberculosis, histoplasmosis, and sarcoidosis. This is particularly common in children with tuberculosis that may result in significant respiratory distress. This process has been referred to as *tuberculosis lymph node compression syndrome*. Treatment consists of antibiotic medication. In an occasional patient, surgical resection of the compressive nodes may be required. Worthington and coworkers (1993) have suggested that when acute airway obstruction occurs, airway decompression may be obtained by incision and curettage of the involved lymph nodes. This precludes major complications when the excision of the lymph node is difficult. Histoplasmosis and sarcoid can likewise cause tracheal, lobar, and segmental compression by enlargement of adjacent lymph nodes, resulting in a bronchocompressive disorder. Discussions of the effect of histoplasmosis have been previously mentioned. Sarcoid frequently responds to corticosteroid therapy.

Mediastinal Tumors

Mediastinal cysts and neoplasms frequently cause respiratory obstruction in children but rarely in adults. A bronchial or an esophageal cyst may occasionally occlude either main bronchus or the trachea. The infant may present with severe respiratory distress and require urgent surgical intervention. Azizkhan and associates (1985) found that of 50 children with mediastinal tumors, nine had significant symptoms of tracheobronchial compression and all nine presented with marked obstruction and required surgical intervention.

In adults, bronchial or tracheal obstruction may occasionally occur from malignant neoplasms. This obstruction is most frequently from bronchial carcinoma occluding a major bronchus by extrinsic compression or from metastatic lymph node disease. In adults, lymphomas and small cell lung cancer also can cause tracheobronchial obstruction resulting in various degrees of respiratory distress.

Miscellaneous Conditions

Esophageal Hiatal Hernia

In an occasional patient, a large paraesophageal hiatal hernia can cause tracheobronchial obstruction of the left main stem bronchus resulting in significant tracheobronchial compression with significant shortness of breath and occasional respiratory distress. Relief of the obstruction by surgical correction of the hiatal hernia is the method of choice.

Acquired Aortic Disease

Traumatic false aneurysms of the descending thoracic aorta and acquired descending thoracic aortic aneurysms can cause significant respiratory compromise by extrinsic compression of the left main stem bronchus. This may result in symptoms of cough, wheezing, dyspnea, and hemoptysis. The diagnosis is suspected on chest radiography by enlargement of the mediastinum. CT scan, magnetic resonance imaging, and aortography confirm the diagnosis. Resection of the aneurysm results in relief of symptoms.

Primary Cardiovascular Disease

Table 84-1 lists some of the cardiac and vascular abnormalities that compress the trachea or main stem bronchi. These abnormalities are frequently a manifestation of airway compression without a history of cardiac or vascular disease. An enlarged left atrium from either acquired mitral valve disease or congenital heart disease can compress or displace the left main stem bronchus. In addition, varieties of vascular rings can cause respiratory obstruction. These include double aortic arch and a right descending thoracic aorta with a left ligamentum arteriosum. These conditions and other vascular rings are discussed in Chapter 78.

REFERENCES

Abati A, et al: Chronic granulomatous disease of childhood: respiratory cytology. Diagn Cytopathol 15:98, 1996.

Abramson SL: Recombinant human interferon-gamma (rIFN-gamma) and interleukin-4 (rIL-4) regulate gene expression of several phagocytic oxidase components. Clin Res 38:236A, 1990.

Annest LS, Kratz JM, Crawford FA Jr: Current results of treatment for bronchiectasis. J Thorac Cardiovasc Surg 83:546, 1982.

Azizkhan RG, et al: Life-threatening airway obstruction as a complication of mediastinal masses in children. J Pediatr Surg 20:816, 1985.

Barker AF: Bronchiectasis: Semin Thorac Cardiovasc Surg 7:112, 1995.

Blades B, Dugan D: Pseudobronchiectasis. J Thorac Surg 13:40, 1944.

Boyden EA: Segmental Anatomy of the Lungs. New York: McGraw-Hill, 1955.

Brock RC: The Anatomy of the Bronchial Tree. 2nd Ed. London: Oxford University Press, 1954.

Brock RC, Cann RJ, Dickinson JR: Tuberculous mediastinal lymphadenitis in childhood; secondary effects on the lungs. Guy Hospital Report 87:295, 1937.

Crouch JD, Keagy BA, Delany DJ: "Pigtail" catheter drainage in thoracic surgery. Am Rev Respir Dis 136:174, 1987.

Culiner MM: The right middle lobe syndrome, a non-obstructive complex. Dis Chest 50:57, 1966.

Dogan R: Surgical treatment of bronchiectasis: a collective review of 487 cases. Thorac Cardiovasc Surg 37:183, 1989.

Geppert EF: Lung abscess and other subacute pulmonary infections. In Niederman MS, Sacosi GA, Glassroth J (eds): Respiratory Infections. Philadelphia: Saunders, 1994.

Graham EA, Burford TH, Mayer JH: Middle lobe syndrome. Postgrad Med 4:29, 1948.

Hodder RV, Cameron R, Todd TRJ: Bacterial infections. In Pearson FG et al (eds): Thoracic Surgery. New York: Churchill Livingstone, 1995.

Hood RM: Bronchial compressive diseases. In Shields TW (ed): General Thoracic Surgery. 4th Ed. Baltimore: Williams & Wilkins, 1994a.

Hood RM: Bacterial infections of the lungs. In Shields TW (ed): General Thoracic Surgery. 4th Ed. Baltimore: Williams & Wilkins, 1994b.

Hovelacque A, Monod O, Eurard H: The Thorax. Anatomie. Paris: Medico-Chirurgicale, 1937.

International Chronic Granulomatous Disease Cooperative Study Group: A controlled trial of interferon gamma to prevent infection in chronic granulomatous disease. N Engl J Med 324:409, 1991.

Lindskog GE: Bronchiectasis revisited. Yale J Biol Med 59:41, 1986.

Lindskog GE, Spear HC: Middle lobe syndrome, a non-obstructive complex. Dis Chest 50:57, 1966.

Margolis DM, et al: Trimethoprim-sulfamethoxazole prophylaxis in the management of chronic granulomatous disease. J Infect Dis 162:723, 1990.

Mathisen DJ, Grillo HC: Clinical manifestation of mediastinal fibrosis and histoplasmosis. Ann Thorac Surg 54:1053, 1992.

Miller JI: The mediastinum. *In* Levine BA, et al (eds): Current Practice of Surgery. Vol. 2. New York: Churchill Livingstone, 1993.

Parker LA, et al: Percutaneous small bore catheter drainage in the management of lung abscesses. Chest *92*:213, 1987.

Paulson DL, Shaw RR: Chronic atelectasis and pneumonitis of the middle lobe. J Thorac Surg *18*:747, 1949.

Pogrebniak HW, et al: Surgical management of pulmonary infections in chronic granulomatous disease of childhood. Ann Thorac Surg *55*:844, 1993.

Rice TW, Ginsberg RJ, Todd TR: Tube drainage of lung abscesses. Ann Thorac Surg *44*:356, 1987.

Roback SA, et al: Chronic granulomatous disease of childhood: surgical considerations. J Pediatr Surg *6*:601, 1971.

Sanderson JM, et al: Bronchiectasis: results of surgical and conservative management. A review of 393 cases. Thorax *29*:407, 1974.

Sealy WC, Bradham RR, Young WG Jr: The surgical treatment of multisegmental and localized bronchiectasis. Surg Gynecol Obstet *123*:80, 1966.

Temeck BK, et al: Thoracotomy for pulmonary mycoses in non-HIV-immunosuppressed patients. Ann Thorac Surg *58*:333, 1994.

Trastek VF, et al: Surgical management of broncholithiasis. J Thorac Cardiovasc Surg *90*:842, 1985.

vanSonnenberg E, et al: Lung abscess: CT-guided drainage. Radiology *178*:347, 1991.

Wagner RB, Johnson MR: Middle lobe syndrome. J Thorac Surg *35*:679, 1983.

Weening RS, Kabel P, Pijman P: Continuous therapy with sulfamethoxazole-trimethoprim in patients with chronic granulomatous disease. J Pediatr Surg *103*:127, 1983.

Weissberg D: Percutaneous drainage of lung abscess. J Thorac Cardiovasc Surg *87*:308, 1984.

White DA: Pulmonary infection in the immunocompromised patient. Semin Thorac Cardiovasc Surg *7*:78, 1995.

Wiedemann HP, Rice TW: Lung abscess and empyema. Semin Thorac Cardiovasc Surg *7*:119, 1995.

Worthington MG, et al: Surgical relief of acute airway obstruction due to primary tuberculosis. Ann Thorac Surg *56*:1054, 1993.

READING REFERENCES

Agasthian T, et al: Surgical management of bronchiectasis. Ann Thorac Surg *62*:976, 1996.

Ashour M: Hemodynamic alternatives in bronchiectasis: a base for a new subclassification of the disease. J Thorac Cardiovasc Surg *112*:328, 1996.

Cole FH, et al: Management of broncholithiasis: is thoracotomy necessary? Ann Thorac Surg *42*:225, 1986.

Dines DR, Bernatz PE, Pairolero PC: Mediastinal granuloma and fibrosing mediastinitis. Chest *73*:320, 1979.

Ferguson TB, Burford TH: Mediastinal granuloma. Ann Thorac Surg *1*:125, 1965.

Harper RR, Condon WB, Wierman WH: Middle lobe syndrome. Arch Surgery *61*:696, 1950.

Inners CR, et al: Collateral ventilation and the middle lobe syndrome. Am Rev Respir Dis *118*:305, 1978.

Kwon KY, et al: Middle lobe syndrome: a clinicopathological study of 21 patients. Hum Pathol *26*:302, 1995.

McLean TR, Beall AC, Jones JW: Massive hemoptysis due to broncholithiasis. Ann Thorac Surg *52*:1173, 1991.

Saha SP, et al: Middle lobe syndrome: diagnosis and management. Ann Thorac Surg *33*:28, 1980.

CHAPTER 85

Pulmonary Tuberculosis and Other Mycobacterial Infections of the Lung

A. *Mycobacterium tuberculosis* and Nontuberculous Mycobacterial Infections of the Lung

Thomas W. Shields

Symptomatic pulmonary disease caused by infections of *Mycobacterium tuberculosis* or, less often, by other mycobacterial organisms continues to be a significant health problem in the United States. It is estimated that 3 to 4% of individuals infected by the organism develop active disease within the first year and thereafter a total of 5 to 15% do so. The incidence of tuberculosis began decreasing after the turn of the 19th century until the late 1980s when a marked increase in incidence occurred, primarily as the result of the widespread occurrence of the disease in immunocompromised hosts with human immunodeficiency virus (HIV) infection and the development of new cases in the immigrant populations from Southeast Asia, Central America, and Eastern Europe. This upward surge continued until 1993, since which time the incidence of new disease again has shown a yearly decline in the number of reported cases. Approximately 10% of the new cases, greater in some urban centers such as Washington, D.C., and New York, are caused by multidrug-resistant tuberculosis organisms (MDRTB) that pose a much greater health hazard than the infections caused by nonresistant organisms. In addition, Frieden and colleagues (1993) noted that as many as 40% of previously treated patients who had recurrent disease had MDRTB. The cause of the emergence of drug-resistant organisms is multifactorial but the commonality is an increase in genetic mutation of *M. tuberculosis* species because of improper drug use. The latter results in modifications of spontaneous, predictable chromosomal muta-

tion of key target genes. According to Telenti (1997), MDRTB reflects the stepwise accumulation of individual gene mutations and not a block acquisition of multiple-drug resistance. Added to this is the occurrence of a greater number of infections caused by drug-resistant nontuberculous mycobacteria in certain population groups.

No age group, race, or sex is exempt from the disease; however, it is clinically manifest at presentation more often in the elderly, minorities, and many of the new immigrant groups. Its emergence as a major public health problem in homeless, prison, and drug-addicted populations is being recognized in most major urban areas. In addition, immunocompromised patients [e.g., those patients receiving various immunosuppressive medications or with severe debilitating disease and those infected by HIV as well as those with the fully developed acquired immunodeficiency disease syndrome (AIDS)] often develop bizarre systemic infections as well as pulmonary infections caused by both *M. tuberculosis* and other nontuberculous mycobacterial (NTM) organisms, primarily the *Mycobacterium avium* complex (MAC). The NTM organisms are also referred to as *mycobacteria other than tuberculosis* (MOTT). Iseman and Huitt (1998) note that these infections are increasing in recognition as well as in absolute numbers.

Most of the clinical infections of *M. tuberculosis*, however, are effectively managed by appropriate antituberculous chemotherapy. However, surgical intervention is required more frequently now than in the past decades to salvage patients with MDRTB who fail to respond to treatment, as well as to manage selected patients with NTM infections.

ETIOLOGY

Pulmonary tuberculosis is caused by the acid-fast organism *M. tuberculosis*. This bacillus produces invasive debilitating infection in humans and is said to be so virulent that infection may be initiated by introduction of a single organism to an alveolar membrane of a susceptible person. Tuberculosis is an infection that necessitates cellular immune response for its control. During the initial few weeks, no immune defense is present, and the *M. tuberculosis* organisms multiply in the alveolar space or within alveolar macrophages. According to Dannenberg (1993), the macrophages have slight if any effect on the rapid multiplication either at the site of the initial focus or in the lymphohematogenous metastatic foci until the development of tissue hypersensitivity and cellular immunity occurs. The indigenous T cells of the CD4+ helper T-cell type react to mycobacterial antigens that have been processed by the macrophages. The CD4+ T cells proliferate, producing a clone of similarly reactive lymphocytes. These cells produce cytokines that activate the macrophages for effective mycobacterial killing. The activated macrophages produce a number of regulatory factors: tumor necrosis factor, platelet-derived growth factor, transforming growth factor-β, and fibroblast growth factor. The CD4+ T cells are also able to directly lyse mononuclear phagocytes infected with *M. tuberculosis* organisms. Dunlap and Briles (1993) note that another T cell (i.e., CD8+ suppressor and cytolytic T cell) becomes activated, and these cells also can release the mycobacteria entrapped in a macrophage that cannot kill the intracellular mycobacteria so that these organisms subsequently can be killed by activated granulocytes. The lymphocytes also secrete additional regulatory proteins, including interferon-γ and migration-inhibiting factor as recorded by Haas and Des Prez (1995). This overall process is the result of the development of both cell-mediated immunity and tissue hypersensitivity to *M. tuberculosis*, and the fate of the infection depends on the effectiveness of these processes and the virulence and number of infecting organisms.

The bacilli responsible for the pulmonary infection are, most often, airborne, and the patient's history usually reveals a close contact with a person or persons having the disease. The disease is highly contagious, and outbreaks often are reported in closed populations of susceptible persons, such as the personnel of naval ships, crowded schools, prisons, and even passengers on long airplane flights.

The initial infection of the lung most often results in the formation of a primary complex (the primary Ghon tubercle with secondary foci of tuberculosis in the hilar lymph nodes) and the development of hypersensitivity to the organism manifested by a cutaneous reaction to tuberculin or its derivatives. Occasionally, the primary infection in children

results in progressive disease, such as the development of extensive pneumonia, granulomatous involvement of the hilar nodes, endobronchial disease, or miliary spread. Primary progressive disease is also recognized in 20 to 30% of the adults who contract the disease. Both Khan and associates (1977) as well as Farman and Speir (1986) have noted this fact, but whether the actual incidence is increasing remains moot.

Most instances of clinical infection caused by the tubercle bacillus, however, are in persons already sensitized to the organism and, thus, represent a postprimary infection, frequently referred to, in the past, as *reinfection tuberculosis*. The postprimary infection may arise in any one of four ways: by direct progression of a primary lesion, by reactivation of a quiescent primary lesion, by hematogenous spread to the lungs, or by exogenous superinfection. Most instances of postprimary pulmonary tuberculosis are thought to arise either as progression of a primary lesion in the young or as reactivation of a dormant lesion, primary or postprimary, in the middle-aged or older person. Thus, most of the infections are considered endogenous rather than exogenous.

The structure and growth characteristics in culture of *M. tuberculosis* are discussed in Chapter 14.

With improved and more sophisticated methods of culture, especially the BACTEC radiometric system with 7H12 broth and other similar liquid cultures, a more rapid identification can occur of *M. tuberculosis* and other NTM organisms that may cause pulmonary disease in a variable percentage of patients thought to have infection caused by *M. tuberculosis*. In the past, these organisms were designated as atypical mycobacteria, but these now have been termed NTM organisms by Heifets (1997). More than 50 species of these organisms have been described, of which one-half, as reviewed by Wayne (1986), are recognized as pathogenic in varying degrees (Table 85-1). The differentiation of these mycobacteria have been expedited by newly developed laboratory techniques: 1) NAP differentiation test (para-nitro-α-acetylamino-β-hydroxypropiophenone) inhibits the growth of *M. tuberculosis* complex but not that of NTM organisms; 2) cell-wall lipid analysis includes three chromatographic methods for speciation of mycobacteria on the basis of their cell wall lipids (i.e., gas-liquid chromatography, high-performance high-pressure liquid, and thin-layer chromatography) as reviewed by Roberts and colleagues (1996); 3) nucleic acid probes involve chemiluminescent acridinium ester-labeled single-stand DNA probe complementary to the ribosomal RNA of the target bacterium; and 4) polymerase chain reaction and other amplification techniques are used, as reviewed by Sandin (1996). The polymerase chain reaction, however, has been found to be limited in its application in the diagnosis of *M. tuberculosis* (see Chapter 14). Heifets (1997) has reviewed in detail the bacteriologic diagnosis and drug susceptibility testing of these mycobacterial organisms as well as that of *M. tuberculosis*. The more important NTM organisms in humans are *Mycobacterium kansasii*, MAC, and *Mycobacterium fortuitum*. In patients with other lung

Table 85-1. Pathogenic and Potential Pathogenic Mycobacteria in Humans

Mycobacterium tuberculosis complex
   M. tuberculosis
   Mycobacterium bovis
   Mycobacterium africanum
Nontuberculous mycobacteria
   Photochromogens
      Mycobacterium kansasii
      Mycobacterium marinum
      Mycobacterium simiae
      Mycobacterium asiaticum
   Scotochromogens
      Mycobacterium scrofulaceum
      Mycobacterium xenopi
      Mycobacterium szulgai
      Mycobacterium gordonae
   Nonchromogens
      Mycobacterium avium
      Mycobacterium intracellulare
      Mycobacterium malmoense
      Mycobacterium ulcerans
      Mycobacterium paratuberculosis
      Mycobacterium haemophilum
      Mycobacterium genavens
   Rapid growers
      Mycobacterium fortuitum
      Mycobacterium peregrinum
      Mycobacterium chelonei

Adapted from Heifets L. Mycobacteriology laboratory. Clin Chest Med *18*:35, 1997.

diseases (e.g., chronic obstructive pulmonary disease, interstitial fibrosis, or pneumoconiosis), superimposed infections caused by *Mycobacterium gordonae*, *Mycobacterium simiae*, *Mycobacterium szulgai*, *Mycobacterium scrofulaceum*, *Mycobacterium xenopi*, and *Mycobacterium chelonei* have occasionally been reported.

Infections caused by *M. kansasii* tend to occur in a distinctly different group of patients than do those infections caused by *M. tuberculosis*. Lichtenstein and colleagues (1965), in summarizing their experience in Chicago, found that patients with infections caused by *M. kansasii* were more likely to be middle-aged men living in good economic surroundings, in contrast to patients with *M. tuberculosis*, who more commonly were living in overcrowded housing under poor economic conditions. In addition, *M. kansasii* does not appear to be contagious from human to human as is *M. tuberculosis*; only rare instances have been reported in which infection has occurred in more than one member of a family. Early experience showed that the highest incidence of *M. kansasii* infection was in Midwestern cities; specifically Kansas City, Dallas, and Chicago. With increased awareness of the organism, isolates are being recognized in many other parts of this country and the world.

Organisms from the scotochromogens group are rarely associated with infection, although in one collected series, Kestle and associates (1967) reported 26 of 50 isolates of *M. scrofulaceum* associated with what was thought to be inva-

sive infection. Gracey and Byrd (1970), however, found only 1 of 71 patients with sputum cultures containing these organisms to have pulmonary disease attributable to the organism. Infection from *M. scrofulaceum* does occur, however, in cervical lymph nodes, particularly in children. Ordinarily, the organism's virulence is considered to be low. A second scotochromogen, *M. gordonae* or the tap water bacillus, which can be confused with *M. scrofulaceum*, is rarely associated with infection in human beings. Perhaps the most important aspect of the scotochromogenic mycobacteria, and particularly *M. scrofulaceum*, is the evidence from skin testing found by Smith (1967), as well as Klare and associates (1967), that inapparent infection has taken place with this organism in approximately one-half of the population of the United States by the time they are in their early 20s. Such evidence was gained by determining skin hypersensitivity by using a specific purified protein derivative made from *M. scrofulaceum* purified protein derivative G, Gause strain. These studies showed that the organism is widely prevalent in the environment and is associated with inapparent infection in a much larger segment of the population than is *M. tuberculosis*. Recognition of a probable previous subclinical infection with *M. scrofulaceum* may explain the increased isolation of this organism from patients who excrete viable organism but show little or no evidence of active infection.

Although as many as seven mycobacterial species have been classified in the nonchromogen group, only two are considered to be a significant cause of infection in humans: MAC and *M. xenopi*. The remaining organisms in the nonchromogen group are important only to the laboratory in the differentiation from the two aforementioned species. Pulmonary infections with MAC are similar to those caused by *M. kansasii* in that they are most common in an older age group and are not as contagious as those caused by *M. tuberculosis*. Like infections from *M. kansasii*, infections from MAC cluster geographically along the southern seaboard of the United States, where apparent prior contact with the organisms, as shown by skin testing, is approximately four times greater in children than is their contact with *M. tuberculosis*. More important, MAC organisms are seen frequently in the immunocompromised patient. *M. xenopi* was first isolated from the South African toad, *Xenopus laevis*. Pulmonary infection with *M. xenopi* has been described in England. Marks and Schwabacher (1965) reported that isolation of the organism from 50 patients was considered clinically significant in 20 and of doubtful significance in an additional six patients. Banks and colleagues (1984) reviewed further experience with the disease in England, and Sors and associates (1979) reported on 50 cases in France, most of the latter occurring in the Ile-de-France region of Paris.

Infections with the rapidly growing mycobacteria are uncommon and, for the most part, are restricted to *M. fortuitum*. As with occasional infections from *M. scrofulaceum* and other weakly pathogenic strains of mycobacteria, *M.*

fortuitum usually is seen as a complication of underlying and, most frequently, severe debilitating disease.

PATHOLOGY

Primary Pulmonary Tuberculosis

The primary infection is located most often in the peripheral portion of the middle zone of the lung. The initial reaction to the invasion of *M. tuberculosis* bacilli is an exudative reaction in the involved, but still intact, alveolar spaces. With the development of hypersensitivity, usually within 6 weeks, caseous necrosis develops in the center of the lesion. At this point, healing is initiated in the lesion by the migration of fibroblasts. Progressive hyalinization and, eventually, calcification occur. Enlargement of the regional lymph nodes draining the primary infection also occurs. As noted, a few persons have progressive disease that, in reality, is a progression directly into postprimary pulmonary tuberculosis.

Postprimary Pulmonary Tuberculosis

Postprimary pulmonary tuberculosis tends to be localized primarily in the apical and posterior segments of the upper lobes and the superior segments of the lower lobes, but other areas are not exempt. The process consists of foci of caseous necrosis with edema, hemorrhage, and mononuclear cell infiltration. These foci may coalesce, and the caseous areas may liquefy and empty into a bronchus. In addition to the caseous necrosis, tubercles continue to develop at the periphery of the necrotic lesions.

The tubercle is composed of a central mass of epithelioid cells in which Langhans' type of giant cells and varying degrees of caseation occur. The periphery is surrounded by lymphocytes, fibroblasts, and fibrous tissue (Fig. 85-1). With appropriate staining techniques, mycobacteria may be demonstrated within the lesion, usually at the junction of the epithelial cells and the caseous necrosis.

With progression of the disease, increased amounts of lung tissue are destroyed and undergo caseation necrosis. Rupture of such large areas of necrosis into a bronchus results in the formation of the characteristic cavities seen in association with the disease. At the same time, attempts at healing take place and are represented by fibrosis and contracture of the involved areas. Depending on the resistance of the host, the virulence of the infecting organisms, and the adequacy of treatment, varying patterns of parenchymal destruction and associated healing may appear.

Early, the exudative, edematous phase is prominent; this stage may go on to complete healing with fibrosis, contracture, and, at times, calcification of the involved areas. In other patients, destruction of lung tissue exceeds the healing process, and caseation and subsequent cavitation are the

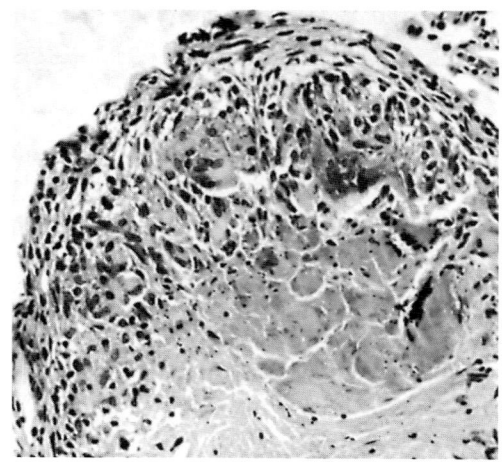

Fig. 85-1. Photomicrograph of tubercle in the lung.

major features. In some patients, the disease shows progression resembling an acute pneumonic process.

Initially, the cavities may be small and multiple, and the walls are irregular, thin, and pliable. These may fuse to form large or even giant cavities (Fig. 85-2). The walls become thick and fibrous, and incomplete septa and trabeculations may appear within the cavities, representing surviving bronchovascular bundles. Because the blood supply of these trabeculae, as well as that of the wall of the cavity, is from the bronchial arterial system, erosion and rupture of these vessels may be the source of frequent hemoptysis. Multiple, bronchial communications are present, and with healing, the cavities become lined by a fibrous membrane. Extensive fibrosis and scarring occur in the adjacent parenchymal tissue (Fig. 85-3).

The tuberculous cavity may become secondarily infected by other bacteria, yeasts, or fungi, and these may contribute to the destructive process. Air trapping may result from stenotic bronchi, now infrequently seen, and

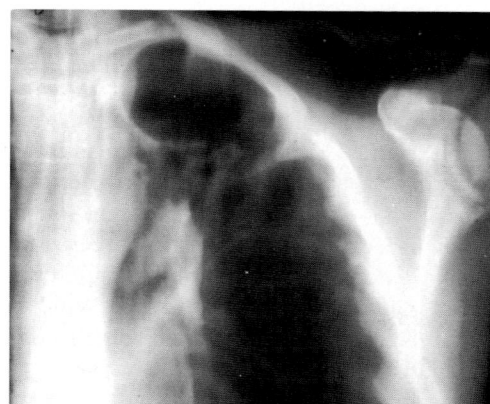

Fig. 85-2. Anteroposterior laminogram of a thin-walled, giant cavity in the left upper lobe. Several small cavities are seen below, extending toward the hilus.

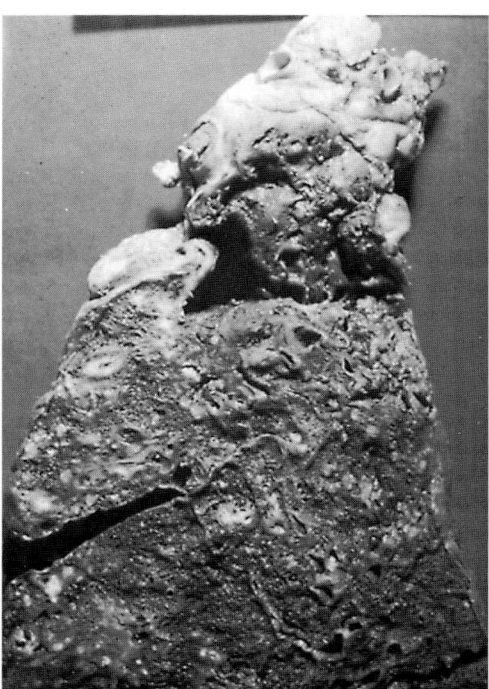

Fig. 85-3. Autopsy specimen of cut lung showing extensive apical pleural involvement, a large cavity in the apical area, plus numerous smaller cavities and fibrocaseous nodules throughout the lung tissue.

tension or giant cavities may develop. Smaller cavities may develop fibrous linings and come to resemble bronchiectatic sacs. Often, if this process does not occur, the cavity may become filled with inspissated caseous material. The lesion, thus, becomes a tuberculoma. The other cause of a tuberculoma (a large, conglomerate tubercle) is a parenchymal focus, either primary or postprimary. The tuberculoma resulting from the accumulation of caseous material in a cavity is associated most often with tuberculous bronchostenosis. The latter, as Lindskog and Liebow (1953) noted, results from one or several mechanisms: many small proliferative tuberculous lesions within the bronchial wall; extensive caseous necrosis within intramucosal tubercles; or necrosis of cartilage resulting from tuberculous chondritis. These processes may occur in bronchi of any caliber, but with modern antituberculous chemotherapy, major bronchial involvement is rare, but a number of cases of major bronchial stenosis have been reported from Japan in the 1980s and 1990s.

Tuberculous bronchiectasis appears in upper lobes extensively involved by the disease process. This condition may result from healing and fibrosis of the tuberculous cavities, but also the pathogenesis may resemble that of nontuberculous bronchiectasis (see Chapter 84). True ectasia can be differentiated from fibrous-lined cavities by the multiple fistulous communications between the sacs in the latter.

Pleural involvement is frequent, and dense, fibrotic pleural adhesions are common. Pleural effusion also is com-

mon, and even so-called idiopathic pleural effusion may be the first clinical manifestation of the disease process.

Nontuberculous Mycobacterial Infections

The pathologic changes observed in pulmonary disease produced by NTM organisms or MOTT are essentially the same as those produced by *M. tuberculosis*. MAC infections are prone to develop (colonize) in previously damaged lungs and to occur as opportunistic infections in immunocompromised hosts. Haque (1990) pointed out that, microscopically, MAC infection in such hosts is different from that seen with *M. tuberculosis*. Caseous necrosis is uncommon, and clusters of histiocytes filled with mycobacteria usually are seen. The granulomatous response to the infection is poor. The infiltration is confined to the interstitium and alveolar walls. Nodules may be seen, but cavitary disease is infrequent.

CLINICAL MANIFESTATIONS

Primary Infection

Most instances of primary infection caused by *M. tuberculosis* have no clinical manifestations and are discovered only at some later date by cutaneous tuberculin sensitivity or indirectly by the finding of a primary Ghon complex on a radiograph of the chest. Various factors influence the course of the initial infection and, of these, age, sex, heredity, race, economic status, intercurrent disease, and psychological factors are believed to be the most important.

Infants are thought to be the least resistant to continued activity of the organism, children from 5 years of age to puberty are apparently the most resistant, and a decrease in resistance extending into adult life appears to occur at puberty. Actually, however, the study of Myers and colleagues (1963) showed that, in many tuberculin reactors between birth and 5 years of age, only 8 to 9% developed clinical evidence of disease. Sixty percent of the patients with active disease recovered, whereas 40%, approximately 3% of the entire group, died because of tuberculosis. These data suggest that young children can resist the disease, although they do seem more prone to develop miliary tuberculosis and tuberculous meningitis than members of any other age group.

Economic conditions, intercurrent disease, and social habits, as these affect the individuals, appear to be more important in the resistance to continued activity of the primary infection as well as to its progression into the postprimary state.

After the development of the primary complex and of tuberculin sensitivity, healing takes place in most persons without the development of any clinical manifestations. The disease in the small remainder progresses into one or more of the fol-

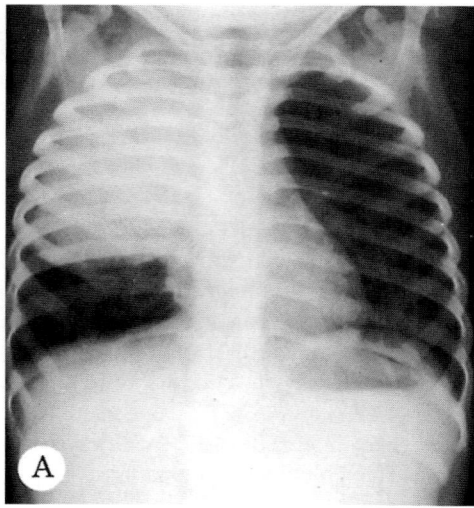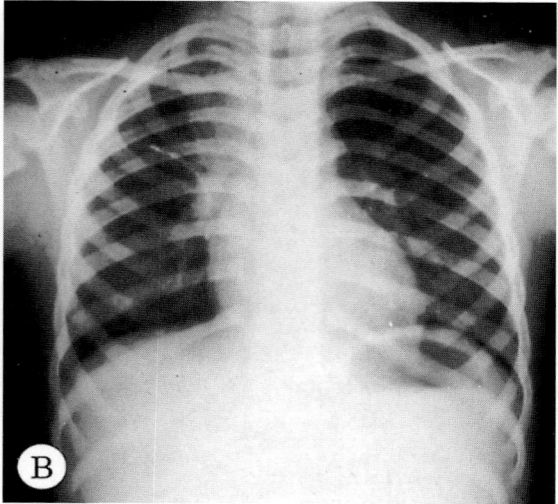

Fig. 85-4. A. Posteroanterior radiograph of an infant with tuberculous pneumonia of the entire right upper lobe. **B.** After medical treatment, the patient at 3 years of age has a right upper lobe that is atelectatic and nonfunctioning.

lowing clinical states: acute hematogenous dissemination with the development of miliary tuberculosis and tuberculous meningitis; extension to the pleura with development of pleurisy and pleural effusion; pulmonary parenchymal spread manifested as tuberculous pneumonia (Fig. 85-4); tracheobronchial tree compression by enlarged lymph nodes causing atelectasis; progression into the postprimary pulmonary disease evidenced by cavitation and extensive parenchymal involvement; or extrathoracic spread to other organ systems.

With pulmonary involvement, fever, cough, anorexia, weight loss, sweating, chest pain, lethargy, and dyspnea are common complaints. In younger patients, erythema nodosum is a frequent finding and may be the initial presenting feature in as many as 12% of those with active disease.

Progressive Primary Infection

As noted, progressive primary infection is seen in young children and in up to 20% of the adult population with newly recognized disease. This is common in the immunocompromised host. The thoracic disease may be manifested by pleural involvement with a symptomatic pleural effusion. Parenchymal disease may occur as miliary spread, lobar pneumonia, or segmental lung collapse from tuberculous lymphadenitis or significant tuberculous endobronchitis. The latter is found commonly in adults who have noncavitary lower lung infiltrates, according to Smith and associates (1987). Bronchopulmonary, as well as mediastinal, lymphadenitis also can be the major manifestation of the disease process.

Postprimary Infection

Many terms, such as *reinfection*, *reactivation*, and *chronic pulmonary tuberculosis*, refer to postprimary tuberculosis.

In many persons, tuberculosis is first discovered in a quiescent phase, an active phase of the postprimary infection having gone undetected. Such persons are asymptomatic and are classified as having inactive disease. However, many patients who have active postprimary disease are also asymptomatic, even in the presence of advanced disease.

Approximately one-half of the new postprimary infections are found on routine radiologic screening of the chest. Of these, an estimated 10 to 30% occur in persons with active disease. The other patients are discovered by investigation of constitutional or respiratory symptoms, or both.

Generalized malaise, lassitude, easy fatigability, anorexia, and weight loss occur early in the course of active infection. Afternoon fever and night sweats are common. Any or all such symptoms are easily attributable to other, less serious diseases. In a susceptible person, such as an alcoholic, drug addict, immunosuppressed, indigent, or diabetic patient, a patient receiving corticosteroid medication, or a patient with AIDS, however, a high index of suspicion should be maintained in the face of such general complaints. The clinical picture of tuberculosis in patients with HIV infection is determined by its degree of immunosuppression, according to Murray (1990) (Table 85-2).

Symptoms and signs referable to the lungs consist of cough, sputum production, hemoptysis, pleuritic chest pain, hoarseness, and shortness of breath.

Cough and sputum production are variable, but most patients with active disease have either one or both during the course of the disease. Hemoptysis is not an early symptom, but occurs in the presence of well-established disease. Actually, it is not a common symptom. The expectoration is seldom profuse, although at times it may be massive and life-threatening. Generally, the hemoptysis is bright red, homogeneous, and self-limited. Persistent blood streaking of the sputum is unusual and should arouse the suspicion of bronchial carcinoma.

Table 85-2. Clinical Manifestations of Active Tuberculosis in Early versus Late Human Immunodeficiency Virus Infections

	Early	Late
Tuberculin test	Usually positive	Usually negative
Adenopathy	Unusual	Common
Pulmonary distribution	Upper lobe	Lower and middle lobes
Cavitation	Often present	Typically absent
Extrapulmonary disease	10–15% of cases	≥50% of cases

Note: For practical purposes, early and late may be defined as CD4$^+$ cell counts greater than 300 cells/µL and less than 200 cells/µL, respectively.
Adapted from Murray JF: Cursed duet: HIV infection and tuberculosis. Respiration 57:210, 1990.

Table 85-3. Risk Factors for Nontuberculous Mycobacteria

Underlying lung disease (33–82%)
    Chronic obstructive pulmonary disease (25–72%)
    Previous tuberculosis (20–24%)
    Cystic fibrosis
    Interstitial lung disease (6%)
        Idiopathic pulmonary fibrosis
        Silicosis
        Asbestosis
Other risk factors
    Smoking (>30 pack years) (46%)
    Alcohol abuse (40%)
    Cardiovascular disease (36%)
    Chronic liver disease (32%)
    Previous gastrectomy (especially *Mycobacterium xenopi*) (18%)
    Achalasia (especially *Mycobacterium fortuitum-chelonei* complex)
    Immunosuppression (corticosteroids, lymphoproliferative disorders, transplantation, acquired immunodeficiency syndrome)

From Patz EF Jr, Swensen SJ, Erasmus J: Pulmonary manifestations of nontuberculous mycobacterium. Radiol Clin North Am 33:719, 1995. With permission.

Chest pain is pleuritic and is affected by deep breathing and cough. It occurs infrequently in postprimary infection and, if the pain is persistent, the presence of carcinoma of the lung involving the pleura should be suspected.

Shortness of breath may result from pleural effusion, the extensive destruction of the lung parenchyma, or even from generalized toxemia with hyperventilation related to a high fever.

Nontuberculous Mycobacterial Infections

The clinical findings in patients with pulmonary infections caused by the pathogenic NTM organisms resemble those present with disease caused by *M. tuberculosis*. The risk factors for these infections are listed in Table 85-3.

Patients with *M. kansasii* infections are more often middle-aged adults with average economic backgrounds. Pleural involvement is infrequent, and the chest radiograph often reveals that the disease is more extensive than the symptoms suggest. Other mycobacterial infections, particularly those caused by MAC, are frequently seen in immunocompromised patients and in older patients with other underlying disease processes. Reich and Johnson (1992) have described the occurrence of isolated lingular or middle lobe infiltrates in elderly women without other pulmonary pathology, which they have termed *Lady Windermere syndrome*. Huang and associates (1999) reviewed 31 HIV-negative patients without preexisting lung disease who were found to have MAC pulmonary infection. Ninety-four percent of the patients were women (90% white) with a median age of 63 years. The disease had no predilection for any specific lobe and consisted of bronchiectasis or multiple small nodules. Drug regimens were poorly tolerated in these patients. In immunocompromised patients, specifically the AIDS patient, MAC is the most common bacterial complication that occurs. More than one-third of these patients have disseminated disease with hepatomegaly, diarrhea, splenomegaly, and abdominal pain. In non-AIDS patients, these complications are seen only infrequently.

RADIOGRAPHIC FEATURES

The radiographic features of *M. tuberculosis* pulmonary infection are influenced by the status of the disease process; it is of either the progressive primary type or the more common postprimary disease state. The manifestations of the latter are more readily recognized, whereas the manifestations of the former may be easily confused with other disease processes. The protean radiographic features have been well described by Fraser and associates (1989), Buckner and Walker (1990), and McAdams and associates (1995).

Primary Pulmonary Tuberculosis

The radiographic manifestations of primary infection with *M. tuberculosis*, as Fraser and Paré (1970) noted, may appear in the pulmonary parenchyma, hilar and mediastinal lymph nodes, tracheobronchial tree, and pleural space. The parenchymal involvement is most often in the middle zone of the lung and resembles a pneumonic consolidation of variable size. The area is homogeneous in density, and the margins are ill defined, although an entire lobe may be involved with resultant sharply defined margins. The anterior segment of the upper lobes and areas of the lower lobes are frequently involved. Cavitation is uncommon in primary tuberculosis. Calcification may occur in the area of parenchymal involvement (Fig. 85-5).

Hilar or paratracheal lymph node enlargement appears in almost all children with primary tuberculosis; it is less common in the adult. Choyke and associates (1983) recorded an incidence of 10%; but Woodring and colleagues (1986) noted an incidence of 32% in adults with progressive primary disease. The enlargement may be bilateral and/or unilateral and hilar and/or paratracheal. Such mediastinal lymph node involvement, even of lymph nodes in the ante-

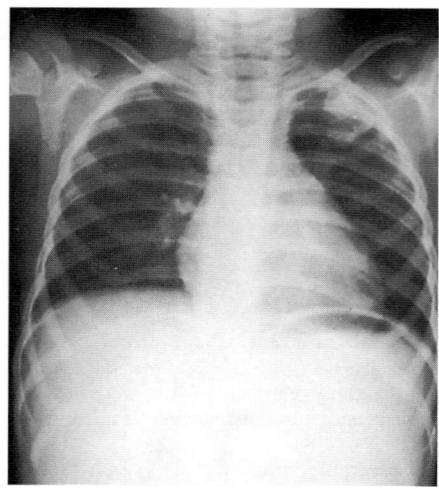

Fig. 85-5. Posteroanterior radiograph of a 3.5-year-old child with calcified residua of a primary infection in the left upper lobe.

rior mediastinal compartment (Fig. 85-6), may be observed in infected AIDS patients.

Tracheobronchial involvement is common and, more often, results from compression by enlarged lymph nodes and, less commonly, from direct involvement of the structure by the disease process (endobronchial tuberculosis). Resultant partial or complete atelectasis of the lung distal to the obstruction occurs, although obstructive emphysema is occasionally present. Any lobe or segment may be involved, but because of the angle of the takeoff of the various segmental bronchi and the distribution of the lymph nodes about them, the anterior segment of the upper lobes, medial segment of the middle lobe, and lower lobes are more likely to be involved.

Endobronchial tuberculosis may be evaluated by computed tomographic scans. Lee and colleagues (1991) reported that the common features are bronchial narrowing associated with bronchial thickening or peribronchial cuff of

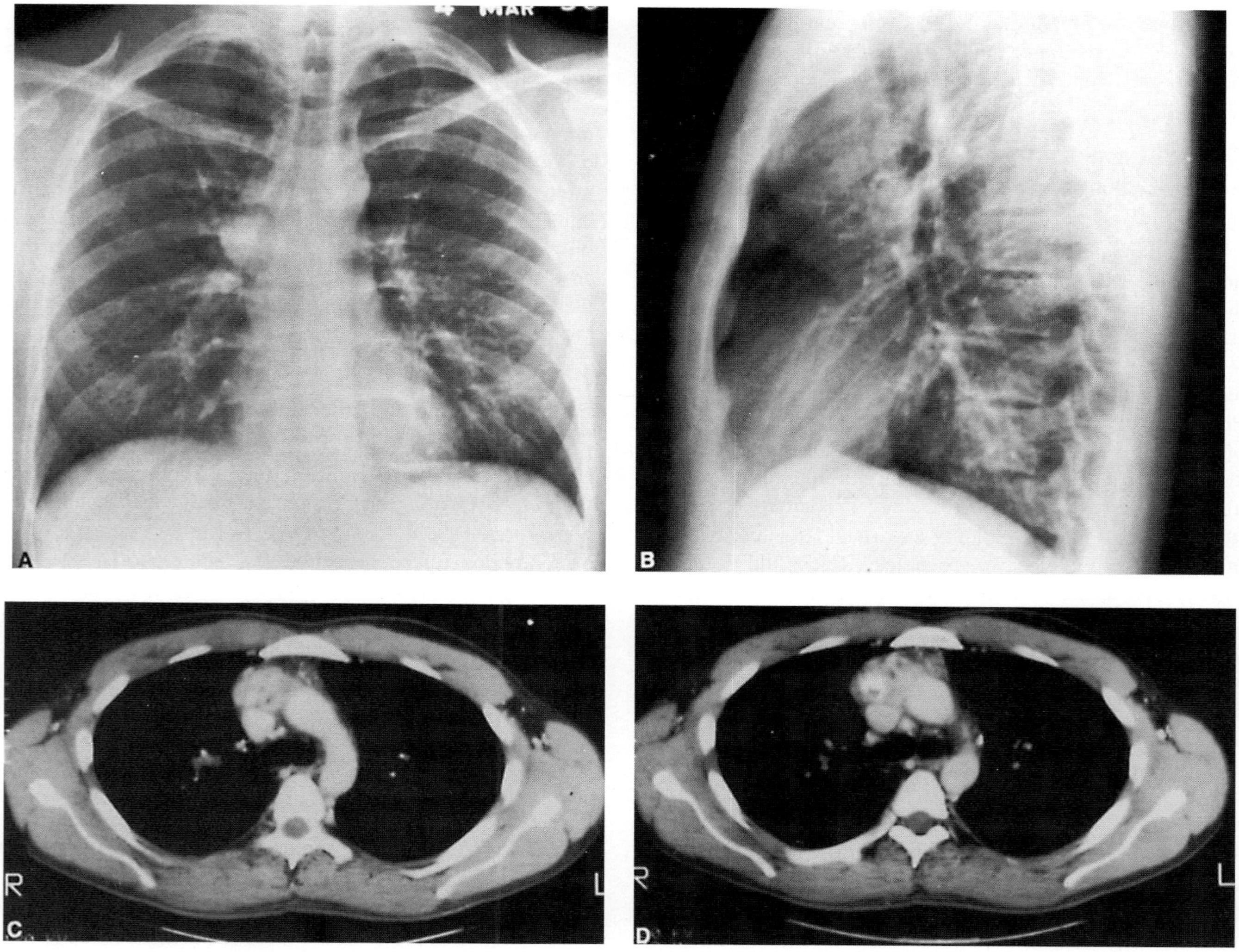

Fig. 85-6. Posteroanterior (**A**) and lateral (**B**) radiographs of a young adult man with acquired immunodeficiency syndrome who developed the anterior mediastinal mass in a 6-month period. Computed tomographic scans (**C, D**) reveal a nonhomogenous anterior mediastinal mass with area of calcification. Biopsy revealed a granulomatous process containing many acid-fast organisms typical of *Mycobacterium tuberculosis*.

soft tissue; bronchial obstruction; enlarged peribronchial lymph nodes; and, rarely, an intraluminal mass. Similar findings are occasionally present in the absence of endoscopically visualized endobronchitis so that such features are not pathognomonic of endobronchitis. The seriousness of this complication, especially in patients with lower lobe involvement, because of resultant bronchial stenosis and collapse of the involved segments, was noted by Ip (1986) and Smith (1987) and their colleagues.

Pleural involvement with the development of an effusion is more common in the young adult than in the child. The volume of the effusion is variable and may be, but usually is not, associated with a demonstrable parenchymal lesion.

Postprimary Pulmonary Tuberculosis

Unlike primary tuberculosis, postprimary pulmonary tuberculosis is identified most often in the apical posterior segments of the upper lobes and less so in the superior segment of the lower lobes. An entire lobe or lung, however, may be involved in extensive disease. Rarely, the inflammatory processes may be isolated in the anterior segment of the upper lobes or in one of the basilar segments of the lung. If this situation occurs, particularly in the older patient, the possibility of carcinoma of the lung must be ruled out.

The radiographic features reflect the pathologic process present in the lung. Although the findings are often characteristic, definitive diagnosis of tuberculosis can be made only by the identification of the organism by culture or by microscopic examination of a specimen of the lung obtained at either operation or autopsy.

Many radiographic patterns can be identified in postprimary tuberculosis; Fraser and Paré (1970) listed local exudative lesions, local fibroproductive lesions, cavitation, bronchial spread and acute tuberculous pneumonia, bronchiectasis, bronchostenosis, and tuberculoma. One or more of these findings are present in two-thirds of all newly diagnosed cases of pulmonary *M. tuberculosis* infections in adults. Both Khan and associates (1977) and Farman and Speir (1986) recorded this observation. Moreover, the latter authors noted that the apical or posterior segment, or both, of the upper lobes were the sites of the radiographic disease. Miliary tuberculosis can occur in postprimary disease, and Grieco and Chmel (1974) and Sahn and Neff (1974) reported that it is more common in the elderly than in any other age group. The typical radiographic features of disseminated, small, discrete opacities may not be observed for as long as 6 weeks after the initial hematogenous dissemination.

Local exudative lesions cause patchy or confluent alveolar consolidation. The lymphatic drainage markings radiating toward the hilus are accentuated.

Local fibroproductive lesions are defined more sharply, although their size and shape may vary. A decrease in lung volume evidences fibrosis and contracture, and the hilus and trachea are sometimes retracted toward the lesion (Fig. 85-7).

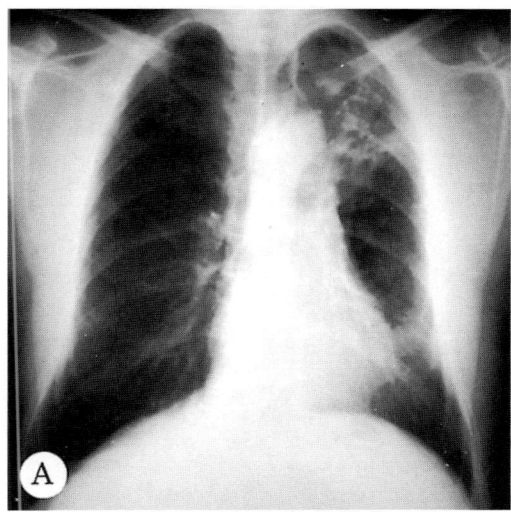

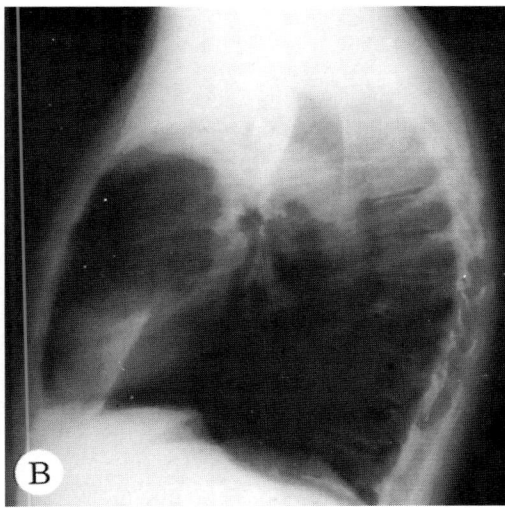

Fig. 85-7. Posteroanterior **(A)** and lateral **(B)** chest radiographs showing fibrosis and contracture of the superior division (apical posterior and anterior segments) of the left upper lobe.

Cavitary lesions have moderately thick walls, but with healing, these tend to become thin; the inner surface linings are smooth, and air-fluid levels are seen only infrequently (Fig. 85-8). The cavities may disappear after adequate therapy, but some persist as open, negative cavities. Computed tomography may be necessary to verify the persistence of some cavities after therapy.

Active tuberculous infection in patients with compromised immune systems, such as those with AIDS, manifest radiographically similar to that seen in children (i.e., primary pulmonary tuberculosis) rather than that normally seen in the adult with postprimary pulmonary tuberculosis, although in most if not all such patients, the infection is a postprimary reactivation. Pitchenik and Rubinson (1985) reviewed the radiographic findings in two groups of Haitian patients, one with and the other without AIDS. Batungwanayo and colleagues (1992) compared the findings in

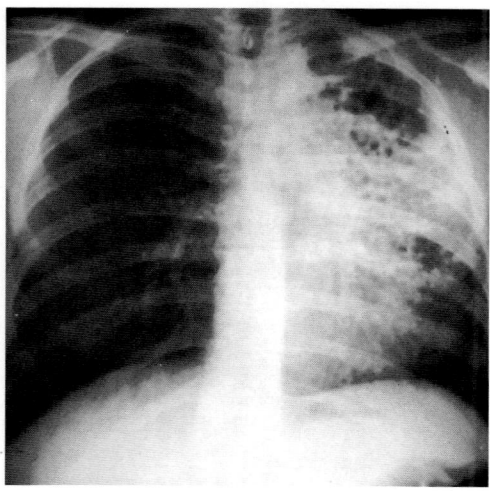

Fig. 85-8. Posteroanterior radiograph shows extensive cavitary disease of the left lung.

similar patients from Rwanda. Table 85-4 summarizes these findings. Thus, in the immunocompromised adult host, atypical radiographic findings should alert the clinician to the possibility of tuberculosis.

Nontuberculous Mycobacterial Infections

The radiographic manifestations of pulmonary disease caused by NTM organisms are generally those of moderate to far advanced parenchymal involvement and may not be differentiated accurately from those with disease caused by *M. tuberculosis.* Patz and coworkers (1995) reviewed the radiologic manifestations of NTM infections. Some features, however, appear to be more characteristic of the infections caused by NTM organisms. Cavitation with multiple, thin-walled cavities is more common than in

infection with the tubercle bacillus; exudative lesions are uncommon, and hematogenous dissemination and pleural effusion are rare. Nonetheless, the diseases rarely can be differentiated by the radiographic features alone. The observation that the patient with infection caused by NTM organisms is often less sick than the extensive radiographic findings suggest is important.

DIAGNOSIS

The diagnosis of pulmonary tuberculosis may be suggested by the history and the clinical and radiographic manifestations, but depends solely on identification of the infecting organism or the histologic features and demonstration of the organism in a specimen of the lung.

Skin testing is important epidemiologically, and the nonreaction to test doses of various strengths, except in certain circumstances, such as immunocompromise, miliary tuberculosis, or severe debilitation from the disease process, excludes the possibility of the disease.

Collection and treatment of material for culture of the organism is outlined in Chapter 14.

Bronchoscopy frequently is indicated, especially if the disease process is not responding well to therapy or if change in therapy is anticipated. The possibility of active endobronchial disease should be ruled out before surgical therapy, especially in those patients who continue to have the causative organisms in their sputum.

Computed tomography is essential in delineating the extent of associated parenchymal disease, particularly in patients with extensive pleural disease before any surgical decision is made.

Because many patients suspected of having tuberculosis are old, special care must be used to rule out the possibility of bronchial carcinoma. Although the risk of bronchial carcinoma in patients with pulmonary tuberculosis may be

Table 85-4. Radiographic Patterns of Pulmonary Tuberculosis in Patients Seropositive for Human Immunodeficiency Virus and Patients with Acquired Immunodeficiency Syndrome

Radiographic Patterns	Incidence (No. of Patients)			
	HIV Positive[a]	AIDS[b]	Non-HIV[a]	Non-AIDS[b]
Hilar or mediastinal adenopathy	31	59	0	3
Pulmonary cavitation	39	0	91	67
Upper lobe infiltrates	16	18	55	97
Middle or lower lobe infiltrates	33	29	8	3
Diffuse infiltrates	20	12	27	0
Miliary infiltrates	25	6	9	0
Pleural effusion	43	12	9	7
No infiltrates	—	35	—	0
Normal radiograph	—	12	—	0

AIDS, acquired immunodeficiency syndrome; HIV, human immunodeficiency virus.
[a]Data from Batungwanayo J, et al: Pulmonary tuberculosis in Kigali, Rwanda. Impact of immunodeficiency virus infection on clinical and radiographic presentation. Am Rev Respir Dis *146*:53, 1992.
[b]Data from Pitchenik AE, Rubinson HA: The radiographic appearance of tuberculosis in patients with the acquired immune deficiency syndrome (AIDS). Am Rev Respir Dis *131*:393, 1985.

increased, the major problem is the coexistence of the two diseases. This problem is perplexing, particularly in the older patient with tuberculosis who has had stable radiographic findings and then manifests a change in chest radiography results. Also troublesome is the older patient who has an area of atelectasis in the basilar portion of either lobe that may be the end result of bronchial stenosis from previous endobronchial disease associated with progressive primary disease. Ip and associates (1986) noted that stenosis occurred in such patients despite adequate antituberculous drug treatment. Consider also the patient who initially presents with radiographic findings that suggest pulmonary tuberculosis and has a positive skin reaction to purified protein derivative but the smear and culture results of the sputum are negative for mycobacteria. A high index of suspicion must be maintained that these radiographic findings represent a bronchial carcinoma, and the patient must be evaluated and managed as if the disease process is carcinoma of the lung. Radiographic findings of unilateral prominence of one hilus; paratracheal node involvement; an atelectatic segment or lobe without mottling, linear streaking, or cavitation; homogeneous spread of the disease under adequate medical management; or a nodular density larger than 2 cm in diameter should suggest the possibility of carcinoma. If doubt remains, exploratory thoracotomy, when feasible, should be carried out after a short, intensive course of antituberculous chemotherapy.

TREATMENT

Medical Therapy of *Mycobacterium tuberculosis*

The primary treatment of pulmonary disease caused by *M. tuberculosis* is medical. Various combinations of the many antituberculous chemotherapeutic drugs are used. The major drugs available are listed in Table 85-5. When a single drug is administered, no matter how specific, early development of bacterial resistance occurs. In contrast, when combinations of two or more agents are used, resistance is postponed or even prevented. In many clinics, these chemotherapeutic agents are divided into first-line and second-line drugs. The first-line drugs are isonicotinic acid hydrazide (INH), ethambutol (EMB), and rifampin (RMP). Streptomycin is used less frequently because its mode of administration by injection necessitates frequent patient visits. Pyrazinamide was not considered a first-line drug, but O'Brien and Snider (1985) noted that when it is added to the initial drug regimen, it can effectively reduce the length of treatment required. For this reason, this drug belongs in the first-line group. Second-line drugs include para-aminosalicylic acid, cycloserine, viomycin, ethionamide, capreomycin, kanamycin, ciprofloxacin, ofloxacin, amikacin, and clofazimine, among others. All of the aforementioned drugs carry some potential toxicity. Demonstra-

Table 85-5. Major Antimycobacterial Drugs

Amikacin (AK)
Aminosalicylic acid (PAS)
Azithromycin (AZI)
Capreomycin (CM)
Ciprofloxacin (CIP)
Clarithromycin (CLAR)
Clofazimine (CFZ)
Cycloserine (CSN)
Ethambutol (EMB)
Ethionamide (ETA)
Isoniazid (INH)
Kanamycin (KM)
Ofloxacin (OFLOX)
Pyrazinamide (PZA)
Rifabutin (RBN)
Rifampin (RIF)
Streptomycin (SM) (STM)
Thiacetazone (Tb1)

tion of individual patient toxicity or intolerance determines the drug regimen to be followed. Table 85-6 details the dosage, toxicity, tests for side effects, and the action of the drugs on the metabolic processes of the tubercle bacillus. For the drugs to have an effect, the organism must be actively metabolizing, although some indication exists that RMP can kill even dormant organisms. Nonetheless, most organisms apparently do metabolize within a 2-year period because active treatment for 18 to 24 months reduces the relapse rate to less than 2%.

Recommended Drug Regimens

Standard Nine-Month Regimens Based on Isonicotinic Acid Hydrazide and Rifampin

The combination of INH (300 mg) plus RMP (600 mg) daily by mouth for 9 months is highly effective for almost all forms of drug-sensitive pulmonary tuberculosis. However, most authorities advise additional pyrazinamide (25 to 35 mg/kg) plus either streptomycin (1 g) or EMB (15 to 25 mg/kg) initially pending sensitivity results for 2 to 8 weeks; the relapse rate is reported to be less than 3%. An intermittent 9-month course is also acceptable. INH and RMP are administered daily as described for 1 to 2 months and twice weekly thereafter with the same dose of RMP but a larger dose of INH (900 mg).

Six-Month Regimens

One of the 6-month regimens uses 2 months of INH, RMP, and pyrazinamide, plus either ethionamide, 25 mg/kg or streptomycin if INH resistance is suspected, followed by INH and RMP daily or two to three times weekly for 4 months.

Table 85-6. Treatment of Mycobacterial Disease

	Daily Dose[a]	Most Common Side Effects	Monitoring	Remarks
Commonly used agents				
Isoniazid	5–10 mg/kg up to 300 mg PO or IM	Peripheral neuritis; hepatitis; hypersensitivity	SGOT/SGPT (not as a routine).	Bactericidal to both extracellular and intracellular organisms; pyridoxine, 10 mg as prophylaxis for neuritis; 50–100 mg as treatment.
Rifampin	10 mg/kg up to 600 mg PO	Hepatitis; febrile reaction; purpura (rare)	SGOT/SGPT (not as a routine).	Bactericidal to all populations of organisms. Orange urine and other body secretions; discoloring of contact lens.
Streptomycin	15–20 mg/kg up to 1 g IM	Eighth nerve damage; nephrotoxicity	Vestibular function, audiograms,[b] BUN and creatinine.	Bactericidal to extracellular organisms. Use with caution in older patients or those with renal disease.
Pyrazinamide	15–30 mg/kg up to 2 g PO	Hyperuricemia; hepatotoxicity	Uric acid, SGOT/SGPT.	Bactericidal to intracellular organisms. Combination with an aminoglycoside is bactericidal.
Ethambutol	15–25 mg/kg	Optic neuritis (reversible with discontinuation of drug; rare at 15 mg/kg); skin rash	Red-green discrimination and visual acuity.[b] Difficult to test in a child younger than 3 years.	Bacteriostatic to both intracellular and extracellular organisms, primarily used to inhibit development of resistant mutants. Use with caution with renal disease or when eye testing is not feasible.
Less commonly used agents[c]				
Capreomycin	15–30 mg/kg up to 1 g IM	Eighth nerve damage; nephrotoxicity	Vestibular function, audiograms,[b] BUN and creatinine.	Bactericidal to extracellular organisms in cavities. Use with caution in older patients. Rarely used with renal disease.
Kanamycin	15–30 mg/kg up to 1 g IM	Auditory toxicity nephrotoxicity; vestibular toxicity (rare)	Vestibular function, audiograms,[b] BUN and creatinine.	Bactericidal to extracellular organisms. Use with caution in older patients. Rarely used with renal disease.
Ethionamide	15–30 mg/kg up to 1 g PO	Gastrointestinal disturbance; hepatotoxicity; hypersensitivity	SGOT/SGPT.	Bacteriostatic to both intracellular and extracellular organisms. Divided dose may help gastrointestinal side effects; has a metallic taste. Avoid use during pregnancy.
Para-aminosalicylic acid (aminosalicylic acid)	150 mg/kg up to 12 g PO	Gastrointestinal disturbance; hypersensitivity; hepatotoxicity; sodium load	SGOT/SGPT.	Bacteriostatic to extracellular organisms only. Gastrointestinal side effects frequent, making cooperation difficult.
Cycloserine	10–20 mg/kg up to 1 g PO	Psychosis; personality changes; convulsions; rash	Psychological testing.	Bacteriostatic to both intracellular and extracellular organisms. Alcohol may aggravate psychiatric problems. Difficult drug to use. Side effects may be blocked by pyridoxine, ataractic agents, or anticonvulsant drugs.
Ciprofloxacin	500–1000 mg/day	Gastrointestinal upset; dizziness; hypersensitivity; drug interactions; headaches; restlessness	Drug interactions.	Not approved by FDA for tuberculosis treatment. Should not be used in children.
Ofloxacin	400–800 mg/day	Gastrointestinal upset; dizziness; hypersensitivity; drug interactions; headaches; restlessness	Drug interactions.	Not approved by FDA for tuberculosis treatment. Should not be used in children. Avoid antacids, iron, zinc, sucralfate.
Amikacin	15 mg/kg	Renal toxicity; vestibular dysfunction; hearing loss; chemical imbalance; dizziness	Assess hearing function. Measure renal function and serum drug levels.	Not approved by FDA for tuberculosis treatment.
Clofazimine	100–300 mg/day	Gastrointestinal upset; discoloration of skin; severe abdominal pain and organ damage caused by crystal deposition	—	—

BUN, blood urea nitrogen; FDA, U.S. Food and Drug Administration; SGOT, serum glutamic-oxaloacetic transaminase; SGPT, serum glutamic-pyruvic transaminase.

[a]Doses for children are the same as for adults. Weight-based dosage should be adjusted as weight changes.

[b]Initial examination should be done at start of treatment.

[c]The less commonly used drugs should be used only in consultation with a clinician experienced in the management of drug-resistant tuberculosis. Other drugs, such as rifabutin and clarithromycin are not FDA-approved for the treatment of *Mycobacterium tuberculosis* complex. However, use as second-line drugs may be helpful in the treatment of multidrug-resistant tuberculosis when drug susceptibility tests demonstrate sensitivity of the infecting *M. tuberculosis* strain.

From Centers for Disease Control and Prevention: Core curriculum in tuberculosis: what a clinician should know. Washington, DC: US Government Printing Office, 1994. With permission.

Table 85-7. A 62-Dose, Four-Drug Regimen for Tuberculosis in Adults

First 2 weeks (once-daily dose for 14 consecutive days)
INH, 300 mg
RMP, 600 mg
PZA, 1.5 g if ≤50 kg body weight, 2.0 g if 51–74 kg, 2.5 g if
≥75 kg
STM, 750 mg if ≤50 kg body weight, 1.0 g if >50 kg
Weeks 3–8 (twice weekly)
INH, 15 mg/kg
RMP, 600 mg
PZA, 3.0 g if ≤50 kg body weight, 3.5 g if 51–74 kg, 4.0 g if
≥75 kg
STM, 1.0 g if ≤50 kg body weight, 1.25 g if 51–74 kg, 1.5 g if
≥75 kg
Weeks 9–26 (twice weekly)
INH, 15 mg/kg body weight
RMP, 600 mg

INH, isoniazid; PZA, pyrazinamide; RMP, rifampin; STM, streptomycin.
From Cohn DL, et al: A 62-dose, 6-month therapy for pulmonary
and extrapulmonary tuberculosis. A twice-weekly, directly observed,
and cost-effective regimen. Ann Intern Med *112*:407, 1990. With
permission.

Directly Observed Therapy in Noncompliant Patients

Directly observed therapy is recommended for the suspected noncompliant patient. Cohn and associates (1990)
have suggested the regimen shown in Table 85-7. EMB may
be substituted for streptomycin without loss of efficacy.

Results of Medical Treatment

Under adequate circumstances in cooperative patients,
most pulmonary infections are controlled by appropriate
medical management. In patients who fail to adhere to the
medical regimen or who have other serious associated disease, however, the failure rate, as Johnston and Wildrick
(1974) noted, is 4 to 7%. Pitchenik and Rubinson (1985), as
well as Dautzenberg and associates (1984), pointed out,
however, that despite immunosuppression from AIDS or
other causes, antituberculous drugs are still effective.

Treatment of Multiple Drug–Resistant Tuberculosis

Many originally noncompliant patients who experience a
relapse, as well as those persons with exposure to patients
with drug-resistant organisms, may have initial drug resistance. The mechanism of drug resistance of *M. tuberculosis*
organisms is shown in Table 85-8. An incidence of primary
drug resistance as high as 10% was recorded by Pomerantz
and associates (1991). As a rule, four or more antimicrobial
drugs are often used, and the duration of treatment is generally 18 to 24 months, depending on individual patient
response and the drug regimen selected. Bacterial sensitivity
studies are made routinely and may indicate the desirability
of switching to other drugs. Conversion rates vary and reactivation rates are high. Iseman (1993) recorded his experience in treating very ill patients with MDRTB in Denver,

Table 85-8. Mechanisms of Drug Resistance in *Mycobacterium tuberculosis*

Antimyco-bacterial Agent	Mechanism of Action	Genes Involved in Resistance	Frequency of Mutations Associated with Resistance	Mechanism of Resistance
Isoniazid	Inhibition of mycolic acid biosynthesis	(i) katG (catalase-peroxidase)	(i) 47–58%	(i) Mutations in katG result in failure to generate an active intermediate of INH
		(ii) inhA (enoyl-ACP reductase)	(ii) 21–34%	(ii) Overexpression of inhA allows continuation of mycolic acid synthesis
		(iii) ahpC (alkyl hydroperoxide reductase)	(iii) 10–15%	(iii) ahpC mutations may just serve as a marker for lesions in katG
Rifampin	Inhibition of transcription	rpoB (β-subunit of RNA polymerase)	96–98%	Mutations in rpoB prevent interaction with rifampin
Streptomycin	Inhibition of protein synthesis	(i) rpsL (ribosomal protein S12)	(i) 52–59%	Mutations prevent interaction with streptomycin.
		(ii) rrs (16S rRNA)	(ii) 8–21%	
Ethambutol	Inhibition of arabinogalac-tan and lipoarabino-mannan biosynthesis	embAB (arabinosyl transferase)	50%	Overexpression or mutation of embAB allows continuation of arabinan biosynthesis
Pyrazinamide	Unknown	pcnA	Unknown	Loss of pyrazinamidase activity results in decreased conversion of pyrazinamide to pyrazinoic acid, the putative active moiety(?)
Fluoroquinolones	Inhibition of the DNA gyrase	gyrA (DNA gyrase subunit A)	75–94%	Mutations in gyrA prevent interaction with fluoroquinolones

From Telenti A: Genetics of drug resistance in tuberculosis. Clin Chest Med *18*:55, 1997. With permission.

and Passannante and colleagues (1994) discussed the use of preventive therapy for contacts of MDRTB. The latter authors noted that many regimens have been used, but none are well accepted by all investigators. However, one of the more common regimens is pyrazinamide and ciprofloxacin for 4 months.

Medical Therapy of Nontuberculous Mycobacterial Infections

The same antituberculous agents are used, with some modifications, to treat NTM infections. RMP and INH are the drugs most commonly used, even though frequently the organisms, particularly *M. kansasii*, have been shown in vitro to be resistant to these drugs. Often, these drugs are augmented by one or more of the second-line drugs. Therapy is given usually for 18 months. Response, as shown by conversion of the sputum and by the radiographic resolution of the parenchymal involvement, occurs slowly; often, conversion of the sputum is more pronounced than is radiographic evidence of resolution. In 20 to 30% of patients with infection caused by *M. kansasii*, the overall response is unsatisfactory. Most of the patients who have disease caused by this organism, however, do not become

surgical candidates. Pulmonary disease caused by MAC responds poorly. Medical therapy usually consists of four or more drugs. The recommended regimen for MAC is RMP (600 mg daily), EMB (25 mg/kg/day for 2 months, then 15 mg/kg/day), and streptomycin (1 g 5 days/week for 6 to 12 weeks then 1 g three times per week). The addition of clarithromycin (50 mg orally twice a day) may be beneficial. Another regimen includes amikacin, ciprofloxacin, EMB, and RMP. Clofazimine may be substituted for amikacin. When the pathologic process is localized, most if not all such patients with the disease are or become surgical candidates despite the use of one of these drug regimens.

Pulmonary infections caused by *M. fortuitum* and *M. chelonei* are usually resistant to the standard antituberculous agents. Young and Bailey (1988) advised medical therapy with cefoxitin and amikacin. Cefoxitin (200 mg/kg/day up to 12 g/day) and amikacin (15 mg/kg/day) are given intravenously and continued for at least 12 weeks.

In patients with AIDS and disseminated MAC infection, Masur and associates (1987) reported that clofazimine and anisomycin may be beneficial, although experience with these drugs is limited. Overall, in NTM infections sputum conversion is seen in only 50 to 80% of cases and relapses occur in up to 20% of cases.

B. Surgery for the Management of *Mycobacterium tuberculosis* and Nontuberculous Mycobacterial Infections of the Lungs

Marvin Pomerantz

In the United States, the most common indication for surgery in patients with tuberculosis is infection with MDRTB. These patients invariably either have thick-walled cavitary disease (Fig. 85-9) or a destroyed lobe or lung (Fig. 85-10). It has been shown by Canetti (1965) that cavities contain from 10^7 to 10^9 organisms compared with 10^2 to 10^4 in nodules. The removal of this heavy bacterial burden is essential in the treatment of MDRTB. A destroyed lobe or lung acts similar to a cavitary disease. In patients with MDRTB, destruction of the left lung that requires a pneumonectomy occurs more frequently than it does in the right lung. As a result, 75% of pneumonectomies in the series reported by Brown and the author (1995) were on the left.

Van Leuven and associates (1997) likewise reported a similar incidence of 80% left-sided pneumonectomies. Earlier, Ashour and colleagues (1990) reported 12 of 13 pneumonectomies were performed on the left side; in a later follow-up by Ashour (1997), 16 of 20 pneumonectomies were done on the left. Ashour and associates (1990) suggested that the propensity for left-sided lung destruction in patients with resistant *M. tuberculosis* infection was possibly related to the smaller caliber of the left main stem bronchus, the tight space surrounding it, and the angle of its takeoff from the trachea. In 172 pneumonectomies performed over the years by the same authors, however, only 63% were on the left side. This latter incidence is not dissimilar to the 57%

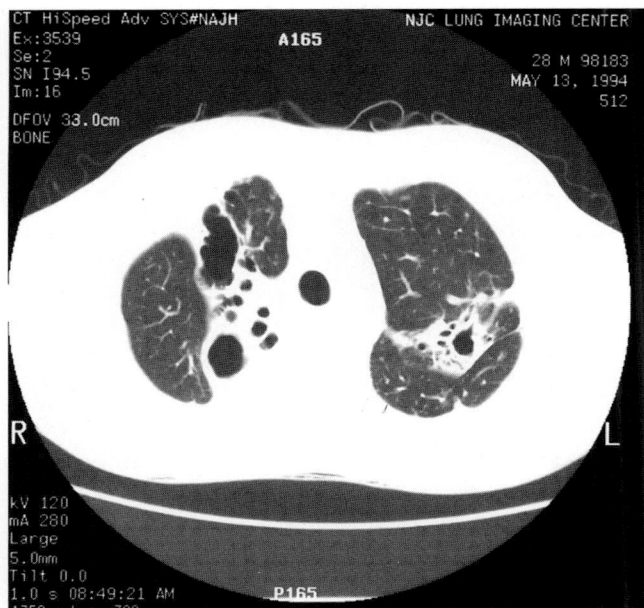

Fig. 85-9. Computed tomographic scan shows bilateral upper lobe cavities.

incidence of left pneumonectomies in 101 patients that Shields and colleagues (1958) had reported earlier. The reasons for this apparent change in incidence remain obscure, and the validity of the postulates advanced by Ashour and colleagues (1990) are as yet unproved. This lateralization does not hold true for NTM (MOTT) infections. Other indications for surgery include massive hemoptysis (greater than 600 mL in 24 hours), bronchopleural fistula (Fig. 85-11), bronchostenosis, to relieve a trapped lung (Fig. 85-12), or to rule out the presence of cancer.

SURGICAL RESECTION OF PARENCHYMAL DISEASE

Preoperative Preparation

Preoperatively, attempts should be made to convert the patient's sputum smear and culture results to negative. However, approximately 50% of the time in patients with MDRTB this is not possible even with appropriate antibiotics. The antituberculous regimen chosen should be given for approximately 3 months before surgery. Several weeks before surgery an additional antibiotic is usually added if the infecting organism is susceptible to it. Clinical judgment is required on the timing of surgery. Mycobacterial patients are usually nutritionally deprived. Few patients requiring surgery are at or above their normal body weight. This is manifested by a low serum albumin. Every effort should be made to supplement oral intake with parenteral nutrition. Appetite stimulation with megestrol acetate (Megace) has been helpful particularly in women.

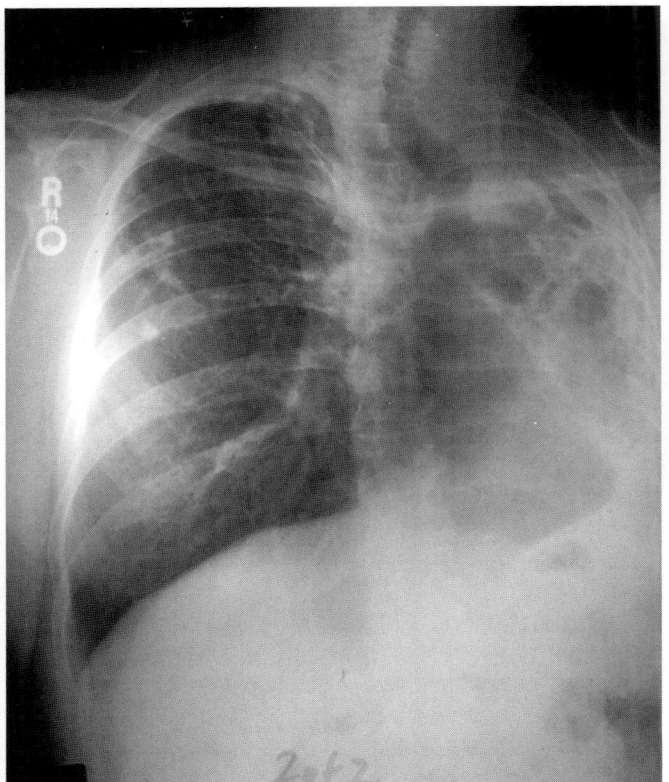

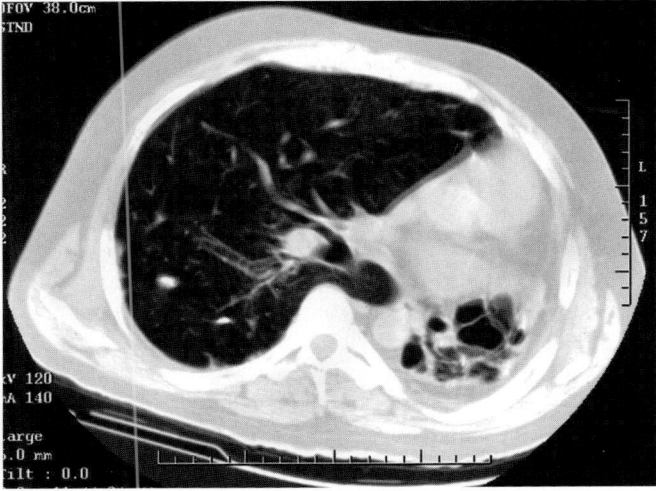

Fig. 85-10. A. Totally destroyed left lung caused by tuberculosis. **B.** Computed tomographic scan demonstrates destroyed left lung.

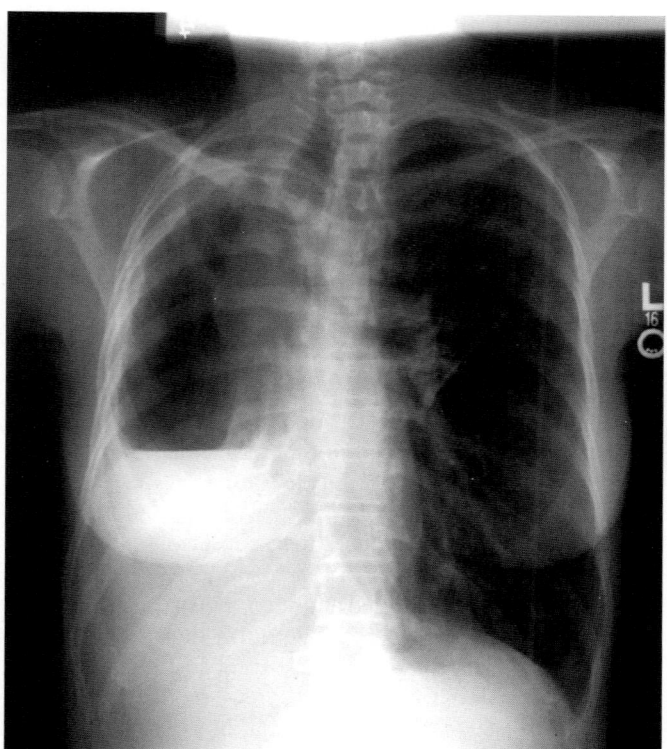

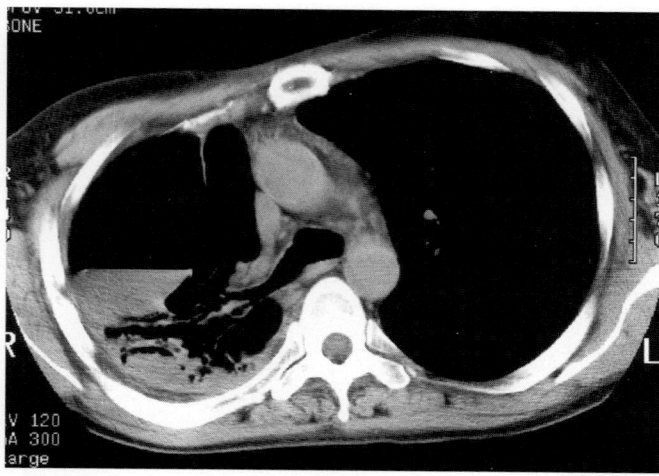

Fig. 85-11. A. Destroyed right lung with air-fluid level indicating a bronchopleural fistula. B. Computed tomographic scan of the destroyed right lung.

The principle of mycobacterial surgery is to remove all gross disease. This requires resection of all cavitary disease as well as destroyed lung. Scattered nodular disease may be left because its mycobacterial burden is low.

Patients with MDRTB and those with NTM (MOTT) infections are prepared similarly. Pulmonary function tests, computed tomography, and ventilation-perfusion scans all contribute to the preoperative evaluation. Based on a 70-kg patient, a calculated forced expiratory volume in 1 second of 1 L should be left after all resections have been completed. Although on chest radiography it may look as if a considerable amount of good lung will be left after lobar resection, a perfusion scan showing only 15% or less going to the remaining lung on that side is an indication for pneumonectomy. This has been particularly useful on the left side. Improvement in pulmonary hygiene is essential in the preoperative management of mycobacterial patients. The remaining lung, although it appears to be normal, usually has some degree of infectious involvement. These patients are more apt to develop atelectasis and other pulmonary complications postoperatively. Ideally, patients should not smoke for 1 month before surgery. Postural drainage, use of the flutter valve, and incentive spirometers should be taught preoperatively.

A specific phenotype has been found in patients with MOTT infections of the right middle lobe, lingula, or both (Fig. 85-13), that may require resection; in a series of 13 patients that I and my associates (1996) reported, 12 MAC and one *M. chelonei* infections occurred. These patients are usually older women with skeletal abnormalities such as pectus excavatum, a straight back or scoliosis, which, as noted previously, has been termed *Lady Windermere syndrome* by Reich and Johnson (1992). Additionally, they often have mitral prolapse. At surgery the major fissure on the right is usually complete with the minor fissure often at least partially complete. This complete fissure results in loss of collateral ventilation, adding to the destructive effects of the infectious process. For lingula disease, the etiology is not as clear, but in many cases the tip of the lingula extends longer, possibly producing the same effect as an isolated middle lobe.

Surgical Technique

Double-lumen endobronchial tubes or a bronchial blocker is used to anesthetically isolate the lungs. At least one large intravenous line is placed to replace blood if needed. An epidural catheter is placed for use postoperatively for pain control. Alternatively, intrathecal one-dose analgesia can be used and then switched to patient-controlled analgesia when the effect wears off.

A posterior lateral thoracotomy incision is routinely used. Muscle flaps have been used for patients who still have positive sputum at the time of surgery, if they have a bronchopleural fistula, if there is polymicrobial contamination, or if there is a need to fill space after a lobectomy as I and my colleagues (1991) have recommended. The latissimus dorsi is

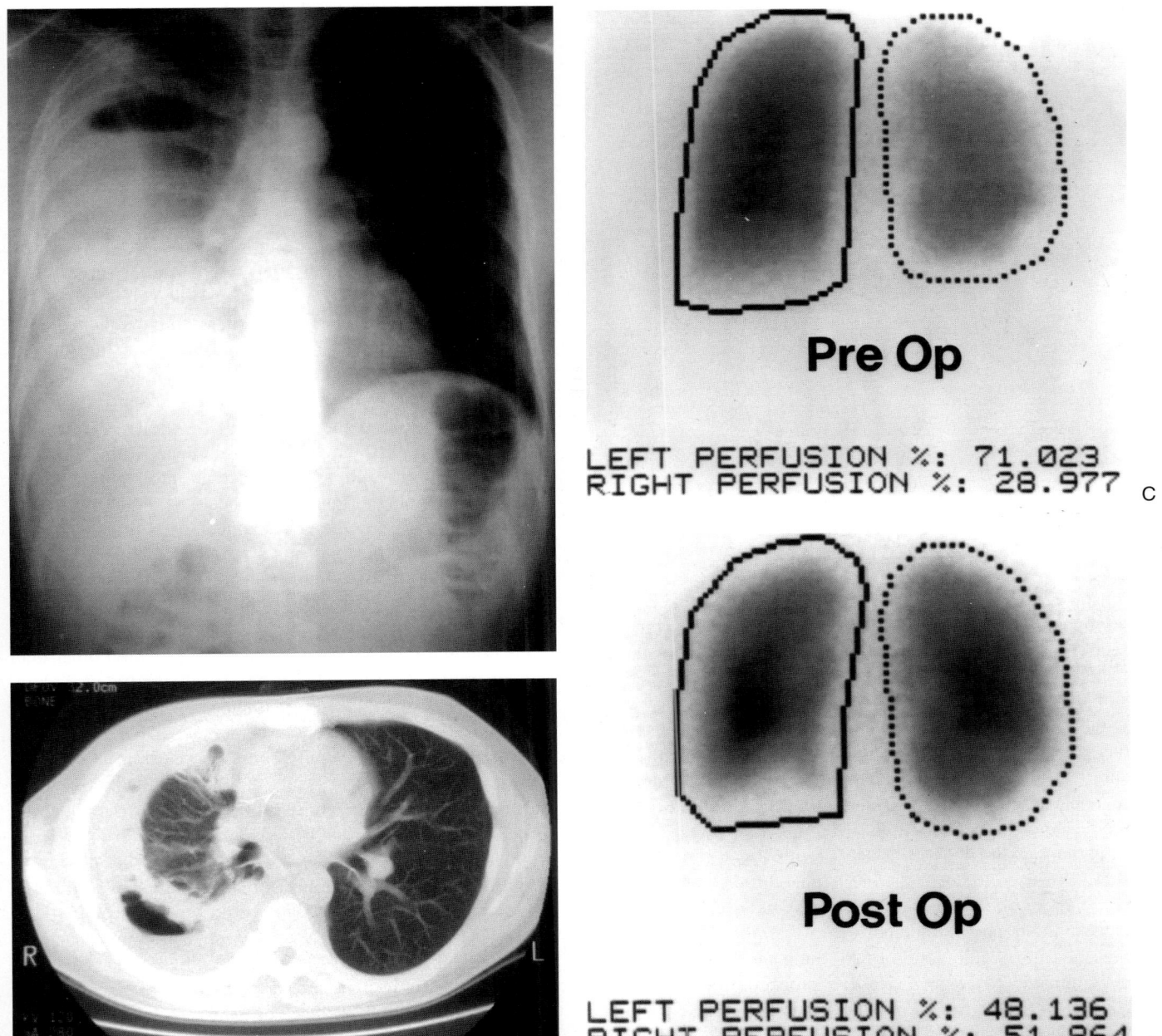

Fig. 85-12. A. Posteroanterior view of the chest with trapped right lung. **B.** Computed tomographic scan of chest demonstrating thick peel and trapped right lung. **C.** Perfusion scan before decortication showing decreased perfuse to right lung. **D.** Perfusion scan after decortication revealing normal perfusion of right lung.

the muscle of choice. Using the serratus anterior produces a winged scapula, which may protrude out the posterior portion of the wound in these usually cachetic patients. The serratus anterior is not divided but is retracted anteriorly. Although no controlled series has been done regarding muscle flaps, it is my impression that fewer bronchopleural fistulas occur in patients when a muscle flap is used for the aforementioned reasons. Muscle flaps are not used for middle lobe and lingula resections, segmental resections, or lower lobectomies. In my experience it is rare to have a bronchial stump break down

with these procedures. However, whenever possible, a pleural flap or pericardial fat pad is used for bronchial stump coverage. When no muscle is available because of previous surgery or when massive contamination has occurred, an omental flap is used. Resectional surgery is often done in the extrapleural plane. Dense adhesions usually are found over the apical and posterior segments of the upper lobe and often over the superior segment of the lower lobes. Often, a free plane of dissection occurs over the aortic arch on the left and the azygos vein on the right. When dissecting in the extrapleural plane, care

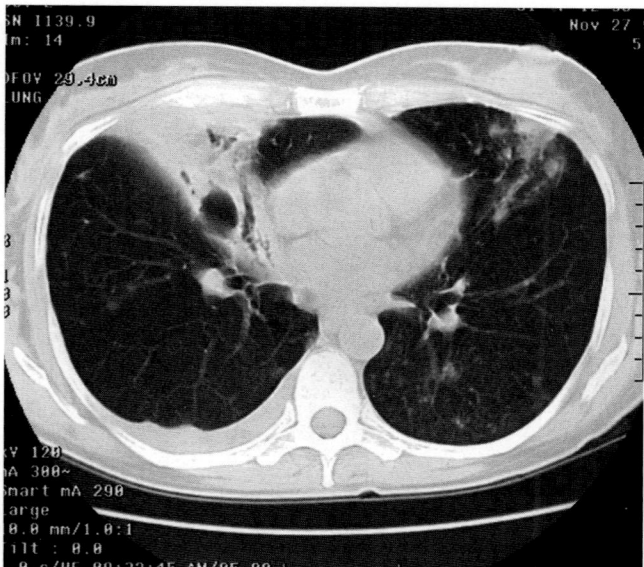

Fig. 85-13. Computed tomographic scan in patient with mycobacteria other than tuberculosis with right middle lobe and lingula disease.

must be taken to avoid the subclavian vessels, recurrent laryngeal nerve, esophagus, or intercostal vessels during dissection posterior to the aorta as emphasized by Brown and me (1995). Frequently, once the lung is freed from its adhesions, the hilum can be isolated without difficulty. However, with completion pneumonectomies, vessel ligations may have to be performed within the pericardium. Bronchial closure can be done either by suture or with staples. In mycobacterial resections, I have found no difference in the incidence of bronchial stump disruption with either closure. In patients with MDRTB or MOTT infection, a muscle flap should be used to cover the bronchial stump closure. At the completion of surgery, bronchoscopy is usually done to cleanse the tracheal bronchial tree of secretions that may be present from manipulation of the lung during resection. In contaminated cases, an Eloesser's procedure (1935) is performed after the resection. The Eloesser is closed 4 to 6 weeks later after daily packing with half-strength Dakin's solution. At the time of closure, a modified Clagett's solution is placed into the pleural cavity.

Postoperative Care

Fluids are restricted for the first 3 to 5 days. After lobectomy, fluids are restricted to 1800 mL/24 hours and after a pneumonectomy to 1500 mL/24 hours. Ambulation is encouraged on the first postoperative day. Compression stockings are used, and pulmonary hygiene is continued. Heparin, 5000 U, is given subcutaneously twice daily until the patient is fully ambulating. Ketorolac is used for several days if renal function is normal. Epidural analgesia is continued for 48 to 72 hours, then patient-controlled analgesia is instituted. Passive

range of motion is begun on the upper extremities to prevent a frozen shoulder. Nutrition is emphasized in the postoperative period as it is preoperatively. Often, when the infected lung is removed, appetite improves and the patient may become anabolic. However, side effects from the antibiotics may continue to negatively affect caloric intake.

Complications

A dreaded complication after mycobacterial surgery is a bronchopleural fistula. This is more common after right pneumonectomies. Some other factors increasing the incidence of bronchopleural fistulae are positive sputum at the time of surgery, significant polymicrobial contamination, diabetes, and prior chest wall irradiation. The incidence of bronchopleural fistula if the previously mentioned factors are present may be as high as 30%. In patients with MAC and positive sputum results plus usually an underlying superinfection undergoing a right pneumonectomy, I and my associates (1991) reported the development of a bronchopleural fistula in seven of nine patients (77%) despite the use of muscle flap reinforcement of the bronchial stump in most patients. Thus, the contemplation of a right-sided pneumonectomy in patients with a destroyed lung associated with polymicrobial infection and a persistent mycobacterial infection other than *M. tuberculosis* must be viewed as a highly morbid procedure. In contrast with middle lobe, lingula, lower lobe, and segmental resection, the incidence is less than 5%.

Postpneumonectomy pulmonary edema is a lethal complication and can occur without fluid overload. It is more common after right pneumonectomy than left. Treatment is supportive with ventilatory assistance, monitoring of pulmonary pressures, diuresis, and other supportive measures. If pulmonary hypertension is present, it is treated with nitroglycerine, nitroprusside sodium (Nipride), or nitric oxide.

Atelectasis and pneumonia are common after mycobacterial surgery. Unlike cancer surgery, in which case the remaining lung may be more normal after resection, the mycobacterial patient usually has other diseased lung remaining. Therefore, pulmonary complications are harder to treat in mycobacterial patients. Prevention using incentive spirometry, the flutter valve, and physiotherapy is essential.

Wound complications are frequent in these catabolic patients. Seromas often form from the latissimus dissection area when muscle flaps are used. Suction drains should be left in these areas until little drainage (less than 25 mL) is collected in a 24-hour period. Infections with *M. chelonei* and *Mycobacterium abscessus* have an increased number of wound problems, which may eventually require revision surgery.

Other complications include postoperative bleeding, often a frequent complication in many of the reported series such as those of Treasure and Seaworth (1995) and van Leuven and associates (1997), among others, injury to the recurrent laryngeal nerve, and empyema. All of these complications occur more commonly in mycobacterial surgery because of the adhesive infected nature of the disease process as well as the debilitated catabolic condition of the patient.

Surgery should be considered an adjunct to medical therapy. Patients are kept on their antibiotic therapy for 12 to 24 months, depending on the bacteriologic and radiographic findings. Stopping antibiotics too soon leads to further resistance or mycobacterial spread.

Results of Surgery

In patients with MDRTB who are good surgical candidates, cure can be obtained in more than 90% of the cases if antibiotics are continued for the appropriate period postoperatively.

In patients with NTM or MOTT, results are more variable than with MDRTB. *Mycobacterium* other than tuberculosis infections are more indolent than those with MDRTB. Therapy is often instituted late and referral to surgery is likewise often delayed. With localized disease, however, results are good, particularly in patients with middle lobe or lingula disease. However, reactivation in other parts of the lung or infection with other organisms because of underlying lung destruction is common. As noted, a high incidence of bronchopleural fistulas occurs after right pneumonectomy in patients infected with MAC organisms. In my experience, these patients invariably have positive sputum results at the time of surgery and frequently are contaminated with other organisms. Diabetic patients also have an increased incidence of postoperative complications.

In my series of more than 325 patients, the operative mortality has been less than 5%. However, complications occur in approximately 25% of the patients. The morbidity and mortality of various series are listed in Table 85-9. Careful

Table 85-9. Mortality and Morbidity of Pneumonectomy and Other Resections for *Mycobacterium tuberculosis* and Nontuberculous Mycobacterial Infections

Reference	No. of Patients	Mortality (%)	Morbidity (%)
Pomerantz et al. (1991)	42	2.4	3.8
Brown and Pomerantz (1995)	61[a,b]	1.6	—
Treasure and Seaworth (1995)	59	0.0	8.4
Conlan et al. (1995)	107	2.4	—
Wu et al. (1996)	126	1.8	16.8
Pomerantz and Brown (1997)	130[b]	2.3	12.3
van Leuven et al. (1997)	62	1.6	—
	35[a]	2.8	23
Ashour (1997)	20[a]	0.0	—
Ono et al. (1997)	8[c]	0.0	0.0
Kir et al. (1997)	27	0.0	14.8

[a]Pneumonectomies.
[b]Multidrug-resistant tuberculosis (MDRTB).
[c]*Mycobacterium avium* complex organisms (MAC).

preparation of the patient undergoing surgery for mycobacterial disease is essential for keeping the morbidity and mortality low.

Other surgical groups in the United States and throughout the world have recorded similar good results with resection of MDRTB and NTM (MOTT) pulmonary infections. These include Treasure and Seaworth (1995), Wu (1996), Mouroux (1996), Kir (1997), Ono (1997), and van Leuven (1997) and their associates.

OTHER SURGICAL INDICATIONS IN PATIENTS WITH MYCOBACTERIAL TUBERCULOSIS*

Mycotic Infection and Life-Threatening Hemoptysis in Patients with Tuberculosis

Superimposed fungal disease is caused most commonly by *Aspergillus fumigatus*, but infections with *Monosporium apiospermum* organisms were reported by Jung and colleagues (1977). Intracavitary mycetoma are seen with either of these infections. Hemoptysis is a common complaint, and massive life-threatening hemorrhage may occur, particularly in those patients in whom the underlying disease process is pulmonary tuberculosis. In a review by Stoller (1992) of 12 series of massive hemoptysis, active tuberculosis was present in 22.5 to 49.0% of the cases and inactive tuberculosis was present in 17 to 51%, with a combined total of 18 to 76% of cases. Although a more conservative approach, as Faulkner (1978) and Jewkes (1983) and their associates suggested, may be appropriate in patients with minor episodes of hemoptysis and mycetoma not associated with underlying tuberculosis, those patients with tuberculosis usually require an eventual resection (elective if possible) to control the problem.

Massive life-threatening hemoptysis in patients with tuberculosis may occur also in the absence of a fungal infection because of erosion into a bronchial artery or, more rarely, because of pulmonary arterial bleeding caused by rupture of a Rasmussen's aneurysm in cavitary tuberculosis.

Management of massive hemoptysis and the timing of surgical intervention pose difficult problems. Initially, the patient should be positioned to minimize as much as possible aspiration of the blood. Bronchoscopy is necessary to identify the site of bleeding, and its role in the management of massive hemoptysis has been stressed by Dweik and Stoller (1999). Gourin and Garzon (1974) recommended prompt surgical resection for any individual who has bled more than 600 mL in 24 hours or less. With such a course of action, the mortality was 18%, as compared with a 75% rate in those treated conservatively after bleeding this amount in 16 hours. When active bleeding is present at the time of operation, these authors recommended single-lung anesthesia with balloon occlusion of the bronchus of the bleeding lung over the use of a double-lumen endotracheal tube for

---

*Addendum by the Senior Editor.

the conduct of anesthesia. Garzon and associates (1982) repeated this recommendation. McCollum and associates (1975), however, stated that the use of the double-lumen tube is satisfactory. Gottlieb and Hillberg (1975) advocated endobronchial tamponade with a Fogarty balloon catheter to control the bleeding, either before surgical intervention or if such intervention is contraindicated.

With the development of the technique of bronchial artery embolization, the necessity of surgical intervention before control of the bleeding site has been reduced. At present, the appropriate therapeutic plan is to identify the side and lobar origin of the bleeding by bronchoscopy; endobronchial tamponade is then established as necessary to prevent flooding of the remaining uninvolved lung. With the bleeding temporarily controlled, bronchial arteriography is performed to identify the bleeding area, and the appropriate vessel is then embolized with Gelfoam. Eckstein and coworkers (1986) and Shetty and Magillijan (1986) reviewed the technique, results, and potential complications of this procedure, such as mediastinal hematoma and neurologic damage. Mal and colleagues (1999) reported immediate control of the bleeding episode in 77% of 56 patients; long-term control was achieved in 45% by embolization alone. In the earlier series reported by Uflacker and associates (1983), bleeding was controlled by embolization alone in 26 of 33 patients (78%); in the remaining seven, surgical resection was required after the embolization. In the presence of a mycetoma and residual pulmonary disease, however, the rebleed rate was high (43%). This was accompanied by a high mortality if interval resection was not or could not be carried out. Thus, even though the bleeding is controlled by the initial embolization, elective resection of the involved area should be carried out when the patient's pulmonary function and the underlying disease are suitable for such a course of action. With this therapeutic approach, Uflacker and associates (1983) reported only an overall 7 to 9% mortality for the management of massive hemoptysis. A modified plombage thoracoplasty with the use of a plastic tissue expander, such as reported by Talamonti and associates (1989), has been suggested as a method of controlling hemoptysis associated with a mycetoma in a patient who is unable to withstand a surgical resection (W. Fry, personal communication, 1991).

Tuberculous Bronchial Stricture

Bronchial stricture associated with previous endobronchial tuberculosis is uncommon. In North America, tuberculous endobronchitis per se, as noted by Matthews and associates (1984), is rare. The incidence of endobronchitis appears somewhat higher in Japan. Ozawa (1981) and Tanaka (1981) and their colleagues reported an incidence of 4.7 to 7.5% of patients with parenchymal tuberculosis. In Hong Kong, So and colleagues (1982) reported an incidence of 18%. With subsequent healing of the area of endobronchitis, stenosis of the involved bronchus can develop as noted in Radiographic

Features. Stricture also can be caused by enlarged granulomatous lymph nodes. Clinical symptoms or radiographic findings resulting from the bronchial obstruction can occur. At times, carcinoma may be considered as the cause of obstruction when evidence of tuberculosis cannot be identified by bronchial biopsy or sputum cultures.

When carcinoma cannot be excluded or when distal parenchymal destruction has occurred, resection of the stenotic bronchus and the distal involved lung parenchyma is necessary. When the stenosis is symptomatic, lung destruction is absent, and the diagnosis of tuberculous stenosis is known, resection of the area of bronchial stenosis with bronchoplastic reconstruction is the preferred method of treatment as noted by Ozawa and associates (1981). Watanabe and colleagues (1988) reported nine operative interventions (i.e., three lobectomies, one pneumonectomy, and five sleeve upper lobectomies) (Fig. 85-14) for these complications with excellent results. Watanabe and coworkers (1997) updated their experience with 19 patients with bronchial stenosis caused by tuberculosis. Twelve patients underwent surgery that included five resections and nine bronchoplastic procedures with either a right or left upper sleeve lobectomy. No deaths or complications were recorded. Han and associates (1992) reported the successful use of a Gianturco self-expanding metallic stent to correct a short but tight stenosis of the left main stem bronchus that was the result of tuberculosis endobronchitis and that had caused a total atelectasis of the left lung. Watanabe and colleagues (1997) had poor results in two patients in whom internal splinting was attempted.

Other Surgical Indications

In patients with known or presumed tuberculosis, the question of the presence of malignant disease poses a problem, especially among patients with peripheral nodules; those who have a radiographic change in previously stable disease but whose sputum results remain negative; and those with an undiagnosed pulmonary lesion but a positive tuberculin test result. The management of these individuals requires appropriate diagnostic investigation, which may include video-assisted thoracic surgical exploration or even a thoracotomy. In the experience of Whyte and associates (1989), suspected malignancy was the most common reason (77%) for resections in 31 patients with subsequently proved or known (16%) pulmonary tuberculosis.

The management of postresectional complications of persistent empyema or a bronchopleural fistula is discussed in Chapters 37, 60, 61, and 62. At times, when the initial operation has been less than a pneumonectomy, a completion pneumonectomy may become the procedure of choice. Although a completion pneumonectomy, when carried out for recurrent or a new pulmonary malignancy, entails low morbidity and mortality, such procedures when done because of extension or recurrent inflammatory disease in the remaining ipsilateral lung tissue have high rates of post-

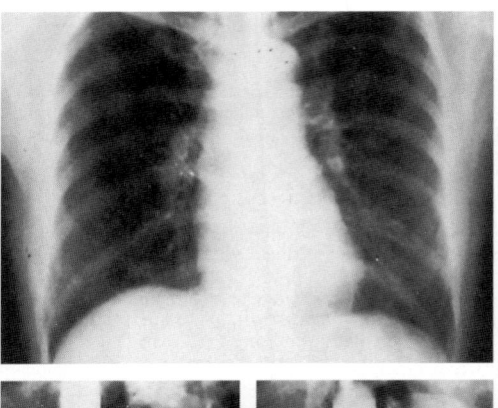

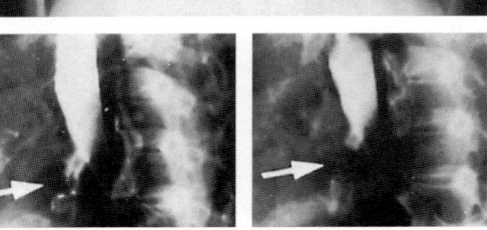

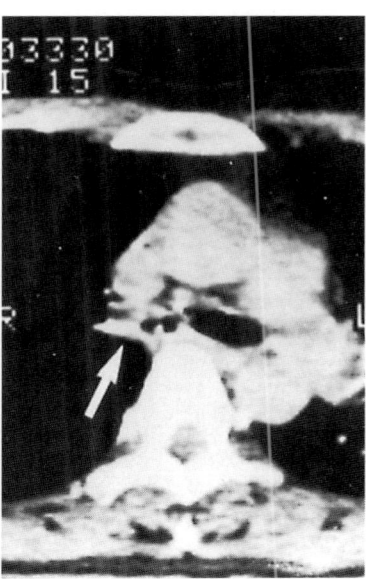

Fig. 85-14. A 50-year-old woman had cough and exertional dyspnea. The chest radiograph was normal, but bronchography and computed tomographic scanning revealed stenosis of the right main stem bronchus (*arrows*) from healed tuberculous endobronchitis. Right upper sleeve lobectomy with bronchoplastic repair resulted in complete relief of symptoms. From Watanabe Y, Murakami S, Iwa T: Bronchial stricture due to endobronchial tuberculosis. Thorac Cardiovasc Surg *36*:27, 1988. With permission.

operative complications and deaths. McGovern and colleagues (1988) noted a mortality of 28% when performed for inflammatory disease versus only 9.2% for lung cancer. Al-Kattan and Goldstraw (1995) also noted a higher mortality after a completion pneumonectomy for benign inflammatory disease, although Gregoire and associates (1993) did not find this difference in mortality in benign versus malignant disease. However, the technical aspects of the procedure are frequently difficult in patients with benign disease, and, at times, intrapericardial ligation of the vascular supply to the remaining lung becomes necessary. Support of the closure of the bronchial stump by a transposed muscle flap or an omental flap is recommended also in those cases with persistent or recurrent MDRTB, NTM disease, or their complications that require a completion pneumonectomy.

Surgery for Pulmonary Tuberculosis in Children

In children, the indications for surgical intervention are few. A caseous pneumonic process may resolve more slowly than in the adult; the decision concerning the advisability of operation frequently should be postponed for many months or years. In children, in addition to the indications as noted in adults, surgical treatment is required in the management of certain complications of progressive primary pulmonary tuberculosis. These complications are an uncontrolled, progressively enlarging primary parenchymal lesion with or without cavitation, persistent distal lobar or segmental atelectasis as the result of postprimary bronchostenosis, and clinically significant bronchiectasis (Fig. 85-15). Infrequently, bronchial obstruction may persist because of enlarged,

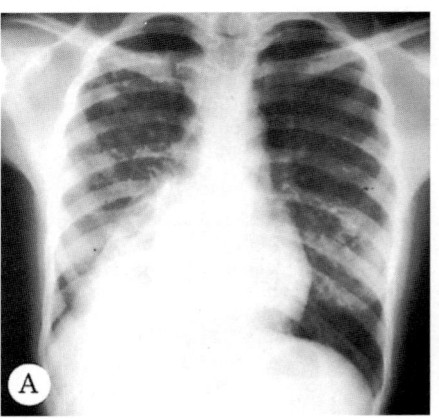

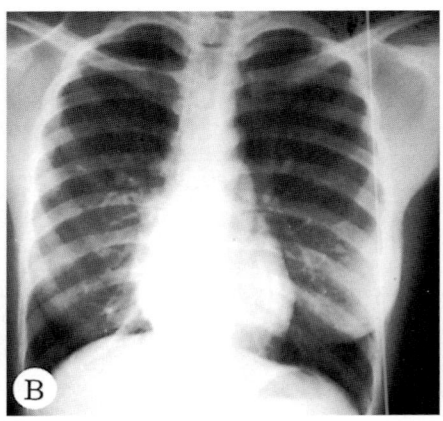

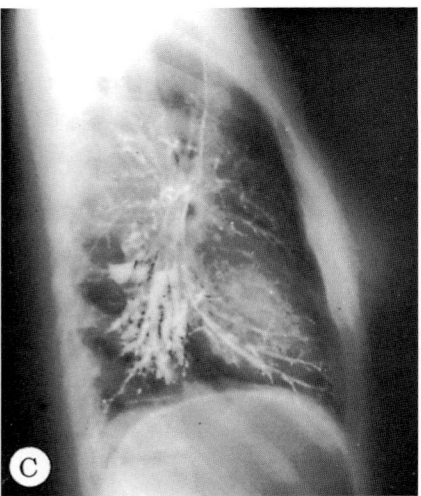

Fig. 85-15. A. Posteroanterior radiograph of a 15-year-old girl with bilateral pulmonary tuberculosis and atelectasis of the right lower lobe. **B.** Same view, after 11 months of treatment, shows clearing of bilateral infiltrate but a completely atelectatic right lower lobe behind the border of the right side of the heart. **C.** Lateral view of the bronchogram showing extensive bronchiectatic changes throughout the entire right lower lobe.

involved peribronchial lymph nodes. With failure of response to medical therapy and persistence of symptoms, particularly respiratory distress, Nakvi and Nohl-Oser (1979) suggested excising or evacuating the caseous material to relieve the obstruction. Worthington and associates (1993) reported this approach in 13 children. Although the incidence of surgical intervention, as Lees and associates (1967) reported, was approximately 5% in children with pulmonary tuberculosis younger than the age of 16 years, at present it is rare. Lowe and associates (1980) reported that in a series of 140 children with pulmonary tuberculosis, surgical intervention was necessary in only two of these individuals for an incidence of only 1.4%. However, Hewiston and Von Oppell (1997) reported on 161 children younger than the age of 13 years in South Africa who underwent 168 procedures for pulmonary tuberculosis or its complications. Surgical decompression of obstructing enlarged lymph nodes (25 acute, 11 chronic) was required and was successful in all but three of the chronic cases. Pulmonary resection was required in 72 patients with postprimary tuberculous parenchymal drainage with a mortality of 2.7% and a morbidity of 16.7%.

REFERENCES

Mycobacterium Tuberculosis and Nontuberculous Mycobacterial Infections of the Lungs

Banks J, et al: Pulmonary infection with *Mycobacterium xenopi*. Review of treatment and response. Thorax 39:376, 1984.

Batungwanayo J, et al: Pulmonary tuberculosis in Kigali, Rwanda. Impact of human immunodeficiency virus infection on clinical and radiographic presentation. Am Rev Respir Dis 146:53, 1992.

Buckner CB, Walker CW: Radiologic manifestations of adult tuberculosis. J Thorac Imaging 5:28, 1990.

Choyke PL, et al: Adult-onset pulmonary tuberculosis. Radiology 148:357, 1983.

Cohn DL, et al: A 62-dose, 6-month therapy for pulmonary and extrapulmonary tuberculosis. A twice-weekly, directly observed, and cost-effective regimen. Ann Intern Med 112:407, 1990.

Dannenberg AM Jr: Immunopathogenesis of pulmonary tuberculosis. Hosp Pract 28:51, 1993.

Dautzenberg B, et al: The management of thirty immunocompromised patients with tuberculosis. Am Rev Respir Dis 129:494, 1984.

Dunlap NE, Briles DE: Immunology of tuberculosis. Med Clin North Am 77:1235, 1993.

Farman DP, Speir WA: Initial radiographic manifestations of bacteriologically proven *Mycobacterium tuberculosis*. Typical or atypical? Chest 89:75, 1986.

Fraser RG, Paré JAP: Diagnosis of Diseases of the Chest. Vol. 2. Philadelphia: WB Saunders, 1970.

Fraser RG, et al: Diagnosis of Diseases of the Chest. 3rd Ed. Philadelphia: WB Saunders, 1989, p. 882.

Frieden TR, et al: The emergence of drug-resistant tuberculosis in New York City. N Engl J Med 328:521, 1993.

Gracey DR, Byrd RB: Scotochromogens and pulmonary disease. Am Rev Respir Dis 101:959, 1970.

Grieco MH, Chmel H: Acute disseminated tuberculosis as a diagnostic problem. Am Rev Respir Dis 109:554, 1974.

Haas DW, Des Prez RM: *Mycobacterium tuberculosis*. In Mandell GL, Bennett JE, Dolin R (eds): Mandell, Douglas and Bennett's Principles and Practice of Infectious Diseases. 4th Ed. New York: Churchill Livingstone, 1995, p. 2213.

Haque AK: The pathology and pathophysiology of mycobacterial infections. J Thorac Imaging 5:8, 1990.

Heifets L: Mycobacteriology laboratory. Clin Chest Med 18:35, 1997.

Huang JH, et al: *Mycobacterium avium-intracellulare* pulmonary infection in HIV-negative patients without preexisting lung disease: diagnostic and management limitations. Chest 115:1033, 1999.

Ip MSM, et al: Endobronchial tuberculosis revisited. Chest 89:727, 1986.

Iseman MD: Treatment of multidrug-resistant tuberculosis. N Engl J Med 329:784, 1993.

Iseman M, Huitt G: Infectious Diseases. 2nd Ed. Philadelphia: WB Saunders, 1998, pp. 1513-1528.

Johnston RF, Wildrick KH: "State of the art" review: the impact of chemotherapy on the care of patients with tuberculosis. Am Rev Respir Dis 109:636, 1974.

Kestle DG, Abbott VD, Kubica GP: Differential identification of mycobacteria: Subgroups of groups II and III (Runyon) with clinical significance. Am Rev Respir Dis 95:1941, 1967.

Khan MA, et al: Clinical and roentgenographic spectrum of pulmonary tuberculosis in the adult. Am J Med 62:31, 1977.

Klare KC, et al: The prevalence of atypical mycobacterial tuberculin sensitivity in a selected population in New York City. Am Rev Respir Dis 95:103, 1967.

Lee KS, et al: Endobronchial tuberculosis: CT features. J Comput Assist Tomogr 15:424, 1991.

Lichtenstein MR, Takamura Y, Thompson JR: Photochromogenic mycobacterial pulmonary infection in a group of hospitalized patients in Chicago, IL. Demographic studies. Am Rev Respir Dis 91:592, 1965.

Lindskog GE, Liebow AA: Thoracic Surgery and Related Pathology. New Haven: Appleton-Century-Crofts, 1953, p. 191.

Marks J, Schwabacher H: Infection due to *Mycobacterium xenopei*. BMJ 1:32, 1965.

Masur H, et al: Effect of combined clofazimine and anisomycin therapy on *Mycobacterium avium-Mycobacterium intracellulare* bacteremia in patients with AIDS. J Infect Dis 155:127, 1987.

McAdams HP, Erasmus J, Winter JA: Radiologic manifestations of pulmonary tuberculosis. Radiol Clin North Am 33:655, 1995.

Murray JF: Cursed duet: HIV infection and tuberculosis. Respiration 57:210, 1990.

Myers JA, Bearman JE, Dixon H: The natural history of tuberculosis in the human body. Am Rev Respir Dis 87:354, 1963.

O'Brien RJ, Snider DE: Tuberculosis drugs—old and new. Am Rev Respir Dis 131:309, 1985.

Passannante MR, Gallagher CT, Reichman LB: Preventive therapy for contacts of multidrug-resistant tuberculosis. A Delphi survey. Chest 106:431, 1994.

Patz EF Jr, Swensen SJ, Erasmus J: Pulmonary manifestations of nontuberculous mycobacterium. Radiol Clin North Am 33:719, 1995.

Pitchenik AE, Rubinson HA: The radiographic appearance of tuberculosis in patients with the acquired immune deficiency syndrome (AIDS). Am Rev Respir Dis 131:393, 1985.

Pomerantz M: Complications of tuberculosis, particularly following thoracoplasty. Proceedings of the Thoracic Surgery Postgraduate Course, American College of Surgeons, Chicago, IL, October 22, 1991, p. 83.

Reich JM, Johnson RE: *Mycobacterium avium* complex pulmonary disease presenting as an isolated lingular or middle lobe pattern. The Lady Windermere syndrome. Chest 101:1605, 1992.

Roberts GD, Böttger EC, Stockman L: Methods for the rapid detection of mycobacterial species. Clin Lab Med 16:603, 1996.

Sahn SA, Neff TA: Miliary tuberculosis. Am J Med 56:495, 1974.

Sandin RL: Polymerase chain reaction and other amplification techniques in mycobacteriology. Clin Lab Med 16:617, 1996.

Smith DT: Diagnostic and prognostic significance of the quantitative tuberculin tests. Ann Intern Med 67:919, 1967.

Smith L, Schillaci RT, Sarlin RF: Endobronchial tuberculosis: Serial fiberoptic bronchoscopy and natural history. Chest 91:644, 1987.

Sors CH, et al: Les mycobactérioses pulmonaires a *M. xenopi*. Á propos de 50 cas. Modalités évolutives et problèmes thérapeutiques. Rev Fr Mal Resp 7:504, 1979.

Telenti A: Genetics of drug resistance in tuberculosis. Clin Chest Med 18:55, 1997.

van Leuven M, et al: Pulmonary resection as an adjunct in the treatment of multiple drug-resistant tuberculosis. Ann Thorac Surg 63:1368, 1997.

Wayne L: The atypical mycobacteria: Recognition and disease association. CRC Crit Rev Microbiol 72:184, 1986.

Woodring JH, et al: Update: The radiographic features of pulmonary tuberculosis. AJR Am J Roentgenol 146:497, 1986.

Young K, Bailey W: Non-TB mycobacterial infections: a rapidly increasing danger. J Resp Dis 9:20, 1988.

Surgery of Mycobacterial Infections

Al-Kattan K, Goldstraw P: Completion pneumonectomy: indications and outcome. J Thorac Cardiovasc Surg 110:1125, 1995.

Ashour M: Pneumonectomy for tuberculosis. Eur J Cardiothorac Surg 12:209, 1997.

Ashour M, et al: Unilateral post-tuberculous lung destruction. The left bronchus syndrome. Thorax 45:210, 1990.

Brown J, Pomerantz M: Extrapleural pneumonectomy for tuberculosis. Chest Surg Clin N Am 5:289, 1995.

Canetti G: Present aspects of bacterial resistance in tuberculosis. Am Rev Respir Dis 92:687, 1965.

Conlan AA: Pneumonectomy for infection. Ann Thorac Surg 60:488, 1995.

Dweik RA, Stoller JK: Role of bronchoscopy in massive hemoptysis. Clin Chest Med 20:89, 1999.

Eckstein MR, Waltman AC, Athanasoulis CA: The management of massive hemoptysis: Control by angiographic methods. In Kittle CF (ed): Current Controversies in Thoracic Surgery. Philadelphia: WB Saunders, 1986, p. 255.

Eloesser L: An operation for tuberculous empyema. Surg Gynecol Obstet 60:1096, 1935.

Faulkner SL, et al: Hemoptysis and pulmonary aspergilloma: Operative versus nonoperative treatment. Ann Thorac Surg 25:389, 1978.

Garzon AA, Cerruti MM, Golding MR: Exsanguinating hemoptysis. J Thorac Cardiovasc Surg 84:829, 1982.

Gottlieb LS, Hillberg R: Endobronchial tamponade therapy for intractable hemoptysis. Chest 67:482, 1975.

Gourin A, Garzon AA: Operative treatment of massive hemoptysis. Ann Thorac Surg 18:52, 1974.

Gregoire J, et al: Indications, risks and results of completion pneumonectomy. J Thorac Cardiovasc Surg 105:918, 1993.

Han JK, et al: Bronchial stenosis due to endobronchial tuberculosis: Successful treatment with self-expanding metallic stint. AJR Am J Roentgenol 159:971, 1992.

Hewiston JP, Von Oppell UO: Role of thoracic surgery for childhood tuberculosis. World J Surg 21:468, 1997.

Jewkes J, et al: Pulmonary aspergilloma: analysis of prognosis in relationship to hemoptysis and survey of treatment. Thorax 38:572, 1983.

Jung JY, et al: The role of surgery in the management of pulmonary monosporosis: a collective review. J Thorac Cardiovasc Surg 73:139, 1977.

Kir A, et al: Role of surgery in multi-drug-resistant tuberculosis: results of 27 cases. Eur J Cardiothorac Surg 12:531, 1997.

Lees WM, Fox RT, Shields TW: Pulmonary surgery for tuberculosis in children. Ann Thorac Surg 4:327, 1967.

Lowe JE, et al: Pulmonary tuberculosis in children. J Thorac Cardiovasc Surg 80:221, 1980.

Mal H, et al: Immediate and long-term results of bronchial artery embolization for life-threatening hemoptysis. Chest 115:996, 1999.

Matthews JI, Matarese SL, Carpenter JL: Endobronchial tuberculosis simulating lung cancer. Chest 86:642, 1984.

McCollum WB, et al: Immediate operative treatment for massive hemoptysis. Chest 67:152, 1975.

McGovern EM, et al: Completion pneumonectomy: indications, complications and results. Ann Thorac Surg 46:141, 1988.

Mouroux J, et al: Surgical management of pulmonary tuberculosis. J Thorac Cardiovasc Surg 111:662, 1996.

Nakvi AJ, Nohl-Oser HC: Surgical treatment of bronchial obstruction in primary tuberculosis in children: report of seven cases. Thorax 34:464, 1979.

Ono N, et al: Surgical management of Mycobacterium avium complex disease. Thorac Cardiovasc Surg 45;311, 1997.

Ozawa K, et al: Bronchial tuberculosis—a clinical study on 26 cases. Jpn J Chest Dis 40:42, 1981.

Pomerantz M, Brown JM: Surgery in the treatment of multidrug-resistant tuberculosis. Clin Chest Med 18:123, 1997.

Pomerantz M, et al: Surgical management of resistant Mycobacterium tuberculosis and other mycobacterial pulmonary infections. Ann Thorac Surg 52:1108, 1991.

Pomerantz M, et al: Resection of the right middle lobe and lingula for mycobacterial infection. Ann Thorac Surg 62:990, 1996.

Reich JM, Johnson RE: Mycobacterium avium complex pulmonary disease presenting as an isolated lingular or middle lobe pattern. The Lady Windermere syndrome. Chest 101:1605, 1992.

Shetty PC, Magillijan DJ: The management of massive hemoptysis: treatment by bronchial artery embolization. In Kittle CF (ed): Current Controversies in Thoracic Surgery. Philadelphia: WB Saunders, 1986, p. 261.

Shields TW, Lees WM, Fox RT: Pneumonectomy in the treatment of pulmonary tuberculosis. Am Rev Tuberc 78:822, 1958.

So SY, Lam WK, Yu DYC: Rapid diagnosis of suspected pulmonary tuberculosis fiberoptic bronchoscopy. Tubercule 63:195, 1982.

Stoller JK: Diagnosis and management of massive hemoptysis: a review. Respir Care 37:564, 1992.

Talamonti MS, et al: A new method of extraperiosteal plombage for atypical pulmonary tuberculosis. Chest 96:237, 1989.

Tanaka K, et al: Tracheo-bronchial tuberculosis. Jpn J Chest Dis 40:1015, 1981.

Treasure RI, Seaworth BJ: Current role of surgery in Mycobacterium tuberculosis. Ann Thorac Surg 59:1405, 1995.

Uflacker R, et al: Management of massive hemoptysis by bronchial artery embolization. Radiology 146:627, 1983.

van Leuven M, et al: Pulmonary resection as an adjunct in the treatment of multiple drug-resistant tuberculosis. Ann Thorac Surg 63:1368, 1997.

Watanabe Y, Murakami S, Iwa T: Bronchial stricture due to endobronchial tuberculosis. Thorac Cardiovasc Surg 36:27, 1988.

Watanabe Y, et al: Treatment of bronchial stricture due to endobronchial tuberculosis. World J Surg 21:480, 1997.

Whyte RI, et al: Recent surgical experience for pulmonary tuberculosis. Respir Med 83:357, 1989.

Worthington MG, et al: Surgical relief of acute airway obstruction due to pulmonary tuberculosis. Ann Thorac Surg 56:1054, 1993.

Wu MH, et al: Results of surgical treatment of 107 patients with complications of pulmonary tuberculosis. Respirology 1:283, 1996.

READING REFERENCES

Anonymous: Diagnosis and treatment of disease caused by nontuberculous mycobacteria. This official statement of the American Thoracic Society was approved by the Board of Directors, March 1997. Medical Section of the American Lung Association. Am J Respir Crit Care Med 156:S1, 1997.

Bates J, Nardell E: Institutional control measures for tuberculosis in the era of multiple drug resistant. Chest 108:690, 1995.

Bradford WZ, Daley CL: Multiple drug-resistant tuberculosis. Infect Dis Clin North Am 12:157, 1998.

Centers for Disease Control and Prevention: Core curriculum in tuberculosis: what a clinician should know. Washington DC: US Government Printing Office, 1994.

Mangura BT, Reichman LB: Prevention and treatment of Mycobacterium avium complex infection. Res Microbiol 145:181, 1994.

Mangura BT, Reichman LB: Nontuberculous mycobacterial pulmonary disease (NTM). In Baum GL, et al (eds): Textbook of Pulmonary Disease. 6th Ed. Philadelphia: Lippincott–Raven, 1998, p. 631.

Mault J, Pomerantz M: Mycobacterium tuberculosis and other mycobacteria. Chest Surg Clin North Am 9:227, 1999.

McDonald RJ, Reichman LB: Tuberculosis. In Baum GL, et al (eds): Textbook of Pulmonary Disease. 6th Ed. Philadelphia: Lippincott–Raven, 1998, p. 603.

Odell JA, Henderson BJ: Pneumonectomy through an empyema. J Thorac Cardiovasc Surg 89:423, 1985.

Orme IM, Andersen P, Boom WH: T cell response to Mycobacterium tuberculosis. J Infect Dis 167:1481, 1993.

Parrot RG, Grosset JH: Post-surgical outcome of 57 patients with Mycobacterium xenopi pulmonary infections. Tubercle 69:47, 1988.

Schluger NW, Rom WN: Current approaches to the diagnosis of active pulmonary tuberculosis. Am J Respir Crit Care Med 149:264, 1994.

Spellman CW, Matty KJ, Weis SE: A survey of drug-resistant Mycobacterium tuberculosis and its relationship to HIV infection. AIDS 12:191, 1998.

CHAPTER 86

Thoracic Mycotic and Actinomycotic Infections of the Lung

John C. Lucke

THORACIC MYCOTIC INFECTIONS

Fungal infections of the lungs are not encountered commonly by most practicing thoracic surgeons. Exceptions are surgeons who practice in the southwestern United States, an area endemic for coccidioidomycosis, or along the Mississippi River Valley, an area endemic for histoplasmosis. But because mycotic lung infections mimic both bronchial carcinoma and tuberculosis, they should be included in the thoracic surgeon's differential diagnoses. Most fungi are opportunistic, causing pulmonary and other systemic infections in humans only when natural host resistance is impaired. Some fungi, however, are true pathogens, causing systemic infections in otherwise healthy patients. These fungi, *Histoplasma*, *Coccidioides*, *Blastomyces*, and *Paracoccidioides*, are endemic. They usually cause only mild infections, and they are dimorphic. In nature, they occur in a mycelial form, but in tissue, they are present as yeast, or yeastlike spherules in the case of *Coccidioides*. These morphologic differences occur in response to changes in temperature. The yeast cells that grow in culture at 37°C, survive and reproduce within tissue macrophages. According to Maresca and Kobayashi (1989), the ability of these fungi to adapt to changing environments through temperature-induced metamorphosis helps to explain their roles as pathogens. Sporothrix is another dimorphic fungus that, although primarily a subcutaneous pathogen, can produce pulmonary and other systemic infections.

In addition to surgeons practicing in endemic areas, surgeons managing organ transplant programs are likely to encounter fungal infections in the lungs of patients whose immune systems have been altered.

Two major considerations are worth noting. First, immunologically compromised patients [i.e., patients undergoing chemotherapy for malignancies, patients receiving corticosteroids or aggressive antibiotic therapy for a wide variety of conditions, very young and very old patients, and patients with acquired immune deficiency syndrome (AIDS)] are more likely to become infected with fungi. Consequently, the incidence of fungal infections has increased significantly (Table 86-1), and many new opportunistic fungi have emerged.

Second, several new antifungal agents have become available that are effective against many fungi and are less toxic to patients (Table 86-2).

In most instances, the role of the thoracic surgeon in the care of patients with fungal infections of the lungs is adjunctive (i.e., consultative and diagnostic). Both roles are important and require close collaboration with the pathologist and internist. Frequently, however, as noted by Godwin (1983) and Lillington (1982), thoracotomy is necessary because of a strong suspicion of carcinoma, especially in men older than 40 years of age.

The laboratory diagnosis of fungal infections is discussed in detail in Chapter 14. The lack of methods for early and accurate diagnosis of many systemic fungal infections is a major concern and frequently the cause of delayed treatment.

Histoplasmosis

Histoplasmosis, probably the most common of all fungal infections of the lungs, is caused by the airborne spore *Histoplasma capsulatum*. Initially, the disease was thought to be rare and almost always fatal. By 1945, however, the relationship between benign pulmonary calcifications and reactivity to skin testing with histoplasmin antigen was established, and widespread, almost universal, subclinical infection with histoplasmosis in certain well-defined geographic areas of the United States was recognized. Some 30 million people were estimated to be infected, mostly along the Mississippi River and its tributaries (Fig. 86-1). Active disease, however, occurs uncommonly, with only 1 in 2000 patients developing chronic pulmonary disease, and dissemination occurs in approximately 1 in 100,000 instances.

Table 86-1. Rank Order of the 10 Most Frequently Isolated Pathogens from Nosocomial Blood Stream Infections in the United States: SCOPE Surveillance Program, April 1995 to June 30, 1996

Rank	Pathogen (No. of Isolates)	Percent[a]
1	Coagulase negative staphylococci (1324)	32.3
2	*Staphylococcus aureus* (787)	16.7
3	*Enterococcus* spp. (553)	11.7
4	*Candida* spp. (379)	8.0
5	*Escherichia coli* (303)	6.4
6	*Klebsiella* spp. (252)	5.3
7	*Pseudomonas* spp. (235)	5.0
8	*Enterobacter* spp. (230)	4.9
9	Viridans group streptococci (139)	2.9
10	*Serratia marcescens* (67)	1.4

[a]Percent of a total of 4725 infections.
From Pfaller MA, Jones RN, Messer ER, Edmond MB, Wenzel RP: National surveillance of nosocomial blood stream infection due to *Candida albicans*: frequency of occurrence and antifungal suceptibility in the SCOPE Program. Diagn Microbiol Inf Dis *31*:327, 1998.

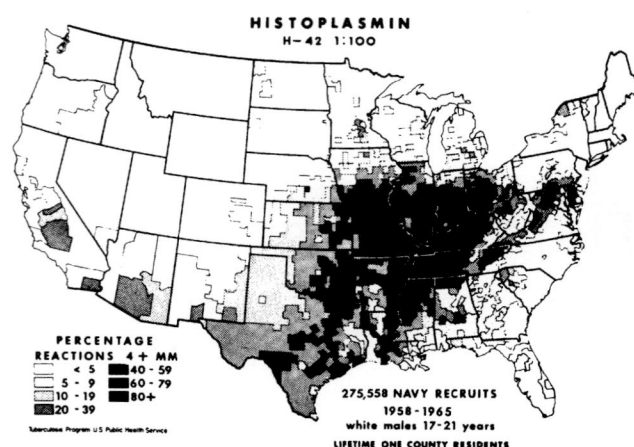

Fig. 86-1. Map of the United States showing areas of endemicity for histoplasmosis, based on county of lifetime residence of naval recruits with positive histoplasmin skin test reactivity, shown as a percent of those treated. From Edwards LB, et al: An atlas of sensitivity to tuberculin, PPD-B, and histoplasmin in the United States. Am Rev Respir Dis *99*:(Suppl)1, 1969. With permission.

The organisms are found in soil, especially that contaminated by the droppings of fowl or bats. In tissue, yeast forms may appear packed in macrophages, or the stained capsules of dead organisms can be identified in the necrotic center of chronic granulomatous lesions (Fig. 86-2).

Goodwin and DesPrez (1978) classified the apparently bewildering variety of clinical presentations of histoplasmosis into three main pathogenetic categories: 1) benign, usu- ally subclinical, infection of millions of otherwise normal people; 2) opportunistic infection; and 3) excessive host response characterized by excessive fibrosis (Table 86-3). The last two categories are of special diagnostic and therapeutic interest to the thoracic surgeon.

Table 86-2. Antifungal Drugs for Pulmonary and Systemic Infections

Disease	Primary Drug and Dosage[a]	Alternatives
Aspergillosis	Amphotericin B, 1–1.5 mg/kg IV	Itraconazole, 200 mg PO bid
Blastomycosis[b]	Itraconazole, 200 mg PO once or bid, or amphotericin B, 0.5–0.6 mg/kg IV	Ketoconazole, 400 mg PO once or bid; fluconazole, 400 mg bid
Candidiasis	Fluconazole,[c] 100–200 mg/day PO	Ketoconazole, 200–400 mg/day PO
Oropharyngeal	—	Itraconazole, 200 mg/day PO
Esophageal	Amphotericin B, 0.5–1.0 mg/kg IV, or fluconazole, 400–800 mg IV or PO qd	—
Invasive	Either plus or minus flucytosine, 100 mg/kg/day PO	—
Coccidioidomycosis[b]	Fluconazole, 400–800 mg/day PO, or amphotericin B, 0.5–1.0 mg/kg IV	Itraconazole, 200 mg PO bid; ketoconazole, 400 mg PO once or bid
Cryptococcosis	Amphotericin B, 0.5–0.7 mg/kg/day IV, plus or minus flucytosine, 100 mg/kg/day PO, followed by fluconazole, 400 mg PO qd chronic suppression; fluconazole, 200 mg/day PO	Itraconazole, 200 mg PO bid; amphotericin B, 0.5–1.0 mg/kg IV weekly
Histoplasmosis[b]	Itraconazole, 200 mg PO bid, or amphotericin B, 0.5–0.6 mg/kg IV chronic suppression; itraconazole, 200 mg PO once or bid	Ketoconazole, 400 mg PO once or bid; fluconazole, 400 mg bid; amphotericin B, 0.5–0.1 mg/kg IVweekly
Mucormycosis	Amphotericin B, 1.0–1.5 mg/kg/day IV	—
Paracoccidioidomycosis[b]	Itraconazole, 100–200 mg/day PO, or itraconazole, 200 mg PO bid	Ketoconazole, 200–400 mg/day PO
Pseudallescheriasis	Ketoconazole, 400–800 mg/day PO, or itraconazole, 200 mg PO bid	—
Sporotrichosis		
Cutaneous	Itraconazole 100–200 mg/day PO	Potassium iodide 1–5 mL PO tid
Systemic[b]	Amphotericin B, 0.5 mg/kg/day IV, or itraconazole, 200 mg PO bid	Fluconazole, 400 mg bid

[a] The optimal duration of treatment with the oral azole drugs is unclear. Depending on the disease, these drugs are continued for weeks or months or, particularly in patients with acquired immunodeficiency syndrome, indefinitely. With ketoconazole and itraconazole, patients with acquired immunodeficiency syndrome may have lower serum concentrations.
[b]Patients with severe illness should receive amphotericin B.
[c]*Candida krusei* infections are usually resistant to fluconazole, *Candida glabrata* infections are often resistant.
From Systemic antifungal drugs. Med Lett *39*:86, 1997. With permission.

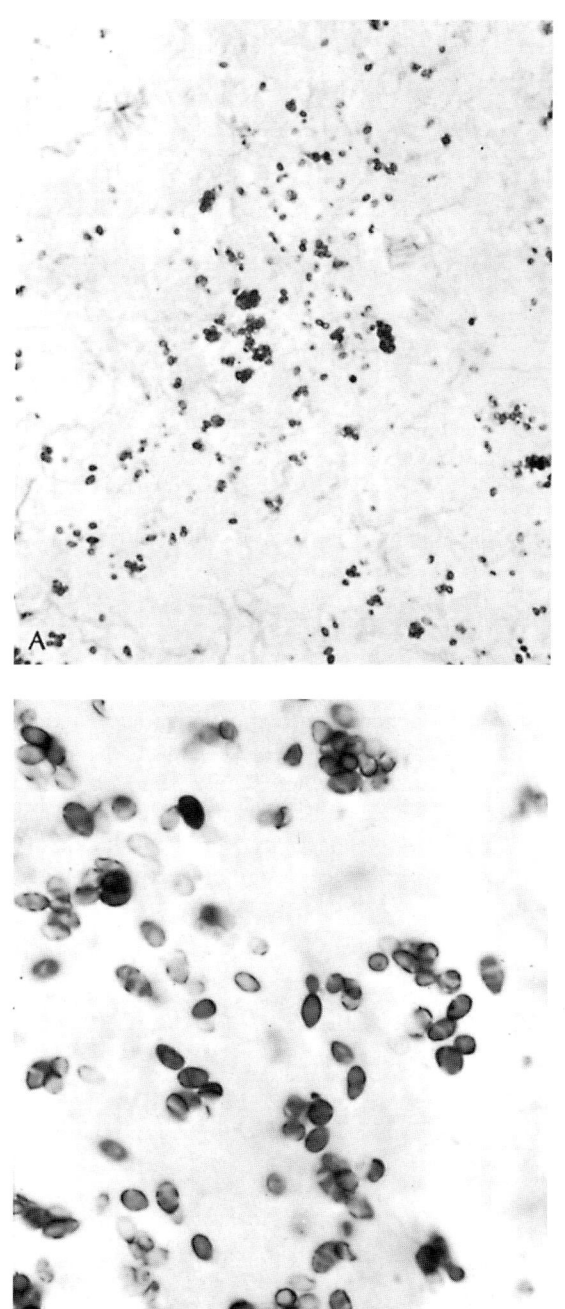

Fig. 86-2. *Histoplasma capsulatum* organisms. **A.** Nonviable capsules in necrotic area of a granuloma (Gomori's stain, ×780). **B.** Viable yeast forms in lymph node (×1300).

Pathogenesis and Symptomatology

Benign Infection of the Normal Host

In highly endemic areas, essentially the entire population becomes infected, without identifiable symptomatology, and often with conversion from a negative to a positive histo-

Table 86-3. Classification of Histoplasmosis

Histoplasmosis in normal hosts, acute pulmonary histoplasmosis
    Usual asymptomatic infection
    Occasional symptomatic infection
    Rare complications
        Pericarditis
        Mediastinal granuloma
        Mediastinal fibrosis
        Histoplasmomas
        Others
Opportunistic infections
    Disseminated histoplasmosis (immune defect)
    Chronic pulmonary histoplasmosis (structural defect)

From Goodwin RA, et al: Histoplasmosis in normal hosts. Medicine *60*:232, 1981. With permission.

plasmin skin test result as the only evidence of infection. Occasionally in infants and children, rarely in adults, cough, fever, and hilar lymphadenopathy mark the episode. Rarely, the process progresses to the second or third categories. After an unusually heavy exposure to dust containing the spores of *H. capsulatum*, however, the clinical entity of acute histoplasmosis of either primary or reinfection types is recognized (Fig. 86-3). Radiographically, the primary type is characterized by scattered, sparse to almost confluent, small pneumonic or nodular infiltrates. The process is self-limiting and may leave multiple nodular or calcific buckshot residues. In fewer than 1% of the infections, dissemination or death occurs. The reinfection type produces a finer, more miliary granulomatous reaction. The radiographic characteristics occurring in an endemic area after exposure to dust contaminated with fowl or bat droppings, a positive skin test result, and positive serologic findings (complement fixation) aid in confirming the diagnosis. Medical treatment is recommended for patients who remain ill more than 10 days to 2 weeks.

Opportunistic Infections

Opportunistic infections occur on two bases: immunologic and structural. Goodwin and DesPrez in 1978 conjectured that disseminated disease occurs as an opportunistic infection in a host with some immunologic deficiency. Since then, Wheat and associates (1990) recorded progressive disseminated disease identified in more than 100 patients with AIDS. This deficiency is identifiable in patients receiving immunosuppressive medications or with lymphatic or hematopoietic malignancies. The pulmonary alveolar macrophage is parasitized by *H. capsulatum* and provides not only nourishment and protection, but also possibly transportation to all parts of the reticuloendothelial system. Progressive disseminated histoplasmosis is a serious condition, for which full courses of medical therapy are mandatory.

Chronic pulmonary histoplasmosis is postulated to occur as an opportunistic infection in an area of lung structurally damaged by centrilobular or bullous emphysema. Substan-

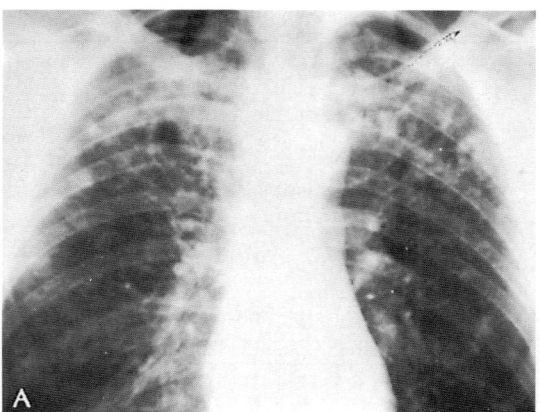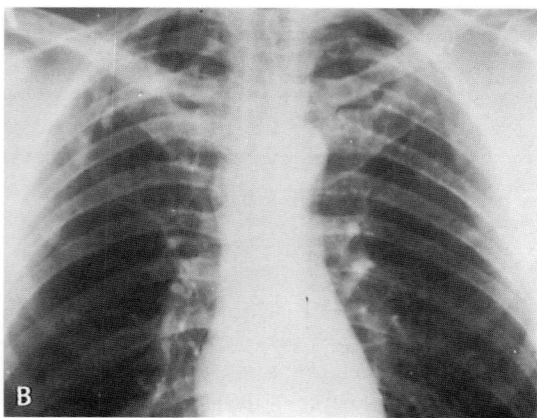

Fig. 86-3. Acute histoplasmosis. **A.** Thoracic radiograph of 48-year-old man who was asymptomatic when this routine radiograph was made. Purified protein derivative and histoplasmin skin test results were both positive. One sputum culture was reported to show *Histoplasma capsulatum*. Radiograph shows bilateral multiple soft infiltrates. No treatment was given. **B.** Thoracic radiograph 2 years later shows minimal residual fibrotic nodules. Patient remained well during the subsequent 5 years.

tial radiologic evidence shows that chronic obstructive pulmonary disease sets the stage for chronic cavitary histoplasmosis. The organisms are found only in effusions in emphysematous spaces or in the necrotic lining of established cavities (Fig. 86-4).

According to this hypothesis, colonization of an emphysematous space, with spillover (i.e., bronchogenic spread) of antigen-laden effusion into adjacent areas of lung, accounts for the recognized interstitial pneumonitis and necrosis

characteristic of this form of the disease. Infection of cavity walls similarly is thought to be secondary to either colonization or to dispersal of the same antigenic material from adjacent colonized spaces that causes, in other areas, pneumonitis and necrosis. Cavitary walls 2 mm or more thick suggest active disease that is likely to persist; thinner walled cavities usually signify inactivity. Persistent thick-walled (4 mm or more) cavities appear to promote continuing necrosis and enlargement, the so-called marching cavities.

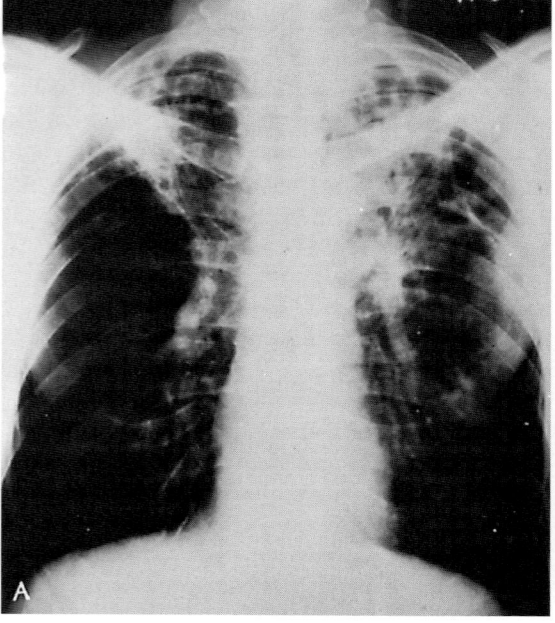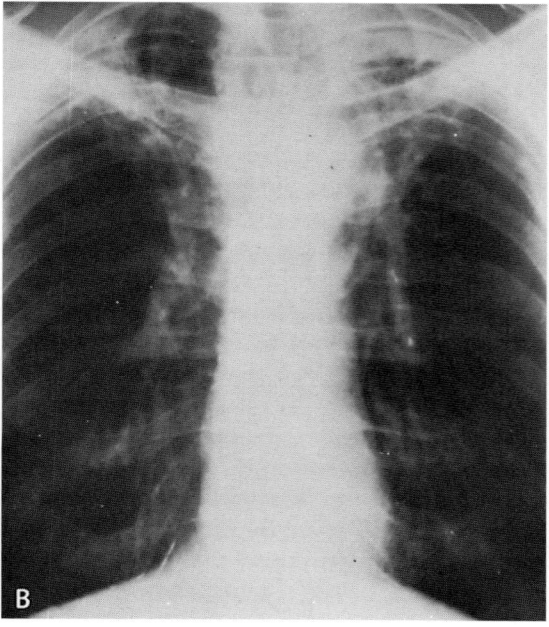

Fig. 86-4. Chronic cavitary histoplasmosis in a 53-year-old man. Initially, pulmonary tuberculosis was suspected; ultimately, sputum cultures and animal innoculation studies proved this to be chronic cavitary histoplasmosis. The patient received 2 g of amphotericin B over a 3-month period; ultimately, the lung lesions cleared. **A.** Thoracic radiograph before treatment. **B.** Appearance 6 months after completed treatment.

Symptomatology is nonspecific, resembling pulmonary tuberculosis as well as chronic obstructive lung disease. Cough, sputum, and hemoptysis are common, as are weight loss, low-grade fever, and weakness. Symptoms of pulmonary insufficiency may be prominent.

Because immunologic testing is unreliable, a positive diagnosis requires the demonstration of *H. capsulatum* in cultures of the sputum, which must be repeatedly and persistently tested for this fungus. The thicker the wall of the cavity, the more readily organisms are identifiable by sputum cultures. In patients with progressive disseminated histoplasmosis, the organism may be seen in circulating phagocytes (buffy coat) or lymph nodes. A bone marrow biopsy and culture often provide the quickest diagnosis. *H. capsulatum* antigen, when positive in blood, urine, or spinal fluid, is of both prognostic and diagnostic value.

Treatment

Chronic cavitary histoplasmosis can be treated with itraconazole or ketoconazole. As noted by Johnson and Sarosi (1991), however, the more severe infection may require amphotericin B. Response rates are 65%; however, the end points are blurred because of the underlying pulmonary disease. Progressive disseminated disease in a normal host may be treated successfully with ketoconazole, itraconazole, or amphotericin B with a response rate of 86%. The immunocompromised patient or the patient with AIDS can be treated with itraconazole or amphotericin B with an 85% response rate.

Progressive disseminated histoplasmosis with prosthetic heart valve involvement has been reported by Kanawaty and associates (1991). Surgical replacement of the diseased valve and high-dose amphotericin B is the treatment of choice.

Goodwin and colleagues (1976) found that treated patients fared better than untreated patients in every category of disease, except the early lesion without persistent cavitation (Table 86-4).

Surgical excision is recommended for localized thick-walled cavities only if no improvement is noted after one or two courses of drug therapy, and if pulmonary function permits. Because chronic obstructive lung disease is almost the sine qua non of opportunistic infection of structurally damaged lung tissue by *H. capsulatum*, however, the risks and benefits of resection in many patients have to be carefully and individually assessed to determine what is in the patient's best interests.

Excessive Fibrosis: Healed Primary Lesion

The solitary pulmonary nodule, one of the most common lesions seen by thoracic surgeons, in endemic areas, is often a histoplasmoma. This benign lesion results from an excessive response to some antigenic stimulus to fibrogenesis in the necrotic center of the small (2 to 4 mm) primary focus containing *H. capsulatum*. Over a period of years, concentric layers of collagen are laid down, approximately 1 to 2 mm/year, resulting in a slowly enlarging and thus ominous-appearing nodular mass. Central or target calcification, however, or concentric laminar calcification that gives unequivocal evidence of the benign nature of the granulomatous reaction, can often be seen radiographically. This calcification is by far most commonly caused by histoplasmosis, but occurs also occasionally with tuberculosis and coccidioidomycosis (Fig. 86-5). Although more than 50% of 1000 solitary pulmonary nodules in adults, mostly men, were benign granulomas, as Steele (1964) reported, 36% were malignant tumors. Therefore, unless the characteristic radiographic findings noted previously are identified by computed tomographic (CT) scan, if not obvious on plain film radiographs of the thorax, exploratory thoracotomy is often indicated, as Godwin (1983) emphasized, especially in men older than 40 years of age (Fig. 86-6). Perioperative drug therapy is not indicated during resection of granulomas. On the other hand, if the diagnosis of a granuloma can

Table 86-4. Results of Treatment in 382 Lesions of Histoplasmosis in 228 Patients[a]

Types of Lesions	No. of Lesions	Conservative Treatment		Amphotericin Therapy		Surgical Resection	
		No. of Lesions	Percent Healed	No. of Lesions	Percent Healed	No. of Lesions	Percent Healed
Early, no persistent cavity	156	139	99+	6	100	11	100
Early, persistent cavity	44	25	16	11	55	8	100
Late, no persistent cavity	41	36	100	0	—	5	100
Late, thin-walled cavity	52	27	63	12	92	13	100
Late, thick-walled cavity	89	53	21	15	63	21	95[a]
Total lesions	**382**	**280**	—	**44**	—	**58**	—

[a]One surgical death.
From Goodwin RA, et al: Chronic pulmonary histoplasmosis. Medicine 55:413, 1976. With permission.

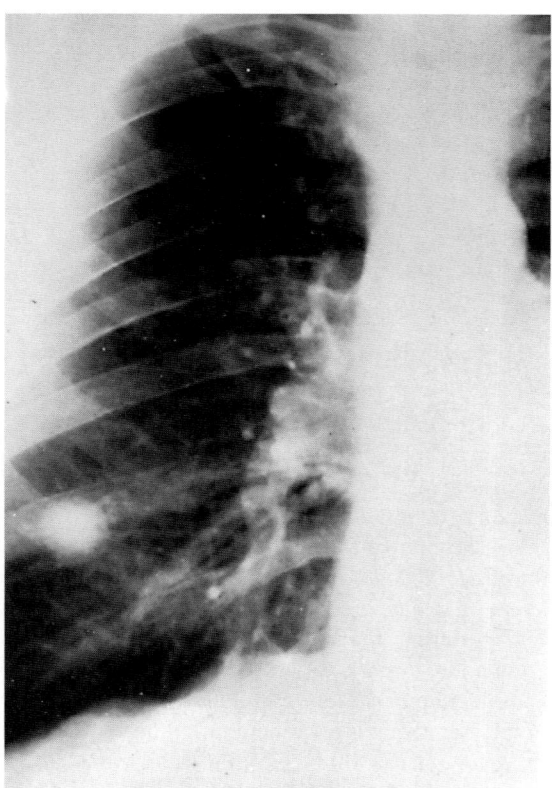

Fig. 86-5. *Histoplasma granuloma* in a male adult. This centrally calcified lesion remained unchanged for 10 years.

be made by the characteristic radiographic findings, or by transbronchial brushing or percutaneous aspiration needle biopsy, or by evidence of an unchanging lesion for a period of several years, neither thoracotomy nor drug therapy may be needed. High-resolution CT, which determines the density of the lesion, may help also. A high Hounsfield unit number (greater than 164) of the lesion, because of microcalcifications, denotes that the lesion is benign and that surgery is unnecessary (see Chapter 91).

In hilar and mediastinal lymph nodes, this excessive encapsulating fibrogenic response to the antigen of *H. capsulatum* may have serious consequences, depending on the region involved. In the right paratracheal region, superior vena caval syndrome or right bronchial stenosis may result; subcarinal lymph node involvement may produce stenosis of either or both main bronchi or the pulmonary veins; hilar lymph nodal involvement may cause either pulmonary arterial or bronchial stenosis. Mediastinal granulomas may be produced by the matting together of several large, caseous lymph nodes, presenting as mass lesions, in addition to giving rise to the aforementioned problems. There has been no proven benefit to antifungal or corticosteroid therapy in patients with mediastinal fibrosis as discussed by Mathisen and Grillo (1992). Because of these serious complications and the difficulties in managing them once they appear, excision of resectable, asymptomatic, mediastinal granulo-

mas to forestall such difficult problems has been advocated by Ferguson and Burford (1965), as well as Dines (1979) and Zajtchuk (1973) and their associates, and is probably appropriate when lymph nodes are heavily calcified. Dunn and colleagues (1990) recommend that surgical reconstruction of mediastinal structures should be attempted whenever possible (see Chapters 165 and 166).

Coccidioidomycosis

Coccidioidomycosis is a suppurative and granulomatous infectious disease that primarily attacks the lungs. The disseminated form of the disease is encountered more frequently than in the past because of the large number of immunocompromised patients.

Coccidioidomycosis bears several resemblances to histoplasmosis. This fungus occurs as a soil contaminant in sharply circumscribed geographic areas, resulting in subclinical infection in one-third of the population who are identifiable by a specific skin test, just as with histoplasmosis.

Drutz and Catanzaro (1978) and Ampel and associates (1989) have presented extensive reviews of this disease.

Epidemiology

Fungal organisms occur in a well-defined area of the southwestern United States, including portions of California, Nevada, Arizona, New Mexico, and Texas (Fig. 86-7), as well as in Mexico and Central and South America. Infection results from the inhalation of spore-laden dust. The estimated average annual incidence of symptomatic coccidioidomycosis among susceptible individuals is 0.439. Agricultural and construction workers and others with similar outdoor pursuits are most likely to become infected. Archeologists are at special risk. Coccidioidomycosis is being diagnosed with increasing frequency in patients with AIDS, mostly among patients residing in endemic areas, as Galgiani and Ampel (1990) have reported.

Unlike most other fungal diseases, infection may be acquired also by inhalation of dust from fomites and from laboratory cultures of *Coccidioides immitis*. Therefore, such materials must be handled with special precautions.

Pathology

Pathologically, coccidioidomycosis resembles pulmonary tuberculosis. The primary complex is composed of a parenchymal pneumonitis and involvement of a regional lymph node or nodes, which may not be detected clinically. Reactivation of the primary complex may result in reinfection, with the development of caseous nodules, effusions, pneumonic areas, cavities, and calcified, fibrotic, or ossified lung lesions (Fig. 86-8).

Extrapulmonary dissemination to lymph nodes, skin, spleen, liver, kidneys, bones, and meninges is more likely to

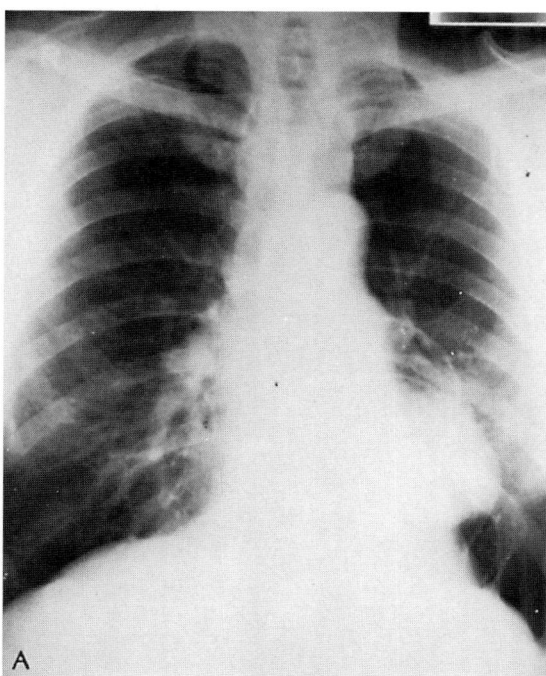
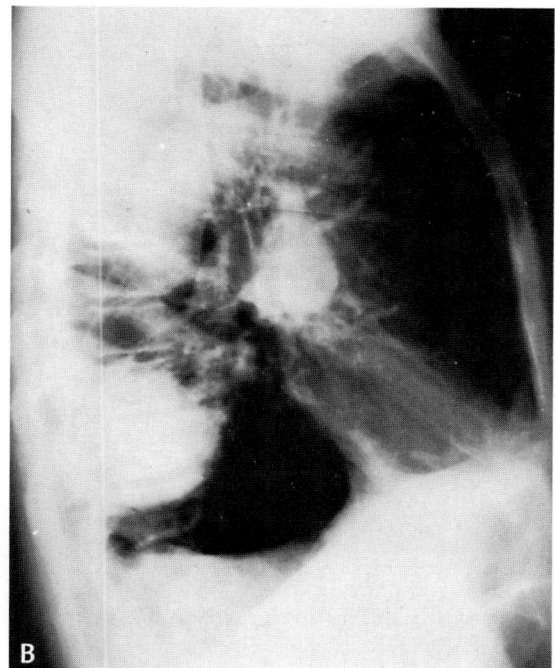

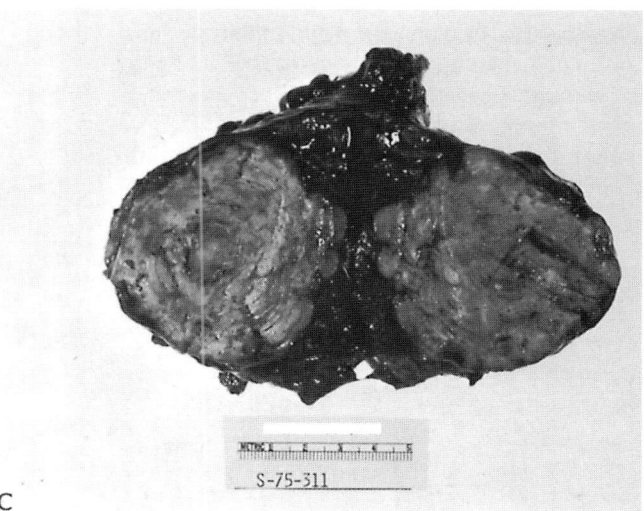

Fig. 86-6. Giant histoplasmoma. Posteroanterior (**A**) and lateral (**B**) radiographs of an asymptomatic 62-year-old man who was having a routine checkup. Diagnostic studies, including pulmonary angiography and thoracic aortography, did not disclose the nature of the lesion. **C.** After exploratory thoracotomy on suspicion of bronchial carcinoma, a left lower lobectomy was performed. A large laminated fibrocollagenous granuloma with a necrotic center containing yeast cells morphologically consistent with *Histoplasma capsulatum* was found. This excessive degree of fibrogenesis is unusual.

occur in the primary than in the reinfection phase of the disease and is more likely to afflict blacks, Filipinos, Native Americans, and Mexicans, by factors of 5 to 10 times the incidence seen in whites.

The histologic characteristics of coccidioidomycosis lesions are those of granuloma formation with suppuration. With special stains, large (e.g., 15 to 80 μm) spherules, packed with tiny endospores when mature, or the endospores themselves can be seen (Fig. 86-9). Rarely, a mycetoma or fungus ball containing hyphae appears, as Bayer (1976), Thadepalli (1977), and Rohatgi (1984) and their associates reported, because *Coccidioides* grows best at body temperature in spherule form.

Symptomatology

Most patients with primary infection have no symptoms. In approximately 25% of patients, either mild or severe symptoms are noted, which are nonspecific, and either referable to the respiratory tract or flulike, with malaise, headaches, and fever. Again, the condition is clustered among blacks and Filipinos. Symptoms may be pleuritic pain and cough productive of mucoid or, rarely, bloody sputum. Erythema multiforme, erythema nodosum, or less specific morbilliform rashes are observed occasionally, especially in women. Mild arthritic manifestations, which are called *desert rheumatism*, also occur sometimes. The radiographic

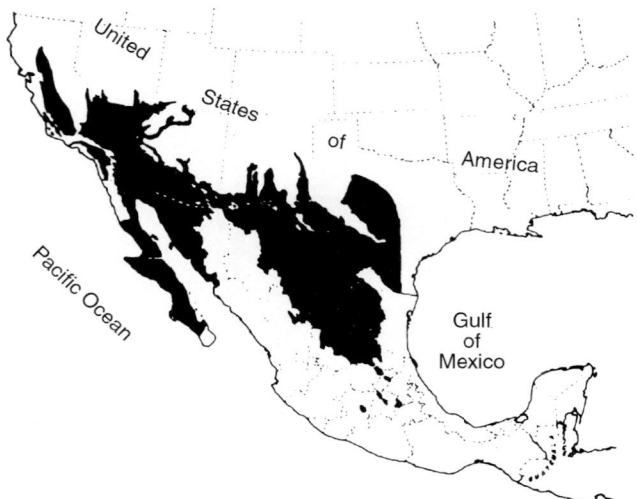

Fig. 86-7. Map showing area of endemicity of coccidioidomycosis in the United States and Mexico. From Ochoa GA: Coccidioidomycosis in Mexico. *In* Ajello CL (ed): Coccidioidomycosis. Tucson: University of Arizona Press, 1967. With permission.

findings are nonspecific. In the acute stage, miliary lesions, pneumonic infiltrates, hilar adenopathy, or pleural and pericardial effusions may appear. With chronic coccidioidomycosis, solitary nodules representing coccidioidal granulomas; chronic, usually, thin-walled cavities, sometimes with a fluid level; pneumothorax; fibrosis; or empyema may be manifestations of the disease.

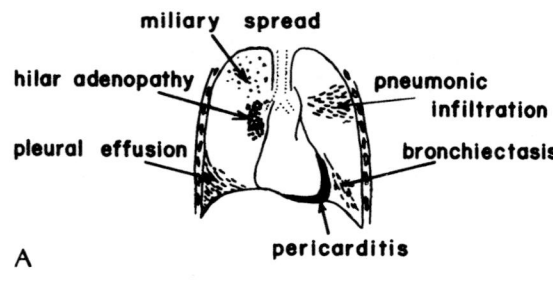

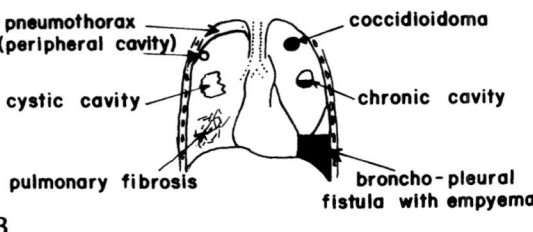

Fig. 86-8. Varieties of pulmonary manifestations of coccidioidomycosis. **A.** Acute stage. **B.** Chronic stage. From Paulsen GA: Pulmonary surgery in coccidioidal infections. *In* Ajello L (ed): Coccidioidomycosis. Tucson: University of Arizona Press, 1967. With permission.

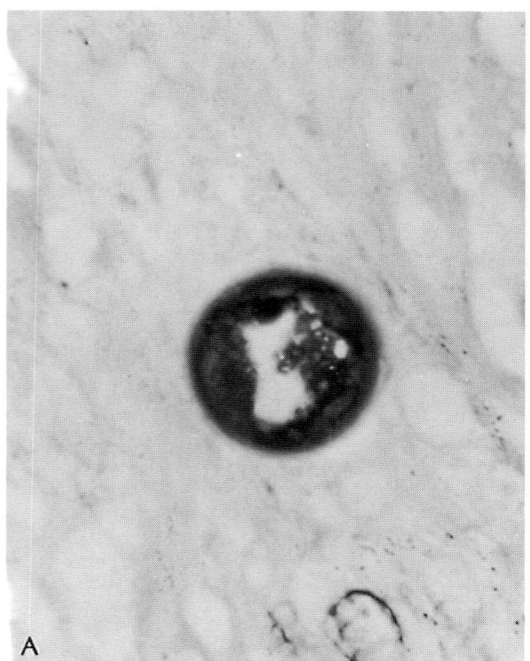

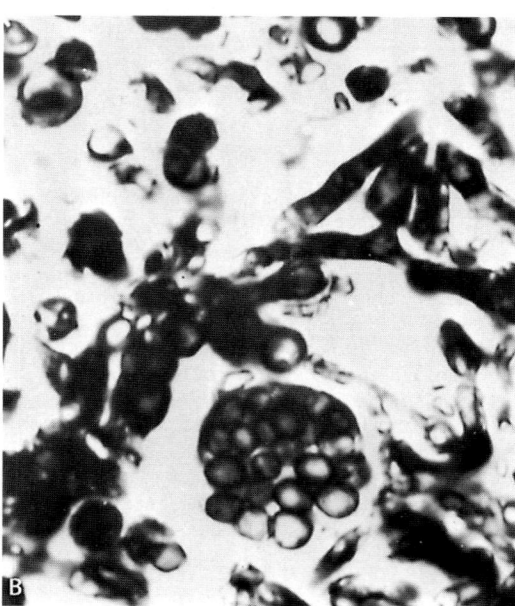

Fig. 86-9. A. Old spherule of *Coccidioides immitis* containing endospores, in an area of pulmonary fibrosis (×1300). **B.** Organisms identified in a coccidioidal fungus ball in a cavitary lesion, showing both hyphae and spore forms (×1300). This patient died of extensive cavitary coccidioidomycosis in spite of amphotericin B therapy 8 years after left pneumonectomy had been performed in an attempt to control his disease.

Diagnosis

A positive culture result of sputum, other body fluid, or tissue is necessary for a definitive diagnosis. In acute coccidioidal pleural effusions, Lonky and associates (1976) noted that cultures of pleural biopsy specimens can be more rewarding than culturing the fluid. Recent conversion of the coccidioidin or Spherulin skin test to positive or positive serology strongly suggests coccidioidomycosis. Although four serologic tests are available, early coccidioidal infection is usually detected only by the tube precipitin or the latex agglutination tests. Chick and coworkers (1973) noted that increasing serial complement fixation test results mean severe disease or even dissemination; a decreasing titer usually indicates regression or improvement.

Treatment

Many patients need no treatment at all. Itraconazole and fluconazole have replaced amphotericin B as the treatment of choice for patients with non–life-threatening coccidioidomycosis. Although these triazoles have never been compared directly with amphotericin B, their response rates are comparable. The majority of patients can be treated as outpatients and the therapy is better tolerated. Fifty-seven percent of patients responded to 400 mg/day of itraconazole treatment as reported by Graybill and associates (1990), whereas 55% of patients with chronic pulmonary coccidioidomycosis responded to 200 to 400 mg/day of fluconazole as reported by Catanzaro and coworkers (1995). Indications for treatment include 1) prevention of dissemination, especially in black patients, Filipinos, Native Americans, and Mexicans, the threat of which may be indicated by continuing elevation of the titer of the complement fixation test (1:64 or higher); 2) control of cavitary disease with sputum culture results positive for *C. immitis*; 3) arrest of dissemination of disease; 4) control of progressive chronic pulmonary lesions; 5) coverage during pulmonary resections; and 6) preventive medical coverage in patients with active coccidioidomycosis that require corticosteroids or during pregnancy. For patients with life-threatening illness (e.g., acute respiratory distress, sepsis, or other evidence of overwhelming infection) amphotericin B remains the treatment of choice. After stabilization, therapy can often be switched to itraconazole or fluconazole.

The indications for resective surgery for coccidioidomycosis include localized granulomatous lesions and cavitary disease (Fig. 86-10). Although most undiagnosed solitary pulmonary nodules occurring in patients in the endemic area are coccidioidomas, Read (1972) and Cohen and associates (1972) found 26 to 35% to be malignant. Therefore, in the endemic area, the indications for resection of undiagnosed solitary pulmonary nodules must be individualized, as for histoplasmosis, because a known granuloma does not ordinarily necessitate resection.

Marks and colleagues (1967) reported that localized resections in more than 700 patients were accompanied by a complication rate of approximately 10%, many of them air leaks or peripheral, small bronchopleural fistulas. Spillage of contaminated material into the pleural cavity is associated with a significant increase in complications. For cavitary lesions, in most patients resection is not indicated. When cavities persist more than 2 to 4 years, however, and are

larger than 2 cm in diameter; when they are rapidly enlarging, thick walled, or ruptured, or contain a fungus ball; when they are associated with severe or recurrent hemoptysis; when they occur in diabetic or pregnant patients; and when they coexist with pulmonary tuberculosis, surgical resection, preferably by lobectomy, is indicated, as Nelson (1974), Baker (1978), and Cunningham (1982) and their colleagues suggested. Some recommend drug coverage with amphotericin B, but it is not clear that the use of amphotericin B has resulted in significantly fewer complications of bronchopleural fistula, empyema, and recurrent cavitation. Intravenous fluconazole may be a reasonable alternative to avoid the potential adverse effects of amphotericin B as described by Johnson and Sarosi (1995). Resection and biopsy of the undiagnosed coccidioidal granuloma may be accomplished thoracoscopically, as shown in Figure 86-10.

North American Blastomycosis

North American blastomycosis is a suppurative and granulomatous infectious disease caused by *Blastomyces dermatitidis*, which is found in tissue as a round, thick-walled single budding yeast cell, 5 to 20 μm in diameter. When originally described by Gilchrist in 1894, it was thought to be a skin disease, but it has since been shown that the lung is the primary site of infection and that skin and other sites are affected because of secondary dissemination.

Epidemiology

North American blastomycosis occurs mostly in the Southeastern, South Central, and Midwestern states, especially in Arkansas, Kentucky, Mississippi, and Wisconsin, according to Klein and associates (1986) (Fig. 86-11). This disease is also an airborne infection of exogenous origin, the fungus having been identified in pigeon manure by Sarosi and Serstock (1976) and in soil by Klein and colleagues (1986). Thus, the incidence in some studies, as Busey and associates (1964) noted, is highest among persons in close contact with the soil. Kitchen and colleagues (1977), however, described an urban epidemic.

Pathology and Microbiology

North American blastomycosis characteristically induces a granulomatous and pyogenic reaction with microabscesses and giant cells and, occasionally, caseation, cavitation, and fibrosis. Primarily, the lungs, skin, bones, and genitourinary tract are affected. Skin lesions exhibit pseudoepitheliomatous squamous cell proliferation with microabscesses between areas of acanthotic epithelium. Special stains reveal the fungal organisms with the characteristic thick refractile walls (Fig. 86-12). Landis and Varkey (1976) as well as Laskey and Sarosi (1977) documented endogenous reinfection, as in pulmonary tuberculosis.

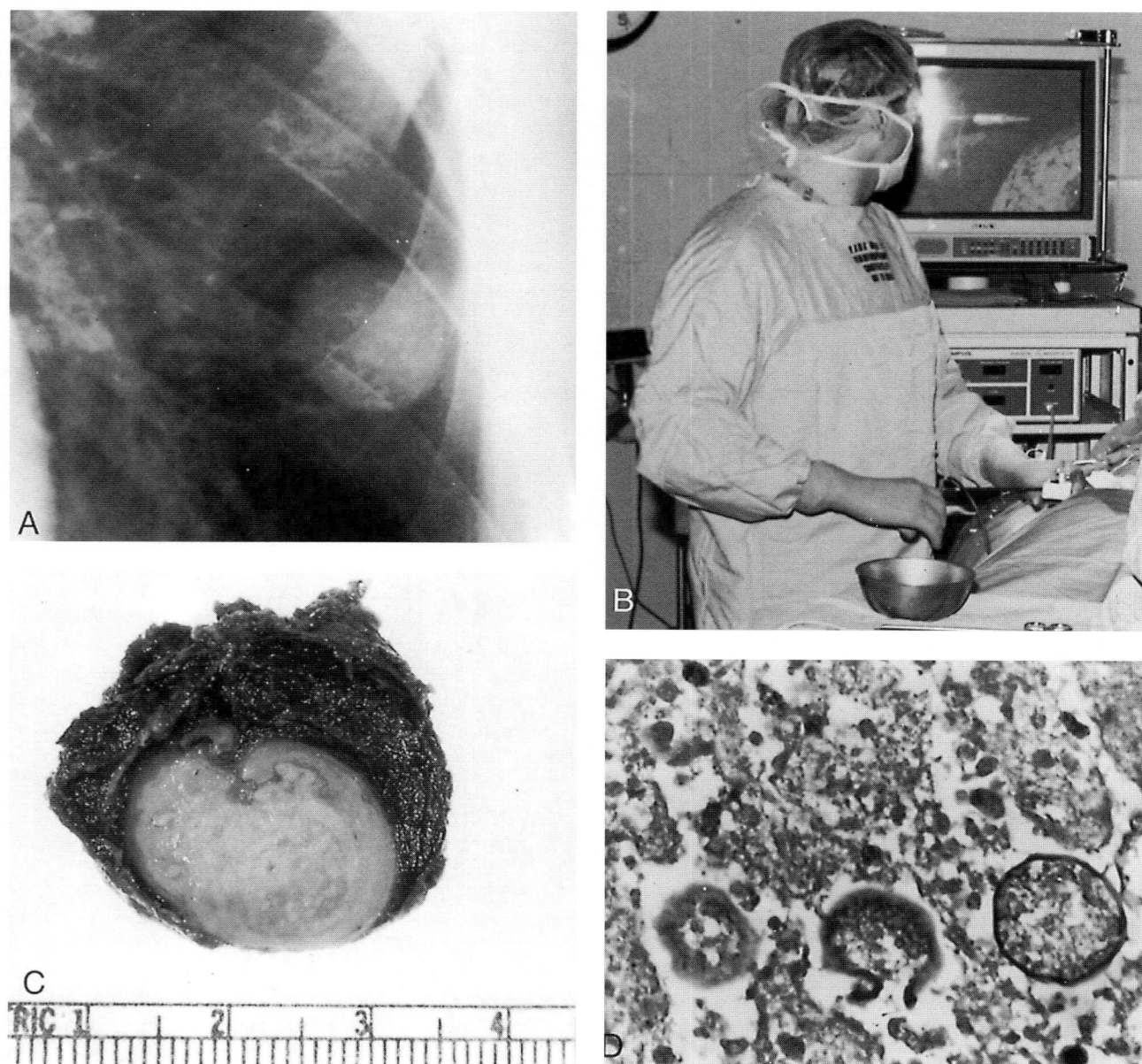

Fig. 86-10. Coccidioidal granuloma. **A.** Thoracic radiograph showing a 2-cm nodule in the left lower lobe of the lung of a 41-year-old man with a 75-pack per year smoking history. He had been stationed in the California desert while in the Army. Bronchoscopy was negative. **B.** The nodule was resected thoracoscopically. Lung and instrument can be visualized on the monitor. **C.** Resected specimen, which was a coccidioidal granuloma. **D.** Microscopic sections (×400) show spherules packed with endospores.

Blastomycosis is not a prevalent disease. It has a long and variable incubation period with a mean of 45 days. Cell-mediated immunity is the major defense against blastomycosis, but as noted by Bradsher (1990), few patients with AIDS have been reported with this disease.

Symptomatology

The patient with blastomycosis is usually first seen because of symptoms referable to the skin or the lungs, or both.

The cutaneous manifestations begin as single and multiple papules or papulopustules that enlarge slowly, ulcerate, and exhibit elevated, cyanotic edges. Biopsies from such areas are more likely than are cultures of sputum to yield the organisms. The lesions may appear anywhere, on both exposed and unexposed portions of the skin, and are characterized by chronicity (Fig. 86-13). The patient may be unaware of the skin lesions. Healing may occur, leaving a soft noncontracting scar. The weight of clinical and pathologic evidence, as Rabinowitz and associates (1976) pointed out, suggests that a primary pul-

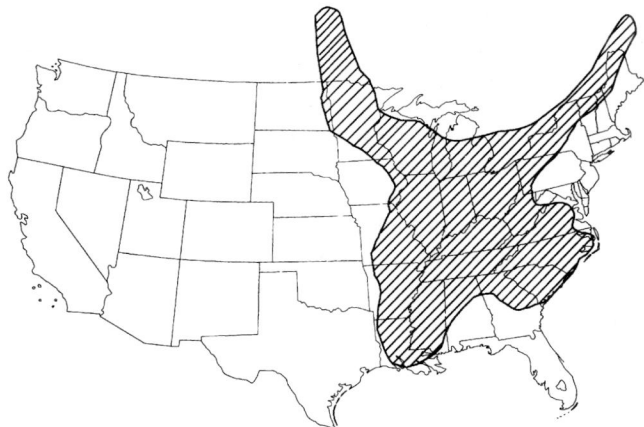

Fig. 86-11. Approximate area of endemicity in the United States for North American blastomycosis. Adapted from Menges RW, et al: Clinical and epidemiological studies on 79 canine blastomycosis cases in Arkansas. Am J Epidemiol *81*:169, 1965. With permission.

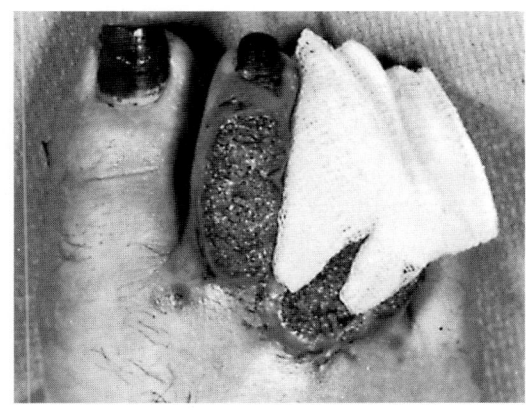

Fig. 86-13. Skin lesions of blastomycosis on dorsum of toes. Biopsy of characteristic raised edges showed multiple microabscesses containing *Blastomyces dermatitidis*. From Takaro T: Thoracic actinomycetic and mycotic infections. *In* Goldsmith HS (ed): Practice of Surgery. Hagerstown, MD: Harper & Row, 1978. With permission.

monary focus is present in practically all instances of both cutaneous and systemic North American blastomycosis.

After the cutaneous form, the next most common manifestations of blastomycosis are caused by pulmonary involvement. Cough, usually productive only of mucoid sputum, chest pain, and hemoptysis may occur, or mild fever, malaise, weight loss, weakness, and other nonspecific symptoms may be the only complaints. Physical signs are not characteristic or particularly helpful.

Thoracic Radiographic Findings

Cush and colleagues (1976) noted that consolidation is characteristic in acute disease but also is common in chronic

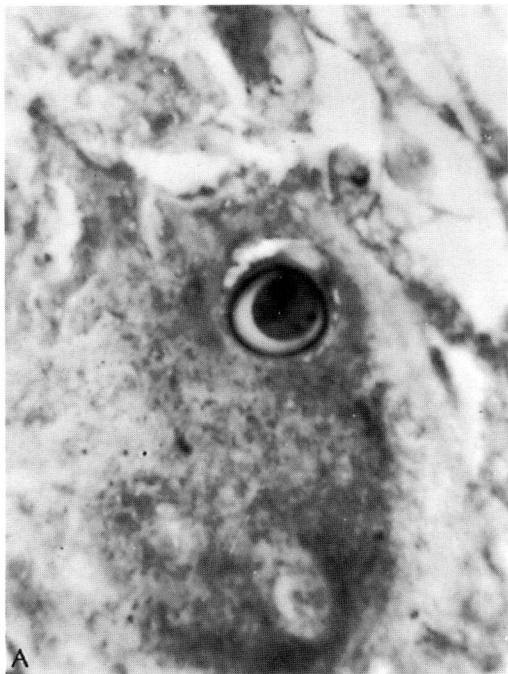
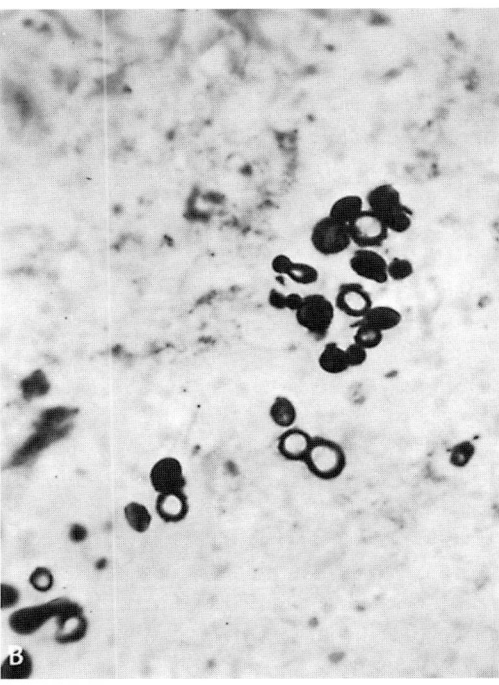

Fig. 86-12. Organisms of *Blastomyces dermatitidis* from resected lung tissue. **A.** Single thick-walled yeast form with refractile cell wall. **B.** Multiple yeast forms with single budding characteristic of this fungus (periodic acid–Schiff stain, ×1100). From Takaro T: Thoracic surgery. *In* Goldsmith HS (ed): Practice of Surgery. Hagerstown, MD: Harper & Row, 1978. With permission.

blastomycosis. Fibronodular lesions, with or without cavitation, reminiscent of pulmonary tuberculosis are also common in chronic disease. Mass lesions, diffuse patterns, pleural involvement, and hilar lymphadenopathy also appear, but less commonly. Kinasewitz and colleagues (1984) recognized that major pleural disease indicates a poor prognosis. Many patients have undergone exploration with the presumptive diagnosis of carcinoma of the lung.

Diagnosis

Most commonly, diagnosis is made by cultural demonstration of the organism in the sputum, in material from skin lesions, or from skeletal lesions: abscesses, sinuses, or biopsy material. Sutliff and Cruthirds (1973) advocated the examination of bronchial washings or sputum cytologic techniques for *B. dermatitidis*; Sanders and associates (1977) confirmed the value of the latter. Several specimens may be required to demonstrate the organisms. Lung biopsy may be necessary to make the diagnosis; however, this procedure is occasionally followed by dissemination of the disease. The major differential diagnostic problem in endemic areas of blastomycosis is carcinoma of the lung, which Poe and associates (1972) emphasized. In patients with unrecognized pulmonary blastomycosis, unnecessarily radical operations may be performed with the mistaken diagnosis of tumor. A preoperative diagnosis is therefore important to avoid an unnecessary operation.

Because skin and complement fixation test results may be negative as often as positive, and because of the close antigenic similarity between coccidioidin, histoplasmin, and blastomycin, these serologic intracutaneous diagnostic tests are inadequate and cannot be relied on for a definitive diagnosis. Turner and Kaufman (1986) reported that serologic tests with improved diagnostic capabilities have been developed.

Treatment

Blastomycosis should be treated whenever the diagnosis can be made unequivocally by identifying the organism. Self-limited disease, however, was described by Sarosi and associates (1986). In any event, a presumptive diagnosis is not an adequate basis for therapy, because the drugs used for treatment are expensive and potentially toxic. Dismukes and coworkers (1992) and Davies and Sarosi (1997) have shown that most patients with pulmonary blastomycosis can be treated with oral itraconazole. The recommended dose is 400 mg orally for 6 months. Response rates with this therapy are 95%, with more than 90% of patients being cured. Ketoconazole and fluconazole are believed to be less active agents. For cavitary lesions or extensive disease or for systemic dissemination, amphotericin B is preferable (Fig. 86-14).

Resection is indicated when bronchial carcinoma is suspected after efforts have been made, especially in endemic areas, to rule out North American blastomycosis. Drug treatment with amphotericin B or itraconazole should follow operation when the diagnosis is made only at the time of the thoracotomy. Resection of known blastomycotic cavitary lesions is indicated if they persist after adequate drug therapy with amphotericin B or itraconazole, or both, because viable organisms are likely to persist in such lesions, even if they cannot be recovered in the sputum.

Pulmonary blastomycosis is still a serious disease, with a 5-year mortality of approximately 20%. Involvement of the genitourinary tract, bones, and nasal and oral mucosa is common.

Cryptococcosis

Definition

Cryptococcosis is a subacute or chronic infection caused by *Cryptococcus neoformans*, formerly known as *Torula histolytica*, which primarily attacks the bronchopulmonary tree but also has a special predilection for the central nervous system. This disease, like blastomycosis, histoplasmosis, and coccidioidomycosis, was formerly thought to be a rare and invariably fatal infection, with meningitis the most prominent feature. Bronchopulmonary manifestations are apparently more common than the dreaded meningeal form, however, and since the introduction of amphotericin B and 5-fluorocytosine, even this form can be controlled. Duperval and colleagues (1977) noted that the number of immunocompromised patients with opportunistic infections with *C. neoformans* had increased; according to Minamoto and Rosenberg (1997), it is presently the fourth most common opportunistic infection in patients with AIDS, with approximately 6 to 10% of patients with AIDS infected.

Epidemiology

Cryptococcosis has no known geographic area of endemicity. Two varieties are found throughout the world. Ellis and Pfeiffer (1990) and Levitz (1991) reviewed the infectious characteristics of the two varieties. *C. neoformans*, serotypes A or D, is most common and is most likely to produce disease in immunodeficient patients. *C. neoformans vargattii*, serotypes B and C, which may have originated in Australia, usually causes disease in normal hosts. Cryptococci may be present in soil and dust contaminated by pigeon droppings; in this regard, it resembles histoplasmosis as well as North American blastomycosis.

Pathology

The organism *C. neoformans* is a round, budding yeast form 5 to 20 μm in diameter (average, 8 to 10 μm) with a sometimes wide gelatinous capsule that surrounds the

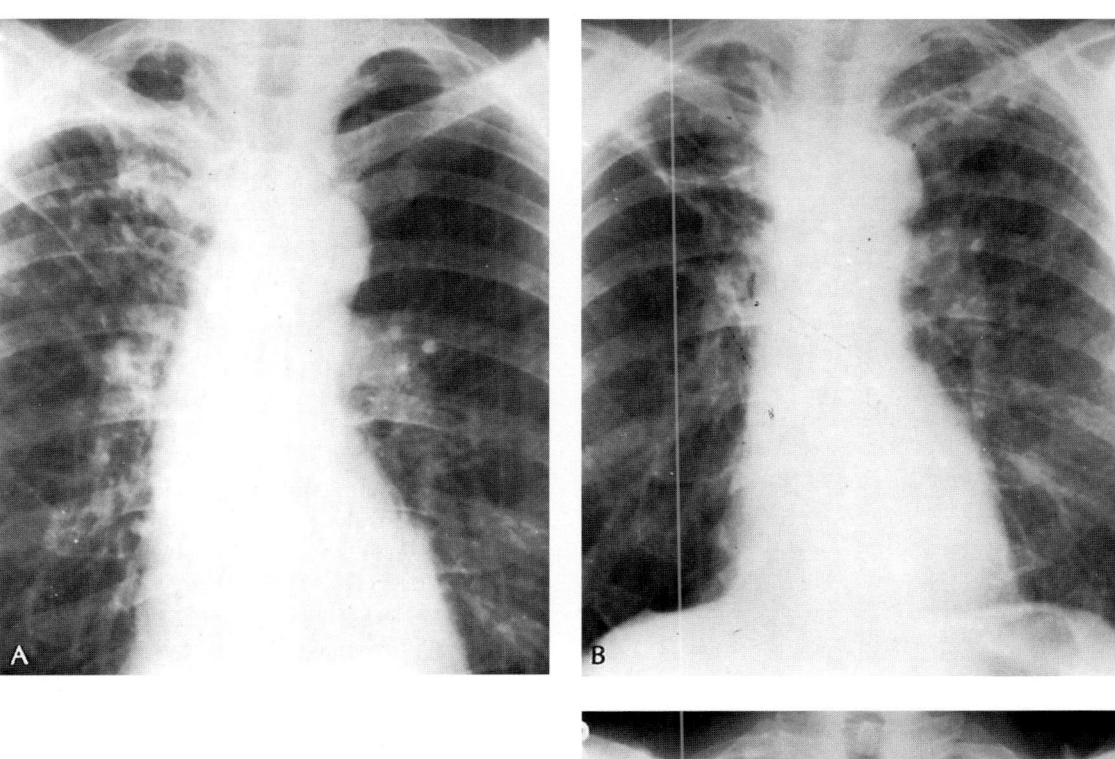

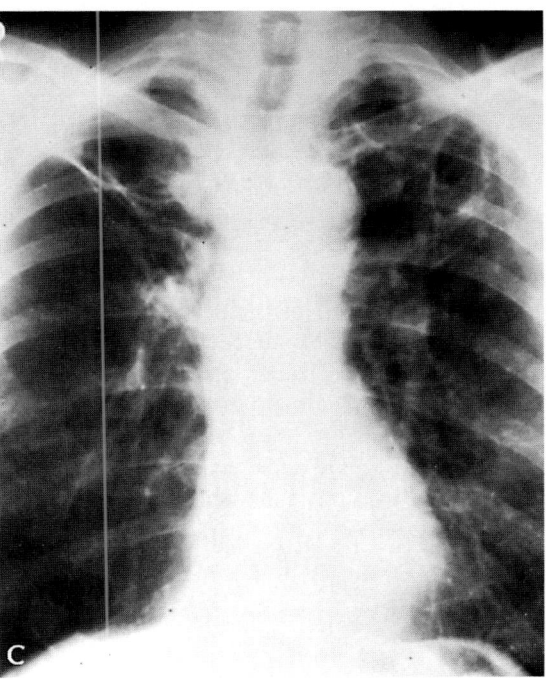

Fig. 86-14. Evolution of chronic pulmonary blastomycosis. **A.** Thoracic radiograph shows extensive right upper lung infiltrative lesion in a man with proven blastomycotic skin lesion of the nostril. Lesion was treated at first with potassium iodide. **B.** Four years later, bilateral cavitary disease is observed, but no organisms were seen in the sputum. **C.** Two and a half years later, two thin-walled cavities in the left upper lobe and an emphysematous bulla in the right upper lobe were noted. A number of sputum specimens showed *Blastomyces dermatitidis.* He was treated with 7 g of 2-hydroxystilbamidine. He has remained well.

organism and remains unstained. The usual special stains for fungi are all effective for demonstrating the organisms. The mucicarmine stain is specific. In fresh material, the capsules can be demonstrated by mounting some of the specimen in a drop of diluted india ink (Fig. 86-15).

This infection is airborne, and the respiratory tract is the portal of entry. McDonnell and Hutchins (1985) described four basic morphologic patterns in the lungs: pulmonary granulomas; granulomatous pneumonias; diffuse alveolar and interstitial cryptococci accompanied by greater or lesser degrees of inflammatory response; and many alveolar and intravascular organisms in the lungs, in which the primary route of infection was uncertain. The lesions are often solid, and the cut surface of the granuloma may be glaring or shiny, as in a mucoid carcinoma. Central necrosis and cavitation may occur but are uncommon, and calcification is rare. Duperval (1977) and Salyer (1974) and their colleagues reported pleural effusions and empyemas, and dis-

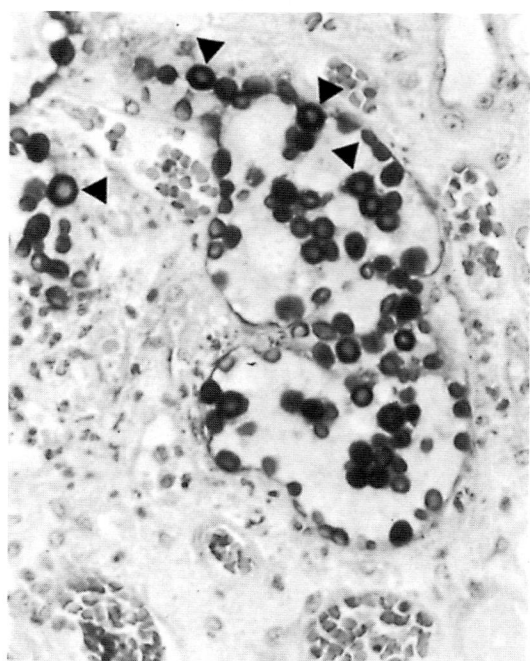

Fig. 86-15. Organisms of *Cryptococcus neoformans* show thick capsules (*arrows*) (periodic acid–Schiff stain, ×780).

semination to parts of the body other than the central nervous system has been described also.

Symptomatology

Pulmonary symptoms are nonspecific, insidious, or absent. Cough, bloody sputum, low-grade fever, weakness, and lethargy sometimes occur. Spontaneous remission may and probably does occur. Because cryptococcosis is often an opportunistic infection, the manifestations of the primary disease may overshadow those of cryptococcosis, and the diagnosis may become apparent only after abnormalities on thoracic radiography call attention to the lungs, or symptoms referable to the central nervous system suggest meningitis.

Diagnosis

Cryptococcus may be isolated from sputum, bronchial washings, bronchial brushing, or percutaneous needle aspiration of the lungs, as well as from cerebrospinal fluid, where it should specifically be sought. Often, the diagnosis is made from a resected lung specimen or at autopsy. No specific skin test for cryptococcosis is available, and serologic tests are of limited value.

The radiographic features of pulmonary cryptococcosis are not sufficiently characteristic to be of diagnostic help. Infiltrative, mass, nodular, and diffuse miliary lesions have all been described (Fig. 86-16). Pleural effusion is unusual, but is recognized more frequently than it once was, as noted

by Epstein (1972) and Littman (1968) and their associates as well as the aforementioned authors.

Kerkering and colleagues (1981) pointed out that the diagnosis of cryptococcosis is often missed because it is not considered often enough in the differential diagnosis of abnormalities found on thoracic radiography.

Treatment

Medical

The specific antifungal agents effective against *C. neoformans* are amphotericin B, 5-fluorocytosine (Ancobon), ketoconazole, and fluconazole. Treatment of pulmonary disease depends on the immune status of the patient. Patients with normal immunity and uncomplicated cryptococcal pneumonia usually require no treatment. Because of the risk of progression to meningitis, however, most patients are treated with a 6-month course of fluconazole and amphotericin B as suggested by Johnson and Sarosi (1995). Before the proven efficacy of the oral azoles, patients were treated with 5-fluorocytosine as described by Minamoto and Rosenberg (1997). Although the Mycoses Study Group and the AIDS clinical trials group found no statistical difference between this therapy and fluconazole (200 to 400 mg/day), patients receiving amphotericin B had a lower mortality and had negative culture results earlier. Fluconazole may be more effective and still well tolerated in these patients when higher doses (800 mg/day) are used as suggested by Duswald and coworkers (1997).

Even the dreaded meningeal form is no longer uniformly fatal. Recovery with drug treatment, sometimes requiring multiple courses, is now the rule rather than the exception.

Surgical

Cryptococcal involvement of the lung in the normal host is often nodular and may resemble pulmonary neoplasm. If the diagnosis is confirmed, a course of medical therapy is warranted, as it will usually be curative. Often, the diagnosis is not established until the time of surgical resection. Once the diagnosis is established, resection is not recommended unless the lesion can be easily removed by wedge resection as discussed by Johnson and Sarosi (1995). Most groups recommend treatment after pulmonary resection unless the lesion was completely resected.

Aspergillosis

Definition

In aspergillosis, the usually saprophytic *Aspergillus fumigatus*, or some other member of the species, has given rise to one of three clinical syndromes: *Aspergillus* hypersensitivity lung disease, aspergilloma (fungus ball), or invasive

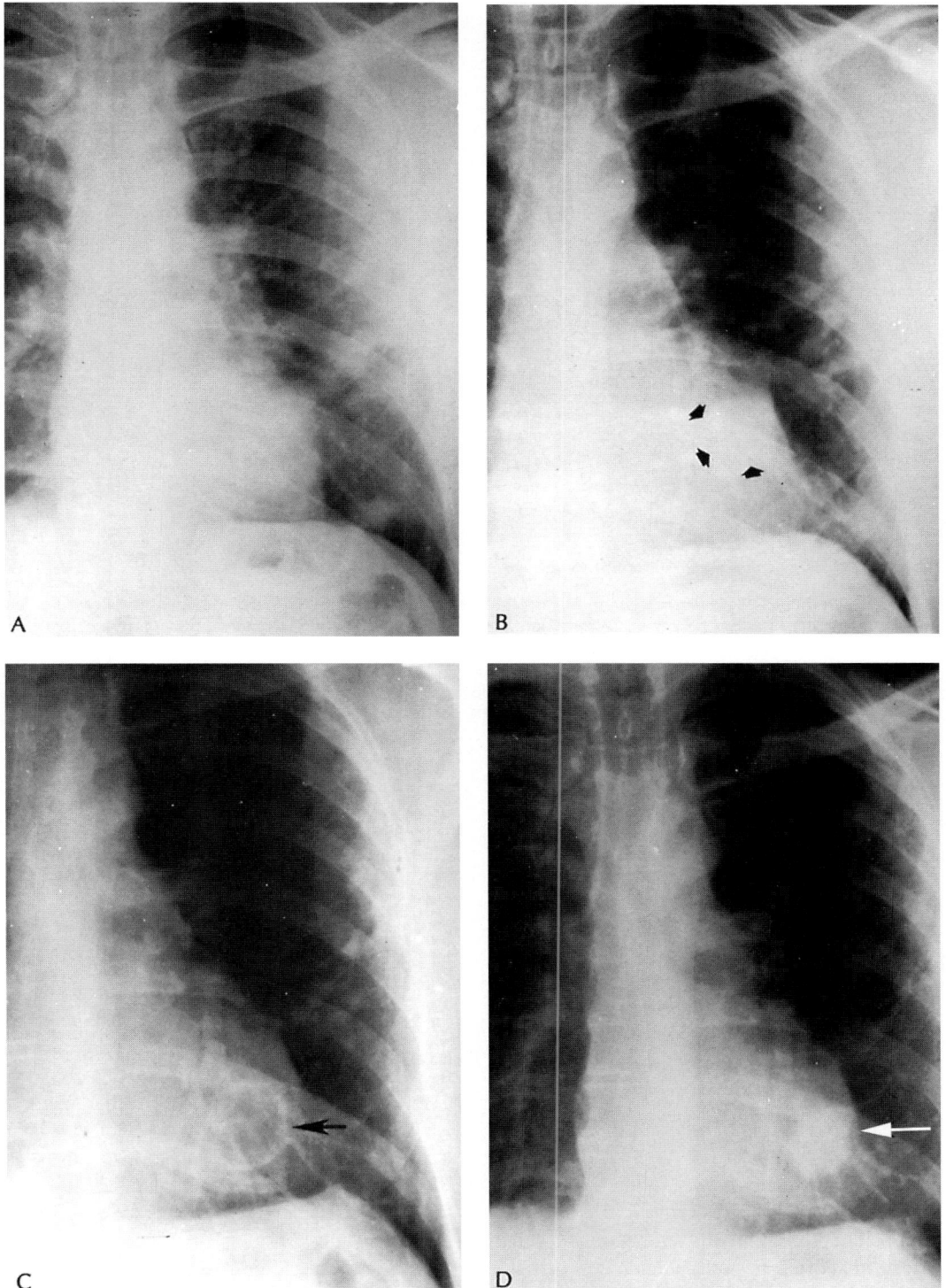

Fig. 86-16. Evolution of a cryptococcoma. **A.** Routine thoracic radiograph of a 54-year-old man with no symptoms referable to the chest shows scattered infiltrative lesions in the left lung. An open lung biopsy was carried out after an unrewarding diagnostic workup; biopsies showed multiple small granulomas containing numerous encapsulated yeast forms characteristic of cryptococci. Mouse virulence tests were confirmatory. Examination of spinal fluid showed no organisms. A course of treatment with amphotericin B was discontinued after 1.5 g had been administered, because of thrombosed veins. **B.** Four months later, a solitary nodule behind the cardiac shadow is seen (*arrows*): The infiltrative lesions have regressed. **C.** Eighteen months later, a thin-walled cavity is seen at the site of the solitary nodule (*arrow*). **D.** Forty months after the process was first noted, a dense, shrunken, irregular nodular lesion is noted (*arrow*). The patient remained without pulmonary symptoms.

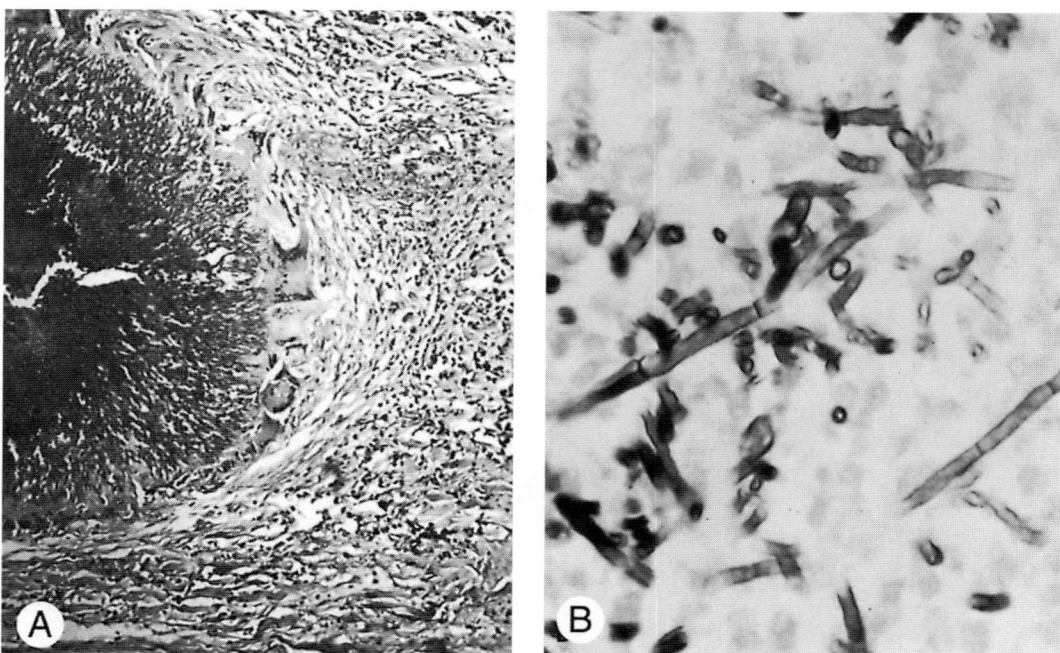

Fig. 86-17. Organisms of *Aspergillus fumigatus* in tissues. **A.** Small colony of aspergilli found in a resected carcinomatous lesion of the lung. Note mycelia radiating outward from the darker center of the colony (×250). From Takaro T: Lung infections and interstitial pneumonopathies. *In* Sabiston DC, Spencer FC (eds): Gibbon's surgery of the chest. Philadelphia: Saunders, 1976. With permission. **B.** Close-up of coarse, septate, fragmented mycelia of *A. fumigatus*. Round bodies are mycelia seen from the end (Gomori's stain, ×950). From Takaro T: Thoracic actinomycotic and mycotic infections. *In* Goldsmith HS (ed): Practice of Surgery. Hagerstown, MD: Harper & Row, 1978. With permission.

pulmonary aspergillosis. Considerable clinical overlap occurs between these syndromes and the clinical manifestations are closely related to the immune status of the patient. In the past, only the aspergilloma was of special interest to surgeons. Because of the extremely poor results of medical therapy, however, several investigators are advocating the benefits of surgical therapy in immunosuppressed patients with invasive pulmonary infections.

Pathogenesis

In the three clinical forms of aspergillosis, *A. fumigatus* is the fungus most commonly isolated, but *Aspergillus flavus*, *Aspergillus niger*, *Aspergillus nidulans*, and *Aspergillus clavatus* are other identified species. These filamentous fungi are found in soil and on decaying vegetation and produce airborne spores that are especially abundant at certain times of the year. Arnow and associates (1978) pointed out that hospital air can become contaminated with *Aspergillus* spores both from within (e.g., false ceilings) and without (e.g., ventilation systems), a serious consideration for immunosuppressed patients. In pathologic materials, usually only the coarse, fragmented, septate, branching hyphae appear either as short strands or as ball-like clusters and can be identified only by isolation and culture (Fig. 86-17).

Because aspergilli are saprophytic and ubiquitous, unless the material has been obtained under aseptic conditions, a diagnosis of aspergillosis cannot safely be made simply by culturing the fungi.

Most of the surgically resected lesions of aspergillosis are aspergillomas. A fungus ball is actually a matted sphere of hyphae, fibrin, and inflammatory cells, which appears grossly as a round or oval, friable, gray, red, brown, or yellow necrotic-looking mass. It is ordinarily found lying in an upper lobe cavity, the wall of which is often smooth and may be thick or thin with relatively little evidence of inflammatory reaction. The cavitary disease results from previous chronic lung disease such as tuberculosis, sarcoidosis, histoplasmosis, bronchiectasis, bronchogenic cyst, chronic lung abscess, or cavitating carcinoma. Rarely, no obvious evidence of preexisting pulmonary damage exists (Fig. 86-18). Robinson and associates (1995) found that resected pulmonary tissue from patients with invasive aspergillosis grossly consisted of hemorrhagic necrosis and varying degrees of cavitation filled with mycotic lung sequestrum and surrounding lung consolidation. This widespread necrosis of the tissue creates multiple wedge-shaped areas of infarction. Microscopically, the specimens showed hemorrhagic infarction with necrotic lung invaded by hyphae. Methenamine silver staining revealed abundant septate hyphae, often with vessel invasion and thrombosis.

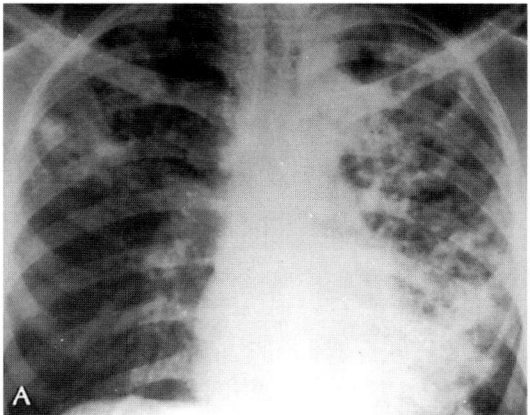

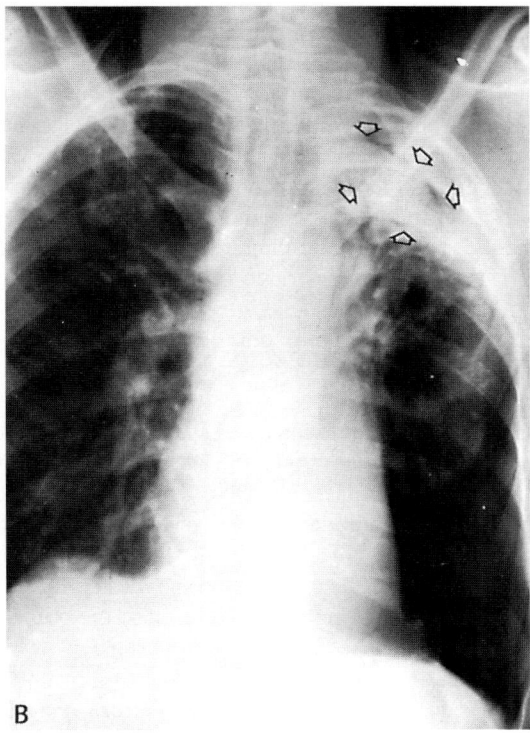

Fig. 86-18. Evolution of an aspergilloma. **A.** Thoracic radiograph in 1959 from a 30-year-old man with advanced cavitary pulmonary tuberculosis. He received multiple drug therapy for many months and sputum was last positive in 1962. **B.** Radiograph obtained in 1973 (14 years later) because of occasional mild hemoptysis shows aspergilloma, or fungus ball. Note radiolucent space between fungus ball and cavity wall (*arrows*). Severe chronic obstructive lung disease precluded resection, although the disease appeared to be localized. Chronic hemoptysis continued. Little change occurred in the patient's condition or the radiographs over a 2-year period. The patient ultimately died 16 years after the radiograph shown in **A** was obtained and 2 years after the discovery of the fungus ball, of "extensive pulmonary infection." Patients with this type of complex aspergilloma often do not do well after surgical therapy, but medical treatment also has little to offer.

Symptomatology

In certain cases, symptoms may be attributable to the aspergilloma. Cough with bloody or blood-streaked sputum, however, frequently occurs, although histopathologic examination of the resected lesion may reveal no bleeding point. Sometimes, hemoptysis is severe to exsanguinating. The first symptoms of the invasive form of aspergillosis usually are those of acute pulmonary infection with fever, cough, dyspnea, and often pleuritic chest pain. Symptoms can initially resemble a pulmonary embolus with a combination of dyspnea, chest pain, and hemoptysis. If not recognized and treated early in the immunosuppressed patient, manifestations of worsening pulmonary function and distant spread may rapidly progress.

Diagnosis

Finding *Aspergillus* in the sputum alone does not justify the diagnosis of aspergillosis. If the clinical picture of aspergilloma is present and sputum culture results are positive for *Aspergillus*, the diagnosis is probable.

Griepp (1975) reported that transtracheal aspirates or direct lung aspirates by thin-walled 18-gauge needles may provide a definitive diagnosis and are especially useful in immunosuppressed patients.

Levitz (1989) has stated that precipitating antibodies against *A. fumigatus* in the serum, skin sensitivity to *Aspergillus* antigen, or characteristic radiographic shadows are confirmatory evidence. An aspergilloma can sometimes be identified radiographically as a mass shifting within a cavity or cyst on changes in position of the patient. Thus, in a radiograph of the thorax exposed in the upright position, a crescentic radiolucency above a rounded radiopaque lesion suggests aspergilloma (Monad's sign) (Fig. 86-19).

Treatment

Medical

Successful medical therapy relies more on the patient's underlying pulmonary disease and immune status than the type of treatment instituted. Isolated cures have been reported after treatment with iodides, nystatin, itraconazole, and with amphotericin B, which is the drug of choice. Hammerman and associates (1974), however, found that intravenous amphotericin B was no more effective than a pulmonary toilet regimen in the treatment of patients with aspergillomas. Some groups have had good results using transthoracic or transbronchial installation of therapeutic agents. Remy and coworkers (1977) reported that embolization of the bronchial arteries in a few patients with massive or repeated hemoptysis caused by aspergilloma resulted in initial remission in four of six cases, but recurrence of bleeding occurred in three of the

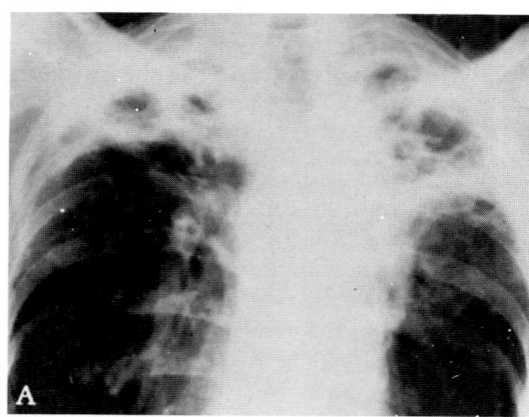

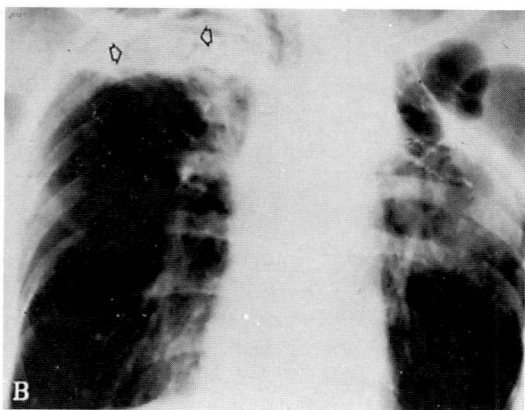

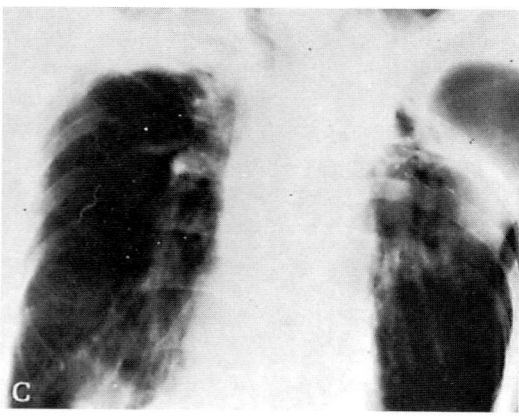

Fig. 86-19. Evolution of bilateral cavitary disease with colonization by aspergilli; surgical treatment. **A.** Thoracic radiograph of a 55-year-old man with symptoms of gradually increasing weakness and weight loss. No positive findings were found on workup other than the destructive lung lesions. Pulmonary ventilatory function was only mildly impaired; segmental resection of the left upper lobe and four-rib thoracoplasty were carried out. Pathologic findings were nonspecific inflammatory disease with a cavity containing soft, brown masses, which proved to be colonies of *Aspergillus*. A chronic bronchocutaneous fistula developed and gradually closed after 3 months. **B.** Two years later, a distinct new fungus ball can be identified in the right upper cavity (*arrows*), with characteristic radiolucent area around the ball. There were few symptoms. **C.** Four years later, radiograph reveals regression of the disease process in the right lung without specific therapy.

four initially controlled. Denning and Stevens (1990) noted that medical treatment has been generally unsatisfactory for invasive aspergillosis and that results may be improved in neutropenic patients when a higher dose of amphotericin B is used (1.0 to 1.5 mg/kg per day). Eastridge (1976) suggested that the definite toxic effects of amphotericin B have been overemphasized, and that treatment failures sometimes are attributable to premature cessation of treatment, rather than lack of efficacy.

Surgical

Surgical treatment is controversial. According to Daly and colleagues (1986), management philosophy is more readily grasped when aspergillomas are classified as either simple (i.e., thin-walled localized cysts with little surrounding parenchymal disease) or complex (i.e., thick-walled cavities associated with gross evidence of parenchymal disease). Because the complication rate after surgery in the latter group is high, symptoms of hemoptysis or cough, or both, should be significant enough to warrant the risk of surgery. On the other hand, patients with simple aspergillomas with even minimal symptoms may be offered surgery because the risk is low and the likelihood of long-term cure is much improved, as Eastridge (1972), Karas (1976), and Daly (1986) and their associates suggested.

Clearly, no unanimity of opinion exists in this regard: Varkey and Rose (1976) and Bower (1977) and Faulkner (1978) and their colleagues, as well as Pennington (1980), take differing views. Individualizing surgical management is clearly critical, as Battaglini (1985) and Butz (1985) and their colleagues emphasized. Allan and colleagues (1986) pointed out that additional surgical measures, short of pulmonary resection, in any event, should be as conservative as possible. Daly and colleagues (1986) suggested, in patients with peripheral and complex aspergillomas, the obliteration of the cavity by transposing muscle from the chest wall into the cavity may be the procedure of choice. Niwa and colleagues (1995) advocate arteriography before resection of aspergillomas and, if indicated, embolization of bronchial arteries or subclavian artery branch ligation to reduce intraoperative blood loss.

Aspergillus empyema, or pleural aspergillosis, was reported by Herring and Pecora (1976) and others and has been treated by intrapleural amphotericin B, or nystatin, and by pleural drainage, pleurectomy, thoracoplasty, and repair of bronchopleural fistulas (see Chapter 60).

Surgery has been suggested by Lupinetti and associates (1992) to have a role in salvaging patients with invasive *Aspergillus* infection after bone marrow transplantation and for other immunodeficient patients. Patients being evaluated for bone marrow transplant, or any procedure that may reduce the patient's immune system, should be screened for possible cavitary lung disease that could be harboring indolent *Aspergillus*. Robinson and colleagues (1995) have had good results operating on immunocompromised patients with hematologic disease or after liver transplantation.

Eleven of 16 patients survived after resection of invasive *Aspergillus*. Temeck and associates (1994) found that angioinvasion in the resected specimen correlated with operative mortality in immunosuppressed patients without human immunodeficiency virus.

Candidiasis (Moniliasis)

Definition

Candidiasis is an acute, subacute, or chronic superficial fungus infection caused by species of *Candida*, usually *Candida albicans*, which commonly affects the skin or the oral, bronchial, or vaginal mucosa. Much less commonly, it can also be a deep or systemic infection, involving the lungs, blood, endocardium, meninges, or almost any other organ. Other fungi of this genus that are occasionally pathogenic to humans are *Candida guiliermondii*, *Candida stellatoidea*, *Candida parakrusei*, *Candida tropicalis*, and *Candida glabrata*.

Epidemiology

Candida occurs in the oropharynx of many normal individuals. It is a common hospital and laboratory contaminant, probably of universal distribution.

Pathogenesis

Candida organisms appear in fresh or potassium hydroxide preparations or on Gram's stain as small (2.5 to 4.0 μm) oval, thin-walled, budding cells with or without mycelial elements (Fig. 86-20). An acute or chronic granulomatous reaction may result. In systemic infections, both mycelial and yeast forms may appear in clusters surrounded by polymorphonuclear leukocytes, forming microabscesses. The fungi also may invade the tissues and blood vessel walls, with little evidence of inflammatory reaction in some instances. Thomas (1977) and Wray (1973) and their associates reported costal chondritis as well as osteomyelitis of the sternum caused by *Candida*.

Clinical Picture and Diagnosis

The importance of this opportunistic fungus infection lies in the slowly but steadily increasing incidence of disseminated disease noted since the 1970s. This phenomenon is essentially iatrogenic, as Louria and colleagues (1962) noted; before the advent of broad-spectrum antibiotics, disseminated disease with invasion of internal organs, septicemia, and endocarditis were almost unheard of.

In the presence of intensive or prolonged antibiotic therapy, especially with multiple drugs, or of immunosuppressive therapy after organ transplantation, the normal bacterial flora of patients may be suppressed, allowing an

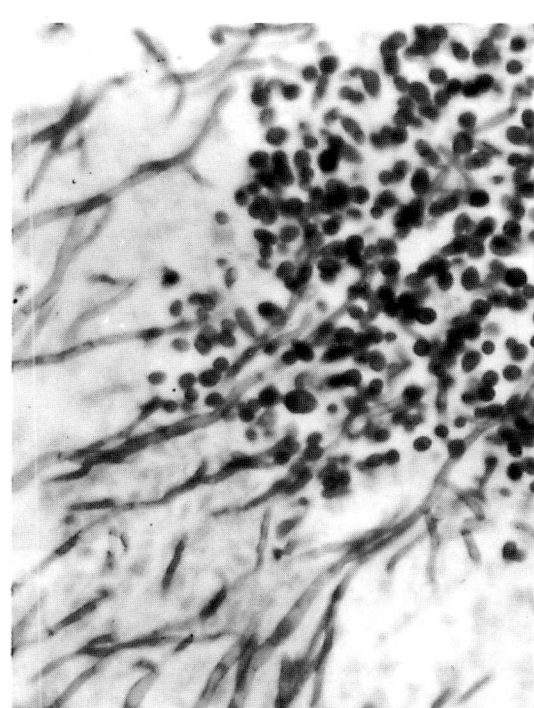

Fig. 86-20. Organisms of *Candida albicans* show both yeast and mycelial forms (Gomori's stain, ×1000). From Takaro T: Thoracic actinomycetic and mycotic infections. *In* Goldsmith HS (ed): Practice of Surgery. Hagerstown, MD: Harper & Row, 1978. With permission.

overgrowth of the often present saprophytic species of *Candida*. This type of superinfection also occurs in patients with AIDS. Invasion then takes place through any portal of entry: the skin, blood (by way of needles or catheters used for intravenous therapy), lungs, or gastrointestinal tract. In the presence of altered host immunity or inhibited inflammatory response for any of various reasons, *Candida* pneumonia, abscess, which Rubin and Alroy (1977) reported, or septicemia and generalized infection may result, often with a fatal outcome. Orringer and Sloan (1978) observed monilial esophagitis with stricture formation, and Spear and colleagues (1976) reported tracheal obstruction associated with *Candida* fungus ball. Thus, although the presence of a species of *Candida* in the sputum of many healthy persons ordinarily is of no diagnostic or prognostic importance, the same cannot be said for the finding of *Candida* in bronchial or lung biopsies, in blood, or in deep tissue spaces. One cannot lightly dismiss such reports as reflecting laboratory contamination, especially not in immunosuppressed or otherwise compromised patients who have symptoms and signs of pneumonia, or of septicemia. Because of the high mortality associated with *Candida* septicemia, Anaissie and Solomkin (1994) recommend early presumptive antifungal therapy for patients with known risk factors who remain febrile despite receiving broad-spectrum antibiotic therapy who are known to have at least one culture showing *Candida* species.

As in the case of the other opportunistic fungi such as *A. fumigatus*, *C. neoformans*, and *Mucor*, the circumstances that place a patient at risk are multiple antibiotics, malignancy, neutropenia, immunosuppressive therapy, urinary catheters, diarrhea, surgical procedures, especially on the gastrointestinal tract, concomitant bacteremia, and extensive burns.

Treatment

The combination of 5-fluorocytosine and amphotericin B is the most proven regimen available for *Candida* tissue infections. Of four patients with *Candida* pneumonias reported by Howard and associates (1978) who were treated with amphotericin B, two of whom received 5-fluorocytosine also, all four made short-term recoveries, with two late deaths unrelated to the *Candida* pneumonia. Early diagnosis and vigorous treatment give these patients a considerably more promising outlook. Dyess and associates (1985) reported that *Candida* septicemia is associated with a mortality of 52%. On the other hand, Strinden and colleagues (1985) reported long-term survival in six of eight patients with septic thrombosis of the central veins caused by *Candida* who had intensive therapy with amphotericin B. Rex and coworkers (1994) from the Mycoses Study Group described a randomized trial comparing amphotericin B and fluconazole in the treatment of candidemia in patients who are not neutropenic. Fluconazole was found to be an equally effective treatment with less toxicity.

Glower and associates (1990) reported that *Candida* mediastinitis is a lethal complication of cardiac surgery (55% mortality) requiring drainage, débridement, vascularized flaps, amphotericin B, and 5-fluorocytosine. *Candida* prosthetic valve endocarditis is difficult to cure even with valve replacement and amphotericin B. Johnson (1991) and Muehrcke (1995) and their coworkers suggested that long-term suppression with fluconazole may be necessary. Acalculous *Candida* cholecystitis is a morbid complication occurring in seriously ill patients after major trauma or surgery. Hiatt and associates (1991) found that cholecystectomy and amphotericin B are necessary.

Sporotrichosis

Sporotrichosis is a mycotic infection caused by *Sporotrichum schenckii*, a cigar-shaped, dimorphic organism that stains bright red with periodic acid–Schiff stains. The disease is characterized by cutaneous and lymphatic involvement ordinarily, and pulmonary disease is relatively rare.

The causative organism is a saprophyte, under normal conditions, and is widely distributed in plants and soil. Thus, florists are especially susceptible. An epidemic involving miners exposed to infested mine timbers in South Africa was reported in 1947. Dixon and colleagues (1991) reported that in 1988, 84 forestry workers exposed to a single source of sphagnum moss were identified in a major epidemic in the United States.

Pulmonary infection produces nonspecific symptoms resembling those of pulmonary tuberculosis: fever, hemoptysis, malaise, and weight loss. Similarly, radiographic findings mimic tuberculosis in the wide variety of presenting patterns, including hilar lymphadenopathy, pleural effusion, lobular consolidation, fibrosis, and multiple nodules. Michelson (1977), Jay (1977), and Jung (1979) and their associates reported localized cavitary disease in more than 50 patients. It is necessary not only to culture the organism from sputum, bronchial washings, or lung tissue, but also to establish its pathogenicity for animals, because the organism is a saprophyte. The diagnostic value of serum agglutination tests for *Sporotrichum* is not established, but direct fluorescent antibody reliably identifies the organisms in specimens and tissue biopsies, according to Rohatgi (1980) (Fig. 86-21).

Responses of patients with pulmonary sporotrichosis have been poor. Initial therapy with itraconazole can be attempted for non–life-threatening infections. Patients who are acutely ill should receive amphotericin B, which can be switched to itraconazole if a good response is obtained. Surgery can play a useful role for localized disease, however, many of these patients have underlying severe obstructive pulmonary disease that precludes operation, as noted by Kauffman (1995). Response rates for both amphotericin B and itraconazole are a disappointing 20 to 50%, as reported by Kauffman (1996). Heller and Fuhrer (1991) reported disseminated sporotrichosis in five patients with AIDS.

Zygomycosis (Mucormycosis)

This rare but potentially lethal fungal infection is caused by genera belonging to the class Zygomycetes. These fungi are characterized structurally by broad (6 to 50 μm) nonseptate but branching hyphae (Fig. 86-22) that are difficult to culture. Among disease-causing organisms in this group are species of *Absidia*, *Rhizopus*, *Mucor*, *Mortierella*, and *Basidiobolus*.

These organisms are generally saprophytes, occurring as molds on manure and foods, and producing spores that can be inhaled. They are not ordinarily pathogenic to humans. Under special conditions of immunosuppression or compromise, they can cause disease. In the lungs, the disease is characterized by blood vessel invasion, thrombosis, and infarction of invaded organs, with marked tissue destruction, cavitation, and abscess formation.

Zygomycosis is usually a rapidly fatal disease, occurring especially in acidotic diabetics, in patients with lymphomas or leukemias, or in persons receiving intensive or prolonged antimetabolite, antibiotic, or corticosteroid therapy. Extensive necrosis of areas around the face (e.g., paranasal sinuses, orbit, mucous membranes) and of the lung and

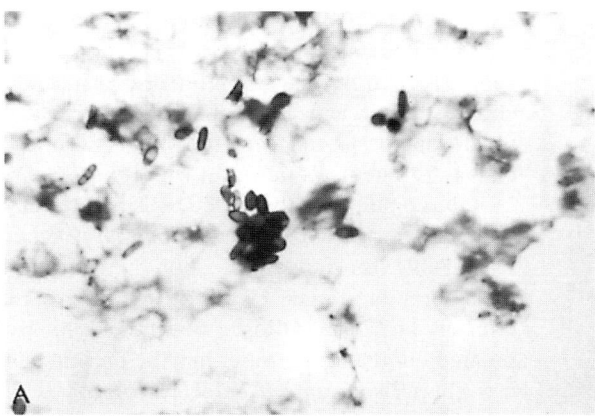

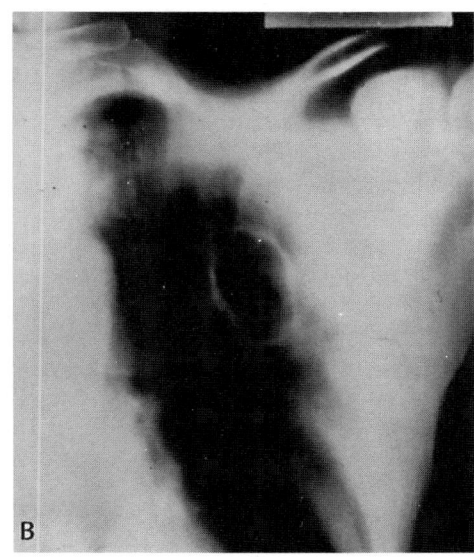

Fig. 86-21. Sporotrichosis. **A.** Cigar-shaped organisms of *Sporothrix schenckii* seen in resected lung specimen (periodic acid–Schiff stain, ×1100). **B.** Thoracic radiograph showing cavitary lesion of pulmonary sporotrichosis. From Scott SM, et al: Pulmonary sporotrichosis. N Engl J Med *265*:453, 1961. With permission.

brain may occur in addition to cutaneous and subcutaneous infection. Murray (1975) reported massive fatal pulmonary hemorrhage. Gartenberg and associates (1978) reported two patients with necrotizing chest wall infections after aorto-coronary bypass operation in which Elastoplast dressings

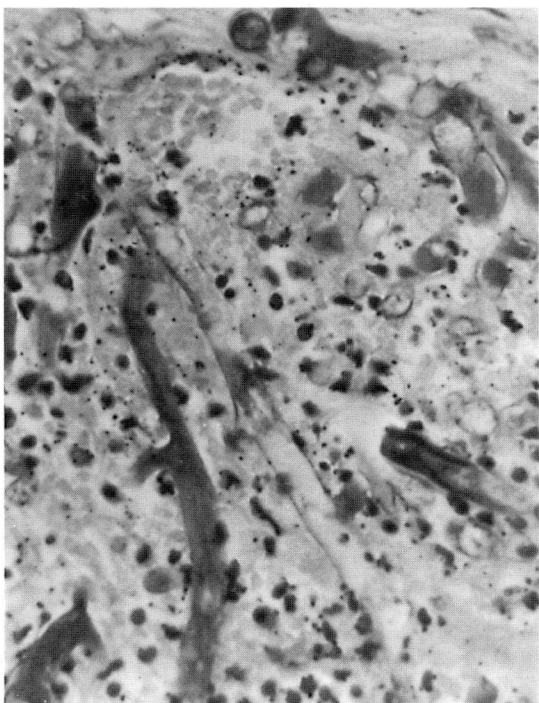

Fig. 86-22. Phycomycosis (mucormycosis). Broad, nonseptate hyphae of a phycomycete, probably *Mucor*, invading thrombosed pulmonary arterial wall (hematoxylin and eosin stain, ×330). From Takaro T: Thoracic actinomycetic and mycotic infections. *In* Goldsmith HS (ed): Practice of Surgery. Hagerstown, MD: Harper & Row, 1978. With permission.

were used; both patients died. Although amphotericin B is the only agent with some evidence of efficacy, of 18 survivors with pulmonary mucormycosis, 11 were managed by surgery alone, according to Bigby and colleagues (1986).

Early recognition, control of diabetes, and termination of antimetabolite, antibiotic, or corticosteroid therapy are all important. Parfrey (1986) noted that, with increasing premortem diagnosis, allowing more vigorous management both surgically and medically, the prognosis of this grave infection is improving. Zygomycosis has occurred after renal, hepatic, and cardiac transplantation. Pulmonary zygomycosis after renal transplantation is a lethal complication, usually associated with corticosteroid-induced diabetes. Tedder and associates (1994) reported the mortality in patients who underwent surgical resection as 11% whereas those treated medically had a 68% mortality. Surgical resection is indicated if the patient can tolerate surgery.

Pulmonary Monosporosis (Pseudallescheriasis)

This rare mycotic infection is caused by *Pseudallescheria boydii* (*Monosporium apiospermum*). This inhabitant of soil appears to act as a secondary invader of previously damaged lung tissue, such as a tuberculous cavity, cyst, or bronchial saccule. Sometimes, but not characteristically, a fungus ball is formed. Amphotericin B has not been effective. Terrell and Hughes (1992) reported miconazole as the drug of choice. Jung and associates (1977) summarized the localized resections that were performed in 10 patients, with two deaths. Conservative management is recommended for asymptomatic patients without cavitary disease or bronchiectasis. Resection is advocated for good-risk patients with localized cavitary disease, or to help make a definitive diagnosis when bronchial carcinoma is suspected.

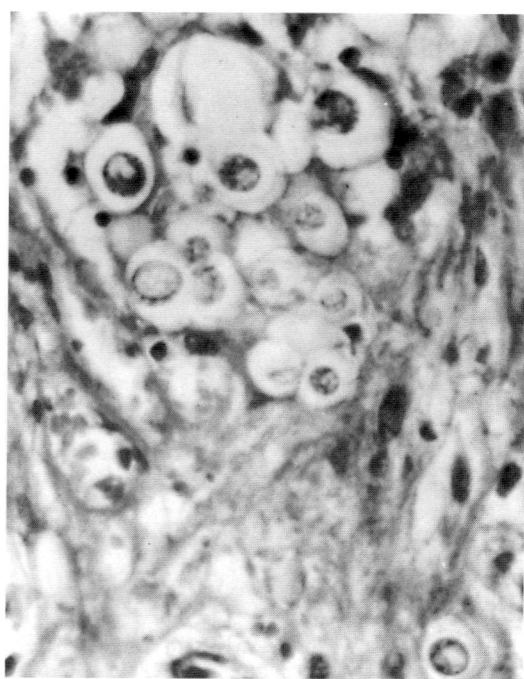

Fig. 86-23. Paracoccidioidomycosis (South American blastomycosis). Organisms of *Paracoccidioides brasiliensis*, in tissue. Note superficial resemblance to *Blastomyces dermatitidis*. From Takaro T: Thoracic actinomycetic and mycotic infections. *In* Goldsmith HS (ed): Practice of Surgery. Hagerstown, MD: Harper & Row, 1978. With permission.

Paracoccidioidomycosis (South American Blastomycosis)

Paracoccidioidomycosis is a chronic granulomatous infection involving the skin, mucous membranes, lymph nodes, and visceral organs, including the lungs; it is caused by *Paracoccidioides brasiliensis*, a soil saprophyte.

Paracoccidioidomycosis is endemic in South and Central America, where it is the most commonly occurring deep systemic fungal infection, and was not recognized outside these areas before the 1970s, as Murray (1974) and Bouza (1977) and their colleagues noted. The organisms resemble *B. dermatitidis* in tissue (Fig. 86-23). Infection results from inhalation of conidia. In one-third of patients, the disease is limited to the lungs and may resolve spontaneously. Cavitary pulmonary disease occurs and is fatal unless treated. The treatment of choice for chronic paracoccidioidomycosis, according to Stamm and Dismukes (1983), is ketoconazole. If therapy is continued for 1 year, the relapse rate is low (less than 10%). Surgical resection apparently has no place in this disease, other than lung biopsy, because bilateral disseminated and polymorphic lung lesions seem to be the rule.

Opportunistic Fungal Infections

Opportunistic infections occur in the lungs of patients receiving cancer chemotherapy, recipients of organ trans-

plants, AIDS patients, and immunocompromised patients. Factors predisposing to fungal infection include immunosuppressive drugs that compromise cell-mediated immunity, corticosteroids and antineoplastic drugs that contribute to myelosuppression and neutropenia, antibiotics, intravenous catheters, parenteral nutrition with lipids, and diabetes.

Neutropenia (less than 1000 cells per µL) associated with corticosteroids and cancer chemotherapy is the major factor responsible for fungal infection in cancer patients. The most common fungal infections in cancer patients are candidiasis and aspergillosis. Anaissie and Bodey (1990) pointed out that other fungi may be present, such as *Fusarium* spp., *Trichosporon beigelii*, *Torulopsis glabrata*, and *Zygomycetes*. The current approach to patients with antibiotic-resistant fever is intravenous amphotericin B. Ellis and coworkers (1995) showed that fluconazole may be a safer alternative; however, it may have inferior results in this patient population.

Pulmonary infections are the most common complications in transplant patients. When the infections are caused by fungi, the mortality is high. The fungi usually associated with organ and bone marrow transplantation are *Aspergillus* spp., *H. capsulatum*, *C. immitis*, *C. neoformans*, *Candida* spp., *P. boydii*, Mucoraceae, and *P. brasiliensis*.

The human immunodeficiency retrovirus, by causing selective depression of T_4 lymphocytes, impairs cell-mediated immunity, but it does not affect neutrophil function or blood monocyte phagocytosis. Because these functions are not impaired, disseminated candidiasis and invasive aspergillosis are uncommon in patients with AIDS. In a review of fungal infections in patients with AIDS, Diamond (1991) noted the following: mucocutaneous candidiasis is present in most patients with AIDS; cryptococcosis is the most common systemic fungal infection and is often the initial manifestation of AIDS; and histoplasmosis and coccidioidomycosis are also commonly encountered in endemic areas. Why blastomycosis is uncommon is unknown.

Emerging Fungal Pathogens

Some fungi previously considered harmless colonizers are now recognized as pathogens that can cause opportunistic infections. Within the Phaeohyphomycoses, the dermatiacious fungi, are the genera *Curvularia*, *Bipolaris*, *Exserohilum*, and *Alternaria*, all of which have caused human infections. The Hyalohyphomycoses are the nondermatiacious molds of which there are three pathogenic genera: *Fusarium*, *Scopulariopsis*, and *Pseudallescheria*. Disseminated *Fusarium* infection resembles that of *Aspergillus*.

Anaissie and Bodey (1989) recorded that among the less common yeasts responsible for opportunistic infection are *T. beigelii*, which causes systemic infections in neutropenic patients, *Malassezia furfur*, which causes infection in debilitated patients receiving intravenous lipids, and *Hansenula* spp., which is associated with intravenous catheter contamination.

Antimycotic Drugs

As stated previously, not all patients with proven infections require treatment with antimycotic agents. Several antifungal agents are available, and others are under study.

Amphotericin B

As shown in Table 86-2, amphotericin B, which was one of the first drugs developed for systemic and deep fungal infections, still has the widest spectrum of effectiveness. Amphotericin A and B are fermentation products of the actinomycete *Streptomyces nodosa*. They are complex lipophilic organic compounds (i.e., polyenes). Only amphotericin B has been developed for clinical use. Polyenes bind to ergosterol, which is present in the cell membranes of fungi, causing disruption and ion leakage.

Amphotericin B is poorly absorbed from the gastrointestinal tract and is effective only by the intravenous route. Because of its toxicity, it should be used only if the diagnosis is reasonably certain and spontaneous cure is unlikely. Suggested modes of administration include giving the patient a test dose of 1 mg of the drug in 250 mL of 5% glucose in water over a 20- to 30-minute period intravenously. On subsequent days, the dose is increased, advancing rapidly to a daily dose of approximately 0.5 to 0.6 mg/kg body weight in 500 mL 5% dextrose in water over a 3- to 4-hour period. Fresh material should be made daily. Drug administration is begun only after obtaining baseline laboratory data (i.e., complete blood cell count, urinalysis, blood urea nitrogen, creatinine, serum potassium, and liver function study results). Hermans (1977) suggested that a flow sheet recording data to be obtained on a continuing basis is helpful. Certain toxic side effects (e.g., headache, nausea, vomiting, fever, hypotension, delirium) may be ameliorated or prevented by adding 25 to 50 mg of hydrocortisone sodium succinate to the infusion bottle, unless the patient is already receiving corticosteroids. Blood pressure and pulse are monitored every half-hour for the duration of the infusion; renal function is monitored twice weekly at first, until azotemia stabilizes, preferably at a level below 50 mg/dL, with serum creatinine below 2 mg/dL. Then, it can be checked once a week; a double dose of drug can be given on alternate days to diminish the patient's discomfort. Pentoxifylline may help to alleviate nephrotoxicity. A total dose of 3 g of amphotericin B is a common goal, but this regimen may be individualized in accordance with the severity of the patient's illness and the known prognosis without therapy of each fungal infection. Hermans (1977) recommended 2.5 g for histoplasmosis, 1.5 g for blastomycosis, and 2 g for nonmeningitic pulmonary coccidioidomycosis. According to Bennett (1974), as well as others, significant permanent reduction of renal function is unlikely in adults at total doses up to 4 g. The use of liposomal amphotericin B allows larger doses of drug to be given with less toxicity. Sorkine and coworkers (1996) found that patients in the intensive care unit had a lower frequency of drug-associated fever, rigors, hypotension, and nephrotoxicity.

Flucytosine

5-Fluorocytosine

Some fungi contain cytosine deaminase, which converts 5-fluorocytosine into 5-fluorouracil, which inhibits DNA and RNA synthesis. The range of effectiveness of flucytosine is narrower than that of amphotericin B, but it provides more effective treatment for pulmonary and meningeal cryptococcosis when used with amphotericin B, and it also allows use of lower doses of the latter. This oral preparation is used in a dose of 150 mg/kg body weight, in divided doses, for several weeks to months. Besides mild side effects similar to those of amphotericin B, 5-fluorocytosine can cause leukopenia, anemia, thrombocytopenia, and occasionally, pancytopenia. Rarely are these side effects serious enough to require discontinuation of treatment. Harder and Hermans (1975), however, noted that when used in combination with amphotericin B, the renal damage caused by 5-fluorocytosine may lead to excessive blood levels of flucytosine.

Azoles

The azole compounds include miconazole, ketoconazole, fluconazole, itraconazole, and the investigational drugs SCH39304 and saperconazole. The azoles, by inhibiting the enzyme cytochrome P450, which converts lanosterol to ergosterol, interfere with fungus cell membrane synthesis.

Miconazole has limited use but is the primary drug for invasive *P. boydii* infections.

Ketoconazole is an oral antifungal agent with relatively low toxicity. Ketoconazole is effective against histoplasmosis and blastomycosis in immunocompetent patients with non–life-threatening disease and against paracoccidioidomycosis. Butman and colleagues (1991) have successfully used ketoconazole prophylactically in heart transplant patients with documented exposure. Because ketoconazole increased cyclosporine levels, the amount of cyclosporine required was reduced significantly, which helped reduce costs.

Fluconazole is a wide-spectrum antifungal agent that can be given orally or intravenously. It is the drug of choice for most *Candida*, cryptococcal, and coccidioidomycosis infections. Indications for use may expand as higher doses are used in clinical trials.

Itraconazole is the drug of choice for paracoccidioidomycosis, sporotrichosis, and blastomycosis. It is useful for treating candidiasis, histoplasmosis, and meningeal cryptococcosis in patients with AIDS. It is also effective against aspergillosis. Itraconazole must be given only orally and adsorption can be erratic, so blood levels should be measured.

THORACIC ACTINOMYCETIC INFECTIONS

Actinomycosis

Actinomycetic infections, including actinomycosis and nocardiosis, have traditionally, albeit mistakenly, been classified and treated along with true fungal infections of the lungs in many textbooks for many years. *Actinomyces* literally means *ray fungus*, for the radiating filaments in microcolonies, the formation of branching hyphae, and the production of spores. The actinomycetes, however, are considered closer to bacteria than to fungi and clearly respond to antibacterial rather than to antifungal agents. In the interests of common usage and expectation, however, they are considered in this chapter.

Actinomycosis is a chronic infectious disease usually caused by *Actinomyces israelii*, rarely by *Actinomyces bovis*, and characterized by chronic suppuration, chronic sinus formation, and the discharge of purulent material containing yellow-brown sulfur granules. These granules are actually microcolonies of the tangled hyphae of actinomycetes (Fig. 86-24). Because the organisms are anaerobic or microaerophilic, they require culturing under anaerobic conditions. They also require culturing of material from closed tissue spaces or from draining sinuses or abscesses; isolation from sputum or secretions from the mouth is not proof of infection, because the organism may reside normally in the oral cavity of humans.

Clinical Features

The clinical syndromes are cervicofacial (55%), thoracic (15%), abdominal (20%), and mixed organs (10%). Thoracic actinomycosis usually results from bronchopulmonary infection after entry of organisms into the lungs through the oropharynx. Characteristically, the pleura and chest wall are involved, but as Eastridge and associates (1972) reported, this is usually preceded by some type of pulmonary infiltrate, or by dense hilar lymphadenopathy. The varieties of lung involvement are nonspecific, although Hsieh and colleagues (1993) emphasized that some of the presentations of actinomycosis may suggest bronchial carcinoma. The disease process may show extensions from one of the anatomic areas to the adjacent area: usually from the cervical or abdominal areas to the thoracic area (Fig. 86-25).

The radiographic manifestations of thoracic actinomycosis, as Balikian and associates (1978a) noted, although nonspecific, often involve the chest wall or pleurae, or both. Thus, pleural effusion or empyema and rib erosion or periosteal involvement occur. Conant and Wechsler (1992) emphasized the usefulness of the thoracic CT evaluation. The CT scan is more sensitive in detecting bone involvement as well as mediastinal and hilar lymphadenopathy. Rarely, as Datta and Raff (1974) reported, the pericardium may be involved.

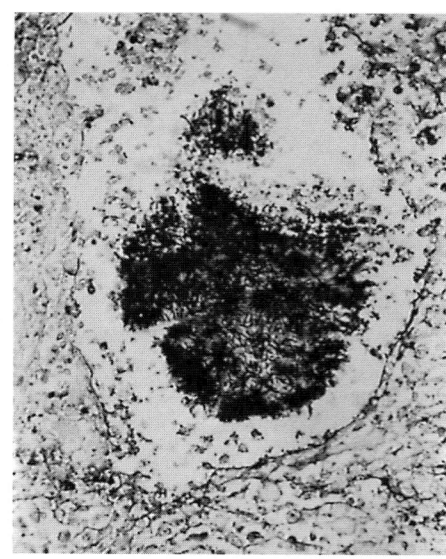

Fig. 86-24. Actinomycotic granule in a microabscess from a patient with actinomycosis. Note branching filaments in center of granule (methenamine silver, ×200).

The diagnosis of actinomycosis is difficult: first, because the disease is uncommon enough that it is not often suspected; second, because, being unsuspected, the anaerobic causative organism is often not given the appropriate cultural conditions; and third, because the radiographic resemblance to bronchial carcinoma often compels exploratory thoracotomy for diagnosis. Thus, in a series of 57 patients reported by Weese and Smith (1975), less than 10% were correctly diagnosed on admission.

Treatment

The drug of choice is penicillin. The dense fibrous tissue surrounding the colonies of organisms requires the use of high doses of antibiotics for long periods. McQuarrie and Hall (1968) recommended 20 million U of penicillin daily for 1 to 3 months. The tetracyclines, as Feingold and coworkers (1985) reported, are generally an adequate substitute when the patient is allergic to penicillin. The prognosis after effective treatment is good, as noted in a case report by Duhra and associates (1992).

Exploratory thoracotomy on suspicion of carcinoma is the most common indication for surgical intervention in patients with actinomycosis. Adequate and prolonged drug therapy is important postoperatively to prevent reactivation of disease or the development of empyema. If a preoperative diagnosis has been made, and excisional surgery is possible, for removal of a destroyed lobe, for example, it should be carried out under adequate drug coverage. Foley and associates (1971) reported that sometimes only drainage of an abscess or empyema may be possible, or necessary, but radical excision of sinus tracts may also sometimes be feasible. Primary

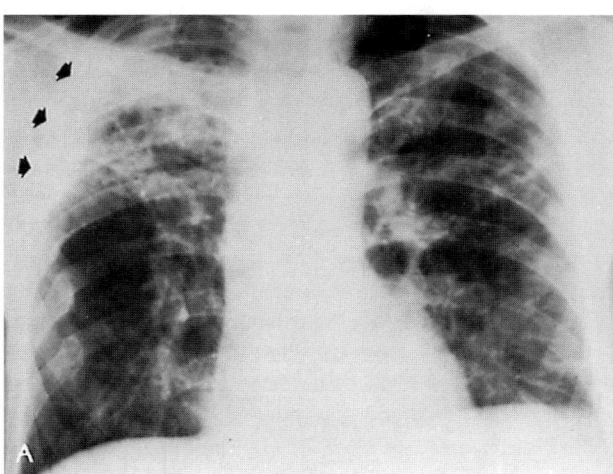
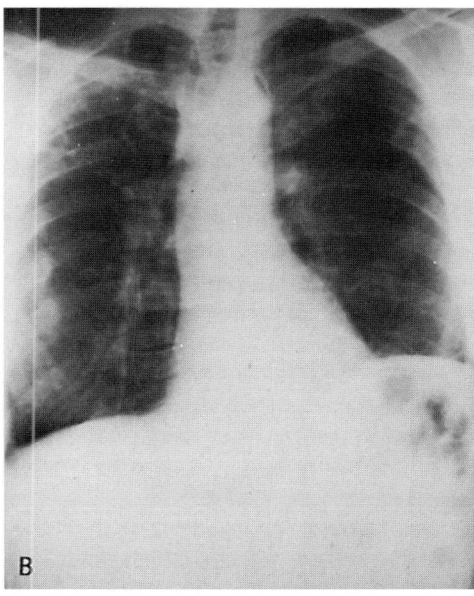

Fig. 86-25. Chronic thoracoabdominal actinomycosis. **A.** Fifty-year-old man with bilateral apical infiltrative disease was treated for presumptive diagnosis of pulmonary tuberculosis until left-sided pain, pleural fluid, and elevated diaphragm led to thoracotomy. A splenic actinomycetic abscess pointing through the diaphragm was removed; lung biopsy of extensive fibronodular disease also showed actinomycosis. Note pleural reaction, right upper lung (*arrows*), and an elevated diaphragm left. The patient was treated with 20 million U of penicillin intravenously for 1 month, followed by 4 weeks of the drug, 2.4 million U daily intramuscularly. **B.** Two years later, the disease process has cleared; except for elevated left diaphragm; chest radiograph is nearly normal. The disease did not recur over a 4-year follow-up period.

actinomycetic empyema is rare, as Harrison (1979) and Merdler (1983) and their associates noted, but George and colleagues (1985) reported that the empyema may require decortication or pleural drainage. On rare occasions, surgery may be required to control massive hemorrhage. Hamer and coworkers (1992), however, reported success with selective bronchial artery embolization.

Nocardiosis

Nocardiosis is a chronic infectious disease usually caused by *Nocardia asteroides*, but occasionally also by *Nocardia brasiliensis* and *Nocardia madurae*. Some clinical features are similar to actinomycosis (e.g., chronic draining sinuses, sulfur granules in the exudate), but some differ, such as hematogenous dissemination from a pulmonary focus or central nervous system involvement, as Frazier (1975) and Krick (1975) and their colleagues pointed out.

The organisms are aerobic and occur not only in microcolonies, but also in coccobacillary or filamentous forms that are acid-fast and gram-positive. The former feature, as well as radiographic similarities, led in the past to confusion with the acid-fast bacilli of *Mycobacterium tuberculosis* (Fig. 86-26A).

Nocardia are widely distributed in soil, grains, and grasses, without a specific area of endemicity. It does not

often occur as a saprophyte in humans; thus, its presence in sputum, together with evidence of lung involvement, is presumptive evidence of disease.

The disease process varies widely, ranging from benign, self-limited suppurative infections of the skin and subcutaneous tissues to pulmonary or generalized systemic infections. Balikian and associates (1978b) reported the radiographic features to be nonspecific pulmonary infiltrates resembling those of pulmonary tuberculosis, including solitary nodules and cavitation (Fig. 86-26B). Empyema caused by *Nocardia* is also not rare. Central nervous system involvement (i.e., brain abscess or meningitis), which is ominous, may be the presenting picture, with minimal pulmonary disease.

The disease occurs primarily in immunosuppressed patients (85% of instances) including patients receiving organ transplants, being treated for malignancies, or those with AIDS. In the compromised host, cavitation or hematogenous dissemination, or both, may be accelerated. In the absence of a predisposing condition leading to the immunosuppressed state, nocardiosis may mimic bronchial carcinoma.

The diagnosis may be difficult to establish short of percutaneous lung aspiration, closed or open lung biopsy, or exploratory thoracotomy. Gomori's stain is useful, and aerobic culture media are necessary.

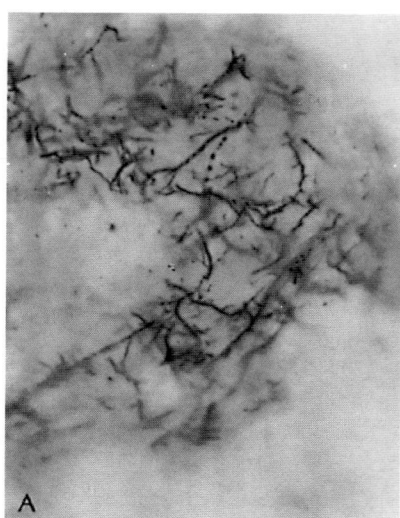 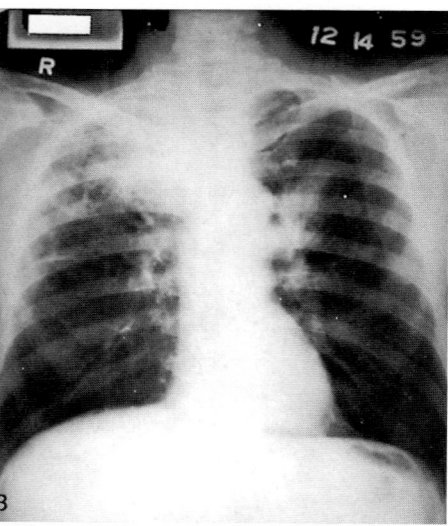

Fig. 86-26. Nocardiosis. **A.** Organisms of *Nocardia asteroides* (Gram's stain, ×1000). **B.** Radiograph of thorax showing bilateral pulmonary pneumonic infiltration. *Nocardia asteroides* was recovered from the sputum. The patient recovered after a course of sulfadiazine. From Takaro T: Thoracic actinomycetic and mycotic infections. *In* Goldsmith HS (ed): Practice of Surgery. Hagerstown, MD: Harper & Row, 1978. With permission.

Treatment is primarily medical, sulfadiazine (4 to 8 g/day) or minocycline (100 mg twice a day) being the mainstays. Prolonged treatment, at least 2 to 3 months, but sometimes longer, may be required. Surgical treatment may be required either to help make the diagnosis or, less frequently, to effect a cure. Drainage of empyemas and abscesses is indicated; with the use of specific drug coverage, this procedure has become safer.

REFERENCES

Allan A, Sethia B, Turner MA: Recent experience of the treatment of aspergilloma with the surgical stapling device. Thorax *41*:483, 1986.

Ampel NM, Wieden MA, Galgiani JN: Coccidioidomycosis: clinical update. Rev Infect Dis *2*:897, 1989.

Anaissie E, Bodey GP: Nosocomial fungal infections. Old problems and new challenges. Infect Dis Clin North Am *3*:867, 1989.

Anaissie EJ, Bodey GP: Fungal infections in patients with cancer. Pharmacotherapy *10*:164S, 1990.

Anaissie EJ, Solomkia JS: Algornion and explanation: approach to the surgical patient at risk for Candidiasis infection IX. *In* Fungal Infection. Scientific American, Inc, 1994.

Arnow PM, et al: Pulmonary aspergillosis during hospital renovation. Am Rev Respir Dis *118*:49, 1978.

Baker EJ, Hawkins JA, Waskow EA: Surgery for coccidioidomycosis in 52 diabetic patients, with special reference to related immunologic factors. J Thorac Cardiovasc Surg *75*:680, 1978.

Balikian JP, et al: Pulmonary actinomycosis. Radiology *128*:613, 1978a.

Balikian JP, Herman PG, Kopit S: Pulmonary nocardiosis. Radiology *126*:569, 1978b.

Battaglini JW, et al: Surgical management of symptomatic pulmonary aspergilloma. Ann Thorac Surg *39*:512, 1985.

Bayer AS, et al: Unusual syndromes of coccidioidomycosis. Diagnostic and therapeutic considerations: a report of 10 cases and review of the English literature. Medicine *55*:131, 1976.

Bennett JE: Chemotherapy of systemic mycoses. Parts I and II. N Engl J Med *290*:30, 320, 1974.

Bigby TD, et al: Clinical spectrum of pulmonary mucormycosis. Chest *89*:435, 1986.

Bouza E, et al: Paracoccidioidomycosis (South American blastomycosis) in the United States. Chest *72*:100, 1977.

Bower GC, et al: Pulmonary aspergilloma: a report of 25 patients. Am Rev Respir Dis *115*:90, 1977.

Bradsher RW: Blastomycosis: fungal infections of the lung update: 1989. Semin Respir Infect *5*:105, 1990.

Busey JF, et al: Blastomycosis. I. A review of 198 collected cases in Veterans Administration Hospitals. Am Rev Respir Dis *89*:659, 1964.

Butman SM, et al: Prospective study of the safety and financial benefit of ketoconazole as adjunctive therapy to cyclosporine after heart transplantation. J Heart Lung Transplant *10*:351, 1991.

Butz RO, Zvetina JR, Leininger BJ: Ten-year experience with mycetomas in patients with pulmonary tuberculosis. Chest *87*:356, 1985.

Catanzaro A, et al: Fluconazole in the treatment of chronic pulmonary and nonmeningeal disseminated coccidioidomycosis. Am J Med *98*:249, 1995.

Chick E, et al: The use of skin tests and serologic tests in histoplasmosis, coccidioidomycosis, and blastomycosis, 1973. Am Rev Respir Dis *108*:156, 1973.

Cohen SL, Gale AM, Liston HE: Report of a pilot study on noncalcified discrete pulmonary coin lesions in a coccidioidomycosis endemic area. Ariz Med *29*:40, 1972.

Conant EF, Wechsler RJ: Actinomycosis and nocardiosis of the lung. J Thorac Imaging *7*:75, 1992.

Cunningham RT, Einstein H: Coccidioidal pulmonary cavities with rupture. J Thorac Cardiovasc Surg *84*:172, 1982.

Cush R, Light RW, George RB: Clinical and roentgenographic manifestations of acute and chronic blastomycosis. Chest *69*:345, 1976.

Daly RC, et al: Pulmonary aspergilloma. Results of surgical treatment. J Thorac Cardiovasc Surg *92*:981, 1986.

Datta JS, Raff MJ: Actinomycotic pleuropericarditis. Am Rev Respir Dis *110*:328, 1974.

Davies SF, Sarosi GA: Epidemiological and clinical features of pulmonary blastomycosis. Semin Respir Infect *12*:206, 1997.

Denning DW, Stevens DA: Antifungal and surgical treatment of invasive aspergillosis: review of 2,121 published cases. Rev Infect Dis *12*:1147, 1990.

Diamond RD: The growing problem of mycoses in patients infected with the human immunodeficiency virus. Rev Infect Dis *13*:480, 1991.

Dines DE, et al: Mediastinal granuloma and fibrosing mediastinitis. Chest *75*:320, 1979.

Dismukes WE, et al: Itraconazole therapy for blastomycosis and histoplasmosis. Am J Med *93*:489, 1992.

Dixon DM, et al: Isolation and characterization of *Sporothrix schenckii* from clinical and environmental sources associated with the largest U.S. epidemic of sporotrichosis. J Clin Microbiol *29*:1106, 1991.

Drutz DJ, Catanzaro A: Coccidioidomycosis. Parts I and II. Am Rev Respir Dis *117*:559, 727, 1978.

Duhra P, Ilchyshyn A, Bell R: Thoracic actinomycosis. J R Soc Med *85*:44, 1992.

Dunn EJ, et al: Surgical implications of sclerosing mediastinitis: a report of six cases and review of the literature. Chest *97*:338, 1990.

Duperval R, et al: Cryptococcosis, with emphasis on the significance of isolation of *Cryptococcus neoformans* from the respiratory tract. Chest *72*:13, 1977.

Duswald KH, Penk A, Pittrow L: High-dose therapy with fluconazole ≥800 mg day-1. Mycoses *40*:267, 1997.

Dyess DL, Garrison RN, Fry DE: Candida sepsis. Arch Surg *120*:345, 1985.

Eastridge CE: Opportunistic infections due to aspergillosis (editorial). Ann Thorac Surg *22*:102, 1976.

Eastridge CE, et al: Pulmonary aspergillosis. Ann Thorac Surg *13*:397, 1972.

Ellis DH, Pfeiffer TJ: Ecology, life cycle, and infectious propagule of *Cryptococcus neoformans*. Lancet *336*:923, 1990.

Ellis ME, et al: Systemic amphotericin B versus fluconazole in the management of antibiotic resistant neutropenic fever—preliminary observations from a pilot, exploratory study. J Infect *30*:141, 1995.

Epstein R, Cole R, Hung KK Jr: Pleural effusion secondary to pulmonary cryptococcosis. Chest *61*:296, 1972.

Faulkner SL, et al: Hemoptysis and pulmonary aspergilloma: Operative versus nonoperative treatment. Ann Thorac Surg *25*:389, 1978.

Feingold SM, George WL, Mulligan ME: Anaerobic Infections. Part II. *In* Cotsonas NJ Jr (ed): Disease-a-Month. Chicago: Year Book, 1985.

Ferguson TB, Burford TH: Mediastinal granuloma 15-year experience. Ann Thorac Surg *1*:125, 1965.

Foley TF, Dines DE, Dolan CT: Pulmonary actinomycosis: report of 18 cases. Minn Med *54*:593, 1971.

Frazier AR, Rosenow EC III, Roberts GD: Nocardiosis: a review of 25 cases occurring during 24 months. Mayo Clin Proc *50*:657, 1975.

Galgiani JN, Ampel NM: *Coccidioides immitis* in patients with human immunodeficiency virus infections. Semin Respir Infect *5*:151, 1990.

Gartenberg G, et al: Hospital-acquired mucormycosis (*Rhizopus rhizopodiformis*) of skin and subcutaneous tissue. N Engl J Med *299*:1115, 1978.

George RB, Penn RL, Kinasewitz GT: Mycobacterial, fungal, actinomycotic and nocardial infections of the pleura. Clin Chest Med *6*:63, 1985.

Glower DD, et al: Candida mediastinitis after a cardiac operation. Ann Thorac Surg *49*:157, 1990.

Godwin JD: The solitary pulmonary nodule. Radiol Clin North Am *21*:709, 1983.

Goodwin RA Jr, DesPrez RM: Histoplasmosis. Am Rev Respir Dis *117*:929, 1978.

Goodwin RA Jr, et al: Chronic pulmonary histoplasmosis. Medicine *55*:413, 1976.

Graybill JR, et al: Itraconazole treatment of coccidioidomycosis. Am J Med *89*:282, 1990.

Griepp RB: *In* discussion of Henderson RD, et al: Surgery in pulmonary aspergillosis. J Thorac Cardiovasc Surg *70*:1088, 1975.

Hamer DH, Schwab LE, Gray R: Massive hemoptysis from thoracic actinomycosis successfully treated by embolization. Chest *101*:1442, 1992.

Hammerman KJ, Sarosi GA, Tosh FE: Amphotericin-B in the treatment of saprophytic forms of pulmonary aspergillosis. Am Rev Respir Dis *109*:57, 1974.

Harder EJ, Hermans PE: Treatment of fungal infections with flucytosine. Arch Intern Med *135*:231, 1975.

Harrison RN, Thomas DJB: Acute actinomycetic empyema. Thorax *12*:406, 1979.

Heller HM, Fuhrer J: Disseminated sporotrichosis in patients with AIDS: case report and review of the literature. AIDS *5*:1243, 1991.

Hermans PE: Antifungal agents used for deep-seated mycotic infections. Mayo Clin Proc *52*:687, 1977.

Herring M, Pecora D: Pleural aspergillosis: a case report. Am Surg *42*:300, 1976.

Hiatt JR, et al: Acalculous Candida cholecystitis: a complication of critical surgical illness. Am Surg *57*:825, 1991.

Howard RJ, Simmons RL, Najarian JS: Fungal infections in renal transplant recipients. Ann Surg *188*:598, 1978.

Hsieh MJ, et al: Thoracic actinomycosis. Chest *104*:366, 1993.

Jay SJ, Platt MR, Reynolds RC: Primary pulmonary sporotrichosis. Am Rev Respir Dis *115*:1051, 1977.

Johnson P, Sarosi G: Current therapy of major fungal diseases of the lung. Infect Dis Clin North Am *5*:635, 1991.

Johnson P, Sarosi G: The endemic mycoses: surgical considerations. Semin Thorac Cardiovasc Surg *7*:95, 1995.

Jung JY, et al: The role of surgery in the management of pulmonary monosporosis: a collective review. J Thorac Cardiovasc Surg *73*:139, 1977.

Jung JY, et al: Role of surgery in the management of pulmonary sporotrichosis. J Thorac Cardiovasc Surg *77*:234, 1979.

Kanawaty DS, Stalker JB, Munt PW: Nonsurgical treatment of histoplasma endocarditis involving a bioprosthetic valve. Chest *99*:253, 1991.

Karas A, et al: Pulmonary aspergillosis: an analysis of 41 patients. Ann Thorac Surg *22*:1, 1976.

Kauffman CA: Old and new therapies for sporotrichosis. Clin Infect Dis *21*:981, 1995.

Kauffman CA: Role of azoles in antifungal therapy. Clin Infect Dis *22*:5148, 1996.

Kerkering TM, Duma RJ, Shadomy S: The evolution of pulmonary cryptococcosis. Ann Intern Med *94*:611, 1981.

Kinasewitz GT, Penn RL, George RB: The spectrum and significance of pleural disease in blastomycosis. Chest *86*:580, 1984.

Kitchen MS, Reiber CD, Eastin GB: An urban epidemic of North American blastomycosis. Am Rev Respir Dis *115*:1063, 1977.

Klein BS, et al: Isolation of *Blastomyces dermatitidis* in soil associated with a large outbreak of blastomycosis in Wisconsin. N Engl J Med *314*:529, 1986.

Krick JA, Stinson EB, Remington JS: Nocardia infection in heart transplant patients. Ann Intern Med *82*:18, 1975.

Landis FB, Varkey B: Late relapse of pulmonary blastomycosis after adequate treatment with amphotericin-B: case report. Am Rev Respir Dis *113*:77, 1976.

Laskey W, Sarosi GA: Endogenous reinfection in blastomycosis. Am Rev Respir Dis *115*:266, 1977.

Levitz SM: Aspergillosis. Infect Dis Clin North Am *3*:1, 1989.

Levitz SM: The ecology of *Cryptococcus neoformans* and the epidemiology of cryptococcosis. Rev Infect Dis *13*:1163, 1991.

Lillington GA: Pulmonary nodules: solitary and multiple. Clin Chest Med *3*:361, 1982.

Littman ML, Walter JE: Cryptococcosis: current status. Am J Med *45*:922, 1968.

Lonky SA, et al: Acute coccidioidal pleural effusion. Am Rev Respir Dis *114*:681, 1976.

Louria DB, Stiff DP, Bennett B: Disseminated moniliasis in the adult. Medicine *41*:307, 1962.

Lupinetti FM, et al: Pulmonary resection for fungal infection in children undergoing bone marrow transplantation. J Thorac Cardiovasc Surg *104*:684, 1992.

Maresca B, Kobayashi GS: Dimorphism in *Histoplasma capsulatum*: a model for the study of cell differentiation in pathogenic fungi. Microbiol Rev *53*:186, 1989.

Marks TS, Spence WF, Baisch BF: Limited resection for pulmonary coccidioidomycosis. *In* Ajello L (ed): Coccidioidomycosis. Tucson: University of Arizona Press, 1967, p. 73.

Mathisen DJ, Grillo HC: Clinical manifestation of mediastinal fibrosis and histoplasmosis. Ann Thorac Surg *54*:1053, 1992.

McDonnell JM, Hutchins GM: Pulmonary cryptococcosis. Hum Pathol *16*:121, 1985.

McQuarrie DG, Hall WH: Actinomycosis of the lung and chest wall. Surgery *64*:905, 1968.

Merdler C, et al: Primary actinomycetic empyema. South Med J *76*:411, 1983.

Michelson E: Primary pulmonary sporotrichosis. Ann Thorac Surg *24*:83, 1977.

Minamoto GY, Rosenberg AS: Fungal infections in patients with acquired immunodeficiency syndrome. Med Clin North Am *81*:381, 1997.

Muehrcke DD, Lytle BW, Cosgrove DM: Surgical and long-term antifungal therapy for fungal prosthetic valve endocarditis. Ann Thorac Surg *60*:538, 1995.

Murray HW: Pulmonary mucormycosis with massive fatal hemoptysis. Chest *68*:65, 1975.

Nelson AR: The surgical treatment of pulmonary coccidioidomycosis. Curr Probl Surg *11*:1, 1974.

Niwa H, et al: Subclavian artery branch ligation reduces hemorrhage during resection of pulmonary aspergilloma. Ann Thorac Surg *59*:1234, 1995.

Orringer MB, Sloan H: Monilial esophagitis. Ann Thorac Surg *26*:364, 1978.

Parfrey NA: Improved diagnosis and prognosis of mucormycosis. A clinicopathologic study of 33 cases. Medicine *65*:113, 1986.

Pennington JE: Aspergillus lung disease. Med Clin North Am *64*:475, 1980.

Poe RH, et al: Pulmonary blastomycosis versus carcinoma—challenging differential. Am J Med Sci *263*:145, 1972.

Rabinowitz JG, Busch J, Buttram WR: Pulmonary manifestations of blastomycosis: radiological support of a new concept. Radiology *120*:25, 1976.

Read CT: Coin lesion, pulmonary, in the Southwest (solitary pulmonary nodules). Ariz Med *29*:775, 1972.

Remy J, et al: Treatment of hemoptysis by embolization of bronchial arteries. Radiology *122*:33, 1977.

Rex JH, et al: A randomized trial comparing fluconazole with amphotericin B for the treatment of Candidemia in patients without neutropenia. N Engl J Med *331*:1325, 1994.

Robinson LA, et al: Pulmonary resection for invasive Aspergillus infections in immunocompromised patients. J Thorac Cardiovasc Surg *109*:1182, 1995.

Rohatgi PK: Pulmonary sporotrichosis. South Med J *73*:1611, 1980.

Rohatgi PK, Schmitt RG: Pulmonary coccidioidal mycetoma. Am J Med Sci *287*:27, 1984.

Rubin AHE, Alroy GG: *Candida albicans* abscess of lung. Thorax *32*:373, 1977.

Salyer WR, Salyer DC: Pleural involvement in cryptococcosis. Chest *66*:139, 1974.

Sanders JS, et al: Exfoliative cytology in the rapid diagnosis of pulmonary blastomycosis. Chest *72*:193, 1977.

Sarosi GA, Serstock DS: Isolation of *Blastomyces dermatitidis* from pigeon manure. Am Rev Respir Dis *114*:1179, 1976.

Sarosi GA, Davies SF, Phillips JR: Self-limited blastomycosis: a report of 39 cases. Semin Respir Infect *1*:40, 1986.

Sorkine P, et al: Administration of amphotericin B in lipid emulsion decreases nephrotoxicity: results of a prospective, randomized, controlled study in critically ill patients. Crit Care Med *24*:1311, 1996.

Spear RK, Walker PD, Lampton LM: Tracheal obstruction associated with a fungus ball. Chest *70*:662, 1976.

Stamm AM, Dismukes WE: Current therapy of pulmonary disseminated fungal diseases. Chest *83*:911, 1983.

Steele JD (ed): Treatment of Mycotic and Parasitic Diseases of the Chest. Springfield, IL: Charles C Thomas, 1964.

Strinden WD, Helgerson RB, Maki DG: Candida septic thrombosis of the great central veins associated with central catheters. Ann Surg *202*:653, 1985.

Sutliff WD, Cruthirds TP: *Blastomyces dermatitidis* in cytologic preparations. Am Rev Respir Dis *108*:149, 1973.

Tedder BK, et al: Pulmonary mucormycosis: results of medical and surgical therapy. Ann Thorac Surg *57*:1044, 1994.

Temeck BK, et al: Thoracotomy for pulmonary mycoses in non-HIV-immunosuppressed patients. Ann Thorac Surg *58*:333, 1994.

Terrell CL, Hughes CE: Antifungal agents used for deep-seated mycotic infections. Mayo Clin Proc *67*:69, 1992.

Thadepalli H, et al: Pulmonary mycetoma due to *Coccidioides immitis*. Chest *71*:429, 1977.

Thomas FE Jr, et al: *Candida albicans* infection of sternum and costal cartilages: combined operative treatment and drug therapy with 5-fluorocytosine. Ann Thorac Surg *23*:163, 1977.

Turner S, Kaufman L: Immunodiagnosis of blastomycosis. Semin Respir Infect *1*:22, 1986.

Varkey B, Rose HD: Pulmonary aspergilloma: a rational approach to treatment. Am J Med *61*:626, 1976.

Weese WC, Smith IM: A study of 57 cases of actinomycosis over a 36-year period. Ann Intern Med *135*:1562, 1975.

Wheat LJ, et al: Disseminated histoplasmosis in the acquired immune deficiency syndrome: clinical findings, diagnosis and treatment, and review of the literature. Medicine *69*:361, 1990.

Wray TM, Bryant RE, Killen DA: Sternal osteomyelitis and costochondritis after median sternotomy. J Thorac Cardiovasc Surg *65*:227, 1973.

Zajtchuk R, et al: Mediastinal histoplasmosis: surgical considerations. J Thorac Cardiovasc Surg *66*:300, 1973.

READING REFERENCES

Bronnimann DA, et al: Coccidioidomycosis in the acquired immunodeficiency syndrome. Ann Intern Med *106*:372, 1987.

Davies SF, Sarosi GA: Blastomycosis. Eur J Clin Microbiol Infect Dis *8*:474, 1989.

Espinel-Ingroff A, Shadomy S: In vitro and in vivo evaluation of antifungal agents. Eur J Clin Microbiol Infect Dis *8*:352, 1989.

Gal AA, et al: The pathology of pulmonary cryptococcal infections in the acquired immunodeficiency syndrome. Arch Pathol Lab Med *110*:502, 1986.

Gale AM, Kleitsch WP: Solitary pulmonary nodule due to phycomycosis (mucormycosis). Chest *62*:752, 1972.

Graybill JR: Azole antifungal drugs in treatment of coccidioidomycosis. Semin Respir Infect *1*:53, 1986.

Hauch TW: Pulmonary mucormycosis: another cure. Chest *72*:92, 1977.

Idigbe EO, Onubogu C, John EKO: Human pulmonary nocardiosis. Microbios *69*:163, 1992.

Johnston PG, et al: Late recurrent *Candida endocarditis*. Chest *99*:1531, 1991.

Murray HW, Littman ML, Roberts RB: Disseminated paracoccidioidomycosis (South American blastomycosis) in the United States. Am J Med *56*:209, 1974.

National Institute of Allergy and Infectious Diseases Mycoses Study Group: Treatment of blastomycosis and histoplasmosis with ketoconazole. Ann Intern Med *103*:861, 1985.

Polak A, Hartman PG: Antifungal chemotherapy—are we winning? *In* Jucker E (ed): Progress in Drug Research. Basel, Switzerland: Hoffmann-La Roche, 1991.

Restrepo A, et al: Itraconazole in the treatment of paracoccidioidomycosis: a preliminary report. Rev Infect Dis *9(Suppl 1)*:S51, 1987.

Rippon JW (ed): Medical Mycology: the Pathogenic Fungi and the Pathogenic Actinomycetes. Philadelphia: WB Saunders, 1988.

Sarosi G, Davies S (eds): Fungal Diseases of the Lung. New York: Grune & Stratton, 1986.

Stansell JD: Fungal disease in HIV-infected persons: cryptococcosis, histoplasmosis, and coccidioidomycosis. J Thorac Imaging *6*:28, 1991.

Wallace RJ Jr, et al: Use of trimethoprim-sulfamethoxazole for treatment of infections due to Nocardia. Rev Infect Dis *4*:315, 1982.

Warnock DW: Amphotericin B: an introduction. J Antimicrob Chemother *28*:27, 1991.

CHAPTER 87

Pleuropulmonary Amebiasis

Mohan Verghese, Rajeev Kapoor, and Forrest C. Eggleston

Pleuropulmonary amebiasis is almost invariably the result of perforation of an amebic liver abscess through the diaphragm. It accounts for 10% of all deaths from amebiasis. To understand its management, the nature of amebiasis and of the liver abscess it produces must be understood.

AMEBIASIS

Amebiasis is caused by the protozoan *Entamoeba histolytica*. The ameba's life cycle has three stages: trophozoite, precyst, and cyst (Fig. 87-1). Infection results from the ingestion of cysts, usually from contaminated food or water. Excystation occurs in the lower ileum. The resulting trophozoites are the active and growing stage of the parasite. Multiplication is by binary fission. The trophozoites can invade the mucosa of the bowel. Invasion is probably the result of physical means combined with production of the lytic substances from which the parasite derives its descriptive name. If the trophozoites do not invade the bowel, they become precysts and then cysts, finally being eliminated in the stool (Fig. 87-2).

According to the World Health Organization, the protozoan *E. histolytica* is present in the gastrointestinal tract of more than 10% of the world's population. However, only approximately 10% of those harboring the parasite develop symptomatic infection. Although amebic infestation occurs throughout the world, clinical infection is far more frequent in tropical and subtropical climates, particularly in areas with inadequate sanitation, poor nutrition, poverty, and overcrowding. Stress, decreased resistance, and the administration of corticosteroids can be important contributing factors.

Morphologic differences distinguish all species in the genus *Entamoeba* except for *E. histolytica* and *Entamoeba hartmanni*, which are identified primarily by size. *E. hartmanni* was formerly known as the "small race" of *E. histolytica*, and is now considered saprophytic. It is the "large race" of *E. histolytica* that produces disease in humans. Several strains or species of ameba, morphologically indistin-

guishable but possibly differing in their pathogenic potential, make up the species complex known as *E. histolytica*. This may account for differences in clinical findings and therapeutic results in geographically separated centers.

Intestinal amebiasis may be acute or chronic. The acute form produces cramping abdominal pain, diarrhea, and tenesmus. The stool frequently contains blood. The chronic form may persist for a long time with alternating bouts of diarrhea and constipation. Many patients who develop liver abscesses, however, give no history of gastrointestinal symptoms.

AMEBIC LIVER ABSCESS

When amebae invade the colonic mucosa, particularly in the cecum, they may be carried to the liver through the portal venous system. There they lodge in the venules, producing thrombosis that is followed by an infarct, necrosis of liver tissue, and a localized abscess. This is not an abscess in the classic sense, but rather a collection of necrotic liver tissue with white blood cells and amebae in the center. The amebae in the periphery multiply, releasing lytic enzymes, resulting in additional necrosis and enlarging the abscess. No fibrous capsule or clear margin exists between the abscess and the surrounding tissue. Although the parasite does not normally stimulate the intense inflammatory response of other infective agents, it may do so under certain conditions, particularly if secondarily infected.

Because of the combination of the laminar flow of the portal venous system and the high incidence of cecal involvement, the right lobe of the liver is most commonly involved. In his review, Grigsby (1969) found that 85% of amebic liver abscesses were in the right lobe and 15% were in the left lobe; both lobes were involved in 15 to 20% of cases. Our own figures are similar.

Although these abscesses may occur at any age, they are most frequent in the third to fifth decade of life. In adults, men are infected seven to nine times as often as women; in children, no sex difference is noted.

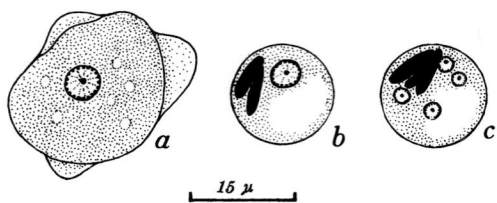

15 μ

Fig. 87-1. *Entamoeba histolytica.* **a.** Trophozoite. **b.** Immature cyst, precystic form. **c.** Cystic or resistant form. Modified from Faust EC, Russell PE: Clinical Parasitology. 7th Ed. Philadelphia: Lea & Febiger, 1964.

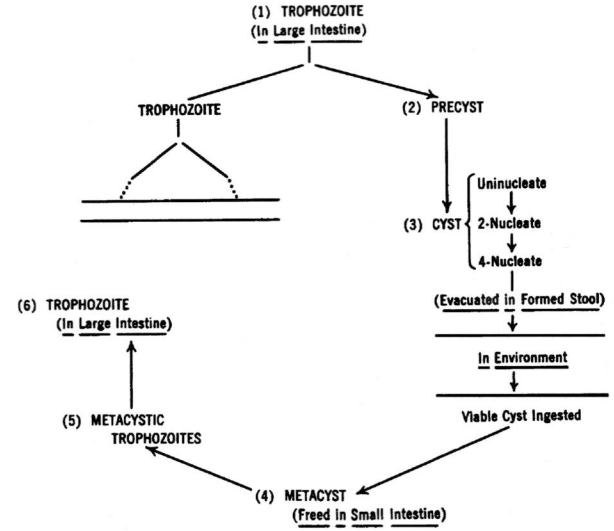

Fig. 87-2. Life cycle of *Entamoeba histolytica.* Modified from Faust EC, Russell PE: Clinical Parasitology. 7th Ed. Philadelphia: Lea & Febiger, 1964.

Symptoms of an amebic liver abscess may be present for a few days to many months before patients seek help. In our and associates' (1978) experience, the average duration was 33 days. Symptoms vary, and as a result, the diagnosis is not clear in one-third of cases.

Virtually all patients have pain, most commonly in the right hypochondrium (73%). Pain also may occur in the epigastrium, left hypochondrium, or right hemithorax. When associated with diaphragmatic irritation, it may be referred to the shoulder. The pain may be mild, moderate, or severe and usually is constant. Many patients complain of a swelling in the upper abdomen. Anorexia, fever, and malaise are usual, and patients whose treatment has been delayed may have profound weight loss.

A history of diarrhea, although helpful in making a diagnosis, is given by less than one-half of all patients. Blood in the stool is noted in only approximately 25% of patients.

Examination of the abdomen shows a large, tender liver. Softening suggests imminent rupture of the amebic liver abscess. In addition, intercostal pressure reveals tenderness. Pleural effusion is common. Jaundice is uncommon, but when present, it is associated with a poor prognosis.

Proctosigmoidoscopy is useful only if punctate lesions are found in the mucosa or amebae are seen on examination of swab material.

Leukocytosis (12,000 to 30,000 cells/μL) is the rule. Liver function test shows moderate elevation of alkaline phosphatase, bilirubin, and transaminases. Serologic test results, if positive, suggest current or previous invasive amebiasis. According to Sharma and colleagues (1988), enzyme-linked immunosorbent assay technique is highly sensitive and easily available, and the test can be completed in approximately 35 minutes. The test result may be negative in the first week; the titer may peak in 3 months and decrease to lower but detectable levels in 9 months. This test may not be useful in endemic areas, where widespread colonic invasion of ameba results in high titers without hepatic involvement. In these areas, its value remains in differentiating it from pyogenic liver abscess and other cystic lesions of the liver.

Chest radiography usually shows an elevated diaphragm, often accompanied by pleural effusion (Fig. 87-3). Computed

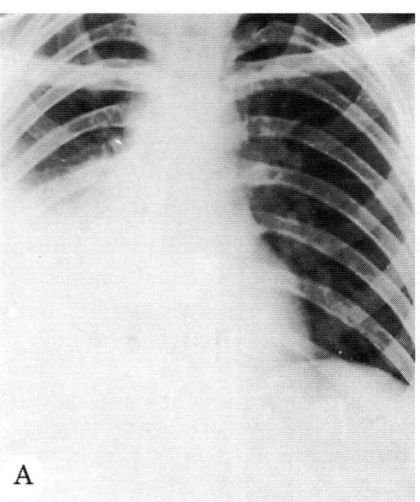

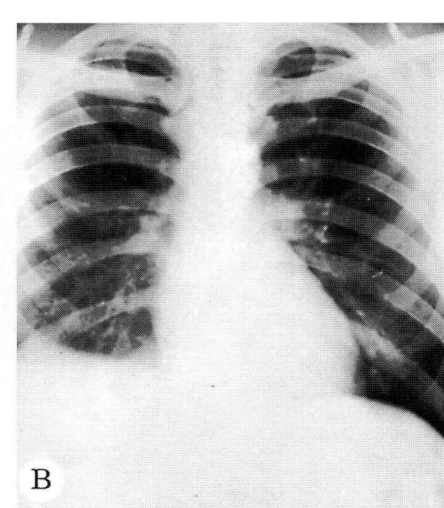

A

B

Fig. 87-3. Simple irritative pleuritis with effusion in the right hemithorax. **A.** Before treatment. **B.** After treatment.

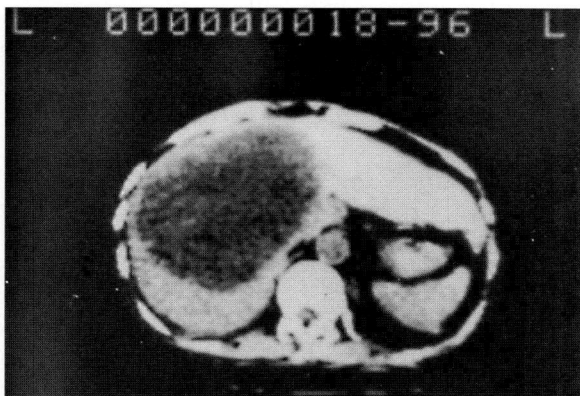

Fig. 87-4. Computed tomographic scan shows a large abscess in the right lobe of the liver.

tomography (Fig. 87-4), ultrasonography (Fig. 87-5), magnetic resonance imaging, and isotopic imaging all demonstrate both the presence and site of liver abscesses. However, in the acute situation, computed tomography, magnetic resonance imaging, and isotope imaging are not any better than ultrasonography. Ultrasound is inexpensive, easy to perform, and has a diagnostic accuracy of 90%. Ultrasound is the best investigation for following up the size of the abscess on treatment. When aspirated, the pus is usually reddish brown or chocolate brown, the so-called anchovy sauce, although initially it may be yellowish or even white. Unless the amebic liver abscess was aspirated previously, it is bacteriologically sterile. Amebae can be demonstrated in only approximately one-half of the abscesses.

Because of the lytic nature of the parasite and the lack of encapsulation of amebic liver abscesses, rupture occurs in from 10 to 30% of patients. The anatomic location of amebic liver abscesses makes upward or transdiaphragmatic rupture more frequent than downward or infradiaphragmatic rupture (Fig. 87-6).

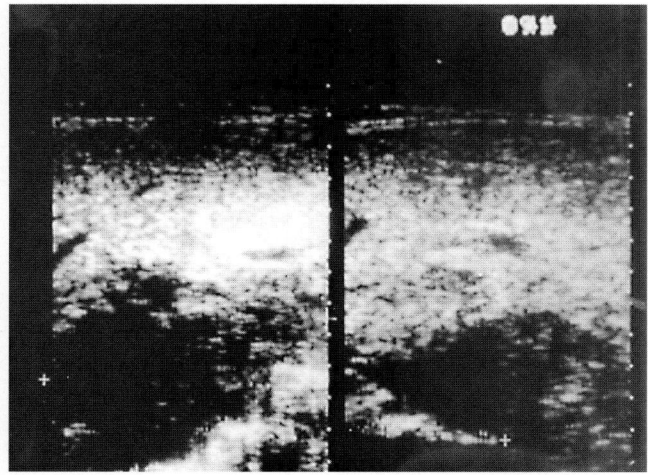

Fig. 87-5. Sonogram. Parasagittal and subcostal sections show a large liver abscess 6 cm below the skin.

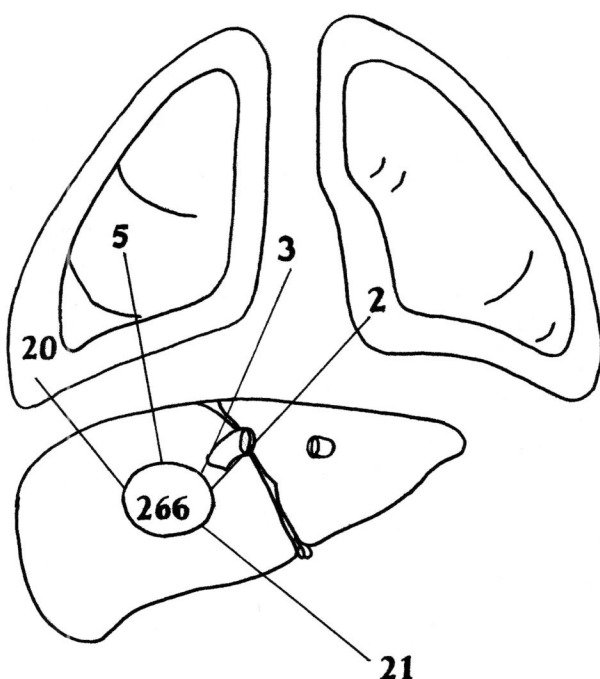

Fig. 87-6. Site of perforation in 266 consecutive patients admitted in our hospital with amebic liver abscess. Thirty (59%) of the perforations were into the thorax and 20 were into the abdomen. A total of 51 perforations were seen in 42 patients.

THORACIC AMEBIASIS

In amebiasis, 70 to 97% of thoracic complications result from extension of an amebic liver abscess through the diaphragm. The type of complication depends on whether the pleural space, lung, or pericardium is involved, either singly or in combination. We shall consider only pleural and pulmonary involvement.

Most patients have the clinical signs of an amebic liver abscess in addition to those related to the thoracic complication.

Pleural Involvement

An amebic liver abscess adjacent to the diaphragm produces irritation and a sympathetic pleural effusion. On chest radiography, the diaphragm is elevated and fixed. The costophrenic angle is obliterated. Sympathetic pleural effusion was present in 15% of cases in our current experience of 266 patients with an amebic liver abscess. Thoracentesis shows that the fluid is clear or serosanguinous and sterile on culture. Amebae are not present. This pleural effusion requires no specific therapy other than that for the causative liver abscess. Should it increase, however, it may presage the rupture of the abscess through the diaphragm and the development of frank empyema. Basal pneumonitis and atelectasis, alone or in combination, are the other complications of an unruptured liver

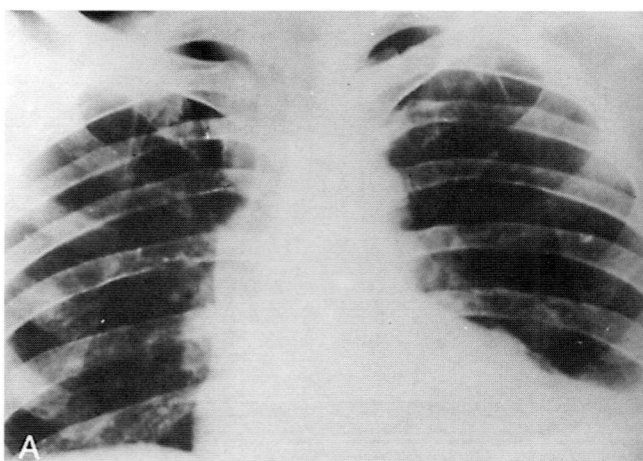

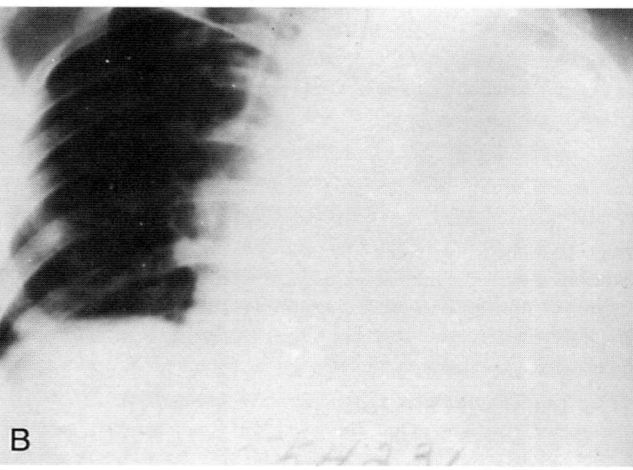

Fig. 87-7. A patient had an acute massive rupture of an amebic liver abscess into the left pleura. **A.** Radiograph taken before rupture. **B.** Radiograph taken 12 hours later. This demonstrates the need for urgent treatment. From Eggleston FC: Pitfalls in the surgical management of ALA. Trop Doc 9:178, 1979. With permission.

abscess. Ten percent of the patients had basal pneumonitis or atelectasis; 22% of our patients with unruptured amebic liver abscess had pleural effusion, pneumonitis, or both.

Amebic Empyema

Excluding sympathetic pleural effusion, amebic empyema is the most common of all the pleuropulmonary complications, occurring in 50 to 75% of patients with thoracic amebiasis. In 95% of patients, the empyema is on the right side. Elevation of the diaphragm, friction rub, and effusion usually precede it. The onset can be either insidious or rapid and overwhelming (Fig. 87-7), depending on the size of the perforation and the volume of the abscess. It is accompanied by pain, dyspnea, and, if massive, shock. Some patients complain of a tearing sensation. Radiography of the chest shows opacification of the ipsilateral lung field (Fig. 87-8).

On thoracentesis, purulent, reddish brown or bile-stained fluid is found. Both in chest aspiration and the establishment of intercostal tube drainage, it is mandatory to go in high on the right lateral intercostal space near the axilla to avoid entry through the already raised diaphragm into the liver. Unless the lung is involved also, the fluid is sterile. Amebae are identified in less than 10% of cases.

Pleural thickening, often out of proportion to the duration of the empyema, follows rapidly, especially in the presence of secondary infection. Accordingly, treatment must be prompt and vigorous to avoid further complications. In addition to specific drug therapy, the purulent exudate must be removed rapidly. Although repeated aspirations, often combined with the instillation of streptokinase, have been recommended, we agree with Ibarra-Pérez (1981) that closed intercostal drainage with the largest cannula possible combined with strong suction offers the best chance for prompt and complete reexpansion of the lung. When carried out promptly, secondary surgical procedures other than an occasional rib resection are rarely required. Le Roux and associ-

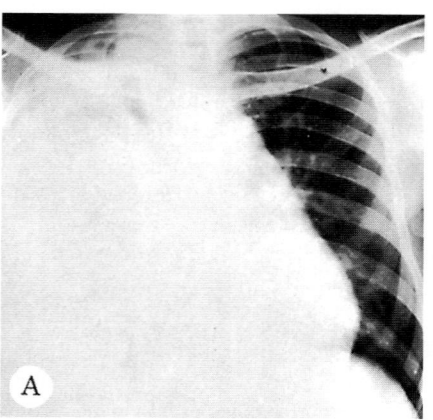

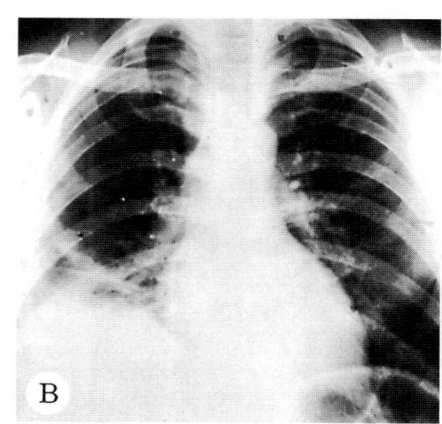

Fig. 87-8. Pure amebic empyema of the right hemithorax. **A.** Before treatment. **B.** After treatment.

ates (1986) pointed out that subcostal drainage of the amebic liver abscess may be necessary when drainage persists or the abscess becomes secondarily infected.

Should initial treatment be delayed or inadequate, reexpansion of the lung may be limited and decortication needed.

Mortality varies from 14 to 40%, depending on the general condition of the patient and the delay in starting treatment.

Pulmonary Amebiasis

Two types of pulmonary amebiasis occur; the first results from rupture of an amebic liver abscess into the lung and the second is metastatic (i.e., with no communication to the liver). The former is by far the more common.

When pleural symphysis precedes the transdiaphragmatic rupture of amebic liver abscess, the lung is directly involved, particularly the basal segments (Fig. 87-9), the middle lobe, or rarely the lingula. After a few days of chest pain and nonproductive cough, the patient complains of expectoration of reddish brown or bile-stained material, sometimes in large quantities. Unless flooding of the tracheobronchial tree is overwhelming, the prognosis is good.

Treatment consists of postural drainage, antibiotics to prevent secondary infection, and most important, specific antiamebic drug therapy. This complication carries the lowest mortality of any of the major complications of amebiasis as the liver abscess is usually well walled off from the peri-

toneal and pleural spaces. In rare cases in which the adhesions are not well formed, rupture of the liver abscess can be into the pleura as well as the bronchi simultaneously. Thoracentesis is required along with the other measures.

Rarely, a persistent bronchobiliary fistula develops. Ragheb and associates (1976) performed lung resection and closure of the fistulous tract. We prefer to drain the liver abscess transabdominally, as one of us (M.V.) and associates (1979) reported. Lung abscess also can occur rarely.

Occasionally, lung involvement is followed by bronchiectasis, usually mild and not severe enough to require resection. Indeed, we have never had to do one.

Metastatic pulmonary amebic lung abscesses are rare and result from hematogenous spread of amebae (Fig. 87-10). Symptoms resemble those of other lung abscesses, with fever, chest pain, cough, and hemoptysis. Occasionally, they rupture into the pleura and produce a localized empyema (Fig. 87-11). Unless amebae can be demonstrated in the sputum or the pleural fluid, diagnosis is difficult and depends on finding evidence of amebiasis elsewhere.

Treatment is like that for any other lung abscess, with the addition of specific antiamebic drug therapy.

Pleural and Pulmonary Amebiasis

In approximately 25% of patients, both the pleura and lungs are involved. Treatment includes intercostal drainage

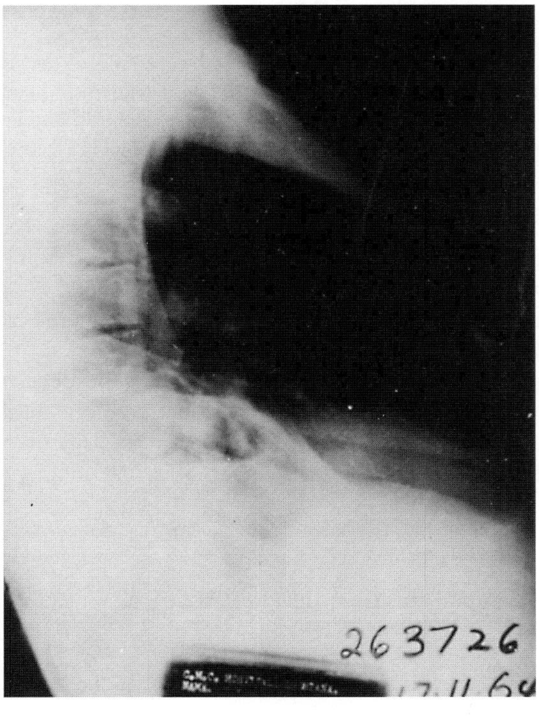

Fig. 87-9. Involvement of the right lower lobe basal segments by amebic abscess extending from the liver.

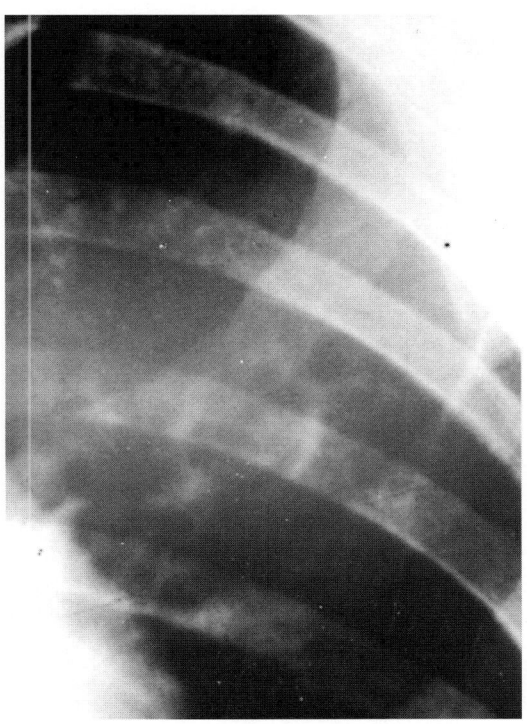

Fig. 87-10. Metastatic amebic lung abscess.

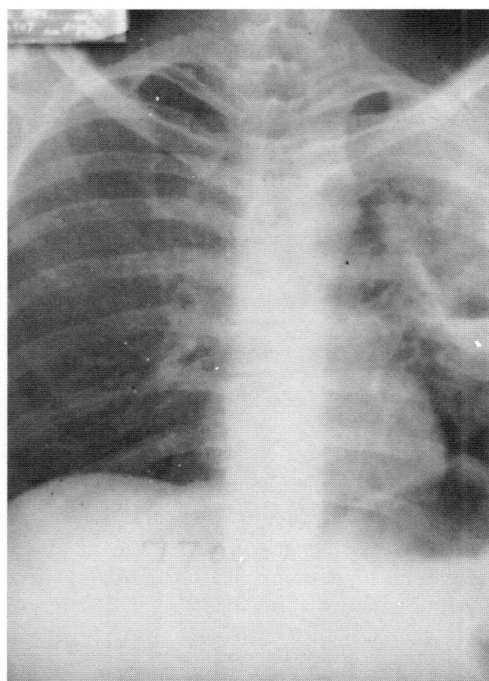

Fig. 87-11. Metastatic amebic lung abscess with rupture and localized empyema and bronchopleural fistula. Amebae were seen on smear of empyema fluid.

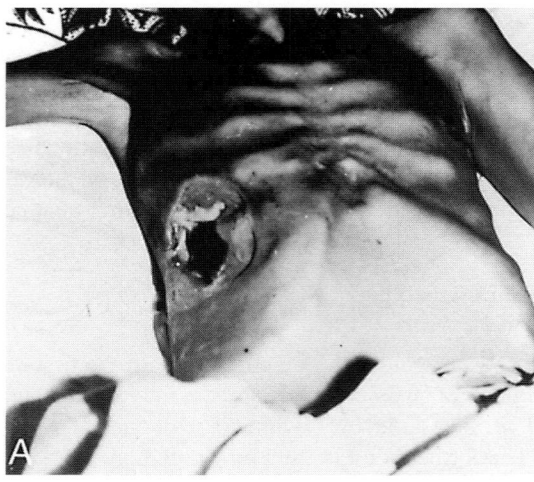

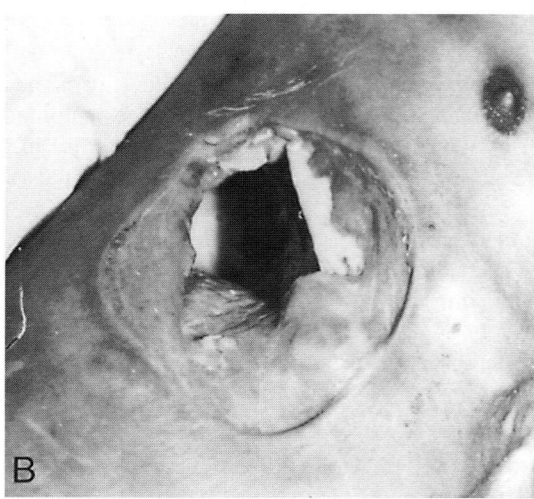

Fig. 87-12. A and B. Necrosis of the chest wall from amebiasis after lung biopsy for suspected malignancy, which resulted in amebic empyema. The patient recovered with antiamebic treatment.

with strong suction, reexpansion of the lung, postural drainage, and appropriate antibiotics.

GENERAL CONSIDERATIONS

Rarely, an amebic liver abscess ruptures transdiaphragmatically after the institution of specific antiamebic therapy. Undoubtedly, this rupture occurs in an already necrotic area of the diaphragm.

We prefer not to routinely drain the liver abscess except for acutely sick patients, patients with pleuropulmonary amebiasis, and patients who have failed to respond to treatment. Drainage of the liver abscess is done through the percutaneous route; laparotomy is only indicated in patients with multiple liver abscesses or in patients in whom percutaneous drainage as well as medical management has failed to improve the condition of the patient. Patients with amebi-

asis, particularly those with pleuropulmonary complications, usually have been sick for a long time and are often economically disadvantaged and malnourished. Consequently, nutritional support is important.

When diagnosis is delayed, results may be devastating (Fig. 87-12). The increasing use of sonography has permitted earlier diagnosis and treatment of amebic liver abscess. As a result, in our experience, the incidence of

Table 87-1. Review of Hospital Admissions for Hepatic Amebiasis from 1980 to Date

Duration	Unruptured Amebic Liver Abscess	Rupture Into the Pleura	Rupture Into the Lungs	Hospital Mortality	Average Hospital Stay (Days)
1980–1984	53	6	3	2	16
1985–1989	42	5	1	1	16
1990–1994	63	9	1	Nil	16
1996 to date	27	2	Nil	Nil	11

Table 87-2. Recommended Antiamebic Drug Schedule

Drug	Route of Administration	Dose	Duration (Days)
Metronidazole	Oral[a]	750 mg tid (children, 35–50 mg/kg in three divided doses for 10 days)	5–10
Chloroquine[b]	Oral	600 mg (base) bid followed by:	2
		300 mg (base) bid	19
Dehydroemetine[c]	Intramuscular	1.0–1.5 mg/kg (maximum of 90 mg)	5–10

[a]Patients unable to tolerate metronidazole orally should receive it intravenously.
[b]For children, 16 mg/kg (salt) daily for 21 days.
[c]The drug should be administered for the least number of days necessary to control severe symptoms (usually 3 to 5 days). For children, the daily dose is divided. Marked toxicity is unlikely if used less than 7 days.

pleuropulmonary complications seems to be decreasing (Table 87-1).

The incidence, clinical manifestations, and therapeutic response of infections with *E. histolytica* do not appear to be influenced by a patient's infection with human immunodeficiency virus infection because the rates of symptomatic infection with this organism do not differ between patients with acquired immunodeficiency syndrome and the general population.

ANTIAMEBIC CHEMOTHERAPY

Metronidazole

Most amebic liver abscesses are cured with a regimen of metronidazole, 750 mg orally or intravenously three times per day. Metronidazole produces little toxicity. Oral administration in high doses may be associated with nausea, anorexia, a metallic taste in the mouth, cramps, and diarrhea, which are less common with the intravenous route. Although metronidazole is carcinogenic in animals when given in large doses, it has not been proved carcinogenic in humans. No evidence that drug resistance develops has yet been demonstrated.

For hepatopulmonary amebiasis, as Jain and coworkers (1990) pointed out, many different acceptable drug regimens are available. Because relapse has been reported after the use of metronidazole alone and because these patients are sicker than patients with uncomplicated amebic liver abscess, we prefer to use a combination of drugs (Table 87-2).

Chloroquine

Chloroquine is generally well tolerated and particularly effective in the amebic liver abscess. It is also effective in pulmonary amebiasis. At the dosage levels used in the treatment of amebiasis, the retinopathy sometimes associated with long-term use of chloroquine does not occur. It should, however, be administered orally, which is not always possible in seriously ill patients.

Dehydroemetine

Dehydroemetine is cardiotoxic, and a careful monitoring of the pulse, blood pressure, and electrocardiography is required. Cardiovascular side effects are characterized by hypotension, tachycardia, chest pain, and dyspnea. Electrocardiography shows T-wave inversion and prolongation of the Q-T interval. It can produce severe myositis at the site of injection. The drug is contraindicated in renal and cardiac disease and must be cautiously used in children and the elderly. We use this drug in patients who are very sick or in patients not responding to a combination of metronidazole and chloroquine. If we see any sign of toxicity, or if the patient has known cardiac problems, we omit it or avoid using it.

Tinidazole

Tinidazole is as effective as metronidazole and can be better tolerated. The recommended dosage in amebic liver abscess is 800 mg three times daily for 5 days or 2 g daily for 3 days. In children, 50 to 60 mg/kg is given up to a maximum of 2 g. Other nitroimidazole derivatives, such as nimorazole, secondizole, and ornidazole, have produced poorer results than metronidazole and tinidazole.

REFERENCES

Eggleston FC, et al: The results of surgery in amebic liver abscess: experiences in 83 patients. Surgery *83*:536, 1978.

Grigsby WP: Surgical treatment of amebiasis. Surg Gynecol Obstet *128*:609, 1969.

Ibarra-Pérez C: Thoracic complications of amebic abscess of the liver: report of 501 cases. Chest *79*:672, 1981.

Jain NK, Madan A, Sharma TN, et al: Hepatopulmonary amebiasis. Efficacy of various treatment regimens containing dehydroemetine and/or metronidazole. J Assoc Physicians India *38*:269, 1990.

Le Roux BT, et al: Pleuropulmonary amebiasis. Diseases of the lung and pleural space. Part I. Empyema thoracis and lung abscess. Curr Probl Surg *23*:73, 1986.

Ragheb MI, Ramadan AA, Khalil MAH: Intrathoracic presentation of amebic liver abscess. Ann Thorac Surg *22*:483, 1976.

Sharma M, Saxena A, Ghosh S, et al: A simple and rapid Dot-ELISA dipstick technique for detection of antibodies to Entamoeba Histolytica in amebic liver abscess. Ind J Med Res *88*:409, 1988.

Verghese M, et al: Management of thoracic amebiasis. J Thorac Cardiovasc Surg 78:757, 1979.

READING REFERENCES

Adams EB, MacLeod IN: Invasive amebiasis. I. Amebic dysentery and its complications. Medicine 56:315, 1977.

Beaver PC, Jung RC, Cupp EW: Clinical Parasitology. 9th Ed. Philadelphia: Lea & Febiger, 1984.

Framm SR, Soave R: Agents of diarrhea. Med Clin North Am 81:427, 1997.

Le Roux BT, et al: Suppurative diseases of the lung and pleural space. Part I. Empyema thoracis and lung abscess. Curr Probl Surg 23:1, 1986.

Markell EK, Voge M, John DT: Medical Parasitology. Philadelphia: WB Saunders, 1986.

Rodriguez C: Pulmonary and pleural amebiasis. In Shields TW (ed): General Thoracic Surgery. 2nd Ed. Philadelphia: Lea & Febiger, 1983.

Wolfe MS: Amebiasis. In Strickland GT (ed): Hunter's Tropical Medicine. 6th Ed. Philadelphia: WB Saunders, 1976.

CHAPTER 88

Hydatid Disease of the Lung

Homeros Aletras and Panagiotis N. Symbas

Hydatid disease, which is caused by the *Echinococcus granulosus* tapeworm and is known as *echinococcosis* or *hydatidosis*, has been acknowledged as a clinical entity since ancient times. Organs of sacrificed animals were described in the Talmud as "bladders full of water," and Hippocrates referred to hydatid disease in the aphorism, "When the liver is filled with water and bursts into the epiploon, the belly is filled with water and the patient dies." Rudolphi (1808) first used the term *hydatid cyst* for the description of echinococcosis in humans.

Echinococcosis is frequently encountered in the sheep- and cattle-raising regions of the world and has been observed most frequently in Australia, New Zealand, South Africa, South America, and the Mediterranean countries of Europe, Asia, and Africa. Although this disease, as Ginsberg and associates (1958) noted, has been rare in the United States and Canada, an increase in the frequency of this clinical entity can be expected in this part of the world with the increase in mobility and migration of people. Therefore, the presence of hydatid disease should be considered in a patient who presents with a well-defined, spherical density of the lung, particularly a patient who has lived or traveled in an endemic area.

PATHOPHYSIOLOGY

The primary hosts for the infecting organism are the members of the Canidae family, usually dogs, wolves, and coyotes. Feline species are seldom naturally infected, but the parasite has been reported in the cat, wild cat, jaguar, and panther. The primary host contracts echinococcosis by ingesting mature and productive echinococcal cysts in the viscera of an intermediate host (e.g., sheep, goats, cattle, hogs, moose, reindeer, deer, elk, and other herbivorous animals). In the intestines of the primary host, the scolices of the hydatid cyst develop into a parasitic worm composed of a scolex, neck, and three proglottids (i.e., segments). The last proglottid, which is approximately one-half the length

of the entire parasite, contains 400 to 800 ova. The proglottid matures and breaks off from the scolex. The ova are released in the feces of the primary host and are then introduced into intermediate hosts by ingestion of contaminated grass, water, vegetables, and such. The larval stage, which cannot occur in the main host, begins in the intermediate host and leads to the development of pulmonary and hepatic hydatid cysts. These organs are then ingested by the primary hosts, and thus the cycle continues (Fig. 88-1).

Saidi (1976) emphasized that the ova are resistant to physical and chemical agents. In the gastrointestinal tract of the intermediate host, however, including humans, the chitinous embryophore that surrounds the hexacanth embryo is lysed and the embryo is released. As Smyth (1968) described, the embryo, with the aid of its hooklets, attaches to and penetrates the mucosa of the duodenum and jejunum, enters the mesenteric venules, and proceeds to the portal vein. From the portal vein, the embryo enters the liver, where it becomes embedded and, if it is not destroyed by phagocytosis, develops into a cyst. In most series of patients, such as that of Toole and associates (1960), the incidence of hepatic involvement in echinococcosis is 50 to 60%; Saidi (1976) reported an incidence of 70 to 80%. In the portal circulation, some embryos whose diameters do not exceed 0.3 mm may pass through the sinus capillaries of the liver and, by way of the hepatic veins and vena cava, proceed to the right side of the heart and the pulmonary capillaries, where they may become embedded. Here, as in the liver, the embryo that survives the phagocytosis hypertrophies, the hooklets disappear, and the embryo enters the larval stage.

The lungs are the second most common site of lodgment of the parasite, as Barrett (1947), Dew (1928), and others noted, with an incidence varying between 10 and 30%. The development of pulmonary echinococcosis presumes hepatic involvement, which is more difficult to diagnose than the pulmonary disease. In some reported cases in which pulmonary cysts were removed, even though an intensive search was made for hepatic cysts, a positive diagnosis of hepatic involvement could not be made, even years later.

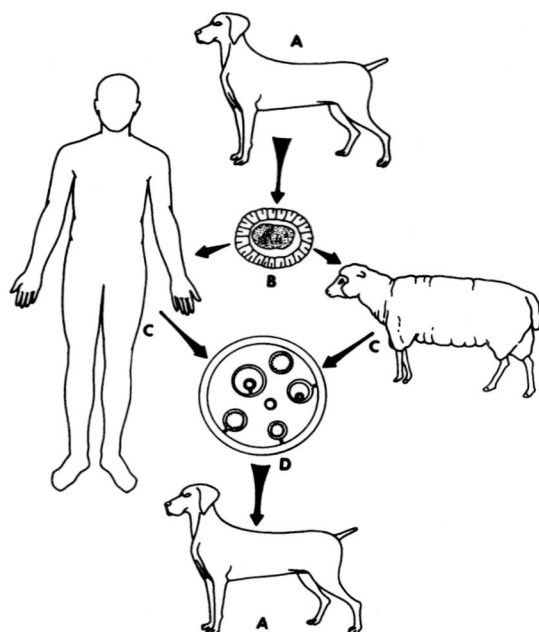

Fig. 88-1. Life cycle of *Echinococcus granulosus*. Primary host A ingests viscera of intermediate host C containing hydatid cyst → development of ova producing parasitic worm in intestine of primary host A → B ova shed with feces from primary host A, contaminating vegetables, grass, etc. → ingestion of contaminated vegetable or grass by intermediate host C → development of hydatid cyst D in viscera of intermediate host C → ingestion of viscera of intermediate host C with hydatid cyst D by primary host A.

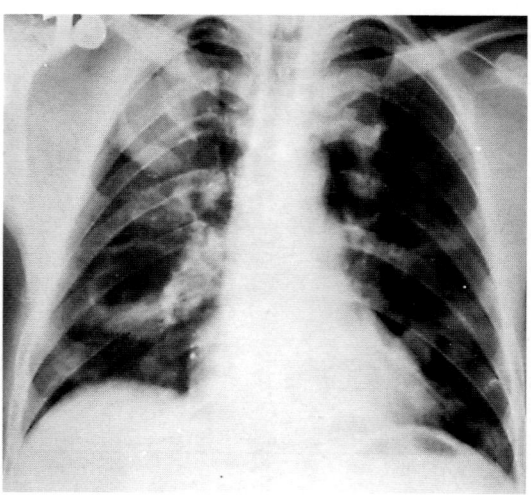

Fig. 88-2. Frontal chest radiograph showing multiple hydatid cysts of the lung.

One alternative pathway of the parasites' entrance into the lung is the lymphatic circulation: The embryo enters the lymphatics of the small intestine, proceeds to the thoracic duct, to the internal jugular vein, to the right side of the heart, and then to the lungs. Another possible route is a venal-venous anastomosis in the liver and the space of Retzius. Some researchers have supported the possibility of direct pulmonary exposure through the inhalation of air contaminated with echinococcus. As Chrysopathis (1966) pointed out, however, it is unclear whether the bronchial secretions can lyse the embryophore of the hexacanth to liberate the embryo. Other investigators, such as Barrett (1960), deny that an inhaled parasite could remain viable in the bronchial tree. Secondary pulmonary cysts may develop when ova enter the venous circulation because of rupture of extrapulmonary cysts. The site of the primary hydatid cysts producing secondary metastatic pulmonary echinococcus cysts in 31 patients was the heart in 64%, the liver in 26%, and the iliac bone in 10%. In such instances, it is difficult to distinguish between primary and secondary cysts.

Peschiera (1964) pointed out that the most common areas of involvement of pulmonary echinococcosis are the right lung and both of the lower lobes. Aletras (1968) and Barrett and Thomas (1952) noted that many cysts have a simultaneous development in either one or both lungs, with a reported

incidence of 14 to 24%. Each cyst grows and matures independently of any developing coexisting cyst (Fig. 88-2).

Tsakayiannis and colleagues (1970) stated that it is unclear whether children are more likely to develop pulmonary than hepatic echinococcus cysts. Some evidence suggests that echinococcus cysts develop more rapidly in the lungs of children than of adults, which may explain the more common appearance of pulmonary echinococcal cysts in children. Sometimes, the entire hemithorax of young children is occupied by parasitic cysts (Fig. 88-3). In these children, either the contamination must have occurred a few months after birth or the cysts grew rapidly.

Two types of hydatid cysts occur in humans, the unilocular and the alveolar. This discussion is limited to the unilocular variety because these are the cysts of clinical importance in the lungs. A hydatid cyst is composed of the wall and the hydatid fluid. The wall of the cyst is composed of three zones, which are constantly present and independent of the shape the cyst finally assumes. Two of these zones, the laminated membrane and the germinal layer or germinative membrane, belong to the parasite, and one zone, the pericyst or adventitia, belongs to the host. The differentiation of these zones begins in the embryo and continues until the three discernible zones develop.

The pericystic zone, also known as the *adventitia* or *ectocyst*, is rarely thicker than a few millimeters and is composed entirely of the host's cells. When the hexacanth embryo embeds in the host's tissue, it causes a local reaction and local migration of mononuclear leukocytes, lymphocytes, and eosinophils into the area. Polymorphonuclear leukocytes are not present, and their presence indicates that the parasite cannot implant at the particular site. The original cells are gradually replaced by fibroblasts so that this zone eventually is transformed into a thin and easily discernible capsule of fibrous matter, connective tissue, and

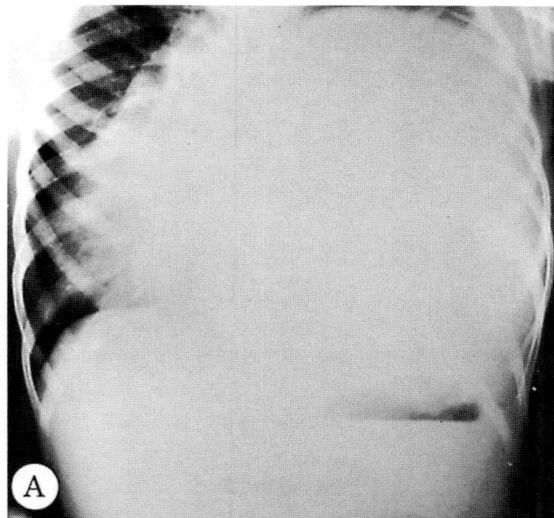

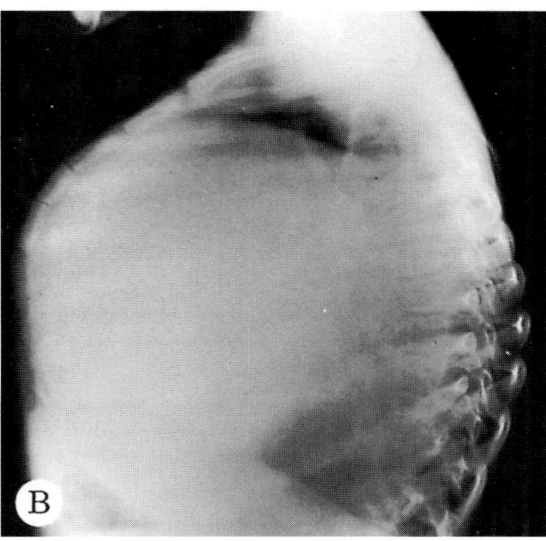

Fig. 88-3. Frontal (**A**) and lateral (**B**) preoperative and postoperative chest radiographs of a 5-year-old boy with a giant left lower lobe hydatid cyst producing chest deformity.

compressed parenchymal cells. Functionally, this layer provides mechanical protection and nutrition to the parasite. Therefore, whenever degenerative changes of the membrane develop, such as calcification, an amorphous degeneration or automatic absorption of the hydatid cysts occurs.

The laminated membrane is 1 to 3 mm thick and is surrounded by a pericystic layer. The membrane is white, gelatinous, rich in polysaccharides, and characteristically laminated, which is often obvious to the naked eye. It is hyaline and elastic, with no host blood vessels entering into it, and it is easily discernible from the pericystic layer, which is vitally important to the surgeon. The laminated membrane, as described by Morseth (1967), is composed of a plexus of fine fibers with a dispersed, thick, reticular substance, which, as Schwabe (1959) noted, is permeable to calcium,

potassium, chlorides, water, and urea. Nutritional and other substances useful to the parasite traverse the membrane by diffusion, but active transport may also play a role. Agosin (1968) suggests that potassium and cyanide ions seem to affect the permeability of this membrane by causing a detachment of the germinal membrane from the rest of the cyst. Physiologic fluids of the host or even purulent fluids do not destroy this membrane, although the smallest break in the membrane may result in total rupture of the cyst and escape of its contents. The large cysts are especially vulnerable to rupture because of an increased pressure exerted by the fluid in the cyst.

The germinal layer, also known as the *germinative membrane* or *endocyst*, is the inner layer of the cystic wall. It is a thin, transparent membrane that is lined with small papillae, which are brood capsules at different stages of development. These capsules, which are formed by the proliferation of the cells of the germinal layer, develop buds of scolices. The scolices have suckers and hooks and represent the mature parasite larvae. The germinative membrane is the living part of the parasite and produces the laminated membrane and reproduces the parasite. Some cysts cannot regenerate, but every undamaged cyst, regardless of size, must be considered capable of reproduction.

The daughter cysts, a rare finding in pulmonary echinococcosis, are produced from the germinal membrane, from the brood capsule, or from the scolices. Daughter cysts vary in size from a few millimeters to a few centimeters; their numbers range from a few to thousands, and they contain viable scolices. Some of the daughter cysts may be degenerated, whereas others may contain their own daughter cysts.

The hydatid vesicle is filled with hydatid fluid, which is colorless and odorless and resembles crystal-clear water. The specific gravity of the fluid is 1.008 to 1.015; the pH is 6.7 to 7.2; and the concentration of sodium, potassium, chloride, and carbon dioxide is approximately that of the host's blood serum. The function of the hydatid fluid is similar to that of amniotic fluid because it suspends the daughter cysts. A large production of hydatid fluid can disrupt the nutrition from the host to the interior of the cyst and cause the death of the parasite.

The parasitic cyst enlarges up to a certain limit, at which time, either accidentally or because of symptoms produced by its presence, it becomes discernible and is removed. The rate of growth of any particular pulmonary cyst varies and may be faster in children than in adults. Their diameter can increase, as Sarsam (1971) and others noted, from a few millimeters up to approximately 5 cm a year. A cyst with a diameter of 10 cm contains approximately 400 mL of hydatid fluid, and any cyst that grows to a diameter of 6 to 7 cm must be removed. Usually, the rate of growth of the echinococcus in the lungs is progressive and constant, but precipitous growth spurts can occur. The growth is rapid, more so than in other organs, mainly because the pulmonary tissue is elastic and shows little resistance to the cyst's expansion.

During the growth period of the cyst, it may rupture spontaneously or during coughing, sneezing, or any other cause of increased intra-abdominal pressure or after injury during diagnostic paracentesis. The rupture may occur within the boundaries of the pericystic layer, into the pleural space, or into a neighboring organ, bronchus, or blood vessel. Rupture of the germinal membrane toward the interior of the cyst may result in the formation of daughter cysts; such formation after a rupture of the laminated membrane is rare. Rupture of the cyst toward the surrounding tissues may be followed by secondary echinococcosis, and rupture into a blood vessel may lead to embolization of a portion of the cyst. Rupture of the cyst and evacuation of the cystic contents into a main bronchus rarely results in spontaneous cure. Suppuration of the cyst can occur after rupture and secondary infection. In the course of their natural evolution, many cysts gradually cease growing and degenerate.

Although hydatid cysts of the liver commonly calcify, calcification of such a cyst in the lung is rare. The calcification, which resembles an eggshell, takes place in the adventitia of complicated cysts and does not always indicate that the hydatid is dead. The calcified lung cyst is almost always in communication with the bronchial tree and is probably infected.

Some investigators, including Bakir (1967), Saidi (1976), and Smyth (1968), contend that the remaining pericystic cavity becomes obliterated after the cystic contents are evacuated through the bronchus or after excision of the cyst. Others, such as Kourias and Tobler (1957), Pérez-Fontana (1948), and Peschiera (1964), contend that the residual cavity persists because of epithelialization of the adventitial sacs.

CLINICAL MANIFESTATIONS

Intact or simple hydatid cysts of the lung produce no characteristic symptoms. Their clinical manifestations depend on the site and size of the cyst. Small, peripherally located cysts are usually asymptomatic, whereas large cysts may manifest with symptoms of compression of adjacent organs. If the patient is symptomatic, the first complaint usually is a nonproductive cough; some patients, particularly those with centrally located cysts, may have blood-streaked sputum, although massive hemoptysis does not occur. Some patients complain of a dull aching pain or the sensation of pressure in the chest with no aggravating or relieving features. In children, who have a supple chest wall, a bulge in the ipsilateral chest may also be observed (see Fig. 88-3).

Rupture of the hydatid cyst into an adjacent bronchus may be manifested by vigorous coughing and expectoration of a large amount of salty sputum, consisting of mucus, hydatid fluid, and, occasionally, fragments of the laminated membrane, generally described as grape skin, or frothy blood. In addition, the patient may develop a severe hypersensitivity reaction manifested by generalized rash, high fever, pulmonary congestion, and severe bronchospasm. Occasion-

ally, the intrabronchial rupture of the cyst manifests with sudden and severe dyspnea, which may lead to suffocation and death from complete tracheal obstruction by fragments from the hydatid membrane. Arce (1941) pointed out that the diagnosis of rupture of the hydatid cyst is unequivocally made when the hooklets of the parasite are found during microscopic examination of sputum. Intrabronchial evacuation of the hydatid cyst contents usually occurs without a catastrophic event. Rather, the patients may complain of repeated febrile episodes, chronic cough, and mucopurulent or dark bloody sputum.

When the hydatid cyst ruptures into the pleural space, the symptoms are usually insidious and moderate; they consist of dry cough, chest pain, moderate dyspnea, generalized malaise, and fever. These relatively mild clinical manifestations result from preexisting pleural adhesions, which prevent the dissemination of the cyst contents into the whole pleural space. In some patients, particularly those without preexisting pleural adhesions, the intrapleural rupture of the cyst produces an acute and dramatic clinical picture consisting of intense chest pain, persistent cough, severe dyspnea, and even cyanosis, shock, and suffocation. Frequently, symptoms of generalized urticaria, intense pruritus, severe anaphylactic shock, and even death can occur. The symptoms of the intrapleural rupture of the hydatid cyst are accompanied by the physical findings of localized or generalized hydropneumothorax.

DIAGNOSIS

Diagnosis of an intact echinococcus cyst is usually based on a suspicion resulting from an unexpected finding on routine chest radiographs. Radiographically, the cyst appears as a smoothly outlined, dense, spherical opacity (Fig. 88-4). Sharma and Eggleston (1969) emphasized that the alteration from a spherical to an oval shape may be observed only during deep inhalation (the Escudero-Nenerow sign). The radiographic picture depends, for the most part, on the size and location of the cyst. The small cyst may appear as a small "vesicle" and is difficult to recognize until it grows large enough to present a clear image on the chest radiograph.

Centrally located cysts may compress the bronchovascular structures, presenting radiographically as a depression or indentation at the site of pressure, the so-called notch sign. The cyst may also have a clear, crescentic shadow on the top or on one side; this type is referred to as a *pneumocyst* by Dévé (1935), *perivesicular pneuma* by Arce (1941), *perivesicular meniscus* by Peschiera (1972), *moon sign* or *crescent sign* by Barrett and Thomas (1952), and *pulmonary meniscus sign* by Saidi (1976). This sign has been attributed to the air that enters the perivesicular space, becoming trapped between the adventitia and the unruptured vesicle after vigorous coughing, straining, or direct trauma to the cyst, and it is the first radiographic sign of impending rupture of the cyst. A *double-dome arch* sign, as Arce (1941) noted, may appear

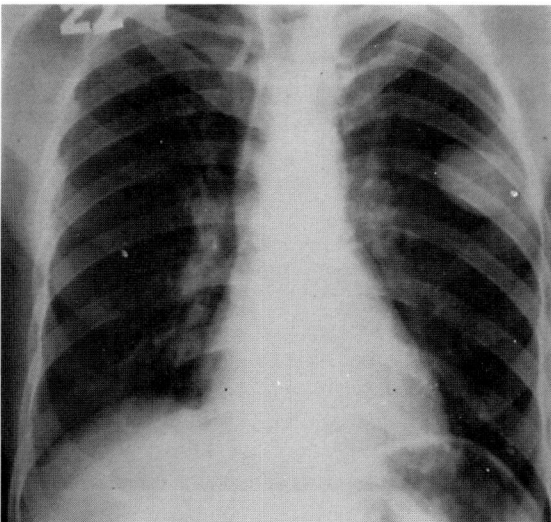

Fig. 88-4. Routine frontal chest radiograph showing a small peripheral hydatid cyst in the left upper lung field.

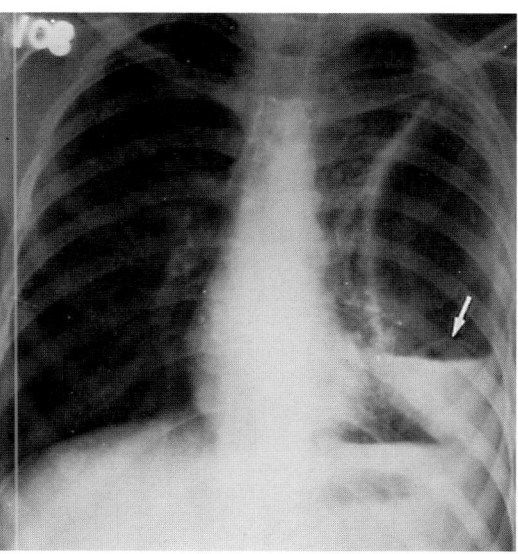

Fig. 88-6. Frontal chest radiograph showing a collapsed echinococcal membrane lying above the air-fluid level (*arrow*), the water lily sign, in a 15-year-old boy admitted with a pyothorax.

when a small additional amount of air further enters the hydatid vesicle. The entrance of free air into the cyst and the perivesicular space after the complete rupture of the laminated membrane displaces the fluid. This finding has been termed a *camalote* sign by Arce (1941) or a *water lily* sign by Lagos Carcia and Segers (1924). It is produced by the floating membrane of the cyst (Fig. 88-5).

These three diagnostic signs, however, are radiographic rarities. Beggs (1985) reviewed the radiographic findings. Most present as a solid mass in the right lower lobe. They are multiple in 30% of patients and bilateral in 20%. Therefore, every discrete radiologic lesion observed in any patient older than 3 years in an endemic area should be considered a hydatid cyst.

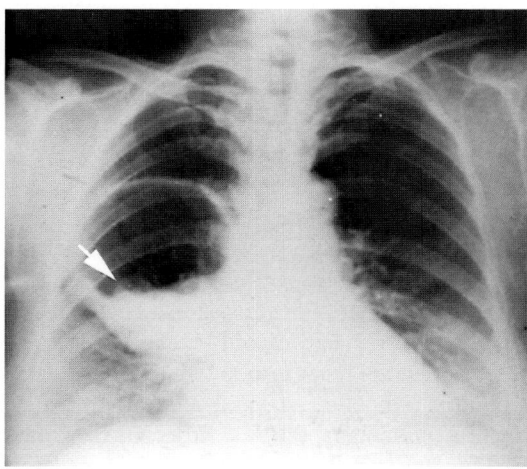

Fig. 88-5. Frontal chest radiograph of a ruptured echinococcal cyst in the right lower lung field, with the cystic membrane floating on the hydatid fluid (*arrow*), the water lily sign.

The radiographic pleural manifestations in the acute stage of rupture of the cyst vary from loculated hydropneumothorax to nonloculated partial, complete, or tension hydropneumothorax. The water lily sign can also be observed in instances of rupture of the cyst into the pleura (Fig. 88-6).

Computed tomography, as Saksouk (1986) and Lewall (1986) and their associates reported, has added to the diagnosis of hydatid disease of the lung, particularly to the early discovery of coexistent small cysts in the lung and of pending or existing rupture of the cyst. Also, as Kalovidouris and colleagues (1984) noted, computed tomography appears to be valuable in the follow-up of patients who have had resection or evacuation of hydatid disease of the lung.

Magnetic resonance imaging may show detached membranes, local host reactions, or communications between the cyst and the bronchial tree in ruptured cysts. It may also show the regression of the cyst during chemotherapy with albendazole, which destroys the germinal layer and accelerates the degeneration of the parasite or increases the local host reaction. Calcifications are not well appreciated on magnetic resonance images.

Sinner (1991) and Sinner and colleagues (1991) reported that the local host reaction is shown as a ring enhancement sign (hypervascularization) or a halo sign (allergic, atelectatic, or inflammatory response).

The diagnosis of echinococcal cyst may also be suspected because of eosinophilia, which, as Faust and Russell (1964) and Aletras (1968) reported, occurred in 20 to 34% of the patients with echinococcosis. Because an increase in eosinophils is also observed in many other pathologic states, this test has little diagnostic value. Tomography and bronchography add little information to the diagnosis and are rarely indicated. Pneumoperitoneum may be used to determine whether the cyst is in the liver or the right lower lobe (Fig. 88-7).

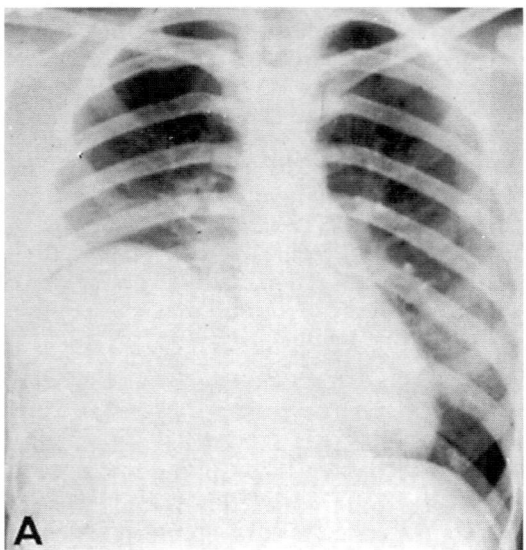

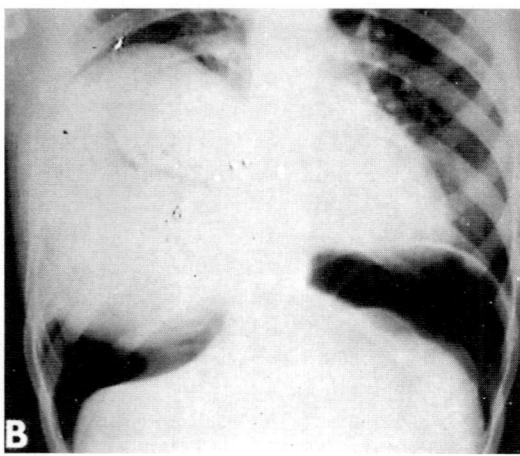

Fig. 88-7. A. Frontal chest radiograph shows radiodensity occupying the right lower lung field and the right upper quadrant. **B.** Pneumoperitoneum shows that the echinococcal cyst involved the right lower lobe rather than the liver.

Several clinical laboratory tests useful in the diagnosis of hydatid disease of the lung include Casoni's intradermal test, the Weinberg complement fixation test, and the indirect hemagglutination test. The latex flocculation (particle-fixation) test, bentonite flocculation (precipitin reaction) test, immunodiffusion test, and immunofluorescence test are, for the most part, used experimentally. Casoni's intradermal test has been the most widely used diagnostic test, but because it lacks specificity, it is no longer recommended.

The Weinberg complement fixation test, used first by Ghedini (1906), is not specific. Its sensitivity rate was reported by Kagan (1968) and coworkers (1966) to vary from 36 to 93%. Gräfe (1964) noted that it has a false-positive rate of 28%, especially in patients with neoplasms.

The indirect hemagglutination test, first used by Garabedian and associates in 1957, is the clinical test of choice.

Kagan and colleagues (1966, 1968) reported that its sensitivity ranges from 66 to 100%, and false-positive results are few (1 to 2%).

TREATMENT

Medical treatment for hydatid disease of the lung was nonexistent until the 1980s. Benzimidazole compounds have shown encouraging results. Gil-Grande and associates (1983) reported the use of mebendazole with a 36 to 94% partial-to-complete response rate. Morris and colleagues (1985) used albendazole (10 mg/kg/day) with some remission in 15 of 22 patients. Aggarwal and Wali (1991), however, used the same agent in 10 patients for 8 weeks with little response. Response to this therapy is apparently related to the thickness of the cyst wall, which the drug must penetrate to reach the germinal layer. Young patients and patients with small cysts, in whom cyst walls are usually thin, respond better to this treatment. The failure rate of this therapy and the recurrence rate after treatment is discontinued are apparently high, and the side effects from the drugs are considerable. As a result, until more data are available, this form of treatment at best may be considered in selected cases under close observation and is mainly recommended for inoperable cysts because of dissemination, difficult location, or contraindication for surgery.

The surgical treatment of hydatid disease of the lung has undergone considerable change since the 1950s. Numerous surgical procedures based on the evacuation of the cyst through the chest wall in one or two stages have been used. These methods, although they may still be practiced, are not applicable when the cysts are near the hilum of the lung and are inadequate because secondary echinococcal cysts may develop in the surgical wound and a chronic bronchocutaneous fistula may be created.

The current treatment of the hydatid cyst of the lung is complete excision of the disease process with maximum preservation of the lung tissue. Peripherally located cysts of any size and small- to medium-sized centrally located cysts should and can be excised without the sacrifice of lung parenchyma. Segmental resection is indicated principally in the treatment of large simple cysts that almost completely occupy the involved segment. It can also be used for complicated cysts of moderate size if the infection does not extend beyond the segmental plane.

Lobectomy should be performed when the size and number of cysts and the degree of infection exclude lesser procedures. The principal indications for lobectomy are large cyst involving more than 50% of the lobe, cysts with severe pulmonary suppuration not responding to preoperative treatment, multiple unilobar cysts, and sequelae of hydatid disease, such as pulmonary fibrosis, bronchiectasis, or severe hemorrhage. Pneumonectomy is rarely indicated for treatment of hydatid disease of the lung, and it should be used only when the whole lung is involved in the disease process, leaving no salvageable pulmonary parenchyma.

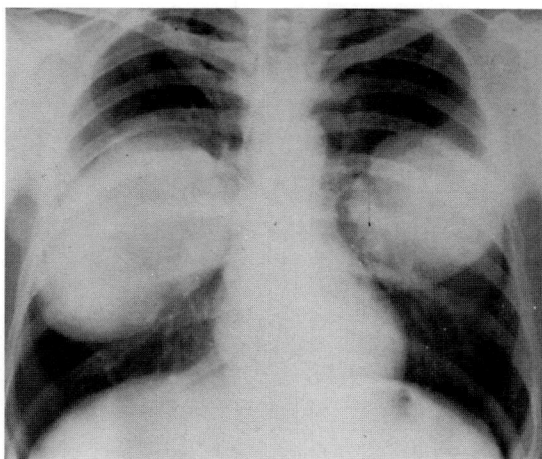

Fig. 88-8. Frontal chest radiograph shows two intact echinococcal cysts, one in each lung. Both were enucleated by separate thoracotomies at a 2-month interval.

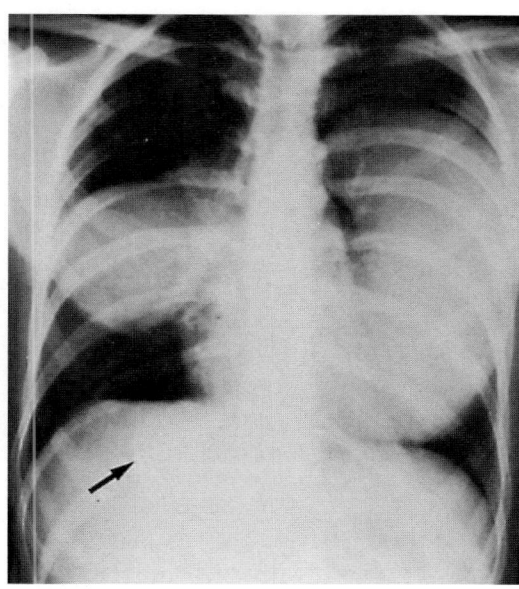

Fig. 88-9. Frontal chest radiograph shows three echinococcal cysts, one in each lung and one in the liver. Left hydatid cyst was removed first. Six weeks later, the cysts (*arrow*) from the right lung and liver were treated simultaneously.

The preoperative preparation of patients with hydatid disease of the lung is similar to the preparation of a patient undergoing thoracotomy for other comparable pulmonary lesions. Patients with small peripheral lesions require limited preparation, but patients with suppurative cysts should be treated with postural drainage, antibiotics, and other supportive measures until the suppurative process is as minimal as possible. Because echinococcal cysts not detected by the preoperative evaluation may exist in the liver or elsewhere, this possibility and the possibility for future surgical interventions should be brought to the patient's attention preoperatively, in addition to all the other information concerning the operative procedure.

Bilateral lung cysts should be resected in two stages (Fig. 88-8). In a patient with uncomplicated lung cysts, the lung with the larger cyst or with the greater number of cysts should be operated on first. In a patient with a lung cyst larger than 4 to 5 cm in one lung and a ruptured cyst in the other lung, the intact cyst should be removed first to eliminate its future rupture. The lesions in the other lung are then resected 2 to 4 weeks after the first operation (Fig. 88-9).

Conventional general anesthesia is used for thoracotomy, and preparation should be made for the management of complications. Complications may include blockage of the tracheobronchial tree by the cyst contents or anaphylactic reaction, which might occur during induction of anesthesia or during the operation from rupture of a hydatid cyst into the bronchus or pleural space.

A posterolateral thoracotomy, through the fifth, sixth, or seventh intercostal space or, rarely, through the bed of the fifth, sixth, or seventh rib, is performed while taking extreme care not to rupture the cyst. The most superficial portion of an intact cyst, which is devoid of pulmonary parenchyma, is a round, grayish white area that is also

devoid of blood vessels (Fig. 88-10A). The perimeter of this area is dark, ill defined, and blends into the normal lung tissue. This appearance, and particularly the elastic feel on palpation of the mass, differentiates the hydatid cyst from a mitotic lesion.

Needle aspiration, for establishing the diagnosis when evidence suggests that the mass lesion is a hydatid cyst, should be avoided because of the danger of spillage of the parasitic material and the subsequent inability to remove the cyst.

Several operative techniques are used to manage hydatid cyst of the lung, and their main objective is resection of the intact or complicated cyst while preserving as much lung as possible.

Intact Cysts

Resection by Enucleation without Needle Aspiration

Excision of the intact hydatid cyst without needle aspiration is accomplished by careful separation of the laminated membrane from the pericystic zone. The separation of these two components of the parasitic cyst is feasible even though they adhere intimately to one another. The enucleation of small cysts can usually be accomplished without difficulty. Large cysts, however, demand greater technical training and patience because of the increased possibility of rupture during the separation of the pericystic zone from the laminated membrane. Because this complication is occasionally unavoidable, the surgical field must be protected from the

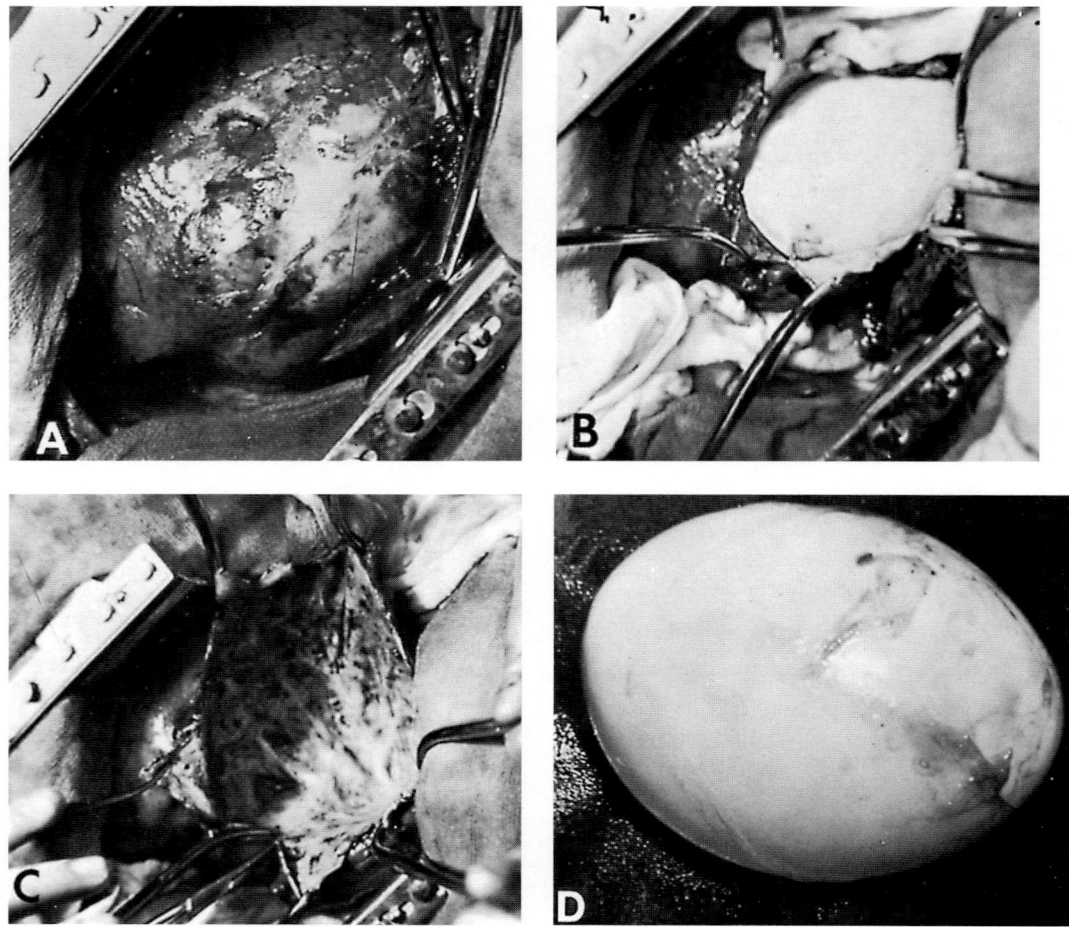

Fig. 88-10. Intraoperative photographs. **A.** The lung containing the hydatid cyst. Note the grayish white surface of the lung where the cyst is located. **B.** The hydatid cyst being dissected. **C.** Residual pericystic cavity after cyst removal. **D.** Hydatid cyst after excision.

possibility of spillage of the parasitic material, with resultant contamination of the pleural space and surgical wound. Therefore, after the hydatid cyst is identified, the surgical wound and adjacent lung tissue are covered with packed gauze steeped in normal saline solution, so that only the area of the lung that contains the cyst is exposed. Because the gauze material filters only macroscopic material, the hydatid fluid may still enter the pleural space and precipitate an allergic reaction. For this reason, before the dissection is begun, two well-functioning suction apparatuses must always be present. After the part of the lung containing the cyst is isolated, the tissue overlying the cyst is incised and the cyst is exposed. A cruciate or stellate incision is then made on the pericystic zone. With blunt dissection, a small space is created between this zone and the laminated membrane. The separation of the two zones is continued with blunt dissection and direct visualization, which is facilitated by traction on Allis clamps applied on the edges of the pericystic zone (Fig. 88-10B). During the dissection, the endopulmonary pressure is lowered by the anesthesiologist to avoid the projection of the laminated membrane through the opening in the pericystic zone. After the two zones are completely separated, the

anesthesiologist increases the endopulmonary pressure. With the current of air coming from the various bronchial openings; the simultaneous even, steady, light pressure on the cyst from the surrounding lung resulting from the increased endopulmonary pressure; and the use of gravity, the cyst pops out into an adjacent kidney basin that contains a small amount of normal saline solution. Before and during the delivery of the cyst, the laminated membrane should never be grasped with an instrument. Significant manual pressure on the pericystic zone should be avoided, and, in general, assistance in the "delivery" of the cyst must be careful to avoid its rupture. After the delivery of the cyst, the residual cavity, which is devoid of epithelium and always has some bronchial openings, must be managed appropriately (Fig. 88-10C).

The management of the residual cavity has historically passed through different stages. In 1899, Posadas advised only suturing of the bronchial openings. This practice, however, did not prevent air leak; thus, fixation of the edges of the sutured pericystic zone to the thoracotomy incision was later added to this method. The same year, Délbét advocated the folding of the pericystic zone by sutures, a method named *capitonnage*. According to Crausaz (1967), purse-string sutures from the base of the pericystic cavity upward were used to obliterate the cavity. Allende and Langer in 1947 supplemented this method with suturing of the individual bronchial openings within the cavity. Chrysospathis (1966) closed the bronchial openings at a more proximal point. To attain this closure, a probe was introduced through the bronchial opening and the surrounding pulmonary tissue was bluntly dissected along its length so that the bronchus could be closed more centrally.

Each of these methods, in the hands of their proponents, yielded good results. One of us (H.A.) favors, especially for a large pericystic cavity, closure of the bronchial openings; partial pericystectomy (i.e., resection of the free portion of the pericystic zone); elimination of the residual cavity by capitonnage; and closure of its edges with continuous sutures. Demirleau and Pernot introduced this method in 1951. Saidi (1976) contended that the approximation and suturing of the edges of the residual cavity are not necessary because the pulmonary parenchyma automatically obliterates the space, and the surface of the lung at the site of the residual cavity is covered by the pleura.

It is generally agreed, however, that the most important point in the management of the residual pericystic cavity is closure of patent bronchial openings. After the grossly evident bronchial openings are closed, smaller openings can easily be detected by filling the residual cavity with normal saline solution. With the application of positive endopulmonary pressure, air escaping through any bronchial openings is visualized by the formation of bubbles. This maneuver must be repeated until sealing of all air leaks is achieved.

Removal of the Intact Cyst After Needle Aspiration

The danger of development of secondary hydatid cysts because of spillage of hydatid fluid as a result of violation of the cyst's integrity by needle aspiration or rupture has led to the development of various chemical substances capable of rendering the hydatid fluid "sterile." These substances generally are used when the surgeon contemplates removing the intact cyst after needle aspiration. Formalin and formaldehyde solutions have mainly been used in the past as scolicidal agents during operation. The escape of these substances into the pericystic space causes irritation of the tissue, which results in impairment of healing and, as Saidi (1976) noted, in the formation of bronchial fistulas. Silver nitrate solution, 0.5%, has scolicidal properties and is used accordingly. Hypertonic saline solution, which is considered to have scolicidal properties, does not affect tissue healing; accordingly, one of us (H.A.) prefers this scolicidal agent.

Before the needle aspiration is begun, four Allis clamps and two suction machines, which are functioning well, should be available. The surgical wound and the lung, except for the segment containing the cyst, are covered with packed gauze, as described previously. The lobe that contains the cyst is immobilized, the lung is maintained inflated, and a 20- or 21-gauge lumbar puncture needle, which is connected to a 20- or 50-mL glass syringe, is inserted into the promi-

nent portion of the cyst and is maintained immobile. The use of plastic syringes is not desirable because their relative opacity does not allow clear observation of the aspirated fluid. The hydatid fluid of the cyst should not be aspirated completely; a small residual amount must always be left in the cyst. The remaining fluid is then removed in one of two ways. First, after withdrawal of the aspirating needle, the wall of the parasitic cyst is incised, a suction tip connected to a suction apparatus is immediately introduced into the cyst, and the remaining contents of the cyst are removed. The suction tip should be of the sump type, with side holes to avoid the blocking of the suction channel by portions of membrane or, rarely, by daughter cysts. While the preceding evacuation is carried out, a second suction apparatus is used to remove any hydatid fluid that may overflow from the cystic cavity, thus avoiding spillage of hydatid material. Second, after most of the hydatid cyst fluid is aspirated, instead of opening the pericystic and cystic walls, a trocar with a side arm connected to a suction apparatus is inserted in the cyst through the same orifice, immediately after the removal of the aspiration needle. The remaining hydatid contents are evacuated, the trocar is removed, the opening of the cyst is enlarged, and a second sump suction tip is introduced to withdraw the remaining contents of the cyst.

Throughout the entire period of evacuation of the parasitic contents of the cyst, the lungs must be kept expanded. This is done by maintaining constant positive pressure because, during the previously described maneuvers, rupture and detachment of the laminated membrane may occur, and a small amount of hydatid fluid may escape into the pericystic space. With the maintenance of constant positive endobronchial pressure, none of the escaped parasitic fluid in the pericystic cavity can advance through the bronchial openings into the bronchial tree. Finally, the remainder of the laminated membrane is removed with sponge forceps, the residual cavity is cleaned, preferably with hypertonic saline solution, and the bronchial openings are closed in the manner described previously.

Pericystectomy

Pérez-Fontana (1951) described removal of the pericystic zone with the intact cyst. The technical difficulty with this method is the creation of an appropriate plane through the pulmonary tissue, near and around the parasitic cyst, with the resulting bleeding and air leak. This method can be easily applied in superficially located small cysts.

Ruptured Cysts

Management of ruptured cyst during the acute stages is mainly directed toward the prevention of major complications resulting from the evacuation of the cystic contents into the tracheobronchial tree or the pleural space. Preventive precautions include the maintenance of the airway free of secretions and cystic tissue by appropriate orotracheal suction or bronchoscopy, evacuation of the hydropneumothorax, and treatment of an anaphylactic reaction. After the acute period, the most conservative treatment should be used to save as much lung tissue as possible.

An infected cyst is opened with minimal damage to the adjacent lung parenchyma, its contents are evacuated, and the cavity is thoroughly irrigated. The bronchial openings, with or without capitonnage of the residual cavity, are then closed, and the pleural space is drained. When the cyst is infected and the lung parenchyma is irreversibly damaged, lobectomy is the operation of choice.

PROGNOSIS

In a series of 115 patients treated by one of us (H.A.), 78 underwent enucleation of the cyst and capitonnage of the remaining cavity, with individual closure of the bronchial openings. Two patients had cystectomy and wedge resection of the surrounding parenchyma; three patients underwent cystectomy according to the Pérez-Fontana method; 14 had enucleation without capitonnage; three patients had partial cystectomy with or without capitonnage; and one patient had enucleation with pleurectomy. Twelve patients underwent lobectomy, and two had segmentectomy. No deaths were encountered. In a follow-up period of 2 to 25 years, no recurrence has been noted. Therefore, with appropriate treatment, the prognosis is excellent.

REFERENCES

Aggarwal P, Wali J Jr: Albendazole in the treatment of pulmonary echinococcosis. Thorax 46:599, 1991.

Agosin M: Biochemistry and Physiology of Echinococcus. Bull World Health Organ 39:115. 1968.

Aletras HA: Hydatid cyst of the lung. Scand J Thorac Cardiovasc Surg 2:218, 1968.

Allende JM, Langer L: Tratamiento de los quistes hidatidicos del pulmon. Boletin Y Trabajos. Academia Argentina di Chirugia 31:539, 1947.

Arce J: Hydatid cyst of the lung. Arch Surg 43:789, 1941.

Bakir F: Serious complications of hydatid cyst of the lung. Am Rev Respir Dis 96:483, 1967.

Barrett NR: Surgical treatment of the hydatid cyst of the lung. Thorax 2:21, 1947.

Barrett NR: The anatomy and the pathology of multiple hydatid cysts in the thorax. Arris and Gale Lecture. Ann Coll Surg Engl 26:362, 1960.

Barrett NR, Thomas D: Pulmonary hydatid disease. Br J Surg 40:222, 1952.

Beggs I: The radiology of hydatid disease. AJR Am J Roentgenol 145:639, 1985.

Casoni T: La diagnosi biologica dell echinococcosi umana medianti l'in-tradermo-reazione. Folia Clinica Chimica et Microscopia Salsomag-giorie 4:5, 1911.

Chrysopathis P: Echinococcus cysts of the lung. Dis Chest 49:278, 1966.

Crausaz PH: Surgical treatment of the hydatid cyst of the lung and hydatid cyst of the liver with intrathoracic evolution. J Thorac Cardiovasc Surg 53:116, 1967.

Délbét P: Kystes hydatiques du foie traités par le capitonnage et al suture sans drainage. Bull Mem Soc chir Paris 25:30, 1899a.

Délbét P: Kystes hydatiques du foie traités par le capitonnage et al suture sans drainage. Semaine Médicale 19:1899b.

Demirleau J, Pernot: Technique et indications therapeutiques de la kystec-tomie pour la traitement du kyste hydatique du poumon. J Chir 67:769, 1951.

Dévé F: Sur la stérilisation du sable hydatique par les solutions formolés et les solutions iodées. CR Soc Biol 119:352, 1935.

Dew H: Hydatid Disease: Its Pathology, Diagnosis, and Treatment. Sydney: Australian Medical Publishing, 1928.

Faust EC, Russell PF: Craig and Faust's Clinical Parasitology. London: Kimpton, 1964, p. 678.

Garabedian GA, Matossian RM, Djanian AY: An indirect hemagglutination test for hydatid disease. J Immunol 78:269, 1957.

Ghedini G: Ricerche sul siero di sangue di individuo affetto da cisti da echinococco e sul liquido in essa contenuto. Gazzetta degli Ospedali e della Cliniche 27:1616, 1906.

Gil-Grande LA, et al: Treatment of liver hydatid disease with mebendazole: a prospective study of thirteen cases. Am J Gastroenterol 78:584, 1983.

Ginsberg M, Miller JM, Surmonte JA: Echinococcus cyst of the lung. Chest 34:496, 1958.

Gräfe HA: Kritscher Beitrag zur Serodiagnostik der Echinokokkose des Menschen. Arch Hyg Bakteriol 148:367, 1964.

Kagan IG: A review of serological tests for the diagnosis of hydatid disease. Bull World Health Organ 39:25, 1968.

Kagan IG, et al: Evaluation of intradermal and serological tests for the diag-nosis of hydatid disease. Am J Trop Med Hyg 15:172, 1966.

Kalovidouris A, et al: Postsurgical evaluation of hydatid disease with CT: Diagnosis pitfalls. J Comput Assist Tomogr 8:1114, 1984.

Kourias B, Tobler AL: L'avenir éloigené des opérés pour kyste hydatique du poumon. Etude de 265 cas sur 305 opérés. Lyon Chir 53:209, 1957.

Lagos Carcia C, Segers A: Consideraciones sobre un caso de quiste hidatico pulmonar abierto in bronquios. Semin Med Bs As 31:271, 1924.

Lewall DB, Bailey TM, McCorkell SJ: Echinococcal matrix: computed tomographic, sonographic, and pathologic correlation. J Ultrasound Med 5:33, 1986.

Morris DL, et al: Albendazole: objective evidence of response in human hydatid disease. JAMA 253:2053, 1985.

Morseth DJ: Fine structure of the hydatid cyst and protoscolex of Echinococcus granulosus. J Parasitol 53:312, 1967.

Pérez-Fontana V: La patologia del guiste hidatico del pulmon. Arch Int Hidatid 8:47, 1948.

Pérez-Fontana V: Traitement chirurgical du kyste hydatique dus poumon. La méthode uruguayenne ou extirpation du perikyste. Arch Int Hydatid 12:469, 1951.

Peschiera CA: Hydatid cyst of the lung. In Steele JD (ed): The Treatment of Mycotic and Parasitic Diseases of the Chest. Springfield, IL: Charles C Thomas, 1964, p. 201.

Peschiera CA: Hydatid cyst of the lung. In Shields TW (ed): General Tho-racic Surgery. Philadelphia: Lea & Febiger, 1972.

Posadas A: Traitement des kystes hydatiques. Rev Chir 19:374, 1899.

Rudolphi KA: Entozoorum Sive Verminum Intestinalium. Historia Natu-ralis, Vol. 2. In Taberna, Libraria et Artinum. Amsterdam: 1808, p. 247. Cited by H. Dew, 1928.

Saidi F: Surgery of Hydatid Disease. Philadelphia: WB Saunders, 1976.

Saksouk FA, Fahl MH, Rizk GH: Computed tomography of pulmonary hydatid disease. J Comput Assist Tomogr 10:226, 1986.

Sarsam A: Surgery of pulmonary hydatid cysts: Review of 55 cases. J Tho-rac Cardiovasc Surg 62:663, 1971.

Schwabe CW: Host-parasite relationship in echinococcosis: Observations on the permeability of the hydatid cyst wall. Am J Trop Med Hyg 8:20, 1959.

Sharma SK, Eggleston FC: Management of hydatid disease. Arch Surg 99:59, 1969.

Sinner WN: New diagnostic signs in hydatid disease: Radiography, ultra-sound, CT and MRI correlated to pathology. Eur J Radiol 12:150, 1991.

Sinner WN, et al: MR imaging in hydatid disease. AJR Am J Roentgenol 157:741, 1991.

Smyth JD: In vitro studies and host-specificity in Echinococcus. Bull World Health Organ 39:5, 1968.

Toole H, et al: Considerations sur la therapie actuelle des kystes hydatiques du poumon. Apprécition des procédés opératoires. Rev Med Moyen Orient 17:358, 1960.

Tsakayiannis E, Pappis C, Moussatos P: Late results of conservative surgi-cal procedures in hydatid disease of the lung in children. Pediatr Surg 68:379, 1970.

CHAPTER 89

Pulmonary Paragonimiasis and Its Surgical Complications

Ronald B. Dietrick

A number of *Paragonimus* species infest humans. According to Nana and Borornkitti (1991), 10 of 43 species do. *Paragonimus westermani* is the most common (Fig. 89-1). The disease is widespread, covering four continents: much of East Asia, including Japan, Asian Russia, the Republic of Korea, the Republic of China, Taiwan, and the Philippines; Southeast Asia, including Indonesia, Thailand, and the Indian subcontinent; Africa, including Nigeria, the Cameroons, Gabon, and Zaire; Honduras; and Venezuela. It does not occur naturally in the United States.

ETIOLOGY

Noble and Noble (1982) described the manner of infestation, which is the same everywhere. Eggs of *P. westermani* lying in moist soil or water hatch as miracidia and enter freshwater snails, from which they are subsequently released as cercariae. These enter freshwater crayfish, probably by ingestion, where they develop into metacercariae. When a human eats the flesh of raw crayfish, the metacercariae enter the gastrointestinal tract. Handling the raw flesh or its juice may result in the metacercariae's transfer from the hand into the mouth. Once in the small intestine, the metacercariae excyst, penetrate the intestine, and pass across the peritoneal cavity into the abdominal wall. There they reside in the muscles for approximately 7 days, only to reenter the peritoneal cavity, migrate upward through the diaphragm, and wander in the pleural space. Here they penetrate the lungs, more on the right than on the left, to develop into mature worms. These become encysted, causing the basic pathologic lesion of the disease. They produce eggs, which enter a bronchus when the cysts rupture, to be coughed up and expectorated or swallowed, thus passing to the outer world in sputum or feces, completing the life cycle of the parasite.

PATHOLOGY

Gross Findings

Multiple cystic lesions form around the mature worms in the lung, as Yokogawa (1965) and Chung (1971) noted. Grossly, the cut surface of the lung shows slightly elevated, oval, firm, resilient, nodular masses varying from yellowish white to gray to reddish brown. Serial section reveals that these masses are cystic, containing one parasite per cyst (Fig. 89-2), although on occasion more than one is found.

Microscopic Findings

Microscopically, a layer of inflammatory cell infiltration, predominantly, polymorphonuclear leukocytes, surrounds the parasites early on. The neutrophils are gradually replaced by eosinophils, and Charcot-Leyden crystals sometimes appear in the necrotic center of the cyst. The eosinophils are gradually replaced by monocytes, lymphocytes, plasma cells, and young fibroblasts. The cyst wall then becomes more fibrotic, and granulomata frequently appear near the cyst along with giant cells of Langhans and foreign-body types. These often contain engulfed ova, but otherwise they closely resemble the tubercle of pulmonary tuberculosis. In later stages, bronchial arteries form a new arteriolar network around the worm cyst, and these vessels may rupture and produce hemoptysis when a cyst communicates with a bronchus. Acute and chronic pathologic changes may coexist in the lung.

CLINICAL FEATURES

Typically, patients infested by *P. westermani* tend to be older children or young adults, predominantly men. A rural

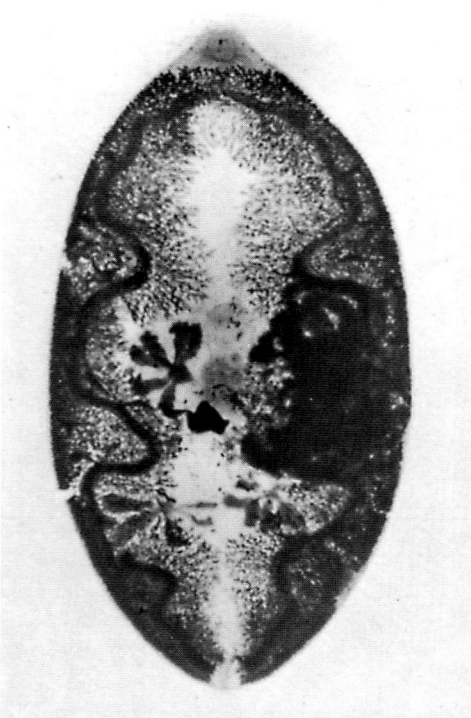

Fig. 89-1. *Paragonimus westermani.* Adult, ventral view. (Courtesy of M. D. Little.) From Beaver PC, Jung RC, Cupp EW (eds): Clinical Parasitology. 9th Ed. Philadelphia: Lea & Febiger, 1984. With permission.

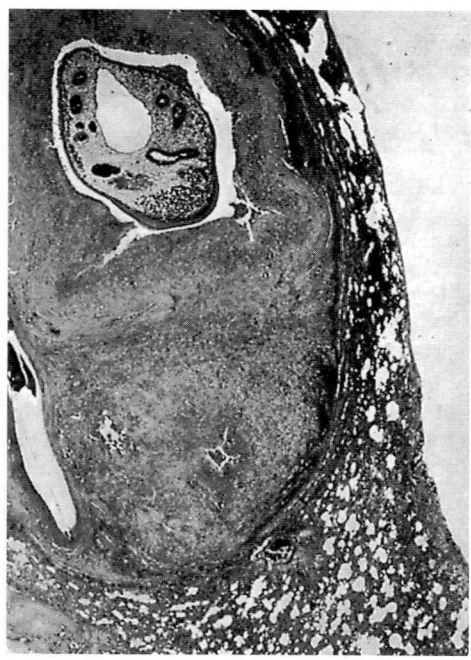

Fig. 89-2. *Paragonimus westermani.* Section of lung showing worm surrounded by infiltration and fibrous encapsulation. From Faust EC (ed): Human Helminthology. Philadelphia: Lea & Febiger, 1929. With permission.

background of poverty is common, and many patients remember handling or eating raw or poorly cooked crayfish, if asked. In past years, crayfish juice was used in Korea to treat measles, causing infestation.

Patients complain of cough productive of thick whitish sputum, very often blood streaked, and some patients volunteer that their sputum smells "fishy." Many complain of pleuritic chest pain, fewer of dyspnea and lassitude. Strikingly, the patient often appears healthy, thus belying the severity of the reported symptoms. Little fever or prostration is reported, and patients remain active. Often, the patient makes the diagnosis in areas where the disease is endemic, coming to the physician for confirmation and treatment. Physical examination is not revealing, usually, although some patients have scattered fine rales and a few rhonchi throughout the chest. The clinical diagnosis depends more on the history than on the physical examination.

DIAGNOSIS

Diagnosis is usually straightforward, provided the possibility is entertained. Many patients are diagnosed and treated for tuberculosis, which is often prevalent in areas where paragonimiasis is endemic, and indeed both diseases may afflict the same patient. A chest radiograph may show typical multiple, small, round, hazy infiltrations, often with tiny lucencies in the centers through both lungs (Fig. 89-3). According to Chung (1971), on the chest radiograph, the disease is indistinguishable from tuberculosis in approximately 40% of patients, and of these, many have been treated for tuberculosis. Im and associates (1992) emphasized the importance of peripheral linear shadows, suggesting that these are worm migration tracts (Fig. 89-4). These shadows were seen in only 41% of their patients, whereas pleural effusion was present in 54%. Paragonimiasis infiltrates are usually poorly defined and change rapidly, whereas infiltrates in tuberculosis tend to be nodular and change slowly. Kaneko and colleagues (1997) noted that a pulmonary infiltrate rarely may persist and even may be observed to enlarge. When the sputum is negative for both acid-fast organisms and *Paragonimus* ova, the persistent mass may be thought to be owing to a carcinoma.

Sputum examination reveals operculated *Paragonimus* eggs in many cases, sometimes with Charcot-Leyden crystals. Eggs may appear in the feces also, so fecal examination is often helpful, especially in children who swallow sputum rather than spitting it out. The number of eggs shed depends on the severity of infestation, so lightly infested patients may have negative sputum and feces. When this is the case, an intradermal skin test is available, at least in Japan and South Korea. Positive reactions produce a wheal within 3 to 5 minutes, reaching a maximum in 15 minutes, according to Yokogawa (1965), so the test may be per-

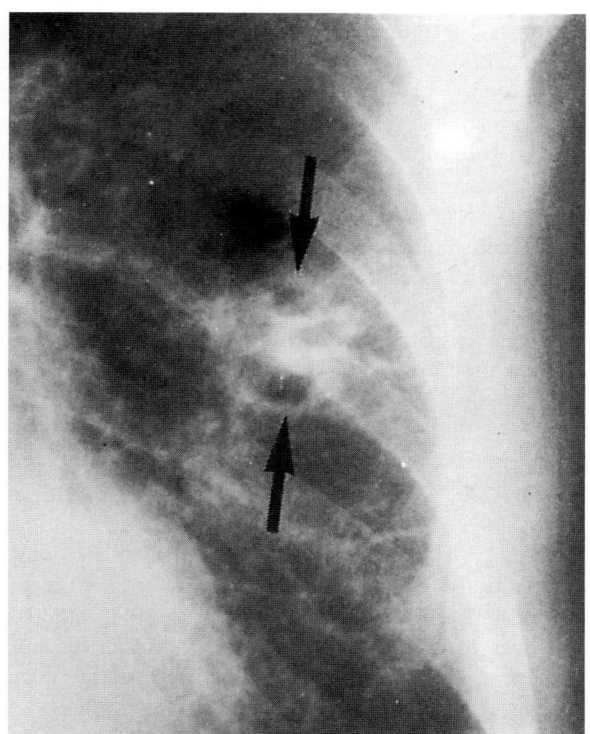

Fig. 89-3. Radiograph of the chest of a patient with paragonimiasis showing aggregated uniform-sized, thin-walled cysts (*arrows*) with soap-bubble appearance of a pulmonary lesion, a characteristic but rather infrequent radiographic finding in the disease. From Im JG, et al: Pleuropulmonary paragonimiasis: radiologic findings in 71 patients. AJR Am J Roentgenol *159*:39, 1992. With permission.

formed in one visit. A minor difficulty is that the antigen may cross-react with antibodies to *Clonorchis sinensis*. In practice, skin tests are done for both diseases concurrently. Because the age groups, history, physical signs, and symptoms are so different in the two diseases, differentiating the two is not difficult.

Further confirmation is available with a complement fixation test or an enzyme-linked immunosorbent assay. Although it is more time consuming, the complement fixation test is more reliable because the skin test may remain positive long after recovery, whereas the complement fixation test correlates with the presence of active disease, as Yokogawa and colleagues (1962) noted. Slemenda and associates (1988) developed an immunoblot assay, which is highly accurate in the diagnosis of paragonimiasis. They reported a sensitivity of 96% and a specificity of 99%. Without a complement fixation test, enzyme-linked immunosorbent assay, or immunoblot assay, a positive skin test is presumptive evidence of disease in the presence of typical symptoms and in the absence of tuberculosis.

Other laboratory tests have little value, except for frequent eosinophilia, but this is seen in many other parasitic infestations. Eosinophilia may be marked, and I saw one patient with eosinophilia greater than 70%. For much of the world where poverty is endemic along with paragonimiasis, the backbone of diagnosis continues to be based on symptoms, chest radiographic findings, sputum or feces examination, or both, and skin testing.

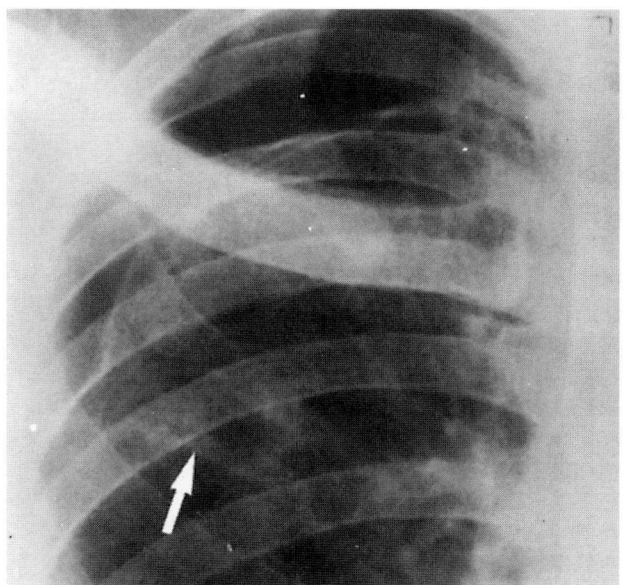
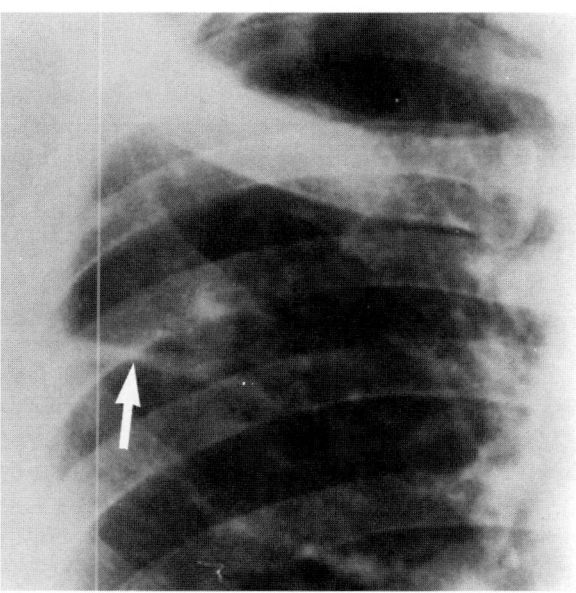

A   B

Fig. 89-4. Pulmonary paragonimiasis in a middle-aged man with pneumothorax and linear opacity. **A.** Initial chest radiograph reveals poorly defined infiltrations (*arrow*) in the right upper lobe. **B.** Subsequent radiograph shows a linear bandlike opacity (*arrow*) abutting the costal pleura, suggesting worm migration tracts. From Im JG, et al: Pleuropulmonary paragonimiasis: radiologic findings in 71 patients. AJR Am J Roentgenol *159*:39, 1992. With permission.

CURRENT MEDICAL THERAPY

Praziquantel is the drug of choice because of effectiveness, short duration of treatment, few and generally mild side effects, and commercial availability. Johnson and associates (1985) used this drug with success, although the numbers were small. Roberts (1988) stated that 90% of patients are cured by a 2-day course of treatment, with 24 mg/kg given three times a day.

Bithionol, for many years the drug of choice in East Asia, is relegated to second choice because of higher toxicity and longer treatment time. It is available from the Centers for Disease Control and Prevention and is 90% effective; gastrointestinal side effects can be decreased by treating on alternate days. It can be used when praziquantel is not appropriate for some reason.

COMPLICATIONS

Complications include pneumothorax, pleural effusion, pleural empyema, and, rarely, a persistent pulmonary infiltrate. The first two occur early; the third is usually late. Only empyema is likely to require major intervention. A critical point in each is that not diagnosing the underlying cause may lead to recurrent difficulty and a poor result.

Pneumothorax

Presumably, pneumothorax occurs when larvae traversing the pleural space penetrate the lung by breaching the visceral pleura. Clinically, pneumothorax is uncommon and occurs early in the disease, approximately the time of pleuritic symptoms. Probably many small pneumothoraces occur, only to resolve without diagnosis, especially in underdeveloped areas where medical care is primitive. Pneumothorax should be treated with a superior-anterior intercostal chest tube connected to underwater drainage on suction until air leakage ceases and the lung reexpands. Small pneumothoraces may be observed a few days to see if they resolve spontaneously. Should fluid be present, or develop, an inferior-posterior tube should be added. The causative disease must be recognized and treated. Any fluid obtained should be examined for *Paragonimus* eggs.

Pleural Effusion

Pleural effusion occurs early but more frequently than pneumothorax. Johnson and associates (1982) found effusion in five of nine patients reported. Im and associates (1992) found pleural effusion in 54% of 71 patients examined radiographically. The early appearance of pleural effusion is not surprising because the larvae wander in the

pleural space before entering the lung and cause an acute reaction. This too is related in time to symptoms of pleurisy. Again, it is likely that many cases of small pleural effusion go undiagnosed. Many patients with well-established paragonimiasis have the haziness of old pleural reaction at the base of the thorax on the chest radiograph. When pleural effusion is diagnosed, it should be treated by drainage with an intercostal chest tube until drainage ceases and the pleural space seals off. Small effusions may be aspirated only. The fluid should be examined for *Paragonimus* eggs, and treatment for the disease given. As noted by Romeo and Pollock (1986), pleural fluid with a low pH, a glucose value below 10 mg/dL, a lactic dehydrogenase level above 1000 IU/L, and eosinophilia are characteristic in paragonimiasis, so testing for these values may be helpful in diagnosis. The danger of not recognizing or not treating the underlying disease is illustrated by Minh and colleagues (1981), who reported a patient with *P. westermani* infection who was tapped for recurrent pleural effusion repeatedly over 24 months before the underlying disease was recognized and treated. Even after treatment, the patient was discharged with a loculated fluid collection in the chest, thus raising the possibility that the lesion was actually an empyema.

Empyema

Empyema often has an insidious onset, indolent nature, and long duration. My associates and I (1981) reported 16 patients with such an empyema, the shortest duration of symptoms being over 6.5 years. The likeliest explanation for the development of *Paragonimus* empyema is that it comes from a long-standing, unresolved, and heretofore undiagnosed pleural effusion. The time between the original symptoms of paragonimiasis and the diagnosis of empyema is so great that their relationship is not suspected. This probably explains why the literature contains so few references to what must be a fairly frequent complication, particularly in endemic areas. A high index of suspicion leads to testing for and treatment of paragonimiasis.

Slowly, over a period of years, an unresolved pleural effusion develops a pleural peel with encapsulation of the fluid, which becomes thick and puslike. Unless secondary infection supervenes or the empyema has been drained with a chest tube, the pus is sterile. The symptoms are caused by restriction of the chest wall from the thick, tight peel and loss of lung capacity from the size of the empyema. The patients are usually young men who complain of mild dyspnea with dull aching in the chest wall overlying the empyema.

If it has not already been done, these patients should not be treated with a chest tube (Fig. 89-5). Rather, a thoracentesis should be performed for bacteriologic studies. The pus obtained is usually moderately thick and yellow or brownish. When a chest tube has been inserted, bacterial

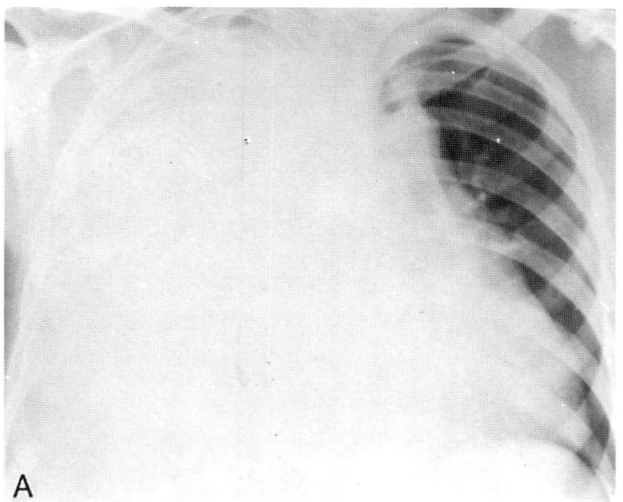

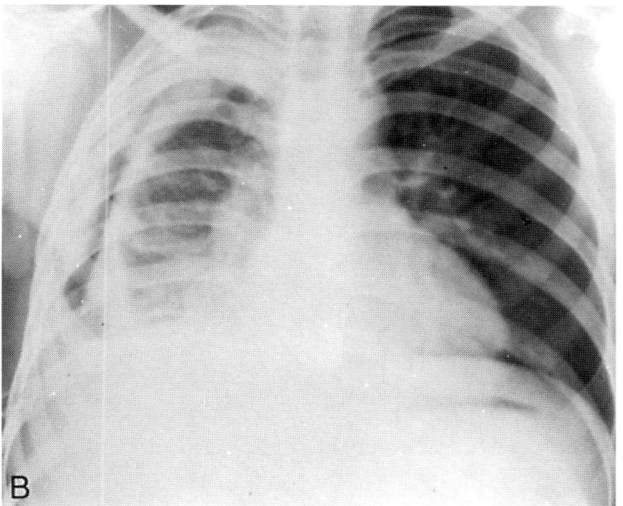

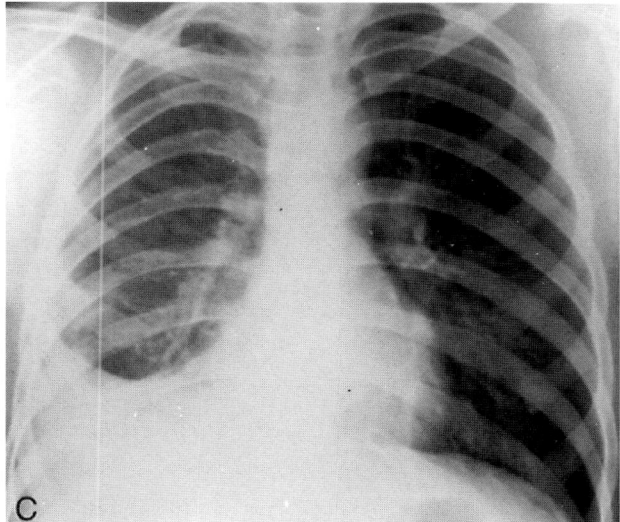

Fig. 89-5. A. Chest radiograph of an 18-year-old Korean man with *Paragonimus* empyema shows complete "white-out" of right thorax and shift of the heart to the left. **B.** After posterior tubing done by the medical service, there is residual space with incomplete expansion of the lung. Note the thick peel over the pleural surface of the lung. **C.** Decortication was delayed for almost 2 months after radiograph shown in **B**. This radiograph, taken approximately 3 weeks after decortication, shows complete reexpansion of the lung but some residual pleural thickening over the diaphragm, which remains slightly elevated.

contamination is common, and a variety of organisms may be cultured.

Treatment is by decortication with reexpansion of the lung (Fig. 89-6). Both parietal and visceral pleural peel should be removed. The peel is often surprisingly thick (up to 1 cm) and amazingly easy to remove. On occasion, operculated *Paragonimus* eggs are found in the surgical specimen. Postoperatively, inferior and superior chest tubes are left in the pleural space until drainage ceases and the space has sealed off with the lung reexpanded. Results are uniformly good in patients who have not had a preoperative chest tube, slightly less so in those who have.

In 16 patients that I and my associates (1981) reported, the results of decortication were good in 14 patients (87.5%), satisfactory in one patient (6.3%), and poor in one patient. This patient subsequently required a thoracoplasty for control of one of the four major complications that occurred in this group of patients. No deaths occurred. Ahn

and associates (1979) reported similar experience, as did Pezzella and colleagues (1981). An important point is that paragonimiasis empyema is much easier to decorticate than is tuberculous empyema, with the results being correspondingly better.

Persistent Pulmonary Infiltrate

When the rare complication of persistent pulmonary infiltrate occurs and a specific diagnosis cannot be made, surgical resection is indicated. Kaneko and colleagues (1997) carried out a right upper lobectomy successfully in one patient. Eggs of paragonimiasis were found within the granulation tissue present in the resected specimen.

If eggs of the organism are found in the sputum or feces, these rare persistent infiltrates disappear rapidly with appropriate medical therapy.

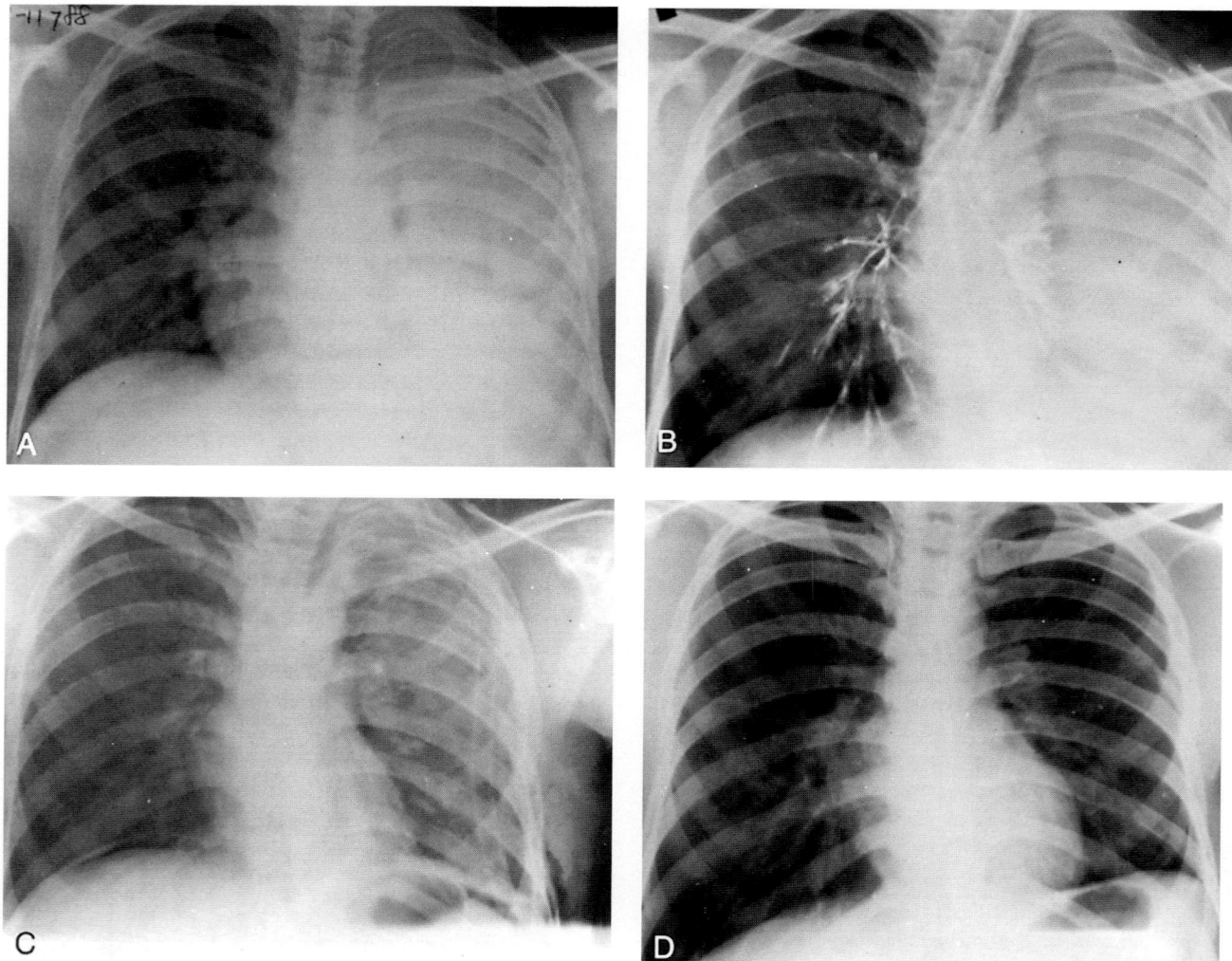

Fig. 89-6. A. Chest radiograph of a 19-year-old man with *Paragonimus* empyema, taken before admission, shows massive empyema causing almost complete "white-out" of the left thorax. **B.** Bronchogram 13 days later reveals complete collapse of the left lung with cutoff of all major bronchi. Note diminution of the left thorax with scoliosis. **C.** Two months later, shortly after left decortication. **D.** Chest radiograph 5 years after decortication shows excellent result. Note regeneration of sixth rib, slight elevation of left diaphragm laterally, and disappearance of scoliosis.

REFERENCES

Ahn WS, et al: Surgical treatment of paragonimiasis. Korean J Thorac Cardiovasc Surg *12*:312, 1979.

Chung CH: Human paragonimiasis (pulmonary distomiasis, endemic hemoptysis). *In* Marcial-Rojas RA (ed): Pathology of Protozoal and Helminthic Diseases. Baltimore: Williams & Wilkins, 1971, p. 531.

Dietrick RB, Sade RM, Pak JS: Results of decortication in chronic empyema with special reference to paragonimiasis. J Thorac Cardiovasc Surg *82*:58, 1981.

Im JG, et al: Pleuropulmonary paragonimiasis: radiologic findings in 71 patients. AJR Am J Roentgenol *159*:39, 1992.

Johnson JR, et al: Paragonimiasis in the United States. A report of nine cases in Hmong immigrants. Chest *82*:168, 1982.

Johnson RJ, et al: Paragonimiasis: diagnosis and the use of praziquantel in treatment. Rev Infect Dis *7*:200, 1985.

Kaneko T, Uemura S, Harada H: Three cases of paragonimiasis including one resected case. J Jpn Assoc Chest Surg *11*:850, 1997.

Minh V, et al: Pleural paragonimiasis in a Southeast Asian refugee. Am Rev Respir Dis *124*:186, 1981.

Nana A, Borornkitti S: Pleuropulmonary paragonimiasis. Semin Respir Med *12*:46, 1991.

Noble RR, Noble GA: Parasitology: The Biology of Animal Parasites. 4th Ed. Philadelphia: Lea & Febiger, 1982, p. 179.

Pezzella AT, Yu HS, Kim JE: Surgical aspects of pulmonary paragonimiasis. Bull Tex Heart Inst *8*:187, 1981.

Roberts PP: Parasitic infections of the pleural space. Semin Respir Infect *3*:362, 1988.

Romeo DP, Pollock JJ: Pulmonary paragonimiasis: diagnostic value of pleural fluid analysis. South Med J *79*:241, 1986.

Slemenda SB, et al: Diagnosis of paragonimiasis by immunoblot. Am J Trop Med Hyg *39*:469, 1988.

Yokogawa M, Tsuji M, Okura T: Studies on the complement fixation test for paragonimiasis as the method of criterion of cure. Jpn J Parasitol *11*:117, 1962.

Yokogawa M: Paragonimus and paragonimiasis. Adv Parasitol *3*:99, 1965.

CHAPTER 90

Solitary Pulmonary Nodule

Ronald B. Ponn

In contrast to diffuse lung disease, discussed in Chapter 91, a single focal pulmonary lesion, usually termed a *solitary pulmonary nodule* (SPN), is frequently asymptomatic and often owing to neoplasm. The vast majority of lung neoplasms are malignant. In this category, the incidence of bronchial carcinoma greatly exceeds that of all other primary and metastatic tumors. Many lung cancers that present as an SPN are early-stage lesions and are potentially curable by resection. Similarly, isolated uncommon primary malignant lung neoplasms, such as carcinoids and salivary gland-type tumors, are associated with a high surgical cure rate. Numerous reports also suggest that there is benefit from resection of tumors metastatic to the lung from a variety of primary sites. Although it is not universally confirmed, patients with single metastases may have a significantly longer disease-free survival after resection than do those with multiple deposits. In contrast to the benefit of resection for localized malignant lung neoplasms, resection of benign tumors and nonneoplastic processes is almost always purely diagnostic, hence "unnecessary," at least from a therapeutic standpoint. When a lung density is detected by radiography, therefore, the clinical imperative is either to establish a specific diagnosis or, in the absence of certainty, to reach a high level of probability that the lesion is benign and that a strategy of periodic follow-up is safe and appropriate. This goal should be accomplished in a timely fashion with the least possible discomfort, morbidity, and cost. The general thoracic surgeon should be familiar with the spectrum of focal lung lesions and their features to participate knowledgeably in the decision pathway about whether, when, and by what means to pursue invasive procedures.

Although approaches to the SPN vary, it is clear that the rate of unnecessary thoracotomy (i.e., open resection for benign disease) has decreased over time. In the era before computed tomography (CT), Steele (1963) reported a cooperative Veterans Administration–Armed Forces study in which only 36% of 941 solitary lung nodules resected between 1958 and 1963 were malignant. Malignancy rates for surgically removed lesions varied from as low as 10 to

68% in contemporaneous series. In a later study, Toomes and associates (1983) found malignancy in just fewer than one-half of 955 nodules resected between 1970 and 1980. Using the same inclusion criteria as the earlier review applied to a similar population of male veterans, Rubins and Rubins (1996) analyzed all solitary lesions resected without a preoperative diagnosis of cancer at their institution between 1981 and 1994. Overall, 79% of the masses were malignant, and 94% of this group were primary lung cancers.

The judicious application of modern imaging technology and newer alternative biopsy modalities should continue to reduce the necessity for major interventions in patients with SPNs, without an increase in missed or delayed detection of cancer arising in or metastatic to the lung. In the past, the options for an SPN were a simple dichotomy: "Watch it or wedge it." In practice, the choices were either 1) a period of observation by serial plain films or linear tomograms and 2) early thoracotomy for diagnosis and possibly treatment or later thoracotomy prompted by radiographic change. Many thoracic physicians and surgeons justifiably advised resection of all SPNs that did not have definitive radiographic signs of benignity or a specific benign histologic diagnosis. Currently, the options have expanded. SPNs can be watched initially and over time by plain film or more sensitive imaging techniques. Similarly, tissue diagnosis no longer always requires wedging by full posterolateral thoracotomy because flexible bronchoscopy, percutaneous transthoracic biopsy, limited incisions, and video-assisted thoracoscopy are often reliable alternatives.

DEFINITION

No universally accepted definition of what constitutes an SPN exists. Variations in nomenclature are based on the size and characteristics of the density and the presence or absence of other radiographic abnormalities. Some authors include lesions as large as 6 cm, but others limit an SPN to 3 or 4 cm in maximum diameter, a larger opacity being a mass. A few series apply a smaller size limit of 1 cm. Some use SPN to denote a small, spherical, mainly smooth-margined density entirely surrounded by lung parenchyma—the classic coin lesion. Nodules with air bronchograms or cavitation are variously included or excluded. The absence of other radiographic abnormalities, such as lymphadenopathy or satellite parenchymal lesions, is variably required for defining an SPN. Some require that an SPN be discovered on a plain chest film rather than other imaging studies, such as CT. Another confounding factor is that sometimes patients with symptoms are included, whereas other reports discuss only the asymptomatic SPN. Clearly, the incidence of malignancy and the conclusions of any series vary depending on the criteria used for definition.

The emphasis of this chapter is on the approach to the patient with a solitary radiographic lung density that may represent cancer and may benefit from thoracic surgical evaluation. Based on these considerations, a narrow definition of SPN would be insufficiently inclusive. SPN is used to encompass lesions that are, or at the time of discovery by any imaging modality appear to be, located in the lung, are predominantly solid (i.e., nodular or masslike rather than infiltrative), and do not have clear-cut signs of malignancy, such as invasion or metastasis to lymph nodes, bone, or other areas on the basis of the presentation radiographs.

An SPN that cannot with certainty be classified as either benign or malignant is an indeterminate nodule. A nodule that is indeterminate at presentation may be diagnosed as benign after additional radiographic studies or review of prior films. If a benign etiology is not proved by imaging criteria or biopsy, the lesion remains indeterminate, even when the suspicion of malignancy is low.

PREVALENCE OF SOLITARY PULMONARY NODULE AND INCIDENCE OF MALIGNANCY

The prevalence of SPNs in the general population is unknown. The reported detection rate varies, depending on the definition of SPN, the study population, and the sensitivity of the imaging modalities used. A higher rate of detection is expected in older people, smokers, people with a current or prior extrapulmonary neoplasm, and those who live in areas where fungal lung infections are common. Good and Wilson (1958) reported finding two SPNs per 1000 chest radiographs. Because of superior contrast resolution, CT is a more sensitive technique than conventional radiography for detecting parenchymal nodules. Edwards and Fry (1982) reviewed 100 consecutive CT scans obtained to evaluate nonpulmonary thoracic abnormalities in patients without known malignant disease. They detected a solitary nodule in two of the 100 studies. In a group of 25 patients with known malignancy, Schaner and associates (1978) found 15 nodules by CT that were not suspected by chest films or conventional tomograms. Because 9 of the 15 lesions turned out to be benign, the authors concluded that

there is an appreciable prevalence of asymptomatic benign nodules in the general population. More recently, Keogan and colleagues (1993) reached a similar conclusion after finding that 16% of 551 lung cancer patients undergoing CT had separate nodules, at least 70% of which were benign. Although the true prevalence of SPNs is uncertain, it is clear that such densities are encountered frequently in clinical practice. Stoller and associates (1988) estimated that in 1987, there were 133,000 newly discovered solitary lung nodules in the United States and emphasized that this figure rivals the annual incidence of other major clinical pulmonary problems, such as lung cancer and adult respiratory distress syndrome. Lillington (1991) estimated that there are 150,000 new SPN cases per year.

Once an SPN has been identified, what is the likelihood that it is malignant? The literature traditionally cites malignancy rates of 30 to 50%. These figures are based on older analyses of resected lesions, such as the aforementioned reports of Steele (1963) and Toomes and colleagues (1983). A selection bias in favor of finding more cancers in patients who have been directed toward resection exists, even during an era when early resection was often the most common approach to SPNs. During a similar period, in contrast, the incidence of malignancy in SPNs in radiographic general population surveys was much lower. Holin and associates (1959) found an incidence of only 3%. Similarly, 6% of nodules were ultimately determined to be malignant in the series collected by McClure and colleagues (1961). The importance of geographic location is emphasized by the experience reported by Trunk and colleagues (1974), who reviewed 137 consecutive nodules resected at a U.S. Air Force hospital in Illinois between 1963 and 1971. Benign lesions were identified in more than 84%, the majority of which (103) were granulomas. In this category, approximately one-half proved to be owing to histoplasmosis, a fungus endemic to the region.

None of these figures represents the current odds of malignancy in the global spectrum of SPNs. Although one might speculate that the lung cancer epidemic in recent decades should increase the likelihood of cancer in solitary lesions, the actual proportion is unknown. The more clinically relevant figure, however, is the incidence of malignancy in a lesion that remains indeterminate after up-to-date imaging, nonsurgical biopsy, or both. In a large cooperative study examining the role of CT, Zerhouni and associates (1986) found malignancy in 56% of nodules ultimately diagnosed by biopsy. The rate of malignancy, however, rose to 77% for nodules that were not called benign by imaging criteria. In the 14-year experience reported by Rubins and Rubins (1996), 90 to 100% of resected nodules were malignant in each of the later years of the study, as opposed to less than 60% in the earlier time period. The lowest current malignancy rates occur in series of thoracoscopic wedge excisions of SPNs. In the reports of Mack (1993), Bernard (1996), and DeCamp (1995) and their colleagues, malignancy was found in 48%, 56%, and 60% of cases, respectively. Lower rates in thoracoscopic series are likely related to the emergence of this technique as an effective method for diagnosing certain SPNs and to the inclusion in these cohorts of patients with smaller lesions and nodules of lower clinical suspicion.

The odds of malignancy in a pulmonary nodule that remains indeterminate after an evaluation that may include combinations of imaging modalities and nonsurgical biopsy are of paramount clinical relevance to thoracic surgeons. This odds ratio is the one that should be used to formulate further recommendations and the one quoted to the patient, who must ultimately decide how to proceed.

ETIOLOGY

The differential diagnostic possibilities for an SPN encompass an extensive list of diverse pathologic processes (Table 90-1). Although the reported frequency of benign versus malignant etiologies is subject to case-selection bias, it is clear that bronchial carcinoma comprises 85 to 90% of malignant lesions, whereas granulomas make up a similar proportion of the benign group. All the cell types of lung cancer can present as an SPN. Although metastatic spread to the lung from extrapulmonary tumors most often manifests as multiple nodules, an isolated deposit is sufficiently common that metastases make up the next most frequent source of malignant SPNs, usually reported in the range of 5 to 10% of resected nodules. Carcinoid tumors account for 1 to 3% of malignant lesions. All other types of malignant primary lung neoplasms are extremely rare.

Benign causes of SPNs include neoplastic and nonneoplastic processes. Benign lung tumors are uncommon. Despite the long list of histologies in this category, hamartomas (see Chapter 111) account for a higher proportion of benign tumors than do bronchial carcinomas among malignant tumors. Fein and coworkers (1998) noted that hamartoma accounted for 192 of 3802 resected nodules (5%) collated from six large series. Nonneoplastic benign nodules are overwhelmingly more common than benign tumors. In the United States, the majority are caused by granulomas from prior infection with the fungal organisms *Histoplasma capsulatum* or *Coccidioides immitis*. In most other parts of the world, granulomatous lesions more commonly represent the residua of pulmonary infection with *Mycobacterium tuberculosis*. Noninfectious granulomas, such as macronodular sarcoidosis and Wegener's granulomatosis, classically occur as scattered multiple lesions, but they may on occasion be confined to a single radiographically evident density. Yousem and Hochholzer (1987) noted that 40% of pulmonary hyalinizing granulomas were solitary. Fichtenbaum and associates (1990) described a case of eosinophilic granuloma, typically a diffuse reticulonodular process, presenting as a solitary nodule on CT.

Table 90-1. Causes of Solitary Pulmonary Nodules

Neoplasms
  Malignant
    Bronchial carcinoma
    Carcinoid tumor
    Metastasis: Carcinoma, sarcoma, melanoma, germ cell
    Uncommon malignant primary lung tumors: Blastoma, carcinosarcoma, lymphoma, melanoma, plasmacytoma, salivary gland–type tumors (adenoid cystic, mucoepidermoid, acinic cell, mixed, oncocytoma), sarcoma, teratoma, thymoma
  Benign
    Hamartoma
    Uncommon benign primary lung tumors: Alveolar adenoma, clear cell tumor (sugar tumor), chondroma, Clara cell adenoma, fibroma, fibromyxoma, glomus tumor, granular cell myoblastoma, hibernoma, leiomyoma, lipoma, mucous gland adenoma, neurogenic tumor, sclerosing hemangioma, squamous papilloma, teratoma, thymoma, xanthoma
Benign nonneoplastic lesions
  Infectious granulomas: Histoplasmosis, tuberculosis, coccidioidomycosis, cryptococcosis, blastomycosis, aspergillosis
  Other: Abscess, arteriovenous malformation, bronchogenic cyst, pulmonary infarction, intrapulmonary lymph node, organizing pneumonia, parasitic lesions (echinococcus, ascaris, Dirofilaria), plasma cell granuloma (inflammatory pseudotumor), postinflammatory fibrosis, rounded atelectasis, sequestration, venous varix
Lesions that are usually multiple but may be solitary: Amyloid nodule, bronchiolitis obliterans-organizing pneumonia (BOOP), endometriosis, eosinophilic granuloma, mucoid impaction, pulmonary hyalinizing granuloma, rheumatoid nodule, sarcoidosis, septic embolus, silicosis, Wegener's granulomatosis
Extrapulmonary densities mistaken for solitary pulmonary nodules by plain film: Blood vessel (dilated or on-end view), bone island, chest wall soft tissue mass, extracorporeal density (e.g., electrocardiographic electrode), overlapping normal structures, nipple shadow, osteophyte, pleural plaque/mass, pseudotumor (fluid in interlobar fissure)

Some apparent SPNs are factitious. Kundel and colleagues (1978) reported that up to 20% of subtle opacities considered lung nodules on chest film turned out to be owing to other causes. Extrapulmonary densities that may simulate nodules include overlapping normal structures, nipple shadows, and soft tissue or osseous lesions of the chest wall. Differentiation from pulmonary nodules is easily accomplished by the use of markers, repeat radiographs, oblique views, fluoroscopy, or spot films. In a series of 502 solitary lung nodules suspected by plain radiography, Huston and Muhm (1987) were able to determine by radiographic means other than CT that 62 opacities (12%) were either nonpulmonary or nonexistent.

CLINICAL EVALUATION

Although a patient's personal profile and medical history may be helpful in the differential diagnosis of an SPN, clinical evaluation alone is not definitive. Older age, male sex, and smoking increase the likelihood that a lesion is a malignant primary lung tumor. Lung cancer is uncommon in people younger than 35 years of age. Cummings and associates (1986a) have shown that the probability of malignancy increases in direct proportion to the number of cigarettes consumed per day. Conversely, the likelihood of lung cancer diminishes in former smokers, concordant with an increasing interval since smoking cessation. Although the changing epidemiology of lung cancer (notably the increasing incidence in women and possibly more cases presenting at an earlier age) may have lessened the importance of age, sex, and smoking habits, these factors remain important in assigning probabilities for clinical decision making. Residence and travel history may raise the possibility of a granulomatous nodule. People who currently reside or have previously lived in the Midwestern and southwestern United States are more likely to have granulomas owing, respectively, to histoplasmosis and coccidioidomycosis. The symptoms that may have occurred during the primary infection are usually mild and nonspecific, temporally remote, and rarely recalled by the patient. A history of exposure to tuberculosis or emigration from countries where mycobacterial infection is endemic may aid in differential diagnosis.

The presence of pulmonary symptoms has been variously reported to correlate with an increased or decreased chance of malignancy. Although some authors believe that a nodule must be unassociated with any symptoms to be classified as an SPN, this limitation seems artificial, because the diagnostic issues are similar in cases with and without symptoms. The presence of symptoms should form part of the clinical synthesis for approaching these lesions. Central masses are more often associated with dyspnea, wheezing, hemoptysis, pneumonia, and sputum production. Very peripheral lesions are most often asymptomatic. The presence of a dry, nonspecific cough, however, and even vague chest pain, in cases of peripheral subpleural masses, is not uncommon in patients who are ultimately found to harbor malignancy. Acute pulmonary symptoms, such as cough productive of purulent sputum, limited hemoptysis and dyspnea, especially when coupled with systemic complaints, such as malaise, fatigue, anorexia, and fever, are more often associated with an acute or subacute infectious process. In this setting, it is reasonable in some cases to follow the patient by plain film for a short period before embarking on more advanced imaging or invasive studies. Although the empiric use of antibiotics is controversial and should be individualized, cultures should be sent and treatment initiated if positive.

A history of prior or synchronous extrapulmonary malignancy is an important consideration. Multiple new nodules most often indicate metastatic disease. Occasionally, multiple densities result from a reaction to chemotherapeutic agents, such as methotrexate, or from infectious processes secondary to immunosuppression from the malignancy or its treatment. Nodules detected synchronously, especially when

found by CT, usually represent metastases but may be benign, especially if they are small. Johnson and associates (1982) noted that fewer than one-third of nodules smaller than 0.5 cm were metastases.

The situation is more complex when a solitary nodule is detected in a cancer patient. Although a history of malignancy increases the chance that the nodule is a metastasis, a large proportion of SPNs in this setting are owing to benign causes or to primary bronchial carcinoma. Overall, as emphasized by Coppage and colleagues (1987) and by Davis (1991), single lung nodules in patients with known extrapulmonary cancers more often represent primary lung carcinoma than metastatic foci. The probability that an SPN in a patient with a cancer history is metastatic depends on the type and extent of the primary neoplasm as well as the individual's risk for primary lung cancer or a benign process. The more advanced the primary, the more likely that an SPN is a metastasis.

The site of origin of the primary neoplasm influences the probability of metastasis, independent of stage. At one extreme, newly detected lung opacities in people with germ cell tumors or sarcomas, as reported by Pass and coworkers (1985), prove to be metastatic deposits in most cases. This high probability results from the biological propensity of these tumors to spread preferentially to the lung combined with a lower risk for lung cancer due to a younger mean age in this population. Similarly, most new SPNs in patients treated for melanoma are metastatic in origin. Although Pogrebniak and associates (1988) found that many SPNs in melanoma cases were benign, the benign causes in their series were rare ones, including hematoma, *Pneumocystis*, histiocytosis, and nonspecific pneumonitis. In contrast to primary sites strongly associated with metastasis in an SPN, squamous cancers of the head and neck have a propensity to precede or appear synchronously with primary malignant lung tumors. Smoking is the common factor that puts these individuals at risk for multiple aerodigestive malignancies. Approximately one-fourth of head and neck cancer patients develop second primary tumors within 8 years of initial treatment, most occurring in the lung. According to Cahan (1977), a new SPN in patients treated for early-stage squamous cancer of the head and neck is a primary bronchial cancer in more than 90% of instances. Malefatto and coworkers (1984) found a lower rate of lung cancer (53%) and a high proportion of benign lesions (28%). The two series are similar in that a minority of the nodules were owing to metastasis. Most of the common extrapulmonary adenocarcinomas, such as those of the breast and colon, are associated with an intermediate likelihood of metastasis in an SPN. Cahan and colleagues (1974) found that slightly less than one-half of synchronous or metachronous SPNs in patients with colon cancer were metastatic deposits, the remainder being primary lung cancers. In a series of patients with breast cancer, Cahan and Castro (1975) noted that 32% of SPNs were metastases, 60% were lung cancer, and 8%

were benign. Casey and associates (1984) reported a similar experience in breast cancer: 43% metastatic, 52% lung cancer, and 5% benign. Although renal cell carcinoma metastasizes to the lung in 30 to 50% of cases, Libby and colleagues (1990) pointed out that synchronous primary lung and kidney cancers are common.

In patients with a history of lung cancer, a new nodule is most often also a bronchial carcinoma. When the histology of the two cancers is the same, and carcinoma in situ is not seen in both lesions, the new lesion is considered either a metastasis or a metachronous primary cancer, depending on the definitions used (see Chapters 96 to 99). Although not an SPN, a nodule separate from the presenting site and usually detected by CT in a patient with a current lung cancer raises similar diagnostic issues. Staging requires determination if the lesion is benign or malignant and, in the latter case, assessment of the often complex question of synchronous primary lung cancer versus metastasis.

In patients without a history of cancer and without symptoms or findings suggestive of an extrapulmonary neoplasm, the chance that an SPN is a metastasis from an occult primary tumor is small (<1%). Extensive evaluation to assess this remote possibility is not warranted. In addition to a complete history and physical examination, however, optimal care of patients older than 50 years of age with suspicious SPNs, especially if a surgical procedure is planned, should include recent mammography, stool testing for blood, and possibly serum prostate-specific antigen. The value of these tests is to identify coincident common cancers rather than to discover an occult primary origin of the lung lesion.

Other elements of the medical history may occasionally be helpful. Ongoing or recently resolved systemic, respiratory, cutaneous, or musculoskeletal symptoms may suggest diagnoses such as bronchiolitis obliterans-organizing pneumonia, sarcoidosis, unresolved pneumonitis, or pulmonary infarction. These are rare causes of SPNs, and in most cases, tissue confirmation is required. The experience reported by Jolles and coworkers (1989) is instructive. Of seven patients with severe rheumatoid arthritis who underwent bronchoscopy during a 4-year period for new SPNs consistent with necrobiotic nodules, all were found to have carcinoma.

An important aspect of the history is the determination of the existence of prior chest radiographs. Although patients are often unsure, a call to their primary physicians and to hospitals to which they have been admitted frequently uncovers these studies. Ideally, any extant films should be obtained and examined in direct comparison with the current studies. If the radiographs are no longer available, the radiologist's report is helpful only if it specifically indicates the size and description of the opacity in question.

Physical findings that may provide a clue to the etiology of an SPN are uncommon. Examples include telangiectases in hereditary cases of arteriovenous malformation (AVM), signs of an asymptomatic extrapulmonary primary cancer (e.g., cutaneous melanoma, breast mass, or abdominal mass), or signs suggesting lung cancer (e.g., clubbing and ipsilateral scalene lymphadenopathy).

RADIOGRAPHIC ASSESSMENT*

Although the clinical evaluation may be helpful on occasion, it is the radiographic assessment of an SPN that most often determines plans to resect, biopsy, observe, or forego any further evaluation. Most solitary nodules are discovered on chest film, but, in the absence of documented chronicity, more sensitive imaging modalities are usually needed for further characterization. The high kilovoltage used for standard chest films limits contrast resolution and the ability to detect subtle calcification. Low-kilovoltage plain tomography and fluoroscopy were for many years the standard technique for assessing lung nodules. Huston and Muhm (1987) showed that conventional tomography combined with fluoroscopy can be used with good results. Classifying 502 nodules on the basis of calcification and shape, they were able to reach a correct benign or malignant diagnosis in 67% of patients. Modifications of the chest radiograph to improve the assessment of SPNs have been described, but they are not widely applied at present. Kelcz and associates (1994) showed improved observer detection and characterization of nodules by using dual-energy radiographs to eliminate rib shadows with tissue-selective images and to enhance calcified areas with bone-selective images. Chiles and Sherrier (1990) reported histogram analysis of digitized plain chest films. Newer imaging methods designed to assess tissue and cellular features have been applied to the evaluation of SPNs. Although magnetic resonance imaging has not generally proved to be valuable, the early experience with positron emission tomography (PET) scanning is promising. In most centers, however, CT is currently the pivotal imaging modality for lung nodules that require further evaluation after review of current and prior chest films. CT has been refined by the development of high-resolution CT (HRCT) and offers superior capability over conventional radiography and tomography to delineate morphologic characteristics, such as size, shape, margins, contours, and internal composition, and to detect unsuspected coexistent nodules or other extrapulmonary thoracic abnormalities. CT also allows precise localization of nodules with respect to the pleura, fissures, blood vessels, and airways, information that is often helpful for planning optimal biopsy approaches. In addition, quantitative CT measurements of the baseline attenuation or contrast-enhanced density of a nodule may suggest a benign or malignant etiology. CT scanning is widely available in the United States. Vock and Soucek (1993) reviewed the advantages of spiral CT in the study of lung nodules; these include rapid study times and the ability to select retrospectively the thin section that represents the center of a nodule. In most cases,

*The author gratefully acknowledges the assistance of Jack L. Westcott, M.D., for providing illustrative radiographs for this section.

a 2-cm nodule can be scanned with 1-mm slices during a single breath-hold, thereby ensuring contiguous sections.

Two radiographic features of an SPN are diagnostic of a benign etiology, namely, certain patterns of calcification and stability over time. In some cases, in addition, baseline density by CT or enhancement by CT or PET can be strongly indicative of a benign or malignant process. In most instances, however, the radiographic appearance alone is not specific enough to exclude malignancy reliably. Nonetheless, the CT features of an SPN, alone or in combination, are often of great value in generating a high, intermediate, or low level of suspicion of a malignant etiology and thereby in planning the optimal diagnostic pathway.

Calcification and Density

Although calcification occurs far more commonly in benign nodules than in malignant lesions, the presence of calcium per se is not definitive. Calcification in malignant tumors can result from neoplastic incorporation of an adjacent granuloma or parenchymal scar, dystrophic calcium deposition in areas of ischemia and necrosis, or calcium production by the cancer. Four patterns of calcium distribution, however, correlate so closely with benignity that their identification is considered diagnostic.

- A laminated pattern results from calcium deposition in concentric, complete, or partial rings and is also referred to as *laminar*, *lamellated*, *target*, or *bull's-eye* calcification.
- A benign central pattern requires identification of a dense nidus of calcium in the center of a nodule (Fig. 90-1). By plain film, the central location of the nidus must be confirmed in two planes.
- The diffuse pattern is a dense homogeneous distribution of calcium throughout the entire nodule.
- The fourth benign pattern is "popcorn" calcification, made up of larger chunks of calcium noted throughout the mass, and is diagnostic of pulmonary hamartoma, although only a minority of hamartomas display this feature.

Calcification that is eccentric or consists of fine scattered flecks (i.e., stippled) can be found in both benign and malignant nodules and cannot be relied on as a sole indicator of a benign process (Fig. 90-2). Stippled calcification may be central but is differentiated from the benign central type by its fine pattern.

As a general rule, benign lesions are associated with more obvious, easily detectable macrocalcifications than are malignant nodules. Malignant lesions rarely contain calcification that is sufficiently extensive or dense to be appreciated on plain chest films. Although calcium was found on radiographs of the resected specimens in 10 of 72 patients (14%) with adenomas, metastatic tumors, or lung cancers studied by O'Keefe and associates (1957), in only one case (1.4%) was calcification noted on the preoperative chest film. In the same study, in contrast, calcium was

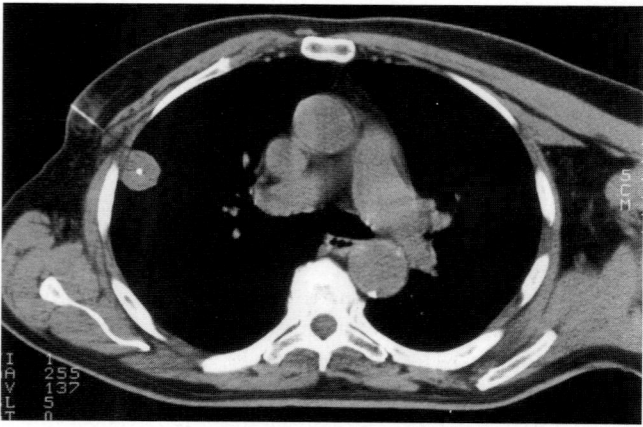

Fig. 90-1. Computed tomographic scan shows a dense central nidus of calcification. Core biopsy documented amyloid.

detected by specimen radiography in one-half of 135 benign lesions and in one-third of the corresponding chest films. The chest film showed calcification in 35 of 90 granulomas (39%) and in 11 of 32 hamartomas (34%). Theros (1977) reported calcification on chest radiographs in only 7 of 1267 (0.5%) cases of primary lung tumors at the Armed Forces Institute of Pathology.

Siegelman and associates (1986a), Proto and Thomas (1985), and others have shown that HRCT is capable of detecting calcification in one-fourth to one-third of nodules that appear uncalcified on plain tomography. In addition, HRCT can detect calcium that is missed by standard 1-cm CT collimation. In cases in which calcification is identified directly by examining thin sections through the nodule, the benign patterns of calcium deposition noted previously are relevant to the evaluation. In other nodules, calcium is not appreciated grossly, but the presence of microcalcification is inferred from the high density of the entire lesion or of its central area. CT densitometry is the measurement of attenuation within a nodule using a computer printout of a matrix of CT numbers. Siegelman and associates (1980) were the first to report application of this approach for identifying benign nodules. In this series, all nodules with a representative CT number greater than 164 Hounsfield units (HU) were reliably confirmed as benign. After these initial promising results could not be universally verified by other investigators, the problem was traced in large measure to variability among CT scanners and reconstruction algorithms and to drift over time in individual machines. Zerhouni and associates (1986) devised and tested a high-density calcium carbonate standard reference nodule simulator, or phantom. In this method, after the clinical nodule is scanned, the phantom model is constructed to simulate the size and location of the nodule and the chest wall thickness of the patient; the phantom is then scanned using the same settings. If the patient's nodule is denser than the phantom, it is likely

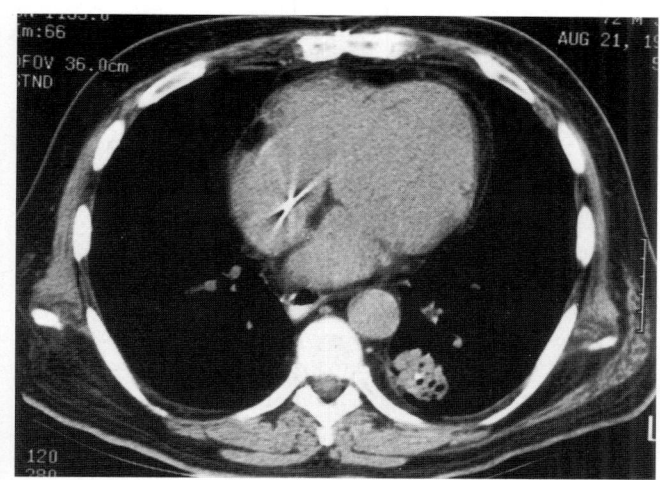

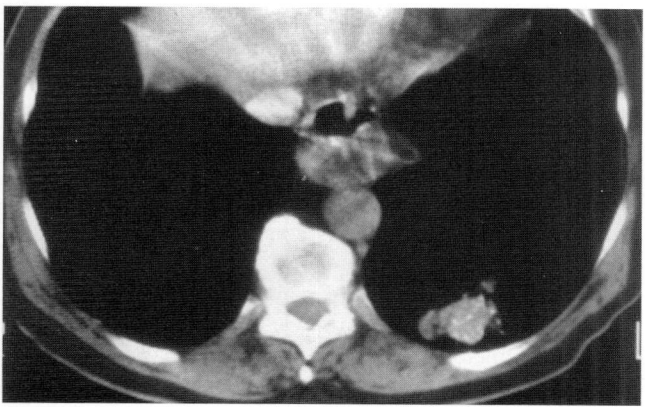

Fig. 90-2. Computed tomographic scans of adenocarcinomas with calcification. **A.** A single eccentric focus. **B.** Scattered or stippled calcification.

benign. If the phantom is denser, the nodule is indeterminate. Subsequent results with the phantom have been variable. Some studies have shown reliability, but others have documented false-negative cases. In a small series reported by Ward and associates (1989), 20 of 50 nodules were diagnosed correctly as benign, whereas 57% of the indeterminate lesions were malignant. Similarly, Huston and Muhm (1989) found that only one of 33 nodules (total series, 112) called benign was actually metastatic uterine cancer. Khan and colleagues (1991) in a series of 62 nodules found that use of the phantom increased sensitivity in detecting benign nodules by 22% over HRCT. However, only nine of the entire group of 62 nodules turned out to be malignant, and two lesions classified as benign by both thin-section CT and phantom were actually malignant (one carcinoid and one bronchial carcinoma). Jones and associates (1989) reported one false-negative diagnosis (an adenocarcinoma) among 11 nodules called benign in a series of 31 nodules. Swenson and associates (1991) also reported a substantial false-negative rate, with 8 of 85 radiographically benign nodules proving to be malignant.

Experience with HRCT has emphasized that cancers contain calcium more often than is appreciated by other techniques. In the series of Siegelman and colleagues (1986a), the rate was 13.4% of malignant lesions, a proportion similar to that noted by O'Keefe and associates (1957) on specimen radiographs and to the estimated histologic incidence of calcification in resected lung cancers. Therefore, radiographic diagnosis must be both quantitative and qualitative. It is suggested that benign calcification must be not only diffuse or central but also must involve more than 10% of the nodule. Exceptions can still be found. Maile and associates (1982) noted that metastatic lesions may contain significant amounts of calcium, including chondrosarcoma, osteogenic sarcoma, thyroid cancer, and mucinous adenocarcinoma of the colon. Zweibel and coworkers (1991) found calcification by CT in 39% of central carcinoids but only 8% (one case) of peripheral carcinoids. Rarely, a primary bronchial carcinoma demonstrates calcification of more than 10% of the lesion. These are generally adenocarcinomas that are 3 cm or larger.

There remains controversy over the role of CT densitometry and especially the need for the phantom in the evaluation of an SPN. The problems of standardization have been largely solved by advances in CT technology. As pointed out by Webb (1990, 1997), newer units provide reproducible and accurate attenuation numbers, thereby obviating the need for the phantom. It is important to note that most calcified lesions can be detected by HRCT. Densitometry may detect a few more. The specificity of densitometry can be enhanced by raising the critical "benign" attenuation level to 200 HU. The technique should be limited to small nodules, preferably 2 cm or smaller, that lack other radiographic features suggesting malignancy, and the results should be interpreted in light of the entire database.

At the opposite end of the attenuation spectrum, very low density by CT indicates the presence of fat. Fat within a pulmonary nodule is diagnostic of a benign process and usually indicates a hamartoma (Fig. 90-3). Lipoid pneumonia or pulmonary lipoma are rare causes of fat density. As noted earlier, the popcorn pattern of calcification is pathognomonic of hamartoma, but only a minority of tumors demonstrate this finding [12% in the series of O'Keefe and associates (1957)]. Using HRCT, however, Siegelman and colleagues (1986b) were able to make a specific diagnosis of hamartoma in 28 of 47 cases (60%). Fat alone was found in 38%, and fat combined with calcification in 21%. The ability of HRCT to diagnose at least one-half of pulmonary hamartomas, and thereby avoid resection or biopsy, is a definite advantage.

In summary, if a nodule exhibits a definitive benign pattern of calcification and has no other features worrisome for malignancy, no further follow-up is indicated. If a benign diagnosis is based on densitometry alone, or if there are any other characteristics of the nodule that arouse suspicion, close observation is mandatory, and early biopsy must be considered.

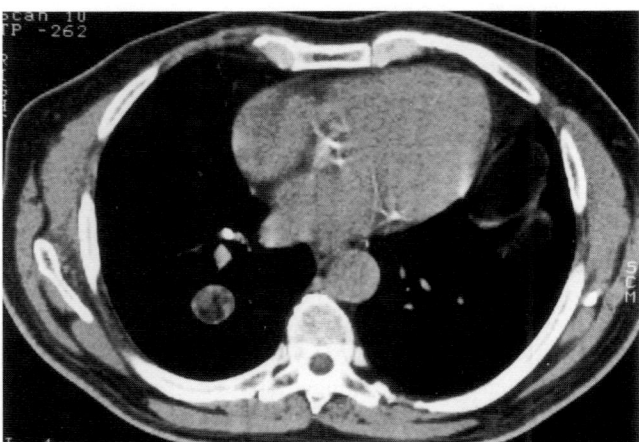

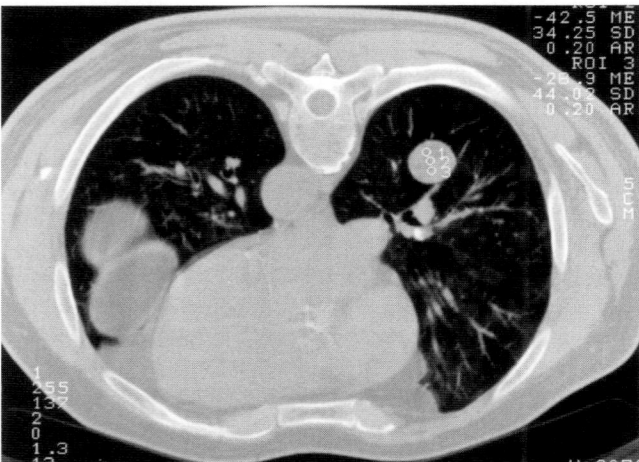

Fig. 90-3. Computed tomographic scan shows smoothly marginated right lower lobe mass. **A.** Inhomogeneous density. **B.** Computed tomographic numbers obtained at the time of planned biopsy (prone position) were negative in all regions of interest, thus confirming a hamartoma. Biopsy was not performed.

Stability and Growth Rate

In addition to fat density or benign calcification, lack of growth over time is commonly accepted as a reliable indication of benignity. The requisite period of stability for a confident benign diagnosis is universally cited as 2 years. Yankelevitz and Henschke (1997) have reviewed this assertion. They confirmed that 2-year stability is accepted as indicative of a benign SPN in textbooks of pulmonary medicine, thoracic surgery, and chest radiology and in major journal articles on the subject. They trace the origin of this dictum to a report by Good and Wilson (1958) but point out that examination of the original data yields a predictive value for benignity based on stability of only 65%. They caution that the current ability to detect smaller nodules casts further doubt on the usefulness of stability. Exceptions to the 2-year rule have been reported. Davis and associates (1956) reported an adenocarcinoma that was unchanged by

chest film for 8 years and suggested that stability for 5 years be required to consider a nodule benign. In a study of 105 surgically treated cases of bronchoalveolar carcinoma, Dumont and colleagues (1998) found that in 12% of the 85 cases presenting as an SPN, the lesion had been radiographically stable for 2 to 7 years. Several of these tumors did not have associated fibrosis, indicating that not all were "scar carcinomas."

The concept that lack of growth over time suggests a benign etiology is based on the fact that malignant neoplasms exhibit cell division and growth. Because some benign lesions also increase in size, the rate of growth of an SPN has been suggested as a means of differentiating benign from malignant processes. Analysis of growth rates is also relevant to the question of how much weight to assign to temporal stability of a nodule. Collins and Loeffler (1956) established the concept of tumor doubling time (DT)—the time it takes for a nodule to increase twofold in volume—as an index of growth rate. Use of DT for determining growth rates is based on three assumptions. First, nodules are assumed to be essentially spherical. The relationship of volume to radius (r), therefore, is volume = $\frac{4}{3}\pi r^3$. Calculation of DT is based on the further assumption that the growth rate of a tumor is either uniformly constant or randomly steady over time. Third, it is assumed that the area or volume of opacity seen radiographically is owing entirely to neoplastic cells. Based on this model, a single cancer cell that measures 10 nm in diameter requires 30 doublings of volume to reach a diameter of 1 cm. Only five more doublings are needed to achieve a diameter of 3 cm. By 40 doublings, the tumor would be 10 cm in diameter. Five more doublings would yield a theoretical tumor of 32 kg. It is assumed that in most cases, death from local invasion or distant metastasis occurs at or before the 10-cm stage. Thus, by the time a tumor is clearly visible by plain film (i.e., 1 cm), at least three-fourths of its natural history have elapsed. For lung nodules, DT can be determined if two radiographs obtained at different times show an increase in nodule diameter. Garland (1966) calculated that the duration of growth from one cell to a 2-cm tumor averaged 8 years for primary squamous and undifferentiated cancers of the lung and 15 years for adenocarcinomas. Masses with very short DT are generally infectious or inflammatory, whereas those with long DT are likely granulomas or benign neoplasms. However, there is much overlap due to wide variations in tumor DT. Nathan (1974) and Nathan and associates (1962) reported that all but three cases in a group of 177 malignant lung nodules had DTs of 280 days or less. The three slowest-growing lesions had DTs of 375, 395, and 465 days. All nodules with DT greater than 465 days were benign. The lower limit of DT consistent with a malignant etiology in these series of primary and metastatic nodules was 7 days. If unusually rapidly progressive (and rare) lesions, such as choriocarcinoma and embryonal cell carcinoma, are excluded, however, a reasonable lower limit of DT for malignant processes is between 30 and 40 days. Mizuno and associates (1984) reported that the mean

DT for adenocarcinoma was 177 days; for large cell carcinoma, 111 days; and for squamous cancer, 102 days. Small cell carcinomas grew considerably faster than non–small cell neoplasms, with a mean DT of only 62 days. There was, however, a wide range of DT within cell types. DT for squamous cancers, for example, ranged from less than 30 days to just longer than 350 days. The fastest-growing adenocarcinomas had DTs similar to those of rapidly doubling squamous cell tumors, but at the opposite extreme, three adenocarcinomas displayed DTs greater than 450 days, with two cases more than 500 days. With the mean DTs in this series, the time from the 1-cm stage to the predicted death of the patient (10 cm) was 4.9 years for adenocarcinoma, 3 years for large cell cancer, 2.8 years for squamous carcinoma, and 1.6 years for small cell tumors. Although for the group as a whole, actual survival time correlated well with predicted survival based on DT, the authors noted that for many resected patients, actual survival far exceeded the interval calculated by DT. Hayabuchi and associates (1983) also emphasized that prolonged DT for lung cancer is not uncommon, especially for adenocarcinomas. They followed people exposed to radiation from the atomic blasts in Japan with biennial chest films. Slow-growing tumors were defined by a DT longer than 5 months. By this definition, 17% of peripheral squamous cancers were slow growing, with a mean DT of 160 days. Forty-two percent of peripheral adenocarcinomas were slow growing, with a mean DT of 367 days. Large cell and small cell anaplastic cancers, in contrast, were all associated with a DT less than 5 months. Among metastases, lung lesions from thyroid cancer and adenoid cystic carcinoma of the salivary glands are often very indolent.

Although growth is universal in malignant pulmonary nodules, benign lesions may increase in size as well. Good and Wilson (1958) found that 4% of hamartomas and 6% of granulomas enlarged over time. In a detailed study, Goodwin and Snell (1969) noted that histoplasmomas could increase in diameter by as much as 1.7 mm per year, a rate that overlaps many cancers. They reported that granulomas owing to tuberculosis and coccidioidomycosis could also enlarge. Opacities caused by rounded atelectasis can also progress, as noted by Silverman and Marino (1987) and Hillerdal (1989). Eschelman and coworkers (1991) reported growth in a case of pulmonary hyalinizing granuloma. AVMs may enlarge over time and, without true progression, may appear radiographically larger or smaller, depending on the respiratory cycle. Conversely, malignant densities sometimes appear to shrink. Garland (1966) reported that 5% of malignant nodules appeared to decrease in diameter temporarily during observation. This phenomenon is probably related to radiographic technique, observer variation, or changes in areas of opacity due to nonneoplastic reaction or obstruction rather than to an actual decline in the volume of cancer cells.

The use of temporal stability and DT for decision making should generally be limited to retrospective applications based on comparison of prior and current radiographs. Except in rare cases, watchful waiting to assess stability or calculate DT prospectively is not prudent. Despite exceptions to the 2-year rule, a lesion that can be confirmed to have been present without change for 2 years by high-quality radiographs (DT >730 days) is very likely benign. In contrast, the vast majority of nodules that have demonstrated any growth should be resected. If, however, review of prior films clearly documents minimal change over a prolonged period, especially if other signs of benignity are present, it may in some cases be reasonable to continue radiographic surveillance. Another problem with using DT for prospectively following SPNs is that small lesions can increase significantly in volume with minimal change in diameter. Recalling the formula volume = $\frac{4}{3}\pi r^3$, a 0.5-cm nodule that doubles in volume increases in diameter by 1.4 mm, and a 1-cm mass increases by only 2.4 mm. Such small increments can be missed by plain radiography and even by CT. This observation indicates that stability over time and prolonged DT carry more clinical weight in the case of larger lesions. It also suggests that CT is generally the imaging modality of choice if one elects to follow a small nodule. Cases in which the concept of DT might have more prospective usefulness are those characterized by very rapid progression (i.e., DT <30 days). In most instances, these are infectious or inflammatory lesions.

Other Radiographic Features

In current practice, the location, size, and morphologic features of an indeterminate SPN are most often defined ultimately by CT. The conventional teaching is that certain internal and edge findings are characteristic of malignant lesions, whereas their opposites are associated with benign nodules. For example, edges with spiculation, notching (Rigler's sign), irregularity, lobulation, or indistinctness are thought of as denoting invasive growth of neoplasms into the adjacent lung parenchyma, as opposed to the smooth or angular margination of a benign nodule. The classic metastatic deposit is generally described as spherical and smoothly marginated. Although these generalizations are basically valid, analysis of large numbers of cases shows that most are insufficiently specific to be of value as univariate predictors. Malignant nodules can be associated with a "pushing" edge as they grow (i.e., the interface between the lesion and the surrounding lung remains radiographically smooth because the tumor is not infiltrating the adjacent parenchyma). Conversely, benign processes may insinuate locally or create a reaction that simulates cancerous infiltration. Although the radiographic features of an SPN, especially in combination, may suggest a malignant or benign etiology, they are only occasionally definitive. Processes that can often be diagnosed radiographically include mucous plugging, AVM, rounded atelectasis, and fungal nodule.

Location of the Solitary Pulmonary Nodule

Nodule location is of little diagnostic value. Primary lung cancers and tuberculous granulomas occur more often in the upper and middle lobes than in the lower lobes, whereas hamartomas show an equal lobar distribution. Metastases most often are located peripherally. In a radiographic-pathologic study by Scholten and Kreel (1977), 92% of metastases were located in the peripheral one-third of the lung fields, and 67% were directly subpleural. Crow and associates (1981) noted that 82% of metastatic deposits were peripheral. Banko and associates (1996) and Yokomise and colleagues (1998) found that intrapulmonary lymph nodes resected for the diagnosis of indeterminate SPNs were located in the lower lobes in 70% and 72% of cases, respectively.

Size of the Solitary Pulmonary Nodule

Larger nodule size correlates with an increased probability of cancer. The converse (i.e., that small lesions are likely benign) is reported in older series. Although more recent studies confirm that larger nodules are overwhelmingly malignant [93 to 99% of resected nodules >3 cm in the reports of Zerhouni (1986) and Siegelman (1986a) and their associates], current experience indicates that small size does not indicate a high probability of a benign process. Steele (1963) found that 80% of nodules larger than 3 cm were malignant, whereas 80% of those smaller than 2 cm and 93% of SPNs 1 cm or smaller were benign. More recently, almost one-half the reported lesions smaller than 2 or 3 cm are malignant. In the aforementioned 1986 studies, 42% of 177 malignant lesions were smaller than 2 cm, and 15% were smaller than 1 cm. In a group of 40 consecutive nodules, all smaller than 3 cm, evaluated between 1990 and 1993 by Libby and coworkers (1995), 53% overall were cancers, as were 80% of those larger than 2 cm and 43% of those 2 cm or smaller. In a group of 65 nodules 1 cm or smaller resected by video-assisted thoracoscopy, Munden and colleagues (1997) found an incidence of malignancy of 58%. The increasing incidence of cancer in smaller histologically confirmed nodules may be the result of improved radiographic detection coupled with a greater willingness to apply a strategy of watchful waiting in low-suspicion cases. The lesson, however, is clear: Small nodules detected by modern imaging are often malignant.

Shape and Margins of the Solitary Pulmonary Nodule

Huston and Muhm (1987) used fluoroscopy and conventional tomography to classify nodules as benign or malignant by shape and edge features (i.e., border, margin, and nodule-lung interface). A lesion with totally circumferential spiculation, known as *corona radiata* or *corona maligna*, was considered malignant; a nodule was called benign if it had a linear or angular shape or was composed of multiple tiny densities. Although all 38 nodules diagnosed as benign

remained stable for 2 years and 31 of 33 lesions classified as malignant proved to be so on biopsy, the limitations of pure morphologic analysis by plain tomography is highlighted by the fact that 70% of all noncalcified lesions in this large series were radiographically indeterminate. Among the indeterminate lesions, 77% were found to be benign and 23% were malignant. In the cooperative CT study of Zerhouni and colleagues (1986), 100 of 178 nodules with smooth or lobulated borders proved to be benign (56%), as opposed to 91 lesions with irregular, spiculated margins, of which only 11 were benign (12%). However, many of these nodules were incorrectly diagnosed by CT criteria. Siegelman and associates (1986a) used a scale of 1 to 4 for edge analysis by CT: 1) sharp and smooth, 2) moderately smooth, 3) showing some undulations or spiculations, and 4) grossly irregular with circumferential spiculations. Although most nodules with smooth margination (type 1) were benign, 20% were malignant. A type 2 edge was common in both categories: 58% were malignant, 42% were benign. Eighty-eight percent of types 3 and 4 lesions were malignant (Fig. 90-4). Zwirewich and associates (1991) correlated edge and internal characteristics determined by HRCT with histology in 93 patients. Although certain features were statistically more common in malignancy, there was much overlap. Spiculation correlated with lymphatic spread and infiltrative tumor growth in some cases but was most often owing to irregular peripheral fibrosis; it was present in 87% of malignant nodules and 55% of benign lesions. Similarly, a pleural tag or pleural tail, due to a desmoplastic reaction extending from the lesion to the visceral pleura and variously cited as indicative of cancer or of a benign process, was present in 58% of malignancies and in 27% of benign nodules (Fig. 90-5). Lobulation was typical of malignancies and represented nodular excrescences of neoplastic growth at the edge of a lesion, but it was seen in 27% of benign nodules as well. In the benign cases, lobulation on HRCT was most often owing to coalescent granulomas. Sone and associates (1997) also emphasized that irregularity, including spiculation, indistinctness, lobulation, and pleural tails, is usually caused by nonmalignant factors, namely, a desmoplastic reaction or scar formation with retraction. They pointed out that a tumor with uniform, solid growth often displays a well-defined, smooth margin.

Internal Composition of the Solitary Pulmonary Nodule

With respect to internal composition, Zwirewich and colleagues (1991) found that homogeneous attenuation correlated more often with benign processes (55%) but was also present in 20% of primary and metastatic growths. The 80% of malignant opacities with inhomogeneous internal findings displayed cavitation, necrosis without cavitation, and air bronchograms or areas of bubblelike low attenuation due to small, patent, air-containing bronchi within the mass. Although considered typical of squamous cell cancer, cavitation can occur in all cell types of lung cancer. The

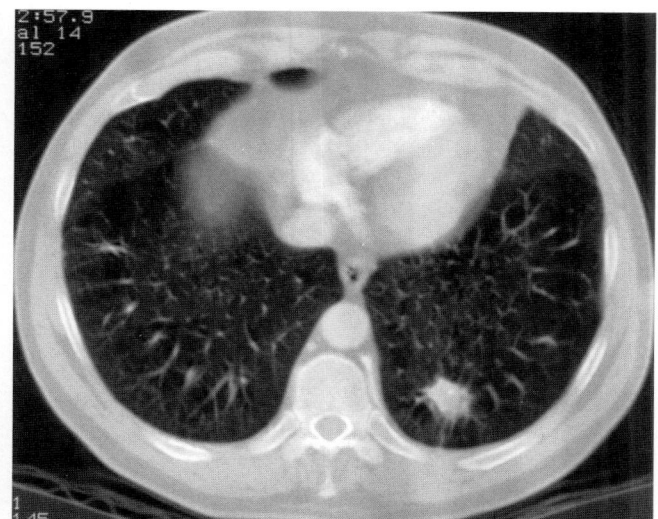

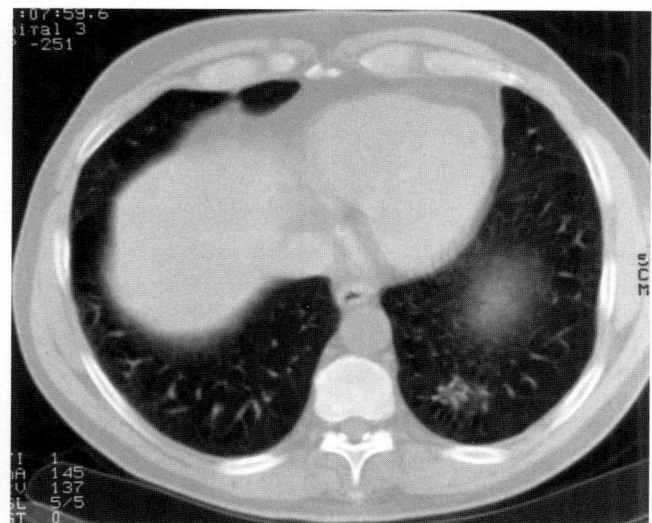

Fig. 90-4. A. Computed tomographic scan shows circumferential spiculation (corona radiata, corona maligna) in a left lower lobe nodule. **B.** Although circumferential spiculation is considered a sign of malignancy, this lesion had regressed 2 weeks later, at the time of planned biopsy, and ultimately resolved entirely.

extremes of wall thickness of a cavitary lesion may be helpful. Malignant lesions tend to have thicker, more irregular walls. In the series of Woodring and Fried (1983), all cavitary masses with a wall thickness less than 1 mm were benign. They also found that 95% of masses smaller than 4 mm were also benign; 27% of masses between 5 and 15 mm were malignant; and 84% of those larger than 15 mm were malignant (Fig. 90-6). Air bronchograms and bubblelike areas, sometimes termed *pseudocavitation*, are typical of bronchoalveolar carcinoma. Kuriyama and coworkers (1991) used HRCT to determine the frequency of air bronchograms or bronchiolograms and the histologic correlate of a patent bronchus or bronchiole in 20 lung cancers smaller than 2 cm compared to 20 benign nodules. The authors con-

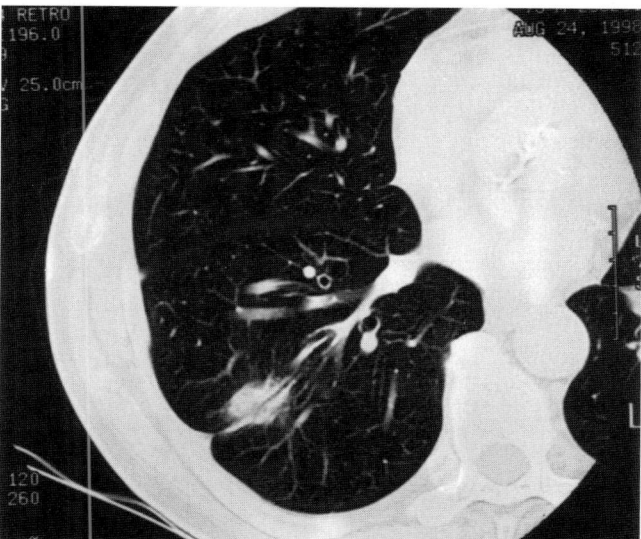

Fig. 90-5. Computed tomographic scan shows a pleural tag in a right lower lobe carcinoma. Benign lesions may also have this feature.

cluded that an air bronchogram should raise a strong suspicion of malignancy because 72% of adenocarcinomas had an air bronchogram, but only 5% of the benign masses demonstrated this feature. Air bronchograms may also be seen in pulmonary lymphoma.

Relationship to Vascular and Airway Structures

The relationship of an SPN to blood vessels or airways may suggest a diagnosis and, in some cases, may be pathognomonic. Naidich and Garay (1991) reviewed angiocentric and bronchocentric focal lung lesions. CT can be helpful in identi-

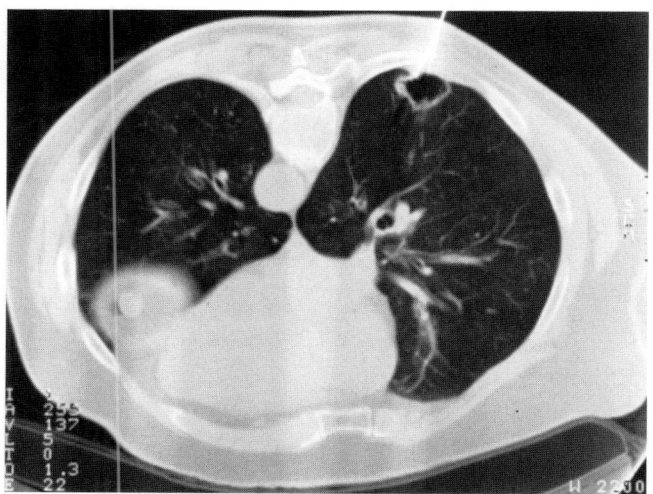

Fig. 90-6. Computed tomographic scan during needle biopsy of wall of right lower lobe cavitary lesion. Biopsy and subsequent resection showed bronchoalveolar carcinoma T_2N_0. Any cell type may be cavitary; thin-walled cavities may be malignant.

fying metastases, septic emboli, and "bland" or noninfectious infarcts, and can be diagnostic for invasive aspergillosis and AVMs. Metastatic deposits, because of their hematogenous mode of dissemination, may be shown on CT to be supplied by a feeding pulmonary artery. Septic pulmonary emboli and noninfected areas of infarction are usually multiple but occasionally solitary. Infarcts are typically wedge shaped and pleura based. The perimeter of an infarct may enhance with intravenous contrast due to collateral bronchial arterial blood supply. A pulmonary artery may be identified at the apex of the triangular infarct. In the case of septic emboli, Huang (1989) and Kuhlman (1990) and their associates found feeding pulmonary vessels by CT in approximately two-thirds of peripheral lesions. Invasive pulmonary aspergillosis, also hematogenously disseminated and rarely solitary, may be associated with an identifiable feeding vessel, as well as with an air-crescent sign (a rim of air surrounding an intracavitary fungus ball). The fungal conglomerate may move with changes in patient position. This constellation of findings in an immunocompromised host is diagnostic, but it is not typical of early lesions before tissue necrosis has occurred. Similarly, in the case of AVMs, plain-film or CT identification of a round or serpiginous density with a feeding and draining vessel is pathognomonic. Although AVMs enhance markedly after administration of intravenous contrast, this finding is often superfluous in the presence of clear-cut vessels and is also nonspecific because some tumors enhance as well. AVMs can be demonstrated to change size with changes in cardiac output induced by Valsalva's maneuver. Rounded atelectasis characteristically appears as a peripheral round or oval mass abutting a thickened pleural surface. Bronchi and blood vessels entering the mass in a curvilinear fashion form a "comet tail" and blur the central margin. Rounded atelectasis is also often associated with volume loss in the affected lobe and with signs of asbestosis or other chronic pleural fibrotic process.

HRCT is particularly suited to demonstrating the relation of a focal lesion to the airways. SPNs caused by lung cancers or carcinoid tumors may have an identifiable endobronchial component, but granulomas do not display this feature. In some cases, the opacity seen on a plain chest film represents an area of consolidation or atelectasis distal to an obstructing endobronchial mass. In these instances, CT may show a small intraluminal mass, raising the possibility of carcinoid, squamous papilloma, and rarer endobronchial lesions. Mucous plugging, usually seen as multiple lesions, may appear as a solitary branching linear opacity with bulges in the expected distribution of the airways. In rare instances, a carcinoid or metastasis may simulate this picture.

Enhancement in Computed Tomography and Positron Emission Tomography

There has been considerable interest in studying and refining methods of separating benign from malignant SPNs, based on their differential uptake of systemically injected substances. Because of quantitative and qualitative differences in vascularity as well as more active metabolism, malignancies generally enhance more than benign processes. Although linear tomography, angiography, and color Doppler ultrasound have been used in this manner, most of the focus has centered on magnetic resonance imaging and contrast enhancement by CT and PET. Although Kono (1993) and Guckel (1996) and their associates reported that malignant nodules assessed by magnetic resonance imaging enhanced significantly more than benign lesions after administration of gadolinium, contrast CT and PET are the techniques most commonly applied clinically at the present time.

Computed Tomography Enhancement

Swenson and colleagues (1996) corroborated their prior extensive work with a prospective study of nonionic contrast CT enhancement of 107 indeterminate SPNs 7 mm to 3 cm in diameter. Malignant nodules enhanced a median of 46 HU from baseline precontrast levels (range, 11 to 110 HU), statistically significantly more than benign neoplasms and granulomas (median 8 HU; range: -10 to 94 HU). Using a cutoff of 20 HU and above to define malignancy, the sensitivity was 98%, specificity was 73%, and accuracy was 85% (Fig. 90-7). Only 1 of 52 primary and metastatic malignant lung neoplasms enhanced less than 20 HU. Combining this series with their prior reports yielded 270 cases with a sensitivity of 99%, specificity of 75%, accuracy of 90%, and, significantly, a negative predictive value of 99%. The authors also showed that enhancement correlated directly with increased central nodule vascularity, as determined by tissue staining with antibody to factor VIII–associated antigen, an endothelial cell marker. Similar results were achieved by Yamashita and associates (1995), who found that all 18 cases of lung cancer studied enhanced 25 or more HU, compared to less than 15 HU for 13 of 14 benign lesions. In a series of 65 indeterminate SPNs, Zhang and Kono (1997) noted significantly more enhancement in malignant nodules (41.9 HU) than in benign, noninflammatory lesions (13.4 HU). They cautioned, however, that active inflammatory processes, such as organizing pneumonia or tuberculosis, can enhance within the range characteristic of malignant neoplasms and thereby yield false-positive tests (Fig. 90-8). Swenson and coworkers (1996) noted similar caveats. The negative predictive value of the test, however, remained acceptable, with only 2 of 42 malignancies enhancing less than 20 HU. False-negative readings were owing to areas of tumor necrosis. The authors point out that careful avoidance of necrotic areas when selecting the region of interest for measurement of baseline and contrast-enhanced attenuation can minimize this potential pitfall. Yamashita and colleagues (1997) emphasized that larger tumors are associated with a higher incidence of necrosis and may be less suitable for this technique. Specifically, lesions of 3 cm or smaller had a 16% incidence of radi-

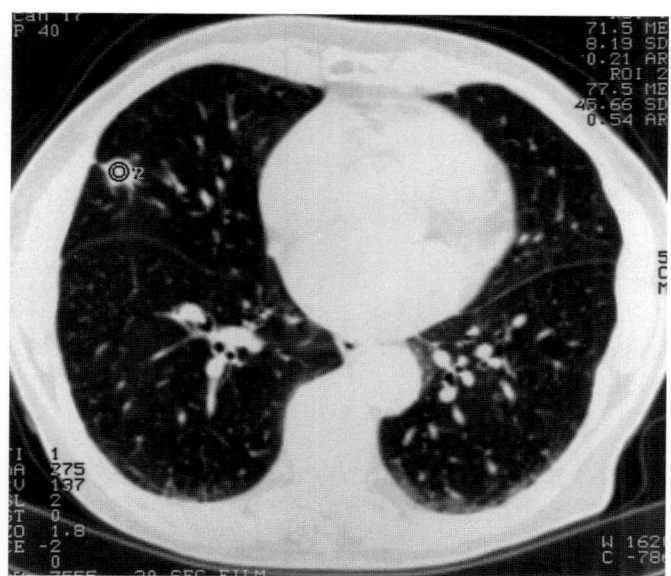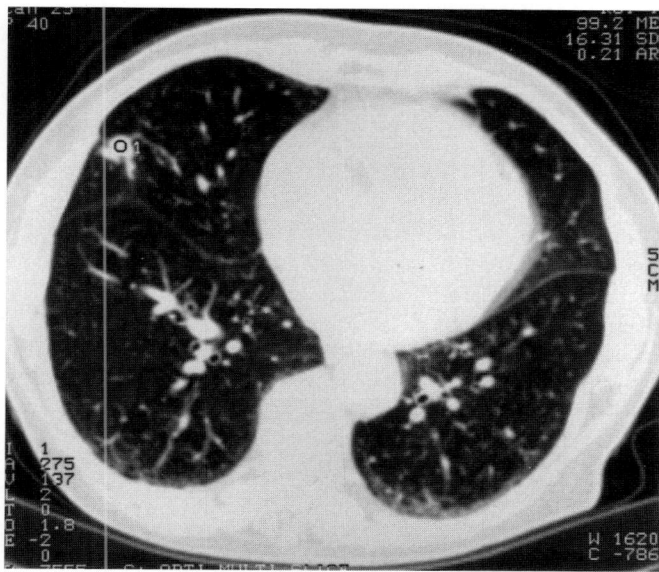

Fig. 90-7. A. "Suspicious" irregular right middle lobe nodule with pleural tail. B. Postcontrast enhancement less than 15 Hounsfield units. Video-assisted thoracic surgery confirmed a granuloma.

ographically evident necrosis, whereas 80% of tumors larger than 3 cm exhibited necrotic regions. Miyake and associates (1995) reported that mucin-producing adenocarcinomas can also contain areas of diminished vascularity that may produce false-negative enhancement studies.

Zhang and Kono (1997) noted two other methods for improving discrimination. First, despite equal peak enhancement for active inflammatory and malignant nodules, time-attenuation curves showed faster washout for the inflammatory processes. Second, the nodule to aorta contrast ratio exceeded 6% for all malignant lesions. By combining this parameter with the 20 HU absolute threshold, there would have been no false-negatives in their series. In addition to quantitative measures, qualitative patterns are

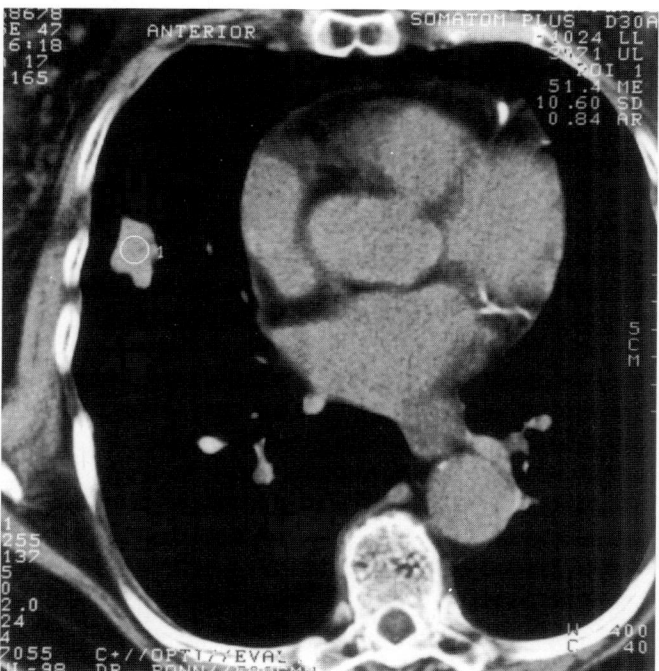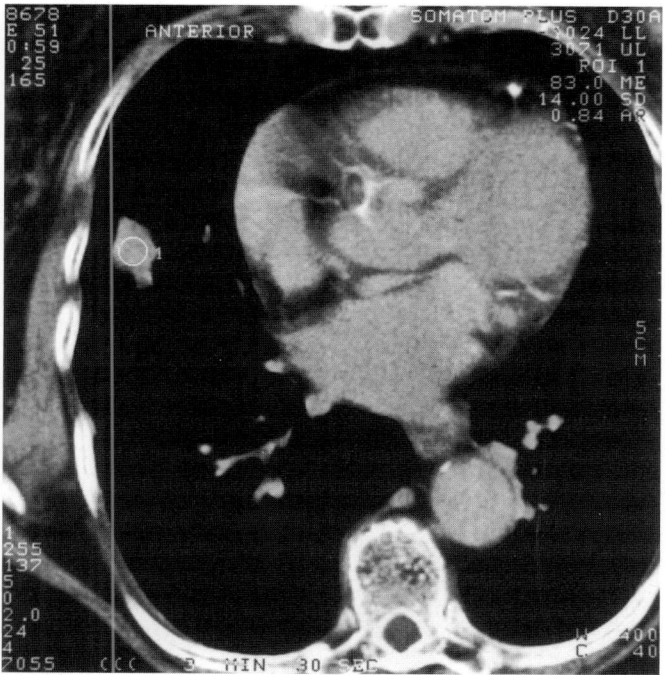

Fig. 90-8. False-positive enhancement study. A. Baseline. B. Postcontrast enhancement by 30 Hounsfield units. Resection documented active tuberculosis.

also being investigated. Benign lesions tend to enhance more peripherally, whereas malignant nodules enhance centrally. Central tumor necrosis, however, can sometimes reverse this pattern and must be taken into account.

Positron Emission Tomography

PET scanning with 2-fluorine-18-fluoro-2-deoxy-D-glucose (FDG) relies on increased metabolic activity measured as augmented glycolysis in malignant cells, compared to normal tissue (see Chapter 12). FDG is a D-glucose analog that enters cells and is phosphorylated by hexokinase. Thereafter, most of the FDG undergoes no further metabolism and is retained in the intracellular space. PET detects the radioactive F-18 positron-emitting label attached to the analog. Scans are interpreted qualitatively as positive (any activity greater than surrounding areas) or semiquantitatively by measurement of the standardized uptake ratio, comparing activity in small regions of interest in the lesion compared to normal tissue. PET has been studied as a diagnostic modality for lung nodules. In an early report, Gupta and associates (1992) found that FDG-PET was completely accurate in 20 patients with indeterminate SPNs. Hypermetabolism by qualitative analysis was detected in all 13 biopsy-proved malignant lesions, but in none of seven benign nodules. The standardized uptake ratio was significantly higher for malignant processes. In a series of 51 patients, Patz and coworkers (1993) found increased uptake in all malignant lesions, but two false-positive studies occurred in cases of active tuberculosis, yielding a sensitivity of 100% and a specificity of 89%. Gupta and colleagues (1996) later reported an expanded series of 61 patients, in which the positive predictive value of PET was 95%, but because of three malignant lesions misinterpreted as benign, the negative predictive value was only 82%. Similarly, Scott and associates (1994) in a cohort of 62 patients noted positive and negative predictive values of 94% and 80%, respectively. These authors also believed that the false-positive cases were owing to active inflammatory processes. The three false-negative studies in the series occurred in two instances of tumors smaller than 1 cm and in one case of bronchoalveolar cancer, a neoplasm that, when focal, is often associated with lower-grade malignant potential and probably less metabolic activity than other histologic types of lung cancer. Higashi and coworkers (1997) found that four of seven bronchoalveolar tumors did not demonstrate increased uptake of FDG by PET scan. In this regard, it is interesting to note that Duhaylongsod and associates (1995) correlated increased FDG activity with more rapid tumor DTs. Knight and colleagues (1996) reported a 100% negative predictive value for lesions larger than 1 cm, but there were six false-positive studies in a series of 48 patients. Lowe and Naunheim (1998) also pointed out that current PET technology may miss small malignant lesions. In a group of 107 patients with sus-

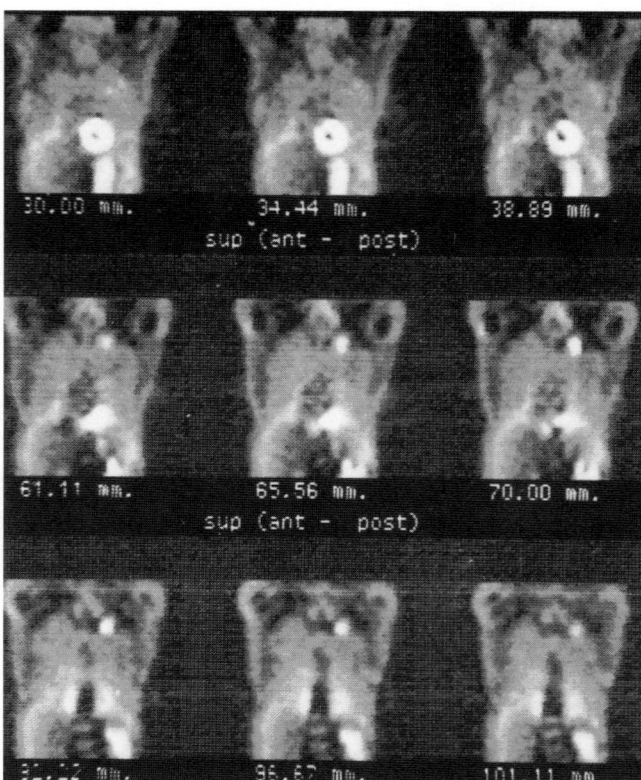

Fig. 90-9. Positron emission tomography scan shows solitary focus of abnormal activity at left pulmonary apex, confirmed by biopsy to be non–small cell carcinoma.

pected lung cancer, Sazon and associates (1996) also found a high sensitivity for detecting malignancy in the lung and mediastinum but a low specificity (52%) because 12 of 25 patients with benign lesions showed FDG uptake. The scans in this study, however, were interpreted qualitatively only. Hagberg and colleagues (1997), in a series of 49 cases with similar entry criteria, achieved a sensitivity of 93% but a specificity of only 70% for pulmonary nodules. Using likelihood ratios, Dewan and coworkers (1997) found that PET was superior to standard radiographic assessment and to formal probabilistic systems as well. In two series, the first retrospective and the second prospective, Lowe and associates (1997, 1998) found a sensitivity of 96 and 92% and an improved specificity of 77 and 90%, respectively (Fig. 90-9).

At present, CT enhancement and PET are promising modalities for the diagnosis of SPNs. In both techniques, active infection or inflammation can cause false positivity. Necrosis can be associated with false-negative studies. Lower-grade tumors are missed in some cases by PET. Future technological refinements, such as manipulation of blood glucose and insulin levels, and ongoing experience likely will improve the accuracy of these tests. For the present, however, enhancement studies should not be considered definitive unless they are corroborated by the entire clinical picture. The results of a multicenter study of CT enhancement in the United States, Canada, and Japan will be available in the near future.

Associated Radiographic Abnormalities

The presence of certain associated radiographic abnormalities may give some clue as to the cause of an SPN. Satellite lesions, which are generally thought of as nodular densities smaller than and in close proximity to the primary nodule, usually indicate malignancy. The coexistence of radiographic hilar or mediastinal lymphadenopathy with an SPN usually indicates primary lung cancer, but they may be seen with other processes, such as metastasis and sarcoidosis. An adrenal mass without characteristics of a benign adenoma on CT or magnetic resonance imaging also increases the odds of malignancy. In both scenarios (i.e., an SPN with signs of regional nodal or distant spread), small cell cancer must be considered a prime possibility. Calcification in the thoracic lymph nodes, liver, or spleen increases the likelihood that an SPN is a granuloma. It must never be assumed a priori, however, that the pulmonary and nodal or extrathoracic findings are necessarily related, especially if the lung mass is known to be a new lesion.

TISSUE SAMPLING OPTIONS

When the clinical evaluation and radiographic assessment are neither confirmatory nor sufficiently suggestive of a benign cause to warrant foregoing further workup or choosing observation only, the next step is either resection or a nonsurgical means to establish a diagnosis.

Sputum Cytology

The simplest approach to tissue sampling is examination of expectorated material: sputum cytology. Much has been written about the value of sputum cytology in focal pulmonary disease. In most cases of classic asymptomatic SPNs, sputum cytology is negative. Indeed, a positive cytology, especially if squamous carcinoma, in the presence of a small peripheral nodule should prompt a search for a large-airway source for the malignant sputum cells. Sputum cytology is of value in the workup of central endobronchial lesions, but its role in the evaluation of larger SPNs remains a subject of controversy. In a decision analysis study of cost-effectiveness, Raab and associates (1997) found that sputum cytology was a worthwhile first test not only for central lesions but also for peripheral masses 3 cm or larger. In contrast, Goldberg-Kahn and colleagues (1997), also using a decision analytical model comparing sputum cytology, transthoracic needle aspiration, bronchoscopy, and open biopsy as the initial approach to central and peripheral

lesions, determined that sputum cytology is not a cost-effective test except when the patient is not a surgical candidate. The authors relate this finding to low sensitivity and the frequent use of other tests after negative sputa. They point out that the increased prevalence of adenocarcinomas compared to squamous cancers, which more often shed cells into the airways, has reduced the sensitivity of sputum cytology in general. The results of the Early Lung Cancer Detection Program reported by Frost and associates (1984) were that sputum analysis is of little value in nonsquamous tumors. In practical terms, sputum cytology in patients with asymptomatic, small, peripheral SPNs is not helpful. For larger lesions, especially if associated with symptoms, cytology may be diagnostic and is risk-free and inexpensive. A negative study, however, should not delay the further expeditious evaluation of an SPN.

Bronchoscopy

Bronchoscopy, like sputum cytology, is limited by the fact that most SPNs do not communicate with an airway visually accessible by fiberoptic endoscopy. Absence of airway communication is especially typical of metastatic malignancies and benign lesions. In practice, however, the flexible bronchoscope in many cases can be directed close to the lesion, and the brush and biopsy forceps often can reach the SPN. Fluoroscopic guidance increases the diagnostic yield, as shown by Fletcher and Levin (1982). The use of a transbronchial aspirating needle catheter may aid in obtaining diagnostic material for cytology and core tissue samples for histology, especially when the lesion is entirely parenchymal. Gasparini and colleagues (1995) achieved a diagnostic yield for malignancy of 54% with bronchoscopic biopsy forceps and 69% with transbronchial needle aspiration. The two techniques in combination resulted in a diagnosis in 75% of malignant lesions. Shure and Fedullo (1983) similarly reported that adding aspiration to biopsy, brushings, and washings increased the yield from 48 to 69%. Overall, however, the reported efficacy of bronchoscopy for SPNs varies widely. As in the case of transthoracic biopsy, bronchoscopy more often confirms malignancy (20 to 80%) than establishes a specific benign diagnosis (0 to 20%). Higher accuracy is achieved with larger lesions and more central location and when CT demonstrates a bronchus leading to or passing through a nodule: a positive bronchus sign (Fig. 90-10). Radke and colleagues (1979) showed that diagnostic material was obtained more than twice as often from nodules larger than 2 cm in diameter (64%) compared to smaller SPNs (28%) and noted a low yield for lesions in the outer one-third of the lung fields. In one review, Mehta and colleagues (1995) found an average yield of 55% for SPNs larger than 2 cm but only 11% for smaller lesions. Naidich and coworkers (1988) established a diagnosis by bronchoscopy in 60% of cases with a positive bronchus sign but in only 30% of cases without bronchial communication by

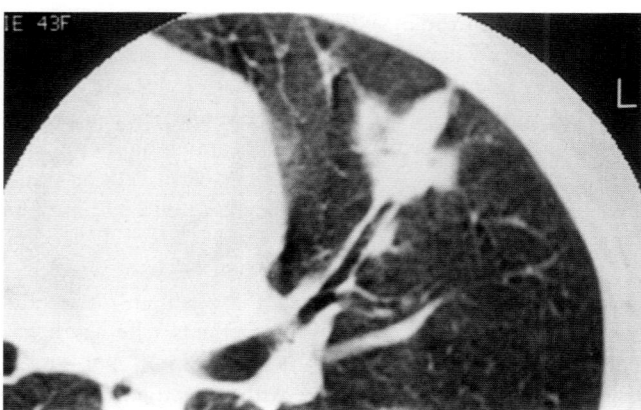

Fig. 90-10. Left upper lobe mass with positive bronchus sign.

standard CT. Furthermore, when HRCT did not show a tumor-bronchial association, endoscopy was diagnostic in only 14% of cases. Gaeta and associates (1993) reported that transbronchial biopsy and brushings were diagnostic in 81% of lesions with a positive bronchus sign but in only 45% of those without this feature. Using biplane fluoroscopy, however, Chechani (1996) reported unusually high diagnostic yields for SPNs without a positive bronchus sign. In this study, nodules located in the basilar segments of the lower lobes or apical segment of the upper lobes were less often diagnosed by bronchoscopy (58%) than were lesions in other areas (83%), likely because of suboptimal radiographic localization.

In summary, although the results of bronchoscopy for SPNs vary, some endoscopists have reported substantial diagnostic usefulness. HRCT can aid in deciding if the lesion is likely to be accessible. Fluoroscopic guidance is helpful, and transbronchial aspiration should be part of the bronchoscopist's expertise. In most instances, the procedure is performed on an outpatient basis. The risks of pneumothorax or significant bleeding are minimal, and mortality should approach zero. Peripheral nodules smaller than 2 cm in diameter are unlikely to be accessible. Finally, as shown by Goldberg and associates (1993) and Torrington and Kern (1993), routine staging bronchoscopy to assess the airways as a separate procedure before resection of an SPN, is unproductive and not warranted.

Transthoracic Needle Biopsy

Transthoracic needle biopsy (TNB) under CT or fluoroscopic guidance is established as a valuable means of assessing a variety of intrathoracic lesions. Westcott (1988) and Klein and Zarka (1997) emphasize that improvements in imaging, biopsy needles, cytopathology, and experience have decreased the risk of TNB while increasing its reliability. Regardless of the imaging modality chosen for TNB, a CT scan is essential for determining the feasibility of TNB,

planning the approach, and assessing the risk. Specially designed needles are currently used that are finer and more versatile than those used in the past. Coaxial needles can obtain multiple samples without reinsertion. In addition, finer-gauge devices increase the safety of multiple passes if needed. In most cases, it is possible to obtain cores or fragments of tissue for histologic study in addition to aspirates for cytologic analysis. Advances in cytopathology have improved the ability to interpret tiny samples. Valuable diagnostic techniques, such as immunohistochemical staining, flow cytometry, DNA probes, and hormone receptor assays, can often be applied to minute amounts of material. The importance of close communication between the radiologist and pathologist involved in TNB is highlighted by one prospective, randomized study reported by Santambrogio and colleagues (1997). These authors achieved an overall accuracy for malignant and benign SPNs of 99% in 110 cases when immediate cytologic evaluation was performed. If the specimen was considered inadequate, more material was obtained. In contrast, diagnostic accuracy was 81% in the control group of 110 patients when the adequacy of the TNB sample was assessed only by its gross characteristics.

As is the case for bronchoscopy, the reported results of TNB for SPNs vary. Although Calhoun and coworkers (1986) found that approximately one-third of resected lesions with a preoperative nondiagnostic aspirate turned out to be cancer, current sensitivity for malignancy should be 90 to 97%, as reported by Khouri (1985) and Caskey (1990) and their coworkers. Although virtually any area of the thorax can be sampled by TNB, the procedure is especially suited for lesions not amenable to bronchoscopic diagnosis (i.e., smaller, peripheral nodules). Although Berquist and associates (1980) reported a yield of only 65% for nodules smaller than 1 cm, more recently Westcott (1997) and Li (1996) and their coworkers achieved a diagnostic accuracy of 95 to 100% for small nodules. Gasparini and colleagues (1995) reported a sensitivity of 95% for malignancy and 59% for benign nodules by integrating into one procedure bronchoscopy, immediate cytology, and TNB if the bronchoscopic sample was not diagnostic.

The most common complications of TNB are pneumothorax and bleeding. Systemic air embolism is exceedingly rare, and malignant seeding of the needle tract is so uncommon since the introduction of finer needles that fear of this problem should not affect the decision process. The incidence of pneumothorax is 15 to 30%, but one-half or fewer of the patients require chest catheters. Severe emphysema, small SPNs, deeper location, and multiple needle passes are among the risk factors. The radiologist performing the biopsy usually treats and follows the pneumothorax. I and my colleagues (1997) have shown that the majority of patients with chest tubes after TNB can be managed with Heimlich valves on an ambulatory basis. Significant hemoptysis, the second most common complication, occurs in approximately 5% of cases and is usually self-limited. Massive intrathoracic bleeding from biopsy of mediastinal masses or vascular pulmonary lesions (e.g., renal cell carcinoma), inadvertent puncture of an intercostal or internal mammary artery, or torn apical adhesions from TNB-induced pneumothorax has been reported but is rare. Overall, the mortality rate of TNB for all thoracic processes is approximately 0.02%.

It is clear that in experienced hands, TNB is effective and safe for establishing malignant diagnoses. The false-negative rate is 5% or less. Two areas of controversy, however, arise from the limitations of TNB. First, the cell type identified by TNB sometimes does not match the histology of the resected lesion. Most often this discrepancy occurs within the subtypes of non–small cell carcinoma, small cell cancers being rarely misinterpreted. DiBonito and associates (1991), comparing cytologic typing of lung cancers with autopsy histology, found that aspiration cytology was accurate in 90% of squamous cancers, 70% of adenocarcinomas, 50% of large cell cancers, and 100% of small cell tumors. Because the treatment for all non–small cell cases is the same, this limitation is of no practical importance at present. A more important issue is a low yield of specific diagnoses and a high incidence of nonspecific findings when a benign lesion is present. To paraphrase Klein and Zarka (1997), a specific benign diagnosis requires the confident identification of a named benign process that renders further evaluation for malignancy unnecessary. Benign lesions that can often be diagnosed with specificity by TNB include hamartoma, chondroma, granuloma, lipoid pneumonia, pulmonary infarct, Wegener's granulomatosis, abscess, and other infectious processes. The yield increases when multiple samples are obtained from representative parts of the nodule (e.g., both the wall and center of a cavitary SPN), core biopsies, expert cytologic input, and liberal use of microbiological cultures and stains. Perhaps in the future, the yield will further increase by applying rapid DNA techniques when fungal or mycobacterial infection is suspected, as reported by Shim and colleagues (1998). The success rate for identifying benign SPNs varies markedly, from 5 to 89%, but the rate for specific diagnosis is in the range of 10 to 20%.

The approach to the large proportion of cases in which TNB is "negative" (i.e., cancer cells are not identified) but nonspecific (i.e., no confirmation of a specific benign process) is the most controversial question about the role of this technique in the evaluation of SPNs. In the past, most authors correctly regarded a nondiagnostic TNB as of insufficient reliability to obviate thoracotomy in the majority of cases. The clinical corollary of this philosophy was that TNB is not helpful in decision making because the ultimate outcome in operable patients is changed only in the minority of cases with a specific benign result. More recently, many clinicians have become willing to follow certain indeterminate SPNs based on radiographic features and nonspecific TNB. This evolution is based on improvements in imaging and sampling techniques noted here. The decision not to resect an SPN after a nondiagnostic TNB must be based on a clinical and radiographic assessment that the likelihood of malignancy is low. In addition, the specifics of the individual TNB are important. A TNB in which the radiologist and pathologist are confident that adequate material has been obtained carries more weight than a suboptimal study. It must be clear that all relevant portions of the lesion have been sampled, that areas of postobstructive pneumonia have not been mistaken for tumor, and that there is no endobronchial component to the lesion. As emphasized by Westcott (1988), a second TNB is often indicated after a nonspecific initial result and can establish a malignant diagnosis in some cases. On the other hand, two or more TNBs yielding sufficient amounts of negative material, especially if core biopsies are obtained, make a malignant process unlikely. Reliability is increased by the repeated demonstration of large numbers of inflammatory cells, histiocytes, or multinucleated giant cells. A factor of great importance in judging the validity of a nonspecific biopsy is the "track record" of the specialists involved—the local expertise. When the clinical and radiographic picture suggests cancer, however, resection is indicated regardless of the results of TNB.

Video-Assisted Thoracic Surgery

In the 1990s, video-assisted thoracoscopy—globally termed *video-assisted thoracic surgery* (VATS) has emerged as an option for diagnosing SPNs and in some instances for treating malignant nodules. The subject of VATS is covered in detail in Chapters 18, 32 and 33. VATS is best suited for peripheral nodules 2 cm or smaller and close to the visceral pleural surface. In such cases, the procedure is expeditious, and an acceptable stapled margin can be achieved. Techniques have been developed for locating deeper lesions, including intrapleural ultrasound and preoperative percutaneous CT-guided marking using mammographic localizing wires, subpleural injection of methylene-blue or colored collagen, and percutaneous intraparenchymal placement of angiographic coils with operative identification by fluoroscopy. Neodymium:yttrium-aluminum-garnet laser alone or in combination with endostaplers has been used for resecting deep SPNs. In all cases, the specimen should be placed in a plastic bag before extraction through the chest wall incision to prevent spillage of neoplastic cells or infected material. As an alternative to wedge excision, Bousamra and Clowry (1997) reported success with VATS needle aspiration and immediate cytology in a small series, emphasizing the rapidity of diagnosis (10 to 20 minutes) and the cost savings realized because staplers are not used for the diagnostic portion of the procedure.

The next step in a VATS procedure for an SPN depends on the frozen-section or cytologic diagnosis and the preoperative clinical evaluation. If the SPN is benign, the procedure is terminated. If the lesion is a solitary metastasis or low-grade primary lung tumor, in many cases the diagnostic wedge resection suffices for therapy. The decision process is more complex in the case of bronchial carcinoma. Although some would not consider a pulmonary density associated with hilar or mediastinal lymph node enlargement an SPN, in practice, VATS may be used in such instances. If the nodes have not been sampled by mediastinoscopy or other means before VATS, ipsilateral nodes may be assessed at the time of VATS. If there is no involvement that would preclude curative resection, the nature of and approach to resection depend on the surgeon's judgment and preference. Most patients are best treated by lobectomy, which can be accomplished either by converting to thoracotomy or by VATS. Alternatively, in certain high-risk cases, the surgeon may believe that wedge resection constitutes optimal treatment. The issue of whether local excision of lung cancer is appropriate for the patient who is able to tolerate anatomic resection remains a subject of controversy (see Chapter 99). Because of the need for general anesthesia for both procedures, the potential for disastrous tumor dissemination after VATS, as reported by Downey and associates (1996), and the absence of equivalent options for treatment of early lesions, definitive resection should be carried out at the time of VATS diagnosis of lung cancer. The various possibilities should be discussed with the patient preoperatively. Practical issues, such as instrument setup, intensive care scheduling, and operative time estimates, must be based on the surgeon's assessment of the likelihood of malignancy in the individual case. Another problem that may arise is the finding in a patient with a prior or synchronous extrapulmonary adenocarcinoma that the SPN is also an adenocarcinoma. The pathologist reading the frozen section should be made aware of the history and ideally should examine the two specimens. The decision to stop or to proceed with lobectomy depends on the pathologic diagnosis of primary or metastatic tumor. Often, a firm differentiation cannot be made, and the surgeon must decide on the basis of the entire clinical synthesis. This dilemma, of course, is not specific to VATS but also occurs with thoracotomy and with nonsurgical biopsy.

The role of VATS in lung cancer treatment remains a subject of controversy. In addition, VATS for therapy in patients with solitary metastases has been criticized for missing other, radiographically occult deposits that would be identified by open operation with bimanual palpation (see Chapter 113). Despite such therapeutic concerns, the diagnostic use of VATS for appropriate SPNs is virtually universally recognized. VATS is versatile, definitive, safe, and probably cost effective in many cases. The sensitivity and specificity of VATS approaches 100% for both benign and malignant SPNs. VATS is associated with lower risk and less pain than thoracotomy. Several groups, including Mack (1993), Hazelrigg (1993), DeCamp (1995), and Bernard (1996) and their colleagues, have reported favorable results with VATS in series devoted to or including large numbers of SPNs. The series of Mack (1993) describes 242 VATS resections for nodules smaller than 3 cm located in the outer one-third of the lung. Fifty-two percent of the lesions were benign and 48% malignant. Only two patients (0.8%) required thora-

cotomy to locate the SPN. In patients with good pulmonary function and a frozen-section diagnosis of lung cancer, open or VATS lobectomy was carried out. There was no mortality. Morbidity was 3.6%, mean hospital stay was 2.4 days for patients having VATS only, and diagnostic accuracy was complete. Although a significantly shorter hospital stay after VATS versus open anatomic resection has not uniformly been reported, wedge resection by VATS should be associated with fewer hospital days. I and my associates (1997) currently perform most VATS pulmonary wedge resections for low-suspicion nodules or diffuse infiltrates on an outpatient basis. The cost of this approach for diagnosing a benign SPN is clearly less than that of thoracotomy and in some cases may be less than the cumulative expense of one or more nonspecific TNBs or bronchoscopic examinations followed by periodic imaging studies for 2 years or more.

Thoracotomy

Thoracotomy remains a reasonable initial approach in operative candidates with lesions that are highly suspicious for malignancy (e.g., older patient, smoking or exposure history, new nodule, growing nodule, size ≥3 cm, or other radiographic features of cancer). In this setting, the chance of obviating resection by nonsurgical sampling is small. Open resection is also often prudent for clinically suspicious lesions even after a nondiagnostic bronchoscopy or TNB, especially if these studies were suboptimal. Thoracotomy as the initial histologic test is also indicated for SPNs with a moderate likelihood of cancer in the increasingly uncommon circumstance of a lesion not accessible by bronchoscopy, TNB, or VATS or undergoing evaluation at an institution without expertise in these modalities. It is instructive to note that in a series (1990 to 1993) of SPNs 3 cm or smaller reported by Libby and colleagues (1995), thoracotomy was the initial method of diagnosis in only 20% of the cases, despite a 53% incidence of malignancy.

DECISION MAKING

The responsible clinician has four options from which to choose as the initial approach to an indeterminate SPN: no further follow-up, periodic radiographic surveillance (watchful waiting or "wait-and-watch" strategy), nonsurgical biopsy (i.e., bronchoscopy, TNB, or both), or resection. Open or VATS resection is a form of biopsy but is considered a separate clinical pathway because of its greater magnitude than nonsurgical tissue acquisition methods as well as its potential role as therapy if the nodule is malignant.

In a minority of cases, a decision for no intervention is straightforward based on clinical grounds, radiography, or patient preference. Severe comorbidity or advanced age may preclude consideration of any treatment modality for malignancy. After discussion of the possibilities and the risks of testing for, treatment of, and failure to diagnose cancer, a patient may refuse intervention. No special follow-up is needed in cases with unequivocal signs of benignity, such as classic benign calcification, fat density, or prolonged radiographic stability. Because of rare exceptions to the 2-year rule, however, most noncalcified lesions should be kept under surveillance for a considerably longer period. Observation without intervention is reasonable in patients whose clinical and radiographic synthesis is highly suggestive of a benign SPN (e.g., young age, nonsmoker, endemic fungal area, radiographic small size, "benign" morphology, high CT numbers, stability ≥2 years, or prolonged DT). It must be emphasized that watchful waiting is an active process that requires periodic reassessment with appropriate imaging at intervals suited to the individual case and early intervention when warranted. If further experience with CT enhancement and PET confirms their reliability, a larger proportion of SPNs may fall into this wait-and-watch category in the future.

In most cases at present, however, the major problem is choosing the initial approach among the invasive options. Sometimes this decision is straightforward. Some patients, for example, may be deemed too tenuous to tolerate general anesthesia and any form of resection but might benefit from nonsurgical therapy if cancer is found. In these instances, diagnostic bronchoscopy or TNB is indicated. The choice of biopsy approach depends on the size and location of the SPN, as discussed earlier. The decision to use nonsurgical versus surgical biopsy in patients who are operative candidates and whose lesions have a moderate-to-high suspicion of malignancy should be based on the factors noted in the previous section (Tissue Sampling Options), the surgeon's preference, and input from the patient. If a high level of expertise in TNB is available, including high diagnostic yields and low complication rates, the surgeon may prefer to obtain a preoperative diagnosis of cancer to expedite resection by obviating the need for frozen section. If the SPN appears likely to be accessible by bronchoscopy, a preoperative endoscopy may achieve the same goal. In addition, some patients are reluctant to proceed directly to resection without a diagnosis. Alternatively, especially for suspicious lesions, the surgeon and patient may prefer to avoid a separate biopsy procedure with its low but finite risks. VATS is an especially useful initial approach in cases suspicious for lung cancer for surgeons who perform lobectomy by this route or when the patient's cardiopulmonary status precludes anatomic resection. Finally, in cases of lower suspicion but without strong benign features, the expert application of TNB or VATS can avoid many thoracotomies for benign SPNs.

As emphasized by Lillington (1991) and Lillington and Caskey (1993), the decision to follow or intervene depends on the probability of cancer (pCA). No infallible systems or clinicians for making this determination exist. In daily practice, the pCA is arrived at nonquantitatively, in large part intuitively, based partly on patient-specific data, but more often on the radiographic features of the lesion. This task can be accomplished equally well by an experienced pulmonologist or thoracic surgeon. The participation of an expert thoracic radiologist is essential. Although much of the SPN literature deals only with plain radiography, it is my opinion that at the present time, CT scan should be part of the initial evaluation for all SPNs that are not definitively benign or factitious on the basis of plain films. If an expectant approach is selected, the imaging modality used for subsequent surveillance (i.e., chest film, CT, or alternating between the two techniques) varies according to individual circumstances. In the few remaining centers with ongoing interest and expertise in linear tomography, this method is also an option. In the future, PET may assume the role of the primary imaging approach to the SPN.

Mathematical models for determining pCA have been reported. Cummings and associates (1986a) first described the use of Bayes' theorem for generating an odds ratio of the pCA by assessing the predictive value of individual clinical and radiographic variables. The prevalence of cancer in the general population may also be considered. Various combinations of patient history are included: age, smoking, prior malignancy, nodule size, edge features, calcification, growth rate, and location. Using decision analysis to compare the life expectancy of patients managed by observation, biopsy, or resection based on the pCA, the same authors (1986b) found that for a pCA of 5% or less, observation was equal or superior to intervention. With increasing pCA, however, intervention became superior to surveillance, and at pCA levels greater than 60%, resection or nonsurgical biopsy were clearly indicated. Edwards and colleagues (1989) validated this approach, although their series was not limited to the classic SPN. Gurney and colleagues (1993) found that radiologists using Bayesian analysis were able to estimate the pCA better than expert radiologists judging the same cases who did not use this methodology. Gurney and Swenson (1995) compared neural network analysis, a nonlinear mathematical model capable of learning from example and identifying relationships among data that are not apparent to human analysis, with the Bayesian method and found the latter superior. Mathematical models for determining the approach to an SPN, however, cannot be accepted in the absence of large prospective studies. In most reports, the input data are limited, and the variables are weighted on the basis of older published series. The conundrum of predicting malignancy is highlighted by the misclassification of 12 of 66 cases (18%), of which 8 of 44 (18%) were false-negative diagnoses, in the series of Gurney and colleagues (1993).

CONCLUSION

The SPN remains a common and challenging problem in thoracic medicine and surgery. Advances in imaging and in surgical and nonsurgical biopsy techniques have improved our ability to diagnose these lesions without missing oppor-

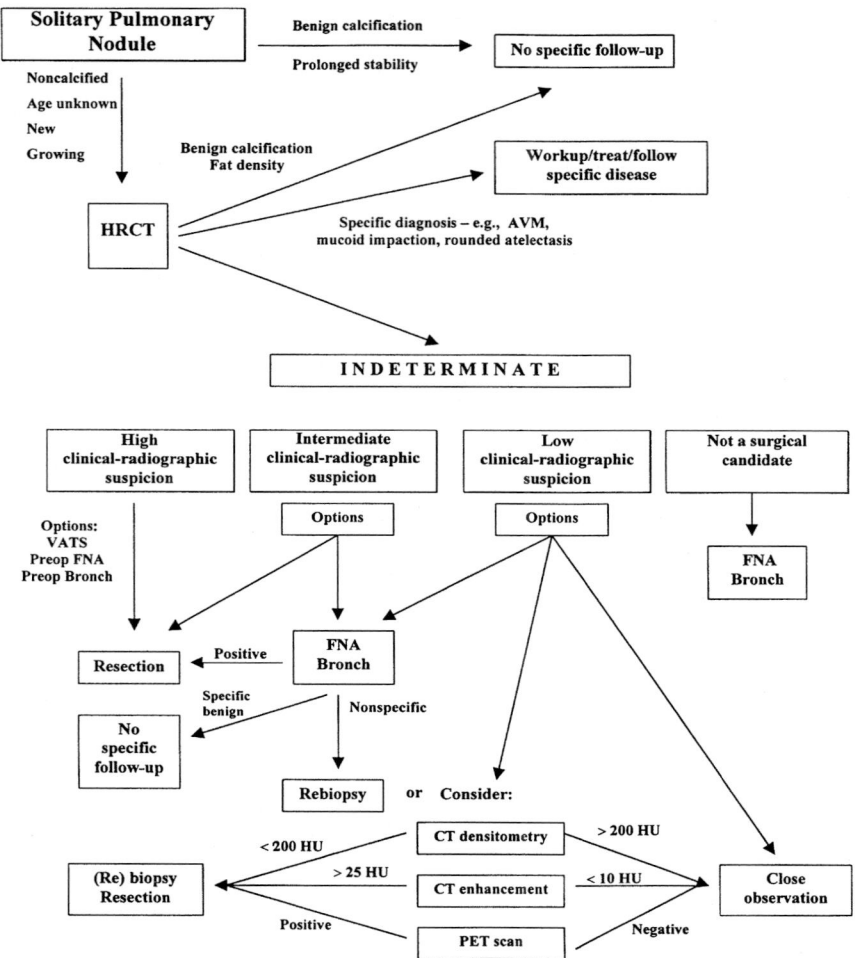

Fig. 90-11. An algorithm for management of a solitary pulmonary nodule. AVM, arteriovenous malformation; Bronch, bronchoscopy; CT, computed tomography; FNA, fine-needle aspiration; HRCT, high-resolution computed tomography; HU, Hounsfield units; PET, positron emission tomography; Preop, preoperative; VATS, video-assisted thoracic surgery.

tunities for treatment of early cancers while minimizing major interventions. Newer promising modalities for the diagnosis of the SPN are undergoing active investigation. At present, the optimal approach to an SPN remains an individualized clinical decision best made by a general thoracic surgeon or pulmonologist, or both, in close collaboration with a thoracic radiologist. A sample algorithm is presented in Figure 90-11.

REFERENCES

Banko MS, et al: Prevalence of pathologically proven intrapulmonary lymph nodes and their appearance on CT. AJR Am J Roentgenol *167*:629, 1996.

Bernard A, et al: Resection of pulmonary nodules using video-assisted thoracic surgery. Ann Thorac Surg *61*:202, 1996.

Berquist TH, et al: Transthoracic needle biopsy: accuracy and complications in relation to location and type of lesion. Mayo Clin Proc *55*:475, 1980.

Bousamra M, Clowry L: Thoracoscopic fine-needle aspiration of solitary pulmonary nodules. Ann Thorac Surg *64*:1191, 1997.

Cahan WG: Multiple primary cancers of the lung, esophagus and other sites. Cancer *40*:Suppl:1954, 1977.

Cahan WG, Castro EB, Hajdu SI: The significance of a solitary lung shadow in patients with colon carcinoma. Cancer *33*:414, 1974.

Cahan WG, Castro EB: Significance of a solitary lung shadow in patients with breast cancer. Ann Surg *181*:137, 1975.

Calhoun P, et al: The clinical outcome of needle aspirations of the lung when cancer is not diagnosed. Ann Thorac Surg *41*:592, 1986.

Casey JJ, et al: The solitary pulmonary nodule in the patient with breast cancer. Surgery *96*:801, 1984.

Caskey CI, Templeton PA, Zerhouni EA: Current evaluation of the solitary pulmonary nodule. Radiol Clin North Am *28*:511, 1990.

Chechani V: Bronchoscopic diagnosis of solitary pulmonary nodules and lung masses in the absence of endobronchial abnormality. Chest *109*:620, 1996.

Chiles C, Sherrier RH: Analysis of the solitary pulmonary nodule by means of digital techniques. J Thorac Imaging *5*:55, 1990.

Collins VP, Loeffler RK: Observations on growth rates of human tumors. Am J Roentgenol Radiat Ther *76*:988, 1956.

Coppage L, Shaw C, Curtis AM: Metastatic disease to the chest in patients with extrathoracic malignancy. J Thorac Imaging *2*:24, 1987.

Crow J, Slavin G, Kreel L: Pulmonary metastasis: a pathologic and radiologic study. Cancer *47*:2595, 1981.

Cummings SR, Lillington GA, Richard RJ: Estimating the probability of malignancy in solitary pulmonary nodules. A Bayesian approach. Am Rev Respir Dis *134*:449, 1986a.

Cummings SR, Lillington GA, Richard RJ: Managing pulmonary nodules. The choice of strategy is a "close call." Am Rev Respir Dis *134*:453, 1986b.

Davis EW, Peabody JW, Katz S: The solitary pulmonary nodule: a 10-year study based on 215 cases. J Thorac Cardiovasc Surg *32*:728,1956.

Davis S: CT evaluation for pulmonary metastasis in patients with extrathoracic malignancy. Radiology *180*:1, 1991.

DeCamp MM, et al: The safety and versatility of video-thoracoscopy: a prospective analysis of 895 consecutive cases. J Am Coll Surg *181*:113, 1995.

Dewan NA, et al: Likelihood of malignancy in a solitary pulmonary nodule: comparison of Bayesian analysis and results of FDG-PET scan. Chest *112*:416, 1997.

DiBonito L, et al: Cytologic typing of primary lung cancer: study of 100 cases with autopsy confirmation. Diagn Cytopathol 7:7, 1991.

Downey RJ, et al: Dissemination of malignant tumors after video-assisted thoracic surgery: a report of twenty-one cases. J Thorac Cardiovasc Surg *111*:954, 1996.

Duhaylongsod FG, et al: Lung tumor growth correlates with glucose metabolism measured by fluoride – 18 fluorodeoxyglucose positron emission tomography. Ann Thorac Surg *60*:1348, 1995.

Dumont P, et al: Bronchoalveolar carcinoma. Histopathological study of evolution in a series of 105 surgically treated patients. Chest *113*:391, 1998.

Edwards FH, et al: Use of artificial intelligence for the preoperative diagnosis of pulmonary lesions. Ann Thorac Surg *48*:556, 1989.

Edwards SE, Fry IK: Prevalence of lung nodules on computed tomography of patients without known malignant disease. Br J Radiol *55*:715, 1982.

Eschelman DJ, et al: Pulmonary hyalinizing granuloma: a rare cause of a solitary pulmonary nodule. J Thorac Imaging 6:54, 1991.

Fein AM, Feinsilver SH, Ares CA: The solitary pulmonary nodule: a systemic approach. *In* Fishman AP (ed): Pulmonary Diseases and Disorders. 3rd Ed. New York: McGraw–Hill, 1998.

Fichtenbaum CJ, Kleinman GM, Haddad RG: Eosinophilic granuloma of the lung presenting as a solitary pulmonary nodule. Thorax *45*:905, 1990.

Fletcher EC, Levin DC: Flexible fiberoptic bronchoscopy and fluoroscopically-guided transbronchial biopsy of solitary pulmonary nodules. West J Med *136*:477, 1982.

Frost JK, et al: Results of the initial (prevalence) radiologic and cytologic screening in the Johns Hopkins study. Am Rev Respir Dis *130*:549, 1984.

Gaeta M, et al: Carcinomatous solitary pulmonary nodules: evaluation of the tumor-bronchi relationship with thin-section CT. Radiology *187*:535, 1993.

Garland LH: The rate of growth and natural duration of primary bronchial cancer. Am J Roentgenol Radium Ther Nucl Med *96*:604, 1966.

Gasparini S, et al: Integration of transbronchial and percutaneous approach in the diagnosis of peripheral pulmonary nodules or masses: experience with 1027 consecutive cases. Chest *108*:131, 1995.

Goldberg-Kahn B, Healy JC, Bishop JW: The cost of diagnosis: a comparison of four different strategies in the workup of solitary radiographic lung lesions. Chest *111*:870, 1997.

Goldberg SK, et al: The role of staging bronchoscopy in the preoperative assessment of a solitary pulmonary nodule. Chest *104*:94, 1993.

Good CA, Wilson TW: The solitary circumscribed pulmonary nodule: study of 705 cases encountered roentgenologically in a period of three and one-half years. JAMA *166*:210, 1958.

Goodwin RA, Snell JD: The enlarging histoplasmoma: concept of a tumor-like phenomenon encompassing the tuberculoma and coccidioidoma. Am Rev Respir Dis *100*:1, 1969.

Guckel C, et al: Solitary pulmonary nodules: MR evaluation of enhancement patterns with contrast-enhanced dynamic snapshot gradient-echo imaging. Radiology *200*:681, 1996.

Gupta NC, Maloof, J, Gunel E: Probability of malignancy in solitary pulmonary nodules using fluorine – 18 – FDG and PET. J Nucl Med *37*:943, 1996.

Gupta NC, et al: Solitary pulmonary nodules: detection of malignancy with PET with 2-(F-18)-fluoro-2-deoxy-D-glucose. Radiology *184*:441, 1992.

Gurney JW, Lyddon DM, McKay JA: Determining the likelihood of malignancy in solitary pulmonary nodules with Bayesian analysis. Radiology *186*:415, 1993.

Gurney JW, Swenson SJ: Solitary pulmonary nodules: determining the likelihood of malignancy with neural network analysis. Radiology *196*:823, 1995.

Hagberg RC, et al: Characterization of pulmonary nodules and mediastinal staging of bronchial carcinoma with F-18 fluorodeoxyglucose positron emission tomography. Eur J Cardiothorac Surg *12*:92, 1997.

Hayabuchi N, Russell WJ, Murakami J: Slow-growing lung cancer in a fixed population sample: radiologic assessments. Cancer *52*:1098, 1983.

Hazelrigg SR, Nunchuck SK, LoCicero J: Video-assisted Thoracic Surgical Study Group data. Ann Thorac Surg *56*:1039, 1993.

Higashi K, et al: Bronchioloalveolar carcinoma: false-negative results on FDG-PET [abstract]. J Nucl Med *38*:79P, 1997.

Hillerdal G: Rounded atelectasis: clinical experience with 74 patients. Chest *95*:836, 1989.

Holin SM, et al: Solitary pulmonary nodules found in a community-wide chest roentgenographic survey: a five-year followup study. Am Rev Tuberc *79*:427, 1959.

Huang RM, et al: Septic pulmonary emboli: CT-radiographic correlation. AJR Am J Roentgenol *153*:41, 1989.

Huston J, Muhm JR: Solitary pulmonary opacities: plain tomography. Radiology *163*:4815, 1987.

Huston J, Muhm JR: Solitary pulmonary nodules: evaluation with a reference phantom. Radiology *170*:653, 1989.

Johnson H, Fatone J, Flye MW: Histologic evaluation of the nodules resected in the treatment of pulmonary metastatic disease. J Surg Oncol *21*:1, 1982.

Jolles H, Moseley, PL, Peterson MW: Nodular pulmonary opacities in patients with rheumatoid arthritis. Chest *96*:1022, 1989.

Jones FA, et al: Computerized tomographic densitometry of the solitary pulmonary nodule using a nodule phantom. Chest *96*:779, 1989.

Kelcz F, et al: Conventional chest radiography vs dual-energy computed radiography in the detection and characterization of pulmonary nodules. AJR Am J Roentgenol *162*:271, 1994.

Keogan MT, et al: The significance of pulmonary nodules detected on CT staging for lung cancer. Clin Radiol *48*:94, 1993.

Khan A, et al: Solitary pulmonary nodules: comparison of classification with standard, thin-section, and reference phantom CT. Radiology *179*:477, 1991.

Khouri NF, et al: Transthoracic needle aspiration biopsy of benign and malignant lung lesions. AJR Am J Roentgenol *144*:281, 1985.

Klein JS, Zarka MA: Transthoracic needle biopsy: an overview. J Thorac Imaging *12*:232, 1997.

Knight SB, et al: Evaluation of pulmonary lesions with FDG-PET: comparison of findings in patients with and without a history of prior malignancy. Chest *109*:982, 1996.

Kono M, et al: Clinical utility of Gd-DTPA-enhanced magnetic resonance imaging in lung cancer. J Thorac Imaging 8:18, 1993.

Kuhlman JE, Fishman EK, Teiger C: Pulmonary septic emboli: diagnosis with CT. Radiology *174*:211, 1990.

Kundel HH, Nodine CF, Carmody D: Visual scanning, pattern recognition and decision-making in pulmonary nodule detection. Invest Radiol *13*:175, 1978.

Kuriyama K, et al: Prevalence of air bronchograms in small peripheral carcinomas of the lung on thin-section CT: comparison with benign tumors. AJR Am J Roentgenol *156*:921, 1991.

Li H, et al: Diagnostic accuracy and safety of CT-guided percutaneous aspiration biopsy of the lung: comparison of small and large pulmonary nodules. AJR Am J Roentgenol *167*:105, 1996.

Libby DM, Henschke CI, Yankelevitz DF: The solitary pulmonary nodule: Update 1995. Am J Med *99*:491, 1995.

Libby DM, et al: Simultaneous pulmonary and renal malignancy. Chest *98*:153, 1990.

Lillington GA: Management of solitary pulmonary nodules. Dis Mon *37*:271, 1991.

Lillington GA, Caskey CI: Evaluation and management of solitary and multiple pulmonary nodules. Clin Chest Med *14*:111, 1993.

Lowe VJ, Naunheim KS: Positron emission tomography in lung cancer. Ann Thorac Surg *65*:1821, 1998.

Lowe VJ, et al: Pulmonary abnormalities and PET data analysis: a retrospective study. Radiology *202*:435, 1997.

Lowe VJ, et al: Prospective investigation of positron emission tomography in lung nodules. J Clin Oncol *16*:1075, 1998.

Mack MJ, et al: Thoracoscopy for the diagnosis of the indeterminate solitary pulmonary nodule. Ann Thorac Surg *56*:825, 1993.

Maile CW, et al: Calcification in pulmonary metastases. Br J Radiol *55*:108, 1982.

Malefatto JP, et al: The clinical significance of radiographically detected pulmonary neoplastic lesions in patients with head and neck cancer. J Clin Oncol 2:625, 1984.

McClure CD, et al: The solitary pulmonary nodule and primary lung malignancy. Arch Environ Health 3:127, 1961.

Mehta AC, et al: Role of bronchoscopy in the evaluation of solitary pulmonary nodules. J Bronchol 2:315, 1995.

Miyake H, et al: Mucin-producing tumor of the lung: CT findings. J Thorac Imaging 10:96, 1995.

Mizuno T, et al: Comparison of actual survivorship after treatment with survivorship predicted by actual tumor-volume doubling time from tumor diameter at first observation. Cancer 53:2716, 1984.

Munden RF, et al: Small pulmonary lesions detected at CT: clinical importance. Radiology 202:105, 1997.

Naidich DP, Garay SM: Radiographic evaluation of focal lung disease. Clin Chest Med 12:77, 1991.

Naidich DP, et al: Solitary pulmonary nodules: CT-bronchoscopic correlation. Chest 93:595, 1988.

Nathan MH: Management of solitary pulmonary nodules. An organized approach based on growth rate and statistics. JAMA 227:1141, 1974.

Nathan MH, Collins VP, Adams RA: Differentiation of benign and malignant pulmonary nodules by growth rate. Radiology 79:221, 1962.

O'Keefe ME, Good CA, McDonald JR: Calcification in solitary nodules of the lung. AJR Am J Roentgenol 77:1023, 1957.

Pass HJ, et al: Detection of pulmonary metastases in patients with osteogenic and soft tissue sarcomas: the superiority of CT scans compared with conventional linear tomograms using dynamic analyses. J Clin Oncol 3:1261, 1985.

Patz EF, et al: Focal pulmonary abnormalities: evaluation with F–18 fluorodeoxyglucose PET scanning. Radiology 188:487, 1993.

Pogrebniak HW, et al: Resection of pulmonary metastases from malignant melanoma: results of a 16-year experience. Ann Thorac Surg 46:20, 1988.

Ponn RB, Silverman H, Federico JA: Outpatient chest tube management. Ann Thorac Surg 64:1437, 1997.

Proto AV, Thomas SR: Pulmonary nodules studied by computed tomography. Radiology 153:149, 1985.

Raab SS, Hornberger J, Raffin T: The importance of sputum cytology in the diagnosis of lung cancer. Chest 112:937, 1997.

Radke JR, et al: Diagnostic accuracy in peripheral lung lesions: factors predicting success with flexible fiberoptic bronchoscopy. Chest 76:176, 1979.

Rubins J, Rubins HB: Temporal trends in the prevalence of malignancy in resected solitary pulmonary lesions. Chest 109:100, 1996.

Santambrogio L, et al: CT-guided fine-needle aspiration cytology of solitary pulmonary nodules: a prospective randomized study of immediate cytologic evaluation. Chest 112:423, 1997.

Sazon DAD, et al: Fluorodeoxyglucose-positron emission tomography in the detection and staging of lung cancer. Am J Respir Crit Care Med 153:417, 1996.

Schaner EG, et al: Comparison of conventional and computed tomography and conventional whole lung tomography in detecting pulmonary nodules: a prospective radiologic-pathologic study. AJR Am J Roentgenol 131:51, 1978.

Scholten ET, Kreel L: Distribution of lung metastases in the axial plane. Radiol Clin (Basel) 46:248, 1977.

Scott WJ, et al: Positron emission tomography of lung tumors and mediastinal lymph nodes using F-18 fluorodeoxyglucose. Ann Thorac Surg 58:698, 1994.

Shim JJ, et al: Nested polymerase chain reaction for detection of mycobacterium tuberculosis in solitary pulmonary nodules. Chest 113:20, 1998.

Shure D, Fedullo PF: Transbronchial needle aspiration of peripheral masses. Am Rev Respir Dis 128:1090, 1983.

Siegelman SS, et al: CT of the solitary pulmonary nodule. AJR Am J Roentgenol 135:1, 1980.

Siegelman SS, et al: Solitary pulmonary nodules: CT assessment. Radiology 160:307, 1986a.

Siegelman SS, et al: Pulmonary hamartoma: CT findings. Radiology 160:313, 1986b.

Silverman SP, Marino L: Unusual cases of enlarging pulmonary mass. Chest 91:457, 1987.

Sone S, et al: Factors affecting the radiologic appearance of peripheral bronchogenic carcinomas. J Thorac Imaging 12:159, 1997.

Steele JD: The solitary pulmonary nodule: report of a cooperative study of resected asymptomatic pulmonary nodules in males. J Thorac Cardiovasc Surg 46:12, 1963.

Stoller JK, Ahmad M, Rice TW: The solitary pulmonary nodule. Cleve Clin J Med 55:68, 1988.

Swenson SJ, et al: CT evaluation of solitary pulmonary nodules: value of 185-H reference phantom, AJR Am J Roentgenol 156:925, 1991.

Swenson SJ, et al: Lung nodule enhancement at CT: prospective findings. Radiology 201:447, 1996.

Theros EG: Varying manifestations of peripheral pulmonary neoplasms: a radiographic-pathologic correlative study. AJR Am J Roentgenol 128:893, 1977.

Toomes H, et al: The coin lesion of the lung: a review of 955 resected coin lesions. Cancer 51:534, 1983.

Torrington KG, Kern JD: The utility of fiberoptic bronchoscopy in the evaluation of the solitary pulmonary nodule. Chest 104:1021, 1993.

Trunk G, Gracey DR, Byrd RB: The management and evaluation of the solitary pulmonary nodule. Chest 66:236, 1974.

Vock P, Soucek M: Spiral computed tomography in the assessment of focal and diffuse lung disease. J Thorac Imaging 8:283, 1993.

Ward HB, et al: The impact of phantom CT scanning on surgery for the pulmonary nodule. Surgery 106:734, 1989.

Webb WR: Radiologic evaluation of the solitary pulmonary nodule. AJR Am J Roentgenol 154:701, 1990.

Webb WR: The solitary pulmonary nodule. In Freundlich IM, Bragg DG (eds): A Radiologic Approach to Diseases of the Chest. Baltimore: Williams & Wilkins, 1997.

Westcott JL: Percutaneous transthoracic needle biopsy. Radiology 169:593, 1988.

Westcott JL, Rao N, Colley DP: Transthoracic needle biopsy of small pulmonary nodules. Radiology 202:97, 1997.

Woodring JH, Fried AM: Significance of wall thickness in solitary cavities of the lung: a follow-up study. AJR Am J Roentgenol 140:473, 1983.

Yamashita K, et al: Solitary pulmonary nodule: preliminary study of evaluation with incremental dynamic CT. Radiology 194:399, 1995.

Yamashita K, et al: Intratumoral necrosis of lung carcinoma: a potential diagnostic pitfall in incremental dynamic computed tomography analysis of solitary pulmonary nodules. J Thorac Imaging 12:181, 1997.

Yankelevitz DF, Henschke CI: Does 2-year stability imply that pulmonary nodules are benign? AJR Am J Roentgenol 168:325, 1997.

Yokomise H, et al: Importance of intrapulmonary lymph nodes in the differential diagnosis of small pulmonary nodular shadows. Chest 113:703, 1998.

Yousem S, Hochholzer L: Pulmonary hyalinizing granuloma. Am J Clin Pathol 87:1, 1987.

Zerhouni EA, et al: CT of the pulmonary nodule: a cooperative study. Radiology 160:319, 1986.

Zhang M, Kono M: Solitary pulmonary nodules: evaluation of blood flow patterns with dynamic CT. Radiology 205:471, 1997.

Zweibel BR, Austin JHM, Grines MM: Bronchial carcinoid tumors: assessment with CT of location and intratumoral calcification in 31 patients. Radiology 179:483, 1991.

Zwirewich CV, et al: Solitary pulmonary nodule: high-resolution CT and radiologic-pathologic correlation. Radiology 179:469, 1991.

CHAPTER 91

Diffuse Lung Disease

Ronald B. Ponn and Herbert Knight

Diffuse parenchymal lung diseases (DPLDs) are characterized by generalized or extreme multifocal involvement of the pulmonary parenchyma. Since Hamman and Rich (1935) described rapidly progressive pulmonary fibrosis, more than 100 disorders have been classified as diffuse diseases. The inclusion of infectious processes raises the number further. Despite variations in etiology, acuity, and outcome, these entities are grouped together because of certain common clinical, histologic, and radiographic features. With the exception of lung transplantation in a small fraction of cases and the treatment of complications, such as pneumothorax or pleural effusion, the role of the thoracic surgeon in DPLD is diagnostic. Although advances in clinicopathologic correlation have lessened the requirement for surgical biopsy, in many instances the need for definitive tissue sampling remains, especially as the limitations of pathologic diagnosis from small specimens are increasingly appreciated. When biopsy is necessary, the surgeon should not function merely as a technician but can play an important role in determining the timing, method, and wisdom of invasive diagnostic efforts.

Diffuse lung diseases are often classified clinically as acute or chronic and pathologically as granulomatous or nongranulomatous, but the overlap is considerable. A simpler approach is to divide the disorders into those of known cause and the larger group in which the cause is unknown (Table 91-1).

PATHOGENESIS: THE LUNG'S RESPONSE TO INJURY

The anatomy and cell populations of the lung are discussed in Chapters 3 and 4. DPLD involves the gas-exchanging structures, including bronchioles, alveolar ducts, alveolar sacs, interstitium, and small vessels. Clinical studies and experimental models induced by radiation therapy, inhaled irritants, immune complexes, and toxins such as bleomycin show similarities in the lung's response to injury.

Crouch (1990) summarized current concepts of pathogenesis, and Rochester and Elias (1993) emphasized the role of cytokines.

Injury produces alveolitis (an accumulation of inflammatory and immune cells in the interstitium and air spaces) (Fig. 91-1). Necrosis of type I epithelial cells results in denuded areas of alveolar wall. Damage to capillary endothelial cells also may occur. Fluid and protein leak into the alveolar space and form fibrin-rich hyaline membranes. After this exudative phase, processes begin that lead either to repair or to further injury and ultimately to fibrosis.

Granulocytes appear early. Activated resident macrophages elaborate cytokines that attract neutrophils, causing them to adhere to capillary endothelium and enter the interstitium and alveoli. Some models suggest that tumor necrosis factor (TNF) is important in the early phase of alveolar injury. Complement activation and platelet products also attract neutrophils. The recruited cells release toxic oxygen products and proteases that break down matrix proteins. Activated macrophages also produce oxidants and proteolytic enzymes.

A mononuclear cell response follows. Macrophages continue to play an important role via chemotaxis for blood monocytes that mature into macrophages. Mediators from activated macrophages also attract and activate T lymphocytes, some of which stimulate eosinophils and mast cells and cause B-cell differentiation into antibody-producing plasma cells. The resultant immune complexes may amplify the inflammatory reaction. In other instances, the balance favors a subpopulation of T lymphocytes that promotes a cell-mediated response. These cells generate cytokines that result in granuloma formation by recruitment of blood monocytes, activation of macrophages, and inhibition of macrophage migration. T cells also enhance injury by stimulation of cytotoxic and killer lymphocytes.

Fibrosis results from an increased number of fibroblasts, their passage into air spaces through damaged alveolar walls, and enhanced collagen synthesis (Fig. 91-2). Cytokine modulation of collagen elaboration is increasingly

Table 91-1. Partial List of Noninfectious Diffuse Lung Diseases

Known cause

Inhalation

Inorganic dusts (pneumoconiosis): asbestos, aluminum, barium, beryllium, cadmium, cerium, hafnium, iron, kaolin, mica, niobium, silica, talc, tin, titanium

Organic dusts (hypersensitivity pneumonitis, extrinsic allergic alveolitis): air-conditioner lung, bagassosis, bird fancier's lung, cheese worker's lung, feather plucker's lung, humidifier lung, malt worker's lung, maple bark stripper's lung, mummy unwrapper's lung, mushroom worker's lung, paprika splitter's lung, sauna lung, sequoiosis, suberosis

Fumes and gases: chlorine, mercury, metals, paraquat, sulfur dioxide

Neoplasm

Lymphangitic carcinoma, bronchoalveolar carcinoma, Kaposi's sarcoma, lymphoma

Drugs

Antibiotics: erythromycin, isoniazid, nitrofurantoin, p-aminosalicylic acid, penicillin, sulfonamides, tetracycline

Chemotherapeutic agents: azathioprine, bleomycin, busulfan, chlorambucil, cyclophosphamide, gemcitabine, melphalan, mercaptopurine, methotrexate, mitomycin, nitrosoureas, procarbazine

Cardiovascular medications: amiodarone, β-blockers, hydralazine, procainamide

Other drugs: allopurinol, carbamazepine, chlorpromazine, chlorpropamide, cromolyn, dantrolene, gold, mecamylamine, methylphenidate, penicillamine, pentolinium, tolbutamide, tricyclic antidepressants

Radiation

Pneumonitis (early), fibrosis (late)

Chronic aspiration

Unknown cause

Idiopathic pulmonary fibrosis (cryptogenic fibrosing alveolitis)

Nonspecific interstitial pneumonia[a]

Bronchiolitis obliterans organizing pneumonia[a]

Collagen vascular disease

Ankylosing spondylitis

Dermatomyositis/polymyositis

Lupus erythematosus

Mixed connective tissue disease

Rheumatoid arthritis

Scleroderma

Sjögren's syndrome

Sarcoidosis

Eosinophilic lung diseases[a]

Acute eosinophilic pneumonia

Chronic eosinophilic pneumonia

Bronchocentric granulomatosis

Churg-Strauss syndrome (allergic angiitis and granulomatosis)[b]

Idiopathic hypereosinophilic syndrome

Simple pulmonary eosinophilia (Löffler's syndrome)

Lymphoid infiltrative disease

Lymphocytic interstitial pneumonia

Pulmonary vasculitis

Wegener's granulomatosis

Lymphomatoid granulomatosis (?neoplasm)

Histiocytosis X (eosinophilic granuloma)

Lymphangioleiomyomatosis

Pulmonary alveolar proteinosis

Diffuse pulmonary hemorrhage

Goodpasture's syndrome

Idiopathic pulmonary hemorrhage

Amyloidosis

Congenital diseases

Gaucher's disease

Hermansky-Pudlak syndrome

Niemann-Pick disease

Neurofibromatosis

Tuberous sclerosis

[a]Some cases are associated with known cause.

[b]May also be classified as a vasculitis.

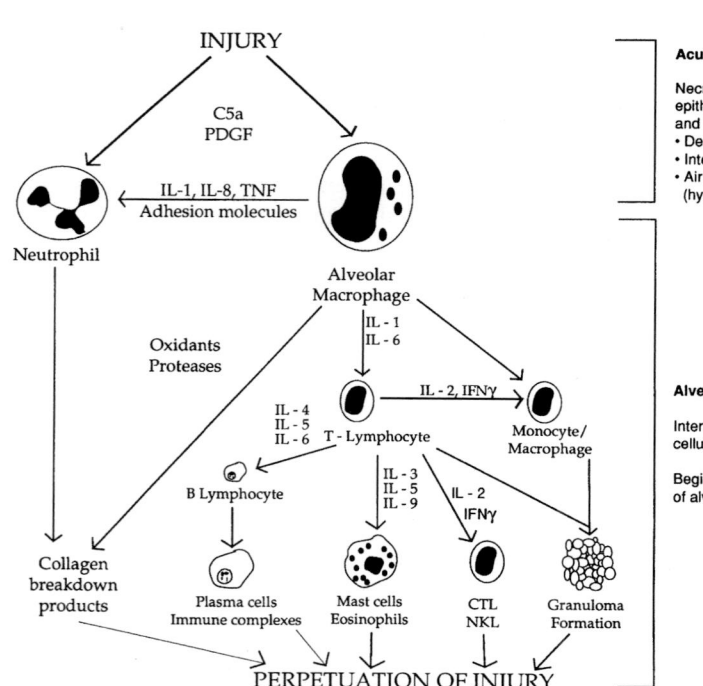

Fig. 91-1. Simplified schema of the cellular and humoral mediators of lung inflammation and injury. Only selected mediators are shown, and normal inhibitory pathways are not demonstrated. C5a, complement; CTL, cytotoxic T lymphocytes; IFNγ, interferon-γ; IL, interleukin; NKL, natural killer lymphocytes; PDGF, platelet-derived growth factor; TNF, tumor necrosis factor.

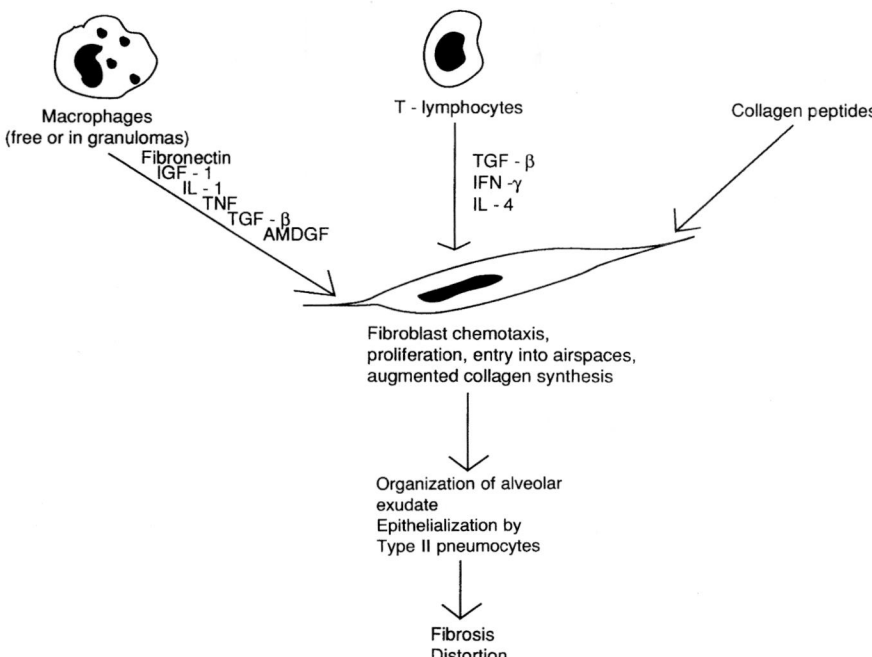

Macrophages
(free or in granulomas)
Fibronectin
IGF - 1
IL - 1
TNF
TGF - β
AMDGF

T - lymphocytes
TGF - β
IFN -γ
IL - 4

Collagen peptides

Fibroblast chemotaxis,
proliferation, entry into airspaces,
augmented collagen synthesis

Organization of alveolar
exudate
Epithelialization by
Type II pneumocytes

Fibrosis
Distortion
Honeycombing

Fig. 91-2. Factors leading to fibroblast stimulation, fibrosis, and lung distortion. AMDGF, alveolar macrophage-derived growth factor; IFN-γ, interferon-γ; IGF, insulinlike growth factor; IL, interleukin; TNF, tumor necrosis factor; TGF-β, transforming growth factor-β.

appreciated, particularly the roles of TNF-α and transforming growth factor-β_1. Macrophages and lymphocytes stimulate fibroblast migration, proliferation, and synthetic activity. Peptides produced by matrix molecule degradation are chemotactic for fibroblasts. Fibronectin, present in the alveolar exudate and produced by activated macrophages, attracts fibroblasts and binds them to fibrin. Organization of the exudate produces accretion of fibrous tissue onto the alveolar wall. Type II pneumocytes proliferate, differentiate into type I cells, and epithelialize the surface of the scar. The result is a widening of the normally thin air–blood interface.

The cells and mediators leading to fibrosis are part of the lung's normal repair mechanisms. Many injuries do not cause histologic or physiologic sequelae. The alveolar exudate is cleared, and the denuded alveolar walls undergo reepithelialization without fibrosis. The outcome in any individual case is determined by the severity of the initial damage, the chronicity or repetition of the injury, the specific toxin or disease, dysregulation and autonomy of the inflammatory reaction, and individual susceptibility, including the age of the patient (i.e., younger people have better reparative capacity). Severe or repetitive insults in the susceptible host ultimately result in the disorderly deposition of collagen, leading to the cystic nonfunctional spaces of the end-stage fibrotic ("honeycomb") lung.

PATHOLOGIC FEATURES

Although some diffuse diseases exhibit unique histologic features, and microorganisms or inhaled irritants are sometimes identified, findings are often nonspecific and reflect a stereotyped response to injury. Pathology reports often describe diffuse alveolar damage (DAD); usual, desquamative, or nonspecific interstitial pneumonia (NSIP); bronchiolitis obliterans; or honeycombing. An expanding array of pathologic labels, used by some to connote specific diseases and by others as purely histologic descriptors, may make clinical correlation difficult. Problems in communication are compounded by the use of different terms to describe identical lesions, especially by authors on different sides of the Atlantic Ocean (Table 91-2; Fig. 91-3).

DAD is typical of severe acute injury. Katzenstein and associates (1976) introduced the term to describe the features of adult respiratory distress syndrome (ARDS). Early cases show interstitial and alveolar edema, epithelial necrosis, and sloughing leading to denuded alveolar walls, acute inflammatory cells, and hyaline membranes. Later, there is organization and repair—the proliferative phase, with proliferation of fibroblasts in the interstitium and air spaces and of type II pneumocytes along the damaged alveolar walls, along with partial or complete resorption of the hyaline membranes seen earlier. The proliferative phase is thought to occur within 1 to 2 weeks after the initial injury. DAD is generally found diffusely throughout the parenchyma and is histologically uniform. These hallmarks suggest a discrete generalized injury. In addition to ARDS, DAD may be seen in other acute syndromes, including acute interstitial pneumonia (Hamman-Rich syndrome), acute radiation pneumonitis, drug reactions, inhalation injury, hypersensitivity pneumonitis (HP), and acute lupus pneumonitis. DAD in immunocompromised patients is often due to infection. Katzenstein and associates (1986) suggested the term *acute interstitial pneumonitis* to describe idiopathic cases, espe-

Table 91-2. Histologic Patterns and Clinical Correlates in Diffuse Lung Diseases

Pattern	Distribution	Histology	Presentation	Idiopathic Syndrome	Selected Associations
Diffuse alveolar damage	Diffuse	Uniform	Acute	Acute interstitial pneumonia (Hamman-Rich)	ARDS, drugs, acute radiation therapy, SLE (acute)
Usual interstitial pneumonia (UIP) [mural fibrosing alveolitis][a]	Patchy	Nonuniform	Chronic	Idiopathic pulmonary fibrosis (IPF) (cryptogenic fibrosing alveolitis)	CVD, inhalation, infections, drugs, other
Desquamative interstitial pneumonia (DIP) [desquamative fibrosing alveolitis][a]	Diffuse	Uniform	Subacute/chronic	DIP or early IPF	Same as UIP
Nonspecific interstitial pneumonia (NSIP)	Patchy	Uniform	Subacute/chronic	NSIP	Immunocompromised CVD, inhalation
Bronchiolitis obliterans organizing pneumonia (BOOP)	Patchy	Uniform	Subacute	BOOP (cryptogenic organizing pneumonia)	Same as UIP, transplant, postinfectious, radiation
Lymphocytic interstitial pneumonia (LIP)	Diffuse	Nonuniform	Variable	LIP	AIDS, Sjögren's, other
Giant cell interstitial pneumonia	Patchy	Uniform	Variable	None	Hard metal inhalation
Honeycombing	Variable	Nonuniform	Variable	NA	Many DPLDs
Honeycomb lung	Diffuse	Uniform	Chronic	NA	IPF, LAM, sarcoidosis, histiocytosis X, asbestosis, scleroderma

AIDS, acquired immunodeficiency syndrome; ARDS, adult respiratory distress syndrome; CVD, collagen vascular disease; DPLD, diffuse parenchymal lung disease; LAM, lymphangioleiomyomatosis; NA, not applicable; SLE, systemic lupus erythematosus.
[a]Synonym.

cially to distinguish this lesion from the more common chronic interstitial pneumonias.

Liebow (1968) described the classic interstitial pneumonias. Usual interstitial pneumonia (UIP) is encountered most frequently. Like DAD, UIP represents a nonspecific response. The clinical syndromes, however, evolve over a longer period. Hyaline membranes, edema, and alveolar exudates are rarely seen. The distribution is patchy and the histology is nonuniform, varying from normal alveoli to inflammation to fibrosis. This pattern suggests repetitive or low-grade chronic injury. Areas of UIP may be seen in idiopathic pulmonary fibrosis (IPF), collagen vascular disease (CVD), chronic HP, some of the pneumoconioses, sarcoidosis, drug-induced DPLD, granulomatous infections, late radiation pneumonitis, healed infections, organized DAD, chronic aspiration, histiocytosis X, and even cases of chronic pulmonary edema due to passive congestion. In desquamative interstitial pneumonia (DIP), the involvement is diffuse and the histology is homogeneous. It was initially believed that the highly cellular histology reflected desquamated alveolar epithelial cells, but it is now known that filling of the alveoli by macrophages is the defining feature. Interstitial monocytic infiltration is also seen, but fibrosis is minimal. A DIP pattern may be found in idiopathic DIP, histiocytosis X, drug reactions (especially amiodarone toxicity), alveolar hemorrhage, pneumoconioses, eosinophilic pneumonias, obstructive pneumonia (in which case the lesion is not diffuse), lipid pneumonia and lipid storage diseases, respiratory bronchiolitis, and infections in the immunosuppressed patient. In Europe,

UIP and DIP are called *mural* and *desquamative fibrosing alveolitis*, respectively.

Carrington and associates (1978) view UIP and DIP as two diseases because of different pathologic findings and because DIP is more amenable to treatment. Other authorities, however, agree with Scadding and Hinson (1967), Patchefsky and colleagues (1973), and Tubbs and colleagues (1977) that DIP is the early cellular phase and UIP the later fibrotic phase of the same reaction. As noted, there is much overlap in clinical processes in which the two patterns may be identified. In addition, areas of DIP can be found in cases of predominant UIP histology, and DIP has been shown to progress to UIP.

Katzenstein and Fiorelli (1994) detailed the features of an additional variant of the interstitial pneumonias of unknown cause, NSIP. Although the characteristic lesion contains varying proportions of interstitial inflammation and fibrosis, NSIP differs from UIP in that all areas appear to be temporally uniform. In addition to an idiopathic form, NSIP also occurs in acquired immunodeficiency syndrome (AIDS), as described by Suffredini and associates (1987), in other immunocompromised patients and in cases of CVD, inhalation of organic antigens, and resolving acute lung injury. In a report of 12 cases, Cottin and associates (1998) found that six were idiopathic, three were associated with CVD, two with organic dust exposure, and one followed an episode of ARDS. The response to treatment is better than for UIP but appears to be more variable than in bronchiolitis obliterans organizing pneumonia (BOOP).

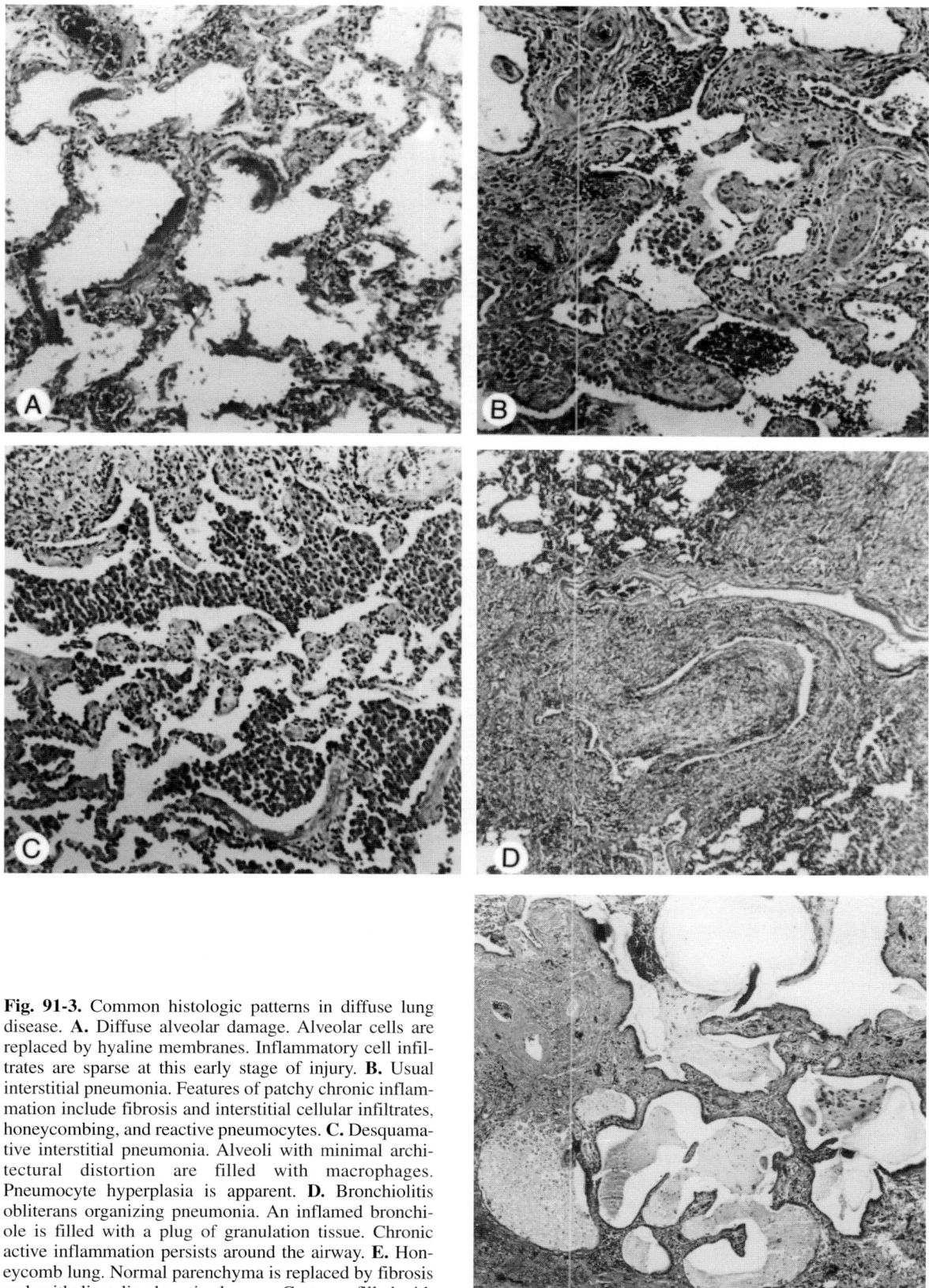

Fig. 91-3. Common histologic patterns in diffuse lung disease. **A.** Diffuse alveolar damage. Alveolar cells are replaced by hyaline membranes. Inflammatory cell infiltrates are sparse at this early stage of injury. **B.** Usual interstitial pneumonia. Features of patchy chronic inflammation include fibrosis and interstitial cellular infiltrates, honeycombing, and reactive pneumocytes. **C.** Desquamative interstitial pneumonia. Alveoli with minimal architectural distortion are filled with macrophages. Pneumocyte hyperplasia is apparent. **D.** Bronchiolitis obliterans organizing pneumonia. An inflamed bronchiole is filled with a plug of granulation tissue. Chronic active inflammation persists around the airway. **E.** Honeycomb lung. Normal parenchyma is replaced by fibrosis and epithelium-lined cystic changes. Cysts are filled with mucus and inflammatory cells.

In BOOP, polypoid plugs of organizing connective tissue partially or totally fill respiratory bronchioles, alveolar ducts, and alveoli. Mononuclear cell infiltrates are seen in the airway walls, and the alveoli often contain lipid-filled macrophages. Fibrosis is absent or minimal. The distribution is patchy but histologically uniform. Similar to other nonspecific reactions, BOOP can be idiopathic or associated with other processes, such as organizing infection, drug reactions, inhalation injury, CVD, HP, and chronic eosinophilic pneumonia.

Lymphocytic interstitial pneumonia (LIP) consists of an interstitial infiltrate of lymphocytes, plasma cells, and macrophages. Granulomas, lymphoid follicles, and amyloid deposits are often present. Although an idiopathic form exists, LIP has a strong association with immunologic diseases, AIDS, and lymphoid malignancies. Giant cell interstitial pneumonia is a rare pattern in which bizarre multinucleated cells fill the air spaces. Ohori and associates (1989) reported that most cases result from inhalation of hard metal particles.

Severe fibrosis results in cyst formation and loss of normal architecture. When this pattern coexists with normal and inflamed areas, as in UIP, it is called *honeycombing*. An etiologic diagnosis can often be made if the histology of the less fibrotic areas is characteristic. *Honeycomb lung* denotes diffuse distortion and represents the potential end stage of any fibrogenic process, but in practice it is seen mainly in IPF, histiocytosis X, scleroderma, rheumatoid lung, asbestosis, lymphangioleiomyomatosis (LAM), and sarcoidosis.

In some DPLDs, necrotizing or nonnecrotizing granulomas are a universal or occasional feature. Processes associated with granuloma formation include sarcoidosis, granulomatous infections, talcosis, berylliosis, Wegener's granulomatosis, necrotizing sarcoid granulomatosis, bronchocentric granulomatosis, certain drug reactions, and hypersensitivity reactions.

RADIOGRAPHIC FEATURES

Despite advances in computed tomography (CT), the chest radiograph remains the basic imaging tool for the initial evaluation and subsequent surveillance of DPLD. Felson (1979) and Fraser and associates (1988) discussed the radiographic features of DPLD. Because the interstitium and air spaces are often affected simultaneously by histology, radiographic division into "interstitial" and "air space" or "alveolar" (acinar) patterns has been criticized as inaccurate. This system, however, is in common usage and serves as a reference point. Predominant interstitial disease produces four patterns: reticular, nodular, reticulonodular, and linear. When filling of the air spaces predominates, an acinar pattern is seen.

Reticular infiltrates appear as a network of curvilinear opacities and are described as fine, medium, or coarse, depending on the size of the mesh. These gradations generally correlate with progression from early alveolitis to advanced fibrosis. Transition over time from fine to medium to coarse patterns has been documented by Wholey and associates (1958) for IPF and by Locke (1963) for rheumatoid lung. Coarse reticulation (i.e., thick-walled cystic spaces at least 5 mm in diameter) indicates severe fibrosis and, like its pathologic counterpart, is termed *honeycombing*. A *nodular* pattern consists of well-circumscribed, small, rounded opacities of varying diameter. More common is a combined *reticulonodular* pattern, which can result from superimposition of nodules and reticulation or from end-on orientation of reticular opacities in the absence of histologic nodules. Thickening of the interlobular septa and perivascular sheaths produces a *linear* pattern, typified by Kerley's B lines. Early *acinar* opacities may simulate nodularity, but the borders are indistinct. Coalescence produces air space consolidation. Patent airways surrounded by opacified acini appear as air bronchograms. Mixed interstitial and air space patterns are common.

Ground-glass opacification results from changes below the resolution of the imaging technique, including fine reticulation, micronodularity, and minimal air space filling. For standard radiographs, this description refers to a generalized, sometimes granular haziness. On CT, ground-glass appearance is often patchy and is defined as an increase in lung density that does not obscure bronchovascular structures.

Table 91-3 lists other features of the chest radiograph, including anatomic distribution, overall lung volume, and extrapulmonary findings, that may aid in diagnosis.

The limitations of conventional radiography in DPLD must be kept in mind. These include limited sensitivity, an incomplete view of the lungs and mediastinum, variability in interpretation, and a lack of specificity of the aforementioned plain film patterns. As much as 40% of the lung parenchyma is obscured by superimposed structures on chest radiographs. The frequent inadequacy of standard radiography was highlighted by McLoud and colleagues (1983). They interpreted films from 365 biopsy-confirmed cases of DPLD and recorded the three most likely diagnoses using a standardized system. Despite a correlation between certain diseases and patterns, the correct diagnosis was included in the first two choices only 50% of the time. Epler and coworkers (1978) found that the chest radiograph was entirely normal in 10% of cases of DPLD.

Chest CT, particularly with high-resolution algorithms (HRCT), is becoming a vital component in assessment of DPLD. The benefits of CT include complete visualization of all lung regions; identification of mediastinal and hilar lymphadenopathy, small effusions, and pleural abnormalities; aid in selecting appropriate sites for biopsy; and, most important, the detection of characteristic and often subtle abnormalities. The resolution of HRCT reliably extends to the anatomic level of the secondary pulmonary lobule. HRCT permits parenchymal visualization in such detail that ground-glass attenuation is increasingly recognized. The degree to which

Table 91-3. Radiographic Features of Noninfectious Diffuse Lung Diseases

Upper lung zone predominance
    Sarcoidosis
    Histiocytosis X
    Silicosis
    Berylliosis
    Chronic hypersensitivity pneumonitis
    Amiodarone toxicity
Increased lung volumes
    Histiocytosis X
    Chronic hypersensitivity pneumonitis
    Lymphangioleiomyomatosis
    Sarcoidosis, stage III
Pleural effusion
    Collagen vascular disease
    Lymphangitic carcinoma/metastatic disease
    Asbestosis
    Lymphangioleiomyomatosis (chylous)
    Radiation fibrosis
Pleural plaques and thickening
    Asbestosis
    Lymphangitic carcinoma/metastatic disease
Pneumothorax
    Lymphangioleiomyomatosis
    Histiocytosis X
    Advanced sarcoidosis
    Pneumocystis carinii pneumonia
Mediastinal or hilar (or both) lymphadenopathy
    Sarcoidosis
    Lymphoma
    Lymphangitic carcinoma/metastatic disease
    Berylliosis
Esophageal dilatation, air-fluid level
    Scleroderma
    Aspiration pneumonitis
Soft tissue calcifications
    Dermatomyositis
    Scleroderma
Skeletal abnormalities
    Lymphangitic carcinoma/metastatic disease (lytic or blastic lesions)
    Rheumatoid lung (humeral or clavicular erosions)

this finding correlates with histopathology is still debated. Colby and Swensen (1996) provided a valuable comprehensive analysis of the HRCT correlates of the histopathologic patterns in DPLD. Mathiesen and coworkers (1989) confirmed the value of HRCT, making a correct first-choice diagnosis in 76% of cases compared to 57% by chest radiographs alone. The highest accuracy was achieved in silicosis (93%), UIP/IPF (89%), lymphangitic carcinoma (85%), histiocytosis X (83%), and sarcoidosis (77%). As with plain radiography, however, a normal HRCT does not eliminate the possibility of DPLD. Orens and associates (1995) found that 12% of dyspneic patients had normal HRCT, despite measured impairment of gas exchange and biopsy-proven IPF, although the false-negative cases had less severe functional and histologic findings than did those with abnormal HRCT. Although HRCT may be nonspecific and sometimes falsely negative, radiographic-clinical correlation is diagnostic in many

instances of lymphangitic carcinoma, IPF, hypersensitivity, among others. CT imaging may also narrow the list of differential diagnoses at presentation and may subsequently aid in assessing disease progression and response to therapy.

Radionuclide scanning with gallium 67 has been studied extensively in DPLD. Because the isotope localizes in areas of inflammation, scintigraphy is abnormal in many cases. Although the intensity of uptake may reflect the degree of alveolitis, the value of scintigraphy for diagnosis, prognosis, and surveillance is limited. Magnetic resonance imaging is not generally useful in DPLD, and positron emission tomography is also unlikely to play a significant role in this area.

CLINICAL FEATURES

Most patients present with shortness of breath. Although dyspnea associated with infections or HP may arise abruptly and progress rapidly, in most processes the clinical syndrome is subacute or chronic. In the pneumoconioses, dyspnea may develop insidiously and may appear many years after exposure. A nonproductive cough is common in both acute and chronic cases. Fever, weight loss, fatigue, and myalgias can occur in infectious and noninfectious disorders. Other nonpulmonary symptoms may be more specific, such as uveitis in sarcoidosis and sinusitis or otitis in Wegener's granulomatosis. Asymptomatic patients with abnormal chest radiographs are most likely to have sarcoidosis or silicosis. Spontaneous pneumothorax may be the presenting event in LAM and histiocytosis X. Hemoptysis is unusual in most DPLD, but it occurs in cases of diffuse pulmonary hemorrhage or advanced lung destruction.

A careful medical, occupational, avocational, and travel history is essential. Drug regimens, prior neoplasm, exposure to dusts or animals, and risk factors for AIDS are examples of information that may suggest a diagnosis.

The physical examination is often normal. Breathlessness and tachypnea may be apparent at rest or provoked by exertion. Jahaveri and Sicilian (1992) demonstrated that ventilation is maintained and hypercapnia is avoided by rapid shallow breathing. Fine crackles reminiscent of the sound of Velcro are the classic finding, occur in late inspiration, and are also called "dry" rales to distinguish them from the "moist" rales of pulmonary edema. Wheezing can occur in DPLD, such as sarcoidosis, histiocytosis X, and lymphangiomyomatosis. Digital clubbing is common in advanced IPF and histiocytosis X but is uncommon in most other disorders. Physical signs of cor pulmonale (peripheral edema, ascites, hepatomegaly, and accentuated pulmonic valve sound) indicate advanced fibrosis. Nonpulmonary physical findings may suggest a diagnosis, as noted with specific diseases.

Arterial oxygen tension can be normal at rest, but exercise-induced hypoxemia is virtually universal. Hypercarbia is a late finding, reflecting respiratory muscle fatigue and end-stage disease. Pulmonary function testing should include spirometry, lung volumes, and diffusion capacity.

Diffusion impairment occurs early and is the most sensitive physiologic sign of DPLD. With advancing fibrosis, pulmonary function tests show a restrictive pattern, with reductions in total lung capacity and its subdivisions. In some cases, however, cystic change, peribronchial fibrosis or granulomas, or bronchiolitis may impair airflow, producing an obstructive or combined pattern.

DIAGNOSIS

A synthesis of the history, physical examination, laboratory data, and radiographs may be diagnostic. A thorough history, including a detailed delineation of current and remote occupational and environmental exposures, as well as hobbies, travel, and pets, is an essential starting point. A history suggestive of active toxic exposure should prompt a trial of avoidance of the suspected toxin. Prior chest radiographs should be examined to date the onset of disease and assess change over time. Invasive approaches are warranted when the clinical synthesis does not produce a confident diagnosis, when the course is atypical, when it is necessary to assess disease activity, and occasionally for legal and compensation purposes. Although biopsy of extrathoracic sites, percutaneous aspiration of the lung or pleura, thoracentesis, or mediastinoscopy may be applicable in some cases, the primary diagnostic methods for DPLD are bronchoalveolar lavage (BAL), transbronchial lung biopsy (TBLB), and surgical lung biopsy. The technical aspects of these procedures are described elsewhere in this text.

BAL is often useful in the evaluation of infectious DPLD in the immunocompromised host and may also be definitive in diffuse bronchoalveolar carcinoma, pulmonary alveolar proteinosis (PAP), and histiocytosis X, but it has a limited role in most other processes. Although analysis of BAL cell types and subsets of T lymphocytes has been suggested to play a role in diagnosis and in following response to therapy in several lesions, Raghu (1995), among others, cautions that this analysis may not differentiate common disorders. In fact, cellular analysis may differ in BAL fluid retrieved at the same time from various lobes in the same patient. Thus, the usefulness of BAL in the global spectrum of DPLD remains controversial at present.

TBLB is a reliable method for detecting processes with characteristic histologic changes concentrated along bronchovascular sheaths, notably sarcoidosis and lymphangitic carcinoma. TBLB can sporadically diagnose many other lesions with distinctive histology but is of little value in diseases with nonspecific features. Reynolds (1998) has observed that overall a confident pathologic diagnosis can be made in only 25% of cases. Coagulopathy and ventilator dependence with high airway pressures are contraindications to TBLB. The procedure may also be poorly tolerated by the very dyspneic patient.

Surgical biopsy encompasses both open and video-assisted thoracic surgery (VATS) procedures for obtaining large samples of lung tissue necessary for diagnosis and staging of disease activity. We consider the latter technique the approach of choice in patients who can tolerate one-lung ventilation because it allows assessment of most of the lung, as opposed to the limited exposure afforded by standard open biopsy by anterior thoracotomy. VATS biopsy is also cost effective. Ponn and colleagues (1997) have shown that, in many cases, VATS lung biopsy can safely be performed on an outpatient basis. In stable chronic DPLD, morbidity and mortality are negligible. Gaensler and Carrington (1980) found a mortality rate of 0.3% for open biopsy. Nonetheless, the benefit of proceeding to surgical biopsy when diagnostic assessment (including bronchoscopy) is inconclusive remains debatable. As with all medical pathways, decisions must fit the individual patient. Elderly patients with clinical and radiographic features typical of IPF, people with systemic disorders frequently associated with DPLD (e.g., connective tissue disease) and those with known neoplasm likely to have lymphangitic dissemination are among the many instances in which management without biopsy is often appropriate. If the subsequent clinical or radiographic course is atypical for the presumed diagnosis, however, definitive tissue sampling should be considered.

Specimens are taken in areas of active disease rather than regions of advanced fibrosis to assess the degree of alveolitis. A ground-glass appearance on HRCT generally denotes active disease and can be helpful in identifying fruitful biopsy sites. Nishimura and associates (1992), however, detected fibrosis in many areas of ground-glass opacity. It was axiomatic in the past that lingular and right middle lobe biopsies are unreliable. Although studies by Wetstein (1986), Miller (1987), and Chechani (1992) and their colleagues in acute and chronic disorders documented the reliability of tissue from these lobes, some authorities continue to advise avoidance of these sites. If feasible, multiple biopsies—from overtly abnormal and adjacent or remote normal-appearing areas—may be helpful. Proper processing of the specimen is crucial. The pathologist is able to render a meaningful interpretation only when apprised of the clinical situation. In addition to light microscopy, samples should be sent for culture with a portion saved for ultrastructural study. Inorganic dust analysis may be indicated for suspected pneumoconiosis. In acute processes, frozen sections and touch preparations are examined and stained for organisms to facilitate early treatment.

SELECTED DIFFUSE LUNG DISEASES

Idiopathic Pulmonary Fibrosis (Cryptogenic Fibrosing Alveolitis)

IPF is a syndrome of unknown etiology that affects men and women equally. Most patients are between ages 40 and 70 years and present with dyspnea and dry cough that progress over months or years. Many recall an antecedent flulike illness; Crystal and associates (1976) reported constitutional symptoms in 50%. "Velcro" rales and digital clubbing are common physical findings. Chest radiographs usually show a reticular or reticulonodular pattern with basilar predominance but are normal in a few early cases. Rarely, a primarily acinar pattern is seen and may correlate with DIP histology. The most prominent changes have a characteristic subpleural location by HRCT (Fig. 91-4). Pleural effusion or adenopathy are rare and should suggest an alternative diagnosis.

Although the initiating factor is unknown, immune mechanisms may be operative in the perpetuation of inflammation. Crystal and associates (1976) found cryoglobulinemia and elevated immunoglobulin A (IgA) in about 40% of patients. Winterbauer and colleagues (1978) reported increased rheumatoid factor and antinuclear antibody in 30 and 15%, respectively. Dreisen and coworkers (1978) detected serum immune complexes in the majority of patients with active inflammation. BAL fluid may also contain immune complexes.

The histology of IPF is most commonly the mixed pattern of UIP; DIP likely represents an early stage. Findings from TBLB and BAL may suggest IPF by the presence of inflammation, fibrosis, or both, but a definitive diagnosis requires a surgical biopsy large enough to encompass the patchy, nonuniform histology. Whether all patients with presumed IPF require biopsy is controversial. Confirmation before therapy is desirable for the reasons outlined by Raghu (1987) and King (1991): 1) to eliminate other possibilities, 2) to obtain prognostic information, and 3) to justify withholding treatment for end-stage disease. In practice, however, many pulmonologists would accept a diagnosis based on firm clinical grounds in a patient who refuses or has a contraindication to biopsy. Winterbauer (1991) described a profile that permits a reliable clinical diagnosis: patient older than 65 years with disease duration of 2 years or more, typical chest film, no extrathoracic symptoms or exposure history, negative evaluation for CVD, and consistent TBLB and BAL findings. Raghu (1995) has elaborated similar criteria for omitting surgical biopsy. HRCT should be included in the evaluation of most cases.

Initial treatment consists of high-dose steroids. Response can be followed by a scoring system devised by Watters and associates (1986), which combines symptomatic, radiographic, and pulmonary function data. Favorable prognostic factors include younger age, duration of less than 1 year, histologic evidence of active alveolitis and inflammation (e.g., cellularity, bronchiolitis, DIP areas, pneumonocyte proliferation), BAL lymphocytosis, and the presence of immune complexes. The overall prognosis of IPF is poor. Only about one-third of patients improve, with most responses apparent within a few weeks. Stack (1972) found a 5-year survival rate of 43% for responders and 20% for nonresponders. Patients who cannot tolerate or do not respond to steroid treatment may benefit from cyclophosphamide or azathioprine. In a randomized trial, Johnson and

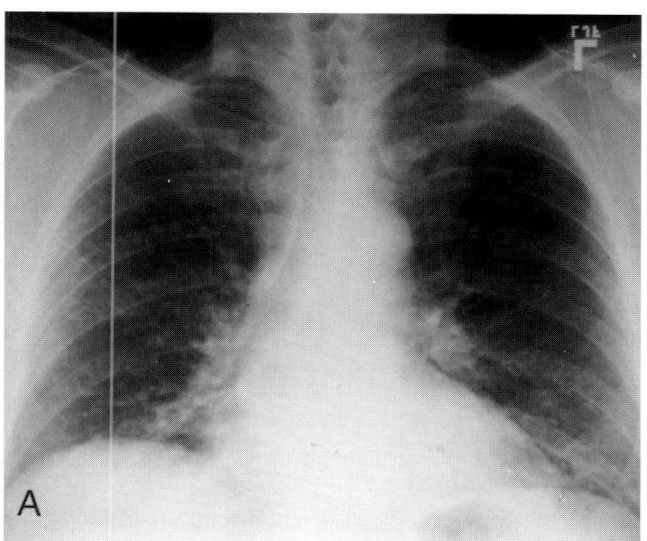

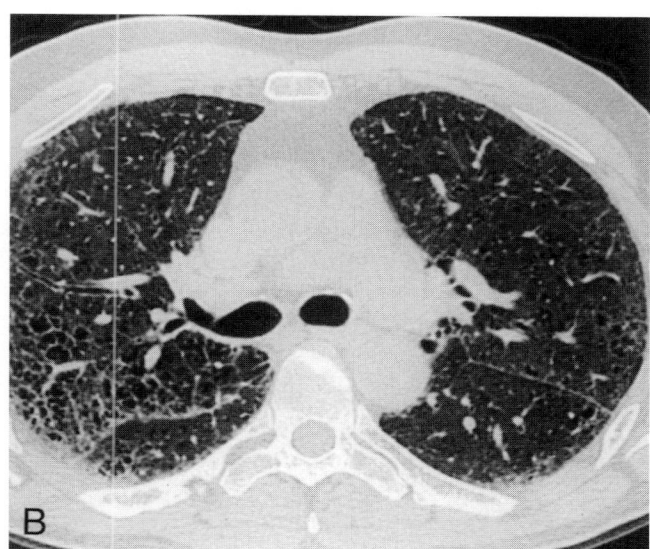

Fig. 91-4. A 59-year-old man with idiopathic pulmonary fibrosis. **A.** Chest radiograph demonstrates mild reticulonodular densities bilaterally. **B.** High-resolution computed tomography reveals extensive honeycombing with a characteristic subpleural distribution.

associates (1989) noted improved survival with steroid-cyclophosphamide therapy versus steroids alone. Some advise early treatment with immunosuppressants in most cases. Peters and colleagues (1993) treated patients with the antifibrogenic agent colchicine and found a response rate similar to other agents but with fewer side effects. Care for advanced IPF is supportive, mainly long-term oxygen therapy. In a minority of younger patients, lung transplantation warrants consideration.

Occasionally, a patient presents with rapidly progressive symptoms, as originally described in Hamman-Rich syndrome. Katzenstein and associates (1986) described eight cases and coined the term *acute interstitial pneumonia*. The absence of an obvious etiology as well as a more prolonged

Table 91-4. Lung Involvement in Collagen Vascular Disease[a]

Usual interstitial pneumonia
Diffuse alveolar damage
Bronchiolitis obliterans with or without organizing pneumonia
Disorders of the small airways
Alveolar hemorrhage
Nodular multifocal involvement
Drug-induced lung disease
Pulmonary hypertension
Infections
Recurrent aspiration pneumonia
Apical fibrobullous disease

[a]Excludes systemic vasculitis.

course separates these patients from those with the usual forms of ARDS. DAD is seen histologically. Acute exacerbation can also occur during the course of otherwise typical IPF and correlates with DAD in a background of chronic change. The outcome is usually fatal.

Collagen Vascular Disease

The reported frequency of lung involvement in CVD depends on the disorder and the method of detection. In general, lung disease presents after or concurrently with CVD and correlates with the severity of the primary process, but it may precede or overshadow other manifestations. Although the clinical, radiographic, and histologic features are often similar to those of IPF, a variety of histologic patterns or predominant sites of pulmonary injury can be observed (Table 91-4).

Scleroderma

DPLD is most common in scleroderma (also known as *systemic sclerosis*). Owens and Follansbee (1987) noted that pulmonary symptoms occur in most patients and that pathologic lung involvement is almost universal. Women are affected more often than are men. Pulmonary vasculopathy may occur alone or in combination with interstitial involvement, especially in patients with the CREST variant of this condition (e.g., *c*alcinosis, *R*aynaud's phenomenon, *e*sophageal dysmotility, *s*clerodactyly, *t*elangiectasia). Symptomatic pleural disease is less common than in other CVD. Chest radiographs typically show fine or coarse reticular markings. Extrapulmonary signs may include cardiomegaly from pulmonary hypertension and esophageal dilation. Aspiration from esophageal dysmotility may produce changing infiltrates. Persistent nodules or infiltrates may indicate adenocarcinoma or bronchoalveolar carcinoma, the incidence of which is increased in scleroderma. Biopsy in cases of diffuse radiographic involvement usually demonstrates UIP with more fibrosis than inflammation. Both the interstitial and vascular involvement are generally resistant to therapy, although penicillamine has been reported to be helpful in some cases.

Rheumatoid Arthritis

Many patients with rheumatoid arthritis (RA) develop DPLD, although symptoms are less frequent than in scleroderma. Although RA is more common in women, most patients with lung disease are men who are seropositive and have erosive nodular RA. Signs of fibrosis are present on chest radiographs in about 5% of cases, usually in the form of bibasilar infiltrates. Using HRCT, however, Fujii and associates (1993) found interstitial disease in 47% overall and in 35% of patients with normal chest radiographs. Pleural effusion may also occur. Frank and colleagues (1973) detected diminished lung volumes and diffusing capacity in 41% of patients with RA, despite normal chest films in 50%. The diffuse involvement is radiographically and histologically similar to IPF but may be more slowly progressive. Rheumatoid (necrobiotic) nodules are sometimes seen radiographically and must be distinguished from carcinoma. Similarly, pathologic specimens, in addition to UIP, may show rheumatoid nodules, pleural fibrosis, or a characteristic bronchovascular lymphoid hyperplasia described by Yousem (1985). Less common causes of DPLD in RA include rheumatoid pneumoconiosis (i.e., Caplan's syndrome), pulmonary vascular disease, and bronchiolitis obliterans. Drug-induced lung disease, in contrast, is a frequent complication of therapy in RA, especially with methotrexate and gold administration.

Systemic Lupus Erythematosus

Although pleural abnormalities are found in more than 70% of patients with systemic lupus erythematosus (SLE), DPLD is uncommon. Haupt (1981) reported an autopsy incidence of only 9%. Women are affected far more often than men. The presentation is generally insidious, with progressive cough, dyspnea and rales. Chest radiographs feature persistent interstitial infiltrates. The UIP of SLE has no pathognomonic histologic features. SLE can also present as an acute pneumonitis, as described by Matthay and associates (1974), with fever, dyspnea, chest pain, and hemoptysis. In this setting, radiographs show acinar opacities and consolidation, and DAD is the most frequent histologic characteristic. DIP and bronchiolitis are also seen. Mortality is high, and survivors often progress to fibrosis. Diffuse alveolar hemorrhage can also occur in SLE and often correlates with histologic evidence of capillaritis.

Polymyositis and Dermatomyositis

DPLD is uncommon in patients with polymyositis and dermatomyositis (PM/DM), with abnormal radiographic findings noted in only 5% of cases reviewed by Frazier and Miller (1974) and 9% in the series of Salmeron and colleagues (1981). Women are affected twice as often as are men. Although the presentation may be indolent, subacute, or rapid, an indolent course predominates, with clinical features similar to IPF. As in scleroderma, the radiographic picture may include signs of aspiration pneumonia, which in PM/DM results from inflammation of pharyngeal striated muscle. Tazelaar and associates (1990) reported that the pathologic findings vary with the presentation and include UIP, DAD, BOOP, and, rarely, LIP. Diagnosis may be difficult because DPLD sometimes antedates other signs of PM/DM.

Other Collagen Vascular Disease

Mixed connective tissue disease combines clinical and serologic features of SLE, RA, PM/DM, and scleroderma. It affects women eight times more often than men. Prakash (1985) and Sullivan (1984) and their colleagues reported a significant incidence of radiographic and functional abnormalities. As an overlap syndrome, the pulmonary manifestations are variable. Lung disease in Sjögren's syndrome, especially the primary type, consists mainly of lymphocytic processes. Although often discussed with CVD-associated DPLD, the apical fibrobullous changes of ankylosing spondylitis—and rarely, RA—are not related to a generalized process. Restriction is present only when there is an extensive thoracic wall deformity.

Diagnosis

The guidelines for biopsy in CVD are similar to those for IPF. When clinical findings are classic, biopsy is unnecessary and is also generally unwarranted in patients already receiving steroid or cytotoxic therapy for extrapulmonary manifestations. If there is suspicion of carcinoma (e.g., rheumatoid nodule), drug-induced injury, or opportunistic infection, and bronchoscopic samples are nondiagnostic, surgical biopsy is indicated.

Despite much variability, CVD lung disease has a more favorable natural history and response to treatment than does IPF. Disease stability is common. Steroids and cyclophosphamide are the mainstays of therapy in cases of progressive disease. Agusti and associates (1992) noted that after 2 years of steroid treatment, pulmonary function deteriorated in IPF patients but remained stable in patients with CVD. Severe lung symptoms, however, are ominous. Hakala (1988) found a 3.5-year median survival and 39% 5-year survival in RA patients requiring hospitalization for interstitial disease. As a general rule, response is best in patients with PM/DM and mixed connective tissue disease and intermediate to poor in those with RA, SLE, and scleroderma. The growing consensus is that early cytotoxic therapy is beneficial.

Sarcoidosis

Sarcoidosis is a multisystem disorder characterized by noncaseating granulomas in various tissues in the absence of an identifiable etiology. The lung is affected in almost all cases (94%). Thomas and Hunninghake (1987) stressed the role of activated T cells in the formation of sarcoid granulomas. Numbers of lung helper T lymphocytes are increased in active cases, and these cells proliferate spontaneously in vitro. Paradoxically, evidence of impaired systemic immunity in the form of cutaneous anergy often accompanies augmented pulmonary cell-mediated reactivity. The cause of sarcoidosis remains unknown, although community and workplace clusters suggest a transmissible agent or environmental agent. This and other aspects of the disease have been recently reviewed by Newman and coworkers (1997).

Most patients present in the third or fourth decade of life. Between 30 and 50% of these individuals are asymptomatic, despite abnormal chest radiographs. Blacks have both a higher prevalence and severity of the disease. When present, symptoms may be systemic or organ specific. The eyes (uveitis, conjunctivitis, retinitis) and skin (nodules, plaques) are the most common symptomatic extrapulmonary sites. Clinical involvement of the liver, synovial joints, central nervous system, larynx, and heart is less frequent. Early pulmonary complaints consist of cough and dyspnea. Wheezing, purulent sputum, and hemoptysis indicate significant lung destruction. The course is usually indolent, but a few patients have an acute multiorgan syndrome (Löfgren's syndrome) that typically includes fever, bilateral hilar lymphadenopathy, polyarthralgias, and erythema nodosum. Of note is that these skin lesions do not contain granulomas.

Physical findings vary from normal breath sounds or dry rales to wheezing and signs of cor pulmonale in advanced cases. Skin and ocular lesions, salivary gland enlargement, hepatosplenomegaly, and peripheral adenopathy may be noted. Laboratory evaluation may show peripheral lymphopenia resulting from lymphocyte accumulation in the lung, polyclonal hypergammaglobulinemia from T cell activation of B lymphocytes, and hypercalcemia secondary to vitamin D produced by macrophages in granulomas. The level of angiotensin-converting enzyme is often elevated in serum and BAL fluid but is nonspecific. Restrictive lung function is typical, but obstructive physiology can result from endobronchial sarcoid, distortion of small airways by granulomas, or airway hyperreactivity.

The chest radiograph is almost always abnormal and defines the stage of sarcoidosis (Table 91-5). Hilar lymphadenopathy with or without mediastinal node enlargement is noted in approximately 80% of patients. Bilateral

Table 91-5. Radiographic Stages of Sarcoidosis

Stage	Chest Radiographic Findings	Frequency at Presentation
0	Normal	8
1	Lymphadenopathy	50
2	Lymphadenopathy and parenchymal infiltrates	30
3	Parenchymal infiltrates only	12
4	End-stage honeycomb lung	Rare

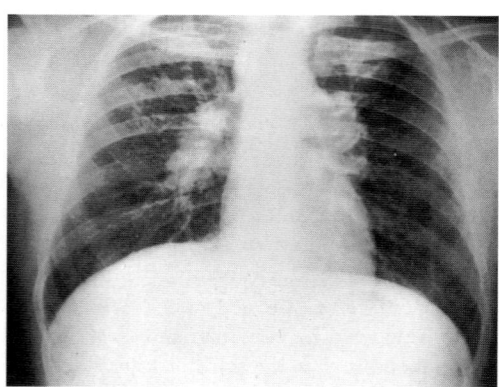

Fig. 91-5. A 21-year-old man with sarcoidosis. Note parenchymal involvement and symmetric bilateral hilar adenopathy (stage 2).

symmetric enlargement is the universal pattern (Fig. 91-5). Unilateral adenopathy warrants consideration of neoplasm or granulomatous infection. Parenchymal findings predominate in the upper lobes and include variable interstitial and acinar lesions. Large nodules are sometimes noted. Honeycombing, increased lung volume, apical bullae, and upward retraction of the hila are late changes. Pleural disease is rare. Pneumothorax can occur in advanced cases. HRCT typically shows small nodules subpleurally and along bronchovascular sheaths. Sulavik and associates (1990) described a pattern of lacrimal, salivary gland, and lymph node activity detected by gallium scintigraphy that is often found in sarcoidosis (Fig. 91-6) but is not entirely specific.

Histologically, in addition to noncaseating granulomas, a mononuclear alveolitis may be seen but is rarely prominent. An inverse relation exists between granulomatous and cellular infiltrates, conforming to the pathogenetic sequence of alveolitis preceding granuloma formation. Granulomas are usually identifiable, even in cases of honeycomb lung and,

at the opposite extreme, in patients with radiographically normal lungs. Because similar granulomas are found in other diseases, most pathology reports describe "noncaseating granulomas consistent with sarcoidosis," emphasizing the necessity of clinicopathologic correlation. Diagnosis depends on exclusion of the spectrum of infectious, neoplastic, environmental, and immunologic conditions associated with granulomatous lung inflammation.

In some cases, biopsy of skin lesions (other than erythema nodosum), lymph nodes, or liver is the simplest approach. The usual source of diagnostic tissue, however, is TBLB, which offers a high yield because of peribronchial clustering of granulomas. Thrasher and Briggs (1982) found granulomas by TBLB in 89% of radiographic stage I lesions, 98% of stage II lesions, and 88% of stage III lesions. Transtracheal lymph node aspiration may be successful. Mediastinoscopy is a safe outpatient procedure with a high diagnostic yield that may be used as an alternative to TBLB. Mediastinoscopy or VATS are also indicated when bronchoscopic methods are nondiagnostic. There is debate about the universal need for tissue confirmation. Some clinicians advocate biopsy in all cases, but others accept a clinical diagnosis in patients with classic features.

Many patients improve or remain stable without treatment. James and associates (1976) reported spontaneous resolution in 65% of those at stage I, 49% at stage II, and 20% at stage III. About 20% have progressive pulmonary impairment, most having presented with stage III disease. When indicated, the current standard treatment is with steroids. Other agents, including methotrexate, cyclosporine, chlorambucil, and antimalarial drugs, have been used, but their role remains uncertain. Because of a high remission rate, patients with stages I and II at presentation who are asymptomatic and have normal lung function are generally followed clinically and radiographically. Treatment is begun if deterioration occurs and is applied at presentation in patients with stage III

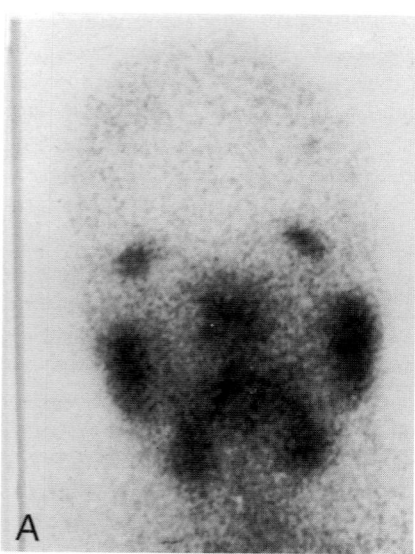

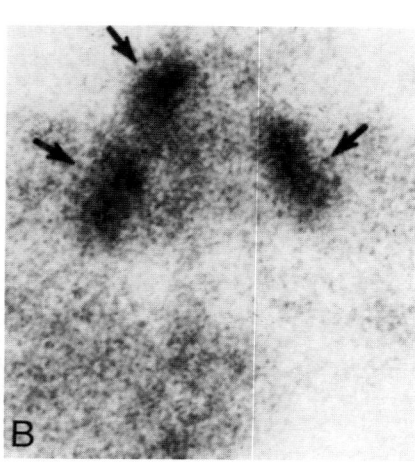

Fig. 91-6. Gallium 67 scan typical of sarcoidosis. **A.** Intense salivary gland uptake ("panda" appearance) coupled with (**B**) hilar and right paratracheal activity (*arrows*) in the shape of the Greek letter lambda. Courtesy of Stephen B. Sulavik, M.D.

sarcoidosis or symptomatic stage II disease and in those with significant extrapulmonary involvement. Baseline function, histology, angiotensin-converting enzyme, and BAL cytology are not accurate predictors of outcome. HRCT may be helpful because response is more likely in patients with signs of active alveolitis (e.g., ground-glass haziness) than in those with radiographic findings of cystic air spaces and advanced fibrosis. The 5-year mortality overall is only 4%, but in most cases death is attributable to pulmonary involvement. As pointed out by Newman and associates (1997), factors associated with a graver prognosis include black race, persistent symptoms for more than 6 months, splenomegaly, involvement of more than three organ systems, absence of erythema nodosum, and radiographic stage III disease. An acute presentation, unlike most other diffuse diseases, has a favorable prognosis with frequent spontaneous resolution and a good response to treatment.

Necrotizing sarcoid granulomatosis is a rare disorder characterized by large granulomas with necrosis, cavitation, and vasculitis. Some consider necrotizing sarcoid granulomatosis a variant of sarcoidosis, whereas others believe it is a hypersensitivity reaction or a type of angiitis.

Bronchiolitis Obliterans Organizing Pneumonia

BOOP is a nonspecific histologic pattern that may occur in many settings, including inhalational lung injury, infection, post-radiation, transplantation, IPF, hypersensitivity, and CVD. The majority of cases, however, are idiopathic. Davison (1983) and Epler (1985) and their associates reported early series of idiopathic BOOP and described the distinctive clinical syndrome.

Most patients have cough, dyspnea, fever, and malaise of 2 to 6 months' duration. Men and women aged 40 to 60 years are affected equally. Most have dry rales, but clubbing is rare. Idiopathic BOOP causes restriction and impaired diffusion. In the series of King and Mortenson (1992), all patients with obstructive findings were current or former smokers. In contrast, bronchiolitis obliterans associated with other diseases is often manifest by airflow obstruction. Although chest radiographic findings are variable, Chandler and associates (1986) stress that, in contrast to IPF, patchy air space disease is common. The CT features of BOOP, reviewed by Muller and associates (1990) and by Nishimura and Itoh (1992), include ground-glass density, small nodules, consolidation, and bronchial wall thickening. Lee and colleagues (1994) found that consolidation is often subpleural or peribronchovascular, or both, in distribution and is less often seen in immunocompromised patients. Unifocal BOOP may simulate bronchial carcinoma.

In general, diagnosis requires a surgical biopsy, but large TBLB specimens are sometimes adequate. The histologic hallmark is occlusion of small airways by connective tissue tufts and inflammatory cells. Steroids effect complete recovery in most cases, but prolonged therapy may be needed.

Some patients improve without treatment. The mortality rate for BOOP is about 12%.

Hypersensitivity Pneumonitis

Also known as *extrinsic allergic alveolitis*, HP is caused by inhalation of organic antigens. Cell-mediated mechanisms with a strong genetic modulation, as discussed by Salvaggio and deShazo (1986), are primary. A long list of antigens has been implicated in specific types of HP, many of which carry unusual occupational or avocational names (see Table 91-1).

The usual presentation is acute, occasionally with cough and wheezing during exposure but more often with dyspnea, myalgias, and fever beginning 4 to 8 hours after contact. Resolution is rapid but symptoms recur, often more intensely, after subsequent exposures. Dry rales may persist after symptoms clear. Decreased lung volumes, impaired diffusion, and hypoxemia are found acutely but resolve between episodes. A mixed obstructive-restrictive pattern is often seen. Continuous exposure causes a chronic illness similar to other fibrogenic diseases. Precipitating antibodies to the offending antigen are found in most cases but are also noted in exposed asymptomatic people. Levels of immunoglobulins other than IgE are elevated. Specific antigens can be used diagnostically for skin testing, in vitro lymphocyte stimulation, or inhalation challenge. Chest radiographic findings vary from normal in mild cases to hyperexpanded honeycomb lung in advanced chronic HP. Severe acute exposure produces transient acinar lesions and consolidation. After repeated exacerbations, a fine nodular or reticulonodular pattern may persist between attacks. The HRCT findings include patchy ground-glass opacity and poorly defined nodules. Adenopathy and pleural disease are not seen in HP.

Coleman and Colby (1988) described an interstitial infiltrate of lymphocytes, plasma cells and macrophages, a similar mononuclear bronchiolitis, and noncaseating granulomas that are less defined and less constant than in sarcoidosis and often are surrounded by a mantle of lymphocytes. Surgical biopsy is rarely necessary. Early diagnosis is of paramount importance to prevent permanent sequelae. Diagnosis is based on recurrent symptoms temporally related to exposure, supportive laboratory data, and improvement after antigen avoidance. Costabel and colleagues (1984) noted that BAL lymphocytosis is higher in HP than in sarcoidosis and that suppressor T cells outnumber helper cells. When used, TBLB is generally insufficient to encompass the triad of lymphocytic pneumonitis, bronchiolitis, and granulomas. Chronic cases without obvious exposure often elude diagnosis until a surgical biopsy suggests HP and the offending antigen is determined retrospectively.

Elimination of contact is the treatment of choice and may entail job relocation, use of air masks or filtering systems, or cessation of a hobby. Steroids are used for patients with severe symptoms or progressive disease.

Pneumoconioses

The pneumoconioses result from inhalation of fibrogenic inorganic particles that reach and are retained in bronchioles and alveoli. The development of fibrosis depends on the duration and intensity of exposure as well as individual sensitivity. Although occupational health measures have decreased the incidence of these diseases, new cases are still seen.

Silicosis

Silicosis is caused by inhalation of silica dust or silicon dioxide in jobs such as sandblasting, mining, foundry casting, glass-making, and ceramic molding. Patients with simple nodular silicosis may have few or no symptoms. The histologic hallmark is a small nodule with a center of whorled fibrous tissue surrounded by macrophages, plasma cells, lymphocytes, and occasionally giant cells. Some cases evolve into "progressive massive fibrosis" or "conglomerate silicosis," resulting from coalescence of nodules to form larger masses. Severe progressive dyspnea is the clinical correlate. In a 9-year, statewide study in Michigan, Roseman and coworkers (1997) give a contemporary view of affected individuals. Most are older men, frequently black, and were exposed from the 1920s through 1960s; 30% have progressive massive fibrosis, 32% have advanced, symptomatic simple nodular disease, and the remainder have normal lung function. Upper lung field rales may be heard; clubbing is uncommon. Radiographs show a nodular pattern, mainly in the upper lobes. Enlarged hilar nodes with peripheral calcium are found in a minority of patients. Although it was once thought to be pathognomonic of silicosis, Parkes (1994) noted that such "eggshell" calcification is occasionally found in sarcoidosis and other granulomatous conditions and after irradiation. Patients with silicosis are at particular risk for infection with both *Mycobacterium tuberculosis* and other mycobacterial organisms, possibly because silica-containing macrophages have impaired phagocytic ability. Secondary mycobacterial infection should be considered when unexpected clinical or radiographic deterioration occurs. On occasion, massive exposure causes acute silicosis, characterized clinically by severe symptoms, radiographically by perihilar air space and ground-glass opacities, and histologically by a reaction with features of DIP and alveolar proteinosis.

Asbestosis

Exposure to asbestos in fields such as welding, pipefitting, boiler making, and insulating is a well-known cause of pulmonary fibrosis. Asbestosis is histologically similar to UIP but with the pathognomonic finding of beaded or dumbbell-shaped asbestos fibers (ferruginous bodies, a translucent fiber core coated by protein and ferritin). The presence of even a few asbestos bodies indicates significant exposure because they are outnumbered by a factor of several thousand by the retained uncoated fibers, which are not seen by light microscopy. Dyspnea and paroxysmal dry cough appear many years after exposure and may progress to respiratory failure. Basilar crackles and clubbing are common. Radiographically, fine reticulation progresses to honeycombing. Staples and colleagues (1989) reported fibrosis demonstrated by HRCT and impaired lung function in exposed workers with normal chest radiographs. Al-Jarad and associates (1992) found HRCT helpful in differentiating IPF and asbestosis. The clinical course of patients with asbestosis may be complicated by benign or malignant pleural disease and by bronchial cancer.

Coal Worker's Pneumoconiosis

Coal worker's pneumoconiosis is uncommon and usually asymptomatic. Cough and expectoration of black sputum in miners is usually due to coal dust bronchitis and does not indicate fibrosis. A minority of patients, however, progress from asymptomatic small nodules (simple pneumoconiosis) to progressive massive fibrosis and respiratory disability.

Beryllium and Other Metals

Inhalation of beryllium can cause an acute illness with DAD histology or a chronic syndrome similar to sarcoidosis, with hilar adenopathy and multiorgan granulomas. Cobalt and tungsten are other heavy metal pulmonary toxins and are associated with a distinctive giant cell reaction.

Diagnosis

Documentation of exposure and typical clinical data generally suffice for the diagnosis of pneumoconiosis for medical and compensation purposes. When surgical biopsy is performed, it is essential to search for retained dusts by light microscopy, electron microscopy, or mineral analysis. There is no primary therapy for the pneumoconioses.

Eosinophilic Lung Disease

A diverse group of disorders are linked by the common finding of DPLD associated with increased tissue or circulating eosinophils, or both. A variety of classification systems have been proposed and were reviewed by Allen and Davis (1994).

Simple Pulmonary Eosinophilia

Patients with simple pulmonary eosinophilia (Löffler's syndrome) have few or no symptoms. Transient migratory infiltrates are noted on serial radiographs, and there is blood and sputum eosinophilia. The syndrome is idiopathic in one-third of cases and drug-induced or caused by parasites (e.g., *Ascaris, Toxocara,* or *Strongyloides*) in the remainder. Rapid resolution is the rule and may be spontaneous or follow treatment of infection or drug avoidance.

Acute Eosinophilic Pneumonia

Patients with acute eosinophilic pneumonia present with rapid progression of fever, myalgia, chest pain, respiratory distress (often severe), and diffuse alveolar infiltrates. Although peripheral eosinophils are usually not increased, significant BAL eosinophilia is universal. Pleural effusions are sometimes seen and also contain large numbers of eosinophils. The cause of acute eosinophilic pneumonia is unknown. Biopsy shows eosinophils in the alveoli and interstitium, without fibrosis or vasculitis. High-dose steroids effect a rapid resolution in most cases.

Chronic Eosinophilic Pneumonia

Chronic eosinophilic pneumonia is also an idiopathic syndrome occurring mainly in women in a ratio of 2:1, up to 50% of whom are past or present asthmatics. Symptoms progress slowly over weeks or months and include fever, cough, dyspnea, wheezing, night sweats, and weight loss. Peripheral eosinophilia may be absent or intermittent. BAL eosinophilia is present during active disease. Serum IgE is usually elevated. Dense peripheral infiltrates (Fig. 91-7), described by Gaensler and Carrington (1977) as the "photographic negative of pulmonary edema," are fairly specific but were present in less than one-half the cases reviewed by Jederlinic and colleagues (1988). Peripheral consolidation, however, was noted on CT scans in all cases reported by Mayo and colleagues (1989). Mediastinal lymphadenopathy is often present. Histologically, interstitial fibrosis is noted in many cases, along with an infiltrate of eosinophils and lymphocytes. Although the response to steroids is excellent, relapses are common, especially early after treatment. Naughton and associates (1993) showed that long-term, and in some cases, lifetime, treatment may be necessary. Progression to diffuse pulmonary fibrosis can occur sporadically or with delayed diagnosis or inadequate treatment.

Idiopathic Hypereosinophilic Syndrome

Idiopathic hypereosinophilic syndrome, once known as eosinophilic leukemia and characterized by extreme BAL and peripheral eosinophilia (30 to 70% of white blood cell count), is a multiorgan disorder associated with DPLD in a minority (40%) of cases. Most patients die from cardiac involvement or thromboembolic complications. Eosinophilic infiltration may also cause symptomatic problems in the gastrointestinal tract, kidneys, skin, and muscles. The hypereosinophilic syndrome occurs more often in men than in women, with a ratio of 7:1.

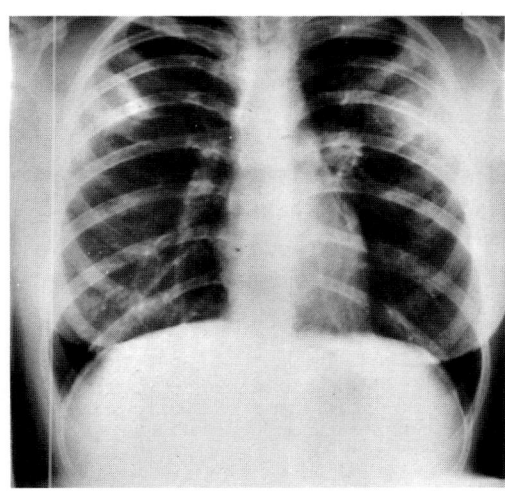

Fig. 91-7. A 21-year-old woman with eosinophilic pneumonia. Chest radiograph shows typical peripheral densities that have been called the photographic negative of pulmonary edema.

Allergic Bronchopulmonary Aspergillosis

Allergic bronchopulmonary aspergillosis is seen in asthmatics and is defined by peripheral and BAL eosinophilia, increased IgE levels and serum, and serum, and BAL precipitins to *Aspergillus.* CT scans show central bronchiectasis, mucus plugging of airways, and consolidation distal to impacted bronchi. The term *toothpaste shadows* has been used for the radiographic appearance of dilated, impacted airways and aptly describes the gross findings of thick mucoid material filling the bronchi. Treatment is with steroids and possibly antifungal agents. Late sequelae of allergic bronchopulmonary aspergillosis include pulmonary fibrosis, irreversible airway obstruction, and aspergilloma.

Churg-Strauss Syndrome

Churg-Strauss syndrome (allergic angiitis and granulomatosis) is another eosinophilic lung disorder that occurs in asthmatics. Men and women are affected equally and usually develop vasculitis months or years after a history of allergic disease. The vasculitis is systemic, with frequent involvement of the nasal passages, sinuses, and skin and the gastrointestinal, central nervous, and musculoskeletal systems. Unlike in Wegener's granulomatosis, significant renal involvement is uncommon. Heart failure from coronary vasculitis, pericarditis, and hypertension are common causes of morbidity and death. Radiographs display patchy infiltrates that may wax and wane, as well as pleural effusions in one-third of cases, and occasionally thoracic lymphadenopathy. Blood and BAL eosinophil counts are markedly elevated, as is serum IgE. The perinuclear form of antineutrophil cytoplasmic antibody (ANCA) may also be elevated. Surgical lung biopsy is generally required for definitive diagnosis and shows a necrotizing giant cell vasculitis involving arteries and veins, along with granulomas and eosinophilic infiltration. Without steroid treatment, approximately 50% of patients die within 3 months of diagnosis.

Bronchocentric Granulomatosis

Bronchocentric granulomatosis is a necrotizing granulomatous inflammation of bronchial epithelium that in some cases (one-third) is similar to allergic bronchopulmonary aspergillosis in that it is seen in asthmatics and is associated with eosinophilic infiltration, blood eosinophilia, and fungal organisms on biopsy or in sputum. The remaining patients have a neutrophilic reaction. Most cases present as a solitary radiographic density rather than as DPLD. Diagnosis usually requires resection.

Diagnosis

The diagnosis of eosinophilic lung disease is most often clinical, based on symptoms, radiographs, serum studies, BAL, assessment for parasitic or fungal infection or drug reaction, and response to therapy. The finding of eosinophilia on BAL may be helpful but is not specific. TBLB sometimes yields a sufficient specimen. Surgical biopsy is indicated before treatment and in patients with atypical features and a nondiagnostic TBLB.

Neoplasms

Lymphangitic Carcinoma

Primary and metastatic malignancies can involve the lung in a diffuse fashion. In lymphangitic carcinoma, tumor cells are found within the peribronchial and perivascular lymphatic channels. The cause is believed to be seeding of lymphatics by hematogenous tumor emboli rather than spread from invaded nodes. Adenocarcinomas of the breast, lung, stomach, and pancreas are the usual sources, but squamous cancer can also cause lymphangitic carcinoma. Pulmonary disease occasionally precedes clinical evidence of the primary tumor. The course may be insidious or rapid. Diffuse microvascular occlusion by tumor emboli can produce early cor pulmonale. Chest radiographs show a nonspecific interstitial pattern. Because of its neoplastic source, associated adenopathy and pleural effusion are common. The CT features of lymphangitic carcinoma are often characteristic (Fig. 91-8). Stein and associates (1987) described nodularity and irregular thickening of bronchovascular sheaths, interlobular septa, and fissures. When tissue confirmation is indicated, TBLB is usually diagnostic because of the peribronchial location of the malignant cells. With few exceptions, the prognosis is dismal.

Bronchoalveolar Carcinoma

Bronchoalveolar carcinoma manifests in a multinodular or diffuse pneumonic form in about 20% of cases. The mode of

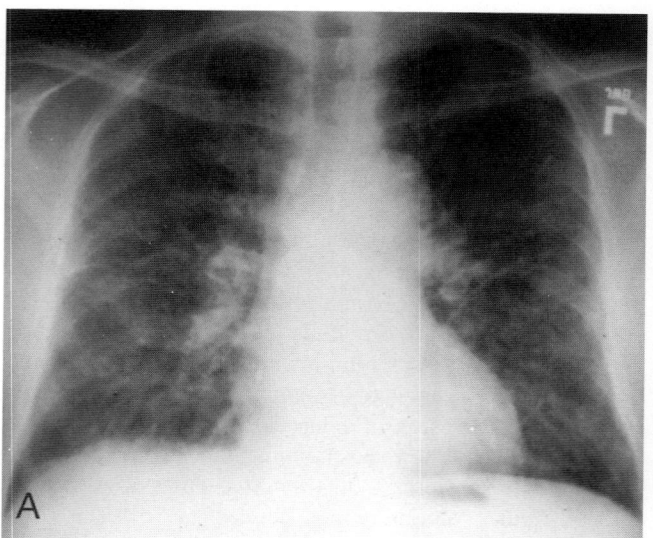

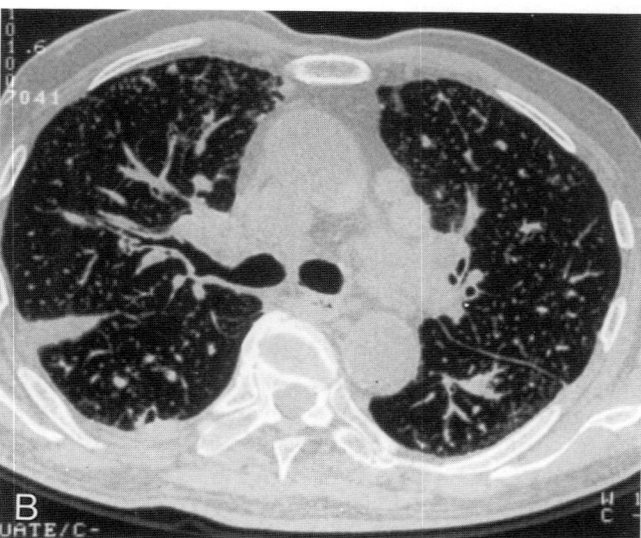

Fig. 91-8. A 70-year-old man with lymphangitic carcinoma. **A.** Chest radiograph demonstrates diffuse irregular and nodular densities with possible hilar and mediastinal adenopathy. **B.** High-resolution computed tomography demonstrates peribronchial and perivascular thickening, scattered nodules, septal thickening, and spiculation of the fissure.

dissemination may be aerogenous. Most patients with diffuse bronchoalveolar carcinoma are dyspneic. Bronchorrhea is rare but may be copious and debilitating. Radiographs demonstrate nodularity or air space opacities, air bronchograms, and consolidation. Im and associates (1990) reported that mucin production by bronchoalveolar carcinoma may result in a lower attenuation on CT scan and helps differentiate this tumor from other consolidative processes. The diagnosis of diffuse bronchoalveolar carcinoma is made on the basis of sputum cytology, bronchoscopy, or transthoracic needle aspiration. On occasion, however, the cellular features are so bland that only a surgical specimen allows recognition of the typical architectural pattern.

Lymphoma and Leukemia

Diffuse lymphomatous infiltration of the lung occurs in patients with known, usually non-Hodgkin's, lymphoma that originated at extrapulmonary sites. Primary pulmonary lymphoma is uncommon and is distinguished by lung involvement in the absence of extrathoracic lymphoma. Small cell lymphoma can present as a diffuse process, but large cell lymphomas more often are focal. Similarly, primary B cell pulmonary lymphoma occurring in AIDS is usually nodular and focal. In leukemia, diffuse neoplastic infiltrates are noted at autopsy in up to 50% of cases but usually do not cause symptoms during life. However, Yoshioka and colleagues (1985) observed that T cell leukemia is often associated with fibrosis, possibly because of fibroblast activation by interaction of malignant T cells and local alveolar macrophages. As in lymphangitic carcinoma, leukemic and lymphomatous infiltrates track along lymphatics, resulting in similar radiographic findings. Despite this location, the yield of TBLB is less than in lymphangitic carcinoma, because, as pointed out by Palosaari and Colby (1986), cytologic atypia may be absent and peribronchial lymphoid infiltrates are found in association with many benign disorders. Newer techniques for establishing monoclonality, however, may improve the yield of BAL, TBLB, fine-needle aspiration biopsy, and pleural fluid, as documented by Keicho and associates (1994), who used gene rearrangement and immunophenotypic analysis to establish both T and B cell monoclonality in BAL fluid. Surgical biopsy, however, remains necessary in most cases.

Kaposi's Sarcoma

The most common AIDS-related neoplasm, Kaposi's sarcoma often affects the lungs diffusely. White and Matthay (1989) reported clinical pulmonary Kaposi's sarcoma in 33% of AIDS patients with systemic Kaposi's sarcoma who had lung lesions and at autopsy in 50% of cases of systemic Kaposi's. Isolated pulmonary Kaposi's sarcoma is rare. Patients have dry cough, dyspnea, and fever. Endobronchial involvement may cause hemoptysis and wheezing. Radiographic findings include bilateral perihilar interstitial and acinar opacities and poorly marginated nodules. Pleural effusion is present in 30% and lymphadenopathy in 8% of patients. Diffuse alveolar hemorrhage can produce rapid changes in the radiographic appearance. Atelectasis may result from endobronchial lesions. Naidich and colleagues (1989) reported that CT scan findings may be similar to those in lymphangitic carcinoma but with a perihilar distribution. Kaposi's sarcoma is not usually gallium-avid, a feature of occasional use in diagnosis.

Histologically, there are nodular foci of plump spindle cells with frequent mitoses and signs of recent or old hemorrhage. In some areas, spindle cells are sparse, and there is a prominent infiltrate of lymphocytes and plasma cells. Endobronchial Kaposi's sarcoma appears grossly as bright red-violet, flat or raised lesions. Because the appearance is characteristic and the yield of biopsy is inconsistent, diagnosis is often made by the gross findings. Surgical biopsy was once considered essential for the diagnosis of parenchymal disease, but Purdy and associates (1986), among others, have shown that TBLB is sufficient in many cases. Fears of excessive bleeding from endobronchial biopsy and TBLB have not been substantiated by experience. A clinical diagnosis may be reasonable in some patients with systemic Kaposi's sarcoma, typical radiographic findings, a negative gallium 67 scan, and no evidence of infection by BAL. Life expectancy in AIDS-associated Kaposi's sarcoma is limited, although some patients survive for several years. Gill and associates (1989) reported prolongation of survival by combination chemotherapy. Local radiation therapy may palliate hemoptysis and airway obstruction.

Lymphomatoid Granulomatosis

Lymphomatoid granulomatosis is an uncommon disorder that has been variously classified as a lymphoid infiltration, a neoplasm, or a vasculitis. Initially described by Liebow and associates (1972), lymphomatoid granulomatosis is marked by a necrotizing angiocentric granulomatous infiltration of small lymphocytes, macrophages, plasma cells, and atypical lymphoreticular cells. Middle-aged men are affected most often and present with cough, chest pain, dyspnea, fever, and malaise. Involvement of other organs occurs in one-third to one-half of cases and may manifest as neurologic symptoms, skin rash, nephropathy, lymphadenopathy, and hepatomegaly. Radiographs show lower lung field nodules of variable size, often with cavitation. Small pleural effusions and hilar lymphadenopathy are seen in some cases. Diffuse infiltrates are uncommon. Initial reports indicated that lymphoma developed in 12% of patients. T cell marker studies and identification of monoclonal atypical cell populations, however, as summarized by Myers (1990), have reclassified most cases as T cell lymphomas. Pisani and DeRemee (1990), on the other hand, consider lymphomatoid granulomatosis a reactive process with a propensity for loss of immunologic control and progression to lymphoma. Despite the etiologic uncertainty, there is clearly a tendency for patients with lymphomatoid granulomatosis to develop diagnosable lymphoma. Although some untreated patients have an indolent course, many die of respiratory failure within 2 years. Fauci and associates (1982) reported long-term remission after treatment with prednisone and cyclophosphamide, but some patients require aggressive chemotherapy. Surgical lung biopsy is usually required for diagnosis, except in patients with accessible cutaneous lesions or peripheral lymphadenopathy.

Lymphocytic Interstitial Pneumonia

Although it is occasionally an isolated DPLD, LIP usually occurs in association with immune disorders, such as

Sjögren's syndrome, SLE, myasthenia, and chronic active hepatitis. It is also found in 50% of human immunodeficiency virus (HIV)-positive children who have pulmonary disease and is considered a criterion for the diagnosis of AIDS in young people. In contrast, only 3% of adults with AIDS and lung disease have LIP. Presentation is similar to other interstitial pneumonias. Clubbing is common in children but infrequent in adults. As reported by Oldham and associates (1989), the radiographic appearance is nonspecific and includes combinations of reticular or reticulonodular opacities and air space consolidation. Pleural effusion and lymphadenopathy are unusual.

The etiology of LIP is unclear. Its associated disorders suggest an autoimmune mechanism. Also, some evidence in AIDS patients suggests that LIP is a response to infection with HIV, Epstein-Barr virus, or both. In AIDS-associated LIP, the infiltrating lymphocytes are T cells, whereas in other forms of LIP, B lymphocytes predominate, suggesting a variable pathogenesis. Similar to the situation with lymphomatoid granulomatosis, the relation between LIP and lymphoma is incompletely understood (see Chapter 112). Differentiation may be difficult in the absence of atypia and invasion. Cellular polyclonality favors LIP, whereas lymphoma is associated with a monoclonal infiltrate. Herbert and associates (1985), however, found that polyclonal populations may exist within malignant lymphomas. These authors, along with Turner and colleagues (1984), believe that many cases are actually well-differentiated lymphomas. Other evidence suggests that LIP is a reactive pneumonitis, including cases of spontaneous regression, an often excellent response to steroids, and documented progression to typical fibrosis. Death occurs in a minority of cases from progressive pulmonary disease. Plasma cell interstitial pneumonia, a rare variant of LIP described by Moran and Totten (1970), does not appear to progress to fibrosis or lymphoma.

Pulmonary Vasculitis

The pulmonary vasculitides are variably classified. Fulmer and Kaltreider (1983) divided these lesions into three categories: the lung as the major affected organ, lung involvement as part of a multiorgan syndrome (e.g., cryoglobulinemia, Henoch-Schönlein purpura, polyarteritis nodosa), and processes in which vasculitis is but one aspect of pulmonary pathology (e.g., CVD, eosinophilic pneumonia). Four processes are often included in the first category: lymphomatoid granulomatosis, necrotizing sarcoid granulomatosis, allergic angiitis and granulomatosis (Churg-Strauss syndrome), and Wegener's granulomatosis. Some recent categorization schemes are based on the size of involved blood vessels (small, medium, and large), but substantial overlap exists within this system and with respect to other features, as emphasized by Jennette and Falk (1997). The variability in classification of these disorders is emphasized by the fact that the first three syndromes are discussed under other headings in this chapter:

lymphomatoid granulomatosis under Neoplasms, necrotizing sarcoid granulomatosis under Sarcoidosis; and Churg-Strauss syndrome under Eosinophilic Lung Disease.

Wegener's granulomatosis, as originally described, is defined by a triad of necrotizing granulomas of the lung and upper respiratory tract, glomerulonephritis, and systemic vasculitis. Carrington and Liebow (1966) later reported a limited form with little or no extrapulmonary involvement. In addition to pulmonary symptoms, sinusitis, epistaxis, rhinitis, fever, and weight loss are frequent complaints. Lung involvement is noted in about 75% of patients at presentation and ultimately in 95%. Proteinuria or hematuria is detected in the majority. Large airway obstruction, "saddle nose" deformity, skin lesions, ocular inflammation, diabetes insipidus, cranial nerve palsy, and coronary vasculitis are seen in some patients. Radiographs typically show multiple, often cavitary nodules of variable size, although Leatherman (1988) reported solitary nodules in many patients. Lesions may resolve and reappear spontaneously. Pleural effusion is noted in 20 to 30% of cases. Atelectasis from large airway Wegener's granulomatosis, air space consolidation from pulmonary hemorrhage, and lymphadenopathy are occasional features. Cordier and associates (1990) found CT scan useful for detecting unsuspected cavitation. Radiographs of the sinuses often show Wegener's granulomatosis lesions or the residua of infection. Rosenberg and colleagues (1980) found that pulmonary function tests demonstrate obstructive more often than restrictive disease. Serum ANCAs are a valuable marker. Approximately 10% of patients, however, are ANCA-negative. Harrison and associates (1989) reported that a positive ANCA is specific for Wegener's granulomatosis in 86% of cases. Histology shows transmural necrotizing granulomatous inflammation of the walls of small and medium arteries and veins. Capillaritis may be found in cases with alveolar hemorrhage and constitutes the most life-threatening manifestation of Wegener's. Because of the sensitivity and specificity of ANCA testing, biopsy is often not required, especially when the history and radiographs are typical. When the clinical synthesis is ambiguous, TBLB is usually inadequate due to the frequent finding of nonspecific necrosis as well as features common to other granulomatous processes, and surgical biopsy may be required for diagnosis. Prolonged therapy with high-dose prednisone and cyclophosphamide achieves 5-year survival rates as high as 90%.

Drug-Induced Lung Disease

The list of drugs that are known to cause DPLD continues to grow. Damage results from direct toxic effects or from induction of the cellular events common to all lung injury. Some agents produce damage in a dose-dependent fashion, whereas the occurrence of DPLD is idiosyncratic with other drugs. The histology is variable and mostly nonspecific. Pietra (1991) provides a comprehensive overview of pathologic patterns and pathogenesis. Histologic variations include DAD, hemorrhage, UIP/DIP, eosinophilic pneumonia, lipid pneumonia, BOOP, and lymphoplasmacytic interstitial pneumonia. The importance of a detailed medical history is obvious. Diagnosis may be complicated by factors such as antecedent or coexisting pulmonary disease, administration of multiple potential toxins, and the possibility of associated diffuse lung infection. Diagnosis is usually clinical. Improvement or resolution after drug withdrawal, of course, supports the diagnosis of drug-induced DPLD. In some cases, bronchoscopic specimens are sufficient for a presumptive diagnosis, but surgical biopsy is sometimes needed. In most cases, drug avoidance is all that is required, but steroids are needed in some instances. Cooper and associates (1986a, 1986b) reviewed the subject, and Rosenow and colleagues (1992) presented an update. A few examples are summarized.

Nitrofurantoin

In addition to an acute eosinophilic pneumonia, nitrofurantoin can cause a syndrome similar to IPF. The acute and chronic reactions are distinct entities and do not overlap. Most patients improve with cessation of the drug, but in a few, the condition progresses, requiring treatment with steroids.

Gold

Gold therapy, used mainly for RA and sometimes for ankylosing spondylitis, psoriatic arthritis, pemphigus, and asthma, can cause DPLD. Distinction of drug toxicity from RA-associated UIP may be difficult. Tomioka and King (1997) suggested clinical features supportive of a diagnosis of gold-induced DPLD, including predominance in women, acute dyspnea, recent dry cough, fever, skin rash, absence of subcutaneous nodules and digital clubbing, crackles on chest examination, and alveolar opacities along bronchovascular bundles on CT scan. Most patients have peripheral eosinophilia and BAL lymphocytosis. ANCA positivity occurs in about 70% of cases, usually in a perinuclear staining pattern, in contrast to the cytoplasmic ANCA associated with Wegener's. Biopsy is usually nonspecific, including the presence of gold within macrophages, because many treated patients have this finding in the absence of DPLD. The key test is drug withdrawal, which usually results in resolution within a few weeks.

Amiodarone

Among cardiovascular drugs, amiodarone is the most common cause of pulmonary toxicity, which occurs in 5 to 10% of patients taking a daily dose of 400 mg or more for two or more months, as reported by Martin and Rosenow (1988). In addition to dyspnea and cough, patients may have fever and pleuritic chest pain without effusion. CT may be helpful because areas of amiodarone accumulation are denser than other soft tissues. The histology is variable and includes UIP, DAD, and BOOP. Foamy macrophages are a nonspecific but characteristic finding and can be retrieved by BAL. In most cases, the diagnosis is based on clinical data and BAL. Resolution usually follows drug withdrawal. A syndrome of fulminant ARDS has been seen in patients currently or previously taking amiodarone who undergo cardiopulmonary bypass or pulmonary angiography. In the former setting, prolonged pump times and exposure to a high inspired oxygen concentration appear to increase the risk.

Chemotherapeutic Agents

Chemotherapeutic agents are a frequent cause of diagnostic difficulty. Although some can produce an acute hypersensitivity reaction or noncardiogenic pulmonary edema, symptoms develop gradually in most cases. Radiographs may be normal, but more often they show nonspecific mixed patterns. The histology usually reflects a subacute process with features of DAD, mononuclear cell infiltrates, and mild fibrosis. Atypia of type II epithelial cells is a distinctive feature and may simulate malignancy. Toxicity from *bleomycin* and *mitomycin* is dose dependent but is enhanced by prior or concurrent thoracic irradiation and by high levels of inspired oxygen. The danger is particularly acute in patients undergoing operation after induction therapy for thoracic tumors. Our current practice is to administer steroids in the perioperative period and to maintain the lowest possible inspired oxygen level because even brief periods of hyperoxia may be detrimental. Although the mortality rate for advanced toxicity is high, high-dose steroids, as reported by Maher and Daly (1993), may effect reversal. *Methotrexate* causes an idiosyncratic reaction in about 5% of patients. Methotrexate pneumonitis has several characteristic features, including peripheral eosinophilia, hilar adenopathy, small pleural effusions, and a characteristic histology (i.e., an intense mononuclear infiltrate of lymphocytes, plasma cells, and eosinophils, along with giant cells and granulomas). The mortality rate is low. Most patients improve after drug withdrawal, but steroids may hasten resolution. Gemcitabine appears to be active against solid tumors, such as lung, breast, pancreas, and ovary. Pavlakis and colleagues (1997) and Vander Els and Miller (1998) reported three cases and one patient, respectively, in whom this drug was associated with DPLD. Two patients in the first report died of respiratory failure and had DAD histology on postmortem examination, whereas the third was treated by drug withdrawal and steroids and survived. The patient in the second report recovered rapidly after institution of prednisone. The increasing use of gemcitabine, especially in lung cancer, warrants recognition of this possible toxicity. Among the many other chemotherapeutic agents that may cause lung damage, busulfan is noteworthy for the often extremely long interval between exposure and the development of symptoms.

Other Drugs

Illicit drugs are usually associated with noncardiogenic pulmonary edema, but cocaine can also cause diffuse alveolar hemorrhage, DAD, eosinophilic infiltrates, and BOOP. Resolution occurs with supportive care and abstention. In contrast, talc (magnesium silicate) particles from intravenous injection of dissolved pills can lead to progressive granulomatous inflammation and fibrosis, resulting in cor pulmonale and death. Radiographic features vary from normal to miliary nodularity to advanced fibrosis. Talc can sometimes be identified by BAL, but TBLB or surgical biopsy may be required.

The herbicide paraquat has received much attention because of frequent fatalities from an acute multisystem syndrome, but DPLD and fibrosis may occur on a more chronic basis.

Radiation Toxicity

Movsas and associates (1997) provided a useful review of radiation toxicity. Radiation lung damage is divided into early (pneumonitis) and late (fibrosis) and depends on the total dose, fractionation, volume-treated, and individual susceptibility (see Chapter 102). The pathogenesis begins with cellular damage and the generation of oxygen radicals. Although only about 10% of patients develop clinical disease, radiographic changes are noted in 40% by plain film and virtually all cases by CT. Pneumonitis usually occurs 2 to 6 months after treatment but can begin within 2 weeks. Ikezoe and associates (1988) found CT scan changes in most patients within 4 weeks. Symptoms vary from mild cough, fever, and dyspnea to ARDS. Radiographs demonstrate ground-glass and acinar opacities that may progress to consolidation and may extend beyond the radiation port. DAD is the major pathologic pattern, along with pneumocyte atypia, scattered small vessel thromboses, and intimal myoepithelial foam cells. High-dose steroids may reverse the process. Late fibrosis usually follows within 6 to 24 months of acute pneumonitis but can develop insidiously without evidence of early reaction. Symptoms vary from slight to severe. Linear opacities conform to the radiation field and may produce a vertical "straight-edge" sign after mediastinal radiation. Upper-zone volume loss and upward hilar retraction are common. When tangential beams are used, the distribution varies. Histologically, vascular changes are prominent and include microvascular obliteration, medial hyperplasia, fibrosis, and foam cell accumulation in larger arterioles. No treatment is effective at this stage. The risk of damage is increased in patients with pre-existing lung disease (e.g., emphysema, asbestosis, pneumoconiosis) and in those treated with agents such as bleomycin, dactinomycin, doxorubicin, cyclophosphamide, and vincristine, especially when administered concomitantly with radiation. The diagnosis is made on the basis of history, review of the radiation details, and absence of evidence of infection or recurrent malignancy.

Radiation-induced lung disease and lymphangitic carcinoma may be difficult to distinguish.

Miscellaneous Diffuse Disorders

Histiocytosis X (Eosinophilic Granuloma)

Pulmonary histiocytosis X is an uncommon idiopathic disorder marked by interstitial infiltration of atypical histiocytes containing intracytoplasmic tennis racket–shaped "X bodies." *Histiocytosis X* is preferable to the term *eosinophilic granuloma* because the process is neither primarily eosinophilic nor granulomatous. Most affected people are young adults, with men predominating. More than 90% are smokers. About 20% are asymptomatic despite an abnormal radiograph. A similar proportion of patients present with or later develop pneumothorax. Constitutional symptoms can accompany cough and dyspnea. Cystic lesions in ribs, skull, and pelvis are found in 20% and may be painful. Diabetes insipidus is noted in 10%. A reticulonodular pattern with cystic honeycombing that spares the bases is the usual radiographic finding. Lung volumes are normal or increased. The additional finding of a solitary lytic rib lesion is highly suggestive of pulmonary histiocytosis X. Brauner and associates (1989) described the HRCT features, which include thin-walled cysts and small, sometimes cavitated nodules (Fig. 91-9). Pulmonary function tests often indicate a mixed obstructive and restrictive process. Histologically, the X cells take up stain with S100 protein and are joined by lymphocytes, fibroblasts, macrophages, and eosinophils to form stellate nodules. Despite advanced fibrosis in later stages, X cells and a stellate pattern may still be found. X cells have been noted in BAL, but they are nonspecific because they can occur in association with other diseases. TBLB may be diagnostic, but surgical biopsy is often required. The disease may resolve, stabilize, or progress to end-stage fibrosis. Steroids may be helpful early in the course of the disease.

Lymphangioleiomyomatosis

LAM is a rare disease resulting from hamartomatous proliferation of smooth muscle cells in airways, lymphatics, and blood vessels (see Chapter 111). Sullivan (1998) has provided a valuable review of the current knowledge about this lesion. LAM occurs only in women, mainly during the childbearing years, and is thought to be hormone related. LAM has been reported, however, in an 11-year-old girl and in postmenopausal women up to age 75 years, most, but not all, of whom were taking estrogens. In addition, onset or exacerbation of LAM has been reported during pregnancy. An interesting and unexplained comorbidity is the occurrence in 44% of LAM patients of an uncommon renal tumor: angiomyolipoma. When present, these tumors are bilateral in 50%.

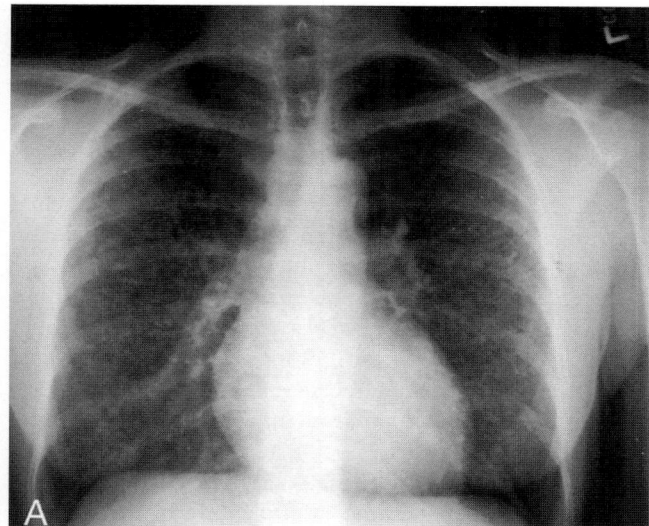

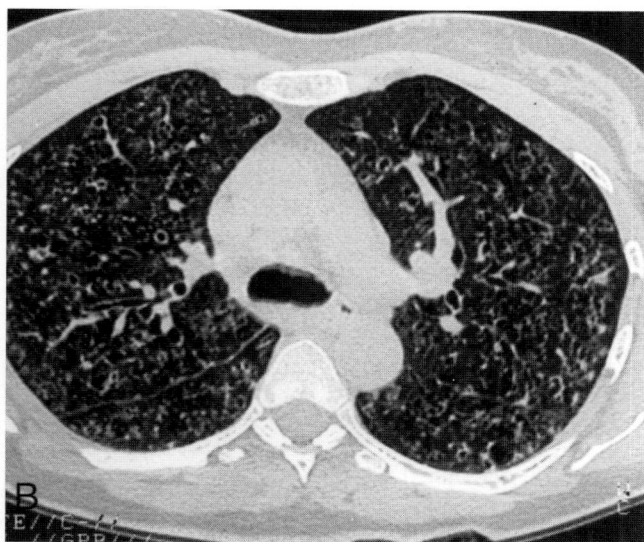

Fig. 91-9. A 45-year-old woman with cough and mild exertional dyspnea. Chest radiograph **(A)** and high-resolution computed tomography **(B)** show multiple nodules, cavities, and thin-walled cysts. Biopsy confirmed histiocytosis X. Courtesy of Jack L. Westcott, M.D.

Patients with LAM present with dyspnea, which may be acute or subacute and result from pneumothorax or chylothorax or slowly progressive from parenchymal infiltration (Fig. 91-10). Alveolar hemorrhage and hemoptysis can occur, as well as cough, chyloptysis, chyluria, chylous ascites, chylous pericardial effusion, and lower extremity lymphedema. In the early stages, radiographs may be normal, but they usually show nonspecific reticulonodular infiltrates. Lung volumes are normal or increased. Alveolar hemorrhage may produce a changing picture. Effusion or pneumothorax may be found on the initial chest film. Disease progression leads to fine interstitial changes followed by honeycombing. HRCT is abnormal in most cases and shows myriad thin-

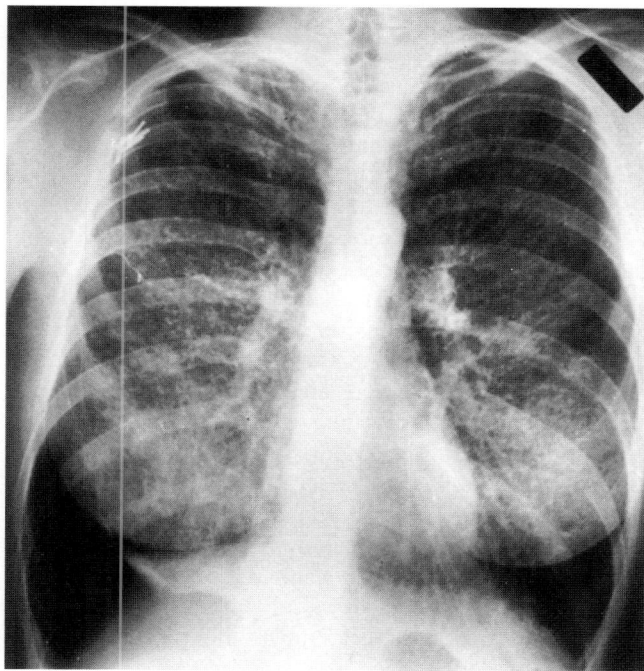

Fig. 91-10. A 35-year-old woman with lymphangioleiomyomatosis, who developed severe dyspnea and chest pain. Radiograph shows right basal pneumothorax under tension (depressed hemidiaphragm). Tube thoracostomy produced immediate relief.

walled cysts similar to pulmonary histiocytosis X but without basilar sparing and without nodules. Abdominal and pelvic lymph nodes may be enlarged. Pulmonary function parameters are variable, showing restrictive, obstructive, or mixed patterns. Although progesterone and tamoxifen may be beneficial, Urban and colleagues (1992) showed eventual deterioration in many cases. Oophorectomy has also been used. The efficacy of treatment is difficult to evaluate because of the rarity of the condition and because the natural history of LAM is not uniform, as emphasized by Sullivan (1998), with 8-year survival varying between 38% and 78%. With respect to diagnosis, surgical biopsy is generally needed, although TBLB may be sufficient in some instances.

Lung disease that is histologically and symptomatically identical to LAM occurs in 1 to 2% of cases of tuberous sclerosis, an inherited disorder with mental retardation, seizures, and tumors of multiple organs. It is noteworthy that, despite the equal sex incidence of tuberous sclerosis, DPLD is found only in women. Lack and associates (1986), among others, reported overlap cases of LAM associated with tumors in other organs but without the other classic features of tuberous sclerosis.

Pulmonary Alveolar Proteinosis

In PAP, the alveoli are filled with a granular, proteinaceous, surfactant-like material. Goldstein and coworkers

(1998) note that only 332 cases have been reported. In contrast to most DPLDs, macrophage number and function are decreased, leading to the hypothesis that PAP results from impaired phagocytic clearance of alveolar debris. Interstitial inflammation and fibrosis are not prominent in early PAP, but late fibrosis may rarely occur. PAP is usually idiopathic, but it can be associated with silicosis, aluminum exposure, fungal or parasitic infection, hematologic malignancies, drug reactions, and immune suppression. Men are affected twice as often as women and present between ages 20 and 50 years. Prakash and colleagues (1987) found that dyspnea, cough, fever, chest pain, and hemoptysis were common symptoms and that 29% of patients had clubbing. Despite the alveolar findings, the cough is usually nonproductive. Bilateral perihilar "bat wing" air space opacities without air bronchograms resemble pulmonary edema but lack Kerley's B lines. According to Godwin and associates (1988), CT demonstrates a sharply demarcated geographic pattern, reflecting juxtaposition of diseased and normal areas. Restrictive pulmonary function is typical. The natural history varies. Opportunistic infection, especially with *Nocardia*, is a common problem and is attributed to impaired macrophage function and the ability of the intra-alveolar lipoprotein to serve as a culture medium. The diagnosis of PAP has been made on the basis of TBLB, BAL, and occasionally sputum examination, but surgical biopsy is often required. Stains and cultures for opportunistic organisms are essential. Progressive symptoms are treated by flushing the alveoli by whole lung lavage, using general anesthesia, selective lung ventilation, and occasionally cardiopulmonary bypass. The procedure is repeated as needed. Steroids are of no benefit in PAP.

Diffuse Pulmonary Hemorrhage

Diffuse pulmonary hemorrhage can complicate many types of DPLD, including CVD, vasculitis, LAM, Kaposi's sarcoma, and drug reactions. Diffuse pulmonary hemorrhage is characterized by hemoptysis, anemia, and changing acinar infiltrates. Goodpasture's syndrome, the most common cause of diffuse pulmonary hemorrhage, includes glomerulonephritis and is marked by immunoglobulin deposition along alveolar and glomerular basement membranes. Most patients are men. Hemoptysis is the usual presentation, but renal insufficiency may be the first manifestation. The diagnosis is usually established by a typical history, elevated antibodies, and renal indices or by renal biopsy. When necessary, TBLB samples are sufficient for demonstrating immunoglobulins. Treatment includes steroids, plasmapheresis, and immunosuppression. Idiopathic pulmonary hemorrhage, sometimes termed *idiopathic pulmonary hemosiderosis*, occurs mainly in children, but young adults are occasionally affected, again with males predominating. The clinical and radiographic picture is similar to Goodpasture's syndrome but without antibodies or renal involvement. BAL may yield hemosiderin-filled macrophages. As a diagnosis of exclusion, idiopathic pulmonary hemorrhage may require surgical biopsy.

Amyloidosis

Amyloidosis may involve the airways (tracheobronchial amyloidosis) or the lung parenchyma. In the latter case, discrete single or multiple nodules (nodular amyloidosis) are seen more often than are diffuse infiltrates (diffuse alveolar amyloidosis). DPLD is part of a systemic syndrome and results from infiltration of alveolar septa and vessel walls with acellular eosinophilic material (amyloid) generated by immunoglobulin light chains κ and λ. Symptoms include dyspnea and cough, and sometimes wheezing and hemoptysis. Signs of pulmonary hypertension may be detected. HRCT may show calcification in micronodules not seen by plain film, as described by Graham and colleagues (1992). The diagnosis is most often made by rectal mucosal or subcutaneous biopsy. TBLB has a high diagnostic yield but may be complicated by bleeding due to pulmonary hypertension. Although colchicine, cytotoxic agents, and dimethyl sulfoxide have been used in treatment, the usual course is one of progressive respiratory failure and death.

DIFFUSE LUNG DISEASE IN THE IMMUNOCOMPROMISED HOST

DPLD is a common problem in immunocompromised people and may result from a broad spectrum of infectious, neoplastic, and inflammatory processes (Table 91-6). Although certain infections in the normal host can present as generalized pneumonias, such as atypical pneumonias and miliary tuberculosis, the immunocompromised person often harbors organisms that are usually not pathogenic (i.e., opportunistic infection). Disseminated presentations of normally localized processes as well as multiorgan and multiorganism infection are more common. Pulmonary infections are discussed in detail in Chapters 84 to 89.

Noninfectious Disorders

Most noninfectious processes occurring in the immunocompromised host are mentioned in previous sections, including drug-induced and radiation pneumonitis; BOOP in bone marrow and lung transplant recipients; lymphoma, LIP, and Kaposi's sarcoma in AIDS patients; lymphangitic cancer; PAP; pulmonary hemorrhage; and recurrence or exacerbation of the primary disorder. In addition, rejection of lung allografts and graft-versus-host reactions in bone marrow recipients may also cause diffuse infiltrates. Tryka and coworkers (1982) reported acute infiltrates in patients treated for leukemia in whom biopsies showed

**Table 91-6. Diffuse Lung Disease
in the Immunocompromised Host**

Noninfectious
  Nonspecific interstitial pneumonitis
  Bronchiolitis obliterans
  Lymphocytic interstitial pneumonia
  Drug-induced
  Radiation-induced
  Kaposi's sarcoma
  Lymphangitic carcinoma
  Pulmonary lymphoma
  Leukemic cell lysis
  Pulmonary alveolar proteinosis
  Diffuse hemorrhage
  Hypersensitivity pneumonitis
  Adult respiratory distress syndrome
  Vasculitis
  Graft-versus-host reaction
  Recurrence of the primary disease, usually neoplasm
Protozoa
  Pneumocystis
  Toxoplasma
Fungi
  Candida
  Aspergillus
  Cryptococcus
  Histoplasma
  Coccidioides
  Blastomyces
  Mucor
Mycobacteria
  Mycobacterium tuberculosis
  Mycobacterium avium-intracellulare and other atypical bacteria
Viruses
  Cytomegalovirus
  Herpes
  Varicella
Bacteria
  Community-acquired (often *Streptococcus pneumoniae, Haemophilus influenzae*)
  Nosocomial (e.g., *Pseudomonas, Escherichia coli, Klebsiella, Serratia*)

DAD and degenerating blast cells. The authors termed the process *leukemic cell lysis pneumonopathy* and postulated that enzyme release from leukemic cell lysis was the initiating injury.

Nonspecific interstitial pneumonia is encountered frequently and was found by Cheson and associates (1985) in 26% of a series of non-AIDS, mixed malignant and nonmalignant immunocompromised hosts, by Crawford and colleagues (1988) in 27% of bone marrow recipients, and by Simmons and coworkers (1987) in 34% of AIDS patients. These proportions likely represent an overestimate because the common denominator consists of patients undergoing biopsy after failure of empiric treatment or less invasive diagnostic approaches. In the series of Potter and associates (1985), however, nonspecific interstitial pneumonia was identified in five of 12 non-neutropenic cancer patients randomized to open biopsy without prior therapy.

Protozoal Infection

Pneumocystis Carinii Pneumonia

Pneumocystis carinii pneumonia (PCP) is the modern epitome of opportunistic infection. Long recognized in malnourished infants and renal transplant recipients, PCP was not a common problem before the AIDS epidemic. PCP afflicts 60 to 80% of people with AIDS, although the incidence is declining due to improved prophylactic regimens. Extrapulmonary disease is rare. The clinical presentation may be acute but more often consists of slowly progressive pulmonary and constitutional symptoms. Pulmonary auscultation may be normal. Pneumothorax with prolonged air leak and failure of lung reexpansion often complicate PCP. Although 10 to 20% of patients have normal chest radiographs, the typical appearance is a diffuse fine reticular, reticulonodular, or ground-glass pattern, sometimes with perihilar accentuation. Sandhu and Goodman (1989) detected pneumatoceles on chest radiographs in 10% of cases. Atypical features include focal consolidation, single or multiple nodules, and upper lobe infiltrates simulating reactivation tuberculosis. Chaffey and associates (1990) found a higher incidence of the last finding in patients treated with aerosolized pentamidine, which may reflect poor drug distribution to the lung apices. Adenopathy and pleural effusion are rare. Bergin and associates (1990) found that ground-glass opacification was the most frequent HRCT feature. Cystic areas are also identified more often by CT than by plain film radiography. Tuazon (1985) and Woolfenden (1987) and their colleagues documented 95 and 100% positivity of gallium scans, respectively. Although gallium uptake is nonspecific, a negative study makes PCP extremely unlikely. Persistent activity after treatment suggests ongoing or new infection. A normal scan despite a diffusely abnormal radiograph raises the possibility of Kaposi's sarcoma. NSIP and PCP have many clinical and radiographic features in common.

The classic finding of a foamy intra-alveolar exudate containing *Pneumocystis* organisms is less common than nonspecific histology, including normal structures, DAD, mild or intense inflammation, fibrosis, and sometimes granulomas. Uncommon histologic findings include LIP-like infiltrates or PAP. Although definitive diagnosis requires microscopic demonstration of the organism in sputum, BAL, or biopsy samples, empiric therapy based on clinical criteria has become increasingly accepted, as noted by Tu and colleagues (1993). Treatment consists of trimethoprim-sulfamethoxazole, pentamidine, or both, and steroids. Because the recurrence rate is high, chronic prophylaxis is indicated. The potential for concurrent infectious or noninfectious lung disease in patients with PCP must always be kept in mind.

Toxoplasmosis

Encephalitis is the predominant feature of toxoplasmosis in the immunocompromised host, but pulmonary infection may coexist. According to Catterall and associates (1986), diffuse infiltrates are seen more frequently than are focal lesions. Brain biopsy is often necessary for diagnosis, but identification of trophozoites by BAL, TBLB, or surgical biopsy may be preferable in patients with pulmonary involvement.

Mycobacterial Infection

M. tuberculosis infection may manifest before the diagnosis of AIDS is made or early in the course, with features similar to standard reactivation cases (upper lobe infiltrates and cavities, positive skin tests). In contrast, later presentations, when immune dysfunction has progressed, are often atypical. Constitutional, neurologic, and gastrointestinal symptoms from disseminated disease may overshadow pulmonary complaints. The purified protein derivative test is rarely positive at this stage. Radiographic patterns are often diffuse and may be accompanied by adenopathy, but cavitation is uncommon. The organisms may not respond to staining, and classic caseating granulomas are usually absent. Triple-drug therapy is generally efficacious. Small and colleagues (1991) found that radiographic deterioration is usually attributed to a different opportunistic infection.

Infection occurs in other immunocompromised hosts as well. The association of *M. tuberculosis* and silicosis noted earlier may be due to locally impaired defenses. Bone marrow transplant recipients are another high-risk group, with a variable reported incidence of *M. tuberculosis* as high as 5%, as noted by Ip and associates (1998).

According to Horsburgh and Selik (1989), only 78 cases of disseminated atypical mycobacterial infection, of which 37 were *Mycobacterium avium-intracellulare*, were reported in the pre-AIDS era. Currently, *M. avium-intracellulare* infection is common and was found in the lung in 34% of AIDS cases in an autopsy series by Wallace and Hannah (1988). *M. avium-intracellulare* infection typically manifests late in the course of AIDS, often in association with other opportunistic infections. Dissemination is the rule. Lung symptoms may be mild or absent. Radiographs show a diffuse reticulonodular pattern but are normal in 20% of patients or occasionally demonstrate focal lesions. The incidence of adenopathy, rarity of cavitation, and absence of classic granulomas are similar in AIDS-associated *M. avium-intracellulare* and *M. tuberculosis* cases. *M. avium-intracellulare* organisms, however, usually can be stained. Treatment response is poor.

Fungal Infection

Fungal pneumonia in the immunocompromised host is often manifest by diffuse air space or micronodular opacities, believed to result from aerogenous and hematogenous dissemination, respectively. Infection is usually disseminated and occurs most often in patients with profound T lymphocyte defects who are often also taking steroids. The ubiquitous *Candida* and *Aspergillus* are the most common pathogens overall, but cryptococcosis is the most frequent AIDS-associated fungal infection, occurring in about 10% of cases. Although meningitis is the predominant feature, concurrent, often asymptomatic, lung disease is noted in many patients. Histoplasmosis occurs in endemic and nonendemic geographic regions. Stansell (1991) reported pulmonary symptoms at presentation in 16 to 53% of AIDS patients with histoplasmosis. Coccidioidomycosis is noted less often, but it predominates in endemic areas. Fish and colleagues (1990) reported pulmonary symptoms in three-fourths of AIDS-associated cases, but plain radiographic abnormalities in only one-third. Reported but less common fungal pneumonias include blastomycosis and mucormycosis. Bigby and associates (1986) noted that pulmonary mucormycosis typically develops in patients with chemotherapy-induced neutropenia who are receiving broad-spectrum antibiotics.

Fungal infection is diagnosed by microscopic or culture evidence of organisms in body fluids or tissues. The source may be skin, lymph nodes, cerebrospinal fluid, sputum, BAL, TBLB, or surgical lung specimens. Serology is rarely useful but may prove helpful in coccidioidomycosis. In addition, serum antigenemia is sensitive and specific in disseminated cryptococcal infection but may not be sensitive in isolated pulmonary involvement. Encouraging results from antigen determination are emerging in aspergillosis and histoplasmosis.

Viral Infection

Cytomegalovirus (CMV) is frequently isolated from respiratory samples in the immunocompromised host, but its pathogenicity is debated. CMV is detected in about 50% of patients with PCP. Wallace and Hannah (1987) found CMV in the lungs of 80% of autopsied AIDS cases, but CMV was an isolated process in only two instances. Waxman and colleagues (1997), in contrast, reported nine AIDS patients with symptomatic DPLD in whom CMV pneumonia was the only active pulmonary process. Three of four untreated patients died within 2 weeks, whereas all five patients who were treated with antiviral therapy (ganciclovir) improved and were free of lung disease 3 months later. When tested, CMV antigen was elevated in all instances. In contrast to AIDS cases, the combination of antigenemia and BAL isolates is diagnostic of CMV pneumonitis in bone marrow recipients. In AIDS, cytopathologic confirmation and strict exclusion of other pathogens are required for diagnosis. TBLB or surgical biopsy accomplishes the cytopathologic confirmation. CMV also causes retinitis, colitis, esophagitis, and encephalitis. Less often noted are herpes simplex and varicella-zoster pneumonia, the latter usually associated with a skin rash. Other viral pneumonias have been described but are uncommon.

Radiographs in viral pneumonitis initially show a diffuse micronodular or reticulonodular pattern that often progresses to diffuse air space opacities and consolidation. Histologic features variably include some degree of DAD, viral inclusion bodies, giant cells, and hemorrhage. Diagnosis depends on typical histology, culture of the virus, and DNA probes or staining with specific antibodies.

Bacterial Infection

Although overshadowed by opportunistic infection, bacterial pneumonia accounts for about 4% of DPLD in people with depressed immunity. According to Murray and Mills (1990), many community-acquired bacterial pneumonias are caused by *Streptococcus pneumoniae* and *Haemophilus influenzae,* but the spectrum of potential pathogens is large. Nosocomial cases are frequently attributable to gram-negative bacteria or *Staphylococcus.* The incidence of associated bacteremia, cavitation, and disseminated tissue infection in all types of bacterial pneumonia is higher in the immunocompromised than in the normal host. Kramer and Uttamchandani (1990) reported that *Nocardia* infection in transplant recipients tends to be focal, but diffuse disease is seen in other immunocompromised hosts. *Legionella* infection may progress from focal to diffuse lung involvement. It afflicts renal transplant patients as both a community-acquired and nosocomial process, but it is uncommon in AIDS. Chastre and colleagues (1987) showed that pulmonary fibrosis can progress even after treatment. Despite its prevalence in the general population, *Mycoplasma* is not a prominent cause of pneumonitis in the setting of impaired immunity.

Diagnostic Approach

Figure 91-11 presents a general approach to the evaluation of DPLD in the immunocompromised patient. It must be stressed that no algorithm is universally applicable. The patient's condition and prognosis, the local experience with diagnostic techniques and epidemiology, and the tempo of the illness are important factors in decision making. The specific immune deficiency and the clinical data often narrow the differential diagnosis. For example, an HIV-positive outpatient with compatible symptoms and radiographic findings and a CD4 count less than 200 cells per μL is very likely to have PCP. Smith and associates (1992) found that an initial episode of PCP could be diagnosed confidently (95% predictive value) on the basis of history, films, absence of prophylaxis, and desaturation with exercise. Leukocytosis, purulent sputum, and a CD4 count greater than 250 cells per μL favor a bacterial process. DPLD developing before chemotherapy in leukemic patients is most often related to bacterial infection or neoplastic infiltration, whereas opportunistic infection is commonly associated with chemotherapy-induced neutropenia in this population. In bone marrow

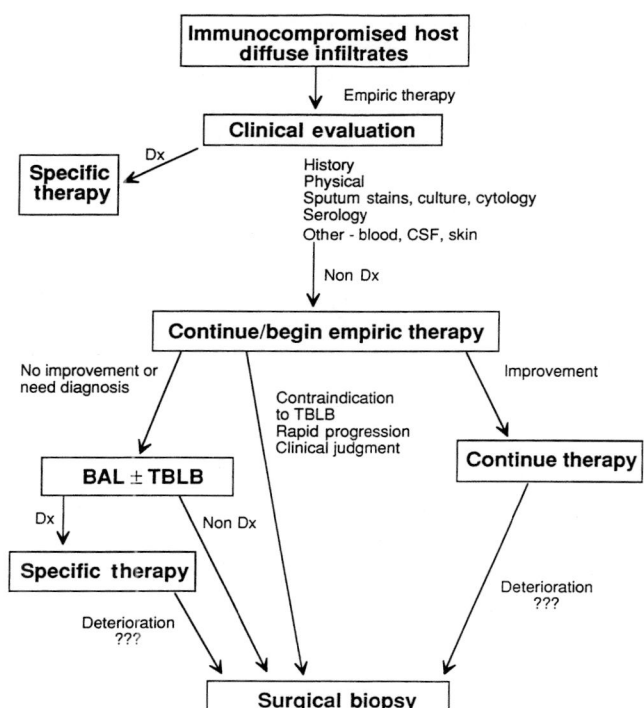

Fig. 91-11. Algorithm for dealing with diffuse lung infiltrates in the immunocompromised host. BAL, bronchoalveolar lavage; CSF, cerebrospinal fluid; Dx, diagnostic; Non Dx, nondiagnostic; TBLB, transbronchial lung biopsy.

recipients, noninfectious causes of diffuse lung disease predominate during the first month.

In most cases, empiric therapy based on the individual context is initiated after appropriate microbiologic and cytologic investigations. Discontinuation of toxic drugs is essential, as is correction of coagulopathy, especially if pulmonary hemorrhage is a consideration. When noninvasive studies are diagnostic or the response to treatment is good, therapy is continued or appropriately modified. Invasive diagnostic methods are indicated when the patient does not improve while receiving empiric or specific therapy. In some instances, confirmation of a suspected diagnosis is needed despite improvement, as in the HIV-positive patient without prior documentation of an index disease. Bronchoscopy with BAL and preferably also TBLB is usually the initial procedure. BAL alone is most successful in the AIDS population, given the high incidence of PCP. In addition, BAL identification of *M. tuberculosis, Histoplasma, Coccidioides, Blastomyces,* or *Legionella* indicates pathogenicity, although concurrent infections may exist. BAL isolation of viruses, atypical mycobacteria, *Cryptococcus, Aspergillus, Candida,* and bacteria, in contrast, usually requires correlative tissue data for a secure diagnosis. Yu and associates (1986), however, believe that in persistently febrile patients with leukemia or neutropenia, the presence of *Aspergillus fumigatus* or *A. flavus* in respiratory secretions often denotes invasive infection. In a study of a large mixed immunocompromised population evaluated by BAL, Pisani and Wright (1992) documented a diagnostic yield of 39%, with a sensitivity of 82% and specificity of 53%. The addition of TBLB to BAL may improve the yield by demonstrating organisms within lung tissue or by providing specimens that document a noninfectious process. Although the complication rate of TBLB is low (at most, bleeding in 3% and pneumothorax in 5%), many clinicians believe that the yield of BAL is sufficiently high that TBLB need not be routine. Others, including Cazzadori and coworkers (1995), advocate TBLB in all bronchoscopies for DPLD in immunosuppressed patients. These authors found an overall diagnostic rate of 67% for TBLB versus 36% for BAL, with TBLB superior in all categories studied: HIV cases, hematologic malignancies, and renal transplant recipients.

Surgical lung biopsy offers the greatest sensitivity and specificity but is less often required than in the past, especially in the AIDS population. In the series of Bonfils-Roberts and associates (1990), 18 of 64 patients with AIDS in 1983 underwent biopsy versus only 2 of 302 in 1987. Surgical biopsy should be considered as the primary invasive procedure in patients with rapidly progressive disease in whom TBLB is relatively or absolutely contraindicated (e.g., ventilator dependence with high airway pressures, coagulopathy) and the clinical suspicion is of a disorder unlikely to be diagnosed by BAL alone and not covered by simple empiric therapy. Occasional patients may be deemed too ill to tolerate bronchoscopy at all. In most cases, however, surgical biopsy is performed after a nondiagnostic bronchoscopy or in patients who do not improve with therapy dictated by the bronchoscopic findings.

Although surgical biopsy almost always produces a definitive diagnosis, the reported benefit in altering therapy and outcome is variable. Studies by Hiatt (1982), Haverkos (1983), and Potter (1985) and their coworkers, among others, found that information obtained by open biopsy did not translate into improved survival in a variety of non-AIDS populations. In contrast, Cheson (1985), Walker (1989), and Robbins (1992) and their associates found that open biopsy was helpful in mixed non-AIDS groups, as did Catterall and associates (1989) in patients with Hodgkin's disease. The data in AIDS cases are also contradictory. Pass and associates (1986) concluded that open biopsy is helpful when TBLB is not diagnostic or is contraindicated and when patients do not improve despite treatment for diagnoses made bronchoscopically. Fitzgerald and associates (1987) also recommended open biopsy when bronchoscopy was nonspecific but found no benefit for patients who did not respond to treatment after diagnostic bronchoscopy. Bonfils-Roberts and colleagues (1990) reported a beneficial therapeutic change in only 1 of 66 AIDS patients who underwent biopsy.

The reported mortality rate of open biopsy is variable. Cheson and associates (1985) had no deaths in 87 procedures, and Robbins and colleagues (1992) noted only one death (1.4%) in 74 cases, despite coagulopathy in many patients. In contrast, Walker and colleagues (1989) reported a mortality of 9% and Potter and coworkers (1985) implicated surgical problems in the deaths of three of 14 biopsy patients (21%). Stover and Kaner (1996) suggest that video-assisted thoracoscopic biopsy in their series of immunosuppressed cancer patients may be less morbid than standard open lung biopsy.

We believe that open or thoracoscopic surgical biopsy can be accomplished safely in most cases and should be performed when a diagnosis eludes less invasive techniques. Surgical biopsy should also be considered in some patients who do not respond to treatment. This bias is based on the frequent coexistence of more than one process, the limitations of BAL or TBLB in the diagnosis of noninfectious lesions, and the occasional gratifying response to therapy for disorders such as Kaposi's sarcoma, diffuse lymphoma, and CMV pneumonia. Surgical biopsy, however, is not likely to alter outcome in patients with respiratory failure despite aggressive specific or empiric treatment. The benefit to individual patients when surgical biopsy yields a specific treatable diagnosis coupled with current low complication rates ensures that this approach will retain a place in the management of subgroups of patients.

REFERENCES

Agusti C, et al: Interstitial pulmonary fibrosis with and without associated collagen vascular disease: results of a two-year follow-up. Thorax 47:1035, 1992.

Al-Jarad N, et al: High resolution computed tomographic assessment of asbestosis and cryptogenic fibrosing alveolitis: a comparative study. Thorax 47:645, 1992.

Allen JN, Davis WB: Eosinophilic lung diseases. Am J Respir Crit Care Med 150:1423, 1994.

Bergin CJ, et al: Pneumocystis carinii pneumonia: CT and HRCT observations. J Comput Assist Tomogr 14:756, 1990.

Bigby TD, et al: Clinical spectrum of pulmonary mucormycosis. Chest 89:435, 1986.

Bonfils-Roberts EA, Nickodem A, Nealon TF: Retrospective analysis of the efficacy of open lung biopsy in acquired immunodeficiency syndrome. Ann Thorac Surg 49:115, 1990.

Brauner MW, et al: Pulmonary histiocytosis X: evaluation with high-resolution CT. Radiology 172:255, 1989.

Carrington CB, Liebow AA: Limited forms of angiitis and granulomatosis of Wegener's type. Am J Med 41:497, 1966.

Carrington CB, et al: Natural history and treated course of usual and desquamative interstitial pneumonia. N Engl J Med 298:801, 1978.

Catterall JR, Hofflin JM, Remington JS: Pulmonary toxoplasmosis. Am Rev Respir Dis 133:704, 1986.

Catterall JR, et al: Open lung biopsy in patients with Hodgkin's disease and pulmonary infiltrates. Am Rev Respir Dis 139:1274, 1989.

Cazzadori A, et al: Transbronchial biopsy in the diagnosis of pulmonary infiltrates in immunocompromised patients. Chest 107:101, 1995.

Chaffey MH, et al: Radiographic distribution of Pneumocystis carinii pneumonia in patients with AIDS treated with prophylactic inhaled pentamidine. Radiology 175:715, 1990.

Chandler PW, et al: Radiographic manifestations of bronchiolitis obliterans with organizing pneumonia versus usual interstitial pneumonia. AJR Am J Roentgenol 147:899, 1986.

Chastre J, et al: Pulmonary fibrosis following pneumonia due to acute Legionaire's disease: clinical, ultrastructural, and immunofluorescent study. Chest 91:57, 1987.

Chechani V, Landrenau RJ, Shaikh SS: Open lung biopsy for diffuse infiltrative lung disease. Ann Thorac Surg 54:296, 1992.

Cheson BD, et al: Value of open-lung biopsy in 87 immunocompromised patients with pulmonary infiltrates. Cancer 55:453, 1985.

Colby TV, Swensen SJ: Anatomic distribution and histopathologic patterns in diffuse lung disease: correlation with HRCT. J Thorac Imaging 11:1, 1996.

Coleman A, Colby TV: Histologic diagnosis of extrinsic allergic alveolitis. Am J Surg Pathol 12:514, 1988.

Cooper JAD, White DA, Matthay RA: Drug-induced pulmonary disease: part 1, cytotoxic drugs. Am Rev Respir Dis 33:321, 1986a.

Cooper JAD, White DA, Matthay RA: Drug-induced pulmonary disease: part 2, noncytotoxic drugs. Am Rev Respir Dis 133:488, 1986b.

Cordier JF, et al: Pulmonary Wegener's granulomatosis: a clinical and imaging study of 77 cases. Chest 97:906, 1990.

Costabel U, et al: T-lymphocytosis in bronchoalveolar lavage fluid of hypersensitivity pneumonitis: changes in profile of T-cell subsets during the course of disease. Chest 85:514, 1984.

Cottin V, et al: Nonspecific interstitial pneumonia: individualization of a clinicopathologic entity in a series of twelve patients. Am J Respir Crit Care Med 158:1286, 1998.

Crawford SW, Hackman RC, Clark JG: Open lung biopsy diagnosis of diffuse pulmonary infiltrates after marrow transplantation. Chest 94:949, 1988.

Crouch E: Pathobiology of pulmonary fibrosis. Am J Physiol 259:L159, 1990.

Crystal RG, et al: Idiopathic pulmonary fibrosis: clinical, histologic, radiographic, physiologic, scintigraphic, cytologic and biochemical aspects. Ann Intern Med 85:769, 1976.

Davison AG, et al: Cryptogenic organizing pneumonitis. Q J Med 52:382, 1983.

Dreisen RB, et al: Circulating immune complexes in the idiopathic interstitial pneumonias. N Engl J Med 298:353, 1978.

Epler GR, et al: Normal chest roentgenograms in chronic diffuse infiltrative lung disease. N Engl J Med 298:934, 1978.

Epler GR, et al: Bronchiolitis obliterans organizing pneumonia. N Engl J Med 312:152, 1985.

Fauci AS, et al: Lymphomatoid granulomatosis: prospective clinical and therapeutic experience over 10 years. N Engl J Med 306:68, 1982.

Felson B: A new look at pattern recognition of diffuse pulmonary diseases. AJR Am J Roentgenol 133:183, 1979.

Fish DG, et al: Coccidioidomycosis during human immunodeficiency virus infection: a review of 77 patients. Medicine 69:384, 1990.

Fitzgerald W, et al: The role of open lung biopsy in patients with the acquired immunodeficiency syndrome. Chest 91:659, 1987.

Frank ST, et al: Pulmonary dysfunction in rheumatoid disease. Chest 63:27, 1973.

Fraser RG, et al: Diagnosis of Diseases of the Chest. 3rd ed. Philadelphia: WB Saunders, 1988.

Frazier AR, Miller RD: Interstitial pneumonitis in association with polymyositis and dermatomyositis. Chest 65:403, 1974.

Fujii M, et al: Interstitial lung disease in rheumatoid arthritis: assessment with high-resolution computed tomography. J Thorac Imaging 8:54, 1993.

Fulmer JD, Kaltreider HB: The pulmonary vasculitides. Chest 82:615, 1983.

Gaensler EA, Carrington CB: Peripheral opacities in chronic eosinophilic pneumonia: the photographic negative of pulmonary edema. AJR Am J Roentgenol 128:1, 1977.

Gaensler EA, Carrington CB: Open biopsy for chronic diffuse infiltrative lung disease: clinical, roentgenographic and physiologic correlations in 502 patients. Ann Thorac Surg 30:411, 1980.

Gill PS, et al: Pulmonary Kaposi's sarcoma: clinical findings and results of therapy. Am J Med 87:57, 1989.

Godwin JD, Muller NL, Takasugi JE: Pulmonary alveolar proteinosis: CT findings. Radiology 169:609, 1988.

Goldstein LS, et al: Pulmonary alveolar proteinosis: clinical features and outcomes. Chest 114:1357, 1998.

Graham CM, Stern EJ, Finkbeiner WE, Webb WR: High-resolution CT appearance of diffuse alveolar septal amyloidosis. AJR Am J Roentgenol 158:265, 1992.

Hakala M: Poor prognosis in patients with rheumatoid arthritis hospitalized for interstitial lung fibrosis. Chest 93:114, 1988.

Hamman L, Rich AR: Fulminating diffuse interstitial fibrosis of the lungs. Trans Am Clin Climatol Assoc 51:154, 1935.

Harrison DJ, Simpson R, Kharbanda R, Abernethy VE, Nimmo G: Antibodies to neutrophil cytoplasmic antigens in Wegener's granulomatosis and other conditions. Thorax 44:373, 1989.

Haupt HM, Moore GW, Hutchins GM: The lung in systemic lupus erythematosus: analysis of the pathologic changes in 120 patients. Am J Med 71:791, 1981.

Haverkos H, et al: Diagnosis of pneumonitis in immunocompromised patients by open lung biopsy. Cancer 52:1093, 1983.

Herbert A, et al: Lymphocytic interstitial pneumonia identified as lymphoma of mucosa-associated lymphoid tissue. J Pathol 146:129, 1985.

Hiatt J, et al: The value of open lung biopsy in the immunocompromised patient. Surgery 92:285, 1982.

Horsburgh CR, Selik RM: The epidemiology of nontuberculous mycobacterial infection in the acquired immunodeficiency syndrome (AIDS). Am Rev Respir Dis 139:4, 1989.

Ikezoe J, et al: CT appearance of acute radiation-induced injury in the lung. AJR Am J Roentgenol 150:765, 1988.

Im JG, et al: Lobar bronchioloalveolar carcinoma: "angiogram sign" on CT scans. Radiology 176:749, 1990.

Ip MSM, et al: Risk factors for pulmonary tuberculosis in bone marrow transplant recipients. Am J Respir Crit Care Med 158:1173, 1998.

Jahaveri S, Sicilian L: Lung function, breathing pattern, and gas exchange in interstitial lung disease. Thorax 47:93, 1992.

James DG, Siltzbach LE, Turiaf A: A worldwide review of sarcoidosis. Ann NY Acad Sci 278:321, 1976.

Jederlinic PJ, Sicilian L, Gaensler EA: Chronic eosinophilic pneumonia: a report of 19 cases and a review of the literature. Medicine 67:154, 1988.

Jennette JC, Falk RJ: Small-vessel vasculitis. N Engl J Med 337:1512, 1997.

Johnson MA, et al: Randomised controlled trial comparing prednisolone alone with cyclophosphamide and low dose prednisolone in combination in cryptogenic fibrosing alveolitis. Thorax 44:280, 1989.

Katzenstein ALA, Bloor CM, Liebow AA: Diffuse alveolar damage: the role of oxygen, shock, and related factors. Am J Pathol 58:210, 1976.

Katzenstein ALA, Myers JL, Mazur MT: Acute interstitial pneumonia: a clinicopathological, ultrastructural, and cell kinetic study. Am J Surg Pathol 10:256, 1986.

Katzenstein ALA, Fiorelli RF: Nonspecific interstitial pneumonia/fibrosis: histologic features and clinical significance. Am J Surg Pathol 18:136, 1994.

Keicho N, et al: Detection of lymphomatous involvement of the lung by bronchoalveolar lavage: application of immunophenotypic and gene rearrangement analysis. Chest 105:458, 1994.

King TE: Diagnostic advances in idiopathic pulmonary fibrosis. Chest 100:238, 1991.

King TE, Mortenson RL: Cryptogenic organizing pneumonitis: the North American experience. Chest 102(Suppl):8, 1992.

Kramer MR, Uttamchandani RB: The radiographic appearance of pulmonary nocardiosis associated with AIDS. Chest 98:382, 1990.

Lack EE, et al: Pulmonary and extrapulmonary lymphangioleiomyomatosis: report of a case with bilateral angiomyolipomas, multifocal lymphangioleiomyomatosis, and a glial polyp of the endocervix. Am J Surg Pathol 10:650, 1986.

Leatherman JW: The lung in systemic vasculitis. Semin Respir Infect 3:274, 1988.

Lee KS, Kullnig P, Hartman TE, Muller NL: Cryptogenic organizing pneumonia: CT findings in 43 patients. AJR Am J Roentgenol 162:543, 1994.

Liebow AA: New concepts and entities in pulmonary diseases. In Liebow AA, Smith DE (eds): The Lung. Baltimore: Williams and Wilkins, 1968.

Liebow AA, Carrington CB, Friedman PJ: Lymphomatoid granulomatosis. Hum Pathol 3:457, 1972.

Locke CB: Rheumatoid lung. Clin Radiol 14:43, 1963.

Maher J, Daly PA: Severe bleomycin lung toxicity: reversal with high dose corticosteroids. Thorax 48:92, 1993.

Martin WJ, Rosenow EC: Amiodarone pulmonary toxicity: recognition and pathogenesis. Chest 93:1067, 1988.

Mathiesen JR, et al: Chronic diffuse infiltrative lung disease: comparison of diagnostic accuracy of CT and chest radiography. Radiology 171:111, 1989.

Matthay RA, et al: Pulmonary manifestations of systemic lupus erythematosus: review of twelve cases of acute lupus pneumonitis. Medicine 54:379, 1974.

Mayo JR, et al: Chronic eosinophilic pneumonia: CT findings in six cases. AJR Am J Roentgenol 153:727, 1989.

McLoud TC, Carrington CB, Gaensler EA: Diffuse infiltrative lung disease: a new scheme for description. Radiology 149:353, 1983.

Miller RR, et al: Lingular and right middle lobe biopsy in the assessment of diffuse lung disease. Ann Thorac Surg 44:269, 1987.

Moran TJ, Totten RS: Lymphoid interstitial pneumonia with dysproteinemia: report of two cases with plasma cell predominance. Am J Clin Pathol 54:747, 1970.

Movsas B, Raffin TA, Epstein AH: Pulmonary radiation injury. Chest 111:1061, 1997.

Muller NL, Staples CA, Miller RR: Bronchiolitis obliterans organizing pneumonia: CT features in 14 patients. AJR Am J Roentgenol 154:983, 1990.

Murray JF, Mills J: Pulmonary infectious complications of human immunodeficiency virus infection. Part 1. Am Rev Respir Dis 141:1356, 1990.

Myers JL. Lymphomatoid granulomatosis: past, present, future? Mayo Clin Proc 65:274, 1990.

Naidich DP, et al: Kaposi's sarcoma: CT-radiographic correlation. Chest 96:723, 1989.

Naughton M, Fahy J, FitzGerald MX: Chronic eosinophilic pneumonia: a long-term follow-up of 12 patients. Chest 103:162, 1993.

Newman LS, Rose CS, Maier LA: Sarcoidosis. N Engl J Med 336:1224, 1997.

Nishimura K, Itoh H: High-resolution computed tomographic features of bronchiolitis obliterans organizing pneumonia. Chest 102 (Suppl):27, 1992.

Nishimura K, et al: Usual interstitial pneumonia: histologic correlation with high-resolution CT. Radiology 182:337, 1992.

Ohori NP, et al: Giant cell interstitial pneumonia and hard metal pneumoconiosis: a clinicopathologic study of four cases and review of the literature. Am J Surg Pathol 13:581, 1989.

Oldham SAA, et al: HIV-associated lymphocytic interstitial pneumonia: radiologic manifestations and pathologic correlation. Radiology 170:83, 1989.

Orens JB, et al: The sensitivity of high-resolution CT in detecting idiopathic pulmonary fibrosis proved by open lung biopsy: a prospective study. Chest 108:109, 1995.

Owens GR, Follansbee WP: Cardiopulmonary manifestations of systemic sclerosis. Chest 91:118, 1987.

Palosaari DE, Colby TV: Bronchiolocentric chronic lymphocytic leukemia. Cancer 58:1695, 1986.

Parkes WR: Occupational Lung Disorders. 3rd Ed. Oxford: Butterworth-Heinemann, 1994.

Pass H, et al. Indications for and diagnostic efficacy of open-lung biopsy in the patient with acquired immunodeficiency syndrome (AIDS). Ann Thorac Surg 41:307, 1986.

Pavlakis N, et al. Fatal pulmonary toxicity resulting from treatment with gemcitabine. Cancer 80:286, 1997.

Patchefsky AS, et al. Desquamative interstitial pneumonia: relationship to interstitial fibrosis. Thorax 28:680, 1973.

Peters SG, et al. Colchicine in the treatment of pulmonary fibrosis. Chest 103:101, 1993.

Pietra GG. Pathologic mechanisms of drug-induced lung disorders: J Thorac Imaging 6:1, 1991.

Pisani RJ, DeRemee RA. Clinical implications of the histologic diagnosis of pulmonary lymphomatoid granulomatosis: Mayo Clin Proc 65:151, 1990.

Pisani RJ, Wright AJ: Clinical utility of bronchoalveolar lavage in immunocompromised hosts. Mayo Clin Proc 67:221, 1992.

Ponn RB, Silverman H, Federico JA: Outpatient chest tube management. Ann Thorac Surg 64:1437, 1997.

Potter D, et al: Prospective randomized study of open lung biopsy versus empirical antibiotic therapy for acute pneumonitis in non-neutropenic cancer patients. Ann Thorac Surg 40:422, 1985.

Prakash UBS, Luthra HS, Divertie MB: Intrathoracic manifestations of mixed connective tissue disease. Mayo Clin Proc 60:813, 1985.

Prakash UBS, et al: Pulmonary alveolar phospholipoproteinosis: experience with 34 cases and a review. Mayo Clin Proc 62:499, 1987.

Purdy LJ, et al: Pulmonary Kaposi's sarcoma: premortem histologic diagnosis. Am J Surg Pathol 10:301, 1986.

Raghu G: Idiopathic pulmonary fibrosis: a rational clinical approach. Chest 92:148, 1987.

Raghu G: Interstitial lung disease: a diagnostic approach. Are CT scan and lung biopsy indicated in every patient? Am J Respir Crit Care Med 151:909, 1995.

Reynolds HY: Diagnostic and management strategies for diffuse interstitial lung disease. Chest 113:192, 1998.

Robbins BE, et al: Diagnosis of acute diffuse pulmonary infiltrates in immunocompromised patients by open biopsy of the lung. Surg Gynecol Obstet 175:8, 1992.

Rochester CL, Elias JA: Cytokines and cytokine networks in the pathogenesis of interstitial and fibrotic lung disorders. Semin Respir Med 14:389, 1993.

Roseman KD, Reilly MJ, Kalinowski DJ, Watt FC: Silicosis in the 1990's. Chest 111:779, 1997.

Rosenberg DM, et al: Functional correlates of lung involvement in Wegener's granulomatosis. Am J Med 69:387, 1980.

Rosenow EC, et al: Drug-induced pulmonary disease: an update. Chest 102:239, 1992.

Salmeron G, Greenberg SD, Lidsky MD: Polymyositis and diffuse interstitial lung disease: a review of the pulmonary histopathologic findings. Arch Intern Med 141:1005, 1981.

Salvaggio JE, deShazo RD: Pathogenesis of hypersensitivity pneumonitis. Chest 89(Suppl):190S, 1986.

Sandhu JS, Goodman PC: Pulmonary cysts associated with Pneumocystis carinii pneumonia in patients with AIDS. Radiology 173:33, 1989.

Scadding JG, Hinson KFW: Diffuse fibrosing alveolitis (diffuse interstitial fibrosis of the lungs). Thorax 22:291, 1967.

Simmons JT, et al: Nonspecific interstitial pneumonitis in patients with AIDS: radiologic features. AJR Am J Roentgenol 149:265, 1987.

Small PM, et al: Course and outcome of tuberculosis in patients who have or subsequently developed AIDS. N Engl J Med 324:289, 1991.

Smith DE, et al: Diagnosis of Pneumocystis carinii pneumonia in HIV antibody-positive patients by simple outpatient assessments. Thorax 47:1005, 1992.

Stack BHR, Choo-Kang YF, Heard BE: The prognosis of cryptogenic fibrosing alveolitis. Thorax 27:535, 1972.

Stansell JD: Fungal disease in HIV-infected persons: cryptococcosis, histoplasmosis, and coccidioidomycosis. J Thorac Imaging 6:28, 1991.

Staples CA, et al: High resolution computed tomography and lung function in asbestos-exposed workers with normal chest radiographs. Am Rev Respir Dis 139:1502, 1989.

Stover DE, Kaner RJ: Pulmonary complications in cancer patients. CA Cancer J Clin 46:303, 1996.

Stein MG, et al: Pulmonary lymphangitic spread of carcinoma: appearance on CT scans. Radiology 162:371, 1987.

Sulavik SB, et al: Recognition of distinctive patterns of gallium-67 distribution in sarcoidosis. J Nucl Med 31:1909, 1990.

Suffredini AF, et al: Nonspecific interstitial pneumonitis: a common cause of pulmonary disease in the acquired immune deficiency syndrome. Ann Int Med 107:7, 1987.

Sullivan EJ: Lymphangioleiomyomatosis: a review. Chest 114:1689, 1998.

Sullivan WD, et al: A prospective evaluation emphasizing pulmonary involvement in patients with mixed connective tissue disease. Medicine 63:92, 1984.

Tazelaar HD, et al: Interstitial lung disease in polymyositis and dermatomyositis. Am Rev Respir Dis 141:727, 1990.

Thomas D, Hunninghake GW: Current concepts of the pathogenesis of sarcoidosis. Am Rev Respir Dis 135:747, 1987.

Thrasher DR, Briggs DD: Pulmonary sarcoidosis. Clin Chest Med 3:537, 1982.

Tomioka H, King TE: Gold-induced pulmonary disease: clinical features, outcome and differentiation from rheumatoid lung disease. Am J Respir Crit Care Med 155:1011, 1997.

Tryka AF, Godleski JJ, Fanta CH: Leukemic cell pneumonopathy: a complication of treated myeloblastic leukemia. Cancer 50:2763, 1982.

Tu JV, Biem J, Detsky AS: Bronchoscopy versus empirical therapy in HIV-infected patients with presumptive Pneumocystis carinii pneumonia: a decision analysis. Am Rev Respir Dis 148:370, 1993.

Tuazon CU, et al: Utility of gallium[67] scintigraphy and bronchial washings in the diagnosis and treatment of Pneumocystis carinii pneumonia in patients with the acquired immune deficiency syndrome. Am Rev Respir Dis 132:1087, 1985.

Tubbs RR, et al: Desquamative interstitial pneumonitis. Chest 72:159, 1977.

Turner RR, Colby TV, Doggett RS: Well-differentiated lymphocytic lymphoma: a study of 47 patients with primary manifestations in the lung. Cancer *54*:2088, 1984.

Urban T, et al: Pulmonary lymphangiomyomatosis: follow-up and long-term outcome with antiestrogen therapy; a report of eight cases. Chest *102*:472, 1992.

Vander Els NJ, Miller V: Successful treatment of gemcitabine toxicity with a brief course of oral corticosteroid therapy. Chest *114*:1779, 1998.

Walker WA, et al: Does open lung biopsy affect treatment in patients with diffuse pulmonary infiltrates? J Thorac Cardiovasc Surg *97*:534, 1989.

Wallace JM, Hannah JB. Cytomegalovirus pneumonitis in patients with AIDS: findings in an autopsy series: Chest *92*:198, 1987.

Wallace JM, Hannah JB. Mycobacterium avium complex infection in patients with acquired immunodeficiency syndrome: a clinicopathologic study: Chest *93*:926, 1988.

Watters LC, et al. A clinical, radiologic and physiologic scoring system for the longitudinal assessment of patients with idiopathic pulmonary fibrosis: Am Rev Respir Dis *133*:97, 1986.

Waxman AB, Goldie SJ, Brett-Smith H, Matthay RA: Cytomegalovirus as a primary pulmonary pathogen in AIDS. Chest *111*:128, 1997.

Wetstein L: Sensitivity and specificity of lingular segmental biopsies of the lung. Chest *90*:383, 1986.

White DA, Matthay RA: Noninfectious pulmonary complications of infection with the human immunodeficiency virus. Am Rev Respir Dis *140*:1763, 1989.

Wholey MH, Good CA, McDonald JR: Disseminated indeterminate pulmonary disease: value of lung biopsy. Radiology *71*:651, 1958.

Winterbauer RH: The treatment of idiopathic pulmonary fibrosis. Chest *100*:233, 1991.

Winterbauer RH, et al: Diffuse interstitial pneumonitis: clinicopathological correlations in 20 patients treated with prednisone/azathioprine. Am J Med *65*:661, 1978.

Woolfenden JM, et al: Acquired immunodeficiency syndrome: Ga-67 citrate imaging. Radiology *162*:383, 1987.

Yoshioka R, et al: Pulmonary complications in patients with adult T-cell leukemia. Cancer *55*:2491, 1985.

Yousem SA, Colby TV, Carrington CB: Lung biopsy in rheumatoid arthritis. Am Rev Respir Dis *131*:770, 1985.

Yu VL, Muder RR, Poorsattar A: Significance of isolation of aspergillus from the respiratory tract in diagnosis of invasive pulmonary aspergillosis. Am J Med *81*:249, 1986.

CHAPTER 92

Lung Transplantation

Bryan F. Meyers and G. Alexander Patterson

HISTORICAL REVIEW

Early Phase

During the early 1950s, Metras (1950) in France and Hardin and Kittle (1954) in the United States reported successful canine lung transplantation. During that decade, many surgical techniques were developed that have proved useful in human lung transplantation. Hardy and associates reported the first human lung transplantation in 1963. Although their patient succumbed after 18 days, their brief success demonstrated the technical feasibility of the operation and stimulated worldwide interest in pulmonary transplantation.

During the next 15 years, approximately 40 clinical lung transplant operations were performed in centers around the world. None of these procedures was successful. Only one recipient was actually discharged from the hospital, a 23-year-old patient of Derom and colleagues (1971). This patient left the hospital 8 months after transplantation but died a short time thereafter as a result of chronic rejection, sepsis, and bronchial stenosis. Most patients died within the first 2 weeks of transplantation as a result of primary graft failure, sepsis, or rejection. The most frequent cause of death beyond the second postoperative week was bronchial anastomotic disruption. This problem of bronchial anastomotic dehiscence stimulated the interest of investigators in a number of surgical laboratories. Lima and colleagues in Toronto demonstrated that high doses of corticosteroids (2 mg/kg per day), which at that time were necessary for adequate immunosuppression, had an adverse effect on bronchial anastomotic healing. The same group, as reported by Morgan and associates (1982), also demonstrated that the ischemic donor bronchus could be revascularized within a few days by a pedicled flap of omentum. Not only did the omental pedicle provide new collateral circulation to the ischemic bronchus but the omentum also provided a potential benefit in containing an anastomotic dehiscence in the event of partial disruption.

During the same interval, it became apparent that the new drug cyclosporine had impressive immunosuppressive properties and could eliminate the routine need for high-dose corticosteroid immunosuppression. Furthermore, it was also demonstrated by the Toronto group and reported by Goldberg and colleagues (1983) that cyclosporine had no adverse effect on bronchial anastomotic healing.

Reitz and associates (1982) of the Stanford group reported their initial clinical experience with combined heart-lung transplantation in a group of patients with pulmonary vascular disease. This experience demonstrated conclusively that the transplanted human lung could provide acceptable long-term function. Yet by 1983, successful isolated lung transplantation had not yet been achieved. Satisfactory patient selection remained the final obstacle to successful clinical lung transplantation. The Toronto group reasoned that end-stage respiratory failure from pulmonary fibrosis would provide the ideal condition for single-lung transplantation. The increased resistance to perfusion and ventilation of the native lung would preferentially direct perfusion and ventilation to the transplanted lung. By careful recipient selection and strict adherence to rigid donor criteria, Cooper and colleagues achieved the first successful single-lung transplantation in 1983 in a 58-year-old man with idiopathic pulmonary fibrosis, as reported by the Toronto Lung Transplant Group (1986).

The subsequent development of an experimental and clinical en bloc bilateral lung replacement technique by Dark (1986) and by us (GAP, 1988) and colleagues, respectively, enabled application of bilateral lung replacement to patients for whom single-lung transplantation was not appropriate. Although this procedure did have the definite attraction of preservation of the recipient heart, it was a technically complex procedure. In addition, it was associated with a high incidence of complications, notably donor airway ischemia, as we described (GAP, 1990), and cardiac denervation, as reported by Schafers and colleagues (1990).

Recent Developments

Lung transplantation was expanded to the pediatric population in a judicious manner in the late 1980s. Its use has expanded to a stable rate of approximately 50 transplants per year over the last 5 years. The primary indications in the pediatric age group (6 to 15 years of age) include cystic fibrosis (CF), congenital heart-lung disease, and primary pulmonary hypertension. In infants and younger children (ages 0 to 5 years), a very small number of transplants have been undertaken, typically performed for congenital disorders. Mendeloff and colleagues (1997) reported a 2-year survival rate of 84% and a 3-year survival rate of 73% for older pediatric patients transplanted for CF, while Sweet and associates (1997) reported a 67% and 60% 2-year and 4-year survival for infants and children under the age of 3 years. As with other groups of lung-transplant recipients, early lung dysfunction and late obliterative bronchiolitis are the greatest impediments to the survival of these young patients. As the pediatric lung transplant experience matures, it is likely that retransplantation will be increasingly considered for the treatment of chronic rejection. Huddleston and coworkers (1998) reported 14 retransplantations with three early deaths and a 2-year survival rate of 58%.

The shortage of donors remains a major threat to progress in lung transplantation. Long waiting lists for organs translate to higher rates of death among potential recipients listed for transplantation. One controversial proposed solution to the critical shortage of cadaveric lung donors has been the concept of living related donors. Starnes and colleagues (1997) have the most extensive experience with living-donor transplantation and have expanded the indications beyond CF to include pulmonary hypertension, pulmonary fibrosis, and assorted other etiologies of pulmonary failure. The reports from this group describe 38 living-donor transplants performed in 27 adults and 10 children with a 38% perioperative mortality rate. Complications resulting from the 76 donor lobectomies included postpericardiotomy syndrome, atrial fibrillation, and surgical re-exploration. Living donors are a rarely used solution to the donor shortage, amounting to 30 to 40 procedures a year for the years 1994 to 1996, and accounting for less than 4% of total recent donors as reported by UNOS (1998). This technique has now been used for over 100 cases with no reports of mortality among the living donors, but the greatest impediment to the expanded use of this strategy is the potential risk of injury or death to a previously healthy donor.

Current Status

As a treatment strategy for end-stage lung disease, transplantation has matured significantly in the past few years. It is now almost 35 years after the first attempted lung transplant procedure. Fourteen years have passed since the first successful single-lung transplantation, and 11 years have passed since the first successful bilateral transplant. A decade ago there were only a handful of lung transplantation programs worldwide. In 1997, more than 1220 lung transplants (625 single, 595 double) were performed worldwide with almost 805 of those cases performed in the United States. Indeed, during 1997 there were 94 United States centers registered as lung transplant programs. Although only six transplant programs performed more than 35 cases annually, some 47 American centers performed at least five lung transplants during the calendar year 1997.

SELECTION OF RECIPIENT

General Considerations

General selection criteria are listed in Table 92-1 and were described in detail in a review by Lynch and Trulock (1996). We maintain a policy of listing for pulmonary transplantation only those patients who we believe have a limited life expectancy (12 to 24 months) as a result of their underlying lung disease. As discussed subsequently, it has become apparent that the time course of deterioration and subsequent death is highly variable depending on the specific disease. With the inherent risk of pulmonary transplantation and the acute shortage of suitable donor lungs, we believe that it is not appropriate to offer pulmonary transplantation to patients who are not in imminent danger of death from their underlying lung disease. Patients who have coexisting dysfunction involving another organ system are not eligible for transplantation, a limitation that especially impacts patients in older age groups. In general, we do not accept a patient over the age of 65 years. In addition, patients with a history of malignant disease within the prior 5 years are generally not eligible for pulmonary transplantation. An exception to this criterion is the patient with bilateral bronchoalveolar carcinoma. Etienne and colleagues (1997) have reported a

Table 92-1. Recipient Selection Criteria

Clinically and physiologically severe disease
Medical therapy ineffective or unavailable
Substantial limitation in activities of daily living
Limited life expectancy
Adequate cardiac function without significant coronary artery
 disease
Ambulatory with rehabilitation potential
Acceptable nutritional status
Satisfactory psychosocial profile and emotional support system

single long-term survivor with this therapy, and Zorn (1998) has reported a favorable experience in a small number of patients. The patient with a more recent malignancy judged to be cured might be considered. Patients with serious psychological dysfunction should not be considered candidates for pulmonary transplantation. We do not evaluate patients who continue to smoke.

A previous thoracotomy is not of itself a specific contraindication to pulmonary transplantation. However, adhesions and anatomic distortion resulting from previous surgery do complicate the conduct of a transplant procedure. Patients receiving high-dose corticosteroid therapy (20 mg prednisone or more per day) are not eligible for pulmonary transplantation. Such high doses of corticosteroid have a well documented negative influence on bronchial healing and lead to susceptibility to postoperative infection. However, patients receiving low- or moderate-dose steroid therapy are candidates and have undergone pulmonary transplantation without an increased incidence of bronchial anastomotic complications. Ventilator dependency is not a contraindication to transplantation, yet most programs have a selective policy concerning such patients lest their waiting list become full of ventilated patients.

We insist that all patients considered for transplantation, except those with primary pulmonary hypertension or Eisenmenger's syndrome, participate in a progressive monitored exercise rehabilitation program while they await transplantation. Virtually all patients experience an improvement in strength and exercise tolerance without any measurable change in pulmonary function. We are convinced that this improved endurance better enables patients to withstand the rigors of a transplant procedure and subsequent convalescence.

Specific Considerations Based on Diagnosis

Obstructive Lung Disease

Obstructive lung disease, notably emphysema and α_1-antitrypsin deficiency, has become the most common indication for pulmonary transplantation, accounting for 55.2% of the adult single-lung transplants and 28.7% of the bilateral-lung transplants reported in the 1998 Registry of the ISHLT, as reported by Hosenpud and colleagues (1998). General criteria for transplantation in these patients have been published by Trulock (1997). Most patients have deteriorated to a point at which oxygen supplementation is required. In our experience, the mean supplemental oxygen requirement is slightly in excess of 4 L per minute. The obstructive physiology in these patients results in an FEV_1 of well under 1 L at approximately 15% of predicted normal values. We and others have found that this patient group usually has a stable course while awaiting pulmonary transplantation. Progressive elevation in P_{CO_2} has been observed in some patients, however, with sev-

eral of these individuals undergoing transplantation with the P_{CO_2} in excess of 100 mm Hg.

Although obstructive lung disease is the most common indication for which single-lung transplantation is performed, the ideal operative procedure for these patients is not yet defined. There are currently two surgical therapies aimed at crippling, end-stage emphysema: lung transplantation and lung volume reduction surgery (see Chapter 83). Early reports of the results of lung volume reduction surgery suggest that this procedure can offer significant improvement in the symptoms of severe emphysema and a measurable improvement in overall functional status. In a retrospective comparison of volume reduction and transplantation for emphysema, Gaissert and associates (1996) reported a lower early and late mortality for patients receiving volume reduction: 3.0% for volume reduction, 10.2% for single-lung transplantation, and 16% for bilateral-lung transplantation. In the same study, the percent improvement of the FEV_1 at 12 months after operation was 83% for the volume reduction group, 212% for the single-lung transplant group, and 518% for the bilateral-lung transplant group. The authors' conclusions were that volume reduction is a suitable alternative for some patients eligible for transplantation; volume reduction may offer earlier therapy for transplant candidates by avoiding the waiting time for organ availability; and volume reduction is the only surgical option for patients not eligible for transplantation.

Lung volume reduction surgery has been proposed by some as a bridge to lung transplantation. It is clear from our own experience, and that of others, that lung transplantation after lung volume reduction surgery, while technically challenging, can be accomplished with good results. However, we favor a meticulous selection process in which both options are considered and the best option selected for each patient. Patients with ideal circumstances for lung volume reduction surgery, such as hyperinflation, heterogeneous distribution of disease, FEV_1 of greater than 20%, and a normal P_{CO_2}, are offered lung volume reduction surgery. Whereas patients with diffuse disease, low FEV_1, hypercapnia, and associated pulmonary hypertension are directed toward transplantation. Lung volume reduction surgery has not been a satisfactory option for patients with α_1-antitrypsin deficiency, and we prefer to transplant in these cases.

The functional outcomes of single- and bilateral-lung transplantation for these patients is discussed subsequently. In general, for young patients, particularly those with α_1-antitrypsin deficiency, we prefer bilateral sequential single-lung transplantation. The bilateral option is also more attractive in larger recipients who will never obtain a sufficiently large single-lung allograft. On the other hand, for smaller recipients, single-lung transplantation offers a more attractive option, particularly when an oversized donor lung can be grafted.

Septic Lung Disease

CF represents the most frequently encountered condition in this category. It is the most common inherited disorder among whites and results in diffuse bronchiectatic destruction of both lungs. Without transplantation, the overwhelming majority of patients die as a result of progressive respiratory failure in the second or third decade of life. The most reliable predictors of life expectancy in CF patients were published by Kerem and associates (1992). An FEV_1 of less than 30% predicted, elevated $Paco_2$, requirement for supplemental oxygen, frequent admissions to the hospital for control of acute pulmonary infection, and failure to maintain weight are reliable predictors of early mortality in these patients. We use these criteria in selecting patients for pulmonary transplantation. Once reaching this stage of disease, patients with CF usually have a rapidly progressive downhill course. Indeed, in the Papworth experience reported by Sharples and coworkers (1993), approximately one-third of CF patients accepted for transplantation died while waiting for a suitable donor. Milla and Warwick (1998) challenged the assertion that an FEV_1 of less than 30% predicted represented an indication for referral for transplantation. In their patient population, patients with FEV_1 less than 30% predicted had a median survival of 3.9 years, and no single-measured parameter was useful in predicting a subset of patients with impending decline causing an urgent need to refer for transplantation. Hayllar and colleagues (1997) constructed a prognostic index based on FEV_1, forced vital capacity (FVC), short stature, elevated white blood cell count, and presence of chronic liver disease to accurately predict mortality in their population of 403 CF patients. Despite these efforts, proper selection of transplant recipients among CF patients remains subjective and based on multiple, diverse criteria.

Fibrotic Lung Disease

Pulmonary fibrosis represents one of the less common indications for single-lung transplantation. Specific selection criteria for patients with pulmonary fibrosis have not changed significantly since originally published by the Toronto Lung Group in 1986. In our experience, candidates for transplantation have had classic restrictive physiology, with mean FVC and FEV_1 of 1.87 and 1.49, respectively, in 47 lung transplant recipients with pulmonary fibrosis. All require supplemental oxygen, show impaired exercise tolerance, and demonstrate oxygen desaturation with minimal exertion. Moderate and occasionally severe pulmonary hypertension is seen in these patients. In contrast to those with obstructive physiology, as Trulock (1997) noted, patients with pulmonary fibrosis who have deteriorated to the point of requiring transplantation generally have a rapid downhill course. Relative indications for early referral for transplantation include

resting hypoxia, worsening desaturation with exercise, failure to respond to medical therapy, and a falling trend in sequential measurements of vital capacity.

Pulmonary Vascular Disease

Patients with pulmonary vascular disease were once thought to require combined heart-lung transplantation. Fremes and colleagues (1990) at the University of Toronto, however, reported the first successful single-lung transplant in a patient with patent ductus Eisenmenger's syndrome. We noted that since this report, Pasque and associates (1995) demonstrated that right ventricular function improves immediately after transplantation and that improvement is maintained with long-term follow-up. D'Alonzo and coworkers (1991) suggest that patients with primary pulmonary hypertension (PPH) unresponsive to systemic vasodilators be listed for transplantation shortly after the diagnosis is established in consideration of the poor prognosis associated with this condition. These patients have elevated pulmonary artery pressures, with mean pressures in excess of 60 mm Hg. Most patients have clinical evidence of right ventricular failure with significant elevation of central venous pressure and depression of cardiac index. Among our first 34 patients undergoing single-lung transplantation for pulmonary vascular disease, the New York Heart Association functional status was class III or IV in every patient. Syncopal episodes are also a predictor of early mortality. The risk of sudden death in this patient population is high. In consideration of this risk, patients with PPH in our program are listed for transplantation and brought to St. Louis as soon as possible after evaluation.

In a report by Gammie and colleagues (1998) from the University of Pittsburgh, the number of patients transplanted for pulmonary hypertension in a 7-year period (58) equaled the number of patients with that diagnosis dying while on the waiting list for the availability of donor lungs. This death rate is higher than that noted in patients with other diseases. Unfortunately, as the number of potential recipients continues to surpass the number of available donors, this problem will remain. At present in the United States, time on the waiting list determines priority for an available donor. No consideration is given to severity of disease or expected survival time.

Observations of our own data reported by Pasque and associates (1995), as well as that of Gammie and colleagues, show a decrease in the use of lung transplantation as a treatment for pulmonary hypertension. This decrease is seen both in absolute terms (number of transplants for pulmonary hypertension) as well as in relative terms (pulmonary hypertension as a fraction of total transplants performed). The reasons for this decrease are unclear. Pulmonary and cardiology specialists may have a reluctance to refer patients for transplantation given the long waiting lists and the likelihood of death while on the waiting list. Other treatment strategies have evolved that improve the prognosis of patients with pulmonary hypertension without subjecting them to the acute risks of lung transplantation and the long-term risks of chronic immunosuppression. Barst and colleagues (1996) reported improvement in symptoms, hemodynamics, and survival in patients with pulmonary hypertension treated with continuous infusion of the potent vasodilator epoprostenol. Adnot and Raffestin (1996), among others, have suggested the potential benefit of chronic ambulatory therapy with inhaled nitric oxide as an alternative to transplantation.

Despite having equivalent degrees of pulmonary hypertension, patients with Eisenmenger's physiology have a less predictable rate of deterioration, and the appropriate timing for transplantation is correspondingly less certain. In these patients, we rely on the development of intractable and progressive symptoms of right ventricular failure as the predominant selection criterion.

DONOR LUNG

Rapid progress in transplantation has resulted in a shortage of suitable allografts for all organs. This problem is particularly significant for lung transplantation insofar as, at most, only 20% of otherwise suitable organ donors have lungs satisfactory for transplantation, according to the criteria listed in Table 92-2. The attrition of lung donors from the general population of multiple organ donors is so steep that in 1996, only 757 lung donors were found among the 5421 multi-organ donors reported by UNOS (1998), a rate of only 14%. Unfortunately, most conditions that result in brain death (trauma, spontaneous intracerebral hemorrhage) lead to significant pulmonary parenchymal pathologic change because of lung contusion, infection, aspiration, or neurogenic pulmonary edema.

Satisfactory gas exchange is imperative for donor lungs. This parameter can be confirmed by noting a PaO_2 greater than 300 mm Hg with an inspired oxygen concentration of 100% and 5 cm H_2O peak end-expiratory pressure (PEEP). A PaO_2 to FiO_2 ratio of 300 or greater provides adequate evidence of satisfactory gas exchange. A donor chest radiograph taken shortly before harvest must reveal clear lung fields. Bronchoscopic assessment at the donor institution often reveals mucopurulent secretions that might contain a variety of micro-organisms. This finding is commonly observed and is not a specific contraindication to pulmonary transplantation if the donor is otherwise suitable. Bronchoscopic evidence of aspiration or frank pus in the airway, however, is a definite contraindication to transplantation of that lung.

Donor and recipient ABO compatibility is essential. Donor and recipient human lymphocyte antigen (HLA) matching is not required. No data in the literature suggest that it may have any impact on subsequent graft function.

Table 92-2. Standard Lung Donor Selection Criteria

Age <55 years
No history of pulmonary disease
Normal serial chest radiographs
Adequate gas exchange—PaO_2 >300 mm Hg on FiO_2 1.0 and PEEP 5 cm H_2O
Normal bronchoscopic examination
Negative serologic screening for hepatitis B and human immunodeficiency virus
Recipient matching for ABO group
Size matching

Furthermore, any delay in donor harvest to conduct such matching places the donor lungs at risk of deterioration. Unfortunately, we do not have at our disposal satisfactory preservation strategies to permit "post-harvest" tissue matching. We prefer to use cytomegalovirus (CMV)-negative donors for CMV-negative recipients whenever possible.

A significant consideration is the matching of size between donor and recipient. Acceptable size matching depends on the nature of the recipient's lung disease and the type of transplant anticipated. Size matching can be achieved by comparison of vertical lung height, transverse chest diameter, and chest circumference. We have found, however, that these donor measurements are sometimes unreliable when made by busy and perhaps inexperienced donor coordinators in the remote donor hospital. More reliable are the predicted donor and recipient lung volumes using standard nomograms based on age, sex, and height, used by all pulmonary function laboratories to obtain predicted lung volumes.

In patients undergoing single-lung transplantation for obstructive lung disease, we attempt to place allografts with 15 to 20% greater volume than the recipient predicted lung volume. Implantation of such a large allograft is easily achieved in a patient with obstructive lung disease because of the enormous size of the recipient pleural space. In patients with pulmonary fibrosis or pulmonary vascular disease, however, the pleural spaces are reduced or normal in size, respectively. It is therefore inadvisable to oversize these patients to an excessive degree. In patients undergoing bilateral lung replacement, we prefer to match the donor lung volumes to the lung volume or anticipated lung dimensions that the recipient would possess in the absence of lung disease. Oversizing a bilateral recipient may produce hemodynamic difficulties on closure of the chest at the termination of the procedure.

In certain circumstances, the donor selection criteria can be somewhat relaxed. A minor degree of pulmonary infiltrate can be accepted in a donor used for a bilateral transplant. On occasion, a donor is identified with marginal gas exchange and radiographic evidence of a unilateral pulmonary infiltrate. In some such situations, we have made an intraoperative assessment with ventilation and perfusion only to the seemingly normal donor lung, judged that lung

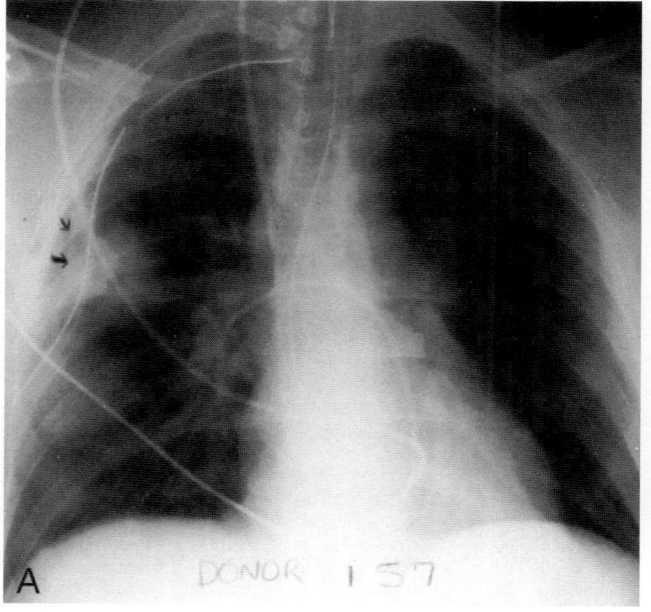

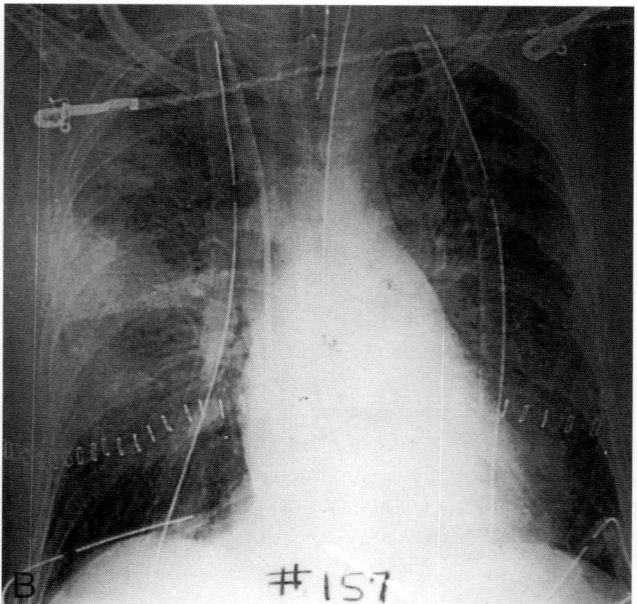

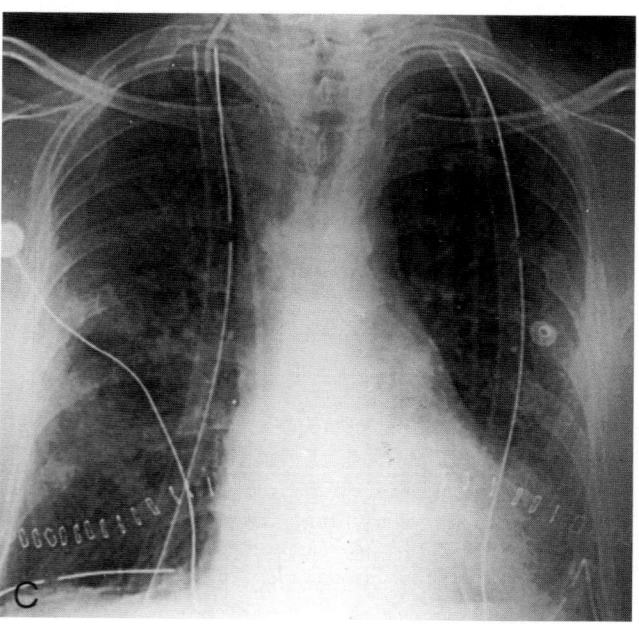

Fig. 92-1. A. Anteroposterior chest radiograph from a patient experiencing brain death as a result of a motor vehicle accident. The right chest tube evacuated a 50% pneumothorax. *Arrows* denote a right upper lobe contusion. Several hours later, both lungs were harvested for use as bilateral sequential allografts in a patient with obstructive lung disease. **B.** Immediate postoperative radiograph of recipient demonstrates some progression of the right upper lobe contusion. **C.** Chest radiograph taken 3 days after transplantation. Note the dramatic clearing of the right upper lobe contusion.

to be acceptable, and conducted a successful unilateral transplant. This procedure has been reported by Puskas and associates (1992a).

Our most recent experience with the use of marginal donors to expand the donor pool was reported by Sundaresan and colleagues (1995a). Of 133 consecutive donors, 44 were considered marginal due to one or more of the standard criteria: age older than 55 years, smoking history greater than 20 pack-years, unsatisfactory chest radiograph, or arterial oxygen tension less than 300 mm Hg. Evaluation of the recipients showed no difference in the median length of mechanical ventilation postoperatively, nor was there a dif-

ference in the mean alveolar-arterial oxygen gradient (Figs. 92-1, 92-2). Immediate and intermediate survival was identical for the two groups.

Finally, we have looked carefully at how the outcome of lung transplantation is affected by various permutations of lung procurement: local procurement by the transplanting team, distant procurement by the transplanting team, and distant procurement by other teams of surgeons. These results, reported by Shiraishi and associates (1997), suggest that the use of donor lungs retrieved by other teams results in transplant outcomes equal to those resulting from local or distant procurement by the transplanting team.

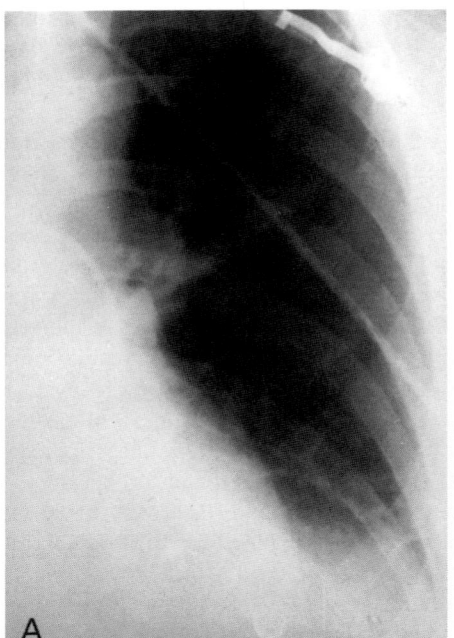 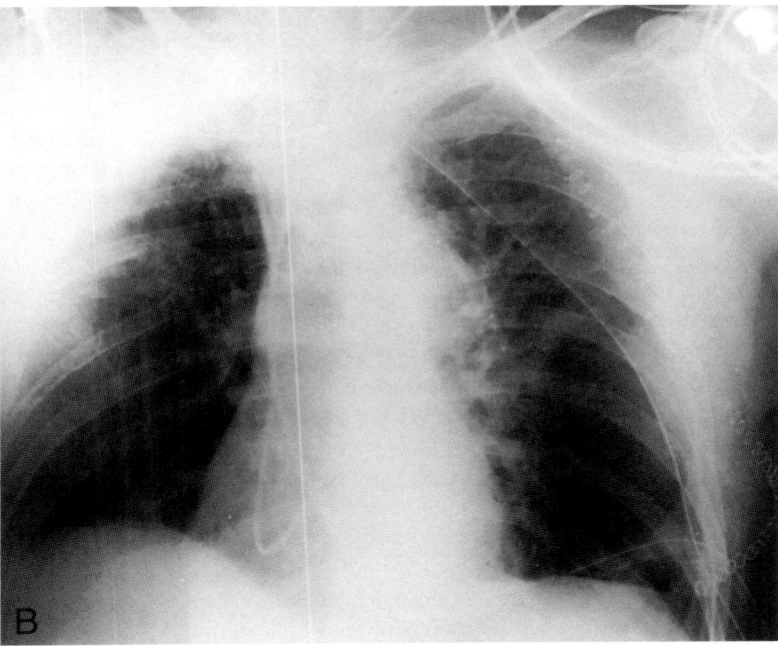

Fig. 92-2. A. Radiographic image of the left lung in a donor with borderline gas exchange. Note the left lower lobe atelectasis. Preharvest fiberoptic bronchoscopy revealed a left lower lobe mucus plug that was evacuated, resulting in satisfactory reexpansion of the left lower lobe. **B.** Postoperative anteroposterior chest radiograph of recipient of the left lung allograft in (**A**) reveals satisfactory expansion of the allograft. The patient obtained an excellent result.

LUNG PRESERVATION

Lung preservation has been the focus of intense laboratory interest since the start of lung transplantation. Many authors have reviewed the current state of the art of lung preservation, including Kirk (1993) and Novick (1996) and their coworkers, as well as Unruh (1995). Clinical pulmonary preservation has progressed considerably since the Toronto Group initially carried out unilateral lung transplantation using donor lungs harvested in an atelectatic state and stored by topical hypothermic immersion, as reported by Todd and associates (1988). Minor differences occur in the preservation strategies of most clinical lung transplant programs, but the basic principles remain the same.

After systemic donor heparinization and just before circulatory arrest, a pulmonary vasodilator is used, usually administered by direct bolus injection into the pulmonary artery. We use 500 μg of prostaglandin E_1 (PGE$_1$). Pulmonary arterial flush is then achieved with the lungs in a state of moderate inflation at an FIO$_2$ greater than room air. In most programs, an intracellular flush solution is used, most commonly modified Euro-Collins solution (4 mg MgSO$_4$), 3% glucose, or University of Wisconsin (UW) solution. After extraction, the lung allograft is immersed in iced crystalloid solution and maintained in a semi-inflated state during transport. This technique results in reliable allograft function with ischemic times of up to 6 hours. We have, on occasion, extended the ischemic time, particularly

for the second lung of a bilateral sequential transplantation, in which the ischemic time has reached 8 to 10 hours with satisfactory subsequent function.

The delivery of the pulmonary flush solution is typically performed in an antegrade manner through the main pulmonary artery. The addition of retrograde perfusion, either before or after antegrade flush, has been described by Varela and colleagues (1997), and this technique has been used in our clinical program with success. There are potential benefits of improved distribution of flush solution with retrograde delivery. In addition, for donors at high risk for acute pulmonary thromboembolism, retrograde flush can identify and remove embolic clot from the pulmonary artery—clot that might otherwise go undetected if flush is delivered only in an anterograde fashion.

A detailed review of experimental pulmonary preservation is beyond the scope of this chapter, but several interesting developments have occurred.

Inflation

We formerly believed that hyperinflation of donor lungs was advantageous, as demonstrated by the work of Puskas and colleagues (1992b). After using this technique in our clinical program and experiencing an increased incidence of reperfusion edema as a result, we have stopped using hyperinflation. We now recommend that lungs be flushed and stored at a moderate stage of inflation consistent with normal end-tidal volumes.

Temperature of Flush and Storage

In virtually all clinical lung transplant programs, pulmonary artery flush temperature is 1° to 4°C. After extraction, lungs are immersed in crystalloid solution and packed in ice, resulting in their storage and transport at approximately 1°C. Some investigators have shown that a more moderate degree of hypothermia (10°C) results in superior lung function. We demonstrated this principle in our own laboratory in an in vitro rabbit lung perfusion model by Wang and coworkers (1993) as well as a standard model of canine left lung allotransplantation and bilateral baboon lung transplantation documented by Sundaresan and associates (1993a). In a previous study, however, Mayer and colleagues (1992) were unable to show a difference between storage at 4°C versus 10°C in canine left lung allografts. The current practice worldwide, as described by Hopkinson and coworkers (1998), is divided, with 70% of programs storing grafts at 0° to 5°C and 30% storing at 5° to 10°C.

Composition of Flush Solution

Considerable controversy has surrounded the optimal composition of pulmonary flush solution. A variety of solutions now are used clinically. Hakim and coworkers (1988) of the Papworth group popularized the use of an extracellular solution supplemented with donor blood to achieve a flush hematocrit of approximately 10%. During the past several years, a number of experimental studies, such as that of Keshavjee and associates (1992), have demonstrated that an extracellular low-potassium dextran (LPD) solution provided superior function over the standard intracellular Euro-Collins solution. It was argued that this low-potassium dextran solution induced less pulmonary vasoconstriction during flush. Puskas and associates (1992a), however, showed that if pulmonary vasodilatation is achieved with PGE_1 before flush, Euro-Collins solution provides preservation equivalent to that achieved with LPD. A commercially available LPD solution (Perfadex) is now in use in a number of Canadian and European transplant programs.

Several groups of investigators have used the intracellular UW solution and observed acceptable results. The Pittsburgh group, as reported by Hardesty and colleagues (1993), conducted a retrospective review of their experience and concluded that UW solution may provide superior preservation to that observed with the more commonly used modified Euro-Collins solution.

Pharmacologic Manipulation

In addition to their apparent benefit when administered before pulmonary artery flush, as documented by Mayer and

coworkers (1992), evidence suggests that vasodilator prostanoids also may have some beneficial effect in the early post-transplant period. Matsuzaki and associates (1993) demonstrated that PGE_1 infusion ameliorated the reperfusion injury after 2 hours of warm ischemia in an in situ rabbit lung model. We continued this work, demonstrating that PGE_1 significantly improves canine lung allograft function after an 18-hour ischemic period, as noted by Aoe and colleagues (1994). We continue to use PGE_1 routinely during the postoperative period in our clinical program. A mounting body of evidence suggests that oxygen-free radicals are important in the genesis of ischemia reperfusion injury in the lung. This subject was concisely reviewed by Christie and Waddell (1993). Other antioxidant interventions including enzymatic (superoxide dismutase, catalase, glutathione peroxidase) as well as nonenzymatic (allopurinol, glutathione, dimethyl-thiourea and lazaroid) have shown impressive results in reducing lung reperfusion injury. Some of these agents have been used with success in clinical lung transplant programs.

The use of inhaled nitric oxide (NO) has been shown to be beneficial in many steps of the lung transplant process. We have demonstrated that inhaled NO administered to the lung recipient is effective in reducing early allograft dysfunction. Date and associates (1996) reported these findings. Fujino and colleagues (1997) reported our work showing that inhaled NO administered to the donor at the time of organ procurement also reduces post-transplantation reperfusion injury. Meyer and colleagues have reviewed the proved and potential applications of NO in the setting of lung transplantation. Yamashita and associates (1996) showed nitroprusside to improve early lung allograft function. We use nitroprusside 1 mg/L in the flush solution in our clinical program, and we are investigating the use of inhaled NO to ameliorate pulmonary hypertension during recipient pneumonectomy and during the early period of graft reperfusion when allograft pulmonary vascular resistance is transiently elevated.

The mechanism of ischemia-reperfusion injury is complex but believed to include activation of leukocytes that eventually produce free radical oxygen species and thereby cause endothelial damage. One approach to minimizing reperfusion injury is to avoid leukocyte activation during initial reperfusion. This goal has been met in several ways, including the inhibition of neutrophil adhesion, as described by Schmid and coworkers (1997), and the complete elimination of leukocytes from the reperfusate solution during the early critical minutes of reperfusion as reported by Shiraishi and colleagues (1998).

In the last 2 years, promising work has been produced on the effects of controlled reperfusion of the lung allograft after implantation. This work is an extension of studies performed originally on ischemic hearts, such as those of Okamoto and colleagues (1986). Bhabra and colleagues (1996) demonstrated improved graft function if the initial 10 minutes of reperfusion were controlled to limit the pulmonary artery pressure to 50% of the physiologic pressure. Halldorsson and colleagues (1998) controlled both the pressure and composition of the perfusate for 10 minutes, using a low-pressure, substrate-enriched, hypocalcemic, hyperosmolar, alkaline solution and demonstrated better lung function in all measured parameters.

TECHNIQUE

Donor Lung Extraction

Our donor extraction technique was reported by Sundaresan and associates (1993b). After the lung extraction team's arrival at the donor hospital, it is important for the team to assess the chest radiographs and to perform fiberoptic bronchoscopy. Final assessment is made by gross inspection of the lungs, which are exposed by median sternotomy performed in conjunction with the midline laparotomy for extraction of abdominal organs.

The abdominal organs are prepared for extraction by the responsible surgical teams. It is important for the liver extraction team to insert a large-caliber cannula in the inferior vena cava for liver flush effluent rather than planning to vent the hepatic flush into the chest through the divided inferior vena cava, thereby obscuring the thoracic organ extraction team's view.

Both venae cavae are encircled within the pericardium. The aorta is mobilized and encircled. Care must be taken to avoid injury to the right main pulmonary artery lying immediately posterior to the superior vena cava and ascending aorta. It is not necessary to dissect the main pulmonary artery.

The donor is heparinized. A cardioplegia cannula is placed in the ascending aorta. A large-bore pulmonary flush cannula then is placed in the main pulmonary artery immediately proximal to its bifurcation. PGE$_1$, 500 µg, is administered directly into the main pulmonary artery, which produces an immediate fall in systemic pressure. At this point, venous inflow occlusion is achieved by double ligation of the superior vena cava and clamping of the inferior vena cava at the diaphragm. The aorta is then cross clamped and cardioplegic solution is initiated. Cardioplegia is vented through the inferior vena cava, which is divided immediately above the previously placed clamp. After cardioplegic arrest has been achieved, lung flush is started. With the lungs maintained in a state of moderate inflation, pulmonary artery flush is achieved with 3 L of modified Euro-Collins solution delivered at a pressure of 30 cm H$_2$O. This solution is vented through the amputated tip of the left atrial appendage (Fig. 92-3). Cold effluent is allowed to collect in both pleural spaces. Topical hypothermia is supplemented by crushed ice.

We prefer to extract the donor heart in situ. It should be stated emphatically that satisfactory cardiac and bilateral lung grafts can be safely extracted in every situation. The superior vena cava is divided between the previously placed

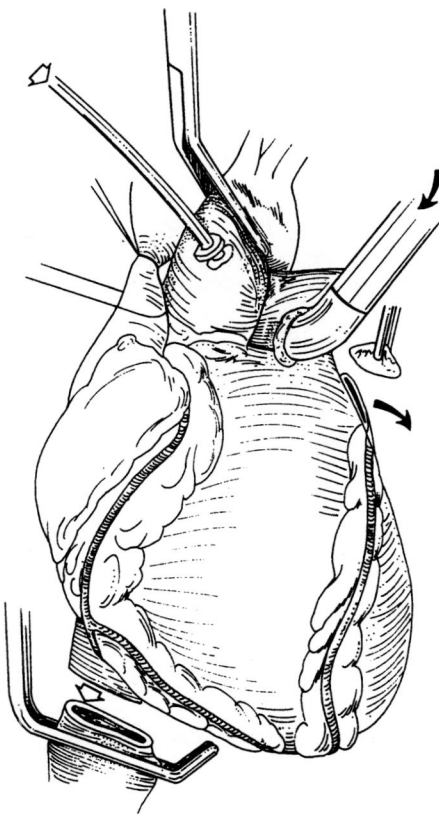

Fig. 92-3. Cardioplegia is administered proximal to an aortic cross clamp and vented through the transected inferior vena cava (*open arrow*). Pulmonary flush solution is administered through the main pulmonary artery and vented through the amputated tip of the left atrial appendage (*solid arrows*).

ligatures, once again taking care not to injure the underlying right main pulmonary artery. The aorta is divided superior to the cardioplegia cannula. The main pulmonary artery then is divided through the cannulation site. The heart then is elevated and retracted to the right. The left atrium is opened midway between the coronary sinus and the inferior pulmonary vein. The left atrial incision is continued toward the right. The right side of the left atrial wall is divided, taking care to preserve a rim of atrial muscle on the pulmonary vein side (Fig. 92-4). This step completes the cardiac excision.

Extraction of the lungs is continued by mobilization and division of the trachea well above the carina. Our preference is to divide the trachea with a stapling instrument at the end of exhalation. The great vessels are divided at the apex of the chest, and the esophagus is transected with a stapling instrument. The entire thoracic contents then are extracted from the spine in a caudal direction. The thoracic aorta and esophagus are transected at the diaphragm. The lung allografts are immersed in cold crystalloid solution and transported semiinflated. Should each lung be used in different transplant centers, they are separated into distinct allografts at the donor hospital. The donor left main bronchus is divided at its origin with a cutting stapling device to leave the airway

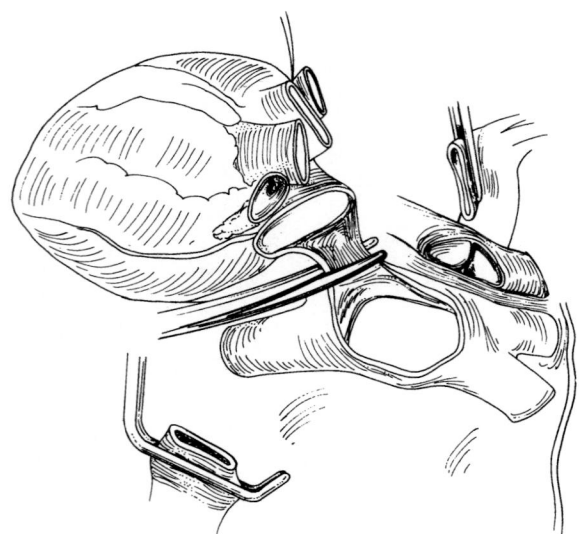

Fig. 92-4. The ascending aorta is divided. The main pulmonary artery has been transected at its bifurcation. The heart is retracted upward and to the right to enable safe division of the left atrium, leaving suitable cuffs on both cardiac and lung allografts.

to both lungs sealed (Fig. 92-5). Otherwise, the grafts should be transported en bloc for separation immediately before implantation. On arrival at the recipient hospital, the graft is exposed and kept cold during the remainder of its preparation. The esophagus and aorta are removed, taking care to leave all other soft tissues on the specimen side to maximize bronchial arterial collateral flow to the donor lung.

Viewing the double-lung block from its anterior aspect, the posterior pericardium is divided from inferior to supe-

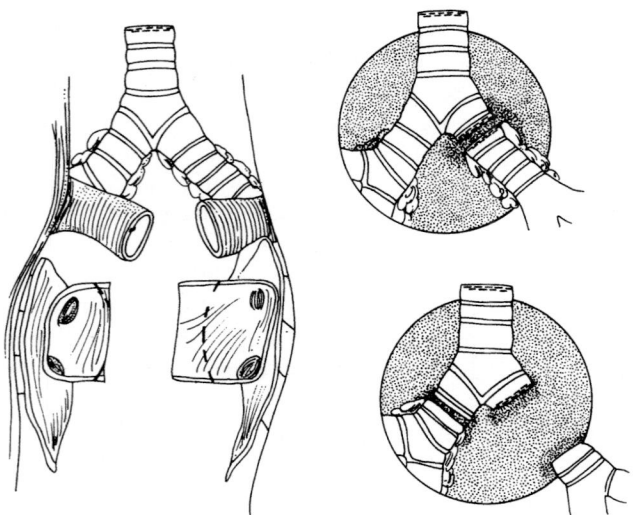

Fig. 92-5. The pericardium and left atrium are divided with the left atrium further trimmed (*dotted lines*). The airway is transected and kept sealed using a GIA stapling device across the proximal left mainstem bronchus. The donor airway is further revised for implantation, as shown at the bottom right.

rior. The posterior wall of the left atrium is divided, leaving equal atrial cuffs on both sides. The remaining pericardium posterior to the left atrium is then divided. The pulmonary artery is divided at its bifurcation (see Fig. 92-5). It is important to separate the pulmonary artery from its pericardial attachments on each side out to the first pulmonary arterial branch. This separation prevents compromise of pulmonary artery caliber distal to the pulmonary artery anastomosis after implantation.

Subcarinal nodes are divided, and the left main bronchus is transected. The left main bronchus is dissected from nodal tissue and divided at a point two rings proximal to the upper lobe orifice. On the right side, excision of the carina usually provides an adequate length (two rings proximal to the upper-lobe origin) for subsequent bronchial anastomosis. It is important during dissection of the bronchus to minimize any nodal dissection at the site of bronchus transection to maximize retrograde bronchial collateral blood flow to the donor bronchus after transplantation.

Recipient Preparation

Anesthesia

A successful lung transplant program requires active involvement of expert anesthesiologists familiar with complex cardiothoracic anesthesia techniques, bronchoscopy, and cardiopulmonary bypass. Full hemodynamic monitoring is required in every patient. We routinely use a Foley catheter, central venous line, pulmonary artery Swan-Ganz catheter, and radial artery catheters. It is often useful to supplement the radial artery catheter with a femoral artery line, especially for cases in which we anticipate a difficult dissection and hemodynamic instability. We also use a transesophageal echocardiographic probe in every patient, but its application is especially critical in patients with severe pulmonary hypertension and coexistent right ventricular dysfunction.

The airway is routinely intubated with a left-sided double-lumen endobronchial tube. In small patients, a single-lumen tube with an endobronchial Fogarty catheter enables independent ventilation; however, this technique does not have the reliability of a double-lumen tube. A single-lumen tube can present difficulties, particularly in a bilateral transplant recipient in whom intraoperative maneuvering of the tube can be troublesome. In patients with cystic fibrosis, thick, tenacious purulent secretions are continuously expressed into the bronchial lumen during manipulation of the lungs for extraction. We generally place a large-caliber, single-lumen tube and, using a flexible fiberoptic bronchoscope, aspirate the airway completely before placement of the double-lumen tube and initiation of the procedure. It is extremely difficult to evacuate secretions from the airway, particularly through a small-caliber double-lumen endotracheal tube. For many patients, it is preferable to use a single-lumen tube and anticipate using cardiopulmonary bypass during extraction and implantation. Spray and associates (1994) reported this approach to be the standard technique for bilateral transplantation in children. It has been our practice to use aprotinin routinely when we anticipate intrapleural adhesions, such as in cystic fibrosis, bronchiectasis, and patients with previous thoracic surgery. This agent, as noted by Westaby (1993), effectively has reduced perioperative blood loss, especially when cardiopulmonary bypass is required in patients with extensive pleural or mediastinal adhesions.

Single-Lung Transplantation

Choice of Side

We prefer to transplant the side having the lesser function as judged by preoperative quantitative nuclear perfusion scans. It was argued previously that the right side was preferable for patients with obstructive lung disease. However, in our experience and that of others, including Levin and coworkers (1994), there is no difference in functional outcome among single-lung recipients regardless of transplant side. If cardiopulmonary bypass is anticipated, as in patients with primary pulmonary hypertension or severe pulmonary fibrosis with associated pulmonary hypertension, the right side is the preferred transplant side. For patients with Eisenmenger's syndrome, we prefer the right side to facilitate closure of the coexisting atrial or ventricular septal defect. A patent ductus arteriosus can be repaired in association with transplantation to either side.

Exposure

A generous posterolateral thoracotomy through the fifth interspace or bed of the excised fifth rib is the preferred approach. However, an anterolateral incision through the fourth interspace with division of the medial fourth costal cartilage provides excellent exposure as well. This muscle-sparing approach has been described by Pochettino and Bavaria (1997) and has been used successfully in our program as well. For right-sided transplants for which cardiopulmonary bypass is anticipated, cannulation of the ascending aorta is facilitated by the use of a fourth interspace incision. Median sternotomy can be used for right-sided transplants, especially if associated cardiac repair dictates an anterior approach permitting access to the left side of the heart. Patients are always positioned with the ipsilateral groin in the operative field for subsequent cannulation if necessary. Femoral partial bypass was formerly our technique of choice; however, intrathoracic cannulation avoids a groin incision and the necessary arterial and venous repairs following decannulation. The ascending aorta and right atrium can be cannulated easily through the right chest. The cannulas are positioned in the anterior aspect of the incision and remain well out of the operative field through-

out the procedure. Through a left posterolateral thoracotomy, the proximal left pulmonary artery and descending aorta can be adequately cannulated, but the aortic cannula can inhibit subsequent placement of the donor lung in the posterior aspect of the left side of the chest.

Recipient Pneumonectomy

After adequate exposure of the pleural space, pleural adhesions are divided. Adhesions can be extensive in patients with fibrotic or septic lung disease but ordinarily are absent in patients with emphysema and primary pulmonary hypertension. Extreme care is taken not to injure the phrenic and recurrent laryngeal nerves. The inferior ligament is divided. The pulmonary veins and main pulmonary artery are encircled outside the pericardium. During this dissection, the need for cardiopulmonary bypass is determined. Ventilation of the contralateral lung and occlusion of the ipsilateral pulmonary artery determine whether the contralateral native lung will provide adequate gas exchange and hemodynamics to tolerate pneumonectomy and implantation without cardiopulmonary bypass. Assessment of right ventricular contractility with the transesophageal echo probe is especially useful at this point.

The first branch of the pulmonary artery then is ligated and divided. The pulmonary artery just distal to this branch is stapled proximally and ligated distally to eliminate back-bleeding after division. The pulmonary veins are divided between staple lines or between silk ligatures placed on each venous branch at the hilum. This latter option increases the size of the subsequent left atrial cuff. Peribronchial nodal tissue is divided, and bronchial arterial vessels are secured with ligatures. The bronchus is transected just proximal to the upper lobe origin and the lung is excised (Fig. 92-6). The recipient bronchus is then trimmed back up into the mediastinum, taking care to avoid any devascularization of the recipient bronchus at the site of anastomosis. The peri-

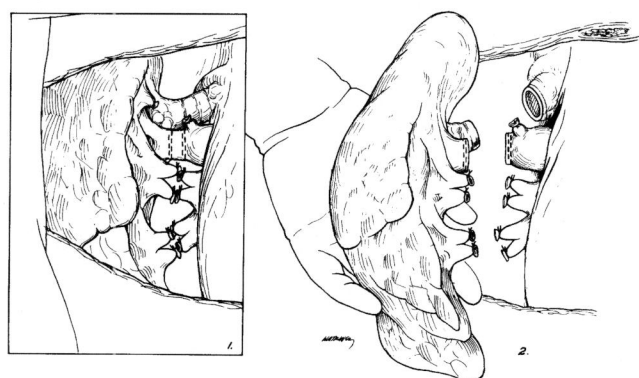

Fig. 92-6. Excision of the native right lung. The pulmonary artery is stapled beyond its first upper lobe branch. Pulmonary veins are divided between ligatures and the bronchus is transected just proximal to the upper lobe orifice.

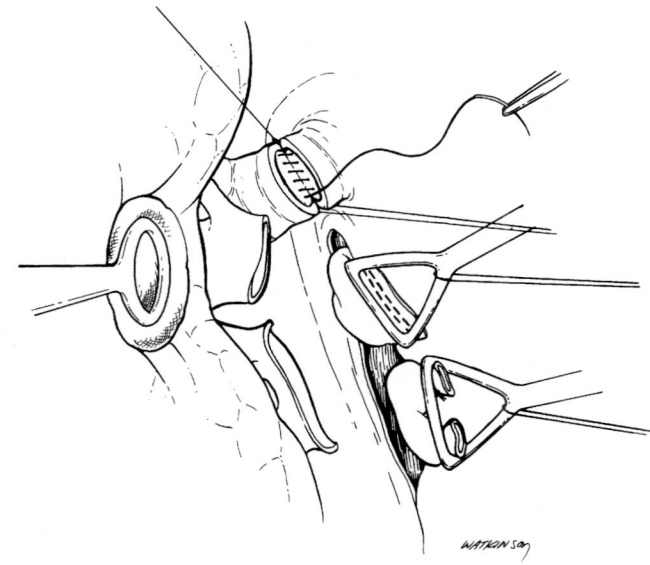

A

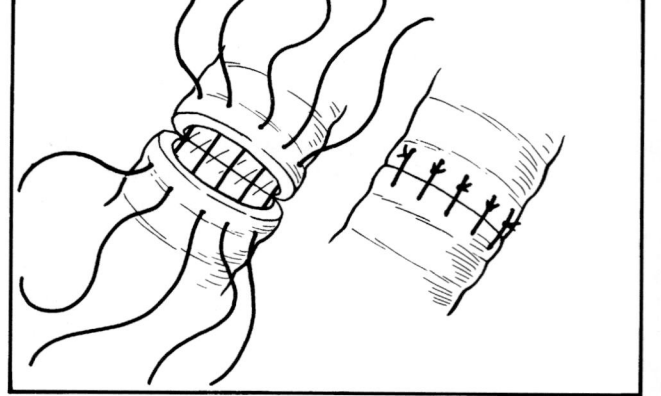

B

C

Fig. 92-7. A right bronchial anastomosis is depicted, with the lung cooled by topical crushed ice. **A.** The membranous wall is closed first. **B.** The cartilaginous wall is closed with interrupted figure-of-eight sutures without any attempt to intentionally telescope one end into another. **C.** Small bronchi are joined with simple interrupted sutures to avoid even the smallest amount of narrowing caused by the figure-of-eight sutures. Peribronchial nodal tissue covers the anastomosis. From Meyers BF, et al: Bilateral sequential lung transplant without sternal division eliminates post-transplant sternal complications. J Thorac Cardiovasc Surg *117*:358, 1999. With permission.

cardium around the vein stumps then is widely opened, and hemostasis is achieved in the mediastinum.

Implantation

The donor lung, wrapped in cold, moist gauze, is placed in the posterior portion of the thorax. In this position, manipulation of the lung can be avoided during the entire implantation. The lung is kept cold by topical application of crushed ice. This topical hypothermia provides an extended period of cold preservation, giving additional time for meticulous anastomoses.

The bronchial anastomosis is performed first (Fig. 92-7). Various techniques have been described. Our preference is to initially close the membranous posterior wall using a continuous suture of 4–0 absorbable monofilament suture. The anterior cartilaginous airway is then closed with four or five interrupted figure-of-eight sutures. In our experience reported by Date and associates (1995), this procedure results in the lowest incidence of anastomotic complications. For small-caliber bronchi, an end-to-end closure is obtained using simple interrupted sutures of monofilament absorbable material. The bronchial anastomosis is always covered using local peribronchial nodal tissue.

A vascular clamp is then placed as proximal as possible on the ipsilateral main pulmonary artery. The donor and recipient

arteries are trimmed to size and an end-to-end anastomosis is created using 5-0 polypropylene sutures (Fig. 92-8). It is important, of course, to maintain proper orientation of donor to recipient artery and to avoid compromising the lumen during creation of the anastomosis. Lateral traction on the pulmonary vein stumps enables central placement of an angled atrial clamp. For right-sided transplants, it is occasionally necessary to open the intra-atrial groove to increase the length of recipient left atrium available for clamp placement. Pulmonary vein stumps are then amputated and the bridge of tissue between the two is incised to create a suitable cuff for the left atrial anastomosis (Fig. 92-9). After completion of this anastomosis but before tying the final stitch, the lung is gently inflated while the pulmonary artery clamp is temporarily removed, enabling the lung to be "de-aired" through the open left atrial anastomosis. All suture lines are then secured and inspected, and the vascular clamps are removed.

If bypass was used, it can be discontinued safely at this point. Our practice is to initiate reperfusion with the recipient receiving a continuous infusion of PGE$_1$. This infusion is continued for at least 24 hours after transplantation, unless the recipient is hypotensive and the pulmonary arterial pressures are correspondingly low. The use of bolus corticosteroid administration during implantation is controversial.

Two drains are left in each pleural space, and routine closure is performed using absorbable suture material. At the

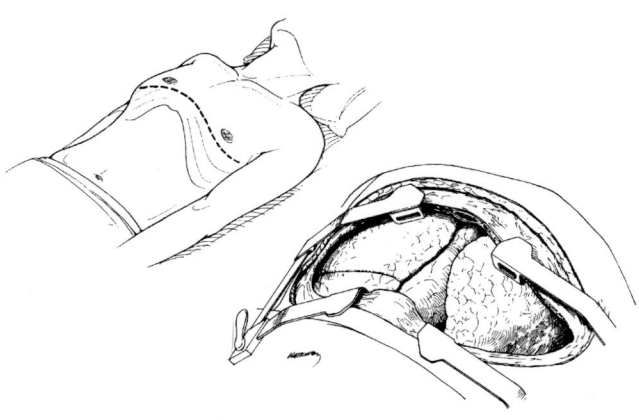

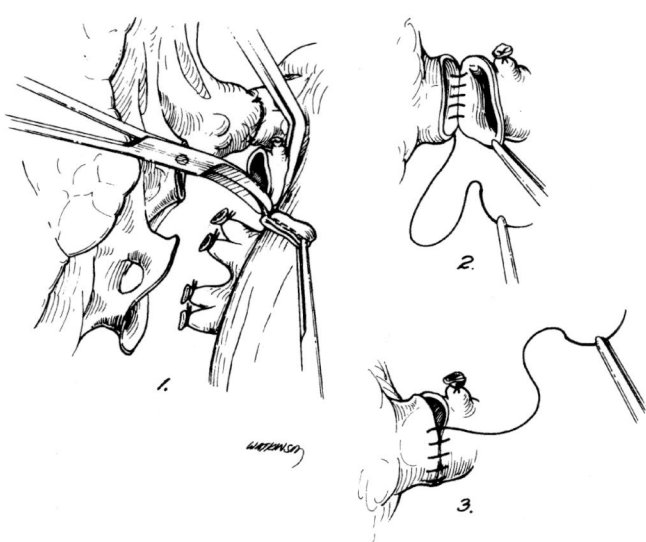

Fig. 92-8. A central pulmonary artery clamp is placed, the staple line is excised, and an end-to-end anastomosis is constructed with 5-0 polypropylene.

termination of the procedure, the double-lumen endotracheal tube is replaced with a large-caliber, single-lumen tube. Flexible bronchoscopy is performed to inspect the bronchial anastomosis and to clear the airway of any blood or secretions.

Bilateral Lung Transplantation

Exposure

Traditionally, bilateral sequential single-lung transplantation is conducted through bilateral anterolateral fourth or

Fig. 92-10. Bilateral anterolateral thoracotomies are performed through the fourth or fifth interspace with transverse division of the sternum.

fifth interspace thoracotomies connected by a transverse sternotomy (Fig. 92-10). This "clamshell" incision as described by Pasque and associates (1990) provides adequate exposure for safe division of pleural adhesions. In patients with cystic fibrosis, adhesions can be particularly dense at the apex and posterior aspect of the chest. In addition, this incision provides satisfactory exposure for institution of cardiopulmonary bypass by ascending aortic and right atrial cannulation. However, we no longer divide the sternum as we have found that adequate exposure (Fig. 92-11) is achieved to conduct a safe transplant procedure while avoiding the complications of sternotomy. Our results as reported by one of us (B.F.M., 1999) demonstrated the safety of a "sternal sparing" approach and the complete avoidance of sternal complications, such as the migration of the stabilizing pin required to maintain sternal alignment after a full clamshell incision (Fig. 92-12).

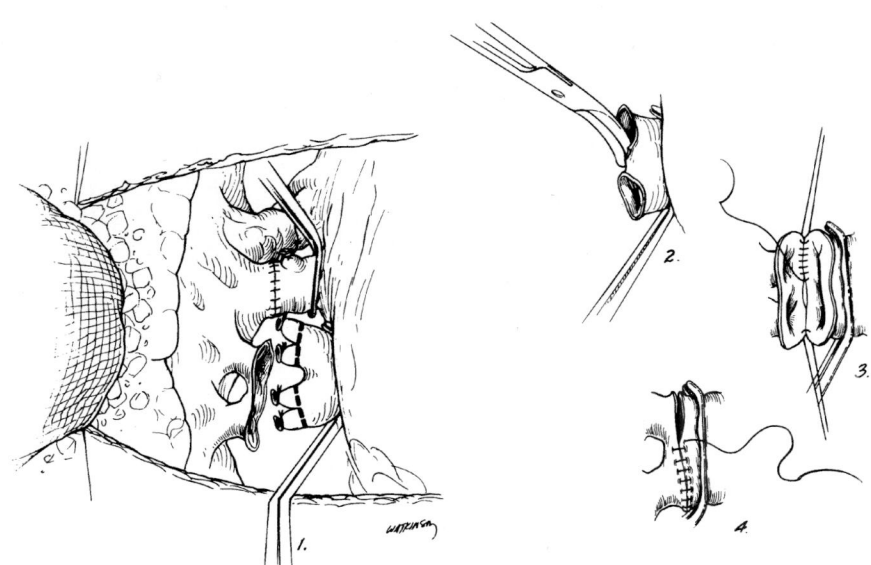

Fig. 92-9. A central left atrial clamp is in place while the vein stumps are amputated and the bridge of atrial muscle is divided. 4-0 polypropylene suture is used to complete the anastomosis.

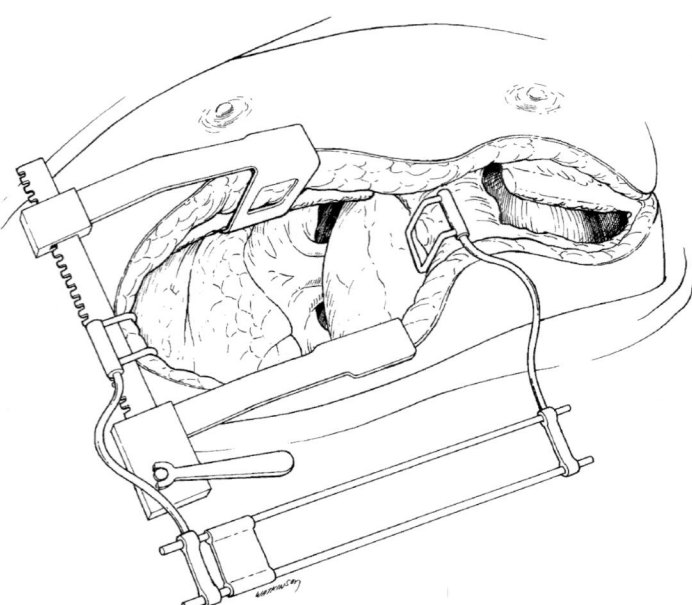

Fig. 92-11. A Finichietto chest retractor is used to spread the ribs vertically, while a Balfour retractor is placed with one jaw on the sternum and one jaw on the muscle and skin of the lateral chest. The intercostal muscle division is carried far more lateral and posterior than the skin incision to maximize rib spreading. The combined effects of these two retractors typically result in excellent exposure without sternal division. From Meyers BF, et al: Bilateral sequential lung transplant without sternal division eliminates post-transplant sternal complications. J Thorac Cardiovasc Surg *117*:358, 1999. With permission.

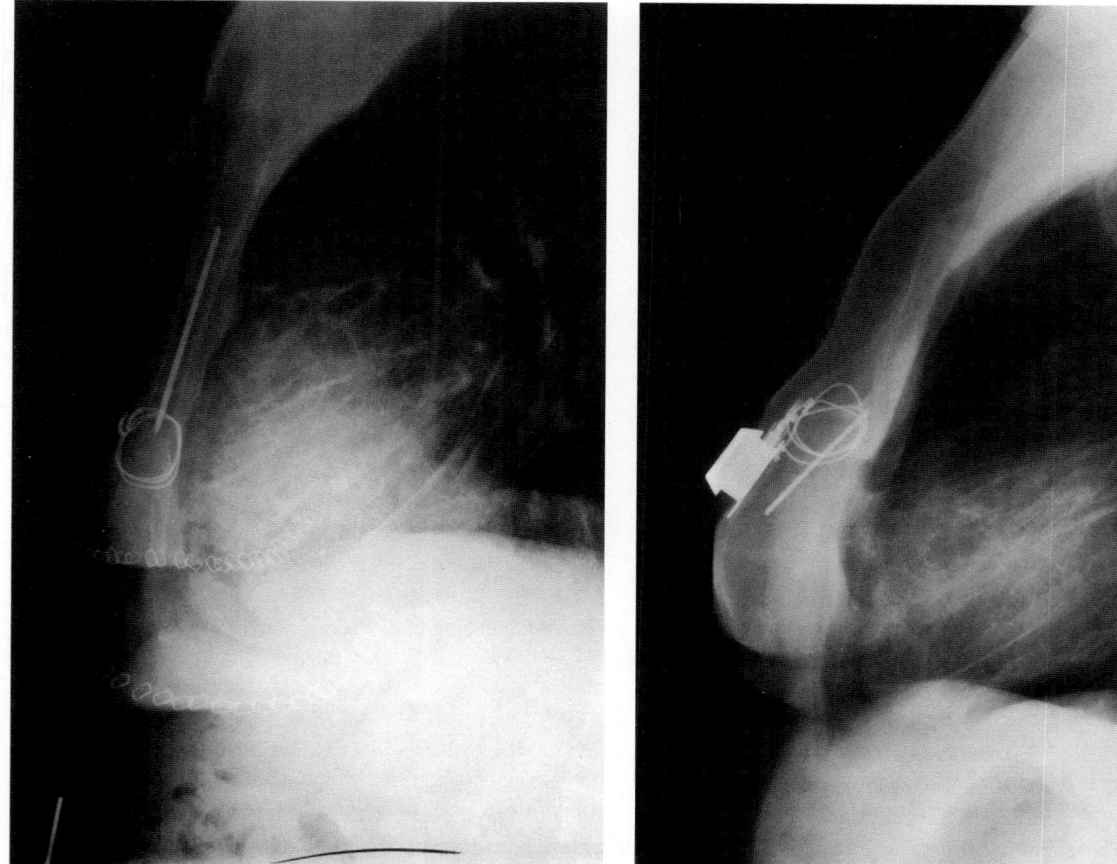

A   B

Fig. 92-12. These lateral radiographs show patients immediately after bilateral sequential lung transplantation using a standard clamshell thoracosternotomy. In the first radiograph (**A**), one of the sternal K-wires has migrated out of the sternum and resides in the anterior abdominal wall. In the second radiograph (**B**), a K-wire has protruded through the anterior sternum, and its sharp end resides just beneath the skin. Both pins required surgical removal. Use of Steinmann pins, or avoidance of transverse sternotomy, will eliminate the possibility of K-wire migration.

Pneumonectomy and Implantation

The techniques of pneumonectomy and implantation are identical to those just described for single-lung transplantation. The side with worse function, as determined by preoperative ventilation and perfusion scans, is replaced first. Cardiopulmonary bypass may prove necessary at several junctures during bilateral sequential transplantation. In patients with small airways not amenable to double-lumen tube placement, cardiopulmonary bypass is instituted after mobilization of both lungs and is maintained during bilateral extraction and implantation. Occasionally, the remaining contralateral native lung does not enable satisfactory gas exchange or hemodynamics during removal or replacement of the first lung. Cardiopulmonary bypass is instituted at that point. The most common situation in which bypass proves necessary occurs after implantation of the first lung. The transplanted lung may not support the recipient's circulation and gas exchange, manifesting as progressive increases in pulmonary artery pressure despite increasing doses of PGE_1. Pulmonary edema develops with associated hypoxemia. Although this clinical phenomenon is typical, its etiology is not well understood. It may occur because of poor preservation or, alternatively, from systemic bacteremia in the recipient because it is observed commonly after implantation of the first lung in cystic fibrosis patients. It is prudent to institute cardiopulmonary bypass as soon as this problem develops rather than waiting until it has become an emergent situation in an unstable patient.

Some authors advocate direct revascularization of the bronchial circulation. In this circumstance, the aortic button previously mentioned in the discussion about donor dissection is identified after reperfusion. A back bleeding orifice is assumed to be of bronchial origin. Alternatively, at the time of allograft preparation, the suspected right bronchial arterial orifice can be marked by a fine suture. Revascularization is then achieved by an anastomosis of the bronchial arterial orifice to one of the internal mammary arteries, as suggested by Daly and colleagues (1993), or by the use of a saphenous vein graft between the orifice and the aorta, as initially recommended by Couraud and associates (1992). Norgaard and colleagues (1997) reported a 2-year patency of 100% in 23 patients revascularized using the internal mammary artery.

POSTOPERATIVE MANAGEMENT

Ventilation

In general, patients are ventilated with standard ventilatory techniques. The F_{IO_2} value is kept at a level so as to maintain the Pa_{O_2} greater than 70 mm Hg. A tidal volume of 10 to 12 mL/kg is usually sufficient, and PEEP of 5.0 to 7.5 cm H_2O is used in most patients. Extubation is performed in accordance with standard requirements of satisfactory gas exchange and mechanics. Most patients are extubated within 24 to 48 hours of transplantation following a standard intermittent mandatory ventilation (IMV) or pressure support wean. This type of ventilatory management is applied in all bilateral lung transplant recipients as well as in single-lung recipients undergoing transplantation because of pulmonary fibrosis.

Patients undergoing single-lung transplantation for chronic obstructive lung disease or pulmonary vascular disease are managed differently, however. In the former condition, we make an effort to avoid the use of PEEP and select tidal volumes that are somewhat lower than would ordinarily be used. These adjustments are made to try to reduce hyperinflation of the contralateral hypercompliant native lung with resultant compression of the less compliant transplanted lung. This situation can be a major problem (Fig. 92-13). In some patients, volume reduction of the native lung by lobectomy has been performed to decompress the contralateral transplanted lung either late postoperatively, as described by Kroshus and associates (1996), or at the time of transplantation, as reported by Todd and colleagues (1997). In patients with pulmonary vascular disease, we use a prolonged period (48 to 72 hours) of elective ventilation. Patients are kept heavily sedated and often paralyzed for that period of time. We choose to maintain these patients in a position with the native lung dependent so as to maintain inflation and appropriate drainage of the transplanted lung. Tidal volumes are standard, but PEEP of 7.5 to 10 cm H_2O is applied.

In some patients, early graft dysfunction, rejection, or infection necessitates a prolonged period of postoperative mechanical ventilation. We have no hesitation to perform tracheostomy in these patients. The procedure facilitates mobilization of the patient, improved oral nutrition, and generally a more positive attitude in the ventilator-dependent patient.

Fluid Management

During the first few postoperative days, fluid management is monitored carefully by determination of pulmonary capillary wedge pressure and daily weight. In spite of the vigilance of our anesthesiology colleagues, most patients return from the operating room with a significant positive fluid balance. Diuretics are used aggressively during the early postoperative period. On occasion, patients having single-lung transplantation for primary pulmonary hypertension develop hemodynamic instability if the filling pressures on the right side of the heart are excessively reduced. These patients do require a higher filling pressure on this side during the first weeks after transplantation.

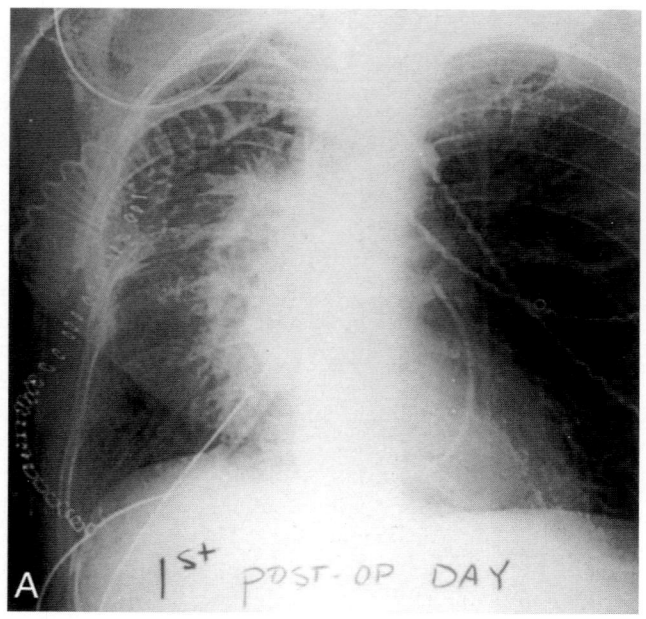

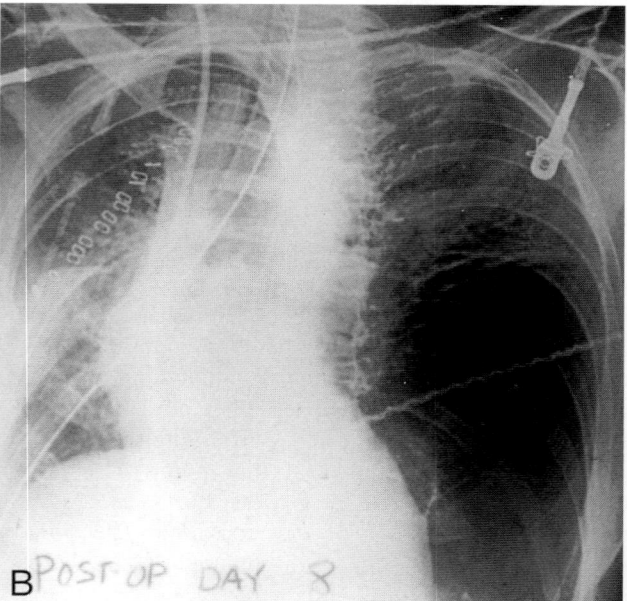

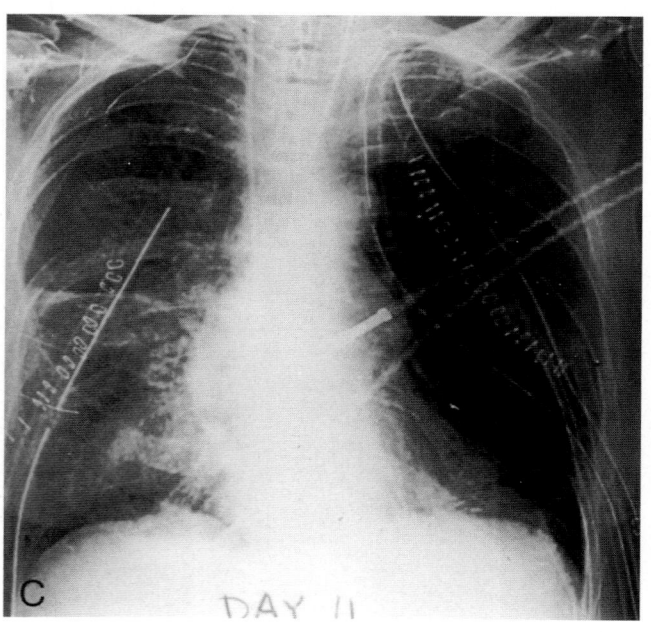

Fig. 92-13. A. Anteroposterior chest radiograph from a patient with obstructive lung disease 1 day after right single-lung transplant. Note a modest perihilar infiltrate in the allograft, presumably from reimplantation edema. Modest mediastinal shift to the allograft side is observed. **B.** One week later. Hyperexpansion of the native left lower lobe is observed, along with further shift of the mediastinum and compression of the allograft. The patient underwent left lower lobectomy on postoperative day 9. **C.** Left lower lobe resection enabled the mediastinum to shift back toward the midline with decompression of the allograft.

Sepsis Prophylaxis

Bacterial Infection

All patients are given routine antibacterial prophylaxis, most often with cefepime and vancomycin. Administration of these agents is continued for several days. Adjustments to these empiric antibiotics are made based on the results of donor and recipient bronchial cultures performed at the time of surgery. In the cystic fibrosis population, aerosolized colistin or tobramycin is also used. In addition to the broad-spectrum antibiotics noted, cystic fibrosis patients also require specific antipseudomonal coverage as dictated by the sensitivities of their preoperative sputum cultures.

Viral Infection

Herpes simplex was formerly a frequent cause of postoperative morbidity because of oral ulcerations as well as occasional pneumonitis. The routine use of acyclovir prophylaxis, however, has eliminated herpes infection as a frequent postoperative complication. CMV remains a significant problem in pulmonary transplant recipients. Most programs have adopted the strategy of matching seronegative donors to seronegative recipients. The highest incidence of severe CMV infection occurs in seronegative recipients receiving lungs from seropositive donors. In these patients, prophylaxis with intravenous ganciclovir is used routinely according to the following protocol: weeks 2 to 8, 5 mg/kg intravenously twice daily; weeks 8 to 12, 5 mg/kg intravenously once daily; weeks 12 to 16, 5 mg/kg intravenously three times weekly. It is reasonable to apply this prophylaxis regimen in any circumstance in which either the donor or the recipient is seropositive.

Fungal Infection

It has not been our practice to use routine fungal prophylaxis. However, in a circumstance in which a heavy growth of yeast is identified post-transplantation in donor bronchial culture, prophylactic low-dose amphotericin is justified. Some anecdotal reports cite early systemic *Candida* septicemia occurring in patients receiving organs from donors whose bronchial cultures grew *Candida*.

Pneumocystis carinii

Pneumocystis carinii parasite was an occasional cause of postoperative pulmonary infection until routine use of trimethoprim-sulfamethoxazole prophylaxis eliminated it as a significant pathogen. Alternative agents, such as inhaled pentamidine, are administered when there is an allergy to sulfa medications.

Immunosuppression

Most clinical lung transplant programs rely on triple-agent immunosuppression consisting of cyclosporine, azathioprine, and corticosteroids. Hosenpud and colleagues (1998) reported the prevalence of various immuno-suppression medications used after lung transplantation. Prednisone was present in more than 90% of the regimens, followed by cyclosporine and azathioprine, each found in more than 80% of the regimens. Newer additions, mycophenolate mofetil and tacrolimus, have shown recent gains but remain second-line agents at this time. In our program, cyclosporine administration typically is delayed until the second postoperative day. By that time, the patient generally is extubated and taking oral medications, and we have found this avoidance of intravenous cyclosporine useful in minimizing or avoiding perioperative renal dysfunction.

Azathioprine therapy also is commenced during the immediate postoperative period. Patients receive 1 to 2 mg/kg intravenously daily. When an oral diet is initiated, the same dose level can be administered orally. The dose must be adjusted to maintain the white blood cell count in excess of 3500.

The use of perioperative corticosteroids is controversial. Most physicians have adopted the use of moderate-dose corticosteroid (methylprednisolone, 0.5 to 1 mg/kg per day intravenously) for several days before initiating an oral dose of prednisone, 0.5 mg/kg per day. However, we have demonstrated, as reported by Miller and coworkers (1993), that withholding the first few days of prednisone has neither an adverse nor a beneficial effect on bronchial healing and may, in fact, lessen the risk of perioperative sepsis. We continue to use the aforementioned moderate doses described, and we begin using them on the day of the transplant.

For most patients, chronic immunosuppression consists of cyclosporin, prednisone, and azathioprine. Doses of cyclosporine are chosen to maintain blood levels in the range of 250 to 300 ng. Prednisone administration is also gradually reduced to minimize the complications of long-term steroid use.

A matter of considerable controversy is the use of postoperative cytolytic therapy (antithymocyte globulin, OKT3). These cytolytic agents are in use in a number of programs. The Pittsburgh group, as reported by Griffith and associates (1992), noted a reduced incidence of acute rejection in patients receiving rabbit antithymocyte globulin (ATG). (We use Atgam in our clinical program.) It has been argued that these agents, particularly OKT3, predispose patients to a higher incidence of CMV infection. This experience was accumulated, however, at a time when CMV matching was not widely practiced and CMV prophylaxis was not routine. It is probable that the early use of cytolytic therapy does reduce the frequency and severity of early postoperative rejection episodes. We also favor early use of Atgam because it allows us to withhold the initial intravenous doses of cyclosporine and thereby enhance early renal function.

Infection-Rejection Surveillance

As discussed by Trulock (1997), the use of radiographic, clinical, and physiological criteria has been insufficient to adequately delineate infection from rejection in the early post-transplant lung recipient. For this reason, it is our approach to perform routine fiberoptic bronchoscopy whenever there is a clinical indication in the absence of recently identified, untreated organisms identified by sputum culture. The advantage of routine flexible bronchoscopy is that it enables performance of bronchoalveolar lavage and transbronchial biopsy. Although bronchoalveolar lavage has not proven useful in the diagnosis of rejection, it is invaluable in the identification of opportunistic infection commonly encountered in transplant recipients. Transbronchial biopsy has proved to be the major tool in the diagnosis of pulmonary rejection. We have used this procedure frequently, both as a routine surveillance and in patients with unexplained pulmonary infiltrates. Routine bronchoalveolar lavage and transbronchial biopsies are performed at 3 weeks; 3, 6, 9, and 12 months; and annually thereafter.

Regardless of the method of diagnosis, if rejection is indeed the problem, a dramatic improvement in clinical findings, radiographic evidence (Fig. 92-14), and PaO_2 value will be observed within 8 to 12 hours after administration of 15 mg/kg of methylprednisolone.

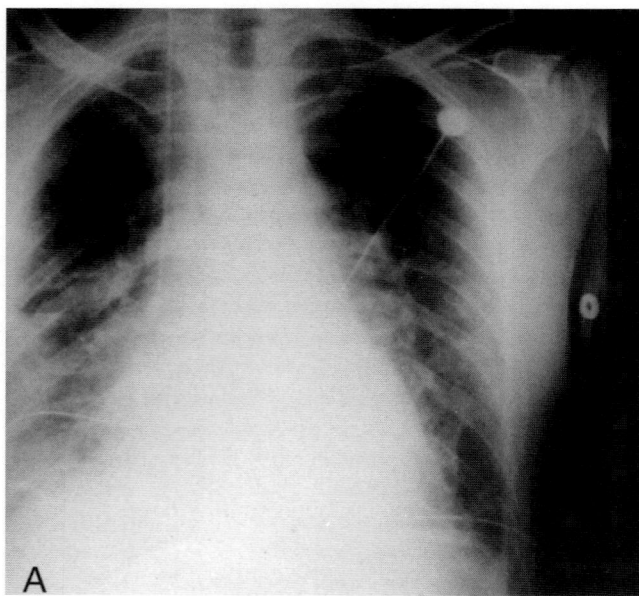

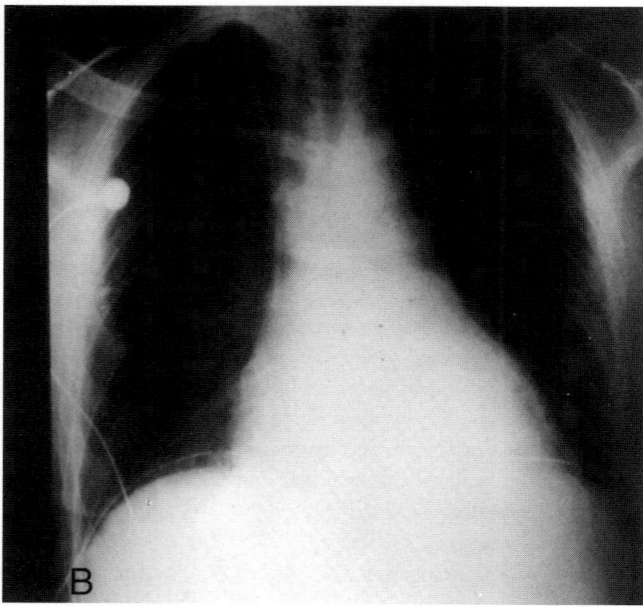

Fig. 92-14. Posteroanterior chest radiographs from a patient 7 days after bilateral sequential single-lung transplantation. **A.** On the morning of postoperative day 7, note bilateral diffuse infiltrate. A diagnosis of rejection was made and the patient received sodium thiopental (Solu-Medrol), 1-g intravenous bolus. **B.** Eight hours later. Dramatic improvement in the infiltrate is consistent with the typical response of acute rejection to steroid bolus therapy.

COMPLICATIONS

Technical Error

As in any major operative intervention, a variety of technical complications may be encountered during the perioperative period.

Postoperative Hemorrhage

Hemorrhage was once a frequent complication. Indeed, in the early experience of some programs undertaking heart-lung and en bloc double-lung transplants, approximately 25% of patients required re-operation for postoperative hemorrhage. With current surgical techniques, however, such as posterolateral thoracotomy for single-lung transplantation and the "clamshell" or "sternal-sparing clamshell" incisions for bilateral lung replacement, surgical exposure is superb. In addition, aprotinin administration has dramatically reduced intraoperative and postoperative bleeding, especially in patients with extensive pleural adhesions requiring cardiopulmonary bypass.

Anastomotic Complications

Anastomotic complications can also occur and result in postoperative graft dysfunction. Date and colleagues (1995) evaluated the clinical factors associated with airway complications after lung transplantation. Griffith and associates (1994) reported their experience with anastomotic complications after lung transplantation and made a number of important technical points. An unsatisfactory bronchial anastomosis is routinely identified in the operating room at postimplantation bronchoscopy. Inadequate anastomotic caliber dictates immediate surgical revision.

Pulmonary Hypertension and Hypoxemia

Persistent pulmonary hypertension and unexplained hypoxemia can occur as a result of stenosis at the pulmonary artery anastomosis. A nuclear perfusion scan that demonstrates less than anticipated flow to a single-lung graft or unequal distribution of flow in a bilateral lung recipient can suggest this problem. Occasionally, transesophageal sonography can visualize a stenotic anastomosis. Contrast angiography, however, should be performed in any patient for whom there is such a concern. At the time of angiography, the pressure gradient across the pulmonary artery anastomosis should be determined. A gradient of 15 to 20 mm Hg commonly is encountered, especially in single-lung recipients in whom most cardiac output is directed to the transplanted lung or in bilateral recipients with a high cardiac output. The need for anastomotic revision is dictated by the clinical situation. Dramatic reduction in flow should not be accepted, however, because the donor bronchus is totally dependent on pulmonary arterial collateral flow.

Compromise in flow across the atrial anastomosis also can occur as a result of unsatisfactory anastomotic technique. Compression of the anastomosis by clot or an omental or pericardial flap brought anterior or posterior to the atrial anastomosis for purposes of bronchial anastomotic cover can also impair ipsilateral pulmonary venous drainage. Impaired venous outflow results in elevated venous pressure and ipsilateral pulmonary edema. Pulmonary artery pressures remain unexpectedly high, and flow through the graft is less than expected. Contrast studies may be helpful in demonstrating a reduced level of flow through the anastomosis. Open exploration occasionally is necessary to confirm the diagnosis and conduct appropriate repair.

Early Graft Dysfunction

According to Haydock and colleagues (1992), approximately 20% of patients have severe early graft dysfunction. Although the prevalence of this problem among lung transplant recipients has certainly decreased in the years since that report, primary graft failure remains one of the most frequent causes of death in the first 30 days post-transplant. Graft failure may arise because of unsuspected pathologic findings in the donor lung, such as aspiration, infection, or contusion. Inadequate preservation can occur because of technical difficulties at the time of harvest or prolonged warm ischemia during implantation. Irrespective of its cause, it is important to establish a diagnosis of early graft dysfunction and rule out other treatable conditions. We adopted an aggressive approach to the diagnosis of this problem using transbronchial biopsy and even open lung biopsy early in the postoperative course in an effort to obtain a conclusive diagnosis. We have performed open lung biopsy at the time of implantation should graft dysfunction be immediately apparent in the operating room.

Typically, these patients exhibit diffuse alveolar damage. In this circumstance, Haydock and colleagues (1992) noted that the patient requires the usual intensive supportive measures with the expectation that the diffuse alveolar damage will ultimately recover and provide satisfactory long-term function. Standard intensive ventilatory and pharmacologic intervention generally suffice, although severe graft dysfunction or coexisting cardiac failure may require extracorporeal membrane oxygenator (ECMO) support. In our entire experience with over 440 lung transplant recipients, only 11 patients have experienced acute allograft dysfunction of such a severity to require ECMO. Three of these patients died while on ECMO, one died after weaning from ECMO, and seven survived to be discharged from the hospital. An alternative approach to severe, reversible allograft dysfunction is reported by Eriksson and Steen (1998), who have successfully used core cooling to avoid ECMO while the lung injury heals.

Infection

Bacterial Infection

Bacterial pneumonia is the most commonly encountered infection after lung transplantation. An aggressive approach is taken to identify the specific organism. Frequent bronchoscopy with protected brush should be undertaken if routine sputum cultures fail to provide an identifiable organism. Routine intravenous antibiotic therapy is used, and in the majority of patients, the pneumonia clears rapidly. Patients with cystic fibrosis present a real management dilemma during the postoperative period as they are susceptible to recurrent pulmonary infections from the same *Pseudomonas* organisms harbored in the airway and upper airway sinuses post transplant. Snell and associates (1993) emphasized that this is particularly true of patients with highly resistant *Pseudomonas cepacia*.

Lung abscess occasionally is encountered in lung transplantation recipients. Patients with cystic fibrosis on occasion develop multifocal lung abscesses, presumably as a result of inhaled contamination from upper airway or sinus infection. In single-lung recipients, the native lung is also susceptible to bacterial infection, which can cavitate and produce a lung abscess. The care of these patients is the same as for any other patient with lung abscess. Appropriate broad-spectrum antibiotic therapy is administered and bronchoscopy is performed to ensure that no airway obstruction is present.

Viral Infection

Viral pneumonitis can occur in the postoperative period. Herpes simplex infection formerly was encountered frequently during the early postoperative phase, although routine use of acyclovir has made it an unusual complication. CMV infection is more commonly encountered when donor or recipient, or both, are CMV seropositive. Ettinger and coworkers (1993) reviewed our experience at Washington University. Ninety-two percent of patients in their report developed CMV infection, with 75% of them having biopsy-proved CMV pneumonitis. Donor-negative/recipient-positive combination resulted in more frequent and severe infection. No donor-negative/recipient-negative patients developed infection or disease. Biopsy-proved CMV pneumonitis was associated with radiographic infiltrate in less than 30% of cases. The detection of CMV in bronchoalveolar lavage was not always predictive of CMV pneumonitis. The high incidence of CMV identification in our experience reflects the aggressive viral surveillance used in our program.

We do not treat CMV infection without biopsy-derived proof of CMV disease. In that circumstance, 5 mg/kg of ganciclovir is administered intravenously twice daily for 2 to 3 weeks. In severe pneumonitis, CMV hyperimmune globulin is also administered. The majority of patients respond promptly to this regimen.

Fungal Infection

The most frequent cause of significant fungal infection after transplantation is *Aspergillus*. Once *Aspergillus* has become a resident organism, it is difficult to clear. In patients without evidence of active invasive infection, we have administered ketoconazole with reasonable success. In patients who fail to clear with ketoconazole or who have developed invasive infection, however, amphotericin is required. *Aspergillus* infection can become a systemic disease involving multiple organs and usually proves to be fatal.

A particularly interesting group of patients are those having undergone single-lung transplantation for pulmonary fibrosis who develop *Aspergillus* in the diseased native lung. These patients should be treated aggressively with the expectation that the *Aspergillus* will not likely clear from the native lung. In this circumstance, contralateral native lung pneumonectomy is warranted.

Pleural Space Complications

Pleural space complications occur frequently after lung transplantation.

Pneumothorax

Pneumothorax is encountered primarily in two circumstances. It can occur as a result of airway dehiscence with communication into the pleural space, although this is not a frequent occurrence and is usually managed readily by intercostal tube drainage with appropriate reexpansion of the underlying lung. A more common circumstance is the development of insignificant pneumothoraces in patients with obstructive lung disease, either emphysema or cystic fibrosis, who have undergone bilateral replacement, receiving lungs much smaller than the pleural space into which they are implanted. Often a minimal degree of bilateral pneumothorax occurs subsequent to chest tube removal. In general, these pneumothoraces can be ignored and the pleural air will eventually resorb and any remaining space will fill with fluid.

Effusion

Pleural effusions are common, particularly in recipients whose lung volume is somewhat smaller than the pleural space. A sympathetic effusion will occur in association with underlying pulmonary infection or rejection. These effusions, as with others, generally clear with appropriate therapy of the underlying parenchymal condition.

Empyema

Empyema is infrequently encountered in lung transplant recipients. Spontaneous development of an empyema is rare. More commonly, an empyema develops after any prolonged air leak as a result of open lung biopsy performed on a patient receiving high-dose corticosteroids. Persistent air leak and failure to achieve reexpansion of the lung and subsequent pleurodesis result in a chronic pleural space that eventually will become infected. A number of these patients have been treated by open drainage by rib resection or by

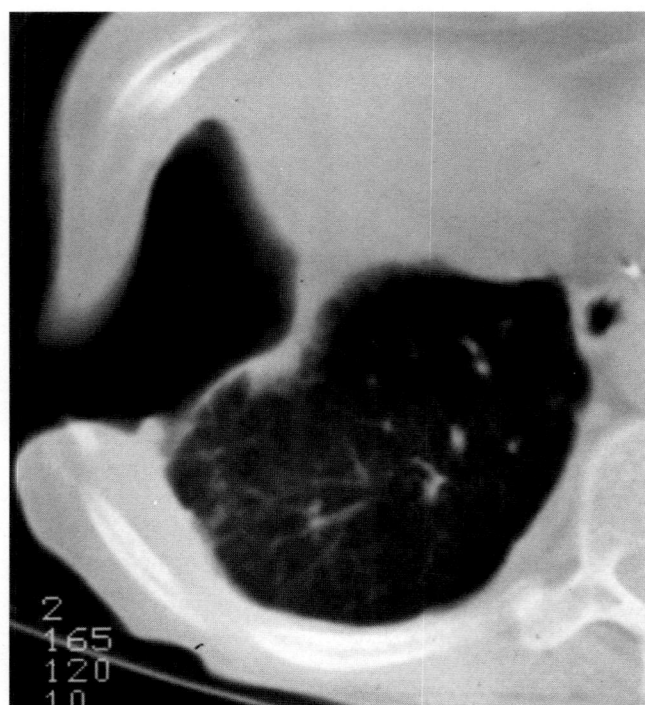

Fig. 92-15. Computed tomographic image of the right chest in a patient 3 years after bilateral sequential single-lung transplant. Previous open lung biopsy resulted in a prolonged bronchopleural fistula and a sizeable residual cavity. A Claggett window was created. Ultimately, the fistula closed. The patient has tolerated the Claggett window for 2.5 years.

creation of a Clagett window or Eloesser flap (Fig. 92-15). Interestingly, an empyema rarely occurs as a result of bronchial dehiscence in communication with the pleural space. As one of us (G.A.P., 1993) has previously noted, in the majority of these latter patients, satisfactory intercostal tube drainage with reexpansion of the underlying lung results in satisfactory anastomotic healing and the absence of any significant pleural space infection.

Airway Complications

Airway complications were formerly a major cause of morbidity and mortality after pulmonary transplantation. Using standard methods of implantation, the donor bronchus is rendered ischemic, without reconstitution of its systemic bronchial artery circulation. The donor bronchus thereby relies on collateral pulmonary flow during the first few days after transplantation. It has been demonstrated that pulmonary collateral flow makes a substantial contribution to bronchial viability at the level of the distal bronchus and lobar origin. A shortened donor bronchial length (two rings proximal to the upper lobe takeoff) reduces the length of donor bronchus dependent on collateral flow. In addition, improved techniques of preservation have resulted in increased bronchial viability after transplantation. Post-transplant pulmonary parenchymal pathologic change also results in decreased collateral flow rendering the ischemic donor bronchus at increased risk of necrosis and subsequent dehiscence. Superior preservation, improved sepsis prophylaxis, and immunosuppression have reduced the incidence of airway complication. In a review of our experience, Date and colleagues (1995) reported a reduction of the prevalence of anastomotic complications from 14% to 4% of anastomoses at risk. The role of perioperative steroids is important in this regard. Davreux and coworkers (1993) reported our work showing that epithelial regeneration and revascularization of rat heterotopic tracheal allografts are improved by postoperative corticosteroid administration. In addition, Inui and associates (1993) of the Hannover group demonstrated that postoperative corticosteroid therapy improves retrograde bronchial blood flow in porcine lung allografts.

Airway complications are identified in a number of ways. Routine postoperative bronchoscopic surveillance, as used in most programs, generally provides early evidence that an anastomotic complication has occurred. On occasion, computed tomography, performed for some other indication, demonstrates an unexpected airway stenosis or dehiscence. In fact, we learned that CT scanning is a useful diagnostic tool in the evaluation of documented or suspected donor airway complications. Late airway stenoses generally manifest with symptoms of dyspnea, wheeze, or decreased FEV_1. Bronchoscopic assessment confirms the diagnosis.

Failure of Normal Bronchial Healing

Most airway complications are identified soon after transplantation. A normal bronchial anastomotic suture line will demonstrate a narrow rim of epithelial slough that ultimately heals. On occasion, one can observe patchy areas of superficial necrosis of donor bronchial epithelium. These areas are also of no concern and ultimately heal causing problems. Minor degrees of bronchial dehiscence are also of little long-term consequence. Membranous wall defects generally heal without any airway compromise, whereas cartilaginous defects usually result in some degree of late stricture. Significant dehiscence (greater than 50% of the bronchial circumference) may result in compromise of the airway. This problem should be managed expectantly by laser or mechanical débridement of the area to maintain satisfactory airway patency. A word of caution should be issued to the laser enthusiasts: Zealous attempts to maintain airway caliber can injure the vital normal distal donor airway. A stent can only be placed if the distal main airway remains intact. Occasionally, a significant dehiscence results in direct communication with the pleural space, resulting in pneumothorax and a significant air leak following chest tube insertion. If the lung remains completely expanded and the pleural space is evacuated, however, the leak will ultimately seal and the airway may heal without significant stenosis. Similarly, a dehiscence may communicate directly with the

mediastinum, resulting in significant mediastinal emphysema. If the lung remains completely expanded and the pleural space is filled, adequate drainage of the mediastinum can be achieved by placing a drain in close proximity to the anastomotic line by mediastinoscopy. This step will also result in satisfactory healing of the anastomosis, often without stricture.

Surgical revision of the anastomosis is only possible if an adequate length of donor airway is available for resuturing. This type of reconstruction has been performed successfully by Kirk and associates (1990). This procedure is rarely possible, however, if the donor bronchus was cut to an appropriate short length at the time of the initial procedure. Massive dehiscence of the airway with uncontrolled leak or mediastinal contamination has been treated by successful retransplantation in a number of programs.

Anastomotic Stenosis

Chronic airway stenoses can present significant management problems. A right main bronchial anastomotic stricture is generally managed easily by repeated dilatation and ultimate placement of an endobronchial stent; there is usually sufficient length for placement of a right main bronchial orifice stent without impingement of the right upper lobe bronchus. On the left side, however, strictures can be somewhat more difficult to manage. Dilatation of the distal left main bronchus is technically more difficult because of the angulation of that bronchus. In addition, the lobar bifurcation immediately distal to the usual site of anastomosis does not provide a suitable length of bronchus distal to the stricture for placement of large-caliber dilating bronchoscopes. Finally, Silastic stents placed across a distal left main bronchial anastomotic stricture may occlude the upper or lower lobe orifice as they bridge the stricture.

Silastic stents are tolerated exceptionally well. Patients do, however, require daily inhalation of N-acetylcystine to keep the stents patent. DeHoyos and Maurer (1992) reported that the stents have resulted in dramatic improvement in pulmonary function. Fortunately, most of these stents have proven to be required only temporarily. After several months, most patients are able to maintain satisfactory airway patency without the stent in place.

Self-expanding metal stents have benefited from impressive technological improvement in recent years. These stents come in a wide variety of lengths and diameters, and they have been exceptionally easy to insert. In rare situations in which the airways distal to an anastomotic stricture are too small to accept a Silastic stent, or when a Silastic stent will obstruct one bronchus while stenting another, the use of a self-expanding metal stent may suit the purpose perfectly. The only caveat is that granulation tissue will rapidly overgrow an uncovered metal mesh stent, sometimes making it impossible to remove.

Finally, distal bronchial strictures can prove unmanageable by dilation or stent insertion. In these patients, retransplantation is an option that has been used successfully by Novick and coworkers (1993, 1998).

Rejection

Insofar as immunologic matching is crude (ABO blood group only) and immunosuppression strategies are imperfect, it is not surprising that post-transplant rejection is a troublesome problem. Acute rejection, as noted by us, is encountered during the early postoperative period in almost all patients. This occurrence rarely presents a significant clinical problem. Chronic rejection, in contrast, is the most common underlying cause of late death following pulmonary transplantation. This problem is particularly vexing because its pathogenesis is poorly understood and no effective means of treatment are known.

Acute Rejection

Acute rejection has a typical clinical presentation including dyspnea, low-grade fever, perihilar interstitial infiltrates (see Fig. 92-14), hypoxia, and increased white blood cell count. Typically, the first episode occurs within the first 5 to 7 postoperative days. Several episodes during the first 2 months are not unusual. In the past, the suspected diagnosis was confirmed by a rapid response to bolus methylprednisolone, typically 500 mg to 1 g. However, the aforementioned clinical scenario can be confused with infection.

At present, the clinical parameters previously described raise the suspicion but are insufficient for the accurate diagnosis of rejection. Intensive laboratory investigations are underway to discover some relatively noninvasive technique by which rejection might be identified. Nuclear scanning has proved to be of little value. A variety of immunologic tests have also been advocated. The University of Pittsburgh group had initial enthusiasm for a primed lymphocyte test, which we found not particularly useful. We demonstrated increased cytotoxicity of bronchoalveolar lavage (BAL) lymphocytes in patients with biopsy-proved rejection. Evidence is mounting that various cytokines are important mediators in the development of rejection and that manipulation of their expression may be of therapeutic importance. The role of NO in the pathophysiology of lung allograft rejection is currently being elucidated, but groups such as Fisher (1998) and Silkoff (1998) and their associates have concluded from preliminary studies that the measurement of exhaled NO may have a role as a noninvasive indicator of pulmonary allograft rejection.

The standard and most useful method for the diagnosis of rejection is transbronchial biopsy performed under fluoroscopic control. The Papworth group, whose work was reported by Higenbottam and coworkers (1988), deserves credit for demonstrating the safety and value of this technique in the lung transplantation population. The typical histologic appearance is that of perivascular lymphocytic

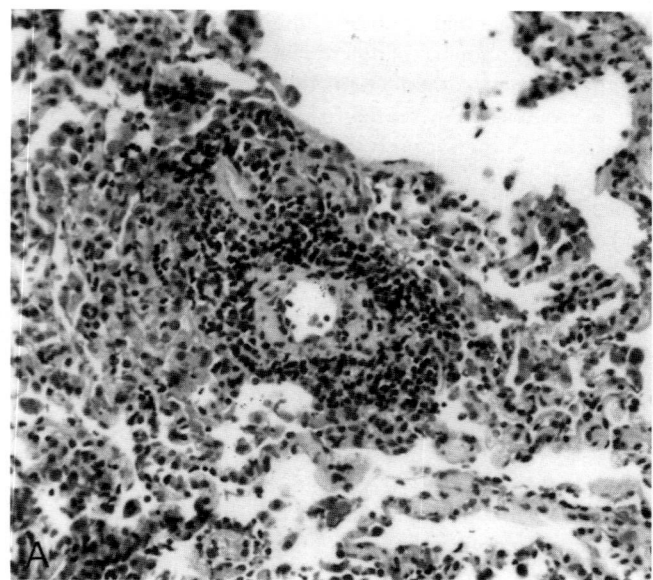

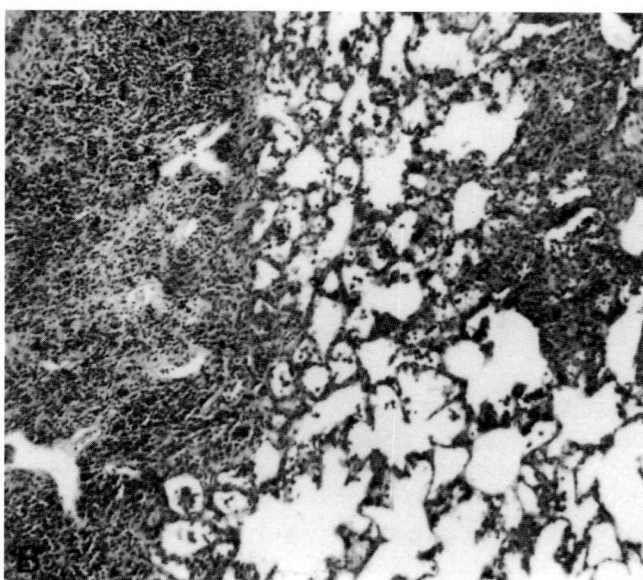

Fig. 92-16. A. Photomicrograph of a transbronchial biopsy specimen showing typical early (A1b) rejection. Isolated perivascular cuffs of lymphocytes are noted. **B.** A more severe degree of rejection is evident in this photomicrograph of a transbronchial biopsy specimen. Perivascular and interstitial lymphoid infiltrates are present, consistent with grade 3 rejection (A3a).

infiltrate (Fig. 92-16). The internationally accepted classification for pulmonary rejection was reported by Yousem and colleagues (1990) and is depicted in Table 92-3.

Factors that predispose patients to an increased incidence of rejection are unclear. Experimental evidence shows that poorly preserved allografts are more likely to suffer subsequent rejection. In addition, expression of major histocompatibility complex (MHC) class II antigens on bronchial epithelium and pulmonary capillary endothelium is increased after extended periods of preservation. We demonstrated

Table 92-3. Working Formulation for Classification and Grading of Pulmonary Rejection

A. Acute rejection
   0. Grade 0: no significant abnormality
   1. Grade 1: minimal acute rejection
      a. With evidence of bronchiolar inflammation
      b. Without evidence of bronchiolar inflammation
      c. With large airway inflammation
      d. No bronchioles are present
   2. Grade 2: mild acute rejection
      a. With evidence of bronchiolar inflammation
      b. Without evidence of bronchiolar inflammation
      c. With large airway inflammation
      d. No bronchioles to evaluate
   3. Grade 3: moderate acute rejection
      a. With evidence of bronchiolar inflammation
      b. Without evidence of bronchiolar inflammation
      c. With large airway inflammation
      d. No bronchioles to evaluate
   4. Grade 4: severe acute rejection
      a. With evidence of bronchiolar inflammation
      b. Without evidence of bronchiolar inflammation
      c. With large airway inflammation
      d. No bronchioles to evaluate
B. Active airway damage without scarring
   1. Lymphocyte bronchitis
   2. Lymphocyte bronchiolitis
C. Chronic airway rejection
   1. Bronchiolitis obliterans: subtotal
      a. Active
      b. Inactive
   2. Bronchiolitis obliterans: total
      a. Active
      b. Inactive
D. Chronic vascular rejection
E. Vasculitis

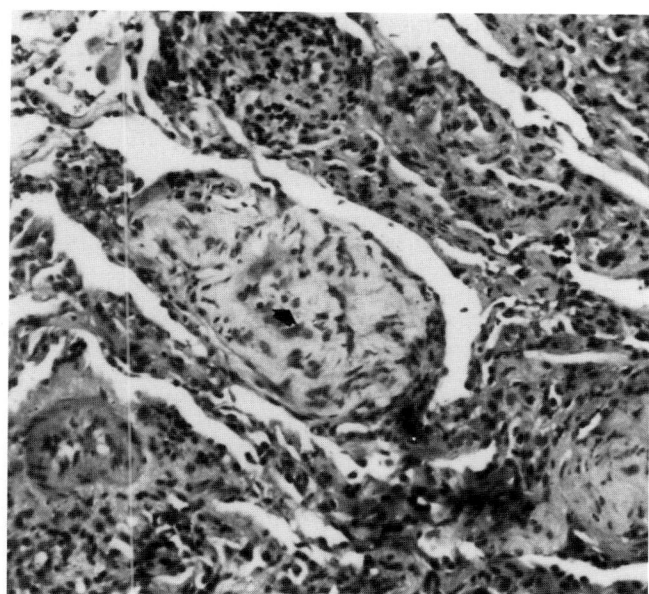

Fig. 92-17. Photomicrograph of a transbronchial biopsy specimen reveals typical findings of bronchiolitis obliterans thought to result from chronic rejection. Mature fibrous obliteration of the bronchiolar lumen is evident (*arrow*).

expression of the adhesion molecule I-CAM after extended preservation of human lung allografts, as reported by Hasagawa and colleagues (1993). Infection may also predispose to subsequent rejection. Serious rejection episodes following close on the heels of established bacterial or viral infection have been reported.

Irrespective of its etiology, acute rejection usually can be controlled effectively. Most patients respond promptly to the first course of methylprednisolone. Occasionally, a second course of steroid may be necessary to control a serious rejection episode. Persistent rejection despite this intervention is distinctly unusual. In this latter circumstance, cytolytic therapy with ATG or OKT3 should be considered. Evidence suggests that alternative immunosuppressants such as FK506 also may be useful in this situation. Increasing experimental evidence as noted by Hirai and associates (1993) shows that FK506 may offer an advantage over cyclosporin as a first-line immunosuppressive agent.

Chronic Rejection-Bronchiolitis Obliterans Syndrome

Unfortunately, chronic rejection remains a major problem. The clinical presentation of chronic rejection is a progressive fall in FEV_1, which may actually precede clinical symptoms of dyspnea and can be detected by the hand-held spirometer used daily by patients in almost all transplant programs. Despite advanced chronic rejection, chest radiographs and CT scans may be normal. They should be performed, however, to rule out other causes of a decreasing FEV_1. Bronchoscopy is necessary to ensure that there is no bronchial anastomotic compromise. Pulmonary function studies reveal obstructive physiologic change. The pathologic hallmark of chronic rejection is obliterative bronchiolitis (Fig. 92-17). Indeed, the term *chronic rejection* is often used interchangeably with bronchiolitis obliterans. The descriptive term *bronchiolitis obliterans syndrome* (BOS) has been used to describe the commonly encountered late decline in graft function which is not attributable to acute rejection, infection, or mechanical obstruction due to a bronchial anastomotic complication. A working formulation has been created by Cooper and colleagues (1993) to characterize and grade BOS (Table 92-4). The histologic diagnosis of obliterative bronchiolitis is a modifier of the classification of stage of disease, but it is not necessary to make the diagnosis.

The prevalence of BOS among lung transplant recipients increases steadily with increasing time since the transplantation. Reichenspurner and the Stanford group (1995) reported an extensive experience with BOS in heart-lung and lung transplant recipients. They reported actuarial freedom from BOS in 72%, 52%, 44%, and 29% of recipients at 1, 2, 3, and 5 years post-transplantation. There was no significant difference between lung transplant recipients and heart-lung transplant recipients in the prevalence of BOS.

Table 92-4. Bronchiolitis Obliterans Syndrome Scoring System

0: No significant abnormality; FEV_1 >80% of baseline value
   a. Without pathologic evidence of obliterative bronchiolitis
   b. With pathologic evidence of obliterative bronchiolitis
1: Mild obliterative bronchiolitis syndrome: FEV_1 66 to 80% of baseline value
   a. Without pathologic evidence of obliterative bronchiolitis
   b. With pathologic evidence of obliterative bronchiolitis
2: Moderate obliterative bronchiolitis syndrome: FEV_1 51 to 65% of baseline value
   a. Without pathologic evidence of obliterative bronchiolitis
   b. With pathologic evidence of obliterative bronchiolitis
3: Severe obliterative bronchiolitis syndrome: FEV_1 50% or less of baseline value
   a. Without pathologic evidence of obliterative bronchiolitis
   b. With pathologic evidence of obliterative bronchiolitis

Multivariate analysis listed CMV infection, acute rejection, and biopsy findings of lymphocytic bronchiolitis as being associated with increased risk of BOS. Similarly, Chaparro and colleagues (1997) from the University of Toronto report a stage I or higher BOS prevalence of 63% for transplant recipients surviving more than 5 years.

Our experience with BOS was reported by Sundaresan and associates (1995b) in a retrospective review of 212 transplant recipients. As a group, 41% had been classified as having BOS while 59% were free of BOS. When grouped as successive quartiles based on time since transplantation, 56% of the longest surviving quartile had BOS while 9.6% of the most recently transplanted quartile had BOS. Mortality was 28.6% in patients with BOS as compared to 7.3% in those without it. Death generally occurred due to primary graft dysfunction, or as a result of infection in the setting of augmented immunosuppression used to treat BOS.

Prevention of BOS depends on preventing those clinical situations which have been shown to be associated with its development. The avoidance of acute rejection episodes and the avoidance of CMV infections through careful clinical monitoring and routine surveillance biopsies are potential approaches. Once BOS is established, intensification of immunosuppression with azathioprine, steroids, Atgam, methotrexate, irradiation, and aerosolized cyclosporine have all been explored as treatments. None has reversed the dysfunction. The goal of present treatment is to arrest the progressive decline. Unfortunately, most patients either develop progressive obliterative bronchiolitis or contract an opportunistic infection that proves lethal.

Retransplantation has been offered to many patients with chronic rejection as noted by Novick and colleagues (1993, 1998). Retransplantation has been explored as therapy for endstage BOS, but results demonstrate significantly worse survival than seen after primary lung transplantation, with 1-year survival rates reported as 48%. Retransplantation remains controversial in the face of ever-increasing waiting lists for first-time transplant recipients. For many of these patients, the process reappears in a short period of time after retransplantation. Nonetheless, a few patients have survived and obtained excellent long-term results after retransplantation for this devastating condition.

RESULTS

Operative Mortality

Improvements in selection, technique, and management have resulted in dramatic reductions in operative mortality. Cooper and coworkers (1994) reported an early mortality of only 8% in 131 consecutive single and bilateral transplants performed in our program. Our updated survival data are illustrated in Table 92-5, with 30-day survival in excess of 90% for all diagnoses. Other large programs have reported equally impressive results. Spray and colleagues (1994) at Washington University reported exciting results of lung transplantation in children. This group of patients, as noted by Spray and associates (1992), represents a particular challenge, especially those with Eisenmenger's syndrome, in whom technically difficult operative procedures were undertaken with success.

Some difference in early mortality apparently depends on the type of procedure or underlying disease. In the early years of bilateral lung transplantation, bilateral procedures were associated with early operative mortality rates, which were higher than those seen after single-lung transplantation. This difference reflects the increase in technical difficulty as well as the enhanced risk of septic complications in the cystic fibrosis group. Ramirez and colleagues (1992) of the Toronto group reported a high incidence of postoperative death from sepsis, particularly in those recipients harboring highly resistant *Pseudomonas cepacia* organisms. In recent years, the mortality of bilateral procedures has decreased,

Table 92-5. Patient Actuarial Survival, Washington University Lung Transplant Program: 1988–1997

Diagnosis	N	1 month (%)	1 year (%)	2 years (%)	3 years (%)	5 years (%)
Chronic obstructive pulmonary disease	128	97	88	86	78	51
α_1-antitrypsin deficiency	70	91	80	77	75	54
Cystic fibrosis	62	94	77	73	58	42
Idiopathic pulmonary fibrosis	42	98	75	72	66	45
Primary pulmonary hypertension	38	90	81	76	73	68
Total	**340**	**94**	**82**	**79**	**71**	**53**

Table 92-6. Cause of Mortality after Lung Transplantation, Grouped by Interval since Transplant

Cause of Death	0–30 days	31 days–1 year	>1 year
Graft failure	23.4	—	—
Infection	16	34.1	15.5
Hemorrhage	3.7	—	—
Acute rejection	4.1	—	—
Bronchiolitis obliterans	—	5.3	33.6
Malignancy	—	—	2.2
Cytomegalovirus	—	4.3	—
Multiorgan failure	—	4.4	2.5
Other thoracic	4.6	4.0	5.2
Other	48.2	47.9	41.0

Modified from Hosenpud JD, et al: The Registry of the International Society for Heart and Lung Transplantation: Fifteenth Official Report—1998. J Heart Lung Transplant 17:656, 1998. With permission.

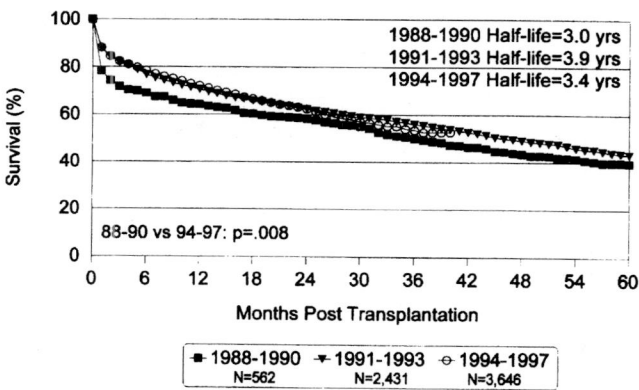

Fig. 92-18. Overall actuarial survival among lung transplant recipients registered in the International Society of Heart and Lung Transplantation. From Hosenpud JD, et al: The Registry of the International Society for Heart and Lung Transplantation: Fifteenth Official Report—1998. J Heart Lung Transplant 17:656, 1998. With permission.

and in our program there is no difference between single-lung transplant and bilateral-lung transplant survival at 1 month (96% versus 95%) or at 1 year (85% versus 83%).

In our program, we noted no difference in perioperative mortality among disease categories for which single-lung transplantation is undertaken. Others, however, have reported increased mortality in patients undergoing single-lung transplantation for primary pulmonary hypertension in comparison with those suffering from emphysema. This finding reflects the difficulties of the postoperative course of patients with pulmonary vascular disease.

The causes of operative mortality as reported by the International Society for Heart and Lung Transplantation (ISHLT) are shown in Table 92-6.

Late Mortality

Only in the last several years have large numbers of patients undergone pulmonary transplantation. Although a few patients have survived 6 to 8 years after lung transplantation, the number of patients is insufficient to have reliable data on long-term survival. In Cooper and associates' (1994) report of our experience, 13 of 131 patients suffered late deaths, and 81% of patients were alive, with a median follow-up of 19 months. The long-term actuarial survival of patients in our program, shown in Table 92-5, demonstrates overall 5-year survival to be better than 50%, with a range of 42 to 68% depending on the underlying diagnosis. In de Hoyos and associates' (1992) report of the Toronto experience, 4-year actuarial survival was 53% and 62% for single and bilateral transplants, respectively.

Survival data from the ISHLT Registry are shown in Figure 92-18. Considering the fact that many of the programs reporting to the registry have limited experience, the overall worldwide results are impressive and are improving steadily. Cause of late deaths as reported to ISHLT are shown in Table 92-6.

Functional Results

Among operative survivors, functional results are excellent. The usual patient is returned to normal levels of exercise tolerance without oxygen supplementation within 6 to 8 weeks after transplantation.

Obstructive Lung Disease

Obstructive lung disease is the most common indication for lung transplantation. Single and bilateral lung transplantation have been used with success. Gas exchange, pulmonary function, and exercise tolerance are dramatically improved, as illustrated in Figures 92-19 to 92-21. Single

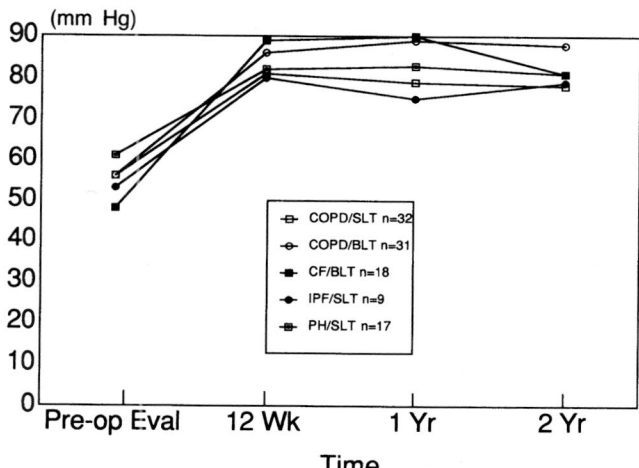

Fig. 92-19. Preoperative and postoperative room air Pao_2 among adult recipients in the Washington University–Barnes Hospital experience according to disease categories. Note the dramatic and sustained increase in oxygenation in all patient groups.

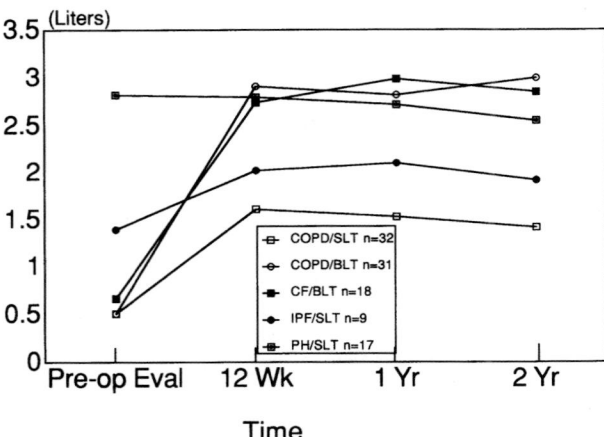

Fig. 92-20. Preoperative and postoperative FEV_1 among adult recipients in the Washington University–Barnes Hospital experience according to disease categories. Dramatic and sustained improvements are noted in bilateral (BLT) recipients having chronic obstructive pulmonary disease (COPD) or cystic fibrosis (CF). Less dramatic improvements in FEV_1 are noted in single-lung recipients (SLT) suffering from COPD or idiopathic pulmonary fibrosis (IPF). Single-lung recipients with pulmonary hypertension (PH) having normal preoperative FEV_1 derive no improvement in that parameter after transplant.

and bilateral recipients achieve satisfactory postoperative lung volume (Figs. 92-22 and 92-23).

Septic Lung Disease

In a number of centers, satisfactory results have been obtained with the application of bilateral-lung transplanta-

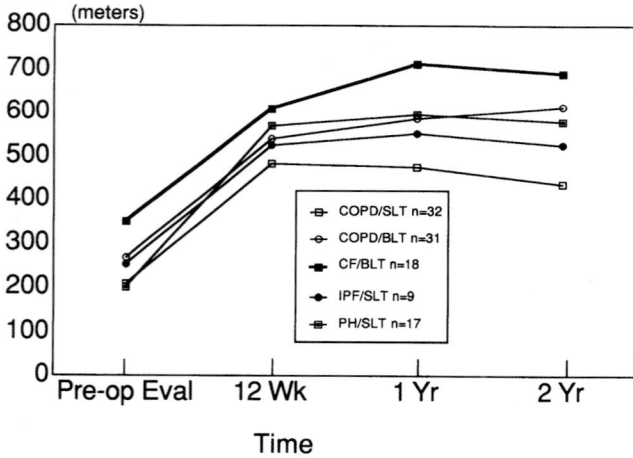

Fig. 92-21. Preoperative and postoperative 6-minute walk distances (meters) for adult recipients in the Washington University–Barnes Hospital program according to various disease and transplant categories. Note the dramatic improvement in exercise tolerance in all patient groups. This improvement appears to be sustained, except perhaps in the chronic obstructive pulmonary disease (COPD) group receiving single-lung transplantation (SLT) where there is a slight decrease noted in late follow-up. BLT, bilateral-lung transplantation; CF, cystic fibrosis; IPF, idiopathic pulmonary fibrosis; PH, pulmonary hypertension.

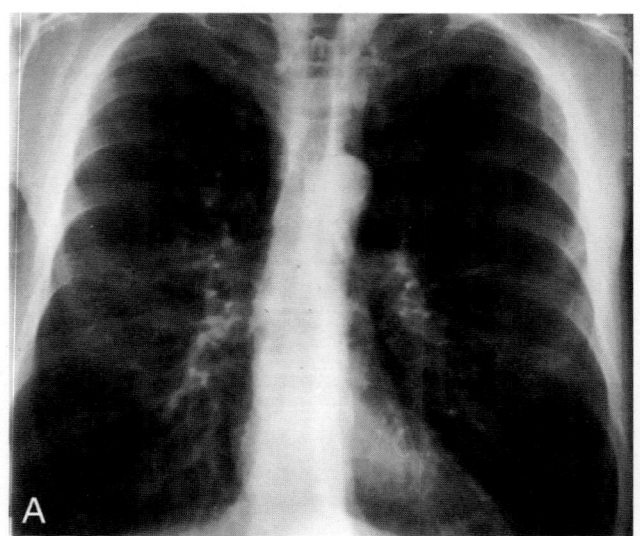

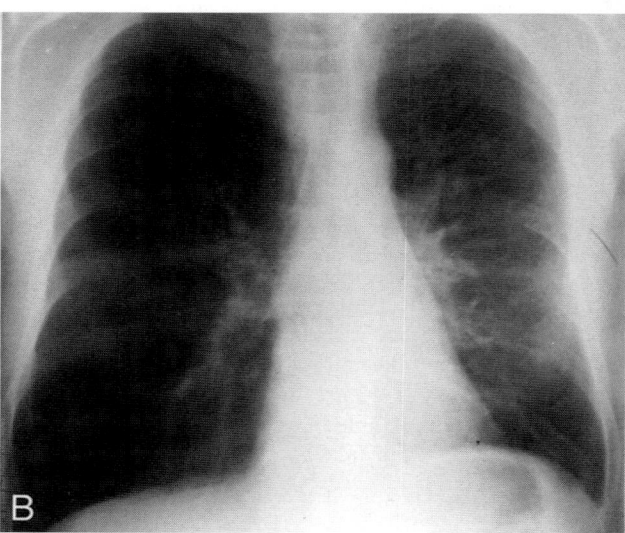

Fig. 92-22. A. Preoperative chest radiograph in a patient with emphysema. **B.** Same patient after left single-lung transplantation. Despite receiving an allograft with greater predicted lung volume than the recipient, the mediastinum is still shifted slightly to the transplanted side.

tion in these patients. Ramirez and colleagues (1992) from Toronto reported excellent gas exchange, pulmonary function, and exercise tolerance among operative survivors. Our experience is similar (see Figs. 92-19 to 92-21). Dramatic improvement in chest contour is apparent (Fig. 92-24).

Fibrotic Lung Disease

Whereas fibrotic lung disease condition was formerly the most frequent indication for pulmonary transplantation, it is now one of the least common indications. Nonetheless, enough data are available to realize that the long-term functional results in this group of patients are excellent. We have

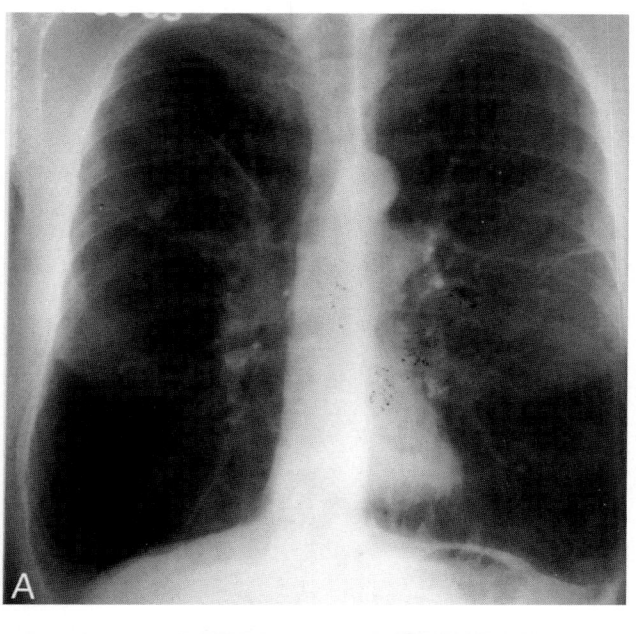

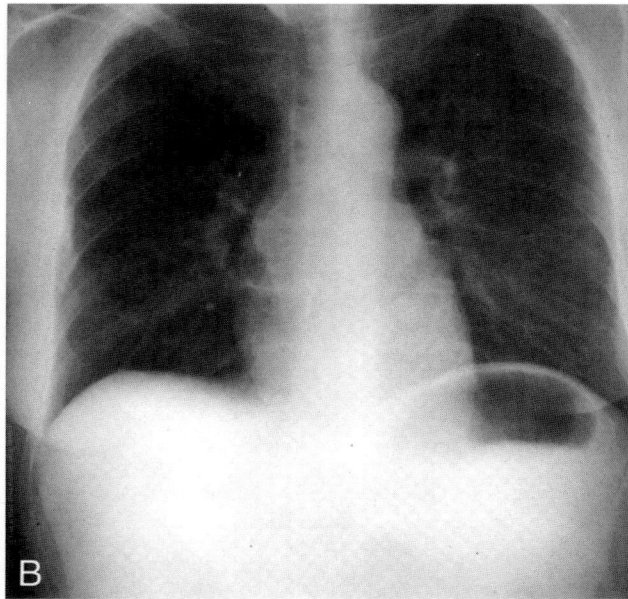

Fig. 92-23. A. Preoperative chest radiograph in a patient with α₁-antitrypsin deficiency emphysema. **B.** After bilateral sequential single-lung transplantation. Note the return to normal chest contour with restoration of a normal cardiac silhouette.

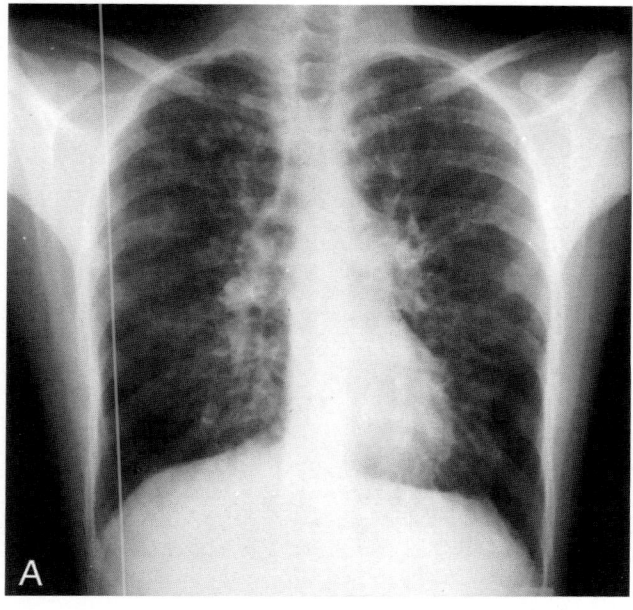

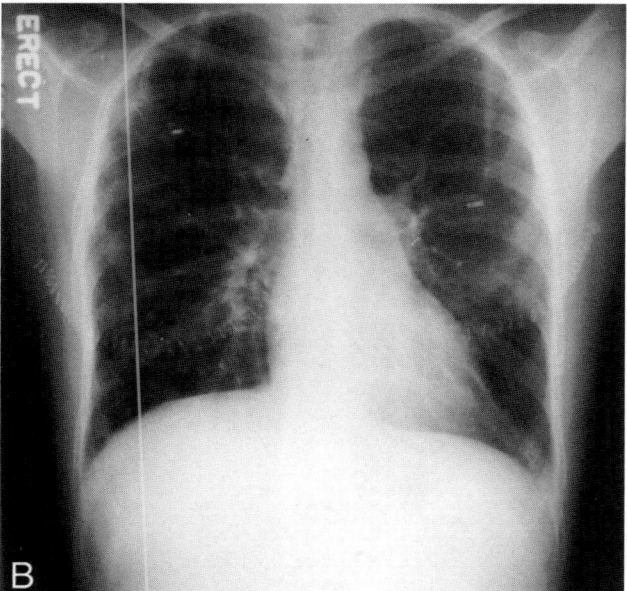

Fig. 92-24. A. Preoperative chest radiograph from a patient with cystic fibrosis. **B.** After bilateral sequential single-lung transplantation. Note the return of normal chest contour.

achieved a 54% survival at 5 years for the fibrotic patients. Single-lung transplantation provides satisfactory lung volume for these patients (Fig. 92-25). Gas exchange and exercise tolerance are maintained during late follow-up (see Figs. 92-19 to 92-21).

Pulmonary Vascular Disease

Our colleagues have been particularly interested in single-lung transplantation for patients with primary pulmonary hypertension and Eisenmenger's syndrome, as reported by Pasque and associates (1995). It is well documented that the cardiac function of these patients recovers promptly with the reduction in right ventricular afterload provided by satisfactory lung allografting. However, the early postoperative course of these patients is complicated because of the impressive ventilation-perfusion mismatch that can occur as 90 to 95% of right ventricular output is directed to the transplanted lung and more than 50% of ventilation is directed to the native lung. Our program has evolved a rigorous protocol for the early postopera-

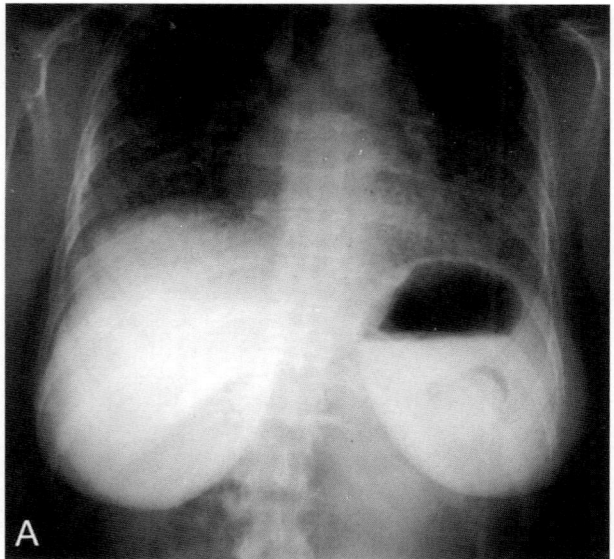

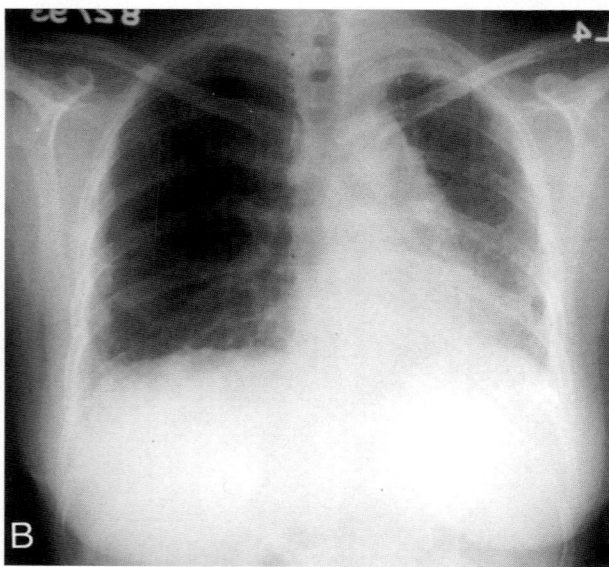

Fig. 92-25. A. Preoperative chest radiograph in a patient with idiopathic pulmonary fibrosis. Note the diffuse interstitial markings and small lung volumes. B. After right single-lung transplantation. With placement of an oversized right lung allograft, the mediastinum has been shifted to the left.

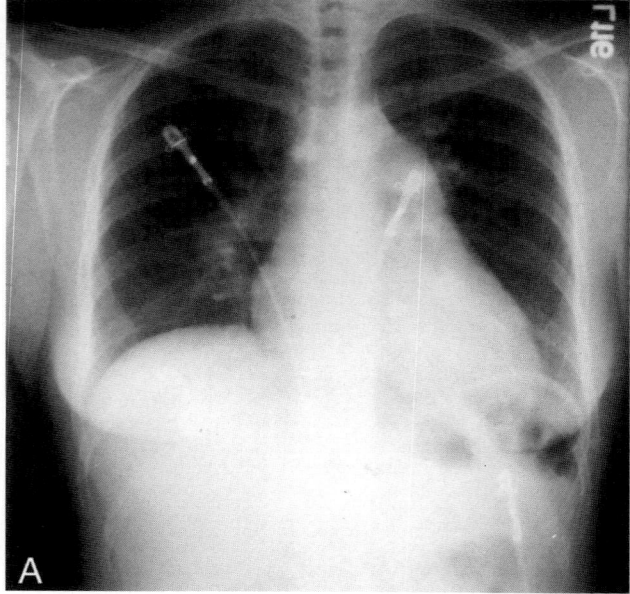

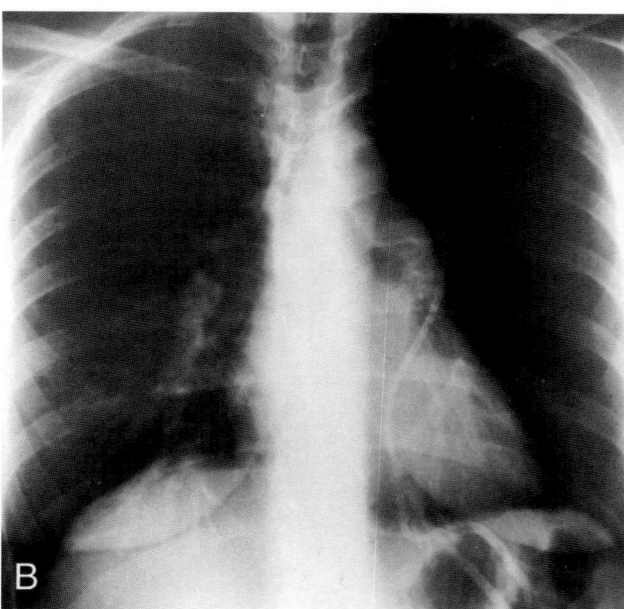

Fig. 92-26. A. Preoperative chest radiograph in a patient with primary pulmonary hypertension. Note the tremendous enlargement of the right ventricle and pulmonary arteries. B. One month after right single-lung transplantation. Note the dramatic reduction in right ventricular and pulmonary arterial size. The relative lack of perfusion to the native lung is apparent from the absence of vascular markings on the left side.

tive management of these patients, and our results have been gratifying. Of 50 patients undergoing transplantation for pulmonary vascular disease, we have had a 1-year survival of 78% and a 5-year survival of 63%. Mean New York Heart Association functional class improved from a pretransplant value of 3.4 to a post-transplant value of 1.3. Gas exchange and exercise tolerance data, depicted in Figures 92-19 to 92-21, demonstrate that these patients have functional results equivalent to any other transplant group in our experience. Postoperative radiographs of the chest illustrate the preponderance of pulmonary artery flow to the transplanted lung (Fig. 92-26).

Follow-up hemodynamic data for the first 34 patients receiving single-lung transplants in our program are depicted in Table 92-7 as reported by Pasque and colleagues (1995). After transplantation, the measured mean PA pressure dropped from 65 mm Hg to 23 mm Hg; the cardiac index (liters/minute/meter^2) improved from 2.2 to 3.4; and the calculated pulmonary vascular resistance decreased

Table 92-7. Mean Hemodynamics Before and After Lung Transplantation for Pulmonary Hypertension

	Pretransplant	3 months to 12 months	2 years	3 years	4 years
PAS (mm Hg)	103 ± 21	36 ± 8	31 ± 6	29 ± 6	31 ± 7
Pulmonary artery diastolic pressure (mm Hg)	46 ± 13	16 ± 4	16 ± 6	14 ± 4	16 ± 6
Pulmonary artery mean pressure (mm Hg)	65 ± 15	23 ± 5	21 ± 6	19 ± 5	21 ± 6
Pulmonary vascular resistance (dyne/sec/cm^{-5})	1361 ± 667	190 ± 84	149 ± 33	200 ± 105	153 ± 68
Central venous pressure (mm Hg)	13 ± 6	4 ± 3	4 ± 4	3 ± 1	4 ± 4
Pulmonary wedge pressure (mm Hg)	9 ± 5	10 ± 4	9 ± 6	7 ± 1	11 ± 5
Cardiac index (L/min/m^2)	2.17 ± 0.72	3.37 ± 0.77	3.66 ± 0.60	3.19 ± 0.55	3.79 ± 1.20

From Pasque MK, et al: Single-lung transplantation for pulmonary hypertension: single-institution experience in 34 patients. Circulation 92:2252, 1995. With permission.

from 1361 to 190. The hemodynamic benefits conferred by single-lung transplantation to recipients with pulmonary hypertension have been shown to be durable for up to 4 years in our cohort of patients.

Other groups have had significant difficulty with the application of single-lung transplantation in these patients. Bilateral lung replacement has been advocated by Bando and colleagues (1994), as well as by individuals in other programs. The standard operation previously offered these patients, combined heart-lung transplantation, is still practiced widely, particularly in the United Kingdom. These bilateral-lung replacement procedures may have a long-term advantage over single-lung transplantation in this patient group. Patients undergoing single-lung transplantation for pulmonary hypertension do exceedingly well as long as bronchiolitis obliterans can be avoided. When BOS develops in PPH or patients with Eisenmenger's syndrome receiving single-lung transplants, the resultant functional impairment is severe. Despite the theoretical early and late advantages of bilateral transplantation, Gammie and colleagues (1998) reviewed 7 years of transplantation for PPH and concluded that there was no measurable survival advantage or functional benefit for bilateral transplants over single-lung transplants.

FUTURE DIRECTIONS

A controversial strategy to increase the supply of donor organs is to expand the use of non–heart-beating donors (NHBDs). These donors can be controlled, meaning death is anticipated and preparations have been made for physiologic management of the donor and extraction of the organs, or uncontrolled, meaning preparations for organ procurement are initiated at some interval after death has occurred. Depending on the degree of control, the organs subject to retrieval are exposed to a variable length of potentially damaging warm ischemic time. The use of NHBDs as a source for lung grafts has been discussed, and we are aware of one case in which Lowe and associates at the University of Wisconsin (personal communication, 1997) used this technique successfully to retransplant a patient with severe reperfusion injury. The physiologic fragility of the ischemic lung has

prevented widespread clinical implementation of this strategy. Egan (1993) and Van Raemdonck (1997) and their colleagues reported experimental evidence that lungs that are kept ventilated or inflated post-mortem maintain physiologic stability despite the warm ischemia for up to 2 hours. Conservative estimates of the future impact of NHBD sources on the nationwide supply of organs predict an expansion of the cadaver organ supply by 25%, while more liberal projections claim a potential donor rate of up to 2.3% of hospital deaths, or in excess of 100 donors per million population per year. Future laboratory and clinical studies will be required to determine what fraction of such donors will provide viable lung allografts.

Another potential avenue of investigation is the ex vivo modification of the lung allograft to improve its function or render it resistant to common post-transplant complications. Boasquevisque and coworkers (1997), working with our group, have demonstrated successful gene transfer into lung isografts using adenoviral-mediated or liposome-mediated gene transfer. This early work shows promise for the eventual ability to insert therapeutic genes into the endothelial cells of a lung graft before surgical implantation into a recipient.

REFERENCES

Adnot S, Raffestin B: Pulmonary hypertension: NO therapy? Thorax 51:762, 1996.

Aoe M, et al: Administration of prostaglandin E$_1$ after lung transplantation improves early graft function. Ann Thorac Surg 58:655, 1994.

Bando K, et al: Indications for and results of single, bilateral and heart-lung transplantation for pulmonary hypertension. J Thorac Cardiovasc Surg 108:1056, 1994.

Barst RJ, et al: A comparison of continuous intravenous epoprostenol (prostacyclin) with conventional therapy for primary pulmonary hypertension. N Engl J Med 334:296, 1996.

Bhabra MS, et al: Critical importance of the first 10 minutes of lung graft reperfusion after hypothermic storage. Ann Thorac Surg 61:1631, 1996.

Boasquevisque CHR, et al: Ex vivo adenoviral-mediated gene transfer to lung isografts during cold preservation. Ann Thorac Surg 63:1556, 1997.

Chaparro C, et al: Status of lung transplant recipients surviving beyond five years. J Heart Lung Transplant 16:511, 1997.

Christie NA, Waddell TK: Lung preservation. Chest Surg Clin North Am 3:29, 1993.

Cooper JD, et al: A working formulation for the standardization of nomenclature and for clinical staging of chronic dysfunction in lung allografts. J Heart Lung Transplant 12:713, 1993.

Cooper JD, et al: Results of single- and bilateral lung transplantation in 131 consecutive recipients. J Thorac Cardiovasc Surg 107:460, 1994.

Couraud L, et al: Bronchial revascularization in double-lung transplantation: a series of 8 patients. Ann Thorac Surg 53:88, 1992.

D'Alonzo GE, et al: Survival in patients with primary pulmonary hypertension: results from a National Prospective Registry. Ann Intern Med 115:343, 1991.

Daly R, et al: Successful double-lung transplantation with direct bronchial artery revascularization. Ann Thorac Surg 56:885, 1993.

Dark JH: Experimental en-bloc double-lung transplantation. Ann Thorac Surg 42:394, 1986.

Date H, et al: Improved airway healing after lung transplantation: an analysis of 348 bronchial anastomoses. J Thorac Cardiovasc Surg 110:1424, 1995.

Date H, et al: Inhaled nitric oxide reduces human lung allograft dysfunction. J Thorac Cardiovasc Surg 111:913, 1996.

Davreux C, et al: Improved tracheal allograft viability in immunosuppressed rats. Ann Thorac Surg 55:131, 1993.

DeHoyos A, Maurer JR: Complications following lung transplantation. Semin Thorac Cardiovasc Surg 4:132, 1992.

de Hoyos AL, et al: Pulmonary transplantation: early and late results. J Thorac Cardiovasc Surg 103:295, 1992.

Derom F, et al: Ten month survival after lung homotransplantation in man. J Thorac Cardiovasc Surg 61:835, 1971.

Egan T, et al: Effect of a free radical scavenger on cadaver lung transplantation. Ann Thorac Surg 55:1453, 1993.

Eriksson LT, Steen S: Induced hypothermia in critical respiratory failure after lung transplantation. Ann Thorac Surg 65:827, 1998.

Etienne B, et al: Successful double-lung transplantation for bronchioalveolar carcinoma. Chest 112:1423, 1997.

Ettinger NA, et al: Cytomegalovirus infection and pneumonitis: impact after isolated lung transplantation. Am Rev Respir Dis 147:1017, 1993.

Fisher AJ, et al: Cross sectional study of exhaled nitric oxide levels following lung transplantation. Thorax 53:454, 1998.

Fremes SE, et al: Single-lung transplantation and closure of patent ductus arteriosus for Eisenmenger's syndrome. J Thorac Cardiovasc Surg 100:1, 1990.

Fujino S, et al: Inhaled nitric oxide at the time of harvest improves early lung allograft function. Ann Thorac Surg 63:1383, 1997.

Gaissert HA, et al: Comparison of early functional results after volume reduction or lung transplantation for chronic obstructive pulmonary disease. J Thorac Cardiovasc Surg 111:296, 1996.

Gammie JS, et al: Single- versus double-lung transplantation for pulmonary hypertension. J Thorac Cardiovasc Surg 115:397, 1998.

Goldberg M, et al: A comparison between cyclosporine A and methylprednisolone plus azathioprine on bronchial healing following canine lung transplantation. J Thorac Cardiovasc Surg 85:821, 1983.

Griffith BP, et al: Acute rejection of lung allografts with various immunosuppressive protocols. Ann Thorac Surg 54:846, 1992.

Griffith BP, et al: Anastomotic pitfalls in lung transplantation. J Thorac Cardiovasc Surg 107:743, 1994.

Hakim M, et al: Selection and procurement of combined heart and lung grafts for transplantation. J Thorac Cardiovasc Surg 85:474, 1988.

Halldorsson A, et al: Controlled reperfusion after lung ischemia: implications for improved function after lung transplantation. J Thorac Cardiovasc Surg 115:415, 1998.

Hardesty R, et al: A clinical trial of University of Wisconsin solution for pulmonary preservation. J Thorac Cardiovasc Surg 105:660, 1993.

Hardin CA, Kittle CF: Experiences with transplantation of the lung. Science 119:97, 1954.

Hardy JD, et al: Lung homotransplantation in man. JAMA 186:1065, 1963.

Hasagawa S, et al: Changes in ICAM-1 expression during human lung preservation. Am Rev Respir Dis 147:A263, 1993.

Haydock DA, et al: Management of dysfunction in the transplanted lung: experience with 7 clinical cases. Ann Thorac Surg 53:635, 1992.

Hayllar KM, et al: A prognostic model for the prediction of survival in cystic fibrosis. Thorax 52:313, 1997.

Higenbottam T, et al: Transbronchial lung biopsy for the diagnosis of rejection in heart-lung transplant patients. Transplantation 46:532, 1988.

Hirai T, et al: Prolonged lung allograft survival with short course of FK 506. J Thorac Cardiovasc Surg 105:1, 1993.

Hopkinson DN, et al: Pulmonary graft preservation - a worldwide survey of current clinical practice. J Heart Lung Transplant 17:525, 1998.

Hosenpud JD, et al: The Registry of the International Society for Heart and Lung Transplantation: Fifteenth Official Report-1998. J Heart Lung Transplant 17:656, 1998.

Huddleston C, et al: Lung retransplantation in children. Ann Thorac Surg 66:199, 1998.

Inui K, et al: Bronchial circulation after experimental lung transplantation. The effect of long term administration of prednisolone. J Thorac Cardiovasc Surg 105:474, 1993.

Kerem E, et al: Prediction of mortality in patients with cystic fibrosis. N Engl J Med 326:1187, 1992.

Keshavjee S, et al: The role of dextran 40 and potassium in extended hypothermic lung preservation for transplantation. J Thorac Cardiovasc Surg 103:314, 1992.

Kirk A, et al: Successful surgical management of bronchial dehiscence after single-lung transplantation. Ann Thorac Surg 49:147, 1990.

Kirk AJB, et al: Lung preservation: a review of current practice and future directions. Ann Thorac Surg 56:990, 1993.

Kroshus TJ, et al: Unilateral volume reduction after single-lung transplantation for emphysema. Ann Thorac Surg 62:363, 1996.

Levin SM, et al: Medium term functional results of single-lung transplantation for endstage obstructive lung disease. Am J Respir Crit Care Med 150:398, 1994.

Lima O, et al: Effects of methylprednisolone and azathioprine on bronchial healing following lung autotransplantation. J Thorac Cardiovasc Surg 82:211, 1981.

Lynch JP, Trulock EP: Recipient selection. Semin Respir Crit Care Med 17:109, 1996.

Matsuzaki Y, et al: Amelioration of post-ischemic lung reperfusion injury by PGE. Am Rev Respir Dis 148:882, 1993.

Mayer E, et al: Reliable eighteen-hour lung preservation at 4°C and 10°C by pulmonary artery flush after high-dose prostaglandin E1. J Thorac Cardiovasc Surg 103:1136, 1992.

Mendeloff EN, et al: Pediatric and adult lung transplantation for cystic fibrosis. J Thorac Cardiovasc Surg 115:404, 1997.

Metras H: Note prelaminar sur la Greeff tootle du pomona cheese le Chiene. C. R. Cad. SCI. (Paris) 231:1176, 1950.

Meyer KC, et al: The therapeutic potential of nitric oxide in lung transplantation. Chest 113:1360, 1998.

Meyers BF, et al: Bilateral sequential lung transplant without sternal division eliminates post-transplant sternal complications. J Thorac Cardiovasc Surg 117:358, 1999.

Milla CE, Warwick WJ: Risk of death in cystic fibrosis patients with severely compromised lung function. Chest 113:1230, 1998.

Miller J, et al: An evaluation of the role of omentopexy and of early perioperative corticosteroid administration in clinical lung transplantation. J Thorac Cardiovasc Surg 105:247, 1993.

Morgan E, et al: Successful revascularization of totally ischemic bronchial autografts with omental pedicle flaps in dogs. J Thorac Cardiovasc Surg 84:204, 1982.

Norgaard MA, et al: Medium-term patency and anatomic changes after direct bronchial artery revascularization in lung and heart-lung transplantation with the internal thoracic artery conduit. J Thorac Cardiovasc Surg 114:326, 1997.

Novick R, et al: Redo lung transplantation: a North American-European experience. J Heart Lung Transplant 12:5, 1993.

Novick RJ, et al: Lung preservation: the importance of endothelial and alveolar type II cell integrity. Ann Thorac Surg 62:302, 1996.

Novick RJ, et al: Pulmonary retransplantation: predictors of graft function and survival in 230 patients. Ann Thorac Surg 65:227, 1998.

Okamoto F, et al: Studies of controlled reperfusion after ischemia. XIV. Reperfusion conditions: importance of ensuring gentle versus sudden reperfusion during relief of coronary occlusion. J Thorac Cardiovasc Surg 92:613, 1986.

Pasque MK, et al: An improved technique for bilateral lung transplantation: rationale and initial clinical experience. Ann Thorac Surg 49:785, 1990.

Pasque MK, et al: Single-lung transplantation for pulmonary hypertension: single-institution experience in 34 patients. Circulation 92:2252, 1995.

Patterson G: Airway complications. Chest Surg Clin North Am 3:157, 1993.

Patterson G, et al: Airway complications after double lung transplantation. J Thorac Cardiovasc Surg 99:14, 1990.

Patterson GA, et al: Technique of successful clinical double-lung transplantation. Ann Thorac Surg 45:626, 1988.

Pochettino A, Bavaria JE: Anterior axillary muscle-sparing thoracotomy for lung transplantation. Ann Thorac Surg 64:1846, 1997.

Puskas J, et al: Equivalent eighteen-hour lung preservation with low-potassium dextran or Euro-Collins solution after prostaglandin E1 infusion. J Thorac Cardiovasc Surg 104:83, 1992a.

Puskas J, et al: Reliable 30 hour lung preservation by donor hyperinflation. J Thorac Cardiovasc Surg 104:1075, 1992b.

Ramirez JC, et al: Bilateral lung transplantation for cystic fibrosis. J Thorac Cardiovasc Surg 103:287, 1992.

Reichenspurner H, et al: Obliterative bronchiolitis after lung and heart-lung transplantation. Ann Thorac Surg 60:1845, 1995.

Reitz B, et al: Heart-lung transplantation: successful therapy for patients with pulmonary vascular disease. N Engl J Med 306:557, 1982.

Schafers HJ, et al: Cardiac innervation after double lung transplant. J Thorac Cardiovasc Surg 99:22, 1990.

Schmid RA, et al: Carbohydrate selectin inhibitor CY-1503 reduces neutrophil migration and reperfusion injury in canine pulmonary allografts. J Heart Lung Transplant 16:1054, 1997.

Sharples L, et al: Prognosis of patients with cystic fibrosis awaiting heart and lung transplantation. J Heart Lung Transplant 12:669, 1993.

Shiraishi Y, et al: Retrieval by other procurement teams provides favorable lung transplantation outcome. Ann Thorac Surg 64:203, 1997.

Shiraishi Y, et al: Use of leukocyte depletion to decrease injury after lung preservation and rewarming ischemia—an experimental model. J Heart Lung Transplant 17:250, 1998.

Silkoff PE, et al: Exhaled nitric oxide in human lung transplantation. Am J Respir Crit Care Med 157:1822, 1998.

Snell G, et al: Pseudomonas cepacia in lung transplant recipients with cystic fibrosis. Chest 103:336, 1993.

Spray T, et al: Pediatric lung transplantation for pulmonary hypertension and congenital heart disease. Ann Thorac Surg 54:216, 1992.

Spray T, et al: Pediatric lung transplantation: indications, techniques and early results. J Thorac Cardiovasc Surg 107:990, 1994.

Starnes VA, et al: Experience with living-donor lobar transplantation for indications other than cystic fibrosis. J Thorac Cardiovasc Surg 114:917, 1997.

Sundaresan S, et al: Lung preservation with low-potassium dextran flush in a primate bilateral transplant model. Ann Thorac Surg 56:1129, 1993a.

Sundaresan S, et al: Donor lung procurement: assessment and operative technique. Ann Thorac Surg 56:1409, 1993b.

Sundaresan S, et al: Successful outcome of lung transplantation is not compromised by the use of marginal donor lungs. J Thorac Cardiovasc Surg 109:1075, 1995a.

Sundaresan S, et al: Prevalence and outcome of bronchiolitis obliterans syndrome after lung transplantation. Ann Thorac Surg 60:1341, 1995b.

Sweet S, et al: Pediatric lung transplantation at St. Louis Children's Hospital. Am J Respir Crit Care Med 155:1027, 1997.

Todd T, et al: Separate extraction of cardiac and pulmonary grafts from a single-organ donor. Ann Thorac Surg 46:356, 1988.

Todd TRJ, et al: Simultaneous single-lung transplantation and lung volume reduction. Ann Thorac Surg 63:1468, 1997.

Toronto Lung Transplantation Group: Unilateral lung transplantation for pulmonary fibrosis. N Engl J Med 314:1140, 1986.

Trulock EP: Lung transplantation. Am J Respir Crit Care Med 155:789, 1997.

UNOS: 1997 Annual Report of the US Scientific Registry for Transplant Recipients and the Organ Procurement and Transplant Network—Transplant Data: 1988–1996. Richmond, VA: US Department of Health and Human Services, Rockville, MD, 1998.

Unruh HW: Lung preservation and lung injury. Chest Surg Clin North Am 5:91, 1995.

Van Raemdonck DEM, et al: Extended preservation of ischemic pulmonary graft by postmortem alveolar expansion. Ann Thorac Surg 64:801, 1997.

Varela A, et al: Early lung allograft function after retrograde and antegrade preservation. J Thorac Cardiovasc Surg 114:1119, 1997.

Wang L, et al: Influence of temperature of flushing solution on lung preservation. Ann Thorac Surg 55:711, 1993.

Westaby S: Aprotinin in perspective. Ann Thorac Surg 55:1033, 1993.

Yamashita M, et al: Nitroprusside ameliorates lung allograft reperfusion injury. Ann Thorac Surg 62:791, 1996.

Yousem SA, et al: A working formulation for the standardization of nomenclature in the diagnosis of heart and lung rejection: Lung Rejection Study Group. J Heart Lung Transplant 9:593, 1990.

Zorn G: Lung transplantation for bronchoalveolar carcinoma of the lung. In Franco KL, Putnam J (eds): Advanced Therapy in Thoracic Surgery. Boston: Blackwell Science, 1998.

SECTION XV

Carcinoma of the Lung

CHAPTER 93

Lung Cancer: Epidemiology and Carcinogenesis

Lynn T. Tanoue and Richard A. Matthay

Carcinoma of the lung is the leading cause of cancer death in the United States. The sheer magnitude of the lung cancer epidemic is staggering. Landis and colleagues (1998) projected that 171,500 new cases of lung cancer would be diagnosed in 1998. At present, more persons succumb annually to lung cancer than die from cancers of the colon, breast, and prostate combined.

Lung cancer mortality in men appears to be plateauing (Fig. 93-1). In 1997 the estimated number of lung cancer deaths was 178,000 while in 1998, 93,100 deaths were projected. However, the mortality from lung cancer in women continues to rise (Fig. 93-2). Lung cancer surpassed breast cancer as the leading cause of cancer death in women in 1987. In 1998 it was estimated to cause 67,000 deaths, accounting for 25% of all cancer mortality in women.

The enormity of the lung cancer problem mandates examination of the epidemiology of the disease. Currently, despite the availability of new diagnostic technologies, advancements in surgical techniques, and the development of nonsurgical treatment modalities, overall 5-year survival rate for lung cancer remains a dismal 14%. Given this, prevention should be a major focus of the efforts now being made in this field. Understanding the epidemiology of lung cancer, including the identification of risk factors, is important because the modification of risks should impact the development of this disease.

This chapter focuses primarily on a discussion of modifiable risk factors, including tobacco smoking, exposure to occupational carcinogens, exposure to ionizing radiation, and diet. The molecular and genetic aspects of carcinogenesis are discussed separately in Chapter 94.

TOBACCO SMOKING

Tobacco has been a part of the cultural and economic structure of this country since the time of Columbus. It was originally chewed or smoked in pipes, and cigarettes became widely available after the development of cigarette wrapping machinery in the mid-1800s. However, before World War I, cigarette use in the United States was modest. Wynder and Hoffman (1950) estimated that in 1900 the average annual adult cigarette consumption was less than 100 cigarettes per person. In 1950 this number rose to approximately 3500 cigarettes per person per year and reached a maximum of approximately 4400 cigarettes per person per year in the mid-1960s. In 1964 the U.S. Public Health Service Surgeon General (1964) published a report on Smoking and Health. The principal findings of this report were as follows: 1) Cigarette smoking was associated with a 70% increase in the age-specific death rates of men and a lesser increase in death rate of women. 2) Cigarette smoking was found to be causally related to lung cancer in men. The magnitude of the effect of cigarette smoking far outweighed all other factors leading to lung cancer. The risk of developing lung cancer increased with duration of smoking and the number of cigarettes smoked per day. The Surgeon General's report estimated that the average male smoker had an approximately ninefold to tenfold risk of developing lung cancer while heavy smokers had at least a 20-fold risk. 3) Cigarette smoking was thought to be much more important than occupational exposures in the causation of lung cancer in the general population. 4) Cigarette smoking was found to be the most important cause of chronic bronchitis in the United States. 5) It was established that male cigarette smokers have a higher death rate from coronary artery disease than nonsmoking men.

At the conclusion of the report, the following judgment was made: "Cigarette smoking is a health hazard of sufficient importance in the United States to warrant appropriate remedial action." Since the submission of the Surgeon General's report, yearly per capita consumption of cigarettes has declined in the United States, although it is estimated that 25% of all Americans continue to smoke (Fig. 43-3).

At the turn of the century, lung cancer was an uncommon disease. In 1912 Adler performed an extensive review of autopsy reports from hospitals in the United States and western European countries and found 374 cases of pri-

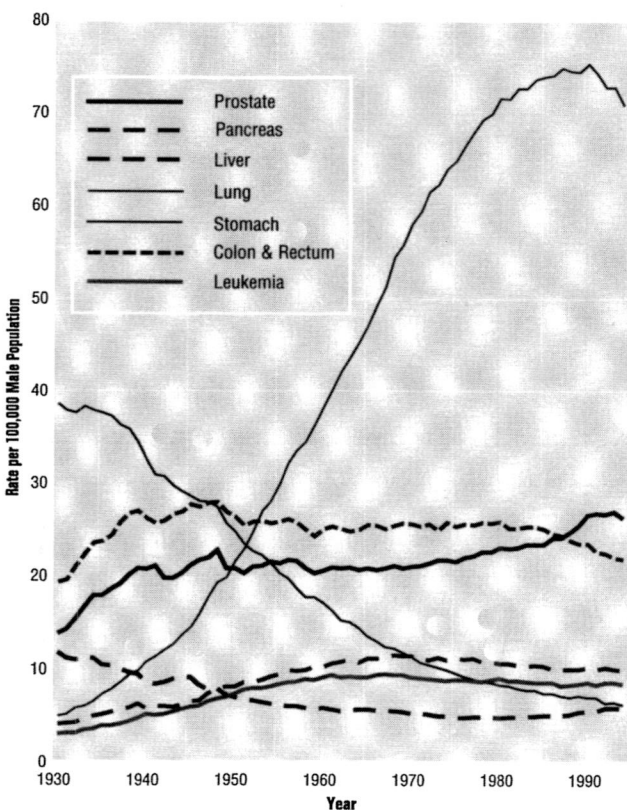

Fig. 93-1. Age-adjusted cancer death rates for males by site, United States, 1930–1994. Rates are per 100,000 population and are age-adjusted to the 1970 U.S. standard population. Note: Because of changes in the *International Classification of Diseases* coding, numerator information has changed over time. Rates for cancer of the liver, lung, and colon and rectum are affected by these coding changes. From Landis SH, et al: Vital statistics of the United States, 1997. CA Cancer J Clin *48*:6, 1998. With permission.

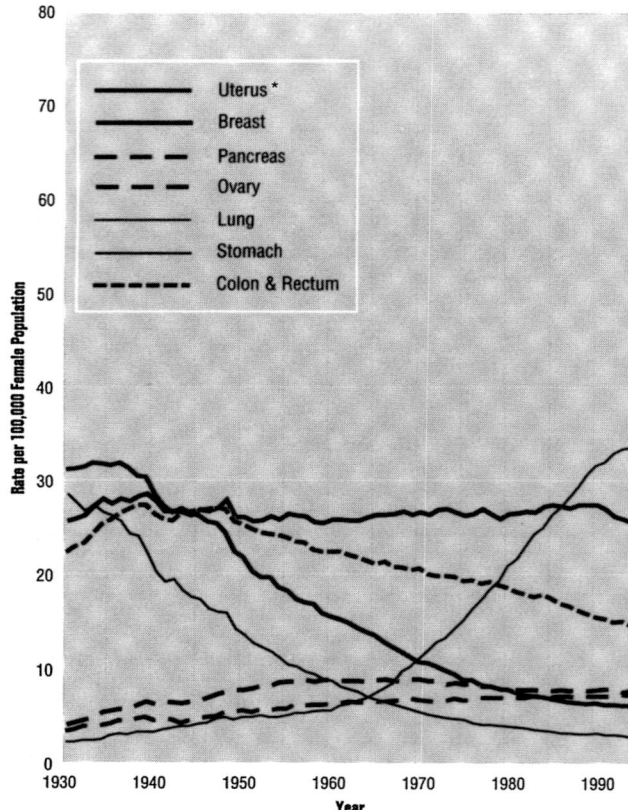

Fig. 93-2. Age-adjusted cancer death rates for females by site, United States, 1930–1994. Rates are per 100,000 population and are age-adjusted to the 1970 U.S. standard population. Note: Because of changes in the *International Classification of Diseases* coding, numerator information has changed over time. Rates for cancer of the liver, lung, and colon and rectum are affected by these coding changes. *Uterine cancer death rates are for cervix (uterus) and endometrium (uterus) combined. From Landis SH, et al: Vital statistics of the United States, 1997. CA Cancer J Clin *48*:6, 1998. With permission.

mary lung cancer. This represented less than 0.5% of all cancer cases. Adler concluded that "primary malignant neoplasms of the lung are among the rarest forms of disease." Over the next several decades a number of authors in the United States and abroad noted an increase in the incidence of carcinoma of the lung. In a series of 185,434 autopsy cases collected between 1897 and 1930, Hruby and Sweany (1933) noted that the incidence of lung cancer had increased disproportionately to the incidence of cancer in general. In the early decades of the century, it was postulated that the observed increase in lung cancer might be due to a variety of etiologies including influenza, tuberculosis, irritating gases, atmospheric pollution from industrial plants and coal fires, and chronic bronchitis. As early as 1930, Roffo concluded from observations made in patients and experimental studies done in animals that tobacco tar liberated from the burning of tobacco was a

carcinogenic agent. By the 1920s and 1930s a number of uncontrolled series called attention to the potential role of cigarette smoking in the observed increase in lung cancer incidence. Fahr (1923), Lickint (1935), McNally (1932), Roffo (1930), Ochsner and DeBakey (1939), Tylecote (1927), and Levin and colleagues (1950), among others, voiced a growing concern that the increase in lung cancer was due to the growing use of cigarettes. In 1941 Ochsner and DeBakey stated in a review of carcinoma of the lung, "It is our definite conviction that the increase in the incidence of pulmonary carcinoma is due largely to the increase in smoking."

In 1950 two landmark epidemiologic studies evaluating the role of tobacco smoking as an etiologic factor in bronchial carcinoma were published. Wynder and Graham (1950) in the United States reported a case-control study examining 605 cases of lung cancer in men compared with a

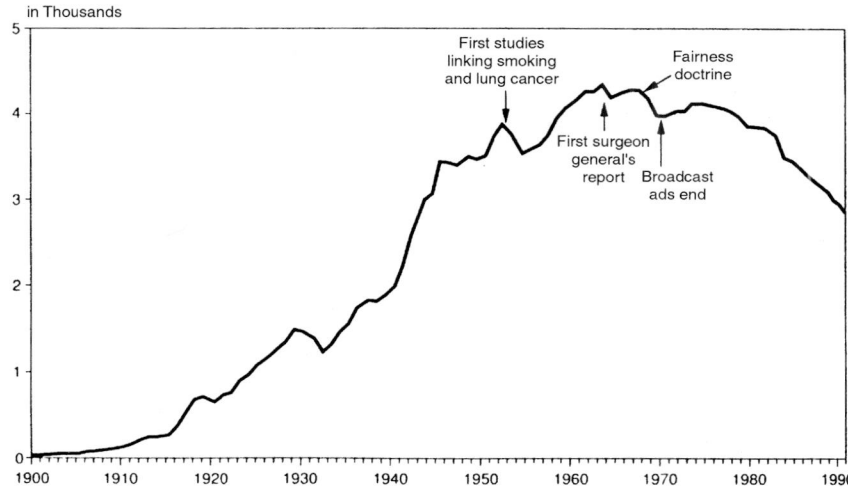

in Thousands

Fig. 93-3. United States adult (ages 18 and older) per capita cigarette consumption during this century, and the influence of select social factors. From Shopland DR: Effect of smoking on the incidence and mortality of lung cancer. *In* Johnson BE, Johnson DH (eds): Lung Cancer. New York: John Wiley & Sons, 1995, pp. 1–14. With permission.

general male hospital population without cancer. The most striking finding was that 96.5% of lung cancers were found in men who were moderate to heavy smokers for many years compared with the general population, which had a smoking rate of 73.7%. Several important conclusions were drawn in this study: 1) Excessive and prolonged use of tobacco was an important factor in the induction of lung cancer, 2) the occurrence of lung cancer in a nonsmoker was a rare phenomenon, and 3) a lag period of 10 years or more between smoking cessation and the clinical onset of carcinoma was observed. This report was closely followed by a similar case-control study done in the United Kingdom by Doll and Hill (1950). Six hundred forty-nine male and 60 female lung cancer subjects were interviewed at 20 London hospitals and compared with 1029 subjects who had cancer in organs other than the lung and 743 general medical and surgical patients matched for age and sex; 0.3% of men and 31.7% of women with lung cancer in this study were nonsmokers compared with 4.2% of men and 53.3% of women without cancer. Like Wynder and Graham, these authors concluded that an association between carcinoma of the lung and cigarette smoking did indeed exist and that the effect on development of lung cancer varied with the amount of cigarette use.

Cigarette smoke is a complex aerosol composed of both gaseous and particulate compounds. It is broken down into mainstream smoke and sidestream smoke components. Mainstream smoke is produced by inhalation of air through the cigarette and is the primary source of smoke exposure for the smoker. Sidestream smoke is produced from smoldering of the cigarette between puffs and is the major source of environmental tobacco smoke. The primary determinant of tobacco addiction is nicotine. *Tar* is defined as the total particulate matter of cigarette smoke after nicotine and water have been removed. Tar exposure appears to be the major link to lung cancer risk. The Federal Trade Commission determines nicotine and tar content of cigarettes by measurements made on standardized smoking machines.

However, it is clear that the composition of mainstream smoke can be quite variable depending on the intensity of inhalation, which differs among individual smokers. While filter tips decrease the amount of nicotine and tar in mainstream smoke, the effect of filter tips can also be variable because compression of the tips by lips or fingers has been shown to affect the composition of inhaled smoke.

More than 4000 individual constituents of cigarette smoke have been identified. Hoffman and Hoffman (1997) and Burns (1994) in extensive reviews of cigarettes and smoke composition noted that 95% of the weight of mainstream smoke comes from 400 to 500 individual gaseous compounds. The remainder of the weight is made up of more than 3500 particulate components. This does not include additives such as flavorings, which are considered trade secrets and often are unknown.

It is clear that mainstream smoke contains a large number of potential carcinogens, including polynuclear aromatic hydrocarbons, aromatic amines, *N*-nitrosamines (TSNA), and miscellaneous organic and inorganic compounds such as benzene, vinyl chloride, arsenic, and chromium (Table 93-1). Furthermore, radioactive materials including radon and its decay products, bismuth and polonium, are also present in tobacco smoke. The agents that appear to be of particular concern in the etiology of carcinoma of the lung are the tobacco specific TSNA formed by nitrozation of nicotine both during tobacco processing and smoking. Eight TSNA have been described, including 4-(methylnitrosamine)-1-(3-pyridyl)-1-butanone (NNK), which is known to induce adenocarcinoma of the lung in experimental animal models. Other TSNA have been linked to cancers of the esophagus, bladder, pancreas, oral cavity, and larynx.

Of the TSNA, NNK appears to the most important inducer of lung cancer. It has carcinogenic effects with both topical and systemic administration. Inhalation of tobacco smoke containing TSNA results in direct delivery of carcinogen to the lungs. As these compounds are also absorbed

Table 93-1. Tumorigenic Agents in Tobacco and Tobacco Smoke

	Processed tobacco (per gram)	Mainstream Smoke (per cigarette)	Evidence for IARC Evaluation of Carcinogenicity	
			In Lab Animals	In Humans
PAH				
Benz(a)anthracene		2–70 ng	Sufficient	NA
Benzo(b)fluorantene		4–22 ng	Sufficient	NA
Benzo(j)fluoranthene		6–21 ng	Sufficient	NA
Benzo(k)fluoranthene		6–12 ng	Sufficient	NA
Benzo(a)pyrene	0.1–90 mg	20–40 ng	Sufficient	Probable
Chrysene		40–60 ng	Sufficient	NA
Dibenz(a,h)anthracene		4 ng	Sufficient	NA
Dibenz(a,i)pyrene		1.7–3.2 ng	Sufficient	NA
Dibenzo(a,l)pyrene		Present	Sufficient	NA
Indeno(1,2,3c,d)pyrene		4–20 ng	Sufficient	NA
S-Methylchrysene		0.6 ng	Sufficient	NA
Aza-arenes				
Quinoline		1 µg	NA	NA
Dibenz(a,h)acridine		0.1 ng	Sufficient	NA
Dibenz(a,j)acridine		3–10 ng	Sufficient	NA
7H-Dibenzo(c,g)carbazole		0.7 ng	Sufficient	NA
N-nitrosamines				
N-Nitrosodimethylamine	ND–215 ng	0.1–180 ng	Sufficient	NA
N-Nitrosoethylmethylamine		3.13 ng	Sufficient	NA
N-Nitrosodiethylamine		ND–25 ng	Sufficient	NA
N-Nitrosopyrrolidine	ND–360 ng	1.5–110 ng	Sufficient	NA
N-Nitrosodiethanolamine	ND–6,900 ng	ND–36 ng	Sufficient	NA
N-Nitrosonornicotine	0.3–89 µg	0.12–3.7 µg	Sufficient	NA
4-(methylnitrosamino)-l-(3-pyridyl)-l-butanone	0.2–7 µg	0.08–0.77 µg	Sufficient	NA
N-Nitrosoanabasine	0.01–1.9 µg	0.14–4.6 µg	Limited	NA
N-Nitrosomorpholine	ND–690 ng		Sufficient	NA
Aromatic amines				
2-Toluidine		30–200 ng	Sufficient	Inadequate
2-Naphthylamine		1–22 ng	Sufficient	Sufficient
4-Aminobiophenyl		2–5 ng	Sufficient	Sufficient
Aldehydes				
Formaldehyde	1.6–7–4 µg	70–100 µg	Sufficient	NA
Acetaldehyde	1.4–7.4 mg	18–1,400 mg	Sufficient	NA
Crotonaldehyde	0.2–2.4 µg	10–20 µg	NA	NA
Miscellaneous organic compounds				
Benzene		12–48 µg	Sufficient	Sufficient
Acrylonitrile		3.2–15 µg	Sufficient	Limited
1,1-Dimethylhydrazine	60–147 µg		Sufficient	NA
2-Nitropropane		0.73–1.21 µg	Sufficient	NA
Ethylcarbamate	310–375 ng	20–38 ng	Sufficient	NA
Vinyl chloride		1–16 ng	Sufficient	Sufficient
Inorganic compounds				
Hydrazine	14–51 ng	24–43 ng	Sufficient	Inadequate
Arsenic	500–900 ng	40–120 ng	Inadequate	Sufficient
Nickel	2,000–6,000 ng	0–600 ng	Sufficient	Limited
Chromium	1,000–2,000 ng	4–70 ng	Sufficient	Sufficient
Cadmium	1,300–1,600 ng	41–62 ng	Sufficient	Limited
Lead	8–10 µg		Sufficient	Inadequate
Polonium-210	0.2–1.2 pCi	0.03–1.0 pCi	NA	NA

IARC, International Agency for Research on Cancer; ND, no data; NA, evaluation has not been done by IARC.
From Burns DM: Tobacco smoking. *In* Samet JM (ed): Epidemiology of Lung Cancer. New York: Marcel Dekker, 1994, pp. 15–49. With permission.

systemically, hematogenous delivery to lung via the pulmonary circulation occurs as well.

The 1989 U.S. Department of Health and Human Services Surgeon General's report on Reducing the Health Consequences of Smoking (1989) stated that 43 chemicals in tobacco smoke have been determined to be carcinogenic. It is important to note that the dosage of smoke constituents to the smoker can be highly variable, depending not just on the cigarette itself but also on the pattern of smoking. Specifically, the duration and intensity of inhalation, the presence and competence of a filter, and the duration of cooling of the smoke before inhalation can all change smoke composition. Over the last several decades the nicotine and tar contents of cigarettes have been lowered. However, the primary factor determining intensity of use of cigarettes is the smoker's nicotine dependence. Thus, though cigarettes now contain less nicotine and tar than before, to satisfy their nicotine need, smokers tend to smoke more intensely with more puffs per minute and deeper inhalations. In such situations the measurements of tar and nicotine cigarette content made by smoking machines may significantly underestimate individual exposure.

Wynder and Hoffman (1994) proposed an intriguing hypothesis as to how low-yield filtered cigarettes might be a contributing factor to the observed increase of adenocarcinoma versus squamous cell carcinoma of the lung over the last several decades. As stated, the nicotine-addicted smoker will smoke low-yield cigarettes far more intensely than older non-filtered higher yield cigarettes. With deeper inhalation, higher order bronchi in the peripheral lung will be exposed to carcinogen-containing smoke as opposed to the major bronchi alone. These peripheral bronchi lack protective epithelium and are being exposed to carcinogens including TSNA, which are linked to induction of adenocarcinoma. Data from several laboratories including those of Hoffman (1993), Belinsky (1988), and Ronan (1993) and their colleagues, have documented that NNK is associated with DNA mutations resulting in the activation of K-*ras* oncogenes. Rodenhuis and Slebos (1992) reported that K-*ras* oncogene activation has been identified in 24% of human lung adenocarcinomas. Of note, Westra and colleagues (1993) have reported that K-ras mutations are present in adenocarcinoma of the lung found in ex-smokers, suggesting that such mutations do not revert with the cessation of tobacco smoking. This may explain in part the persistent elevation in lung cancer risk in ex-smokers even years after discontinuing cigarette use.

There is no doubt that tobacco smoking is the most important modifiable risk factor for lung cancer. However, it is clear that individual susceptibility is also a factor in carcinogenesis. While more than 80% of lung cancers occur in persons with tobacco exposure, less than 20% of smokers will ever develop lung cancer. The variability seen in susceptibility presumably must be influenced by other environmental factors or by genetic predisposition.

Spitz and associates (1998) reviewed markers of susceptibility in lung cancer. They pointed out that factors that affect the absorption, metabolism, and accumulation of tobacco or other carcinogens in lung tissue will also affect cancer susceptibility. For example, the cytochrome P450 multigene family, glutathione S-transferase gene families, and the genes determining N-acetylation (rapid, intermediate, or slow acetylator phenotypes) may all be involved in activation or detoxification of tobacco carcinogens. These genes themselves are subject to genetic polymorphisms, which may alter the levels of these metabolizing/detoxifying enzymes, thus impacting relative risks for cancer. Furthermore, susceptibility to carcinogenic agents may also be affected by individual differences in mutagen sensitivity. Mutagen sensitivity can be measured by assaying the frequency of bleomycin-induced chromosomal aberrations in lymphocytes, as outlined by Hsu and colleagues (1989). Wu and associates (1995) demonstrated that the presence of mutagen sensitivity is associated with an increased risk of lung cancer. Furthermore, Spitz's group (1998) demonstrated that the combined risk for lung cancer was greater in individuals with mutagen sensitivity and who smoked compared with individuals with either smoking or mutagen sensitivity, and greater than in nonsmokers with mutagen sensitivity alone. Alterations in cytogenetics as well as variability in the ability of the individual to monitor and repair DNA damage may also impact cancer susceptibility.

Smoking has been shown to be associated with mutations in the p53 tumor suppressor gene. Mutations in this gene are the most common genetic alterations seen in human cancers. Work by a number of investigators, including Ryberg (1994), Field (1991), Koch (1995), Wang (1995), and Kawajiri (1996) and their colleagues, has demonstrated that specific exposures may be associated with specific mutations, thus establishing a link between environmental agents and chromosomal abnormalities. In particular, p53 mutations have been associated with a history of heavy tobacco use. Work by several groups demonstrated increased frequencies of p53 mutations in heavy smokers as compared with persons with lower levels of tobacco exposure or nonsmokers. However, as noted by Brennan and associates (1995), endogenous, or at least nontobacco-related p53 mutations have also been identified, underscoring the point that tobacco is only one of multiple factors leading to lung cancer.

Lung cancer susceptibility is thus determined at least in part by host genetic factors. Persons with genetic susceptibility therefore might be at even higher risk if they also smoke cigarettes. As technology advances, it may be possible to target subgroups identified as genetically at high risk for lung cancer for specific interventions, including intensive efforts at smoking cessation, screening, and prevention programs.

Airways Obstruction

Tobacco smoking is the primary cause of both lung cancer and chronic obstructive pulmonary disease (COPD). A study by Wu, Fontham, and Reynolds (1995) of women with lung cancer who had never smoked demonstrated a statistically significant association between the presence of air flow obstruction and the development of lung cancer. A number of other groups including Skillrud (1986) and Tockman (1987) and their colleagues, as well as Cohen (1980), have also presented evidence that air-flow obstruction itself constitutes a risk for lung cancer. This conclusion was further supported by the outcomes observed by Anthonisen and coworkers in the Lung Health Study (1994), in which a total of 5887 male and female smokers with spirometric evidence of mild to moderate COPD were monitored over a 5-year period with or without intervention of smoking cessation or bronchodilator therapy. One of the notable findings from this study was that mortality from lung cancer exceeded that from cardiovascular disease by nearly 50%. Lung cancer was the most common cause of death, accounting for 38% of all deaths among study participants.

Gender

Since 1950 a more than 500% increase in lung cancer mortality has been noted in women. While most of this increase is attributed to the dramatic increase in the prevalence of smoking among women since the 1940s, several disturbing facts have emerged. The first is that dose for dose, women appear to have an enhanced susceptibility to carcinogens in cigarettes when compared with men. This may translate into an increased risk for lung cancer. A number of studies, including those by Zang and Wynder (1996), Risch (1993), Brownson (1992), and McDuffie (1987) and their colleagues, as well as Lubin and Blot (1984), suggested that women may be more vulnerable to tobacco carcinogens than men. Specifically, in a case-control study of male-female differences in lung cancer covering the period 1981 to 1985 in Ontario, Canada, Risch and associates (1993) demonstrated that with a history of 40 pack years of cigarette smoking relative to lifelong nonsmoking, the odds ratio for women developing lung cancer was 27.9 versus 9.6 in men. Similarly, another large case-control study by Zang and Wynder (1996) showed that dose-response-odds ratios for the development of lung cancer in women were 1.2-fold to 1.7-fold higher in women than men. In both studies the increase in lung cancer risk was true for all major histologic types of cancer. The observed gender difference in susceptibility may be related to a number of factors including hormonal effects and sex-related differences in nicotine metabolism, metabolic activation, or detoxification of lung carcinogens.

The second issue is that cigarette smoking may also be associated with a higher risk of the development of non-cancer lung disease in women than men, including obstructive airway disease. Studies by Chen and colleagues (1991) suggested that cigarette smoking may be more harmful in terms of its effects on pulmonary function in women than men. In their studies, changes in forced expiratory volume in one second (FEV_1) and maximal mid-expiratory flow rate (MMFR) and the slope of phase III of the single-breath nitrogen test increased with increasing pack years more rapidly in female smokers than in their male counterparts. These changes were independent of age, height, and weight. Similar results have been reported by Buist (1979) and Detels (1981) and their coworkers. Furthermore, Beck and colleagues (1981), in a study of 4690 whites, found that for a given level of smoking, female subjects demonstrated changes in FEV_1 and MMFR at 25% and 50% of vital capacity at a younger age (15 to 24 years) than male subjects (40 to 45 years). Because people with tobacco exposure and

spirometric evidence of airway obstruction are at higher risk for developing lung cancer, the suggestion that women may have increased susceptibility to cigarette-induced airway disease may be important in the consideration of their risk for lung cancer as well.

Last, although women may have enhanced susceptibility to the carcinogenic effects of tobacco, it also appears that lung cancer occurs more commonly in nonsmoking women than in nonsmoking men. In their early report of tobacco smoking as a possible etiologic factor in lung cancer, Wynder and Graham (1950) noted that a greater percentage of cancers in nonsmokers occurred in women than men. However, the number of women in that study was relatively small, and few women had at that time smoked for a duration of decades. Thus no definite conclusion regarding an altered risk of lung cancer related to tobacco smoking in women could be made on the basis of their observations. Subsequently, however, it has become clear that women never-smokers are more likely than male never-smokers to develop lung cancer. In a case control study by Zang and Wynder (1996) of 1889 lung cancer subjects and 2070 control subjects, the proportion of never-smoking lung cancer patients was more than twice as high in women than men. The reasons for this are not clear, but speculation has been raised regarding the potential for women having greater susceptibility to nontobacco environmental carcinogens, having increased exposure to environmental tobacco smoke, or to sex-linked differences in the metabolism of nontobacco environmental carcinogens.

Environmental Factors

A tremendous amount of epidemiologic work has been directed toward understanding the effects of lung carcinogenesis resulting from environmental factors other than tobacco, as well as interactions between them. In particular, the combined effects of tobacco smoke with occupational carcinogens has received much attention. An additive or multiplicative risk of lung cancer has been demonstrated when cigarette smoking is present in the setting of exposure to asbestos, radon, arsenic, silica, and nickel, among others. The role of nutrition in cancer development has also received more attention. The carcinogenic potential of occupational exposures including asbestos and radon and the influence of diet are discussed separately in this chapter.

Environmental Tobacco Smoke

The 1964 U.S. Public Health Service Surgeon General's report on the Health Consequences of Smoking (1964) did not address the issue of environmental tobacco smoke (ETS). However, because nonsmoking persons exposed to ETS are observed to have an increased rate of smoke-related problems including upper respiratory symptoms, eye irritation, and an observed increased frequency of respiratory illnesses in children, it logically follows that the acknowledged carcinogenic effect of active tobacco smoking might also be present in those involuntarily exposed. A 1972 Surgeon General's report raised concerns about involuntary smoke exposure, as did reports by Hirayama (1981) and Trichopoulos and colleagues (1981). The reports demonstrated an increased risk of lung cancer in nonsmoking women married to smoking men. In 1986 the National Research Council commissioned a review of the effects of ETS as a potential causal agent of lung cancer in nonsmokers exposed to household cigarette smoke. Review of all available evidence yielded an overall odds ratio of 1.34. In nonsmokers this translates into an approximately 30% increase of risk in lung cancer. This should be interpreted in the perspective that the background risk of lung cancer in a nonsmoker is very low and contrasted appropriately with the 1000% increase of lung cancer in lifelong active smokers. In 1986 the U.S. Department of Health and Human Services released a report on the Health Consequences of Involuntary Smoking. On the basis of prior evidence, this report concluded that involuntary smoking is a cause of disease including lung cancer in healthy nonsmokers.

The Environmental Protection Agency (1993) now classifies ETS as a lung carcinogen. A study by Cardenas and colleagues (1997) examined lung cancer mortality and ETS within the context of the American Cancer Society's Cancer Prevention Study. These authors performed a prospective comparative evaluation of 133,835 never-smokers with smoking spouses versus 154,000 never-smokers with nonsmoking spouses. These authors concluded that the relative risk of lung cancer in women with smoking husbands was 1.2, which represents an increase in lung cancer incidence of 20%. The relative risk in nonsmoking men with smoking wives was somewhat less but still elevated at 1.1. These figures are in agreement with data from prior studies evaluating lung cancer risk due to ETS. Pershagen (1994) evaluated pooled data from eight such studies in the United States from 1981 to 1991 and found a relative risk of lung cancer in nonsmokers living with smokers of 1.23.

The exact impact of ETS on lung cancer is still not clear. However, with 25% of the American adult population still smoking, it should be obvious that ETS is a major public health issue. Though the exact number of cases of lung cancer due to involuntary smoking is difficult to calculate, Beckett (1993) estimated that the number of lung cancer deaths in the United States attributable to ETS is comparable to the annual number caused by asbestos or radon.

OCCUPATIONAL CARCINOGENS

Several workplace substances have been implicated as or proven potential carcinogens in the lung. The International Agency for Research on Cancer (IARC) has identified a number of such agents, including arsenic, asbestos, beryllium,

Table 93-2. Occupational Carcinogens and Associated Occupational Exposures

Agent	Occupational Exposure
Arsenic	Copper, lead, or zinc ore smelting
	Manufacture of insecticides
	Mining
Asbestos	Asbestos mining
	Asbestos textile production
	Brake lining work
	Cement production
	Construction work
	Insulation work
	Shipyard work
Beryllium	Ceramic manufacture
	Electronic and aerospace equipment manufacture
	Mining
Cadmium	Electroplating
	Pigment production
	Plastics industry
Chloromethyl ethers	Chemical manufacturing
Chromium	Chromate production
	Chromium electroplating
	Leather tanning
	Pigment production
Nickel	Nickel mining, refining, electroplating
	Production of stainless and heat-resistant steel
Polycyclic aromatic compounds	Aluminum production
	Coke production
	Ferrochromium alloy production
	Nickel-containing ore smelting
	Roofers
Radon	Mining
Silica	Ceramics and glass industry
	Foundry industry
	Granite industry
	Metal ore smelting
	Mining and quarrying
Vinyl chloride	Plastic production
	Polyvinyl chloride production

cadmium, chloromethyl ethers, chromium, nickel, radon, silica, and vinyl chloride. The occupations associated with exposure to these agents are outlined in Table 93-2.

Asbestos

Asbestos has historically been the most widely appreciated and most common occupational cause of lung cancer. Asbestos is a class of naturally occurring fibrous minerals consisting primarily of two groups: serpentine (chrysotile) and amphibole (amosite, crocidolite, tremolite, and others). Used commercially since the late 1800s, their fire-retarding qualities and strength have made them useful in construction and insulating materials. Hughes and Weill (1994) pointed out that asbestos was noted to be a lung carcinogen as early as 1943 in Germany. However, the wide recognition of its carcinogenicity dates to reports in the United Kingdom in the 1950s including that by Doll (1955). It is recognized widely that asbestos exposure can result in a number of pleural and pulmonary manifestations.

Asbestos-related pleural disease may present as effusion, pleurisy, or both. Chronic pleural involvement is seen as areas of pleural thickening known as pleural plaques, usually involving the parietal pleura and often calcified. The presence of pleural plaques is not believed to herald development of mesothelioma and has not been definitively proved to be a marker of increased risk for lung cancer.

Inhalation of asbestos fibers can result in parenchymal lung disease, specifically interstitial lung disease (asbestosis). All the major types of asbestos can cause interstitial lung disease, though amphibole fibers may be more fibrogenic than chrysotile. The presentation of asbestosis is essentially identical to nonspecific interstitial lung disease as well as idiopathic pulmonary fibrosis. Symptoms typically include dry cough and dyspnea. Physical examination and chest radiograph are consistent with a bilateral basilar distribution of fibrotic changes. The distinction between asbestosis and nonspecific interstitial lung disease lies in a history of heavy occupational asbestos exposure. In a statement by the American Thoracic Society on the diagnosis of nonmalignant diseases related to asbestosis (1986) the following were considered necessary to the clinical diagnosis of asbestosis: 1) a reliable history of exposure, 2) an appropriate time interval between exposure and detection, and 3) clinical evidence of interstitial lung disease including chest radiographic abnormality, restrictive pulmonary physiology, abnormal diffusing capacity, and abnormal physical examination consistent with fibrosis. In a review of the pathogenesis of asbestosis and silicosis, Mossman and Churg (1998) noted that the development of asbestosis occurs above a threshold fiber dose of approximately 25 to 105 fibers per mL per year. This threshold dose is usually reached only in workers with heavy occupational exposure, including asbestos insulators, miners, millers, and textile workers. As is the case with other inorganic dusts including silica, the development of interstitial fibrosis usually requires prolonged exposure over months to years. Disease can also follow shorter, more intense exposure, such as occurred in shipyard workers employed inside ship compartments during and after World War II. The latency period from exposure to presentation of disease is inversely proportional to exposure level. Thus, the less the exposure, the longer the latency period. It is important to note that most persons with occupational asbestos exposure never manifest any evidence of interstitial lung disease.

The distinction between asbestos exposure and asbestosis becomes extremely important because of controversy as to which represents the actual risk factor for lung cancer. Two recent reviews discussing the extensive available epidemiologic data illustrated this controversy. Jones and colleagues (1995) in an extensive literature review highlighted several important points. First, it is widely recognized that lung fibrosis of many causes is associated with an increased risk

of lung cancer. This is true of idiopathic pulmonary fibrosis as well as interstitial lung disease associated with connective tissue diseases. Secondly, these authors pointed out animal experiments in which asbestos-exposed animals who developed lung cancer did so only when they also developed pulmonary fibrosis. Thirdly, pleural plaques, a marker for asbestos exposure, have not proved a reliable marker for increased risk of lung cancer. These authors concluded that the issue of whether asbestosis is a necessary precursor to asbestos-attributable lung cancer cannot be definitively settled. However, their assessment was that the available data strongly support that hypothesis. In contrast, another review of the available medical literature by Egilman and Reinert (1996) arrived at the opposite conclusion. In their extensive assessment of the available epidemiologic data, these authors concluded that "asbestos meets accepted criteria for causation of lung cancer in the absence of clinical or histologic parenchymal asbestosis." Their evaluation of pathologic and epidemiological studies resulted in the conclusion that asbestos can act as a carcinogen independent of the presence of asbestosis.

The question of whether asbestos exposure alone or asbestosis per se represents the risk factor for lung cancer remains an area of debate. However, from a public health perspective, the issue is of particular significance because of concern about lung cancer risk related to asbestos in the general environment. As noted by Hughes and Weill (1994), all persons living in industrialized countries have accumulated asbestos fibers in their lungs; in adults the number of fibers is estimated to be in the millions. However, as stated, asbestosis requires prolonged and intense exposure to asbestos and is not observed with the level of asbestos fibers encountered from everyday exposure. It should be firmly stated that the risk of developing lung cancer from nonoccupational asbestos exposure in the general environment is extremely low. Moreover, as pointed out by Hughes and Weill, if as postulated asbestosis is a necessary prerequisite to the development of cancer, the extrapolation of risk of lung cancer related to occupational asbestos exposure to risk from exposure to asbestos in the general environment would substantially overestimate that risk.

Another area of controversy in the area of asbestos and lung cancer is whether all types of fibers are carcinogenic. Epidemiologic and experimental data have suggested that amphibole fibers are more carcinogenic than chrysotile. In the United States, chrysotile has been by far the most commonly used type of asbestos. Thus, though all fibers may be carcinogenic, public concern about low-level asbestos exposure and lung cancer should be appropriately tempered.

Whether asbestos exposure alone or asbestosis is the actual risk factor for lung cancer, and whether or not all types of asbestos fibers are carcinogens, tobacco smoking clearly potentiates the observed carcinogenic effect. The magnitude of the combined effect of asbestos and cigarette smoking is, however, not clear. Whether the interaction of these two agents results in an additive or multiplicative

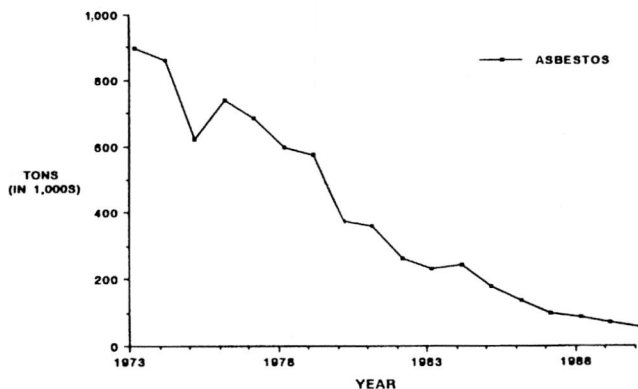

Fig. 93-4. United States asbestos use, 1973–1990. From Hughes J, Weill H: Asbestos and man-made fibers. *In* Samet JM (ed): Epidemiology of Lung Cancer. New York: Marcel Dekker, 1994, pp. 185–205.

Table 93-3. Radium: Principal Decay Products

Decay Product	Half-Life
Radium 226 ↓	1620 yrs
Radon 222 ↓	3.82 days
Polonium 218 ↓	3.05 mos
Lead 214 ↓	26.8 mos
Bismuth 214 ↓	19.7 mos
Polonium 214 ↓	0.000164 secs
Lead 210	22 yrs

From Samet JM: Radon and lung cancer. J Natl Cancer Inst *81*:745, 1989. With permission.

increase in the risk of lung cancer is debated. The increase in relative risk of lung cancer in smokers is approximately 10-fold. Hammond and colleagues (1979) estimated that the relative risk of lung cancer among smoking asbestos workers increases by a factor of at least 15, but that the increase may be as much as 50-fold. Thus, the exact nature of the interaction in terms of relative risk is not defined. What is clear is that most lung cancers occur in asbestos-exposed workers who smoke. Smoking cessation should therefore be the most important goal of cancer prevention programs in this population, with particular targeting of the subgroup of workers with asbestosis.

With recognition of health risks related to asbestos, its use has precipitously declined in the United States since the 1970s (Fig. 93-4). Assuming that occupational exposure continues to decline, in future years the risk of asbestos-related lung cancer will become increasingly small.

Radon

Mining

Mining is the oldest identified occupation associated with lung cancer. Agricola (1950) in the 1500s described a wasting pulmonary disease of miners and metal smelters associated with early mortality. Known as miners' pthisis, the cause of this illness was variably attributed to dust or metal exposure, tuberculosis, or even to inbreeding among mining communities. However, in 1879 Harting and Hesse performed an autopsy study of miners exposed to ores in the central European mines of Schneeberg and Joachimstahl in the Erz Mountains and documented that the process was actually neoplastic. Of note, Frank (1979) pointed out that these same mines produced the material from which Marie Curie later isolated radium. While the etiologic factors causing the increased lung cancer risk were originally speculated to be dust-related pneumoconioses, arsenic, or cobalt, the

actual carcinogens have been identified as radioactive materials, primarily radon and its decay products.

Radon (radon-222) is a naturally occurring decay product of radium-226, itself a decay product of uranium-238 (Table 93-3). Uranium and radium are ubiquitously present in soil and rock although in highly variable concentration. At usual temperatures, radon is released as a radium decay product as an inert radioactive gas. Radon itself decays with a half-life of 3.82 days into a series of radioisotopes known as radon decay products (or radon daughters), which have half-lives measured in seconds to minutes. These products include polonium-218 and polonium-214, which emit alpha particles. Alpha radiation is highly damaging to tissues. Inhalation of these radon decay products and subsequent alpha-particle emission in the lung may cause damage to cells and genetic material. Ultimately, radon decay produces lead-210, which has a half-life of 22 years.

The concentration of radon gas in an environment will vary depending on two factors: 1) the richness of the source of radium and 2) the degree to which the air around that source is ventilated. Thus, while the gas is present in ubiquitous fashion in the general environment, certain sites may be more likely to have high radon concentration with the prototypical situation being underground mines with poorly ventilated passageways.

Since Harting and Hesse's (1879) description of lung neoplasm in miners, an increased risk of lung cancer associated with exposure to radon decay products has been demonstrated in a number of different population studies of underground miners. These have included studies based in the United States by Samet (1989), Hornung and Meinhardt (1987), and Archer and colleagues (1974, 1976); in Sweden by Radford and associates (1984); in Canada by Howe and colleagues (1986); in China by Lubin and coworkers (1990); and in Czechoslovakia by Sevc and associates (1988). While not all miners will have increased risk of lung cancer, both uranium and nonuranium mines may have high radon concentrations, and the risk of lung cancer in such a setting is raised. Samet (1989) and Samet and Hornung (1990) in reviews of these studies emphasized the following points: 1) In general, the relative risk of lung cancer increases with estimated cumulative exposure to radon. The occupational measure of cumulative exposure to radon decay products is the working level month (WLM). The working level (WL) is any combination of radon decay products in 1 L of air that results in the release of 1.3×105 mV of potential alpha energy. The number of hours worked in a month is defined as 170 hours. The WLM is a product of radon decay product concentration in WL and the duration of working months. In miners with cumulative exposures of 0 to 500 WLM, excess relative risks of lung cancer increases in approximately linear fashion to the amount of exposure. In miners with cumulative exposure of over 1000 WLM, the excess relative risk becomes nonlinear and decreases. Darby and Samet (1994) suggested this decrease in excess risk at high cumulative radon exposure may reflect cell sterilization as opposed to genetic mutation. 2) Excess relative risk reaches a maximum about a decade after exposure and then declines with time. 3) The rate of exposure to radon affects lung cancer risk. Higher excess relative rates per unit exposure are associated with lower average exposure rates. In other words, among miners with equivalent cumulative exposure to radon, those exposed to lower levels for longer periods of time have a higher risk for lung cancer (Table 93-4). 4) An increased risk of lung cancer is seen in smoking miners compared to nonsmoking miners. The Committee on Biologic Effects of Ionizing Radiation (BEIR IV) concluded in 1988 that radon and smoking increased lung cancer risk in multiplicative fashion. However, a more recent review by Darby and Samet (1994) suggested that the two act only additively. Regardless, the combination of exposure to the two carcinogens is clearly worse than exposure to either alone.

It should be noted that the number of lung cancer cases reported in nonsmoking miners is small due to a high prevalence of cigarette smoking in this working population. However, in a study of white underground uranium miners from Colorado by Waxweiler and colleagues (1981), nonsmoking miners had a higher relative risk for lung cancer as compared to all miners. This finding was also seen in a study of fluorspar miners in Newfoundland reported by Morrison and colleagues (1988). Such work emphasizes the potential importance of radon as a carcinogen in the nonsmoking population at large.

Uranium mining has now ceased in the United States. However, radon exposure continues to be an occupational concern in nonuranium mining and underground work in this country as well as in uranium and nonuranium mines around the world. In the United States, occupational exposure to radon is legislatively controlled. Individual exposure records are mandated for all workers in areas where concentration of radon exceeds 0.3 WL, with an annual cumulative exposure limit of 4 WLM. The BEIR IV (1988) study estimated that a 40-year exposure at this level would increase a person's lifetime risk of lung cancer twofold. However, this is at best a rough estimate. Continued longitudinal evaluation of occupationally exposed persons is clearly necessary to improve our understanding of the carcinogenic effects of radon.

General Environment

The National Council on Radiation Protection and Measurements (1984) identified radon and its decay products as the largest component of environmental radiation to persons living in the United States. Furthermore, radon is now recognized as the primary source of natural radiation to the bronchial epithelium (Table 93-5). These findings in conjunction with extrapolation of data collected in groups with high occupational radon exposure have escalated concern about the risks of lung cancer related to domestic radon.

The concentration of radon gas in the environment is usually expressed as the number of disintegrations of radon gas in a given volume of air over a given time period. This is usually expressed in becquerels per cubic meter (Bq/m^3), where 1 Bq/m^3 = 1 disintegration per second per cubic meter of air. Alternatively, radon concentration also can be expressed in picocuries per liter (pCi/L). One pCi/L is equal to 37 Bq/m^3. The average concentration of radon gas in the environment is 0.2 pCi/L. In a 1991 survey of homes in the United States, Samet and colleagues (1991) reported a mean indoor radon level of approximately 1.25 pCi/L. In this survey, the range of indoor radon levels was quite broad. Most homes had levels only slightly higher than outdoor environmental levels, but a few had levels ranging in excess of 100 pCi/L. The primary factor determining radon gas concentration in homes is the concentration of radium in the soil and

Table 93-4. Relative Risks and Average Exposure Rates in Miners Exposed to Radon

Mining Cohort	Average Radon Exposure Rate (WLM/Year)	Relative Risk of Lung Cancer (% per WLM)	References
Malemberget, Sweden (iron)	5	3.6	Radford (1984)
Ontario, Canada (uranium)	10	1.3	Muller (1983)
Eldorato Port, Northwest Territories, Canada (uranium)	109	0.27	Howe (1986)

WLM, working level month.
From Darby SC, Samet JM: Radon. *In* Samet JM (ed): Epidemiology of Lung Cancer. New York: Marcel Dekker, 1994, p 223. With permission.

Table 93-5. Estimated Annual Average Dose Equivalents from Natural Radiation in the United States

Source of Radiation	Average Annual Dose Equivalent (mSv) to				Annual Effective Dose Equivalent Whole Body (mSv)
	Bronchial Epithelium	Other Soft Tissues	Bone Surface	Bone Marrow	
Cosmic	0.27	0.27	0.27	0.27	0.27
Terrestrial gamma	0.28	0.28	0.28	0.28	0.28
Cosmic radionuclides	0.01	0.01	0.01	0.03	0.01
Inhaled radionuclides (mainly radon)	24.00	—	—	—	2.00
Other radionuclide in the body	0.36	0.36	1.10	0.50	0.39
All sources	~25.0	0.9	1.7	1.1	~3.0

From Darby SC, Samet JM: Radon. *In* Samet JM (ed): Epidemiology of Lung Cancer. New York: Marcel Dekker, 1994, p. 230. With permission.

rock beneath those structures. Building materials, well water, and natural gas are less common sources, usually contributing only minimally to indoor radon concentrations. Indoor to outdoor air exchange may also affect radon concentration within the home.

Broad concern for the public health implications of domestic radon exposure has been heightened by the documented carcinogenic effect of radon in miners. However, the potential for mutagenic and carcinogenic effects of low-level alpha radiation has been an area of controversy. A number of studies examining lung cancer risks from domestic exposure have been performed. A meta analysis of eight such studies was reported by Lubin and Boice (1997). This analysis included 4263 lung cancer and 6612 control subjects. These authors concluded that greater residential exposure levels were associated with an increased relative risk of lung cancer. The overall estimated relative risk with exposure of 150 Bq/m³ was 1.14. This is consistent with extrapolation of risk from studies performed in miners as well as with actual calculated risks in miners with low cumulative radon exposure. Importantly, this meta-analysis did not demonstrate any greater increase in lung cancer risk than what would be extrapolated from radon exposure in miners. This is important in that an inverse exposure-rate effect has been reported in miners by a number of groups including Lubin and colleagues (1995), Darby and Doll (1990), Hornung and Meinhardt (1987), and Sevc and colleagues (1988). This effect describes the observation that for a given total radon exposure, lung cancer risk in miners increases as the duration of exposure increases and the exposure rate decreases. However, based on the results reported by Lubin and Boice, concern that the exposure-rate effect might cause a relative increase in the carcinogenic effect of long-term, low-level domestic radon exposure appears to be unfounded.

Using miner-based risk models, it is now estimated that domestic radon may account for 7000 to 36,000 lung cancer deaths in the United States each year. However, studies disputing this projection or demonstrating no increased risk even with high indoor domestic radon levels have also been reported, including those by Auvinen (1996), Blot (1990), Letourneau (1994), and Alavanja (1994) and their colleagues. Cohen (1995) concluded that use of a theoretic, lin-

ear, no-threshold relationship to extrapolate known risks in miners with high radon exposure levels to risk in persons with residential radon exposure grossly overestimates lung cancer risk. Cohen pointed out that the effects of low-dose, low-rate radiation have never been adequately evaluated, and he contested the assumptions inherent in extrapolation of high radon exposure to domestic situations.

An important recent study by Hei and coworkers (1997) addressed this issue. Using a novel and unique technique of microbeam irradiation of cell nuclei, the biological effects of a single or known number of alpha particle traversals on genetic mutation and cytotoxicity were evaluated in single cells. Heretofore, the effect on cells of a traversal by a single alpha particle has been controversial, as pointed out by Cohen (1995). Hei's group pointed out that a single alpha particle hit to a cell is the most relevant to the general population, as environmental radon exposure levels make the probability of multiple traversals in a single cell very low. In their study, this group made several important observations. The first was that 80% of cells traversed by a single alpha particle survive that exposure. This answered earlier speculation that a single alpha particle traversal would likely cause cell death rather than result in genetic mutations. Hei and colleagues (1997) were able to show that 10% of cells survived even up to 8 alpha particle traversals. The second important observation was that in cells surviving alpha particle exposure, the frequency of gene mutation after a single traversal was enhanced twofold. The third was that the frequency of mutation was further increased in cells traversed by up to eight alpha particles although multiple hits were associated with higher cytotoxicity.

The National Research Council Committee on Health Risks of Exposure to Radon (1994) estimated that 1 in 107 bronchial cells will be subject to alpha particle exposures per year. Given this, the results of the work by Hei and colleagues would indicate that a small number of bronchial epithelial cells are at significant risk of radiation-induced mutation. Assuming that genetic mutation may be an early step in induction of cancer, these data suggest that environmental and indoor radon exposure does indeed constitute a significant public health problem in its potential contribution to the development of lung cancer. Thus, further evaluation of the effects of domestic radon on the lung cancer epidemic would appear to be justified and warranted.

DIET

It is generally accepted that diet may be a significant cofactor in the development of cancer. Retinoids, including retinol (vitamin A) and its precursor carotenoids, including beta-carotene, have been the most intensively studied. One of the most widely cited reports of the effect of diet on the development of cancer was a prospective survey performed by Shekelle and colleagues (1981) of 2080 men aged 40 to 55 employed by the Western Electric Company. Detailed dietary histories of these men were taken in 1957. The cohort was then followed over 19 years. In this study beta-carotene intake was inversely related to lung cancer incidence. Subsequent studies, including those by Cade and Margetts (1991) and Stryker and colleagues (1988), demonstrated that smokers have lower serum beta-carotene levels than nonsmokers. These and other studies have suggested that vitamin A and beta-carotene may have a protective effect against lung cancer. Byers (1994) evaluated 27 such studies published before 1994 and concluded that persons in the lowest quartile of carotene intake had an approximately 50 to 100% increase in lung cancer risk as compared with persons in the highest quartile. Thus, by 1994 the cumulative information suggested that beta-carotene and vitamin A might be useful as cancer chemopreventive agents.

Three important large-scale epidemiologic studies were recently performed to address this possibility. The Alpha-Tocopherol, Beta-Carotene Cancer Prevention (ATBC) Study (1994) was a randomized, double-blind, placebo-controlled trial designed to determine whether daily supplementation of alpha-tocopherol, beta-carotene, or both could reduce the incidence of cancers, including cancer of the lung. The study enrolled 29,133 male smokers age 50 to 60 in Finland. Unexpectedly, a higher than expected mortality, primarily due to lung cancer and heart disease, was observed in the group receiving beta-carotene. Omenn and colleagues (1996a,b) then reported results of the Beta-Carotene and Retinol Efficacy Trial (CARET), also a randomized, double-blind, placebo-controlled study. The study was intended to determine whether dietary supplementation with beta-carotene, vitamin A, or both would decrease the incidence of lung cancer. It enrolled 18,314 men and women believed to be at increased risk of lung cancer. The CARET study (1996) was stopped 21 months early because of "clear evidence of no benefit and substantial benefit of harm." As compared with placebo, the group that received both vitamin A and beta-carotene experienced a 17% increase in mortality and a 28% increase in the number of lung cancers.

A third randomized, double-blind, placebo-controlled trial, the Physicians Health Study reported by Hennekens and colleagues (1996), evaluated the effect of beta-carotene in 22,071 male physicians. Eleven percent were current smokers and 39% former smokers at the onset of the trial. Over 12 years of follow-up, neither benefit nor harm in terms of malignancy or cardiovascular disease was demonstrated. Of note, the dose of beta-carotene in this trial was lower than both the ATBC trial and the CARET study.

Based on a large body of epidemiologic studies, a balanced dietary intake of fruits and vegetables, including those containing beta-carotene, should be encouraged. On the basis of the findings of the ATBC and CARET trials, the use of supplemental beta-carotene and vitamin A should be discouraged. The final word about the role of dietary supplementation in cancer chemoprevention is not out. However, these studies should serve as a reminder that indiscreet and excessive intake of vitamins or other chemicals can be potentially harmful.

CONCLUSION

At present, the 5-year survival rate for lung cancer is only 14%. This is in stark contrast to the 5-year survival rates for the other leading causes of cancer death in the United States including cancers of the colon (63%), breast (86%), and prostate (90%). The absolute number of lung cancer cases continues to be alarming, with the continued rise of lung cancer in women a particularly disturbing feature. The role of tobacco as an etiologic factor in lung cancer has been convincingly established. Likewise, ionizing radiation and certain occupational exposures have been recognized as carcinogenic. The challenge in the future will be to modify the impact of these identified external sources of risk while continuing to expand our knowledge of the genetic and molecular basis of carcinogenesis.

Early diagnosis of lung cancer should be considered imperative as the 5-year survival rate for treated stage I lung cancer is substantially better than for stages II to IV. The issue of lung cancer screening deserves to be revisited. The American Cancer Society (1994) does not now recommend routine screening for lung cancer. Prior trials from the 1970s and 1980s demonstrating no reduction in cancer mortality despite screening effectively eliminated such testing. Petty (1997) points out that groups at high risk, specifically heavy smokers with spirometric and clinical evidence of air flow obstruction, can be easily identified. Screening with chest radiograph and sputum cytology in such a group might be justifiable. Moreover, the development of new technologies, including identification of markers of cellular transformation in exfoliated bronchial cells present in sputum, may increase the accuracy of sputum examination as part of the screening process.

At present, with one-fourth of the American population still smoking cigarettes, continued efforts must be directed at smoking cessation and at preventing persons from becoming addicted to smoking. While work in the field of lung cancer treatment remains extremely important, the dismal mortality associated with this disease demands that the medical profession contribute to efforts aimed at limiting its primary cause. If tobacco smoking could be eliminated, or at least severely curtailed, we might then be able to return lung cancer to what Adler at the turn of the century designated as "among the rarest forms of disease."

REFERENCES

Adler I: Primary Malignant Growth of the Lung and Bronchi. New York: Longman, Green and Company, 1912.

Agricola G: De Re Metallica. Basel, New York: Dover Publications, English reprint, 1950.

Alavanja M, et al: Residential radon exposure and lung cancer among non-smoking women. J Natl Cancer Inst 86:1829, 1994.

Alpha-Tocopherol Beta Carotene Cancer Prevention Study Group: The effect of vitamin E and beta carotene on the incidence of lung cancer and other cancers in male smokers. JAMA 330:1029, 1994.

American Cancer Society: Cancer facts and figures; 1994, CA Cancer J Clin 44:1, 1994.

American Thoracic Society. Medical Section of the American Lung Association. The diagnosis of non-malignant diseases related to asbestos. Am Rev Respir Dis 134:363, 1986.

Anthonisen N, et al: Effects of smoking intervention and the use of an inhaled anticholinergic bronchodilator on the rate of decline of FEV_1. JAMA 272:1497, 1994.

Archer V, Gillam J, Wagoner J: Respiratory disease mortality among uranium miners. Ann N Y Acad Sci 271:280, 1976.

Archer V, Sacconianno G, Jones J: Frequency of different histologic types of bronchogenic carcinoma as related to radiation exposure. Cancer 34:2056, 1974.

Auvinen A, et al: Indoor radon exposure and the risk of lung cancer: a nested case control study in Finland. J Natl Cancer Inst 88:966, 1996.

Beck G, Doyle C, Schachter E: Smoking and lung function. Am Rev Respir Dis 123:149, 1981.

Beckett W: Epidemiology and etiology of lung cancer. Clin Chest Med 14:1, 1993.

Belinsky S, et al: Activation of the K-ras protooncogene in lung tumors of mice treated with 4(methyl-N-nitrosamines)-1pyridyl-1. Cancer Res 48:5303, 1988.

Blot W, et al: Indoor radon and lung cancer in China. J Natl Cancer Inst 82:1025, 1990.

Brennan JA, Boyle JO, Koch WK: Association between cigarette smoking and mutation of the p53 gene in squamous cell CA of the head and neck. N Engl J Med 332:712, 1995.

Brownson R, Chang J, David J: Gender and histologic type variations in smoking-related risk of lung cancer. Epidemiology 3:61, 1992.

Buist A, Ghezzo H, et al: Relationship between the single breath N2 test and age, sex, and smoking habits in three North American cities. Am Rev Respir Dis 120:305, 1979.

Burns D: Tobacco smoking. In Samet JA (ed): Epidemiology of Lung Cancer. New York: Marcel Dekker, 1994, pp. 15-49.

Byers T: Diet as a factor in the etiology and prevention of lung cancer. In Samet JA (ed): Epidemiology of Lung Cancer. New York: Marcel Dekker, 1994, pp. 335-352.

Cade J, Margetts B: Relationship between diet and smoking: is the diet of smokers different? J Epidemiol Community Health 45:270, 1991.

Cardenas V, et al: Environmental tobacco smoke and lung cancer mortality in the American Cancer Society's Cancer Prevention Study. Cancer Causes Control 8:57, 1997.

Chen Y, Horne S, Dosman J: Increased susceptibility to lung function in female smokers. Am Rev Respir Dis 143:1224, 1991.

Cohen B: Chronic obstructive pulmonary disease: a challenge in genetic epidemiology. Am J Epidemiol 112:274, 1980.

Cohen B: How dangerous is low level radiation? Risk Anal 15:645, 1995.

Committee on Biologic Effects of Ionizing Radiation (BEIR IV): Health risks of radon and other internally deposited alpha-emitters. Committee on Biological Effects of Ionizing Radiation (BEIR IV). Washington, DC: National Academy Press, 1988.

Darby S, Doll R: Radiation and exposure rate. Nature 344:824, 1990.

Darby S, Samet T: Radon in epidemiology of lung cancer. In Samet JA (ed): Epidemiology of Lung Cancer. New York: Marcel Dekker, 1994, pp. 219-243.

Detels S, et al: The UCLA population studies of chronic obstructive respiratory disease IV: respiratory effect of long term exposure to four chemical oxidants, nitrogen, dioxide and sulfates on current and never smokers. Am Rev Respir Dis 124:673, 1981.

Doll R: Mortality for lung cancer in asbestos workers. Br J Ind Med 12:81, 1955.

Doll R, Hill A: Smoking and carcinoma of the lung. BMJ 2:739, 1950.

Egilman D, Reinert A: Lung cancer and asbestos exposure: asbestosis is not necessary. Am J Ind Med 30:398, 1996.

Environmental Protection Agency: Respiratory Health Effects of Passive Smoking: Lung Cancer and other Disorders. NIH Publication No. 93, 1993.

Fahr in Discussion on Teutschlaender: Bronchialkrebs, Verhandi. d. deutsch. path. Gesellsch 10:191, 1923.

Field J, et al: Elevated p53 expression correlates with a history of heavy smoking in squamous cell cancer of the head and neck. Br J CA 64:573, 1991.

Frank AL: The epidemiology and etiology of lung cancer. Clin Chest Med 3:219, 1982.

Hammond E, Selilcott I, Seidman H: Asbestos exposure, cigarette smoking, and death rates. Ann NY Acad Sci 33:473, 1979.

Harting F, Hesse W: Der Lungenkrebs, die Bergkrankheit in den Schneeberger Gruben. Gesundheitswesen 31:102-105, 313-337, 1879.

Hei T, et al: Mutagenic effects of a single and an exact number of alpha particles in mammalian cells. Proc Natl Acad Sci 94:3765, 1997.

Hennekens C, et al: Lack of effect of long-term supplementation with beta carotene on the incidence of malignant neoplasms and cardiovascular disease. N Engl J Med 334:1145, 1996.

Hirayama, T: Nonsmoking wives of heavy smokers have a higher risk of lung cancer: a study from Japan. BMJ 282:183, 1981.

Hoffman D, Hoffman I: The changing cigarette, 1950 to 1995. J Toxicol Environ Health 50:307, 1997.

Hoffman D, et al: Cigarette smoking and adenocarcinoma of the lung: the relevance of nicotine-derived N-nitrosamines. J Smoking Related Disorders 4:165, 1993.

Hornung R, Meinhardt T: Quantitative risk assessment of lung cancer in US uranium miners. Health Phys 52:417, 1987.

Howe G, et al: Lung cancer mortality (1950-80) in relation to radon daughter exposure in a cohort of workers at the Eldorado Beaverlodge Uranium Mine. J Natl Cancer Inst 77:357, 1986.

Hruby A, Sweany H: Primary carcinoma of the lung. Arch Intern Med 52:497, 1933.

Hsu T, Johnston D, Cheny L: Sensitivity to genotoxic events of Bleomycin in humans: possible relationship to environmental carcinogens. Int J Cancer 43:403, 1989.

Hughes J, Weill H: Asbestos and man made fibers. In Samet JA (ed): Epidemiology of Lung Cancer. New York: Marcel Dekker, 1994.

Jones RN, Hughes JM, Weill H: Asbestos exposure, asbestosis, and asbestos-attributable lung cancer. Lancet 345:1074, 1995.

Kawajiri K, Ejuchi H, Nakachi U: Association of CYP1A1 germlike polymorphisms with mutations of the p53 gene in lung cancer. Cancer Res 56:72, 1996.

Koch W, Patel H, Brennan J: Squamous cell carcinoma of the head and neck in the elderly. Arch Otolaryngol Head Neck Surg 121:262, 1995.

Landis S, et al: Cancer statistics, 1998. CA Cancer J Clin 48:6, 1998.

Letourneau E, et al: Case-control study of residential radon and lung cancer in Winnipeg, Manitoba, Canada. Am J Epidemiol 140:310, 1994.

Levin M, Goldstein H, Gerhardt P: Cancer and tobacco smoking. JAMA 143:336, 1950.

Lickint F: Der bronchialkrebs der raucher. Munchen Med Wehnschr 82:1232, 1935.

Lubin J, Blot W: Assessment of lung cancer risk factors by histologic category. J Natl Cancer Inst 73:383, 1984.

Lubin J, Boice J: Lung cancer risk from residential radon: meta-analysis of eight epidemiologic studies. J Natl Cancer Inst 89:49, 1997.

Lubin J, et al: Lung cancer in radon-exposed miners and estimation of risk from indoor exposure. J Natl Cancer Inst 87:817, 1995.

Lubin J, et al: Quantitative evaluation of the radon and lung cancer association in a case control study of Chinese tin miners. Cancer Res 50:174, 1990.

McDuffie H, Klaassen D, Dosman J. Female-male differences in patients with primary lung cancer. Cancer 59:1825, 1987.

McNally W: The tar in cigarette smoke and its possible effects. Am J Cancer 16:1502, 1932.

Morrison H, et al: Cancer mortality among a group of fluorspar miners exposed to radon progeny. Am J Epidemiol *128*:1266, 1988.

Mossman B, Churg A: Mechanisms in the pathogenesis of asbestos and silicosis. Am J Respir Crit Care Med *157*:1666, 1998.

Muller J, Wheeler W, Gentleman J: Study of mortality of Ontario miners, 1955-57. Part 1. Report to Ontario Ministry of Labour, Ontario Workers' Compensation Board and Atomic Energy Control Board of Canada, 1983.

National Council on Radiation Protection and Measurements: Report No. 79. Washington, DC: National Academy of Sciences, 1984.

National Research Council. Committee on Health Risks of Exposure to Radon (BEIR VI) Health Effects of Exposure to Radon: Time for Reassessment. Washington, DC: National Academy of Sciences, 1994.

National Research Council: Environmental Tobacco Smoke: Measuring Exposures and Assessing Health Effects. US National Research Council. Washington DC: National Academy Press, 1986.

Ochsner A, DeBakey M: Primary pulmonary malignancy: treatment of total pneumonectomy: analysis of seventy-nine collected cases and presentation of seven personal cases. Surg Gynecol Obstet *68*:435, 1939.

Ochsner A, DeBakey M: Carcinoma of the lung. Arch Surg *42*:209, 1941.

Omenn G, et al: Effects of a combination of beta carotene and vitamin A on lung cancer and cardiovascular disease. N Engl J Med *334*:1150, 1996a.

Omenn G, et al: Risk factors for lung cancer and for intervention effects in CARET, the beta-carotene and retinol efficacy trial. J Natl Cancer Inst *88*:1550, 1996b.

Pershagen G: Passive smoking and lung cancer. *In* Samet JA (ed): Epidemiology of Lung Cancer. New York: Marcel Dekker, 1994, pp. 109–130.

Petty T: The predictive value of spirometry. Postgrad Med *101*:128, 1997.

Radford E, St. Clair Renard K: Lung cancer in Swedish iron miners exposed to low doses of radon daughters. N Engl J Med *310*:1485, 1984.

Risch H, et al: Are female smokers at higher risk for lung cancer than male smokers? A case-control analysis by histologic type. Am J Epidemiol *138*:281, 1993.

Rodenhuis S, SleboS R: Clinical significance of K-ras oncogene activation in human lung cancer. Cancer Res *52*:2668, 1992.

Roffo A: Leucoplasia tabaquica experimental. Bol Inst de med experi para el estud y trat del cancer *7*:501, 1930.

Ronan Z, et al: G to T transversion in codon 12 of the K-ras oncogene isolated from mouse lung tumors. Induced and related DNA methylating and pyridyloxobutylating agents. Carcinogenesis *14*:2419, 1993.

Ryberg D, Kure E, Lystad E: p53 mutations in lung tumors: relationship to putative susceptibility markers for cancer. J Cancer Res *54*:1551, 1994.

Samet J: Radon and lung cancer. J Natl Cancer Inst *81*:745, 1989.

Samet J, Hornung R: Review of radon and lung cancer risk. Risk Anal *10*:65, 1990.

Samet J, Stolwijk J, Rose S: Summary: International Workshop on Residential Radon Epidemiology. Health Phys *60*:223, 1991.

Samet J, et al: Radon progeny exposure and lung cancer risk in New Mexico U miners: a case-control study. Health Phys *56*:415, 1989.

Sevc J, et al: Cancer in man after exposure to radon daughters. Health Phys *54*:27, 1988.

Shekelle R, Liu S, Raynor W: Dietary vitamin A and risk of cancer in the Western Electric Study. Lancet *2*:1185, 1981.

Skillrud D, Offord K, Miller R: Higher risk of lung cancer in chronic obstructive pulmonary disease. A prospective, matched, controlled study. Ann Intern Med *105*:503, 1986.

Spitz MR, Wu X, Lippman S: *In* Roth JA, Cox JD, WK Hong (eds): Markers of Susceptibility in Lung Cancer. 2nd Ed. Malden, MA: Blackwell Science, 1998, pp. 1–24.

Stryker W, Kaplan L, Stein E: The relation of diet, cigarette smoking and alcohol consumption to plasma beta carotene and alpha tocopherol levels. Am J Epidemiol *127*:283, 1988.

Tockman M, et al: Airways obstruction and the risk for lung cancer. Ann Intern Med *106*:512, 1987.

Trichopoulos D, et al: Lung cancer and passive smoking. Int J Cancer *27*:1, 1981.

Tylecote F: Cancer of the lung. Lancet *2*:256, 1927.

US Department of Health and Human Services Public Health Service, Center for Disease Control: Reducing the Health Consequences of Smoking: 25 Years of Progress. Report of the Surgeon General. DHHS Publication No. (CDC) 89-8411, 1989.

US Department of Health and Human Services Public Health Service, Center for Disease Control: The Health Consequences of Involuntary Smoking. A Report of the Surgeon General. DHHS Publication No. (CDC) 87-88398, 1986.

US Department of Health, Education and Welfare, Public Health Service, Health Services and Mental Health Administration: The Health Consequences of Smoking. A Report of the Surgeon General. DHEW Publication No. (HSM) 72-7516, 1972.

US Public Health Service: Smoking and Health. Report of the Advisory Committee to the Surgeon General of the Public Health Services, Washington, DC. Public Health Service Publication No. 1103, 1964.

Wang X, Christiani D, Wienche J. Mutations in the p53 gene in lung cancer as associated with cigarette smoking and asbestos exposure. Cancer Epidemiol Biol Markers *4*:543, 1995.

Waxweiler RJ, et al: Mortality follow-up through 1977 of the white underground uranium miners cohort examined by the United States Public Health Service. *In* International Conference on Radiation Hazards in Mining: Control, Measurement, and Medical Aspects, 1981.

Westra W, et al: K-ras oncogene activation in lung adenocarcinoma from former smokers. Cancer *72*:432, 1993.

Wu A, Fontham E, Reynolds P: Previous lung disease and risk of lung cancer among lifetime nonsmoking women in the United States. Am J Epidemiol *141*:1023, 1995.

Wu X, Delclos G, Annyers F: A case-control study of wood dust exposure mutagen sensitivity, and lung cancer risk. Cancer Epidemiol Biomarkers *4*:583, 1995.

Wynder E, Graham E: Tobacco smoking as a possible etiologic factor in bronchiogenic carcinoma. JAMA *143*:329, 1950.

Wynder E, Hoffmann D: Smoking and lung cancer: scientific challenges and opportunities. Cancer Res *54*:5284, 1994.

Zang E, Wynder E: Differences in lung cancer risk between men and women: examination of the evidence. J Natl Cancer Inst *88*:183, 1996.

CHAPTER 94

Screening for Lung Cancer

Gary R. Epler

Lung cancer continues to be a major cause of death in the United States in both men and women. Cancer statistics according to Parker and associates (1997) indicate 160,000 deaths from lung cancer in the United States. This is more than the deaths from colon, breast, and prostate cancers combined. Although the 5-year survival rate for breast and prostate cancers approaches 80 to 90%, the 5-year survival rate for lung cancer remains dismal at 10 to 15%. The search for an appropriate screening method continues at a vigorous pace. The risk factors for developing lung cancer, the different types of screening tests available, and current recommendations for lung cancer screening are discussed in this chapter.

RISK FACTORS

Cigarette smokers are at the highest risk for developing lung cancer (Table 94-1). The risk increases dramatically with the number of cigarettes smoked—more than 20 times higher in smokers who smoke two packs or more per day than in nonsmokers. Smokers younger than 40 years of age are at risk. Studies, including the one by Mor and associates (1988), have shown an inverse relationship between age and extent of lung cancer at the time of detection—that is, cancer in younger patients may be more extensive, and less curable, than in older patients. According to the Surgeon General's report (1989), by 1986 lung cancer caught up with breast cancer as the leading cause of cancer death in women. One-fourth of high school seniors who have ever smoked had their first cigarette by sixth grade, one-half by eighth grade. Thus, smoking prevention education must begin in elementary school, and smoking cessation programs are needed in high school. The 1964 Surgeon General's report indicated that tobacco use was habit forming. The 1988 report indicated that cigarettes were addicting. Although cigarette use and lung-cancer rates are increasing in many countries of the world, findings in the United States are encouraging. The prevalence of smoking among adults decreased from 40% in 1965 to 29% in 1985. Quitting and

noninitiation of smoking during the same 20-year period have been or will be associated with the avoidance of almost 3 million smoking-related deaths.

Individuals with previous lung cancer are at high risk of developing a new lung cancer. Thomas and Piantadosi (1987) reported that among 572 patients with lung cancer, 27% were found to have a second lung cancer within 3 to 5 years.

Preexisting lung disease is a risk factor. Patients with giant bullous emphysema who smoke have a higher risk of lung cancer compared with smokers who do not have bullous lesions. Such individuals are younger, and the cancer is often contiguous with the bulla. In patients aged 40 to 59 years, Goldstein and associates (1968) noted that bullous disease occurred six times more frequently in patients with lung cancer. Stoloff and colleagues (1971) calculated a risk that is 32 times higher among smokers with bullous disease compared with a healthy population. The increased risk may be attributed to poor clearance mechanisms and trapping of carcinogenic agents in the large cysts.

Airway obstruction in smokers is associated with increased risk of lung cancer. Tockman and associates (1987) observed that among 1031 smokers with airway obstruction, 27 (2.6%) had lung cancer compared with 14 (0.4%) among 3364 smokers without airway obstruction. Furthermore, airway obstruction was more of an indicator for the development of lung cancer than age or amount of smoking. The lung-cancer risk also increased in proportion to the degree of airway obstruction. Petty (1991) suggested documentation of airflow obstruction by physical examination, peak flow meter, and spirometry as a selective screening approach. Large-scale testing of this approach is needed to confirm decreased mortality rates and determine impact of false-positive findings.

Specific occupational exposures can lead to lung cancer. Asbestosis as a result of asbestos exposure is a risk factor for increased lung cancer. For example, a 1955 study by Doll found a 10-fold increase in lung cancer among asbestos-exposed workers who had asbestosis. The increased risk of lung cancer is limited to individuals with asbestosis. Churg

Table 94-1. Risk Factors for Lung Cancer
Cigarette smoking
Prior lung cancer
Preexisting lung disease
Giant bullous emphysema
Chronic airflow obstruction
Occupational exposures

Table 94-2. Screening Tests for Lung Cancer
Chest radiograph
Sputum cytology
Bronchoalveolar lavage biomarkers
Serum serology testing

(1993) reported that the only scientifically established association of lung cancer and asbestos exposure is the association of asbestosis and lung cancer. Among asbestos-exposed smokers, cigarette smoking acts synergistically to produce a higher risk than that among nonexposed cigarette smokers. Camus and associates (1998) found an increased risk of lung cancer from exposure to chrysotile asbestos in a nonoccupational setting and no measurable increased risk of death due to lung cancer among women in two mining regions.

Radon gas has a half-life of 4 days and is a naturally occurring decay product of radium that is found in most soil and rock. Samet (1989) suggested that the alpha-particle emissions from radon decay, polonium 218, and polonium 214 can damage cells lining airways, possibly resulting in lung cancer. A study published by Roscoe and colleagues (1989) of 516 nonsmoking miners indicated a 12-fold increased risk: 14 deaths occurred from lung cancer with only one expected. In addition, Samet (1989) noted that smoking and radon exposures combine synergistically. Exposures to certain alkylating compounds, chromates, nickel, and specific halo ethers in an occupational setting can result in an increased risk for lung cancer.

Genetic events also may result in an increased risk for lung cancer. Viallet and Minna (1990) hypothesized that genetic events may be involved in the pathogenesis of lung cancer. For example, lung cancer cells may be able to activate dominantly acting cellular proto-oncogenes and inactivate recessive tumor-suppresser genes. Sellers and colleagues (1992) conducted a generational study of families of patients with lung cancer and suggested there may be a genetic predisposition to lung cancer that is expressed in the presence of an environmental stimulus such as smoking.

SCREENING TESTS

Chest Radiograph

The chest radiograph as a screening test has been studied extensively (Table 94-2). In the early 1970s, the National Cancer Institute sponsored a large lung-cancer screening project at three hospitals in the United States for 31,000 men who were aged 45 years or older and who smoked at least one package of cigarettes per day. The trials at The Johns Hopkins Hospital and Memorial Sloan-Kettering Cancer Center included the "single-screen" group that had an annual chest radiograph, and the "dual-screen" group that had the annual chest radiograph and submitted sputum samples for cytologic testing every 4 months. The trial at Mayo Clinic had both a chest film and sputum cytologic screening every 4 months for 6 years.

The first part was a prevalence study. At The Johns Hopkins Hospital, Frost and associates (1984) reported 79 cancers were found among 10,000 subjects. Fewer lung cancers were found at Memorial Sloan-Kettering Cancer Center. Flehinger and colleagues (1984) found 53 cases in total, 23 in those who received a screening chest radiograph and 30 among subjects receiving the dual screen of sputum cytology and chest radiography. Among the 53 patients, 22 (40%) had cancer detected early at stage I with an 85% 5-year survival rate. The cancers detected by sputum cytology were squamous cell carcinomas, and two-thirds of cancers detected radiographically were adenocarcinoma. In the Mayo Clinic study published by Fontana and coworkers (1984), the highest number of cancers were found—91 in total. Of the early detected cancers among those found by the chest radiograph, 50% were resected, whereas among the 20% detected solely by sputum cytology, all were resected. This large-scale prevalence screening program resulted in identification of earlier cancers, but it had no impact on overall survival, leading to the abandonment of the recommendation by the American Cancer Society for annual chest radiographic examinations in asymptomatic persons.

The second part of these studies involved an ongoing screening program. Analysis of the data from the Mayo Clinic study by Woolner and associates (1981) indicated that chest radiography surpassed sputum cytology as a means of early detection of lung cancer, although sputum cytology was effective in early detection of squamous carcinoma. In small cell lung cancer lesions, neither screening method was of value. Additional analysis by Muhm and colleagues (1983) indicated that 50 of 92 subjects during 6 years of monitoring had a peripheral nodule that was surprisingly visible in retrospect in 90% of patients for months or even years earlier. The centrally located cancers grew rapidly, usually manifesting as hilar or mediastinal enlargements in patients who had normal findings on radiographs obtained 4 months earlier; most were at an incurable stage.

The Mayo Clinic ongoing program also indicated a better 5-year survival rate. The survival rate was more than 80% among cytologically detected cases and 40% among patients with radiographically detected lesions. Symptomatic patients had a 5-year survival rate of less than 10%. Thus, the cancers were detected earlier, and the 5-year survival rate was better, but Fontana and associates (1991) found that the death rate from lung cancer was slightly higher in the 4-month dual-screened group (122 lung cancer deaths) compared to the control group (115 lung cancer deaths).

Wilde (1989) recorded similar findings in a European study. Among 40,000 men who received chest fluorography every 6 months and 100,000 men who received chest fluorography every 18 months, Wilde reported earlier detection in the former group with a 28% resection rate compared with 19% resection rate in the latter group. The 5-year survival rate was 52% among those who received chest fluorography every 6 months and 27% among those who had the test every 18 months. The 10-year survival rate was 39% in those tested every 6 months compared with 19% in the group tested every 18 months. Wilde noted no reduction of lung cancer mortality.

Since the 1950s, mass screening for lung cancer has been performed in more than 500,000 people in approximately 80% of the local communities in Japan every year. A case-control study by Sobue and associates (1992) indicated a better risk ratio in the cohort that underwent annual screening for lung cancer. Kaneko (1996) and associates compared low-dose spiral computed tomography (CT) with chest radiography. In this comparison study, posteroanterior and lateral radiographs and low-dose spiral CT scans were obtained twice a year in 1369 individuals who were at high risk for lung cancer. Fifteen cancers were detected during a 2-year period, 11 had negative chest radiography and were detected only by spiral CT. Detection rates were 0.43% for the spiral CT and 0.12% for chest radiography. Fourteen (93%) of the 15 lung cancers were stage I. These investigators suggested that large-scale studies were warranted to clarify the efficacy and cost-effectiveness of low-dose spiral CT.

Walter and colleagues (1992) used the results from the randomized, controlled study of 6364 high risk men in Czechoslovakia, aged 40 to 64 years, screened with chest radiographs and sputum cytology every 6 months, to develop a model of the natural history of the disease process. These investigators noted that there are three methods to determine the natural history of lung cancer. First, the radiologic method suggests that 75% of the tumor has elapsed before radiographic detection. The final radiologically visible quarter of the natural history theoretically lasts less than 2.5 to 3.0 years. In an actual study of 17 men with lung cancers and serial film measurements, Weiss (1971) estimated median doubling time to be 4.3 months and the median lead-time to be 11.7 months. Second, serial cytologic studies of sputum suggest that there is a progression from squamous cell metaplasia to mild, moderate, and marked atypia ending with carcinoma in situ and invasive carcinoma. The stages follow each other in an orderly manner with 2 or 3 years as the average duration of each. Third, the mathematical model used for this analysis indicated 0.7 years as the average duration of the detectable preclinical phase of lung cancer. The results from this model suggest that because of the short time period in the detectable phase, very frequent screening would be required. To gain an overall advance of 6 months in diagnosis of all lung cancers, the entire population at risk would need to be screened at 6-month intervals. It is not known whether this 6-month gain in lead-time would result in a decrease in the mortality rate.

Sputum Cytology

Fewer cases are detected by sputum cytology alone than radiography alone, but sputum cytology is useful in detecting squamous cell carcinoma at an early stage and that is radiographically occult. A review of the National Cancer Institute studies by Midthun and Jett (1998) indicated that 94 patients with non–small cell lung cancer (73 stage I and 14 stage III) were detected by sputum cytology alone, and 426 patients by chest radiographs alone—226 stage I, 55 stage II, and 125 stage III.

Investigations have shown that monoclonal antibodies can be attached to cells for an improved yield. Tockman and associates (1988) used monoclonal antibodies to a glycolipid antigen of a small cell carcinoma and a protein antigen of non–small cell lung cancer and applied them to sputum specimens from 5000 men who participated in the Johns Hopkins Lung Project. During the next 8 years, 12% of subjects showed definite atypia. Among the 62 subjects who had monoclonal antibody testing, specimens from 14 of the 22 patients who subsequently developed lung cancer stained positively, and those from 35 of the 40 who did not progress to lung cancer stained negatively. Furthermore, samples from the 14 with positive results were collected 24 months in advance of the detection of lung cancer, and the 8 specimens that were negative were collected 57 months in advance, suggesting that the antigen may be expressed within 2 but not 4 years in advance.

Bronchoalveolar Lavage Biomarkers

The ras oncogene family consists of three functional genes, N-*ras*, K-*ras*, and H-*ras*. Detectable ras mutations occur frequently in non–small cell lung cancer. This finding can be applied to early detection. Jacobson and colleagues (1995) found that the ras assay was more sensitive than routine cytology. Telomerase is a ribonucleoprotein that is related to chromosomal stability. Arai and colleagues (1998) used telomerase activity as a marker of lung cancer in lavage fluid and found it to be more sensitive than sputum cytology.

Serum Serology

Serologic testing is useful for monitoring therapeutic response, but it has no value as a screening test to distinguish localized from advanced cancer. For example, Gail and colleagues (1988) tested sera from 127 patients with localized lung cancer, 341 with advanced lung cancer, 148 with benign lung disease, and 145 healthy subjects for 10 markers: ferritin, lipid-bound sialic acid (LSA), total sialic acid (TSA), microglobulin, lipotropin, human chorionic gonadotropin (HCG), two assays of calcitonin, parathyroid hormone, and carcinoembryonic antigen (CEA). Only CEA and ferritin seemed potentially valuable for detecting localized lung cancer. Furthermore, age and CEA together did as well as more elaborate combinations. A statistical review noted by Ruckdeschel (1988) indicated that the positive predictive value is too low; that is, if lung cancer occurred in 1% of a clinic population, only 7% of the patients that tested positively would have cancer. These markers are too nonspecific to be considered for use in an effective screening program.

IS SCREENING FOR LUNG CANCER RECOMMENDED?

Screening can result in earlier detection and improved 5-year survival rates but without a reduction in mortality. Lead-time bias is the major reason. Eddy (1989) believes lead-time bias occurs because screening allows earlier diagnosis without necessarily delaying the time of death; that is, an earlier diagnosis increases the 5-year survival rate but does not necessarily change the mortality rate. Patients and their physicians may have known about the cancer longer, but the mortality rate did not change.

A false-positive result is also a factor in weighing the benefits of earlier detection and better 5-year survival rate. Detection of noncancerous lesions results in patient inconvenience, discomfort, anxiety, and expense. For example, about 10% of patients may have abnormal chest radiographs leading to additional studies to rule out cancer, and 5% of these individuals may require bronchoscopy, needle aspiration, or thoracotomy. Eddy (1989) pointed out that about 100 patients are evaluated for every one cancer that is found.

In a review of early detection of lung cancer, Wolpaw (1996) noted that the following organizations do not recommend routine chest radiographic screening: American Cancer Society, American College of Radiology, National Cancer Institute, U.S. Preventive Services Task Force, and the Canadian Task Force on the Health Examination.

Some individuals have suggested the reconsideration of periodic chest radiographic screening. Strauss and associates (1997) reviewed the Mayo Lung Project and the Czechoslovakian study and concluded that periodic screening chest radiographs lead to clinically meaningful improvements in stage distribution, resectability, survival, and fatality in lung cancer.

PREVENTION AND AN APPROACH TO EARLY DETECTION OF LUNG CANCER

Prevention remains the best means of eliminating lung cancer. Every effort should be spent to get the adolescent population not to smoke and to get all patients to stop smoking. A computerized simulation model developed by Yamaguchi and coworkers (1992) indicated that a 0.5% annual smoking-cessation rate would have a minimal impact of a 13% reduction in lung-cancer deaths, but a 5% annual smoking-cessation rate would result in a 66% reduction in lung-cancer deaths.

There are smokers who will not quit, and those who do quit remain at high risk for several years. Community-based chest radiographic screening is not recommended; however, Midthun and Jett (1998) suggest case finding as an appropriate alternative. Case finding occurs when a patient seeks care about a disease or symptoms. Testing is individualized. For example, a 60-year-old smoker or recent ex-smoker with airflow obstruction is seen for a comprehensive evaluation. A chest film and sputum cytology might be appropriate. A cost and risk benefit study is needed to explore this alternative.

CONCLUSION

High-risk individuals include smokers of all ages, even those aged 40 years or younger; individuals with a previous lung cancer; patients with bullous emphysema; patients with asbestosis; and patients with pulmonary function showing chronic airflow obstruction. Although radiographic lung-cancer screening may lead to earlier cancer detection and result in an increased 5-year survival rate, lung cancer mortality is not reduced. Prevention remains the single most effective weapon against lung cancer.

REFERENCES

Arai T, et al: Application of telomerase activity for screening of primary lung cancer in bronchoalveolar lavage fluid. Oncol Rep 5:405, 1998.

Camus M, Siemiatycki J, Meek B: Nonoccupational exposure to chrysotile asbestos and the risk of lung cancer. N Engl J Med 338:1565, 1998.

Churg A: Asbestos, asbestosis, and lung cancer. Mod Pathol 6:509, 1993.

Doll R: Mortality from lung cancer in asbestos workers. Br J Ind Med 12:81, 1955.

Eddy DM: Screening for lung cancer. Ann Intern Med 111:232, 1989.

Flehinger BJ, et al: Early lung cancer detection: results of the initial (prevalence) radiologic and cytologic screening in the Memorial Sloan-Kettering study. Am Rev Respir Dis 130:555, 1984.

Fontana RS, et al: Early lung cancer detection: results of the initial (prevalence) radiologic and cytologic screening in the Mayo Clinic study. Am Rev Respir Dis 130:561, 1984.

Fontana RS, et al: Screening for lung cancer. Cancer 67:1155, 1991.

Frost JK, et al: Early lung cancer detection: Results of the initial (prevalence) radiologic and cytologic screening in the Johns Hopkins study. Am Rev Respir Dis 130:549, 1984.

Gail MH, et al: Multiple markers for lung cancer diagnosis: validation of models for localized lung cancer. J Natl Cancer Inst 80:97, 1988.

Goldstein MJ, et al: Bronchogenic carcinoma and giant bullous disease. Am Rev Respir Dis 97:1062, 1968.

Jacobson DR, Fishman CL, Mills NE: Molecular genetic tumor markers in the early diagnosis and screening of non-small cell lung cancer. Ann Onc 6(Suppl):S3-S8, 1995.

Kaneko M, et al: Peripheral lung cancer: screening and detection with low-dose spiral CT versus radiography. Radiology 201:798, 1996.

Midthun DE, Jett JR. Early detection of lung cancer: today's approach. J Respir Dis 19:59, 1998.

Mor V, et al: Lung, breast, and colorectal cancer: the relationship between extent of disease and age at diagnosis. J Am Geriatr Soc 36:873, 1988.

Muhm JR, et al: Lung cancer detected during a screening program using four-month chest radiographs. Radiology *148*:609, 1983.

Parker SL, et al. Cancer statistics, 1997. Cancer J Clin *47*:5, 1997.

Petty TL: Time to rethink lung cancer screening. J Respir Dis *12*:403, 1991.

Roscoe RJ, et al: Lung cancer mortality among nonsmoking uranium miners exposed to radon daughters. JAMA *262*:629, 1989.

Ruckdeschel JC: Whither screening for lung cancer? J Natl Cancer Inst *80*:78, 1988.

Samet JM: Radon and lung cancer: How great is the risk? J Respir Dis *10*:73, 1989.

Sellers TA, et al: Lung cancer detection and prevention: evidence for an interaction between smoking and genetic predisposition. Cancer Res *52*(Suppl):2693s, 1992.

Sobue T, Suzuki T, Naruke T: The Japanese Lung-Cancer Screening Research Group: a case-control study for evaluating lung cancer screening in Japan. Int J Cancer *50*:230, 1992.

Stoloff IL, Kanofsky P, Magilner L: The risk of lung cancer in males with bullous disease of the lung. Arch Environ Health *22*:163, 1971.

Strauss GM, Gleason RE, Sugarbaker DJ: Screening for lung cancer: another look, a different view. Chest *111*:754, 1997.

Thomas PA, Piantadosi S: Postoperative T1 N0 non-small cell lung cancer. J Thorac Cardiovasc Surg *94*:349, 1987.

Tockman MS, et al: Airways obstruction and the risk for lung cancer. Ann Intern Med *106*:512, 1987.

Tockman MS, et al: Sensitive and specific monoclonal antibody recognition of human lung cancer antigen on preserved sputum cells: a new approach to early lung cancer detection. J Clin Oncol *6*:1685, 1988.

US Department of Health and Human Services Public Health Service, Center for Disease Control: Reducing the Health Consequences of Smoking: 25 Years of Progress. Report of the Surgeon General. DHHS Publication No. (CDC) 89-8411, 1989.

Viallet J, Minna JD: Dominant oncogenes and tumor suppressor genes in the pathogenesis of lung cancer. Am J Respir Cell Mol Biol *2*:225, 1990.

Walter SD, et al: The natural history of lung cancer estimated from the results of a randomized trial of screening. Cancer Causes Control *3*:115, 1992.

Weiss W: Peripheral measurable bronchogenic carcinoma. Am Rev Respir Dis *103*:198, 1971.

Wilde J: A 10-year follow-up of semi-annual screening for early detection of lung cancer in the Erfurt County, GDR. Eur Respir J *2*:656, 1989.

Wolpaw DR: Early detection in lung cancer: case finding and screening. Med Clin N Am *80*:63, 1996.

Woolner LB, et al: Evaluation of lung cancer screening through December 1979. Mayo Clin Proc *56*:544, 1981.

Yamaguchi N, et al: A 50-year projection of lung cancer deaths among Japanese males and potential impact evaluation of anti-smoking measures and screening using a computerized simulation model. Jpn J Cancer Res *83*:251, 1992.

READING REFERENCES

Berndt R, Nichan P, Ebeling K: Screening for lung cancer in the middle-aged. Int J Cancer *45*:229, 1990.

Kubik A, Polak J: Lung cancer detection: results of a randomized prospective study in Czechoslovakia. Cancer *57*:2427, 1986.

Kubik A, et al: Lack of benefit from semi-annual screening for cancer of the lung: follow up report of a randomized controlled trial on a population of high-risk males in Czechoslovakia. Int J Cancer *45*:26, 1990.

Mulshire JL, Tockman MS, Smart CR: Considerations in the development of lung cancer screening tools. J Natl Cancer Inst *81*:900, 1989.

Nash FA, Morgan JM, Tomkins JG: South London lung cancer study. Br Med J Clin Res *2*:715, 1968.

CHAPTER 95

Lung Cancer

A. Present Concepts in the Molecular Biology of Lung Cancer

Gregory P. Kalemkerian and Harvey I. Pass

MOLECULAR BIOLOGY OF LUNG CANCER

Since the 1980s, dramatic advances in cellular and molecular biology have led to an exponential increase in our understanding of the pathophysiologic events underlying the development and progression of lung cancer. On a molecular level, these events involve not only the dysregulation of proto-oncogenes and tumor-suppressor genes that regulate cellular proliferation and differentiation, but also the disruption of physiologic cell death pathways that regulate the life span of normal bronchial epithelial cells. In addition, the metastatic potential of lung cancer cells depends on their ability to produce and secrete a variety of growth factors and angiogenic factors. The identification of the cellular and molecular derangements involved in the pathogenesis and progression of lung cancer has encouraged the development of novel biologically rational diagnostic and therapeutic approaches directed at specific molecular targets. We review the most important aspects of the biology of both small cell lung cancer (SCLC) and non–small cell lung cancer (NSCLC) and emphasize the potential effect that these advances will have on the clinical management of patients with lung cancer.

Proto-oncogenes

Proto-oncogenes encode for proteins that serve as major components of the signal transduction pathways regulating cellular growth and differentiation in normal cells. The proteins encoded by proto-oncogenes fall into several discrete functional categories, including growth factors, receptors, membrane-bound and cytoplasmic second messengers, and transcription factors. In nonneoplastic cells the expression of these proto-oncogenes is tightly regulated in order to maintain normal homeostatic control of cellular proliferation and differentiation. Oncogenic events induce mutations, amplifications, and translocations of various proto-oncogenes, resulting in either the overexpression of a normal proto-oncogene product or the expression of an overactive protein. These alterations lead to an overall increase in proto-oncogene function and, because most proto-oncogene products are positive mediators of proliferative pathways, this functional amplification results in inappropriate activation of these pathways and uncontrolled neoplastic growth. Such proto-oncogene abnormalities are a common finding in all malignancies, including lung cancer (Table 95-1).

myc *Oncogenes*

The *myc* proto-oncogenes were discovered because of their homology to the *v-myc* gene in the acute-transforming avian myelocytomatosis virus. The *myc* family consists of at least three functional genes—c-*myc*, L-*myc* and N-*myc*—that encode nuclear phosphoproteins with DNA-binding capability. Although the exact functions of the *myc* proteins are unknown, ample evidence suggests that they are transcription factors that are important mediators of proliferation, differentiation, and cell death. All three *myc* genes complement activated *ras* resulting in malignant transformation, and Birrer and colleagues (1988) noted that c-*myc* exhibits significantly more transforming potency than N-*myc* or L-*myc*. In general, the transforming capacity of the *myc* genes is directly related to their degree of dysregulation and overexpression. In the normal bronchial epithelium, Broers and colleagues (1993) reported that c-*myc* expression is limited to basal cells and alveolar type II pneumocytes, whereas N-*myc* and L-*myc* are not expressed.

Table 95-1. Proto-oncogenes Implicated in Lung Cancer

	Mechanism	Histology
Nuclear transcription factors		
c-*myc*	A/OE	S, N
N-*myc*	A/OE	S
L-*myc*	A/OE	S
c-*jun*	IE	S, N
c-*fos*	IE	N
c-*erbA*	LOH/?	S
c-*myb*	IE	S
Membrane-associated G protein		
K-*ras*	M	N
Growth factor receptor kinases		
c-*erbB-2* (*HER2/neu*)	OE	N
c-*fms*	IE	N
c-*kit*	IE	S, N
c-*met*	OE	S, N
Cytoplasmic kinases		
c-*raf-1*	LOH/?	S
c-*src*	IE	S
Apoptosis inhibitor		
bcl-2	IE	S, N

A, amplification; IE, inappropriate expression; LOH, loss of heterozygosity; M, mutation; N, non–small cell lung cancer; OE, overexpression; S, small cell lung cancer; ?, unknown.

In NSCLC, 8% of tumors have c-*myc* gene amplification and 50% exhibit c-*myc* overexpression, but the dysregulation of N-*myc* or L-*myc* is rare. In SCLC, overexpression of c-*myc*, L-*myc*, or N-*myc* occurs in up to 80% of cell lines and primary tumors. Takahashi and colleagues (1989a) and Bergh (1990) reported that *myc* gene amplification occurs in 40 to 50% of SCLC cell lines and 20 to 30% of tumors, but the mechanism of *myc* overexpression remains unknown in the remainder of cases. C-*myc* is the most commonly dysregulated of the *myc* genes in SCLC cell lines and primary tumors, and several studies, including that of Gazdar and colleagues (1985), have reported that c-*myc* gene amplification is associated with prior chemotherapy and tumors of the variant SCLC phenotype with a relatively low level of neuroendocrine differentiation. Further support for the association of c-*myc* overexpression with the variant phenotype comes from the work of Johnson and colleagues (1986) in which the heterologous expression of c-*myc* in a classic SCLC cell line resulted in transition to a partial variant phenotype. Brennan and colleagues (1991) have reported that amplification, overexpression, or both of c-*myc*, but not of L-*myc* or N-*myc*, is associated with a poor prognosis. In addition, amplification was more frequent in patients who had previously received chemotherapy (28%) than in untreated patients (8%), and appeared to correlate with the administration of alkylating agents. These results suggest that *myc* gene amplification is not an early event in the development of SCLC but that it may play an important role in tumor progression.

Dysregulation of N-*myc* gene expression has been reported primarily in neuroendocrine tumors, such as neu-roblastoma, and SCLC. In SCLC, Ibson (1987) and Takahashi (1989a) and their associates found that N-*myc* overexpression is associated with the classic phenotype and a greater degree of neuroendocrine differentiation. As is the case with c-*myc*, Wong (1986) and Nau (1986) and their associates showed that N-*myc* overexpression can occur in the presence or absence of gene amplification. However, in contrast to c-*myc*, N-*myc* overexpression is seen in a considerable number of samples from untreated patients and therefore may represent an early oncogenic event. Although Funa (1987) and Brooks (1987) and their coworkers have suggested an association between N-*myc* overexpression and poor prognosis, the largest such series by Brennan and colleagues (1991) revealed no correlation.

The L-*myc* proto-oncogene was initially described in SCLC cell lines by Nau and colleagues (1985), and its expression is highly specific for lung tissue. Rygaard and associates (1993a) and others have reported that amplification and overexpression of L-*myc* are seen predominantly in SCLC tumors with a classic phenotype and a relatively low proliferative index, but that these molecular derangements do not correlate with stage or clinical outcome. Analysis of the L-*myc* locus on chromosome 1 has revealed a restriction fragment length polymorphism (RFLP) resulting in two distinct DNA fragments, S (6.6 kb) and L (10 kb). However, the RFLP phenotype is not tumor specific and is not associated with lung cancer risk. Although, some studies, such as that of Kawashima and colleagues (1988), have suggested that the L-L and S-S phenotypes predict a poorer prognosis in patients with SCLC or NSCLC, these associations remain controversial. Makela and associates (1991) identified a chromosomal rearrangement on 1p in some SCLC cell lines that joins the L-*myc* and *RLF* genes, resulting in the expression of a fusion protein that may play a role in the pathogenesis of SCLC.

The high rate of *myc* oncogene dysregulation in lung cancer has led to a variety of novel therapeutic strategies targeting the *myc* genes, including the use of antisense technology. The expression of any gene depends on the transcription of gene-specific DNA into single-stranded messenger RNA (mRNA) followed by the translation of this mRNA into the functional protein. Determination of the mRNA nucleotide sequence that encodes for protein (the sense sequence) allows for the synthesis of a complementary, antisense oligonucleotide sequence that can specifically bind to the mRNA of interest. The creation of a double-stranded segment of mRNA effectively blocks the progression of the translational complex and inhibits the expression of functional protein. Robinson and colleagues (1995) have shown that c-*myc* antisense oligonucleotides can block the expression of c-*myc* and inhibit the proliferation of NSCLC cells in culture, whereas Van Waardenburg and coworkers (1997) reported that transfection of a c-*myc* antisense expression construct into a platinum-resistant SCLC cell line inhibited proliferation through the induction of apoptosis and potentiated the activity of cisplatin. Similarly, Dosaka-Akita and associates (1995) found that anti-sense oligonucleotides targeting L-*myc* mRNA inhibited L-*myc* expression and SCLC cell growth.

One molecular chemotherapeutic approach involves the selective transfection of cancer cells with a suicide gene that interacts with a specific pharmacologic agent to induce the death of the transfected cancer cell. In one study evaluating this strategy, Kumagai and colleagues (1996) inserted an expression construct containing a herpes simplex virus–thymidine kinase gene under the control of a *myc*-responsive promoter into SCLC cells that overexpressed either c-*myc*, N-*myc*, or L-*myc* resulting in high levels of herpes simplex virus–thymidine kinase expression specifically in these *myc* overexpressing cancer cells. Subsequent treatment with ganciclovir inhibited the growth of these transfected cells, as well as the growth of untransfected cells added to the transfected cell cultures, suggesting a therapeutic bystander effect, in which dying transfected cells emit signals that activate cell death pathways in adjacent untransfected cells. Another potential therapeutic strategy involves the direct modulation of specific proto-oncogene expression by selective pharmacologic agents. The retinoids are vitamin A analogues that are natural mediators of proliferation, differentiation, and death in many normal and malignant cell types. Many epidemiologic and molecular studies have suggested that dysregulation of retinoid signaling pathways may play a significant role in the development of upper aerodigestive tract cancers, including lung cancer. Based on these findings, one of us (G.P.K., 1994) evaluated the effects of all-trans-retinoic acid in an in vitro model of SCLC and found that retinoic acid inhibited c-*myc* expression and induced L-*myc* expression resulting in increased neuroendocrine differentiation and the inhibition of proliferation and progression events.

ras *Oncogenes*

The *ras* oncogenes encode for three proteins (H-*ras*, K-*ras*, and N-*ras*) that are membrane-associated G-proteins linking tyrosine-kinase growth factor receptors to the cascade of cytoplasmic second messenger molecules. Normal *ras* proteins possess GTPase activity and their activation depends on the binding of either guanosine diphosphate (inactive) or guanosine triphosphate (active), allowing for tight control of signal transduction. The *ras* proteins become oncogenic through mutations at codons 12, 13, or 61 that ablate GTPase activity, resulting in persistence of the activated GTP-bound state and unregulated cellular proliferation.

Mutations that activate the *ras* oncogene have been identified in up to one-third of NSCLCs. These mutations primarily involve the K-*ras* gene and Slebos and colleagues (1991) found that they occur almost exclusively in adenocarcinomas from patients with a history of tobacco use. The most common *ras* mutation in human NSCLC is a G-T transversion at codon 12, which is the same mutation noted by You and colleagues (1989) in benzo(a)pyrene-induced

murine adenomas, suggesting a direct molecular effect of cigarette smoke in human lung carcinogenesis.

The clinical implications of *ras* mutations in NSCLC have been extensively evaluated, but these studies have yielded some conflicting results. The association between the presence of K-*ras* mutation and poor prognosis in patients with NSCLC has been documented by Mitsudomi and colleagues (1991a) and others and is most evident in patients with early-stage adenocarcinoma. In a study of 69 patients undergoing curative resections reported by Slebos and associates (1990), 5-year survival was 37% in patients whose tumors exhibited a *ras* mutation and 56% in those without a mutation. However, Siegfried and colleagues (1997a) reported conflicting data suggesting that the presence of K-*ras* mutations did not have prognostic significance in 181 patients with early-stage adenocarcinomas. Although initial studies in animal cells by Sklar (1988) suggested that *ras* mutations induced resistance to cytotoxic therapy, subsequent work in human NSCLC cell lines by Tsai and coworkers (1993) failed to identify a correlation between the presence of *ras* mutations and chemosensitivity. In addition, Rodenhuis and colleagues (1997) reported that *ras* mutations did not correlate with chemoresistance nor survival in patients with advanced-stage adenocarcinoma.

Despite the frequency of activating *ras* mutations in NSCLC, Mitsudomi and colleagues (1991b) and others have not detected *ras* mutations in SCLC cell lines or tumors. This genetic difference between SCLC and NSCLC has been exploited by Mabry and associates (1988) to develop an in vitro model of phenotypic transition that mimics clinical SCLC progression. In this model, the expression of heterologous activated v-H-*ras* in variant SCLC cells that overexpress c-*myc* or N-*myc* resulted in transition to a phenotype consistent with large cell undifferentiated cancer, suggesting that cooperation between the *ras* and *myc* oncogenes may play a role in the progression of SCLC to a more treatment-resistant phenotype.

A variety of pharmacologic and molecular strategies targeting activated *ras* have been developed in an attempt to inhibit NSCLC growth. Promising results have been reported by Georges and colleagues (1993), who implanted NSCLC cells that possess activating K-*ras* mutations into the trachea of nude mice. Intratracheal injection of a retroviral construct expressing K-*ras* antisense was then performed to investigate the effect of *ras* inhibition on subsequent tumor growth. Ninety percent of control animals developed tumors, compared with only 13% of antisense-treated animals. This approach is currently being evaluated in patients with endobronchial non–small cell tumors. A second therapeutic strategy targeting *ras* is based on the finding that the attachment of a farnesyl group is required for *ras* localization and activation. Numerous farnesyl transferase inhibitors, such as the one reported by Sun and associates (1995), can preferentially block the farnesylation of mutant *ras* proteins and can selectively inhibit the growth of human NSCLC cells and xenografts with activating *ras* mutations.

HER2/neu

The *HER2/neu* (c-*erbB*-2) oncogene encodes p185[HER2], a transmembrane growth factor receptor with tyrosine-kinase activity that has significant homology to the epidermal growth factor receptor (EGF-R). In breast cancer and other tumors, gene amplification is the primary mode of *HER2/neu* dysregulation. However, although Kern and colleagues (1990) and others have reported overexpression of *HER2/neu* in 30 to 60% of NSCLCs, gene amplification appears to be a rare event. Moreover, several groups have consistently found that SCLC does not express p185[HER2]. Studies with immortalized human bronchial epithelial cells by Noguchi and coworkers (1993) and with transgenic mice by Stocklin and colleagues (1993) have suggested that over-expression of *HER2/neu* may be involved in the development of preneoplastic lung lesions but is not sufficient for malignant transformation. *HER2/neu* has become a popular target for novel therapeutic strategies because of reports by Kern (1990) and Tsai (1993) and their associates that identified an association between *HER2/neu* overexpression and advanced stage disease, chemoresistance, and poor prognosis in patients with NSCLC. Among the preclinical approaches that have resulted in growth inhibition or increased chemosensitivity in lung cancer cells are anti-sense *HER2/neu* cDNA constructs reported by Casalini and colleagues (1997); monoclonal anti-p185[HER2] antibodies conjugated to gelonin, a potent ribosomal inhibitor, reported by Snider and associates (1996); and tyrphostin AG825, a p185[HER2]-selective tyrosine kinase inhibitor, reported by Tsai and colleagues (1996). In addition, the significant clinical activity of Herceptin, a monoclonal antibody targeting p185[HER2], as a single agent and in combination with chemotherapy in patients with breast cancer, as reported by Cobleigh (1998) and Slamon (1998) and their coworkers, has led to interest in applying this approach to patients with NSCLC.

c-jun and c-fos

The AP-1 transcription factor that stimulates the expression of numerous genes involved in cellular proliferation is comprised of the products of the c-*jun* and c-*fos* proto-oncogenes. Because AP-1 is a positive regulator of proliferative pathways, inappropriate expression of c-*jun*, c-*fos*, or both may result in chronic activation of this pathway and neoplastic growth. Szabo and colleagues (1996) and others have reported that c-*jun* is expressed in 31 to 51% of NSCLCs, as well as many bronchial and alveolar preneoplastic lesions, but not in normal lung epithelium. Similarly, Schuette and associates (1988) found that approximately one-half of SCLC cell lines express c-*jun*. Volm (1992) and Wodrich (1993) and their colleagues showed that 41 to 60% of NSCLCs express c-*fos*, and that the expression of c-*fos* and c-*jun* is more common in lung cancers of smokers than non-smokers. Heintz and associates (1993) reported that

Table 95-2. Tumor-Suppressor Genes Implicated in Lung Cancer

	Mechanism	Histology
p53	I/D/M	S, N
RB1	I	S, N
p16	D/M/HM	N
APC	LOH/?	S, N
hMLH1	LOH/?	N
FHIT	LOH/?	S, N
nm23	LOH/LE	N

D, deletion; HM, hypermethylation; I, inactivation; LE, low expression; LOH, loss of heterozygosity; M, mutation; N, non–small cell lung cancer; S, small cell lung cancer; ?, unknown.

asbestos, a known lung carcinogen, induces the expression of c-*jun* in rat mesothelial and hamster tracheal epithelial cells, and increases cellular growth in both cell types. These studies suggest that tobacco carcinogens and asbestos may activate cellular oncogenes, such as c-*jun* and c-*fos*, leading to dysregulated neoplastic proliferation.

Tumor-Suppressor Genes

In contrast to the proto-oncogenes that encode positive regulators of cellular proliferation, the prototypical tumor-suppressor genes—*p53*, *RB1*, and *p16*—encode negative regulators of the cell cycle. Therefore, malignant transformation can occur through the loss or inactivation of tumor-suppressor gene function, as well as through the gain of proto-oncogene function. This inactivation requires that both alleles of the specific tumor-suppressor gene undergo genetic or epigenetic alterations resulting in lack of gene expression or loss of protein function, as initially proposed by the two-hit hypothesis of Knudson (1971). The characterization of non-random loss of heterozygosity, the selective deletion of one allele, at specific chromosomal regions in familial and sporadic cancers has led to the identification of several tumor-suppressor genes, some of which are relatively tumor-specific (*RB1*, retinoblastoma; *WT1*, Wilms' tumor; *NF1*, neurofibromatosis), whereas others are involved in a wide variety of human malignancies (*p53*, *p16*). Not surprisingly, a number of tumor-suppressor genes have been found to be inactivated in both SCLC and NSCLC (Table 95-2).

p53

The *p53* tumor-suppressor gene encodes a transcription factor with diverse biological functions, including the mediation of cell cycle arrest and cell death after DNA damage. The loss of wild-type (normal) *p53* activity is the most common genetic abnormality thus far identified in human cancer and can occur through allelic deletions and point mutations that result in amino acid substitutions that alter the protein's functional characteristics. Abnormalities in *p53* are also the most frequent genetic alterations in lung cancer, occurring in 90% of SCLCs and 60% of NSCLCs. These alterations primarily involve inactivating point mutations, but deletions, rearrangements, and splicing mutations also have been described by Takahashi and colleagues (1989b) and others. Interestingly, most of the *p53* mutations in SCLC are guanine to thymine transversions similar to those found in activated *ras* genes in NSCLC, but distinct from the usual guanine to adenine transitions that affect *p53* in other tumor types. Site-specific carcinogen exposure may account for the high incidence of this particular mutation in oncogenes associated with lung cancer. Denissenko and associates (1996) reported that benzo(a)pyrene, a major carcinogen in tobacco smoke, preferentially forms adducts at the guanine positions in *p53* that are most frequently mutated in human lung cancer. A functional role for *p53* inactivation in the pathogenesis of lung cancer has been suggested by Takahashi and colleagues (1992), who reported that the induction of expression of heterologous wild-type *p53* via gene transfection suppressed in vitro and xenograft growth of NSCLC cells, which lack endogenous wild-type *p53*. Further support for the role of *p53* mutations in the progression of lung cancer comes from a study by Mabry and coworkers (1990) in which the expression of heterologous mutant *p53* in an SCLC cell line resulted in increased growth and decreased neuroendocrine differentiation, changes that mimic those occurring during the clinical course of SCLC.

These and other studies also suggest that the manipulation of *p53* expression or activity is a rational therapeutic strategy. Fujiwara and colleagues (1993, 1994a,b) have demonstrated that a retroviral vector expressing wild-type *p53* can infect human lung cancer cells and induce cell death in vitro and in an orthotopic lung cancer xenograft model. In addition, they reported that infection of NSCLC cells and xenografts with an adenovirus vector expressing wild-type *p53* augments the cytotoxic activity of cisplatin. Roth and associates (1996) subsequently tested this approach in humans, demonstrating evidence of response in four of nine endobronchial NSCLC tumors after intratumoral injections of an adenovirus vector that expressed wild-type *p53*.

The prognostic significance of *p53* abnormalities in lung cancer remains controversial. Since the half-life of mutant *p53* protein is usually significantly longer than that of the wild-type protein, the detection of *p53* by immunohistochemistry is considered a marker for *p53* mutation. Quinlan and colleagues (1992) reported that immunohistochemical accumulation of *p53* was predictive of poor prognosis in early stage patients, whereas Horio (1993) and Mitsudomi (1993) and their associates found that the presence of *p53* mutations was a negative prognostic factor in early and advanced stage NSCLC. In contrast, several studies in both NSCLC and SCLC have reported no association between *p53* mutations and survival. In a study of 85 patients with early-stage NSCLC, Carbone and colleagues (1994) found that the concordance between positive *p53* immunostaining and the presence of a *p53* mutation was only 67%, and that neither positive *p53* immunostaining nor the presence of a

p53 mutation had a significant effect on survival in a multivariate analysis. These latter data imply that the effect, if any, of *p53* alterations on the survival of patients with lung cancer is small.

The central role that *p53* occupies in the control of DNA damage-induced cell death suggests that the loss of *p53* function could abrogate the activity of many cytotoxic agents. Lowe and colleagues (1994) were the first to show that defects in cell death caused by the inactivation of *p53* resulted in in vivo resistance of tumor cells to both gamma irradiation and doxorubicin. In a small series of patients with advanced NSCLC, Kawasaki and coworkers (1996) reported that *p53*-positive tumors were significantly more resistant to platinum-based therapy.

More recent work has suggested that the mutant *p53* protein that is commonly found in tumors, but not in normal tissue, may be a useful target for immunotherapy, which requires the identification of tumor-specific antigens to serve as targets for immunologic interventions. Winter and colleagues (1992) reported that 13% of lung cancer patients produced anti-*p53* antibodies, and these patients all harbored tumors containing missense *p53* mutations. In a study of 170 patients with SCLC, Rosenfeld and associates (1997) detected anti-*p53* antibodies in the serum of 16% of patients, but the presence of antibodies did not correlate with clinical characteristics or survival. Yanuck and colleagues (1994) demonstrated that immunization of mice with mutant *p53* protein from a lung carcinoma induced specific CD8+ cytotoxic T lymphocytes that were capable of killing cells expressing mutant *p53*, but not cells expressing wild-type *p53* protein.

RB1

The *RB1* tumor-suppressor gene encodes a 105-kd protein that plays a central role in the regulation of cell cycle progression (Fig. 95-1). Unphosphorylated *RB1* acts as an inhibitor of cellular proliferation by binding to the E2F transcription factor and inhibiting its ability to stimulate the expression of a variety of factors required for progression through the G_1/S boundary. The phosphorylation of *RB1* by G_1 cyclin:cyclin-dependent kinase (cdk) complexes, such as cyclin D1:cdk4, results in the release of E2F and the expression of genes required for cell cycle progression. Therefore, the loss of *RB1* expression, function, or both during carcinogenesis results in uncontrolled proliferation through the loss of a major cell cycle checkpoint. The seminal finding by Friend and colleagues (1986) that retinoblastoma is caused by the inactivation of both *RB1* alleles through deletions or mutations provided the first evidence for a human tumor-suppressor gene. The high frequency of cytogenetic abnormalities at the *RB1* locus in chromosomal band 13q14 in lung tumors led investigators to evaluate the integrity of the *RB1* in lung cancer. Overall, over 90% of SCLC cell lines and tumors exhibit defects in *RB1* gene expression or protein function. Although Harbour (1988) and Gouyer (1998)

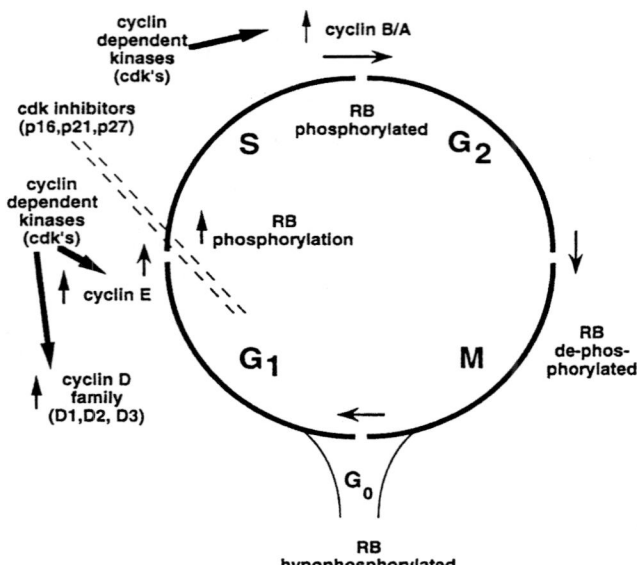

Fig. 95-1. The cell cycle. RB1 protein remains unphosphorylated and bound to E2F transcription factors in quiescent cells (G_0/G_1). In response to growth stimulatory signals, cyclin D levels rise and cyclin D-associated cyclin-dependent kinases (cdk4, cdk6) mediate RB1 phosphorylation and the release of E2F, allowing entry into the proliferative phases of the cell cycle. Further RB1 phosphorylation by cyclin E:cdk2 complexes commits the cell to DNA replication (S phase). RB1 remains phosphorylated until late in G_2, when specific phosphatase activity leads to RB1 dephosphorylation. The cdk inhibitors (p16, p21, p27) repress cdk kinase activity, thereby inhibiting cell cycle progression. Adapted from Carbone D, Kratzke R: RB1 and p53 genes. *In* Pass HI, Mitchell JB, Johnson DH, et al. (eds): Lung Cancer: Principles and Practice. Philadelphia: Lippincott–Raven, 1996.

and their colleagues have reported that *RB1* rearrangements are rare, Yokota (1988) and Hensel (1990) and their associates have identified loss of heterozygosity at the *RB1* locus in nearly all SCLCs. Several groups, including Mori and colleagues (1990), reported that the majority of SCLCs express aberrant *RB1* transcripts that lead to the expression of an *RB1* protein that is incapable of being phosphorylated or to the production of no *RB1* protein at all. Leonard and coworkers (1988) and others have described patients with inherited germ-line abnormalities of *RB1* who have developed SCLC at an early age after having been cured of retinoblastoma. In addition, Sanders and colleagues (1989) found that heterozygous relatives of patients with retinoblastoma have a markedly increased risk of developing lung cancer, predominantly of the small cell type.

Abnormalities of *RB1* expression and function are far less common in NSCLC cell lines and tumors than in SCLC. A review by Carbone and Kratzke (1996) determined that 30 to 40% of NSCLC samples failed to express functional *RB1* protein, caused by a variety of defects at the DNA, RNA, and protein levels. Studies by Shimizu (1994) and Reissmann (1993) and their associates found aberrant *RB1* protein expression in 15% of NSCLC cell lines and 32% of tumors,

respectively, and both groups failed to identify any correlation between *RB1* expression and clinical response or survival. However, Dosaka-Akita and colleagues (1997) reported that the lack of *RB1* expression had a significant negative effect on survival in patients with NSCLC whose tumors expressed either *ras* or *p53*. Kratzke (1993) and Ookawa (1993) and their coworkers transfected wild-type *RB1* into *RB1*-deficient NSCLC and SCLC cells, respectively, and noted partial suppression of growth and tumorigenicity.

The retinoblastoma gene family includes two homologues of *RB1*, *p107* and *p130*, that have also been implicated in the regulation of the cell cycle. However, despite strong structural and functional similarities with *RB1*, few alterations of *p107* and *p130* have been identified in human cancers. Helin and colleagues (1997) reported the loss of *p130* expression caused by a point mutation at a splice acceptor site in one SCLC cell line, suggesting that genetic alterations in other retinoblastoma gene family members may contribute to lung carcinogenesis.

p16

Cytogenetic studies have identified chromosomal region 9p21 as one of the most commonly affected loci in human cancers, including lung cancer. The *p16* (*MTS1*, *INK4a*, *CDKN2A*) gene, located at 9p21, has been characterized as a tumor-suppressor gene based on the high frequency of *p16* mutations and deletions present in a wide variety of human tumors and the presence of germ line mutations in families with hereditary cutaneous melanoma. The *p16* protein product is one of a family of cyclin-dependent kinase inhibitors that regulate progression through the cell cycle by inactivating cdk4 or cdk6, thereby inhibiting the phosphorylation of *RB1* by cyclin D:cdk4/6 complexes. The maintenance of *RB1* in the unphosphorylated state allows *RB1* to remain bound to E2F, resulting in cell cycle arrest at the G_1/S boundary. The nature of these interactions dictates that the loss of *p16* function or the overexpression of cyclin D1 would have the same net effect as the loss of *RB1* function—namely, unregulated passage through the G_1/S checkpoint and neoplastic proliferation. At least one of these three abnormalities, *RB1* loss, *p16* loss, or cyclin D1 overexpression, occurs in most, if not all, human cancers, suggesting that dysregulation of the cyclin D:cdk4/6-p16-RB pathway controlling the G_1/S transition may be a necessary step during malignant transformation. In NSCLC, Tanaka (1998) and Betticher (1997) and their colleagues have reported that at least 90% of tumors exhibit inactivation of *p16* or *RB1* or overexpression of cyclin D1.

A review by Liggett and Sidransky (1998) calculated that inactivation of *p16* is present in 30% of NSCLCs and 5% of SCLCs. The low incidence of *p16* inactivation in SCLC can be explained by the fact that over 90% of SCLCs have lost expression or function of *RB1* and that the additional loss of *p16* would offer no further advantage to the tumor cell because passage through the G_1/S boundary had already been ensured. In support of this theory, Otterson and associates (1994) reported that all six SCLC cell lines that they identified as *p16*-negative expressed wild-type *RB1*, whereas all 48 *RB1*-negative cell lines had detectable levels of *p16*. In NSCLC, several mechanisms of *p16* inactivation have been identified, including homozygous deletion, point mutation, and promoter methylation, resulting in aberrant transcription. Evaluation of a large series of lung cancer cell lines by Kelley and colleagues (1995) identified homozygous deletions of *p16* in 23% of NSCLC lines and only 1% of SCLC lines. The clinical effect of *p16* inactivation in early stage NSCLC has been addressed by several groups. Kratzke (1996) and Taga (1997) and their coworkers reported that the loss of *p16* was associated with a poor prognosis, whereas Kinoshita and colleagues (1996) found that inactivation of *p16* or *RB1* was associated with an increased proliferative index in tumors lacking *p53* activity. The potential utility of *p16* gene therapy has been explored by Shapiro and associates (1995) who demonstrated that the expression of heterologous *p16* resulted in growth inhibition and G_1 arrest only in NSCLC cells that expressed *RB1*.

nm23-H1

Reduced expression of the nucleoside diphosphate kinase gene, *nm23-H1*, has been associated with increased metastatic potential and poor prognosis in patients with breast cancer and other solid tumors, leading to its characterization as a metastasis-suppressor gene. Although allelic loss of *nm23-H1* is infrequent in NSCLC, nucleoside diphosphate kinase expression is low or absent in 35 to 82% of these tumors according to the work of Higashiyama and colleagues (1992) and others. However, the effect of *nm23-H1* inactivation in NSCLC remains unclear because some studies, such as that of Kawakubo and associates (1997), have found that low *nm23-H1* expression correlated with advanced-stage disease and poor prognosis in patients with pulmonary adenocarcinoma, supporting a metastasis-suppressor role, whereas others, such as that of Huwer and colleagues (1994), reported that high levels of *nm23-H1* expression were associated with poor prognosis in patients with squamous cell carcinoma.

Cytogenetic Abnormalities

Complex karyotypic alterations have been described in nearly all human malignancies, including lung cancer, suggesting that genomic instability is an inherent characteristic of cancer cells. Flow cytometry studies have revealed broad variations in DNA content, not only between tumors and normal tissue samples but also between different cells within the same tumor. Approximately 75% of lung cancers have an abnormal number of chromosomes, or aneuploidy, but studies by Bunn and colleagues (1983) and others have failed to identify any consistent associations between aneuploidy and clinical features or survival. Cytogenetic and RFLP studies have identified numerous nonrandom chromosomal abnormalities in both SCLC and NSCLC. These abnormalities include gains or losses of entire chromosomes, unbalanced translocations, and internal and terminal deletions that suggest the inactivation of unidentified tumor-suppressor genes. Chromosomal structures known as *double minutes* and homogenous staining regions are commonly seen in SCLC and are associated with amplification of gene copy number. Loss of heterozygosity of regions on chromosome arms 3p, 5q, 9p, 13q, or 17p are present in many SCLC and NSCLC specimens, and the tumor-suppressor genes *APC* (5q21), *p16* (9p21), *RB1* (13q14), and *p53* (17p13) have been mapped to the most commonly affected loci.

Repetitive DNA sequences known as microsatellites are distributed throughout the human genome and instability of these microsatellites is a marker for DNA repair defects that are characteristic of many cancer cells. Several genes, including *hMLH1* at 3p21, encode mismatch repair enzymes that are involved in the maintenance of genomic integrity. Shridhar (1994) and Merlo (1994) and their associates have shown that microsatellite instability is present in at least 34% of NSCLCs and 45% of SCLCs, respectively. Subsequently, Wieland and colleagues (1996) demonstrated that 82% of NSCLCs with microsatellite instability exhibited loss of heterozygosity of *hMLH1*, suggesting that 3p deletions may result in inactivation of mismatch repair mechanisms, genomic instability, and malignant transformation.

3p Deletions

Karyotypic and RFLP analyses by Yokota (1987) and Johnson (1988) and their coworkers, as well as others, have demonstrated that interstitial or terminal deletions of 3p occur in all SCLC, and most NSCLC, cell lines and tumors, regardless of phenotype or treatment status. In the initial report by Whang-Peng and colleagues (1982), all 16 SCLC cell lines examined had 3p deletions, with 3p14-23 being the region of common overlap. Normal lymphoid cells from the patients from whom these cell lines were established failed to reveal any 3p abnormalities, implying that the loss of 3p is an acquired somatic mutation and not a germ line anomaly. Brauch (1987) and Kok (1987) and their associates reported that 3p deletions in NSCLC commonly involved the same region. Data from Wu and colleagues (1998) suggest that 3p is particularly sensitive to the mutagenic effects of benzo(a)pyrene diol epoxide, a metabolite of tobacco smoke carcinogens, and that benzo(a)pyrene diol epoxide–induced 3p alterations may be a marker for lung cancer risk.

Extensive RFLP mapping has identified three regions of 3p that are likely to house tumor-suppressor genes: 3p14, 3p21.3, and 3p25. Strong evidence for the presence of at least one tumor-suppressor gene on chromosome 3 comes from the work of Satoh and colleagues (1993), who reported that the introduction of a normal chromosome 3 into a lung adenocarcinoma cell line that exhibited loss of heterozygosity on 3p resulted in a complete loss of tumorigenicity.

Although Latif and associates (1993) identified the von Hippel-Lindau (*VHL*) gene at 3p25 and associated its loss with hereditary renal cell carcinoma, subsequent work has shown that *VHL* inactivation is not a common event in lung cancer. The identification of relatively small deletions at 3p12-14 and 3p21 should facilitate the isolation of tumor-suppressor genes at these loci. Several other candidate genes have been mapped to the deleted regions of 3p, including retinoic acid receptor β (RARβ), c-*erbA*, and c-*raf-1*. Loss of heterozygosity of c-*erbA*, a proto-oncogene that encodes a thyroid hormone receptor, has been found in over 90% of SCLC cell lines by Dobrovic and colleagues (1988). The c-*raf-1* oncogene maps to 3p25 and encodes a second messenger protein with serine/threonine kinase activity involved in proliferative signal transduction pathways. Work by Ravi and associates (1998) demonstrated that transfection of SCLC cells with an activated form of c-*raf-1* induced growth inhibition through cell cycle arrest, suggesting that c-*raf-1* may have tumor-suppressor activity. However, Sithanandam and colleagues (1989) reported that although all SCLC cell lines examined had lost one allele at the c-*raf-1* locus, these cells continued to express c-*raf-1* kinase activity. In addition, Pfeifer and coworkers (1989) demonstrated that cotransfection of c-*raf-1* and c-*myc* into immortalized bronchial epithelial cells results in transformation to a large cell carcinoma phenotype with neuroendocrine features, suggesting that c-*raf-1* has the functional characteristics of a proto-oncogene, rather than a tumor-suppressor gene. Jensen and colleagues (1998) identified a novel gene, *BAP1*, on 3p21.3 that encodes a ubiquitin hydrolase that enhances *BRCA1*-mediated growth inhibition. They also reported homozygous rearrangements and deletions of *BAP1* in lung cancer cell lines, suggesting that *BAP1* is a candidate tumor-suppressor gene in lung cancer.

The *FHIT* gene, which encodes an enzyme involved in adenosine metabolism, has been mapped to 3p14.2 and contains the most fragile breakpoint region in the human genome. Sozzi and associates (1996) found allelic loss of *FHIT* in 79% of 59 primary lung tumors and aberrant *FHIT* transcripts in 80% and 40% of SCLCs and NSCLCs, respectively. In a follow-up study, Sozzi and colleagues (1997) reported that 73% of SCLCs and 39% of NSCLCs also failed to express FHIT protein and that such loss was also evident in preneoplastic bronchial lesions. Although subsequent studies have confirmed these findings, they have also shown that 1) aberrant transcripts are frequently found by normal, as well as malignant, cells; 2) many tumors also express wild-type *FHIT* transcripts; and 3) point mutations in the *FHIT* gene are rare. These findings suggest that *FHIT* is not a typical tumor-suppressor gene. Studies to evaluate the functional role of *FHIT* in lung cancer by Siprashvili (1997) and Otterson (1998) and their coworkers have failed to settle the question. Although both of these studies reported that heterologous expression of *FHIT* in cancer cells lacking endogenous *FHIT* expression did not significantly alter cellular proliferation, the former group found that *FHIT* expres-

sion decreased tumorigenicity, whereas the latter group did not. One explanation for these disparate findings would be that although the loss of *FHIT* expression does not appear to play a role in the dysregulation of proliferation in lung cancer cells, it may be an important factor in tumor progression. In support of this possibility, Burke and colleagues (1998) reported that the inactivation of *FHIT* is an independent poor prognostic factor in patients with NSCLC.

Other Cytogenetic Abnormalities

Deletions involving 5q13-21 were found by Miura and associates (1992) in all 13 SCLC samples examined, including some newly diagnosed primary tumors. Hosoe and colleagues (1994) identified 5q deletions in 81% of lung tumors of all histologic types and suggested that 5q may contain two separate tumor-suppressor loci. The *APC* tumor-suppressor gene, which is involved in familial polyposis coli, localizes to 5p21, and D'Amico and coworkers (1992) have reported loss of heterozygosity of *APC* in 80% of SCLCs and 40% of NSCLCs. However, studies, including that of Cooper and colleagues (1996), failed to identify *APC* mutations in lung tumors, leaving the role of *APC* allelic loss in lung cancer open to debate.

Center and colleagues (1993) have described cytogenetic abnormalities of the short arm of chromosome 9 that occur in 85% of NSCLCs, but only in a few SCLCs. These abnormalities primarily involve the 9p21-22 region that contains the *p16* tumor-suppressor gene. Olopade and colleagues (1993) also reported that deletions involving the interferon gene cluster at 9p22 occurred in 25 to 44% of lung cancer cell lines.

Deletions involving 18q have been reported frequently in NSCLC but appear to be rare in SCLC. Shiseki and colleagues (1994) found that although allelic losses at 3p, 13q, and 17p were common in both early stage NSCLCs and brain metastasis from patients with advanced NSCLC, deletions of 18q were significantly more frequent in brain metastases, suggesting that loss of a tumor-suppressor gene in this locus may be involved in lung cancer progression. Although *DPC* and *DCC* are candidate tumor-suppressor genes that map to 18q, deletions and mutations of these genes occur infrequently in NSCLCs, as reported by Nagatake (1996) and colleagues and Fong (1995) and their colleagues, respectively.

Apoptosis

Although the concept of apoptosis, or programmed cell death, has been recognized by pathologists for many years, its importance in a wide variety of physiologic and pathologic processes was first noted by Kerr and associates (1972). *Apoptosis* refers to the morphologic and biochemical features that define one particular type of cell death. The morphologic criteria of apoptosis include membrane ruffling, cytoplasmic shrinkage, chromatin margination and condensation with resultant nuclear pyknosis, and nuclear fragmentation into apoptotic bodies, which are then phagocytosed by neighboring cells. Because the integrity of the cell membrane is maintained, intracellular contents are not extruded and inflammation is not induced. The biochemical features of apoptosis include new protein synthesis, use of cellular energy stores, and activation of specific proteases and endonucleases resulting in intracellular proteolysis and intranucleosomal cleavage of DNA, respectively.

Apoptosis is a tightly regulated process that can be triggered by a variety of intracellular and extracellular signals that activate a final common cell death pathway. The molecular pathways that regulate apoptosis are highly evolutionarily conserved and involve interactions between numerous stimulators and inhibitors, some of which are also mediators of cellular proliferation and differentiation. The protein product of the *bcl-2* oncogene serves as a major inhibitor of the final common apoptotic pathway in mammalian cells, inhibiting cell death induced by a variety of signals. Several homologues of *bcl-2* have been identified that also function as mediators of apoptosis. The *bcl-x* gene encodes two proteins via alternative mRNA splicing. The long-form, $bcl-x_L$, inhibits apoptosis, whereas the short-form, $bcl-x_S$, antagonizes *bcl-2* and promotes apoptotic cell death. The *bcl-2* homologues *bax*, *bad*, and *bak* also encode proteins that promote apoptosis through interactions with *bcl-2* and $bcl-x_L$. In addition, the *p53* and c-*myc* oncogenes act as stimulators of apoptotic pathways under a variety of conditions.

For well over a century, cancer has been viewed primarily as a disease of increased cellular proliferation. However, it is now clear that disturbances in cell death pathways are also involved in carcinogenesis. The discovery of *bcl-2* overexpression in follicular B-cell lymphomas illustrated for the first time that the disruption of apoptotic pathways can result in neoplasia and malignant transformation. Overexpression of *bcl-2* is now being found in an increasing number of solid tumors and malignant cell lines. One of the functions of the protein product of the *p53* tumor-suppressor gene is the induction of apoptosis in the face of DNA damage and other oncogenic stimuli, perhaps through direct regulation of *bcl-2* and *bax* gene expression as reported by Miyashita and colleagues (1994). Harris and Hollstein (1993) have noted that the loss of *p53* function is the most common molecular abnormality thus far identified in human tumors and has been found also in a variety of premalignant lesions. These findings suggest that suppression of physiologic cell death through alterations in oncogenes that mediate apoptosis, such as *bcl-2* and *p53*, may represent a common theme in carcinogenesis.

The activation of apoptotic pathways also has been recognized by Fisher (1994) and others as an important mechanism by which radiation therapy and many chemotherapeutic agents exert their cytotoxic activities. Therefore, molecular alterations that result in suppression of apoptosis also may play a significant role in resistance to standard anticancer therapy. This novel mechanism of drug resistance has now

been demonstrated in numerous experimental tumor models, as reviewed by Reed (1995), suggesting that the modulation of apoptotic pathways in tumor cells is a rational strategy for augmenting the effectiveness of anticancer therapy.

bcl-2

In the normal bronchial epithelium, *bcl-2* expression is limited to basal cells, which comprise the renewable stem cell compartment of the pulmonary mucosa. In NSCLC, most studies, including those of Pezzella (1993), Pastorino (1997), and Flemming (1998) and their associates, have suggested significant *bcl-2* expression in 15 to 40% of primary tumors, with a higher rate of positivity in squamous cell than in adenocarcinoma. Brambilla and colleagues (1996) have reported that the expression of *bcl-2* is also more frequent in NSCLCs with neuroendocrine features. Although several investigators, including Pezzella (1993) and Ishida (1997) and their coworkers, have suggested that the overexpression of *bcl-2* is associated with improved survival in patients who underwent resection for early stage NSCLC, a large study of patients with stage I disease by Pastorino and colleagues (1997) failed to identify *bcl-2* as an independent prognostic factor in a multivariate analysis considering a variety of clinical features and molecular markers. In SCLC, numerous reports, including those by Ikegaki (1994), Kaiser (1996), and Brambilla (1996) and their associates, have noted that over 80% of cell lines and 70 to 90% of primary tumors overexpress *bcl-2*. A role for *bcl-2* in chemoresistance was suggested by Ohmori and colleagues (1993), who demonstrated that a SCLC cell line engineered to express heterologous *bcl-2* exhibited greater resistance to several cytotoxic agents than the non–*bcl-2*-expressing parental line. However, although a clinical study by Takayama and associates (1996) suggested that *bcl-2* overexpression resulted in increased treatment resistance, a larger analysis by Kaiser and colleagues (1996) failed to identify *bcl-2* as an independent prognostic factor in patients with SCLC. Among the other known apoptotic mediators, Reeve and coworkers (1996) reported that both $bcl-x_L$ and *bax* are overexpressed in most SCLC and NSCLC cell lines relative to their expression in normal lung tissue. These data suggest that the modulation of apoptotic pathways is a rational strategy for novel anti-SCLC therapy. One promising approach is the use of antisense oligonucleotides that inhibit the expression of *bcl-2* by specifically interfering with *bcl-2* mRNA. Ziegler (1997) and Zangemeister-Wittke (1998) and their associates demonstrated that *bcl-2* antisense oligonucleotides inhibit the growth of SCLC cells through the induction of apoptosis and augment the activity of chemotherapy in both SCLC cell lines and xenografts.

Fas:Fas-Ligand

The ability of cancers to avoid immune surveillance also may be dependent on the modulation of apoptotic pathways.

In T lymphocytes, the binding of Fas-ligand (FasL) to its receptor, Fas, activates cell death pathways and serves as a major negative regulator of the immune response. Studies have shown that the expression of FasL by cells in the eye and testis is responsible for maintaining the immune privileged status of these organs. Several reports have suggested that the production of FasL by tumor cells may also protect a variety of cancers from immune attack. Niehans and colleagues (1997) reported that all SCLC and NSCLC cell lines, 80% of SCLC tumors, and 93% of NSCLC tumors express FasL, and that in co-culture experiments, FasL-producing lung cancer cells could induce apoptosis in human T lymphocytes. In addition, Nambu and associates (1998) found that NSCLC cells fail to exhibit surface expression of Fas, enabling them to resist autocrine-induced Fas-mediated cell death.

Telomerase

Telomeres are structures at the ends of chromosomes that are composed of tandem hexameric DNA repeat sequences and are necessary for the maintenance of chromosomal integrity. Telomere length also appears to be an important mediator of cellular aging and survival. In normal mortal cells, the telomere shortens with each cellular division, because of the inability of common DNA polymerases to fully replicate chromosomal ends, until a critical length is reached that signals cell cycle arrest and senescence. Cellular immortalization requires the acquisition of the ability to maintain telomere integrity in the face of ongoing cellular division, and the potential role of telomeres in cancer has been concisely reviewed by Morin (1996). The telomerase enzyme is a specialized ribonucleoprotein that can maintain telomere length in long-lived proliferating cells, such as germ cells. It has now been clearly demonstrated by Kim and colleagues (1994) and others that many cancer cells express telomerase and that inappropriate telomerase activity plays a major role in the immortalization associated with malignant transformation. Hiyama (1995) and Albanell (1997) and their coworkers have shown that over 80% of resected lung cancers, both small cell and non–small cell, express telomerase activity, whereas such activity is limited to basal cells in the normal bronchial mucosa. In addition, Yashima and colleagues (1997) identified telomerase in most preneoplastic lung lesions, ranging from hyperplasia to carcinoma in situ, suggesting that telomerase dysregulation is an early event in lung carcinogenesis. These findings have led to efforts to use telomerase activity as a diagnostic or surveillance marker for lung cancer. In clinical trials by Yahata (1998) and Arai (1998) and their associates, the presence of telomerase activity in bronchoscopic washing and lavage specimens identified 80% of patients with known lung cancer and was significantly more sensitive than traditional cytologic evaluation, suggesting a possible role in screening of high-risk populations.

Table 95-3. Growth Factors and Receptors Implicated in Lung Cancer

Growth Factor/Receptor	Histology
Gastrin-releasing peptide/GRP receptor	S
Vasopressin/V1 receptor	S
Neuromedin B/NMB receptor	S
Neurotensin/NT receptor	S
Nerve growth factor/NGF receptors	S
Insulinlike growth factors/IGF receptors	N, S
Vasoactive intestinal peptide/VIP receptor	N, S
Opioids-endorphins/opioid receptors	N, S
Nicotine/nicotinic receptors	N, S
Stem cell factor/SCF receptor (c-*kit*)	N, S
Hepatocyte growth factor/HGF receptor (c-*met*)	N, S
Transforming growth factor-β/TGF-β receptors	N, S
Transferrin/TF receptor	N, S
Epidermal growth factor/EGF receptor (c-*erbB-1*)	N
Transforming growth factor-α/EGF receptor (c-*erbB-1*)	N
Amphiregulin/EGF receptor (c-*erbB-1*)	N
Colony-stimulating factor 1/CSF-1 receptor (c-*fms*)	N
Platelet-derived growth factor	N
Parathyroid hormone-related peptide	N

N, non–small cell lung cancer; S, small cell lung cancer.

Growth Factors

Most growth factors act through binding to specific membrane-associated receptors. This interaction activates signal transduction pathways that carry growth stimulatory signals to the nucleus where cell cycle activation results in cellular proliferation. Dysregulation of the expression or function of growth factors, receptors, or signal-transduction pathways can result in uncontrolled proliferation and malignant transformation. Although most growth factors implicated in cancer are stimulators of proliferation, a variety of growth inhibitory factors have been identified also. Growth factors secreted by cancer cells can participate in both autocrine and paracrine loops by interacting with specific receptors on their own cell membranes or on the surfaces of nearby cells, respectively. The ability of malignant cells to produce autocrine growth factors plays an important role in the establishment and survival of both primary tumors and metastatic deposits. A wide variety of growth factors and growth factor receptors have been implicated in the pathogenesis and progression of lung cancer (Table 95-3). Many of these are preferentially expressed by either SCLC or NSCLC cells, and their proliferative effects are similarly cell-type specific.

Neuropeptides

The proliferation of most SCLC cells is enhanced by a network of autocrine and paracrine pathways involving multiple neuropeptides and their receptors. Gastrin-releasing peptide (GRP) is the mammalian homologue of the amphibian neuropeptide bombesin. Moody and colleagues (1981, 1985) were the first to identify the expression of GRP and high-affinity GRP receptors in SCLC, and Sausville and associates (1986) later showed that nearly all SCLC cell lines and tumors produce and secrete GRP. Carney and colleagues (1987) subsequently reported that GRP selectively stimulates the growth of SCLC, but not NSCLC, cells in vitro. Further evidence that GRP is an autocrine growth factor in SCLC came from Cuttitta and coworkers (1985), who demonstrated that an antibombesin monoclonal antibody blocked the GRP to GRP receptor interaction, inhibited the growth of SCLC cell lines, and induced regression of human SCLC xenografts. A role for inappropriate GRP expression in lung carcinogenesis was suggested by Willey and colleagues (1984), who found that GRP induces the proliferation of normal human bronchial epithelial cells, and by Aguayo and associates (1989), who identified high levels of bombesinlike immunoreactivity in bronchoalveolar lavage fluid from smokers. GRP has also been evaluated as a clinical tumor marker for SCLC. Although most studies have found that serum levels of GRP have low sensitivity and specificity for SCLC, Maruno and colleagues (1989) reported high plasma GRP levels in 76% of patients with SCLC, and Pedersen and coworkers (1986) noted that 75% of SCLC patients with carcinomatous meningitis had high cerebrospinal fluid GRP levels.

In addition to GRP, the effects of numerous other neuropeptides on SCLC cells have been examined. Although many of these molecules induce biochemical evidence of activation of signal-transduction pathways, including intracellular calcium ion mobilization, relatively few have been shown to enhance the proliferation of SCLC cells. Among this latter group are bradykinin, vasopressin, cholecystokinin, gastrin, galanin, and neurotensin. Missale and colleagues (1998) reported that SCLC cells can produce nerve growth factor and express nerve growth factor receptors and that nerve growth factor inhibits both the growth and tumorigenicity of SCLC cells.

The profound effect of neuropeptides on SCLC proliferation has led to the evaluation of neuropeptide antagonists as therapeutic agents. Stemming from the work of Woll and Rozengurt (1988), a number of investigators have synthesized substance P analogues that inhibit basal and neuropeptide-stimulated growth of SCLC cell lines and xenografts, and at least one of these compounds has entered into clinical trials. Another therapeutic strategy aimed at interrupting autocrine growth loops in SCLC was reported by Kelley and colleagues (1997), who used an anti-GRP monoclonal antibody to induce a complete response in a patient with SCLC.

Insulinlike Growth Factors

The insulinlike growth factors, IGF-I and IGF-II, are polypeptides that are closely related to insulin in both structure and biological activity. IGF-I and IGF-II are predominantly produced in the liver but also appear to be expressed by many cell types and to have paracrine functions in most organs, including the lung. The ability of IGF-I to act as an autocrine growth factor in SCLC cell lines and primary tumor cells has been demonstrated by Nakanishi (1988) and Macaulay (1990) and their associates. However, Quinn and colleagues (1996) reported that although nearly all SCLC and NSCLC cell lines express IGF-I, IGF-II, and high-affinity IGF-I receptors, IGF-II represents the major secreted product, suggesting that the IGF-II/IGF-1 receptor pathway may be more important in the development of all types of lung cancer. IGF activity is regulated by specific binding proteins that are differentially expressed by SCLC and NSCLC and may serve as useful tumor markers as reported by Reeve and coworkers (1990), who found that 93% of patients with lung cancer had elevated plasma IGF binding protein levels. The apparent importance of IGF pathways in lung cancer led Lee and colleagues (1996) to develop an adenoviral IGF-I receptor antisense vector that has been shown to inhibit receptor expression and proliferation in NSCLC cells and to improve survival in mice with human NSCLC xenografts.

Colony-Stimulating Factors

Although many SCLC cells express receptors for hematopoietic colony-stimulating factors (CSFs), few proliferate in response to granulocyte (G)-CSF or granulocyte-macrophage (GM)-CSF. However, Young and colleagues (1993) reported that GM-CSF enhanced in vitro cellular motility and invasiveness of murine Lewis lung carcinoma cells, suggesting that CSFs may regulate biological properties other than proliferation. Despite the concerns raised by these findings, clinical trials have not revealed adverse consequences resulting from the use of G-CSF or GM-CSF in patients with SCLC. CSF-1 (macrophage CSF) and its receptor, CSF-1R, the product of the c-fms oncogene, mediate normal macrophage invasiveness. Filderman and associates (1992) showed that CSF-1R is expressed on some NSCLC cells and that exposure of these cells to CSF-1 increased basement membrane invasiveness, suggesting a potential role for CSF-1:CSF-1R in the metastatic cascade.

Epidermal Growth Factor Receptor and Its Ligands

Epidermal growth factor receptor (EGF-R), a tyrosine kinase receptor encoded by the c-erbB-1 oncogene, can be activated by several ligands including EGF and transforming growth factor-α (TGF-α). Rusch and colleagues (1993) documented the overexpression of EGF-R, and TGF-α in over 80% of NSCLCs when compared with normal lung tissue but did not detect any expression of EGF. In contrast to NSCLC, several series have failed to show significant expression of TGF-α, EGF, or EGF-R in SCLC cell lines or tumors. The prognostic value of EGF-R remains unclear despite the findings of Volm and associates (1992), who found that EGF-R expression correlated with drug resistance and short survival, and Fontanini and coworkers (1995), who reported that high levels of EGF-R expression were predictive of lymph node metastases. Evidence that EGF-R and TGF-α participate in an autocrine growth loop in NSCLC comes from the work of Rabiasz (1992) and Lee (1992) and their colleagues who have reported that the growth of NSCLC cell lines is inhibited by monoclonal antibodies directed against EGF-R or TGF-α. In addition, Hamburger and associates (1998) showed that TGF-α enhances tumorigenicity in lung epithelial cells expressing EGF-R and p185[HER2]. These studies have led to the development of numerous therapeutic approaches that target the EGF-R pathway in NSCLC. Modjtahedi and colleagues (1996) reported that an anti-EGF-R rat monoclonal antibody that inhibited growth of EGF-R–positive xenografts could be administered safely to humans and localized to EGF-R–expressing lung tumors. Suarez-Pestana and colleagues (1997) augmented the growth inhibitory activity of an anti-EGF-R monoclonal antibody against NSCLC cells by adding GM3, an antityrosine kinase ganglioside that inhibits the activation of EGF-R. Cristiano and Roth (1996) took advantage of the relatively high expression of EGF-R in NSCLC cells to develop an efficient gene therapy delivery system in which the gene of interest was conjugated to EGF and this EGF-DNA conjugate was then specifically taken up by EGF-R–expressing cells resulting in efficient heterologous gene expression.

Transforming Growth Factor-β

The transforming growth factor-β (TGF-β) family consists of several growth factors and associated receptors with pleiotropic effects on growth and differentiation in a variety of normal and malignant cell types. Jetten and colleagues (1990) have demonstrated that TGF-β inhibits growth and regulates normal mucoepithelial differentiation in tracheobronchial epithelial cells. Dysregulation of TGF-β pathways has been implicated in the pathogenesis of lung cancer by the work of Bottinger and associates (1997), who found an increased rate of lung tumors after exposure to chemical carcinogens in transgenic mice expressing dominant-negative mutant TGF-β. Jakowlew and coworkers (1995) reported that TGF-β1 and TGF-β2 are both secreted by some SCLC and NSCLC cell lines, that most of these lines express TGF-β receptors, and that TGF-β1 inhibits lung cancer cell growth. Others have also shown that TGF-β can inhibit the growth of lung cancer cells, and Norgaard and colleagues (1996) reported that resistance to TGF-β1 correlated with the loss of TGF-β receptor expression in SCLC cells. In addition, Inoue and associates (1995) found that high levels of TGF were associated with better survival in patients with adenocarcinoma, whereas Raynal and colleagues (1997) noted that TGF-β1 enhances the apoptotic effects of DNA-damaging agents in NSCLC cells.

Other Growth Factors

The production of platelet-derived growth factor (PDGF) has been demonstrated in most NSCLCs by Kawai and col-leagues (1997) and appears to be associated with a poor prognosis. However, conflicting data regarding the expression of PDGF receptors in NSCLCs and tumor stromal cells has left some question as to whether PDGF serves as an autocrine growth factor or mediates stromal reactions. In contrast, PDGF expression has not been found in SCLC cells.

Rygaard and coworkers (1993b), among others, have reported that over 70% of SCLC cell lines and tumors coexpress stem cell factor and its receptor, the product of the c-kit proto-oncogene. Subsequently, Krystal and colleagues (1996, 1997) demonstrated that the coexpression of stem cell factor and c-kit constitutes an autocrine growth pathway in SCLC cells, and that AG1296, a tyrosine kinase inhibitor that is relatively selective for c-kit, induced apoptosis in these cells. In another study of a potential therapeutic intervention, DiPaola and associates (1993) inhibited the growth of NSCLC cells that coexpress c-kit and stem cell factor with an antisense c-kit oligonucleotide.

Hepatocyte growth factor (HGF), the ligand for the receptor product of the c-met proto-oncogene, plays a physiologic role in angiogenesis, cell motility, and invasion. In the lung, HGF is primarily expressed by fibroblasts, whereas the expression of c-met has been demonstrated in nearly all lung cancer cells by Rygaard and colleagues (1993b). Singh-Kaw and associates (1995) reported that HGF induced proliferation, motility, and invasiveness in c-met–expressing lung cancer and normal bronchial epithelial cells. Siegfried and colleagues (1997b) showed that high tumor levels of HGF were a strong negative prognostic factor in patients with resected early stage NSCLC.

Maneckjee and Minna (1990) reported that some SCLC and NSCLC cells express opioid and nicotinic acetylcholine receptors and that exogenous opioids inhibited the growth of these cells. In addition, they found that nicotine reversed opioid-induced growth inhibition and suggested that in normal bronchial epithelium the endogenous opioid system may act as a natural tumor-suppressor pathway that can be disabled by chronic exposure to tobacco smoke.

Angiogenesis

The ability of tumors to stimulate the directed growth of new blood vessels to support their nutritional needs is a primary requirement for the development of clinically relevant primary tumors and the establishment of distant metastatic foci. Most human cancers secrete a variety of angiogenic factors that stimulate the proliferation and motility of endothelial cells, leading to the formation of a tumor-specific vascular system. Blood vessel invasion by tumor cells and the density of vessels within a tumor may be indicators of metastatic potential. In NSCLC, many, but not all, reports, such as that of Fontanini and associates (1997a), demonstrated that high microvessel density is an independent indicator of metastatic disease and poor prognosis in patients with stage I to IIIa disease undergoing potentially curative resection. Angiogenic factors that have been implicated in lung cancer include vascular endothelial growth factor, basic fibroblast growth factor, platelet-derived endothelial cell growth factor, and interleukin 8 (IL-8). Vascular endothelial growth factor and its receptor, flt-1, are expressed by over 50% of squamous cell carcinomas, and vascular endothelial growth factor positivity has been associated with high microvessel density, lymph node metastasis, and poor prognosis by Fontanini (1997b), Ohta (1997), and Volm (1997a) and their coworkers, respectively. In patients with SCLC, Salven and colleagues (1998) reported that high serum levels of vascular endothelial growth factor correlated with chemoresistance and poor survival. Although nearly all NSCLCs express both basic fibroblast growth factor and its receptor, fibroblast growth factor R1, Volm and associates (1997b) found that their levels of expression were not independent predictors of survival. Koukourakis and colleagues (1997) noted high levels of platelet-derived endothelial cell growth factor expression in a third of early stage NSCLCs, but in none of the SCLCs evaluated, and correlated high expression of platelet-derived endothelial cell growth factor with increased tumor vascularity, but not with survival. The inhibition of angiogenesis has become a popular experimental strategy for inhibiting the growth and spread of many types of cancer. Angiostatin, a fragment of plasminogen that potently inhibits endothelial cell proliferation, was reported by Sim and coworkers (1997) to inhibit 90% of Lewis lung carcinoma metastases. The work of Smith and associates (1994), who showed that IL-8 is produced by and induces angiogenesis in lung cancer, led to a study by Arenberg and colleagues (1996) in which an IL-8 neutralizing antibody decreased angiogenesis and tumor size in NSCLC xenografts. These promising studies have led to widespread interest in the clinical development of antiangiogenic interventions for the treatment of patients with lung cancer.

Preneoplasia

The seminal work of Saccomanno and associates (1974) on sputum cytology in patients at high risk for lung cancer led to the identification of a series of nonmalignant lesions occurring predominantly in the epithelium of central bronchi. Pathologically, these lesions have been categorized as hyperplasia; squamous metaplasia; mild, moderate, and severe dysplasia; and carcinoma in situ, and are associated with a progressively increasing risk of lung cancer, primarily of the squamous cell subtype. Studies of peripheral airways have also identified histopathologic lesions, such as atypical adenomatous and alveolar hyperplasia, that appear to be precursors of adenocarcinoma. The prognostic significance of preneoplastic lung lesions remains controversial because 1) they can be identified in most smokers, even those that never develop lung cancer; 2) even severe dysplasia can spontaneously regress; and 3) most lung cancers arise in histopathologically normal mucosa. To more accurately predict a patient's risk of malignant transformation, intense research has been focused on the molecular events that trigger the progression of preneoplastic lesions to invasive cancer. The identification of specific genetic derangements that can define a high-risk population will facilitate the development of strategies designed to inhibit preneoplastic progression or detect lung cancer at an early stage.

Chromosomal abnormalities have been identified not only in cells from preneoplastic lesions, but also in normal appearing bronchial epithelial cells from current and former smokers. Sundaresan and colleagues (1992) reported loss of heterozygosity of 3p in most dysplastic lesions from smokers with and without lung cancer, and Hung and associates (1995) identified similar lesions in 76% of hyperplastic lesions. These findings suggest that 3p deletion is a relatively ubiquitous response to lung injury that probably does not correlate with lung cancer risk. Similarly, Miozzo and colleagues (1996) detected microsatellite alterations in normal-appearing bronchial mucosa from one-third of patients with early-stage NSCLC. Both Mao (1997) and Wistuba (1997) and their coworkers reported that loss of heterozygosity of 3p, 9p, and 17p was common in normal-appearing bronchial cells from both current and former smokers but was not present in the airway epithelial cells of nonsmokers. In addition, they found that these genetic abnormalities persisted for many years in former smokers despite continued abstinence.

Specific oncogene abnormalities have been detected also in preneoplastic bronchial lesions. Sozzi and colleagues (1991) detected the overexpression of HER-2/neu or EGF-R in normal bronchial epithelium from one-half of lung cancer patients, whereas Rusch and associates (1995) found that EGF-R expression was common in all levels of preneoplastic lesions. Several studies, as summarized by Vermylen and colleagues (1997), have reported evidence of p53 mutation in most dysplastic lesions but in only a few samples of normal or metaplastic epithelium. Mutations of p53 have also been found in many atypical adenomatous hyperplasias. These findings suggest that p53 mutation is a relatively late event that may be associated with progression to both squamous cell and adenocarcinoma. K-ras mutations were also frequently detected in atypical alveolar hyperplasia from patients with adenocarcinoma by Westra and associates (1996). Although current evidence suggests that several molecular derangements can be detected in preneoplastic and normal bronchial epithelial cells from patients exposed to lung carcinogens, the natural history of these abnormalities has not been well defined, and their clinical usefulness as predictors of malignant transformation remains unproved.

As noted earlier, retinoids are important mediators of normal bronchoepithelial differentiation and, in animals, retinoid deficiency results in reversible preneoplastic changes. The biological activity of retinoids is mediated through nuclear retinoic acid and retinoid X receptors (RARs and RXRs) that act as transcriptional activating factors when bound to the appropriate ligand. Therefore, alterations in retinoid receptor expression can simulate retinoid deficiency, allowing affected cells to stray from normal differentiation pathways. Gebert (1991) and Geradts (1993) and their associates among others have demonstrated that most lung cancer cell lines exhibit abnormal expression of the *RAR*-β gene. Other receptor- and non–receptor-associated defects in retinoid signaling pathways have also been identified in lung cancer cells. In addition, Houle and colleagues (1993) reported that the expression of heterologous *RAR*-β in NSCLC cells lacking endogenous *RAR*-β expression inhibited growth and tumorigenicity, suggesting that *RAR*-β may possess tumor-suppressor activity. These findings suggest that derangements of retinoid signaling pathways represent early, reversible events in the pathogenesis of lung cancer.

Clinical Implications

Advances in our understanding of the cellular and molecular events involved in the pathogenesis and progression of lung cancer allow the development of rational diagnostic, prognostic, and therapeutic strategies that favorably affect the overall survival of patients with this disease. Long-term survival rates in SCLC and NSCLC remain poor, with 5-year survival of only 5 to 10% and 10 to 15%, respectively. Because most eventual long-term survivors present with limited stage SCLC or stage I to II NSCLC, the development of effective early diagnostic strategies increases the percentage of patients with curable, early-stage disease. However, because many early-stage patients relapse and die of lung cancer despite undergoing potentially curative therapy, it also would be useful to identify prognostic factors that define subgroups of patients with relatively poor prognoses who would benefit from aggressive adjuvant therapy. In light of the high incidence of primary and secondary resistance to standard cytotoxic treatment in NSCLC and SCLC, respectively, novel therapeutic strategies are required to improve the clinical outcome of patients with both advanced and early stage disease.

Molecular Diagnostics

Conventional screening techniques, including chest radiography and sputum cytology, have not improved overall survival rate in lung cancer. However, the identification of tumor-specific molecular abnormalities has led to renewed interest in screening using molecular techniques to identify patients with early-stage disease. Mao and colleagues (1994) retrospectively analyzed sputum samples acquired before the diagnosis of NSCLC from 10 patients whose tumors harbored *p53* or *ras* mutations. They reported that the same mutation was detectable in the sputum from 8 of these 10 patients up to 13 months prior to the clinical diagnosis of lung cancer. Others have reported that a variety of oncogene and chromosomal abnormalities can be detected in sputum and bronchoalveolar lavage samples from patients with pre-neoplastic and malignant lung lesions. However, most of these studies were performed retrospectively in preselected populations with known bronchial lesions and thus, they do not directly address the utility of such techniques for mass screening. In a prospective study, Ahrendt and associates (1998) reported that *p53* or K-*ras* mutations or microsatellite alterations were detectable in bronchoalveolar lavage fluid from 37% of patients with early stage NSCLC whose tumors were subsequently found to harbor at least one of these genetic alterations. Although the low sensitivity is disappointing, this study did demonstrate that molecular techniques can prospectively detect tumor cells in patients with peripheral, early-stage NSCLC.

Molecular Prognostic Markers

Many studies have identified that tumor stage and performance status are the strongest clinicopathologic prognostic determinants in patients with lung cancer. Unfortunately, because of the lack of curative therapy for patients with advanced stage disease, the clinical usefulness of prognostic factors in this setting remains limited. However, the ability to select early-stage patients with a high risk for relapse and death would be useful in planning novel adjuvant treatment trials. Throughout this chapter, numerous studies evaluating the prognostic potential of individual molecular markers, such as c-*myc*, K-*ras*, and *p53*, have been discussed. The fact that most of these studies are retrospective analyses of single biomarkers in relatively small cohorts of patients severely limits their clinical applicability. Two groups have sought to develop a prognostic model in patients with stage I NSCLC by evaluating the relationships between an array of biomarkers and clinicopathologic features. Harpole and colleagues (1995) analyzed the prognostic significance of several clinicopathologic features, as well as the immunohistochemical overexpression of *p53*, *HER2/neu*, and Ki-67, a proliferative marker, in 271 patients with stage I NSCLC. By multivariate analysis, they identified the presence of symptoms, *HER2/neu* overexpression, T_2 tumor size, vascular invasion, and *p53* overexpression as significant negative prognostic factors. In addition, they reported 5-year survival of 72% in patients with tumors that had negative results for both *p53* and *HER2/neu* expression but only 38% in patients with tumors that were positive for both markers. In the second study, Pastorino and associates (1997) performed a multivariate analysis using a variety of clinicopathologic and immunohistochemical parameters, including *p53*, *bcl-2*, *HER2/neu*, EGF-R, and vessel density, on 515 patients with stage I NSCLC and identified T-stage as the strongest prognostic variable. However, none of the molecular markers emerged as independent predictive factors for survival. A review of prognostic factors in early-stage NSCLC by Strauss and colleagues (1995) concluded that although a reliable model integrating clinical and biological parameters to predict prognosis has not yet been developed, such a model based on prospective studies would greatly facilitate future trials of postresection therapy in high-risk patients.

Molecular Therapeutics

Insights into the cellular and molecular events involved in the pathogenesis and progression of lung cancer have led to myriad novel therapeutic strategies, many of which have been discussed in this chapter and are summarized in Table 95-4. Many of these approaches are currently being evaluated in early-phase clinical trials, and several have already yielded promising results. However, because of the genetic and phenotypic heterogeneity of malignant cells, it is unlikely that any one of these strategies will be the final solution for the treatment of lung cancer. Nevertheless, it is now reasonable to envision a scenario in which cancer patients can be effectively treated with a specific combination of molecular therapies based on the particular cellular and genetic derangements present in their tumor. In addition to having intrinsic anticancer activity, some molecular modalities also potentiate the activity of traditional cytotoxic agents. For example, although the inhibition of bcl-2 expression may not completely eradicate tumors exhibiting bcl-2 overexpression, it can lower the apoptotic threshold of malignant cells and enhance the activity of standard chemotherapeutic agents that act through apoptotic pathways. Similarly, combinations

Table 95-4. Molecular Therapeutic Approaches in Lung Cancer

Inhibition of growth factor production or availability (e.g., anti-gastrin-releasing peptide antibodies)
Antagonism of growth factor binding (e.g., neuropeptide antagonists)
Inhibition of proto-oncogene expression or function (e.g., ras-directed farnesyl transferase inhibitors)
Reconstitution of tumor-suppressor gene function (e.g., wild-type p53 gene therapy)
Immunotherapy targeting mutant oncogene or tumor-suppressor gene products (e.g., cytotoxic T cells specific for mutant p53 or ras protein)
Stimulation of apoptotic pathways (e.g., antisense bcl-2 oligonucleotides)
Manipulation of signal transduction components (e.g., tyrosine kinase inhibitors)
Inhibition of angiogenesis (e.g., angiostatin, endostatin)
Inhibition of invasion/metastatic factors (e.g., metalloprotease inhibitors)

of molecular treatments can be devised to take advantage of synergistic interactions resulting in complete inhibition of tumor cell proliferation. Although traditional cancer treatment approaches clearly benefit some patients with lung cancer, most still die within 1 year of diagnosis. Further advances in the clinical management of these patients will depend on our ability to translate our understanding of the biology of lung cancer into effective therapeutic strategies.

B. Pathology of Carcinoma of the Lung

Thomas W. Shields

CARCINOGENESIS

Mechanisms

According to Farber (1984), the process of carcinogenesis is complicated, with multiple steps. The exact cellular events or cellular alterations that take place at each point of the malignant transformation are unclear. The neoplastic transformation can be subdivided into three steps: 1) initiation, 2) promotion, and 3) progression. *Initiation* is the interaction of the cell with the carcinogen, resulting in some type of cellular injury that may or may not be repaired. In *promotion*, the initiated cells proliferate and become nodules, papillomas, or polyps. The precise mech-

anism by which these cells expand is not understood. *Progression* is the final step, in which the initiated cells have undergone promotion and become malignant. Whether this experimental model of carcinogenesis with initiation, promotion, and progression remains a viable concept requires further time and investigation.

Derivation of Tumor Cell Types

In the normal lung, stem cell activity, according to Otto and Wright (1997), involves three cell types: 1) the basal cell of the bronchi and trachea, 2) the Clara cell of the bronchioles, and 3) the type II pneumocyte of the alveoli. These authors further note that stem cell activity of secretory cells remains unproved and that this is likewise true of the neuroendocrine cells. In tumor histogenesis, the role of one or more of these aforementioned cells remains unanswered. Many investigators have implicated one or more of these cell types, but no unified concept has evolved. At present, two main hypotheses of lung cancer pathogenesis exist. The first hypothesis is that of a pluripotent stem cell from which the various tumor phenotypes arise by differentiation. The second is the multiple primary hypothesis in which the various phenotypes arise from different cells of origin. No universal acceptance of either hypothesis has occurred. Brambilla (1997), in reviewing the basaloid carcinomas of the lung, has noted that "basaloid carcinoma cells show the morphological, immunophenotypical, and ultrastructural features of totipotent reserve or basal cells, which have the propensity for further multi-directional differentiation among squamous, glandular, or even neuroendocrine pathways." This observation, if confirmed by others, would help to explain the heterogenicity of tumor cell types within a given tumor. Actually, heterogenicity is the rule rather than the exception in most lung tumors. Yesner (1977, 1983) reported the frequent finding of areas of non–small cell tumor phenotypes in SCLCs, as well as the presence of neuroendocrine differentiation in NSCLs. Roggli and colleagues (1985) observed that only 34% of tumors studied in their investigation were homogenous for one cell type of cancer and that 45% of tumors contained two major histologic cell types. Of the SCLCs reviewed, at least one-half contained an area of another major histologic type. What triggers the basal (indifferent/indeterminate basal or suprabasal intermediate cells, the small mucous granule cells) cell in the tracheobronchial epithelium to differentiate into one or more of the multiple tumor phenotypes is unknown. Minna (1993), however, has suggested that malignant transformation under various stimuli may result in different phenotypes depending on the type of mutation acquired on key genes that control proliferation, differentiation, and apoptosis.

PATHOLOGY

Gross Characteristics

Bronchial carcinoma occurs more frequently in the right lung than in the left lung, in a ratio of approximately 6 to 4. The upper lobes are involved more often than the lower lobes, and the middle lobe is involved the least frequently of all. In the upper lobes, the tumor is most likely located in the anterior segment, although the other segments are not spared as the site of origin.

The anatomic site of origin of the tumor may be classified as 1) the central zone, including the main stem, lobar bronchi, and primary segmental bronchi of the lower lobe; 2) the segmental or intermediate zone, including the third-, fourth-, and possibly the fifth-order segmental bronchi; and 3) the peripheral zone, which includes the remainder of the distal bronchi, bronchioles, and alveoli. In the radiographic localization of lung tumors, zones 1 and 2 may be considered the central area and zone 3 is the peripheral area.

According to Meyer and Liebow (1965), approximately 50 to 60% of carcinomas of the lung originate in the peripheral area. Of those carcinomas that arise in the central and segmental zones (the central area), 20 to 40% arise in the former and 60 to 80% in the latter.

Grossly, the tumors in the central and segmental zones appear as a firm, irregular mass of varying size. Intraluminal growth may occlude the bronchial lumen partially or completely, although obstruction also may be caused by circumferential narrowing of the lumen. Extrabronchial spread may extend for a variable distance into the adjacent lung parenchyma. The tumor is generally homogeneous, with a whitish gray cut surface. The endobronchial surface typically is ulcerated. Atelectasis or secondary inflammatory change, including secondary bronchiectasis, pneumonitis, or lung abscess distal to the site of the tumor, is frequently present.

The peripherally located tumors are firm and irregular and may or may not appear to be demarcated from the surrounding lung tissue. The cut surface is homogeneous. The smaller lesions are usually solid, although the larger ones may reveal central necrosis with cavitation. Umbilication or puckering of the overlying adjacent visceral pleura is often present. The blood supply of both the centrally and the peripherally located bronchial carcinomas is from the bronchial arteries.

Histologic Classification

Many histologic classifications of lung tumors have been suggested. The modified classification suggested by Moori (1996) is shown in Table 95-5. In clinical practice it is common to separate these tumor types into either SCLC or NSCLC. Furthermore, the SCLC belong to the spectrum of neuroendocrine tumors of the lung. Azzopardi (1959) and Bensch and associates (1968) were among the early investigators who established the recognition of the neuroendocrine features of these tumors. Subsequently, over the last 40 years the initial classification has undergone numerous modifications, with better delineation and characterization of the various subtypes in the neuroendocrine tumor classification (Table 95-6). Arrigoni and colleagues (1972) identified the atypical carcinoid tumors. Gould and coworkers (1983a,b), incorporating the increased knowledge concerning these tumors, suggested that the atypical carcinoid tumors be termed *well-differentiated neuroendocrine carcinomas*. They further suggested the term *neuroendocrine carcinoma of the intermediate cell type* be applied to all types of poorly differentiated neuroendocrine tumors that were distinct from either the atypical carcinoids or the small cell type of neuroendocrine tumors. Travis and associates

Table 95-5. Modified Classification of Lung Carcinoma[a]

Squamous cell carcinoma[b]
Small cell carcinoma
    Pure small cell carcinoma
    Small cell–large cell carcinoma
    Combined small cell carcinoma (with areas of squamous or glandular differentiation)
Adenocarcinoma
    Variant: bronchioloalveolar carcinoma
Large cell carcinoma[c]
Adenosquamous carcinoma

[a]Basaloid tumors may be regarded as a distinct subtype of non–small cell carcinoma.
[b]Presence of spindle cell tumor may be seen.
[c]Tumors may be of a giant cell or clear cell variety but this does not alter the diagnosis.
Modified from Moori WJ. Common lung cancers. *In* Hasleton PS (ed): Spencer's Pathology of the Lung. 5th Ed. New York: McGraw-Hill, 1996, p. 1009. With permission.

(1991) proposed a new category of these tumors, the large cell neuroendocrine tumors. The latter author and colleagues (1998a,b) have further defined the criteria for the classification of the large cell neuroendocrine tumors.

Non–Small Cell Tumors

Squamous Cell Carcinoma

Gross Features

The squamous cell tumors constitute approximately 20 to 35% of all lung carcinomas. In the early period of the last half of the twentieth century, squamous cell carcinoma was the most common cell type of lung cancer throughout the world, but in the United States and Japan, this cell type is now less common than adenocarcinomas of the lung. However, squamous cell tumors remain the most common lung cancer in Europe and most other countries of the world. The cause of

Table 95-6. Comparison of Classifications of Neuroendocrine Tumors of the Lung

World Health Organization (1982)	Gould et al. (1983)	Travis et al. (1998a)
Carcinoid	Carcinoid	Carcinoid
Atypical carcinoid	Well-differentiated neuroendocrine	Atypical carcinoid
	Neuroendocrine carcinoma of intermediate cell type	Large cell neuro-endocrine carcinoma
Small cell carcinoma, oat cell type	Neuroendocrine carcinoma of small cell type	Small cell neuro-endocrine carcinoma
Intermediate cell type		
Combined type		

the changing incidence in the United States and Japan is obscure but is most likely the change in smoking habits and the demographics of smoking in these two countries.

The squamous cell carcinomas may occur in either the central or peripheral areas of the lung, although two-thirds are found in the central area. Squamous cell tumors grow relatively slowly and tend to metastasize late. The centrally located lesions tend to extend both intrabronchially as well as peribronchially, so frequently, the lumen is constricted by extrinsic pressure but has a grossly normal appearing mucosal pattern. The obstructing tumors are often associated with obstructive pneumonitis, distal pulmonary collapse, and consolidation. The peripherally located squamous cell tumors as they enlarge tend to undergo central necrosis with resultant cavitation. This may occur in 10 to 20% of the peripheral lesions. Small, superficial squamous cell tumors of the bronchial mucosa, although not a separate variety, deserve mention. These tumors are radiographically occult and may occur in both the larger main stem and lobar bronchi as well as in the more distal divisions of the bronchial tree. The more proximal lesions may be identified by bronchoscopic examination as abnormal areas in the otherwise normal-appearing bronchial mucosa. Some of these tumors are only carcinoma in situ, but many are invasive lesions, most of which do not extend beyond the bronchial wall. The length, the gross area of involvement, and the depth of extension determine whether these are aggressive lesions (see Lymphatic Metastasis, later in this chapter).

Microscopic Features

The well-differentiated squamous cell tumors have polygonal or prickle-type cells, stratification, and intercellular bridge formation (Fig. 95-2). Individual cells keratinize or tend to form epithelial pearls or both; the nuclei may be uniform, pleomorphic, or giant. The moderately differentiated

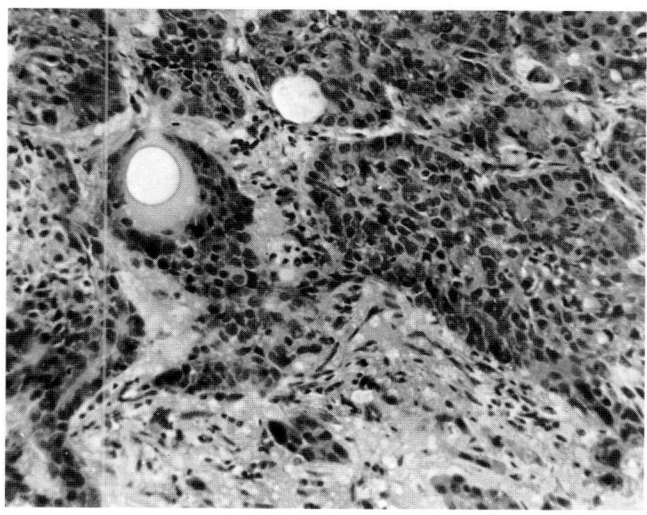

Fig. 95-2. Photomicrograph of squamous cell carcinoma of the lung.

tumors have polygonal or prickle-type cells, stratification, intercellular bridge formation, and some keratinization. Rarely, squamous cells can take on a spindle shape, which makes the tumor look sarcomatous histologically. The poorly differentiated tumors are composed predominantly of anaplastic cells, with little but still distinct evidence of intercellular bridge formation or individual cell keratinization, or both. A tumor without these latter features should not be placed in this category. Some squamous cell carcinomas may be composed of small cells resembling basal cells. These tumors may be confused with small cell carcinoma, but these tumors have been placed in a separate non–small cell category called *basaloid cancers* by Brambilla and associates (1992). These tumors are described in Chapter 112.

Electron Microscopic Features

Tumor cells frequently have degenerated and bizarre mitochondria and have more free ribosomes, fewer profiles of granular endoplasmic reticulum, and more lipid than normal cells. The Golgi apparatus is usually poorly developed. Squamous cell carcinomas are composed mainly of polygonal cells with distinct cell membranes and numerous desmosomes between adjacent cells. Tonofilaments, keratohyalin granules, and some keratin pearls are dominant features. No neuroendocrine granules as a rule or mucin are seen.

Immunohistochemical Features

Squamous cell carcinomas are readily stained by polyclonal antibodies to epidermal-type cytokeratin, as noted by Blobel (1984) and Gould (1992) and their associates. Schaafsma and Ramaekers (1994) identified that keratins 4, 8, 13, 14, 15, 16, 17, and 18 of Moll's (1982) catalog are present. Many of these keratins are found in other lung tumors, but keratin 14 is found in all squamous cell tumors but not in pulmonary adenocarcinomas or in any of the neuroendocrine tumors. L1 antigen is also strongly associated with a squamous phenotype. Also, these tumor cells are stained with antibodies to epithelial membrane antigen, carcinoembryonic antigen (CEA), and desmosomal plaque proteins, but these are not unique to squamous cell differentiations. Berendsen and colleagues (1989) observed that neuroendocrine differentiation status could be identified by monoclonal antibody–based immunohistologic procedures in a small percentage of squamous cell carcinoma cells.

Exophytic Endobronchial Carcinoma

Sherwin (1992) and Dulmet-Brender (1986) and their coworkers described exophytic endobronchial squamous carcinoma as an uncommon type of squamous lung cancer with a papillomatous, polypoid, or verrucous growth pattern. This tumor has a gray-white granular to papillary appearance. It tends to fill and obstruct the bronchus. Microscopically, these tumors have a verrucous, papillary, or poly-poid growth pattern with an underlying fibrovascular stalk. The epithelial cells are malignant squamous cells with intercellular junctions (prickle cells) and possible keratinization. A lymphoplasmacytic reaction may be present in the underlying connective tissue. The squamous cells usually show superficial, focal invasion into the bronchial wall, but some may be only in situ carcinoma. The electron microscopic and immunohistochemical findings in these tumors are similar to those of the typical squamous cell carcinomas.

Spindle Cell Variant

Although the spindle cell variant, a rare tumor, is listed by the World Health Organization (1981) under the squamous cell category, the true nature of the lesion—sarcomatous or epithelioid—is often in doubt. The use of the various immunohistochemical staining techniques for epidermal-type cytokeratin, epithelial membrane antigen, and desmosomal proteins may be helpful in this regard. The prognosis of the epithelial variant is believed to be better than that of the sarcomatous spindle cell lesion (see Chapter 112).

Adenocarcinoma

Gross Features

Adenocarcinomas account for approximately 30 to 50% of all carcinomas of the lung. Vincent and associates in 1977 reported an increasing incidence of adenocarcinoma; they identified more adenocarcinomas than squamous cell tumors in 1682 lung tumors studied. This observation was confirmed by numerous investigators, including Yesner and Carter (1982), who reported that in an all male population of veterans in a two-decade period, a 7% increase in adenocarcinomas of the lung and an associated decrease of 4% in squamous cell tumors and a 3% decrease in small cell carcinomas occurred. Amemiya and Oho (1982) noted a similar preponderance of adenocarcinoma in the Japanese.

The usual glandular variety of adenocarcinoma arises in the peripheral area of the lung, although one-fourth or even more may occur in the central area. Many of the tumors are thought to arise in areas of chronic interstitial fibrosis and in conjunction with lung scars—the so-called scar carcinoma. The carcinoma is presumed to arise from or in the scar. The studies of Barsky (1986) and Madri (1984) and their coworkers, however, suggest that the scars are secondary to the desmoplastic properties of the carcinoma, and in most cases these tumors do not represent an adenocarcinoma arising in a scar. Clinically, these so-called scar carcinomas behave as typical adenocarcinomas.

The growth rate of the adenocarcinomas is intermediate between that of the squamous cell and the undifferentiated small cell types. The peripheral tumors may become large. In contrast to the peripheral squamous cell tumors, necrosis with cavitation is rarely observed. These tumors tend to spread early by way of the vascular system. Lymphatic

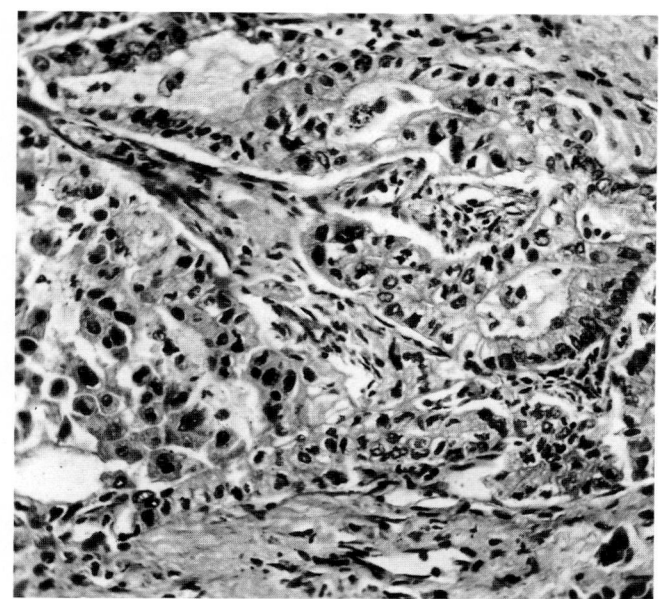

Fig. 95-3. Photomicrograph of adenocarcinoma of the lung.

metastases are also common early in the course of the disease, and small lesions appear to have a greater propensity to do so than similarly sized squamous cell tumors. Sagawa and associates (1990) reported an incidence of mediastinal node metastasis of 20% in patients with adenocarcinoma 3 cm or smaller in size as compared with a 10% incidence in small squamous cell lesions.

Microscopic Features

The well-differentiated tumors are composed of cuboidal to columnar epithelial cells with fairly uniform round nuclei, have adequate pink or vacuolated cytoplasm, are arranged in distinct acinar or glandular patterns, and are supported by a fibrous stroma. The cells may show papillary intraluminal growth and may contain mucicarmine-positive vacuoles or secretions. The moderately differentiated tumors are composed of nests, cords, or isolated cells, occasionally arranged in an acinar or glandular pattern (Fig. 95-3). The cytoplasm is supported by a fibrous or desmoplastic stroma, and the cells may contain mucicarmine-positive vacuoles or secretions. The poorly differentiated tumors are composed predominantly of anaplastic cells of variable size and shape, with minimal but distinct evidence of acinar formation. Mucicarmine-positive vacuoles may be present. It has been suggested that tumors without distinct acinar formation should not be placed in the category of adenocarcinomas.

The current classification of the World Health Organization lists four subtypes of adenocarcinoma: acinar adenocarcinoma, papillary adenocarcinoma, bronchioloalveolar carcinoma, and solid carcinoma with mucus formation. The degree of differentiation may vary in each subgroup.

Sørensen and Olsen (1989), Sørensen and Badsberg (1990), and Sørensen and colleagues (1988, 1989) noted prognostic implications of this histologic subtyping. Not all investigators agree that the aforementioned subtypes are of necessary importance. Moori (1996) believes that only the bronchioloalveolar variant needs to be considered separately among the four subtypes. Edwards (1987) has even suggested from a review of 106 cases that the adenocarcinomas should simply be classified into parenchymal adenocarcinomas, bronchial adenocarcinomas, and adenocarcinomas of uncertain origin, representing 67, 13, and 20%, respectively, of the total cases in his study.

Electron Microscopic Features

Adenocarcinomas are composed of cuboidal or columnar cells. Aggregates of chromatin are dispersed inside the nuclei. Well-developed apparatuses are often missing or poorly formed in many of the tumor cells. Intracellular or intercellular lumina are present. Mucin production is evident, and Clara cell or type II pneumocyte differentiation may be identified. The tumor cells show the presence of *straight microvilli*. Desmosomes and terminal bars may be identified.

Immunohistochemical Features

According to Lee and associates (1985, 1987) and summarized by Gould and Warren (1989), adenocarcinomas of the lung are readily immunostained with monoclonal antibodies that recognize either a membrane-associated glycoprotein molecule or the specific sugar sequence found in lacto-N-fucopentose III. Of particular interest is that these reactions, according to Gould and Warren (1995), are either absent or weakly expressed in diffuse mesotheliomas and thus may be a differentiating feature when, histologically, a mesothelioma may present as a glandular and papillary structure. Adenocarcinomas also immunostain for epithelial keratins CK7, 8, 18, and 19. According to van de Molengraft and associates (1993), CK7 antibody (OV-TL 12/30) is a marker for glandular differentiation in lung cancer. CK14, found in all squamous cell tumors, is not present. Asada and colleagues (1993) has noted further that in most adenocarcinomas (26 of 29 tumors in his study), dipeptidyl aminopeptidase IV activity is expressed. Other markers may be identified, including CEA, found in approximately 75% of adenocarcinomas, and Leu M1, Ber-Ep4, β 72.3, and vimentin, found in a minority of tumors. Surfactant apoproteins (PE-10 immunoreactivity or Clara cell protein) may be demonstrated in approximately 50% of tumors according to Mizutani and colleagues (1988). The latter investigators did not identify PE-10 activity by pulmonary tumors of other cell types; however, Nicholson and associates (1995) have described the presence of PE-10 reactivity in both small cell carcinomas and atypical carcinoids. Lastly, occasional neuroendocrine differentiation features can be identified by monoclonal antibody–staining techniques.

Bronchioloalveolar Carcinoma

Bronchioloalveolar carcinoma represents highly differentiated adenocarcinoma, but many pathologists have considered it a separate and distinct tumor. Nonetheless Moori (1996), as previously noted, believes these tumors represent a unique subset of adenocarcinoma. These tumors constitute 1.5 to 7.0% of all bronchial carcinomas, with an average incidence of 2.5%. However, Barsky and colleagues (1994a) have noted an increasing incidence of these tumors; in 1955 the bronchioloalveolar carcinomas accounted for only 5% of the resected lung cancer specimens, whereas in 1990 these tumors made up 25% of the resected lung cancers. Grossly, these tumors may occur in one of three forms: solitary, multinodular, and diffuse or pneumonic type. The first is the most common and accounts for slightly less than one-half to almost two-thirds of the tumors of this subclassification. In the series reported by Hill (1984), the percentage of a solitary mass or nodule was 43%, and in the series reported by Harpole (1988) and Daly (1991) and their colleagues, the percentages were 59 and 69%, respectively. Approximately 66% of the solitary tumors in Daly and associates (1991) series were 3 cm or less in diameter. Only a small number of these, however, fit the criterion of a solitary pulmonary nodule (i.e., a well-demarcated lesion less than 3 cm in diameter completely surrounded by pulmonary parenchyma). In the aforementioned series of 184 bronchioloalveolar carcinomas, only an 11.2% incidence of "solitary pulmonary nodules" was recorded. The vast majority of the small lesions were ill-defined infiltrates. The larger diffuse tumors may appear as a mass, an infiltrate, or even consolidation of an entire lobe. The multinodular, unilateral, or bilateral lesions make up just less than 10% of the total. Direct extension beyond the lung is uncommon and lymph node metastasis is likewise infrequent. Daly and associates (1991) recorded only a 7.5% incidence of lymph node metastasis in tumors of this type.

Singh and associates (1981) described the criteria for the diagnosis of bronchioloalveolar carcinoma as follows: 1) absence of primary adenocarcinoma elsewhere in the body, 2) absence of a central bronchial adenocarcinoma, 3) a peripheral location, 4) growth using the alveolar septa as supporting structures (lepidic growth), and 5) a characteristic histologic appearance different from other lung tumors.

Microscopically, the alveolar spaces are lined by malignant cuboidal or nonciliated columnar epithelium in layers or in papillary formation (Fig. 95-4). The alveolar spaces may be filled, or even distended, with this proliferating epithelium. Occasionally, single cells or clusters containing large multinucleated giant cells may appear lying free. The nuclei are hypochromatic, but mitoses are not common. The cytoplasm is acidophilic and abundant, or the cells may be mucous cells with extensive amounts of mucus filling the alveolar spaces. The lung architecture is most often preserved, although a few show diffuse malignant invasion. Scar formation is seen in approximately one-half of the tumors.

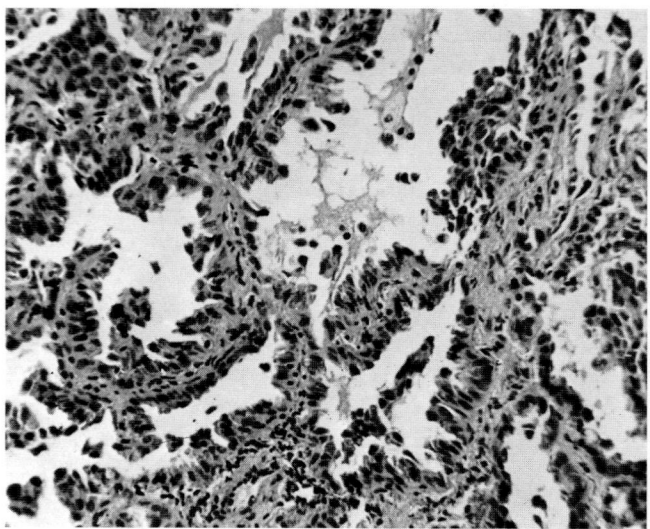

Fig. 95-4. Photomicrograph of bronchioloalveolar cell carcinoma.

Also, in approximately one-half of tumors, mucin-producing cells are observed as the dominant cell type. Clayton (1986) initially separated bronchioloalveolar carcinomas into two cell types: mucinous and nonmucinous (i.e., Clara cells and type II pneumocytes). Aerogenous spread of the tumor within the lung is believed to be important. Clayton (1988) subsequently has divided the bronchioloalveolar carcinomas into three subgroups. Histologically, the first group is those tumors composed of high columnar, mucin-producing cells with little nuclear atypia; in Clayton's series this group made up approximately one-fourth of all bronchioloalveolar tumors. The second subgroup is made up of tumors composed of cuboidal or low columnar cells with a high degree of atypia and producing little or no mucin; psammoma bodies are frequently present. The third subgroup is formed by those tumors that have a central area of necrosis and that are often termed *sclerosing bronchioloalveolar tumors*. Barsky and associates (1994a) reported the incidences of the three subtypes as nonmucinous in 48%, mucinous in 42%, and sclerotic in 10%, respectively. Of possible prognostic significance was that areas of dedifferentiation of this tumor into solid areas of moderately or poorly differentiated adenocarcinoma were seen in 10, 27, and 42% of the nonmucinous, mucinous, and sclerotic types, respectively.

Clayton (1986) had earlier shown by electron microscopy that the bronchioloalveolar carcinomas may be composed of Clara type cells, type II-granular pneumocytes, or mucous cells. Barsky and colleagues (1994b) also identified these three phenotypes in the bronchioloalveolar tumors and have suggested that these findings, as well as the multifocality of these cancers, are evidence of a multiclonal origin of these tumors. This conclusion was supported to some extent by the study of *p53* mutations in primary and secondary lung cancers by Mitsudomi and associates (1997). However, Holst and coworkers (1998), in a study of eight multifocal cases of bronchioloalveolar carcinoma by using topographic genotyping, used to define the spectrum of point mutational changes in K-ras-2 and *p53* oncogenes, showed that, although no commonality existed between the two gene mutations, the primary tumor and the satellite and intrathoracic metastases showed the same point mutations of either oncogene when present. These authors concluded that their findings support a monoclonal origin of multifocal bronchioloalveolar carcinoma; the multifocal disease being the result of intra-alveolar, lymphatic, and aerosol spread.

Immunohistochemical studies by Lee and colleagues (1987) have shown that antibodies used to detect exocrine features that depend on sugar or glycolipid epitopes immunostain alveolar carcinomas regardless of mucin production. These tumor cells also immunostain for high- and low-molecular-weight keratin, epithelial membrane antigen, CEA, and Leu M1.

Undifferentiated Large Cell Carcinoma

Gross Features

Because of the lack of uniformity in the criteria for the histologic diagnosis of these lesions, their actual incidence is unknown, but it probably is between the 4.5% recorded by Shinton (1963) and the 15.0% recorded by Yesner and associates (1965). These tumors may occur in either the central or the peripheral zone, although the latter site is somewhat more common. They spread earlier and have a relatively poorer prognosis than that associated with the more differentiated non–small cell types. The peripherally located tumors may cavitate, but the incidence is less than that seen in peripheral squamous cell tumors (6% versus 15 to 20%, respectively).

Microscopic Features

These heterogeneous tumors, which cannot be classified readily either as squamous cell carcinomas or as adenocarcinomas, are considered anaplastic tumors that show no apparent evidence of squamous or glandular differentiation (Fig. 95-5). Tumors composed of stratifying cells without evidence of intercellular bridge formation or keratin production are included in this group. Individual cells have enlarged, irregular vesicular or hyperchromatic nuclei that may have prominent nucleoli. The cells have abundant cytoplasm and may show a high mitotic rate.

Electron Microscopic and Immunohistochemical Features

Undifferentiated large cell carcinomas show marked variation in cell shape. Cell membranes are often indistinct. Large nuclei with abundant cytoplasm and numerous organelles are present. Occasionally, tonofilaments are identified, but no distinctive features are present to permit categoric determination of cell type. Warren and associates

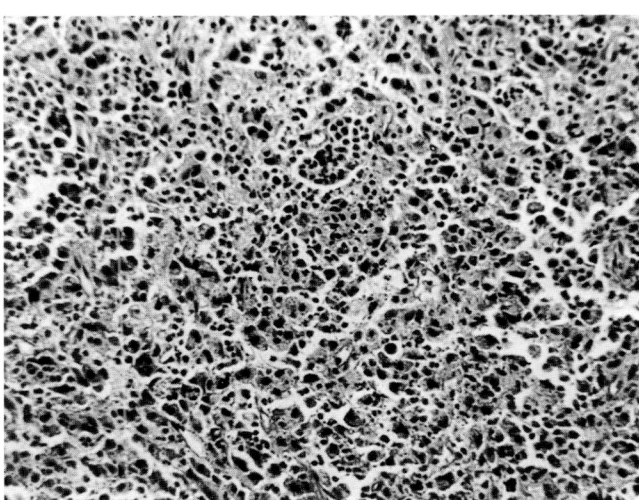

Fig. 95-5. Photomicrograph of undifferentiated large cell carcinoma of the lung.

(1985) noted that dense-core granules and predominantly neuroendocrine differentiation appear in 40% of the so-called large cell tumors; such tumors are now classified as large cell neuroendocrine carcinomas.

Piehl and associates (1988) suggested that approximately 50% of undifferentiated large cell carcinomas could be regarded as poorly differentiated adenocarcinomas given their expression of exocrine phenotype antigens. Also, Gould and colleagues (1992) reported that most of these large cell undifferentiated carcinomas express cytokeratin polypeptides of the simple epithelial type shown by adenocarcinomas and neuroendocrine neoplasms, and only a small number display cytokeratin of the epidermal type that is characteristic of squamous cell carcinoma.

Giant Cell Tumors

The so-called giant cell tumor is considered a variety of the undifferentiated large cell carcinoma. A varying combination of cell types may occur in this lesion: pleomorphic, anaplastic-multinucleated cells, and spindle cells. The clinical course of these lesions is rapidly fatal. Fortunately, this variety is uncommon and constitutes less than 1% of all lung tumors.

Clear Cell Carcinoma

Clear cell carcinoma is considered a subtype of large cell anaplastic lung cancer. Histologically, these tumors are composed of malignant cells in nests, sheets, or clusters with large vesicular nuclei and abundant clear cytoplasm, which may or may not contain glycogen. Edwards and Carlyle (1985) reviewed six cases of clear cell lung carcinoma. On further analysis of the tissue by both light and electron microscopy, they found glandular differentiation in three cases and squamous differentiation in two. They concluded

Table 95-7. Clear Cell Tumors of the Lung

Benign clear cell tumor (sugar tumor)
Clear cell acinic cell carcinoma
Clear cell large cell anaplastic carcinoma
Clear cell change in squamous cell carcinoma or adenocarcinoma
Clear cell carcinoid tumor
Metastatic renal cell carcinoma
Tumors showing focal clear cell change
Granular cell tumor
Bronchioloalveolar carcinoma
Oncocytoma
Mucoepidermoid carcinoma
Various miscellaneous primary and metastatic tumors

From Leong AS-Y, Meredith DJ: Clear cell tumors of the lung. *In* Pathology of Lung Tumors. New York: Churchill Livingstone, 1998, p. 172. With permission.

that clear cell carcinoma should not be considered a separate entity. Katzenstein and colleagues (1980) reviewed 348 cases of lung cancer and found 15 tumors with clear cells. Ten of these tumors showed foci of epidermoid differentiation and four had glandular differentiation. Only one lesion qualified as a true clear cell carcinoma. In summary, these two reports question the validity of having a separate category of clear cell anaplastic carcinoma, given that these tumors really appear to be poorly differentiated epidermoid carcinomas or adenocarcinomas. Even when one is attempting to classify a lesion as a clear cell carcinoma, other pathologic diagnostic possibilities must be considered (Table 95-7). Gaffey and coworkers (1998) note that immunohistochemical and electron microscopic features are necessary to establish the proper diagnosis. The features of the benign clear cell tumor (sugar tumor) are discussed in detail in Chapter 111, especially its uniqueness in its reactivity to HMB45, a melanogenesis-related marker.

Adenosquamous Carcinoma

Adenosquamous carcinomas are defined as tumors composed of an admixture of squamous cell carcinoma and adenocarcinoma. At least 5% of the tumor should be composed of the minority cell type according to the criterion of Takamori (1991) and Shimizu (1996) and their coworkers; although the World Health Organization (1982) gives no reference to the actual ratio. The Japan Lung Cancer Society (1987) stated that at least 20% of the tumor should be formed by the less dominant variety; this group also notes that the tumors should be categorized as 20 to 40%, 40 to 60%, and 60 to 80% of either one of the cell types. The overall incidence of adenosquamous carcinoma is between 0.4 and 4.0%; in the surgical series reported by of Takamori (1991) and Shimizu (1996) and their associates, the incidence was 2.6% and 3.4%, respectively. These tumors are more often peripheral rather than central in location. Although Ishida and coworkers (1992) reported an almost equal occurrence in men and women, Shimizu and associates (1996), in a much

larger series (44 patients versus 11 patients), reported a marked preponderance of men (35:9). Three-fourths of these tumors were greater than 3 cm in size with a range of 1.5 to 6.0 cm. Microscopically, either component may be well, moderately, or poorly differentiated. The squamous cell component was the dominant tumor in the majority of cases in Shimizu and associates' (1996) report.

Ichinose and associates (1993) reported that the DNA ploidy patterns of both components showed, despite the different phenotypes, that in 67% of the specimens examined, similar biological characteristics were present. These findings support the theory of Steele and Nettesheim (1981) that these tumors arise from instability of differentiation. Immunohistochemically, the pan keratin stained both the squamous and glandular components. The high-molecular-weight keratin stained mostly the squamous component and not the glandular one. The low-molecular-weight keratin stained the glandular component slightly more often than the squamous component, but in most cases, it did not stain either component to any great extent. The CEA and epithelial membrane antigen stained both elements of most tumors with relatively high frequency.

Blood vessel invasion is common, and lymph node metastasis occurs in over 50% of patients. The latter was present in 61% of the specimens in Takamori and associates' (1991) series. The incidence of lymphatic metastasis appears to be greater in patients with a higher percentage of adenocarcinoma present in the tumor. The cell type of the metastatic disease can vary, as shown in Table 95-8. Overall, the prognosis is poorer than that of either a squamous cell carcinoma or adenocarcinoma of a similar stage. Likewise, a greater number of patients have a higher stage of disease when initially identified. The studies of the aforementioned authors, as well as the observations of Fitzgibbons and Kern (1985) and Naunheim and colleagues (1987), support this conclusion, although it should be noted that Sridhar and associates (1990) found that no significant difference existed in the survival rates of patients with adenosquamous carcinomas and those patients with other non–small cell cancers.

Table 95-8. Comparison of Histologic Types Between the Primary Adenosquamous Lesions of the Lung and Lymph Node Metastasis

Primary Lesion	No. of Cases	Lymph Node Metastasis			Lymph Node Metastasis Absent
		Ad	Ad-Sq	Sq	
Ad > Sq	8	3	2	1	2
Ad = Sq	5	4	0	0	1
Ad < Sq	29	3	9	2	15
	42	10	11	3	18

Ad, adenocarcinoma; Ad-Sq, adenosquamous carcinoma; Sq, squamous cell carcinoma.
From Shimizu J, et al: A clinicopathologic study of resected cases of adenosquamous carcinoma of the lung. Chest *109*:989, 1996. With permission.

Small Cell Lung Cancers

Small cell lung cancers are aggressive, highly malignant lesions. Only a few patients with these tumors are considered surgical candidates. The origin of these lesions, as previously noted, is debated and as yet unsettled. Yesner (1977, 1986) believes these tumors arise from the same stem cells that give rise to the NSCLCs, whereas other authors think they arise from basally located neuroendocrine cells (endodermal Kulchitsky's cells) or their precursors.

The cells of these tumors have the features of neuroendocrine cells, including common expression of amine precursor uptake and decarboxylation cell properties. Many investigators including Gould and colleagues (1983a,b), Travis (1994), and Gould and Warren (1995), categorize these tumors as one of the neuroendocrine tumors of the lung. However, in this chapter the SCLCs are considered separately from the other tumors in this category. According to Moori (1996) and others, the World Health Organization classification is not appropriate because both the typical oat cell tumors and the intermediate small cell tumors behave essentially in a similar manner clinically. Hirsch and colleagues (1988) and, more recently, Moori (1996) have suggested that their reported pathologic differences may only be artifacts caused by variations in processing of these tumors for histologic examination. As shown in Table 95-9, Moori (1996) alternatively has classified these tumors as 1) pure small cell carcinoma, 2) mixed small cell–large cell carcinoma, and 3) combined small cell carcinoma with areas of squamous or glandular differentiation. Each of these types make up approximately 90%, 4 to 6%, and 6 to 4%, respectively.

Gross Features

The various types of small cell tumors constitute approximately 15 to 35% of all bronchial carcinomas. Approximately four-fifths of these arise in the central area, and the remainder arise in the peripheral area of the lung. The mucosa overlying the tumor in the bronchus is frequently uninvolved, although the normal furrowing of the mucosa may be obliterated. Tumors arising in either region involve the hilar and mediastinal lymph nodes early. Central necrosis with cavitation within the tumor or changes in the parenchyma of the lung distal to the tumor occur less frequently than do such changes in squamous cell carcinomas.

Table 95-9. Classification of Small Cell Lung Carcinoma

Pure small cell carcinoma
Mixed small cell–large cell carcinoma
Combined small cell carcinoma admixed with either squamous cell or adenocarcinoma

Adapted from Hirsch FR, et al: Histopathologic classification of small cell lung cancer. Changing concepts and terminology. Cancer 62:973, 1988.

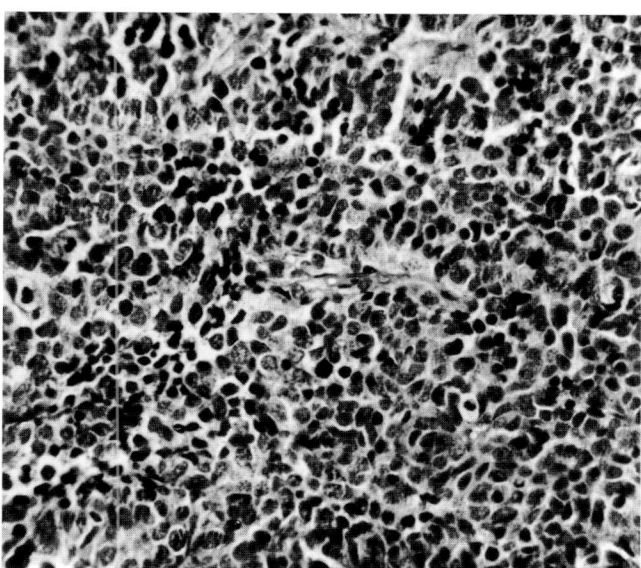

Fig. 95-6. Photomicrograph of undifferentiated small cell carcinoma of the lung.

Microscopic Features

Pure Small Cell Carcinomas

The histologic features may be either those of the typical or intermediate cell type. The first type is characterized by clusters, nests, or sheets of small, round, oval, or spindle-shaped cells with small, dark, round nuclei, with delicate chromatin and without prominent nucleoli (Fig. 95-6). Cytoplasm is scanty and the cells are supported by a vascular fibrous stroma. The second type, the intermediate small cell carcinomas, are composed of clusters or sheets of slightly larger size than the typical small cell and are fusiform or polygonal in shape. The cytoplasm, although still scanty, is more distinct. The central nuclei tend to have peripheral aggregations of clumped chromatin material. This form of pure small cell tumor is occasionally misclassified as undifferentiated large cell carcinoma.

Mixed Small Cell–Large Cell Carcinomas

Histologically, mixed small cell–large cell tumors present varying combinations of areas of pure small cells, often of the fusiform or polygonal type, and large cells in an organized, trabecular, or palisading pattern. The latter cells have a low nuclear cytoplasmic ratio, and mitotic figures are frequently seen.

Combined Small Cell Carcinoma Admixed with Either Squamous Cell Carcinoma or Adenocarcinoma

In these tumors, areas of either typical squamous cell carcinoma or adenocarcinoma are readily identified within the small cell carcinoma. Adelstein and colleagues (1986) noted that 10% of their patients with SCLC had another major type of NSCLC present. Baker (1987) and Shepherd (1989) and their associates, as well as others, have observed that the incidence of the presence of areas of non–small cell carcinoma in small cell tumors is increased following chemotherapy. In fact, at times only non–small cell cancer cells can be identified in a tumor that was a pure small cell cancer on the original biopsy specimen.

Electron Microscopic Features

Undifferentiated small cell carcinoma reveals cellular pleomorphism, but the shape of the cell is usually round to ovoid in transection. Some cells adjacent to the basement membrane possess *pseudopodlike* processes extending between adjacent cells. Cell membranes are often indistinct. The nuclei are large, often with eccentric nucleoli, and are surrounded by a narrow zone of cytoplasm. Bensch and coworkers (1968) identified neurosecretory granules in the undifferentiated small cell tumors, which many authors, including Warren and associates (1985), subsequently have confirmed. According to Moori and colleagues (1986), the neuroendocrine granules can almost always be found in the cells of the pure small cell tumors as well as in the cells of the mixed small cell–large cell tumors.

Biological Behavior

The small cell tumors have been studied extensively in cell cultures, and such cultures can be established in 75% of small cell cancers. The cultures can be separated into two cell lines: the classic cell line and the variant lines. The former is characterized by tight spherical aggregates and has a doubling time of 50 hours and low colony-forming efficiency, whereas the latter grows in looser aggregates of floating cell lines and has a faster doubling time and a greater colony-forming efficiency. The classic line corresponds to the pure small cell carcinoma, expresses the usual production of the various biological substances, and contains many dense granules. The variant lines have few granules, produce fewer biologically active substances, such as adrenocorticotropic hormone, and resemble the combined cell types clinically. The production of peptides is characteristic of small cell carcinoma. Classic small cell lines produce L-dopa decarboxylase, adrenocorticotropic hormone, bombesin or its mammalian analogue GRP, neuron-specific enolase, and creatine kinase. The variant lines do not produce L-dopa decarboxylase or bombesin and the level of neuron-specific enolase is usually significantly lower.

Immunohistochemical Features

The SCLC cells react positively to neuron-specific enolase, creatine kinase, synaptophysin, chromogranin, and occasionally to serotonin. Positivity is often shown to EGF and to cytokeratins 8 and 18 of Moll's catalog.

Large Cell Neuroendocrine Carcinomas

Travis and coworkers (1991) described the identification of a fourth subset of neuroendocrine tumors of the lung: the large cell neuroendocrine carcinoma.

Histologic Features

Microscopically, the cells of these tumors have an organoid, trabecular, or palisading pattern. The tumor cells are large with a low nuclear cytoplasmic ratio and eosinophilic cytoplasm. Saldiva and associates (1997) describe the nuclei as showing peripheral clumping of chromatin and a prominent nucleolus. Halseton (1996) reported similar findings, but Travis (1998a,b) has reported the nucleoli to often be absent or faint at best. Mitotic activity is high, and often extensive necrosis is present. Travis and associates (1998a) have used these two features to aid in the differentiation of the large cell tumors from the atypical carcinoids (Table 95-10). Lastly, foci of adenomatous or squamous differentiation may be present.

Electron Microscopic and Immunohistochemical Features

Travis and colleagues (1991) described the electron microscopic and immunohistochemical features of these tumors. Electron microscopy revealed that these tumor cells contain neurosecretory granules and occasionally a suggestion of granular differentiation or intercellular junctions suggestive of squamous differentiation. Immunohistochemically, these tumor cells stained for neuron-specific enolase, CEA, and keratin and stain variably for chromogranin, Leu 7, synaptophysin, and adrenocorticotropic hormone. Wick and associates (1992) have confirmed these findings.

Clinical Features

The clinical course, response to treatment, and prognosis of large cell neuroendocrine tumors of the lung is yet to be determined. Only small numbers of cases have been

Table 95-10. Modified Diagnostic Criteria for Neuroendocrine Lung Tumors

Tumor	Mitotic Activity	Necrosis
Typical carcinoid	<2 per 10 HPF	Absent
Atypical carcinoid	>2 <10 per 10 HPF	Punctate
Large cell neuroendocrine	>11 per 10 HPF[a]	Extensive
Small cell neuroendocrine	>11 per 10 HPF[b]	Extensive

HPF, high power field.
[a]Median number of 70 per 10 HPF.
[b]Median number of 80 per 10 HPF.
Adapted from data from Travis WD, et al: Survival analysis of 200 pulmonary neuroendocrine tumors with classification of criteria for atypical carcinoid and its separation from typical carcinoids. Am J Surg Pathol 22:934, 1998.

reported, but the majority view suggests that these patients on the whole respond poorly to treatment and have a poor prognosis. The report of Dresler and colleagues (1997) on 40 cases cites a 13% 5-year survival despite early-stage disease in many patients that supports the aforementioned statements; however, this latter report has been criticized by Travis and associates (1998a) because they believe the diagnostic criteria were not strict enough to ensure a true representation of this tumor's true clinical behavior. Obviously, additional studies are necessary.

METASTASIS OF BRONCHIAL CARCINOMA

Carcinoma of the lung has three modes of spread. Its dissemination occurs by direct extension and by lymphatic and hematogenous metastases.

Direct Extension

A lung tumor may extend directly into the adjacent pulmonary parenchyma, across the fissure, along the bronchus of origin, and also into adjacent structures in the thorax. Commonly, tumors situated in the central area extend directly along the bronchus.

Cotton (1959) studied this bronchial extension and noted five important factors in this type of spread, as follows: 1) direct extension continuous with the tumor in the bronchial wall and the adjacent peribronchial tissues; 2) direct extension into bronchi other than the bronchus of origin, particularly by tumors arising close to a segmental or a major lobar bronchial orifice; 3) invasion of the submucosal lymphatics in the bronchial wall; 4) extension of the tumor proximally along the lumen of the bronchus by papillary or polypoid process without further attachment to the bronchial wall; and 5) the presence of epithelial metaplasia, particularly if the epithelial change shows atypical proliferative features. Cotton (1959) found spread into the bronchial wall beyond the palpable mass occurred in 12% of patients with lung cancer, and the maximum distance of the spread was three-fourths of an inch (1.9 cm). This extent of spread essentially agrees with findings reported by Griess and colleagues (1945), who found that the proximal extension of tumor in the bronchial wall could be removed satisfactorily if the line of resection included 1.5 cm of grossly normal bronchus. Polypoid extension of the tumor into the lumen of the bronchus without bronchial wall involvement was observed as far as 2.5 to 3.2 cm. Submucosal lymphatic spread was noted in only 6% of the tumors, and these specimens had extensive lymph node involvement. Cotton (1959) found epithelial metaplasia beyond the tumor in 31 of 100 specimens, but it was extensive in only eight specimens. In these eight, it extended as far as 5 cm. All the aforementioned factors are important considerations in the surgical treatment of carcinoma of the lung.

Most important, however, is that direct extension occurs into adjacent structures within the thorax. The sites commonly involved are the pleura, pulmonary vessels, chest wall, superior sulcus area and its adjacent neurogenic and bony structures, diaphragm, pericardium, and heart and great vessels. Although direct extension from the tumor may involve the superior vena cava, contiguous nerves (i.e., the recurrent laryngeal and phrenic nerves), and esophagus, these structures more frequently are invaded by secondary extension from metastatic disease within the mediastinal lymph nodes.

Lymphatic Metastasis

Lymphatic metastasis is common in patients with carcinoma of the lung. Ochsner and DeBakey (1942) reported regional node metastases in 72.2% of 3047 lung cancer patients studied. Cell type, as noted, affects the rate of incidence; it occurs in undifferentiated small cell carcinoma, undifferentiated large cell carcinoma, adenocarcinoma, and squamous cell carcinoma, in the order of decreasing frequency. According to Martini and Ginsberg (1990), approximately one-half of patients with NSCLC have mediastinal lymph node involvement at the time of presentation; this, of course, is not reflected in the surgical series reported in the literature.

In many patients, the initial lymphatic metastases are either to the lobar or hilar nodes of the ipsilateral lung but in some, as is noted, the mediastinal lymph nodes may be the initial site. The sites of potential involvement from each lobe are described in detail in Chapter 6. The most important intrapulmonary area is the lymphatic sump of each lung, as defined by Borrie (1952). With progression of the lymphatic spread of the tumor, the various lymph node groups of the mediastinum become involved. However, lymph node involvement is not systematically progressive from the tumor to the most adjacent node group and then successively to the next higher lymph node level(s). Instead, any given lymph node level (segmental, bronchial, hilar, or mediastinal) associated with the lymphatic drainage pattern of each lobe (described in Chapter 6) may be bypassed in the lymphatic metastasis of the tumor. Lymphatic spread, however, is most often regional (i.e., upper lobe tumors metastasize to the superior mediastinal node levels and the lower lobe tumors metastasize to the inferior lymph node groups). Nonregional metastases do occur (i.e., upper lobe tumors to inferior mediastinal nodes and lower lobe tumors to superior mediastinal nodes). Watanabe (1996) observed that in 182 patients with mediastinal node metastases resected at operation, 77 with a single level of metastasis and 105 with multilevel metastasis, most of the metastases were noted in the regional lymph nodes. The upper lobe lesions primarily involved the upper, superior, mediastinal node levels (levels 4, 3, and 2 on the right and levels 6, 5, 4, 3, and 2 on the left). The lower lobe tumors mostly involved the levels in the inferior mediastinum (7, 8, and 9 on both the right and left). It was also noted that tumors in the right and left lower lobes involved the nonregional superior mediastinal nodes and tumors of the right upper lobe involved the nonregional inferior nodes more frequently than tumors of the left upper lobe involved the nonregional inferior mediastinal nodes. A variable number of patients—approximately 29% of patients who undergo resection of lung tumors with involved mediastinal lymph nodes—have no metastatic involvement of either the hilar or lobar nodes. Such metastatic mediastinal disease is referred to as *skip metastases* by Libshitz (1986), Martini (1983, 1987), and Ishida (1990b) and their associates. The probable pathways of these skip metastases have been described by many of the early investigators of the lymphatic drainage of the lungs, as well as more recently by Riquet and colleagues (1989) (see Chapter 6). Clinically, skip metastases are seen more commonly in patients with peripheral adenocarcinomas located in either upper lobe. Watanabe and associates (1990) reported a higher frequency of metastatic involvement of lower, inferior, mediastinal lymph nodes in patients with right upper lobe lesions than was recorded in most earlier studies. These authors noted that in 11% of the patients with right upper lobe primary lesions, metastasis to the inferior mediastinal nodes (i.e., subcarinal nodes) was the only mediastinal lymph node involvement present. This finding supports the recommendation of the Lung Cancer Study Group reported by Thomas and colleagues (1988) that the subcarinal lymph nodes be evaluated in all patients regardless of the primary site of the tumor.

The spread of tumor from the various lobes of the lung to the tracheobronchial and other mediastinal lymph nodes is usually ipsilateral. Contralateral spread, however, does occur. From the right side, such contralateral spread is unusual; Nohl-Oser (1989) (see Chapter 6) reported this spread in only 4% of patients with right upper lobe tumors and 5% of those with right lower lobe tumors. On the left side, however, patients with upper lobe lesions had a 9.3% incidence of contralateral spread, and those with lower lobe tumors had a 28% incidence. Greschuchna and Maassen (1973) also reported a high incidence of bilateral or contralateral spread (a total of 21% in 540 patients with nodal metastases from bronchial carcinoma routinely investigated by mediastinoscopy). In an update of his continuing experience, Maassen (1985) noted that 30% of his patients had locally advanced stage III disease, and that the incidence of positive mediastinal nodes was 71% in this group. The high incidence of advanced disease obviously influenced the high rate of contralateral spread originally reported. Hata and colleagues (1990) reported contralateral spread from the left lung to the right side of the mediastinum was affected by the cell type of the primary lung tumor. Contralateral spread was more common with adenocarcinoma than with squamous cell carcinoma (Table 95-11) and, in fact, contralateral spread rarely is seen in early clinical stage I squamous cell tumors.

The size of the primary non–small cell carcinoma also affects the incidence of mediastinal lymph node metastasis. Ishida and associates (1990a) reported no positive mediasti-

Table 95-11. Influence of Cell Type and Contralateral Lymph Node Metastasis (Left Lung)

Primary Site	Cell Type (%)		Total
	Squamous Cell	Adenocarcinoma	
Left upper lobe	12	37.5	18.2
Left lower lobe	20	50	28.6
Total	14.3	41.7	21.3

From Hata E, et al. Rationale for extended lymphadenectomy for lung cancer. Theor Surg 5:19, 1990. With permission.

nal nodes in any tumor less than 1 cm in diameter, a 12% incidence in tumors ranging from 1.1 to 2.0 cm, and a 25% incidence of involvement in tumors 2.1 to 3.0 cm in diameter in a series of 221 patients with tumors 3 cm or less in diameter. Sagawa and colleagues (1990) reported similar data in tumors 3 cm or less in size; 8.9 and 24.5%, respectively, for lesions 2 cm or less versus tumors 2.1 to 3.0 cm. The overall incidence of 19% of mediastinal lymph node involvement in patients with T_1 tumors in the two aforementioned series is similar to the 17% incidence reported by Vallieres and Waters (1987). In the latter series, such metastases were most common in patients with large cell carcinomas (33%), less so in patients with adenocarcinoma (17%), and infrequently in patients with squamous cell tumors (10%). Watanabe (1996) reported that in 1053 patients with resected and nonresected lung cancers (875 were peripheral in location and 178 were hilar in location) the incidence of N_1, N_2, and N_3 metastatic disease was 14, 27, and 4%, respectively. The incidence of N_2 disease, as in the aforementioned series, increased as the tumor size increased. Patients with tumors of less than 10 mm had an incidence of less than 2%; when the tumor size was 11 to 20 mm, the incidence was 15%; when the size was 21 to 30 mm, the incidence was 24%; and when the size was greater than 30 mm, more than 30% of the patients had N_2 disease (Fig. 95-7). Comparable data are not

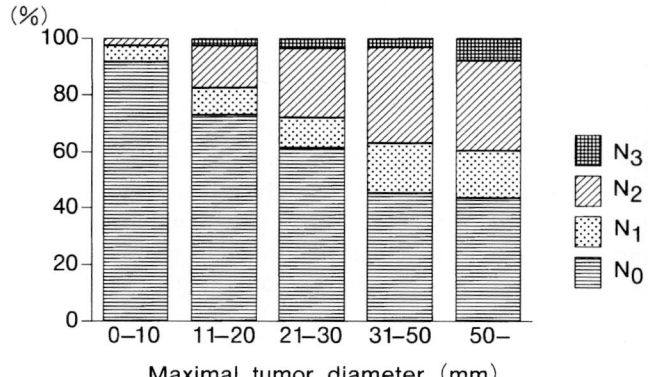

Fig. 95-7. Incidence of lymph node metastasis in relation to tumor diameter. From Watanabe Y: Results of surgery for N2 non–small cell lung cancer. J Thorac Cardiovasc Surg 2:85, 1996. With permission.

available for tumors of larger size, but in most surgical series, such as those of Martini and Flehinger (1987) and Naruke (1978, 1988), Watanabe (1990), and Ishida (1990b) and their colleagues, mediastinal lymph node involvement is three or more times more common with lesions greater than 3 cm in diameter than with smaller primary lesions.

In patients with radiographically occult tumors that are localized only by bronchoscopy, Nagamoto and associates (1989) reported a zero incidence of lymph node metastasis if the tumor was only a carcinoma in situ or if the longitudinal length of an invasive lesion was less than 20 mm. If the length of involvement was greater, as was noted in a total of 25 patients, a 24% incidence of hilar/lobar lymph node invasion was observed, as was a 4% incidence of mediastinal node invasion. In each of these cases, the tumor had extended beyond the bronchial wall.

Lymph nodes beyond the thorax may become involved with metastatic disease. Supraclavicular and, infrequently, other cervical lymph node metastasis occurs in approximately 16% of all lung cancer patients. The incidence of involvement of the scalene (supraclavicular) lymph nodes is affected by the location, in the right or left lung, of the primary tumor according to Kiricuta and colleagues (1994). In assessing 266 patients for irradiation, these authors found that in 105 patients with tumors in the left lung, scalene node involvement was present in 13.3% (9.5% of the nodes were ipsilateral and 3.8% were contralateral in location). In 161 patients with tumors in the right lung, the incidence was 10.3% (8.5% were ipsilateral and 1.8% were contralateral, respectively). The overall incidence was slightly greater than 11%. Lee and Ginsberg (1996) also noted that the extent and location of intrathoracic mediastinal lymph node involvement also affected the incidence of scalene lymph node disease. In a small series of patients with right-sided tumors undergoing mediastinoscopy, they found that 15.4% of patients with N_2 disease had occult scalene node metastases, whereas those with intrathoracic N_3 disease (contralateral mediastinal lymph node metastases) had an incidence of 68.4%. No patient with either N_0 or N_1 disease had scalene node involvement. Lymph nodes in the para-aortic region below the diaphragm are involved in approximately 8% of patients. Riquet and colleagues (1988, 1990) demonstrated direct connection to these lymph nodes from the lungs in a small percentage of patients. Axillary lymph nodes are involved rarely. Although, over 50 years ago Ochsner and DeBakey (1942) reported an incidence of 6.6% in a collective review, Riquet and associates (1998) reported an incidence of less than 1%. In 1233 patients resected for cure, these latter authors observed the presence of axillary lymph node involvement at the time of operation in one patient with chest wall involvement (1 in 147 patients with such disease, an incidence of 0.6%) and in eight other patients during subsequent follow-up. The overall incidence was 0.7% in this select group of patients. The commonly held concept that chest wall

involvement is a major factor in the occurrence of axillary node metastases is not supported by Riquet and colleagues' (1998) findings. A second hypothesis is that of retrograde spread from involved supraclavicular lymph nodes as suggested by Marcantonio and Libshitz (1995) from their observations of computed tomographic findings in 17 patients (the total patient base not stated). These latter authors also noted in support of their hypothesis that M. M. Lindell, in a personal communication, had recorded a 2% incidence of retrograde lymphatic flow from the supraclavicular nodes to the axillary nodes in 200 bipedal lymphangiograms. However, Riquet and associates (1998) refute this hypothesis from their own observations and suggest that the most likely route of spread is hematogenous in nature. This certainly is true for the rare occurrence of inguinal lymph node involvement (0.08% in Riquet and associates' [1998] series).

Hematogenous Spread

Blood-borne metastases are common in patients with bronchial carcinoma. Direct invasion of the smaller branches of the pulmonary veins occurs in many of the patients with these tumors. At times, a major vein may be filled with tumor, which may extend even as far as the left atrium. Invasion of the pulmonary artery also occurs.

Detectable blood vessel invasion on histologic examination of the tumor has been documented in most surgical series to portend an unfavorable prognosis; although in reviewing data from the Veterans Administration Surgical Oncology Group's lung studies, one of the authors (T.S.) (1983) did not find that parenchymal blood vessel invasion had prognostic significance. Interestingly, however, parenchymal lymphatic vessel invasion, even in the absence of lymph node metastases, suggested a poor prognosis.

The finding of tumor cells in the circulation has not been well correlated with prognosis. The fate of these circulating cells is undetermined in the individual patient, but these cells are certainly responsible for the development of metastatic deposits in distal organs at one time or another in the host-tumor relationship.

The size of the lesion, as well as its histology as noted, affects the initial incidence of distant metastatic spread. Hematogenous metastasis is rare in lesions less than 1 cm in diameter and, in fact, Ishida and associates (1990a) recorded no occurrences of this type of spread in their experience in patients with small (less than 1 cm) NSCLCs. They did note, however, a 4 and 5% incidence of hematogenous metastasis, respectively, in lesions 1.1 to 2.0 cm and 2.1 to 3.0 cm in diameter. In larger lesions, both occult and clinically manifest distant metastases are more common. Accurate data, however, are not readily available.

The organs and structures most commonly involved by hematogenous spread are the brain, liver, lungs, skeletal system, adrenal glands, kidneys, and pancreas (Table 95-12).

Table 95-12. Incidence of Organ Involvement by Metastatic Disease from Carcinoma of the Lung

	Liver (%)	Lung (%)	Skeleton (%)	Adrenals (%)	Kidneys (%)	Brain (%)	Pancreas (%)
Ochsner and DeBakey (1942), 3047 autopsies	33.3	23.3	21.3	20.3	17.5	16.5[a]	7.3
Galluzzi and Payne (1955), 741 autopsies	39.0	—	15.0	33.0	15.0	—	—
Spencer (1968), 1000 autopsies	38.5	—	15.5	26.4	14.3	18.4[a]	—

[a]Brain examination not done in all autopsies.

The incidence of brain metastasis varies with the cell type, the extent of disease at time of presentation, and duration of the patient's survival after appropriate treatment of the primary lesion. Salbeck and associates (1990) reported that in a total of 271 patients with lung cancer who underwent computed tomographic scans of the brain during initial staging, metastatic disease was present in 11% of the asymptomatic patients and in 33% of the patients with symptoms of possible brain involvement. Asymptomatic patients with SCLC had an incidence of 11.9%, whereas asymptomatic patients with NSCLC had an incidence of 17.5%. However, the incidence was zero in all stage I and II NSCLC patients and all occult metastases were identified in stage III patients: squamous cell carcinoma, 4.9%; adenocarcinoma, 12.1%; and large cell undifferentiated carcinoma, 38.5%. In symptomatic patients the incidences were 37.5%, 66.7%, and 40.0%, respectively. In symptomatic patients with SCLC the incidence was 21.1%. The overall incidence was highest in patients with large cell carcinoma followed in the order of decreasing frequency by those with adenocarcinoma, small cell carcinoma, and squamous cell carcinomas. No brain metastases were recorded in patients with mixed cell histology. Furthermore, it is to be noted that in almost all surgical series, such as those of Martini (1983), Feld (1984), Pairolero (1984), and Ichinose (1989) and their associates, the brain is the most common site of initial failure caused by metastatic disease. Skeletal metastases are usually osteolytic; they occur most commonly in the ribs, spine, femur, humerus, and pelvis. Metastatic deposits distal to the knee or elbow are rare. Although, as Clain (1965) noted, the incidence of bony metastasis from carcinoma of the lung is less than that from four other primary sites (i.e., prostate gland, breast, kidney, and thyroid gland), the lung is second only to the breast as the most common primary site of metastases to bone.

Metastatic deposits may occur in the skin and subcutaneous tissue, myocardium, thyroid gland, small intestine, spleen, and ovary. Although deposits in these locations are uncommon, the lung is the most common primary site responsible for secondary metastases in the heart. After carcinoma of the breast and melanoma, the lung is the next most common primary site for metastases to the skin and subcutaneous tissue. Rosen (1980) reported that cutaneous metastases occur in 2.8 to 7.5% of lung cancer patients and, as noted by Coslett and Katlic (1990), it may be the initial manifestation in a small number of patients.

REFERENCES

Molecular Biology of Lung Cancer

Aguayo SM, et al: Increased levels of bombesin-like peptides in the lower respiratory tract of asymptomatic cigarette smokers. J Clin Invest 84:1105, 1989.

Ahrendt SA, et al: Molecular detection of tumor cells in bronchoalveolar lavage fluid from patients with early-stage non–small cell lung cancer. Proc Am Assoc Cancer Res 39:410, 1998.

Albanell J, et al: High telomerase activity in primary lung cancers: association with increased cell proliferation rates and advanced pathologic stage. J Natl Cancer Inst 89:1609, 1997.

Arai T, et al: Application of telomerase activity for screening of primary lung cancer in broncho-alveolar lavage fluid. Oncol Rep 5:405, 1998.

Arenberg D, et al: Inhibition of interleukin-8 reduces tumorigenesis of human non–small cell lung cancer in SCID mice. J Clin Invest 97:2792, 1996.

Bergh JCS: Gene amplification in human lung cancer. Am Rev Respir Dis 142:S20, 1990.

Betticher DC, et al: G1 control gene status is frequently altered in resectable non–small cell lung cancer. Int J Cancer 74:556, 1997.

Birrer MJ, et al: L-myc cooperates with ras to transform primary rat embryo fibroblasts. Mol Cell Biol 8:2668, 1988.

Bottinger EP, et al: Transgenic mice overexpressing a dominant-negative mutant type II transforming growth factor beta receptor show enhanced tumorigenesis in the mammary gland and ling in response to the carcinogen 7,12-dimethylbenz-[a]-anthracene. Cancer Res 57:5564, 1997.

Brambilla E, et al: Apoptosis-related factors p53, bcl-2 and bax in neuroendocrine lung tumors. Am J Pathol 149:1941, 1996.

Brauch H, et al: Molecular analysis of the short arm of chromosome 3 in small cell and non–small cell carcinoma of the lung. N Engl J Med 317:1109, 1987.

Brennan J, et al: Myc family DNA amplification in 107 tumors and tumor cell lines from patients with small cell lung cancer treated with different combination chemotherapy regimens. Cancer Res 51:1708,1991.

Broers JL, et al: Expression of c-myc in progenitor cells of the bronchopulmonary epithelium and in a large number of non–small cell lung cancers. Am J Respir Cell Mol Biol 9:33, 1993.

Brooks BJ, et al: Amplification and expression of the myc gene in small cell lung cancer. Adv Viral Oncol 7:155, 1987.

Bunn PA, et al: Diagnostic and biologic implications of flow cytometric DNA content analysis in lung cancer. Cancer Res 43:5026, 1983.

Burke L, et al: Allelic deletion analysis of the FHIT gene predicts poor survival in non–small cell lung cancer. Cancer Res 58:2533, 1998.

Carbone DP, et al: p53 immunostaining positivity is associated with reduced survival and is imperfectly correlated with gene mutations in resected non–small cell lung cancer. Chest 106:377S, 1994.

Carbone D, Kratzke R: RB1 and p53 genes. In Pass HI, Mitchell JB, Johnson DH, Turrisi AT (eds). Lung Cancer: Principles and Practice. Philadelphia: Lippincott-Raven, 1996.

Carney DN, et al: Selective stimulation of small cell lung cancer clonal growth by bombesin and gastrin-releasing peptide. Cancer Res 47:821, 1987.

Casalini P, et al: Inhibition of tumorigenicity in lung adenocarcinoma cells by c-erbB-2 antisense expression. Int J Cancer 72:631, 1997.

Center R, et al: Molecular deletion of 9p sequences in non–small cell lung cancer and malignant mesothelioma. Genes Chromosomes Cancer 7:47, 1993.

Cobleigh MA, et al: Efficacy and safety of Herceptin as a single agent in 222 women with HER2 overexpression who relapsed following chemotherapy for metastatic breast cancer. Proc Am Soc Clin Oncol 17:97a, 1998.

Cooper CA, et al: Loss of heterozygosity at 5q21 in non–small cell lung cancer: a frequent event but without evidence of APC mutation. J Pathol 180:33, 1996.

Cristiano RJ, Roth JA: Epidermal growth factor mediated DNA delivery into lung cancer cells via the epidermal growth factor receptor. Cancer Gene Ther 3:4, 1996.

Cuttitta F, et al: Bombesin-like peptides can function as autocrine growth factors in human small cell lung cancer. Nature 316:823, 1985.

D'Amico D, et al: Polymorphic sites within the MCC and APC loci reveal very frequent loss of heterozygosity in human small cell lung cancer. Cancer Res 52:1996, 1992.

Denissenko MF, et al: Preferential formation of benzo(a)pyrene adducts at lung cancer mutational hotspots in p53. Science 274:430, 1996.

DiPaola RS, et al: Growth inhibition of non–small cell lung cancer with c-kit antisense oligodeoxynucleotides. Proc Am Assoc Cancer Res 34:389, 1993.

Dobrovic A, et al: ErbA-related sequence coding for DNA-binding hormone receptor localized to chromosome 3p21-3p25 and deleted in small cell lung carcinoma. Cancer Res 48:682, 1988.

Dosaka-Akita H, et al: Inhibition of proliferation by L-myc antisense DNA for the translational initiation site in human small cell lung cancer. Cancer Res 55:1559, 1995.

Dosaka-Akita H, et al: Altered retinoblastoma protein expression in non–small cell lung cancer: its synergistic effects with altered ras and p53 protein status on prognosis. Cancer 79:1329, 1997.

Filderman AE, et al: Macrophage colony-stimulating factor (CSF-1) enhances invasiveness in CSF-1 receptor-positive carcinoma cell lines. Cancer Res 52:3661, 1992.

Fisher DE: Apoptosis in cancer therapy: crossing the threshold. Cell 78:539, 1994.

Flemming MV, et al: Bcl-2 immunohistochemistry in a surgical series of non–small cell lung cancer patients. Hum Pathol 29:60, 1998.

Fong KM, Zimmerman PV, Smith PJ: Tumor progression and loss of heterozygosity at 5q and 18q in non–small cell lung cancer. Cancer Res 55:220, 1995.

Fontanini G, et al: Epidermal growth factor receptor expression in non–small cell lung carcinomas correlates with metastatic involvement of hilar and mediastinal lymph nodes in the squamous subtype. Eur J Cancer 31A:178, 1995.

Fontanini G, et al: Angiogenesis as a prognostic indicator of survival in non–small cell lung carcinoma: a prospective study. J Natl Cancer Inst 89:881, 1997a.

Fontanini G, et al: Neoangiogenesis and p53 protein in lung cancer: their prognostic role and their relation with vascular endothelial growth factor expression. Br J Cancer 75:1295, 1997b.

Friend SH, et al: A human DNA segment with properties of the gene that predisposes to retinoblastoma and osteosarcoma. Nature 323:643, 1986.

Fujiwara T, et al: A retroviral wild-type p53 expression vector penetrates human lung cancer spheroids and inhibits growth by inducing apoptosis. Cancer Res 53:4129, 1993.

Fujiwara T, et al: Induction of chemosensitivity in human lung cancer cells in vivo by adenovirus-mediated transfer of the wild-type p53 gene. Cancer Res 54:2287, 1994a.

Fujiwara T, et al: Therapeutic effect of a retroviral wild-type p53 expression vector in an orthotopic lung cancer model. J Natl Cancer Inst 86:1458, 1994b.

Funa K, et al: Increased expression of N-myc in human small cell lung cancer biopsies predicts lack of response to chemotherapy and poor prognosis. Am J Clin Pathol 88:216, 1987.

Gazdar AF, et al: Characterization of variant subclasses of cell lines derived from small cell lung cancer having distinctive biochemical, morphological and growth properties. Cancer Res 45:2924, 1985.

Gebert JF, et al: High frequency of retinoic acid receptor β-abnormalities in human lung cancer. Oncogene 6:1859, 1991.

Georges RN, et al: Prevention of orthotopic human lung cancer growth by intratracheal instillation of a retroviral antisense K-ras construct. Cancer Res 53:1743, 1993.

Geradts J, et al: Human lung cancer cell lines exhibit resistance to retinoic acid treatment. Cell Growth Differ 4:799, 1993.

Gouyer V, et al: Mechanism of retinoblastoma gene inactivation in the spectrum of neuroendocrine lung tumors. Am J Respir Cell Mol Biol 18:188, 1998.

Hamburger AW, et al: The role of transforming growth factor alpha pro-

duction and erbB-2 overexpression in induction of tumorigenicity of lung epithelial cells. Br J Cancer 77:1066, 1998.

Harbour JW, et al: Abnormalities in structure and expression of the human retinoblastoma gene in SCLC. Science 241:353, 1988.

Harpole DH, et al: A prognostic model of recurrence and death in stage I non–small cell lung cancer utilizing presentation, histopathology, and oncoprotein expression. Cancer Res 55:51, 1995.

Harris CC, Hollstein M: Clinical implications of the p53 tumor-suppressor gene. N Engl J Med 329:1318, 1993.

Heintz NH, Janssen YM, Mossman BT: Persistent induction of c-fos and c-jun expression by asbestos. Proc Natl Acad Sci U S A 90:3299, 1993.

Helin K, et al: Loss of retinoblastoma protein-related p130 protein in small cell lung carcinoma. Proc Natl Acad Sci U S A 94:6933, 1997.

Hensel CH, et al: Altered structure and expression of the human retinoblastoma susceptibility gene in small cell lung cancer. Cancer Res 50:3067, 1990.

Higashiyama M, et al: Immunohistochemical analysis of nm23 gene product/NDP kinase expression in pulmonary adenocarcinoma: lack of prognostic value. Br J Cancer 66:533, 1992.

Hiyama K, et al: Telomerase activity in small cell and non–small cell lung cancers. J Natl Cancer Inst 87:895, 1995.

Horio Y, et al: Prognostic significance of p53 mutations and 3p deletions in primary resected non–small cell lung cancer. Cancer Res 53:1, 1993.

Hosoe S, et al: A frequent deletion of chromosome 5q21 in advanced small cell and non–small cell carcinoma of the lung. Cancer Res 54:1787, 1994.

Houle B, Rochette-Egly C, Bradley WE: Tumor-suppressive effect of the retinoic acid receptor beta in human epidermoid lung cancer cells. Proc Natl Acad Sci U S A 90:985, 1993.

Hung J, et al: Allele-specific chromosome 3p deletions occur at an early stage in the pathogenesis of lung cancer. JAMA 273:558, 1995.

Huwer H, et al: Squamous cell carcinoma of the lung: does the nm23 gene expression correlate to the tumor stage? Thorac Cardiovasc Surg 42:298, 1994.

Ibson JM, et al: Oncogene amplification and chromosomal abnormalities in small cell lung cancer. J Cell Biochem 33:267, 1987.

Ikegaki N, et al: Expression of bcl-2 in small cell lung carcinoma cells. Cancer Res 54:6, 1994.

Inoue T, et al: The relationship between the immunodetection of transforming growth factor-beta in lung adenocarcinoma and longer survival rates. Surg Oncol 4:51, 1995.

Ishida H, et al: The prognostic significance of p53 and bcl-2 expression in lung adenocarcinoma and its correlation with Ki-67 growth fraction. Cancer 80:1034, 1997.

Jakowlew SB, et al: Expression of transforming growth factor beta ligand and receptor messenger RNAs in lung cancer cell lines. Cell Growth Differ 64:465, 1995.

Jensen DE, et al: BAP1: a novel ubiquitin hydrolase which binds to the BRCA1 RING finger and enhances BRCA1-mediated cell growth suppression. Oncogene 16:1097, 1998.

Jetten AM, et al: Positive and negative regulation of proliferation and differentiation in tracheobronchial epithelial cells. Am Rev Respir Dis 142:S36, 1990.

Johnson BE, et al: Changes in the phenotype of human small cell lung cancer cell lines after transfection and expression of the c-myc proto-oncogene. J Clin Invest 78:525, 1986.

Johnson BE, et al: Restriction fragment length polymorphism studies show consistent loss of chromosome 3p alleles in small cell lung cancer patients' tumors. J Clin Invest 82:502, 1988.

Kaiser U, et al: Expression of bcl-2 protein in small cell lung cancer. Lung Cancer 15:31, 1996.

Kalemkerian GP, et al: All-trans-retinoic acid alters myc gene expression and inhibits in vitro progression of small cell lung cancer. Cell Growth Differ 5:55, 1994.

Kawai T, et al: Expression in lung carcinomas of platelet-derived growth factor and its receptors. Lab Invest 77:431, 1997.

Kawakubo Y, et al: Expression of nm23 protein in pulmonary adenocarcinomas: inverse correlation to tumor progression. Lung Cancer 17:103, 1997.

Kawasaki M, et al: p53 immunostaining predicts chemosensitivity in non–small cell lung cancer: a preliminary report. Cancer J Sci Am 2:217, 1996.

Kawashima K, et al: Close correlation between restriction fragment length polymorphism of the L-myc gene and metastasis of human lung cancer to the lymph nodes and other organs. Proc Natl Acad Sci U S A 85:2353, 1988.

Kelley MJ, et al: Differential inactivation of CDKN2 and Rb protein in non–small cell and small cell lung cancer cell lines. J Natl Cancer Inst 87:756, 1995.

Kelley MJ, et al: Antitumor activity of a monoclonal antibody directed against gastrin-releasing peptide in patients with small cell lung cancer. Chest 112:256, 1997.

Kern JA, et al: p185neu expression in human lung adenocarcinomas predicts shortened survival. Cancer Res 50:5184, 1990.

Kerr JFR, Wyllie AH, Currie AR: Apoptosis: a basic biologic phenomenon with wide-ranging implications in tissue kinetics. Br J Cancer 26:239, 1972.

Kim NW, et al: Specific association of human telomerase activity with immortal cells and cancer. Science 266:2011, 1994.

Kinoshita I, et al: Altered p16INK4 and retinoblastoma protein status in non–small cell lung cancer: potential synergistic effect with altered p53 protein in proliferative activity. Cancer Res 56:5557, 1996.

Knudson AG: Mutation and cancer: statistical study of retinoblastoma. Proc Natl Acad Sci U S A 68: 820, 1971.

Kok K, et al: Deletion of a DNA sequence at the chromosomal region 3p21 in all major types of lung cancer. Nature 330:578, 1987.

Koukourakis MI, et al: Platelet-derived endothelial cell growth factor expression correlates with tumor angiogenesis and prognosis in non–small cell lung cancer. Br J Cancer 75:477, 1997.

Kratzke RA, et al: RB-mediated tumor suppression of a lung cancer cell line is abrogated by an extract enriched in extracellular matrix. Cell Growth Differ 4:629, 1993.

Kratzke RA, et al: Rb and p16INK4a expression in resected non–small cell lung tumors. Cancer Res 56:3415, 1996.

Krystal GW, Hines SJ, Organ CP: Autocrine growth of small cell lung cancer mediated by coexpression of c-kit and stem cell factor. Cancer Res 56:370, 1996.

Krystal GW, Carlson P, Litz J: Induction of apoptosis and inhibition of small cell lung cancer growth by the quinoxaline tyrphostins. Cancer Res 57:2203, 1997.

Kumagai T, et al: Eradication of myc-overexpressing small cell lung cancer cells transfected with herpes simplex thymidine kinase gene containing myc-max response elements. Cancer Res 56:354, 1996.

Latif F, et al: Identification of the von Hippel-Lindau disease tumor suppressor gene. Science 260:1317, 1993.

Lee CT, et al: Antitumor effects of an adenovirus expressing antisense insulin-like growth factor I receptor on human lung cancer cell lines. Cancer Res 56:3038, 1996.

Lee M, et al: Epidermal growth factor receptor monoclonal antibodies inhibit the growth of lung cancer cell lines. Monogr Natl Cancer Inst 13:117, 1992.

Leonard RCF, et al: Small cell lung cancer after retinoblastoma. Lancet 2:1503, 1988.

Liggett WH, Sidransky D. Role of the p16 tumor suppressor gene in cancer. J Clin Oncol 16:1197, 1998.

Lowe SW, et al: p53 status and the efficacy of cancer therapy in vivo. Science 266:807, 1994.

Mabry M, et al: v-Ha-ras oncogene insertion: a model for tumor progression of human small cell lung cancer. Proc Natl Acad Sci U S A 85:6523, 1988.

Mabry M, et al: Introduction of a mutated p53 gene results in increased growth and reduced hormone production in human small cell lung cancer. Proc Am Assoc Cancer Res 31:313, 1990.

Macaulay VM, et al: Autocrine function for insulin-like growth factor I in human small cell lung cancer cell lines and fresh tumor cells. Cancer Res 50:2511, 1990.

Makela TP, et al: Intrachromosomal rearrangements fusing L-myc and rlf in small cell lung cancer. Mol Cell Biol 11:4015, 1991.

Maneckjee R, Minna JD: Opioid and nicotine receptors affect growth regulation of human lung cancer cell lines. Proc Natl Acad Sci U S A 87:3294, 1990.

Mao L, et al: Detection of oncogene mutations in sputum precedes diagnosis of lung cancer. Cancer Res 54:1634, 1994.

Mao L, et al: Clonal genetic alterations in the lungs of current and former smokers. J Natl Cancer Inst 89:857, 1997.

Maruno K, et al: Immunoreactive gastrin-releasing peptide as a specific tumor marker in patients with small cell lung carcinoma. Cancer Res 49:629, 1989.

Merlo A, et al: Frequent microsatellite instability in primary small cell lung cancer. Cancer Res 54:2098, 1994.

Miozzo M, et al: Microsatellite alterations in bronchial and sputum specimens of lung cancer patients. Cancer Res 56:2285, 1996.

Missale C, et al: Nerve growth factor abrogates the tumorigenicity of human small cell lung cancer cell lines. Proc Natl Acad Sci U S A 95:5366, 1998.

Mitsudomi T, et al: Ras gene mutations in non–small cell lung cancers are associated with shortened survival irrespective of treatment intent. Cancer Res 51:4999, 1991a.

Mitsudomi T, et al: Mutations of ras genes distinguish a subset of non–small cell lung cancer cell lines from small cell lung cancer cell lines. Oncogene 6:1353, 1991b.

Mitsudomi T, et al: Mutations of the p53 gene as a predictor of poor prognosis in patients with non–small cell lung cancer. Proc Am Assoc Cancer Res 34:516, 1993.

Miura I, et al: Chromosome alterations in human small cell lung cancer: frequent involvement of 5q. Cancer Res 52:1322, 1992.

Miyashita T, et al: Tumor suppressor p53 is a regulator of bcl-2 and bax gene expression in vitro and in vivo. Oncogene 9:1799, 1994.

Modjtahedi H, et al: Phase I trial and tumor localisation of the anti-EGFR monoclonal antibody ICR62 in head and neck and lung cancer. Br J Cancer 73:228, 1996.

Moody TW, et al: High levels of intracellular bombesin characterize human small cell lung carcinoma. Science 214:1246, 1981.

Moody TW, et al: High affinity receptors for bombesin/GRP-like peptides on human small cell lung cancer. Life Sci 37:105, 1985.

Mori N, et al: Variable mutations of the RB gene in small cell lung carcinoma. Oncogene 5:1713, 1990.

Morin GB: Telomere integrity and cancer. J Natl Cancer Inst 88:1095, 1996.

Nagatake M, et al: Somatic in vivo alterations of the DPC4 gene at 18q21 in human lung cancer. Cancer Res 56:2718, 1996.

Nakanishi Y, et al: Insulin-like growth factor-I can mediate autocrine proliferation of human small cell lung cancer cell lines in vitro. J Clin Invest 82:354, 1988.

Nambu Y, et al: Lack of cell surface fas/apo-1 expression in pulmonary adenocarcinomas. J Clin Invest 101:1102, 1998.

Nau MM, et al: L-myc, a new myc-related gene amplified and expressed in human small cell lung cancer. Nature 318:69, 1985.

Nau MM, et al: Human small cell lung cancers show amplification and expression of the N-myc gene. Proc Natl Acad Sci U S A 83:1092, 1986.

Niehans GA, et al: Human lung carcinomas express fas ligand. Cancer Res 57:1007, 1997.

Noguchi M, et al: Biological consequences of overexpression of a transfected c-erbB-2 gene in immortalized human bronchial epithelial cells. Cancer Res 53:2035, 1993.

Norgaard P, Spang-Thomsen M, Poulsen HS: Expression and autoregulation of transforming growth factor beta receptor mRNA in small cell lung cancer cell lines. Br J Cancer 73:1037, 1996.

Ohmori M, et al: Apoptosis of lung cancer cells caused by some anti-cancer agents is inhibited by bcl-2. Biochem Biophys Res Comm 192:30, 1993.

Ohta Y, et al: Vascular endothelial growth factor and lymph node metastasis in primary lung cancer. Br J Cancer 76:1041, 1997.

Olopade OI, et al: Homozygous loss of the interferon genes defines the critical region on 9p that is deleted in lung cancers. Cancer Res 53:2410, 1993.

Ookawa K, et al: Reconstitution of the RB gene suppresses the growth of small cell lung carcinoma cells carrying multiple genetic alterations. Oncogene 8:2175, 1993.

Otterson GA, et al: Absence of p16INK4 protein is restricted to the subset of lung cancer lines that retains wildtype RB. Oncogene 9:3375, 1994.

Otterson GA, et al: Protein expression and functional analysis of the FHIT gene in human tumor cells. J Natl Cancer Inst 90:426, 1998.

Pastorino U, et al: Immunohistochemical markers in stage I lung cancer: relevance to prognosis. J Clin Oncol 15:2858, 1997.

Pedersen AG, et al: Cerebrospinal fluid bombesin and calcitonin in patients with central nervous system metastases from small cell lung cancer. J Clin Oncol 4:1620, 1986.

Pezzella F, et al: Bcl-2 protein in non–small cell lung carcinoma. N Engl J Med 329:690, 1993.

Pfeifer AMA, et al: Cooperation of c-raf-1 and c-myc proto-oncogenes in the neoplastic transformation of simian virus 40 large tumor antigen-immortalized human bronchial epithelial cells. Proc Natl Acad Sci U S A 86:10075, 1989.

Quinlan DC, et al: Accumulation of p53 protein correlates with a poor prognosis in human lung cancer. Cancer Res 52:4828, 1992.

Quinn KA, et al: Insulin-like growth factor expression in human cancer cell lines. J Biol Chem 271:11477, 1996.

Rabiasz GJ, et al: Growth control by epidermal growth factor and transforming growth factor-α in human lung squamous carcinoma cells. Br J Cancer 66:254, 1992.

Ravi RK, et al: Activated raf-1 causes growth arrest in human small cell lung cancer cells. J Clin Invest 101:153, 1998.

Raynal S, et al: Transforming growth factor-beta enhances the lethal effects of DNA-damaging agents in a human lung-cancer cell line. Int J Cancer 72:356, 1997.

Reed, JC: Bcl-2: prevention of apoptosis as a mechanism of drug resistance. Hematol Oncol Clin North Am 9:451, 1995.

Reeve JG, Payne JA, Bleehan NM: Production of insulin-like growth factor-I (IGF-I) and IGF-I binding proteins by human lung tumors. Br J Cancer 62:504, 1990.

Reeve JG, et al: Expression of apoptosis-regulatory genes in lung tumour cell lines: relationship to p53 expression and relevance to acquired drug resistance. Br J Cancer 73:1193, 1996.

Reissmann PT, et al: Inactivation of the retinoblastoma susceptibility gene in non–small cell lung cancer. The Lung Cancer Study Group. Oncogene 8:1913, 1993.

Robinson LA, et al: C-myc antisense oligodeoxyribonucleotides inhibit proliferation of non–small cell lung cancer. Ann Thorac Surg 60:1583, 1995.

Rodenhuis S, et al: Mutational activation of the K-ras oncogene and the effect of chemotherapy in advanced adenocarcinoma of the lung: a prospective study. J Clin Oncol 15:285, 1997.

Rosenfeld MR, et al: Serum anti-p53 antibodies and prognosis of patients with small cell lung cancer. J Natl Cancer Inst 89:381, 1997.

Roth JA, et al: Retrovirus-mediated wild-type p53 gene transfer to tumors of patients with lung cancer. Nat Med 2:985, 1996.

Rusch V, et al: Differential expression of the epidermal growth factor receptor and its ligands in primary non–small cell lung cancers and adjacent benign lung. Cancer Res 53:2379, 1993.

Rusch V, et al: Aberrant expression of p53 or the epidermal growth factor receptor is frequent in early bronchial neoplasia and coexpression precedes squamous cell carcinoma development. Cancer Res 55:1365, 1995.

Rygaard K, Vindelov LL, Spang-Thomsen M: Expression of myc family oncoproteins in small cell lung cancer cell lines and xenografts. Int J Cancer 54:144, 1993a.

Rygaard K, Nakamura T, Spang-Thomsen M: Expression of the proto-oncogenes c-met and c-kit and their ligands hepatocyte growth factor/scatter factor and stem cell factor, in SCLC cell lines and xenografts. Br J Cancer 67:37, 1993b.

Saccomanno G, et al: Development of carcinoma of the lung as reflected in exfoliated cells. Cancer 33:256, 1974.

Salven P, et al: High pre-treatment serum level of vascular endothelial growth factor is associated with poor outcome in small cell lung cancer. Int J Cancer 79:144, 1998.

Sanders BM, et al: Non-ocular cancer in relatives of retinoblastoma patients. Br J Cancer 60:358, 1989.

Satoh H, et al: Suppression of tumorigenicity of A549 lung adenocarcinoma cells by human chromosomes 3 and 11 introduced via microcell-mediated chromosome transfer. Mol Carcinog 7:157, 1993.

Sausville EA, et al: Expression of the gastrin-releasing peptide gene in human small cell lung cancer. J Biol Chem 261:2451, 1986.

Schuette J, et al: Constitutive expression of multiple mRNA forms of the c-jun oncogene in human lung cancer cell lines. Proc Am Assoc Cancer Res 29:455, 1988.

Shapiro GI, et al: Multiple mechanisms of p16INK4A inactivation in non–small cell lung cancer cell lines. Cancer Res 55:6200, 1995.

Shimizu E, et al: RB protein status and clinical correlation from 171 cell lines representing lung cancer, extrapulmonary small cell carcinoma and mesothelioma. Oncogene 9:2441, 1994.

Shiseki M, et al: Frequent allelic loss on chromosome 2q, 18q and 22q in advanced non–small cell lung carcinoma. Cancer Res 54:5643, 1994.

Shridhar V, et al: Genetic instability of microsatellite sequences in many non–small cell lung carcinomas. Cancer Res 54:2084, 1994.

Siegfried JM, et al: Prognostic value of specific K-ras mutations in lung adenocarcinoma. Cancer Epidemiol Biomarker Prev 6:841, 1997a.

Siegfried JM, et al: Association of immunoreactive hepatocyte growth factor with poor survival in resectable non–small cell lung cancer. Cancer Res 57:433, 1997b.

Sim BKL, et al: A recombinant human angiostatin protein inhibits experimental primary and metastatic cancer. Cancer Res 57:1329, 1997.

Singh-Kaw P, Zarnegar R, Siegfried JM: Stimulatory effects of hepatocyte growth factor on normal and neoplastic human bronchial epithelial cells. Am J Physiol 268:L1012, 1995.

Siprashvili Z, et al: Replacement of Fhit in cancer cells suppresses tumorigenicity. Proc Natl Acad Sci U S A 94:13771, 1997.

Sithanandam G, et al: Loss of heterozygosity at the c-raf locus in small cell lung carcinoma. Oncogene 4:451, 1989.

Sklar MD: Increased resistance to cis-diamine-dichloroplatinum(II) in NIH 3T3 cells transformed by the ras oncogene. Cancer Res 48:793, 1988.

Slamon D, et al: Addition of Herceptin to first line chemotherapy for HER2 overexpressing metastatic breast cancer markedly increases anticancer activity. Proc Am Soc Clin Oncol 17:98a, 1998.

Slebos RJC, et al: K-ras oncogene activation as a prognostic marker in adenocarcinoma of the lung. N Engl J Med 323:561, 1990.

Slebos RJC, et al: Relationship between K-ras oncogene activation and smoking in adenocarcinoma of the lung. J Natl Cancer Inst 83:1024, 1991.

Smith DR, et al: Inhibition of interleukin 8 attenuates angiogenesis in bronchogenic carcinoma. J Exp Med 179:1409, 1994.

Snider JM, et al: C-erbB-2/p185-directed therapy in human lung adenocarcinoma. Ann Thorac Surg 62:1454, 1996.

Sozzi G, et al: Cytogenetic abnormalities and overexpression of receptors for growth factors in normal bronchial epithelium and tumor samples of lung cancer patients. Cancer Res 51:400, 1991.

Sozzi G, et al: The FHIT gene 3p14.2 is abnormal in lung cancer. Cell 85:17, 1996.

Sozzi G, et al: Absence of Fhit protein in primary lung tumors and cell lines with FHIT gene abnormalities. Cancer Res 57:5207, 1997.

Stocklin E, Botteri F, Groner B: An activated allele of the c-erbB-2 oncogene impairs kidney and lung function and causes early death in transgenic mice. J Cell Biol 122:199, 1993.

Strauss GM, et al: Molecular and pathologic markers in stage I non–small cell carcinoma of the lung. J Clin Oncol 13:1265, 1995.

Suarez-Pestana E, et al: Growth inhibition of human lung adenocarcinoma cells by antibodies against epidermal growth factor receptor and by ganglioside GM3: involvement of receptor-directed protein tyrosine phosphatase(s). Br J Cancer 75:213, 1997.

Sun J, et al: Ras CAAX peptidomimetic FTI 276 selectively blocks tumor growth in nude mice of a human lung carcinoma with K-ras mutation and p53 deletion. Cancer Res 55:4243, 1995.

Sundaresan V, et al: p53 and chromosome 3 abnormalities, characteristic of malignant lung tumours, are detectable in preinvasive lesions of the bronchus. Oncogene 7:1989, 1992.

Szabo E, et al: Altered c-jun expression: an early event in human lung carcinogenesis. Cancer Res 56:305, 1996.

Taga S, et al: Prognostic value of the immunohistochemical detection of p16INK4 expression in non–small cell lung carcinoma. Cancer 80:389, 1997.

Takahashi T, et al: Expression and amplification of myc gene family in small cell lung cancer and its relation to biological characteristics. Cancer Res 49:2683, 1989a.

Takahashi T, et al: p53: a frequent target for genetic abnormalities in lung cancer. Science 246:491, 1989b.

Takahashi T, et al: Wild-type but not mutant p53 suppresses the growth of human lung cancer cells bearing multiple genetic lesions. Cancer Res 52:2340, 1992.

Takayama K, et al: Bcl-2 expression as a predictor of chemosensitivity and survival in small cell lung cancer. Cancer J Sci Am 2:212, 1996.

Tanaka H, et al: Disruption of the RB pathway and cell-proliferative activity in non–small cell lung cancers. Int J Cancer 79:111, 1998.

Tsai CM, et al: Correlation of intrinsic resistance of non–small cell lung cancer cell lines with HER-2/neu gene expression but not with ras gene mutations. J Natl Cancer Inst 85:897, 1993.

Tsai CM, et al: Enhancement of chemosensitivity by tyrphostin AG825 in high-p185(neu) expressing non–small cell lung cancer cells. Cancer Res 56:1068, 1996.

Van Waardenburg RC, et al: Effects of an inducible anti-sense c-myc gene transfer in a drug-resistant human small cell-lung-carcinoma cell line. Int J Cancer 73:544, 1997.

Vermylen P, et al: Biology of pulmonary preneoplastic lesions. Cancer Treat Rev 23:241, 1997.

Volm M, Efferth T, Mattern J: Oncoprotein (c-myc, c-erbB1, c-erbB2, c-fos) and suppressor gene product (p53) expression in squamous cell carcinomas of the lung: clinical and biological correlations. Anticancer Res 12:11, 1992.

Volm M, Koomagi R, Mattern J: Prognostic value of vascular endothelial growth factor and its receptor Flt-1 in squamous cell lung cancer. Int J Cancer 74:64, 1997a.

Volm M, et al: Prognostic value of basic fibroblast growth factor and its receptor (FGFR-1) in patients with non–small cell lung carcinomas. Eur J Cancer 33:691, 1997b.

Westra WH, et al: K-ras oncogene activation in atypical alveolar hyperplasias of the human lung. Cancer Res 56:2224, 1996.

Whang-Peng J, et al: Specific chromosome defect associated with human small cell lung cancer: deletion 3p(14-23). Science 215:181, 1982.

Wieland I, et al: Microsatellite instability and loss of heterozygosity at the hMLH1 locus on chromosome 3p21 occur in a subset of nonsmall cell lung carcinomas. Oncology Res 8:1, 1996.

Willey JC, Lechner JF, Harris CC: Bombesin and the C-terminal tetradecapeptide of gastrin-releasing peptide are growth factors for normal human bronchial epithelial cells. Exp Cell Res 153:245, 1984.

Winter SF, et al: Development of antibodies against p53 in lung cancer patients appears to be dependent on the type of p53 mutation. Cancer Res 52:4168, 1992.

Wistuba II, et al: Molecular damage in the bronchial epithelium of current and former smokers. J Natl Cancer Inst 89:1366, 1997.

Wodrich W, Volm M: Overexpression of oncoproteins in non–small cell lung carcinomas of smokers. Carcinogenesis 14:1121, 1993.

Woll PJ, Rozengurt E: [D-Arg¹,D-Phe⁵,D-Trp⁷,⁹,Leu¹¹]substance P, a potent bombesin antagonist in murine Swiss 3T3 cells, inhibits the growth of human small cell lung cancer cells in vitro. Proc Natl Acad Sci U S A 85:1859, 1988.

Wong AJ, et al: Gene amplification of c-myc and N-myc in small cell carcinoma of the lung. Science 233:461, 1986.

Wu X, et al: Benzo(a)pyrene diol epoxide-induced 3p21.3 aberrations and genetic predisposition to lung cancer. Cancer Res 58:1605, 1998.

Yahata N, et al: Telomerase activity in lung cancer cells obtained from bronchial washings. J Natl Cancer Inst 90:684, 1998.

Yanuck M, et al: A mutant p53 tumor suppressor protein is a target for peptide-induced CD8+ cytotoxic T-cells. Cancer Res 53:3257, 1993.

Yashima K, et al: Telomerase expression in respiratory epithelium during multistage pathogenesis of lung carcinomas. Cancer Res 57:2373, 1997.

Yokota J, et al: Loss of heterozygosity on chromosomes 3, 13, and 17 in small cell carcinoma and on chromosome 3 in adenocarcinoma of the lung. Proc Natl Acad Sci U S A 84:9252, 1987.

Yokota J, et al: Altered expression of the retinoblastoma (RB) gene in small cell carcinoma of the lung. Oncogene 3:471, 1988.

You M, et al: Activation of the K-ras proto-oncogene in spontaneously occurring and chemically induced lung tumors of the strain A mouse. Proc Natl Acad Sci U S A 86:3070, 1989.

Young MR, et al: Granulocyte-macrophage colony-stimulating factor stimulates the metastatic properties of Lewis lung carcinoma cells through a protein kinase A signal-transduction pathway. Int J Cancer 53:667, 1993.

Zangemeister-Wittke U, et al: Bcl-2 antisense oligonucleotide 2009 synergizes with chemotherapy on lung cancer cell lines and has antitumor activity against lung cancer xenografts. Proc Am Assoc Cancer Res 39:417, 1998.

Ziegler A, et al: Induction of apoptosis in small cell lung cancer cells by antisense oligonucleotide targeting the bcl-2 coding sequence. J Natl Cancer Inst 89:1027, 1997.

Pathology of Lung Tumors

Adelstein DJ, et al: Mixed small cell and non–small cell lung cancer. Chest 89:699, 1986.

Amemiya R, Oho K: X-ray diagnosis of lung cancer. In Hayata Y (ed): Lung Cancer Diagnosis. Tokyo: Igaku-Shoin, 1982, p. 4.

Arrigoni MG, et al: Atypical carcinoid tumors of the lung. J Thorac Cardiovasc Surg 64:413, 1972.

Asada Y, et al: Expression of dipeptidyl aminopeptidase IV activity in human lung carcinoma. Histopathology 23:265, 1993.

Azzopardi JG: Oat-cell carcinoma of the bronchus. J Pathol Bacteriol 78:513, 1959.

Baker RR, et al: The role of surgery in the management of selected patients with small cell carcinoma of the lung. J Clin Oncol 5:697, 1987.

Barsky SH, Huang SJ, Bhuta S: The extracellular matrix of pulmonary scar carcinomas is suggestive of a desmoplastic origin. Am J Pathol 124:412, 1986.

Barsky SH, et al: Rising incidence of bronchioloalveolar lung carcinoma and its unique clinicopathologic features. Cancer 73:1163, 1994a.

Barsky SH, et al: The multifocality of bronchioloalveolar carcinoma: evidence and implications of a multiclonal origin. Mod Pathol 7:633, 1994b.

Bensch KG, et al: Oat-cell carcinoma of the lung. Cancer 22:1163, 1968.

Berendsen HH, et al: Clinical characteristics of non–small cell lung cancer tumors showing neuroendocrine differentiation features. J Clin Oncol 17:1614, 1989.

Blobel GA, et al: Cytokeratins in normal lung and lung carcinomas: I. Adenocarcinomas, squamous cell carcinoma and cultured cell lines. Virchows Arch 45:407, 1984.

Borrie J: Pulmonary carcinoma of the bronchus. Ann R Coll Surg Engl 10:165, 1952.

Brambilla E: Basaloid carcinoma of the lung. In Corrin B (ed): Pathology of Lung Tumors. New York: Churchill Livingstone, 1997, p. 71.

Brambilla E, et al: Basal cell (basaloid) carcinoma of the lung: a new morphologic and phenotypic entity with separate prognostic significance. Hum Pathol 23:993, 1992.

Clain A: Secondary malignant disease of bone. Br J Cancer 19:15, 1965.

Clayton F: Bronchoalveolar carcinomas: Cell types, patterns of growth, and prognostic correlates. Cancer 57:1555, 1986.

Clayton F: The spectrum and significance of bronchioloalveolar carcinomas. Pathol Annu 23:361, 1988.

Coslett LM, Katlic MR: Lung cancer with skin metastasis. Chest 97:757, 1990.

Cotton, RE: The bronchial spread of lung cancer. Br J Dis Chest 53:142, 1959.

Daly RC, et al: Bronchoalveolar cell carcinoma: Factors affecting survival. Ann Thorac Surg 51:368, 1991.

Dresler CM, et al: Clinical-pathologic analysis of 40 patients with large cell neuroendocrine carcinoma of the lung. Ann Thorac Surg 63:180, 1997.

Dulmet-Brender E, Jaubert F, Hunchon G: Exophytic endobronchial epidermoid carcinoma. Cancer 57:1358, 1986.

Edwards C, Carlyle A: Clear cell carcinoma of the lung. J Clin Pathol 38:880, 1985.

Edwards CW: Pulmonary adenocarcinoma: review of 106 cases and proposed new classification. J Clin Pathol 40:125, 1987.

Farber E: The multistep nature of cancer development. Cancer Res 44:4217, 1984.

Feld R, et al: Site of recurrence in resected stage I non–small cell lung cancer: a guide for future studies. J Clin Oncol 2:1352, 1984.

Fitzgibbons PL, Kern WH: Adenosquamous carcinoma of the lung: a clinical and pathologic study of seven cases. Hum Pathol 16:463, 1985.

Gaffey MJ, et al: Pulmonary clear cell carcinoid tumor: another entity in the differential diagnosis of pulmonary clear cell neoplasia. Am J Surg Pathol 22:1020, 1998.

Gould VE, Warren WH: Epithelial neoplasms of the lung. In Roth JA, Ruckdeschel JC, Weisenburger TH (eds): Thoracic Oncology. Philadelphia: WB Saunders, 1989, p. 77.

Gould VE, Warren WH: Epithelial neoplasms of the lung. In Roth JA, Ruckdeschel JC, Weisenburger TH (eds): Thoracic Oncology. 2nd Ed. Philadelphia: WB Saunders, 1995, p. 49.

Gould VE, et al: Neuroendocrine cells and neuroendocrine neoplasms of the lung. Pathol Annu 18:287, 1983a.

Gould VE, et al: Neuroendocrine components of the bronchopulmonary tract: hyperplasia, dysplasia, and neoplasms. Lab Invest 49:519, 1983b.

Gould VE, et al: Cytoskeletal characteristics of epithelial neoplasm of the lung. In Lenfant C, et al (eds): Biology of Lung Cancer. New York: Marcel Dekker,1992.

Greschuchna D, Maassen W: Die lymphogenen Absiedlungswege des Bronchialkarzinoms. Stuttgart: Thieme, 1973.

Griess DF, McDonald JR, Clagett OT: The proximal extension of carcinoma of the lung in the bronchial wall. J Thorac Surg 14:362, 1945.

Harpole DH, et al: Alveolar cell carcinoma of the lung. A retrospective analysis of 205 patients. Ann Thorac Surg 46:502, 1988.

Hasleton PS: Benign lung tumors and their malignant counterparts. *In* Hasleton PS (ed): Spencer's Pathology of the Lung. 5th Ed. New York: McGraw-Hill, 1996, p. 66.

Hata E, et al: Rationale for extended lymphadenectomy for lung cancer. Theor Surg 5:19, 1990.

Hill CA: Bronchioloalveolar carcinoma: a review. Radiology 150:15, 1984.

Hirsch FR, et al: Histopathologic classification of small cell lung cancer. Changing concepts and terminology. Cancer 62:973, 1988.

Holst VA, Finkelstein S, Yousem SA: Bronchioloalveolar adenocarcinoma of the lung: monoclonal origin for multifocal disease. Am J Surg Pathol 22:1343, 1998.

Ichinose Y, et al: Preoperative examination to detect distant metastasis is not advocated for asymptomatic patients with stages 1 and 2 non–small cell lung cancer. Preoperative examination for lung cancer. Chest 96:1104, 1989.

Ichinose Y, et al: DNA ploidy pattern of each carcinomatous component in adenosquamous lung carcinoma. Ann Thorac Surg 55:593, 1993.

Ishida T, et al: Strategy for lymphadenectomy in lung cancer three centimeters or less in diameter. Ann Thorac Surg 50:708, 1990a.

Ishida T, et al: Surgical treatment of patients with non–small cell lung cancer and mediastinal lymph node involvement. J Surg Oncol 43:161, 1990b.

Ishida T, et al: Adenosquamous carcinoma of the lung: clinicopathologic and immunohistochemical features. Am J Clin Pathol 97:678, 1992.

Katzenstein AA, Prioleau PG, Askin FB: The histologic spectrum and significance of clear-cell change in lung carcinoma. Cancer 45:943, 1980.

Kiricuta IC, et al: The lymphatic pathways of non–small cell lung cancer and their implications in curative irradiation treatment. Lung Cancer 11:71, 1994.

Lee I, et al: Immunohistochemical analyses of pulmonary carcinomas using monoclonal antibody 44-3A6. Cancer Res 45:5813, 1985.

Lee I, et al: Immunohistochemical demonstration of lacto-N-fucopentose III in lung carcinomas with monoclonal antibody 624A12. Pathol Res Pract 182:40, 1987.

Lee JD, Ginsberg RJ: Lung cancer staging: the value of ipsilateral scalene lymph node biopsy performed at mediastinoscopy. Ann Thorac Surg 62:338, 1996.

Libshitz HI, et al: Patterns of mediastinal metastases in bronchogenic carcinoma. Chest 90:229, 1986.

Maassen W: The staging issue—problems: accuracy of mediastinoscopy. *In* Delarue NC, Eschapasse H (eds): Lung Cancer. Philadelphia: WB Saunders, 1985, p. 42.

Madri JA, Carter D: Scar cancers of the lung: origin and significance. Hum Pathol 15:625, 1984.

Marcantonio DR, Libshitz HI: Axillary lymph node metastases of bronchogenic cancer. Cancer 76:803, 1995.

Martini N, Flehinger BJ: The role of surgery in N2 lung cancer. Surg Clin North Am 67:1037, 1987.

Martini N, Ginsberg RJ: Surgical approach to non–small cell lung cancer stage IIIa. Hematol Oncol Clin North Am 6:1121, 1990.

Martini N, et al: Results in resection in non-oat cell carcinoma of the lung with mediastinal lymph node metastases. Ann Surg 198:386, 1983.

Meyer EC, Liebow AA: Relationship of interstitial pneumonia honeycombing and atypical epithelial proliferation to carcinoma of the lung. Cancer 18:322, 1965.

Minna JD: The molecular biology of lung cancer pathogenesis. Chest 103:449, 1993.

Mitsudomi T, et al: Mutations of the *p53* tumor suppressor gene as a clonal marker for multiple primary lung cancers. J Thorac Cardiovasc Surg 114:354, 1997.

Mizutani Y, et al: Immunohistochemical location of pulmonary surfactant apoproteins in various lung tumors. Special reference to nonmucous producing lung adenocarcinomas. Cancer 61:532, 1988.

Moll R, et al: The catalog of human cytokeratins: patterns of expression in normal epithelia, tumors and cultured cells. Cell 31:11, 1982.

Moori WJ: Common lung cancers. *In* Hasleton PS (ed): Spencer's Pathology of the Lung. 5th Ed. New York: McGraw-Hill, 1996, p. 1009.

Moori WJ, Dingemans KP, Van Zandwijk N: Prevalence of neuroendocrine granules in small cell lung carcinoma. Usefulness of electron microscopy in lung cancer classification. J Pathol 149:41, 1986.

Nagamoto N, et al: Relationship of lymph node metastases to primary tumor size and microscopic appearance of roentgenographic occult lung cancer. Am J Surg Pathol 13:1009, 1989.

Naruke T, Suemasu K, Ishikawa S: Lymph node mapping and curability at various levels of metastasis in resected lung cancer. J Thorac Cardiovasc Surg 76:832, 1978.

Naruke T, et al: The importance of surgery to non–small cell carcinoma of the lung with mediastinal lymph node metastasis. Ann Thorac Surg 46:603, 1988.

Naunheim KS, et al: Adenosquamous lung carcinoma: clinical characteristics, treatment, and prognosis. Ann Thorac Surg 44:462, 1987.

Nicholson AG, et al: The value of PE-40, a monoclonal antibody against pulmonary surfactant, in distinguishing primary and metastatic lung tumors. Histopathology 27:57, 1995.

Nohl-Oser HC: Lymphatics of the lung. *In* Shields TW (ed): General Thoracic Surgery. 3rd Ed. Philadelphia: Lea & Febiger, 1989.

Ochsner A, DeBakey M: Significance of metastasis in primary carcinoma of the lungs: report of two cases with unusual site of metastasis. J Thorac Surg 11:357, 1942.

Otto WR, Wright NA: Stem cells of the lung. *In* Corrin B: Pathology of Lung Tumors. New York: Churchill Livingstone, 1997.

Pairolero PC, et al: Postsurgical stage I bronchogenic carcinoma: morbid implications of recurrent disease. Ann Thorac Surg 38:331, 1984.

Piehl MR: Immunohistochemical identification of exocrine and neuroendocrine subsets of large cell lung carcinomas. Pathol Res Pract 183:675, 1988.

Riquet M, Hidden G, Debasse B: Abdominal nodal connections of the lymphatics of the lung. Surg Radiol Anat 10:251, 1988.

Riquet M, Hidden G, Debasse B: Direct lymphatic drainage of lung segments to the mediastinal nodes. An anatomic study on 260 adults. J Thorac Cardiovasc Surg 97:623, 1989.

Riquet M, Le Pimpec-Barthes F, Danel D: Axillary lymph node metastases from bronchogenic carcinoma. Ann Thorac Surg 66:920, 1998.

Riquet M, et al: Direct metastases to abdominal lymph nodes in bronchogenic carcinoma (Letter to the Editor). J Thorac Cardiovasc Surg 100:153, 1990.

Rodenhuis S, et al: Incidence of possible clinical significance of K-ras oncogene activation in adenocarcinoma of the human lung. Cancer Res 48:5738, 1988.

Roggli VL, et al: Lung cancer heterogeneity: A blinded and randomized study of 100 consecutive cases. Hum Pathol 16:569, 1985.

Rosen T: Cutaneous metastases. Med Clin North Am 64:885, 1980.

Sagawa M, et al: Clinical and prognostic assessment of patients with resected small peripheral lung cancer lesions. Cancer 66:2653, 1990.

Salbeck R, Grau HC, Artmann M: Cerebral tumor staging in bronchial carcinoma by computed tomography. Cancer 66:2007, 1990.

Saldiva PHN, Capelozzi VL, Battlehner CN: Neuroendocrine tumors of the lung. *In* Corrin B: Pathology of Lung Tumors. New York: Churchill Livingstone, 1997, p. 55.

Schaafsma HE, Ramaekers FCS: Cytokeratin subtyping in normal and neoplastic epithelium: basic principles and diagnostic application. Pathol Annu 29:21, 1994.

Shepherd FA, et al: A prospective study of adjuvant surgical resection after chemotherapy for limited small cell lung cancer. A University of Toronto Lung Oncology Group study. J Thorac Cardiovasc Surg 97:177, 1989.

Sherwin RP, Laforet EG, Strider JW: Exophytic endobronchial carcinoma. J Thorac Cardiovasc Surg 43:716, 1992.

Shields TW: Prognostic significance of parenchymal lymphatic vessel and blood vessel invasion in carcinoma of the lung. Surg Gynecol Obstet 157:185, 1983.

Shimizu T, et al: A clinicopathologic study of resected cases of adenosquamous carcinoma of the lung. Chest 109:989, 1996.

Shinton NK: The histologic classification of lower respiratory tract tumors. Br J Cancer 17:1, 1963.

Singh G, Katyal SL, Torikata C: Carcinoma of type II pneumocytes: Immunodiagnosis of a subtype of "bronchoalveolar carcinomas." Am J Pathol 102:195, 1981.

Sørensen JB, Badsberg JH: Prognostic factors in resected stages I and II adenocarcinoma of the lung. A multivariate regression analysis of 137 consecutive patients. J Thorac Cardiovasc Surg 99:218, 1990.

Sørensen JB, Olsen JE: Prognostic implications of histologic subtyping in patients with surgically treated stage I or II adenocarcinoma of the lung. J Thorac Cardiovasc Surg 97:245, 1989.

Sørensen JB, Badsberg JH, Olsen J: Prognostic factors in inoperable adenocarcinoma of the lung: a multivariate regression analysis of 259 patients. Cancer Res 49:5798, 1989.

Sørensen JB, Hirsch FR, Olsen J: The prognostic implications of histopathologic subtyping of pulmonary adenocarcinoma according to the classification of the World Health Organization. An analysis of 259 consecutive patients with advanced disease. Cancer 62:361, 1988.

Sridhar KS, et al: Clinical features of adenosquamous lung carcinoma in 127 patients. Am Rev Respir Dis 142:19, 1990.

Steele VE, Nettesheim P: Unstable cellular differentiation in adenosquamous cell carcinoma. J Natl Cancer Inst 67:149, 1981.

Takamori S, et al: Clinicopathologic characteristics of adenosquamous carcinoma of the lung. Cancer 67:649, 1991.

The Japan Lung Cancer Society: General rules for clinical and pathological recording of lung cancer. 3rd Ed. Tokyo: Kanehara, 1987.

The World Health Organization: Histologic Typing of Lung Tumors. 2nd Ed. Geneva: World Health Organization, 1981.

The World Health Organization: Histological typing of lung tumours. Am J Clin Pathol 77:123, 1982.

Thomas PA, Piantadosi S, Mountain CF: Should subcarinal lymph nodes be routinely examined in patients with non–small cell lung cancer. J Thorac Cardiovasc Surg 95:883, 1988.

Travis WD: Classification of neuroendocrine tumors of the lung. Lung Cancer 11(Suppl 2):197, 1994.

Travis WD, et al: Neuroendocrine tumors of the lung with proposed criteria for large-cell neuroendocrine carcinoma: An ultrastructural, immunohistochemical, and flow cytometric study of 35 cases. Am J Surg Pathol 15:529, 1991.

Travis WD, et al: Survival analysis of 200 pulmonary neuroendocrine tumors with classification of criteria for atypical carcinoid and its separation from typical carcinoids. Am J Surg Pathol 22:934, 1998a.

Travis WD, et al: Reproducibility of neuroendocrine lung tumor classification. Hum Pathol 29:272, 1998b.

Vallieres E, Waters PF: Incidence of mediastinal node involvement in clinical T$_1$ bronchogenic carcinoma. Can J Surg 30:341, 1987.

van de Molengraft FJJM, et al: OV-TL 12/30 (keratin 7 antibody) is a marker of glandular differentiation in lung cancer. Histopathology 22:35, 1993.

Vincent RG, et al: The changing histopathology of lung cancer: A review of 1682 cases. Cancer 39:1647, 1977.

Warren WH, et al: Neuroendocrine neoplasms of the bronchopulmonary tract: a classification of the spectrum of carcinoid to small cell carcinoma and intervening variants. J Thorac Cardiovasc Surg 89:819, 1985.

Watanabe Y, et al: Mediastinal spread of metastatic lymph nodes in bronchogenic carcinoma. Mediastinal nodal metastases in lung cancer. Chest 97:1059, 1990.

Watanabe Y: Results of surgery for N2 non–small cell lung cancer. J Thorac Cardiovasc Surg 2:85, 1996.

Wick MR, Berg LC, Hertz MI: Large cell carcinoma of the lung with neuroendocrine differentiation: a comparison with large cell "undifferentiated" pulmonary tumors. Am J Clin Pathol 97:796, 1992.

Yesner R: A unified concept of lung cancer. In Proceedings of the Veterans Administration Third Diagnostic Electron Microscopy Conference. Washington, DC: Veterans Administration, 1977, p. 29.

Yesner R: Small cell tumors of the lung. Am J Surg Pathol 7:775, 1983.

Yesner R: Heterogenicity of small cell carcinoma of the lung. In Mountain CF, Carr DT (eds): Lung Cancer: Current Status and Prospects for the Future. Austin: University of Texas Press, 1986, p. 3.

Yesner R: Classification of lung-cancer histology. N Engl J Med 312:652, 1985.

Yesner R, Carter D: Pathology of carcinoma of the lung: Changing patterns. Clin Chest Med 3:257, 1982.

Yesner R, Gerstl B, Auerbach O: Application of the World Health Organization classification of lung carcinoma to biopsy material. Ann Thorac Surg 1:33, 1965.

CHAPTER 96

Clinical Presentation of Lung Cancer

Gail Darling and Carolyn M. Dresler

Lung cancer is the leading cause of cancer deaths in both men and women. The prognosis is related to stage; thus, early detection and treatment are key to improved survival. Unfortunately, most lung cancer is asymptomatic in the early stages. By the time the patient experiences symptoms and seeks medical attention, the disease is often advanced and may be incurable. Based on work reported by Geddes (1979), a 1-cm tumor that is detectable on a plain chest radiograph contains 1 billion cells and represents 30 doublings. Depending on the cell type, that tumor may have been present for 20 years.

The clinical presentation of lung cancer is quite variable, depending on the location of the primary tumor or any metastatic disease, because any body system may be affected. Clinicians must be aware of the many presentations of lung cancer and have a high index of suspicion because of the frequency of this disease. Loeb and associates (1984) reported that 80 to 90% of lung cancer cases are attributed to smoking. Other people at increased risk of developing lung cancer include patients with chronic obstructive pulmonary disease; miners of uranium, gold, asbestos, nickel, and chromium; and people exposed to secondhand smoke, as found by Janerich and colleagues (1990), Repace and Lowery (1985), and Weiss (1986), but no one is immune. The risk of developing lung cancer increases with age, as noted by O'Rourke and Crawford (1987). Several authors, however, including Antkowiak and coworkers (1989), DeCaro and Denfield (1982), Putnam (1977), and Pemberton and associates (1983), have found lung cancer in patients less than 40 years of age and even in patients as young as 19. Wells and Feinstein (1988) and McFarlane and colleagues (1986) have noted a detection bias that favors older male smokers (i.e., these patients are more likely to be evaluated for lung cancer). Younger patients, women, and nonsmokers are more likely to have their symptoms attributed to benign disease, which leads to a delay in diagnosis and possibly adverse affect on outcome. Epidemiologic evidence reported by Risch and colleagues (1993) found that the odds ratio for lung cancer

risk for women who smoked between 30 and 60 pack years was 26.7 versus 11.0 for men. This evidence suggests that women smokers are at increased risk of developing lung cancer for the same level of tobacco consumption.

Of all patients with lung cancer, 5 to 20% are asymptomatic at the time of detection. In patients detected in screening programs up to 60% are asymptomatic. However, in the absence of screening, the majority of patients present with symptoms that may be considered local or bronchopulmonary; locally advanced (e.g., extrapulmonary intrathoracic, metastatic, or paraneoplastic), or nonspecific.

BRONCHOPULMONARY SYMPTOMS

Local or bronchopulmonary symptoms include cough, hemoptysis, wheezing, stridor, chest pain, and dyspnea (Table 96-1). They are often caused by the primary tumor, and their presence does not necessarily preclude curable or resectable disease. However, they may indicate locally advanced (extrapulmonary intrathoracic) or even metastatic disease and should be evaluated carefully.

Cough

Cough is caused by irritation of the bronchial wall by disease within the bronchial lumen or extrinsic compression or invasion of the bronchial wall. Cough is such a common symptom that it is easily dismissed by both doctor and patient. This is especially true in smokers, many of whom experience some daily cough. Cough may be associated with acute respiratory tract infections, bronchiectasis, chronic lung diseases, post-nasal drip, asthma, and gastroesophageal reflux as well as lung cancer. The features of cough that should arouse suspicion are a new cough, change in the nature of the cough, or nocturnal or positional cough, which is typically worse when the patient is recumbent. Smokers who seek medical attention because of cough usually have

Table 96-1. Intrathoracic Signs and Symptoms of Lung Cancer

Cough	29–87%
Hemoptysis	9–57%
Chest pain	6–60%
Dyspnea	3–58%
Wheezing or stridor	2–14%
Hoarseness	1–18%
Pleural effusion	7%
Dysphagia	2%
Superior vena cava syndrome	4–11%
Pancoast's syndrome	3–5%
Phrenic nerve paralysis	1%

Data from Chute et al. (1985), Hyde and Hyde (1974), Rahim and Sarma (1984), Lam et al. (1983), Hopwood et al. (1995), Cohen (1974), LeRoux (1968), and Chernow and Sahn (1977).

experienced a change in their cough because most are so accustomed to their daily cough that they frequently deny its existence. Cough is the most common presenting complaint in patients with lung cancer, occurring in 29 to 87%, as reported by Weiss (1978), Lam (1983), Chute (1985), and Hopwood (1995) and their colleagues, as well as by Hyde and Hyde (1974) and Rahim and Sarma (1984). However, in a review by Irwin and associates (1990), of all patients presenting with cough, less than 2% had lung cancer.

Hemoptysis

Hemoptysis occurs as a presenting symptom in 9 to 57% of patients with lung cancer reported by LeRoux (1968), Hyde and Hyde (1974), and Chute (1985), Lam (1983), and Weiss (1978) and their coworkers. Although Hyde and Hyde (1974) found that it occurs some time in the course of the disease in 43 to 63%, more recent reports indicate that hemoptysis is the presenting complaint in one-fourth of patients. Hemoptysis is less easily ignored by patients and should never be dismissed by doctors. Lung cancer is increasing as a cause of hemoptysis. Santiago and associates (1991) reported that in patients undergoing bronchoscopy for hemoptysis, 29% were found to have lung cancer. Tuberculosis is now a relatively rare cause, occurring in 6% of these patients. Plaza (1995) and Hirshberg (1997) and their colleagues reported similar results. In the presence of a normal chest radiograph, O'Neil and Lazarus (1991), Lederle and associates (1989), and Schraufnagel and Margolis (1990) found that hemoptysis is due to lung cancer in 2.5 to 9% of cases. However, a negative chest radiograph should be followed by a chest CT and bronchoscopy. In 67 patients with a negative chest radiograph and negative bronchoscopy reported by Adelman and colleagues (1985), who were followed for a mean of 38 months, only one patient (<1%) was subsequently found to have lung cancer.

Hemoptysis associated with lung cancer typically varies from minimally blood-streaked sputum to 5 to 30 mL of bloody clot. Massive hemoptysis is more commonly associ-

ated with inflammatory lung diseases but is caused by lung cancer in 20% of cases. Because such massive bleeding is caused by erosion of the tumor into a major vessel, such as the pulmonary artery or even the aorta, Corey and Hla (1987) found that approximately 50% of patients with massive hemoptysis due to lung cancer die compared to 28% from other causes.

Wheezing and Stridor

Wheezing or, less often, stridor, is caused by tumor occluding or compressing a bronchus or trachea. It is a relatively rare presenting symptom of lung cancer, occurring in only 2 to 14% of patients reported by Hyde and Hyde (1974) and Oschner (1956). Wheezing is monophonic and is loudest centrally over the affected airway, compared to asthmatic wheezing, which is polyphonic and is often best appreciated over the lung periphery. These differences are often not clinically appreciated. A diagnosis of adult-onset "asthma" should be viewed with suspicion, particularly if the expected response to bronchodilators is poor.

Stridor is always pathologic and always requires further investigation. Stridor occurs when the lumen of the airway is compromised by more than 75% of the cross-sectional diameter. Stridor is usually associated with tracheal compromise but may occur with bronchial obstruction if central and severe. Stridor may be due to either endobronchial tumor or from extrinsic compressive disease.

Dyspnea

Dyspnea may be caused by primary obstructing tumors causing atelectasis of a lobe or an entire lung or by obstruction of pulmonary artery but more often it is the result of a malignant pleural effusion. It occurs in 3 to 58% of patients reported by Hyde and Hyde (1974) and Chute and colleagues (1985). Less common causes include pericardial effusion, phrenic nerve paralysis, or direct involvement of the diaphragm itself. Piehler and associates (1982) reported that in patients with unilateral diaphragmatic paralysis in whom a cause could be determined, one-third of patients were found to have lung cancer. Patients with postobstructive pneumonia may experience dyspnea but usually have associated cough, fever, and sputum. These patients may also experience pleuritic chest pain. Dyspnea may also be caused by lymphangitic carcinomatosis, tumor, or thromboemboli or rarely by pneumothorax. Pneumothorax is a rare presentation of lung cancer and was found in 0.003% of patients reported by Dines and coworkers (1973). Concurrent disease, such as chronic obstructive lung disease or congestive heart failure, may cause dyspnea unrelated to the tumor. Although some causes of dyspnea are due to local disease, more often it is a symptom of locally advanced or even metastatic disease.

Infectious Symptoms

Lung cancers may cause pulmonary infections with fever, chills, and productive cough, usually from obstruction of a bronchus causing postobstructive pneumonitis or even abscess. More often, symptoms of lung cancer are interpreted as caused by pneumonia or bronchitis and treated as such, and it is only when symptoms or radiographic changes do not resolve that the true etiology of the symptoms is discovered. Similarly, patients with cavitating tumors found on radiographs are frequently treated for lung abscess with similar lack of success.

EXTRAPULMONARY INTRATHORACIC SYMPTOMS

Extrapulmonary intrathoracic symptoms include hoarseness, pain, dysphagia, dyspnea, and the symptoms and signs of Horner's syndrome, Pancoast's syndrome, and superior vena cava (SVC) syndrome. These symptoms suggest locally advanced intrathoracic disease, which require combined modality therapy or complex resections or may be incurable.

Hoarseness

Hoarseness is caused by involvement of the recurrent laryngeal nerve and occurs in 1 to 18% of patients with lung cancer as reported by Hyde and Hyde (1974), Chute and associates (1985), and LeRoux (1968). Most often, the left recurrent nerve is affected during its intrathoracic course, most commonly by lymph node metastases near its origin from the left vagus nerve as it passes through the subaortic space or aortopulmonary window. The presence of hoarseness has been accepted as an indication of inoperability and usually incurability. However, the left recurrent nerve may be involved by the primary tumor, as opposed to lymph node metastases, along its course through the chest, in which case the tumor may be resectable and possibly curable.

The right recurrent laryngeal nerve is less commonly affected by lung cancer but may be involved by a primary apical tumor rather than nodal disease, where it courses around the right subclavian artery, and may be amenable to treatment with curative intent.

Chest Pain

Chest pain may be associated with lung cancer, but it varies, depending on the site of disease. Central tumors may cause vague, dull aching or central or retrosternal pain, whereas peripheral tumors may cause localized pain. Invasion of the pleura typically causes pleuritic pain, whereas constant, gnawing pain occurs with invasion of the inter-costal muscles or ribs. Radicular pain occurs with involvement of intercostal nerves. Involvement of the vertebra, either by the primary tumor or by metastatic disease, causes back or posterior chest pain with or without a radicular component. Pain often indicates locally advanced or metastatic disease; however, intermittent aching pain does not have the same implications as constant, well-localized pain. As reported by Hyde and Hyde (1974) and Chute and colleagues (1985), chest pain is a presenting complaint in 6 to 60% of patients but occurs in 28 to 60% during the course of their illness.

Pleural Effusion

Chernow and Sahn (1977) reported that 7% of patients with bronchial cancer are found to have a pleural effusion at the time of diagnosis. About one-fourth of these patients are asymptomatic. The finding of cancer cells in pleural fluid defines a malignant pleural effusion and indicates a T_4 tumor. One of us (C.D.) and associates (1999) found that in 14% of patients with stage I lung cancer, a lavage of the pleural space at the time of thoracotomy was positive for malignant cells. Kondo (1989, 1993), Buhr (1990), and Okumura (1991) and their colleagues reported similar findings. In an autopsy study reported by Matthews (1976), the pleura was involved in 34 to 67%, with adenocarcinoma and large cell carcinomas having the highest incidence. However, not all pleural effusions in patients with lung cancer are due to involvement of the pleura by tumor. They may be caused by lymphatic obstruction, postobstructive pneumonitis, or atelectasis. The majority of patients with lung cancer and a pleural effusion, however, are found inoperable: 69 of 73 patients in a series reported by Decker and coworkers (1978) and 70 of 78 patients in a series reported by Canto and associates (1985).

Dysphagia

Dysphagia is a rare presenting complaint, but Hyde and Hyde (1974) reported that it occurs in 2 to 6% of patients sometime over the course of their disease, most commonly caused by nodal disease in the subcarinal space compressing or invading the esophagus. Occasionally, it is caused by direct invasion of the esophagus by the primary tumor or by paraesophageal lymph nodes. Progressive growth may lead to the development of a tracheoesophageal fistula, but this is rare compared to that caused by primary esophageal cancer.

Horner's Syndrome

Horner's syndrome, consisting of ptosis, miosis, and anhidrosis on the affected side, is usually associated with a superior sulcus tumor and usually occurs as part of Pancoast's syndrome. It is caused by invasion of the stellate ganglion by the tumor and indicates locally invasive disease.

Pancoast's Syndrome

The uncommon tumors of Pancoast's syndrome, as reported by Miller and associates (1979) and Johnson and Goldberg (1997), occur in 3 to 5% of patients with lung cancer. Pancoast (1932) described the syndrome, which consists of a Horner's syndrome, pain (usually in the shoulder or forearm), and atrophy of the intrinsic muscles of the hand associated with a tumor in the superior sulcus. Symptoms are due to invasion of adjacent structures, including the brachial plexus, particularly the lower cords; hence involvement of structures innervated by C7, C8, and T1. Neural invasion may manifest as weakness and wasting of the intrinsic muscles of the hand. The tumor may invade the adjacent proximal ribs and associated intercostal muscles or adjacent vertebrae. Pain may be due to chest wall invasion, vertebral destruction, or involvement of nerves, either intercostal nerves or the lower cords of the brachial plexus. The location and nature of the pain varies depending on the structures involved. Watson and Evans (1987) reported that the pain is most commonly located in the shoulder, medial forearm, and scapula and less commonly in the fourth and fifth fingers and medial upper arm. Pain in the inner aspect of the arm is due to involvement of the intercostal brachial branch of the second intercostal nerve. Because pain is often the predominant complaint in these patients, they are often first referred to chiropractors, physiotherapists, orthopedic surgeons, or neurosurgeons.

Pancoast's tumors are locally invasive but may be amenable to resection alone or in combination with other therapeutic modalities.

Superior Vena Cava Syndrome

SVC syndrome is usually readily diagnosed by the clinical presentation of the patient. It is caused by obstruction of venous return from the head, neck, and arms. Patients describe tearing and facial swelling initially appearing around the eyes in the morning that regresses over the day but may progress to involve the entire face, resulting in a swollen face with a plethoric complexion. Patients describe a sensation that their head is "full" or "going to burst," dizziness, headaches, and tinnitus. They may also complain of dyspnea and vague, aching chest pain. As time passes, they develop dilated venous collaterals visible on their upper anterior chest wall. Venous hypertension may produce cerebral edema, vascular thrombosis, or hemorrhage. Rarely, extreme edema of the skin may result in the appearance of peau d'orange of the breast. SVC syndrome occurs in 4 to 11% of patients with lung cancer, as reported by Cohen (1974), Hyde and Hyde (1974), Lam (1983), and Chute (1985) and their associates as well as Rahim and Sarma (1984). SVC syndrome was previ-

ously considered a radiation oncology emergency, but there is usually sufficient time to obtain a tissue diagnosis by mediastinoscopy, anterior mediastinotomy, or needle biopsy. Although SVC syndrome is considered a contraindication to mediastinoscopy, it is a relative one, and if necessary, mediastinoscopy can be accomplished safely with attention paid to hemostasis. The correct diagnosis has significant implications because, as reported by Parish (1981) and Bell (1986) and their colleagues, lung cancer causes 65 to 85% of cases, but other malignancies may cause it [e.g., lymphoma or benign diseases, such as fibrosing mediastinitis, thrombosis secondary to indwelling central venous lines, aneurysms, or radiation effects (see Chapter 164)]. Obstruction of the SVC may be caused by either the primary tumor or by nodal disease. It is most often associated with a right upper lobe tumor, most commonly due to small cell lung cancer. Chan and associates (1997) reported that the incidence of SVC syndrome in patients with newly diagnosed small cell lung cancer is 11%. Even if due to non–small cell lung cancer, the presence of SVC syndrome is usually considered a sign of inoperability and, in most cases, incurability. Rarely, patients with involvement of the SVC by primary tumor only may be resected with concomitant resection of the SVC.

METASTATIC DISEASE

The symptoms of metastatic disease are as variable as the potential sites of involvement. The most common sites of metastatic disease are lymph nodes, pleura, lung, brain, spinal cord, liver, adrenal gland, and bones, but any organ system can be involved (Table 96-2). In autopsy series, the

Table 96-2. Frequency (%) of Metastatic Disease at Autopsy

Site	Small Cell	Adeno-carcinoma	Large Cell	Squamous
Hilar or mediastinal lymph nodes	96	80	84	77
Contralateral lung	34	60	34	21
Pericardium	18	25	25	20
Liver	74	41	48	25
Adrenal	55	50	59	23
Bone	37	36	30	20
Central nervous system	29	37	25	18
Meninges	3	10	9	0
Gastrointestinal tract	14	5	20	12
Pancreas	41	12	22	4
Spleen	10	6	13	3
Thyroid	18	2	6	4
Abdominal lymph nodes	52	24	30	10
Skin	0	0	6	0

Modified from Matthews MJ: Problems in morphology and behaviour of bronchopulmonary malignant disease. *In* Israil L, Chahanien P (eds): Lung Cancer: Natural History, Prognosis and Therapy. New York: Academic Press, 1976, p. 23. With permission.

highest incidence of metastatic disease is found with small cell cancer, followed by large cell anaplastic, adenocarcinoma, and squamous cell carcinoma.

Not all metastatic disease is symptomatic. In a series reported by Matthews and coworkers (1973) of autopsy results on patients dying within 1 month of supposedly curative lung cancer surgery, 17% of patients with squamous cell carcinoma were found to have undetected metastases versus 40% of patients with adenocarcinoma. In small cell carcinoma, 80% of patients have metastatic disease at the time of diagnosis. Kato and colleagues (1969) found similar results.

Neurologic Metastases

Merchut (1989) found that symptomatic brain metastases from an unknown primary tumor are most often due to lung cancer. Lung cancer is also the most common tumor to cause extradural spinal cord compression, accounting for 19 to 33% of cases reported by Stark (1982), Kim (1990), and Sørensen (1990) and their associates.

In patients with a new diagnosis of lung cancer, Newman and Hansen (1974) found that 10% have central nervous system (CNS) metastases, most of which are clinically apparent. In a study of 50 asymptomatic patients, however, Jacobs and associates (1977) reported that 6% had occult brain metastases. Meyer and Reach (1953), Galluzzi and Payne (1956), Halpert and colleagues (1960), and Newman and Hansen (1974) report that 15 to 38% of patients develop CNS metastases over the course of the disease. In small cell lung cancer, the incidence of brain metastases at the time of diagnosis is 23%, as reported by Giannone (1987) and Nugent (1979) and their associates and by Pedersen (1986), and up to 80% of patients develop CNS metastases by the time of death. Newman and Hansen (1974) also observed that up to 3% of patients have cord compression at the time of diagnosis, most of whom were found to have small cell lung cancer by Nugent (1979), Pedersen (1985), and Goldman (1989) and their colleagues.

Symptoms of brain metastases are most commonly secondary to increased intracranial pressure (e.g., headache, nausea, diplopia, blurred vision, and changes in level of consciousness or mentation) and are less commonly focal in nature.

Carcinomatous meningitis occurs rarely (<1% at diagnosis) but more commonly with small cell lung cancer. Pedersen (1986) reports that it develops in 5 to 18% of cases during therapy. These patients present with symptoms of changes in mental status, seizures, headache, cranial neuropathies, weakness or sensory changes, bowel or bladder dysfunction, or back pain but have a normal computed tomographic (CT) scan of the brain. Cerebrospinal fluid (CSF) cytology is usually diagnostic. Magnetic resonance imaging is often helpful in confirming the diagnosis.

Vertebral metastases extending into the epidural space are the most common cause of extradural spinal cord compression. Bach and colleagues (1992) report that metastases occur in the thoracic spine in more than two thirds of cases. They also found that in a series of consecutive lung cancer patients with spinal metastases, 40% had small cell lung cancer, 26% had adenocarcinoma, and 18% had squamous cell carcinoma. Rarely, tumors may extend through the neural foramen, causing cord compression without vertebral destruction. The first symptom is back pain in 95% of patients. Rodichok and colleagues (1981) found that patients presenting with back pain, a normal neurological examination, and demonstrable vertebral body destruction on radiography have an incidence of spinal cord compression in more than 50%. The radiographic changes may be minimal or absent, however, as reported by Schiff and coworkers (1997). Neurologic findings, such as weakness, sensory loss, and bowel and bladder dysfunction, are late findings.

It must be remembered, however, that neurologic symptoms in lung cancer patients may be due to causes other than metastatic disease (Table 96-3). Thus, metastasis must be confirmed by the appropriate studies.

Bone Metastases

Hyde and Hyde (1974) found that bone pain due to metastases is a presenting symptom in 22% of patients, but metastases were present in the autopsy series reported by Matthews and associates (1973) in up to 37% of cases. The most common sites involved are the spine (70%), pelvis (40%), and femur (25%). Most metastases are osteolytic, but Beer and colleagues (1964) observed that osteoblastic lesions may occur in small cell or adenocarcinoma. Lesions occurring in the juxta-articular bone or synovium may present as arthritis. In cases presenting as arthritis, Murray and Persellin (1980) report finding malignant cells in the joint effusion.

Table 96-3. Etiology of Neurologic Symptoms Associated with Metastasis

Central nervous system metastases
Spinal cord compression secondary to epidural or vertebral metastases
Leptomeningeal carcinomatosis
Hyponatremia secondary to syndrome of inappropriate antidiuretic hormone
Hypercalcemia
Embolic infarction secondary to marantic endocarditis
Embolic infarction secondary to tumor emboli
Thrombotic infarction secondary to disseminated intravascular coagulation or superior sagittal sinus thrombosis
Intracranial hemorrhage due to coagulopathy secondary to tumor or treatment (chemotherapy)
Central nervous system infections
Paraneoplastic syndromes

Liver

Liver metastases are rarely symptomatic and are usually detected on staging CT scan. Sparup and colleagues (1990) reported occult liver metastases in 5% of patients with presumed operable disease. But in small cell lung cancer, Mirvis and coworkers (1987) reported that 26% of patients have liver metastases at the time of initial staging. In autopsy series, Matthews and associates (1973) and Hyde and Hyde (1974) found that 25 to 48% of patients with non–small cell lung cancer and 78% of those with small cell lung cancer have liver metastases. Liver metastases may present with anorexia and abdominal pain, but as the disease progresses, patients may develop jaundice, ascites, hepatomegaly, and liver failure. However, the last four findings occur very late and are unusual.

Adrenal Glands

Adrenal metastases are usually asymptomatic unless more than 90% of the gland is replaced. Metastases tend to occur in the medulla, causing symptoms of Addison's disease. Lung cancer is the most common tumor that causes adrenal dysfunction. With routine CT scanning, adrenal enlargement or masses are detected more frequently. The incidence of adrenal enlargement in patients with presumed operable lung cancer varies from 4.1%, reported by Ettinghausen and Burt (1991), to 7.5%, reported by Oliver and colleagues (1984), and up to 15%, as reported by Dunnick and coworkers (1979). However, Oliver and associates (1984) and Ettinghausen and Burt (1991) found that only approximately one-half of the adrenal abnormalities identified on CT are proved to be due to metastatic disease. The sensitivity of CT scanning in detecting adrenal metastases has been reported at only 40%, based on a study by Allard and colleagues (1990) of patients having a CT within 90 days of death from lung cancer. However, Silverman and colleagues (1993) found that once an adrenal lesion is detected, CT-guided needle biopsy has an accuracy of 96%. At autopsy, Matthews and associates (1973), Hansen (1983), and Karolyi (1990) found that 23 to 55% of patients have adrenal metastases.

Other Sites

Reingold (1966) reported that skin and soft tissue metastases occur in 1% of patients, and Matthews and colleagues (1973) found them in 6% of patients at autopsy. Matthews (1973) and Bisel (1953) and their associates, as well as Adenle and Edwards (1982), noted that cardiac metastases are found in 8 to 30% of patients in autopsy series. Series reported by Matthews (1973), Burbige (1980), and Winchester (1977) and their coworkers and by Morton and Tedesco (1974), found intra-abdominal metastases in stomach (2 to 4%), intestine (5 to 33%), spleen (3 to 13%), pancreas (4 to 41%), and intra-abdominal lymph nodes (10 to 52%). Renal metastases are identified in 15 to 28% of cases. Other endocrine organ metastases, including thyroid, parathyroid, and pituitary, also occur (1 to 6%) and, as with other organ sites, the incidence with small cell lung cancer is higher (10 to 41%).

PARANEOPLASTIC SYNDROMES

Paraneoplastic syndromes refer to those remote effects of a tumor not due to direct invasion or metastases. They occur in 10 to 20% of patients with lung cancer and are most commonly associated with small cell lung cancer. Some syndromes are due to the secretion of biologically active peptides or antibodies, but others are still unexplained. The paraneoplastic syndromes may be categorized as endocrine-metabolic, neurologic, skeletal, hematologic, dermatologic, and miscellaneous (Table 96-4).

Endocrine-Metabolic

The best-recognized endocrine syndromes are hypercalcemia, the syndrome of inappropriate antidiuretic hormone (SIADH), and Cushing's syndrome (Table 96-5). Less common endocrine abnormalities include gynecomastia secondary to secretion of beta–human chorionic gonadotropin, carcinoid syndrome, galactorrhea secondary to prolactin, excess growth hormone, increased calcitonin, increased thyroid-stimulating hormone, and hyper- or hypoglycemia.

Syndrome of Inappropriate Antidiuretic Hormone

The symptoms of SIADH include nausea, altered mental status, confusion, and lethargy progressing to coma. These symptoms occur in 1 to 27% of patients, as reported by Lees (1975), Odell and Wolfsen (1978), Fichman and Bethune (1974), and Bliss (1990) and List (1986) and their associates. However, elevated levels of ADH (arginine vasopressin) have been detected in 70% or more of patients with lung cancer, depending on the technique of measurement. De Troyer and Demanet (1976) and List and colleagues (1986) found that SIADH is more common in small cell lung cancer, which accounts for 75% of all tumors associated with SIADH, and in women (Table 96-6). SIADH also occurs in association with infectious processes, such as empyema, other tumors, drugs, and CNS disorders. The diagnosis is based on the findings of hyponatremia, inappropriately elevated urine osmolality in the presence of low serum osmolality, and increased urinary sodium. Shimizu and colleagues (1991) reported that SIADH may be associated with ectopic production of atrial natriuretic factor, and Bliss and coworkers (1990) identified the gene for atrial natriuretic factor in small cell lung cancer cells and tumor cell lines.

Table 96-4. Paraneoplastic Syndromes in Lung Cancer Patients

Metabolic
    Hypercalcemia
    Cushing's syndrome
    Inappropriate antidiuretic hormone production
    Carcinoid syndrome
    Gynecomastia
    Hypercalcitoninemia
    Elevated growth hormone level
    Elevated prolactin, follicle-stimulating hormone, luteinizing
        hormone levels
    Hypoglycemia
    Hyperthyroidism
Neurologic
    Encephalopathy
    Subacute cerebellar degeneration
    Peripheral neuropathy
    Polymyositis
    Autonomic neuropathy
    Lambert-Eaton syndrome
    Opsoclonus and myoclonus
Skeletal
    Clubbing
    Pulmonary hypertrophic osteoarthropathy
Hematologic
    Anemia
    Leukemoid reactions
    Thrombocytosis
    Thrombocytopenia
    Eosinophilia
    Pure red cell aplasia
    Leukoerythroblastosis
    Disseminated intravascular coagulation
Cutaneous and muscular
    Hyperkeratosis
    Dermatomyositis
    Acanthosis nigricans
    Hyperpigmentation
    Erythema gyratum repens
    Hypertrichosis lanuginosa acquisita
Other
    Nephrotic syndrome
    Hypouricemia
    Secretion of vasoactive intestinal peptide with diarrhea
    Hyperamylasemia
    Anorexia-cachexia

Table 96-5. Frequency of Paraneoplastic Endocrine Syndromes

Syndrome of inappropriate antidiuretic hormone	1–27%
Hypercalcemia	1.0–12.5%
Cushing's syndrome	2–6%
Elevated β–human chorionic gonadotropin level	0.5–2.0%

(1981) reported hypercalcemia in only 3% of patients with small cell lung cancer. Most cases of small cell cancer with hypercalcemia are associated with bone or bone marrow metastases.

The symptoms of hypercalcemia include nausea, constipation, anorexia, polydipsia, polyuria, irritability, or lethargy and confusion. Examination of the patient may reveal decreased deep tendon reflexes, cardiac dysrhythmias, decreased level of consciousness, or coma. The treatment of hypercalcemia has improved with the use of biphosphonates, but Campbell and associates (1991) found that the prognosis for lung cancer patients with associated hypercalcemia is poor, with a median survival of 30 to 45 days, unless the tumor is resectable.

Hypocalcemia may occur with osteoblastic metastases but is rarely symptomatic. It is associated with elevated levels of calcitoninlike hormone.

Ectopic Adrenocorticotropic Hormone

Ectopic adrenocorticotropic hormone or corticotropin-releasing hormone production causes 15 to 20% of cases of Cushing's syndrome, of which one-half are associated with small cell lung cancer, as reported by Howlett and colleagues (1986). Gropp (1980) and Howlett (1986) and their associates reported that fewer than 2% of lung cancer patients have symptoms of Cushing's syndrome, although 70% have elevated levels of corticotropin. Cushing's syndrome is most often associated with small cell lung cancer, but Richardson (1978), Shepherd (1992), and Delisle (1993) and their coinvestigators, as well as Lees (1975), noted that it occurs in only 0.8 to 6% of these patients. Hypokalemic alkalosis is present, but Odell and Wolfsen (1978) observed that the clinical course of these patients is so fulminant that patients rarely have the physical stigmata of hypercortisolism.

Hypercalcemia

Hypercalcemia occurs in 10.0 to 12.5% of all patients with lung cancer and most frequently is caused by bone metastases, but Cryer and Kissaine (1979) and Bender and Hansen (1974) found that 10 to 15% of cases are caused by secretion of parathyroid hormone–related protein. Mundy (1989) reported that, rarely, other substances may cause hypercalcemia, including interleukin-1, tumor necrosis factor, transforming growth factor-α, lymphotoxin, and prostaglandins of the E series. In contrast to all the other paraneoplastic syndromes, it is more common with squamous cell lung cancer and is rare in small cell lung cancer (see Table 96-6). Hayward and coworkers

Table 96-6. Frequency of Paraneoplastic Endocrine Syndromes Relative to Cell Type of Lung Cancer

	Small cell	Adenocarcinoma/ large cell	Squamous cell
Cushing's syndrome	+++	±	±
Syndrome of inappropriate antidiuretic hormone	++++	±	±
Tumor hypercalcemia	+	+	++++
Gynecomastia	++	+	±

Ectopic Gonadotropin Production

Gonadotropin production has been recorded in some men with tender gynecomastia; the gynecomastia is often associated with hypertrophic pulmonary osteoarthropathy (HPO). Faiman and associates (1967) documented increased levels of gonadotropin in the blood after passage through a lung containing a bronchial carcinoma; increased gonadotropic activity was also noted in the tumor tissue in this case. Gonadotropin is produced by all types of lung tumor cells, but clinically, gynecomastia is seen most often in patients with small cell lung cancers.

Musculoskeletal Syndromes

HPO is found in 2 to 12% of patients with lung cancer reported by Lam (1983) and Stenseth (1967) and their associates, as well as by Yacoub (1965). It is more common in adenocarcinoma but is rare in small cell lung cancer. Patients experience pain affecting the long bones and joints and may have clubbing of the fingers and toes.

The most common bones affected are the tibia, radius, ulna, and fibula, but the femur, humerus, metacarpals, and metatarsals may also be affected. The bone pain is due to symmetric, proliferating periostitis of the distal ends of the long bones. On examination, there is tenderness and swelling over the affected bones, and the pain may improve when the patient is placed in Trendelenburg's position. Schumacher (1976) reported that the associated polyarthritis and synovitis are similar to rheumatoid arthritis, are usually symmetric, and affect the knees, ankles, elbows, and wrists. Fever and toxicity may be present.

The bone scan in affected patients shows symmetric, markedly increased uptake in typical locations secondary to osteoid deposition along the inner aspect of the periosteum (Fig. 96-1). Plain radiographs show periosteal elevation with new bone formation (Fig. 96-2). The clinical presentation, bone scan, and radiographs are sufficient to make the diagnosis and should not be confused with metastatic disease.

Clubbing may occur alone. Hyde and Hyde (1974) and LeRoux (1968) found clubbing in 21% of patients with lung cancer at the time of diagnosis (Fig. 96-3). It also occurs in patients with cyanotic heart disease and in chronic lung diseases. Thus the presence of clubbing, although it may raise the suspicion of lung cancer, is not pathognomonic of the disease. HPO is almost always associated with lung cancer but rarely may occur in patients with chronic lung disease, such as bronchiectasis, tuberculosis, or lung abscess and with various pleural tumors (see Chapter 64). It is unusual to see these conditions today of such chronicity and severity as to produce associated clubbing, but when it does occur, it develops more slowly and is much less painful than that associated with lung cancer.

HPO may precede the discovery of cancer by months and may lead to the discovery of the tumor. The etiology of HPO

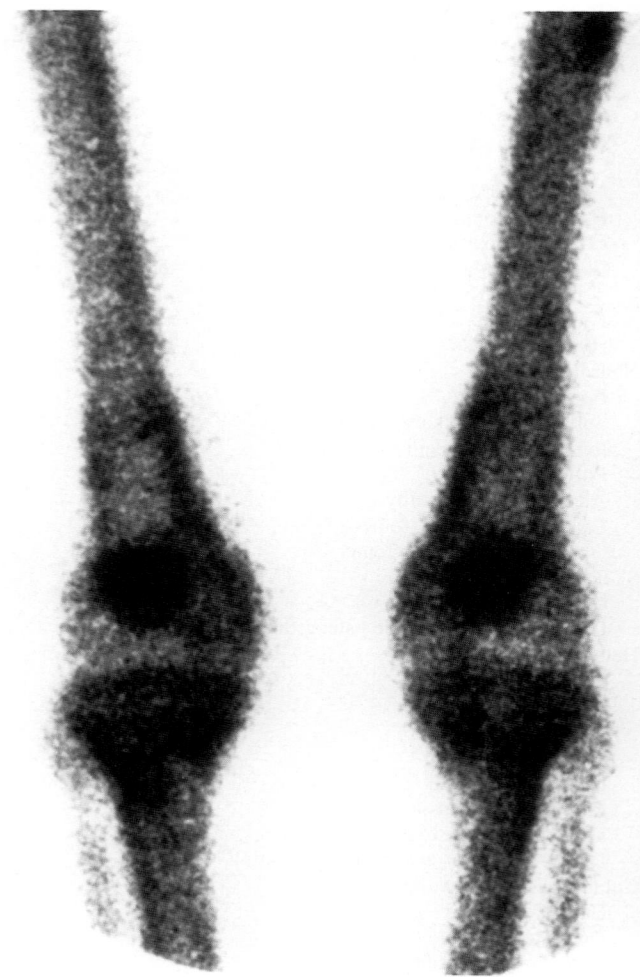

Fig. 96-1. Bone scan of a patient with lung cancer illustrating the classic appearance of symmetric increased uptake of the radioisotope in the periosteum of the distal femur and proximal tibia.

is not known but may be related to secretion of estrogens or growth factor or due to vagal stimulation or other neural signals (see Chapter 64). Knowles and Smith (1960) found that resection of the tumor results in resolution of HPO. In unresectable tumors, Carroll and Doyle (1974) report that vagotomy has been useful in relieving the pain due to HPO.

Neuromuscular Syndromes

The neuromuscular syndromes are the most common paraneoplastic syndromes but are usually underdiagnosed. Croft and Wilkinson (1965) reported that 16% of patients with lung cancer have a paraneoplastic neuromuscular syndrome and that more than one-half of these are associated with small cell lung cancer. They are more common late in the course of disease and are rare at the time of presentation, although they may predate the diagnosis of lung cancer by months or years. The neuromuscular syndrome does not

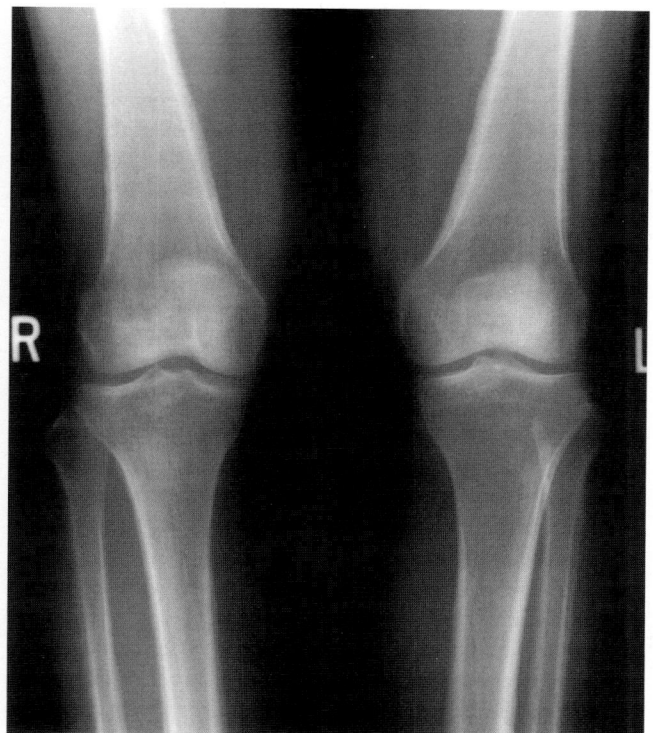

Fig. 96-2. Radiograph of the distal femur of a patient with lung cancer presenting with hypertrophic pulmonary osteoarthropathy, illustrating periosteal elevation and new bone formation.

necessarily respond to treatment of the lung tumor, although some may respond to steroids. These syndromes may affect the CNS or peripheral nerves or muscles. Neuropathies, other than pure motor neuropathies, are most common. The symptoms of these syndromes may mimic those due to metastatic disease or electrolyte abnormalities, such as

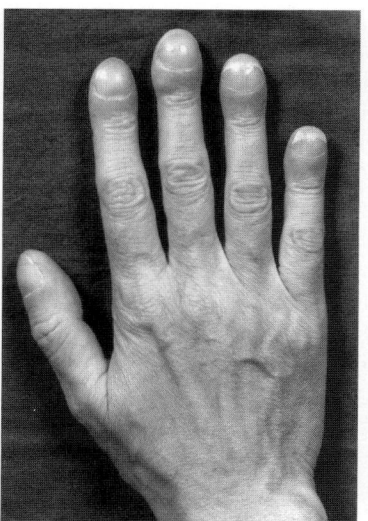
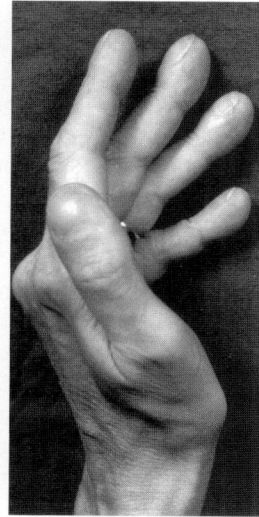

Fig. 96-3. Hands of patient with lung cancer illustrating clubbing, with increased nail base angle to 180 degrees and fusiform enlargement of the distal digit ("drumstick fingers").

hypercalcemia or hyponatremia. In contrast to neurologic deficits caused by metastatic disease, paraneoplastic syndromes present with several symmetric deficits involving different parts of the nervous system.

These syndromes are thought to be due to the secretion of brain-gut peptides, as reported by Gropp and associates (1980), or due to autoantibodies. Bell and Seltharam (1979) found that small cell lung cancer cells share antigens with neural tissue. The antineuronal nuclear antibody type I (ANNA-1) or anti-Hu selectively bind to neuronal elements. Moll and colleagues (1990) and Wilkinson and Zeronski (1965) reported that ANNA-1 has been identified in the serum and spinal fluid of patients with small cell lung cancer and sensory neuropathies or encephalomyelitis. Antineuronal antibodies were identified in 38% of patients with paraneoplastic syndromes.

In a study of 162 patients who were positive for ANNA-1, Lucchinetti and coworkers (1998) reported that 142 had cancer (88%), 132 of whom had small cell lung cancer. Pathologic studies reported by Antoine (1998) and Eggers (1998) and their associates found demyelination, axonal degeneration, microvasculitis, and inflammation. Anderson (1989) reported that anti-Purkinje cell or anti-Yo antibodies have been identified in patients with cerebellar degeneration (Table 96-7).

The CNS syndromes include cortical cerebellar degeneration, subacute or spinal cerebellar degeneration, dementia, limbic encephalitis, internuclear ophthalmoplegia, and cancer-associated retinopathy (CAR). These may present alone or as part of a wider neurologic disorder called *paraneoplastic encephalomyelitis*. The peripheral manifestations include sensory or sensorimotor polyneuropathy, subacute necrotic myelopathy, autonomic and gastrointestinal neuropathy, dermatomyositis or polymyositis, and Lambert-Eaton syndrome (Table 96-8).

Patients with cortical cerebellar degeneration develop intention tremor, ataxia, vertigo, and dysarthria (which is rapidly progressive and develops over a few weeks). Hyde and Hyde (1974) reported that neurologic findings are symmetric. CSF and CT scans are normal. Morton and colleagues (1966) and Anderson (1989) report that at autopsy, there is degeneration of the cerebellar Purkinje's cells and brainstem nuclei. A subacute presentation of cerebellar dysfunction, termed *spinal cerebellar degeneration*, was reported by Brain and Wilkinson (1965) and is associated with weakness, muscle wasting, and paresthesia. There are no changes in higher cortical function.

Brennan and Craddock (1983) reported that limbic encephalitis may present with dementia, inappropriate affect, psychosis, loss of short- and long-term memory, depression, agitation, hallucinations, and seizures but no focal abnormalities. The CSF may show elevated protein and cell count, but cytology is negative for malignant cells, thus differentiating it from meningeal carcinomatosis. The electroencephalogram shows focal involvement of the temporal lobes, as does magnetic resonance imaging. Anderson (1989) reported that

Table 96-7. Autoantibodies Associated with Neurologic Paraneoplastic Syndromes and Lung Cancer[a]

Syndrome	Tumor	Antibody	Antigen
Encephalomyelitis and sensory neuropathy	SCLC	Anti-Hu	35- to 40-kD neuronal nucleoprotein found throughout the CNS
Subacute cerebellar degeneration	Lung	Anti-Yo	34- to 40-kD protein in Purkinje cell cytoplasm (ribosomes and granular endoplasmic reticulum)
Cancer-associated retinopathy	SCLC	Cancer-associated retinopathy autoantibodies	23-kD retinal nuclear protein in both rods and cones
Opsoclonus and myoclonus	SCLC	Anti-Ri[b]	55- and 75-kD nuclear proteins
Lambert-Eaton syndrome	SCLC	Anti-VGCC	VGCCs on presynaptic membrane of peripheral cholinergic nerve terminals

CNS, central nervous system; SCLC, small cell lung cancer; VGCC, voltage-gated calcium channels.
[a]See original report for reference.
[b]Has not been identified in patients with SCLC to date.
From Richardson GE, Johnson BE: Paraneoplastic syndromes in lung cancer. Curr Opin Oncol 4:323, 1992. With permission.

it is associated with the presence of ANNA-1 or anti-Hu. However, Alamowitch and associates (1997) found that only 50% of patients with small cell lung cancer and limbic encephalitis have antibodies to Hu. Autopsy findings reported by Corsellis and colleagues (1968) include degenerative changes and inflammation in the limbic system. It is almost always associated with small cell lung cancer.

CAR presents with photosensitivity, ring scotomata, and rapid loss of binocular vision. It is usually associated with small cell lung cancer but is rare even in these patients. Similarly, internuclear ophthalmoplegia has been reported only in patients with small cell lung cancer. Thirkell (1989) and Jacobson (1990) and their coworkers reported that CAR may be related to an autoantibody to a photoreceptor protein.

The peripheral neurologic manifestations include sensorimotor and isolated sensory neuropathy, as reported by Horwich (1977) and Croft (1977) and their associates. Isolated motor neuropathy does not occur. In the more common sensorimotor neuropathy, patients present with distal sensory loss and lower extremity weakness, which may progress to paralysis and areflexia. Ataxia may occur. Mancall and Rosales (1964) reported on a combined motor and sensory loss, which ascends rapidly to the thoracic level, associated with lung cancer; it is termed *subacute necrotic myelopathy*. It is rapidly fatal over days to weeks. Destruction of gray and white matter is found at autopsy. Isolated sensory neuropathy may occur and is associated with degeneration in the dorsal root ganglia with loss of proprioception and reflexes. Paresthesias do not follow the distribution of a single nerve. In isolated sensory neuropathy, muscle strength is normal, as is motor nerve conduction velocity. The symptoms in these syndromes may vary over time. CSF protein is elevated. ANNA-1 has been detected in both sera and CSF of patients with peripheral neuropathies, including necrotizing myelopathy, as reported by Schuller-Petrovic (1983), Dalmau (1990), and Altermatt (1991) and their colleagues.

Muscle weakness may be secondary to a carcinomatous myopathy. Croft and Wilkinson (1965) and Wilkinson and Zeronski (1965) found that these occur in 6.4% of lung cancer patients and are strongly associated with small cell lung cancer. In patients with carcinomatous myopathy, Morton and coworkers (1966) reported that 56% had small cell lung cancer. Myopathies are divided into myositis, in which there is primary degeneration of the muscle fibers, and myasthenic-like syndrome, in which the defect is in neuromuscular transmission. Both myopathies are characterized by proximal muscle weakness, with the thigh and pelvic girdle muscles most severely affected. Muscle wasting is more prominent in myositis. The most well-known syndrome is Lambert-Eaton myasthenic syndrome, which is usually associated with small cell lung cancer, whereas myositis may be seen with all histologies of lung cancer.

The myasthenic syndrome presents with weakness and fatigability of proximal muscles but differs from myasthenia gravis in that muscle strength improves with exercise. First described by Lambert and colleagues (1956), patients with this syndrome may experience blurred vision, ptosis, dysarthria, and autonomic dysfunction. Elrington and associates (1991) found that it is present at the time of diagnosis in 1% of patients with small cell lung cancer. Spiro and colleagues (1991) noted that 44% of patients with small cell lung cancer had neuromuscular or autonomic defects, and there was an overall prevalence of Lambert-Eaton syndrome of 3%. Clamon (1984) and Chalk (1990) and their associates found that there is a poor response to anticholinesterase inhibitors and a variable response to antitumor therapy.

Table 96-8. Paraneoplastic Neuromuscular Syndromes

Limbic encephalitis
Cortical cerebellar degeneration
Spinal cerebellar degeneration
Dementia
Subacute necrotic myelopathy
Peripheral neuropathies (cranial nerves, sensory-motor, sensory)
Cancer-associated retinopathy
Internuclear ophthalmoplegia
Autonomic neuropathy
Gastrointestinal neuropathy
Polymyositis or dermatomyositis
Lambert-Eaton syndrome

McEnvoy and associates (1989) reported that 3,4-diaminopyridine in doses up to 100 mg per day may be effective in treating this syndrome. Antibodies to the voltage-gated calcium channels and synaptotagmin of the peripheral cholinergic nerve terminals have been implicated in this syndrome by Roberts (1985) and Takamori (1995) and their coworkers, as well as by Lennon and Lambert (1989). Lennon and Lambert implicate a specific subtype of voltage-gated calcium channel that is labeled by ⍵-conotoxin.

Polymyositis is characterized by muscle weakness and wasting, most marked in the extensors of the arm, associated with an elevated sedimentation rate and necrosis on muscle biopsy, as described by DeVere and Bradley (1976). Sigurgeirsson and colleagues (1992) have suggested an association between polymyositis-dermatomyositis and lung cancer, but this was not supported by work done by Lakhanpal and associates (1986). Whether a blind search for an underlying malignancy is justified in a patient with newly diagnosed dermatomyositis is controversial. A report by Callen (1982) suggests that 90% of associated malignancies are not found by a blind search but become apparent over the course of the disease.

Autonomic and gastrointestinal dysfunction may also occur. Schuffler and colleagues (1983) reported intestinal pseudo-obstruction (Ogilvie's syndrome) in association with small cell lung cancer and found degeneration of the myenteric plexus, lymphocytic infiltration, and neuronal loss. Lennon and associates (1991) found enteric antineuronal antibodies in association with Ogilvie's syndrome. Roberts and colleagues (1997) reported finding granulomatous inflammation centered on the myenteric plexus and nerves. Ahmed and Carpenter (1975) reported that postural hypotension, neurogenic bladder, excessive sweating, and ejaculatory dysfunction may be associated with lung cancer.

Hematologic and Vascular Abnormalities

Hematologic abnormalities associated with lung cancer are common and generally occur late in the course of the disease. Zucker and coworkers (1974) reported that the most common of these is a normochromic, normocytic anemia occurring in 20% of lung cancer patients secondary to decreased iron use and blocking of reticuloendothelial iron release. There is moderate shortening of red cell survival. Investigations show decreased serum iron, decreased total iron-binding capacity, and increased marrow iron stores. Even more common is thrombocytosis, which was reported in 60% of lung cancer patients in a paper by Silvis and colleagues (1970). Less common abnormalities include sideroblastic anemia, hemolytic anemia, red cell aplasia, erythrocytosis, leukoerythroblastic changes, granulocytic or eosinophilic leukemoid reactions, eosinophilia, thrombocytopenia, idiopathic thrombocytopenic purpura, and disseminated intravascular coagulation.

Thrombophlebitis occurs in 1% of patients with lung cancer and predates the malignancy in one-third of cases. It is typically resistant to treatment with warfarin but responds to heparin. Recurrent or migratory thrombophlebitis or unusual sites of thrombophlebitis, such as inferior vena cava, jugular vein, or arm veins, should raise the suspicion of an underlying malignancy. Of all cases of thrombophlebitis, Sack and associates (1977) reported that 3% are related to cancer. Thromboses may be recurrent or simultaneous, as reported by Byrd and colleagues (1967). Several mechanisms may contribute to the development of deep venous thrombosis in cancer patients, including thrombocytosis, platelet activation, dysfibrinogenemia, and release of procoagulant substances from the tumor.

Nonbacterial thrombotic endocarditis is present in 7% of patients with carcinoma of the lung at autopsy, reported by Fayemi and Deppisch (1979) and Rosen and Armstrong (1973). It is more common with adenocarcinoma. Patients usually have advanced disease and present with symptoms of systemic emboli. Less than one-third of patients have systolic murmurs, and few are febrile. McDonald and Robbins (1957) found that the vegetations are small and are difficult to diagnose with echocardiography.

Embolic disease in lung cancer patients may be due to thromboemboli from venous sources or systemic emboli from marantic endocarditis or from tumor emboli. Tumor emboli typically affect the pulmonary and cerebral circulation. Goldhaber and colleagues (1987) found that the tumor was the source of embolism in 23% of patients with solid tumors dying from pulmonary embolism.

Dermatologic Manifestations of Lung Cancer

Many skin conditions are associated with lung cancer, including dermatomyositis, erythema gyratum, lanuginosa acquisita, acanthosis nigricans, pruritus, tylosis, urticaria, angioedema, acquired ichthyosis, Bazex's disease, Leser-Trelat syndrome, pachydermoperiostosis, hyperpigmentation, scleroderma, and exfoliative dermatitis. The onset of these conditions is more rapid when associated with malignancy. Dermatomyositis, erythema gyratum, and lanuginosa acquisita are frequently associated with cancer, and the presence of these conditions should arouse the suspicion of malignant disease.

Barnes (1976) reported that 7 to 50% of patients with dermatomyositis have an associated malignancy. A blind search for malignancy is not generally recommended, however. Most cancers are suspected based on history, although on average, the skin condition precedes the diagnosis of cancer by 6 months. It is more common with adenocarcinoma than other lung cancers.

Miscellaneous

Other paraneoplastic syndromes include renal paraneoplastic syndromes, the most common of which is nephrotic syndrome. da Costa and colleagues (1974) found that nephrotic syndrome is most commonly due to membranous glomerulonephritis with subepithelial and capillary deposits of immunoglobulin G. There may be glomerular deposition of antigen-antibody complexes. Moorthy (1983) reported that the renal abnormalities often respond to treatment of the lung tumor.

Other common symptoms occurring in lung cancer patients are anorexia, fatigue, and weight loss. These symptoms usually occur late in the course of disease but are often unexplained based on known sites of disease and disease burden. Nevertheless, 10 to 33% of patients report these symptoms at the time of their first assessment.

REFERENCES

Adelman M, et al: Cryptogenic hemoptysis clinical features, bronchoscopic findings and natural history in 67 patients. Ann Intern Med 102:829, 1985.

Adenle AD, Edwards JE: Clinical and pathological features of metastatic neoplasms of the pericardium. Chest 81:166, 1982.

Ahmed MN, Carpenter S: Autonomic neuropathy and carcinoma of the lung. Can Med Assoc J 113:410, 1975.

Alamowitch S, et al: Limbic encephalitis and small cell lung cancer: clinical and immunologic features. Brain 120:923, 1997.

Allard P, et al: Sensitivity and specificity of computed tomography for the detection of adrenal metastatic lesions among 91 autopsied lung cancer patients. Cancer 66:457, 1990.

Altermatt HJ, et al: Paraneoplastic anti-Purkinje and type I anti neuronal nuclear auto antibodies bind selectively to central, peripheral and autonomic nervous system cells. Lab Invest 65:412, 1991.

Anderson NE: Antineuronal autoantibodies and neurological paraneoplastic syndromes. Aust N Z J Med 19:379, 1989.

Antkowiak JG, Regal AM, Takita H: Bronchogenic carcinoma in patients under age 40. Ann Thorac Surg 47:391, 1989.

Antoine JG, et al: Paraneoplastic demyelinating neuropathy, subacute sensory neuropathy and anti-Hu antibodies, clinicopathological study of an autopsy case. Muscle Nerve 21:850, 1998.

Bach F, et al: Metastatic spinal cord compression secondary to lung cancer. J Clin Oncol 10:1781, 1992.

Barnes BE: Dermatomyositis and malignancy: a review of the literature. Ann Intern Med 84:68, 1976.

Beer OT, Dubowy J, Jimenez FA: Osteoblastic metastases from bronchogenic carcinoma. AJR Am J Roentgenol 91:161, 1964.

Bell CE, Seltharam S: Expression of endodermally derived and neural crest derived differentiation antigens by human lung and color tumors. Cancer 44:12, 1979.

Bell DR, Woods RL, Levi JA: Superior vena caval obstruction: a ten year experience. Med J Aust 145:566, 1986

Bender RA, Hansen H: Hypercalcemia in bronchogenic carcinoma. A prospective study of 200 patients. Ann Intern Med 80:205, 1974

Bisel FH, Wroblewski F, Ladue SJ: Incidence and clinical manifestations of cardiac metastases. JAMA 153:712, 1953.

Bliss DP, et al: Expression of the atrial natriuretic factor gene in small cell lung cancer tumors and tumor cell lines. J Natl Cancer Inst 82:305, 1990.

Brain L, Wilkinson M: Subacute cerebellar degeneration associated with neoplasms. Brain 88:465, 1965.

Brennan LV, Craddock PR: Limbic encephalopathy as a non metastatic complication of oat cell lung cancer. Am J Med 75:518, 1983.

Buhr J, et al: Tumor cells in intraoperative pleural lavage. An indicator for poor prognosis of bronchogenic carcinoma. Cancer 65:1801, 1990.

Burbige EJ, Radigan N, Belber JP: Metastatic lung carcinoma involving the gastrointestinal track. Am J Gastroenterol 74:504, 1980.

Byrd RB, Divertie MB, Spittell JA: Bronchogenic carcinoma and thromboembolic disease. JAMA 202:1019, 1967.

Callen JP: The value of malignancy evaluation in patients with dermatomyositis. J Am Acad Dermatol 6:253, 1982.

Campbell JH, et al: Symptomatic hypercalcemia in lung cancer. Respir Med 85:223,1991.

Canto A, et al: Lung cancer and pleural effusions: clinical significance and study of pleural metastatic locations. Chest 87:649, 1985.

Carroll KB, Doyle L: A common factor in hypertrophic osteoarthropathy. Thorax 29:262, 1974.

Chalk CH, et al: Response of the Lambert Eaton myasthenic syndrome to treatment of associated small cell lung carcinoma. Neurology 40:1552, 1990.

Chan RH, et al: Superior vena cava obstruction in small cell lung cancer. Int J Radiat Oncol Biol Phys 38:513, 1997.

Chernow B, Sahn S: Carcinomatous involvement of the pleura: an analysis of 96 patients. Am J Med 63:695, 1977.

Chute CG, et al: Presenting condition of 1539 population based lung cancer patients by cell type and stage in New Hampshire and Vermont. Cancer 56:2107, 1985.

Clamon GH, et al: Myasthenic syndrome and small cell cancer of the lung. Arch Intern Med 144:999, 1984.

Cohen MH: Signs and symptoms of bronchogenic carcinoma. Semin Oncol 1:183, 1974.

Corey R, Hla KM: Major and massive hemoptysis: reassessment of conservative management. Am J Med Sci 294:301, 1987.

Corsellis JAN, Goldberg GH, Norton AR: Limbic encephalitis and its association with carcinoma. Brain 91:481, 1968.

Croft PB, Urich H, Wilkinson M: Peripheral neuropathy of the sensorimotor type associated with malignant disease. Brain 90:31, 1977.

Croft PB, Wilkinson M: The incidence of carcinomatous neuromyopathy in patients with various types of carcinoma. Brain 88:427, 1965.

Cryer PE, Kissaine JM: Clinicopathologic conference: malignant hypercalcemia. Am J Med 65:486, 1979.

da Costa RC, et al: Nephrotic syndrome in bronchogenic carcinoma: report of two cases with immunochemical studies. Clin Nephrol 2:245, 1974.

Dalmau J, et al: Detection of anti-Hu antibody in the serum of patients with small cell lung cancer—a quantitative Western blot analysis. Ann Neurol 27:544, 1990.

DeCaro L, Denfield JR: Lung cancer in young persons. J Thorac Cardiovasc Surg 83:372, 1982.

Decker DA, et al: The significance of a cytologically negative pleural effusion in bronchogenic carcinoma. Chest 74:640, 1978.

Delisle L, et al: Ectopic corticotropin syndrome and small cell carcinoma of the lung, clinical failures, outcome and complications. Arch Intern Med 153:746, 1993.

De Troyer A, Demanet SC: Clinical, biological and pathogenic features of the syndrome of inappropriate secretion of antidiuretic hormone. QJM 45:521, 1976.

DeVere R, Bradley WG: Polymyositis: its presentation, morbidity and mortality. Brain 98:637, 1976.

Dines DE, et al: Malignant pulmonary neoplasms predisposing to spontaneous pneumothorax. Mayo Clinic Proc 48:541, 1973.

Dresler C, Fratelli C, Babb J: Prognostic value of positive pleural lavage in patients with lung cancer resection. Ann Thorac Surg 67:1435, 1999.

Dunnick NR, Ihde DC, Johnston-Early A: Abdominal CT in the evaluation of small cell carcinoma of the lung, AJR Am J Roentgenol 133:1085, 1979.

Eggers C, Hazel C, Pfeiffer G: Anti-Hu associated paraneoplastic sensory neuropathy with peripheral nerve demyelination and microvasculitis. J Neurol Sci 155:178, 1998.

Elrington GM, et al: Neurological paraneoplastic syndrome in patients with small cell lung cancer: a prospective survey of 150 patients. J Neurol Neurosurg Psychiatry 54:764, 1991.

Ettinghausen SE, Burt ME: Prospective evaluation of unilateral adrenal masses in patients with operable non-small cell lung cancer. J Clin Oncol 9:1462, 1991.

Faiman C, et al: Gonadotropic secretion from a bronchogenic carcinoma. N Engl J Med 227:1395, 1967.

Fayemi AO, Deppisch LM: Nonbacterial thrombotic endocarditis and myocarditis infarction. Am Heart J 97:405, 1979.

Fichman M, Bethune J: Effects of neoplasms on renal electrolyte function. Ann NY Acad Sci 230:448, 1974.

Galluzzi S, Payne PM: Brain metastases from primary bronchial carcinoma: a statistical study of 741 necropsies. Br J Cancer 10:408, 1956.

Geddes DM: The natural history of lung cancer: a review board on rates of tumor growth. Br J Dis Chest 73:1, 1979.

Giannone L, et al: Favorable prognosis of brain metastasis in small cell lung cancer. Ann Intern Med 106:386, 1987.

Goldhaber SZ, et al: Clinical suspicion of autopsy proven thrombotic and tumor pulmonary embolism in cancer patients. Am Heart J *114*:1432, 1987.

Goldman JM, et al: Spinal cord compression in small cell lung cancer: a retrospective study of 610 patients. Br J Cancer *59*:591, 1989.

Gropp C, Havemann K, Scheuer A: Ectopic hormone in lung cancer patients at diagnosis and during therapy. Cancer *46*:347, 1980.

Halpert B. Erickson EE, Fields WS: Intracranial involvement from carcinoma of the lung. Arch Pathol *69*:93, 1960.

Hansen HH: Diagnosis in metastatic sites. *In* Strano M (ed): Lung Cancer: Clinical Diagnosis and Treatment. 2nd Ed. Philadelphia: Grune & Stratton, 1983, p. 185.

Hayward ML, et al: Hypercalcemia complicating small cell carcinoma. Cancer *48*:1643, 1981.

Hirshberg B, et al: Hemoptysis: etiology, evaluation, and outcome in a tertiary referral hospital. Chest *112*:440, 1997.

Hopwood P, et al: Symptoms at presentation for treatment in patients with lung cancer: implications for the evaluation of palliative treatment. Br J Cancer *71*:633, 1995.

Horwich MS, et al: Subacute sensory neuropathy: a remote effect of cancer. Ann Neurol *1*:7, 1977.

Howlett TA, et al: Diagnosis and management of ACTH dependent Cushing's syndrome: comparison of the features in ectopic and pituitary ACTH production. Clin Endocrinol *24*:699, 1986.

Hyde L, Hyde CI: Clinical manifestations of lung cancer. Chest *65*:299, 1974.

Irwin RS, Curley FJ, French CL: Chronic cough: the spectrum and frequency of causes, key components of the diagnostic evaluation and outcome of specific therapy. Am Rev Respir Dis *141*:640, 1990.

Jacobs L, Kinkel WR. Vincent RG: Silent brain metastases from lung carcinoma determined by computerized tomography. Arch Neurol *34*:690, 1977.

Jacobson DM, Thirkhill CE, Tipping SJ: A clinical triad to diagnose paraneoplastic retinopathy. Ann Neurol *28*:162, 1990.

Janerich DT, et al: Lung cancer and exposure to tobacco smoke in one household. N Engl J Med *323*:632, 1990.

Johnson DE, Goldberg M: Management of carcinoma of the superior pulmonary sulcus. Oncology *11*:981, 1997.

Karolyi P: Do adrenal metastases from lung cancer develop by lymphogenous or hematogenous route? J Surg Oncol *43*:154, 1990.

Kato Y, et al: Oat cell carcinoma of the lung. Cancer *23*:517, 1969.

Kim RY, et al: Extradural spinal cord compression: analysis of factors determining functional prognosis—prospective study. Radiology *176*:279, 1990.

Knowles JH, Smith LH: Extrapulmonary manifestations of bronchogenic carcinoma. N Engl J Med *263*:506, 1960.

Kondo H, et al: Pleural lavage cytology immediately after thoracotomy as a prognostic factor for patients with lung cancer. Jpn J Cancer Res *80*:233, 1989.

Kondo H, et al: Prognostic significance of pleural lavage cytology immediately after thoracotomy in patients with lung cancer. J Thorac Cardiovasc Surg *106*:1092, 1993.

Lakhanpal S, et al: Polymyositis-dermatomyositis and malignant lesions: does an association exist? Mayo Clin Proc *61*:645, 1986.

Lam WK, So SY, Yu DYC: Clinical features of bronchogenic carcinoma in Hong Kong: review of 480 patients. Cancer *53*:369, 1983.

Lambert EH, Eaton LM, Rooke ED: Defect of neuromuscular conduction associated with malignant neoplasms. Am J Physiol *187*:612, 1956.

Lederle FA, Nichol KL, Parenti CM: Bronchoscopy to evaluate hemoptysis in older men with nonsuspicious chest roentgenogram. Chest *95*:1043, 1989.

Lees LH: The biosynthesis of hormone by nonendocrine tumors—a review. J Endocrinol *67*:143, 1975.

Lennon VA, Lambert EH: Autoantibodies bind solubilized calcium channel-ω-conotoxin complexes from small cell lung cancer: a diagnostic aid for Lambert-Eaton myasthenic syndrome. Mayo Clin Proc *64*:149, 1989.

Lennon VA, et al: Enteric neuronal autoantibodies in pseudoobstruction with small cell lung carcinoma. Gastroenterology *100*:137, 1991.

LeRoux BT: Bronchial carcinoma. Thorax *23*:136, 1968.

List AF, et al: The syndrome of inappropriate secretion of antidiuretic hormone in small cell lung cancer. J Clin Oncol *4*:1191, 1986.

Loeb LA, et al: Smoking and lung cancer: an overview. Cancer Res *44*:5940, 1984.

Lucchinetti CF, Kimmel DW, Lennon VA: Paraneoplastic and oncologic profile of patients seropositive for type 1 antineuronal antibodies. Neurology *150*:652, 1998.

Mancall EL, Rosales RK: Necrotizing myelopathy associated with visceral carcinoma. Brain *87*:636, 1964.

Matthews MJ: Problems in morphology and behaviour of bronchopulmonary malignant disease. *In* Israil L, Chahanien P (eds): Lung Cancer: Natural History, Prognosis and Therapy. New York: Academic Press, 1976, p. 23.

Matthews MJ, et al: Frequency of residual and metastatic tumor in patients undergoing curative surgical resection for lung cancer. Cancer Chemother Rep *4*:63, 1973.

McDonald RA, Robbins SG: The significance of nonbacterial thrombotic endocarditis: autopsy and clinical study of 78 patients. Ann Intern Med *46*:255, 1957.

McEnvoy KM, et al: 3;4 Diaminopyridine in the treatment of Lambert-Eaton myasthenic syndrome. N Engl J Med *321*:1567, 1989.

McFarlane MJ, Feinstein AR, Wells CK: Necropsy evidence of detection bias in the diagnosis of lung cancer. Arch Intern Med *146*:1695, 1986.

Merchut MP: Brain metastases from undiagnosed systemic neoplasms. Arch Intern Med *149*:1076, 1989.

Meyer PC, Reach TG: Secondary neoplasms of the central nervous system and meninges. Br J Cancer *7*:438, 1953.

Miller JL, Mansour KA, Hatcher JR: Carcinoma of the superior pulmonary sulcus. Ann Thorac Surg *28*:44, 1979.

Mirvis SE, et al: Abdominal CT in the staging of small cell carcinoma of the lung: incidence of metastases and effect on prognosis. AJR Am J Roentgenol *148*:845, 1987.

Moll JWR, et al: Diagnostic value of anti-neuronal antibodies for paraneoplastic disorders of the nervous system. J Neurol Neurosurg Psychiatry *53*:940, 1990.

Moorthy AV: Minimal change glomerular disease: a paraneoplastic syndrome in two patients with bronchogenic carcinoma. Am J Kidney Dis *3*:58, 1983.

Morton DL, Itabashi HH, Gromes OF: Nonmetastatic neurological complications of bronchogenic carcinoma: the carcinomatous myopathies. J Thorac Cardiovasc Surg *51*:14, 1966.

Morton WJ, Tedesco FJ: Metastatic bronchogenic carcinoma seen as a gastric ulcer. Am J Dig Dis *19*:766, 1974.

Mundy GR. Hypercalcemic factors other than prethyroid related protein. Endocrinol Metab Clin North Am *18*:795, 1989.

Murray GC, Persellin RH: Metastatic carcinoma presenting as monoarticular arthritis: a case report and review of the literature. Arthritis Rheum *23*:95, 1980.

Newman SJ, Hansen HH: Frequency, diagnosis and treatment of brain metastases in 247 consecutive patients with bronchogenic carcinoma. Cancer *33*:492, 1974.

Nugent JL, et al: CNS metastases in small cell lung carcinoma: increasing frequency and changing pattern with lengthening survival. Cancer *44*:1885, 1979.

Odell WD, Wolfsen AR: Humoral syndromes associated with cancer. Ann Rev Med *29*:379, 1978.

Okumura M, et al: Intraoperative pleural lavage cytology in lung cancer patients. Ann Thorac Surg *51*:599, 1991.

Oliver TW, et al: Isolated adrenal masses in non-small cell bronchogenic carcinoma. Radiology *153*:217, 1984.

O'Neil KM, Lazarus AA: Hemoptysis: indication for bronchoscopy. Arch Intern Med *151*:2449, 1991.

O'Rourke MA, Crawford J: Lung cancer in the elderly. Clin Geriatr Med *3*: 595, 1987.

Oschner A: Surgery for diseases of the lung. Post Grad Med *19*:584, 1956.

Pancoast HK: Superior sulcus tumor: tumor characterized by pain, Horner's syndrome, destruction of bone and atrophy of hand muscles. JAMA *99*:1391, 1932.

Parish JM, et al: Etiologic considerations in superior vena cava syndrome. Mayo Clin Proc *56*:407, 1981.

Pedersen AG: Diagnostic procedures in the detection of CNS metastases from small cell lung cancer. *In* Hansen HH (ed): Lung Cancer: Basic and Clinical Aspects. Boston: Martinus Nijhoff, 1986, p. 153.

Pedersen AG, Bach F, Melgaard B: Frequency, diagnosis and prognosis of spinal cord compression in small cell bronchogenic carcinoma. Cancer *55*:1818, 1985.

Pemberton JH, et al: Bronchogenic carcinoma in patients younger than 40 years. Ann Thorac Surg *36*:509, 1983.

Piehler JM, et al: Unexplained diaphragmatic paralysis: a harbinger of malignant disease. J Thorac Cardiovasc Surg *84*:861, 1982.

Plaza V, et al: Have the causes of hemoptysis changed? An analysis of 213 patients undergoing fiber bronchoscopic exploration. Arch Bronchopneumol *31*:323, 1995.

Putnam JS: Lung cancer in young adults. JAMA *238*: 35, 1977.

Rahim MA, Sarma SK: Pulmonary and extrapulmonary manifestations in delayed diagnosis of lung cancer in Bangladesh. Cancer Detect Prev *7*:31, 1984.

Reingold IM: Cutaneous metastases from internal carcinoma. Cancer *19*:162, 1966.

Repace JL, Lowery AH: A quantitative estimate of nonsmokers' lung cancer risk from passive smoking. Environ Int *1*:3, 1985.

Richardson RI, et al: Tumor products and potential markers in small cell lung cancer. Semin Oncol *5*:253, 1978.

Risch HA, et al: Are female smokers at higher risk for lung cancer than male smokers: a case control analysis by histologic type. Am J Epidemiol *138*: 281, 1993.

Roberts A, et al: Paraneoplastic myasthenic syndrome IgG inhibits Ca^{2+} flux in a human small cell carcinoma line. Nature *317*:737, 1985.

Roberts PF, Stebbing WSL, Kennedy HJ: Granulomatous visceral neuropathy of the colon with non-small cell lung cancer. Histology *30*:588, 1997.

Rodichok LD et al: Early diagnosis of spinal epidural metastases. Am J Med *70*:1181, 1981.

Rosen P, Armstrong D: Nonbacterial thrombotic endocarditis in patients with malignant neoplastic diseases. Am J Med *54*:231, 1973.

Sack GH, Levin J, Bell WR: Trousseau's syndrome and other manifestations of chronic disseminated coagulopathy in patients with neoplasms. Medicine *56*:1, 1977.

Santiago S, Tobias J, Williams AJ: A reappraisal of the causes of hemoptysis. Arch Intern Med *151*:2449, 1991.

Schiff D, O'Neill BP, Suman VJ: Spinal epidural metastases as the initial manifestation of malignancy. Neurology *49*:452, 1997.

Schraufnagel D, Margolis B: Bronchoscopy for hemoptysis. Chest *97*:1502, 1990.

Schuffler MD, Baird HW, Fleming CR: Intestinal pseudo-obstruction as the presenting manifestation of small cell lung cancer. Ann Intern Med *98*:129, 1983.

Schuller-Petrovic S, et al: A shared antigenic determinant between natural killer cells and nervous tissue. Nature *306*:179, 1983.

Schumacher HR: Articular manifestations of hypertrophic pulmonary osteoarthropathy in bronchogenic carcinoma. Arthritis Rheum *19*:629, 1976.

Shepherd FA, Laskey J, Evans WK: Cushing's syndrome associated with ectopic corticotropin production and small cell lung cancer. J Clin Oncol *10*:21, 1992.

Shimizu K, et al: Ectopic atrial natriuretic peptide production in small cell lung cancer with the syndrome of inappropriate antidiuretic hormone secretion. Cancer *68*:2284, 1991.

Sigurgeirsson B, et al: Risk of cancer in patients with dermatomyositis or polymyositis: a population based study. N Engl J Med *326*:363, 1992.

Silverman SG, et al: Predictive value of image-guided adrenal biopsy: analysis of results of 101 biopsies. Radiology *187*:715, 1993.

Silvis SE, Turkbas N, Doscherhdmen A: Thrombocytosis in patients with lung cancer. JAMA *211*:1852, 1970.

Sørensen PS, et al: Metastatic epidural spinal cord compression: results of treatment and survival. Cancer *65*:1502, 1990.

Sparup J, et al: Computed tomography and the TNM classification of lung cancer. Scand J Thorac Cardiovasc Surg *24*:207, 1990.

Spiro SG, et al: Neurological paraneoplastic syndrome in patients with small cell lung cancer. A prospective study of 150 patients. J Neurol Neurosurg Psychiatry *54*:764, 1991.

Stark RJ, Hensen RA, Evans SJW: Spinal metastases: a retrospective survey from a general hospital. Brain *105*:189, 1982.

Stenseth JH, Clagett OT, Woolner LB: Hypertrophic pulmonary osteoarthropathy. Dis Chest *52*:62, 1967.

Takamori M, et al: Antibodies to recombinant synaptotagmin and calcium channel subtypes in Lambert-Eaton myasthenic syndrome. J Neurol Sci *133*:95, 1995.

Thirkell CE, et al: Cancer associated retinopathy (CAR syndrome) with antibodies reacting with retinal, optic nerve and cancer cells. N Engl J Med *321*:1589, 1989.

Watson PN, Evans RJ: Intractable pain with lung cancer. Pain *29*:163, 1987.

Weiss ST: Passive smoking and lung cancer. What is the risk? Am Rev Respir Dis *133*:1, 1986.

Weiss W, Seidman H, Boucto KR: The Philadelphia pulmonary neoplasm research project: symptoms in occult lung cancer. Chest *73*:57, 1978.

Wells CK, Feinstein AR: Detection bias in the diagnostic pursuit of lung cancer. Am J Epidemiol *128*:1016, 1988.

Wilkinson PC, Zeronski J: Immunofluorescent detection of antibodies against neurons in sensory carcinomatous neuropathy. Brain *88*:529, 1965.

Winchester DP, et al: Small bowel perforation secondary to metastatic carcinoma of the lung. Cancer *40*:410, 1977.

Yacoub MH: Relation between the histology of bronchial carcinoma and hypertrophic pulmonary osteoarthropathy. Thorax *20*:537, 1965.

Zucker S, Friedman S, Lysik RM: Bone marrow erythropoiesis in the anemia of the infection, inflammation and malignancy. J Clin Invest *53*:1132, 1974.

CHAPTER 97

Radiologic Evaluation of Lung Cancer

Patrick J. Fultz and Richard H. Feins

The radiologic evaluation of lung cancer is directed at determining the best means for diagnosing and staging lung cancer and the best method of treating patients with that diagnosis. Although both the standard chest radiograph and computed tomography (CT) of the chest are the mainstays of radiologic evaluation, neither, alone or in combination, can make a definitive diagnosis of lung cancer. Such a diagnosis requires cytologic or histologic study. Similarly, except for the size criteria (T), neither study can very often stage a given lung cancer definitively. Such staging usually requires either direct operative examination or cytologic or histologic proof. Yet, all too often patients are told they have lung cancer or are assigned to a specific treatment based on radiologic evidence alone. This has been true even of some large-scale cooperative trials. This "leap of faith" is not only unfounded but also unnecessary, given today's variety of relatively minimally invasive diagnostic procedures.

ROUTINE SCREENING FOR LUNG CANCER

With lung cancer being the most common cause of death by cancer in both men and women and with the belief that the earlier the stage of the tumor, the more curable it is, screening for lung cancer by routine chest radiographs or, more recently, CT has appeared very attractive. Indeed, several studies have been done to test the hypothesis that routine chest radiographs, especially in a high-risk population, lead to earlier discovery of the disease and more curative treatment. Unfortunately, this has not proved to be the case. Studies were done of large numbers of cigarette-smoking men at the Mayo Clinic by Fontana and associates (1986), at Memorial–Sloan Kettering Cancer Center by Melamed and colleagues (1984), at Johns Hopkins University by Tockman and coworkers (1986), and in Czechoslovakia by Kubik and coinvestigators (1990). All studies found that although screening did indeed lead to earlier detection of tumors, increased resectability, and improved length of survival,

overall mortality was not decreased from that of controls. Salomaa and colleagues (1998) found only 93 men to have lung cancer out of 33,743 male cigarette smokers screened as part of the screening process for the Alpha Tocopherol, Beta-Carotene Cancer Prevention Study. While Strauss (1998) has argued that the "significant stage distribution, resectability, and long-term survival advantages" in this study proves that chest radiographic screening can save lives, the current guidelines for cancer screening do not recommend routine screening chest radiographs for lung cancer.

Advances in low-dose spiral CT scanning have led to several small studies of the ability of these techniques to detect early tumors. Lung cancers were discovered more frequently with spiral CT than with chest radiographs; the radiographs missed 73% of the lesion. However, again only a small number of tumors were discovered in a large number of examinations in the report of Kaneko and associates (1996). Studies of the overall effect on mortality have yet to be done. Given the higher cost of spiral CT versus chest radiography, it seems unlikely that this modality will be shown to be an effective screening tool under current circumstances.

DIAGNOSING LUNG CANCER

Although definitive diagnosis of lung cancer requires histologic or cytologic confirmation, several aspects of a given radiographic finding may lead one to be more suspicious of lung cancer. The most important of these is probably the radiographic history of the lesion. Lesions that can be shown on older studies (either chest radiographs or CT) to be completely stable in size and shape are unlikely to be cancerous. A search for old films should be one of the first steps toward diagnosis. Most films are destroyed after 7 years, however, which makes it difficult to confirm stability. It is hoped that digital archiving of radiographic studies will eliminate the need to purge studies and will make obtaining them for comparison easier. It should be remembered, however, that a change in a lesion, even after a long period of documented stability, could be an indicator of a scar carcinoma or a particularly slow-growing tumor.

Radiographic Features

The radiographic findings caused by carcinoma of the lung may result from the tumor itself, from changes in the pulmonary parenchyma distal to a bronchus obstructed by the tumor (atelectasis, infection, or both), and from spread of the tumor to extrapulmonary intrathoracic sites (e.g., hilar and mediastinal lymph nodes, pleura, chest wall, and other mediastinal structures). The findings vary with location, cell type, and length of time the tumor has been present.

Garland (1966) estimated that when a lung tumor is first detectable on a chest radiograph, it has completed three-fourths of its natural history. Rigler (1957) observed that the radiographic abnormality frequently antedates the first symptoms or signs of the disease by 7 months or more. These early features are subtle and often are appreciated only in retrospect.

Early Radiographic Features

The early signs visible in the radiographs of the chest, as Rigler (1966) noted, are produced directly by the tumor itself. The limit of visibility of a single, solitary lesion is approximately 7 mm in diameter, although multiple smaller lesions (diffuse lung lesions) may be recognized. The single lesion frequently is not identified until it is at least 10 mm in diameter; a smaller lesion may be obscured by overlying or adjacent structures. Muhm and associates (1983) studied lung cancer in 92 patients in a chest radiographic lung cancer screening study, where at least two observers initially reviewed all radiographs, and found that 90% of the peripheral lung cancers were visible in retrospect on prior radiographs.

The early signs of a lung tumor are as follows:

- A density within the lung parenchyma
- A cavitary mass
- A segmental, indistinct, poorly defined dense area
- A nodular streaked, local infiltration along the course of a blood vessel
- Segmental consolidation
- A roughly triangular lesion arising in the apex and extending toward the hilus
- A mediastinal mass (an uncommon early sign)
- An enlargement of one hilus
- Segmental or lobar obstructive emphysema (a rare finding in carcinoma of the lung)
- Segmental atelectasis

The relative incidences of these various early changes are difficult, if not impossible, to discern, because most patients have more advanced disease when first examined. Weiss and

associates (1982), however, recorded the incidences of these early features in a screening program to detect lung cancer. A peripheral nodule or mass occurred in 33%, a peripheral "infiltrate" in 25%, and hilar enlargement in 28% of patients who developed a lung cancer. Atelectasis and a pleural effusion each occurred in 3%, and obstructive emphysema was seen in only 1%.

Usual Radiographic Manifestations

Byrd and associates (1969) classified the radiographic features as hilar, pulmonary parenchymal, and intrathoracic extrapulmonary. In their review of the chest radiographs of 600 patients with carcinoma of the lung, a hilar abnormality either alone or associated with other abnormalities was present in 41% of the patients. Obstructive pneumonitis, collapse, or consolidation was also present in 41%. A large parenchymal mass was present in 21.7%, and a small mass was evident in 20.3%; multiple masses were present in only 1.1%. An apical mass was found in 2.6% of the patients, and in no patient was hypertranslucency seen. The various extrapulmonary intrathoracic manifestations were present in 11%, mediastinal widening and pleural effusion being the more common. Table 97-1 lists the usual radiographic findings. Amemiya and Oho (1982) (Table 97-2) and Swett and associates (1982) have noted that a peripheral nodular mass is now the most common radiographic presentation of bronchial carcinoma. Many, if not most of these, are 3 cm or smaller and fall into the category of solitary pulmonary nodule.

Uncommon Radiographic Manifestations

Woodring (1990a) reviewed the uncommon radiologic presentations of a lung cancer. The more important of these were 1) spontaneous regression after initial recognition (extremely rare) or an observed decrease in size of the tumor mass, 2) calcification in psammoma bodies in the tumor or dystrophic calcification in areas of tumor infection or necrosis, and 3) a tumor presenting as a thin-walled cavity (Fig. 97-1). Woodring and Fried (1983) had reported a 6% inci-

---

Table 97-1. Chest Radiographic Presentations of Lung Cancer

Pulmonary nodule <3 cm in size
Pulmonary or hilar mass
Pulmonary opacities (lobar, segmental, subsegmental)
Tracheal or bronchial intraluminal opacity, luminal narrowing, or wall thickening
Atelectasis (lung, lobar, segmental, subsegmental)
Pulmonary cavitary lesion
Air trapping (hyperinflation)
Mediastinal mass
Pleural lesion
Pleural effusion
Pericardial effusion (enlarged cardiac silhouette)
Elevated hemidiaphragm (paralysis or paresis)
Chest wall mass or bone metastases

Table 97-2. Radiographic Findings in 200 Patients with Lung Cancer

Findings	Percentage of Patients
Tumor in the periphery of the lung	39.5
Hilar tumor	19.5
Atelectasis	13.5
Pleural effusion	7.0
Hilar invasion	5.0
Normal	4.0
Infiltrative shadow in the periphery	3.0
Other	8.5

Adapted from Amemiya R, Oho K: X-ray diagnosis of lung cancer. *In* Hayata Y (ed): Lung Cancer Diagnosis. Tokyo: Igaku-Shoin, 1982, p. 4.

dence of primary carcinoma in a series of solitary cavities with a wall thickness of 4 mm or less. Other unusual findings were the radiologic presence of satellite nodules or the occurrence of two separate synchronous primary tumors, one being a possible metastasis of the other, in 1% of the initial radiographs, respectively. Other rare findings were the presence of a meniscus or "crescent sign" within the tumor mass and the occurrence of two anatomically separated areas of atelectasis or pulmonary consolidation, which is by far more typical of an inflammatory disease process. Of passing interest also is the occurrence of a spontaneous pneumothorax as the initial radiographic feature of a lung cancer. Steinhauslin and Cuttat (1985) reported this occurrence in 0.46% of lung cancer cases. Although dystrophic calcification is considered uncommon, Mahoney and

coworkers (1992) identified it on CT scans in 13% of lesions that were subsequently proved to be cancer.

Influence of Cell Type

Certain radiographic patterns are characteristic of the various cell types. From the studies of Byrd and associates (1969) and that of Theros (1977), as well as the review by Sider (1990), several generalities can be made.

Squamous cell carcinoma most often presents a picture of obstructive pneumonitis, pulmonary collapse, or parenchymal consolidation because 65% of these tumors occur in a central location in the bronchial tree. A hilar abnormality is often present. Approximately one-third of the squamous cell tumors appear as a peripheral mass. Many are small lesions (3 cm or less in diameter), but in previous decades, up to two-thirds of the peripheral squamous cell tumors were larger than 4 cm. Cavitation is more common in peripheral squamous cell carcinomas than in other lung carcinomas, occurring in approximately 10 to 20% of patients with these peripheral tumors. Cavitation in this instance results from necrosis in the tumor mass. Cavitation and abscess formation also may occur distal to a bronchus obstructed by tumor. When both types of cavities are combined, they constitute approximately 50% of all lung abscesses seen in patients older than 50. In 3 to 4% of patients with squamous cell tumors, the radiograph of the chest may show no abnormality, the tumor being located in a main stem bronchus and producing no changes in the parenchyma distal to it.

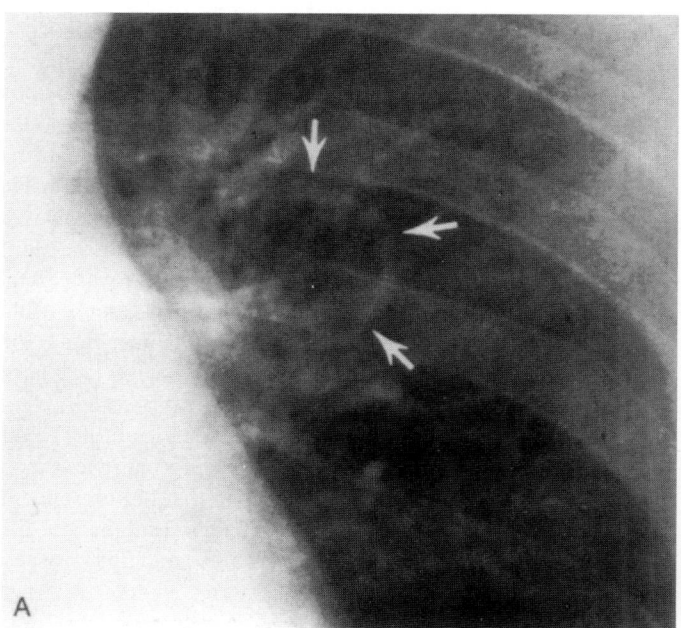
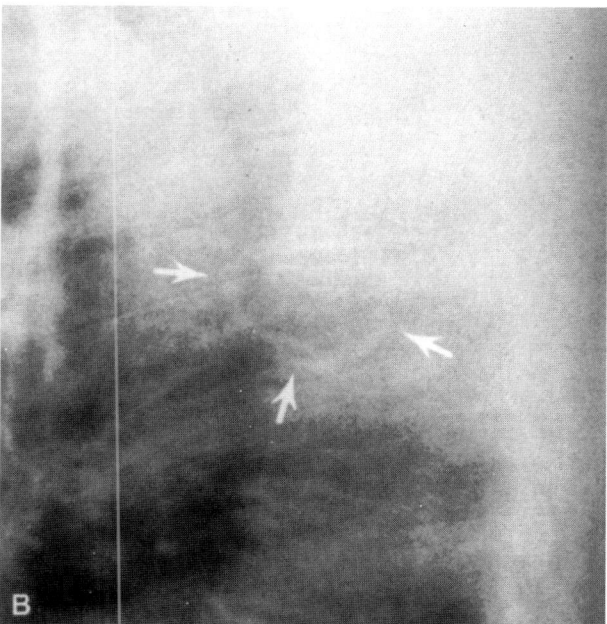

Fig. 97-1. Posteroanterior (**A**) and lateral (**B**) radiographs reveal a smooth, thin-walled carcinomatous cavity in a 43-year-old man with hypertrophic pulmonary osteoarthropathy with positive sputum cytology. Maximum wall thickness was 2 mm. From Woodring JH: Unusual radiographic manifestations of lung cancer. Radiol Clin North Am *28*:599, 1990. With permission.

Adenocarcinomas are most often peripheral masses and, as with the peripheral squamous cell tumors, a great percentage of these lesions are initially recognized when they are 3 cm or less in diameter. Many still are not discovered, however, until the tumor is larger than 4 cm. Cavitation is rare. These peripheral lesions represent 60 to 70% of all the primary adenocarcinomas of the lung. The lesion most often has a nodular or ill-defined border. A *corona radiata*, as it was termed by Heitzman and colleagues (1982), or sunburst appearance of the border, is often readily appreciated on the standard radiographs and may represent local lymphatic spread. Eccentric calcification may be present within the mass. A hilar abnormality or an obstructive parenchymal lesion is less common than the peripheral mass, but it appears to be increasing in frequency. Woodring and Stelling (1983) reported that 28% of adenocarcinomas presented solely as a central mass, and 51% of all patients had some degree of central involvement: hilar or mediastinal node adenopathy.

A subtype of adenocarcinoma, bronchioloalveolar carcinoma, may present as a solitary peripheral mass. It represents approximately 35% of all small peripheral masses, a localized area of pneumonic infiltrate that may extend to involve an entire lobe or even more of the lung, or less commonly as multiple unilateral or bilateral coalescent multinodular infiltrates. In a study of 136 patients with this tumor, Hill (1984) reported that the presenting radiographic findings were 1) a solitary nodule less than 4 cm in diameter in 23%, 2) a mass in 20%, 3) a localized area of consolidation (less than one lobe) in 7%, 4) diffuse coalescent consolidation in 23%, and 5) diffuse nodules in 27%. Unlike tumors of other cell types, the presence of air bronchograms in the areas of involvement is common. Less frequently, an interstitial pattern of involvement of the lung is noted, which Berkman (1977) reported to be the result of secondary lymphatic spread of the tumor. According to Sider (1990), pleural effusion may be present in 8 to 10% of patients and, rarely, a pneumothorax can occur.

Large cell undifferentiated carcinomas are most likely to be peripheral lesions (approximately 60%), and two-thirds of these are larger than 4 cm. Cavitation occurs in approximately 6% of these peripheral large cell tumors. A hilar abnormality and parenchymal changes are each present in association with approximately one-third of these tumors. Ten percent of the patients with this type of tumor have mediastinal widening as one of the presenting features.

Small cell undifferentiated tumors appear primarily as hilar abnormalities (78%), which usually represent hilar or mediastinal lymph node metastases. These tumors are associated with mediastinal widening in more than 13% of patients, and in some of the patients with this finding, a parenchymal abnormality cannot be recognized. Parenchymal obstructive lesions occur as the result of extrinsic compression of a bronchus in slightly less than 40% of patients. A peripheral mass may occur in somewhat less than one-

third of the patients; Carter and Eggleston (1980) reported that a peripheral mass occurred in only 14%. Three-fourths of the peripheral small cell tumors may be smaller than 4 cm in diameter. This cell type represents the least common cause of a peripheral solitary pulmonary nodule of all cell types of bronchial carcinoma and the reported incidence, as reviewed by Kreisman and associates (1992), varied between 4 and 12%.

Despite these generalizations, no radiographic feature is diagnostic of the cell type or even of the presence of carcinoma. Nonetheless, these features should alert one's suspicion as to the possibility of a malignancy so that proper cytologic or histologic material is obtained to make a diagnosis.

Special Radiographic Studies

In addition to the routine posteroanterior and lateral radiographs, other radiographs of the chest can be obtained with the patient in the right or left anterior oblique, lordotic, or other special positions to delineate further any suspected lesion. Contrast-enhanced study of the esophagus may be helpful at times. Other radiographic studies (e.g., laminography, 55-degree oblique tomography, bronchography, angiography, azygography, and pneumomediastinography) can be obtained but are rarely indicated in the evaluation of lung cancer patients at present. These techniques are noted mainly for historic interest.

Computed Tomography of Lung Cancer

CT has become a routine examination for patients suspected of having lung cancer. Like any other noninvasive examination, however, it cannot distinguish inflammatory tissue from cancer tissue. In patients with central lesions, CT is useful for demonstrating enlarged hilar lymph nodes, but this finding in itself is not of great import because it does not disqualify the patient for surgical exploration. The demonstration of enlarged nodes may suggest, however, the need for a pneumonectomy as the surgical procedure. The caliber, distortion, and thickening of the wall of the proximal bronchi also can be discerned. Involvement of the pulmonary vessels, even with contrast enhancement, is difficult to determine at times. In patients with peripheral lesions, the margins, presence of calcification, and cavitation can be elicited. Zwirewich and associates (1991) evaluated high-resolution CT in distinguishing malignant from benign peripheral nodules. They found that the presence of spiculation of the borders, pleural tags, and bubble-like areas of low attenuation were 87%, 58%, and 25%, respectively, in malignant lesions; in benign lesions, these percentages were 55%, 27%, and 9%, respectively. Thus, none of these criteria can be used as unequivocal signs of malignancy. Im and associates (1990) described the CT angiogram sign in patients with bronchioloalveolar carcinoma. With contrast enhancement in patients with segmented or lobar consolidation, enhanced branching pulmonary vessels are seen in areas of homogeneous low attenuation when the consolidation is related to the presence of this tumor. Air bronchograms may also be seen. With high-resolution CT and spiral CT, numerous investigators, including Jang and associates (1996), have described a ground-glass appearance as typical of small peripheral nodules that are early bronchioloalveolar carcinomas. This haziness is thought to be due to the lepidic growth pattern of these tumors. In addition, bubble-like hyperlucency or pseudocavitation (representing patent airways) can also be present. With growth, areas of consolidation with high attenuation values may be seen; these areas represent so-called scar or sclerotic areas within the tumor. According to Noguchi (1995), Eto (1996), and Yamashiro (1995) and their colleagues, an increasing size of the scar within the tumor portends a worse prognosis.

Calcification occurs as often as 13% of the time in lung cancer, as shown by Mahoney and coworkers (1990) in a CT study of lesions subsequently proved to be cancer. This calcification is most often eccentric. Concentric laminated calcification centered on the middle of a mass, however, is virtually diagnostic of a tuberculous or fungal granuloma, whereas diffuse calcification throughout the mass ("popcorn" calcifications) is the hallmark of the benign hamartoma.

However, the most important aspect of the radiologic diagnosis of lung cancer is that radiologic studies alone cannot make the diagnosis. Definitive diagnosis can be made only by cytology or histology. Therefore, the chest radiograph and CT scan should be used primarily to raise the level of suspicion and to direct diagnostic procedures, such as bronchoscopy, for central lesions or removal for peripheral lesions. It has been our practice not to do needle biopsies on new peripheral lesions in otherwise operable candidates without an alternative reason for having a lung mass. This is based on a personal review by one of us (R.H.F. in 1989, unpublished) of 2 years of fine-needle aspirations in this population; in it, only 3% of patients had a definitive benign diagnosis, thus saving the patient an operation. It has far more often been the case that patients, falsely believing that a negative diagnosis meant benignity, were lost to follow-up until such time as they reappeared, only to find themselves inoperable. Criticism is also warranted for the practice of "following" new lesions radiographically for any significant length of time to avoid operation. This is particularly unwarranted in face of the development of thoracoscopic removal of these lesions, which makes definitive diagnosis possible. Indeed, if one believes that the degree of lymphatic invasion can be correlated with curability, allowing lung lesions to grow radiographically in an attempt to show them benign may be ill advised. Ichinose and coworkers (1994) showed that local lymphatic vessel invasion was 25% for tumors less than 1 cm in diameter but rose to 40% in tumors 1.1 to 2.0 cm in

diameter. Although the hypothesis that tumors less than 1 cm in diameter are more curable than those 1 to 2 cm in diameter will never be subjected to a prospective randomized trial, it seems far better to remove a lesion and find it benign than to leave in a lesion and find it malignant.

STAGING OF LUNG CANCER BY RADIOGRAPHIC TECHNIQUES

Accurate staging of lung cancer is essential to proper treatment. Just as chest radiographs and CT imaging should be used only as guides to obtaining definitive diagnosis of lung cancer, so too should they be used only as guides to staging. With the possible exception of the size criteria for the T classification of a cancer, neither modality is capable of determining reliable TNM classification and therefore staging. The TNM staging criteria, as updated by Mountain (1997), are now universally accepted by those treating patients with lung cancer (see Chapter 98). Certain specific radiologic findings should lead the clinician to the appropriate steps to maximize the accuracy of clinical TNM staging.

Primary Tumor (T)

Lesion size can be reliably measured on chest radiograph and CT; therefore, the differentiation between T_1 lesions (≤ 3 cm) and T_2 lesions (>3 cm) is most often straightforward (Fig. 97-2). Invasion of the visceral pleura, another criterion for upstaging to T_2, is more difficult to recognize radiographically but is rarely a criterion of operability. The same is true for associated atelectasis or obstructive pneumonia that does not involve the entire lung. This level of clinical staging however, although not necessary in the decision to resect a given tumor, may be important for clinical trials of stage IB (T_2N_0) tumors.

Non–small cell cancers that contiguously invade the chest wall (T_3) are potentially resectable. In a CT study by G. M. Glazer (1985) using various combinations of criteria for assessing parietal pleural and chest wall invasion, the sensitivity for chest wall invasion was 87% and the specificity was 59%. It is interesting that, although CT had limited predictive value, clinical symptoms of focal pain yielded a sensitivity of 67% and a specificity of 94% for parietal pleural or chest wall invasion. Webb and associates (1991) in the Radiology Diagnostic Oncology Group (RDOG) study compared CT with magnetic resonance (MR) imaging for assessing chest wall invasion and found no statistically significant differences between the two modalities. Because surgical resection is the treatment of choice for tumors that locally abut and for those that actually invade the chest wall, making the radiologic distinction between the two probably is not critical for proper treatment.

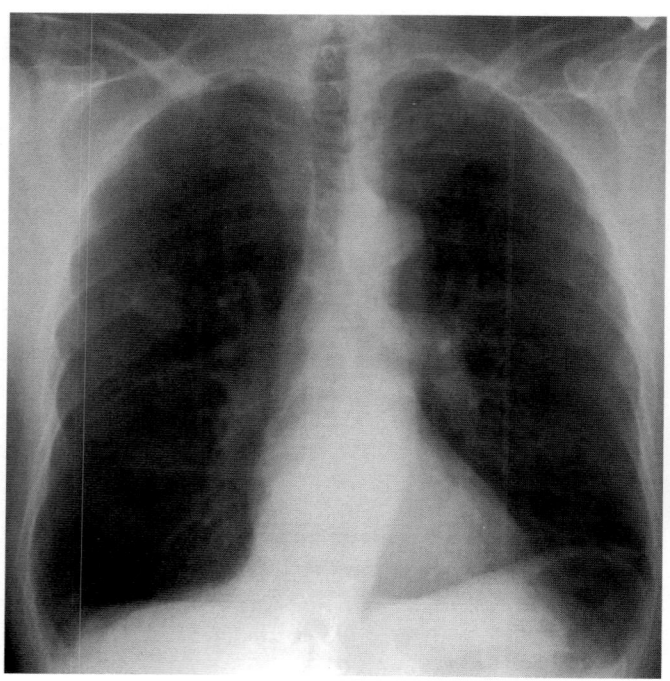

A

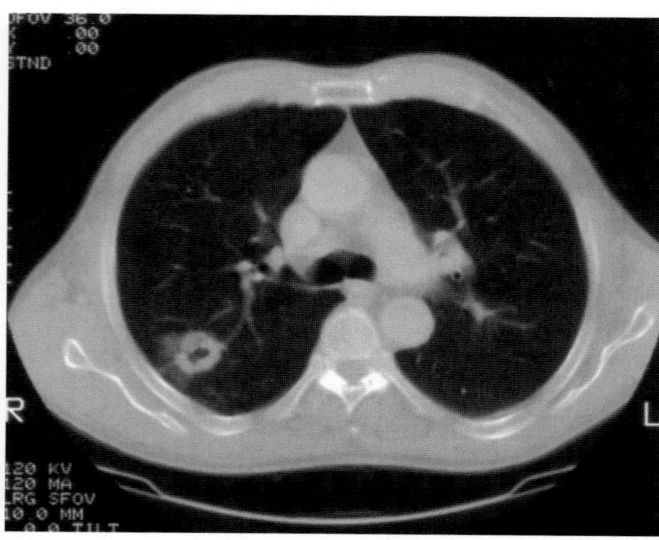

Fig. 97-2. T$_2$ disease. **A.** Chest radiographic demonstrates a 4-cm cavitary spiculated right upper lobe mass. **B.** Corresponding computed tomographic image in the center of this non–small cell lung cancer also shows the irregular, thick-walled cavitary lesion.

Perhaps the most important distinction in terms of the T status of a tumor is between T$_3$ (Fig. 97-3) and T$_4$ (Fig. 97-4) because the former (stage IIB) could potentially be resected, whereas the latter (stage IIIB) usually should not be resected. In the absence of gross tumor invasion of the mediastinum or chest wall, these lesions present the greatest challenge because the distinction between tumor abutment and invasion of vital structures is often subtle. Several investigators, including Herman (1994), Glazer (1989), and Webb (1991) and their associates, have indicated that CT is generally insensitive for detecting mediastinal invasion. However, after assessing a number of CT criteria in a limited number of patients, Herman and colleagues (1994) suggested that a mediastinal structure with more than one-half its circumference in contact with the tumor was likely to be invaded. Webb and associates' (1991) study did show however that MR imaging was significantly more accurate than CT for assessing mediastinal invasion.

Patients with more than one lesion in a given lobe are now more commonly identified preoperatively with the use of spiral CT scans. Under the new staging criteria, if the lobe contains two or more metastatic sites of the same tumor, the lesion is categorized as a T$_4$ lesion. Confirmation of the histology of the second lesion is important to differentiate a T$_4$ tumor from concurrent benign disease or a second early-stage lung cancer. If the chest radiograph or CT demonstrates a pleural effusion in the presence of a suspected or known lung cancer, the possibility exists for the effusion to be malignant and the tumor to be stage T$_4$. It is important to confirm malignant cells cytologically in the fluid before concluding inoperability because benign effusions can accompany malignant tumors. If questions still exist about

the cause of a given effusion, a prethoracotomy thoracoscopic evaluation is probably warranted. CT evidence of a pericardial effusion could be indicative of a malignant pericardial effusion (T$_4$) and should be further investigated.

Finally, chest radiographic evidence of an elevated diaphragm can be an indication of phrenic nerve involvement (T$_4$). Many thoracic surgeons, however, believe that isolated invasion of the phrenic nerve in the absence of mediastinal lymph node involvement does not necessarily preclude curative resection.

Lymph Nodes (N)

The American Thoracic Society/European Respiratory Society (ATS/ERS) (1997) recommendations for assessment of patients with suspected lung cancer includes the use of chest CT for evaluation of mediastinal lymph node enlargement. In patients with possible or proved lung cancer, the generally accepted threshold for suspecting metastatic nodal involvement is a lymph node 10 mm or greater. Sensitivity and specificity vary, depending on whether one chooses to apply that measurement to the long or short axis of a lymph node. In addition, G. M. Glazer and coworkers (1985) showed that variations in size threshold may be applicable based on nodal locations. In the study by G. M. Glazer and coworkers (1985) of CT examinations of 100 patients (excluding those with conditions that may enlarge mediastinal lymph nodes), the short-axis threshold for normal lymph nodes varied from 7 to 11 mm. Many clinical studies have simplified these variable size criteria by using a 10-mm lymph node short-axis threshold. In another study by Glazer

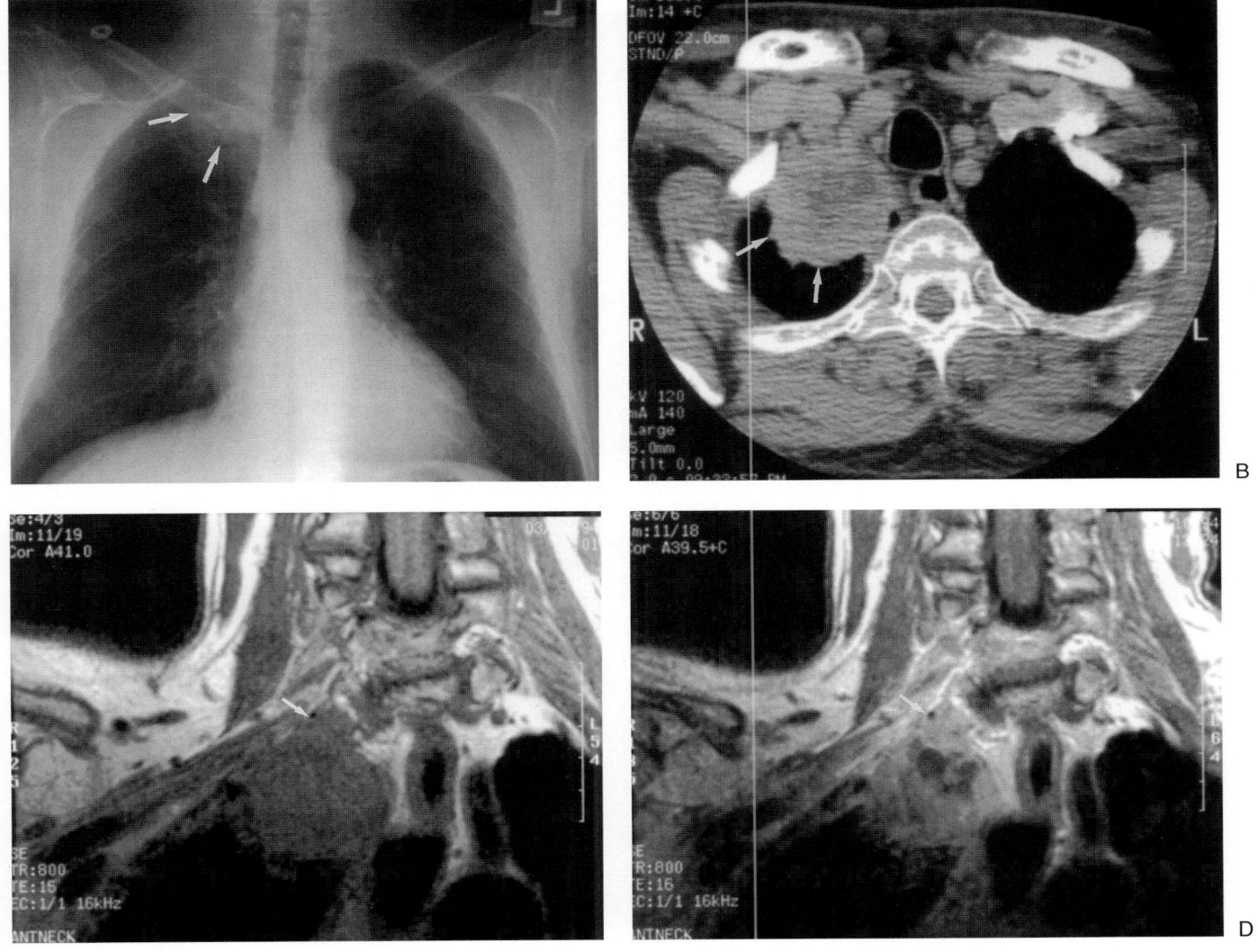

Fig. 97-3. T$_3$ disease: Chest wall invasion. **A.** Chest radiograph demonstrates a right apical mass (*arrows*). **B.** Axial computed tomographic image identifies the lesion (*arrows*), but details regarding possible chest wall involvement are limited. **C.** Pre- and (**D**) postgadolinium contrast-enhanced coronal magnetic resonance images show lobular protrusion of the mass into the apical right chest wall (*arrows*).

and colleagues (1984) using receiver operating characteristic analysis, a short-axis mediastinal lymph node dimension of 10 mm was most efficacious for recognition of nodal metastases in non–small cell lung cancers. It should also be noted that enlarged lymph nodes are by no means necessarily involved by metastatic disease. In the RDOG study findings reported by McCloud and coworkers (1992), 37% of the 19 lymph nodes that measured 2 to 4 cm in their short-axis dimension were benign hyperplastic lymph nodes.

Recent CT-surgical correlative studies by McCloud (1992) and Seely (1993) and their associates in staging mediastinal nodal metastases have highlighted some limitations and the relatively low levels of sensitivity and specificity for recognition of metastatic mediastinal lymph nodes by CT. In the study by McCloud and coworkers (1992), intravenous iodinated contrast-enhanced CT was performed with 10-mm slice thickness, and a lymph node short-axis size threshold of 10 mm was used. The CT sensitivity for metastases in that study on a per-patient basis was 64%, and the specificity was 62%. Seely and associates (1993) used a similar CT protocol and the same size criteria for short-axis lymph node measurements in group of 104 patients with T$_1$ lesions; the CT sensitivity was 59% and specificity was 91%. As we noted previously, when criteria are switched from short- to long-axis lymph node measurement in that same study, CT sensitivity increases (77%) and specificity correspondingly decreases (73%). Previous authors, including Glazer and colleagues (1984), have reported CT sensitivities for lymph node involvement using a 1-cm short-axis dimension as high as 93 to 95%. Although it is generally accepted that there are limitations in the sensitivity and specificity of CT for detecting mediastinal lymph node

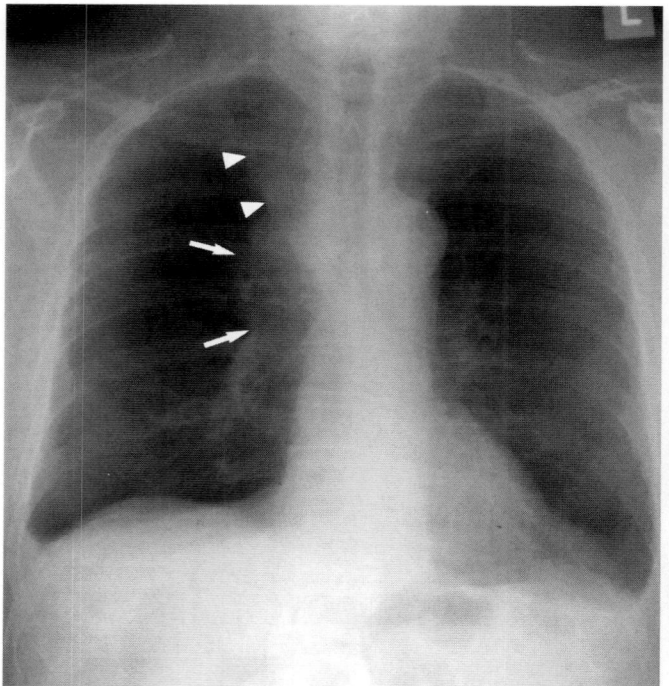

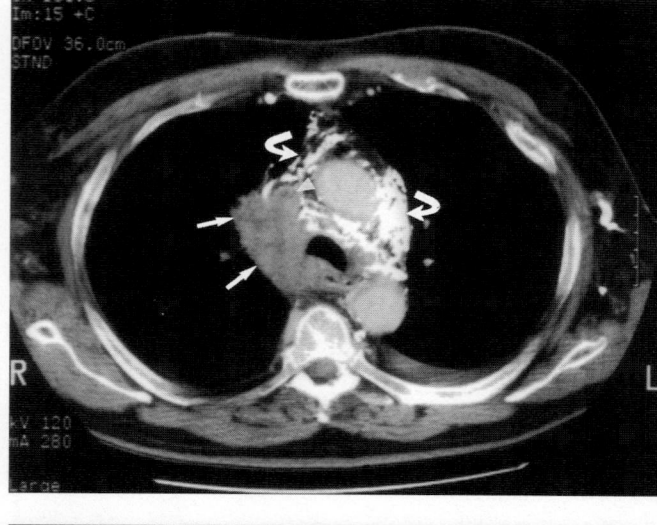

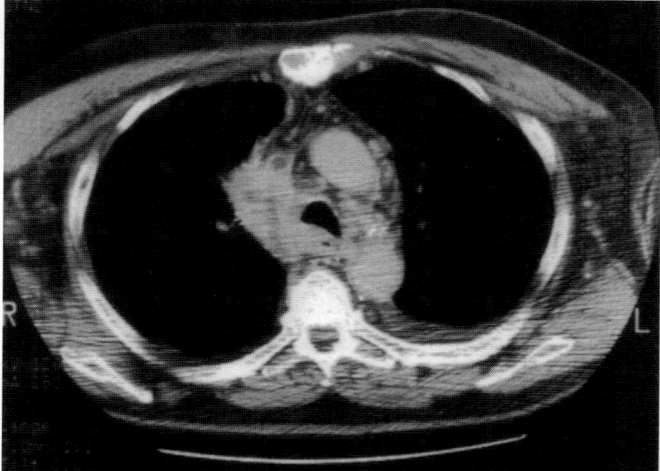

Fig. 97-4. T_4 disease: Mediastinal invasion. **A.** Chest radiograph shows a right hilar (*arrows*) and right upper mediastinal mass (*arrowheads*). There are also small bilateral pleural effusions in this patient with non–small cell lung cancer. **B.** Initial contrast-enhanced computed tomography (CT) shows the right mediastinal tumor mass (*arrows*) with obliteration of the superior vena cava, focal luminal thrombus (*arrowhead*), and numerous iodinated contrast-filled collateral veins (*curved arrows*) due to the superior vena caval obstruction. **C.** A 6-minute–delay post–contrast-enhanced CT scan illustrates clearing of the dense intravenous contrast from the collateral mediastinal vessels in this patient with mediastinal invasion.

metastases, this modality does provide a guide to the appropriate invasive method for definitive diagnostic procedures used in the staging of non–small cell lung cancer.

In the RDOG study results reported by McCloud and coworkers (1992) of CT and MR imaging for staging of non–small cell lung cancer, the sensitivity and specificity of CT for distinguishing N_0 or N_1 disease (Fig. 97-5) from N_2 or N_3 mediastinal nodal disease (Figs. 97-6 to 97-8) was 52% and 69%, respectively. In the same study, there was no statistically significant difference in accuracy between CT and conventional MR imaging for recognizing mediastinal lymph node metastases. As suggested by Jelink and associates (1990), there may be a role for MR imaging in the global assessment at initial staging for small cell lung cancer with the Veterans Administration Lung Study Group simplified dichotomous staging system for both recognition of disease and efficient distinction of localized from extensive disease.

Additional sites of potential metastatic lymph node involvement by non–small cell lung cancer that are not usually addressed in the CT literature are the supraclavicular and upper abdominal lymph nodes. Once they are palpable, supraclavicular lymph nodes are usually involved by metastatic disease in patients with lung cancer; a cytologic diagnosis can be obtained with fine-needle aspiration biopsy. Nonpalpable supraclavicular lymph nodes have a variable prevalence reported in the literature. Brantigan and associates (1973), for example, reported that in their series of 341 consecutive patients with lung cancer, 286 had nonpalpable scalene lymph nodes. Approximately 24% of these 286 patients with pulmonary tumors greater than 3 cm and no palpable scalene lymph nodes had positive scalene lymph node surgical biopsies. The validity of this study, however, must be questioned because this represents a higher incidence of involvement of these nodes than is normally found in lung cancer patients at autopsy. In a study of 47 lung cancer patients with nonpalpable scale lymph nodes, Shields and Shocket (1958) found an incidence of only 6.3%. In another report by Shields and colleagues (1958), one or more of these

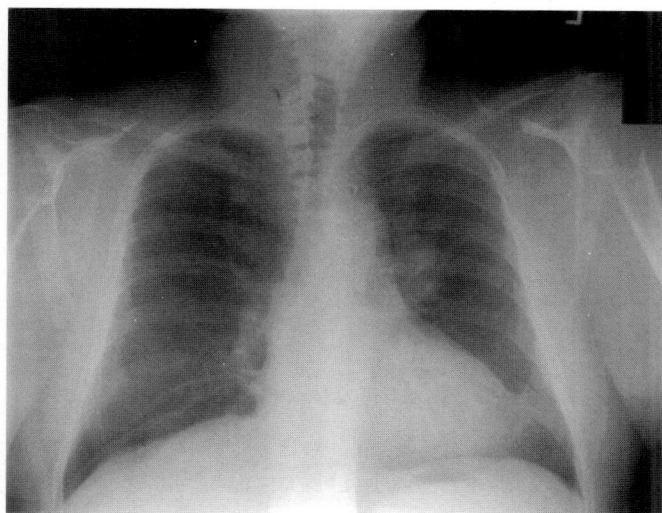 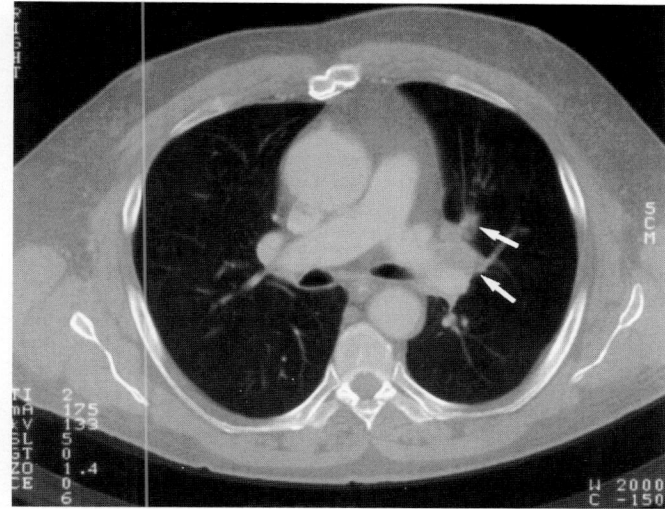

Fig. 97-5. N_1 disease: Ipsilateral hilar involvement by the left upper lobe tumor. **A.** Chest radiograph demonstrates a left hilar mass. **B.** Computed tomographic scan of left hilar involvement by tumor (*arrows*) also revealed left upper lobe air trapping due to bronchial luminal narrowing.

clinical findings appeared in all patients with positive nodes: 1) superior mediastinal lymph node enlargement, 2) a large hilar mass, and 3) a diagnosis of small cell carcinoma. More recently, Lee and Ginsberg (1996) identified positive involvement of the scalene lymph nodes in 15.4% of patients with centrally located, nonsquamous, non–small cell carcinoma with proved N_2 disease and in 63% with N_3 disease—a highly select group of patients. Directing further attention to this area at the time of the

initial chest CT evaluation will likely aid in the initial staging of patients with central lesions.

Ultrasound and ultrasound-guided fine-needle aspiration biopsies may ultimately prove to have a role in assessment of patients with nonpalpable supraclavicular nodes. In a series of 79 patients reported by Monso and coworkers (1992), ultrasound detected an additional 16.7% of patients with enlarged (>1 cm) nonpalpable supraclavicular lymph nodes when compared with physical examination findings.

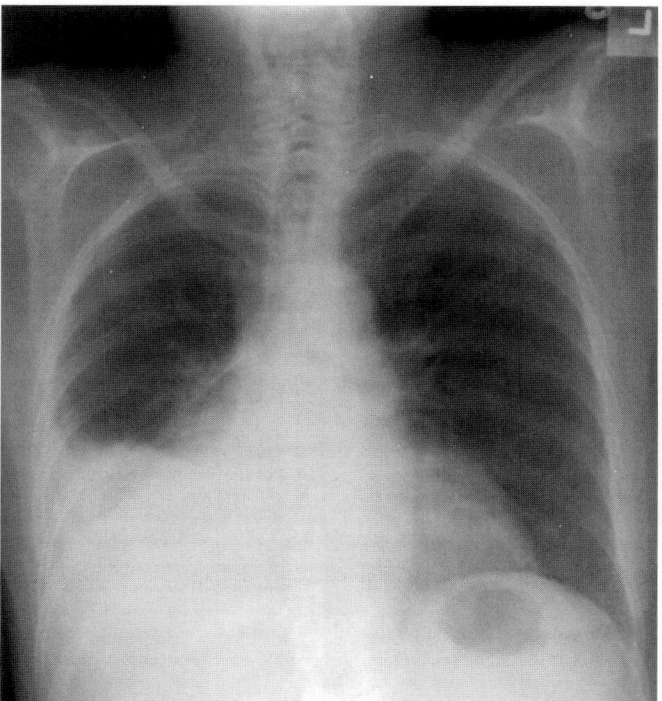 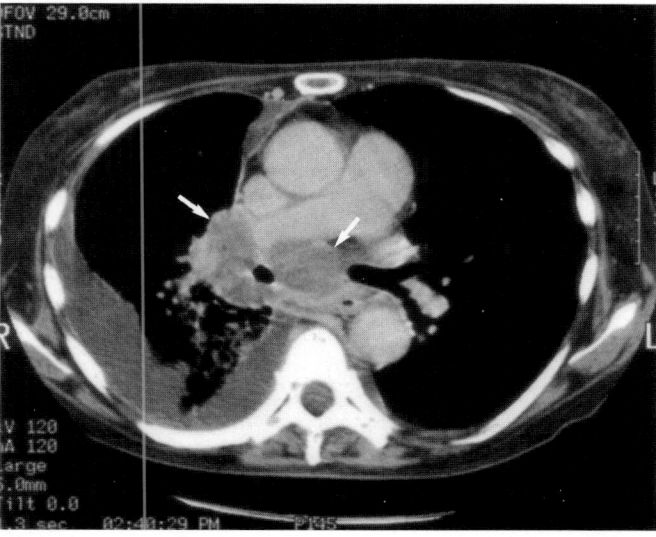

Fig. 97-6. N_2 disease: Ipsilateral hilar and subcarinal nodal disease. **A.** Chest radiograph reveals a right hilar mass and large right pleural effusion. **B.** Large right hilar and subcarinal lymph nodes (*arrows*) are present in this patient who also has a malignant right pleural effusion (T_4).

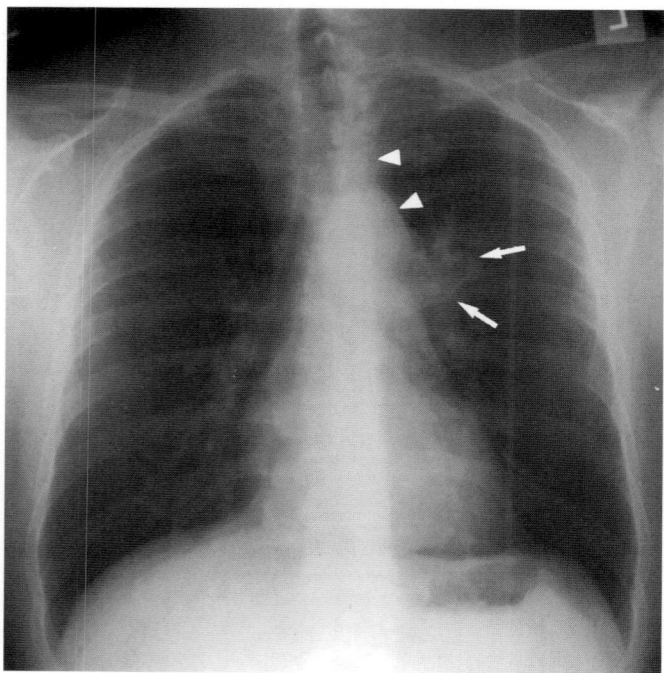

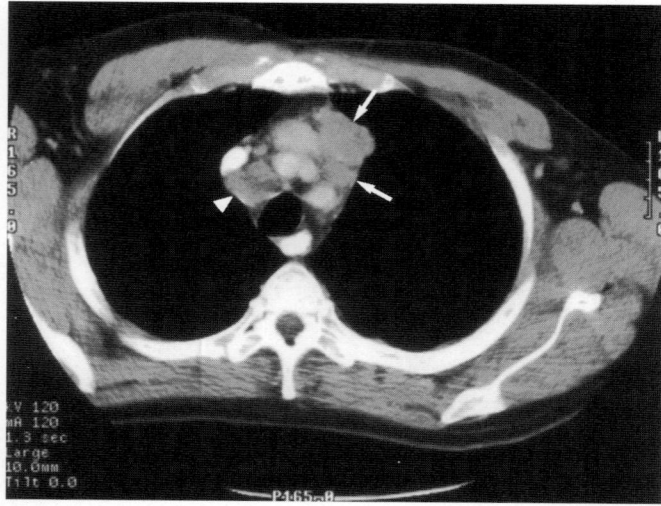

Fig. 97-7. N_3 disease: Contralateral mediastinal lymph nodes. **A.** Chest radiograph of a left hilar mass (*arrows*) and left mediastinal mass (*arrowheads*) displaying tracheal deviation to the right in this patient with non–small cell lung cancer. **B.** Computed tomographic image in the upper chest demonstrates anterior mediastinal mass (*arrows*) by the tumor (*arrowhead*).

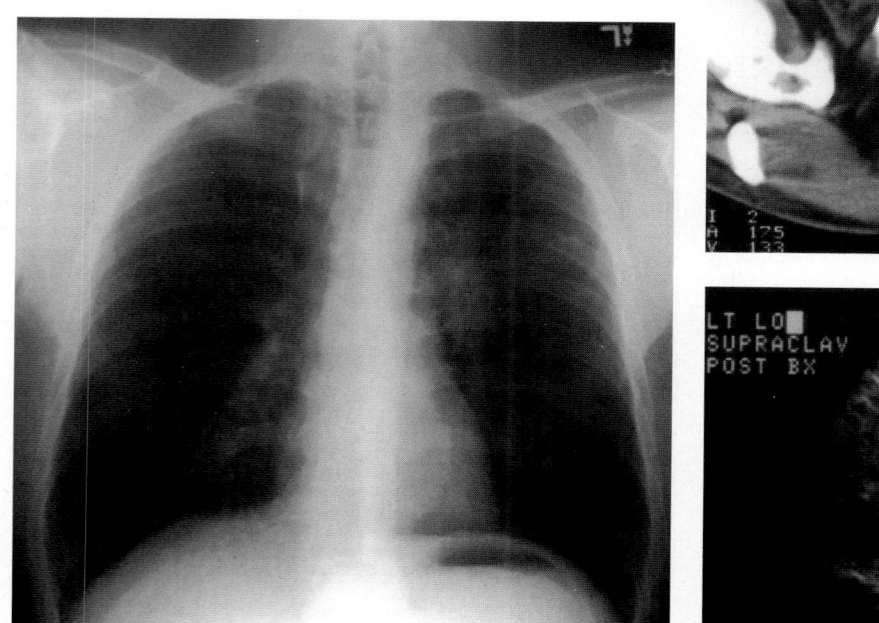

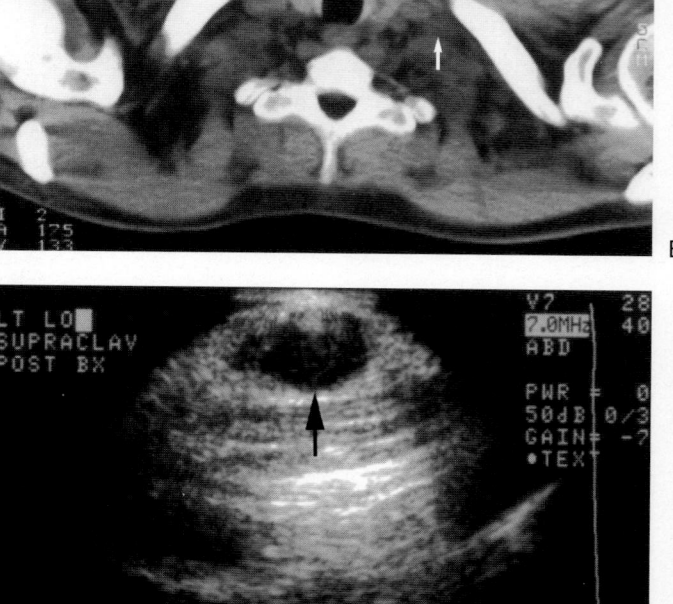

Fig. 97-8. N_3 disease: Supraclavicular lymph node. **A.** Chest radiograph of an irregular left hilar mass. **B.** Computed tomography showed an enlarged left supraclavicular lymph node (*arrow*) that was not palpable in this patient. **C.** Ultrasound was used to guide the fine-needle aspiration biopsy of the nonpalpable left supraclavicular lymph node (*arrow*). The aspiration yielded the diagnosis of non–small cell lung cancer.

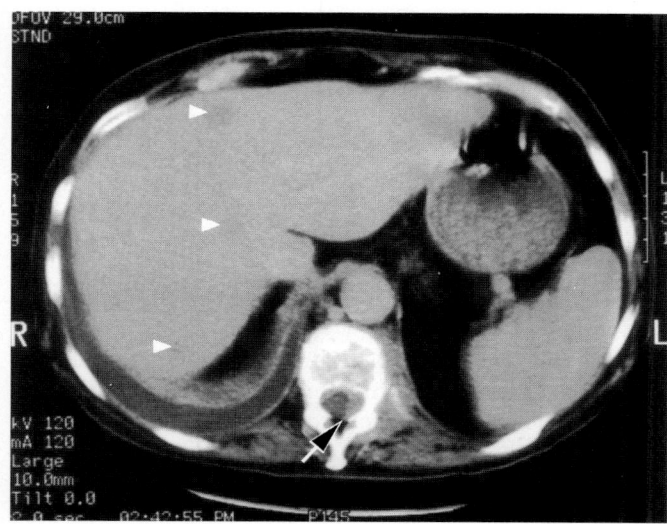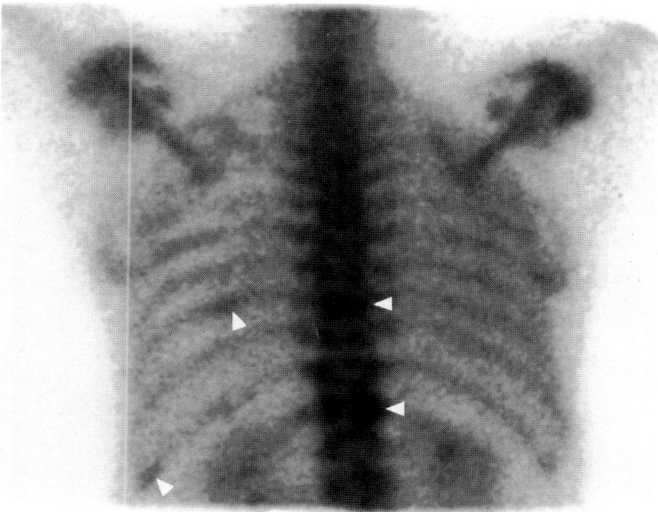

A   B

Fig. 97-9. M$_1$ disease: Liver and bone metastasis (same patient as in Fig. 97-6). **A.** Computed tomographic image in the upper liver and lower thoracic spine shows at least three liver metastasis (*arrowheads*) and a left T12 bony metastasis with extraosseous tumor invading the spinal canal (*arrow*). **B.** Nuclear medicine bone scan (posterior image of chest) shows abnormal activity in T12, T9, and in two left ribs (*arrowheads*) consistent with metastasis.

Using a combination of ultrasound and ultrasound-guided fine-needle biopsy techniques, Chang and colleagues (1992) found that six of 51 patients (12%) had metastatic nonpalpable supraclavicular lymph nodes from non–small cell lung cancer.

Because the status of mediastinal lymph nodes is so critical to proper staging and treatment, it is sometimes more expedient to biopsy them even before the main lesion itself because a positive finding not only provides a diagnosis but also stages the patient at the same time.

Metastatic Disease (M)

CT is the mainstay for initially directing the workup for M$_1$ metastatic disease (Fig. 97-9). In addition, a tumor with multiple foci of lung cancer involving more than one lobe is now staged as metastatic disease (M$_1$) because of Mountain's 1997 revision of the staging system and therefore is believed to be inoperable. There is, however, some question about the validity of this point of view. The histology of a second lung lesion in another lobe must, of course, be definitely determined, as mentioned in the previous discussion of multiple lesions in the same lobe (T$_4$).

With high-speed intravenous contrast-enhanced spiral CT, it is now also possible to scan the thorax and upper abdomen, including the liver and adrenal glands. With this capability has come the identification of a large number of lesions in the adrenal glands. The differentiation of benign versus malignant adrenal lesions is critical to proper staging. The relative proportion of benign versus metastatic adrenal lesion in patients with lung cancer varies with the patient series. In a study by Oliver and associates (1984) of patients

with non–small cell lung cancer with isolated adrenal lesions, fewer than 50% of these lesions were actually metastases.

For purposes of our discussion, the more proper distinction is between adrenal adenoma and nonadenoma (i.e., the nonadenoma is potentially, but not necessarily a metastatic lesion). Noninvasive assessment of the adrenal glands appears to be able to accurately characterize many of these lesions (Fig. 97-10). Dunnick and colleagues (1996) have outlined noninvasive adrenal imaging options that include non–contrast-enhanced and contrast-enhanced CT, MR imaging, and nuclear medicine studies. Currently, the most widely available options are CT and MR imaging.

An extensive review by Boland and colleagues (1998) pooled data from 10 previous studies comprising 495 adrenal lesions (272 benign and 223 malignant) studied by non–contrast-enhanced CT for characterization of adrenal lesions. They correlated the use of various threshold CT Hounsfield unit (HU) values of the adrenal lesions and found that a threshold CT number of 0 HU yielded a sensitivity of 41% and a specificity of 100%. When the threshold was raised to 10 HU, the sensitivity increased to 71%, with a specificity of 98%, and at 20 HU, the sensitivity was 88% but the specificity dropped to 84%. For adrenal lesions between 0 and 20 HU, McNicholas (1995) and Mayo-Smith (1995) and their colleagues have reported the use of chemical shift MR. This technique uses a form of MR that enables recognition of most adenomas because of their higher lipid content. Patients with lesions greater than 20 HU on non–contrast-enhanced CT should undergo an invasive diagnostic procedure because chemical shift MR has not differentiated lesions in this setting. Some concerns with chemical shift MR have been expressed by Reinig (1992) that some

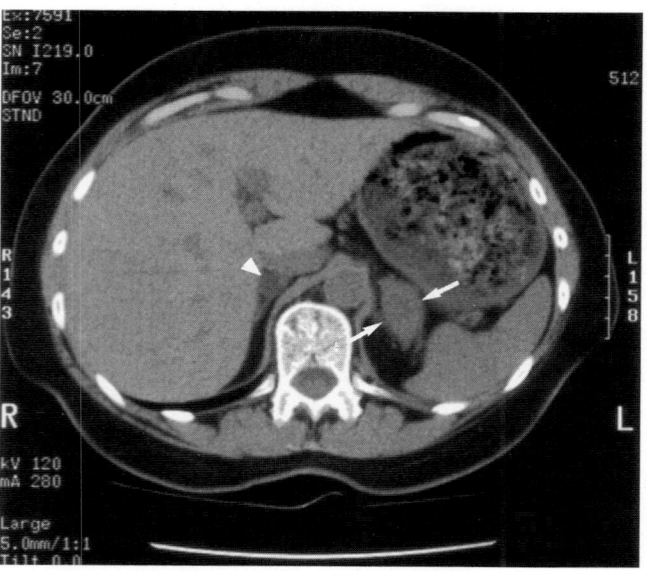

Fig. 97-10. M$_1$ disease: Synchronous adrenal metastasis and adrenal adenoma. Non–contrast-enhanced computed tomographic (CT) image shows a biopsy-proved large left adrenal metastasis from non–small cell lung cancer (*arrows*) with a CT density of 23 Hounsfield units (HU). There is also a typical right adrenal adenoma (*arrowhead*) with a CT density measurement of 0 HU.

unknown percentage of nonedematous lesions could contain lipid, but this is likely to be the case in only a small minority of instances.

Identification of distant metastasis is a critical part of preoperative evaluation. Sider and Horejs (1988) found that metastasis can be present in 25% of patients, even with preoperative CT scans showing only a solitary mass and no recognizable hilar or mediastinal lymph nodes greater than 1 cm. Routine scanning of bone, brain, and liver in the absence of symptoms and abnormal blood laboratory values, however, has not been found worthwhile. Silvestri and associates (1995), in a multivariant analysis, determined criteria for scanning for metastatic disease. They identified specific parts of the patient history and specific laboratory tests that, when normal, made the yield from a radiologic search for metastasis scans very low. That has also been our experience, but one must be careful to cover all the points detailed in the study.

FUTURE DIRECTIONS IN IMAGING PATIENTS WITH LUNG CANCER

Endeavors to improve imaging of patients with lung cancer should include efforts to optimize both observer performance and performance of the primary imaging modalities currently in use (i.e., chest radiography and chest CT examinations). Woodring (1990b) indicated that there can be significant limitations and variability in radiologic interpretations. This can occur even among expert readers. A variety of methods to improve observer performance have been proposed by Metz

and Shen (1992) and Hessel (1978), Hillman (1976, 1977), Curtis (1988), and Seltzer (1997) and their coworkers with variable degrees of success. Uniform adherence to the American College of Radiology (1995) and ATS/ERS guidelines for performance of chest CT in this setting should be a goal. In a survey by Chen and colleagues (1997), 13% of U.S. hospitals with at least 300 beds do not routinely carryout CT examinations through the adrenal glands. Improved CT protocols, including thinner slices and uniform delivery of intravenous iodinated contrast via a power injector, may also improve preoperative staging accuracy. With the arrival of helical (spiral) CT technology, inclusion of the supraclavicular lymph node region and liver in standard staging CT examinations may ultimately prove to be efficacious.

In addition, our ability to determine the etiology of solitary pulmonary nodules may be improved by comparing pre– and post–contrast-enhanced CT, as proposed by Swensen and colleagues (1996). This group ran a multicenter trial of evaluating nodules by this technique.

As with CT, MR technology continues to improve. Use of intravenous contrast-enhanced MR sequences and the development of new MR pulse sequences may provide a growing role for MR imaging in patients with suspected lung cancer. Furthermore, MR lymph node contrast imaging agents are under development, and testing and may affect the detection of nodal metastases. One such agent is a form of superparamagnetic iron oxide that is phagocytized by the reticuloendothelial system in the lymph nodes, bone marrow, liver, and spleen, as described by Anzai and colleagues (1994). Normal lymph nodes change on certain imaging sequences performed before and after administration of this contrast agent, but metastatic nodes do not. Van den Brekel and colleagues (1994) were able to recognize some tumor-bearing lymph nodes by MR imaging using this technique.

Advances in imaging are paralleled by advances in image-guided needle biopsy techniques. All major radiologic modalities, including fluoroscopy, CT, ultrasound, and MR imaging as well as nuclear medicine, have the potential to serve as guidance for pathologic confirmation of disease in and outside of the chest.

When feasible, real-time ultrasound guidance for biopsy has similar advantages to CT fluoroscopy and is more convenient. In addition, ultrasound guidance for biopsy allows greater flexibility in angled approaches (e.g., at the thoracic inlet). Furthermore, Rubens and associates (1997a, b) emphasized that many lesions that were traditionally sampled using fluoroscopy or CT guidance (e.g., mediastinal and skeletal lesions) are sometimes readily accessible to ultrasound-guided needle biopsy.

CONCLUSIONS

A patient's presenting symptoms and signs and chest radiographic findings, or both, prompt the initial evaluation of patients with suspected lung cancer. The chest radiograph is usually followed by chest CT, which aids in characterization of abnormalities noted on the radiographs (e.g., lung nodule assessment). CT also defines the extent of possible disease and directs invasive procedures to obtain pathologic confirmation of cell type and maximal extent of disease. Further evaluation with MR imaging, nuclear medicine bone scan, or other imaging modalities is currently believed to be most optimally guided by results of history, physical, and clinical laboratory evaluations, as per the ATS/ERS guidelines.

In patients for whom a diagnosis has been established, chest CT is an adjunct to directing the final determination of the stage of disease at presentation. It is for patients whose history, physical, and laboratory evaluations suggest that they are potential surgical candidates that CT has had great impact in patient management. When potential sites of disease that would contraindicate surgery are identified on CT, a minimally invasive radiology-guided biopsy can frequently be performed to confirm a diagnosis. If that is not the case, initial surgical staging procedures can usually be directed to such sites of concern.

Continuing challenges in the radiologic diagnosis and staging of lung cancer include earlier recognition of disease and minimizing errors in perception and interpretation of radiologic studies. Another challenge is to standardize radiologic techniques and noninvasive characterizations of incidental benign lesions that complicate preoperative staging studies (e.g., benign pulmonary nodules, benign enlarged lymph nodes, and benign adrenal lesions).

Ongoing and future directions of study include radiologic screening of high-risk patients and optimization of observer performance for interpretation of examinations. Future and ongoing research in expanding the use of CT (e.g., noninvasive characterization of indeterminate pulmonary nodules based on pre– and post–contrast-enhanced scanning and positron emission tomography scanning for patients with possible lung cancer) will further enhance the accuracy of patient staging evaluations.

REFERENCES

Amemiya R, Oho K: X-ray diagnosis of lung cancer. *In* Hayata Y (ed): Lung Cancer Diagnosis. Tokyo: Igaku-Shoin, 1982, p. 4.

American College of Radiology Task Force on Appropriateness Criteria: Staging of bronchogenic carcinoma, non-small cell lung carcinoma. American College of Radiology Appropriateness Criteria For Imaging and Treatment Decisions, TH2-1, 1995.

American Thoracic Society/European Respiratory Society: Pretreatment evaluation of non-small-cell lung cancer. Am J Respir Crit Care Med *156*:320, 1997.

Anzai Y, et al: Initial clinical experience with dextran-coated superparamagnetic iron oxide for detection of lymph node metastases in patients with head and neck cancer. Radiology *192*:709, 1994.

Berkman YM: The many facets of bronchioloalveolar cell carcinoma. Semin Roentgenol *12*:207, 1977.

Boland GWL, et al: Characterization of adrenal masses using unenhanced CT: an analysis of the CT literature. AJR Am J Roentgenol *171*:201, 1998.

Brantigan JW, Brantigan CO, Brantigan O: Biopsy of nonpalpable scalene lymph nodes in carcinoma of the lung. Am Rev Respir Dis *107*:962, 1973.

Byrd RB, et al: Radiographic abnormalities in carcinoma of the lung as related to histological cell type. Thorax *124*:573, 1969.

Carter D, Eggleston JC: Tumors of the lower respiratory tract. *In* Atlas of Tumor Pathology. 2nd Series. Fasc 17. Washington DC: Armed Forces Institute of Pathology, 1980, pp. 113–160.

Chang D-B, et al: Ultrasonography and ultrasonographically guided fine-needle aspiration biopsy of impalpable cervical lymph nodes in patients with non-small cell lung cancer. Cancer *70*:1111, 1992.

Chen MYM, et al: Bronchogenic carcinoma: a survey of CT protocols for staging disease. Acad Radiol *4*:687, 1997.

Curtis PB, Ferrell WR, Hillman BJ: Improved imaging diagnosis by sequentially combined confidence judgments. Invest Radiol *23*:342, 1988.

Dunnick NR, Korobkin M, Francis I: Adrenal radiology: distinguishing benign from malignant adrenal masses. AJR Am J Roentgenol *167*:861 1996.

Eto T, et al: The changes of the stromal elastotic framework in the growth of peripheral lung adenocarcinomas. Cancer *77*:646, 1996.

Fontana RS, et al: Lung cancer screening: the Mayo program. J Occup Med *28*:746, 1986.

Garland LH: The rate of growth and natural duration of primary bronchial cancer. AJR Am J Roentgenol *96*:604, 1966.

Glazer GM, et al: The mediastinum in non-small cell lung cancer: CT-surgical correlation. AJR Am J Roentgenol *142*:1101, 1984.

Glazer GM, et al: Normal mediastinal lymph nodes: number and size according to American Thoracic Society mapping. AJR Am J Roentgenol *144*:261, 1985.

Glazer HS, et al: Pleural and chest wall invasion in bronchogenic carcinoma: CT evaluation. Radiology *157*:191, 1985.

Glazer HS, et al: Indeterminate mediastinal invasion in bronchogenic carcinoma: CT evaluation. Radiology *173*:37, 1989.

Heitzman ER, et al: Pathways of tumor spread through the lung: radiologic correlation with anatomy and pathology. Radiology *144*:3, 1982.

Herman SJ, et al: Mediastinal invasion by bronchogenic carcinoma: CT signs. Radiology *190*:841, 1994.

Hessel SJ, Herman PG, Swensson RG: Improving performance by multiple interpretations of chest radiographs: effectiveness and cost. Radiology *127*:589, 1978.

Hill CA: Bronchioloalveolar carcinoma: a review. Radiology *150*:15, 1984.

Hillman BJ, et al: The value of consultation among radiologists. AJR Am J Roentgenol *127*:807, 1976.

Hillman BJ, et al: Improving diagnostic accuracy: a comparison of interactive and Delphi consultations. Invest Radiol *12*:112, 1977.

Ichinose Y, et al: The correlation between tumor size and lymphatic vessel invasion in resected peripheral stage I non-small-cell lung cancer. A potential risk of limited resection. J Thorac Cardiovasc Surg *108*:684, 1994.

Im JG, et al: Lobar bronchioloalveolar carcinoma: "Angiogram sign" on CT scans. Radiology *176*:749, 1990.

Jang HJ, et al: Bronchioloalveolar carcinoma: focal areas of ground-glass attenuation at thin-section CT as an early sign. Radiology *199*:485, 1996.

Jelink JS, et al: Small cell lung cancer: staging with MR imaging. Radiology *177*:837, 1990.

Kaneko M, et al: Peripheral lung cancer: screening and detection with low-dose spiral CT versus radiography. Radiology *201*:798, 1996.

Kreisman H, Wolkove N, Quoix E: Small cell lung cancer presenting as a solitary pulmonary nodule. Chest *101*:225, 1992.

Kubik A, et al: Lack of benefit from semi-annual screening for cancer of the lung: follow-up report of a randomized controlled trial on a population of high-risk males in Czechoslovakia. Int J Cancer *45*:26, 1990.

Lee JD, Ginsberg RJ: Lung cancer staging: the value of ipsilateral scalene lymph node biopsy performed at mediastinoscopy. Ann Thorac Surg *62*:338, 1996.

Mahoney MC, et al: CT demonstration of calcification in carcinoma of the lung. AJR Am J Roentgenol *154*:255, 1990.

Mahoney MC, et al: Computed tomography of the thorax. Chest Surg Clin N Am *2*:465, 1992.

Mayo-Smith WW, et al: Characterization of adrenal masses (<5 cm) by use of chemical shift MR imaging: observer performance versus quantitative measures. AJR Am J Roentgenol *165*:91, 1995.

McCloud TC, et al: Bronchogenic carcinoma: analysis of staging in the mediastinum with CT by correlative lymph node mapping and sampling. Radiology *182*:319, 1992.

McNicholas MJ, et al: An imaging algorithm for the differential diagnosis of adrenal adenomas and metastases. AJR Am J Roentgenol *165*:1453, 1995.

Melamed MR, et al: Screening for early lung cancer: results of the Memorial-Sloan Kettering study in New York. Chest *86*:44, 1984.

Metz CE, Shen J-H: Gains in accuracy from replicated readings of diagnostic images: prediction and assessment in terms of ROC analysis. Med Decis Making *12*:60, 1992.

Monso E, et al: Usefulness of supraclavicular ultrasonography in the staging of lung cancer. Lung *170*:243, 1992.

Mountain CF: Revisions in the international system for staging lung cancer. Chest *111*:1710, 1997.

Muhm JR, et al: Lung cancer detected during a screening program using four-month chest radiographs. Radiology *148*:609, 1983.

Noguchi M, et al: Small adenocarcinoma of the lung. Histologic characteristics and prognosis. Cancer *75*:2844, 1995.

Oliver TW Jr, et al: Isolated adrenal masses in nonsmall-cell bronchogenic carcinoma. Radiology *153*:217, 1984.

Reinig JW: MR imaging differentiation of adrenal masses: has the time finally come? Radiology *185*:339, 1992.

Rigler LG: A roentgen study of the evolution of carcinoma of the lung. J Thorac Cardiovasc Surg *34*:283, 1957.

Rigler LG: The earliest roentgenographic signs of carcinoma of the lung. JAMA *195*:655, 1966.

Rubens DJ, et al: Effective ultrasonographically guided intervention for diagnosis of musculoskeletal lesions. J Ultrasound Med *16*:831, 1997a.

Rubens DJ, et al: Sonographic guidance of mediastinal biopsy: an effective alternative to CT guidance. AJR Am J Roentgenol *169*:1605, 1997b.

Salomaa ER, et al: Prognosis of patients with lung cancer found in a single chest radiograph screening. Chest *114*:1514, 1998.

Seely J, et al: T1 lung cancer: prevalence of mediastinal nodal metastases (diagnostic accuracy of CT). Radiology *186*:129, 1993.

Seltzer SE, et al: Staging prostate cancer with MR imaging: a combined radiologist-computer system. Radiology *202*:219, 1997.

Shields TW, Lees WM, Fox R: The diagnostic value of nonpalpable lymph nodes in chest diseases. Ann Surg *148*:184, 1958.

Shields TW, Shocket E: Preoperative evaluation of patients with clinically resectable bronchogenic carcinoma. A role of biopsy of nonpalpable scalene nodes. AMA Arch Surg *76*:707, 1958.

Sider L: Radiographic manifestations of primary bronchogenic cancer. Radiol Clin North Am *28*:583, 1990.

Sider L, Horejs D: Frequency of extrathoracic metastases from bronchogenic carcinoma in patients with normal-sized hilar and mediastinal lymph nodes on CT. AJR Am J Roentgenol *151*:893, 1988.

Silvestri GA, Littenberg B, Colice GL: The clinical evaluation for detecting metastatic lung cancer. A meta-analysis. Am J Respir Crit Care Med. *152*:225, 1995.

Steinhauslin CA, Cuttat JF: Spontaneous pneumothorax a complication of lung cancer? Chest *88*:709, 1985.

Strauss GM: The ABCs of lung cancer screening. Chest *114*: 1502, 1998.

Swensen SJ, et al: Lung nodule enhancement at CT: prospective findings. Radiology *201*:447, 1996.

Swett HA, Nagel JS, Sostman HD: Imaging methods in primary lung carcinoma. Clin Chest Med *3*:331, 1982.

Theros EG: Varying manifestations of peripheral pulmonary neoplasms: a radiologic-pathologic correlative study. AJR Am J Roentgenol *128*:893, 1977.

Tockman MS: Survival and mortality from lung cancer in a screened population. The Johns Hopkins Study. Chest *89*:325s, 1986.

Van den Brekel MWM, Castelijns JA, Snow GB: Detection of lymph node metastases in the neck: radiologic criteria. Radiology *192*:617, 1994.

Webb WR, et al: CT and MR imaging in staging non-small cell bronchogenic carcinoma: report of the radiologic diagnostic oncology group. Radiology *178*:705, 1991.

Weiss W, Bouocot KR, Seidman H: The Philadelphia pulmonary neoplasm research project. Clin Chest Med *3*:243, 1982.

Woodring JH: Unusual radiologic manifestations of lung cancer. Radiol Clin North Am *28*:599, 1990a.

Woodring JH: Pitfalls in the radiologic diagnosis of lung cancer. AJR Am J Roentgenol *154*:1165, 1990b.

Woodring JH, Fried AM: Significance of wall thickness in solitary cavities of the lung: a follow-up study. AJR Am J Roentgenol *140*:473, 1983.

Woodring JH, Stelling CB: Adenocarcinoma of the lung: a tumor with a changing pleomorphic character. AJR Am J Roentgenol *140*:657, 1983.

Yamashiro K, et al: Prognostic significance of an interface pattern of central fibrosis and tumor cells in peripheral adenocarcinoma of the lung. Hum Pathol *26*:67, 1995.

Zwirewich CV, et al: Solitary pulmonary nodule: high-resolution CT and radiologic-pathologic correlation. Radiology *179*:469, 1991.

CHAPTER 98

Diagnosis and Staging of Lung Cancer

Carolyn E. Reed and Gerard A. Silvestri

Once the radiographic (see Chapter 97) or clinical presentation (see Chapter 96) raises the possibility of lung cancer, the physician must proceed in an expeditious manner to confirm a diagnosis. The choice of approach is influenced by lesion characteristics (e.g., size, location), presence or absence of symptoms (e.g., hemoptysis or obstructive phenomena), and evidence of extrathoracic disease. The evaluation should establish the diagnosis as well as determine the extent or stage of the cancer. This information is critical for treatment decisions and discussion of prognosis with the patient. At times, the diagnosis and stage can be determined by a single test (e.g., liver biopsy or thoracentesis of a pleural effusion). In most cases, careful evaluation of the tumor status (T), nodal status (N), and evidence of metastatic disease (M) requires consideration of a variety of noninvasive and invasive procedures. The staging should be performed in a cost-effective manner.

DIAGNOSIS OF LUNG CANCER

Sputum Cytology

Since the advent of fiberoptic bronchoscopy, the use of sputum cytology for diagnosis of lung cancer has declined dramatically. However, this diagnostic technique should be considered in certain cases because it has no risk to the patient and is inexpensive. Sputum cytology is most beneficial when the lesion is central or the patient presents with hemoptysis. Travis and colleagues (1996) have reviewed the literature and suggest that the diagnostic yield of sputum cytology increases from 52 to 87% when the sample is an induced collected sputum sample rather than spontaneous expectoration and when three samples are obtained rather than one.

Fiberoptic Bronchoscopy

Fiberoptic bronchoscopy is used to diagnose, stage, and, in some cases, treat lung cancer. It is the procedure of choice for patients with centrally located lung masses. The diagnostic yield of fiberoptic bronchoscopy for centrally located lung masses presumed to be cancer is approximately 70% and increases to greater than 90% when the lesion is visualized in the airway. The addition of bronchial brushings increases the diagnostic yield over biopsy alone, but Arroglia and Matthay (1993) reported that the addition of bronchial washing may not further improve the diagnostic accuracy. If washing is performed, it should be done after biopsy and brushing.

The use of bronchoscopy for peripheral lesions is less well validated. In the review by Arroglia and Matthay (1993), the diagnostic yield of transbronchial biopsy, brush, and washing with the use of biplane fluoroscopy varied between 40 and 80%. Success is most dependent on the size of the lesion. Transbronchial biopsy of lesions that are greater than 4 cm in diameter has a diagnostic yield of approximately 80%, whereas lesions less than 2 cm in diameter have a yield of approximately 30%. Torrington and Kern (1993) evaluated 91 patients with solitary pulmonary nodules (clinical stage I) and found that the diagnostic yield of fiberoptic bronchoscopy was low. Shure and Fedullo (1983) reported an increase in the diagnostic yield of peripheral lesions from 48 to 69% by the addition of transbronchial needle aspirate to routine fiberoptic bronchoscopy. Pirozynski (1992) and de Gracia and associates (1993) assessed the addition of bronchoalveolar lavage to fiberoptic bronchoscopy for the diagnosis of peripheral pulmonary nodules. They did not show a significant increase in diagnostic yield and did not recommend routine bronchoalveolar lavage. It is our recommendation that patients with a mass that is less than 3 cm and lateral to the midclavicular line should not undergo fiberoptic bronchoscopy because the diagnostic yield is too low compared to that of transthoracic needle aspiration.

The complication rate of fiberoptic bronchoscopy is low and includes cough, bleeding, pneumothorax, and iatrogenic infection. Major bleeding (>50 mL) occurs in approximately 2% of patients. Pneumothorax after biopsy of a central lesion is extremely rare.

Table 98-1. Characteristics of Solitary Pulmonary Nodules Predicting Malignancy

Radiologic characteristics
Diameter >2 cm
Spiculation present
Upper lobe location
Clinical characteristics
Age >40 years
Positive smoking history
History of other cancer

Transthoracic Needle Aspiration

Transthoracic needle aspiration has been the procedure of choice for the diagnosis of peripheral pulmonary nodules measuring less than 3 cm in diameter. Salazar and Westcott (1993) reported an accuracy between 80 and 95%. The presence of an on-site cytopathologist improves the diagnostic yield. The use of a core needle biopsy can sometimes yield a definitive benign diagnosis. Unfortunately, a negative or nondiagnostic fine-needle aspiration (FNA) does not reassure the clinician that the patient does not have cancer because up to 30% of these patients have malignant lesions discovered at surgery. A repeat transthoracic FNA is diagnostic in 35 to 65% of these patients.

If the lesion is amenable to video-assisted thoracoscopic surgery (VATS), and the probability of malignancy is high, VATS should be considered. Swensen and colleagues (1997) identified three clinical characteristics and three radiologic characteristics that were independent predictors of malignancy (Table 98-1). In patients who have these clinical characteristics, transthoracic needle aspirate is unlikely to provide additional information and only delays surgery.

An FNA can also be useful in the diagnosis of mediastinal masses and in the staging of cancers that extend to the mediastinum, chest wall, or pleura. Transthoracic FNA also can be useful after a nondiagnostic bronchoscopy. We recommend transthoracic needle aspirate in the diagnosis of a solitary pulmonary nodule for the following scenarios: 1) the patient is a high operative risk, 2) the patient has a low risk of malignancy based on clinical and radiologic characteristics, 3) a definite benign diagnosis is considered, 4) the patient prefers to have a definite diagnosis of cancer before proceeding to the operating room, or 5) the patient is not an operative candidate, but tissue confirmation is needed before definitive treatment with chemotherapy or radiation therapy.

Positron Emission Tomography

Positron emission tomography (PET) is discussed in detail in Chapter 12. A brief summary of its diagnostic value is presented here. PET is a noninvasive tool that can be used to evaluate indeterminate pulmonary lesions. It depends on the detection of specific radioactive isotopes that decay by positron emission and are detected by specific radioactive isotopes. The most widely used PET tracer for the detection of malignancy is fluoride-18-fluorodeoxyglucose (FDG). A high rate of glycolysis is a biochemical feature of malignancy; FDG competes with glucose for uptake in the cell. FDG is phosphorylated and then accumulates in the cell because it cannot be further metabolized. The amount of FDG that accumulates in the cell over a fixed period is proportional to the rate of cellular glucose metabolism, and the differences in glucose metabolism between benign and malignant tissues are the basis for the use of PET in the diagnosis and staging of lung cancer. PET imaging provides numeric data for each pixel of an image that accurately reflects the amount of FDG accumulating in a selected region. The standardized uptake ratio (SUR) is an uptake value normalized for patient body weight and imaging dose that provides a means of comparison of FDG uptake between patients. It is calculated as follows: SUR = mean selected region activity (mCi/mL)/injected dose – mCi per body weight (kg). SUR values 2.5 or higher or slightly different values have been considered indicative of malignancy. Other investigators have considered abnormal any visual FDG uptake greater than mediastinal uptake.

Lowe and Naunheim (1998) summarized the use of PET in the diagnosis of pulmonary abnormalities (Table 98-2). Overall, there was an average sensitivity of 94% and specificity of 82% for the detection of malignancy.

False-positive PET scans are usually the result of active infectious or inflammatory lesions. False-negative PET scans have been documented in tumors with relatively low metabolic activity. Higashi and colleagues (1997) noted four false-negative scans in seven patients with bronchoalveolar carcinoma. Carcinoid tumors are another example of a malignancy that may have a low level of FDG accumulation. Size of the lesion is also an important factor in the accuracy of PET scanning. At present, sensitivity is much lower for lesions less than 1 cm in diameter.

The clinical application of PET for indeterminate pulmonary nodules is still controversial. A positive PET scan helps the physician in recommending further invasive testing or resection options, depending on further anatomic factors, patient factors, and so forth. A negative PET scan can prompt the physician to recommend observation with follow-up imaging. Weber and colleagues (1997) used cost-effectiveness analysis to show that such an approach resulted in a significant cost reduction per patient.

Bolus Contrast Computed Tomography

Another modality for evaluation of solitary pulmonary nodules currently undergoing scrutiny is the use of bolus contrast computed tomographic (CT) scan. This technology relies on the fact that malignant tumors are highly vascularized and therefore are enhanced by intravenous contrast material. It can be performed in most hospitals in the United States with

Table 98-2. FDG PET Studies of Pulmonary Opacities or Solitary Pulmonary Nodules

Author	Lesions (malignant/benign)	Indication	PET Criteria (SUV or visual)	Sensitivity (%)	Specificity (%)
Kubota et al. (1990)	12/10	Opacity	→ 2.0	83	90
Duhaylongsod et al. (1995)	59/28	Opacity	→ 2.5	97	81
Bury et al. (1996a)	33/17	SPN	Visual	100	88
Knight et al. (1996)	32/16	Opacity	>2.5	100	63
Gupta et al. (1996)	45/16	SPN	Visual	93	88
Lowe et al. (1997)	120/77	Opacity	→ 2.5	96	77
PIOPLIN (1998)	60/30	SPN	→ 2.5	92	90
Totals	361/194			94	82

FDG, fluoride-18-fluorodeoxyglucose; PET, positron emission tomography; PIOPLIN, prospective investigation of PET in lung nodules; SPN, solitary pulmonary nodules; SUV, standardized uptake value.
From Lowe VJ, Naunheim KS: PET in lung cancer. Ann Thorac Surg *65*:1821, 1998. With permission.

a little extra time and expense. Swensen and colleagues (1995) reported that malignant tumors enhanced with a median of 40 Hounsfield units (HU) (range 20 to 108 HU) compared to benign tumors, which only enhanced with a median of 12 HU (range 2 to 58 HU) on CT scan. Using 20 HU as a cutoff, the sensitivity (100%) and specificity (76.9%) of bolus contrast CT rivals that reported with PET scan.

Video-Assisted Thoracoscopic Surgery

For patients with peripheral indeterminate pulmonary nodules, wedge excision via VATS offers an alternative to transthoracic needle biopsy. In lesions less than 2 cm in diameter, Berquist and associates (1980) noted that the transthoracic needle biopsy yield of a positive diagnosis in the presence of malignancy was only 60%. Mack and colleagues (1993a) reported the results of 242 patients undergoing thoracoscopic excisional biopsy as the primary diagnostic method for indeterminate solitary pulmonary nodules. Such lesions were defined as less than 3 cm in diameter, noncalcified, and located in the outer one-third of the lung parenchyma. Only two patients required thoracotomy to locate the nodule; a definitive diagnosis was obtained in all other patients. Data from the VATS Study Group, reported by Hazelrigg and colleagues (1993), support the very low morbidity of thoracoscopy.

Before VATS, the CT scan should be carefully examined to determine the likelihood that the nodule can be located at thoracoscopy. If the nodule is based in the pleura and larger than 1 cm, visualization of the nodule can be anticipated. If the nodule is immediately subpleural, effacement of the lung parenchyma around the nodule as the lung collapses aids in detection. For nodules deeper than 1 cm below the pleural surface or less than 1 cm in diameter, the techniques described by Mack and associates (1993b) are helpful. The CT scan may indicate subtle pleural puckering, or soft tissue windows may reveal the nodule adjacent to the fissure. A blunt grasping instrument may be used for palpation of the lung and give the surgeon a partial tactile sense. A finger can be inserted through a port site initially

placed over the lesion and the lung palpated by partial insufflation. If it is anticipated preoperatively that the nodule will not be found at thoracoscopy, Mack and colleagues (1993b) suggest a technique of needle localization consisting of a CT-guided 20-gauge needle from a localizer system placed percutaneously into the nodule. After needle localization, 0.05 mL of diluted methylene blue is injected through the needle to stain the subpleural area overlying the lesion. Shennib and Bret (1992) reported the use of intraoperative transthoracic ultrasonography to locate lung lesions during VATS.

Allen and associates (1993) from the Mayo Clinic showed that total hospital charges for VATS resection of an indeterminate nodule did not differ significantly from excision via thoracotomy. Although VATS shortened the hospital stay, there were higher operating room costs. However, time to full recovery status was not assessed. Once a diagnosis of malignancy is confirmed by VATS, conversion to an open thoracotomy depends on the patient's pulmonary status and the surgeon's experience with extended VATS resection versus standard open resection of the carcinoma.

Thoracotomy

When other noninvasive diagnostic techniques have been unsuccessful and the lesion has features suggestive of malignancy, open thoracotomy should be performed. If the lesion is deep within a lobe and cannot be removed easily and completely by a wedge excision, Tru-Cut needle biopsy should be performed.

ASYMPTOMATIC SOLITARY PULMONARY NODULE

One of the most difficult dilemmas for a physician is the indeterminate pulmonary nodule. It is a significant problem because approximately 150,000 new nodules are detected each year in the United States. Although the traditional definition of a solitary pulmonary nodule includes a size range from 1 to 6 cm, the designation of a T_1 lesion (<3 cm) is more appropriate. Westcott (1988) and Zerhouni and colleagues (1986) reported that a nodule 3 cm or greater in diameter has a likelihood of malignancy of 93 to 99%. The indeterminate nodule should be surrounded by lung parenchyma and relatively well demarcated. In addition to size, contour, calcification, and growth rate of a nodule are useful criteria in the assessment of potential malignancy. Patient characteristics, such as age, smoking history, and prior history of malignancy, also play a role.

One should start with the least invasive method of evaluation. Swensen and colleagues (1990) suggest that if prior roentgenograms demonstrate a stable lesion over a 2-year period or if a particular pattern of calcification (diffuse, central, laminar, or "popcorn") exists, a benign diagnosis can be affirmed, and an "observation only" approach is justified. If the patient is less than 30 to 35 years old, has no previous history of malignancy, and is a nonsmoker, an observation only approach is also appropriate. If chest films indicate growth, the doubling time of the volume of the mass may yield useful information. Nathan and associates (1962) reported that in patients older than 40 years, a doubling time of a solitary nodule of less than 37 days or greater than 465 days represented a benign lesion. A 25% increase in the diameter of a nodule represents approximately a doubling of the volume of the mass.

High-resolution CT scan can be helpful in determining calcium content, contour, and internal characteristics. Zwirewich and colleagues (1991) compared edge and internal composition of benign nodules with those of malignant nodules. Spiculation of the margin was present in 55% of the benign and 87% of the malignant nodules; pleural tags were present in 27% and 58%, respectively; and bubblelike areas of low attenuation (air bronchograms, cavitation, or tumor necrosis) were observed in 25% of the malignant and only 9% of the benign nodules.

When a solitary noncalcified nodule less than 3 cm in diameter is found in a patient 25 years or older with no current or past evidence of extrapulmonary malignancy and with no knowledge of prior films documenting stability of the lesion, the burden is on the physician to disprove malignancy. If the patient is high risk for surgery or wants to avoid any invasive procedure, we suggest PET or bolus contrast CT scan as the next step. A negative scan would help the physician to recommend observation and follow-up imaging. If the nodule is amenable to thoracoscopic resection, this procedure has 100% sensitivity and 100% specificity. As Mack and colleagues (1993a) have demonstrated, operative mortality should be zero and the complication rate should be under 5%. Most patients have already had a CT scan for evaluation, and if thoracoscopy demonstrates malignancy, definitive therapy can be undertaken. A cost-effective analysis of the role of PET versus thoracoscopy or thoracotomy needs further study.

We rarely perform transthoracic needle aspiration for a solitary pulmonary nodule, except in special circumstances

previously discussed. In the series by Calhoun and associates (1986) of 397 consecutive patients undergoing transthoracic needle aspiration, 132 patients had a "no cancer" diagnosis, and 29% were subsequently found to have a malignancy. Because of such a high yield of nondiagnostic results, we favor a more aggressive approach.

DIAGNOSTIC APPROACH TO OCCULT LUNG CANCER

Occasionally, patients present with hemoptysis and a negative chest radiograph. If they have a significant smoking history and are older than 40, Colice (1997) estimates that 6% will eventually have the diagnosis of lung cancer established. The diagnostic strategy that uses the least number of tests to diagnose the lung cancer begins with sputum cytology. Colice (1997) reported little role for CT scan as an initial test in patients with hemoptysis and a normal chest radiograph. If sputum cytology is positive for malignant cells, fiberoptic bronchoscopy with airway inspection should be performed. If a visible endobronchial lesion is not identified for biopsy, the patient should have the bronchoscopy performed under general anesthesia so that cytologic brushing of each subsegment of the lungs can be undertaken. When a positive cytologic brush is obtained, the procedure should be repeated in the affected area. Surgical resection is recommended when two positive results are obtained from the same lobe.

STAGING OF LUNG CANCER

The staging of lung cancer is critical to the planning of treatment strategies, defining prognostic subgroups, and comparing research data and the results of clinical trials. Staging provides a common language of communication between physicians caring for the patient. The staging process should be accurate and reproducible.

Over the last two decades, the staging system for non–small cell lung cancer (NSCLC) has undergone significant changes in an attempt to minimize variability of prognosis within each group and correlate different treatment strategies for groups at different stages. Mountain (1997) has refined the TNM staging system to increase specificity in stage classification and decrease the heterogeneity of end results that exist for the TNM categories within stage groups. This system used a database of 5319 patients with primary lung cancer treated at the M. D. Anderson Cancer Center from 1975 to 1988 and by the North American Lung Cancer Study Group from 1977 to 1982.

The TNM descriptors are detailed in Table 98-3. Most components are unchanged, but the problem of satellite nodules is addressed in the new system. Any synchronous satellite pulmonary nodule situated in the same lobe as the primary is considered T_4 (stage IIIB), whereas tumor nod-

Table 98-3. TNM Definitions

Primary tumor (T)

T_X Primary tumor cannot be assessed, or tumor proved by the presence of malignant cells in sputum or bronchial washings but not visualized by imaging or bronchoscopy

T_0 No evidence of primary tumor

T_{is} Carcinoma in situ

T_1 Tumor >3 cm in greatest dimension, surrounded by lung or visceral pleura, without bronchoscopic evidence of invasion more proximal than the lobar bronchus[a] (i.e., not in the main bronchus)

T_2 Tumor with any of the following features of size or extent:
>3 cm in greatest dimension
Involves main bronchus, → 2 cm distal to the carina
Invades the visceral pleura
Associated with atelectasis or obstructive pneumonia that extends to the hilar region but does not involve the entire lung

T_3 Tumor of any size that directly invades any of the following: chest wall (including superior sulcus tumors), diaphragm, mediastinal pleura, parietal pericardium; or tumor in the main bronchus <2 cm distal to the carina, but without involvement of the carina; or associated atelectasis or obstructive pneumonitis of the entire lung

T_4 Tumor of any size that invades any of the following: mediastinum, heart, great vessels, trachea, esophagus, vertebral body, carina; or tumor with a malignant pleural or pericardial effusion,[a] or with satellite tumor nodule(s) within the ipsilateral primary-tumor lobe of the lung

Regional lymph nodes (N)

N_X Regional lymph nodes cannot be assessed

N_0 No regional lymph node metastasis

N_1 Metastasis to ipsilateral peribronchial and/or ipsilateral hilar lymph nodes, and intrapulmonary nodes involved by direct extension of the primary tumor

N_2 Metastasis to ipsilateral mediastinal and/or subcarinal lymph node(s)

N_3 Metastasis to contralateral mediastinal, contralateral hilar, ipsilateral or contralateral scalene, or supraclavicular lymph node(s)

Distant metastasis (M)

M_X Presence of distant metastasis cannot be assessed

M_0 No distant metastasis

M_1 Distant metastasis present[a]

[a]From Mountain CF: Revisions in the international system for staging lung cancer. Chest *111*:1710, 1997. With permission.

ules in the ipsilateral non–primary tumor lobe are classified as M_1 disease.

Mountain and Dresler (1997) recommended a classification of regional lymph node stations that unified the system developed and reported by Naruke and colleagues (1978) and the system advocated by the American Thoracic Society and the North American Lung Cancer Study Group (1983). The schema was adopted by the American Joint Committee on Cancer and the Prognostic Factors TNM Committee of the Union Internationale Contre le Cancer at the 1996 annual meeting. The regional lymph node stations are illustrated in Figure 98-1 (see Color Fig. 98-1) and defined in Table 98-3. All N_2 nodes are contained within the mediastinal (parietal) pleural envelope and are designated by single-digit numbers.

According to the location of the primary tumor, ipsilateral N_2 nodes are designated right or left. Midline prevascular and retrotracheal lymph nodes are considered ipsilateral. All N_1 nodes (numbered 10 through 14) lie distal to the mediastinal pleural reflection and are within the visceral pleural envelope.

Stage grouping in Mountain's (1997) revised system is shown in Table 98-4. New features include 1) the division of stage I into IA and IB, 2) the division of stage II into IIA and IIB, and 3) the designation of $T_3N_0M_0$ as stage IIB.

The separation of $T_1N_0M_0$ from $T_2N_0M_0$ highlights the prognostic differences between the two groups and facilitates different therapeutic approaches to their management. Patients with $T_1N_0M_0$ lesions have a significantly better survival after complete resection than do patients who have tumors larger than 3 cm, and increasing tumor size seems to have a continuous deleterious impact on survival. Williams and associates at the Mayo Clinic (1981) observed a 5-year survival of 80% in patients with $T_1N_0M_0$ disease compared to 62% in $T_2N_0M_0$ disease. Harpole and colleagues (1995) confirmed these results with a difference in 5-year survival of 70% and 50% for $T_1N_0M_0$ and $T_2N_0M_0$ disease, respectively.

Mountain's 1997 database supports from a prognostic standpoint the separation of $T_1N_1M_0$ from $T_2N_1M_0$. The improved survival of patients with completely resected $T_3N_0M_0$ lesions compared to other subgroups placed in the stage IIIA category was confirmed in a large study by McCaughan and associates (1985) at Memorial Sloan-Kettering Cancer Center. Movement of $T_3N_0M_0$ disease to stage IIB reflects the appropriateness of these patients as candidates for primary surgical therapy.

Noninvasive Intrathoracic Staging

Computed Tomography

CT of the chest is the most widely used imaging modality for staging lung cancer. CT scan is almost always obtained after an abnormality is discovered on plain chest radiograph. In some clinical scenarios, chest radiograph alone may suffice (e.g., multiple metastatic pulmonary nodules in a patient with a poor performance status or gross rib destruction with chest wall invasion). However, because plain chest radiograph is not sensitive enough to detect mediastinal lymphadenopathy or chest wall or pleural invasion, CT scan of the chest carried down through the level of the adrenal glands is almost always necessary.

For evaluation of the primary tumor CT scan has difficulty distinguishing between T_3 and T_4 tumors, as well as T_1 and T_2 tumors. In fact, in a study by Webb and colleagues (1991), CT was only able to discriminate between advanced chest wall tumors and primary tumors in 62% of the cases. When rib destruction was present or there was a definite chest wall mass, the CT had a better predicted value. The surgeon cannot rely solely on the CT scan for central tumors that may invade the mediastinum. The sensitivity of CT for

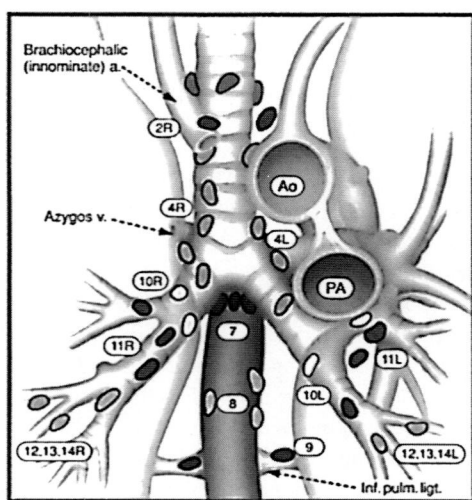

Superior Mediastinal Nodes

● **1** Highest Mediastinal

● **2** Upper Paratracheal

● **3** Pre-vascular and Retrotracheal

● **4** Lower Paratracheal
(including Azygos Nodes)

N₂ = single digit, ipsilateral
N₃ = single digit, contralateral or supraclavicular

Aortic Nodes

● **5** Subaortic (A-P window)

● **6** Para-aortic (ascending
aorta or phrenic)

Inferior Mediastinal Nodes

● **7** Subcarinal

● **8** Paraesophageal
(below carina)

● **9** Pulmonary Ligament

N₁ Nodes

○ **10** Hilar

● **11** Interlobar

● **12** Lobar

● **13** Segmental

● **14** Subsegmental

Fig. 98-1. Regional lymph node stations. (See Color Fig. 98-1.) Ao, aorta; PA, pulmonary artery.

Table 98-4. Revised Stage Grouping for Lung Cancer

Stage	TNM Subset
0	Carcinoma in situ
IA	$T_1N_0M_0$
IB	$T_2N_0M_0$
IIA	$T_1N_1M_0$
IIB	$T_2N_1M_0$
	$T_3N_0M_0$
IIIA	$T_3N_1M_0$
	$T_1N_2M_0$
	$T_2N_2M_0$
	$T_3N_2M_0$
IIIB	$T_4N_0M_0$
	$T_4N_1M_0$
	$T_4N_2M_0$
	$T_1N_3M_0$
	$T_2N_3M_0$
	$T_3N_3M_0$
	$T_4N_3M_0$
IV	Any T, any N, M_1

From Mountain CF: Revisions in the international system for lung staging cancer. Chest *111*:1710, 1997. With permission.

invasion of the mediastinum is low, in the range of 60 to 75%. Occasionally, CT scan can detect invasion of a vessel. Given this low sensitivity, there are occasions when surgical exploration is the only way to definitively stage for tumor invasion into the mediastinum (T_4 disease). It was initially thought that magnetic resonance (MR) imaging would be useful in detecting mediastinal and chest wall invasion, as reported by Webb (1988, 1989) and associates (1991). However, the sensitivity and specificity of this technique are not significantly higher than CT scan alone. MR imaging is useful in evaluating superior sulcus (Pancoast's) tumors for involvement of the brachial plexus, spinal cord, chest wall, and subclavian artery.

The use of CT scan to detect mediastinal lymphadenopathy is fraught with difficulties. Although CT scan is an excellent tool for detecting most enlarged lymph nodes, it cannot differentiate benignity from malignancy. Also, CT examination is of little or no value in the identification of enlarged nodes in stations 8 and 9. CT scans also frequently do not identify enlarged nodes in station 7 as well as a percentage of enlarged nodes in station 6. Lymph nodes in the mediastinum are considered enlarged if they are greater than 1 cm in short-axis diameter. The finding of an enlarged lymph node in the mediastinum in patients with a known primary lung cancer does not ensure that those lymph nodes have metastatic deposits. False-positive lymph nodes are especially common in patients with postobstructive pneumonia secondary to their primary lung cancer. Patients with other underlying diseases, such as sarcoidosis, may have abnormally enlarged mediastinal lymph nodes. When lymph node enlargement is detected by CT scan, the onus is on the clinician to prove that the lymph node has a metastatic deposit. It must be emphasized that enlarged lymph glands on CT alone should not preclude a patient from a potentially curative resection. In addition, a CT scan of the chest can be helpful in directing the clinician to the most appropriate staging procedure for lymph node biopsy.

In patients with no evidence of mediastinal lymphadenopathy by CT scan, there is some controversy as to whether an invasive mediastinal staging study (i.e., mediastinoscopy) should be performed before surgery. Although up to 15% of these patients with negative CT do have microscopic deposition in a lymph node at surgery, this group generally has up to a 30% 5-year survival rate when completely resected.

Transesophageal Ultrasonography

Soga (1987), Kondo (1990), and Lee (1992) and their associates have reported that transesophageal ultrasonography may be particularly valuable in the identification of enlarged nodes in the inferior mediastinum (levels 7, 8, and 9) and in the para-aortic region (level 5). The criteria for metastatic involvement have been suggested but not agreed on. At present, endoscopic ultrasonography (EUS) combined with FNA of identified nodes in levels 5 and 7 is its

major application. This invasive technique is discussed later in this chapter, under Endoscopic Ultrasonography.

Positron Emission Tomography for Intrathoracic Staging

PET scanning does not replace the CT scan for assessment of the tumor and has poor accuracy in determining structural invasion. In several studies, PET has shown improved sensitivity and specificity in mediastinal lymph node staging compared to CT scanning (Table 98-5). Because nodal enlargement seen on CT can be due to reactive hyperplasia, a negative PET could potentially reduce the need for invasive staging, provided specificity approaches 100%. A positive PET scan in the light of a negative CT scan would prompt more invasive staging (e.g., mediastinoscopy, mediastinotomy).

Vansteenkiste and associates (1997) have emphasized the complementary features of the CT and PET scans. PET scans lack anatomic information. The difficulty of distinguishing hilar and adjacent N_2 stations may be resolved with the evaluation of both scans. The presence of a large tumor near the hilum or mediastinum is another case in which caution must be exercised.

Detection of Metastatic Disease

As is often the case, a careful history and physical examination provide valuable information that may guide the physician in locating metastatic disease. For example, the recent onset of severe pain in the midhumerus may prompt a bone scan that reveals uptake in the area of the pain consistent with metastasis. A more difficult decision arises when the patient has a negative clinical evaluation, and the clinician must consider the likelihood that metastatic disease will be discovered by CT or radionuclide scan if the

Table 98-5. Studies Comparing PET and CT in Mediastinal Staging of Lung Cancer

Author	No. of Patients	Nodal Status: Malignant/Benign (Type of Evaluation)	PET Sensitivity (%)	PET Specificity (%)	CT Sensitivity, % (Size Criteria)	CT Specificity (%)
Chin et al. (1995)	30	9/21 (patients)	78	81	56 (1.5 cm)	86
Wahl et al. (1994)	23	11/16 (sides)	82	81	64 (1.0 cm)	44
Patz et al. (1995)	42	23/39 (stations)	83	82	43 (1.0 cm)	85
Scott et al. (1996)	62	10/65 (stations)	100	98	60 (1.0 cm)	93
Sasaki et al. (1996)	29	17/54 (stations)	76	98	65 (1.0 cm)	87
Steinert et al. (1997)	47	58/133 (stations)	93	99	72 (0.7–1.1 cm)	94
Sazon et al. (1996)	37	16/16 (patients)	100	100	81 (1.0 cm)	56
Valk et al. (1995)	74	24/52 (sides)	83	94	63 (1.0 cm)	73
Vansteenkiste et al. (1997)	50	14/36 (patients)	67 / 93[a]	97 / 97[a]	67 (1.5 cm)	63
Guhlman et al. (1997)	32	20/12 (patients)	80	100	50 (1.0 cm)	75
Bury et al. (1996b)	50	21/19 (patients)	90	86	72 (1.0 cm)	81

CT, computed tomography; PET, positron emission tomography.
[a]PET plus CT.
Adapted from Lowe VJ, Naunheim KS: PET in lung cancer. Ann Thorac Surg 65:1821, 1998.

Table 98-6. Extended Clinical Evaluation Suggesting Metastatic Disease in Patients with Lung Cancer

Symptoms elicited in history
    Constitutional: weight loss
    Musculoskeletal: focal skeleton pain, chest pain
    Neurologic: headaches, syncope, seizures, extremity weakness, recent change in mental status
Signs found on physical examination
    Lymphadenopathy (<1 cm)
    Hoarseness
    Superior vena cava syndrome
    Bone tenderness
    Hepatomegaly
    Focal neurologic signs, papilledema
    Soft tissue mass
Routine laboratory tests
    Hematocrit <40% in males
    Hematocrit <35% in females
    Elevated alkaline phosphatase, γ-glutamyltransferase, serum glutamic-oxaloacetic transaminase, calcium

Adapted from Silvestri GA, Littenberg B, Colice GL: The clinical evaluation for detecting metastatic lung cancer: a meta-analysis. Am J Respir Crit Care Med *152*:225, 1995.

clinical evaluation is normal. This introduces the concept of negative predictive value (NPV) of a test which, in the context of the clinical evaluation, is defined as the probability of a negative scan for metastatic disease, given a negative clinical evaluation. A high NPV of the clinical evaluation in patients with newly diagnosed lung cancer implies that if the clinical evaluation were normal, the probability of a positive CT or radionuclide scan for metastatic disease is low. One of us (G.A.S.) and colleagues (1995) found that the NPV of the clinical evaluation is quite high compared to subsequent staging scans of the head, abdomen, and radionuclide bone scan. This is particularly true if an extensive clinical evaluation was performed (Table 98-6). The most common metastatic sites for NSCLC include the brain, bone, liver, and adrenal glands. Table 98-7 compares the NPV of the clinical evaluation to staging examinations of these metastatic sites. Individual discussion of these organ systems is warranted.

Table 98-7. Comparison of Negative Clinical Evaluation and Staging Examinations for Metastatic Disease

Staging Examination	Negative Predictive Value of Clinical Examination	
	Median	Mean
Brain CT	94	94
Abdominal CT	97	95
Bone scan	92	89

CT, computed tomography.
Adapted from Silvestri GA, Littenberg B, Colice GL: The clinical evaluation for detecting metastatic lung cancer. Am J Respir Crit Care Med *152*:225, 1995.

Cranial Metastases

The finding of brain metastases is frequent in patients with lung cancer. They are present in 10% of patients at the time of diagnosis and in up to 30 to 50% of patients by autopsy series. When a comprehensive clinical evaluation is performed, the median NPV of the clinical evaluation was 94% when studies were pooled in nearly 1400 patients. If the clinical evaluation were comprehensive, the finding of asymptomatic brain metastases in a patient with primary lung cancer was 3% or less. Two subgroups of asymptomatic patients may have a higher incidence of cranial metastases. Kormas and associates (1992) found that patients with known N$_2$ disease detected on chest CT or at the time of surgery had a higher incidence of clinically silent cranial metastases. In addition, Silvestri and colleagues (1995) reported in the meta-analysis that the incidence of adenocarcinoma carries a higher likelihood of asymptomatic brain metastases than does squamous cell carcinoma. A cost-effectiveness study by Colice and colleagues (1995) found that overall, it was not cost effective to perform a CT scan if the clinical evaluation was negative. A positive clinical finding on cranial CT does not necessarily equate with true metastases. Patchell and associates (1990) studied 54 patients with known primary cancers elsewhere and presumed cranial metastases seen by CT scan; six (11%) studied were indeed false-positive scans. The patient that has a solitary brain lesion discovered on cranial CT may warrant biopsy or total excision of this lesion before exclusion from potentially curative thoracotomy. With the reported increased sensitivity of MR imaging, investigators have hypothesized that clinically silent cranial metastases would be discovered more frequently using this modality. Cole and colleagues (1994) performed preoperative cranial CT scans in 42 patients with lung cancer and normal neurologic examinations. The scans were followed by MR imaging for comparison. Neither modality detected a metastatic lesion, but MR imaging detected benign pathology more frequently than CT did. Currently, the consensus is to perform a cranial CT during the staging evaluation if the patient has positive findings that suggest the presence of cranial disease (e.g., headaches, seizures). Cranial CT should also be performed before thoracotomy in patients with nonspecific findings that suggest widespread disease (e.g., weight loss, anemia), if metastatic disease has not been documented elsewhere. Patients with adenocarcinoma who have N$_2$ disease documented before surgery may warrant a head CT scan.

Bone Metastases

Lung cancer metastasis to the bone occurs frequently and is found in up to 30% of patients at autopsy. Radionuclide bone scan is often positive in patients with bone metastases. Only 5 to 15% destruction of bone is necessary before neoplastic deposits are detected by bone scanning, according to Rogers (1993). However, false-positive bone scan or radionuclide bone scans also occur because patients in this age group can have a history of coexistent trauma, osteoporosis, or benign lesions. The clinical evaluation is useful in deciding whether to order a radionuclide bone scan. Common clinical findings of bone metastases include bone pain, pathologic fracture, and an elevated alkaline phosphatase or serum calcium. Silvestri and associates (1995) found that the median NPV for the clinical evaluation was 92%. This included data from more than 600 patients. Of the seven studies included in that meta-analysis, several made note of the fact that false-positive scans were common.

The radionuclide bone scan has its greatest use in patients who have a positive clinical evaluation. The patient who has multiple areas of uptake consistent with metastases needs no further evaluation. However, an isolated area of uptake may require further evaluation, including plain radiographs to assess for pathologic fracture. In the absence of plain radiographic abnormality or local signs of symptoms, biopsy of a suspected osseous metastasis becomes a challenging problem.

Robinson and associates (1998) reported on the use of an intraoperative gamma probe-directed biopsy of ribs and sternum in 10 patients after a standard dosage of technetium 99m oxidronate 6 to 12 hours before surgery. The technique proved to be easy and highly accurate (100% sensitivity) to localize areas of abnormal radioisotope uptake. Of note is that in only one of five asymptomatic patients with known lung cancer did biopsy confirm metastasis. This low yield of positivity is confirmed by Ichinose and associates (1989), who found a 55% false-positive rate in routine bone scans in asymptomatic patients with lung cancer.

Abdominal Metastases

Lung cancer may metastasize to both the adrenal gland and the liver. Because adrenal metastases are generally considered clinically silent, it has been common practice to extend the chest CT through the adrenal gland to evaluate them for the presence of metastatic disease. However, an abnormally enlarged adrenal gland does not necessarily represent metastatic disease.

Adrenal adenomas occur in 2 to 10% of the general population. Oliver and colleagues (1984) showed that an enlarged adrenal gland was more likely to be an adenoma than metastatic disease in the preoperative patient with NSCLC. One of us (G.A.S.) and associates (1992) discovered that the likelihood of adrenal metastases noted on abdominal CT was zero in patients with a normal clinical evaluation. All patients who ultimately had adrenal metastases had findings that suggested the presence of metastatic disease.

The recurring problem of false-positive scans occurs in patients who have liver abnormalities noted on CT scan. Liver metastases occur in up to 5% of patients with lung cancer. However, a benign pathology of the liver is common, and abnormalities visualized in the liver during abdominal CT are more likely to be benign than malignant. Thus, additional studies to rule out the presence of metastases may become necessary, including ultrasound to evaluate cystic lesions and bolus contrast CT to establish the presence of a hemangioma. Occasionally, a CT-guided percutaneous liver biopsy may be performed.

Combining patients from 10 studies with a total of more than 1000 patients in which a clinical evaluation was performed before the abdominal CT scan, the clinical evaluation performed well, with a median NPV of 97%. It can therefore be argued that because the likelihood of abdominal metastases in patients who have a negative clinical evaluation is low and testing may result in a false-positive abdominal CT scan, routine CT scans through the abdomen should not be performed in patients with NSCLC and a negative clinical evaluation. Any abnormal finding suggestive of metastatic disease discovered during the clinical evaluation should be followed by a chest CT that is extended through the abdomen unless the symptoms are referent to a specific organ system (e.g., severe headache). A complete staging algorithm for the evaluation of metastatic disease is shown in Figure 98-2.

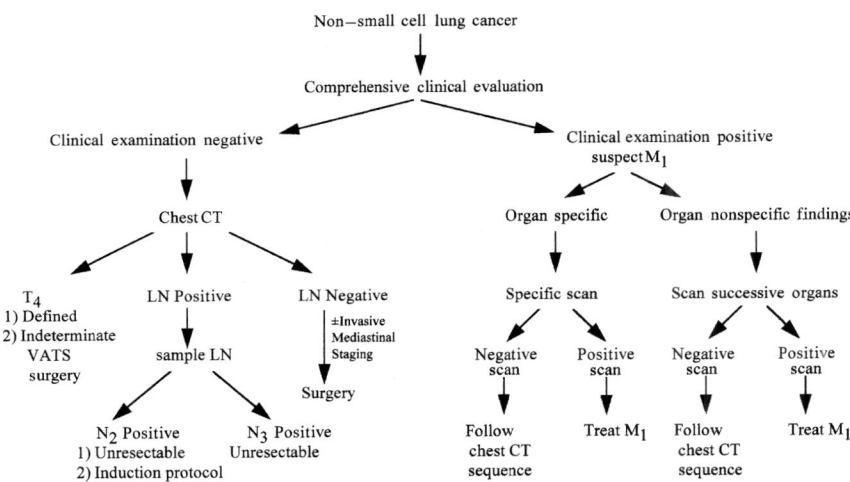

Fig. 98-2. Staging algorithm for lung cancer. CT, computed tomography; LN, lymph node.

Positron Emission Tomography for Metastatic Disease

PET may find its greatest use in the evaluation of metastatic disease. PET has detected unsuspected metastasis in 10 to 20% of patients. Saunders and colleagues (1999) reported that PET detected unsuspected distant metastases and prevented inappropriate surgery in 16.5%. These authors found that PET was least accurate in identifying cerebral metastasis, probably secondary to high FDG uptake in normal brain.

Invasive Staging of the Mediastinum

Because disparate results have been reported on the accuracy of CT scanning to evaluate mediastinal lymph node metastases, the surgeon must consider the use of invasive biopsy techniques. The need to perform invasive mediastinal staging on every patient remains controversial. It is accepted that histologic evaluation of enlarged lymph nodes identified by CT is required to confirm staging. McCloud and associates (1992) found that 37% of nodes 2 to 4 cm in diameter did not contain metastatic disease at thoracotomy.

On the other hand, peripheral $T_1N_0M_0$ tumors with a negative mediastinum by CT (short-axis diameter <1 cm) are unlikely to have mediastinal metastases. Positivity in this setting has been variably reported as between 5 to 15%. In a prospective trial conducted and reported by the Canadian Lung Cancer Oncology Group (1995), patients in one group underwent mediastinoscopy if lymph nodes by CT scan were larger than 1 cm but proceeded directly to thoracotomy if lymph nodes were smaller than 1 cm on CT. All patients in another group underwent mediastinoscopy. CT evaluation alone led to similar rates of thoracotomy without cure. Selective mediastinoscopy in patients with enlarged nodes only was more cost effective. Daly and colleagues (1993) reported overall projected 2-year and 5-year survival rates for 37 patients with false-negative CT results of 40% and 28%, respectively.

Other predictors of N_2 disease may be useful in making a decision to perform invasive mediastinal staging in the setting of a CT-negative scan. For patients with T_3 tumors or central adenocarcinomas, Daly and colleagues (1993) reported a high incidence of positive mediastinal lymph nodes and a low NPV for CT. Jolly and associates (1991) found that 35% of patients with adenocarcinoma, 46% with large cell carcinoma, and 65% with small cell lung cancer had N_2 involvement versus 19% of patients with squamous histology. If resection is contemplated for a peripheral clinical $T_1N_0M_0$ small cell carcinoma, mediastinoscopy is warranted because of the propensity of early spread to mediastinal lymph nodes. Accurate evaluation of the outcomes of clinical trials using adjuvant therapy for patients with N_2 disease requires invasive staging for pathologic confirmation.

Transbronchial Needle Aspiration

Transcarinal needle aspiration (Wang needle) offers the opportunity to stage the mediastinum at the time of diagnostic bronchoscopy. Transcarinal needle aspiration can easily reach station 7 lymph nodes. Using selective criteria of a visualized widened carina or CT evidence of subcarinal adenopathy provides the greatest specificity. Shure and Fedullo (1984) reported an association between malignant carinal aspirates and the presence of an endobronchial tumor (24%) or an abnormal-appearing carina (widening or mucosal erythema) at bronchoscopy (38%). Caution must be exercised with paratracheal tumors with possible mediastinal extension because false-positive biopsies can occur. A study by Schenk and colleagues (1993) found that transbronchial needle aspiration with a 19-gauge needle compared with a 22-gauge needle increased diagnostic yield from 53 to 86%.

Mediastinoscopy

Cervical mediastinoscopy allows exploration of lymph nodes in the paratracheal and pretracheal regions, in the tracheobronchial angles, and the anterior aspect of the subcarinal space. It is the most accurate method of assessing superior mediastinal lymph node metastases. Ginsberg (1987) reported that in two analyses of 2259 mediastinoscopies, the total complication rate was 2.0%. There were no deaths. Only 0.3% of life-threatening complications (hemorrhage, tracheal injury, or esophageal injury) required surgical intervention, consisting of thoracotomy or sternotomy. Recurrent nerve injury and pneumothorax occurred in 0.9% of mediastinoscopies. The false-negative rate of mediastinoscopy is generally less than 10%, and there should be no false-positives.

Funatsu and colleagues (1992) reported that the sensitivity of mediastinoscopy was lowest for subcarinal lymph nodes (64.0%). The false-negative results were low for the paratracheal regions (1 to 2%) but were 6.1% for the subcarinal lymph nodes sampled.

Mediastinoscopy can be "extended" to evaluate the subaortic (level 5) and para-aortic (level 6) regions. This extension is created by finger dissection in the space superolateral to the aorta between the innominate artery and left common carotid artery. Lopez and colleagues (1994) reported 100% specificity and 83.3% sensitivity, which is similar to the data obtained by Ginsberg and associates (1984).

Anterior Mediastinotomy

For left upper lobe tumors, evaluation of the subaortic and lateral aortic areas for N_2 disease is required for complete staging. As a more frequent alternative to extended mediastinoscopy, biopsy can be achieved using an anterior mediastinotomy (the Chamberlain procedure). The technique may include a vertical parasternal incision, as originally described by McNeil and Chamberlain (1966), an excision of the second intercostal cartilage, or an intercostal exploration. Biopsy of stations 5 and 6 lymph nodes is achieved by inserting the mediastinoscope in the extrapleural plane. For left upper lobe tumors, a cervical mediastinoscopy is performed in addition to the Chamberlain procedure to rule out contralateral disease.

Video-Assisted Thoracoscopy

Video-assisted thoracoscopy is an alternative to the Chamberlain procedure. Not only does it allow biopsy of lymph nodes in levels 5 and 6, but it also allows access to paraesophageal (level 8) and inferior pulmonary ligament (level 9) lymph nodes. On the right side, video-assisted thoracoscopy permits exploration of upper and lower paratracheal lymph nodes, subcarinal nodes, and paraesophageal and inferior pulmonary lymph nodes. Landreneau and associates (1993) reported the use of thoracoscopic mediastinal exploration in 40 patients with CT-enlarged aortopulmonary window or right periazygos or subcarinal lymph nodes. Thoracoscopic nodal sampling was 100% sensitive and 100% specific in diagnosing the mediastinal adenopathy.

An added benefit to using video-assisted thoracoscopy to stage the mediastinum is the ability to view the tumor and explore the pleural cavity. Unsuspected pleural seeding may be discovered. As noted by Roviaro and associates (1995), dissection maneuvers can allow evaluation of operability when a lesion is suspected of contacting, compressing, or invading hilar or mediastinal structures. In their experience, video-assisted thoracoscopy revealed causes of inoperability and avoided unnecessary thoracotomy in 8.3% of cases.

Endoscopic Ultrasonography

EUS allows the depiction of lesions in and around the gastrointestinal tract, including adjacent lymph nodes. With the development of the linear array echoendoscope, EUS/FNA of lymph nodes became possible. One of us (G.A.S.) and colleagues (1996) demonstrated an accuracy of 89% when assessing subcarinal, aortopulmonary, or inferior mediastinal lymph nodes designated by the radiologist as abnormal. Figure 98-3 shows an EUS/FNA of an enlarged subcarinal lymph node. Gress and colleagues (1997) reported an accuracy of 96% in 24 patients who underwent EUS/FNA. The accuracy of EUS alone was 84% for predicting metastasis to lymph nodes.

At our institution, more than 140 patients with a lung mass and mediastinal adenopathy have now been evaluated by EUS and FNA. Both the radiographically designated abnormal lymph nodes in the aortopulmonary window and subcarinal region are now preferentially evaluated by EUS/FNA. The sensitivity for the diagnosis of malignancy is 88%, and specificity is 100%. There have been no observed complications.

EUS with needle biopsy is meant to complement cervical mediastinoscopy and thoracoscopy. In our hands, EUS/FNA is less invasive and more cost effective when applied to the correct situation.

Intraoperative Staging

Presurgical staging must be confirmed by intraoperative staging. The tumor is usually easily assessed on opening the chest. Extrapleural dissection should be performed if there is adhesion to the parietal pleura. If the plane is not clearly

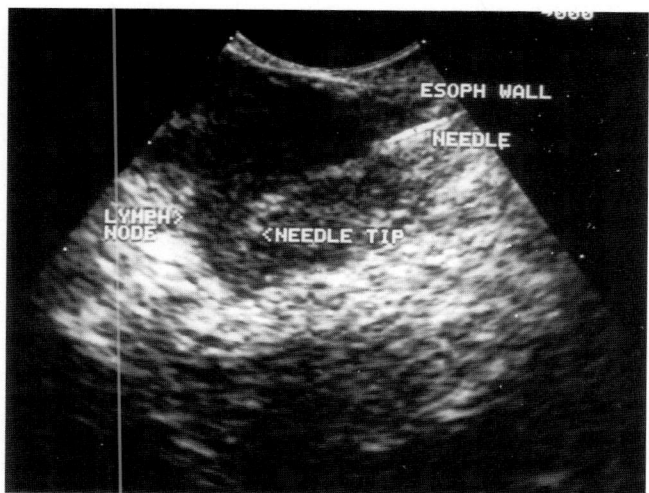

Fig. 98-3. Fine-needle aspiration guided by endoscopic ultrasonography of an enlarged subcarinal lymph node. The needle is shown entering the lymph node.

defined, assumption of chest wall or mediastinal invasion beyond parietal pleura must be assumed.

Careful assessment of the parietal pleura for tumor "studding" should be done immediately after opening the chest. Palpation of the non–tumor-bearing lobes should be performed to assess for satellite tumor nodules. Suspicious lesions are sent for frozen section.

Palpation of the mediastinal lymph nodes should precede resection. Although mediastinal node dissection or systemic sampling is usually performed at the completion of pulmonary resection, it should be done first if positive mediastinal nodes will alter treatment plans. Gaer and Goldstraw (1990) reported that intraoperative palpation of lymph nodes had a positive predictive value of only 64.1% but an NPV of 96.0%.

Prediction of disease recurrence and survival after surgical resection of NSCLC remains imprecise, despite improvements in staging. Cytologic analysis of cells obtained at intraoperative pleural lavage may be a valuable adjunct to current staging techniques. Studies by Eagan and associates (1984) and Kondo and colleagues (1993) found that detection of malignant cells in the lavage liquid correlated with a worse survival. These studies prompted the prospective study by Buhr and associates (1997) of pleural lavage in 342 patients with NSCLC undergoing curative resection. The pleural surfaces were lavaged before and after resection, and cytologic evaluation of the cells in the lavage was performed. Malignant cells were found in the first pleural lavage in 38% of patients, and the presence of malignant cells in the lavage fluid correlated with a significantly worse 4-year survival (69% for lavage-negative stage I versus 35% for lavage-positive stage I patients). Additional studies may improve the sensitivity of pleural lavage analysis Biomarkers associated with lung cancer, such as k-*ras* mutations and telomerase activity, may be useful adjuncts to cytology.

REFERENCES

Allen MS, et al: Video-assisted thoracoscopic stapled wedge excision for indeterminate pulmonary nodules. J Thorac Cardiovasc Surg *106*:1048, 1993.

American Thoracic Society: Clinical staging of primary lung cancer. Am Rev Respir Dis *1271*:1, 1983.

Arroglia AC, Matthay RA: The role of bronchoscopy in lung cancer. Clin Chest Med *14*:87, 1993.

Berquist TH, et al: Transthoracic needle biopsy accuracy and complications in relation to location and type of lesion. Mayo Clin Proc *55*:475, 1980.

Buhr J, et al: The prognostic significance of tumor cell detection in intra-operative pleural lavage and lung tissue cultures for patients with lung cancer. J Thorac Cardiovasc Surg *113*:683, 1997.

Bury T, et al: Evaluation of the solitary pulmonary nodule by positron emission tomography imaging. Eur Respir J *9*:410, 1996a.

Bury TH, et al: Staging of the mediastinum: value of positron-emission tomography imaging in non-small cell lung cancer. Eur Respir J *9*:2560, 1996b.

Calhoun P, et al: The clinical outcome of needle aspirations of the lung when cancer is not diagnosed. Ann Thorac Surg *41*:592, 1986.

Canadian Lung Oncology Group: Investigation for mediastinal disease in patients with apparently operable lung cancer. Ann Thorac Surg *60*:1382, 1995.

Chin RJ, et al: Mediastinal staging of non-small-cell lung cancer with positron emission tomography. Am J Respir Crit Care Med *152*:2090, 1995.

Cole FH, et al: Cerebral imaging in the asymptomatic preoperative bronchogenic carcinoma patient: is it worthwhile? Ann Thorac Surg *57*:838, 1994.

Colice GL: Detecting lung cancer as a cause of hemoptysis in patients with a normal chest radiograph: bronchoscopy vs CT. Chest *111*:877, 1997.

Colice GL, et al: Cost-effectiveness of head CT in patients with lung cancer and no clinical evidence of metastases. Chest *108*:1264, 1995.

Daly BOT, et al: N2 lung cancer: outcome in patients with false-negative computed tomographic scans of the chest. J Thorac Cardiovasc Surg *105*:904, 1993.

de Gracia JC, et al: Diagnostic value of bronchoalveolar lavage in peripheral lung cancer. Am Rev Respir Dis *147*:649, 1993.

Duhaylongsod FG, et al: Detection of primary and recurrent lung cancer by means of F-18 fluorodeoxyglucose positron emission tomography (FDG PET). J Thorac Cardiovasc Surg *110*:130, 1995.

Eagan RT, et al: Pleural lavage after pulmonary resection for bronchogenic carcinoma. J Thorac Cardiovasc Surg *88*:1000, 1984.

Funatsu T, et al. The role of mediastinoscopic biopsy in preoperative assessment of lung cancer. J Thorac Cardiovasc Surg *104*:1688, 1992.

Gaer JAP, Goldstraw P: Intraoperative assessment of nodal staging at thoracotomy for carcinoma of the bronchus. Eur J Cardiothorac Surg *4*:207, 1990.

Ginsberg RJ: Evaluation of the mediastinum by invasive techniques. Surg Clin North Am *67*:1025, 1987.

Ginsberg RJ, et al: Extended cervical mediastinoscopy. A single procedure for bronchogenic carcinoma of the left upper lobe. J Thorac Cardiovasc Surg *94*:673, 1984.

Gress FG, at al: Endoscopic ultrasonography, fine-needle aspiration biopsy guided by endoscopic ultrasonography and computed tomography in the preoperative staging of non-small cell lung cancer: a comparison study. Ann Intern Med *127*:604, 1997.

Guhlman A, et al: Lymph node staging in non-small cell lung cancer: evaluation by [^{18}F] FDG positron emission tomography (PET). Thorax *52*:438, 1997.

Gupta NC, Maloof J, Gunel E. Probability of malignancy in solitary pulmonary nodules using fluorine-18-FDG and PET. J Nucl Med *37*:943, 1996.

Harpole DH, et al: A prognostic model of recurrence and death in stage I non-small cell lung cancer utilizing presentation, histopathology, and oncoprotein expression. Cancer Res *55*:51, 1995.

Hazelrigg SR, et al: Video assisted thoracic surgery study group data. Ann Thorac Surg *56*:1039, 1993.

Higashi K, et al: Bronchioalveolar carcinoma: false-negative results on FDG-PET. J Nucl Med *38*:79P, 1997.

Ichinose Y, et al: Preoperative examination to detect distant metastasis is not advocated for asymptomatic patient with stages 1 and 2 non-small cell lung cancer. Chest *96*:1104, 1989.

Jolly PC, et al: Routine computed tomographic scans, selective mediastinoscopy, and other factors in evaluation of lung cancer. J Thorac Cardiovasc Surg *102*:266, 1991.

Knight SB, et al: Evaluation of pulmonary lesions with FDG-PET. Comparison of findings in patients with and without a history of prior malignancy. Chest *109*:982, 1996.

Kondo D, et al: Endoscopic ultrasound examination for mediastinal lymph node metastases of lung cancer. Chest *98*:586, 1990.

Kondo H, et al: Prognostic significance of pleural lavage cytology immediately after thoracotomy in patients with lung cancer. J Thorac Cardiovasc Surg *106*:1092, 1993.

Kormas P, Bradshaw JR, Jeyasingham K: Preoperative computed tomography of the brain in non-small cell bronchogenic carcinoma. Thorax *47*:106, 1992.

Kubota K, et al: Differential diagnosis of lung tumor with positron emission tomography: a prospective study. J Nucl Med *31*:1927, 1990.

Landreneau RJ, et al: Thoracoscopic mediastinal lymph node sampling: useful for mediastinal lymph node stations inaccessible by cervical mediastinoscopy. J Thorac Cardiovasc Surg *106*:554, 1993.

Lee N, et al: Patterns of internal echoes in lymph nodes in the diagnosis of lung cancer metastasis. World J Surg *16*:986, 1992.

Lopez L, et al: Extended cervical mediastinoscopy: prospective study of fifty cases. Ann Thorac Surg *57*:555, 1994.

Lowe VJ, Naunheim KS: PET in lung cancer. Ann Thorac Surg *65*:1821, 1998.

Lowe VJ, et al: Pulmonary abnormalities and PET data analysis: a retrospective study. Radiology *202*:435, 1997.

Mack MJ, et al: Thoracoscopy for the diagnosis of the indeterminate solitary pulmonary nodule. Ann Thorac Surg *56*:825, 1993a.

Mack MJ, et al: Techniques for localization of pulmonary nodules for thoracoscopic resection. J Thorac Cardiovasc Surg *106*:550 1993b.

McCaughan BC, et al: Chest wall invasion in carcinoma of the lung: therapeutic and prognostic implications. J Thorac Cardiovasc Surg *89*:836, 1985.

McCloud TC, et al: Bronchogenic carcinoma: analysis of staging in the mediastinum with CT by correlative lymph node mapping and sampling. Radiology *182*:319, 1992.

McNeil TM, Chamberlain JM: Diagnostic anterior mediastinotomy. Ann Thorac Surg *2*:532, 1966.

Mountain CF: Revisions in the international system for staging lung cancer. Chest *111*:1710, 1997.

Mountain CF, Dresler CM: Regional lymph node classification for lung cancer staging. Chest *111*:1718, 1997.

Naruke T, Suemasu K, Ishikawa S: Lymph node mapping and curability of various levels of metastasis in resected lung cancer. J Thorac Cardiovasc Surg *76*:832, 1978.

Nathan MH, Collins VP, Adams RA: Differentiation of benign and malignant pulmonary nodules by growth rate. Radiology *79*:221, 1962.

Oliver TWJ, et al: Isolated adrenal masses in non small-cell bronchogenic carcinoma. Radiology *153*:217, 1984.

Patchell PA, et al: A randomized trial of surgery in the treatment of single brain metastases. N Engl J Med *322*:494, 1990.

Patz EJ, et al: Thoracic nodal staging with PET imaging with 18 FDG in patients with bronchogenic carcinoma. Chest *108*:1671, 1995.

Pirozynski M: Bronchoalveolar lavage in the diagnosis of peripheral, primary lung cancer. Chest *102*:372, 1992.

Robinson LA, et al: Intraoperative gamma probe-directed biopsy of asymptomatic suspected bone metastases. Ann Thorac Surg *65*:1426, 1998.

Rogers LF: Secondary malignancies in bone. *In* Juhl JH, Crummy AB (eds): Paul and Juhl's Essentials of Radiologic Imaging. Philadelphia: JB Lippincott, 1993, p. 164.

Roviaro GC, et al: Videothoracoscopic staging and treatment of lung cancer. Ann Thorac Surg *59*:971, 1995.

Salazar AM, Westcott JL: The role of transthoracic needle biopsy for the diagnosis and staging of lung cancer. Clin Chest Med *14*:99, 1993.

Sasaki M, et al: The usefulness of FDG positron emission tomography for the detection of mediastinal lymph node metastases in patients with non-small cell lung cancer: a comparative study with X-ray computed tomography. Eur J Nucl Med *23*:741, 1996.

Saunders CAB, et al: An evaluation of fluorine-18-fluorodeoxyglucose whole body positron emission tomography imaging in the staging of lung cancer. Ann Thorac Surg *67*:790, 1999.

Sazon DA, et al: Fluorodeoxyglucose-positron emission tomography in the detection and staging of lung cancer. Am J Respir Crit Care Med *153*:417, 1996.

Schenk PA, et al: Comparison of the Wang 19-gauge and 22-gauge needle in the mediastinal staging of lung cancer. Am Rev Respir Dis *147*:1251, 1993.

Scott WJ, et al: Mediastinal lymph node staging of non-small cell lung cancer: a prospective comparison of computed tomography and positron emission tomography. J Thorac Cardiovasc Surg *111*:642, 1996.

Shennib H, Bret P: Intraoperative transthoracic ultrasonography: a useful tool to localize a lung lesion during video assisted thoracic surgery. Ann Thorac Surg *55*:767, 1992.

Shure D, Fedullo PF: Transbronchial needle aspiration of peripheral masses. Am Rev Respir Dis *128*:1090, 1983.

Shure D, Fedullo PF: The role of transcarinal needle aspiration in the staging of bronchogenic carcinoma. Chest *86*:693, 1984.

Silvestri GA, et al: The relationship of clinical findings to CT evidence of adrenal metastases in the staging of bronchogenic carcinoma. Chest *102*:1748, 1992.

Silvestri GA, et al: The clinical evaluation for detecting metastatic lung cancer: a meta-analysis. Am J Respir Crit Care Med *152*:225, 1995.

Silvestri G, et al: Endoscopic ultrasound with fine-needle aspiration in the diagnosis and staging of lung cancer. Ann Thorac Surg *61*:1441, 1996.

Soga H, et al: Ultrasonic examination of mediastinal lymph node metastasis especially to subcarinal node in lung cancer by trans-esophageal radial scan. Rinsho Gekka *42*:1405, 1987.

Steinert HC, et al: Non-small cell lung cancer: nodal staging with FDG PET versus CT with correlative lymph node mapping and sampling. Radiology *202*:441, 1997.

Swensen SJ, et al: An integrated approach to evaluation of the solitary pulmonary nodule. Mayo Clin Proc *65*:173, 1990.

Swensen SJ, et al: Pulmonary nodules. CT evaluation of enhancement with iodinated contrast material. Radiology *194*:393, 1995.

Swensen SJ, et al: The probability of malignancy in solitary pulmonary nodules. Arch Int Med *157*:849, 1997.

Torrington KG, Kern JD: The utility of fiberoptic bronchoscopy in the evaluation of the solitary pulmonary nodule. Chest *104*:1021, 1993.

Travis WD, Linden J, MacKay B. Classification histology, cytology and electron microscopy. *In* Pass HI, Mitchell JB, Johnson DH, Turrisi AJ (eds): Lung Cancer Principles and Practice. Philadelphia: Lippincott–Raven, 1996, p. 361.

Valk PE, et al: Staging non-small cell lung cancer by whole-body positron emission tomographic imaging. Ann Thorac Surg *60*:1573, 1995.

Vansteenkiste JF, et al: Mediastinal lymph node staging with FDG-PET scan in patients with potentially operable non-small cell lung cancer. Chest *112*:1480, 1997.

Wahl RL, et al: Staging of mediastinal non-small cell lung cancer with FDG PET, CT, and fusion images: preliminary prospective evaluation. Radiology *191*:371, 1994.

Webb WR: Magnetic resonance imaging of the chest. Curr Opin Radiol *1*:40, 1987.

Webb WR: MR imaging in the evaluation and staging of lung cancer. Semin Ultrasound CT MR *9*:53, 1988.

Webb WR, et al: CT and MR imaging in staging non-small cell bronchogenic carcinoma: report of the Radiologic Diagnostic Oncology Group. Radiology *178*:705, 1991.

Weber W, et al: FDG-PET in solitary pulmonary nodules: a German cost-effectiveness analysis. J Nucl Med *38*:245P, 1997.

Westcott JL. Percutaneous transthoracic needle biopsy. Radiology *169*:593, 1988.

Williams DE, et al: Survival of patients surgically treated for stage I lung cancer. J Thorac Cardiovasc Surg *82*:70, 1981.

Zerhouni EA, et al: CT of the pulmonary nodule: a cooperative study. Radiology *160*:319, 1986.

Zwirewich CV, et al: Solitary pulmonary nodule: high resolution CT and radiologic-pathologic correlation. Radiology *179*:469, 1991.

CHAPTER 99

Surgical Treatment of Non–Small Cell Lung Cancer

Joseph LoCicero III, Ronald B. Ponn, and Benedict D. T. Daly

Of the 160,000 new cases of lung cancer discovered each year in the United States, many present with distant metastasis. Pulmonary resection as the primary or the sole treatment in such cases is not beneficial. For the minority of patients with non–small cell lung carcinoma (NSCLC) limited to the lung, however, resection alone is the most effective therapy. For those with more advanced locoregional disease, many current clinical trials include operation as part of a multimodality approach. Some of these trials are showing promising early results. This chapter focuses on the role of primary resection in the management of NSCLC and the indications, surgical options, and results. The growing experience with combining operation with other treatment (i.e., adjuvant and induction therapy) is discussed in detail in Chapter 106. A thorough understanding of staging (as presented in Chapter 98) is presumed.

HISTORICAL ASPECTS

Surgical resection for lung cancer began with the first successful pneumonectomy, reported by Graham and Singer (1933). Subsequent advances have led to smaller resections, while improving mortality. Bronchoplastic procedures were developed during the late 1940s, culminating in Allison's successful sleeve lobectomy for a bronchial carcinoma in 1952, as reported by Price-Thomas (1960). Lesser resections such as lobectomy and segmentectomy were also pioneered in the 1940s. Churchill and Belsey (1939) demonstrated the feasibility of segmentectomy in a patient with bronchiectasis. These techniques were developed and popularized by Overholt (1946) and Jensik (1973) and their colleagues, as well as by Shields and Higgins (1974). The introduction and refinement of surgical staplers have made lung resection safer, faster, and less traumatic, while maintaining surgical oncologic principles. All of the modern trials in lung cancer therapy use resection as the

accepted standard therapy control arm for study of new experimental treatments.

OVERVIEW OF RESECTION FOR NON–SMALL CELL LUNG CANCER

Every patient with locoregional NSCLC should be approached as a potential candidate for resection. At present, all patients with clinical stage I and most with clinical stage II should undergo resection as the definitive primary therapy. The majority of patients with clinical stage IIIA or IIIB should not be resected primarily, but should be considered for multimodality therapy, ideally as part of a clinical trial. Only under exceptional circumstances should patients with stage IV NSCLC be considered for resection. Certain anatomic or physiologic considerations may make an individual patient a poor candidate for resection.

Anatomic Considerations

Complete resection is the goal of all operations for lung cancer. There should be a logical progression from chest radiography to computed tomographic (CT) scanning of the chest and abdomen and other imaging, to invasive assessment (most commonly surgical mediastinal evaluation and, occasionally, biopsy of extrathoracic sites), and, if indicated, to thoracotomy. A detailed discussion of radiologic evaluation appears in Chapters 9 to 13 and in Chapter 97. In patients in whom the tumor is deemed resectable, the appropriate procedure is carried out. If a tissue diagnosis is not made preoperatively, an operative biopsy is desirable, particularly if more than a lobectomy is required. When the clinical and imaging data indicate that a complete resection cannot be achieved or that the clinical tumor stage is associated with a poor long-term outcome even with complete resection, operation is not indicated, and induction therapy before an attempted resection should be considered, or resection should be abandoned as an option. Tumors that present as T_4 lesions are almost uniformly unresectable. Pleural effusion positive for malignant cells is an example of a categorically unresectable T_4 lesion. NSCLC invading the superior vena cava, main pulmonary vessels, aorta, vertebral bodies, esophagus, or heart is not considered resectable, despite occasional reports of success. Patients with phrenic or recurrent laryngeal nerve invasion, once considered an absolute contraindication to resection, are being included in multimodality protocols leading to operation. Many patients with T_3N_0 NSCLC because of chest wall invasion are candidates for complete resection. In addition, a small number of centers have accumulated substantial experience with the extensive operations required for complete resection of central bronchial (T_3) cancers and also some cases with tracheal invasion (T_4).

The optimal initial management of NSCLC with clinically proven lymph node dissemination is also generally nonsurgical. N_3 disease remains out of bounds for resection. This was pointed out by Watanabe and colleagues (1991c) who support the position that even the anterior mediastinal nodes (station 3) have a poor prognosis. In addition, little disagreement remains for patients with N_2 nodal disease documented before thoracotomy. In patients discovered to have N_2 disease at thoracotomy after a negative clinical evaluation, in contrast, resection should usually proceed. Resection as primary treatment in this group carries a better prognosis than for patients with prethoracotomy N_2 status, with late survivals between 17 and 28%, as reported by Pearson (1982), Daly (1993), and Miller (1994) and their colleagues.

Metastatic Disease

The presence of multiple extrathoracic metastases is an absolute contraindication to pulmonary resection. When a solitary metastasis is thought to be present, resection of the primary lung cancer should be considered only in occasional cases of cerebral metastasis and only after thorough imaging and invasive assessment has confirmed the absence of other sites of disease. Multiple series have shown compelling evidence of the efficacy of complete resection, when possible, of both the cranial and intrathoracic sites. In contrast, median survival with no treatment, corticosteroids only, or cranial radiation therapy is approximately 1 month, 2 months, and 6 to 9 months, respectively. Although a handful of solitary adrenal metastases synchronous with NSCLC have been treated by combined resections, experience with this approach is extremely limited, and an initial nonsurgical plan is preferable. Primary lung resection is not indicated in the presence of other sites of dissemination, even if clinically thought to be isolated. In all cases of suspected single metastasis associated with limited intrathoracic disease, in addition to ensuring that a distant lesion is solitary before

embarking on combined resection, it is also important to reach a secure diagnosis that the abnormal focus is malignant before deciding against primary pulmonary resection. Brain metastases are usually diagnosed reliably by imaging and rarely require invasive confirmation. If an apparently solitary cerebral metastasis is identified by CT scan, however, it is prudent to obtain a magnetic resonance (MR) scan of the brain before resection, because of the superior sensitivity of the latter technique. Additional imaging is also often required after abnormalities are detected on bone scan or an adrenal, renal, hepatic, or other mass is identified by CT. In most instances, a synthesis of the data provided by an appropriate combination of plain films, CT, MR imaging, ultrasound, and positron emission tomography combined with staging of the thorax as indicated, reliably confirm or rule out distant metastasis. In the few patients with solitary lesions that remain equivocal, percutaneous or open biopsy may be indicated before pulmonary resection is denied. The importance of securing a reliable radiographic or tissue diagnosis in this setting is exemplified by the findings of Porte and associates (1998), who found that nearly one-half of all adrenal masses detected during the evaluation of NSCLC patients were benign. Ettinghausen and Burt (1991) also stressed the frequency of coexistent benign adenomas in patients with operable NSCLC. Other radiographic and scintigraphic abnormalities identified during staging are also frequently unrelated. Although its role in diagnosing and staging NSCLC remains under study, positron emission tomography may prove helpful in assessing such findings or may ultimately replace other imaging in initial evaluation (see Chapter 12).

Physiologic Considerations

Traditionally established physiologic barriers to surgical resection have been falling steadily. Centers with a strong commitment to aggressive preoperative and postoperative care are reporting mortality and morbidity equal to series with limited patient entry. Kirsch and associates (1976) noted that age per se is not a contraindication to resection but cautioned against pneumonectomy in patients older than 70 years of age. However, Naunheim and associates (1994) reported good survival among octogenarians having a pneumonectomy. Pagni and colleagues (1998) performed 24 pneumonectomies in patients older than 70 years with a 12.5% mortality compared with a 4.3% mortality for pneumonectomies in younger individuals. Nugent and coworkers (1997) point out that they screen many more elderly than they eventually operate on, with only 6% of patients 80 years and older versus 32% of those 45 years and younger undergoing thoracotomy. Long-term survival after resection is not different for elderly patients, as pointed out by Harviel (1978) and Ishida (1990b) and their colleagues. However, there tends to be a decreased survival in patients younger than 40 years of age, as noted by Pemberton and coworkers

(1983). Jubelirer and Wilson (1991) attribute this difference to more advanced disease at the time of diagnosis rather than to a differential response to treatment.

Despite the fact that most patients with lung cancer are older and have a significant smoking history that can lead to coronary artery disease, significant cardiac morbidity is rare in patients undergoing a thoracotomy for carcinoma. Recent myocardial infarction within 3 months of surgery carries some risk for reinfarction. However, Rao and associates (1983) found this rate to be only 5.7%. A full discussion of the appropriate cardiac evaluation for thoracotomy is covered in Chapter 20. If significant disease is identified, many patients can still undergo pulmonary resection, as reported by Piehler (1985) and Canver (1990) and their associates. Successful resections have been performed after angioplasty, concomitantly with coronary artery bypass surgery, or sequentially within 2 weeks after bypass.

Poor pulmonary function has been a formidable barrier to resection. Based on old, unconfirmed data, elaborate schemata were established to filter only the best candidates for resection. In the experience of lung volume reduction surgery, surgeons have learned that nearly all patients tolerate a pulmonary resection. In general, individuals who function daily at a normal activity level, regardless of their measured parameters, do well. A report by Korst and coworkers (1998) showed that after 6 months, patients who underwent a lobectomy had measured pulmonary function that was not statistically different from their preoperative values. In fact, some patients who had upper lobectomies actually had better postoperative function.

Assessment of pulmonary function testing (PFT) remains the best objective evaluation of a patient's ability to tolerate resection. However, no single parameter has proven to be reliably prognostic, and strict interpretation could deny resection to many physiologically eligible patients. As many as 60% of patients identified as high risk by PFT criteria did well with surgery, according to Boushy and associates (1971). Several prospective studies have found no correlation between PFT and postoperative complications. Gerson and colleagues (1990), studying elderly patients, and Milledge and Nunn (1975), studying patients with emphysema, found that neither PFTs nor arterial blood gases correlated with postoperative problems. This lack of correlation led Kohman and colleagues (1986) to conclude that the majority of postthoracotomy deaths are unpredictable and random. Ferguson and coworkers (1991) have suggested that a predicted postoperative diffusion capacity of less than 20% was correlative with mortality, but such patients now routinely undergo lung volume reduction surgery with little trouble. However, Ninan and coworkers (1997) found a highly significant correlation between exercise desaturation and postpneumonectomy morbidity.

Algorithms for preoperative pulmonary evaluation are presented in Chapter 19. Briefly, assessment begins with the patient's history. An assessment of the patient's physical activity should be elicited. Specifically, attention should be paid to the ability to climb one or more flights of stairs, walk more than a block without stopping, and perform house or yard work without difficulty. Office assessment may include a modified 6-minute walk test. Standard PFT should be performed and include the following: 1) spirometry, including forced vital capacity, forced expiratory volume in 1 second, and forced expiratory flow rate; and 2) lung volumes, including total lung capacity, residual volume, functional residual capacity, and diffusion capacity. The predicted postoperative parameters (e.g., predicted postoperative forced expiratory volume in 1 second) can be estimated by multiplying the measured forced expiratory volume in 1 second by the expected number of segments remaining after resection, each of which is assigned a contribution to overall pulmonary function of 5%. A predicted postoperative forced expiratory volume in 1 second of less than 30% of the patient's expected value may be cause for concern. Additional testing that may be helpful in equivocal situations includes quantitative ventilation-perfusion scanning, and exercise testing, as reviewed in Chapter 19.

DEFINITIVE SURGICAL RESECTION

As noted, the goal of surgical treatment of lung cancer is complete resection. Incomplete resection not only confers no therapeutic advantage, but may also temporarily postpone and physiologically limit any potential benefit of subsequent radiation therapy or chemotherapy, as well as impair the patient's postoperative quality of life. With currently available staging modalities, the incidence of nonresective thoracotomy or grossly incomplete resections should be low and never unanticipated. In contrast, a microscopically positive resection margin, usually involving the bronchial margin, a finding of subclinical parenchymal sites of cancer, or, most commonly, the pathologic documentation of unsuspected malignant lymphadenopathy, is often unavoidable, despite appropriate preoperative assessment. The absence of gross residual tumor and microscopically negative surgical margins define a complete resection, and, when either is present, the resection must be considered as incomplete, as pointed out by Shields (1989). In addition, however, the presence of metastatic involvement of the highest or most distant resected lymph node has been included in many lung cancer trials as one of the criteria of an incomplete resection. Although, such patients as a rule do not do well, few, if any, data actually support this conclusion (see Chapter 95). The failure to do a complete mediastinal lymph node dissection (MLD) is considered by most Japanese surgeons likewise to render a resection as incomplete. This too is an assumption that remains unproven; of course, we believe that either a complete lymph node dissection or, less satisfactory, lymph node sampling of each ipsilateral lymph node station is mandatory for appropriate intraoperative staging of the lung cancer.

Every operation for lung cancer has three essential parts: establishment or confirmation of the diagnosis and the intrathoracic stage, complete resection of the tumor, and the systematic sampling or complete dissection of every lymph node station potentially draining the primary tumor. In addition, when complex resections are performed, appropriate reconstruction may be necessary.

Intraoperative Diagnosis and Surgical Staging

Depending on the specifics of each case and the surgeon's preferred approach, a diagnosis of NSCLC will have been made preoperatively in many patients by bronchoscopy or transthoracic needle biopsy, less commonly by thoracoscopy, and rarely by mediastinoscopy in cases of primary resection. When a diagnosis of cancer has not been secured before thoracotomy, either intentionally or because of inconclusive attempts, it is advisable to establish a diagnosis intraoperatively before proceeding with resection. Stapled wedge resection and frozen section most often accomplish this goal. Frozen section assessment for NSCLC is generally straightforward and essentially totally accurate. For lesions that are central or otherwise not amenable to a nontraumatic wedge resection, sampling can be carried out by thin needle aspiration cytology or core needle biopsy. Incisional biopsy may occasionally be needed, but is less desirable because it requires macroscopic violation of a potential neoplasm. For the same reason, stapling across abnormal tissue for diagnostic assessment is especially discouraged. In the rare instance of a suspicious tumor not amenable to wedge resection and in which aspiration or core biopsy is nondiagnostic, a lobectomy may be required. Pneumonectomy and extended lobar resections, however, should not be performed in the absence of a firm confirmation of malignancy.

In addition to confirming the diagnosis of cancer when necessary, thoracotomy for NSCLC includes an assessment of the hemithorax for other sites of disease, whether suggested by preoperative imaging or not. The entire lung is palpated and inspected for other masses. The hilar and mediastinal nodes are examined, as is the pleura and any fixation of the primary tumor to adjacent structures. Although it is currently rare to abandon a planned resection based on totally unexpected intraoperative findings, an occasional seemingly straightforward case may be found at thoracotomy to be unresectable, based on the intraoperative finding of multiple undetected, usually subpleural lesions, noneffusive pleural dissemination, or a small malignant pleural effusion. More often, nonresective thoracotomy occurs in the setting of suspected, but clinically unproven, invasion of vital structures that is confirmed and deemed unresectable at the time of operation. When unsuspected lymphadenopathy is found at operation, resection should generally proceed. As discussed subsequently, the presence of N_2 disease discovered at operation after an appropriate invasive and noninvasive staging evaluation does not per se preclude a definitive resection. Exceptions include the unusual finding of unexpected extensive, fixed, and bulky adenopathy or the pres-

ence of positive interlobar nodes, or transfissural direct tumor extension, that would mandate a pneumonectomy in a patient with insufficient pulmonary reserve. In any case, there should be no hesitation to sample and assess by frozen section or cytologic analysis any nodal, pleural, or parenchymal tissue or pleural fluid that, if positive, would render resection inappropriate. Special care is warranted in cases that require a pneumonectomy. The potential for nonresective thoracotomy is generally known preoperatively and should be clearly discussed with the patient. The incidence of nonresective thoracotomy in older series was as high as 20%, but should currently be 5% or less, although no specific modern benchmark exists. Despite appropriate clinical staging, a small number of patients with locally advanced lesions still require exploratory operation to ascertain resectability with certainty.

In addition to standard surgical staging by gross inspection and frozen section, a number of authors, including Kondo (1993), Okada (1999), and Dresler (1999) and their associates, have suggested that intraoperative pleural lavage be performed in all cases without obvious pleural effusion, before resection or before chest closure, or both. The rationale for this procedure is to detect the presence of malignant cells in the pleural cavity and thereby identify patients at higher risk for recurrence. Although the volume of lavage fluid used varies from 50 to 500 mL of physiologic saline solution, all protocols require that the preresection sample be obtained immediately on entry into the chest, before any manipulation of the tumor. When obtained, the postresection sample is taken just before closure of the thoracotomy, with some protocols requiring prior copious pleural irrigation. At present, it is not suggested that the results of pleural lavage be used to affect intraoperative decisions regarding resectability. In addition, positive lavage cytology does not currently alter the stage of the tumor or the definition of complete resection, nor have recommendations for adjuvant treatment been based on this finding. Although worthy of further study, pleural lavage is not presently considered a standard component of resection for lung cancer.

Resection

Once a diagnosis of cancer has been made and resectability established, the appropriate pulmonary or extended resection is carried out. For patients with adequate lung function, the current standard cancer resections include lobectomy, bronchoplastic lobectomy, bilobectomy, and pneumonectomy, based on the extent of disease. In some cases, an anatomic segmentectomy may be appropriate. At present, nonanatomic or wedge resection should only be considered as definitive therapy in the minority of patients whose cardiac or pulmonary status mandates a limited operation and conservation of pulmonary parenchyma or in certain cases of synchronous or metachronous multiple tumors, as discussed later in this section.

Lobectomy

Lobectomy is the ideal operation for resection of a lung cancer confined to the parenchyma of a single lobe. It permits removal of the tumor along with the associated peripheral (pleural) and central lymphatic drainage pathways. Lobectomy is generally well tolerated, usually leaves sufficient lung volume to fill the pleural void left by resection, and avoids some of the short-term and late complications of pneumonectomy. Lobectomy is associated with approximately one-half the operative mortality of pneumonectomy (approximately 2% versus 4%) as reported by Ginsberg (1983) and Wada (1998) and their colleagues (see Chapter 37). In the elderly, the risk is higher, but in more recent series is acceptable, as demonstrated by Naunheim (1994), Damhuis (1996), and Wada (1998) and their associates. Pagni and coworkers (1997, 1998) showed an operative mortality for lobectomy of 2.4% in 293 patients older than 70 years of age and of 4.4% in 45 octogenarians.

A bilobectomy involves resection of the right upper and middle lobes or of the right lower and middle lobes. The former operation is indicated when a tumor located in the anterior segment of the right upper lobe or in the right middle lobe has spread across the minor fissure or approximates an incomplete fissure. Failure to perform a bilobectomy in this setting may result in a positive or unacceptably close parenchymal resection margin. When a tumor in the right lower lobe is central, a bilobectomy may be required because of the proximity of the origins of the superior segmental and middle lobe bronchi. Other indications may include certain cases of interlobar vascular or nodal involvement, but a pneumonectomy should be considered in most such instances. In a series of 166 bilobectomies reported by Keller and colleagues (1988a), the indications for this procedure were tumor extending across a fissure in 45%, absent fissure in 21%, endobronchial tumor in 14%, external or nodal invasion of the bronchus intermedius in 10%, vascular invasion in 5%, and miscellaneous reasons in 5%. The operative mortality for bilobectomy is generally reported as slightly higher than for lobectomy, but lower than the risk of pneumonectomy (see Chapter 37).

A sleeve lobectomy consists of the resection of a lobe along with a circumferential segment of the adjacent main stem bronchus and is generally an alternative to pneumonectomy. Bronchial continuity is restored and lung parenchyma preserved by anastomosis of the proximal and distal bronchial resection edges. Bronchoplastic lobectomy is discussed in Chapter 28. This operation is most often indicated for endobronchial tumors at the origins of the right upper or left upper lobe bronchi. Occasionally, sleeve lobectomy is suitable for patients with limited nodal disease affixed to the bronchial wall at the orifices of these lobes. Nodal disease of this type was the indication in 21% of the cases reported by Deslauriers and associates (1993). Overall, these authors achieved a complete resection in 87% of 142 sleeve lobectomies, with an operative mortality of only

2.5%. Five- and 10-year survivals were 63% and 52% for stage I tumors. Local recurrence ultimately occurred in 23% overall and in 17% of completely resected cases. The success of bronchoplastic resection in properly selected patients is also shown in the extensive series reported by Watanabe and colleagues (1990), with late survival in 79% of stage I, 55% of stage II, 30% of stage III, and 45% overall.

A bronchoplastic resection is less often appropriate when bronchi other than those of the upper lobes are involved by NSCLC, but is occasionally undertaken in oncologically favorable situations or as an alternative to pneumonectomy in patients with limited lung function. Sleeve resection of the pulmonary artery can be accomplished with or without a bronchial sleeve resection, but most cases with this degree of local invasion are inoperable or are treated by pneumonectomy. Although the use of sleeve lobectomy varies widely among institutions, in most centers it averages 5% or less of lung cancer resections.

Chapter 28 presents in detail the techniques, indications, and results of sleeve lobectomy and its variations, including associated sleeve resection of the pulmonary artery. Although concern has been raised that the local recurrence rate is higher after bronchoplastic lobectomy than after pneumonectomy, reports from centers with significant experience with this approach, including those of Faber (1987), Vogt-Moykopf (1986), Watanabe (1990), Newton (1991), Tedder (1992), and Deslauriers (1993) and their associates, show an acceptable operative mortality, a high rate of complete resection, and a late survival that is generally comparable, stage for stage, with other types of complete resection in NSCLC.

Pneumonectomy

A pneumonectomy is required when a lobectomy or one of its modifications is not sufficient to remove all locoregional disease. It must be kept in mind that a pneumonectomy is a radical procedure that can result in the loss of more than 50% of a patient's lung function and pulmonary vascular bed. It is most often indicated in patients with central tumors that involve the main stem bronchus, large parenchymal cancers that violate the fissures or invade the interlobar vessels or lymph nodes, and in some cases of lymph node involvement at the level of the main stem bronchus. Pneumonectomy in the latter situation should be reserved for cases in which higher stations are benign, and a complete resection is possible. The operative mortality for pneumonectomy is approximately twice that of lobectomy (see Chapter 37). Ginsberg and colleagues (1983) reported a 6.2% operative mortality among 2220 cases of the Lung Cancer Study Group (LCSG), and Wada and associates (1998) noted a rate of 3.2% among 7099 patients undergoing resection for lung cancer in Japan during 1994. Right pneumonectomy carries a higher risk than does removal of the left lung. An increasing number of patients with N_2 disease or central, locally invasive cancers, are being treated by induction therapy. Because of the extent of their disease, a high percentage of them require pneumonectomy (23% to as high as 53%). Despite the frequent technical difficulty posed by postinduction peribronchial and perivascular fibrosis, operative mortality in this group can be as low as 5%, but ranges up to 15%, as reported by Faber (1989), Strauss (1992), Rusch (1993, 1994), Mathisen (1996), and Weiden (1994) and their coworkers.

Three types of extended pneumonectomy exist (see Chapter 29). The most commonly used variation is an intrapericardial pneumonectomy, necessitated by encroachment of a central tumor at or near the entry of the pulmonary vessels, most often the artery central to its branches, into the pericardium. Ligation within the pericardium may provide both a greater margin of resection and a longer segment for safe division of the vessel. Although this approach may be associated with a higher incidence of postoperative arrhythmias, the operative risk is not higher than for standard pneumonectomy. Another modification is a supra-aortic pneumonectomy and involves transecting the left main stem bronchus more proximal than in a standard left pneumonectomy, close to the trachea, above the aortic arch. This approach is occasionally needed for tumors originating high in the bronchus. The third variation is the carinal or sleeve pneumonectomy, consisting of resection of the lower trachea, the carina, and a main stem bronchus and its associated lung, usually the right, with a tracheobronchial anastomosis of the remaining lung. This procedure is indicated for central lesions approximating or involving the carina that appear totally resectable by this approach and is discussed in detail in Chapter 30. Although some series have reported operative mortality in as many as one-fourth to one-third of cases, reports by Dartevelle (1995) and Mitchell (1998) and their colleagues have achieved rates of 7% and 16%, respectively. The risk of the less often performed left carinal pneumonectomy is higher than that for the right lung.

Segmentectomy

When a patient has limited pulmonary reserve and a small peripheral tumor confined to an anatomic segment, a segmentectomy is an acceptable operation for NSCLC. Although any segment can be removed by anatomic dissection, resections of the upper lobe segments or the superior segments of the lower lobes are performed most commonly. Lingulectomy, although encompassing two segments, is also a form of segmentectomy and is often feasible for peripheral NSCLC. Jensik and colleagues (1973) reported the first large series of segmental resection for lung cancer. Among 123 patients, 5- and 10-year survivals were 56% and 27%, respectively. In an instructive analysis, Kodama and colleagues (1997) compared three groups of patients with T_1N_0 NSCLC, 46 undergoing segmentectomy as an intentional procedure, 17 in whom segmental resection was viewed as a compromise because of limited lung function, and 77 treated by lobectomy and lymph node dissection. No significant dif-

ference occurred in late survival between the lobectomy group (88%) and the intentional segmentectomy patients (93%). However, the difference in survival between these two groups and patients undergoing segmentectomy as a compromise procedure (48%) was significant. In a report by Warren and Faber (1994) comparing 68 patients with $T_{1-2}N_0$ tumors treated by segmental resection with 105 similar patients undergoing lobectomy, an overall survival difference favored the lobectomy group, but the differential was not significant for tumors 3 cm or less in size. For the total series, however, the rate of locoregional recurrence was 23% after segmentectomy as contrasted to 5% after lobectomy. Similarly, the only prospective experience, collected by the LCSG and reported by Ginsberg and Rubinstein (1995), indicates that local recurrence after limited resection for T_1N_0 NSCLC, including segmentectomy and wedge excision, is threefold higher than for lobectomy, although ultimate survival is less dramatically affected. Despite an increased risk of local recurrence, anatomic segmental resection remains an appropriate option in patients with limited lung function and also in patients with small peripheral tumors.

Wedge Resection

In contrast to segmentectomy, wedge resection is a nonanatomic operation that should be considered as definitive therapy only in poor-risk patients. Despite a higher risk of local recurrence when compared with anatomic resection, however, wedge excision may still be preferable to alternative treatments when applied appropriately. In an early nonrandomized series reported by Errett and associates (1985), wedge resection was performed as a compromise operation in 97 patients with pulmonary impairment and compared with 100 patients treated by lobectomy. Despite higher predicted risk, the wedge resection group incurred only a 3% operative mortality, as compared with 2% in the lobectomy group, and late survival was not statistically different. In patients with T_1N_0 NSCLC, Landreneau and colleagues (1996) retrospectively compared 42 cases treated by open wedge resection, 60 by video-assisted thoracic surgery (VATS) wedge, and 117 by standard lobectomy. Despite reduced pulmonary function and older age, there was no mortality in the combined wedge groups versus 3% for the lobectomy group. However, as in the LCSG experience, local recurrence rates were higher in the open and VATS wedge patients (24% and 16%, respectively) than in the cases treated by lobectomy (9%). Although 5-year survival was significantly lower in the open wedge cohort than for the lobectomy patients (58% versus 70%) survival for the VATS cases was similar to lobectomy at 65%. The authors point out that the minimum requirements for an appropriate wedge resection for NSCLC include the following: a tumor smaller than 3 cm in diameter, a location in the outer third of the lung and technically amenable to adequate local excision, absence of endobronchial extension, clear margins by frozen section, and mediastinal and hilar lymph node sampling. When these criteria are met, wedge resection is an acceptable option in the few patients unable to tolerate an anatomic operation. Local excision by cautery or laser has been performed, but the late benefit is unknown, and this approach cannot be recommended.

Video-Assisted Resection

VATS has been successfully used for lobectomy, pneumonectomy, and local resection of NSCLC. For surgeons with experience and skill with this approach, VATS may be an acceptable alternative to open operation. It is essential that the same principles of lung cancer surgery that guide standard resection be maintained when VATS is applied. This topic is addressed fully in Chapters 32 and 33.

Evaluation of the Lymph Nodes

The single most important prognostic factor in bronchial carcinoma is the status of the mediastinal lymph nodes. Evaluation begins preoperatively with a CT scan of the chest. Although controversy exists regarding the need for routine mediastinoscopy, all accessible nodes that are enlarged should be biopsied before thoracotomy. In addition, invasive mediastinal node assessment should be considered in all patients at high risk of metastasis, such as those with central tumors, especially when known to be adenocarcinoma. In addition to mediastinoscopy, extended mediastinoscopy and anterior mediastinotomy (see Chapter 17), transthoracic needle biopsy is often useful, especially for the subaortic and posterior subcarinal nodes. Roviaro (1995) and DeGiacomo (1997) and their associates, among others, have proposed thoracoscopy as a method of nodal and tumor staging (see Chapter 18).

At thoracotomy, lymph node assessment has been performed by examining only those nodes attached to the resected specimen, sampling only nodes that appear abnormal, systematic biopsy of each node station, and complete lymph node dissection. It is clear that the first two approaches are insufficient, because N_2 nodes can be involved in the presence of benign N_1 levels (i.e., skip metastases) and even small, normal appearing nodes may harbor metastasis, as shown by one of us (B.D.T.D.) and colleagues (1993), among others.

The minimum standard is a systematic sampling of each lymph node station draining a tumor. For right-sided resections, nodes should be taken from mediastinal levels 2, 4, 7, 8, and 9, as well as from the tracheobronchial angle and interlobar area (levels 10 and 11). On the left, the subaortic and anterior mediastinal nodes (levels 5 and 6) should be biopsied as well. Systematic sampling is required because of the frequent finding of pathologic N_2 disease that was unsuspected by clinical staging and the prognostic and therapeutic implications of this situation, as discussed later in the section on stage IIIA lung cancer in this chapter. The incidence of

unsuspected N_2 after various staging pathways using modern imaging and routine or selective mediastinoscopy is approximately 10%. Goldstraw and colleagues (1994) found pathologic N_2 in 24% of clinical $N_{0/1}$ cases.

Some surgeons believe that complete MLD is indicated for therapeutic reasons in all resections for NSCLC. In the prospective randomized series reported by Sugi and associates (1998) and by Izbicki and colleagues (1998), however, MLD did not increase overall survival in patients without overt N_2 disease. Although also therapeutically unproven, we believe that it is reasonable to perform MLD in patients found at thoracotomy to have N_2 disease. In addition, operations after induction therapy for N_2 NSCLC should include MLD in virtually all cases. Although improved survival with routine MLD has not been documented, this approach does minimize sampling error by identifying N_2 metastases that otherwise might have been missed, as shown by Graham and associates (1999). In the aforementioned study by Izbicki and coworkers (1998), N_2 disease in 5.5% of the MLD group would have been missed by sampling. This figure may be high, because in their sampling cohort only levels 4, 5, and 7 were routinely biopsied, whereas nodes were taken from other mediastinal areas only when suspicious. The use of routine MLD remains controversial and is discussed in detail in Chapter 100. The American College of Surgeons is conducting a randomized study to address this question. At present, either MLD or a complete systematic sampling is acceptable as a routine approach. There should be a low threshold to proceed to MLD, however, in the presence of intraoperatively documented N_2 disease.

Selection of the Operative Procedure

The appropriate operation depends on the clinical and surgical stage of the tumor and an accurate assessment of the structures involved. Unless all gross tumor can be encompassed in the resection, operation should not be undertaken. With rare exceptions, therefore, T_4 NSCLC is not suitable for resection.

Tumors can be classified as occult, peripheral, or central. Occult lesions are not seen radiographically, but their presence has been detected by sputum cytology or bronchoscopy. Central lesions are located radiographically within the central third of the hemithorax or bronchoscopically within or proximal to a segmental bronchus. Peripheral tumors are located beyond a segmental bronchus and in the outer two-thirds of the lung.

Occult Tumors

Most cases of occult NSCLC are brought to attention in screening programs for high-risk people or present with hemoptysis. Lobectomy is most often required [70% in the experience of Cortese and colleagues (1983)] because the lesion cannot be further localized anatomically or because of a documented location in a lobar or segmental bronchus. Because of a more central location, some require bilobectomy or pneumonectomy. In a report of 94 cases by Saito and associates (1992), there were 58 lobectomies, 12 bilobectomies, 11 sleeve lobectomies, and 12 pneumonectomies. In a small number of patients, when the radiographically occult NSCLC is confined to the bronchial mucosa or is an in situ carcinoma covering less than 3 cm of the mucosal surface, or in medically inoperable cases, photodynamic therapy has been used successfully as primary treatment, as reported by Lam (1994), as well as by Kato (1996) and Cortese (1997) and their associates. Alternatively, brachytherapy can be delivered via bronchoscopically placed catheters, as reported by Taulelle and colleagues (1998). Chapter 101 reviews endobronchial techniques for lung cancer treatment. In most patients, however, the depth of invasion cannot be determined with certainty and some have associated lymph node involvement (see Chapter 95). Resection, therefore, remains the most common approach.

Peripheral Tumors

The major considerations in the surgical evaluation of a peripheral tumor are its location within the lobe and its relationship to other structures. Lesions that are clearly surrounded by parenchyma and confined to a single lobe are treated by lobectomy and, occasionally, by lesser resections. If a tumor abuts the chest wall on CT, the possibility of at least visceral pleural invasion should be entertained, especially if the patient has associated pain. If the tumor approximates an interlobar fissure, the possibility of extension into an adjacent lobe should be considered. In all such cases, the operation should be planned and discussed with the patient by including the possibility of chest wall resection, bilobectomy, or pneumonectomy, as appropriate. When peripheral tumors invade other structures, en bloc resection is often necessary.

Chest Wall

Tumors invading the chest wall are often resectable. The involved rib(s) should be transected several centimeters beyond the margin of gross involvement. In most cases, one rib and intercostal tissue above and below the tumor also should be included in the resection. Chest wall reconstruction is carried out as needed to prevent physiologic impairment because of paradoxical chest wall function or for cosmetic reasons (see Chapter 46). For posterior defects, support by the remaining chest wall muscles and scapula is usually sufficient, whereas anterior and lateral defects more often require prosthetic reconstruction. Although full-thickness resection is mandatory for tumors invading the osseous and muscular structures of the chest wall, controversy exists regarding the necessity of chest wall resection when invasion is confined to the parietal pleura. McCaughan and associates (1985) reported good results in such cases treated by

the development of an extrapleural dissection plane when possible, stripping away the lung and parietal pleura from the endothoracic fascia, and proceeding to a full-thickness resection only if the margin was positive on frozen section. Albertucci and associates (1992), in contrast, found that a histologic complete resection was achieved in only one-third of their patients treated by extrapleural dissection versus all of those undergoing a standard chest wall resection. The experience of Trastek and colleagues (1984) also suggests that chest wall resection is preferable even when invasion is confined to the parietal pleura. We agree with Ratto and associates (1991), who suggest that when a tumor is firmly affixed to the parietal pleura, no attempt be made to strip it away, and that an en bloc resection be carried out. However, extrapleural dissection may be appropriate in patients in whom the risk of an extended resection is high, in those treated with preoperative radiation therapy, or if intraoperative brachytherapy is applied, although the overall role of external and interstitial radiation therapy for fully resectable chest wall T_3 NSCLC is unknown.

Diaphragm

The diaphragm is rarely involved by direct extension of NSCLC. When invaded, it should be resected with a wide margin of normal tissue, without regard to the extent of the defect. Although unlikely to be helpful for NSCLC, it is feasible to resect and replace an entire hemidiaphragm. Unless the defect is small and can be closed primarily without tension, it should generally be replaced with a prosthetic material. Alternatively, a variety of muscle flaps can be used. When a large area of diaphragm has been resected or when the phrenic nerve has been sacrificed, it is important that the diaphragm be reconstructed near the position of full inspiration, to avoid paradoxical motion. When the defect is peripheral, it may be possible to reinsert the remaining cut edge at a higher level on the chest wall and thereby obviate the need for prosthetic material, as described by Daly and Feins (1998).

Pericardium

Total resection of the pericardium on the left can be performed without reconstruction. Partial defects should be closed to prevent herniation and strangulation of the left ventricle. On the right side, all pericardial defects, regardless of size, require repair. The potential problem if the pericardium remains open after right pneumonectomy is torsion of the heart into the chest along the axis of the venae cavae, with consequent total occlusion of venous inflow. Large defects can be closed with the pericardial fat pad, a pleural flap, or nonautologous material such as bovine pericardium or polytetrafluoroethylene. Many surgeons suggest that a small opening be left in the repair or that the prosthetic material be perforated to prevent intrapericardial fluid accumulation and cardiac tamponade.

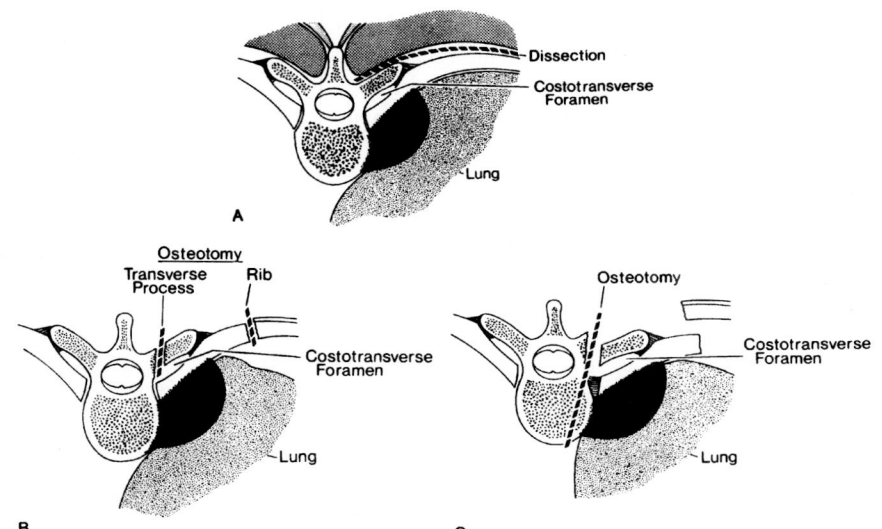

Fig. 99-1. Technique of removing part of the vertebral body when a tumor has become attached to the overlying parietal pleura. The costotransverse foramen must be free of disease. **A–C.** Sequential steps in resection. From DeMeester TR, et al: Management of tumor adherent to the vertebral column. J Thorac Cardiovasc Surg 97:373, 1989. With permission.

Vertebrae

Tumors invading the vertebral bodies are rarely cured and under most circumstances are considered unresectable. DeMeester and colleagues (1989) described a technique of partial vertebral resection for tumors fixed to the paravertebral fascia, involving a tangential osteotomy through the transverse process, costotransverse foramen, and superficial vertebral body (Fig. 99-1). The authors emphasize that this approach is not suitable for patients with radiographic evidence of bone destruction. Grunenwald and associates (1996), however, reported a small group of patients with radiographic evidence of osseous invasion who were treated by en bloc pulmonary resection and complete vertebrectomy with reconstruction by a combined thoracic and posterior approach. This technique should be limited to rare cases in which the tumor extent is completely delineated, node-negative, totally resectable, and, after careful evaluation with MR imaging, does not involve the spinal canal.

Superior Sulcus Tumors

Peripheral tumors involving the apex of the chest or the lower portion of the brachial plexus (superior sulcus or Pancoast's tumors) are discussed in depth in Chapters 35 and 36. In most instances, resection is preceded by radiation therapy and, in some centers, by chemotherapy as well. Resection involves removal of the involved portions of the apical chest wall, typically including the first, second, and third ribs, and the T1 nerve root, along with lobectomy or lesser pulmonary resection. Although invasion of the vertebral body or of the subclavian vessels, clinical N_2 disease, or the presence of a Horner's syndrome generally contraindicate primary operation, a more aggressive approach may be indicated in selected cases, especially after induction therapy. These tumors can be resected through a high postero-lateral thoracotomy or by an anterior approach using a cervical incision with extension down to the second intercostal space and resection of the first and second costal cartilages. Dartevelle and colleagues (1993) have used the anterior approach alone to perform extensive vascular resection along with lobectomy in this setting.

Central Tumors

Central tumors are more likely to be associated with malignant lymphadenopathy and to involve mediastinal structures. Accordingly, careful imaging and invasive evaluation is mandatory before consideration of thoracotomy. By definition, complete resection requires at least a lobectomy, and often a pneumonectomy or more extended procedure. Central bronchial T_3 lesions and some T_4 cancers involving the carina can be treated successfully by primary operation, in the latter situation usually by a carinal pneumonectomy. The selection, techniques, and results of resection in this setting are discussed in Chapter 30. The decreasing mortality associated with these extensive procedures has been noted previously. Infrequently, for a small lesion in the left main stem bronchus, a localized bronchial sleeve resection with pulmonary conservation can be carried out, as reported by Newton and associates (1991). Localized tumors involving the pulmonary veins, even with extension into the pericardium and left atrium, may be amenable to resection by excision of a contiguous cuff of the atrium, using vascular clamps and sutured closure or vascular staplers. Central NSCLC with local invasion limited to the mediastinal pleura and adipose tissue, but not involving deeper structures, is also often suitable for total resection. With exceedingly rare exceptions, in contrast, tumors invading the superior vena cava or the aorta or its branches should not be addressed by primary operation, but should be considered for resection in a few cases only after postinduction reassessment. It cannot be overemphasized that, in all cases of locally invasive NSCLC considered for resection, the absence of N_2 lymphadenopathy should be confirmed by rigorous preoperative staging.

Simultaneous Cardiac Operation and Pulmonary Resection

When a patient requires myocardial revascularization or other cardiac procedure and also has a resectable lung cancer, the question of simultaneous versus staged procedures arises. This clinical situation can arise during the physiologic assessment of a lung cancer patient being considered for resection or in the preoperative radiographic evaluation of a cardiac patient. When the lung cancer can be resected via a median sternotomy, the timing of the procedures is largely a matter of the surgeon's preference and patient-specific factors. The experience reported by Canver (1990), Terzi (1994), and Danton (1998) and their colleagues, support the safety and efficacy of simultaneous operations. The cardiac procedure should be performed first and without complications. Pulmonary resection is carried out after reversal of anticoagulation and confirmation of hemodynamic and hemostatic stability. Because cardiac retraction required during trans-sternal left lower lobectomy may cause hemodynamic problems, many left lower lobe tumors should be resected at a separate session. Combined procedures have the advantage of a single operation and recovery, as well as absence of delay in cancer treatment. In addition, concerns have been raised about the adverse oncologic effect of immunosuppression and the possibility of tumor dissemination associated with cardiopulmonary bypass, if the cardiac operation is performed before the pulmonary resection. Generally, a lobectomy is carried out, although pneumonectomy has been reported by Piehler (1985) and Danton (1998) and their associates. Limited resections should be used only with the appropriate indications. In all cases except emergent cardiac surgery, a full staging evaluation of the lung tumor should be carried out before operation.

Synchronous Lung Cancers

Although the incidence of a second primary lung cancer in patients previously treated for NSCLC may be as high as 10%, the prevalence of synchronous primary lung cancers has generally been placed at approximately 1% of surgical cases. Evidence suggests, however, that the incidence of this problem is increasing. In addition, the nature of multiple primary sites of involvement appears to have changed coincident with the rise in the proportion of adenocarcinomas among NSCLC. Multiple sites of parenchymal adenocarcinoma at presentation are now more commonly encountered than multiple sites of squamous cancer in the airways. Both the diagnosis of synchronous lesions, as opposed to metastasis, and the optimal surgical and nonsurgical treatment of such lesions represent a

challenge. The criteria for differentiating between synchronous and metastatic lesions established by Martini and Melamed (1975) are accepted by most surgeons. For lesions to be considered synchronous primaries, they must be physically distinct and separate. The histology must be different or, if similar, the neoplasms must have an origin from carcinoma in situ, or be located in different pulmonary segments, and have no carcinoma in the lymphatic vessels and nodes common to both lesions and no extrapulmonary metastasis. Antakli and associates (1995) modified the criteria for tumors of similar histology, regarding them as separate primaries if two or more of the following five conditions were met: anatomically distinct, presence of associated premalignant lesions, absence of systemic metastasis, no mediastinal disease, and different DNA ploidy. Ichinose and colleagues (1991) reported on the use of flow cytometry to differentiate metastatic from synchronous lesions and recurrent NSCLC from a metachronous new primary.

As reviewed by Adebonojo and associates (1997), the incidence of multiple NSCLC in surgical series varies widely from 0.8 to 14.0%. Ohada and coworkers (1998) noted a 3.2% incidence of synchronous cancers among 908 consecutive resections. McElvaney and colleagues (1989) reported the disturbing finding that, on careful pathologic examination, 12 of 62 consecutive resections for adenocarcinoma (19%) were found to have multiple sites of cancer that met the criteria for separate primary lesions. In only two cases were the additional lesions suspected preoperatively, despite CT scanning in all cases.

In practice, resection for synchronous primary NSCLC is largely confined to patients with two lesions. The presence of three or more sites strongly suggests metastatic disease or, at least, a patient unlikely to benefit by primary operation. Selection of the appropriate surgical approach depends on the size and location of the tumors and the patient's pulmonary function. In general, anatomic resection should be carried out, especially for the larger or more central tumor. The specifics of each case dictate whether sternotomy with bilateral resections or staged thoracotomies are preferable when the lesions are bilateral. Although extensive anatomic parenchymal resection, including pneumonectomy, may be indicated when a high degree of certainty exists that the tumors are separate primaries without lymph node spread, the difficulty in distinguishing intrapulmonary metastasis often makes lesser resection of the smaller lesion prudent. Similar guidelines should be followed when dealing with metachronous NSCLC, although surgical options for new cancers after prior pneumonectomy are markedly limited, as noted by Westermann and associates (1993).

Incomplete Surgical Resection

Incomplete resection of NSCLC, with rare exceptions, does not result in long-term survival. With current staging methods, complete resection should be achieved in 95% or

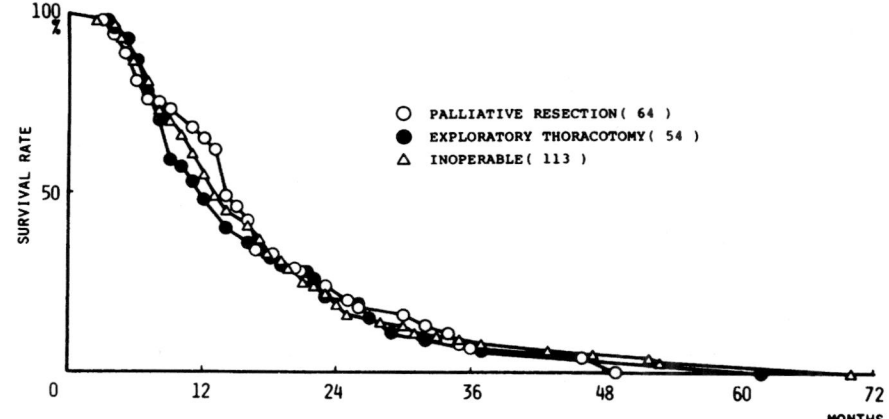

Fig. 99-2. Survival curves of patients with stage III carcinoma of the lung after palliative resection, exploratory thoracotomy only, or no surgical therapy. From Hara N, et al: Assessment of the role of surgery for stage III bronchogenic carcinoma. J Surg Oncol 25:153, 1984. With permission.

more of operated patients. When a patient is found at thoracotomy to have disease that cannot be removed completely, resection should be carried out only if it can be accomplished with low risk and with the expectation that it will prevent or reduce the likelihood of complications in the future. Only under unusual circumstances, when infection, bleeding, or pain cannot be palliated by other means, should an incomplete resection be intentionally considered. Patients who have an incomplete resection, whether of the primary tumor or metastatic lymph nodes, have a clinical course identical to those who undergo nonresective exploration or no operation, as shown by Hara and associates (1984), among others (Fig. 99-2). Furthermore, patients who undergo incomplete resection may have a poorer quality of remaining life than those treated by other modalities or by supportive care.

Patients with microscopic invasive residual tumor in the mucosa and submucosa of the bronchial resection margin appear to have an unexpectedly favorable late survival, despite incomplete resection. Most such cases involve squamous histology. Shields (1974) described three categories of positive bronchial margins: gross disease, microscopic tumor in the peribronchial tissue, and microscopic mucosal or submucosal residual cancer. Although the first two findings portend a prognosis similar to other incomplete resections, late survival without adjuvant therapy occurs in approximately one-fourth of patients in the third group. Similar findings were reported by Soorae and Stevenson (1979). More recently, Gebitekin and colleagues (1994) noted that a microscopically positive margin adversely affected survival only in stage III cases. Snijder and associates (1998), however, found that among 23 of 834 resections for stage I NSCLC found to have a bronchial margin that has positive test results, survival was significantly worse in patients with either peribronchial or mucosal involvement versus those with clear margins or positive results limited to carcinoma in situ. Nonetheless, late survival in the positive margin group was 27%, with adjuvant radiation used in only a minority of cases. Intraoperatively, frozen section assessment of the airway margin should be used frequently, and more proximal resection carried out if indicated. When an involved margin is detected only on final

pathologic review, especially when peribronchial cancer is noted and N_2 disease is absent, reoperation to achieve more proximal airway resection should be considered, as reported by Kaiser (1989), Liewald (1992), and Snijder (1998) and their coworkers.

In patients treated with induction therapy for advanced stage NSCLC, incomplete resection may be unavoidable, because treatment effects may render precise intraoperative staging difficult. In some cases, the completeness of resection can only be determined after histopathologic examination of the resected specimen, because extensive fibrosis and necrosis may render intraoperative gross and microscopic evaluation difficult. Although a survival advantage for incomplete resection after aggressive induction as compared with historical controls has been suggested, with some protocols for N_3 disease not requiring resection of known preinduction malignant sites, to date no conclusive evidence exists that this approach is superior to nonsurgical treatment.

Although external radiation therapy has not been shown to prolong survival in the overall spectrum of incompletely resected NSCLC, adjuvant radiation therapy should be used in most such cases, because local control may be enhanced. The role of brachytherapy is unclear, because no randomized studies have been done, and experience is limited. As a practical matter, however, because the risk of this local treatment is minimal and the rationale is sound, it should be considered in cases of intraoperatively confirmed or suspected positive or close resection margins. Permanently implanted radioactive seeds, available incorporated into absorbable suture material that can be placed directly into tissue or first arranged in an absorbable mesh, or various afterloaded catheters can be placed simply and expeditiously during operation, as described in Chapter 103.

RESULTS OF SURGICAL TREATMENT

The results of surgical treatment of NSCLC are assessed based on the risk of death or significant complications and the long-term survival realized after resection, as measured

Table 99-1. Five-Year Survival by TNM Classification and by Stage According to the 1997 System

TNM	Stage (1997 System)	Naruke (1988)		Mountain (1997)	
		No.	5-Year Survival (%)	No.	5-Year Survival (%)
$T_1N_0M_0$	IA	245	75	511	67
$T_2N_0M_0$	IB	291	57	549	57
$T_1N_1M_0$	IIA	66	52	76	55
$T_2N_1M_0$	IIB	153	38	288	39
$T_3N_0M_0$	IIB	106	33	87	38
$T_3N_1M_0$	IIIA	85	39	55	25
$T_{1-3}N_2M_0$	IIIA	368	15	344	23
$T_{1-3}N_3M_0$	IIIB	55	0	572	3
T_4 any N M_0	IIIB	104	8	458	6
Any T any N M_1	IV	293	7	1427	1

TNM, tumor, node, metastasis.
Note: Classification is postsurgical except in Mountain's IIIB and IV, which is clinical.
From Naruke T, et al: Prognosis and survival in resected lung carcinoma based on the new international staging system. J Thoracic Cardiovasc Surg *96*:440, 1988; and Mountain CF: Revisions in the international system for staging lung cancer. Chest *111*:1710, 1997. With permission.

by prolongation of life or by cure. The acute risk is dependent mainly on patient-specific factors, such as comorbidity and age. Tumor-related factors are important insofar as they dictate the extent of the required resection. Mortality and morbidity are addressed earlier in this chapter and in detail in Chapters 19, 20, and 37.

Long-term survival is determined by multiple factors. At present, the most valuable predictors are the tumor stage and the tumor, node, metastasis (TNM) subsets within each stage. As emphasized, the ability to accomplish a complete resection is also paramount and largely depends on the tumor stage. In assessing surgical results, the concept of clinical stage versus pathologic stage must be clearly appreciated (see Chapter 98). The clinical stage is based on the synthesis of all invasive and noninvasive studies short of resection. The pathologic stage is determined from the resected tissue and may or may not coincide with the clinical stage. Discordance is often caused by clinical understaging of malignant lymphadenopathy. Clinical assessment of the T descriptor, as shown by Bulzebruck and associates (1991), among others, often overstages the primary site. Fernando and Goldstraw (1990) found that clinical and pathologic stage coincided in only 47% of cases. Clinically undocumented node involvement was found in 23% of patients. In a prospective study comparing clinical staging by CT and mediastinoscopy with pathologic stage, Gdeedo and colleagues (1997) found that the T factor was overstaged in 27% and understaged in 18% of cases, whereas adenopathy was clinically overstaged by imaging in 45% and understaged in 20% of patients. Newer modalities, such as positron emission tomography, may increase the concordance between clinical and pathologic stages.

The vast literature on the surgical treatment of NSCLC can be confusing. A few general principles for assessing individual reports may facilitate comparison with other material. Of obvious importance is the time period encompassed, not only because of variations in imaging, but also evolution of surgical philosophy. It is similarly imperative to be clear regarding

the clinical staging methods applied. Of utmost importance is recognition of the subset of patients on which the conclusions are based, whether the entire group, all operated patients, or only those who had a complete resection. Some series eliminate from survival calculations cases of operative mortality or late noncancer deaths. Perspective may be enhanced by noting the actual number of long-term survivors, in addition to the actuarial probability of survival. Although the latter is the most valid figure for statistical reporting, the methodology is such that a small surviving cohort may yield a surprisingly favorable actuarial survival. Another variable requiring attention is the use of preoperative and postoperative adjuvant treatments that in many surgical reports are not factored into the conclusions. Finally, it must be recognized that results vary from institution to institution, and that, especially in cases of advanced NSCLC, results in a small number of patients from centers of excellence cannot routinely be translated to the larger cohort of similar stage.

This discussion focuses on surgical results based on TNM staging, with brief reviews of other prognostic factors. The type of resection and the management of the mediastinal lymph nodes has been addressed previously in the section on resection in this chapter. Although the new staging system proposed by Mountain (1997) remains the subject of some controversy and virtually all extant data are reported according to the prior iterations, the material is presented largely according to the new system. Table 99-1 presents survival by stage and TNM subsets from the reports of Mountain (1997) and Naruke and associates (1988a).

Occult Lung Cancer

Although occult NSCLC does not constitute a specific stage, many of the least advanced tumors are detected in this manner, and the results of resection in this group are excellent. Most occult cancers are squamous cell lesions, and many involve the large airways. Saito and colleagues (1992) reported 94 patients with occult squamous lung cancer who were treated by resection. Although all were clinical stage I lesions, pathologic staging showed 16 $TisN_0$ (stage 0), 72 T_1N_0 (stage IA, and 6 stage IIA and B), four T_1N_1, and two T_2N_1. Five-year actuarial survival overall was 80.4%, and when noncancer deaths were eliminated survival was 93.5%. Cortese and associates (1983) reported on 54 patients and postresection staging including 19 cases of $TisN_0$, 25 T_1N_0, five T_1N_1, four T_2N_1, and one T_3N_0. All were squamous cancers, some with large cell features. The overall 5-year survival was 74%, with 90% survival when only lung cancer deaths were included. Survival was 91% for the $TisN_0$ and T_1N_0 patients. Likewise, Martini and Melamed (1980), in a series of 47 cases, reported a high incidence of low-stage cancers and a high surgical cure rate. All three reports, however, noted a disturbing incidence of both synchronous and metachronous multiple aerodigestive squamous cancers in this patient population. Saito and coworkers (1992) noted an incidence of 9.6% synchronous and 7.4% metachronous lesions; Martini and Melamed (1980) ultimately found new cancers in 45%; and Cortese and colleagues (1983) calculated an incidence of 5% per postoperative year, a rate that did not decrease over time.

Stage I: Localized Node-Negative Lung Cancer

Because of an often striking and usually statistically significant difference in survival between tumors 3 cm or smaller that are entirely parenchymal (T_1) as opposed to those that are larger, invade the visceral pleura, are located in a main bronchus more than 2 cm from the carina, or cause lobar atelectasis (T_2), the 1997 system divides stage I into two subsets (Table 99-2). Postsurgical 5-year survival rates in the T_1N_0 group are uniformly excellent, whereas postresection survival in IB disease is less satisfactory. In both categories, the efficacy of resection is not matched by any other treatment modality. In addition, presently no evidence exists that additional therapy, as induction or postoperative adjuvant, offers benefit over resection alone, although trials of postresection chemotherapy for stage IB are in progress.

In the databases of Naruke (1988a) and Mountain (1997), 5-year postsurgical survival for IA cases is 61 to 65% for clinical IA tumors (cT_1N_0) and 67 to 76% for pathologic IA (pT_1N_0). Table 99-2 shows that surgeons worldwide have confirmed these results, and some have reported higher survival rates, up to 85%, in cooperative and single-center series spanning three decades. The LCSG noted a median survival of 8 years for 907 pT_1N_0 cancers resected between 1977 and 1988, as reported by Thomas and colleagues (1990). Pairolero and associates (1984) reported their experience as rates of recurrence at 5 years (29% for T_1N_0 and 40% for T_2N_0).

Factors that have been shown to affect survival in cases of limited NSCLC include tumor size, cell type, and location. Among these variables, the size of the primary lesion has most consistently been found to influence the prognosis. Read and associates (1990) noted significantly better survival for T_1N_0 tumors 2 cm or smaller than for T_1 lesions between 2 and 3 cm. Similarly, Ishida and coworkers (1990a) found a less favorable prognosis for tumors 2 to 3 cm compared with those smaller than 1 cm, but no difference between T_1N_0 cancers 1 cm or smaller as compared with 1.1 to 2.0 cm (Fig. 99-3). Padilla and colleagues (1997) reported markedly better late survival for smaller diameter pT_1N_0 tumors (87% at 5 years and 74% at 10 years for 2 cm or smaller versus 65% at 5 years and 49% at 10 years for 2.1 to 3.0 cm). Koike and associates (1998), among others, have shown that the incidence of pathologic N_2 adenopathy rises with increasing tumor diameter in cases clinically staged as T_1N_0. In a multivariate analysis of stage IA NSCLC, Harpole and associates (1995a,b) also correlated larger primaries with diminished long-term survival.

Although not as consistently important as tumor size, some series note a difference in late survival based on cell type, with T_1N_0 squamous histology conferring an improved

Table 99-2. Selected Series Reporting Postresection 5-Year Survival for Pathologic Stage IA (T_1N_0) and Stage IB (T_2N_0) Non–Small Cell Lung Carcinoma

Report	Dates	T_1N_0 IA		T_2N_0 IB	
		No.	5-Year Survival (%)	No.	5-Year Survival (%)
Williams et al. (1981)	1972–1978	225	80	236	62
Little et al. (1986)[a]	1974–1984	44	72	47	68
Martini et al. (1986)	1973–1976	50	83	78	65
Roeslin et al. (1987)	1977–1982	108	71	121	43
Naruke et al. (1988a)	1962–1986	245	76	327	57
Read et al. (1990)	1966–1988	214	73	158	49
Shimizu et al. (1993)	1973–1989	228 total	75	—	54
Ichinose et al. (1993)	1981–1988	71	85	80	67
Padilla et al. (1997)	1969–1993	109	76	45	78
Mountain (1997)	1975–1988	511	67	549	57
Inoue et al. (1998)	1980–1993	480	80	271	65

[a]Series limited to complete resection.

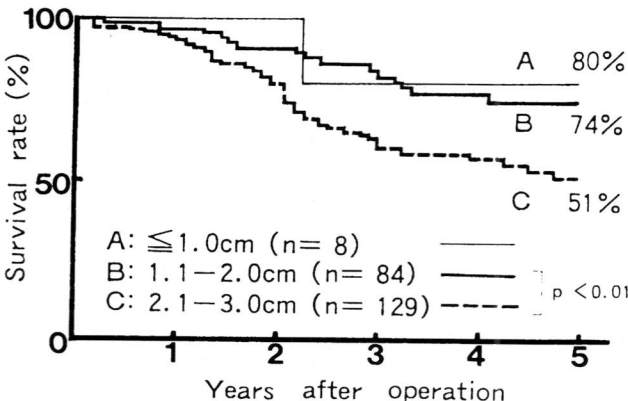

Fig. 99-3. Survival curves of T_1N_0 lesions based on size of the lesion. From Ishida T, et al: Strategy for lymphadenectomy of lung cancer less than 3 cm in diameter. Ann Thorac Surg 50:708, 1990a. With permission.

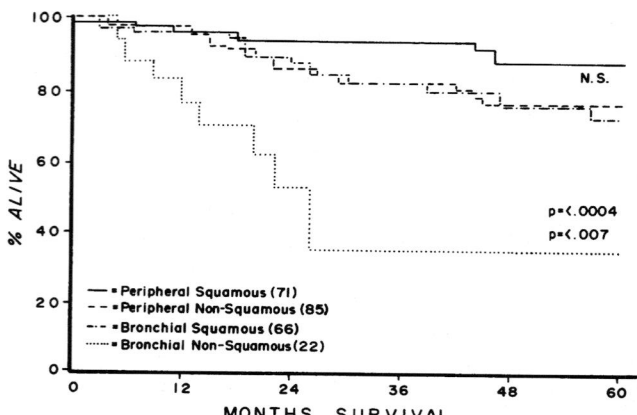

Fig. 99-4. T_1N_0 lesions that communicate with a segmental of subsegmental bronchus have a worse prognosis than more peripheral tumors in both squamous and nonsquamous cases. Bronchial nonsquamous cancers do particularly poorly. From Read RC, et al: Survival after conservative resection for T1N0M0 non-small cell lung cancer. Ann Thorac Surg 49:391, 1990. With permission.

prognosis over adenocarcinomas, large cell lesions, and mixed cancers of comparable extent. Gail and associates (1984), reporting for the LCSG, showed significantly lower recurrence and death rates per patient per year for squamous versus nonsquamous or mixed histologies, noting that at 3 years, 90% of resected patients with T_1N_0 squamous cancer were free of recurrence, as opposed to only 62% of those with nonsquamous histology. Similarly, Read and colleagues (1988) concluded that 5-year postresection survival is more often realized for T_1N_0 squamous tumors than for comparable adenocarcinomas. Macchiarini (1993) and Kodama (1997) and their coworkers, in contrast, did not detect a significant difference in outcome for T_1N_0 disease based on the subsets of non–small cell histology. In addition, many series combining T_1N_0 and T_2N_0, such as those reported by Shields (1975), Pairolero (1984), Little (1986), Ichinose (1993), and Harpole (1995a,b) and their associates, have not established a statistically significant difference in survival based on cell type, although absolute long-term survival is often better in squamous cases.

The location of the primary lesion may influence the results of resection. Peripheral T_1N_0 tumors have a better prognosis than central lesions. Although Read and colleagues (1990) found that nonsquamous T_1N_0 patients fared worse overall after resection than did squamous cases, the difference was largely confined to central lesions. When the tumor did not communicate with a segmental or subsegmental bronchus, the effect of cell type was negated. The presence of airway communication for both cell types conferred a significantly poorer outlook, dramatically so for nonsquamous histology (Fig. 99-4). Likewise, the influence of peripheral versus central location negated the effect of tumor size in the experience reported by Sagawa and colleagues (1990). Assessing only NSCLC arising in or peripheral to a subsegmental bronchus, they recorded similar 5-year survival for smaller or larger T_1N_0 lesions (80% for tumors 2 to 3 cm in diameter and 83% for smaller cancers).

The favorable influence of parenchymal location is also emphasized by the report of Kodama and associates (1997), who achieved a 5-year survival of 93% in 77 patients with peripheral pT_1N_0 NSCLC treated by lobectomy and 88% in 46 cases after intentional lesser resection.

In the databases of Naruke and associates (1988a) and Mountain (1997) postresection survival for clinical T_2N_0 cancer is only 36 to 42%, and 57% for pathologic IB. It is striking that the most optimistic upper limit of late survival for IB disease in these series falls below the lower limit for IA lesions. As for stage IA, however, Table 99-2 shows that some authors report better results. The differences for IB, however, are small; most series note survival of 62 to 65% for pT_2N_0 cases. The 78% survival reported by Padilla and colleagues (1997) is confined to small lesions.

Specific variables within stage IB that influence prognosis have not been as clearly elucidated as have those for IA disease, because the subsets are new and most prior reports in this area have focused on T_1N_0 cases, especially on favorable small peripheral lesions. Larger tumor diameter and nonsquamous histology probably correlate with a poorer prognosis, but the data are sparse. Although noting a highly significant adverse effect of increasing size within IA, Read and associates (1988) found no significant difference between cancers equal to or smaller than 5 cm versus those larger than 5 cm in IB cases. Harpole and colleagues (1995a), in contrast, found that larger tumors were associated with a more limited survival than smaller cancers, but the groupings were 2 to 4 cm versus tumors larger than 4 cm, so some cases were likely IA. Involvement of a main bronchus further than 2 cm from the carina or a lesion causing lobar atelectasis, both defining features of some T_2 primaries, are not clearly negative prognostic indicators. In fact, central T_2 cancers limited to the bronchial wall, and often occult, as noted by Naruke (1988a) and Watanabe

Table 99-3. Selected Series Reporting Postresection 5-Year Survival for Pathologic Stage IIA (T_1N_1) and Stage IIB (T_2N_1, T_3N_0) Non–Small Cell Lung Carcinoma

Report	Dates	T_1N_1 IIA		T_2N_1 IIB		T_3N_0 IIB	
		No.	5-Year Survival (%)	No.	5-Year Survival (%)	No.	5-Year Survival (%)
Williams et al. (1981)	1972–1978	30	50	—	—	—	—
Holmes (1987)	NS	NS	75 squamous 52 adenocarcinoma	NS	53 squamous 25 adenocarcinoma	—	—
Roeslin et al. (1987)	1977–1982	50	45	All 113	37	—	—
				Lobar 79	41		
				Hilar 34	14		
Naruke et al. (1988a)	1962–1986	48	44	118	38	147	32
Martini et al. (1992)[a]	1973–1989	35	40	179	38	—	—
van Velzen et al. (1996, 1997)	1977–1994	All 57	46	All 369	38	—	—
		Lobar 25	57	Lobar 57	57		
		Hilar 32	23	Hilar 161	30		
Mountain (1997)	1975–1988	76	55	288	39	87	38
Inoue et al. (1998)[a]	1980–1993	57	57	141	42	46	34
Nakahashi et al. (1996)	1974–1994	—	—	—	—	15	Complete resection, 44
						8	Incomplete resection, 30

NS, not stated.
[a]Series limited to complete resections.

(1991a) and their colleagues among others, have an excellent postresection survival. Direct invasion of the visceral pleura, another defining feature of T_2 lesions, correlates with a poorer prognosis than comparably sized T_2 cancers without pleural involvement, as noted early by Brewer (1977) and also by Merlier and colleagues (1985). Harpole and colleagues (1995a) found that visceral pleural invasion was a significant predictor of poor outcome on both univariate and multivariate analysis, with 5-year survivals of 44% for invasive lesions versus 67% for those without pleural transgression, and respective 10-year survivals of 62% and 37%. Ichinose and colleagues (1993) reported similar findings. The LCSG, reported by Gail and associates (1984), noted a 1.66-fold increase in recurrence rates in stage I patients when the visceral pleura was involved by cancer.

Stage II: Lung Cancer with N_1 Adenopathy or Resectable Local Invasion

The 1997 system divides stage II lung cancer into two subsets. Stage IIA is limited to $T_1N_1M_0$ lesions, whereas IIB includes both node-positive ($T_2N_1M_0$) and node-negative ($T_3N_0M_0$) cases (Table 99-3). All three subsets of the current stage II, especially T_1N_1 and T_3N_0, include small numbers of patients. This problem may account for some of the reported discrepancies regarding prognostic factors.

Stage IIA represents a small proportion of patients based on clinical staging. Pathologic T_1N_1 is more common, but remains a small group. The 5-year survival for the few patients with cT_1N_1 cancer is only 34% in the databases of both Naruke and associates (1988a) and Mountain (1997), and for pT_1N_1 cases is 53% and 55%, respectively. The Lud-

wig Cancer Study Group (1987) reported their results as median survival time: 4.8 years for resected T_1N_1 patients, significantly longer than the median of 2.3 years for T_2N_1.

As in stage I, variables that may affect prognosis include tumor size, histology, and location. In addition, in stage II and above, lymph node metastases come into play. The effect of any single non-nodal factor is less clear than in stage I. Holmes (1987), reporting the LCSG experience, confirmed a significant difference favoring squamous T_1N_1 cancers at 5 years (75% versus 52% for nonsquamous histology). In a mixed group of $T_{1-2}N_1$ cases, Ichinose and coworkers (1995) also found better results with squamous lung cancers. In contrast, Martini (1992) and Yano (1994) and their colleagues did not find a significant histologic variance, although squamous cases had an 8 to 10% absolute survival advantage over other cell types. The data with respect to tumor size are also limited, conflicting, and not focused by stage II subset. Within stage II, however, Martini and associates (1992) found that tumors smaller than 3 cm had a higher survival than those larger than 5 cm, but other series have not found an effect of size. The influence of central versus peripheral location has not been studied sufficiently to allow firm conclusions.

Variables related to the nature of the N_1 lymphadenopathy in stage II appear to be important. Martini and colleagues (1992) found that patients with a single malignant node had a 5-year survival of 45%, as opposed to 31% for those with multiple N_1 metastases. Of note was that one-half of their patients had only a single cancerous node and 86% had spread to only one N_1 nodal level. In a study focused on N_1 disease and including T_{1-3} cases, but only three with T_3, Yano and colleagues (1994) achieved a postresection survival of 65% in patients with "lobar" nodal disease (levels

Table 99-4. Selected Series Reporting Postresection 5-Year Survival for Tumors Classified as T$_3$ Because of Invasion of the Parietal Pleura or Chest Wall

Report	Dates	Chest Wall Overall		Chest Wall T$_3$N$_0$ IIB		Chest Wall T$_3$N$_1$/N$_2$ H1A		Chest Wall CR/IR	
		No.	5-Year Survival (%)	No.	5-Year Survival (%)	No.	5-Year Survival (%)	No.	5-Year Survival (%)
Piehler et al. (1982)[a]	1960–1980	56	33	26	54	19	7	—	—
Allen et al. (1991)	1973–1988	52	26	43	29	N$_1$ 9	11	—	—
Casillas et al. (1989)	1969–1986	97	23	58	34	N$_1$ 16	8	—	—
Mountain (1990)	1965–1982	31	39	—	—	—	—	—	—
Watanabe et al. (1991b)[a]	1973–1989	24	43	—	—	—	—	—	—
Ratto et al. (1991)	1983–1988	—	—	14	47	N$_1$ 19	22	CR 45	16
						N$_2$ 22	0	IR 10	0
Albertucci et al. (1992)[a]	1976–1988	37	30	21	41	N$_1$ 9	29	—	—
						N$_2$ 7	0		
McCaughan (1994)	1974–1983	125	NS	45	56	N$_1$ 17	35	CR 77	40
						N$_2$ 42	16	IR 48	0

CR, complete resection; IR, incomplete resection; NS, not stated.
[a]Series limited to complete resections.

12 and 13) versus only 40% when the "hilar" nodes (levels 10 and 11) contained metastatic cancer. Van Velzen and colleagues (1996) reported a late overall survival of 46%, and also noted that lobar N$_1$ portended a better outcome than hilar N$_1$ (57% versus 23%). They also found that node involvement by direct extension carried a markedly more favorable surgical prognosis than noncontiguous metastasis (69% versus 30%). Naruke and associates (1988a) and Mountain (1997) report postresection survival at 5 years for the T$_2$N$_1$ subset of clinical stage IIB of 32% and 24%, respectively, with corresponding success for pathologic T$_2$N$_1$ of 38% and 39%. These figures suggest that current clinical modalities overstage this cohort. Little information is available specifically relating to prognostic factors in this group, likely for the reasons noted for IIA disease. In fact, some series have not detected a survival difference between T$_1$N$_1$ and T$_2$N$_1$ at all. Roeslin and coworkers (1987) found a dramatic difference between lobar and hilar N$_1$ disease in patients with T$_2$ tumors (41% versus 14% late survival). In their experience, the latter group did as poorly as patients with N$_2$ lymphadenopathy. Van Velzen and associates (1997) also detected a differential favoring lobar over hilar N$_1$ and direct invasion over metastasis. It is interesting that the survival for lobar T$_2$N$_1$ was identical to that for lobar T$_1$N$_1$ in their earlier study (57%), whereas hilar T$_2$N$_1$ had a slightly better survival rate than hilar T$_1$N$_1$ (30% versus 23%). In the presence of nodal spread, the prognostic significance of the T factor is diminished. The influence of visceral pleural extension, for example, remains unclear in the presence of N$_1$ disease. Van Velzen and associates (1997) determined that such local invasion in T$_2$N$_1$ unfavorably affected outcome. Although the initial report of Martini and colleagues (1983) found that pleural invasion was associated with a significantly worse prognosis, their updated series (1992) negated this factor in mixed T$_{1-2}$N$_1$.

Stage IIB also includes node-negative tumors that invade resectable structures (T$_3$N$_0$M$_0$). Naruke and coworkers

(1988a) reported a 22% 5-year survival for clinical T$_3$N$_0$ and 32% for pathologic T$_3$N$_0$; the corresponding rates calculated by Mountain (1997) were 22% and 38%. The largest surgical experience involves tumors invading the chest wall or the superior sulcus. Data in other T$_3$ categories are limited. Detterbeck and Socinski (1997) have provided a comprehensive review of this subject.

The results of resection for chest wall T$_3$ cancers are summarized in Table 99-4. The major correlates of long-term survival are node negativity and complete resection. When both criteria are met, the outlook is excellent: late survival of 29% to 56%, averaging 42%. When malignant lymphadenopathy accompanies chest wall invasion (T$_3$N$_1$ or T$_3$N$_2$, both subsets now stage IIIA) the efficacy of resection is markedly limited. Five-year survival in the presence of N$_1$ metastasis ranges from 8 to 35%, with an average of 19%. When metastases reach N$_2$ nodes, the outcome is dismal, with no survivors in many series to a maximum of 16% in one report. Incomplete resection is also a strong negative prognostic factor. With both lymphadenopathy and incomplete resection, operation alone results in no late survival.

The extent of invasion, divided pathologically into parietal pleural involvement versus extension into muscle and bone, and surgically into those amenable to extrapleural dissection versus those requiring chest wall resection, may influence resectability. Deep invasion portends a more limited survival. In T$_3$N$_0$ disease, McCaughan and associates (1985) achieved a 5-year survival of 62% for parietal pleural T$_3$, as opposed to 35% for deeper invasion, but the difference was not statistically significant. Likewise, Casillas and colleagues (1989) noted no difference between cases treated by extrapleural dissection versus full-thickness chest wall resection. In contrast, Albertucci and associates (1992), among others, stress the importance of en bloc chest wall resection for all peripheral tumors densely adherent to the chest wall. These authors found a significant incidence of incomplete resection and lower survival (33% versus 50%)

Table 99-5. Selected Series of Postresection 5-Year Survival for Superior Sulcus Tumors

Report	Dates	Overall		CR		Incomplete Resection		T_3N_0 IIB		N_2 IIIA		T_4 Vertebrae IIIB		T_4 Subclavian Vessels IIIB	
		No.	5-Year Survival (%)	No.	5-Year Survival (%)	No.	5-Year Survival (%)	No.	5-Year Survival (%)	No.	5-Year Survival (%)	No.	5-Year Survival (%)	No.	5-Year Survival (%)
Miller et al. (1979)	1971–1977	26	31	—	—	—	—	20	40	5	0	—	—	—	—
Stanford et al. (1980)	1962–1977	—	—	—	—	—	—	16	50	—	—	—	—	—	—
Paulson (1985)	1956–1983	78	31	—	—	—	—	56	44	17	0	—	—	—	—
Anderson et al. (1986)	1956–1983	28	34	—	—	—	—	—	—	—	—	—	—	—	—
Wright et al. (1987)	1976–1985	21	27	—	—	—	—	—	—	—	—	—	—	—	—
Sartori et al. (1992)	1981–1990	42	25	—	—	—	—	37	30	5	0	NS	0	5	0
Dartevelle et al. (1993)	1980–1991	29	31	—	—	—	—	—	—	—	—	—	—	—	—
Ginsberg et al. (1994a)[a]	1974–1991	All 124	26	69	41	55	9	All 96	33	All 8	4	22	9	NS	0
		Resected cases, 100	30					CR 60	46	CR 9	15				
Maggi et al. (1994)	1982–1990	60	17	36	24	24	0	—	—	—	—	NS	0	NS	0
Muscolino et al. (1997)	1984–1988	15	27	11	40	4	0	CR 6	57	4	0	—	—	—	—

CR, complete resection; NS, not stated.

[a] Series includes use of interstitial brachytherapy in some cases.

for extrapleural dissection. It appears that NSCLC involving limited areas of the parietal pleura may be treated adequately by pulmonary resection combined with extrapleural dissection, but any degree of deeper invasion requires full-thickness chest wall resection. The practical challenge is the definitive identification of the extent of invasion by preoperative and intraoperative assessment. When doubt exists, a low threshold to proceed with en bloc resection is prudent. Superior sulcus tumors also have been the focus of much surgical attention. Pancoast's tumors may be staged locoregionally as IIB (T_3N_0), IIIA (T_3N_{1-2}), or IIIB (T_4N_{1-3}, T_3N_3). Chapters 35 and 36 review the techniques and results of resection of these challenging lesions. Apical lung cancer invading the thoracic inlet was considered unresectable and uniformly fatal, until Shaw and colleagues (1961) demonstrated that radiation therapy followed by radical resection could yield long-term survival. Although the optimal approach (radiation therapy alone, irradiation followed by operation, preoperative and postoperative "sandwich" radiation therapy, induction chemoradiotherapy, brachytherapy) is not established, many patients with clinical $T_3N_{0-1}M_0$ superior sulcus cancers are treated currently with initial radiation therapy followed by resection (Table 99-5). As for chest wall lesions, the major surgical correlates of cure are the associated lymph node status and the completeness of

resection. Complete resection in the absence of adenopathy offers significant late survival (40 to 50%), with a range of 30 to 57%. When N_2 dissemination has occurred, in contrast, resection is not helpful, with most series reporting no late survivors. In addition to N_2 status, T_4 disease is overwhelmingly inoperable. In a few cases, however, an anterior approach, as noted earlier and detailed in Chapter 36, may allow a complete resection and reconstruction. Confirmation of an oncologic benefit from radical surgical approaches must await broader experience. Vertebral body invasion precludes surgical cure. Sartori and associates (1992) noted that patients who experienced pain relief from radiation therapy fared better than those with ongoing symptoms. Anderson and colleagues (1986) noted that durable pain relief after resection portended a favorable outlook of 73% 5-year survival for patients who experienced pain relief, in contrast to no long-term survivors among those with persistent discomfort. The presence of Horner's syndrome is also a negative prognostic factor.

Despite good results in favorable subsets, the large series reported by Ginsberg and colleagues (1994) emphasizes the challenging nature of superior sulcus cancers. Resection was not possible in 24 of 124 operated patients and was incomplete in 31 other cases, overall 44%. As in other NSCLC, incomplete resection was associated with the same dismal 5-

Table 99-6. Selected Series Reporting Postresection 5-Year Survival for Tumors Classified as T_3 Because of Invasion of the Mediastinum or Diaphragm or Because of Proximal Main Bronchial Location

Report	Dates	Mediastinum		Proximal Bronchus		Diaphragm	
		No.	5-Year Survival (%)	No.	5-Year Survival (%)	No.	5-Year Survival (%)
Burt et al. (1987)	1974–1984	All 225	7	—	—	—	—
		CR 49	9				
		N_0 57	10				
		N_1 30	9				
		N_2 38	8				
Watanabe et al. (1991b,c)[a]	1973–1989	17	43	—	—	—	—
Martini et al. (1994)	1974–1992	All 102	19	—	—	—	—
		T_3 CR 38	36				
		T_4 CR	12				
Pitz et al. (1996)	1977–1993	All 40	25	75	40	—	—
		N_2 9	0				
Vogt-Moykopf et al. (1986)	—	—	—	97	12	—	—
Deslauriers et al. (1993)	—	—	—	31	14	—	—
Weksler et al. (1997)[a]	1974–1995	—	—	—	—	8 (see text)	0

CR, complete resection.
[a]Series limited to complete resections.

year survival as nonresective thoracotomy. The extensive earlier experience of Paulson (1985) also highlights the limitations of surgery, because only 60% of patients presenting with Pancoast's tumors were deemed suitable for treatment pathways that included resection. It is parenthetically noteworthy that, in the series of Ginsberg and colleagues (1994), a better outcome occurred after lobectomy, as compared with nonanatomic resection, which approached statistical significance for superior sulcus tumors, often cited as the paradigm of peripheral lesions and treated by extensive operations with minimal lung resection.

Data are limited regarding the results of resection in other types of T_3 disease (Table 99-6). Mediastinal invasion portends a poorer surgical outcome than does chest wall involvement, with late survival in one-fourth to one-third of completely resected cases versus more than one-half of similarly staged and treated chest wall T_3 cancers. An early large series from Memorial reported by Burt and colleagues (1987) found that complete resection was possible in 49 of 225 patients (22%) and that even in this subset, 5-year survival was only 9%, but this report included many cases now classified as T_4. In an update, however, Martini and associates (1994) reviewed 102 surgical patients with mediastinal invasion, excluding N_2 disease, superior vena cava obstruction, superior sulcus cancers, and malignant pleural effusion, and applying current criteria for T_3 and T_4. Of 58 patients with T_3 lesions, complete resection was possible in 38 cases (66%) and late survival was 36%. In contrast, resectability for T_4 tumors was 18%, and 5-year survival was 12% after complete resection. Pitz and colleagues (1996) noted a 25% postoperative 5-year survival in 40 patients with T_3 cancers invading the mediastinum, but no

late survival in those with N_2 disease. Watanabe and associates (1991b) reported excellent results of 43% late survival in a small group of patients after complete resection in the presence of limited pericardial invasion.

Survival for main bronchial cancers classified as T_3 because of carinal proximity varies widely from 12 to 46%. The highest reported survival, however, was based on only 11 patients, all of whom had complete resection, and was calculated exclusive of operative mortality. Detterbeck and Socinski (1997) determined from the literature an average of 24%, a figure similar to T_3 mediastinal invasion. Although Pitz and associates (1996) reported 40% survival for proximal bronchial T_3 versus 25% for mediastinal T_3, the difference was not statistically significant. Firm conclusions regarding the incidence and outcome of proximal bronchial T_3 NSCLC are hampered by problems of definition, largely because lesions at the right upper lobe origin may variably be classified as T_1, T_2, or T_3, based on subjective assessment of the radiographic and bronchoscopic features and interpretation of the staging criteria. By extrapolation from the considerable literature on bronchoplastic and carinal resection (see Chapters 28 and 30), however, it appears that complete resection of node-negative main bronchial T_3 cancers yields late survival in one-fourth to one-third of cases. N_2 disease is a strong negative factor, whereas the data with respect to N_1 metastasis versus N_0 are conflicting.

Despite the fact that the hemidiaphragms abut a large surface of lung parenchyma and that direct invasion in this area is potentially resectable, a paucity of reported surgical experience exists. Weksler and associates (1997) found only eight cases in a review spanning two decades at Memorial. All four patients with N_2 disease died of their lung cancers, with a mean survival of only 92 weeks. Although a single N_0 patient was alive at 70 weeks at the time of the report, the remaining three died of nonmalignant causes between 5 and 17 weeks after surgery. The diaphragmatic lesions also differed from the usual spectrum of T_3 NSCLC, in that seven were squamous cancers, and the eighth had adenosquamous histology. Inoue and associates (1998) also reported no 3-year survival in five operated patients with diaphragmatic invasion, despite complete resection and N_{0-1} status.

In contrast to lower stage lesions, tumor size and histology are less predictive for T_3 cancers. In general, invasive squamous cancer is more favorable than adenocarcinoma. Although most reports indicate no significant difference, Mountain (1990) found a trend in favor of squamous histology, and Ratto and associates (1991) reported that patients with squamous cancer invading the chest wall fared better with both complete and incomplete resection than did those with adenocarcinoma. In T_3 with either mediastinal invasion or carinal proximity, Pitz and coauthors (1996) also achieved better results in squamous cases. The experience reported by Martini and colleagues (1994) is unusual, because T_3 adenocarcinomas with mediastinal infiltration were more favorable.

Although complete resection of T_3N_0 NSCLC yields late survival in one-fourth to two-thirds of cases, depending on the structures invaded, it remains unknown whether the addition of adjuvant therapy is helpful. Postoperative radiation therapy is used frequently, but sporadically. Interstitial brachytherapy and systemic chemotherapy are applied less often.

Stage IIIA: Lung Cancer with Mediastinal Lymph Node Involvement

The T_3N_1 subset of stage IIIA represents a minority of cases. Results in this group have been discussed and are presented in Tables 99-4 to 99-6. N_2 disease comprises the majority of stage IIIA and has been the subject of much debate with respect to the role of primary resection. The concept of resectable N_2 disease is based on reports documenting late survival in 20 to 30% of patients with various combinations of favorable features: complete resection; single-node or single-level, microscopic metastasis; N_2 confined to lower stations; and left upper lobe cancers with N_2 limited to the subaortic level. The problem with clinical application of this concept is that these results are based on retrospective pathologic staging in patients who were considered preoperatively by a variety of staging pathways either to be clinical N_0 or N_1 or, less often, to be good candidates for resection despite suspected or documented N_2 metastasis. As pointed out by Shields (1990) and by Goldstraw (1992), among others, the number of patients in the spectrum of N_2 NSCLC who benefit from operation is low. Even with careful selection for minimal N_2 disease, patients whose malignant N_2 lymphadenopathy is diagnosed preoperatively rarely benefit from surgery. The rate of incomplete

resection or nonresective exploration is high, whereas the 5-year survival is low. In contrast, those whose N_2 disease is not apparent by clinical staging, but is diagnosed only by surgical or pathologic staging, have a markedly better postoperative outlook. Retrospective outcome in the latter setting cannot be generalized to clinical N_2 lung cancer.

Table 99-7 summarizes selected reports of operation in N_2 disease. The seminal modern study is the series of Pearson and associates (1982), who found that resection in mediastinoscopy-positive cases, with adjuvant radiation in most, was associated with a 5-year survival of only 9%. In contrast, survival in mediastinoscopy-negative, pathologically positive cases ($cN_{0/1}$-pN_2) was almost threefold higher (24%). The operated cN_2 patients represented only one-fifth of all such cases evaluated during the period and were deemed to have surgically favorable N_2 disease. Nonetheless, only 64% had a complete resection, with 15% 5-year survival. There were no late survivors in the 36% who had incomplete resections. These authors also noted that there was no survival with surgery alone in five prior reports of mediastinoscopy-positive patients. No subsequent series has negated these conclusions.

Vansteenkiste and colleagues (1997) also reported a significant survival difference for mediastinoscopy-negative versus mediastinoscopy-positive patients (32% and 15%, respectively), despite strict criteria for exploring only those thought to have minimal N_2 metastasis. The authors emphasize that the few late survivors in the clinical N_2 group had truly minimal N_2 disease pathologically. In a distinctly unusual but instructive experience, Funatsu and coworkers (1992) performed mediastinoscopy in 619 patients and proceeded to thoracotomy in virtually all cases. Among 117 instances of positive mediastinoscopy complete resection was possible in only 13 instances (11%). In the remainder, resection was either incomplete (78 cases, 67%) or not possible (26 nonresective explorations, 22%). Although late survival was 28% for the small group of completely resected patients, when incomplete resections are included, even eliminating nonresective operations, survival was only 6%.

In addition to mediastinoscopy-proven N_2 cases, true-positive N_2 results in patients staged clinically by pathways using only noninvasive modalities or selective mediastinal exploration also fare poorly with primary exploration. Martini and Flehinger (1987) reviewed a large experience with N_2 cancers in which clinical staging was based on radiography and bronchoscopy, with few mediastinoscopies. Of 706 patients with N_2 disease, 404 were considered operable. Of these, 224 were $cN_{0/1}$ and 179 cN_2. The survival analysis is limited to complete resections, which were possible in 53% of the former group but only 18% of the cN_2 cases, with corresponding 5-year survivals of 34% and 9%. Stated numerically, among 179 cN_2 cases deemed operable, complete resection was possible in only 32 instances, and only a few of this highly selected group enjoyed late postoperative survival. Using CT scan as the primary staging modality, Watanabe and associates (1991d) similarly found that only one-half

Table 99-7. Selected Series Reporting Postsurgical Survival in Patients with Involvement of N_2 Lymph Nodes

Report	Dates	Staging	All Operated pN_2		$cN_{0/1}$ to pN_2		cN_2 to pN_2		Comments
			No.	5-Year Survival (%)	No.	5-Year Survival (%)	No.	5-Year Survival (%)	
Pearson et al. (1982)	1964–1980	M-scopy	—	—	62	24	All 79 CR 51 IR 28	9 15 0	Preoperative and postoperative RT in majority
Martini and Flehinger (1987)	1974–1981	Radiography Bronch Few m-scopy	404	NS	All 224 CR 119 IR 105	NS 34 NS	All 179 CR 32 IR 147	NS 9 NS	Presents only CR (18% of cN_2); postoperative RT in 90%
Naruke (1988a)	1962–1986	Variable	All 426 CR 242 IR 184	NS 19 7	—	—	—	—	—
Ishida et al. (1990a)	1974–1988	Radiography Bronch CT scan Selective m-scopy	All 115 CR 63 IR 52	18 27 9	—	—	—	—	Nonresective thoracotomies eliminated; postoperative RT in 56%; IR includes patients without mediastinal lymph node dissection
Watanabe et al. (1991d)	1980–1990	Mainly CT scan	153	17	All 47 CR 31 IR 16	20 33 0	All 106 CR 53 IR 53	16 20 0	Nonresective thoracotomies eliminated (8% of cN_2-pN_2)
Regnard et al. (1991)	1982–1988	CT scan Few m-scopy	All 254 CR 191 IR 63	18 23 0	—	—	—	—	93% adj rx 19 small cell
Funatsu et al. (1992)	1970–1990	M-scopy	—	—	46	14	All 91 CR 13 IR 78	6 28 2	Nonresective thoracotomies eliminated (22% of cN_2-pN_2)
Daly et al. (1993)	1979–1991	CT scan Bronch Selective m-scopy	—	—	All 37 CR 31	28 31	—	—	Adj rx in most
Maggi et al. (1993)	1980–1990	CT scan Bronch Selective m-scopy	—	—	All 278 CR 236 IR 42	14 19 0	—	—	—
van Klaveren et al. (1993)	1975–1985	Radiography CT scan Selective m-scopy	—	—	All 48	10	—	—	—
Goldstraw (1994)	1979–1989	Radiography CT scan Selective m-scopy	—	—	All 149 CR 127	17 20	—	—	No adj rx in CR cases
Miller (1994)	1982–1986	CT scan Bronch M-scopy in 28%	—	—	All 167 CR 147 IR 20	21 24 5	—	—	Adj rx in 80%
Vansteenkiste et al. (1997)	1985–1993	CT scan Bronch Selective m-scopy	140	21	All 121 Med (−) 68	22 32	Med (+)	15	Postoperative RT in 50% CR ($n = 113$), 25% year IR ($n = 27$), 4% 5 year
Mountain (1997)	1975–1988	Variable	—	—	344	23	471	13	—

adj rx, postoperative adjuvant therapy; Bronch, bronchoscopy; CR, complete resection; CT, computed tomography; IR, incomplete resection; m-scopy, cervical mediastinoscopy, and anterior mediastinoscopy, mediastinotomy, or both; RT, radiation therapy.

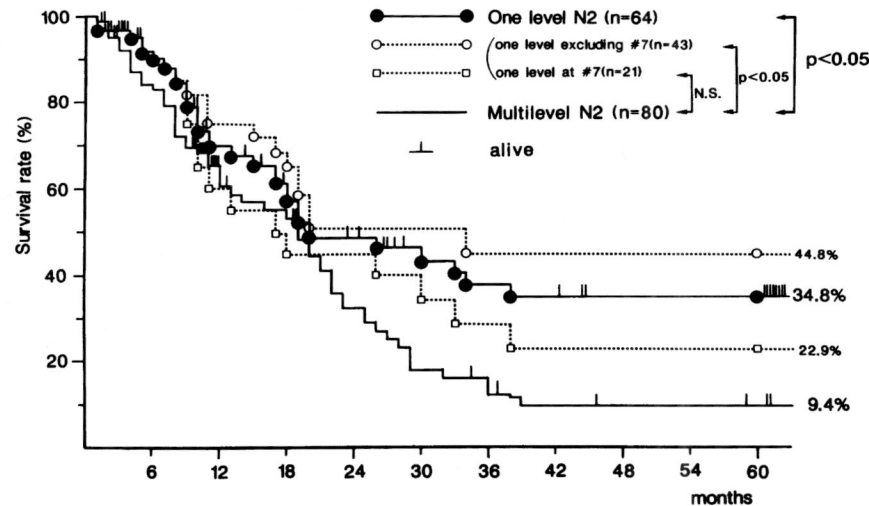

Fig. 99-5. Survival curves among N_2 patients undergoing curative resection with single level, multiple levels, single station exclusive of station 7, and single station involvement. From Watanabe Y, et al: Mediastinal nodal involvement and the prognosis of non–small cell lung cancer. Chest *100*:422, 1991d. With permission.

of cN_2-pN_2 cancers could be resected completely, with a late survival of 20%. In the remaining 50% of patients undergoing subtotal tumor removal there were no late survivors. In contrast, complete resection was possible in two-thirds of $cN_{0/1}$-pN_2 cases and yielded a 33% long-term survival.

Numerous studies using CT scan and selective invasive mediastinal staging, have confirmed high complete resection rates and reasonable survival in $cN_{0/1}$-pN_2 lung cancer. Goldstraw and colleagues (1994) emphasize that clinically unsuspected N_2 disease is common. These authors found that a quarter of $cN_{0/1}$ patients staged by CT scan and by mediastinoscopy in 48% were found to have pN_2. Complete resection was possible in 85% and yielded late survival in 20%, with no adjuvant treatment. Although Daly and colleagues (1993), also using CT and selective mediastinoscopy, found only a 7% incidence of unsuspected N_2, they likewise noted respectability and late survival in 89% and 28%, respectively. Similarly, Maggi (1993) and Miller (1994) and their coworkers were able to accomplish complete resection in 85% and 88% of such cases, with late survival in 19% and 24%, respectively. Incomplete resection in this group, as in cN_2 patients, however, is of no benefit, with only a rare patient surviving 5 years. Although the actuarial survival for incomplete resection in unsuspected N_2 in the series of Miller and colleagues (1994) is 5%, for example, this figure is based on a single case. The remaining patients all died within 3 years of operation. In summary, primary resection is useful only in patients with limited N_2 NSCLC. Current methods of clinical assessment are inadequate for reliably identifying this group.

Despite the difficulty of prospectively identifying prognostic indices in individual cN_2 cases, multiple factors have been extensively analyzed in postresection N_2 disease. Incomplete resection, as in other subsets of NSCLC, is the most powerful negative prognostic factor. The extent of N_2 metastases also appears to be a predictor of prognosis. Other factors that have been variably reported to be significant

include the anatomic location of N_2, the presence or absence of associated N_1 lymphadenopathy, the T classification, and the cell type.

Watanabe and associates (1991d) found that with only one nodal station involved the 5-year survival was 35%, as opposed to 9% when more than one level was affected (Fig. 99-5). Regnard (1991) and Maggi (1993) and their colleagues confirmed this finding (24% versus 9%, and 30% versus 19%, respectively). Miller and associates (1994) reported a dramatic difference between the extremes of node station involvement: 30% late survival in patients with single level N_2, but no survival when four or five levels harbored cancer. Goldstraw and associates (1994), however, reported that single-level N_2 metastasis was associated with improved survival only for the first 3 postoperative years, with no advantage beyond that point. In the report by Vansteenkiste and colleagues (1997), the negative effect of multilevel metastases was limited to cases of nonsquamous histology.

In some series, such as that of Martini and Flehinger (1987), the number of involved nodes correlated directly with a worsened prognosis. Ishida (1990a) and Vansteenkiste (1997) and their associates, among others, have also shown that gross replacement of nodes by malignant cells, especially when disruption of the nodal capsule occurs, presages a poorer postresection result than does the presence of intranodal or microscopic metastasis. Five-year survival in these studies for gross versus intranodal disease were 16% versus 23%, and 11% versus 34%, respectively. Although also not universally confirmed, the anatomic site of N_2 adenopathy may influence surgical curability. Metastasis to the subcarinal nodes (level 7) is often associated with lower survival than other sites, as reported by Pearson (1982), Regnard (1991), Watanabe (1991d), and Miller (1994) and their coworkers. Also, when N_2 disease is divided into inferior (levels 7, 8, and 9) and superior mediastinal categories (all other levels) survival in the former group is comparatively limited. In the series of Maggi (1993) and associates survival rates for N$_2$ in an inferior or superior location were 8% versus 25%. Nakanishi and coworkers (1997) reported a more marked difference, with no late survivors when inferior stations were involved, in contrast to survival in approximately one-third of patients with superior mediastinal N$_2$. Miller and colleagues (1994) also identified metastasis to inferior mediastinal nodes as a negative prognostic index. In contrast to the finding that N$_1$ disease defined by direct extension is more favorable than N$_1$ anatomically separate from the primary site, Regnard and associates (1991) achieved better late survival in patients with separate N$_2$ lymphadenopathy compared with those with direct invasion. This finding, however, has not been noted by others. The coexistence of N$_1$ metastasis along with N$_2$ disease is another node-specific factor that has occasionally been designated as a negative predictor. Although skip metastases, N$_2$ disease in the presence of benign N$_1$ stations, occurs in approximately one-fourth of all pathologic N$_2$ cases, the prognostic implication of this finding is not addressed in most analyses.

The primary tumor classification (T stage) in the presence of N$_2$ disease overall appears less prognostically important than in lower stages. As noted earlier, however, the coexistence of N$_2$ metastasis from a T$_3$ NSCLC generally precludes surgical cure. In contrast, although a trend exists toward better results in T$_1$N$_2$ compared with T$_2$N$_2$ cases, most series do not report a statistically significant difference when other factors coincide. The effect of histology is similar, in that squamous cell cancers appear to have a slightly more favorable outlook, but the difference is usually not dramatic. Naruke and associates (1988b), however, calculated a statistically significant, approximately double, better survival for T$_1$N$_2$ versus T$_2$N$_2$ cases and for squamous cancers versus adenocarcinomas: 30% versus 15% by T factor, and 31% versus 16% by cell type. Maggi (1993) and Regnard (1991) and colleagues also showed longer survival with T$_1$ lesions. In their series of

patients with unexpected pathologic N$_2$, Goldstraw and colleagues (1994) found a markedly more favorable outcome for squamous cancer compared to adenocarcinoma (29% and 5%, respectively).

Left upper lobe NSCLC with N$_2$ metastasis confined to the subaortic (aortopulmonary, level 5) nodes has been suggested as a uniquely favorable subset (Table 99-8). Patterson and associates (1987) brought this area to attention in a review of 35 patients with isolated level 5 N$_2$, in which they reported late survival in 28%. Two-thirds underwent complete resection, with a 5-year survival of 42%. Watanabe (1991d) and Cybulsky (1992) and their colleagues noted 20% and 21% survival, respectively. In the latter series, late survival was only 10% for the entire N$_2$ group. Although one-half of the left upper lobe patients in this report had positive CT scans (cN$_2$), survival in this subset is not reported separately. In the experience reported by Nakanishi and associates (1997) surgical survival was markedly better (80%) among patients with single-level N$_2$ disease when localized to the subaortic area, but there were only six patients. In a study limited to skip metastasis (pathologic N$_2$ with negative N$_1$ nodes) Tateishi and coworkers (1994) also noted a numerically striking but statistically borderline better surgical prognosis in isolated level 5 N$_2$ disease than in the total group (50% versus 24%). The reports of Goldstraw (1994) and Vansteenkiste (1997) and their associates, among others, however, do not confirm an advantage in this setting.

Although isolated pathologic level 5 N$_2$ may be more favorable than other single level N$_2$, firm conclusions regarding operation in patients with clinical N$_2$ are hampered by the absence of clearly stated clinical staging in most reports. Two practical issues are related. First, inclusion of such patients in induction or adjuvant trials along with other N$_2$ cases is problematic if their prognosis is inherently superior. Second is the question of clinical staging of the subaortic nodes in patients

Table 99-8. Series Reporting Postsurgical Results in Patients with Left Upper Lobe Tumors Associated with N$_2$ Lymphadenopathy Confined to the Subaortic Station Level 5

Report	Dates	Staging	Operated Left Upper Lobe N$_2$		Comment
			No.	5-Year Survival (%)	
Patterson et al. (1987)	1968–1985	M-scopy	All 35	28	Two cases of small cell, one a long-term survivor; radiation therapy in 57%
			Complete resection, 23	42	
			Incomplete resection, 12	NS	
Watanabe et al. (1991d)	1973–1990	Variable	38	21	Limited to complete resection
Cybulsky et al. (1992)	1982–1988	CT scan	All 32	20	Postoperative adjuvant therapy in most
			cN$_2$ 16	NS	
Nakanishi et al. (1997)	1979–1994	Radiography CT scan Bronchoscopy M-scopy	6	80	21% 5-year survival for unsuspected pN$_2$; for cN$_2$-pN$_2$, 25%

cN$_2$, clinical N$_2$; CT, computed tomography; m-scopy, cervical mediastinoscopy, and anterior mediastinoscopy, mediastinotomy, or both.

with left upper lobe tumors and no other evidence of metastasis, a subject discussed by Ginsberg (1994).

Stage IIIB: Lung Cancer with Unresectable Local Invasion or N_3 Adenopathy

Although IIIB is defined as unresectable disease, an exceptional T_4 case may be suitable for operation. In the overwhelming majority, however, primary operation is of no oncologic value and operative mortality is high. Any benefit with respect to local control is offset by early distant metastasis. In the series of Mountain (1997) 5-year survival is 6% for clinical T_4 and 3% for N_3. In the database of Naruke and associates (1988a), only 8% of a small group of pathologic T_4 patients enjoyed late survival, and no patient with N_3 disease lived for 5 years. The role of induction therapy in rendering IIIB NSCLC resectable is discussed in Chapter 106. A new factor complicating surgical consideration of stage IIIB as a homogeneous group is the inclusion in the 1997 staging system of patients with more than one parenchymal site of cancer within a single lobe. Although these cases overall have survival after clinical staging similar to T_4 and N_3, the place of operation in this setting is presently not at all as clear as in other IIIB. Multiple tumors are discussed separately.

With respect to T_4 lesions, the only patients who should be considered for primary operation are those few whose tumors, after rigorous imaging and invasive assessment, appear to be totally and safely resectable. The extensive disappointing experience in T_3N_2 disease is compounded in the lesser experience with T_4 primaries associated with nodal metastasis. Initial exploration is never indicated in clinical T_4N_2 disease. Martini and colleagues (1994) noted that complete resection was possible in only 18% (8 of 44 cases) of T_4 tumors with mediastinal invasion that were selected for operation. Among the eight complete resections, only one survived 5 years. Applying a policy of more aggressive extended resection, Tsuchiya and associates (1994) noted a complete resection rate of 66% by gross inspection, but a histologic rate of 30%, because of microscopically positive margins. The 5-year survival in this series was 13% for the entire group, 19% after complete resection, and 0% after incomplete resection. Although Fukuse and colleagues (1997a) reported complete resection in 35% of 42 cases with atrial, great vessel, or both kinds of invasion, only 3-year survival is specified (17%).

Variation exists in surgical results within the T_4 category. The grave prognostic implication of T_4 invasion in superior sulcus tumors has been noted. Likewise, T_4, because of a pleural effusion containing malignant cells, is never resectable. If the effusion is not malignant, however, but is caused by atelectasis secondary to an obstructing cancer or other etiology, the usefulness of operation is dependent on other clinical staging factors. Earlier, Decker (1978) noted that resectable cases in this setting were few in number (only 5% of operated patients with cytologically negative effusions

had limited disease and were late survivors). Although the significance of cytologically negative effusions has been the subject of much debate, the clinical dilemma is largely resolved, because a combination of modern imaging, thoracoscopy, and other modalities establishes the benign or malignant etiology of the pleural fluid with a high degree of accuracy.

The largest surgical experience with T_4 NSCLC encompasses tumors involving the carina (see Chapter 30). In properly selected cases treated at centers with experience, late survival can be realized in up to 20%, as reported by Faber (1987), Mathisen and Grillo (1991), and by Watanabe (1990), Deslauriers (1993), and Roviaro (1994) and their colleagues.

Reports of resection in other T_4 subsets are confined to case presentations or small series. Tangential resection and primary closure or patching of the superior vena cava, as well as circumferential resection requiring graft reconstruction, has been reported by Dartevelle (1991), Nakahara (1989), and Tsuchiya (1994) and their coworkers. Late survival, however, is limited to a few cases, one reported by Inoue and associates (1990) and 2 of 30 cases in the series of Tsuchiya and associates (1994). In the experience of Burt and associates (1987), no late survival occurred among 18 cases of NSCLC invading the superior vena cava and treated by pulmonary resection, brachytherapy, or both. The rarity of lung cancers suitable for caval resection is underscored by the reports of Dartevelle and colleagues (1987, 1991). In their earlier paper, 4 of 13 superior vena cava resections (31%) were performed for lung cancer. In the subsequent 4 years encompassed in the updated series, only two cases of NSCLC were added. All six patients had malignant adenopathy, and four received adjuvant radiation therapy. Neither of the two cases with N_2 disease survived beyond 8 months, whereas two of four N_1 patients died at 1 month and 38 months and two were alive at 16 and 52 months.

Operation for tumors invading the aortic arch and its branches or the descending thoracic aorta has been performed in even fewer instances. Klepetko and associates (1999) reported five cases of combined left lung and aortic resection. Three with N_2 disease died between 17 and 27 months, and two with pathologic T_4N_1 were alive at 14 and 50 months. Nakahara (1989), Horita (1993), and Tsuchiya (1994) and their colleagues also reported aortic resection for T_4 lung cancer, but the long-term results of this aggressive approach, usually requiring cardiopulmonary bypass, are not specified. In the aforementioned report of Burt and colleagues (1987), there were no late survivors among 19 patients with aortic involvement. In summary, resection of the great vessels for NSCLC, even when surgically possible, is of unproven therapeutic value and should be considered only in exceptional circumstances.

T_4 cancers involving the main pulmonary artery trunk have rarely been approached surgically. In a report by Ricci and associates (1994), among 17 resections involving pulmonary arterial reconstruction, 14 had extrapericardial invasion. Among the three cases requiring cardiopulmonary bypass for intrapericardial repair, one operative death occurred, and the other two patients died from metastases at 3 and 25 months after operation. Similarly, there were no late survivors among seven patients in the series of Tsuchiya and colleagues (1994) who underwent main pulmonary arterial resection. In contrast, some localized cancers with direct invasion of the left atrium at the junction with the pulmonary veins can be resected and closed primarily, without the need for cardiopulmonary bypass. In the report of Tsuchiya and associates (1994), 5-year survival in this group was 22%, and 7 of 13 absolute late survivors in the entire series of 101 cases of mediastinal invasion had undergone left atrial resection.

Although technically feasible in a few instances, the usefulness of total vertebrectomy is unknown. Combined pulmonary and esophageal resection for invasive lung cancer, another occasionally reported surgical feat, must also be viewed in the global context of T_4 disease.

Resection of N_3 disease has been carried out via sternotomy, bilateral thoracotomy, or cervical dissection combined with thoracotomy, and in a few instances has achieved complete removal of all known neoplasm. However, this approach has not been shown to result in long-term survival. Primary operation in clinical N_3 lung cancer is never indicated. The usefulness of induction therapy followed by resection [including all sites of original disease or addressing only ipsilateral metastasis, essentially a postinduction staging operation, as in the Southwest Oncology Group series reported by Rusch and colleagues (1993)] remains unknown and is discussed in Chapter 106.

Stage IV: Lung Cancer with Distant Metastases

Although dissemination of NSCLC can occur to virtually any organ, the most common sites are the brain, bone, liver, and adrenal glands. Only in cases of solitary cerebral metastasis has a combination of metastasectomy and lung resection been shown to be beneficial. Adrenal metastases from NSCLC have been resected in a few instances, but the effect on survival is questionable. No long-term benefit occurs by a surgical approach to the primary site in the presence of other areas of nonpulmonary disease. Although 5-year survival for surgical patients with M_1 disease in the series of Naruke and associates (1988a) was 7%, more than one-half the patients were classified as M_1 because of pulmonary metastases (PM). In Mountain's database (1997) the cumulative survival for M_1 was 1%.

Solitary Brain Metastasis

Several series have shown improved survival with removal of a synchronous solitary brain metastasis (SBM) and pulmonary resection for otherwise limited NSCLC. As many as one-third of patients with brain metastasis at presentation have a solitary lesion, but most also have extracerebral distant foci or advanced locoregional disease. Although resection of the cranial lesion may frequently offer

optimal neurologic palliation, pulmonary resection should be undertaken only in cases that would have been suitable for primary resection in the absence of M_1 disease. The first large experience was reported and later updated by Magilligan and colleagues (1986), who found a 5-year survival of 21% and 10-year survival of 15% in 41 synchronous and metachronous cases of SBM. Burt and associates (1992) reported 185 consecutive patients who underwent craniotomy for NSCLC (65 synchronous and 120 metachronous). The frequency of otherwise advanced NSCLC in the setting of cerebral M_1 disease is emphasized by the fact that 37% of the 65 synchronous cases were not considered for pulmonary resection and that, among the 41 thoracotomies, incomplete or no resection occurred in 22%. Overall late survival was 13% at 5 years and 7% at 10 years, with a median of 14 months. Complete resection of the primary site was a significant favorable prognostic factor, whereas stage per se, synchronous versus metachronous presentation, and the application of whole brain radiation were not significant. In a randomized trial, however, Patchell and associates (1998) found that the addition of whole brain radiation after complete resection of SBM significantly decreased brain recurrences and death from neurologic causes. In a series of synchronous and metachronous cases, Read and associates (1989) reported a 21% 5-year survival after complete resection of both the SBM and the primary site in 27 cases as compared with a median survival of only 6.4 months in patients who underwent noncurative resection of either or both sites. Although a report by Mussi and colleagues (1996) notes only a 6.6% 5-year survival for combined resection in synchronous SBM, their figure was 19% for metachronous lesions. In summary, in selected patients with SBM and resectable primary sites of NSCLC, a surgical approach to both areas is warranted and can result in late survival in up to 20%. Further experience with stereotactic radiosurgery as an alternative to craniotomy or in cases of surgically inaccessible lesions may increase the proportion of patients suitable for pulmonary resection in this setting.

Solitary Adrenal Metastasis

The importance of documenting the nature of a solitary adrenal mass in patients with otherwise resectable lung cancer has been noted earlier. Experience with resection of both synchronous and metachronous adrenal metastases from NSCLC is limited. Ayabe and associates (1995) summarized the literature and added three cases. Among 12 cases, documented late survival occurred in three cases at 6, 9, and 14 years. Two of these were synchronous and one metachronous. Luketich and Burt (1991) reported on 14 patients with synchronous NSCLC and solitary adrenal metastasis, all treated initially with cisplatinum-based chemotherapy. Eight patients ultimately underwent resection and had a median survival of 31 months as compared with 8 months for those treated with chemotherapy alone. Porte and colleagues (1998) identified 11 cases of solitary adrenal metastases in

598 consecutive patients with otherwise operable or resected NSCLC. Among eight patients with synchronous disease treated by resection, the median survival was only 10 months, although one patient remained free of cancer at 66 months. Of the three patients with metachronous lesions, two died at 6 and 14 months, and one was alive at 6 months. Although these reports suggest that a tiny subset of patients demonstrate late survival after primary resection, the majority of operated patients experience rapid dissemination of their disease.

Other Metastatic Sites

Late survival has rarely been reported in any of the few reports of resection of other presumed solitary sites of metastatic NSCLC, including splenic resection as reported by Macheers and Mansour (1992) and hepatic resection, as reported by Hughes and Sugarbaker (1987). Burt (1996), however, reported a unique experience showing late survival in 14 cases of metachronous solitary metastases from NSCLC to a variety of sites, 13 of whom were treated by resection.

Multiple Tumors

Although the 1997 staging system classifies PM as T_4 or M_1, depending on relative location, the role of resection in these groups is not as clearly limited as in other subsets of T_4 and M_1 NSCLC. In addition, as noted earlier, it is often not possible to determine with certainty whether two lesions are separate primaries, or if one is metastatic from the other. Deslauriers and associates (1989) noted that the presence of satellite nodules, malignant foci close to, but separate, from the dominant tumor, halved the late survival after resection. Nonetheless, survival was 22% in patients with such nodules. A more favorable prognosis than other T_4 or M_1 NSCLC treated by primary operation has been confirmed by others. Fukuse and colleagues (1997b) reported a 5-year survival of 26% in 41 cases of resected ipsilateral PM, with no significant difference between unilobar or multilobar PM. Yoshino and coworkers (1997) found a similar late survival in resected unilobar PM. In a series of 36 cases, Deschamps and colleagues (1990) reported survival of 16% and 14% at 5 and 10 years, respectively. If both tumors were stage I, survival was 25% at both 5 and 10 years. Rosengart (1991), Pommier (1996), and Okada (1998) and their associates also noted varying, but favorable results, with late survivals of 44%, 24%, and 70%, respectively. These authors also emphasized that low stage correlates with improved results. In contrast, Ribet and Dambron (1995) and Adebonojo and colleagues (1997) had no 5-year survivors among synchronous cases, although each series consisted of only 15 patients and each had a high proportion of bilateral resections. In addition, it is noteworthy that in the latter series median survival was excellent (43 months) despite absence of 5-year survival.

Although now classified with unresectable NSCLC, resection should be considered in patients thought to have limited, node-negative PM, especially when unilateral. It is possible that some of the discrepancy among series of PM and synchronous primaries results from unavoidably inaccurate classification, thereby improving results for proposed PM and worsening results for multiple primaries. More accurate differentiation by DNA studies in future reports may help clarify this important surgical issue. The role of systemic treatment as induction or adjuvant therapy requires further study.

Other Prognostic Factors

Although the TNM stage is the most clinically useful determinant of outcome and the basis of most surgical decisions and reporting in NSCLC, numerous other factors have been variably shown to affect prognosis. Multivariate analysis, including both clinical and biological factors, as reported by Harpole and colleagues (1995a,b), will likely become increasingly applied and prospectively more helpful as further data are accumulated. At present, however, the practical implications of individual factors other than TNM predictors and the obvious issue of performance status are limited. The effect of the extent of resection, with the exception of lesser resection versus lobectomy, as discussed previously, is related to the completeness of resection and the TNM stage. Without these specifics, general comparisons of lobectomy to pneumonectomy are not useful.

Sex and Age

Despite occasional reports noting a better prognosis for women than for men with stage I disease, especially for adenocarcinoma, sex is not a prognostic factor in most series. Albain (1998) has commented on the lack of current evidence of a differential outcome by gender in NSCLC. With respect to age, it has been claimed that patients older than 70 years of age have a poorer late outcome than younger patients. Ishida and associates (1990b), however, showed similar survival stage for stage. Current attention has shifted to the role of resection in octogenarians. The acute risk of operation is higher in people older than 80 years of age, but octogenarians who have undergone resection have an acceptable late outcome, with 5-year survival in stage I cases ranging from 30% to as high as 79% (Table 99-9), as summarized by Pagni and colleagues (1997).

Histologic and Molecular Biological Factors

The influence of cell type has been discussed within TNM stage (see also Chapter 95). When matched for other variables, squamous histology appears to have a slightly more favorable prognosis than the collective group of nonsquamous NSCLC, but the differential is usually not statistically

Table 99-9. Reported Experience with Pulmonary Resection for Lung Cancer in Octogenarians

Report	No. of Years (Dates)	No. of Resections	Postoperative Stay (Days)	Major Morbidity (%)	Operative Mortality[a] (%)	5-Year Survival in All Patients (%)	5-Year Survival, Stage I (%)
Ginsberg et al. (1983)	3 (1979–1981)	37	NS	NS	8.1	NS	NS
Shirakusa et al. (1989)	10 (1978–1987)	33	NS	51	13	55	79
Osaki et al. (1994)	17 (1974–1991)	31	NS	67	21	32	38
Naunheim et al. (1994)	10 (1981–1991)	37	14 ± 8.8	30	16	30	NS
Riquet et al. (1994)	6 (1984–1990)	11	NS	NS	12.1	16[b]	30.1[b]
Harvey et al. (1995)	9 (1985–1994)	17	NS	NS	17.6	42[c]	65[c]
Pagni et al. (1997)	16 (1980–1995)	54	8.1 ± 3.5	11	3.7	43	57

NS, not stated.
[a]Operative mortality reflects all deaths within 30 days or same hospitalization for resected patients, as determined from the data reported.
[b]Long-term survival for all patients older than 75 years.
[c]Long-term survival for all patients older than 70 years.
From Pagni S, et al: Pulmonary resection for lung cancer in octogenarians. Ann Thorac Surg 63:785, 1997. With permission.

significant, especially in higher stages, and rarely affects therapeutic decisions. Bronchoalveolar carcinoma (BAC) is a subset of adenocarcinoma that, despite its well-differentiated cytologic features, is often associated with lobar, single lung, or bilateral multifocality or with local aerogenous and vascular dissemination. The reported results of surgical treatment of BAC encompass the extremes. Late survival for resected unifocal BAC is excellent: 90% for T_1N_0 and 55% for T_2N_0, according to Daly and colleagues (1991). These authors, however, found no late survival in bilateral cases. The limitations of resection in multifocal and diffuse BAC are also emphasized in the series reported by Hsu (1995), Albertine (1998), Dumont (1998), and Regnard (1998) and their associates. Although BAC is associated with a varied complex of radiographic and clinical presentations, as well as distinct histologic subsets such as mucinous, Clara cell, and alveolar epithelial cell types, the major predictors of surgical outcome for these lesions remain TNM classification and resectability. Large cell and giant cell undifferentiated variants of NSCLC have been noted to predict a poor surgical outcome, as reported by Razzuk (1976) and Downey (1989) and their colleagues. Reassessment by immunohistochemical techniques, as in the study of Wertzel and colleagues (1997), however, has reclassified many of these tumors to a more differentiated category and in many instances has identified neuroendocrine expression (see Chapter 95). In summary, cell type is not a univariate major prognostic factor in surgical results for NSCLC and rarely should influence surgical decision pathways.

Lung cancer made up of more than one cell type is occasionally recognized by standard light microscopy, but is more often identified when special studies of differentiation are applied. The histogenesis of these tumors is a subject of active investigation. Although the common belief is that mixed tumors behave according to the more aggressive or the more prominent cellular component, documentation is lacking, and the clinical implication of mixed histology is unclear. Naunheim and associates (1987) reported that the

prognosis for stage III adenosquamous carcinomas was worse than that for either of the components alone and even for small cell cancers. Takamori and colleagues (1991) also found an adverse effect of adenosquamous histology that was most pronounced in stages I and II. Intermingling of small cell elements and NSCLC occurs in less than 1% of surgical cases. The surgical prognosis for these lesions is similar to that for pure small cell cancers, as discussed by Hage and colleagues (1998). Patients found to have mixed histology after resection should be treated with adjuvant chemotherapy (see Chapter 107).

Simple histopathologic features presumed to be associated with clinical neoplastic aggressiveness (i.e., lesser degree of differentiation, high mitotic index, vascular or lymphatic invasion) variably have been correlated directly with a poor prognosis. Other histopathologic findings, including necrosis, the presence of fibrosis (scar carcinoma), and local infiltration by plasma cells or lymphocytes have been suggested as influencing prognosis. In practice, the prevalence of any of these features is low, and histologic grading of tumor virulence by light microscopy is largely subjective. When more sophisticated assays of tumor behavior, such as cell proliferative activity, DNA content, and angiogenesis, are applied, clinical correlation is improved. Molecular biological markers are receiving increasing attention as potential indices of prognosis. This area is discussed fully in Chapter 95. An example of this approach is the report by D'Amico and associates (1999), who assessed a panel of 10 markers in resected stage I NSCLC, reflecting all phases of tumor growth and spread (i.e., growth regulation, cell cycle regulation, apoptosis, angiogenesis, and cellular adhesion). Five markers were shown on multivariate analysis to be independent predictors of recurrence. In decreasing order of predictive value, with 5-year survivals for positive versus negative cases in parentheses, these included $p53$ mutation (52% versus 70%), hot-area angiogenesis factor VIII (56% versus 70%), the proto-oncogene erb-b2 (47% versus 67%), and

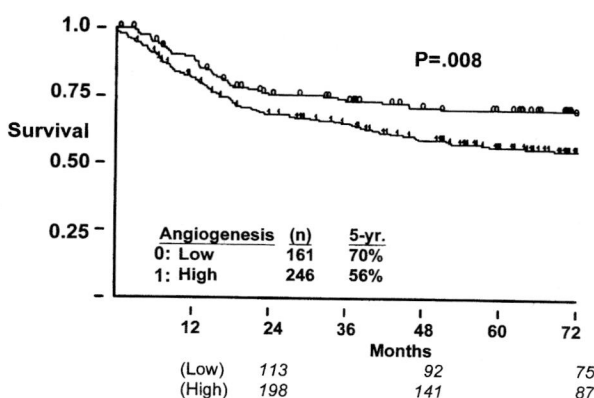

Fig. 99-6. Cancer-specific survival among patients with T₁ tumors according to the involvement of the five molecular markers that were significant in the multivariate analysis. From D'Amico TA, et al: A biologic risk model for stage I human lung cancer: immunohistochemical analysis of 408 patients with use of ten molecular markers. J Thorac Cardiovasc Surg *117*:736, 1999. With permission.

the adhesion protein CD-44 (54% versus 67%). Presence of the fifth marker (rb, a cell cycle regulator) was a positive predictor, with 63% late survival for positive cases and 55% when absent. The number of markers in each case also affected survival. Survival for those with zero to three, four to five, and six to nine markers was 76%, 62%, and 48%, respectively. When only the five independently predictive markers were included, survival for zero to one, two, and three to five markers was 80%, 63%, and 50%, respectively (Fig. 99-6). It is likely that, with further experience, information of this type will help identify patients at high risk of recurrence who might benefit from adjuvant therapy or, at least, require special surveillance.

Miscellaneous Prognostic Factors

Trotter and associates (1984) first reported an adverse effect on survival of perioperative blood transfusion in patients with stage I disease, and Hyman and colleagues (1985) supported this observation. Moores and colleagues (1989) also found a deleterious effect of blood transfusion in the data of the LCSG. Little and associates (1990) also provided supportive data. The series reported by Pastorino (1986) and Keller (1988b) and their coworkers, however, showed no correlation between blood transfusion and its amount and late survival in limited lung cancer. Elevation of the white blood cell count, serum lactic dehydrogenase, and carcinoembryonic antigen, as well as decreased hemoglobin level, are among basic blood tests that have been proposed to affect prognosis, but the data are sparse. Positive pleural lavage cytology has correlated with increased recurrence, as reported by Kondo (1993), Higashiyama (1997), Dresler (1999), and Okada (1999) and their colleagues. In the latter study, 5-year survival among a group of mixed stages was

54% for patients with negative lavage results versus 15% when malignant cells were identified.

RECURRENCE AFTER RESECTION

Much has been written about recurrence rates and locations after surgical treatment of NSCLC. In brief, surgical patients with NSCLC remain at risk for recurrence of the original tumor and development of new primary lung cancers. Although the rate of recurrence decreases over time, metastasis can appear many years after initial diagnosis and treatment. Among 62 patients who were found to have new lesions 5 or more years after resection, Martini and associates (1999) noted that 26 experienced recurrence of the original tumor, and 36 cases represented new primaries. Lifelong surveillance is mandatory. Most treatment failures occur within the first 3 years. These cases, especially those with early clinical recurrence, likely represent instances of failure of the initial staging evaluation to detect the true extent of disease, unconfirmed incomplete resection, or both. In older series, between 10 and 30% of operated patients who died soon after surgery had unsuspected grossly evident metastases identified at autopsy. Although Stenbygaard and associates (1995), found no postmortem evidence of distant disease in eight patients who died within 30 days of resection for stage I or II adenocarcinoma performed between 1981 and 1985, data in this area are limited, and the incidence of micrometastasis in this group is unknown. Maruyama and colleagues (1997) found that in patients with resected pathologic stage I NSCLC unsuspected micrometastases to the N₁ and N₂ lymph nodes can often be found by monoclonal antibody stains, and that this finding correlates with early relapse.

Locoregional recurrence is less common than the appearance of distant metastasis in patients with lower stage NSCLC after complete resection. The sites of first failure were distant metastases to the brain, bone, liver, or contralateral lung in most of the patients reported by Mountain (1980), Immerman (1981), Martini (1983), Feld (1984), Pairolero (1984), and Ichinose (1989) and their associates. In each, the brain was the most common site. In contrast, the Ludwig Lung Cancer Study Group (1987) reported the highest initial failure rate in patients with stage I disease to be in the ipsilateral hemithorax, as did Iascone and associates (1986).

REFERENCES

Adebonojo SA, Moritz DM, Danby CA: The results of modern surgical therapy for multiple primary lung cancers. Chest *112*:693, 1997.

Albain K: Invited commentary. *In* Ouellette D, et al: Lung cancer in women compared with men: stage, treatment and survival. Ann Thorac Surg *66*:1140, 1998.

Albertine KH, et al: Analysis of cell type and radiographic presentation as predictors of the clinical course of patients with bronchioloalveolar cell carcinoma. Chest *113*:997, 1998.

Albertucci M, et al: Surgery and the management of peripheral lung tumors adherent to the parietal pleura. J Thorac Cardiovasc Surg 103:8, 1992.

Allen MS, et al: Bronchogenic carcinoma with chest wall invasion. Ann Thorac Surg 51:948, 1991.

Anderson TM, May PM, Holmes EC: Factors affecting survival in superior sulcus tumors. J Clin Oncol 4:1598, 1986.

Antakli T, et al: Second primary lung cancer. Ann Thorac Surg 59:863, 1995.

Ayabe H, et al: Surgical management of adrenal metastasis from bronchogenic carcinoma. J Surg Oncol 58:149, 1995.

Boushy SF, et al: Clinical course related to preoperative and postoperative pulmonary function in patients with bronchogenic carcinoma. Chest 59:383, 1971.

Brewer LA: Patterns of survival in lung cancer. Chest 71:644, 1977.

Bulzebruck H, et al: Validation of the TNM classification for lung cancer: first results of a prospective study of 1086 patients with surgical treatment. Eur J Cardiothorac Surg 5:356, 1991.

Burt ME: Role of surgery in the treatment of patients with solitary metastasis from non-small cell lung cancer. In Aisner J, et al (eds): Comprehensive Textbook of Thoracic Oncology. Baltimore: Williams & Wilkins, 1996, p. 416.

Burt ME, et al: Results of surgical treatment of Stage III lung cancer invading the mediastinum. Surg Clin North Am 67:987, 1987.

Burt ME, et al: Resection of brain metastases from non-small cell lung carcinoma: results of therapy. J Thorac Cardiovasc Surg 103:399, 1992.

Canver CC, et al: Pulmonary resection combined with cardiac operations. Ann Thorac Surg 50:796, 1990.

Casillas M, et al: Surgical treatment of lung carcinoma involving the chest wall. Eur J Cardiothorac Surg 3:325, 1989.

Churchill ED, Belsey R: Segmental pneumonectomy in bronchiectasis; lingula segment of left upper lobe. Ann Surg 109:481, 1939.

Cortese DA, et al: Roentgenographically occult lung cancer: ten-year experience. J Thorac Cardiovasc Surg 86:373, 1983.

Cortese DA, Edell ES, Kinsey JH: Photodynamic therapy for early-stage squamous carcinoma of the lung. Mayo Clin Proc 72:595, 1997.

Cybulsky IJ, et al: Prognostic significance of computed tomography in resected N2 lung cancer. Ann Thorac Surg 54:533, 1992.

Daly BDT, Feins NR: The diaphragm. In Kaiser LR, Kron IL, Spray Tl (eds.): Mastery of Cardiothoracic Surgery. Philadelphia: Lippincott–Raven. 1998, p. 196.

Daly BDT, et al: N2 lung cancer: outcome in patients with false-negative computed tomographic scans of the chest. J Thorac Cardiovasc Surg 105:904, 1993.

Daly RC: Bronchoalveolar carcinoma: factors affecting survival. Ann Thorac Surg 51:368, 1991.

Damhuis RA, Schutte PR: Resection rates and postoperative mortality in 7,899 patients with lung cancer. Eur Respir J 9:7, 1996.

D'Amico TA, et al: A biologic risk model for stage I lung cancer: immunohistochemical analysis of 408 patients with the use of ten molecular markers. J Thorac Cardiovasc Surg 117:736, 1999.

Danton MH, et al: Simultaneous cardiac surgery with pulmonary resection: presentation of a series and review of the literature. Eur J Cardiothorac Surg 13:667, 1998.

Dartevelle PG, et al: Replacement of the superior vena cava with polytetrafluoroethylene grafts combined with resection of mediastinal-pulmonary malignant tumors: report of thirteen cases. J Thorac Cardiovasc Surg 94:361, 1987.

Dartevelle PG, et al: Long-term follow-up after prosthetic replacement of the superior vena cava combined with resection of mediastinal-pulmonary malignant tumors. J Thorac Cardiovasc Surg 102:259, 1991.

Dartevelle PG, et al: Anterior transcervical-thoracic approach for radical resection of lung tumors invading the thoracic inlet. J Thorac Cardiovasc Surg 105:1025, 1993.

Dartevelle PG, et al: Tracheal-sleeve pneumonectomy for bronchogenic carcinoma: update 1995. Ann Thorac Surg 60:1854, 1995.

Decker DA: The significance of cytologically negative pleural effusion in bronchogenic carcinoma. Chest 74:640, 1978.

DeGiacomo T, et al: Thoracoscopic staging of IIIB non-small cell lung cancer before neoadjuvant therapy. Ann Thorac Surg 64:1409, 1997.

DeMeester TR, et al: Management of tumor adherent to the vertebral column. J Thorac Cardiovasc Surg 97:373, 1989.

Deschamps C, et al: Multiple primary lung cancers: results of surgical treatment. J Thorac Cardiovasc Surg 99:769, 1990.

Deslauriers J, et al: Carcinoma of the lung: evaluation of satellite nodules as a factor influencing prognosis after resection. J Thorac Cardiovasc Surg 97:504, 1989.

Deslauriers J, et al: Staging and management of lung cancer: sleeve resection. World J Surg 17:712, 1993.

Detterbeck FC, Socinski MA: IIB or not IIB: the current question in staging non-small cell lung cancer. Chest 112:229, 1997.

Downey RS, Sewell CW, Mansour KA: Large cell carcinoma of the lung: a highly aggressive tumor with dismal prognosis. Ann Thorac Surg 47:806, 1989.

Dresler CM, Fratelli C, Babb J: Prognostic value of positive pleural lavage in patients with lung cancer resection. Ann Thorac Surg 67:1435, 1999.

Dumont P, et al: Bronchoalveolar carcinoma: histopathologic study of evolution in a series of 105 surgically treated patients. Chest 113:391, 1998.

Errett LE, et al: Wedge resection as an alternative procedure for peripheral bronchogenic carcinoma in poor-risk patients. J Thorac Cardiovasc Surg 90:656, 1985.

Ettinghausen S, Burt ME: Prospective evaluation of unilateral adrenal masses in patients with operable non-small cell lung cancer. J Clin Oncol 9:1462, 1991.

Faber LP: Results of surgical treatment of stage III lung carcinoma with carinal proximity: the role of sleeve lobectomy versus pneumonectomy and the role of sleeve pneumonectomy. Surg Clin North Am 67:1001, 1987.

Faber LP, et al: Preoperative chemotherapy and irradiation for stage III non-small cell lung cancer. Ann Thorac Surg 47:669, 1989.

Feld R, et al: Site of recurrence in resected stage I non-small cell lung cancer: a guide for future studies. J Clin Oncol 2:1352, 1984.

Ferguson MK, et al: Diffusion capacity predicts morbidity and mortality after pulmonary resection. J Thorac Cardiovasc Surg. 96:894, 1991.

Fernando HC, Goldstraw P. The accuracy of clinical evaluative intrathoracic staging in lung cancer as assessed by postsurgical pathologic staging. Cancer 65:2503, 1990.

Fukuse T, Wada H, Hitomi S: Extended operation for non-small cell lung cancer invading great vessels and left atrium. Eur J Cardiothorac Surg 11:664, 1997a.

Fukuse T, et al: Prognosis of ipsilateral intrapulmonary metastases in resected non-small cell lung cancer. Eur J Cardiothorac Surg 12:218, 1997b.

Funatsu T, et al: The role of mediastinoscopic biopsy in preoperative assessment of lung cancer. J Thorac Cardiovasc Surg 104:1688, 1992.

Gail MH, et al: Prognostic factors in patients with resected Stage I non-small cell lung cancer. Cancer 54:1802, 1984.

Gdeedo A, et al: Comparison of imaging TNM (iTNM) and pathological TNM (pTNM) in staging of bronchogenic carcinoma. Eur J Cardiothorac Surg 12:224, 1997.

Gebitekin C, et al: Fate of patients with residual tumor at the bronchial resection margin. Eur J Cardiothorac Surg 8:339, 1994.

Gerson MC, et al: Prediction of cardiac and pulmonary complications related to abdominal and noncardiac thoracic surgery in geriatric patients. Am J Med 88:101, 1990.

Ginsberg RJ: The role of preoperative surgical staging in left upper lobe tumors. Ann Thorac Surg 57:526, 1994.

Ginsberg RJ, Rubinstein LV: Randomized trial of lobectomy versus limited resection for T1N0 non-small cell lung cancer: Lung Cancer Study Group. Ann Thorac Surg 60:615, 1995.

Ginsberg RJ, et al: Modern 30-day operative mortality for surgical resections in lung cancer. J Thorac Cardiovasc Surg 86:654, 1983.

Ginsberg RJ, et al: Influence of surgical resection and brachytherapy in the management of superior sulcus tumor. Ann Thorac Surg 57:1440, 1994.

Goldstraw P: Mediastinoscopy 1992: is it still essential? Lung Cancer 8:79, 1992.

Goldstraw P, et al: Surgical management of non-small cell lung cancer with ipsilateral mediastinal node metastasis (N2 disease). J Thorac Cardiovasc Surg 107:19, 1994.

Graham ANJ, et al: Systematic nodal dissection in the intrathoracic staging of non-small cell lung cancer. J Thorac Cardiovasc Surg 117:246, 1999.

Graham EA, Singer JJ: Successful removal of the entire lung for carcinoma of the bronchus. JAMA 101:1371, 1933.

Grunenwald D, et al: Total vertebrectomy for en bloc resection of lung cancer invading the spine. Ann Thorac Surg 61:723, 1996.

Hage R, et al: Surgery for combined type small cell lung carcinoma. Thorax 53:450, 1998.

Hara N, et al: Assessment of the role of surgery for stage III bronchogenic carcinoma. J Surg Oncol 25:153, 1984.

Harpole DH, et al: Stage I non-small cell lung cancer: a multivariate analysis of treatment methods and patterns of recurrence. Cancer 76:787, 1995a.

Harpole DH, et al: A prognostic model of recurrence and death in Stage I non-small cell lung cancer utilizing presentation, histopathology and oncoprotein expression. Cancer Res 55:51, 1995b.

Harviel JD, McNamara JJ, Straehley CJ: Surgical treatment of lung cancer in patients over the age of 70 years. J Thorac Cardiovasc Surg 75:802, 1978.

Harvey JC, et al: Surgical treatment of non-small cell lung cancer in patients older than seventy years. J Surg Oncol 60:247, 1995.

Higashiyama M, et al: Pleural lavage cytology immediately after thoracotomy and before closure of the thoracic cavity for lung cancer without pleural effusion and dissemination: clinicopathologic and prognostic analysis. Ann Surg Oncol 4:409, 1997.

Holmes EC: Treatment of Stage II lung cancer. Surg Clin North Am 67:945, 1987.

Horita K, Itho T, Ueno T: Radical operation using cardiopulmonary bypass for lung cancer invading the aortic wall. Thorac Cardiovasc Surg 41:130, 1993.

Hsu C, Chen C, Hsu N: Bronchioloalveolar carcinoma. J Thorac Cardiovasc Surg 110:374, 1995.

Hughes KS, Sugarbaker PH: Treatment of metastatic liver tumors. In Rosenberg SA (ed): Surgical Cure of Metastatic Cancer. Philadelphia: Lippincott, 1987.

Hyman NH, et al: Blood transfusions and survival after lung cancer resection. Am J Surg 149:502, 1985.

Iascone C, et al: Local recurrence of resectable non-small cell carcinoma of the lung. Cancer 57:471, 1986.

Ichinose Y, Hara N, Ohta M: Synchronous lung cancers defined by deoxyribonucleic acid flow cytometry. J Thorac Cardiovasc Surg 102:418, 1991.

Ichinose Y, et al: Preoperative examination to detect distant metastasis is not advocated for asymptomatic patients with stages 1 and 2 non-small cell lung cancer. Chest 96:1104, 1989.

Ichinose Y, et al: Is T factor of the TNM staging system a predominant prognostic factor in pathologic stage I non-small cell lung cancer? J Thorac Cardiovasc Surg 106:90, 1993.

Ichinose Y, et al: Prognostic factors obtained by a pathologic examination in completely resected non-small cell lung cancer: an analysis in each pathologic stage. J Thorac Cardiovasc Surg 110:601, 1995.

Immerman SC, et al: Site of recurrence with stage I and II carcinoma of the lung resected for cure. Ann Thorac Surg 32:23, 1981.

Inoue H, et al: Resection of the superior vena cava for primary lung cancer: 5 years' survival. Ann Thorac Surg 50:661, 1990.

Inoue H et al: Prognostic assessment of 1310 patients with non-small cell lung cancer who underwent complete resection from 1980 to 1993. J Thorac Cardiovasc Surg 116:407, 1998.

Ishida T, et al: Strategy for lymphadenectomy of lung cancer less than 3 cm in diameter. Ann Thorac Surg 50:708, 1990a.

Ishida T, et al: Long-term results of operation for non-small cell lung cancer in the elderly. Ann Thorac Surg 50:919, 1990b.

Izbicki JR, et al: Effectiveness of radical systematic mediastinal lymphadenectomy in patients with resectable non-small cell lung cancer: results of a prospective randomized trial. Ann Surg 227:138, 1998.

Jensik RJ, et al: Segmental resection for lung cancer. A 15 year experience. J Thorac Cardiovasc Surg 66:563, 1973.

Jubelirer S, Wilson RA: Lung cancer in patients younger than 40 years of age. Cancer 67:1436, 1991.

Kaiser LR, et al: Significance of extramucosal residual tumor at the bronchial resection margin. Ann Thorac Surg 47:265, 1989.

Kato H, Okunaka T, Shimatani H: Photodynamic therapy for early stage bronchogenic carcinoma. J Clin Laser Med Surg 14:235, 1996.

Keller SM, Kaiser LR, Martini N: Bilobectomy for bronchogenic carcinoma. Ann Thorac Surg 45:62, 1988a.

Keller SM, et al: Blood transfusion and lung cancer recurrence. Cancer 62:606, 1988b.

Kirsch MM, et al: Major pulmonary resections for bronchogenic carcinoma in the elderly. Ann Thorac Surg 22:369, 1976.

Klepetko W, et al: T4 lung tumors with infiltration of the thoracic aorta: is an operation reasonable? Ann Thorac Surg 67:340, 1999.

Kodama K, et al: Intentional limited resection for selected patients with T1N0M0 non-small cell lung cancer: a single institution study. J Thorac Cardiovasc Surg 114:347, 1997.

Kohman LJ, et al: Random versus predictable risks of mortality after thoracotomy for lung cancer. J Thorac Cardiovasc Surg 91:551, 1986.

Koike T, et al: Clinical analysis of small-sized peripheral lung cancer. J Thorac Cardiovasc Surg 115:1015, 1998.

Kondo H, et al: Prognostic significance of pleural lavage cytology immediately after thoracotomy in patients with lung cancer. J Thorac Cardiovasc Surg 106:1092, 1993.

Korst RJ, et al: Lobectomy improves ventilatory function in selected patients with severe COPD. Ann Thorac Surg 66:898, 1998.

Lam S: Photodynamic therapy of lung cancer. Semin Oncol 21:15, 1994.

Landreneau RJ, et al: Wedge resection versus lobectomy for stage I (T1N0M0) non-small cell lung cancer. J Thorac Cardiovasc Surg 113:691, 1996.

Liewald F, et al: Importance of microscopic residual disease at the bronchial margin after resection of non-small cell carcinoma of the lung. J Thorac Cardiovasc Surg 104:408, 1992.

Little AG, et al: Modified stage I (T1N0M0, T2N0M0) non-small cell lung cancer: treatment results, recurrence patterns and adjuvant immunotherapy. Surgery 100:621, 1986.

Little AG, et al: Perioperative blood transfusion adversely affects prognosis of patients with stage I non-small cell lung cancer. Am J Surg 160:630, 1990.

Ludwig Lung Cancer Study Group: Patterns of failure in patients with resected Stage I and II non-small cell carcinoma of the lung. Ann Surg 205:67, 1987.

Luketich JD, Burt ME: Does resection of isolated adrenal metastases in non-small cell lung cancer (NSCLC) improve survival? Lung Cancer 10:53, 1991.

Macchiarini P, et al: Blood vessel invasion by tumor cells predicts recurrence in completely resected T1N0M0 non-small cell lung cancer. J Thorac Cardiovasc Surg 106:80, 1993.

Macheers SK, Mansour KA: Management of isolated splenic metastases from carcinoma of the lung: a case report and review of the literature. Am Surgeon 58:683, 1992.

Maggi G, et al: Results of surgical resection of Stage IIIa (N2) non-small cell lung cancer, according to the site of the mediastinal metastases. Int Surg 78:213, 1993.

Maggi G, et al: Combined radiosurgical treatment of Pancoast tumor. Ann Thorac Surg 57:198, 1994.

Magilligan DJ, et al: Surgical approach to lung cancer with solitary cerebral metastasis: twenty-five years experience. Ann Thorac Surg 42:360, 1986.

Martini N, Flehinger BJ: The role of surgery in N2 lung cancer. Surg Clin North Am 67:1037, 1987.

Martini N, Melamed MR: Multiple primary lung cancers. J Thorac Cardiovasc Surg 70:606, 1975.

Martini N, Melamed MR: Occult carcinomas of the lung. Ann Thorac Surg 30:215, 1980.

Martini N, et al: Prognostic significance of N1 disease in carcinoma of the lung. J Thorac Cardiovasc Surg 86:646, 1983.

Martini N, et al: Lobectomy for stage I lung cancer. In Kittle CF (ed): Current Controversies in Thoracic Surgery. Philadelphia: WB Saunders, 1986, pp. 171–174.

Martini N, et al: Survival after resection of Stage II non-small cell lung cancer. Ann Thorac Surg 54:460, 1992.

Martini N, et al: Management of non-small cell lung cancer with direct mediastinal involvement. Ann Thorac Surg 58:1447, 1994.

Martini N, et al: Factors influencing ten-year survival in resected stages I to IIIA non-small cell lung cancer. J Thorac Cardiovasc Surg 117:32, 1999.

Mathisen DJ, Grillo HC: Carinal resection for bronchogenic carcinoma. J Thorac Cardiovasc Surg 102:16, 1991.

Mathisen DJ, et al: Assessment of preoperative accelerated radiotherapy and chemotherapy in stage IIIA (N2) non-small cell lung cancer. J Thorac Cardiovasc Surg 111:123, 1996.

McCaughan BC: Primary lung cancer invading the chest wall. Chest Surg Clin North Am 4:17, 1994.

McCaughan BC, et al: Chest wall invasion in carcinoma of the lung: therapeutic and prognostic implications. J Thorac Cardiovasc Surg 89:836, 1985.

McElvaney G, et al: Multicentricity of adenocarcinoma of the lung. Chest 95:151, 1989.

Merlier M, et al: The staging issue: unification of criteria. In Delarue NC, Eschapasse H (eds): International Trends in General Thoracic Surgery. Philadelphia: WB Saunders, 1985, pp. 27–36.

Milledge JS, Nunn JF: Criteria of fitness for anesthesia in patients with chronic obstructive lung disease. BMJ 3:670, 1975.

Miller DL, et al: Results of surgical resection in patients with N2 non-small cell lung cancer. Ann Thorac Surg 57:1095, 1994.

Miller JI, Mansour KA, Hatcher CR: Carcinoma of the superior pulmonary sulcus. Ann Thorac Surg 28:44, 1979.

Mitchell JD, et al: Proceedings of the American Association for Thoracic Surgery (abstr), 1998, p. 46.

Moores DWO, Piantadosi S, McKneally MF: Effect of perioperative blood transfusions on the outcome in patients with surgically resected lung cancer. Ann Thorac Surg 47:346, 1989.

Mountain CF: Expanded possibilities for surgical treatment of lung cancer: survival in stage IIIA disease. Chest 97:1045, 1990.

Mountain CF: Revisions in the international system for staging lung cancer. Chest 111:1710, 1997.

Mountain CF, et al: Present status of postoperative adjuvant therapy for lung cancer. Cancer Bull 32:108, 1980.

Maruyama R, et al: Relationship between early recurrence and micrometastases in the lymph nodes of patients with stage I non-small cell lung cancer. J Thorac Cardiovasc Surg 114:535, 1997.

Muscolino G, Valente M, Andreani S: Pancoast tumours: clinical assessment and long-term results of combined radiosurgical treatment. Thorax 52:284, 1997.

Mussi A, et al: Resection of single metastasis in non-small cell lung cancer: prognostic factors. J Thorac Cardiovasc Surg 112:146, 1996.

Nakahara K, et al: Extended operation for lung cancer invading the aortic arch and superior vena cava. J Thorac Cardiovasc Surg 97:428, 1989.

Nakahashi H, Yasumoto K, Sugimachi K: Results of surgical treatment of patients with T3 non-small cell lung cancer—update. Ann Thorac Surg 61:273, 1996.

Nakanishi R, et al: Treatment strategy for patients with surgically discovered N2 stage IIIA non-small cell lung cancer. Ann Thorac Surg 64:342, 1997.

Naruke T, et al: Prognosis and survival in resected lung carcinoma based on the new international staging system. J Thorac Cardiovasc Surg 96:440, 1988a.

Naruke T, et al: The importance of surgery to non-small cell carcinoma of the lung with mediastinal lymph node metastasis. Ann Thorac Surg 46:603, 1988b.

Naunheim KS, et al: Adenosquamous lung carcinoma: clinical characteristics, treatment and prognosis. Ann Thorac Surg 44:462, 1987.

Naunheim KS, et al: Lung cancer surgery in the octogenarian. Eur J Cardiothorac Surg 8:453, 1994.

Newton JR, Grillo HC, Mathisen DJ: Main bronchial sleeve resection with pulmonary conservation. Ann Thorac Surg 52:1272, 1991.

Ninan M, et al: Standardized exercise oximetry predicts postpneumonectomy outcome. Ann Thorac Surg 64:323, 1997.

Nugent WC, et al: Non-small cell lung cancer at the extremes of age: impact on diagnosis and treatment. Ann Thorac Surg 63:193, 1997.

Ohada M, et al: Operative approach for multiple primary lung carcinomas. J Thorac Cardiovasc Surg 115:836, 1998.

Okada M, et al: Operative approach for multiple primary lung carcinomas. J Thorac Cardiovasc Surg 115:836, 1998.

Okada M, et al: Role of pleural lavage cytology before resection for primary lung cancer. Ann Surg 229:579, 1999.

Osaki T, et al: Surgical treatment of lung cancer in the octogenarian. Ann Thorac Surg 57:188, 1994.

Overholt RH, et al: A new technique for pulmonary segmental resection: its application in the treatment of bronchiectasis. J Thorac Surg 15:384, 1946.

Padilla J, et al: Surgical results and prognostic factors in early non-small cell lung cancer. Ann Thorac Surg 63:324, 1997.

Pagni S, Federico JA, Ponn RB: Pulmonary resection for lung cancer in octogenarians. Ann Thorac Surg 63:785, 1997.

Pagni S, et al: Pulmonary resection for malignancy in the elderly: is age still a risk factor? Eur J Cardiothorac Surg 14:40, 1998.

Pairolero P, et al: Postsurgical stage I bronchogenic carcinoma: morbid implications of recurrent disease. Ann Thorac Surg 38:332,1984.

Pastorino U, et al: Perioperative blood transfusion and prognosis if resected stage Ia lung cancer. Eur J Clin Oncol 22:1375, 1986.

Patchell RA, et al: Postoperative radiotherapy in the treatment of single metastases to the brain. JAMA 280:1485, 1998.

Patterson GA, et al: Significance of metastatic disease in subaortic lymph nodes. Ann Thorac Surg 43:155, 1987.

Paulson DL: The "superior sulcus" lesion. In Delarue N, Eschapasse H (eds): International Trends in General Thoracic Surgery. Philadelphia: WB Saunders, 1985, pp. 121–131.

Pearson FG, et al: Significance of positive mediastinal nodes identified at mediastinoscopy in patients with resectable cancer of the lung. J Thorac Cardiovasc Surg 83:1, 1982.

Pemberton JH, et al: Bronchogenic carcinoma in patients younger than 40 years. Ann Thorac Surg 36:509, 1983.

Piehler JM, et al: Bronchogenic carcinoma with chest wall invasion: factors affecting survival following en bloc resection. Ann Thorac Surg 34:684, 1982.

Piehler JM, et al: Concomitant cardiac and pulmonary operations. J Thorac Cardiovasc Surg 90:662, 1985.

Pitz CCM, et al: Results of resection of T3 non-small cell lung cancer invading the mediastinum or main bronchus. Ann Thorac Surg 62:1016, 1996.

Pommier RF, et al: Synchronous non-small cell lung cancers. Am J Surg 171:521, 1996.

Porte HL, et al: Adrenalectomy for a solitary adrenal metastasis from lung cancer. Ann Thorac Surg 65:331, 1998.

Price-Thomas C: Lobectomy with sleeve resection. Thorax 15:9, 1960.

Rao TH, Jacobs KH, Err EL: Reinfarction following anesthesia in patients with myocardial infarction. Anesthesiology 54:449, 1983.

Ratto GB, et al: Chest wall involvement by lung cancer: computed tomographic detection and results of operation. Ann Thorac Surg 51:182, 1991.

Razzuk MA, et al: Pulmonary giant cell carcinoma. Ann Thorac Surg 21:540, 1976.

Read RC, Yoder G, Schaeffer RC: Survival after conservative resection for T1N0M0 non-small cell lung cancer. Ann Thorac Surg 49:391, 1990.

Read RC, et al: Diameter, cell type, and survival in Stage I primary non-small cell lung cancer. Arch Surg 123:446, 1988.

Read RC, et al: Management of non-small cell carcinoma with solitary brain metastasis. J Thorac Cardiovasc Surg 98:884, 1989.

Regnard JF, et al: Results of resection for bronchogenic carcinoma with mediastinal lymph node metastases in selected patients. Eur J Cardiothorac Surg 5:583, 1991.

Regnard JF, et al: Bronchioloalveolar lung carcinoma: results of surgical treatment and prognostic factors. Chest 114:45, 1998.

Ribet M, Dambron P: Multiple primary lung cancers. Eur J Cardiothorac Surg 9:231, 1995.

Ricci C, et al: Reconstruction of the pulmonary artery in patients with lung cancer. Ann Thorac Surg 57:627, 1994.

Riquet M, et al: Operation for lung cancer in the elderly. What about octogenarians? Letter to the Editor. Ann Thorac Surg 58:916, 1994.

Roeslin N, et al: A better prognostic value from a modification of lung cancer staging. J Thorac Cardiovasc Surg 94:504, 1987.

Rosengart TK, et al: Multiple primary lung carcinomas: prognosis and treatment. Ann Thorac Surg 52:773, 1991.

Roviaro G, et al: Tracheal sleeve pneumonectomy for bronchogenic carcinoma. J Thorac Cardiovasc Surg 107:13, 1994.

Roviaro G, et al: Videothoracoscopic staging and treatment of lung cancer. Ann Thorac Surg 59:971, 1995.

Rusch VW, et al: Surgical resection of stage IIIA and stage IIIB non-small cell lung cancer after concurrent induction chemoradiotherapy. J Thorac Cardiovasc Surg 105:97, 1993.

Rusch VW, et al: Neoadjuvant therapy: a novel and effective treatment for stage IIIB non-small cell lung cancer. Ann Thorac Surg 58:290, 1994.

Sagawa M, et al: Clinical and prognostic assessment of patients with resected small peripheral lung cancer lesions. Cancer 66:2653, 1990.

Saito Y, et al: Results of surgical treatment for roentgenographically occult bronchogenic squamous cell carcinoma. J Thorac Cardiovasc Surg 104:401, 1992.

Sartori F, et al: Carcinoma of the superior pulmonary sulcus: results of irradiation and radical resection. J Thorac Cardiovasc Surg 104:679, 1992.

Shaw RR, Paulson DI, Kee JL: Treatment of the superior sulcus tumor by irradiation followed by resection. Ann Surg 154:29, 1961.

Shields TW: The fate of patients after incomplete resection of bronchial carcinoma. Surg Gynecol Obstet 139:569, 1974.

Shields TW: The "incomplete" resection. Ann Thorac Surg 47:487, 1989.

Shields TW: The significance of ipsilateral mediastinal lymph node metastasis in non-small cell lung cancer. J Thorac Cardiovasc Surg 99:48, 1990.

Shields TW, Higgins GA: Minimal pulmonary resection. Arch Surg 108:420, 1974.

Shields TW, et al: Relationship of cell type and lymph node metastases to survival after resection of bronchial carcinoma. Ann Thorac Surg 20:501, 1975.

Shimizu J, et al: Results of surgical treatment of stage 1 lung cancer. Nippon Geka Gakkai Zasshi 94:505, 1993.

Shirakusa T, et al: Results of resection for bronchogenic carcinoma in patients over the age of 80. Thorax *44*:189, 1989.

Snijder RJ, et al: Survival in resected stage I lung cancer with residual tumor at the bronchial resection margin. Ann Thorac Surg *65*:212, 1998.

Soorae AS, Stevenson JM: Survival with residual tumor on the bronchial margin after resection for bronchogenic carcinoma. J Thorac Cardiovasc Surg *78*:175, 1979.

Stanford W, Barnes RP, Tucker AR: Influence of staging in superior sulcus (Pancoast) tumors of the lung. Ann Thorac Surg *29*:406, 1980.

Stenbygaard LE, Sorensen JB, Olsen JE: Metastatic pattern of adenocarcinoma of the lung: an autopsy study from a cohort of 137 consecutive patients with complete resection. J Thorac Cardiovasc Surg *11*:1130, 1995.

Strauss GM, et al: Neoadjuvant chemotherapy and radiotherapy followed by surgery in stage IIIA non-small cell carcinoma of the lung: report of a Cancer and Leukemia Group B phase II study. J Clin Oncol *10*:1237, 1992.

Sugi K, et al: Systematic lymph node dissection for clinically diagnosed peripheral non-small cell lung cancer less than 2 cm in diameter. World J Surg *22*:290, 1998.

Takamori S, et al: Clinicopathologic characteristics of adenosquamous carcinoma of the lung. Cancer 67:649, 1991.

Tateishi M, et al: Skip mediastinal lymph node metastasis in non-small cell lung cancer. J Surg Oncol 57:139, 1994.

Taulelle M, et al: High dose rate endobronchial brachytherapy: results and complications in 189 patients. Eur Respir J *11*:162, 1998.

Tedder M, et al: Current morbidity, mortality and survival after bronchoplastic procedures for malignancy. Ann Thorac Surg *54*:387, 1992.

Terzi A, et al: Lung resections concomitant to coronary artery bypass grafting. Eur J Cardiothorac Surg 8:580, 1994.

Thomas P, Rubinstein L, and the Lung Cancer Study Group: Cancer recurrence after resection: T1N0 non-small cell lung cancer. Ann Thorac Surg *49*:242, 1990.

Trastek VF, et al: En bloc (non-chest wall) resection for bronchogenic carcinoma with parietal fixation. J Thorac Cardiovasc Surg *87*:352, 1984.

Trotter PI, Burrow L, Kirschner P: Perioperative blood transfusion adversely affects prognosis after resection of stage I non-oat cell lung cancer. J Thorac Cardiovasc Surg *88*:659, 1984.

Tsuchiya R, et al: Extended resection of the left atrium, great vessels, or both for lung cancer. Ann Thorac Surg *57*:960, 1994.

van Klaveren RJ, et al: Prognosis of unsuspected but completely resectable N2 non-small cell lung cancer. Ann Thorac Surg *56*:300, 1993.

Vansteenkiste JF, et al: Survival and prognostic factors in resected N2 non-small cell lung cancer: a study of 140 cases. Ann Thorac Surg *63*:1441, 1997.

van Velzen E, et al: Type of lymph node involvement influences survival rates in T1N1M0 non-small cell lung carcinoma. Chest *110*:1469, 1996.

van Velzen E, et al: Lymph node type as a prognostic factor for survival in T2N1M0 non-small cell lung carcinoma. Ann Thorac Surg *63*:1436, 1997.

Vogt-Moykopf I, et al: Bronchoplastic and angioplastic operation in bronchial carcinoma: long-term results of a retrospective analysis from 1973 to 1983. Int Surg *71*:211, 1986.

Wada H, et al: Thirty-day operative mortality for thoracotomy in lung cancer. J Thorac Cardiovasc Surg *115*:70, 1998.

Warren WH, Faber LP: Segmentectomy versus lobectomy in patients with stage I pulmonary carcinoma. J Thorac Cardiovasc Surg *107*:1087, 1994.

Watanabe Y, et al: Results in 104 patients undergoing bronchoplastic procedures for bronchial lesions. Ann Thorac Surg *50*:607, 1990.

Watanabe Y, et al: Early hilar lung cancer: its clinical aspect. J Surg Oncol *48*:75, 1991a.

Watanabe Y, et al: Results of surgical treatment in patients with stage IIIA non-small cell lung cancer. Thorac Cardiovasc Surg *39*:44, 1991b.

Watanabe Y, et al: Results of surgical treatment of patients with stage IIIb non-small cell lung cancer. Thorac Cardiovasc Surg *39*:50, 1991c.

Watanabe Y, et al: Mediastinal nodal involvement and the prognosis of non-small cell lung cancer. Chest *100*:422, 1991d.

Weiden PL, et al: Preoperative chemotherapy (cisplatin and fluorouracil) and radiation therapy in stage III non-small cell lung cancer: a phase II study of the LCSG 773. Chest *106*(Suppl):297s, 1994.

Weksler B, et al: Resection of lung cancer invading the diaphragm. Ann Thorac Surg *114*:500, 1997.

Wertzel H, et al: Results after surgery in undifferentiated large cell carcinoma of the lung: the role of neuroendocrine expression. Eur J Cardiothorac Surg *12*:698, 1997.

Westermann CJJ, et al: Pulmonary resection after pneumonectomy in patients with bronchogenic carcinoma. J Thorac Cardiovasc Surg *106*:868, 1993.

Wright CD, et al: Superior sulcus lung tumors: results of combined treatment (irradiation and radical resection). J Thorac Cardiovasc Surg *94*:69, 1987.

Williams DE, et al: Survival of patients surgically treated for stage I lung cancer. J Thorac Cardiovasc Surg *82*:70, 1981.

Yano T, et al: Surgical results and prognostic factors of pathologic N1 disease in non-small cell carcinoma of the lung. J Thorac Cardiovasc Surg *107*:1398, 1994.

Yoshino I, et al: Postoperative prognosis in patients with non-small cell lung cancer with synchronous ipsilateral intrapulmonary metastasis. Ann Thorac Surg *64*:809, 1997.

CHAPTER 100

Mediastinal Lymph Node Dissection

Tsuguo Naruke

The basic controversy surrounding the necessity of complete mediastinal lymph node dissection or systematic nodal dissection for lung cancer is similar to the controversy related to the need for and efficacy of lymph node dissection in tumors of other organ systems. The resection of the primary lesion, including the regional lymph nodes en bloc—systematic nodal dissection—is the universally accepted surgical treatment for patients with potentially curable localized lung cancer.

The four major arguments against complete mediastinal lymph node dissection are as follows: 1) systemic nature of the cancer (cancer has spread outside of the thoracic cavity), 2) complete dissection (difficulty of 100% removal of all lymph nodes), 3) effect on the immune system (removal of normal lymph nodes may reduce normal immunologic resistance), and 4) surgical risk (increased surgical risk has not been justified by improved patient prognosis).

The four basic arguments supporting complete dissection are as follows: 1) microscopic identification—the only method to verify the true stage of the lung cancer; 2) postoperative treatment plan; reliable staging information produces a more effective treatment plan; 3) surgical risk—complete lymph node dissection does not always increase operative risk, operative mortality, or postoperative quality of life; and 4) survival rates—many surgeons report increased survival rates when complete dissection is performed. Reports on the results in patients with N_2 non–small cell lung cancers that have undergone complete resection have been published by the following authors: Naruke (1967, 1976, 1993), Smith (1978), Kirschner (1981), Mountain (1985), Goldstraw (1994), Levasseur and Regnard (1990), Pearson (1982), Martini (1983), Rubinstein (1979), Watanabe (1991a, 1991b), Maggi (1993), Miller (1994), Izbicki (1994, 1995, 1998), and Riquet (1995) and their colleagues.

The standard surgical procedure for patients with lung cancer is either lobectomy or pneumonectomy combined with mediastinal lymph node dissection. Cases in which the lobe or lung containing the primary lesion has been resected and mediastinal lymph nodes have been dissected are termed by the author as *radical* or complete operations. A term of systematic nodal dissection was recommended for use and accepted in the International Workshop on Intrathoracic Staging. Cases in which mediastinal lymph node resection has been performed incompletely are termed *palliative* or noncurative operations.*

With a complete mediastinal lymph node dissection, not only ipsilateral mediastinal lymph nodes but also the contralateral lymph nodes can be dissected on the right side by a standard right posterolateral thoracotomy. A bilateral lymph node resection cannot be performed on the left side by standard left thoracotomy; it is necessary, depending on the site and presence of ipsilateral mediastinal lymph node metastases, to perform a contralateral lymph node dissection by mobilization of the aortic arch or with an additional median sternotomy in selected cases.

SITES AND NOMENCLATURE OF LYMPH NODES

Although many reports have been presented in the past on the topography of the mediastinal lymph nodes and on the usual routes of lymphatic spread, no standard terminology had been accepted for the location of the various mediastinal and bronchopulmonary lymph nodes, and thus it was difficult to clinically record the sites of nodal metastases. The author (1967), based on a large number of lymph node dissections combined with lung resection for lung cancer and using the many basic studies of Rouviére (1932), Borrie (1952), Nohl (1956, 1962), and Cahan (1960), among others, suggested a nomenclature for the mapping of the sites of the intrathoracic lymph nodes. This system of lymph node mapping was subsequently recommended by the American Joint Committee (AJCC) in 1976, and its use has been sup-

---

*Senior Editor's Note: This terminology is used widely in Japan for complete and noncurative (incomplete) resections. As I have noted (1989), however, a resection should be termed *incomplete* only if histologic proof has been obtained that residual disease remains in the hemithorax.

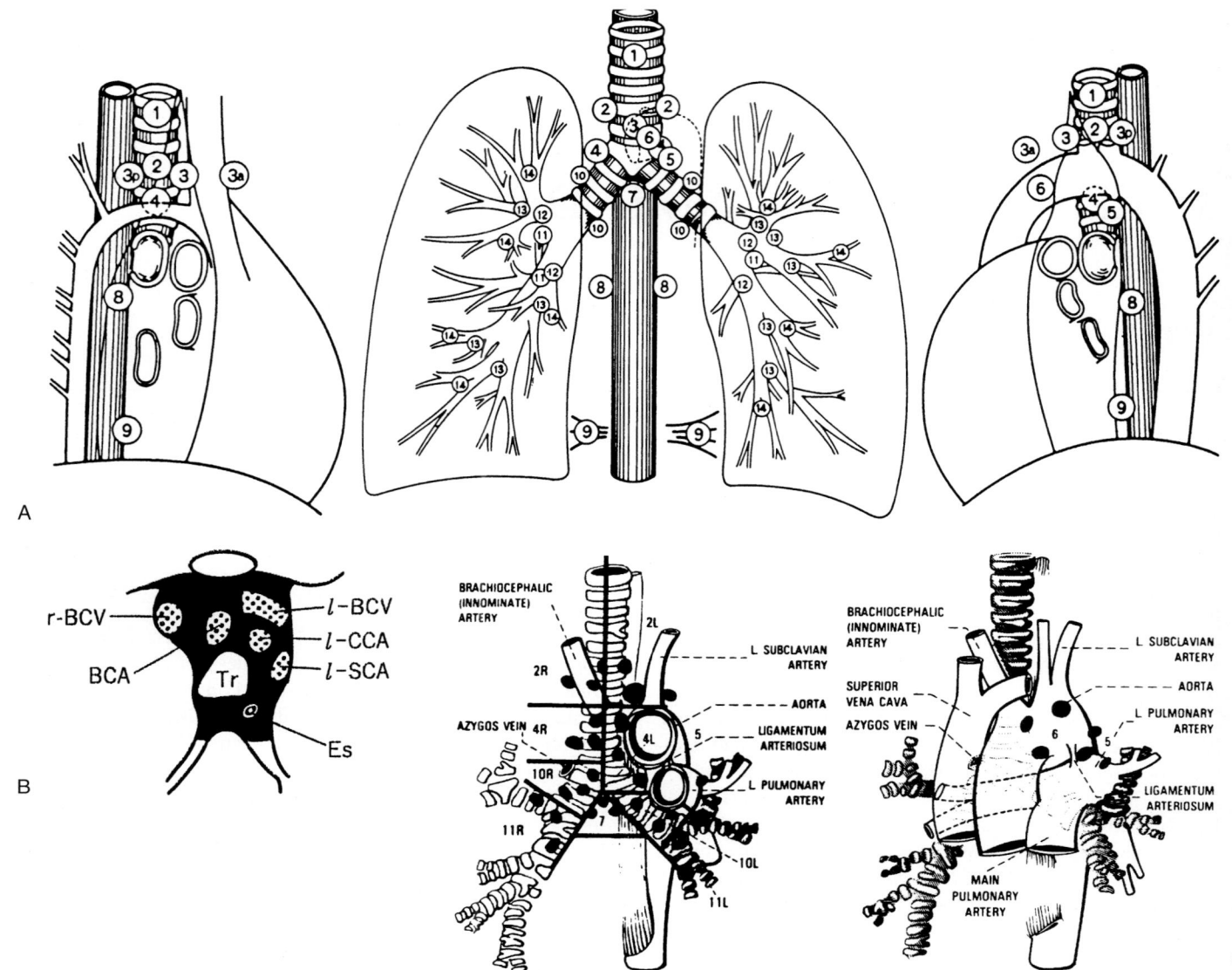

Fig. 100-1. A. Lymph node map (American Joint Committee/Union Internationale Contre le Cancer/Japan Lung Cancer Society) and numeric designations for the mediastinal and bronchopulmonary stations. 1, Superior mediastinal or highest mediastinal; 2, paratracheal; 3, pretracheal, retrotracheal, or posterior mediastinal (3p), and anterior mediastinal (3a); 4, tracheobronchial; 5, subaortic or Botello's; 6, para-aortic, ascending aorta; 7, subcarinal; 8, paraesophageal below carina; 9, pulmonary ligament; 10, hilar; 11, interlobar; 12, lobar, upper lobe middle lobe and lower lobe; 13, segmental; 14, subsegmental. **B.** Sites of lymph nodes on computed tomographic scan (American Joint Committee/Union Internationale Contre le Cancer/Japan Lung Cancer Society). BCA, brachiocephalic artery; BCV, brachiocephalic vein; CCA, common carotid artery; ES, esophagus; l, left; r, right; SCA, subclavian artery; Tr, trachea. **C.** Lymph node map (American Thoracic Society/Lung Cancer Study Group of North America) recommended by the Lung Cancer Study Group of North America.

ported by the reports of Mountain (1976) and Martini (1976). These reports of the classification of lung cancer were in agreement for the graphic representation of the operative findings with the suggested TNM classification of malignant tumors by Union Internationale Contre le Cancer (UICC). The mediastinal lymph node map used here has been authorized and used by the Committee of the Japan

Lung Cancer Society (JLCS) in accordance with the General Rule for Clinical and Pathological Record of Lung Cancer (1987) since 1980 (Fig. 100-1).

On the other hand, the American Thoracic Society (ATS), using transverse section anatomy as defined by computed tomography and viewed at thoracotomy, developed a regional lymph node staging map reported by Tisi and associates (1983) that modified the AJCC/UICC/JLCS map, which was further revised by the Lung Cancer Study Group of North America (LCSG) (Fig. 100-1C). The important difference between the two classifications exists in recognizing the location of station 10. In the ATS/LCSG map, station 10 represents mediastinal lymph nodes. In the AJCC/UICC/JLCS map, station 10 represents hilar lymph nodes. Therefore, when labeling station 10 lymph nodes, it is important to specify whether the ATS/LCSG map or the AJCC/UICC/JLCS map is being used. Station 10 should be recognized as hilar lymph node and belongs to the N_1 group, as clearly indicated in a prognostic study of the National Cancer Center Hospital. A modified map has been introduced by Mountain (1997); however, its final approval is still to be obtained.

The sites of mediastinal lymph node stations and their designation as used by the author are as follows:*

No. 1, the superior mediastinal lymph nodes: The superior nodes are present about the upper third of that part of the trachea within the thorax. These include the nodes located around the trachea, the site of which is defined by a horizontal line at the height of the upper rim of the subclavian artery and a horizontal line at the center point of the trachea, where the upper rim of the brachiocephalic vein ascends to the left, crossing in front of the trachea. Thus, they are located from the level of the apex of the lung along the level where the left brachiocephalic vein intersects the tracheal midsagittal line.

No. 2, the paratracheal lymph nodes: The nodes located between stations 1 and 4 lateral to the trachea, and caudal to station 1, excluding the intersection of the left brachiocephalic vein and the tracheal midline, and cranial to the azygos vein, excluding the section around the azygos vein, where the center of the lymph nodes is located between the anterior and posterior wall lines of the trachea.

No. 3a, the anterior mediastinal lymph nodes: The nodes located caudal to station 1 while the center of the lymph nodes is located on the front side of the superior vena cava, the anterior wall line of the ascending aorta.

No. 3, the pretracheal lymph nodes: The nodes are located caudal to station 1 and cranial to the right main pulmonary artery, which is on the right side of the left line of the aorta where the center of the lymph nodes is located either on the front side of the tracheal anterior wall line or behind the anterior wall line of the superior vena cava. Within this area, the lymph nodes above the aortic arch and on the left of the left subclavian artery as well as the left common carotid artery are classified as No. 6.

No. 3p, the retrotracheal lymph nodes: The nodes are located caudal to station 1 and cranial to the tracheal bifurcation, and the center of lymph nodes is located behind the tracheal posterior line.

No. 4, the tracheobronchial lymph nodes: The nodes located along the angle between the trachea and the main bronchus, and caudal to the arch of the azygos vein, including the area around the arch of the azygos vein, and the center of lymph nodes is located between the anterior and posterior wall lines of the trachea, and similarly, on the right side of the left line of the aorta, which is on the left side of the arch of azygos vein, and adjacent to the carina. Note that although the center of lymph node is located within the area of the left No. 4, those nodes located obviously away from the trachea are classified as No. 5.

No. 5, the subaortic lymph nodes: The nodes are located between the aortic arch and the left pulmonary artery, which is behind the posterior wall line of the ascending aorta where the center of lymph nodes is located on the left side of the left line of aorta.

No. 6, the para-aortic lymph nodes: The nodes are located on the left side of the ascending aorta and the aortic arch where the center of lymph nodes is located between the anterior, posterior wall lines of the ascending aorta, and anterior to the vagus nerve.

No. 7, the subcarinal lymph nodes: The nodes are located adjacent to the lower part of the tracheal bifurcation, and the center of lymph nodes is located behind the anterior wall line of the main bronchus. Those adjacent to either the left and the right main bronchus, or the mediastinal aspect of the intermediate bronchus, and those without a relationship to the lower part of the tracheal bifurcation are classified as No. 10.

No. 8, the paraesophageal lymph nodes: The nodes are located caudad to the tracheal bifurcation (i.e., the area where the right and the left main bronchi are apart), and adjacent to the esophagus but away from the bronchus.

No. 9, the pulmonary ligament lymph nodes: The nodes located caudal to the inferior pulmonary vein.

No. 10, lymph nodes just distal to the trachea and extending along the length of the main stem bronchi: These nodes are also referred to as hilar lymph nodes.

No. 11, interlobar lymph nodes and those present between the lobar bronchi: On the right side, when these nodes have to be specified, these nodes are classified as existing between the upper and middle lobes (11s) and as existing between the middle and lower lobes (11i).

No. 12, lymph nodes present around a lobar bronchus.

No. 13, lymph nodes are located along a segmental bronchus.

No. 14, lymph nodes present around a subsegmental bronchus or distal to this site.

ANESTHESIA

General anesthesia using a double-lumen endobronchial tube is the standard procedure for pulmonary resections with

---

*When unsure whether a lymph node should be placed into either one or two contiguous lymph node stations, classify it as being located in the station with the smaller numerical number (e.g., in the case of either station 2 or 3, categorize it as being a No. 2 node, in the case of station 7 or 8 place it in station 7, or in the case of station 3a or 3, classify it as being a No. 3 node. In determining whether a node is on the right or left in station 1, use the tracheal midsagittal line. In station 3a, use the anterior mediastinal midline. In stations 3p and 3, use the esophageal midline. The nodes along the left main pulmonary artery are classified as station left 10.

mediastinal lymph node dissection. After the endotracheal tube has been inserted into the trachea, the position of the tube is confirmed by visualization with the bronchofiberscope (3.0-mm diameter Olympus Bf type 3C), and the tube is then fixed in place. Whenever the patient's position is changed, the location of the endotracheal tube is rechecked for proper positioning.

POSITION OF PATIENT

The patient is placed in the appropriate complete lateral decubitus position and a standard posterolateral thoracotomy is carried out. The skin incision is started at the midpoint between the thoracic vertebral column and the medial edge of the scapula at the level of the third rib. It is extended to the point at the inferior angle of the scapula in a loose arc, continued as far as the fifth costal cartilage, and extended to the anterior axillary line or farther forward. The chest wall muscles are incised by electroknife in the same line as the skin incision. The pleural space is entered through the fourth intercostal space. The fourth and fifth ribs are partially dissected for a length of 1.5 to 2.0 cm just proximal to the vertebrae, and a section of each rib is excised. The fifth rib is also cut at its junction with the anterior cartilage.

In patients with cancer in the right lung, it is possible to perform a dissection of the potentially involved left contralateral mediastinal lymph nodes combined with a complete dissection of the right ipsilateral mediastinal lymph nodes with the standard right posterolateral thoracotomy. In patients with cancer in the left lung, however, a contralateral lymph node dissection cannot be performed by the standard left thoracotomy for anatomic reasons.

As a standard approach in patients with cancer in the left lung, a left posterolateral thoracotomy may be used if only an ipsilateral mediastinal lymph node dissection is contemplated. A median sternotomy also may be used, but it has disadvantages, as is noted. If a bilateral lymph node dissection is indicated, a median sternotomy with a left anterior intercostal incision may be used or the sternotomy may be combined with a standard left posterolateral thoracotomy.

When a left lung resection is combined with mediastinal lymph node dissection by a median sternotomy only, the disadvantage is that a complete dissection of the subcarinal lymph nodes and of the posterior mediastinal lymph nodes can be difficult to perform. Likewise, a left lower lobectomy is difficult to accomplish readily. Therefore, this incision alone is not recommended.

In patients with cancer in the left lung, frequent metastases are found in the subaortic (No. 5) and the para-aortic (No. 6) lymph nodes. Therefore, the initial procedure to perform for the mediastinal lymph node dissection is a standard left posterolateral thoracotomy with the patient in the right lateral decubitus position. In patients with metastases present in either the tracheobronchial (No. 4) or the subcarinal (No. 7) lymph nodes, or both, however, it is logical to assume the potential presence of metastases in the lymph nodes in the contralateral mediastinum. Because squamous cell carcinomas have a tendency toward localized locoregional growth only, in some cases, the lymphatic route is the major source of spread of disease. Therefore, it is essential to identify possible metastases to the tracheobronchial (No. 4) and the subcarinal (No. 7) lymph nodes by frozen section diagnosis during the operation. When metastases have been identified in these areas, it is then important to perform a more complete contralateral lymph node dissection by the addition of a median sternotomy in these selected cases. In cases in which systematic lymph node dissection is to be performed, the alternative methods to a standard posterolateral thoracotomy include muscle-sparing posterolateral thoracotomy as recommended by Bethencourt and Holmes (1988), modified muscle-sparing posterolateral thoracotomy as described by Ashour (1990), lateral thoracotomy, or video-assisted thoracic surgical lobectomy.

MEDIASTINAL LYMPH NODE DISSECTION

Timing

A principle of lung cancer surgery should be the ligation of the pulmonary vein first, followed by en bloc dissection of the mediastinum and hilum together with the lung, without interrupting lymphatic channels during the dissection. Particularly in cases in which nodal enlargement suggests metastases extending from the hilar lymph nodes to mediastinal lymph nodes, the lymphatic channels should not be incised during the dissection. The order of the operative procedure should be changed appropriately during the operation, however, depending on the site and size of the tumor as well as its extent. When the pulmonary lobes in the diseased lung obscure the visual field, the accuracy of dissection is lowered. The basic rule is to vary the standard procedure as necessary, but nonetheless perform a complete dissection even though it may take longer to complete the operation than is usually required.

Technique

Dissection of the mediastinal lymph nodes is carried out with scissors and electroknife to excise en bloc the fatty tissues of the hilum and mediastinum that contain the lymph nodes while completely exposing all structures and walls of the organs present within the hilum and mediastinum. As noted, the lung, including the fatty alveolar tissues and lymph nodes, are to be dissected en bloc.

Before starting the mediastinal dissection, the pulmonary ligament is separated from the mediastinal pleura adjacent anteriorly and posteriorly to it. The mediastinal pleura inferior to the hilum is then separated from the fatty tissue adjacent to the esophagus. For the dissection of the superior mediastinum, the mediastinal pleura is incised vertically from the upper edge of the hilar pleura, just below the azygos vein, to the apex of the thorax and opened and retracted away from the mediastinal structures by retraction sutures. The vagus and phrenic nerves are identified, taped, and preserved carefully.

Fatty tissues including the lymph nodes, held by a lymph node forceps or Allis' intestinal forceps, are separated gently to expose the arteries, veins, trachea, bronchi, esophagus, and the aforementioned nerves. At all times, it is necessary to be careful not to damage the lymph nodes but to dissect free the adipose tissue enclosing the lymph nodes. The adipose tissues are grasped by the forceps without grasping the lymph nodes. When lymph nodes are squeezed, cancer cells can spread into the operated field; therefore, the nodes should not be grasped during the procedure. It is necessary to ligate any small blood vessels and to cauterize small lymphatic channels by electroknife to prevent postoperative bleeding and exudation of lymphatic fluid into the hemithorax postoperatively.

Patients with Carcinoma of the Right Lung

Right Upper Lobectomy

When a right upper lobectomy is performed, I prefer initially to stand at the back of the patient and to move to the front after the thoracotomy incision has been completed. The hilar pleura is opened anteriorly just posterior to the phrenic nerve and the phrenic nerve is then isolated, taped, and retracted to prevent injury to it. Next, the fatty tissues and contained lymph nodes are dissected off of the pericardium from the site of the pleural incision toward the hilum to expose the superior pulmonary vein. The superior pulmonary vein, except for its branch from the middle lobe, is isolated, ligated, and divided. After this maneuver, the azygos vein can be divided, or this step can be done after the upper mediastinal dissection has been completed, depending on feasibility at the respective times.

The tracheobronchial lymph nodes (No. 4) are present on the medial side, the undersurface, of the azygos vein, and when the cancer is located in the right upper lobe, these No. 4 nodes, as well as the pretracheal lymph nodes (No. 3), are frequently involved by metastatic disease. When it is suspected by the gross appearance of these nodes that they are involved, the azygos vein is not divided at its middle but is divided proximally as it enters the superior vena cava and distally as it turns anteriorly from its location on the vertebral bodies. That portion of the azygos vein overlying the tracheobronchial lymph nodes (No. 4) is thus left attached to this nodal group, and a combined excision of the azygos vein and tracheobronchial lymph nodes is performed.

The lung is next retracted anteriorly to expose the posterior aspect of the hilum and the pleura is incised posterior to the hilar structures. The vagus nerve is exposed and taped.

The pulmonary branch or branches of the vagus nerve are divided. Next, an intestinal flexible ribbon retractor is placed beneath the bifurcation of the trachea and the area is exposed, taking care to avoid injury to the descending aorta. The contralateral left main stem bronchial lymph nodes (No. 10, left) are brought to the midline by the use of a lymph node forceps and dissection of the subcarinal lymph nodes (No. 7) is started. A branch of the bronchial artery, which runs from the tracheal bifurcation to the posterior wall of the right main bronchus, is ligated and divided. The medial side of the left main stem bronchus is exposed as it ascends toward the tracheal bifurcation. Along with the contralateral left main stem bronchial lymph nodes (No. 10, left), the subcarinal lymph nodes (No. 7), the right main stem bronchial lymph nodes (No. 10, right), and the right upper lobe bronchial lymph nodes (No. 12) are dissected en bloc from the surrounding structures. It is readily seen during the dissection that these lymph nodes are in direct continuity with each other (Figs. 100-2 and 100-3).

The next step is separation of the interlobar fissure, and then the posterior ascending artery is isolated, ligated, and divided. The lymph nodes present between the lobes are dissected free from the pulmonary artery in continuity with the upper lobe. The lymphatic sump area located in the area

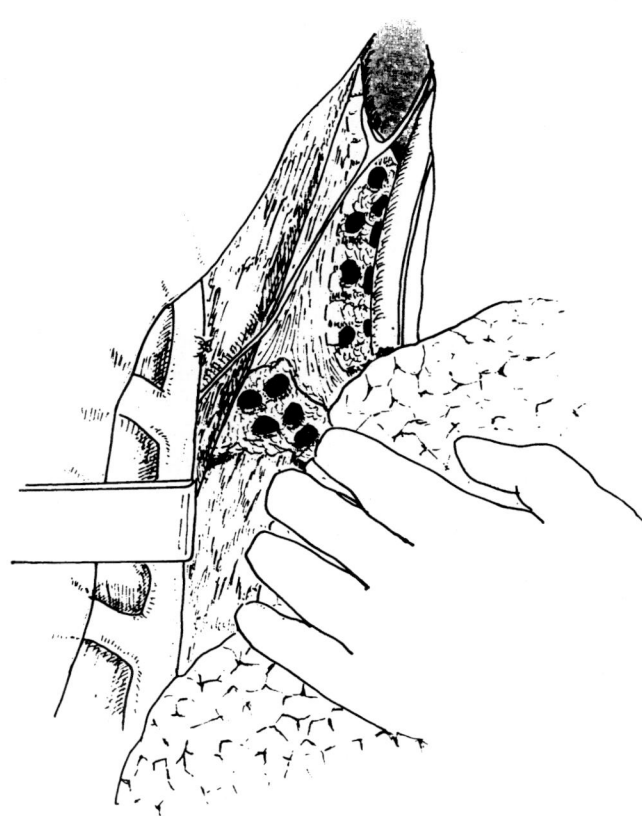

Fig. 100-2. Exposure of the subcarinal area during a right upper lobectomy by retraction of lung toward the operator at the front of the patient.

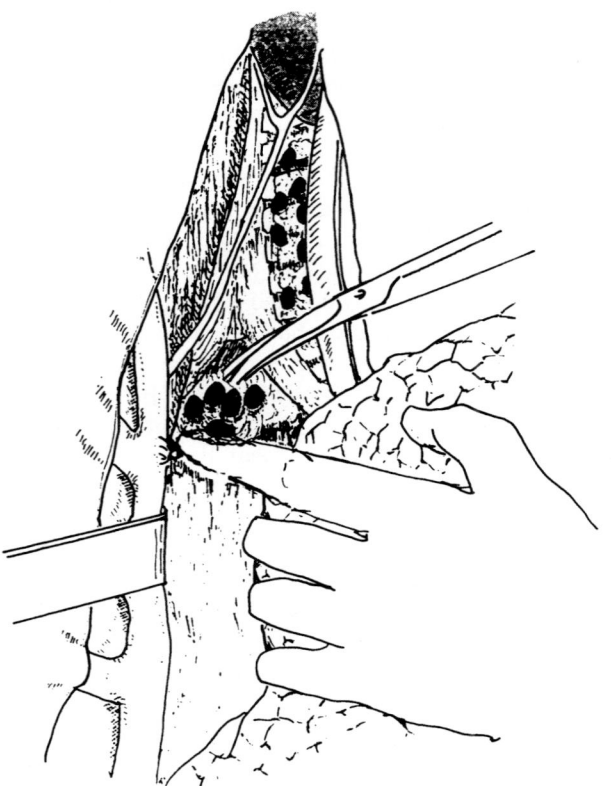

Fig. 100-3. Sharp scissors dissection of the subcarinal fat pad containing the subcarinal (No. 7) lymph nodes.

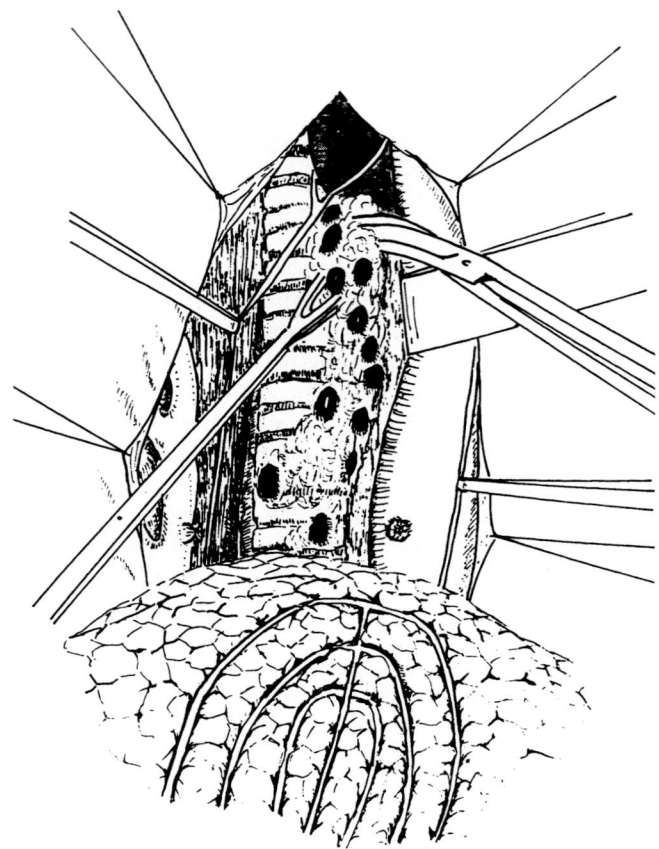

Fig. 100-4. Beginning dissection of the superior mediastinal lymph nodes at the level of the right subclavian artery.

between the upper lobe bronchus, middle lobe bronchus, and the superior segmental branch of the lower lobe bronchus contains regional lymph nodes (No. 11s) that receive lymphatic drainage from the upper lobe. It is necessary to dissect and to remove these nodes as completely as possible together with the peribronchial lymph nodes (No. 12) of the upper lobe bronchus.

When it is suspected that the dissection of superior interlobar lymph nodes (No. 11s) might be incomplete when only a right lobectomy is carried out in some cases of a right upper lobe tumor, a more complete dissection of these nodes, as well as of the peribronchial lymph nodes (No. 12), may be accomplished by a right upper and middle bilobectomy. Furthermore, if the sump area contains large, involved lymph nodes and the bronchus or pulmonary artery, or both, have been infiltrated by metastatic disease from the involved lymph nodes or by the tumor itself, a pneumonectomy is indicated.

When the dissection of the subcarinal, hilar, and peribronchial lymph nodes is completed, the surgeon should move to the opposite (back) side of the patient. When division of the azygos vein has not been performed previously, it is now exposed and ligated. The vein is then transfixed and divided. As noted previously, a part of the azygos vein may be left attached to underlying tracheobronchial lymph nodes (No. 4) and removed together with the lymph nodes at the completion of the dissection.

The mediastinal pleura is then opened from the upper edge of the hilar pleura upward toward the apex of the thorax. Sutures are placed through either edge of the opened upper mediastinal pleura at four points, and the pleural incision is held open by traction on these sutures to expose the superior aspect of mediastinum above the hilum.

The pleura is incised further cephalad to the level of the upper edge of the subclavian artery. The right recurrent nerve is identified and protected from injury. The wall of the subclavian artery is exposed and the superior mediastinal lymph nodes (No. 1) and the adjacent fatty tissue are dissected free from the mediastinal structures. The right brachiocephalic vein is retracted anteriorly with an intestinal flexible ribbon retractor. The adipose tissues located at the highest level of the anterior and the right lateral surfaces of the trachea are grasped with lymph node forceps or Allis' intestinal forceps and retracted toward the operator, and sharp dissection is performed to free this tissue and any contained lymph nodes from this portion of the trachea (Figs. 100-4 and 100-5). To prevent postoperative lymphatic leaks or bleeding, ligation or electrocauterization of all cut vascular or lymphatic vessels is done as completely as possible. The right vagus nerve is exposed, starting at the level of the takeoff of the recurrent nerve. Then, the right lateral wall of the esophagus and right

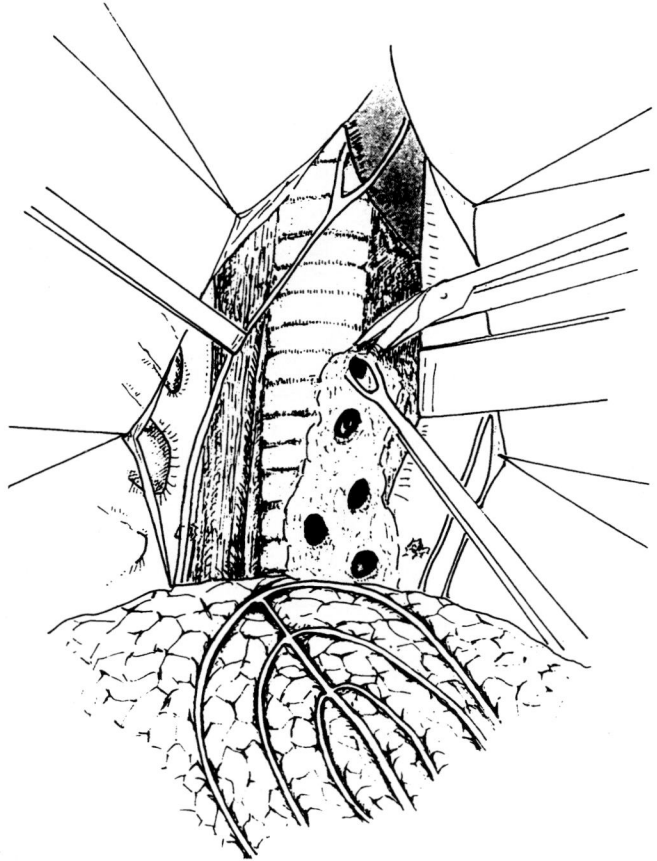

Fig. 100-5. Continued downward dissection along the anterolateral wall of the trachea with the retraction of the superior vena cava anteriorly to free the paratracheal (No. 2) lymph nodes.

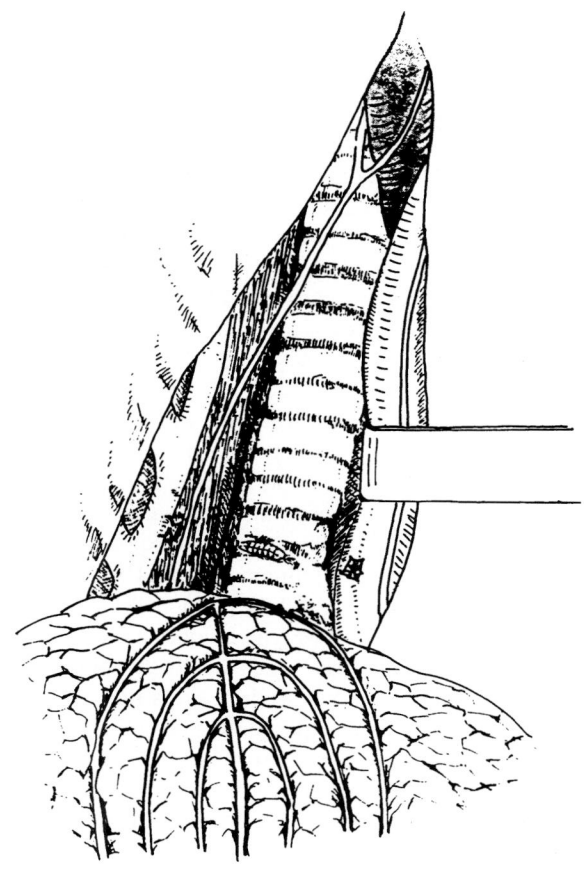

Fig. 100-6. Status of the superior mediastinal area after complete dissection and removal of the right upper lobe. Proximal and distal ligated ends of the azygos vein are clearly seen.

lateral wall of the trachea are exposed. The adipose tissue, including the contained lymph nodes existing at the highest site (No. 1), are held by lymph node forceps and the dissection is continued downward toward the hilum. A few thin venous branches from the right brachiocephalic vein and superior vena cava are usually present; these branches are ligated and divided. The intestinal flexible ribbon retractor is slid downward a little and inserted between the trachea and the right brachiocephalic vein near its junction with the superior vena cava. At the bottom of this site, the ascending brachiocephalic artery is identified. Because the right wall of the ascending aorta is further caudal, the dissection is carried down along the aforementioned arterial branch until the wall of the aorta is exposed.

The pretracheal lymph nodes (No. 3), which, as noted, are located where the upper edge of the left brachiocephalic vein crosses the anterior aspect of the trachea, are then dissected in continuity with the tissues already freed from above. The lymph nodes at this site are numerous and metastasis to these nodes in patients with cancer in the right upper lobe occurs frequently; only the tracheobronchial lymph nodes (No. 4) and the paratracheal lymph nodes (No. 2) are more prone to metastatic involvement.

The retrotracheal (No. 3p) lymph nodes are then freed and the paratracheal (No. 2) nodes along with previously dissected fatty tissue and lymph nodes from above are dissected away from the tracheal wall and the posterior wall of the lower portion of the superior vena cava. The dissection is continued down to and including the superior tracheobronchial (No. 4) lymph nodes and attached section of the azygos vein when these latter lymph nodes are enlarged, thus completing the superior mediastinal lymph node dissection.

Next, the right pulmonary artery is exposed and the upper lobectomy combined with dissection of the mediastinal lymph nodes is completed by the following procedure. The right upper lobe artery (the truncus anterior) is isolated, ligated, and divided. The lymph nodes attached to the anterior aspect of the upper lobe bronchus are dissected in continuity with the tracheobronchial lymph nodes (No. 4), which have been freed previously (Fig. 100-6). The dissection is completed by isolation, division, and closure of the right upper lobe bronchus. In patients with cancer in the upper lobe, it is not necessary to perform a dissection of the paraesophageal (No. 8) lymph nodes, but the pulmonary ligament lymph nodes (No. 9) are removed with the specimen.

Middle Lobectomy

In patients with a cancer in the middle lobe, a bilobectomy of the middle and upper lobes or of the middle and lower lobes is performed, depending on the extent of metastasis to the interlobar lymph nodes (No. 11s or 11i). Pneumonectomy is carried out as necessitated by the extent of the spread of metastasis to the lymph nodes or the direct extent of the primary tumor. The mediastinal lymph node dissection is essentially the same as that carried out for upper lobe tumors.

Right Lower Lobectomy

For excision of the right lower lobe, the author stands at the back of the patient. After opening the right side of the chest and freeing any adhesions as necessary, the mediastinal pleura is incised just anterior to the pulmonary ligament, as well as posterior to it. The esophagus is exposed from the diaphragm up to the inferior pulmonary vein. Dissection continues in a superior direction and the pulmonary ligament and paraesophageal (Nos. 9 and 8) lymph nodes are dissected en bloc with the adjacent fatty tissue up to the inferior pulmonary vein. The pleura behind the vein is incised and the inferior pulmonary vein is exposed, ligated, and divided.

The surgeon now moves to the front of the patient and the esophagus is retracted posteriorly by an intestinal flexible ribbon retractor placed at the level of the bifurcation of the trachea. The lung is retracted anteriorly toward the surgeon's side and the bifurcation of the trachea is exposed. Dissection of lymph nodes at the bifurcation of the trachea (No. 7) is performed first and then the nodes present along the right main stem bronchus (No. 10, right) are dissected down to the lower lobe. Next, the major interlobar fissure is opened using an electroknife to expose the bronchovascular structures. The interlobar lymph nodes (Nos. 11s and 11i) and the lymph nodes clustered around the lower lobe bronchus are dissected free, along with the previously dissected lymph nodes at the bifurcation of the trachea and the peribronchial lymph nodes of the right main bronchus. The pulmonary artery branch or branches to the lower lobe are isolated, ligated, and divided. Next, the lower lobe bronchus is divided and the proximal stump is closed. Then, the lymph node dissection of the upper mediastinum is performed as previously described.

Right Pneumonectomy

The technical steps of a right pneumonectomy are taken in the order of the dissection of the inferior mediastinum, ligation and division of the inferior and superior pulmonary veins, dissection of the bifurcation of the trachea, dissection of the upper mediastinum, ligation and division of the pulmonary artery, and finally the division and closure of the right main stem bronchus. The area of dissection of the lymph nodes present in the hilum and mediastinum when a right pneumonectomy is performed is shown in Figure 100-7.

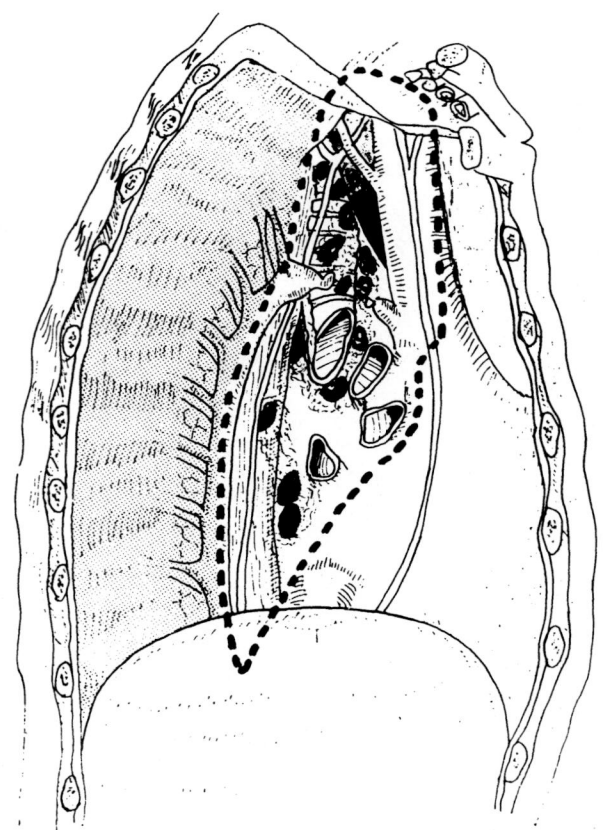

Fig. 100-7. View of the right side of the mediastinum. Outline denotes the region of dissection of the right hilum and mediastinum with contained hilar and mediastinal structures exposed during right pneumonectomy.

Patients with Carcinoma of the Left Lung

Left Upper Lobectomy

For a left upper lobectomy, the surgeon moves to the front side of the patient after performing the thoracotomy incision into the pleural space. The mediastinal pleura is incised anterior to the hilum. The phrenic nerve is identified and taped. Lymph nodes in the region of the pulmonary vein are dissected from the anterior aspect of the pericardium toward the pulmonary side of the superior pulmonary vein. The superior pulmonary vein is isolated, ligated, and divided.

The lung is retracted anteriorly toward the surgeon, and dissection of subcarinal lymph nodes (No. 7) is started. First, the vagus nerve is isolated and taped. The descending aorta and esophagus are retracted posteriorly by an intestinal flexible ribbon retractor and the bifurcation of the trachea is exposed (Fig. 100-8). The bronchus is exposed from the inferior border of the upper lobar bronchus toward the main bronchus. Lymph nodes about the left upper lobar bronchus are mobilized and the dissection is continued distally on the bronchus to the area of the bifurcation of the bronchus

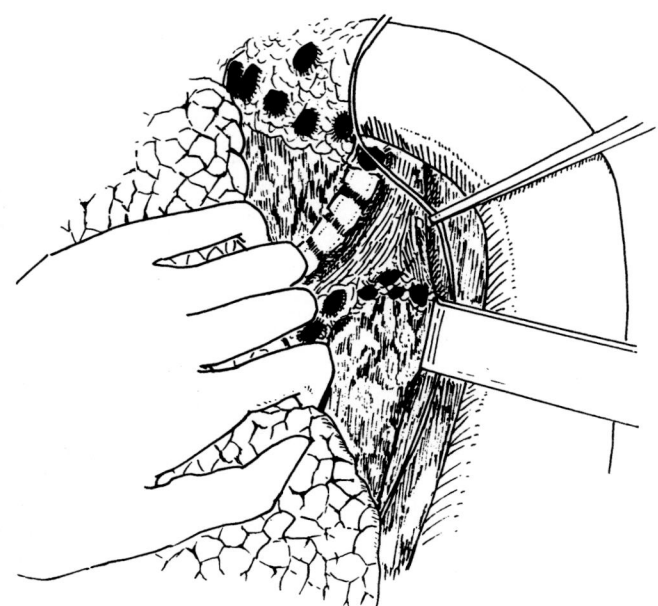

Fig. 100-8. Exposure of the subcarinal area from the left side after division of the inferior pulmonary vein. Retraction of the left lung anteriorly and the esophagus posteriorly permits the operative exposure of the carina and both the right and left main stem bronchi.

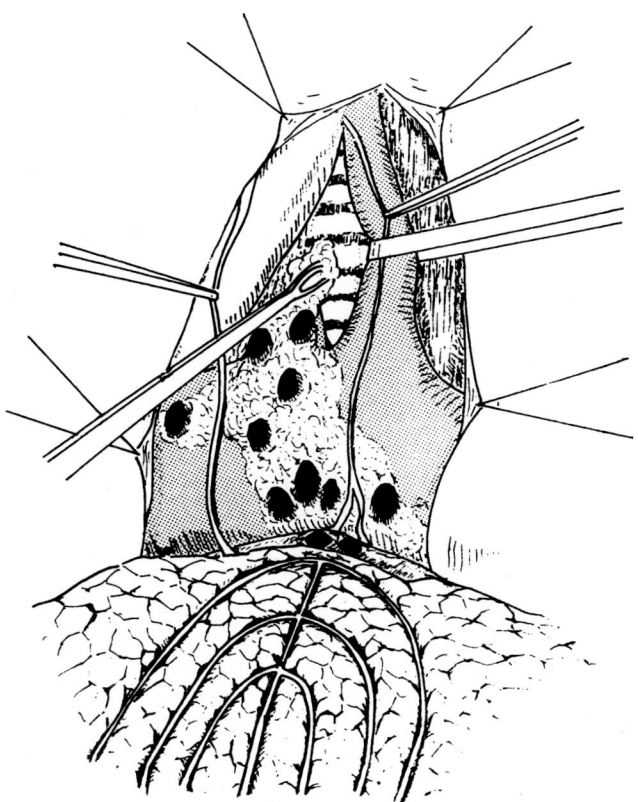

Fig. 100-9. Exposure of the left superior mediastinal and paratracheal lymph nodes during a standard left thoracotomy by retraction of the left common carotid artery posteriorly and the left brachiocephalic vein anteriorly.

between the upper and lower lobes (the left lymphatic sump). The pulmonary branches of the vagus nerve are ligated and divided. With completion of these steps, the visual field of the tracheal bifurcation is increased by further retraction of the left lung toward the surgeon by use of the left hand or a lung retractor. Lymph nodes are dissected away from the inferior surface of the right main bronchus (No. 10, right), then the subcarinal lymph nodes (No. 7) are dissected free, and lastly, the left bronchial hilar lymph nodes (No. 10, left) are mobilized. It is necessary at the site of the bifurcation of the trachea to ligate and divide the branch of the left bronchial artery. The dissection of the sump lymph nodes between the upper lobe and lower lobe bronchus is completed after division of the interlobar fissure and the lobes have been separated. The branches of the pulmonary artery are ligated and divided from below upward, but all of the arterial branches may not be divided at this stage.

Next, the upper mediastinal pleura is incised as far as the apex of the thorax, and the phrenic and vagus nerves are identified and taped. Four retraction sutures are placed in the cut edges of the mediastinal pleura. The hemiazygos vein is identified, isolated, ligated, and divided. Anteriorly, the thymic fatty tissue is identified and the pericardium is reached when this adipose tissue is dissected free. The ascending aorta is exposed and the para-aortic (No. 6) lymph nodes are dissected from the aortic wall. The dissection is carried toward the main pulmonary artery in the hilum. The left brachiocephalic vein is also exposed. Now, a portion of the anterior mediastinal fat pad containing the anterior mediastinal (No. 3a) lymph nodes can be dissected.

The left common carotid and the left subclavian arteries are exposed at the apex of the thorax and caudad dissection of the fatty tissue containing the lymph nodes is carried out. The superior mediastinal (No. 1) and paratracheal (No. 2) lymph nodes are dissected as shown in Figure 100-9. The left superior mediastinal lymph nodes (No. 1), as on the right, are the nodes present at the apex to the level where the upper edge of the brachiocephalic vein crosses the midline of the trachea; the lymph nodes present below this level on the side of the trachea are the paratracheal lymph nodes (No. 2). The lymph nodes located on the frontal aspect of the left common carotid artery are pretracheal (No. 3) and are also dissected at this time.

The thoracic duct is in the deepest area between the left common carotid artery and the left subclavian artery; however, the thoracic duct, as a rule, cannot be identified. Damage to mediastinal branches of the thoracic duct can result in a postoperative chylothorax. Therefore, all lymphatic channels and fine blood vessels should be ligated and divided. When the left subclavian artery is taped, paratracheal lymph nodes (No. 2) can be dissected more easily. Lymph nodes in the deeper area between the left brachiocephalic vein and left common carotid artery are pretracheal lymph nodes (No. 3). It is impossible to dissect all the nodes on the anterior surface of the trachea with the standard operative procedure of a left thoracotomy; therefore, when dissection in this area is necessary, the aorta should be mobilized and retracted or the dissection of the superior mediastinum should be performed through a median sternotomy. After dissection of the paratracheal and pretracheal nodes, attention is turned to the dissection of the remaining para-aortic and subaortic nodes.

In patients with cancer in the left upper lobe, it is most important to dissect the para-aortic lymph nodes (No. 6) as well as the subaortic lymph nodes (No. 5). The tracheobronchial lymph nodes (No. 4) are located at the medial side of the subaortic lymph nodes, and these nodes can be dissected easily after Botallo's ligament has been ligated and divided.

The remaining, ordinarily the more proximal, pulmonary arteries of the upper lobe, are now isolated, ligated, and divided. After exposing the left upper lobe bronchus together with the dissected nodes, the bronchus is divided. By this procedure, left upper lobectomy combined with mediastinal lymph node dissection has been completed.

When metastases are identified in the subcarinal lymph nodes (No. 7) or the tracheobronchial lymph nodes (No. 4), or both, it is necessary to perform a complete dissection of the superior mediastinal (No. 1), paratracheal (No. 2), pretracheal (No. 3), and posterior mediastinal (No. 3p) lymph nodes. This may be accomplished by one of two procedures. The steps of one of the procedures are to tape the subclavian artery, incise the pleura at the posterior side of the aorta, ligate and divide a few intercostal arteries, and tape the descending aorta. The left subclavian artery and aorta are retracted anteriorly and the left wall of the trachea and esophagus are exposed. The superior mediastinal (No. 1), paratracheal (No. 2), pretracheal (No. 3), and retrotracheal (No. 3p) lymph nodes are more readily dissected with this maneuver (Fig. 100-10). At this time, it is necessary to pay careful attention to avoid damaging the recurrent nerve, which runs upward along the left lateral wall of the trachea. By incision of Botallo's ligament, the tracheobronchial (No. 4) lymph nodes can be dissected easily as previously described. The other option is to move the patient to a supine position and to perform a median sternotomy to carry out a more complete mediastinal lymph node dissection. This operative approach is described subsequently.

Left Lower Lobectomy

When a left lower lobectomy is performed in patients with the primary lesion in the left lower lobe, the surgeon moves to the front of the patient. The pulmonary ligament lymph nodes (No. 9) are freed and the paraesophageal (No. 8) lymph nodes are dissected from about the esophagus from the anterior surface of the descending aorta posteriorly to the pericardial surface anteriorly. These nodes are dissected upward and the inferior pulmonary vein is exposed. The inferior pulmonary vein is then isolated, ligated, and divided. The lung is further retracted anteriorly toward the surgeon

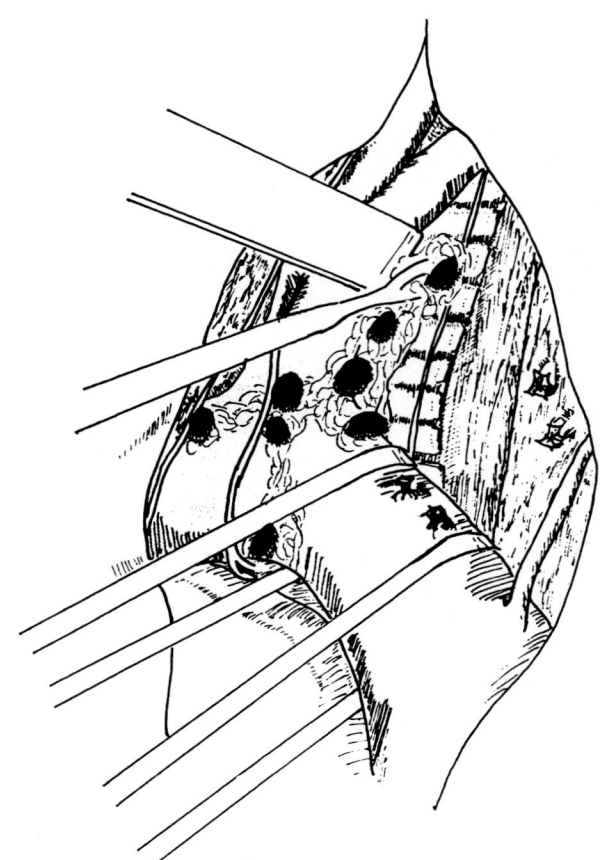

Fig. 100-10. Upper intercostal arteries have been divided and the aorta and the left subclavian and common carotid arteries have been retracted anteriorly to give more complete access to the superior mediastinal (No. 1), the left paratracheal (No. 2), the pretracheal (No. 3), and the retrotracheal (No. 3p) lymph nodes during a standard left thoracotomy incision.

and dissection of the contralateral hilar lymph nodes (No. 10, right), subcarinal lymph nodes (No. 7), and ipsilateral hilar lymph nodes (No. 10, left) is performed. After opening the interlobar fissure, the dissection of the interlobar lymph nodes (No. 11) is accomplished. The lower lobectomy is completed by ligation and division of the pulmonary arterial branches to the lobe and division and closure of the bronchus. In patients with cancer in the left lower lobe, as well as in those patients with metastases to subaortic lymph nodes (No. 5), the subcarinal lymph nodes (No. 7) are frequently involved and must be included in the dissection.

Left Pneumonectomy

When a left pneumonectomy is indicated, the operative steps for dissection of mediastinal lymph nodes are started by the surgeon moving to the front side of the patient after the pleural space is entered. The area of dissection of the hilar and the mediastinal lymph nodes during a left pneumonectomy is shown in Figure 100-11. The pulmonary lig-

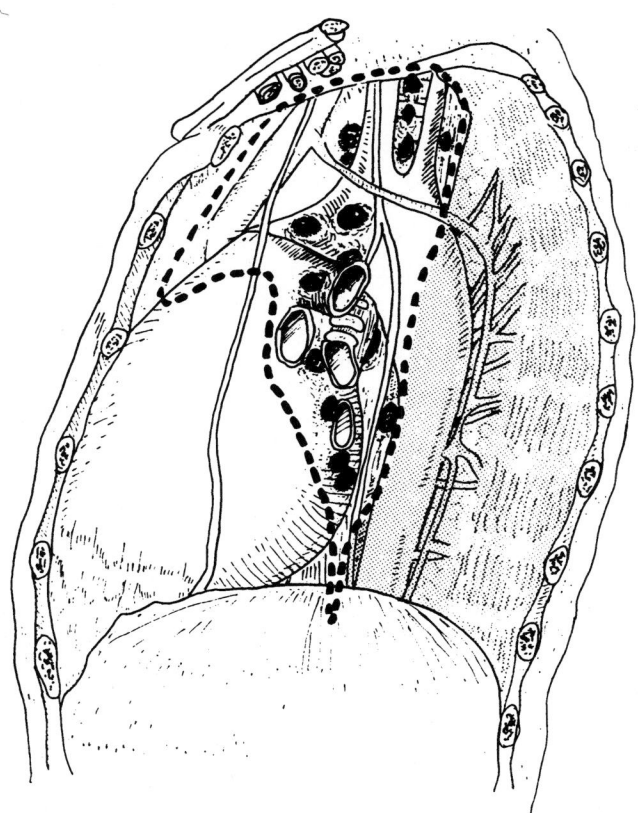

Fig. 100-11. The mediastinum as viewed during a standard left thoracotomy. Outline denotes the region of hilar and mediastinal dissection with contained exposed hilar and mediastinal structures during a left pneumonectomy.

ament lymph nodes (No. 9) and the paraesophageal (No. 8) lymph nodes, as for a lower lobectomy, are dissected and the dissection is continued superiorly as far as the inferior pulmonary vein. This vein is ligated and divided. Next, the superior pulmonary vein is ligated and divided. The mediastinal dissection is then continued as described for a left upper lobectomy. As noted previously, the area of the left upper mediastinum is narrow and its borders are not defined as clearly as are the borders of the right upper mediastinum. The superior mediastinal (No. 1), pretracheal (No. 3), and paratracheal (No. 2) lymph nodes are covered by the aorta and its branches. Therefore, it is not possible to perform a complete dissection of these nodes unless the brachiocephalic vein, aorta, and carotid arteries are retracted. With the nodal dissection completed, the main pulmonary artery is exposed, ligated, and divided. By dividing the left main bronchus, the left pneumonectomy has been accomplished with dissection of the mediastinal lymph nodes en bloc. Of course, the mediastinal lymph node dissection can be performed after the pulmonary resection has been performed. As a rule, however, the lung can usually be collapsed easily, and therefore the operation is not difficult with the lung in place and is recommended as the procedure of choice.

Upper Mediastinal Dissection Via a Median Sternotomy

In patients with cancer of the left lung and metastases in the subcarinal lymph nodes (No. 7) or in the tracheobronchial lymph nodes (No. 4), particularly those persons with squamous cell carcinoma, a more complete dissection of the mediastinum is indicated. This may be performed by accomplishing the dissection via a median sternotomy. In a case of cancer invading from the left main bronchus into the tracheal carina, for which carinal resection should be done, this and the mediastinal lymph node dissection should be performed via a median sternotomy.

The patient is placed supine and a median sternotomy is carried out to improve the dissection of the upper mediastinal lymph nodes. The left brachiocephalic vein is exposed and taped. The right brachiocephalic artery and common carotid artery are taped. Care is needed to avoid damaging the recurrent nerve that is present at the left side of the trachea. Dissection is started precisely underneath the thyroid gland, and the superior mediastinal lymph nodes (No. 1), paratracheal lymph nodes (No. 2) bilaterally, and any pretracheal lymph nodes (No. 3) are dissected en bloc (Fig. 100-12). To expose lymph nodes in the inferior portion of the trachea, the pericardium between the superior vena cava and ascending aorta is incised. The aorta is retracted out of the way by using an intestinal flexible ribbon retractor, and the posterior wall of

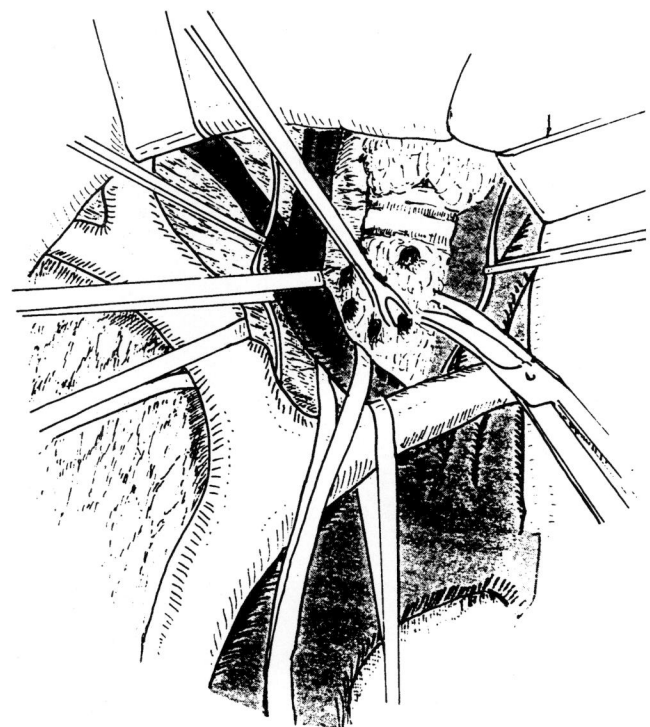

Fig. 100-12. Upper mediastinal lymph node dissection through a median sternotomy. The superior portion of the trachea is exposed by downward retraction of the innominate artery and left brachiocephalic vein.

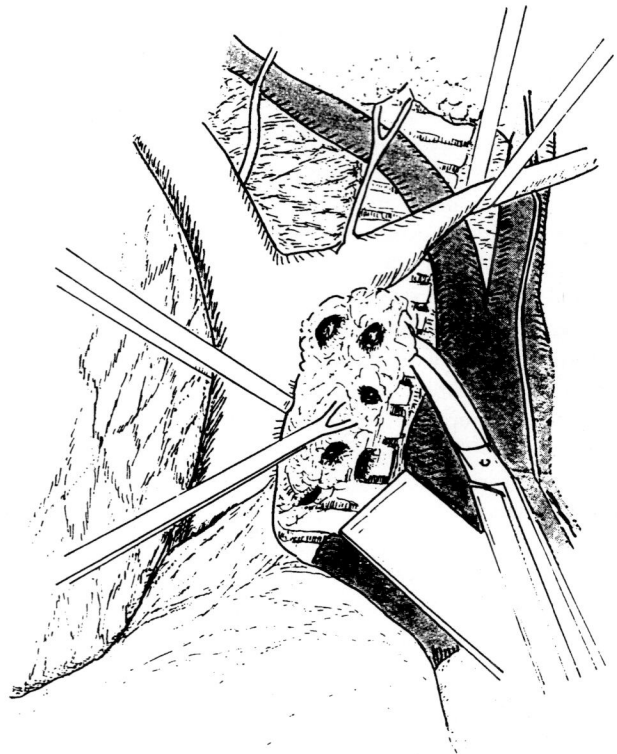

Fig. 100-13. Dissection of the pretracheal (No. 3) and paratracheal (No. 2) lymph nodes through a median sternotomy. The superior vena cava is retracted to the right and the aorta to the left after division of the upper anterior and posterior layers of the pericardial sac.

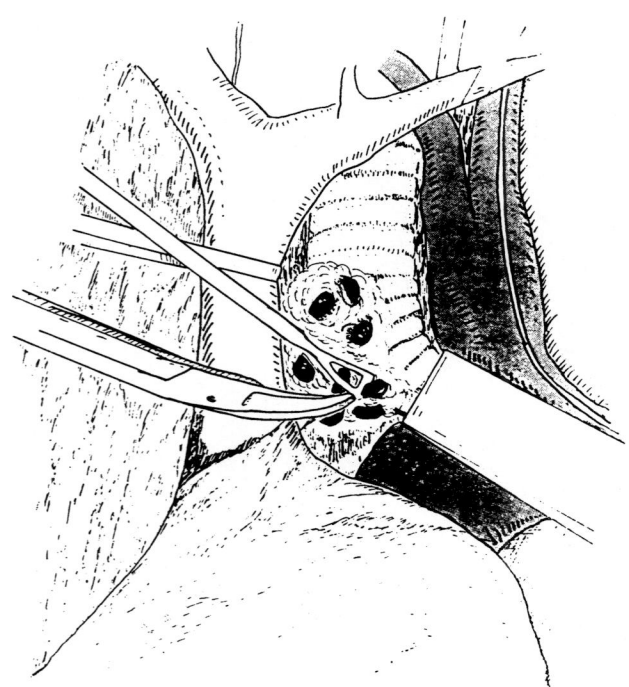

Fig. 100-14. Continued dissection of pretracheal (No. 3) and subcarinal (No. 7) lymph nodes through the median sternotomy incision described in Figure 100-13.

the pericardium is incised medial to the superior vena cava and as far inferiorly as the lower edge of the pulmonary artery. The superior vena cava is retracted to the right side and the brachiocephalic artery is retracted upward. The superior mediastinal lymph nodes (No. 1), which already have been dissected, the left and right paratracheal lymph nodes (No. 2), and the pretracheal lymph nodes (No. 3) are dissected downward, going underneath the brachiocephalic artery. The dissection is then carried downward to the level of the tracheal bifurcation by retraction of the superior vena cava to the right and the ascending aorta to the left (Figs. 100-13 and 100-14). The superior tracheobronchial (No. 4) lymph nodes on the right, as well as any tissue on the left that remains despite the previous dissection of the area during the initial standard left thoracotomy, are removed. During the left-sided dissection, care is needed to protect the left recurrent nerve. The subcarinal (No. 7) area is further inspected, although this area should be clear as a result of the dissection accomplished during the left thoracotomy.

LYMPH NODE INVOLVEMENT INCIDENCE AND SENTINEL LYMPH NODE FOR SYSTEMATIC NODAL DISSECTION

Oncologic systematic nodal dissection in the radical operation for lung cancer is one that is designed to obtain the most complete local control of the lung cancer. Lobectomy or pneumonectomy combined with complete oncologic nodal dissection is standard procedure. It requires dissection, in a minimally invasive way, of those lymph nodes with a possibility of metastasis, but is not necessary for those without metastasis.

A study was done by our group for the purpose of determining the sentinel lymph node while seeking to practice systematic nodal dissection rationally with regard to each location invaded by lung cancer. We recorded each lymph node station as described in the AJCC/UICC/JLCS map where there were lymph nodes with positive histologic metastasis in the 1815 cases of non–small cell lung cancer that underwent complete nodal dissection and complete resection (pN_0: 974/53.7%; pN_1: 430/23.7%; pN_2: 407/22.4%, and pN_3: 4/2.2%). A lobectomy was done in 1546 cases and a pneumonectomy in 269. The tumor was in the right upper lobe in 648 cases, the right middle lobe in 79, the right lower lobe in 380, the left upper lobe in 489, and the left lower lobe in 219 cases. The study indicates the probability of lymph node metastasis by each lymph node station, as well as each area invaded by cancer.

The majority of right upper lobe tumor metastases can be found in station Nos. 12 (24.4%), 11 (18.2%), 10 (10.7%), 3 (14.6%), and 4 (14.4%), but not often in 7 (only 4.9%). Similarly, the right middle lobe metastases were found in Nos. 12 (30.6%), 11 (34.6%), 10 (16.3%), to either 7 (17.3%) or 3 (20.0%). In right lower lobe tumors, metastases can be found mostly in Nos. 12 (15.5%), 11 (27.2%), 10 (19.7%), and 7 (15.2%), but less often in 1 (6.3%) through 4 (8.3%). Furthermore, left upper lobe tumor metastases can be found in stations 12 (26.6%), 11 (18.0%), 10 (13.5%), 5 (16.0%), and 6 (10.5%), but not often in 7 (3.9%). Left lower lobe tumors had metastases in 12 (16.5%), 11 (27.6%), 10 (19.4%), and 7 (13.8%), but infrequently in 5 (6.7%) and 6 (1.7%). When right upper lobe tumor metastasis is found in station 3, this means a 20% chance of metastasis exists in station 7, and similarly, when found in station 4 a 13.5% possibility of metastasis exists in 7. When right middle lobe tumor metastasis is found in station 7, the possibilities of 1, 2, 3, and 4 metastases are 53.8%, 15.4%, 53.8%, and 30.8%, respectively. Moreover, when found in station 3, the possibilities of station 1, 2, 4, or 7 metastases are 53.8%, 30.8%, 30.8%, and 53.8%, respectively. In right lower lobe tumor metastases, a station 7 metastasis implies possible metastases in 1, 2, 3 or 4 of 21.2%, 17.3%, 19.2%, and 17.3%, respectively. Furthermore, when left lower lobe tumor metastasis is found in station 7, the possibilities of metastases in 1, 2, 3, 4, 5, or 6 were 3.8%, 3.8%, 11.5%, 15.4%, 23.1%, and 3.8%, respectively.

On the other hand, among the 279 cases of right upper lobe tumor of less than 3 cm in size, 249 were without metastasis in stations 3, 4, or both. The occurrence of N_2 level lymph node metastasis, other than to 3 and 4, were 1 and 2 (1 case), 3 (1 case), and 7 (2 cases) for a total of 4 cases (1.6%). Among the 49 cases of right middle lobe tumor, 38 were without metastasis in stations 7 or 3, and in the 11 patients with involvement of N_2 level(s) 7, 3, or both, no other levels were found to be involved. In right lower lobe tumor, 147 cases out of 164 were without metastasis in level 7, but one case each was seen in levels 1 and 3, level 2, level 3, level 4, and in levels 1, 3, and 4, and two cases in level 9, for a total of seven cases (4.8%) of metastasis other than to level 7. Furthermore, 186 cases of 205 of left upper lobe tumor had no metastasis in 5 and 6, but metastases in 1 (one case), 2 (two cases), 4 (five cases), and 7 (three cases), for a total of 11 cases (5.9%) of metastasis other than to levels 5 and 6. Among the 220 cases of left lower lobe tumor, 75 had level 7 metastasis; in addition there was one case each of metastasis in levels 1, 4, and 5 and 6, for a total of three cases (2.0%); 3 of 145 of lymph node metastasis other than to level 7 was found. The possibility of N_2 metastasis when N_1 metastasis is found in 10, 11, or 12 was 44.6% (241 of 540).

The sentinel lymph node is uniformly identified as a mediastinal lymph node, but with differing numeric orders of the lymph node station(s) for each lobe. That is to say, in right upper lobe tumor the sentinel node stations are 3 and 4, in right middle lobe tumor 3 and 7, in right lower lobe tumor 7, in left upper lobe tumor 5 and 6, and in left lower lobe tumor 7, respectively. When metastasis is found in any of these nodes, it should be seen as a sign indicating possibilities of other metastasis and, therefore, complete systematic lymph node dissection should be undertaken. However, in T_1 lung cancer of less than 3 cm, when the sentinel lymph node sampling indicates no sign of metastasis, the chance of N_2 level

metastasis other than the sentinel node is only 5.9%. Moreover, in both right and left upper lobe tumors, No. 7 lymph node metastasis is rarely present when the sentinel node sampling proved that no metastasis was present in the nodes of the aforementioned sentinel lymph node station(s).

A systematic, oncologic lymph node dissection is to effectively perform a minimally invasive lymph node dissection and should be recognized as an operative procedure to improve local control of lung cancer. Therefore, an effective operation requires an oncologically performed lymph node dissection with a thorough understanding of the anatomic and pathologic characteristics of the lymphatic spread in each lobe.

REFERENCES

Ashour M: Modified muscle sparing posterolateral thoracotomy. Thorax 45:935, 1990.
Bethencourt DM, Holmes EC: Muscle-sparing posterolateral thoracotomy. Ann Thorac Surg 45:337, 1988.
Borrie J: Primary carcinoma of the bronchus: prognosis following surgical resection. Ann R Coll Surg Engl 10:165, 1952.
Cahan WG: Radical lobectomy. J Thorac Cardiovasc Surg 39:555, 1960.
Goldstraw P: Surgical management of non-small-cell lung cancer with ipsilateral mediastinal node metastasis (N_2 disease). J Thorac Cardiovasc Surg 107:19, 1994.
International Union Against Cancer—Union Internationale Contre le Cancer TNM: Atlas Illustrated Guide to the TNM/pTNM-Classification of Malignant Tumors. 3rd Ed. Genera: Union Internationale Contre le Cancer, 1989, p. 134.
Izbicki JR, et al: Radical systematic mediastinal lymphadenectomy in non-small cell lung cancer: a randomized controlled trial. Br J Surg 81:229, 1994.
Izbicki JR, et al: Impact of radical systematic mediastinal lymphadenectomy on tumor staging in lung cancer. Ann Thorac Surg 59:209, 1995.
Izbicki JR, et al: Effectiveness of radical systematic mediastinal lymphadenectomy in patients with resectable non-small cell lung cancer: results of a prospective randomized trial. Ann Surg 227:138, 1998.
Kirschner PA: Lung cancer. Preoperative radiation therapy and surgery. NY State Med J 81:339, 1981.
Levasseur PH, Regnard JF: Surgery of primary bronchial cancer. Helv Chir Acta 56:711, 1990.
Maggi G, et al: Results of surgical resection of stage IIIa (N_2) non small cell lung cancer, according to the site of the mediastinal metastases. Int Surg 78:213, 1993.
Martini N: Improved methods of recording data in lung cancer. Clin Bull Memorial Sloan-Kettering Cancer Center 6:93, 1976.
Martini N, et al: Results of resection in non-oat cell carcinoma of the lung with mediastinal lymph node metastases. Ann Surg 198:386, 1983.
Miller DL, et al: Results of surgical resection in patients with N_2 non-small cell lung cancer. Ann Thorac Surg 57:1096, 1994.
Mountain CF: "Cancer of the Lung" Classification and Staging of Cancer by Site. Chicago: American Joint Committee on Cancer, 1976, p. 95.
Mountain CF: The biological operability of stage III non-small cell lung cancer. Ann Thorac Surg 40:60, 1985.
Mountain CF, Dresler CM: Regional lymph node classification for lung cancer staging. Chest 111:1718, 1997.
Naruke T: Significance of lymph node metastases in lung cancer. Semin Thorac Cardiovasc Surg 5:210, 1993.
Naruke T: The spread of lung cancer and its relevance to surgery. J Jpn Surg Soc 68:1607, 1967.
Naruke T, Suemasu, Ishikawa S: Surgical treatment for lung cancer with metastasis to mediastinal lymph nodes. J Thorac Cardiovasc Surg 71:2, 1976.
Nohl HC: An investigation into the lymphatic and vascular spread of carcinoma of the bronchus. Thorax 11:172, 1956.
Nohl HC: The Spread of Carcinoma of the Bronchus. London: Lloid-Luke, Ltd, 1962, p. 37.

Pearson FG, et al: Significance of positive superior mediastinal nodes identified at mediastinoscopy in patients with resectable cancer of the lung. J Thorac Cardiovasc Surg *83*:1, 1982.

Riquet M, et al: Factors determining survival in resected N$_2$ lung cancer. Eur J Cardiothorac Surg *9*:300, 1995.

Rouviére H: Anatomie des Lymphatiques de l'Homme. Paris: Masson et Cie, 1932.

Rubinstein I, et al: Resectional surgery in the treatment of primary carcinoma of the lung with mediastinal lymph node metastases. Thorax *34*:33, 1979.

Shields TW: The incomplete resection. Ann Thorac Surg *47*:487, 1989.

Smith PA: The importance of mediastinal lymph node invasion by pulmonary carcinoma in selection of patients for resection. Ann Thorac Surg *25*:5, 1978.

The Japan Lung Cancer Society: General Rule for Clinical and Pathological Record of Lung Cancer. 3rd Ed. Tokyo: Kanehara Syuppann, 1987, p. 69.

Tisi GM, et al: Clinical staging of primary lung cancer. Am Rev Respir Dis *127*:659, 1983.

Watanabe Y, et al: Aggressive surgical intervention in N$_2$ non-small cell cancer of the lung. Ann Thorac Surg *51*:253, 1991a.

Watanabe Y, et al: Mediastinal nodal involvement and the prognosis of non-small cell lung cancer. Chest *100*:422, 1991b.

READING REFERENCES

Carr DT: Staging of Lung Cancer. Chicago: American Joint Committee for Cancer Staging and End-Results Reporting: Task Force on Lung, 1979.

Glazer GM, et al: Normal mediastinal lymph nodes: number and size according to American Thoracic Society mapping. AJR Am J Roentgenol *144*:261, 1985.

Hata E, et al: The efficiency of systematic mediastinal dissection for survival and investigation into lymph node metastasis in patients of non–small cell lung cancer. Lung Cancer *18*(Suppl 1):373, 1997.

Hirono T, et al: Surgical treatment of N2 non-small cell lung cancer. Lung Cancer *4*(Suppl):A90, 1988.

Kirsh MM, Sloan H: Mediastinal metastases in bronchogenic carcinoma: influence of postoperative irradiation, cell type, and location. Ann Thorac Surg *33*:459, 1982.

Naruke T, et al: Lymph node mapping and curability at various levels of metastasis in resected lung cancer. J Thorac Cardiovasc Surg *76*:832, 1978.

Nohl HC: The spread of carcinoma of the bronchus. London: Lloid-Luke, Ltd, 1962.

Sellers AH: A Brochure of Checklists. Geneva: UICC, 1980.

CHAPTER 101

Endoluminal Management of Malignant Airways Disease

Joseph LoCicero III

Because patients with endobronchial tumor obstruction often present with acute and dramatic symptoms, they have been the subject of considerable investigation during the last quarter of the century. Many physicians and surgeons developed innovative methods to relieve the acute symptoms. Now, most patients present with symptoms of obstruction after some initial therapy for lung cancer. Yet approximately 7% of all newly diagnosed lung cancers still present with primary obstruction.

Despite presentation with dyspnea, hemoptysis, or obstructive pneumonia, the care of most patients can be managed conservatively. Hospitalization and initiation of oxygen therapy, sedation, and antibiotics often ameliorate the acute symptoms, allowing completion of medical evaluation and staging of the tumor. Approximately 20% of patients with newly discovered lung cancer still have early stage disease and will be candidates for surgical resection. In such patients, pulmonary function testing, nuclear perfusion scanning, and accurate surgical mediastinal exploration may be necessary. The best form of treatment for most of the late-stage or medically inoperable patients having no previous therapy is palliative external beam radiation therapy. Endobronchial management thus becomes a secondary palliative method for those patients who remain acutely ill with initial unabated symptoms or those who fail following or progress during palliative radiation therapy.

METHODS OF EVALUATION

Several investigators have attempted to objectify pretreatment and posttreatment signs and symptoms (Table 101-1). Subjective criteria include nebulous symptoms such as fatigue, cough, wheezing, or stridor. Semiquantitative signs and symptoms include shortness of breath, hemoptysis, and fever. Quantitative signs and symptoms include segmental, lobar, or lung collapse evident on radiography of the chest, changes in spirometry or flow-volume loop on pulmonary function testing, and changes in oxygenation status. Bronchoscopic documentation of percent obstruction is the most objective value and is the easiest to estimate.

According to Schray and colleagues (1988), 68% of patients present with dyspnea, 37% with hemoptysis, 28% with cough without hemoptysis, and 14% with no subjective symptoms. Walsh and associates (1990) attempted to quantify the symptoms for better pretherapy and posttherapy comparisons. They used a dyspnea scale; evaluation of segmental collapse on chest radiography; pulmonary function testing, including forced expiratory volume in 1 second, the ratio of this value to forced vital capacity, and the midexpiratory flow rate; and arterial oxygenation. They added a 6-minute walk test performed on level ground to assess the endurance of the patients and their potential for oxygen desaturation.

Despite careful evaluation, functional tests correlate poorly with symptomatic improvement. My colleagues and I (1990) confirmed this fact. Most patients achieve symptomatic improvement with little change in objective numbers, with the exception of the chest radiography. Radiographic evaluation of improvement in collapse also gives an excellent and easily evaluable criterion (Fig. 101-1). Because oxygen desaturation is linked to the amount of ventilation-perfusion mismatch caused by segmental collapse, peripheral saturation and the radiographic picture together are excellent predictors of the potential effectiveness of the therapy. Cough and hemoptysis are present in many patients and are often relieved by noninvasive therapy. Improvement in the 6-minute walk test is usually but not always accompanied by symptomatic relief.

Table 101-1. Measures of Obstruction

Nebulous symptoms
 Fatigue
 Cough
 Wheezing
 Stridor
Semiquantitative symptoms
 Shortness of breath
 Hemoptysis
 Fever
Quantitative symptoms
 Percent endobronchial obstruction
 Radiographic evidence of pulmonary collapse
 Oxygenation/ventilation
 Pulmonary function testing
  Changes in functional capacity
  6-minute talk test
  Dyspnea scale

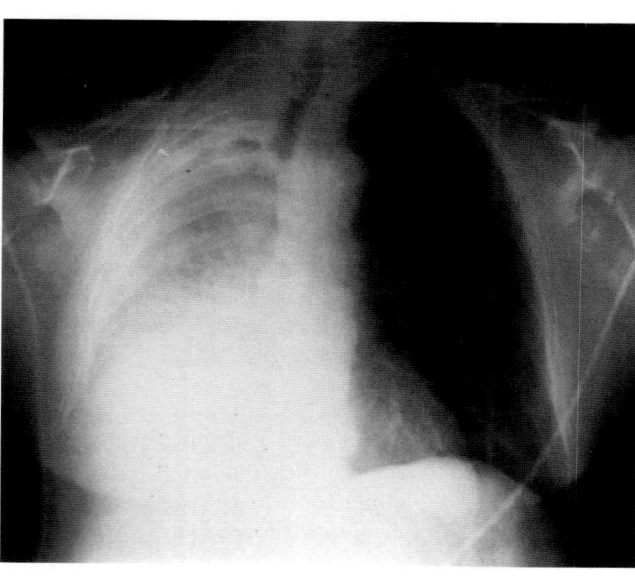

Fig. 101-1. Chest radiograph of a patient with near total obstruction of the right main stem bronchus. This patient presented with severe shortness of breath. Predictably, early reestablishment of a patent airway ameliorated all symptoms.

Table 101-2. Dyspnea Scale

0	No restrictions
1	Dypsnea only with strenuous activity
2	Dyspnea with moderate daily activity
3	Dyspnea with minimal exertion
4	Dyspnea at rest
5	Ventilator dependency

Another attempt at objective evaluation is the simple dyspnea scale (Table 101-2). This takes the rather subjective symptom of shortness of breath and makes it quantifiable. Some investigators add general functional evaluation, such as the physical status scale (0 to 4) or Karnofsky's scale (0 to 100) to their pretherapy evaluation.

Table 101-3. Endoluminal Tumor Management

Mechanical débridement
Electrosurgery
Cryosurgery
Carbon dioxide laser
Neodymium:yttrium-aluminum-garnet laser
Endobronchial brachytherapy
Photodynamic therapy
Endoluminal stent

MANAGEMENT STRATEGIES

Table 101-3 lists the wide variety of techniques available to manage tumor obstruction of the trachea and bronchi. Each has advantages and disadvantages. Sometimes, a combination of techniques may be used to minimize the disadvantages of any one therapy.

Mechanical Débridement

The earliest method of endobronchial tumor management was simple mechanical removal. Jackson (1943) reported reasonable success with this technique. Later, in 1959, he reported establishment of a patent airway simply by mechanical débridement, noting that with the use of a large rigid bronchoscope and adequate suctioning, many tumors could be débrided with minimal airway compromise. He noted that tumors of this size lack much vascularity, and bleeding could be controlled through patience and persistence. Despite these reports, most tumor excision is combined with some method for control of hemorrhage.

Electrosurgery

Endoscopic electrosurgery has been used safely for many years. Its principal use has been in removing colon polyps. More recently, it has achieved widespread use in fulguration of various bleeding lesions of the upper gastrointestinal tract. It has been one of the resources of the thoracic surgeon to remove obstructing lesions from the airways, but few major reports of its use have been published.

Hooper and Jackson (1985) cited eight previously reported cases and added four of their own. Methodology was rather straightforward and involved passing a probe through the aspiration port of the bronchoscope. They found cautery sectioning most easily accomplished for removal of a polypoid lesion. The alternate approach is vaporization using the closed wire snare as a cautery probe. In 1988, these authors extended their experience to 32 procedures on 18 patients of whom 13 had primary malignancy. In the 13 patients, 11 had successful airway palliation. Similarly, Girasin and Shafirovsky (1988) used a diathermic snare inserted through a fiberoptic bronchoscope in 14 patients.

They believed that the snare was more effective than electrodestruction alone.

With the proliferation of laparoscopic and thoracoscopic instrumentation specifically designed for use with the electrocautery, further interest in this technique may be generated. Because of the size of these instruments (5 mm), only a rigid bronchoscope may be used. Because the bronchoscope is 40 cm long, only the nondisposable 45-cm instruments are usable.

Cryosurgery

Cryosurgery involves the use of a low-temperature probe that induces coagulation necrosis generally limited to the immediate area of the probe. Liquid nitrogen is fed into a cannula that has an inner tube and an outer tube attached to a specifically designed interchangeable tip. Except for the tip, the cannula is insulated. Liquid nitrogen is fed under pressure and delivered to the tip, where it expands and escapes through the outer tube. Profound cooling occurs at the tip because of rapid gas expansion. Intracellular and extracellular ice crystal formation injures cells and reduces their survival by disrupting membranes. It has a profound effect on decreasing blood supply.

In animal experiments laying the groundwork for this therapy, Carpenter and associates (1977) noted complete necrosis of the mucosa and thrombosis of vessels, with relatively well-preserved basic bronchial architecture. Surrounding areas of necrosis within the lung itself subsequently healed by fibrosis. The bronchi appeared to heal without stricture. They later applied the technique in eight patients with good results.

Homasson and associates (1986) used a cryoprobe through a rigid bronchoscope for 27 patients. The cryoprobe itself was flexible and could reach into the right upper lobe bronchus. For malignant tumors, they achieved airway palliation in 13 of 21 patients. They also easily ablated five small granulomas without complications. They recommended using flexible endoscopy 4 to 6 weeks after cryotherapy to aspirate and remove the slough. They noted that because it took several days for necrosis to occur, immediate palliation of the airway was not obtained. With more experience, another group headed by Mathur (1996) was able to completely remove the obstructions in 18 of 20 patients (90%). Now, miniaturized flexible probes can be used through a flexible bronchoscope.

Carbon Dioxide Laser

Shapsay and Simpson (1983) used the carbon dioxide laser 59 times on 34 patients with malignant airway disease. They achieved airway palliation in 30 of these patients. McElvein and Zorn (1986) used this laser to treat 89 patients from 1979 to 1983. Of this group, 51 had malignant lesions;

46 of these patients achieved an immediate good result. Five patients became worse.

Ossoff and colleagues (1985) surveyed their use of the carbon dioxide laser and its attendant problems. Because of potential fires, the inability of laser light to be bent, poor hemorrhage control, the need for an absolutely dry field, and poor depth of penetration, they recommended limiting the use of this laser to relatively avascular lesions of the trachea. They now favor the neodymium:yttrium-aluminum-garnet (Nd:YAG) laser for all cancer applications. Most bronchoscopists have abandoned this modality because of its limited usefulness and the need for rigid instruments and delivery systems.

Neodymium:Yttrium-Aluminum-Garnet Laser

When the Nd:YAG laser became available for clinical use, it revolutionized the endobronchial management of tumor. The laser source is a crystal of neodymium-doped yttrium-aluminum-garnet powered by a xenon flash lamp. It presented immediate advantages over the carbon dioxide laser. It can be delivered through a flexible quartz fiber, thus allowing use with fiberoptic bronchoscopy. It causes coagulation necrosis that can control vascular lesions. It also produces a 4- to 5-mm zone of necrosis beyond the visualized destruction that the endoscopist observes, which allows débridement of avascular tissue immediately after treatment. The early disadvantages were the high level of power and the need for water cooling, which limited the location of the laser. These problems have now been addressed and resolved.

Dumond and colleagues (1984) emphasized some important safety features. These included low-laser power levels (below 50 watts), short pulses (under 3 seconds), and a maximum inspiratory oxygen content of 50%. They advised mechanical removal of necrotic debris as early as possible to reestablish the airway.

Cavaliere and colleagues (1996) have the largest recent series. They reported on 3069 procedures on 2008 patients. They used the rigid bronchoscope for 96% of the procedures. They used the laser in 91% of the patients with an average of 1.4 applications per case (mean time between procedures, 102 days). They also used other modalities such as brachytherapy (3.3% of cases) and stents (19.5% of cases) with good results. Early mortality now is an acceptable 0.4%. Although rigid instrumentation was used in this series, many endoscopists use flexible bronchoscopes for all but the most proximal lesions.

Endobronchial Brachytherapy

Henschke (1958) described interstitial radiation therapy with permanently implantable sources for unresectable or residual lung cancer. Using these techniques, Hilaris and Martini (1979) reported their sizable 20-year experience showing that local control was better if brachytherapy was added to surgical resection when residual disease was present. Lewis and colleagues (1990) suggested that brachytherapy should be an available technique for all patients found to have unresectable disease at the time of thoracotomy.

In 1979, Hilaris and colleagues began endobronchial implantation. The major advance in this field came with the refinement of flexible systems that could be placed in the patient using flexible bronchoscopy. Mittal and associates (1984) placed a catheter into which radon, gold, or other radioactive sources could be injected for therapy. Patients tolerated these catheters well during the 3 to 5 days required for therapy.

The next advancement came with the ultrafast, high-dose remote afterloading techniques using iridium 192. Miller and Phillips (1990) described this technique. They used the Nucleotron (Leersum, The Netherlands) selectron high-dose system, which is a three-channel remote afterloading system. It consists of a treatment unit that stores the sources within a lead-shielded safe and can be controlled remotely. The unit can store 100 sources that could be individually programmed for different treatment times. These sources are automatically corrected for source decay. The treatment time and number of positions of sources can be programmed independently for each channel to give the required dose distribution for a particular patient or tumor geometry. The sources are placed into a No. 5F catheter. The dose levels within 1 cm of the source range from 30 to 60 Gy.

Table 101-4 shows the results with this technique. In comparison with the Nd:YAG laser in a large series of patients, endobronchial brachytherapy showed equal survival with similar symptom palliation. If the laser was used to open the airway to allow better implantation of the seeds, the results were improved to 95% survival at 6 months. A series from Hernandez and colleagues (1996) prospectively evaluated 29 patients. They found a 25% improvement in symptoms related to pneumonitis, a 69% improvement in hemoptysis, and a 24% improvement in performance status.

Photodynamic Therapy

Photo-activation of light-sensitive compounds to produce chemical reactions, first recognized around 1900, was applied to human cancers beginning in 1966, according to Carruth (1986). Patients receive a purified derivative of the hemoglobin molecule diethyl ether hematoporphyrin. This drug circulates in all cells, but in experiments by Doiron and Keller (1986), it clears normal cells faster than tumors. Photo-activation by light at 630 nm causes apoptosis, presumably by toxic oxygen metabolites. The therapy is approved for both lung cancer and esophageal cancer. However, it remains expensive. A single therapy dose costs the pharmacy $2000. The laser approved by the U.S. Food and Drug Administration (FDA) for use with this drug has a purchase price of $110,000 and is available from at least two laser companies. Other light sources are used in Europe that are considerably cheaper, but they are not approved for human use by the FDA.

Results often are dramatic with minimal morbidity to the patient (Figs. 101-2 and 101-3). Edell and colleagues (1993) suggested that there may be a bimodal use for photodynamic therapy. It has a role in the early superficial squamous cell carcinoma, which it can eradicate. Its usefulness at the other end of the disease with tumor obstruction may be less because of the other available technologies.

McCaughan and Williams (1997) showed that patients could undergo frequent and repeated treatments. They treated a series of 175 patients, many receiving multiple treatments. At 1 month, 96% experienced either complete or partial response. In their overall series, the mean survival rate by stage of disease was stage I (not yet reached), stage II (22.5 months), stage IIIA (5.7 months), stage IIIB (55 months), and stage IV (5.0 months). They treated 16 stage I patients with photodynamic therapy as primary therapy, only achieving a 93% estimated 5-year survival rate.

In my experience (1990) with medically inoperable and late-stage patients in whom life expectancy is short, the photosensitivity may interfere with reasonable quality of life. These patients must remain out of any sunlight for up to 6 weeks, a significant amount of time out in a patient with limited survival. Physicians must weigh the potential side effects against any expected short-term benefits.

Endobronchial Stents

For many years, surgeons have used silicone stents to keep open the airway in cases of benign and malignant stenosis or obstruction. These stents were of value when there were no alternatives. Because of the difficulty in anchoring the stents, the use was confined to the trachea and main stem bronchi. T-shaped stents were used for the upper trachea and are anchored in the site of a new or previous tracheostomy. Y-shaped stents were used for the lower trachea and proximal bronchi. These required rigid bronchoscopy for placement. Short, straight stents are available and depend on a tight stenosis to keep them in position.

Silicone stents may play an important role in the management of bronchoesophageal fistulas. After the esophagus is

Table 101-4. Survival Comparison of Neodymium:Yttrium-Aluminum-Garnet Laser and Endobronchial Brachytherapy

Treatment	No. of Patients	6 Months	Percent Survival
Nd:YAG	130	110	85
EB	67	60	90
Nd:YAG + EB	21	20	95

EB, endobronchial brachytherapy; Nd:YAG, neodymium:yttrium-aluminum-garnet laser.
Adapted from Miller JI, Phillips TW: Neodymium:YAG laser and brachytherapy in the management of inoperable bronchogenic carcinoma. Ann Thorac Surg 50:190, 1990.

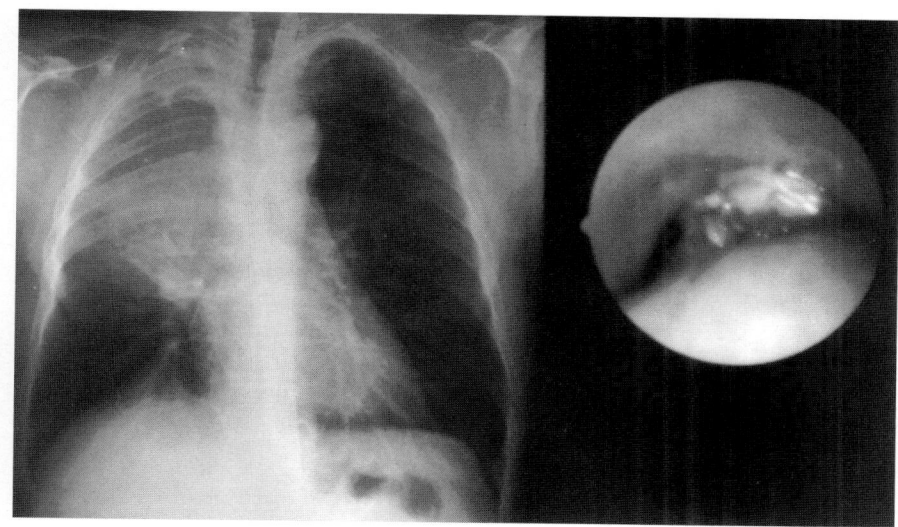

Fig. 101-2. Chest radiograph and corresponding view of a large endobronchial squamous carcinoma at the orifice of a right main stem bronchus in a 61-year-old smoker. The computed tomographic scan demonstrated bulky mediastinal disease.

stented, Yim and colleagues (1997) used 17 silicone stents in 15 patients to restore airway integrity. All patients noted a significant improvement in dyspnea, although they did not report on other signs or symptoms.

Through the late 1980s and early 1990s, radiologists gained experience with the use of metallic endovascular and endobiliary prostheses. Rosch and coworkers (1987) used one of the more successful stents, the Gianturco stent, for superior vena cava syndrome after radiation therapy. David and colleagues (1992) performed a randomized trial comparing polyethylene versus metallic stents for biliary stenosis. They found the expandable capability of the metallic stents was a distinct advantage in maintaining patency. In 1990, Varela and associates placed Gianturco stents in three patients with endobronchial stenosis attributable to cancer in one patient. All of the patients had good results. The current stent models include the Wallstent (Schneider, Inc., Minneapolis, MN) and the Microvasive stent (Boston Scientific, Natick, MA). Boston Scientific has acquired Schneider, Inc., so all the expandable stents for the airway will be under one management. Figure 101-4 demonstrates the new silicone-covered Wallstent that can be deployed, sheathed, and redeployed off the delivery device. This new feature is helpful in the airway where placement around other lobar orifices is critical.

Endobronchial stents have found usefulness for the vexing problem of extrinsic compression secondary to malignant disease. Dilation of the stenosis lasts only a short time, leaving no permanent solution. Lasering of an extrinsic compression can produce an open airway but replaces the malignant obstruction with a cicatrix that requires repeated lasering approximately every 3 weeks, adding expense and risk to the patient. Nomori and associates (1993) presented successful stent placements in a series of patients in which over 70% of the stenoses were caused by extrinsic compression.

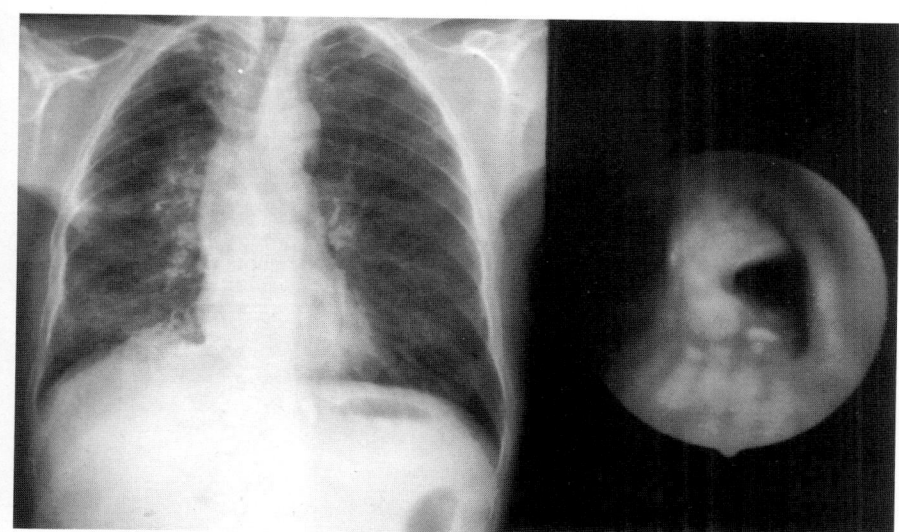

Fig. 101-3. Same patient as seen in Figure 101-2. Chest radiograph and corresponding bronchoscopy 6 weeks after photodynamic therapy. The right lung is expanded and biopsy revealed no evidence of residual cancer in the right main stem.

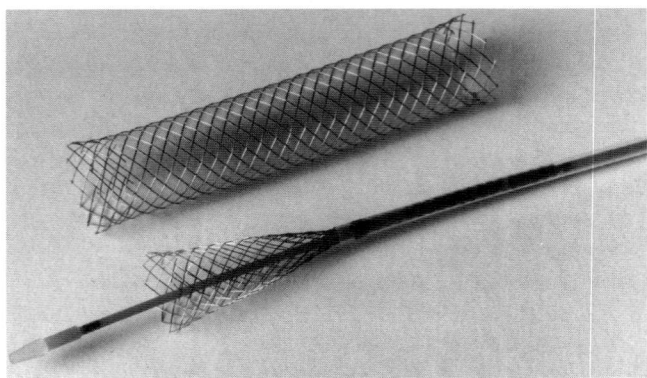

Fig. 101-4. One of the most popular stents in use is the Wallstent (Schneider, Inc.). The stent is covered with silicone and can be reconstrained for repositioning during deployment.

Another situation in which endobronchial stents have been useful is as a temporary solution for a patient presenting with a malignant obstruction. A stent can be used to open an obstruction acutely to allow expansion of atelectatic lung and drainage of postobstructive pneumonia prior to the start of radiation therapy, chemotherapy, or both. Witt and associates (1997) reported a series of 22 patients who presented with acute blockage. After the start of definitive therapy, 50% of the stents could be removed.

Special Endoluminal Stents

Malignant disease can cause obstruction of other intrathoracic structures that could be handled with an endoluminal stent. The most notable situation is superior vena cava obstruction. Gross and colleagues (1997) successfully dilated and stented 13 patients with malignant superior vena cava syndrome. One patient died of a cardiac arrhythmia 1 day after placement, but the rest of the patients had no recurrence of the syndrome.

A more difficult problem that is amenable to stent management is the malignant esophagorespiratory fistula. This devastating situation has foiled many attempts at surgical resolution. The innovative development of silicone-covered esophageal stents can allow closure of the fistula from the esophageal side. Nelson and colleagues (1997) placed 23 stents in 21 patients, with sealing of the fistula in 87% and improvement in more than one-half of the cases. Sometimes the placement of an endoesophageal stent adds to the respiratory compromise in a patient because of airway compression. In such cases, placement of an airway stent can be beneficial. I have had experience with three such patients. In each case the relief was immediate and the airway stent provided considerable palliation for a desperate situation. Takamori and associates (1996) placed stents in 12 patients with acute respiratory compromise from esophageal cancer, achieving immediate relief in eight patients without complications.

COMPLICATIONS

Sufficient data are available for most endobronchial methods to compare complications. The incidence of complications overall is approximately 10%; approximately one-half are life-threatening. Table 101-5 lists the major complications.

The methods associated with the most acute complications are cautery and the Nd:YAG laser. Endobronchial fires can be fatal, particularly because of the carbonaceous smoke plume from the standard endotracheal tubes (Fig. 101-5). Several companies now make special tubes that retard the initiation of a fire. The best way to prevent a fire is to keep the power below 40 watts and to limit exposure time to 3 seconds or less.

Hemorrhage is also a potentially fatal complication. Cautery and the laser most often cause bleeding acutely as a result of perforation through the bronchial wall. For the Nd:YAG laser, the risk is ever present because of the depth of penetration of the laser injury. The beam should be kept as coaxial as possible with the lumen to decrease the occurrence of this complication. Delayed hemorrhage may occur with any form of therapy, but it happens most often when the pulmonary artery is involved by the tumor. When the tumor becomes necrotic and sloughs at approximately 14 to 21 days, hemorrhage ensues. Most of these patients are out of the hospital and exsanguinate before medical assistance is available.

Table 101-5. Complications of Endoluminal Tumor Management

Complication	Cautery	Cryosurgery	Neodymium:Yttrium-Aluminum-Garnet Laser	Photodynamic Therapy	Endobronchial Brachytherapy	Stent
Endobronchial fire	X		X			
Immediate hemorrhage	X		X			
Delayed hemorrhage	X	X	X	X	X	X
Pneumothorax	X		X			
Bronchoesophageal fistula	X	X	X	X	X	
Bronchial stenosis	X	X	X	X	X	X
Occlusion (secretions/debris)						X
Photosensitivity				X		

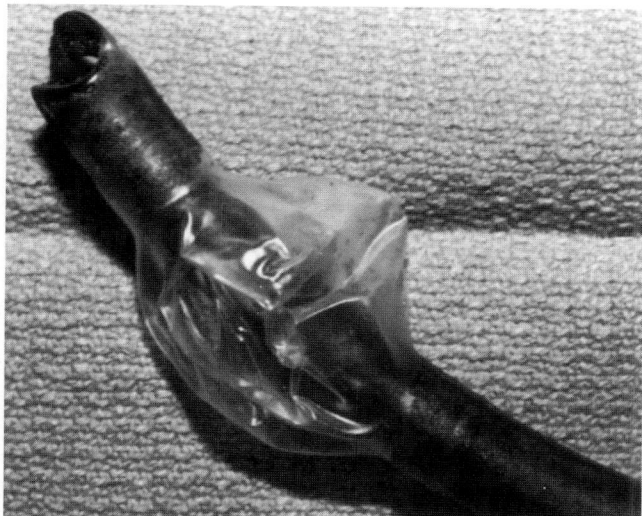

Fig. 101-5. Tip of an endotracheal tube after a laser fire. Note that only the tip is damaged, but the entire tube is filled with deposits from the carbonaceous plume.

Few complications have been reported with expandable stents. The most common problem is inspissated secretions in the stent causing obstruction. Stents can be replaced but because they are designed to become incorporated into the mucosa, they cause hemorrhage when removed and can lead to bronchostenosis if not replaced within a short period of time. Most bronchoscopists have limited their use to malignant obstructions or benign conditions that are considered short-term or for which a stent is a temporizing maneuver until a more definitive solution can be employed.

Of special note is the unique complication of photosensitivity with photodynamic therapy. The chemical used for photodynamic therapy is a derivative of the hemoglobin molecule. The exogenous porphyrin produces the same photosensitivity found in patients with porphyria. Although most of the drug is cleared from the body within 1 week, the photosensitivity may persist for 4 to 6 weeks. Patients must remain out of even minimal sunlight. Even after this time, patients should wear a sunscreen. Any patient who may be a candidate for this type of therapy should carefully consider this limitation.

REFERENCES

Carpenter RJ III, et al: Cryosurgery of bronchopulmonary structures. Chest 72:279, 1977.

Carruth JA: Photodynamic therapy: state of the art. Lasers Surg Med 6:404, 1986.

Cavaliere S, et al: Endoscopic treatment of malignant airway obstructions in 2008 patients. Chest 110:1536, 1996.

David S, et al: Randomized trial of self expanding metal stents versus poly-ethylene stents for distal malignant biliary obstruction. Lancet 340:1488, 1992.

Doiron DR, Keller GS: Porphyrin photodynamic therapy: principles and clinical applications. Curr Probl Dermatol 15:85, 1986.

Dumond JF, et al: Principles for safety in application in neodymium:YAG laser in bronchoscopy. Chest 86:163, 1984.

Edell S, Cortese DA, McDougall JC: Ancillary therapies in the management of lung cancer: photodynamic therapy, laser therapy and endobronchial prosthetic devices. Mayo Clin Proc 68:685, 1993.

Girasin VA, Shafirovsky BB: Endobronchial electrosurgery. Chest 93:270, 1988.

Gross, CM et al: Stent implantation in patients with superior vena cava syndrome. Am J Roentgenol 169:429, 1997.

Henschke UK: Interstitial implantation in the treatment of primary bronchogenic carcinoma. AJR Am J Roentgenol 79:981, 1958.

Hernandez P et al: High dose rate brachytherapy for the local control of endobronchial carcinoma following external irradiation. Thorax 51:354, 1996.

Hilaris BS, Martini N: Interstitial brachytherapy in cancer of the lung: a twenty year experience. Int J Radiat Oncol Biol Phys 5:1951, 1979.

Hilaris BS, et al: A new endobronchial implanter. Clin Bull 9:21, 1979.

Homasson JP, et al: Bronchoscopic cryotherapy for airway strictures caused by tumors. Chest 87:705, 1986.

Hooper RG, Jackson FN: Endobronchial electrocautery. Chest 87:712, 1985.

Jackson CL, Kozelman FW: Bronchial carcinoma. J Thorac Surg 4:165, 1943.

Jackson CL: Diseases of the Nose, Throat and Ear. 2nd Ed. Philadelphia: WB Saunders, 1959.

Lewis JW, et al: Role of brachytherapy in the management of pulmonary mediastinal malignancy. Ann Thorac Surg 49:728, 1990.

LoCicero J, Metzdorff M, Almgren C: Photodynamic therapy in the palliation of late stage obstructing non small cell lung cancer. Chest 98:97, 1990.

Mathur PN, et al: Fiberoptic bronchoscopic cryotherapy in the management of tracheobronchial obstruction. Chest 110:718, 1996.

McCaughan JS, Williams TE: Photodynamic therapy for endobronchial malignant disease: a prospective fourteen-year study. J Thorac Cardiovasc Surg 114:940, 1997.

McElvein RB, Zorn GL: The use of lasers for tracheal bronchial lesions. In Kittle CF (ed): Controversies in Thoracic Surgery. Philadelphia: WB Saunders, 1986.

Miller JI, Phillips TW: Neodymium:YAG laser and brachytherapy in the management of inoperable bronchogenic carcinoma. Ann Thorac Surg 50:190, 1990.

Mittal BB, Matuschak G, Culpepper J: Endobronchial interstitial brachytherapy using bronchofiberscope with a flexible injector system. Radiology 152:219, 1984.

Nelson DB et al: Silicone-covered Wallstent prototypes for palliation of malignant esophageal obstruction and digestive-respiratory fistulas. Gastrointest Endosc 45:31, 1997.

Nomori H, et al: Indications for an expandable metallic stent for tracheobronchial stenosis. Ann Thorac Surg 56:1324, 1993.

Ossoff RH, et al: Limitations of bronchoscopic carbon dioxide laser surgery. Ann Otol Rhinol Laryngol 94:498, 1985.

Rosch J, et al: Gianturco expandable wire stents in the treatment of superior vena cava syndrome recurring after maximum tolerance radiation. Cancer 60:1243, 1987.

Schray MF, et al: Management of malignant airway compromise with laser and low dose rate brachytherapy. Chest 93:264, 1988.

Shapsay SM, Simpson GT: Lasers in bronchology. Otolaryngol Clin North Am 16:819, 1983.

Takamori, S et al: Expandable metallic stents for tracheobronchial stenoses in esophageal cancer. Ann Thorac Surg 62:844, 1996.

Varela A: The use of Gianturco self expandable stents in the tracheal bronchial tree. Ann Thorac Surg 49:806, 1990.

Walsh DA, et al: Bronchoscopic cryotherapy for advanced bronchial carcinoma. Thorax 45:509, 1990.

Witt, C et al: Temporary tracheobronchial stenting in malignant stenoses. Eur J Cancer 33:204, 1997.

Yim APC, Abdullah, VJ, Izzat, MB: Comment on Takamori, S et al: Expandable metallic stents for tracheobronchial stenoses in esophageal cancer. Ann Thorac Surg 63:1511, 1997.

CHAPTER 102

Basic Principles of Radiation Therapy in Carcinoma of the Lung

Bahman Emami and Carlos A. Perez

PHYSICAL ASPECTS OF IONIZING RADIATION

Ionizing radiations are part of the spectrum of electromagnetic or particle energy that produce physical and biochemical events when they interact with atoms of irradiated materials. The different types of ionizing rays differ in the size and charge of the particles involved, or, in the case of x-rays and gamma rays, in their wavelength, frequency, and velocity of propagation in air or tissues. The several types of ionizing rays are alpha and beta particles, gamma rays, neutrons, and negative pi-mesons.

Units of Radiation

A roentgen is a unit of radiation exposure. Rad is the unit of absorbed dose equal to the amount of ionizing radiation that delivers 100 ergs per g of absorber. The Gray is equivalent to 100 rad: 1 cGy = 1 rad, which is the most widely used unit. Another unit of radiation is the curie. The curie, which is used to describe the activity of any radioactive isotope, is approximately the equivalent of the number of disintegrations per second undergone by 1 g of radium, as Johns and Cunningham (1983) noted. A practical unit frequently used is the millicurie, 1/1000 of a curie.

Nomenclature

The International Commission of Radiation Units and Measurements has recommended definitions of important concepts in treatment planning in radiation therapy (International Commission of Radiation Units and Measurements Report 50). The *gross tumor volume* refers to the actual physical dimensions of tumor determined by either palpation or imaging. The *clinical target volume* refers to the gross tumor volume plus regions of presumed occult spread of malignancy. The *planning target*

volume, defined arbitrarily by the radiation oncologist, represents the tumor volume, including potential areas of local and regional spread, and a margin of surrounding normal tissue, to allow for patient movement and positioning errors (Fig. 102-1). This target volume is to be irradiated to a specified absorbed dose in a specified time-dose pattern.

EQUIPMENT USED IN CLINICAL RADIATION THERAPY

External beam therapy units are designed to deliver gamma rays, x-rays, or electrons. Electron beams have special physical characteristics (e.g., the depth of penetration can be controlled by energy used) and are used in the treatment of relatively localized lesions.

Currently Used Equipment in Clinical Practice

For a detailed review of the physical aspect of ionizing radiation, the reader is referred to more comprehensive textbooks on this subject.

Orthovoltage X-Ray Unit

The main disadvantages of this type of equipment are the relative lack of penetration and maximum ionization occurring at the skin level, so that erythema and either dry or moist desquamation appear rapidly, even with moderate doses of radiation.

Cobalt 60 Teletherapy Units

The basic cobalt 60 machine consists of a shielded head in which the radioactive source is housed, a collimating

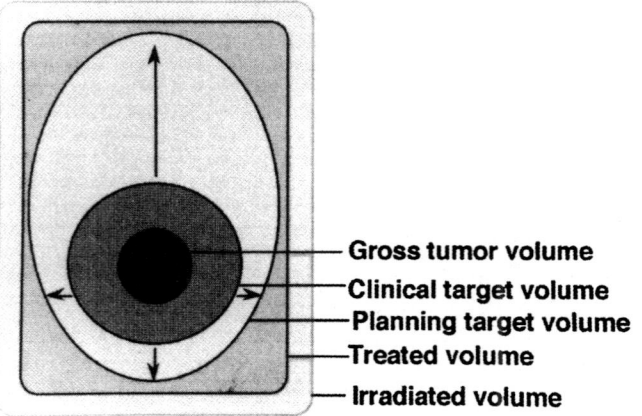

Fig. 102-1. Schematic illustration of the different volumes as defined by ICRU Report 50. From ICRU Report No 50—Prescribing, Recording, and Reporting Photon Beam Therapy. Bethesda, MD: International Commission on Radiation Units and Measurements, 1993, p. 5. With permission.

device, an on-off system, and an electric circuit. These machines produce more penetrating radiation than conventional x-ray machines; the skin is therefore less affected and higher doses can be delivered to deeper tissues than with conventional x-rays.

Linear Accelerators

Linear accelerators are high-energy electron accelerators that can be used to produce either electron or x-ray beams. The usual energies for electrons are 4, 6, 8, 10, 12, 18, and

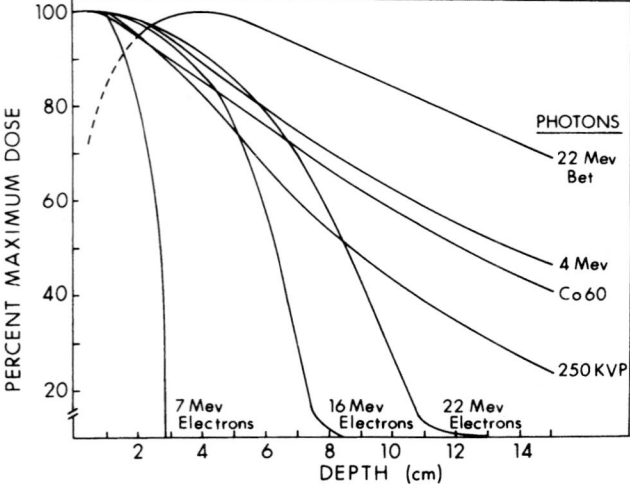

Fig. 102-2. Depth dose curves for a variety of photon and electron beams. Notice the higher doses delivered by 22 meV betatron photons and the sharp decrease in dose delivered by electron beams. From Perez CA: Principles of radiation therapy. *In* Horton J, Hill GJ (eds): Clinical Oncology. Philadelphia: WB Saunders, 1977, p. 131. With permission.

20 meV. The main feature of the electrons is that in tissues, they have a definite range that depends on their energy (Fig. 102-2). Linear accelerators have a high output (200 to 1000 rad per minute at the center of rotation), depending on the type of unit. The beam provides excellent skin-sparing effect and depth of penetration; the dose is more homogeneous than with the cobalt 60 unit because of the small focal spot, which generates little penumbra at the edge of the beam.

Radioactive Sources and Internally Administered Isotopes

It is sometimes appropriate to treat a tumor with a source of radiation directly implanted into the tumor: interstitial therapy with ^{125}I. Likewise, intracavitary administration of radioisotopes (e.g., ^{32}P) is sometimes used to treat malignant pleural effusions.

BIOLOGICAL EFFECTS OF IONIZING RADIATIONS AND BIOLOGICAL BASIS OF RADIATION THERAPY

The critical target in cell death is in the nucleus and is probably DNA. Ionizing radiation damages DNA in at least four different ways: double-helix strand breaks, single-strand breaks, base damage, and damage to cross-links in which both DNA-DNA and DNA-protein cross-links are involved.

These physical and biochemical phenomena take place in fractions of a second at the time of the radiation exposure. Various nuclear and cytoplasmic molecular changes then follow, leading to loss of reproductive ability, cell cycle delays, somatic transformation, and mutations, among others.

Chromosomes may be damaged by ionizing radiation, as Little (1968) noted. Classically, the damage is not detected in interphase and only appears as the cells go through cell division. Kaplan (1963) reported that the frequency of mutations produced by the single- or double-strand breaks on the DNA molecule depends on not only the number of initial breaks but also the adequacy of the repair mechanisms.

Carcinogenesis

Ionizing radiation can induce carcinoma of the skin, leukemia, thyroid cancer, osteosarcoma of bone, fibrosarcomas of soft tissues, and other disorders. The instances of leukemia that have reportedly been caused by prior exposure to radiation include acute leukemias of all types and chronic granulocytic leukemias. The adult thyroid gland may tolerate as much as 4000 rad without significant changes, but in children who received between 200 and 800 rad to the neck for thymic enlargement, the development many years later of thyroid carcinoma, usually of the papillary type, has been reported.

Cell Kill by Ionizing Radiation

When a cell is hit by an ionizing particle, different kinds of damage may take place. Lethal damage occurs when the cell loses its ability for unlimited proliferation. After radiation exposure, the cell and its progeny die, although Dogget and associates (1967) noted that as many as five to six cell divisions may occur. Potentially lethal damage consists of slightly less severe impairment of the proliferative ability of the cell from which it may recover, but any modification in its environment interferes with repair and causes the cell to die. Stewart and Fajardo (1972) reported that in humans, this happens, for instance, when certain drugs such as hydroxyurea are administered.

Sublethal damage occurs, as Elkind and colleagues (1967) noted, when the injury induced by the ionizing radiation can be repaired by the cell. After exposure to ionizing radiation, the cells exhibit changes in their growth rate, including prolongation of the generation time and mitotic delay.

Cell Survival Curves

A cell survival curve, such as that Hewitt and Wilson (1959) described, represents the probability of cell death after various doses of radiation. In biological terms, cell kill is the loss of unlimited proliferative capacity. It is the inability of the cell to proliferate in an unlimited clonogenic manner. Thus, it is important in radiation therapy. As Puck and Marcus (1956) pointed out, however, a cell may appear to be morphologically intact after exposure to radiation, and it may even undergo several more divisions before lysis. Mathematically speaking, cell survival can be expressed as a modified exponential function in which the fraction of cells killed is independent of the number of cells irradiated. The exponential shape of the cell survival curve indicates that cell kill is a probable event. If this curve is a decreasing straight line (i.e., an unmodified exponential function), a single hit must affect a single target to kill the cell. Most cell survival curves, however, have an *initial shoulder* (i.e., a modified exponential function), suggesting that more than one target must be inactivated by an ionizing event or that one target must be hit several times before the cell is lethally affected. The shoulder seen in the initial portion of the survival curve suggests the presence of sublethal damage, but it also reflects the progression of some cells through the cell cycle. For the survival curves with a shoulder, the projection of the straight exponential portion of the curve to dose 0 represents the extrapolation number (Fig. 102-3) or the number of targets previously mentioned.

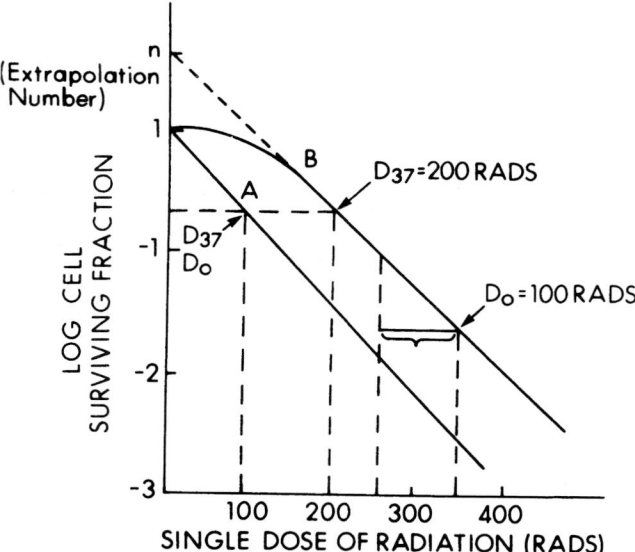

Fig. 102-3. Theoretic cell survival curves. Single-hit curve (A) is represented by the equation $SF = 1 - e^{D/DO}$. Multiple-hit survival curve (B) with an initial shoulder is represented by the equation $SF = 1 - (1 - e^{D/DO})^n$. See text for explanation of DO, D37, and extrapolation number. From Perez CA: Principles of radiation therapy. *In* Horton J, Hill GJ (eds): Clinical Oncology. Philadelphia: WB Saunders, 1977, p. 131. With permission.

Factors Affecting the Biological Effects of Ionizing Radiation

Cell Sensitivity to Radiation

Bergonie and Tribondeau (1906) stated that "cells with greater mitotic activity are more sensitive to radiation." It is not necessary, however, for the cells to be in mitosis at the time of radiation. Terasima and Tolmach (1963) and other investigators demonstrated in cell cultures and experimental animals that the sensitivity of cells to ionizing radiation and to most chemotherapeutic agents varies according to the phase of the cell cycle in which exposure of the cell to the physical or chemical event occurs.

In clinical practice, a distinction must be made between cell sensitivity to radiation on the one hand and tumor response and curability on the other. Some tumors, such as seminomas, dysgerminomas, lymphomas, and small cell undifferentiated lung carcinoma, are sensitive to radiation and may disappear after low or moderated doses, but the patient may not necessarily be cured and eventually dies of disseminated disease. Epidermoid carcinoma requires higher doses (6500 to 7500 rad or higher) for tumor control. On the other hand, some individuals thought for a long time that the adenocarcinomas of the breast and prostate were resistant to radiation. The concept is incorrect. Adenocarcinomas are as curable with irradiation as squamous cell carcinomas.

Oxygen Enhancement Effect (Reoxygenation)

With sparsely ionizing radiation, such as x-rays or gamma rays, a given biological effect produced by a given dose is two to three times greater in the presence of oxygen than if it is absent. This augmentation is called the *oxygen enhancement ratio*. Oxygen must be present during the radiation exposure. The oxygen enhancement effect is lessened or absent in high linear energy transfer (LET) radiations, such as alpha particles, fast neutrons, and pi-mesons. Although increasing concentrations of oxygen result in more sensitization to radiation, Gray (1961) reported that no significant gain is observed when the oxygen pressure is over 30 mm Hg. The exact mechanism of the oxygen effect has not been fully elucidated, although it is generally agreed that oxygen at the level of the free radicals combines to cause less repairable forms of DNA damage in specimens of bronchial carcinoma. Thomlinson (1967) reported no evidence of necrosis pathologically in any tumor with a radius of less than 160 μm; tumors with radii of over 200 μm always had necrotic centers. Suit and Shalek (1963) suggested that the hypoxic cell populations determine the response of a tumor to and probability of control of a tumor by radiation (Fig. 102-4). Fractionated radiation causes a decrease in the size of the tumor and the initial number of cells, as well as new blood vessel proliferation and reoxygenation. Kallman (1972) noted that these changes result in a transfer of hypoxic tumor cells to a more oxygenated compartment, and this transfer in turn eventually leads to complete sterilization of the tumor without significant injury to the surrounding normal tissues. The lack of oxygen enhancement effect in the biological events induced by high LET particles, as noted by Bond (1971), has resulted in renewed interest in the clinical applications of these radiations. Kolstad (1979) summarized several clinical trials with hyperbaric oxygen and radiation in tumors of the head and neck, cervix, and urinary bladder.

Linear Energy Transfer

LET represents the energy transferred by an ionizing particle per unit length of pathway. Because most ionizing particles are not energetic, the LET that results from a beam of energy is an average of all the particles or photons in the beam. In addition, at the molecular level, the energy per unit length of track varies. So the LET of an ionizing particle depends in a complex way on the energy and charge of the particle: The greater the charge and the smaller the velocity, the higher the LET.

Because of these varying amounts of energy released in an absorber, equal doses of various types of radiation do not produce the same biological effects on the absorber, or patient. The term *relative biological effect* was established to compare the biological effectiveness of a given ionizing radiation with a certain standard, which is 250-kV x-rays. For instance, Hall (1976) recorded that cobalt 60 has a relative biological effect of approximately 0.95, and neutrons have a relative biological effect of between 2.0 and 2.5, depending on their energy.

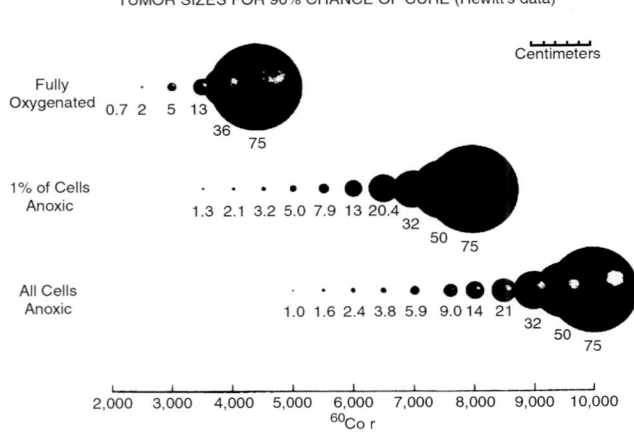

Fig. 102-4. Effect of hypoxic cells on curability of tumors. A tumor with hypoxic cells, regardless of the proportion, needs a dose of radiation two to three times greater to achieve the same control rate. Tumor sizes for a 90% chance of cure are illustrated. From Fowler J, Morgan RL, Wood CA: Pre-therapeutic experiments with the fast neutron beam from the Medical Research Council Cyclotron. I. The biological and physical advantages and problems of neutron therapy. Br J Radiol *36*:77, 1963. With permission.

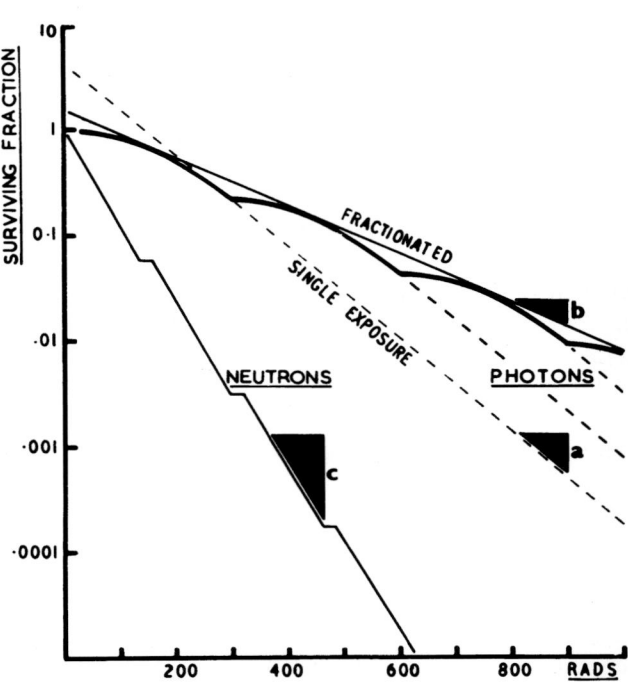

Fig. 102-5. Cell survival curves showing repair with fractionated doses using photons and absence of repair with neutrons. From Perez CA: Principles of radiation therapy. *In* Horton J, Hill GJ (eds): Clinical Oncology. Philadelphia: WB Saunders, 1977, p. 131. With permission.

Repair of Radiation Damage (Dose Fractionation)

Radiation therapy is given in daily fractions, four or five per week, on the presumption, as noted by Withers (1970), that normal cells generally have a greater and faster capacity to repair sublethal damage and cell repopulation between fractions. Ellis (1969) suggested that a patient's chances of survival are greater when the doses of radiation are fractionated, except in the case of high LET particles (Fig. 102-5). This time-dose relation depends on individual sensitivity of the cells and their repair ability, size of the radiation fractions, total dose given, time between fractions and of overall treatment, initial hypoxic subpopulation and reoxygenation that takes place throughout the fractionated therapy, and the type of ionizing radiation used.

In analyzing the treatment of the patient, the specifications should include not only the volume of tissue treated and the total dose given but also the number of fractions and the overall period of time in which they are administered.

PROCESS OF RADIATION THERAPY

The process of radiation therapy is initiated with evaluation and staging of the patient, both anatomically and pathologically. Comprehensive evaluation of the physiologic and functional status of the normal tissue organs such as lungs, heart, and spinal cord are an essential part of this evaluation. After the decision is made on the regimen to be used (e.g., conventional fractionation, hyperfraction, radiation-chemotherapy), the technical process of administering radiation therapy initiates with simulation. In the past this planning process was with a single radiograph, called *simulator film*. On obtaining the simulation film, which is usually in anteroposterior or lat-

eral projection, a portal would be outlined by the radiation oncologist that presumably contained the area of gross tumor as well as areas of subclinical disease and outlined the area to be radiated. After appropriate measurements of the dimensions of this area of the film and the separation of the patient, calculations would have been carried out and the delivery of treatment would commence. This technique is currently labeled *1D radiation therapy*.

Introduction of computed tomographic (CT) scanning to the practice of radiation oncology in the 1970s was an important step, not only for evaluation of the patients but also for planning purposes. This technique of planning, which is currently used in many radiation therapy departments around the world, is labeled *2D treatment planning*. In this technique one slice of CT scan, usually from the central axis of the radiation therapy or from the areas of gross tumor, is chosen and calculated isodoses are superimposed on this slice, in order to depict the doses received by the target volume as well as surrounding normal tissue surface (Fig. 102-6). Moving from the 1D to the 2D technique, as noted by one of us (B.E.) and colleagues (1978), was a major improvement. Nevertheless, even after two decades of use of 2D technology, serious limitations exist with this technique that are listed as follows.

Problems with Current 2D Treatment Planning and Delivery of External Beam Radiation Therapy

The problems with current treatment planning are 1) lack of realistic appreciation of gross tumor volume and clinical target volume, 2) lack of appreciation of real volume of normal tissue and organs irradiated to various doses, 3) deficiencies in the algorithms for computing dose, 4) failure to

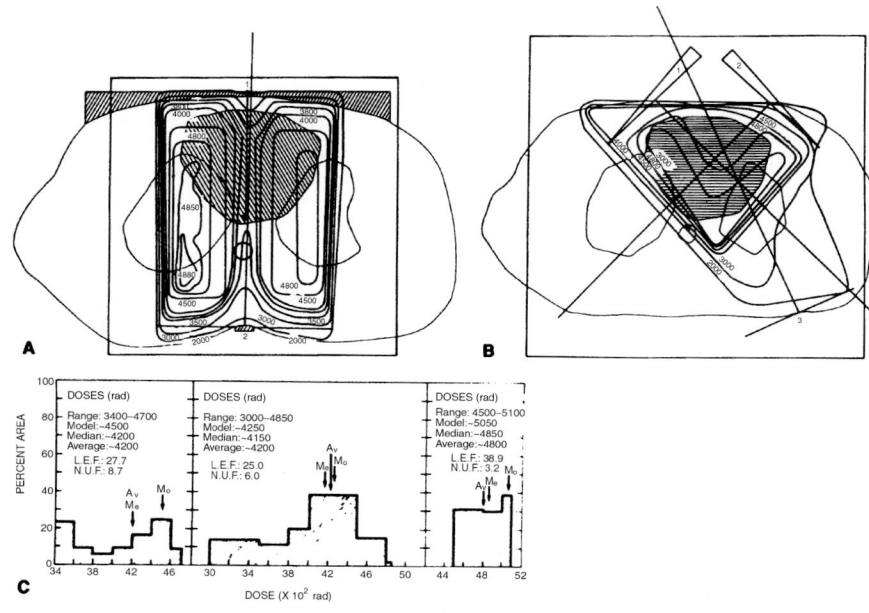

Fig. 102-6. A. Computed tomographic (CT) unoptimized treatment plan with lung transmission correction. Beam configuration and weights were identical to those in the conventional plan. Hatched area within patient's contour represents the target area as defined by a CT scan. Accurate lung transmission correction could be made because of the lung outline and density could be obtained directly from CT scans. Hatched area outside the patient's contour represents the compensating filter and spinal cord block. B. CT optimized plan with lung transmission correction. Wedged beams improved the uniformity of dose and reduced the dose to normal structures. C. Doses and local efficiency and nonuniformity factors for each plan. Notice the decreased mediastinal dose resulting from the posterior spinal cord block. From Prasad S, Pilepich MV, Perez CA: Contribution of CT to quantitative radiation therapy planning. AJR Am J Roentgenol *136*:123, 1981. With permission.

compute dose throughout the volume of interest, 5) restriction of treatment of coplanar beams, 6) failure to provide estimates of error, 7) unavailability of tools to compare and judge rival plans, 8) inadequate definition of geometric coverage of anatomic structures by external beams, and 9) failure to provide tools for specifying and verifying the accuracy of treatment delivery.

Review of the list reveals that with current practice of radiation therapy (i.e., 2D: simulation film and one slice of CT scan), it is impossible to accurately delineate the target volume that needs to be treated nor is it possible to accurately assess the true volume of normal tissues at risk that are radiated to various doses of radiation therapy and how these two relate to clinical success or complications. Other major drawbacks of 2D technology are limitations of beam arrangements of coplanar beams and significant difficulty in judgment of rival survival plans.

Technological advances in the areas of computers, faster CT scans, and graphics during the last decade have given birth to three-dimensional conformal radiation therapy (3D CRT). Enhanced capabilities of 3D CRT are superior, and more accurate delineation of target volumes and normal tissue structures, along with advanced dose calculations algorithm, have allowed clinicians to accurately conform the dose of radiation therapy to the target volume (tumor volume) and created a new opportunity to search for improved therapeutic outcome in radiation therapy in lung cancer.

To review the current status of 3D CRT in lung cancer, a review of various stages and procedures involved in 3D CRT is described (Table 102-1).

Patient immobilization in the treatment position is the first step of the planning process. This step, which was not paid adequate attention in 2D technology, is absolutely essential for 3D CRT.

CT scanning, for planning, is done either by specialized CT scans within radiation therapy departments or carried out with diagnostic CT scans with some connections to treatment planning systems of radiation therapy. These scans are used for contouring of desired target volumes and normal tissue structures. In contouring of target volumes, the recommendations of the International Commission of Radiation Units and Measurements Report 50 is usually followed. After contouring these volumes on every one of the CT scan slices, the data are transferred to specialized computers for 3D reconstruction of the anatomy and the desired target volumes. Virtual simulation and design of portals and initial beam arrangements are done after transferring data to 3D CRT planning systems. The next step is to design radiation entry portals using a specific tool—namely beams' eye view. Beam arrangements are usually done using the tool called room view. Radiation oncologists are no longer limited to anteroposterior/posteroanterior or lateral beams as was the case with the rotation of 2D technology. Three-dimensional dose calculations and plan evaluation and optimization of 3D beam arrangements are done through specialized tools. For plan evaluation, display tools such as

Table 102-1. Three-Dimensional Radiation Therapy Planning and Conformal Radiation Therapy

I. Delineation of target volumes
  Evaluation of patient, tumor (staging), and normal tissue and organs
  Patient immobilization
  Computed tomographic scanning
  Contouring of target volumes and normal organs
  Volumetric computed tomography data transfer to radiation treatment planning system
II. Planning and optimization
  Virtual simulation: design of portals and initial beam arrangement
  Three-dimensional dose calculations and display (dose-volume histogram, dose surface, dose statistics)
  Plan evaluation and optimization of three-dimensional beam arrangement
III. Predelivery preparation
  Digitally reconstructed radiograph
  Block template
  Verification of portals
  Marking of patient
  Radiographic verification
  Block making (Cerrobend) and block check
  Multileaf collimation
IV. Treatment delivery
V. Treatment verification and documentation
  Portal films
  On-line imaging
  Record and verifying system

dose volume histograms, dose cloud, and dose statistics are used (Fig. 102-7). Currently, many commercial systems provide most of these tools. After the final plan is decided on, the delivery of these complicated plans is carried out via sophisticated and modern linear accelerators equipped with specialized tools such as multileaf collimators, dynamic wedges, asymmetric jaws, and so forth. Verification of the delivery of these complicated plans is usually done through on-line imagining systems.

Clinical Experience with Three-Dimensional Conformal Radiation Therapy

For the majority of patients with unresectable non–small cell lung cancer referred for radiation therapy, local control and survival remains poor. As reported by Arriagada and associates (1991) in a randomized study of over 350 patients, the local control at 2 years with or without chemotherapy was 10%. Reports from the Radiation Therapy Oncology Group by Komaki (1998) and Sause (1998) and their coworkers, in which over 452 patients were randomized to conventional radiation therapy, radiation therapy and chemotherapy, and hyperfractionated radiotherapy, the 5-year survival was 5%, 8%, and 6%, respectively. These extremely poor results may be attributed to extremely poor local control. One of the possible reasons for the poor local

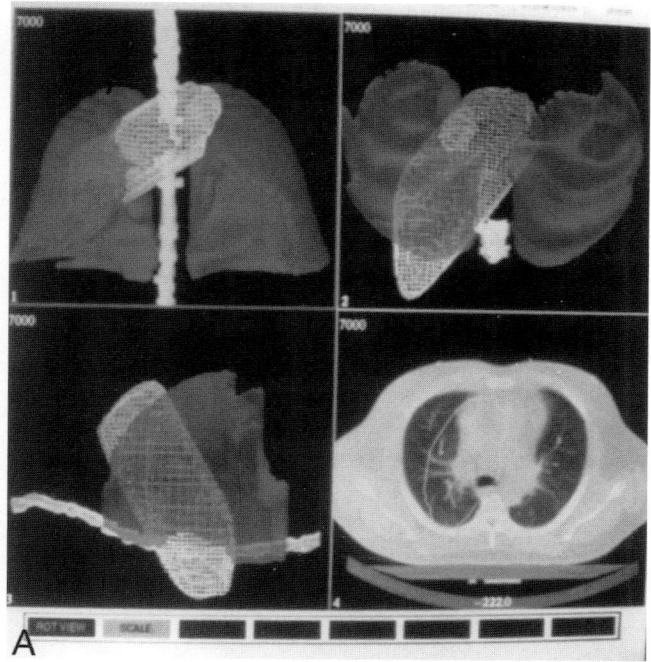

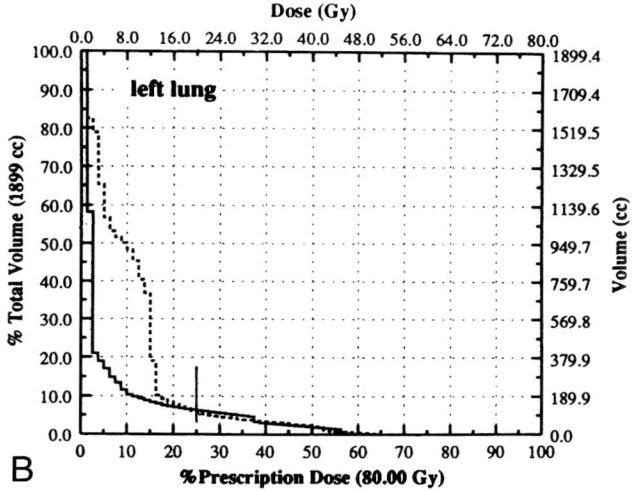

Fig. 102-7. A. Display on viewing monitor shows the various capabilities of three-dimensional radiation treatment planning system developed at the Radiation Oncology Center at Washington University. Representative views of anteroposterior, transverse, and lateral orientation of the patient's anatomy as well as the tumor volume and the dose of radiation (7000 cGy) covering the intended target volume are shown. A representative slice of CT scan at the level of the target volume is also shown. This interactive system enables radiation therapists to evaluate the true relationship between the radiation dose, intended target volume, and normal anatomic structures in a three-dimensional fashion. **B.** Cumulative dose volume histogram for the left lung of a patient with right lung cancer compares the dose received with the contralateral lung volume with two different treatment plans. As for volume of the contralateral lung, as well as the dose of radiation to normal tissue, the plan represented with solid lines shows more sparing of the opposite lung than the plan represented with the dash line. The dose-volume histogram provides a tool for quick viewing of the volumetric information on the dose of radiation to any tumor volume or normal organ.

control and poor survival may be the use of traditional large volumes in combination with the use of inferior 2D technology that precludes delivering a tumoricidal dose to the primary lung cancers commensurate with the tumor volume. From the original teaching of Fletcher (1973), it is generally accepted that for epithelial tumors, the dose for eradicating microscopic disease is 50 to 60 Gy and for gross disease of 1- to 3-cm dimension is approximately 75 Gy. On the other hand, the significant majority of patients seen with inoperable lung cancer in radiation therapy clinics have an average tumor size of 4 to 6 cm. Even with knowledge of the aforementioned facts, in most centers patients with inoperable lung cancer, irrespective of the size of the tumor, are treated with doses of 50 to 60 Gy. One of the possible reasons for using this low dose has been the limited tolerance of normal tissue to radiation and the inability of 2D technology to adequately protect normal tissues from high doses of radiation and thus avoid unacceptable complications.

After almost a decade of research, such as that by one of us (B.E.) (1996, 1998) and colleagues (1991b) and by Purdy and one of us (B.E.) (1991) on the application of 3D CRT in the treatment of patients with lung cancer, significant progress has been made. Superiority of 3D technology over 2D in precise and more accurate delineation of target volumes has already been proven. It is clearly shown that using 3D CRT tools, the delineation of treatment volume is more accurate and superior in avoidance of geographic misses. The therapeutic value of inclusion of subclinical disease, in view of poor local tumor control at the primary site, has been seriously questioned by investigators using 3D CRT, such as by one of us (B.E.) (1998), as well as by Leibel (1996), Armstrong (1997), and Martel (1997) and their colleagues. It is suggested that these large volumes have significantly contributed to the complication rates that can and should be avoided. Many investigators who currently use 3D CRT in the treatment of lung cancer have omitted the subclinical disease of various volumes to be irradiated in the treatment of lung cancer. Thus, this process has allowed radiation oncologists to initiate dose-escalating studies that, it is hoped, will result in higher tumor control rates, eventually contributing to survival, and lowering complication rates. Currently, several institutions have ongoing clinical trials using this new modality in treatment of patients with lung cancer, which includes a national multicenter study by a radiation therapy oncology group.

RADIOSENSITIZERS AND RADIOPROTECTIVE AGENTS

Radiation is a physical event that damages cells through biochemical mechanisms. The biochemical effects depend on cellular physiology (e.g., oxygen, cell cycle) and may be modifiable through biochemical additives (e.g., sensitizers, protectors). Berry (1965) and Doggett and colleagues (1967) noted that numerous drugs, including halogenated pyrimidines, dactinomycin, alkylating agents, and others, augment the effect of radiation on some tumors and normal tissues. The therapeutic aim of radiosensitizers may be additive or synergistic, depending on the degree of enhancement of effects.

Hypoxic sensitizers have been introduced in clinical trials. These drugs, which potentiate the effects of radiation on hypoxic cells, must be present at the time of irradiation. Phillips (1978) and Simpson (1987) and their colleagues reported the results of clinical trials with radiosensitizers. In randomized trials, no significant improvement in tumor control or survival was noted when compared with radiation alone. Significant peripheral neuropathy was the main toxicity associated with these drugs. Even newer compounds, such as SR-2508, with less lipophilicity, allowing larger doses to be administered with the same peripheral neuropathy, have failed to show any improvement in randomized clinical trials reported by Brown (1984) and Chassagne and associates (1992).

EFFECTS OF RADIATION ON NORMAL TISSUES

Esophagus

The effects of radiation on the esophagus are caused by damage to the germinal cell layers of the epithelium and the muscular layers and by vascular changes in the underlying tissues. Acute radiation esophagitis usually begins in the third week of radiation therapy, at the dose level of approximately 3000 to 4000 cGy. After 4000 cGy, a brisk mucositis and fibrinous exudate appear. These changes frequently are reversible. From the Radiation Therapy Oncology Group trials, the incidence of acute esophagitis was approximately 12% for grade II and 3% for grade III. With the current dose used (i.e., 6000 to 6500 cGy), the incidence of long-term sequelae such as esophageal stricture is rare. As one of us (B.E.) and associates (1991a) reported in the Radiation Therapy Oncology Group trials, this incidence was approximately 1%.

Lung

The most frequently reported sequela in the radiation therapy of thoracic neoplasms is pneumonitis. One of us (B.E.) and colleagues (1991a) noted that the incidence of grade II pneumonitis is approximately 10% and that of grade III pneumonitis is approximately 4.6%. Graham and associates (1994, 1995) reported the incidence and grade of pneumonitis after radiation therapy on 99 patients treated with 3D CRT. The incidence of a grade II pneumonitis was 14%, grade III pneumonitis was 2%, and grade IV was 2%. The threshold dose for radiation pneumonitis is 2000 cGy. The incidence and degree of radiation pneumonitis depends on the total dose, fractionation, and volume of lung irradiated.

The maximum lung volume that can be included in a high-dose zone of radiation therapy without significant clinical symptoms is 25% of the total lung volume. Use of 3D CRT in the management of lung cancer has given us significant insight to the volumetric radiation tolerance of lungs. Based on published information by Graham (1995) and Martel (1994) and their coworkers, it is generally agreed that if less than 25% of the total lung volume receives 2000 cGy, the patient is considered at low risk for the development of pneumonitis. If a radiation therapy plan shows 25 to 37% of the total lung volume is receiving more than 2000 cGy, then the patient is considered at medium risk for the development of pneumonitis. An attempt should be made to develop alternative plans in order to reduce the risk of pneumonitis. If the treatment plan includes over 37% of total lung volume receiving more than 2000 cGy, then we do not recommend that plan for the treatment of patients, because such patients are considered high risk for development of pneumonitis. When more than 75% of the pulmonary tissue is radiated with doses over 2000 cGy, patients may develop severe and sometimes fatal pneumonitis. The radiation-induced pneumonitis is usually manifested by respiratory distress, temperature peaks, and shortness of breath, and the patient may even die of acute respiratory insufficiency and cor pulmonale. Sputum culture result is negative unless a bacterial infection is superimposed, which is common and may be life-threatening. Radiography of the chest shows diffuse pulmonary infiltrates that may coalesce and may be associated with pleural or interlobar effusions. The underlying pathologic damage consists of alveolar degeneration and hyaline membrane formation, followed by fibrosis of the alveolar wall and interlobar septa as well as capillary thrombosis and fibrinoid degeneration of the small arterioles. Many of these acute changes are reversible after 3 to 4 weeks with moderate doses of radiation therapy. After larger doses, however, the chronic changes become permanent and can be seen as early as 3 months after radiation treatment. Substantial function impairment ensues. Decreased pulmonary blood flow can be demonstrated in nuclide ventilation-perfusion scanning. Pulmonary function studies in patients with lung cancer receiving radiation therapy demonstrated decreased compliance, diffusing capacity, and lung volumes. The decreased ventilatory and diffusing capacity results from alveolar cell degeneration and interstitial fibrosis.

Heart

The probability of radiation-induced cardiac disease after radiation therapy for lung cancer is relatively rare and depends on the volume irradiated, the size of the fraction, and the total dose of radiation. Transient, subacute, or chronic pericarditis is the most common form of clinical cardiac damage caused by radiation and may appear with doses over 5000 cGy. Stewart and Fajardo (1972) reported an incidence of cardiac complications of 6.6% after a mean dose of 4281 cGy. It is important to note that these patients were treated at the fractionation of 225 cGy/day, and in most of them, almost the entire volume of the heart was radiated.

Spinal Cord

Acute radiation effects in the spinal cord are usually of minimal clinical significance and are caused mostly by transient edema. A transient radiation effect on the spinal cord is known as Lhermitte's syndrome. It occurs a few weeks after exposure and is characterized by some electric shock-like sensations that radiate along the spinal cord and spinal nerves into the extremities. In most instances, the syndrome is reversible and does not correlate with subsequent permanent radiation myelopathy. A more severe type of brainstem or spinal cord injury appears after 6 months or as late as several years after radiation. Radiation myelopathy causes motor and sensory changes referable to the injured segment. If the entire width of the cord is irradiated, complete paraplegia and anesthesia occur as a result of a total physiologic transection of the spinal cord. If only one-half of the cord is irradiated, the neurologic picture is that of Brown-Séquard syndrome. These permanent changes are secondary to severe capillary degeneration, fibrinoid necrosis of the small arterioles, and necrosis of neurons and other oligodendrocytes, accompanied by demyelination of the white matter.

Small segments of brainstem or spinal cord may tolerate doses of more than 5000 cGy, given in weekly increments of 1000 cGy. With doses of 6000 cGy in 6 weeks, the probability of radiation myelitis is 10 to 15%. A strong probability exists that higher doses induce radiation myelopathy more frequently. Also, the greater the length of segment of the spinal cord being irradiated, the more likely the possibility of developing permanent myelopathy.

Table 102-2 presents the accepted tolerated doses for intrathoracic structures in the absence of chemotherapy.

Bone Marrow

The acute effects of radiation on the bone marrow, mostly caused by direct cell killing, are related to the volume irradiated and the dose and fractions given. Usually, a reduction in the number of lymphocytes occurs; a reflection on the extreme sensitivity of circulating lymphocytes to interphase death. The lymphocyte count remains low for weeks or months; gradually repopulation occurs. The granulocytes decrease 1 to 2 weeks after segmental irradiation, with recovery taking weeks or up to 18 months. Moderate thrombocytopenia is common; if the platelets decrease to less than 20,000, hemorrhages with ecchymosis, hematemesis, and melena, which complicate the fluid and electrolyte imbalance, may occur. The circulating red cells are extremely radioresistant, but chronic irradiation may cause protracted anemia.

Knospe (1966) and Rubin (1973) and their colleagues noted that when the bone marrow is irradiated with over 4000 rad, more permanent chronic changes occur. Vascular degeneration, as pointed out by Rubin and Cassarett (1968), and fibrosis, as Lejar and associates (1966) noted, occur, preventing repopulation. These changes are more severe in patients who previously received bone marrow–depressing chemotherapeutic agents or in patients who were treated with these drugs after radiation therapy. Special care should be exercised for patients receiving combination therapy or re-treatment after radiation therapy or chemotherapy, and frequent leukocyte and platelet counts are necessary, particularly if the bone marrow is infiltrated with malignant cells.

EFFECT OF ADJUVANT CHEMOTHERAPY ON COMPLICATIONS

Chemotherapy significantly enhances the effect of irradiation. Phillips and Margolis (1972) reported a 50% incidence of radiation pneumonitis in patients treated with radiation alone (approximately 2650 rad in 20 fractions). When dactinomycin was added, the incidence of pneumonitis was 50% with delivery of 2050 rad in 20 fractions. Patients receiving bleomycin may develop interstitial pulmonary fibrosis, which can accentuate the similar effects of irradiation.

Johnson and associates (1976) reported instances of severe esophageal fibrosis with stenosis after the administration of 3000 rad in 2 weeks combined with intensive triple-agent chemotherapy (doxorubicin, vincristine, and cyclophosphamide) given the same day every 3 to 4 weeks. Also, the well-known cardiotoxicity of doxorubicin coupled

Table 102-2. Normal Tissue Tolerance to Therapeutic Irradiation

Organ	Tolerated Doses 5/5 Volume			Tolerated Doses 50/5 Volume			Selected End Point
	1/3	2/3	3/3	1/3	2/3	3/3	
Spinal cord (cm)	5	10	20	5	10	20	Myelitis necrosis
	5000	5000	4700	7000	7000	—	
Lung	4500	3000	1750	6500	4000	2450	Pneumonitis
Heart	6000	4500	4000	7000	5500	5000	Pericarditis
Esophagus	6000	5800	5500	7200	7000	6800	Clinical stricture/perforation

Modified from Emami B, et al: Tolerance of normal tissue to therapeutic irradiation. Int J Radiat Oncol Biol Phys *21*:109, 1991.

with the effects of radiation on the heart makes this combination more toxic. When these two agents are combined, Chan and colleagues (1976) recommended that no more than a total of 4000 rad be given to the entire heart, or that a maximum of 450 mg/m^2 total dose of doxorubicin be administered. Also, the two agents should not be administered simultaneously.

The effects of combined irradiation and chemotherapy on the spinal cord have not been evaluated properly, but it is reasonable to believe that an additive or potentiating effect is present.

REFERENCES

Armstrong J, et al: Promising survival with three-dimensional conformal radiation therapy for non-small cell lung cancer. Radiother Oncol *44*:17, 1997.

Arriagada R, et al: ASTRO (American Society for Therapeutic Radiology and Oncology) plenary: Effect of chemotherapy on locally advanced non-small cell lung carcinoma: a randomized study of 353 patients. Int J Radiat Oncol Biol Phys *20*:183, 1991.

Bergonie J, Tribondeau L: De quesques resultats de la radiotherapie et essai de fization d'une technique rationelle. CR Acad Sci *143*:983, 1906.

Berry RJ: Modification of radiation effects. Radiol Clin North Am *3*:249, 1965.

Bond VP: Negative pions: their possible use in radiotherapy. AJR Am J Roentgenol *111*:9:1971.

Brown JM: Clinical trials of radiosensitizers. What should we expect? Int J Radiat Oncol Biol Phys *10*:425, 1984.

Chan YM, et al: Co-incident Adriamycin (A) and x-ray therapy (XRT) in bronchogenic carcinoma (BC): response and cardiotoxicity (CT). Proc AACR ASCO *17*:276, 1976.

Chassagne D, et al: First analysis of tumor regression for the European randomized trial of etanidazole combined with radiotherapy in head and neck carcinomas. Int J Radiat Oncol Biol Phys *22*:581, 1992.

Doggett R, et al: Combined therapy using chemotherapeutic agents and radiotherapy. *In* Wood C, Deeley TJ (eds): Modern Trends in Radiotherapy. Vol. 1. New York: Appleton-Century-Crofts, 1967, p. 107.

Elkind MM, et al: Sub-lethal and lethal radiation damage. Nature *214*:1088, 1967.

Ellis F: Dose-time and fractionation: a clinical hypothesis. Clin Radiol *20*:1. 1969.

Emami B, et al: The current status of 3D conformal radiotherapy in lung cancer. *In* Mornex F, Van Houtte P (eds): Treatment optimization for lung cancer from classical to innovative procedure. ISALC International Workshop. Annecy, France: Elsevier, 1998, pp. 81–88.

Emami B, et al: Three-dimensional conformal radiotherapy in bronchogenic carcinoma: considerations for implementation. Lung Cancer *11*(Suppl 3):117, 1994.

Emami B, et al: Three dimensional treatment planning for lung cancer. Int J Radiat Oncol Biol Phys *21*:217, 1991b.

Emami B, et al: Tolerance of normal tissue to therapeutic irradiation. Int J Radiat Oncol Biol Phys *21*:109. 1991a.

Emami B: Optimization of volume in radiotherapy of non-small cell lung cancer; small volume. *In* Mornex F, Van Houtte P (eds): Treatment optimization for lung cancer from classical to innovative procedure. ISALC International Workshop. Annecy, France: Elsevier, 1998, pp. 59–66.

Emami B, Melo A, Carter B: Value of computed tomography in radiotherapy of lung cancer. AJR Am J Radiol *131*:63, 1978.

Fletcher GH: Clinical dose-response curves of human malignant epithelial tumors. Br J Radiol *46*:1, 1973.

Graham M, et al: 3-D radiation treatment planning study for patients with carcinoma of the lung. Int J Radiat Oncol Biol Phys *29*:1105, 1994.

Graham M, et al: Preliminary results of a prospective trial using three-dimensional radiotherapy for lung cancer. Int J Radiat Oncol Biol Phys *33*:993, 1995.

Gray LH: Radiobiologic basis of oxygen as modifying factor in radiation therapy. AJR Am J Roentgenol *85*:803, 1961.

Hall EJ: Radiobiology for the Radiologist. 2nd Ed. New York: Harper & Row, 1976.

Hewitt HB, Wilson CW: Survival curve for mammalian leukemia cells irradiation in vivo. Br J Cancer *13*:69, 1959.

Johns HE, Cunningham JR: The Physics of Radiology. 4th Ed. Springfield IL: Charles C Thomas, 1983.

Johnson RE, Brereton HD, Kent CH: Small cell carcinoma of the lung: attempt to remedy causes of past therapeutic failure. Lancet 2:289.1976.

Kallman RF: The phenomenon of reoxygenation and its implications for fractionated radiotherapy. Radiology *105*:135, 1972.

Kaplan HS: Biochemical basis of reproductive death in irradiated cells. AJR Am J Roentgenol *909*:907, 1963.

Knospe WH, Blom J, Crosby WH: Regeneration of locally irradiated bone marrow. I. Dose-dependent long-term changes in the rat, with particular emphasis upon vascular and stomal reaction. Blood *28*:308, 1966.

Kolstad P: Oxygen tension and radiocurability. *In* Deeley T (ed): Modern Radiotherapy-Gynecological Cancer. New York: Appleton-Century-Crofts, 1979, p. 155.

Komaki R, et al: Failure patterns by prognostic group determined by recursive partitioning analysis (RPA) of 1547 patients on four Radiation Therapy Oncology Group (RTOG) studies in inoperable non-small cell lung cancer (NSCLC). Int J Radiat Oncol Biol Phys *42*:263, 1998.

Leibel SA, et al: 3-D conformal radiation therapy for non–small cell lung carcinoma. Clinical experience at the Memorial Sloan-Kettering Cancer Center. Front Radiat Ther Oncol *29*:199, 1996.

Lejar TJ, et al: Effects of focal irradiation on human bone marrow. AJR Am J Roentgenol *96*:183, 1966.

Little JB: Cellular effects of ionizing radiation. N. Engl J Med *278*:308, 1968.

Martel MK, et al: Dose-volume histogram and 3D treatment planning evaluation of patients with pneumonitis. Int J Radiat Oncol Biol Phys *28*:575, 1994.

Martel MK, et al: Volume and dose parameters for survival of non-small cell lung cancer patients. Radiother Oncol *44*:23, 1997.

Perez CA: Principles of radiation therapy. *In* Horton J, Hill GJ (eds): Clinical Oncology. Philadelphia: WB Saunders, 1977, p. 131.

Phillips T, Margolis L: Radiation pathology and the clinical response of lung and esophagus. *In* Vaeth JM (ed): Frontiers of Radiation Therapy and Oncology. Vol 6. Baltimore: University Park Press, 1972, p. 254.

Phillips TL, et al: The hypoxic cell sensitizer program in the United States. Br J Cancer *37*(Suppl III):276, 1978.

Prasad S, Pilepich MV, Perez CA: Contribution of CT to quantitative radiation therapy planning. AJR Am J Roentgenol *136*:123, 1981.

Puck TT, Marcus PI: Action of x-rays on mammalian cells. J Exp Med *103*:653, 1956.

Purdy JA, Emami B: Computed tomography and three dimensional approaches to radiation therapy I treatment planning. *In* Levitt S, Tapley N (eds): Technological Basis of Radiation Therapy: Practical Clinical Applications. Philadelphia: Lea & Febiger, 1991, pp. 56–66.

Rubin P, Cassarett G: Clinical Radiation Pathology. Philadelphia: WB Saunders, 1968.

Rubin P, et al: Bone marrow regeneration and extension after extended field irradiation in Hodgkin's disease. Cancer *32*:699, 1973.

Sause W, et al: Five-year results: phase III trial of regionally advanced unresectable non-small cell lung cancer, RTOG 8808, ECOG 4588, SWOG 8992. Presented at the ASCO 34th Annual Meeting, Los Angeles, May 1998.

Simpson JR, et al: Large fraction irradiation with or without misonidazole in advanced non-oat cell carcinoma of the lung: a phase III randomized trial of the RTOG. Int J Radiat Oncol Biol Phys *13*:861, 1987.

Stewart JR, Fajardo LF: Radiation-induced heart disease. *In* Vaeth JM (ed): Frontiers of Radiation Therapy and Oncology. Vol 6. Baltimore: University Park Press, 1972, p. 274.

Suit HD, Shalek RJ: Response of anoxic C3H mouse mammary carcinoma isotransplants (1-25 MM3) to x-irradiation. J Natl Cancer Inst *31*:479, 1963.

Terasima T, Tolmach LJ: Variations in several responses of hela cells to x-irradiation during division cycle. Biophys J *3*:11, 1963.

Thomlinson RH: Oxygen therapy-biological considerations. *In* Wood C, Deeley TJ (eds): Modern Trends in Radiotherapy. Vol 1. New York: Appleton-Century-Crofts, 1967.

Withers HR: Capacity for repair in cells of normal and malignant tissues. *In* Time and Dose Relationships in Radiation Biology as Applied to Radiotherapy. Upton, NY: Brookhaven National Laboratory Associated Universities, 1970, p. 54.

READING REFERENCES

Cox JD, et al: Dose-time relationships and the local control of small cell carcinoma of the lung. Radiology *128*:205, 1978.

Eichorn HJ, Lessel A, Matschke S: Comparison between neutron therapy and ^{60}CO gamma ray therapy of bronchial, gastric and oesophagus carcinomata. Eur J Cancer *10*:361, 1974.

Emami B, Graham MV: Lung. *In* Principles and Practice of Radiation Oncology. Philadelphia: JB Lippincott, 1998, pp. 1181–1220.

Emami B, Perez CA: Lung. *In* Perez CA, Brady L (eds): Principles and Practice of Radiation Oncology. Philadelphia: JB Lippincott, 1992, pp. 806–836.

Emami B, et al: Three-dimensional conformal radiation therapy: clinical aspects. *In* Principles and Practice of Radiation Oncology. Philadelphia: JB Lippincott, 1998, pp. 371–386.

Hall EJ: Radiobiology for the Radiologist. 4th Ed. Lippincott–Raven, 1993.

Purdy JA, Emami B: 3D radiation treatment planning and conformal therapy. International Symposium Proceedings, April 21–23, 1993.

Prescribing, Recording, and Reporting Photon Beam Therapy (ICRU report, No. 50). International Commission on Radiation, Nov. 1993.

CHAPTER 103

Radiation Therapy for Carcinoma of the Lung

Ritsuko Komaki and James D. Cox

Carcinoma of the lung encompasses a group of diseases that require the collaboration of the thoracic surgeon, radiation oncologist, medical oncologist, pathologist, and diagnostic radiologist. Unless dramatic accomplishments in prevention are made in the next decade, the effective interplay of these specialists represents the best hope for the millions of patients worldwide who will develop cancer of the lung.

Radiation therapy, like surgical resection, is a technically complex local-regional treatment that can be used with curative intent. The results depend on the experience of the physician-led team and appropriate application to patients whose disease is confined to a primary tumor and regional lymph node metastasis. In patients with disease too advanced to be considered potentially curable, radiation therapy also can be used to relieve symptoms from the intrathoracic tumor and discrete metastases, especially in the brain or bones.

The end points used to evaluate the effectiveness of surgery, radiation therapy, and chemotherapy have differed historically. In surgical management of lung cancer, the focus has been on the curability of the patient, and the end point has usually been survival, and less frequently relapse-free survival, at 3 or 5 years. The most common end points used in evaluating chemotherapy alone for lung cancer have been complete and partial response rates and median survival. These are, for practical purposes, palliative end points. Two-year survival or relapse-free survival has widely been used to assess the results of treatment of patients with small cell carcinoma of the lung (SCCL) with chemotherapy alone or chemotherapy combined with radiation therapy.

Radiotherapeutic effectiveness has been assessed using both sets of end points. The palliative contribution has been reported in terms of response rates and median survival. The lack of sensitive indicators of recurrence after radiation therapy, however, and the recognition that the treatment can cause changes in the irradiated volume that obscure response, raise questions as to the value of *response* as a useful end point. Median survival has no necessary relationship to long-term survival.

The standards of treatment for most patients with carcinoma of the lung without distant metastasis have changed in recent years. Integration of two or all three therapeutic modalities is advantageous for most patients rather than a single approach. Combinations of resection and irradiation improve local tumor control and may decrease the risk of distant metastasis. Increasingly, chemotherapy is effective in eradicating subclinical metastases; it also may improve local control if used concurrently with radiation therapy.

One of the challenges is proper application of the treatments to groups of patients most likely to benefit. Pretreatment prognostic variables probably outweigh treatment factors in short-term survival of patients with inoperable squamous cell carcinoma, adenocarcinoma, and large cell carcinoma [non–small cell carcinoma (NSCCL)] of the lung. At least 20% of all patients with NSCCL have unresectable tumors without distant metastasis, little loss of weight (less than 5%), and mild to moderate symptoms (Karnofsky's performance status scores of 70 to 100). One of the authors (R.K.) and associates (1985) showed that these patients were potentially curable with radiation therapy alone. The outlook for these relatively favorable inoperable patients is better with induction chemotherapy followed by radiation therapy as demonstrated by Dillman (1990), Le Chevalier (1991), and Sause (1995) and their colleagues.

SCCL, heretofore considered the most malignant form of cancer of the lung, is more highly curable than NSCCL when the tumor is limited to the primary site and regional lymph nodes. Radiation therapy to these regions concurrent with combination chemotherapy has been shown by Turrisi and coworkers (1990, 1992) to cure more than 20% of patients with limited SCCL.

INDICATIONS FOR RADIATION THERAPY FOR BRONCHIAL CARCINOMA BASED ON FAILURE ANALYSES

Failure pattern analyses by Shields (1983) of patients with resectable carcinoma of the lung suggest that a group of patients with squamous cell carcinoma, adenocarcinoma, and large cell carcinoma of the lung could benefit from irradiation of the mediastinum and hila. Patients with $T_1N_0M_0$ and $T_2N_0M_0$ fail infrequently in the thorax after complete resection. The presence of regional lymph node metastasis increases considerably the risk of local failure, and it also portends a higher rate of distant metastasis, especially to the brain.

Failure pattern analyses by one of the authors (J.D.C.) (1983) of patients with inoperable or unresectable carcinoma of the lung showed that the intrathoracic tumor is a major determinant of survival after palliative irradiation or single-agent chemotherapy, especially in patients with squamous cell carcinoma. Saunders and associates (1984) studied the causes of death in patients with unresectable NSCCL who were treated with a few large fractions of irradiation to a modest total dose of 35 Gy. They showed that 72% of their patients died of complications of the intrathoracic disease and only 15% died from distant metastasis. Arriagada and coworkers (1997) analyzed the effects of local failure relative to distant metastasis in a large prospective trial of induction chemotherapy. The local failure rate was 92% at 5 years, the reason for the small survival benefit of induction chemotherapy even though there was a highly significant reduction in distant metastasis.

EVALUATION BEFORE RADIATION THERAPY

The evaluation of patients with carcinoma of the lung apparently confined to the thorax differs little whether the patient is to be treated with surgical resection or with definitive radiation therapy. The intent of the pretreatment evaluation is to determine the extent of the local and regional manifestations of the intrathoracic tumor and to investigate the most likely sites of distant metastasis. With rare exceptions, it is inappropriate to undertake a long course of radiation therapy to high total doses if distant metastasis is recognized.

A complete blood count, biochemical survey, and posteroanterior and lateral chest radiographs are performed routinely. The intrathoracic tumor can be assessed well by high-resolution computed tomography (CT) with intravenous contrast administration. Multiple parenchymal lesions, pericardial involvement with effusion, and pleural effusion are signs of intrathoracic dissemination and are contraindications to aggressive local-regional therapy. Magnetic resonance (MR) imaging has not been found to be more sensitive or accurate than CT by Webb and colleagues (1991), although apical sulcus (Pancoast's) tumors are well demonstrated by MR imaging, especially in parasagittal planes (Fig. 103-1). The liver, adrenal glands, and kidneys, all common sites of distant metastasis at autopsy, can be assessed by high-resolution, contrast-enhanced CT of the upper abdomen.

The diagnosis of adenocarcinoma, large cell carcinoma, or small cell carcinoma justifies contrast-enhanced CT or

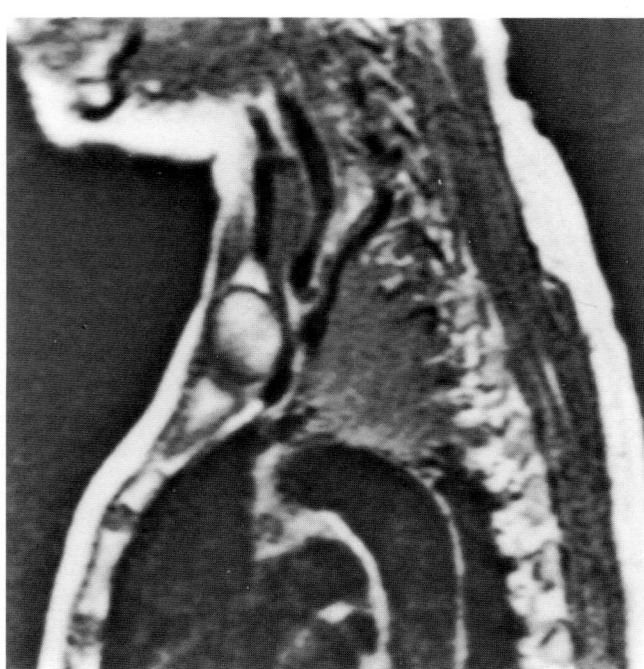

Fig. 103-1. Magnetic resonance image reconstruction in the parasagittal plane showing superior extensions of adenocarcinoma of the left apical sulcus.

MR imaging of the head to look for occult cerebral metastasis. In patients with no neurologic symptoms, the frequency of occult cerebral metastasis recorded by Jacobs (1977) and Tarver (1984) and their associates ranged from 10 to 20%. The finding of cerebral metastasis, of course, profoundly affects the prognosis as well as the plan of therapy.

SURGICAL ADJUVANT RADIATION THERAPY

Radiation therapy is clearly of benefit in a subset of patients with resectable carcinomas of the lung. The indications for adjuvant irradiation, the timing (whether preoperative or postoperative), and the use of chemotherapy in conjunction with radiation therapy are being refined by clinical investigations.

Radiation therapy can have an adverse effect on pulmonary function among patients who have had major resections of the lung, so only those patients at high risk for regional recurrence should be treated. Preoperative or postoperative radiation therapy has no role among patients without surgical pathologic evidence of metastasis to regional lymph nodes (pN_0). A meta-analysis of clinical trials of postoperative irradiation by the PORT Meta-analysis Trialist Group (1998) found no value for patients with hilar lymph node involvement (pN_1).

The excellent review by Van Houtte and Henry (1985) summarized trials of both preoperative and postoperative radiation therapy. They concluded that preoperative irradiation has no benefit in patients with clearly operable tumors. Patients with marginally resectable tumors, especially those with spread to mediastinal lymph nodes, continue to be studied. Chemotherapy concurrent with radiation therapy followed by thoracotomy and resection, as reported by Albain (1991), is being compared with chemotherapy and radiation therapy alone in a prospective intergroup trial.

Van Houtte and Henry (1985) concluded that a suggestion of benefit existed from postoperative irradiation for patients with hilar or mediastinal lymph node involvement. Three- and 5-year survival rates in these studies ranged from 16 to 33% in patients with squamous cell carcinoma treated with surgical resection alone versus survival rates of 21 to 52% for those treated with surgery plus radiation therapy. The data were even more striking for adenocarcinoma with hilar or mediastinal lymph node involvement: 0 to 8% 5-year survival with surgery alone versus 12 to 62% survival with surgery and postoperative irradiation. The meta-analysis showed no value of surgical adjuvant radiation therapy for pN_1 tumors, but insufficient data existed to draw conclusions concerning patients with mediastinal lymph node metastasis.

Two prospective randomized trials of postoperative radiation therapy have been conducted. An European Organization for Research on the Treatment of Cancer trial reported by Israel and associates (1979) suggested a survival benefit of the same order of magnitude as the retrospective studies (i.e., 20 to 25%), but the results were preliminary and not statistically significant. The Lung Cancer Study Group (1986) conducted a trial of postoperative radiation therapy versus surgery alone for patients with stage III squamous cell carcinoma of the lung. They found a striking reduction in the frequency of local recurrence within the thorax but no survival benefit.

DEFINITIVE RADIATION THERAPY FOR SQUAMOUS CELL CARCINOMA, ADENOCARCINOMA, AND LARGE CELL CARCINOMA OF THE LUNG

Radiation therapy is the mainstay of treatment for patients with inoperable squamous cell carcinoma, adenocarcinoma, and large cell carcinoma of the lung (NSCCL). Once the determination has been made that such patients' disease is inoperable or unresectable and a thorough evaluation has shown no evidence of distant metastasis, technically sophisticated, high-dose radiation therapy offers the best opportunity for long-term, disease-free survival.

Admittedly, as pointed out by Arriagada and colleagues (1991), standard radiation therapy is far from sufficient local treatment. Moreover, effective thoracic irradiation does not contribute to control of already established subclinical extrathoracic metastases. The evolution of more effective systemic therapy reinforces the importance of local-regional control; the actual cause of death is the result more often of intrathoracic complications than distant organ involvement.

Determination of the Treatment Volume

Definitive irradiation for lung cancer is predicated on irradiation of the primary tumor and involved lymph nodes with adequate margins. Ipsilateral hilar and mediastinal lymph node regions must also be treated.

No systematic study of supraclavicular irradiation has been performed, but data from biopsy studies suggest that at least one-fourth of patients with upper lobe tumor have spread to the scalene or supraclavicular nodes, whereas this risk is less than 10% for tumors arising in the lower lobes. Systematic irradiation of the ipsilateral supraclavicular nodes is considered standard for upper lobe or middle lobe tumors.

Treatment Planning

Treatment planning to achieve permanent control of the intrathoracic tumor has increased in sophistication and complexity. This is an area of intensive research and is changing rapidly. Chapter 102 by Emami complements the following brief description.

The process of planning definitive treatment for carcinoma of the lung, after complete assessment of the diagnostic studies, especially the CT scan of the thorax, starts with simulation. The treatment planning simulator is a diagnostic x-ray unit, usually with fluoroscopy, in which the focal spot for diagnostic radiographs is set exactly at the same point as the source or target that emits high-energy photons. The image intensifier can be moved independently to assess the margins of the field to determine that they adequately encompass the entire volume to be treated.

A radiograph of diagnostic quality that shows the intrathoracic anatomy sharply is obtained; the photons from the actual treatment machine are so penetrating that anatomic distinctions between bone and soft tissues are obscured. Correlation of the anatomy displayed on the simulation image with that apparent from the CT of the chest serves as the basis for defining the exact margins of the volume to be treated. A treatment planning CT scan of the entire thorax permits definition of all known tumor in each axial slice as well as delineation of critical normal structures (i.e., both lungs, spinal cord, heart, and esophagus). Multiple fields may be used with individualized external blocks or machine-based collimation, which encompass the tumor but exclude all normal tissue possible. Increasingly, three-dimensional treatment planning is used with the goals of increasing doses to the tumor while sparing normal tissues.

Sophisticated treatment planning has become standard. There is no reason any longer to consider unshaped, square, or rectangular fields the norm, or to base treatment only on posteroanterior and lateral chest films. Careful blocking must be undertaken if the high doses thought necessary to control common epithelial tumors, including those arising in the lung, are to be achieved.

Dose-Time Relationships

The interplay of the individual dose of irradiation (fraction size), the frequency of delivery of the individual dose or fraction, the total dose to the tumor and to normal tissues, and the overall time of treatment are encompassed by the terms *dose-time relationships* or *fractionation*. In the 1960s and 1970s, it was assumed that outcome in the radiation therapy of carcinomas of the lung was not greatly influenced by differing fractionation schemes. Low total doses were used with the rationale that adequate palliation could be achieved without recourse to high doses that might injure normal structures, especially the lung parenchyma. Because the total doses were low, changing the fractionation to a smaller number of large fractions led to the same poor result. Deeley (1967) reported a prospective clinical trial that compared 30 with 40 Gy, both given in 20 fractions in 4 weeks: 12- and 18-month survival data convinced him that the lower dose was at least as effective. A subsequent comparison by Deeley (1974) of 40 Gy in 20 fractions in 4 weeks with 32 Gy in eight fractions (two fractions per week) in 4 weeks confirmed his expectation that both regimens were equal. Thus, a school of thought prevailed that irradiation to low total doses, with or without large fractions, was sufficient to relieve distressing symptoms and would cause few deleterious effects on the normal lung.

The Radiation Therapy Oncology Group (RTOG) conducted a landmark study in which a multicenter, prospective, centrally randomized trial compared the effectiveness of 40, 50, and 60 Gy, delivered as 2.0-Gy per fraction, five fractions per week, for 4, 5, or 6 weeks, respectively. Early analyses of this trial by Perez and associates (1980) revealed a dose-response relationship for tumor control with lower failure rates resulting from higher total doses. Long-term follow-up of the patients in this study, although showing no difference in median survival, showed a highly significant direct relationship between 2- and 3-year survival and total dose. As noted by the authors (1989), these differences have been discounted because the 5-year survival rates did not differ. Nonetheless, a total dose of at least 60 Gy in 30 fractions in 6 weeks became a standard for RTOG studies and in many institutions in the United States.

Higher total doses might be used, and they are currently being explored in prospective studies using three-dimensional conformal radiation therapy.

A large body of data from the radiation therapy of common epithelial tumors of many sites suggests that fractions larger than 2.0 Gy and treatments less frequent than 5 days per week are disadvantageous. As one of the authors (J.D.C.) observed (1985b), large-dose fractionation can include hypofractionation (fewer than five treatments per week, rapid fractionation), large doses 5 days per week for only 3 or 4 weeks, and split-course radiation therapy (interruption of 1 week or more during the course of radiation therapy) with fractions of 2.0 Gy or less, or larger fractions attempting to compensate for the split, thus combining the split with rapid fractionation. Based on a review of RTOG studies over 15 years, Perez and associates (1989) reported a significantly higher rate of late reactions in normal tissues with larger fractions, compared with 2.0 Gy or less.

Studies of hypoxic cell sensitizers that, theoretically, would produce the most effective result from combination with a few large fractions of radiation therapy have provided important information on the results of hypofractionation. Saunders and colleagues (1984) randomly assigned 62 patients to receive 35 Gy in six fractions in 3 weeks with and without the nitrofuran misonidazole. Their careful assessment based on a high autopsy rate showed the fractionation regimen to be ineffective; the overwhelming cause of death was progression of the local-regional tumor. Fewer than 5% of patients had control of the tumor within the irradiated volume. Also, misonidazole proved to be of no benefit.

Proliferation of Tumor Cells During Treatment

An expanding body of data suggests that failure to control common epithelial tumors results, in part, from continued proliferation of surviving tumor cells during treatment. Fowler and Lindstrom (1992) reviewed 12 sets of data from radiation therapy for carcinomas of the upper respiratory and digestive tracts and concluded that interruptions of treatment reduced tumor control by approximately 14% per extra week of prolongation. Adverse consequences of prolonging treatment time in NSCCL have been shown by one of the authors (J.D.C.) and associates from the RTOG (1993). Withers and associates (1988) found evidence that proliferation actually accelerated approximately 3 to 4 weeks after the start of irradiation.

Several means of overcoming proliferation of clonogenic cells during treatment are being investigated. Diener-West and colleagues (1991) noted that hyperfractionation (i.e., giving larger numbers of smaller than standard fraction of irradiation) permits higher total doses to be delivered in the same overall treatment time. The RTOG showed, in a report by one of the authors (J.D.C.) and colleagues (1990), a higher survival rate with 69.6 Gy using 1.2 Gy twice daily, compared with lower total doses (Fig. 103-2). This study led to a randomized comparison of hyperfractionation with 69.6 Gy at 1.2 Gy twice daily to 60 Gy at 2.0 Gy daily (RTOG 88-08/Eastern Cooperative Oncology Group 4588). Sause and colleagues (1995) reported no improvement in this randomized trial, although longer follow-up reported by one of the authors (R.K.) (1997) showed that 3-year survival rates were higher in the hyperfractionated irradiation arm. Lee and associates (1998) combined this fractionation schedule with concurrent cisplatin and oral etoposide, resulting in 5-year survival of 22% among a small group of patients with inoperable NSCCL.

Accelerated fractionation seeks to avoid the effects of proliferation of residual tumor cells by completing the total course of treatment in the shortest period of time. It is achieved by delivering more than one fraction per day for all

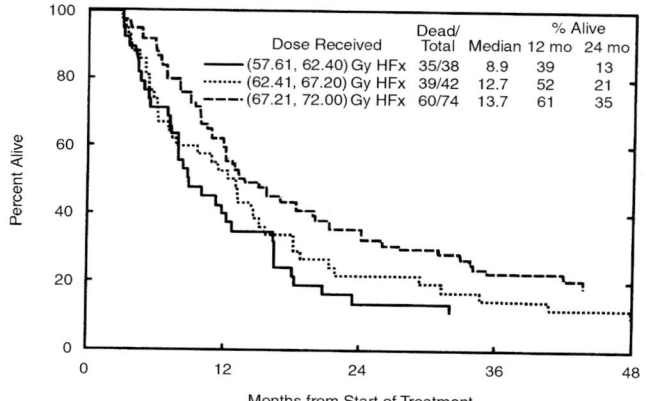

Fig. 103-2. RTOG 83-11 trial of non–small cell carcinoma of the lung. Survival by dose received for Cancer and Leukemia Group B patients, lower three doses. From Cox JD, et al: A randomized phase I/II trial of hyperfractionated (HFx) radiation therapy with total doses of 60.0 Gy to 79.2 Gy: possible survival benefit with 69.6 Gy in favorable patients with Radiation Therapy Oncology Group stage III non-small cell carcinoma of the lung. Report of RTOG 83-11. J Clin Oncol 8:1543, 1990. With permission.

or part of the therapeutic regimen: Each fraction is close to the same size as that used with a single treatment per day, and the total dose is similar to that with standard fractionation. The most accelerated regimen was studied at the Mount Vernon Hospital in the United Kingdom by Saunders and Dische (1992). Continuous hyperfractionated accelerated radiation therapy used 1.5 Gy delivered three times daily with 6-hour interfraction intervals, with no interruption for the weekend, to achieve 54 Gy in 36 fractions in 12 days. Saunders and her colleagues (1996) reported a significant improvement in survival among patients receiving continuous hyperfractionated accelerated radiation therapy com-

pared with standard fractionation. Because most of their patients had squamous cell carcinoma, the relevance of continuous hyperfractionated accelerated radiation therapy for patients with adenocarcinoma and large cell carcinoma remains to be determined.

Finally, concurrent chemotherapy and radiation therapy is a means of accelerating treatment. Schaake-Koning and colleagues (1992) studied cisplatin, administered weekly or daily during radiation therapy, and found significant improvement in local-regional tumor control (Fig. 103-3A) and survival (Fig. 103-3B). Induction chemotherapy and standard radiation has not improved local control, although Arriagada and colleagues (1991) observed apparent elimination of distant metastasis. The possibility of increasing local control and decreasing distant metastasis by using concurrent combination chemotherapy and radiation therapy is being explored with the hope of clear improvements in survival for patients with unresectable NSCCL.

RESULTS OF RADIATION THERAPY FOR INOPERABLE NON–SMALL CELL CARCINOMA OF THE LUNG

Palliation

Slawson and Scott (1979) suggested that symptomatic relief by radiation therapy for local-regional manifestations of squamous cell, adenocarcinoma, and large cell carcinomas of the lung can be predicted fairly accurately. Superior vena caval obstruction can be relieved in more than three-fourths of patients. Hemoptysis can be eliminated with similar consistency. Pain in the chest, shoulder, and arm can usually be decreased or eliminated: the more vague and nonspecific the discomfort, the less predictable the relief. By contrast,

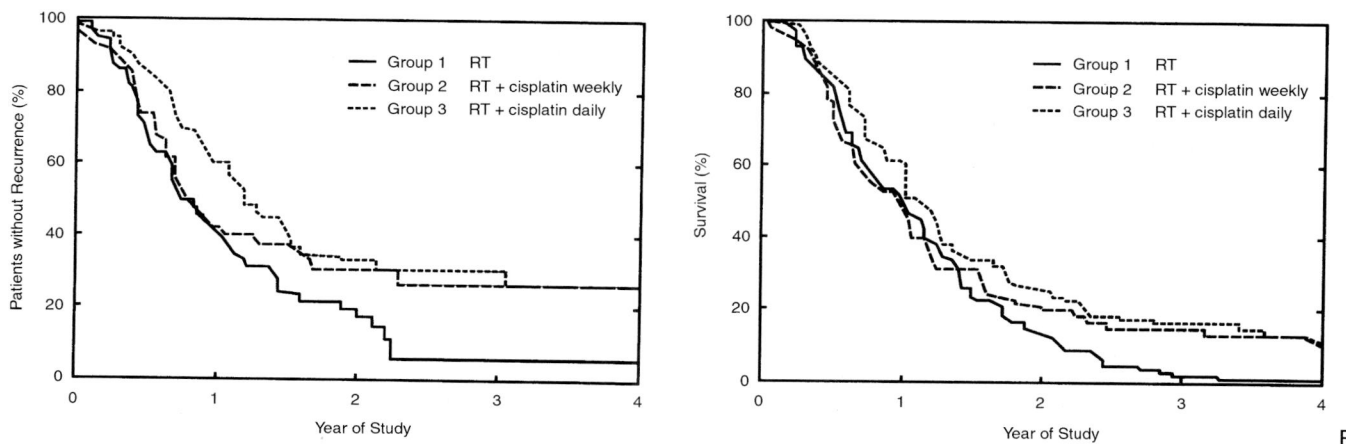

Fig. 103-3. Effects of concomitant cisplatin and radiation therapy (RT) on inoperable non–small cell lung carcinoma. **A.** Survival without local recurrence. Comparison of group 1 with groups 2 and 3 ($P = .009$). **B.** Overall survival in treatment groups. Comparison of group 1 with groups 2 and 3 ($P = .04$). From Schaake-Koning C, et al: Effects of concomitant cisplatin and radiotherapy on inoperable non-small cell lung cancer. N Engl J Med 326:524, 1992. With permission.

bronchial obstruction with established atelectasis, usually complicated by obstructive pneumonitis, can be ameliorated in only one-fourth of patients. The longer the atelectasis has been established, the greater the opportunity for infectious complications and the less the possibility of effective relief by local radiation therapy. Paralysis of the vocal cord resulting from involvement of the recurrent laryngeal nerve at the aorticopulmonary window is rarely relieved despite long-term control of the tumor. Whether this paralysis is caused by destruction of the nerve by direct invasion or entrapment of the nerve in the tumor and subsequently fibrosis is not clear.

Prolongation of Survival

Radiation therapy of the intrathoracic tumor prolongs survival, even of patients who will eventually die of lung cancer. In a retrospective series of radiation therapy for inoperable or unresectable carcinoma of the lung, Eisert and associates (1976) showed a prolongation of survival for patients whose intrathoracic tumors were controlled with radiation therapy compared with those whose tumors were not controlled. Various fractionation schemes have been used, including common or standard fractionation and hypofractionation. Perez and associates (1986) corroborated this prolongation of survival in a prospective trial conducted by the RTOG. In addition, a dose response was demonstrated for 2- and 3-year survival. By contrast, one of the authors (J.D.C.) and associates (1983) reported that patients with tumors limited to the thorax who received no definitive treatment rarely lived 3 years, and fewer than 5% were alive at 2 years.

The value of chemotherapy in prolonging survival in patients with NSCCL is discussed elsewhere (see Chapter 105). Dillman and colleagues from the Cancer and Leukemia Group B (1990) demonstrated prolongation of survival when chemotherapy with cisplatin and vinblastine was administered for 6 weeks before radiation therapy. Sause and associates from the RTOG and the Eastern Cooperative Oncology Group (1995) confirmed the Cancer and Leukemia Group B findings. Le Chevalier and associates (1991) from France also found survival to be prolonged when cisplatin-based combination chemotherapy was given before thoracic irradiation. Arriagada and colleagues (1991) showed that this benefit resulted from decreased distant metastasis (Fig. 103-4A), and no improvement occurred in local tumor control from induction chemotherapy (Fig. 103-4B). One of the authors (R.K.) and colleagues from the RTOG and Eastern Cooperative Oncology Group (1997) reported data supporting the value of induction chemotherapy in eliminating distant metastasis and no effect on local tumor control (Fig. 103-5).

Potential for Cure by Radiation Therapy

The most important role for radiation therapy is its potentially curative use in patients who have few or mild

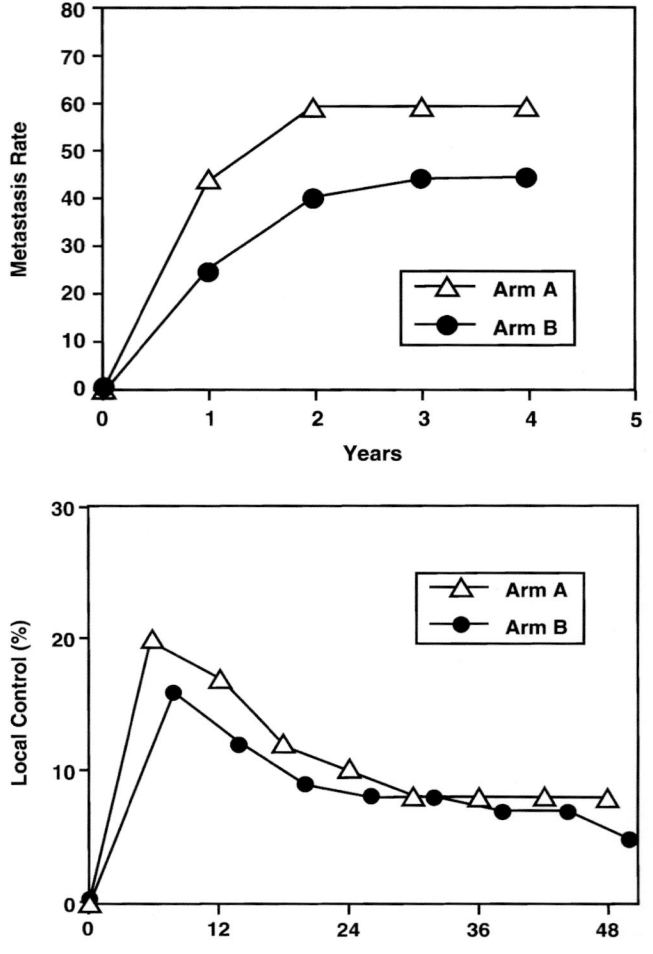

Fig. 103-4. A. Distant metastasis rate by treatment arm: arm A, standard radiation therapy; arm B, induction chemotherapy plus radiation therapy plus adjuvant chemotherapy. **B.** Local control by treatment group. arm A, standard radiation therapy; arm B, induction chemotherapy plus radiation therapy plus adjuvant chemotherapy. From Arriagada R, et al: ASTRO Plenary: effect of chemotherapy on locally advanced non-small cell lung carcinoma: a randomized study of 353 patients. Int J Radiat Oncol Biol Phys 20:1183, 1991. With permission.

symptoms. One of the authors (R.K.) and associates (1985) reported the change in 3-year survival rates among patients with inoperable carcinoma of the lung treated at the Medical College of Wisconsin from 1971 to 1978. Of patients treated with radiation therapy alone between 1971 and 1975, 7% of 197 were alive at 3 years, a figure similar to many reports of the results of megavoltage radiation therapy. Of 213 patients treated between 1975 and 1978, 14% (29 patients) were alive after 3 or more years. Long-term observations of the 3-year survivors showed that 80% (23 patients) were still alive at 5 years (11% of entire group), and two-thirds lived 10 years. No patient in this series died of lung cancer after 54 months.

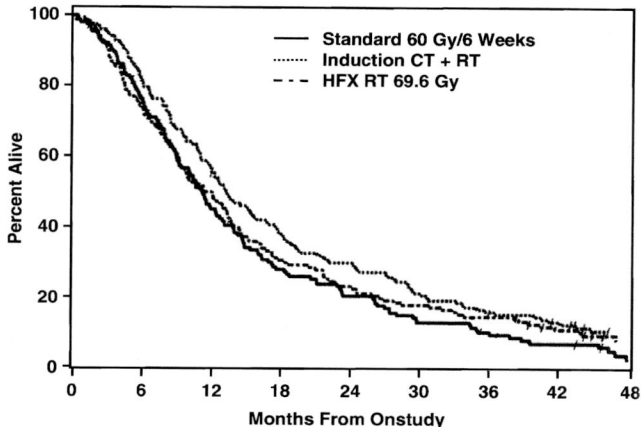

Fig. 103-5. Survival by treatment groups: standard radiation therapy (RT), induction chemotherapy plus radiation therapy (CT + RT), and hyperfractionated radiation therapy (HFX RT). From Komaki R, et al: Induction cisplatin/vinblastine and irradiation vs. irradiation in unresectable squamous cell lung cancer: failure patterns by cell type in RTOG 88-08/ECOG 4588. Int J Radiat Oncol Biol Phys *39*:537, 1997. With permission.

The important gains between the earlier and later time periods were not the result of the treatment of more favorable patients with less extensive disease. Indeed, the patients with more advanced tumors provided the additional long-term survivors (Table 103-1). Only 1% of patients with stage III tumors lived 3 or more years in the earlier time period, compared with 11% of those treated between 1975 and 1978. Most of the improvement in survival was found in patients with mediastinal lymph node involvement.

No patient with the performance status less than 80 on the Karnofsky's scale survived 3 years, compared with 7% whose performance status was 80 to 89, 25% with a performance status 90 to 99, and 70% (7 of 10 patients) who were truly asymptomatic (i.e., had a performance status of 100). The

Table 103-1. Percentage of Patients Surviving 36 or More Months by Extent of Tumor, Medical College of Wisconsin: 1971–1978

Extent of Tumor	1971–1975		1975–1978	
	No. of Patients	Percent	No. of Patients	Percent
Stage				
I	36	33.3	48	20.8
II	21	4.8	33	18.2
III	140	1.4	132	10.6
Nodal involvement				
None	72	18.2	81	8.0
Hilar	21	14.3	33	15.2
Mediastinal	86	1.2	82	12.2
Supraclavicular	18	5.6	17	17.6

Modified from Komaki R, et al: Characteristics of long-term survivors after treatment of inoperable carcinoma of the lung. Am Clin Oncol *8*:362, 1985.

patients studied from 1971 through 1978 did not have the benefit of pretreatment evaluation by CT and other sophisticated imaging procedures. This experience should be considered only a baseline for what can be accomplished with contemporary treatment methods and pretreatment selection.

We have been most impressed with the effectiveness of concurrent chemotherapy and radiation therapy. Lee (1999) reported our long-term results with cisplatin, oral etoposide, and hyperfractionated radiation therapy: 5 of 23 patients whom we treated in this manner were living and well more than 5 years later.

SPECIAL CONSIDERATIONS

Several special circumstances may be encountered among patients with lung cancer that appropriately might lead to the use of radiation therapy.

Apical Sulcus (Pancoast's) Tumors

Tumors in the extreme apex of either lung may cause shoulder or arm pain; sensory and motor dysfunction, especially along the distribution of the ulnar nerve; destruction of ribs or, less frequently, vertebral bodies; and Horner's syndrome. Paulson's (1966, 1968) recommendations have been followed for more than two decades: A brief course of preoperative radiation therapy is followed by thoracotomy, mediastinal exploration, and definitive resection if regional lymph node metastasis was not evident (see Chapter 35). This was a justifiable approach when surgical resection was the only tenable treatment. Several series have now demonstrated the efficacy of definitive radiation therapy for these tumors, which seem to have a lesser propensity for extrathoracic dissemination than other presentations of lung cancer. The disadvantages of hypofractionation or split-course radiation therapy have been noted previously. Those patients who receive preoperative irradiation and then are found to have unresectable tumors are placed at a great disadvantage; subsequent radiation therapy with such a long interruption is of little use and frequently is applied to an already progressing tumor. Martini and McCormack (1983) reported that fewer than 20% of patients who underwent exploration at the Memorial Sloan-Kettering Cancer Center were able to have complete surgical resection. Preoperative selection by contemporary imaging with CT and MR imaging permits a higher rate of complete resection.

One of the authors (R.K.) and associates (1990) studied, retrospectively, all patients with superior sulcus tumors who fulfilled the original criteria of Pancoast, seen at the M. D. Anderson Cancer Center between 1977 and 1987. Adenocarcinoma was found in one-half the 85 patients studied. A favorable outlook for survival was associated with high performance status, 5% or less weight loss, lack of vertebral involvement, and control of the primary tumor and its extensions. A higher probability of local control was associated with treatment with surgical resection. No advantage was noted from preoperative compared with postoperative irradiation. For unresectable patients, high total doses (more than 65 Gy) with radiation therapy resulted in better local control.

Therefore, the most appropriate approach to permit benefit for the entire spectrum of patients with apical sulcus tumors is immediate exploration for those thought to have resectable tumors. If the tumors prove unresectable, the patients can still benefit from the most effective type of radiation therapy.

Superior Vena Cava Obstruction

Obstruction of the superior vena cava usually results from a malignant neoplasm. Lung cancer is, by far, the most frequent neoplasm encountered. Approximately 5% of all patients with carcinoma of the lung present with superior vena caval obstruction. The frequent presentation with dyspnea and swelling of the face, neck, and upper extremities with collateral venous circulation on the upper thorax may be a radiotherapeutic emergency. This presentation, however, is rarely ominous enough to preclude cytologic diagnosis by needle aspirate or even fiberoptic bronchoscopy. The finding of a neoplasm other than lung cancer may change both the therapeutic options and the prognosis. If small cell carcinoma is identified, the treatment programs are different than that for superior vena caval obstruction from NSCCL and are described subsequently.

The finding of squamous cell carcinoma, adenocarcinoma, or large cell carcinoma of the lung justifies immediate treatment with a few large fractions (3.5 to 4.0 Gy per fraction), followed by common fractionation with 1.8 to 2.0 Gy per fraction. The additional destruction of tumor cells with the initial large fractions is associated with more immediate relief of symptoms than with smaller fractions. The number of such large fractions is sufficiently small that the late effects on normal tissues do not become a serious problem. A common approach is the use of three or four large fractions and then a continuation of common fractionation. Over 80% of patients with superior vena caval obstruction experience rapid relief of symptoms. Unfortunately, the remaining patients probably do not benefit because of thrombosis of the superior vena cava.

Treatment of Metastases

Radiation therapy is frequently useful for the palliation of symptoms from distant metastasis in patients with carcinoma of the lung. Relief of the various symptoms resulting from the intrathoracic tumor has already been reviewed. The most frequent extrathoracic symptoms that can be alleviated by radiation therapy are neurologic dysfunction resulting from

Table 103-2. Frequency of Brain Metastasis at Autopsy by Histopathologic Type of Lung Cancer

Histopathologic Type	Patients with Metastasis/ Patients Autopsied	Percent
Squamous cell	16/123	13
Adenocarcinoma	69/129	54
Large cell	28/54	52
Combined	3/12	25
Non–small cell	116/318	36
Small cell	37/82	45

metastasis involving the central nervous system and pain from metastasis to bones or, less frequently, soft tissues.

Central Nervous System Metastasis

Approximately 10% of all patients with cancer of the lung present with cerebral metastasis. Most of these metastases result in neurologic symptoms and signs that suggest the need for further evaluation. Small cell carcinoma, adenocarcinoma, and large cell carcinoma of the lung cause cerebral metastasis so frequently (Table 103-2) that CT or MR imaging of the brain is worthwhile even in asymptomatic patients. The yield of occult metastasis is approximately 10%.

Borgelt and associates (1980) suggested that relief of symptoms from brain metastasis by radiation therapy is reasonably consistent and predictable. Seizures and impaired mentation are reversible more frequently than are specific motor deficits.

At least one-half of all patients who develop brain metastasis from carcinoma of the lung die as a direct result of central nervous system involvement. The median survival is little more than 3 months. Patients who have cerebral metastasis at the time of initial diagnosis have a somewhat worse prognosis. Patients who develop cerebral metastasis after initial surgical resection or radiation therapy of the intrathoracic tumor have a slightly better prognosis. Indeed, as one of the authors (R.K.) and associates (1983) suggested, a few of these patients live for years after aggressive surgical intervention or irradiation for the cerebral metastasis, undoubtedly the result of single-organ brain metastasis (i.e., metastasis exclusively to the brain in the absence of other extrathoracic dissemination). This phenomenon is more frequent with adenocarcinoma and large cell carcinoma than with squamous cell carcinoma or small cell carcinoma.

Skeletal Metastases

One of the authors (R.K.) and associates (1977) reported that at least one-third of patients with disseminated lung cancer have symptomatic involvement of the skeletal system, usually manifested as pain. A high probability of pain relief can be expected from palliative irradiation of symptomatic bony metastasis, but complete relief of pain is less frequent than partial relief. Tong and associates (1982) and

Blitzer (1985) concur that brief but intensive courses of radiation therapy are indicated for the palliation of pain because it is desirable to reduce as much as possible the amount of time patients spend undergoing treatment when their life expectancy is short. For the uncommon situation in which multiple sites of symptomatic metastases are present simultaneously, single-dose, hemibody irradiation can be considered. Treatment of the upper one-half of the body with 600 or 700 rad in a single fraction or treatment of the lower hemibody with 800 rad in a single fraction produces remarkable, if short-lived, palliation.

Paraneoplastic Syndromes

Radiation therapy, like surgical resection, can diminish or eliminate paraneoplastic effects. Some paraneoplastic syndromes are more readily reversible than others. Endocrinologic syndromes, including adrenocorticotropic hormone and antidiuretic hormone production, can be reduced or eliminated by local-regional radiation therapy. Hypercalcemia is more complex and less predictably reversible with radiation therapy. Paraneoplastic neurologic symptoms and signs are infrequently altered by radiation therapy, and hypertrophic pulmonary osteoarthropathy is rarely affected.

Chronic Obstructive Pulmonary Disease and Pulmonary Infection

Chronic obstructive pulmonary disease is rarely a contraindication to radiation therapy for inoperable cancer of the lung. Choi and associates (1985) showed by serial pulmonary function studies that judiciously applied radiation therapy rarely causes acute or late pulmonary effects greater than those already caused by the malignant tumor. Effective radiation therapy involves doses higher than those tolerated by the normal lung, so the high-dose area must be minimized and confined to a volume that sharply circumscribes the intrathoracic tumor. With careful treatment planning using individualized blocks and multiple sets of fields as described, the primary tumor and regional lymph nodes can be irradiated adequately with few serious effects in the adjacent lung. Three-dimensional conformal radiation therapy may permit higher total doses of radiation to be delivered while protecting normal lung in patients with limited pulmonary reserve.

Many pulmonary tumors with a significant endobronchial component result in obstruction, distal atelectasis, and subsequent bacterial infection. This condition is, indeed, an indication for urgent radiation therapy; once atelectasis is well established, reversal is not achieved readily.

Active tuberculosis in a patient with carcinoma of the lung has been considered a contraindication to radiation therapy. With current antituberculous drug therapy, however, treatment for tuberculosis and radiation therapy can both be initiated immediately, if indicated. No evidence shows that radiation therapy diminishes the effectiveness of antimicrobial therapy. Anecdotes suggest that radiation therapy has reactivated tuberculosis; this phenomenon, if real, is so rare that it has little practical consequence.

RADIATION EFFECTS ON NORMAL TISSUES OF THE THORAX

A detailed description of radiation effects on normal tissues that might be included during high-dose, definitive radiation therapy of lung cancer is discussed in Chapter 102. One of the authors (J.D.C.) and associates reviewed this subject in 1986.

The most sensitive structure irradiated with the treatment of bronchopulmonary carcinomas is the lung itself. With single doses, 8 to 10 Gy predictably produce radiation pneumonitis. Common fractionation with 1.5 to 1.8 Gy/day permits some repair of radiation effects; pneumonitis occurs in fewer than 5% of patients with total doses of 18 to 20 Gy. As noted, irradiation for lung cancer, which incidentally treats some normal lung, usually results in improvement in pulmonary function because of the response of the tumor, followed by some degradation in function resulting from radiation pneumonitis and subsequent scarring. Prior, concurrent, or even subsequent chemotherapy may enhance or recall radiation effects and lower the total dose for radiation-induced inflammation and scarring. Drugs that notably increase radiation effects in the lung include dactinomycin, bleomycin, carmustine, cyclophosphamide, and methotrexate. To limit the adverse effects of radiation therapy on the lung, the volume irradiated must be limited. Techniques that use multiple field arrangements, *shrinking fields*, and individualized blocking are essential. Geara and associates (1998) reported our data suggesting that variations in late effects of treatment, at least in the lungs, could be related to inherent differences in individual sensitivities.

The normal tissue that most frequently gives rise to symptoms during the course of irradiation is the esophagus. The germinal layer of the squamous epithelium lining the esophagus is affected by doses between 15 and 20 Gy. A pseudomembranous inflammation results in symptoms of dysphagia 10 to 14 days after the start of treatment. The symptoms improve even though the treatments continue, but they increase during the fourth week and again during the sixth week because of the cyclic nature of the reaction, resulting from accelerated proliferation of the viable germinal cells. Dietary recommendations and analgesics usually prevent significant weight loss. Late effects of the irradiation on the esophagus (i.e., stenosis or complete obstruction) are rare with common fractionation, unless one or more of the aforementioned chemotherapeutic agents is combined with the radiation therapy. Radiation myelopathy is, unquestionably, the most serious potential result of radiation therapy. Experiences with large-dose fractionation by Hatlevoll (1983) and Dische (1981) and their associates resulted in many reported cases of radiation myelopathy. Symptoms consist of weakness of the lower extremities and a Brown-Séquard syndrome beginning 6 to 36 months after completion of radiation therapy. Wollin and Kagan (1976) suggested that this grave, late effect of radiation therapy can be avoided entirely by careful attention to individual fraction size and overall treatment time.

Finally, some of the heart must be included within the field of irradiation, with rare exceptions. Stewart and Fajardo (1971) reported that when the entire heart is treated with doses of 40 Gy in 4 to 5 weeks, symptomatic radiation pericarditis is seen in approximately 5% of patients. Because most pulmonary neoplasms arise in the upper lobes, it is usually only necessary to treat the atria and great vessels. When a significant amount of the ventricles must be included within the field of irradiation, the dose must be limited, and treatment plans that sharply confine high doses to a minimal volume must be sought.

RECURRENT CANCER OF THE LUNG

Lung cancer may recur in the thorax after definitive surgery or definitive radiation therapy performed with the intent of complete eradication. In many cases, the recurrence may take the form of diffuse parenchymal metastases or pleural involvement with effusion. Radiation therapy has little, if anything, to offer patients with these manifestations of intrathoracic progression of tumor.

Infrequently, the tumor may progress in the lung or mediastinum adjacent to the site of the primary tumor or in the regional lymph nodes. This appearance is an indication for local-regional radiation therapy, but the expectations, necessarily, are limited. A tumor that regrows within an operative bed rarely can be controlled. This circumstance is similar to that of macroscopic residual tumor after subtotal resection. The precise reasons for a limited effect of external radiation therapy are not known, but they presumably relate to altered vasculature with broad areas of hypoxia resulting in a tumor less sensitive to the effects of ionizing radiations. Interestingly, Green and Melbye (1982) reported that postirradiation recurrences have a somewhat less grave outlook, and limited success has been achieved with repeat irradiation. Hilaris and Martini (1979) suggested that operative intervention with implants (i.e., brachytherapy) may rarely result in benefit.

Patients in whom tumor growth recurred after external irradiation with high total doses may be offered palliation by endobronchial irradiation. This procedure is indicated only if the patient has a significant endobronchial or endotracheal component determined bronchoscopically. We require that there be no bleeding disorder and no plan for systemic chemotherapy for at least a month. If sufficient occlusion is present, laser resection may be indicated, because attempts to force a catheter through an obstructing tumor may risk uncontrolled bleeding. We use a high-dose rate afterloading unit with a single, highly specific activity iridium 192 source, permitting the use of a dose rate of 15 Gy at a distance of 6

mm from the source in less than 15 minutes. Often, a second and occasionally a third procedure are used, unless striking relief of symptoms occurred with the first application. Our experience with 81 patients, reported by Delclos and colleagues (1996), has been extended to over 100 patients. At least 75% of patients had evidence of response to treatment radiographically or bronchoscopically, and the same proportion had symptomatic improvement.

RADIATION THERAPY FOR SMALL CELL CARCINOMA

The consistency of overt or subclinical dissemination of SCCL was previously noted. Radiation therapy and cytotoxic drugs, administered individually, resulted in frequent responses but little long-term benefit. Combination chemotherapy was demonstrably superior, when measured by rate of response and median survival, and radiation therapy temporarily was thought no longer necessary. Retrospective studies suggested that survival at 2 years or more was superior when radiation therapy of the intrathoracic tumor was integrated with combination chemotherapy. Several prospective, randomized trials were launched to assess the role of thoracic irradiation. Pignon and coworkers (1992) performed a meta-analysis of 2140 patients enrolled in 13 prospective, randomized trials initiated between 1976 and 1986 designed to compare chemotherapy alone with chemotherapy plus thoracic irradiation. The 14% reduction in mortality with the combination of the two methods was highly significant ($P = .001$).

The role of radiation therapy was obscured, not just by selection of end points such as response rates and median survival but also by assessment of intrathoracic failure rates that seemed to differ little in studies that compared chemotherapy and integrated radiation therapy and chemotherapy. One of the authors (J.D.C.) (1985a) suggested that it is now more widely recognized that intrathoracic failures are of three types: 1) failure within the irradiated volume is truly a failure of the dose-time relationships used; 2) failure at the margin of the irradiated volume may represent insufficient appreciation of the extent of the original tumor; and 3) failure in the periphery of the pulmonary parenchyma or the pleura represents failure of the systemic regimen, not the radiation therapy.

Quality control in radiation therapy of SCCL profoundly influences the results of treatment. White and colleagues (1982) assessed the importance of compliance with protocol specifications in Southwestern Oncology Group trials; they showed that full compliance with radiation therapy specifications was the single most important prognostic factor. Failure to mandate rigorous protocol compliance with regard to radiation therapy is the likely reason some studies have shown little effect of thoracic irradiation combined with chemotherapy.

The optimal means of integrating radiation therapy into the management of small cell carcinoma remains to be defined. Perry and associates (1987) reported results of studies of the Cancer and Leukemia Group B that suggested that radiation therapy after three or more cycles of chemotherapy was associated with a lesser toxicity and better long-term outcome than when radiation therapy was used with chemotherapy immediately after diagnosis. Bunn (1987) found, in studies at the National Cancer Institute of the United States, that maximal initial therapy with radiation therapy and simultaneous chemotherapy was superior to chemotherapy alone. McCracken and colleagues (1990) from the Southwest Oncology Group combined intravenous etoposide and vincristine in two 4-week cycles with concurrent radiation therapy (45 Gy at 1.8 Gy per fraction once a day for 5 weeks); prophylactic cranial irradiation was given with a third cycle of cisplatin and etoposide, followed by cycles of methotrexate, doxorubicin, and cyclophosphamide for 12 weeks. Among 154 patients treated, 42% were alive at 2 years, and 30% lived 4 years.

Turrisi and Glover (1990) treated 32 patients with intravenous cisplatin and etoposide concurrent with accelerated radiation therapy (45 Gy at 1.5 Gy twice daily for 3 weeks). Initially, two cycles of chemotherapy were given at 3-week intervals, and then these two drugs were alternated with cyclophosphamide, doxorubicin, and vincristine, for six additional cycles. Prophylactic cranial irradiation was given to complete responders after chemotherapy was completed. Turrisi and associates (1992) recorded that the 2-year survival rate was 54% and the 4-year survival rate was 36%. A phase III intergroup trial coordinated by the Eastern Cooperative Oncology Group compared once daily versus twice daily radiation therapy concurrent with cisplatin and etoposide. Turrisi and associates (1999) reported the best short-term survival achieved to date in a multi-institutional trial: 44% at 2 years. The patients treated twice daily had significantly higher survival at the cost of increased transient esophagitis.

Radiation therapy is thus an important element in management of SCCL clinically confined to the intrathoracic primary tumor and regional lymph nodes. Patients with disseminated disease at presentation respond less favorably to systemic chemotherapy than those with more limited disease, and they have not been shown to benefit from the addition of radiation therapy. Livingston and associates (1984) showed that a subset of these patients—those who have clinical complete responses to combination chemotherapy—fail often enough in the thorax that they constitute an appropriate group for further study of thoracic irradiation with systemic therapy.

CLINICAL RESEARCH IN RADIATION THERAPY OF CANCER OF THE LUNG

The aforementioned results described are encouraging. Patients with cancer of the lung have often been considered curable only if they had resectable tumors. Reports from large cooperative trials show clear improvements in survival for patients with inoperable NSCCL as well as SCCL. These improvements are limited, however, to subsets of all patients

with cancer of the lung. Clearly, radiation therapy, as currently used, addresses only part of the multifaceted problem of lung cancer. Efforts are underway to enhance the effectiveness of local radiation therapy in eradication of the intrathoracic tumor. These efforts included intensification of treatment by means of concurrent chemotherapy. Roth and colleagues (1996) have reported the use of gene therapy to correct acquired genetic abnormalities of lung cancer cells. New studies are underway by our team to combine such gene therapy with radiation therapy. Mauceri and associates (1998) have studied the combination of antiangiogenesis factors with radiation therapy. Clinical cancer research in lung cancer has an exciting future. Finally, systemic chemotherapeutic agents, when optimally combined with radiation therapy, not only may enhance tumor control within the irradiated volume but also may reduce or eliminate disease that has disseminated beyond the irradiated volume. Biological response modifiers, similarly, may enhance effects on the local tumor and simultaneously enhance host defenses to permit eradication of subclinical disease.

REFERENCES

Albain KS: Concurrent cisplatin, VP-16, and chest irradiation followed by surgery for stages IIIA and IIIB non-small cell lung cancer: a Southwest Oncology Group Study (number 8805) [abstract]. Proc Am Soc Clin Oncol 10:244,1991.
Arriagada R, et al: ASTRO Plenary: effect of chemotherapy on locally advanced non-small cell lung carcinoma: a randomized study of 353 patients. Int J Radiat Oncol Biol Phys 20:1183, 1991.
Arriagada R, et al: Cisplatin-based chemotherapy (CT) in patients with locally advanced non-small cell lung cancer (NSCLC): late analysis of a French randomized trial. Proc ASCO 16:446a, 1997.
Blitzer PH: Reanalysis of the RTOG study of the palliation of symptomatic osseous metastasis. Cancer 55:1468, 1985.
Borgelt B, et al: The palliation of brain metastases: final result of the first two studies by the Radiation Therapy Oncology Group. Int J Radiat Oncol Biol Phys 6:1,1980.
Bunn PAJ: Chemotherapy alone or chemotherapy with chest radiation therapy in limited stage small cell lung cancer. Ann Intern Med 106:655, 1987.
Choi NC, et al: Physiologic changes in pulmonary function after thoracic radiotherapy for patients with lung cancer and role of regional pulmonary function studies in predicting postradiotherapy pulmonary function before radiotherapy. Cancer Treat Symp 2:119, 1985.
Cox JD: Failure analysis of inoperable carcinoma of the lung of all histopathologic types and squamous cell carcinoma of the esophagus. Cancer Treat Symp 2:77, 1983.
Cox JD: Importance of endpoints in determining effectiveness of thoracic irradiation for small cell carcinoma of the lung. Cancer Treat Symp 2:31, 1985a.
Cox JD: Large dose fractionation (hypofractionation). Cancer 55:2105, 1985b.
Cox JD, et al: A randomized phase I/II trial of hyperfractionated radiation therapy with total doses of 60.0 Gy to 79.2 Gy: possible survival benefit with greater than or equal to 69.6 Gy in favorable patients with Radiation Therapy Oncology Group stage III non-small-cell lung carcinoma: report of Radiation Therapy Oncology Group 83-11. J Clin Oncol 8:1543, 1990.
Cox JD, et al: Complications of radiation therapy and factors in their prevention. World J Surg 10:171, 1986.
Cox JD, et al: Is immediate chest radiotherapy obligatory for any or all patients with limited-stage non-small cell carcinoma of the lung? Yes. Cancer Treat Rep 67:327, 1983.
Cox JD, et al: Interruptions of high-dose radiation therapy decrease long-term survival of favorable patients with unresectable non-small cell carcinoma of the lung: analysis of 1244 cases from three Radiation Therapy Oncology trials. Int J Radiat Oncol Biol Phys 27:493,1993.
Cox JD, et al: Radiation therapy is indicated for asymptomatic inoperable

lung cancer. *In* Gitnicket F, et al (eds): Debates in Medicine. Chicago: Year Book Medical Publishers, 1989, p. 245.

Deeley TJ: Radiotherapy for carcinoma of the bronchus. Cancer Treat Rev *1*:39,1974.

Deeley TJ: The treatment of carcinoma of the bronchus. Br J Radiol *40*:801, 1967.

Delclos ME, et al: Endobronchial brachytherapy with high-dose-rate remote afterloading for recurrent endobronchial lesions. Radiology *201*:279, 1996.

Diener-West M, et al: Randomized dose searching phase ILK/II trials of fractionation in radiation therapy for cancer. J Natl Cancer Inst *83*:1065, 1991.

Dillman RO, et al: A randomized trial of induction chemotherapy plus high-dose radiation versus radiation alone in stage III non-small-cell lung cancer. N Engl J Med *323*:940, 1990.

Dische S, et al: Radiation myelopathy in patients treated for carcinoma of bronchus using a six-fraction regime of radiotherapy. Br J Radiol *54*:29, 1981.

Eisert DR, et al: Irradiation for bronchial carcinoma: reasons for failure. 1. Analysis as a function of dose-time-fractionation. Cancer *37*:2665, 1976.

Fowler JF, Lindstrom MJ: Loss of local control with prolongation in radiotherapy. Int J Radiat Oncol Biol Phys *23*:457, 1992.

Geara FB, et al: Factors influencing the development of lung fibrosis after chemoradiation for small cell carcinoma of the lung: evidence for inherent interindividual variation. Int J Radiat Oncol Biol Phys *41*:279,1998.

Green N, Melbye RW: Lung cancer: retreatment of local recurrence after definitive irradiation. Cancer *49*:865, 1982.

Hatlevoll R, et al: Myelopathy following radiotherapy of bronchial carcinoma with large single fractions: a retrospective study. Int J Radiat Oncol Biol Phys *9*:41, 1983.

Hilaris BS, Martini N: Interstitial brachytherapy in cancer of the lung: a 20 year experience. Int J Radiat Oncol Biol Phys *5*:1951,1979.

Israel L, et al: Controlled study with adjuvant radiotherapy, chemotherapy, immunotherapy, and chemoimmunotherapy in operable squamous carcinoma of the lung. *In* Muggis F, et al (eds): Lung Cancer. Progress in Therapeutic Research. New York: Raven Press, 1979, p. 443.

Jacobs L, et al: Silent brain metastasis from lung carcinoma determined by computerized tomography. Arch Neurol *34*:690, 1977.

Karnofsky DA, Burchenal JH: The clinical evaluation of chemotherapeutic agents in cancer. *In* Macleod CM (ed): Evaluation of Chemotherapeutic Agents. New York: Columbia University Press, 1949, p. 191.

Komaki R, et al: Characteristics of long-term survivors after treatment of inoperable carcinoma of the lung. Am J Clin Oncol *8*:362, 1985.

Komaki R, et al: Frequency of brain metastasis in adenocarcinoma and large cell carcinoma of the lung: correlation with survival. Int J Radiat Oncol Biol Phys *9*:1467, 1983.

Komaki R, et al: Induction cisplatin/vinblastine and irradiation vs irradiation in unresectable non-small cell lung cancer: failure patterns by cell type in RTOG 88-08/ECOG 4588. Int J Radiat Oncol Biol Phys *39*:537,1997.

Komaki R, et al: Irradiation of bronchial carcinoma. II. Pattern of spread and potential for prophylactic irradiation. Int J Radiat Oncol Biol Phys *2*:441, 1977.

Komaki R, et al: Superior sulcus tumors: treatment selection and results for 85 patients without metastasis (Mo) at presentation. Int J Radiat Oncol Biol Phys *19*:31, 1990.

Le Chevalier T, et al: Radiotherapy alone versus combined chemotherapy and radiotherapy in nonresectable non-small cell lung cancer. First analysis of a randomized trial in 353 patients. J Natl Cancer Inst *83*:417,1991.

Lee JS, et al: A pilot trial of hyperfractionated thoracic radiation therapy with concurrent cisplatin and oral etoposide for locally advanced inoperable non-small cell lung cancer: a 5-year follow-up report. Int J Radiat Oncol Biol Phys *42*:479, 1998.

Livingston RB, et al: Combined modality treatment of extensive small cell lung cancer: a Southwest Oncology Group study. J Clin Oncol *2*:585, 1984.

The Lung Cancer Study Group: Effects of postoperative mediastinal radiation on completely resected stage II and stage III epidermoid cancer of the lung. N Engl J Med *315*:1377, 1986.

Martini N, McCormack P: Therapy of stage III (nonmetastatic disease). Semin Radiat Oncol *10*:95, 1983.

Mauceri HJ, et al: Combined effects of angiostatin and ionizing radiation in antitumour therapy. Nature *394*:287, 1998.

McCracken JD, et al: Concurrent chemotherapy/radiotherapy for limited small cell lung carcinoma: a Southwest Oncology Group study. J Clin Oncol *8*:892, 1990.

Paulson DL: The survival rate in superior sulcus tumors treated by presurgical irradiation. JAMA *196*:342, 1966.

Paulson DL: Treatment of superior sulcus tumors. *In* Rush BF, et al (eds): Cancer Therapy by Integrated Radiation and Operation. Springfield, IL: Charles C Thomas, 1968.

Perez CA: Sequelae of definitive irradiation in the treatment of carcinoma of the lung. *In* Motta G (ed): Lung Cancer. Advanced Concepts and Present Status. Genoa: Grafica LP, 1989, p. 237.

Perez CA, et al: Impact of tumor control on survival in carcinoma of the lung treated with irradiation. Int J Radiat Oncol Biol Phys *12*:539, 1986.

Perez CA, et al: Patterns of tumor recurrence after definitive irradiation for inoperable non-oat cell carcinoma of the lung. Int J Radiat Oncol Biol Phys *6*:987, 1980.

Perry MC, et al: Chemotherapy with or without radiation therapy in limited small-cell carcinoma of the lung. N Engl J Med *316*:912, 1987.

Pignon JP, et al: A meta-analysis of thoracic radiotherapy for small cell lung cancer. N Engl J Med *327*:1618, 1992.

PORT Meta-analysis Trialists Group: Postoperative radiotherapy in non-small-cell lung cancer: systematic review and meta-analysis of individual patient data from nine randomised controlled trials. Lancet *352*:257,1998.

Roth JA, et al: Retrovirus-mediated wild-type p53 gene transfer to tumors of patients with lung cancer. Nature Med *2*:985, 1996.

Saunders MI, Dische S: Continuous, hyperfractionated, and accelerated radiotherapy. Semin Radiat Oncol *2*:41, 1992.

Saunders MI, et al: Primary tumor control after radiotherapy for carcinoma of the bronchus. Int J Radiat Oncol Biol Phys *10*:499, 1984.

Saunders MI, et al: Randomised multicentre trials of CHART vs conventional radiotherapy in head and neck and non-small-cell lung cancer: an interim report. Br J Cancer *73*:1455, 1996.

Sause WT, et al: RTOG 88-08 and ECOG 4588: preliminary results of a phase III trial in regionally advanced unresectable non-small cell lung cancer. J Natl Cancer Inst *87*:198, 1995.

Schaake-Koning C, et al: Effects of concomitant cisplatin and radiotherapy on inoperable non-small cell lung cancer. N Engl J Med *326*:524, 1992.

Shields TW: Treatment failures after surgical resection of thoracic tumors. Cancer Treat Symp *2*:69, 1983.

Slawson RG, Scott RM: Radiation therapy in bronchogenic carcinoma. Radiology *132*:175, 1979.

Stewart JR, Fajardo LF: Radiation-induced heart disease. Clinical and experimental aspects. Radiol Clin North Am *9*:511,1971.

Tarver RD, et al: Cerebral metastases from lung carcinoma: neurological and CT correlation. Work in progress. Radiology *153*:689, 1984.

Tong D, et al: The palliation of symptomatic osseous metastases: final results of the study by the Radiation Therapy Oncology Group. Cancer *50*:893, 1982.

Turrisi AT: Long-term results of platinum etoposide + twice-daily thoracic radiotherapy for limited small cell lung cancer: results on 32 patients with 48 month minimum followup [abstract]. Proc Am Soc Clin Oncol *11*: 292, 1992.

Turrisi AT, Glover D: Thoracic radiotherapy variables: influences on local control in small cell lung cancer limited disease. Int J Radiat Oncol Biol Phys *19*:1473, 1990.

Turrisis AT, et al: Twice-daily compared with once-daily thoracic radiotherapy in limited small cell lung cancer treated concurrently with cisplatin and etoposide. N Engl J Med *340*:265, 1999.

Van Houtte P, Henry J: Preoperative and postoperative radiation therapy in lung cancer. Cancer Treat Symp *2*:57, 1985.

Webb WR, et al: CT and MR imaging in staging non-small cell bronchogenic carcinoma: report of the Radiologic Diagnostic Oncology Group. Radiology *178*:705, 1991.

White JE, et al: The influence of radiation therapy quality control on survival, response, and sites of relapse in oat cell carcinoma of the lung: preliminary report of a Southwest Oncology Group study. Cancer *50*:1084, 1982.

Withers HR, et al: The hazard of accelerated tumor clonogen repopulation during radiotherapy. Acta Oncol *27*:131, 1988.

Wollin M, Kagan AR: Modification of biological dose to normal tissue by daily fractionation. Acta Radiol *15*:481, 1976.

CHAPTER 104

Principles of Chemotherapy

Przemek W. Twardowski, Christiana M. Brenin, and Merrill S. Kies

Modern cytotoxic chemotherapy originated with the serendipitous observation during World War II that human exposure to nitrogen mustard results in hypoplasia of bone marrow and lymphoid tissues. In the 1940s, nitrogen mustard and other alkylating compounds were shown to induce remission in patients with Hodgkin's disease and lymphoid malignancies. Another pivotal discovery from that era was an observation that folic acid accelerates the growth of leukemic cells. That led to the development of the inhibitor of folic acid metabolism, methotrexate. In the 1960s, combination chemotherapy became an effective treatment for selected hematologic malignancies, thus proving that some disseminated neoplasms can be cured with drug therapy. Recent decades have witnessed a dramatic expansion of the applications of chemotherapy for solid tumors. Despite some spectacular successes, such as effective treatment for germ cell tumors and the benefits of adjuvant chemotherapy in breast and colon cancer, the cure for the majority of metastatic solid malignancies remains elusive. There are many reasons for the inability to eradicate malignant neoplasms by conventional cytotoxic drugs. Chemotherapy is not specific against cancer but targets all proliferating cells by inhibiting DNA synthesis or interfering with different pathways of cell division and metabolism. It is frequently associated with significant dose-limiting side effects related to toxicity to normally dividing cells in the bone marrow, skin, and gastrointestinal mucosa. In addition, neoplastic cells exhibit profound genetic instability, and over time, accumulate genetic mutations that enhance their metastatic potential and render them resistant to chemotherapeutic agents, as noted by Simon and Schinder (1994). In addition to discovery of novel, more active chemotherapeutic agents, intense research efforts focus on the improvements in applications of existing therapies, reducing toxicity, and circumventing drug resistance.

CELL CYCLE AND TUMOR GROWTH KINETICS

To comprehend the principles that guide the use of cytotoxic chemotherapy in cancer, it is important to understand the basic biological features of malignant neoplasms and the kinetics of tumor growth and cell cycle.

Cell division is a complex, tightly regulated process with identifiable steps within the cell's life cycle. The critical period of DNA replication takes place in the S, or synthesis, phase. The physical division of the cell into two progenies occurs in the M (mitosis) phase. These periods are separated by G (gap) phases, during which the enzymes and proteins used in subsequent phases are synthesized. G_1 precedes the S phase, and G_2 precedes the M phase. G_0 denotes the resting state of the cell, during which cells are not committed to division. The duration of specific phases of the cell cycle vary between cell types and also between cells within a particular tumor. S phase lasts from 10 to 20 hours, and M phase lasts from 0.5 to 1.0 hour. G phases are highly variable, ranging from 2 to 10 hours (Fig. 104-1).

Malignant transformation of normal cells results from the dysfunction of genes regulating cellular growth, differentiation, and cell death. This transformation is usually the effect of activation of proto-oncogenes (i.e., *ras, myc*), or inactivation of tumor suppressor genes, such as *p53, rb, dcc*, and *BRCA*. The resulting malignant phenotype is characterized by uncontrolled cell proliferation, decreased cell differentiation and death, enhanced ability to invade surrounding tissues, and ability to grow at ectopic sites, or metastasis. Even though increased cell proliferation is an important feature of numerous malignant tumors, the other characteristics listed above are equally significant. For example, many normal cells exhibit a high rate of proliferation (e.g., gonads, gastrointestinal epithelium, and bone marrow), but this is balanced by a higher rate of maturation and programmed cell death (apoptosis).

Tumor growth depends on several interrelated factors that include cell cycle time (i.e., average time between mitosis of dividing cancer cells), growth fraction (i.e., proportion of actively dividing cancer cells), total number of cancer cells, and intrinsic tumor cell death rate. The observed growth pattern of solid tumors is described by a gompertzian growth curve (Fig. 104-2), which shows an initial rapid exponential growth phase and a terminal phase of slowing growth. In the

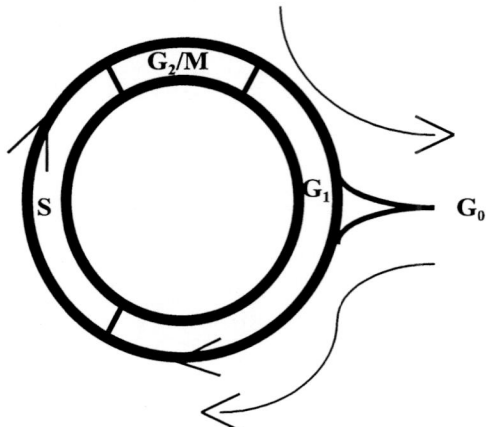

Fig. 104-1. Cell cycle.

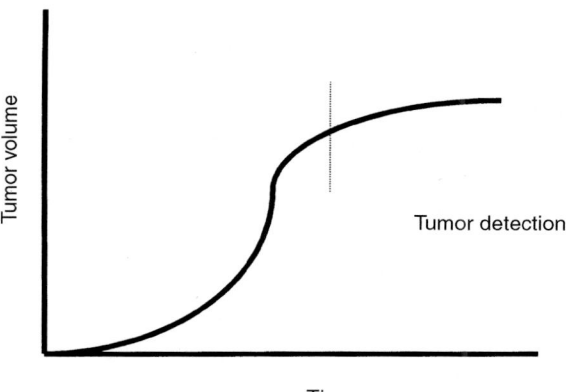

Fig. 104-2. Gompertzian growth curve.

early part of the curve, most cells are in the division cycle, but by the time of the tumor detection, growth has usually begun to slow, and only a small fraction of cells may be dividing. This has important therapeutic implications because slowly dividing cancer cells tend to be less responsive to chemotherapeutic agents. In the early portion of the

curve (i.e., clinically undetectable disease), the fraction of dividing cells is larger and the cells may be more susceptible to chemotherapy (see Fig. 104-2).

GENERAL MECHANISMS BY WHICH CHEMOTHERAPY DRUGS CONTROL CANCER

Anticancer chemotherapy drugs inhibit cell proliferation, either by blocking the synthesis of nucleic acids or proteins or by interfering with different metabolic pathways of cellular division. Generally, they are most effective against rapidly dividing cells. Cancer cells may die as a direct result of toxicity of the chemotherapeutic agent, but sometimes DNA damage caused by chemotherapy triggers the cell's own mechanism of apoptosis. Therefore, cell death may take place at the time of exposure to the drug, but frequently, a cancer cell must undergo several divisions before the lethal event that took place earlier finally results in the death of the cell.

PHASE AND CELL CYCLE SPECIFICITY OF CHEMOTHERAPEUTIC COMPOUNDS

Chemotherapeutic agents can be grouped according to whether their action depends on cells being in the division cycle (cycle specific) or not (cycle nonspecific). Cycle-specific drugs can be further divided into compounds that are most active in specific phases of cell cycle or are independent of the phase of the cycle. Cycle-nonspecific and phase-nonspecific compounds generally have a linear dose-response curve. The greater the amount of drug administered, the greater the fraction of cells killed. The effect of phase-specific drugs is a function of the dose as well as the duration of exposure. Above a certain dose level, further increases in dosage do not result in more cell killing. However, if the drug concentration is maintained over a longer period, more cells enter the specific, susceptible phase of the cycle and are killed. These drug characteristics are used in the design of dosing schedules of chemotherapy regimens. Examples of chemotherapy drugs are listed in Table 104-1.

Table 104-1. Common Chemotherapy Drugs

Cycle Specific					
Phase Specific				Phase Nonspecific	Cycle Nonspecific
G_1	S	G_2	M		
L-asparaginase Prednisone	Methotrexate Cytarabine 5-FU Fludarabine Hydroxyurea	Bleomycin Etoposide Teniposide Taxol	Vincristine Vinblastine Vindesine	Chlorambucil Cyclophosphamide Melphalan Busulfan Cisplatinum Doxorubicin Daunorubicin Idarubicin	Mechlorethamine Carmustine Lomustine

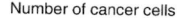

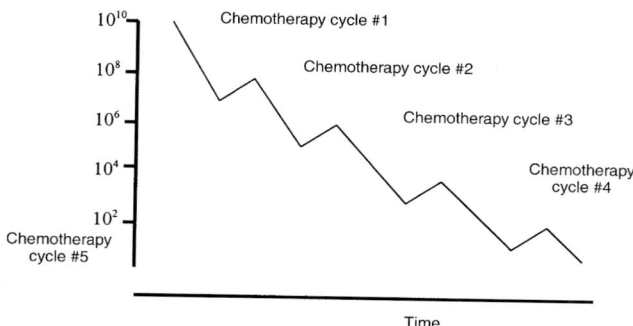

Fig. 104-3. Effect of chemotherapy on cancer cell numbers.

KINETICS OF CANCER CHEMOTHERAPY

Because only a fixed proportion of cancer cells die after a single exposure to chemotherapeutic compound, repeated doses of chemotherapy must be given to continue to reduce the cell number. Each time the dose is repeated, the same proportion of cells is killed—not the absolute number. In the example shown in Figure 104-3, 99.9% (3 logs) of cancer cells are killed with each treatment, and there is a 10-fold (1 log) growth between treatments, for a net reduction of 2 logs with each treatment. Starting at 10^{10} cells (approximately 10 g), it would take five treatments to reach fewer than 10^0, or one cell, resulting in likely cure. This model is helpful in explaining basic kinetics of the effect of chemotherapy on cancer, but it does not account for many important variables. Not all cells in a tumor population are equally sensitive to a drug; delivery of a drug is variable and depends on local host factors, including blood supply and surrounding fibrosis; and tumor sensitivity changes during therapy as cells acquire new mutations.

COMBINATION CHEMOTHERAPY

Combination of chemotherapy agents is usually more effective in inducing responses and prolonging life than single compounds are. By using drugs with different mechanisms of action, it is possible to generate the synergistic effect and decrease the likelihood of the emergence of resistant clones. By choosing drugs without overlapping side-effect profiles, doses can be maximized for improved efficacy without encountering prohibitive toxicity. However, not all human cancers have been shown to clearly benefit from combination therapies (e.g., low-grade lymphomas and colon cancer). In addition, one must be very careful with combining multiple compounds because of the necessity to reduce the doses of the most effective drugs to levels at which antitumor effects are not seen.

GENERAL APPLICATIONS OF CHEMOTHERAPY

- *Neoadjuvant chemotherapy* is used as induction therapy before definitive treatment (radiation or surgery). Examples include locally advanced esophageal and head and neck cancers. Chemotherapy may convert locally advanced, inoperable cancers to smaller, potentially resectable tumors.
- *Adjuvant chemotherapy* is used as an adjunct to local therapy to eliminate micrometastases. Examples include chemotherapy treatment of breast and colon cancers after surgical resection. Implementation of chemotherapy reduces mortality by about 30% in patients at high risk of recurrence.
- *Primary chemotherapy* is used in a variety of localized and advanced cancers. Primary chemotherapy is a potentially curative treatment for a variety of hematologic malignancies and germ cell tumors. It can prolong survival and improve quality of life in many advanced malignancies, including breast, prostate, colon, and pancreas.
- *Radiosensitization* combines chemotherapy with radiation to improve the effectiveness of radiation therapy and to provide systemic antitumor activity. It is used in rectal, esophageal, head and neck, pancreatic, and lung cancers.

MECHANISMS OF CHEMOTHERAPY RESISTANCE

The development of resistance to chemotherapeutic drugs by neoplastic cells is one of the major obstacles to the cure of many malignancies. Some malignant cells may be intrinsically resistant to chemotherapy, whereas others may become resistant by acquiring various detoxification pathways that enable them to survive the exposure to chemotherapy.

Transmembrane glycoprotein P, which is the product of the *MDR-1* gene, is present in many cells that are resistant to vinca alkaloids and doxorubicin. Glycoprotein P functions as a pump that is capable of removing cytotoxic agents from inside the cell. The type of drug resistance that is associated with glycoprotein P expression has been called *typical multidrug resistance* (MDR). The hallmark of MDR is cross-resistance to several drugs after exposure to a single drug, such as vinca alkaloid, dactinomycin, or anthracycline, but not to an alkylating agent. The activity of the glycoprotein P pump can be inhibited in the laboratory by several compounds, including verapamil, cyclosporine, cyclosporine analogs, and phenothiazines. Clinical trials are ongoing to investigate circumventing MDR by using some of these compounds.

Atypical MDR is associated with abnormal DNA topoisomerases, which are the enzymes that catalyze conformational changes of chromosomal DNA during replication. Several antineoplastic drugs exert their effect by inhibiting topoisomerases. Topoisomerase I is blocked by topotecan and irinotecan, and topoisomerase II is blocked by etoposide, teniposide, and doxorubicin. Alterations in topoisomerase structure and activity have been shown in cells resistant to topoisomerase inhibitors.

Glutathione is a thiol that accounts for the majority of intracellular nonprotein sulfhydryl content. Glutathione plays an important role in detoxifying toxins, scavenging free radicals, and repairing DNA damage. Glutathione S-transferase (GST) joins toxins, including chemotherapeutic drugs, with glutathione, forming less toxic metabolites. Increased amounts of GST have been found in cancers of the head and neck, lung, and colon. High GST and glutathione expression play a role in resistance to melphalan and other alkylating agents. Drugs that inhibit activity of GST, such as buthionine sulfoximine and ethacrynic acid, are being tested clinically for use in reversing resistance to alkylating agents.

ADVERSE EFFECTS OF CHEMOTHERAPY

Myelosuppression

One of the most common and important side effects of chemotherapy is suppression of the bone marrow, resulting in leukopenia, thrombocytopenia, and anemia. Myelosuppressive drugs generally should not be administered to patients with solid tumors who have an absolute neutrophil count less than 2000/μL or a platelet count less than 120,000/μL. For such a patient, increasing the interval between the doses is preferable to decreasing the dosage. The length of time it takes after treatment to reach the nadir is different for various agents. Most myelotoxic agents result in a nadir at 10 days, with recovery in 3 to 4 weeks. For busulfan, melphalan, dacarbazine (DTIC), and procarbazine, the nadir develops in 2 to 4 weeks, with recovery in about 6 weeks. For nitrosoureas, the nadir develops in 4 to 5 weeks, with resolution of neutropenia in 6 to 8 weeks, and the time to recovery usually lengthens with each course of treatment. Patients with neutropenia (i.e., absolute neutrophil count <500/μL) who develop temperature greater than 100.5°F should be hospitalized and treated promptly with broad-spectrum antibiotics. The recovery from neutropenia can be accelerated by the use of granulocyte colony-stimulating factors (GCSF or GMCSF), but their routine use is not cost-effective. Chemotherapy-induced anemia can be managed by administration of erythropoietin or periodic blood transfusions, or both. It is imperative to rule out other treatable causes of anemia. Patients with severe, persistent chemotherapy-induced thrombocytopenia present a difficult management problem because the effectiveness of platelet transfusions is usually brief. The newly developed megakaryocyte-stimulating cytokines, such as interleukin-11 and thrombopoietin, will improve the ability to treat chemotherapy-associated thrombocytopenia.

Alimentary Tract Toxicity

Chemotherapy-induced nausea and vomiting are mediated primarily by stimulation of serotonin and other receptors in the central nervous system. Highly emetogenic chemotherapy drugs include cisplatin, anthracyclines, dactinomycin, dacarbazine, and nitrosoureas. Acute chemotherapy-induced vomiting occurs usually 1 to 2 hours after treatment and typically resolves in 24 hours. Subacute and chronic vomiting occurs 8 to 18 hours and 48 to 72 hours, respectively, after chemotherapy. Delayed vomiting is most common after treatment with cisplatin at doses greater than 100 mg/m^2 and diminishes in 1 to 3 days. Anticipatory vomiting occurs before chemotherapy and is psychological in nature. There has been a significant improvement in the prevention of chemotherapy-induced nausea and vomiting with the introduction of serotonin-receptor antagonists, such as ondansetron and granisetron. These drugs bind to type 3 serotonin receptors and are very effective in preventing nausea induced by the most emetogenic chemotherapy drugs, including cisplatin. Serotonin-receptor antagonists are frequently used in combination with other antiemetics that have a different mode of action. These include phenothiazines (prochlorperazine, butyrophenones), haloperidol, droperidol, corticosteroids, and benzodiazepines.

Mucositis and diarrhea are most commonly associated with the use of fluorouracil (5-FU). Treatment is supportive, and chemotherapy is usually interrupted until symptoms resolve and is then followed by dose reduction. Paralytic ileus can occur as the result of autonomic neuropathy associated with the use of vinca alkaloids.

Renal and Urinary Tract Toxicity

Chemotherapy drugs that cause renal toxicity include cisplatin, methotrexate, and streptozocin. Aggressive hydration is used before administration of these compounds to prevent renal toxicity. Nephrotoxic drugs should not be administered unless the creatinine clearance exceeds 55 mL/minute. Amifostine is an organic sulfhydryl compound that was recently approved as a treatment to reduce the nephrotoxicity of cisplatin in patients with ovarian carcinoma and non–small cell lung cancer. Patients with underlying renal dysfunction who are treated with renally excreted chemotherapeutic agents require appropriate dose reductions. Acrolein (a metabolite of cyclophosphamide and ifosfamide) is responsible for hemorrhagic cystitis. This toxicity can be prevented by maintenance of high urine output and the use of the cytoprotective compound mesna, which binds and inactivates acrolein.

Cardiac Toxicity

Cardiomyopathy may occur with repetitive administration of anthracyclines, such as doxorubicin. Monitoring of the left ventricular ejection fraction with radionuclide techniques is mandatory in patients treated with anthracyclines. Maximum total cumulative dose of doxorubicin is 550 mg/m^2 or 450 mg/m^2 in patients who received mediastinal irradiation. Chemotherapy must be discontinued in case of documented decrease in ejection fraction or new electrocardiographic changes. Dexrazoxane is an intracellular chelating agent that prevents iron from combining with doxorubicin to form cardiotoxic free oxygen radicals. It was approved for use in patients with metastatic breast cancer who have received a total cumulative doxorubicin dose of at least 300 mg/m^2 and who would benefit from additional treatment with anthracyclines.

Neurologic Toxicity

Peripheral and cranial neuropathy can occur with administration of vinca alkaloids, cisplatin, paclitaxel (Taxol), and procarbazine. This complication may not be reversible and frequently necessitates interruption of treatment with the offending drug. Cerebellar toxicity is associated with high doses of cytarabine, procarbazine, 5-FU, and nitrosoureas. Seizures are very rare but have been reported after administration of procarbazine, ifosfamide, cisplatin, hydroxyurea, and L-asparaginase.

Hair Loss

Hair loss or thinning is a common result of treatment with most chemotherapeutic agents. It usually begins about 2 weeks after the initiation of chemotherapy and is reversible on the discontinuation of the drug.

More detailed discussion of toxicities of chemotherapy is included with the description of specific chemotherapeutic compounds.

CHEMOTHERAPY DRUGS

Alkylating Agents

Alkylating agents are antitumor drugs that act through the covalent bonding of alkyl groups (one or more saturated carbon atoms) to cellular molecules under physiologic conditions. The reaction proceeds through the formation of carbonium ion intermediates or of transition complexes with target molecules, usually having phosphate, amino, sulfhydryl, hydroxyl, carboxyl, imidazole, or other nucleophilic groups. Alkylating agents can react with a variety of cellular components, including DNA, RNA, protein, and phospholipids. However, reaction with DNA appears to be the prime event leading to either cell death or the cell's inability to reproduce, making these agents cytotoxic, mutagenic, and carcinogenic. The strongly nucleophilic 7-nitrogen of guanine, a purine base, appears to be the most susceptible group on DNA to the alkylating

agents, although other areas of nucleophilic attack exist. The activity of most alkylating agents is enhanced by hyperthermia, nitroimidazoles, and glutathione depletion. Their toxicity profile and antitumor activity differ greatly, which is undoubtedly the result of differences in pharmacokinetic features, lipid solubility, ability to penetrate the central nervous system, membrane transport properties, detoxification reactions, and specific enzymatic reactions capable of repairing alkylation sites on DNA. In general, cells that are resistant to one alkylating agent will be resistant to other alkylating agents and to other drugs that cross-link DNA, such as cisplatin. However, clinically, it has been shown that tumor cells resistant to one alkylating agent may be sensitive to another.

The active site in classic alkylators is chloroethylamine, with the following structure: (N)-CH$_2$-CH$_2$-Cl. Most of the biologically active alkylating agents are at least bifunctional (i.e., two chloroethyl groups on the molecule are bound to nitrogen and capable of alkylation). Although monofunctional agents (one chloroethyl group bound to nitrogen) are capable of producing irreversible damage to DNA, agents that are bifunctional can cause greater damage by interstrand or intrastrand cross-links. Atypical alkylators contain other moieties capable of binding DNA.

Nitrogen Mustards

The most clinically useful alkylating agents have been the bischloroethylamines or nitrogen mustards. The prototype antitumor alkylating agent is mechlorethamine, a bifunctional alkylator, also known as Mustargen, HN$_2$, or nitrogen mustard. This agent is now rarely used in the clinic except as a component in standard treatment regimens for Hodgkin's disease, but even this use is now becoming less frequent due to the mutagenic potential of mechlorethamine. Another potential application of this compound has been in the form of a topical solution in patients with mycosis fungoides. When administered systemically, myelosuppression is its principal dose-limiting toxicity.

Several analogs of mechlorethamine have been synthesized in which the methyl group has been replaced by a variety of chemical groups. Four such derivatives have been discovered, with higher therapeutic indices and a broader range of clinical activity. These agents, which can be administered both orally and intravenously, are melphalan (Alkeran), chlorambucil (Leukeran), cyclophosphamide (Cytoxan), and ifosfamide (Ifos). The latter two must be metabolized to produce alkylating compounds. Cyclophosphamide has been the most widely used of these agents due to its activity in a wide range of tumors. High-dose cyclophosphamide (up to 120 mg/kg) is also used as part of combination chemotherapy in bone marrow transplantation. Ifosfamide, an isomer of cyclophosphamide, was brought into clinical use in 1972 and has activity in testicular cancer and sarcomas. Melphalan is most active in ovarian cancer and multiple myeloma, and chlorambucil has mostly been used for the treatment of chronic lymphocytic leukemia and indolent lymphoma.

Estramustine (Emcyt) is a nitrogen mustard derivative of estradiol used in the treatment of advanced prostate cancer refractory to hormonal therapy. Theoretically, the estrogen component carries the nitrogen mustard moiety to the tumor site, where alkylation occurs. In addition, the estradiol metabolite has a cytostatic effect and decreases testosterone levels. Bone marrow suppression is the principal dose-limiting toxicity.

Alkyl Alkane Sulfonates

Busulfan (Myleran) is the only member of this group of compounds in common clinical use. It is an atypical bifunctional alkylator and was prepared in an attempt to produce a less toxic alkylating agent than nitrogen mustard. In contrast to the nitrogen mustards and the nitrosoureas, busulfan displays a more marked effect on myeloid cells than on lymphoid cells, making it a potent agent against chronic myelogenous leukemia (CML). As predicted, its dose-limiting toxicity is bone marrow suppression to a possible prolonged aplasia, given its equally toxic effect on hematopoietic stem cells. Interstitial pulmonary fibrosis ("busulfan lung") is a complication primarily associated with long-term use. This condition is irreversible and usually fatal within 6 months of onset.

Aziridines

The aziridine moiety is a three-membered ring in which one atom is nitrogen. Aziridine compounds were originally tested for antitumor activity because they are analogs of the ring-closed intermediates of the nitrogen mustards, and they alkylate in a similar fashion, through opening of the aziridine rings. Three of the most active compounds in this category include thiotepa, mitomycin-C (described under Antitumor Antibiotics, later in this chapter), and AZQ.

Triethylene-thiophosphoramide (Thiotepa) has been effective in breast cancer, ovarian cancer, and as a component of high-dose combination regimens in the treatment of lymphoma, breast cancer, and pediatric solid tumors. It has also been used intrathecally for the treatment of meningeal carcinomatosis, intravesically for the treatment of superficial bladder cancer, and intrapleurally for controlling malignant effusions. Its dose-limiting toxicity is myelosuppression.

Di-aziridinyl benzoquinone (diaziquone or AZQ) contains two aziridine moieties and is thus believed to be a bifunctional alkylator. This drug was designed and synthesized specifically to cross the blood-brain barrier, with brain-tumor levels reaching 48 to 85% of concurrent plasma levels. It is active alone and in combination with carmustine in tumors of the central nervous system. The dose-limiting toxicity of AZQ is myelosuppression, with a potential cumulative effect after several cycles of therapy.

Nitrosoureas

The nitrosoureas are alkylating compounds that were developed as anticancer agents, based on the fact that agents containing the nitroso functionality had activity in mouse tumor models. The nitrosoureas in common clinical use include carmustine (BCNU), lomustine (CCNU), and streptozocin (streptozotocin). The alkylating activity of these agents leads to interstrand DNA cross-links, which are believed to mediate the antitumor effects; the carbamoylating activity is associated with toxic side effects. Like other alkylating agents, the nitrosoureas appear to kill cells equally well in all phases of the cell cycle. Inhibition of DNA synthesis occurs. Carmustine and lomustine, two chloroethyl nitrosoureas, are lipid soluble and cross the blood-brain barrier. Streptozocin, a glycosylated nitrosourea, is specifically taken up by the beta cells of the islets of Langerhans, making the drug particularly useful in the therapy of metastatic pancreatic islet cell carcinoma.

The major adverse reaction encountered with nitrosourea is a delayed-onset dose-dependent depression of the hematopoietic system. Severe nausea and vomiting may also be dose limiting. With streptozocin, nephrotoxicity occurs instead of myelotoxicity, and this is cumulative and may be life threatening.

Platinum Complexes

The development of cisplatin (Platinol) encompassed a very interesting series of events. In 1965, Rosenberg observed that an electric current passing through platinum electrodes could inhibit *Escherichia coli* bacterial cell division. Chemical analysis showed that this inhibition was due to a hydrolysis product of the platinum electrodes, *cis*-diamine dichloroplatinum, or cisplatin. This discovery was confirmed by the subsequent testing of platinum complexes in murine tumor model systems.

Inside a cell, the two chloride atoms in cisplatin are displaced by two water molecules, yielding an aquated complex, which can react bifunctionally with DNA, RNA, or protein molecules to form cross-linked species. Platination (DNA/platinum adduct formation, commonly referred to as *alkylation*) is thought to be the cytotoxic event. Both intrastrand and interstrand DNA cross-links are formed. Cytotoxicity appears to be cell cycle phase independent, but some types of cells may be more sensitive in the G_1 phase.

Cisplatin has become the primary building block for regimens that cure patients with testicular carcinoma and produces high response rates in patients with small cell lung cancer, bladder cancer, and ovarian cancer. Toxic effects associated with cisplatin administration include renal damage, which is preventable with mannitol diuresis; nausea and vomiting, which can be severe; and peripheral neuropathy, with mild-to-moderate myelosuppression.

Carboplatin (Paraplatin) is a second-generation platinum complex. Although it is quite myelosuppressive, with platelets being most affected, it has a lower potential for nephrotoxicity, neurotoxicity, and emesis. Doses, however, must be adjusted in the setting of renal failure because approximately 90% of a given dose is excreted in the urine in 24 hours. Because efficacy is comparable to cisplatin in many settings, it is commonly used instead of cisplatin, especially in the elderly and otherwise compromised patients, to minimize the toxicity of a palliative regimen.

Nonclassic Alkylators

Procarbazine (Matulane), dacarbazine, and altretamine (hexamethylmelamine, or Hexalen) are structurally unrelated agents requiring metabolic activation to exert cytotoxic effects. They are all believed to act via alkylation, but the chemical intermediates have not been precisely characterized, and the mechanism of action is not clearly understood. They have mild bone marrow toxicity compared with other alkylating agents. They are therefore frequently used in combination with other agents because they can be administered at full therapeutic doses. Nausea and vomiting are common side effects. Procarbazine can also cause central and peripheral neurotoxicity.

Antitumor Antibiotics

Bleomycin is an antitumor antibiotic produced by a strain of *Streptomyces verticillus* and is purified by ion-exchange chromatography. Many of its effects are related to its ability to degrade preformed DNA. Subsequent to binding, free bases are released, and DNA is degraded. In vitro, it has also been found to produce a rapid and significant DNA synthesis inhibition but very little inhibition of RNA or protein synthesis. Bleomycin is most active in the G_2 and M phases of the cell cycle and least active in G_1. The dose-limiting toxicity of bleomycin is delayed-onset pulmonary fibrosis, occurring in 10% of patients, mostly past the age of 70. A history of chest radiation therapy, postoperative exposure, and a dose of more than 400 U increase the risk of pulmonary fibrosis. Chest radiographs may reveal increased interstitial markings, patchy reticulonodular infiltrates, consolidation, or nodules indistinguishable from metastatic lesions that may cavitate. Biopsy findings are nonspecific. Reversal may take months after the drug is discontinued, and fibrosis may be fatal. There is no known therapy, and the role of steroids is questionable. Fevers occur in 20 to 50% of patients. Mucocutaneous toxicities are also common, with mucositis, hyperpigmentation, and peeling that may progress to ulceration. The areas most likely to be affected are the digits, hands, joints, and areas of prior radiation therapy or surgery.

Mitomycin-C (MMC), an atypical alkylating antibiotic, is a natural product isolated from *Streptomyces caespitosus* as blue-violet crystals. In its parent form, MMC is inactive. Two mechanisms of activation have been identified that provide MMC with its alkylating effects. After reductive activation (chemical or enzymatic) to the semiquinone or hydroquinone species, anaerobic or aerobic activation of these intermediates can take place. The principal cell target for MMC is DNA, to which it binds by either monofunctional or bifunctional alkylation. Bifunctional alkylation, representing 10% of the covalent interactions, is thought to lead to cross-linking of strands of double-helical DNA. Monofunctional alkylation is by far the most frequently observed interaction.

The initial experience with this agent in the United States was quite poor because it was characterized by serious myelosuppression and responses of very brief duration. In 1974, the potential for this agent to induce delayed cumulative myelosuppression was recognized, and more rational dosage schedules were developed. Pharmacologically, MMC is absorbed erratically after oral administration. Intravesical and intraperitoneal administration, however, result in a significant local exposure advantage and very low plasma levels. This yields its activity in the treatment of recurrent superficial bladder carcinoma. Other cancers with demonstrated sensitivity to MMC include adenocarcinoma of the stomach, pancreas, colon, and breast. MMC is also used in combination chemotherapy regimens in non–small cell lung cancer (NSCLC). The most significant toxicity of MMC is delayed, cumulative myelosuppression, which seems to be directly related to schedule and dose. Other potentially lethal side effects include hemolytic-uremic syndrome, interstitial pneumonitis, and cardiac failure.

Additional antitumor antibiotics are described under Intercalating Topoisomerase II Inhibitors, later in this chapter.

Antimetabolites

Antimetabolites have been used over the past 40 years for the treatment of cancer. These compounds are structural analogs of the naturally occurring metabolites involved in DNA and RNA synthesis. As the constituents of these metabolic pathways have been understood, a large number of structurally similar drugs have been developed that alter the critical pathways of nucleotide synthesis.

Antimetabolites exert their cytotoxic activity by either competing with normal metabolites for the catalytic or regulatory site of a key enzyme or by substituting for a metabolite that is normally incorporated into DNA and RNA. Because of this mechanism of action, the antimetabolites are most active when the cells are in S phase, thus affecting mostly tumors that have a high growth fraction. Unlike the alkylating agents, the antimetabolites uncommonly produce severe, prolonged myelosuppression, and they do not increase the risk of secondary malignancies.

Folate Analogs

Methotrexate (MTX) is the 4-amino-4-deoxy-*N*-methyl analog of folic acid and is the principal folate antagonist used clinically. It exerts its cytotoxic effect by binding tightly to the enzyme dihydrofolate reductase, thereby blocking the reduction of folate to its active form. Synthesis of thymidine and purine is stopped, thus arresting DNA and RNA synthesis. For maximum cytotoxic effect, the intracellular levels of methotrexate must be sufficiently high to bind essentially all the dihydrofolate reductase. Currently, MTX has a broad range of clinical applications and is used most frequently in combination with other chemotherapeutic agents.

MTX normally enters the cell through an active, carrier-mediated cell membrane transport system. Some tumors lack or have reduced transport capabilities. In such tumors, very high extracellular levels of MTX must be achieved to effect transport into the cells by passive diffusion. High-dose MTX regimens can achieve such a goal and can also improve drug penetration into "sanctuary sites": the testis and the brain. The toxic effect of such high doses of MTX can be minimized by the rescue of normal cells with reduced folates, such as folinic acid and calcium leucovorin-citrovorum factor. Other rescuing agents, such as thymidine, carboxypeptidase G_1, and L-asparaginase, have a different mechanism of action.

A small fraction of an administered dose of MTX is conjugated intracellularly to a polyglutamate form with a prolonged biochemical effect in vivo. This results either from the preferential binding of the polyglutamate form to dihydrofolate reductase or from lengthy retention within cells. This polyglutamation may contribute to the enhanced toxicity of MTX in patients with ascites and pleural effusions. The length of "rescue" must therefore be extended in patients with third-space effusions to minimize the nephrotoxicity of MTX, especially when used in high-dose regimens. Other toxicities of MTX include myelosuppression with a predictable nadir at 1 to 2 weeks, and gastrointestinal endothelium damage resulting in diarrhea, mucositis, ulceration, and bleeding.

Purine Analogs

Fludarabine (Fludara) is a fluorinated nucleotide analog that interferes with DNA synthesis by inhibiting ribonucleoside reductase. It is indicated in the treatment of chronic lymphocytic leukemia and has activity in other lymphoproliferative disorders. Its dose-limiting toxic effect is myelosuppression. Possibly irreversible or lethal neurotoxicity has been observed but it occurs with extremely anti-leukemic doses of the drug administered by a continuous infusion.

Mercaptopurine (6-MP) and thioguanine (6-TG) are S phase–specific cytotoxic analogs of the natural purines hypoxanthine and guanine, respectively, acting as false metabolites. Both agents must be activated to the nucleotide form before being incorporated into the DNA and blocking DNA synthesis. Mercaptopurine can also be metabolized to a form that is itself a potent inhibitor of purine synthesis, thus interfering with RNA synthesis as well. Mercaptopurine is active in the treatment of acute lymphocytic leukemia (ALL). Thioguanine is used primarily with ara-C for acute myelocytic leukemia. Doses should be reduced in patients with renal and liver impairment. The side effects of

these two drugs are similar, with myelosuppression being the dose-limiting toxicity. Allopurinol, when given concomitantly with mercaptopurine, may significantly block its metabolism, necessitating a dose reduction of 66 to 75%.

Adenosine Analogs

Deoxycoformycin (Pentostatin) is structurally similar to adenosine and is a potent and irreversible inhibitor of adenosine deaminase, resulting in the accumulation of adenosine metabolites, which inhibit DNA synthesis. Initial trials demonstrated that pentostatin has profound lymphocytotoxic effects. Hairy-cell leukemia has shown exceptionally dramatic responses, with most patients achieving durable remissions with short courses of therapy. Toxic effects of pentostatin include neutropenia and increased risk of infection unrelated to myelosuppression, in addition to renal and central nervous system effects, skin rash, nausea and vomiting, conjunctivitis, and lethargy.

Cladribine (2-CdA, Leustatin) is an adenosine antimetabolite that is resistant to metabolic inactivation by adenosine deaminase. The accumulated drug is incorporated into DNA, creating DNA strand breaks. It is highly effective in lymphoid malignancies, such as hairy-cell leukemia, Waldenström's macroglobulinemia, chronic lymphocytic leukemia, and low-grade lymphomas. Myelosuppression is one of its major toxicities, with CD4 and CD8 counts also declining with therapy. Resulting infections reflect impaired cellular immunity and may include atypical bacteria (i.e., *Legionella*) and viruses.

Pyrimidine Analogs

Cytarabine (ara-C) is an analog of deoxycytidine that is phosphorylated to its active metabolite, ara-CTP. Ara-CTP inhibits DNA polymerase and is incorporated into DNA, resulting in strand breaks. Ara-C is most active in hematologic malignancies, being commonly used in combination with an anthracycline (daunorubicin or idarubicin) in the remission, induction, and consolidation therapy of acute myelocytic leukemia, resulting in a 60 to 80% remission rate. It is also used in several multidrug regimens in the treatment of non-Hodgkin's lymphoma (NHL). High-dose ara-C can be used in consolidating and inducing remissions in relapsed patients. Because the central nervous system can be a sanctuary site for leukemia, ara-C is effectively used intrathecally as a prophylactic agent. The toxic side effects include myelosuppression and gastrointestinal symptoms. High-dose regimens are associated with a significant incidence of cerebral and cerebellar neurotoxicity. Methotrexate combined with cytarabine enhances toxicity, so concurrent use of these drugs should be undertaken cautiously.

Floxuridine (FUDR), the chemically prepared nucleoside of 5-FU that undergoes rapid metabolism to 5-FU, inhibits thymidylate synthetase (TS). It is used primarily in continuous regional intra-arterial infusion therapy of cancers metastatic to the liver. It is more soluble than 5-FU, thus allowing administration of smaller volumes by means of portable infusion pumps. Another advantage over 5-FU is significant first-pass extraction by the liver. During infusional therapy, a chemical hepatitis is seen, as well as frequent fever. Numerous catheter-related problems can occur. Long-term complications include sclerosing cholangitis.

Fluorouracil (5-FU) is a fluorinated pyrimidine antimetabolite of uracil. It is activated by enzymatic conversion to 5-fluorouracil deoxyuridine 5' monophosphate (5FdUMP), after which it acts as a "false" antimetabolite. It interrupts DNA synthesis by inhibiting TS and by incorporating itself into DNA and RNA. Fluorouracil has maximal effect on cells in the S phase of the cell cycle. It is used primarily in gastrointestinal malignancies but is effective in the treatment of many different solid tumors. It can be given by a wide variety of routes and dosing schedules. Gastrointestinal toxicities, such as stomatitis, esophagitis, and diarrhea, are common and are dose limiting. These are more common with the continuous infusion of 5-FU, whereas myelosuppression occurs with the bolus injection.

Gemcitabine (Gemzar) is an antimetabolite structurally similar to ara-C. It was originally developed as an antiviral agent. Gemcitabine is triphosphorylated by the tumor cell and accumulates in high intracellular concentrations. It acts by inhibiting DNA polymerase and ribonucleotide reductase. It is approved for first-line therapy for locally advanced and metastatic pancreatic cancer but is also active in other tumors, including bladder cancer and NSCLC. Myelosuppression is the dose-limiting toxicity. Transient fever and flulike syndrome can occur but are usually relieved by acetaminophen. A reversible skin rash may appear and can be ameliorated with corticosteroids.

Substituted Urea

Hydroxyurea (Hydrea) is a DNA-selective antimetabolite that interferes with the enzymatic conversion of ribonucleotides to deoxyribonucleotides. It therefore causes immediate inhibition of DNA synthesis without interfering with the synthesis of RNA or protein. It may also inhibit the incorporation of thymidine into DNA and directly damage DNA. Hydroxyurea is most commonly used to manage myeloproliferative disorders, especially CML, polycythemia vera, and essential thrombocytosis. It is also used in acute leukemias to rapidly reduce high circulating blast counts. Its dose-limiting toxicity is bone marrow suppression. Gastrointestinal symptoms also occur, with nausea, vomiting, diarrhea, and constipation occurring in most patients receiving a higher dose of this drug.

DNA Topoisomerase Inhibitors

Topoisomerases constitute a group of enzymes that regulate the three-dimensional conformation of chromosomal DNA in cells by unwinding or unlinking coiled DNA double-strand molecules. They play critical roles in DNA replication and transcription. They act by breaking and rejoining one or both strands of the phosphodiester backbone. Topoisomerase I relaxes supercoiled DNA. Topoisomerase II mediates the passage of one double-strand DNA segment through another by formation of a temporary gate through both strands of one segment. Topoisomerase inhibitors trap the covalent complex formed between DNA and the enzyme, thereby causing DNA breaks.

Intercalating Topoisomerase II Inhibitors

DNA intercalation, inhibition of topoisomerase II, and free radical formation all contribute to the antitumor efficacy of intercalating topoisomerase II inhibitors. Such agents in clinical use include the anthracyclines: doxorubicin (Adriamycin), daunorubicin (Cerubidine), and idarubicin (Idamycin), dactinomycin (Actinomycin D), mitoxantrone (Novantrone), and amsacrine (m-AMSA).

The anthracycline antibiotics are derived from cultures of various strains of *Streptomyces*. Idarubicin is a synthetically prepared analog of daunorubicin. Doxorubicin is generally considered the most effective antitumor agent, with life-extending or palliative activity in a broad range of malignancies. Daunorubicin and idarubicin are used mostly for the acute leukemias, with idarubicin being orally bioavailable. The dose-limiting acute side effect is myelosuppression. In addition, the cumulative use of an anthracycline can lead to an irreversible cardiomyopathy, leading to congestive heart failure. This toxicity therefore limits the lifetime exposure of a patient to such an agent. Extravasation at the injection site can lead to tissue necrosis. A central line or a secure peripheral intravenous line is critical for the administration of these agents.

Dactinomycin, the first approved antitumor drug of natural origin, is derived from *Streptomyces parvulus* or can be synthesized chemically. Intercalation of this compound with DNA blocks the ability of DNA to act as a template for RNA and DNA synthesis in a concentration-dependent manner. It is believed to act in the G_1 phase of the cell cycle. Dactinomycin can also cause topoisomerase-mediated single-strand DNA breaks. It is highly effective in the treatment of Wilms' tumor, Ewing's sarcoma, embryonal rhabdomyosarcoma, and gestational choriocarcinoma. The dose-limiting toxicity is myelosuppression. As for the anthracyclines, extravasation can lead to severe soft tissue damage and necrosis. Previous radiation exposure can lead to enhanced toxicity, even if the two modalities are separated by months in time.

Plicamycin (Mithramycin), an antitumor antibiotic isolated from *Streptomyces plicatus*, possesses a cytotoxic action similar to that of dactinomycin. It has its greatest antitumor activity in disseminated embryonal cell carcinoma of the testis or germ cell tumor. Its major clinical use, however, is in the treatment of hypercalcemia of malignancy unresponsive to other methods of treatment. The major toxic consideration for this agent is hemorrhage secondary to a combination of drug-induced thrombocytopenia and simultaneous drug-induced decreases of clotting factors II, V, VII, and X. This syndrome may ensue rapidly and is typically heralded by epistaxis, ecchymoses, facial flushing, and prolonged coagulation times.

Mitoxantrone, a synthetic DNA intercalator and topoisomerase II inhibitor, was clinically designed based on the structure of anthracyclines. Despite a mechanism of action similar to the anthracyclines, free radical formation is not as profound and therefore cardiac toxicity is less common. In addition, it has a diminished potential for extravasation injury and for causing nausea and vomiting. Its narrow spectrum of antitumor activity is confined to the treatment of breast cancer and leukemia.

Nonintercalating Topoisomerase II Inhibitor: Epipodophyllotoxins

The two podophyllotoxin derivatives currently in use are etoposide (VP-16) and teniposide (VM-26). These are semisynthetic compounds derived from the mandrake plant. Podophyllotoxin is an antimitotic agent that binds to tubulin. Its two clinically useful synthetic derivatives (epipodophyllotoxins) do not affect microtubular assembly but cause DNA damage (primarily strand breakage) through formation of a ternary complex with DNA and topoisomerase II. Maximum cell kill occurs in late S or G_2 phase. Etoposide is more widely used and has activity in testicular cancer, lung cancer, and lymphoma. Teniposide is efficacious in the treatment of relapsed ALL in children and in small cell lung cancer metastatic to brain. Therapy-related ANLL has been described with epipodophyllotoxin-containing therapy. Other toxicities include dose-limiting leukopenia, alopecia, and peripheral neuropathy.

Topoisomerase I Inhibitor: Camptothecin Analogs

Camptothecin is isolated from *Camptotheca acuminata*, an ornamental tree found in the People's Republic of China. Irinotecan (CPT-11, Camptosar) is a semisynthetic, water-soluble analog of camptothecin. It induces protein-linked DNA single-strand breaks that are dependent on topoisomerase I. This ultimately blocks both DNA and RNA synthesis in dividing cells. This cytotoxic activity prevents cells from entering mitosis. In June of 1996, irinotecan was approved for use in patients with colon cancer refractory or progressive after fluorouracil-based therapy. It is now being investigated as a first-line agent in patients with metastatic colorectal cancer. Treatment may continue indefinitely in patients with a response or stable disease. Dose-limiting side effects include leukopenia on the single-dose schedule and diarrhea with the 5-day continuous infusion schedule.

Topotecan (Hycamtin), a selective inhibitor of topoisomerase I, is another camptothecin analog, which has increased aqueous solubility compared to camptothecin and

fewer toxic side effects. It was approved for use in patients with advanced ovarian cancer refractory to standard therapy, although significant responses have been observed in lung cancer, myelodysplastic syndrome, and chronic myelomonocytic leukemia. Its dose-limiting toxicity is neutropenia. Hemorrhagic cystitis, a dose-limiting toxic effect of camptothecin, has not been observed, but microscopic hematuria can be seen in a small fraction of patients.

Tubulin Interactive Agents

Vinca Alkaloids

The vinca alkaloids are derived from the periwinkle plant, *Vinca rosea*. On entering the cell, these agents bind rapidly to the tubulin. This occurs in the S phase of the cell cycle at a site different from that associated with paclitaxel and colchicine. As a consequence, the polymerization of microtubules is blocked, resulting in impaired mitotic spindle formation in the M phase.

Vincristine (Oncovin) has broad-spectrum antitumor activity in human cancer. Its major clinical indication is in acute lymphoblastic leukemia, usually in combination with prednisone, occasionally with asparaginase and an anthracycline. It has also been used in breast carcinoma, sarcomas, Wilms' tumor, Hodgkin's disease, and NHL. Its dose-limiting toxicity is the occurrence of significant neuropathies, which manifest as paresthesias of the hands and feet, foot drop, constipation, and paralytic ileus.

Vinblastine (Velban) is used for the treatment of Hodgkin's disease, NHL, testicular cancer, choriocarcinoma, and breast cancer, in combination with other drugs. It has also been used in mycosis fungoides and acquired immunodeficiency syndrome (AIDS)-related Kaposi's sarcoma. Dose-related bone marrow depression is the major toxic effect associated with this agent, more frequently and severely than with vincristine.

Vinorelbine (Navelbine) is a new semisynthetic vinca alkaloid derived from vinblastine. It has recently been approved for the treatment of NSCLC as a single agent or in combination with cisplatin. Local tissue necrosis can occur with extravasation. Just like vinblastine, granulocytopenia is the major dose-limiting toxicity. Clinically significant peripheral neuropathy is rarely observed.

Taxanes

Paclitaxel (Taxol) is derived from the pacific yew, *Taxus brevifolia*. Unlike the vinca alkaloids, which cause microtubule disassembly, paclitaxel promotes microtubule assembly and stability. It has shown activity in refractory ovarian cancer and is currently approved for use in this malignancy. Considerable antitumor effects have also been observed in metastatic breast cancer, NSCLC, and locoregionally recurrent squamous cell carcinoma of the head and neck. Administration of paclitaxel has been associated with a severe acute hypersensitivity reaction, manifested by hypotension, dyspnea, bronchospasm, and urticaria. This reaction may be attributable to the polyoxyethylated castor oil (Cremophor EL) vehicle used to solubilize paclitaxel. Premedicating patients with corticosteroids, diphenhydramine, and an H_2-antagonist prevents this reaction.

Docetaxel (Taxotere) is a semisynthetic derivative from the leaf extracts of *Taxus baccata*. It is more potent than paclitaxel in enhancing microtubule assembly. It is approved for the treatment of breast cancer in patients who relapse after anthracycline-based therapy, but clinical responses have been noted in ovarian cancer, pancreatic cancer, and NSCLC. The toxicity profile is similar to paclitaxel, including myelosuppression, except that hypersensitivity reactions have not been reported as commonly and that some patients have developed edema and effusions.

Enzymes

Asparaginase (Elspar) is an enzyme isolated from a number of natural sources (*E. coli, Serratia marcescens, Erwinia carotovora,* and guinea pig serum), but clinically useful antitumor preparations are only derived from *E. coli* and from the plant parasite *E. carotovora*. Asparaginase acts indirectly to inhibit protein synthesis in certain tumor cells dependent on exogenous asparagine, a nonessential amino acid in humans. Normal cells have the ability to synthesize asparagine intracellularly; however, some tumors, such as ALL, do not have this capability and therefore are quite sensitive to asparaginase, which blocks the external supply of asparagine. Asparaginase is therefore indicated for the induction treatment of ALL and is conventionally used in combination with other cytotoxic drugs. Bone marrow suppression is not usually significant with asparaginase. Hypersensitivity or anaphylactoid reactions, however, are common, occurring in 20 to 35% of patients. An intradermal skin test is recommended before therapy. Asparaginase alters the clearance of vincristine, and therefore, when administered in combination, should follow vincristine by 12 to 24 hours. Asparaginase can affect the synthesis of coagulation factors. Fibrinogen and antithrombin III may be depressed, and disseminated intravascular coagulation associated with bleeding and thrombosis can occur.

Biological Agents

Biological therapy refers to antitumor treatment using the actions of natural host defense mechanisms or mammalian-derived substances, or both. The most promising agents in this category of drugs include interferons, interleukins, and monoclonal antibodies. Although many interferons have obtained approval by the U.S. Food and Drug Administration (FDA), only interferon-α has a cancer indication. Interferon-α is used in hairy-cell leukemia, AIDS-related Kaposi's sarcoma, and CML. Interleukin-2 is the most widely studied interleukin, and it has achieved efficacy in the treatment of metastatic renal cell carcinoma. Monoclonal antibodies are being tested in clinical trials in patients with lymphomas, colorectal cancer, lung cancer, breast cancer, and leukemia. IDEC C2B8 (Rituximab) was the first monoclonal antibody approved by the FDA for the treatment of cancer. In November of 1997, this agent was approved for the treatment of refractory NHL. These observations provide the foundation for extensive further investigation of biological response modifiers.

Retinoids

Retinoids induce cellular differentiation or suppress proliferation in a number of cell lines, and they suppress carcinogenesis in various model systems. These findings have generated widespread interest in these agents for cancer treatment and prevention. The agent 13-cis retinoic acid has undergone the most extensive clinical testing. Although its activity as a single agent in established cancer is limited, it is being explored in combination with other drugs, particularly interferon-α. Enthusiasm also exists for exploration of this agent as a means of primary or secondary cancer prevention. It has been found to reverse oral leukoplakia (a known precursor to squamous carcinoma of the oral cavity) in heavy tobacco users and to reduce the incidence of second primary tumors of the aerodigestive tract when used in the adjuvant setting in head and neck cancer patients. All-trans-retinoic acid has achieved a clinical remission in a very high proportion of patients with acute promyelocytic leukemia. This activity has not been replicated in other diseases, although minor activity has been reported in gliomas and AIDS-related Kaposi's sarcoma.

Investigational Agents

New Antifolates

Raltitrexed (Tomudex) is a quinazoline folate analog that has a mechanism of action similar to that of 5-FU: potent and specific inhibition of TS. Unlike 5-FU, Tomudex is a pure TS inhibitor, and its metabolite inhibits TS for long periods to achieve a greater cytotoxic effect. It is currently undergoing phase II and III testing and has activity in breast cancer, colorectal cancer, and pancreatic cancer. Tomudex has less severe toxicities than 5-FU does, probably due to its more selective action. The major toxicities reported include an anorexia-fatigue syndrome, diarrhea, myelosuppression, and reversible transaminasemia.

Trimetrexate (TMTX, Neurexin) differs from MTX by not requiring the reduced folate carrier system for cellular transport and by lacking the potential for polyglutamation. It therefore has a shorter intracellular half-life than does MTX, necessitating frequent or continuous dosing schedules. Like MTX, it is a potent inhibitor of dihydrofolate reductase and produces metabolic inhibition through mechanisms similar to MTX. TMTX has been approved by the FDA for the treatment of *Pneumocystis carinii* pneumonia in patients infected with human immunodeficiency virus (HIV) refractory to trimethoprim-sulfamethoxazole. Its antitumor activity includes cancer of the head and neck and NSCLC. The dose-limiting toxicity has been myelosuppression.

Antiangiogenic Agents

It is now generally accepted that solid tumor growth and metastases depend on the acquisition of an adequate blood supply. Pharmacological targeting of the microvasculature in patients with malignant neoplasms represents an attractive therapeutic approach because inhibitors of angiogenesis are less likely to have the hematopoietic and gastrointestinal toxicity of standard antiproliferative therapies, and they appear not to induce acquired drug resistance.

Clinical experience with antiangiogenic compounds, although limited to phase I and II studies, is beginning to accumulate. Several agents, such as Marimastat, TNP-470, and suramin, have exhibited promising antitumor activity and are being evaluated in large comparative phase III trials in the setting of a variety of malignancies. Even more important, dozens of compounds that interfere with different steps of the angiogenic cascade are currently in preclinical development. One report suggests that at least some of these agents, such as endostatin, may circumvent the acquired drug resistance that is so common to cancer therapy. It appears increasingly possible that inhibition of angiogenesis will become a useful addition to anticancer treatment. The strategies that use antiangiogenic compounds may include combination with chemotherapy or radiation therapy (or both); this has proved synergistic in some animal studies. Other such strategies are prolonged administration of the antiangiogenic agent as an adjuvant therapy, use of angiogenesis inhibitors in the perioperative period of cancer surgery, and the use of a combination of inhibitors of angiogenesis acting at different steps of the angiogenic pathway.

Miscellaneous Drugs

Suramin is a polysulfonated napthylurea that has been used for many years as an antitrypanosomal agent. It was also shown to have anti-HIV activity, and during these trials, it was found to have activity against AIDS-related lymphomas. Suramin acts at numerous cellular sites to exert effects on growth factors, surface receptors, signal transduction, cell-adhesion molecules, and migration. It appears to interact at many levels to stop cell growth and inhibit angiogenesis. It is being studied in metastatic prostate cancer, in which 40% of patients have shown an objective tumor response. It is a toxic drug, however, with the most serious side effect being a polyneuropathy, which may begin within several weeks of therapy. Other common toxicities include myelosuppression, renal dysfunction, transaminase elevations, and coagulopathy.

Homoharringtonine (HHT) is an alkaloid derived of the needles and bark of the Chinese evergreen *Cephalotoxus fortueni*. It inhibits protein synthesis by altering chain elongation. Early results suggest that HHT may be a promising drug for CML, producing some durable responses, but no significant activity has been seen in solid tumors. Myelosuppression and cardiovascular hemodynamic instability are the major dose-limiting toxicities.

UFT is a combination of uracil and ftorafur (Tegafur). As an oral prodrug, it is metabolized to 5-FU. Preliminary results show that it produces a response rate in colorectal cancer similar to that of 5-FU. Its toxicity profile is milder than that of 5-FU, with reduced neutropenia and mucositis.

The agent 9-aminocamptothecin (9-AC) is a camptothecin analog that inhibits normal topoisomerase I function. Compared to the other camptothecins, it has been late getting into clinical trials because of formulation problems. Phase II trials have shown some activity in refractory metastatic breast cancer and lymphoma. Myelosuppression has been the major dose-limiting toxicity.

Capecitabine (Xeloda) is an oral fluoropyrimidine carbamate that is activated by tumor cells into 5-FU. In phase II trials, it has shown efficacy in advanced colorectal cancer. In April 1998, the FDA approved it as the first oral chemotherapy for the treatment of patients with metastatic breast cancer resistant to standard chemotherapies. The most frequently reported side effect was gastrointestinal toxicity.

Dolastatin-10 is a potent antimitotic peptide isolated from the marine mollusk, *Dolabella auricularia*, which inhibits tubulin polymerization. It is the first antimitotic natural product from an animal source, with a tubulin-binding site different from that of the vinca alkaloids. Phase I trials have revealed a mild peripheral sensory neuropathy occurring in 40% of patients. Myelosuppression is the dose-limiting toxicity. Phase II studies are under way.

REFERENCES

Rosenberg B: Fundamental studies with cisplatin. Cancer 55:2303, 1985.

Simon SM, Schinder M: Cell biological mechanisms of multidrug resistance in tumors. Proc Natl Acad Sci U S A 91:3497, 1994.

READING REFERENCES

Brown JM, Giaccia AJ: The unique physiology of solid tumors: opportunities (and problems) for cancer therapy. Cancer Res 58:1408, 1998.

Chabner, BA: Biological basis for cancer treatment. Ann Intern Med 118:633, 1993.

DeMario MD, Ratain MJ: Oral chemotherapy: rationale and future directions. J Clin Oncol 16:2557, 1998.

Frei E, et al: The relationship between high-dose treatment and combination chemotherapy: the concept of summation dose intensity. Clin Cancer Res 4:2027, 1998.

Principles of cancer management: chemotherapy in cancer. *In* Cancer Principles & Practice of Oncology. 5th Ed. Philadelphia: Lippincott-Raven, 1997.

Seminars in Oncology. Vol. 25. October 1998.

CHAPTER 105

Chemotherapy of Non–Small Cell Lung Cancer

Martin H. Cohen

Non–small cell lung cancer chemotherapy has been the subject of several reviews, including those of Buccheri and Ferrigno (1996), Langer and Rosvold (1996), Ramanthan and Belani (1997), Vokes and Green (1998), Goss and colleagues (1996), and Herbst and colleagues (1997). These reviews uniformly suggest that progress is being made, that active chemotherapy drugs and drug combinations continue to be identified, and that combined chemotherapy and radiation therapy may produce better outcomes than either method alone. They also show that patients benefit from treatment, as evidenced by symptom relief, tumor shrinkage, and increased disease-free and overall survival, and that the future can be viewed optimistically. My purpose is to present treatment results in a way that permits the reader to decide the merits of these conclusions. My approach to the use of chemotherapy is organized on the basis of tumor burden, starting with advanced metastatic disease and ending with surgical adjuvant chemotherapy. Because of the many manuscripts and abstracts that might be cited in a review of this type, all abstracts were excluded (insufficient information and short follow-up), as were all studies with a median follow-up of less than 1 year (imprecise survival estimates) and, whenever possible, nonrandomized trials.

ADVANCED (METASTATIC) DISEASE

Advanced metastatic disease provides the setting for the initial evaluation of new chemotherapy drugs and new chemotherapy regimens. Practical as well as ethical reasons justify this practice. Practically, the population of lung cancer patients at most centers forms a pyramid, with a relatively small percentage of favorable stage I patients at the apex of the pyramid and relatively large numbers of patients with a poorer prognosis and unresectable and metastatic disease at the pyramid base. Because of the poor prognosis and the symptomatic nature of advanced disease, treatment is readily justified. Furthermore, patients with advanced disease have measurable disease, a requirement for chemotherapy efficacy studies.

From an ethical standpoint, it is appropriate to establish the safety and efficacy of a new treatment in a poor prognosis group before taking the regimen to a population with a better prognosis. Although neoadjuvant (protochemotherapy, induction chemotherapy, preoperative chemotherapy) treatment patients have measurable disease, they are not appropriate candidates for previously untested drug regimens because of their potential resectability and long-duration survival.

Must some minimal response rate be achieved in patients with advanced disease before a regimen is deemed sufficiently active to be used in patients with less advanced disease? This question has no definitive answer. On the basis of breast cancer results reported by Tormey and associates (1982) and Tranum and associates (1982), however, it appears that regimens active in the adjuvant setting have achieved overall response rates of about 50%, with complete response rates of 10 to 15% in patients with advanced disease.

Chemotherapy results in patients with advanced non–small cell lung cancer are strongly influenced by patient prognostic factors. Using data obtained from placebo-treated patients enrolled in Veterans Administration Lung Study Group trials, Zelen (1973) demonstrated that performance status was a major prognostic factor for survival. Patients with good performance status in whom disease was confined within an acceptable thoracic radiation therapy portal (i.e., limited disease) had a median survival of 28 weeks versus 7 weeks for individuals with poor performance status. Corresponding survivals for patients with extensive disease were 26 and 1.4 weeks, respectively. Nearly every study since then has confirmed or extended this observation, including, most recently, Muers (1996), Paesmans (1995), and Takigawa (1996) and their associates. Other important clinical prognostic factors for response and survival are listed in Table 105-1.

The evolution of non–small cell lung cancer combination chemotherapy trials has proceeded through three generations. The first, the 1970s generation, evaluated non–cisplatin-containing regimens; the second, the 1980s to early 1990s generation, evaluated cisplatin or a cisplatin derivative with chemotherapy drugs available in that decade. The third (pres-

Table 105-1. Advanced Non–Small Cell Lung Cancer: Clinical Prognostic Factors

Parameter	Good Prognosis	Reference
Performance status	Eastern Cooperative Oncology Group 0–1 Karnofsky 100–80	Stanley (1980)
Stage	Lower stage	Green et al. (1971)
Gender	Female	Palomares et al. (1996)
Weight loss	None or slight	Palomares et al. (1996)
Bone, skin, brain metastases	None	Paesmans et al. (1995)
Hemoglobin level	Normal	Takigawa et al. (1996)
White blood cell count	Normal	Paesmans et al. (1995)
Lactate dehydrogenase level	Normal	O'Connell et al. (1986)
Albumin level	Normal	Fatzinger et al. (1984)
Calcium level	Normal	Paesmans et al. (1995)
Sodium level	Normal	Muers et al. (1996)
Treatment response	Yes	O'Connell et al. (1986)

ent) generation is evaluating newer chemotherapy agents, including paclitaxel (Taxol), docetaxel (Taxotere), vinorelbine (Navelbine), gemcitabine (Gemzar), and two semisynthetic camtothecin derivatives, Irinotecan and Topotecan, with or without cisplatin or a cisplatin derivative. In addition to different drug regimens, the three generations also differ in criteria for patient eligibility into clinical trials (Tables 105-2 and 105-3). Thus, the Eastern Cooperative Oncology Group trials, from 1978 to the present, included only ambulatory [performance status (PS) 0–2] patients and excluded patients with brain metastases. The Southwest Oncology Group similarly adopted more stringent performance status eligibility criteria by 1980 and, in 1993, further limited study entry to PS 0–1 patients. It is uncertain whether the modest improvement in median survival seen in the more recent trials listed in Tables 105-2 and 105-3 is a result of better treatment or better patient selection.

Results with newer chemotherapy agents seem somewhat more promising. Studies of paclitaxel and carboplatin by Langer (1995) and Johnson (1996) and their associates, the former including only PS 0–1 patients, the latter including PS 0–3 patients, reported median survivals of 53 weeks and 38 weeks, respectively. Vinorelbine plus cisplatin proved to be the best arm of a European multicenter randomized trial reported by Le Chevalier and associates (1994). This treatment of PS 0–2, stage III–IV patients resulted in a median survival of 40 weeks versus 32 weeks in the vindesine-cisplatin arm and 31 weeks in the vinorelbine-alone arm. Combinations of docetaxel-cisplatin and gemcitabine-cisplatin, as summarized by Natale (1997), are currently being evaluated in randomized, multi-institution national and international clinical trials.

Stage migration is another factor that may improve current chemotherapy results. Over the past 25 years, new diagnostic technology has greatly increased our ability to detect otherwise occult disease. As described by Black and Welch (1993), the resulting upward stage migration improves survival of all disease stages and makes stage-specific historic comparisons invalid.

One way to gauge the efficacy of non–small cell lung cancer chemotherapy is to analyze trials that randomized patients to chemotherapy or supportive care, the latter consisting of no cytotoxic treatment or low-dose, presumably ineffective, chemotherapy. Nine trials of this design are listed in Table 105-4. Three of these trials, reported by Rapp (1988), Cartei (1993), and Cormier (1982) and their associates, demonstrated that the median survival of chemotherapy-treated patients was significantly longer than that of the supportive care control group. In two other trials, described by Luedke and colleagues (1990) and by Ganz and associates (1989), median survival results approached statistical significance in favor of the chemotherapy-treated group. In three of the four remaining studies, a trend was noted toward improved survival of chemotherapy-treated patients, the exception being the study of Lad and associates (1981). These results strongly suggest that chemotherapy has activity in advanced non–small cell lung cancer, with some exceptions. In three of these trials, by Rapp (1988), Woods (1990), and Luedke (1990) and their associates, nearly identical vindesine-cisplatin (120 mg/m^2) treatment schedules were used in relatively prognostically comparable patients. Median survival of chemotherapy-treated patients in these studies varied from 24.7 to 32.6 weeks. This 8-week median survival difference is comparable to the difference generally seen between the chemotherapy and supportive care study arms. The one outlying study in Table 105-4 is the trial of Cormier and colleagues (1982). That trial demonstrated a highly statistically significant median survival difference between treated and control patients. The 8.5-week median survival of the supportive care group, however, is shorter than the 16.6- to 25-week median survivals reported for other supportive care groups in Table 105-4.

In analyzing survival differences between chemotherapy and supportive care patients in Table 105-4, it is also important to look at chemotherapy response rates. Only two trials had a response rate above 30%—both non–cisplatin-containing regimens. The median response rate for cisplatin-containing combinations was 22%. Because response rates were less than 50%, median survival was determined by the survival of nonresponding patients. This observation does not negate a possible benefit of chemotherapy; rather, it suggests that response rate may not be a sensitive measure of chemotherapy effectiveness.

Randomized trials of chemotherapy versus supportive care have been evaluated in four meta-analyses, including those of Grilli (1993), Marino (1994), Souquet (1993) and their associates and the Non–Small Cell Lung Cancer Collaborative Group (1995). Each study demonstrated a significant, although modest, benefit of chemotherapy. Perhaps the best of these studies was that of the Non–Small Cell Lung Cancer Collaborative Group. This meta-analysis, using updated data on individual patients, demonstrated that

Table 105-2. Non–Small Cell Lung Cancer Eastern Cooperative Oncology Group Advanced Disease Trials: Patient Eligibility

Eligibility Criteria	Activation Year					
	1975	1976	1978	1979	1981	1984–Present
Performance status	0–3	0–3	0–2	0–2	0–2	0–2
Central nervous system metastases	Yes	Yes	No	No	No	No
Cisplatin regimens[a]	0/7	2/10	0/2	0/2	3/4	5/5
Median survival (weeks)	13–34	12–27	20–21	18	21–29	23–32
Reference	Creech et al. (1981)	(1981a)	Ruckdeschel et al. (1981b) (1984) (1985)			Bonomi et al. (1989)

[a]Number of cisplatin-containing regimens/total number of regimens.

Table 105-3. Non–Small Cell Lung Cancer Southwest Oncology Group Advanced Disease Trials: Patient Eligibility

Eligibility Criteria	Activation Year				
	1974	1979	1980	1983	1993
Performance status	0–4	0–4	0–3	0–3	0–1
Central nervous system metastases	Yes	Yes	Yes	Yes	?
Cisplatin regimens	0/2	0/1	2/3	5/5	2/2
Median survival (weeks)	16	23	20–24	21–26	26–34
Reference	Livingston et al. (1977)	Miller et al. (1982)	Miller et al. (1986)	Weick et al. (1991)	Wozniak et al. (1998)

Table 105-4. Advanced Non–Small Cell Lung Cancer: Combination Chemotherapy versus Supportive Care or Suboptimal Single-Agent Chemotherapy

Chemotherapy Regimen (P dose, mg/m)	No. of Patients	PS 0–1 (%)	Limited Stage (%)	% Response (CR/CR+PR)	Median Survival (weeks)			Reference
C, A, P (40)	43	58	14	0/15	24.7			Rapp et al. (1988)
Vn, P (120)	44	57	18	2/25	32.6	0.01	0.05	
SC	50	60	10	—	17.0			
Vl, P (120)	22	73	0	0/22	20.4	0.09		Ganz et al. (1989)
SC	26	69	0	4/12[a]	16.6			
Vn, P (120)	97	73	27	6/28	27.0	0.33		Woods et al. (1990)
SC	91	73	41	—	17.0			
C, E, P/M, VP, CC (80)	62	65	40	0/21	34.3	0.15		Cellerino et al. (1991)
SC	61	62	43	—	21.1			
Vn, M	143	58	43	1/23	20.4			Luedke et al. (1990)
Vn, P (120)	150	56	39	2/16	24.7	0.06		
Vn	141	57	43	0/1	14.8			
C, A, M, P	37	73	59	3/44	27.4	0.26		Lad et al. (1981)
CC	35	74	41	0/0	25			
Mx, A, C, CC	20	70	45	0/35	30.5	0.0005		Cormier et al. (1982)
SC	17	53	53	—	8.5			
VP, P (70)	44	59	—	0/11	21.7	NS		Kaasa et al. (1991)
SC	43	60	—	—	16.5			
C, M, P (75)	52	48	0	—	37	0.0001		Cartei et al. (1993)
SC	50	50	0	—	17			

A, adriamycin; C, cyclophosphamide; CC, lomustine; CR, complete response; E, epirubicin; M, mitomycin C; Mx, methotrexate; NS, not stated; P, cisplatin; PR, partial response; PS, performance status; SC, supportive care; Vl, vinblastine; Vn, vindesine; VP, etoposide.
[a]After radiation therapy.

Table 105-5. Advanced Non–Small Cell Lung Cancer: Combination Chemotherapy versus Single-Agent Chemotherapy

Chemotherapy Regimen (P dose, mg/m)	No. of Patients	PS 0–1 (%)	Limited Stage (%)	% Response (CR/CR+PR)	Median Survival (weeks)			Reference
Vn, P (100)	43	80	69	0/33	47.7	0.008		Elliott et al. (1984)
Vn	45	79	69	0/7	17.4			
Nvb, P (120)	206	80	39	—/30	40.0	0.04	0.01	Le Chevalier et al. (1994)
Vn, P	200	82	35	—/19	32.0			
Nvb	206	77	41	—/14	31.0			
5FU, L	68	72	0	0/3	22.0	0.03		Crawford et al. (1996)
Nvb	143	79	0	0/12	30.0			
Vn, P (120)	41	44	17	0/27	26.0			Einhorn et al. (1986)
Vn, P, M (60)	41	46	5	0/20	17.0	0.03		
Vn	42	45	10	0/14	18.0			
Vn, P (80)	77	47	48	0/29	45.0	NS		Kawahara et al. (1991)
P (80)	78	43	46	0/12	39.0			
VP, P (120)	103	79	49	5/26	34.7	0.87		Rosso et al (1990)
VP	113	86	45	1/7	26.0			
VP, P (120)	81	52	33	0/26	22.0	0.33		Klastersky et al. (1989)
P	81	62	35	0/19	26.0			
M, Vl, P (40)	176	76	0	1/20	22.7			Bonomi et al. (1989)
Vl, P (60)	175	76	0	1/13	25.1			
M, Vl, P/C, A, Mx, Pr	172	77	0	2/13	25.0	0.008		
I	88	79	0	1/6	26.1			
CP	88	82	0	0/9	31.7			
M, Vl, P, Mx (40)	52	—	21	0/25	27.2	> 0.5		Niell et al. (1989)
M	53	—	19	0/19	23.6			
C	41	29	0	0/5	20.8			Davis et al. (1980)
C, CC	47	19	0	0/8	17.1	> 0.3		
C, CC, A	36	25	0	0/6	19.3			

A, adriamycin; C, cyclophosphamide; CC, lomustine; CP, carboplatin; CR, complete response; E, epirubicin; 5FU, 5-fluorouracil; I, iproplatin; L, leukovorin; M, mitomycin C; Mx, methotrexate; NS, not stated; Nvb, Navelbine; P, cisplatin; Pr, procarbazine; PR, partial response; PS, performance status; Vl, vinblastine; Vn, vindesine; VP, etoposide.

cisplatin-based chemotherapy combinations were associated with a hazard ratio of 0.73, equivalent to an absolute improvement in survival of 10% [confidence interval (CI) 5% to 15%] at 1 year or to an increased median survival of 1.5 months (CI 1.0 to 2.5 months).

A second test of chemotherapy efficacy in patients with advanced non–small cell lung cancer comes from randomized trials of combination versus single-agent chemotherapy. Ten trials with this design are listed in Table 105-5. Four of these trials demonstrated a statistically significant median survival advantage, the studies by Elliott (1984) and Le Chevalier (1994) and their colleagues favoring combination chemotherapy and the trials of Bonomi (1989) and Crawford (1996) and their associates favoring single-agent treatment. Navelbine and carboplatin were the single agents used in the aforementioned trials. Both of these agents have known activity in patients with non–small cell lung cancer. The combination regimens that significantly increased survival were vindesine-cisplatin and navelbine-cisplatin. None of the drug combinations using three or more drugs was associated with significant survival improvement. This is a potentially important observation because the optimal number of drugs to be used in a treatment regimen has not been rigorously defined. First-generation chemotherapy regimens often included four or five drugs [e.g., COMB (cyclophosphamide, vincristine, MeCCNU, bleomycin), CAMP (cyclophosphamide, Adriamycin, methotrexate, procarbazine), MACC (methotrexate, Adriamycin, cyclophosphamide, CCNU), and BACON (bleomycin, Adriamycin, cyclophosphamide, vincristine, nitrogen mustard)]. More recent investigators favor two-drug regimens. Advantages of the latter approach are that each drug can be used at doses closer to its optimal single dose and that toxicity is more predictable when chemotherapy is combined with radiation therapy.

Design of several of the studies listed in Table 105-5 called for patients who received single-agent chemotherapy to receive additional therapy (combination regimens or new single agents) at disease stabilization or progression. Similarities of survival between patients receiving initial combination or single-agent chemotherapy might then be a result of second-line therapy in the latter group. Generally, however, fewer than one-half of the single-agent–treated patients actually received second-line therapy. Responses to second-line therapy were infrequent, and no survival differences were noted between individuals receiving and not receiving that therapy. Consequently, single-agent survival results likely reflect the efficacy of that drug.

In the vindesine-cisplatin studies listed in Table 105-5, as opposed to those in Table 105-4, there was considerable

Table 105-6. Patients with Advanced Non–Small Cell Lung Cancer Who Are Performance Status 0 at Presentation

No. of Patients	Percentage Performance Status 0	Reference
486	19	Ruckdeschel et al. (1986)
432	21	Ruckdeschel et al. (1984)
203	9	Fukuoka et al. (1991)
699	19	Bonomi et al. (1989)
216	18	Rosso et al. (1990)
160	3	Kawahara et al. (1991)
105	13	Elliott et al. (1984)

Table 105-7. Presenting Symptoms in Patients with Advanced Non–Small Cell Lung Cancer

Symptom	Percentage of Patients
Pain	
Chest	33
Bone	30
Shoulder/arm	17
Respiratory	
Cough	46
Dyspnea	39
Hemoptysis	17
Other	
Anorexia	36
Hoarseness	10

variability in the cisplatin dose (40 to 120 mg/m^2). Median survival rates varied from 25.1 to 47.7 weeks. Because of differences in patient prognostic factors from study to study and because of differences in data analysis, including exclusion of early treatment failures in the study of Elliott and colleagues (1984), these reports cannot be used to determine a cisplatin dose effect on median survival.

The focus of the previous discussion on chemotherapy efficacy was median survival. Also important is whether chemotherapy produces any long-term survivors. This information is hard to discern. Many trials are reported too early to have accurate long-term survival information, and results typically are not updated. One study specifically addressing the issue of prolonged survival after chemotherapy was by Finkelstein and colleagues (1986). They reviewed 893 cases of metastatic disease treated according to Eastern Cooperative Oncology Group protocols. Overall, 168 of 893 patients (19%) survived for more than 1 year and 36 (4%) survived for more than 2 years. As expected, the majority of long-term survivors were patients with favorable pretreatment prognostic factors who responded to therapy. Small percentages of unfavorable patients, however (i.e., with performance status of 2, >10% weight loss, large primary tumors, multiple metastatic sites, and no response to chemotherapy) were included in the long-surviving group.

If, as indicated in Tables 105-4 and 105-5, survival gains with combination chemotherapy are modest, at best, should patients with advanced non–small cell lung cancer be offered treatment? This question is irrelevant at research centers where patients are offered research protocols seeking better therapy. In nonprotocol settings, the question is probably also irrelevant because the main rationale for chemotherapy is symptom palliation. Patients with advanced non–small cell lung cancer are generally symptomatic. Table 105-6 indicates that fewer than 20% of such patients are performance status 0 (i.e., normal activity and asymptomatic) at presentation. Common symptoms, based on data from Ruckdeschel and associates (1986), are listed in Table 105-7. Chemotherapy treatment often results in palliation of symptoms. Table 105-8 summarizes three studies that demonstrate this effect by Hardy (1989), Gridelli (1997), and Thatcher (1995) and their colleagues. As evident from the Hardy study, symptomatic improvement may occur in the absence of chemotherapy response. This finding was reported in regard to breast cancer treatment by Brunner (1975), Coates (1987), and Tannock (1988) and their colleagues. It might be expected that symptomatic improvement would lead to improved quality of life. Quality-of-life data are sparse to date, but they should be collected with increasing frequency in future studies.

In deciding whether to recommend chemotherapy for a patient with advanced disease, risk–benefit considerations should be used. Generally, only ambulatory patients should be considered for treatment because risk more often exceeds benefit in nonambulatory individuals. As summarized by Simes (1985), risks of treatment include treatment toxicities up to and including death, cost and inconvenience of receiving chemotherapy, and the possibility of increased hospitalization. Benefits include symptom palliation, increased survival, psychological benefits of knowing everything was done, and the altruistic benefit of possibly helping future patients.

If a decision is made to use chemotherapy, how long is the course of treatment? In responding patients, chemotherapy is generally continued for the duration of response unless toxicity is severe. In patients with stable disease, duration of

Table 105-8. Advanced Non–Small Cell Lung Cancer: Symptom Palliation with Chemotherapy

No. of Patients	Impact on Cancer		Symptom Benefit			Reference
	Response (%)	Median Survival (wks)	Cough	Dyspnea	Pain	
24	21	24	71	65	63	Hardy et al. (1989)
43	23	36	43	28	42	Gridelli et al. (1997)
332	20	35–40	44	26	32	Thatcher et al. (1995)

Table 105-9. Alternating Combination Chemotherapy

Chemotherapy Regimen	No. of Patients	Performance Status 0–1 (%)	Limited Stage (%)	Response Rate (CR/CR+PR)	Median Survival (wks)	Reference
C, E, P/M, VP, CC	62	65	40	0/21	34.3	Cellarino et al. (1991)
M, Vl, P/C, A, Mx, Pr	172	77	0	2/13	25.0	Bonomi et al. (1989)
P, Vl/M, Vl	125	56[a]	38[b]	4/17	21.6	Weick et al. (1991)
F, O, M/C, A, P	114	55[a]	39[b]	1/10	21.6	Weick et al. (1991)

A, adriamycin; C, cyclophosphamide; CC, lomustine; CR, complete response; E, epirubicin; F, 5-fluorouracil; M, mitomycin C; Mx, methotrexate; O, vincristine; P, cisplatin; Pr, procarbazine; PR, partial response; CS, supportive care; Vl, vinblastine; Vn, vindesine; VP, etoposide.
[a]Percentage of patients with performance status 0–1 may be higher because patients with that performance status but with weight loss >10% are excluded.
[b]Percentage of limited disease patients may be lower as only patients with bone, brain, or lung metastases were excluded.

treatment is less clear. A randomized trial by Buccheri and associates (1989) addressed this issue. After two or three cycles of treatment with methotrexate, Adriamycin, cyclophosphamide, and lomustine (MACC), patients with stable disease were randomized to either continue or discontinue therapy. Time to progression and median survival were similar for both groups. Although a slight improvement in physical symptoms was noted in the continued treatment group, this was partially or wholly negated by increased chemotherapy toxicity.

Two other chemotherapy concepts have been tested in patients with advanced non–small cell lung cancer. The first involves the use of alternating, non–cross-resistant drug combinations. The purpose of this therapy, based on the Goldie and Coldman (1979) mathematical model, is to delay or prevent the emergence of drug-resistant clones of cancer cells. Table 105-9 summarizes the alternating combination chemotherapy arms from four randomized trials comparing that therapy to either supportive care or a single drug combination. In no case did the alternating non–cross-resistant drug combination produce statistically significant survival improvement.

A second strategy to improve chemotherapy results involves the use of high dose intensity (mg/m^2 per week) regimens. As documented by Frei and Canellos (1980), many chemotherapy drugs, especially alkylating agents, have a steep dose-response relationship. An early study demonstrating the importance of dose was done by Gralla and associates (1981). These investigators randomly selected patients to receive vindesine plus high-dose (120 mg/m^2) or low-dose (60 mg/m^2) cisplatin therapy. Median duration of response and median survival of responding patients were both significantly longer with high-dose cisplatin treatment (Table 105-10). Results of this trial provided impetus for two studies of high-dose chemotherapy

with autologous bone marrow support by Williams (1989) and Gomm (1991) and their colleagues. Both studies yielded disappointing results with response rates and survival durations similar to those seen with conventional chemotherapy. Because of the availability of bone marrow colony-stimulating factors, which, as demonstrated by Lieschke and Burgess (1992), decrease the duration of chemotherapy-induced myelotoxicity, additional trials testing the dose intensity hypothesis are likely.

INOPERABLE OR UNRESECTABLE M_0 DISEASE: CHEMOTHERAPY PLUS RADIATION THERAPY VERSUS RADIATION THERAPY ALONE

Chemotherapy has three potential roles in combined chemotherapy-radiation therapy treatment: When given simultaneously with radiation therapy, it might act as a radiation sensitizer. When given before radiation therapy, it might decrease tumor size, rendering the lesion more amenable to sterilization by an achievable radiation dose. When given after radiation therapy, it might kill surviving cells within the radiation port. In all three scenarios, chemotherapy would also be expected to have an adjuvant effect on subclinical metastatic disease. It follows that combined chemotherapy-radiation therapy, as summarized by Arriagada (1997), should increase the complete response rate and delay both local and systemic recurrence compared to radiation therapy alone.

Table 105-11 summarizes results of nine randomized trials comparing combined chemotherapy-radiation therapy to radiation therapy alone. Three of these trials involved a chemotherapy regimen that did not include cisplatin, whereas cisplatin- or carboplatin-containing regimens were used in all the other trials. Studies reported by Schaake-Koning (1992),

Table 105-10. Vindesine-Platinum Treatment of Advanced Non–Small Cell Lung Cancer: Effect of Cisplatin Dose Intensity

Cisplatin Dose (mg/m^2)	Percentage Response Rate	Median Response Duration (months)	Responders Median Survival (months)
60	46	5.5	10.0
120	40	12.0	21.7

Table 105-11. Randomized Trials of Chemotherapy-Radiation Therapy Compared to Radiation Therapy Only

Disease Stage	Radiation Therapy (Gy/schedule/fractions)	Chemotherapy (mg/m²)	No. of Patients	Treatment Outcome		Reference
				CR (%)	Survival Benefit	
I–III	55/Split/20	P 30 day 1&8	79	23	Yes	Schaake-Koning et al. (1992)
		P 6 daily	79	28		
		None	88	22		
I–III	60/Cont/30	Vl, P 100	78	19	Yes	Dillman et al. (1990)
		None	77	16		
II–III	60/Cont/30	Vl,P 100	151	—	Yes	Sause et al. (1995)
		None	149	—		
	69.6/Hfx/58	None	152	—		
III	64.8/Hfx/54	VP, CBDCA (w)	52	37	Yes	Jeremic et al. (1995)
		None	61	25		
I–III	60–65/Cont/≥30	P 70	104	—	No	Blanke et al. (1995)
		None	111	—		
III	50/Cont/20	Vn, P 100	39		No	Gregor et al. (1993)
		None	39	7		
III	50.4/Cont/28	P 15 weekly	45	9	No	Soresi et al. (1988)
		None	50	2		
I–III	65/Cont/26	Vn, C, CC, P 100	165	16	No	Le Chevalier et al. (1991)
		None	167	20		
I–III	55/Split/20	C, A, P40	119	15	No	Mattson et al. (1988)
		None	119	11		
I–III	40/Split/10	C, A, P 40	78	—	No	Lad et al. (1988)
		None	86	—		
I–III	60/Cont/30	M, A, C, CC	56	14	No	Morton et al. (1991)
		None	58	17		
III	45/Cont/15	C, A, Mx, Pr	49	6	No	Trovo et al. (1990)
		None	62	10		
I–III	60/Cont/33	Vn	87	2	No	Johnson et al. (1990)
		None	87	5		
		Vn alone	98	1		

A, adriamycin; C, cyclophosphamide; CBDCA, carboplatin; CC, lomustine; Cont, continuous; CR, complete response; Hfx, hyperfractionated radiation therapy; Mx, methotrexate; P, cisplatin; Pr, procarbazine; Vl, vinblastine; Vn, vindesine.

Johnson (1990), Lad (1988), Jeremic (1995), and Blanke (1995) and their associates used simultaneous chemotherapy-radiation therapy, with Lad and associates continuing chemotherapy after completion of the radiation therapy. Morton (1991), Dillman (1990), Le Chevalier (1991), Gregor (1993), and Sause (1995) and their associates gave chemotherapy before radiation therapy. Mattson and associates (1988) gave chemotherapy before, between, and after courses of radiation therapy, and Trovo and associates (1990) gave chemotherapy after radiation therapy was completed.

A first, somewhat disappointing observation from these trials is that combined-method therapy did not produce a striking increase in the complete response rate compared to radiation therapy alone. In four studies, however, investigators did observe prolonged survival in patients treated with a combined method. These data are summarized in Table 105-12. In the studies by Schaake-Koning (1992) and Jeremic (1995) and their associates, the increased survival appeared to result primarily from a delayed local recurrence in patients receiving low-dose, daily cisplatin. The study of Dillman and associates (1990) revealed an apparent delay in both local and systemic recurrence in the combined-method arm. The former outcome suggests a radiosensitizing effect

of low-dose daily cisplatin, whereas the latter suggests that a high-dose cisplatin regimen is active against both local and metastatic disease. Failure patterns were not reported by Sause and colleagues (1995).

Further suggestive evidence of activity of a high-dose cisplatin-containing regimen against subclinical metastatic disease comes from the study of Le Chevalier and associates (1991). In this trial, survival results approached statistical significance ($P = .08$) in favor of the combined-method arm (median survival of 10 months versus 8 months and 2-year survival of 21% versus 14%). Although local recurrence was comparable in the two arms, the distant recurrence rate was significantly decreased in the combined method arm.

Two meta-analyses of randomized trials comparing chemotherapy and radiation therapy to radiation therapy alone have been reported by Pritchard and Anthony (1996) and by the Non–Small Cell Lung Cancer Collaborative Group (1995). Pritchard and Anthony reviewed 14 studies, reporting on a total of 2589 patients. The addition of chemotherapy to radiation therapy resulted in a 1.7-month improvement in median survival. The relative risk of death for each 6-month interval, up to 36 months from onset of

Table 105-12. Randomized Trials with Significantly Increased Survival with Chemotherapy-Radiation Therapy versus Radiation Therapy Alone

Reference	Treatment Regimens	Survival			
		Median (months)	1 yr (%)	2 yrs (%)	3–5 yrs (%)
Schaake-Koning et al. (1992)	CT (d) + RT	—	54	26	16 (3 yrs)
	CT (w) + RT	—	44	19	13
	RT	—	46	13	2
Dillman et al. (1990, 1996)	CT + RT	13.8	55	26	17 (5 yrs)
	RT	9.7	40	13	6
Sause et al. (1995)	CT + RT	13.8	60	—	—
	RT	11.4	46	—	—
	RT (Hfx)	12.3	51	—	—
Jeremic et al. (1995)	CT (w) + RT (Hfx)	18.0	73	35	23 (3 yrs)
	RT (Hfx)	8.0	39	25	6.6

CT, chemotherapy; Hfx, hyperfractionated radiation therapy; RT, standard radiation therapy; d, daily; w, weekly.

treatment, decreased 12 to 17% in the combined-modality arm compared to radiation therapy alone. Comparable results were obtained when chemotherapy and radiation therapy were administered sequentially or simultaneously and when cisplatin or non–cisplatin-containing chemotherapy regimens were used.

The Non–Small Cell Lung Cancer Collaborative Group (1995) meta-analysis reviewed data from 22 trials with a total of 3033 patients. Eleven of these trials, including a majority of the total patients analyzed, used cisplatin-based chemotherapy. These regimens produced a 13% reduction in the risk of death, equivalent to an absolute benefit of 4% (CI 1 to 7%) at 2 years and 2% (CI 1 to 5%) at 5 years.

The cost of the modest survival increase associated with high-dose cisplatin-containing regimens is increased treatment-related toxicity. In the study of Schaake-Koning and associates (1992), two deaths occurred among patients receiving the weekly cisplatin regimen. Hematologic toxicity was increased in patients receiving daily cisplatin, although it was rarely severe or life threatening. Nausea and vomiting was also more common and more severe in chemotherapy-treated patients. Dillman and associates (1990) found a similar toxicity profile. In their trial, infection requiring hospitalization occurred in 7% of patients treated with the combined method versus 3% of those receiving radiation therapy. Similarly, nausea and vomiting and weight loss were more severe when chemotherapy was added to radiation therapy. In their trial, Le Chevalier and associates (1991) reported eight treatment-related deaths, five in the combined-method arm.

To gain greater perspective on the combined effect of chemotherapy and radiation therapy on small volume thoracic and subclinical metastatic disease, the study of Lad and associates (1988) is instructive. Patients in this study had pulmonary resections, with the majority of study participants (84%) having only microscopic residual cancer within the chest. Compared with the aforementioned studies, this trial evaluated a low-dose cisplatin chemotherapy regimen. Of interest in this trial is a low rate of local recurrence. Only 20 study patients (12%) had local recurrence, with no difference between the two treatment arms. Chemotherapy resulted in a significant delay in systemic recurrence during the first year of follow-up but not thereafter. A trend toward increased survival favoring combined-method treatment was evident (median survival of 20 months versus 13 months, and 1-year survival of 68% versus 54%; $P = 0.113$).

LOCOREGIONAL NON–SMALL CELL LUNG CANCER: NEOADJUVANT THERAPY

The rationale for presurgical, neoadjuvant induction chemotherapy or chemotherapy-radiation therapy in patients with local or regionally advanced disease is to permit the resection of disease that initially was unresectable, to initiate treatment of subclinical metastatic disease at the earliest possible time, to reduce toxicity from that expected to occur if treatment was given postoperatively, and to prolong the survival of treated patients. To date, all published studies of neoadjuvant therapy, except two, are phase II feasibility trials. These trials clearly indicate that neoadjuvant therapy is feasible. Evaluation and comparison of these nonrandomized studies is complicated, however, by the absence of common criteria for patient selection, staging procedures, determination of operability, and resectability and by whether or not the patient received postoperative therapy. Another complicating factor is that study results are subject to changing denominators. Consequently, individual studies are difficult to evaluate, and it is impossible to compare studies to determine a "best" treatment program.

Table 105-13 provides an overview of 14 chemotherapy and combined chemotherapy–radiation therapy neoadjuvant trials. Of the 14 trials, only five included more than 50 patients. All involved cisplatin-containing chemotherapy regimens. The cisplatin dose was 100 mg/m^2 or higher in seven of the trials and ranged from 50 to 80 mg/m^2 in the others. Preoperative radiation therapy was given concur-

Table 105-13. Locoregional Non–Small Cell Lung Cancer: Neoadjuvant Trials

No. of Patients	Stage		Preoperative Therapy	Complete Response				Reference
	T	N		Clinical		Pathologic		
				No.	%	No.	%	
136	1–3	2	C	13	10	19/98	21	Martini (1983)
58	1–3	2	C	7	12	9/28	32	Gralla (1988)
32	1–3	0–2	C	4	13	3/29	10	Raut et al. (1984)
11	2	2	C	0	0	1/11	9	Pass et al. (1992)
20	3	2–3	C	0	0	1/2	50	Bitran et al. (1986)
13	1–3	0–2	C	1/11	9	0/9	0	Dautzenberg et al. (1990)
39	1–4	2	C	3	8	3/39	8	Burkes et al. (1992)
126	1–4	0–3	C+RT	2	2	19/89	21	Albain et al. (1995)
64	1–3	0–2	C+RT	5	8	9/39	23	Taylor et al. (1987)
24	1–3	0–3	C+RT	0	0	4/8	50	Bonomi et al. (1986)
36	2–3	2	C+RT	—	—	10/31	32	Yashar et al. (1992)
39	1–3	1–2	C+RT	2	5	—	—	Eagan et al. (1987)
85	1–4	2	C+RT	2	2	8/35	23	Weiden and Piantadosi (1991)
41	1–3	0–2	C+RT	0	0	7/31	23	Strauss et al. (1992)

C, chemotherapy; RT, radiation therapy.

rently with chemotherapy (five trials) or was delayed until the completion of three cycles of chemotherapy (one trial). In several of the trials, additional chemotherapy or radiation therapy, or both, was given postoperatively as well. As implied in Table 105-13, a heterogeneous patient population was studied. Primary tumor stage (T stage) was determined by physical examination, CT of the chest, and bronchoscopy. Mediastinal node status (N_2 disease) was defined by chest radiographic or bronchoscopic findings or results of chest CT or surgical biopsy. Although not specifically stated in the table, tumor stage in these patients ranged from $T_1N_0M_0$ to $T_4N_3M_0$.

Neoadjuvant treatment response rates—complete and partial—were from 50 to 70%. The majority of responses were less than complete. As noted in Table 105-13, clinical complete response rates after chemotherapy alone or chemotherapy plus radiation therapy were between 0 and 13%. Significantly,

pathologic complete responses outnumbered clinical complete responses. Whereas the majority of pathologic complete responders were also clinical complete responders, partial responders or patients with stable disease occasionally had no evidence of cancer in their resected tissues.

Table 105-14 analyzes sites of recurrence after completion of the treatment protocol. In general, the denominator for these calculations is the number of patients who had a surgical resection. Local or regional failure, or both, occurred in 27 to 63% of postresection patients who received neoadjuvant chemotherapy and in 0 to 40% of patients treated with the combined method. A common site for systemic failure was the brain. This finding led several authors to suggest that prophylactic cranial radiation be evaluated in this patient group.

Roth (1994) and Rosell (1994) and their colleagues reported two randomized chemotherapy neoadjuvant stud-

Table 105-14. Locoregional Non–Small Cell Lung Cancer Neoadjuvant Trials: Patterns of Recurrence

Therapy	No. of Patients	Sites of Recurrence[a]						Reference
		None		Locoregional		Systemic		
		No.	%	No.	%	No.	%	
C	41	10/21	48	8/21	31	14/21	67	Martini et al. (1988)
C	11	3/11	27	5/8	63	3/8	37	Pass et al. (1992)
C	13	4/13	31	3/11	27	6/11	55	Dautzenberg et al. (1990)
C	39	10/22	45	6/22	27	7/22	32	Burkes et al. (1992)
C + RT	136	33/82	40	14/82	17	31/82	38	Martini (1983)
C + RT	126	61/126	48	25/89	30	58/89	65	Albain (1995)
C + RT	85	26/85	31	17/43	40	26/43	61	Faber et al. (1989)
C + RT	36	—	—	1/29	3	7/29	24	Yashar et al. (1992)
C + RT	39	5/13	38	0/13	0	8/13	61	Eagan et al. (1987)
C + RT	85	8/35	23	11/32	34	27/32	84	Weiden and Piantadosi (1991)
C + RT	41	13/35	38	12/35	34	12/35	34	Strauss et al. (1992)

C, chemotherapy; RT, radiation therapy.
[a]Patients with both locoregional and systemic recurrence are counted twice.

Table 105-15. Locoregional Non–Small Cell Lung Cancer: Randomized Neoadjuvant Trials

No. of Patients	Treatment	Stage T	Stage N	Survival (%) Median (months)	Survival (%) 2 year	Reference
28	C + S	1–4	0–3	64	60	Roth et al. (1994)
32	S	2–3	0–2	11	25	
30	C + S	1–3	0–2	26	30	Rosell et al. (1994)
30	S	1–3	0–2	8	0	

C, chemotherapy; S, surgery.

ies. Both trials were terminated early when scheduled interim analyses demonstrated a significant survival advantage for combined-modality treatment. Trial results are summarized in Table 105-15.

A problem with accepting the results of the studies by Roth (1994) and Rosell (1994) and colleagues is that the combined-modality and surgery-alone treatment groups may not have been comparable for prognostic factors influencing survival. In the former study, the surgery-alone arm had a higher percentage of patients 60 years of age or older, a smaller percentage of women, and a smaller percentage of patients with clinical stage N_0 or N_1 disease. Except for performance status, other clinical prognostic factors listed in Table 105-1 were not mentioned. In the Rosell study, the treatment groups were unbalanced for K-*ras* oncogene mutation and tumor cell ploidy. The prevalence of mutated K-*ras* oncogenes was 42% and 15% in the surgery and combined-modality treatment groups, respectively. The prevalence of flow cytometry demonstrated aneuploidy was 70% and 29% in the surgery and combined-modality treatment groups, respectively.

Mountain (1995) has reviewed biological lung cancer prognostic factors, including aberrant gene expression, tumor-associated antigens, tumor cell DNA content, growth factors, proliferation markers, basement membrane deposition, and soluble interleukin-2 receptor. Focusing on K-*ras* mutations, Mountain summarizes several studies that demonstrate that the presence of mutation is associated with a worse outcome. In the study by Rosell and colleagues (1994), all 13 patients with the mutation died, whereas seven of 33 patients (21%) who were completely resected and who did not have the mutation survived.

What are the implications of these neoadjuvant results? From one perspective, results are encouraging in that chemotherapy response rates are considerably higher in this patient population than in patients with metastatic disease. In addition, clinical and pathologic complete responses occur, but not necessarily in the same patient. If chemotherapy is sufficiently active to produce complete responses of bulky intrathoracic disease, it presumably should be even more effective against subclinical metastatic disease. If both local-regional and systemic disease is controlled, survival should be prolonged. Depending on the complete response rate, one might see either prolongation of median survival or a tail on the survival curve.

In fact, long-duration survivors have been noted in nearly every combined-modality study report. The question is, who are these long survivors? Are they patients with minimal mediastinal disease, or are patients with bulky, multistation mediastinal disease included in the group? It is evident from the reports of Shields (1990) and by Vansteenkiste (1997) and Goldstraw (1994) and their associates that stage IIIA patients with minimal N_2 disease have 5-year survival rates of 15 to 30% after surgery alone. These results are in the same ballpark as the combined-modality results, which emphasizes the need for future authors of neoadjuvant trials to carefully document the characteristics of long-duration survivors. This means that surgeons must obtain and label lymph nodes from as many mediastinal lymph node stations as possible, as described by Mountain and Dresler (1997), and that pathologists, as discussed by Jett (1997), examine and fully report on each node.

If extent of mediastinal disease determines prognosis it may be necessary to further modify the TNM staging classification, as suggested by Ruckdeschel (1997). The current, revised lung cancer staging system has been described by Mountain (1997) (see Chapter 98).

Before numerous randomized neoadjuvant therapy trials are initiated, however, it is necessary to ask whether there is rationale for this strategy. The fact remains that the majority of responses to neoadjuvant therapy are less than complete. Because no evidence shows that cancers have elastic qualities that enable them to collapse inward during treatment, clonogenic cancer cells likely remain at the periphery of the original tumor mass. If the tumor is unresectable initially, and if the patient does not attain a complete clinical or pathologic response, cancer cells will likely remain at or beyond the margin of resection.

Another question relating to the rationale for neoadjuvant therapy is whether there is urgency to begin treatment of subclinical metastatic disease a month or so earlier than would occur if the patient received adjuvant (postoperative) rather than neoadjuvant therapy. Geddes (1979) reported, on the basis of literature review, that the mean doubling time for squamous cell carcinoma, adenocarcinoma, and undifferentiated bronchial carcinoma was 88, 161, and 86 days, respectively. Friberg and Mattson (1997) confirmed these data. Given these relatively long doubling times, a 1-month delay in the start of chemotherapy would not have a great effect on tumor burden or on the chance of a spontaneous mutation to drug resistance.

A second potential problem of neoadjuvant therapy is increased frequency of surgical complications. Several authors comment that combined-method therapy makes dissection more difficult. In addition, there is an increased risk of pulmonary complications, especially when mitomycin C is part of a combined-method chemotherapy regimen. Bilfinger and Hartman (1991), on the basis of their own experience with two patients and a survey of other institutions, documented that neoadjuvant combined method therapy with mitomycin C–containing drug regimens was associated with acute, fatal, postoperative respiratory insufficiency. Burkes and colleagues (1992) reported similar experience.

SURGICAL ADJUVANT THERAPY

A meta-analysis using updated data in individual patients has been reported by the Non–Small Cell Lung Cancer Collaborative Group (1995). This meta-analysis included five trials using long-duration alkylating agent therapy, eight trials using cisplatin-based chemotherapy, and three trials using noncisplatin drug regimens. The long-term alkylating agent trials all favored the surgery-alone arm. Alkylating agent therapy, primarily cyclophosphamide and lomustine (CCNU), was associated with an absolute detriment of chemotherapy of 4% at 2 years and 5% at 5 years. By contrast, cisplatin-based chemotherapy adjuvant trials generally favored chemotherapy with an absolute benefit of 3% at 2 years and 5% at 5 years. CIs of these values were broad, however, consistent with a 0.5% detriment to a 7% benefit of chemotherapy at 2 years and a 1.0% detriment to a 10% benefit at 5 years.

A possible reason why better results have not been obtained from adjuvant trials is treatment compliance. In a study reported by Holmes and Gail (1986), 15 of the 62 eligible patients assigned to CAP chemotherapy did not receive that treatment. For the entire CAP population, only 58% of protocol-prescribed CAP dosage was actually received. Dose modification for treatment toxicity and discontinuation of therapy because of tumor progression accounted for some of this shortfall, but it did not account for all of it.

Similarly, an adjuvant vindesine-cisplatin trial, in completely resected stage III non–small cell lung cancer, reported by Ohta and associates (1993), called for three cycles of chemotherapy over 3 months. In fact, only 41% of patients received three cycles, with 44% receiving two cycles, and 16% receiving only one cycle.

In contrast to the above studies, the Cancer and Leukemia Group B, as reported by Sugarbaker and associates (1995), conducted a phase II trimodality study for PS 0–1 patients with stage IIIA disease. Study design called for both preoperative and postoperative treatment. Patients received two preoperative cycles of vindesine-cisplatin at higher dose than the Ohta and associates (1993) trial. Postoperatively, they received an additional two cycles of identical chemotherapy

followed by radiation therapy. In this study, 69% of patients undergoing resection completed the full adjuvant therapy, and 95% completed planned irradiation.

SUMMARY

In conclusion, I offer my view of the state of the art of non–small cell lung cancer chemotherapy. It appears that our current drug regimens are sufficiently active to palliate symptoms during the limited life span of most patients with newly diagnosed, disseminated disease and good performance status. Survival benefit from chemotherapy is modest in this group of patients. In patients with less advanced disease, current chemotherapy regimens produce clinically or pathologically complete responses (or both) in a minority of patients. Members of this group, to be defined, may have prolonged survival. For patients presenting with locoregional disease, the two competing approaches are neoadjuvant and adjuvant therapy. Both of these approaches still have major unanswered questions. For neoadjuvant therapy, there is a need to more precisely define the patient population that will benefit from this approach. This definition will require patients to have their mediastinal node status determined either by surgical staging or by newer diagnostic radiology procedures. For surgical adjuvant therapy, there is a need to determine whether chemotherapy and radiation therapy prescriptions can be delivered, in full dose, in the postoperative setting.

Summing up all the studies discussed here and acknowledging the many thousands of patients who have participated in the various trials, it can be stated that all the treatment approaches evaluated to date are feasible. Efficacy is harder to define: Patient populations differ, follow-up is often too short to determine survival accurately, and other efficacy parameters, such as quality of life, are rarely analyzed. Because several new chemotherapy drugs have been identified as active in non–small cell lung cancer, it is likely that several more years will be required to sort out the most active drug combinations. Similar advances in radiation oncology leave the best radiation therapy prescription also in doubt. As these issues are sorted out, properly designed, randomized trials can be initiated to determine efficacy, in broadest terms, and to define subsets of patients that might benefit from specific approaches. This strategy does not preclude simultaneous phase II testing of new drugs and new drug combinations in patients with disseminated disease and a good prognosis. It is hoped that additional active drugs and drug combinations will be discovered.

REFERENCES

Albain KS, et al: Concurrent cisplatin/etoposide plus chest radiotherapy followed by surgery for stages IIIA (N2) and IIIB non-small cell lung cancer: mature results of Southwest Oncology Group phase II study 8805. J Clin Oncol 13:1880, 1995.

Arriagada R: Optimizing chemotherapy and radiotherapy in locally advanced non-small cell lung cancer. Hematol Oncol Clin North Am 11:461, 1997.

Bilfinger TV, Hartman AR: Acute pulmonary failure with neoadjuvant protocol including mitomycin C and surgical therapy [letter]. J Thorac Cardiovasc Surg 102:935, 1991.

Bitran JD, et al: Protochemotherapy in non-small cell lung carcinoma. An attempt to increase surgical resectability and survival. A preliminary report. Cancer 57:44, 1986.

Black WC, Welch HG: Advances in diagnostic imaging and overestimations of disease prevalence and the benefits of therapy. N Engl J Med 328:1237, 1993.

Blanke C, et al: Phase III trial of thoracic irradiation with or without cisplatin for locally advanced unresectable non-small cell lung cancer: a Hoosier Oncology Group protocol. J Clin Oncol 13:1425, 1995.

Bonomi P, et al: Phase II trial of etoposide, cisplatin, continuous infusion 5-fluorouracil, and simultaneous split-course radiation therapy in stage III non-small-cell bronchogenic carcinoma. Semin Oncol 13(Suppl 3):115, 1986.

Bonomi PD, et al: Combination chemotherapy versus single agents followed by combination chemotherapy in stage IV non-small-cell lung cancer. A study of the Eastern Cooperative Oncology Group. J Clin Oncol 7:1602, 1989.

Brunner KW, et al: A controlled study in the use of combined drug therapy for metastatic breast cancer. Cancer 36:1208, 1975.

Buccheri GF, et al: Continuation of chemotherapy versus supportive care alone in patients with inoperable non-small cell lung cancer and stable disease after two or three cycles of MACC. Results of a randomized prospective study. Cancer 63:428, 1989.

Buccheri G, Ferrigno F: Therapeutic options for regionally advanced non-small cell lung cancer. Lung Cancer 14:281, 1996.

Burkes RL, et al: Induction chemotherapy with mitomycin, vindesine and cisplatin for stage III unresectable non-small-cell lung cancer: results of the Toronto phase II trial. J Clin Oncol 10:580, 1992.

Cartei G, et al: Cisplatin-cyclophosphamide-mitomycin combination chemotherapy with supportive care versus supportive care alone for treatment of metastatic non-small cell lung cancer. J Natl Cancer Inst 85:794, 1993.

Cellerino R, et al: A randomized trial of alternating chemotherapy versus best supportive care in advanced non-small-cell lung cancer. J Clin Oncol 9:1453, 1991.

Coates A, et al: Improving the quality of life during chemotherapy for advanced breast cancer. A comparison of intermittent and continuous treatment strategies. N Engl J Med 317:1490, 1987.

Cormier Y, et al: Benefits of polychemotherapy in advanced non-small-cell bronchial carcinoma. Cancer 50:845, 1982.

Crawford J, et al: Randomized trial of vinorelbine compared with fluorouracil plus leukovorin in patients with stage IV non-small cell lung cancer. J Clin Oncol 14:2774, 1996.

Creech RH, et al: Results of a phase II protocol for evaluation of new chemotherapeutic regimens in patients with inoperable non-small cell lung carcinoma (EST-2575, Generation I). Cancer Treat Rep 65:431, 1981.

Dautzenberg B, et al: Failure of perioperative PCV neoadjuvant polychemotherapy in resectable bronchial non-small cell carcinoma. Results of a randomized phase II trial. Cancer 65:2435, 1990.

Davis S, Pandya MR, Rambotti P: Single-agent and combination chemotherapy for extensive non-small cell carcinomas of the lung. Cancer Treat Rep 64:685, 1980.

Dillman RO, et al: A randomized trial of induction chemotherapy plus high-dose radiation versus radiation alone in stage III non-small-cell lung cancer. N Engl J Med 323:940, 1990.

Dillman RO, et al: Improved survival in stage III non-small cell lung cancer: seven-year follow-up of Cancer and Leukemia Group B (CALGB) 8433 trial. J Natl Cancer Inst 88:1210, 1996.

Eagan RT, et al: Pilot study of induction therapy with cyclophosphamide, doxorubicin and cisplatin (CAP) and chest irradiation prior to thoracotomy in initially inoperable stage III M0 non-small cell lung cancer. Cancer Treat Rep 71:895, 1987.

Einhorn LH, et al: Random prospective study of vindesine versus vindesine plus high-dose cisplatin versus vindesine plus cisplatin plus mitomycin C in advanced non-small-cell lung cancer. J Clin Oncol 4:1037, 1986.

Elliott JA, et al: Vindesine and cisplatin combination chemotherapy compared to vindesine as a single agent in the management of non-small cell lung cancer: A randomized study. Eur J Cancer Clin Oncol 20:1025, 1984.

Faber LP, et al: Preoperative chemotherapy and irradiation for stage III non-small cell lung cancer. Ann Thorac Surg 47:669, 1989.

Fatzinger P, et al: The use of serum albumin for further classification of stage III non-oat cell lung cancer and its therapeutic implications. Ann Thorac Surg 37:115, 1984.

Finkelstein DM, Ettinger DS, Ruckdeschel JC: Long term survivors in metastatic non-small-cell lung cancer: an Eastern Cooperative Oncology Group study. J Clin Oncol 4:702, 1986.

Frei E, Canellos GP: Dose: a critical factor in cancer chemotherapy. Am J Med 69:585, 1980.

Friberg S, Mattson S: On the growth rates of human malignant tumors: implications for medical decision making. J Surg Oncol 65:284, 1997.

Fukuoka M, et al: A randomized trial in inoperable non-small cell lung cancer: vindesine and cisplatin versus mitomycin, vindesine and cisplatin versus etoposide and cisplatin alternating with vindesine and and mitomycin. J Clin Oncol 9:606, 1991.

Ganz P, et al: Supportive care versus supportive care and combination chemotherapy in metastatic non-small cell lung cancer. Does chemotherapy make a difference? Cancer 63:1271, 1989.

Geddes DM: The natural history of lung cancer: a review based on rates of tumour growth. Br J Dis Chest 73:1, 1979.

Goldie JH, Coldman AJ: A mathematical model relating drug sensitivity of tumors to their spontaneous mutation rate. Cancer Treat Rep 63:1727, 1979.

Goldstraw P, et al: Surgical management of non-small cell lung cancer with ipsilateral mediastinal node metastasis (N2 disease). J Thorac Cardiovasc Surg 107:19, 1994.

Gomm SA, et al: High dose combination chemotherapy with ifosfamide, cyclophosphamide or cisplatin, mitomycin C and mustine with autologous bone marrow support in advanced non-small cell lung cancer. A phase I/II study. Br J Cancer 63:293, 1991.

Goss GD, Dahrouge S, Lochrin CA: Recent advances in the treatment of non-small cell lung cancer. Anticancer Drugs 7:363, 1996.

Gralla RJ: Preoperative and adjuvant chemotherapy in non-small cell lung cancer. Semin Oncol 15(Suppl 7):8, 1988.

Gralla RJ, et al: Cisplatin and vindesine combination chemotherapy for advanced carcinoma of the lung: a randomized trial investigating two dosage schedules. Ann Intern Med 95:414, 1981.

Green N, Kurohara S, George F: Cancer of the lung. An in-depth analysis of prognostic factors. Cancer 28:1229, 1971.

Gregor A, et al. Radical radiotherapy and chemotherapy in localized non-small cell lung cancer: a randomized trial. J Natl Cancer Inst 85:997, 1993.

Gridelli C, et al: Vinorelbine is well tolerated and active in the treatment of elderly patients with advanced non-small cell lung cancer. A two-stage phase II study. Eur J Cancer 33:392, 1997.

Grilli R, Oxman AD, Julian JA: Chemotherapy for advanced non-small cell lung cancer: how much benefit is enough? J Clin Oncol 11:1866, 1993.

Hardy JR, Noble T, Smith IE: Symptom relief with moderate dose chemotherapy (mitomycin C, vinblastine and cisplatin) in advanced non-small cell lung cancer. Br J Cancer 60:764, 1989.

Herbst RS, Dang NH, Skarin AT: Chemotherapy for advanced non-small cell lung cancer. Hematol Oncol Clin North Am 11:473, 1997.

Holmes EC, Gail M: Surgical adjuvant therapy for stage II and stage III adenocarcinoma and large-cell undifferentiated carcinoma. J Clin Oncol 4:710, 1986.

Jeremic B, et al: Randomized trial of hyperfractionated radiation therapy with or without concurrent chemotherapy for stage III non-small cell lung cancer. J Clin Oncol 13:452, 1995.

Jett JR: What's new in staging of lung cancer. Chest 111:1486, 1997.

Johnson DH, et al: Thoracic radiotherapy does not prolong survival in patients with locally advanced, unresectable non-small cell lung cancer. Ann Intern Med 113:33, 1990.

Johnson DH, et al: Paclitaxel plus carboplatin in advanced non-small cell lung cancer: a phase II trial. J Clin Oncol 14:2054, 1996.

Kaasa S, et al: Symptomatic treatment versus combination chemotherapy for patients with extensive non-small cell lung cancer. Cancer 67:2443, 1991.

Kawahara M, et al: A randomized study of cisplatin versus cisplatin plus vindesine for non-small cell lung carcinoma. Cancer 68:714, 1991.

Klastersky J, et al: Cisplatin versus cisplatin plus etoposide in the treatment of advanced non-small-cell lung cancer. J Clin Oncol 7:1087, 1989.

Lad TE, et al: Immediate versus postponed combination chemotherapy

(CAMP) for unresectable non-small cell lung cancer: A randomized trial. Cancer Treat Rep 65:973, 1981.

Lad T, Rubinstein L, Sadeghi A: The benefit of adjuvant treatment for resected locally advanced non small-cell lung cancer. J Clin Oncol 6:9, 1988.

Langer CJ, et al: Paclitaxel and carboplatin in combination in the treatment of advanced non-small cell lung cancer: a phase II toxicity, response, and survival analysis. J Clin Oncol 13:1860, 1995.

Langer CJ, Rosvold E: Newer aspects in the diagnosis, treatment, and prevention of non-small cell lung cancer. Part II. Curr Probl Cancer 20: 221, 1996.

Le Chevalier T, et al: Radiotherapy alone versus combined chemotherapy and radiotherapy in nonresectable non-small-cell lung cancer: first analysis of a randomized trial in 353 patients. J Natl Cancer Inst 83:417, 1991.

Le Chevalier T, et al: Randomized study of vinorelbine and cisplatin versus vindesine and cisplatin versus vinorelbine alone in advanced non-small cell lung cancer: results of a European multicenter trial including 612 patients. J Clin Oncol 12:360, 1994.

Lieschke GJ, Burgess AW: Granulocyte colony-stimulating factor and granulocyte-macrophage colony-stimulating factor. N Engl J Med 327:28, 99, 1992.

Livingston RB, et al: Comparative trial of combination chemotherapy in extensive squamous carcinoma of the lung: a Southwest Oncology Group study. Cancer Treat Rep 61:1623, 1977.

Luedke DW, et al: Randomized comparison of two combination regimens versus minimal chemotherapy in non-small cell lung cancer: a Southeastern Cancer Study Group trial. J Clin Oncol 8:886, 1990.

Marino P, et al: Chemotherapy vs supportive care in advanced non-small cell lung cancer. Results of a meta-analysis of the literature. Chest 106:861, 1994.

Martini N, et al: Results of resection in non-oat cell carcinoma of the lung with mediastinal lymph node metastases. Ann Surg 198:386, 1983.

Martini N, et al: The effects of preoperative chemotherapy in the resectability of non-small cell lung carcinoma with mediastinal lymph node metastases (N2M0). Ann Thorac Surg 45:371, 1988.

Mattson K, et al: Inoperable non-small cell lung cancer: radiation with and without chemotherapy. Eur J Cancer Clin Oncol 24:477, 1988.

Miller TP, et al: Extensive adenocarcinoma and large cell undifferentiated carcinoma of the lung treated with 5-FU, vindesine and mitomycin (FEMi): a Southwest Oncology Group study. Cancer Treat Rep 66:563, 1982.

Miller TP, et al: Effect of alternating combination chemotherapy on survival of ambulatory patients with metastatic large cell and adenocarcinoma of the lung. A Southwest Oncology Group study. J Clin Oncol 4:502, 1986.

Morton RF, et al: Thoracic radiation therapy alone compared with combined chemoradiotherapy for locally unresectable non-small cell lung cancer. A randomized, phase III trial. Ann Intern Med 115:681, 1991.

Mountain CF: New prognostic factors in lung cancer. Biologic prophets of cancer cell aggression. Chest 108:246, 1995.

Mountain CF. Revisions in the international system for staging lung cancer. Chest 111:1710, 1997.

Mountain CF, Dresler CM: Regional lymph node classification for lung cancer staging. Chest 111:1718, 1997.

Muers MF, et al: Prognosis in lung cancer: physicians' opinions compared with outcome and a predictive model. Thorax 51:894, 1996.

Natale RB: Overview of current and future chemotherapeutic agents in non-small cell lung cancer. Semin Oncol 24(Suppl 7):S7-29, 1997.

Niell HB, et al: Combination versus sequential single-agent chemotherapy in the treatment of patients with advanced non-small cell lung cancer. Med Pediatr Oncol 17:69, 1989.

Non–small Cell Lung Cancer Collaborative Group: Chemotherapy in non-small cell lung cancer: a meta-analysis using updated data on individual patients from 52 randomized clinical trials. BMJ 311:899, 1995.

O'Connell JP, et al: Frequency and prognostic importance of pretreatment clinical characteristics in patients with advanced non-small-cell lung cancer treated with combination chemotherapy. J Clin Oncol 4:1604, 1986.

Ohta M, et al: Adjuvant chemotherapy for completely resected stage III non-small-cell lung cancer. Results of a randomized prospective study. J Thorac Cardiovasc Surg 106:703, 1993.

Paesmans M, et al: Prognostic factors for survival in advanced non-small cell lung cancer: univariate and multivariate analyses including recur-

sive partitioning and amalgamation algorithms in 1,052 patients. J Clin Oncol 13:1221, 1995.

Palomares MR, et al: Gender influence on weight loss pattern and survival of non-small cell lung carcinoma patients. Cancer 789:2119, 1996.

Pass HI, et al: Randomized trial of neoadjuvant therapy for lung cancer: interim analysis. Ann Thorac Surg 53:992, 1992.

Pritchard RS, Anthony SP: Chemotherapy plus radiotherapy compared with radiotherapy alone in the treatment of locally advanced, unresectable non-small-cell lung cancer. A meta-analysis. Ann Intern Med 125:723, 1996.

Ramanthan RK, Belani CP: Chemotherapy for advanced non-small cell lung cancer: past, present, and future. Semin Oncol 24:440, 1997.

Rapp E, et al: Chemotherapy can prolong survival of patients with advanced non-small-cell lung cancer—report of a Canadian multicenter randomized trial. J Clin Oncol 6:663, 1988.

Raut Y, et al: Surgery and chemotherapy. A new method of treatment for squamous cell bronchial carcinoma. J Thorac Cardiovasc Surg 88:754, 1984.

Rosell R, et al: A randomized trial comparing preoperative chemotherapy plus surgery with surgery alone in patients with non-small-cell lung cancer. N Engl J Med 330:153, 1994.

Rosso R, et al: Etoposide versus etoposide plus high-dose cisplatin in the management of advanced non-small-cell lung cancer. Results of a prospective randomized FONICAP trial. Cancer 66:130, 1990.

Roth JA, et al: A randomized trial comparing perioperative chemotherapy and surgery with surgery alone in resectable stage IIIA non-small-cell lung cancer. J Natl Cancer Inst 86:673, 1994.

Ruckdeschel JC, et al: Chemotherapy for inoperable, non-small cell bronchial carcinoma: EST 2575, Generation II. Cancer Treat Rep 65:965, 1981a.

Ruckdeschel JC, et al: Chemotherapy for metastatic, non-small cell bronchial carcinoma: EST 2575, Generation III, HAM versus CAMP. Cancer Treat Rep 65:959, 1981b.

Ruckdeschel JC, et al: Chemotherapy for metastatic, non-small cell bronchial carcinoma: Cyclophosphamide, doxorubicin and etoposide versus mitomycin and vinblastine: EST 2575, Generation IV. Cancer Treat Rep 68:1325, 1984.

Ruckdeschel JC, et al: Chemotherapy for metastatic, non-small cell bronchial carcinoma: EST 2575, Generation V, a randomized comparison of four cisplatin-containing regimens. J Clin Oncol 3:72, 1985.

Ruckdeschel JC, et al: A randomized trial of the four most active regimens for metastatic non-small cell lung cancer. J Clin Oncol 4:414, 1986.

Ruckdeschel JC: Combined modality therapy of non-small cell lung cancer. Semin Oncol 24:429, 1997.

Sause WT, et al: Radiation Therapy Oncology Group (RTOG) 88-08 and Eastern Cooperative Oncology Group (ECOG) 4588: preliminary results of a Phase III trial in regionally advanced, unresectable non-small-cell lung cancer. J Natl Cancer Inst 87:198, 1995.

Schaake-Koning C, et al: Effects of concomitant cisplatin and radiotherapy on inoperable non-small-cell lung cancer. N Engl J Med 326:524, 1992.

Shields TW: The significance of ipsilateral mediastinal lymph node metastasis (N2 disease) in non-small cell carcinoma of the lung. A commentary. J Thorac Cardiovasc Surg 99:48, 1990.

Simes RJ: Risk-benefit relationships in cancer clinical trials: The ECOG experience in non-small-cell lung cancer. J Clin Oncol 3:462, 1985.

Soresi E, et al: A randomized clinical trial comparing radiation therapy vs radiation therapy plus cis-dichloramine platinum (II) in the treatment of locally advanced non-small cell lung cancer. Semin Oncol 15(Suppl 7):20, 1988.

Souquet PJ, et al: Polychemotherapy in advanced non small cell lung cancer: a meta-analysis. Lancet 342:19, 1993.

Stanley KE: Prognostic factors for survival in patients with inoperable lung cancer. J Natl Cancer Inst 65:25, 1980.

Strauss GM, et al: Neoadjuvant chemotherapy and radiotherapy followed by surgery in stage IIIA non-small-cell carcinoma of the lung: report of a Cancer and Leukemia Group B phase II study. J Clin Oncol 10:1237, 1992.

Sugarbaker DJ, et al: Results of Cancer and Leukemia Group B protocol 8935. A multiinstitutional phase II trimodality trial for stage IIIA (N2) non-small-cell lung cancer. J Thorac Cardiovasc Surg 109:473, 1995.

Takigawa N, et al: Prognostic factors for patients with advanced non-small cell lung cancer: univariate and multivariate analyses including recursive partitioning and amalgamation. Lung Cancer 15:67, 1996.

Tannock I, et al: A randomized trial of two dose levels of cyclophosphamide, methotrexate and fluorouracil chemotherapy for patients with metastatic breast cancer. J Clin Oncol 6:1377, 1988.

Taylor SG IV, et al: Simultaneous cisplatin, fluorouracil infusion and radiation followed by surgical resection in regionally localized stage III, non-small cell lung cancer. Ann Thorac Surg 43:87, 1987.

Thatcher N, et al: Symptomatic benefit from gemcitabine and other chemotherapy in advanced non-small cell lung cancer: changes in performance status and tumour related symptoms. Anticancer Drugs 6(Suppl 6):39, 1995.

Tormey DC, et al: Comparison of induction chemotherapies for metastatic breast cancer. An Eastern Cooperative Oncology Group trial. Cancer 50:1235, 1982.

Tranum BL, et al: Adriamycin combinations in advanced breast cancer. A Southwest Oncology Group study. Cancer 49:835, 1982.

Trovo MG, et al: Combined radiotherapy and chemotherapy versus radiotherapy alone in locally advanced epidermoid bronchial carcinoma. Cancer 65:400, 1990.

Vansteenkiste JF, et al: Survival and prognostic factors in resected N2 non-small cell lung cancer. A study of 140 cases. Ann Thorac Surg 63:1441, 1997.

Vokes EE, Green MR: Clinical studies in non-small cell lung cancer: the CALGB experience. Cancer Invest 16:72, 1998.

Weick JK, et al: A randomized trial of five cisplatin-containing treatments in patients with metastatic non-small cell lung cancer: A Southwest Oncology Group study. J Clin Oncol 9:1157, 1991.

Weiden PL, Piantadosi S: Preoperative chemotherapy (cisplatin and fluorouracil) and radiation therapy in stage III non-small cell lung cancer: A phase II study of the Lung Cancer Study Group. J Natl Cancer Inst 83:266, 1991.

Williams SF, et al: High-dose, multiple-alkylator chemotherapy with autologous bone marrow reinfusion in patients with advanced non-small cell lung cancer. Cancer 63:238, 1989.

Woods RL, et al: A randomized trial of cisplatin and vindesine versus supportive care only in advanced non-small cell lung cancer. Br J Cancer 61:608, 1990.

Yashar J, et al: Preoperative chemotherapy and radiation therapy for stage IIIa carcinoma of the lung. Ann Thorac Surg 53:440, 1992.

Wozniak AJ, et al. Randomized phase III trial of cisplatin vs CDDP plus Navelbine in treatment of advanced non-small cell lung cancer: an update of Southwest Oncology Group study (SWOG-9308). Proc ASCO 17:453a, 1998.

Zelen M: Keynote address on biostatistics and data retrieval. Cancer Chemother Rep 4:31, 1973.

CHAPTER 106

Multimodality Therapy for Non–Small Cell Lung Cancer

Sunil Singhal and Larry R. Kaiser

Historically, management of non–small cell lung cancer (NSCLC) has been the center of debate. Experience has demonstrated that the only curative treatment is surgical resection for early and localized disease. However, fewer than 15% of all NSCLC patients are candidates for surgical resection. Extrathoracic recurrence has continued to be a significant problem. Autopsy studies by Martini and Flehinger (1987), as well as Gail (1984), Matthews (1973), and Feld (1984) and their colleagues have shown that more than one-half of first recurrences tend to be systemic. Feld and associates (1984) reported 43 recurrences in 162 patients with T_1N_0 lesions, 65% of which were extrathoracic sites. Fifty-nine of the 81 recurrences in 196 patients with T_2N_0 disease were extrathoracic. Clearly, other methods of therapy in addition to surgical resection should be considered. Adjuvant and neoadjuvant therapy has the potential to improve the overall management for NSCLC. Staging techniques have matured so that fewer patients with inoperable disease are subjected to operation. Adjuvant and neoadjuvant therapies have in many cases permitted patients who previously were considered nonsurgical candidates to be considered for resection.

INDICATIONS FOR MULTIMODALITY TREATMENT

Stages I and II NSCLC have traditionally been managed by operation alone. Complete surgical resection, as noted by Mountain (1983), still carries the best chance of long-term survival and cure for NSCLC if the tumor is confined to the chest. According to Vansteenkiste and colleagues (1997) and others, the 5-year survival rate for clinical stages I and II ranges from 50 to 80%. The role of postoperative adjuvant therapy for stage II (N_1) disease is controversial but has been recommended by Sawyer (1997b) and Bunn (1994) and their coworkers, as well as by Mountain (1986) because of

the 50% failure rate with surgery alone. A locoregional intrathoracic failure rate of 31% was observed by the Ludwig Lung Cancer Group (1987) for completely resected stage II patients. For medically inoperable cases, stage I and II tumors also are potentially curable with radiation therapy alone. For such patients, radiation therapy yields an average 5-year survival rate of 15 to 20% and local control rate that usually is less than satisfactory as noted by Jeremic (1997), Graham (1995), and Slotman (1994) and their colleagues.

Stage IV metastatic disease traditionally has been managed by supportive care alone, chemotherapy, or radiation therapy alone as reported by the American Society of Clinical Oncology (1997) and Livingston (1994), as well as by Flaherty (1991) and Johnson (1990) and their associates. Median survival is approximately 4 months, with essentially no 5-year survivors, as pointed out by Dosoretz and coworkers (1993). In 1997, the American Society of Clinical Oncology adopted practical clinical guidelines for the treatment of unresectable NSCLC. It was recommended that chemotherapy, ideally a platinum-based regimen, should be administered for no more than eight cycles. Definitive dose thoracic irradiation should be no less than 60 Gy in 1.8- to 2.0-Gy fractions. In patients with controlled disease except for isolated cerebral metastases in an unresectable area, the American Society of Clinical Oncology (1997) believes that resection followed by radiation therapy is superior to radiation therapy alone. New evidence will be evaluated by annual updates of these guidelines.

Although surgery is the treatment of choice for stage I and II disease, and surgery can offer little for stage IV disease, considerable controversy exists regarding the appropriate management of locally advanced NSCLC [stage III as discussed by Lee and Ginsberg (1997) and Lilenbaum and Green (1994)]. The former international staging system created by a collaboration of the American Joint Committee on Cancer Staging and International Union Against Cancer as reported by Mountain (1986) divided stage III lung cancer into two distinct groups. Stage IIIA comprises those lesions that are potentially resectable and includes any N_2 disease, any T_3 primary tumors, or both. Stage IIIB designates those patients with disease that involves structures that usually preclude resection. These include T_4 primary tumor and N_3 nodal disease. The international staging system published in 1997 by Mountain has changed the categories in IIIA disease (see Chapter 98), but almost all of the studies to be quoted in this chapter have used the former international staging system and this system, albeit outdated, is used throughout this chapter. Certain patients with stage IIIB disease may be amenable to resection, especially with the advent of multimodality therapy. According to Bulzebruck and coworkers (1992), approximately 20% of patients with NSCLC present with stage IIIA disease at diagnosis, and another 20% are stage IIIB at presentation. The overall median and 5-year survival for stage IIIA disease is 12 months and 15 to 20%, respectively, and for stage IIIB, 8 months and 0 to 5% as documented by Saijo (1998), Yoshino and associates (1997), and Albain (1993). Now that a precise surgical staging system has been in place since 1986, adjuvant and neoadjuvant therapies can be more critically compared, as suggested by Bonomi (1993).

Patients with T_3N_0 disease, usually those with chest wall invasion, are considered stage IIb in the revised classification published by Mountain (1997) because their survival is significantly better than patients who present with N_2 disease. Martini and Flehinger (1987) reported that 5-year survival in this group approximates 60%.

Management of N_2 disease continues to be controversial as noted in the aforementioned report of Lee and Ginsberg (1997) and those of Brundage and Mackillop (1996) and Strauss and colleagues (1992a, 1992b). Until recently, patients who presented with involved mediastinal lymph nodes were considered inoperable and usually were treated with radiation therapy alone. This treatment nihilism evolved from the recognition that many of these patients, if explored, were found to be unresectable because of the bulky disease, and even if resected, the long-term outlook was poor. However, Mirimanoff (1994) and Damstrup and Poulsen (1994) note that radiation therapy has a modest, but definitive curative potential, with a 1-, 2-, and 5-year survival of approximately 40%, 20%, and 5%, respectively, and median survival of 9 to 12 months. Collective results of operation alone for N_2 disease demonstrate 5-year survival rates ranging from 14 to 30% as recorded by Ginsberg (1993) and van Klaveren and coworkers (1993). Even in patients thought to have N_0 disease after preoperative staging, including mediastinoscopy, Goldstraw and associates (1994) noted that up to 25% may have N_2 disease identified at the time of thoracotomy when mediastinal lymph nodes are sampled. Any chance at long-term survival in patients found to have N_2 disease at the time of thoracotomy according to Nakanishi and colleagues (1997) is dependent on achieving a complete resection. Some, including Vansteenkiste and associates (1997), argue resection should be limited only to cases of minimal N_2 disease, and

Shields (1990) has presented a detailed discussion of the significance of N_2 disease in NSCLC.

Using mediastinoscopy, mediastinal lymph node involvement may be detected before thoracotomy, allowing the patient to be treated with combination therapy in a protocol setting. In general, single modality therapy produces modest results, at best, when used for patients with locally advanced disease, in particular, N_2 disease. The recognition of this prompted numerous investigators to look at combination therapy in the hope of improving resectability rate and survival. Especially in patients with bulky N_2 disease, the idea of reducing the tumor burden before attempting resection was particularly appealing, recognizing the low resectability rate of these patients when subjected to operation alone. Patients with N_2 disease are at significant risk for developing disseminated disease, and it is likely that many of them have metastatic disease at the time of presentation, although it cannot be detected because of the limitations in the resolution of currently available imaging modalities. It is attractive to think that chemotherapy given up front might be more effective in reducing this micrometastatic tumor burden and thus lead to long-term survival. One should look carefully at the studies of combined modality therapy, particularly because no rigorous definition of *unresectable* or *marginally resectable* exists, terms often used to describe patients entered onto a clinical trial. Failure to specify performance status before therapy also may limit the ability to interpret the result of a clinical trial. A number of trials, especially ones in which surgery was not involved, failed to establish histologic evidence of N_2 disease and assumed staging based on the appearance on computed tomographic scan. These trials clearly are flawed by this lack of precise histologic staging. A patient who is assumed to have N_2 disease but who actually has N_0 disease obviously will do well, and several of these patients can alter significantly the results of a clinical trial.

Surgery may either follow an induction regimen (e.g., chemotherapy or combined chemoradiation therapy); precede chemotherapy, irradiation, or both; or be sandwiched between some combination of chemotherapy and radiation therapy. Many of these trials involved patients with bulky N_2 disease but also included other patients with locally advanced disease such as those involving chest wall (T_3) or locally invading the mediastinum. Including patients with T_3N_0 chest wall disease would tend to improve overall survival in a trial because these patients, as a rule, have a better long-term outlook than patients with N_2 disease, and these now are staged as IIb. Other trials included patients with stage IIIB disease (T_4 primary tumor, contralateral mediastinal lymph nodes). As noted by Macchiarini and associates (1991), not all trials included rigorous staging of the mediastinum in the form of a mediastinal lymph node dissection.

A variety of therapeutic modalities have been compiled in review articles. One review by Brundage and Mackillop (1996) examined 441 phase II studies and 108 phase III reports that enrolled stage III patients between 1966 and

1993. Review of the literature demonstrated significant diversity in research practices. Analysis of trials for stage III management found five major types of variation between studies: 1) selection of control arms, 2) selection of study investigational arms, 3) choice of eligibility criteria, 4) outcomes measures selected for study, and 5) magnitude of benefit sought in the primary outcome measure. This diversity of research studies has made it increasingly difficult to definitively decide what is the best treatment option.

As studies are reviewed, what parameters are truly reflective of clinical benefit to the patients should be considered. Median survival is not a particularly useful indicator. The aim as clinicians is to increase the number of long-term survivors. Also, another parameter to consider is response to induction therapy and adjuvant therapy. Grading of response, according to Milano and colleagues (1996), is a valid parameter to evaluate standard regimens and novel drug associations.

ADJUVANT THERAPY

Adjuvant therapy refers to postoperative treatment, usually specific for chemotherapy, radiation therapy, immunotherapy, or some combination of these. Distant metastatic disease is the dominant form of relapse after surgical resection. Adjuvant therapy is aimed at those patients deemed to be at increased risk of local or distant relapse after surgical resection.

Adjuvant therapy was first used in the 1970s. Physicians were optimistic that cure was forthcoming because adjuvant therapy was able to stop NSCLC recurrences in animal models. Until the mid-1980s, however, analysis of various adjuvant therapies was difficult because of the differences in staging across various trials. In the early 1980s, with the advent of computed tomography and advances in imaging techniques, patients were more accurately classified, treated, and results recorded. Since then, initial optimism has been tempered by the demonstration of only modest improvement in survival rates, as discussed by Turrisi (1992). Currently,

no convincing evidence exists that patients who have undergone complete surgical resection benefit from postoperative treatment [i.e., currently no postoperative adjuvant therapy regimen exists that has been shown to prolong survival as noted by Livingston (1997) and Johnson (1997) and their coworkers].

The first advance in structured adjuvant therapy came in the late 1970s and early 1980s. McKneally and colleagues (1976a, 1976b) compared a randomized group of 39 patients with stage I NSCLC who received 107 viable units of the Tice strain of bacillus Calmette-Guérin (BCG) to no further treatment. BCG treatment prolonged survival and time to recurrence in these patients. McKneally and associates (1981) in a 4-year follow-up reported that the recurrence rate in the control population was high, 62% at 3 years, whereas the recurrence rate was 33% at 3 years in the BCG-treated group. The National Institutes of Health funded a consortium of institutions, the Lung Cancer Study Group (LCSG), to verify the results of this trial and to investigate other treatment modalities in separate trials. The LCSG was a collaboration of thoracic surgeons, medical and radiation oncologists, and pathologists who conducted clinical trials based on rigid standards of staging and follow-up as outlined by Holmes (1994b) and Lad (1990). This group routinely and systematically required assessment of mediastinal lymph nodes and helped establish the revised international staging system for NSCLC. During the 12 years of its existence, before being disbanded in 1989, the LCSG focused its attention on those patients who had disease localized to the thorax that was potentially resectable as reported by Lad (1990) and Holmes (1992). This group made significant advances in the multimodality management of NSCLC, eventually completing nine studies before being disbanded (Table 106-1).

The first trial started by this group, LCSG 771, was a randomized double-blind comparison of postoperative intrapleural BCG with isoniazid versus saline solution with isoniazid. Between 1977 and 1980, 473 patients were enrolled and followed until 1990 as reported by Feld (1984) and Gail (1984) and their colleagues. No evidence

Table 106-1. Lung Cancer Study Group (LCSG) Multimodality Trials for Non–Small Cell Lung Cancer (NSCLC)

LCSG	Phase	Study	Reference
771	III	Adjuvant immunotherapy with bacillus Calmette-Guérin in patients with stage I disease	Mountain (1983); Gail (1994)
772	III	Adjuvant CAP chemotherapy in patients with stage II/III nonsquamous disease	Holmes (1986)
773	III	Adjuvant thoracic radiation therapy in patients with stage II/III squamous disease	Weisenburger (1994)
791	III	Adjuvant CAP chemotherapy/radiation therapy in stage IIIA NSCLC	Lad et al. (1988)
801	III	Adjuvant chemotherapy with CAP in patients with completely resected stage I NSCLC	Feld et al. (1993, 1994)
831	II	Neoadjuvant CAP and radiation therapy in patients before thoracotomy in initially inoperable stage III disease	Eagan et al. (1987)
852	II	Neoadjuvant cisplatin, 5-fluorouracil, and radiation therapy in stage III NSCLC	Weiden and Piantadosi (1991, 1994)
853	III	Immediate versus delayed adjuvant CAP for stage II/III NSCLC	Figlin and Piantadosi (1994)
881	II	Neoadjuvant mitomycin C, vindesine or vinblastine, and cisplatin versus radiation therapy for stage III NSCLC	Wagner et al. (1994)

CAP, cyclophosphamide, doxorubicin, and cisplatin.

existed of improved survival or time to recurrence among patients given BCG in the group's report published by Gail (1994). The only differences between McKneally and associates' (1976a) study and the LCSG 771 was the LCSG required lymph node biopsies for pathologic staging, injecting intrapleural saline solution in the control group, and using isoniazid placebo instead of isoniazid in the control group beginning 14 days after instillation. Review of the data surrounding these two studies demonstrates that positive results, ultimately found to be caused by chance, are not uncommon in small preliminary studies, further underscoring the need for larger confirmatory trials. This experience convincingly demonstrated to investigators the importance of rigid, well-conducted clinical trials. Over the years since this trial, a number of adjuvant chemotherapy and radiation therapy regimens have been attempted. Many of these trials are summarized subsequently to provide an historical perspective. Currently, according to Johnson and coinvestigators (1997), at least seven adjuvant trials are ongoing worldwide, some of which are nearing their accrual goals.

Adjuvant Radiation Therapy

As noted by Curran (1995), since the 1960s postoperative irradiation often has been used in the management of NSCLC (Table 106-2). It has been well demonstrated that radiation therapy is capable of sterilizing carcinoma of the lung at the primary site and the regional lymph nodes when the radiation dose is significantly high (i.e., 50 to 64 Gy). However, no definitive study has demonstrated any correlation with improved survival. Theoretically, postoperative radiation therapy should be beneficial. Whereas surgery fails at the margins of disease, radiation therapy fails centrally where hypoxic conditions exist. Some studies, such as those of Israel (1978), Van Houtte (1980), Choi (1990), and Bleehen (1994) and their coworkers, have been able to show there is a dose-response relationship. However, pulmonary

tolerance to adjuvant radiation therapy continues to be a major concern.

One of the earliest studies came from San Diego Naval Hospital. Investigators reported a total of 219 patients with proven lung cancer. There were 66 patients with positive nodes who were treated with a radiation dose of 30 to 60 Gy radiation after surgery. Green and Kern (1978) and Green and associates (1975) reported the 5-year survival of these patients approximated 35%; in contrast, only 3% of 30 patients treated with surgery alone survived for 5 years.

The European Organization for Research and Treatment of Cancer (EORTC) conducted two prospective trials of postoperative radiation therapy. In the first trial, 230 of 392 patients with squamous cell carcinoma were evaluated, 88 of whom had regional lymph node metastases. Israel and coworkers (1978) reported the 3-year tumor-free survival rate was 70% in 104 patients given postresection radiation therapy compared with 50% in 126 treated with resection without postoperative irradiation. This result must be treated with caution because of the large and unbalanced numbers of patients excluded.

In the second EORTC trial, Van Houtte and colleagues (1980) in Brussels, Belgium, studied 224 patients without lymph node involvement (T_1, T_2, or T_3 for main stem bronchus involvement) and with complete resection of tumor. This trial included 14 patients with small cell lung cancer and two with pulmonary sarcoma. A postoperative radiation dose of 60 Gy in 6 weeks decreased the number of locoregional recurrences within the treatment field from 13% to 8%. In an analysis of 175 of 224 patients randomized with no intraoperative evidence of lymph node metastases, survival was better in the nonirradiated group. The 5-year survival rate was 45% in this group as opposed to 24% in the irradiated group. Although the survival difference was not statistically significant, the results suggested that adjuvant mediastinal radiation therapy may be harmful in patients with N_0 or N_1 disease.

In 1986, the LCSG reported on 230 completely resected patients with stage II and III squamous cell lung carcinoma

Table 106-2. Adjuvant Radiation Therapy

Group	N	Stage	Postoperative Radiation Dose	Survival Benefit	Reference
San Diego Naval Hospital	66	N_2	30–60 Gy	5-year survival (35%)	Green et al. (1975)
EORTC 08741	230	N_0,N_1,N_2	45–55 Gy	3-year survival (70%)	Israel et al. (1978)
EORTC	75	N_0	60 Gy	5-year survival (20%)	Van Houtte et al. (1980)
LCSG 773	110	II,III	50 Gy	5-year survival (38%)	Weisenburger (1994)
LCSG 791	83	IIIA	40 Gy	1-year survival (54%)	Lad et al. (1988)
British Medical Research Council	154	N_1,N_2	40 Gy	5-year survival (6%)	Bleehen et al. (1994)
Memorial Sloan-Kettering	318	III	30–40 Gy	5-year survival (22%)	Hilaris et al. (1985)
University of Michigan	110	N_2	50–60 Gy	5-year survival (26%)	Kirsh and Sloan (1982)
Barcelona, Spain	86	IIIA	45–50 Gy	5-year survival (19%)	Astudillo and Conill (1990)
Mayo Clinic	88	N_2	45–55 Gy	4-year survival (43%)	Sawyer et al. (1997a,b)
Washington University, St. Louis	173	I,II,III	50–60 Gy	5-year survival (22%)	Emami et al. (1997)
Graz Medical School, Austria	83	I,II,III	50–56 Gy	5-year survival (30%)	Mayer et al. (1997)

EORTC, European Organization for Research and Treatment of Cancer; LCSG, Lung Cancer Study Group.

treated between 1978 and 1985 (LCSG 773). No patients with adenocarcinoma were included. A dose of 50 Gy was delivered over 5 weeks to 110 randomized patients. The locoregional failure rate was reduced from 41% to 3% with irradiation for all node-positive patients. In the control (no treatment) group ($n = 108$), 21 (19%) developed a first recurrence at a local site. Conversely, the radiation therapy group ($n = 102$) had only one (1%) local recurrence as the first site of disease ($P <.001$). However, as noted by Weisenburger (1994), the increase in locoregional control with irradiation did not translate into a survival benefit for stage II patients because more than two-thirds of the failures were secondary to distant metastasis. The LCSG did not separate patients with N_1 and N_2 disease. Instead, they reported them as a single group.

This study has been criticized by radiation oncologists such as Choi (1991) for using a radiation dose that many thought was too low. The study also did not contain a sufficient number of patients with mediastinal lymph node disease (N_2) to detect a survival difference with any power. It has also been suggested by Cox (1991) and Choi (1991) that only 76% of the patients received within 5% of the dose, and the study included 12 control patients who received radiation therapy after having local recurrence without distant metastases. However, follow-up subset analysis of the survival of those patients who received within 5% of the protocol dose compared with those control patients who did not receive initial or delayed radiation therapy revealed no significant benefit in survival. The data generated by the LCSG 773, as noted by Weisenburger (1994), indicated that postoperative irradiation significantly reduced local recurrence in patients with resected squamous cell carcinoma, but that benefit did not result in increased survival in the population studied because of the large percentage of patients who had recurrences outside the locoregional area. A similar trial, as documented by Curran (1995), was conducted by the EORTC (EORTC 08861) and was closed with incomplete accrual in 1992.

Bleehen and associates (1994) on behalf of the British Medical Research Council reported on 308 patients with T_{1-2}, N_{1-2} NSCLC. A dose of 40 Gy was delivered in 3 weeks to 308 patients. One hundred thirty-six patients received their complete course of postoperative irradiation. The median survival was 19 months in the surgery alone group versus 17.5 months in the surgery and radiation therapy arm. The 1-, 3-, and 5-year survival was 68%, 16%, and 5% for surgery only arm versus 61%, 21%, and 6% for the combined modality group, respectively. Stephens and colleagues (1996) concluded that this trial did not provide any convincing evidence that postoperative radiation therapy affects survival, local recurrence, or development of metastases.

The randomized trials have consistently demonstrated decreased locoregional recurrence; however, this has not translated to any significant survival advantage. Other trials have demonstrated some added advantage of irradiation in selected subsets of patients. In patients with advanced disease (T_3 or N_{1-3}), radiation therapy may help control local relapse.

Kirsh and Sloan (1982) reported that at the University of Michigan, mediastinal lymph node dissection in conjunction with pulmonary resection was performed on 690 patients with bronchial carcinoma from 1959 through 1975. One hundred thirty-six of these patients had mediastinal lymph node metastases found at resection. One hundred ten patients who survived operation were treated with 50 to 60 Gy of postoperative irradiation. Of the patients who underwent irradiation, 18 of the 50 patients (36%) with squamous cell carcinoma survived 5 years, whereas only 7 of 55 (13%) with adenocarcinoma survived 5 years. In addition to demonstrating better local control by radiation therapy, this study suggested that histologic cell type in patients with mediastinal metastases is an important factor in prognosis. These investigators also postulated a relationship between prognosis and the level of mediastinal lymph node metastases, with patients with subcarinal disease (level VII) having a poorer outcome than those with metastases to the paratracheal area. Patients with superior mediastinal lymph node involvement had a 33% 5-year survival; with subcarinal involvement there was only a 16% 5-year survival. These results remain controversial.

From 1977 to 1980 at Memorial Sloan-Kettering Cancer Center, Hilaris and associates (1985) reported on 318 patients with stage III disease who underwent thoracotomy. After resection, all patients received external beam irradiation consisting of 30 to 40 Gy given over 2 to 4 weeks. One hundred of these patients were treated with intraoperative brachytherapy, the criteria for this being either the presence of residual gross disease or close resection margins. The local control in those patients with gross residual disease treated with brachytherapy and postoperative external beam irradiation was 72%. The overall 5-year survival was 22%. The 5-year survival was better in patients who had all gross disease removed compared with patients who had gross residual disease (30% versus 13%). The disease-free survival in these two groups was 27% and 12%, respectively.

At the Radiation Oncology Center at Washington University, St. Louis, Emami and colleagues (1987) reported on 173 patients with stage I, II, and III NSCLC who were treated with surgery and postoperative radiation therapy between 1974 and 1989. All patients were retrospectively reviewed and restaged according to the 1986 American Joint Committee staging classification. All patients were treated with a continuous course of radiation therapy with conventional fractionation of 180 to 200 cGy/day, the average receiving between 50 and 60 Gy over the course of their therapy. Seventy-four patients were stage IIIA and two were stage IIIB. Locoregional control for stages I, II, and IIIA was 85%, 75%, and 85%, respectively. Five-year actuarial survival was 35% for stage I and 20% for stage II and IIIA. In a follow-up report, Emami and associates (1997) noted that patients with N_0 disease had 5-year survival of 25%, whereas patients with N_1 and N_2 disease had 5-year survival of 20%. Although the authors did not demonstrate a survival advantage with this treatment, they concluded that the minimum recommended target dose to positive margins is 60 Gy and the minimum recommended dose for microscopic nodal metastases is 50 Gy.

In a report from Barcelona by Astudillo and Conill (1990), 146 patients with pathologic stage IIIA NSCLC were retrospectively analyzed to determine whether postoperative radiation therapy (45 to 50 Gy) improved survival and reduced locoregional recurrences. The survival rates of the untreated group ($n = 60$) at 3 and 5 years was 28% and 12%, respectively. The 3- and 5-year survival in the radiated arm ($n = 86$) was 20% and 19%, respectively, failing to show any statistically significant differences. Patients with N_0 and N_1 disease were grouped and survival at 3 and 5 years was 41% and 27%, respectively, for the T_3N_{0-1} group 17% and 15%, respectively, and for the T_3N_2 group the survival was significantly worse, $P < .001$ and $P > .05$, respectively. Median survival was 6 months for patients without irradiation and 15 months for those with irradiation ($P = .071$). A slightly decreased incidence of locoregional recurrence was observed in the group receiving postoperative radiation therapy.

Two studies of adjuvant radiation therapy have shown mixed results for survival benefit. A retrospective review by Sawyer and coworkers (1997b) was performed at the Mayo Clinic to determine the local recurrence and survival rates for 124 patients with N_2 disease undergoing complete surgical resection with or without adjuvant radiation therapy. More than one mediastinal lymph node station was sampled in 98% of patients; 88 patients then received adjuvant radiation therapy (range, 45 to 55 Gy; median 50.6 Gy). After treatment with surgery alone, the 4-year local recurrence rate was 60%, compared with 17% for treatment with adjuvant radiation therapy ($P < .0001$). The 4-year survival rate was 22% for treatment with surgery alone, compared with 43% for treatment with adjuvant radiation therapy ($P = .005$). On multivariate analysis, the addition of thoracic irradiation was associated with an improved survival rate.

Conversely, a study from the University Medical School of Graz, Austria, reported by Mayer and associates (1997), randomized 155 stage I, II, and III patients to adjuvant radiation therapy of 50 to 56 Gy ($n = 83$) or no treatment ($n = 72$). The overall 5-year survival was 29.7% for the irradiated group and 20.4% for the control group ($P > .05$, not significant). The rate of local recurrence was significantly smaller in the irradiated group than the control arm but the incidence of distant metastases was slightly, but not significantly, higher in patients without irradiation. Thus, again, although local disease was better controlled, no survival advantage was demonstrated.

Also of note, a retrospective analysis of 340 patients by Wurschmidt and colleagues (1997) studied the issue of time interval between surgery and initiation of radiation therapy to assess whether this is important in resected NSCLC. Shortening the time interval to less than 6 weeks, even in patients with positive nodes, does not seem to be necessary. Survival of patients with a long interval between surgery and start of radiation therapy actually was better in this retrospective analysis as compared with patients with shorter intervals.

The PORT Meta-analysis Trialists Group (1998) looked at individual patient data from nine randomized trials (2128 patients) of postoperative radiation therapy versus surgery alone. The mean follow-up was 3.9 years for the survivors, and the results showed a significant adverse effect of postoperative radiation therapy on survival with a 21% relative increase in the risk of death. This adverse effect was greatest in patients with stage I/II, N_0, N_1 disease, but for those with N_2 disease no clear evidence of adverse effect existed. They concluded that postoperative radiation therapy should not be used routinely in patients with early stage disease and its role in patients with N_2 disease remains unclear. This study is somewhat misleading because few patients with N_0 disease are irradiated routinely and some selection factors must have been operable. Any meta-analysis, of course, is only as good as the data on which it draws and the quality of several of the studies included in the analysis is questionable.

As noted by Stewart and Burdett (1997), in patients with early stage tumor without positive lymph nodes, few clinical trials have demonstrated any survival advantage when postoperative radiation therapy is given. In patients with advanced disease, however, Sawyer and colleagues (1997b) noted that postoperative radiation therapy has demonstrated some added benefit of local control of disease in uncontrolled retrospective data. Improvement in locoregional control with radiation therapy does not translate into improved long-term survival, as disseminated disease continues to be the main problem. All of these trials have been plagued with problems related to interpretation caused by heterogeneity of stage and inability to make conclusions based on each stage. The imaging methods used for determining local control are far from precise and various studies have used different means to make this assessment. Differentiating "scar" from active tumor can be problematic, although one would also like to call a remaining mass *scar*. The use of positron emission tomography, an imaging modality that relies on the differential handling of glucose between tumors and normal tissue, has the potential to improve the ability to distinguish active tumor from scar tissue. The fact that many of these studies were retrospective introduces the variable of selectivity into the equation; why were certain patients selected for postoperative radiation therapy? Were they the worst patients who were not expected to do well and thus were given radiation therapy as attempted salvage after an incomplete surgical resection and staging, or were they patients with the better prognosis in whom radiation therapy was used as "icing on the cake"? Even prospective randomized trials must be looked at with caution, especially if it is not known how many patients were excluded from the study or chose not to participate.

Adjuvant Chemotherapy

The role of adjuvant chemotherapy in NSCLC remains controversial. This uncertainty persists despite more than 30 years of research involving more than 10,000 patients in more than 50 randomized clinical trials such as those conducted by the Non–small Cell Lung Cancer Collaborative Group in Britain (1995) and the Study Group of Adjuvant Chemotherapy for Lung Cancer (Chubu, Japan, 1995), as well as the studies noted in the reviews of Bunn (1994), Marangolo and Fiorenti (1988), and Kris (1987) and Haraf (1992) and their colleagues, examining the efficacy of chemotherapy when combined with local treatment or best supportive care. Theoretically, postoperative adjuvant chemotherapy is an attractive concept because this should be a time of minimal tumor burden. Adjuvant chemotherapy has been demonstrated to increase the disease-free interval after surgical resection in breast cancer and osteogenic sarcoma. Preclinical studies by Schabel (1977) in mice have demonstrated surgical adjuvant chemotherapy for lung cancer increases the long-term cure rate and significantly increases the life span of treatment failures.

Two phases of adjuvant chemotherapy have occurred since the 1950s. In the 1960s and 1970s, trials of various drugs, chiefly alkylating agents, were highly ineffective. Not until the early 1980s, particularly from the experience of the LCSG, did the use of platinum-based chemotherapy usher in the most effective management of NSCLC. Current evidence suggests platinum-based agents may be the most effective single drug for the management of NSCLC patients, though newer agents such as paclitaxel, gemcitabine, irinotecan, and vinorelbine (Navelbine) all show significant activity, as noted by Greco and Hainsworth (1997) and Tan and Ang (1996). Now the more active combinations include cisplatin and can produce a response rate between 20% and 60%, although responses are higher in previously untreated patients given higher doses, as noted by the aforementioned British (1995) and Japanese (1995) group studies and the trials reported by Cullen (1995a, 1995b).

Saijo (1998), in discussing new chemotherapeutic agents, raises the fundamental question of whether combination chemotherapy makes a difference, which remains to be seen. A meta-analysis demonstrated that combination chemotherapy increases survival at 3, 6, and 9 months, but not at 12 months. For the Eastern Cooperative Oncology Group trials, according to Bonomi (1998) and Natale (1998), two-drug combinations with a *Vinca* alkaloid or etoposide consistently have provided the best overall survival with acceptable toxicity. As noted by Bonomi (1998) and Natale (1998), combination cisplatin and etoposide produced the highest 1-year survival rates when compared with several combined chemotherapy regimens (25% versus less than 19%) and served as the group's standard reference regimen until 1997. Factors that can affect the achievement of an objective response include the initial performance status, stage of disease, weight loss, and prior treatment. It has not yet been clearly established whether regimens with cisplatin at doses of approximately 100 to 120 mg/m^2 are more effective than regimens with a lower dosage of 50 to 60 mg/m^2. Trodella (1997) and Paccagnella (1996) and their associates point out

that it appears that combinations higher than 100 to 120 mg/m^2 cannot further increase the response rate.

The third-generation of chemotherapeutic agents for NSCLC are arriving, namely paclitaxel and paclitaxel-based combinations. Many other single agents (e.g., docetaxel, irinotecan, gemcitabine, and topotecan) and combinations are just beginning to enter clinical trials as reported by Greco and Hainsworth (1997), Natale (1997), Saijo (1998), Natale (1998), Bonomi and colleagues (1996), and Tan and Ang (1996).

Until fairly recently, NSCLC has been regarded as a chemoresistant tumor, mainly on the basis that the older established drugs (i.e., doxorubicin, methotrexate, cyclophosphamide) are ineffective. As noted by Cullen (1995a, 1995b), only five drugs (i.e., ifosfamide, mitomycin, cisplatin, vinblastine, and vindesine), when tested as single agents on large numbers of patients, produce major responses in 15% or more of cases. Two of the most frequently used drug regimens in the management of NSCLC are mitomycin C, vindesine or vinblastine, and cisplatin (MVP) and cyclophosphamide, doxorubicin, and cisplatin (CAP). The MVP combination originally was developed by Gralla (1990) at Memorial Sloan-Kettering Cancer Center. According to Bonomi (1998) and Spain (1993) this regimen can produce a response rate between 20 and 75%. The activity of mitomycin in NSCLC has been well documented, as noted by Spain (1993), in both single-institution pilot and multi-institution randomized trials. Mitomycin is associated with excessive pulmonary toxicity, however, making the thoracic surgeon reluctant to use mitomycin-based regimens. The CAP regimen avoids the pulmonary toxicity of mitomycin but has a lower overall response rate.

Clinical trials with adjuvant chemotherapy before the 1980s were plagued by many shortcomings in methodology. Often, the trials failed to differentiate between small cell and NSCLC. Nodal status was rarely assessed and clinical staging was inadequate. Only a limited number of trials were randomized or properly designed during this period. The most commonly used chemotherapeutic agent during this phase was cyclophosphamide because of its low toxicity, easy oral administration, and preliminary positive results in other lung cancer studies. Other agents considered during this period included nitrogen mustard, methotrexate, and hydroxyurea.

The earliest and largest randomized, controlled postoperative lung cancer trial was started in 1957 by the Veterans Administration Surgical Adjuvant Lung Cancer Chemotherapy Cooperative Group that involved 22 hospitals. In this trial, reported by Hughes and Higgins (1962), 1002 patients were randomized to receive either intrapleural saline or nitrogen mustard, 0.1 mg/kg, immediately postoperatively on day 1 and postoperative day 2. Because the 30-day mortality was significantly increased, the initial drug dose was reduced to 0.3 mg/kg. After a 55-month follow-up, this trial failed to show any survival advantage over the control group. In a similar trial by the same group, 1008 patients were randomized to receive placebo or short-term intravenous cyclophosphamide. Although there was less toxicity, the report by Higgins and coinvestigators (1969) failed to demonstrate any survival advantage.

Slack (1970) reported the experience of the University Surgical Adjuvant Lung Project, which randomized 1192 patients to receive placebo or nitrogen mustard, 0.4 mg/kg intrapleurally and intravenously in the same manner as the VA experience. This study also failed to demonstrate any survival advantage. Postoperative complications were frequent in the control series (33%) but were significantly higher (45%) in the treatment series. There was 14% perioperative mortality.

The last large studies of the 1970s were those reported by Shields and colleagues (1974, 1977) conducted by the Veterans Administration Surgical Adjuvant Group. In one trial, 909 patients were randomized to receive either placebo or cyclophosphamide, 6 mg/kg intrapleurally postoperatively, followed by 4 days of intravenous treatment, and concluded with 8 mg/kg intravenously 5 days during the fifth postoperative week. Again, there was no survival advantage associated with this approach. Numerous prospective randomized trials were undertaken to evaluate the single-drug chemotherapy after resection of bronchial carcinoma, which often included small cell lung cancers. The drugs studied were mechlorethamine, cyclophosphamide, and methotrexate. In one of the largest of these studies reported by Shields and associates (1982), 865 patients were assigned to lomustine (CCNU) and hydroxyurea ($n = 432$) or no treatment. In all, a total of 2348 curative resections were carried out; 1172 patients received adjuvant therapy after the resection, and 1176 underwent operation alone. The accumulated 5- and 10-year survival rates were 24.8% and 13.5%, respectively, for the treatment group and 26.2% and 16.3% for the control group. The differences were not significant. These survival figures further underscore the primitive nature of knowledge of staging in the early years of clinical trials.

The British Medical Research Council reported a long follow-up series in NSCLC, one in 1971 and one in 1985. The first report described 735 patients with bronchial carcinoma admitted between 1966 and 1968 who were treated postoperatively with long-term busulphan, oral cyclophosphamide, or placebo. The 2-year survival was 49% for busulphan, 50% for the cyclophosphamide arm, and 50% for the placebo arm. No statistically significant differences in survival existed. The 15-year follow-up reported by Girling and coinvestigators (1985) revealed 8% alive of the 243 allocated to busulphan, 9% in the cyclophosphamide group, and 10% of the 249 who received placebo.

By the mid-1980s two advances had changed the direction of adjuvant chemotherapy. The introduction of the 1986 staging system by Mountain and the use of platinum-based agents shifted the direction of adjuvant therapy as discussed by Tan and Ang (1996). Some of the first postoperative platinum-based adjuvant chemotherapy trials were conducted by the LCSG, as reported by Holmes (1989). Study 772

reported by Holmes (1986) and Holmes and Gail (1986) included 141 patients with resected stage II (T_2N_1) and stage III (any T_3 or N_2) adenocarcinoma and large cell undifferentiated carcinoma randomized to receive either immunotherapy with BCG/levamisole or CAP. All patients underwent a prescribed, rigorous, intraoperative lymph node staging procedure. Patients were stratified by stage, weight loss, cardiac function, and institution, and prognostic variables were equally divided between the two groups. The chemotherapy protocol consisted of cyclophosphamide, 400 mg/m^2, doxorubicin, 40 mg/m^2, and cisplatin, 40 mg/m^2 once a month for 6 months beginning 1 month postoperatively. Holmes (1989) recorded that the average cumulative dose of CAP received was 58% of the calculated full protocol dosages. At a median follow-up of 7.5 years, the median time to recurrence was 15 months for the chemotherapy group compared with 8 months for the immunotherapy arm ($P = .032$). The median survival was 23 months for the chemotherapy group compared with 16 months for the immunotherapy group ($P = .113$), and the long-term survival at 2 years was 42% for the chemotherapy group versus 32% for the immunotherapy group. Holmes (1993) pointed out that if one excludes the 15 patients in the treatment group who did not receive the CAP therapy, the recurrence rates and survival rate become even more statistically significant: $P = .005$ and $P = .013$, respectively. The main criticism of this trial was the lack of an adequate control. However, as noted by Holmes (1994a), the LCSG was reluctant to use a no-treatment arm in these patients in view of their perceived poor prognosis after surgery. This study suggested that CAP chemotherapy might have an effect on disease-free survival and death from cancer in patients with advanced, resectable NSCLC. This trial provided the impetus for a number of future clinical trials.

LCSG Study 801 reported by Feld and colleagues (1993) consisted of 269 stage I (T_1N_1 and T_2N_0) patients, who were randomized to receive four cycles of CAP chemotherapy administered every 3 weeks starting within 1 month of surgery. The dose of cisplatin was 60 mg/m^2, significantly higher than LCSG trial 772, however, as noted by Feld and associates (1994) only 53% of patients received all four cycles and only 57% of those were administered at the prescribed time. There were 101 recurrences, most of which were extrathoracic. No difference in time to recurrence or overall survival occurred between the treatment group and the no treatment control arm even when the analysis was adjusted for specific prognostic variables. The LCSG investigators concluded, as reported by Johnson (1994), that better systemic therapy was needed for completely resected stage I patients and because some of the recurrences were local, thoracic irradiation was believed to be needed "where appropriate."

The LCSG 853 reported by Figlin and Piantadosi (1994) randomly assigned 188 patients with completely resected stage II (41%) and stage III (59%) NSCLC to receive either immediate or delayed CAP chemotherapy administered at the time of first systemic relapse. Despite the prior trials with CAP chemotherapy, both the median time to recurrence

(19.5 months) and overall survival (32.7 months) did not differ significantly between the two groups. These authors also reported that immediate combination chemotherapy was associated with a 12% reduction in risk of recurrence and an 18% reduction in the risk of death, although these rates were not statistically significant.

Niiranen and colleagues (1992) subsequently reported a randomized CAP regimen from the Helsinki University Central Hospital in which CAP was given monthly for six cycles to a group of 110 patients with stages I to II tumor (N_0). Five-year survival was 67% versus 56%, 10-year survival was 61% versus 48%, and recurrence rate was 48% versus 31% for the chemotherapy and control groups, respectively. The investigators concluded that patients with NSCLC of pathologic stage I who undergo radical surgery benefit from adjuvant chemotherapy. Of note, patients in the chemotherapy arm who completed six cycles had a slightly better 5-year survival compared with those who discontinued (72.5% versus 50.3%, $P = .15$). However, this study suffers from a disparity in the distribution of prognostically important clinical characteristics between the two arms despite the randomization.

The Japanese have also contributed significantly to the knowledge regarding adjuvant chemotherapy for NSCLC. A number of the studies, such as those by the group from Chubu, Japan (1995), and those of Ohta (1993) and Wada (1997) and their coinvestigators using cisplatin-based regimens, have shown significantly enhanced 5-year survivals.

Ohta and colleagues (1993), reporting for the Japan Clinical Oncology Group, reported on 209 patients with completely resected stage III NSCLC who were randomized to receive postoperative cisplatin and vindesine chemotherapy or no further treatment. No statistically significant difference existed in disease-free and overall survival between the chemotherapy ($n = 90$) and control ($n = 91$) arms. In the chemotherapy group, the median survival time and the 3- and 5-year survivals were 31 months and 48% and 35%, respectively. Those of the control group were 37 months and 51% and 41%, respectively. The multivariate prognostic factor analyses in this trial demonstrated that pathologic nodal disease had a significant effect on survival of patients with stage III disease. The 5-year survivals were 62% for pathologic N_0, 44% for N_1, and 29% for N_2. This observation confirms that patients with stage III tumors should be stratified according to pathologic nodal stage disease before randomization.

The Study Group of Adjuvant Chemotherapy for Lung Cancer in Chubu, Japan (1995), randomized 333 stage I, II, and III NSCLC patients to either adjuvant cisplatin, doxorubicin (Adriamycin), and uracil-FT ($n = 155$) or surgery only ($n = 154$). The 5-year survival in the therapy group was 61.8% versus 58.1% in the no adjuvant treatment arm. No statistically significant difference existed in the survival between these two groups ($P > .2$).

An encouraging randomized trial from the West Japan Study Group for Lung Cancer Surgery, reported by Wada and associates (1996), examined patients with all stages of NSCLC, allocating 323 patients into one of three different treatment arms: surgical resection alone, resection followed by three courses of cisplatin and vindesine with 1 year of oral tegafur and uracil or resection followed by 1 year of oral uracil. Uracil inhibits 5-fluorouracil degradation and has antitumor activity as well. Wada and coinvestigators (1997) noted that 5-year follow-up was completed successfully on all patients. Both chemotherapy treatment groups had improved 5-year survival (60.6% oral tegafur and uracil, $P = .08$; versus 64.1% uracil, $P = .02$) as compared with the surgery alone groups (49.0%). The investigators noted good compliance and acceptable toxicity. Most of the patients had stage I disease and another 36 had stage III disease. However, only 62 of the 310 patients (20%) in this study had locally advanced disease (stages IIIA, IIIB); therefore, the results of this subset were not presented individually, and the usefulness of this adjuvant regimen for locally advanced lesions remains unclear.

In conclusion, no group or subset of patients has been demonstrated to definitively benefit from postoperative chemotherapy (Table 106-3). The use of active single agents or combinations was tested early in the 1960s and the 1970s. The observation that these were ineffective is not surprising in view of the relative inactivity of most chemotherapeutic agents in advanced NSCLC. With the introduction of cisplatin-based regimens, considerable enthusiasm for postoperative adjuvant chemotherapy developed. Nevertheless, after all the years and all the trials, postoperative chemotherapy still should be confined to clinical trials and no justification exists for its use outside of a protocol setting. It is also not clear whether the small benefit derived from therapy justifies the treatment. Feld (1996) and Johnson (1994) have pointed out that the possible reasons for the failure of clinical trials to show reproducible benefit include the following: 1) inadequate sample size to detect small survival benefits as was required to establish the place of adjuvant therapy in breast cancer, 2) inadequate drug delivery, and, probably most important, 3) lack of chemotherapeutic agents with sufficient antitumor activity. Furthermore, a full course of therapy can require 6 months, a period equal to the survival benefit of patients treated with postoperative chemotherapy. Quality of life studies in patients undergoing postoperative adjuvant chemotherapy are woefully lacking.

Adjuvant Chemoradiation Therapy

Given the results obtained with either adjuvant chemotherapy or radiation therapy, a number of studies, as noted by Bonomi and colleagues (1990), have tried using combined postoperative chemoradiation therapy to assess whether the combination might provide a greater benefit (Table 106-4). Use of chemotherapy and radiation therapy potentially offers a number of advantages. Ideally, chemotherapeutic agents used simultaneously with radiation therapy should enhance the effects of radiation therapy on tumor

Table 106-3. Adjuvant Chemotherapy for Non–Small Cell Lung Cancer

Group	N	Stage	Postoperative Chemotherapy	Survival Benefit	Reference
Veterans Administration	1002	NS	Nitrogen mustard	No benefit	Hughes and Higgins (1962)
Veterans Administration	1008	NS	Cyclophosphamide	No benefit	Higgins et al. (1969)
University Surgical Adjuvant Group	1192	I,II,III	Nitrogen mustard	No benefit	Slack (1970)
Veterans Administration	909	I,II,III	Cyclophosphamide	No benefit	Shields et al. (1974)
Veterans Administration	417	I,II,III	Cyclophosphamide + methotrexate	No benefit	Shields et al. (1977)
Veterans Administration	865	I,II,III	Lomustine + hydroxyurea	No benefit	Shields et al. (1982)
British Medical Research Council	243	NS	Busulphan	No benefit	Girling et al. (1985)
British Medical Research Council	234	I,II,III	Cyclophosphamide	No benefit	Girling et al. (1985)
LCSG 772	141	II,III	CAP	2-year survival (42%)	Holmes and Gail (1986)
Helsinki University	54	$T_{1-3}N_0$	CAP	5-year survival (67%); 10-year (61%)	Niiranen et al. (1992)
LCSG 801	269	I	CAP	5-year survival (55%)	Feld et al. (1993)
LCSG 853	188	II,III	CAP	2.6-year survival (50%)	Figlin and Piantadosi (1994)
Japan Clinical Oncology Group	90	III	PVn	3-year survival (48%); 5-year survival (35%)	Ohta et al. (1993)
Study Group (Chubu, Japan)	155	I,II,III	PAUft	3-year survival (76%); 5-year survival (62%)	Study Group of Adjuvant Chemotherapy for Lung Cancer (1995)
West Japan Study Group	115	I,II,III	CVUft	5-year survival (61%)	Wada et al. (1996)
West Japan Study Group	108	I,II,III	Uft	5-year survival (64%)	Wada et al. (1996)

CAP, cyclophosphamide, doxorubicin, and cisplatin; CVUft, cisplatin, vindesine, and uracil; LCSG, Lung Cancer Study Group; NS, not staged; PAUft, cisplatin, doxorubicin, and uracil; PVn, cisplatine, vindesine; Uft, uracil.

without producing excessive toxicity. Using chemotherapy before radiation therapy allows the opportunity to give chemotherapeutic agents at full-dose intensity, whereas using radiation therapy before chemotherapy has the potential advantage of being able to use continuous thoracic irradiation at full dose. The optimal sequence for chemotherapy and radiation therapy in stage III NSCLC has not been determined.

Lad and associates (1988) reported the Lung Cancer Study Group trial 791, which was the first LCSG study to include all non–small cell histologies in an adjuvant chemotherapy study. This study looked at 172 patients with incompletely resected tumors, as defined by the presence of residual tumor at the margins or the presence of metastatic tumor in the highest paratracheal lymph nodes sampled.* The study randomized patients to postoperative radiation

---
*No proof exists that tumor in the highest paratracheal lymph node sampled actually defines the presence of residual tumor.—The Senior Editor

therapy (40 Gy) alone or radiation therapy with six cycles of cyclophosphamide, 400 mg/m^2 + doxorubicin 40 mg/m^2 + cisplatin 40 mg/m^2. No untreated control arm was used. The study differed from LCSG trial 771 in that it included patients with squamous cell carcinoma. Although only 51% of the patients completed the prescribed chemoradiation therapeutic regimen, Lad (1994) was able to show a statistically significant survival advantage. Median survival in the chemoradiation therapeutic group was 20 months compared with 13 months ($P = .13$) with radiation therapy alone. Median time to recurrence was 14 months and 8 months ($P = .004$) in the chemoradiation therapy and radiation therapy groups, respectively. LCSG 791 built on the results of study 773. Study 773 demonstrated the ability of adjuvant irradiation to prevent local recurrence in squamous cell carcinoma. The patients in LCSG study 791 additionally received chemotherapy that did not affect local control of disease. Twenty patients experienced local relapse, nine of which were confined to the mediastinum. However, patients in

Table 106-4. Adjuvant Chemoradiation Therapy for Non–Small Cell Lung Cancer

Group	N	Stage	Postoperative Chemoradiation	Median Survival (mos)	Survival Benefit	Reference
University of Chicago	16	N_1	30 Gy + CAMtxPe	45.5	5-year survival (46%)	Ferguson et al. (1986)
Lung Cancer Study Group 791	78	IIIA	40 Gy + PACtx	20	1-year survival (68%); 2-year survival (22%)	Lad et al. (1988)
Memorial Sloan-Kettering	36	III	40 Gy + PVn	16.3	2-year survival (31%); 5-year survival (17%)	Pisters et al. (1994)

CAMtxPe, cyclophosphamide, doxorubicin, methotrexate, procarbazine; PACtx, cisplatin, doxorubicin, cyclophosphamide; PVn, cisplatine, vindesine.

LCSG 791 receiving chemotherapy had a favorable, albeit modest, effect on recurrence and survival rates. Simultaneous irradiation and chemotherapy were able to be delivered without untoward local toxic reactions. Recurrences were more common in the patients who had radiation therapy compared with those given CAP plus radiation therapy and were usually extrathoracic (66 versus 50, P = .001).

At the University of Chicago, Ferguson and coinvestigators (1986) reported a nonrandomized, retrospective study of 34 patients with stage II disease. Patients were treated with resection alone or with resection followed by radiation therapy, chemotherapy, or both. Chemotherapy involved cyclophosphamide, doxorubicin, and methotrexate, on days 1 to 8, followed by oral procarbazine on days 3 to 13. These cycles were repeated monthly for 1 year. Median survival in the chemoradiation therapy arm was increased to 45.5 months compared with 19.2 months in the radiation therapy group and 13 months in the control groups (P <.005). The 5-year survival in this group was 45.9%, compared with 28.6% in the radiation therapy only group. The investigators concluded in this special subset of patients with N_1 tumor that adjuvant radiation therapy and chemotherapy offered an improved median survival over resection alone.

At Memorial Sloan-Kettering Cancer Center, a prospective randomized trial was performed to determine whether postoperative chemotherapy with vindesine and cisplatin could lengthen time to progression and overall survival in 72 patients with stage III disease. All had surgery and mediastinal irradiation for 6 to 7 weeks postthoracotomy. Incompletely resected patients had intraoperative ^{125}I implantation, ^{192}Ir implantation, or both. Vindesine and cisplatin were planned for the 36 patients randomized to additional chemotherapy. No difference in time to progression (median, 9.2 months for radiation therapy and chemotherapy versus 9.0 months for radiation therapy alone, P = .35) or overall survival (16.3 months for radiation therapy and chemotherapy versus 19.1 months for radiation therapy alone, P = .42) was found by Pisters and associates (1994).

Compared with LCSG 772 and LCSG 791, this trial differed in that all patients had mediastinal lymph node involvement. In addition, the planned cisplatin dose intensity was roughly twice that of the other LCSG studies. Despite the differences among the three studies, Pisters and colleagues (1994) noted that if one examines the survival difference at 2 years between patients receiving postoperative cisplatin-based chemotherapy and controls, the 95% confidence intervals for the difference overlap. Although the authors concluded that an important survival advantage is not gained by adjuvant cisplatin chemotherapy, these results are difficult to assess because of the small numbers. The Memorial Sloan-Kettering experience had only 13 of the 30 patients who received all four planned doses of cisplatin. LCSG 772 and LCSG 791 only looked at another 60 to 80 patients.

Currently, thoracic surgeons, medical oncologists, radiation oncologists, and pathologists have joined forces to determine the most effective management of NSCLC. Since the last LCSG 791 trial, an Intergroup trial has been underway that calls on the collaborative effort of the Cancer and Leukemia Group B (CALGB), Eastern Cooperative Oncology Group 3590, the Southwest Oncology Group (SWOG), the North Central Cancer Therapy Group 91-24-51, and the Radiation Therapy Oncology Group 9105. This Intergroup INT-0115 trial is trying to determine whether chemotherapy plus radiation therapy improves survival compared with radiation therapy alone in patients with completely resected stage II and IIIA NSCLC. CAP has been replaced by cisplatin-etoposide as a frontline cancer combination. This trial randomizes patients to thoracic irradiation (50.4 Gy in 5 weeks) or concomitant cisplatin (60 mg/m²) and etoposide with thoracic irradiation. Chemotherapy is administered beginning shortly after surgery and is continued for four courses. The target accrual was 462 patients, a number that has been reached and the study has been closed. We await the final results but the preliminary report by Rusch and Feins (1994) did not suggest a benefit for the chemoradiation therapy arm.

Of note in this large intergroup trial is the lack of a no treatment arm despite the evidence that radiation therapy is of no benefit in prolonging survival. Despite the evidence there remains, a built-in bias that patients with stages II and IIIA disease should get some postoperative treatment, so the radiation therapy only arm is the control arm in this trial.

NEOADJUVANT THERAPY

In the early 1980s, *neoadjuvant therapy*, a term that implied treatment given before definitive local management, began to be used in the treatment of NSCLC. Previously, patients with bulky tumor or extensive nodal involvement usually were not considered surgical candidates and were treated with radiation therapy as definitive treatment.

With the introduction of the concept of neoadjuvant therapy, chemotherapy and radiation therapy were given to reduce bulky tumor in an attempt to convert marginally or unresectable disease to resectable disease. As suggested by Shepherd (1993) and reemphasized by Green and Barkley (1997), preoperative or induction therapy theoretically may have advantages in being used before resistant clones of cells have the opportunity to develop. Also, treatment before resection allows the clinician to assess tumor responsiveness, helping to identify patients who may benefit from continuation of postoperative adjuvant chemotherapy. Finally, neoadjuvant therapy in concept might lessen the incidence of later distant disease when given at a time when only micrometastatic disease may be present. The control of distant disease likely also is influenced by the effectiveness of local therapy in obtaining local control.

A number of contrary positions exist regarding neoadjuvant therapy. Tumors might progress during the delay to the time of operation and a previously resectable tumor can become unresectable. Preoperative therapy is associated with systemic toxicity that might cause difficulty during the postoperative recuperation. Several chemotherapeutic agents are associated with pulmonary toxicity and can result in reduced pulmonary function. In addition to the usual toxicities of antitumor drugs, they also may be a factor in decreasing wound healing capability. Resections after postoperative therapy can be extremely difficult and potentially hazardous because of the fibrosis that often results as a response to the therapy. Tissue planes may be obliterated because of mediastinal fibrosis. Patients should be taken to the operating room 2 to 4 weeks after the completion of induction therapy before the development of fibrosis occurs. This is especially significant when there has been a response in the lymph nodes, because the nodes are intimately associated with the pulmonary artery and its branches, often making resection quite challenging. It is particularly important to have proximal control of the pulmonary artery before undertaking a resection in a patient with N_2 disease who has received preoperative therapy. Resections of this type ideally should be undertaken by a surgeon experienced in dealing with complex resections so as to avoid an unnecessary pneumonectomy.

Evidence exists, as noted by Livingston and associates (1997), that neoadjuvant therapy results in improved survival when compared with surgery alone; however, this has not been confirmed in a large phase III randomized, multiinstitutional trial reported by Perry and colleagues (1997). It is difficult to assess the various trials for neoadjuvant therapy. Staging criteria have differed widely as have inclusion criteria. The criteria used to determine mediastinal lymph node involvement has varied from simple radiologic evidence to pathologic confirmation. The majority of studies do report a 50 to 60% objective response rate, although the complete remission rate tends to be less than 15%. The overall response rate is significantly higher as when these same agents are used in patients with disseminated disease. In the reports of Blanke and Johnson (1995), Pujol and associates (1995), Holmes and Ruckdeschel (1994), and Shepherd (1993), the vast majority of responders and approximately one-half the patients overall are able to go on to surgical resection. In the reports of Pujol and colleagues (1995), Blanke and Johnson (1995), Albain (1993), and Murren and associates (1991), among others, approximately 10% of patients treated with neoadjuvant therapy attain complete histologic clearance of disease. Median survival is approximately 18 months for patients receiving combined modality treatment, including induction chemotherapy (ranging from 8 to 30 months) with 2- to 3-year survival ranging from 25 to 30%. Although it may seem that the median survival of approximately 18 months is superior to that of surgery or radiation therapy alone, one must remember that the patients in these trials represent a select subgroup of stage III patients overall, usually patients with the best performance status and minimal weight loss, and that this survival advantage may reflect better patient selection rather than actual improvement with therapy. Neoadjuvant chemotherapy

alone has not been associated with increased morbidity after operation except when it is combined with preoperative radiation therapy.

Neoadjuvant Radiation Therapy

Neoadjuvant radiation therapy at one time was an appealing concept. Preoperative radiation may reduce the tumor size, facilitating resection or possibly even downstaging the tumor. It may also minimize seeding of tumor cells by surgical manipulation and sterilize the tumor bed, but evidence for this is lacking. Faber (1994) has pointed out that tumor cells are particularly sensitive to radiation therapy at higher oxygen tensions, therefore preoperative use would be expected to be most effective on the highly vascularized peripheral border of the invasive tumor. Depending on the total dose of radiation delivered preoperatively, investigators, including Reddy (1990), Sherman (1978), and Shields (1970) and their associates, as well as Warram (1975) and Bloedorn (1964), have reported a range of 20 to 50% of patients having no persistent tumor or only microscopic disease in the resected specimen. One of the problems with preoperative radiation therapy, however, is a tendency for significant fibrosis and loss of distinct tissue planes, making resection challenging, but this should not be interpreted as a limitation. The doses required to obtain a response when given as a single agent, however, are associated with decreased healing of the bronchial stump.

The first use of neoadjuvant radiation therapy dates back to 1955 when Bromley and Szur (1955) at the Hammersmith Hospital used a dose of 45 Gy before surgical resection (Table 106-5). Sixty-six of 573 patients were resected. At operation, no viable tumor was found in 47% of the patients. Ten of the patients died of complications within the first month and only two patients were alive 5 years later. This trial did demonstrate that 47% of the patients had no histologically demonstrable tumor in the surgical specimen. Subsequently in 1964, Bloedorn used a radiation dose of 60 Gy preoperatively to treat 109 patients with presumed unresectable lung cancer. The postoperative mortality was approximately 35% and the 1-year survival approached 20%. Bloedorn (1964) reported that tumor sterilization rates of 54% at the primary site and 92% at the mediastinal lymph nodes were obtained by preoperative radiation therapy using 60 Gy/25 fractions/6 weeks but the status of the mediastinal nodes was not histologically documented before initiation of the preoperative regimen. Thus, potentially, carefully planned irradiation at a moderately high dose (50 to 60 Gy) should be able to convert a surgical resection from incomplete to complete by sterilization of residual microscopic carcinoma in the tumor bed and regional lymph nodes, but this concept is difficult to prove. What is unresectable in one surgeon's hands may be eminently resectable in another's.

In the 1960s and 1970s, the Veterans Administration and the National Cancer Institute performed two large-scale tri-

Table 106-5. Neoadjuvant Radiation Therapy for Non–Small Cell Lung Cancer

Group	N	Stage	Postoperative Radiation Dose	Survival Benefit	Reference
Hammersmith Hospital	66	NS	45 Gy	5-year survival (3%)	Bromley and Szur (1955)
University of Maryland	192	I,II,III,IV	55–60 Gy	1-year survival (23%)	Bloedorn (1964)
Veterans Administration	166	NS	30–60 Gy	5-year survival (7%)	Shields (1972)
National Cancer Institute	290	NS	37–60 Gy	5-year survival (14%)	Warram (1975)
Harvard Medical School	38	NS	30–40 Gy	5-year survival (27%)	Sherman et al. (1978)
Rush-Presbyterian	74	III	40 Gy	5-year survival (23%)	Reddy et al. (1990)
Lung Cancer Study Group 881	—	III	44 Gy	4-year survival (27%)	Wagner et al. (1994)

NS, not staged.

als that randomized patients to immediate surgery versus preoperative 40- to 50-Gy radiation. In the Veterans Administration study reported by Shields and associates (1970), 331 male patients with biopsy-proven bronchial carcinoma were randomized to one of two groups: 166 patients received preoperative radiation therapy and subsequent surgery and the other 165 patients underwent surgery alone. No statistically significant increase in survival was noted in the pretreatment group (12.5% versus 21.0%). In fact, as noted by Shields (1972), the survival rate in the preoperative treatment group was significantly less during the first 12 postoperative months than in those patients who only underwent resection.

In the National Cancer Institute study (1969), patients thought to be resectable at the time of diagnosis were randomly assigned to receive either immediate surgery ($n = 278$) or preoperative irradiation followed by surgery ($n = 290$). The 3-year survival rates for these two groups were nearly identical. At 5 years, Warram (1975) reported that the survival rate was 14% after preoperative radiation therapy and 16% after immediate surgery. The preoperative radiation therapy was believed not to improve the resectability or survival rates in either study. Long-term survival was not improved even though local control was enhanced. Operative mortality was 12% in both groups. These trials clearly did not resolve the issue of the benefit, or lack thereof, of neoadjuvant radiation therapy. These trials lacked pretreatment histologic staging and there was significant variation in the amount of radiation therapy delivered and excessively long intervals between radiation therapy and surgery. Furthermore, the trials did not exclude patients with small cell histology.

Soon afterward, a phase II trial was reported from the Harvard Medical School, suggesting a benefit for preoperative radiation therapy followed by surgical resection. Fifty-three patients with marginally resectable NSCLC were treated with 30 to 40 Gy of preoperative radiation therapy followed by resection and postoperative radiation therapy. Thirty-eight (72%) patients were resected. Sherman and colleagues (1978) reported that the 5-year survival for the 38 resected patients was 27%, whereas it was 18% for all 53 patients.

At Rush-Presbyterian-St. Luke's Medical Center, 74 patients with clinical stage III NSCLC were treated with a 40-Gy preoperative radiation dose to the primary tumor in the lung and regional lymph node areas. Fifteen patients (20%) did not undergo operation because of tumor progression, patient refusal, or death. At the time of surgery, two patients had histologically negative specimens, nine patients had microscopic disease only, and 37 patients had gross residual disease. The 5-year survival and recurrence-free survival rates for the entire group were 20% and 24%, respectively. Patients with a pathologic response had a recurrence-free survival rate of 53% at 5 years, whereas only 17% of those with gross residual disease at surgery remained recurrence free at 5 years. Reddy and coworkers (1990) noted that one-half of the patients with clinically uninvolved nodes were living recurrence free at 5 years, compared with only 20% of the patients with N_2 disease.

By the late 1980s, no definitive work had come out in favor of neoadjuvant chemotherapy over neoadjuvant radiation therapy. A phase II clinical trial was started by LCSG to determine whether either one was sufficiently active and safe. Each arm was to be evaluated for its ability to induce an approximate 15% incidence of complete histologic clearance. Sixty-seven patients with stage III NSCLC were enrolled to receive either preoperative MVP chemotherapy (cisplatin, 120 mg/m^2; mitomycin, 8 mg/m^2; vinblastine 4.5 mg/m^2) or preoperative radiation therapy (44 Gy). All patients had systematic surgical staging of the mediastinum. Radiologic response to treatment was virtually identical for the two approaches (54% and 48%), with 29 of the 57 available patients achieving objective responses. Twenty-three of the 57 (40%) patients eventually underwent complete tumor resection. Wagner and associates (1994) recorded that median survival for the entire group was 12 months, with a 4-year survival rate of 27%. Thus, despite rigorous staging and excellent quality control, a more favorable stage III subset had a disappointing result.

Neoadjuvant Chemotherapy: Unrandomized Trials

Pastorino (1996), Cullen (1995b), Vokes (1990), and Kris and colleagues (1987) have shown that neoadjuvant chemotherapy also may offer benefits in the management of NSCLC. It has the potential of reducing tumor size, may prevent tumor progression caused by perioperative immuno-suppression and release of growth factors related to wound healing, and theoretically may eliminate clinically occult micrometastases. As suggested by a mathematical model, chemotherapy can eradicate a neoplastic subclone if the number of cells is less than 106. Neoadjuvant chemotherapy gives the oncologist an opportunity to assess individual tumor sensitivity. The degree of response can be assessed histologically from the surgically resected specimen. From these results, Pujol and associates (1995) suggest that it may be possible to individualize postsurgical treatment.

Many reviews, such as those by Tonato (1996), Shepherd (1993), Ginsberg (1993), and Ihde (1988), have taken the position that neoadjuvant chemotherapy is beneficial in patients with inoperable stage IIIA NSCLC. Side effects are tolerable, and a high resection rate occurs after neoadjuvant chemotherapy and median survival can increase up to 8 months as noted by Tonato (1996), as well as by Fossella (1996) and Murren (1991) and their coworkers. The long-term survival in phase II studies has reached 18%, compared with 9% of historic control subjects, as reported by Pastorino (1996). However, many remain skeptical about neoadjuvant chemotherapy because of the inadequacy of many phase II trials to date and lack of convincing phase III randomized trials. Many of these studies have poorly defined eligibility criteria, poor pretreatment staging sys-

tems, or lack of adequate numbers to draw a definitive conclusion. However, efforts continue to define the role of neoadjuvant chemotherapy in the management of stage IIIA disease (Table 106-6).

Perhaps the prototype phase II trial of neoadjuvant therapy was begun by investigators at Memorial Sloan-Kettering Cancer Center in 1986 and reported by Kris (1995) and Martini (1993) and their associates. A preliminary phase I/II clinical trial conducted between 1984 and 1986 on 41 patients with bulky N_2 disease set the stage for this trial. The preliminary trial reported by Armstrong and coworkers (1992) demonstrated that a treatment program that consisted of induction chemotherapy, operation, and postoperative radiation therapy (reserved for patients with residual disease at thoracotomy) yielded acceptable and perhaps improved median survival and long-term survival for some patients. In the subsequent study, again trying to keep the patient population as homogeneous as possible, only patients with bulky N_2 disease were entered. Thus, only patients with clinical evidence of extensive mediastinal lymph node involvement, as defined by lymph node enlargement seen on plain chest radiography or with marked widening of the carina noted at bronchoscopy, were included. Patients received two to three cycles of mitomycin C, vindesine or vinblastine, and high-dose cisplatin (120 mg/m²). Four to six weeks later, patients underwent surgery even if no radiologic response could be

Table 106-6. Neoadjuvant Chemotherapy for Non–Small Cell Lung Cancer, Unrandomized Studies

Group	N	Stage	Preoperative Chemotherapy	Postoperative Chemotherapy	Postoperative Response (%)	Complete Resection (%)	Median Survival (mos)	Survival Benefit	Reference
Memorial Sloan-Kettering	136	IIIA	MVP	MVP ± XRT	77	65	19	3-year survival (28%); 5-year survival (17%)	Martini et al. (1993)
Memorial Sloan-Kettering	68	N_2	MVP			13	20	1-year survival (68%)	Pisters et al. (1993)
University of Toronto	55	IIIA	MVP	MVP ± XRT	71	51	21	6-year survival (29%)	Burkes et al. (1992)
Memorial Sloan-Kettering	41	N_2	MVP	Brachytherapy	73	59	19	3-year survival (27%); 5-year survival (12%)	Armstrong et al. (1992)
University of Miami	35	III	PEF	± XRT	69	74	19		Sridhar et al. (1993)
Lung Cancer Study Group 881	24	III	MVP		54	46	12	4-year survival (27%)	Wagner et al. (1994)
Pujol and colleagues	33	III	PEIMe	PEI ± XRT	70	55	11	3-year survival (19%)	Pujol et al. (1995)
Perugia Group	46	IIIA	PE	± XRT	82	73	25	2-year survival (53%)	Darwish et al. (1995)
University of Pisa, Italy	36	N_2	MVP	MVP ± 50 Gy	78	10	31	3-year survival (49%)	Chella et al. (1995)
Cancer and Leukemia Group B 8935	74	IIIA	PV	PV + 54–60 Gy	88	31	15	1-year survival (63%) 3-year survival (23%)	Sugarbaker et al. (1995)
Dana-Farber	34	N_2	PFL	54–60 Gy	65	75	18	4-year survival (23%)	Elias et al. (1997)
University of Navarra	62	III	MVP	45 Gy	64		10		Aristu et al. (1997)

I, ifosfamide; L, leucovorin; Me, mesna; MVP, mitomycin C, vindesine or vinblastine, and cisplatin; PE, cisplatin, etoposide; PEF, 5-fluorouracil, etoposide, and cisplatin; PFL, cisplatin, 5-fluorouracil, leucovorin; PV, cisplatin and vinblastine; XRT, radiation therapy.

shown as long as no progression of disease occurred. This experimental design, with a few variations, became the model for numerous other studies, including those at the cooperative group level, which followed. A 77% "major radiographic response" rate to the chemotherapy occurred (105 of 136 patients) with a 10% (13 of 136) incidence of complete response. Of these patients, 98 had a thoracotomy. Complete resection was achieved in 65% of patients, and no histologic evidence of tumor was found in 19 (21.3%) completely resected patients. Median survival for the completely resected group was 27 months, with a 3- and 5-year survival of 44% and 26%, respectively. For the entire group, overall survival at 1, 3, and 5 years was 72%, 28%, and 17%, respectively. In patients in whom a pathologic complete response was achieved, survival was 95%, 71%, and 61% at 1, 3, and 5 years, respectively. Median survival was 64 months in this group. Also of note, 78 of 136 patients received postoperative radiation therapy to the mediastinum.

This trial, as reported by Kris (1995) and Martini (1993, 1997) and their associates, demonstrated that with a combined chemotherapy and surgery approach, survival in stage IIIA patients with the worst prognosis (those with bulky N_2 disease) could approximate that observed in patients with the best prognosis (microscopic N_2 disease discovered at the time of thoracotomy in a patient in whom it was not suspected). This represents a significant advance when one realizes that with surgery alone, essentially a 0% survival at 3 years exists in the group of patients with bulky mediastinal nodal disease and less than a 10% rate of resectability.

A number of other phase II trials conducted by Burkes (1992), Elias (1994), Skarin (1989), and Kirn (1993) and their colleagues using preoperative chemotherapy have confirmed the previously mentioned results, but the optimal induction regimen has yet to be determined because of the heterogeneity of the patients entered in these trials. Among the various trials, the response rates to induction chemotherapy varied from 60 to 77%, and resectability rates ranged from 56 to 90%. The percentage of patients able to undergo complete resection ranged from 46 to 76%, and approximately 10% were found to have a pathologic complete response.

The University of Toronto study by Burkes and coworkers (1992) and the LCSG 881 trial reported by Wagner and associates (1994) tried to reproduce the results from the Memorial Sloan-Kettering Cancer Center experience by using a similar MVP induction regimen. All of the patients in these two trials had N_2 disease proven by mediastinoscopy. The LCSG also included a few patients who were designated stage IIIB by virtue of T_4 disease. In the Toronto trial, the overall response rate was 65% and the complete resection rate was 46%. The overall survival at 3 years was 26% and the median survival was 18.6 months for all 35 patients studied. A 17.9% treatment-related mortality occurred, two from bronchopleural fistula, one from mitomycin pulmonary toxicity, and four from septic deaths in

patients with postobstructive pneumonitis. In a preliminary report of the LCSG trial, the overall response rate was 46%, the complete resection rate was 36%, and the treatment related mortality was 12.5%.

These various trials with MVP demonstrate the high major response and resectability rates. Some groups, such as Lee and Ginsberg (1997), advocate, before the administration of MVP chemotherapy, complete resolution of tumor obstruction by either rigid bronchoscopy and débridement or laser ablation. Clearly, the Sloan-Kettering experience has been the most promising and effective. Oncologists are concerned about the perceived risk of mitomycin-induced pulmonary toxicity, however, especially postoperative adult respiratory distress syndrome. An 11% mitomycin-associated pulmonary toxicity occurred in the Memorial Sloan-Kettering experience in patients who received a cumulative dose of 24 mg/m².

Another similar trial from Memorial Sloan-Kettering, reported by Pisters and colleagues (1993), involved 68 patients treated with mitomycin, high-dose cisplatin, and either vinblastine or vincristine for two or three cycles before surgery. Study patients did not have preoperative radiation therapy and all were defined as having clinical N_2 disease by the presence of mediastinal adenopathy on chest radiography. Sixty-nine percent went on to surgery, with 19% of the resected patients (13% of the total patients) demonstrating complete histologic clearance of tumor. The median length of survival for these patients was 19.5 months, and the 1-year survival rate was 68%.

The results obtained from the CALGB protocol 8935, a multi-institutional phase II trimodality study for stage IIIA disease reported by Kumar and coinvestigators (1996), are illustrative both from the standpoint of the magnitude of the therapy and the patterns of recurrent disease. This study enrolled patients only with N_2 disease documented by mediastinoscopy who subsequently received two cycles of preoperative chemotherapy consisting of cisplatinum, 100 mg/m², and vinblastine, 5 mg/m². Sugarbaker and associates (1995) emphasized that the surgery included resection of the primary tumor and a complete mediastinal lymph node dissection. Patients who could be completely resected received an additional two cycles of postoperative chemotherapy and 5400 cGy of radiation therapy. Patients with unresectable disease received postoperative radiation therapy only to a dose of 5940 cGy.

Only 63 of 74 (85%) patients entered in the trial were able to complete the induction chemotherapy regimen as planned. Forty-six of the 63 (73% but only 62% of those originally enrolled in the trial) patients underwent resection, of whom only 23 of these were complete resections, whereas 17 (27%) were unresectable. Thirty-three of the 46 (72% but only 44% of those originally enrolled in the study) resected patients completed the postoperative chemotherapy and radiation therapy as planned. Overall survival at 3 years was 23% for all 74 eligible patients. Survival rates at 3 years for completely resected, incompletely resected, and unresectable patients were 46% (median, 20.9 months), 25% (median, 17.8 months), and 0% (median, 8.5 months), respectively. Of the resected patients, 28 recurred, with all but one having distant disease. In 12 of the 28 patients (43%), brain metastases occurred, as noted by Sugarbaker (1995) and Kumar (1996) and their colleagues.

These data demonstrate that trimodality therapy, although seemingly well-tolerated, is a difficult regimen to complete even for patients in optimal shape with minimal or no weight loss. Granted, some of the patients progressed during the induction regimen, resulting in their failure to complete the protocol, but of those who underwent operation only approximately two-thirds completed the postoperative therapy. Distant failure remains the major limitation despite the intuitive notion that treating distant micrometastatic disease should be advantageous. The use of preoperative chemotherapy presupposes that micrometastatic disease likely is present, although not detectable by current imaging technology, and, it is hoped, will be eliminated by the induction chemotherapy regimen. The success in controlling local disease has not translated into prevention of distant disease, which likely is present early in the course of disease but only comes to attention later in the course. Again, this begs the question regarding the contribution toward long-term survival made by the operation over and above the selection factor.

At the University of Miami, an intensive multimodality therapy protocol incorporating neoadjuvant chemotherapy was initiated in July 1985 for patients with either borderline resectable or unresectable stage III NSCLC. All patients tolerated chemotherapy with 5-fluorouracil, etoposide, and cisplatin (PEF). The combination PEF appears to yield results similar to MVP. The advantage of PEF over MVP are a lower incidence of myelosuppression and the inclusion of two radiosensitizers, namely cisplatin and 5-fluorouracil. Also, mitomycin, with its potential for pulmonary toxicity, is avoided in the PEF regimen. A complete response to the induction regimen occurred in two patients (6%) and a partial response in 22 (63%). Thirty-two patients underwent surgery and 26 patients were rendered disease free, including two found disease free at operation. The median survival for all patients was 19 months, with those undergoing incomplete surgical resection achieving 12 months and patients rendered disease free at operation achieving 21 months.

The Perugia group in 1988 tried to improve the curative potential of surgery. They enrolled 46 patients with clinical N_2 disease and gave two to three cycles of neoadjuvant cisplatin and etoposide. Darwish and associates (1994) reported that the overall response rate was 37 of 45 (82%). Surgical exploration was carried out in 35 patients with complete resections possible in 28 (62%) patients. Median survival for the entire group was 24.5 months, with a 2-year survival of 53%, similar to previously reported studies. However, unlike these studies, pathologic documentation of N_2 involvement was not required in this trial, leaving some question regarding the true stage of disease in each patient.

Between September 1987 and September 1989, Pujol and colleagues (1990) enrolled 33 patients with $T_3N_2M_0$ ($n = 32$) and T_4N_2 ($n = 1$) NSCLC were enrolled in a phase II trial. Chemotherapy consisted of three cycles of preoperative etoposide, cisplatin, ifosfamide, and mesna for 4 days. Responding patients underwent thoracotomy and then received 45 Gy of thoracic irradiation. Chemotherapy induced a 55% partial response rate, and a 15% complete response rate and complete resection were achieved in 55% of patients. Complete response was histologically confirmed for the five of the complete responders. Pujol and coworkers (1994, 1995) reported that the median survival was 11 months, although six patients were long-term survivors (3-year survival rate, 19%).

At the University of Navarra, Aristu and associates (1997) reported on 62 patients with histologically confirmed stage III NSCLC who were treated with neoadjuvant chemotherapy of cisplatin, mitomycin, and vindesine. Each cycle was repeated every 4 weeks for one to six cycles. Resection was attempted 4 to 5 weeks after the last course of chemotherapy. Intraoperative radiation therapy of 1000 to 1500 cGy was delivered and postoperative external beam radiation therapy of 4500 cGy was begun 4 weeks after surgery. Only partial responses were seen (64%), and 29 patients (53%) underwent resection. The median survival time was 10 months, and the 5-year survival rate was 29% and 7% for stage IIIA and stage IIIB, respectively. In spite of the similar response rates for stages IIIA and IIIB in this study, differences exist in complete resection (86% versus 40%), and disease-free and local disease-free survival (50 to 70% versus 28 to 36%, $P = .15$ and .55, respectively).

At the University of Pisa, from 1990 to 1993, 36 patients were enrolled by Chella and colleagues (1995) in a phase II study aimed at determining the feasibility of surgery, patterns of disease recurrence, and survival after neoadjuvant and adjuvant MVP in NSCLC. Cisplatin was administered at a dose of 90 mg/m^2. The overall objective response was 78.1%. Three histologically complete responses and 22 partial responses occurred. Patients with histologically proven lymph node involvement at the time of surgery underwent radiation therapy of 50 Gy to the mediastinum and supraclavicular fossae. Three postoperative deaths occurred, two caused by empyema and one caused by pulmonary embolism. Median survival was 31 months, with a 3-year survival rate of 49%.

A report by Elias and coworkers (1997) from the Brigham and Women's Hospital describes the use of cisplatin, 5-fluorouracil, and leucovorin before thoracotomy followed by thoracic irradiation of 54 to 60 Gy. Thirty-four patients with N_2 disease were treated, 28 patients received a thoracotomy, and complete resection was obtained in 21 patients (75%). Mean survival time was 18 months and six patients remain alive and disease free with a median follow-up of 47 (range, 33 to 50) months.

From these phase II trials, it is safe to conclude that the neoadjuvant regimens are well tolerated and produce meaningful response rates. A suggestion of improved long-term survival exists in this group of patients after surgical resection and especially in the subset of patients who achieve a pathologic complete response. This further underscores the importance of better chemotherapeutic agents that can achieve a higher percentage of responses.

Based on the feasibility of neoadjuvant therapy and the encouraging results obtained in patients with locally advanced disease, it was only logical to try this regimen in patients with a less advanced stage of disease, specifically stage IIB disease. These patients, though a more favorable group than patients with stage IIIA disease, still have less than a 50% 5-year survival and thus a multimodality approach can be justified. The Bimodality Lung Oncology Team (BLOT) trial is a multi-institutional trial looking at neoadjuvant chemotherapy in stage IIB disease. The phase III trial that will follow completion of the BLOT trial will randomize these patients with early stage disease to preoperative chemotherapy or surgery alone. This should provide the definitive answer as to whether preoperative chemotherapy increases overall survival enough to justify the delay in operation in a group classically treated with operation alone.

Neoadjuvant Chemotherapy: Randomized Trials

The most compelling data in support of induction chemotherapy come from two randomized phase III trials; these have been conducted by Rosell (1994a, 1994b) and Roth (1994) and their associates. These two studies evaluated 60 patients each with stage IIIA NSCLC. Both studies included patients with clinical N_2 disease as well as those with T_3N_0 or N_1 lesions. All patients were randomly selected to receive either surgery alone or three cycles of platinum-based chemotherapeutic regimens followed by surgery.

The M. D. Anderson study by Roth and colleagues (1994) compared 60 patients randomized to perioperative chemotherapy followed by operation, and then three more cycles of chemotherapy versus surgery alone. The chemotherapy consisted of cyclophosphamide, etoposide, and cisplatin. A significant improvement in survival occurred in those patients randomized to the combined therapy regimen. Results indicated a response rate of 35% in the perioperative chemotherapy arm and 56% survival at 3 years. The 3-year survival rate in the surgical arm of the study was 15%, with six patients surviving to 3 years or more in the chemotherapy arm. Median survival in the surgery only group was 11 months versus 64 months in the combined therapy group (P >.008). This is all the more interesting considering that less than 40% of the patients in each group underwent complete resection (39% combined therapy versus 31% surgery alone). This trial is notable for several reasons. It clearly showed an advantage to neoadjuvant therapy in a group of patients with locally advanced disease. Survival in the surgery only group was significantly shorter than what would be expected, however, making the survival difference between the groups seems more striking. Excluded from the trial were patients with left lung tumors and left paratracheal disease, because these patients' tumors were thought to be unresectable. The numbers are small, and all of the patients, before entry, had to be judged to be potentially resectable, thus, some selection bias is inherent in the study. What is not known is how many patients were screened to find the 60 patients who were ultimately randomized.

Rosell and colleagues (1994a, 1994b) in Barcelona randomized 60 patients with stage IIIA disease, 44 of whom had N_2 disease. One group was treated with operation and postoperative radiation therapy of 50 Gy, whereas the other group received neoadjuvant chemotherapy consisting of mitomycin, ifosfamide, and cisplatin. Median survival was 26 months in patients treated with the combination preoperative regimen compared with 8 months in patients undergoing operation and radiation therapy alone (P <.001). The median period of disease-free survival was 20 months in the former group, as compared with 5 months in the latter (P <.001. In each group, 90% of the patients underwent resection. The rate of recurrence was 56% in the group treated with chemotherapy and 74% in the group without chemotherapy. This trial also showed, as reported by Rosell and associates (1996), a significant (P <.001) improvement in survival for the groups receiving induction chemotherapy. The preoperative regimen was well tolerated with no chemotherapy-related mortality, although two patients in each treatment group died postoperatively.

The aforementioned study by Rosell and associates (1994a, 1994b) was terminated early when an interim analysis demonstrated a highly significant difference in survival. This trial is difficult to analyze because the control group seemed to have an unexpectedly short survival time, even for patients with stage IIIA disease. Rosell and coworkers (1995) analyzed the tumor specimens for the presence of mutated K-*ras* oncogenes as a marker of poor prognosis. The investigation suggested that mutated K-*ras* constitutes an additional prognostic factor that deserves to be included together with the tumor, node, metastasis (TNM) classification. The surgery/radiation therapy group had tumors with a higher incidence of K-*ras* (42% versus 15%) and aneuploid cellular content (70% versus 29%). Rosell and associates in 1996 and 1997 suggest this may be a treatment effect of the chemotherapy by destruction of those tumor cells with aneuploid content. Alternatively, there may have been inhomogeneity between the two patient groups, as suggested by Lee and Ginsberg (1997).

Prospective, randomized trials that have been completed show the superiority of preoperative neoadjuvant chemotherapy followed by operation compared with operation alone in patients with N_2 disease. Both trials were terminated early when interim analysis indicated a survival advantage in the chemotherapy arm. However, both of these trials are flawed in that they included a heterogeneous patient population comprised of those with N_2 disease and with T_3N_0 disease, the numbers were small, and the control

Table 106-7. Neoadjuvant Chemotherapy for Non–Small Cell Lung Cancer, Randomized Trials

	Rosell et al. (1994b)		Roth et al. (1994)		Pass et al. (1992)	
	Surgery	Chemotherapy	Surgery	Chemotherapy	Surgery	Chemotherapy
Patients	30	30	32	28	13	14
Chemotherapy arm		MIP		CEP		PE
Squamous histology (%)	37	17	34	39	—	—
Resection rate (%)	90	85	66	61	86	85
Response rate (%)	—	60	—	35	—	62
Disease-free survival (mos)	5	20	9	NR	5.8	12.7
Median survival (mos)	8	26	11	64	15.6	28.7
2-year survival (%)	0	25	25	60	—	—
3-year survival (%)	—	—	19	56	23	50

CEP, cyclophosphamide, etoposide, cisplatin; MIP, mitomycin, ifosfamide, cisplatin; NR, not reported; PE, cisplatin, etoposide.

groups had a shorter survival than what would ordinarily be expected (Table 106-7).

Another earlier attempt at a randomized trial that was reported by Dautzenberg and coworkers (1990) was also stopped early but for other reasons. In 1985, investigators in France began to assess cisplatin, cyclophosphamide, and vindesine (PCV) preoperative chemotherapy in patients with resectable NSCLC. Patients were randomized to receive either two preoperative courses of PCV chemotherapy, operation, and two postoperative courses of PCV or immediate surgery. There were 26 randomized patients, 13 in each group. In the chemotherapy arm, 11 patients agreed to receive the two preoperative courses of chemotherapy. The results were disappointing, however, because despite the 16% reduction in tumor volume in the PCV group as compared with the control group, this value did not reach statistical significance. A response was observed in five patients (45%), and a progression was observed in four patients, leading to a cancellation of operation in two of them. Although no death could be related to the chemotherapy, it was decided to stop entering new patients into this trial because of the rate of preoperative progression in the PCV group. The authors concluded that in future trials of perioperative or preoperative chemotherapy, medical staging should be planned after the first cycle and after the second cycle of chemotherapy to monitor progression early enough so that surgical resection is still feasible.

At the National Institutes of Health, Pass and associates (1992) have attempted to randomize 27 stage IIIA patients with documented mediastinal adenopathy to two treatment arms. Thirteen patients were treated with preoperative platinum and etoposide, followed by surgery, and a postoperative course of the same chemotherapy. The other 14 patients received only 54 to 60 Gy of postoperative irradiation. The resectability rate was approximately 85% in both groups, with no operative mortality. Eight of the 13 patients receiving platinum and etoposide responded as evidenced by a 50% or greater radiographic tumor shrinkage after two cycles with one histologically confirmed complete response. The median survival and disease-free interval for the induc-

tion chemotherapy arm was 28.7 months and 12.7 months, respectively, versus 15.6 months and 5.8 months for the control arm. The differences were not statistically significant, however, perhaps because of the small number of patients. Because the original study was meant to accrue 148 patients to detect a 20% improvement in 5-year survival caused by chemotherapy, the power of the study was reduced when the trial was closed early with only 27 patients. Again, the study demonstrated the feasibility of this approach, as noted by Belani and Ramanathan (1998).

Neoadjuvant Chemoradiation Therapy

Although a standard induction regimen remains to be defined, a number of studies have been performed in which preoperative radiation therapy has been used in addition to chemotherapy to improve response rates (Table 106-8). The rationale for chemotherapy alone is that it potentially allows greater dose intensity, as well as the use of some drugs such as mitomycin, which cannot be administered with radiation therapy. As expected, the more aggressive trimodality strategy of chemoradiation therapy followed by surgery can be more toxic, as noted by Reboul and associates (1996) and Lilenbaum and Green (1994).

One of the earliest experiences with neoadjuvant chemoradiation therapy was reported by Spain (1988, 1993) from the Penrose Hospital in Colorado Springs. From 1981 to 1985, 31 patients with locoregionally advanced disease were enrolled in a study of neoadjuvant therapy with MVP and continuous thoracic irradiation (n = 26). Spain (1993) reported that a median follow-up from the initiation of therapy was 81 months; median survival was 19 months with 3- and 6-year survival of 33% and 23%, respectively.

Between 1981 and 1984, investigators at the Dana-Farber Cancer Institute treated 41 patients with pathologically determined marginally resectable stage IIIA disease. Included within this group were patients with T_3N_0 disease and patients with N_2 mediastinal metastases. Patients received two cycles of perioperative CAP chemotherapy fol-

Table 106-8. Neoadjuvant Chemoradiation Therapy for Non–Small Cell Lung Cancer

Group	N	Stage	Preoperative Chemoradiation therapy	Postoperative Chemotherapy	Postoperative Response (%)	Complete Resection (%)	Median Survival (mos)	Survival Benefit	Reference
Penrose Hospital	31	III	MVP + XRT	None	73	23	19	3-year survival (33%); 6-year survival (23%)	Spain (1988)
LCSG 831	39	IIIA	CAP + 30 Gy	± XRT	51	33	11	2-year survival (8%)	Eagan et al. (1987)
LCSG 852	85	IIIA	PF + 30 Gy	± XRT	56	34	13	2-year survival (22%)	Weiden and Piantadosi (1991)
Dana-Farber	41	IIIA	CAP + 30 Gy	CAP + 25 Gy	29	88	32	1-year survival (75%); 5-year survival (31%)	Skarin (1989)
Cancer and Leukemia Group B 8634	41	IIIA	PVF + 30 Gy	± XRT	46	62	16	1-year survival (58%); 2-year survival (35%)	Strauss et al. (1992b)
Southwest Oncology Group 8805	126	III	PE + 45 Gy	PE ± XRT	59	86	13	2-year survival (40%); 3-year survival (26%)	Rusch et al. (1993)
Rush-Presbyterian	64	III	PF + 40 Gy	None	56	23	16	1-year survival (61%); 5-year survival (30%)	Taylor et al. (1987)
Rush-Presbyterian	64	III	PEF + 40 Gy	None	84	36	13	3-year survival (30%)	Recine et al. (1990)
Roger Williams Cancer Center	53	III	PE + 56 Gy	None	89	51	24	2-year survival (50%)	Weitberg et al. (1993)
Favaretto and colleagues	39	III	CE + 52 Gy	CE	67	51	16	3-year survival (18%); 5-year survival (13%)	Favaretto et al. (1996)
Massachusetts General Hospital	42	IIIA	PVF + 42 Gy	PVF + 15 Gy	74	81	25	2-year survival (66%); 5-year survival (37%)	Choi et al. (1997)

CAP, cyclophosphamide, doxorubicin, and cisplatin; CE, cyclophosphamide, etoposide; LCSG, Lung Cancer Study Group; MVP, mitomycin C, vindesine or vinblastine, and cisplatin; PE, cisplatin, etoposide; PEF, 5-fluorouracil, etoposide, and cisplatin; PF, cisplatin, 5-fluorouracil; PVF, cisplatin, vinblastine, 5-fluorouracil; XRT, radiation therapy.

lowed by a radiation dose of 30 Gy. A complete resection was accomplished in 36 of 41 patients (88%). Postoperative radiation therapy and four more cycles of CAP were used in all cases. Tumor shrinkage was observed in 53% of patients after neoadjuvant CAP, and 90% of potentially operable patients were resected. Skarin and associates (1989) reported that the median survival was 32 months and the 1-year and 5-year survivals were 75% and 31%, respectively. Eighteen of 36 patients failed systemically (66%) and four patients failed locally.

A second trial at Dana-Farber was begun in 1983 that attempted better systemic treatment before locoregional therapy. A total of 54 patients were treated, with 39% showing some response to neoadjuvant chemotherapy. Thirty-one patients went to the operating room, of whom 24 (44%) were completely resected. The median survival time was 17.9 months overall and 33.5 months for completely resected patients; an overall 5-year survival of approximately 22% was observed by Elias and coworkers (1994).

One of the first trials of combined chemoradiation therapy came from the LCSG. LCSG 831 treated 39 patients with clinical stage III disease. The patients received three cycles of chemotherapy with CAP and 30 Gy of irradiation in 300-cGy fractions. The overall response rate to induction therapy was 51%. Thirty-three percent of patients subsequently were able to undergo a complete resection. Eagan and associates

(1987) reported an overall survival of 8% at 2 years with a median survival of 11 months. No statistically significant survival differences between patients not having thoracotomy and those who had thoracotomy or even those with complete tumor excision occurred. The patients who received chemotherapy, chest irradiation, and surgical resection had a low incidence of local or regional failure (5%), but distant disease remained problematic.

The difference in patient outcome in this trial compared with the Dana-Farber trial may be caused primarily by patient selection; the latter trial included T_3 (chest wall) cases and excluded patients with extracapsular N_2 disease. Thus, the Dana-Farber trial had a more favorable stage III subset mix than the LCSG trial. Furthermore, according to Albain (1993), the LCSG trial did not allow resection for postinduction stable disease; the surgical resection possibly had a favorable effect on this subgroup in the Dana-Farber trial.

Compared with the Dana-Farber experience and LCSG 831, the next three trimodality trials used higher cisplatin doses and enrolled more patients. The LCSG trial 852, reported by Weiden and Piantadosi (1991, 1994), used neoadjuvant cisplatin, 5-fluorouracil, and partially concurrent low-dose radiation therapy (3000 cGy in 15 fractions) in 85 patients with stage IIIA (80%) or stage IIIB (13%) disease. Only two patients achieved a complete response, and 46 achieved a partial response, with an overall response rate of 56%. Fifty-four (64%) underwent thoracotomy, but only 34% had complete resections. Median survival of all patients was 13 months. The investigators concluded that this neoadjuvant regimen did not provide major benefit in patients with advanced but potentially resectable NSCLC. What became apparent from this study, however, was that neoadjuvant chemoradiation therapy altered the usual pattern of disease recurrence. Patients whose tumors were completely resected were less likely to have isolated local recurrences initially (17% versus 46%) and were more likely to have metastatic disease in the brain (17% versus 5%) than were patients whose tumors could not be completely resected.

Strauss and associates (1992b) reported the treatment and results of the CALGB 8634 study of neoadjuvant treatment on 41 patients with mediastinoscopically confirmed stage IIIA NSCLC (80% N_2; 20% T_3N_0 or T_3N_1). The patients received two cycles of preoperative chemotherapy with cisplatin, vinblastine, and 5-fluorouracil along with concurrent 30-Gy chest irradiation in 15 fractions. Resection was performed in 76% of the patients followed by another cycle of chemotherapy and 30-Gy chest irradiation. A total of 61% of patients had resectable disease. Three treatment-related deaths occurred. Median survival was 15.5 months and 1-year survival was 58%.

In one of the largest phase II trials, the SWOG 8805 study, published by Albain (1995) and Rusch (1993) and their colleagues, used concurrent induction chemotherapy and radiation therapy in 154 patients with stage IIIA and IIIB disease. Cisplatin was administered on days 1, 8, 29, and 36, etoposide on days 1 to 5, 29 to 33, and 45 Gy of radiation therapy given over 5 weeks. Two notable differences between the SWOG trial and early neoadjuvant trials were the use of higher dose, continuous radiation therapy and the concurrent administration of the chemotherapy and the radiation therapy. All patients had pathologically confirmed N_2 or N_3 disease (IIIA, $n = 75$; and IIIB, $n = 51$). Surgical resection was performed 2 to 4 weeks after completion of the induction therapy in patients demonstrating tumor regression or stable disease. Of the 154 patients, 127 were eligible for resection. Complete resection was accomplished in 74% of patients taken to the operating room. Although there was an 8% incidence of postoperative death, no tumor was found in 22% of the resections. A clinical response or stable disease was verified in 87% of the patients. Complete surgical resection was accomplished in 86% of the 100 patients who underwent exploration. Median survival in stages IIIA and IIIB was essentially the same at 13 and 16 months, respectively. Three-year survival was 26% and 24% in these groups. Patients with a pathologic complete response in the lymph nodes had a 30-month median survival compared with 10 months for those with persistent lymph node disease ($P <.0005$). Of no surprise, according to Albain and coworkers (1995), the strongest predictor of long-term survival was lack of positive mediastinal nodes at surgery, with a 3-year survival of 44% versus 18%, in those who had persistent nodal disease ($P = .0005$). The SWOG investigators noted substantial toxicity. Two treatment-related deaths (1.6%) occurred during the induction therapy period. During the postoperative period, 11 (8.4%) additional deaths occurred. Most of the lethal toxicities were drug related. Rusch and Feins (1994) concluded the feasibility of instituting neoadjuvant therapy in patients with stage IIIB NSCLC and recommended that future clinical trials should evaluate combined modality approaches in this subset of patients as well.

The Rush-Presbyterian group, as reported by Bonomi (1993), has performed two sequential neoadjuvant trials of low-dose cisplatin, chemotherapy, and concurrent radiation therapy in patients with clinical stage III disease. In the first 64 patients reported by Taylor and associates (1987), 5-fluorouracil was added to the cisplatin. In the second trial, 64 patients also received etoposide, as recorded in the publications of Reddy (1992), Recine (1990), Faber (1989), Bonomi (1986), and Pincus (1988) and their coworkers. All patients received 40 Gy of split-course radiation therapy administered concurrently with the four cycles of induction chemotherapy. Bonomi (1993) recorded that the toxicity of the induction regimen was significant. The third trial ($n = 45$) used the same dosages of chemotherapy, but the radiation dosage was altered to 150-cGy fractions given twice daily. Of the 128 patients entered into the first two studies, 85 were considered potential candidates for surgical resection, and 73% ultimately went to thoracotomy. The complete resection rate was 68% and the operative mortality was 5%. The overall survival rate for all 85 patients was 40% at 3 years, with a median survival of 21 months. The addition of etoposide to the induction regimen in the second trial ($n = 29$) did not increase the response or resectability rates significantly.

The overall response rate, complete and partial, was 67% (86 of 128). Histologic absence of tumor was observed in 22% of resected specimens, and this did not correlate with disappearance of disease documented by imaging studies. Complete resection of gross disease was accomplished in 77% (99 of 128) of patients who were initially considered eligible for surgery. Overall surgical mortality was 5% (5 of 102) and there was a 4% (4 of 102) bronchopleural fistula rate. The Kaplan-Meier survival estimate for all 128 patients revealed a median survival of 22 months and a projected 5-year survival rate of 34%.

Despite the relatively encouraging results observed with preoperative chemoradiation therapy, the majority of patients eventually died of metastatic disease. Investigators at Rush-Presbyterian initiated a subsequent trial building on the etoposide/platinum and radiation regimen by adding paclitaxel. Bonomi (1998) has noted that this agent has produced a 40% 1-year survival in two phase II trials. In addition, it has been shown by Natale (1997, 1998) to enhance the effect of radiation therapy in vitro. Bunn (1997) and Bonomi and associates (1995) have enrolled all stage IIIA and selected stage IIIB patients considered eligible for pulmonary resection after two courses of chemoradiation therapy (40 Gy). Preliminary results demonstrate that pulmonary resection is feasible after treatment with radiation therapy and concurrent paclitaxel-containing chemotherapy. Patient accrual by Bonomi (1998) and Bonomi and colleagues (1996) is ongoing to determine the ensuing efficacy. The relatively high incidence of postoperative bronchopulmonary complications, as noted by Bonomi and associates (1997), suggests however that the use of preoperative paclitaxel-containing chemotherapy and simultaneous thoracic irradiation should be looked at closely. Other groups, such as those of Pisters (1997) and Palackdharry (1997) and their coworkers, are exploring the use of paclitaxel in the neoadjuvant setting either as a single agent or in combination. As the data mature, they may provide the basis for intergroup randomized trials comparing neoadjuvant paclitaxel regimens.

A trial presented by Favaretto and colleagues (1996) enrolled 39 patients with stage III disease. Treatment consisted of two courses of cisplatin and etoposide plus radiation therapy delivered in two cycles of 2560 cGy each. After operation, three additional chemotherapy courses were planned. The complete response rate was 67% and a resection was completed in 20 (51%) patients. Of the 23 patients who attained a complete response, five relapsed locally and 11 only with distant disease. Median survival was 16 months with 18% 3-year survival and 13% 5-year survival. Resected patients had a median survival of 21 months, versus 10 months for unresected patients ($P = .01$). No significant difference was evident between stage IIIA and stage IIIB disease.

At the Massachusetts General Hospital, 42 biopsy-proven patients with N_2 disease were treated by Choi and associates (1997) with two courses of cisplatin, vinblastine, 5-fluorouracil, and 42-Gy radiation therapy followed by operation followed by another course of twice daily chemoradiation therapy. The study was used to evaluate tumor response, resection rate, and pathologic tumor downstaging. Treatment-related mortality was noted in 7% of patients. Mean survival was 25 months with an actuarial 5-year survival of 37%. Importantly, concurrent chemoradiation therapy resulted in 67% tumor downstaging, compared with 13.5% in the CALGB 8935 reported by Sugarbaker and associates (1995), 28% in the University of Toronto experience reported by Burkes and colleagues (1992), and 30% in the Memorial Sloan-Kettering Cancer Center experience reported by Martini and coworkers (1993). Results are difficult to interpret because of small patient numbers. However, Choi and associates' (1997) study suggested the possible added benefit of twice daily radiation therapy given with concurrent chemotherapy.

Bedini and associates (1993) in Italy reported on a phase II study of 38 patients, 27 of whom had "nonresectable" stage IIIB disease. They used concurrent continuous infusion of cisplatin given at a daily dose of 6 mg/m², plus radiation therapy of 50 Gy. Treatments were given on an outpatient basis by means of a central venous catheter and a portable infusion pump. Thoracotomy was carried out in 18 patients. Partial or complete locoregional response at 4 weeks after treatment completion was 83%. Eighteen patients were

resected. Overall 1-, 2-, and 3-year progression-free survival probabilities were 42%, 24%, and 21%, respectively.

Another use of continuous infusion cisplatin involved 53 patients with stage IIIA disease treated with a multimodality approach consisting of induction radiation therapy (55.8 Gy) and two cycles of concurrent chemotherapy with cisplatin for 4 days given by continuous infusion and bolus etoposide, on days 2 and 4 of each cycle, followed by operation and additional adjuvant chemotherapy that was reported by Weitberg and coworkers (1993). Of the 53 evaluable patients, 47 achieved clinical responses after induction therapy, and complete surgical resection was accomplished in 27 patients. The median survival of the entire group was 24 months; the median survival of the resected patients had not been reached; however, their 6-year survival rate was 55%.

In a retrospective analysis, Yoneda and colleagues (1993) reported on 25 patients with stage III NSCLC who were treated with cisplatin-based chemotherapy and thoracic irradiation (50 to 75 Gy) followed by surgery. Eighteen patients underwent curative resection. Severe postoperative complications occurred in five patients (20%), with one death reported. Disease recurred in 5 of the 18 patients who underwent a curative resection. The estimated 3-year survival was 67% for all patients. The treatment-related morbidity in this study seems excessive.

It is difficult to draw conclusions based on these trials because considerable differences in eligibility criteria exist. The LCSG and SWOG trials included both stage IIIA and IIIB, whereas the Rush-Presbyterian trial included patients with stage IIIA (now IIB) but not N_2, and a few patients had stage IIIB tumors. Another difficulty involves the measurement of response. Certain investigators determine response based on radiologic appearance whereas others base it on pathologic response. They are not necessarily equivalent and are not even always stated.

In an attempt to definitively determine if adding chemotherapy to surgery and radiation therapy improves survival compared with radiation therapy and surgery alone, CALGB 9134 has been undertaken, as noted by Rusch and Feins (1994). A target of 250 patients with stage IIIA disease will be randomized to two possible treatment strategies. The first will receive a radiation dose of 40 Gy followed by surgery and adjuvant 20 Gy of irradiation. The other arm will receive preoperative and postoperative cisplatin, etoposide, and granulocyte-colony stimulating factor immunotherapy in addition to 40 Gy adjuvant radiation therapy.

A large National Cancer Institute trial, described by Green and Barkley (1997), currently is attempting to determine the role of surgical resection in the combined modality treatment of patients with stage IIIA biopsy-proven $T_{1-3}N_2$ disease. All patients will receive induction radiation therapy of 45 Gy over 5 weeks and concurrent cisplatin and etoposide for two cycles 28 days apart. Before this induction therapy, patients will be randomized to receive either surgical resection afterward, if feasible, plus two additional cycles of chemotherapy or additional radiation therapy (60 Gy total) plus two additional cycles of chemotherapy. Finally, there is an ongoing North American Intergroup 0139 trial (Radiation Therapy Oncology Group, SWOG, Eastern Cooperative Oncology Group, CALGB, North Central Cancer Treatment Group, and National Cancer Institute of Canada), as reported by Martini (1997) and Albain (1995) and their associates and also recorded by Albain (1997), of chemoradiation therapy with a target enrollment of 512 patients. This is one of the largest trials in this field to date, testing the trimodality program developed by SWOG.

CONCLUSION

The optimal and definitive management of patients with early stage NSCLC, stages I and II, consists of surgical resection. Currently, stage IV patients usually are not curable with any available therapy and the only issue is palliation.

The entire group of stage III tumors remains an arena of debate. This accounts for a large group because approximately 40% of patients fit into this group at the time of presentation. The treatment, however, for locally advanced NSCLC remains controversial despite the large number of trials of adjuvant and neoadjuvant therapy that have been completed. Concurrent chemotherapy and radiation therapy have become the most common form of treatment for stage IIIA NSCLC when it is believed to be unresectable. Usually, this type of combination therapy is the definitive treatment recommended for most patients with stage IIIB disease, when operation usually has little role in management. However, it has been difficult to define the best regimen because considerable differences exist among the completed clinical trials with respect to eligibility criteria, accuracy of pretreatment staging, and induction regimens. The criteria for taking patients to thoracotomy after induction treatment also vary among these trials but usually rely more on the absence of documented progression and the absence of disseminated disease than on response gauged by imaging studies.

Despite all of the clinical trials that have used cisplatin-containing regimes, the agent currently favored is carboplatin. This agent, when combined with paclitaxel, is the current regimen of choice for patients with disseminated disease and undoubtedly will be used in phase II neoadjuvant trials as well. At present, despite considerable optimism regarding some of the newer agents, one must conclude that neither radiation therapy nor chemotherapy nor a combination of the two can be recommended as standard treatment after a complete resection for lung cancer even with locally advanced disease. Currently, no evidence exists that any of these regimens when used in the adjuvant setting has been definitively shown to improve survival. Outside of a clinical trial, postoperative adjuvant therapy cannot be recommended at this time. In patients with NSCLC the role of induction chemotherapy has been established in bulky mediastinal lymph node (N_2) as well as in patients with potentially resectable N_2 disease, though the two positive

randomized trials by Rosell (1994a, 1994b) and Roth (1994) and their colleagues remain controversial. It remains difficult to define the optimal regimen for neoadjuvant therapy as the standard combination regimen has changed, as pointed out by Feld (1996), Johnson (1994), and Lee and Ginsberg (1997) since most of the phase II trials and both of the phase III trials have been reported. Even the current intergroup trial that is looking at the role that operation plays in the management of patients with N_2 disease uses a chemotherapy regimen, cisplatin and etoposide, that currently is no longer in favor. Different chemotherapy regimens have been used, with either low-dose cisplatin alone or with other agents in a multidrug regimen. The role of paclitaxel (Taxol) and carboplatin in the neoadjuvant setting either alone or combined with radiation therapy remains to be determined.

Cisplatin-based regimens, the gold standard of NSCLC chemotherapy since the mid-1980s, ultimately may not be as active as other regimens that include agents such as epirubicin, docetaxel, irinotecan, topotecan, gemcitabine, vinorelbine (taxoid) (Navelbine), and edatrexate as suggested by many investigators such as Saijo (1998), Natale (1997, 1998), Greco and Hainsworth (1997), Tan and Ang (1996), as well as by Bonomi (1996) and Cerny (1994) and their associates, and Bunn (1994), Livingston (1994), Murphy and colleagues (1993), Green (1993), and Gralla (1990). Various combinations of these agents, some without a platinum compound but often with paclitaxel, are currently in clinical trial.

The results of a meta-analysis by the Non–Small Cell Lung Cancer Collaborative Group (1995) looking at 52 randomized clinical trials using cisplatin-based chemotherapeutic regimens demonstrated that the cumulative survival benefit was small, approximately 3% at 2 years. Johnson (1994) suggests that the chemotherapeutic trials could have failed to demonstrate survival advantage because of failure to commit to a single regimen by various intergroup trials, inadequate doses and dose intensity of active agents, or inadequacy of trial design.

One of the main problems with many of the chemotherapeutic regimens is patient compliance. As observed by Feld (1994) and Niiranen (1992) and their coinvestigators, chemotherapy-induced nausea has consistently been a source of problems in enforcing treatments. The use of new antiemetics may improve compliance and consequently improve survival statistics.

Future studies will attempt to incorporate novel schemes for the treatment of locally advanced NSCLC. Novel radiation therapy fractionation regimens have been an area of continued investigation. The Radiation Therapy Oncology Group published a randomized trial of hyperfractionated radiation therapy showing some improved survival at higher doses. Continuous hyperfractionated accelerated radiation therapy is another novel regimen in which multiple fractions of irradiation are given each day, and the entire course is completed over a shorter period. It remains to be seen how operation and these new radiation therapy techniques are combined.

Induction radiation therapy alone likely is not indicated in the treatment of NSCLC. No survival benefit has ever been demonstrated. Preoperative radiation therapy given before operation in patients with so-called Pancoast's tumors has classically been used but has never been subjected to a prospective trial to assess its efficacy. Currently, an intergroup phase II nonrandomized trial is attempting to assess the feasibility of combined chemotherapy and radiation therapy as a preoperative regimen for this subset of apical lung tumors that involve the thoracic inlet.

Dillman and associates (1990) have predicted that in combination with chemotherapy, radiation therapy likely will find a role within an effective induction regimen, particularly in stage IIIA disease. Postoperative radiation therapy has been shown to reduce locoregional relapse rates in completely resected disease, but no demonstrable survival benefit has ever been convincingly shown. In incompletely resected disease, usually more advanced initially, there may be a similar effect of smaller magnitude, as suggested by Payne (1994). Despite these data, postoperative radiation therapy continues to be recommended almost as a routine in patients with N_1 or N_2 resected disease. The authors tend to avoid routine postoperative radiation therapy outside of a protocol setting, recognizing that it is without survival benefit. Close postoperative follow-up should avoid a situation in which a local recurrence would become problematic and if a local or regional recurrence is detected it may be promptly treated with a course of radiation therapy. As well, radiation therapy is useful for the palliation of symptoms in patients with metastatic disease.

Of great importance is the consideration of quality of life in patients undergoing these combined regimens, an area that has not been adequately addressed up to the present time. Quality-of-life measurement tools are available to incorporate into future studies so that additional information should be forthcoming. Toxicity from these preoperative regimens can be substantial, especially if an element of post-obstructive pneumonia exists. In the SWOG trial, as noted by Albain and colleagues (1995), there were two deaths that resulted from the preoperative regimen, and 13% of patients experienced grade 4 or greater acute toxicity. An overall treatment-related mortality of 15% occurred in the neoadjuvant study by Burkes and associates (1992) from Toronto. This further underscores the importance of confining multimodality therapy for N_2 disease to a protocol setting as opposed to routine community use, despite the current enthusiasm, until such time that definitive evidence of efficacy has been established.

In an interesting review by Mackillop and coworkers (1987), 118 Canadian physicians who treat lung cancer were asked how they would wish to be managed if they had NSCLC. Although opinion was divided as to the role of immediate radiation therapy in inoperable cancer and the role of postoperative radiation therapy followed by incomplete surgery, there was little controversy as to the role of chemotherapy. Three percent of doctors wanted adjuvant chemotherapy after surgery for early disease, 9% wanted chemotherapy for advanced disease confined to the chest, and 15% wanted chemotherapy for symptomatic metastatic disease. Another similar questionnaire by Palmer and associates (1990) was sent to 461 American and Canadian physicians. This series reported no evidence of a consensus as to preferred treatment in clinical situations. Perhaps with the better regimens available today, the answers might be different.

REFERENCES

Albain KS: Induction therapy followed by definitive local control for stage III non–small-cell lung cancer. A review, with a focus on recent trimodality trials. Chest *103*(Suppl):43S, 1993.

Albain KS: Induction chemotherapy with/without radiation followed by surgery in stage III non–small-cell lung cancer. Oncology *11*(Suppl 9):51, 1997.

Albain KS, et al: Concurrent cisplatin/etoposide plus chest radiotherapy followed by surgery for stages IIIA (N2) and IIIB non–small-cell lung cancer: mature results of Southwest Oncology Group phase II study 8805. J Clin Oncol *13*:1880, 1995.

The American Society of Clinical Oncology: Clinical practice guidelines for the treatment of unresectable non–small-cell lung cancer. Adopted on May 16, 1997. J Clin Oncol *15*:2996, 1997.

Aristu J, et al: Cisplatin, mitomycin, and vindesine followed by intraoperative and postoperative radiotherapy for stage III non–small cell lung cancer: final results of a phase II study. Am J Clin Oncol *20*:276, 1997.

Armstrong JG, et al: Induction chemotherapy for non–small cell lung cancer with clinically evident mediastinal node metastases: the role of postoperative radiotherapy. International J Radiat Oncol Biol Phys *23*:605, 1992.

Astudillo J, Conill C: Role of postoperative radiation therapy in stage IIIa non–small cell lung cancer. Ann Thorac Surg *50*:618, 1990.

Bedini AV, et al: Non-resectable stage IIIa-b lung carcinoma: a phase II study on continuous infusion of cisplatin and concurrent radiotherapy (plus adjuvant surgery). Lung Cancer *10*:73, 1993.

Belani CP, Ramanathan RK: Combined-modality treatment of locally advanced non–small cell lung cancer: incorporation of novel chemotherapeutic agents. Chest *113*(Suppl):53S, 1998.

Blanke CD, Johnson DH: Combined modality therapy in non–small cell lung cancer. Curr Opin Oncol *7*:144, 1995.

Bleehen NM, et al: Combined radiation and chemotherapy for unresectable non–small cell lung carcinoma. Lung Cancer *10*(Suppl 1):S19, 1994.

Bloedorn FG: The value of preoperative radiation in the treatment of lung cancer: results of a preliminary study. Proc Natl Cancer Conf *5*:475, 1964.

Bonomi P: Radiation and simultaneous cisplatin in non–small cell lung cancer. Int J Radiat Oncol Biol Phys *27*:739, 1993.

Bonomi P: Eastern Cooperative Oncology Group experience with chemotherapy in advanced non–small cell lung cancer. Chest *113*(Suppl):13S, 1998.

Bonomi P, Reddy S, Faber LP: Concurrent chemotherapy and thoracic irradiation in non–small cell lung cancer. Hematol Oncol Clin North Am *4*:1143, 1990.

Bonomi P, et al: Phase II trial of etoposide, cisplatin, continuous infusion 5-fluorouracil, and simultaneous split-course radiation therapy in stage III non–small-cell bronchogenic carcinoma. Semin Oncol *13*(Suppl 3):115, 1986.

Bonomi P, et al: Carboplatin/etoposide/radiation plus escalating doses of paclitaxel in stage III non–small cell lung cancer: a preliminary report. Semin Oncol *22*(Suppl 9):42, 1995.

Bonomi P, et al: Escalating paclitaxel doses combined with carboplatin/etoposide and thoracic radiotherapy as preoperative or definitive treatment for stage III non–small cell lung cancer. Semin Oncol *23*(Suppl 16):102, 1996.

Bonomi P, et al: Postoperative bronchopulmonary complications in stage III lung cancer patients treated with preoperative paclitaxel-containing chemotherapy and concurrent radiation. Semin Oncol *24*(Suppl 12):123, 1997.

Bromley L, Szur L: Combined radiotherapy and resection for carcinoma of the bronchus: experience with 66 patients. Lancet 2:937, 1955.

Brundage MD, Mackillop WJ: Locally advanced non–small cell lung cancer: do we know the questions? A survey of randomized trials from 1966–1993. J Clin Epidemiol 49:183, 1996.

Bulzebruck H, et al: New aspects in the staging of lung cancer. Prospective validation of the International Union Against Cancer TNM classification. Cancer 70:1102, 1992.

Bunn PA Jr: The treatment of non–small cell lung cancer: current perspectives and controversies, future directions. Semin Oncol 21(Suppl 6):49, 1994.

Bunn PA Jr: Defining the role of paclitaxel in lung cancer: summary of recent studies and implications for future directions. Semin Oncol 24(Suppl 12):153, 1997.

Burkes RL, et al: Induction chemotherapy with mitomycin, vindesine, and cisplatin for stage III unresectable non–small-cell lung cancer: results of the Toronto Phase II Trial. J Clin Oncol 10:580, 1992.

Cerny T, et al: Docetaxel (Taxotere) is active in non–small-cell lung cancer: a phase II trial of the EORTC Early Clinical Trials Group (ECTG) [see comments]. Br J Cancer 70:384, 1994.

Chella A, et al: Pre-operative chemotherapy for stage IIIa (N2) non–small cell lung cancer. Eur J Surg Oncol 21:393, 1995.

Choi NC: Controversies in the role of postoperative radiotherapy in stages II and IIIA resected non–small cell lung carcinoma [editorial comment] [see comments]. Int J Radiat Oncol Biol Phys 20:1137, 1991.

Choi NC, Kanarek DJ, Grillo HC: Effect of postoperative radiotherapy on changes in pulmonary function in patients with stage II and IIIA lung carcinoma. Int J Radiat Oncol Biol Phys 18:95, 1990.

Choi NC, et al: Potential impact on survival of improved tumor downstaging and resection rate by preoperative twice-daily radiation and concurrent chemotherapy in stage IIIA non–small-cell lung cancer. J Clin Oncol 15:712, 1997.

Cox JD: Induction chemotherapy for non–small cell carcinoma of the lung: limitations and lessons [editorial comment]. Int J Radiat Oncol Biol Phys 20:1375, 1991.

Cullen MH: Adjuvant and neo-adjuvant chemotherapy in non–small cell carcinoma. Ann Oncol 6(Suppl 1):43, 1995a.

Cullen MH: Trials with mitomycin, ifosfamide and cisplatin in non–small cell lung cancer. Lung Cancer 12(Suppl 1):S95, 1995b.

Curran WJ Jr: New therapeutic strategies involving radiation therapy for patients with non–small cell lung cancer. Chest 107(6 Suppl):302S, 1995.

Damstrup L, Poulsen HS: Review of the curative role of radiotherapy in the treatment of non–small cell lung cancer. Lung Cancer 11:153, 1994.

Darwish S, et al: Neoadjuvant cisplatin and etoposide for stage IIIA (clinical N2) non–small cell lung cancer. Am J Clin Oncol 17:64, 1994.

Darwish S, et al: A phase II trial of combined chemotherapy and surgery in stage IIIA non–small cell lung cancer. Lung Cancer 12(Suppl 1):S71, 1995.

Dautzenberg B, et al: Failure of the perioperative PCV neoadjuvant polychemotherapy in resectable bronchogenic non–small cell carcinoma. Results from a randomized phase II trial. Cancer 65:2435, 1990.

Dillman RO, et al: A randomized trial of induction chemotherapy plus high-dose radiation versus radiation alone in stage III non–small-cell lung cancer [see comments]. N Engl J Med 323:940, 1990.

Dosoretz DE, et al: Local control in medically inoperable lung cancer: an analysis of its importance in outcome and factors determining the probability of tumor eradication. Int J Radiat Oncol Biol Phys 27:507, 1993.

Eagan RT, et al: Pilot study of induction therapy with cyclophosphamide, doxorubicin, and cisplatin (CAP) and chest irradiation prior to thoracotomy in initially inoperable stage III M0 non–small cell lung cancer. Cancer Treat Res 71:895, 1987.

Elias AD, et al: Neoadjuvant treatment of stage IIIA non–small cell lung cancer. Long-term results. Am J Clin Oncol 17:26, 1994.

Elias AD, et al: Neoadjuvant therapy for surgically staged IIIA N2 non–small cell lung cancer (NSCLC). Lung Cancer 17:147, 1997.

Emami B, et al: Postoperative radiation therapy in the management of lung cancer. Radiology 164:251, 1987.

Emami B, et al: Postoperative radiation therapy in non–small cell lung cancer. Am J Clin Oncol 20:441, 1997.

Faber LP: Current status of neoadjuvant therapy for non–small cell lung cancer. Chest 106(6 Suppl):355S, 1994.

Faber LP, et al: Preoperative chemotherapy and irradiation for stage III non–small cell lung cancer. Ann Thorac Surg 47:669, 1989.

Favaretto A, et al: Pre-operative chemoradiotherapy in non–small cell lung cancer stage III patients. Feasibility, toxicity and long-term results of a phase II study. Eur J Cancer 32A:2064, 1996.

Feld R: Chemotherapy as adjuvant therapy for completely resected non–small-cell lung cancer: have we made progress? [editorial comment]. J Clin Oncol 14:1045, 1996.

Feld R, Rubinstein L, Thomas PA: Adjuvant chemotherapy with cyclophosphamide, doxorubicin, and cisplatin in patients with completely resected stage I non–small-cell lung cancer. The Lung Cancer Study Group. J Natl Cancer Inst 85:299, 1993.

Feld R, Rubinstein L, Thomas PA: Adjuvant chemotherapy with cyclophosphamide, doxorubicin, and cisplatin in patients with completely resected stage I non–small cell lung cancer. An LCSG Trial. Chest 106(6 Suppl):307S, 1994.

Feld R, Rubinstein LV, Weisenberger TH: Sites of recurrence in resected stage I non–small-cell lung cancer: a guide for future studies. J Clin Oncol 2:1352, 1984.

Ferguson MK, et al: The role of adjuvant therapy after resection of T1 N1 M0 and T2 N1 M0 non–small cell lung cancer. J Thorac Cardiovasc Surg 91:344, 1986.

Figlin RA, Piantadosi S (Piantodosi): A phase 3 randomized trial of immediate combination chemotherapy vs delayed combination chemotherapy in patients with completely resected stage II and III non–small cell carcinoma of the lung. Chest 106(6 Suppl):310S, 1994.

Flaherty L, et al: 5-Fluorouracil, etoposide, and cisplatin in the management of metastatic non–small cell lung cancer. Cancer 68:944, 1991.

Fossella FV, Rivera E, Roth JA: Preoperative chemotherapy for stage IIIa non–small cell lung cancer. Curr Opin Oncol 8:106, 1996.

Gail MH: A placebo-controlled randomized double-blind study of adjuvant intrapleural BCG in patients with resected T1N0, T1N1, or T2N0 squamous cell carcinoma, adenocarcinoma, or large cell carcinoma of the lung. LCSG Protocol 771. Chest 106(Suppl):287S, 1994.

Gail MH, et al: Prognostic factors in patients with resected stage I non–small cell lung cancer. A report from the Lung Cancer Study Group. Cancer 54:1802, 1984.

Ginsberg RJ: Multimodality therapy for stage IIIA (N2) lung cancer. An overview. Chest 103(4 Suppl):356S, 1993.

Girling DJ, et al: Fifteen-year follow-up of all patients in a study of postoperative chemotherapy for bronchial carcinoma. Br J Cancer 52:867, 1985.

Goldstraw P, et al: Surgical management of non–small-cell lung cancer with ipsilateral mediastinal node metastasis (N2 disease). J Thorac Cardiovasc Surg 107:19, 1994.

Graham PH, Gebski VJ, Langlands AO: Radical radiotherapy for early non–small cell lung cancer. Int J Radiat Oncol Biol Phys 31:261, 1995.

Gralla RJ: New directions in non–small cell lung cancer. Semin Oncol 17(4 Suppl 7):14, 1990.

Greco FA, Hainsworth JD: Multidisciplinary approach to potentially curable non–small cell carcinoma of the lung. Oncology 11:27, 1997.

Green MR: New directions for chemotherapy in non–small-cell lung cancer. Chest 103(Suppl):370S, 1993.

Green MR, Barkley JE: Intensity of neoadjuvant therapy in resectable non–small cell lung cancer. Lung Cancer 17(Suppl 1):S111, 1997.

Green N, Kern W: The clinical course and treatment results of patients with postresection locally recurrent lung cancer. Cancer 42:2478, 1978.

Green N, et al: Postresection irradiation for primary lung cancer. Radiology 116:405, 1975.

Haraf DJ, et al: The evolving role of systemic therapy in carcinoma of the lung. Semin Oncol 19(Suppl 11):72, 1992.

Higgins GA, et al: Cytoxan as an adjuvant to surgery for lung cancer. J Surg Oncol 1:221, 1969.

Hilaris BS, et al: Combined surgery, intraoperative brachytherapy, and postoperative external radiation in stage III non–small cell lung cancer. Cancer 55:1226, 1985.

Holmes EC: Surgical adjuvant therapy of non–small cell lung cancer. Chest 89(Suppl):295S, 1986.

Holmes EC: Surgical adjuvant therapy of non–small-cell lung cancer. J Surg Oncol Suppl 1:26, 1989.

Holmes EC: Adjuvant therapy of non–small cell lung cancer. Hematol Oncol 10:21, 1992.

Holmes EC: Postoperative chemotherapy for non–small-cell lung cancer. Chest 103(Suppl):30S, 1993.

Holmes EC: Surgical adjuvant therapy for stage II and stage III adenocarcinoma and large cell undifferentiated carcinoma. Chest 106(Suppl):293S, 1994a.

Holmes EC: Historic background of the Lung Cancer Study Group. Chest 106(Suppl):280S, 1994b.

Holmes EC, Gail M: Surgical adjuvant therapy for stage II and stage III adenocarcinoma and large-cell undifferentiated carcinoma. J Clin Oncol 4:710, 1986.

Holmes EC, Ruckdeschel JC: Preoperative chemotherapy for locally advanced non–small cell lung cancer. Semin Oncol 21(Suppl 6):97, 1994.

Hughes FA, Higgins G: Veterans Administration Surgical Adjuvant Lung Cancer Chemotherapy Study: Present Status. J Thorac Cardiovasc Surg 44:295, 1962.

Ihde DC: Neoadjuvant chemotherapy for non–small cell lung cancer: current North American experience. Semin Oncol 15(Suppl 7):3, 1988.

Israel L, Depierre A, Sylvester R: Influence of postoperative radiotherapy on local recurrence and survival of bronchial epidermoid carcinoma with regard to nodal status: preliminary results of the EORTC protocol 08741. Recent Results Cancer Res 68:242, 1978.

Jeremic B, et al: Hyperfractionated radiotherapy alone for clinical stage I non–small cell lung cancer. Int J Radiat Oncol Biol Phys 38:521, 1997.

Johnson DH: Adjuvant chemotherapy for non–small cell lung cancer. Chest 106(Suppl):313S, 1994.

Johnson DH, et al: Thoracic radiotherapy does not prolong survival in patients with locally advanced, unresectable non–small cell lung cancer [see comments]. Ann Intern Med 113:33, 1990.

Johnson D, et al: Post-operative adjuvant therapy for non–small-cell lung cancer. Lung Cancer 17(Suppl 1):S23, 1997.

Kim DH, et al: Multimodality therapy of patients with stage IIIA, N2 non–small-cell lung cancer. Impact of preoperative chemotherapy on resectability and downstaging. J Thorac Cardiovasc Surg 106:696, 1993.

Kirsh MM, Sloan H: Mediastinal metastases in bronchogenic carcinoma: influence of postoperative irradiation, cell type, and location. Ann Thorac Surg 33:459, 1982.

Kris MG, et al: Preoperative and adjuvant chemotherapy in locally advanced non–small cell lung cancer. Surg Clin North Am 67:1051, 1987.

Kris MG, et al: Effectiveness and toxicity of preoperative therapy in stage IIIA non–small cell lung cancer including the Memorial Sloan-Kettering experience with induction MVP in patients with bulky mediastinal lymph node metastases (Clinical N2). Lung Cancer 12(Suppl 1):S47, 1995.

Kumar P, et al: Patterns of disease failure after trimodality therapy of non–small cell lung carcinoma pathologic stage IIIA (N2). Analysis of Cancer and Leukemia Group B Protocol 8935. Cancer 77:2393, 1996.

Lad T: The comparison of CAP chemotherapy and radiotherapy to radiotherapy alone for resected lung cancer with positive margin or involved highest sampled paratracheal node (stage IIIA). LCSG 791. Chest 106(Suppl):302S, 1994.

Lad T, Rubinstein L, Sodeghi A: The benefit of adjuvant treatment for resected locally advanced non–small-cell lung cancer. J Clin Oncol 6:9, 1988.

Lad T, et al: A prospective randomized trial to determine the benefit of surgical resection of residual disease following response of small cell lung cancer to combination chemotherapy. Chest 106(Suppl):320S, 1994.

Lad TE: Postsurgical adjuvant therapy in stages I, II, and IIIA non–small cell lung cancer. Hematol Oncol Clin North Am 4:1111, 1990.

Lee JD, Ginsberg RJ: The multimodality treatment of stage III A/B non–small cell lung cancer. The role of surgery, radiation, and chemotherapy. Hematol Oncol Clin North Am 11:279, 1997.

Lilenbaum RC, Green MR: Multimodality therapy for non–small-cell lung cancer. Oncology 8:25, 1994.

Livingston RB: Current management of unresectable non–small cell lung cancer. Semin Oncol 21(Suppl 10):4, 1994.

Livingston RB, et al: Summary of the proceedings of the United States-Japan lung cancer clinical trials summit. Maui, Hawaii, 24–25 February 1996. J Cancer Res Clin Oncol 123:461, 1997.

Ludwig Lung Cancer Study Group: Adverse effect of intrapleural Corynebacterium parvum as adjuvant therapy in resected stage I and II non–small cell carcinoma of the lung. J Thorac Cardiovasc Surg 89:842, 1985.

The Ludwig Lung Cancer Study Group (LLCSG): Immunostimulation with intrapleural BCG as adjuvant therapy in resected non–small cell lung cancer. Cancer 58:2411, 1986.

The Ludwig Lung Cancer Study Group: Patterns of failure in patients with resected stage I and II non–small-cell carcinoma of the lung. Ann Surg 205:67, 1987.

The Lung Cancer Study Group: Effects of postoperative mediastinal radiation on completely resected stage II and stage III epidermoid cancer of the lung. N Engl J Med 315:1377, 1986.

Macchiarini P, et al: Results of treatment and lessons learned from pathologically staged T4 non–small cell lung cancer. J Surg Oncol 47:209, 1991.

Mackillop WJ, O'Sullivan B, Ward GK: Non–small cell lung cancer: how oncologists want to be treated. Int J Radiat Oncol Biol Phys 13:929, 1987.

Marangolo M, Fiorentini G: Adjuvant chemotherapy of non–small cell lung cancer: a review. Semin Oncol 15(Suppl 7):13, 1988.

Martini N, Flehinger BJ: The role of surgery in N2 lung cancer. Surg Clin North Am 67:1037, 1987.

Martini N, Kris MG, Ginsberg RJ: The role of multimodality therapy in locoregional non–small cell lung cancer. Surg Oncol Clin North Am 6:769, 1997.

Martini N, et al: Preoperative chemotherapy for stage IIIa (N2) lung cancer: the Sloan-Kettering experience with 136 patients. Ann Thorac Surg 55:1365, 1993.

Matthews MJ, et al: Frequency of residual and metastatic tumor in patients undergoing curative surgical resection for lung cancer. Cancer Chemother Rep 4:63, 1973.

Mayer R, et al: Postoperative radiotherapy in radically resected non–small cell lung cancer. Chest 112:954, 1997.

McKneally MF, Maver C, Kausel HW: Regional immunotherapy of lung cancer with intrapleural BCG. Lancet 1:377, 1976a.

McKneally MF, et al: Regional immunotherapy with intrapleural BCG for lung cancer. J Thorac Cardiovasc Surg 72:333, 1976b.

McKneally MF, et al: Four-year follow-up on the Albany experience with intrapleural BCG in lung cancer. J Thorac Cardiovasc Surg 81:485, 1981.

Milano S, et al: Histopathological grading of response to induction chemotherapy in non–small cell lung cancer: a preliminary study. Lung Cancer 15:183, 1996.

Mirimanoff RO: Concurrent chemotherapy (CT) and radiotherapy (RT) in locally advanced non–small cell lung cancer (NSCLC): a review. Lung Cancer 11(Suppl 3):S79, 1994.

Mountain CF: Therapy of stage I and stage II non–small cell lung cancer. Semin Oncol 10:71, 1983.

Mountain CF: A new international staging system for lung cancer. Chest 89(Suppl):225S, 1986.

Mountain CF: Revisions in the International Staging System for Lung Cancer. Chest 111:1710, 1997.

Murphy WK, et al: Phase II study of Taxol in patients with untreated advanced non–small-cell lung cancer [see comments]. J Natl Cancer Inst 85:384, 1993.

Murren JR, Buzaid AC, Hait WN: Critical analysis of neoadjuvant therapy for Stage IIIa non–small cell lung cancer [corrected] [published erratum appears in Am Rev Respir Dis 143:1473, 1991]. Am Rev Respir Dis 143:889, 1991.

Nakanishi R, et al: Treatment strategy for patients with surgically discovered N2 stage IIIA non–small cell lung cancer. Ann Thorac Surg 64:342, 1997.

Natale RB: Overview of current and future chemotherapeutic agents in non–small cell lung cancer. Semin Oncol 24(Suppl 7):S29, 1997.

Natale RB: Experience with new chemotherapeutic agents in non–small cell lung cancer. Chest 113(Suppl):32S, 1998.

National Cancer Institute Study: Preoperative irradiation of cancer of the lung. Preliminary report of a therapeutic trial. A collaborative study. Cancer 23:419, 1969.

Niiranen A, et al: Adjuvant chemotherapy after radical surgery for non–small-cell lung cancer: a randomized study. J Clin Oncol 10:1927, 1992.

Non–small Cell Lung Cancer Collaborative Group: Chemotherapy in non–small cell lung cancer: a meta-analysis using updated data on individual patients from 52 randomised clinical trials. BMJ 311:899, 1995.

Ohta M, et al: Adjuvant chemotherapy for completely resected stage III non–small-cell lung cancer. Results of a randomized prospective study. The Japan Clinical Oncology Group. J Thorac Cardiovasc Surg 106:703, 1993.

Paccagnella A, et al: Mitomycin C, vinblastine, and carboplatin regimen in patients with non–small cell lung cancer. A phase II trial. Cancer 78:1701, 1996.

Palackdharry CS, et al: Preliminary results of neoadjuvant paclitaxel and carboplatin in the treatment of early stage non–small cell lung cancer. Semin Oncol 24(Suppl 12):S12-34, 1997.

Palmer MJ, et al: Controversies in the management of non–small cell lung cancer: the results of an expert surrogate study [see comments]. Radiother Oncol 19:17, 1990.

Pass HI, et al: Randomized trial of neoadjuvant therapy for lung cancer: interim analysis. Ann Thorac Surg 53:992, 1992.

Pastorino U: Benefits of neoadjuvant chemotherapy in NSCLC. Chest 109(Suppl):96S, 1996.

Payne DG: Is preoperative or postoperative radiation therapy indicated in non–small cell cancer of the lung? Lung Cancer 10(Suppl 1): S205, 1994.

Perry MC, et al: Induction treatment for resectable non–small-cell lung cancer. Lung Cancer 17(Suppl 1):S15, 1997.

Pincus M, et al: Preoperative combined modality therapy for stage III M0 non–small cell lung carcinoma. Int J Radiat Oncol Biol Phys 15:189, 1988.

Pisters KM, et al: Pathologic complete response in advanced non–small-cell lung cancer following preoperative chemotherapy: implications for the design of future non–small-cell lung cancer combined modality trials. J Clin Oncol 11:1757, 1993.

Pisters KM, et al: Randomized trial comparing postoperative chemotherapy with vindesine and cisplatin plus thoracic irradiation with irradiation alone in stage III (N2) non–small cell lung cancer. J Surg Oncol 56:236, 1994.

Pisters KM, et al: Induction paclitaxel/carboplatin in early stage non–small cell lung cancer. Bimodality Lung Oncology Team. Semin Oncol 24(Suppl 12):41, 1997.

PORT Meta-analysis Trialists Group: Postoperative radiotherapy in non–small-cell lung cancer: systematic review meta-analysis of individual patient data from none randomised controlled trials. Lancet 352:257, 1998.

Pujol JL, et al: Pilot study of neoadjuvant ifosfamide, cisplatin, and etoposide in locally advanced non–small cell lung cancer. Eur J Cancer 26:798, 1990.

Pujol JL, et al: Long-term results of neoadjuvant ifosfamide, cisplatin, and etoposide combination in locally advanced non–small-cell lung cancer. Chest 106:1451, 1994.

Pujol JL, et al: Neoadjuvant chemotherapy of locally advanced non–small cell lung cancer. Lung Cancer 12(Suppl 1):S107, 1995.

Reboul F, et al: Concurrent cisplatin, etoposide, and radiotherapy for unresectable stage III non–small cell lung cancer: a phase II study. Int J Radiat Oncol Biol Phys 35:343, 1996.

Recine D, et al: Combined modality therapy for locally advanced non–small cell lung carcinoma. Cancer 66:2270, 1990.

Reddy S, et al: Preoperative radiation therapy in regionally localized stage III non–small cell lung carcinoma: long-term results and patterns of failure. Int J Radiat Oncol Biol Phys 19:287, 1990.

Reddy S, et al: Combined modality therapy for stage III non–small cell lung carcinoma: results of treatment and patterns of failure. Int J Radiat Oncol Biol Phys 24:17, 1992.

Report by a Medical Research Council Working Party: Study of cytotoxic chemotherapy as an adjuvant to surgery in carcinoma of the bronchus. BMJ 2:421, 1971.

Rosell R, et al: A randomized trial comparing preoperative chemotherapy plus surgery with surgery alone in patients with non–small-cell lung cancer [see comments]. N Engl J Med 330:153, 1994a.

Rosell R, et al: A randomized trial of mitomycin/ifosfamide/cisplatin preoperative chemotherapy plus surgery versus surgery alone in stage IIIA non–small cell lung cancer. Semin Oncol 21(Suppl 4):28, 1994b.

Rosell R, et al: Mutated K-ras gene analysis in a randomized trial of preoperative chemotherapy plus surgery versus surgery in stage IIIA non–small cell lung cancer. Lung Cancer 12(Suppl 1):S59, 1995

Rosell R, et al: The role of induction (neoadjuvant) chemotherapy in stage IIIA NSCLC. Chest 109(Suppl):102S, 1996.

Rosell R, Lopez-Cabrerizo MP, Astudillo J: Preoperative chemotherapy for stage IIIA non–small cell lung cancer [see comments]. Curr Opin Oncol 9:149, 1997.

Roth JA, et al: A randomized trial comparing perioperative chemotherapy and surgery with surgery alone in resectable stage IIIA non–small-cell lung cancer [see comments]. J Natl Cancer Inst 86:673, 1994.

Rusch VW, Feins RH: Summary of current cooperative group clinical trials in thoracic malignancies. The Thoracic Intergroup [see comments]. Ann Thorac Surg 57:102, 1994.

Rusch VW, et al: Surgical resection of stage IIIA and stage IIIB non–small-cell lung cancer after concurrent induction chemoradiotherapy. A Southwest Oncology Group trial. J Thorac Cardiovasc Surg 105:97, 1993.

Saijo N: New chemotherapeutic agents for the treatment of non–small cell lung cancer: the Japanese experience. Chest 113(Suppl):17S, 1998.

Sawyer TE, et al: Effectiveness of postoperative irradiation in stage IIIA non–small cell lung cancer according to regression tree analyses of recurrence risks. Ann Thorac Surg 64:1402, 1997a.

Sawyer TE, et al: The impact of surgical adjuvant thoracic radiation therapy for patients with non–small cell lung carcinoma with ipsilateral mediastinal lymph node involvement. Cancer 80:1399, 1997b.

Schabel FM Jr: Rationale for adjuvant chemotherapy. Cancer 39(Suppl):2875, 1977.

Shepherd FA: Induction chemotherapy for locally advanced non–small cell lung cancer. Ann Thorac Surg 55:1585, 1993.

Sherman DM, et al: An aggressive approach to marginally resectable lung cancer. Cancer 41:2040, 1978.

Shields TW: Preoperative radiation therapy in the treatment of bronchial carcinoma. Cancer 30:1388, 1972.

Shields TW: The significance of ipsilateral mediastinal lymph node metastasis (N2 disease) in non–small cell carcinoma of the lung. A commentary. J Thorac Cardiovasc Surg 99:98, 1990.

Shields TW, Robinette CD, Keehn RJ: Bronchial carcinoma treated by adjuvant cancer chemotherapy. Arch Surg 109:329, 1974.

Shields TW, et al: Preoperative x-ray therapy as an adjuvant in the treatment of bronchogenic carcinoma. J Thorac Cardiovasc Surg 59:49, 1970.

Shields TW, et al: Adjuvant cancer chemotherapy after resection of carcinoma of the lung. Cancer 40:2057, 1977.

Shields TW, et al: Prolonged intermittent adjuvant chemotherapy with CCNU and hydroxyurea after resection of carcinoma of the lung. Cancer 50:1713, 1982.

Skarin A, et al: Neoadjuvant chemotherapy in marginally resectable stage III M0 non–small cell lung cancer: long-term follow-up in 41 patients. J Surg Oncol 40:266, 1989.

Slack NH: Bronchogenic carcinoma: nitrogen mustard as a surgical adjuvant and factors influencing survival. University surgical adjuvant lung project. Cancer 25:987, 1970.

Slotman BJ, Njo KH, Karim AB:. Curative radiotherapy for technically operable stage I non–small cell lung cancer. Int J Radiat Oncol Biol Phys 29:33, 1994.

Spain RC: Neoadjuvant mitomycin C, cisplatin, and infusion vinblastine in locally and regionally advanced non–small cell lung cancer: problems and progress from the perspective of long-term follow-up. Semin Oncol 15(Suppl 4):6, 1988.

Spain RC: The case for mitomycin in non–small cell lung cancer. Oncology 50(Suppl 1):35, 1993.

Sridhar KS, et al: Multidisciplinary approach to the treatment of locally and regionally advanced non–small cell lung cancer: University of Miami experience. Semin Surg Oncol 9:114, 1993.

Stephens RJ, et al: The role of post-operative radiotherapy in non–small-cell lung cancer: a multicentre randomised trial in patients with pathologically staged T1-2, N1-2, M0 disease. Medical Research Council Lung Cancer Working Party. Br J Cancer 74:632, 1996.

Stewart L, Burdett S: Post-operative radiotherapy in NSCLC [letter comment]. Br J Cancer 75:1224, 1997.

Strauss GM, et al: Multimodality treatment of stage IIIA non–small-cell lung carcinoma: a critical review of the literature and strategies for future research. J Clin Oncol 10:829, 1992a.

Strauss GM, et al: Neoadjuvant chemotherapy and radiotherapy followed by surgery in stage IIIA non–small-cell carcinoma of the lung: report of a Cancer and Leukemia Group B phase II study. J Clin Oncol 10:1237, 1992b.

The Study Group of Adjuvant Chemotherapy for Lung Cancer (Chubu, Japan): A randomized trial of postoperative adjuvant chemotherapy in non–small cell lung cancer (the second cooperative study). Eur J Surg Oncol 21:69, 1995.

Sugarbaker DJ, et al: Results of cancer and leukemia group B protocol 8935. A multiinstitutional phase II trimodality trial for stage IIIA (N2) non–small-cell lung cancer. Cancer and Leukemia Group B Thoracic Surgery Group. J Thorac Cardiovasc Surg 109:473, 1995.

Tan EH, Ang PT: Chemotherapy in non–small cell lung cancer: a review. Ann Acad Med Singapore 25:570, 1996.

Taylor SG, et al: Simultaneous cisplatin fluorouracil infusion and radiation followed by surgical resection in regionally localized stage III, non–small cell lung cancer. Ann Thorac Surg 43:87, 1987.

Tonato M: The role of neoadjuvant chemotherapy in NSCLC. Chest 109(Suppl):93S, 1996.

Trodella L, et al: Phase I-II trial of concomitant continuous carboplatin (CBDCA) infusion and radiotherapy in advanced non–small cell lung cancer with evaluation for surgery: final report. Int J Radiat Oncol Biol Phys 37:93, 1997.

Turrisi AT 3rd: The sound and fury about postoperative therapy for lung cancer [editorial comment]. Mayo Clin Proc 67:1197, 1992.

Van Houtte P, et al: Postoperative radiation therapy in lung cancer: a controlled trial after resection of curative design. Int J Radiat Oncol Biol Phys 6:983, 1980.

van Klaveren RJ, et al: Prognosis of unsuspected but completely resectable N2 non–small cell lung cancer. Ann Thorac Surg 56:300, 1993.

Vansteenkiste JF, et al: Survival and prognostic factors in resected N2 non–small cell lung cancer: a study of 140 cases. Leuven Lung Cancer Group. Ann Thorac Surg 63:1441, 1997.

Vokes EE: Sequential combined modality therapy for stage III non–small cell lung cancer. Hematol Oncol Clin North Am 4:1133, 1990.

Wada H, Hitomi S, Teramatsu T: Adjuvant chemotherapy after complete resection in non–small-cell lung cancer. West Japan Study Group for Lung Cancer Surgery. J Clin Oncol 14:1048, 1996.

Wada H, Tanaka F, Hitomi S: Postoperative adjuvant chemotherapy for non–small-cell lung cancer. West Japan Study Group for Lung Cancer Surgery. The Japan Lung Cancer Research Group on Postsurgical Adjuvant Chemotherapy. Oncology 11(Suppl 10):98, 1997.

Wagner H Jr, et al: Randomized phase 2 evaluation of preoperative radiation therapy and preoperative chemotherapy with mitomycin, vinblastine, and cisplatin in patients with technically unresectable stage IIIA and IIIB non–small cell cancer of the lung. LCSG 881. Chest 106(6 Suppl):348S, 1994.

Warram J: Preoperative irradiation of cancer of the lung: final report of a therapeutic trial. A collaborative study. Cancer 36:914, 1975.

Weiden PL, Piantadosi S: Preoperative chemotherapy (cisplatin and fluorouracil) and radiation therapy in stage III non–small-cell lung cancer: a phase II study of the Lung Cancer Study Group. J Natl Cancer Inst 83:266, 1991.

Weiden PL, Piantadosi S: Preoperative chemotherapy (cisplatin and fluorouracil) and radiation therapy in stage III non–small cell lung cancer. A phase 2 study of the LCSG. Chest 106(Suppl):344S, 1994.

Weisenburger TH: Effects of postoperative mediastinal radiation on completely resected stage II and stage III epidermoid cancer of the lung. LCSG 773. Chest 106(Suppl):297S, 1994.

Weitberg AB, et al: Combined modality therapy for stage IIIA non–small cell carcinoma of the lung. Eur J Cancer 29A:511, 1993.

Wurschmidt F, et al: Is the time interval between surgery and radiotherapy important in operable non–small cell lung cancer? A retrospective analysis of 340 cases. Int J Radiat Oncol Biol Phys 39:553, 1997.

Yoneda S, et al: Induction chemoradiotherapy followed by surgery for stage III non–small cell lung cancer. Jpn J Clin Oncol 23:173, 1993.

Yoshino I, et al: Postoperative prognosis in patients with non–small cell lung cancer with synchronous ipsilateral intrapulmonary metastasis. Ann Thorac Surg 64:809, 1997.

READING REFERENCES

Anonymous: Effects of postoperative mediastinal radiation on completely resected stage II and stage III epidermoid cancer of the lung. The Lung Cancer Study Group. N Engl J Med 315:1377, 1986.

Bitran JD, et al: Protochemotherapy in non–small cell lung carcinoma. An attempt to increase surgical resectability and survival. A preliminary report [published erratum appears in Cancer 1558:1377, 1986]. Cancer 57:44, 1986.

Bonomi P, et al: Phase II trial of therapy with etoposide, 5-fluorouracil by continuous infusion, cisplatin, and simultaneous split-course radiation in stage III non–small cell bronchogenic carcinoma. Monogr Natl Cancer Inst 6:331, 1988.

Buccheri G, Ferrigno D: Therapeutic options for regionally advanced non–small cell lung cancer. Lung Cancer 14:281, 1996.

Bunn PA Jr: The expanding role of cisplatin in the treatment of non–small-cell lung cancer. Semin Oncol 16(Suppl 6):10, 1989.

Carretta A, et al: Surgery following neoadjuvant MPV chemotherapy (mitomycin, cisplatin, vinblastine) in locally advanced (IIIa and IIIb) non–small cell lung cancer. Eur J Cardiothorac Surg 8:457, 1994.

Choi NC: Basis for new strategies in postoperative radiotherapy of bronchogenic carcinoma. Int J Radiat Oncol Biol Phys 6:31, 1980.

Cvitkovic E, Wasserman E: Role of vindesine as neoadjuvant chemotherapy for non–small cell lung and head and neck cancers. Anticancer Drugs 8:734, 1997.

Debevec M, et al: Postoperative radiotherapy for radically resected N2 non–small-cell lung cancer (NSCLC): randomised clinical study 1988-1992. Lung Cancer 14:99, 1996.

Depierre A, et al: An ongoing randomized study of neoadjuvant chemotherapy in resectable non–small cell lung cancer. Semin Oncol 21(Suppl 4):16, 1994.

Deutsch MA, et al: Carboplatin, etoposide, and radiotherapy, followed by surgery, for the treatment of marginally resectable non–small cell lung cancer. Cancer Treat Rev 19(Suppl C):53, 1993.

Durci ML, et al: Comparison of surgery and radiation therapy for non–small cell carcinoma of the lung with mediastinal metastasis. Int J Radiat Oncol Biol Phys 21:629, 1991.

Eagan RT: Management of regionally advanced (stage III) non–small cell lung cancer. LCSG 831. Chest 106(Suppl 6):340S, 1994.

Folman RS: Multidisciplinary management of non–small cell lung cancer in the community. Semin Oncol 17:30, 1990.

Fram R, et al: Combination chemotherapy followed by radiation therapy in patients with regional stage III unresectable non–small cell lung cancer. Cancer Treat Rep 69:587, 1985.

Frontini L, et al: Cisplatin-vinorelbine combination chemotherapy in locally advanced non–small cell lung cancer. Tumori 82:57, 1996.

Goss GD, Dahrouge S, Lochrin CA: Recent advances in the treatment of non–small cell lung cancer. Anticancer Drugs 7:363, 1996.

Gradishar WJ, et al: The impact on survival by adjuvant chemotherapy and radiation therapy in stage II non–small-cell lung cancer. Am J Clin Oncol 15:405, 1992.

Gridelli C, et al: Neoadjuvant chemotherapy with cisplatin, epirubicin and VP-16 for stage IIIA-IIIB non–small-cell lung cancer: a pilot study. Tumori 78:377, 1992.

Hilaris BS, Nori D, Martini N: Intraoperative radiotherapy in stage I and II lung cancer. Semin Surg Oncol 3:22, 1987.

Ichinose Y, et al: Postoperative adjuvant chemotherapy in non–small cell lung cancer: prognostic value of DNA ploidy and post-recurrent survival. J Surg Oncol 46:15, 1991.

Kaiser LR, Friedberg JS: The role of surgery in the multimodality management of non–small cell lung cancer. Semin Thorac Cardiovasc Surg 9:60, 1997.

Kaiser LR, Friedberg JS: Adjuvant therapy of lung cancer: introduction. Semin Thorac Cardiovasc Surg 9:55, 1997.

Kayser K, et al: Changes during the last decade in clinical parameters of operated lung carcinoma patients of a center for thoracic surgery and the prognostic significance of TNM, morphometric, cytometric, and glycohistochemical properties. Thorac Cardiovasc Surg 45:196, 1997.

Kupelian PA, Komaki R, Allen P. Prognostic factors in the treatment of node-negative non–small cell lung carcinoma with radiotherapy alone. Int J Radiat Oncol Biol Phys 36:607, 1996.

Lee JS, et al: Concurrent chemoradiation therapy with oral etoposide and cisplatin for locally advanced inoperable non–small-cell lung cancer: radiation therapy oncology group protocol 91-06. J Clin Oncol 14:1055, 1996.

Leung J, et al: Survival following radiotherapy for post-surgical locoregional recurrence of non–small cell lung cancer. Lung Cancer 13:121, 1995.

Lokich J, Chaffey J, Neptune W: Concomitant 5-fluorouracil infusion and high-dose radiation for stage III non–small cell lung cancer. Cancer 64:1021, 1989.

Martini N, et al: The effects of preoperative chemotherapy on the resectability of non–small cell lung carcinoma with mediastinal lymph node metastases (N2 M0). Ann Thorac Surg 45:370, 1988.

McKneally MF, Maver C: Regional immunotherapy using intrapleural BCG and isoniazid for resectable lung cancer: results in the first 100 cases. In Salmon SE, Jones SE (eds): Adjuvant Therapy of Cancer. Amsterdam: North Holland Publ, 1977, pp. 207–215.

Palazzi M, et al: Preoperative concomitant cisplatin/VP16 and radiotherapy in stage III non–small cell lung cancer. Int J Radiat Oncol Biol Phys 27:621, 1993.

Rossi NP, Zavala DC, VanGilder JC: A combined surgical approach to non-oat-cell pulmonary carcinoma with single cerebral metastasis. Respiration 51:170, 1987.

Ruckdeschel JC: Future directions in non–small cell lung cancer. A personal view. Lung Cancer 12(Suppl 2):S147, 1995.

Rusch VW, et al: Neoadjuvant therapy: a novel and effective treatment for stage IIIb non–small cell lung cancer. Southwest Oncology Group. Ann Thorac Surg 58:290, 1994.

Slater JD, et al: Radiation therapy following resection of non–small cell bronchogenic carcinoma [see comments]. Int J Radiat Oncol Biol Phys 20:945, 1991.

Splinter T, et al: A multicenter phase II trial of cisplatin and oral etoposide (VP-16) in inoperable non–small-cell lung cancer. Semin Oncol 13(Suppl 3):97, 1986.

Splinter TA: Paclitaxel and carboplatin as neoadjuvant chemotherapy in operable (stage I and II) and locally advanced (stage IIIA-N2) non–small cell lung cancer. Semin Oncol 23(Suppl 16):59, 1996.

Sridhar KS, et al: Multimodality treatment of non–small cell lung cancer: response to cisplatin, VP-16, and 5-FU chemotherapy and to surgery and radiation therapy. J Surg Oncol 38:193, 1988.

Stockler M, et al: Combination chemotherapy with cisplatin, vindesine and mitomycin-C for advanced, inoperable non–small-cell lung cancer. Med J Aust 156:698, 1992.

Taylor SG, et al: Concomitant therapy with infusion of cisplatin and 5-fluorouracil plus radiation in stage III non–small cell lung cancer. Monogr Natl Cancer Inst 6:327, 1988.

Tomirotti M, et al: Concurrent carboplatin (CBDCA), vindesine (VDS) and radiotherapy in stage III non small cell lung cancer (NSCLC). Tumori 79:49, 1993.

Treat J, Kaiser LR: The role of chemotherapy in the treatment of non–small cell carcinoma of the lung. Semin Thorac Cardiovasc Surg 9:90, 1997.

Vokes EE, et al: Neoadjuvant vindesine, etoposide, and cisplatin for locally advanced non–small cell lung cancer. Final report of a phase 2 study. Chest 96:110, 1989.

Yang SC, et al: Combination immunotherapy for non–small cell lung cancer. Results with interleukin-2 and tumor necrosis factor-alpha. J Thorac Cardiovasc Surg 99:8, 1990.

Yang SC, Grimm EA, Roth JA: Combination immunotherapy for advanced lung cancer. Monogr Natl Cancer Inst 13:197, 1992.

CHAPTER 107

Small Cell Lung Cancer

Ronald Feld, David Payne, and Frances A. Shepherd

According to Ihde (1984), small cell lung cancer (SCLC) accounts for approximately 15 to 20% of all cases of lung cancer worldwide. Minna and associates (1985) and Aisner and Matthews (1985) reported that the classic oat cell or lymphocyte tumor is composed of cells with small, round or spindle-shaped, darkly staining nuclei and scant cytoplasm. Neurosecretory granules are often found in electron micrograph studies. The intermediate subtype of small cell carcinoma has cells with more fusiform or polygonal nuclei, and the cytoplasm is often more distinct (see Chapter 95).

SCLC, as discussed by Bergsagel and one of us (R.F.) (1984) as well as Davis and colleagues (1985), differs in several biological and clinical respects from other types of lung cancer in that it has a large growth fraction, grows rapidly, and usually is widely disseminated at diagnosis. It is dissimilar to non–SCLC (NSCLC) in that SCLC is responsive to single-agent and combination chemotherapy and that more than two-thirds of patients, even those with advanced disease, achieve at least a partial response. Ihde (1984) as well as Shank (1985) and Stevens (1979) and their colleagues reported that intensive early treatment can evoke complete responses in 25 to 60% of patients with limited disease and in 10 to 40% of those with extensive disease. Hyde and colleagues (1965, 1973) and Zelen (1973) noted that untreated patients have median survivals of only 6 to 17 weeks. As Davis (1985), Hansen (1980), Livingston (1984), and Sorensen (1986) and their colleagues point out, however, even with optimum treatment, fewer than 10% of patients are alive 5 years from the start of treatment. Improved integration of chemotherapy and radiation therapy has produced high survival rates in certain subsets of patients with this once rapidly fatal disease. This clinical experience served as a model for the combined method approach to these tumors.

CELL BIOLOGY

Carney (1991, 1992) reported that it was possible to establish lung cancer cell lines from tumors obtained from both newly diagnosed, previously untreated patients and from patients who have relapsed after therapy. The cell lines could be established readily from various sites, including the primary tumor as well as specific metastatic sites. In 68 patients with untreated SCLC, Stevenson and associates (1989) found no difference in the response rate or survival probabilities of patients in whom tumor cell lines were established compared to those in whom in vitro growth of tumor could not be accomplished.

The two types of lung cancer, SCLC and NSCLC, as reported by Carney (1991), are thought to come from a single stem cell. Carney (1986) suggests that a "common" stem cell may exist for all lung tumors, thus adding weight to the theory presented by Cutitta (1981), Whang-peng (1982), and Little (1983) and their colleagues that individual lung tumors may spontaneously change from one histologic type to another. This concept derives from clinical reports on mixed cell types as well as from autopsy series in which up to 40% of patients may have mixed histologic findings. In addition, the overlapping expression of endocrine biomarkers in small cell and non–small cell tumors may reflect this fact biologically. Differences are noted in the markers produced by the two types of cancer cells, but, nonetheless, there is some overlap. Carney (1986), Bunn and Rosen (1985), as well as Carney (1985), Gazdar (1985), Cutitta (1981), and Little (1983) and their coworkers looked at a number of cell lines from patients with SCLC and separated these lines into two major categories: classic and variant. Classic cell lines express elevated levels of biomarkers, including L-dopa decarboxylase, bombesin, neuron-specific enolase, and the brain isoenzyme of creatinine kinase. The variants express elevated levels of neuron-specific enolase and creatinine kinase only. Patients with the variant cell line have a less optimistic clinical prognosis. Amplification of C-*myc* has been associated with the variant class of SCLC, which may clarify the more malignant clinical behavior of variant tumors. Significantly, NSCLC lines only infrequently express any of the markers, allowing one to distinguish the tumor types using biological testing. This area has proved to be one of great interest that may lead to new approaches in treatment.

Also of interest is whether neuroendocrine properties of lung cancer cells have any prognostic significance. These characteristics have been seen in NSCLC as well as SCLC tumors. It may be that NSCLC tumors with neuroendocrine differentiation may represent a distinct biological subset. Various studies reported by Skov (1991) and Sundaresan (1991) and their associates recounted data on the prognostic significance of neuroendocrine differentiation in clinical trials. Conflicting findings suggest that further studies are needed to establish conclusively the importance of this parameter.

Interest has been expressed in relating the results of in vitro drug sensitivity testing with response to chemotherapy in patients with SCLC. Studies by Tsai (1990), Gazdar (1990a), and Johnson (1991a) and their colleagues confirmed that selection of individualized chemotherapy based on drug sensitivity testing is possible, but at the present time it is not considered useful in the management of SCLC patients. Although evaluations continue in the endeavor to recognize the mechanisms of resistance in patients with lung cancer, Carney (1992) notes that it is relatively clear that the multidrug-resistant phenotype is not a major determinant in this disease.

According to Brennan and colleagues (1991), C-*myc*, M-*myc*, and L-*myc* have been observed primarily in SCLC cell lines and fresh biopsy specimens. Carney (1991) found that amplification of C-*myc* has also been noted in variant SCLC cell lines, whereas both M-*myc* and L-*myc* have been demonstrated in classic cell types. Studies of large panels of cell lines reveal that amplification of oncogenes is more apt to be observed in cell lines established from heavily pretreated patients and is seen more frequently in established cell lines than in fresh biopsy specimens. Subsequently, Carney (1992) observed that *myc* amplification is seen more frequently in pretreated patients. The frequency of amplification was similar from fresh specimens and from cell lines in the same patient, suggesting that the *myc* family of oncogenes may accompany the more aggressive growth behavior observed at relapse. The clinical relevance of amplification of the *myc* oncogenes has not yet been demonstrated in prospective clinical trials.

Several studies undertaken by Weiner (1990) and Kern (1990) and their colleagues have provided evidence that cell lines from primary tumors that express c-*erb*-b2 genes in SCLC have shorter survival.

Cytogenetic abnormalities have been demonstrated in lung cancer cells. Carney (1991) found that lesions occur in the chromosome region 3p (14-23) in almost all cases of SCLC and have been shown in both primary and metastatic specimens, which suggests that it is a preliminary event in the biology of lung cancer. Of potential importance, as well, is the fact that the 3p deletion has not been demonstrated in extrapulmonary SCLC. Allele loss from chromosomes 13 and 17 has also been demonstrated. Some evidence also suggests that the expression of the *p53* oncogene in lung cancer

may be abnormal. Although other chromosomal abnormalities have been noted, Carney (1991) as well as Iggo and coworkers (1990) report that the mutation of this gene is the most commonly identified genetic change in human lung cancer. This area certainly demands more study.

Panels of monoclonal antibodies for identifying different types of lung cancer, including SCLC and NSCLC, may be feasible because many of the antibodies identified in lung cancer are under study by Boerman and associates (1991) for use in imaging, diagnosis, and target-directed therapy with toxins, as discussed by Carney (1992). Gazdar and colleagues (1990b) reported that monoclonal antibodies were used effectively for early detection and management of lung cancer using a sputum immunocytologic approach. This method was associated with 90% diagnostic accuracy 2 years before the ensuing diagnosis of cancer using orthodox techniques. Of significance, according to Carney (1991) and Woll and Rozengurt (1989), growth factors have been identified, at least in cell lines of lung cancer. These growth factors include bombesin (gastrin-releasing peptide), transferrin, and insulinlike growth factor. As reported by Macauley (1990) and Sausville (1990) and their colleagues, the latter may be an autocrine growth factor for SCLC. Interpreting how these factors function may be important in helping design a specific growth factor antagonist for therapeutic strategies, particularly in the treatment of SCLC. In studies of SCLC lines by Avalos and associates (1990), SCLC colony formation was enhanced by granulocyte colony-stimulating factor (G-CSF). Granulocyte colony-stimulating receptors were also shown on SCLC cells, which raises concern about the possible negative effects of using therapeutic G-CSF preparations in this patient population. This has not been a primary issue to date, however, and Crawford and colleagues (1991) have shown that G-CSF preparations have, in fact, been used successfully to lessen the myelosuppressive toxicity of chemotherapy in this disease with no apparent negative effect on survival. On the other hand, no survival advantage was observed in this landmark study and in a similar European study undertaken by Green and associates (1991), which creates uncertainty about whether the growth factors might be negatively affecting the outcome.

STAGING

Staging holds a key position in the choice of therapeutic treatment modalities for SCLC. Although chemotherapy is undoubtedly the main form of therapy used in SCLC, thoracic irradiation, and, rarely, even surgery may also be helpful, depending on tumor stage before treatment. The most fundamental purpose for staging, however, is its potential effect on prognosis. As one would expect, patients with less advanced SCLC have better long-term survival than do those with more advanced tumors.

Although tumor, node, metastasis (TNM) staging with the relatively recent Union Internationale Contre le Cancer-

American Joint Committee on Cancer classification as defined by Mountain (1997) is now used routinely in NSCLC (see Chapter 98), this approach has not proven to be very useful for staging in SCLC. Most patients with this disease have stage III or IV disease at the time of diagnosis, thereby making the TNM staging system less likely to predict long-term survival. Most therapeutic trials in the treatment of SCLC have used the simple two-stage system originally suggested by the Veterans Administration Lung Cancer Study Group (VALG), which classifies patients into those with limited and those with extensive disease. *Limited disease* is described as a tumor confined to one hemithorax and its regional lymph nodes, including the ipsilateral mediastinal, ipsilateral supraclavicular, and contralateral hilar nodes. These sites should all be easily encompassed within a tolerable radiation therapy portal, as noted by Zelen (1973). Ipsilateral pleural effusions, left laryngeal nerve involvement, and superior vena cava (SVC) obstruction are judged limited, whereas pericardial involvement and bilateral pulmonary involvement are considered extensive because they would necessitate the use of too large a radiation therapy portal. Some difficulty occurs when staging patients with contralateral mediastinal or supraclavicular lymph node metastases and patients with ipsilateral pleural effusions. These situations are often managed differently by different investigators. Some confusion exists about the lack of strict adherence to the VALG definition of limited disease. According to Ihde (1985), some investigators exclude ipsilateral pleural effusions and ipsilateral supraclavicular nodes, whereas others include contralateral supraclavicular nodes. For the most part, however, most groups adhere reasonably closely to the definition. In a consensus report prepared for the International Association for the Study of Lung Cancer Workshop on SCLC, Stahel and colleagues (1989) suggested that limited disease should include patients with disease restricted to one hemithorax with regional lymph node metastases (including hilar, ipsilateral, and contralateral mediastinal nodes and ipsilateral and contralateral supraclavicular nodes) and with ipsilateral pleural effusions, independent of whether cytology is positive or negative. The inclusion of contralateral mediastinal and supraclavicular metastases and ipsilateral pleural metastases in limited disease is recommended because the prognosis of patients with these sites of disease, which includes ipsilateral pleural effusions, is superior to that of patients with distant sites of metastases.

Variability in staging among investigators can also affect the number and type of staging procedures performed. If one investigator conducts more comprehensive staging than another does, a higher yield of patients with extensive disease results, but, surprisingly, the results in both groups of patients (limited and extensive disease) improve although not influencing overall survival. As discussed by Pfister and colleagues (1990), this has usually been termed *stage migration* or the *Will Rogers phenomenon*. Although it is virtually impossible to correct for this effect, one must be aware of its possibility when unusually good results are reported.

The two-stage system generally separates patients with disparate outcomes well. Those with limited disease have a higher objective regression rate and a higher complete response rate, as well as notably longer disease-free and long-term survival, than do patients who have extensive disease. Patients who attain complete response in either stage do relatively well.

The University of Toronto group has identified a subgroup called *very limited disease*. This designation arose during a retrospective study of 180 limited-stage patients undertaken by one of us (F.A.S.) and associates (1993). They found that the 33 patients without mediastinal involvement, supraclavicular node involvement, or pleural effusions had a projected 25% 5-year survival rate. If these data are confirmed by others in future trials, the status of the mediastinum may need to be specifically investigated in patients with limited SCLC. In addition, it should be noted that this is the exact patient population that frequently is chosen for trials of intensive locoregional therapy, such as hyperfractionated radiation therapy or even surgery. Thus, favorable results in phase II trials may result in part from patient selection for study rather than to superior therapy.

Even within extensive disease, some subgroups of patients may have better prognosis. Ihde and coworkers (1971) report that patients with single sites of extensive disease have longer survival than do patients with multiple sites of metastases and, in fact, are not distinct from limited-disease patients. As well, Ihde (1985) found that patients with specific sites of involvement, including liver and brain, do particularly poorly. In most series, 50 to 65% of patients who ultimately have extensive disease are, to some degree, reliant on how inclusive the staging is at a specific center.

Staging Procedures

The staging procedures that are most appropriate and essential for patients who are not participants in clinical trials are listed in Table 107-1. Extensive staging procedures in this setting may be difficult for some patients and can also needlessly escalate the cost of medical care. Extrathoracic staging is important, however, because the decision to incorporate radiation therapy into the overall treatment plan is based on confirmation of a limited-stage tumor. All patients must have a chest radiographic examination, physical examination, and simple blood tests before starting therapy. It has been suggested by the Memorial Sloan Kettering Cancer Center that a certain order for the subsequent examinations be established and that the cost of staging could be reduced by canceling further investigation once a positive test was obtained. Although, in theory, this approach seems logical, it may not be practical because staging procedures, particularly computed tomographic (CT) scans, usually are done all at the same time, and sequential booking of tests and the waiting time for reporting may cause unnecessary delays in the time before initiating treatment. For patients entering a

Table 107-1. Staging Procedures for Patients with Small Cell Lung Cancer Not Participating in Clinical Trials

Complete physical examination
Chest radiograph
Routine hematology: complete blood cell count, differential, and platelet count
Liver function tests
Alkaline phosphatase (for bony metastases)
Serum electrolytes, looking for low sodium
Sonography or computed tomography (CT) of abdomen, for liver and adrenals
Radionuclide bone scan
Skeletal radiographic examinations if bone scan is not definite
CT or magnetic resonance imaging of the brain, if symptomatic
Bone marrow aspiration and biopsy (only if abnormal hematology)

clinical trial, pretherapy staging must be more extensive (Table 107-2), and these procedures are comparable to those noted in a review by Stahel (1991) on the staging of patients with SCLC.

During treatment, patients should undergo physical examination and have a chest radiograph and blood work to evaluate response. More extensive staging, as shown in Table 107-2, during therapy is probably indicated only in clinical trials. A study conducted by Richardson and colleagues (1991) proposes that a simpler approach to staging may be as good and economical.

At the completion of therapy, it is appropriate to repeat known positive studies at designated intervals to document the completeness of response. This is important because the decision to offer prophylactic cranial irradiation (PCI) is often based on confirmation of complete response. As reported by one of us (R.F.) and colleagues (1993), little evidence supports duplicating all pretherapy studies in patients with limited disease who seem to have attained a complete response based on the results of a radiograph of the chest. Although bronchoscopy may identify areas of occult resid-

Table 107-2. Possible Staging Procedures for Patients with Small Cell Lung Cancer Participating in Clinical Trials

Computed tomography (CT) of thorax, for mediastinum and measurement of primary lesion
Sonography or CT of abdomen, for liver and adrenals
Routine bone marrow aspiration and biopsy (?), multiple sites
Liver biopsy, by peritoneoscopy or possibly with ultrasound guidance
Routine CT scans of brain [? magnetic resonance (MR) imaging]
Total-body MR imaging, including bone marrow
Fiberoptic bronchoscopy
Mediastinoscopy (rarely necessary)
Gallium 67 scanning of mediastinum
Serum carcinoembryonic antigen
Serum lactate dehydrogenase
Neuron-specific enolase (serum and ? cerebrospinal fluid)
Serum arginine-vasopressin
Lumbar puncture for cytology
Growth pattern of tumor cells in culture (i.e., classic vs. variant)

ual disease, it is not necessary for the majority of patients or outside the clinical trial setting.

Areas of Controversy

Intrathoracic Tumor

Although chest radiographs are worthwhile for the evaluation of disease in the lungs, chest wall, and mediastinum, they may still underestimate the degree of disease in these sites. According to Hirsch (1989) as well as Lewis and colleagues (1990), CT scanning of the thorax is more precise in detecting tumors within the lung itself, and it is considered essential for radiation therapy planning. In up to 15% of patients, enlarged nodes in the mediastinum may not contain tumor and may misdirect the investigator into raising the stage of the patient being evaluated. The impact of incorrectly up-staging a patient with SCLC is minimal because this tumor is seldom treated surgically, however, and the mediastinum is always included in the radiation treatment field. CT scans of the thorax should be extended to include the abdomen, which, of course, may assist in defining metastases in the liver or the adrenals. Abnormalities in the adrenals are fairly common, but available data have not clearly established that a patient with abnormalities (metastases or adenoma) at this site has a worse outcome than does a patient with limited disease. Hirsch (1989) reports that magnetic resonance (MR) imaging shows no benefit over CT in patients with SCLC. Although fluorodeoxyglucose positron emission tomography (FDG PET) has not often been used in patients with SCLC, it could prove to be useful in staging mediastinal and supraclavicular nodal involvement in patients with very limited intrathoracic disease on the chest radiograph. According to Erasmus and associates (1998), the accuracy of FDG PET in demonstrating intrathoracic metastatic nodal disease in NSCLC is greater than either that of CT or MR imaging, and this probably would be the same in SCLC patients. Fiberoptic bronchoscopy is not necessarily useful unless surgery is contemplated, as discussed by Ginsberg (1989) and Ginsberg and Karrer (1989), although Stahel (1991) finds that a baseline may be useful if reevaluation is considered after possible response to therapy.

Liver Metastases

Liver metastases are extremely common in patients with SCLC. Hirsch (1989) notes that liver function tests alone are not useful for detection unless results are entirely normal, in which case tumor is rarely evident at this site. Sonography and CT of the liver are the favored approaches because both techniques may also detect adrenal metastases. Some investigators also suggest the addition of an ultrasound-guided needle biopsy or peritoneoscopy. However, these invasive tests are associated with potential morbidity and are probably superfluous because, as discussed by Ihde (1985), virtually all patients are treated with combination chemotherapy, which should treat any occult microscopic liver metastases that might be present. Again, whole-body FDG PET scanning might prove to be useful in demonstrating liver and adrenal gland involvement because FDG uptake is noted in metabolically active metastatic disease, as shown in the study of Rege and associates (1993) as well as others.

Bone Marrow

One of us (R.F.) and associates (1988) reported that a standard practice during clinical trials is to do bone marrow aspirates and biopsies in patients with SCLC, although its value is now questioned outside the clinical trial setting. Single iliac crest aspirations and biopsies are usually performed, but in some series, they have been done bilaterally. Stahel (1985) and Berendsen (1988) and their colleagues report that even more refined techniques increase the potential for finding bone marrow involvement by tumor (e.g., using specific monoclonal antibodies). The latter approach may be important for the evaluation of the small subgroup of patients who may be assessed for autologous bone marrow transplantation, but it is likely of far less importance for patients who are not undergoing this type of aggressive therapy. Carney and colleagues (1989) note that MR imaging of the marrow has been used, with early data suggesting that this procedure may be more sensitive. The data of Layer and Jarosch (1992), as well as that of Hochstenbag (1996), Trillet-Lenoir (1994), and Seto (1997) and their coworkers demonstrate that MR imaging for detection of bone marrow metastasis is superior to that of either bone marrow biopsy or bone scintigraphy. However, whether identifying such metastasis in patients with limited disease influences the therapeutic approach is as yet unresolved.

A more controversial issue is whether bone marrow involvement should be sought at all. Studies reported by Hirsch (1989) and by Campling and colleagues (1986) showed that few patients (<10%) have metastases at this site; even less frequently is the bone marrow the only site that classifies the patient as having extensive disease. Hirsch (1989) and Sagman and associates (1991a) found that lactate dehydrogenase (LDH) might also provide comparable information without the need for this relatively uncomfortable invasive procedure. This theory is still controversial; therefore, at this time, bone marrow aspiration and biopsy should be undertaken only in patients who are potential candidates for clinical trials of limited stage disease.

Central Nervous System Metastases

Hirsch (1989) and Klastersky (1990) report that brain metastases are seen at presentation in approximately 10% of patients with SCLC, but they may be present at autopsy in up to 65%. The standard investigation for this site has been CT scanning, although MR imaging is probably superior to CT, as it is for most brain abnormalities. The role of FDG PET scans for identifying brain metastases is limited at best owing to the increased metabolism of normal brain tissue.

Carcinomatous meningitis is an infrequent presenting characteristic of this disease. As shown by one of us (R.F.) and colleagues (1988), meningeal involvement may be confirmed by microscopic examination of the cerebrospinal fluid. According to Bunn (1978), Rosen (1982), and Aisner (1981) and their colleagues, however, several lumbar punctures may be required to demonstrate meningeal involvement. Nodular filling defects along the root sleeves may be seen at myelography or with MR imaging of the vertebral column when spinal cord compression is present.

Biomarkers

Many biomarkers have been studied in patients with this disease, and their expression may correlate with response to treatment. Adrenocorticotropic hormone, calcitonin, neuron-specific enolase, plasma neurophysin, and antidiuretic hormone have not, as discussed by one of us (R.F.) and coworkers (1988) and Hansen (1990), been conclusively useful prognostic factors in these patients. Pretreatment levels of carcinoembryonic antigen (CEA) correlate with the stage of the disease and, as proposed by Sculier and associates (1985a) may actually be an independent prognostic factor. However, levels are elevated only in approximately one-third of patients, thereby making CEA a less valuable indicator. According to Rawson and Peto (1990), as well as Albain (1990), Stahel (1991) and their coworkers, pretreatment LDH values may be a useful pretreatment prognostic factor. Values often return to normal if the patient responds to therapy.

As noted by one of us (R.F.) and coworkers (1988), as well as by Biran and colleagues (1991), several investigative groups have reported that rising levels of biomarkers sometimes precede clinical evidence of tumor relapse by weeks or months. Because of the lack of effective therapy at the time of relapse, as discussed by Boyer and associates (1992), the benefit of early knowledge of relapse of tumors is debatable. Combinations of markers may better predict early relapse. The consensus at the moment is that biomarkers other than LDH, perhaps, are of little value for pretreatment prognosis or as early evidence of relapse, although additional research continues on the subject. A relatively new biomarker, noted by Holst and colleagues (1989), is the C-terminal flanking peptide of human gastrin-releasing peptide, which may indicate a worse prognosis. Giovanella and associates (1997) reported that the tumor marker neuron-specific enolase may be useful in monitoring therapy and in patient follow-up.

Restaging

Restaging is a distinct area of debate. In a retrospective study conducted by the National Cancer Institute of Canada (NCIC), one of us (R.F.) and colleagues (1992) found that routine restaging in patients with limited disease who had responded was probably of little value. Although a small survival benefit was demonstrated in a subgroup of patients who had negative posttreatment bronchoscopy compared to patients with positive bronchoscopic findings, the investigators suggested considering this approach only in a clinical trial. Economic analysis also supported the concept of not proceeding with restaging, although Stahel and coworkers (1989) and Stahel (1991) still encourage restaging, particularly repeat bronchoscopy.

New Staging Systems

Although the simple VALG two-stage system for SCLC has been worthwhile for many years, it may soon be time for necessary changes to this strategy. The newer methods currently available may identify more subgroups at high and low risk. They may have to be assimilated into future staging systems, but at present the overall significance of staging small subsets of SCLC patients can be questioned. As previously mentioned, however, one of us (F.A.S.) and colleagues (1993) studied 130 patients with very limited SCLC who did not have a peripheral nodule and had not had definitive surgery. Thirty-three patients had no evidence of mediastinal involvement; findings in two-thirds of these patients were based on mediastinoscopy, the rest on chest radiography. They had a projected 25% 5-year survival rate, which is notably higher than that of all other patients with limited disease. Comparable findings were observed by Osterlind and colleagues (1985), although these conclusions were not clearly expressed in their report. Our patients progressed favorably despite having had no surgical intervention. Because this group of patients accounts for most, if not all, of the 5-year survivors seen with this disease, an imbalance of this group in a clinical trial could have major consequences on interpretation of outcome. As remarked previously, we also noted the apparent influence of markers, such as LDH and CEA, which may additionally subdivide this group of patients without mediastinal disease and identify the best candidates for long-term survival. Patients with liver and brain metastases seem to be among those with the poorest results in the category of extensive disease, whereas patients with isolated bone metastases seem to do well. Therefore, it may be necessary to divide the clinical trial population into a reasonably large number of groups, possibly using TNM staging to develop a more workable staging system in the 21st century for future clinical trials. At present, these subdivisions can only be considered hypotheses, and until proved valuable, they will not become part of the standard staging system for this disease.

Prognostic Factors

Prognostic factors may be useful for individual patient prognosis as well as for accurate stratification in clinical tri-

Table 107-3. Possible Prognostic Factors for Survival in Treated Patients with Small Cell Lung Cancer

Prognostic Factors	Positive Effect	Negative Effect
Increasing stage (limited vs. extensive)		X
Worsening, poorer performance status		X
Weight loss		X
Prior treatment		X
Sex (women do better)	X	
Increased number of sites of distant metastases		X
Site of metastases (liver or brain vs. others)		X
Site of primary tumor (TNM staging) smaller	X	
Age 70 years		X
Mediastinal involvement (TNM staging)		X
Increased serum CEA, LDH, neuron-specific enolase		X
Histologic subtypes intermediate vs. other		?X
Hypouricemia		X
Alkaline phosphatase increased		X
Hypoalbuminemia		X
Immune defects		X
Classic growth patterns vs. variant	X	
Pericardial involvement		X

CEA, carcinoembryonic antigen; LDH, lactate dehydrogenase; TNM, tumor, node, metastasis.

als. The factors documented as important by Stahel (1991) and Rawson and Peto (1990), as well as by Ihde (1971), Albain (1990), and Stahel (1989) and their colleagues, encompass the following: 1) stage of disease (limited versus extensive), 2) performance status, and 3) whether patients have received previous chemotherapy. Various investigators have found additional prognostic factors (Table 107-3). Female sex is an accepted good prognostic factor, as noted by a number of investigators, including Stahel (1992) and Ferguson and coworkers (1990). Consensus has not yet been reached as to which factors are most significant; the knowledge gleaned from staging and prognostic factors must be considered carefully when comparing results of therapy in reports of clinical trials in this disease. Newer statistical methods, such as recursive partitioning and amalgamation, may prove useful, as evidenced by two articles by Albain (1990) and Sagman (1991b) and their coworkers.

EVOLUTION OF THERAPY

Although chemotherapy is the predominant form of treatment and is addressed in detail, it is useful to review how treatment of SCLC developed to its present approach. Initially, surgery was the treatment of choice for patients with all types of lung cancer, but it was abandoned after the results of a randomized trial carried out in the United Kingdom by the Medical Research Council comparing radiation therapy alone to surgery alone in patients with limited disease. The 5- and 10-year results of this study were reported by Miller and colleagues (1969) and Fox and Scadding (1973), respectively. Even though the mean survival time for all these patients was short (10 months, with only 5% of patients alive at 5 years), the fact that all surviving patients were on the radiation arm made radiation therapy the standard form of treatment from that point on.

Green and coworkers (1969) demonstrated the activity of cyclophosphamide against SCLC compared to placebo. They showed that the median survival for patients with extensive disease receiving placebo was approximately 6 weeks and that for patients with limited disease who received the placebo was only 12 weeks. These data must be recognized when endeavoring to put into perspective the modest improvements observed in the treatment of this disease between the 1970s and 1990s.

One of us (R.F.) and colleagues (1988) reported that many single agents in patients with SCLC yield response rates of 20% and higher. In a review of all studies from 1970 to 1990, Grant and coworkers (1992) identified 11 active drugs. Newer agents shown to be active have since been added to initial lists. Minna and colleagues (1989) report that when active drugs were combined, an improved response rate was observed, with complete response rates ranging from 20 to 50% and rising even higher in patients with limited disease. Retrospective reviews of the median survival of patients treated with either single agents or combination chemotherapy showed that individuals receiving combinations survived longer. Randomized trials comparing single agents with combination chemotherapy with or without chest irradiation demonstrated benefit to the combinations, as emphasized by Ihde and associates (1991).

Bergsagel and colleagues (1972) showed that the addition of cyclophosphamide to conventional thoracic irradiation in patients with limited disease resulted in a survival benefit. This result was confirmed by Smyth (1984) and led to the use of combined-method treatment in the early 1970s. Most frequently, thoracic irradiation is added to combination chemotherapy in patients with limited disease, but it is not routinely given to patients with extensive disease. Some medical groups are adding thoracic irradiation to the treatment plan for patients with extensive disease who achieve complete response.

When it was observed that in many patients, relapse involved the central nervous system (CNS), Hansen and colleagues (1980) suggested that the brain was a potential sanctuary from chemotherapy. Subsequently, it became routine to administer PCI to all patients with SCLC, regardless of stage. One of us (R.F.) and colleagues (1988) reviewed the results of PCI as investigated in randomized trials: Its use reduced the failure rate in the brain but did not result in any survival benefit. In the 1980s, signs of neurologic toxicity were identified with either radiation therapy or combined treatment (radiation therapy and chemotherapy) and more rigorous criteria for the use of PCI have been advocated since then. In particular, it has been recommended that

application of PCI be confined to patients who have shown a complete response because they are the most liable to benefit. According to Lishner and coworkers (1990), the possible disadvantage of PCI in this subpopulation (i.e., CNS toxicity, which was not observed in all studies) is probably worth risking (see Elective Brain Irradiation).

Although still debated in some circles, it seems that on the basis of a meta-analysis of randomized trials conducted by Arriagada and associates (1991a) and by Warde and one of us (D.P.) (1992), thoracic irradiation adds to combination chemotherapy in patients with limited SCLC. Accordingly, most physicians treat patients who achieve a complete response, and many treat patients who achieve at least a partial response with this method of therapy. Controversy also surrounds how best to give thoracic irradiation. The issues include dose, fractionation, portal size, and at what point the radiation therapy should be given in reference to the beginning of combination chemotherapy. These questions are examined in more detail later in this chapter under Radiation Therapy

Significant interest has also been generated in the use of surgery in this disease. Most groups advise operating on peripheral lesions in early-stage disease (stages I and II). Frequently, these patients receive thoracic irradiation and possibly PCI with or without chemotherapy along with their surgery. In patients with more advanced disease, the only well-designed randomized trial, reported by Lad and associates (1991) for the Lung Cancer Study Group, did not show benefit associated with the addition of surgery to radiation and chemotherapy. Consequently, this approach is not standard, although it is still a component of therapy in selected patients in some centers around the world.

In general, immunotherapy (biological responsive modifiers) has not proved to be of any superior benefit in this disease. One study by Cohen and colleagues (1979), who used thymosin fraction V, did show a survival benefit, but this effect was not validated in a study undertaken by Shank and coworkers (1985). In a study in Finland by Mattson and colleagues (1991), results suggested a benefit to maintenance therapy with α-interferon in patients responding to standard methods of treatment. Cooperative groups in the United States have endeavored to corroborate this information, but conclusive analysis of these data is not yet available. A trial piloted by Jett and colleagues (1992) in the North Central Group using interferon maintenance showed no benefit. At present, this form of therapy should not be considered standard.

CHEMOTHERAPY

Single Agents

Chemotherapy is currently the mainstay of treatment for all stages of SCLC. In the 1960s, Green and associates (1969) demonstrated improved survival in patients with extensive SCLC after three courses of cyclophosphamide compared to placebo. Since that time, many active drugs

Table 107-4. Established Active Single Agents in the Treatment of Small Cell Lung Cancer

Active Single Agents	Approximate Single-Agent Activity (%)
Bischloroethylnitrosourea (carmustine)	20
Carboplatin	40
Chloroethylcyclohexylnitrosourea (lomustine[a])	15
Cisplatin[a]	15
Cyclophosphamide[a]	40
Doxorubicin[a]	30
Epirubicin (high-dose)	50
Etoposide (VP-16) intravenous	40–50
Etoposide oral	50
Gemcitabine	27
Hexamethylmelamine (altretamine)	30
Ifosfamide	40–50
Methotrexate[a]	35
Nitrogen mustard	35
Paclitaxel (Taxol)	35–50
Teniposide (VM-26)	40–50
Topotecan	—
Vincristine[a]	35
Vindesine	30

[a]Agents most commonly used today.

Table 107-5. Activity of Recently Tested Single Agents in Small Cell Lung Cancer

Active agents[a]
  Carboplatin
  Epirubicin (high-dose)
  Hexamethylmelamine
  Ifosfamide
  Teniposide (VM-25)
  Vindesine
Possibly active agents[b]
  Gemcitabine
  Iproplatin
  Irinotecan
  Lonidamine
  Taxol
  Topotecan
Inactive agents[c]
  Aclarubicin
  Bisantrene
  Cytarabine
  Diaziquone
  Esorubicin
  Idarubicin
  Mitoguazone
  Mitomycin C
  Mitoxantrone
  PCNU
  Vinblastine

[a]At least 20% single-agent activity.
[b]10 to 20% single agent activity.
[c]<10% single-agent activity. Data for this table were collected from multiple sources.

have been identified. A partial list of the most active single agents in SCLC is shown in Table 107-4. The agents used most frequently include etoposide (VP-16), cisplatin, cyclophosphamide, doxorubicin (Adriamycin), and vincristine. Promising new agents include gemcitabine, which has single-agent activity with a response rate of 27%, as reported by Cormier and colleagues (1994). Gemcitabine also has been the focus of a phase II study by Eisenhauer and colleagues (1992). Other agents are CPT-11, for which Masuda and colleagues (1992) have undertaken a study, and paclitaxel (Taxol) and its derivatives. Paclitaxel has shown single-agent activity with a 31 to 50% response, as pointed out by Ettinger (1993), Hainsworth and Greco (1995), and Bunn (1997). Other new agents include irinotecan, topotecan, and docetaxel, which are being studied in phase I and II trials. Topotecan, a new non–cross-resistant chemotherapeutic agent, is a topoisomerase I inhibitor, and early studies by Schiller (1996), Perez-Soler (1996) and Ardizzoni (1997) and their associates have shown that it has significant activity in SCLC.

Single-agent chemotherapy produces objective responses but seldom produces complete regression, even in previously untreated patients with SCLC. On the basis of studies carried out by Ettinger (1990) for the Eastern Cooperative Oncology Group (ECOG) and Evans and coworkers (1990) for NCIC, it seems both ethical and appropriate to treat previously untreated patients with extensive SCLC using an experimental agent. Evaluation should occur early in this case, and if no response is observed, the patient should be shifted to an active regimen before the disease is irretrievable. Expectation of response rates of 70% or greater should be used to estimate sample sizes in this population. Black-

stein and coworkers (1990) note that less difficulty may be associated with use of derivatives of known active agents, such as anthracyclines; this is also true of new platinum compounds. Both ECOG and NCIC have had experiences with active and inactive agents and have observed reasonable response rates and survival, regardless of the action of the new drug. Treating previously treated patients may result in artificial negative data, which may then not identify potentially useful drugs. Grant and colleagues (1992) suggested that using a lower response rate (10%) as an indication of activity in previously treated patients may still be a useful approach. In addition to the active agents mentioned, Grant and colleagues (1992) note that phase II trials have found that many agents show little or no activity (Table 107-5) in patients with SCLC.

Combination Chemotherapy

In spite of partial responses and occasional complete responses, the relatively poor results with single-agent chemotherapy led to efforts at combining these agents in patients with SCLC, as had been done with other malignancies. Less than 20% of 753 patients given single-agent chemotherapy had an objective response, and less than 3% obtained a complete response in a retrospective review carried out by Bunn and Ihde (1981). In contrast, among 1236 patients receiving combination chemotherapy, a 70% objective response rate was seen, 31% being complete. Those receiving combination chemotherapy survived longer than did those receiving single agents. Authors of randomized trials have compared single agents and combination chemotherapy with or without chest irradiation and demonstrated a slight benefit from combination chemotherapy in objective tumor response and median survival. Bunn and Ihde (1981) and Minna and colleagues (1989) also reviewed the literature about the appropriate number of drugs to be included in combination for this disease. They found no significant difference in the complete response rate or long-term, disease-free survival when more than three drugs were used in patients with limited disease.

Table 107-6 shows the most traditionally used and highly active combinations for treatment of this disease worldwide. Although these are among the most conventional, virtually any combination of the most active agents has achieved reasonable results. As discussed by one of us (R.F.) and colleagues (1988), any of these regimens should result in response rates in excess of 80% (50 to 60% complete response) in patients with limited disease and 65 to 70% in patients with extensive disease (10 to 20% complete response). If appropriate staging procedures are carried out, the median survival for patients with limited disease should be 12 to 15 months or more. In trials undertaken by Murray (1991b), Johnson (1987a,b), and Tourani (1991) and their colleagues on combined-method treatment, median survivals of 18 to 20 months or more were observed for patients with limited disease. Ihde (1991) and Kristjansen (1991) and their colleagues found that the median survival for patients with extensive disease is still roughly 10 months or less, with a range of 8 to 12 months. Approximately 15 to 20% of patients with limited disease and less than 5% of those with extensive disease remain disease free for more than 2 years. Patients who achieve a complete response usually live longer than those who show only a partial response, the former being the only group with the potential for long-term,

disease-free survival. Patients with limited disease usually live significantly longer than do those with extensive disease, as do patients who have a superior performance status at presentation.

Proper Dosing of Available Drugs

Diverse pharmacologic approaches with known active drugs may be illustrated by interest in the use of relatively low-dose oral etoposide (VP-16) on a continuous 14- or 21-day schedule, with approximately 1 week off, followed by restarting this therapy. This regimen was developed by Johnson and colleagues (1991b) from Vanderbilt University and Slevin and associates (1989), as well as by Einhorn and coworkers (1990) from Indiana University and Clark and coworkers (1990, 1991) from the United Kingdom. Carney and colleagues (1990) note that toxicity in formerly untreated patients seems tolerable and makes this a sound approach for elderly patients in whom an aggressive approach with a more conventional regimen is contraindicated or declined by the patient. Some patients also responded to injectable etoposide who had either responded in the past or did not respond at all. Oral etoposide has also been combined with cisplatin and carboplatin, but preliminary data presented by Murphy (1991) and Evans (1991) and their colleagues did not suggest a significant benefit over oral etoposide alone by continuous daily treatment. A randomized trial reported by Souhami and coworkers (1997), however, did not confirm the findings of benefit of the use of oral etoposide; in fact, its use was inferior to the use of intravenous chemotherapy.

Dose Intensification

Dose Intensification by Increasing Chemotherapy Dose

Despite initial response rates of 80 to 90% to conventional chemotherapy, most patients experience relapse within 2 years and die with disseminated malignancy. Improvements in local control and the metastatic disease are required, but it is likely that any substantial improvement or increases in cure rate are secondary to the development of more effective systemic treatment. The concept of dose intensity in cancer chemotherapy has been reviewed by Dodwell and associates (1990). Although convincing evidence of a steep dose-response curve for most chemotherapeutic agents when they are studied in vitro or in animal model systems exists, the clinical evidence is considerably less compelling when the randomized trials with SCLC are examined (Table 107-7).

In an older trial reported by Cohen and colleagues (1977), patients in the higher dose arm demonstrated superior overall response rates and median survival. O'Donnell and coworkers (1985) undertook a similar study using higher

Table 107-6. Frequently Used Chemotherapy Combinations for Small Cell Lung Cancer

Chemotherapy Combination	Possible Abbreviation
Cyclophosphamide, doxorubicin (Adriamycin), etoposide (VP-16)	CAV$_P$P V$_P$P
Etoposide, cisplatin	V$_P$P
Cyclophosphamide, doxorubicin, vincristine, etoposide	CAVE
Cyclophosphamide, doxorubicin, vincristine	CAV
Etoposide, carboplatin	V$_P$CP*
Etoposide, ifosfamide, cisplatin	ICE (VIP)
Cisplatin, vincristine (Oncovin), doxorubicin, etoposide	CODE

Note: All regimens give response rates of 70 to 90% in patients with limited disease and 55 to 75% in patients with extensive disease.

Table 107-7. Prospective Randomized Trials of the Importance of Dose in Small Cell Lung Cancer

Author	Drug and Dose (mg/m²)	Patients	Overall Response Rate (%)	Median Survival Rate (Months)	Comments
Cohen et al., 1977	C 1000, MTX 15, CCNU 100	23	96 (P <.05)	(P <.05)	Inadequate doses in low-dose arm
	C 500 MTX 10, CCNU 50	9	46	5.0	
Mehta and Vogl, 1982	C 1500, MTX 15, CCNU 70	175	64 (P = .04)	(P = .04)	
	C 700, MTX 15, CCNU 70	174	54	9	Inadequate cyclophosphamide dose in low-dose arm
Figueredo et al., 1985	C 1500, A 60, VCR 2	52	71 (ns)	14 (ns)	—
	C 1000, A 50, VCR 2	51	61	12	
Johnson et al., 1987a	C 1200, A 70, VCR 1	101	63 (P = .04)	7	
	C 1000, A 40, VCR 1	146	53	8	High doses only for first 9 weeks
Ihde et al., 1991	E 80 x 5, P 27 x 5	39	85 (ns)	12	—
	E 80 x 3, P 80 x 1	42	42	11	
Arriagada et al., 1993	C 1200, A 40, P 100, E 75 x 3	55	67 (CR) (P = .16)	43%	High dose only for cycle 1
	C 900, A 40, P 80, E 75 x 3	40	54 (CR)	26%	Survival reported at 2 years (P = .02)

A, doxorubicin; C, cyclophosphamide; CR, complete response; E, etoposide; MTX, methotrexate; ns, not significant; P, cisplatin; VCR, vincristine.

doses of the same drugs and demonstrated a higher response rate but no significant prolongation of survival. This was a small trial of only 32 patients, however, and the cyclophosphamide dose of only 500 mg/m² in the low-dose arm would be considered inadequate treatment today. Mehta and Vogl (1982) performed a larger trial using the same agents with the same results. Once again, though, the cyclophosphamide dose would be considered too low by today's standards. Figueredo and coworkers (1985) compared standard-dose cyclophosphamide, doxorubicin, and vincristine (CAV) to higher doses of the same drugs (i.e., doxorubicin, 20% increase; cyclophosphamide, 50% increase). No difference in complete response rate or duration of response could be identified. Johnson and colleagues (1987a, 1987b) also reported a higher response rate with higher doses of cyclophosphamide and doxorubicin but no improvement in survival. In a similar trial evaluating the usefulness of high-dose etoposide and cisplatin reported by Ihde and colleagues (1991), no difference in complete response rate or overall survival was seen for patients in the high-dose arm (i.e., 67% increase for both drugs). In the last study of dose, Arriagada and colleagues (1993) gave higher doses of cyclophosphamide and cisplatin only in cycle 1. Surprisingly, median and 2-year survival rates were both significantly higher in the high-dose arm.

Despite the relatively negative results of most of these initial trials, considerable interest was generated in the 1990s in dose intensification for SCLC. Even though the differences demonstrated in most of the trials did not reach statistical significance, each study did show a trend toward improved response and prolonged survival in the high-dose arm. In the assessment of dose intensity, the dosage of individual drugs as well as the duration of treatment and the interval between individual drug administrations should be

taken into consideration, as discussed by Bonomi and coworkers (1985). Hryniuk and Levine (1986) and Hryniuk and associates (1987) define *dose intensity* as the amount of drug administered per unit of time, expressed for a single drug regimen as milligrams per square meter per week. For a multiple-drug regimen, they recommend definition of an average relative dose intensity by comparison with a standard regimen and by giving a relative weight to each drug. In an analysis of 67 published studies, Klasa and associates (1991) attempted to correlate response and median survival time with dose intensity over the first 6 weeks of chemotherapy for SCLC. They identified a trend (P = .07) toward a positive correlation between dose intensity and median survival time for patients with extensive disease treated with CAV. When only randomized studies were considered, they noted a positive correlation (P = .001) for the relative dose intensity of doxorubicin with total response rate but not with overall survival. A similar correlation was also seen for etoposide-containing regimens for response rate and survival in patients with extensive disease.

On the basis of these observations, individual investigators and cooperative groups have continued to assess new chemotherapy strategies aimed at increasing the dose intensity of the regimen, either through alteration in the scheduling of drug delivery or by increasing the actual doses of chemotherapeutic agents.

Acceleration of Chemotherapy Delivery to Increase Dose Intensity

The mathematical model for the development of chemotherapy-resistant clones in malignancies proposed by Goldie and Coldman (1984) suggests that the number of drug-resistant clones of cells within the tumor is most likely at its lowest at the time of diagnosis. As tumor size increases, the number of drug-resistant clones also increases, either as a spontaneous event or in response to exposure to chemotherapeutic agents. This finding suggests that a potential therapeutic advantage may be gained by the early introduction of as many active agents (drugs or irradiation) as possible in the treatment protocol. Klimo and Connors (1985) first evaluated an intensive weekly chemotherapy protocol with the rapid alternation of myelosuppressive and nonmyelosuppressive agents over a short 9- to 12-week course for patients with diffuse large cell lymphoma. The favorable results achieved in lymphoma patients led Murray and coworkers (1991b) to develop a similar protocol for patients with extensive SCLC. Their CODE regimen [*c*isplatin, vincristine (*O*ncovin), *d*oxorubicin, and *e*toposide]; a supportive care program of prednisone and cimetidine on alternate days; and daily cotrimoxazole and ketoconazole resulted in an overall response rate of 94%, a complete response rate of 40%, and a survival time of 61 weeks in 48 patients with extensive-stage SCLC. The authors emphasized that the main toxicity for this regimen was constitutional, and they recommended administering 9 rather than 12 weeks of therapy, which resulted in a dose intensity that was almost twice as great as that achieved with standard 18-week protocols using the same drugs. Miles and colleagues (1991) reported another study using similar chemotherapeutic agents but substituted ifosfamide for vincristine. They also achieved a high overall response rate of 92%, a complete response rate of 48%, and median survivals of 58 weeks for limited disease and 42 weeks for extensive disease.

The regimens piloted by Murray (1991b) and Miles (1991) and their associates both contained four chemotherapeutic agents. In a Southwest Oncology Group (SWOG) pilot study reported by Taylor and coworkers (1990), six agents were alternated weekly for a total of 16 weeks. The overall response rate was 82%, and 38% of patients with extensive disease achieved complete remission. The median survivals for limited and extensive disease were 16.6 and 11.4 months, respectively. The Lung Group at the Institut Jules Bordet went one step further and tested a seven-drug combination. Sculier and colleagues (1988) reported an overall response rate of 78% for limited- and extensive-disease patient groups combined. Based on results of this pilot study, this regimen is to be compared to standard therapy in a European Organization for Research and Treatment of Cancer (EORTC) prospective randomized trial. However, the phase II study of Murray and associates (1991b) noted previously was followed by a randomized phase III trial undertaken by NCIC and SWOG. Patients with extensive-stage SCLC were randomized to receive either the CODE regimen or standard chemotherapy (alternation of CAV with etoposide and cisplatin). The study closed early when an excessive toxic death rate was observed in the CODE arm, with no evidence of a survival benefit from the dose-intensive treatment (N. Murray, personal communication, 1999). Thus,

the question of the value of the acceleration of delivery to increase dose intensity remains unresolved.

Colony-Stimulating Factors to Increase or Maintain Dose Intensity

Myelosuppression is the dose-limiting toxicity for most chemotherapeutic agents that are active against SCLC. Several clinical studies have revealed that the recombinant CSFs, G-CSF, and granulocyte-macrophage CSF (GM-CSF) can accelerate the recovery of myelopoiesis after cytotoxic chemotherapy. In two similar randomized trials reported by Crawford (1991) and Green (1991) and their associates, patients were treated with cyclophosphamide, doxorubicin, and etoposide. They were randomized either to receive or not to receive G-CSF on the first cycle. Both trials showed that the incidence of febrile neutropenia and hospital admission was substantially reduced in the G-CSF arms. Although these trials were not designed to evaluate response and survival, no overall improvement in either outcome could be identified in the groups receiving G-CSF.

The primary objective of these two trials was to ameliorate toxicity by reducing the period of absolute neutropenia and the incidence of neutropenia-associated sepsis. These efforts led to pilot studies to determine whether CSF would allow repeated administrations of higher doses of chemotherapy in an attempt to improve response rate and survival rate without an unacceptable increase in toxic effects. In a study undertaken by the Cancer and Acute Leukemia Group B, Mitchell and coworkers (1988) reported that the maximum tolerated doses of etoposide and cisplatin without CSF support were 200 mg/m^2 etoposide and 35 mg/m^2 cisplatin given intravenously daily for 3 days. In a dose-escalation study of the Cancer and Acute Leukemia Group B, three of six patients developed dose-limiting toxic effects with 200 mg/m^2 per day etoposide for 3 days and 125 mg/m^2 per day carboplatin with 10 µg/kg of GM-CSF for 3 days. A greater degree of myeloprotection was achieved by increasing the dose of GM-CSF to 20 µg/kg, but it was not possible to escalate chemotherapy doses further. Greater bone marrow protection was seen in a small cohort of patients treated with 5 µg/kg of GM-CSF every 12 hours compared with either 10 or 20 µg/kg once daily. In a similar trial reported by Mitchell and colleagues (1988), the addition of GM-CSF to etoposide and cisplatin at the maximum tolerated doses did not allow further dose escalation. Four of six patients developed febrile neutropenia or infections, and only one of six patients was able to tolerate six cycles of chemotherapy, and that patient required one dose reduction for hematologic toxicity. Furthermore, all patients who received more than one course of high-dose chemotherapy required blood product support (packed red blood cells and platelets).

Significant myelosuppression occurred in all the aforementioned weekly intensive chemotherapy protocols discussed. This result has led investigators to assess the role of CSF in accelerated chemotherapy programs. Ardizzoni and coworkers (1990) reported the results of a small nonrandomized pilot study of GM-CSF in which five patients received GM-CSF when grade IV leukopenia occurred and five patients received no growth factor support. The mean interval between chemotherapy courses and the mean duration of therapy were 10 and 57 days, respectively, in patients treated with GM-CSF compared with 13 and 72 days in the control group. Overall, chemotherapy dose intensity was increased twofold in the patients given GM-CSF compared with a 1.5-fold increase in the control patients. Other studies continue with GM-CSF, but at this time, as noted by Bishop (1991) and Anderson (1991a) and their associates, data are not as good as those observed with G-CSF.

The only reported prospective randomized trial of intensive weekly chemotherapy and G-CSF was undertaken by Fukuoka and colleagues (1991b). These investigators compared CODE alone to CODE with a small dose (50 µg/m²) of G-CSF given daily on the nonchemotherapy days. The complete remission rate was similar in both arms, but the median survival in the G-CSF arm was 59 weeks compared to 35 weeks in the control arm. The total dose delivered in the G-CSF arm was 85% of predicted compared to 76% of predicted in the control arm. The median number of days of neutropenia was 1.33 in the G-CSF arm compared to 3.31 in the control arm, and febrile episodes were seen in only 13 patients compared to 36 patients in the group receiving no treatment. This degree of marrow protection was achieved despite a low dose of G-CSF. It is important, however, that these patients remained in the hospital throughout the 9-week course of therapy. It is also critical that the response rates and survival rates in the G-CSF arm are not superior to those reported by Murray and associates (1991b) for CODE given with alternate-day prednisone and prophylactic antibiotics and without CSF support.

In a randomized trial of dose intensity reported by Pujol and colleagues (1995), the addition of GM-CSF to the high-dose arm did not allow higher doses of drugs to be delivered. In fact, after the first dose, patients frequently required dose reduction for toxicity, and only 75% of intended doses could be administered despite the use of growth factors.

In a randomized trial of standard-dose vincristine, ifosfamide, carboplatin, etoposide (V-ICE) versus intensified V-ICE, reported by Steward and associates (1995), there was a second randomization in each arm to either GM-CSF or placebo. No differences in dose delivery, dose intensity, remission rate, or survival were detected between the GM-CSF and placebo arms. Woll and colleagues (1995) reported the results of a similar trial that used the same drugs and G-CSF. They found no differences in the response rates or survival, and lethal toxicity was actually higher in the G-CSF arm.

Clearly, CSFs can reduce the degree and duration of neutropenia after standard-dose chemotherapy, but they do not seem to allow repeated administration of higher doses of chemotherapy or dosing at significantly shorter intervals. If CSFs allow only modest dose escalation, their costs and tox-

icity likely are not justified. In summary, CSFs have very little role to play in the routine management of patients with SCLC who are receiving standard doses of chemotherapy either in classic 3- to 4-week intervals or in more dose-intense weekly schedules.

Bone Marrow Transplantation

High-dose chemotherapy followed by autologous bone marrow transplantation in patients with SCLC has been under investigation since the 1980s and it is probably safe to say that this form of treatment is not appropriate for most patients with this tumor. Of necessity, almost all trials have been small phase I to II pilot studies, and diverse patient populations make comparisons between studies almost impossible. Some trials focused only on patients with limited disease, whereas others included those with extensive disease as well. Furthermore, high-dose therapy has been studied as initial induction treatment, as intensification after induction at standard doses, or as salvage at the time of relapse.

High-Dose Induction Chemotherapy

Several trials of high-dose induction chemotherapy are summarized in Table 107-8. The trial of Johnson and colleagues (1987a) is interesting because patients with extensive disease were treated with two courses of high-dose cyclophosphamide and etoposide plus high-dose cisplatin without bone marrow transplantation. Although myelosuppression was severe, 17 of 20 patients were able to receive their second course of high-dose chemotherapy. The complete response rate was 65%, but the median survival was only 41 weeks, and 2-year survival was approximately 20%.

Several London hospitals evaluated intensive chemotherapy with autologous bone marrow transplantation, and Souhami and coworkers (1989) reviewed the results of four sequential trials undertaken by their group. Most patients in their studies had limited disease. In the first study, patients received cyclophosphamide alone, and in study II, etoposide was added. In studies III and IV, patients were treated with multidrug combinations consisting of cyclophosphamide, etoposide, doxorubicin, and vincristine or carboplatin, etoposide, and either melphalan or cyclophosphamide. Once again, high response rates were observed, but the 2-year survival was only 20% (data were available only for studies I, II, and III). Of interest, the highest response rate, median survival, and 2-year survival rate were seen in study I, in which only high-dose cyclophosphamide was used.

Late Intensification with High-Dose Chemotherapy and Autologous Bone Marrow Transplantation

The disappointing long-term results achieved with high-dose chemotherapy as initial induction treatment led several investigators to offer such treatment as late intensification

Table 107-8. Trials of High-Dose Induction Chemotherapy for Small Cell Lung Cancer

Author	Number	Drugs	Median (wks)	Survival (2 yrs)	Comments
Littlewood et al., 1986	2 limited, 5 extensive	Etoposide 1.2–2.4 g/m^2	42–50	14%	No patient achieved complete response
Johnson et al., 1987a	20 extensive	Etoposide 1.2 g/m^2 Cisplatin 120 mg/m^2 Cyclophosphamide 100 mg/kg	41	20%	No ABMT; two treatment-related deaths
Souhami et al., 1989	70 limited, 5 extensive	Four different protocols	43–74	20%	Five treatment-related deaths; primary was most frequent site of relapse
Nomura et al., 1990	6 limited	Varying doses of cyclophosphamide, etoposide, cisplatin, and vincristine	41	?	Only two patients achieved complete response; all patients now dead

ABMT, autologous bone marrow transplantation.

only to patients who responded well to standard-dose induction therapy (Table 107-9).

Cunningham and associates (1985) treated 22 patients (16 with limited and six with extensive disease) with high-dose chemotherapy consisting of 180 mg/kg cyclophosphamide and 1 g/m^2 etoposide after induction with standard doses of cyclophosphamide, doxorubicin, methotrexate, etoposide, and vincristine. Autologous bone marrow was reinfused 36 hours after the beginning of high-dose chemotherapy. Eight patients with limited disease were in complete remission at the time of late intensification, and three (40%) achieved long-term survival. Ihde and colleagues (1986) reported the experience of the U.S. NCI in a small study of eight patients with extensive disease who also were treated with high-dose cyclophosphamide and etoposide and irradiation to the chest. The median survival was less than 1 year, and there

were no 2-year survivors. Somewhat more encouraging results were reported by Goodman and coworkers (1991) for SWOG and by Elias and colleagues (1992) for the Dana Farber Cancer Institute. In the SWOG trial, 58 patients with limited disease were assessed for induction chemotherapy and late intensification. Only 21 patients received high-dose chemotherapy, which consisted of 150 mg/kg cyclophosphamide without autologous bone marrow transplantation. Of the 21 patients, five relapsed, four died as a result of toxicity from intensification, and three died of other causes but were in complete remission at the time of death. Nine of the 21 patients remain in complete remission with a median survival greater than 27 months. Elias and colleagues (1992) also studied 17 patients with limited disease who had responded to induction therapy (12 complete responses and five partial responses). Late intensification consisted of 5.6

Table 107-9. Late Intensification Therapy for Small Cell Lung Cancer

Author	Number	Remission Status Preintensification	Drugs	Survival Median (wks)	Survival 2 yrs	Comments
Cunningham et al., 1985	16 limited, 6 extensive	11 CR, 11 PR	Cyclophosphamide 180 mg/kg Etoposide 1 g/m^2	?	?	40%+ long-term survival for limited-stage patients in CR after induction
Ihde et al., 1986	8 extensive	9 CR, 14 CR	Cyclophosphamide 120 mg/kg Etoposide 600 mg/m^2 20 Gy XRT	47	None	Two treatment-related deaths
Humblet et al., 1987	16 limited, 7 extensive	9 CR, 14 PR	Bischloroethylnitrosourea 300 mg/m^2 Cyclophosphamide 6 g/m^2	68	20%	Part of a randomized trial
Marangolo et al., 1989	10 limited, 5 extensive	8 CR, 7 CR	Etoposide 500 mg/m^2 Etoposide 18 g/m^2	?	20%	Nine of 11 patients relapsed in the chest
Goodman et al., 1991	21 limited	?	Cyclophosphamide 150 mg/kg	116+	43%	No ABMT; 4 treatment-related deaths
Elias et al., 1992	17 limited	12 CR, 5 PR	Cyclophosphamide 5.6 g/m^2 Bischloroethylnitrosourea 480 mg/m^2 Cisplatin 165 mg/m^2	?	75%	—
Sculier et al., 1985b	11 limited, 4 extensive	3 CR, 10 PR	Cyclophosphamide 200 mg/kg etoposide 1.0–3.5 g/m^2	?	None	One treatment-related death

ABMT, autologous bone marrow transplantation; CR, complete remission; PR, partial remission; XRT, radiation therapy.

g/m^2 cyclophosphamide, 480 mg/m^2 bischloroethylni-trosourea (carmustine), and 165 mg/m^2 cisplatin followed by autologous bone marrow transplantation. The projected 2-year survival rate for that study is 75%.

Results from the two studies just mentioned are encouraging and suggest that further investigation should focus on eligible patients with limited disease of good performance status who have demonstrated an excellent response to standard-dose induction chemotherapy. It must be remembered, however, that this population represents less than one-half of patients with limited SCLC and a small percentage of the entire SCLC population. Certainly, randomized controlled trials testing this hypothesis are required. Does this review leave any room for optimism for high-dose therapy and autologous bone marrow transplantation? Although the long-term survival in most of the studies is disappointing, findings of three studies suggest that further investigation in this area is warranted. The early study of Cunningham and associates (1985) and the more recent study of Elias and coworkers (1992) both demonstrated that a significant proportion of patients with limited disease who underwent intense chemotherapy at the time of complete remission achieved long-term survival. Of even greater importance is a study of Humblet and colleagues (1987), which was part of a randomized trial in which patients underwent induction chemotherapy and were then randomized to late intensification with bone marrow transplantation or crossover to standard doses of the same drugs. The median relapse-free survival after randomization for the intensified group was 28 weeks compared to only 10 weeks for the standard-dose group ($P = .002$). The median overall survival was also longer for the intensified group despite four treatment-related deaths in that arm of the study. Relapse occurred frequently at the primary site, suggesting that local radiation therapy should be included in any further trials.

High-Dose Chemotherapy for Salvage

The very low response rate to standard-dose chemotherapy for patients with recurrent or refractory SCLC led some investigators to evaluate the role of very high-dose chemotherapy in this patient population. Lazarus (1990) and Postmus (1985) and their colleagues demonstrated that response could be achieved by dose intensification, but the response duration was short, toxicity was considerable, and few patients achieved long-term survival. For these reasons, high-dose chemotherapy is not appropriate for patients with resistant SCLC.

Alternating Non–Cross-Resistant Chemotherapy

According to Goldie and Coldman (1984), tumor resistance to chemotherapy is likely a significant cause of treatment failure in SCLC. This resistance may exist at the start of therapy or it may be acquired during treatment. During the 1980s, the Goldie-Coldman hypothesis, an approach to early

resistance, had become popular. The authors proposed a mathematical model based on the hypothesis that tumor cell kill displays a logarithmic pattern and tumors continuously develop resistant mutations during treatment. The conjecture of Goldie and coworkers (1982) and Goldie and Coldman (1984) is that alternating two combinations of non–cross-resistant drugs early in the course of treatment might lessen the development of drug-resistant clones and increase the chance of cure. In their model, it is essential that the combinations tested be truly clinically non–cross-resistant and that both non–cross-resistant combinations be active as initial treatment for the disease being evaluated. Bonadonna (1982) described the benefit of this approach, seen most often in the treatment of Hodgkin's disease, in which it appeared that treatment with MOPP [mechlorethamine (nitrogen mustard), vincristine (Oncovin), procarbazine, and prednisone] alternating with ABVD [doxorubicin (Adriamycin), bleomycin, vinblastine, and dactinomycin (DTIC)] was superior to MOPP alone. Studies by Santoro and colleagues (1987), however, show that ABVD may be superior to MOPP, which may mean that another explanation for the observation is still necessary. Preliminary data presented by Canellos and associates (1992) suggest that ABVD is equivalent to alternating MOPP and ABVD, again emphasizing the difference in the two regimens rather than the superiority of the alternating approach.

Because of the promising results in Hodgkin's disease and the availability of many active agents, resulting in possible non–cross-resistant combinations to test, this method has been used frequently in the treatment of patients with SCLC. A review by Elliott and colleagues (1984) pointed out shortfalls in some of the trial designs but also showed few clearly positive studies. In a Canadian study, CAV therapy alone was compared to alternating CAV with etoposide and cisplatin for a total of six courses in previously untreated patients with extensive SCLC. In this large trial, Evans and colleagues (1987) observed a 6-week difference in median survival and, as noted by Goodwin and coworkers (1988), the treatment was cost effective. A second study in Canadian patients with limited disease compared three courses of CAV followed by three courses of etoposide and cisplatin with six courses of the alternating regimen. As reported by one of us (R.F.) and associates (1987), no difference in outcome was found. It may be that etoposide and cisplatin is a superior combination, which could explain the positive result obtained in the Canadian limited-stage study but not that of the extensive-stage trial. Other studies, such as those carried out by Roth and colleagues (1992) and Fukuoka and associates (1991a), do not totally advocate the concept that alternating combination chemotherapy is superior to standard regimens, although Fukuoka's group showed a significant survival advantage to alternation in patients with limited disease. In the Roth study, survival of patients treated with only four courses of etoposide and cisplatin was the same as that of patients treated with longer courses of alternating regimens. A review by Havemann (1990) upholds the opinion that results in the literature are conflicting, and no clear superiority to alternating chemotherapy can be proved.

Some authors believe that the results from the Canadian study undertaken by Evans and colleagues (1987) indicate that alternating chemotherapy should be standard treatment, at least in extensive disease, but with etoposide and cisplatin added to CAV rather than the alternation, as suggested by Ihde (1992). The consensus of investigators worldwide is that the alternating approach is sound but not necessarily superior to other approaches, such as four to six courses of etoposide and cisplatin alone.

Duration

Until the middle or late 1980s, it was not unusual to treat patients with chemotherapy for a minimum of 12 to 24 months.

Results of retrospective studies, including a large one from the University of Toronto undertaken by one of us (R.F.) and colleagues (1984), suggested no benefit to prolonged therapy. A large randomized trial carried out by Splinter (1989) and colleagues (1986, 1988) in the EORTC Lung Group revealed no benefit in survival, at least in patients with limited disease, although there may have been the suggestion of benefit in patients with extensive disease. Ettinger (1990) from ECOG also showed no benefit to maintenance therapy. An update of a French trial by LeBeau and coworkers (1991a) that also tested this theory does show a small survival benefit in maintained patients with SCLC. Few studies promote the use of prolonged therapy in this disease. An update by Girling and associates (1991) of the Medical Research Council trial shows no benefit of six courses of therapy over three courses.

At this point, it seems that four to six courses of chemotherapy for patients who show a response should be sufficient, and presently available maintenance chemotherapy is of no added benefit.

New Drug Development

Clearly, one of the most important approaches in the treatment of SCLC is the procurement of new active agents for managing the disease as well as defining better ways of using presently available therapy. One has to reemphasize the concept of using new agents in previously untreated patients. This practice seems to be safe as long as a crossover design is used, with early crossover to an established regimen to avoid patients being too ill to receive potentially valuable treatment after waiting too long. Grant and colleagues (1992) also looked for lower response rates in previously treated patients in studies conducted from 1970 to 1990.

Although a large number of new agents have become available for testing in this disease, few look promising, but as emphasized in a review by Ihde (1992), new drugs

should be sought to try to improve the survival of these patients. High-dose epirubicin has been found by a number of groups, including Blackstein (1990), Meyer (1982a, 1982b), Banham (1990), Johnson (1989), one of us (R.F.) (1992), Eckhardt (1990), Wils (1990) and colleagues, to be active in both SCLC and NSCLC. Although not used routinely, as noted by Grant (1992), Johnson (1989), Thatcher and Lind (1990) and their coworkers, carboplatin has been established as an active agent in this disease. It is unclear whether it is quite as active as cisplatin, but it is certainly a reasonable alternative to prevent or reduce neurotoxicity and nephrotoxicity in selected patients at high risk (e.g., patients with preexisting kidney or hearing problems). According to Johnson (1989, 1990), ifosfamide is also active in SCLC and is relatively nonmyelosuppressive compared to cyclophosphamide. Loehrer (1996) has shown that VIP (ifosfamide combined with etoposide and cisplatin) proved to be superior to etoposide plus cisplatin in patients with extensive SCLC. Expense, the required use of mesna, and its usual requirement for in-hospital administration all make ifosfamide a somewhat more difficult agent to use in SCLC than most other available active agents. The only other agents that look promising at this stage of development are gemcitabine, paclitaxel (Taxol), topotecan, and irinotecan (CPT-11). According to Anderson (1991b) and Lund (1991) and their colleagues, gemcitabine may be active in NSCLC. In preliminary data, gemcitabine appears active in SCLC. Earle and associates (1998), in a phase I study of gemcitabine-cisplatin-etoposide in the treatment of SCLC found that the response rate was 54 to 75%. The recommended dose of gemcitabine was 800 mg/m^2 intravenously on days 1 and 8. Further trials are indicated. Paclitaxel has undergone extensive phase I and II studies. The dose-limiting toxicity is leukopenia; Ettinger and colleagues (1995) noted a 58% development of grade 4 leukopenia; other toxic effects included involvement of the liver, lung, and heart. Perez and coworkers (1996) suggested a dose of 150 mg/m^2 intravenously over 3 hours. Greco and Hainsworth (1996) conducted a phase II study of paclitaxel, carboplatin, and etoposide with an 83% response rate and complete response rate of 24%. Median survival was 7 months for patients with extensive disease and 17 months for those with limited disease. Neill and coworkers (1997) reported a response in seven of eight patients when paclitaxel was added to the carboplatin and etoposide regimen. Gatzemeier and associates (1997) reported a complete response rate of 37.1% and a partial response rate of 51.4%. In 117 patients, Hainsworth and colleagues (1998) used paclitaxel, carboplatin, and extended-schedule oral etoposide plus radiation therapy and found that median survival rates in patients with limited and extensive disease compared favorably with other accepted chemotherapy regimens. Finally, Birch and coworkers (1997) conducted a randomized study to evaluate etoposide and carboplatin with or without paclitaxel. Bunn (1996) has reviewed the North American experience with paclitaxel.

Another drug that has received great attention is topotecan, a topoisomerase I inhibitor that leads to a break in the DNA strand resulting in apoptosis and cell death. Lilenbaum (1998) and Kollmannsberger (1999) and their associates have reported phase I studies evaluating dosage and toxicity of this potent antitumor agent. Future phase II and III trials, such as those discussed by Schiller (1997) and Takimoto and Arbuck (1997), are needed to define the role of topotecan in the treatment of SCLC. Masuda and coworkers (1992) also reported activity in a small group of 16 refractory patients (47%) with another new agent, irinotecan (CPT-11); these data have been confirmed. Other chemotherapeutic agents on the horizon for this disease are 254-S, vinorelbine, and docetaxel (Taxotere), as noted by Ariyoshi and Sugiura (1994). Figueredo and (1990) and Milroy (1991) and their colleagues have found that agents that attempt to bypass established drug resistance, such as verapamil, have to date not proved to be clearly helpful in patients with SCLC. Correlation of in vitro drug sensitivity with potentially active agents may turn out to be useful. Preliminary data from Gazdar and coworkers (1990a) at the NCIC are not overly encouraging but do show that this approach is feasible.

RADIATION THERAPY

Radiation therapy has been an important method of treatment of SCLC for many years, and it continues to play a vital role in the management of this disease. It has not been recommended as sole therapy since the British 5-year follow-up trial conducted by Miller and colleagues (1969) and the 10-year follow-up trial undertaken by Fox and Scadding (1973) and Fox and coworkers (1980, 1981) comparing it to surgery 30 years ago. It is, however, widely used in combination with chemotherapy for curative approaches and for palliation, usually alone. The last decade in particular has seen advances in the knowledge about radiation therapy in SCLC and its more effective administration, both with and without associated chemotherapy. In this discussion, the role of radiation therapy in the routine management of the SCLC patient is considered and areas of recent progress are identified, emphasizing controversies in management and future directions of research in this field.

Radiation and Combined-Modality Therapy

The absorption of radiation by cells results in reproductive cell death in a proportion of the cell population. As discussed by Hall (1988), this proportion increases exponentially with dose, except for doses smaller than approximately 2 to 3 Gy, for which cell killing is somewhat less efficient. Thus, the cycling population tends to be progressively reduced as treatments are continued or the dose is increased. Malignant cells are distinguished by their ability to reproduce indefinitely and often rapidly; they therefore tend to be susceptible to this type of injury. When cell populations can be reduced to relatively low numbers by irradiation, host defenses may eliminate the survivors, resulting in a cure. Normal tissues are also injured, however; depletion of the stem cells of various tissue populations results in chronic tissue damage. Ideally, one seeks to maximize tumor cell kill while minimizing normal tissue damage. In practice, cells may survive the irradiation for various reasons, including intrinsic radioresistance, technical error, or underdosage because of the need to protect critical structures.

The response of a tumor, in terms of volume change measured at some time after treatment, is not an important end point of treatment. It may be influenced by the intrinsic cell kinetics (rapidly cycling tumors may respond quickly, then regrow with similar speed), the proportion of cells actively cycling, and the response of associated tissues. More important end points of treatment after suitable periods of follow-up are locoregional control of tumor, survival without relapse, and overall survival.

In determining the radiation dose to be delivered to the intended volume, past experience of tissue tolerance to irradiation is of great value. Tolerance in general depends on the tissue type, notably its normal cell kinetics (rapidly proliferating epithelial tissues differ from slow or nonproliferating vascular, connective, or nervous tissues), the volume irradiated, and the presence of other conditions, such as diabetes. It was determined long ago that radiation therapy is more effective when administered over multiple treatment sessions, or fractions. According to Thames and Hendry (1987) and Arriagada and colleagues (1989), the radiobiological reasons relate to cellular repair, oxygenation of the cellular environment, and cell cycle responses, which are beyond the scope of this discussion. Many years of clinical-biological experience and insights have led to the development of dose fractionation schemes that tend to enhance antitumor effect while preserving, at least relatively, vital tissues. Important determinants of biological effect are the total dose, the dose per fraction (individual treatment session), the number of fractions into which the total dose is divided, the frequency of fractions, and the overall time required to administer all of the prescribed dose.

In particular, the understanding of the role of fraction size has advanced greatly since the late 1980s, as discussed by Fowler (1989) and Withers (1988). Many critical normal tissues, such as the nervous system and the microvasculature that supports function in all tissues, are characterized by cells that regenerate over long cycle times (months or years). Their response to radiation injury is related to this regeneration time. These tissues tend to manifest clinical damage after a latent period of months and slowly progress over a time scale of years. These changes are the so-called late effects seen in irradiation (e.g., myelopathy), in contrast to the acute effects of tissues that normally regenerate rapidly (e.g., mucosa) but are correspondingly rapidly depleted, hence manifesting injury early, such as with mucositis. Important investigations have shown that these late effects are sensitive to the size of the dose per fraction. The acutely responding tissues are less sensitive, and hence the severity of late injury cannot be predicted from the degree of early injury seen at or shortly after the time of treatment. Because the late effects on normal tissues are usually those that limit the ability to deliver radiation dose to the tumor, it should be possible to increase the biological dose to the tumor while continuing to respect the tolerance of critical normal tissues by designing regimens with smaller doses per fraction. A related observation suggests that small cell cancer cells may be particularly susceptible to small doses per fraction, which would also be tolerable by late-responding tissues. These insights from the 1980s are being subjected to clinical testing in a number of areas, usually with positive or promising results. These ideas may have profound effects on radiation therapy practice in the future. The application of these ideas to lung cancer is considered subsequently.

In a discussion of the concepts of dose, time, and fractionation, it is useful to define certain terms that relate to various schedules of fractionation (i.e., the partitioning of the total radiation dose into individual treatment sessions or fractions) (Table 107-10). In a course of treatment, the fractions are usually, but not always, of equal dose. Fractionation is described as conventional when it is given in a single daily fraction of 1.8 to 2.0 Gy per day, 5 days per week. Typical courses given with curative intent administer 60 to 65 Gy over 6.0 to 6.5 weeks using this fractionation. Treatment is termed *hypofractionation* when fraction sizes larger than 2 Gy (typically 3 to 8 Gy) are given, usually on a less frequent basis, such as once per week. An example might be 5-Gy fractions given once weekly for 12 weeks to a total of 60 Gy. *Hyperfractionation*, a more common unconventional program, refers to smaller fraction sizes, usually 1.0 to 1.5

Gy, which are typically given two or even three times per day, again normally 5 days per week. Small fraction sizes confer biological advantages, but for similar antitumor effect, the total dose usually must be increased over a comparable conventional schedule and the number of individual treatments then becomes larger. This means that multiple fractions per day must be given to maintain the overall time of treatment similar to that of a course of conventional fraction size. Administration of radiation therapy is accelerated when the total dose is delivered in a shorter overall time. Accelerated administration may be achieved by using hypofractionation techniques, by using multiple fractions per day and conventional fraction sizes, or by treating the patient 7 days per week. Some experimental regimens may be described by more than one of these terms.

The manner in which chemotherapy and radiation therapy are combined temporally may have important effects on the outcome. Arriagada and associates (1988) recommend that the integration of the two methods be described as follows. When chemotherapy and irradiation are given on days of the chemotherapy cycle in which no chemotherapy is administered, without any delay in chemotherapy beyond that which would normally occur if chemotherapy were being given alone, this is called *alternating therapy*. If the administration of chemotherapy and radiation therapy occur separately in time, it is *sequential* (e.g., chemotherapy followed by radiation therapy, or a delay in chemotherapy administration to permit delivery of radiation therapy). Finally, chemotherapy and irradiation may be administered *concurrently*, with both treatment methods given on the same day for some or even all of the cycle (Table 107-11).

Clinical Considerations

SCLC typically presents with locally advanced disease not suitable for surgery. The greatest burden of disease is found in the thorax, which requires a correspondingly intense locoregional therapy, but disease confined to the thorax is at least potentially curable. Cancer in the lymph nodes of the mediastinum often indicates systemic disease, which is either occult or obviously evident by current clinical methods. The simple classification *limited* (to one hemitho-

Table 107-10. Typical Methods of Radiation Therapy Fractionation

"Conventional"   lllll___lllll___lllll___...
  Dose per fraction = 1.8–2.0 Gy
  Fractions per day = 1
  Continuous (rarely interrupted)
  Duration 4–7 wks
"Hypofractionated"   l___l___l___l___l___l...
  Dose per fraction = >2 Gy
  Fractions per day = 1
  Continuous or interrupted
  Duration variable
"Hyperfractionated"   ll ll ll ll ll___ll ll ll ll ll___...
  Dose per fraction = 1.0–1.5 Gy
  Fractions per day = 2–3
  Continuous
  Duration 4–7 wks
"Accelerated"   lll lll lll lll lll___ lll lll lll lll lll___...
  Dose per fraction = 1.8–2.0 Gy
  Fractions per day = 2–3
Continuous
Duration <4 wks

Table 107-11. Combined-Method Radiation and Chemotherapy Regimens

Exclusive chemotherapy (CT)
  CT-CT-CT-CT-CT
Concomitant radiation (RT) therapy
  CT-CT-CT-CT-CT
  RT—RT
  Simultaneous
Alternating RT and CT
  CT-RT-CT-RT-CT-RT-CT
  RT alternating between cycles of CT with no delay of CT

-, 1-week intervals; —, daily.

rax, mediastinum, or ipsilateral supraclavicular fossa, or both, but without malignant effusion) or *extensive* (metastatic disease, after standard staging procedures) has proved useful in identifying a group of potentially curable patients with small cell histology. As already discussed, these definitions may vary in detail between different studies, which may influence results. Survival longer than 2 years may be found in more than 20% of patients with limited disease, many of whom may indeed be cured. Metastatic disease cannot be cured by any known regimen, although chemotherapy, radiation therapy, or both, often give excellent short-term palliation.

Many of the "limited" patients in fact have occult systemic disease, undetectable at diagnosis, which subsequently appears as distant metastases. This tendency for occult metastatic disease to develop accounts in large measure for the poor results obtained with locoregional treatments, such as radiation therapy or surgery. It is also true that the inability of irradiation, with or without chemotherapy, to control all local disease in many cases is important. Although the understanding of the capabilities of available therapies has improved greatly since the early 1980s, the need for more effective locoregional and systemic agents for SCLC must be acknowledged.

The task of the radiation oncologist is to assess the patient and the tumor, determine appropriate therapy in light of available alternatives, and, if radiation therapy is indicated, prescribe and deliver an appropriate dose of irradiation to the tumor while minimizing the dose to normal tissues. This approach exploits the technical ability to focus radiation therapy beams on the tumor tissue and thus achieve a therapeutic advantage. For this reason, radiation oncologists make extensive use of advanced imaging techniques, including CT scanning, supplemented by computerized dose calculations and diagrams of distribution of radiation dose within the tissues.

The primary decision after assessment of the patient is whether to offer treatment with palliative or curative intent. For SCLC, radiation therapy is usually given in association with chemotherapy, although various temporal relations are possible. A target volume for treatment is determined from the diagnostic studies available, such as the chest radiograph and CT scans, and includes the known disease extent and the possible routes of spread. The possible routes of spread are considered significant and normally include the primary tumor and some or all of the mediastinal lymph nodes. The dose fractionation scheme reflects the goal of treatment and the tolerance of other organs. The target volume is identified radiologically at the time of treatment simulation, and skin reference points are established. A CT scan of the thorax in the treatment position permits visualization of the target volume in conjunction with treatment beams and computerized dose distributions. Shielding of nearby organs is implemented. The final step is verification by making radiographic portal images from each therapy beam, using the therapy treatment machine. Posttherapy radiographs may show tumor regression and radiation pulmonary fibrosis within the treatment volume.

Thoracic Irradiation in Limited Disease

Early reports by Watson and Berg (1962) of radiation therapy for this disease demonstrated its tendency to respond dramatically ("melt away") only to recur in a short period, often at a distant site. Subsequently, Bergsagel and coworkers (1972) noted the activity of chemotherapy in this disease, which led to two decades of investigations into combined-method treatments. One might anticipate that the addition of intense local therapy directed at the region of clinically evident disease might improve local control, which in turn might lead to an increased survival rate, even in a systemic disease such as limited-stage SCLC. This is the rationale for thoracic irradiation, at least for patients who have no occult metastases or those who might have them but whose metastases are curable by the chemotherapy regimen.

The best results for limited-stage disease are obtained using a carefully integrated regimen of chemotherapy and thoracic irradiation. Ample evidence shows that radiation treatment produces objective responses, but its impact on survival has been difficult to demonstrate. The simple question of the benefit of thoracic irradiation combined with chemotherapy compared to administration of the same chemotherapy alone has been studied in many randomized trials. The drug regimens have been different among the various trials, as have the radiation therapy details of dose, fractionation, and sequencing with respect to the chemotherapy. Such trials may be "falsely" negative by chance, due to a low statistical power of finding a positive result when it truly exists, especially in the smaller trials, or the irradiation may be truly without benefit. Some of these trials, although not all, have shown a survival benefit, notably in the more recent trials of greater numbers of patients. A set of randomized trials may be analyzed collectively by the method of meta-analysis, as undertaken by Sacks and colleagues (1987), which analyzes the set of trial results together and effectively increases the chance of identifying a difference that exists but is modest in size. Another meta-analysis by Warde and one of us (D.P.) (1992) of 11 SCLC trials (with adequate reporting, consisting of 1911 randomized patients) was undertaken to determine the distribution of outcomes of these trials, such as improvements in survival rates and local control rates. The trials conducted by Bunn (1987), Osterlind (1986), Kies (1987), Ohnoshi (1986, 1987), Souhami (1984), Birch (1988), Perry (1987), Creech (1987), Nou (1988), Carlson (1991), and Rosenthal (1991) and their colleagues are listed in Table 107-12. The additional study by Rosenthal and coworkers (1991) shows a trend to prolonged survival in the irradiated group, reporting 10-year follow-up of a study completed in 1979. The analysis showed a modest but significant improvement in 2-year survival of approximately 5 to 6% (from approximately 17 to 23%) and a larger effect of approximately 25% (from approximately 23 to 48%)

Table 107-12. Randomized Trials of Thoracic Irradiation with Chemotherapy

Author	No.	Chemotherapy	Dose/Fractions/Time	Timing	EBI
Bunn et al., 1987	91	CML/VAP	40 Gy/15 f/3 wks	With first chemotherapy	Y
Osterlind et al., 1986	145	CMVL	40 Gy/10 f/4 wks–split	Days 43–47, days 71–75	N
Kies et al., 1987	93	CMVEA	48 Gy/22 f/6.5 wks–split	Days 85–99	Y
Birch et al., 1988 (study 328)	291	CAV	40 Gy/14 f/7 wks–split	Wks 5, 8, 11	Y
Birch et al., 1988 (study 81343)	369	CML	40 Gy/20 f/4 wks	Wks 1, 2, 7	Y
Ohnoshi et al., 1987	52	CMVP/EAN	40 Gy/20 f/4 wks	Between first two chemotherapy sets	NS
Souhami et al., 1984	130	AV/MC	40 Gy/20 f/4 wks	After four chemotherapy sets CR + PR	N
Perry et al., 1987	299	CVEA	50 Gy/25 f/5 wks	Cycles 1–4	Y
Creech et al., 1987	232	CMLAE	50 Gy/25 f/5 wks	Day 43 after chemotherapy	Y
Nou et al., 1988	56	CMAV/CMLV	40 Gy/20 f/4 wks	After three chemotherapy sets	Y
Carlson et al., 1991	48	CLVP/EAM	55 Gy/30 f/5–7 wks	After 6–9 months	Y
Rosenthal et al., 1991	91	VCA	40 Gy/20 f/4 wks	After three chemotherapy sets	N

A, doxorubicin; C, cyclophosphamide; CR, complete response; E, etoposide; EBI, elective brain irradiation; f, fractions; L, lomustine; M, methotrexate; N, mustine; NS, not significant; No., number of randomized patients; V, vincristine; P, procarbazine; PR, partial response.

in local control at 2 years, associated with a small increase (1%) in treatment-related mortality. A more detailed meta-analysis by Pignon and colleagues (1992) as well as Joss (1985) and LeBeau (1991b) and their associates, with additional verification and follow-up, has been published and confirms these conclusions. This effect is real—that is, the results are statistically significant ($P <.01$); therefore, thoracic irradiation truly does impart benefit.

In the meta-analysis of Pignon and colleagues (1992), it was noted that only younger patients achieved longer survival with radiation. In fact, the addition of radiation to chemotherapy in patients older than age 70 years resulted in poorer survival, such that the overall risk of death actually increased. Quon and associates (1999), who reviewed the results of two NCIC trials of combined modality therapy for limited SCLC, did not observe a negative impact of age. In their review, response rates, local relapse rates, and survival were the same for patients younger and older than 70 years of age. Furthermore, the elderly patients did not experience greater early or late toxicity from radiation therapy, nor did they require more frequent treatment delays or longer time to complete treatment.

A large study piloted by Perry and associates (1987) is another trial of this type involving 399 patients. The chemotherapy was CAV, used every 21 days for up to 18 months. The thoracic radiation therapy used was 50 Gy in 2-Gy fractions (40 Gy to the primary and mediastinum followed by 10 Gy to the primary, given with either the first cycle, the fourth cycle, or not at all, in this three-arm study). All patients received elective brain irradiation to a dose of 30 Gy in 10 fractions. This study showed a doubling of the 2-year disease-free survival from 15 to 30%, and a doubling of local control from 26 to 58% (first failure in the chest) in favor of those patients receiving thoracic irradiation. In an update, Perry and associates (1998) reported that the advantage of the combined-modality regimens was maintained in 10 years of follow-up. A second study from the U.S. NCI by Bunn and coworkers (1987) randomized 74 patients to receive irradiation, 40 Gy in 15 fractions over 3 weeks given concurrently with the first cycle. This regimen resulted in an unacceptable

mortality rate from pulmonary toxicity. In spite of this negative finding, a small but statistically significant survival benefit was seen for patients in the combined-method treatment arm. Although it is acknowledged that other studies have not shown a survival benefit, these results illustrate the modest impact identified by the more comprehensive meta-analysis.

Improvements of this magnitude are important, but because these gains are modest, either a large trial or, as discussed by Sacks and colleagues (1987), a meta-analysis is required. Why have the results of these combined-method trials been so disappointing? First, the chemotherapy used in many of these trials was not optimal by today's standards and did not always contain active agents, such as cisplatin, etoposide, or doxorubicin. Second, the radiation therapy may have been suboptimal with regard to dose, fractionation, or timing with respect to chemotherapy. Only one study of randomized doses of irradiation, undertaken by Coy and the NCIC (1988), has been attempted; the doses used are generally considered low and were not sufficiently different to determine an optimum. Optimal volume prescriptions are unknown; however, Liengswangwong and colleagues (1994) in a retrospective analysis from the Mayo Clinic concluded that use of postchemotherapy volumes in treatment planning did not increase the risk of marginal failures. This issue becomes less relevant with the use of early concurrent therapy regimens. Further advances may be anticipated as these problems are addressed. In fact, as systemic therapy improves, the control of local disease to achieve overall cure becomes ever more important. It is accepted, however, that thoracic irradiation, carefully integrated with chemotherapy, has well-demonstrated benefits by the standards prevailing in lung cancer therapy and is well tolerated. It should therefore be adopted as proper routine management for the patient with limited-stage SCLC.

Innovations in Combined-Modality Approaches

Results of combined-modality approaches are modest and require further improvement. New insights from the clinic and from biology have suggested innovations, including timing of radiation therapy with respect to chemotherapy, the use of small doses per fraction, and the intercalation of chemotherapy and the irradiation.

In Canada, Goldie and associates (1988) used drug-resistance data and mathematical modeling to develop the hypothesis that using multiple anticancer agents of different mechanisms of action so as to be non–cross-resistant to each other was required to prevent the emergence of resistant cell clones during treatment. This suggested the clinical hypothesis that concurrent early administration of multiple agents might be advantageous. There have been several formal tests of this idea. Murray and colleagues (1991a, 1993) of the NCIC randomized 308 patients to receive thoracic irradiation (40 Gy in 15 fractions) administered concurrently with etoposide and cisplatin either early (with the second cycle of chemotherapy) or late (with the sixth cycle of chemotherapy). The early administration of radiation therapy significantly improved survival at 5 years from 13 to 22%, compared to giving it 12 weeks later. This finding suggests that the cancer may be developing drug-resistant cell clones within the chest, which can then metastasize to distant sites if radiation therapy is delayed or withheld. The tumor thus needs an aggressive early approach with all methods of treatment, including radiation therapy. On the other hand, the CALGB trial reported by Perry and associates (1987, 1988)included a randomized comparison of thoracic irradiation given with either the first or fourth cycle (a 9-week delay) and found no effect of the delay on survival. Delivery of chemotherapy was compromised by toxicity in the early radiation therapy arm of this study, which may account for the result. Another negative trial from Denmark by Work and colleagues (1997) randomized 199 patients to early radiation (40 to 45 Gy in split-course fashion, not concurrent with chemotherapy) or similar treatment 18 weeks later. The chemotherapy doses and nonoptimal radiation therapy administration raise questions about this trial. More recently, trials from Japan and Yugoslavia have both found 5-year survival rates in the range of 30% compared to approximately 15% in favor of early concomitant administration of radiation therapy and chemotherapy. The Japanese trial of Takada and associates (1996) used twice-daily fractions of 1.5 Gy, as did that of Jeremic and colleagues (1997). In the Jeremic study, the radiation therapy regimen was 54 Gy in 18 days over 3.6 weeks, commencing on day 1 or day 43 (a 6-week delay). All patients received elective brain irradiation. Both local control and survival rates were superior with the early combination. It appears that in a well-staged population of patients with limited disease and good prognostic factors, there is an advantage to early administration of radiation therapy. This practice, although not universal, is becoming widespread.

The shape of the cell survival curve for irradiated SCLC suggests sensitivity to irradiation with small doses per fraction. Because a large number of small fractions is required to obtain adequate total dose, regimens of hyperfractiona-

tion (1.5 Gy given two fractions per day, to 45 Gy total) have been evaluated in the United States by Turrisi and Glover (1990). Administration of this form of chest radiation therapy was concurrent with the first cycles of chemotherapy (cisplatin and etoposide). Similar pilot studies recorded by Mornex and coworkers in France (1990) and Johnson and colleagues (1991a,b) at the American NCI were promising, with 2-year survivals of approximately 44% and a low rate of local failure (<16%). As a result, Turrisi and associates (1999) carried out a large randomized trial of the hyperfractionation approach. A total of 417 patients were treated with four cycles of chemotherapy (cisplatin and etoposide) together with several weeks of daily (5 treatment days/month) chest irradiation, commencing on the first day of chemotherapy. They were randomized to receive 5 weeks of 1.8-Gy fractions given daily (total 45 Gy/25 fractions) or 3 weeks of 1.5-Gy fractions given twice daily, 6 hours apart (total 45 Gy/30 fractions). Treatment was safe and well tolerated, although esophagitis was more severe in the twice-daily group. The median survivals were similar in the two groups (19 and 23 months), but a significant advantage in survival emerged in favor of the twice-daily group ($P = .04$). With a median follow-up of 8 years, the survival advantage is 26% versus 16%, associated with significant reductions in both local and distant failure. This suggests that an important subgroup of potentially curable patients exists who may be more responsive to a strategy of hyperfractionation.

After a study by Seydel and associates (1983), the desire to integrate all methods early in the course of treatment while controlling toxicity prompted Arriagada and colleagues (1985) of the Institut Gustave Roussy group to develop the alternating method. This approach has experimental support in observations by Looney and coworkers (1985) that the radiation therapy, if added after chemotherapy at approximately the time of chemotherapy-induced tumor repopulation between cycles, could produce tumor control that was not possible with either method alone. The clinical trials followed the general chemotherapy (CT)-radiation therapy (RT) schema CT-CT-RT-CT-RT-CT-RT-CT-CT-CT in which "-" indicates a 1-week interval. In a series of trials with somewhat varying doses but using the same overall scheme of alternating therapies, Looney and colleagues have also achieved 3-year disease-free survivals in the range of 20 to 30%. Gregor and associates (1997a) tested this approach in a randomized clinical trial for the EORTC. They gave 50 Gy in 20 fractions at the end of a course of chemotherapy (cyclophosphamide, doxorubicin, etoposide) as the sequential arm, compared with an alternating arm that integrated 10 Gy in four fractions over 1 week alternating with the same chemotherapy over four treatment cycles. This direct comparison of alternating and sequential approaches randomized 335 patients, but there was no evidence of superiority of either; the alternating regimen was characterized by severe hematologic toxicity, which compromised delivery of the treatment.

A logical extension of this approach combines the hyperfractionation procedure with the alternation of chemotherapy and radiation therapy. In the United States, the ECOG in a small trial conducted by Johnson and coworkers (1991) gave cisplatin and etoposide chemotherapy in four cycles of 3 weeks each. In each of the first three cycles, 1 week of hyperfractionated thoracic irradiation was administered (1.5 Gy twice daily to 15 Gy total in 1 week). In a similar fashion, Arriagada and colleagues (1991b) of the Institut Gustave Roussy group in Paris used doxorubicin, etoposide, cyclophosphamide, and cisplatin, together with three intercalated courses of radiation therapy. They gave the first irradiation doses as 1.4 Gy three times per day to a total of 21 Gy. Mornex and associates (1990) of the Lyon group reported on their experience with an alternating bifractionated regimen. No large randomized trial experience is available, so definite conclusions about this approach cannot be made.

All regimens that combine radiation and chemotherapy, particularly when closely associated in time, are somewhat more toxic than single-modality or sequential protocols. Authors of most pilot studies of these approaches revealed some severe morbidity and even mortality. In a meta-analysis of 11 randomized trials by Warde and one of us (D.P.) (1992), the addition of thoracic irradiation therapy produced a significant but small increase (1%) in treatment-related fatality. This change was substantially less than the overall survival gain produced by this treatment. Significantly, a review of 88 elderly patients (age 80 years or older) in combined modality trials of the NCIC reported by Quon and associates (1999) showed that their compliance with, tolerance of, and response to the thoracic irradiation were similar to that of the younger patients.

In summary, combined-method therapies in patients with limited disease produce modestly superior rates of survival and tumor control in the chest, with some increase in toxicity associated with the concurrent administration of both methods early in the chemotherapy cycles. However, both theoretical considerations and clinical results support the use of early and concurrent combinations. Chest irradiation appears to be well tolerated when given concurrently with etoposide-cisplatin regimens, but extensive concurrent experience with newer agents is not yet available. The use of a small dose per fraction seems to be beneficial, even if the result is the requirement of giving multiple fractions per day. In the only large randomized test so far, this method showed a significant improvement in survival at 5 years.

No reason for complacency exists. Arriagada and colleagues (1991a) have shown that local failure is still frequent, with 33% of failures local only, 25% distant only, and 9% local and distant simultaneously. The state of current practice with respect to radiation therapy and directions of future research is evolving. Patients with limited SCLC should be referred to radiation oncology centers that conduct this research, if possible. Alternatively, they should be referred to the local radiation oncologist for an opinion on thoracic irradiation, preferably at the outset of chemotherapy administration.

Elective Brain Irradiation

Elective brain irradiation is the practice of irradiating the entire brain electively on the principle that the patient is at risk for the development of brain metastases even if clinical tests do not demonstrate them. (It is also known less accurately as *PCI*.) Elective irradiation is recommended because chemotherapy alone often does not prevent the development of symptomatic brain metastases in approximately 25% of patients. Tumor cells in the brain "sanctuary" may be protected from chemotherapy by physiologic factors peculiar to the CNS. Kristjansen (1989) reported that this brain failure rate can be reduced to 5% if elective irradiation is given. This policy, however, results in approximately 75% of patients receiving a treatment that they may not need and that may harm them. It is important to remember that the results from clinical trials depend on factors such as the length of follow-up, the criteria required for diagnosing relapse, and whether isolated brain relapses are distinguished from those occurring in the setting of failure at multiple sites. Investigations tend to be performed reluctantly in terminally ill patients, so such data are not readily available.

There is general agreement about the aforementioned figures, as found by Jackson (1977, 1983), Cox (1978, 1980), Beiler (1979), Maurer (1980), Hansen (1980), Eagen (1981), Katsenis (1982), Seydel (1985), Aroney (1983) and their colleagues. This is especially important when combined with the evidence from randomized trials that overall survival is not improved (Table 107-13). Some large trials from groups in France, as reported by Arriagada (1995) and Laplanche (1998), and elsewhere in Europe, as reported by Gregor (1997b) (see Table 107-13), have confirmed these earlier conclusions. The trials by Gregor (1997b) and Arriagada (1995), however, included prospective neuropsychiatric evaluations and found no significant adverse effects in the treated group compared to the untreated patients. An interesting literature analysis by Suwinski and colleagues (1998) suggested that a threshold in dose-response for prevention of brain relapse was evident if treatment was delayed. They suggested that optimum control is achieved with doses of 30 to 35 Gy at 2 Gy/fraction, administered early in the overall treatment regimen. Many of these conclusions have been further supported by the meta-analysis presented in abstract form by Arriagada and an international collaborative group (1998). Elective brain irradiation was associated with an improvement in survival rate at 3 years from 15.3 to 20.7%.

Advocates argue that the morbidity of a brain relapse compared to that of the treatment justifies the practice and improves overall quality of life in these patients. The degree to which patients are actually harmed by the procedure is controversial, however, as is the optimal dose. Newer prospective randomized trials of therapy with and without elective brain irradiation are in progress in Europe and the United States, including prospective neuropsychiatric evalu-

Table 107-13. Randomized Trials of Elective Brain Irradiation

Author	No.	Gy/f/Time	CNS Relapse	Survival
Jackson et al., 1983	29	30/10 wk 1	S	NS
Cox et al., 1980	45	20/10 wk 1	NS	NS
Beiler et al., 1979	54	24/8 wk 3	S	NS
Maurer et al., 1980	163	30/10 wk 9	S	NS
Hansen et al., 1980	109	40/20 wk 12	NS	NS
Eagen et al., 1981	30	36/10 wk 20	S	NS
Katsenis et al., 1982	35	40/25 wk 1	S	NS
Seydel et al., 1985	219	30/10 wk 1	S	NS
Aroney et al., 1983	32	30/10 at complete response	NS	NS
Arriagada et al., 1995	294	24/12[a] at complete remission	S	NS
Gregor et al., 1997b	314	30/10[a] at complete remission	S	NS
Laplanche et al., 1998	211	24–30/3 weeks at complete remission	NS	NS

CNS, central nervous system; f, number of fractions; No., number of patients randomized; NS, not significant; S, significant $P < .05$.
[a]Fractions.

ations in some trials, to compare brain morbidity from relapse and from treatment, taking into account the patient's condition at the onset of treatment. In this elderly, tobacco-abusing group, prior neurologic morbidity frequently exists, and, as suggested by Lishner and coworkers (1990), can cloud the interpretation of subsequent events. Whether long-term toxicities are a serious and typical problem is a controversial issue. The Toronto experience with PCI in SCLC, as reported by Lishner and colleagues (1990), has been relatively positive, with a low incidence of notable abnormalities not unlike those found in patients who do not receive PCI. The same issue of the *Journal of Clinical Oncology* in which the Lishner study appeared includes a study by Fleck and associates (1990) from Indiana University with extremely grave long-term complications. In a companion editorial, Turrisi (1990) endeavors to account for this result, and indicates that it may be associated with the fractionation schemes used.

Many questions in this area are unanswered. It is not known whether treatment failure occurs as a result of inadequate treatment of occult metastases or as a result of reseeding of the brain by cells from a persistent primary or other metastatic sites. Some clinicians believe that only patients exhibiting a complete response to treatment have the potential for cure and hence benefit from elective irradiation of a brain sanctuary site. One trial randomized only such patients, but other randomized trials have included patients with partial responses.

An alternative approach is to offer palliative therapeutic brain irradiation to patients only if and when they exhibit relapse in the brain. This treatment is generally thought to produce symptomatic improvement in up to 70% of patients. The available studies are retrospective, however, and have the methodologic difficulties of addressing this population, particularly in assessing their quality of life, so it must be stated that reliable data on valid end points of treatment are not available. Nevertheless, a policy of therapeutic brain irradiation given only at the time of relapse

would spare approximately 60% of responding patients from brain irradiation, which was of no benefit to them because they were not destined to relapse in the brain in any case.

On the other hand, the elective administration of cranial irradiation may prolong the duration of life without brain metastases, and because these lesions usually cause significant morbidity, this may be a worthwhile goal. Judging whether it is worthwhile depends on the morbidity of the treatment itself. In dose ranges from 20 to 40 Gy, using fraction sizes from 2 to 4 Gy, patients may experience nausea, headaches, and, occasionally, vomiting along with alopecia and scalp erythema. The use of 20 Gy in five fractions produced nausea in up to 15% of patients, but this effect may be controlled by steroids and antinauseants. Of greater concern are the long-term effects on the neurologic status of survivors. Clinical and anatomic lesions evident by CT have been noted. In general, these patients are in the seventh decade and have had many years of tobacco use. Neurologic problems may thus be attributed to coexisting morbidity or to cytotoxic therapies, chemotherapy, or irradiation. A retrospective review of late survivors by Lishner and colleagues (1990) revealed that most observed neurologic problems had other plausible explanations besides the radiation therapy; indeed, some occurred in nonirradiated patients. This and other studies are not adequately controlled, however, and cannot be considered definitive. As noted, some prospective randomized trials with neurologic and neuropsychiatric evaluations by Arriagada (1995) and the EORTC, as reported by Gregor (1997b), strongly suggest that the concerns about adverse effects of elective brain irradiation have been overestimated.

At present, elective brain irradiation is standard at many centers, although certainly not all. Some centers offer treatment of complete responders only as an option and therapeutic brain irradiation for all others at the time of relapse; this policy is probably also widespread. On the other hand, the trials of the late 1990s have led to general acceptance that elective brain irradiation for complete responses with limited disease is appropriate treatment.

Extensive-Stage Small Cell Lung Cancer

When small cell cancer is metastatic at diagnosis, the prognosis is poor, with a median survival of 8 to 10 months. The amount of disease is usually great and difficult to control at multiple sites. The Medical Research Council (1991) reports that radiation therapy for extensive disease should, therefore, be directed only at symptomatic sites and not controlled by chemotherapy. The palliative benefit is often good, especially for bone pain, venous obstruction, cerebral metastases, and so forth. Elective irradiation of chest or brain would normally be considered only for the rare complete responder to chemotherapy or for patients who responded completely at distant sites and who had only minimal residual thoracic disease. Because of the poor prognosis, no active investigation of the role of radiation therapy in extensive disease has been undertaken. The effort must await the development of more effective systemic chemotherapy, which, by prolonging survival, might demonstrate a more compelling need for aggressive local palliation.

Palliation of Lung Cancer

The lung cancer patient has a wide variety of symptoms caused by the tumor or its metastases. Common symptoms of the primary tumor are hemoptysis, cough, dyspnea (especially if obstruction of significant airways exists), chest pain, hoarseness from vocal cord palsy, and sometimes SVC obstruction. Systemic effects are weight loss, anorexia, lethargy, and anemia. Localized metastases may produce bone pain, mediastinal compression with venous obstruction or esophageal compression, brain involvement with neurologic deficit, and spinal cord compression leading to paralysis. Radiation therapy often benefits patients because it can be directed to the site of the problem without causing side effects outside the field, and it is simple and painless to deliver, as described by Barkley (1986). Table 107-14 illustrates the expected response rates for various symptoms based on a retrospective evaluation by Slawson and Scott (1979). Trials

Table 107-14. Relief of Symptoms in 330 Patients with Metastatic Non–Small Cell Lung Cancer Using Radiation Therapy

Symptom	Response (%)
Hemoptysis	84
Chest pain	61
Superior vena cava obstruction	86
Dyspnea	60

From Slawson R, Scott R: Radiation therapy in bronchogenic carcinoma. Radiology *132*:175, 1979. With permission.

undertaken by Grafton (1991) and Simpson (1985) and their colleagues randomized patients to different dose levels in an attempt to assess the need for long treatment regimens in patients with a short expected survival. Results of these trials have shown little advantage to longer schedules, but the assessment of benefit in such trials poses many difficulties, and treatment decisions are usually individualized. The short overall survival of these patients means that duration of response is an important consideration, and modern trials now try to assess this interval. However, several randomized trials done by the Medical Research Council in the United Kingdom (1991, 1992, 1996) have consistently shown the usefulness of short, convenient fractionation schedules.

Major airway obstruction is an important problem, particularly for tumors involving the carina or trachea, especially after relapse. Whenever possible, endobronchial tumors should be treated by endoscopic débridement by mechanical or laser methods. New therapy technology permits endoscopic placement of a catheter across the area of involvement. A wire provided with a 2.5-mm radioactive source at its tip may then be inserted. This source has high activity and delivers its dose rapidly to the region of the tumor. By retracting it in a series of 2.5-mm steps, under precise computer control of both position and duration, any desired portion of endobronchial wall can be irradiated selectively in a brief outpatient procedure using local anesthesia. Early experience with this device, as noted by Grafton and colleagues (1991), is promising, although the technique does not treat the deeper extent of the tumor. Endobronchial treatment modalities are discussed in Chapter 101.

Bone lesions from metastatic cancer are an important cause of morbidity in cancer patients and a frequent challenge to the radiation oncologist. Their frequency in lung cancer, their tendency to disable rather than kill, and their presence in patients refractory to therapy pose significant management problems. In addition, they are a common problem in patients who already have other lesions and a poor prognosis. The ability of irradiation to reach specific local sites with minimal adverse effects has made it an attractive mode of therapy in these situations. Although irradiation remains a mainstay of the palliative care of these patients, important questions remain about its optimal use. The major indications for irradiation of bone metastases are the need to 1) alleviate or abolish pain, 2) prevent impending fracture or treat malignancy in conjunction with orthopedic fixation, 3) maintain activity and function, and 4) prevent or alleviate compression syndromes, especially of the spinal cord. Prolongation of survival is not usually a realistic goal of therapy.

Findings of prospective and retrospective studies suggest that common regimens ranging from 8 Gy in 1 fraction to 40 Gy in 20 fractions produce improvement in 70 to 80% of patients and result in sustained relief in 60% of patients surviving 1 year. A series of randomized trials undertaken by Price and colleagues (1986) showed that most bony sites can be treated effectively with a single dose of approximately 8

Gy. More fractionated courses do not appear to confer additional benefit. Many radiation oncologists prefer to administer larger doses to bones that bear weight or are close to the spinal cord, in the belief that patients should have the benefit of the small improvement in disease control that might arise from a higher dose.

Although maximal pain relief is usually achieved by 3 months, the time of onset of relief varies considerably, and the precise mechanisms involved in relief of pain are uncertain. Because late normal-tissue effects are not usually a limiting consideration, experience with small dose-per-fraction, multiple-fraction-per-day regimens is minimal. Other experimental techniques include half-body radiation therapy in patients with widely metastatic disease. Studies by Salazar and associates (1986) have shown that prompt and meaningful responses are found in one-half or more of patients. This method may be associated with increased toxicity when combined with systemic agents because there may be shared adverse effects.

The syndrome of compression of the SVC is well-known in lung cancer patients. Sculier and one of us (R.F.) (1985) have made recommendations for its management. Although SVC compression is sometimes considered an emergency, Ahmann (1984) suggests that a tissue diagnosis should always be obtained to guide treatment, particularly because in chemosensitive tumors, such as small cell carcinoma, chemotherapy may be equally effective. Many series have shown the palliative benefit of radiation therapy. Patients often experience rapid subjective relief (1 to 2 days) long before radiologic improvement is seen. Nieto and Doty (1986) reported that, when thrombotic occlusion is present, response is poor. On the other hand, a multivariate analysis of 408 cases by Wurschmidt and colleagues (1995) in Germany concluded that the syndrome might in fact be favorable prognostically, perhaps as an early symptom. They recommend a curative approach to such patients with otherwise limited disease.

Brain metastases are an important cause of morbidity, but they can be palliated successfully. As discussed by Kurtz (1981) and Mornex (1991) and their colleagues, typical regimens are well within brain tolerance and may make it possible for the patient to discontinue the use of steroids. The optimum regimen is unknown; doses usually range from 20 to 40 Gy over 1 to 4 weeks. A randomized trial of therapy, piloted by Patchell and colleagues (1990), for solitary brain metastases (by CT scan; mostly lung primaries) demonstrated better survival and function if the lesion was resected before irradiation; both groups received whole-brain irradiation (36 Gy in 12 fractions). Most patients with extensive SCLC, however, are not suitable for this combined approach because of multiple metastases or poor general condition.

Epidural metastases producing compression of the spinal cord is an oncologic emergency. Rodichok and associates (1981) note that early diagnosis is essential because most patients have long-standing warning symptoms and the onset of paresis may herald rapid development of paralysis.

Paralysis may also occur, and some radiotherapists recommend the prophylactic use of steroids for these patients. According to Pedersen (1985) and Constans (1983) and their colleagues, as well as Byrne (1992), laminectomy or irradiation can produce relief of compression and symptoms; there are no standard indications for the use of both together.

Adverse Effects

Radiation effects on normal tissues are confined to the irradiated volume, especially the volume receiving doses intended for the tumor. The adverse effects depend on the nature of tissues within the irradiated volume, the intrinsic tolerance of the tissues to the dose fractionation scheme administered, and the degree to which the tissues have already been compromised by the malignancy, other treatment methods, or other nonmalignant disease processes. The clinical importance of radiation injury is influenced greatly by the proportion of the functional capacity of the organ that incurs the injury. Thus, severe fibrosis of a lobe of the lung caused by treatment may be acceptable, whereas the same therapy would be lethal if administered to a whole lung.

According to Maasilta (1991), McDonald and colleagues (1989), and Rubin and Casarett (1972), radiation injury to lung is primarily mediated by damage to alveolar pneumocytes and vascular endothelial cells. The dose required to produce loss of function within the treated volume is equivalent to approximately 20 Gy in 10 fractions, an amount well below the doses usually required for treatment of cancer. Reactions considered early (within 2 to 3 months) are only rarely symptomatic, but a clinical syndrome is sometimes observed when large volumes of lung are treated. Symptoms include cough, dyspnea, and a low-grade fever. Hemoptysis and progressive pulmonary failure can develop. Characteristically, the involved portion of the lung corresponds to the treated volume. Infectious causes must be ruled out. Diffuse infiltrates develop over the next 2 weeks and then resolve. With or without clinical symptoms in the few months after treatment, progressive fibrotic change within the irradiated volume is invariable. This development constitutes the pattern of late pulmonary injury and is permanent. Although in general they correspond to the treatment changes in lung fields, secondary retraction of lung tissue may modify this pattern somewhat. Mah and Van Dyk (1988) as well as Brooks (1986) and Van Dyk (1989) and their colleagues noted that density changes in lung display a definite dose-response relationship, as measured by CT methods. The combination of radiation therapy with chemotherapy, notably drugs such as doxorubicin and bleomycin, may result in more severe injury at the same level of radiation dose as the injury seen with radiation therapy alone.

The esophagus is usually included in the treatment volume for lung cancer. The early epithelial reaction results in dysphagia for solid food and sometimes liquids in many patients. This effect is transient and resolves shortly after the end of treatment. The later development of stricture is rare for doses up to 60 Gy, but more so when chemotherapy is also used, especially doxorubicin.

Cardiac toxicity may occur when large volumes of the heart are irradiated to 40 Gy or more. The usual manifestation is that of late pericardial problems, usually constriction. Patients with pacemakers may be treated safely. Lewin and colleagues (1984) recommend that the device not be directly irradiated, and cardiology consultation should be sought to assess pacemaker function after the use of linear accelerators because of their associated electromagnetic fields.

As noted by Dische and colleagues (1988), the most feared complication of thoracic radiation therapy is myelopathy. The doses required for lung cancer are well in excess of the tolerance of the spinal cord (45 to 50 Gy at 1.8 to 2.0 Gy per fraction). Much of the detailed treatment planning and shielding undertaken in a lung cancer patient is directed at limiting dose to this critical organ to less than 46 Gy. As a result, this complication is rare. When a previously treated patient develops signs of cord dysfunction at the upper thoracic level, it is imperative to investigate for spinal metastases, which are a more common cause of myelopathy.

Patients sometimes complain of fatigue or lethargy during thoracic irradiation, but this condition is rarely severe, unless liver is included in the irradiated volume. Greenberg and coworkers (1992) observed a similar syndrome in patients receiving localized breast irradiation, and it may be a systemic adaptation to the stress of being treated for cancer.

SURGERY

The initial optimism engendered by the success of combination chemotherapy in the 1970s has been tempered in the 1990s by the observation that cure still remains an elusive goal for most patients with SCLC, and less than 20% of patients with limited disease survive more than 2 years. The poor survival rate for patients in the surgical arm of the British Medical Research Council Study reported by Fox and Scadding (1973) led most investigators to abandon surgery as the initial treatment for bronchial neoplasms of this type. Nonetheless, almost all surgical series from the precombination chemotherapy era reported a small percentage of patients who achieved 5-year survival with surgical treatment alone. This observation led Shields and coworkers (1982) to review the Veterans Administration Surgical Oncology Group (VASOG) results of surgical therapy for SCLC in an attempt to identify a subgroup of patients with limited disease who might benefit from surgical resection. They made the important observation that TNM staging, which has long been recognized to have prognostic importance for NSCLC, could also define prognostic subgroups for patients undergoing surgery for SCLC. Perhaps of even greater importance was Shields' observation of possible prolongation of survival

in the patients who had received adjuvant chemotherapy in these early VASOG trials. The number of patients in these trials was insufficient for the results to achieve statistical significance, and the chemotherapy they received would certainly be considered inadequate by today's standards.

The poor survival of patients with SCLC who are treated by surgery alone is undoubtedly attributable to the presence of occult micrometastatic disease that cannot be detected by current clinical staging techniques. For patients who have undergone surgical resection of the primary tumor, it should theoretically be possible to eradicate this small bulk of micrometastatic disease with chemotherapy. On the basis of Shields' observations from the VASOG studies, several groups initiated prospective trials of adjuvant chemotherapy after surgery for limited SCLC. One of us (F.A.S.) and colleagues (1988) for the University of Toronto Lung Oncology Group reported a median survival of 83 weeks and projected 5-year survival of 31% for 63 patients who received adjuvant chemotherapy after surgical resection. Patients with pathologic stage I tumors had a projected 5-year survival of 48%. Karrer (1990) and Karrer and Shields (1991) reported similar results for the International Society of Chemotherapy Small Cell Program in Europe and in Asia. The projected 4-year survival rate for their patients with pathologic stage I tumors was 61%.

Elliott and colleagues (1987) have shown that the primary tumor bed and hilar or mediastinal lymph node areas are the most frequent single sites of failure after chemotherapy for limited disease. Despite the addition of thoracic irradiation, relapse occurs at the primary site in one-fourth to one-third of patients. In the early 1980s, investigators postulated that it might be possible to improve control at the primary site by the addition of surgery to standard combined-method therapy, which included chemotherapy and radiation therapy for patients with limited SCLC. Two small retrospective reviews suggested that indeed this might be possible, at least in patients whose condition permitted selection for surgery before the definitive histologic diagnosis was made. One of us (F.A.S.) and coworkers (1983) noted relapse at the primary site in only two of 35 patients who had undergone surgical resection, and similar results were reported by Comis and colleagues (1982), who identified no local relapses after surgical treatment in their feasibility study of 22 patients.

During the 1980s, several groups initiated prospective feasibility studies of adjuvant surgical treatment after remission induced by chemotherapy for patients with limited SCLC. Surgery was usually offered only to responding patients, and on average, approximately 50% of the patients identified initially were considered candidates for surgery after induction chemotherapy. Surgical eligibility rates ranged from a low of 27% reported by Prager and colleagues (1984) to 79% reported by one of us (F.A.S.) and associates (1989) for the University of Toronto Group. All groups have reported favorable median survivals of up to 2 years and projected 5-year survivals of 60 to 80% for patients with pathologic stage I tumors.

These phase II trials led to observations that were important in the design of subsequent randomized trials of surgery for limited SCLC. They demonstrated that combined-method treatment was feasible and that chemotherapy did not result in unacceptable postoperative morbidity or mortality. They emphasized the importance of TNM staging. Reviews by one of us (F.A.S.) and associates (1991b,c) and Karrer (1990) suggested that combined-method treatment that included both systemic chemotherapy and surgery resulted in 5-year survival for small cell patients that was almost indistinguishable from that of patients with NSCLC of similar stage (Fig. 107-1A). They also identified the difficulties associated with clinical staging for patients with SCLC. Clinical TNM stage correlated with final pathologic TNM stage in less than 50% of patients, and the survival differences identified by pathologic stage were not seen when the same patients were analyzed by clinical pretreatment stage (Fig. 107-1B). Most authors also reported a small number (approximately 10 to 15%) of patients with mixed histology tumors that included a non–small cell component.

Because these feasibility studies were all nonrandomized trials, it was not possible to state that the favorable survival achieved was related to surgery rather than patient selection. In an attempt to answer this question, the Lung Cancer Study Group initiated a prospective randomized trial in 1983 in which all patients were treated initially with induction chemotherapy consisting of CAV and responding patients were randomized to surgical resection and radiation therapy or to radiation alone. Lad presented preliminary results of this trial on behalf of the Lung Cancer Study Group (1988). Three hundred forty patients were registered on this trial, but only 144 (42%) were randomized: 68 to surgery and 76 to no surgery. Attrition related to progression in nonresponders or to reluctance of some patients to accept a randomization to receive or not receive a thoracotomy after several months of chemotherapy. Of the 68 patients randomized to surgery, six did not undergo operation, but a further eight patients had off-study surgery, for a total of 70 thoracotomies. Fifty-eight patients underwent resection (83%) of which 54 were thought to be complete (77%). A complete pathologic response of 18% was seen, and non–small cell pathologic change occurred in 11% of patients. The results of this trial were disappointing in that no difference in survival was seen between randomized patients in the surgical and nonsurgical arms (Fig. 107-2). Because only one-half of the randomized patients (one-fourth of all patients) in this study underwent surgical stag-

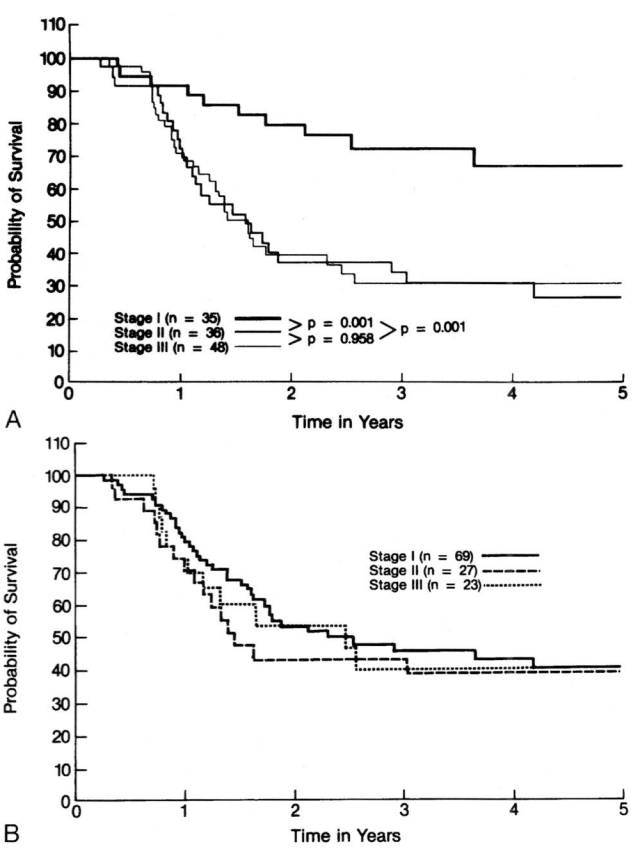

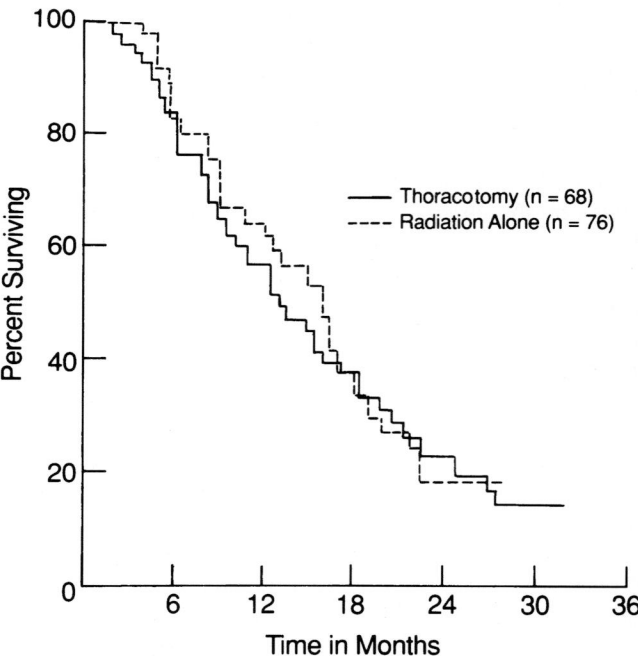

Fig. 107-1. A. Comparison of survival by pathologic stage for 119 patients who underwent surgery for limited small cell lung cancer. **B.** Comparison of survival by pretreatment clinical stage for 119 patients who underwent surgery for limited small cell lung cancer. From Shepherd FA, et al: Surgical treatment for limited small-cell lung cancer. J Thorac Cardiovasc Surg *101*:385, 1991. With permission.

Fig. 107-2. Survival curves of the randomized patients with limited small cell lung cancer treated with initial chemotherapy and irradiation alone or with the addition of surgical resection after chemotherapy and irradiation in the North American Lung Cancer Study reported by Lad and coworkers (1991).

ing, it is not possible to compare survival based on stage or TNM subgroups. Within the surgical group, no difference in resectability could be identified for patients in any T or N subgroup, although there seemed to be a trend toward unresectability for patients with T_3 tumors ($P = .08$).

How should the results of this Lung Cancer Study Group Trial be interpreted? It is clear that surgical resection does not benefit the majority of patients with limited SCLC and that its future role will be minor in the management of this disease. Nonetheless, a small subgroup of patients (likely less than 10%) may benefit from combined-method therapy, with a significant chance of prolonged disease-free survival and even cure. It is essential, therefore, for medical oncologists and thoracic surgeons to identify such patients from the larger group of limited-disease SCLC overall. In general, the aforementioned phase II studies suggest that the criteria of operability applied to NSCLC are equally valid for SCLC. Surgery should be considered for all patients with $T_{1-2}N_0$ tumors. Whether surgery is offered as initial therapy or after induction chemotherapy is probably not important, as shown in Figure 107-3, from the review by one of us (F.A.S.) and coworkers (1991a). With respect to stage II disease, it is not possible to make firm generalizations about surgery, and treatment decisions should be individualized. Chemotherapy should be offered as initial treatment, and surgery may be considered for patients with an excellent performance status who have responded well to induction therapy. If a small cell tumor is identified unexpectedly at thoracotomy, complete resection and mediastinal node dissection should be undertaken whenever possible and chemotherapy should be administered postoperatively, even to patients with stage I tumors.

Surgery plays a very limited role for patients with stage III tumors. Although most investigators have reported long-term survival for a small number of stage III patients, most of these patients had only microscopic involvement of medi-

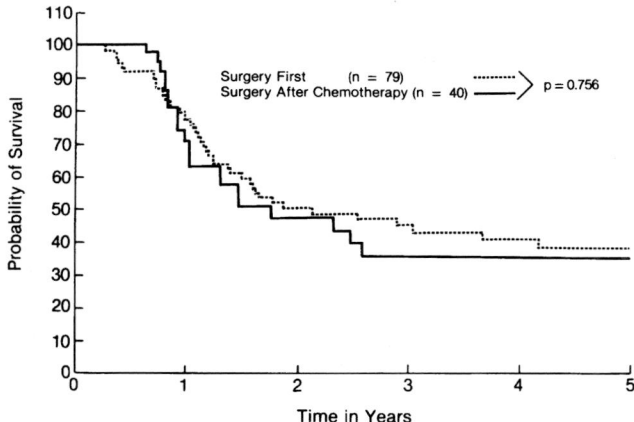

Fig. 107-3. Comparison of the survival of patients with small cell lung cancer who had surgery first or surgery after chemotherapy. From Shepherd FA, et al: Surgical treatment for limited small-cell lung cancer. J Thorac Cardiovasc Surg *101*:390, 1991. With permission.

astinal lymph glands or T_3N_0 tumors. Even though chemotherapy can result in dramatic resolution of bulky mediastinal disease, the addition of surgical resection does not contribute significantly to long-term survival for most of these patients.

Another group who may benefit from surgical resection are the 10 to 15% of patients with combined small cell and non–small cell tumors. When such patients are identified at diagnosis, initial treatment should be chemotherapy to control the small cell component of the disease. Surgery should then be considered for the more chemotherapy-resistant non–small cell component. For patients who demonstrate an unexpectedly poor response to chemotherapy or patients who experience localized late relapse after treatment for pure small cell tumors, a repeat biopsy should be performed to rule out non–small cell pathology. In a small study of 28 patients who underwent salvage operations, one of us (F.A.S.) and colleagues (1991b) identified 10 patients who had non–small cell pathologic findings. Four of these patients achieved long disease-free survival from 2 to 6 years after surgery. Although it is recognized that only a minority of patients fall into this favorable subgroup, it is important to take steps to identify them because curative therapy may be available. Shields and Karrer (1998) reviewed all the various aspects of the role of surgery in managing patients with SCLC. Their views are essentially the same as ours, although they prefer initial resection followed by chemotherapy in most of the highly selected patients that are surgical candidates.

BIOLOGICAL RESPONSE MODIFIERS

Induction Therapy

In general, Shank and colleagues (1985) report that numerous agents, including bacille Calmette-Guérin, its methanol-extractive residue, and *Corynebacterium parvum*, have been investigated in all types of lung cancer with no definitive evidence that they are beneficial. The only encouraging study was conducted by Cohen and associates (1979) from the U.S. NCI, who initiated a randomized trial using thymosin fraction V. A notable increase in survival was seen by Shank and coworkers (1985), with the highest dose (60 mg/m²), but this has not been corroborated. Woll and Rozengurt (1989) reviewed the literature on this subject.

Antibodies directed against bombesin (a gastrinlike peptide hormone) have been evaluated in phase I studies. Additional work is being performed with this approach, as reviewed by Carney (1991, 1992), but these antibodies so far are not clinically usable. Interferons and interleukins have not been found to be useful as therapy in lung cancer. Therefore, to date, it can be said that biological response modifiers alone are not part of the standard induction therapy of patients with SCLC. Aisner and coauthors (1992) reported on a pilot study showing an apparent improved response rate (survival compared to historic data) with warfarin added to standard therapy in patients with SCLC. This finding forms the basis for an ongoing effort by the Cancer and Leukemia Group. Future agents to be investigated could turn out to be useful, but only time will tell.

Maintenance Therapy

The only significantly positive study using maintenance therapy is the one by Mattson and colleagues (1991) from Finland, who appear to have shown a survival advantage with long-term α-interferon maintenance. This study was reproduced by SWOG, but the results were negative, and compliance with treatment was poor. The use of maintenance γ-interferon has been tested by Jett and the North Central Oncology Group (1992) but has not yet been found beneficial.

Combination with Other Therapies

The foremost example of using biological response modifiers in combination with other therapy is using growth factors such as G-CSF and GM-CSF (see section on colony-stimulating factors). In summary, G-CSF seems to decrease myelosuppression, febrile episodes, and days of hospitalization, but to date, it has no proven survival benefit. It is possible that GM-CSF also has such an effect, but it has other inherent toxicity, including the possibility of enhanced thrombocytopenia. In fact, thrombocytopenia not dealt with by either G-CSF or GM-CSF may present serious difficulties. When using myelosuppressive therapy, the dose-limiting hematologic toxicity is thrombocytopenia rather than granulocytopenia, as is the case when the presently available CSF preparations are used. New growth factors, such as interleukin-3, as reported by Postmus and coworkers (1992), alone or in combination, may be able to circumvent this problem in the future. It can be stated, however, that CSFs are not a required part of therapy in patients with SCLC treated with moderate-dose chemotherapy.

Another potential use for one type of biological response modifier—monoclonal antibodies to small cell cancer tumor antigens—is the staging of these tumors. Imaging techniques are already available and look promising. The same monoclonal antibodies may turn out to be useful as viable therapeutic interventions in the future, as considered in a review by Stahel (1992), but clinical studies are still preliminary.

Other important new molecular biological therapeutic developments that include antigrowth factors (antagonists G and D), antimetastatic agents [matrix metalloproteinase (MMP) inhibitors], and other genetic products have been reviewed by Smyth (1996). The MMP inhibitors are believed to be associated with cellular metastatic potential and the development of tumor angiogenesis. Szabo (1998), Gonzalez-Avila (1998), and Okamoto (1999) and their col-

leagues, among others, have carried out many basic microbiological molecular investigations relating to the inhibition of the activity of MMP inhibitors. The activity of the MMP inhibitors is thought to have an anticancer effect in three ways: 1) inhibition of local and regional tumor growth, 2) inhibition of the formation of metastatic deposits, and 3) restriction of tumor angiogenesis. Marimastat, an MMP inhibitor, has been studied in a phase I trial by Wojtowicz-Praga and associates (1998) to evaluate the safety and pharmacokinetics of various doses of the drug in humans. Marimastat is well absorbed from the GI tract, with detectable drug levels in the plasma within hours after drug administration. Dose levels of 50 to 100 mg orally twice daily achieve plasma concentrations that are substantially higher than those required for MMP inhibition in vitro. The dose-limiting toxicity is severe inflammatory polyarthritis. One of us (F.A.S.) (1997) has recorded that the NCIC and the EORTC have initiated a trial to evaluate the value of adjuvant Marimastat for SCLC patients who have responded to induction chemotherapy, this being the first adjuvant antiangiogenesis factor trial to be initiated for any tumor type. Other studies include monoclonal antibodies, which may inhibit tumor cell growth by binding to growth factors or may be conjugated to toxins or other chemotherapeutic agents, which results in tumor cell death. The success of our attempts to manipulate abnormal genes in malignant cells has yet to be resolved. However, our increasing knowledge and understanding of the regulation of normal and neoplastic cell growth at the molecular level may prove to be the key. Except for CSF preparations to attempt to reduce myelosuppression and its complications, however, biological response modifiers at present have no established role in patients with SCLC.

Carcinomatous Meningitis

Several studies by Aisner (1979), Aroney (1981), Brereton (1978), and Wasserstrom (1982) and their colleagues, as well as by Greco and Fer (1978) and Oster and Fetell (1982), stressed that carcinomatous leptomeningitis may be more frequent in SCLC than was thought previously. Rosen and colleagues (1982) from the U.S. NCI observed that 60 of 526 (11%) of their patients who entered various protocols between August 1969 and June 1980 developed this complication; most arose after the time of presentation. Bunn and Rosen (1985) submit that the condition reaches an incidence of approximately 25% during the first 3 years and then plateaus. Only approximately 1% of patients relapse from a complete response in this way; the majority are discovered to have carcinomatous leptomeningitis concurrent with finding other progressive systemic disease.

The NCI review conducted by Rosen and associates (1982), using a multivariate analysis, indicated that liver metastasis was the element most strongly associated with the development of this complication, followed by bone and other CNS metastases. Because patients with CNS metastases (e.g., epidural, brain) are at high risk for developing carcinomatous leptomeningitis, they should probably have a lumbar puncture. Looking for tumor cells by means of standard methodology warrants cytocentrifuge examination. If the initial CSF examination is abnormal but cytologically negative, repeat lumbar punctures should be carried out. A more detailed description of the clinical picture and of the evidence of this problem at autopsy is beyond the range of this chapter. These topics are well discussed by Bunn and Rosen (1985).

The fundamental issue is whether treatment is useful. The best treatment is clearly not established. Often, intrathecal drug therapy is administered, most often with methotrexate, combined with irradiation to the sites of bulk or systemic disease in the CNS. According to Rosen and colleagues (1982), combined treatment seemed to improve the symptomatology better than intrathecal treatment alone, at least in the U.S. NCI series. Because it is difficult to continue giving intrathecal medication without a catheter permanently in place, a subcutaneous (Ommaya) reservoir with a ventricular channel is placed. Use of this device ensures that all the injected drug enters the CNS, permits uniform dose distribution, and eliminates the requirement for repeated lumbar punctures. No comparative study in patients with solid tumors has been undertaken, but as discussed by Bleyer and Poplack (1979), this routine certainly seems preferable in patients with acute leukemia with leptomeningeal involvement.

Bunn and Rosen (1985) also noted that the only agents that seem active when given intrathecally or intraventricularly are methotrexate and thiotepa. Trump and colleagues (1981) propose that a combination of intrathecal methotrexate and thiotepa may be superior to methotrexate alone. In spite of all these treatments, the median survival appears to be only approximately 7 weeks. The patients typically deteriorate as a result of concurrent progressive systemic tumor in addition to the leptomeningeal involvement. Therefore, newer methods of treatment for this complication are unquestionably in demand. With the high drug levels observed in the brain with the use of high-dose etoposide, perhaps this regimen can be used as an adjunct in the future. Trials are essential, however, before this treatment is acceptable, and further research in this area is clearly in order.

COMPLICATIONS OF TREATMENT

Early Complications and Toxicities of Chemotherapy

All methods of therapy can effect significant individual toxicities. Those associated with individual types of therapy, as shown in Table 107-15, are classified into those that occur early and those that occur late after treatment. These toxicities must be considered when offering such treatment to patients who have SCLC and should be discussed with the patient in detail. One of us (R.F.) (1981, 1989a,b, 1994) has provided a

Table 107-15. Early and Possible Late Toxicities in Patients with Small Cell Lung Cancer

Therapy	Early Toxicities	Possible Late Toxicities
Chemotherapy	Nausea and vomiting	Unusual infections (e.g., herpes zoster)
	Alopecia	Anthracycline-induced cardiomyopathy
	Peripheral neuropathy	Pulmonary fibrosis
	Myelosuppression with possible resulting bleeding (cisplatin)	Central nervous system toxicity, especially in conjunction with PCI
	Anemia	Second malignancies
	Constipation	Second lung primaries
	Electrolyte disturbances	Other solid tumors
	Cardiotoxicity	Acute leukemia
	Nephrotoxicity and ototoxicity	
	Hemorrhagic cystitis	
	Mucositis	
	Hypotension or hypertension (etoposide)	
	Bronchoesophageal fistulae	
Radiation therapy		
Thoracic	Esophagitis ± stricture	Pulmonary fibrosis
	Pneumonitis	Late cardiac effects
	Cardiac toxicity	Myelitis
		? Predisposition to second primary
Cranial	Erythema of the scalp	Somnolence, confusion, problems with concentration and memory deficits
	Otitis externa	Tremor, dysarthria, slurred speech, and ataxia
	Prolongation of chemotherapy-induced myelosuppression	Frank dementia
Surgery	Immediate postoperative problems can be fatal	Continued long-term pain at incision site
	Pain at thoracotomy incision site	Bronchopleural fistulae
	Bronchopleural fistulae	Respiratory failure secondary to removal of functioning lung

PCI, prophylactic cranial irradiation.

detailed description of these problems, but it is beyond the range of this chapter and can be found elsewhere.

Of significance is that new approaches and supportive care may well counter many of these toxicities. For example, nausea and vomiting cause frequent and serious distress in patients with SCLC because cisplatin is frequently used along with other agents that cause moderate emesis. In an overview by Aapro (1991), the use of dexamethasone in combination with 5-hydroxytryptamine antagonists, as exemplified by ondansetron and granisetron, have improved the situation substantially. Nausea in the early posttreatment period is essentially eliminated, although delayed onset of nausea remains a possible issue for some patients.

Myelosuppression, with its capacity for infection, has been a potential serious problem in the treatment of SCLC. A common regimen used in the 1980s was CAE (cyclophosphamide, doxorubicin, and etoposide). This combination led to severe and prolonged myelosuppression, with a hospital admission rate as high as 40 to 50% for febrile neutropenia for these patients. Therapeutic results were reasonable, but the complication rate was likely unacceptable. This usage has been superseded by regimens such as etoposide and cisplatin, which are associated with less than 5% admission rates for this complication. Another approach to this problem has been the use of growth factors, particularly G-CSF, to lessen the extent and duration of neutropenia and thereby reduce the infection and hospitalization rate. Consequently, patients in the hospital are also discharged sooner. In a review by Crawford and associates (1991), the addition of G-CSF to CAE considerably reduced myelosuppressive and subsequent infectious complications. A similarly designed European study by Green and colleagues (1991) confirmed this result. This approach, however, is extremely costly. Alternate choices include less myelosuppressive but equally effective chemotherapy, as already proposed, or perhaps using oral prophylactic antibiotics, such as cotrimoxazole or various marketed fluoroquinolones.

Blackstein (1990) and Eckhardt (1990) and their colleagues observed that cardiotoxicity usually can be avoided by using less cardiotoxic anthracyclines, such as epirubicin, which is active in both SCLC and NSCLC, as reported by one of us (R.F.) and coworkers (1992). In addition, the use of only four to six courses of therapy, which is now standard throughout the world, decreases the recurrence of this problem and many of the other side effects, thereby enhancing the quality of life of these patients. Johnson (1990) found that Mesna, especially when combined with ifosfamide, has essentially eradicated the problem of hemorrhagic cystitis with the latter agent. Mesna also can be used with high-dose cyclophosphamide to avoid hemorrhagic cystitis. If nephrotoxicity, ototoxicity, or emesis is a concern, one can switch the cisplatin-containing regimen to carboplatin, which usually either averts or stabilizes these side effects but also causes more myelosuppression. Carboplatin, as discussed

by Green and associates (1992), may be more expensive and possibly less active in this disease.

Late Complications of Chemotherapy

Peripheral neuropathy remains a frequent problem. Of specific concern is the late-onset neuropathy identified with cisplatin. This condition can begin even a few months after the final course of cisplatin and can be disabling. New approaches to this dilemma are needed.

Although many of the late complications of therapy are shown in Table 107-15, the one that is potentially of most concern is the formation of second malignancies in potentially cured patients. In a study by Sagman and colleagues (1992), second lung primaries in patients with SCLC are relatively frequent complications if patients survive long enough. A review by Heyne and associates (1992) from M. D. Anderson Hospital also revealed cases involving second primaries. Perhaps these complications can be prevented in future by the use of agents such as retinoids, as suggested by Ihde (1992). These lesions may be overlooked and presumed to be a relapse of the original tumor, thereby precluding possible surgical removal with the potential for cure. A second primary must always be contemplated when new lesions are observed in patients, undoubtedly beyond 2 years from diagnosis and even less in some cases. Other solid tumors also occur with reasonable frequency as second primaries, probably related in part to treatment but more likely associated with the patients' age (median 60+ years). Acute leukemia is an unusual occurrence and will become less typical with the discontinued use of nitrosurea and procarbazine for SCLC and the considerably shorter span of treatment involved. Second lung primaries and, indeed, acute leukemia are sometimes seen in patients with NSCLC, but they are less of a problem.

REFERENCES

Aapro MS: 5-HT receptor antagonists—an overview of their present status and future potential in cancer therapy-induced emesis. Drugs 42:551, 1991.

Ahmann F: A reassessment of the clinical implications of the superior caval syndrome. J Clin Oncol 2:961, 1984.

Aisner SC, Matthews MJ: The pathology of lung cancer. In Aisner J (ed): Contemporary Issues in Clinical Oncology. Vol 3. Lung Cancer. New York: Churchill Livingstone, 1985.

Aisner J, et al: Meningeal carcinomatosis from small cell carcinoma of the lung. Acta Cytol 23:292, 1979.

Aisner J, et al: Leptomeningeal carcinomatosis in small cell carcinoma of the lung. Med Pediatr Oncol 9:47, 1981.

Aisner J, et al: Intensive combination chemotherapy, concurrent chest irradiation, and warfarin for the treatment of limited-disease small-cell lung cancer: a Cancer and Leukemia Group B pilot study. J Clin Oncol 10:1230, 1992.

Albain KS, et al: Determinants of improved outcome in small-cell lung cancer: an analysis of the 2,580-patient Southwest Oncology Group data base. J Clin Oncol 8:1563, 1990.

Anderson H, et al: Recombinant human GM-CSF in small cell lung cancer: a phase I/II study. Recent results. Cancer Res 121:155, 1991a.

Anderson H, et al: Phase II study of Gemcitabine in non small cell lung cancer (NSCLC). Proc Am Soc Clin Oncol 10(abstr 848):247, 1991b.

Ardizzoni A, Sertoli MR, Corcione A: Accelerated chemotherapy with or without GM-CSF for small cell lung cancer: a non-randomized pilot study. Eur J Cancer 26:937, 1990.

Ardizzoni A, et al: Topotecan, a new active drug in the second-line treatment of small-cell lung cancer: a phase II study in patients with refractory and sensitive disease. The European Organization for Research and Treatment of Cancer Early Clinical Studies Group and New Drug Development Office, and the Lung Cancer Cooperative Group. J Clin Oncol 15:2090, 1997.

Aroney RS, et al: Meningeal carcinomatosis in small cell carcinoma of the lung. Am J Med 71:26, 1981.

Aroney RS, et al: Value of prophylactic cranial irradiation in prevention of central nervous system metastases in small cell lung cancer. Potential benefit restricted to patients with complete response. Cancer Treat Rep 67:675, 1983.

Arriagada R, Pignon JP, Le Chevalier TL: Thoracic radiation therapy in small cell lung cancer: rationale for timing and fractionation. Lung Cancer 5:237, 1989.

Arriagada R, et al: Alternating radiation therapy and chemotherapy schedules in small cell lung cancer, limited disease. Int J Radiat Oncol Biol Phys 11:1461, 1985.

Arriagada R, et al: Consensus report on combined radiation therapy and chemotherapy modalities in lung cancer. Antibiot Chemother 41:232, 1988.

Arriagada R, et al: Meta-analysis of randomized trials evaluating the role of thoracic radiation therapy in limited small cell lung carcinoma (SCLC). 6th World Conference on Lung Cancer, Melbourne, November 10–14. Lung Cancer 7(Suppl)(abstr 359):98, 1991a.

Arriagada R, et al: Initial high dose chemotherapy and multifractionated radiation therapy in limited small cell lung cancer. Lung Cancer 7:159, 1991b.

Arriagada R, et al: Initial chemotherapy doses and survival in limited small cell lung cancer. N Engl J Med 329:1848, 1993.

Arriagada R, et al: Prophylactic cranial irradiation for patients with small-cell lung cancer in complete remission. J Natl Cancer Inst 87:183, 1995.

Arriagada R, et al: Prophylactic cranial irradiation overview (PCIO) in patients with small cell lung cancer (SCLC) in complete remission. Proc Am Soc Clin Oncol 17(abstr 1758):450, 1998.

Ariyoshi Y, Sugiura T: New promising anticancer drugs for lung cancer (article in Japanese). Gan To Kagaku Ryoho 21:2578, 1994.

Avalos BR, et al: Human granulocyte colony-stimulating factor: biologic activity and receptor characterization of hematopoietic cells and small cell lung cancer cell lines. Blood 75:851, 1990.

Banham SW, et al: High dose epirubicin chemotherapy in untreated poorer prognosis small cell lung cancer. Respir Med 84:241, 1990.

Barkley H (ed): Radiation therapy for relief of intrathoracic symptoms arising from unresectable bronchial carcinoma. University of Texas System Cancer Center. Annual Clinical Conference on Cancer. Vol. 28. Houston: University of Texas Press, 1986, p. 191.

Beiler DD, et al: Low volume elective brain irradiation in small cell carcinoma of the lung. Int J Radiat Oncol Biol Phys 5:941, 1979.

Berendsen HH, et al: Detection of small cell lung cancer metastases in bone marrow aspirates using monoclonal antibody directed against neuroendocrine differentiation antigen. J Clin Pathol 41:273, 1988.

Bergsagel D, Feld R: Small cell lung cancer is still a problem (editorial). J Clin Oncol 2:1189, 1984.

Bergsagel DE, et al: Lung cancer: clinical trial of radiation therapy alone vs. radiation therapy plus cyclophosphamide. Cancer 30:621, 1972.

Biran H, Feld R, Malkin A: Circulating arginine-vasopressin, calcitonin, carcinoembryonic antigen, neuron-specific enolase, and beta-2 microglobulin fluctuations during combined modality induction therapy for small-cell bronchial carcinoma. Association of postchemotherapy AVP surge with high tumor response rate and durable remission. Tumour Biol 12:131, 1991.

Birch R, et al: Patterns of failure in combined chemotherapy and radiation therapy for limited small-cell lung cancer: South Eastern Chemotherapy Group experience. J Natl Cancer Inst Monogr 6:265, 1988.

Birch R, et al: A randomized study of etoposide and carboplatin with or without paclitaxel in the treatment of small cell lung cancer. Semin Oncol 12:S12–135, 1997.

Bishop JF, et al: Dose and schedule of granulocyte macrophage colony

stimulating factor (GM-CSF) carboplatin and etoposide in small cell lung cancer (SCLC). Proc Am Soc Clin Oncol 10(abstr 820):240, 1991.

Blackstein M, et al: Epirubicin in extensive small-cell lung cancer: a phase II study in previously untreated patients: a National Cancer Institute of Canada Clinical Trials group study. J Clin Oncol 8:385, 1990.

Bleyer WA, Poplack DG. Intraventricular versus intralumbar methotrexate for central nervous system leukemia: prolonged remission with the Ommaya reservoir. Med Pediatr Oncol 6:207, 1979.

Boerman OC, et al: Biodistribution of a monoclonal antibody (RnH-1) against the neural cell adhesion molecule (WCAM) in athymic mice bearing human small-cell lung-cancer xenografts. Int J Cancer 48:457, 1991.

Bonadonna G: Chemotherapy strategies to improve the control of Hodgkin's disease: The Richard and Hinda Rosenthal Foundation Award Lecture. Cancer Res 42:4309, 1982.

Bonomi P, et al: Intensive induction treatment of small cell bronchogenic carcinoma with cyclophosphamide, methotrexate and etoposide. Cancer Treat Rep 69:1007, 1985.

Boyer M, Feld R, Warr D: LDH alone does not predict relapse of small cell lung cancer (SCLC) (abstr 1223). Proc Am Assoc Cancer Res 33:204, 1992.

Brennan J, et al: myc family DNA amplification in 107 tumors and tumor cell lines from patients with small cell lung cancer treated with different combination chemotherapy regimens. Cancer Res 51:1708, 1991.

Brereton HD, et al: Spinal meningeal carcinomatosis in small cell carcinoma of the lung. Ann Intern Med 88:517, 1978.

Brooks BJ Jr, et al: Pulmonary toxicity with combined modality therapy for limited stage small-cell lung cancer. J Clin Oncol 4:200, 1986.

Bunn PA Jr: The North American experience with paclitaxel combined with cisplatin or carboplatin in lung cancer. Semin Oncol 23:18, 1996.

Bunn PA Jr: Defining the role of paclitaxel in lung cancer: summary of recent studies and implications for future directions. Semin Oncol 24:S12–153, 1997.

Bunn PA Jr, Ihde DC: Small cell bronchogenic carcinoma: a review of therapeutic results. In Livingston RB (ed): Lung Cancer. Vol. 1. Boston: Martinus Nijhoff, 1981, p. 169.

Bunn PA Jr, Nugent JL, Matthews MJ: Central nervous system metastases in small cell bronchogenic carcinoma. Semin Oncol 5:314, 1978.

Bunn PA Jr, Rosen ST. Central nervous system manifestation of small cell lung cancer. In Aisner J (ed): Contemporary Issues in Clinical Oncology. Vol. 3. Lung Cancer. New York: Churchill Livingstone, 1985, p. 287.

Bunn PA, et al: Chemotherapy alone or chemotherapy with chest radiation therapy in limited stage small-cell lung cancer. Ann Intern Med 106:655, 1987.

Byrne T: Spinal cord compression from epidural metastases. N Engl J Med 327:614, 1992.

Campling B, et al: Is bone marrow examination in small-cell lung cancer really necessary? Ann Intern Med 105:508, 1986.

Canellos GP, Anderson JR, Propert KJ: Chemotherapy of advanced Hodgkin's disease with MOPP, ABVD, or MOPP alternating with ABVD. N Engl J Med 327:1478, 1992.

Carlson R, et al: Late consolidative radiation therapy in the treatment of limited stage small cell lung cancer. Cancer 68:948, 1991.

Carney DN: Recent advances in the biology of small cell lung cancer. Chest 89(Suppl):253S, 1986.

Carney D: Lung cancer biology. Curr Opin Oncol 3:288, 1991.

Carney DN: The biology of lung cancer. Curr Opin Oncol 4:292, 1992.

Carney DN, et al: Establishment and identification of small cell lung cancer cell lines have classic and variant features. Cancer Res 45:2913, 1985.

Carney DN, et al: Bone marrow involvement (BMI) by small cell lung cancer (SCLC) using magnetic resonance imaging (MRI). Proc Am Soc Clin Oncol 9(abstr 889):228, 1989.

Carney DN, et al: Single-agent oral etoposide for elderly small cell lung cancer patients. Semin Oncol 17(Suppl 2):49, 1990.

Clark PI, et al: Prolonged administration of single-agent oral etoposide in patients with untreated small cell lung cancer (SCLC). Proc Am Soc Clin Oncol 9(abstr 874):226, 1990.

Clark P, et al: Two prolonged schedules of single-agent oral etoposide of differing duration and dose in patients with untreated small cell lung cancer (SCLC). Proc Am Soc Clin Oncol 10(abstr 931):268, 1991.

Cohen MH, et al: Intensive chemotherapy of small cell bronchogenic carcinoma. Cancer Treat Rep 61:349, 1977.

Cohen MH, et al: Thymosin fraction V and intensive combination chemotherapy. Prolonging the survival of patients with small cell lung cancer. JAMA 241:1813, 1979.

Comis R, et al: The current results of chemotherapy (CTH) plus adjuvant surgery (AS) in limited small cell anaplastic lung cancer (SCALC). Proc Am Soc Clin Oncol 1(abstr C-571):147, 1982.

Constans J, et al: Spinal metastases with neurological manifestations. Review of 600 cases. J Neurosurg 59:111, 1983.

Cormier Y, et al: Gemcitabine is an active new agent in previously untreated extensive small cell lung cancer (SCLC). A study of the National Cancer Institute of Canada Clinical Trials Group. Ann Oncol 5:283, 1994.

Cox JD, et al: Prophylactic cranial irradiation in patients with inoperable carcinoma of the lung. Preliminary report of a cooperative trial. Cancer 42:1135, 1978.

Cox J, et al: Results of whole brain irradiation for metastases from small cell carcinoma of the lung. Cancer Treat Rep 64:957, 1980.

Coy P, et al: The effect of dose of thoracic irradiation on recurrence in patients with limited stage small cell lung cancer. Initial results of a Canadian multicenter randomized trial. Int J Radiat Oncol Bio Phys 14:219, 1988.

Crawford J, et al: Reduction by granulocyte colony-stimulating factor of fever and neutropenia induced by chemotherapy in patients with small-cell lung cancer. N Engl J Med 325:164, 1991.

Creech R, Richter M, Finkelstein D: Combination chemotherapy with or without consolidation radiation therapy for regional small-cell carcinoma of the lung. Proc Am Soc Clin Oncol 6:66A, 1987.

Cunningham D, et al: High-dose cyclophosphamide and VP 16 as late dosage intensification therapy for small cell carcinoma of lung. Cancer Chemother Pharmacol 15:303, 1985.

Cutitta F, et al: Monoclonal antibodies that demonstrate specificity for several types to human lung cancer. Proc Natl Acad Sci U S A 78:4591, 1981.

Davis S, et al: Long-term survival in small cell carcinoma of the lung: a population experience. J Clin Oncol 3:80, 1985.

Dische S, Warburton M, Saunders M: Radiation myelitis and survival in the radiation therapy of lung cancer. Int J Radiat Oncol Biol Phys 15:75, 1988.

Dodwell DJ, Gurney H, Thatcher N: Dose intensity in cancer chemotherapy. Br J Cancer 61:789, 1990.

Eagen RT, et al: A case for preplanned thoracic and prophylactic whole brain irradiation therapy in limited small cell lung cancer. Cancer Clin Trials 4:261, 1981.

Earle CC, et al: A phase I study of gemcitabine/cisplatin/etoposide in the treatment of small cell lung cancer. Lung Cancer 22:235, 1998.

Eckhardt S, et al: Phase II study of 4'-epi-doxorubicin in patients with untreated extensive small cell lung cancer. Med Oncol Tumor Pharmacother 7:19, 1990.

Einhorn LH, Pennington K, McClean J: Phase II trial of daily oral VP-16 in refractory small cell lung cancer: a Hoosier Oncology Group study. Semin Oncol 17(Suppl 2):32, 1990.

Eisenhauer E, et al: Gemcitabine is active in patients (pts) with previously untreated extensive small cell lung cancer (SCLC)—a phase II study of the National Cancer Institute of Canada Clinical Trials Group (NCIC CTG). Proc Am Soc Clin Oncol 11(abstr 1043):309, 1992.

Elias AD, et al: High dose combination alkylating agents supported by autologous marrow (ABMT) with chest radiation therapy for responding limited stage (LD) small cell lung cancer (SCLC). Proc Am Soc Clin Oncol 11(abstr 991):296, 1992.

Elliott JA, Osterlind K, Hansen HH: Cyclic alternating "non-cross resistant" chemotherapy in the management of small cell anaplastic carcinoma of the lung. Cancer Treat Rev 11:103, 1984.

Elliott JA, et al: Metastatic patterns in small-cell lung cancer: correlation of autopsy findings with clinical parameters in 537 patients. J Clin Oncol 5:246, 1987.

Erasmus JJ, et al: Thoracic FDG PET: state of the art. Radiographics 18:5, 1998.

Ettinger DS: Evaluation of new drugs in untreated patients with small-cell lung cancer: its time has come. J Clin Oncol 8:374, 1990.

Ettinger DS: Taxol in the treatment of lung cancer. J Natl Cancer Inst Monogr 15:177, 1993.

Ettinger DS, et al: Phase II study of paclitaxel in patients with extensive-disease small cell lung cancer: an Eastern Cooperative Oncology Group study. J Clin Oncol 13:1430, 1995.

Evans WK, et al: Superiority of alternating non-cross-resistant chemotherapy in extensive small cell lung cancer. A Multicenter Randomized Clinical Trial by the National Cancer Institute of Canada. Ann Intern Med 107:451–458, 1987.

Evans WK, et al: Phase II study of amonafide: results of treatment and

lessons learned from the study of an investigational agent in previously untreated patients with extensive small-cell lung cancer. J Clin Oncol 8:390, 1990.

Evans WK, et al: Oral VP-16 and carboplatin for small cell lung cancer. Proc Am Soc Clin Oncol 10(abstr 847):247, 1991.

Feld R: Complications in the treatment of small cell carcinoma of the lung. Cancer Treat Rev 8:5, 1981.

Feld R: Late complications associated with the treatment of small-cell lung cancer. Cancer Treat Res 45:301, 1989a.

Feld R: Long term complications in small cell lung cancer. In Hansen HH (ed): Basic and Clinical Concepts of Lung Cancer. Boston: Kluwer, 1989b, pp. 301–323.

Feld R: Complications associated with the treatment of small cell lung cancer. Lung Cancer 10:S307, 1994.

Feld R, Ginsberg R, Payne DG: Treatment of small cell lung cancer. In Roth JA, Ruckdeschel JC, Weisenburger TH (eds): Thoracic Oncology. Philadelphia: WB Saunders, 1988, p. 229.

Feld R, et al: Combined modality induction therapy without maintenance chemotherapy for small cell carcinoma of the lung. J Clin Oncol 2:294, 1984.

Feld R, et al: Canadian multicentre randomized trial comparing sequential and alternating administration of two non-cross resistant chemotherapy combinations in patients with limited small cell carcinoma of the lung. J Clin Oncol 5:1401, 1987.

Feld R, et al: Phase I-II study of high dose epirubicin in advanced non-small cell lung cancer. J Clin Oncol 20:297, 1992.

Feld R, et al: The restaging of responding patients with limited small cell lung cancer—is it really useful? Chest 103:1010, 1993.

Ferguson MK, et al: Sex-associated differences in presentation and survival in patients with lung cancer. J Clin Oncol 8:1402, 1990.

Figueredo A, et al: Addition of verapamil and tamoxifen to the initial chemotherapy of small cell lung cancer. A phase I/II study. Cancer 65:1895, 1990.

Figueredo AT, et al: Co-trimoxazole prophylaxis during high dose chemotherapy of small cell lung cancer. J Clin Oncol 3:54, 1985.

Fleck JF, et al: Is prophylactic cranial irradiation indicated in small-cell lung cancer? J Clin Oncol 8:209, 1990.

Fowler J: The linear-quadratic formula and progress in fractionated radiation therapy. Br J Radiol 62:679, 1989.

Fox RM, Tattersall MHN, Woods RL: Radiation therapy as an adjuvant in small cell lung cancer treated by combination chemotherapy: a randomized study. Proc Am Soc Clin Oncol 22(abstr 661):502, 1981.

Fox RM, et al: A randomized study: small cell anaplastic lung cancer treated by combination chemotherapy and adjuvant radiation therapy. Int J Radiat Oncol Biol Phys 6:1083, 1980.

Fox W, Scadding JG: Medical Research Council comparative trial of surgery and radiation therapy for primary treatment of small celled or oat celled carcinoma of the bronchus. Ten year follow-up. Lancet 2:63, 1973.

Fukuoka M, et al: Randomized trial of cyclophosphamide, doxorubicin and vincristine versus cisplatin and etoposide versus alternation of these regimens in small cell lung cancer. J Natl Cancer Inst 83:855, 1991a.

Fukuoka M, et al: Dose intensive weekly CODE chemotherapy (CT) with or without recombinant human granulocyte colony-stimulating factor (rhG-CSF) in extensive-stage (ES) small cell lung cancer (SCLC). Lung Cancer 7:123, 1991b.

Gatzemeier U, et al: Paclitaxel, carboplatin, and oral etoposide: a phase II trial in limited-stage small cell lung cancer. Semin Oncol 24:S12-149, 1997.

Gazdar AF, Mulshine JL, Kramer BS: Biological, molecular, and clinical markers for the diagnosis and typing of lung cancer. Immunol Series 53:453, 1990b.

Gazdar AF, et al: Characterization of variant subclasses of cell lines derived from small cell lung cancer having distinctive biochemical, morphological and growth properties. Cancer Res 45:2924, 1985.

Gazdar AF, et al: Correlation of in vitro drug-sensitivity testing results with response to chemotherapy and survival in extensive-stage small cell lung cancer: a prospective clinical trial. J Natl Cancer Inst 82:117, 1990a.

Ginsberg RJ: Surgery and small cell lung cancer—an overview. Lung Cancer 5:232, 1989.

Ginsberg RJ, Karrer K: Surgery in small cell lung cancer. Lung Cancer 5:139, 1989.

Giovanella L, et al: Immunoassay of neuron-specific enolase (NSE) and serum fragments of cytokeratin 19 (CYFRA 21.1) as tumor markers in small cell lung cancer: clinical evaluation and biological hypothesis. Int J Biol Markers 12:22, 1997.

Girling DJ: Prospective randomised trial of 3 or 6 courses of etoposide, cyclophosphamide, methotrexate and vincristine and of 6 courses of etoposide and ifosfamide in small cell lung cancer (SCLC). For the British Medical Research Council Lung Cancer Working Party, 6th World Conference on Lung Cancer, Melbourne. Lung Cancer 7(Suppl):103, 1991.

Goldie JH, Coldman AJ: The genetic origin of drug resistance in neoplasms: implications for systemic therapy. Cancer Res 44:3643, 1984.

Goldie JH, Coldman AJ, Gudavskas GA: Rationale for the use of alternating non-cross resistant chemotherapy. Cancer Treat Rep 66:439, 1982.

Goldie J, et al. A mathematical and computer-based model of alternating chemotherapy and radiation therapy in experimental neoplasms. Antibiot Chemother 41:11, 1988.

Gonzalez-Avila G, et al: 72-kD (MMP-2) and 92-kD (MMP-9) type IV collagenase production and activity in different histologic types of lung cancer cells. Pathobiology 66:5, 1998.

Goodman GE, et al: Treatment of limited small cell lung cancer with concurrent CP-16/cisplatin radiation therapy followed by intensification with high-dose cyclophosphamide. A Southwest Oncology Group Study. J Clin Oncol 9:453, 1991.

Goodwin PJ, Feld R, Evans WK: Cost-effectiveness of cancer chemotherapy: an economic evaluation of a randomized trial in small cell lung cancer. J Clin Oncol 6:1537, 1988.

Grafton C, et al: High dose rate endobronchial brachytherapy using the MicroSelectron. Lung Cancer 7(Suppl):97, 1991.

Grant SC, et al: Single-agent chemotherapy trials in small-cell lung cancer, 1970 to 1990: the case for studies in previously treated patients. J Clin Oncol 10:484, 1992.

Greco FA, Fer MF: Oat-cell carcinoma of the lung with carcinomatosis in small cell carcinoma of the lung. Ann Intern Med 88:517, 1978.

Greco FA, Hainsworth JD: Paclitaxel, carboplatin, and oral etoposide in the treatment of small cell lung cancer. Semin Oncol 23:7, 1996.

Green JA, Trillet VN, Manegold C: 4-metHuG-Csf (G-CSF) with CDE chemotherapy (CT) in small cell lung cancer (SCLC): interim results from a randomized, placebo controlled trial. For The European G-CSF Lung Cancer Study Group. Proc Am Soc Clin Oncol 10(abstr 832):243, 1991.

Green M, et al: Carboplatin in non-small cell lung cancer: an update on the Cancer and Leukemia Group B experience. Semin Oncol 19(Suppl 2):44, 1992.

Green RA, et al: Alkylating agents and bronchogenic carcinoma. Am J Med 46:516, 1969.

Greenberg D, et al: Fatigue syndrome due to localized radiation. J Pain Symptom Management 7:38, 1992.

Gregor A, et al: Randomized trial of alternating versus sequential radiation therapy/chemotherapy in limited-disease patients with small cell lung cancer: a European Organization for Research and Treatment of Cancer Lung Cancer Cooperative Group study. J Clin Oncol 15:2840, 1997a.

Gregor A, et al: Prophylactic cranial irradiation is indicated following complete response to induction therapy in small cell lung cancer: results of a multicentre randomised trial. United Kingdom Coordinating Committee for Cancer Research (UKCCCR) and the European Organization for Research and Treatment of Cancer (EORTC). Eur J Cancer 33:1752, 1997b.

Hainsworth JD, Greco FA: Paclitaxel in lung cancer: 1-hour infusions given alone or in combination chemotherapy. Semin Oncol 22:45, 1995.

Hainsworth JD, et al: Paclitaxel, carboplatin, and extended-schedule oral etoposide for small cell lung cancer. Oncology (Huntingt) 12(Suppl 2):31, 1998.

Hall E: Radiobiology for the Radiologist. 3rd Ed. Philadelphia: Lippincott, 1988.

Hansen HH, et al: Prophylactic irradiation in bronchogenic small cell anaplastic carcinoma. Cancer 46:279, 1980.

Hansen M: Paraneoplastic syndrome and tumor markers for small cell and non-small cell lung cancer. Curr Opin Oncol 2:345, 1990.

Havemann MWK: Alternating chemotherapy in small cell lung cancer. Onkologie 13:157, 1990.

Heyne KH, et al: The incidence of second primary tumors in long-term survivors of small cell lung cancer. J Clin Oncol 10:1519, 1992.

Hirsch F: Staging and prognostic factors: 1. Staging procedures. Lung Cancer 5:152, 1989.

Hochstenbag MM, et al: Detection of bone marrow metastases in small cell lung cancer: comparison of magnetic resonance imaging with standard methods. Eur J Cancer 32:779, 1996.

Holst JJ, et al: Elevated plasma concentration of C-flanking gastrin-releasing peptide in small cell lung cancer. J Clin Oncol 7:1831, 1989.

Hryniuk W, Levine MN: Analysis of dose intensity for adjuvant chemotherapy trials. J Clin Oncol 4:1161, 1986.

Hryniuk WM, Figueredo A, Goodyear M: Applications of dose intensity to problems of chemotherapy of breast and colorectal cancer. Semin Oncol 14:3, 1987.

Humblet Y, Symann M, Bosly A: Late intensification chemotherapy with autologous bone marrow transplantation in selected small cell carcinoma of the lung: a randomized study. J Clin Oncol 5:1864, 1987.

Hyde L, et al: Cell type and the natural history of lung cancer. JAMA 193:140, 1965.

Hyde L, et al: Natural course of inoperable lung cancer. Chest 64:309, 1973.

Iggo R, et al: Increased expression of mutant forms of p53 oncogene in primary lung cancer. Lancet 335:675, 1990.

Ihde DC: Current status of therapy for small cell cancer of the lung. Cancer 54:2722, 1984.

Ihde DC: Staging evaluation and prognostic factors in small cell lung cancer. In Aisner J (ed): Contemporary Issues in Clinical Oncology. Vol 3. Lung Cancer. New York: Churchill Livingstone, 1985, p. 241.

Ihde DC: Chemotherapy of lung cancer. Review article. N Engl J Med 327:1434, 1992.

Ihde DC, Deisseroth AB, Lichter AS: Late intensive combined modality therapy followed by autologous bone marrow infusion in extensive-stage small-cell lung cancer. J Clin Oncol 4:1433, 1986.

Ihde DC, et al: Prognostic implications of stage of disease and sites of metastases in patients with small cell carcinoma of the lung treated with intensive combination chemotherapy. Am Rev Respir Dis 123:500, 1971.

Ihde DC, et al: Randomized trial of high vs. standard dose etoposide (VP16) and cisplatin in extensive small cell lung cancer (SCLC). For the 6th World Conference on Lung Cancer, Melbourne. Proc Am Soc Clin Oncol 10(abstr 819):240, 1991.

Jackson DV, et al: Prophylactic cranial irradiation in small cell carcinoma of the lung. A randomized study. JAMA 237:2730, 1977.

Jackson D, et al: Prophylactic cranial irradiation in small cell carcinoma of the lung. JAMA 237:2730, 1983.

Jeremic B, et al: Initial versus delayed accelerated hyperfractionated radiation therapy and concurrent chemotherapy in limited small cell lung cancer: a randomized study. J Clin Oncol 15:893, 1997.

Jett JR, Su JQ, Maksymiuk AW: Phase III trial of recombinant interferon gamma (IFN-γ) in complete responders (CR) with small cell lung cancer (SCC). Proc Am Soc Clin Oncol 11(abstr 956):287, 1992.

Johnson BE, et al: Limited (Ltd) stage small cell lung cancer (SCLC) treated with concurrent BID chest radiation therapy (RT) and etoposide cisplatin (VP/PT) followed by chemotherapy (CT) selected by in vitro drug sensitivity testing (DST). For the 6th World Conference on Lung Cancer, Melbourne. Lung Cancer 7(Suppl):152, 1991a.

Johnson BE, et al: Limited (Ltd) stage small cell lung cancer treated with concurrent bid chest radiation therapy and etoposide/platinum followed by chemotherapy selected by in vitro drug sensitivity testing. Proc Am Soc Clin Oncol 10:240, 1991b.

Johnson DH: New drugs in the management of SCLC. Lung Cancer 5:221, 1989.

Johnson DH: Overview of Ifosfamide in small cell and non-small cell lung cancer. Semin Oncol 17(Suppl 4):24, 1990.

Johnson DH, et al: High-dose induction chemotherapy with cyclophosphamide, etoposide, and cisplatin for extensive-stage small-cell lung cancer. J Clin Oncol 5:703, 1987a.

Johnson DH, et al: A randomized comparison of high-dose versus conventional-dose cyclophosphamide, doxorubicin and vincristine for extensive-stage small cell lung cancer. J Clin Oncol 5:1731, 1987b.

Johnson DH, et al: Alternating chemotherapy (CT) and thoracic radiation therapy (TRT) in limited small cell lung cancer (LSCLC): a test of the Looney hypothesis. For the Eastern Cooperative Oncology Group. Proc Am Soc Clin Oncol 10(abstr 829):243, 1991.

Joss R, et al: Combined modality treatment of small cell lung cancer (SCLC): randomized comparison of induction chemotherapy with or without radiation therapy to the chest (RT). Proc Fourth World Conference on Lung Cancer (abstr 141). Toronto: International Association for the Study of Lung Cancer, 1985.

Karrer K: Is the progress in cancer treatment results adequate or are we confronted with a more or less world wide stagnation? J Cancer Res Clin Oncol 116:1, 1990.

Karrer K, Shields T: The importance of complete resection in the multimodality treatment of SCLC. For ISC-Lung Cancer Study Group, 6th World Conference on Lung Cancer, Melbourne. Lung Cancer 7(Suppl):71, 1991.

Katsenis AT, et al: Elective brain irradiation in patients with small-cell carcinoma of the lung: preliminary report. Tokyo: Lung Cancer International Congress Series, Excerpta Medica, 1982, p. 277.

Kern JA, et al: p185neu expression in human lung adenocarcinoma predicts shortened survival. Cancer Res 50:5184, 1990.

Kies M, et al: Multimodal therapy for limited small cell lung cancer: a randomized study of induction combination chemotherapy with or without thoracic radiation in complete responders; and with wide-field versus reduced field radiation in partial responders: a South West Oncology Group study. J Clin Oncol 5:592, 1987.

Klasa RJ, Murray N, Colman AJ: Dose intensity meta-analysis of chemotherapy regimens in small-cell carcinoma of the lung. J Clin Oncol 9:499, 1991.

Klastersky J: Diagnosis and staging in small cell lung cancer. Curr Opin Oncol 2:331, 1990.

Klimo P, Connors JM: MACOP-B chemotherapy for the treatment of diffuse large-cell lymphoma. Ann Intern Med 102:596, 1985.

Kollmannsberger C, et al: Topotecan—a novel topoisomerase I inhibitor: pharmacology and clinical experience. Oncology 56:1, 1999.

Kristjansen PEG: The role of cranial irradiation in the management of patients with SCLC. Lung Cancer 5:264, 1989.

Kristjansen PEG, et al: A three-armed randomized trial in small cell lung cancer (SCLC) of two induction regimens with teniposide and cisplatin or carboplatin followed by alternating chemotherapy versus alternating chemotherapy. Lung Cancer 7(Suppl):121, 1991.

Kurtz J, et al: The palliation of brain metastases in a favourable patient population: a randomized clinical trial by the RTOG. Int J Radiat Oncol Biol Phys 7:891, 1981.

Lad T: The role of surgery in small cell lung cancer (SCLC): an intergroup prospective randomized trial. Lung Cancer 4:A83, 1988.

Lad T, et al: Thoracotomy staging of small cell lung cancer. For the 6th World Conference on Lung Cancer, Melbourne. Lung Cancer 7(Suppl):(abstr 205), 1991.

Laplanche A, et al: Controlled clinical trial of prophylactic cranial irradiation for patients with small-cell lung cancer in complete remission. Lung Cancer 21:193, 1998.

Layer G, Jarosch K: Magnetic resonance tomography of the bone marrow for the detection of metastases of solid tumors (article in German). Radiologe 32:502, 1992.

Lazarus HM, Spitzer TR, Creger RJ: Phase I trial of high-dose etoposide, high-dose cisplatin and reinfusion of autologous bone marrow for lung cancer. Am J Clin Oncol 13:110, 1990.

LeBeau B, Chastang CL, Brechot JM: Small cell lung cancer (SCLC): long term results of a randomized trial assessing chemotherapy continuation in patients reaching complete remission after six courses. For the "Petites Cellules" Group (02PC 83 Protocol), 6th World Conference on Lung Cancer, Melbourne. Lung Cancer 7(Suppl):130, 1991a.

LeBeau B, et al: Small cell lung cancer (SCLC): negative results of a randomized trial on delayed thoracic radiation therapy administered to complete responders (CR) patients. Lung Cancer 7:94, 1991b.

Lewin A, et al: Radiation-induced failures of complementary metal oxide semiconductor containing pacemakers: a potentially lethal complication. Int J Radiat Oncol Biol Phys 10:1967, 1984.

Lewis JW Jr, et al: Can computed tomography of the chest stage lung cancer? Yes and no. Ann Thorac Surg 49:591, 1990.

Liengswangwong V, et al: Limited-stage small-cell lung cancer: patterns of intrathoracic recurrence and the implications for thoracic radiation therapy. J Clin Oncol 12:496, 1994.

Lilenbaum RC, et al: Phase I and pharmacologic study of continuous infusion topotecan in combination with cisplatin in patients with advanced cancer: a Cancer and Leukemia Group B study. J Clin Oncol 16:3302, 1998.

Lishner M, et al: Late neurological complications after prophylactic cranial irradiation in patients with small-cell lung cancer: the Toronto experience. J Clin Oncol 8:215, 1990.

Little CD, et al: Amplification and expression of the C-myc oncogene in human lung cancer cell lines. Nature 306:194, 1983.

Littlewood TJ, Bentley DP, Smith AP: High-dose etoposide with autologous bone marrow transplantation as initial treatment of small cell lung cancer—a negative report. Eur J Respir Dis 68:370, 1986.

Livingston RB, et al: Long-term survival and toxicity in small cell lung cancer. Am J Med 77:415, 1984.

Loehrer PJ Sr: The role of ifosfamide in small cell lung cancer. Semin Oncol 23:40, 1996.

Looney WB, Hopkins HA, Carter WH Jr: Solid tumour models for the assessment of different treatment modalities. XXIII. A new approach to the more effective utilization of radiation therapy alternating with chemotherapy. Int J Radiat Oncol Biol Phys 11:2105, 1985.

Lund B, et al: Phase II study of Gemcitabine in non-small cell lung cancer

(NSCLC). For the 6th World Conference on Lung Cancer, Melbourne. Lung Cancer 7:121, 1991.

Maasilta P: Radiation-induced lung injury. From the chest physician's point of view. Lung Cancer 7:367, 1991.

Macauley VM, et al: Autocrine insulin-like growth factor 1 in human small cell lung cancer cell lines and fresh tumor cells. Cancer Res 50:2511, 1990.

Mah K, Van Dyk J: Quantitative measurements of change in human lung density following irradiation. Radiother Oncol 11:169, 1988.

Marangolo M, et al: High-dose etoposide and autologous bone marrow transplantation as intensification treatment in small cell lung cancer: a pilot study. Bone Marrow Transplant 4:405, 1989.

Masuda N, et al: CPT-11: a new derivative of camptothecin for the treatment of refractory or relapsed small-cell lung cancer. J Clin Oncol 10:1225, 1992.

Mattson K, et al: Natural alpha interferon as maintenance therapy for small cell lung cancer. For the 6th World Conference on Lung Cancer, Melbourne. Lung Cancer 7(Suppl):127, 1991.

Maurer LH, et al: A randomized combined modality trial in small cell carcinoma of the lung. Comparison of combination chemotherapy-radiation therapy versus cyclophosphamide-radiation therapy: effects of maintenance chemotherapy and whole brain irradiation. Cancer 45:30, 1980.

McDonald S, Rubin P, Maasilta P: Response of normal lung to irradiation: tolerance doses/tolerance volumes in pulmonary radiation syndromes. Front Radiat Ther Oncol 23:255, 1989.

Medical Research Council Lung Cancer Working Party: Inoperable non-small-cell lung cancer (NSCLC): a Medical Research Council randomised trial of palliative radiation therapy with two fractions or ten fractions. Report to the Medical Research Council by its Lung Cancer Working Party. Br J Cancer 63:265, 1991.

Medical Research Council Lung Cancer Working Party: A Medical Research Council (MRC) randomised trial of palliative radiation therapy with two fractions or a single fraction in patients with inoperable non-small-cell lung cancer (NSCLC) and poor performance status. Br J Cancer 65:934, 1992.

Medical Research Council Lung Cancer Working Party: Randomised trial of palliative two-fraction versus more intensive 13-fraction radiation therapy for patients with inoperable non-small cell lung cancer and good performance status. Clin Oncol 8:167, 1996.

Mehta C, Vogl SE: High-dose cyclophosphamide in the induction therapy of small cell lung cancer. Minor improvements in rate of remission and survival. Proc Am Soc Cancer Res 23:155, 1982.

Meyer JA, Comis RL, Ginsberg RJ: Selective surgical resection in small cell carcinoma of the lung. J Thorac Cardiovasc Surg 84:641, 1982a.

Meyer JA, et al: Phase II trial of extended indications for resection in small cell carcinoma of the lung. J Thorac Cardiovasc Surg 83:12, 1982b.

Miles DW, et al: Intensive weekly chemotherapy for the treatment of extensive-stage small cell lung cancer. J Clin Oncol 9:280, 1991.

Miller AB, Fox W, Tall R: Five-year follow-up of the Medical Research Council's comparative trial of surgery and radiation therapy for the primary treatment of small celled carcinoma or oat celled carcinoma of the bronchus. Lancet 12:501, 1969.

Milroy R, et al: Randomised clinical study of Verapamil in addition to chemotherapy in small cell lung cancer (SCLC). For the 6th World Conference on Lung Cancer, Melbourne. Lung Cancer 7(Suppl):114, 1991.

Minna JD, Higgins GA, Glatstein EJ: Cancer of the Lung. In DeVita VT Jr, Hellman S, Rosenberg S (eds): Cancer Principles and Practice of Oncology. Philadelphia: JB Lippincott, 1985, p. 507.

Minna JD, et al: Cancer of the Lung. In De Vita VT Sr, Hellman S, Rosenberg S (eds): Cancer Principles and Practice of Oncology. 3rd Ed. Philadelphia: JB Lippincott, 1989, p. 591.

Mitchell EP, et al: Etoposide (VP-16) and Cisplatin (DDP) in untreated extensive small cell lung cancer (SCLC): a dose-escalation study. Proc Am Soc Clin Oncol 7(abst 796):206, 1988.

Mornex F, Nayel H, Videira A: Efficacy of radiation therapy in 79 patients with brain metastases from primary lung cancer. Lung Cancer 7:98, 1991.

Mornex F, et al: Hyperfractionated radiation therapy alternating with multidrug chemotherapy in the treatment of limited small cell lung cancer (SCLC). Int J Radiat Oncol Biol Phys 19:223, 1990.

Mountain C: Revisions in the International System for Staging Lung Cancer. Chest 111:1710, 1997.

Murphy PB, et al: Cisplatin (P) & prolonged administration of oral etoposide (E) in extensive small cell lung cancer (ESCLC) patients (PT): a phase II trial. Proc Am Soc Clin Oncol 10(abstr 886):257, 1991.

Murray N, et al: The importance of timing for thoracic irradiation (TI) in the combined modality treatment of limited stage small cell cancer (LSCLC). Proc Am Soc Clin Oncol 10(abstr 831):243, 1991a.

Murray N, et al: Intensive weekly chemotherapy for the treatment of extensive-stage small-cell lung cancer. J Clin Oncol 9:1632, 1991b.

Murray N, et al: The importance of timing for thoracic irradiation in the combined modality treatment of limited stage small cell lung cancer. The National Cancer Institute of Cancer Clinical Trials Group. J Clin Oncol 11:336, 1993.

Neill HB, et al: A phase II study evaluating the efficacy of carboplatin, etoposide, and paclitaxel with granulocyte colony-stimulating factor in patients with stage IIIB and IV non-small cell lung cancer and extensive small cell lung cancer. Semin Oncol 24:S12-130, 1997.

Nieto A, Doty D: Superior vena cava obstruction: clinical syndrome, etiology, and treatment. Curr Probl Cancer 10:442, 1986.

Nomura F, et al: High dose chemotherapy with autologous bone marrow transplantation for limited small cell lung cancer. Jpn J Clin Oncol 20:94, 1990.

Nou E, Brodin O, Bergh J: A randomized study of radiation treatment in small cell bronchial carcinoma treated with two types of four drug chemotherapy regimens. Cancer 62:1079, 1988.

O'Donnell MR, et al: Intensive induction chemotherapy for small-cell anaplastic carcinoma of the lung. Cancer Treat Rep 69:571, 1985.

Ohnoshi T, Hiraki S, Kimura I: Randomised trial of chemotherapy alone or with chest irradiation in limited-stage small-cell lung cancer. Lung Cancer International Congress Series, 1987, p. 186.

Ohnoshi T, et al: Randomized trial comparing chemotherapy alone and chemotherapy plus chest irradiation in limited stage small cell lung cancer: a preliminary report. Jpn J Clin Oncol 16:271, 1986.

Okamoto I, et al: CD-44 cleavage induced by a membrane-associated metalloproteinase plays a critical role in tumor cell migration. Oncogene 18:1435, 1999.

Oster MW, Fetell M: Meningeal carcinomatosis in small cell carcinoma of the lung. Med Pediatr Oncol 10:157, 1982.

Osterlind K, et al: Treatment policy of surgery in small cell carcinoma of the lung: retrospective analysis of a series of 874 consecutive patients. Thorax 40:272, 1985.

Osterlind K, et al: Chemotherapy versus chemotherapy plus irradiation in limited small cell lung cancer. Results of a controlled trial with 5 years follow-up. Br J Cancer 54:7, 1986.

Patchell R, Tibbs P, Walsh J: A randomized trial of surgery in the treatment of single metastases to the brain. N Engl J Med 322:494, 1990.

Pedersen A, Bach F, Melgaard B: Frequency, diagnosis and prognosis of spinal cord compression in small cell bronchogenic carcinoma. A review of 817 patients. Cancer 55:1818, 1985.

Perez EA, Buckwalter CA, Reid JP: Combinations of paclitaxel and etoposide in the treatment of lung cancer. Semin Oncol 223(Suppl 15):21, 1996.

Perez-Soler R, et al: Treatment of patients with small cell lung cancer refractory to etoposide and cisplatin with the topoisomerase I poison topotecan. J Clin Oncol 14:2785, 1996.

Perry M, et al: Chemotherapy with or without radiation therapy in limited small cell carcinoma of the lung. N Engl J Med 316:912, 1987.

Perry MC, et al: Thoracic radiation therapy added to chemotherapy for small cell lung cancer: an update of Cancer and Leukemia Group B Study 8083. J Clin Oncol 16:2466, 1998.

Pfister DG, et al: Classifying clinical severity to help solve problems of stage migration in nonconcurrent comparisons of lung cancer therapy. Cancer Res 50:4664, 1990.

Pignon J-P, et al: A meta-analysis of thoracic radiation therapy for small-cell lung cancer. N Engl J Med 327:1618, 1992.

Postmus PE, et al: High-dose cyclophosphamide and high-dose VP-16-213 for recurrent or refractory small cell lung cancer. A Phase II study. Eur J Cancer Clin Oncol 21:1467, 1985.

Postmus PE, et al: Effects of recombinant human interleukin-3 in patients with relapsed small cell lung cancer treated with chemotherapy: a dose-finding study. J Clin Oncol 10:1131, 1992.

Prager RL, et al: The feasibility of adjuvant surgery in limited-stage small cell carcinoma: a prospective evaluation. Ann Thorac Surg 88:495, 1984.

Price P, et al: Prospective randomized trial of single and multifraction radiation therapy schedules in the treatment of painful bony metastases. Radiother Oncol 6:247, 1986.

Pujol JL, et al: Dose intensive chemotherapy in patients with advanced small cell lung cancer. Eur J Cancer 31:S21, 1995.

Quon H, et al: The influence of age on the delivery, tolerance and efficacy of thoracic irradiation in the combined modality treatment of limited stage small cell lung cancer. Int J Radiat Oncol Biol Phys 43:39, 1999.

Rawson NSB, Peto J: An overview of prognostic factors in small cell lung cancer: a report of prognostic factors in small cell lung cancer. A Report of the Subcommittee for the Management of Lung Cancer in the United Kingdom, Coordinating Committee on Cancer Research. Br J Cancer 61:597, 1990.

Rege SD, et al: Imaging of pulmonary mass lesions with whole-body positron emission tomography and fluorodeoxyglucose. Cancer 72:82, 1993.

Richardson GE, et al: An algorithm for staging patients (PTS) with small cell lung cancer (SCLC) can save 40% of the initial evaluation costs. Proc Am Soc Clin Oncol 10(abstr 828):242, 1991.

Rodichok L, et al: Early diagnosis of spinal epidural metastases. Am J Med 70:1181, 1981.

Rosen ST, et al: Carcinomatous leptomeningitis in small cell lung cancer: a clinicopathologic review of the National Cancer Institute experience. Medicine (Baltimore) 61:45, 1982.

Rosenthal M, et al: Adjuvant thoracic radiation therapy in small cell lung cancer: ten year follow-up of a randomized study. Lung Cancer 7:235, 1991.

Roth BJ, et al: Randomized study of cyclophosphamide, doxorubicin, and vincristine versus etoposide and cisplatin versus alternation of these two regimens in extensive small cell lung cancer: a Phase III trial of the Southeastern Cancer Study Group. J Clin Oncol 10:282, 1992.

Rubin P, Casarett GI: A direction for clinical radiation pathology. Front Radiat Ther Oncol 6:1, 1972.

Sacks H, et al: Meta-analyses of randomized controlled trials. N Engl J Med 326:450, 1987.

Sagman U, et al: The prognostic significance of pretreatment serum lactate dehydrogenase in patients with small-cell lung cancer. J Clin Oncol 9:954, 1991a.

Sagman U, et al: Small cell carcinoma of the lung: derivation of a Prognostic Staging System. J Clin Oncol 9:1639, 1991b.

Sagman U, et al: Second primary malignancies following the diagnosis of small cell lung cancer. J Clin Oncol 10:1525, 1992.

Salazar O, et al: Single-dose half-body irradiation for palliation of multiple bone metastases from solid tumours. Cancer 58:29, 1986.

Santoro A, et al: Long-term results of combination chemotherapy-radiation therapy approach in Hodgkin's disease: superiority of ABVD plus radiation therapy versus MOPP plus radiation therapy. J Clin Oncol 5:27, 1987.

Sausville EA, Trepel JB, Moyer JD: Inhibitors of bombesin-stimulated intracellular signals: interruption of an autocrine pathway as a therapeutic strategy in small cell lung carcinoma. Clin Biol Res 354A:193, 1990.

Schiller JH: Topotecan in small cell lung cancer. Semin Oncol 24:S20–S27, 1997.

Schiller JH, et al: Phase II study of topotecan in patients with extensive-stage small cell carcinoma of the lung: an Eastern Cooperative Oncology Group trial. J Clin Oncol 14:2345, 1996.

Sculier J, Feld R: Superior vena cava obstruction syndrome: recommendations for management. Cancer Treat Rev 12:209, 1985.

Sculier JP, Klastersky J, Strickmans P: Late intensification in small cell lung cancer: a Phase I study of high doses of cyclophosphamide and etoposide with autologous bone marrow transplantation. J Clin Oncol 3:184, 1985b.

Sculier JP, et al: Carcinoembryonic antigen: a useful prognostic marker in small cell lung cancer. J Clin Oncol 3:1349, 1985a.

Sculier JP, et al: A 7-drug combination polychemotherapy for small cell lung cancer (SCLC): report of a Phase-II study. Proc Am Soc Clin Oncol 7(abst 832):215, 1988.

Seto T, et al: Effect on prognosis of bone marrow infiltration detected by magnetic resonance imaging in small cell lung cancer. Eur J Cancer 33:2333, 1997.

Seydel H, et al: Prophylactic versus no brain irradiation in regional small cell lung carcinoma. Am J Clin Oncol 8:218, 1985.

Seydel JG, et al: Combined modality treatment of regional small cell undifferentiated carcinoma of the lung. A cooperative study of the RTOG and ECOG. Int J Radiat Oncol Biol Phys 9:1135, 1983.

Shank B, et al: Increased survival with high-dose multifield radiation therapy and intensive chemotherapy in limited small cell carcinoma of the lung. Cancer 56:2771, 1985.

Shepherd FA: Alternatives to chemotherapy and radiotherapy as adjuvant treatment for lung cancer. Lung Cancer 17(Suppl 1):S121, 1997.

Shepherd FA, Ginsberg R, Patterson GA: Is there ever a role for salvage operations in limited small cell lung cancer? J Thorac Cardiovasc Surg 101:196, 1991b.

Shepherd FA, et al: Reduction in local recurrence and improved survival in surgically treated patients with small cell carcinoma of the lung. J Thorac Cardiovasc Surg 86:498, 1983.

Shepherd FA, et al: Adjuvant chemotherapy following surgical resection for small cell carcinoma of the lung. J Clin Oncol 6:832, 1988.

Shepherd FA, et al: A prospective study of adjuvant surgical resection after chemotherapy for limited small cell lung cancer. J Thorac Cardiovasc Surg 97:177, 1989.

Shepherd FA, et al: Surgical treatment for limited small-cell lung cancer. J Thorac Cardiovasc Surg 101:385, 1991a.

Shepherd FA, et al: Surgical treatment for limited small-cell lung cancer: the University of Toronto Lung Oncology Group experience. J Thorac Cardiovasc Surg 1091:385, 1991c.

Shepherd FA, et al: Importance of clinical staging in limited small-cell lung cancer: a valuable system to separate prognostic subgroups. J Clin Oncol 11:1592, 1993.

Shields TW, Karrer K: Surgery for small cell lung cancer. In Roth JA, Cox JD, Hong WK (eds): Lung Cancer. 2nd Ed. Cambridge, MA: Blackwell Science, 1998, pp 115–134.

Shields TW, et al: Surgical resection in the management of small-cell carcinoma of the lung. J Thorac Cardiovasc Surg 84:481, 1982.

Simpson J, et al: Palliative radiation therapy for inoperable carcinoma of the lung: final report of a RTOG multi-institutional trial. Int J Radiat Oncol Biol Phys 11:751, 1985.

Skov BG, et al: Prognostic impact of histologic demonstration of chromogranin A and neuron-specific enolase in pulmonary adenocarcinoma. Ann Oncol 2:355, 1991.

Slawson R, Scott R: Radiation therapy in bronchogenic carcinoma. Radiology 132:175, 1979.

Slevin ML, et al: A randomized trial to evaluate the effect of schedule on the activity of etoposide in small cell lung cancer. J Clin Oncol 7:1333, 1989.

Smyth JF: The management of small cell anaplastic lung cancer. In Smyth JF (ed): The Management of Lung Cancer. London: Edward Arnold, 1984, pp. 115–131.

Smyth JF: Cancer genetics and cell and molecular biology. Is this the way forward? Chest 109(5 Suppl):125S, 1996.

Sorensen HR, Lund·C, Alstrup P: Survival in small cell lung carcinoma after surgery. Thorax 41:479, 1986.

Souhami RL, et al: Radiation therapy in small cell cancer of the lung treated with combination chemotherapy: a controlled trial. BMJ 288:1643, 1984.

Souhami RL, et al: Intensive chemotherapy with autologous bone marrow transplantation for small cell lung cancer. Cancer Chemother Pharmacol 24:321, 1989.

Souhami RL, et al: Five-day oral etoposide treatment for advanced small cell lung cancer: randomized comparison with intravenous chemotherapy. J Natl Cancer Inst 89:577, 1997.

Splinter TAW: Chemotherapy of SCLC: duration of treatment. Lung Cancer 5:186, 1989.

Splinter TAW: EORTC 08825 induction versus induction plus maintenance chemotherapy in small cell lung cancer: definitive evaluation. For the EORTC Lung Co-operative Group. Proc Am Soc Clin Oncol 7(abstr 779):202, 1988.

Splinter T, et al: EORTC 08825 induction versus induction plus maintenance chemotherapy (CT) in small cell lung cancer. Proc Am Soc Clin Oncol 5(abstr 739):188, 1986.

Stahel RA: Diagnosis, staging and prognostic factors of small cell lung cancer. Curr Opin Oncol 3:306, 1991.

Stahel RA: Morphology, surface antigens, staging and prognostic factors of small cell lung cancer. Curr Opin Oncol 4:308, 1992.

Stahel RA, et al: Detection of bone marrow metastasis in small cell lung cancer by monoclonal antibody. J Clin Oncol 3:455, 1985.

Stahel R, et al: Staging and prognostic factors in small cell lung cancer. Lung Cancer 5:119, 1989.

Stevens E, Einhorn L, Sohn R: Treatment of limited small cell lung cancer. Proc Am Assoc Cancer Res 20(abstr C–599):435, 1979.

Stevenson BC, et al: Lack of relationship between in vitro tumour cell growth and prognosis in extensive-stage small-cell lung cancer. J Clin Oncol 113:923, 1989.

Steward W, et al: Dose intensification of V-ICE chemotherapy with GM-CSF in small cell lung cancer—a prospective randomized study of 301 patients. Eur J Oncol 31:S18, 1995.

Sundaresan V, et al: Neuroendocrine differentiation and clinical behaviour in non-small cell lung tumours. Br J Cancer 64:333, 1991.

Suwinski R, Lee S, Withers HR: Dose-response relationship for prophylactic cranial irradiation in small cell lung cancer. Int J Radiat Oncol Biol Phys 40:797, 1998.

Szabo E, et al: Overexpression of CC10 modifies neoplastic potential in lung cancer cells. Cell Growth Differ 9:475, 1998.

Takada M, et al: Phase III study of concurrent versus sequential thoracic radiation therapy in combination with cisplatin and etoposide for limited-stage small cell lung cancer: preliminary results of the Japan Clinical Oncology Group Proc Am Soc Clin Oncol 15(abstr):1103, 1996.

Takimoto CH, Arbuck SG: Clinical status and optimal use of topotecan. Oncology (Huntingt) 11:1635, 1997.

Taylor CW, et al: Treatment of small-cell lung cancer with an alternating chemotherapy regimen given at weekly intervals: a Southwest Oncology Group pilot study. J Clin Oncol 8:1811, 1990.

Thames H, Hendry J: Fractionation in Radiation Therapy. Philadelphia: Taylor & Francis, 1987, p. 297.

Thatcher N, Lind M: Carboplatin in small cell lung cancer. Semin Oncol 17(Suppl 2):40, 1990.

Tourani JM, et al: Short intensive five drug chemotherapy (CT) followed by intensive irradiation for limited small cell lung cancer (LSCLC). Improved response rate and survival. A pilot study. Proc Am Soc Clin Oncol 10(abstr 838):245, 1991.

Trillet-Lenoir VN, Arpin D, Brune J: Bone marrow metastases detection in small cell lung cancer: a review. Anticancer Res 14:2795, 1994.

Trump D, et al: Treatment of neoplastic meningitis with intrathecal methotrexate and thiotepa. Proc Am Soc Clin Oncol 22(abstr 633):160, 1981.

Tsai CM, et al: Correlation of in vitro sensitivity testing of long-term small cell lung cancer cell lines with response and survival. Eur J Cancer 26:1148, 1990.

Turrisi AT: Brain irradiation and systemic chemotherapy for small-cell lung cancer: dangerous liaisons? J Clin Oncol 8:196, 1990.

Turrisi A, Glover D: Thoracic radiation therapy variables: influence on local control in small cell lung cancer limited disease. Int J Radiat Oncol Biol Phys 19:1473, 1990.

Turrisi AT III, et al: Twice-daily compared with once-daily thoracic radiation therapy in limited small cell lung cancer treated concurrently with cisplatin and etoposide. N Engl J Med 340:265, 1999.

Van Dyk J, Mah K, Keane T: Radiation-induced lung damage: dose-time-fractionation considerations. Radiother Oncol 14:55, 1989.

Warde P, Payne D: Does thoracic irradiation improve survival or local control in limited-stage small-cell carcinoma of the lung? A meta analysis. J Clin Oncol 10:890, 1992.

Wasserstrom WR, Glass JP, Posner JB: Diagnosis and treatment of leptomeningeal metastases from solid tumors: experience with 90 patients. Cancer 49:759, 1982.

Watson W, Berg J: Oat cell lung cancer. Cancer 15:759, 1962.

Weiner DB, et al: Expression of the new gene-encoded protein (p185neu) in human non-small carcinoma of the lung. Cancer Res 50:421, 1990.

Whang-peng J, et al: A specific chromosome defect associated with human small cell lung cancer detection, 3p (14–23). Science 215:181, 1982.

Wils J, et al: Phase II study of high dose epirubicin in non-small cell lung cancer. Eur J Cancer 26:1140, 1990.

Withers H: Some changes in concepts of dose fractionation over 20 years. Front Radiat Ther Oncol 22:1, 1988.

Wojtowicz-Praga S, et al: Phase I trial of Marimastat, a novel matric metalloproteinase inhibitor, administered orally to patients with advanced lung cancer. J Clin Oncol 16:2150, 1998.

Woll PJ, Rozengurt E: Therapeutic implications of growth factors in small cell lung cancer. Lung Cancer 5:287, 1989.

Woll PJ, et al: Can cytotoxic dose-intensity be increased by using granulocyte colony-stimulating factor? A randomized controlled trial of lenograstim in small cell lung cancer. J Clin Oncol 13:652, 1995.

Work E, et al: Randomized study of initial versus late chest irradiation combined with chemotherapy in limited-stage small cell lung cancer. Aarhus Lung Cancer Group. J Clin Oncol 15:3030, 1997.

Wurschmidt F, et al: Small cell lung cancer with and without superior vena cava syndrome: a multivariate analysis of prognostic factors in 408 cases. Int J Radiat Oncol Biol Phys 33:77, 1995.

Zelen M: Keynote address on biostatistics and data retrieval. Cancer Chemother Rep 4:31, 1973.

READING REFERENCE

Arriagada R, Kramar A, Le Chevalier T: The competing risk approach in determining relapse-free survival in limited small cell lung carcinoma. J Clin Oncol 10:447, 1992.

CHAPTER 108

Immunology and Immunotherapy of Lung Cancer

David S. Schrump and Dao M. Nguyen

Clinical observations linking bacterial sepsis and spontaneous tumor regression dating back to the 1800s, as noted by Nauts (1980) and reviewed by Old (1992), prompted administration of heat-killed bacteria (Coley's toxins) to hundreds of cancer patients before the modern era of chemotherapy. Subsequently, Old and associates (1959) reported that bacillus Calmette-Guérin enhanced resistance of animals to challenge with tumor cells, thereby validating these clinical efforts, and prompting a series of trials using nonspecific immune stimulants in cancer patients. Although bacillus Calmette-Guérin and levamisole, as well as interleukin-2 in the study of Kradin and colleagues (1987), and lymphokine-activated killer (LAK) cells had no significant effect in patients with lung cancer, as recorded in the review of Fishbein (1993), advances in tumor immunology suggest that effective and specific immunotherapy of this disease may ultimately be possible. This chapter focuses on the evidence for antitumor immunity, candidate tumor antigens, and strategies to augment immune-mediated tumor regression in lung cancer patients.

EVIDENCE FOR IMMUNE RESPONSE TO TUMOR ANTIGENS IN LUNG CANCER PATIENTS

Observations of clonal expansion of lymphocytes derived from primary tumors and regional lymph nodes, and the isolation of tumor-reactive monoclonal antibodies as well as HLA-restricted cytolytic T cells (CTL) confirm that serologic and cell-mediated antitumor responses occur in lung cancer patients. One of the authors (D.S.S.) and coinvestigators (1990) analyzed over 16,500 supernatants from Epstein-Barr virus–transformed lymphocytes derived from regional lymph nodes of 22 lung cancer patients for serologic activity against a large panel of allogeneic cancer cell lines. Overall, 8% (range: 1 to 33%) of these Epstein-Barr virus supernatants contained antibodies reactive with sur-

face antigens on cancer cells, and recurrent reactivity patterns were observed, suggesting recognition of shared tumor antigens in lung cancer patients. Biochemical analyses by one of the authors (D.S.S.) and associates (1988) revealed that one of the immunogenic shared tumor antigens was the stage-specific embryonic antigen 3 carbohydrate structure present on poorly differentiated lung cancers and embryonal carcinomas, but not normal lung tissue. A second shared antigen that appeared to be immunogenic in these patients, as noted by one of the authors (D.S.S.) and colleagues, as well as by Yoda (1979), was a sulfated carbohydrate epitope (SO_3-gal) aberrantly expressed in approximately 30% of pulmonary adenocarcinomas and large cell carcinomas.

Hirohashi and associates (1986) isolated a monoclonal antibody from regional lymph node lymphocytes of a lung cancer patient that recognized the i blood group antigen present in the autologous primary cancer but not the adjacent normal lung epithelium. Winter and colleagues (1993) detected serum antibodies against autologous tumor cell lysates in 21% of 36 individuals with small cell lung cancer (SCLC), noting that patients with serologic response to autologous tumor cell lysates tended to have improved survival compared with individuals without such antitumor reactivity. Collectively, these data provide the most convincing biochemical evidence for specific serologic immune response to tumor-associated antigens in lung cancer patients.

Several studies have demonstrated recognition of lung cancer antigens by CTLs derived from cancer patients. Nakao and coworkers (1995) isolated a CTL from an esophageal cancer patient that recognized a peptide sequence expressed on esophageal and pulmonary squamous cell carcinomas in an HLA-restricted manner. Slingluff (1994) and Takenoyama (1998) and their associates also observed recognition of autologous and HLA-matched allogeneic cancer cells by tumor-specific CTL clones isolated from patients with pulmonary adenocarcinomas and squamous cell carcinomas.

Although the epitopes recognized by these CTLs have not been fully characterized, the aforementioned data indicate that shared tumor antigens are recognized in lung cancer patients and suggest that strategies designed to enhance cell-mediated antitumor responses may be efficacious in these individuals. Vanky and colleagues (1983) observed that lung cancers were nearly as immunogenic as melanomas and renal cell carcinomas, and that immune recognition of autologous tumor cells enhanced survival in lung cancer patients. Uchida and coinvestigators (1990) examined autologous antitumor responses in 50 lung cancer patients undergoing curative resection. Autologous tumor killing was observed in 19 of 32 patients with stage I lung cancer and 8 of 18 individuals with stage II disease. Interestingly, 23 of 27 patients with autologous tumor killing were alive at 5 years, whereas all patients without such reactivity had recurrences within 18 months and succumbed to their disease within 42 months. T-cell mediated, but not natural killer, response to autologous tumor correlated in a statistical manner with disease-free interval and overall survival in these individuals.

Hollinshead and associates (1987, 1988) vaccinated lung cancer patients with autologous tumor cell extracts after curative resection. Delayed-type hypersensitivity and serologic responses to autologous tumor extracts were induced in these vaccinated patients. Seventy-five percent of patients receiving adjuvant specific immunotherapy survived 5 years compared with only 30% of control patients; the favorable effect of immunotherapy was most apparent for individuals with stage I disease.

According to Rosenberg and colleagues (1998), approximately 15% of individuals with metastatic melanoma can be cured by interleukin-2 (IL-2)–based regimens, and several studies suggest that similar treatments may be efficacious in lung cancer patients. Kimura and Yamaguchi (1995) randomized 105 lung cancer patients undergoing noncurative resections to receive either adjuvant chemotherapy with radiation therapy, or chemotherapy, radiation therapy, and IL-2 with LAK cells. Survival at 7 years was 12.1% for the control group versus 39% for the experimental group. Although no difference in survival was noted for individuals with squamous cell cancers, patients with adenocarcinomas had significantly improved survival if they received chemoimmunotherapy. Additional analysis revealed that adjuvant immunotherapy appeared most beneficial for those individuals with pulmonary parenchymal or nodal metastases but did not appear to improve survival of patients with residual tumor in chest wall, pleura, or diaphragm.

In a subsequent trial, Kimura and Yamaguchi (1996) prospectively randomized 82 lung cancer patients undergoing curative resection to receive either chemotherapy with IL-2/LAK, chemotherapy alone, or no adjuvant therapy. Survival rates were 58% for patients receiving chemoimmunotherapy versus 31% for those receiving either chemotherapy alone or no treatment. Chemotherapy

alone had no effect on outcome in these individuals. Post-surgical survivals for stage II and III patients receiving chemoimmunotherapy were 69% and 37%, respectively. In contrast, survival rates for similarly staged control patients were 46% and 15%, respectively. Multivariate analysis revealed that IL-2/LAK therapy was the only significant independent variable correlating with prolonged survival in these patients.

Ratto and associates (1998) conducted a randomized trial of adoptive immunotherapy with tumor-infiltrating lymphocytes and IL-2, versus "standard therapy" as adjuvant treatment of 113 patients undergoing resection for non–small cell lung cancer (NSCLC). Fifty-six patients received an intravenous infusion of autologous tumor-infiltrating lymphocytes, expanded in vitro for approximately 6 to 8 weeks, in combination with subcutaneous IL-2. Stage II patients in the control arm received no additional therapy; stage III patients in both groups received adjuvant radiation therapy. Median survival was approximately 22.4 months for the immunotherapy group versus 14 months for the control group. Survival of patients with stage II lung cancers who received adoptive immunotherapy was not significantly improved compared with similarly staged control patients. A tendency for improved survival was noted for patients with stage III disease who received immunotherapy relative to controls ($P = .06$), with median survivals being 22 months and 9.9 months, respectively. Survival for stage IIIB patients who received adoptive immunotherapy was significantly improved relative to similarly staged controls (median survivals, 24 months and 7 months, respectively). Interestingly, adoptive immunotherapy appeared to reduce local but not distant relapse rates in patients with stage III cancers. Collectively, these studies warrant additional well-designed trials evaluating the efficacy of IL-2 alone or in combination with LAK or tumor antigen vaccines in lung cancer patients.

Mechanisms of Antitumor Immunity

Schreiber (1999), as well as Farah and colleagues (1998), note that regression of solid tumors in humans occurs primarily, but not exclusively, by T-cell mediated mechanisms. As such, appreciation of how T cells recognize tumor antigens enables a more comprehensive understanding of the obstacles that must be overcome in order to develop effective and specific immunotherapy of lung cancer.

T cells can be broadly subdivided into two major classes, namely, CD4+ (T helper) cells, and CD8+ (suppressor and cytolytic) T cells. These subsets are distinguished by their specific interactions with major histocompatibility complex (MHC) antigens and their effector functions. CD4+ T-helper cells recognize peptide antigens presented in the context of class II MHC molecules typically expressed by professional antigen-presenting cells (APCs) such as dendritic cells, macrophages, and B cells. T-helper cells are critical for initiating and perpetuating T-cell reactivity to viral, tissue allograft, and autologous tumor antigens. These cells also secrete cytokines required for immunoglobulin class switch in activated B cells. In contrast, CTLs recognize peptide antigens in the context of class I MHC molecules typically expressed on epithelial cells. According to Hellstrom and Hellstrom (1998), as well as Sherman and coworkers (1998), CTLs participate in killing virally infected cells, as well as epithelia expressing transplantation or tumor-associated antigens.

The class I HLA molecule is a heterodimer consisting of a highly polymorphic alpha chain having three regions (i.e., alpha 1, alpha 2, and alpha 3) and β_2-microglobulin; the CD8 molecule on the CTL binds to the alpha 3 domain to stabilize interaction between the T-cell receptor and the MHC-peptide complex on the target cell. The class II HLA molecule is also a heterodimer consisting of an alpha chain, containing alpha-1 and alpha-2 subunits, and a beta chain consisting of beta-1 and beta-2 subunits; the CD4 molecule on the T-helper cell binds to the beta-2 domain to stabilize interaction between the T-cell receptor and MHC-peptide complex on the surface of the professional APCs as noted by Restifo and Wunderlich (1997). According to Pichler and Wyss-Coray (1994) and Peace and associates (1991), although the overall architecture of the peptide-binding sites for class I and class II MHC molecules are relatively similar, class I molecules present peptides containing 8 to 10 amino acids, whereas class II MHC molecules usually present peptides containing 12 to 20 residues often nested within a larger sequence.

Pichler and Wyss-Coray (1994) note that class I MHC molecules generally present peptides derived from intracellular proteins such as mutant or overexpressed oncoproteins, as well as normal tissue-differentiation antigens. Gaczynska and colleagues (1994) have shown that these peptides are generated within proteasomes composed of low-molecular-weight proteins (LMPs), including LMP2 and LMP7, and then transferred to newly synthesized class I molecules in the endoplasmic reticulum by an ATP-dependent mechanism requiring several proteins including TAP (transporter associated with antigen binding) 1 and 2 according to Ortmann and associates (1994). β_2-microglobulin is critical for the folding and stability of the class I MHC complex at the cell surface, and deficiencies of β_2-microglobulin expression, as noted by Restifo and colleagues (1996), result in markedly reduced MHC expression in a variety of human cancers. Expression of LMP, TAP, class I heavy chain, and β_2-microglobulin can be induced by interferon-γ (IFN-γ), the significance of which is discussed later in this chapter. In contrast, as recorded by Chicz and Urban (1994), class II molecules are generally involved in the presentation of soluble antigens that are endocytosed by professional APCs and subsequently bound to class II MHC molecules as they recycle to the cell surface.

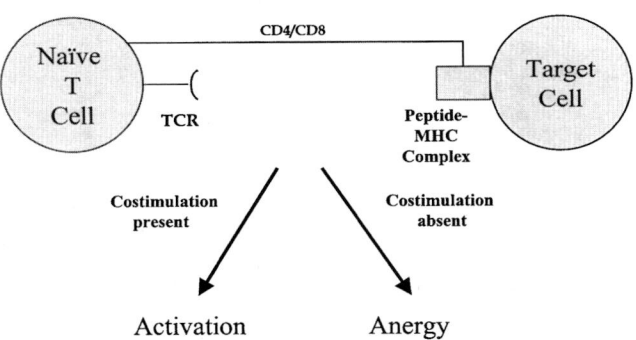

Fig. 108-1. Mechanisms of T-cell activation or anergy after interaction with target cell. MHC, major histocompatibility complex; TCR, T-cell receptor.

Hellstrom and Hellstrom (1998) have recorded that T-cell activation requires high-affinity interaction between the T-cell receptor and the appropriate MHC peptide complex on the target cell as well as the presence of a variety of adhesion molecules and ligands such as B7.1 and B7.2, which provide costimulatory signals. In the presence of high-affinity interaction and appropriate costimulation, T-helper cells proliferate in response to antigen and secrete a variety of cytokines, particularly IL-2 and IFN-γ, which provide costimulation required to activate CTLs. As noted by Seder and Mosmann (1999), interaction between T cells and their respective targets in the absence of appropriate costimulation results in antigen-specific unresponsiveness (anergy) (Fig. 108-1).

It is apparent from this brief overview that antigen recognition by T cells is highly complex, and a number of potential mechanisms exist whereby a transformed cell may escape immune surveillance (Table 108-1). Lack of antigen presentation because of the absence of epitopes that can bind MHC motifs, or deficiencies in antigen processing or class I MHC expression, may result in impaired recognition of tumor cells. Interaction of initiator (T helper) or effector (cytolytic) T cells with antigens in the tumor site or shed into the circulation in the absence of costimulation may inhibit response despite antigen recognition. Antitumor immunity also may be inhibited by soluble factors secreted by cancer cells, or by FAS-mediated depletion of activated T cells interacting with tumor cell targets. Each of these

Table 108-1. Mechanisms of Impaired Immune Response to Cancer

Lack of tumor antigens
Deficient processing and presentation of tumor antigens
Lack of major histocompatibility complex expression
Lack of costimulation
Clonal deletion or anergy of tumor-reactive T cells
Secretion of immunosuppressive factors by tumor cells

complex issues must be simultaneously considered as we attempt to develop strategies for lung cancer therapy.

POTENTIAL TARGETS FOR LUNG CANCER IMMUNOTHERAPY

Ras

The N-, R-, and K-*ras* genes encode 21-kilodalton proteins that are integral membrane components of mitogen signal cascades. Mutations involving *ras* genes have been observed in 20% of all solid malignancies, including nearly 40% of pulmonary adenocarcinomas as observed by Rodenhuis and Slebos (1992). Somatic mutations involving *ras* genes that typically occur in codons 12, 13, or 61 create tumor-specific antigens that may be exploited for lung cancer immunotherapy as suggested by Abrams and associates (1996).

In 1991 Peace and colleagues reported that mice immunized with mutant *ras* peptides developed CD4+ MHC class II restricted T cells that proliferated in response to syngeneic APCs expressing these mutant peptides. Subsequently, Fenton and coinvestigators (1993) demonstrated that mice immunized with peptides containing the gly→arg alteration corresponding to a frequently observed codon 12 (arg 12) mutation generated CD8+ T cells that lysed tumor cells expressing arg 12 *ras*; no reactivity was observed when splenocytes from immunized mice were exposed to val 12 or wild type gly 12 peptides. Vaccination with mutant *ras* peptides rendered animals free from challenge with cells expressing mutant, but not wild-type *ras* genes. Subsequent studies by Abrams and associates (1995) revealed that mice immunized with peptide corresponding to the gly to val mutation at position 12 generated CD4+ T cells that proliferated and expressed a variety of cytokines including IL-2, IFN-γ, tumor necrosis factor, and granulocyte-monocyte colony stimulating factor (GM-CSF) in response to mutant but not wild-type *ras* peptides.

The exquisite specificity of *ras* immunity demonstrated in animal models has been observed in cancer patients. Jung and Schluesener (1991) isolated CD4+ T-cell lines from peripheral blood of normal individuals following in vitro exposure to val 12 *ras* peptides, demonstrating the capacity of these individuals to recognize mutant *ras* proteins. In a series of experiments, Fossum and colleagues (1994, 1995) isolated CD4+ and CD8+ cells from colorectal cancer patients, specific for mutant K-*ras*→gly 13 to asp, and demonstrated that the CD8+ cells were cytotoxic toward an HLA-matched cancer cell line containing this *ras* mutation. Collectively, these data indicate that mutant *ras* proteins can be recognized in normal and tumor-bearing individuals. Given the immunogenicity of mutant *ras* peptides, it is somewhat surprising that tumors expressing *ras* mutations are not eradicated in cancer patients. Normal *ras* peptides do not bind to HLA motifs and therefore are not immunogenic. However, mutations at codons 12 or 13 result in amino acid

substitutions that enable HLA binding by anchoring the peptide in the HLA motif, thereby enhancing peptide presentation. However, interaction between mutant peptides and class I MHC molecules is still quite weak, and maximal killing of tumor cells by *ras*-specific CTL in vitro often requires IFN-γ, which enhances HLA and adhesion molecule expression on tumor targets as pointed out by Bergmann-Leitner and associates (1998). Hence, naturally occurring mutant *ras* epitopes may be relatively weak immunogens because of their inefficient binding to HLA molecules. In support of these observations are studies by Bristol and coworkers (1998) demonstrating that *ras* 4-12 (val 12) peptide induced only a weak *ras*-related CTL response in mice. Substitution of valine at position 12 with a more dominant anchor residue, such as leucine or isoleucine, improved the binding of the *ras* peptide to MHC class I, and enhanced proliferation and cytotoxic responses of anti-*ras* CTL relative to the original *ras* (val 12) peptide. Interestingly, mice immunized with *ras* 4-12 (leu 12) peptide exhibited cytolytic activity against tumor cells endogenously expressing *ras* (val 12) epitopes. In similar studies, Yokomizo and colleagues (1997) demonstrated that replacement of tyrosine residue by tryptophan at position 4 of *ras* 3-17 peptide enhanced the recognition of *ras* (val 12) by a CD4+ T-cell line isolated from a gastric cancer patient. Collectively these data suggest that 1) mutant *ras* peptides can be processed by cancer cells for recognition by CD4 and CD8+ T cells specific for mutant epitopes; 2) immunogenicity of these peptide sequences can be augmented by alterations in anchor residues that enhance peptide binding to MHC molecules; and 3) cytotoxicity of *ras*-specific CTL against tumor cells expressing mutant peptides can be augmented by cytokines such as IFN-γ, which enhance antigen processing and MHC expression.

Abrams and associates (1997) vaccinated cancer patients with a 13 mer sequence (*ras* 5-17) reflecting tumor-specific substitutions of gly 12 to asp, cys, or val. One of these patients was a 58-year-old woman with a poorly differentiated pulmonary adenocarcinoma. After three immunizations with 500 μg peptide in Detox adjuvant, a CD4+ T-cell line was isolated that proliferated in response to mutant but not wild-type *ras* peptide sequences. Additional studies revealed that this T-cell line recognized HLA-matched allogenic tumor cells endogenously expressing K-*ras* protein containing the gly 12 to cys mutation. No reactivity was observed against control peptides or wild-type *ras* proteins, demonstrating the specificity of this immune recognition, and no such reactivity was detected in lymphocytes harvested before vaccination.

The previously mentioned experience was derived from a larger phase I trial using peptides reflecting *ras* mutations in cancer patients reported by Khleif and coworkers (1999). Preliminary studies revealed that all patients were immunologically competent before and after three vaccinations with peptide sequences corresponding to K-*ras* mutations observed in their tumors. Overall, 3 of 10 available patients had evidence of immunization after three vaccinations. Two individuals, including the lung cancer patient previously described, developed CD4+ T-cell responses, whereas one patient developed a CD8+ T-cell response to mutant *ras* peptides; the CD8+ T-cell line specifically recognized an HLA-matched allogeneic tumor line expressing the appropriate *ras* mutation. No severe or delayed systemic toxicity was noted in this phase I study, and response to vaccination was not dose dependent. Although no major therapeutic responses were observed in these patients, all of whom had advanced bulky disease, this clinical trial demonstrates the ability to generate CD4+ and CD8+ T cells specific for mutant *ras* epitopes in cancer patients; conceivably, high-affinity *ras*-reactive T cells could be expanded ex vivo for adoptive immunotherapy of lung cancer patients in future clinical trials.

p53

The *p53* gene encodes a 53-kilodalton protein that is intimately involved in cell cycle regulation, DNA repair, and programmed cell death. Mutations involving *p53* have been observed in nearly 75% of lung cancers irrespective of histology by Mitsudomi (1992) and D'Amico (1992) and their associates. Although the *p53* gene contains 10 exons spanning an open reading frame of approximately 20 kilobases, the majority of mutations occur in evolutionarily conserved regions within exons 5 to 8, which encode the DNA-binding domain of the *p53* molecule as noted by Hollstein and colleagues (1991). Most of these mutations are missense mutations that alter the conformation of the *p53* protein and stabilize it against ubiquitin-mediated degradation. According to Kirsch and Kastan (1998), the prolonged half-life of mutant *p53* accounts for the increased immunoreactivity observed in cancers relative to adjacent normal tissues in which *p53* levels are barely detectable.

Accumulating evidence suggests that both mutant as well as wild-type *p53* sequences can be recognized as immunogenic in cancer patients. In initial studies, Winter and associates (1992) detected *p53* reactive autoantibodies in the sera of 13% of lung cancer patients including 4 of 40 individuals with SCLC and 2 of 6 patients with NSCLC. All patients with *p53* autoantibodies expressed *p53* containing missense mutations in their primary tumors; no anti-*p53* reactivity was observed in individuals whose tumors had stop, splice, or frame shift mutations involving this oncoprotein. Considerable cross-reactivity was observed for *p53* reactive sera against tumor cell lysates containing a variety of missense *p53* mutations.

Whereas mutant, but not wild-type *ras*, sequences are immunogenic, the epitopes recognized by *p53* autoantibodies are wild-type sequences located in the amino terminus and the carboxy terminus of the *p53* molecule as shown by Lubin and coworkers (1993); hence, overexpressed wild-type peptides can be as immunogenic in lung cancer patients, and the presence of *p53* autoantibodies may predate the diagnosis of lung cancer in high-risk individuals,

according to Lubin and colleagues (1995). In a large prospective study, Trivers and associates (1996) detected *p53* autoantibodies in the sera of 5 of 23 individuals with chronic obstructive pulmonary disease who developed carcinomas, two of which were lung cancers.

Iizasa and colleagues (1998) evaluated the correlation between *p53* autoantibodies, *p53* expression in tumor tissue, and clinical characteristics of 62 lung cancer patients undergoing curative resection. *p53* autoantibodies were detected preoperatively in 13 patients (21%); these autoantibodies were observed more frequently in individuals with large cell lung carcinomas relative to those with either squamous cell or adenocarcinomas. Overall, 40% of patients whose tumors exhibited *p53* immunoreactivity had *p53* autoantibodies compared with only 3 of 37 patients whose tumors lacked detectable *p53* expression. No correlation between *p53* autoantibodies and clinical stage was observed, and *p53* autoantibodies had no prognostic significance in this study.

In an additional clinical study, Bergqvist and associates (1998) evaluated sera from 67 lung cancer patients undergoing radiation therapy. *p53* autoantibodies were detected in 18 patients (27%). A statistically significant improvement in survival was noted in those patients who exhibited *p53* autoantibodies before radiation therapy relative to those who did not (median survival time: 543 days versus 304 days, respectively). In a separate study, Lai and coworkers (1998) detected *p53* autoantibodies in 10 of 125 lung cancer patients; no such antibodies were detected in sera collected from normal individuals or patients with benign pulmonary disease. The presence of *p53* autoantibodies correlated with malignant effusions and diminished survival in these individuals.

In another extensive analysis, Mitsudomi and associates (1998) evaluated the frequency of *p53* autoantibodies in 188 consecutive lung cancer patients undergoing curative resection. Overall, 38% of individuals had *p53* autoantibodies detectable preoperatively. The presence of *p53* autoantibodies correlated significantly with squamous cell histology, advanced stage of disease, and *p53* overexpression in the primary tumor. Postoperatively, *p53* autoantibody titers were diminished in virtually all patients who exhibited reactivity preoperatively; however, no correlation between change in antibody titer and clinical course was observed. Although no relationship between *p53* autoantibodies and overall survival was detected in these individuals, patients with antibody reactivity to amino terminus epitopes appeared to have diminished survival, suggesting that the type of *p53* mutations that induced the reactivity also may have influenced the aggressiveness of the primary cancers. Collectively, these data indicate that *p53* autoantibodies can be detected in 10 to 20% of lung cancer patients, the presence of which correlates with missense mutations and overexpression of *p53* in the primary tumor; the epitopes typically recognized by *p53* autoantibodies are normal sequences generated by overexpression of the mutant protein, and these autoantibodies may predate the diagnosis of lung cancer patients in high-risk individuals.

A number of investigators have isolated HLA-restricted CTLs recognizing mutant as well as wild-type *p53* epitopes in transgenic mice, as well as normal and tumor-bearing individuals. Houbiers and colleagues (1993) isolated a CTL line specifically recognizing a *p53* peptide representing a single-point mutation, demonstrating the fine specificity of T-cell immunity to *p53* epitopes, analogous to what has been observed for *ras*-specific CTLs. Ropke and coinvestigators (1995), evaluated the precursor frequency of *p53* reactive lymphocytes in peripheral blood of healthy volunteers using bulk and limiting dilution methods. Of 15 wild-type sequences and 29 mutant peptides predicted to bind to HLA-A2, 4 wild-type sequences and 3 mutant peptides exhibited high-affinity binding to HLA-2. Interestingly, peptide-specific responses were generated against two of the wild-type peptide sequences, the frequency of which correlated with their relative binding affinities to HLA-2, demonstrating the capacity of normal individuals to recognize these *p53* epitopes. Subsequent limiting dilution analysis revealed no difference between precursor frequencies for mutant versus wild-type *p53* epitopes, suggesting that mutant *p53* peptides are no more immunogenic than wild-type sequences in normal individuals. Although tolerance to *p53* antigens may occur against peptides with high-affinity binding to MHC motifs, a T-cell repertoire exists that is reactive with peptides exhibiting lower-affinity MHC interactions. Whereas *ras* mutations produce only a limited number of tumor-specific epitopes, *p53* mutations generate many epitopes, the vast majority of which are wild-type sequences, because of over-expression of this oncoprotein. The fact that wild-type sequences are immunogenic suggests that these epitopes may be useful for cancer immunotherapy.

Restifo and associates (1993) pointed out that a critical issue regarding use of *p53* as a target for cancer immunotherapy concerns the extent to which *p53* epitopes are recognized on lung cancer cells, which frequently exhibit deficiencies regarding antigen presentation. Ciernik and colleagues (1996) demonstrated that human lung cancer cells can process and present mutant *p53* epitopes for recognition by HLA-restricted CTLs specific for these peptides. Ropke and coinvestigators (1996) generated a CTL clone specific for a wild-type *p53* sequence from peripheral blood of a normal individual. Subsequent analysis revealed that this CTL could recognize and kill oropharyngeal carcinoma cells expressing mutant *p53* in an HLA-restricted manner. Collectively, these data demonstrate that tolerance to endogenously processed *p53* protein epitopes can be broken by peptide-specific in vitro priming, and that overexpression of mutant *p53* in human carcinoma cells results in the presentation of wild-type *p53* epitopes that can be recognized by CTL specific for these peptide sequences.

A second critical issue regarding *p53*-directed immunotherapy concerns the tumor specificity of CTL response directed at wild-type *p53* sequences. To examine this issue, Vierboom and associates (1997) generated CTL specific for a wild-type *p53* peptide sequence by immunizing *p53*-deficient mice with syngeneic tumor cells overexpressing *p53*. Adoptive transfer of *p53*-specific CTL into *p53*+/+ mice resulted in complete eradication of tumors, demonstrating that CTL specific for wild-type *p53* peptides can discriminate between tumor cells overexpressing *p53* and normal tissues in which *p53* expression is much lower.

If *p53* peptide sequences can be recognized as immunogenic in normal and tumor-bearing individuals, why, then, are tumors that express *p53* not eradicated by immune surveillance mechanisms in humans? Possible causes of nonreactivity to *p53* antigens in tumor-bearing individuals include 1) clonal deletion of high-affinity CTL recognizing *p53* epitopes, 2) anergy or suppression of established CTLs against these epitopes, and 3) insufficient antigen processing and presentation. In all likelihood, each of these mechanisms contributes to the lack of a robust immune response to *p53*, as well as other self-antigens in solid tumors. However, observations by Ropke and colleagues (1995) that tolerance to *p53* epitopes can be broken by in vitro priming with *p53* peptides, and that cytokines such as IFN-γ, as shown by Singal and associates (1996), can enhance antigen presentation in cancer cells, suggest that *p53*-directed antitumor immunity may eventually be efficacious in cancer patients.

CANCER TESTIS ANTIGENS

The cancer testis antigens MAGE and NY-ESO-1 belong to a growing class of T cell–defined antigens encoded on chromosome X that are typically expressed only on normal testis and ovary yet are apparently expressed in a variety of malignancies. Because testes do not express HLA class I molecules as demonstrated by Haas and colleagues (1988), MAGE and NY-ESO-1 gene products represent bona fide rejection antigens that may be exploited for cancer immunotherapy.

The MAGE genes were initially identified by van der Bruggen and associates (1991) during molecular analysis of tumor antigens recognized by CTL from a melanoma patient (MZ2) receiving an autologous tumor vaccine. The MZ2E gene encoded a peptide—designated MAGE-1—which could be presented in an HLA-restricted manner to autologous CTL. An additional CTL clone derived from the same patient recognized a second peptide subsequently shown by van der Bruggen (1994) and Gaugler (1994) and their colleagues to be encoded by a gene designated MAGE-3 having 75% sequence homology to MAGE-1. To date, 16 closely related MAGE genes have been identified, six of which (MAGE-1, -2, -3, -4, -6, and -12) are expressed in a significant percentage of tumors of diverse histologies and, as pointed out by Chen and Old (1999), may be future targets for cancer immunotherapy.

Using reverse transcriptase-polymerase chain reaction techniques, Sakata (1996) detected expression of MAGE-1, -2, and -3 in 70% of lung cancer cell lines, and nearly 30% of primary lung cancer specimens. Using similar techniques, Weynants and associates (1994) confirmed expression of MAGE-1, -2, and -3 genes in 35% of primary lung tumors irrespective of histology. Yoshimatsu and coworkers (1998) detected expression of MAGE-1, -2, and -3 in 21%, 30%, and 46% of 57 primary lung cancer specimens, respectively; no expression of MAGE genes was observed in normal lung tissues.

Gotoh and associates (1998) analyzed the frequency of MAGE-3 expression in lung cancer patients of HLA-A2 genotype, the most common class I MHC allele. Reverse transcriptase-polymerase chain reaction analyses revealed that MAGE-1 and -3 were expressed in 33 and 42% of lung cancer specimens, respectively. Of 22 patients with HLA-A2 genotype, 5 (23%) had absent class I MHC expression in their tumors. The frequency of MAGE-3 expression in HLA-A2 patients was 29%, whereas the frequency of MAGE-3 expression in individuals without the HLA-A2 genotype was 42%, a difference that did not reach statistical significance. No evidence of eradication of tumors simultaneously expressing MAGE-3 and HLA-A2 was observed, and no correlation between MAGE-3 expression and survival was noted in this study.

The inability to detect antitumor immune responses in patients whose neoplasms simultaneously expressed MAGE-3 and HLA-A2 may have been because lung cancer cells, particularly those derived from SCLC, frequently exhibit decreased expression of TAP-1, TAP-2, LMP-2, and LMP-7 genes encoding proteins involved in the processing of endogenous tumor antigen, as well as diminished HLA class I expression as noted by Doyle and colleagues (1985); all of these can be induced with IFN-γ, according to the studies of Restifo and coworkers (1993). Traversari and associates (1997) observed that transfection of SCLC cells with an IFN-γ construct increased TAP-1 and LMP-2 transcription, enhanced class I expression, and enabled recognition by an HLA-restricted CTL specific for MAGE-3 that did not react with nontransfected cells. These experiments suggest that strategies designed to enhance cancer testis antigen presentation in lung cancer tissues may be efficacious in clinical settings.

The production of high-titered IgG antibodies reactive with autologous tumor requires antigen recognition by CD4+ T-helper cells, and several groups have used serologic techniques to identify T cell–defined tumor antigens. Chen and colleagues (1997) isolated the NY-ESO-1 gene from a complementary DNA library established from an esophageal cancer. Soon thereafter, Jager and associates (1998) isolated an HLA-A2 restricted CTL clone reactive with NY-ESO-1 from a melanoma patient having high-titered antibody reactivity to this cancer testis antigen, and further analysis revealed that three peptides derived from NY-ESO-1 could induce CTL activity in vitro. Wang and coworkers (1998) isolated an HLA-A31–restricted CTL specific for NY-ESO-1 reactive with melanoma and breast cancer cells. Collectively, these data demonstrate that NY-ESO-1 induces humoral as well as cell-mediated antitumor reactivity in cancer patients. The epitopes recognized by NY-ESO-1 antibodies in these individuals have not been characterized.

Lee and colleagues (1999) used reverse transcriptase-polymerase chain reaction techniques to evaluate NY-ESO-1 expression in a panel of lung cancer cell lines. Expression of NY-ESO-1 was observed in 11 of 16 (69%) SCLC lines, and this expression was pronounced in 8 of these lines. In contrast, NY-ESO-1 expression was detected in three of seven (43%) NSCLC lines. Additional experiments using similar techniques revealed expression of MAGE-3 in 14 of 17 (82%) SCLC lines and four of seven (57%) NSCLC lines; a high concordance was noted for NY-ESO-1 and MAGE-3 expression in lung cancer cells. To date, expression of NY-ESO-1 in SCLC specimens has not been systematically evaluated; however, Chen and Old (1999) observed that expression of this tumor antigen in primary NSCLC specimens appears comparable with that observed in established cell lines. Additional experiments by Lee and associates (1999) revealed that lung cancer cells expressing NY-ESO-1 can process and present NY-ESO-1 for recognition by an HLA-restricted CTL specific for this antigen.

Previous studies by De Smet and colleagues (1996) revealed that MAGE gene expression in lung cancer cells occurs in the context of genome-wide demethylation, and that the demethylating agent 5-aza-2'-deoxycitidine (DAC) could induce expression of this cancer testis gene in cultured lung cancer cells. Lee and associates (1999) observed that DAC induced expression of NY-ESO-1 in four of four lung cancer lines, three of which were negative before treatment; expression was enhanced in one cell line that expressed NY-ESO-1 before DAC exposure. Additional analysis by Lee and colleagues (personal communication, 1999) revealed that expression of MAGE-3 could be induced in a similar manner. In an attempt to further define the kinetics of NY-ESO-1 induction by DAC, these investigators exposed lung cancer cells to 4 μM DAC × 8 hours, 2 μM DAC × 24 hours, and 1 μM DAC × 24 hours. NY-ESO-1 expression was readily induced by DAC under all conditions in lung cancer cells, but not in normal human bronchial epithelial cells nor Epstein-Barr virus–transformed lymphocytes. Serum concentrations of 4 μM were achieved in lung cancer patients during an 8-hour DAC infusion in a phase I to II study conducted by Momparler and associates (1997). Collectively, these data suggest that tumor-specific induction of cancer testis antigens may be feasible in lung cancer patients.

Stockert and colleagues (1998) used enzyme-linked immunosorbent assay techniques to analyze the humoral immune response to a panel of human tumor antigens. None of 70 samples of normal sera had detectable antibody reactivity to MAGE-3 or NY-ESO-1. None of 24 lung cancer patients had detectable antibody reactivity to MAGE-3, whereas 1 individual had high-titered antibody reactivity to NY-ESO-1. In contrast, 2 of 127 melanoma patients had high-titered antibody reactivity to MAGE-3, and 12 individuals had high-level reactivity to NY-ESO-1. Expression of NY-ESO-1 was evaluated in biopsy specimens from 62 melanoma patients; 15 individuals had tumors that were positive for NY-ESO-1, and 8 of these patients had NY-

ESO-1 antibodies. No NY-ESO-1 antibodies were detected in patients whose tumors were negative for NY-ESO-1. Interestingly, seven patients had tumors positive for NY-ESO-1 but no detectable NY-ESO-1 antibodies, possibly related to low-level NY-ESO-1 expression in their tumors. These data confirm that NY-ESO-1, and to a lesser extent MAGE-3, are immunogenic in cancer patients, and suggest that strategies to augment expression of cancer testis antigens may prove efficacious for lung cancer immunotherapy.

FUTURE DIRECTIONS

A variety of normal tissue differentiation antigens, such as gp-100, MART-1, TRP-1, TRP-2, and tyrosinase, all involved in melanin biosynthesis, as well as MAGE and NY-ESO-1 cancer testis antigens, have been identified by Kawakami and Rosenberg (1997) as targets for immunotherapy of melanoma patients. Significant correlation between clinical response after transfer of autologous tumor–infiltrating lymphocytes and recognition of gp-100 peptides in vitro has been observed in clinical trials. Binding of an immunogenic peptide derived from gp-100, designated g209-217, to HLA-A2 can be enhanced by substitution of a threonine at position 2 with methionine, resulting in increased generation of tumor-specific CTL from peripheral blood lymphocytes of melanoma patients. Rosenberg and associates (1998) reported that 13 of 31 (42%) melanoma patients receiving this modified peptide in conjunction with systemic IL-2 had objective clinical responses; four additional patients experienced mixed or partial responses. Previous trials by these investigators have shown that only 15% of melanoma patients receiving IL-2 alone achieve objective clinical tumor responses. Current trials are underway to evaluate the efficacy of simultaneous immunization with synthetic peptides derived from several different melanoma tumor antigens, and additional trials are in progress to evaluate adoptive transfer of lymphocytes expanded in vitro from patients receiving these peptide vaccines.

Data from Khleif and colleagues (1999) suggest that lung cancer patients can be immunized with mutant ras peptides, and additional studies by Yokomizo and associates (1997) have shown that the immunogenicity of these peptides can be enhanced by modifications that facilitate MHC binding. Because MHC binding affinity correlates with immunogenicity of tumor-derived peptides, administration of modified ras sequences, particularly in conjunction with IL-2, may enhance the efficacy ras peptide vaccines in lung cancer patients. Furthermore, synthetic wild-type p53 peptides capable of inducing antitumor responses in vitro, as well as peptides corresponding to MAGE and NY-ESO-1 tumor antigens, some of which have already been shown by Marchand and coworkers (1999) to mediate tumor regression in melanoma patients, should be evaluated in a similar context in lung cancer patients. Conceivably, a combination of synthetic peptides derived from immunogenic sequences pertaining to multiple different tumor antigens could be used for adjuvant therapy

Table 108-2. Strategies to Enhance Immune Response to Lung Cancer

Active immunization with tumor antigens (i.e., ras, p53, MAGE, or NY-ESO-1 with interleukin-2)
Adoptive therapy using high-affinity lymphokine-activated killer cells expanded in vitro using synthetic targets
Induction of tumor antigen expression by demethylation agents
Cytokine-mediated augmentation of antigen presentation in tumor cells

following resection or in combination with conventional therapies for inoperable lung cancer patients (Table 108-2).

Another strategy for the generation of autologous tumor immunity involves the use of dendritic cells to present tumor antigens in vitro and in vivo. Dendritic cells exhibit extremely high-level MHC expression, which enhances antigen presentation; these APCs also express a variety of adhesion molecules and costimulatory ligands that optimize T-cell activation as noted in the studies of Nair and associates (1997). Clinical trials using dendritic cells pulsed with melanoma antigen are currently underway, and similar strategies could be used to immunize lung cancer patients with peptides derived from ras, p53, or cancer testis antigens. Furthermore, the use of recombinant viral vectors expressing tumor antigens alone, or in conjunction with cytokines such as IL-12 and B7.1, may be useful for inducing prolonged and specific antitumor immunity in lung cancer patients as suggested by the works of Reed (1997), Putzer (1997), and Carroll (1998) and their colleagues.

A variety of cytokines including IL-2, GM-CSF, IL-12, and B7.1 are known to modulate and potentiate antitumor immunity, and these cytokines will in all likelihood constitute important components of future immunotherapy regimens for lung cancer. The studies of Ohe and associates (1993) have shown that IL-2 secreted from activated $CD4^+$ cells induces proliferation and activation of CTLs, and transduction of tumor cells with IL-2 provides the necessary costimulation to activate both $CD4^+$ and $CD8^+$ cells in the absence of professional APCs. GM-CSF is extremely potent with regard to enhancing tumor immunity because of its ability to induce differentiation of dendritic cells and macrophages from hematopoietic precursor cells. Lee and colleagues (1997) reported that the transduction of Lewis lung carcinoma cells with a recombinant adenoviral vector expressing GM-CSF inhibits the tumorigenicity of these otherwise highly malignant and poorly immunogenic cells.

IL-12 enhances differentiation of T-helper cells and activates CTLs as well as natural killer cells, in part via IFN-γ pathways; in addition, this cytokine enhances the potency of p53 peptide vaccines. Guo and associates (1999) observed that inoculation of mice with Lewis lung carcinoma cells transduced with IL-12 and B7.1 protected them from challenge with parental lung carcinoma cells. These experiments are highly relevant to human lung cancer immunotherapy in that the cytokine-mediated effects observed in the Lewis lung carcinoma model were achieved after viral transduction of only 1 to 2% of the tumor cells; hence, expression of appropriate cytokines from a small percentage of lung cancer cells can mediate significant tumor regression and induce systemic immunity against highly lethal lung cancer cells. Conceivably, direct intratumoral injection of recombinant viruses expressing cytokines such as IL-2, GM-CSF, IFN-g, and IL-12, as well as costimulatory molecules such as B7.1, will enhance antigen processing and presentation, facilitate MHC class I expression, and provide sufficient costimulation to enable immunologically mediated tumor regression in lung cancer patients.

Although the aforementioned strategies may enhance local antitumor responses, they may be impractical for eradication of metastatic disease involving cells with deficient antigen presentation. Induction of cancer testis antigen expression in lung cancer cells is a potentially novel strategy to enhance systemic antitumor immunity, and a trial of DAC-mediated induction of tumor antigen expression in lung cancer patients is scheduled to commence in the Thoracic Oncology Section, Surgery Branch, National Cancer Institute, in the near future. Because DAC also enhances MHC class I expression in vitro, as reported by Coral and colleagues (1999), this agent may simultaneously facilitate de novo expression and presentation of cancer testis antigens in lung cancer patients. During this trial, experiments will be performed to analyze levels of MAGE-3 and NY-ESO-1 expression and extent of immune recognition of these tumor antigens in lung cancer patients before and after DAC exposure. If antigen induction and immune recognition can be documented, additional trials will be undertaken to determine if antitumor responses can be boosted with peptide vaccines in conjunction with systemic cytokines.

The focus of tumor immunology has shifted from the esoteric quest to define unique tumor antigens to a more practical search for shared tumor antigens and the evaluation of mechanisms that augment antitumor immunity. The extensive clinical experience regarding melanoma immunotherapy may hasten the development of immunotherapy of epithelial tumors. It remains to be seen if these efforts will culminate in specific and efficacious immunotherapy for lung cancer.

REFERENCES

Abrams SI, et al: Peptide-specific activation of cytolytic CD4[+] T lymphocytes against tumor cells bearing mutated epitopes of K-ras p21. Eur J Immunol 25:2588, 1995.

Abrams SI, et al: Mutant ras epitopes as targets for cancer vaccines. Semin Oncol 23:118, 1996.

Abrams SI, et al: Generation of stable CD4[+] and CD8[+] T cell lines from patients immunized with ras oncogene-derived peptides reflecting codon 12 mutations. Cell Immunol 182:137, 1997.

Bergmann-Leitner ES, et al: Identification of a human CD8[+] T lymphocyte neo-epitope created by a ras codon 12 mutation which is restricted by the HLA-A2 allele. Cell Immunol 187:103, 1998.

Bergqvist M, et al: P53 auto-antibodies in non-small cell lung cancer patients can predict increased life expectancy after radiotherapy. Anticancer Res 18:1999, 1998.

Bristol JA, Schlom J, Abrams SI: Development of a murine mutant Ras CD8+ CTL peptide epitope variant that possesses enhanced MHC class I binding and immunogenic properties. J Immunol 160:2433, 1998.

Carroll MW, et al: Construction and characterization of a triple-recombinant vaccinia virus encoding B7-1, interleukin 12, and a model tumor antigen. J Natl Cancer Inst 90:1881, 1998.

Chen Y-T, Old LJ: Cancer-testis antigens: targets for cancer immunotherapy. Cancer J Sci Am 5:16, 1999.

Chen Y-T, et al: A testicular antigen aberrantly expressed in human cancers detected by autologous antibody screening. Proc Natl Acad Sci U S A 94:1914, 1997.

Chicz RM, Urban RG: Analysis of MHC-presented peptides: applications in autoimmunity and vaccine development. Immunol Today 15:155, 1994.

Ciernik IF, Berzofsky JA, Carbone DP: Human lung cancer cells endogenously expressing mutant p53 process and present the mutant epitope and are lysed by mutant-specific cytotoxic T lymphocytes. Clin Cancer Res 2:877, 1996.

Coral S, et al: Prolonged upregulation of the expression of HLA class I antigens and costimulatory molecules on melanoma cells treated with 5-aza-2-deoxycytidine (5-AZA-CdR). J Immunother 22:16, 1999.

D'Amico D, et al: High frequency of somatically acquired p53 mutations in small-cell lung cancer cell lines and tumors. Oncogene 7:339, 1992.

De Smet C, et al: The activation of human gene MAGE-1 in tumor cells is correlated with genome-wide demethylation. Proc Natl Acad Sci U S A 93:7149, 1996.

Doyle A, et al: Markedly decreased expression of class I histocompatibility antigens, protein, and mRNA in human small-cell lung cancer. J Exp Med 161:1135, 1985.

Farah RA, et al: The development of monoclonal antibodies for the therapy of cancer. Crit Rev Eukaryot Gene Expr 8:321, 1998.

Fenton RG, et al: Cytotoxic T-cell response and in vivo protection against tumor cells harboring activated ras proto-oncogenes. J Natl Cancer Inst 85:1294, 1993.

Fishbein GE: Immunotherapy of lung cancer. Semin Oncol 20:351, 1993.

Fossum B, et al: p21 ras peptide specific T-cell responses in a patient with colorectal cancer. CD4[+] and CD8[+] T cells recognized a peptide corresponding to a common mutation (13Gly→Asp). Int J Cancer 56:40, 1994.

Fossum B, et al: CD8[+] T cells from a patient with colon carcinoma, specific for a mutant p21-Ras-derived peptide (Gly13→Asp), are cytotoxic towards a carcinoma cell line harbouring the same mutation. Cancer Immunol Immunother 40:165, 1995.

Gaczynska M, et al: Peptidase activities of proteasomes are differentially regulated by the major histocompatibility complex-encoded genes for LMP2 and LMP7. Proc Natl Acad Sci U S A 91:9213, 1994.

Gaugler B, et al: Human gene MAGE-3 codes for an antigen recognized on a melanoma by autologous cytolytic T lymphocytes. J Exp Med 179:921, 1994.

Gotoh K, et al: Frequency of MAGE-3 gene expression in HLA-A2 positive patients with non-small cell lung cancer. Lung Cancer 20:117, 1998.

Guo ZS, et al: Interleukin 12 and B7.1 costimulatory molecules coexpressed from an adenoviral vector act synergistically to induce antitumor response and suppress tumor formation in Lewis lung carcinoma model. Proc ASCO 40:255, 1999.

Haas GJ, D'Cruz O, DeBault L: Distribution of human leukocyte antigen-ABC and -D/DR antigens in the unfixed human testis. Am J Reprod Immunol Microbiol 18:47, 1988.

Hellstrom I, Hellstrom KE: T cell immunity to tumor antigens. Crit Rev Immunol 18:1, 1998.

Hirohashi S, et al: A human monoclonal antibody directed to blood group i antigen: heterohybridoma between human lymphocytes from regional lymph nodes of a lung cancer patient and mouse myeloma. J Immunol 136:4163, 1986.

Hollinshead A, et al: Adjuvant specific active lung cancer immunotherapy trials. Cancer 60:1249, 1987.

Hollinshead A, et al: Specific active lung cancer immunotherapy. Immune correlates of clinical responses and an update of immunotherapy trials evaluations. Cancer 62:1662, 1988.

Hollstein M, et al: p53 mutations in human cancers. Science 253:49, 1991.

Houbiers JGA, et al: In vitro induction of human cytotoxic T lymphocyte responses against peptides of mutant and wild-type p53. Eur J Immunol 23:2072, 1993.

Iizasa T, et al: Serum anti-*p53* autoantibodies in primary resected non-small-cell lung carcinoma. Cancer Immunol Immunother *46*:345, 1998.

Jager E, et al: Simultaneous humoral and cellular immune response against cancer testis antigen NY-ESO-1: definition of human histocompatibility leukocyte antigen (HLA)-A2-binding peptide epitopes. J Exp Med *187*:265, 1998.

Jung S, Schluesener HJ: Human T lymphocytes recognize a peptide of single point-mutated, oncogenic ras proteins. J Exp Med *173*:273, 1991.

Kawakami Y, Rosenberg SA: Human tumor antigens recognized by T-cells. Immunol Res *16*:313, 1997.

Khleif SN, et al: A Phase I vaccine trial with peptides reflecting ras oncogene mutations of solid tumors. J Immunother *22*:155, 1999.

Kimura H, Yamaguchi Y: Adjuvant immunotherapy with interleukin 2 and lymphokine-activated killer cells after noncurative resection of primary lung cancer. Lung Cancer *13*:31, 1995.

Kimura H, Yamaguchi Y: Adjuvant chemo-immunotherapy after curative resection of Stage II and IIIA primary lung cancer. Lung Cancer *14*:301, 1996.

Kirsch DG, Kastan MB: Tumor-suppressor *p53*: implications for tumor development and prognosis. J Clin Oncol *16*:3158, 1998.

Kradin RL, et al: Tumor-derived interleukin-2 dependent lymphocytes in adoptive immunotherapy of lung cancer. Cancer Immunol Immunother *24*:76, 1987.

Lai C-L, et al: Presence of serum anti-*p53* antibodies is associated with pleural effusion and poor prognosis in lung cancer patients. Clin Cancer Res *4*:3025, 1998.

Lee C-T, et al: Genetic immunotherapy of established tumors with adenovirus-murine granulocyte-macrophage colony-stimulating factor. Hum Gene Ther *8*:187, 1997.

Lee L, et al: NY-ESO-1 may be a potential target for lung cancer immunotherapy. Cancer J Sci Am *5*:20, 1999.

Lubin R, et al: Analysis of *p53* antibodies in patients with various cancers define B-cell epitopes of human *p53*: distribution on primary structure and exposure on protein surface. Cancer Res *53*:5872, 1993.

Lubin R, et al: Serum *p53* antibodies as early markers of lung cancer. Nat Med *1*:701, 1995.

Marchand M, et al: Tumor regressions observed in patients with metastatic melanoma treated with an antigenic peptide encoded by gene MAGE-3 and presented by HLA-A1. Int J Cancer *80*:219, 1999.

Mitsudomi T, et al: *p53* gene mutations in non-small-cell lung cancer cell lines and their correlation with the presence of ras mutations and clinical features. Oncogene *7*:171, 1992.

Mitsudomi T, et al: Clinical implications of *p53* autoantibodies in the sera of patients with non-small-cell lung cancer. J Natl Cancer Inst *90*:1563, 1998.

Momparler RL, et al: Pilot phase I-II study on 5-aza-2'-deoxycytidine (Decitabine) in patients with metastatic lung cancer. Anti-Cancer Drugs *8*:358, 1997.

Nair SK, et al: Antigen-presenting cells pulsed with unfractionated tumor-derived peptides are potent tumor vaccines. Eur J Immunol *27*:589, 1997.

Nakao M, et al: HLA A2601-restricted CTLs recognize a peptide antigen expressed on squamous cell carcinoma. Cancer Res *55*:4248, 1995.

Nauts HC: The beneficial effects of bacterial infections on host resistance to cancer end results in 449 cases. New York: Cancer Research Institute, 1980.

Ohe Y, et al: Combination effect of vaccination with IL2 and IL4 cDNA transfected cells on the induction of a therapeutic immune response against Lewis lung carcinoma cells. Int J Cancer *53*:432, 1993.

Old LJ: Tumor immunology: the first century. Curr Opin Immunol *4*:603, 1992.

Old LJ, Clarke DA, Banaceraff B: Effects of bacillus Calmette-Guérin on transplanted tumors in the mouse. Nature *184*:291, 1959.

Ortmann B, Androlewicz MJ, Cresswell P: MHC class I/beta 2-microglobulin complexes associate with TAP transporters before peptide binding. Nature *368*:864, 1994.

Peace DJ: T cell recognition of transforming proteins encoded by mutated ras proto-oncogenes. J Immunol *146*:2059, 1991.

Pichler WJ, Wyss-Coray T: T cells as antigen-presenting cells. Immunol Today *15*:312, 1994.

Putzer BM, et al: Interleukin 12 and B7-1 costimulatory molecule expressed by an adenovirus vector act synergistically to facilitate tumor regression. Proc Natl Acad Sci U S A *94*:10889, 1997.

Ratto GB, et al: A randomized trial of adoptive immunotherapy with tumor-infiltrating lymphocytes and interleukin-2 versus standard therapy in the postoperative treatment of resected non-small cell lung cancer carcinoma. Cancer *78*:244, 1998.

Reed DS, et al: Construction and characterization of a recombinant adenovirus directing expression of the MAGE-1 tumor-specific antigen. Int J Cancer *72*:1045, 1997.

Restifo NP, Wunderlich JR: Essentials of immunology. *In* DeVita VT Jr, et al (eds): Cancer: Principles and Practice of Oncology. Philadelphia: Lippincott–Raven, 1997, pp. 47–75.

Restifo NP, et al: Identification of human cancers deficient in antigen processing. J Exp Med *177*:265, 1993.

Restifo NP, et al: Loss of functional beta 2-microglobulin in metastatic melanomas from five patients receiving immunotherapy. J Natl Cancer Inst *88*:100, 1996.

Rodenhuis S, Slebos RJ: Clinical significance of ras oncogene activation in human lung cancer. Cancer Res *52*:2665, 1992.

Ropke M, Regner M, Claesson MH: T cell-mediated cytotoxicity against *p53*-protein derived peptides in bulk and limiting dilution cultures of healthy donors. Scand J Immunol *42*:98, 1995.

Ropke M, et al: Spontaneous human squamous cell carcinomas are killed by a human cytotoxic T lymphocyte clone recognizing a wild-type *p53*-derived peptide. Proc Natl Acad Sci U S A *93*:14704, 1996.

Rosenberg S, et al: Immunologic and therapeutic evaluation of a synthetic peptide vaccine for the treatment of patients with metastatic melanoma. Nat Med *4*:321, 1998.

Sakata M: Expression of MAGE gene family in lung cancers. Kurume Med J *43*:55, 1996.

Schreiber H: Tumor immunology. *In* Paul WE (ed): Fundamental Immunology. Philadelphia: Lippincott–Raven, 1999, pp. 1237–1270.

Schrump DS, et al: Recognition of galactosylgloboside by monoclonal antibodies derived from patients with primary lung cancer. Proc Natl Acad Sci U S A *85*:4441, 1988.

Schrump DS, et al: Generation of monoclonal antibodies from patients with primary lung cancer. J Cell Biochem Suppl *14B*:92, 1990.

Seder RA, Mosmann TM: Differentiation of effector phenotypes of CD4+ and CD8+ cells. *In* Paul WE (ed): Fundamental Immunology. Philadelphia: Lippincott–Raven, 1999, pp. 879–902.

Sherman LA, et al: Strategies for tumor elimination by cytotoxic T lymphocytes. Crit Rev Immunol *18*:47, 1998.

Singal DP, Ye M, Qiu X: Molecular basis for lack of expression of HLA class I antigens in human small-cell lung carcinoma cell lines. Int J Cancer *68*:629, 1996.

Slingluff CL Jr, et al: Cytotoxic T-lymphocyte response to autologous human squamous cell cancer of the lung: epitope reconstitution with peptides extracted from HLA-Aw68. Cancer Res *54*:2731, 1994.

Stockert E, et al: A survey of the humoral immune response of cancer patients to a panel of human tumor antigens. J Exp Med *187*:1349, 1998.

Takenoyama M, et al: Autologous tumor-specific cytotoxic T lymphocytes in a patient with lung adenocarcinoma: implications of the shared antigens expressed in HLA-A24 lung cancer cells. Jpn J Cancer Res *89*:60, 1998.

Traversari C, et al: IFN-γ gene transfer restores HLA-class I expression and MAGE-3 antigen presentation to CTL in HLA-deficient small cell lung cancer. Gene Ther *4*:1029, 1997.

Trivers GE, et al: Anti-*p53* antibodies in sera from patients with chronic obstructive pulmonary disease can predate a diagnosis of cancer. Clin Cancer Res *2*:1767, 1996.

Uchida A, et al: Prediction of postoperative clinical course by autologous tumor-killing activity in lung cancer patients. J Natl Cancer Inst *82*:1697, 1990.

van der Bruggen P, et al: A gene encoding an antigen recognized by cytolytic T lymphocytes on a human melanoma. Science *254*:1643, 1991.

van der Bruggen P, et al: A peptide encoded by human gene MAGE-3 and presented by HLA-A2 induces cytolytic T lymphocytes that recognize tumor cells expressing MAGE-3. Eur J Immunol *24*:3038, 1994.

Vanky JF, et al: Correlation between lymphocyte-mediated auto-tumor reactivities and the clinical course. Cancer Immunol Immunother *16*:17, 1983.

Vierboom MPM, et al: Tumor eradication by wild-type *p53*-specific cytotoxic T lymphocytes. J Exp Med *186*:695, 1997.

Wang R-F, et al: A breast and melanoma shared tumor antigen: T cell responses to antigenic peptides translated from different open reading frames. J Immunol *161*:3598, 1998.

Weynants P, et al: Expression of MAGE genes by non-small-cell lung carcinomas. Int J Cancer *56*:826, 1994.

Winter SF, et al: Development of antibodies against *p53* in lung cancer patients appears to be dependent on the type of *p53* mutation. Cancer Res *52*:4168, 1992.

Winter SF, et al: Antibodies against autologous tumor cell proteins in patients with small-cell lung cancer: association with improved survival. J Natl Cancer Inst *85*:2012, 1993.

Yoda Y: Study on glycolipids in human lung carcinoma of histologically different types [author's translation]. Hokkaido Igaku Zasshi *54*:355, 1979.

Yokomizo H, et al: Augmentation of immune response by an analog of the antigenic peptide in a human T-cell clone recognizing mutated Ras-derived peptides. Hum Immunol *52*:22, 1997.

Yoshimatsu T, et al: Expression of the melanoma antigen-encoding gene in human lung cancer. J Surg Oncol *67*:126, 1998.

READING REFERENCES

Panelli CM, Marincola FM: Immunotherapy update: from IL-2 to antigen specific therapy. *In* Anonymous: American Society of Clinical Oncology Educational Book, 1998, pp. 467–473.

Traversari C, et al: A nonapeptide encoded by human gene MAGE-1 is recognized on HLA-A1 by cytolytic T lymphocytes directed against tumor antigen MZ2-E. J Exp Med *176*:1453, 1992.

Visseren MJ, et al: Identification of HLA-A*0201-restricted CTL epitopes encoded by the tumor-specific MAGE-2 gene product. Int J Cancer *73*:125, 1997.

SECTION XVI

Other Tumors of the Lung

SECTION XVI

Other Types of the Lens

CHAPTER 109

Carcinoid Tumors

Robert J. Ginsberg

Carcinoid tumors are the second most common tumor type arising in the tracheobronchial tree and account for 0.5 to 1.0% of all tumors of bronchial origin. They are an interesting group of malignant growths originally described in the 1800s and coined "Karzinoid" in 1907 by Oberndorfer because of their resemblance to lung cancer. Until recently, these tumors were grouped with cylindromas (adenoid cystic carcinoma) and mucoepidermoid tumors as "bronchial adenomas" because of their relatively benign course. It has since become apparent that they represent a spectrum of neuroendocrine tumors of varying malignant potential, depending on their differentiation (typical versus atypical) and stage at presentation. Although reports have proffered other descriptive nomenclatures, including "Kulchitsky cell tumor" (KCT) or "neuroendocrine carcinoma," the original term, *carcinoid tumor*, remains commonly accepted and serves to differentiate them from lung cancers with neuroendocrine features, which have a much more ominous prognosis, as recorded by Dresler and associates (1997).

CLINICAL FEATURES

McCaughan and associates (1985) identified 124 carcinoid tumors in a review of the experience at Memorial Sloan-Kettering Cancer Center. The patient population consisted of 68 women and 56 men ranging in age from 12 to 82 years with a median age of 55 years. These demographic features reflect the experience of other large series in the literature.

Signs and Symptoms

The symptoms and physical findings associated with these tumors depend on their location (central or peripheral). The peripheral tumors are most often asymptomatic, presenting as solitary pulmonary nodules on radiographic studies of the chest (Fig. 109-1). The proximally located tumors grow partially or wholly within a bronchus. Partial or complete endobronchial obstruction and its sequelae, as well as the vascularity of the tumor, account for the symptoms. Cough, hemoptysis, and recurrent infection constitute the classic triad of symptoms (Table 109-1). A history of smoking is unusual.

Because of the small size and slow growth of these tumors, symptoms may persist for many years before the underlying cause is discovered. A history of wheezing or recurrent infection dating back many years is common (Fig. 109-2). One patient in the Memorial Sloan-Kettering series had recurrent hemoptysis for 40 years before diagnosis and treatment of a carcinoid tumor of the bronchus. These tumors frequently masquerade clinically as bronchial asthma, chronic bronchitis, or bronchiectasis, particularly if the tumor produces incomplete obstruction and is located in the trachea or proximal portions of the bronchial tree.

Incomplete obstruction leads to cough, wheezing, or recurrent distal infection with its sequelae. On occasion, a unilateral hyperlucent segment, lobe, or lung is identified on the chest radiograph because of a ball-valve mechanism. Complete obstruction may result in obstructive pneumonitis with pain, fever, and dyspnea. Bronchiectasis or chronic lung abscesses are found in patients with longstanding undiagnosed tumors, eventually resulting in total destruction of lung tissue distal to the obstruction (Fig. 109-3).

Stridor can be the presenting symptom in tracheal or main stem bronchial tumors. Occasionally, this high airway obstruction becomes life-threatening. Recurrent hemoptysis, another frequent symptom, results from ulceration of the mucosa overlying the tumor or simply from chronic inflammation distally. In women, it has been noted to be accentuated during times of menstrual flow. Occasionally, a patient with an atypical carcinoid presents initially with metastatic disease.

The carcinoid syndrome occurs infrequently (a 2% incidence) and exclusively in patients with large primary tumors or extensive hepatic metastases.

Carcinoid Syndrome

Carcinoid syndrome is a clinical entity consisting of well-described cutaneous, cardiovascular, gastrointestinal, and

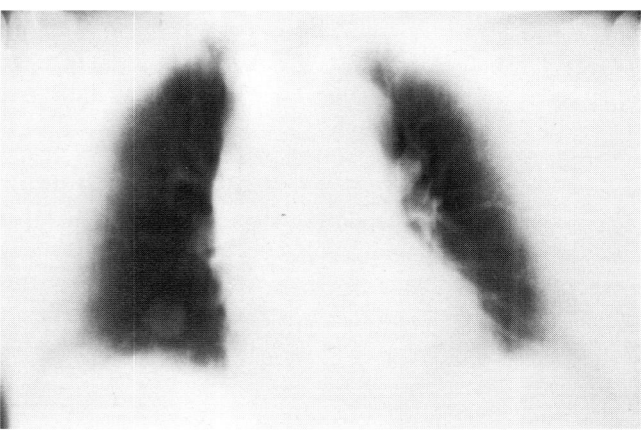

Fig. 109-1. Tomogram of an asymptomatic peripheral carcinoid adenoma.

Table 109-1. Clinical Presentation in 124 Patients at Memorial Sloan-Kettering Cancer Center

Presenting Features	No. of Patients	Percent
Asymptomatic	74	60
Hemoptysis	22	18
Recurrent infection and cough	21	17
Dyspnea or wheeze	3	2
Metastatic disease	3	2
Carcinoid syndrome	1	1

respiratory manifestations. It was first described in and most commonly occurs with metastatic carcinoid tumors of the gastrointestinal tract, but this syndrome occasionally occurs in association with bronchial carcinoids and was the presenting symptom in one patient in McCaughan and colleagues' (1985) series. Harpole and associates (1992) reported a high incidence of the syndrome of 12%. The carcinoid syndrome occurs in bronchial tumors only when the primary tumor is large or when liver metastases have occurred, often many years after removal of the primary tumor. An interesting phenomenon is the left-sided cardiac valvular abnormalities reported in the carcinoid syndrome associated with large primary tumors of the lung, unlike the right-sided valvular lesions found with hepatic metastases.

The rarity of this syndrome in carcinoids of pulmonary origin may be because they reportedly contain less serotonin per gram of tissue than do intestinal carcinoids. It is possible that this level is reduced because of the lung's high content of monoamine oxidase that can detoxify serotonin.

Other Endocrinopathies

Like small cell carcinoma, bronchial carcinoids have also been associated with various other endocrine disorders (including Cushing's syndrome) as the result of increased adrenocorticotropic hormone (ACTH) production, excessive pigmentation from melanophore-stimulating hormone (MSH), inappropriate antidiuretic hormone (ADH) secretion, and hypoglycemia. In addition, the multiple endocrine adenomatosis syndrome (MEA) has been reported in association with these tumors.

Cushing's Syndrome

Limper and colleagues (1992) reviewed 15 cases of a bronchial carcinoid tumor associated with Cushing's syndrome. The latter condition was the presenting clinical feature in each patient. The bronchial carcinoids were of the typical type in 10 patients, three patients had atypical carcinoids, and metastatic disease was present in three. Almost all of the tumors were nodules located in the periphery of the lungs. Ten of the 15 tumors were radiographically occult initially; of these, five subsequently were discovered radiographically over long periods of observation, and five (after 1980) were discovered by computed tomography (CT) scans. Resection resulted in 10 complete and two partial remissions. The three patients with metastatic disease continued to have hypersecretion of ACTH and remained symptomatic. The experience of Pass and associates (1990) at the National Cancer Institute with 13 patients with bronchial carcinoids associated with Cushing's syndrome is not dissimilar. Although 12 of the tumors in this series were typical carcinoids and only one was atypical, lymph node metastases were present in 50% of the patients in this series. An additional seven patients with bronchial carcinoid tumors associated with Cushing's syndrome were reported by Shrager and associates (1997) from the Massachusetts General Hospital. Five of the tumors were

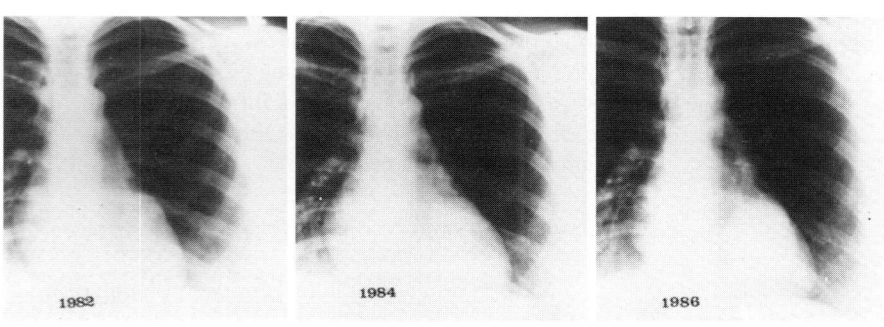

Fig. 109-2. Serial radiographs of a retrocardiac bronchial adenoma demonstrating slow growth over a 4-year period.

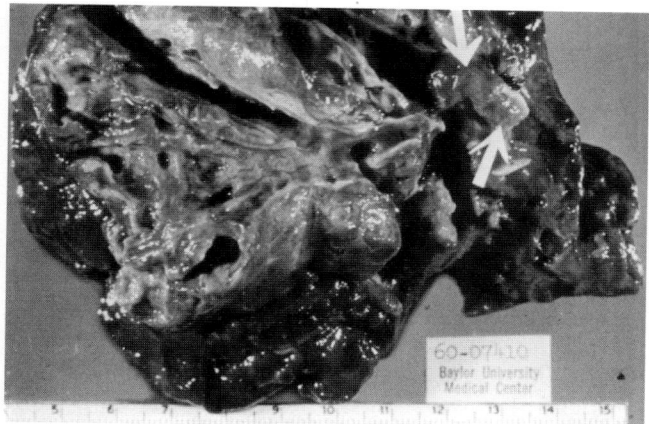

Fig. 109-3. Gross specimen of a typical polypoid bronchial carcinoid (*arrows*) resected by superior segmentectomy of the right lower lobe, wedge resection of the bronchus intermedius, and bronchoplasty. Note the bronchiectasis and abscesses distally.

histologically of the typical type, but two of these showed local invasion and two were associated with lymph node metastases (43%). Both of the atypical carcinoid tumors had involved lymph nodes. The overall incidence of lymph node invasion was 57%. In these two aforementioned series, the high incidence of lymph node involvement is in contrast with only a 20% incidence of metastases in Limper and colleagues' (1992) collected series and a 24% incidence of lymph node metastases in 72 patients collected by Pass and associates (1990) from the literature (1957 to 1989).

Although Cushing's disease occurs in no more than 1% of patients with bronchial carcinoid, it is the second most commonly observed paraneoplastic syndrome associated with these tumors. Any patient who presents with Cushing's disease, par-

ticularly with prominent hypokalemic alkalosis, and who has no evidence of either adrenal or pituitary disease should undergo a search for an occult bronchial carcinoid. The other two thoracic diseases that must also be considered are small cell cancer of the lung and carcinoid tumor of the thymus.

DIAGNOSIS

No single investigative method is sufficient to diagnose the presence of a bronchial carcinoid in all patients, but by various radiographic techniques and bronchoscopy, most tumors can be located and correctly identified. Fine-needle aspiration biopsy of peripheral lesions can be accurate, but they may be mistaken for a small cell carcinoma. Histologic examination of tumor tissue is the only completely reliable means of diagnosis.

Radiographic Studies

Standard radiographs of the chest may reveal a tumor mass or changes in pulmonary parenchyma caused by tracheobronchial obstruction. Frequently, a standard radiograph will detect no abnormality (Fig. 109-4A). Oblique views may detect an otherwise undetectable central lesion and may delineate an endobronchial component of the tumor not readily apparent on routine studies. CT scan can further delineate the endobronchial and parenchymal component of the tumor (Fig. 109-4B), although this examination is not essential in most patients. In the past, hilar tomography and bronchography were used frequently to outline the endobronchial obstruction and to demonstrate irreversible bronchiectasis in the bronchial tree distally.

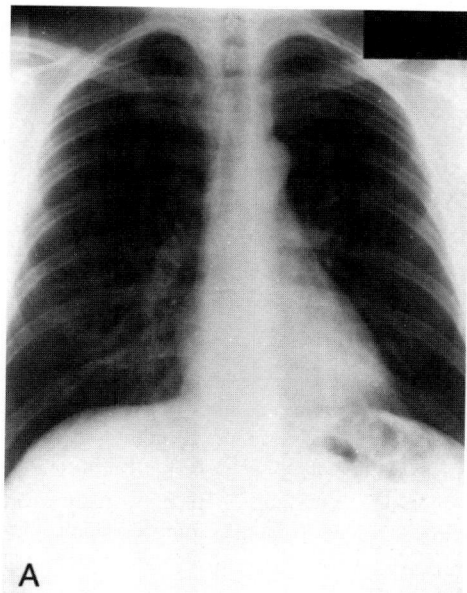

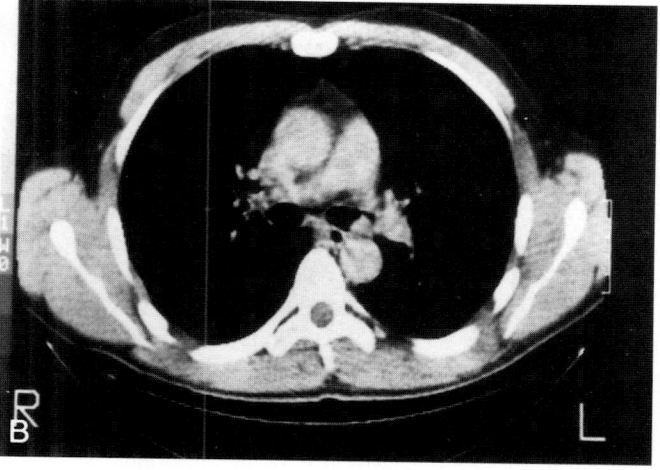

Fig. 109-4. A. A chest radiograph called "normal." An endobronchial carcinoid is in the distal left main stem bronchus. **B.** An endobronchial carcinoid of the left main stem bronchus demonstrated by computed tomography. Note the minimal involvement of the bronchial wall.

With current, more sophisticated techniques, such as CT scan, these examinations are now rarely, if ever, indicated.

CT scan of centrally located lesions reveals the presence of a well-defined mass that narrows, deforms, or obstructs an adjacent airway. Diffuse or punctate calcifications can be identified in approximately 30% of lesions. According to Magid and associates (1989), this finding should suggest that the tumor is a carcinoid. High-resolution CT scan, as reported by Sutedja and associates (1996), may be used effectively to demonstrate bronchial wall irregularities, bronchial wall thickening, and peribronchial tumor invasion in patients with central endobronchial lesions. When such findings are absent, it may be surmised that no bronchial wall infiltration by the tumor is present. High-resolution CT is also of value in revealing the presence of enlarged hilar and peribronchial lymph nodes. Peripheral parenchymal changes such as atelectasis or bronchiectatic changes of the distal airways may be demonstrated. Peripheral lesions usually lie adjacent to an airway. Lastly, using CT scan, homogeneous contrast enhancement of a typical carcinoid is observed after intravenous administration of a bolus of contrast media. Atypical carcinoids show less contrast enhancement and frequently have irregular contours. Regional adenopathy is often seen in association with the atypical lesions.

None of these radiologic techniques accurately differentiates these tumors from other benign and malignant neoplasms, although one may suspect their nature by the radiographic appearance of an obstructive lesion or peripheral tumor in a young, nonsmoking person.

Bronchoscopy

Bronchoscopy should be successful in identifying all tumors situated within and proximal to the segmental orifices. Approximately 75% of all carcinoid tumors are visible endoscopically.

Accurate identification of the tumors requires bronchial biopsy. Wilkins (1963) and Donahue (1968) and their associates, among others, reported massive bleeding after biopsies of carcinoid tumors. Indeed, these highly vascular tumors do tend to bleed, but almost all severe postbronchoscopic hemorrhages result from endoscopic attempts at partial or complete removal of the tumor. These tumors present submucosally and do require deeper biopsies than are necessary for other malignant bronchial neoplasms. Care must be taken in performing such biopsies. As also suggested by Rozenman and colleagues (1987), I continue to perform bronchoscopic biopsies of these tumors using a dilute epinephrine solution for vasoconstriction before and after biopsy. Some authors recommend general anesthesia and rigid bronchoscopy for airway control in case uncontrollable hemorrhage occurs during fiberoptic bronchoscopic examination. I have not found this necessary.

Transbronchoscopic fine-needle aspiration biopsy of the submucosal tumor for cytologic examination may help in diagnosing carcinoid tumors when biopsy is unwarranted or unhelpful and should be included as a routine part of the bronchoscopic examination when a submucosal lesion is apparent.

Frozen section examination of the biopsy material may be misleading. Because of their similarity to small cell carcinomas, carcinoid tumors have occasionally been misdiagnosed as this more aggressive tumor. Examination of permanent hematoxylin and eosin preparations usually leads to an accurate diagnosis, although mistaken diagnoses (especially atypical carcinoids versus small cell carcinoma) have unfortunately been made by this method as well.

Staging

Because of the adverse prognostic effect of lymph node metastases in this disease, authors reporting results of treatment have used the American Joint Committee on Cancer/International Union Against Cancer Lung Cancer Staging criteria for carcinoid tumors as well. Despite this effort, there has been no disease-free survival correlation found for the various tumor, node, metastasis (TNM) subsets, prognosis being dependent on histology, lymph node involvement (positive or negative), and the presence or absence of distant metastases at the time of presentation. Most typical carcinoid tumors present as stage I lesions, whereas over 50% of atypical carcinoids present as stage II or III with bronchopulmonary or mediastinal lymph node involvement.

Preoperative nodal staging by mediastinoscopy has little value in typical carcinoid tumors unless mediastinal involvement is suspected, although, it may be useful in the rare case that an atypical carcinoid tumor is present and complete unresectability by virtue of mediastinal spread is suspected on imaging studies.

Biochemical Studies

Unless the carcinoid syndrome is suspected, screening patients with suspected bronchial carcinoids for serotonin and its breakdown product (5-hydroxyindoleacetic acid) in blood or urine has no diagnostic value, although Harpole and associates (1992) found elevated levels to be an adverse prognostic variable on univariate analysis.

Nuclear Scanning

Reubi and colleagues (1990) have shown that 54 of 62 (87%) carcinoid tumors could be labeled by the autoradiographic technique of somatostatin analog binding. This has led to the use of anatomic localization by somatostatin-receptor scintigraphy (octreotide scanning) in patients with Cushing's syndrome caused by an occult ectopic corticotropin-producing tumor by de Herder (1994) and Dewey (1996) and their associates, among others. When metastatic disease is suspected,

Matte and colleagues (1998) also have suggested that this type of scanning by a somatostatin analogue can be diagnostic. The role of positron emission tomography (PET) scanning in suspected metastatic disease is also being investigated, but its value is as yet undetermined.

Pathology

Experimental evidence reported by Churg (1988) suggested that these tumors arise from stem cells of the bronchial epithelium rather than from amine precursor uptake and decarboxylation (APUD) cells that migrated from the neural crest. A review by Gould and associates (1983) of the histogenesis and differentiation of bronchial carcinoids and their proposed relationship with other pulmonary tumors with neuroendocrine features is provocative.

Some tumor markers can be identified in carcinoid tumors of the lung. These markers include the following: the polypeptide hormones ACTH, arginine vasopressin (ADH), calcitonin, and bombesin (gastrin-releasing peptides), the enzymes neuron-specific enolase and synaptophysin, and the aforementioned biogenic amine serotonin. All of these markers can also be identified in small cell cancer cells, and thus their presence is of no differential diagnostic value between these two tumor cell types.

"Typical" Carcinoids

Most of these tumors are situated centrally; 20% are located in the main stem bronchi, approximately 60% in the lobar and segmental bronchi, and another 20% are located peripherally. Data reported from Memorial Sloan-Kettering Cancer Center as to location are different from the norm, most likely the result of the pattern of patient referral (Table 109-2). Carcinoid tumors infrequently involve the main carina or trachea (Fig. 109-5), and multiple or multicentric tumors rarely are discovered in one patient.

Bronchoscopically, typical carcinoids appear as highly vascularized pink to purplish soft tumors, covered by intact epithelium (Fig. 109-6). Large areas of ulceration are rare. A few tumors are polypoid with a definite stalk, but most are sessile. Because the bulk of the tumor is usually extraluminal, they have been called "iceberg tumors." They penetrate

Table 109-2. Location of Tumor in 124 Carcinoid Tumors at Memorial Sloan-Kettering Cancer Center

Site	Right	Left
Main bronchus	7	7
Upper lobe bronchi	7	7
Bronchus intermedius	5	—
Middle lobe bronchus	2	—
Lower lobe bronchi	3	8
Peripheral	41	37

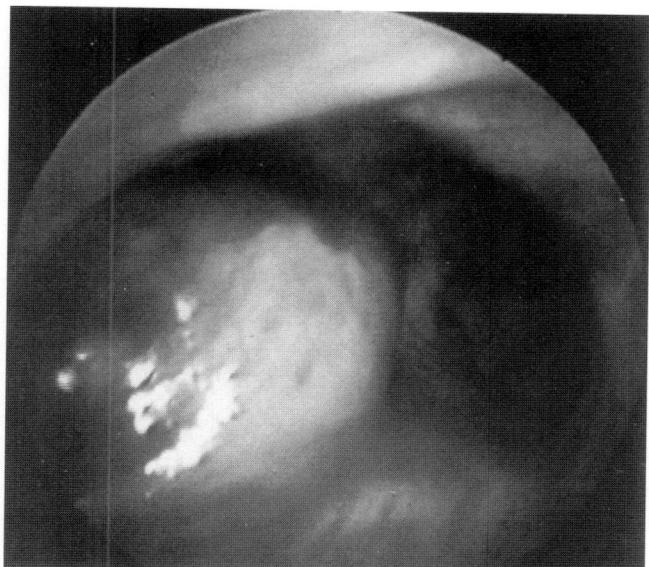

Fig. 109-5. An unusual carcinoid tumor presenting in the left main stem bronchus and extending to the carina. This lesion required carinal resection for management.

the bronchial wall and may directly extend into the pulmonary parenchyma and peribronchial lymph nodes.

Microscopically, the tumor consists of uniform round to polygonal cells with small oval nuclei and finely granular chromatin, but cells may be spindle-shaped, particularly in peripherally located tumors. The cytoplasm is abundant and eosinophilic. Mitoses are infrequent. The cells are arranged in small clusters or interlacing cords, or both, separated by highly vascular connective tissue (Fig. 109-7). The stroma may show osseous metaplasia, which may be secondary to necrosis within the tumor or necrosis of compressed bronchial cartilage with secondary ossification (Fig. 109-8). As previously noted, this may be seen as calcification within the tumor on CT scans. The overlying bronchial epithelium can undergo squamous metaplasia, but frank ulceration or invasion by tumor is rare. As Bertelsen and colleagues

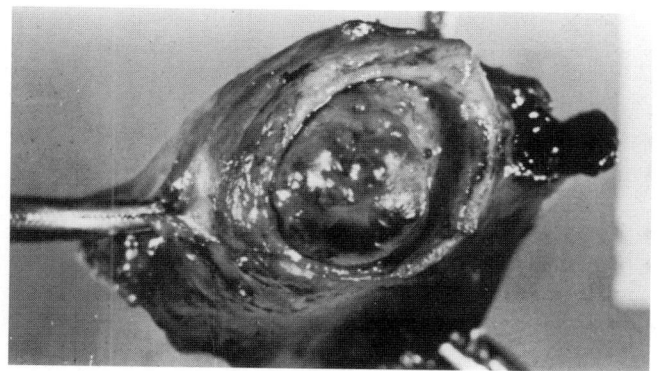

Fig. 109-6. "Bronchoscopic" view of a carcinoid adenoma.

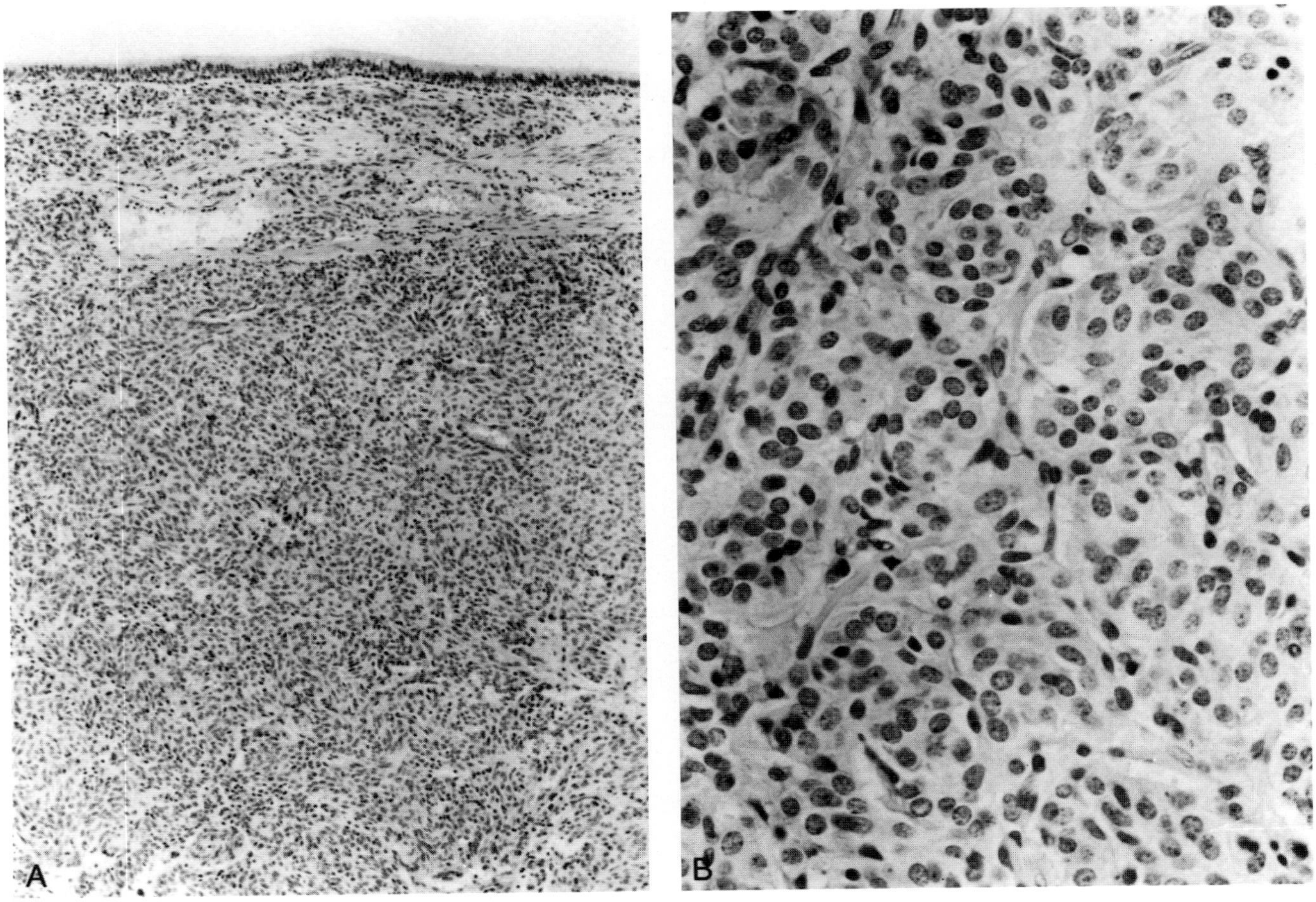

Fig. 109-7. **A.** Low-power photomicrograph of a typical carcinoid with intact overlying bronchial epithelium. **B.** High-power photomicrograph of a typical carcinoid tumor comprised of nests of regular polygonal cells separated by a network of capillary vessels reflecting the vascularity of the tumor.

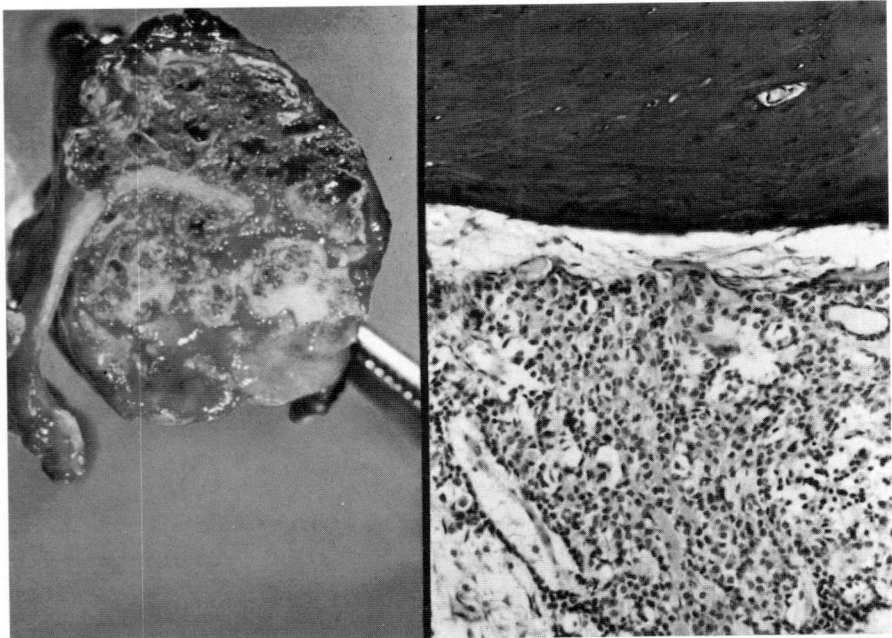

Fig. 109-8. Gross (**A**) and microscopic (**B**) appearance of a carcinoid adenoma with osseous metaplasia. Note the large, extrabronchial component of this tumor.

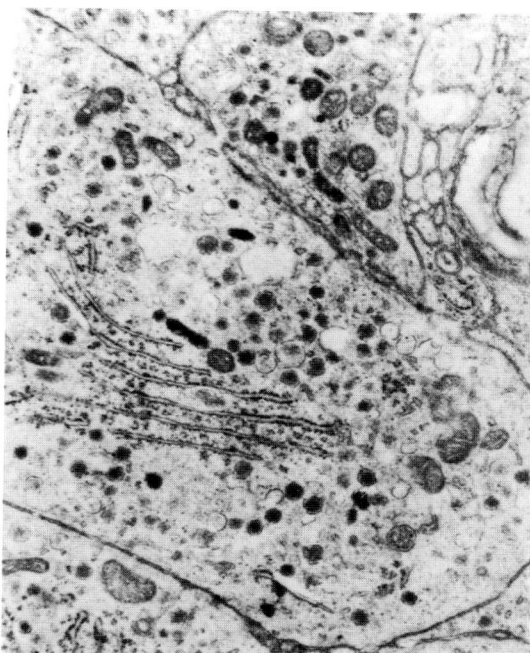

Fig. 109-9. High-power electron photomicrograph (×2300) of a carcinoid adenoma reviewing secretion granules, typical of neurosecretory cells. From Toker C: Observations on the ultrastructure of a bronchial adenoma (carcinoid-type). Cancer *19*:1943, 1966. With permission.

(1985) reported, only 10 to 15% of patients with typical carcinoid tumors present with lymph node metastases.

Ultrastructurally, Bensch and associates (1965) were the first to describe that these tumors consist of closely packed cells with small but well-formed desmosomes and numerous neurosecretory granules. The neurosecretory granules (Fig. 109-9) are large, heterogeneous, and numerous.

Atypical Carcinoids

Atypical carcinoids, which display both malignant histologic features and aggressive behavior, were described by Englebreth-Holm (1944–1945) and Von Albertini (1951), but most accurately by Arrigoni and associates (1972). The average age of patients with atypical carcinoids is 55 years, compared to 45 years for patients with typical carcinoids. Warren and colleagues (1985) referred to these tumors as "well-differentiated neuroendocrine carcinomas." They have also been referred to as a "Kultchitsky cell II tumor"; Kultchitsky I is a typical carcinoid and Kultchitsky III is a small cell carcinoma. In contrast to typical carcinoids, more than 50% of these tumors are located peripherally, the age of onset is later, and 50 to 70% of patients present with lymph node or distant metastases. In some instances, it is difficult to differentiate an atypical carcinoid from a small cell undifferentiated carcinoma. Despite the pathologic similarities, it

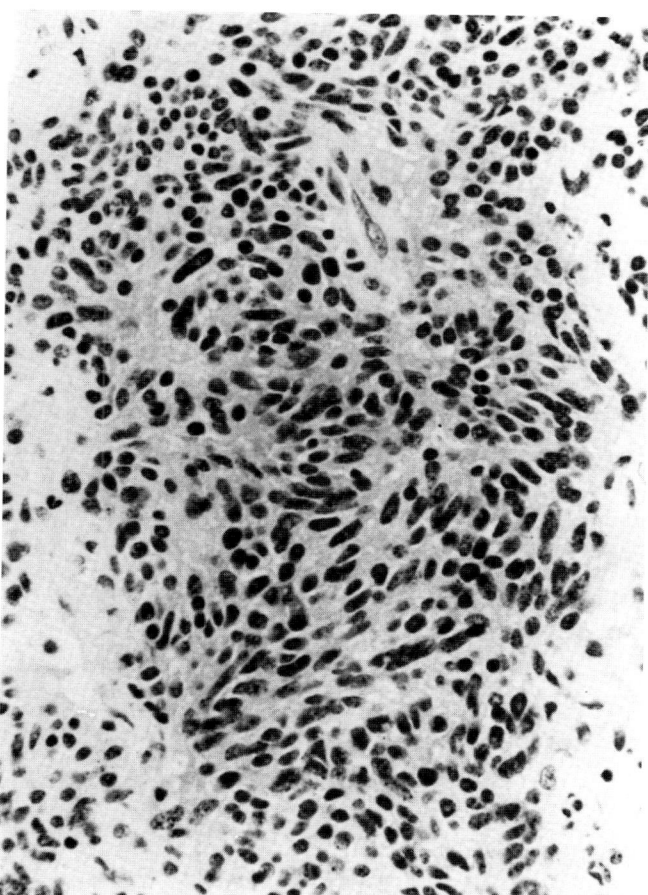

Fig. 109-10. High-power photomicrograph of an atypical carcinoid tumor consisting of ribbons of polygonal cells that show greater pleomorphism and mitotic activity than those seen in a typical carcinoid tumor.

is interesting to note the absence of a history of smoking with carcinoid tumors and the invariable smoking history in patients with small cell carcinomas, as well as the relatively poor response of atypical carcinoids to chemotherapy.

Histologically, while retaining a carcinoid-like pattern, they display unmistakable pleomorphism with mitotic activity, nuclear abnormalities, prominent nucleoli, peripheral palisading, and necrosis (Fig. 109-10). Neurosecretory granules are present but are of small size—that is, typical carcinoid. In any series, about 10% of carcinoids are atypical, and this is reflected in my own experience.

Unlike small cell lung cancers, genetic abnormalities are infrequently found in typical and atypical carcinoid tumors; a p53 mutation is found in about 20% of cases. On the other hand, with small cell lung cancer, 3p deletions, p53 mutations, RB deletions, and *myc* oncogene overexpression are found frequently.

Salgia (1997) has conveniently summarized the differences between typical and atypical carcinoids versus small cell lung cancer (Table 109-3).

Table 109-3. Selected Histopathologic and Molecular Features of Pulmonary Neuroendocrine Tumors

	Typical Carcinoid	Atypical Carcinoid	Small Cell Lung Cancer
Morphology			
N/C ratio	Moderate	Moderate	High
Mitoses	<1/10 hpf	1–10/10 hpf	>20/10 hpf
Necrosis	Absent	Present	Present
Nuclear	Absent/rare	Present	Present
Pleomorphism	—	—	—
DNA encrustation of vessel walls (Azzapardie effect)	Rare	Mild	Moderate
Vascular invasion	Absent	Present	Present
Chemical analysis			
Chromogranin A	Positive	Positive	Positive (20–50%)
NSE	Positive	Positive	Positive
CEA	Positive/negative	Positive/negative	Positive
Synaptophysin	Positive/negative	Positive/negative	Positive
MAb 735	Negative	Negative	Positive
Topolysialic acid	—	—	—
Electron microscopy	Large, numerous	Small, moderate	Small, occasional
Molecular analysis			
3p deletion	Not present	Not present	Positive (90%)
7q deletion	Not present	Not present	?
p53 mutation	Infrequent (20%)	Infrequent (20%)	Present (80%)
Rb deletion	Present	Present	Present (>90%)
Myc oncogenes	?	?	Amplified/overexpressed (10–40%)

CEA, carcinoembryonic antigen; hpf, high power field; MAb, monoclonal antibody; N/C, nuclear/cytoplasmic; NSE, neuron-specific enolase; ? = no data.

Pathologists have identified a group of large cell tumors with neuroendocrine features. These tumors are indeed lung cancers, have prognoses similar to those seen with small cell lung cancer, and must be differentiated from atypical carcinoids. The criteria of differentiating large cell neuroendocrine tumors from atypical carcinoids, as suggested by Travis and associates (1998), are presented in detail in Chapter 95. Like small cell lung cancers, these neuroendocrine large cell tumors have been shown to have mutations in p53 exons, and immunohistochemistry for p53 may be required to differentiate these tumors from atypical carcinoids. According to Przygodzki and associates (1996), these large cell neuroendocrine tumors are more akin genetically and immunohistochemically to small cell cancers and also behave like them.

Melanocytic Carcinoid

The rare pigmented carcinoid has been reported by Cebelin (1980) and by Grazer (1982) and Gal (1993) and their colleagues. Its differentiation from a pulmonary melanoma is discussed in Chapter 112.

Oncocytic Carcinoid

Oncocytic carcinoid is a rare subtype of the typical carcinoid tumor. It is composed of a variable admixture of large eosinophilic oncocytes and cells characteristic of the typical carcinoid tumor. Ghadially and Block (1985), among others,

have described this tumor and its differentiation as a true oncocytic tumor.

Clear Cell Carcinoid Tumors

According to Leong and Meredith (1997) a carcinoid tumor very infrequently may exhibit extensive clear cell change and thus require differentiation from other clear cell tumors of the lung. Differentiation requires immunohistochemical stains and ultrastructural examination. Clear cell tumors are discussed in Chapters 95 and 111.

Tumorlets and Multiple Peripheral Carcinoids

Whitwell (1955) coined the term *pulmonary tumorlet* to describe isolated foci of atypical hyperplastic bronchial epithelium. Tumorlets were initially regarded as forms of early invasive or in situ small cell carcinoma. They are usually an incidental finding at autopsy or in a lung resected for infection or tumor. Miller and coworkers (1978) described them particularly in patients with restrictive pulmonary disease.

Immunohistochemical staining has demonstrated differences in secretory products between tumorlets and typical carcinoids. Because of the similarity in staining patterns between tumorlets and normal bronchial epithelium, Cutz and associates (1982) suggested that tumorlets are hyperplastic proliferations of neuroendocrine cells rather than neoplasms, although D'Agati and Perzin (1985) described

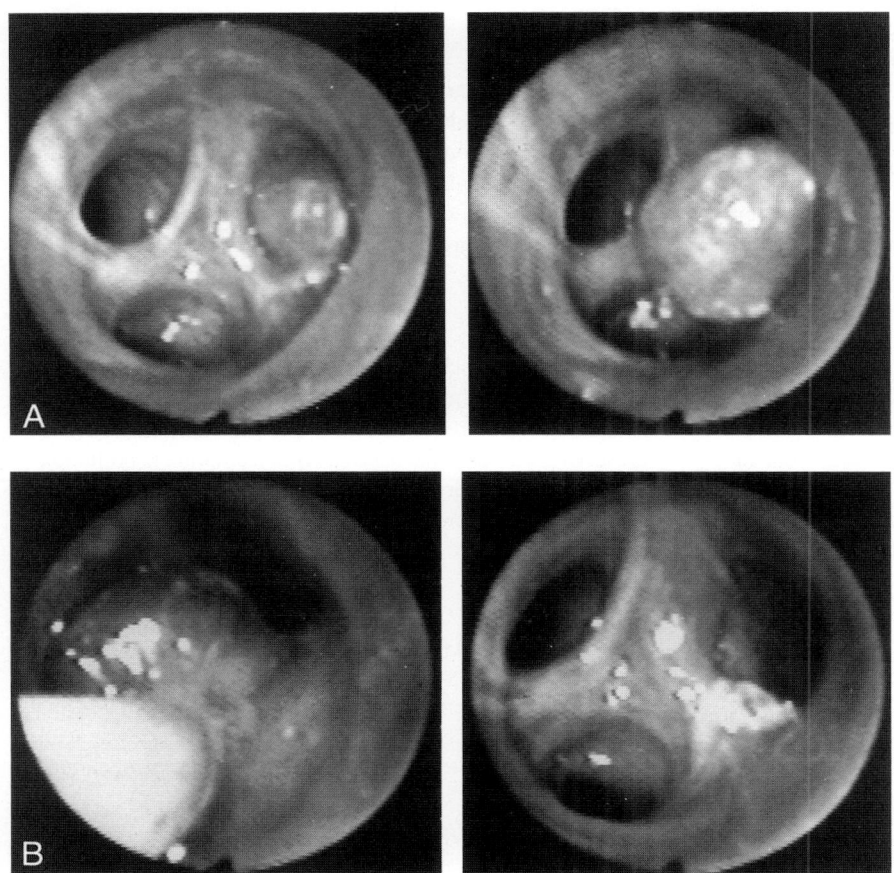

Fig. 109-11. A. A polypoid carcinoid tumor arising in the apical segment of the right upper lobe. Note that on exhaling (right), the tumor protrudes out of the orifice. This lesion was found to have a definite uninvolved stalk. **B.** The polypoid tumor in **A** was smeared (left) and removed with the base coagulated using an Nd:YAG laser (right). The stalk was uninvolved with tumor. Two-year follow-up has failed to reveal any local recurrence. Courtesy of M. Burt.

one case with peribronchial lymph node metastases. Aguayo and associates (1992) implicated a diffuse form as an etiologic mechanism in small airway obliterative disease.

TREATMENT

Unless distant metastatic disease is evident, the principles of treatment of carcinoid tumors include complete removal of the primary lesion with preservation of as much normal lung tissue as possible. Because most of these tumors are only locally invasive, the most conservative resection that allows complete removal of the tumor is indicated when possible. Surgical lymph node staging is mandatory and regional lymphadenectomy is advised in all patients with positive nodes or atypical carcinoids.

Endoscopic Resection

Endoscopic removal of carcinoid tumors was a frequent mode of treatment before the advent of modern techniques in surgery, anesthesia, and postoperative care, which has permitted removal of pulmonary tissue with low morbidity and mortality. Because most of these tumors are also extralumi-

nal, and frequently only a small part of the tumor is visible and accessible to the rigid bronchoscope, incomplete removal with recurrence was common. The highly vascular connective tissue within the tumor made this mode of therapy fraught with dangers, including exsanguinating hemorrhage. Personne (1986) and Diaz-Jimenez (1990) and their colleagues reported that the advent of the neodymium: yttrium-aluminum-garnet (Nd:YAG) laser has reduced the risk of hemorrhage in endoscopic removal of these tumors by photocoagulation. This technique is not recommended as the primary form of treatment of carcinoids, however, because local recurrence is inevitable, except for the rare occasion when a polypoid tumor, easily accessible, is on a narrow, uninvolved stalk (Fig. 109-11). Sutedja and associates (1995) described 11 patients with endobronchial carcinoids treated endoscopically by Nd:YAG laser plus photodynamic therapy or mechanical removal. In six patients, subsequent resection demonstrated no residual tumor, and in five patients, not surgically treated, follow-up between 27 and 246 months demonstrated no sign of recurrence. Van Boxem and colleagues (1998) of Sutedja's group have attempted to better define the role of endoscopic treatment of intraluminal typical carcinoid tumors by a prospective study. Only patients who met the criteria of accessibility of the tumor by fiberoptic bronchoscopy and, more important, the absence of any signs of bronchial wall infiltration on high-resolution CT scan and the absence of any enlarged lymph nodes were included in the study. Endoscopic resection was carried out by the use of Nd:YAG laser or bronchoscopic electrocautery. Complete response was obtained in 14 of 19 patients. In the five patients who did not respond completely, the distal margin of the tumor could not be determined because of its location in a segmental bronchus. Thus, they now believe that patients in whom the distal margin cannot be adequately visualized are not candidates for this type of therapy. Furthermore, they suggested that when subsequent resection was required in such patients, a less extensive procedure could be performed after preoperative bronchoscopic treatment. Although additional experience must be reported before this therapeutic approach is fully accepted, it appears that in a highly selected subset of patients, definitive endoscopic therapy is possible. Before definitive thoracotomy, these techniques can be helpful in relieving distal obstructive symptoms and controlling infection.

When thoracotomy is contraindicated for other reasons, transbronchoscopic removal of the tumor may be warranted to alleviate bronchial obstruction and perhaps to provide long-term asymptomatic management. The use of Nd:YAG, photodynamic laser therapy, or electrocautery may well augment this approach.

Surgical Resectional Therapy

Keeping in mind the locally invasive nature of this tumor, complete removal with preservation of as much normal lung as possible is the goal of treatment. Destroyed, functionless lung tissue distal to the lesion should also be removed. The types of procedures performed in the Memorial Sloan-Kettering Cancer Center series are listed in Table 109-4. The high incidence of pneumonectomy reflects earlier management efforts in patients who now would commonly be treated by sleeve resection, when possible.

Surgical staging is a necessary adjunct to any thoracotomy. Biopsies of the lymph nodes located in the bronchopulmonary segment, lobar areas, and hilum should be performed. Frozen section analysis is required. In those patients who have nodal metastases, a more extensive cancer operation (with complete lymph-node dissection, including all accessible mediastinal lymph nodes) is required.

Table 109-4. Treatment of Carcinoid Tumors at Memorial Sloan-Kettering Cancer Center (101 Operations)

Procedure	No. of Patients
Pneumonectomy	14
Bilobectomy	9
Lobectomy (with sleeve resection)	52 (5)
Segmentectomy or wedge	15
Endobronchial resection (palliative)	6

Bronchotomy

Bronchotomy and simple wedge excision of the affected bronchial wall can be used on occasion. Polypoid tumors accessible by bronchotomy thus can be removed with the attached bronchial wall, ensuring a complete resection, in comparison to endoscopic removal. However, this simple bronchotomy approach is rarely applicable.

Sleeve Resection

Main stem bronchial tumors or, occasionally, tumors located in the bronchus intermedius, as Frist and associates (1987) described, can be removed by sleeve resection of the bronchus, preserving all pulmonary tissue. This technique is preferable to pneumonectomy or bilobectomy. On occasion, carinal resection is required, as reported by Stamatis and coworkers (1990).

Wedge Resection

Wedge resection is appropriate only in dealing with the occasional small peripheral, typical carcinoid tumor and should be accompanied by lymph node sampling and frozen section analysis of proximal (segmental and hilar) lymph nodes as well as the primary tumor to confirm that it is truly a typical carcinoid.

Segmental Resection

Segmental resection is the procedure of choice for selected tumors arising distal to the origin of the tertiary bronchi. For example, tumors originating in the orifice of the superior segment of the lower lobes can be treated by segmental resection combined with sleeve resection of the lower lobe bronchus, preserving all basal segments, assuming frozen section analysis reveals regional lymph nodes are uninvolved and bronchial resection margins are clear.

Lobectomy

Lobectomy, with or without a bronchoplastic procedure, is the most common operation because most tumors occur in or near the origins of the lobar bronchi. A concomitant sleeve resection of the main stem bronchus is required if the orifice of the lobar bronchus or the adjacent main stem bronchus is involved by tumor. Addition of the bronchoplastic procedure permits preservation of distal normal lung tissue that otherwise would have to be sacrificed and is preferable to pneumonectomy. In this regard, preoperative endoscopic removal of tumor can allow time for recovery of concomitant pneumonia and assessment of the reversibility of the damage to the distal lung parenchyma before definitive therapy.

Pneumonectomy

Since the advent of bronchoplastic procedures, pneumonectomy is rarely required in the treatment of this tumor. Only in the unusual instances of destruction of all lobes by a proximal tumor, or an unusually positioned tumor not permitting a sleeve resection, should pneumonectomy be considered.

When resecting these endobronchial lesions, the margin of the bronchial resection must be examined by frozen section at the time of operation. If microscopic tumor is found at the margin of resection, a more proximal resection is required. With typical carcinoids, a negative resection margin, only millimeters away from the tumor, is sufficient. Although some surgeons, such as Smith (1969) and some of my colleagues, including McCaughan and associates (1985), advocate a complete mediastinal node dissection in all patients because of the possibility of occult microscopic involvement, I prefer nodal staging by frozen section at the time of surgery. I only prefer the more extensive node dissection when an atypical carcinoid is present or nodal involvement is identified at frozen section analysis.

Radiation Therapy

Bronchial carcinoids are resistant to irradiation, so this type of therapy should not be considered the primary treatment when surgical resection can be performed. However, Baldwin and Grimes (1967) and others have reported cases of an inoperable lesion that responded to such treatment. Postoperative irradiation has been recommended for patients with atypical carcinoids and lymph node metastases when a complete surgical resection has not been accomplished or mediastinal lymph nodes are involved. The benefit of this treatment has not been documented, although in our own institution, as reported by Martini and colleagues (1994), only one local recurrence was seen in this group of patients treated with postoperative radiation therapy.

Chemotherapy

Combination chemotherapy similar to that used in small cell carcinoma, especially etoposide (VP-16) and cisplatin, has been effective in managing metastatic carcinoid tumors, although the response rate to this chemotherapy is not as high as that seen in small cell carcinoma, with only 50% or less of patients demonstrating a major response. Some authors advocate adjuvant chemotherapy for atypical carcinoids that have been associated with mediastinal nodal spread at the time of surgery, usually in combination with mediastinal radiation therapy. The value of this therapy has never been assessed.

Carcinoid Syndrome

Total removal of large primary tumors associated with the carcinoid syndrome ablates the symptoms of the syndrome. However, once hepatic metastases have occurred, the man-

agement of the syndrome can become more difficult. Karmy-Jones and Vallieres (1993) describe the successful use of a somatostatin analogue (octreotide) in preventing a carcinoid crisis at the time of resection of an active bronchial carcinoid tumor in a patient that had developed a carcinoid crisis after biopsying this tumor. These somatostatin analogues also have been demonstrated to be effective in treating patients with metastases suffering from the carcinoid syndrome.

PROGNOSIS

Carcinoid tumors grow slowly, and the natural history is prolonged. I have seen one patient with symptoms of 40 years duration without treatment, and a second patient, who refused surgical treatment, alive and well 20 years later.

Five-year survival rates after resection depend on the aggressiveness of the tumor. Almost all typical carcinoid tumors with or without lymph node metastases are cured by adequate surgical treatment. One should expect a 90% or greater 5-year survival rate in this group of patients, as Hurt and Bates (1984), Wilkins (1984), Brandt (1984), Okike (1976), Martensson (1987), Rea (1989), Harpole (1992), and Deschamps (1992) and their associates have reported. The Memorial Sloan-Kettering Cancer Center series confirms these excellent results.

Once lymph node metastases have occurred with typical carcinoids, complete excision with lymph node dissection still allows an excellent prognosis. In a series reported by Martini and colleagues (1994) involving 12 typical carcinoids with lymph node metastases (N1 or N2) the 5-year disease-free survival rate was 100%. One patient only had a recurrence after 8 years.

Atypical carcinoids, with their frequent incidence of lymph node and distant metastases, are associated with a lower 5-year, disease-free survival rate (no greater than 60%). Of 13 patients with atypical carcinoids with nodal involvement at our institution, the 5-year disease-free survival rate was only 57%, but 73% of all patients were still alive with lymph node dissection and postoperative radiation therapy; most patients in whom the carcinoid recurred had distant metastases only, with only one local recurrence identified. In this latter group of tumors, the role of postoperative adjuvant chemotherapy and irradiation has not been adequately assessed, although standard chemotherapy has yet to achieve greater than 50% response rate. More aggressive management (e.g., postoperative chemoradiation) is worthy of this study.

REFERENCES

Aguayo SM, et al: Brief report: Idiopathic diffuse hyperplasia of pulmonary neuroendocrine cells and airways disease. N Engl J Med 327:1285, 1992.

Arrigoni MG, Woolner LB, Bernatz TE: Atypical carcinoid tumors of the lung. J Thorac Cardiovasc Surg 64:413, 1972.

Baldwin JN, Grimes OF: Bronchial adenomas. Surg Gynecol Obstet *124*:813, 1967.

Bensch KG, Gordon GB, Miller LR: Electron microscopic and biochemical studies on the bronchial carcinoid tumour. Cancer *18*:592, 1965.

Bertelsen S, et al: Bronchial carcinoid tumours: a clinical pathologic study of 82 cases. Scand J Thorac Cardiovasc Surg *19*:105, 1985.

Brandt B, et al: Bronchial carcinoid tumours. Ann Thorac Surg *38*:63, 1984.

Cebelin MS: Melanocytic bronchial carcinoid tumor. Cancer *46*:1843, 1980.

Churg A: Tumors of the lungs. *In* Thurlbeck WM (ed): Pathology of the Lung. Stuttgart, Germany: Thieme Medical Publishers, 1988.

Cutz E, et al: Immunoperoxidase staining for serotonin, bombesin, calcitonin, and leu-n-enkephalin in pulmonary tumorlets, bronchial carcinoids, and oat cell carcinomas. Lab Invest *46*:16A, 1982.

D'Agati V, Perzin KA: Carcinoid tumorlets of the lung with metastases to a peribronchial lymph node: report of a case and review of the literature. Cancer *55*:2472, 1985.

de Herder WW, et al: Somatostatin receptor scintigraphy: its value in tumor localization in patients with Cushing's syndrome caused by ectopic corticotropin or corticotrypin-releasing hormone stimulation. Am J Med *96*:305, 1994.

Deschamps CR, et al: Bronchial carcinoid: effects of staging on late survival. Chest *102*:103s, 1992.

Dewey TM, Yeung H, Downey RJ: Localization of adrenocorticotropic hormone-producing pulmonary carcinoid by somatostatin receptor scintigraphy. J Thorac Cardiovasc Surg *112*:832, 1996.

Diaz-Jimenez JP, Canela-Cardona M, Maestre-Alcacer J: Nd Yag laser photo-resection of low-grade malignant tumors of the tracheobronchial tree. Chest *97*:920, 1990.

Donahue JK, Weichert RR, Ochsner JL: Bronchial adenoma. Ann Surg *167*:873, 1968.

Dresler CM, et al: Clinical-pathologic analysis of 40 patients with large cell neuroendocrine carcinoma of the lung. Ann Thorac Surg *63*:180, 1997.

Englebreth-Holm J: Benign bronchial adenomas. Acta Chir Scand *90*:383, 1944–1945.

Frist WH, et al: Bronchial sleeve resection with and without pulmonary resection. J Thorac Cardiovasc Surg *93*:350, 1987.

Gal AA, et al: Pigmented pulmonary carcinoid tumor. An immunohistochemical and ultrastructural study. Arch Pathol Lab Med *117*:832, 1993.

Ghadially FN, Block HJ: Oncocytic carcinoid of the lung. J Submicrosc Cytol Pathol *17*:435, 1985.

Gould VE, et al: Neuroendocrine components of the bronchopulmonary tract: hyperplasias, dysplasias, and neoplasms. Lab Invest *48*:519, 1983.

Grazer R, et al: Melanin-containing peripheral carcinoid of the lung. Am J Surg Pathol *6*:73, 1982.

Harpole DH Jr, et al: Bronchial carcinoid tumors: a retrospective analysis of 126 patients. Ann Thorac Surg *54*:50, 1992.

Hurt R, Bates M: Carcinoid tumours of the bronchus: a 33-year experience. Thorax *39*:617, 1984.

Karmy-Jones R, Vallieres E: Carcinoid crisis after biopsy of a bronchial carcinoid. Ann Thorac Surg *56*:1403, 1993.

Leong A S-Y, Meredith DJ: Clear cell tumors of the lung. *In* Corrin B (ed): Pathology of Lung Tumors. New York: Churchill Livingstone, 1997, p. 159.

Limper AH, et al: The Cushing's syndrome induced by bronchial carcinoid tumors. Ann Intern Med *117*:209, 1992.

Magid D, et al: Pulmonary carcinoid tumors. CT assessment. J Comput Assist Tomogr *13*:244, 1989.

Martensson H, et al: Bronchial carcinoid: an analysis of 91 cases. World J Surg *II*:356, 1987.

Martini N, et al: Treatment and prognosis in bronchial carcinoids involving regional lymph nodes. J Thorac Cardiovasc Surg. *107*:1, 1994.

Matte J, et al. Ectopic Cushing's syndrome and pulmonary carcinoid tumor identified by octreotide. Postgrad Med J *74*:l08, 1998.

McCaughan BC, Martini N, Bains MJ: Bronchial carcinoids: review of 124 cases. J Thorac Cardiovasc Surg *89*:8, 1985.

Miller M, Mark G, Kanarek D: Multiple peripheral pulmonary carcinoid and tumorlets of carcinoid type with restrictive and obstructive lung disease. Am J Med *65*:373, 1978.

Oberndorfer S: Karzinoide. Ergebnisse der allgemeinen Pathologie und pathologischen Anatomie des Menschen und der Tiere *13*:527, 1907.

Okike N, Bernatz P, Woolner LB: Carcinoid tumours of the lung. Ann Thorac Surg *22*:270, 1976.

Pass HI, et al: Management of the ectopic ACTH syndrome due to thoracic carcinoids. Ann Thorac Surg *50*:52, 1990.

Personne C, et al: Indications and technique for endoscopic laser resection in bronchology. J Thorac Cardiovasc Surg *91*:710, 1986.

Przygodzki RM, et al: Analysis of p53, K-ras-2, and C-raf-1 in pulmonary neuroendocrine tumors. Correlation with histological subtype and clinical outcome. Am J Pathol *148*:1531, l996.

Rea F, et al: Bronchial carcinoids: a review of 60 patients. Ann Thorac Surg *47*:412, 1989.

Reubi JC, et al: Detection of somatostatin receptors in surgical and percutaneous needle biopsy samples of carcinoids and islet cell carcinomas. Cancer Res *50*:5960, 1990.

Rozenman J, et al: Bronchial adenoma. Chest *92*:145, 1987.

Shrager JB, et al: Bronchopulmonary carcinoid tumors associated with Cushing's syndrome: a more aggressive variant of typical carcinoid. J Thorac Cardiovasc Surg *114*:367, 1997.

Smith RA: Bronchial carcinoid tumours. Thorax *24*:98, 1969.

Stamatis G, Freitag L, Greschuchna D: Limited and radical resection for tracheal and bronchopulmonary carcinoid tumors: report on 227 cases. Eur J Cardiothorac Surg *4*:527, 1990.

Sutedja G, Golding RP, Postmus PE: High resolution computed tomography in patients referred for intraluminal typical carcinoid: with curative intent. Eur Respir J *9*:1020, 1996.

Sutedja G, et al: Bronchoscopic therapy in patients with intraluminal typical bronchial carcinoid. Chest *107*:556, 1995.

Travis WD, et al: Survival analysis of 200 pulmonary neuroendocrine tumors with clarification of criteria for atypical carcinoid and its separation from typical carcinoids. Am J Surg Pathol *22*:934, 1988.

Van Boxem TJ, et al: Bronchoscopic treatment of intraluminal typical carcinoid: a pilot study. J Thorac Cardiovasc Surg *116*:402, 1998.

Von Albertini A: Patholisch-anatomisches Kurzreferat zum Thema Lungenkrebs. Schweiz Med Wochensch *81*:659, 1951.

Warren WH, et al: Neuroendocrine neoplasms of the bronchopulmonary tract. J Thorac Cardiovasc Surg *89*:819, 1985.

Whitwell F: Tumourlets of the lung. J Pathol *70*:529, 1955.

Wilkins EW, et al: A continuing clinical survey of adenomas of the tracheum bronchus in a general hospital. J Thorac Cardiovasc Surg *46*:279, 1963.

Wilkins EW, et al: Changing times and surgical management of bronchopulmonary carcinoid tumor. Ann Thorac Surg *38*:339, 1984.

READING REFERENCES

Davila DG, et al: Bronchial carcinoid tumors. Proc Mayo Clin *68*:795, 1993.

Kincaid-Smith P, Brossy J-J: A case of bronchial adenoma with liver metastasis. Thorax *11*:36, 1956.

Knott-Craig CJ, et al: Carcinoid disease of the heart: surgical management of ten patients. J Thorac Cardiovasc Surg *104*:475, 1992.

Ricci C, et al: Carcinoid syndrome in bronchial adenoma. Am J Surg *126*:671, 1973.

CHAPTER 110

Adenoid Cystic Carcinoma and Other Primary Salivary Gland–Type Tumors of the Lung

Richard S. D'Agostino and Ronald B. Ponn

The submucosal serous and mucous glands of the tracheo-bronchial tree are similar to those of the major and minor salivary glands and can give rise to morphologically and biologically analogous tumors. Adenoid cystic carcinoma, mucoepidermoid carcinoma, mixed tumors of salivary gland type, acinic cell carcinoma, and oncocytoma have been included with carcinoid tumors under the misleading rubric "bronchial adenomas." However, in contrast with true adenomas, adenoid cystic carcinoma, mucoepidermoid carcinoma, and acinic cell carcinoma are malignant lesions. Although their growth rate is often indolent, local invasion and lymph node metastases ultimately may occur, and, in some cases, biological behavior is aggressive. Mixed tumors and oncocytoma can behave in a benign or malignant fashion. These noncarcinoid, salivary gland–type tumors of the lung are uncommon and constitute less than 1% of all primary lung neoplasms.

ADENOID CYSTIC CARCINOMA

Adenoid cystic carcinoma, also called *cylindroma*, most often arises in the salivary glands. Less frequent primary sites include the lung, breast, skin, uterine cervix, esophagus, and prostate.

Pathology

The majority of pulmonary adenoid cystic carcinomas develop centrally in the trachea and major bronchi. These otherwise uncommon tumors account for 20 to 30% of all primary tracheal malignancies. Dalton and Gatling (1990) and Inoue and colleagues (1991), among others, reported instances of primary adenoid cystic carcinoma arising peripherally and suggested that this may be the case in approximately 10% of patients. Hatton and colleagues

(1993) reported a singular case of peripheral right upper lobe adenoid cystic carcinoma presenting with Pancoast syndrome. Peripheral lesions, however, are more likely to represent metastases from an extrathoracic primary site. In a review of their own experience and previously reported series, Goldstraw and associates (1976) noted local invasion in up to 29% of cases. Hematogenous metastases at the time of presentation are rarely encountered. However, Maziak and coworkers (1996) noted metachronous hematogenous metastases in 44% of their patients.

On macroscopic inspection, adenoid cystic carcinoma appears white, pink, or light tan and is either polypoid or annular. The overlying mucosa is usually intact, although ulceration may occur. Direct transluminal extension is the rule. Malignant submucosal and perineural infiltration is common and often extends a considerable distance proximally and distally from the main tumor mass (Fig. 110-1).

Adenoid cystic carcinomas are histologically similar regardless of their primary site. The following three patterns are recognized: cribriform, tubular, and solid. The cribriform or cylindromatous subtype is the classic finding (Fig. 110-2). Nests and columns of small rounded or polyhedral cells arranged in a sieve-like pattern surround gland-like spaces filled with periodic acid–Schiff (PAS)-positive material. The tubular pattern is defined by cords of polygonal cells containing central ducts that are separated from surrounding stroma. The solid or basaloid pattern is morphologically the least differentiated and consists of sheets of small cuboidal cells with prominent mitoses and occasional small clusters of larger polygonal cells. Nomori and associates (1988) found that tumors with solid elements are associated with an aggressive clinical course and found the appearance of distant metastases more often than other patterns. An individual tumor can display more than one pattern (Fig. 110-3).

By electron microscopy, Balazs (1986) showed that most tumors are dimorphous and contain both mature ductal cells and immature myoepithelial cells. A high proportion of

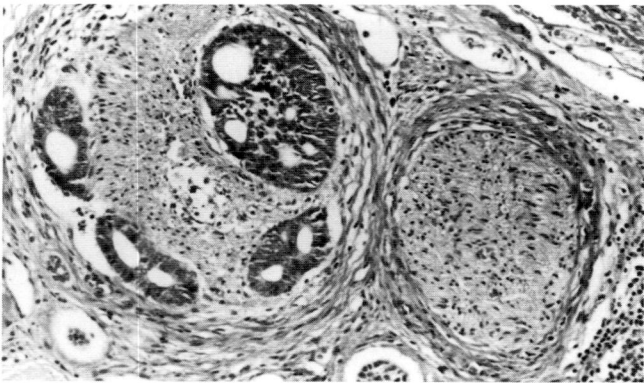

Fig. 110-1. Perineural infiltration of adenoid cystic carcinoma is characteristic of this tumor and is the route of extension toward the mediastinum. Courtesy of Darryl Carter.

immature elements correlated with increased infiltrative potential, whereas more circumscribed tumors had equal populations of ductal and myoepithelial cells. Moran (1995) noted that the immunohistochemical profile of adenoid cystic carcinoma is dominated by the myoepithelial cell proliferation. These tumor cells showed positive staining with both wide-spectrum and low-molecular-weight keratin as well as with vimentin and actin antibodies. Reactivity to S-100 protein has been variable. Staining for glial fibrillary acidic protein was uniformly negative. This latter finding can be used to distinguish adenoid cystic carcinoma from pleomorphic adenoma, a tumor that also has a prominent myoepithelial cell component. Although the histopathologic features of adenoid cystic carcinoma are usually distinctive enough to allow for definitive diagnosis by routine light microscopy, this tumor can be confused with adenocarcinoma, especially when faced with a small biopsy specimen. In such situations, the demonstration of a myoepithelial cell immunophenotype supports the diagnosis of adenoid cystic carcinoma.

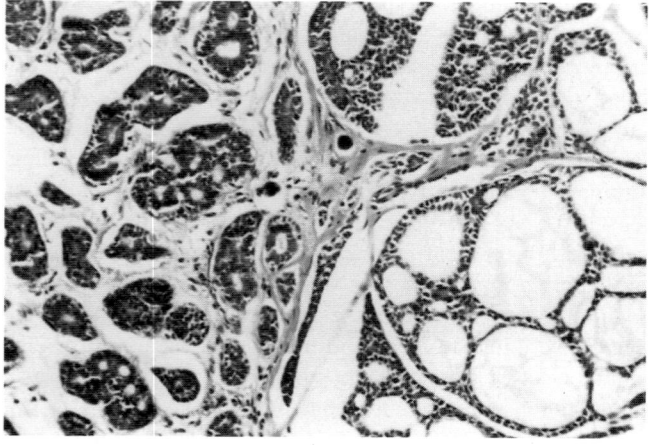

Fig. 110-2. Adenoid cystic carcinoma with the typical cribriform or cylindromatous pattern.

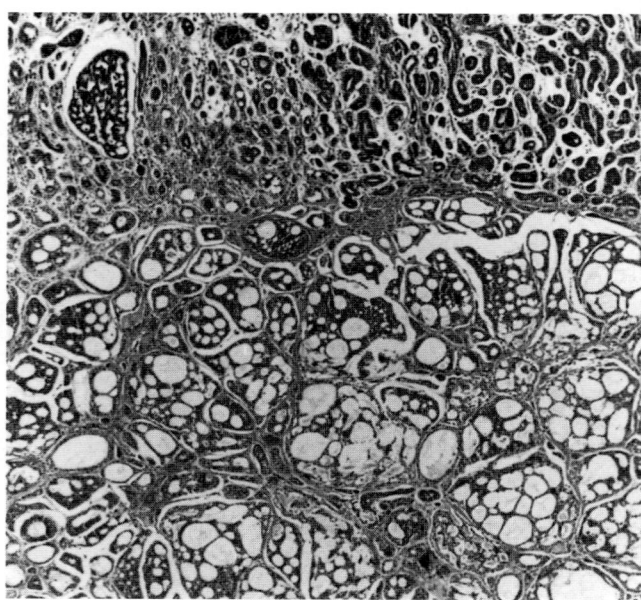

Fig. 110-3. Adenoid cystic carcinoma in the bronchial submucosa. The tumor is growing in a basaloid pattern beneath the intact ciliated epithelium. In the deeper zone, it displays the classic cribriform appearance.

Clinical Features

Adenoid cystic carcinoma typically occurs in patients aged 40 to 50 years, but it has been reported in persons ranging in age from 18 to 82 years. Men and women are affected equally. There is no known association with tobacco use or environmental toxins. Because they are located centrally and are often not apparent on chest radiographs, most tumors are detected only after they produce symptoms. Patients generally describe one or more of the following problems: cough, dyspnea, sputum production, hemoptysis, wheezing, or recurrent pneumonias. In some cases, significant tracheal or main bronchial obstruction occurs early and can be life-threatening. However, in many instances the intraluminal component is relatively small despite extensive submucosal and extraluminal spread. This pattern, coupled with typically slow growth, can produce an insidious presentation. An interval of several months to years may elapse between the onset of symptoms and the establishment of a diagnosis. Some patients are treated for prolonged periods for an erroneous diagnosis of asthma. The physical examination may demonstrate abnormal findings generally limited to the chest and include diminished or absent breath sounds because of complete obstruction of a lobe or an entire lung, a unilateral wheeze from partial blockage of a main bronchus, or stridor produced by tracheal involvement, but may be negative. Peripheral adenopathy and clubbing are not features of adenoid cystic carcinoma.

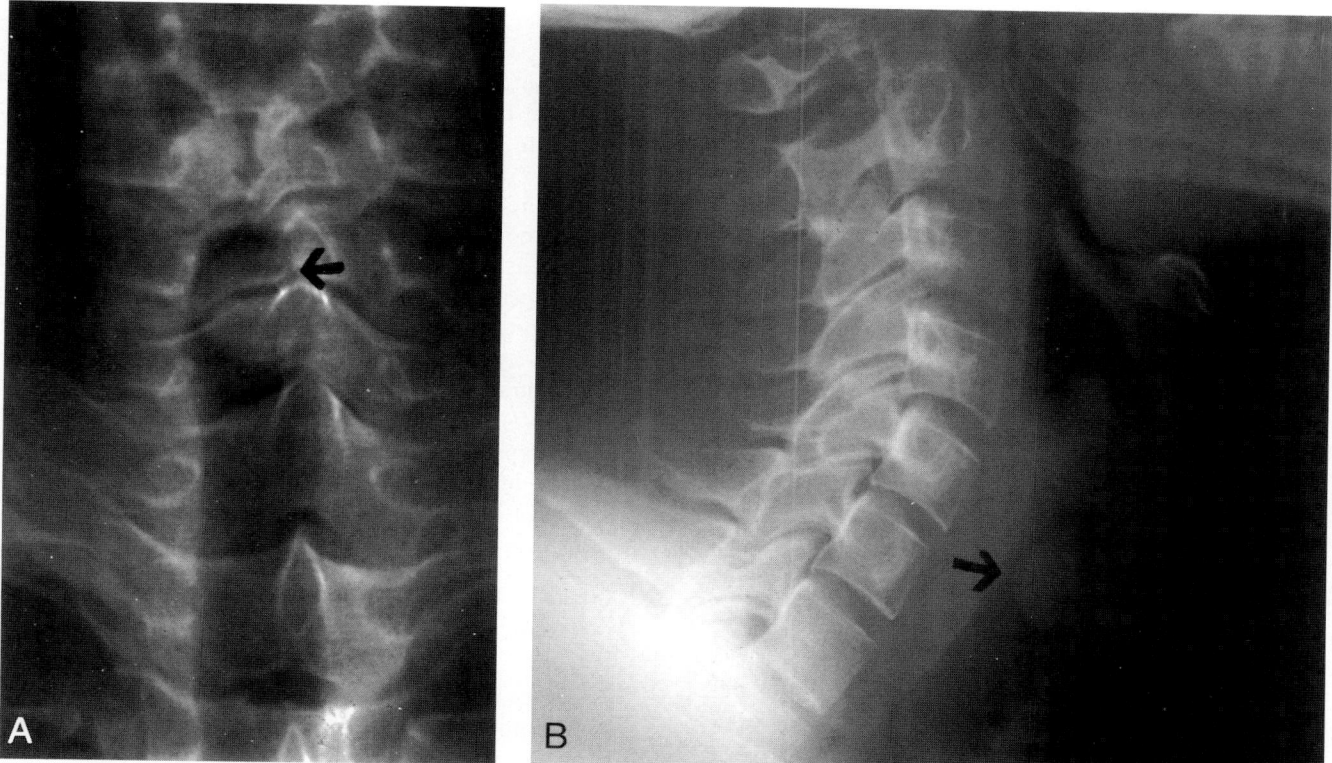

Fig. 110-4. Anteroposterior **(A)** and lateral **(B)** neck radiographs show an endotracheal mass (*arrows*). Biopsy confirmed adenoid cystic carcinoma.

Radiographic Features

The standard chest radiograph results may be normal, but often it shows atelectasis of a lobe or an entire lung. A hilar or mediastinal mass may be present. Subtle changes in airway contour occasionally are noted, particularly with lesions of the intrathoracic trachea. On the other hand, tumor masses in the cervical trachea are often easily appreciated on plain neck radiographs (Fig. 110-4). Spizarny (1986) and Wei (1990) and their colleagues showed that computed tomography (CT) scan accurately defines both intraluminal and transverse extraluminal tumor and is helpful in detecting metastases to the lung or pleura. As with other malignancies, the obliteration of fat planes is not a reliable predictor of local invasion. However, CT scan usually underestimates the longitudinal extent of airway involvement because of partial volume averaging and the tendency for submucosal tumor extension. Although rarely used, conventional tomography offers an excellent assessment of the intraluminal length of gross tumor because it yields images in the coronal and sagittal planes; it is inferior, however, for demonstrating extraluminal tumor mass (Fig. 110-5). Shanley and associates (1991) found magnetic resonance imaging, with its ability to image multiple anatomic

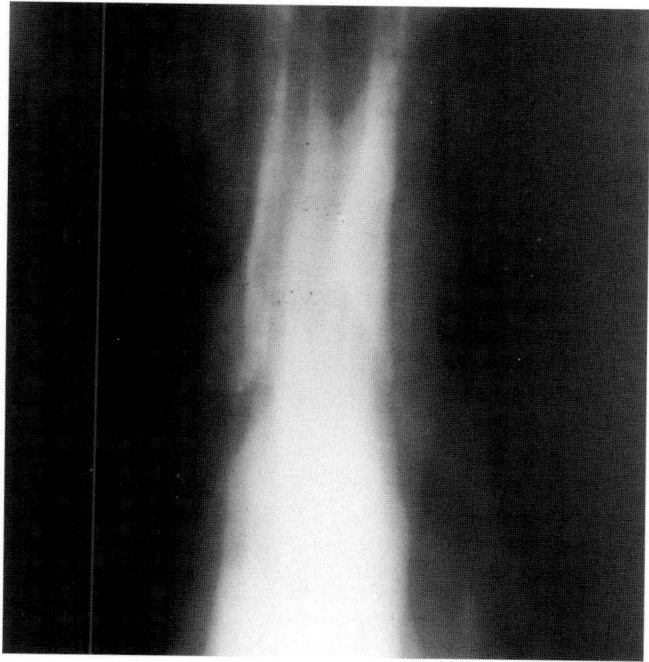

Fig. 110-5. Anteroposterior tomogram shows an adenoid cystic carcinoma involving the lateral wall of the distal trachea and right main stem bronchus.

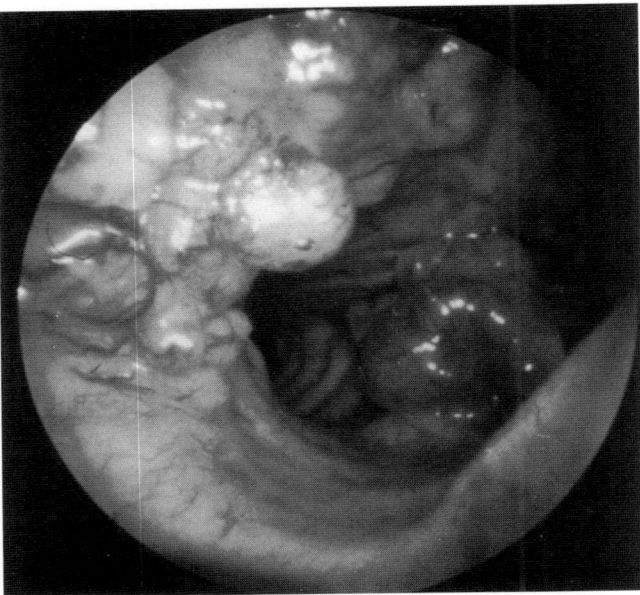

Fig. 110-6. Bronchoscopic view of an extensive polypoid adenoid cystic carcinoma of the distal trachea, the larger component of which obstructs the left bronchial orifice. Courtesy of John Beamis.

planes and to provide variably weighted images, superior to CT for delineating the extent of both submucosal infiltration and mediastinal involvement. In some cases, contrast esophograms may be helpful by showing esophageal compression or invasion.

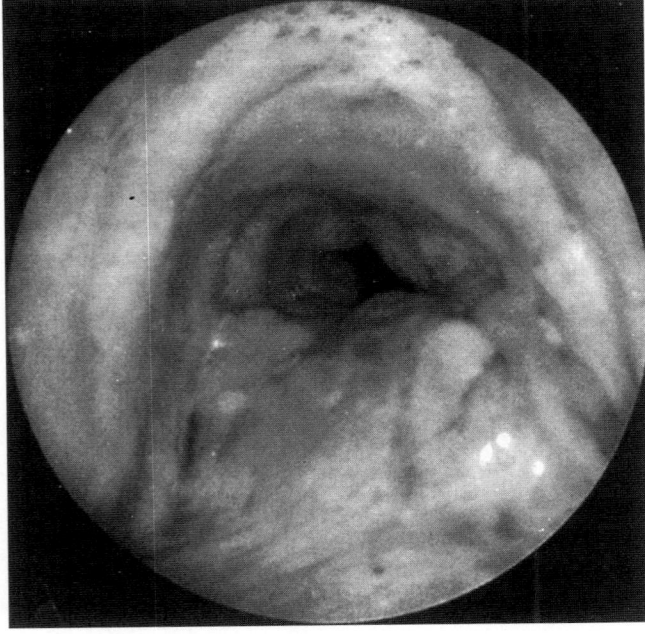

Fig. 110-7. Bronchoscopic appearance of an infiltrating adenoid cystic carcinoma causing distortion and partial obstruction of the distal trachea. Courtesy of John Beamis and Sergio Cavaliere.

Diagnosis

Because adenoid cystic carcinomas usually are covered by normal bronchial epithelium, cytologic examination of the sputum is generally unrewarding unless the overlying respiratory epithelium has been eroded. Except for the unusual circumstance of a peripherally situated lesion, these tumors are identified at bronchoscopy, and the diagnosis is established by transmucosal biopsy. The typical bronchoscopic appearance is that of a broad-based polypoidal mass partially or completely obstructing the airway (Fig. 110-6). Alternatively, the tumor may appear as a diffuse, submucosal infiltration causing luminal distortion and obstruction (Fig. 110-7). Although Attar and associates (1985), among others, reported substantial bleeding after biopsy of bronchial tumors in some patients, hemorrhage appears to be more of a problem with carcinoid and mucoepidermoid tumors than with adenoid cystic carcinomas.

Treatment

The treatment of choice is resection when feasible. It cannot be overemphasized that submucosal and perineural infiltration commonly extends beyond macroscopic tumor boundaries. Intraoperative frozen section examination of resection margins should be performed routinely as a method of ensuring adequate tumor clearance. Conlan and associates (1978) and Grillo and Mathisen (1990) found that tumor spread to hilar and mediastinal lymph nodes does not preclude long-term survival. In the case of adenoid cystic carcinoma of the trachea, Grillo and Mathisen stress that lymph nodes adjacent to the tumor should be resected and distant nodes sampled, but that extensive dissection should be avoided because it may jeopardize anastomotic healing. They also point out that, in some cases, one must accept a microscopically positive margin rather than extend the resection and produce tension on the suture line.

Tumors involving a lobar bronchus can often be managed with lobectomy, using bronchoplastic techniques where applicable. However, submucosal spread in the main stem bronchus may mandate a pneumonectomy. Extensive tracheal or carinal involvement present more complex situations. Maziak and colleagues (1996) noted carinal involvement in 13 of 38 patients. In such situations, the risks of resection must be considered carefully because nonresectional treatment methods can provide effective palliation for long periods. Perelman and Koroleva (1987) recommended preoperative transmucosal bronchoscopic biopsies at different levels above and below an obvious tumor as a guide to therapeutic planning. Pearson and associates (1984), Grillo and Mathisen (1990), and Perelman and Koroleva (1987) described their extensive experience with these situations. The techniques of bronchial sleeve lobectomy and tracheal and carinal resections are discussed in Chapters 28, 30, and 75.

Many patients with adenoid cystic carcinoma are not candidates for resection, and others are at high risk for postoperative local recurrence because of incomplete resection. Most adenoid cystic carcinomas are radiosensitive. Therefore, radiation therapy is the primary treatment for extensive inoperable cancers and for patients in whom resection carries an unacceptable risk. Fields and associates (1989) noted that in patients treated with radiation therapy alone, the rate of complete response was significantly related to a tumor dose of 6000 cGy or more. Conventional low linear energy transfer radiation therapy (photons or electrons) has also been applied as an adjunct to resection. Pearson and colleagues (1984) administered 3000 to 3500 cGy preoperatively. Patients with incomplete resection received additional treatment within 1 to 2 months of operation. Similarly, Perelman and Koroleva (1987) delivered preoperative and postresection irradiation in doses ranging from 3000 to 6500 cGy. Grillo and Mathisen (1990) referred most patients in their large series for postoperative irradiation (4500 to 6500 cGy) and noted a low incidence of local recurrence. However, it is worth noting that the results of treatment for incompletely resected or inoperable salivary gland adenoid cystic carcinoma with conventional radiotherapy have been suboptimal. Douglas and associates (1996), among others, have used high linear energy transfer forms of radiation, such as fast neutrons, for advanced or inoperable head and neck adenoid cystic carcinoma with an apparent two to threefold increase in locoregional control over conventional radiotherapy. Although Batterman and Mijnheer (1986), in an investigational trial of neutron radiation therapy for lung metastases of varying primary histologies, found one of the highest relative biological effectiveness ratios for adenoid cystic carcinoma, there has been no subsequent reported experience with this modality for primary pulmonary adenoid cystic carcinoma.

For many patients with unresectable or recurrent disease, tumor debulking by Nd:YAG laser ablation may provide satisfactory palliation. Diaz-Jimenez and colleagues (1990) reported laser treatment in five patients with unresectable adenoid cystic carcinoma causing tracheal and main stem bronchial obstructions of 75 to 90% of luminal diameter. One to two laser applications provided palliation for up to 33 months in four cases. The remaining patient was treated on multiple occasions over the course of 49 months before dying of hemoptysis. Brutinel and associates (1987) found that four of their eight patients treated with Nd:YAG laser were asymptomatic at 6 months, and Huber and coworkers (1986) reported a single patient treated with laser and radiation therapy who was symptom-free 1 year later. Treatment may be affected with either the fiberoptic or rigid bronchoscope, although the latter is favored by most clinicians because it allows easier tumor debulking by morcellation, rapid control of hemorrhage, and protection of the contralateral airway if so needed.

As reported by Personne and associates (1986), laser photocoagulation and radiation therapy are often used in combination for the palliation of symptoms related to adenoid cystic carcinoma. Laser ablation should be considered before radiation therapy in patients with critical proximal airway obstruction because irradiation in this setting may produce enough edema to cause asphyxia. Munsch and colleagues (1987) reported the dramatic case of a young woman with extensive unresectable tracheal involvement who developed life-threatening respiratory distress after the start of radiation therapy. Oxygenation was maintained by partial cardiopulmonary bypass during which time the tracheal tumor was sufficiently debulked through the rigid bronchoscope to allow tracheal stenting with a silicone prosthesis. Endoluminal brachytherapy is another method that appears to have a palliative role. Ryan and associates (1986) reported prolonged survival with combinations of Nd:YAG laser, external beam irradiation, and endobronchial brachytherapy. Chin and associates (1991) also reported a favorable result in a patient treated with laser and brachytherapy.

We are aware of no published data regarding the efficacy of systemic chemotherapy for pulmonary adenoid cystic carcinoma. Chemotherapy is used for the palliative treatment of salivary gland adenoid cystic carcinoma. However, since this tumor is generally slow-growing, the response rates are frequently disappointing. Methotrexate, cyclophosphamide, bleomycin, vincristine, cisplatin, 5-fluorouracil, adriamycin, and epirubicin have all shown some degree of activity when used as single agents. Dimery and colleagues (1990) and Licitra and associates (1996), among others, have reported the use of combination chemotherapy in salivary gland adenoid cystic carcinomas. The combination regimens have generally consisted of cyclophosphamide, doxorubicin, and cisplatin, with or without 5-fluorouracil. Objective response rates range from 18 to 40%, and the median duration of response is generally less than 12 months.

Prognosis

Because adenoid cystic carcinoma tends to grow slowly and recur locally, prolonged survival with persistent disease is not unusual. As noted, purely palliative therapy may offer long-term, symptom-free survival. Carter and Eggleston (1979) compiled the results of several studies including patients who were treated both definitively and palliatively and noted that the 5-year, 10-year, and 20-year survival rates were 85%, 55%, and 20%, respectively. Studies of patients who have undergone resection for central adenoid cystic carcinomas, often with adjuvant radiation therapy, document favorable results. Perelman and Koroleva (1987) reported a 66% survival rate at 5 years and a 56% survival rate at 15 years. Pearson and associates (1974) reported that 8 of 14 patients (57%) were free of recurrent tumor from 2 to 18 years after therapy. In an update of that experience, Maziak and associates (1996) reported a 79% 5-year and a 51% 10-year survival rate for 32 patients treated with primary resection. Twenty-six of these patients received adjuvant radiation therapy. These investigators found a statistically nonsignificant trend for increased 10-year survival rate in those patients who underwent complete resection—69% versus 39% for incomplete resection. Grillo and Mathisen (1990) reported that only 7 of 60 operated patients (12%) had died of their tumors during the 26-year study period and that 75% of those who survived operation were alive and tumor-free at varying postoperative intervals. However, local recurrence can occur many years after complete resection.

MUCOEPIDERMOID CARCINOMA

Mucoepidermoid carcinoma, first reported by Smetana and associates (1952), is an uncommon lesion that accounts for approximately 1% of primary malignant bronchial gland tumors and less than 0.2% of all lung neoplasms. It is morphologically similar to the mucoepidermoid tumor of the salivary glands.

Pathology

Like their salivary gland counterparts, bronchial mucoepidermoid carcinomas are classified as high grade or low grade on the basis of their histologic appearance. Most mucoepidermoid carcinomas arise beyond the carina, usually main stem bronchi, but occasionally in lobar or segmental airways. Unlike adenoid cystic carcinoma, tracheal involvement is uncommon. Most tumors appear grossly as intrabronchial polypoid masses without a significant extraluminal component. Penetration of the bronchial wall and a more infiltrative growth pattern are usually associated with the high-grade malignant tumors.

Histologically, mucoepidermoid carcinomas comprise varying mixtures of clear non–mucus-secreting columnar cells and mucus-rich goblet cells (Fig. 110-8), along with basaloid, transitional, and epidermoid cells. Although low-grade malignant tumors can have mixed cystic and solid histologic characteristics, the cystic component usually predominates. Microscopic invasion of the bronchial submucosa is common, but extension into pulmonary parenchyma is unusual. Although mild cytologic atypia can be seen, mitoses are rare. Metastasis to hilar or mediastinal lymph nodes is distinctly unusual.

High-grade tumors more commonly show areas of solid growth, but mixed solid and cystic or predominantly glandular growth can be seen (Fig. 110-9). Cellular atypia, mitotic activity, areas of necrosis, and abrupt transition from one cell type to another are characteristic. The high-grade variant of mucoepidermoid carcinoma occasionally can be difficult to distinguish from adenosquamous carcinoma of the lung. Klacsmann and colleagues (1979) proposed several criteria by which this differentiation can be made. The diagnostic confusion is compounded by infrequent reports, such as that of Barsky and associates (1983), of mucoepi-

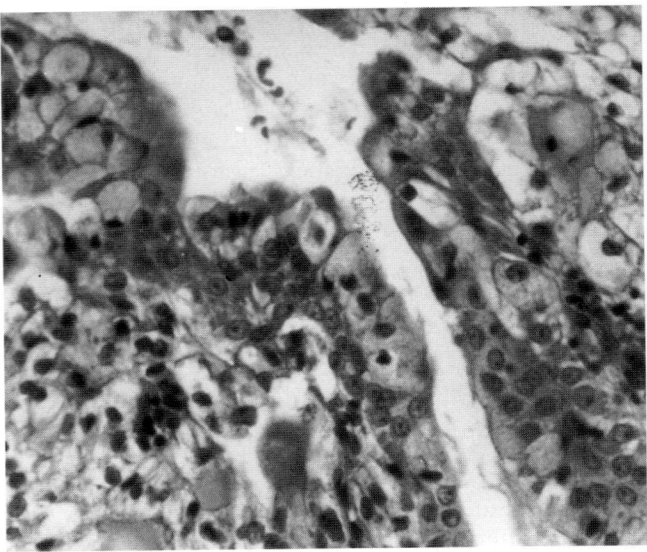

Fig. 110-8. High-power photomicrograph shows clear cells and mucin-secreting cells in a low-grade mucoepidermoid carcinoma. Courtesy of Irwin Nash.

dermoid tumors with low-grade histologic features that clinically behave in an aggressive fashion.

Clinical Features

Although Turnbull and colleagues (1971) reported that men are affected three times as frequently as women, other investigators have noted an equal dispersion among sexes.

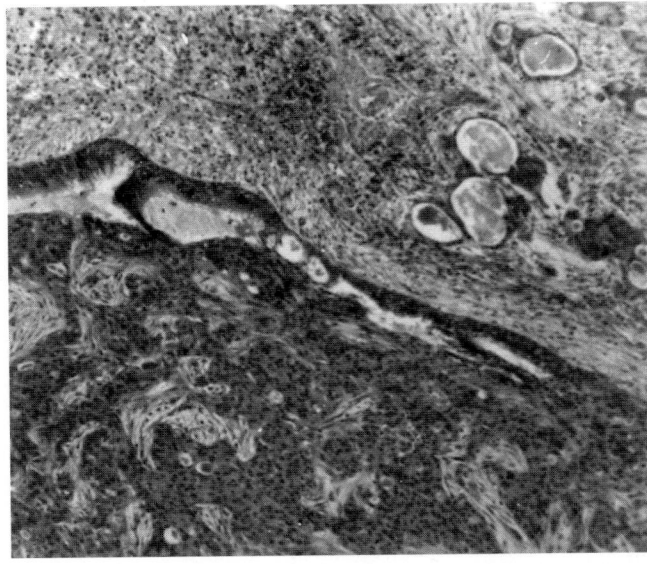

Fig. 110-9. Mucoepidermoid carcinoma consisting predominantly of solid nests of squamous cells with foci of glandular elements and mucin production (upper right).

The average age of patients is between 35 and 45 years, but patients as young as 6 years and as old as 75 years have been reported. Yousem and Hochholzer (1987) found that more than 50% of low-grade lesions occurred in patients younger than 30 years of age, whereas the majority of high-grade tumors were found in people older than 30 years. As with adenoid cystic carcinoma, there is no apparent relationship to tobacco use or exposure to environmental toxins.

Most patients present with cough, dyspnea, wheezing, hemoptysis, or obstructive pneumonia. The average duration of symptoms is between 8 and 18 months, but some individuals report symptoms for many years. An occasional patient is asymptomatic. The occurrence of pain, weight loss, or other constitutional symptoms suggests a more aggressive or disseminated tumor. The results of physical examination may be normal or signs of partial or total airway obstruction may be noted.

Radiographic Features

The radiographic appearance of mucoepidermoid carcinoma is similar to that described for adenoid cystic tumors. The chest radiograph results may be normal or may show signs of whole lung, lobar, or segmental obstruction with or without an associated proximal mass. A distinct intraluminal tumor, however, is generally identified by CT scan (Fig. 110-10), which may also demonstrate significant destruction of chronically obstructed parenchymal areas (Fig. 110-11). CT scan is also valuable for assessing local invasion and nodal metastases in cases of high-grade tumors. Mucoepidermoid carcinoma rarely presents as an isolated peripheral pulmonary nodule or mass.

Diagnosis

As with adenoid cystic tumors, the diagnosis of mucoepidermoid carcinoma is made most often by bronchoscopic

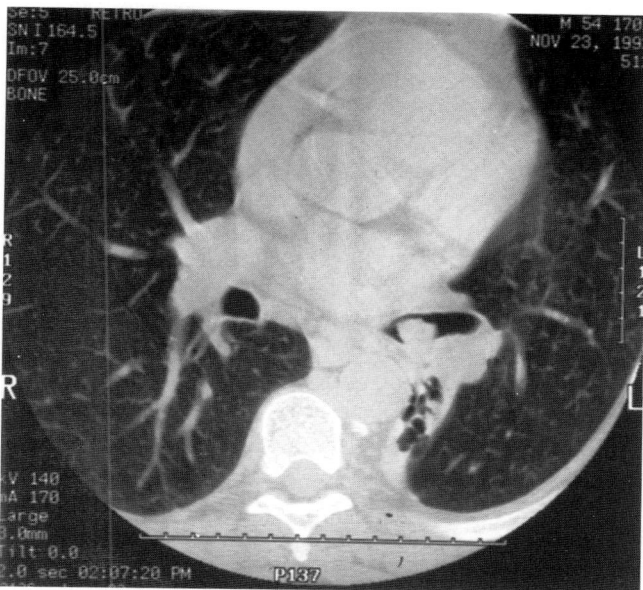

Fig. 110-11. Computed tomogram shows a polypoid mass arising from the left lower lobe bronchus and extending into but not invading the distal main stem bronchus. The lower lobe is destroyed and shrunken. Biopsy showed a mucoepidermoid carcinoma.

biopsy. The tumors appear as soft, well-demarcated polypoid masses and generally have a small base (Fig. 110-12). Conlan and associates (1978) reported hemorrhage following biopsy in two of 12 patients in their series, but neither required special measures for control. Because the overlying

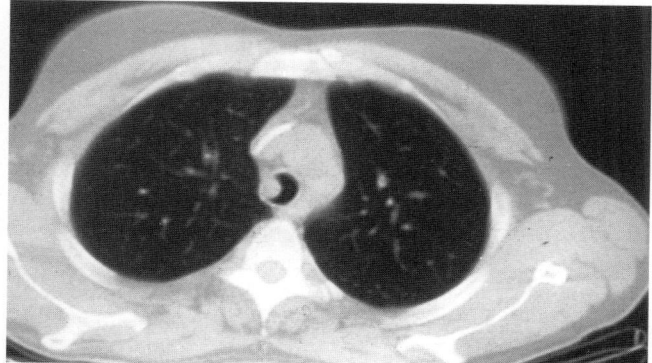

Fig. 110-10. Computed tomogram shows a well-circumscribed mass arising from the lateral tracheal wall with no apparent extraluminal component. Biopsy documented a low-grade mucoepidermoid carcinoma.

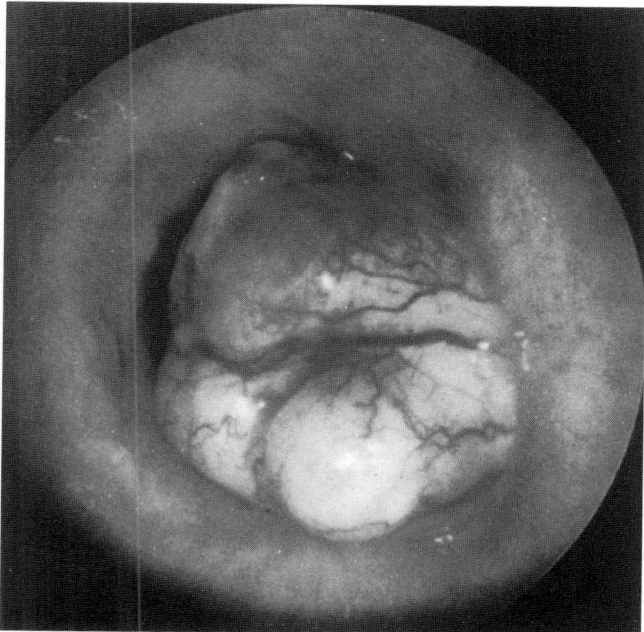

Fig. 110-12. Endoscopic view of a well-circumscribed polypoid mucoepidermoid carcinoma incompletely obstructing the left main stem bronchus.

mucosa is usually intact, sputum cytology results are negative in most cases.

Treatment

Most patients present with low-grade tumors that are either localized or minimally invasive. These lesions are best treated by complete resection, often using bronchoplastic techniques to conserve as much normal lung as possible. Hilar and mediastinal node sampling is also performed. Patients with the high-grade variant should be managed similarly, but they frequently have unresectable disease attributable to extensive local invasion. Occasionally, patients with low-grade tumors are found to have microscopically positive margins after resection. The management and ultimate fate of such patients is uncertain at this time. Heitmiller and associates (1989) have used reoperation and resection successfully in such instances.

The role of radiation therapy, either as the primary therapy or as preoperative or postoperative adjuvant treatment, is undefined. Turnbull and colleagues (1971), as well as Heitmiller and associates (1989), noted radiation therapy to be ineffective in altering the course of high-grade tumors. However, Leonardi and associates (1978) reported one patient who had sufficient regression of an endobronchial tumor after treatment with 3000 cGy to allow resection by pneumonectomy. As with adenoid cystic carcinoma, no data are available concerning the efficacy of chemotherapy. Endobronchial laser and brachytherapy should be considered for palliation of obstructive symptoms in some patients, but clinical experience with these methods in mucoepidermoid carcinoma is minimal.

Prognosis

Patients with low-grade tumors who undergo complete resection can be expected to be cured of their disease. In contrast, Turnbull (1971), Leonardi (1978), and Heitmiller (1989) and their associates all reported 100% mortality rates between 11 and 28 months in cases of high-grade mucoepidermoid carcinoma. The prognosis is intermediate for patients with low-grade tumors who have undergone operation but have microscopically involved bronchial resection margins. The role of adjuvant treatment in this group is unknown. Serial radiographic and bronchoscopic surveillance is indicated to detect local recurrence.

MIXED TUMOR OF SALIVARY GLAND TYPE

Mixed tumor of salivary gland type, also known as *pleomorphic adenoma*, is rarely encountered in the lung and tracheobronchial tree. Payne and associates (1965) were the first to report two cases of mixed tumors arising in bronchial glands. In a literature review, Moran (1995) could identify only 16 reported instances of this tumor. Patients range in age from 35 to 74 years, and there is no apparent gender predilection. Symptoms of bronchial obstruction such as cough, dyspnea, and wheezing are most common, but some patients have had fever, weight loss, and pleural effusion. Other patients are asymptomatic, and the lesion is discovered incidentally. Chest radiographs can show a pulmonary mass, post-obstructive atelectasis or pneumonitis, or an associated pleural effusion. Reported tumors have ranged in size from 2 to 16 cm. Macroscopically, these tumors are soft to rubbery in texture and have a gray-white myxoid appearance. Most parenchymal tumors are well circumscribed. Endobronchial tumors present as a polypoid mass with some degree of bronchial obstruction.

Histologically, these are biphasic neoplasms showing admixtures in varying proportions of epithelial and stromal elements. Moran and colleagues (1994) have identified three distinct histologic patterns: 1) the "classical" mixed tumor with prominent glandular component and chondromyxoid stroma, 2) the solid variant with few glandular structures and predominant solid sheets of myoepithelial cells set against a myxoid background, and 3) obvious cytologic features of malignancy with trabeculae of myoepithelial cells set in a prominent myxoid background. Immunohistochemically, these tumors react strongly with low-molecular-weight keratin antibodies and with antibodies against muscle-specific actin.

Because mixed tumors of the lung can be either benign or malignant, careful histopathologic evaluation is mandatory. The therapeutic goal is complete surgical resection. Most of the reported patients were treated with lobectomy, bilobectomy, or pneumonectomy. Patients with small circumscribed and completely resected lesions have done well. However, two reported patients with large poorly circumscribed masses and histologic features of malignancy have developed recurrent disease despite resection. For such patients the role of adjuvant therapy needs to be defined.

ACINIC CELL CARCINOMA

Fechner and coworkers (1972) were the first to report a primary pulmonary neoplasm that was histologically and ultrastructurally identical to acinic cell carcinomas arising in the salivary glands. Since then, only 14 other instances of this entity have been reported. These tumors usually occur in adults, but reported ages of patients range from 12 to 75 years. There is no apparent sex predilection. These lesions can present as an endobronchial or endotracheal mass or as a peripheral nodule and range in size between 1 and 4.5 cm. Presenting symptoms correspond to the size and location of the tumor. Endobronchial lesions produce symptoms of bronchial obstruction such as cough or wheezing. Peripheral lesions may be totally asymptomatic and discovered as incidental radiographic findings. Macroscopically, these tumors are usually well circumscribed, although not encapsulated, and tan-white or yellow in color.

Histologically, four different growth patterns are recognized: solid, acinar, microcystic, and papillary-cystic. Additionally, oncocytic, clear, and vacuolated cell populations are observed. In a detailed pathologic analysis of five pulmonary acinic cell carcinomas, Moran and colleagues (1992) found these lesions to stain positively with low-molecular-weight and broad-spectrum keratin antibodies as well as epithelial membrane antigen antibodies. Stains for vimentin, S-100 protein, chromogranin, and lysozyme were uniformly negative. Electron microscopy shows abundant zymogen-type cytoplasmic granules characteristic of acinar-type secretory cells. These ultrastructural and immunohistochemical characteristics can be of use in differentiating pulmonary acinic cell carcinomas from other morphologically similar primary and metastatic lung tumors.

Most reported cases have been managed by primary surgical resection including segmentectomy, lobectomy, bilobectomy, and tracheal resection. The results of treatment appear to be excellent because there have been no reported deaths from this lesion. Ansari and associates (1996) reported endoscopic laser tumor ablation to improve airway patency before tracheal resection. Horowitz and Kronenberg (1994) reported a case of tracheal acinic cell carcinoma removed through the bronchoscope with electrocauterization of the tumor base. This patient has been followed for 8 years without evidence of recurrence. Ukoha and colleagues (1999) have reported the only documented case of primary pulmonary acinic cell carcinoma metastatic to interlobar lymph nodes. Their patient was treated with lobectomy, mediastinal lymphadenectomy, and adjuvant radiation therapy and remained without recurrence 20 months postoperatively.

ONCOCYTOMA

Oncocytoma is the most infrequent of all salivary gland–type pulmonary neoplasms, and only a handful of cases have been documented. This tumor is composed of *oncocytes*, a descriptive term for epithelial cells with abundant granular eosinophilic cytoplasm and relatively small nuclei. A variety of organelles can impart an eosinophilic granular appearance to the cytoplasm by light microscopy, and a true oncocytoma is defined by the sole ultrastructural criterion of marked mitochondrial hyperplasia. The cause of the mitochondrial hyperplasia is unknown. Oncocytes are normally found in mature organs forming part of the lining epithelium of glandular ducts and acini. They have been found in the salivary glands, thyroid, buccal mucosa, breast, trachea, kidney, and gastrointestinal tract, as well as in other locations. According to Hamperl (1962), oncocytes represent a special metaplastic transformation of epithelial cells and their numbers increase in frequency with the advancing age of the individual. Tashiro and associates (1995) demonstrated immunoreactivity to cytokeratin and vimentin but

not to α-actin. Oncocytomas are different from oncocytic carcinoids, which demonstrate biphasic populations of oncocytic and carcinoid cells or the presence of neurosecretory granules by electron microscopy.

Fechner and Bentinck (1972) reported the first case of a true pulmonary oncocytoma confirmed by electron microscopy. Subsequent isolated instances of pulmonary oncocytoma have been reported by Santos-Briz and colleagues (1977), Fernandez and Nyssen (1982), Cwierzyk and associates (1985), and Tesluk and Dajee (1985). Patients range in age from 22 to 68 years, and most are men. The presenting symptoms have been cough, pneumonitis, or chest discomfort. One patient's tumor was discovered as an incidental radiographic finding. Chest radiographs can show a well-circumscribed parenchymal mass or an area of infiltrate distal to an obstructed bronchus. These tumors are yellowish tan or reddish brown in color. Patients were treated with local excision or with lobectomy, and there have been no reported instances of recurrence. Nielsen (1985) reported the only case of bronchial oncocytoma with an infiltrative growth pattern and a microscopic metastasis to a parabronchial lymph node. The patient underwent lobectomy and remained without recurrence 2 years later.

REFERENCES

Ansari MA, et al: Upper airway obstruction secondary to acinic cell carcinoma of the trachea: use of Nd:YAG laser. Chest *110*:1120, 1996.
Attar S, et al: Bronchial adenoma: a review of 51 patients. Ann Thorac Surg *40*:126, 1985.
Balazs M: Adenoid cystic (cylindromatous) carcinoma of the trachea: an ultrastructural study. Histopathology *10*:425, 1986.
Barsky SH, et al: "Low-grade" mucoepidermoid carcinoma of the bronchus with "high-grade" biological behavior. Cancer *51*:1505, 1983.
Batterman JJ, Mijnheer BJ: The Amsterdam fast neutron radiotherapy project: a final report. Int J Radiat Oncol Biol Phys *12*: 2093, 1986.
Brutinel WM, et al: A two-year experience with the neodymium-YAG laser in endobronchial obstruction. Chest *91*:159, 1987.
Carter D, Eggleston J: Fascicle 17. *In* Tumors of the Lower Respiratory Tract. Washington, DC: Armed Forces Institute of Pathology, 1979.
Chin HW, et al: Endobronchial adenoid cystic carcinoma. Chest *100*:1464, 1991.
Conlan AA, et al: Adenoid cystic carcinoma (cylindroma) and mucoepidermoid carcinoma of the bronchus—factors affecting survival. J Thorac Cardiovasc Surg *76*:369, 1978.
Cwierzyk TA, et al: Pulmonary Oncocytoma: report of a case with cytologic, histologic and electron microscopic study. Acta Cytol *29*:620, 1985.
Dalton L, Gatling RR: Peripheral adenoid cystic carcinoma of the lung. South Med J *83*:577, 1990.
Diaz-Jiminez JP, Canela-Cardona M, Maestre-Alcacer J: Nd:YAG laser photoresection of low-grade malignant tumors of the tracheobronchial tree. Chest *97*:920, 1990.
Dimery I, et al: Fluorouracil, doxorubicin, cyclophosphamide and cisplatin combination chemotherapy in advanced or recurrent salivary gland carcinoma. J Clin Oncol *8*:1056, 1990.
Douglas JG, et al: Neutron radiotherapy for adenoid cystic carcinoma of minor salivary glands. Int J Radiat Oncol Biol Phys *36*:87, 1996.
Fechner RE, Bentinck BA: Ultrastructure of bronchial oncocytoma. Cancer *31*:1451, 1973.
Fechner RE, Bentinck BA, Askew JB: Acinic cell tumor of the lung: A histologic and ultrastructural study. Cancer *29*:501, 1972.
Fernandez MA, Nyssen: Oncocytoma of the Lung. Can J Surg *25*:332, 1982.
Fields JN, Rigaud G, Emani BN: Primary tumors of the trachea. Results of radiation therapy. Cancer *63*:2429, 1989.

Goldstraw P, et al: The malignancy of bronchial adenoma. J Thorac Cardiovasc Surg 72:309, 1976.

Grillo HC, Mathisen DJ: Primary tracheal tumors: treatment and results. Ann Thorac Surg 49:69, 1990.

Hamperl H: Benign and malignant oncocytoma. Cancer 15:1019, 1962.

Hatton MQF, Allen MB, Cooke NJ: Pancoast syndrome: an unusual presentation of adenoid cystic carcinoma. Eur Respir J 6:271, 1993.

Heitmiller RF, et al: Mucoepidermoid lung tumors. Ann Thorac Surg 47:394, 1989.

Horowitz Z, Kronenberg J: Acinic cell carcinoma of the trachea. Auris Nasus Larynx 21:193, 1994.

Huber RM, et al: Adenoid cystic carcinoma masquerading as asthma: Resection by laser. J Respir Dis 69:195, 1986.

Inoue H, et al: Peripheral pulmonary adenoid cystic carcinoma with substantial submucosal extension to the proximal bronchus. Thorax 46:147, 1991.

Klacsmann PG, Olson JL, Eggleston JC: Mucoepidermoid carcinoma of the bronchus. Cancer 43:1720, 1979.

Leonardi HK, et al: Tracheobronchial mucoepidermoid carcinoma: Clinicopathological features and results of treatment. J Thorac Cardiovasc Surg 76:431, 1978.

Licitra L, et al: Cisplatin, doxorubicin and cyclophosphamide in advanced salivary gland carcinomas. Ann Oncol 7:640, 1996.

Maziak DE, et al: Adenoid cystic carcinoma of the airway: thirty-two-year experience. J Thorac Cardiovasc Surg 112:1522, 1996.

Moran CA: Primary salivary gland-type tumors of the lung. Semin Diagn Pathol 12(2):106, 1995.

Moran CA, Suster S, Koss MN: Acinic cell carcinoma of the lung ("Fechner tumor"): a clinicopathologic, immunohistochemical and ultrastructural study of five cases. Am J Surg Pathol 16:1039, 1992.

Moran CA, et al: Benign and malignant salivary gland-type mixed tumors of the lung: clinicopathologic and immunohistochemical study of eight cases. Cancer 73:2481, 1994.

Munsch C, Westaby S, Sturridge M: Urgent treatment for a nonresectable, asphyxiating tracheal cylindroma. Ann Thorac Surg 43:663, 1987.

Nielsen AL: Malignant bronchial oncocytoma: case report and review of the literature. Hum Pathol 16:852, 1985.

Nomori H, et al: Adenoid cystic carcinoma of the trachea and mainstem bronchus. J Thorac Cardiovasc Surg 96:271, 1988.

Payne WS, Schier J, Woolner LB: Mixed tumors of the bronchus (salivary gland type). J Thorac Cardiovasc Surg 49:663, 1965.

Pearson FG, Todd TRJ, Cooper JD: Experience with primary neoplasms of the trachea and carina. J Thorac Cardiovasc Surg 88:511, 1984.

Pearson FG, et al: Adenoid cystic carcinoma of the trachea. Ann Thorac Surg 18:16, 1974.

Perelman MI, Koroleva NS: Primary tumors of the trachea. In Grillo H, Eschapasse H (eds): International Trends in General Thoracic Surgery. Vol. 2. Philadelphia: WB Saunders, 1987.

Personne C, et al: Indications and technique for endoscopic laser resections in bronchology: a critical analysis based upon 2,284 resections. J Thorac Cardiovasc Surg 91:710, 1986.

Ryan KL, Lowy J, Harrell JH: Management of adenoid cystic carcinoma. Chest 89(Suppl):503, 1986.

Santos-Briz A, et al: Oncocytoma of the lung. Cancer 40:1330, 1977.

Shanley DJ, Daum-Kowalski R, Embry RL: Adenoid cystic carcinoma of the airway: MR findings. AJR Am J Roentgenol 156:1321, 1991.

Smetana HF, Iverson L, Swann LL: Bronchogenic carcinoma, an analysis of 100 autopsy cases. Milit Surg 111:335, 1952.

Spizarny DL, et al: CT of adenoid cystic carcinoma of the trachea. AJR Am J Roentgenol 146:1129, 1986.

Tashiro Y, et al: Pulmonary oncocytoma: report of a case in conjunction with an immunohistochemical and ultrastructural study. Pathol Int 45:448, 1995.

Tesluk H, Dajee A: Pulmonary Oncocytoma. J Surg Oncol 29:173, 1985.

Turnbull AD, et al: Mucoepidermoid tumors of bronchial glands. Cancer 28:539, 1971.

Ukoha OO, et al: Acinic cell carcinoma of the lung with metastasis to lymph nodes. Chest 115:591, 1999.

Wei L, Ellerbroek NA, Libshitz HI: Primary malignant tumors of the trachea: A radiologic and clinical study. Cancer 66:894, 1990.

Yousem SA, Hochholzer L: Mucoepidermoid tumors of the lung. Cancer 60:1346, 1987.

CHAPTER 111

Benign Tumors of the Lung

Thomas W. Shields and Philip G. Robinson

Benign tumors of the lung are infrequently encountered. Martini and Beattie (1983) reported that less than 1% of the lung tumors resected at Memorial Sloan-Kettering Hospital were benign. Benign tumors may be derived from all cell types present in the lung and may be parenchymal or endo-bronchial in location. A review by Kuda and associates (1990) of 35 benign tumors removed at the Kyushu Cancer Center revealed 23 hamartomas, four sclerosing hemangiomas, three benign mesotheliomas (solitary fibrous tumors), and one each of the following: plasma cell granuloma, fibroma, lipoma, and pseudolymphoma. The various lesions are listed in Table 111-1, which includes the common as well as the rare benign pulmonary tumors.

HAMARTOMA

The most common benign tumor is the hamartoma; Arrigoni and associates (1970) reported that hamartomas account for 77% of all benign tumors of the lungs. Bateson (1973) described this lesion as a benign true neoplasm of fibrous connective tissue of the bronchi encased by a passively included lining of respiratory epithelium. Most often, hamartomas contain cartilage (Fig. 111-1), and the tumor is frequently referred to as a *chondroma* or *chondromyxoid hamartoma*. Fatty tissue is also a frequent component.

Ninety percent of these lesions manifest as a solitary peripheral mass (Fig. 111-2A, B); Khouri and associates (1987) reported that hamartomas represent 4% of all solitary pulmonary nodules. Rarely, multiple lesions are observed as one of us (T.W.S.) encountered and as recorded by Bennett and associates (1985). The rare cystic pulmonary hamartoma has been reported in the literature at least nine times. A few of these reports were by Jackson (1956), Demos (1983), and Miura (1990) and their colleagues. The remaining 8 to 10% of all hamartomas are endobronchial lesions.

Hamartomas are most common in the middle-aged adult, although no age group is exempt. Arrigoni and associates (1970) reported that pulmonary hamartomas are observed twice as often in men as in women. Slow growth of the lesion may be observed (Fig. 111-2C, D), but the doubling time usually is well above that of malignant lesions (see Chapter 90). Hansen and colleagues (1992) reported the size of the hamartoma could increase by an average of 3.2 ± 2.6 mm/year.

Most patients with peripherally located lesions are asymptomatic. Only those few patients who have an endobronchial lesion have symptoms that include cough, hemoptysis, and, frequently, repeated or persistent pulmonary infection.

Radiographically, the peripheral lesion, most often located in the lower lung fields, appears as a smooth and well-circumscribed mass; at times, the margins appear lobulated or, more specifically, bosselated (Fig. 111-3). The usual size is 1 to 2 cm, but larger lesions occasionally are observed. Calcifications have been noted in 10 to 30% of these lesions. On computed tomographic (CT) examination, however, Ledor and associates (1981) found identifiable calcification in less than 5% of these tumors. When present, the calcification occurs most often in a diffuse or popcorn distribution. This calcification can be seen on a standard tomogram, but high-resolution CT scans may demonstrate it more readily (Fig. 111-4). Siegelman and colleagues (1984) also reported that fatty tissue was identified in 50% of the hamartomas evaluated by CT. Because of the fat content, the CT number (Hounsfield unit) is most often low and is generally of no diagnostic significance. The presence of a fat density identified by the CT scan (Fig. 111-5) in a peripheral solitary lesion, however, is strong presumptive evidence that the lesion is a benign hamartoma and excision can be deferred.

The endobronchial lesions per se are undetectable radiographically, except that distal parenchymal lung changes (e.g., atelectasis, obstructive pneumonia, or abscess formation) may suggest an obstructing, endobronchial lesion.

Bronchoscopy and biopsy are indicated in any patient with pulmonary symptoms: cough, hemoptysis, repeated pulmonary infection, or atelectasis. Endoscopy is not an essential diagnostic step in patients with a peripheral lesion.

Table 111-1. Benign Tumors of the Lung

Epithelial tumors
    Alveolar adenoma
    Mucinous cystadenoma
    Papillary adenoma of type II cells, Clara cell adenoma
    Salivary gland type
        Pleomorphic adenoma
        Mucous gland adenoma
        Myoepithelioma
    Squamous papilloma
Mesenchymal tumors
    Benign endobronchial fibrous histiocytoma
    Chondroma
    Fibroma (solitary fibrous tumor, localized fibrous mesothelioma)
    Fibrous polyp
    Glomus tumor
    Hamartoma
    Hemangioma
    Inflammatory pseudotumor (plasma cell granuloma, fibrous
        histiocytoma)
    Leiomyoma
    Lipoma
    Lymphatic lesions
    Meningioma
    Neurilemoma and neurofibroma
Miscellaneous tumors
    Granular cell tumor
    Pulmonary paraganglioma
    Nodular pulmonary amyloidosis
    Pulmonary hyalinizing granuloma
    Sclerosing hemangioma
    Sugar tumor (clear cell tumor)
    Teratoma
    Thymoma
Multiple tumors
    Benign metastasizing leiomyomas
    Pulmonary lymphangioleiomyomatosis
    Capillary hemangiomatosis
    Cystic fibrohistiocytic tumor (mesenchymal cystic hamartoma)

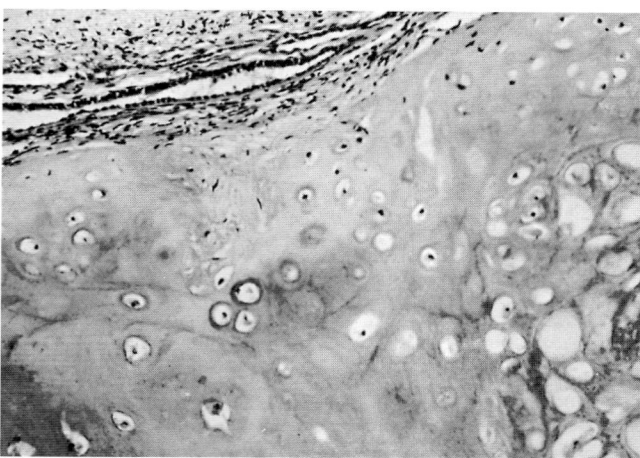

Fig. 111-1. Photomicrograph of a hamartoma. Note the predominance of cartilage cells.

Hamper and colleagues (1985) reported that percutaneous, transthoracic needle aspiration biopsy yields diagnostic information in 85% of hamartomas. Care must be taken when aspirating these peripheral lesions because of their firm consistency; the aforementioned authors reported a 50% incidence of postaspiration pneumothorax, which is twice the incidence after biopsy of other peripheral nodules. The histologic examination of the aspiration has higher diagnostic yield than cytologic examination of the aspirated specimen. One may suspect that the lesion is a hamartoma when fibromyxomatous tissue, which stains metachromatically with Giemsa or Wright's stain, and fragments of low columnar epithelium are present. When fragments of cartilage are present cytologically, the aspiration is diagnostic of a hamartoma. Cartilage is more often demonstrated by standard histologic examination of the aspirated material. Therefore, if the diagnosis of a hamartoma is suspected from the standard radiographic, tomographic, or CT studies but doubt still remains as to the diagnosis, a needle aspiration biopsy is indicated, particularly in a patient who is a poor candidate for a major operation. A positive result negates the necessity of a thoracotomy.

When the diagnosis is known in a patient with a peripherally located hamartoma, Nili and associates (1979) reported that the patient may be observed without surgical intervention. De Rooij and coworkers (1988) concur with this suggestion, but they do believe if the mass is larger than 2.5 cm it should be removed. We believe that clinical judgment should be the final determinant as to whether lesions larger than 2.5 cm should be removed. Minimal growth over time may be noted. Unless the growth rate becomes excessive, excision remains unnecessary. In a patient in whom the diagnosis has been established by histologic evaluation of a needle biopsy, the necessity of resection, except under unusual circumstances, can be questioned.

If a prethoracotomy diagnosis has not been made, thoracotomy and excision are indicated. The least possible amount of normal pulmonary tissue should be excised. At times, when a suspected hamartoma is palpated within the lung, the mass is readily moved and may be advanced to just beneath the visceral pleural surface. Incision of the pleura and enucleation of the mass can then be readily carried out. Any fixation of the mass within the parenchyma of the lung necessitates a standard resection (wedge resection), segmentectomy, or even at times a lobectomy. A pneumonectomy should be avoided if at all possible. Video-assisted thoracoscopic removal of small, peripherally located hamartomas is an acceptable approach. Recurrence after excision of a hamartoma is practically unknown. A second, separate primary hamartoma rarely occurs later.

When the hamartoma is endobronchial, a lobectomy or segmentectomy, as one of us (T.W.S.) and Lynn reported (1958), is most often required to remove the tumor as well as the chronically infected pulmonary parenchyma distal to the lesion.

Carney (1979) reported an infrequent association of a gastric epithelioid leiomyosarcoma, a functioning extra-adrenal paraganglioma, and a pulmonary hamartoma (chon-

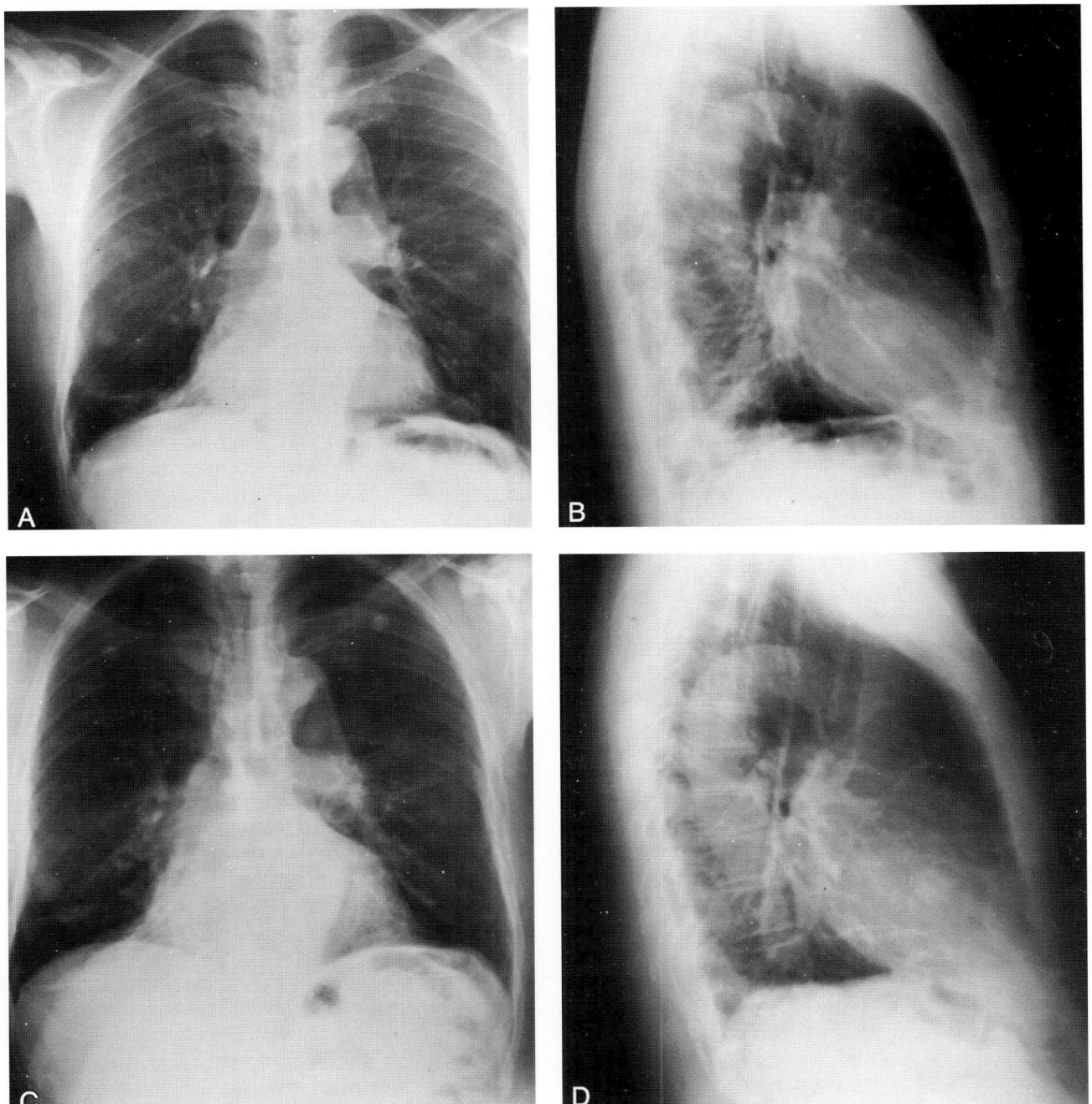

Fig. 111-2. Hamartoma demonstrated on posteroanterior (**A**) and lateral (**B**) radiographs of the chest, presenting as a peripheral mass in the middle lobe. Posteroanterior (**C**) and lateral (**D**) radiographs of the chest of the peripheral hamartoma show slow growth of the mass over a 4-year period.

droma) and suggested that this triad could be considered a syndrome (Carney's triad). Including his cases and those he found in the literature, 15 patients were identified who had two or more of these three lesions. All but one of the patients were young women who ranged in age from 9 to 24 years. In a follow-up publication, Carney (1983) stated that at the Mayo Clinic, the only pulmonary "chondromas" on file

were from these patients. The chest radiographs of these patients showed calcified and noncalcified nodules that could be solitary or multiple. In only 1 of his 24 patients was the pulmonary lesion the presenting manifestation. The most common presenting symptoms were from the gastric lesion and then the functioning extra-adrenal paraganglioma. The pulmonary chondromas were removed by enucleation or by

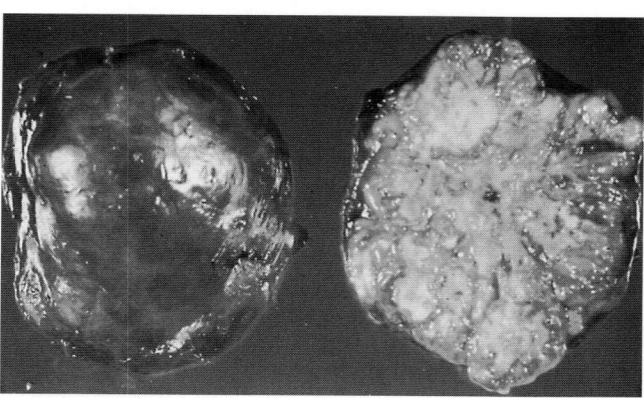

Fig. 111-3. Gross specimen of a resected hamartoma showing typical bosselated appearance.

segmental resection. On microscopic examination, the chondromas were composed mostly of cartilage and sometimes showed bone formation. The most mature bone and cartilage were at the periphery of the lesion, with the central part usually showing degenerative changes. Lancha (1994), Argos (1993), and Acha (1994) and their coworkers have all described additional cases of Carney's triad. Ribet and associates (1994) in a series of 65 patients with a hamartoma identified two patients with incomplete Carney's triad. The diagnostic and prognostic aspects of this triad were considered significant with regard to management and the long-term evaluation of young women with hamartomas.

There have been several reports of malignancy occurring in a hamartoma. Hayward and Carabasi (1967) presented a patient in whom an adenocarcinoma was believed to have

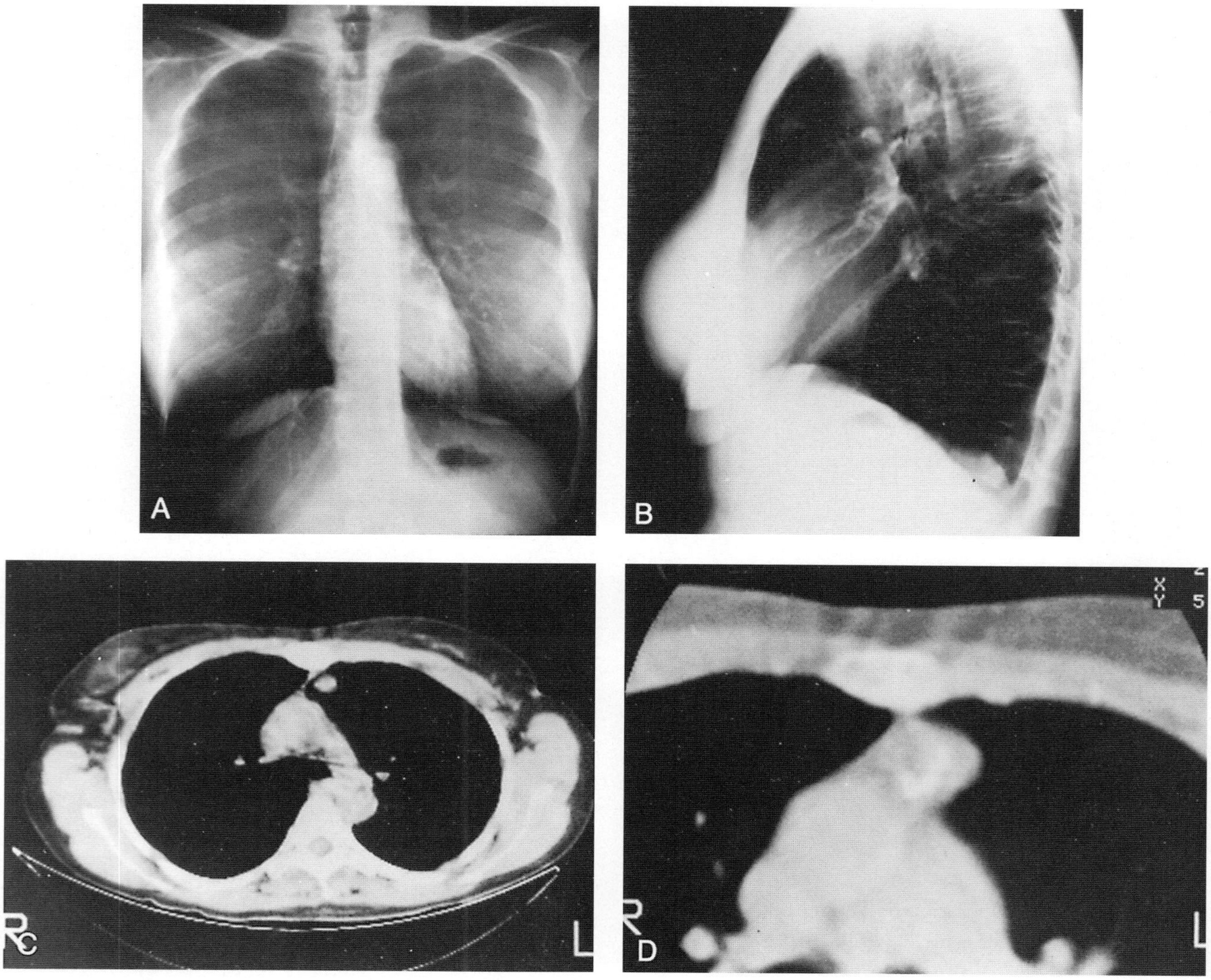

Fig. 111-4. A. Posteroanterior radiograph of calcified lesion overlying aortic knob on the left. **B.** Lateral radiograph shows the lesion to be in the anterior segment of the left lung. **C.** Computed tomographic scan shows calcification within the mass. **D.** Enhanced computed tomographic scan revealing popcornlike calcifications in the mass, typical of a hamartoma.

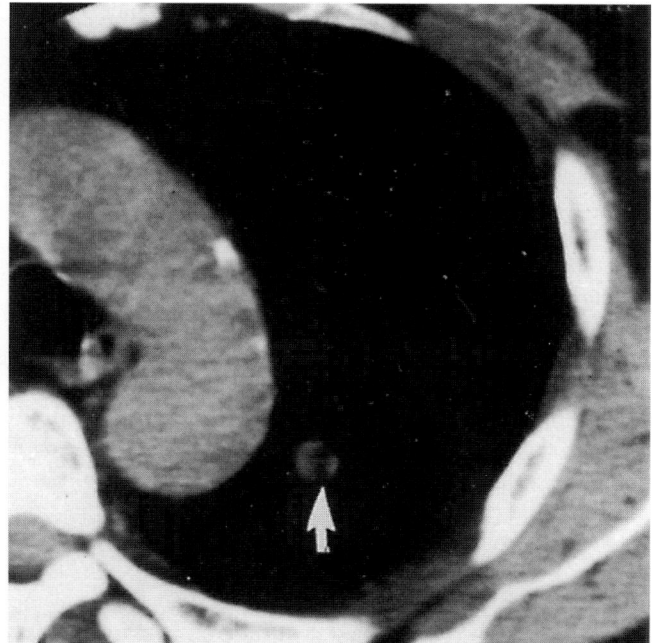

Fig. 111-5. Thin-section computed tomographic scan demonstrates a 1.0-cm pulmonary nodule with fat density material within (*arrow*). Lesion has the appearance consistent with a hamartoma. From Swensen SJ, et al: An integrated approach to evaluation of the solitary pulmonary nodule. Mayo Clin Proc 65:173, 1990. With permission.

developed from a hamartoma, and Basile and associates (1989) recorded a sarcoma that developed promptly at the site of a resected benign hamartoma. Neither of these events is convincing on close scrutiny, and no real evidence exists that either tumor actually arose from an underlying hamartoma. One may be as critical of these reports as were Hayward and Carabasi (1967) of the 12 cases of possible malignancy they reviewed in their own publication. However, of interest in this regard is the possible potential of malignant change. Okabayashi and colleagues (1993) reported a giant hamartoma associated with a high production of carbohydrate antigen 19-9. The significance of this is unknown, but the source of the antigen was demonstrated to be the epithelial component and not from the mesenchymal component. Further investigations such as those of Fletcher and coworkers (1991) might provide insight as to any possible malignant potential of these two components of this normally benign biphasic tumor.

Karasik and associates (1980) reported that a bronchial carcinoma (synchronous or metachronous) was identified 6.3 times more often in patients with a hamartoma than would be expected in the normal population. They suggested an etiologic relationship was present. Van den Bosch and colleagues (1987), however, who identified six synchronous and five metachronous bronchial carcinomas in a series of 154 patients with a hamartoma (an incidence of 7%) believed the association was essentially coincidental. In a more recent series of 65 patients with a hamartoma, Ribet

and associates (1994) recorded that three patients had an associated bronchial carcinoma, a 6.6-fold increase in the number of cases normally expected. These authors came to the same conclusion that there was an etiologic relationship present as had Karasik and colleagues (1980). However, in nine other series of a total of 598 patients with hamartomas, the rate of occurrence of a lung cancer was only 5.8%. The question of the nature of the relationship between these two lesions remains unresolved.

OTHER SOLITARY BENIGN TUMORS

Benign tumors of epithelial, mesenchymal, or lymphoid origin are rare. Many of these tumors may be either endobronchial or peripheral in location but generally have a greater predilection for one of the two locations. The symptomatology depends on whether a bronchus is irritated or a bronchial lumen is occluded partially or completely by an endobronchial lesion. The peripherally located tumors usually are asymptomatic.

Primarily Endobronchial Tumors

Benign Endobronchial Fibrous Histiocytoma

A fibrous histiocytoma is a benign lung tumor that is composed of collagen, inflammatory cells, and mesenchymal cells. It has been called by a variety of names, the most common of which are *inflammatory pseudotumor*, *plasma cell granuloma*, and *fibroxanthoma*. We have chosen to discuss the endobronchial lesion separately from the peripheral lesion (see Inflammatory Pseudotumor, later in this chapter).

Duncan and associates (1986) described a patient with endobronchial fibrous histiocytoma that revealed no clinical evidence of malignant behavior. This rare endobronchial lesion has been noted in at least 13 patients; one-third of whom were children. The other patients were generally young adults. Tagge and coworkers (1991) described two cases of this lesion and they advocated a combination of tumor resection with lavage and selective ventilation to salvage the distal lung as an alternative to pneumonectomy, even if the lung appears to be unsalvageable. Aisner and colleagues (1995) suggested that a wide local excision (i.e., a lobectomy or a bronchial sleeve lobectomy) should be carried out because of the low-grade malignant potential of these tumors. Bueno and coworkers (1996) at the Massachusetts General Hospital concur with this approach and have carried out bronchoplastic resections of five endobronchial fibrous histiocytomas.

Fibrous Polyps and Squamous Papillomas

Drennan and Douglas (1965) divided bronchial papillomas into three groups: 1) multiple papillomatosis, 2) inflammatory polyps, and 3) solitary papilloma. Multiple papillomatosis is usually a disease of children in which the patients develop multiple papillomas of the vocal cords and trachea. These papillomas are thought to be caused by the human papilloma virus. This lesion is discussed in Chapter 77.

Fibrous polyps are in the second group and they can be solitary or multiple. They are polypoid areas of bronchial mucosa that have a fibrous stalk and are covered by ciliated columnar epithelium with possible areas of squamous metaplasia. The stalk is usually composed of loose connective tissue with capillaries and an infiltrate of plasma cells, lymphocytes, and eosinophils. These polyps are thought to be secondary to a chronic inflammatory process. They are always benign, but they may cause bronchial obstruction. Arguelles and Blanco (1983) described an asthmatic, 10-year-old boy who had multiple bronchial polyps.

Solitary squamous papillomas are in the third group. They are defined as a benign neoplasm of squamous epithelium. Histologically, they have a thin central fibrovascular core that is covered by stratified squamous epithelium and they form multiple papillary fronds. They occur in adults as solitary lesions rather than the multiple lesions seen in children, although adults may have multiple lesions. Miura (1993) and Popper (1994) and their colleagues, as well as Katial and associates (1994), have all reviewed cases of bronchial squamous papillomas. The patients range in age from 22 to 85 years, with men being affected more commonly than women. The most common symptom is cough, but patients may have hemoptysis as well as symptoms secondary to obstruction. Chest radiography may show a lesion or atelectasis. The papillomas are usually located in segmental or more proximal bronchi. They do not have a predilection for either the right or left lung. The human papilloma virus is probably the cause for most of these lesions. Popper and colleagues (1994) demonstrated that human papilloma virus types 11 and 6 were associated with benign papillomas, whereas types 16 or 18, sometimes in combination with type 31, 33, or 35, were found in papillomas of patients who developed squamous cell carcinoma.

Miura and colleagues (1993) pointed out that treatment should be conservative but patients may require further surgery if they develop a malignancy. They suggested that if the lesion is limited to a small area it could be treated with photodynamic therapy, yttrium-aluminum-garnet laser, or both; these patients should be followed. These aforementioned lesions are usually removed endoscopically, or occasionally, a bronchotomy or sleeve resection may be necessary. When irreversible parenchymal damage distal to the lesion is present, surgical resection of the destroyed lung tissue also is required.

Granular Cell Tumors (Myoblastoma)

Granular cell tumors are rare, benign tumors that used to be called *granular cell myoblastomas*, because they were thought to be derived from skeletal muscle. Fisher and Wechsler (1962) were among the first investigators to suggest these tumors are of Schwann cell origin. Oparah and Subramanian (1976) and Lui and associates (1989) reviewed the features of the endobronchial granular cell tumors. Deavers (1995) and coworkers reviewed a series of 20 cases. The patients ranged in age from 20 to 57 years and were evenly divided between men and women. In approximately one-half of the patients, the tumors were incidental findings. The other patients had symptoms secondary to obstruction, which included postobstructive pneumonia and atelectasis. A few patients had hemoptysis. The chest radiographs showed lobar infiltration, coin lesions, and lobar atelectasis. Some patients had findings caused by other diseases. Solitary lesions were present in 75% of the patients. Multiple pulmonary lesions were present in 10% (two patients). Three other patients (15%) had a solitary pulmonary lesion in addition to the presence of multiple skin tumors.

On gross examination, the tumors ranged in size from 0.3 to 5.0 cm. They are usually located in an endobronchial position in a large bronchus but occasionally may occur in the pulmonary parenchyma. The cut surfaces of the tumor may be tan-white, pink, or yellow. They are usually circumscribed, but not encapsulated. On microscopic examination, the tumors are composed of large cells with an abundant pink granular cytoplasm. The treatment is conservative resection. Complete resection is curative, although these tumors may recur. Asymptomatic patients may be followed. Epstein and Mohsenifar (1993) used neodymium:yttrium-aluminum-garnet laser to treat an obstructing granular cell tumor and suggested this might be an effective tool for treating these cases in certain instances. Surgical resection of the tumor and any associated damaged lung tissue may be required.

Mucous Gland Adenomas

Mucous gland adenoma, also known as *bronchial cyst adenoma*, is a benign tumor of the bronchus that is derived from the mucous glands of the bronchus. The tumor must be composed of cystic glands, be above the cartilaginous plate, be in the bronchus, and have some normal bronchial seromucous glands. It is rare and has been described by Weinberger (1955), Gilman (1956), Weiss (1961), Kroe (1967), and Emory (1973) and their associates, as well as by Edwards and Matthews (1981). England and Hochholzer (1995) reported another 10 cases and reviewed the subject. Their patients ranged in age from 25 to 67 years, with a mean of 52 years. Historically, this lesion tends to occur twice as often in men as in women, but these authors found only a slight predominance of women. The symptoms are cough, fever, recurrent pneumonia, and hemoptysis. The chest radiograph may also show obstructive pneumonitis, postobstructive atelectasis, and on rare occasions, a coin lesion. The lesion occurs equally between the right and left sides, and more often is found in the major bronchi of the middle and lower lobes. On gross examination, the tumors varied in size from 0.8 to 6.8 cm, with a mean of 1.8 cm. The

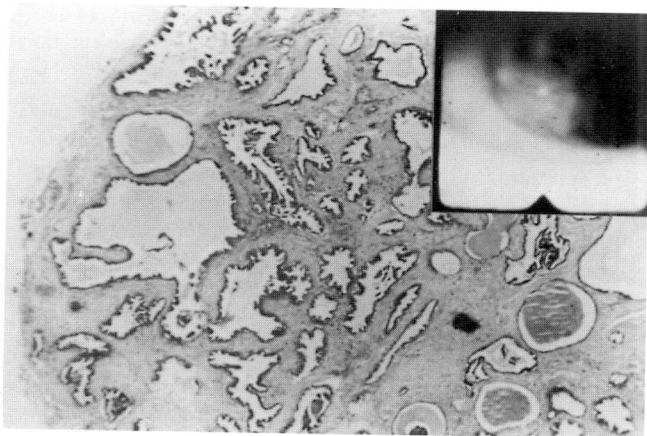

Fig. 111-6. Low-power photomicrograph of a mucous gland adenoma. Inset shows the endoscopic appearance (upper right).

tumors projected into the lumen of the bronchus. They were usually encapsulated by a thin membrane and easily separated from the bronchus. The cut surface is cystic with mucus within the cystic space.

Endoscopically, they appear as firm pink masses with intact overlying epithelium (Fig. 111-6). Histologically, they are composed of numerous small mucus-filled cysts lined by well-differentiated mucous epithelium (Fig. 111-7). The major differential diagnosis is low-grade mucoepidermoid carcinoma. Even though these lesions rarely have a stalk, they can be completely removed endoscopically by curettage, cryotherapy, or laser ablation, as reported by Ishida and colleagues (1996). Thoracotomy and surgical resection is indicated only when distal lung has been destroyed or endoscopic removal is contraindicated or incomplete. Complete removal of these tumors endoscopically or surgically results in a permanent cure.

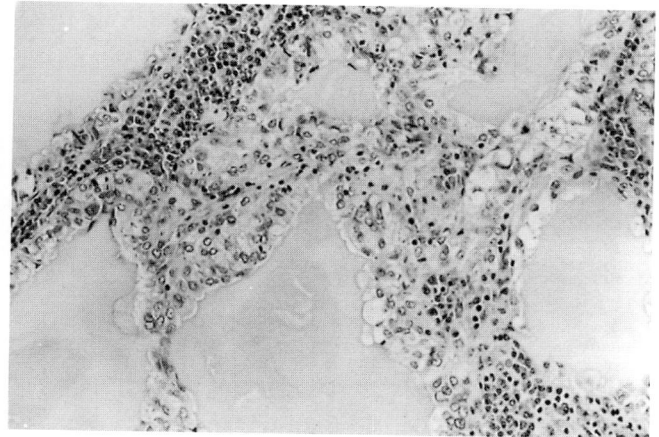

Fig. 111-7. High-power photomicrograph of a mucous gland adenoma consisting of cysts of various diameters lined by columnar mucous cells. A chronic inflammatory reaction separates the tubules.

Lipoma

Lipomas arise most often from the wall of the tracheobronchial tree (80%). The lesion is more common in men than in women. Local resection by bronchotomy or sleeve resection should be done whenever possible if the parenchyma distal to the lesion is normal. They may cause obstruction with pulmonary complications. Bango (1993) and Yokozaki (1996) and their colleagues have urged CT examination to determine the extent of pulmonary involvement. They also suggest bronchoscopic laser vaporization of the tumor as the treatment of choice.

Primarily Benign Parenchymal Tumors

Myoepithelioma

Myoepithelial cells are flat cells that lie between the epithelial cells of a gland and the basement membrane. They are usually found in the salivary glands and are thought to have contractile properties. Myoepitheliomas are benign tumors of these cells that are usually found in the salivary glands or the breast. Strickler (1987) and Tsuji (1995) and their coworkers have described this tumor in the lung. In both instances, the patients were men in their 60s with a mass on chest radiography; one was discovered incidentally. On gross examination, one lesion was 3.3 cm and the other was 16 cm. Both had well-demarcated margins with tan-yellow-white surfaces. On microscopic examination, both tumors were composed of spindle-shaped cells, but the patient reported by Tsuji and coworkers (1995) also showed areas composed of polygonal cells and others with papillary features and a two-cell layer. In both cases the cells immunostained for S-100, which is consistent with a myoepithelioma, and also demonstrated the presence of smooth muscle actin; the tumor also had a glandular component that stained with epithelial membrane antigen and carcinoembryonic antigen. In view of this admixture of cells, the authors called the tumor an *adenomyoepithelioma*. On electron microscopy, Strickler and associates (1987) were able to demonstrate myofilaments, but Tsuji and coworkers (1995) could not. Both groups concluded that the tumors were of myoepithelial origin. The patients were followed for 1 to 3 years without evidence of recurrence. Surgery appears to be curative, but clinical follow-up is advised.

Mucinous Cystadenoma

According to Colby and colleagues (1995) a mucinous cystadenoma is a "unilocular cystic lesion whose fibrous wall is lined by well-differentiated, presumably benign columnar mucinous epithelium." This lesion was first described by Sambrook Gowar (1978) and later by Dail and Hammar (1988). Kragel (1990), Dixon (1993), and Roux

(1995) and their colleagues, as well as Graeme-Cook and Mark (1991), have further described this entity. These lesions occur in both men and women, who are usually in their 50s and 60s and are smokers. Most of these tumors are discovered as an asymptomatic mass on routine chest radiography. The mass is usually located at or toward the periphery of the lung.

On gross examination, the mass is a unilocular cyst filled with clear gelatinous material. On microscopic examination, a fibrous cyst wall is lined by mucinous epithelium. Occasionally, the wall is thinned and the mucin extravasates into the adjacent pulmonary parenchyma. The cysts should be examined completely, because they may have areas of borderline malignancy or adenocarcinoma. The differential diagnosis ranges from bronchogenic cysts to bronchoalveolar carcinoma. The treatment for these lesions is complete resection, and the prognosis of the benign tumors is excellent.

Alveolar Adenoma

Yousem and Hochholzer (1986) reported six patients with alveolar adenomas. These tumors are a proliferation of benign alveolar epithelium and septal mesenchyme. The patients were mostly women and ranged in age from 45 to 74 years. Most of the lesions were found on routine chest radiography. On excision, the tumors averaged 2 cm in diameter and were easily shelled out from the adjacent pulmonary parenchyma. Five of the patients were alive and well at the end of a 12-month follow-up period, with one patient lost to follow-up.

Since the description of Yousem and Hochholzer (1986), Bohm and colleagues (1997), as well as Oliveira and associates (1996), have each described an additional case. Both groups believe this is a distinct benign neoplasm of the lung. Oliveira and colleagues (1996) speculate the lesion is derived from a primitive mesenchymal cell with the capacity to differentiate toward a type II pneumocyte lineage. In contrast, Bohm and associates (1997) believe the neoplasm is derived from a benign proliferation of both the type II pneumocytes and the septal mesenchyme. Both groups conclude that alveolar adenoma is a distinct, rare, benign pulmonary neoplasm.

Papillary Adenoma of Type II Cells (Clara Cell Adenoma)

Papillary adenoma of type II cells is a rare benign papillary neoplasm of type II cell origin that may have admixed Clara cells. This lesion may also be called a *Clara cell adenoma*, *bronchiolar papilloma*, or a *papillary adenoma of type II pneumocytes*. Spencer and colleagues (1980) described two cases. Fantone (1982) and Noguchi (1986) and their associates described papillary adenomas of the lung that had ultrastructural differentiation toward type II pneumocytes (lamellar bodies) and Clara cells (membrane-bound, electron-dense granules). Hegg (1992), Sanchez-Jimenez (1994),

Fukuda (1992), as well as Mori (1996), and their colleagues have all added additional cases to the literature.

The patients range in age from 2 months to 60 years, and the tumor may occur in either sex. The lesions are usually detected in asymptomatic patients as a result of mass radiologic screening. On gross examination, the tumors are usually described as well-demarcated white nodules in the pulmonary parenchyma. Microscopic examination shows a papillary architecture with prominent fibrovascular cores. The epithelial cells, lining the cores, are predominantly cuboidal with basal nuclei and eosinophilic cytoplasm. Ultrastructurally, Clara cells and type II pneumocytes are identified. The differential diagnosis includes alveolar adenoma, papillary bronchioalveolar carcinoma, sclerosing hemangioma, papillary variant of carcinoid tumor, and metastatic carcinoma. Resection appears to be curative with all of the patients surviving for at least 2 to 10 years. Mori and coworkers (1996), using morphometry with 12-dimensional cluster analysis, found a resemblance of some of the cells to type II pneumocyte adenocarcinoma, but their patient was alive with no evidence of recurrence at 3 years.

Leiomyoma

Leiomyomas account for approximately 2% of the benign tumors of the lung. They may occur in the trachea, bronchus, or pulmonary parenchyma (Table 111-2). As Hurt (1984), as well as Arrigoni (1970), Yellin (1984), and White (1985) and their colleagues, noted, the distribution is approximately equal between a tracheobronchial and a parenchymal location. The tumor is most often discovered in young and middle-aged adults and is more common in women than in men. The parenchymal lesions are solitary masses of varying size. Gotti and associates (1993) described one that was a multiloculated mass associated with a large pedunculated cyst that occupied the upper third of the left pleural space. These authors also noted other reports of "leiomyomas" associated with cyst formation, but most if not all of these were in patients with leiomyomatosis (see later in this chapter in the section Multiple Benign Tumors). Surgical resection is the treatment of choice. In selected patients with endobronchial lesions without distal destroyed lung tissue, laser resection of the tumor may be possible. Archambeaud-Mouveroux and associates (1988) reported successful management of a benign bronchial leiomyoma by endoscopic use of a neodymium:yttrium-aluminum-garnet laser. Endobronchial

Table 111-2. Leiomyoma of the Lower Respiratory Tract

Site	No. of Cases	Percent
Trachea	12	16
Bronchus	22	33
Parenchyma	34	51

From White SH, et al: Leiomyomas of the lower respiratory tract. Thorax *40*:306, 1985. With permission.

resection without the use of laser is also satisfactory. Kim and colleagues (1993) reported two such cases.

Benign Neurogenic Tumor

Benign neurogenic tumors [neurilemoma (neurinoma, schwannoma) or neurofibroma] may occur in the lung, but nothing distinctive is evident in these tumors. Yamakawa and colleagues (1993) reviewed 20 examples of a neurilemoma in the Japanese literature. The sex distribution was equal and the tumor could occur at any age. Six were in a major bronchus and the other 14 were located within the lung parenchyma. Sugita and coworkers (1996) performed a sleeve resection on a neurilemoma to preserve lung capacity. McCluggage and Bharucha (1995) pointed out that the neurogenic tumor may be difficult to classify because of degenerative changes. In this case, a special stain for S-100 may be helpful because the neurogenic tumor stains positively.

Cavernous Hemangioma

Yousem (1989) reviewed the pulmonary vascular lesions and believed that benign ones include cavernous hemangiomas, arteriovenous malformations (see Chapter 81), capillary hemangiomas, and pulmonary telangiectasia. Cavernous hemangiomas are rare lung tumors that in reality are pulmonary arteriovenous malformations. Early on, Wodehouse (1948) described four patients with pulmonary hemangiomas, and Forsee and associates (1950) described this tumor in a 20-year-old man with cyanosis. Galliani and colleagues (1992) described a cavernous hemangioma in a 10-week-old male infant. They emphasized that if the lesion is a true arteriovenous malformation, the possibility of hereditary hemorrhagic telangiectasia (Rendu-Osler-Weber disease) should be considered. Silverman and colleagues (1994) studied patients with pulmonary venous malformations by magnetic resonance imaging. They concluded that by using their criteria, magnetic resonance imaging was an excellent noninvasive modality for evaluating these lesions. Pulmonary telangiectasia is usually associated with Rendu-Osler-Weber disease or is found in individuals with cirrhosis of the liver. Solitary cavernous hemangiomas are excised surgically. Paul and associates (1991) and Cohen and Kaschula (1992) have described capillary hemangiomas in infants. Paul and associates (1991) described how their patient developed a bronchial obstruction, and they performed a successful sleeve resection of the right main stem bronchus.

Lymphatic Lesions

Lymphatic lesions of the lung are rare and can be divided into lymphangiomas and diffuse lymphangiomatosis. A pulmonary lymphangioma has been described by Kim and coworkers (1995). Their case involved a 6-month-old infant with a cystic pulmonary lesion. The patient underwent surgery for dyspnea. On gross examination, the lung had

cystic spaces that on microscopic examination had the features of a cystic lymphangioma.

Pleomorphic Adenoma (Mixed Tumor)

Pleomorphic adenomas or mixed tumors are benign tumors composed of epithelial and myoepithelial cells, usually set in a cartilaginous stroma. Sakamoto and colleagues (1991) reported one case of pleomorphic adenoma in the lung and reviewed six other reported cases. The patients ranged in age from 47 to 74 years, with an average age of 57 years. Both sexes were equally affected by these tumors. The clinical symptoms included pneumonia and cough; one patient was asymptomatic. Moran (1995) also summarized 16 patients with pleomorphic adenomas. His patients ranged in age from 35 to 74 years and had a predominance in women. The tumors could be either endobronchial or parenchymal in location, but no predilection occurred for a particular lung or segment. On microscopic examination, Moran points out that the pulmonary tumors do not have as prominent a cartilaginous stroma as do the salivary gland tumors. Treatment is surgical excision. These tumors can also occur in the trachea.

Nodular Amyloid

Hui and colleagues (1986) reported 48 cases of amyloid involving the upper and lower respiratory tracts. They divided their cases into three types: 1) tracheobronchial, 2) nodular pulmonary, and 3) diffuse (interstitial) pulmonary. We focus on the nodular form. Nodular pulmonary amyloidosis is a focal collection of amyloid in the lung, usually with a surrounding giant cell reaction. It can occur as either a solitary nodule or multiple nodules. Desai (1979), Hayes (1969), and Laden (1984) and their colleagues described cases of nodular pulmonary amyloidosis. The patients range in age from young to old, but most patients tend to be in their sixth and seventh decades of life, and both sexes are affected equally. Higuchi and associates (1997) collected 34 cases of primary nodular pulmonary amyloidosis from the Japanese literature and added one of their own. Sixteen of the patients had single lesions and 19 had multiple lesions. The majority of the patients, as in the aforementioned series, were middle-aged or older adults. Patients are usually asymptomatic and the amyloid tumors are discovered on incidental chest radiography. Surgical resection is considered curative. Multiple myeloma does not appear to be frequently associated with these lesions, but the patients should be evaluated for the possibility of this disease. Also, these patients should undergo long-term follow-up because the occasional association with macroglobulinemia and malignant lymphoma occurs as noted by Kyle and Garton (1987).

Inflammatory Pseudotumor

Inflammatory pseudotumors are benign tumors that have a wide histologic spectrum and, over the years, they have been called *fibroxanthoma, histiocytoma, xanthofibroma, xanthoma, xanthogranuloma, mast cell granuloma, plasma cell granuloma,* and, incorrectly, a *sclerosing hemangioma.* Colby and coworkers (1995) divide the inflammatory pseudotumors into two major groups, according to their histology: fibrohistiocytic and plasma cell granuloma. Berardi and associates (1983) reviewed this subject and found that these tumors could occur in patients of any age, with an average age of 29.5 years. No predilection for either sex was evident. Most (74%) of the patients were asymptomatic. Patients may have obstructive symptoms if the lesion is located in the bronchus. Cohen and Kaschula (1992) described these lesions as the most common lung tumor of childhood. Matsubara and coworkers (1988) postulated that these tumors originate as an organizing intra-alveolar pneumonia. Ishida and colleagues (1989) reported seven patients with this lesion and described its clinicopathologic features. Agrons and associates (1998) described the chest radiographs as showing a solitary, peripheral, sharply circumscribed mass usually in one of the lower lobes. Diagnosis and treatment are often made by resection of the mass. Fine-needle aspiration may yield confusing results because many malignancies may be surrounded by reactive connective tissue. These lesions are best treated by a conservative surgical excision, but with the realization that they may recur if they are not completely excised. Doski and colleagues (1991) used corticosteroids to lessen infiltration in an unresectable plasma cell granuloma. Imperato and coworkers (1986) used radiation therapy to treat lesions that could not be completely resected. Gal and associates (1994) addressed the problem of tumor extension into the mediastinum, recurrence, and blood vessel invasion. They believed there was an intermediate form between malignant fibrous histiocytoma and inflammatory pseudotumors that could be locally recurrent.

Sclerosing Hemangioma

Sclerosing hemangioma, originally described by Liebow and Hubbell (1956), is a benign lung tumor of undetermined histogenesis. Katzenstein and associates (1982) described 51 cases Liebow saw after his initial description in 1956. These authors noted that the patients ranged in age from 15 to 69 years, with an average age of 42 years. Eighty-four percent of the patients were women. Most (78%) of the patients were asymptomatic. Those who were symptomatic complained of hemoptysis, vague chest pain, or both. On radiographic study, the sclerosing hemangioma appears as a solitary nodule that is found more often in one of the lower lobes (Fig. 111-8). Sugio and coworkers (1992) described an additional 10 cases of this tumor with similar clinical and pathologic findings to those of Katzenstein and associates (1982). The former authors also cited new studies that suggest the tumor may be derived from type II alveolar pneumocytes. One of these studies was reported by Yousem and colleagues (1988). These investigators performed immuno-

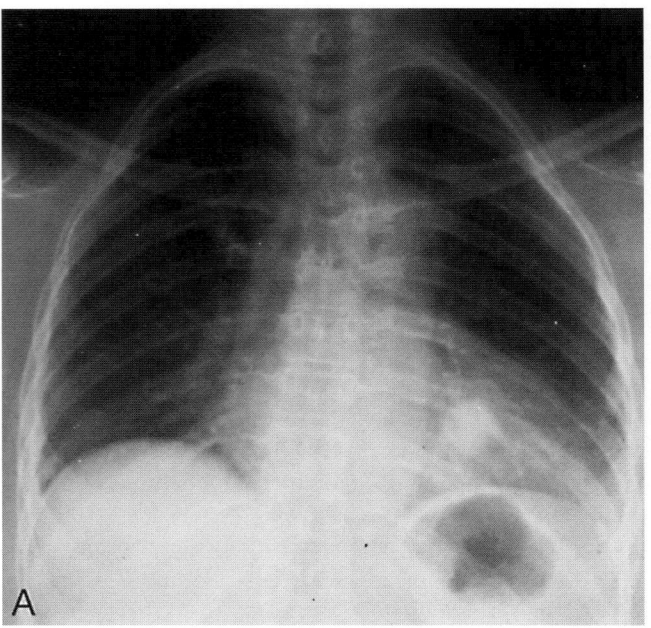

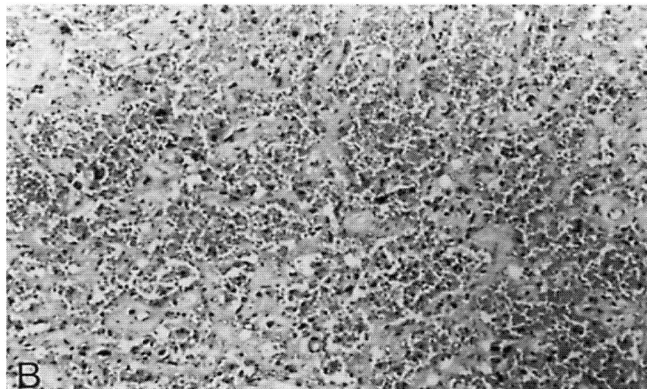

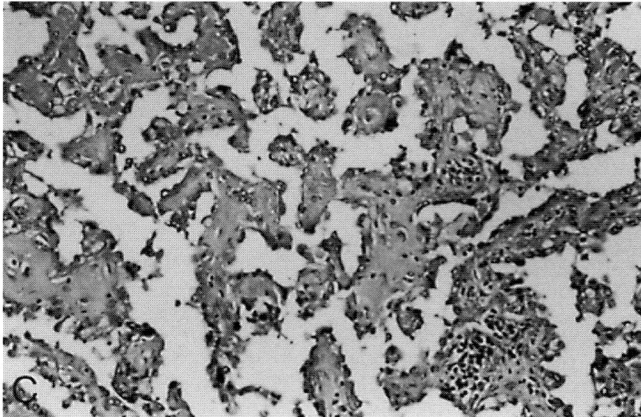

Fig. 111-8. A. Radiograph of the chest of an asymptomatic 63-year-old woman with a mass in the left lower lung field that had been present for more than 5 years. Recent growth was noted. Removal and histologic examination of the mass revealed a sclerosing hemangioma. **B.** Low-power photomicrograph of the sclerosing hemangioma. Dense solid areas contain typical polygonal cells. **C.** High-power photomicrograph shows papillary areas with the fibrovascular cores lined by cuboidal cells.

Table 111-3. Immunophenotype of Common Clear Cell Tumors of the Lung

	Broad-Spectrum Cytokeratin	Vimentin	Chromogranin	Melanosome-Associated Protein	S-100 Protein
Sugar tumor	−	+	−	+	+
Clear cell carcinoma	+	±	−	−	−
Clear cell carcinoid	+	−	+	−	−
Renal cell carcinoma	+	+	−	−	±

From Leong AS-Y, Meredith DJ: Clear cell tumors of the lung. *In* Corrin B (ed): Pathology of Lung Tumors. New York: Churchill Livingstone, 1997, p. 159. With permission.

histochemical studies on eight sclerosing hemangiomas and concluded that the tumor was of epithelial origin, with evidence of both bronchiolar and alveolar pneumocyte differentiation. Despite these aforementioned studies, Leong and associates (1995), from an extensive immunohistochemical and ultrastructural analysis of 25 sclerosing hemangiomas, concluded that although the tumor cells are of epithelial origin, they believe these cells do not clearly correspond to any cell currently recognized in the periphery of the lung. They strongly believe no good evidence exists of pneumocyte origin. In a subsequent publication, Leong and Meredith (1997) listed three reasons for their aforementioned conclusion: 1) by light microscopy the pneumocytes are morphologically different than the tumor cells, 2) by electron microscopy the pneumocytes are clearly separated from the underlying tumor cells, and 3) the immunophenotype expressed by pneumocytes differs from that of the tumor cells. These authors further opine that the name of this tumor "is inappropriate as there is no evidence to implicate endothelial differentiation."

Regardless of the controversy as to the origin of a sclerosing hemangioma or as to the correctness of its name, surgical excision of the tumor is indicated and is curative in nature.

Sugar Tumor (Clear Cell Tumor) of the Lung

Benign clear cell or sugar tumor of the lung is a benign lung lesion of unknown histogenesis. The tumor was first reported by Liebow and Castleman (1963), who later described a series of 12 cases (1971). Seventy-five percent of the lesions occurred in patients between 45 and 59 years of age. The tumors were equally distributed between men and women. All of the patients were asymptomatic. Similar age and sex distribution were noted in the 14 cases in the Japanese literature reviewed by Miura and associates (1993). Radiographically, the lesions were solitary and peripheral and ranged in size from 1.5 to 3.0 cm. Excision is curative. From their light microscopic, histochemical, and ultrastructural study of the tumor, Andrion and colleagues (1985) suggested it is derived from either epithelial nonciliated bronchiolar (Clara cells) epithelium or epithelial serous cells. Gaffey and coworkers (1990) studied eight clear cell tumors of the lung by electron microscopy and immunohistochemistry. They found some evidence of neuroendocrine differentiation in some of the tumor cells, but

they could not be certain as to the cell of origin for this tumor. In a subsequent report, Gaffey and colleagues (1991) noted that the sugar tumor cells were uniformly negative for epithelial features, but were strongly reactive for human melanin black or melanosome-associated protein and positive for S-100 protein.

Leong and Meredith (1997) have not only extensively discussed the possible histogenesis of the benign sugar tumor but also have stressed the necessity of differentiating these benign lesions from the numerous malignant "clear cell" tumors that can be encountered in the lung. Metastatic renal cell carcinoma or a primary clear cell carcinoma of the lung are the most troubling that are encountered. The aforementioned authors suggest that the immunohistochemical features are most important in distinguishing these various tumors (Table 111-3). Searching for an asymptomatic primary tumor is most often fruitless.

Pulmonary Paraganglioma

Primary pulmonary paraganglioma or chemodectoma are rare. Singh and colleagues (1977) reported one case and reviewed the literature, finding only 11 cases up to that time. Tanimura and associates (1993) found a total of 23 case reports and added one case of their own. One of the major problems with this tumor has been the inability to distinguish it from a carcinoid tumor. Tanimura and colleagues (1993) suggested the use of immunohistochemical staining techniques to aid in this differentiation. They noted that Googe and coworkers (1988) reported that paragangliomas had a positive reaction to S-100 protein and were negative for cytokeratin and serotonin, whereas carcinoid tumors were negative for S-100 protein but were positive for cytokeratin and serotonin. Therefore, results of these studies should be used when considering the cellular origin of a tumor that histologically simulates a possible paraganglioma. Rarely, a pulmonary paraganglioma, although its histologic features are those of a benign lesion, may metastasize to the regional lymph nodes; such a tumor must be considered malignant. Hangartner (1989) and Lemonick (1990) and their colleagues each reported such a case. Pulmonary paragangliomas should not be confused with the so-called minute chemodectoma of the lung described by Torikata and Mukai (1990). These are multiple minute tumors that are usually found incidentally on microscopic examination of the tissue. The origin of these tumors is obscure.

Glomus Tumor

According to Marchevsky (1995), a glomus tumor (glomangioma) is derived from the cells of a special arteriovenous shunt, the Suquet-Hoyer canal. They are generally located in the nail beds as well as the pads of the fingers and toes. They are involved in temperature control. On chest radiography, pulmonary glomus tumors appear as solitary nodules. They should be distinguished from hemangiopericytomas, carcinoids, paragangliomas, and smooth muscle tumors.

Teratoma

Teratomas occur rarely as primary lung tumors (see Reading References). More than 20 cases have been reported, but many of the early reports may have represented anterior mediastinal teratomas that had extended into the lung. Most that do occur in the lung are found in the anterior segment of the left upper lobe. Resection is curative.

Pulmonary Meningioma

Meningiomas in the pulmonary parenchyma can be primary or metastatic. One of us (P.G.R.) (1992), as well as Flynn and Yousem (1991) and Drlicek and coworkers (1991) described primary pulmonary meningiomas. Lockett and associates (1997) and Kaleem and coworkers (1997) have reviewed and described primary pulmonary meningiomas. Patients with this tumor are mostly women and they range in age from 19 to 74 years, with a mean age of 61 years. The patients generally present with an asymptomatic nodule on chest radiography. Grossly, the tumor is usually a well-circumscribed, round, gray-to-white nodule ranging in size from 1.7 to 6.0 cm in greatest dimension. Microscopically, the tumors are composed of meningothelial cells with psammoma bodies. Electron microscopically, the tumors contain interdigitating cell membranes and desmosomes. The tumor cells immunohistochemically stain consistently with vimentin and variably with epithelial membrane antigen, but not with keratin, S-100, or neuron-specific enolase. Moran and coworkers (1996) concluded that vimentin and epithelial membrane antigen are the most reliable immunologic markers of these tumors. The treatment is surgical excision and the prognosis is excellent.

Wende (1983), Miller (1985), and Kodama (1991) and their colleagues reported cases of metastatic meningioma from the cranium to the lung. A patient in whom a pulmonary meningioma is diagnosed should be examined to exclude an intracranial lesion.

Hyalinizing Granuloma

Pulmonary hyalinizing granuloma is a tumor of dense hyalinized connective tissue that occurs in the lung as a result of inflammatory or postinflammatory changes. Engleman and associates (1977) first described the lesion.

Yousem and Hochholzer (1987) summarized 24 cases. The tumor occurs in patients between 24 and 77 years of age, with an average age of 42.3 years. The lesions are equally distributed between men and women. Patients may be asymptomatic or complain of cough, shortness of breath, chest pain, or weight loss. The lesions are nodular and vary from a few millimeters to 15 cm in greatest dimension. Many of the patients have multiple lesions, with most being bilateral. More than one-half of the patients who develop hyalinizing granulomas have a history of an autoimmune disorder or a past history of fungal or mycobacterial disease. John and associates (1995) described a case in a patient with multiple sclerosis and Kuramochi and colleagues (1991) described one in a patient with systemic idiopathic fibrosis.

Fibroma (Solitary Fibrous Tumor and Localized Fibrous Mesothelioma)

A fibroma is known by a variety of names. Colby and associates (1995) prefer the term *intrapulmonary localized fibrous tumor*, but this lesion has also been called *solitary fibrous tumor*, *intraparenchymal localized fibrous mesothelioma*, *intrapulmonary fibrous mesothelioma*, and *inverted fibrous tumor of the pleura*. These benign tumors have a histologic appearance that is identical to that of a localized fibrous tumor of the pleura (see Chapter 64). These tumors are most commonly found on the visceral pleura of the lung, but occasionally they are intrapulmonary. They also may be found in the mediastinum, retroperitoneum, and external surface of the stomach and small intestine. Rarely, as reported by Yousem and Flynn (1988), a fibrous tumor can occur in the lung tissue without any connection to the visceral pleural layer. Histologically, the tumors are composed of spindle cells with dense bundles of collagen. According to a review by Khalifar and associates (1997) the cells immunostain for vimentin and CD34. A malignant variant of this tumor exists. Adequate resection is curative.

Primary Pulmonary Thymoma

A primary thymoma may occur in the lung. In all such cases, the mediastinal thymus gland must be normal and a thymoma in the mediastinal gland or the history of a previous resection of a thymoma must be absent. Kalish (1963) divided the primary intrapulmonary thymomas as either peripheral or hilar in location. In the latter instance, the thymoma must be inside the visceral pleura, because ectopic mediastinal thymic tissue can be found in the aortopulmonary window as well as in the aortocaval groove (Chapter 149). Twenty cases have been reported in the literature, with a preponderance of the cases in women. Two patients had myasthenia gravis.

The tumor is usually found in older individuals. The location of the hilar or the peripheral tumors may be in either lung. The more recent cases have been described by James

(1992), Moran (1995), and Veynovich (1997) and their colleagues. Fukayama (1988) and Veynovich (1997) and coworkers used immunohistochemical techniques to identify thymic T lymphocytes in the tumor to differentiate the tumor from lymphoepithelial-like carcinoma of the lung and from primary lymphomas of the lung. Moran and associates (1995) used different immunohistochemical studies to determine the nature of the epithelial cells in six of their eight cases. These cells had positive results for keratin and the epithelial membrane antigen, but negative results for vimentin, desmin, actin, and S-100 protein. Although these studies per se do not differentiate the cells from being squamous in origin, the benign appearance and the absence of mitotic activity of these epithelial cells rule out the possibility of an undifferentiated squamous cell tumor. When localized, as most of these primary thymomas of the lung are, surgical resection appears to be curative. When the tumor is extensive with involvement of the pleura and is thought not to be resectable, which is rare, therapeutic radiation therapy has resulted in long-term survival.

MULTIPLE BENIGN TUMORS

Benign Metastasizing Leiomyoma

Rare, multiple benign peripheral lesions, such as the benign metastasizing leiomyoma, may be seen. The exact nature of the lesions remains undetermined. These tumors occur in young women and frequently are associated with a leiomyoma of the uterus. The lesions may grow. Regression of these tumors can occur after oophorectomy. Winkler and colleagues (1987) suggested resection of the pulmonary lesions when feasible. Gal and coworkers (1989) described a series of 12 patients with smooth muscle tumors of the lung. In five of these patients, the tumors were thought to be from the uterus, and four of these patients died of their disease.

Parenti and colleagues (1992) reported a case and reviewed the subject. These authors point out no standard of treatment exists for benign metastasizing leiomyoma. Patients are usually managed with a combination of surgery, hormonal manipulation, and chemotherapy. Jautzke and colleagues (1996) tested five benign metastasizing leiomyomas for estrogen and progesterone receptors. All had a high content of progesterone receptors and four of five had a high content of estrogen receptors. These findings give a scientific basis for treating patients with hormonal manipulation. Jacobson and associates (1995) treated a patient with goserelin, a luteinizing hormone-releasing hormone analogue, and showed improvement in the patient's blood gasses and chest radiograph. The exact etiology of this disease is unknown, but Takemura and colleagues (1996) pointed out that this condition could be the result of multicentric benign leiomyomatous growths rather than metastases.

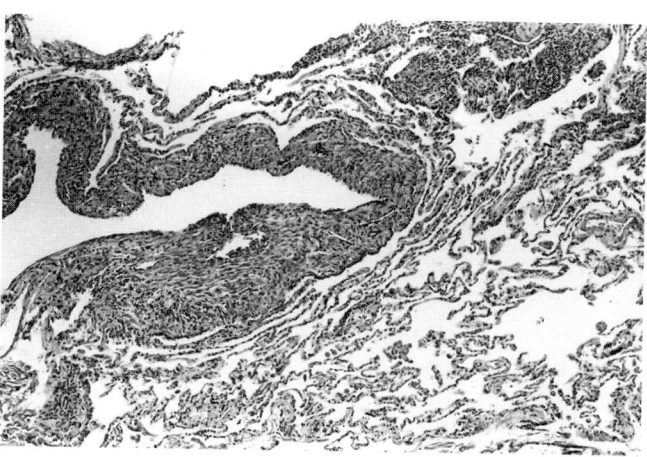

Fig. 111-9. Photomicrograph of a section of lung in a patient with lymphangioleiomyomatosis. Note the accumulation of muscle cells that appear immature and are clustered randomly in the alveolar walls and about the small bronchi and blood vessels.

Pulmonary Lymphangioleiomyomatosis

Pulmonary lymphangioleiomyomatosis (LAM), as recorded by Bonetti and Chiodera (1997), was first reported by Leutenbacher (1918) in a woman with tuberous sclerosis (Fig. 111-9). As subsequently observed, the pulmonary involvement accompanying tuberous sclerosis was only seen in women. At times there may be no other manifestation of tuberous sclerosis; when other organ involvement is absent, Valensi (1973) as well as others consider LAM as a forme fruste of tuberous sclerosis.

The pulmonary disease (LAM) is seen almost exclusively in women during their reproductive years. Numerous cases of women with LAM have been reported by Corrin (1975), Taylor (1990), Tazelaar (1993), and Kitaichi (1995) and their colleagues. Single case reports abound in the literature. The average age of the women is approximately 40 years; although a few cases have been reported in postmenopausal women by Sinclair (1985) and Baldi (1994) and their associates. Because of LAM's almost exclusive incidence in women during their reproductive years, it has been assumed that the disease has a hormonal basis as well as its association with tuberous sclerosis. The hormonal relationship is unclear. However, it has been observed that LAM does not develop in women with low levels of estrogen and that the disease process, as reported by Shen (1987), is exacerbated by exogenous estrogens. Likewise the disease is worsened during the menstrual periods.

Clinically, the patient frequently presents initially with an episode of spontaneous pneumothorax with marked dyspnea. The history, however, reveals antecedent shortness of breath for a variable period. Pulmonary hemorrhage with hemoptysis, chylothorax, and increasing respiratory insufficiency occurs over time. Death occurs in many within 10 years of diagnosis.

The radiographic findings are those of a reticulonodular pattern throughout the lung fields. In late cases, a honeycomb appearance may be, and in fact is, usually present. The CT findings have been described by Swensen and colleagues (1995).

Pathologically, Corrin and associates (1975) describe the process to be "an irregular, nodular or laminar 'irrational' proliferation of smooth muscle within all portions of the lungs." The accumulation of the smooth muscle cells is progressive. As the smooth muscle cells proliferate, they produce secondary obstruction of the small airways, small veins, and lymphatic of the lung parenchyma. Cystic changes within the lung parenchyma occur as the process progresses. The cystic spaces throughout the lungs are characteristic CT features in advanced cases. Immunohistochemical studies, as noted by Bonetti and Chiodera (1997), reveal the smooth muscle cells in cases of LAM to have a distinctive phenotype (in addition to the presence of muscle deviation, such as muscle-specific actin, the cells are consistently positive for human melanin black, the marker for melanogenesis). The significance of the presence of this marker has not been resolved.

Hormonal therapy (i.e., the use of oophorectomy, antiestrogen agents, and progesterone therapy, alone or in combination) has been used with equivocal results. Banner (1981), Adamson (1985), and Urban (1992) and their associates, among others, have reported varying success rates with such medical intervention. Yet meta-analysis of many small series by Eliasson and colleagues (1989) suggests that some stabilization of the disease process and longer survival was observed. It is generally agreed that at present medroxyprogesterone acetate is the drug of choice with or without oophorectomy. The role of the use of tamoxifen is unsettled. In unresponsive patients, Klein and coworkers (1992) suggested the alternative use of oophorectomy, interferon-α_{2b}, and tamoxifen. The value of this regimen is unknown.

In patients who have failed to respond to the aforementioned medical regimens and continue to show increasing pulmonary insufficiency, bilateral or unilateral lung transplantation has been carried out. The early experience has been noted by Marchevsky and colleagues (1991). Wellens and associates (1985) successfully used combined heart-lung transplantation. Nine (1994) and O'Brien (1995) and their colleagues used a single lung transplantation. In each of the patients, however, LAM subsequently developed in the allograft; the donors for both allografts were men, which is of some interest. Thus, the use of a single lung transplant in patients with end-stage LAM may not be a suitable solution. Without further information, bilateral lung transplantation would appear to be the surgical procedure of choice.

Pulmonary Capillary Hemangiomatosis

Pulmonary capillary hemangiomatosis is an aggressive benign tumor of the lung that according to Tron and col-

leagues (1986) is formed by numerous cytologically benign thin-walled capillary-sized vessels proliferating diffusely through the pulmonary interstitium, in and around the pulmonary vessels and small airways. The clinical course is characterized by pulmonary hypertension. Hemoptysis may be present. The process is slowly progressive and leads to right-sided heart failure. Radiographic examination of the lung reveals a reticulonodular pattern. Fewer than 20 cases have been recorded in the literature. The only successful treatment has been bilateral lung transplantation as reported by Faber and associates (1989). Eltorky and colleagues (1994) reported single lung transplantation was unsuccessful in this condition.

Cystic Fibrohistiocytic Tumor

Joseph and colleagues (1990) described two cases of cystic fibrohistiocytic tumors of the lungs. These tumors are histologically identical to benign fibrous histiocytomas (dermatofibromas) in the skin and other sites. Leroyer and colleagues (1993) described a similar lesion that they thought was better termed a *mesenchymal cystic hamartoma*. In the lung, the tumor proliferation is interstitial and is associated with microscopic and macroscopic cyst formation. The lesions, as described by Joseph and colleagues (1990), were bilateral and nodular, cystic, or both, in appearance. Slow growth of the lesions was observed. Clinically, one patient was asymptomatic and the other experienced episodes of pneumothorax and shortness of breath. No specific treatment is indicated other than to control any complications that arise.

REFERENCES

Acha T, et al: Carney's triad: apropos of a new case. Med Pediatr Oncol 22:216, 1994.
Adamson D, et al: Successful treatment of pulmonary lymphangiomyomatosis with oophorectomy and progesterone. Am Rev Respir Dis 132:916, 1985.
Agrons GA, et al: Pulmonary inflammatory pseudotumor: radiologic features. Radiology 206:511, 1998.
Aisner SC, et al: Endobronchial fibrous histiocytoma. Ann Thorac Surg 60:710, 1995.
Andrion A, et al: Benign clear cell ("sugar") tumor of the lung: a light microscopic, histochemical, and ultrastructural study with a review of the literature. Cancer 56:2657, 1985.
Archambeaud-Mouveroux F, et al: Bronchial leiomyoma. Report of a case successfully treated by endoscopic neodymium-yttrium aluminum garnet laser. J Thorac Cardiovasc Surg 95:536, 1988.
Argos MD, et al: Gastric leiomyoblastoma associated with extra-adrenal paraganglioma and pulmonary chondroma: a new case of Carney's triad. J Pediatr Surg 28:1545, 1993.
Arguelles M, Blanco I: Inflammatory bronchial polyps associated with asthma. Arch Intern Med 143:570, 1983.
Arrigoni MG, et al: Benign tumors of the lung: a ten-year surgical experience. J Thorac Cardiovasc Surg 60:589, 1970.
Baldi S, et al: Pulmonary lymphangioleiomyomatosis in postmenopausal women: report of two cases and review of the literature. Eur Respir J 7:1013, 1994.
Bango A, et al: Endobronchial lipomas. Respiration 60:297, 1993.
Banner AS, et al: Efficacy of oophorectomy in lymphangioleiomyomatosis and benign metastasizing leiomyoma. N Engl J Med 305:204, 1981.

Basile A, et al: Malignant change in a benign pulmonary hamartoma. Thorax 44:232, 1989.

Bateson EM: So-called hamartoma of the lung: a true neoplasm of fibrous connective tissue of the bronchi. Cancer 31:1458, 1973.

Bennett LL, Lesar MJ, Tellis CJ: Multiple calcified chondrohamartomas of the lung: CT appearance. J Comput Assist Tomogr 9:180, 1985.

Berardi RS, et al: Inflammatory pseudotumors of the lung. Surg Gynecol Obstet 156:89, 1983.

Bohm J, et al: Pulmonary nodule caused by an alveolar adenoma of the lung. Virchows Arch 430:181, 1997.

Bonetti F, Chiodera P: The lung in tuberous sclerosis. In Corrin B (ed): Pathology of Lung Tumors. New York: Churchill Livingstone, 1997, p. 225.

Bueno R, et al: Bronchoplasty in the management of low-grade airway neoplasms and benign bronchial stenoses. Ann Thorac Surg 62:824, 1996.

Carney JA: The triad of gastric epithelioid leiomyosarcoma, functioning extra-adrenal paraganglioma, and pulmonary chondroma. Cancer 43:374, 1979.

Carney JA: The triad of gastric epithelioid leiomyosarcoma, pulmonary chondroma, and functioning extra-adrenal paraganglioma: a five year review. Medicine 62:159, 1983.

Cohen MC, Kaschula ROC: Primary pulmonary tumors in childhood: a review of 31 years experience and the literature. Pediatr Pulmonol 14:222, 1992.

Colby TV, Koss MN, Travis WD: Atlas of Tumor Pathology: tumors of the Lower Respiratory Tract. Washington, DC: Armed Forces Institute of Pathology, 1995, p. 61, 338.

Corrin B, Liebow AA, Friedman PJ: Pulmonary lymphangiomyomatosis. A review. Am J Pathol 79:348, 1975.

Dail DH, Hammar SP (eds): Pulmonary Pathology. New York: Springer-Verlag, 1988.

Deavers M, et al: Granular cell tumors of the lung: clinicopathologic study of 20 cases. Am J Surg Pathol 19:627, 1995.

Demos TC, et al: Cystic hamartoma of the lung. J Can Assoc Radiol 34:149, 1983.

De Rooij PD, et al: Solitary hamartoma of the lung: is thoracotomy still mandatory. Neth J Surg 40:145, 1988.

Desai RA, et al: Pulmonary amyloidoma and hilar adenopathy. Rare manifestations of primary amyloidosis. Chest 76:170, 1979.

Dixon AY, et al: Pulmonary mucinous cystic tumor: case report and review of the literature. Am J Surg Pathol 17:722, 1993.

Drennan JM, Douglas AC: Solitary papilloma of a bronchus. J Clin Pathol 18:401, 1965.

Drlicek M, et al: Pulmonary meningioma: immunohistochemical and ultrastructural features. Am J Surg Pathol 15:455, 1991.

Duncan JD, et al: Benign fibrous histiocytoma: a rare endobronchial neoplasm. Int Surg 71:110, 1986.

Edwards CW, Matthews HR: Mucous gland adenoma of the bronchus. Thorax 36:147, 1981.

Eliasson AH, Phillips YY, Tenholder MF: Treatment of lymphangioleiomyomatosis. A meta-analysis. Chest 96:1352, 1989.

Eltorky MA, et al: Pulmonary capillary hemangiomatosis: a clinicopathological review. Ann Thorac Surg 57:772, 1994.

Emory WB, Mitchell WT, Hatch HB Jr: Mucous gland adenoma of the bronchus. Am Rev Respir Dis 108:1407, 1973.

England DM, Hochholzer L: Truly benign "bronchial adenoma." Report of 10 cases of mucous gland adenoma with immunohistochemical and ultrastructural findings. Am J Surg Pathol 19:887, 1995.

Engleman P, et al: Pulmonary hyalinizing granuloma. Am Rev Respir Dis 115:997, 1977.

Epstein LJ, Mohsenifar Z: Use of Nd:YAG laser in endobronchial granular cell myoblastoma. Chest 104:958, 1993.

Faber CN, et al: Pulmonary capillary hemangiomatosis. A report of three cases and a review of the literature. Am Rev Respir Dis 140:808, 1989.

Fantone JC, Geisinger KR, Appelman HD: Papillary adenoma of the lung with lamellar and electron dense granules: an ultrastructural study. Cancer 50: 2939, 1982.

Fisher ER, Wechsler H: Granular cell myoblastoma—a misnomer. Electron microscopic and histochemical evidence concerning its Schwann cell derivation and nature. Cancer 15:936, 1962.

Fletcher JA, et al: Lineage-restricted clonality in biphasic solid tumors. Am J Pathol 138:1199, 1991.

Flynn SD, Yousem SA: Pulmonary meningiomas: a report of two cases. Hum Pathol 22:469, 1991.

Forsee JH, Mahon HW, James LA: Cavernous hemangioma of the lung. Ann Surg 131:418, 1950.

Fukayama M, et al: Pulmonary and pleural thymoma. Diagnostic application of lymphocyte markers to the thymoma of unusual site. Am J Clin Pathol 89:617, 1988.

Fukuda T, et al: Papillary adenoma of the lung: Histological and ultrastructural findings in two cases. Acta Pathol Jpn 42:56, 1992.

Gaffey MJ, et al: Clear cell tumor of the lung: a clinicopathologic, immunohistochemical, and ultrastructural study of eight cases. Am J Surg Pathol 14:248, 1990.

Gaffey MJ, et al: Clear cell tumor of the lung. Immunohistochemical and ultrastructural evidence of melanogenesis. Am J Surg Pathol 15:644, 1991.

Gal AA, Brooks JS, Pietra GG: Leiomyomatous neoplasms of the lung: a clinical, histologic, and immunohistochemical study. Mod Pathol 2:209, 1989.

Gal AA, et al: Prognostic factors in pulmonary fibrohistiocytic lesions. Cancer 73:1817, 1994.

Galliani CA, Beatty JF, Grosfeld JL: Cavernous hemangioma of the lung in an infant. Pediatr Pathol 12:105, 1992.

Gilman RA, Klassen KP, Scarpelli DG: Mucous gland adenoma of the bronchus. Am J Clin Pathol 26:151, 1956.

Googe PB, et al: A comparison of paraganglioma, carcinoid tumor, and small-cell carcinoma of the larynx. Arch Pathol Lab Med 112:908, 1988.

Gotti G, et al: Pedunculated pulmonary leiomyoma with large cyst formation. Ann Thorac Surg 56:1178, 1993.

Graeme-Cook F, Mark EJ: Pulmonary mucinous cystic tumors of borderline malignancy. Hum Pathol 22:185, 1991.

Hamper UM, et al: Pulmonary hamartoma: diagnosis by transthoracic needle aspiration biopsy. Radiology 155:15, 1985.

Hangartner JRW, et al: Malignant primary pulmonary paraganglioma. Thorax 44:154, 1989.

Hansen CP, et al: Pulmonary hamartoma. J Thorac Cardiovasc Surg 104:674, 1992.

Hayes WT, Bernhardt H: Solitary amyloid mass of the lung: report of a case with 6-year follow-up. Cancer 24:820, 1969.

Hayward RH, Carabasi RJ: Malignant hamartoma of the lung: fact or fiction? J Thorac Cardiovasc Surg 53:457, 1967

Hegg CA, et al: Papillary adenoma of the lung. Am J Clin Pathol 97:393, 1992.

Higuchi M, et al: A case of primary nodular pulmonary amyloidosis. J Jpn Assoc Chest Surg 11:34, 1997.

Hui AN, et al: Amyloidosis presenting in the lower respiratory tract: clinicopathologic, radiologic, immunohistochemical, and histochemical studies on 48 cases. Arch Pathol Lab Med 110:212, 1986.

Hurt R: Benign tumours of the bronchus and trachea: 1951–1981. Ann R Coll Surg Engl 66:22, 1984.

Ishida T, et al: Inflammatory pseudotumor of the lung in adults: radiographic and clinicopathological analysis. Ann Thorac Surg 48:90, 1989.

Ishida T, et al: Mucous gland adenoma of the trachea resected with an endoscopic neodymium:yttrium aluminum garnet laser. Intern Med 35:890, 1996.

Jackson RC et al: Massive cystic hamartoma. A report of two cases. J Thorac Surg 31:504, 1956.

Jacobson TZ, Rainey EJ, Turton CWG: Pulmonary benign metastasizing leiomyoma: response to treatment with goserelin. Thorax 50:1225, 1995.

Jautzke G, Muller-Ruchholtz E, Thalman U: Immunohistochemical detection of estrogen and progesterone receptors in multiple and well differentiated leiomyomatous lung tumors in women with uterine leiomyomas (so-called benign metastasizing leiomyomas). Pathol Res Pract 192:215, 1996.

James CL, Iyer PV, Leong AS: Intrapulmonary thymoma. Histopathology 21:175, 1992.

John PG, Rahman J, Payne CB: Pulmonary hyalinizing granuloma: an unusual association with multiple sclerosis. South Med J 88:1076, 1995.

Joseph MG, et al: Multiple cystic fibrohistiocytic tumors of the lung: report of two cases. Mayo Clin Proc 65:192, 1990.

Kaleem Z, Fitzpatrick MM, Ritter JH: Primary pulmonary meningioma. Report of a case and review of the literature. Arch Pathol Lab Med 121:631, 1997.

Kalish PE: Primary intrapulmonary thymoma. NY State J Med. 63:1705, 1963.

Karasik A, et al: Increased risk of lung cancer in patients with chondromatous hamartoma. J Thorac Cardiovasc Surg 80:217, 1980.

Katial RK, Ranlett R, Whitlock WL: Human papilloma virus associated with solitary squamous papilloma complicated by bronchiectasis and bronchial stenosis. Chest 106:1887, 1994.

Katzenstein AL, Gmelich JT, Carrington CB: Sclerosing hemangioma of the lung: a clinicopathologic study of 152 cases. Am J Surg Pathol 4:343, 1982.

Khalifa MA, et al: Solitary fibrous tumors: a series of lesions, some in unusual sites. South Med J 90:793, 1997.

Khouri NF, et al: The solitary pulmonary nodule. Assessment, diagnosis, and management. Chest 91:128, 1987.

Kim KH, Suh JS, Han WS: Leiomyoma of the bronchus treated by endoscopic resection. Ann Thorac Surg 56:1164, 1993.

Kim WS, et al: Cystic intrapulmonary lymphangioma: HRCT findings. Pediatr Radiol 25:206, 1995.

Kitaichi M, et al: Pulmonary lymphangioleiomyomatosis: a report of 46 patients including a clinicopathologic study of prognostic factors. Am J Respir Crit Care Med 151:527, 1995.

Klein MO, et al: Treatment of lymphangioleiomyomatosis by ovariectomy, interferon alpha 2b and tamoxifen—a case report. Arch Gynecol Obstet 252:99, 1992

Kodama K, et al: Primary and metastatic pulmonary meningioma. Cancer 67:1412, 1991.

Kragel PJ, et al: Mucinous cystadenoma of the lung. A report of two cases with immunohistochemical and ultrastructural analysis. Arch Pathol Lab Med 114:1053, 1990.

Kroe DJ, Pitcoc JA: Benign mucous gland adenoma of the bronchus. Arch Pathol Lab Med 84:539, 1967.

Kuda T, et al: Clinical analysis of benign tumors and tumor-like lesions of the lung. J Jpn Assoc Chest Surg 4:416, 1990 (English abstract).

Kuramochi S, et al: Multiple pulmonary hyalinizing granulomas associated with systemic idiopathic fibrosis. Acta Pathol Jpn 41:375, 1991.

Kyle RA, Garton JP: The spectrum of IgM monoclonal gammopathy in 430 cases. Mayo Clin Proc 62:719, 1987.

Laden SA, Cohen ML, Harley RA: Nodular pulmonary amyloidosis with extrapulmonary involvement. Hum Pathol 15:594, 1984.

Lancha C, et al: A case of complete Carney's syndrome. Clin Nucl Med 19:1008, 1994.

Ledor K, et al: CT diagnosis of pulmonary hamartomas. J Comput Assist Tomogr 5:343, 1981.

Lemonick DM, Pai PB, Hines GL: Malignant primary pulmonary paraganglioma with hilar metastasis. J Thorac Cardiovasc Surg 99:563, 1990.

Leong AS-Y, Chan KW, Leong FJ W-N: Sclerosing hemangioma. In Corrin B (ed): Pathology of Lung Tumors. New York: Churchill Livingstone, 1997, p. 175.

Leong AS, Chan KW, Seneviratne HS: A morphological and immunohistochemical study of 25 cases of so called "sclerosing hemangioma" of the lung. Histopathology 27:121, 1995.

Leong AS-Y, Meredith DJ: Clear cell tumors of the lung. In Corrin B (ed): Pathology of Lung Tumors. New York: Churchill Livingstone, 1997, p. 159.

Leroyer C, et al: Mesenchymal cystic hamartoma of the lung. Respiration 60:305, 1993.

Liebow AA, Castleman B: Benign "clear cell" tumors of the lung (abstract). Am J Pathol 43:13a, 1963.

Liebow AA, Castleman B: Benign clear cell ("sugar") tumors of the lung. Yale J Biol Med 43:213, 1971.

Liebow AA, Hubbell DS: Sclerosing hemangioma (histiocytoma xanthoma) of the lung. Cancer 9:53, 1956.

Lockett L, Chiang V, Scully N: Primary pulmonary meningioma: report of a case and review of the literature. Am J Surg Pathol 21:453, 1997.

Lui RC, et al: Primary endobronchial granular cell myoblastoma. Ann Thorac Surg 48:113, 1989.

Lutenbacher R: Dysembryomes metatypique des reins. Carcinose submiliare aigue poumon avec emphysème generalisé et double pneumothorax. Ann Med Intern (Paris) 5:435, 1918.

Marchevsky A, et al: Lung transplantation: the pathologic diagnosis of pulmonary complications. Mod Pathol 4:133, 1991.

Marchevsky AM: Lung tumors derived from ectopic tissues. Semin Diagn Pathol 12:172, 1995.

Martini N, Beattie EJ Jr: Less common tumors of the lung. In Shields TW (ed): General Thoracic Surgery. 2nd Ed. Philadelphia: Lea & Febiger, 1983, p. 780.

Matsubara O, et al: Inflammatory pseudotumors of the lung: progression from organizing pneumonia to fibrous histiocytoma or to plasma cell granuloma in 32 cases. Hum Pathol 19:807, 1988.

McCluggage WG, Bharucha H: Primary pulmonary tumours of nerve sheath origin. Histopathology 26:247, 1995.

Miller DC, et al: Benign metastasizing meningioma. Case report. J Neurosurg 62:763, 1985.

Miura H, et al: Asymptomatic solitary papilloma of the bronchus: review of occurrence in Japan. Eur Respir J 6:1070, 1993.

Miura K, et al: Cystic pulmonary hamartoma. Ann Thorac Surg 49:828, 1990.

Miura K, et al: Benign clear cell tumor of the lung: a case report. J Jpn Assoc Chest Surg 7:95, 1993 (In Japanese with English abstract.)

Moran CA: Primary salivary gland-type tumors of the lung. Semin Diagn Pathol 12:106, 1995.

Moran CA, et al: Primary intrapulmonary thymoma. A clinicopathologic and immunohistochemical study of eight cases. Am J Surg Pathol 19:304, 1995.

Moran CA, et al: Primary intrapulmonary meningiomas. A clinicopathologic and immunohistochemical study of ten cases. Cancer 78:2328, 1996.

Mori M, et al: Papillary adenoma of type II pneumocytes might have malignant potential. Virchows Arch 428:195, 1996.

Nili M, et al: Multiple pulmonary hamartomas: a case report and review of the literature. Scand J Thorac Cardiovasc Surg 13:157, 1979.

Nine JS, et al: Lymphangioleiomyomatosis recurrence after lung transplantation. J Heart Lung Transplant 13:714, 1994.

Noguchi M, et al: Papillary adenoma of type 2 pneumocytes. Am J Surg Pathol 10:134, 1986.

O'Brien JD, et al: Lymphangioleiomyomatosis recurrence in the allograft after single-lung transplantation. Am J Respir Crit Care Med 151:2033, 1995.

Okabayashi K, et al: Giant hamartoma of the lung with a high production of carbohydrate antigen 19-9. Ann Thorac Surg 55:511, 1993.

Oliveira P, et al: Alveolar adenoma of the lung: further characterization of this uncommon tumour. Virchows Arch 429:101, 1996.

Oparah SS, Subramanian VA: Granular cell myoblastoma of the bronchus: report of 2 cases and review of the literature. Ann Thorac Surg 22:199, 1976.

Paul KP, et al: Capillary hemangioma of the right main bronchus treated by sleeve resection in infancy. Am Rev Respir Dis 143:876, 1991.

Popper HH, et al: Prognostic importance of human papilloma virus typing in squamous cell papilloma of the bronchus: comparison of in situ hybridization and the polymerase chain reaction. Hum Pathol 25:1191, 1994.

Ribet M, Jaillard-Thery S, Nuttens MC: Pulmonary hamartoma and malignancy. J Thorac Cardiovasc Surg 107:611, 1994.

Robinson PG: Pulmonary meningioma: Report of a case with electron microscopic and immunohistochemical findings. Am J Clin Pathol 97:814, 1992.

Roux FJ, et al: Mucinous cystadenoma of the lung. Cancer 76:1540, 1995.

Sakamoto H, et al: Pleomorphic adenoma in the periphery of the lung: report of a case and review of the literature. Arch Pathol Lab Med 115:393, 1991.

Sambrook Gowar FJ: An unusual mucous cyst of the lung. Thorax 33:796, 1978.

Sanchez-Jimenez J, et al: Papillary adenoma of type 2 pneumocytes. Pediatr Pulmonol 17:396, 1994.

Shen A, et al: Exacerbation of pulmonary lymphangioleiomyomatosis by exogenous estrogens. Chest 91:782, 1987.

Shields TW, Lynn TE: Endobronchial hamartoma: a case report. Arch Surg 76:358, 1958.

Siegelman SS, et al: CT of pulmonary hamartoma. Presented at the 84th Annual Meeting of the American Roentgen Ray Society, Las Vegas, NV, April 1984.

Silverman JM, et al: Magnetic resonance imaging evaluation of pulmonary vascular malformations. Chest 106:1333, 1994.

Sinclair W, Wright JL, Churg A: Lymphangioleiomyomatosis presenting in postmenopausal women. Thorax 40:475, 1985.

Singh G, Lee RE, Brooks DH: Primary pulmonary paraganglioma: report of a case and review of the literature. Cancer 40:2286, 1977.

Spencer H, Dail DH, Arneaud J: Non-invasive bronchial epithelial papillary tumors. Cancer 45:1486, 1980.

Strickler, JG et al: Myoepithelioma of the lung. Arch Pathol Lab Med 111:1082, 1987.

Sugio K, et al: Sclerosing hemangioma of the lung: radiographic and pathological study. Ann Thorac Surg 53:295, 1992.

Sugita M, et al: Sleeve superior segmentectomy of the right lower lobe for endobronchial neurinoma. Report of a case. Respiration 63:191, 1996.

Swensen SJ, et al: Diffuse pulmonary lymphangiomatosis. CT findings. J Comput Assist Tomogr 19:348, 1995.

Tagge E, et al: Obstructing endobronchial fibrous histiocytoma: potential for lung salvage. J. Pediatr Surg 26:1067, 1991.

Takemura G, et al: Metastasizing uterine leiomyoma. A case with cardiac and pulmonary metastasis. Pathol Res Pract 192:622, 1996.

Tanimura S, et al: Primary pulmonary paraganglioma: a report of a case and review of the literature. J Jpn Assoc Chest Surg 7:88, 1993 (In Japanese with English abstract).

Taylor JR, et al: Lymphangioleiomyomatosis. Clinical course in 32 patients. N Engl J Med 323:1254, 1990.

Tazelaar HD, et al: Diffuse pulmonary lymphangiomatosis. Hum Pathol 24:1313, 1993.

Torikata C, Mukai M: So-called minute chemodectoma of the lung. An electron microscopic and immunohistochemical study. Virchows Arch Pathol Anat Histopathol 417:113, 1990.

Tron V, et al: Pulmonary capillary hemangiomatosis. Hum Pathol 17:1144, 1986.

Tsuji N, et al: Adenomyoepithelioma of the lung. Am J Surg Pathol 19:956, 1995.

Urban T, et al: Pulmonary lymphangiomyomatosis. Follow-up and long-term outcome with antiestrogen therapy: a report of eight cases. Chest 102:472, 1992.

Valensi QJ: Pulmonary lymphangiomyoma, a probable forme fruste of tuberous sclerosis. A case report and survey of the literature. Am Rev Respir Dis 108:1411, 1973.

Van den Bosch JM, et al: Mesenchymoma of the lung (so-called hamartoma): a review of 154 parenchymal and endobronchial cases. Thorax 42:790, 1987.

Veynovich B, et al: Primary pulmonary thymoma. Ann Thorac Surg 64:1471, 1997.

Weinberger MA, Katz S, Davis EW: Peripheral bronchial adenoma of mucus gland type. J Thorac Cardiovasc Surg 29:626, 1955.

Weiss L, Ingram M: Adenomatoid bronchial tumors: a consideration of the carcinoid tumors and salivary tumors of the bronchial tree. Cancer 14:161, 1961.

Wellens F, et al: Combined heart-lung transplantation for terminal pulmonary lymphangioleiomyomatosis. J Thorac Cardiovasc Surg 89:872, 1985.

Wende S, et al: Lung metastasis of a meningioma. Neuroradiology 24:287, 1983.

White SH, et al: Leiomyomas of the lower respiratory tract. Thorax 40:306, 1985.

Winkler TR, Burr LH, Robinson CLN: Benign metastasizing leiomyoma. Ann Thorac Surg 43:100, 1987.

Wodehouse GE: Hemangioma of the lung: a review of four cases. J Thorac Cardiovasc Surg 17:408, 1948.

Yamakawa T, et al: Intrapulmonary schwannoma: a case report. J Jpn Assoc Chest Surg 7:165, 1993 (In Japanese with English summary).

Yellin A, Rosenman Y, Lieberman Y: Review of smooth muscle tumours of the lower respiratory tract. Br J Dis Chest 78:337, 1984.

Yokozaki M, et al: Endobronchial lipoma: a report of three cases. Jpn J Clin Oncol 26:53, 1996.

Yousem SA: Pulmonary vascular neoplasia. Prog Surg Pathol 10:27, 1989.

Yousem SA, Flynn DS: Intrapulmonary localized fibrous tumor: intraparenchymal so-called localized fibrous mesothelioma. Am J Clin Pathol 89:365, 1988.

Yousem SA, Hochholzer L: Alveolar adenoma. Hum Pathol 17:1066, 1986.

Yousem SA, Hochholzer L: Pulmonary hyalinizing granuloma. Am J Clin Pathol 87:1, 1987.

Yousem SA, et al: So-called sclerosing hemangiomas of the lung: an immunohistochemical study supporting a respiratory epithelial origin. Am J Surg Pathol 12:582, 1988.

READING REFERENCES

General

Carter D, Eggleston JC: Tumors of the lower respiratory tract, Series 2. Washington, DC: Armed Forces Institute of Pathology, 1980, p. 221.

Churg A: Tumors of the Lung. In Thurlbeck W (ed): Pathology of the Lung. New York: Thieme, 1988, p. 311.

Dail DH, Hammar SP: Pulmonary Pathology. New York: Springer, 1987.

Dunnill MS: Rare Pulmonary Tumors. In Dunnill MS (ed): Pulmonary Pathology. 2nd Ed. New York: Churchill Livingstone, 1987, p. 413.

Mackay B, Lukeman JM, Ordonez NG: Tumors of The Lungs. Philadelphia: WB Saunders, 1991.

Madewell JE, Feigin DS: Benign tumors of the lung. Semin Roentgenol 12:175, 1977.

Marchesky AM (ed): Surgical Pathology of Lung Neoplasms. New York: Marcel Dekker, 1990.

Spencer H: Rare pulmonary tumors. In Spencer H (ed): Pathology of the Lung. 4th Ed. New York: Pergamon Press, 1985, p. 933.

Connective Tissue Tumors, Benign

Orlowski TM, Stasiak K, Kolodziej J: Leiomyoma of the lung. J Thorac Cardiovasc Surg 76:257, 1978.

Schraufnagel DE, Morin JE, Wang NS: Endobronchial lipoma. Chest 75:97, 1979.

Epithelial Tumor

Spencer H, Dail DH, Arneaud J: Noninvasive bronchial epithelial papillary tumors. Cancer 45:1486, 1986.

Fibrous Histiocytoma, Benign

Viguera JL, et al: Fibrous histiocytoma of the lung. Thorax 31:475, 1976.

Granular Cell Myoblastoma—Granular Cell Tumor

O'Connell DJ, MacMahon H, DeMeester TR: Multicentric tracheobronchial and oesophageal granular cell myoblastoma. Thorax 33:596, 1978.

Valenstein SL, Thurer RJ: Granular cell myoblastoma of the bronchus: case report and literature review. J Thorac Cardiovasc Surg 76:465, 1978.

Hamartoma

Becker RM, ViLorio J, Chiu C: Multiple pulmonary myomatous hamartomas in women. J Thorac Cardiovasc Surg 71:631, 1976.

Bennett LL, Lesar MS, Tellis CJ: Multiple calcified chondrohamartomas of the lung: CT appearance. J Comput Assist Tomogr 9:180, 1985.

Hansen CP, et al: Pulmonary hamartoma. J Thorac Cardiovasc Surg 104:674, 1992.

Koutras P, Urschel HC Jr, Paulson DL: Hamartoma of the lung. J Thorac Cardiovasc Surg 61:768, 1971.

Minasian H: Uncommon pulmonary hamartomas. Thorax 32:360, 1977.

Petheram IS, Heard BE: Unique massive pulmonary hamartoma: case report with review of hamartoma treated at Brompton Hospital in 27 years. Chest 75:95, 1979.

Ramzy I: Pulmonary hamartomas: cytologic appearances of fine-needle aspiration biopsy. Acta Cytol 20:15, 1976.

Shah JP, et al: Hamartomas of the lung. Surg Gynecol Obstet 136:406, 1973.

Spencer H: Hamartomas, Blastoma and Teratoma of the Lung. In Spencer H (ed): Pathology of the Lung. 4th Ed. New York: Pergamon Press, 1985, p. 1061.

Tomashefski JF Jr: Benign endobronchial mesenchymal tumors: their relationship to parenchymal pulmonary hamartomas. Am J Surg Pathol 6:531, 1982.

Lymphangioleiomyomatosis

Graham ML, et al: Pulmonary lymphangiomyomatosis: with particular reference to steroid-receptor assay studies and pathologic correlation. Mayo Clin Proc 59:3, 1984.

Luna CM, et al: Pulmonary LAM associated with tuberous sclerosis: treatment with tamoxifen and tetracycline pleurodesis. Chest 88:473, 1985.

Pseudotumors

Bahadori H, Liebow AA: Plasma cell granulomas of the lung. Cancer *31*:191, 1973.
Graham ML, et al: Pulmonary lymphangiomyomatosis: with particular attention to steroid-receptor assay studies and pathologic correlation. Mayo Clin Proc *59*:3, 1984.
Spencer H: The pulmonary plasma cell/histiocytoma complex. Histopathology *8*:903, 1984.
Spoto G Jr, Rossi NP, Allsbrook WC: Tracheobronchial plasma cell granuloma. J Thorac Cardiovasc Surg *73*:804, 1977.

Warter A, Satge D, Roeslin N: Angioinvasive plasma cell granuloma of the lung. Cancer *59*:435, 1987.

Teratomas, Benign

Ali MY, Wong PK: Intrapulmonary teratoma. Thorax *19*:228, 1964.
Holt S, Peverall PB, Boddy JE: A teratoma of the lung containing thymic tissue. J Pathol *126*:85, 1978.
Spencer H: Hamartomas, Blastoma and Teratoma of the Lung. *In* Spencer H (ed): Pathology of the Lung. 4th Ed. New York: Pergamon Press, 1985, p. 1061.

CHAPTER 112

Uncommon Primary Malignant Tumors of the Lung

Philip G. Robinson and Thomas W. Shields

Most of the uncommon primary malignant tumors of the lungs are sarcomas, but they also include pulmonary blastomas, carcinosarcomas, primary pulmonary lymphomas, and various other malignancies, including the rare primary malignant melanoma, primary teratoma, and malignant ependymoma (Table 112-1). In an 11-year review (1980 through 1990) of 80 rare pulmonary neoplasms seen at the Mayo Clinic, Miller and Allen (1993) reported that 41% were non-Hodgkin's lymphomas, 20% were carcinosarcomas, 15% were mucoepidermoid carcinomas (these tumors are discussed in Chapter 110), and 18% were sarcomas; the remainder were either malignant melanomas or blastomas. The patients had a median age of 60 years. In contrast, Hancock and colleagues (1993) described the distribution of lung tumors in children. They added nine cases to the literature and summarized a total of 383 cases. Most of the tumors (76%) were malignant. Of these, 40.5% were bronchial "adenoma," and 16.8% were bronchial carcinomas. The remaining malignant tumors were pulmonary blastomas (15.5%), lymphomas or plasmacytomas (2.4%), and malignant teratomas (1%). Benign tumors made up 24% of the cases, with the majority of these being inflammatory pseudotumors.

SOFT TISSUE SARCOMAS

Primitive mesenchymal cells are present in every organ of the human body. In the lung, tumors of mesenchymal origin may arise from the stromal elements of the bronchial or vascular wall or from the interstices of lung parenchyma. These tumors usually expand toward the lung parenchyma; occasionally, they extend into the lumen of a bronchus. Only rarely do they invade and break through the bronchial epithelium. As a result, these tumors do not exfoliate cells, and diagnosis by cytologic examination of expectorations or of tracheobronchial washings is uncommon. Grossly, the tumor usually appears as a well-circumscribed and encapsulated mass in the lung parenchyma (Fig. 112-1). They generally spread by local invasion. Peripheral lesions may invade the adjacent pleura and chest wall; only rarely do they cavitate. They can metastasize by way of the circulation and rarely by lymphatic invasion. As Watson and Anlyan (1954) noted, metastases to distant organs are usually late manifestations of the disease process. Microscopically, these tumors present a wide range of cellular differentiation.

Primary pulmonary sarcomas occur at almost any age, with equal frequency in either sex. Fadhli and colleagues (1965) reported an age range of 4 to 83 years. The tumors occur with equal frequency in either lung. Many patients are asymptomatic, and lesions are detected only on a routine radiograph of the chest. Symptomatic patients most commonly experience chest pain, cough, dyspnea, and hemoptysis. Fever, fatigue, anorexia, and weight loss usually are late manifestations. On radiographs of the chest, the tumor usually appears as a sharply demarcated mass density within the lung substance at the hilus or in the lung periphery. The lesions are usually solitary. Martini and associates (1971) reported that these tumors vary in diameter from 1 to 15 cm or more, with an average diameter of 6 to 7 cm. Peripheral tumors invading the chest wall may be associated with varying degrees of pleural effusion. Tumors obstructing a bronchus (approximately 15%) may result in distal parenchymal changes (Fig. 112-2).

Dail (1988) categorized the soft tissue sarcomas arising within the lung into three groups: 1) parenchymal and bronchial-endobronchial sarcomas, 2) sarcomas of large vessel origin, and 3) sarcomas of small vessel origin.

Parenchymal and Bronchial-Endobronchial Sarcomas

Fibrosarcoma, leiomyosarcoma, rhabdomyosarcoma, neurogenic sarcoma, chondrosarcoma, osteosarcoma, mono-

Table 112-1. Less Common Malignant Tumors of the Lung

Soft tissue sarcomas
    Parenchymal and bronchial sarcomas
    Sarcomas of large vessel origin
    Sarcomas of small vessel origin
Carcinosarcoma
Pulmonary blastoma (embryoma), including pleuropulmonary
    blastomas and well-differentiated fetal adenocarcinomas
Basaloid carcinoma
Primary pulmonary choriocarcinoma
Lymphoepithelioma-like carcinoma
Primary malignant melanoma
Primary malignant teratoma
Malignant ependymoma
Primary pulmonary lymphoma
    Non-Hodgkin's lymphoma
    Small cell lymphocytic lymphoma (BALT lymphoma)
    Large cell "histocytic" lymphoma
    Lymphomatoid granulomatosis
    Intravascular lymphomatosis
    Plasma cell disorders
    Primary pulmonary Hodgkin's disease

BALT, bronchial-associated lymphoid tissue.

phasic synovial sarcoma, malignant mesenchymoma, liposarcoma, and malignant fibrous histiocytoma are included in this category. These sarcomas may occur in either an endobronchial or a parenchymal location; however, the occurrence of any of these sarcomas as primary lesions in the lung is rare. Table 112-2 is a list of the distribution of some of these lesions in adults and children in the series reported by Nascimento (1982), Hartman (1983), McCormack (1988), Janssen (1994) and their associates.

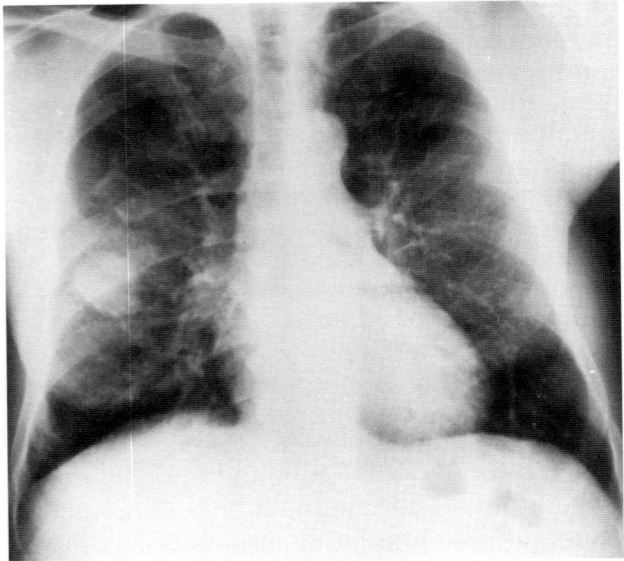

Fig. 112-1. Posteroanterior chest radiograph reveals recurrent fibrosarcoma of the right lung after previous wedge resection of a "fibromatous" tumor from the middle lobe.

Pulmonary Fibrosarcoma

Combining the patients in the series of Guccion and Rosen (1972) and Nascimento and colleagues (1982) yields a total of 22 cases of primary pulmonary fibrosarcomas. The patients ranged in age from 23 to 69 years with an average age of 47 years. There were 16 (72%) men and 6 (27%) women. This bias might exist because one of the studies is from the Armed Forces Institute of Pathology. These fibrosarcomas may occur in either an endobronchial or a parenchymal location. The endobronchial tumors were almost always symptomatic. The symptoms ranged from none to chest pain, cough, hemoptysis, and shortness of breath. McLigeyo (1995) and associates reported a pulmonary fibrosarcoma in a 50-year-old woman who presented with hypoglycemia and hypertrophic pulmonary osteoarthropathy. Most patients were treated mainly by surgical excision. A few patients received radiation therapy and chemotherapy. In Guccion and Rosen's (1972) series, several patients were lost to follow-up, but the majority of the followed patients died of their disease. Those patients with endobronchial lesions seemed to survive longer. In the nine cases of Nascimento and colleagues (1982), seven died from their disease within 3 months to 18 years after treatment. Two were alive at 7 and 18 years following treatment. The patient who survived 18 years had an endobronchial lesion. The one who survived 7 years had a parenchymal tumor.

In a case report Goldthorn and colleagues (1986) described a cavitating fibrosarcoma in an 11-year-old girl who underwent a resection followed by chemotherapy. She had a 36-month disease-free survival.

Pulmonary Leiomyosarcoma

Guccion and Rosen (1972), Nascimento (1982), and Moran and colleagues (1997) have reported a total of 41 cases of pulmonary leiomyosarcomas. These patients ranged in age from a newborn to 91 years, with an average of 51

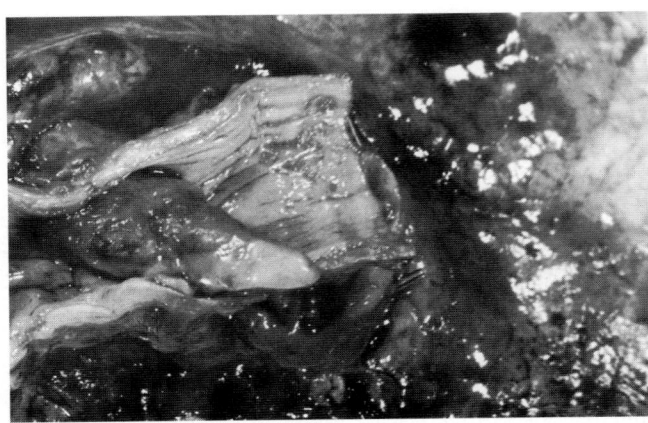

Fig. 112-2. Malignant endobronchial sarcoma.

Table 112-2. Distribution of Soft Tissue Sarcomas

	Nascimento et al. (1982) (Adults)	McCormack and Martini (1988) (All Age Groups)	Janssen et al. (1994) (All Age Groups)	Hartman and Shochat (1983) (Children)
Pulmonary blastoma	—	1	—	14
Fibrosarcoma	9	2	4	—
Leiomyosarcoma	4	16	9	9
Rhabdomyosarcoma	—	5	1	6
Hemangiopericytoma	3	1	—	3
Osteosarcoma	2	—	—	—
Myxosarcoma	—	—	—	1
Spindle cell sarcoma	—	13	—	—
Angiosarcoma	—	2	1	—
Malignant fibrous histiocytoma	—	3	—	—
Malignant schwannoma	—	—	5	—
Undifferentiated sarcoma	—	—	2	—
Total	**18**	**43**	**22**	**33**
Total Number of Cases				**116**

years. There were 29 men and 12 women for a gender ratio of 2.4:1.0. The symptoms ranged from none to cough, chest pain, dyspnea, and hemoptysis. The chest radiographs usually showed a solitary homogenous density with sharply lobulated borders. Cavitation was observed in some of the leiomyosarcomas, as noted by Lillo-Gil and associates (1985). The tumors were randomly distributed to all the lobes of both lungs. On gross examination, the leiomyosarcoma may be in an endobronchial, parenchymal, or subpleural location and is usually well-circumscribed, firm, and gray-white. Areas of necrosis or hemorrhage may exist. Microscopically, the tumor comprises spindle cells with broad fascicles that intersect at right angles.

Moran and colleagues (1997) divided the pulmonary leiomyosarcomas into low-grade malignancy, intermediate-grade malignancy, and high-grade malignancy. The low-grade neoplasms have a well-developed fascicular pattern. The cells have "cigar-shaped" nuclei without much atypia, eosinophilic cytoplasm, and one to three mitoses per 10 high power fields (HPFs). The intermediate-grade tumors have a fairly well-preserved fascicular pattern but are more cellular. The cells have slightly more atypical hyperchromatic nuclei. Mitoses are slightly increased to three to eight per 10 HPFs. Areas of hemorrhage and necrosis are not apparent. High-grade tumors show a more solid cellular proliferation with less of a fascicular pattern. The cells are markedly pleomorphic with large hyperchromatic nuclei and prominent nucleoli. Mitoses are increased to 8 to 12 per 10 HPFs, and areas of hemorrhage and necrosis are present. Immunostaining shows that most of the tumors (75%) stain for smooth muscle actin.

Treatment is surgical removal of the tumor. The prognosis is poor, with the majority of the patients dying of the disease, although a few patients have survived for 15 to 20 years. Moran and colleagues (1997) concluded the grade of the tumor was important in determining prognosis. Patients with low-grade to intermediate-grade tumors had a better prognosis than patients with high-grade tumors.

Pulmonary Rhabdomyosarcoma

Rhabdomyosarcomas are malignant tumors of skeletal muscle and can occur in various age groups and in either sex. The majority of the cases occur in infants and children from the ages of 1.5 years to 14.0 years, but Przygodzki and associates (1995) described three cases in men ranging in age from 57 to 78 years. The symptoms depend on whether the lesion is endobronchial or parenchymal. According to d'Agostino and colleagues (1997) many of the rhabdomyosarcomas that arise in children are associated with cystic adenomatoid malformations. The chest radiographs usually show a tumor that may have cysts. The computed tomographic (CT) scan shows a soft tissue mass that may be cystic. Pathologically, the tumors have reddish gray surfaces with hemorrhagic and necrotic areas. On microscopic examination, the cells may be arranged in fascicles or be randomly organized. The nuclei are hyperchromatic with a nucleolus and eosinophilic cytoplasm. Cross striations within the cytoplasm can be demonstrated with a phosphotungstic acid hematoxylin (PTAH) stain. The cells will immunostain for desmin, myoglobin, and vimentin. Treatment is surgical resection, and according to Schiavetti and colleagues (1996), it is usually combined with chemotherapy and radiation therapy. McDermott and colleagues (1993) pointed out that these patients were predisposed to develop cerebral metastases. In the younger age group, approximately one-third of patients died or were living with disease, and approximately two-thirds were alive with no evidence of disease at varying periods of follow-up. Noda and coworkers (1995) noted that serum neuron specific enolase (NSE) was helpful in detecting metastasis and disease recurrence in a patient with alveolar rhabdomyosarcoma of the lung.

Malignant Fibrous Histiocytoma

A malignant fibrous histiocytoma is usually found in the extremities or retroperitoneum in adults. It occurs infrequently in the lung and is less common than pulmonary fibrosarcomas and leiomyosarcomas. Yousem and Hochholzer (1987a) reviewed 22 cases that they identified from the files of the Armed Forces Institute of Pathology. McDonnell and colleagues (1988) reported one case of pulmonary malignant fibrous histiocytoma and reviewed 15 other cases they found in the literature. Halyard and colleagues (1996) reported four cases and reviewed 49 cases that have appeared in the English literature. The patients in these three reports ranged in age from 18 to 80 years with an average age of 55. There was a slight preponderance of men to women (30:23). The most common clinical symptoms were cough, chest pain, weight loss, and hemoptysis. Hypoglycemia and hypertrophic pulmonary osteoarthropathy also were observed in a few patients. In most instances, the chest radiograph showed a mass lesion, usually a large solid noncavitary mass. Calcification in the mass is rarely seen. The tumors appear to be distributed randomly between both lungs. Microscopically, most of the tumors were storiform (pleomorphic), and a few were of the myxoid or inflammatory type. Tian and associates (1997) reported seven cases seen in 11 years in their thoracic unit in Shanyang, China. The findings were similar in all respects to those in the aforementioned reports.

The primary therapeutic approach to these tumors is complete surgical excision followed by radiation therapy or chemotherapy, if either is clinically indicated. Poor prognostic indicators are an advanced stage at the time of diagnosis, such as extension of the tumor into the chest wall or mediastinum; metastasis beyond the thorax; or incomplete excision. Halyard and associates (1996) reported that eight patients in their report had survived more than 5 years after surgical excision with or without adjuvant therapy for a survival rate of 15%.

Pulmonary Chondrosarcoma

Morgan and Salama (1972) reported a case of pulmonary chondrosarcoma, an extremely rare tumor, and reviewed the literature. The eight patients identified with primary pulmonary chondrosarcoma ranged in age from 23 to 73 years, with an average age of 46 years. The lesions were distributed equally between the sexes. The clinical symptoms in the order of frequency were cough, chest pain, and dyspnea. The tumor seemed to be more common in the left lung. Radiologically, these tumors may have shown areas of calcification or ossification. These tumors were solid masses, but Parker (1996) and coworkers described a patient in whom the CT scan and magnetic resonance (MR) imaging findings mimicked a bronchogenic cyst. Grossly, these tumors had a gray surface, were circumscribed, and appeared to have a capsule. Microscopically, the tumors contained areas of malignant cartilage with calcification or ossification. Three of the patients in the aforementioned review died of their tumor, two were lost to follow-up, and three others who had smaller resectable lesions were doing

well; their follow-up ranged from 15 months to 4 years. Morgenroth and colleagues (1989) reported an additional patient in whom the lesion arose in the left inferior lobar bronchus. This patient underwent a left pneumonectomy but died 8 months later with recurrent disease. Hayashi and associates (1993) reported another case; the patient developed metastases first to the skull and then to the kidneys.

Pulmonary Osteosarcoma

Primary pulmonary osteosarcoma is rare. Loose and colleagues (1990) reported two cases and found nine other cases in the literature. For the lesion to be considered an extraosseous osteosarcoma, they adhered to the following criteria: 1) the tumor must be composed of a uniform pattern of sarcomatous tissue that excludes the possibility of a malignant mixed mesenchymal tumor, 2) osteoid or bone must be formed by the sarcoma, and 3) a primary osseous tumor can be excluded. The patients ranged in age from 35 to 83 years with a mean of 61 years. The tumors were seen equally in men and women. The most common clinical symptom was chest pain. The sarcomas approximately were distributed equally in the right and left lungs. When possible, the tumor should be resected. The prognosis is poor. Seven patients in the collected series died of their disease, two patients died of other diseases, and three patients were alive within 2 to 14 months of follow-up. Several additional case reports of osteosarcomas have appeared in the literature in the early 1990s, but none since then. Petersen (1990) reported a 70-year-old man with a large lung mass. A technetium-99m-methylene diphosphonate bone scan revealed an abnormal area in the left lower lung, but not in the skeleton. After lobectomy, the lesion was diagnosed as an osteosarcoma. Connolly and associates (1991) described a 93-year-old man whose chest radiograph showed a densely calcified lung lesion. On needle biopsy it was an osteosarcoma. The patient died at home, and the family refused an autopsy. Lastly, Bhalla and colleagues (1992) described a 58-year-old man with a cavitary lesion that was thought to be an abscess. The CT scan showed an irregular cavity with a partially calcified thick wall. A repeat scan, 3 weeks later, showed increasing calcifications and a marked increase in size. The patient was treated with drainage and antibiotics but without improvement. At autopsy, the mass was a pulmonary osteosarcoma.

Pulmonary Liposarcoma

A primary liposarcoma is one of the rarer sarcomas that occur in the lung. Krygier and associates (1997) described a patient with a pleomorphic liposarcoma whose disease ran a rapidly fatal course despite aggressive treatment. These authors also noted 11 other cases of primary liposarcomas of the lung that had been reported in the literature. The most common type of liposarcoma was the myxomatous variety as reported by Hochberg and Crastnopol (1956) and others.

The most successful treatment is complete surgical resection when possible.

Synovial Sarcoma

Zeren and associates (1995) reported a study of 25 cases of primary pulmonary sarcomas with features of monophasic synovial sarcoma. These tumors were seen slightly more often in women than in men. The majority of patients were middle-aged adults (30 to 50 years old). The clinical symptomatology consisted of chest pain, cough, dyspnea, and hemoptysis. The tumors varied in size with a median of 4.2 cm. The tumors were either peripheral or central in location and appeared to be well circumscribed but were not encapsulated. The tumors had histologic and ultrastructural features of monophasic synovial sarcoma. Immunohistochemical studies revealed the tumor cells to react positively to vimentin, cytokeratins, and epithelial membrane antigen (EMA). Kaplan and colleagues (1996) presented two similar cases. However, in each (one a 12-year-old girl and the other a 40-year-old woman) the authors described the presence of a specific chromosome translocation t(x; 18) that is associated with synovial sarcoma of other sites. In all patients surgical removal is suggested as the treatment of choice. The prognosis of the patients with this rare tumor is undetermined but is suspected to be poor.

Neurogenic Sarcoma

A neurogenic sarcoma is a malignant proliferation of Schwann cells. Other synonyms for this lesion include malignant schwannoma and neurofibrosarcoma. McCluggage and Bharucha (1995) reported two cases and reviewed the literature. Their patients were 34 and 45 years old; one was a man and the other a woman. Both presented with dyspnea and chest pain. On gross examination, one tumor was 8 cm in size and the other 10 cm in size. One was a white, circumscribed mass that had a whirled appearance on cut section. The other was white but contained necrotic areas. On microscopic examination, the smaller tumor had a benign appearance with a fibrous capsule and spindle cells with irregular wavy nuclei. The larger tumor was highly cellular with necrosis. It had pleomorphic cells and multinucleated giant cells with easily identified mitotic figures. Immunostaining revealed that both tumors were focally positive for S-100 protein and diffusely positive for vimentin. They were negative for desmin, carcinoembryonic antigen, and CAM 5.2, a keratin. The tumor was resected in both patients, but each patient subsequently developed metastatic disease.

Malignant Mesenchymoma

Malignant mesenchymoma is a sarcoma composed of two or more cellular elements, excluding fibrous tissue. Domizio and colleagues (1990) reported a case in a 4-year-old boy arising from a cyst. The boy had a history of pulmonary cyst in the right lower lobe diagnosed when he was 6 months old by chest radiograph, and he had a clinical history of anorexia, recurrent dry cough, and night sweats. He was anemic with an elevated sedimentation rate. At the time of admission, the chest radiograph showed an opaque right hemithorax with an air fluid level in the right mid lung field and the mediastinum shifted to the left. He underwent a right lower lobectomy. On gross examination, the lobe was replaced by a necrotic tumor. The viable outer rim was composed of yellowish-gray gelatinous nodules with an area of central necrosis. Microscopically, the tumor was composed of large anaplastic cells with numerous multinucleate giant cells. There were areas of rhabdomyosarcoma and chondrosarcoma. A cystic lesion was also present with multiple cystic spaces lined by epithelial cells. The patient was treated with chemotherapy and radiation therapy and was free of disease at short-term follow-up.

Sarcomas of Large Vessel Origin

A pulmonary trunk sarcoma is a primary lesion arising within the pulmonary artery or, as Mandelstramm (1923) described, from the pulmonary valve of the heart. In reviews by Wackers (1969), Bleisch (1980), Baker (1985), Emmert-Buck (1994), and Nonomura (1988) and their associates, as well as Goldblum and Rice (1995), undifferentiated sarcoma, leiomyosarcoma, and fibrosarcoma make up the majority of the cell types of these intravascular tumors but also include pleomorphic rhabdomyosarcoma and epithelioid angiosarcoma. Burke and Virmani (1993), after doing immunohistochemistry, concluded that most pulmonary artery sarcomas were derived from intimal cells with myofibroblastic differentiation. Ko (1996) and Leone (1996) and their coworkers both described leiomyosarcomas in the pulmonary vein.

The large-vessel sarcomas may spread distally within the vascular tree or extend outside the vessel to invade the lung tissue. The patients may be of any age. In reported cases, the age range was from 21 to 81 years, with an average age of 50 years. There is a slight predominance of these large-vessel sarcomas in women. The patients present with chest pain and dyspnea, and one-third may also have cough, hemoptysis, and palpitations. A systolic heart murmur may be present. Pulmonary hypertension with proximal dilation of the vessels is a constant feature. A late manifestation is right-sided heart decompensation. Moffat and colleagues (1972) reported the radiographic features, as did Britton (1990). The lesion manifests most often as a lobulated perihilar mass. Angiography may reveal multiple defects within the pulmonary artery. CT scanning and MR imaging may help to determine the extent of the disease. Mader and colleagues (1997) believe that MR imaging is the imaging modality of choice for these lesions because it is noninvasive and gives an excellent definition of the heart, pericardium, mediastinum, and lungs. MR imaging can also delineate both the extent and location of the lesion. Cox and colleagues (1997) agree with this assessment and believe the imaging findings are quite specific. Parish and associates (1996), in addition to discussing the MR imaging and CT scan features of nine cases, suggested that transesophageal echocardiography might also be useful in evaluating pulmonary trunk sarcomas. Treatment is resection. Head (1992) and Redmond (1990) and their coworkers, among others, reported cases in which these tumors were successfully resected. Kruger and associates (1990) reported prolonging survival with resection followed by adjuvant therapy; however, the prognosis for long-term survival is poor.

Sarcomas of Small Vessel Origin

Angiosarcoma, epithelioid hemangioendothelioma, and hemangiopericytoma are malignant vascular tumors that occasionally may occur in the lung but are very rare in this location. Kaposi's sarcoma, a vascular neoplasm, is not discussed here because it has not been described as having a primary pulmonary origin. Lastly, according to Enzinger and Weiss (1983), the term *hemangioendothelioma* should be used only to designate a group of vascular tumors that cannot be accurately classified histologically as to their ultimate biological behavior.

Angiosarcoma

An angiosarcoma is a malignant neoplasm of endothelial cells. They have also been called *malignant hemangiomas* or *malignant hemangioendotheliomas*. When the neoplastic endothelial cells have an epithelial appearance, the sarcomas are referred to as *epithelioid angiosarcomas*. Spragg and associates (1983) reviewed the literature and presented 10 possible cases of angiosarcoma arising in the lung, but some doubts exist about whether these cases were all true pulmonary angiosarcomas. Yousem (1986) believes that these tumors are most likely metastases from an angiosarcoma of the right ventricle, pulmonary arterial trunk, or an extrathoracic site. Patel and Ryu (1993) reviewed the files of the Mayo Clinic from 1950 to 1990, and they could not identify any primary pulmonary angiosarcomas. They identified 15 patients with metastatic angiosarcoma and discussed the single case reports of so-called primary angiosarcoma. Sheppard and colleagues (1997) described an epithelioid angiosarcoma of the lung in a 65-year-old man who presented with pulmonary hemorrhage. At autopsy, the lungs were hemorrhagic with multiple nodules of tumor. An angiosarcoma can be associated with a hemothorax, hypertrophic pulmonary osteoarthropathy, or both. The prognosis is poor.

Epithelioid Hemangioendothelioma

Epithelioid hemangioendothelioma is a low-grade sclerosing angiosarcoma that occurs in the lung as well as the liver, bone, soft tissue, and other sites. This vascular lesion was first described by Dail and Liebow in 1975. Dail and colleagues (1983) reviewed an additional 19 cases. They initially called this tumor an *intravascular bronchioloalveolar tumor* (IVBAT), but they now prefer the term *sclerosing endothelial tumor* (SET). Weiss and Enzinger (1982) described 41 cases of an identical tumor occurring in soft tissue and proposed the name *epithelioid hemangioendothelioma*, which has become widely accepted. Weiss and colleagues (1986) published a combined review of lesions in soft tissue, lung, liver, and bone. Wenisch and Lulay (1980) reported that, in the lung, these tumors occur in patients from 4 to 70 years of age, with one-third of the patients aged less than 30 years. The tumor occurs four times more frequently in women than in men. Most of the patients are asymptomatic or complain of a nonproductive cough. According to Ross and associates (1989), the chest radiographs and CT scans reveal many small (i.e., 1 cm in diameter) nodular densities in both lung fields. The average survival after diagnosis is 4.6 years, but Miettinen and associates (1987) reported a patient who survived for 24 years with repeated surgical excisions. Kawashima and colleagues (1995) reported a case and suggested that aggressive surgical intervention is the treatment of choice for these lesions. Death from pulmonary insufficiency is the usual course of this disease.

Hemangiopericytomas

Hemangiopericytomas are unusual sarcomas derived from the ubiquitous capillary pericytic cell and are commonly located in the soft tissues of the thigh and retroperitoneum. Yousem and Hochholzer (1987b) found that pulmonary hemangiopericytomas occurred with equal frequency in men and women; the average age of patients was 46.1 years. Approximately one-third of the patients were asymptomatic. Those with symptoms complained of chest pain, hemoptysis, dyspnea, and cough. One patient had pulmonary osteoarthropathy. Radiographs of the chest usually show a lobulated, well-circumscribed, homogenous soft tissue density, but other findings may be present (Fig. 112-3). Rusch and colleagues (1989) found that MR imaging was critical in the preoperative evaluation of these patients because of its ability to delineate the anatomic extent of the lesion. Treatment is surgical excision. Prognosis is variable; indicators of a poor prognosis are chest symptoms, size of the tumor more than 8 cm, pleural and bronchial wall invasion, tumor giant cells, greater than three mitoses per 10 HPFs, and tumor necrosis. Shinn and Ho (1979) noted that tumors 5 cm or larger had metastasis in 33% of the cases, and tumors 10 cm or larger had metastasis in 66% of the cases. Davis and coworkers (1972) demonstrated that most recurrences took place within 2 years of diagnosis. Enzinger and Smith (1976) and Feldman and Seaman (1964) reported that chemotherapy and radiation therapy do not consistently help the patient. In separate case reports, Wu (1997),

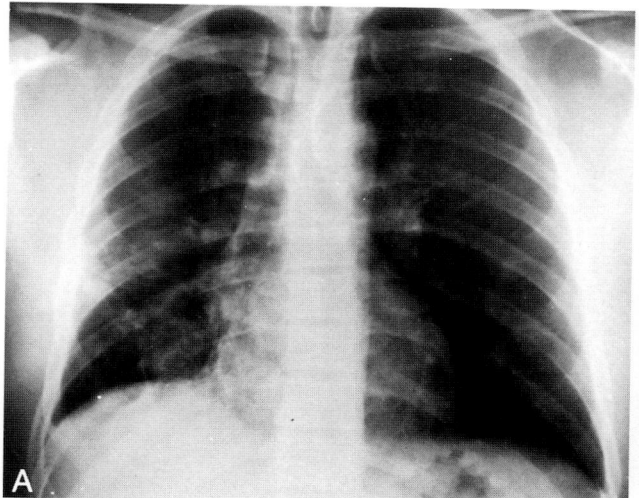
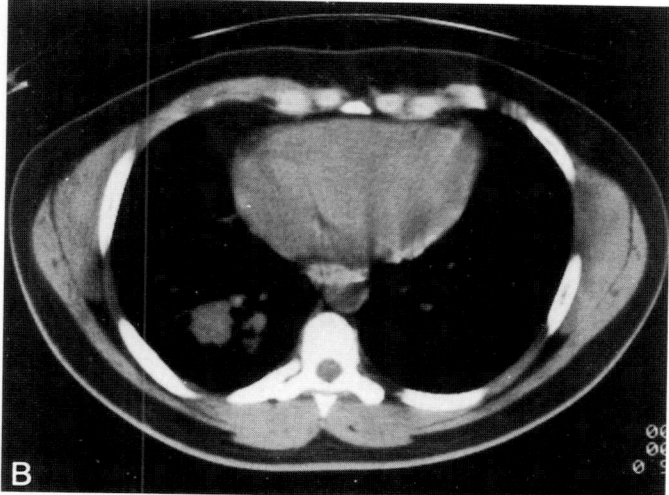

Fig. 112-3. A. Posteroanterior radiograph of the chest reveals a 5-cm mass in the right lower lobe. Suggestion of additional masses evident on the levels of the second and third anterior interspaces. **B.** CT scan reveals a mass in the right lower lobe with multiple satellite lesions. Histologic examination of the resected specimen revealed a poorly differentiated hemangiopericytoma.

Shimizu (1993), Kiefer (1997), Van Damme (1990), Rusch (1989), and Hansen (1990) and their colleagues described their experience with pulmonary hemangiopericytomas. The patients described by Van Damme and coworkers (1990) died within several months of their operation. In contrast, the patient of Rusch and associates (1989) was disease-free 28 months after surgical excision. Wu and colleagues (1997) described a patient who had an associated coagulopathy which recurred when the tumor recurred.

CARCINOSARCOMA

The terminology of carcinosarcoma has been changing as pathologists examine these neoplasms more closely. A *carcinosarcoma* is defined as a malignant neoplasm composed of both malignant epithelium and mesenchymal elements. The mesenchymal component should show differentiation into specific heterologous mesenchymal tissues, such as bone, cartilage, or striated muscle, but not fibroblasts. The purpose of this definition is to separate carcinosarcoma from spindle cell carcinoma. A spindle cell carcinoma is a type of squamous cell carcinoma with spindling of the squamous cells and the presence of squamous islands. Heterologous sarcomatous elements, such as osteosarcoma, are not identified in these spindle cell carcinomas. Nappi and associates (1994) reviewed 21 cases of carcinosarcomas and spindle cell carcinomas. They believed these two neoplasms were merely part of a spectrum and suggested adopting the name *biphasic sarcomatoid carcinoma* for carcinosarcoma and *monophasic sarcomatoid carcinoma* for spindle cell carcinoma. They noted that both of these tumors tended to behave in an aggressive fashion, with 20 of their patients dying within 2 years and only one patient alive with no evi-

dence of disease at 21 months. Finally, Wick and colleagues (1997) went on to place both these tumors under the designation *sarcomatoid carcinoma*.

Ishida and colleagues (1990) described five cases of carcinosarcoma and three cases of spindle cell carcinoma. Kimino and coworkers (1996) described a case in which the sarcomatous component was positively stained by the EMA, suggesting a sarcomatous transformation of the carcinomatous component of the tumor. Grahmann and coworkers (1993) reported three cases of carcinosarcoma and reviewed the literature, as did Berho (1995) and Wick (1997) and their colleagues.

Carcinosarcomas account for 0.3% of all pulmonary neoplasms and are found most often in a proximal bronchus, although they may arise in the parenchyma (Fig. 112-4). They occur more often in men than in women (5:1). Approximately 87% of carcinosarcomas develop in patients more than 50 years of age. These tumors frequently have a slow rate of growth. Much of the growth can be endobronchial with little propensity to infiltrate the bronchial wall, but extensive invasion into the surrounding lung does occur. Metastases to the regional lymph nodes and to distant organs, especially to the brain, are common. The more common symptoms are cough and hemoptysis. Chest pain and malaise may occur. Meade and coworkers (1991) described a patient with associated pulmonary osteoarthropathy. Patients with a peripheral tumor may be asymptomatic. Bronchial biopsy may be followed by excessive hemorrhage but is nonetheless indicated for the preoperative evaluation of an endobronchial lesion. Surgical resection, when possible, is the indicated treatment. In most series, 75 to 80% of the patients die within the first year of resection. Approximately 16% of patients survive 5 years or longer. In the series reported by Miller and Allen (1993), a 5-year survival

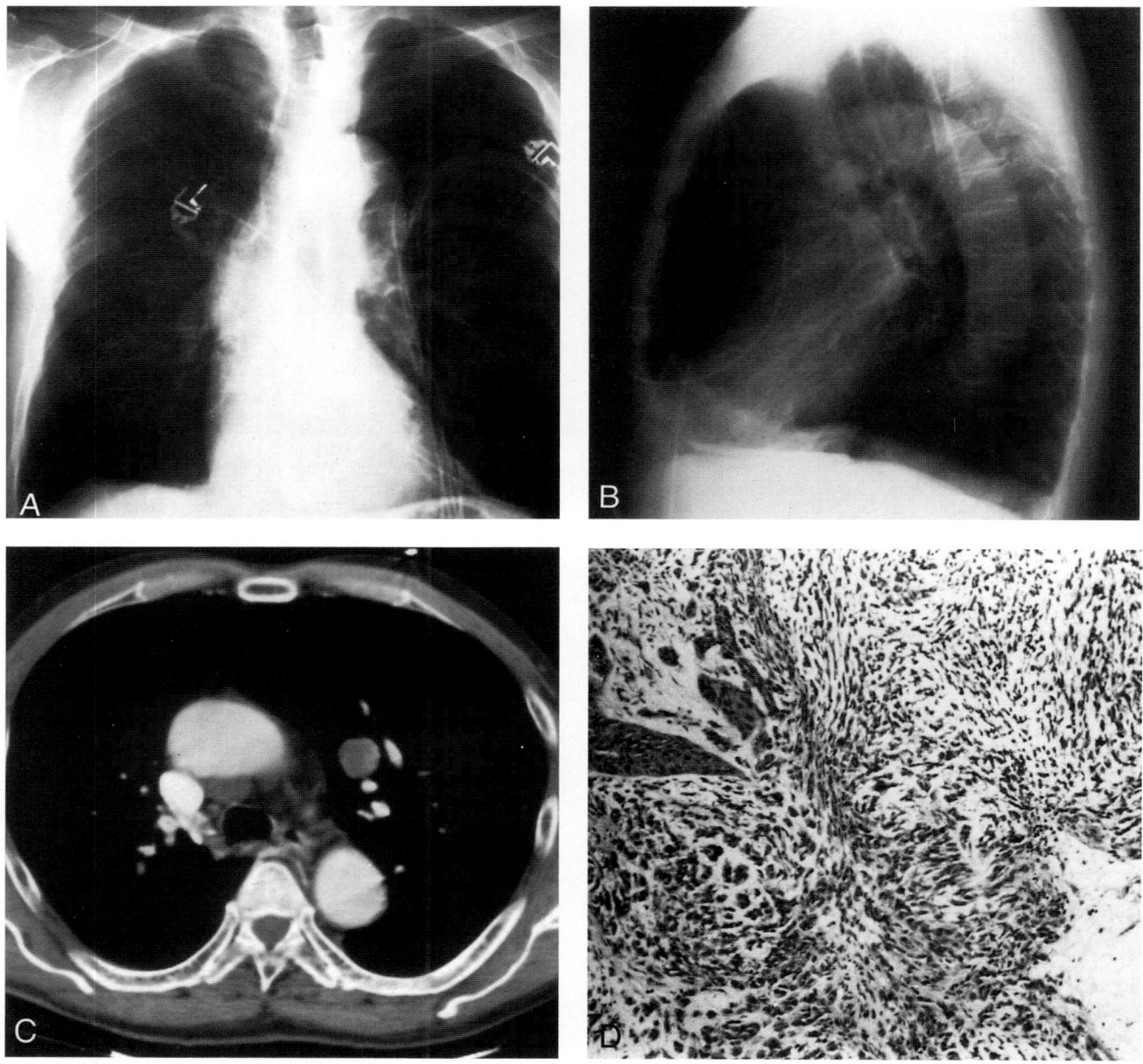

Fig. 112-4. Posteroanterior (**A**) and left lateral (**B**) chest radiographs of a 75-year-old man with suspected myocardial infarction. An asymptomatic 3×2-cm mass is identified just below the aortic arch. CT (**C**) demonstrates a solitary parenchymal lung mass. Photomicrograph (**D**) shows the lesion is a carcinosarcoma of the lung after its removal by a left upper lobectomy.

rate of only 6% was recorded. However, survival as long as 10 to more than 20 years has been recorded.

PULMONARY BLASTOMA

Barnard (1952) first reported a pulmonary blastoma but called it an embryoma. Spencer (1961) reviewed Barnard's case, added three cases of his own, and renamed the tumor a *pulmonary blastoma*. These tumors comprise both malig-

nant mesenchymal stroma and epithelial components that resemble the lung at 3 months' gestation—primitive blastoma and epithelial tubules. The two malignant components make the pulmonary blastoma conceptually similar to the carcinosarcoma.

Kradin and associates (1982) reported a histologic variant that contained malignant fetal-type glands but not a malignant stroma. They called this neoplasm a pulmonary endodermal tumor resembling fetal lung. It later came to be known as a *well-differentiated fetal adenocarcinoma*

(WDFA). Maniveland coworkers (1988) described a neoplasm in children that they termed the *pleuropulmonary blastoma*. In contrast to the WDFA, this neoplasm comprises malignant mesenchyme and blastema but no malignant glands. In summary, a pulmonary blastoma has both malignant mesenchymal and epithelial tissue, the pleuropulmonary blastoma has malignant mesenchyme and blastema, and the WDFA has only malignant epithelial cells.

Pulmonary Blastoma and Well-Differentiated Fetal Adenocarcinoma

Larsen and Sorensen (1996) reviewed the subject of pulmonary blastomas, and they estimated their incidence to be only 0.5% of all pulmonary neoplasms. Francis and Jacobsen (1983) reviewed 72 cases and added another 11 of their own. Koss and associates (1991) reviewed 52 cases and divided them into WDFAs and pulmonary blastomas. In the review of Larsen and Sorensen (1996), the authors described 156 cases of pulmonary blastoma with a median age of 40 years and an age range of newborn to 80 years. The ratio of men to women was approximately 2:1. They described 23 cases of WDFA with a median age of 40 years and an age range of 12 to 73 years, with this tumor being approximately divided evenly between men and women. In Koss and associates' (1991) study, the average age at the time of diagnosis was 35 years, although the range was from less than 1 year to 72 years of age. The tumor occurred slightly more frequently in women than in men. Twenty-one of 52 patients (41%) were asymptomatic, and the tumors were discovered on routine chest radiographs. They did not separate the WDFA from the pulmonary blastomas when they described the patient demographics. The most common clinical complaints were cough, hemoptysis, and dyspnea. In a large percentage of cases, the chest radiographs revealed a unilateral pulmonary mass randomly located in the lung. The tumors were peripheral or hilar, and some involved both regions. Results of clinical laboratory tests were nonspecific. Sputum cytology was negative in the six patients from whom it was obtained. Bronchoscopy and fine-needle aspiration were variably helpful in the diagnosis of the tumor.

Twenty-eight of the 52 tumors (54%) were classified as WDFA; the other 24 (46%) were biphasic blastomas. The WDFAs ranged in size from 1 to 10 cm with a mean of 4.5 cm. Histologically, they were malignant glands composed of pseudostratified columnar epithelium and benign stroma. The biphasic blastomas ranged in size from 2 to 27 cm with a mean of 10.2 cm. Histologically, these were malignant glands and either an adult sarcomatous or embryonic mesenchyme. Bodner and Koss (1996) studied nine pulmonary blastomas and 12 WDFAs for mutations in the p53 gene. They found a mutation in five out of nine (42%) pulmonary blastomas but none in the WDFAs. In the pulmonary blastomas, both the epithelial and mesenchymal components showed the mutation, suggesting they both came from a single clone of cells.

The treatment was surgical removal of the tumor sometimes followed by chemotherapy. Postoperatively, the patients with the WDFA type of pulmonary blastoma had better survival than those with the biphasic type. Nakatani and associates (1990) also noted that those patients with a low-grade malignant fetal adenocarcinomatous type tumor had a better prognosis than those with high-grade malignant features. In the series by Koss and colleagues (1991), tumor metastases and recurrence were poor prognostic signs. In patients with biphasic pulmonary blastoma, tumors less than 5 cm in greatest dimension carried a prognosis that was more favorable than that noted with the larger tumors.

Pleuropulmonary Blastoma

Priest and colleagues (1997) reported 50 cases of pleuropulmonary blastomas. Their report included the 11 cases previously reported by Manivel and coworkers (1988). They classified the lesions as types I, II, and III based on whether the lesions were cystic (type I), cystic and solid (type II), or solid (type III). Their patients ranged in age from a newborn to 12 years. They found that each type tended to occur at a different age. Type I (7 patients) presented at an average age of 10 months. Type II (24 patients) presented at an average age of 34 months. Type III (19 patients) presented at an average age of 44 months. There were 24 boys and 26 girls. Their symptoms included respiratory distress, fever, chest or abdominal pain, and malaise. The chest radiographs showed densities, sometimes with cystic formation. On gross examination, the tumors ranged in size from 2 to 28 cm and weighed up to 1100 g. The appearance ranged from cystic to solid with gray, soft surfaces. On microscopic examination, the type I tumors had multiloculated cysts separated by thin septa and lined by respiratory mucosa. Beneath the epithelium, there were round to spindle-shaped immature cells. Some of these cells had the appearance of rhabdomyoblasts. The type II and III tumors had mixed sarcomatous and blastomatous elements. Rhabdomyoblasts and chondroblasts could be identified in the sarcomatous areas. The immunohistochemical studies showed the rhabdomyoblasts to stain for muscle-specific actin and desmin. Electron microscopy studies also supported the presence of skeletal muscle and cartilage.

The treatment for these lesions is surgical excision followed by chemotherapy and rarely by radiation therapy. The thorax was a common site of recurrence. The central nervous system and bone were common metastatic sites. At the last follow-up, 26 of the patients were disease free, 23 had died of their disease, and 1 was alive with disease. Although statistically there did not seem to be a survival advantage of one type over another, the data seemed to suggest that patients with the type I tumor may have a survival advantage over those with a type II or III tumor. The 2-year survival rate was 80% for type I, 73% for type II, and 48% for type III.

BASALOID CARCINOMA OF THE LUNG

Basaloid carcinoma of the lung may be considered as one variety of the non–small cell, non-neuroendocrine lung carcinomas. It was initially described by Brambilla and associates in 1992 as a separate entity from a group of poorly differentiated squamous cell and undifferentiated large cell carcinomas. Grossly these tumors are located in the lobar or segmented bronchi in 88% of the cases; 15% are located more distally. The tumor is usually exophytic but is associated with bronchial wall invasion. Brambilla (1997) and associates (1992) have described the histologic features of this tumor: small moderately pleomorphic cuboidal to fusiform cells with hyperchromatic nuclei with granular dense chromatin and a scanty amount of cytoplasm. The mitotic index is high. Immunohistochemically, the basaloid carcinomas express low-molecular-weight cytokeratins, and in 90% of cases neuroendocrine markers are absent. Genetic studies have shown *p53* is stabilized in 85% of these tumors. The origin of the tumor is thought to be from the basal, pluripotent reserve cells of the bronchial mucosa.

The basaloid carcinomas of the lung are highly aggressive, and despite resection of even early stage lesions, with or without subsequent irradiation, the 5-year survival rate has been reported to be zero by Moro and colleagues (1994).

PRIMARY PULMONARY CHORIOCARCINOMA

Primary pulmonary choriocarcinoma is a rare tumor first described by Hayakawa and colleagues in 1977. This tumor is discovered almost exclusively in men; only one of the fewer than 20 reported cases has been in a woman. Uwatoko and Kajita (1997) reported an additional case in a man and reviewed five other cases that were reported in the Japanese literature. The two cases reported by Hayakawa and colleagues (1977) have been included in most reviews. The other two cases reported by Nakamura (1982) and Endo (1988) and their associates, as well as that of Uwatoko and Kajita (1997) and the Russian report by Uspenski and colleagues (1982), have been missed in most English reviews. Thus, the total number of reported cases is probably 24.

The tumor may present as a peripheral nodule, as in the case reported by Canver and Voytovich (1996), but in most of the patients the tumor is far advanced locally and accompanied by distant metastases at the time of diagnosis. The serum beta-human chorionic gonadotropin (β-HCG) level is elevated well above normal in most cases. Gynecomastia is a common finding in these men.

Histologically the tumor has the appearance of a typical choriocarcinoma (an admixture of anaplastic cytotrophoblastic cells and syncytiotrophoblastic cells). The anaplastic cytotrophoblastic cells exhibit immunohistochemical reactivity to HCG antigen. Most patients have been managed by a combination of radiation therapy and chemotherapy, as noted by Sridher (1989) and Tanimura (1985) and their associates. The recommended chemotherapy of a choriocarcinoma at the present time as suggested by Ghosen (1988) and Garris (1995) and their coworkers is a combination of etoposide, ifosfamide, and cisplatin. Uwatoko and Kajita (1997) added surgical resection of the primary tumor in addition to chemotherapy. With rare exception, however, survival is recorded in months despite aggressive therapy, and long-lasting control of the tumor remains elusive.

LYMPHOEPITHELIOMA-LIKE CARCINOMA OF THE LUNG

The first patient with a lymphoepithelioma-like carcinoma of the lung was described by Begin and associates (1987). To date there have been 27 case reports in the literature. Most of the reported lymphoepithelioma-like carcinomas of the lung have occurred in patients of Asian descent, especially those from South Eastern China. Previous exposure to the Epstein-Barr (EB) virus has been documented in these Asian patients. In the small number of non-Asian patients in whom this tumor has occurred, previous exposure to the EB virus has not been documented. The histologic features of the tumor in both Asians and non-Asians are typical of the lymphoepithelioma-like carcinomas seen in the nasopharynx and those occasionally seen in the thymus (see Chapter 167). Most of the lung lesions are solitary masses; occasionally lymph node metastases may be present as in the patient reported by Frank and colleagues (1998) of our group. These authors, as well as Curcio and associates (1997), have reviewed the literature on this subject. The usual therapy for these unusual tumors has been surgical resection. Curcio (1997) and Frank (1998) and their coworkers added intensive chemotherapy after the initial resection. The rationale of adding adjuvant chemotherapy is based on the study of Al-Sarraf and associates (1996), who reported the superiority of chemotherapy versus radiation therapy with locally advanced nasopharyngeal lymphoepithelioma-like carcinoma. With surgery alone, in early-stage pulmonary disease the short-term survival rate has been satisfactory, but the long-term prognosis is yet unknown. Likewise, the value of chemotherapy as an adjunct in patients with resected pulmonary lymphoepithelioma-like carcinoma remains unknown.

MALIGNANT MELANOMA OF THE BRONCHUS

Miller and Allen (1993) reviewed 80 patients over a 10-year span with rare pulmonary neoplasms at the Mayo Clinic. Only three patients had pulmonary melanoma, which represents 0.03% of their 10,134 patients with lung

Table 112-3. Differentiation of a Primary Melanoma of the Lung and a Melanin-Containing Carcinoid

Primary Melanoma		Melanin-Containing Carcinoid
Ultrastructural features		
Cytoplasmic organelles		Abundant mitochondria
Smooth endoplastic reticulum		Desmosomes
Pigment-laden bodies		
No neurosecretory granules		Neurosecretory granules present
Immunohistochemical features		
+++	S-100 protein	±
—	Neuron-specific enolase	+++
—	Calcitonin	++
—	Keratin	+
—	Epithelial membrane antigen	+
—	Chromogranin A	++
+++	HMB-45	NR

±, present or absent; +++, strongly positive; ++, moderately positive; +, present; NR, not recorded.

cancer. Jennings and colleagues (1990) described a primary malignant melanoma of the lower respiratory tract and summarized another 19 cases in the literature. They used the following criteria to exclude other possible primary sites: 1) no previously removed skin lesion, particularly pigmented; 2) no ocular tumors removed and no enucleation; 3) solitary tumor; 4) morphologic tumor characteristics compatible with a primary tumor; 5) no demonstrable melanoma in other organs at the time of removal; and 6) autopsy without primary melanoma demonstrated elsewhere, especially the skin or the eyes. The differentiation of a primary melanoma from a melanin-containing carcinoid tumor is necessary in all cases. The immunohistochemical and ultrastructural differences between these two tumors (Table 112-3) may be helpful in this regard. In the 20 reported cases reviewed by Jennings and colleagues (1990), the patients ranged in age from 29 to 80 years, with almost equal distribution between men and women. In four patients, the melanoma arose in either the trachea or the tracheal carina, whereas in the remaining 16 patients, the melanoma arose in bronchial sites involving any one of the lobes of the lungs. The clinical symptoms, physical findings, and radiographic features were not described for many of these patients, although melanomas arising in the bronchus behave clinically like a primary lung carcinoma with resulting bronchial obstruction. Marchevsky (1995) pointed out that bronchial melanomas are morphologically similar to those of the skin and mucosa. These melanomas, as noted in Table 112-3, also immunostain for S-100 protein and HMB-45 but not for neuroendocrine markers, which helps separate them from carcinoids. If a melanoma is encountered and no history or evidence of a simultaneous or previous primary lesion can be elicited, resection should be carried out if possible. Treatment instituted in the cases reported in the literature ranged from no therapy to resection of the entire lung. Eight patients died of their disease. Six were free of disease for as long as 11 years, and two other patients were free of disease at 12 and 19 months.

MALIGNANT TERATOMAS

Intrapulmonary teratomas are uncommon; one-half of these tumors may be malignant. Day and Taylor (1975) reviewed the available literature and noted that for some unexplained reason, most malignant teratomas occurred in the left upper lobe. In the past, some malignant lesions have been confused with the pulmonary blastomas. The prognosis of a malignant teratoma is poor. Kakkar and associates (1996) described a pulmonary teratoma with a yolk sac tumor. The patient was a 20-year-old man who presented with a history of fever, chest pain, dry cough, and a recent onset of hemoptysis. The chest radiograph showed a consolidation in the right middle lobe. He died 4 days after admission. Grossly, the right middle and upper lobes were involved with a tumor that showed necrosis and hemorrhage. Microscopically, the tumor showed benign elements from all the germ layers. It also contained malignant glands and areas of yolk sac tumor. The immunostain for α-fetoprotein was focally positive. In addition, this patient had myeloid metaplasia with atypical megakaryocytes in the liver, spleen, hilar lymph nodes, and the left adrenal gland as well as myelofibrosis in the marrow. Kakkar and associates (1996) note this is the first described malignant teratoma of the lung associated with a hematologic malignancy.

MALIGNANT EPENDYMOMA

A case report of a possible primary malignant ependymoma of the lung was reported by Crotty and associates (1992). This heretofore unreported pulmonary lesion occurred in a patient previously treated for small cell lung cancer. The ultrastructural and immunohistochemical features of the solitary peripheral ependymoma and the original small cell tumor were remarkably dissimilar. It was hypothesized that a metaplastic event related to therapy may have caused an unexplained alteration of the original tumor phenotype. The importance of this observation remains to be determined.

PULMONARY LYMPHOMA

Lymphomas of the lung can be divided into Hodgkin's lymphoma and non-Hodgkin's lymphoma. Primary lymphomas of the lung are rare. L'hoste and colleagues (1984) reported that these tumors represented 0.5% of all lung tumors, and Miller and Allen (1993) recorded a 0.33% incidence. Secondary involvement of the lung by lymphoma, however, is common and is the result of spread of original mediastinal disease, especially Hodgkin's disease.

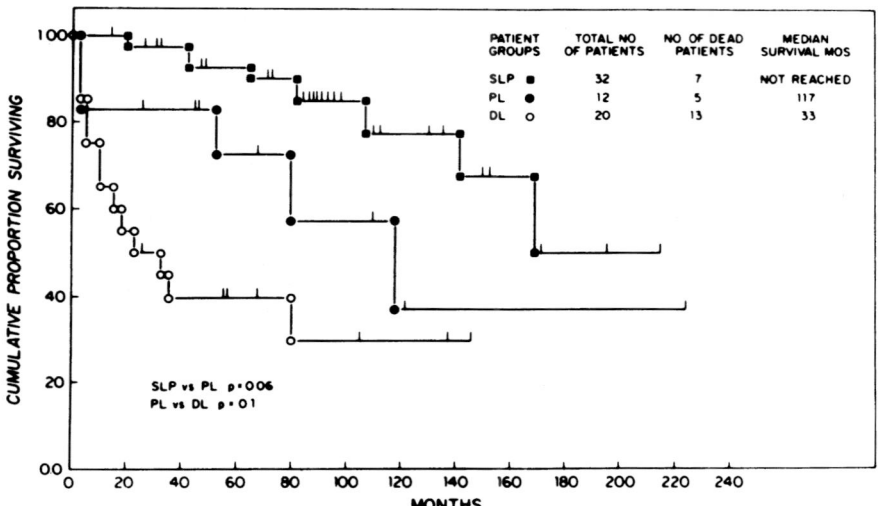

Fig. 112-5. Survival curves of patients with primary and secondary lymphoma of the lung. SLP: Survival curve of patients with small lymphocytic proliferation including those with small cell lymphocytic lymphoma as well as pseudolymphoma or lymphocytic interstitial pneumonia. PL: Survival curve of patients with presumed primary lymphoma of the lung, limited to one or both lungs, exclusive of primary Hodgkin's disease. DL: Survival curve of patients with disseminated lymphoma of extrapulmonary origin involving the lungs. From Kennedy JL, et al: Pulmonary lymphomas and other pulmonary lymphoid lesions: a clinicopathologic and immunologic study of 64 patients. Cancer 56:539, 1985. With permission.

Secondary Pulmonary Lymphomas

Kern and associates (1961) reported secondary involvement to be as high as 40%, but Fisher and associates (1962) believed it was less. Berkman and associates (1996) noted that pulmonary parenchymal involvement occurred in 38% of Hodgkin's disease and 24% of non-Hodgkin's lymphoma. In a review of 108 patients with newly diagnosed Hodgkin's disease, in whom the extent of the thoracic disease was evaluated by CT scans, Diehl and coworkers (1991) found thoracic involvement in 77. In these patients, they observed a pattern of contiguous spread from the anterior mediastinal or paratracheal areas, to adjacent mediastinal lymph node groups, to the hilar nodes, and lastly into the lungs. The pulmonary involvement was present as either direct extension or discrete nodules. Only when bulk disease—with an anterior mediastinal or paratracheal mass greater than 30% of the thoracic diameter—was present was involvement noted in the pleura, pericardium, or chest wall. Any exception to these patterns suggests the presence of a disease process other than Hodgkin's disease. In non-Hodgkin's lymphoma, Risdall and associates (1979) found lung involvement at autopsy in 39 of 72 patients. Most of these lymphomas that involved the lung were of the large cell type.

After treatment of an initial thoracic lymphoma, recurrent or secondary involvement of the lungs and thorax may have manifestations entirely different from those seen with original disease. Lewis and colleagues (1991) reported that in 31 patients with recurrent or secondary lymphoma of the lungs—15 with Hodgkin's disease and 16 with non-Hodgkin's lymphoma—CT scans identified the following findings: 1) pulmonary nodules of less than 1 cm; 2) mass or mass-like consolidations of more than 1 cm, with or without cavitation; 3) alveolar or interstitial infiltrates; 4) masses of pleural origin; 5) peribronchial or perivascular thickening,

with or without atelectasis; 6) pleural effusions; and 7) hilar or mediastinal adenopathy. In most patients (68%), three or more of these CT abnormalities were present simultaneously. Unfortunately, whether these CT findings, especially multiple simultaneous findings, can effectively differentiate secondary pulmonary parenchymal lymphoma from other pathologic processes without invasive confirmation remains to be seen. Of note is the observation that the prognosis of primary lymphoma of the lung is better than that of secondary involvement of the lung (Fig. 112-5).

Primary Pulmonary Lymphoma

Non-Hodgkin's Lymphoma

The multiple classification schemes for non-Hodgkin's lymphoma have confused clinicians and pathologists alike. These schemes are those of Jackson and Parker (1947), Rappaport (1966), Lukes and Collins (1975), the Kiel classification reported by Lennert (1978), and the Working Formulation of the Non-Hodgkin's Lymphoma Pathologic Classification Project (1982). Costa and Martin's (1985) classification of pulmonary lymphoid disorders is both practical and useful. However, several new entities, such as the mucosa-associated lymphoid tissue (MALT) lymphoma, have been described in recent years, and a new classification system has been proposed: the Revised European-American Lymphoma (REAL) classification. Chan and colleagues (1995), as well as Harris and associates (1994), have described this new classification, and it is listed and compared with the Rappaport classification and the Working Formulation in Table 112-4. Table 112-5 shows the clinical stage grouping of primary pulmonary non-Hodgkin's lymphoma as modified from the original Ann Arbor classification.

The rare primary pulmonary lymphoma may occur in any of the deposits of lymphoid elements normally present in the

Table 112-4. Pulmonary Lymphoreticular Disorders

Benign primary pulmonary lymphoproliferative lesions
    Pseudolymphoma (PSL)[a]
    Lymphocytic interstitial pneumonia (LIP)[b]
Non-Hodgkin's lymphoma of the lung

Rappaport Classification	Working Formulation	Revised European-American Classification of Lymphoid Neoplasm (R.E.A.L.)	
		B-cell Neoplasms	T-cell Neoplasms
	Low grade		
Well-differentiated lymphocytic (WDL)	Small lymphocytic	B-cell CLL/PLL/SLL Marginal zone/MALT Mantle cell	T-cell CLL/PLL LGL ATL/L
	Small lymphocytic, plasmacytoid	Lymphoplasmacytoid Marginal zone/MALT B-cell CLL/PLL/SLL	—
Nodular, poorly differentiated lymphocytic (PDL)	Follicular, predominantly small cleaved cells	Follicle center, follicular, grade I Marginal zone/MALT Mantle cell	—
	Intermediate grade		
Nodular histiocytic	Follicular, predominantly large cells	Follicle center, follicular, grade III	—
Diffuse, poorly differentiated lymphocytic	Diffuse, small cleaved cells	Mantle zone Follicle center, diffuse small cell Marginal zone/MALT	T-cell CLL/PLL LGL ATL/L Angioimmunoblastic Angiocentric
Diffuse, mixed lymphocytic and histiocytic	Diffuse, mixed small and large cells	Large B-cell lymphoma (rich in T cells) Follicle center, diffuse small cell Lymphoplasmacytoid Marginal zone/MALT Mantle cell	Peripheral T-cell, unspecified ATL/L Angioimmunoblastic Angiocentric Intestinal T-cell lymphoma
Diffuse, histiocytic	Diffuse, large cell	Diffuse large B-cell lymphoma	Peripheral T-cell, unspecified ATL/L Angioimmunoblastic Angiocentric Intestinal T-cell lymphoma
	High grade		
Diffuse histiocytic	Large cell immunoblastic	Diffuse large B-cell lymphoma	Peripheral T-cell, unspecified ATL/L Angioimmunoblastic Angiocentric Intestinal T-cell lymphoma Anaplastic large cell
Lymphoblastic	Lymphoblastic, convoluted cells	Precursor B-lymphoblastic	Precursor T-lymphoblastic
Diffuse, undifferentiated			
Burkitt's	Burkitt's		
Non-Burkitt's	Small non-cleaved cell		

Other non-Hodgkin's lymphomas
Angiocentric immunoproliferative lesions (AIL)
    Lymphocytic vasculitis
    Lymphomatoid granulomatosis (LYG)
    Angiocentric large cell lymphoma
Plasma cell disorders
    Waldenstrom's macroglobulinemia
    Plasmacytoma
    Multiple myeloma
Hodgkin's disease

ATL/L, adult T-cell leukemia/lymphoma, which is associated with HTLV 1 infection; CLL, chronic lymphocytic leukemia; LGL, large granulated lymphocyte leukemia; MALT, mucosa-associated lymphoid tissue; PLL, prolymphocytic leukemia; SLL, small lymphocytic lymphoma.
[a]Pseudolymphoma is also known as nodular lymphoid hyperplasia.
[b]Lymphocytic interstitial pneumonia is also known as diffuse lymphoid hyperplasia. In some instances, these two lesions have been reported to progress lymphoma.
Modified from Jaffe ES: An overview of the classification of Non-Hodgkin's lymphoma. *In* Jaffe ES (ed): Surgical Pathology of the Lymph Nodes and Related Organs. 2nd Ed. Philadelphia: Saunders, 1995, p. 193; and Harris NL: Lymphoma classification presented at the Tutorial on Neoplastic Hematopathology, February 1998, Miami, Florida. With permission.

Table 112-5. Clinical Staging Grouping of Pulmonary Non-Hodgkin's Lymphoma

Stage	Extent of Disease
IE	Lung only involved
II1E	Lung and hilar nodes involved
II2E	Lung and mediastinal nodes involved
II2EW	Lung and adjacent chest wall or diaphragm involved
III and IV	Disseminated disease

Note: Modified Ann Arbor classification.
From L'hoste RJ, et al: Primary pulmonary lymphomas. Cancer *54*:1397, 1984. With permission.

lung: 1) in the bronchial-associated lymphoid tissue (BALT), which represents MALT; 2) in the interstices of the lung parenchyma; or 3) in the intrapulmonary and subpleural lymph nodes (intrapulmonary and subpleural lymph nodes are normally present, particularly in persons more than 25 years of age). Using pulmonary lymphangiography, Trapnell (1964) demonstrated that 18% of normal persons had intrapulmonary nodes within the lung parenchyma (see Chapter 6).

Primary non-Hodgkin's pulmonary lymphoma develops from B lymphocytes predominantly. Husband and Gowans (1978) reported that the primary lymphoma develops from centrocyte-like cells, that in turn develop from parafollicular B lymphocytes. These B lymphocytes express either κ- or λ-immunoglobulin light chains—so-called light chain restriction—and imply a clonal proliferation derived from a single B cell. Although the tumor is often referred to as a B-cell lymphoma, as in the report of Uppal and Goldstraw (1992), these tumors more frequently are referred to as small cell lymphocytic lymphomas or as large cell (histocytic) lymphomas.

It is difficult for the pathologist to separate benign lymphoid lesions, lymphocytic interstitial pneumonia (LIP), and pseudolymphoma (PSL) of the lung from primary pulmonary lymphocytic lymphomas (PPL). Addis and coworkers (1988) studied 15 cases of pulmonary lymphoid lesions with immunohistochemical staining for various B-cell markers. They concluded that cases of PSL and LIP required careful evaluation because many of them are really primary pulmonary lymphomas (PPL). Bragg and colleagues (1994) emphasized that with monoclonal antibodies and molecular biology, it is possible to establish whether a group of lymphocytes is monoclonal or polyclonal in origin. This distinction is important because monoclonal proliferations are considered malignant and polyclonal ones are considered benign. Kradin and Mark (1983) applied the term *nodular lymphoid hyperplasia* to PSL, and *diffuse lymphoid hyperplasia* to LIP. These terms may be better for describing these two lesions. Until they are used more widely, they unfortunately confuse clinicians.

Saltzstein (1963) addressed the problem of separating benign from malignant lymphoid lesions by proposing three criteria for primary pulmonary lymphomas. His criteria were: 1) "immature" lymphocytes, 2) absence of germinal centers, and 3) involvement of hilar lymph nodes. Despite these criteria for differentiating benign from malignant lymphoid lesions, there are reports of LIP and PSL progressing to PPL. Turner and associates (1984) tried to clarify the situation with regard to pulmonary lymphoid lesions by proposing that a pattern of lymphangitic spread and a monomorphic cell population could be used to separate the malignant and benign lesions. With regard to Saltzstein's criteria, they pointed out that germinal centers could be seen with lymphomas and that hilar lymph nodes are not always involved when a lymphoma is present. Hence, the lack of hilar lymph node involvement should not be used to support the diagnosis of a benign lymphoid process. In conclusion, truly benign lymphoid lesions of the lung—LIP and PSL—probably exist, but unfortunately, the current histologic criteria do not always allow for a clear distinction of LIP and PSL from PPL. Therefore, LIP and PSL must be viewed as potentially premalignant lesions.

Lymphocytic Interstitial Pneumonia

Carrington and Liebow (1966) first described LIP, and Liebow and Carrington (1973) further defined LIP as widespread pulmonary interstitial infiltrates composed of lymphocytes, plasma cells, and histiocytes. In some cases, germinal centers are present, and the term *diffuse lymphoid hyperplasia* has been applied to this condition. Colby and Carrington (1983) and Turner and colleagues (1984) believed that some cases reported in the past actually represented diffuse, well-differentiated lymphocytic lymphomas arising in the lung. Saldana and Mones (1992) believe that LIP is best considered a prelymphomatous state frequently associated with other immune dysfunction, such as dysgammaglobulinemia. Most patients with LIP are adult women, usually in their fifth through seventh decades of life. These patients have nonspecific symptoms, such as dry cough, dyspnea, weight loss, and fever. Typical radiographic features are diffuse bilateral lower lobe reticular infiltrates. Small (1 cm) or large (1 to 3 cm) nodules or patchy consolidations may be present on the chest radiograph. Koss (1995) described the lung as showing angiocentric and bronchocentric lymphoid nodules with germinal centers. The interstitium may show granulomas and giant cells. The cells should be polyclonal in origin. Patients with LIP can have diseases with immunologic abnormalities such as Sjögren's syndrome (one-third of cases), collagen vascular diseases, autoimmune diseases, and immunodeficiency diseases, including acquired immunodeficiency syndrome (AIDS). Whether LIP in AIDS patients is a prelymphomatous lesion remains to be demonstrated. Pitt (1991) noted that LIP is more common in the pediatric AIDS population than in the adult counterpart. The course of LIP varies. Patients have been treated with corticosteroids and immunosuppressive drugs, but the response is difficult to judge because of the occurrence of spontaneous remissions. Fishback and Koss (1996) pointed out that LIP sometimes evolves into lymphoma, but the frequency of this transformation is difficult to assess because low-grade lymphomas may mimic LIP.

Pseudolymphoma

As noted, Saltzstein (1963) attempted to establish histologic criteria to separate malignant from benign lymphocytic pulmonary infiltrates. He termed the benign lymphocytic proliferations *pseudolymphomas* (PSLs), or, as they were later called, *nodular lymphoid hyperplasias of the lung*. Koss (1983), Herbert (1984), and Weiss (1985) and their colleagues, as well as others, reinterpreted many of the lesions that were called PSL as well-differentiated lymphocytic lymphoma (PPL). True PSLs are reactive lymphoid proliferations that manifest in the lung as one or several masses or as localized infiltrates, as noted by Holland and coworkers (1991). Koss and associates (1983) reviewed 23 pseudolymphomas and found that the lesions were usually discovered in asymptomatic patients on routine radiographs of the chest. The patients ranged in age from the third to the eighth decade of life, with a mean age of 51 years. Many of the few symptomatic patients had fever. Microscopically, it is a lymphoid lesion with well-defined germinal centers separated by plasma cells. Koss (1995) re-emphasized that the cells should be polyclonal and not monoclonal. Shiota and colleagues (1993) described two cases of pseudolymphoma that showed monoclonality by gene rearrangement studies. Monoclonality indicates these lesions are lymphomas. Resection of a true PSL is both diagnostic and curative. The lesion has a low rate of recurrence at the original surgical site. The prognosis is excellent, provided the pathologist has made the correct diagnosis.

Small Cell Lymphocytic Lymphoma (Bronchus-associated Lymphoid Tissue Lymphoma)

According to Koss (1995), the majority of the non-Hodgkin's lymphomas that originate in the lung are low grade and are derived from B cells. They are thought to be derived from the BALT, which is composed of lymphoid tissue within the bronchial mucosa. This system is thought to have a role in dealing with inhaled antigens. In various series, the low-grade lymphomas constitute the majority (50 to 70%) of the primary pulmonary lymphomas. In Fiche and associates' (1995) study, 61of the 69 (88%) primary pulmonary lymphomas were low grade. Of the low-grade lymphomas, 54 (88%) were BALT lymphomas. These lesions are proliferations of small lymphocytes or lymphocytes with plasmacytoid features. Wotherspoon and coworkers (1990) studied the immunohistochemistry, molecular biology, and cytogenetics of a primary small cell lymphoma of the lung. Presence of λ light chains and gene rearrangement demonstrated that the clonality of these proliferations was B cells. A translocation between the short arm of chromosome 1 and the long arm of chromosome 14, t (1;14) (p 22; q 32), was also present. This translocation is characteristically found in

B-cell lymphomas. Patients with pulmonary small cell lymphocytic lymphomas range in age from the second to the ninth decade of life, with a peak at the sixth decade. Distribution between men and women is equal. One-third of patients are asymptomatic, and their lesions are found on routine chest radiographs. Symptomatic patients complain of cough, dyspnea, chest pain, and hemoptysis. BALT lymphoma, LIP, and atypical lymphoproliferative disorders (ALD) can occur in HIV-positive and AIDS patients. *Atypical lymphoproliferative disorder* is defined as a diffuse moderate to heavy infiltrate of atypical lymphoid cells. McGuinness and colleagues (1995) described the radiographic and CT findings of these lesions. The chest radiographs may be normal or may reveal reticulonodular interstitial markings present in the lower portions of the lungs. On CT scan, all three entities have a similar appearance of small nodules scattered throughout the lung fields. In LIP and ALD the nodules are 2 to 4 mm in size. In the BALT lymphomas the nodules are 2 to 4 mm, but larger nodules—5 to 6 mm—are also present. The nodules are mostly in a peribronchial distribution, except in a few cases of LIP. The differentiating clinical, pathologic, and radiographic features of LIP, PSL, and small cell lymphocytic lymphoma are presented in Table 112-6. Treatment may be limited to surgical removal of the mass or additional radiation therapy, chemotherapy, or both, if other factors suggest the need. The prognosis of small cell lymphocytic (BALT) lymphomas of the lung is excellent. Koss and associates (1983) reported a 5-year survival rate of 70%, and L'hoste and coworkers (1984) cited a survival rate of 83%. Miller and Allen (1993) recorded a similar 86% 5-year survival rate in their series of 22 patients with small cell lymphomas of the lung. Kennedy and colleagues (1985) reported a 9.75-year median survival rate for a group of 12 patients, and Turner and associates (1984) reported a median 4-year survival rate for a group of 33 patients of whom only one died of lymphoma. In the series of Fiche and coworkers (1995), the patients with small cell lymphomas had a 93.6% survival at 5 years and a 60% survival at 10 years.

Large Cell (Histiocytic) Lymphoma

A primary large cell (histiocytic) lymphoma of the lung is extremely uncommon. In the series of primary pulmonary lymphoma reported by Toh and Ang (1997), two out of 11 patients (18%) had a large cell lymphoma; Tamura and coworkers (1995), reporting a similar study, found three out of 24 (12.5%) were large cell lymphomas. Polish (1989) and Poelzleitner (1989) and their coworkers have described large cell lymphoma originating in the lungs of patients with AIDS.

Patients without AIDS are usually in their fifth and sixth decades of life, and men and women are affected almost equally. Symptoms include cough, chest pain, dyspnea, fever, and weight loss. The tumors tend to occur in the upper lobes but also may be found in the other lobes, and even the entire lung may be involved. The chest radiographs show an

Table 112-6. Differentiation of Lymphoma, Lymphocytic Interstitial Pneumonia, and Pseudolymphoma

	Lymphoma (Small Lymphocytes)	Lymphocytic Interstitial Pneumonia	Pseudolymphoma
Clinical			
Pulmonary symptoms	+	+++	+
Systemic symptoms	++	+	+
Adenopathy (when present)	++++	0	0
Histologic			
Pleomorphic infiltrate	0	++	+++
Germinal centers	+	++	++
Node involvement	++++	0	0
Cartilage destruction	+++	0	±
Pleural invasion	+++	0	±
Immunologic stain			
Monoclonal cells	+	0	0
Polyclonal cells	0	+	+
Radiographic			
Solitary lesion	++	0	++
Multiple lesions	+++	0	+
Adenopathy	++++	0	+
Effusion	+++	0	+
Diffuse lesion	+	+++	0

+, present; ++, more frequent; +++, very frequent; ++++, almost always present; 0, absent.
From Seminar in Pulmonary and Mediastinal Diagnosis. Given by the Armed Forces Institute of Pathology in October 1986. With permission.

infiltrate. On histologic examination, the tumors are composed of cells with large nuclei and prominent nucleoli. Hilar lymph nodes are always involved. Chest wall and pleural involvement have been noted. Cavitation may occur with the mixed (large and small) cell types. When feasible, surgical resection should be attempted. When the hilar nodes are positive, postoperative radiation therapy is indicated. In patients with widespread disease, chemotherapy is the treatment of choice. These large cell tumors are more aggressive than the small cell lymphocytic lymphomas, and the prognosis is correspondingly poorer, although the survival data for large cell (histiocytic) lymphomas of the lung is less clear because fewer cases have been reported (see Fig. 112-5). L'hoste and colleagues (1984) reported late recurrence in 53% of their patients. Recurrences can occur within months or many years after the initial treatment. Cordier and associates (1993) reported no survivors out of nine patients by the end of 4 years. In general, these patients do not survive as long as patients with small cell lymphocytic lymphomas. Patients with AIDS and primary large cell lymphoma have a poor prognostic outlook, despite an initial response to appropriate therapy. The presence of prior or concurrent opportunistic infection is particularly harmful in these patients.

Lymphomatoid Granulomatosis

Lymphomatoid granulomatosis is an atypical lymphoreticular infiltrate that involves the vessels of the lung and other organs (skin and brain). Lymphomatoid granulomatosis (LYG) was first described in 1972 by Liebow and colleagues. The lesion had certain histologic features of lymphoma and Wegener's granulomatosis—hence the name *lymphomatoid*

granulomatosis. Since the original description, the knowledge of extranodal lymphomas has grown considerably. Weis and associates (1986) examined the subject of peripheral T-cell lymphomas and concluded from their cases and the existing literature that LYG is an example of a peripheral T-cell lymphoma. Koss (1995) reviewed the subject of LYG and its histogenesis. The histogenesis is unclear, although it may be related to infection by Epstein-Barr virus (EBV). He postulated that LYG might represent a T-cell reaction to B cells infected with EBV or it could be a T-cell–rich analogue of the EBV-associated B-cell lymphoproliferative disorders that occur in immunosuppressed individuals.

Lymphomatoid granulomatosis usually affects middle-aged adults with a slight predominance in men. Patients present with cough, shortness of breath, chest pain, fever, malaise, and weight loss. The disease also involves the skin, central nervous system, and sometimes upper respiratory tract. Staples (1991) described the radiographic findings as multiple small pulmonary nodules ranging from 0.6 to 0.8 cm in size. These nodules tend to be ill defined and are usually present in the lower lung fields. On microscopic examination, there is an atypical polymorphous lymphoid infiltrate around pulmonary blood vessels with necrosis. In a study of 15 patients, Fauci and colleagues (1982) found that cyclophosphamide and prednisone could be beneficial in these patients. However, Katzenstein and coworkers (1979) reported that two-thirds of patients died despite treatment with corticosteroids, chemotherapy, or both; the median survival was 14 months. Koss and colleagues (1986) reported that 38% of patients with LYG died within 1 year of diagnosis. Pisani and DeRemee (1990) found that 16 of 28 patients with LYG had an average survival of 23.8

months. In summary, this disease should be viewed as a form of malignant lymphoma that primarily involves the lung and has a poor prognosis.

Intravascular Lymphomatosis

Intravascular lymphomatosis is a neoplastic proliferation of lymphoid cells within vascular spaces. The lymphocytes are usually of B-cell origin, but a few cases have been reported to be of T-cell origin. This entity was originally described by Pfleger and Tappeiner (1959), who called it angioendotheliomatosis proliferans systemisata. Other names include malignant *angioendotheliomatosis* and *angiotropic lymphoma*. This entity usually presents with cutaneous infiltrates and central nervous system symptoms. Gabor (1997), Demirer (1994), Stroup (1990) and their colleagues, as well as Yousem and Colby (1990), have all described pulmonary presentations of this type of lymphoma. Combining all of these reports, seven patients have been recorded with a primary pulmonary presentation. The patients were between 40 and 71 years with an average of 56 years. One patient had a past history of a lymphoma in the breast. The presenting symptoms included fever, cough, night sweats, and progressive shortness of breath. The chest radiographs showed bilateral reticular and reticulonodular infiltrates. Some patients showed hypoxia on analysis of their blood gases. The biopsy specimens showed dilated vessels filled with aggregates of large atypical lymphoid cells. The immunohistochemical staining of these cells showed they were positive for leukocyte common antigen (LCA). A biopsy is necessary to establish the diagnosis. The treatment is chemotherapy and possibly radiation therapy. Of the seven patients with primary pulmonary presentation, three died from their disease, one is alive with disease, and three are alive without disease at 8 months, 8 years, and 9 years, respectively, after diagnosis.

Plasma Cell Disorders

Waldenström's macroglobulinemia, plasmacytoma, and multiple myeloma originate in the lung in rare instances. Noach (1956) first reported Waldenström's macroglobulinemia involving the lung. Systemic manifestations, such as lymphadenopathy, splenomegaly, and weight loss, may be present in these patients. Plasmacytomas rarely occur in the lung. Roikjaer and Thomsen (1986) described a patient with pulmonary plasmacytoma that recurred after surgical removal. The patient was well 4 years after the second removal of recurrent tumor. The plasma cells immunostained for κ-light chains in both resected specimens. Kazzaz and colleagues (1992) described a multifocal plasmacytoma in the lung of a 60-year-old man. The plasmacytoma demonstrated κ-light chain on immunostaining, but there was no paraprotein in either the serum or urine. Nine years after surgery, the patient was well with no evidence of multiple myeloma. In 1993, Joseph and colleagues described an addi-

tional case of primary pulmonary plasmacytoma; they reviewed the literature and found a total of 19 cases. The patients ranged in age from 3 to 72 years with a median age of 42.3 years. Men and women were equally affected. On microscopic examination, these tumors comprised sheets of plasma cells. The cells in the case reported by Joseph and colleagues immunostained for lambda, but not κ-light chains. This is in contrast to the cases reported by Roikjaer and Thomsen (1986) and Kazzaz and associates (1992) in which κ-light chains were found. These lesions are usually treated surgically, and radiation therapy may be added. Chemotherapy is now not indicated. In the follow-up period, these patients must be evaluated for multiple myeloma. Of the cases reviewed, three out of eight patients developed myeloma within 2 years, and they all died of the disease. Thus, the pulmonary lesion may be a forerunner of disseminated disease. Excision of a solitary extrapulmonary lesion is recommended when possible; however, in most instances, chemotherapy is the therapeutic method of choice for patients with disseminated disease. Occasionally, multiple myeloma may involve the lung as a solitary mass or as part of a systemic disease process. Shin and colleagues (1992) described two patients with rare secondary pulmonary involvement by myeloma.

Primary Pulmonary Hodgkin's Disease

Primary Hodgkin's disease of the lung is infrequent; no cases were observed in the Mayo Clinic series recorded by Miller and Allen (1993). Radin (1990) reported one case of primary pulmonary Hodgkin's disease and summarized an additional 60 cases in the literature. Chetty and colleagues (1995) added three cases; two of Chetty and colleagues' patients had very aggressive disease and died within 6 to 21 months of presentation.

The patients with primary pulmonary Hodgkin's disease have an average age of 42.5 years, with an age range from 12 to 82 years. The peak occurrence of the disease is bimodal, with the first peak between 21 and 30 years of age and the second between 60 and 80 years of age. Women are affected slightly more frequently than men (1.4:1.0). The most common symptoms are cough, weight loss, chest pain, dyspnea, hemoptysis, fatigue, and rash. Physical examination of the chest usually reveals signs of pulmonary consolidation, but abnormal physical findings may be absent. Other findings include paradoxical movement of the thorax, rash, edema, and lymphadenopathy. Radiographically, most patients show nodular or mass lesions in their lungs, as well as cystic lesions, infiltrates, atelectasis, and effusions. Results of bronchoscopic examination in most patients are normal, and rarely do they yield the diagnosis. This lack of bronchoscopic specificity indicates that most patients require an open lung biopsy for diagnosis. The histologic types most commonly seen are the nodular sclerosing and the mixed cellularity forms of Hodgkin's disease. Chetty and colleagues (1995) pointed out the importance of separating Hodgkin's disease from pleomorphic T-cell, large B-cell, and anaplastic large cell lymphomas. They stressed the immunohistochemical staining of Reed-Sternberg cells for CD15 and CD30. Patients are treated with a variety of regimens that include surgery, chemotherapy, and radiation therapy. Patients with the poorest outcome are those with involvement of more than one lobe or of a single lung, those with bilateral lung disease, and those with a high clinical stage. Other factors indicative of a poor prognosis are the presence of B symptoms—fever, night sweats, loss of 10% or more of body weight, penetration of the pleura, and cavitary disease.

Summary of Lymphoid Lesions of the Lung

Pulmonary lymphoid lesions can be either primary or secondary. Primary lesions include both non-Hodgkin's lymphoma and Hodgkin's disease. Lymphocytic interstitial pneumonia, pseudolymphoma, and BALT lymphoma are the most difficult to evaluate because separating the reactive lesions from the neoplastic ones is difficult. Many studies cited have shown LIP and pseudolymphoma to be low-grade lymphoma by immunohistochemical staining and gene rearrangement studies. The primary large cell lymphoma is easier to diagnose, because it resembles its nodal counterparts. LYG has the appearance of a vasculitis with pulmonary necrosis. It is considered to be a peripheral T-cell lymphoma, but studies have questioned this concept. Intravascular lymphomatosis does not usually present in the lung, but when it does, diagnosis may be difficult. It does not present as a mass but rather as an intravascular proliferation of lymphoid cells. Primary pulmonary plasmacytomas are extremely rare. They are easy to diagnose since they comprise plasma cells.

In view of the pathologist's difficulty in interpreting lymphoid lesions of the lung, the surgeon should take extra steps if a lymphoid tumor is suspected. Touch preparations should be made from the cut surface of the lesion. These preparations can be air dried and stained with Wright's or Giemsa stain. Some part of the tumor should be fixed in B-5 solution or some equivalent solution that provides better nuclear detail than formalin. The hilar lymph nodes should be sampled for both diagnosis and staging, and some of the tumor should be frozen for immunologic markers and gene rearrangement studies. Fresh tissue may also be submitted for cytogenetic studies because many lymphoid markers are destroyed in paraffin-embedded tissue. Marker studies on true PSL and LIP demonstrate polyclonal staining for heavy chains (IgG, IgA, IgM) and light chains (κ, λ) of immunoglobulins; B-cell lymphomas show monoclonal staining. Also, some of the fresh, unfixed tissue should be sent for flow cytometric studies in RPMI medium. These studies will produce information about the cell cycle, the DNA content of the cells, and immunologic markers. The S phases of the cell cycle reveal how rapidly the cells are proliferating. The DNA content differentiates diploid from aneuploid cell populations. Aneuploid tumors have an increased or decreased amount of DNA, and they generally are more aggressive than diploid tumors. Flow cytometry can give a percentage distribution of immunologic markers, whereas frozen sections give only an architectural distribution of the markers. These two ways of performing immunologic markers complement each other. The flow cytometry is very helpful in establishing the presence of a monoclonal population of cells. In conclusion, new scientific techniques are offering more ways for the surgeon and the oncologist to evaluate pulmonary lymphoid lesions of the lung. The crucial step is to consider the possibility of a lymphoid lesion and then collect the appropriate fresh, frozen, B-5, and formalin-fixed tissue.

REFERENCES

Addis BJ, Hyjek E, Isaacson PG: Primary pulmonary lymphoma: a reappraisal of its histogenesis and its relationship to pseudolymphoma and lymphoid interstitial pneumonia. Histopathology 13:1, 1988.

Al-Sarraf M, et al: Superiority of chemoradiation vs. radiotherapy in patients with locally advanced nasopharyngeal cancer. Proc ASCO 15:313, 1996.

Baker PB, Goodwin RA: Pulmonary artery sarcoma: a review and report of a case. Arch Pathol Lab Med 109:35, 1985.

Barnard WG: Embryoma of lung. Thorax 7:299, 1952.

Begin LR, et al: Epstein-Barr virus related lymphoepithelioma-like carcinoma of the lung. J Surg Oncol 36:280, 1987.

Berho M, Moran CA, Suster S: Malignant mixed epithelial/mesenchymal neoplasms of the lung. Semin Diagn Pathol 12:123, 1995.

Berkman N, et al: Pulmonary involvement in lymphoma. Leuk Lymphoma 20:229, 1996.

Bhalla M, et al: Primary extraosseous pulmonary osteogenic sarcoma: CT findings. J Comput Assist Tomogr 16:974, 1992.

Bleisch VR, Kraus FT: Polypoid sarcoma of the pulmonary trunk: analysis of the literature and report of a case with leptomeric organelles and ultrastructural features of rhabdomyosarcoma. Cancer 46:314, 1980.

Bodner SM, Koss MN: Mutations in the p53 gene in pulmonary blastomas: immunohistochemical and molecular studies. Hum Pathol 27:1117, 1996.

Bragg DG, et al: Lymphoproliferative disorders of the lung: histopathology, clinical manifestations, and imaging features. AJR Am J Roentgenol 163:273, 1994.

Brambilla E: Basaloid carcinoma of the lung In Corrin B (ed): Pathology of Lung Tumors. New York: Churchill Livingstone, 1997, p. 71.

Brambilla E, et al: Basal cell (basaloid) carcinoma of the lung; a new morphologic and phenotypic entity with separate prognostic significance. Hum Pathol 23:993, 1992.

Britton PD: Primary pulmonary artery sarcoma—a report of two cases, with special emphasis on the diagnostic problems. Clin Radiol 41:92, 1990.

Burke AP, Virmani R: Sarcomas of the great vessels. A clinicopathologic study. Cancer 71:1761, 1993.

Canver CC, Voytovich MC: Resection of an unsuspected primary pulmonary choriocarcinoma. Ann Thorac Surg 61:1249, 1996.

Carrington CB, Liebow AA: Lymphocytic interstitial pneumonia [abstract]. Am J Pathol 48:36a, 1966.

Chan JKC, et al: A revised European American classification of lymphoid neoplasms proposed by the international lymphoma study group. A summary version. Am J Clin Pathol 103:543, 1995.

Chetty R, et al: Primary Hodgkin's disease of the lung. Pathology 27:111,1995.

Colby TV, Carrington CB: Lymphoreticular tumors and infiltrates of the lung. Pathol Annu 18:27, 1983.

Connolly JP, et al: Intrathoracic osteosarcoma diagnosed by CT scan and pleural biopsy. Chest 100:265, 1991.

Cordier J, et al: Primary pulmonary lymphomas. A clinical study of 70 cases in nonimmunocompromised patients. Chest 103:201, 1993.

Costa J, Martin S: Pulmonary lymphoreticular disorders. In Jaffee E (ed): Surgical Pathology of the Lymph Nodes and Related Organs. Philadelphia: Saunders, 1985, p. 289.

Cox JE, et al: Pulmonary artery sarcomas: a review of clinical and radiologic features. J Comput Assist Tomogr 21:750, 1997.

Crotty TB, et al: Primary malignant ependymoma of the lung. Mayo Clin Proc 67:373, 1992.

Curcio LD, et al: Primary lymphoepithelioma–like carcinoma of the lung in a child. Chest 111:250, 1997.

d'Agostino, et al: Embryonal Rhabdomyosarcoma of the lung arising in cystic adenomatoid malformation. Case report and review of the literature. J Pediatr Surg 32:1381, 1997.

Dail DH: Uncommon tumors. In Dail DH, Hammar SP (eds): Pulmonary Pathology. New York: Springer, 1988, p. 847.

Dail D, Liebow AA: Intravascular bronchioalveolar tumor [abstract]. Am J Pathol 78:6, 1975.

Dail DH, et al: Intravascular, bronchiolar, and alveolar tumor of the lung (IVBAT): an analysis of twenty cases of a peculiar sclerosing endothelial tumor. Cancer 51:452, 1983.

Davis Z, et al: Primary pulmonary hemangiopericytoma. J Thorac Cardiovasc Surg 64:882, 1972.

Day DW, Taylor SA: An intrapulmonary teratoma associated with thymic tissue. Thorax 30:582, 1975.

Demirer T, Dail DH, Aboulafia DM: Four varied cases of intravascular lymphomatosis and literature review. Cancer 73:1738, 1994.

Diehl LF, et al: The pattern of intrathoracic Hodgkin's disease assessed by computed tomography. J Clin Oncol 9:438, 1991.

Domizio P, et al: Malignant mesenchymoma associated with a congenital lung cyst in a child: case report and review of the literature. Pediatr Pathol 10:785, 1990.

Emmert-Buck MR, et al: Pleomorphic rhabdomyosarcoma arising in association with the right pulmonary artery. Arch Pathol Lab Med 118:1220, 1994.

Endo, et al: (1988). (See reference list of Uwatoko K, Kajita M: Primary choriocarcinoma of the lung: a case report involving a male. J Jpn Assoc Chest Surg 11:662, 1997.)

Enzinger FM, Smith BH: Hemangiopericytoma. Hum Pathol 7:61, 1976.

Enzinger FM, Weiss SW: Soft Tissue Tumors. St. Louis: Mosby, 1983, p. 409.

Fadhli HA, Harrison AW, Shaddock SH: Primary pulmonary leiomyosarcoma. Dis Chest 48:431, 1965.

Fauci AS, et al: Lymphomatoid granulomatosis: Prospective clinical and therapeutic experience over 10 years. N Engl J Med 306:68, 1982.

Feldman F, Seaman WB: Primary thoracic hemangiopericytoma. Radiology 82:998, 1964.

Fiche M, et al: Primary pulmonary non-Hodgkin's lymphoma. Histopathology 26:529, 1995.

Fishback N, Koss MN: Update on lymphoid interstitial pneumonitis. Curr Opin Pulm Med 2:429, 1996.

Fisher AMH, Kendall B, Van Leuven BD: Hodgkin's disease: a radiologic survey. Clin Radiol 13:115, 1962.

Francis D, Jacobsen M: Pulmonary blastoma. Curr Top Pathol 73:265, 1983.

Frank MW, et al: Lymphoepithelioma-like carcinoma of the lung. Ann Thorac Surg 64:1162, 1998.

Gabor EP, Sherwood T, Mercola KE: Intravascular lymphomatosis presenting as adult respiratory distress syndrome. Am J Hematol 56:155, 1997.

Garris PD, Gallup DG, Melton K: Long-term remission of previously resistant choriocarcinoma with a combination of etoposide, ifosfamide and cisplatin. Gynecol Oncol 57:252, 1995.

Ghosen M, et al: Salvage chemotherapy in refractory germ cell tumors with etoposide (VP-16) plus ifosfamide plus high dose cisplatin. Cancer 62:24, 1998.

Goldblum JR, Rice TW: Epithelioid angiosarcoma of the pulmonary artery. Hum Pathol 26:1275, 1995.

Goldthorn JF, et al: Cavitating primary pulmonary fibrosarcoma in a child. J Thorac Cardiovasc Surg 91:932, 1986.

Grahmann PR, et al: Carcinosarcoma of the lung. Three case reports and literature review. Thorac Cardiovasc Surg 41:312, 1993.

Guccion JG, Rosen SH: Bronchopulmonary leiomyosarcoma and fibrosarcoma: a study of 32 cases and review of the literature. Cancer 30:836, 1972.

Halyard MY, et al: Malignant fibrous histiocytoma of the lung. Report of four cases and review of the literature. Cancer 78:2492, 1996.

Hancock BJ, et al: Childhood primary pulmonary neoplasms. J Pediatr Surg 28:1133, 1993.

Hansen CP, Francis D, Bertelsen S: Primary hemangiopericytoma of the lung. Case report. Scand J Thorac Cardiovasc Surg 24:89, 1990.

Harris, NL et al: A revised European-American classification of lymphoid neoplasms: a proposal from the international lymphoma study group. Blood 84:1361, 1994.

Hartman GE, Shockat SJ: Primary pulmonary neoplasms of childhood: a review. Ann Thorac Surg 36:108, 1983.

Hayakawa K, et al: Primary choriocarcinoma of the lung. Acta Pathol Jpn 27:123, 1977.

Hayashi T, et al: Primary chondrosarcoma of the lung. A clinicopathologic study. Cancer 72:69, 1993.

Head HD, et al: Long-term palliation of pulmonary artery sarcoma by radical excision and adjuvant therapy. Ann Thorac Surg 53:332, 1992.

Herbert A, Wright DH, Isaacson PG: Primary malignant lymphoma of the lung: Histopathologic and immunologic evaluation of nine cases. Hum Pathol 15:415, 1984.

Hochberg L, Crastnopol P: Primary sarcoma of the bronchus and lung. Arch Surg 73:74, 1956.

Holland EA, et al: Evolution of pulmonary pseudolymphomas: clinical and radiologic manifestations. J Thorac Imaging 6:74, 1991.

Husband AJ, Gowans JL: The origin and antigen-dependent distribution of IgA-containing cells in the intestine. J Exp Med 148:1146, 1978.

Ishida T, et al: Carcinosarcoma and spindle cell carcinoma of the lung: clinicopathologic and immunohistochemical studies. J Thorac Cardiovasc Surg 100:844, 1990.

Jackson H, Parker F: Hodgkin's Disease and Allied Disorders. New York: Oxford University Press, 1947.

Janssen JP, et al: Primary sarcoma of the lung: a clinical study with long-term follow-up. Ann Thorac Surg 58:1151, 1994.

Jennings TA, et al: Primary malignant melanoma of the lower respiratory tract. Report of a case and literature review. Am J Clin Pathol 94:649, 1990.

Joseph G, Pandit M, Korfliage L: Primary pulmonary plasmacytoma. Cancer 71:721, 1993.

Kakkar N, et al: Primary pulmonary malignant teratoma with yolk sac element associated with hematologic neoplasia. Respiration 63:52, 1996.

Kaplan MA, et al: Primary pulmonary sarcoma with morphologic features of monophasic synovial sarcoma and chromosome translocation t(x; 18). Am J Clin Pathol 105:195, 1996.

Katzenstein AL, Carrington C, Liebow AA: Lymphomatoid granulomatosis: a clinicopathologic study of 152 cases. Cancer 43:360, 1979.

Kawashima O, et al: Pulmonary epithelioid hemangioendothelioma: a case report. Jpn J Clin Oncol 25:278, 1995.

Kazzaz B, Dewar A, Corrin B: An unusual pulmonary plasmacytoma. Histopathology 21:285, 1992.

Kennedy JL, et al: Pulmonary lymphomas and other pulmonary lymphoid lesions: a clinicopathologic and immunologic study of 64 patients. Cancer 56:539, 1985.

Kern WH, Crepeau AG, Jones JC: Primary Hodgkin's disease of the lung: report of 4 cases and review of the literature. Cancer 14:1151, 1961.

Kiefer T, et al: Long-term survival after repetitive surgery for malignant hemangiopericytoma of the lung with subsequent systemic metastases: case report and review of the literature. Thorac Cardiovasc Surg 45:307, 1997.

Kimino K, Nakasone T, Kishikawa M: A case of so called pulmonary carcinosarcoma. J Jpn Assoc Chest Surg 10:833, 1996.

Ko TM, et al: Leiomyosarcoma of the pulmonary vein. J Cardiovascular Surg 37:421, 1996.

Koss M, et al: Lymphomatoid granulomatosis: a clinicopathologic study of 42 patients. Pathol (Sydney) 18:283, 1986.

Koss MN, Hochholzer L, O'Leary T: Pulmonary blastomas. Cancer 67:2368, 1991.

Koss MN, et al: Primary non-Hodgkin's lymphoma and pseudolymphoma of the lung: A study of 161 patients. Hum Pathol 14:1024, 1983.

Koss MN: Pulmonary lymphoid disorders. Semin Diagn Pathol 12:158, 1995.

Kradin R, et al: Pulmonary blastoma with argyrophil cells and lacking sarcomatous features (pulmonary endodermal tumor resembling fetal lung). Am J Surg Pathol 6:165, 1982.

Kradin RL, Mark EJ: Benign lymphoid disorders of the lung, with a theory regarding their development. Hum Pathol 14:857, 1983.

Kruger I, et al: Symptoms, diagnosis, and therapy of primary sarcomas of the pulmonary artery. Thorac Cardiovasc Surg 38:91, 1990.

Krygier G, et al: Primary lung liposarcoma. Lung Cancer 17:271, 1997.

Larsen H, Sorensen JB: Pulmonary blastoma: a review with special emphasis on prognosis and treatment. Cancer Treat Rev 22:145, 1996.

Lennert K: Malignant Lymphomas Other Than Hodgkin's Disease. New York: Springer, 1978.

Leone O, et al: Leiomyosarcoma of the pulmonary vein: case report with immunohistochemical and ultrastructural findings. Gen Diagn Pathol 142:235, 1996.

Lewis ER, Caskey CI, Fishman EK: Lymphoma of the lung: CT findings in 31 patients. AJR Am J Roentgenol 156:711, 1991.

L'hoste RJ, et al: Primary pulmonary lymphomas. Cancer 54:1397, 1984.

Liebow AA, Carrington CB: Diffuse pulmonary lymphoreticular infiltration associated with dysproteinemia. Med Clin North Am 57:809, 1973.

Liebow AA, Carrington C, Friedman P: Lymphomatoid granulomatosis. Hum Pathol 3:457, 1972.

Lillo-Gil R, Albrechtsson U, Jakobsson B: Pulmonary leiomyosarcoma appearing as a cyst. Report of one case and review of the literature. Thorac Cardiovasc Surg 33:250, 1985.

Loose JH, et al: Primary osteosarcoma of the lung. Report of two cases and review of the literature. J Thorac Cardiovasc Surg 100:867, 1990.

Lukes RJ, Collins RD: New approaches to the classification of lymphomata. Br J Cancer 2(Suppl):1, 1975.

Mader MT, Poulton TB, White RD: Malignant tumors of the heart and great vessels: MR imaging appearance. Radiographics 17:145, 1997.

Mandelstramm M: Über primary Neubildung des Herzens. Virchows Arch [A] 245:43, 1923.

Manivel JC, et al: Pleuropulmonary blastoma: The so-called pulmonary blastoma of childhood. Cancer 62:1516, 1988.

Marchevsky AM: Lung tumors derived from ectopic tissues. Semin Diagn Pathol 12:172, 1995.

Martini N, Hajdu SI, Beattie EJ Jr: Primary sarcoma of lung. J Thorac Cardiovasc Surg 61:33, 1971.

McCluggage WG, Bharucha H: Primary pulmonary tumors of nerve sheath origin. Histopathology 26:247, 1995.

McCormack PM, Martini N: Primary Sarcomas and Lymphomas of Lung. In Martini N, Vogt-Moykopf I (eds): International Trends in General Thoracic Surgery. Vol. 5. St. Louis: Mosby, 1988.

McDermott VG, Mackenzie S, Hendry GM: Case report: primary intrathoracic rhabdomyosarcoma: a rare childhood malignancy. Br J Radiol 66:937, 1993.

McDonnell T, et al: Malignant fibrous histiocytoma of the lung. Cancer 61:37, 1988.

McGuinness G, et al: Unusual lympho-proliferative disorders in nine adults with HIV or AIDS: CT and pathologic findings. Radiology 197:59, 1995.

McLigeyo SO, et al: Fibrosarcoma of the lung with extrapulmonary manifestations: case report. East Afr Med J 72:465, 1995.

Meade P, et al: Carcinosarcoma of the lung with hypertrophic pulmonary osteoarthropathy. Ann Thorac Surg 51:488, 1991.

Miettinen M, et al: Intravascular bronchioloalveolar tumor. Cancer 60:2471, 1987.

Miller DL, Allen MS: Rare pulmonary neoplasms. Mayo Clin Proc 68:492, 1993.

Moffat RE, Chang CHJ, Slaven JE: Roentgen considerations in primary pulmonary artery sarcoma. Radiology 104:283, 1972.

Moran CA, et al: Primary leiomyosarcoma of the lung: a clinicopathologic and immunohistochemical study of 18 cases. Mod Pathol 10:121, 1997.

Morgan AD, Salama FD: Primary chondrosarcoma of the lung: case report and review of the literature. J Thorac Cardiovasc Surg 64:460, 1972.

Morgenroth A, et al: Primary chondrosarcoma of the left inferior lobar bronchus. Respiration 56:241, 1989.

Moro D, et al: Basaloid bronchial carcinoma a histological group with a poor prognosis. Cancer 73:2734, 1994.

Nakamura M, et al: Case of pulmonary choriocarcinoma in a 59-year-old man. Nippon Naika Gakkai Zasshi 71:1445, 1982 (in Japanese).

Nakatani Y, Dicersin GR, Mark EJ: Pulmonary endodermal tumor resembling fetal lung: a clinicopathologic study of five cases with immunohistochemical and ultrastructural characterization. Hum Pathol 21:1097, 1990.

Nappi O, et al: Biphasic and monophasic sarcomatoid carcinomas of the lung: A reappraisal of 'carcinosarcomas' and 'Spindle-cell carcinomas.' Am J Clin Pathol 102: 331, 1994.

Nascimento AG, Unni KK, Bernatz PE: Sarcomas of the lung. Mayo Clin Proc 57:355, 1982.

Noach AS: Pulmonary involvement in Waldenström's macroglobulinemia. Ned Tijdschr Geneeskd 100:3881, 1956.

Noda T, et al: Alveolar rhabdomyosarcoma of the lung in a child. J Pediatr Surg 30:1607, 1995.

The Non-Hodgkin's Lymphoma Pathologic Classification Project: National Cancer Institute-sponsored study of classification on non-Hodgkin's lymphoma. Cancer 49:2112, 1982.

Nonomura A, et al: Primary pulmonary artery sarcoma: report of two autopsy cases studied by immunohistochemistry and electron microscopy, and review of 110 cases reported in the literature. Acta Pathol Jpn 38:883, 1988.

Parish JM, et al: Pulmonary artery sarcoma. Clinical features. Chest 110: 1480, 1996.

Parker LA, et al: Primary pulmonary chondrosarcoma mimicking bronchogenic cyst on CT and MRI. Clin Imaging 20:181, 1996.

Patel AM, Ryu JH: Angiosarcoma in the lung. Chest 103:1531, 1993.

Petersen M: Radionuclide detection of primary pulmonary osteogenic sarcoma: A case report and review of the literature. J Nucl Med 31:1110, 1990.

Pfleger L., Tappeiner J: Zur Kenntnis der Systemisienten Endotheliomatose der Cutanen Blutegefasse (Reticuloendotheliose) Hautarzt 10:359, 1959.

Pisani RJ, DeRemee RA: Clinical implications of the histopathologic diagnosis of pulmonary lymphomatoid granulomatosis. Mayo Clin Proc 65:151, 1990.

Pitt J: Lymphocytic interstitial pneumonia. Pediatr Clin North Am 38:89, 1991.

Poelzleitner D, et al: Primary pulmonary lymphoma in a patient with the acquired immune deficiency syndrome. Thorax 44:438, 1989.

Polish LB, et al: Pulmonary non-Hodgkin's lymphoma in AIDS. Chest 96:1321, 1989.

Priest J, et al: Pleuropulmonary blastoma: a clinicopathologic study of 50 cases. Cancer 80:147, 1997.

Przygodzki RM, et al: Primary pulmonary rhabdomyosarcomas: a clinicopathologic and immunohistochemical study of three cases. Mod Pathol 8:658, 1995.

Radin AI: Primary pulmonary Hodgkin's disease. Cancer 65:550, 1990.

Rappaport H: Tumors of the hematopoietic system. In Atlas of Tumor Pathology, Fascicle 8. Washington DC: Armed Forces Institute of Pathology, 1966.

Redmond ML, et al: Primary pulmonary artery sarcoma: a method of resection. Chest 98:752, 1990.

Risdall R, Hoppe TR, Warnke R: Non-Hodgkin's lymphoma: a study of the evolution of the disease based upon 92 autopsied cases. Cancer 44:529, 1979.

Roikjaer O, Thomsen JK: Plasmacytoma of the lung: a case report describing two tumors of different immunologic type in a single patient. Cancer 58:2671, 1986.

Ross GJ, et al: Intravascular bronchioloalveolar tumor: CT and pathologic correlation. J Comput Assist Tomogr 13:240, 1989.

Rusch VW, et al: Massive pulmonary hemangiopericytoma: an innovative approach to evaluation and treatment. Cancer 64:1928, 1989.

Saldana MJ, Mones JM: Lymphoid interstitial pneumonia in HIV-infected individuals. Prog Surg Pathol 12:181, 1992.

Saltzstein SL: Pulmonary malignant lymphomas and pseudolymphomas. Classification, therapy and prognosis. Cancer 16:928, 1963.

Schiavetti A, et al: Primary pulmonary rhabdomyosarcoma in childhood: clinico-biologic features in two cases with review of the literature. Med Pediatr Oncol 26:201, 1996.

Sheppard MN, et al: Primary epithelioid angiosarcoma of the lung presenting as pulmonary hemorrhage. Hum Pathol 27:383, 1997.

Shimizu J, et al: Primary pulmonary hemangiopericytoma: a case report. Jpn J Clin Oncol 23:313, 1993.

Shin MS, Carcelen MF, Ho K: Diverse roentgenographic manifestations of the rare pulmonary involvement in myeloma. Chest 102:946, 1992.

Shinn MS, Ho KJ: Primary hemangiopericytoma of lung: Radiography and pathology. AJR Am J Roentgenol 133:1077, 1979.

Shiota T, et al: Gene analysis of pulmonary pseudolymphoma. Chest 103:335, 1993.

Spencer H: Pulmonary blastoma. J Pathol 82:161, 1961.

Spragg RG, et al: Angiosarcoma of the lung with fatal pulmonary hemorrhage. Am J Med 74:1072, 1983.

Sridher KS, et al: Primary choriocarcinoma of the lung: report of a case treated with intensive multimodality therapy and review of the literature. J Surg Oncol 41:93, 1989.

Staples CA: Pulmonary angiitis and granulomatosis. Radiol Clin North Am 29:973, 1991.

Stroup RM, et al: Angiotropic (intravascular) large cell lymphoma. A clinicopathologic study of seven cases with unique clinical presentations. Cancer 66:1781, 1990.

Tamura A, et al: Primary pulmonary lymphoma: relationship between clinical features and pathologic findings in 24 cases. Jpn J Clin Oncol 25:140, 1995.

Tanimura A, et al: Primary choriocarcinoma of the lung. Hum Pathol 16:1281, 1985.

Tian D, et al: Results of surgical treatment of primary pulmonary malignant fibrous histiocytoma. J Jpn Assoc Chest Surg 11:631, 1997.

Toh HC, Ang PT: Primary pulmonary lymphoma—clinical review from a single institution in Singapore. Leuk Lymphoma 27:153, 1997.

Trapnell DH: Recognition and incidence of intrapulmonary lymph nodes. Thorax 19:44, 1964.

Turner RR, Colby TV, Doggett RS: Well-differentiated lymphocytic lymphoma: a study of 47 cases with primary manifestation of the lung. Cancer 54:2088, 1984.

Uppal R, Goldstraw P: Primary pulmonary lymphoma. Lung Cancer 8:95, 1992.

Uspenski LV, et al: Primary lung chorioepithelioma in a male. Khirurgiia (Mosk) 5:1065, 1982 (in Russian).

Uwatoko K, Kajita M: Primary choriocarcinoma of the lung: a case report involving a male. J Jpn Assoc Chest Surg 11:662, 1997.

Van Damme H, et al: Primary pulmonary hemangiopericytoma: Early local recurrence after perioperative rupture of the giant tumor mass (two cases) Surgery 108:105, 1990.

Wackers FJ, van der Schoot JB, Hamper JR: Sarcoma of the pulmonary trunk associated with hemorrhagic tendency: a case report and review of the literature. Cancer 23:339, 1969.

Watson WL, Anlyan AJ: Primary leiomyosarcoma: A clinical evaluation of six cases. Cancer 7:250, 1954.

Weis JW, et al: Peripheral T-cell lymphomas: histologic, immunologic, and clinical characterization. Mayo Clin Proc 61:411, 1986.

Weiss LM, Yousem SA, Warnke RA: Non-Hodgkin's lymphomas of the lung. Am J Surg Pathol 9:480, 1985.

Weiss SW, Enzinger FM: Epithelioid hemangioendothelioma: a vascular tumor often mistaken for a carcinoma. Cancer 50:970, 1982.

Weiss SW, et al: Epithelioid hemangioendothelioma and related lesions. Semin Diagn Pathol 3:259, 1986.

Wenisch HJC, Lulay M: Lymphogenous spread of an intravascular bronchioloalveolar tumour: case report and review of the literature. Virchows Arch [A] 387:117, 1980.

Wick MR, et al: Sarcomatoid carcinomas of the lung: a clinicopathologic review. Am J Clin Pathol 108:40, 1997.

Wotherspoon AC, et al: Low-grade primary B-cell lymphoma of the lung: an immunohistochemical, molecular, and cytogenetic study of a single case. Am J Clin Pathol 94:655, 1990.

Wu Y, et al: Primary pulmonary malignant hemangiopericytoma associated with coagulopathy. Ann Thorac Surg 64:841, 1997.

Yousem SA: Angiosarcoma presenting in the lung. Arch Pathol Lab Med 110:112, 1986.

Yousem SA, Colby TV: Intravascular lymphomatosis presenting in the lung. Cancer 65: 349,1990.

Yousem SA, Hochholzer L: Malignant fibrous histiocytoma of the lung. Cancer 60:2532, 1987a.

Yousem SA, Hochholzer L: Primary pulmonary hemangiopericytoma. Cancer 59:549, 1987b.

Zeren H, et al: Primary pulmonary sarcomas with features of monophasic synovial sarcoma. A clinicopathologic, immunohistochemical and ultrastructural study of 25 cases. Human Pathol 26:474, 1995.

READING REFERENCES

Malignant Fibrous Histiocytoma

Bedrossian CWM, et al: Pulmonary malignant fibrous histiocytoma: light and electron microscopic studies of one case. Chest 75:186, 1979.

Silverman JF, Coalson JJ: Primary malignant myxoid fibrous histiocytoma of the lung: light and ultrastructural examination with review of the literature. Arch Pathol Lab Med 108:49, 1984.

Lymphomas

Freeman C, Berg JW, Cutler SJ: Occurrence and prognosis of extranodal lymphoma. Cancer 29:252, 1972.

Gibbs AR, Seal RME: Primary lymphoproliferative conditions of lung. Thorax 33:140, 1978.

Greenberg SD, Jenkins DE: Xanthomatous inflammatory pseudotumors of the lung. South Med J 68:754, 1975.

Greenberg SD, et al: Pulmonary lymphoma versus pseudolymphoma: a perplexing problem. South Med J 65:775, 1972.

Hurt RL, Kennedy WPU: Primary lymphosarcoma of the lung. Thorax 29:258, 1974.

Rubin M: Primary lymphoma of lung. J Thorac Cardiovasc Surg 56:293, 1968.

Pulmonary Blastoma

Ashworth TG: Pulmonary blastomas: a true congenital neoplasm. Histopathology 7:585, 1983.

Gibbons JRP, McKeown F, Field TW: Pulmonary blastoma with hilar lymph node metastases: survival for 24 years. Cancer 47:152, 1981.

Kodama T, et al: Six cases of well-differentiated adenocarcinoma simulating fetal lung tubules in pseudoglandular stage. Comparison with pulmonary blastoma. Am J Surg Pathol 8:735, 1984.

Spencer H: Hamartomas, Blastoma and Teratoma of the Lung. In Spencer H (ed): Pathology of the Lung. 4th Ed. New York: Pergamon Press, 1985, p. 1061.

Tomashefski JF Jr: Fetal (endometroid) adenocarcinomas of the lung. In Corrin B (ed): Pathology of Lung Tumors. New York: Churchill Livingstone, 1997, p. 149.

Pulmonary Rhabdomyosarcoma

Avignina A, et al: Pulmonary rhabdomyosarcoma with isolated small bowel metastases: a report of a case with immunohistological and ultrastructural studies. Cancer 53:1948, 1984.

Lee SH, Reganchary SS, Paramesk J: Primary pulmonary rhabdomyosarcoma: a case report and review of the literature. Hum Pathol 12:92, 1981.

Luck SR, Reynolds M, Raffensperger JG: Congenital bronchopulmonary malformations. Curr Probl Surg 23:251, 1986.

Shariff S, et al: Primary pulmonary rhabdomyosarcoma in a child, with review of the literature. J Surg Oncol 38:261, 1988.

Pulmonary Sarcoma

Cameron EWJ: Primary sarcoma of the lung. Thorax 30:516, 1975.

Ramanathan T: Primary leiomyosarcoma of the lung. Thorax 29:482, 1974.

Sawamura K, et al: Primary liposarcoma of the lung: report of a case. J Surg Oncol 19:243, 1982.

Wick MR, et al: Primary pulmonary leiomyosarcomas: a light and electron microscopic study. Arch Pathol Lab Med 106:510, 1982.

Sarcomas of Large Vessel Origin

Anderson MD, et al: Primary pulmonary artery sarcoma: a report of six cases. Ann Thorac Surg 59:1487, 1995.

Johansson L, Carlen B: Sarcoma of the pulmonary artery: report of four cases with electron microscopic and immunohistochemical examinations, and review of the literature. Virchows Arch 424:217, 1994.

Tanaka I, et al: Primary pulmonary artery sarcoma. Report of a case with complete resection and graft replacement, and review of 47 surgically treated cases reported in the literature. Thorac Cardiovasc Surg 42:64, 1994.

Velebit V, et al: Preoperative diagnosis of a pulmonary artery sarcoma. Thorax 50:1014, 1995.

Yamada N, et al: Primary leiomyosarcoma of the pulmonary artery confirmed by catheter suction biopsy. Chest 113:555, 1998.

Teratomas (Benign and Malignant)

Ali MY, Wong PK: Intrapulmonary teratoma. Thorax 19:228, 1964.

Gantam HP: Intrapulmonary malignant teratoma. Am Rev Respir Dis 200:863, 1969.

Holt S, Peverall PB, Boddy JE: A teratoma of the lung containing thymic tissue. J Pathol 126:85, 1978.

Spencer H: Hamartomas, Blastoma and Teratoma of the Lung. In Spencer H (ed): Pathology of the Lung. 4th Ed. New York: Pergamon Press, 1985, p. 1061.

CHAPTER 113

Secondary Tumors of the Lung

Joe B. Putnam, Jr.

Pulmonary metastases represent a particular manifestation of systemic metastases from primary malignant tumors. Although primary tumors can be locally controlled with surgery or radiation, the optimal treatment of systemic metastases remains elusive. Most commonly, metastases are treated with chemotherapy as a systemic treatment modality. Radiation therapy may be used to treat or palliate the local manifestations of metastatic disease, particularly when metastases occur within the bony skeleton causing significant pain. Frequently, the systemic spread of metastases represents uncontrolled tumor and heralds a rapid course of disease progression and eventual death. In contrast, patients with metastases isolated within the lungs may have biology more amenable to local or local and systemic treatment options than do other patients with multiorgan metastases. Isolated pulmonary metastases, therefore, should not be viewed as untreatable. Patients who have complete resection of all metastases have associated longer survival than do those patients who are unresectable. Long-term survival (>5 years) may be expected in approximately 20 to 30% of all patients with resectable pulmonary metastases. Optimal—and more consistent—survival awaits improvements in local control, systemic therapy, or regional drug delivery to the lungs.

HISTORIC PERSPECTIVE

Early resection of pulmonary metastases has been described by Meade (1961) and Martini and McCormack (1998). Weinlechner (1882) and Kronlein (1884) reported early resections of pulmonary metastasis as incidental procedures while resecting primary chest wall tumors. The first resection of a pulmonary metastasis as a planned procedure was described by Divis (1927) and Torek (1930). Barney and Churchill (1939) reported one of the first long-term survivors of pulmonary metastasectomy after resection of a metastasis from a patient with hypernephroma. After local control of the primary tumor and resection of the metastasis, the patient survived for 23 years and died from unrelated causes. Alexander

and Haight (1947) reviewed the first large series (25 patients) of patients who had resection of metastases from carcinoma and sarcoma. They noted that patients generally did well, and a survival advantage was possible. Mannix (1953) described for the first time resection of multiple pulmonary metastases from a patient with osteochondromas. Few attempts were made at multiple resections for pulmonary metastases until Martini and associates (1971) described the value of resecting multiple metastases and multiple resections (multiple sequential operations) in the treatment of osteogenic sarcoma (OST). In the past 20 years, resection of solitary and multiple pulmonary metastases from numerous primary neoplasms have been performed with good long-term survival in 20 to 40% of patients, as shown by Pastorino and colleagues (1997).

Autopsy studies have demonstrated that about one-third of patients with cancer die with pulmonary metastases and a small percentage die with metastases confined solely to the lungs. Metastases from osteogenic and soft tissue sarcomas commonly occur only in the lungs. Patients with other solid organ neoplasms from melanoma, breast, or colon have isolated pulmonary metastases less commonly, but these metastases may represent favorable tumor biology and a treatable subset of such patients. In the absence of extrathoracic metastases, patients with isolated and resectable pulmonary metastases should undergo complete resection for treatment and possible cure of their disease. Even in the presence of extrathoracic metastases, selected individual patients with complete resection may have a survival advantage. Limitations on the number of metastases have not as yet been determined; however, the greater the number of metastases, the greater likelihood that micrometastases may exist that the surgeon cannot see or feel. These micrometastases continue to grow and will require additional surgery or systemic therapy on diagnosis.

PATHOLOGY

Neoplasms may metastasize in four ways: hematogenous, lymphatic, direct invasion, and aerogenous. Underlying tumor

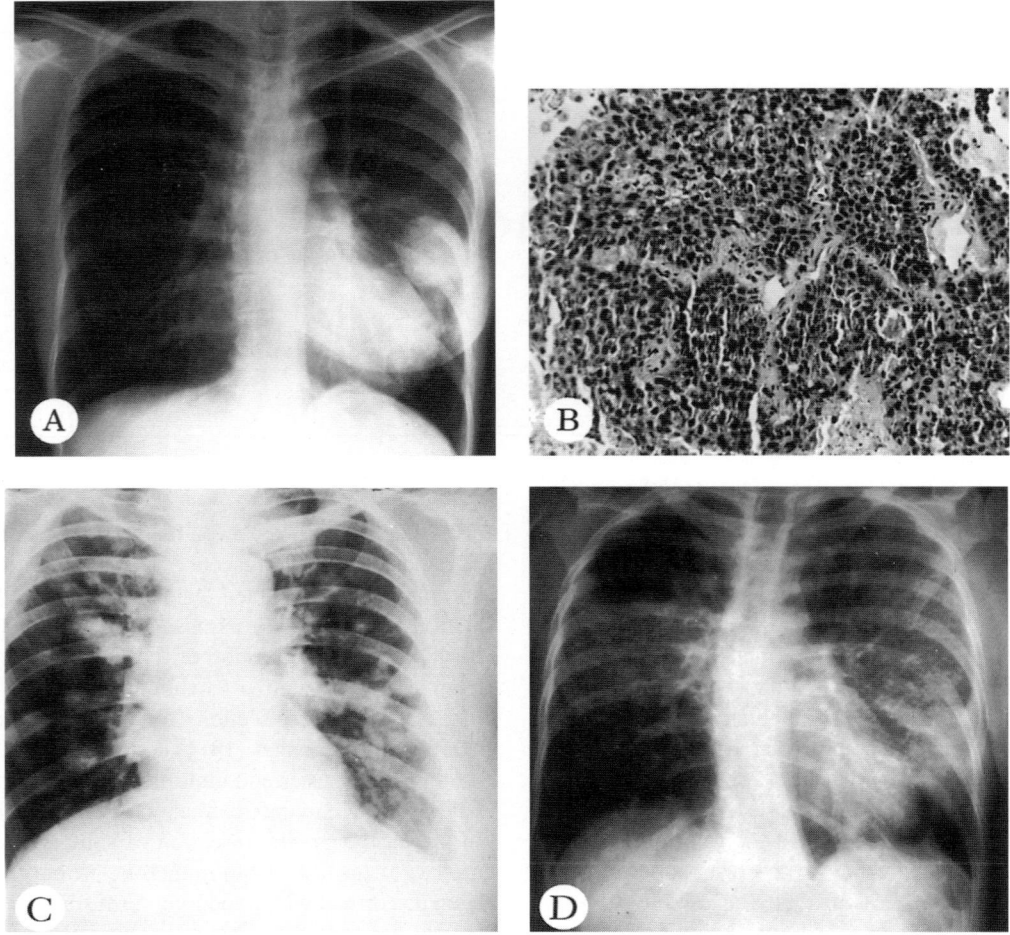

Fig. 113-1. A. Posteroanterior radiograph of the chest shows solitary metastasis in the left lung from a primary breast carcinoma. **B.** Photomicrograph of metastatic carcinoma of the breast in the lung. **C.** Posteroanterior radiograph of the chest shows bilateral metastases to the lungs from a primary carcinoma of the breast. **D.** Posteroanterior radiograph of the chest shows lymphangitic carcinomatosis from breast carcinoma.

biology and host resistance determine mechanisms of spread, location of metastases, and extent of growth. Hematogenous metastases are most frequently found in the lung, liver, brain, and bone. Clumps of tumor cells filtered out in the lungs may preferentially adhere to the underlying capillary endothelium. Tumor cells may travel by lymphatics and occupy a discrete position within the lung or may diffusely involve the entire lung (e.g., lymphangitic spread of breast carcinoma or other metastatic adenocarcinomas) (Fig. 113-1). Pulmonary metastases may metastasize to other organs. Depending on the primary histology, metastases can develop in draining pulmonary lobar, hilar, or mediastinal nodes. Direct invasion of metastases into other structures may occur as the metastasis grows. Thus, extended resection may still be possible and benefit obtained if complete resection of metastases can be achieved with negative margins. Aerogenous spread of tumor from one site within the tracheobronchial tree to another site is rare if it occurs at all.

SYMPTOMS

Symptoms rarely occur from pulmonary metastases, therefore, diagnosis of metastases is routinely made on chest radiographs after primary tumor resection. Palliation for pain is rarely needed because the pleura is infrequently involved. Few (<5%) patients with metastases present with symptoms of dyspnea, pain, cough, or hemoptysis. Rarely, patients with peripheral sarcomatous metastases may develop pneumothorax from disruption of the peripheral pulmonary parenchyma.

DIAGNOSIS

Chest radiographs obtained after primary tumor resection may demonstrate pulmonary parenchymal changes consistent with metastases. Metastases may appear as solitary or multiple nodules, well-circumscribed or diffuse opacities, and be miliary or massive in appearance. Routine chest radiographs represent an effective means of screening patients for pulmonary metastases. Patients without evidence of metastases on chest radiograph may have metastases demonstrated by tomography. Today's high-resolution computed tomography (CT) may achieve resolution of pulmonary abnormalities of 2 to 3 mm in diameter. Metastases may appear at this size, but more commonly sequelae of infections, granulomas, or other pulmonary parenchymal changes may produce these small indeterminate lesions. Resection may provide the most direct way to evaluate histology; however, the surgeon must be able to palpate the 2-mm lesion, which may lie deep within the lung parenchyma. Most commonly, physicians at this institution have followed these indeterminate lesions. If they enlarge in size on subsequent high-resolution or spiral CT, then resection or other treatment is planned.

Patients with known metastases on chest radiographs should undergo CT to identify other smaller metastases. CT of the chest demonstrates nodules as small as 3 mm. When clinically correlated with the patient's age, prior history of malignancy, and prior treatment, a diagnosis of pulmonary metastases can be made. Lien and coworkers (1988) showed that approximately one-half of patients with nonseminomatous testicular tumors have negative chest radiographs but have abnormalities identified on CT scans. Chang and colleagues (1979) at the National Cancer Institute prospectively evaluated linear tomograms and CT for pulmonary metastases. They found metastases in only 20% of nodules greater than 3 mm, which were identified by CT and not by linear tomograms. CT provided a more sensitive but less specific examination than chest radiographs for identifying metastatic lesions. CT of the chest provides a consistent anatomic reference for resection of pulmonary metastases.

Magnetic resonance (MR) imaging may be as sensitive as CT scans for identifying pulmonary metastases but adds little information, as observed by Feuerstein and associates (1992). A short inversion time inversion-recovery sequence provided the best sensitivity for individual nodules (82%). MR imaging is not routinely recommended for evaluation of patients with pulmonary metastases limited to the pulmonary parenchyma. MR imaging may provide complementary information to CT in planning resection for metastases involving the posterior mediastinum, neural foramina, or great vessels.

One prospective study of 19 patients by Pass and colleagues (1985) evaluated CT and full lung linear tomograms (FLT) to detect pulmonary metastases from osteogenic or soft tissue sarcomas. These authors noted that CT was significantly better than FLT in detecting metastatic nodules when they were early (56 by CT vs. 7 by FLT, $P = 0.001$) and small (7.6 mm by CT vs. 13.2 mm by FLT, $P < .05$). They recommended that surgical decisions for resection of pulmonary metastases be based on CT findings rather than FLT.

Benign granulomatous diseases may mimic metastases; however, in patients with a prior diagnosis of malignancy, nodules in the lung parenchyma are most likely metastases. Clinical stage I or II primary lung carcinoma may be indistinguishable from a solitary metastasis, particularly if the original tumor was squamous cell carcinoma (SCCA) or adenocarcinoma. For the two histologies specifically, thoracotomy and lobectomy would be a procedure of choice. Mediastinal lymph node dissection would complete the staging. Fine-needle aspiration or thoracoscopic wedge excision may be helpful for diagnosis or staging of pulmonary nodules in high-risk patients. In patients with lymphangitic spread of cancer, biopsy may be required to differentiate neoplasm from infection.

Other diagnostic modalities, such as whole-body ^{18}F-fluorodeoxyglucose positron emission tomography (FDG PET), can be used to identify pulmonary metastases in patients with soft tissue tumors after treatment. One study by Lucas and coworkers (1998) evaluated the results of FDG PET and chest CT in 62 patients who had been treated for pulmonary metastases (mean age was 51 years) with 15 types of soft tissue sarcoma. Local recurrence, distant recurrence, and pulmonary metastases were evaluated. The mean follow-up was 3 years. For local disease, FDG PET was 73.7% sensitive and 94.3% specific (14 true positive, five false negative). MR imaging was 88.2% sensitive and 96.0% specific. When FDG PET was used to identify lung metastases in 70 comparisons, sensitivity was 86.7% and specificity was 100% (13 true positive, two false negative). CT of the chest had 100% sensitivity and 96.4% specificity. Other metastases (n = 13) were identified by FDG PET. The authors concluded that FDG PET can identify local and distant recurrence of tumor and other metastases and recommend that all three methods be used in a complementary fashion to identify the extent of disease initially and during follow-up.

TREATMENT OF PULMONARY METASTASES

The majority of patients with pulmonary metastases have multiple sites of metastases or unresectable pleural or pulmonary metastases. In these patients, treatment is directed systemically for control of the disease and to palliate symptoms. Although radiation therapy or chemotherapy is frequently used, little hope exists for cure. In patients with control of the primary tumor and metastases confined to the lungs, resection of all visualized or palpable metastases may be considered. Complete resection of pulmonary metastases is generally associated with improved patient survival, regardless of primary histology.

Chemotherapy

The value of chemotherapy for treatment of pulmonary metastases that develop after treatment of the primary is controversial. The incidence of pulmonary metastases in patients with primary OST treated with surgical resection and adjuvant chemotherapy has dramatically declined compared to treatment with surgery alone, as shown by Skinner (1992), Goorin (1991), Pastorino (1991), and Yamaguchi (1988) and their coworkers. Bacci and associates (1988) found that in patients who receive adjuvant chemotherapy for primary OST, surgical resection of pulmonary metastases may be accomplished in a larger proportion of patients (51%) than in those who did not receive chemotherapy (29%). Salvage chemotherapy with resection may be effective in prolonging survival in patients who develop pulmonary metastases from OST, as described by Marina (1992) and Pastorino (1992) and their colleagues. The results of preoperative chemotherapy (high-dose methotrexate, cisplatin, doxorubicin, and ifosfamide) followed by surgery and additional chemotherapy have been examined. Bacci and coworkers (1997) noted that in 23 patients with OST of the extremity who presented with pulmonary metastases treated in this manner, three patients had complete response and in four patients, the metastases remained unresectable. Only the primary tumor was resected in these patients. In the 16 other patients, chemotherapy was given, followed by simultaneous resection of the primary and metastatic tumors. Complete resection was accomplished in 15 patients. The five unresectable (metastatic) patients died within a few months. Eighteen patients survived 30 months (78%) and 10 (55%) remained disease free. Survival was strongly correlated to the chemotherapy effects (necrosis) in the primary tumor and metastasis. Improved survival with combined-modality therapy (chemotherapy followed by salvage surgery) was achieved compared to historic results.

Glasser and associates (1992) noted that histologic response to chemotherapy (percent necrosis) was the only independent predictor of enhanced survival in a study of 279 patients with stage II OST.

Completeness of resection after chemotherapy significantly affects subsequent survival. Kim and Louie (1992) treated patients with metastatic renal cell carcinoma with interleukin-2 before surgical resection of residual tumor. Nine of 11 patients were alive with no evidence of disease at a median follow-up of 21 months. Lanza and associates (1991) examined the response of soft tissue sarcoma metastases that were treated with chemotherapy before surgery. Patients were graded as having complete, partial, or no response or progression from the chemotherapy. Survival could not be predicted on the basis of response to chemotherapy alone. One prospective randomized trial comparing chemotherapy followed by resection to resection alone for pulmonary metastases of soft tissue sarcomas is being conducted in Europe by the European Organisation for Research and Treatment of Cancer (1996).

The current practice at M. D. Anderson Cancer Center is to consider patients with soft tissue sarcomas, one or two lesions, and a long disease-free survival for immediate surgery. For patients with more than two lesions, chemotherapy (Adriamycin, ifosfamide) to assess a biological response, followed by surgery, and then additional chemotherapy (if response was noted) is usually planned in a multidisciplinary setting. For unresectable metastases, chemotherapy may provide a response sufficient for surgical resection, after which additional chemotherapy may be considered. If chemotherapy is unsuccessful, surgery may be considered for palliation of symptoms. In marginal patients in whom chemotherapy provided only a minimal response or no change, surgery may be considered for local control of the metastases. Occasionally, metastases may grow to enormous size, compressing the heart and mediastinum (a "tumor-thorax") with the same consequences of tension pneumothorax or tension hemothorax on the heart and pulmonary function. Chemotherapy is not commonly effective here, and a heroic attempt at resection may be required. Cardiopulmonary bypass for cardiac decompression, and circulatory and pulmonary support may be required simply to manipulate the tumor within the thorax or mediastinum.

Radiation Therapy

Currently, radiation therapy is used for palliation of symptoms of advanced metastases (e.g., extensive pleural involvement, bone metastases). Radiation therapy is rarely used for treatment of pulmonary metastases. Prophylactic lung radiation has been performed for OST. Patients with prophylactic lung radiation for primary OST had similar recurrence of pulmonary metastases to patients having adjuvant chemotherapy, as observed by Burgers and colleagues (1988).

Surgery

In selected patients with resectable pulmonary metastases and absence of extrathoracic metastases, complete resection is generally associated with improved long-term survival regardless of histology. In even more highly selected patients with extrathoracic metastases controlled or resected, resection of isolated pulmonary metastases may be considered to remove all known disease. An example of such a patient is one with colorectal carcinoma who has had previously resected hepatic metastases and is now discovered to have pulmonary metastases. In these patients, the thoracic surgeon may take advantage of the tumor biology, limiting metastases to the liver and lung. These patients have enhanced long-term survival compared to those with unresectable metastases.

Selection of Patients for Resection

Takita (1992), Morrow (1980), McCormack (1978), Mountain (1984), and Pastorino (1997) and their coworkers have described criteria for selecting patients with isolated pulmonary metastases for resection in an attempt to quantitate the tumor biology of the metastases and to identify patients who would benefit from surgical resection. Criteria

Table 113-1. Excision of Pulmonary Metastases

Criteria for resection of pulmonary metastases
  Pulmonary nodules consistent with metastases
  Control of primary tumor
  All nodules potentially resectable with planned surgery
  Adequate postoperative pulmonary reserve anticipated
  No extrathoracic metastases
Other indications for partial or complete resection of pulmonary
    metastases
  Need to establish a diagnosis
  Remove residual nodules after chemotherapy
  Obtain tissue for tumor markers or immunohistochemical studies
  Decrease tumor burden

have been proposed to identify and select patients who can benefit optimally from resection of their pulmonary metastases (Table 113-1).

Most patients with metastases do not benefit from surgery because of a biologically aggressive tumor characterized by extensive disease, a short disease-free interval (DFI) between control of their primary tumor and identification of multiple and unresectable pulmonary metastases, and rapid metastatic growth.

Surgical Techniques and Incisions

Surgical procedures for resection include single thoracotomy, staged bilateral thoracotomies, median sternotomy, or the "clamshell" incision. These procedures have almost no mortality and minimal morbidity. Patients with bilateral metastases may be safely explored with either a median sternotomy or staged bilateral thoracotomies, as noted by Johnston (1983) and Roth and associates (1986). The incisions chosen do not influence patient survival if all metastases are resected; various advantages and disadvantages are unique to each approach (Table 113-2).

Patients with sarcomas and unilateral nodules often have multiple and bilateral metastases discovered during the operation. Bilateral metastases may occur in 38 to 60% of patients with preoperative unilateral sarcomatous metastasis. Postresection survival after median sternotomy or bilateral staged thoracotomies and complete resection is similar.

A median sternotomy is most frequently performed for the initial exploration and resection in patients with unilateral or bilateral nodules and in patients with pulmonary metastases from osteogenic or soft tissue sarcomas. It should be considered the procedure of choice in patients with suspected bilateral metastases from any primary neoplasm in which wedge resections may be required. An exploration for unilateral or bilateral nodules as well as resection of these nodules may be accomplished through a median sternotomy incision. Before surgery, the patient is examined thoroughly for the extent of metastases and to see if an operation can be safely performed. Standard radiographic and physiologic studies are requested and reviewed. In the operating room, the chest radiographs and chest CT scans are displayed prominently. After bronchoscopy, a double-lumen endotracheal tube is placed. A median sternotomy incision is used, and sequential deflation of each lung aids in exposure and palpation of the pulmonary nodules. All nodules are resected with a margin of normal tissue. Nodules should not be "shelled out" as viable tumor cells remain on the periphery of the resected area. Often the decision of adequacy of margin is the surgeon's alone because lung parenchyma may become distorted around the nodule after resection, thereby giving the illusion of a positive or close margin. Mediastinal lymph node metastases rarely occur from pulmonary metastases, as I and my colleagues (1984) and Udelsman and coworkers (1986) showed.

Laser-assisted pulmonary resection, described by Kodama (1991), Branscheid (1992), Miyamoto (1992), and Landreneau (1991) and their associates, using the neo-

Table 113-2. Advantages and Disadvantages of Various Surgical Resections

Procedure	Advantages	Disadvantages
Median sternotomy	Bilateral thoracic explorations with one incision Less patient discomfort	Resection of lesions posterior and medial (near the hila) may be difficult Difficult exposure to the left lower lobe in patients with obesity, congestive heart failure, or chronic obstructive pulmonary disease (increased thoracic anteroposterior diameter)
Transverse sternotomy or clamshell sternotomy	Bilateral thoracic explorations with one incision Good exposure to all aspects of both right and left thoraces Access to both right and left hila and to left lower lobe	Larger incision Patient discomfort
Posterolateral thoracotomy	"Standard" approach Excellent exposure of the hemithorax	Patient discomfort Only one hemithorax may be explored per operation A second operation is needed for bilateral metastases Unable to fully evaluate metastases in the lung parenchyma Chest wall recurrences
Video-assisted thoracic surgery	Potentially less immunosuppressive Excellent visualization Minimal morbidity and discomfort Excellent exposure for visceral pleural metastases May identify unresectable metastases, pleural studding, etc.	Does not identify occult nodules

XVI. Other Tumors of the Lung

dymium:yttrium-aluminum garnet laser may provide a better means of resecting pulmonary metastases than the surgical stapler. Disadvantages of laser resection may include longer operating time and potential for prolonged postoperative air leaks; however, use of the laser may enhance preservation of lung parenchyma with less distortion. Bovie electrocautery may also spare lung parenchyma by removing the metastases with minimal distortion of remaining lung. Air leaks, if they occur, can be sealed by oversewing the parenchymal defect or the use of fibrin glue.

Median Sternotomy and Clamshell Incision

The patient is positioned supine with the entire anterior thorax exposed from the neck to the umbilicus and laterally to each anterior axillary line. The sternum is divided. The pulmonary ligament is divided on each side to mobilize the lung completely. The lungs are sequentially deflated and palpated. Metastases are identified and resected, and then the deflated lung is reinflated. The deflated right lung may be brought completely into the field, attached by only the hilar structures. Exposure of the left lower lobe may be more difficult than exposure of the other lobes because of the overlying heart. With appropriate gentle traction on the pericardium, the left lower lobe can be exposed quite readily and brought into the operative field. Various techniques to better visualize the lung may be used, such as surgical packs behind the hilum of the deflated lung to elevate the parenchyma or an internal mammary artery retractor to expose basilar tumors or posterior hilar left lower lobe masses.

The clamshell incision, as described by Bains (1998) and coworkers (1994) is a modification of the median sternotomy incision. Originally, this approach developed from the early days of cardiac surgery and was later rediscovered for access to enhance bilateral sequential single lung transplantation. A curvilinear incision is made under the breasts or pectoral muscles, and the pectoral muscles are mobilized (Fig. 113-2A). The pectoral muscles are elevated to gain access to the fourth intercostal space bilaterally, whereupon the chest is entered and the incision carried to the sternum bilaterally. The most lateral aspect of the incision may curve superiorly toward the axilla (Fig. 113-2B). The sternum is divided transversely at the level of the fourth intercostal space with a Gigli or oscillating saw. After placement of a chest retractor for both the right and left thorax, the chest is opened, giving excellent exposure to right and left thorax, hilum, and mediastinum. Advantages of this approach include better exposure of the left hilum posteriorly and the left lower lobe. Disadvantages include a large, painful incision and some difficulty with sternal reconstruction and stabilization.

Posterolateral Thoracotomy

The posterolateral thoracotomy is a familiar and standard approach to pulmonary resection for carcinoma of the lung, although Urschel and Razzuk (1986) have advocated

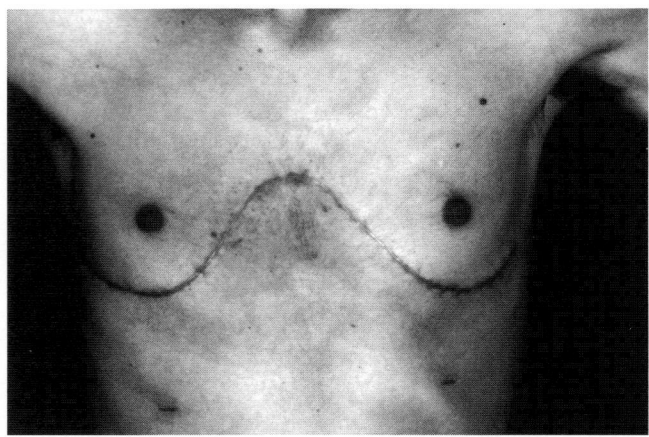

A

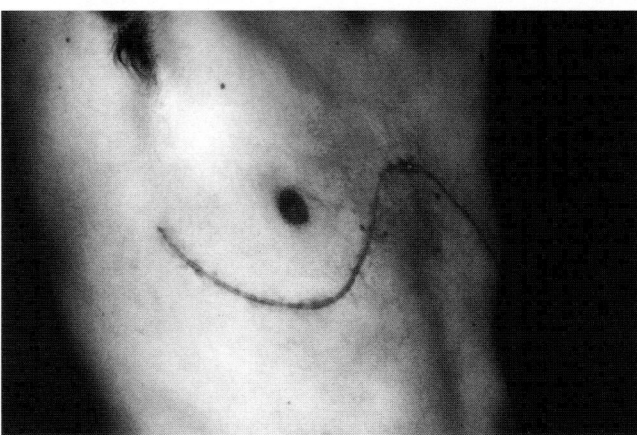

B

Fig. 113-2. A. Transverse sternotomy or clamshell sternotomy. The incision shown begins at the inferior-lateral aspect of the pectoral major and travels superiorly and medially to allow transverse division of the sternum in the fourth intercostal space. The pectoral major muscle is detached from its inferior and medial attachments and lifted up with overlying skin and soft tissue. This maneuver exposes the underlying chest wall. To close the wound, pericostal stitches are placed, pectoralis major muscles are reattached, and subcutaneous tissues and skin are closed. **B.** Oblique view of transverse sternotomy. To gain additional exposure by opening the chest wider, it is helpful to curve the incision up toward the axilla.

median sternotomy for resection of lung carcinoma. Posterolateral thoracotomy may provide better exposure for metastases located posteriorly near the hilum on the left side. In addition, for patients with bulky metastases, a posterolateral thoracotomy provides good access for faster resection and optimal sparing of lung parenchyma. The surgeon is limited to operating in one hemithorax. Bilateral thoracotomies are rarely performed in the same patient at the same operation, although left thoracotomy after median sternotomy may be performed safely in selected patients.

Video-Assisted Thoracic Surgery

Video-assisted thoracoscopic resection using high-resolution video imaging may be helpful for diagnosis, staging, and resection of metastases, as suggested by Kodama (1991), Miller (1992), and Amos (1997) and their colleagues. Its usefulness is limited, however, because metastases can be identified only on the surface of the lung or the outer 10 to 20%, depending on size. Metastases within the lung parenchyma may be undetectable with this technique. Landreneau and associates (1992) have described minimal morbidity and no mortality in 61 patients who underwent 85 thoracoscopic pulmonary resections. Lesions were small (<3 cm) and in the outer one-third of the lung parenchyma. Metastases in 18 patients were resected via thoracoscopy in this series. Video-assisted thoracic surgery (VATS) was the only procedure performed in these patients.

The limitations of thoracoscopy continue to evolve as more experience with the technique is obtained and prospective studies mature. Thoracoscopy may readily be used for diagnosis of metastatic disease, as stated by McCormack

and coworkers (1993), but its use in treatment of metastatic disease is more controversial. In an elegant study, McCormack and colleagues (1996) prospectively evaluated VATS resection for treatment of pulmonary metastases. Patients were screened with CT, and VATS was performed on all patients. Under the same anesthetic, thoracotomy or median sternotomy was performed. The authors found more nodules by thoracotomy and noted that VATS did not identify all nodules. Limitations of the study were the inclusion of patients with multiple metastases or prior sarcoma histology and screening with older CT scans. VATS is not the standard approach for resection in patients with pulmonary metastases. However, VATS may be considered in highly selected patients with a solitary nodule and nonsarcomatous histology on high-resolution (spiral) chest CT scan. Patients with sarcomatous histology frequently (40 to 60%) have occult metastases, which may be palpated and resected with open

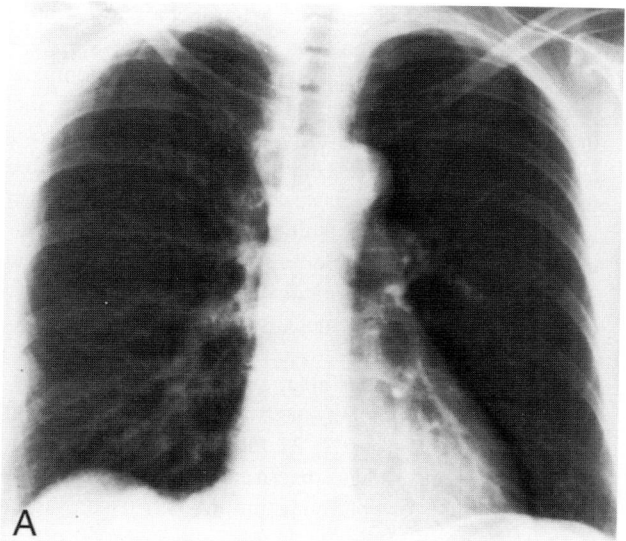
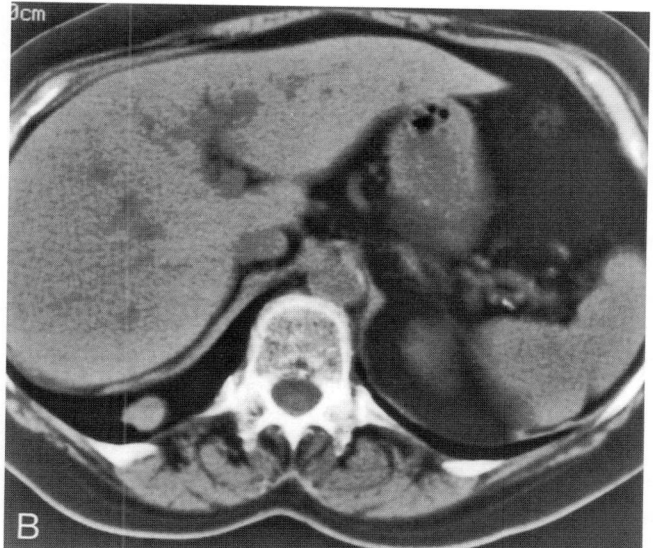
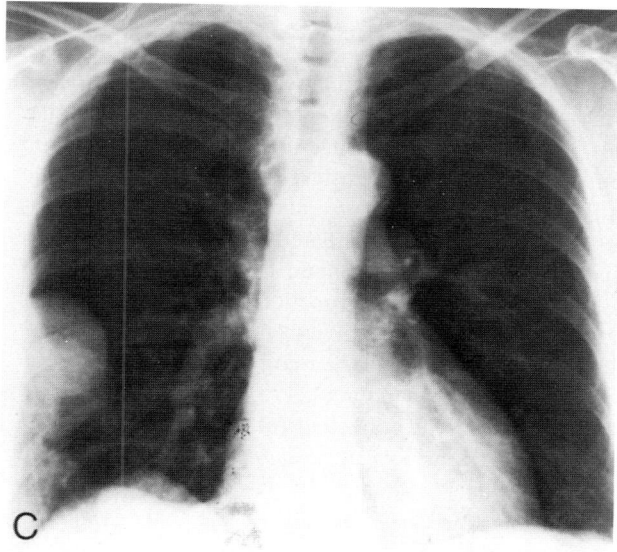

Fig. 113-3. A 61-year-old woman with pleomorphic malignant fibrous histiocytoma of the proximal right femur. **A.** Eight months after resection. A nodule was noted in the periphery of the right lung field. **B.** Computed tomographic scan confirmed the presence of a solitary nodule. Video-assisted thoracic surgery was used to resect the nodule. All parenchymal margins were negative for tumor; the tumor did extend to the pleural surface. **C.** Two months later, multiple metastases were identified.

thoracotomy. In patients with solitary metastasis from solid tumor adenocarcinoma or SCCA, careful consideration must be given to excluding primary lung carcinoma, which would require lobectomy and mediastinal lymph node dissection for optimal care.

At present, VATS can be advocated only for diagnosis or staging of the extent of metastases or in highly selected patients (i.e., those with solitary, nonsarcomatous histology on high-resolution spiral CT scan and peripheral location). Complications of VATS may include not resecting all metastases, positive margins, or pleural seeding with extraction of the metastasis (Fig. 113-3). Follow-up on all patients is necessary at regular intervals because the likelihood of recurrence remains for a period of years.

RESULTS OF RESECTION OF PULMONARY METASTASES

The results of resection for pulmonary metastasectomy require critical analysis of factors that may potentially influence survival. Results should be based on single primary histology (breast, colon, melanoma) or similar histology (e.g., soft tissue sarcomas) and sufficient numbers of patients. Prognostic indicators have been reviewed to assess their influence singularly and in combination on postresection survival in patients with pulmonary metastases and to assist clinically in describing appropriate patients for resection of pulmonary metastases. Age, gender, histology, grade and location of the primary tumor, stage of primary tumor, disease-free survival, number of nodules on preoperative radiologic studies, unilateral or bilateral metastases, tumor doubling time (TDT), and synchronous or metachronous metastases may be evaluated preoperatively. Postoperatively, extent of resection, technique of resection, nodal spread, number of metastases and location, re-resection, postthoracotomy disease-free survival, and overall survival may also be considered in selecting patients for resection of pulmonary metastasis.

In 1997, Pastorino and associates reviewed the long-term results of resection of pulmonary metastasis based on an International Registry of Lung Metastases. This International Registry was established in 1991 based on 5206 patients with pulmonary metastases and treatment collected from Europe, the United States, and Canada. Various clinical characteristics were compared in a retrospective yet consistent and controlled manner. Eighty-eight percent of these patients had complete resection. A solitary metastasis was resected in 2383 patients; multiple lesions were resected in 2726. Epithelial histology predominated (2260 patients), followed by sarcoma (2173), germ cell (363), and melanoma (328). With a median follow-up of 46 months, actuarial survival was 36% at 5 years, 26% at 10 years, and 22% at 15 years. For incomplete resection, actuarial survival was 15% at 5 years. The multivariate analysis showed several favorable prognostic indicators: resectable metas-

tases, germ cell tumors, DFIs of 36 months or greater, and a solitary metastasis. In this international and multiinstitutional study, the overall operative mortality was 1%; mortality was 2.4% after incomplete resections and 0.8% after complete resections.

The most frequently performed operation was unilateral thoracotomy (58% of patients). Bilateral exploration was performed through either bilateral synchronous or staged thoracotomy (11%) or median sternotomy (27%). Thoracoscopy was only performed in 2% of patients. Wedge resections (67%), segmentectomy (9%), lobectomy or bilobectomy (21%), and pneumonectomy (4%) also were performed. Only 26% of patients had four or more metastases. Only 9% had 10 or more metastases, and 3% had 20 or more. Multiple metastases were most commonly resected in sarcomas (64%), germ cell tumors (57%), epithelial tumors (43%), and melanoma (39%). Metastases to the mediastinal lymph nodes were uncommon. Three percent had redo surgery. Fifteen percent had two operations, 4% three operations, and 1% had four or more operations. The maximum number of resections performed on a single patient was seven.

The authors proposed a system by which patients can be grouped into prognostic categories. These would include three parameters: resectability, DFI, and number of metastases. In patients with resectable lesions, a DFI less than 36 months and multiple metastases were found to be independent risk factors. In resectable patients, therefore, three clinically distinct groups could be identified: 1) no risk factors, DFI ≥36 months, single metastasis; 2) one risk factor, DFI <36 months, or multiple metastases; and 3) two risk factors, DFI <36 months, and multiple metastases.

Group 4 consisted of all the unresectable patients. The authors noted that median survival was 61 months for group 1, 34 months for group 2, 24 months for group 3, and 14 months for group 4. The discriminant power of the model was appropriate for epithelial tumors, soft tissue sarcomas, and melanomas.

The value of this International Registry of Lung Metastases lies in its large collection of patient characteristics. These clinically identifiable characteristics may be reexamined and analyzed for various hypotheses. The limitations of such a registry lie in not accounting for variables in the biological behavior of these metastases. This variable behavior may be explained by molecular characteristics on which the clinical characteristics are based. This clinical database will be invaluable in the years ahead as the applicability of molecular characteristics is tested to optimally select patients for therapy for their pulmonary metastasis.

Extended Resection of Pulmonary Metastases

Pneumonectomy or other extended resection of pulmonary metastases may be performed safely in selected patients with associated long-term disease-free survival. Less than 3% of all patients undergoing resection of pulmonary metastases require an extended resection. Pneumonectomy or en bloc resection of pulmonary metastases with chest wall or other thoracic structures, such as diaphragm, pericardium, or superior vena cava, have been performed in a small number of patients with good results, as noted by the author and associates (1993). Nineteen patients had a pneumonectomy, and 19 patients had other extended resection. The 5-year actuarial survival was 25%. Mortality was 5% and occurred in patients having pneumonectomy, often after multiple prior wedge resections for metastases.

Pneumonectomy is rarely performed for resection of pulmonary metastases. In a French study by Spaggiari and colleagues (1999) of 42 patients treated over 10 years, 29 patients underwent pneumonectomy for sarcoma, 12 for carcinoma, and one for a lipoma. Most tumors were centrally located. Two postoperative deaths occurred. Four patients had major complications. Five patients (12%) had recurrences in the residual lung. The median survival was only 6.25 months, and 5-year survival was 16%. Given that the standard surgical mortality for operations for pulmonary metastases is less than 1%, mortality for pneumonectomy should be considered in planning operations for patients with large, centrally located metastases. Although mortality for pneumonectomy for pulmonary metastases corresponds to mortality for other histologies, the 5-year survival of only 16% should prompt strict preoperative selection criteria. The authors suggest that young patients, those with a long DFI, and those with normal carcinoembryonic antigen (CEA) levels (for patients with metastases from colorectal carcinoma) be considered for pneumonectomy for pulmonary metastases.

Koong and coworkers (1999) also examined the value of pneumonectomy by retrospective review of the International Registry of Lung Metastases. Of the 5206 patients who were enrolled, 133 patients (2.6%) had undergone pneumonectomy for pulmonary metastases between 1962 and 1994. Eighty-four percent of these patients underwent complete resection, and 30-day mortality was 3.6%. Five-year survival was 20% with complete resection. For incomplete resection, the perioperative mortality was 19%, and the majority did not survive beyond 5 years. The authors identified favorable prognostic factors of single metastasis, negative mediastinal lymph nodes, and R0 resection. The authors concluded that pneumonectomy may be performed safely with adequate long-term survival.

Intraatrial extension of sarcoma through the pulmonary vein is rare but may be also safely treated with pulmonary resection (pneumonectomy and resection of the tumor from the left atrium). Extracorporeal cardiopulmonary support is required, as noted by Heslin (1998) and Shuman (1984) and their associates.

Osteogenic Sarcoma

Pulmonary metastases from OST may occur in up to 80% of patients who relapse after treatment for their primary neo-plasm, whether or not they receive adjuvant chemotherapy, as described by Goorin (1991) and Al Jilaihawi (1988) and their associates, as well as by Huth and Eilber (1989). Because these metastases are often isolated to the lungs, resection may render a significant number of patients disease free and enhance long-term survival, as described by Meyer and colleagues (1987). Five-year survival may range up to 40%, as shown by Snyder (1991) and Belli (1989) and their coworkers.

Carter (1991), Jaffe (1983), the author (1983), and Rosen (1978) and coworkers have evaluated survival and prognostic factors in patients with pulmonary metastases from OST. In a series from the National Institutes of Health, the author and associates (1983) evaluated 80 patients with OST of the extremity. Forty-three patients developed pulmonary metastases, and 39 patients underwent one or more thoracic explorations for resection of their metastases. Five-year survival was 40%. Various prognostic factors were analyzed. Fewer number of nodules (≤3 nodules), longer DFI, resectable metastases, and the fewer metastases identified and resected were associated with longer postthoracotomy survival. Resection was not possible if more than 16 nodules were identified on preoperative tomograms. A multivariate analysis did not find any combination of factors to be more predictive than the number of nodules identified on preoperative tomograms. In a more recent study, a review of 40 children with OST found that incomplete excision, lack of primary tumor control, and progression and development of metastases during treatment were all negative prognostic factors. Surprisingly, in resectable patients, the number of metastases, DFI, unilateral versus bilateral metastases, preoperative and postoperative adjuvant treatment, and the number of thoracotomies performed were not significant prognostic factors, as described by Heij and colleagues (1994).

Beattie and coworkers (1991) evaluated four long-term survivors who had lived more than 19 years, even after multiple resections for multiple metastases. Surgical resectability was the only predictive factor associated with prolonged survival for recurrent OST. Chemotherapy had no effect on the postthoracotomy survival after complete resection of pulmonary metastases from OST. However, it did prolong the DFI between the surgical treatment of the primary and the appearance of pulmonary metastases. Chemotherapy may prevent or cure micrometastatic disease not amenable to surgery, as stated by Belli and associates (1989).

Soft Tissue Sarcomas

Soft tissue sarcomas comprise a family of nonossifying malignant neoplasms arising from mesenchymal connective tissues. Potter and colleagues (1985) demonstrated that, as with OSTs, local recurrence is common (20%) and metastases are predominantly to lungs. Casson and coworkers (1992) evaluated determinants of 5-year survival in 58 patients who had complete resection and who were followed until death or for a minimum of 5 years. Absolute 5-year survival was 25% (15/58 patients). Favorable prognostic factors included TDT greater than 40 days, unilateral disease, three or fewer nodules identified on preoperative tomograms, two or fewer metastases resected, and tumor histology (median survival 33 months for malignant fibrous histiocytoma vs. 17 months for all others). Using multivariate analysis, number of nodules (≥4) was the most significant prognostic indicator. The addition of tumor histology (malignant fibrous histiocytoma) improved the predictive ability of this model.

In patients with histologically documented pulmonary metastases from soft tissue sarcomas treated at the National Cancer Institute, Jablons (1989) and the author (1984) and associates showed that significant preoperative predictors of enhanced survival included TDT (>20 days), number of metastases on preoperative tomograms (≤4 nodules), and DFI (>12 months). Predictive ability for better survival was improved when all three prognostic factors were combined. These patients represent the patients who will have the best response (i.e., prolonged postresection survival) to pulmonary metastasectomy.

Resection of recurrent pulmonary metastases also improves postresection survival, as shown by Rizzoni and colleagues (1986). Pogrebniak and coworkers (1991) presented 43 patients with two or more resections; in 31 completely resectable patients (72%), median survival was 25 months compared to not completely resectable or unresectable patients, who had a median survival of only 10 months. A longer DFI (≥18 months) was also associated with prolonged disease-free survival. Increased age and female sex were associated with an increased risk of death from disease in resected patients with recurrent pulmonary metastases, in contrast to initial isolated pulmonary metastases. Casson and associates (1991) noted that in 39 patients with recurrent pulmonary metastases from adult soft tissue sarcomas, resectable patients and those with only one metastasis had the best postresection survival. Chemotherapy for metastatic soft tissue sarcoma remains poor. Median survival ranges from 13 to 16 months, as described by Weh (1990) and Elias (1989) and their colleagues, although a multidisciplinary treatment plan of combination chemotherapy, surgery, and additional chemotherapy may provide improved survival over single-modality care, as noted by Rosen and coworkers (1994).

Colorectal Neoplasms

Colorectal metastases commonly spread to local or regional nodes or are trapped in the liver through the portal venous drainage. Patients with prior colorectal neoplasms have had pulmonary metastases resected with prolonged postresection survival. An absolute distinction cannot be made between a single carcinomatous metastasis and a primary bronchial carcinoma except by direct visual comparison of the two. Molecular markers specific for metastases or lung carcinoma may aid in distinguishing metastatic tumor from a primary lung carcinoma.

As with other isolated pulmonary metastases, patients with pulmonary metastases from colorectal carcinoma may be resected safely with low morbidity and mortality and long-term survival. Reports by Murray (1991) and Brister (1988), Roberts (1989), Scheele (1990), Goya (1989), and Mansel (1986) and their associates describe 5-year survival from 21% up to 50% after resection of pulmonary metastases from colon carcinoma. Differences in age, gender, location, grade, and stage of the primary colorectal cancer are not associated with either improved or worsened survival after resection of these metastases. Patients with metachronous liver lesions excised for cure may also be candidates for resection of pulmonary metastases. Sauter and colleagues (1990) evaluated 49 patients with isolated pulmonary metastases (18) and hepatic metastases (31). Patients with pulmonary metastases had a 47% 5-year survival compared to patients with hepatic metastases (5-year survival of 19%). Of 1578 patients treated for colon and rectal cancer and reported by Pihl and coworkers (1987), 117 of 1013 patients with rectal carcinoma (11.5%) and 20 of 565 patients with colon cancer (3.5%) had recurrence in the lungs. In 66 patients who underwent resection of pulmonary metastases from colorectal adenocarcinoma, patients with solitary metastasis had a longer postresection survival than did others, as described by Mansel and associates (1986). Five-year survival was 38% in both studies. In another study of 62 patients by Goya and colleagues (1989), metastases less than 3 cm in diameter were associated with improved survival.

In a large series from the Mayo Clinic, McAfee and associates (1992) presented 139 patients who underwent resection of pulmonary metastases from colorectal carcinoma with an operative mortality of 1.4%. Overall 5-year survival was 30.5%, and the median follow-up was 7 years. Patients with a solitary pulmonary metastasis and those with a preoperative CEA level less than 4.0 ng/mL had better postthoracotomy survival than others. Longer DFI and diameter of metastases of less than 3 cm were not associated with improved survival.

Patients with resection of colon metastases from the lung and the liver have a survival advantage with complete resection, as suggested by Murata (1998) and McCormack (1992) and their coworkers. Robinson and colleagues (1999) noted that in 48 patients with both liver and lung metastasis, 25 patients underwent resection and 23 patients did not. Median survival was longer after resection of the last metastasis (either lung or liver) than in those individuals who did not undergo resection (16 months to 6 months; $P < .001$). They also noted that patients with metachronous resections survived longer than did patients with synchronous resections (70 months median compared to 22 months, $P < .001$). The authors noted that the ideal candidate for resection was less than 50 years of age, had a solitary liver metastasis, and had had a 4-year interval between the colorectal cancer resection and occurrence of the pulmonary metastasis. The worst patients for resection included those aged 70 years or older, those with multiple liver metastases, and those with synchronous disease. In a French study by Regnard and associates (1998), the authors examined 43 patients who had undergone complete resection of hepatic metastasis and then developed pulmonary metastases. The median survival was 19 months, and 5-year survival was estimated to be 11%. Patients with a CEA exceeding 0.5 ng/mL had a significantly lower probability of survival than did those with lower levels [>0.5 ng/mL ($P = .0018$)].

In patients with colorectal metastases to both liver and lung, complete resection is generally associated with improved survival. Whether the liver metastases occur first and then lung metastases, or whether lung metastases occur first and then liver metastases, complete surgical resection tends to be associated with longer survival. Poorer survival is found in patients who cannot be completely resected or who are deemed unresectable without operation. Of the total population of patients with colorectal metastases, those with completely resectable lung and or hepatic metastases represent a small percentage and one with the most favorable "biology" of the tumor. The surgeon can take advantage of this biologically favorable subset of patients. With complete resection of both lung and hepatic metastases, survival may be enhanced.

Breast Carcinoma

Patients with metastases from breast carcinoma usually do poorly because metastases occur in multiple sites. Patanaphan and colleagues (1988) described 145 patients with metastatic breast carcinoma (145/558, or 26%); the major sites of metastases were bone (51%), lung (17%), brain (16%), and liver (6%). Overall median survival was 12 months for patients with lung metastases, who were mostly treated with palliative chemotherapy or irradiation, or both. Lanza and coworkers (1992) noted that in 44 women with a prior history of breast cancer who underwent pulmonary resection for new pulmonary lesions, seven patients were excluded who had benign nodules (n = 3) or unresectable metastases (n = 4). In 37 resectable patients, actuarial 5-year survival was 50% (Fig. 113-4). DFI exceeding 12 months was associated with a longer median survival (82 months) and 5-year survival (57%) compared to patients with a DFI of less than 12 months (15 months median, 0% 5-year survival; $P = .004$). Estrogen receptor–positive status tended to be associated with a longer postthoracotomy survival ($P = .098$). Other favorable prognostic factors included positive receptor status of the primary tumor (improved 3-year survival: 61%) compared to negative receptor status (38% 3-year survival). Resection of solitary metastasis, according to Friedel and associates (1994) provided a 35% 5-year survival compared to 0 for resection of five or more metastases. Simpson and colleagues (1997) noted that favorable selection of patients has enabled survival to increase up to 62% at 5 years.

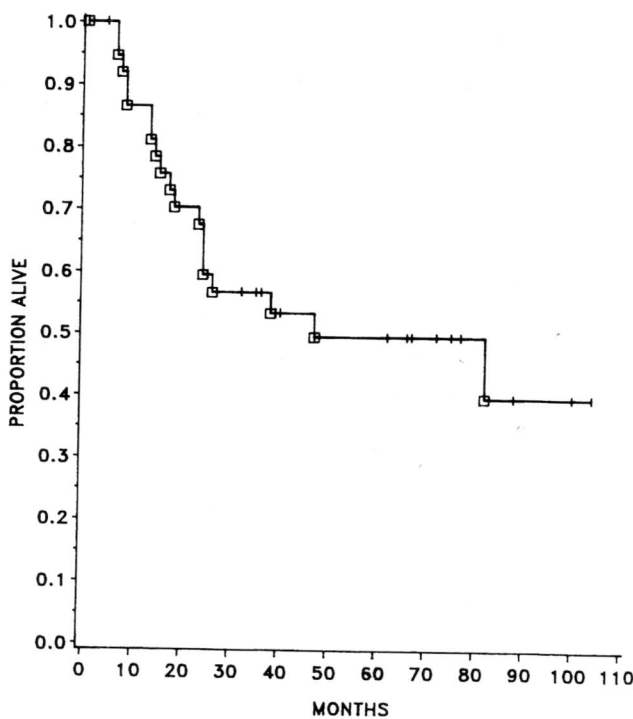

Fig. 113-4. Overall survival of patients with pulmonary metastases from carcinoma of the breast (n = 39). Median survival was 47 months. From Lanza LA, et al: Long-term survival after resection of pulmonary metastases from carcinoma of the breast. Ann Thorac Surg 54:244, 1992. With permission.

Staren and coworkers (1992) evaluated 33 patients treated with surgical resection of pulmonary metastases from breast carcinoma and compared the results to that of 30 patients treated primarily with systemic chemotherapy and hormonal therapy. Patients having complete resection of metastases had a better median survival than did patients with medical therapy, particularly when single nodules were compared (58 months median survival vs. 34 months). Five-year survival in patients treated with some surgical resection was 36%, compared to 11% in patients treated with other than surgical treatment. A review by Bodzin and associates (1998) confirms these findings.

Testicular Neoplasms

Nonseminomatous testicular tumors can be diagnosed by the occurrence of new pulmonary nodules identified on chest radiograph or by CT scan, as described by Lien (1988) and Tesoro-Tess (1987) and their colleagues. Metastatic testicular seminoma most commonly is identified as mediastinal nodal enlargement. CT scan therefore is more accurate in diagnosis of seminomatous metastases than are plain chest radiographs, as suggested by Williams and coworkers (1987).

Cytoreductive surgery for disseminated nonseminomatous germ cell tumors of the testis may be performed after chemotherapy for removal of residual metastatic disease. The response to chemotherapy may be assessed when there is no further reduction in size of the nodules. The majority of patients require retroperitoneal lymph node dissections (69%), although thoracotomies may be required in 18% of patients. Kulkarni (1991), Van Schil (1989), and Carsky (1992) and their associates evaluated 80 patients with germ cell tumors and lung metastases treated with chemotherapy and subsequent surgery. In this series, 35% (n = 28) achieved complete response after chemotherapy, 36 patients with partial response underwent surgery for resection of metastases in the abdomen (n = 17), the lungs (n = 15), or both (n = 4); 27 of 36 patients achieved complete response after both chemotherapy and surgery. Carter and colleagues (1987) noted that extensive pulmonary metastases (unresectable metastases) are a predictor of ultimate treatment failure.

Liu and colleagues (1998) evaluated the role of pulmonary metastasectomy for testicular germ cell tumors over a 28-year period. The typical patient was young (median age 27 years) and complete resection was generally possible. Most of these patients had already undergone chemotherapy. Viable metastasis was present in 44% of the patients; 25% had metastasis to other sites after resection of their pulmonary metastasis. Overall 5-year survival was 68%, and for the patients diagnosed after 1985, the survival was 82%. The authors noted that extrathoracic metastasis (nonpulmonary visceral sites) as well as the presence of viable tumor in the resected specimens were adverse prognostic indicators. Preoperative tumor markers were normal in majority of the patients, and patients with multiple metastases predominated. About one-half the patients had synchronous presentation of their metastases, and 66% of patients had no viable tumor. Mature teratoma and fibrosis or necrosis were equally represented. Patients with metastases outside the pulmonary parenchyma, elevated tumor markers, and a viable tumor had a worse prognosis. Parenchymal resection not only removed all identifiable disease but also provided a measure of the effectiveness of their chemotherapy treatment.

Schnorrer and coworkers (1996) described 28 patients with pulmonary metastases from germ cell or testicular neoplasms who were treated with bleomycin, etoposide, and cisplatin. An overall complete response was achieved in 21 patients (75%); in 11 of them, a complete response was achieved after chemotherapy alone. Resection of residual mass was necessary in 12 patients with normalized serum markers. Resection of the residual mass was recommended for histology and may modify subsequent treatment. The overall cure rate was 89.3%.

Gynecologic Neoplasms

Fuller and colleagues (1985) from the Massachusetts General Hospital reviewed a 40-year experience of treating 15 patients with pulmonary metastases from gynecologic cancer. Six patients had primary tumors involving the cervix;

the remainder had primary tumors of the endometrium (three patients), ovary (two patients), uterine sarcomas (two patients), and choriocarcinomas (two patients). Five-year survival was 36%. Lesions less than 4 cm in diameter and a DFI exceeding 36 months were associated with prolonged survival. Levenback and coworkers (1992) reviewed 45 patients with pulmonary metastases from uterine sarcomas. Most patients (71%) had unilateral lesions, and 51% had only one lesion. Five-year survival was 43%. Unilateral metastases or fewer numbers of metastases were not significantly associated with prolonged survival.

Kumar and colleagues (1988) reviewed 97 patients with metastatic gestational trophoblastic disease; chemotherapy was the treatment of choice. Selective thoracotomy in patients with solitary lung metastases reduced the treatment time and need for further aggressive chemotherapy. Overall 2-year survival after diagnosis was 65%. A DFI less than 1 year was associated with poorer survival.

Barter and associates (1990) studied 2,116 patients with primary cervical malignancy between 1969 and 1984 and found 88 patients (88/2116, or 4.16%) with pulmonary lesions consistent with metastases. Prognosis was poor with chemotherapy only (median survival 8 months), and only 2 of 88 were long-term survivors. Imachi and colleagues (1989) identified 50 patients out of 817 patients (6.1%) treated for carcinoma of the uterine cervix who developed pulmonary metastases; 81% of these patients had local recurrence or other metastases, and chemotherapy was given. The authors suggest that surgery may be considered for patients with pulmonary metastases without extrathoracic metastases.

Resection of pulmonary metastases from SCCA of the uterine cervix has also been described by Fuller (1985) and Seki (1992) and their coinvestigators.

Renal Cell Carcinoma

Various series have examined the value of resection of pulmonary metastases from renal cell carcinoma. Five-year survival has ranged from 21%, as noted by Dernevik and coworkers (1985), to 60%, as found by Pogrebniak and associates (1992). Schott and colleagues (1988) reported 39 patients with pulmonary metastases after nephrectomy for renal carcinoma in 938 patients (38/938, or 4.1%). Patients with pulmonary metastases less than 2 cm in diameter and limited to one site had prolonged survival and DFI compared to other patients. Dernevik and colleagues (1985) resected 33 patients for pulmonary metastases, with a minimum follow-up period of 5 years or until death. Longer DFI (>1 year) was better than a shorter DFI (<1 year). Pogrebniak and associates (1992) from the National Cancer Institute reported 23 patients who underwent resection of pulmonary metastases from renal cell carcinoma, of which 18 had previous interleukin-2–based immunotherapy. Resectable patients (15/23, or 65%) had a longer survival (mean 49 months; median not yet reached) than did unresectable patients (median 16 months, $P = .02$). Postresection survival did not depend on the number of nodules seen on CT, resected nodules, or the DFI. Five-year survival after complete resection was 44% in one study of 50 patients undergoing resection of metastases from renal cell carcinoma. Twelve patients had repeat resection, achieving a 42% 5-year survival rate after second resection. Complete resection was the most important factor associated with 5-year survival, as described by Fourquier and associates (1997).

Melanoma

The overall biological behavior of melanoma cannot be predicted. Most commonly, pulmonary metastases occur in addition to other visceral sites, and overall long-term survival is poor. Immunotherapy has been used with some favorable results. In the rare patient who presents with isolated pulmonary metastases, resection may be associated with long-term survival, as noted by Ollila and Morton (1998). Current 5-year survival ranges from 4.5 to 25%. In a large series of 1521 patients with American Joint Committee on Cancer stage IV melanoma, 5-year survival was only 4% (median survival 8.3 months), as described by Barth (1995) and Pogrebniak (1988) and their coworkers.

Gorenstein and colleagues (1991) evaluated 56 patients with histologically proved pulmonary metastases from melanoma. The overall postresection survival was 25% at 5 years (Fig. 113-5). Patients with earlier primary stage melanoma and patients with metastases to the lungs as the first site of metastases had longer postresection survival than did other patients. Neither location of the primary tumor, histology, thickness, Clark level, nodal metastases, metastasis doubling time, nor type of resection of the primary tumor was associated with improved postresection survival.

Harpole and associates (1992) evaluated pulmonary metastases in 945 patients with melanoma in a population of 7564 melanoma patients. Bilateral as well as multiple metastases were present in the majority of these patients. Multivariate predictors of survival included complete resection, DFI, chemotherapy, two or fewer metastases, negative lymph nodes, and histologic type. Five-year survival for all 7564 patients was 4%, in contrast to 20% 5-year survival in patients with resection of pulmonary metastases.

Squamous Cell Carcinoma

Patients with primary SCCA outside the lungs frequently have metastases to the lungs. These secondary lung neoplasms may be resected with subsequent survival benefit, as emphasized by Nibu and colleagues (1997). With solitary pulmonary lesions after treatment of primary SCCA elsewhere in the body, the origin of the lesion is uncertain. The lesion may represent a solitary metastasis, a primary bronchial carcinoma, or a benign process. The recommended treatment for such a solitary lesion is bronchoscopy, thoracic exploration, and excisional biopsy. If an SCCA is identified, a lobectomy and mediastinal lymph node dissection should be performed, as treatment would be if the lesion were a second primary neoplasm. Less desirous would be a generous wedge excision and mediastinal lymph node dissection because local control may be limited.

Finley and coworkers (1992) described factors associated with improved survival in patients with SCCA metastases

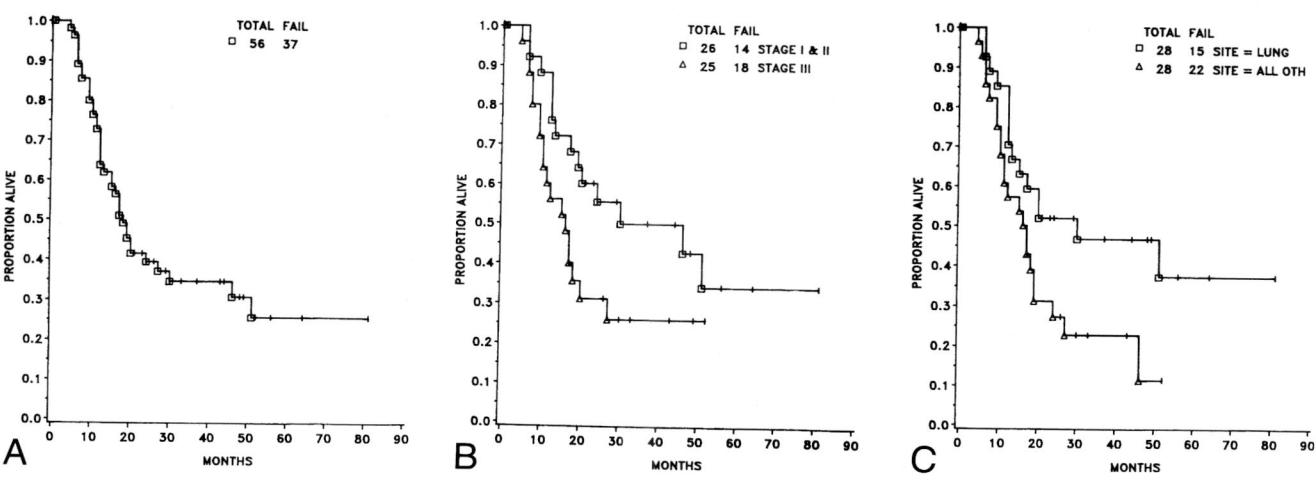

Fig. 113-5. Survival after resection of pulmonary metastases from melanoma. **A.** Five-year survival was 25%, median survival 18 months. **B.** Patients with early-stage melanoma (stage I, II) had median survival of 30 months compared to 16 months with later-stage melanoma (stage III) ($P = .04$). **C.** Patients with the lung as the site of first recurrence had a median survival of 30 months versus 17 months for all other patients ($P = .03$). From Gorenstein LA, et al: Improved survival after resection of pulmonary metastases from malignant melanoma. Ann Thorac Surg *52*:204, 1991. With permission.

from head and neck cancers. These included complete resection, control of primary, early stage of head and neck primary, one nodule on chest radiograph, and longer DFI (>2 years) from primary resection. Complete resection of all malignant disease was associated with 5-year survival of 29%. The number of nodules was not significantly associated with survival. In eight patients with more than one nodule, median survival was 2 years, and there were no 5-year survivors. Therefore, the benefits of resection of multiple pulmonary metastases from head and neck primary SCCA are not completely clear. In another study of 44 patients, 5-year survival after pulmonary resection was 43%. Mazer and associates (1988) noted that single nodules, primary tumor stage, or absence of locoregional recurrence were not associated with enhanced survival. The presence of mediastinal disease was associated with the worst outcome.

Lefor and colleagues (1986) attempted to correlate primary carcinomas of the head and neck with subsequent development of pulmonary metastases or second primary lung carcinomas. They used an algorithm that considered the DFI, histology, radiographic findings, and characteristics of the lung lesion as well as the identification of mediastinal lymphadenopathy. The authors recommended that indeterminate lesions be treated as primary lung carcinomas (e.g., lobectomy and mediastinal lymph node dissection) because this provides best local control of the disease as well as the potential for cure.

Childhood Tumors

Primary tumors of childhood, such as hepatoma, neuroblastoma, hepatoblastoma, Ewing's sarcoma, and rhabdomyosarcoma, commonly spread to the lungs; however, other sites of metastasis are frequent, with the exception of OST. Chemotherapy remains the major treatment modality for metastases in multiple sites. Pulmonary resection for metastases may be required to document metastases in the lungs, to assess the tumor's response to chemotherapy or the viability of the remaining tumor, or to enhance postresection survival in these children with resectable metastases.

Wilms' Tumor

Patients with Wilms' tumor may present with pulmonary metastases at diagnosis or relapse after initial treatment, as noted by Macklis and colleagues (1991). Early diagnosis using CT may identify metastases in up to 36% of patients, as shown by Wilimas and coworkers (1988). Pulmonary metastases may be resected safely from children with Wilms' tumor, as emphasized by de Kraker and associates (1990) and Di Lorenzo and Collin (1988). In contrast, Green and colleagues (1991) described 211 patients entered in one of the three National Wilms' Tumor Studies whose initial relapse was in the lungs and who showed no survival advantage to resection of pulmonary metastases over treatment with chemotherapy and whole-lung irradiation.

Ewing's Sarcoma

Ewing's sarcoma metastasizes preferentially to the lungs in children and may be resected. Lanza and coworkers (1987) examined patients with resectable pulmonary metastases from Ewing's sarcoma. These patients had prolonged survival (actuarial 5-year survival 15%, median 28 months) compared to patients who were explored but found to have unresectable metastases (no survivors beyond 22 months, median survival 12 months; $P = .0047$). Patients with four nodules or fewer had better survival than patients with more than four nodules. Lung irradiation may aid in prolonging survival, according to Dunst and associates (1993). In the European Intergroup Cooperative Ewing's Sarcoma Studies, 114 patients with Ewing's sarcoma underwent perioperative chemotherapy and local treatment for the primary tumor. Whole-lung radiation (15 to 18 Gy) was given to 75 patients; 63% of first relapses involved the lung. Adverse risk factors included poor chemotherapy response of the primary tumor, bilateral metastases, and no lung irradiation, as reported by Paulussen and colleagues (1998a, 1998b).

Osteogenic Sarcoma

OST metastasizes preferentially to the lungs. Resection of pulmonary metastases from OST is associated with prolonged postresection survival, as noted by La Quaglia (1998) and Bacci (1997), Beattie (1991), Goorin (1991), Pastorino (1991), and Snyder (1991) and their coworkers. Adjuvant therapy, such as chemotherapy, as proposed by Yamaguchi (1988) and Al Jilaihawi (1988) and their associates, or lung irradiation, as proposed by Burgers (1988) and Zaharia (1986) and their associates, may also be valuable, particularly for micrometastases. Snyder and coworkers (1991) suggested that postresection survival may be as high as 39% at 5 years. La Quaglia (1998) found that 80% of patients without distant metastases at presentation had long-term survival with treatment including chemotherapy compared to only 20% before 1970. For long-term survival, it is necessary to completely resect both the primary and metastatic disease.

Recurrent Pulmonary Metastases

If pulmonary metastases recur in the lungs, Groeger and associates (1997) note that resection can again be accomplished safely, with prolonged postthoracotomy survival. Patients are screened by the criteria presented in Table 113-1. Patients with pulmonary metastases may undergo multiple procedures for re-resection of metastases with prolonged survival after complete resection. In one report by Kandioler and colleagues (1998) of 396 operations in 330 patients, the authors identified a subgroup of 35 patients who had undergone reoperation for pulmonary metastasis. In this group, 5- and 10-year survival rates were 48% and 28%, respectively. The favorable prognostic factors included a DFI greater than 1 year. There was no survival advantage associated with histology, whether epithelial carcinoma, osteosarcoma, or soft tissue sarcoma. In this patient population, successful repeat surgical resection of pulmonary metastasis and survival advantage are probably related to a favorable biological behavior. The specific criteria for this favorable behavior are not yet known.

Several studies have reviewed results of multiple resections for recurrent pulmonary metastases. Rizzoni and associates (1986) described 29 patients with recurrent pulmonary metastases from soft tissue sarcomas with two or more resections of pulmonary metastases. Patients with favorable tumor biology (resectable metastases, longer TDT, ≤3 nodules, and DFI >6 months) had longer survival. There was no operative mortality, and complications occurred in only 7.5%. Median survival was 14.5 months, and overall 5-year survival was 22%. Resectable patients had a median survival of 24 months. Casson and colleagues (1991) confirmed these findings in 39 patients with adult soft tissue sarcomas. Thirty-four patients were resectable (median survival 28 months; 5-year survival approximately 32%). Unresectable patients had a median survival of 7 months. Median survival after resection of a solitary recurrent metastasis was 65 months compared to patients with two or more nodules (14 months median; $P = .01$).

Repeat resection of pulmonary metastasis may salvage a subset of pediatric patients with sarcomatous histologies. These pediatric sarcomas include OST, nonrhabdomyosarcoma soft tissue sarcoma, and Ewing's sarcoma. At the National Cancer Institute, Temeck and coworkers (1999) described 70 patients who underwent at least one reoperation between 1965 and 1995. Osteosarcoma predominated, with 36 patients. Single-wedge resection was the most common operation performed (84%). The authors noted that complete resection was the most important and favorable prognostic factor: Patients with complete resection had improved survival compared to those who were incompletely resected. Median survival was 2.25 years. In resectable patients, median survival was 5.6 years compared to 0.7 year in unresectable patients ($P < .0001$). From this review, the authors concluded that an aggressive surgical approach in patients with small numbers of lesions, longer DFI, and the ability to obtain a complete resection is warranted and is associated with prolonged survival.

Metastasis or Primary Bronchial Carcinoma

Pulmonary metastases from sarcomas or other distinctive nonpulmonary neoplasms are easy to diagnose. Solitary carcinomatous metastasis from breast or colon and SCCA metastasis from head and neck primary tumors are difficult to distinguish from primary lung carcinoma. Patients with

two or more pulmonary nodules can be considered to have metastases. Treatment may be similar. In tumors without a propensity for bilaterality (e.g., nonsarcomatous histology), a solitary pulmonary nodule may be approached through a lateral thoracotomy incision. A generous wedge excision or lobectomy and mediastinal lymph node dissection should be performed. The final pathology may suggest histology amenable to adjuvant therapy.

Traditionally, a comparison of the primary neoplasm and the lung nodule using light microscopy has been the only method for determining origin of the lung nodule or neoplasm. Electron microscopy, as studied by Herrera and associates (1985), or specific molecular or genetic characteristics may identify more precisely the origin of these neoplasms. Monoclonal antibodies may assist in discriminating between primary bronchial adenocarcinoma and colon carcinoma metastatic to the lung, as described by Ghoneim and colleagues (1990). Amplified K-ras oncogene expression in a pulmonary metastasis from colon adenocarcinoma primary was noted by Slebos and coworkers (1991) and was also present in the primary tumor. A monoclonal antibody to identify colorectal carcinoma in 46 patients has been used by Flint and Lloyd (1992). Cytology samples from patients with metastatic colon carcinoma and primary lung adenocarcinoma were examined. The monoclonal antibody was not sufficient to discriminate primary lung cancer from metastatic adenocarcinoma. Flow cytometry and DNA analysis have been used by Nomori (1991), Sauter (1990), and Salvati (1989) and their colleagues to describe primary carcinomas of the lung and to distinguish them from metastases. Lefor and coworkers (1986) developed algorithms for patients with SCCAs of the head and neck who developed pulmonary nodules after treatment. Characteristics of metastases and of primary lung carcinoma were examined in an attempt to better direct subsequent therapy.

SURVIVAL ANALYSIS

Survival may be absolute or actuarial and is usually calculated from the time the surgical procedure is performed until death or until the date of last follow-up, as noted by Toledano and Olak (1998). For example, patients followed for a minimum of 5 years (survivors) or until death provide an absolute 5-year survival rate (patients alive/all patients studied); patients followed for varying periods of time (i.e., 2 to 7 years) may be evaluated by using an actuarial survival curve. Actuarial survival and disease-free survival may be estimated using the method of Kaplan and Meier (1958). Patients grouped into two or more populations are defined as meeting or not meeting objective criteria and compared to evaluate differences in survival. Univariate analysis (comparisons between groups) may be made using the generalized Wilcoxon test of Gehan (1965) or log-rank test; if sample sizes are small, Thomas's exact text (1975) may be used. Cox's proportional hazards model (1972) is used to determine the relative effect of various prognostic indicators on survival. Univariate analysis identifies the most important prognostic indicators. Multivariate analysis evaluates the predictive ability of two or more prognostic indicators to provide additional prognostic value.

PROGNOSTIC INDICATORS

Predictors for improved survival have been studied retrospectively for various tumor types to identify selected patients who will benefit from pulmonary metastasectomy. These prognostic indicators are clinical, biological, and molecular criteria that describe the biological interaction between the metastases and the patient and their association with prolonged survival. These prognostic indicators may be used to identify patients who are most likely to benefit from resection of pulmonary metastases.

Analysis of prognostic indicators in groups of patients with pulmonary metastases from heterogeneous tumors describes prolonged survival in patients with resectable metastases. Resectable patients, longer DFI, longer TDT, fewer numbers of metastases, or solitary metastasis are prognostic indicators generally associated with prolonged postresection survival. Prognostic indicators should be studied in patients with the same primary tumor to define their association with postresection survival. A wide variability exists in the characteristics of pulmonary metastases from different primary neoplasms and the subsequent survival of patients with these metastases. The study of prognostic indicators from the same primary neoplasm yields the most precise information on association with postresection survival. Age or gender do not usually influence postthoracotomy survival and generally should not be considered prognostic factors.

Location and Stage of Primary Tumor

Postresection survival is not usually influenced by the specific anatomic location of the primary tumor. Postresection survival in patients with more advanced primary neoplasms does not usually differ from patients with earlier-stage disease. Still, initial or primary stage may suggest the biological aggressiveness of the tumor. Schlappack and associates (1988) found that a negative nodal status predicted improved postresection survival for patients with breast cancer. McCormack and Attiyeh (1979) found better postthoracotomy survival in patients with Dukes' stage A colorectal carcinoma (5-year survival 37.5%) compared to patients with Dukes' stage C tumor (5-year survival 15%), although this was not confirmed in the recent study by McAfee and colleagues (1992).

Disease-Free Interval

The initial DFI extends from resection of the primary tumor until pulmonary metastases or other metastases are detected. A short DFI may indicate a more virulent tumor with a poor prognosis. Metastases may be multiple and grow rapidly. A longer DFI may represent a less biologically aggressive tumor and correlates with a longer postresection survival. The DFI may also be defined as the time between resection of the pulmonary metastases and recurrence of metastases in the lungs or elsewhere. DFIs of greater than 12 months are usually associated with improved survival in patients with breast carcinoma, as noted by Schlappack and coworkers (1988). Brister (1988) and Mansel (1986) and their associates found the same to be true in colorectal carcinoma, as did Pastorino and colleagues (1988) for OST, Roth (1985) and the author (1984) and coinvestigators for soft tissue sarcomas, and Jett and coworkers (1983) for renal cell carcinoma. A DFI longer than 36 months was an independent predictor of survival in the International Registry of Lung Metastases, as shown by Pastorino and colleagues (1997).

Number of Nodules on Preoperative Radiographic Studies

High-resolution CT has replaced linear tomograms as the examination of choice in patients with suspected pulmonary metastases. CT of the chest provides a sensitive and specific study for patients with pulmonary metastases. CT of the chest is quite sensitive but less specific than conventional linear tomography or chest radiograph. Nodules may or may not represent metastases. Theoretically, earlier detection and treatment of metastases could improve survival. Laterality (unilateral or bilateral) of pulmonary metastases does not directly influence postresection survival; the number of nodules is a more precise prognostic indicator.

Number of Metastases Resected

Nodules on preoperative chest radiographic studies usually correspond to the number of metastases present; however, not all nodules are malignant, as noted by Pogrebniak and associates (1988). Usually, fewer pulmonary metastases at the time of resection means better postresection survival. Postresection survival after complete resection of pulmonary metastases has been examined in patients with pulmonary metastases from multiple histologies to evaluate the influence of number of metastases resected.

Tumor Doubling Time

TDT is based on original observations by Collins and coworkers (1956), as calculated by Joseph and colleagues (1971a, 1971b), and has been analyzed for multiple tumor types. TDT is calculated by measuring the same metastasis on similar studies (e.g., serial chest radiographs), which are separated by a minimum of 10 to 14 days. The most rapidly growing nodule is selected. The TDT can be easily calculated by plotting changing diameters of pulmonary metastases on semilogarithmic paper; however, graphical error may be present. A mathematical formula may be used to precisely calculate TDT:

$$TDT = \frac{time^a \times 0.231}{\ln^b (second\ diameter \div first\ diameter)}$$

[a]time is the difference in days between the first diameter measurement and the second diameter measurement
[b]natural logarithm

Example: If, on the basis of a chest radiograph, a nodule grows from 1.0 to 1.5 cm in diameter in 22 days, what is the TDT?

$$TDT = \frac{22\ days \times 0.231}{\ln (1.5\ cm/1.0\ cm)} = \frac{5.082}{0.405} = 12.5\ days$$

Errors may occur in the calculation of TDT. All metastases do not grow at the same rate. In general, homogeneous metastases from the same primary neoplasm may grow at similar rates. Different growth rates between tumor nodules may reflect heterogeneity of metastases from the primary. The TDT may indirectly reveal the underlying biological nature of the metastases and, as such, influence the patient's postresection survival.

Pulmonary metastases initially grow exponentially, and with increased size, the growth rate diminishes. Gompertz (1825) described growth kinetics [expanded by Laird (1960)], which considered a gradual diminution in TDT with time and increased size of the metastasis. Whether the growth rate is linear, exponential, or "gompertzian" may be difficult to evaluate because a chest radiograph shows a three-dimensional structure in two dimensions. In addition, the growth rate measured over a few weeks represents only a brief period in the lifetime of the metastasis. Although this growth rate is presumed to be linear, it may not always be linear, and TDT only reflects growth during the interval measured. Rooser and associates (1987) suggest that differences in tumor growth rates may be explained in part by tumor cell polyclonality.

Resectability

Complete resection consistently correlates with improved postthoracotomy survival for patients with pulmonary metastases. If pulmonary metastases cannot be completely removed, the postthoracotomy survival is shortened for patients with most tumors compared to those who were completely resected.

Endobronchial or Nodal Metastases

Involvement of mediastinal lymph nodes from pulmonary metastases is rare. Udelsman and colleagues (1986) noted that patients with endobronchial metastases from adult soft tissue sarcomas have a short postresection survival. Seven of 11 patients with endobronchial metastases lived 6 months or less. Jablons and coworkers (1989) found that survival is poor (5 months) in patients with mediastinal lymph node involvement from soft tissue sarcomas compared to patients without nodal metastases (31 months).

Multivariate Analysis of Prognostic Factors

Use of multivariate analysis may allow more accurate prediction of postresection survival and allow better patient selection. Separate prognostic variables may be combined to enhance the predictive value for survival. Jablons and associates (1989) found the DFI, gender, resectability, and truncal location in patients with pulmonary metastases from soft tissue sarcomas to be the best predictor of postthoracotomy survival. The author and colleagues (1984) noted that DFI greater than 12 months, TDT greater than 20 days, and four nodules or fewer on preoperative full lung tomograms as a multivariate prognostic indicator was the best predictor of postthoracotomy survival in patients with pulmonary metastases from soft tissue sarcomas. Roth and coworkers (1985) compared prognostic indicators in patients with OST and soft tissue sarcoma. The TDT, number of metastases on preoperative full lung tomograms, and DFI when combined improved predictive ability over any single indicator or pair of indicators.

NOVEL TREATMENT STRATEGIES

Molecular Events

Molecular events associated with pulmonary metastases have been identified in patients with OST. Amplification of the *MDM2* gene (the human homologue of a murine p53 binding protein) may regulate p53 protein function by inactivating the protein and deregulating or enhancing tumor growth. In one study, Ladanyi and associates (1993) noted no detectable *MDM2* gene amplification in primary OST compared to 14% of metastases (three pulmonary metastases, one local metastasis). Amplification of *MDM2* may be associated with metastases and tumor progression in OST.

Pollock and colleagues (1998) noted that in soft tissue sarcomas, alterations (mutations of the *p53* gene, a tumor-suppressor gene) may provide for uncontrolled cell growth. Restoration of normal *p53* ("wild-type") in soft tissue sarcomas may provide for more controlled cell growth or even programmed cell death (apoptosis). In one in vitro study, transduction of wild-type p53 into soft tissue sarcomas bearing mutated *p53* genes altered the malignant potential of the tumor. After transduction, transfected cells expressed wild-type *p53*, decreased cell proliferation, and decreased colony formation in soft agar and demonstrated decreased tumor formation in severe combined immunodeficient mice in vivo. The ability to restore wild-type *p53* function in soft tissue sarcoma in vitro and in these mice may ultimately be considered as future therapy for patients with soft tissue sarcomas.

Other investigations by Pollock and colleagues (1996) have shown that pulmonary metastases from soft tissue sarcoma can develop from clonal expansion of primary tumor cells bearing *p53* mutations. Use of specific molecular markers may provide better stratification of patients who will and who will not optimally benefit from surgery, chemotherapy, or other treatment modalities.

Other targets of gene therapy may include chemotherapy-resistant tumors or tumors with greater propensity for metastatic spread. Scotlandi and associates (1996) noted that overexpression of the *MDR1* gene product P-glycoprotein is an important predictor of poor prognosis in osteosarcoma patients treated with chemotherapy. In these patients, the MDR phenotype is not de novo more aggressive (i.e., more metastatic); however, the poor outcome of patients with the MDR phenotype related to P-glycoprotein overexpression is related to the cells' lack of response to cytotoxic drugs. In another study, by Onda and colleagues (1996), 42% of patients with OSTs had metastases that expressed ErbB-2 and correlated with early development of pulmonary metastasis and poor survival. ErbB-2 therefore may enhance tumor growth and promote metastases. These authors recommended that ErbB-2 may be considered a prognostic factor for patients with osteosarcoma.

Regional Drug Delivery to the Lung (Lung Perfusion)

Novel drug delivery systems may enhance chemotherapy treatment effects by increasing drug concentration in lung tissues and minimizing systemic effects of such treatment. In many patients, surgery has been used as salvage treatment after maximal chemotherapy response has been achieved. Systemic toxicity may limit the amount of chemotherapy given to an individual patient. Regional drug delivery to the lungs minimizes systemic drug delivery, preventing systemic toxicity; however, this technique dramatically increases the drug delivered to the lung over a short period.

Preclinical studies by Weksler and coinvestigators (1993a,b, 1994) in rodents with experimental pulmonary metastases from a methylcholanthrene-induced syngeneic sarcoma have shown that chemotherapy may be delivered regionally to pulmonary tissue in significantly higher concentrations than by systemic delivery. Minimal to no systemic toxicity was noted. In this model, isolated single lung perfusion with doxorubicin (Adriamycin) was safe and effective.

This simple microsurgical technique was performed in rats. After left thoracotomy, the pulmonary artery and pulmonary vein were isolated and clamped. The lung was flushed before infusing doxorubicin. The infusion occurred over 10 minutes. Then, the drug was flushed out before

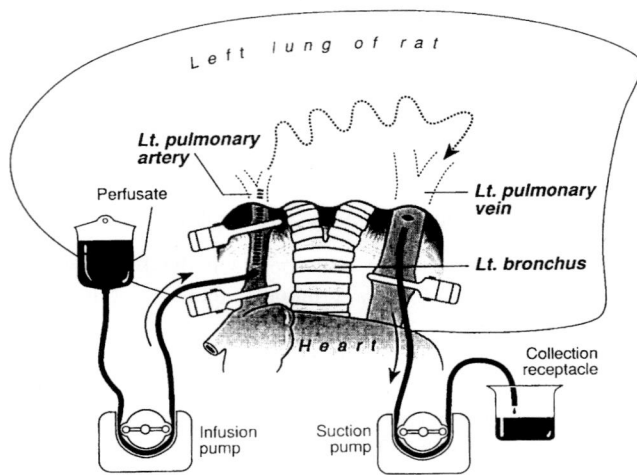

Fig. 113-6. Rodent model for isolated single-lung perfusion. After intubation and left thoracotomy, and using microvascular techniques, isolated single-lung perfusion can be performed. In this diagram, isolation of the pulmonary hilum and perfusion is shown. The bronchus is not occluded. The pulmonary artery is clamped and perfused. The left pulmonary vein is also clamped and vented, and effluent is collected and removed. Regional drug delivery is effectively accomplished using this technique. From Weksler B, Burt M: Isolated lung perfusion with antineoplastic agents for pulmonary metastases. Chest Surg Clin North Am 8:157, 1998. With permission.

removing the cannulas and restoring circulation (Fig. 113-6). A perfusion concentration of 255 mg/L caused less general toxicity than a systemic dose equivalent to 75 mg/m^2. The extraction ratio was 58%, and pulmonary tissue concentration of doxorubicin was 25-fold higher than with the systemic dose. The technique was also effective: 9 of 10 animals treated at 320 mg/L had complete eradication of metastases from an implanted methylcholanthrene-induced sarcoma.

Previous clinical studies of lung perfusion by Pass (1996) and Johnston (1995) and their associates have shown higher drug concentrations in pulmonary tissue, although clinical tumor response has been mixed. Johnston and colleagues (1995) described a continuous perfusion of the lungs with Adriamycin (single lung, continuous perfusion) as a safe technique and subsequently applied their technique clinically. Drug concentrations in normal lung and tumor generally increased with higher drug dosages. Two of eight patients had major complications: one patient developed pneumonia and sternal dehiscence; one patient developed respiratory failure 4 days after lung perfusion. No objective responses occurred (0/4 patients with sarcomas). Although continuous perfusion with a pump circuit offers some theoretical advantages, the technique is cumbersome, equipment intensive, and time consuming, and has the inherent problem of the incompatibility of Adriamycin and heparin. Pass and coworkers (1996) examined isolated single-lung perfusion with tumor necrosis factor-α, interferon-γ, and moderate hyperthermia for patients with unresectable pulmonary metastases. No hospital deaths occurred, and a short-term (<6-month) decrease in nodule size was noted in three of 15 patients.

Phase I studies in patients with unresectable pulmonary metastases from soft tissue sarcomas are ongoing at the University of Texas M. D. Anderson Cancer Center in Houston. A paucity of effective treatment and the potential for high drug concentrations for pulmonary metastases by regional lung perfusion warrants further clinical study.

CONCLUSIONS

Isolated and resectable metastases to the lungs represent a unique biology between the host, the primary neoplasm, and the metastases. Patients may have long-term survival associated with complete resection of all pulmonary metastases. Is the associated long-term survival the result of surgery or the result of the unique biology of the tumor and its metastases? This question remains unanswered. Complete resection is the crucial characteristic associated with long-term survival, regardless of the primary tumor histology. Patients with resectable pulmonary metastases should undergo resection to render them disease free with the potential for long-term survival and cure.

Various prognostic indicators may define the biological nature of the metastases, predict postresection survival, and assist the clinician in selecting patients who will benefit from surgery. Prognostic factors are heterogeneous among different tumor histologies. Factors predictive of improved survival for one type of tumor may not be predictive for another. Combining prognostic indicators together may be better than any single prognostic indicator. Multivariate analyses of combinations of prognostic indicators in patients with osteogenic or soft tissue sarcomas may be helpful in deciding which patients would benefit from surgery but should not be used to deny a potentially resectable patient the benefits of resection. Groupings of prognostic indicators for a particular tumor histology may facilitate selection of patients for investigational therapies. Further and more detailed analyses of prognostic factors from larger populations of patients with single tumor histologies will better define the value of surgical resection in patients with pulmonary metastases and the value of prognostic indicators to select these patients. No single criterion in resectable patients consistently and reliably predicts which patients will have enhanced long-term survival after resection; however, unresectable patients do poorly, despite adjuvant therapy. The presence of bronchial carcinoma often cannot be excluded in patients with solitary metastasis and prior adenocarcinoma or SCCA. Radiographic appearance of the nodule or mass should be considered. If a question exists as to the etiology of the mass, it should be treated congruent with the clinical stage of primary lung cancer. Current molecular biological techniques may improve the ability to select patients for surgery or other treatment based on observations of survival in patients with certain molecular char-

acteristics. Use of additional adjuvant therapy may allow for prolonged survival or cure.

Surgery for treatment of pulmonary metastases will not benefit a significant number of patients. Surgery attempts to control mechanically the biological sequelae of the primary malignancy. Surgical resection still remains the best means of local control and the best way to render the patient disease free. Patients with complete resection of pulmonary metastases have associated long-term survival, in contrast to patients with unresectable metastases. Nonetheless, surgery remains unsuccessful in obtaining long-term survival, disease-free survival, or cure in 60 to 80% of patients with resectable metastases. The fundamental biology of the neoplastic and metastatic process is unchanged by surgery. Other novel therapies, such as identification of molecular events for therapy and gene transfer or regional delivery of drug via the isolated pulmonary vasculature, may provide better and more directed therapy to the patients. Cure in most patients represents a serendipitous occasion in which the host biology, spread of tumor, and surgical resection remove all tumor, including micrometastases. The best results of treatment of pulmonary metastases await improved adjuvant therapies directed at biological and molecular events in the life cycle of the metastatic cell.

REFERENCES

Alexander J, Haight C: Pulmonary resection for solitary metastatic sarcoma and carcinoma. Surg Gynecol Obstet 85:129, 1947.

Al Jilaihawi AN, et al: Combined chemotherapy and surgery for pulmonary metastases from osteogenic sarcoma. Results of 10 years experience. Eur J Cardiothorac Surg 2:37, 1988.

Amos AM, Kim FH, McRoberts JW: The utility of video-assisted thoracic surgery in the diagnosis of pulmonary metastases from renal cell carcinoma. Urology 49:123, 1997.

Bacci G, et al: Metastatic patterns in osteosarcoma. Tumori 74:421, 1988.

Bacci G, et al: Osteogenic sarcoma of the extremity with detectable lung metastases at presentation. Results of treatment of 23 patients with chemotherapy followed by simultaneous resection of primary and metastatic lesions. Cancer 79:245, 1997.

Bains MS: Thoracic surgery via clamshell or median sternotomy incision. In Franco KL, Putnam JB Jr (eds): Advanced Therapy in Thoracic Surgery. Hamilton, BC: Decker, 1998, p. 54.

Bains MS, et al: The clamshell incision: an improved approach to bilateral pulmonary and mediastinal tumor. Ann Thorac Surg 58:30, 1994.

Barney JD, Churchill EJ: Adenocarcinoma of the kidney with metastasis to the lung cured by nephrectomy and lobectomy. J Urol 42:269, 1939.

Barter JF, et al: Diagnosis and treatment of pulmonary metastases from cervical carcinoma. Gynecol Oncol 38:347, 1990.

Barth A, Wanek LA, Morton DL: Prognostic factors in 1,521 melanoma patients with distant metastases. J Am Coll Surg 181:193, 1995.

Beattie EJ, et al: Results of multiple pulmonary resections for metastatic osteogenic sarcoma after two decades. J Surg Oncol 46:154, 1991.

Belli L, et al: Resection of pulmonary metastases in osteosarcoma. A retrospective analysis of 44 patients. Cancer 63:2546, 1989.

Bodzin GA, Staren ED, Faber LP: Breast carcinoma metastases. Chest Surg Clin North Am 8:145, 1998.

Branscheid D, et al: Does ND-YAG laser extend the indications for resection of pulmonary metastases? Eur J Cardiothorac Surg 6:590, 1992.

Brister SJ, et al: Contemporary operative management of pulmonary metastases of colorectal origin. Dis Colon Rectum 31:786, 1988.

Burgers JM, et al: Osteosarcoma of the limbs. Report of the EORTC-SIOP 03 trial 20781 investigating the value of adjuvant treatment with chemotherapy and/or prophylactic lung irradiation. Cancer 61:1024, 1988.

Carsky S, et al: Germ cell testicular tumours with lung metastases: chemotherapy and surgical treatment. Int Urol Nephrol 24:305, 1992.

Carter GE, et al: Reassessment of the role of adjunctive surgical therapy in the treatment of advanced germ cell tumors. J Urol 138:1397, 1987.

Carter SR, et al: Results of thoracotomy in osteogenic sarcoma with pulmonary metastases. Thorax 46:727, 1991.

Casson AG, et al: Efficacy of pulmonary metastasectomy for recurrent soft tissue sarcoma. J Surg Oncol 47:1, 1991.

Casson AG, et al: Five-year survival after pulmonary metastasectomy for adult soft tissue sarcoma. Cancer 69:662, 1992.

Chang AE, et al: Evaluation of computed tomography in the detection of pulmonary metastases: a prospective study. Cancer 43:913, 1979.

Collins VP, Loeffler RK, Tivey H: Observations on growth rates of human tumors. AJR Am J Roentgenol 76:988, 1956.

Cox DR: Regression models and life-tables. J R Stat Soc B 34:187, 1972.

de Kraker J, et al: Wilms tumor with pulmonary metastases at diagnosis: the significance of primary chemotherapy. International Society of Pediatric Oncology Nephroblastoma Trial and Study Committee. J Clin Oncol 8:1187, 1990.

Dernevik L, et al: Surgical removal of pulmonary metastases from renal cell carcinoma. Scand J Urol Nephrol 19:133, 1985.

Di Lorenzo M, Collin PP: Pulmonary metastases in children: results of surgical treatment. J Pediatr Surg 23:762, 1988.

Divis G: Ein Beitrag zur operativen Behandlung der Lungengeschwulste. Acta Chir Scand 62:329, 1927.

Dunst J, Paulussen M, Jurgens H: Lung irradiation for Ewing's sarcoma with pulmonary metastases at diagnosis: results of the CESS-studies. Strahlenther Onkol 169:621, 1993.

Elias A, et al: Response to mesna, doxorubicin, ifosfamide, and dacarbazine in 108 patients with metastatic or unresectable sarcoma and no prior chemotherapy. J Clin Oncol 7:1208, 1989.

European Organisation for Research and Treatment of Cancer: Phase III Randomized Study of Neoadjuvant High-Dose DOX/IFF with or without G-CSF Followed by Metastasectomy vs Metastasectomy Alone for Lung Metastases in Patients with Soft Tissue Sarcoma. EORTC-62933, 1996.

Feuerstein IM, et al: Pulmonary metastases: MR imaging with surgical correlation—a prospective study. Radiology 182:123, 1992.

Finley RK III, et al: Results of surgical resection of pulmonary metastases of squamous cell carcinoma of the head and neck. Am J Surg 164:594, 1992.

Flint A, Lloyd RV: Colon carcinoma metastatic to the lung. Cytologic manifestations and distinction from primary pulmonary adenocarcinoma. Acta Cytol 36:230, 1992.

Fourquier P, et al: Lung metastases of renal cell carcinoma: results of surgical resection. Eur J Cardiothorac Surg 11:17, 1997.

Friedel G, Linder A, Toomes H: The significance of prognostic factors for the resection of pulmonary metastases of breast cancer. Thorac Cardiovasc Surg 42:71, 1994.

Fuller AF Jr, Scannell JG, Wilkins EW Jr: Pulmonary resection for metastases from gynecologic cancers: Massachusetts General Hospital experience, 1943–1982. Gynecol Oncol 22:174, 1985.

Gehan EA: A generalized Wilcoxon test for comparing arbitrarily singly-censored samples. Biometrika 522:203, 1965.

Ghoneim AH, et al: Monoclonal anti-CEA antibodies in the discrimination between primary pulmonary adenocarcinoma and colon carcinoma metastatic to the lung. Mod Pathol 3:613, 1990.

Glasser DB, et al: Survival, prognosis, and therapeutic response in osteogenic sarcoma. The Memorial Hospital experience. Cancer 69:698, 1992.

Gompertz B: On the nature of the function expressive of the law of human mortality, and on a new mode of determining the value of life contingencies. Philos Trans 513, 1825.

Goorin AM, et al: Changing pattern of pulmonary metastases with adjuvant chemotherapy in patients with osteosarcoma: results from the multi-institutional osteosarcoma study. J Clin Oncol 9:600, 1991.

Gorenstein LA, et al: Improved survival after resection of pulmonary metastases from malignant melanoma. Ann Thorac Surg 52:204, 1991.

Goya T, et al: Surgical resection of pulmonary metastases from colorectal cancer: 10-year follow-up. Cancer 64:1418, 1989.

Green DM, et al: The role of surgical excision in the management of relapsed Wilms' tumor patients with pulmonary metastases: a report from the National Wilms' Tumor Study. J Pediatr Surg 26:728, 1991.

Groeger AM, et al: Survival after surgical treatment of recurrent pulmonary metastases. Eur J Cardiothorac Surg 12:703, 1997.

Harpole DH Jr, et al: Analysis of 945 cases of pulmonary metastatic melanoma. J Thorac Cardiovasc Surg 103:743, 1992.

Heij HA, et al: Prognostic factors in surgery for pulmonary metastases in children. Surgery 115:687, 1994.

Herrera GA, Alexander CB, Jones JM: Ultrastructural characterization of pulmonary neoplasms. II. The role of electron microscopy in characterization of uncommon epithelial pulmonary neoplasms, metastatic neoplasms to and from lung, and other tumors, including mesenchymal neoplasms. Surv Synth Pathol Res 4:163, 1985.

Heslin MJ, et al: Preoperative identification and operative management of intraatrial extension of lung tumors. Ann Thorac Surg 65:544, 1998.

Huth JF, Eilber FR: Patterns of recurrence after resection of osteosarcoma of the extremity. Arch Surg 124:122, 1989.

Imachi M, et al: Pulmonary metastasis from carcinoma of the uterine cervix. Gynecol Oncol 33:189, 1989.

Jablons D, et al: Metastasectomy for soft tissue sarcoma. Further evidence for efficacy and prognostic indicators. J Thorac Cardiovasc Surg 97:695, 1989.

Jaffe N, et al: Osteogenic sarcoma: alterations in the pattern of pulmonary metastases with adjuvant chemotherapy. J Clin Oncol 1:251, 1983.

Jett JR, et al: Pulmonary resection of metastatic renal cell carcinoma. Chest 84:442, 1983.

Johnston MR: Median sternotomy for resection of pulmonary metastases. J Thorac Cardiovasc Surg 85:516, 1983.

Johnston MR, Minchen RF, Dawson CA: Lung perfusion with chemotherapy in patients with unresectable metastatic sarcoma to the lung or diffuse bronchioloalveolar carcinoma. J Thorac Cardiovasc Surg 110:368, 1995.

Joseph WL, Morton DL, Adkins PC: Prognostic significance of tumor doubling time in evaluating operability in pulmonary metastatic disease. J Thorac Cardiovasc Surg 61:23, 1971a.

Joseph WL, Morton DL, Adkins PC: Variation in tumor doubling time in patients with pulmonary metastatic disease. J Surg Oncol 3:143, 1971b.

Kandioler D, et al: Long-term results after repeated surgical removal of pulmonary metastases. Ann Thorac Surg 65:909, 1998.

Kaplan EL, Meier P: Nonparametric estimation from incomplete observations. J Am Stat Assoc 53:457, 1958.

Kim B, Louie AC: Surgical resection following interleukin 2 therapy for metastatic renal cell carcinoma prolongs remission. Arch Surg 127:1343, 1992.

Kodama K, et al: Surgical management of lung metastases. Usefulness of resection with the neodymium:yttrium-aluminum-garnet laser with median sternotomy. J Thorac Cardiovasc Surg 101:901, 1991.

Koong HN, Pastorino U, Ginsberg RJ: Is there a role for pneumonectomy in pulmonary metastasis? Program Book, Annual Meeting of the Society of Thoracic Surgeons, San Antonio, TX, 1999, p. 210.

Kronlein RU: Ueber Lungenchirirugie. Berlin Klin Wschr 9:129, 1884.

Kulkarni RP, et al: Cytoreductive surgery in disseminated non-seminomatous germ cell tumours of testis. Br J Surg 78:226, 1991.

Kumar J, Ilancheran A, Ratnam SS: Pulmonary metastasis in gestational trophoblastic disease: a review of 97 cases. Br J Obstet Gynecol 95:70, 1988.

Ladanyi M, et al: MDM2 gene amplification in metastatic osteosarcoma. Cancer Res 53:16, 1993.

Laird AK: Dynamics of tumor growth. Br J Cancer 18:490, 1960.

Landreneau RJ, et al: Thoracoscopic neodymium:yttrium-aluminum garnet laser-assisted pulmonary resection. Ann Thorac Surg 52:1176, 1991.

Landreneau RJ, et al: Thoracoscopic resection of 85 pulmonary lesions. Ann Thorac Surg 54:415, 1992.

Lanza LA, et al: The role of resection in the treatment of pulmonary metastases from Ewing's sarcoma. J Thorac Cardiovasc Surg 94:181, 1987.

Lanza LA, et al: Response to chemotherapy does not predict survival after resection of sarcomatous pulmonary metastases. Ann Thorac Surg 51:219, 1991.

Lanza LA, et al: Long-term survival after resection of pulmonary metastases from carcinoma of the breast. Ann Thorac Surg 54:244, 1992.

La Quaglia MP: Osteosarcoma. Specific tumor management and results. Chest Surg Clin North Am 8:77, 1998.

Lefor AT, et al: Multiple malignancies of the lung and head and neck. Second primary tumor or metastasis? Arch Surg 121:265, 1986.

Levenback C, et al: Resection of pulmonary metastases from uterine sarcomas. Gynecol Oncol 45:202, 1992.

Lien HH, et al: Computed tomography and conventional radiography in intrathoracic metastases from non-seminomatous testicular tumor. Acta Radiol 29:547, 1988.

Liu D, et al: Pulmonary metastasectomy for testicular germ cell tumors: a 28-year experience. Ann Thorac Surg 66:1709, 1998.

Lucas JD, et al: Evaluation of fluorodeoxyglucose positron emission tomography in the management of soft-tissue sarcomas. J Bone Joint Surg Br 80:441, 1998.

Macklis RM, Oltikar A, Sallan SE: Wilms' tumor patients with pulmonary metastases. Int J Radiat Oncol Biol Phys 21:1187, 1991.

Mannix: Resection of multiple pulmonary metastases fourteen years after amputation for osteochondroma of tibia: apparent freedom for recurrence three years later. J Thorac Surg 26:544, 1953.

Mansel JK, et al: Pulmonary resection of metastatic colorectal adenocarcinoma. A ten year experience. Chest 89:109, 1986.

Marina NM, et al: Improved prognosis of children with osteosarcoma metastatic to the lung(s) at the time of diagnosis. Cancer 70:2722, 1992.

Martini N, et al: Multiple pulmonary resections in the treatment of osteogenic sarcoma. Ann Thorac Surg 12:271, 1971.

Martini N, McCormack PM: Evolution of the surgical management of pulmonary metastases. Chest Surg Clin N Am 8:13, 1998.

Mazer TM, et al: Resection of pulmonary metastases from squamous carcinoma of the head and neck. Am J Surg 156:238, 1988.

McAfee MK, et al: Colorectal lung metastases: results of surgical excision. Ann Thorac Surg 53:780, 1992.

McCormack PM, Attiyeh FF: Resected pulmonary metastases from colorectal cancer. Dis Colon Rectum 22:553, 1979.

McCormack PM, et al: Pulmonary resection in metastatic carcinoma. Chest 73:163, 1978.

McCormack PM, et al: Lung resection for colorectal metastases. 10-year results. Arch Surg 127:1403, 1992.

McCormack PM, et al: Accuracy of lung imaging in metastases with implications for the role of thoracoscopy. Ann Thorac Surg 56:863, 1993.

McCormack PM, et al: Role of video-assisted thoracic surgery in the treatment of pulmonary metastases: results of a prospective trial. Ann Thorac Surg 62:213, 1996.

Meade RH: A History of Thoracic Surgery. Charles C. Thomas 1:194, 1961.

Meyer WH, et al: Thoracotomy for pulmonary metastatic osteosarcoma. An analysis of prognostic indicators of survival. Cancer 59:374, 1987.

Miller DL, et al: Videothoracoscopic wedge excision of the lung. Ann Thorac Surg 54:410, 1992.

Miyamoto H, et al: Application of the Nd-YAG laser for surgical resection of pulmonary metastases. Kyobu Geka 45:56, 1992.

Morrow CE, Vassilopoulos PP, Grage TB: Surgical resection for metastatic neoplasms of the lung: experience at the University of Minnesota Hospitals. Cancer 45:2981, 1980.

Mountain CF, McMurtrey MJ, Hermes KE: Surgery for pulmonary metastasis: a 20-year experience. Ann Thorac Surg 38:323, 1984.

Murata S, et al: Resection of both hepatic and pulmonary metastases in patients with colorectal carcinoma. Cancer 83:1086, 1998.

Murray KD: Excision of pulmonary metastasis of colorectal cancer. Semin Surg Oncol 7:157, 1991.

Nibu K, et al: Surgical treatment for pulmonary metastases of squamous cell carcinoma of the head and neck. Am J Otolaryngol 18:391, 1997.

Nomori H, et al: Tumor cell heterogeneity and subpopulations with metastatic ability in differentiated adenocarcinoma of the lung. Histologic and cytofluorometric DNA analyses. Chest 99:934, 1991.

Ollila DW, Morton DL: Surgical resection as the treatment of choice for melanoma metastatic to the lung. Chest Surg Clin North Am 8:183, 1998.

Onda M, et al: ErbB-2 expression is correlated with poor prognosis for patients with osteosarcoma. Cancer 77:71, 1996.

Pass HI, et al: Detection of pulmonary metastases in patients with osteogenic and soft-tissue sarcomas: the superiority of CT scans compared with conventional linear tomograms using dynamic analysis. J Clin Oncol 3:1261, 1985.

Pass HI, et al: Isolated lung perfusion with tumor necrosis factor for pulmonary metastases. Ann Thorac Surg 61:1609, 1996.

Pastorino U, et al: Lung resection as salvage treatment for metastatic osteosarcoma. Tumori 74:201, 1988.

Pastorino U, et al: The contribution of salvage surgery to the management of childhood osteosarcoma. J Clin Oncol 9:1357, 1991.

Pastorino U, et al: Primary childhood osteosarcoma: the role of salvage surgery. Ann Oncol 3(Suppl 2):S43, 1992.

Pastorino U, et al: Long-term results of lung metastasectomy: prognostic analyses based on 5206 cases. The International Registry of Lung Metastases. J Thorac Cardiovasc Surg 113:37, 1997.

Patanaphan V, Salazar OM, Risco R: Breast cancer: metastatic patterns and their prognosis. South Med J 81:1109, 1988.

Paulussen M, et al: Primary metastatic (stage IV) Ewing tumor: survival analysis of 171 patients from the EICESS studies. European Intergroup Cooperative Ewing Sarcoma Studies. Ann Oncol 9:275, 1998a.

Paulussen M, et al: Ewing's tumors with primary lung metastases: survival analysis of 114 (European Intergroup) Cooperative Ewing's Sarcoma Studies patients. J Clin Oncol 16:3044, 1998b.

Pihl E, et al: Lung recurrence after curative surgery for colorectal cancer. Dis Colon Rectum 30:417, 1987.

Pogrebniak HW, et al: Resection of pulmonary metastases from malignant melanoma: results of a 16-year experience. Ann Thorac Surg 46:20, 1988.

Pogrebniak HW, et al: Reoperative pulmonary resection in patients with metastatic soft tissue sarcoma. Ann Thorac Surg 52:197, 1991.

Pogrebniak HW, et al: Renal cell carcinoma: resection of solitary and multiple metastases. Ann Thorac Surg 54:33, 1992.

Pollock R, et al: Wild-type p53 and a p53 temperature-sensitive mutant suppress human soft tissue sarcoma by enhancing cell cycle control. Clin Cancer Res 4:1985, 1998.

Pollock RE, et al: Soft tissue sarcoma metastasis from clonal expansion of p53 mutated tumor cells. Oncogene 12:2035, 1996.

Potter DA, et al: Patterns of recurrence in patients with high-grade soft-tissue sarcomas. J Clin Oncol 3:353, 1985.

Putnam JB Jr, et al: Survival following aggressive resection of pulmonary metastases from osteogenic sarcoma: analysis of prognostic factors. Ann Thorac Surg 38:516, 1983.

Putnam JB Jr, et al: Analysis of prognostic factors in patients undergoing resection of pulmonary metastases from soft tissue sarcomas. J Thorac Cardiovasc Surg 87:260, 1984.

Putnam JB Jr, et al: Extended resection of pulmonary metastases: is the risk justified? Ann Thorac Surg 55:1440, 1993.

Regnard JF, et al: Surgical treatment of hepatic and pulmonary metastases from colorectal cancers. Ann Thorac Surg 66:214, 1998.

Rizzoni WE, et al: Resection of recurrent pulmonary metastases in patients with soft-tissue sarcomas. Arch Surg 121:1248, 1986.

Roberts DG, et al: Long-term follow-up of operative treatment for pulmonary metastases. Eur J Cardiothorac Surg 3:292, 1989.

Robinson BJ, et al: Is resection of pulmonary and hepatic metastases warranted in patients with colorectal cancer? J Thorac Cardiovasc Surg 117:66, 1999.

Rooser B, Pettersson H, Alvegard T: Growth rate of pulmonary metastases from soft tissue sarcoma (published erratum appears in Acta Oncol 26:496 1987) Acta Oncol 26:189, 1987.

Rosen G, et al: Chemotherapy and thoracotomy for metastatic osteogenic sarcoma. A model for adjuvant chemotherapy and the rationale for the timing of thoracic surgery. Cancer 41:841, 1978.

Rosen G, et al: Thoracotomy in the management of metastatic soft-tissue sarcomas in adults. Chest Surg Clin North Am 4:67, 1994.

Roth JA, et al: Comparison of median sternotomy and thoracotomy for resection of pulmonary metastases in patients with adult soft-tissue sarcomas. Ann Thorac Surg 42:134, 1986.

Roth JA, et al: Differing determinants of prognosis following resection of pulmonary metastases from osteogenic and soft tissue sarcoma patients. Cancer 55:1361, 1985.

Salvati F, et al: DNA flow cytometric studies of 66 human lung tumors analyzed before treatment. Prognostic implications. Chest 96:1092, 1989.

Sauter ER, et al: Improved survival after pulmonary resection of metastatic colorectal carcinoma. J Surg Oncol 43:135, 1990.

Scheele J, et al: Pulmonary resection for metastatic colon and upper rectum cancer. Is it useful? Dis Colon Rectum 33:745, 1990.

Schlappack OK, et al: The clinical course of lung metastases from breast cancer. Klin Wochenschr 66:790, 1988.

Schnorrer M, et al: Management of germ cell testicular cancer with pulmonary metastases. Neoplasma 43:47, 1996.

Schott G, Weissmuller J, Vecera E: Methods and prognosis of the extirpation of pulmonary metastases following tumor nephrectomy. Urol Int 43:272, 1988.

Scotlandi K, et al: Multidrug resistance and malignancy in human osteosarcoma. Cancer Res 56:2434, 1996.

Seki M, et al: Surgical treatment of pulmonary metastases from uterine cervical cancer. Operation method by lung tumor size. J Thorac Cardiovasc Surg 104:876, 1992.

Shuman RL: Primary pulmonary sarcoma with left atrial extension via left superior pulmonary vein. En bloc resection and radical pneumonectomy on cardiopulmonary bypass. J Thorac Cardiovasc Surg 88:189, 1984.

Simpson R, et al: Pulmonary resection for metastatic breast cancer. Aust N Z J Surg 67:717, 1997.

Skinner KA, et al: Surgical treatment and chemotherapy for pulmonary metastases from osteosarcoma. Arch Surg 127:1065, 1992.

Slebos RJ, et al: Allele-specific detection of K-ras oncogene expression in human non-small-cell lung carcinomas. Int J Cancer 48:51, 1991.

Snyder CL, et al: A new approach to the resection of pulmonary osteosarcoma metastases. Results of aggressive metastasectomy. Clin Orthop 270:247, 1991.

Spaggiari L, et al: Pneumonectomy for lung metastases: indications, risks, and outcome. Ann Thorac Surg 66:1930, 1999.

Staren ED, et al: Pulmonary resection for metastatic breast cancer. Arch Surg 127:1282, 1992.

Takita H, et al: The surgical management of multiple lung metastases. Ann Thorac Surg 24:359, 1992.

Temeck BK, et al: Reoperative pulmonary metastasectomy for sarcomatous pediatric histologies. Ann Thorac Surg 66:908, 1999.

Tesoro-Tess JD, et al: Reliability of diagnostic imaging after orchiectomy alone in follow-up of clinical stage I testicular carcinoma: excessive cost with potential risk. Lymphology 20:161, 1987.

Thomas DG: Exact and asymptotic methods for the combination of 2×2 tables. Comput Biomed Res 8:423, 1975.

Toledano AY, Olak J: Statistical Techniques and Analysis in Thoracic Surgery. In Franco KL, Putnam JB Jr (eds): Advanced Therapy in Thoracic Surgery. Hamilton, ONT: BC Decker, 1998, p. 146.

Torek F: Removal of metastatic carcinoma of the lung and mediastinum: suggestions as to technic. Arch Surg 21:1416, 1930.

Udelsman R, et al: Endobronchial metastases from soft tissue sarcoma. J Surg Oncol 32:145, 1986.

Urschel HC Jr, Razzuk MA: Median sternotomy as a standard approach for pulmonary resection. Ann Thorac Surg 41:130, 1986.

Van Schil P, et al: Surgical excision of pulmonary metastases from primary testicular cancer—case reports. Acta Chir Belg 89:175, 1989.

Weh HJ, et al: Chemotherapy of metastatic soft tissue sarcoma with a combination of adriamycin and DTIC or adriamycin and ifosfamide. Onkologie 13:448, 1990.

Weinlechner JW: Zur Kasuistik der Tumoren an der Brustwand und deren Behandlung (Resektion der rippen, Eroffnung der Brusthohle, partielle Entfernung der Lungen). Wein Med Wochenschr 32:589, 1882.

Weksler B, et al: Isolated single-lung perfusion with doxorubicin is pharmacokinetically superior to intravenous injection. Ann Thorac Surg 56:209, 1993a.

Weksler B, et al: Isolated single lung perfusion in the rat: an experimental model. J Appl Physiol 74:2736, 1993b.

Weksler B, et al: Isolated single lung perfusion with doxorubicin is effective in eradicating soft tissue sarcoma lung metastases in a rat model. J Thorac Cardiovasc Surg 107:50, 1994.

Wilimas JA, et al: Significance of pulmonary computed tomography at diagnosis in Wilms' tumor. J Clin Oncol 6:1144, 1988.

Williams MP, Husband JE, Heron CW: Intrathoracic manifestations of metastatic testicular seminoma: a comparison of chest radiographic and CT findings. AJR Am J Roentgenol 149:473, 1987.

Yamaguchi H, et al: The alteration in the pattern of pulmonary metastasis with adjuvant chemotherapy in osteosarcoma. Int Orthop 12:305, 1988.

Zaharia M, et al: Postoperative whole lung irradiation with or without adriamycin in osteogenic sarcoma. Int J Radiat Oncol Biol Phys 12:907, 1986.

CHAPTER 114

Lung Tumors in the Immunocompromised Host

Joseph LoCicero III and Philip G. Robinson

Several situations may lead to the development of an immunocompromised state that could last for life or for extended periods of time. Iatrogenic immunosuppression, such as solid organ transplantation or autoimmune diseases; chronic infections, such as human immunodeficiency virus (HIV); and even other malignancies or anticancer therapy may cause altered immunocompetence (Table 114-1). Patients with these altered states have a greater incidence of certain malignancies than does the general population. In some cases, immunocompromised patients may develop pulmonary neoplasms that are not necessarily related to their immune status but may be the result of other influences. Autoimmune diseases do not cause immunosuppression, but many of these patients are treated with immunosuppressive agents to control the inflammatory response. Each specific situation has been analyzed individually by various investigators. Some of the mechanisms of malignancy development now appear to be similar. To show the significance of lung tumors in the immunocompromised host, we review the broader spectrum of tumor biology in these patients.

POSTTRANSPLANT MALIGNANCIES

Patients on immunosuppression drugs for organ transplantation have a higher incidence of certain malignancies. This observation was made within a few years of the routine use of cadaver renal transplantation for renal failure. Since then, multiple reports have confirmed this fact. Penn (1988) noted the staggering increase in transplant cancers compared to that in the general population (Table 114-2). He found that uterine cervical cancers increased 14 times, skin cancers increased 21 times, lung cancers increased 29 times, non-Hodgkin's lymphoma increased 50 times, carcinoma of the anus and vulva increased 100 times, and Kaposi's sarcoma increased up to 500 times over expected rates. Penn (1994) pointed out that these neoplasms may develop a short time after transplantation. Kaposi's sarcoma appeared at an average of 21 months after transplantation, and non-Hodgkin's

lymphomas appeared at an average of 32 months. The International Society of Heart and Lung Transplantation (1998) listed cumulative 15-year data from the International Transplant Registry. In 1,728 lung transplant recipients who have been followed for at least 1 year, the incidence of new malignancies is 4.5%. The majority of these tumors (57.6%) were labeled lymphoproliferative disorders or T-cell lymphomas. Skin tumors were the second most common, at 20.5%. A variety of other tumors accounted for 18% of the cancers. In a single-institution series, Mihalov and associates (1996) reported on 674 recipients, including 305 renal, 307 heart, 54 lung, and eight heart and lung transplants. They noted a 3.7% incidence of cancer in lung transplants. They also noted that thoracic organ transplant recipients, in contrast to renal transplant recipients, had a significantly higher rate of lymphomas. Spiekerkoetter and colleagues (1998) reported one patient who developed pulmonary squamous cell carcinoma out of 219 patients who underwent lung transplantation.

Approaching this problem from a different perspective, End and associates (1995) looked at pulmonary nodules in 64 lung transplant recipients. Nodules developed in eight patients (12.5%) an average of 5.8 months after transplant. In two patients, the nodules spontaneously resolved over 3 weeks. Of the remaining six patients, three had posttransplant lymphoproliferative disorder (PTLD), two had aspergillosis, and one had a mixed bacterial abscess. Diagnoses were made by CT-directed needle aspiration.

Proposed Causal Mechanisms of Posttransplant Malignancies

Concepts about the development of posttransplant tumors have varied over the years. Penn (1977) described the early theories. Tumors were thought either to be carried into the host in the transplanted tissue or to develop de novo in patients who were cancer free at the time of their transplant. The tumors in the latter scenario were thought to result in some way from the immunosuppression.

Table 114-1. Common Thoracic Malignancies in Immunocompromised Hosts

Immunocompromised states	Cancers
Transplant	Lymphoproliferative disorders, lymphoma, Kaposi's sarcoma, lung cancer
Human immunodeficiency virus infection	Lymphoma, Kaposi's sarcoma, lung cancer
Previous neoplasms	Lung cancer
Autoimmune disorders	Lymphoma, lung cancer

As more experience was gained over the years and immunosuppression became better understood, theories became more focused. One popular theory was that the immune system provides a feedback loop to regulate the production of lymphoid tissue. When this loop is suppressed, there could be uncontrolled lymphoid proliferation. Chronic antigenic stimulation by the graft could cause lymphoid hyperplasia and somehow lead to lymphomas. A possibility also considered was that the immunosuppressive drugs might have a direct oncogenic effect on the host.

Speculation on analysis of anogenital cancers in transplant recipients has led to the development of one current theory about at least some posttransplant malignancies. Penn (1986) noted that among 65 women transplant patients with cancers of the vulva, vagina, uterine cervix, or anus, several had a history of condyloma acuminatum or herpes genitalis. He suggested that these viruses might be contributing to cancer development. Subsequently, other viruses were implicated (Table 114-3): Epstein-Barr virus (EBV) and lymphoma; papillomavirus and carcinoma of the vulva, perineum, and uterine cervix; human herpesvirus and carcinoma of the vulva, uterine cervix, lips, and skin; human herpesvirus 8 (HHV-8) and Kaposi's sarcoma; and hepatitis and hepatocellular carcinoma.

A concentrated effort has been made to delineate the role of the EBV in the collection of lymphoid conditions now known as PTLDs. Although the B lymphocyte is the usual host for EBV, T lymphocytes also may become infected. Infections in either cell line may lead to PTLD. The exact

Table 114-2. Incidence of De Novo Tumors in Transplant Patients Compared to General Population

Cancer	Increase over expected[a] incidence
Uterine cervix (carcinoma in situ)	14-fold
Skin	21-fold
Lung	29-fold
Non-Hodgkin's lymphoma	49-fold
Vulva and anus	100-fold
Kaposi's sarcoma	500-fold

[a]Incidence in general population.

Table 114-3. Viruses Implicated in the Development of Cancers in Transplant Recipients

Virus	Potential cancers
Epstein-Barr virus	Lymphoproliferative disorders
Hepatitis B and C virus	Hepatoma
Human herpesvirus	Lips, skin, perineum, uterine cervix, vulva
Human herpesvirus 8	Kaposi's sarcoma
Papillomavirus	Perineum, uterine cervix, vulva

mechanism for the development of PTLD from EBV is unclear. In the next paragraph, we discuss the thoughts of Mathur (1994) and Birkeland (1995) and their associates about the role of cytokines in the pathogenesis of PTLD. Most PTLDs contain the EBV genome. Berger and Delecluse (1993) have postulated that PTLD is the result of the interaction between the virus and the host cells. After infection, there is a primary response, which is initially mediated by natural killer cells and CD4 suppressor T cells. Later, the secondary immune response is mediated by HLA-restricted CD8 cytotoxic T cells, which are specific for EBV. Also, there is an immunoglobulin M (IgM) and later an IgG response to the viral capsid antigen, early antigen, and EBV nuclear antigens. When the EBV-infected B cells escape the cytotoxic T cells, other EBV products, such as EBV nuclear antigens and latent membrane proteins, upregulate a series of genes, leading to proliferation and transformation of EBV-infected cells. This enlarged pool of proliferating cells carries an additional risk for mutation of an oncogene or a tumor-suppressor gene. In an immunosuppressed patient, the EBV-infected cells are not controlled; this leads to the spectrum of PTLD, which ranges from hyperplasia to lymphoma (Fig. 114-1). The pathologic classification of PTLD is discussed later in this chapter.

Mathur and associates (1994) contend that unbalanced lymphokine production contributes to the development of

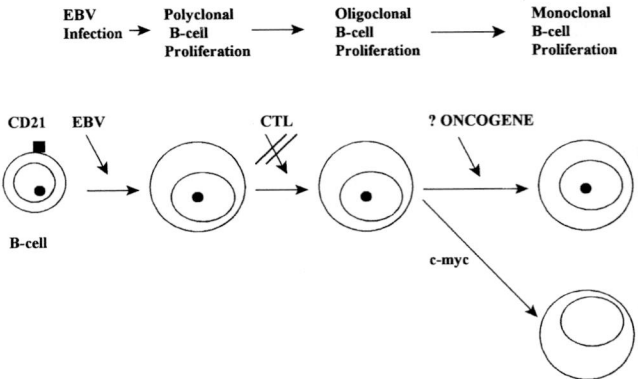

Fig. 114-1. A schematic representation of the multiple steps for B-cell lymphomagenesis in immunodeficient hosts. Epstein-Barr virus (EBV) most likely plays a direct role in the proliferation of B cells, which leads to additional mutations or oncogene activation. CD21, EBV receptor; CTL, cytotoxic T cell.

PTLD. They found that levels of interleukin-4 (IL-4) were significantly elevated in patients with PTLD and in healthy immunosuppressed organ transplant recipients compared with normal healthy individuals. They also found that patients with PTLD exhibited significantly lower levels of interferon-α (INF-α) and higher levels of IgE than either healthy EBV-seropositive individuals or healthy immuno-suppressed organ recipients. These findings suggest that a circulating imbalance of cytokines may contribute to PTLD. Along similar lines, Birkeland and coworkers (1995) described four patients with elevated levels of IL-10 in patients with PTLD. In one patient, the level decreased to zero after treatment with acyclovir. They also pointed out that the coding sequence for the IL-10 gene is highly homol-ogous to the EBV open reading frame, *BCRF1*. Expression of this gene produces a viral IL-10, which has the same activities as IL-10. This cytokine, IL-10, is a potent sup-pressor of macrophages. These articles raise important ques-tions about the pathogenesis of PTLD.

Both Montone and Mentzer and their colleagues in 1996 reported PTLD in lung transplant recipients. Montone's group found the incidence of PTLD in lung transplant to be an astonishing 20%. Using in situ hybridization techniques, they found that all patients had EBV-related polymorphous B-cell lesions. Most lesions were hyperplasia, but two of nine had lymphoma. Schwend and associates (1994) described a non-Hodgkin's lymphoma occurring in the lung of a patient 8 weeks after undergoing heart transplantation. Immunostaining of the high-grade B-cell lymphoma revealed the latent membrane protein of EBV in the tumor cells. They suggested that immunosuppression permits an uncontrolled proliferation of EBV-infected B lymphocytes, resulting in a lymphoma. Marchioli and colleagues (1996) also have implicated HHV-8 in body cavity lymphomas.

Dockrell and colleagues (1998) examined their series at the Mayo Clinic, noting that only one of 61 cases of PTLD were restricted to the T lymphocyte line. They specifically studied 21 cases, finding 38% to be induced by EBV. Haque and associates (1996) found that EBV-seronegative recipi-ents can develop PTLD from a seropositive organ.

Boyle and colleagues (1997) studied 120 children receiv-ing thoracic organ transplants and found a 19.5% incidence of PTLD in heart-lung and lung recipients and only a 7.7% incidence in heart recipients. They also discovered that recipients who were EBV positive before transplant did not develop PTLD. Only those who developed a primary EBV infection developed PTLD.

AUTOIMMUNE DISEASES

Autoimmune diseases do not produce a compromised immune system until they are treated. Patients with these dis-eases are usually treated with steroids and anticancer agents, such as azathioprine or cyclophosphamide. Mellemkjaer (1997) and Ramsey-Goldman (1998) and their associates have

both reported an increased incidence of the usual types of lung carcinomas in patients with systemic lupus erythematosus. Mellemkjaer and colleagues (1996) also described a similar increase of lung carcinomas in patients with rheumatoid arthri-tis. Quismorio (1996) reviewed the subject of pulmonary com-plications in Sjögren's syndrome. He found an increased risk of pulmonary lymphomas. In a study from the Mayo Clinic, Hansen and coworkers (1989) described 10 of 50 patients with Sjögren's syndrome who had pulmonary lymphomas. The lymphomas ranged from low- to high-grade, with the high-grade ones being associated with increased mortality. Nichol-son and coworkers (1996) described six cases of primary pulmonary B-cell non-Hodgkin's lymphomas in patients with autoimmune diseases who were receiving immunosuppressive drugs. The patients had rheumatoid arthritis, polymyositis, cryptogenic fibrosing alveolitis, mixed connective tissue dis-ease, and Sjögren's syndrome. Only the patient with Sjögren's syndrome was not receiving immunosuppressive therapy. He developed a low-grade lymphoma. The other five patients were receiving immunosuppressive therapy, and they all devel-oped high-grade lymphomas. In conclusion, patients with autoimmune diseases who may be immunosuppressed can develop carcinomas and lymphomas of the lung. The relation-ship between these autoimmune diseases and pulmonary neo-plasms is unclear.

Kamel (1997) reviewed iatrogenic lymphoproliferative disorders. The most frequent setting is in patients with rheumatoid arthritis who are receiving methotrexate. He did not specifically discuss lung involvement. He cited a case of a 15-year-old girl with juvenile dermatomyositis being treated with methotrexate who developed a lymphoprolifer-ative disorder in the lung and died. Consequently, the diag-nosis of a lymphoproliferative disorder should be considered in patients with autoimmune diseases who are receiving immunosuppressive therapy.

HUMAN IMMUNODEFICIENCY VIRUS–RELATED MALIGNANCIES

Patients with the archetypal infectious immunodeficiency, acquired immunodeficiency syndrome (AIDS), have an increased incidence of three malignancies: Kaposi's sar-coma, intermediate- or high-grade lymphoma, and uterine cervical cancer. Within the very recent past, there has been speculation that primary lung cancer also may have an increased incidence in patients infected with HIV. Alshafie and associates (1997) reviewed the patients with lung cancer at the Harlem Hospital in New York. Eleven patients had HIV infection, and 116 cases were classified as HIV inde-terminate. The HIV patients were younger and had shorter life expectancies than those without HIV but no conclusion could be reached. Parker and colleagues (1998) discovered a more convincing link when they evaluated the state of Texas database of patients with HIV-AIDS and lung cancer diag-nosed between 1990 and 1995. Of 26,181 HIV-positive patients with or without AIDS, they found 76 cases of lung cancer. This was a 6.5-fold increased incidence over the general U.S. population. Further data are necessary to establish a firm link.

In 1992, Fraire and Awe reported a case of pulmonary adenocarcinoma occurring in a 34-year-old, HIV-positive man with a past history of intravenous drug abuse and smoking. At the time of diagnosis, he was at stage IV and was treated with radiation therapy. He was alive 17 months after diagnosis but had progressive disease. In their review of the literature, Fraire and Awe found 22 patients who had lung cancer and were HIV positive. In general, the patients were young, with a median age of 38 years. There were 20 men and two women, for a male-to-female ratio of 10:1, in contrast to the usual ratio of 2:1. Most patients were smokers. Eleven of the patients had adenocarcinomas (50%), six had small cell carcinomas (27.3%), three had squamous cell carcinomas (13.5%), and one had adenosquamous carcinoma (4.5%). They pointed out that, in general, younger patients tend to have adenocarcinomas more frequently than do older patients, which may partly explain the high percentage of adenocarcinomas in this population.

In 1993, Karp and colleagues described seven HIV-positive patients with lung adenocarcinoma and compared them to a control group. Their findings were similar to those of Fraire and Awe (1992), except that they described their patients as having a rapidly progressive course. In 1995, Flores and associates reported another 19 patients. Vyzula and Remick (1996) reported another 16 patients and reviewed the literature. In summary, HIV-positive patients with lung cancer tend to be younger and have a higher percentage of adenocarcinomas than do other patients. Most of them have a history of smoking. They usually present at a higher stage and have a more rapidly progressive course than do control groups. Whether there is a true increased incidence of lung cancer in HIV-positive patients is not clear, although the report of Parker and colleagues (1998) suggests that there is. As better treatments become available to prolong the life of patients infected with HIV, it may become more apparent that these patients are susceptible to other diseases. Another possibility is that the occurrence of the diseases together may be coincidence.

Proposed Causal Mechanisms of Human Immunodeficiency Virus–Related Malignancies

The HIV-infected patient has disease-related mechanisms that increase the risk of cancer. In the case of Kaposi's sarcoma, several mechanisms may be at work. Beral and associates (1992) noted an increased incidence of Kaposi's sarcoma among homosexual and bisexual men. Lassoued and colleagues (1991), however, found a low incidence of Kaposi's sarcoma in HIV-infected women. In Africa, where HIV is spread mainly by heterosexual contact, the incidence among the sexes is more closely aligned. Regulatory pro-

teins, such as oncostatin M and HIV-TAT, may play a role. Vogel and coworkers (1988) demonstrated that HIV-TAT can initiate cell transformation and stimulate the proliferation of Kaposi's sarcoma spindle cells. Miles and associates (1992) discovered that oncostatin M functions as both a primary growth factor and a stimulator of IL-6, which serves the same purpose.

Speculation about the etiology of Kaposi's sarcoma has abounded over the years. In Africa, it has a similar distribution to Burkitt's lymphoma, which suggests viral origin. Cytomegalovirus and HIV have been suggested as etiologic agents. In 1994, Chang and colleagues described DNA sequences in Kaposi's sarcoma tissue that were similar to herpesvirus. This virus is now known as HHV-8, or Kaposi's sarcoma-associated herpesvirus. A subsequent study by Moore and Chang (1995) found the HHV-8 DNA sequence in 20 of 21 tissue samples (95%) of Kaposi's sarcoma but in only one of 21 control samples (5%). The same sequence was identified from Kaposi's sarcoma tissue in AIDS patients (the "classic" patient) and in HIV-negative homosexual men. Kennedy and associates (1998) detected HHV-8 in early lesions of Kaposi's sarcoma. They concluded this virus had a role in the pathogenesis of Kaposi's sarcoma, although the exact mechanism is not clear. In 1995, Karcher and Alkan confirmed this finding in several of their patients and also noted an association in Castleman's disease. In 1998, Jones and associates discovered an associated HHV-8 infection in an immunosuppressed, HIV-negative cardiac transplant patient who developed Kaposi's sarcoma. This strong association suggests that human herpesvirus is an initiator of the process leading to the development of Kaposi's sarcoma. In addition, Cesarman and coworkers (1995) identified an HHV-8 DNA sequence in eight of eight effusion lymphomas, which strongly suggests a link between HHV-8 and effusion lymphomas (effusion lymphomas are discussed in greater detail under Primary Effusion Lymphomas, later in this chapter).

Besides the EBV theory of the etiology of lymphoma described previously, HIV itself exerts a strong influence on the lymphatic system. In Knowles' (1997) review of HIV lymphomagenesis, he concluded that HIV is not directly involved in the malignant transformation of B cells nor, consequently, in the induction of B-cell lymphomas. Both functional and quantitative defects can be measured in the CD4 T cells. Pantaleo and colleagues (1993) described the expansion of the B-cell population induced by a variety of factors, including IL-1, IL-2, IL-4, IL-6, IL-7, IL-10, and tumor necrosis factor-α. This stimulation leads to generalized lymphadenopathy and monoclonal hypergammaglobulinemia. Such intense stimulation magnifies the DNA rearrangements. Pelicci and associates (1986) reported on the multiple clonal rearrangements, espousing the theory that subsequent selection and growth advantage goes to the eventual development of a monoclonal B-cell malignancy. Finally, translocations, particularly of t(8;14), t(8;2), and t(8;22) result in the deregulation of *c-myc* present on chromosome 8. Laurence and Astrin (1991) showed that HIV infection of immortalized B-cell lines results in upregulation of *c-myc*. Lombardi and associates (1987) demonstrated that increased activity of *c-myc* resulted in transformation of B cells.

Chronic B-cell stimulation is present in HIV-infected patients, as manifest by polyclonal hypergammaglobulinemia and the persistent generalized lymphadenopathy syndrome. This may be another factor contributing to the development of lymphomas in HIV-positive patients. Pelicci and colleagues (1986) postulated that HIV immunosuppression allows an EBV infection, which results in polyclonal B-cell activation. Because the B-cell regulation is now aberrant, it allows some EBV-infected, immortalized B cells to undergo *c-myc* gene rearrangement and become lymphomas. This does not completely explain the pathogenesis of their lymphomas because, as Hamilton-Dutoit and coworkers (1989, 1991) have pointed out, only about one-half of AIDS lymphomas contain EBV.

Similar mechanisms are at work in the development of uterine cervical cancer. HIV and human papillomavirus are both sexually transmitted diseases and may have a synergistic influence on the development of cervical epithelial neoplasia.

SECOND NEOPLASM SYNDROMES

During the 1970s, transplantation was offered to patients who had a history of a malignancy or who were receiving chemotherapy for existing cancers. Penn (1976) found that there was a 4% incidence of new malignancies in the group with a preexisting malignancy, which was not different from the 6% incidence of de novo cancer development in patients with no evidence of cancer before transplantation. However, he found that 166 new malignancies began in 160 patients receiving chemotherapy for 161 tumors. This striking occurrence was blamed directly on the combination of immunosuppression and anticancer chemotherapy. Today, strict criteria are used for selecting cancer patients for possible transplantation; cancers must have been low-grade malignancies, and the patients must be disease-free for at least 5 years.

A special group of patients is the group who survived aggressive chemotherapy 20 or more years previously only to develop second cancers. The patients who have received recent attention are survivors of Hodgkin's disease. Most of these patients were children treated between 1970 and 1990. This was first reported by Sont and colleagues (1992) from Leiden, the Netherlands. Tucker, of the United States National Cancer Institute, acknowledged this serious problem in 1993. In a follow-up study, van Leeuwen and associates (1994) reviewed the statistics from the Netherlands Cancer Center, discovering a 3.5-fold increased rate of cancer among 1939 Hodgkin's patients over that expected in the general population. They found that the second cancers, in decreasing frequency, were leukemia, non-Hodgkin's lymphoma, lung cancer, gastrointestinal cancers, urogenital cancers,

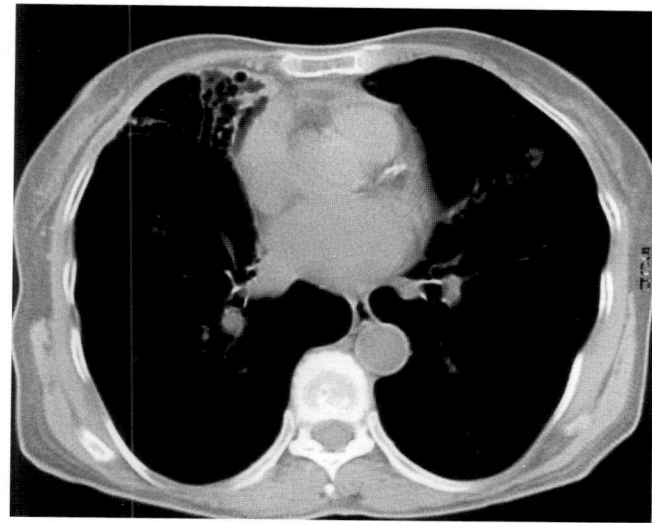

Fig. 114-2. Radiograph of a patient with lung cancer that developed 20 years after mantle radiation therapy for Hodgkin's lymphoma. The lesion appears as a deepening density in the area of the scar from the previous irradiation.

melanoma, and soft tissue sarcoma. By contrast, Wolden and colleagues (1998) of Stanford studied 694 treated patients, finding that the most common solid tumors were breast cancer and sarcoma. Oddou and associates (1998) described six patients (of 171) who developed second neoplasms after treatment of their lymphomas with chemotherapy and autologous stem cell transplantation. One of these patients was a 55-year-old man who developed a squamous cell carcinoma of the lung. He was a cigarette smoker.

Analysis by van Leeuwen's group found that risk factors for the development of second cancers in Hodgkin's disease included chemotherapy during the first year, follow-up chemotherapy, age greater than 40 at first diagnosis, splenectomy, and advanced stage. Earlier forms of chemotherapy led to a higher risk of developing leukemia. Women less than 20 years of age when treated with mantle radiation had a 40-fold increase in breast cancer. Risk of lung cancer was strongly related to treatment with thoracic irradiation (Fig. 114-2). These patients usually have lesions in the apex of the lung, which could be bilateral in those who had mantle radiation.

PULMONARY TUMORS PRODUCED BY IMMUNOSUPPRESSION

In HIV-positive patients, the most common tumors are non-Hodgkin's lymphomas and Kaposi's sarcoma. Transplant patients develop PTLD. More recently, smooth muscle tumors have been described as a rare complication after transplantation. Many tumors presenting in immunosuppressed patients look and act the same as they would in an immunocompetent patient, but stage for stage, the prognosis is worse.

Pham and colleagues (1995) evaluated 608 cardiac transplant recipients, of whom 10 developed lung cancer. Eight of the 10 patients had stage III disease at the time of diagnosis. All patients had a poor prognosis. Taniguchi and coworkers (1997) subsequently reported on four patients with bronchial carcinoma. The morphologies were diverse. Three patients died at 1, 6, and 11 months after diagnosis. Only one survived to live 15 months after multimodality therapy.

Kaposi's Sarcoma

Recognized and studied most thoroughly in the AIDS population, Kaposi's sarcoma is of uncertain cellular origin and does not fulfill all the criteria for a true cancer. As reviewed by Levine (1993), it has not been demonstrated that this sarcoma possesses clonality or clonal chromosomal abnormalities.

Mitchell (1992) and Miller (1992) and their associates reviewed the subject of pulmonary involvement by Kaposi's sarcoma. All 48 of their patients were men with ages ranging from 24 to 55 years. Their main presenting symptoms were cough and shortness of breath. A rare patient complained of chest pain or hemoptysis. On physical examination, all patients had cutaneous Kaposi's sarcoma, and most also had oral lesions. Pulmonary function studies showed normal values for peak flow, forced expiratory volume in 1 second, and functional vital capacity in patients with localized disease but reduced values in patients with widespread disease. In both groups of patients, the carbon monoxide transfer factor and the transfer factor were reduced.

Clinical presentation varies with the organ system involved. The incidence of pulmonary Kaposi's sarcoma is difficult to determine. The autopsy study of Meduri and associates (1986) found Kaposi's sarcoma in the lungs of 47% of patients with cutaneous lesions. The lesions are purple, reddish, or brown macules or patches. The most common presenting lesions are in the genital area, followed by the gastrointestinal tract. When the gastrointestinal tract is involved, the oral cavity is involved 50% of the time. Occasionally, patients develop involvement of lymph nodes and may present with lymphedema. Pulmonary or pleural involvement, or both, is serious and is a harbinger of short life expectancy.

Radiographically, pleural effusions are common. The chest radiographs vary in their findings, depending on whether the lesions are localized or widespread. In localized disease, they may be normal or they may show bilateral interstitial patterns and, rarely, a bilateral coarse reticulonodular pattern or lobar consolidation. Patients with widespread disease can have chest radiographs that show a normal pattern, perihilar infiltrates, bilateral interstitial shadows, bilateral coarse reticulonodular shadows, or lobar consolidation. Parenchymal lesions are best seen on CT scan and appear as discrete, low-attenuation nodules or as an infiltrate.

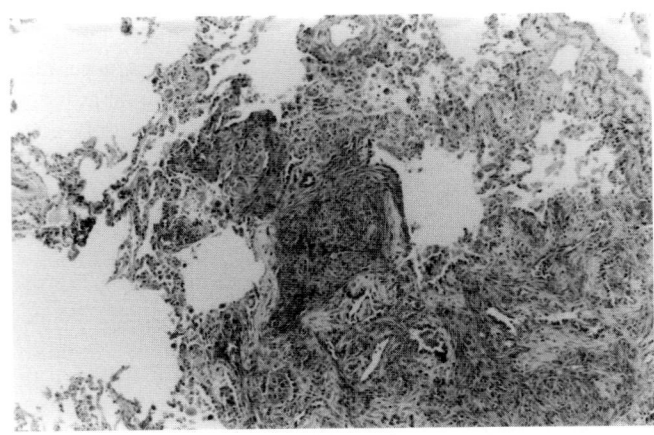

Fig. 114-3. Kaposi's sarcoma in the lung. The interstitial and peri-bronchial areas of the lung are thickened by cells with bland spindle-shaped nuclei.

Pulmonary Kaposi's sarcoma is usually diagnosed bronchoscopically. However, lesions can be seen on the visceral or parietal pleura. In the airway, the lesions may be submucosal patches or heaped-up mucosa with a red color. They may be friable and bleed when biopsied. The patients in both studies were not biopsied because of the concern about bleeding. Intrathoracic lesions look like skin lesions and are usually limited in size.

On microscopic examination, the early stage of the disease shows a proliferation of thin-walled vessels around larger vessels (Fig. 114-3). They also usually have a sparse surrounding infiltrate of lymphocytes and plasma cells (Fig. 114-4). The more mature lesions are composed of plump, bland spindle cells with slitlike spaces filled with red blood cells (Fig. 114-5). Hemosiderin as well as some lymphocytes and plasma cells are seen around the periphery of the lesion.

Although single-agent chemotherapy has been used, combination therapy is best for patients with pulmonary Kaposi's sarcoma. Gill and colleagues (1991) gave what is now known

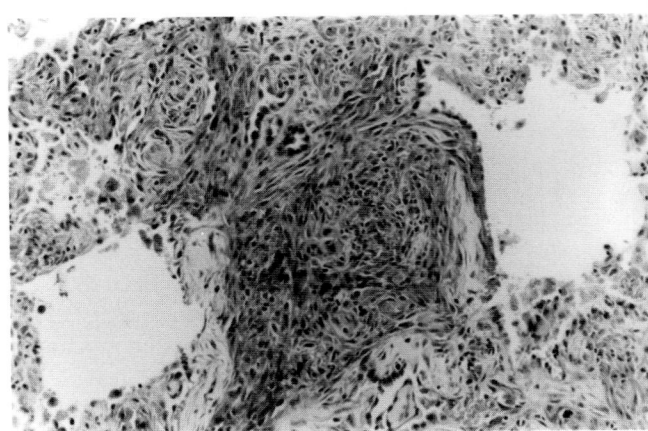

Fig. 114-4. Kaposi's sarcoma in the lung. In the center and the lower right, the interstitium is thickened by abundant spindle cells.

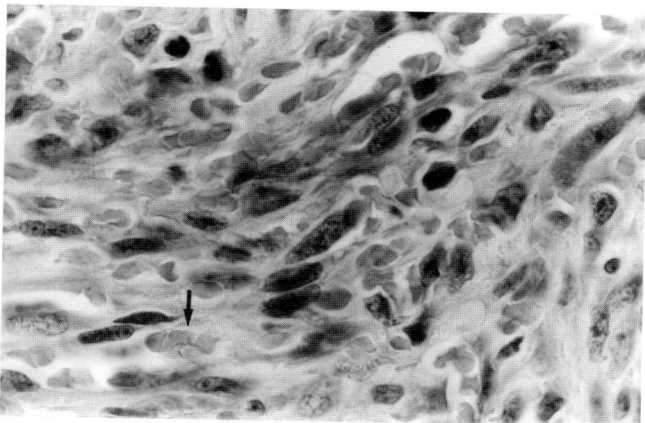

Fig. 114-5. Kaposi's sarcoma in the lung. The bland spindle-shaped nuclei of Kaposi's sarcoma with adjacent slitlike spaces containing red blood cells (*arrow*).

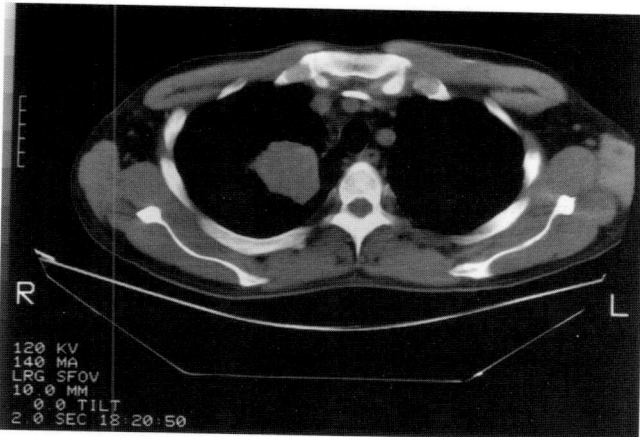

Fig. 114-6. Solitary nodular lymphoma in the right upper lobe of a patient with acquired immunodeficiency syndrome. This lesion is irregularly convex and homogeneous.

as ABV chemotherapy [doxorubicin (20 mg/m^2), bleomycin (10 mg/m^2), and vincristine (2 mg)] every 2 weeks to patients with widely disseminated gastrointestinal Kaposi's sarcoma. They observed an 88% response rate with ABV chemotherapy, a 38% response rate with Adriamycin alone, and a 20% opportunistic infection rate.

Shepherd and associates (1997) at Toronto Hospital treated biopsy-proven Kaposi's sarcoma in 12 transplant patients. They initially reduced or withdrew immunosuppression and used local radiation therapy. This was sufficient therapy in seven of the patients. They gave ABV therapy to the remaining five, who either had disseminated Kaposi's sarcoma or who did not respond to immunomodulation. Four of five responded, two with complete remission. The last patient was given third-line chemotherapy of cisplatin and etoposide, with a response. Only grade 1 toxicities were encountered. In the report of Mitchell and coworkers (1992), all 19 of their patients died, with a median survival of 7 months.

Lymphoma

Non-Hodgkin's lymphomas occur in all groups of immunosuppressed patients. As a whole, the lymphomas are very different from the non-Hodgkin's lymphomas found in the general population (Fig. 114-6). B-cell lymphomas are the most common and are intermediate or high grade in type. Some large cell types have been reported in transplant and AIDS patients. T-cell lymphomas also have been encountered. Kohler and colleagues (1995) described an HIV-positive patient with a primary T-cell lymphoma of the lung. The patient was an HIV-positive, 32-year-old man. He presented with a right upper lobe mass that, on histologic examination, was an intermediate-grade, mixed small and large cell lymphoma of T-cell type. The patient refused treatment and died

19 months after diagnosis. Today, after histologic confirmation of lymphoma is made, the tumor is further classified by immunohistochemistry, flow cytometry, and DNA extraction to detect gene rearrangements.

Any anatomic site may be involved with non-Hodgkin's lymphoma. Extranodal disease occurs in 75% of patients. The central nervous system (CNS) is involved nearly 50% of the time. Other areas include the gastrointestinal tract (40%), the bone marrow (33%), and the liver (26%). Involvement of the lung is unusual but significant.

In HIV-positive patients, the incidence of both non-Hodgkin's and Hodgkin's lymphoma is greater than that in the general population. The non-Hodgkin's lymphomas, according to Said (1997), are 70 to 90% high-grade immunoblastic or small noncleaved (Burkitt's-like). In AIDS-associated pulmonary lymphomas, the distinction must be made between a primary pulmonary lymphoma and secondary pulmonary involvement by a disseminated lymphoma.

Primary Pulmonary Lymphoma

Ray and associates (1998) described 11 men and one woman with AIDS who had primary pulmonary lymphomas. They ranged in age from 32 to 56 years. The main risk factors were homosexuality, with a few patients being intravenous drug users and one patient having had a blood transfusion. Most had a history of opportunistic infections or Kaposi's sarcoma. The interval from the diagnosis of HIV disease until the diagnosis of lymphoma ranged from 1 to 8 years, with an average of 5 years. The symptoms of these patients included cough, dyspnea, and chest pain, with most of them having systemic symptoms (B symptoms), including fever, weight loss, and, less commonly, night sweats. The mean CD4 cell count was 17/μL, with a range from 4 to 50/μL. The serum lactate dehydrogenase was 1.5 times normal in four patients. The most common finding on the chest radiographs was a well-defined nodule (≤2 cm) or a mass (>2 cm) in the subpleural area. Occasionally, cavitary lesions developed. Lee and colleagues (1997) reviewed the chest radiographic findings in primary pulmonary lymphomas. Their most common finding was an area of opacification with poorly defined margins and an air bronchogram. Less common findings were nodules, diffuse bilateral air space consolidation, and segmental or lobar atelectasis. The chest CT scans showed no mediastinal lymph nodes exceeding 1 cm in diameter. Five of the patients showed cavitary lesions.

On gross examination, the lesions were white to yellow solid nodules that sometimes had soft central areas of necrosis. On microscopic examination, six cases were diagnosed as high-grade lymphoma, not otherwise specified. The others were mostly immunoblastic and centroblastic (large noncleaved cell) lymphomas. On immunophenotyping, 11 cases were B cell and one was null cell. All 12 cases had EBV latent membrane protein-1 by immunohistochemistry. Eleven patients, with one not tested, had EBV-encoded RNA transcripts by in situ hybridization. These findings strongly implicate EBV in the pathogenesis of these lymphomas. All except one patient were treated. The untreated patient died before therapy began. The other patients received various combinations of agents, which included CHOP (cyclophosphamide, Adriamycin, vincristine, prednisone) or parts of CHOP as well as etoposide, bleomycin, cisplatinum, and Novantrone. All patients died either from their lymphoma or intercurrent conditions. The median survival after diagnosis was 4 months, with a range of less than 1 month to 17 months.

Teruya-Feldstein and associates (1995) described a lymphoma of mucosa-associated lymphoid tissue (MALT) in the lung of a 7-year-old girl who had been HIV positive since she was 2 years old. In February 1992, she developed enlarged submandibular and submental lymph nodes. The following month, a chest radiograph showed a left upper lobe lung lesion. In August 1993, the patient's mother consented to removal of the lesion after it had grown on two consecutive computed tomographic (CT) scans. Grossly, it was a solid, white-tan mass that measured 4 cm in greatest dimension. On microscopic examination, the lesion was composed of a dense lymphoid infiltrate with germinal centers surrounded by monocytoid cells, small lymphocytes, and plasma cells. Lymphoepithelial lesions were present. The remaining lung tissue showed pulmonary lymphoid hyperplasia and lymphocytic interstitial pneumonitis. Immunohistochemical stains showed staining for λ light chains but not for κ light chains. EBV in situ hybridization was positive in a few background cells, thus suggesting that EBV was not an important factor in the development of this MALT lymphoma. Southern blot studies showed clonal immunoglobulin gene rearrangements. All these findings are consistent with a MALT lymphoma. The patient received no further treatment, and a CT scan done in December 1993 showed no evidence of recurrent tumor.

Secondary Pulmonary Lymphoma

In contrast to primary lymphomas, the lung frequently is involved secondarily by lymphomas in AIDS patients. Eisner and colleagues (1996) reviewed 38 HIV-infected patients with pulmonary or pleural involvement by non-Hodgkin's lymphoma. Their 38 patients were all men, with a mean age of 40.5 years and a range from 28 to 61 years. The main risk factors were homosexuality and intravenous drug use, with a small percentage of patients having no known risk factors. Approximately one-third of the patients had a history of an opportunistic infection, and one-fourth had a history of Kaposi's sarcoma. Most had cough, dyspnea, or chest pain, and almost all had systemic symptoms (B symptoms), such as fever, weight loss, or night sweats. On physical examination, the patients had tachypnea (74%), crackles (37%), dullness to percussion (26%), decreased breath sounds (26%), and bronchial breath sounds (24%). Laboratory examination showed low CD4 counts (67 ± 6.5 cells/μL). The sedimentation rate and serum lactate dehydrogenase were usually elevated.

Almost all the chest radiographs were abnormal. The most common patterns were lobar consolidation (40%), nodules (40%), reticular infiltrates (24%), and masses (24%). Dodd and associates (1992) reviewed the chest radiographs of patients with AIDS-related lymphoma. Their most common abnormalities were pleural effusions (47%), reticulonodular infiltrates and alveolar consolidation (22%), hilar and mediastinal adenopathy (22%), pulmonary nodules or masses (17%), and pericardial effusions or masses (13%). Pleural effusions were present in many patients (44%). Lee and coworkers (1997) also reviewed the chest radiographic findings in AIDS patients with secondary pulmonary involvement. Their most common findings were thickening of bronchovascular bundles (41%), discrete pulmonary nodules (39%), and areas of consolidation (14%). Other findings include cavitated masses and bronchial masses. They also described CT scan findings of masses or masslike areas of consolidation larger than 1 cm (68%) and nodules smaller than 1 cm (61%). The CT scans described by Eisner and colleagues (1996) showed parenchymal nodules (50%), lobar consolidations (27%), and masses (19%). Pleural effusions were also present in many of the patients.

On microscopic examination, the lymphomas of Eisner and colleagues (1996) were immunoblastic (61%), large cell (18%), Burkitt's (5.3%), small noncleaved (2.6%), and undifferentiated high-grade lymphomas (13%). They found the lungs to be the most common extranodal site (71%) of involvement in patients with non-Hodgkin's lymphoma. Unfortunately, studies for EBV were not reported for these cases. They suggested transbronchial biopsy, pleural fluid cytology, pleural biopsy, transthoracic needle biopsy, and open lung biopsy as the most useful methods of obtaining a diagnosis. In their series, they did not discuss treatment or survival of these patients. In additional studies by Hamilton-Dutoit and associates (1989, 1991), EBV was detected only in approximately 50% of these patients. Other studies have lower rates. This is in contrast to PTLD, in which EBV is detected in about 95% of cases.

The best therapy for lymphoma in patients who are not infected with HIV is CHOP chemotherapy. Attempts at more aggressive therapy did not result in greater response, as noted by Fisher and coworkers (1993). For HIV-associated lymphomas, various therapies have been tried. No specific regimen has emerged as the best. However, two seem to have a good response rate with fewer side effects. Kaplan and colleagues (1991) used CHOP with granulocyte-macrophage colony-stimulating factor, which kept the nadir granulocyte counts higher, thus decreasing the complication rate. Levine and associates (1991) used methotrexate, bleomycin, doxorubicin, cyclophosphamide, vincristine, and dexamethasone (M-BACOD) as a "less is more" therapy with success. Walsh of their group (1993) later reported use of M-BACOD with granulocyte-macrophage colony-stimulating factor, with a 67% complete response rate and only a 10% opportunistic infection rate.

Said (1997) discussed the relationship between Hodgkin's disease and HIV-positive patients. The incidence of Hodgkin's disease is increased in HIV-positive patients, but Hodgkin's disease is not a defining criterion for AIDS. Hodgkin's disease has a more aggressive course in HIV-positive individuals. A definite causal link between HIV, EBV, and Hodgkin's disease has not been established.

Summary

HIV-positive patients have a high incidence of non-Hodgkin's lymphoma. The lymphomas are usually of high grade and stage when they are diagnosed, and the patients have a short survival. The lymphomas may be primary pulmonary lymphomas or, more frequently, represent secondary pulmonary involvement. EBV may be detected in approximately 50% of these patients. This is in contrast to CNS lymphomas, which are almost all associated with EBV. MALT lymphomas, T-cell lymphomas, and Hodgkin's disease may occur in HIV-positive patients, but they are far less common.

POSTTRANSPLANT LYMPHOPROLIFERATIVE DISORDERS

Thoracic organ transplant patients seem particularly susceptible to PTLD. The presentation ranges from asymptomatic pulmonary nodules to multiorgan failure. Symptoms are usually associated with enlarged lymph nodes.

PTLDs occur more frequently in patients who have lung, liver, and heart transplants than in those with kidney transplants. In kidney transplants, the clinician is more likely to temper the immunosuppression because the patient can always be returned to dialysis. With other organ transplants, this is not a viable alternative, and when rejection occurs, immunosuppression is usually increased. Morrison and col-

leagues (1994) described 26 patients with PTLD, some of whom had pulmonary involvement. Ferry and associates (1989) described a clinical series of PTLD, although none of her patients had pulmonary involvement. Hsi and coworkers (1998) described a patient with a PTLD of the natural killer cell type. Basgoz and Preiksaitis (1995) reviewed the subject of PTLD and described the clinical characteristics of the disease.

Clinical Presentation

The age and sex of the patients would depend on the transplantation recipient. The risk factors for the development of PTLD are listed in Table 114-4. They include the type of organ transplant, primary EBV infection, the type of immunosuppression (e.g., antilymphocyte antibody, cyclosporin A, FK 506), HLA mismatch, and cytomegalovirus disease. Kidney transplant recipients have a less than 1% chance of developing PTLD, whereas liver transplant recipients have a 4% chance, and heart-lung recipients have a 10% chance. The greater the degree of immunosuppression, the greater the risk of developing a PTLD. A patient with a primary EBV infection after transplantation is more at risk than is a person who was EBV seropositive before receiving the organ. In bone marrow transplant recipients, the greatest incidence of PTLD occurred among patients with HLA mismatching. Patients with previous symptomatic infections of cytomegalovirus are also at increased risk for PTLD.

PTLDs may present in a variety of ways. Newly transplanted patients who develop a primary EBV infection may present with an infectious mononucleosislike illness. They have a febrile illness with leukopenia, pharyngitis, fevers, lymphadenopathy, and hepatosplenomegaly. Laboratory testing may not show atypical lymphocytosis, heterophile antibodies, or antibodies to specific EBV antigens. Patients who develop PTLD months or years after transplantation may present with persistent fever, malaise, and leukopenia without localizing signs. Therefore, any long-term transplant patient should be evaluated for PTLD as well as a variety of infectious agents, if they develop generalized symptoms. The CNS is a favored site. These patients may present with subtle alterations of mental status or advanced neurologic findings. If the gastrointestinal tract is involved,

Table 114-4. Risk Factors for the Development of Posttransplant Lymphoproliferative Disorders

Type of organ transplant
Primary Epstein-Barr virus infection
Type and intensity of immunosuppression
    Antilymphocyte antibody
    Cyclosporin A
    FK 506
HLA mismatch
Cytomegalovirus disease

patients may present with abdominal pain, gastrointestinal bleeding, obstruction, or bowel perforation. PTLD may involve such organs as the lung, liver, kidney, allograft, lymph nodes, and bone marrow.

Radiographic Features

Rappaport and colleagues (1998) reviewed radiographic images of lymphoproliferative disorders in lung transplant patients. They presented data on nine patients who developed PTLD of 246 transplant patients. Eight of the nine had only intrathoracic disease. The most common presentation was multiple, well-defined nodules with a basilar and peripheral prominence. Other presentations were mediastinal adenopathy, upper lobe consolidation, and a pleural mass. Dodd (1992) and Lee (1997) and their associates reviewed the radiologic manifestations of thoracic PTLD. The radiologic findings are nonspecific and varied. They include multiple nodules scattered throughout the lungs ranging from 0.5 to 2.0 cm, solitary masses ranging up to 5 cm, an interstitial pattern of disease, and an alveolar disease pattern. These patients may or may not have hilar adenopathy (Fig. 114-7). Pleural effusions are common.

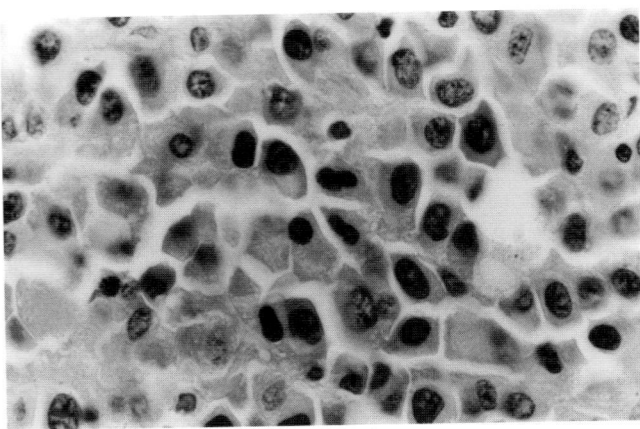

Fig. 114-8. Posttransplant lymphoproliferative disorder. This lesion is composed of a sheet of plasma cells with eccentrically placed nuclei.

Pathology

Because PTLD is a recently described disease, the pathology and nomenclature are undergoing an evolution. The origin of the disease appears to be an infection of lymphocytes by EBV that develops into a lymphoid proliferation (Fig. 114-8). The exact mechanism by which the transformation takes place is not completely understood, although various explanations have been put forward. Chadburn and associates (1995), using molecular analysis of involved and uninvolved recipient tissue, were able to determine that PTLD in solid organ transplant patients derives from the recipients' tissue. This is in contrast to bone marrow transplants, in whom the majority of PTLDs are of donor origin.

PTLD is the catch-all phrase used to describe a variety of lymphoid lesions, ranging from benign lymphoid proliferations to malignant lymphomas. Swerdlow (1992, 1997) reviewed the various classifications, and Harris and colleagues (1997) reviewed the morphology for the different categories of PTLD. Three published classifications exist for PTLD. The first is the one by Frizzera and colleagues (1981), which was later modified by Shapiro and coworkers (1988) with the help of Frizzera. The second is the one by Nalesnik and associates (1988), which was later modified by Wu and colleagues (1996). Knowles and coworkers (1995) published the third classification.

All three classifications have distinct merits, but the nomenclature is confusing. One reason for a classification is to determine treatment. In some cases, PTLD regresses if immunosuppression is stopped, whereas in others, PTLD progresses in spite of therapy. All three of these classifications use one or more of the terms *atypical, polymorphic,* and *monomorphic.* Before discussing the classifications, it is appropriate to define these terms. *Atypical* is defined as irregular or not conforming to type. In terms of a pathologic description, it can mean: 1) a certain cell that is not in its

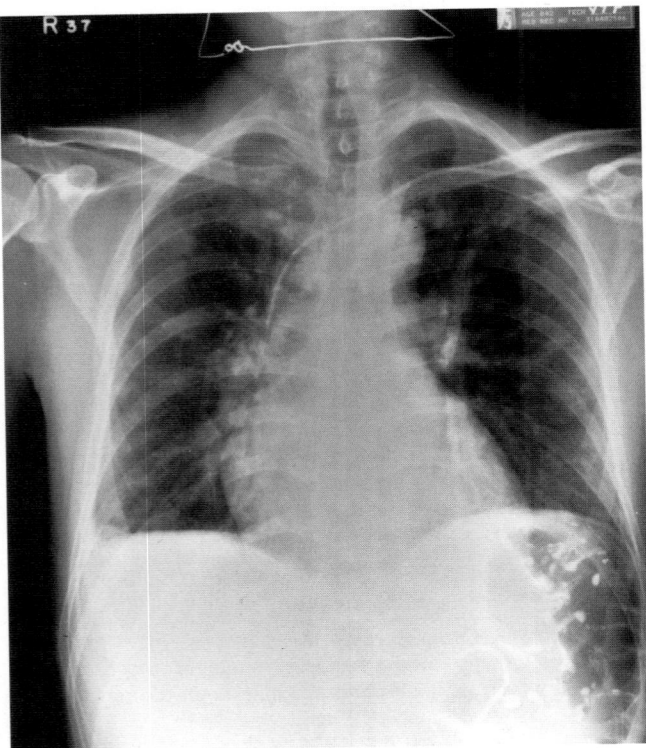

Fig. 114-7. Chest radiograph of a liver transplant patient with posttransplant lymphoproliferative disorder. Lesions are finely nodular and are present mainly in the lower lobe.

Table 114-5. Frizzera's Classification of Posttransplant Lymphoproliferative Disorders, as Modified by Shapiro

Atypical lymphoid hyperplasia
Polymorphic diffuse B-cell hyperplasia
Atypical polymorphic diffuse B-cell hyperplasia
Polymorphic diffuse B-cell lymphoma
Immunoblastic sarcoma of B cells

Reproduced with slight modifications from Swerdlow SH: Classification of the post-transplant lymphoproliferative disorders: from the past to the present. Semin Diagn Pathol *14*:2, 1997.

Table 114-6. Nalesnik's Classification of Posttransplant Lymphoproliferative Disorders, as Modified by Wu

Epstein-Barr virus–positive lymphadenitis resembling infectious mononucleosis
Polymorphic posttransplant lymphoproliferative disorder
Monomorphic posttransplant lymphoproliferative disorder

Reproduced with slight modifications from Swerdlow SH: Classification of the post-transplant lymphoproliferative disorders: from the past to the present. Semin Diagn Pathol *14*:2, 1997.

proper location in the lymph node, 2) an abnormal increase of a certain type of cell, or 3) cells with an irregular nucleus, which gives them an "atypical" appearance. *Polymorphous* means that many different cell types are present, such as lymphocytes, plasma cells, and immunoblasts. It also suggests that, because the lesion is composed of different cell types, it is not yet a lymphoma. *Monomorphic* means only one cell type is present, such as immunoblasts. Because these lesions are of the same cell type, they are consistent with a lymphoma.

Shapiro and coworkers (1988) modified the earliest classification of Frizzera and colleagues (1981) (Table 114-5). These authors described five types of PTLD, which included atypical lymphoid hyperplasia, polymorphic diffuse B-cell hyperplasia, atypical polymorphic diffuse B-cell hyperplasia, polymorphic diffuse B-cell lymphoma, and immunoblastic sarcoma of B cells. They distinguished PTLD from reactive lymph nodes by their invasiveness, diffuse distribution of follicular center cells, architectural effacement, and a prominent large cell component mimicking malignant lymphoma. *Invasiveness* refers to infiltration of the vessel walls, nodal fibrous trabeculae, capsule, and extranodal tissues by lymphoid cells. Atypical lymphoid hyperplasia shows a polymorphic paracortical or interstitial proliferation that lacks invasiveness but has an abundance of immunoblasts as well as small lymphocytes with irregular nuclei. Polymorphic diffuse B-cell hyperplasia shows a diffuse proliferation of cells, resembling cleaved and noncleaved follicular center cells, small lymphocytes, plasma cells, and immunoblasts. Atypical polymorphic diffuse B-cell hyperplasia is similar to polymorphic diffuse B-cell hyperplasia, except that it has nuclear atypia and multinucleation of large cells. Polymorphic diffuse B-cell lymphoma shows extensive coagulative necrosis and atypical immunoblasts. The immunoblasts are atypical because of their nuclei. These nuclear changes include bilobulation or multilobulation, deep grooves, and irregular borders. The immunoblastic sarcoma of B cells is composed of cells that have enlarged oval nuclei with a vesicular appearance and nucleoli.

Wu and associates (1996) modified the second classification of Nalesnik and coworkers (1988) (Table 114-6). Their three categories are EBV-positive lymphadenitis resembling infectious mononucleosis, polymorphic PTLD, and monomorphic PTLD. EBV-positive lymphadenitis resembling infectious

mononucleosis has polymorphic cells, but it lacks an invasive growth pattern, and there is partial or complete architectural retention. The cells are composed of a scattering of follicular cells with lymphocytes and plasma cells. Polymorphic PTLD includes both polymorphic B-cell hyperplasia and polymorphic B-cell lymphoma of Frizzera and coworkers (1981). Monomorphic PTLD shows a population of lymphoid cells that are all at the same stage of differentiation. They can be either small or large noncleaved lymphocytes.

Knowles and coworkers' (1995) classification of PTLD correlated morphology and clonality of the cells, clonality of EBV, and alterations in oncogenes or tumor-suppressor genes (Table 114-7). Their first category is plasmacytic hyperplasia. It is most commonly located in the oropharynx or the lymph nodes. It consists of an expansion of the interfollicular area of a lymph node by plasmacytoid lymphocytes, plasma cells, and sparse immunoblasts. Germinal centers may be hyperplastic, involuted, or absent. These are polyclonal, have only a minor cell population infected by a single form of EBV, and lack oncogene and tumor-suppressor gene alterations. The second category, polymorphic B-cell hyperplasia and polymorphic B-cell lymphoma, is the morphologic equivalent of polymorphic B-cell hyperplasia and lymphoma of Frizzera and coworkers (1981) and the polymorphic PTLD of Nalesnik and associates (1988). These PTLDs may arise in nodal and extranodal sites. They are monoclonal, contain a single form of EBV, but lack oncogene or tumor-suppressor gene alterations. The last category is immunoblastic lymphoma or multiple myeloma. Immunoblastic lymphomas are composed of a monomorphic cell population that have either enlarged, bizarre pleomorphic nuclei or plasmacytoid nuclei. Multiple myeloma is composed of a dense infiltrate of atypical plasma cells. Both are generally widely disseminated at the time of presenta-

Table 114-7. Knowles' Classification of Posttransplant Lymphoproliferative Disorders

Plasmacytic hyperplasia
Polymorphic B-cell hyperplasia and polymorphic B-cell lymphoma
Immunoblastic lymphoma or multiple myeloma

From Swerdlow SH: Classification of the post-transplant lymphoproliferative disorders: from the past to the present. Semin Diagn Pathol *14*:2, 1997. With permission.

Table 114-8. Recognized Patterns of Posttransplant Lymphoproliferative Disorders (PTLDs)

Plasma cell hyperplasia
Infectious mononucleosislike PTLD
Plasma cell–rich PTLD
Polymorphic PTLD
Monomorphic PTLD
    Small noncleaved–like
    Immunoblastic B cell–like
Polymorphic with predominantly transformed cells
Not otherwise specified
Multiple myelomalike PTLD
T cell–type PTLD
Hodgkin's disease–like PTLD
Composite PTLD
Not otherwise specified PTLD
Other

From Swerdlow SH: Classification of the post-transplant lympho-proliferative disorders: from the past to the present. Semin Diagn Pathol *14*:2, 1997. With permission.

tion. They are monoclonal, contain a single form of EBV, and have alterations in one or more oncogenes (N-*ras* gene codon 61 point mutation, or *c-myc* gene rearrangement) or tumor-suppressor genes (*p53* mutation).

Swerdlow (1997) summarized all the categories of PTLD (Table 114-8). In addition to the histology, these lesions should be evaluated for cellular monoclonality and oncogene or tumor-suppressor gene mutations.

Treatment

Basgoz and Preiksaitis (1995) point out that the treatment varies for PTLD. It includes reduction in immunosuppression, surgical resection, antiviral treatment, radiation therapy, cytotoxic chemotherapy, IFN, and gamma globulin as well as a variety of experimental treatments. In 1984, Starzl and coworkers reported a regression of PTLD with a decrease in immunosuppression. Regression has been observed in localized or polyclonal lesions as well as some multifocal or monoclonal cases. Therefore, decreased immunosuppression is the first step in treatment. The next step may include resection or irradiation of a localized lesion. According to Morrison and coworkers (1994), more extensive disease may be treated with standard combination chemotherapy regimens, which include CHOP; CHOP-bleomycin; cyclophosphamide, vincristine methotrexate, leucovorin, cytosine, and arabinoside; cyclophosphamide, vincristine, prednisone; M-BACOD; etoposide, doxorubicin, cyclophosphamide, vincristine, bleomycin, and prednisone; and ifosfamide and etoposide. Antiviral agents, such as acyclovir and ganciclovir, have been used to stop the replication of EBV. Their value in treating PTLD is in patients with polyclonal lesions rather than those with monoclonal ones.

Mentzer and associates (1998) used a unique way to achieve success in controlling this disease. They began with the usual therapy for one of their lung transplant patients with posttransplant lymphoma. As in other series, the therapy was ineffective. They established a cell line from the lymphoma and "activated" the virus by inducing the enzyme thymidine kinase with arginine butyrate. With this combination, the ganciclovir was effective and seemed to work synergistically with the chemotherapy to produce tumor necrosis.

Prognosis

In the study by Morrison and associates (1994), eight of 26 patients (31%) were rendered disease free by surgery or radiation therapy, or they achieved complete remission by chemotherapy. The remission duration ranged from 8 to 122 months. Of the 26 patients, 21 (81%) died. Their survival ranged from less than 1 month to 122 months, with a median of 14 months. In summary, the survival for patients who develop PTLD is not very good.

At this point, a strategy to prevent PTLD would be helpful. The objective would be to minimize the previously discussed risk factors associated with PTLD. Other strategies involve vaccinating EBV-seronegative recipients. The development of methods to determine viral load may indicate the patients who are more susceptible to developing PTLD and who may benefit from antiviral chemotherapy. Finally, because the EBV latency gene products play a major role in the transformation of cells, a method to inactivate these proteins might be useful in preventing PTLD.

POSTTRANSPLANT LYMPHOPROLIFERATIVE DISORDERS OF T-CELL ORIGIN

PTLDs of T-cell origin have also been described. Hsi and colleagues (1998) described the case of a 42-year-old man who underwent a cadaveric renal transplant for complete renal failure of unknown etiology. His immunosuppressive therapy consisted of cyclosporine, azathioprine, and prednisone. Eight years after transplantation, he developed a PTLD, which was diagnosed as a large cell malignant lymphoma. The immunophenotyping was consistent with a T-cell origin. The Southern blot studies did not show rearrangements of the heavy or light immunoglobulin genes or the T-cell receptor beta or gamma genes. The in situ hybridization for EBV-encoded RNA was negative. The polymerase chain reaction for detecting EBV genome was also negative.

The patient underwent an allograft nephrectomy as well as a nephrectomy of both native kidneys. Postoperatively, the patient was treated by a withdrawal of immunosuppression, acyclovir, and a single cycle of CHOP. The patient had a rapidly progressive disease and died 4 weeks after surgery. This case illustrates that not all PTLDs are of EBV-infected B-cell origin.

PRIMARY EFFUSION LYMPHOMA

Another lymphoma that occurs in HIV-positive patients is body cavity-based lymphoma or, as it is now called, *primary effusion lymphoma*. These lymphomas were probably first described by Knowles and colleagues (1989). They occur in both HIV-positive patients and transplant recipients. Jones and associates (1998) reported on this entity, as have Karcher and Alkan (1997). Primary effusion lymphomas are defined as lymphoma cells in body cavity effusions (pleural, pericardial, and peritoneal) with no identifiable contiguous tumor mass, lymphadenopathy, or organomegaly. These neoplasms are interesting because many of them contain both EBV and HHV-8. Cesarman and Knowles (1997) found HHV-8 in a significant proportion of patients with AIDS and in those with non–AIDS-related multicentric Castleman's disease.

Nador and colleagues (1996) described 19 cases of primary effusion lymphoma. Seventeen were in HIV-positive homosexual men who ranged in age from 31 to 58 years with a median age of 41 years; the other two were in HIV-negative men aged 79 and 85 years. Of the effusions, eight were in the pleural cavity, two in the pericardial cavity, seven in the peritoneal cavity, and one in both pleural and peritoneal cavities. The clinical symptoms of these patients are not described in the report. Morassut and coworkers (1997) described the radiologic findings in six patients with effusion lymphomas. The chest radiographs showed bilateral or unilateral pleural effusions with no evidence of pulmonary infiltrates or mediastinal enlargement. The CT scans confirmed the findings of the chest radiographs and also revealed a slight thickening of the parietal pleura in all patients and a pericardial thickening in four patients. They also revealed five patients with pericardial effusions and two patients with peritoneal effusions.

The pathologic features of these cases varied. In 15 cases, the malignant cells contained HHV-8, and in four they did not. Microscopic examination of the cells from the 15 HHV-8–positive cases revealed polymorphic large cells, which had features between a large cell immunoblastic lymphoma and an anaplastic large cell lymphoma. The four HHV-8–negative cases consisted of monomorphic medium-sized cells with round regular nuclei that resembled the cells of Burkitt's lymphoma. On immunophenotyping, five of the 19 cases had B-cell markers. The remaining 14 cases were indeterminate. The gene rearrangement studies were not performed on all cases. Sixteen of 17 cases had clonal heavy immunoglobulin gene rearrangement, 14 of 16 cases had clonal κ light-chain gene rearrangement, and four of 11 cases had clonal λ light-chain gene rearrangement. One case exhibited bigenotypism with clonal markers for both B and T cells. EBV was present in 18 of 19 cases, the exception being an HIV-negative, but HHV-8–positive 85-year-old man. HIV was not detected in any of the 19 effusions. The *c-myc* proto-oncogene was germline in the 12 HHV-8–positive cases tested. In contrast, the four HHV-8–negative lymphoma effusions displayed a rearrangement of *c-myc*. No other consistent genotypic changes were detected in these neoplasms.

Nine of the patients were treated with chemotherapy, three patients received supportive care, and the treatment for six patients is unknown. All patients had a poor prognosis, with 18 of 19 patients dying between 12 days and 14 months (median 5 months) after their diagnosis.

SMOOTH MUSCLE TUMORS

Benign and malignant smooth muscle tumors have been documented in posttransplant patients by Penn (1995) as well as by Lee (1995) and Timmons (1995) and their associates. In addition, these tumors have been reported in HIV-infected patients by van Hoeven and colleagues (1993). McClain and colleagues (1995) reported EBV infection in seven smooth muscle tumors (leiomyomas and leiomyosarcomas) from six children with HIV infection. In contrast, they found no evidence of EBV infection in normal muscle or tumors from HIV-negative children. They concluded that EBV had a role in the development of smooth muscle tumors in HIV-infected children.

Similar smooth muscle tumors have been described in liver transplant patients. Timmons (1995) and Lee (1995) and their coworkers found latent EBV in the neoplastic smooth muscle cells of transplant patients. One of the patients described by Lee and associates (1995) had multiple nodules of smooth muscle in the lung at the time of autopsy. In 1998, Somers and associates described a heart-lung transplant patient who developed multiple leiomyosarcomas in both the lung transplant and the host liver. The patient was a 15-year-old boy who underwent heart-lung transplantation for primary pulmonary hypertension at the age of 11 years. He was treated with cyclosporine, azathioprine, and prednisolone as well as a course of antithymocyte globulin to prevent rejection. He developed a chronic pulmonary infection with *Pseudomonas aeruginosa* that quickly became resistant to antibiotics. At 41 months after transplantation, he underwent a thoracic CT scan to evaluate bronchiectasis. He had multiple solid nodules approximately 0.5 cm in diameter throughout both lung fields. A CT scan of the abdomen did not show any abdominal disease. The patient was treated with decreased immunosuppression and intravenous ganciclovir, which was later changed to oral acyclovir. He eventually developed pneumonia and died 43 months after transplant. At autopsy, the patient had multiple nodules in both lungs as well as extensive suppurative bronchopneumonia. Two nodules were present in the liver. On histologic examination, the pulmonary and liver nodules were leiomyosarcomas. EBV DNA was extracted from lung tumor biopsy specimens but not from the autopsy lung and liver specimens. Somers and colleagues performed DNA amplification of microsatellite repeat polymorphisms. By this technique, they were able to demonstrate that the lung tumors arose from the donor tissue, whereas the liver lesions arose from host tissue. They postulated that the lack of detectable EBV DNA in the autopsy specimens was because of the treatment with ganciclovir and acyclovir. In conclusion, immunosuppressed patients can develop smooth muscle tumors of the lung. The evidence suggests these smooth muscle tumors develop in a manner analogous to PTLD.

REFERENCES

Alshafie MT, et al: Human immunodeficiency virus and lung cancer. Br J Surg 84:1068, 1997.

Basgoz N, Preiksaitis JK: Post-transplant lymphoproliferative disorder. Infect Dis Clin North Am 9:901, 1995.

Beral V, et al: Risk of Kaposi's sarcoma and sexual practices associated with fecal contact in homosexual or bisexual man with AIDS. Lancet 339:632, 1992.

Berger F, Delecluse HJ: Lymphomas in immunocompromised hosts. Rev Prat 43:1661, 1993.

Birkeland SA, et al: EBV-induced post-transplant lymphoproliferative disorder. Transplant Proc 27:3467, 1995.

Boyle GJ, et al: Posttransplantation lymphoproliferative disorders in pediatric thoracic organ recipients. J Pediatr 131:309, 1997.

Cesarman E, Knowles DM: Kaposi's sarcoma-associated herpesvirus: a lymphotropic human herpesvirus associated with Kaposi's sarcoma, primary effusion lymphoma and Castleman's disease. Semin Diagn Pathol 14:54, 1997.

Cesarman E, et al: Kaposi's sarcoma-associated herpesvirus-like DNA sequence are present in AIDS-related body cavity-based lymphomas. N Engl J Med 332:1186, 1995.

Chadburn A, et al: Post-transplantation lymphoproliferative disorders arising in solid organ transplant recipients are usually of recipient origin. Am J Pathol 147:1862, 1995.

Chang Y, et al: Identification of herpesvirus-like DNA sequences in AIDS-associated Kaposi's sarcoma. Science 266:1865, 1994.

Dockrell DH, et al: Epstein Barr virus induced T cell lymphoma in solid organ transplant recipients. Clin Infect Dis 26:180, 1998.

Dodd GD, Greenler DP, Confer SR: Thoracic and abdominal manifestations of lymphoma occurring in the immuno-compromised patient. Radiol Clin North Am 30:597, 1992.

Eisner MD, et al: The pulmonary manifestations of AIDS-related non-Hodgkin's lymphoma. Chest 110:729, 1996.

End A, et al: The pulmonary nodule after lung transplantation. Cause and outcome. Chest 107:1317, 1995.

Ferry JA, et al: Lymphoproliferative disorders and hematologic malignancies following organ transplantation. Mod Pathol 2:583, 1989.

Fisher RI, et al: Comparison of a standard regimen (CHOP) with three intensive chemotherapy regimens for advanced non-Hodgkin's lymphoma. N Engl J Med 328:1002, 1993.

Flores MR, et al: Lung cancer in patients with human immunodeficiency virus infection. Am J Clin Oncol 18:59, 1995.

Fraire AE, Awe RJ: Lung cancer in association with human immunodeficiency virus infection. Cancer 70:432, 1992.

Frizzera G, et al: Polymorphic diffuse B-cell hyperplasias and lymphomas in renal transplant recipients. Cancer Res 41:4262, 1981.

Gill PS, et al: A systemic treatment of AIDS-related Kaposi's sarcoma: results of a randomized trial. Am J Med 90:427, 1991.

Hamilton-Dutoit SJ, et al: Identification of EBV-DNA in tumour cells of AIDS-related lymphomas by in-situ hybridization. Lancet 1:554, 1989.

Hamilton-Dutoit SJ, et al: AIDS-related lymphoma: histopathology, immunophenotype, and association with EBV as demonstrated by in situ nucleic acid hybridization. Am J Pathol 138:149, 1991.

Hansen LA, Prakash UB, Colby TV: Pulmonary lymphoma in Sjögren's syndrome. Mayo Clin Proc 64:920, 1989.

Haque T, et al: Transmission of donor Epstein Barr virus (EBV) in transplanted organs causes lymphoproliferative disease in EBV seronegative recipients. J Gen Virol 77:1169, 1996.

Harris NL, Ferry JA, Swerdlow SH: Post-transplant lymphoproliferative disorders: summary of Society for Hematopathology Workshop. Semin Diagn Pathol 14:8, 1997.

Hsi ED, Pickens MM, Alkan S: Post-transplant lymphoproliferative disorder of the NK cell type: a case report and review of the literature. Mod Pathol 11:479, 1998.

International Society of Heart and Lung Transplantation: Fifteenth Annual Data Report. V. Post transplant events (US: April 1994–Dec 1997). ISHLT *Web site 1998.

Jones D, et al: Primary-effusion lymphoma and Kaposi's sarcoma in a cardiac-transplant recipient. N Engl J Med 339:444, 1998.

Kamel OW: Iatrogenic lymphoproliferative disorders in nontransplantation settings. Semin Diagn Pathol 14:27, 1997.

Kaplan LD, et al: Clinical and virologic effects of recombinant human granulocyte-macrophage colony-stimulating factor in patients receiving chemotherapy for human immunodeficiency virus-associated non-Hodgkin's lymphoma: results of a randomized trial. J Clin Oncol 9:929, 1991.

Karcher DS, Alkan S: Herpes-like DNA sequences, AIDS-related tumors and Castleman's disease. N Engl J Med 333:797, 1995.

Karcher DS, Alkan S: Human Herpesvirus-8 associated body cavity-based lymphoma in human immunodeficiency virus-infected patients: a unique B-cell neoplasm. Hum Pathol 28:801, 1997.

Karp J, et al: Lung cancer in patients with immunodeficiency syndrome. Chest 103:410, 1993.

Kennedy MM, et al: Identification of HHV8 in early Kaposi's sarcoma: implications for Kaposi's sarcoma pathogenesis. Mol Pathol 51:14, 1998.

Knowles DM: Molecular pathology of acquired immunodeficiency syndrome-related non-Hodgkin's lymphoma. Semin Diagn Pathol 14:67, 1997.

Knowles DM, et al: Molecular genetic analysis of three AIDS-associated neoplasms of uncertain lineage demonstrates their B-cell derivation and the possible pathogenetic role of Epstein-Barr virus. Blood 73:792, 1989.

Knowles DM, et al: Correlative morphologic and molecular genetic analysis demonstrates three distinct categories of posttransplantation lymphoproliferative disorders. Blood 85:552, 1995.

Kohler KA, et al: Primary pulmonary T-cell lymphoma associated with AIDS: the syndrome of the indolent pulmonary mass lesion. Am J Med 99:324, 1995.

Lassoued K, et al: AIDS-associated Kaposi's sarcoma in female patients. AIDS 5:877, 1991.

Laurence J, Astrin SM: Human immunodeficiency virus induction of malignant transformation in human B lymphocytes. Proc Natl Acad Sci U S A 88:7635, 1991.

Lee ES, et al: The association of Epstein-Barr virus with smooth muscle tumors occurring after organ transplantation. N Engl J Med 332:19, 1995.

Lee KS, Kim Y, Primack SL: Imaging of pulmonary lymphomas. Am J Radiol 168:339, 1997.

Levine AM: AIDS-related malignancies: the emerging epidemic. J Natl Cancer Inst 85:1382, 1993.

Levine AM, et al: Low-dose chemotherapy with central nervous system prophylaxis and azidothymidine maintenance in AIDS-related lymphoma: a prospective multiinstitutional trial. JAMA 266:84, 1991.

Lombardi L, Newcomb EW, Dalla-Favera R: Pathogenesis of Burkitt's lymphoma: expression of an activated c-myc oncogene causes the tumorigenic conversion of EBV-infected human B lymphoblasts. Cell 46:161, 1987.

Marchioli CC, et al: Prevalence of human herpesvirus 8 DNA sequences in several patient populations. J Clin Microbiol 34:2635, 1996.

Mathur A, et al: Immunoregulatory abnormalities in patients with Epstein-Barr virus-associated B-cell lymphoproliferative disorders. Transplantation 57:1042, 1994.

McClain KL, et al: Association of Epstein-Barr virus with leiomyosarcomas in children with AIDS. N Engl J Med 332:12, 1995.

Meduri GU, et al: Pulmonary Kaposi's sarcoma in acquired immunodeficiency syndrome. Am J Med 81:11, 1986.

Mellemkjaer L, et al: Rheumatoid arthritis and cancer risk. Eur J Cancer 32A:1753, 1996.

Mellemkjaer L, et al: Non-Hodgkin's lymphoma and other cancers among a cohort of patients with systemic lupus erythematosus. Arthritis Rheum 40:761, 1997.

Mentzer SJ, et al: Immunoblastic lymphoma of donor origin in the allograft after lung transplantation. Transplantation 61:1720, 1996.

Mentzer SJ, et al: Arginine butyrate induced susceptibility to ganciclovir in an Epstein Barr virus associated lymphoma. Blood Cells Mol Dis 24:114, 1998.

Mihalov ML, et al: Incidence of post-transplant malignancy among 674 solid-organ-transplant recipients at a single center. Clin Transplant 10:248, 1996.

Miles SA, et al: Oncostatin M as a potent mitogen for AIDS-Kaposi's sarcoma derived cells. Science 255:1432, 1992.

Miller RF, et al: Bronchopulmonary Kaposi's sarcoma in patients with AIDS. Thorax 47:721, 1992.

Mitchell DM, et al: Bronchopulmonary Kaposi's sarcoma in patients with AIDS. Thorax 47:726, 1992.

Montone KT, et al: Analysis of Epstein Barr virus associated post transplantation lymphoproliferative disorder after lung transplantation. Surgery 119:544, 1996.

Moore PS, Chang Y: Detection of herpesvirus-like DNA sequences in Kaposi's sarcoma in patients with and without HIV infection. N Engl J Med 332:1181, 1995.

Morassut S, et al: HIV-associated human herpesvirus 8-positive primary lymphomatous effusion: radiologic findings in six patients. Radiology 205:459, 1997.

Morrison VA, et al: Clinical characteristics of post-transplant lymphoproliferative disorders. Am J Med 97:14, 1994.

Nador RG, et al: Primary effusion lymphoma: a distinct clinicopathologic entity associated with Kaposi's sarcoma-associated herpes virus. Blood 88:645, 1996.

Nalesnik MA, et al: The pathology of post-transplant lymphoproliferative disorders occurring in the setting of cyclosporine A-prednisone immunosuppression. Am J Pathol 133:172, 1988.

Nicholson AG, et al: Pulmonary B-cell non-Hodgkin's lymphoma associated with autoimmune disorders: a clinicopathological review of six cases. Eur Respir J 9:2022, 1996.

Oddou S, et al: Second neoplasms following high-dose chemotherapy and autologous stem cell transplantation for malignant lymphomas: a report of six cases in a cohort of 171 patients from a single institution. Leuk Lymphoma 31:187, 1998.

Pantaleo G, Graziosi C, Fauci AS: Mechanisms of disease: the immunopathogenesis of human immunodeficiency virus infection. N Engl J Med 328:327, 1993.

Parker MS, et al: AIDS related bronchogenic carcinoma: fact or fiction? Chest 113:154, 1998.

Pelicci PG, et al: Multiple monoclonal B cell expansions and c-myc oncogene rearrangements in acquired immunodeficiency syndrome-related lymphoproliferative disorders: implications for lymphomagenesis. J Exp Med 164:2049, 1986.

Penn I: Cancers of the anogenital region in renal transplant recipients. Analysis of 65 cases. Cancer 58:611, 1986.

Penn I: Development of new tumors after transplantation. In Cerilli (ed): Transplantation. 1988, p. 825.

Penn I: Horizons in organ transplantation. Malignancy. Surg Clin North Am 74:1247, 1994.

Penn I: Malignancies associated with renal transplantation. Urology 10:57, 1977.

Penn I: Sarcomas in allograft recipients transplantation. Transplantation 60:1485, 1995.

Penn I: Second malignant neoplasms associated with immunosuppressive medications. Cancer 37(2 Suppl):1024, 1976.

Pham SM, et al: Solid tumors after heart transplantation: lethality of lung cancer. Ann Thorac Surg 60:1623, 1995.

Quismorio FP: Pulmonary involvement in primary Sjögren's syndrome. Curr Opin Pulm Med 2:424, 1996.

Ramsey-Goldman R, et al: Increased risk of malignancy in patients with systemic lupus erythematosus. J Invest Med 46:217, 1998.

Rappaport DC, et al: Lymphoproliferative disorders after lung transplantation: imaging features. Radiology 206:519, 1998.

Ray P, et al: AIDS-related primary pulmonary lymphoma. Am J Respir Crit Care Med 158:1221, 1998.

Said JW: Human immunodeficiency virus-related lymphoid proliferations. Sem Diagn Pathol 14:48, 1997.

Schwend M, et al: Rapidly growing Epstein-Barr virus-associated pulmonary lymphoma after heart transplantation. Eur Respir J 7:612, 1994.

Shapiro RS, et al: Epstein-Barr virus associated B-cell lymphoproliferative disorders following bone marrow transplantation. Blood 71:1223, 1988.

Shepherd FA, et al: Treatment of Kaposi's sarcoma after solid organ transplantation. J Clin Oncol 15:2371, 1997.

Somers GR, et al: Multiple leiomyosarcomas of both donor and recipient origin arising in a heart-lung transplant patient. Am J Surg Pathol 22:1423, 1998.

Sont JK, et al: Increased risk of second cancers in managing Hodgkin's disease: the 20-year Leiden experience. Ann Hematol 65:213, 1992.

Spiekerkoetter E, et al: Prevalence of malignancies after lung transplantation. Transplant Proc 30:1523, 1998.

Starzl TE, et al: Reversibility of lymphomas and lymphoproliferative lesions developing under cyclosporine-steroid therapy. Lancet 1:583, 1984.

Swerdlow SH: Post-transplant lymphoproliferative disorders: a morphologic, phenotypic and genotypic spectrum of disease. Histopathology 20:373, 1992.

Swerdlow SH: Classification of the post-transplant lymphoproliferative disorders: from the past to the present. Semin Diagn Pathol 14:2, 1997.

Taniguchi S, et al: Primary bronchogenic carcinoma in recipients of heart transplants. Transpl Int 10:312, 1997.

Teruya-Feldstein J, et al: Pulmonary malignant lymphoma of mucosa-associated lymphoid tissue (MALT) arising in a pediatric HIV-positive patient. Am J Surg Pathol 19:357, 1995.

Timmons CF, et al: Epstein-Barr virus associated leiomyosarcomas in liver transplantation recipients. Origin from either donor or recipient tissue. Cancer 76:1481, 1995.

Tucker MA: Solid second cancers following Hodgkin's disease. Hematol Oncol Clin North Am 7:389, 1993.

van Hoeven KH, et al: Visceral myogenic tumors. A manifestation of HIV infection in children. Am J Surg Pathol 17:1176, 1993.

van Leeuwen FE, et al: Second cancer risk following Hodgkin's disease: a 20-year follow-up study. J Clin Oncol 12:312, 1994.

Vogel J, et al: The HIV tat gene induces dermal lesions resembling Kaposi's sarcoma in transgenic mice. Nature 335:606, 1988.

Vyzula R, Remick SC: Lung cancer in patients with HIV-infection. Lung Cancer 15:325, 1996.

Walsh C, et al: Phase I study of M-BACOD and GM-CSF in AIDS associated non-Hodgkin's lymphoma. J AIDS 6:265, 1993.

Wolden SL, et al: Second cancers following pediatric Hodgkin's disease. J Clin Oncol 16:536, 1998.

Wu T-T, et al: Recurrent Epstein-Barr-virus associated lesions in organ transplant recipients. Hum Pathol 27:157, 1996.

Index

Page numbers followed by *f* indicate figures; numbers followed by *t* indicate tables.

Candida esophagitis, 1801–1802, 1802f
Candidiasis, 1095f, 1095–1096
  treatment of, 1078t, 1096
Cantrell's pentalogy, 554–555, 554f, 555t,
  556f, 557t
Capecitabine (Xeloda), for lung cancer,
  1400
Capillary(ies)
  alveolar, fine structure of, 39
  number and size of, 42
Capillary hemangiomatosis, of lungs, 1528
Capnography, in neonatal anesthesia moni-
  toring, 358
Capnometry, in neonatal anesthesia moni-
  toring, 358
Capreomycin, in tuberculosis, 1064t
Carbohydrate antigen 19-9, in hamartoma,
  1519
Carbon dioxide
  arteriovenous, removal of, 527–528
  properties of, 93, 94f
Carbon dioxide laser, for malignant airways disease, 1359
Carbon monoxide, 94
  in inhalation injuries, 836t, 836–837
Carboplatin, for lung cancer, 1394
Carcinoembryonic antigen, in small cell
  lung cancer, 1447
Carcinogenesis, multiple genetic hits of,
  56–57, 57f
Carcinoid syndrome, 1493–1494, 1503
Carcinoid tumor, 1493–1503
  atypical, 1499f, 1499–1500, 1500t
    vs. large cell neuroendocrine tumors,
    1500
  clear cell, 1500
  clinical features of, 1493–1495, 1494f,
    1494t
  diagnosis of, 1495–1501
    biochemical studies in, 1496
    bronchoscopy in, 1496, 1497f
    CT in, 1495f, 1496
    nuclear scanning in, 1496–1497
    radiographic studies in, 1495f,
     1495–1496
  genetic factors in, 1499
  lung abscess and, 1493, 1495f
  melanocytic, 1500
    vs. melanoma, 1543, 1543t
  microscopic findings in, 1497–1499,
    1498f, 1499f
  neurosecretory granules of, 1499, 1499f
  octreotide imaging in, 2046–2047,
    2047f
  oncocytic, 1500
  pathology of, 1497
  prognosis for, 1503
  signs and symptoms of, 1493–1495,
    1494f, 1494t
  staging of, 1496
  thymic, 2013, 2200f, 2200–2202
    markers of, 2060t, 2060–2062
  of trachea, 901f, 908
  treatment of, 1501–1503
    chemotherapy in, 1503
    endoscopic resection in, 1501f,
     1501–1502

    radiation therapy in, 1503
    surgical resection in, 1502t,
     1502–1503
  typical, 1497f, 1497t, 1497–1499,
    1498f, 1499f, 1500t
  vs. tumorlets, 1500–1501
Carcinosarcoma, of lungs, 1539–1540,
  1540f
Cardiac arrhythmias, after pulmonary
  resection, 481, 486–488
Cardiac complications, after thoracic procedures, 322–323, 323t
Cardiac gating, in MRI of thorax,
  167–168
Cardiac herniation, after pulmonary resection, 485–486
Cardiac injury syndrome, pleural effusions
  after, 695
Cardiac tamponade, after pulmonary
  resection, 486
Cardiac transplantation, in mediastinal
  pheochromocytoma manage-
  ment, 2348–2349
Cardial incompetence, gastroesophageal
  reflux associated with,
  1819–1821
  diagnosis of, 1819
  symptoms of, 1819
  treatment of, 1819–1821, 1820f,
    1821f
Cardiovascular disease
  primary, bacterial infections and, 1051
  thoracic surgical patients with
    arrhythmias, management of,
     309–311
    bradyarrhythmias, management of,
     310
    congestive heart failure in, 309
     acute, management of, 312–313
    hypertension in, management of,
     307–308
    low cardiac output syndrome, man-
     agement of, 311–312
    management of, 307–313
     ACE inhibitors in, 308–309
     adrenergic blockers in, 308–309
     diuretics in, 308
     vasodilators in, 308
    pulmonary edema, management of,
     312–313
    supraventricular tachyarrhythmias,
     management of, 310–311
Cardiovascular studies, in pectus excava-
  tum, 537, 537f
Cardiovascular system, in neonates, 353,
  354f, 355f, 355t
Carmustine, for lung cancer, 1394
Carney's heritable disorder, 2316
Carney's triad, 1516–1518
Carotid artery, left, anomalous, 932
Cartilage, chest wall, infections of,
  564–568, 565f–568f. *See
  also specific infection*
Castleman's disease, 2254–2255, 2255t
  diagnosis and treatment of, 2273
Catecholamine(s)
  in ganglionic tumors, 2063

  in mediastinal pheochromocytoma diag-
    nosis, 2337
  in pheochromocytoma, 2064
Cavernous hemangioma, of lungs, 1523
Cavitary lung disease, CT of, 151
CD5, in thymic carcinoma, 2059
CD30, in mediastinal germ cell tumors,
  2058
Cell(s). *See specific types*
Cell cycle, and tumor growth kinetics,
  1389–1390, 1390f
Cell death, programmed, in lung cancer,
  1242–1244
Cellular schwannomas, in adults, 2315
Cell-wall lipid analysis, in mycobacteria
  detection, 234
Central alveolar hypoventilation,
  diaphragm pacing in,
  624–625
Central nervous system (CNS)
  lung cancer metastasis to, 1384, 1384t
  metastatic tumors of, small cell lung
    cancer and, 1447
Central sleep apnea, vs. obstructive sleep
  apnea, 624
Central tumors, non–small cell lung cancer, surgical resection for,
  1319–1320
Central venous pressure (CVP), measurement of, 328–329
Centriacinar emphysema, terminology
  associated with, 1002
c-erbB2/HER-2/neu, 247
Cerebrovascular accident, after pneumonectomy, 500
Cervical infection, mediastinitis and,
  2094–2097, 2095f, 2096f
Cervical mediastinal thymic parathyroid
  cyst, 2128
Cervical mediastinoscopy, 2069–2071,
  2070f, 2071f
  in superior vena cava obstruction, 2101
Cervical mediastinotomy, in descending
  necrotizing mediastinitis,
  2096
Cervical perforation, 1769–1770, 1770f
Cervicothoracic region, anatomy of, 579,
  580f
Cervix, cancer of, pulmonary metastases
  from, 1566
c-fos oncogenes, in lung cancer, 1236t,
  1238
Chagas' disease, 1836–1837
  of esophagus, 1807–1817
    causes of, 1807
    clinical features of, 1808–1809
    diagnosis of, 1809–1812
     endoscopy in, 1811
     laboratory tests in, 1811–1812,
      1812t
     manometric studies in, 1811, 1811f
     radiography in, 1809, 1809f
     radiologic studies in, 1810, 1810f
     scintigraphy in, 1810–1811
    pathophysiology of, 1807–1808
    treatment of, 1812–1816, 1812t, 1813f,
     1815f, 1813t, 1816f, 1816t

in mediastinal pheochromocytoma diagnosis, 2341
in pectus excavatum, 537–538
ECMO. *See* Extracorporeal membrane oxygenation
Ectopia cordis, 552–555
  causes of, 552
  thoracic, 552–554, 552f, 553t, 554f, 554t
  thoracoabdominal, 554–555, 554f, 554t, 555f, 555t
Ectopic adrenocorticotropic hormone, lung cancer and, 1275
Ectopic gonadotropin production, lung cancer and, 1276
Edema, pulmonary. *See* Pulmonary edema
Edrophonium chloride, in myasthenia gravis, 2209
Effusion
  parapneumonic, vs. empyema, CT of, 156
  pericardial. *See* Pericardial effusion
  pleural. *See* Pleural effusion
EGF-R, in lung cancer, 1244t, 1245–1246
Elastofibrolipoma(s), 2375
Electrocardiography, in neonatal anesthesia monitoring, 357
Electrocautery, in VATS, 441–443, 442f
Electron microscopy, for poorly differentiated carcinoma of mediastinum, 2297–2298, 2298t
Electron-beam CT, of lungs, pleura, and chest wall, 147
Electrophrenic respiration, 623–636. *See also* Diaphragm pacing
Electrosurgery, for malignant airways disease, 1358–1359
Eloesser's flap, 710
Embolic disease, lung cancer and, 1279
Embolism
  after pneumonectomy, 499
  air, post-traumatic, 823–824
  pulmonary. *See* Pulmonary embolism
Embolization
  bronchial artery
    in hemoptysis, 966–967
    in tuberculosis, 1072
  of esophageal varices, 1660
  therapeutic, in pulmonary arteriovenous fistula, 980f, 981f, 981–983, 982f, 983f
Embolus(i)
  peripheral tumor, after pulmonary resection, 499
  septic, radiographic appearance of, 139f
Emphysema
  centriacinar, terminology associated with, 1002
  cicatricial, terminology associated with, 1002, 1003f
  congenital lobar, in neonates, thoracotomy for, 359–360
  CT of, 153, 153f
  diffuse
    historical background of, 1021–1023, 1022f
    surgical management of, 1021–1035
     airflow obstruction and, 1023

cardiovascular hemodynamics and, 1023–1024
    lung volume reduction, current status of. *See* Lung volume reduction surgery
    rationale for, 1023–1024
    ventilation-perfusion mismatch and, 1023–1024
  lobar
    acquired, in hyaline membrane disease, 941, 941f
    congenital, 940–941, 941f
    mediastinal, thoracic trauma and, 817–818
  panacinar, terminology associated with, 1002
  paraseptal, terminology associated with, 1002
  subcutaneous
    after pulmonary resection, 497–498
    thoracic trauma and, 817–818, 818f
  terminology associated with, 1001–1002, 1002f
  variety of, surgical management of, 1024
Empyema, 731f
  after lung transplantation, 1200, 1200f
  after pulmonary resection, 495–496
  in amebiasis, 1108f, 1108–1109
  Aspergillus, 722–725
    acute, 723–724
    chronic, 724–725, 724f, 725f
  in children, treatment of, 707–708, 707t
  chronic, 707
  complex, VATS for, 449–450, 449f
  fungal, 501
  hemorrhagic, after pulmonary resection, 500–501
  late, after pulmonary resection, 500–501
  lobectomy, postresectional, 714–715, 714f, 715f
  and loculated pleural effusion, radiographic appearance of, 140f
  in paragonimiasis, 1126–1127, 1127f, 1128f
  parapneumonic. *See* Parapneumonic empyema
  postpneumonectomy, 710–711, 711f
    muscle flap closure in, 711–712
  postsurgical, 709–715
    defined, 709
    incidence of, 709
    nonresectional, 709, 710t
    omentum transposition in, 712f
    single-stage complete muscle flap closure in, 713–714, 713f, 714f
    timing of, 709–710
    transposition in, 712–713, 712f
    treatment of, general principles in, 710, 711f
  post-traumatic, 827–828, 828f
  pyogenic, after pulmonary resection, 500
  thoracic, causes of, 699
  tuberculous, 719–720, 719t, 731f
  vs. abscess, CT of, 156, 156f

vs. parapneumonic effusion, CT of, 156
Empyema necessitatis, 564
Empyemectomy, for paraneumonic empyema, 707
Encephalomyelitis, paraneoplastic, 1277
Endobronchial brachytherapy, for malignant airways disease, 1359–1360, 1360t
Endobronchial stents, for malignant airways disease, 1360–1362, 1362f
Endobronchial tubes
  double-lumen, in one-lung ventilation. *See* Double-lumen endobronchial tubes
  single-lumen, in one-lung ventilation, 329
Endobronchial tumors, 1519–1521
EndoGIA, 443, 443t
Endoluminal stents, for malignant airways disease, 1362
Endometrium, cancer of, pulmonary metastases from, 1566
Endonucleases, restriction, defined, 244
Endoscopic ultrasonography
  in esophageal squamous cell carcinoma, 1915–1917, 1916f
  of esophagus, 1678f, 1678–1679, 1679f
  for mediastinal lymph node metastases, 1307, 1307f
Endoscopic variceal sclerotherapy, pleural effusions after, 696
Endoscopy
  in Chagas' disease of esophagus, 1811
  esophageal perforation with, 1868
  in gastroesophageal reflux, 1856
Endostatin, for lung cancer, 1400
Endothelial cells, in lung, 54–55, 54t
Endothelium
  of alveoli, 38, 38f
  injury to, in acute respiratory distress syndrome, 845
Endotracheal intubation, for mediastinal video-assisted surgery, 2081–2082, 2082f
Endovascular stents, in superior vena cava syndrome, 2161
Entamoeba histolytica
  infection with, 1105–1111. *See also* Amebiasis
  life cycle of, 1105, 1106f
Enteric cysts, in infants and children, 2397–2398, 2397f, 2398f
Environmental factors, in lung cancer due to tobacco smoking, 1220–1221
Enzyme(s), for lung cancer, 1399
Eosinophilia
  in echinococcosis, 1117
  in paragonimiasis, 1125
Eosinophilic granuloma, 1170, 1171f
Eosinophilic lung disease, 1164–1166
Eosinophilic pneumonia, 1165, 1165f
Ependymoma, 2375
  of lungs, 1543
Epidermal growth factor receptor (EGF-R), in lung cancer, 1244t, 1245–1246

idiopathic, 1630, 1631f
laryngitis due to, 1855
management of, 1857–1862, 1857t,
1859f–1862f
Belsey Mark IV operation in,
1859–1860, 1860f, 1861f
Hill antireflux repair in, 1860, 1861f,
1862f
laparoscopic antireflux repair in,
1860–1861
medical, 1857–1858
Nissen fundoplication in, 1859,
1859f
standard transthoracic approach in,
1861–1862
surgical, 1858–1862
transthoracic video-assisted antireflux
repair in, 1861
manometry in, 1856–1857
motility studies in, 1631
mucosal assessment in, 1856
pathogenesis of, 1852–1853
pH studies in, 1856–1857
potential difference measurements
in, 1632
pulmonary aspiration due to, 1855
radiography in, 1856
radionuclide scintigraphy in,
1666–1669, 1668f, 1669f,
1670f
respiratory symptoms in, 1642–1644,
1643f, 1644f
in scleroderma, 1631, 1631f
sequelae of, 1853–1855, 1854t
symptoms of, 1855–1856
tracheoesophageal fistula without
esophageal atresia and,
1793–1794
upper esophageal sphincter in,
1627–1628
Gastrointestinal hemorrhage, massive,
after pneumonectomy, 500
Gastrointestinal tract, diseases of, pleural
effusions due to,
694–695
Gemcitabine (Gemzar), for lung cancer,
1169, 1397
Gender
as factor in lung cancer due to tobacco
smoking, 1220
as factor in non–small cell lung cancer
resection, 1335, 1336t
Gene(s). See specific types
Gene therapy, in pulmonary disease,
254–255
Genetic(s), in lung regulation, 56–59, 57f,
57t–59t, 59f
Genetic polymorphism, defined, 244
Germ cell tumors
benign, of mediastinum. See Mediastinum, benign germ cell
tumors of
malignant, nonseminomatous, of
mediastinum. See Medi-
astinum, nonseminomatous
malignant germ cell
tumors of

mediastinal, 2013, 2055f, 2056f. See
also Mediastinum, benign
germ cell tumors of; Mediastinum, nonseminomatous
malignant germ cell tumors of
CD30 in, 2058
classification of, 2054t
cytogenetic markers in, 2058
α-fetoprotein in, 2053t, 2053–2055,
2054t
β-human chorionic gonadotropin in,
2053t, 2054t, 2055–2057
lactic acid dehydrogenase in, 2057
markers of, 2051–2058, 2053t, 2054t
neuron-specific enolase in, 2058
placental alkaline phosphatase in,
2057
TRA-1–60 in, 2057–2058
MRI of, 171–172
superior vena cava syndrome and, 2153,
2153f
Gestational trophoblastic disease, pulmonary metastases from,
1566
Ghon tubercle, 1054
Gianturco Z-stent, in inoperable
esophageal carcinoma, 1952,
1952f
Gibbus deformity, 2030
Glomus tumors, 2367–2368
of lungs, 1526
of trachea, 905
Glucagon, with esophagography, 1656
Glucocorticoid(s), fetal lung differentiation affected by, 23f
Glucose, pleural fluid, 690–691
Goblet cells, in large airways, 51–52
Goiter
intrathoracic, 2115–2125
airway obstruction in, 2118
anatomic features of, 2115–2117,
2116f
blood supply of, 2117
contrast studies of, 2120, 2123f
CT of, 2119f, 2119–2120, 2120f,
2121f, 2122f
defined, 2115
diagnosis of, 2119f, 2119–2123,
2120f, 2121f, 2122f
incidence of, 2115
MRI of, 2120, 2122f
needle biopsy of, 2123
occult tumor in, 2118
pathology of, 2117–2118
radiographic features of, 2119, 2119f,
2120f
symptoms and signs of, 2118
thyroid scintigraphy of, 2121
treatment of, 2123–2125, 2124f,
2125f
ultrasonography of, 2120
iodine-131 imaging of, 2038, 2038f
multinodular, 2011
tracheal compression by, 889
Goitre plongeaut, 2118
Gold, lung disease with, 1169
Gompertzian growth curve, 1390f

Gradient, defined, 166
Gradient moment nulling, 169
Granular cell tumors
in adults, 2317, 2317f
of esophagus, 1896, 1896f
of lung, 1520
of trachea, 904
Granulocyte colony-stimulating factor, in
small cell lung cancer,
1453–1454, 1470
Granulocyte-macrophage colony-stimulating factor, in small cell
lung cancer, 1453–1454,
1470
Granuloma(s)
eosinophilic, 1170, 1171f
hyalinizing, of lungs, 1526
pulmonary, radiographic findings in,
115, 116f
Granulomatosis
bronchocentric, 1166
lymphomatoid, 1167
of lungs, 1548–1549
Wegener's, 1168, 2254
of trachea, 890
Granulomatous disease
chronic, in children, pulmonary infections in, 1047–1048
mediastinal, 2251–2254
Grasshead, aspiration of, 860
Great vessels, abnormalities of, 2018–2021,
2019f, 2020f, 2021f
Ground-glass opacity, defined, 150
Growth factors, in lung cancer,
1244–1246, 1244t
colony-stimulating factors, 1244t, 1245
EGF-R, 1244t, 1245–1246
insulin-like growth factors, 1244t, 1245
neuropeptides, 1244–1245
platelet-derived growth factor, 1244t,
1246
transforming growth factor-β, 1244t,
1246
Guardian of the genome, 247–248
Gunshot injury, to chest wall, 821

Hair loss, chemotherapy and, 1393
Halothane, in neonatal anesthesia, 356
Hamartoma
of esophagus, 1897
of lungs, 1515–1519, 1516f, 1517f,
1518f, 1528
malignant tumor in, 1518–1519
of trachea, 900f, 906, 906f
Hamman-Rich syndrome, 1159
Hansenula infection, 1098
Harmonic Scalpel, in VATS, 442, 442f
Hassall's corpuscles, of thymus, 1991,
1991f
Head and neck cancer, solitary pulmonary
nodule in, 1132
Heart
radiation effects on, 1372–1373
radiation injury to, in small cell lung
cancer treatment, 1467
snowman, 1243f, 2140
tumors of, imaging studies of, 2027

in rheumatoid arthritis, 1160
right, lymphatic drainage of, to medi-
    astinal lymph nodes, 87–88
in sarcoidosis, 1161t, 1161–1163,
    1162f
schwannoma of, 1535t, 1537
in scleroderma, 1160
sclerosing hemangioma of, 1524f,
    1524–1525
sequestration of, 945f, 945–947
    extralobar, 945f, 945–946, 946f
    intralobar, 945f, 946f, 946–947, 947f,
    948f
silica-induced disease of, 1164
in SLE, 1160
small cell lymphocytic lymphoma of,
    1547
small conducting airways of, 52–53
soft tissue sarcoma of, 1533–1539,
    1534f, 1535t, 1563–1564
solitary nodule of, 1129–1148. *See also*
    Solitary pulmonary nodule
spindle cell sarcoma of, 1535t
Sporotrichum schenckii infection of,
    1096
squamous papilloma of, 1519–1520
sugar (clear cell) tumor of, 1525, 1525t
surface relations of
    anterior view of, 14f
    lateral view of, 14f
synovia sarcoma of, 1537
teratoma of, 1526, 1543
thymoma of, 1526–1527
tissue of, 31
transplantation of. *See* Lung transplan-
    tation
trauma to. *See* Thorax, trauma to
in tuberous sclerosis, 1171
tumors of, in immunocompromised
    hosts, 1577–1590. *See also*
    Immunocompromised
    patients, lung tumors in
type II epithelial cell from, 23f
ultrastructure of, 31–41
vasculitis of, 1168
venous system of, anatomy of, surgical
    anatomy of, 71–72, 71f
ventilation-perfusion scintigraphy of,
    2034f–2035f, 2034–2036
viral infections of, infectious pulmonary
    diseases due to, 238–239,
    239f
vital capacity of, 106
Zygomycetes infection of, 1096–1097,
    1097f
Lung biopsy
    in carcinoid tumor, 1496
    in diffuse lung disease, 1158
    in hamartoma, 1516
    in immunocompromised host, 1046,
        1077, 1175–1176
    open, in pulmonary disease diagnosis,
        225
    percutaneous. *See* Percutaneous lung
        biopsy
    site of, in pulmonary disease diagnosis,
        225–226

transbronchial, in pulmonary disease
    diagnosis, 226
VATS, in pulmonary disease diagnosis,
    225
Lung cancer, 115, 116f, 119f, 1213–1490
adenocarcinoma, 1252–1253, 1253f
adenoid cystic. *See* Adenoid cystic car-
    cinoma
adenosquamous carcinoma, 1256, 1256t
in AIDS, 1579–1580
asymptomatic solitary pulmonary nod-
    ule, diagnosis of, 1299–1300
biopsy of, VATS in, 290–292, 291f
bronchioloalveolar carcinoma,
    1254–1255, 1254f
bronchoalveolar, 1166
bronchoplastic and angioplastic proce-
    dures for, 407, 407t
calcification in, 1134–1135, 1135f
carcinogenesis of, 1215–1228,
    1249–1250
chemotherapy for. *See* Chemotherapy,
    in lung cancer
clinical presentation of, 1269–1282
    bronchopulmonary symptoms in,
        1269–1271, 1270t
    chest pain in, 1271
    cough in, 1269–1270, 1270t
    dermatologic, 1279
    dysphagia in, 1270t, 1271
    dyspnea in, 1270, 1270t
    ectopic adrenocorticotropic hormone,
        1275
    ectopic gonadotropin production,
        1276
    endocrine-metabolic, 1274–1276,
        1275t
    extrapulmonary intrathoracic symp-
        toms in, 1270t, 1271–1272
    hematologic abnormalities in, 1279
    hemoptysis in, 1270, 1270t
    hoarseness in, 1270t, 1271
    Horner's syndrome in, 1271–1272
    hypercalcemia in, 1275
    infectious symptoms in, 1271
    in metastatic disease, 1272–1274,
        1272t, 1273t
    musculoskeletal syndromes, 1276,
        1276f, 1277f
    neuromuscular syndromes,
        1276–1279, 1278t
    Pancoast's syndrome in, 1270t, 1272
    paraneoplastic syndromes. *See* Para-
        neoplastic syndromes
    pleural effusions in, 1270t, 1271
    SIADH and, 1274, 1275t
    stridor in, 1270, 1270t
    superior vena cava syndrome in,
        1270t, 1272
    vascular abnormalities in, 1279
    wheezing in, 1270, 1270t
CNS metastasis of, 1384, 1384t
CT of, 149–150, 185–186, 1286–1287
cytogenetic abnormalities in,
    1241–1242
death due to, 1215, 1216t
diagnosis of, 1283–1287, 1297–1300

CT in, 1298–1299
PET in, 1298, 1299t, 1303, 1303t
sputum cytology in, 1297
thoracotomy in, 1299
transthoracic needle aspiration in,
    1298, 1298t
VATS in, 1298, 1299
diet and, 1226
with distant metastases, surgical treat-
    ment of, results of,
    1334–1335
doubling time of, 1136–1137
early detection of, approach to, 1232
enhanced CT in, 1140–1142
epidemiology of, 1215–1228
general features of, 1283–1284
gross characteristics of, 1250
hamartoma and, 1519
hilar and mediastinal lymph node
    involvement in, PET of,
    196–197, 197f
histologic classification of, 1250–1251,
    1251t
immune response in, 1479–1482, 1481f
    T cells in, 1480–1482, 1481f
immunotherapy in, 1482–1484
    cytokines in, 1486–1487
    MAGE genes in, 1484–1486
    NY-ESO-1 genes in, 1485–1486
    p53 genes in, 1483–1484
    ras genes in, 1482–1483, 1486
inherited predisposition to, 246–247
large cell neuroendocrine carcinomas,
    1258–1259, 1258t
of left lung, mediastinal lymph node
    dissection for, 1350–1354,
    1351f–1354f
localized node–negative, surgical treat-
    ment of, results of,
    1323–1325, 1323t
location of, 1138
lymphangitic, 1166, 1166f
mechanisms of, 1249
with mediastinal lymph node involve-
    ment, surgical treatment of,
    results of, 1329–1333, 1330t,
    1331f, 1332t
mediastinal metastases from,
    2016–2017
metastasis of, 1259–1262
    to adrenal gland, symptoms of, 1274
    bone, symptoms of, 1273
    direct extension, 1259
    to liver, symptoms of, 1274
    lymphatic, 1259–1261, 1260f, 1260t
    neurologic, symptoms of, 1273,
        1273t
    to skin, symptoms, 1274
    to soft tissue, symptoms of, 1274
    symptoms of, 1272–1274, 1272t,
        1273t
molecular biology of, 1235–1249
    3p deletions in, 1241–1242
    angiogenesis in, 1246–1247
    apoptosis in, 1242–1244
    bcl-2 expression in, 1243
    clinical implications of, 1248–1249